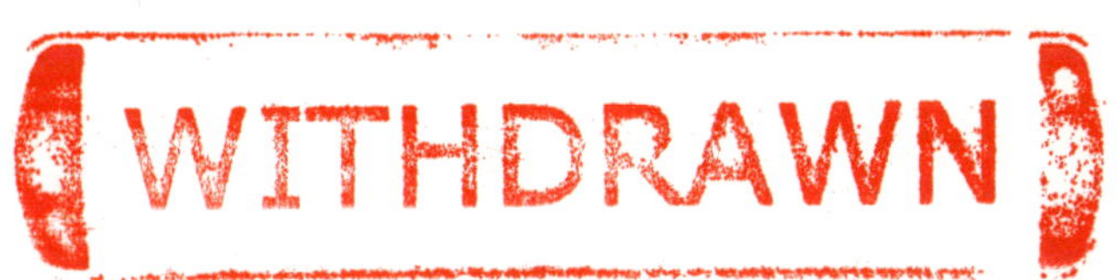

WILLIAM F. MAAG LIBRARY
YOUNGSTOWN STATE UNIVERSITY

WILDERNESS MEDICINE

Management of Wilderness and Environmental Emergencies

WILDERNESS MEDICINE

Management of Wilderness and Environmental Emergencies

Edited by

PAUL S. AUERBACH, M.D., M.S., F.A.C.E.P.

Chief Operating Officer
Sterling Healthcare Group
Coral Gables, Florida
Formerly, Professor and Chief, Division of Emergency Medicine
Department of Surgery, Stanford University Medical Center
Stanford, California

THIRD EDITION

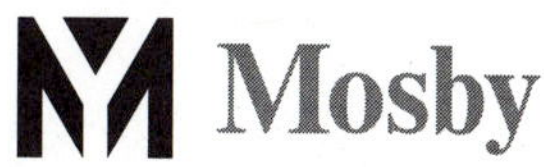

St. Louis Baltimore Boston Carlsbad Chicago Naples New York Philadelphia Portland
London Madrid Mexico City Singapore Sydney Tokyo Toronto Wiesbaden

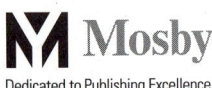

A Times Mirror Company

Publisher: Anne Patterson
Acquisition Editor: Laurel Craven
Managing Editor: Kathryn H. Falk
Project Manager: Patricia Tannian
Senior Book Designer: Gail Morey Hudson
Cover Designer: Teresa Breckwoldt
Manufacturing Supervisors: Betty Richmond, Tim Stringham

THIRD EDITION

Copyright © 1995 by Mosby–Year Book, Inc.

Copyright © 1995 Chapter 16 by John B. Walden.

Previous editions copyrighted 1983 and 1989.

All rights reserved. No part of this publication may be reproduced, stored in a retrieval system, or transmitted, in any form or by any means, electronic, mechanical, photocopying, recording, or otherwise, without prior written permission from the publisher.

Permission to photocopy or reproduce solely for internal or personal use is permitted for libraries or other users registered with the Copyright Clearance Center, provided that the base fee of $4.00 per chapter plus $.10 per page is paid directly to the Copyright Clearance Center, 27 Congress Street, Salem, MA 01970. This consent does not extend to other kinds of copying, such as copying for general distribution, for advertising or promotional purposes, for creating new collected works, or for trade.

Printed in the United States of America
Composition by Clarinda Company
Printing/binding by Maple Vail Book Mfg Group

Mosby–Year Book, Inc.
11830 Westline Industrial Drive
St. Louis, Missouri 63146

Library of Congress Cataloging in Publication Data

Wilderness medicine: management of wilderness and environmental emergencies/edited by Paul S. Auerbach.—3rd ed.
p. cm.
Rev. ed. of: Management of wilderness and environmental emergencies. 2nd ed. 1989.
Includes bibliographical references and index.
ISBN 0-8016-7044-6
1. Outdoor life—Accidents and injuries. 2. Medical emergencies. 3. Mountaineering injuries. 4. Environmentally induced diseases. I. Auerbach, Paul S. II. Management of wilderness and environmental emergencies.
[DNLM: 1. Recreation. 2. Emergencies. 3. Environmental Exposure. QT 250 W673 1995]
RC88.9.095M36 1995
616.9′8—dc20
DNLM/DLC
for Library of Congress

94-12663
CIP

95 96 97 98 9 8 7 6 5 4 3 2

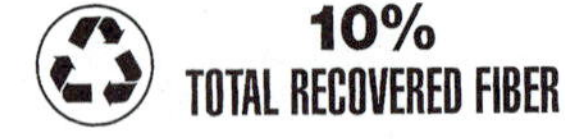

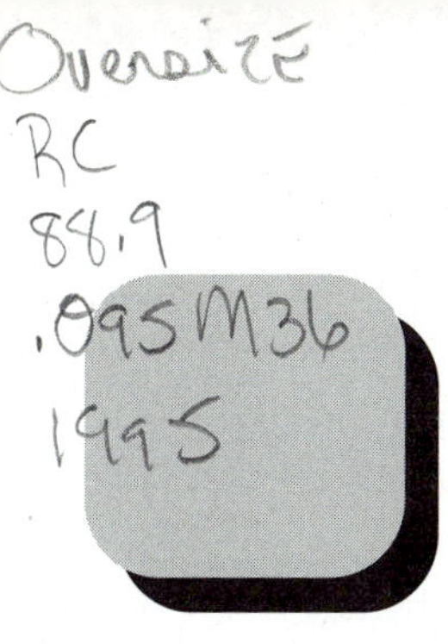
Oversize
RC
88.9
.O95M36
1995

ABOUT THE ARTIST

CHRISTINE GRALAPP, M.A., CMI
Christine graduated from the master's degree program in medical/biological illustration at the University of California–San Francisco in 1984. She is a Certified Medical Illustrator, as well as an active member of the Association of Medical Illustrators. When not creating scientific artwork, she can be found in the Southwest deserts searching for Native American rock art. Christine lives and works in Fairfax, California.

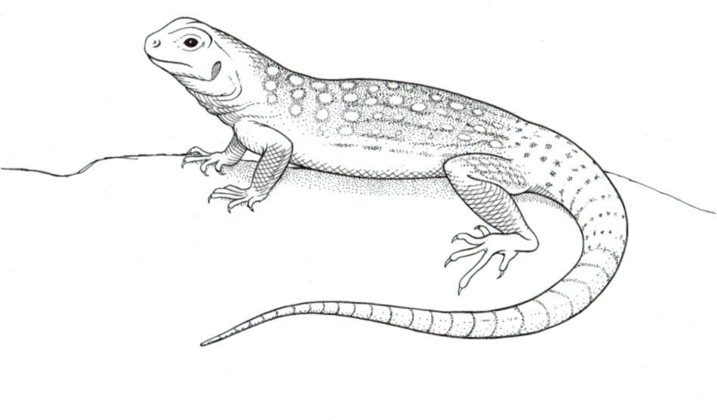

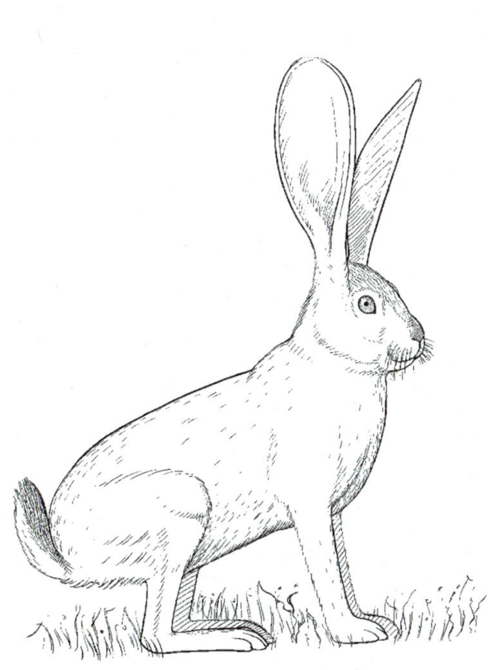

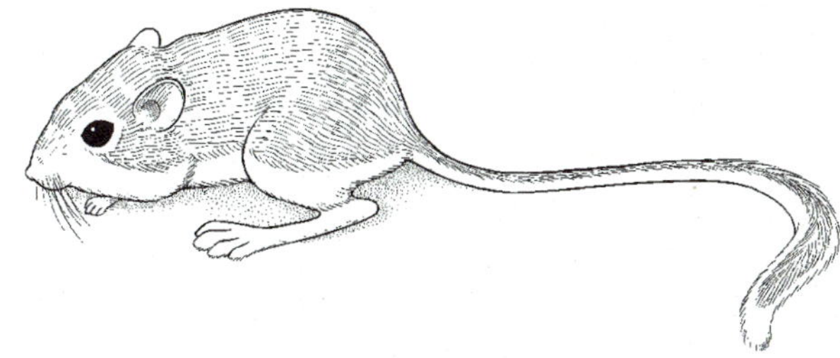

WILLIAM F. MAAG LIBRARY
YOUNGSTOWN STATE UNIVERSITY

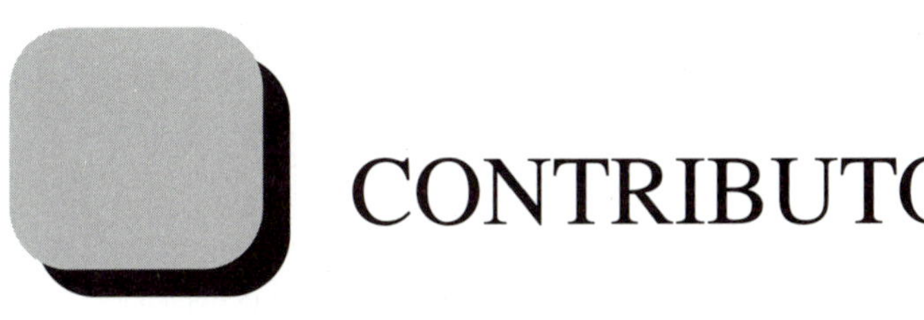

CONTRIBUTORS

Michele Adler, B. Pharm., Cert. Hoft. Hons., Post. Grad. Dip. Ed.

Lecturer in Horticulture,
Horticultural Consultant,
Victorian College of Agriculture and Horticulture (VCAH),
Richmond, Victoria, Australia

Christopher J. Andrews, B.E., M.B.B.S., M.Eng.Sc., Ph.D., Grad. Dip. Comp. Sc., E.D.I.C.

Registrar, Department of Anaesthesiology and Intensive Care,
University of Queensland and Royal Brisbane Hospital;
University of Queensland,
Brisbane, Australia

Betsy R. Armstrong, M.A.

Publications Director, Denver Museum of Natural History,
Denver, Colorado

Richard L. Armstrong

Cooperative Institute for Research in Environmental Sciences,
University of Colorado,
Boulder, Colorado

Paul S. Auerbach, M.D., M.S., F.A.C.E.P.

Professor and Chief, Division of Emergency Medicine,
Department of Surgery,
Stanford University School of Medicine,
Stanford, California

Howard D. Backer, M.D.

Lecturer, International Health,
University of California, San Francisco,
San Francisco, California;
Emergency Department, Kaiser Permanente Hospital,
Hayward, California

H. Bernard Bechtel, M.D.

Private Practice
Valdosta, Georgia

Warren D. Bowman, M.D.

Clinical Associate Professor of Medicine,
University of Washington, Seattle;
National Medical Advisor, National Ski Patrol System, Inc.;
President, Wilderness Medical Society;
Department of Hematology and Oncology, Billings Clinic,
Billings, Montana

George Braitberg, M.B., B.S., F.A.C.E.M.

Fellow in Medical Toxicology, Department of Medical Toxicology,
Good Samaritan Regional Medical Center,
Phoenix, Arizona

Christopher J. Brooks, M.D.

Winnipeg, Manitoba

Gunhilde M. Buchsbaum, M.D.

Instructor in Gynecology,
Fellow in Urogynecology, Plastic and Reconstructive Surgery,
Department of Obstetrics and Gynecology,
University of Rochester School of Medicine,
Rochester, New York

Robert K. Bush, M.D.

Professor of Medicine (CHS), Chief of Allergy,
William S. Middleton VA Hospital;
Department of Medicine,
University of Wisconsin–Madison,
Madison, Wisconsin

Michael L. Callaham, M.D., F.A.C.E.P.

Chief, Division of Emergency Medicine,
Professor of Emergency Medicine,
University of California, San Francisco,
San Francisco, California

David A. Connor, M.D.

Medical Toxicology Fellow,
Department of Medical Toxicology,
Good Samaritan Regional Medical Center,
Phoenix, Arizona

Donald C. Cooper, M.S.

Captain, Cuyahoga Falls Fire Department;
President, National Rescue Consultants;
Associate, Emergency Response Institute;
Cuyahoga Falls, Ohio

Mary Ann Cooper, M.D., F.A.C.E.P.

Associate Professor and Deputy Head for Academic Affairs,
Director, Lightning and Electrical Injury Evaluation Program,
Department of Emergency Medicine,
University of Illinois at Chicago College of Medicine,
Chicago, Illinois

Larry I. Crawshaw, Ph.D.

Professor of Biology,
Director, Environmental Sciences and Resources Doctoral Program,
Portland State University;
Adjunct Professor of Medical Psychology,
Oregon Health Sciences University,
Portland, Oregon

Daniel F. Danzl, M.D.

Professor and Chair, Department of Emergency Medicine,
University of Louisville School of Medicine,
Louisville, Kentucky

Richard C. Dart, M.D., Ph.D.

Director, Rocky Mountain Poison Center;
Assistant Professor, Department of Surgery,
University of Colorado Health Sciences Center,
Denver, Colorado

Kathleen Mary Davis, B.S. Forestry, M.S. Forestry

Chief of Resources Management,
U.S. Department of the Interior,
Southern Arizona Group, National Park Service,
Phoenix, Arizona

Kevin Jon Davison, N.D., L.Ac.

Maui East-West Clinic, Ltd.,
Kahului, Hawaii

Arthur L. Dickinson, Ph.D., F.A.C.S.M.

Human Performance Laboratory,
Department of Kinesiology, University of Colorado,
Boulder, Colorado

Howard J. Donner, M.D.

Telluride Medical Center,
Telluride, Colorado

Herbert L. DuPont, M.D.

Mary W. Kelsey Professor and Director,
Center for Infectious Diseases,
The University of Texas–Houston,
Medical School/School of Public Health,
Houston, Texas

Bruno Dürrer, M.D.

Allgemeine Medizin FMH,
Air Rescue Doctor/Mountain Guide,
Swiss Air Rescue/Air REGA,
Lauterbrunnen, Switzerland

John H. Epstein, M.D.

Clinical Professor, Department of Dermatology,
University of California, San Francisco,
San Francisco, California

William L. Epstein, M.D.

Professor, Department of Dermatology,
University of California, San Francisco,
San Francisco, California

Murray E. Fowler, D.V.M.

Professor Emeritus, Department of Medicine and Epidemiology,
School of Veterinary Medicine,
University of California, Davis,
Davis, California

Steven P. French, M.D.

Co-Director, Yellowstone Grizzly Foundation;
Member, I.V.C.N. Bear Specialists Group;
Adjunct Assistant Professor, Montana State University;
Director of Emergency Medical Services,
IHC Evanston Regional Hospital,
Evanston, Wyoming

Josiah Friedlander, M.D.

Clinical Research Fellow,
Skin Research Foundation of California,
Santa Monica, California

Stephen L. Gaffin, Ph.D.

Comparative Physiology Division,
Environmental Pathophysiology Directorate,
U.S. Army Research Institute of Environmental Medicine,
Natick, Massachusetts

Edward C. Geehr, M.D.

Senior Vice President for Medical Affairs, UniHealth America,
Burbank, California

Douglas A. Gentile, M.D.

Attending Physician, Department of Emergency Medicine,
Medical Center Hospital of Vermont,
Burlington, Vermont

Philip H. Goodman, M.D., M.S.

Associate Professor of Medicine,
Chief, Division of General Internal Medicine,
University of Nevada School of Medicine,
Reno, Nevada

Peter H. Hackett, M.D.

Director, Denali Medical Research Project;
Adjunct Associate Professor,
College of Nursing and Health Sciences,
University of Alaska Anchorage,
Anchorage, Alaska;
Affiliate Associate Professor, Department of Medicine,
University of Washington School of Medicine,
Seattle, Washington

Bruce W. Halstead, M.D.

World Life Research Institute,
Colton, California

Murray P. Hamlet, D.V.M.

Director, Research Programs and Operations Division,
U.S. Army Research Institute of Environmental Medicine,
Natick, Massachusetts

Keith Harrington

Doctoral Candidate, Department of Geography,
Rutgers University,
New Brunswick, New Jersey

Leslie V. Boyer Hassen, M.D.

Medical Director, Arizona Poison and Drug Information Center,
University of Arizona Health Sciences Center,
Tucson, Arizona

John S. Hayward, Ph.D.

Department of Biology, University of Victoria,
Victoria, British Columbia

Susan L. Hefle, M.S., Ph.D.

Research Associate, Allergy and Immunology Section,
Department of Medicine, University of Wisconsin–Madison,
Madison, Wisconsin

John P. Heggers, Ph.D.

Professor of Surgery (Plastic), Microbiology, and Immunology,
University of Texas Medical Branch;
Director, Clinical Microbiology, Shriners Burns Institute,
Galveston, Texas

David M. Heimbach, M.D.

Professor of Surgery, University of Washington School of Medicine;
Director, University of Washington Burn Center,
Department of Surgery, University of Washington,
Seattle, Washington

Gregory L. Henry, M.D., F.A.C.E.P.

Clinical Associate Professor,
Department of Surgery, Section Emergency Medicine,
The University of Michigan,
CEO Medical Practice Risk Assessment,
Ann Arbor, Michigan;
President, American Physician Assurance Society, Limited;
Vice President Emergency Physician Medical Group

Henry J. Herrmann, D.M.D.

Falls Church, Virginia

Rivka S. Horowitz, M.D., Ph.D.

Rocky Mountain Poison Center;
Clinical Instructor, Department of Surgery,
University of Colorado Health Sciences Center,
Denver, Colorado

Roger W. Hubbard, Ph.D.

Director, Environmental Pathophysiology Directorate,
U.S. Army Research Institute of Environmental Medicine,
Natick, Massachusetts

Franklin R. Hubbell, D.O.

Executive Director, SOLO, Inc.;
Member, Mountain Rescue Service,
Conway, New Hampshire

S. Marshal Isaacs, M.D., F.A.C.E.P.

San Francisco Department of Public Health, Paramedic Division;
Assistant Clinical Professor of Surgery,
University of California, San Francisco;
Emergency Services, San Francisco General Hospital,
San Francisco, California

Kenneth V. Iserson, M.D., M.B.A., F.A.C.E.P.

Director, Arizona Bioethics Program;
Professor of Surgery, University of Arizona Health Sciences Center;
Medical Director, Southern Arizona Rescue Association,
Tucson, Arizona

Elaine C. Jong, M.D.

Clinical Professor of Medicine,
Co-Director, Travel Medicine Service,
Director, University of Washington Student Health Center,
Department of Medicine,
University of Washington School of Medicine,
Seattle, Washington

James W. Kazura, M.D.

Chief, Division of Geographic Medicine,
Professor of Medicine and International Health,
Case Western Reserve University School of Medicine,
Cleveland, Ohio

Barbara C. Kennedy, M.D.

Pediatrician, Community Health Plan,
Attending Physician,
Medical Center Hospital of Vermont,
Burlington, Vermont

Kenneth W. Kizer, M.D., M.P.H., F.A.C.E.P.

Undersecretary for Health,
Department of Veterans Affairs,
Washington, D.C.

Donald B. Kunkel, M.D.

Medical Director, Samaritan Regional Poison Center,
Department of Medical Toxicology,
Good Samaritan Medical Center,
Phoenix, Arizona

Patrick H. LaValla

Emergency Response Institute,
Olympia, Washington

Nicholas J. Lowe, M.D., F.R.C.P., F.A.C.P.

Clinical Professor, Department of Dermatology,
UCLA School of Medicine;
Director, Skin Research Foundation of California,
Santa Monica, California

Roberta Mann, M.D.

Assistant Professor of Surgery,
University of Washington School of Medicine;
Assistant Director, University of Washington Burn Center,
Department of Surgery, University of Washington,
Seattle, Washington

Leonard C. Marcus, V.M.D., M.D.

Consultant in Travel Medicine and in Tropical, Parasitic, and Zoonotic Diseases,
Travelers' Health and Immunization Services,
Newton, Massachusetts

Robert L. McCauley, M.D.

Associate Professor of Surgery and Pediatrics,
University of Texas Medical Branch;
Chief, Plastic and Reconstructive Surgery,
Shriners Burns Institute,
Galveston, Texas

Jude T. McNally, R.Ph.

Assistant Director, College of Pharmacy,
University of Arizona Health Sciences Center,
Tucson, Arizona

Sherman A. Minton, M.D.

Professor Emeritus,
Department of Microbiology and Immunology,
Indiana University School of Medicine,
Indianapolis, Indiana

James K. Mitchell, Ph.D.

Professor of Geography, Rutgers University,
New Brunswick, New Jersey

John A. Morris, Jr., M.D.

Associate Professor of Surgery,
Director, Division of Trauma,
Vanderbilt University School of Medicine,
Nashville, Tennessee

Joseph F. Mortola, M.D.

Associate Professor of Obstetrics, Gynecology, and Reproductive Biology,
Harvard Medical School,
Boston, Massachusetts

Robert W. Mutch, B.A. Biology, M.S. Forestry

Research Application Leader,
U.S. Department of Agriculture–Forest Service,
Intermountain Fire Sciences Laboratory,
Missoula, Montana

Andrew B. Newman, M.D., F.C.C.P.

Clinical Assistant Professor of Medicine,
Division of Pulmonary and Critical Care,
Stanford University School of Medicine,
Stanford, California

Eric K. Noji, M.D., M.P.H.

Chief, Disaster Assessment and Epidemiology Section, Health Studies Branch,
Division of Environmental Hazards and Health Effects,
National Center for Environmental Health,
Centers for Disease Control and Prevention,
Atlanta, Georgia

Robert L. Norris, Jr., M.D., F.A.C.E.P.

Assistant Professor of Surgery and Associate Chief,
Division of Emergency Medicine, Department of Surgery,
Stanford University School of Medicine,
Stanford, California

Scott A. Oslund, M.D.

Division of Emergency Medicine,
Department of Surgery,
Stanford University Medical Center,
Stanford, California

Edward J. Otten, M.D.

Professor of Emergency Medicine and Pediatrics,
Director, Division of Toxicology,
Department of Emergency Medicine, University of Cincinnati,
Cincinnati, Ohio

Robert S. Pozos, Ph.D.

Head, Department of Applied Physiology,
Naval Health Research Center,
San Diego, California

Sheila B. Reed

Consultant, InterWorks (Supporting Development and Disaster Management);
Disaster Management Center,
University of Wisconsin,
Madison, Wisconsin

Robert C. Roach, Ph.D.

Physiologist, Cardiopulmonary Physiology Program,
Lovelace Institute of Basic and Applied Medical Research,
Albuquerque, New Mexico

Martin C. Robson, M.D.

Professor of Surgery, Division of Plastic Surgery,
Department of Surgery, University of South Florida,
Tampa, Florida

Charles E. Saunders, M.D., F.A.C.E.P., F.A.C.P.

Associate Professor of Medicine,
University of California, San Francisco;
Emergency Services, San Francisco General Hospital,
San Francisco, California

Sandra M. Schneider, M.D.

Professor and Chair, Department of Emergency Medicine,
University of Rochester/Strong Memorial Hospital,
Rochester, New York

Carl E. Schreck, B.S.

Research Entomologist, U.S. Department of Agriculture,
Agricultural Research Service,
Medical and Veterinary Entomology Research Laboratory,
Gainesville, Florida

Brad S. Selden, M.D.

Department of Emergency Medicine,
Maricopa County Medical Center,
Phoenix, Arizona

Bern Shen, M.D.

Assistant Professor of Emergency Medicine,
University of California, San Francisco;
Research Scientist,
Hewlett Packard Laboratories,
Palo Alto, California

David J. Smith, Jr., M.D.

Professor of Surgery,
Section Head, Plastic and Reconstructive Surgery,
Surgery Department, Section of Plastic and Reconstructive Surgery,
University of Michigan Medical Center,
Ann Arbor, Michigan

Deborah L. Squire, M.D.

Division of General Pediatrics,
Duke University Medical Center,
Durham, North Carolina

Edward R. Stein, J.D.

Attorney at Law, Stein, Moran, Raimi & Goethel, P.C.,
Ann Arbor, Michigan

Alan M. Steinman, M.D., M.P.H., R.A.D.M.

Chief, Office of Health and Safety,
U.S. Coast Guard Surgeon General,
U.S. Coast Guard,
Washington, D.C.

Robert C. Stoffel

Emergency Response Institute,
Olympia, Washington

John B. Sullivan, Jr., M.D.

Associate Professor, Emergency Medicine,
University of Arizona Health Sciences Center,
Tucson, Arizona

Marc F. Swiontkowski, M.D., F.A.C.S.

Professor of Orthopaedics, University of Washington;
Chief, Department of Orthopaedics,
Harborview Medical Center,
Seattle, Washington

John B. Walden, M.D.

Professor, Department of Family and Community Health,
Associate Dean, Medical School Development and Outreach,
Marshall University School of Medicine,
Huntington, West Virginia

Eric A. Weiss, M.D.

Assistant Professor, Division of Emergency Medicine,
Department of Surgery,
Stanford University School of Medicine,
Stanford, California

Jay D. Wenger, M.D.

Chief, Childhood and Respiratory Diseases Branch,
Division of Bacterial and Mycotic Diseases,
Centers for Disease Control and Prevention,
Atlanta, Georgia

Knox Williams, M.S. Atmospheric Science

Director, Colorado Avalanche Information Center,
Colorado Geological Survey,
Denver, Colorado

Willis A. Wingert, M.D.

Claremont, California

Steven C. Zell, M.D., F.A.C.P.

Associate Professor of Medicine,
Division of General Internal Medicine and Health Care Research,
University of Nevada School of Medicine,
Reno, Nevada

FOREWORD

In September 1970, my friend Gert Judmaier fell for at least 15 vertical meters close to the summit of Mount Kenya. Among other injuries he suffered an open tibia fracture. The chances for rescue and survival were grim. I had accompanied him on the climb, and my knowledge of wilderness medicine and the therapeutic options was meager. Furthermore, we were the only men on the mountain, we had no radiotransmitter with which to call for help, and there were no organized rescue groups in Africa. I somehow succeeded in stopping the bleeding from my friend's shattered leg and provided him with all of our fluids, which consisted of a can of plums and 100 ml of whiskey. I encouraged him to stay alive until I had organized a rescue and we descended. Miraculously he survived. This was due to his determination and a rescue effort that ultimately involved a hundred people and lasted for 7 days.

Not so lucky were four mountaineers who attempted the unclimbed Eiger North Face in 1937. Although seasoned by many alpine ascents and despite the heroic efforts of local rescue squads, they all perished. Some were within a few meters of the rescuers—it just took too long to reach them. Today a climber who is hurt or who is too tired to continue climbing can call for an air rescue on the walkie-talkie and may be in the closest hospital within 30 minutes. In Nepal the helicopter has replaced the yak as the means of transportation for victims of high-altitude mishaps. Furthermore, medical posts are located at remote places in the Himalaya where in earlier times travelers died of easily treatable illnesses. The technology facilitating rescue, as well as the medical knowledge of the management of wilderness and environmental emergencies, has changed dramatically during the last few decades. Once it was left to the victim and his or her friends to improvise a way out of such dilemmas as negotiating crevasses, procuring insulation when hypothermic, and performing "load and go" with the recipient of a spine fracture. These days powerful helicopters guided by experienced and daring pilots, sophisticated field devices to deliver heat to the hypothermic victim, and endotracheal intubation and supervision during transport have turned wilderness medicine into a technologic art and science. All these advances have also reduced the risk and the spirit of adventure.

The number of people who play potentially dangerous games in the wilderness has increased exponentially. On any given day a dozen or more adventurers may be enjoying the ascent of Mount Kenya or the slopes of Denali. Others shoot the rapids of the Colorado River or explore the undersea canyons of the Pacific Ocean. However, the excitement of the finest recreation may suddenly turn into tragedy, although most accidents are preventable. Many tourists are not well prepared and are naive about the risks of visiting remote areas in the Himalaya, the Sahara, the Amazon basin, or the Grand Canyon. Therefore the environments that have been designated "hostile" are so mainly because of human arrogance, ignorance, and failures caused by irresponsible behavior. However, natural hazards such as lightning, wildland fires, or unpredictable avalanches cause the death of some of the most experienced and safety-conscious guides. We should always be aware of the potential price of our desire to experience permanently uninhabited areas. Every wilderness user has to decide whether the rewards outweigh the risks and how best to adapt to the fact that where there is no risk, there may be less fun.

In the past few decades the management and teaching related to wilderness medical emergencies have come a long way. It was not until 1983 that a comprehensive textbook became available. Therefore the enormous efforts of Paul Auerbach and his colleagues to produce the greatly revised and expanded third edition of *Wilderness Medicine: Management of Wilderness and Environmental Emergencies* are greatly appreciated. From the first to the current edition the number of chapters has increased from 27 to 56, providing a thorough reference for physicians and allied health care professionals who treat victims of injuries and illnesses that originate in wilderness environments. The spectrum of topics is impressive and reflects the diversity of medical problems caused by such forces as cold, heat, wild animals, marine microbes, snakes, sharks, and earthquakes. In a time when the administrators of wilderness areas are increasingly sued for mishaps and accidents, the chapter on legal issues is particularly appropriate.

Ethical issues are daunting and are also addressed. Is there a "right for rescue"? What is the ethical solution if someone leaves a dying friend behind to save his or her own life? These issues extend to the wider issues of risking lives in principle as conquistadores of the useless or as unveilers and destroyers of the last secrets of our planet. If we are to invoke wilderness medicine, let us do so because we are exploring for the challenge and in harmony, not to plunder.

Oswald Oelz, M.D.

PREFACE to the third edition

Since the first edition of this text was published 12 years ago, a tremendous amount of information on wilderness medicine has accumulated. Furthermore, advances in information technology and the increased interest in wilderness recreation have resulted in centralized sources of data about wilderness medicine. The explosion of knowledge is reflected in this textbook.

Any of the chapters that appear in this third edition could have been expanded into a book in its own right, and some undoubtedly will be. There are institutes devoted to diving medicine, high-altitude physiology, search and rescue, natural disaster management, venomous creatures, and so forth. Without creating an encyclopedia, I have attempted to assemble in this volume much more than a cursory approach to the field, so that the reader will have a solid framework on which to venture into the more esoteric literature.

Wilderness Medicine has evolved from *Management of Wilderness and Environmental Emergencies* in response to the comments of readers and reviewers of the previous editions. While much of the medicine practiced in remote areas or under environmental extremes is emergency in nature, the field of wilderness medicine has rapidly grown beyond the exciting rescues of extreme alpinists and intrepid ocean explorers. Although we may find it hard to muster the same excitement about physiology and biochemistry that we have about a caged descent into shark-filled waters or an Eskimo roll through a mammoth standing wave on the Colorado River, knowledge of the basic science is crucial and so these subjects are presented. However, the wilderness medical setting also calls for action, so this book is imbued with "how to" information on approaching difficult clinical situations. Whenever possible, practical discourse on preparation and injury prevention is provided.

The contributors poured themselves into this project. The writing styles and content reflect their expertise and passion for their work, which ranges from firsthand observation of grizzly bear behavior in the wild to laboratory elucidation of the fundamental molecular changes associated with heatstroke. In addition to updated chapters from the last edition, there are new chapters dealing with taking children into the wilderness, special concerns of women, Arctic medicine, thermoregulation, travel medicine, survival at sea, the changing environment, antivenins, natural plant-derived medicines, and many other subjects. Chapters that had become too long, such as the old "Hazardous Aquatic Life," have been divided to help the reader more easily find the topic of interest. The publisher has allowed a doubling of the number of color plates, for which I am grateful. Kathy Falk was a diligent and compassionate editor.

In the decade since its founding, the Wilderness Medical Society (WMS) has become the glue that holds together adventurers, scientists, scholars, authors, and doctors (Color Plate 1). This book would not have been possible had I not been able to call on the incredible talent that resides within the society. Five years ago the WMS began publication of the *Journal of Wilderness Medicine* (Color Plate 2), which has now become *Wilderness and Environmental Medicine,* an important forum for original research reports, cases, and reviews of wilderness medical phenomena. The mission of the WMS (Color Plate 3) continues to evolve as the membership grows and more health professionals seek to combine their love of the outdoors with their calling as healers.

As they have time and again, my friends and family carried me through this project. The world needs more Barb Kennedys, Doug Gentiles, Ken Kizers, and Peter Hacketts. I am a lucky person to have chosen an area of study that is populated with so many fascinating and generous individuals. What next? Surely a fourth edition, perhaps in a format that will sustain this project into the next century. To paraphrase one reviewer of the second edition, I'll have to figure out a way to do it so that a pack animal won't be needed to carry the book into the wilderness.

For the time being, however, the book has grown and so has my family. Now there are three little people to whom I would like to dedicate the work. I hope that Brian, Lauren, and Dan enjoy the wilderness as much as their mother and I have enjoyed it and that they learn in time the importance of keeping it whole for *their* children.

P.S.A.

PREFACE to the second edition

The last 10 years have witnessed an upward spiral of interest in wilderness and wildland medicine. Since publication of the first edition of *Management of Wilderness and Environmental Emergencies* in 1983, many textbooks on selected topics, such as hypothermia, heat-related illnesses and snake envenomations, have been written; a Wilderness Medical Society has grown to include participants from every state and many foreign countries; the *Journal of Wilderness Medicine* is poised for its inaugural issue; continuing medical education seminars on wilderness medicine topics have proliferated; and international symposia that integrate physicians, paramedical personnel, and medical students increasingly continue to define the broad base of research and enthusiasm that support the field.

It is with a great deal of satisfaction that we offer the second edition of this text. Recognizing the limitations of attempting to please everyone on the first go-round, we previously included a number of topics that were a bit peripheral to medical considerations of man in the natural environment. Despite an overwhelming positive response in reviews and private comments, we were the first to identify the first edition's shortcomings, and hope that we have attained a more accurate focus in this new version. Although we recognize the impact of man, chemicals, and machines upon our natural resources, discussions of nuclear war and toxic spills are beyond the scope of what we have intended from the start. This is a book about the environment, the way it sits without our intrusion, and how it can create medical emergencies for persons who confront by intention or are caught unaware of its behavior and extremes of temperature, toxins, and elemental forces.

The book is longer, as there is a considerable amount of original and updated material that we needed to include. Seventeen new chapters have been created; some are related to revised organization, while others support an expanded range of topics. The color supplement offers the reader an appreciation of some of the more classic visual presentations of wilderness hazards. A single chapter on hypothermia would not do justice to this rapidly evolving field, so there are separate expanded discussions of cold water immersion and frostbite. The concept of wilderness survival spawned new presentations of search and rescue, wilderness equipment and medical supplies, and wilderness trauma emergencies. Many explorers and recreational travelers are required to use pack animals, hence the chapter on emergency veterinary medicine. The therapies and related discussions of many topics, such as high altitude medicine and hazardous marine animals, have been vastly expanded and could be published as smaller books in their own right. We asked each contributor to spare no detail, and did not attempt to edit away complicated concepts for the sake of brevity, to allow the full expression of our contributors' expertise.

We are enormously grateful to all of our current contributors, and equally appreciative of our other colleagues' previous efforts. In most cases, the first edition chapters precisely illuminated the needs of the revised chapters, and we therefore offer thanks to their authors. The editorial and production staffs at the C.V. Mosby Company were efficient and kind, and we are grateful for their support. As was the case with the previous edition, our families demonstrated superhuman tolerance, and allowed us the inordinate amount of time necessary to complete this project.

It is our hope that perpetuation of *Management of Wilderness and Environmental Emergencies* in this and future editions will serve as further impetus for medical student curriculum development in this extremely vital area of medicine. In no other conceptual area of medicine is there such an obvious integration of wellness with disease and surgical illness. Wilderness and environmental emergencies follow forays into precisely the sorts of activities that men and women should pursue with regularity: adventure, exercise, and outdoor exploration. In an era of catastrophic infectious disease, constant debate over entitlement of health care, and a waning enrollment in graduate medical education, we find wilderness medicine refreshing and relevant.

Our final comment is that we hope that this book will become a banner for the concept of education as a form of injury prevention. As practitioners and teachers of wilderness medicine, we are quite comfortable with treating victims of rock-climbing accidents, decompression sickness, high altitude cerebral edema, and poisonous mushroom ingestions. Still, we are constantly reminded of the avoidable nature of most trauma and adverse environmental exposures. Implicit in the management of every variety of wilderness emergency is the message of prevention. We cannot and should not take all of the risk out of the wilderness, but we certainly can strive to eliminate the uninformed and foolish risks. This edition of *Management of Wilderness and Environmental Emergencies* is dedicated to every individual who takes the time to position a warning rope near hazardous water or a caution sign on a dangerous slope. We applaud health professionals and laypersons alike who have committed themselves to the safe enjoyment of wilderness and wildland areas.

P.S.A.
E.C.G.

PREFACE to the first edition

Emergency and primary care physicians, unpredictably confronted with disorders of every variety, need access to descriptions of and therapeutic guidelines for common and uncommon diseases. Our purpose is to provide the clinician with a body of knowledge concerned with the interactions between people and the natural environment.

What some may consider peripheral, we see as mainstream and vital for spiritual and recreational health. Environmental encounters, however, are not without risk, even for the prepared. As increased wilderness activity leads to a rising incidence of misfortune, medical personnel must sharpen their awareness of environmental hazards. Competitive athletics, and underwater and aerospace exploration have engendered medical subspecialities. Because wilderness and environmental medicine are poorly organized in the medical literature, we direct this book toward defining the field and gathering the best available information. We have solicited contributions from experts in diverse specialties who have a common bond of recreational and wilderness pursuits. Their vast experience and irrepressible enthusiasm are evident in this work.

The chapters that discuss wilderness rescue, forest fires, aerospace medicine, and disaster planning are designed as a primer to introduce the reader to unfamiliar terminology and equipment, define resources, and explore emergency management strategies. More detailed clinical information is included in the chapters that address the commonly encountered physical forces such as sun, heat, cold, lightning, altitude, and barotrauma and the biologic toxins such as plant poisons, animals bites, insect stings, and marine envenomations. In addition, because industry and nuclear technology threaten the environment in every-increasing fashion, we have added a chapter on inhalation injuries and an appendix on the management of radiation incidents. The true focus of our work and space limitations prevent us from fully exploring the environmental and health impact of modern technology.

The text is intended to serve emergency and primary care physicians as a definitive therapeutic guide, to provide residents in training and medical students with an authoritative reference source, and to offer nurses and paramedic personnel a background in the health consequences of environmental stress.

The need for medical education is self-evident. A larger issue is that of conservation and the environment. Sadly, much of our land and resources have been exploited, polluted, and consumed. This book is a plea for thoughtful management and preservation of the wildernesses of the world. The harvesting of wildlife and elimination of ecosystems for economic gain threaten to be the undoing of the wilderness as we know it. What we do not actively protect will be endangered by those unconcerned with or unaware of the history, fragility, and natural order of things. It is our wish to make the wildlands safer through greater awareness and to foster the spirit of conservation. We encourage our colleagues to encounter the wildlands, and wish them safe expeditions.

P.S.A.
E.C.G.

CONTENTS

WILDERNESS MEDICINE

Management of Wilderness and Environmental Emergencies

1 HIGH-ALTITUDE MEDICINE

Peter H. Hackett
Robert C. Roach

Millions of persons annually visit recreation areas above 2400 m in the American West. Hundreds of thousands visit central and south Asia, Africa, and South America, many traveling to altitudes over 4000 m.[191] Increasingly, physicians and other health care providers are confronted with questions of prevention and treatment of high-altitude medical problems (Box 1-1), as well as the effects of altitude on preexisting medical conditions. Despite advances in high-altitude medicine, significant morbidity and mortality persist (Table 1-1). Clearly, better education of the population at risk and those advising them is essential. This chapter reviews the basic physiology of ascent to high altitude, as well as the pathophysiology, recognition, and management of medical problems associated with high altitude.

BOX 1-1

POTENTIAL MEDICAL PROBLEMS OF LOWLANDERS ON ASCENT TO HIGH ALTITUDE

- Acute hypoxia
- Acute mountain sickness
- High-altitude cerebral edema
- Cerebrovascular syndromes
- High-altitude pulmonary edema
- Peripheral edema
- Retinopathy
- Thromboembolism
- Disordered sleep
- Sleep periodic breathing
- High-altitude pharyngitis and bronchitis
- Ultraviolet keratitis (snowblindness)
- Exacerbation of preexisting illness

Table 1-1 Incidence of Altitude Illness in Various Groups

Study Group	Number at Risk per Year	Sleeping Altitude (m)	Maximum Altitude Reached (m)	Average Rate of Ascent*	Percent with AMS	Percent with HAPE and/or HACE	Reference
Western State visitors	30 million	~2000	3500	1-2	18-20	0.01	105, 190
		~2500			22		105
		~≥3000			27-42		43, 105
Mt. Everest trekkers	6000	3000-5200	5500	1-2 (fly in)	47	1.6	84
				10-13 (walk in)	23	0.05	
Mt. McKinley climbers	800	3000-5300	6194	3-7	30	2-3	89
Mt. Rainier climbers	6000	3000	4392	1-2	67	—	154
Indian soldiers	Unknown	3000-5500	5500	1-2	†	2.3-15.5	255, 256

AMS, Acute mountain sickness; *HAPE,* high-altitude pulmonary edema; *HACE,* high-altitude cerebral edema.
*Days to sleeping altitude from low altitude.
†Reliable estimate unavailable.

BOX 1-2

GLOSSARY OF PHYSIOLOGIC TERMS

P_B Barometric pressure (torr)
Po_2 Partial pressure of oxygen
PIo_2 Inspired Po_2 [$0.21 \times P_B - 47$ torr (vapor pressure of H_2O at 37° C)]
PAo_2 Po_2 in alveolus
$PAco_2$ Pco_2 in alveolus
Pao_2 Po_2 in arterial blood
$Paco_2$ Pco_2 in arterial blood
$Sao_2\%$ Arterial oxygen saturation (%HbO_2/total Hb)
R Respiratory quotient (CO_2 produced/O_2 consumed)

Alveolar gas equation: $PAo_2 = PIo_2 - PAco_2/R$

Table 1-2 Altitude Conversion and Barometric Pressure

Meters	Feet	P_B*	Meters	Feet	P_B*
Sea level		760	5486	18000	380
1000	3281	670	5500	18045	380
1219	4000	651	5791	19000	366
1524	5000	627	6000	19685	356
1829	6000	603	6096	20000	352
2000	6562	591	6401	21000	339
2134	7000	581	6500	21326	335
2438	8000	559	6706	22000	326
2500	8202	554	7000	22966	314
2743	9000	538	7010	23000	314
3000	9843	520	7315	24000	302
3048	10000	517	7500	24606	295
3353	11000	497	7620	25000	291
3500	11483	489	7925	26000	279
3658	12000	479	8000	26247	277
3962	13000	462	7230	27000	269
4000	13123	460	8500	27887	260
4267	14000	445	8534	28000	259
4500	14764	431	8839	29000	249
4572	15000	426	9000	29528	244
4877	16000	410	9144	30000	240
5000	16404	404	9500	31168	229
5182	17000	395	10000	32808	215

*Barometric pressure is approximated by the equation $P_B = 760(e^{-a/7924})$, where P_B = barometric pressure in torr, a = altitude above sea level in meters, and e = natural antilog. Feet ~ meters × 3.28.

Definitions

HIGH ALTITUDE (1500 TO 3500 M)

The onset of physiologic effects of diminished PIo_2 includes decreased exercise performance and increased ventilation (lower arterial Pco_2) at rest (Box 1-2). Minor impairment exists in arterial oxygen transport (Sao_2 at least 90%), but high-altitude illness is common with rapid ascent above 2500 m (Table 1-2).

VERY HIGH ALTITUDE (3500 TO 5500 M)

Maximum arterial oxygen saturation falls below 90% as the arterial Po_2 falls below 60 mm Hg (Table 1-3; Fig. 1-1). Extreme hypoxemia may occur during exercise, sleep, and high-altitude illness. This is the most common range for severe altitude illness.

EXTREME ALTITUDE (OVER 5500 M)

Marked hypoxemia and hypocapnia exist at extreme altitude. Progressive deterioration of physiologic function eventually outstrips acclimatization. These altitudes are above the highest permanent human habitation. Abrupt ascent to this altitude without supplemental oxygen for other than brief exposures is very dangerous.

High-Altitude Medical Research

Much of the information presented in this chapter is drawn from major high-altitude physiology and medical studies of the last 35 years, including the work of Carlos Monge in South America,[186] the 1960-1961 Himalayan Silver Hut expedition, the Arctic Institute Mt. Logan laboratory (1967-1979), the 1981 American Medical Research Expedition to Mt. Everest (AMREE), the Denali Medical Research Project (on Mt. McKinley, 1982-1990), Operation Everest II (1985), and the Capanna Margharita Hut, 1986 to the present. The Silver Hut expedition, led by Sir Edmund Hillary and the physiologist Griffith Pugh, studied acclimatization and exercise and made careful measurements up to 7440 m on Makalu. They wintered for 9 months in a hut at 5800 m on the slopes of Ama Dablam and determined that prolonged stay at that altitude resulted in steady, gradual deterioration, rather than improved acclimatization.[209,212,291]

On Mt. Logan, Dr. Charles Houston and colleagues focused on acclimatization and high-altitude illness, describing changes in retinal circulation and retinal hemorrhage, pulmonary changes in acute mountain sickness (AMS), fluid and electrolyte disturbances, and the effects of acetazolamide.* Twenty years later, continuing in the Silver Hut tradition, Dr. John West and colleagues returned to the Himalaya (Mt. Everest) with a team determined to "climb

*References 59, 60, 68, 82, 109, 163, 177, 265, 266, 268, 270.

Table 1-3 Blood Gases and Altitude*

Altitude					
Meters	**Feet**	**P_B (mm Hg)**	**Pa_{O_2} (mm Hg)**	**Sa_{O_2} (%)**	**Pa_{CO_2} (mm Hg)**
1646	5400	630	73.0 (65.0-83.0)	95.1 (93.0-97.0)	35.6 (30.7-41.8)
2810	9200	543	60.0 (47.4-73.6)	91.0 (86.6-95.2)	33.9 (31.3-36.5)
3660	12020	489	47.6 (42.2-53.0)	84.5 (80.5-89.0)	29.5 (23.5-34.3)
4700	15440	429	44.6 (36.4-47.5)	78.0 (70.8-85.0)	27.1 (22.9-34.0)
5340	17500	401	43.1 (37.6-50.4)	76.2 (65.4-81.6)	25.7 (21.7-29.7)
6140	20140	356	35.0 (26.9-40.1)	65.6 (55.5-73.0)	22.0 (19.2-24.8)

*Data for 1646 m from Loeppky et al.[162]; other altitude data from McFarland et al.[179] Data are mean values and (range). All values are for subjects age 20 to 40 years who were acclimatizing well.

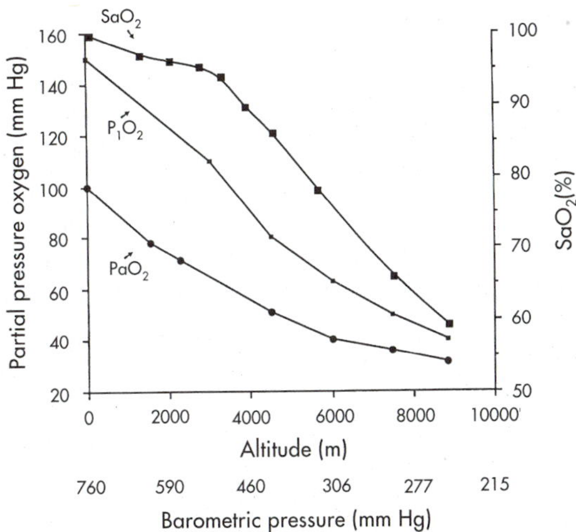

Fig. 1-1 Increasing altitude results in decrease in inspired P_{O_2} (PI_{O_2}), arterial P_{O_2} (Pa_{O_2}), and arterial oxygen saturation (Sa_{O_2}). Note that difference between inspired and arterial P_{O_2} narrows at high altitude because of increased ventilation and that Sa_{O_2} is well maintained while person is awake until over 3000 m. *BTPS*, Body temperature pressure saturated. (Data from Morris A: *Clinical pulmonary function tests: a manual of uniform laboratory procedures*, Salt Lake City, 1984, Intermountain Thoracic Society; and Sutton JR et al: *J Appl Physiol* 64[4]:1309, 1988.)

for science." The American Medical Research Expedition to Mt. Everest (AMREE) measured barometric pressure and alveolar gases on the summit and performed extensive studies on acclimatization and exercise.* In 1985, to eliminate the confounding variables of field studies, eight men were gradually decompressed to a PI_{O_2} equivalent to that at the summit of Mt. Everest. The study was titled Operation Everest II (OEII), after Operation Everest I conducted in 1946 by Houston and Riley.[106] Twenty-two scientists participated in this ambitious project, which included complex studies using Swan-Ganz catheterization, inert gas measurements of ventilation-perfusion inequalities, extensive exercise and muscle biopsy tests, and metabolic studies and ventilatory responses, on participants both awake and asleep.* OEII offered an opportunity to study acclimatization to extreme altitude to a degree never before attained in a laboratory. The Denali Medical Research Project and the Capanna Margharita group have focused on clinical high-altitude illness, unraveling the complex relationships of pulmonary, circulatory, and central nervous system function in acclimatization and illness at high altitude.† The current explosion in the number of high-altitude visitors has sparked new altitude research efforts around the world.‡

*References 28, 242, 286, 288-290, 298, 299.

Environment at High Altitude

Barometric pressure falls with increasing altitude in a logarithmic fashion (Table 1-2). Therefore the partial pressure of oxygen (21% of barometric pressure) also decreases, resulting in the primary insult of high altitude: hypoxia. At approximately 5500 m, barometric pressure is one half that at sea level, and on the summit of Mt. Everest (8848 m) the inspired pressure of oxygen is approximately one third that at sea level (Fig. 1-1).

The relationship of barometric pressure to altitude changes with the distance from the equator. Thus polar regions afford greater hypoxia at high altitude, as well as extreme cold. West[287] has calculated that the barometric pressure on the summit of Mt. Everest (27° N latitude) would be about 222 torr instead of 253 torr if Everest were located at the latitude of Mt. McKinley (62° N). Such a difference, he claims, would be sufficient to render an ascent without supplemental oxygen impossible.

In addition to the role of latitude, fluctuations related to

*References 2, 113, 168, 199, 216, 217, 264, 271.
†References 13, 14, 17, 18, 20, 77, 85, 87, 89-92, 201, 202, 240, 241, 243.
‡References 114, 197, 221-223, 229, 301.

season, weather, and temperature affect the pressure-altitude relationship. Pressure is lower in winter than in summer. A low-pressure trough can reduce pressure 10 mm Hg in one night on Mt. McKinley, making climbers awaken "physiologically higher" by 200 m. The degree of hypoxia, then, is directly related to the barometric pressure, not solely to geographic altitude.[287]

Temperature decreases with altitude (average of 6.5° C per 1000 m), and the effects of cold and hypoxia are generally additive in provoking both cold injuries and altitude problems.[35,215,219,269,282] Ultraviolet light penetration increases approximately 4% per 300 m gain in altitude, increasing the risk of sunburn, skin cancer, and snowblindness. Reflection of sunlight in glacial cirques and on flat glaciers can cause intense radiation of heat in the absence of wind. We have observed temperatures of 40° to 42° C in tents on both Mt. Everest and Mt. McKinley. Heat problems, primarily heat exhaustion, are often unrecognized in this usually cold environment. Dark clothing on still, sunny days increases heat absorption. Physiologists have not yet examined the consequences of heat stress or rapid, extreme changes in environmental temperature combined with the hypoxia of high altitude.

Above the snow line is the "high-altitude desert," where water can be obtained only by melting snow or ice. This factor, combined with increased water loss through the lungs from increased respiration and through the skin, commonly results in dehydration that may be debilitating. Thus the high-altitude environment imposes multiple stresses, some of which may contribute to or be confused with high-altitude illnesses.

Acclimatization to High Altitude

Rapid ascent and exposure to the altitude at the summit of Mt. Everest (8848 m) cause loss of consciousness in a few minutes and death shortly thereafter. Yet climbers ascending Mt. Everest over a period of weeks, without supplemental oxygen, have experienced only minor symptoms of illness. The process by which individuals gradually adjust to hypoxia and enhance survival and performance is termed acclimatization. A complex series of physiologic adjustments increases oxygen delivery to cells and improves their hypoxic tolerance. The severity of hypoxic stress, rate of onset, and individual physiology determine whether the body successfully acclimatizes or is overwhelmed.

Individuals vary in their ability to acclimatize; some adjust quickly, without discomfort, while AMS develops in others, who go on to recover. A small percentage fail to acclimatize even with gradual exposure over weeks. The tendency to acclimatize well or to become ill is consistent on repeated exposure if rate of ascent and altitude gained are similar.[231] Successful initial acclimatization protects against altitude illness and improves sleep. Longer term acclimatization (weeks) primarily improves aerobic exercise ability. These adjustments disappear at a similar rate on descent to low altitude. A few days at sea level may be sufficient to render a person susceptible to altitude illness, especially high-altitude pulmonary edema (HAPE), on reascent. The improved ability to do physical work at high altitude, however, persists for weeks.[164] Persons who live at high altitude during growth and development appear to realize the maximum benefit of acclimatization changes; for example, their exercise performance matches that of persons at sea level.[31,192] No genetic adaptation to high altitude in humans has yet been confirmed, but a recent report of normal pulmonary artery pressures in Tibetans, unlike those of all other high-altitude peoples studied, is intriguing.[194]

VENTILATION

By reducing alveolar carbon dioxide, increased ventilation raises alveolar oxygen, improving efficiency of delivery (Fig. 1-1). This response starts at an altitude as low as 1500 m (PIO_2 = 122 mm Hg)[195] and within the first few hours of high-altitude exposure. The carotid body, sensing a decrease in arterial PO_2, signals the central respiratory center in the medulla to increase ventilation. This carotid body function (hypoxic ventilatory response or HVR) may be genetically determined but is influenced by a number of extrinsic factors.[225,284] Respiratory depressants such as alcohol and soporifics, as well as fragmented sleep, depress the HVR. Agents that increase general metabolism, such as caffeine and coca, as well as specific respiratory stimulants, such as progesterone[149] and almitrine,[87] also increase the HVR. (Acetazolamide, a respiratory stimulant, acts on the central respiratory center rather than on the carotid body.) Physical conditioning apparently has no effect on the HVR. Numerous studies have shown that a good ventilatory response enhances acclimatization and performance* and that a low HVR may contribute to illness (see "Acute Mountain Sickness" and "High-Altitude Pulmonary Edema").

Other factors influence ventilation on ascent to high altitude. As ventilation increases, hypocapnia produces alkalosis, which acts as a braking mechanism on the central respiratory center and limits a further increase in ventilation.[116] To compensate for the alkalosis, within 24 to 48 hours of ascent the kidneys excrete bicarbonate, decreasing the pH toward normal; ventilation increases as the negative effect of the alkalosis is removed. Ventilation continues to increase slowly, reaching a maximum only after 4 to 7 days at the same altitude (Fig. 1-2).[45] The plasma bicarbonate concentration continues to drop and ventilation to increase with each successive ascending altitude. This process is greatly facilitated by acetazolamide (see "Acetazolamide Prophylaxis").

A way to appreciate the importance of the ventilatory pump at increasing altitude is to plot values for alveolar oxy-

*References 173, 174, 193, 238, 241, 242.

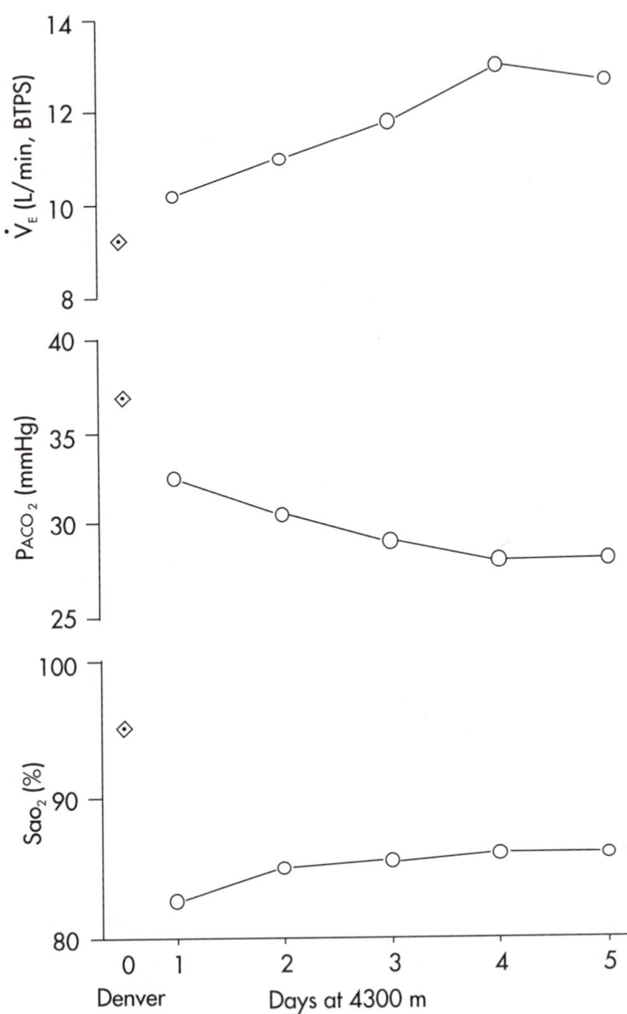

Fig. 1-2 Change in minute ventilation, end-tidal carbon dioxide (P_{ACO_2}), and arterial oxygen saturation (Sa_{O_2}) during 5 days' acclimatization to 4300 m. (Modified from Huang SY et al: *J Appl Physiol* 56[3]:602, 1984.)

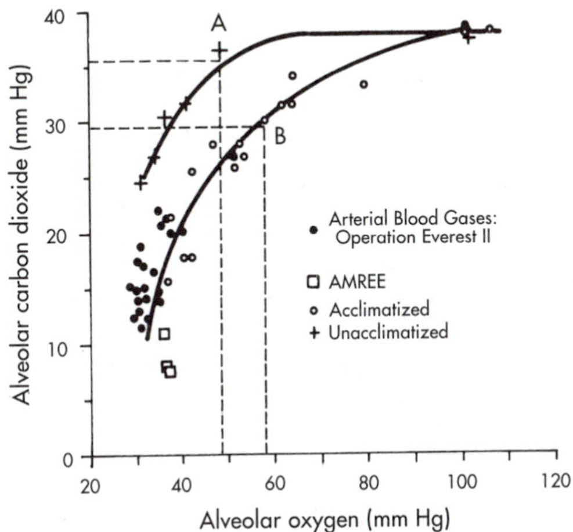

Fig. 1-3 Rahn-Otis diagram, with recent data from extreme high altitude. Note that after acclimatization, alveolar oxygen is higher because of lower alveolar carbon dioxide. Point *A* is average alveolar gases in unacclimatized subjects (1 hour's exposure) to 3800 m. Point *B* is after acclimatization to 3800 m. (Data from Malconian MK et al: *Aviat Space Environ Med* 63:37, 1993; Rahn H, Otis AB: *Am J Physiol* 157[2]:445, 1949; and West JB et al: *J Appl Physiol* 55[3]:678, 1983.)

gen and carbon dioxide on the Rahn and Otis diagram (Fig. 1-3). This approach clearly contrasts the effects of acute and chronic hypoxic exposure and can be used to assess the degree of ventilatory acclimatization.[213] As ventilation increases, the decrease in alveolar carbon dioxide allows an equivalent increase in alveolar oxygen. The level of ventilation (~P_{ACO_2}) is therefore what determines alveolar oxygen for a given inspired oxygen tension, according to the alveolar gas equation: $P_{AO_2} = P_{IO_2} - P_{ACO_2}/R$. The paramount importance of hyperventilation is readily apparent from the following calculation: the alveolar P_{O_2} on the summit of Mt. Everest (about 33 mm Hg) would be reached at only 5000 m if alveolar P_{CO_2} stayed at 40 mm Hg, limiting an ascent without supplemental oxygen to near this altitude. Table 1-3 gives the measured arterial blood gases resulting from short-term acclimatization to various altitudes.[247]

CIRCULATION

The circulatory pump is the next step in the transfer of oxygen, moving oxygenated blood from the lungs to the tissues.

Systemic Circulation

Increased catecholamine activity on ascent causes an initial mild increase in blood pressure, a moderate increase in heart rate and cardiac output, and an increase in venous tone. Stroke volume is low because of decreased plasma volume, which drops as much as 15% over 1 to 3 days[96] as a result of the bicarbonate diuresis and a fluid shift from the intravascular space. Resting heart rate returns to near sea level values with acclimatization, except at extremely high altitude. Maximum heart rate follows the decline in maximal oxygen uptake with increasing altitude. As the limits of hypoxic acclimatization are approached, maximum and resting heart rates converge. During OEII, cardiac function was appropriate for the level of work performed and cardiac output was not a limiting factor for performance.[216,264] Interestingly, myocardial ischemia at high altitude has not been reported in healthy persons, despite marked hypoxemia. This is partly because of the reduction in myocardial oxygen demand from reduced maximal heart rate and cardiac output.[71] Pulmonary capillary wedge pressures are low, and there has been no evidence of left ventricular dysfunction or abnormal filling pressures in humans at rest.[75,126] On echocardiography the left ventricle is smaller than normal because of decreased stroke volume, while the right ventricle may become enlarged.[123,264]

Pulmonary Circulation

A prompt but variable increase in pulmonary vascular resistance occurs on ascent to high altitude as a result of hypoxic pulmonary vasoconstriction. This increases pulmonary artery pressure.[161] Mild pulmonary hypertension is greatly augmented by exercise, with pulmonary pressure reaching near-systemic values,[75] especially in persons with a previous history of high-altitude pulmonary edema.[131,138,303] During OEII, Groves and colleagues[75] demonstrated that even when associated with a mean pulmonary artery pressure of 60 mm Hg, cardiac output remained appropriate and right atrial pressure did not rise above sea level values. This suggested that right ventricular function was intact in spite of extreme hypoxemia and hypertension.

Administration of oxygen at high altitude does not completely restore pulmonary artery pressure to sea level values, which indicates that increased pulmonary vascular resistance may not result solely from hypoxic vasoconstriction.[75,124,125] Obstructive pulmonary vascular lesions such as microemboli or microthrombi, endothelial cell swelling, or remodeling with medial hypertrophy have been hypothesized.[118,248]

Cerebral Circulation

Cerebral oxygen delivery is the product of arterial oxygen content and cerebral blood flow (CBF) and depends on the net balance between hypoxic vasodilation and hypocapnia-induced vasoconstriction. CBF is thought to increase, despite the hypocapnia, when Pa_{O_2} is less than 60 mm Hg (altitude greater than 2800 m). CBF increased 24% on abrupt ascent to 3810 m and then returned to normal over 3 to 5 days.[249] More recent studies have shown considerable individual variation,[117,218] but overall, cerebral oxygen delivery is thought to be well maintained with moderate hypoxia.[42] As cerebral oxygen delivery starts to decrease, the extraction fraction of the brain increases to compensate (see "Acute Mountain Sickness").

BLOOD

Hemopoietic Responses to Altitude

Ever since the observation in 1890 by Viault[275] that hemoglobin concentration was higher than normal in animals living in the Andes, scientists have regarded the hemopoietic response to increasing altitude as an important component of the acclimatization process.[34,209,297] Interestingly, hemoglobin concentration has no relationship to susceptibility to high-altitude illness.

In response to hypoxemia, erythropoietin is secreted and stimulates bone marrow production of red blood cells. The hormone is detectable within 2 hours of ascent, nucleated immature red blood cells can be found on a peripheral blood smear within days, and new red blood cells are in circulation within 4 to 5 days. Over a period of weeks to months, red blood cell mass increases in proportion to the degree of hypoxemia. Women who take supplemental iron have a greater increase in hematocrit than those who do not (Fig. 1-4).[95] Recent studies during OEII suggest that the maximum erythropoietic stimulation may occur at modest rather than extreme altitudes.[267]

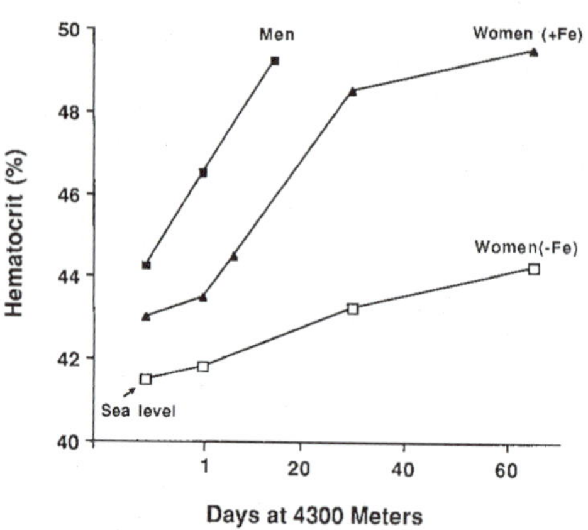

Fig. 1-4 Hematocrit changes on ascent to altitude in men and in women with and without supplemental iron. (Modified from Hannon JP, Chinn KS, Shields JL: *Fed Proc* 28[3]:1178, 1969.)

Overshoot of the hemopoietic response causes excessive polycythemia, which may actually impair oxygen transport because of increased blood viscosity. Although the "ideal" hematocrit at high altitude is not established, phlebotomy is often recommended when hematocrit values exceed 60% to 65%.[296,297] During AMREE, hematocrit was reduced by hemodilution from 58% ± 1.3% to 50.5% ± 1.5% at 5400 m with no decrement in maximum oxygen uptake and an increase in cerebral functioning.[237] The increase in hemoglobin concentration seen 1 to 2 days after ascent is due to hemoconcentration secondary to decreased plasma volume, rather than a true increase in red blood cell mass. This effects a higher hemoglobin concentration at the cost of decreased blood volume, a trade-off that may impair exercise performance. Longer term acclimatization leads to an increase in plasma volume as well as in red blood cell mass, thereby increasing total blood volume.

Oxyhemoglobin Dissociation Curve

The oxygen dissociation curve plays a crucial role in oxygen transport. Because of the sigmoidal shape of the curve, Sa_{O_2}% is well maintained up to 3000 m, despite a significant decrease in arterial P_{O_2} (Fig. 1-1). Above that altitude, small changes in arterial P_{O_2} result in large changes in arterial oxygen saturation (Fig. 1-5).

In 1936, Ansel Keys and colleagues[7,141] demonstrated an in vitro right shift in the position of the oxyhemoglobin dissociation curve at high altitude, a shift that favors the release of oxygen from the blood to the tissues. This change occurs because of the increase in 2,3-diphosphoglycerate

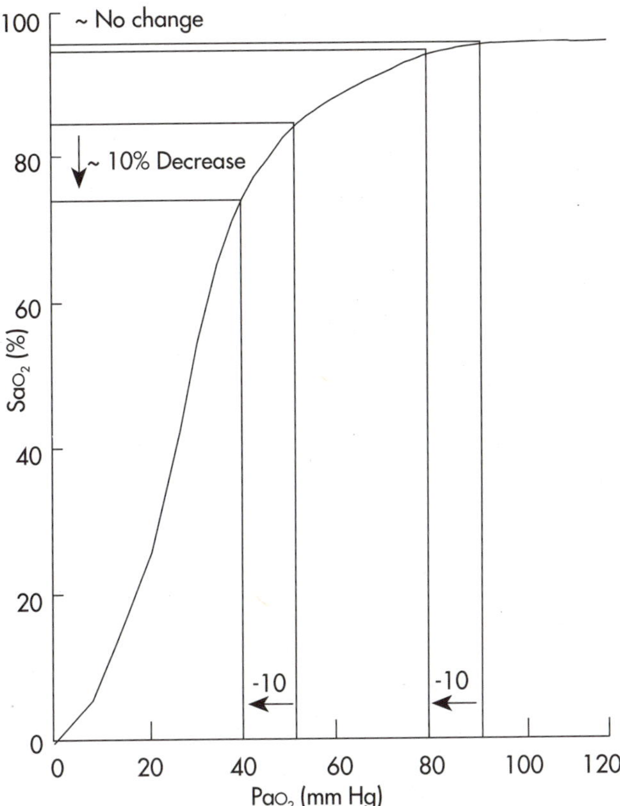

Fig. 1-5 Oxygen-hemoglobin dissociation curve showing effect of 10 torr decrement in PaO_2 on arterial oxygen saturation at sea level and near 4400 m. (Modified from Severinghaus JW et al: *Circ Res* 19:274, 1966.)

(2,3-DPG), which is proportional to the severity of hypoxemia. In vivo, however, this is offset by the alkalosis, and at moderate altitude little net change occurs in the position of the oxygen dissociation curve. On the other hand, the marked alkalosis of extreme hyperventilation, as measured on the summit and simulated summit of Mt. Everest (PCO_2 8 to 10 mm Hg, pH greater than 7.5), shifts the oxygen-hemoglobin dissociation curve to the left, which facilitates oxygen-hemoglobin binding in the lung, raises SaO_2%, and is thought to be advantageous.[236,286] This concept is further supported by observing that when persons with a very left-shifted oxygen-hemoglobin curve, caused by an abnormal hemoglobin (Andrew-Minneapolis), were taken to moderate (3100 m) altitude, they had less tachycardia and dyspnea and remarkably had no decrease in exercise performance.[103]

TISSUE CHANGES

The next link in the oxygen transport chain is tissue oxygen transfer, which depends on capillary perfusion, diffusion distance, and driving pressure of oxygen from the capillary to the cell. The final link, then, is use of oxygen within the cell. Banchero[11] has shown that capillary density in dog skeletal muscle doubled in 3 weeks at a barometric pressure of 435 mm Hg. A recent study in humans noted higher than normal muscle capillary density, although it was impossible to determine whether this was an adaptation to high altitude or to physical training.[200] Ou and Tenney[205] revealed a 40% increase in mitochondrial number but no change in mitochondrial size, while the study of Oelz and colleagues[200] showed that high-altitude climbers had normal mitochondrial density. During OEII a significant reduction in muscle size was noted, and although no de novo synthesis of capillaries or mitochondria occurred, capillary density and the ratio of mitochondrial volume to contractile protein fraction increased, primarily as a result of the atrophy.[165] Nevertheless, this change decreased the diffusion distance for oxygen.

SLEEP AT HIGH ALTITUDE

Disturbed sleep is common at high altitude.[208,220,268,270,285] Reite and colleagues[220] studied six men during a 12-day stay at 4300 m. All subjects complained of disturbed sleep. Compared with sea level control studies, in stages 3 and 4 sleep time decreased significantly, stage 1 time increased, and stage 2 did not change. More time was spent awake, with a significant increase in arousals and slightly less rapid eye movement (REM) time. The subjective complaints of poor sleep were out of proportion to the small reduction in total sleep time. Five of the six had periodic breathing. Interestingly, the arousals were not necessarily related to periodic breathing. One subject had periodic breathing for 90% of the night and no recorded arousals. With more extreme hypoxia, sleep time was dramatically shortened and arousals increased, without a change in ratio of sleep stages but with a reduction in REM sleep.[4] Presumably the mechanism of the arousals is cerebral hypoxia.

Periodic Breathing

Periodic breathing is primarily a nocturnal phenomenon, characterized by hyperpnea followed by apnea (Fig. 1-6). Respiratory alkalosis during hyperpnea acts on the central respiratory center, causing apnea. During apnea, SaO_2% decreases, carbon dioxide level increases, and the carotid body is stimulated, causing a recurrent hyperpnea and apnea cycle. Persons with a high hypoxic ventilatory response have more periodic breathing, with mild oscillations in SaO_2%,[151] while persons with a low hypoxic ventilatory response have more even breathing but may suffer periods of extreme hypoxemia not related to periodic breathing.[85,87] As acclimatization progresses, periodic breathing lessens but does not disappear and arterial oxygen saturation increases (Fig. 1-7).[208,263,268] Periodic breathing has not been associated with high-altitude illness, but a chaotic pattern without apparent periodicity was found in HAPE-susceptible subjects.[63]

WILLIAM F. MAAG LIBRARY
YOUNGSTOWN STATE UNIVERSITY

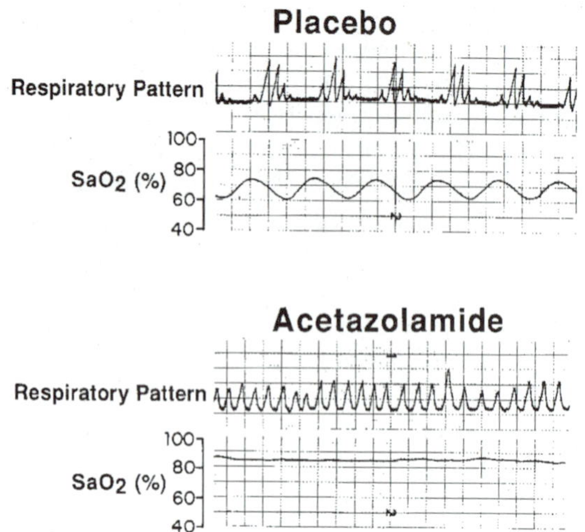

Fig. 1-6 Respiratory patterns and arterial oxygen saturation (Sao_2) with placebo and acetazolamide in two sleep studies of subject at 4200 m. Note pattern of hyperpnea followed by apnea during placebo treatment, which is changed with acetazolamide. (Modified from Hackett PH et al: *Am Rev Respir Dis* 135:896, 1987.)

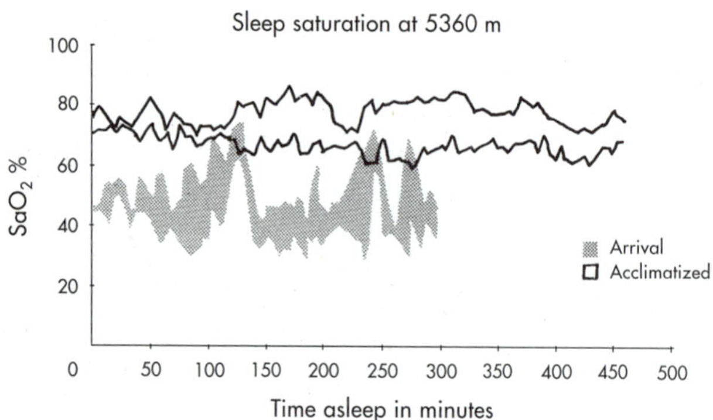

Fig. 1-7 Sleep oxygenation improves with acclimatization to same altitude. Top line is maximum and bottom line is minimum Sao_2 in acclimatized person. Shaded area is maximum and minimum Sao_2 values for new arrival at 5360 m. (Modified from Sutton JR et al: *N Engl J Med* 301[24]:1329, 1979.)

Acetazolamide, 125 mg at bedtime, diminishes periodic breathing, improves oxygenation, and is a safe and superior agent to use as a sleeping aid (Figs. 1-6 and 1-7).[87] If insomnia is due to causes other than periodic breathing, diphenhydramine (Benadryl, 50 to 75 mg) or the short-acting benzodiazepines such as triazolam (Halcion, 0.125 to 0.25 mg) and temazepam (Restoril, 15 mg) can be used. However, these are potentially dangerous in ill persons at high altitude because of resulting respiratory depression, and they may decrease oxygenation even in persons who are acclimating well.[208] Bradwell and colleagues[30] showed that acetazolamide (500 mg slow-release orally) given with temazepam (10 mg orally) improved sleep and maintained arterial oxygen saturation, counteracting a 20% decrease in arterial oxygen saturation when temazepam was given alone.

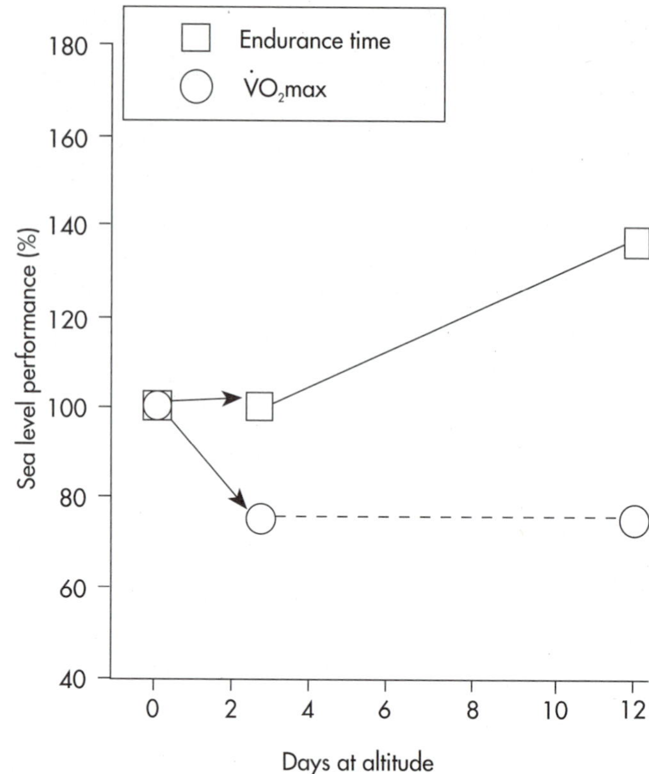

Fig. 1-8 On ascent to altitude, $\dot{V}o_2$max decreases and remains suppressed. In contrast, endurance time (minutes to exhaustion at 75% of altitude-specific $\dot{V}o_2$max) increases with acclimatization. (Modified from Maher JT, Jones LG, Hartley LH: *J Appl Physiol* 37[6]:895, 1974.)

EXERCISE

Maximal oxygen consumption drops dramatically on ascent to high altitude. Data from the Andes,[62,273] the Himalaya,[209] and the Colorado Rocky Mountains[72] indicate a decrease in maximal oxygen uptake ($\dot{V}o_2$max) from sea level of approximately 10% for each 1000 m of altitude gain above 1500 m.[31] Those with the highest sea level $\dot{V}o_2$max values had the greatest decrement in $\dot{V}o_2$max at high altitude, but overall performance at high altitude is not consistently related to sea level $\dot{V}o_2$max.[200,222] In fact, many of the world's elite mountaineers have quite average $\dot{V}o_2$max values, in contrast to other endurance athletes.[200] If a person remains at a constant moderate altitude, such as 4300 m, many of the processes associated with acclimatization will occur, enhancing submaximal endurance time 62% in 12 days,[166] but an increase in maximal oxygen uptake will not be seen (Fig. 1-8).[235]

Oxygen transport during exercise at high altitude becomes increasingly dependent on the ventilatory pump. The marked rise in ventilation produces a sensation of breathlessness, even at low work levels. The following quotation is from a high-altitude mountaineer:

> After every few steps, we huddle over our ice axes, mouths agape, struggling for sufficient breath to keep our muscles going. I have the feeling I am about to burst apart. As we get higher, it becomes necessary to lie down to recover our breath.[183]

In contrast to the increase in ventilation with exercise, at increasing altitudes in OEII, cardiac function and cardiac output were maintained at or near sea level values for a given oxygen consumption (workload). Although related to decreased oxygen transport, the exact limiting factors to exercise at high altitude remain elusive. Wagner[280] has proposed that the pressure gradient for diffusion of oxygen from capillaries to the working muscle cells may be inadequate.

Training at High Altitude

Optimal training for increased performance at high altitude depends on the altitude of residence and the athletic event. For aerobic activities (events lasting more than 3 or 4 minutes) at altitudes above 2000 m, acclimatization for 10 to 20 days is necessary to maximize performance.[8] For events occurring above 4000 m, acclimatization at an intermediate altitude is recommended. Highly anaerobic events at intermediate altitudes require only arrival at the time of the event, although mountain sickness may become a problem. At higher altitudes time must be allowed for acclimatization.

The benefits of training at high altitude for subsequent performance at or near sea level depend on choosing the training altitude that maximizes the benefits and minimizes the "detraining" inevitable when maximal oxygen uptake is limited (altitude greater than 1500 to 2000 m). Hence, data from training above 2400 m have shown no increase in subsequent sea level performance. Balke, Nagle, and Daniels[10] returned subjects to sea level after 10 days' training at 2000 m and demonstrated an increase in aerobic power, plasma volume, and hemoglobin concentration, with faster running times. More recent work suggests training benefits from intermittent altitude exposure[157] and from training at low altitude while sleeping at high altitude.[159] Whatever the mechanism of performance enhancement, coaches and endurance athletes from around the world are convinced of the benefits of training at moderate altitude for sea level performance.[46]

HIGH-ALTITUDE DETERIORATION

On the International High Altitude Expedition to Chile in 1935, Ansel Keys[140] reported that residents who lived at an altitude of 5340 m and worked in the mines approximately 500 m higher preferred to live low and work high. Apparently they could not live and work at the higher altitude because of weight loss, increasing lethargy, very poor quality sleep, weakness, and headache. This was taken as good evidence that altitudes of approximately 5800 m were probably the upper limit for long-term human habitation. Although considerable interindividual variation is to be expected above such altitudes, mountaineers also report that prolonged stays result in their deterioration rather than further acclimatization.

In persons with chronic lung disease the point of deterioration may be as low as 1750 m. The higher above the maximum point of acclimatization, the more rapid the deterioration. Above 8000 m, deterioration is so rapid that without supplemental oxygen death can occur in a matter of days. Life-preserving tasks such as melting snow for water may become too difficult and death may result from dehydration, starvation, hypothermia, and perhaps high-altitude illness.

Body weight is progressively lost because of anorexia and malabsorption during expeditions to extreme high altitude. Pugh[210] reported a 14 to 20 kg body weight loss in climbers on the 1953 British Mt. Everest Expedition. Nearly 30 years later, with improvement in food and cooking techniques, climbers on the American Medical Research Expedition to Mt. Everest still lost an average of 6 kg.[28] This was due in part to a 49% decrease in fat absorption and a 24% decrease in carbohydrate absorption. During OEII, in which the "climbers" were allowed to eat foods of their choosing ad libitum, they still suffered large weight losses: 8 kg overall, including 3 kg of fat and 5 kg of lean body weight (muscle).[113] At 4300 m, weight loss was attenuated by adjusting caloric intake to match caloric expenditure.[32] Thus significant weight loss with prolonged exposure to high altitude may be overcome with adequate caloric intake, but decreased appetite is a problem.[139]

High-Altitude Syndromes

High-altitude syndromes are illnesses attributed directly to hypobaric hypoxia. Exact mechanisms, however, are unclear. For example, all persons at high altitude are hypoxic and those with AMS are barely more hypoxemic than those who are well.[56,57] Also, there is a delay from the onset of hypoxia to the onset of high-altitude illness. These two facts have led to the conclusion that hypoxia induces time-dependent processes that are responsible for AMS, in contrast to the syndrome of acute hypoxia.[73]

Considerable overlap exists among the high-altitude syndromes, and terminology and classification of high-altitude illness remain somewhat confusing. Sudden exposure to extreme altitude may result in death from acute hypoxia (asphyxia), while more gradual ascent to the same altitude may result in AMS or no illness at all. Where "acute hypoxia" ends and AMS begins is vague, as reflected in the classic experiments of Bert.[25] Nevertheless, the general concept of a spectrum of altitude illness with a common underlying pathogenesis is well accepted and provides a useful framework for discussion. Acute hypoxia is one end of the spectrum, followed by AMS, with pulmonary and cerebral edema at the severe end of the spectrum. These illnesses all occur within the first few days of ascent to a higher altitude, have many common features, and respond to descent and oxygen. Longer term problems of altitude exposure include high-altitude deterioration and chronic mountain sickness.

ACUTE HYPOXIA

Acute, profound hypoxia, although of greatest interest in aviation medicine, may also occur on terra firma when ascent is too rapid or when hypoxia abruptly worsens. Carbon monoxide poisoning, pulmonary edema, overexertion, sleep apnea, or a failed oxygen delivery system may rapidly exaggerate hypoxemia. In an unacclimatized person, loss of consciousness from acute hypoxia occurs at an Sao_2% of 40% to 60% or at an arterial Po_2 of less than about 30 mm Hg.[24] A graphic description of the effects of acute hypoxia was given in 1875 by Tissandier, the sole survivor of the flight of the balloon *Zenith:*

> But soon I was keeping absolutely motionless, without suspecting that perhaps I had already lost use of my movements. Towards 7,500 m, the numbness one experiences is extraordinary. The body and the mind weakens little by little, gradually, unconsciously, without one's knowledge. One does not suffer at all; on the contrary. One experiences inner joy, as if it were an effect of the inundating flood of light. One becomes indifferent; one no longer thinks of the perilous situation or of the danger; one rises and is happy to rise. Vertigo of the lofty regions is not a vain word. But as far as I can judge by my personal impression, this vertigo appears at the last moment; it immediately precedes annihilation—sudden, unexpected, irresistible. I wanted to seize the oxygen tube, but could not raise my arm. My mind, however, was still very lucid. I was still looking at the barometer; my eyes were fixed on the needle which soon reached the pressure number of 280, beyond which it passed. I wanted to cry out "We are at 8,000 meters." But my tongue was paralyzed. Suddenly I closed my eyes and fell inert, completely losing consciousness.[25]

The ascent to over 8000 m took 3 hours, and the descent less than 1 hour. When the balloon landed, Tissandier's two companions were dead.

The prodigious work that Paul Bert conducted in an altitude chamber during the 1870s showed that lack of oxygen, rather than an effect of isolated hypobaria, explained the symptoms experienced during rapid ascent to extreme altitude.

> [T]here exists a parallelism to the smallest details between two animals, one of which is subjected in normal air to a progressive diminution of pressure to the point of death, while the other breathes, also to the point of death, under normal pressure, an air that grows weaker and weaker in oxygen. Both will die after having presented the same symptoms.[25]

Bert goes on to describe the symptoms of acute exposure to hypoxia:

> [I]t is the nervous system which reacts first. The sensation of fatigue, the weakening of the sense perceptions, the cerebral symptoms, vertigo, sleepiness, hallucinations, buzzing in the ears, dizziness, pricklings . . . are the signs of insufficient oxygenation of central and peripheral nervous organs. . . . The symptoms of decompression disappear very quickly when the balloon descends from the higher altitudes, very quickly also . . . the normal proportion of oxygen reappears in the blood. *There is an unfailing connection here.*[25]

Bert was also able to prevent and immediately resolve symptoms by breathing oxygen.

Acute hypoxia can be quickly reversed by immediate administration of oxygen, rapid pressurization or descent, or correction of an underlying cause, such as relief of apnea, removal of a carbon monoxide source, repair of an oxygen delivery system, or cessation of overexertion. Hyperventilation increases time of useful consciousness.

ACUTE MOUNTAIN SICKNESS

Although the syndrome of AMS has been recognized for centuries, modern rapid transport and the proliferation of participants in mountain sports have increased the number of victims and therefore public awareness (Table 1-1). The incidence and severity of AMS depend on the rate of ascent and the altitude attained (especially the sleeping altitude), length of altitude exposure, level of exertion, and inherent physiologic susceptibility. For example, AMS is more common on Mt. Rainier because of the rapid ascent, while high-altitude pulmonary edema is uncommon because of the short stay (less than 36 hours). Age has a small influence on incidence.[84] Women apparently have the same or a slightly greater incidence of AMS[84,100] but may be less susceptible to pulmonary edema.[260] It is useful clinically to classify AMS as mild, moderate, or severe on the basis of symptoms (Table 1-4). The primary significance of AMS is that it may progress to life-threatening pulmonary or cerebral edema.

Diagnosis

The diagnosis of AMS is based on setting, symptoms, physical findings, and exclusion of other illnesses. The setting is generally rapid ascent of unacclimatized persons to 2500 m or higher from altitudes below 1500 m. For partially acclimatized persons, abrupt ascent to a higher altitude, overexertion, and use of respiratory depressants are common contributing factors.

The cardinal symptoms of AMS are headache, fatigue, dizziness, and anorexia.[84,226,256] The headache is usually throbbing, bitemporal or occipital, typically worse during the night and on awakening, and made worse by Valsalva's maneuver or stooping over. A good appetite is distinctly uncommon. Nausea is common. These initial symptoms are strikingly similar to an alcohol hangover. Sleep may be fragmented by frequent awakening, and periodic breathing often produces a feeling of suffocation. Although sleep disorder is

Table 1-4 Distribution of Symptoms and Signs in 154 Trekkers in Nepal with Acute Mountain Sickness

Severity	Percent	Symptoms
Mild	65	Headache, anorexia, nausea, malaise
Moderate	30	Unrelieved headache, vomiting, reduced urine output
Severe	5	Altered consciousness, ataxia, rales, cyanosis, dyspnea at rest, possibly papilledema

Modified from Hackett PH, Rennie ID: *Am J Med* 67:214, 1979.

nearly universal at high altitude, these symptoms may be exaggerated during AMS. Affected persons commonly complain of a deep inner chill, unlike mere exposure to cold temperature, accompanied by facial pallor. Other symptoms may include vomiting, dyspnea on exertion, and irritability. Lassitude can be disabling, with the victim too apathetic to contribute to his or her own or the group's basic needs. Any symptom suggestive of AMS should be considered caused by altitude unless proven otherwise.

Pulmonary symptoms vary considerably. Everyone experiences dyspnea on exertion at high altitude; it may be difficult to distinguish normal from abnormal. Dyspnea at rest is distinctly abnormal and presages HAPE. Dry cough is common in AMS. Any pulmonary symptom mandates a careful examination for pulmonary edema.

Specific physical findings are lacking in mild AMS. Early authors described tachycardia, but Singh and associates[256] noted bradycardia (heart rate less than 66 beats/min) in two thirds of 1975 soldiers with AMS. Blood pressure is normal, but postural hypotension may be present. Rales localized to one area of the chest are common (25% to 35% incidence) and probably represent pulmonary vascular congestion.[81,108] No fever is present unless the individual has pulmonary edema. Funduscopic examination reveals venous tortuosity and dilation; retinal hemorrhages may or may not be present and are not diagnostic. Absence of the normal altitude diuresis, evidenced by lack of increased urine output and retention of fluid, is an early finding in AMS.[21,83,256]

Physical findings develop if AMS worsens. Ataxia is the single most useful sign for recognizing the progression of AMS from mild to severe. Lassitude may progress to the point of inability to perform perfunctory activities such as eating and dressing. Typically, as AMS progresses to cerebral edema, the victim wants to be left alone, declines to eat or drink, is ataxic, and finally has changes in consciousness with confusion, disorientation, and impaired judgment. Coma may ensue within 24 hours of the onset of ataxia.

Differential Diagnosis

AMS is most commonly misdiagnosed as a viral flulike illness, hangover, exhaustion, or dehydration. Unlike an infectious illness, uncomplicated AMS is not associated with fever and myalgias. Hangover is excluded by the history. A common misconception is that alcohol is more toxic at high altitude. The effects of alcohol on the brain are the same at low and high altitude.[61] Alcohol may actually potentiate the effects of altitude (not vice versa) because of dehydration, respiratory depression, increased pulmonary artery pressure, and hangover.

Exhaustion may cause lassitude, weakness, irritability, and headache and may therefore be difficult to distinguish from AMS. Dehydration, which causes weakness, decreased urine output, headache, and nausea, is commonly confused with AMS. Response to fluids helps to differentiate the two. AMS is not improved by fluid administration alone, nor does body hydration influence susceptibility to AMS.[5] Hypothermia may be manifested as ataxia and mental changes. Sleeping medication may also cause ataxia and mental changes without high-altitude illness the following day, but soporifics may also precipitate high-altitude illness because of increased hypoxemia during sleep.

Carbon Monoxide

Carbon monoxide poisoning is a danger at high altitude, where field shelters are designed to be small and windproof. Cooking inside closed tents and snow shelters during storms is a particular hazard, recently highlighted by two deaths on Mt. McKinley.[274] The effects of carbon monoxide and high-altitude hypoxia are additive. A reduction in oxyhemoglobin caused by carbon monoxide increases hypoxic stress, rendering a person at a "physiologically higher" altitude, which may precipitate AMS. Because of preexisting hypoxemia, smaller amounts of carboxyhemoglobin produce symptoms of carbon monoxide poisoning. These two problems may coexist. Immediate removal of the victim from the source of carbon monoxide and forced hyperventilation, preferably with supplemental oxygen, rapidly reverse carbon monoxide poisoning. Persistent unconsciousness in the setting of carbon monoxide exposure at high altitude can be caused by either severe carbon monoxide poisoning or high-altitude cerebral edema. The management is nearly the same and includes coma care, oxygen, descent, and evacuation to a hospital.

Pathophysiology

Although the basic cause of AMS is hypobaric hypoxia (Fig. 1-9), the syndrome is different from acute hypoxia. Because of a lag time in onset of symptoms after ascent and a lack of immediate reversal of all symptoms with oxygen, AMS is thought to be secondary to the body's responses to modest hypoxia. Indeed, an altitude of 2500 to 2700 m presents only a minor decrement in arterial oxygen transport (Sao_2% is still above 90%), but certain individuals may

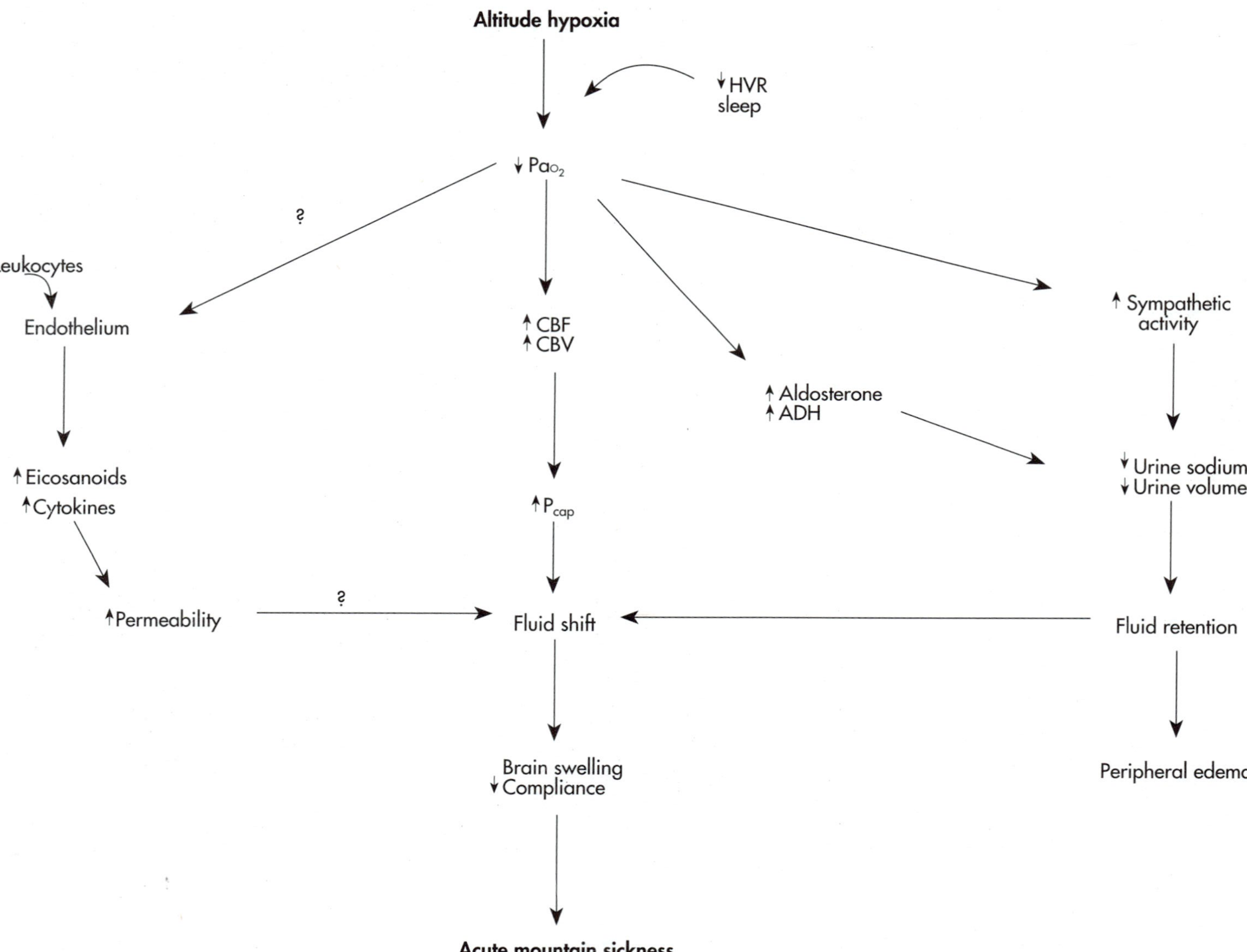

Fig. 1-9 Proposed pathophysiology of acute mountain sickness. *HVR,* Hypoxic ventilatory response; *CBF,* cerebral blood flow; *CBV,* cerebral blood volume; P_{cap}, capillary pressure; *ADH*, antidiuretic hormone.

nonetheless become desperately ill. Clearly, some persons are particularly susceptible, while others are relatively immune; the most predictive factor is previous history of AMS.

Findings documented in moderate to severe AMS that relate to pathophysiology include relative hypoventilation,* fluid retention and redistribution,[21,83,256] increased intracranial pressure,[112,147,256,295] and impaired gas exchange and pulmonary mechanics (interstitial edema).†

Relative hypoventilation may be due primarily to a decreased drive to breathe (low hypoxic ventilatory response) or may be secondary to ventilatory depression associated with AMS or HAPE.[225] Persons with quite low hypoxic ventilatory response are more likely to suffer AMS than are those with a high ventilatory drive.‡ For persons with intermediate hypoxic ventilatory response values (the majority of people), ventilatory drive probably has no predictive value.[185,225] Relative hypoventilation increases cerebral blood flow on the basis of both increased hypoxemia and relative hypercapnia. The protective role of the hypoxic ventilatory response most likely results from increased oxygen transport, with less cerebral hypoxia and less cerebral vasodilation.

The mechanism of fluid retention may be multifactorial. Renal responses to hypoxia are variable and depend on plasma arginine vasopressin (AVP) concentration.[104] Persons with AMS (and HAPE) had elevated plasma or urine AVP levels in some studies,[18,125,256] but cause and effect could not be established. Other studies showed no AVP elevation.[21,99] The usual decrease in aldosterone on ascent to altitude does not occur in persons with AMS, and this may contribute to the antidiuresis.[21] The renin-angiotensin system, although suppressed compared with its activity at sea level in both AMS and non-AMS groups, was more active in persons with AMS.[20] Claybaugh and colleagues[37] reported an actual increase in plasma renin activity. Atrial natriuretic peptide (ANP) is elevated in AMS. Although this is most likely compensatory,[20] data indicate that elevated plasma ANP level may contribute to microvascular permeability.[20,294] Delamere and Jones[44] reported decreased urine output in persons with AMS, resulting in part from decreased glomerular filtration rate, the reasons for which were elusive.[44] One factor that may explain many of these changes is increased sympathetic stimulation, which reduces renal blood flow, glomerular filtration rate, and urine output and suppresses renin; increased sympathetic nervous system activity is consistent with the greater rise in norepinephrine noted in subjects with AMS.[18] In any event it seems that renal water handling switches from net loss or no change to net gain of water as persons become ill with AMS. In addition to fluid retention, redistribution of fluid into the intracellular space takes place within 3 days, within the same time frame as the development of AMS.[60,96] Presumably the net water retention seen in AMS exaggerates the intracellular shift and could contribute to brain overhydration.[97] The effectiveness of diuretics in treating AMS supports a pivotal role for fluid retention and fluid shifts in the pathology of AMS.[256]

The increase in intracranial pressure known to occur in more advanced cases of AMS may be due either to cytotoxic edema with a shift of fluid into the cells, as mentioned previously, or to vasogenic (interstitial) edema from increased permeability of the blood-brain barrier, or both.[94] The classic view that hypoxia causes failure of the adenosine triphosphate (ATP)-dependent sodium pump and subsequent intracellular edema[110] is untenable, given the newer understanding of brain energetics. ATP levels are maintained in moderate and even severe hypoxemia.[252] Hackett and colleagues[93] recently reported magnetic resonance imaging (MRI) findings of white matter edema in high-altitude cerebral edema (HACE), and Levine[160] noted the same on a computed tomographic (CT) scan of one subject with moderately severe AMS. White matter edema, with sparing of the gray matter, supports vasogenic edema.[93] The fact that dexamethasone improves both AMS and vasogenic cerebral edema, but not other types of cerebral edema, also suggests that the edema in AMS is vasogenic. Although cell swelling may contribute in part, and would certainly exacerbate cerebral edema, the predominant mechanism seems to be vasogenic. The pathophysiology may be similar to hypertensive encephalopathy, in which loss of vascular autoregulation results in increased pressures transmitted to the capillaries with resultant white matter edema.[155,156,193]

The vasogenic brain swelling hypothesis is supported by a model of AMS in conscious sheep exposed to 10% oxygen for several days. Krasney and associates[146] have shown that cerebral capillary pressure rises, which causes filtration of fluid across the blood-brain barrier and an increase in wet to dry cerebral tissue ratio. Interestingly, cerebral oxygen delivery is maintained by increased cerebral blood flow, as in humans, and the cerebral metabolic rate for oxygen ($CMRO_2$) remains at stable normoxic levels after an initial transient increase. In fact, cerebral blood flow is apparently much greater than necessary for the $CMRO_2$, resulting in "luxury perfusion."

If cerebral oxygen consumption is constant, what causes the well-documented, albeit mild, cognitive changes at high altitude, and what causes vasogenic edema? The cognitive changes may be related to specific neurotransmitters that are affected by mild hypoxia; for example, tryptophan hydroxylase in the serotonin synthesis pathway has a high requirement for oxygen (Km = 37 mm Hg).[38,64] The edema may be due to dysfunction of oxygen-sensitive pathways regulating the blood-brain barrier, or more likely is due to changes in intracranial dynamics,[101] as in the sheep model (Fig. 1-9).[145]

Pulmonary dysfunction in AMS includes decreased vital capacity and peak expiratory flow,[3,135,154,256] increased alve-

*References 27, 68, 83, 142, 176, 193, 266.
†References 70, 135, 147, 154, 256, 266.
‡References 80, 115, 142, 174, 176, 193.

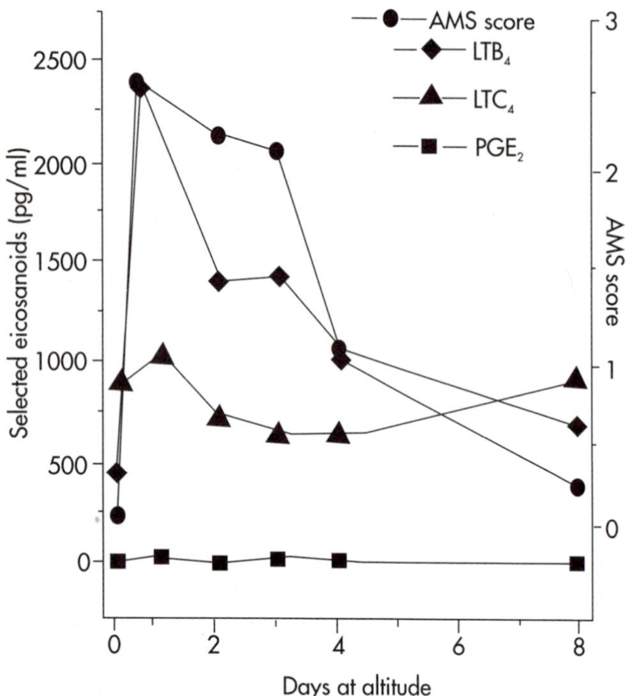

Fig. 1-10 Mean values for AMS score, leukotriene B_4 (LTB_4), leukotriene C_4 (LTC_4), and prostaglandin E_2 (PGE_2) over 8 days at high altitude in 10 subjects with acute mountain sickness. See text for explanation. (Modified from Richalet JP et al: *Respir Physiol* 85:205, 1991.)

olar-arterial oxygen difference,[70,91,266] decreased transthoracic impedance,[132,234] and a high incidence of rales.[81] These findings are compatible with interstitial edema, that is, increased extravascular lung water. Recent careful measurements of ventilation/perfusion ratios in the lung at various altitudes (4500 to 8800 m) have confirmed gross inequalities consistent with increased lung water in subjects without clinical evidence of pulmonary edema or AMS.[281] Accumulation of interstitial fluid is most likely minor or low-grade pulmonary edema, with a mechanism similar to that of HAPE.

A final consideration in the pathophysiology of AMS (and other high-altitude illnesses) is the concept of a primary dysfunction of the vascular endothelium leading to generalized increased vascular permeability. Preliminary data in humans with AMS showed increased eicosanoid LTB_4, favoring increased permeability, which paralleled the time course of AMS symptoms (Fig. 1-10).[221] Similar endothelial modulators were also found in lavage fluid of HAPE.[244] Whether this and other vasoactive mediators are primarily involved in the pathogenesis or are present as a secondary phenomenon remains unanswered.

Natural Course of Acute Mountain Sickness

The natural history of AMS varies with the initial altitude and rate of ascent and the clinical severity. Singh and associates[256] followed the illness in soldiers airlifted to altitudes of 3300 to 5500 m. Incapacitating illness lasted 2 to 5 days, but 40% still had symptoms after 1 week and 13% after 1 month. Nine soldiers failed to acclimatize in 6 months and were considered unfit for duty at high altitude.[256] Chinese investigators report that a percentage of lowland Han Chinese stationed on the Tibet Plateau cannot tolerate the altitude because of persistent symptoms and must be relocated to the plains. Persistent anorexia, nausea, and headache may afflict climbers at extreme altitude for weeks and can be considered a form of persistent AMS. The natural history of AMS in tourists who sleep at more moderate altitudes is much more benign. Duration of symptoms at 2700 m was 15 hours, with a range of 6 to 94 hours.[190] Most individuals treat or tolerate their symptoms as the illness resolves over 1 to 3 days while acclimatization improves, but some persons with AMS seek medical treatment or are forced to descend if symptoms persist. A small percentage (8% at 4243 m)[54] of those with AMS go on to develop cerebral or pulmonary edema, especially if ascent is continued in spite of illness.

Treatment

The proper management of AMS is based on early diagnosis and acknowledgment that initial clinical presentation does not predict eventual severity (Box 1-3). Therefore *proceeding to a higher sleeping altitude in the presence of symptoms is contraindicated.* The victim must be carefully monitored for progression of illness. If symptoms worsen despite an extra 24 hours of acclimatization or treatment, descent is indicated. The two indications for immediate descent are abnormal neurologic changes (ataxia or change in consciousness) and pulmonary edema.

Mild AMS can be treated by halting the ascent and waiting for acclimatization to improve, which can take from 12 hours to 3 or 4 days. Acetazolamide (125 to 250 mg twice a day orally) speeds acclimatization and thus terminates the illness if given early.[70] Symptomatic therapy includes analgesics such as aspirin (650 mg) or acetaminophen (650 to 1000 mg) for headache. Prochlorperazine (Compazine, 5 to 10 mg intramuscularly) can be given by an appropriate route for nausea and vomiting and has the advantage of augmenting the HVR.[204] Promethazine (Phenergan, 50 mg by suppository or ingestion) is also useful. Persons with AMS should avoid alcohol and sedative-hypnotics because of the danger of respiratory depression during sleep.

Descent to an altitude lower than where symptoms began effectively reverses AMS. Although the person should descend as far as necessary for improvement, descending 500 to 1000 m is usually sufficient. Exertion should be minimized. Oxygen, if available, is particularly effective (and supply is conserved) if given in low flow (0.5 to 1 L/min by mask or cannula) during the night. Oxygen usually, but not always, relieves a high-altitude headache. Experienced physicians and lay mountaineers have consistently noted that descent seems more effective than oxygen.

BOX 1-3

FIELD TREATMENT OF HIGH-ALTITUDE ILLNESS

MILD ACUTE MOUNTAIN SICKNESS

Stop ascent, rest, acclimatize at same altitude
Acetazolamide, 125 to 150 mg bid, to speed acclimatization
Symptomatic treatment as necessary with analgesics and antiemetics
or Descend 500 m or more

MODERATE ACUTE MOUNTAIN SICKNESS

Low-flow oxygen, if available
Acetazolamide, 125 to 250 mg bid, with or without dexamethasone, 4 mg po, IM, or IV q6h
Hyperbaric therapy
or Immediate descent

HIGH-ALTITUDE CEREBRAL EDEMA

Immediate descent or evacuation
Oxygen, 2 to 4 L/min
Dexamethasone, 4 mg po, IM, or IV q6h
Hyperbaric therapy

HIGH-ALTITUDE PULMONARY EDEMA

Minimize exertion and keep warm
Oxygen, 4 to 6 L/min until improving, then 2 to 4 L/min
Nifedipine, 10 mg po q4h by titration to response, or 10 mg po once, followed by 30 mg extended release q12 to 24h
Hyperbaric therapy
or Immediate descent

PERIODIC BREATHING

Acetazolamide, 62.5 to 125 mg at bedtime as needed

The use of diuretics has a sound basis because of fluid retention associated with AMS. Improvement with any therapy, as well as descent, is associated with a noticeable diuresis. Acetazolamide is of unquestionable prophylactic value and is now commonly and successfully used to treat AMS as well. Acetazolamide may be helpful in part because of its diuretic action; its multiple modes of action are discussed later. Singh and colleagues[256] successfully used furosemide (80 mg twice a day for 2 days) to treat 446 soldiers with all degrees of AMS; it has not been studied for treatment since.[256] Furosemide induced a brisk diuresis, relieved pulmonary congestion, and improved headache and other neurologic symptoms. Spironolactone, hydrochlorothiazide, and other diuretics have not yet been evaluated for treatment.

The steroid betamethasone was initially reported by Singh and associates[256] to improve symptoms of soldiers with severe AMS and to promote diuresis. Since then, dexamethasone, usually in combination with descent and oxygen, has been used routinely to treat HACE, without benefit of controlled study. Recently dexamethasone was found effective for treatment of moderate AMS. Hackett and colleagues[92] used 4 mg orally or intramuscularly every 6 hours, and Ferrazinni and associates[53] gave 8 mg initially, followed by 4 mg every 6 hours. Both studies reported marked improvement within 12 hours, with no significant side effects. Symptoms increased when dexamethasone was discontinued after 24 hours.[92,232] In light of these studies the indications for dexamethasone should be expanded to include treatment of moderate to severe AMS. The drug should probably be reserved for patients with progressive neurologic symptoms or ataxia, started in conjunction with descent if possible, and continued until the victim is down to low altitude. Although the mechanism of action of dexamethasone is not clear, it probably acts by improving brain capillary integrity and diminishing vasogenic edema. Dexamethasone seems not to improve acclimatization, since symptoms recur when the drug is withdrawn. Therefore an argument could be made for using dexamethasone to relieve symptoms and acetazolamide to speed acclimatization.

Hyperbaric chambers have been used to treat AMS and aid acclimatization in India, Tibet, China, and Nepal, mostly by the military. Pressurization simulates descent; it is thus effective and requires no supplemental oxygen. Lightweight (less than 7 kg) fabric pressure bags inflated by manual air pumps are now being used on mountaineering expeditions and in mountain clinics (Fig. 1-11). An inflation of 2 PSI is roughly equivalent to a drop in altitude of 1600 m; the exact equivalent depends on initial altitude.[130,227] A few hours of pressurization results in symptomatic improvement and can be an effective temporizing measure while awaiting descent or the benefit of medical therapy.[137,227] Long-term (12 hours or more) use of these portable devices would be necessary to resolve AMS completely but has not yet been reported.

Prevention

Graded ascent is the surest and safest method of prevention, although particularly susceptible individuals may still become ill (see Box 1-3). Current recommendations for persons without altitude experience are to avoid abrupt ascent to sleeping altitudes greater than 3000 m and to spend 2 to 3 nights at 2500 to 3000 m before going higher, with an extra night for acclimatization every 600 to 900 m if continuing ascent. Abrupt increases of more than 600 m in sleeping altitude should be avoided when over 2500 m. Day trips to higher altitude, with a return to lower altitude for sleep, aid acclimatization. Alcohol and sedative-hypnotics are best avoided on the first 2 nights at high altitude. A diet high in carbohydrates (greater than 70%) reduced AMS symptoms by 30% in soldiers taken quickly to near the summit of Pike's Peak (4300 m).[39,98] Overexertion is thought to con-

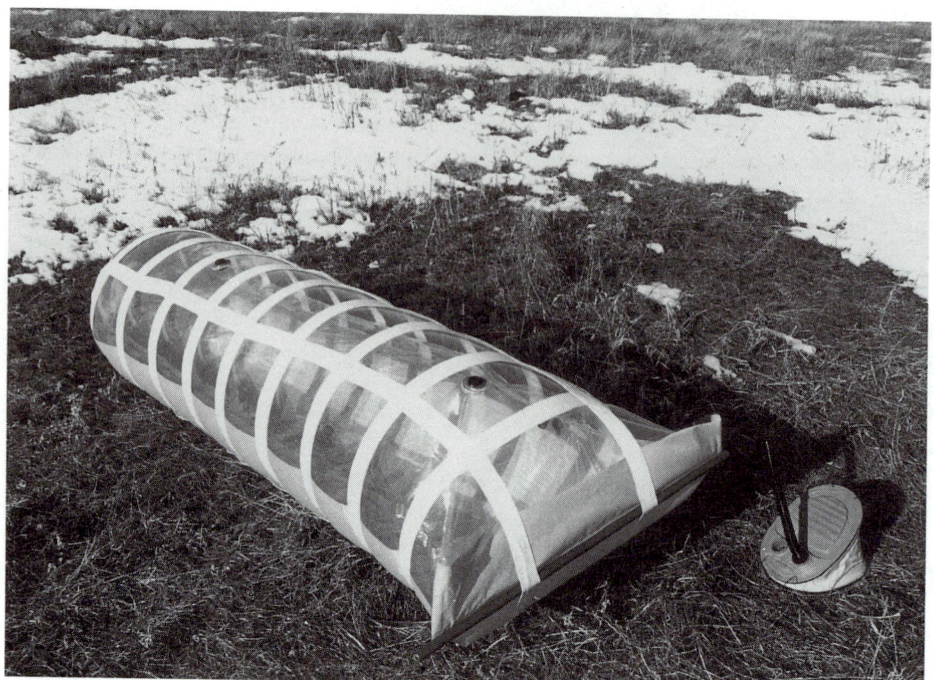

Fig. 1-11 The HELP System (Live High, Boulder, Colo.) uses breathing bladder technology to minimize the pumping necessary to circulate air in the hyperbaric compartment.

tribute to illness, while mild exercise seems to aid acclimatization.

Acetazolamide Prophylaxis. Acetazolamide is the drug of choice for prophylaxis of AMS. A carbonic anhydrase (CA) inhibitor, acetazolamide slows the hydration of carbon dioxide:

$$CO_2 + H_2O \overset{CA}{\Longleftrightarrow} H_2CO_3 \Longleftrightarrow H^+ + HCO_3^-$$

The effects are protean, involving particularly the red blood cells, brain, lungs, and kidneys. By inhibiting renal carbonic anhydrase, acetazolamide reduces reabsorption of bicarbonate and sodium and thus causes a bicarbonate diuresis and metabolic acidosis starting within 1 hour after ingestion. This rapidly enhances ventilatory acclimatization. Perhaps most important, the drug maintains oxygenation during sleep and prevents periods of extreme hypoxemia (Fig. 1-6).[87,270,272] Because of acetazolamide's diuretic action, it counteracts the fluid retention of AMS. It also diminishes nocturnal ADH secretion[37] and decreases cerebrospinal fluid (CSF) production and volume and possibly CSF pressure.[246] Which of these effects is most important in preventing AMS is unclear. Numerous studies taken together indicate that acetazolamide is approximately 75% effective in preventing AMS in persons rapidly transported to altitudes of 4000 to 4500 m.[33,54,57,69,154]

Indications for acetazolamide prophylaxis include rapid ascent (1 day or less) to altitudes over 3000 m; a rapid gain in sleeping altitude, for example, moving camp from 4000 m to 5000 m in a day; and a past history of recurrent AMS or HAPE. Numerous dosage regimens have been effective.[48,50] Smaller doses (125 to 250 mg twice a day) starting 24 hours before ascent work as well as higher doses started earlier. A 500 mg sustained action capsule of Diamox taken every 24 hours is probably equally effective and results in fewer side effects because of lower peak serum levels.[299] Most authors recommend continuing for the first day or two at high altitude, and some suggest daily acetazolamide the entire time at high altitude.[29] This hardly seems necessary once acclimatization is established and the danger of AMS has passed. Spironolactone[133,153] and other diuretics have shown equivocal results for AMS prevention.

Acetazolamide has side effects, most notably peripheral paresthesias and polyuria, and less commonly nausea, drowsiness, impotence, and myopia. Since it inhibits the instant hydration of carbon dioxide on the tongue, acetazolamide allows carbon dioxide to be tasted and can ruin the flavor of carbonated beverages, including beer. A sulfa drug, acetazolamide carries the usual precautions about hypersensitivity, crystalluria, and bone marrow suppression.

Dexamethasone. Dexamethasone is also useful for prevention of AMS. The initial chamber study in 1984 was with sedentary subjects.[134] The drug reduced the incidence of AMS from 78% to 20%, comparable to previous studies with acetazolamide. Dexamethasone was not as effective in exercising subjects on Pike's Peak,[232] but subsequent work has shown effectiveness comparable to acetazolamide.[52,160,305] The combination of acetazolamide and dexamethasone proved superior to dexamethasone alone.[305] Because of potential serious side effects and the rebound phenomenon, dexamethasone is best reserved for treatment rather than for prevention of AMS, or used for prophylaxis when necessary in persons intolerant of or allergic to acetazolamide.

NEUROLOGIC SYNDROMES

The neurologic syndromes of high altitude encompass multiple pathologic diagnoses. Because of the remote location of these events, few reliable clinical and experimental data are available to document exact diagnoses. Cerebral edema, however, is well described in animals and was well documented in humans by Singh and associates,[256] who considered it the end stage of AMS. Since their description, most neurologic problems at high altitude have been diagnosed as high-altitude cerebral edema, which has clearly not always been appropriate. Other syndromes now recognized on clinical or pathologic grounds include cerebrovascular spasm, cerebral arterial or venous thrombosis, transient ischemic attacks, and hemorrhage from aneurysms, arterial venous malformations, or other causes. Cerebral edema is characterized by generalized encephalopathy, while the other syndromes are more often characterized by focal lesions.

High-Altitude Cerebral Edema

HACE is characterized clinically by a progression to encephalopathy in the setting of AMS or HAPE. As discussed previously, AMS is essentially a neurologic disorder, probably related to brain swelling, and HACE appears to be the extreme form of AMS; the distinction between AMS and HACE is inherently blurred.

Clinical Presentation. The hallmarks of HACE are ataxic gait, severe lassitude, and altered consciousness, including confusion, impaired mentation, drowsiness, stupor, and coma. Headache, nausea, and vomiting are frequently, but not always, present. Hallucinations, cranial nerve palsy, hemiparesis, hemiplegia, seizures, and focal neurologic signs have also been reported.[94,112,256] Retinal hemorrhages are common but not diagnostic. The progression from mild AMS to unconsciousness may be as fast as 12 hours but usually requires 1 to 3 days. Cyanosis or a gray pallor is common. Arterial blood gas study or pulse oximetry reveals exaggerated hypoxemia. Clinical examination, chest radiography, and autopsy have often demonstrated pulmonary edema; indeed, isolated HACE without HAPE is uncommon.[76,93]

The following case report from Mt. McKinley illustrates a clinical course of HACE, in conjunction with HAPE:

H.E. was a 26-year-old German lumberjack with extensive mountaineering experience. He ascended to 5200 m from 2000 m in 4 days and attempted the summit (6194 m) on the fifth day. At 5800 m he turned back because of severe fatigue, headache, and malaise. He returned alone to 5200 m, stumbling on the way because of loss of coordination. He had no appetite and crawled into his sleeping bag too weak, tired, and disoriented to undress. He recalled no pulmonary symptoms. In the morning H.E. was unarousable, slightly cyanotic, and noted to have Cheyne-Stokes respirations. After 10 minutes on high-flow oxygen H.E. began to regain consciousness, although he was completely disoriented and unable to move. A rescue team lowered him down a steep slope, and on arrival at 4400 m 4 hours later he was conscious but still disoriented, able to move extremities but unable to stand. Respiratory rate was 60 breaths/min and heart rate was 112 beats/min. Papilledema and a few rales were present. $Sao_2\%$ was 54% on room air (normal is 85% to 90%). On a nonrebreathing oxygen mask with 14 L/min oxygen, the $Sao_2\%$ increased to 88% and the respiratory rate decreased to 40 breaths/min. Eight milligrams of dexamethasone was administered intramuscularly at 4:20 PM and continued orally, 4 mg every 6 hours. At 5:20 PM H.E. began to respond to commands. The next morning H.E. was still ataxic but was able to stand, take fluids, and eat heartily. He was evacuated by air to Anchorage (sea level) at 12:00 PM. On admission to the hospital at 3:30 PM, roughly 36 hours after regaining consciousness, H.E. was somewhat confused and mildly ataxic. Arterial blood gas studies on room air showed a Po_2 of 58 mm Hg, pH of 7.5, and Pco_2 of 27 mm Hg. Bilateral pulmonary infiltrates were present on the chest radiograph. Magnetic resonance imaging of the brain revealed white matter edema, primarily of the corpus callosum (Fig. 1-12). On discharge the next morning H.E. was oriented, bright, and cheerful and had very minor ataxia and clear lung fields.

Pathophysiology. The pathophysiology of HACE is probably a progression of the same mechanism as in AMS (see "Acute Mountain Sickness" and Fig. 1-8). The early brain swelling of AMS becomes much more severe. In cases similar to this, lumbar punctures have revealed elevated CSF pressures, often more than 300 mm H_2O,[23,112,295] evidence of cerebral edema on CT scan and MRI,[93,144] and gross cerebral edema on necropsy.[47,49] Small petechial hemorrhages were also consistently found on autopsy, and venous sinus thromboses were occasionally seen.[47,49] Well-documented cases have often included pulmonary edema, which was not clinically apparent.

Whereas the mild brain swelling of AMS and reversible HACE is most likely vasogenic, as the spectrum shifts to severe, end-stage HACE, culminating in death, gray matter and presumably cytotoxic edema develops as well. As Klatzo[143] has pointed out, as vasogenic edema progresses, the distance between brain cells and their capillaries increases so that nutrients and oxygen eventually fail to diffuse and the cells are rendered ischemic, leading to intracellular (cytotoxic) edema. Raised intracranial pressure produces many of its effects by decreasing cerebral blood flow, and brain tissue becomes ischemic on this basis also.[180] Focal neurologic signs caused by brainstem distortion and by extraaxial compression, as in third and sixth cranial nerve palsies, may develop,[233] making cerebral edema difficult to differentiate from primary cerebrovascular events. The most common clinical presentation, however, is change in consciousness associated with ataxia, without focal signs.

Treatment. Successful treatment of HACE requires early recognition. At the first sign of ataxia or change in consciousness, descent should be started, dexamethasone (4 to 8 mg intravenously, intramuscularly, or orally initially, followed by 4 mg every 6 hours) administered, and oxygen (2 to 4 L/min by mask or nasal cannula) applied if available (Box 1-3). Oxygen can be titrated to maintain Sa_{O_2} at greater than 90% if oximetry is available. Comatose patients require additional airway management and bladder drainage. Attempting to decrease intracranial pressure by intubation and hyperventilation is a reasonable approach, although these patients are already alkalotic and overhyperventilation could result in cerebral ischemia. Loop diuretics such as furosemide (40 to 80 mg) or bumetanide (1 to 2 mg) may reduce brain hydration, but an adequate intravascular volume to maintain perfusion pressure is critical. Hypertonic solutions of saline, mannitol, or urea have been suggested but rarely are used in the field. Controlled studies are lacking, but empirically the response to steroids and oxygen seems excellent if they are given early in the course of the illness and disappointing if they are not started until the patient is unconscious. Coma may persist for days, even after evacuation to low altitude, but other causes of coma must be considered and ruled out by appropriate evaluation.[112] Prevention of HACE is the same as for AMS. Sequelae lasting weeks are common[93,112]; longer term follow-up has been limited.

Focal Neurologic Conditions Without Cerebral Edema

Various localizing neurologic signs, transient in nature and not necessarily occurring in the setting of AMS, suggest cerebrovascular spasm, transient ischemic attack, local hypoxia without loss of perfusion (watershed effect), or focal edema. Cortical blindness is one such condition. Hackett and colleagues[77] reported six cases of transient blindness in climbers or trekkers with intact pupillary reflexes, which indicated that the condition was due to a cortical process. Treatment with breathing of either carbon dioxide (a potent cerebral vasodilator) or oxygen resulted in prompt relief, suggesting that the blindness was due to inadequate regional circulation or oxygenation. Descent effected relief more slowly. Other conditions that could be attributed to spasm or "transient ischemic attack" have included transient hemiplegia or hemiparesis, unilateral paresthesia, aphasia, and scotomas.[300]

The occurrence of stroke in a young, fit person at high altitude is uncommon but tragic. A number of case reports have described climbers with resultant permanent dysfunction.[36,111,259] Factors contributing to stroke may include polycythemia, dehydration, increased intracranial pressure if AMS is present, increased cerebrovenous pressure, cerebrovascular spasm, and perhaps coagulation abnormalities. Stroke may be confused with HACE. Neurologic symptoms, especially focal abnormalities without AMS or HAPE or in the setting of high-altitude illness that persists despite treatment with oxygen, steroids, and descent, suggest a cerebrovascular event and mandate careful evaluation.

Clinical Presentation

E.H., a 42-year-old male climber on a Mt. Everest expedition, awoke at 8000 m with dense paralysis of the right arm and weakness of the right leg. On descent the paresis cleared, but at base camp (5000 m) severe vertigo developed, along with extreme ataxia and weakness. Neurologic consultation on return to the United States resulted in a diagnosis of multiple small cerebral infarcts, but none was visible on CT scan of the brain. The hematocrit value 3 weeks after descent from the mountain was 70%. Over the next 4 years signs gradually improved, but mild ataxia, nystagmus, and dyslexia persist. The focal and persistent nature of the cerebral symptoms and signs, although multiple, indicates a cerebrovascular, rather than an intracranial pressure, etiology. The hematocrit value on the mountain was greater than 70%, high enough for increased viscosity and microcirculatory sludging to contribute to ischemia and infarction.

Treatment of stroke is simply supportive. Oxygen and steroids may be worthwhile to treat any AMS or HACE component. Immediate evacuation to a hospital is indicated. Patients with transient ischemic attacks at high altitude should probably be started on aspirin therapy and proceed to a lower altitude. Oxygen may quickly abort cerebrovascular spasms and will improve watershed hypoxic events. When oxygen is not available, rebreathing to raise alveolar P_{CO_2} may be helpful by increasing cerebral blood flow.

HIGH-ALTITUDE PULMONARY EDEMA

The most common cause of death related to high altitude, HAPE, is completely and easily reversed if recognized early and treated properly. Undoubtedly HAPE was misdiagnosed for centuries, as evidenced by frequent reports of young, vigorous men suddenly dying of "pneumonia" within days of arriving at high altitude. The death of Dr. Jacottet, "a robust, broad-shouldered young man," on Mt. Blanc in 1891 (he refused descent so that he could "observe the acclimatization process" in himself) may have provided the first autopsy of HAPE. Angelo Mosso wrote,

> [F]rom Dr. Wizard's post-mortem examination . . . the more immediate cause of death was therefore probably a suffocative catarrh accompanied by acute edema of the lungs. . . . I have gone into the particulars of this sorrowful incident because a case of inflammation of the lungs also occurred during our expedition, on the summit of Monte Rosa, from which, however, the sufferer fortunately recovered.[196]

On an expedition to K2 (Karakorum Range, Pakistan) in 1902, Alistair Crowley[41] described a climber "suffering from edema of both lungs and his mind was gone." In the Andes, Hurtado[130] reported a case of pulmonary edema peculiar to high altitude. In 1960 Houston[107] made the English-speaking world aware of pulmonary edema as a complication of high-altitude exposure when he reported the condition in a well-trained, healthy cross-country skier and presented four other case reports. The next year Hultgren[128] published hemodynamic measurements in persons with HAPE, demonstrating that it was a noncardiogenic type of edema. Since then many studies and reviews have been published,[86,239] but HAPE is still something of a medical curiosity; the exact cause of the leak in the lung is unknown.

The incidence of HAPE varies from less than 1 in 10,000 skiers in Colorado to 1 in 50 climbers on Mt. McKinley and was higher (15%) in some regiments in the Indian Army (Table 1-1). Individual susceptibility, rate of ascent, altitude reached, degree of cold,[219] physical exertion, and use of sleeping medications are all factors implicated in its occurrence. Younger persons seem more susceptible.[127,128,261] Although HAPE occurs in both sexes, it is perhaps less common in women.[260]

Clinical Presentation

D.L., a 34-year-old man, was in excellent physical condition and had been on numerous high-altitude backpacking trips, occasionally suffering mild symptoms of AMS. He drove from sea level to the trailhead and hiked to a 3050 m sleeping altitude the first night of his trip in the Sierra Nevada. He proceeded to 3700 m the next day, noticing more dyspnea on exertion when walking uphill, a longer time than usual to recover when he rested, and a dry cough. He complained of headache, shivering, dyspnea, and insomnia the second night. The third day the group descended to 3500 m and rested, primarily for D.L.'s benefit. That night D.L. was unable to eat, noted severe dyspnea, and suffered coughing spasms and headache. On the fourth morning D.L. was too exhausted and weak to get out of his sleeping bag. His companions noted that he was breathless, cyanotic, and ataxic but had clear mental status. A few hours later he was transported by helicopter to a hospital at 1200 m. On admission he was cyanotic, oral temperature was 37.8° C, blood pressure 130/76 mm Hg, heart rate 96 beats/min, and respiratory frequency 20 breaths/min. Bilateral basilar rales were noted up to the scapulae. Findings of the cardiac examination were reported as normal. Romberg and finger-to-nose tests revealed 1+ ataxia. Arterial blood gas studies on room air revealed Po_2 24 mm Hg, Pco_2 28 mm Hg, and pH 7.45. The chest radiograph showed extensive bilateral patchy infiltrates (Fig. 1-13, *C*). D.L. was treated with bed rest and supplemental oxygen. On discharge to his sea level home 3 days later, his pulmonary infiltrates and rales had cleared, although his blood gas levels were still abnormal: Po_2 76 mm Hg, Pco_2 30 mm Hg, and pH 7.45. He had an uneventful, complete recovery at home. D.L. was advised to ascend more slowly in the future, staging his ascent with nights spent at 1500 m and 2500 m. He was taught the early signs and symptoms of HAPE and was advised about pharmacologic prophylaxis.

This case illustrates a number of typical aspects of HAPE. Victims are frequently young, fit males who ascend rapidly from sea level and may not have previously suffered HAPE even with repeated altitude exposures.

HAPE usually occurs within the first 2 to 4 days of ascent to higher altitudes (above 2500 m), most commonly on the second night.[76] The earliest indications of the illness are decreased exercise performance and increased recovery time from exercise. The victim usually notices fatigue, weakness, and dyspnea on exertion, especially when he or she is trying to walk uphill; he or she often ascribes these nonspecific symptoms to various other causes. Signs of AMS such as headache, anorexia, and lassitude are often present. A persistent dry cough develops. Nailbeds and lips become cyanotic. The condition typically worsens at night, and tachycardia and tachypnea develop at rest. Dyspnea at rest and audible congestion (rales) in the chest herald to the victim the development of a serious pulmonary problem. In contrast to the usual 1- to 2-day gradual onset, HAPE may strike abruptly, especially in a sedentary person who may not notice the early stages.[276] Orthopnea is common. Pink or blood-tinged, frothy sputum is a very late finding. Severe hypoxemia (or cerebral edema) may produce mental changes, ataxia, decreased level of consciousness, and coma.

On admission to the hospital the victim does not generally appear as ill as would be expected based on arterial blood gas and radiographic findings. A temperature of up to 38.5° C is common. Tachycardia correlates with respiratory rate and severity of illness (Table 1-5).[128] Rales may be unilateral or bilateral and usually originate from the right middle lobe. Concomitant respiratory infection is sometimes present.

Pulmonary edema may have the atypical initial features of predominantly neurologic manifestations and minimal pulmonary symptoms and findings. Coma or cerebral edema may obscure the diagnosis of HAPE.[86] Pulse oximetry, sometimes available in the field, or chest radiography confirms the diagnosis. The differential diagnosis includes pneumonia, pulmonary embolism or infarct, and sometimes asthma. Complications include infection, cerebral edema, pulmonary embolism or thrombosis, and such injuries as frostbite or trauma secondary to incapacitation.[86]

Hemodynamic measurements show elevated pulmonary artery pressure and pulmonary vascular resistance, a low to normal pulmonary wedge pressure, and low to normal cardiac output and systemic arterial blood pressure (Table 1-6).[60,126] Echocardiography demonstrates high estimated pulmonary artery pressures, tricuspid regurgitation, normal left ventricular function, and variable right-sided heart findings of increased atrial and ventricular size.[88,202]

The electrocardiogram usually reveals sinus tachycardia. Changes consistent with acute pulmonary hypertension have been described, such as right axis deviation, right bundle branch block, voltage for right ventricular hypertrophy, and P wave abnormalities.[107,129,182,255] Atrial flutter has been reported, but ventricular arrhythmias have not.

Table 1-5 Severity Classification of High-Altitude Pulmonary Edema

Grade	Symptoms	Signs	Chest Film
1 Mild	Dyspnea on exertion, dry cough, fatigue while moving uphill	HR (rest) < 90-100; RR (rest) < 20; dusky nailbeds; localized rales, if any	Minor exudate involving less than 25% of one lung field
2 Moderate	Dyspnea, weakness, fatigue on level walking; raspy cough; headache; anorexia	HR 90-100; RR 16-30; cyanotic nailbeds; rales present; ataxia may be present	Some infiltrate involving 50% of one lung or smaller area of both lungs
3 Severe	Dyspnea at rest, productive cough, orthopnea, extreme weakness	Bilateral rales; HR > 110; RR > 30; facial and nailbed cyanosis; ataxia; stupor; coma; blood-tinged sputum	Bilateral infiltrates > 50% of each lung

Modified from Hultgren HN: High altitude pulmonary edema. In Staub NC, editor: *Lung water and solute exchange,* New York, 1978, Dekker.
HR, Heart rate; *RR,* respiratory rate.

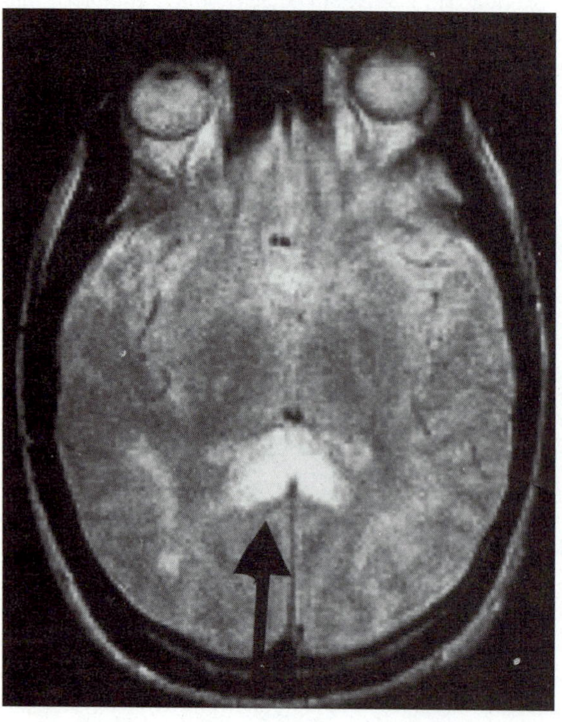

Fig. 1-12 Magnetic resonance image of patient with high-altitude cerebral edema. Increased T2 signal in splenium of corpus callosum *(arrow)* indicates edema.

Table 1-6 Hemodynamic Measurements During High-Altitude Pulmonary Edema (HAPE) and After Recovery in Two Subjects and in a Group of 31 Control Subjects

	HAPE*	Recovery*	Controls†
Sao_2%	58.0	84.0	89.0
Mean pulmonary artery pressure (mm Hg)	63.0	18.0	21.3
Wedge pressure (mm Hg)	1.5	3.5	7.1
Cardiac index (L/m^2)	2.5	4.4	4.1
Pulmonary vascular resistance ($dyne/cm^{-5}$)	1210.0	169.0	169.0
Mean arterial blood pressure (mm Hg)	82.0	—	96.0

*HAPE and recovery values from Penaloza and Sime.[207]
†Mean values from 31 normal subjects studied at 3700 m.[123]

Laboratory Studies

Kobayashi and colleagues[144] reported clinical laboratory values in 27 patients with HAPE. This report confirms typical mild elevations of hematocrit and hemoglobin, probably secondary to intravascular volume depletion and perhaps plasma leakage into the lung. Elevation of the peripheral white blood cell count is common, but rarely is it above 14,000 cells/ml^3. The serum concentration of creatinine phosphokinase (CPK) is increased. Most of the rise in CPK has been attributed to skeletal muscle damage, although in two patients CPK isoenzymes showed brain fraction levels of 1% of the total, which according to the authors may have indicated brain damage.[144]

Arterial blood gas studies consistently reveal respiratory alkalosis and marked hypoxemia, more severe than expected for the patient's clinical condition and radiologic findings. Respiratory or metabolic acidosis related to hypoxemia has not been reported. Therefore arterial blood gas studies are not essential if noninvasive pulse oximetry is available to measure arterial oxygenation. At 4200 m on Mt. McKinley the mean value of arterial Po_2 in HAPE was 28 ± 4 mm Hg. Values as low as 24 mm Hg in HAPE are not unusual here and at other altitudes as well. Arterial oxygen saturation values in our HAPE subjects ranged from 40% to 70%, with a mean of 56% ± 8%.[244] Arterial acid-base values may be misleading in patients taking acetazolamide, since this drug produces significant metabolic acidosis.

Radiologic Findings

The radiologic findings in HAPE have been described in original reports.[128,169,278,279] Findings are consistent with noncardiogenic pulmonary edema, with generally normal heart size and left atrial size and no evidence of pulmonary venous prominence, such as Kerley lines. The pulmonary arteries increase in diameter.[279] Infiltrates are commonly described as fluffy and patchy with areas of aeration between infiltrates and in a peripheral location rather than central. Infiltrates may be unilateral or bilateral, with a predilection for the right middle lung field, which corresponds to the usual area of rales. Pleural effusion is quite rare. The x-ray findings generally correlate with the severity of the illness and degree of hypoxemia. A small right hemithorax, absence of pulmonary vascular markings on the right, and edema confined to the left lung are the basis for a diagnosis of unilateral absent pulmonary artery syndrome.[79] The x-ray findings of HAPE are presented in Fig. 1-13.

Clearing of infiltrates is generally rapid once treatment, especially descent, is initiated. Depending on severity, complete clearing may take from one to several days. Infiltrates are likely to persist longer if the patient remains at high altitude, even if confined to bed and receiving oxygen therapy. Radiographs taken within 48 hours of return to low altitude may confirm a diagnosis of HAPE.

Pathologic Findings

More than 20 autopsy reports of persons who died of HAPE have been published.* Of those whose cranium was opened, more than half had cerebral edema. All lungs showed extensive and severe edema, with bloody, foamy fluid in the airways. Lung weights were two to four times normal. The left side of the heart was normal. The right atrium and main pulmonary artery were often distended. Proteinaceous exudate with hyaline membranes was characteristic. All lungs had areas of inflammation with neutrophil accumulation. The diagnosis of bronchopneumonia was common, although bacteria were not noted. Pulmonary veins, the left ventricle, and the left atrium were generally not dilated, in contrast to the right ventricle and atrium. Most reports mention capillary and arteriolar thrombi and alveolar fibrin deposits, as well as microvascular and gross pulmonary hemorrhage and infarcts. The autopsy findings thus suggest a protein-rich, permeability-type edema, with thrombi or emboli. Confirmation of HAPE as a permeability edema was obtained by analysis of alveolar lavage fluid by Schoene and associates.[243,244] These authors found a 100-fold increase in lavage fluid protein levels in patients with HAPE compared with well control subjects and patients with AMS.[244] The lavage fluid also had a low percentage of neutrophils, in contrast to findings in adult respiratory distress syndrome. Further evidence for a permeability edema was a 1:1 ratio of aspirated edema fluid protein to plasma protein level found by Hackett and colleagues.[78] In addition, the lavage fluid contained vasoactive eicosanoids and complement proteins, indicative of endothelium-leukocyte interactions.[244]

*References 6, 49, 198, 255, 257, 295.

Mechanisms of High-Altitude Pulmonary Edema

The search continues for the mechanism triggering the pulmonary vascular leak. An acceptable explanation for HAPE must take into account three well-established facts: excessive pulmonary hypertension; high-protein permeability leak; and normal function of the left side of the heart. One mechanism that is consistent with the facts is overperfusion edema (Fig. 1-14).

Role of Pulmonary Hypertension. Excessive pulmonary artery pressure (PAP) is the sine qua non of HAPE; no cases of HAPE have been reported without pulmonary hypertension. All persons ascending to high altitudes or otherwise enduring hypoxia, however, have some elevation of PAP. The hypoxic pulmonary vasoconstrictor response (HPVR) is thought to be useful in humans at sea level because it helps match perfusion with ventilation. When local areas of the lung are poorly ventilated because of infection, atelectasis, or some other cause, the HPVR directs blood away from those areas to well-ventilated regions. In the setting of global hypoxia as occurs with ascent to high altitude, HPVR is presumably diffuse and all areas of the lung constrict, causing a restricted vascular bed and an increase in PAP, which is of little if any value for ventilation-perfusion matching at high altitude. The degree of HPVR varies widely among individuals (as well as among species). Presumably those with a greater HPVR have a greater percentage of muscularized arterioles, constrict more units (a greater amount) of the circulation, and have a more restricted vascular bed and a greater rise in PAP. Although other factors, such as the vigor of the ventilatory response and subsequent arterial Po_2, may help to determine the ultimate degree of pulmonary hypertension, the HPVR appears the dominant factor. The distribution of mean PAP values, as estimated by Doppler echocardiography at 4200 m on Mt. McKinley, is shown in Fig. 1-15. All HAPE subjects are at one end of the curve, but there is no bimodal distribution and some subjects with a degree of pulmonary hypertension similar to that in HAPE do not have HAPE. Therefore pulmonary hypertension is a necessary factor but in itself is not the cause of HAPE.

Overperfusion. Hultgren suggested that in those who

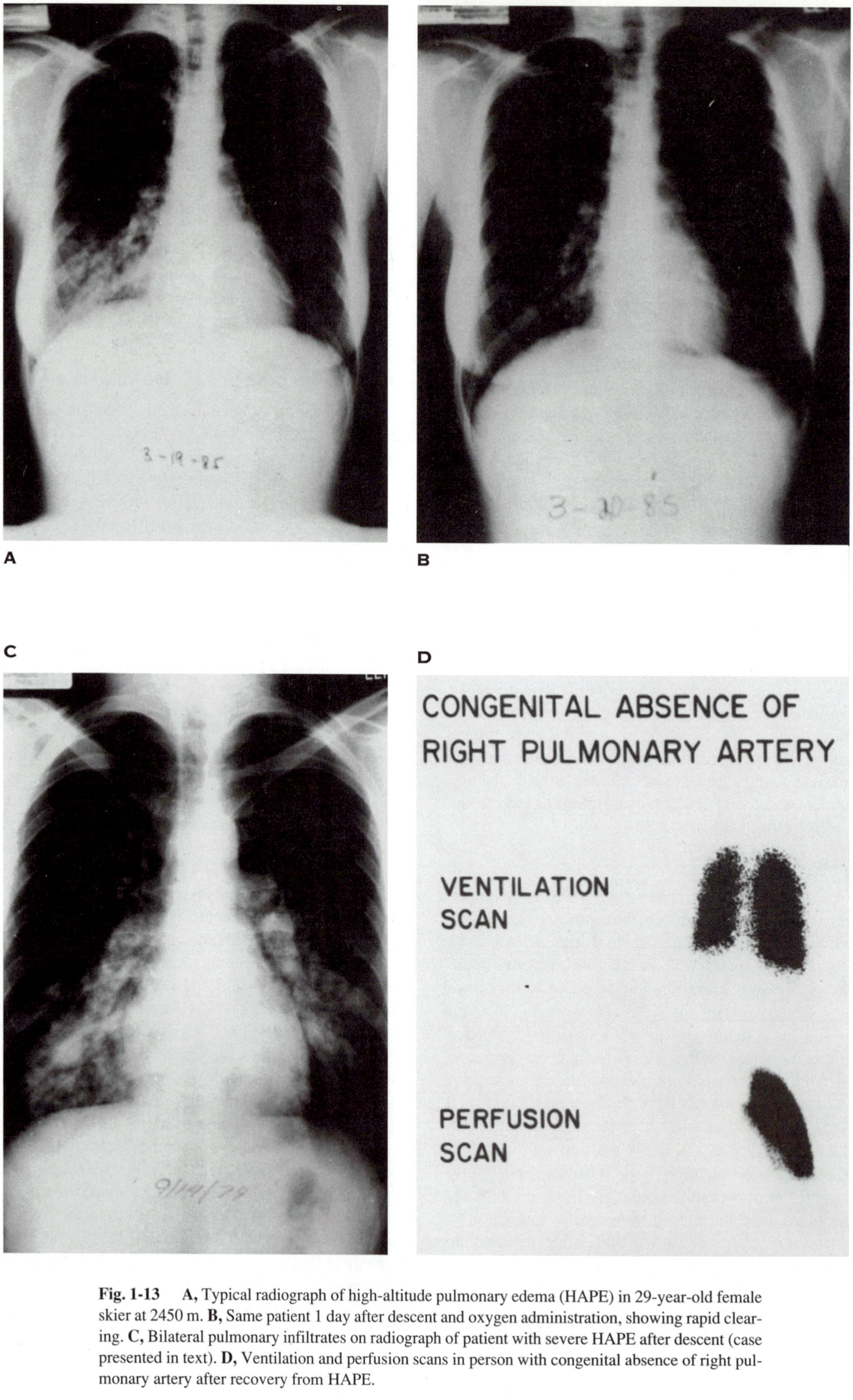

A

B

C

D

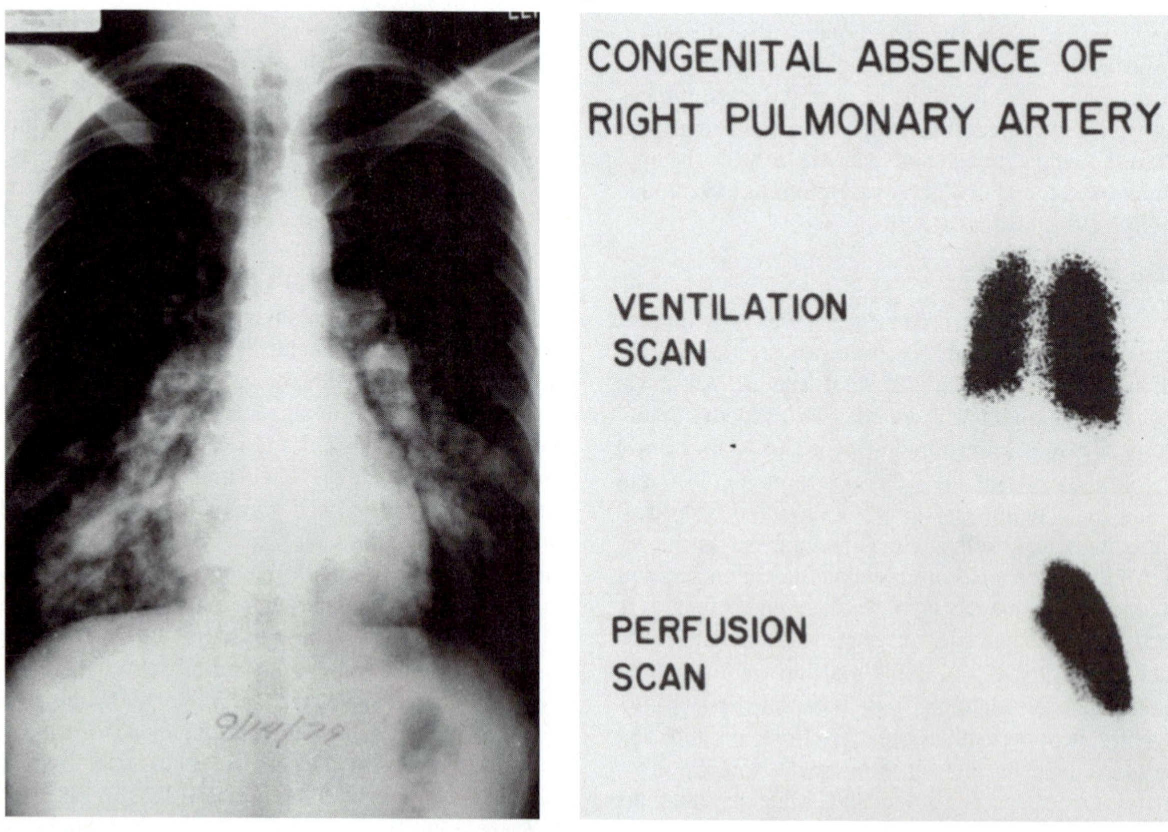

Fig. 1-13 **A,** Typical radiograph of high-altitude pulmonary edema (HAPE) in 29-year-old female skier at 2450 m. **B,** Same patient 1 day after descent and oxygen administration, showing rapid clearing. **C,** Bilateral pulmonary infiltrates on radiograph of patient with severe HAPE after descent (case presented in text). **D,** Ventilation and perfusion scans in person with congenital absence of right pulmonary artery after recovery from HAPE.

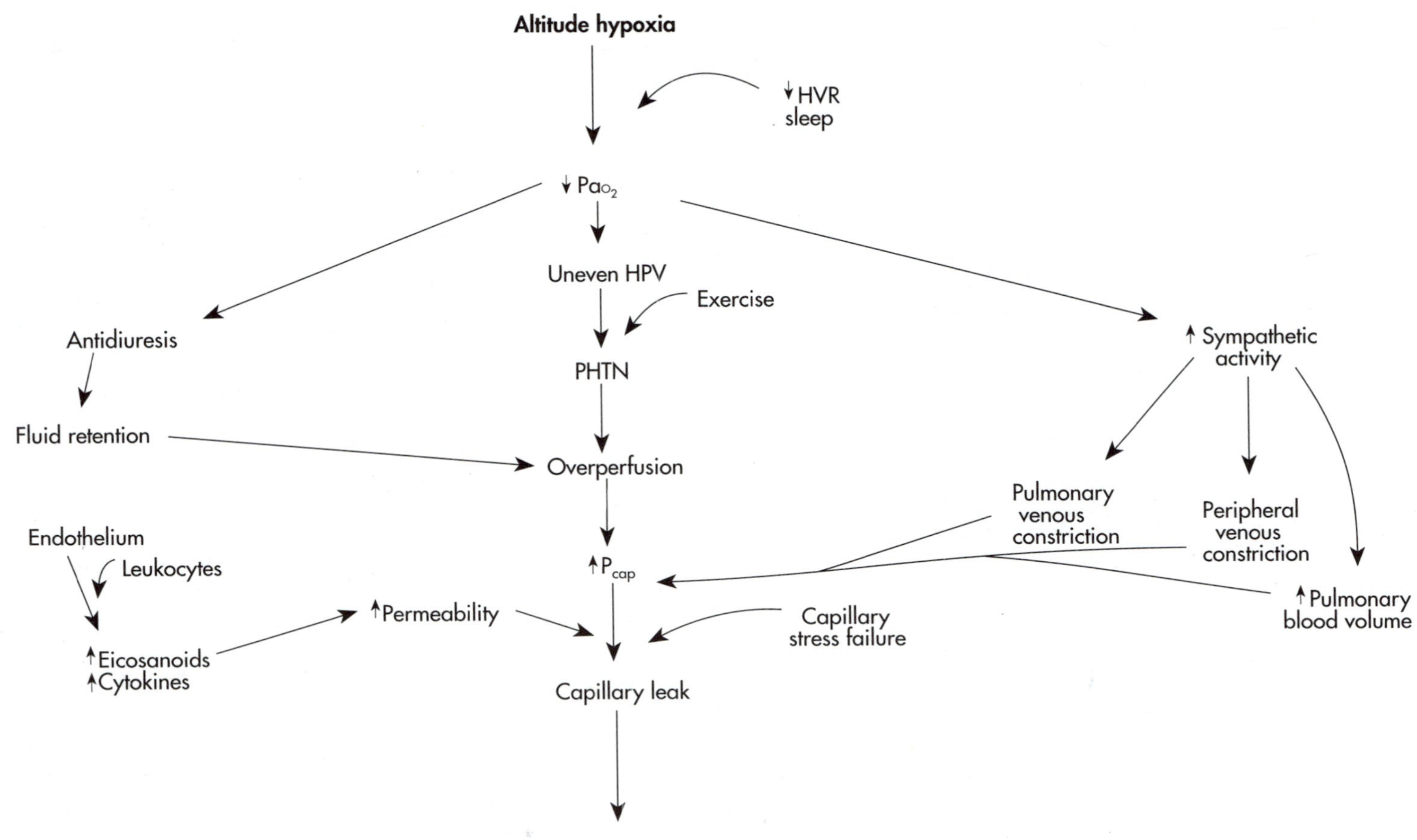

Fig. 1-14 Proposed pathophysiology of high-altitude pulmonary edema. *HVR*, Hypoxic ventilatory response; *HPV*, hypoxic pulmonary vasoconstriction; *PHTN*, pulmonary hypertension; P_{cap}, capillary pressure.

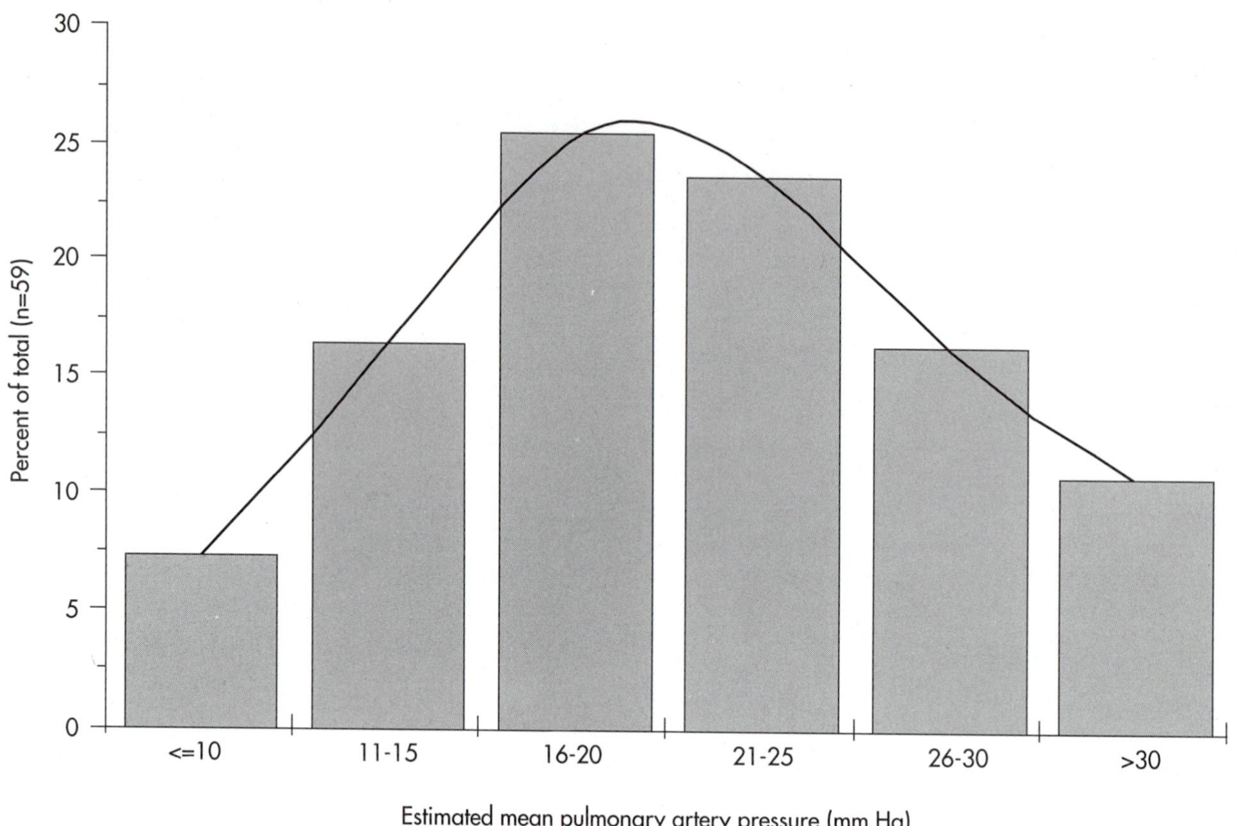

Fig. 1-15 Distribution of mean pulmonary artery pressure estimated by Doppler echocardiography in well-acclimatized mountaineers at 4200 m on Mt. McKinley.

develop HAPE the hypoxic pulmonary vasoconstriction is uneven and the microcirculation in an unconstricted (relatively dilated) area is subjected to high pressure and flow, leading to edema. The unevenness could be due to anatomic characteristics, such as distribution of muscularized arterioles, or to functional factors, such as loss of HPVR in severely hypoxic regions.[118] Uneven perfusion is suggested clinically by the typical patchy x-ray appearance and is supported by lung scans during acute hypoxia that show uneven perfusion in persons susceptible to HAPE.[277] Persons born without a right pulmonary artery are highly susceptible to HAPE (Fig. 1-13, *D*),[79] supporting the concept of overperfusion of a restricted vascular bed as a cause of edema, since the entire cardiac output flows into one lung. Staub,[262] in an accompanying editorial, supported the concept of overperfusion edema and pointed out that hydrostatic edema generally produces a low-protein transudate. Endothelial damage from shear forces,[230] as well as stress failure of the capillary membrane,[292,293] has therefore been invoked to explain the high-protein permeability leak from overperfusion. A recent preliminary study has found activity of adhesion molecules on ascent to high altitude,[51] which indicates interaction of leukocytes and endothelium. The lavage fluid findings of inflammatory mediators also point to the possible endothelial involvement, as do a number of animal studies that failed to produce permeability edema with overperfusion alone but succeeded when the pulmonary vascular bed was embolized with microspheres.[67]

The overperfusion hypothesis is consistent with recent clinical trials of vasodilators intended for prevention and treatment of HAPE. Presumably, when pulmonary vasoconstriction is relieved, flow becomes more homogeneous, and since overall PAP is reduced, microvascular pressure also drops. The rapid reversibility of the illness is also consistent with this mechanism.

Other factors contributing to increased hydrostatic pressure, such as exercise or a high salt load with subsequent hypervolemia, could also play a role in HAPE. The effective use of diuretics and vasodilators also supports a rationale for reducing hydrostatic pressure. A recent study found that an intravenous α-adrenergic blocker, phentolamine, was effective in reducing PAP in HAPE,[88] which raises the possibility that pulmonary venous constriction, which is sympathetically mediated, could be a factor. Any degree of venous constriction could significantly contribute to increased microvascular pressure.

Experiments that convincingly demonstrate the validity of the preceding hypotheses are obviously difficult to perform in humans and await a successful animal model of HAPE. For now, the exact site and mechanism of the leak in HAPE remain enigmatic.

Control of Ventilation. As in AMS, control of ventilation may play a role in the pathophysiology of HAPE. Victims have been shown to have a lower hypoxic ventilatory response (HVR) than persons who acclimatized well,[90,175] but not all persons with a low HVR become ill. Thus a low HVR appears to play a permissive, rather than a causative, role in the development of HAPE. A brisk HVR, and therefore a large increase in ventilation, appears to be protective. Persons who tend to hypoventilate are more hypoxemic and presumably suffer greater pulmonary hypertension. Possibly more important, a low HVR may permit episodes of extreme hypoxemia during sleep (Fig. 1-6). Supporting this concept is the frequency with which the onset of HAPE occurs during sleep, especially in persons who have ingested sleep medications.[76,90] In addition, a HAPE victim with a low HVR does not mount an adequate ventilatory response to the severe hypoxemia of the illness and may suffer further ventilatory depression through CNS suppression. Such persons, when given oxygen, show an increase in ventilation.[90]

Treatment

Early recognition is the key to successful outcome, as with other high-altitude illnesses (Box 1-3). The therapy for HAPE depends on the severity of the illness and on the environment. In the wilderness, where oxygen and medical expertise may not be available, persons with HAPE should be evacuated to a lower altitude as soon as possible. However, because of augmented pulmonary hypertension and greater hypoxemia with exercise, exertion must be minimized. If the disorder is diagnosed early, recovery is rapid with a descent of only 500 to 1000 m and the victim may be able to reascend slowly 2 or 3 days later. In high-altitude locations with oxygen supplies, bed rest with supplemental oxygen may suffice,[171] but severe HAPE may require high-flow oxygen (4 to 6 L/min or more until the patient improves) for more than 24 hours. Hyperbaric therapy is equivalent to low-flow oxygen and can help conserve oxygen supplies.[227]

Oxygen immediately increases arterial oxygenation and reduces pulmonary artery pressure, heart rate, respiratory rate, and symptoms. When descent is not possible, oxygen (or a hyperbaric bag) can be lifesaving. Rescue groups should make delivery of oxygen to the victim, by air drop if necessary, the highest priority if descent is slow or delayed. If oxygen is not available, immediate descent is lifesaving. Waiting for a helicopter or rescue team has too often proved fatal. Since cold stress elevates PAP, the patient should be kept warm.[35] Recently the use of a mask providing pressure (resistance) on expiration was shown to improve gas exchange in HAPE, and this may be useful as a temporizing measure.[242] The same is accomplished with pursed-lip breathing. An unusual case report suggested that a climber may have saved his partner's life by postural drainage to expel airway fluid.[26]

Drugs are of limited value in HAPE, since oxygen and descent are so effective. Medications that reduce pulmonary blood volume, PAP, and pulmonary vascular resistance are physiologically rational. Singh and associates[256] reported good results with furosemide (80 mg every 12 hours), and greater diuresis and clinical improvement occurred when 15 mg parenteral morphine was given with the first dose of furosemide. Hultgren[120] raised concerns about hypovolemia and hypotension with this regimen, but no case reports or studies have documented untoward effects with these drugs for treatment (in contrast to prevention). There are no reports of the use of other diuretics. Morphine sulfate (used only when CNS function is intact) reduces dyspnea, improves oxygenation and comfort, and reduces heart and respiratory rates.[55,256] Furosemide and morphine, through peripheral venodilation, decrease central blood volume, pulmonary congestion, and hydrostatic capillary pressure. However, their use has been eclipsed by recent results with vasodilators. The calcium channel blocker nifedipine (30 mg slow release every 12 to 24 hours or 10 mg sublingually repeated as necessary) has proved effective in reducing pulmonary vascular resistance and PAP, as have hydralazine and phentolamine.[88,201,202] The vasodilators can cause hypotension, but they avoid the danger of CNS depression from morphine and the possible hypovolemia from diuretics. Clinical improvement, however, is much better with oxygen and descent than with any of these drugs. Nifedipine, and perhaps other vasodilators, appears to be useful adjunctive therapy but is no substitute for definitive treatment (see Box 1-3).

After evacuation of the victim to a lower altitude, hospitalization may be warranted for severe cases. Treatment consists of bed rest and oxygen (sufficient to maintain $Sao_2\%$ greater than 90%), and rapid recovery is the rule. A rare instance of progression to adult respiratory distress syndrome has been reported, but it was impossible to exclude other diagnoses completely.[306] Antibiotics are indicated for infection documented by Gram stain or culture. Occasionally, pulmonary artery catheterization is necessary to differentiate cardiogenic from high-altitude pulmonary edema. Rarely are endotracheal intubation and mechanical ventilation needed. Hospitalization until blood gases are completely normal is not warranted; all persons returning from high altitude are at least partially acclimatized to hypoxemia, and hypocapnic alkalosis persists for days after descent. Distinct clinical improvement, radiographic improvement over 24 to 48 hours, and an arterial Po_2 of 60 mm Hg or an $Sao_2\%$ greater than 90% are adequate discharge criteria. Patients are advised to resume normal activities gradually and are warned that they may require up to 2 weeks to recover complete strength. Physicians should recommend preventive measures, including graded ascent with adequate time for acclimatization, and should provide instruction on the use of acetazolamide or nifedipine for future ascents. An episode of HAPE is not a contraindication to subsequent high-altitude exposure, but education to ensure proper preventive measures and recognition of early symptoms is essential.

Prevention

The preventive measures previously described for AMS also apply to HAPE: graded ascent, time for acclimatization, low sleeping altitudes, and avoidance of alcohol and sleeping pills (Box 1-3). The role of exertion in HAPE may be overemphasized. Reports from North America have included hikers, climbers, and skiers, all of whom were exercising vigorously. Menon and colleagues[182] clearly showed that sedentary men taken abruptly to high altitude were just as likely to become victims of HAPE. Nonetheless, since pulmonary artery pressure rises with increasing level of exercise, prudence dictates no overexertion for the first day or two at altitude. Considerable clinical experience (but no data) suggests that acetazolamide prevents HAPE in persons with a history of recurrent episodes. Nifedipine (20 mg slow release every 8 hours) prevented HAPE in subjects with a history of repeated episodes.[17] The drug should be carried by such individuals and started at the first signs of HAPE or, for an abrupt ascent, started when leaving low altitude.

REENTRY PULMONARY EDEMA

In some persons who have lived for years at high altitude, HAPE develops on reascent from a trip to low altitude. Authors have suggested that the incidence of HAPE on reascent may be higher than that during initial ascent by flatlanders,[20,121] but data on true incidence are difficult to obtain. Children and adolescents are more susceptible than adults. Hultgren[119] found a prevalence of HAPE in Peruvian natives of 6.4 per 100 exposures in the 1 to 20 age group, and 0.4 per 100 exposures in persons over 21 years. The phenomenon has been observed most often in Peru, where high-altitude residents can return from sea level to high altitude quite rapidly. Cases have also been reported in Leadville, Colorado,[245] but reports are conspicuously absent from Nepal and Tibet, perhaps because such rapid return back to high altitude is not readily available. Severinghaus[248] has postulated that increased muscularization of pulmonary arterioles that develops with chronic high-altitude exposure generates an inordinately high pulmonary artery pressure on reascent, causing the edema.

SUBCLINICAL PULMONARY EDEMA

On ascent to high altitude, many persons, especially those with AMS, have evidence of increased extravascular lung water. This is evidenced by a widened alveolar-arterial oxygen tension difference (especially in those with AMS symptoms)[17,70,218,248,266] and decreased transthoracic impedance.[234] Persons with AMS also frequently have rales.[22,81] The dynamic balance between fluid production and lymphatic clearance is apparently tilted so that fluid accumulates in the perivascular and interstitial spaces. Subclinical pulmonary edema undoubtedly occurs much more often than does clinical HAPE. Rest, extra time acclimatizing, temporary descent, or drug therapy may help stop progression to HAPE.

THROMBOSIS: COAGULATION AND PLATELET CHANGES

A higher than expected incidence of venous thrombosis, pulmonary embolism, and stroke in mountaineers,[102,283] as well as autopsy findings of widespread thrombi in the brain and lungs, has led to investigations of the clotting mechanism at high altitude. Changes in platelets and coagulation have been observed in rabbits, mice, rats, calves, and humans on ascent to high altitude.[102] A report from OEII found no changes in concentration or inhibition of coagulation factors,[2] nor did significant altitude illness develop in OEII subjects. A remarkable case illustrating coagulation abnormalities at high altitude was reported by O'Brodovich and associates.[199] In one of the women in this chamber study, disseminated intravascular coagulation developed within 1½ hours of exposure to hypobaric hypoxia (P_B = 410 mm Hg, about 4600 m). The platelet count had decreased by 93,000/mm^3, and the activated partial thromboplastin time (aPTT) had shortened by 10 seconds. When symptoms of AMS developed, the study was discontinued. The exact mechanism is unknown. The woman and other subjects showed a shortening of the aPTT, perhaps secondary to the increase in procoagulant VII:C.

Singh and colleagues[254] reported that patients with HAPE had increased fibrinogen levels and prolonged clot lysis times, attributed to a breakdown of fibrinolysis. These authors also reported thrombotic, occlusive hypertensive pulmonary vascular disease in soldiers who had recently arrived at high altitude.[253] These findings, plus autopsy data, prompted Dickinson and associates[49] to conclude that "hypercoagulability of the blood and sequestration of platelets in the pulmonary vascular bed provoke pulmonary thrombosis, and may contribute to the pathogenesis of HAPE."

A recent series of experiments by Bärtsch and colleagues,[14-16] however, carefully examined this issue in well subjects and in those with AMS and HAPE. They concluded that HAPE is not preceded by a prethrombotic state and that only in "advanced HAPE" is there fibrin generation, which abates rapidly with oxygen treatment. They considered the coagulation and platelet activation as an epiphenomenon rather than as an inciting pathophysiologic factor. Fibrin formation would, however, contribute to worsening of edema caused by vascular obstruction, increased vascular permeability, and derangement of surfactant function.[15]

Thrombotic and embolic events in mountaineers may be explained on the basis of dehydration, polycythemia, cold, constrictive clothing, and venous stasis from prolonged periods of weather-imposed inactivity. The role of abnormal clotting in the pathogenesis of these events, especially stroke, warrants further investigation.

PERIPHERAL EDEMA

Edema of the face, hands, and ankles at high altitude is common, especially in females. Incidence of edema in at least one area of the body in trekkers at 4200 m was 18% overall, 28% in females, 14% in males, 7% in asymptomatic trekkers, and 27% in those with AMS.[81] Although not a serious clinical problem, edema can be bothersome. The presence of peripheral edema demands an examination for pulmonary and cerebral edema. In the absence of AMS, peripheral edema is effectively treated with a diuretic. Treatment of accompanying AMS by descent or medical therapy also results in diuresis and resolution of peripheral edema. The mechanism is presumably similar to fluid retention in AMS but may also be merely due to exercise.[184]

HIGH-ALTITUDE RETINOPATHY

A number of retinal abnormalities have been identified.[59,256,265] These include tortuosity and dilation of retinal veins and disc hyperemia (Color Plate 4). Retinal hemorrhages are common at altitudes over 5200 m, are not necessarily related to AMS, and usually are not symptomatic (Color Plate 5).[265] The precipitating stress is apparently hypoxemia, so that blood Po_2 rather than absolute altitude is a better predictor of occurrence; the hemorrhages are more common with HAPE. Hemorrhages have been induced by strenuous exercise, which increases blood pressure and decreases $Sao_2\%$.[265] Below 5200 m, hemorrhages are more likely to be associated with high-altitude illness. Hemorrhages resolve spontaneously in 7 to 14 days. The only pathologic specimen reported was from a physician who died of pulmonary and cerebral edema in Nepal. Microscopy showed hemorrhage from veins and capillaries, but not from arteries.[163] The hemorrhages were similar to those seen in the brain, and it is sobering to think that the presence of retinal hemorrhages may reflect a similar pathologic process behind the retina. Cotton-wool exudates, thought to be due to vascular obstruction and ischemia rather than hypoxemia, have also been reported (Color Plate 6).[82,177]

IMMUNOSUPPRESSION

Mountaineers have observed that infections are common at high altitude, are slow to resolve, and are often resistant to antibiotics. On the American Medical Research Expedition to Mt. Everest in 1981, serious skin and soft tissue infections developed. "Nearly every accidental wound, no matter how small, suppurated for a period of time and subsequently healed slowly."[237] A suppurative hand wound and septic olecranon bursitis did not respond to antibiotics but did respond to descent to 4300 m from the 5300 m base camp. Nine of 21 persons had significant infections not related to the respiratory tract. Most high-altitude expeditions report similar problems.

Data from OEII indicated that healthy individuals are more susceptible to infections at high altitude as a result of impaired T lymphocyte function; this is consistent with previous Russian studies in humans and animals.[181] In contrast, B cells and active immunity are not impaired. Therefore resistance to viruses may not be impaired, while susceptibility to bacterial infection is increased. The degree of immunosuppression is similar to that seen with trauma, burns, emotional depression, and space flight. The mechanism is thought to be related at least in part to release of adrenocorticotropic hormone, cortisone, and β-endorphins, all of which modulate the immune response. Intense ultraviolet exposure has also been shown to impair immunity. Persons with serious infections at high altitude may need oxygen or descent for effective treatment. Impaired immunity because of altitude should be anticipated in situations where infection could be a complication, such as trauma, burns, and surgical and invasive procedures.

HIGH-ALTITUDE FLATUS EXPULSION

High-altitude flatus expulsion (HAFE) is the unwelcome spontaneous passage of colonic gas at altitudes above 3000 m.[9] The mechanism has been postulated to relate to the expansion of intraluminal bowel gas at the decreased atmospheric pressure of altitude. Affected individuals may benefit from the oral administration of digestive enzymes or simethicone and a preferential carbohydrate diet.

HIGH-ALTITUDE PHARYNGITIS AND BRONCHITIS

Sore throat, chronic cough, and bronchitis are nearly universal in persons who spend more than 2 weeks at an extreme altitude (over 5500 m). All 21 members of the 1981 American Medical Research Expedition to Mt. Everest suffered these problems. Only two of eight subjects in OEII (where the temperature was greater than 21° C and relative humidity was greater than 80%) developed cough, and only above 6500 m. Only four had sore throat. Obviously factors other than hypoxia are involved. In the field these problems usually appear without fever or chills, myalgias, lymphadenopathy, exudate, or other signs of infection. Whether these are infections is debatable. The increase in ventilation, especially with exercise, forces obligate mouth breathing at altitude, bypassing the warming and moisturizing action of the nasal mucous membranes and sinuses. The movement of large volumes of dry, cold air across the pharyngeal mucosa can cause marked dehydration, irritation, and pain, similar to pharyngitis. Vasomotor rhinitis, quite common in cold temperatures, aggravates this condition by necessitating mouth breathing during sleep. For this reason, decongestant nasal spray is one of the most coveted items in an expedition medical kit. Other countermeasures include forced hydration, hard candies, lozenges, and steam inhalation.

High-altitude bronchitis can be disabling because of severe coughing spasms. Cough fractures of one or more ribs are not rare; two climbers on the 1981 American Medical Research Expedition to Mt. Everest had such fractures. Purulent sputum is common. Response to antibiotics is poor; most victims resign themselves to taking medications such as codeine and do not expect a cure until descent. A recent study of high-altitude bronchitis on Aconcagua revealed that bronchitis developed in 13 of 19 climbers above 4300 m.[214] Mean sputum production was 6 teaspoons per day. All reported that onset was after a period of excessive hyperventilation associated with strenuous activity. Although an infectious etiology is possible, especially in light of impaired immune response to bacterial infection, experimental evidence suggests that respiratory heat loss results in purulent sputum and sufficient airway irritation to cause persistent cough.[178] This is supported by the beneficial effect of steam inhalation and the lack of response to antibiotics. Many climbers find that a silk balaclava or similar material that is porous enough to breathe through but traps some moisture and heat effectively prevents or ameliorates the problem.

CHRONIC MOUNTAIN POLYCYTHEMIA

In 1928 Carlos Monge[188] described a syndrome in Andean high-altitude natives that was characterized by headaches, insomnia, lethargy, plethoric appearance, and polycythemia greater than expected for the altitude. Known variously as Monge's disease, chronic mountain polycythemia, or chronic mountain sickness, the condition has now been recognized in all high-altitude areas of the world.[148,189,206] Both lowlanders who relocate to high altitude and native residents are susceptible. Chinese investigators reported that 13% of lowland Chinese males and 1.6% of females who had relocated to Tibet developed excessive polycythemia (hemoglobin level greater than 20 g/dl blood).[302] The incidence in Leadville, Colorado, is also high in men over 40 and distinctly low in women.[150] The increased hemopoiesis is apparently related to greater hypoxic stress, which may be due to a number of causes, such as lung disease, sleep apnea syndromes, and idiopathic hypoventilation. A diagnosis of true chronic mountain polycythemia excludes lung disease and is characterized by relative alveolar hypoventilation and respiratory insensitivity to hypoxia.[189] Some studies suggest that even for the degree of hypoxemia, the red blood cell mass is excessive, implying overproduction of erythropoietin.[297] Increasing age is also an important factor.[187]

Regardless of the exact mechanism, therapy is routinely successful. Descent to a lower altitude is the definitive treatment. Supplemental oxygen during sleep is valuable. Phlebotomy is a common practice, provides subjective improvement (without significant objective changes), and is generally recommended when hematocrit is greater than 60% or hemoglobin level is greater than 20 g/dl blood.[297] The respiratory stimulants medroxyprogesterone acetate (20 to 60 mg/day) and acetazolamide (250 mg twice a day) have also been shown to reduce the hematocrit value by improving oxygenation.[149] The response to respiratory stimulants emphasizes the contribution of hypoventilation to chronic mountain polycythemia.

ULTRAVIOLET KERATITIS (SNOWBLINDNESS)

Ultraviolet (UV) radiation increases roughly 4% for every 300 m gain in altitude, attributable to decreased cloudiness, dust, and water vapor at higher altitudes. Ultraviolet (UVA and UVB) is reflected back from snow (75%), further increasing UV exposure. Significant UV radiation may strike the eye, even on cloudy days. The cornea absorbs UV radiation below 300 nm (UVB). Radiation of wavelengths greater than 300 nm is transmitted to the lens and in time can cause yellowing and cataracts. High exposure levels can cause corneal burns in 1 hour, although symptoms do not become apparent for 6 to 12 hours. Symptoms of keratitis are pain, which can be severe, a gritty sensation in the eyes, light sensitivity, tearing, marked conjunctival erythema, chemosis, and eyelid swelling. Although spontaneous healing generally occurs in 24 hours, steps can be taken to minimize pain and disability. Contact lenses must be removed. A single dose of a topical anesthetic such as tetracaine helps control pain initially, but systemic narcotic analgesics may be necessary. Antiinflammatory drugs such as aspirin or ibuprofen may be helpful. Cold compresses provide some relief. Mydriatic-cycloplegic agents reduce ciliary spasm. Ophthalmologists do not recommend topical steroids.

Affected eyes should be patched for 12 hours, and the patient should rest. Patches can be removed at 12 hours, and if total resolution has not occurred, they can be replaced for another 12 hours. The condition is so painful and disabling and potentially dangerous in rugged terrain that prevention is of utmost importance.

Sunglass lenses should transmit less than 10% of UVB light. A dark tint is usually necessary to reduce glare and brightness but has no effect on UV absorption. Side shields are necessary, and polarizing lenses help by absorbing glare from reflective surfaces such as snow. Goggles do not obstruct peripheral vision as much as do the side shields of glasses. They should be practically unbreakable and secured with a neck loop. Since climbers often have glasses blown off by a sudden wind gust or lose glasses during a fall, spares should always be carried. When a climber is stranded without glasses or goggles, makeshift shields can be fashioned by cutting narrow horizontal slits for essential vision in a piece of cardboard, foam padding, or similar material and securing it over the eyes with a string or strap around the head. Most expedition and trip leaders consider snowblindness a "demerit offense," since the condition is entirely preventable.

Illnesses Aggravated by High Altitude

Illnesses that are aggravated by high-altitude exposure are listed in Box 1-4.

CHRONIC LUNG DISEASE

Patients with chronic obstructive lung disease may have hypoxemia, pulmonary hypertension, disordered control of ventilation, and sleep-disordered breathing at sea level. All of these conditions can reasonably be expected to worsen on ascent to high altitude, although the problem has not received much attention.

Oxygen saturation remains above 90% in a normally acclimatizing, healthy, awake person until an altitude over 3000 m (Fig. 1-1). Patients with hypoxemic lung disease reach this threshold at a lower altitude. Gong and colleagues[65] studied such patients by acute hypoxia testing at sea level and found that sea level Po_2 values of 68 and 72 mm Hg successfully classified more than 90% of the subjects with a Pao_2 greater than 55 mm Hg while breathing 17% O_2 (1525 m) and a Pao_2 greater than 55 mm Hg while breathing 15% O_2 (2440 m), respectively. A Pao_2 of 55 mm Hg results in a saturation of 90% at high altitude, where there is slight alkalosis.

Nearly all patients with chronic obstructive pulmonary disease (COPD) who venture to high altitude report reduced exercise ability. Patients with predicted arterial oxygen saturation less than 85% should probably be given supplemental oxygen for use at high altitude. Since these patients are at a "physiologically higher" altitude, altitude syndromes might be expected more frequently or sooner. On the other hand, these patients are already partially acclimatized to hypoxia. Graham and Houston[66] found that eight subjects with COPD tolerated 1920 m altitude quite well. High-altitude pulmonary edema in a patient with chronic lung disease has not been reported.

Symptomatic pulmonary hypertension may be a contraindication to high-altitude exposure because of exacerbation of the primary disease and also because it increases susceptibility to HAPE. Patients with sleep apnea syndrome who become mildly hypoxemic at sea level may become severely hypoxemic at high altitude, which contributes to high-altitude illness and aggravates attendant problems such as polycythemia, pulmonary hypertension, or insomnia. Airway heat loss may aggravate asthma at extreme altitude, as it does at sea level,[178] but reports of high-altitude illness in asthmatic persons or of asthma being aggravated by altitude are conspicuously absent. In the past, moderate altitude was considered an advantage for asthmatic patients because of decreased air density and lower concentration of pollutants and pollens.[258] Physicians experienced in high-altitude medicine do not consider asthma a contraindication for ascent to high altitude but caution that appropriate medications must be taken along.

BOX 1-4

ADVISABILITY OF EXPOSURE TO HIGH AND VERY HIGH ALTITUDE FOR COMMON CONDITIONS (WITHOUT SUPPLEMENTAL OXYGEN)

PROBABLY NO EXTRA RISK

Young and old
Fit and unfit
Obesity
Diabetes
After coronary artery bypass grafting (without angina)
Mild chronic obstructive pulmonary disease (COPD)
Asthma
Low-risk pregnancy
Controlled hypertension
Controlled seizure disorder
Psychiatric disorders
Neoplastic diseases
Inflammatory conditions

CAUTION

Moderate COPD
Compensated congestive heart failure (CHF)
Sleep apnea syndromes
Troublesome arrhythmias
Stable angina/coronary artery disease
High-risk pregnancy
Sickle cell trait
Cerebrovascular diseases
Any cause for restricted pulmonary circulation
Seizure disorder (not on medication)

CONTRAINDICATED

Sickle cell anemia (with history of crises)
Severe COPD
Pulmonary hypertension
Uncompensated CHF

ARTERIOSCLEROTIC HEART DISEASE

The healthy heart tolerates even extreme hypoxia quite well, all the way to the summit of Mt. Everest (Pa_{O_2} less than 30 mm Hg). Numerous electrocardiograms (ECGs), echocardiograms, heart catheterizations, and exercise tests have failed to demonstrate any evidence of cardiac ischemia or cardiac dysfunction in healthy persons at high altitudes.

Persons with arteriosclerotic heart disease (ASHD), however, might not have the same compensatory capacities. Surprisingly little literature is available on the effects of acute high-altitude exposure on persons with ASHD. No evidence from state or county mortality statistics suggests an increased prevalence of acute coronary events in visitors to high-altitude locations. Migration to lower altitude of persons with heart and lung disease may partly explain the reported reduced mortality.[191] To assess risk from altitude exposure, Okin[203] performed a pilot study with 11 patients; 7 had previous myocardial infarctions, 2 had angina, and 2 had both previous myocardial infarctions and stable exercise-induced angina. Stress ECGs were completed in Denver (1600 m), at 2500 m, and at 3170 m. No patient who had a normal test in Denver had a positive test at higher altitudes, and no patient had symptoms at high altitude who did not have them in Denver. Likewise, Grover and associates[74] found that skiing at high altitude produced considerable cardiac stress but did not produce evidence of ischemia on ECG tracings in middle-aged men.

A large group of elderly people, many of whom had ASHD and abnormal ECGs, was found to exhibit no evidence of new or increased myocardial ischemia at 2500 m.[228,304] Furthermore, 7 elderly subjects with coronary artery disease, as well as 13 other elderly without coronary artery disease (CAD), showed no changes in signal-averaged ECG, despite an increase in norepinephrine and an elevation in blood pressure.[158] Maximum work performance, however, was low in the elderly with CAD.[158] The lesson for the physician advising such persons is that ascent to moderate altitude seems to have little or no deleterious effect on CAD, but that patients should be cautioned to reduce exercise levels. Patients with multiple-vessel bypass grafts for arteriosclerotic heart disease who were asymptomatic and with normal exercise tests at sea level have successfully visited altitudes as high as 4600 to 5200 m.

Despite the lack of evidence for increased risk, the general absence of information causes many physicians to caution their patients to avoid high-altitude exposure. A stress ECG to screen for ascent to high altitude is not indicated in a healthy person (of any age) who regularly exercises. The level of exercise appears to be a more significant stress than is high altitude. The usual admonition for sedentary persons to train (increase aerobic conditioning) before an event requiring rigorous exercise is especially applicable to high-altitude events, such as a Himalayan trek or skiing.

Increased catecholamine levels at high altitude would be expected to increase the risk of arrhythmias, but again, evidence is lacking. Both tachycardia and bradycardia have been described in healthy climbers at extreme altitude, with a degree of hypoxemia not likely to be experienced by older persons unless they have lung disease. No dangerous arrhythmias have ever been reported in high-altitude studies. Patients whose arrhythmias are well controlled on antidysrhythmic medication should certainly continue the medication at altitude, while those with poorly controlled arrhythmias should probably forgo visits to high altitude. The same may be said of congestive heart failure; marginally compensated patients frequently decompensate at high-altitude ski resorts.

HYPERTENSION

In healthy persons rapidly ascending to high altitude, blood pressure increases mildly because of increased catecholamine activity and increased sympathetic tone.[215] One well-controlled study showed an increase in blood pressure at 3500 m from a mean of 105/66 mm Hg at sea level to 119/77 mm Hg at 3 days, 111/75 mm Hg at 3 weeks, and back to 102/65 mm Hg on return to sea level.[170] Pugh[211] reported transient increases in blood pressure in athletes at the Olympics in Mexico City. Whether or when the blood pressure returns to normal is unclear. Arterial hypertension develops in 10% of lowland Chinese who move to Tibet.[250] The authors consider this a form of mountain sickness and treat the condition by returning the affected individuals to low altitude. Twenty-five percent of 243 Indian soldiers residing for a few months at altitudes of 2500 to 4000 m had blood pressure equal to or greater than 140 mm Hg systolic or 100 mm Hg diastolic.[136] Long-term residents of high altitude have lower blood pressure than their sea level counterparts.[122,172]

The effect of altitude on preexisting hypertension was recently evaluated in a group of the elderly.[228] After ascent to 2500 m, blood pressure increased in hypertensive subjects to the same small, but significant degree as seen in normotensive control subjects.[228] Patients receiving antihypertensive treatment should continue their medications while at high altitude. Hypertension in short-term high-altitude sojourners should be considered transient and should not be treated, since it rarely reaches dangerously high levels and will resolve on descent. There is no evidence to suggest that hypertensive patients are more likely to develop high-altitude illnesses. Hypertension does not seem to be a contraindication to high-altitude exposure.

SICKLE CELL DISEASE

Sickle cell crisis is a well-recognized complication of high-altitude exposure.[58] Even the modest altitude of a pressurized aircraft (1500 to 2000 m) causes 20% of persons with hemoglobin SC and sickle-thalassemia genetic configuration to have a vasoocclusive crisis.[167] High-altitude exposure may precipitate the first vasoocclusive crisis in persons previously unaware of their condition. Patients with sickle cell anemia and a history of vasoocclusive crises are advised to avoid altitudes over 1800 m unless they are taking supplemental oxygen.[251] Persons with sickle cell disease who live at high altitude in Saudi Arabia have twice the incidence of crises, hospitalizations, and complications as do Saudis at low altitude.[1] Splenic infarction syndrome has been reported more commonly in those with sickle cell trait than in those with sickle cell anemia, probably because sickle cell disease produces autosplenectomy early in life. Frequent reports in the literature emphasize the need to consider splenic syndrome caused by sickle cell trait in any person with left upper quadrant pain, even at an altitude of only 1500 m.[152,167,251] A number of authors have suggested that nonblack persons with the trait may be at greater risk for splenic syndrome at high altitude than are black persons.[152] Treatment of splenic syndrome consists of intravenous hydration, oxygen, and removal to a lower altitude. The overall incidence of problems in persons with the trait is low, however, and no special precaution other than recognition of the splenic syndrome is recommended.

PREGNANCY

Essentially no data exist on the influence of a high-altitude visit during pregnancy. The fact that pregnancy-induced hypertension is four times more common in women living at high altitude and that the preeclampsia syndrome is more common may warrant caution in some pregnant women visiting high-altitude areas.[191] However, there is no evidence that increased spontaneous abortion, abruptio placentae, placenta previa, or other such problems are related to high altitude. A number of studies of acute hypoxia in human pregnancy have shown no fetal heart rate change or slight tachycardia in response to mild hypoxia, while severe hypoxia can cause bradycardia.[40] Such severe hypoxemia (PIo_2 of 60 to 90 mm Hg at 4500 m to 7500 m) is encountered only at extreme altitudes or accompanying HAPE. Women with complicated pregnancies are more likely to have abnormal fetal heart rate response to hypoxia, and one study even suggested that an acute hypoxia test may be of value in assessing placental reserve.[224] The advice given to near-term women not to travel by air is based on the airlines' fear of in-flight labor and delivery, not on physiologic data that such flights may be harmful or may induce labor. The hypoxia of cabin altitudes of 1500 m to 2400 m is well tolerated by the fetus.[12] Until more data become available, it seems prudent to advise against unnecessary altitude exposure for complicated pregnancies and against excessively high (greater than 4000 m) or prolonged exposures for lowland women with normal pregnancy. When considering wilderness travel, especially in the developing countries, pregnant women should be informed that remoteness from medical care should problems develop is more important than the mild hypoxemia of altitude. A recommendation to avoid trekking above 2100 m (about 7000 feet) was based on the fact that high-altitude babies are small for gestational age,[12] a finding irrelevant for the tourist or trekker.

REFERENCES

1. Adzaku F et al: Clinical features of sickle cell disease at altitude, *J Wilderness Med* 3:260, 1992.
2. Andrew M, O'Brodovich H, Sutton JR: Operation Everest II: coagulation system during prolonged decompression to 282 torr, *J Appl Physiol* 63(3):1262, 1987.
3. Anholm JD, Houston CS, Hyers TM: The relationship between acute mountain sickness and pulmonary ventilation at 2,835 meters (9,300 feet), *Chest* 75(1):33, 1979.
4. Anholm JD et al: Operation Everest II: arterial oxygen saturation and sleep at extreme simulated altitude, *Am Rev Respir Dis* 145(4):817, 1992.
5. Aoki VS, Robinson SM: Body hydration and the incidence and severity of acute mountain sickness, *J Appl Physiol* 31(3):363, 1971.
6. Arias-Stella J, Kryger H: Pathology of high altitude pulmonary edema, *Arch Pathol Lab Med* 76:43, 1963.
7. Aste-Salazar H, Hurtado A: The affinity of hemoglobin for oxygen at sea level and at high altitudes, *Am J Physiol* 142:733, 1944.
8. Åstrand PO, Rodahl K: *Textbook of work physiology,* New York, 1977, McGraw-Hill.
9. Auerbach PS, Miller EY: High altitude flatus expulsion (HAFE) (letter), *West J Med* 134:173, 1981.
10. Balke B, Nagle FJ, Daniels JT: Altitude and maximum performance in work and sports activity, *JAMA* 194(6):176, 1965.
11. Banchero N: Capillary density of skeletal muscle in dogs exposed to simulated altitude, *Proc Soc Exp Biol Med* 148:435, 1975.
12. Barry M, Bia F: Pregnancy and travel, *JAMA* 261(5):728, 1989.
13. Bärtsch P et al: Comparison of carbon-dioxide enriched, oxygen-enriched, and normal air in treatment of acute mountain sickness, *Lancet* 336:772, 1990.
14. Bärtsch P et al: Coagulation and fibrinolysis in acute mountain sickness and beginning pulmonary edema, *J Appl Physiol* 66(5):2136, 1989.
15. Bärtsch P et al: High altitude pulmonary edema: blood coagulation. In Sutton JR, Houston CS, Coates G, editors: *Hypoxia and molecular medicine,* Burlington, Vt, 1993, Queen City Press.
16. Bärtsch P et al: Contact phase of blood coagulation is not activated in edema of high altitude, *J Appl Physiol* 67(4):1336, 1989.
17. Bärtsch P et al: Prevention of high-altitude pulmonary edema by nifedipine, *N Engl J Med* 325:1284, 1991.
18. Bärtsch P et al: Enhanced exercise-induced rise of aldosterone and vasopressin preceding mountain sickness, *J Appl Physiol* 711(1):136, 1991.
19. Bärtsch P et al: Effects of slow ascent to 4559 m on fluid homeostasis, *Aviat Space Environ Med* 62:105, 1991.
20. Bärtsch P et al: Atrial natriuretic peptide in acute mountain sickness, *J Appl Physiol* 65(5):1929, 1988.
21. Bärtsch P et al: Aldosterone, antidiuretic hormone and atrial natriuretic peptide in acute mountain sickness. In Sutton JR, Coates G, Houston CS, editors: *Hypoxia and mountain medicine,* Burlington, Vt, 1992, Queen City Press.
22. Bärtsch P et al: Respiratory symptoms, radiographic and physiologic correlations at high altitude. In Sutton JR, Coates G, Remmers JE, editors: *Hypoxia: the adaptations,* Philadelphia, 1990, BC Decker.
23. Beall CM: Tibetans adapt to high altitude without high hemoglobin levels (abstract). In Sutton JR, Houston CS, Jones NL, editors: *Hypoxia, exercise and altitude,* New York, 1983, AR Liss.
24. Berry CA, Berry MA: Aerospace medicine: the vertical frontier. In Auerbach PS, Geehr EC, editors: *Management of wilderness and environmental emergencies,* New York, 1983, Macmillan.

25. Bert P: *Barometric pressure: researches in experimental physiology,* Bethesda, Md, 1978, Undersea Medical Society.
26. Bock J, Hultgren HN: Emergency maneuver in high altitude pulmonary edema (letter), *JAMA* 255(23):3245, 1986.
27. Boycott AE, Haldane JS: The effects of low atmospheric pressures on respiration, *J Physiol* 37:355, 1908.
28. Boyer SJ, Blume FD: Weight loss and changes in body composition at high altitude, *J Appl Physiol* 57(5):1580, 1984.
29. Bradwell AR, Burnett D, Davies F: Acetazolamide in control of acute mountain sickness, *Lancet* 1(8213):180, 1981.
30. Bradwell AR et al: The effect of temazepam and diamox on nocturnal hypoxia at altitude (abstract). In Sutton JR, Houston CS, Coates G, editors: *Hypoxia and cold,* New York, 1987, Praeger.
31. Buskirk ER et al: Maximal performance at altitude and return from altitude in conditioned runners, *J Appl Physiol* 23(2):259, 1967.
32. Butterfield GE et al: Increased energy intake minimizes weight loss in men at high altitude, *J Appl Physiol* 72(5):1741, 1992.
33. Cain SM, Dunn JE: Low doses of acetazolamide to aid accommodation of men to altitude, *J Appl Physiol* 21(2):1195, 1965.
34. Cerretelli P: Limiting factors to oxygen transport on Mount Everest, *J Appl Physiol* 40(5):658, 1976.
35. Chauca D, Bligh J: An additive effect of cold exposure and hypoxia on pulmonary artery pressure in sheep, *Res Vet Sci* 21:123, 1976.
36. Clarke CR: Cerebral infarction at extreme altitude (abstract). In Sutton JR, Houston CS, Jones NL, editors: *Hypoxia, exercise and altitude,* New York, 1983, AR Liss.
37. Claybaugh JR, Brooks DP, Cymerman A: Hormonal control of fluid and electrolyte balance at high altitude in normal subjects. In Sutton JR, Coates G, Houston CS, editors: *Hypoxia and mountain medicine,* Burlington, Vt, 1992, Queen City Press.
38. Cone JB: Cellular oxygen utilization. In Snyder JV, Pinsky MR, editors: *Oxygen transport in the critically ill,* St Louis, 1987, Mosby.
39. Consolazio CF et al: Effects of a high-carbohydrate diet on performance and clinical symptomology after rapid ascent to high altitude, *Fed Proc* 28(3):937, 1969.
40. Copher DE, Huber CP: Heart rate response of the human fetus to induced maternal hypoxia, *Am J Obstet Gynecol* 98:320, 1967.
41. Crowley A: *The confessions of Alistair Crowley: an autobiography,* New York, 1971, Bantam Books.
42. Curran-Everett DC et al: Intracranial pressures and O_2 extraction in conscious sheep during 72 h of hypoxia, *Am J Physiol* 261(1):H103, 1991.
43. Dean AG, Yip R, Hoffman R: An epidemic of acute mountain sickness among epidemiologists: high attack rate at moderate altitude (abstract). In Sutton JR, Coates G, Remmers JE, editors: *Hypoxia: the adaptations,* Philadelphia, 1990, BC Decker.
44. Delamere JP, Jones GT: Birmingham Medical Research Expedition Society 1977 expedition: changes in renal function observed during a trek to high altitude, *Postgrad Med J* 55:487, 1979.
45. Dempsey JA et al: Regulation of CSF [HCO^{-3}] during long-term hypoxic hypocapnia in man, *J Appl Physiol* 44(2):175, 1978.
46. Dick FW: Training at altitude in practice, *Int J Sports Med* 13(suppl 1):S203, 1992.
47. Dickinson JG: High altitude cerebral edema: cerebral acute mountain sickness, *Semin Respir Med* 5(2):151, 1983.
48. Dickinson JG: Acetazolamide in acute mountain sickness, *Br Med J* 295:1161, 1987.
49. Dickinson JG et al: Altitude-related deaths in seven trekkers in the Himalayas, *Thorax* 38:646, 1983.
50. Editorial: Acetazolamide prophylaxis for acute mountain sickness, *Drug Ther Bull* 25(12):45, 1987.
51. Eldridge MW et al: Evidence of immunological mediator activation with exposure to high altitude (abstract). Presented at ALA/ATS International Conference, Boston, 1994.
52. Ellsworth AJ, Meyer EF, Larson EB: Acetazolamide and dexamethasone use versus placebo to prevent acute mountain sickness on Mount Rainier, *West J Med* 154:289, 1991.
53. Ferrazzini G et al: Successful treatment of acute mountain sickness with dexamethasone, *Br Med J* 294:1380, 1987.
54. Fishman RA: Brain edema, *N Engl J Med* 293(14):706, 1975.
55. Flynn WJ et al: Contact lens wear at altitude: subcontact lens bubble formation, *Aviat Space Environ Med* 58(11):1115, 1987.
56. Forster PJ: Effect of different ascent profiles on performance at 4200 m elevation, *Aviat Space Environ Med* 56:758, 1985.
57. Forwand SA et al: Effect of acetazolamide on acute mountain sickness, *N Engl J Med* 279(16):839, 1968.
58. Franklin V: Sickle cell crisis. In Sutton JR, Jones NL, Houston CS, editors: *Hypoxia: man at altitude,* New York, 1982, Thieme-Stratton.
59. Frayser R et al: Retinal hemorrhage at high altitude, *N Engl J Med* 282:1183, 1970.
60. Frayser R et al: Hormonal and electrolyte response to exposure to 17,500 ft, *J Appl Physiol* 38(4):636, 1975.
61. Freedman R et al: Electrophysiological effects of low dose alcohol on human subjects at high altitude, *Alcohol Drug Res* 6(4):289, 1986.
62. Frisancho AR: Perspectives on functional adaptation of the high altitude native. In Sutton JR, Houston CS, Jones NL, editors: *Hypoxia, exercise and altitude,* New York, 1983, AR Liss.
63. Fujimoto K et al: Irregular nocturnal breathing patterns at high altitude in subjects susceptible to high-altitude pulmonary edema (HAPE): a preliminary study, *Aviat Space Environ Med* 60:786, 1989.
64. Gibson GE, Blass JP: Impaired synthesis of acetylcholine in brain accompanying mild hypoxia and hypoglycemia, *J Neuro Chem* 27:37, 1976.
65. Gong H et al: Hypoxia-altitude simulation test: evaluation of patients with chronic airway obstruction, *Am Rev Respir Dis* 130:980, 1964.
66. Graham WG, Houston CS: Short-term adaptation to moderate altitude: patients with chronic obstructive pulmonary disease, *JAMA* 240(14):1491, 1978.
67. Gray GW: High altitude pulmonary edema, *Semin Respir Med* 5(2):141, 1983.
68. Gray GW et al: Control of acute mountain sickness, *Aerospace Med* 42(1):81, 1971.
69. Greene MK et al: Acetazolamide in prevention of acute mountain sickness: a double blind controlled cross-over study, *Br Med J* 283:811, 1981.
70. Grissom CK et al: Acetazolamide in the treatment of acute mountain sickness: clinical efficacy and effect on gas exchange, *Ann Intern Med* 116(6):461, 1992.
71. Grover RF, Lufschanowski R, Alexander JK: Decreased coronary blood flow in man following ascent to high altitude, *Adv Cardiol* 5:72, 1970.
72. Grover RF et al: Muscular exercise in young men native to 3100 meter altitude, *J Appl Physiol* 22(3):555, 1967.
73. Grover RF, Tucker A, Reeves JT: Hypobaria: an etiologic factor in acute mountain sickness. In Loeppky JA, Riedesel ML, editors: *Oxygen transport to human tissue,* New York, 1982, Elsevier/North Holland.
74. Grover RF et al: The coronary stress of skiing at high altitude, *Arch Intern Med* 150:1205, 1990.
75. Groves BM et al: Operation Everest II: elevated high altitude pulmonary resistance unresponsive to oxygen, *J Appl Physiol* 63(2):521, 1987.
76. Hackett PH: *Mountain sickness: prevention, recognition and treatment,* New York, 1980, American Alpine Club.
77. Hackett PH: Cortical blindness in high altitude climbers and trekkers—a report on six cases (abstract). In Sutton JR, Houston CS, Coates G, editors: *Hypoxia and cold,* New York, 1987, Praeger.

78. Hackett PH et al: Pulmonary edema fluid protein in high altitude pulmonary edema (letter), *JAMA* 256(1):36, 1986.
79. Hackett PH et al: High altitude pulmonary edema in persons without the right pulmonary artery, *N Engl J Med* 302(19):1070, 1980.
80. Hackett PH et al: Ventilation in human populations native to high altitude. In West JB, Lahiri S, editors: *High altitude and man,* Bethesda, Md, 1984, American Physiological Society.
81. Hackett PH, Rennie ID: Rales, peripheral edema, retinal hemorrhage and acute mountain sickness, *Am J Med* 67:214, 1979.
82. Hackett PH, Rennie ID: Cotton-wool spots: a new addition to high altitude retinopathy. In Brendel W, Zink RA, editors: *High altitude physiology and medicine,* New York, 1982, Springer-Verlag.
83. Hackett PH et al: Fluid retention and relative hypoventilation in acute mountain sickness, *Respiration* 43:321, 1982.
84. Hackett PH, Rennie ID, Levine HD: The incidence, importance, and prophylaxis of acute mountain sickness, *Lancet* 2(7995):1149, 1976.
85. Hackett PH, Roach RC: Medical therapy of altitude illness, *Ann Emerg Med* 16(9):980, 1987.
86. Hackett PH, Roach RC: High altitude pulmonary edema, *J Wilderness Med* 1:3, 1990.
87. Hackett PH et al: Respiratory stimulants and sleep periodic breathing at high altitude: almitrine versus acetazolamide, *Am Rev Respir Dis* 135:896, 1987.
88. Hackett PH et al: The effect of vasodilators on pulmonary hemodynamics in high altitude pulmonary edema: a comparison, *Int J Sports Med* 13(suppl 1):S68, 1992.
89. Hackett PH et al: The Denali Medical Research Project, 1982-1985, *Am Alpine J* 28(60):129, 1986.
90. Hackett PH et al: Abnormal control of ventilation in high-altitude pulmonary edema, *J Appl Physiol* 64(3):1268, 1988.
91. Hackett PH et al: Subclinical pulmonary edema in acute mountain sickness (abstract). In Sutton JR, Houston CS, Coates G, editors: *Hypoxia: the tolerable limits,* Indianapolis, 1988, Benchmark Press.
92. Hackett PH et al: Dexamethasone for prevention and treatment of acute mountain sickness, *Aviat Space Environ Med* 59:950, 1988.
93. Hackett PH, Yarnell P, Hill RP: MRI in high altitude cerebral edema: evidence for vasogenic edema (abstract). In Sutton JR, Coates G, Remmers JE, editors: *Hypoxia: the adaptations,* Philadelphia, 1990, BC Decker.
94. Hamilton AJ, Cymerman A, Bloch M: High altitude cerebral edema, *Neurosurgery* 19(5):841, 1986.
95. Hannon JP: Comparative altitude adaptability of young men and women. In Folinsbee LJ et al, editors: *Environmental stress: individual human adaptations,* New York, 1978, Academic Press.
96. Hannon JP, Chinn KS, Shields JL: Effects of acute high altitude exposure on body fluids, *Fed Proc* 28(3):1178, 1969.
97. Hansen JE, Evans WO: A hypothesis regarding the pathophysiology of acute mountain sickness, *Arch Environ Health* 21:666, 1970.
98. Hansen JE, Hartley LH, Hogan RP: Arterial oxygen increased by high-carbohydrate diet at altitude, *J Appl Physiol* 33(4):441, 1972.
99. Harber MJ, Williams JD, Morton JJ: Antidiuretic hormone excretion at high altitude, *Aviat Space Environ Med* 52(1):38, 1981.
100. Harris CW, Shields JL, Hannon JP: Acute altitude sickness in females, *Aerospace Med* 37(11):1163, 1966.
101. Hartig GS, Hackett PH: Cerebral spinal fluid pressure and cerebral blood velocity in acute mountain sickness. In Sutton JR, Coates G, Houston CS, editors: *Hypoxia and mountain medicine,* Burlington, Vt, 1992, Queen City Press.
102. Heath D, Williams DR: *Man at high altitude,* Edinburgh, 1989, Churchill Livingstone.
103. Hebbel RP et al: Human llamas: adaptation to altitude in subjects with high hemoglobin oxygen affinity, *J Clin Invest* 62:593, 1978.
104. Heyes MP, Sutton JR: High altitude ills: a malady of water, electrolyte, and hormonal imbalance? *Semin Respir Med* 5(2):207, 1983.
105. Honigman B et al: Acute mountain sickness in a general tourist population at moderate altitudes, *Ann Intern Med* 118(8):587, 1993.
106. Houston CS: Operation Everest, *U.S. Naval Med Bull* 46:1783, 1946.
107. Houston CS: Acute pulmonary edema of high altitude, *N Engl J Med* 263(10):478, 1960.
108. Houston CS: Altitude illness, *Proc Mountain Med Symp, 1975,* Yosemite, Calif, 1975, Yosemite Institute.
109. Houston CS: *High altitude physiology study—collected papers,* Burlington, Vt, 1980, Queen City Press.
110. Houston CS: Altitude illness: manifestations, etiology and management. In Loeppky JA, Riedesel ML, editors: *Oxygen transport to human tissue,* New York, 1982, Elsevier/North Holland.
111. Houston CS: *Going higher: the story of man at high altitude,* Boston, 1987, Little, Brown.
112. Houston CS, Dickinson JG: Cerebral form of high altitude illness, *Lancet* 2(7938):758, 1975.
113. Houston CS, Sutton JR, Cymerman A: Operation Everest II: man at high altitude, *J Appl Physiol* 63:877, 1987.
114. Hu ST: Hypoxia research in China: an overview. In Sutton JR, Houston CS, Coates G, editors: *Hypoxia, exercise and altitude,* New York, 1983, AR Liss.
115. Hu XC, Huang SY, Zhu ZF: Peripheral chemoresponsiveness at sea level and susceptibility of acute mountain sickness. In *Proceedings of a Symposium on the Tibet Plateau,* New York, 1981, Gordon & Breach.
116. Huang SY et al: Hypocapnia and sustained hypoxia blunt ventilation on arrival at high altitude, *J Appl Physiol* 56(3):602, 1984.
117. Huang SY et al: Internal carotid and vertebral arterial flow velocity in men at high altitude, *J Appl Physiol* 63(1):395, 1987.
118. Hultgren HN: High altitude pulmonary edema. In Hegnauer A, editor: *Biomedical problems of high terrestrial elevations,* Springfield, Va, 1967, Federal Scientific Technical Information Service.
119. Hultgren HN: High altitude pulmonary edema, *Adv Cardiol* 5:24, 1970.
120. Hultgren HN: Furosemide for high altitude pulmonary edema (letter), *JAMA* 234(6):589, 1975.
121. Hultgren HN: High altitude pulmonary edema. In Staub NC, editor: *Lung water and solute exchange,* New York, 1978, Marcel Dekker.
122. Hultgren HN: Reduction of systemic arterial blood pressure at high altitude, *Adv Cardiol* 5:49, 1979.
123. Hultgren HN, Grover RF: Circulatory adaptations to high altitude, *Annu Rev Med* 19:119, 1968.
124. Hultgren HN, Grover RF, Hartley LH: Abnormal circulatory responses to high altitude in subjects with a previous history of high altitude pulmonary edema, *Circulation* 54:759, 1971.
125. Hultgren HN, Kelly J, Miller H: Effect of oxygen upon pulmonary circulation in man acclimatized at high altitude, *J Appl Physiol* 20(2):239, 1965.
126. Hultgren HN et al: Physiologic studies of pulmonary edema at high altitude, *Circulation* 29:393, 1964.
127. Hultgren HN, Marticorena E: High altitude pulmonary edema: epidemiologic observations in Peru, *Chest* 74(4):372, 1978.
128. Hultgren HN et al: High altitude pulmonary edema, *Medicine* 40:289, 1961.
129. Hultgren HN, Spickard WB, Lopez C: Further studies of high altitude pulmonary edema, *Br Heart J* 24:95, 1962.
130. Hurtado A: *Aspectos fisiologicos y patologicos de la vida en las Alturas,* Lima, 1937, Imprenta Rimac.
131. Hyers TM et al: Accentuated hypoxemia at high altitude in subjects susceptible to high-altitude pulmonary edema, *J Appl Physiol* 46(1):41, 1979.
132. Jaeger JJ et al: Evidence for increased intrathoracic fluid volume in man at high altitude, *J Appl Physiol* 47(4):670, 1979.
133. Jain SC et al: Amelioration of acute mountain sickness: comparative study of acetazolamide and spironolactone, *Int J Biometeolor* 30(4):293, 1986.
134. Johnson TS et al: Prevention of acute mountain sickness by dexamethasone, *N Engl J Med* 310(11):683, 1984.

135. Kamat SR, Banerji BC: Study of cardiopulmonary function on exposure to high altitude: acute acclimatization to an altitude of 3500 to 4000 meters, *Am Rev Respir Dis* 106:404, 1972.
136. Kamat SR et al: A study of some cardiorespiratory parameters in newcomers to high altitude. In Malhotra MS, editor: *Human adaptability to environments and physical fitness,* Madras, India, 1966, Defence Institute of Physiology and Allied Sciences.
137. Kasic JF et al: Treatment of acute mountain sickness: hyperbaric versus oxygen therapy, *Ann Emerg Med* 20:1107, 1991.
138. Kawashima A et al: Hemodynamic responses to acute hypoxia, hypobaria, and exercise in subjects susceptible to high-altitude pulmonary edema, *J Appl Physiol* 67(5):1982, 1989.
139. Kayser B: Nutrition and high altitude exposure, *Int J Sports Med* 13(suppl 1):S129, 1992.
140. Keys A: The physiology of life at high altitude, *Sci Monthly* 43:289, 1936.
141. Keys A, Hall FG, Barron ES: The position of the oxygen dissociation curve of human blood at high altitude, *Am J Physiol* 115:292, 1936.
142. King AB, Robinson SM: Ventilation response to hypoxia and acute mountain sickness, *Aerospace Med* 43(4):419, 1972.
143. Klatzo I: Pathophysiological aspects of brain edema, *Acta Neuropathol (Berl)* 72:236, 1987.
144. Kobayashi T et al: Clinical features of patients with high altitude pulmonary edema in Japan, *Chest* 92(5):814, 1987.
145. Krasney JA, Curran-Everett DC, Iwamoto J: High altitude cerebral edema: an animal model. In Sutton JR, Coates G, Remmers JE, editors: *Hypoxia: the adaptations,* Philadelphia, 1990, BC Decker.
146. Krasney JA, Jensen JB, Lassen NA: Cerebral blood flow does not adapt to sustained hypoxia, *J Cerebral Blood Flow Metab* 10(6):759, 1990.
147. Kronenberg RS et al: Pulmonary artery pressure and alveolar gas exchange in man during acclimatization to 12,470 ft, *J Clin Invest* 50:827, 1971.
148. Kryger MH, Grover RF: Chronic mountain sickness, *Semin Respir Med* 5(2):164, 1983.
149. Kryger M et al: Treatment of excessive polycythemia of high altitude with respiratory stimulant drugs, *Am Rev Respir Dis* 117:455, 1978.
150. Kryger M et al: Excessive polycythemia of high altitude: role of ventilatory drive and lung disease, *Am Rev Respir Dis* 118:659, 1978.
151. Lahiri S, Maret KH, Sherpa MG: Dependence of high altitude sleep apnea on ventilatory sensitivity to hypoxia, *Respir Physiol* 52:281, 1983.
152. Lane PA, Githens JH: Splenic syndrome at mountain altitudes in sickle cell trait: its occurrence in nonblack persons, *JAMA* 253:2252, 1985.
153. Larsen RF et al: Effect of spironolactone on acute mountain sickness (abstract). In Sutton JR, Houston CS, Coates G, editors: *Hypoxia and cold,* New York, 1987, Praeger.
154. Larson EB et al: Acute mountain sickness and acetazolamide: clinical efficacy and effect on ventilation, *JAMA* 288:328, 1982.
155. Lassen NA: Increase of cerebral blood flow at high altitude: its possible relation to AMS, *Int J Sports Med* 13(suppl 1):S47, 1992.
156. Lassen NA, Harper AM: High altitude cerebral oedema (letter), *Lancet* 2(7945):1154, 1975.
157. Leadbetter G et al: The effect of intermittent altitude exposure on acute mountain sickness (abstract), San Diego, 1992, Southwest Chapter of American College of Sports Medicine.
158. Levine BD et al: High altitude exposure in the elderly. In Sutton JR, Coates G, Houston CS, editors: *Proceedings of the 8th International Hypoxia Symposium,* Burlington, Vt, 1993, Queen City Press.
159. Levine BD, Stray-Gundersen J: A practical approach to altitude training: where to live and train for optimal performance enhancement, *Int J Sports Med* 13(suppl 1):S209, 1992.
160. Levine BD et al: Dexamethasone in the treatment of acute mountain sickness, *N Engl J Med* 321:1707, 1989.
161. Lockhart A, Saiag B: Altitude and human pulmonary circulation, *Clin Sci* 60:599, 1981.
162. Loeppky JA, Caprihan A, Luft UC: VA/Q inequality during clinical hypoxemia and its alterations. In Shiraki K, Yousef MK, editors: *Man in stressful environments,* Springfield, Ill, 1987, Charles C Thomas.
163. Lubin JR et al: High altitude retinal hemorrhage: a clinical and pathological case report, *Ann Ophthalmol* 14(11):1071, 1982.
164. Lyons TP et al: Prior acclimatization to 4300 m reduces acute mountain sickness symptomatology with reinduction. In Sutton JR, Coates G, Houston CS, editors: *Proceedings of the 8th International Hypoxia Symposium,* Burlington, Vt, 1993, Queen City Press.
165. MacDougall JD et al: Operation Everest II: structural adaptations in skeletal muscle in response to extreme simulated altitude, *Acta Physiol Scand* 142:421, 1991.
166. Maher JT, Jones LG, Hartley LH: Effects of high altitude exposure on submaximal endurance capacity of men, *J Appl Physiol* 37(6):895, 1974.
167. Mahoney BS, Githens JH: Sickling crisis and altitude: occurrence in the Colorado patient population, *Clin Pediatr* 18:431, 1979.
168. Malconian MK et al: Operation Everest II: gas tensions in expired air and arterial blood at extreme altitude, *Aviat Space Environ Med* 64:37, 1993.
169. Maldonado D: High altitude pulmonary edema, *Radiol Clin North Am* 16(3):537, 1978.
170. Malhotra MS et al: Responses of the autonomic nervous system during acclimatization to high altitude in man, *Aviat Space Environ Med* 47(10):1076, 1976.
171. Marticorena E, Hultgren HN: Evaluation of therapeutic methods in high altitude pulmonary edema, *Am J Cardiol* 43:307, 1979.
172. Marticorena E, Severino J, Chavez A: Presion arterial sistemica en al nativo de altura, *Arch Inst Biol Andina* 2:18, 1967.
173. Masuyama S et al: Control of ventilation in extreme-altitude climbers, *J Appl Physiol* 61(2):500, 1986.
174. Mathew L et al: Chemoreceptor sensitivity and maladaptation to high altitude in man, *Eur J Appl Physiol* 51:137, 1983.
175. Matsuzawa Y et al: Blunted hypoxic ventilatory drive in subjects susceptible to high-altitude pulmonary edema, *J Appl Physiol* 66(3):1152, 1989.
176. Matsuzawa Y et al: Low hypoxic ventilatory response and relative hypoventilation in acute mountain sickness, *Jpn J Mountain Med* 10:151, 1990.
177. McFadden DM et al: High altitude retinopathy, *JAMA* 245(6):581, 1981.
178. McFadden ER: The lower airway. In Sutton JR, Houston CS, Coates G, editors: *Hypoxia and cold,* New York, 1987, Praeger.
179. McFarland RA, Dill DB: A comparative study of the effects of reduced oxygen pressure on man during acclimatization, *J Aviat Med* 9:18, 1938.
180. McGillicudy JE: Cerebral protection: pathophysiology and treatment of increased intracranial pressure, *Chest* 87(1):85, 1985.
181. Meehan RT: Immune suppression at high altitude, *Ann Emerg Med* 16(9):974, 1987.
182. Menon ND: High altitude pulmonary edema, *N Engl J Med* 273(2):66, 1965.
183. Messner R: *Everest: expedition to the ultimate,* London, 1979, Kay & Ward.
184. Milledge JS: Salt and water control at altitude, *Int J Sports Med* 13(suppl 1):S61, 1992.
185. Milledge JS et al: Acute mountain sickness susceptibility, fitness and hypoxic ventilatory response, *Eur Respir J* 4:1000, 1991.
186. Monge CC: Medical research in the Andes, *Ann Sports Med* 4(4):245, 1989.
187. Monge CC, Leon-Velarde F, Arregui A: Increasing prevalence of excessive erythrocytosis with age among healthy high-altitude miners (letter), *N Engl J Med* 321(18):1271, 1989.

188. Monge CM: La enfermedad de las Andes: sindromes eritremicos, *Ann Fac Med (Lima)* 11(1):75, 314, 1928.
189. Monge CC, Arregui A, Leon-Velarde F: Pathophysiology and epidemiology of chronic mountain sickness, *Int J Sports Med* 13(suppl 1):S79, 1992.
190. Montgomery AB, Mills J, Luce JM: Incidence of acute mountain sickness at intermediate altitude, *JAMA* 261(5):732, 1989.
191. Moore LG: Altitude aggravated illness: examples from pregnancy and prenatal life, *Ann Emerg Med* 16(9):965, 1987.
192. Moore LG et al: Are Tibetans better adapted? *Int J Sports Med* 13(suppl 1):S86, 1992.
193. Moore LG et al: Low acute hypoxic ventilatory response and hypoxic depression in acute altitude sickness, *J Appl Physiol* 60(4):1407, 1986.
194. Moore LG et al: Genetic adaptations to high altitude. In Wood SC, Roach RC, editors: *Modern topics in sports medicine,* New York, 1993, Marcel Dekker.
195. Morris A: *Clinical pulmonary function tests: a manual of uniform lab procedures,* Salt Lake City, 1984, Intermountain Thoracic Society.
196. Mosso A: *Life of man in the high alps,* London, 1898, T Fisher Unwin.
197. Nakashima M: High altitude medical research in Japan. In Sutton JR, Houston CS, Jones NL, editors: *Hypoxia, exercise and altitude,* New York, 1983, AR Liss.
198. Nayak NC, Roy S, Narayaran TK: Pathologic features of altitude sickness, *Am J Pathol* 45(1):381, 1964.
199. O'Brodovich H et al: Hypoxia alters blood coagulation during acute decompression in humans, *J Appl Physiol* 56(3):666, 1984.
200. Oelz O et al: Physiological profile of world-class high altitude climbers, *J Appl Physiol* 60(5):1734, 1986.
201. Oelz O et al: Prevention and treatment of high altitude pulmonary edema by a calcium channel blocker, *Int J Sports Med* 13(suppl 1):S65, 1992.
202. Oelz O et al: Nifedipine for high altitude pulmonary edema, *Lancet* 2:1241, 1989.
203. Okin JT: Response of patients with coronary heart disease to exercise at varying altitudes, *Adv Cardiol* 5:92, 1970.
204. Olson LG, Hensley MJ, Saunders NA: Augmentation of ventilatory response to asphyxia by prochlorperazine in humans, *J Appl Physiol* 53(3):637, 1982.
205. Ou LC, Tenney SM: Properties of mitochondria from hearts of cattle acclimatized to high altitude, *Respir Physiol* 8:151, 1970.
206. Pei SX et al: Chronic mountain sickness in Tibet, *Q J Med* 71(266):555, 1989.
207. Peñaloza D, Sime F: Circulatory dynamics during high altitude pulmonary edema, *Am J Cardiol* 23:369, 1969.
208. Powles AP, Sutton JR: Sleep at altitude, *Semin Respir Med* 5(2):175, 1983.
209. Pugh LG: Physiological and medical aspects of the Himalayan scientific and mountaineering expedition, 1960-61, *Br Med J* 2(5305):621, 1962.
210. Pugh LG: Metabolic problems of high altitude operations. In Vaughan L, editor: *Proceedings Symposia Arctic Biology and Medicine V: nutritional requirements for survival in the cold and at altitude,* Ft Wainwright, Alaska, 1966, Arctic Aeromedical Laboratory.
211. Pugh LG: Report of medical research project into effects of altitude in Mexico City. In Astrand PO, Rodahl K, editors: *Textbook of work physiology,* New York, 1977, McGraw-Hill.
212. Pugh LG et al: Muscular exercise at great altitude, *J Appl Physiol* 19(3):431, 1964.
213. Rahn H, Otis AB: Man's respiratory response during and after acclimatization to high altitude, *Am J Physiol* 157(2):445, 1949.
214. Rebold MB: *High altitude bronchitis on Cerro Aconcagua* (abstract), Aspen, Colo, 1987, Wilderness Medical Society.
215. Reeves JT: Sympathetics and hypoxia: a brief overview. In Sutton JR, Houston CS, Coates G, editors: *Hypoxia and molecular medicine,* Burlington, Vt, 1993, Queen City Press.
216. Reeves JT et al: Operation Everest II: preservation of cardiac function at extreme altitude, *J Appl Physiol* 63(2):531, 1987.
217. Reeves JT et al: Oxygen transport during exercise at extreme altitude: Operation Everest II, *Ann Emerg Med* 16(9):993, 1987.
218. Reeves JT et al: Headache at high altitude is not related to internal carotid arterial blood velocity, *J Appl Physiol* 59(3):909, 1985.
219. Reeves JT et al: Seasonal variation in barometric pressure and temperature in Summit County: effect on altitude illness. In Sutton JR, Houston CS, Coates G, editors: *Hypoxia and molecular medicine,* Burlington, Vt, 1993, Queen City Press.
220. Reite M et al: Sleep physiology at high altitude, *Electroencephalogr Clin Neurophysiol* 38:463, 1975.
221. Richalet JP et al: Plasma prostaglandins, leukotrienes and thromboxane in acute high altitude hypoxia, *Respir Physiol* 85:205, 1991.
222. Richalet JP et al: Physiological characteristics of high altitude climbers, *Science and Sports* 3:89, 1988.
223. Richalet JP et al: Plasma volume, body weight and acute mountain sickness, *Lancet* 1(8323):525, 1983.
224. Ritchie K: The fetal response to changes in the composition of maternal inspired air in human pregnancy, *Semin Perinatol* 4(4):295, 1980.
225. Roach RC: The role of the hypoxic ventilatory response in performance at high altitude. In Wood SC, Roach RC, editors: *Modern topics in sports medicine,* New York, 1994, Marcel Dekker.
226. Roach RC et al: The Lake Louise acute mountain sickness scoring system. In Sutton JR, Houston CS, Coates G, editors: *Hypoxia and molecular biology,* Burlington, Vt, 1993, Queen City Press.
227. Roach RC, Hackett PH: Hyperbaria and high altitude illness. In Sutton JR, Coates G, Houston CS, editors: *Hypoxia and mountain medicine,* Burlington, Vt, 1992, Queen City Press.
228. Roach RC et al: How well do the elderly tolerate moderate altitudes? Presented at the Eighth International Hypoxia Symposium, Lake Louise, Canada, 1994.
229. Roach RC et al: Fluid balance in humans at high altitude: does hypobaria play a role? (abstract), *FASEB J* 8(4):A553, 1994.
230. Robin ED: Permeability pulmonary edema. In Fishman AP, Renkin EM, editors: *Pulmonary edema,* Bethesda, Md, 1979, American Physiological Society.
231. Robinson SM, King AB, Aoki VS: Acute mountain sickness: reproducibility of its severity and duration in an individual, *Aerospace Med* 42:706, 1971.
232. Rock PB et al: Effect of dexamethasone on symptoms of acute mountain sickness at Pike's Peak, Colorado (4,300), *Aviat Space Environ Med* 58(11):668, 1987.
233. Ropper AH: Raised intracranial pressure in neurologic diseases, *Semin Neurol* 4(4):397, 1984.
234. Roy SB et al: Transthoracic electrical impedance in cases of high-altitude hypoxia, *Br Med J* 3:771, 1974.
235. Saltin B et al: Maximal oxygen uptake and cardiac output after 2 weeks at 4,300 m, *J Appl Physiol* 25(3):400, 1968.
236. Samaja M, di Prampero PE, Cerretelli P: The role of 2,3-DPG in the oxygen transport at altitude, *Respir Physiol* 64:191, 1986.
237. Sarnquist FH: Physicians on Mount Everest, *West J Med* 139:480, 1983.
238. Schoene RB: Control of ventilation in climbers at extreme altitude, *J Appl Physiol* 53(4):886, 1982.
239. Schoene RB: Pulmonary edema at high altitude: review, pathophysiology and update, *Clin Chest Med* 6(3):491, 1985.
240. Schoene RB, Hackett PH, Roach RC: Blunted hypoxic chemosensitivity at altitude and sea level in an elite high altitude climber (abstract). In Sutton JR, Houston CS, Coates G, editors: *Hypoxia and cold,* New York, 1987, Praeger.

241. Schoene RB et al: The relationship of hypoxic ventilatory response to exercise performance on Mount Everest, *J Appl Physiol* 56(6):1478, 1984.
242. Schoene RB et al: High altitude pulmonary edema and exercise at 4400 meters on Mt McKinley: effect of expiratory positive airway pressure, *Chest* 87(3):330, 1984.
243. Schoene RB et al: High altitude pulmonary edema: characteristics of lung lavage fluid, *JAMA* 256(1):63, 1986.
244. Schoene RB et al: The lung at high altitude: bronchoalveolar lavage in acute mountain sickness and pulmonary edema, *J Appl Physiol* 64(6):2605, 1988.
245. Scoggin CH et al: High altitude pulmonary edema in the children and young adults of Leadville, Colorado, *N Engl J Med* 297:1269, 1977.
246. Senay LC, Tolbert DL: Effect of arginine vasopressin, acetazolamide and angiotensin II on CSF pressure at simulated altitude, *Aviat Space Environ Med* 55:370, 1984.
247. Severinghaus JW: Blood gas calculator, *J Appl Physiol* 21(3):1108, 1966.
248. Severinghaus JW: Transarterial leakage: a possible mechanism of high altitude pulmonary edema. In Porter R, Knight J, editors: *High altitude physiology: cardiac and respiratory aspects,* London, 1971, Churchill-Livingstone.
249. Severinghaus JW et al: Cerebral blood flow in man at high altitude: role of cerebrospinal fluid pH in normalization of flow in chronic hypoxia, *Circ Res* 19:274, 1966.
250. Shinfu S: Epidemiology of hypertension on the Tibetan Plateau, *Hum Biol* 58(4):507, 1986.
251. Sickle Cell Treatment and Research Center, University of Colorado Health Sciences Center (personal communication), Denver, 1987.
252. Siesjo BK, Ingvar M: Ventilation and brain metabolism. In Cherniack NS, Widdicombe JG, editors: *Handbook of physiology: the respiratory system,* Bethesda, Md, 1986, American Physiological Society.
253. Singh I: Pulmonary hypertension in new arrivals at high altitude, *Proceedings of World Health Organization Meeting on Primary Pulmonary Hypertension, 1973,* Geneva, 1974, World Health Organization.
254. Singh I, Chohan IS, Mathew NT: Fibrinolytic activity in high altitude pulmonary oedema, *Ind J Med Res* 57(2):210, 1969.
255. Singh I, Roy SB: High altitude pulmonary edema: clinical, hemodynamic, and pathologic studies. In Hegnauer A, editor: *Biomedical problems of high terrestrial elevations,* Springfield, Va, 1962, Federal Scientific and Technical Information Service.
256. Singh I et al: High altitude pulmonary oedema, Lancet 1(7379):229, 1965.
257. Singh I et al: Acute mountain sickness, *N Engl J Med* 280(4):175, 1969.
258. Smith JM: The use of high altitude treatment for childhood asthma, *Practitioner* 225:1663, 1981.
259. Song SY et al: Cerebral thrombosis at altitude: its pathogenesis and the problems of prevention and treatment, *Aviat Space Environ Med* 57:71, 1986.
260. Sophocles AM: High-altitude pulmonary edema in Vail, Colorado, 1975-1982, *West J Med* 144:569, 1986.
261. Sophocles AM, Bachman J: High altitude pulmonary edema among visitors to Summit County, Colorado, *J Fam Pract* 17(6):1015, 1983.
262. Staub NC: Pulmonary edema-hypoxia and overperfusion (editorial), *N Engl J Med* 302(19):1085, 1980.
263. Strohl KP, Fouke JM: Periodic breathing at altitude, *Semin Respir Med* 5(2):169, 1983.
264. Suarez J, Alexander JK, Houston CS: Enhanced left ventricular systolic performance at high altitude during Operation Everest II, *Am J Cardiol* 60:137, 1987.
265. Sutton JR: High altitude retinal hemorrhage, *Semin Respir Med* 5(2):159, 1983.
266. Sutton JR et al: Pulmonary gas exchange in acute mountain sickness, *Aviat Space Environ Med* 47(10):1032, 1976.
267. Sutton JR et al: Increased erythropoietin and hemoglobin with exposure to extreme altitude (abstract). In Sutton JR, Houston CS, Coates G, editors: *Hypoxia: the tolerable limits,* Indianapolis, 1988, Benchmark Press.
268. Sutton JR et al: Effects of acclimatization on sleep hypoxemia at altitude. In West JB, Lahiri S, editors: *High altitude and man,* Bethesda, Md, 1984, American Physiological Society.
269. Sutton JR, Houston CS, Coates G, editors: *Hypoxia and cold,* new York, 1987, Praeger.
270. Sutton JR et al: Effect of acetazolamide on hypoxemia during sleep at high altitude, *N Engl J Med* 301(24):1329, 1979.
271. Sutton JR et al: Operation Everest II: oxygen transport during exercise at extreme simulated altitude, *J Appl Physiol* 64(4):1309, 1988.
272. Swenson ER et al: Renal carbonic anhydrase inhibition reduces high altitude sleep periodic breathing, *Respir Physiol* 86:333, 1991.
273. Tufts DA et al: Distribution of hemoglobin and functional consequences of anemia in adult males at high altitude, *Am J Clin Nutr* 42:1, 1985.
274. Turner WA et al: Carbon monoxide exposure in mountaineers on Denali, *Alaska Med* 30(3):85, 1988.
275. Viault F: On the large increase in the number of red cells in the blood of the inhabitants of the high plateaus of South America. In West JB, editor: *High altitude physiology,* Stroudsburg, Pa, 1981, Hutchinson Ross.
276. Viswanathan R, Subramanian S, Radha TG: Effect of hypoxia on regional lung perfusion, by scanning, *Respiration* 37:142, 1979.
277. Viswanathan R et al: Further studies on pulmonary oedema of high altitude, *Respiration* 36:216, 1978.
278. Vock P et al: Variable radiomorphologic data of high altitude pulmonary edema: features from 60 patients, *Chest* 100(5):1306, 1991.
279. Vock P et al: High-altitude pulmonary edema: findings at high-altitude chest radiography and physical examination, *Radiology* 170(3):661, 1989.
280. Wagner PD: Gas exchange and peripheral diffusion limitation, *Med Sci Sports Exerc* 24(1):54, 1992.
281. Wagner PD et al: Operation Everest II: pulmonary gas exchange during a simulated ascent of Mt. Everest, *J Appl Physiol* 63(6):2348, 1987.
282. Ward MP: *Mountain medicine: a clinical study of cold and high altitude,* London, 1975, Crosby, Lockwood, Staples.
283. Ward MP, Milledge JS, West JB: *High altitude medicine and physiology,* Philadelphia, 1989, University of Pennsylvania Press.
284. Weil JV et al: Hypoxic ventilatory drive in normal man, *J Clin Invest* 49(6):1061, 1970.
285. Weil JV, Kryger MH, Scoggin CH: Sleep and breathing at high altitude. In Guilleminault C, Dement WC, editors: *Sleep apnea syndromes,* New York, 1978, AR Liss.
286. West JB: Human physiology at extreme altitudes on Mt Everest, *Science* 223:784, 1984.
287. West JB: "Oxygenless" climbs and barometric pressure, *Am Alpine J* 226(58):126, 1984.
288. West JB, Lahiri S: *High altitude and man,* Washington, DC, 1984, American Physiological Society.
289. West JB, Mathieu-Costello O: High altitude pulmonary edema is caused by stress failure of pulmonary capillaries, *Int J Sports Med* 13(Suppl 1):S54, 1992.
290. West JB et al: Arterial oxygen saturation during exercise at high altitude, *J Appl Physiol* 17(4):617, 1962.
291. West JB et al: Maximal exercise at extreme altitudes on Mount Everest, *J Appl Physiol* 55(3):688, 1983.
292. West JB et al: Pulmonary gas exchange on the Summit of Mount Everest, *J Appl Physiol* 55(3):678, 1983.
293. West JB et al: Stress failure in pulmonary capillaries, *J Appl Physiol* 70(4):1731, 1991.
294. Westendorp RG et al: Atrial natriuretic peptide improves pulmonary gas exchange in subjects exposed to hypoxia, *Am Rev Respir Dis* 148:304, 1993.

295. Wilson R: Acute high altitude illness in mountaineers and problems of rescue, *Ann Intern Med* 78(3):421, 1973.
296. Winslow RM: Hypoxia and polycythemia: the "optimal" hematocrit. In Sutton JR, Jones NL, Houston CS, editors: *Hypoxia: man at altitude,* New York, 1982, Thieme-Stratton.
297. Winslow RM: High altitude polycythemia. In West JB, Lahiri S, editors: *High altitude and man,* Bethesda, Md, 1984, American Physiological Society.
298. Winslow RM, Samaja M, West JB: Red cell function at extreme altitude on Mt. Everest, *J Appl Physiol* 56(1):109, 1984.
299. Wistrand PJ: The use of carbonic anhydrase in ophthalmology and clinical medicine, *Ann NY Acad Sci* 429:609, 1984.
300. Wohns RN: Transient ischemic attacks at high altitude, *Crit Care Med* 14(5):517, 1986.
301. Wu TY: An epidemiological study on high altitude disease, *Chung-Hua Liu Hsing Ping Hsueh Tsa Chih* 8(2):65, 1987.
302. Xie CF, Pei SX: Some physiological data on sojourners and native highlanders at three different altitudes on Xizang. In *Proceedings of a Symposium on the Tibet Plateau,* New York, 1981, Gordon & Breach.
303. Yagi H et al: Doppler assessment of pulmonary hypertension induced by hypoxic breathing in subjects susceptible to high altitude pulmonary edema, *Am Rev Respir Dis* 142:796, 1990.
304. Yaron M, Alexander J, Hultgren H: Low risk of myocardial ischemia in the elderly at moderate altitude. In Sutton JR, Coates G, Houston CS, editors: *Proceedings of 8th International Hypoxia Symposium,* Burlington, Vt, 1993, Queen City Press.
305. Zell SC, Goodman PH: Acetazolamide and dexamethasone in the prevention of acute mountain sickness, *West J Med* 148:541, 1988.
306. Zimmerman GA, Crapo RO: Adult respiratory distress syndrome secondary to high altitude pulmonary edema, *West J Med* 133:335, 1980.

2 THERMOREGULATION

Larry I. Crawshaw

A warm body has long been recognized as one of the primary conditions for, and signs of, life. Under primitive circumstances the maintenance of body temperature can require great ingenuity. Three thousand years ago, King David was old, stricken in years, and a bit hypothermic. Ministrations included covering him with clothes and finding a "fair damsel" to cherish him and lie in his bosom such that he might "gat heat." Unfortunately, these attempts to decrease heat loss, increase heat production, and increase heat transfer were not successful.[38] In 1993 the efficacy of body-to-body contact was assessed in a more quantitative manner: immersion hypothermia "victims" were placed in a sleeping bag alone or with male or female "heat donors." Surprisingly, the "victims" who were supplied with "donors" exhibited a blunted shivering thermogenesis and rewarmed at a lower rate.[26]

Because the thermal environment can be extremely complicated and the thermoregulatory system of humans is complex and only partially understood, decisions about body temperature maintenance in the field can be difficult. This chapter is designed to aid in the decision process by providing a basic understanding of the relationships among the ambient thermal environment, the thermal characteristics of the body, and the thermoregulatory system. First, the heat balance equation is used to quantify the thermal nature of the environment. Then peripheral neuronal inputs and the nature of the central regulator are elucidated. After this the various organ systems that the body uses as effectors to regulate body temperature are outlined. Finally, a number of special circumstances that affect temperature regulation are noted.

Physical Factors Governing Heat Exchange

The physical laws governing heat transfer determine the net energy flux into or out of the body. Useful treatments of this subject can be found in Hardy,[31] Cossins and Bowler,[12] Schmidt-Nielsen,[64] Nobel,[57] and Mount[49]; these sources were used in the formulation of much of the material in this section.

HEAT BALANCE EQUATION

The heat balance equation is a convenient method for partitioning and quantifying the flow of energy between the environment and the body. Because the high metabolic heat production of mammals is critical for maintaining a constant body temperature, total heat production by the organism is represented on the left side of the equation. For a person whose body is at thermal equilibrium,

$$H_{tot} = \pm H_d \pm H_c \pm H_r \pm H_e$$

where

H_{tot} = total metabolic heat production
H_d = conductive heat exchange
H_c = convective heat exchange
H_r = radiative heat exchange
H_e = evaporative heat exchange

H_{tot} is always positive. The various channels of heat exchange can be positive or negative, depending on the situation. Positive values refer to net heat loss from the body. If the sum of the net heat exchange through the various channels exceeds H_{tot}, the heat content of the body will decrease and mean body temperature will fall. On the other hand, if H_{tot} is greater than the net heat exchange, the heat content of the body will increase and mean body temperature will rise.

CONDUCTIVE HEAT EXCHANGE (H_D)

Heat transfer between objects in direct contact is termed conduction. The direction of heat flow is always from the higher to the lower temperature. Since conduction involves a direct interaction between molecules (contact), this type of heat transfer is minimal except under certain circumstances such as sitting on a cold rock with little insulation. Under such conditions the heat loss to the rock per unit area would be similar to that lost from the remainder of the body surface by radiation and convection.[48] The equation governing heat exchange by conduction is

$$H_d = \frac{k\,A\,(T_{sk} - T_a)}{1}$$

where

k = thermal conductivity
A = area of contact
T_{sk} = skin temperature
T_a = ambient temperature
1 = distance between the two surfaces

The thermal conductivity of a number of substances is given in Table 2-1. Note that water has 25 times the conductivity of air but only one-fifth that of granite. Muscle tissue has about twice the conductivity of fat. The conduction of heat through a tissue is termed thermal diffusivity. This expression is obtained by dividing the thermal conductivity by the product of the density and the specific heat. The specific heat of various substances is also given in Table 2-1. Water and muscle tissue (mostly water) have particularly high values. Specific heats can be misleading, however, so the volumetric heat capacities are also listed in Table 2-1. Although the specific heat of water is four times that of air, it takes about 3500 times as much heat to raise the temperature of a given volume of water 1° C as it does to accomplish the same feat with a similar volume of air.

Table 2-1 Thermal Characteristics of Selected Substances

Substance	Conductivity ($cal \cdot s^{-1} \cdot cm^{-1} \cdot C^{-1}$)	Specific Heat ($cal \cdot g^{-1} \cdot °C^{-1}$)	Volumetric Heat Capacity ($cal \cdot l^{-1} \cdot °C^{-1}$)
Air	0.000057	0.24	0.29
Water	0.0014	1.0	1000
Granite	0.007	0.2	540
Muscle tissue	0.0011	0.8	850
Fat	0.00051	0.5	460

Data from Schmidt-Nielsen K: *Animal physiology: adaptation and environment,* ed 4, Cambridge, 1990, Cambridge University Press; Cossins AR, Bowler K: *Temperature biology of animals,* New York, 1987, Chapman & Hall; and Hodgman CD, editor: *Handbook of chemistry and physics: a ready-reference book of chemical and physical data,* ed 43, Cleveland, 1962, Chemical Rubber.

CONVECTIVE HEAT EXCHANGE (H_C)

Convection can be seen as a facilitation of conduction caused by the movements of molecules in a gas or liquid. This movement decreases 1 in the conduction equation. Convection can be either forced or natural (free). Forced convection results from gas or liquid movement caused by the application of an external force, such as the movement of a fan or the pumping of a heart. Natural convection occurs from density changes that are produced by heating or cooling molecules adjacent to the body. These density changes cause the molecules to either rise or fall, moving them away from the body. For humans natural convection predominates at air speeds below 0.2 m sec^{-1}, whereas forced convection is more important at air speeds above this level.[49]

The relationships defining heat exchange resulting from convection can be complicated and depend on surface temperature profiles, surface shape, flow dynamics, density, conductivity, and specific heat. Any factor that impedes movement of the boundary layer (the molecules immediately adjacent to the body) greatly retards convective heat transfer.

Brengelmann and Brown[4] have noted that under relatively neutral conditions (T_a = 29° C, wind velocity = 0.9 m sec^{-1}) about 40% of the heat loss from a nude human is mediated by convection. Increases in air or fluid velocity greatly increase convective heat transfer.

RADIATIVE HEAT EXCHANGE (H_R)

All objects at temperatures above absolute zero emit electromagnetic radiation. This energy transfer occurs through space and does not require an intervening medium. In any given situation the body is both transmitting and receiving infrared thermal radiation. In some cases the body also receives solar radiation. The net heat transfer depends on the absolute temperatures, the nature of the surfaces involved, and solar input. Surfaces that are effective absorbers of radiation are also effective emitters of radiation. The idealized "black body" illustrates this property; such bodies absorb all and reflect none of the incident radiation. Conversely, poor absorbers (such as a polished silver surface) are also poor emitters. The exchange of heat resulting from infrared (first-term) and solar (second-term) radiation is given by:

$$H_r = \sigma\,\varepsilon_{sk}\,\varepsilon_a\,(T_{sk}^4 - T_a^4) + a(1 + r)s$$

where

σ = Stefan-Boltzmann proportionality constant
ε_{sk} = emissivity of the skin
ε_a = emissivity of the environment
T_{sk} = skin temperature (K)
T_a = ambient temperature (K)
a = absorptance
r = reflectance
s = solar radiation

For temperatures in the physiologic range, and where ($T_{sk} - T_a$) is less than 20° C, several authors have noted that infrared radiation heat exchange is roughly proportional to

$T_{sk} - T_a$.[5,64] Also of note is that the spectrum of emitted radiation depends on the temperature of the object. At physiologic temperatures the wavelengths of the emitted radiation are longer (infrared), while at higher temperatures, like that of the sun's surface, the emissions are shorter (visible radiation) and can be detected by the human eye. This difference leads to some important consequences. The middle infrared radiation that is emitted by mammals is maximal regardless of the pigmentation of the skin or the color of clothing. Solar radiation, however, peaks in the visible portion of the spectrum and is absorbed to a significantly greater extent by darker clothes or skin.

Incident radiation can vary drastically under different environmental conditions and may severely tax the body's ability to respond. Heat input from solar radiation on a cloudless day may exceed by several times the heat produced by basal metabolism; on a cloudless night there is a significant net loss of radiation to the sky. Under the conditions noted earlier by Brengelmann and Brown,[4] radiant heat loss accounts for about 45% of the total.

EVAPORATIVE HEAT EXCHANGE (H_E)

When water changes state, a large amount of energy is either absorbed or given off. Evaporation of 1 g of water at 35° C, the usual skin temperature of a person sweating,[64] requires the input of 0.58 kcal of thermal energy. In a neutral thermal environment, sweating does not occur and evaporation accounts for about 15% of the total heat loss. Of this, slightly more than half is due to evaporation from the respiratory tract, with the remainder coming from water that passively diffuses through the skin and evaporates.[4]

Although it is unusual, the evaporation term (H_e) of the heat balance equation can become negative (meaning that heat is being introduced into the body). This occurs during airway rewarming when water-saturated oxygen is introduced into the respiratory system at about 43° C. Since the victim's body is considerably colder than 43°, water condenses in the airways. For every gram of liquid water that is formed, the body heat content increases by 0.58 kcal.

Thermoregulatory Network

A regulatory system requires sensing the controlled variable, comparing it with an ideal value, and producing an appropriate output signal. In this section the role of the nervous system in the maintenance of a stable body temperature is outlined.

PERIPHERAL THERMAL SENSORS

The entire outer surface of the body is well supplied with sensitive thermoreceptive structures. Since information from these receptors travels to the sensory cortex, many properties of the receptors can be gleaned from direct experience. The afferent thermal information produces both hot and cold sensations and is particularly rate sensitive. In addition to the cortical input that arrives via the medial lemniscus and ventrobasal thalamus, the brain receives a large amount of thermal information from pathways that synapse in the reticular area.[6] Although the cortical thermal input is probably part of the sensory information that is used to reconstruct the external thermal environment, the reticular inputs are more important in the behavioral and autonomic regulation of body temperature.[15] This distinction was pointed out by Cabanac,[9] who found that internal body temperature determined whether a particular surface temperature was perceived as pleasant or unpleasant. However, the altered body temperature did not affect the discriminative (cortically mediated) aspects of the thermal stimulus: the subjects had no problem in correctly identifying the actual peripheral temperature. This study also confirms the intimate relationship between the thermoregulatory network and the pleasure-pain system.[60]

Although the structure, location, and properties of peripheral thermoreceptors are well documented, the transduction mechanism is poorly understood. Thermal sensors are free nerve endings and are categorized as either warm or cold. Cold receptors are found immediately beneath the epidermis, while warm receptors are located slightly deeper in the dermis. The hallmark of both types of receptors is their extremely high rate sensitivity (Fig. 2-1).[34] Although the static firing rate of cold receptors is usually less than 10 impulses per second, under conditions of rapid temperature change the firing rates are often an order of magnitude higher. Cold receptors are excited by cooling, are inhibited by warming, and have static maxima at about 25° C. These receptors are active from about 10° to 40° C. Warm receptors are excited by warming, inhibited by cooling, and have static maxima above 40° C. They are active from about 30° to 45° C.[33] Studies on the mechanism underlying peripheral cold sensitivity have implicated thermal effects on the electrogenic Na^+,K^+ pump.[3]

Psychophysical and physiologic studies indicate that thermal receptors are not uniformly distributed and that there are far more cold receptors.[33] Since peripheral thermal input is intimately involved in the regulation of body temperature, the body site that is heated or cooled can have a definite effect on the magnitude of the response produced. In one study, for example, cooling the forehead was more than three times as effective (per unit area) in decreasing ongoing sweating as was cooling the lower leg.[14] A separate study evaluated regional trunk and appendage sensitivity to cooling by assessing the magnitude of the gasping response that occurs at the onset of immersion. In this case, exposing various parts of the body to 15° C water indicated that the upper torso had the greatest cold receptor density or sensitivity or both. The lower torso was somewhat less sensitive, with the arms and legs exhibiting similar but considerably lower sensitivity.[8]

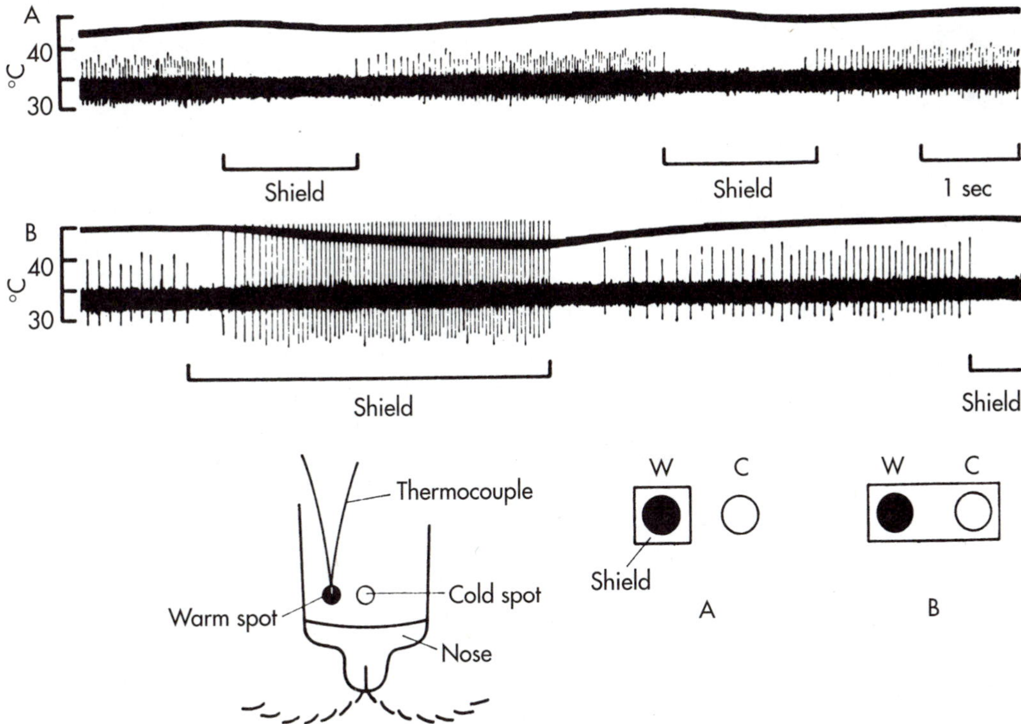

Fig. 2-1 Impulses from a recording that includes a single warm fiber and a single cold fiber. In recording *A* a shield was periodically placed in front of and then moved away from the skin site that was innervated by the warm fiber. The discharge stops immediately when the skin is shielded from the radiation source. In recording *B* the shield was simultaneously placed in front of the skin site innervated by both the warm fiber and the cold fiber. This caused excitation of the cold fiber and inhibition of the warm fiber. (From Hensel H, Kenshalo DR: *J Physiol [Lond]* 204:99, 1969.)

The extremes of the thermal spectrum are sensed by a separate set of receptors, the hot-pain and cold-pain endings.[28] Evidence provided by intradermal and intravenous temperature profiles, as well as intravenous nerve block, indicates that the cold-pain receptors may be the nociceptors of the cutaneous veins.[44]

CENTRAL THERMAL SENSORS

Many sites within the body are capable of eliciting generalized thermoregulatory responses. Such areas include the abdominal viscera, spinal cord, hypothalamus, and lower portions of the brainstem.[3,31] In general, the genesis of input to the regulator resulting from heating or cooling these areas is poorly understood. Some of the effects may be due to the modulation of synaptic connections, rather than an effect on specific thermodetectors per se. Input from central detectors is not rate sensitive but rather is a direct reflection of the actual temperature. The area with the highest thermal sensitivity, and that has received the greatest amount of experimental attention, is the preoptic nucleus–anterior hypothalamic area (PO/AH). Heating and cooling this portion of the brainstem elicit the entire array of autonomic and behavioral heat loss and heat gain responses, respectively.[29] Neurons in this portion of the brain exhibit both warm sensitivity and cold sensitivity.[3] Recent work on hypothalamic slice preparations using synaptic blockers has indicated that warm sensitivity may be an inherent property of some of the PO/AH neurons, while cold sensitivity in this area of the brain requires synaptic input.[3,17] Work using hypothalamic slices has also established that about half of the thermosensitive neurons also respond to nonthermal stimuli such as osmotic pressure, glucose concentration, or steroid hormone concentration. Such neurons could form the basis for the interactions between homeostatic systems described subsequently. Fig. 2-2 illustrates the response of a warm-sensitive PO/AH neuron in a slice preparation. This cell is excited by increased temperature, low glucose, and increased osmotic pressure.[2]

REGULATOR

The neuroanatomic structures that establish the regulated body temperature include portions of the spinal cord,

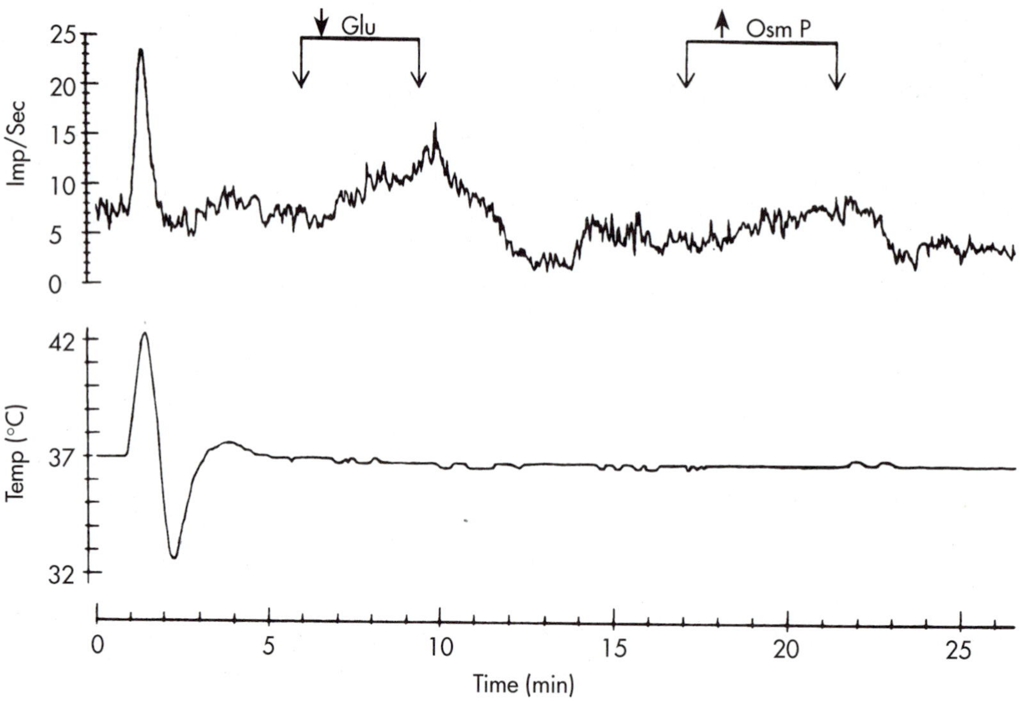

Fig. 2-2 The response of a warm-sensitive preoptic nucleus–anterior hypothalamic area neuron to changes in temperature, glucose concentration, and osmotic pressure. The large downward arrows indicate media changes. (From Boulant JA, Silva NL: *Brain Res Bull* 20[6]:871, 1988.)

lower brainstem, hypothalamus, and septum. The PO/AH and the caudal hypothalamus, in particular, are recognized as important integrating areas.[30] The PO/AH has been assigned a unique role as the center of central nervous thermosensitivity and thermointegration,[29] but other sites are also involved. As noted by Blatteis,[1]

> autonomic thermoregulatory functions may be attributed to brain areas outside of the PO/AH. These mechanisms appear to be subsidiary controls, may have their own (direct?) links to thermoeffectors, and are capable of operating independently of the PO/AH, although they normally may be influenced by it through ascending and/or descending connections. Thus, the role of the PO/AH in temperature regulation may be seen as not essential, but nevertheless pre-eminent in the control of appropriate, coordinated, and low-threshold thermoregulatory responses. In this role, it receives afferent information from thermosensitive regions throughout the body, and is connected with all the thermoeffectors.

A model for the regulation of body temperature is depicted in Fig. 2-3. This network is based on the work of Hammel[29] but also incorporates other sources.[3,6] This system depends on input from peripheral warm and cold receptors and central thermodetectors. Input arising from cold-sensitive peripheral neurons impinges on cells that excite noradrenergic neurons projecting to cold-sensitive neurons in the PO/AH. Peripheral warm-sensitive neurons provide input to serotonergic cells in the nucleus raphe magnus, which project to warm-sensitive cells in the PO/AH. The warm- (*W* in Fig. 2-3) and cold- (*C* in Fig. 2-3) sensitive neurons of the PO/AH provide the reciprocal innervation that forms the basis for the thermostat. In this scheme the central cold sensitivity is postulated to be derived from inhibitory input via inherently warm-sensitive PO/AH cells. The interconnections of these neurons are shown in Fig. 2-3, *B*.

The firing characteristics of the warm *(W)* and cold *(C)* cells are illustrated in Fig. 2-3, *C*. At 37° C the firing rate of warm and cold cells is balanced and there is no net output to either the heat loss or the heat gain effectors. If internal temperature increases, the warm cells fire faster and vasodilation, sweating, and seeking of a cool environment are stimulated. On the other hand, if the internal temperature falls below 37° C, the cold cells predominate and vasoconstriction, shivering, and seeking of a warm environment are stimulated.

Without the aforementioned peripheral input, body temperature would have to change considerably in order to create the error signal necessary to compensate for varying ambient thermal conditions. This does not occur; core temperature remains remarkably constant under most climatic conditions. This is accomplished by incorporating information from the peripheral thermodetectors. As illustrated in Fig. 2-3, *C*, if an animal moves into a cold environment, the pe-

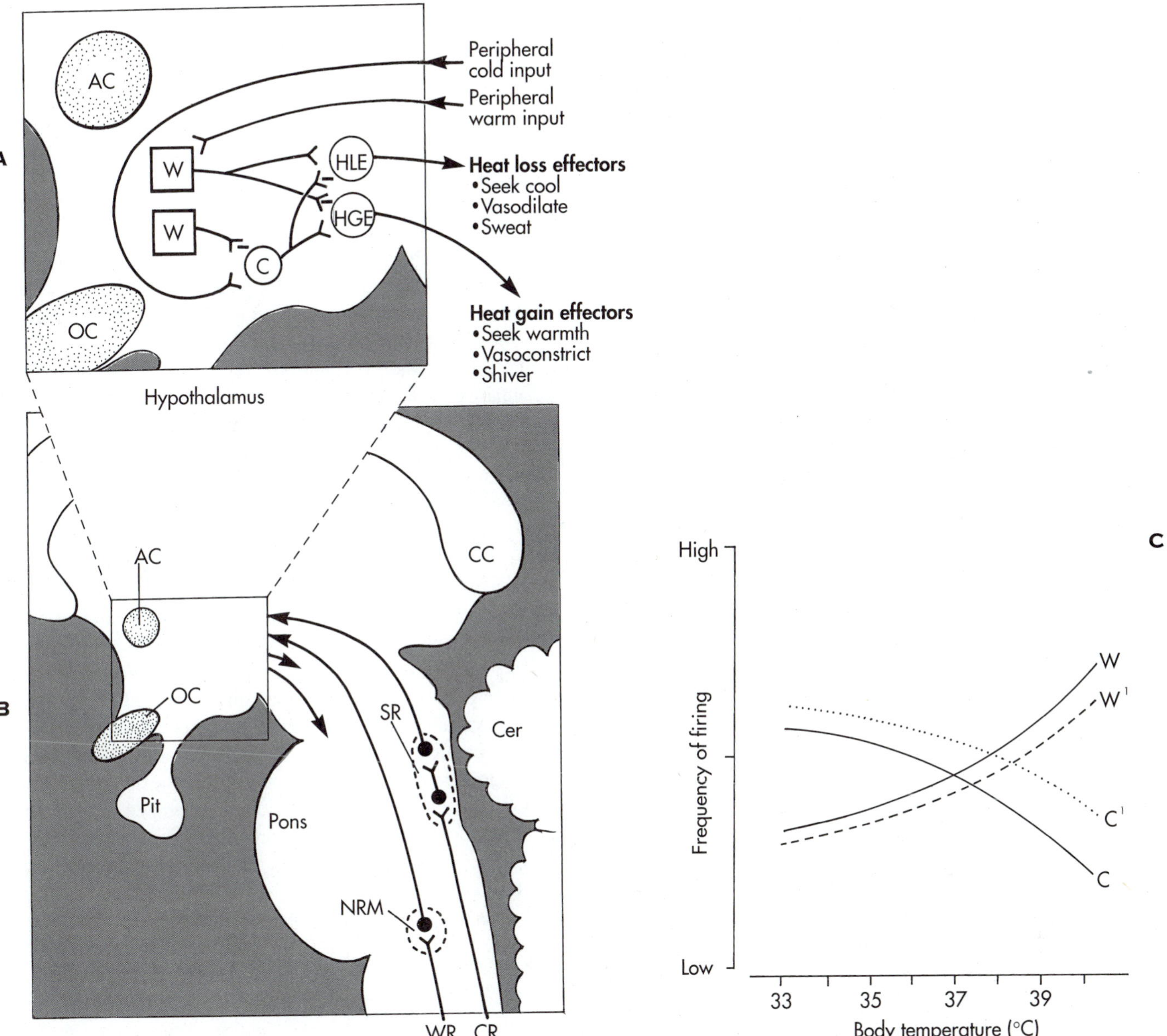

Fig. 2-3 A schematic diagram denoting a suggested neuronal network to account for thermoregulation. **A,** The peripheral inputs and the site of the preoptic nucleus–anterior hypothalamic area (PO/AH)—the rectangle. **B,** Neuronal connections in the PO/AH. **C,** The firing rates of the warm *(W)* and cold *(C)* sensitive PO/AH neurons at different body (brain) temperatures. Synapses not shown as inhibitory are assumed to be excitatory. Details about the functioning of this system are in the text. *AC,* Anterior commissure; *CC,* corpus callosum; *Cer,* cerebellum; *CR,* relays input from peripheral cold receptor; *NRM,* nucleus raphe magnus; *OC,* optic chiasm; *Pit,* pituitary; *SR,* subceruleus region; *WR,* relays input from peripheral warm receptor. (Concepts and information for this figure from Boulant JA, Curras MC, Dean JB: Neurophysiological aspects of thermoregulation. In Wang LCH, editor: *Advances in comparative and environmental physiology,* vol 4, Berlin, 1989, Springer-Verlag; Brück K, Hinckel P: Thermoafferent networks and their adaptive modifications. In Schönbaum E, Lomax P, editors: *Thermoregulation: physiology and biochemistry,* New York, 1990, Pergamon Press; and Hammel HT: *Annu Rev Physiol* 30:641, 1968.)

ripheral cold receptors are stimulated and the peripheral warm receptors are inhibited. This produces the altered firing rates shown by the W′ and C′ curves. Now, even though the body temperature is still at 37° C, the hypothalamic cold cells are firing faster than the hypothalamic warm cells. This leads to the activation of the heat gain effectors. If the system is properly designed (it is), the augmentation of vasoconstriction and metabolism is just sufficient to match the increased heat loss caused by the new, cooler thermal environment. The reverse occurs when a warmer environment is encountered. Peripheral warm receptors are stimulated and peripheral cold receptors are inhibited; the greater firing rate of the hypothalamic warm cells initiates sweating and vasodilation even though the body temperature remains at 37° C. In this way the regulator is able to maintain a remarkably constant internal temperature despite wide variations in the ambient temperature.

Effector Responses

This section examines the properties of the response systems that heat or cool the body according to the output demands of the regulator as described previously. These effectors are influenced both by the output of the thermoregulatory network and by the temperature of the effector organ itself. Since patients away from medical facilities often exhibit whole body or regional hyperthermia or hypothermia, both central outputs and local effects are relevant; these factors are discussed separately.

VASCULAR ADJUSTMENTS

Grayson[27] has produced a useful overview of the role of the vasculature in coping with thermal stresses. One of the primary functions of the circulatory system is to maintain a relatively homogeneous internal body temperature. Heat from metabolically active organs is convectively distributed to portions of the body where less heat is being produced. More commonly appreciated are the alterations of blood flow that increase or decrease the overall thermal conductivity of the body to deal with hot or cold environments, respectively. Some of these alterations in conductivity result from preferentially shunting peripheral blood flow externally and internally to the subcutaneous fat layer. Indeed, fat has about half the tissue conductivity of muscle. Nevertheless, shunting of blood away from major portions of the body is at least as important in determining overall conductivity as is the conductive property of the tissue itself. For example, during immersion in cold water, muscle accounts for about 90% of the total tissue insulation of the forearm.[18]

In addition to capillaries, microcirculatory units contain arterioles, metarterioles, and arteriovenous anastomoses. Flow through all of these vessels is under the control of smooth muscle. Capillary smooth muscle is largely influenced by local factors, while the other vessels are well supplied with adrenergic receptors that respond to both neuronal and endocrine inputs.

Operation of the vasomotor effector system is affected by excessive exposure to ultraviolet B radiation. A moderate sunburn impairs the vasoconstrictor response to cold; the associated, uncontrolled increase in thermal conduction is still present 1 week after the exposure, although the associated erythema has disappeared.[59]

Central Signal

Vascular changes are bioenergetically the least costly autonomic effector response. Because of the high sensitivity of the vasomotor system, ambient temperatures between the thresholds for sweating and shivering are often referred to as being in the zone of vasomotor regulation. If a particular vascular bed is kept at a relatively constant temperature, output from the central nervous regulator can be assessed. Under these conditions, in dogs, manipulations of hypothalamic temperature confirm a high level of vasomotor activity between the thresholds for the activation of panting and shivering.[32] In humans forearm blood flow increases rapidly as core temperature rises; a sixfold increase in blood flow can occur with a core temperature that has risen to only 38° C.[73] Altering the mean skin temperature (while holding the forearm temperature constant) alters the circulatory response at a given core temperature. Under normal conditions core and peripheral temperatures are used to produce an appropriate output as outlined in the section on the regulator. Although most peripheral arterioles are well supplied with adrenergic receptors, the output from the thermoregulatory centers is not homogeneously distributed. Extensive nervous inputs from the thermoregulator occur only in the lips, ears, and distal extremities. Thus immersing the feet in cold water leads to marked vasoconstriction in the hands and forearms but not in the abdomen or upper arms.[27]

Local Modulation

Local temperature has a great effect on the vasomotor status of the peripheral vessels and in some cases may be largely responsible for observed thermal conductivities. Although heat is generally considered a vasodilator,[27] this is true only for cutaneous vascular beds; many other vascular beds dilate when cooled.[21] The specific response to cold shown by cutaneous vessels follows from the observed distribution and properties of the α-adrenergic vascular receptors. Although in most of the vasculature there is a great predominance of α_1-receptors, in the superficial cutaneous areas α_2-receptors constitute a clear majority. The usual predominance of α_1-receptors is found in the deeper blood vessels. Local temperature affects the α_2- and α_1-receptors in a reciprocal manner. While cooling augments the response of the α_2-receptors, it either inhibits or does not affect the response of the α_1-receptors. Cooling the skin, then, not only constricts the superficial vessels, but also concomitantly dilates any underlying vessels. The ensuing flow pattern increases tissue insulation and augments countercurrent exchange between incoming cool blood and outgoing warm blood.[21,22] Although the initial work was done on canine vessels, subsequent studies using α-adrenergic agonists and antagonists have demonstrated that a similar mechanism exists in human fingers.[19,23]

EVAPORATIVE RESPONSES

At high workloads and at environmental temperatures approaching 37° C, the only way to maintain thermal balance is to augment evaporative cooling by mobilizing the eccrine sweat glands. This sympathetic, cholinergically innervated organ system is spread over the entire body surface but is more profuse in some areas than in others. High rates of sweating occur on the forehead, neck, anterior and posterior portions of the trunk, and dorsal parts of the hand and forearm. Low rates occur on the medial femoral regions, lateral trunk areas, palms, and soles.[55] Sweat is secreted in these latter two areas in response to emotional, but not thermal, inputs.[4] Sweat gland activity interacts with the regional vasculature; cholinergic receptors on local vessels and the metabolic products of active sweat glands both increase blood flow in areas of active sweating.[27]

Central Signal

By control of the local milieu at different skin sites, it has been possible to separate the central thermoregulatory drive to sweat glands from local effects on the glands themselves. The central thermoregulatory system provides a proportional output that is influenced by both internal and whole body skin temperatures. Per degree increase above thermoneutral values, internal temperature is about 10 times as important as mean skin temperature in eliciting an output to the sweat glands.[51,52]

Local Modulation

Local effects are important in determining the output of sweat glands. Temperature exerts a multiplicative effect on sweat secretion; the temperature coefficient (Q_{10}) for this augmentation is about 3.[70] Skin wetness also has an important local effect on sweat glands. The wetter the skin, the greater the suppression of sweating.[53]

A moderate sunburn disrupts evaporative cooling. The effect is locally mediated and involves decreases in both the responsiveness and the capacity of the sweat glands.[58]

METABOLIC RESPONSES

Increased metabolism in cold environments is critical for the maintenance of body temperature. The elevated heat production is derived largely from the simultaneous rhythmic excitation of agonistic and antagonistic skeletal muscles (shivering), but other domains such as the gastrointestinal tract or adipose tissue[27,68] may be involved to some degree. There is evidence that both epinephrine and thyroid hormones are released in humans following cold exposure.[24] Since these hormones augment overall tissue metabolism, they may be components of the response to cold environments.

Central Signal

Of the various thermoregulatory output responses, metabolism is the easiest to evaluate quantitatively; the most complete information is available for this response and most models of the thermoregulatory system are based on this information. Experiments on medium-sized mammals have allowed the separate thermal manipulation of various parts of the brain, body core, and skin temperature. This work has made it clear that the thermoregulatory centers act as a proportional controller and that skin temperature provides a feed-forward input to the system.[29,41] Thus greater decreases of both core and skin temperature below neutral values elicit progressively larger compensatory increases in metabolism.

Evidence indicates that humans have a similar control system. In a summary of their data and of that collected previously, Hong and Nadel[39] noted that the central output for shivering is augmented by an increased rate of cooling. They also concluded that a given decrease in core temperature elicits 10 to 20 times the metabolic response of an equivalent decrease in mean skin temperature. Although exercise is not incompatible with shivering, increased levels of exercise exert increasing degrees of suppression of the shivering response, possibly as a consequence of an increased arousal response.[39]

Local Modulation

Although the central and local effects of decreased core temperature on shivering have not been directly partitioned, it appears likely that the central effects are far more important. Slight decreases in core temperature create large compensatory responses, as delineated previously. However, even moderate hypothermia decreases the metabolic response to cold, and at about 30° C the shivering response is lost.[5] This decrement must involve nervous system malfunction, since the muscles themselves are quite responsive below 30° C. Limb muscles and diaphragm muscles develop peak tensions that are not greatly affected by temperatures down to 25° C, and fatigue resistance is considerably increased at 25° C.[61,65]

BEHAVIORAL RESPONSES

In most wilderness situations a variety of ambient temperatures are available and external insulation is easily adjusted. Under these conditions the choice of thermal microenvironment and clothing provides a far higher gain than do any of the autonomic effector systems discussed previously. These whole body adjustments are achieved by all motile animals and are particularly well developed in vertebrates.[13] In addition to moving the body, the somatic effectors are important for optimizing the autonomic responses to thermal stress. Thus spreading out the arms and legs during heat stress increases the surface area available for autonomic augmentation of conductive, convective, evaporative, and radiative heat losses.

Central Signal

Available evidence indicates that behavioral responses are elicited by the thermoregulatory controller by outputs similar to those delivered to the autonomic effector organs.[13,15] Severe deviations of core temperature disrupt this system; when this occurs, the person no longer feels too hot or too cold and the desire to take corrective action is lost.

Local Modulation

As with shivering, most problems involving behavioral temperature regulation probably emanate from a disruption of the centrally generated output. The muscles used to move the body are fairly resistant to thermal incapacitation (see previous discussion), but if this occurs, a major disruption of the body's thermal defenses ensues.

Important Modifications of Thermoregulatory Responses

In addition to the importance of a stable body temperature for normal physiologic function, monitoring body temperature provides a significant diagnostic indicator for many pathologic conditions. Whether the goal is to stabilize or to monitor body temperature, it is necessary to understand the many conditions that affect both the level and effectiveness of the thermoregulatory system. In this section these circumstances are elucidated.

NORMAL VARIATION IN THE REGULATED TEMPERATURE AND IN THE ABILITY TO MAINTAIN BODY TEMPERATURE

The same body temperature can represent a different state of affairs even under regularly encountered circumstances. Some of these conditions are noted in the following paragraphs.

Level of Activity

Activity normally leads to increases in body temperature. Unlike peripheral temperature, the level of activity does not appear to provide direct input to the regulator of body temperature.[70] Rather, the magnitude of the error signal for increased heat dissipation is determined simply by the increase in body temperature. Thus someone exercising heavily (or having just exercised) in a neutral environment has an unusually high body temperature, while someone sleeping or resting quietly has a relatively low body temperature.

Circadian Changes

Body temperature shows cyclic changes throughout the day. Some of this variation is due to the daily cycle of activity, as described earlier. However, there also exists a circadian rhythm for the body temperature set point. This sinusoidal rhythm accounts for much of the observed variation in body temperature. The mean oral reading is about 37° C (98.6° F), but this is only a midpoint; the early morning low is around 36.6° C (97.9° F) and the late afternoon high is approximately 37.4° C (99.3° F). These changes definitely reflect alterations in the controller, since the body temperature thresholds for the elicitation of sweating and peripheral vasodilation are significantly lower in the early morning than in the afternoon.[74] Melatonin may be an important factor in the rhythm of body temperature; light exposure produces similar shifts in both temperature and melatonin rhythms,[67] and artificial reductions in melatonin levels attenuate the circadian decline in body temperature.[10] A thorough, current review of body temperature cycles is available.[62]

Interindividual Differences

Normally, individuals display surprisingly little interindividual variability in core body temperature. At a particular time the internal temperature of most individuals differs by less than 0.5° C.[5] On the other hand, it is important to be aware of exceptions. In one person the core temperature was consistently 35.5° C to 36° C. He mentioned that on one occasion he had felt chills and malaise but was told that his temperature of 37° C was normal. It was not; for this person a core temperature of 37° C represented a febrile state.

Age

The circadian rhythm of body temperature develops soon after birth. Although newborns display small-amplitude rhythms, the patterns are not circadian. Circadian rhythmicity begins to develop during the second and third weeks of life, and following a progressive increase in amplitude, the typical adult temperature rhythms are reached at 2 years of age.[62]

Thermoregulatory capacities show a similar progressive increase but are not fully developed until after puberty. Effectors more important to infants than adults include certain behavioral responses (call for help) and the ability to activate thermogenic brown adipose tissue. Although brown adipose tissue is of little consequence in adults, it may aid in the production of heat in infants; adults may have the capacity to develop brown adipose tissue if subjected to chronic cold stress.[36] Shivering is not present in infants and develops fully only after several years as the nervous system matures. Metabolism in infants is increased to some degree by an increase in motor activity, which accompanies cold stress.[43]

Sweating is present and effective in children, but increases in sweat gland output during puberty lead to the typical high capacity for evaporative heat loss present in adults.[20] The factors affecting heat loss from cold stress during the adult years have been investigated by using a multiple regression analysis to evaluate fitness, fatness, and age (from the twenties to the early fifties).[7] Fitness has no effect, while fatness retards heat loss. Aging during this period is correlated with a progressive weakening of the vasoconstrictor response to cold.

Individuals in the late sixties and beyond have a definite decrease in thermoregulatory capacity. Sweating is lessened in response to passive heating,[40] the vasoconstrictor response to cold stress is significantly reduced,[42] and a distinct shivering tremor is rarely observed.[43]

Gender

Although less work has been done on thermoregulation in females, evidence indicates that their thermoregulatory responses are qualitatively similar to those of males. Taken as a group, females have a number of physiologic and morphologic characteristics that produce subtle differences in the regulation of body temperature.[47] Such attributes include a

> smaller blood volume, lower hemoglobin concentration, smaller heart, smaller lean body mass, greater percent of subcutaneous and total body fat, greater surface area-to-mass ratio, higher set point for cutaneous vasodilation and sweating onset, greater resting vasoconstriction in hands and feet, geometrically thinner extremities, and cyclic hormonal changes.[2]

The menstrual cycle, pregnancy, and menopause are all associated with important effects on the thermoregulatory system. During menstrual cycling the core temperature is typically 0.5° C lower in the follicular phase than in the luteal phase. Increased progesterone levels are implicated in the higher temperatures seen in the luteal phase.[72]

During pregnancy the thermoregulatory system is far more sensitive to the heat produced by continuous exercise. The effector responses are initiated sooner and are more vigorous, so that toward the end of pregnancy the steady-state core temperature during exercise is about 1° C lower than before conception. This adjustment is seen as an adaptation that reduces possible thermal stress on the embryo and fetus.[11]

During menopause women often experience thermoregulatory and cardiovascular irregularities. Heat and exercise may also be particularly stressful during and after this phase. Estrogen therapy, often employed to alleviate various symptoms of menopause, also affects the responsiveness of the thermoregulatory system. This replacement therapy increases activity-induced peripheral vasodilation and sweating and significantly decreases steady-state core temperature during exercise in the heat.[72]

INDUCED ALTERATIONS OF THE REGULATED TEMPERATURE

The optimal body temperature is not always 37° C. In certain conditions of stress or vulnerability the regulated temperature of the body may be altered. This is assumed to be an adaptive response to the particular predicament. Some of these situations are delineated in the following paragraphs. In such circumstances altered body temperatures may be beneficial and should not necessarily be manipulated until the underlying condition is improved.

Fever

Increased body temperatures have been associated with illness for thousands of years. Pathogens, however, do not directly cause the increased body temperature. Rather, they interact with portions of the immune system such as macrophages, Kupffer's cells, and glial cells to produce an endogenous fever-producing protein, interleukin-1.[45] Interleukin-1 acts on cells in or near the PO/AH to cause the release of E series prostaglandins, which leads to an increase in the regulated temperature, that is, a fever. Aspirin and related drugs block fevers by inhibiting prostaglandin synthesis.[69] Interleukin-1 has many other effects, including decreased appetite, hypoferremia, activation of B and T lymphocytes, and increased slow wave sleep.[45] The increase in body temperature during a fever provides a major stimulus for immune functions: neutrophil migration, the secretion of antibacterial chemicals, and interferon production are all augmented. The presence and beneficial effects of fever have been documented in a variety of cold- and warm-blooded vertebrates and even in some invertebrates. Thus under most conditions it is not advisable to alleviate a fever. Obvious exceptions include malignant hyperthermia, particularly high fevers during pregnancy, and any situation in which weakness makes the thermally induced increase in metabolic demands dangerous.[45]

Alcohol, Anesthetics, and Toxins

Increases in the blood concentration of ethanol, anesthetics, and a number of toxic substances lead to substantial decrease in body temperature.[16,66] In many cases this fall in core temperature is due to a decrease in the regulated temperature. In the case of alcohol and certain toxins the reduction appears to be an adaptive adjustment that promotes survival. These chemicals disrupt the cell membrane and alter its physiologic function, in part by decreasing the viscosity of the phospholipid bilayer. This effect is counteracted by a lowered temperature, which increases membrane viscosity. Indeed, studies of mice have shown that a decreased body temperature counteracts ethanol toxicity.[46]

An excellent overview of the thermal effects of general

anesthetics is available.[66] Substances tested to date (halothane, fentanyl–nitrous oxide, enflurane, and isoflurane) act in a consistent manner. Heat loss thresholds are increased by about 1° C, and heat maintenance thresholds are lowered by approximately 2.5° C. Interestingly, in the typical clinical dose range the gain (sensitivity) of the effector responses is nearly normal. In the conditions under which general anesthetics are normally administered, body temperature decreases significantly. An initial rapid drop is due to redistribution of heat; cool blood from the periphery lowers the central core temperature. A second, slower decrease results from a fall in body heat content. Finally, a plateau is reached, either because heat production and heat loss are passively balanced or because the heat maintenance thresholds are reached. During postanesthetic recovery there is vigorous shivering. This can be avoided by cutaneous warming before and during anesthesia.[66]

Severe Hypoxia

When the inspired oxygen falls to 10% to 12%, a substantial decrease in the regulated temperature occurs. This reaction has been documented, using behavioral responses, in fish, amphibians, and reptiles.[75] It also occurs in mammals.[25] The value of the resultant lowered body temperature is clear: the affinity of hemoglobin for oxygen is increased and the overall metabolic rate is decreased. The mechanism underlying the change in the regulated temperature may involve differential sensitivities of central neurons; hypoxia specifically increases the activity of the warm-sensitive neurons (the cells denoted by *W* in Fig. 2-3) in the PO/AH.[71]

ALTERED SYSTEM RESPONSIVENESS

A number of situations alter the responsiveness of the thermoregulatory system. An awareness of these conditions is important in assessing the thermoregulatory capabilities of a particular person and determining possible causes for hyperthermia or hypothermia.

Thermal Acclimation

Thermoregulation is affected by chronic exercise in cool or warm environments as well as by chronic exposure to very cold environments. Such exercise in a cool environment greatly increases the responsiveness of the sweat glands; if the exercise is in the heat, the central temperature at which sweating is initiated is also lowered. The net consequence of these adjustments is that a heat- and exercise-acclimated individual can work at a given level with far less increase in core temperature.[54]

Conversely, repeated exposure to very cold environments (for example, 80 30-minute sessions at 5° C) decreases the metabolic response to a standard cold air test, often leading to lower internal temperatures in the cold-acclimated individuals.[35]

Competition with Other Homeostatic Systems

In addition to a constant core temperature, the body has many alternative requirements. When certain of these other needs are not met, thermoregulatory response can be compromised. For heat production and heat conservation an adequate energy supply, a patent nervous system, and functional effector organs are critical. For maintaining exercise performance and body temperature in a warm environment, body water status is also critical. This subject is covered in an excellent review by Sawka.[63] It is common for a person working in the heat to lose 1 L of water per hour, and even when fluids are readily available, maintaining a euhydrated state may be difficult. For hypohydration during activity, each percent decrease in body weight leads to a core temperature increase of about 0.15° C. This decreased ability to dissipate heat is mediated by two mechanisms. At a given core temperature, hypertonicity decreases the sweating response and hypovolemia reduces skin blood flow.[63]

Alcohol, Drugs, Anesthetics, and Toxins

Although moderate doses of many substances elicit adaptive changes in the regulated body temperature, elevated doses impair or abolish thermoregulation. Body temperature then changes passively, depending on the thermal environment. This can be particularly dangerous when elevated levels of alcohol or similar substances are combined with heat stress. An impaired ability to dissipate heat is then combined with the enhanced toxicity of increased tissue temperature.

Acknowledgments

During the preparation of this chapter, the author was partially supported by NIAAA Grant 1-PO1-AA08621-03. Helpful suggestions were made by Dr. Stanley Hillman, Dr. Randy Zelick, Mr. Richard Rausch, Mr. Amish Desai, and Ms. Ruth Baecker. Mr. Rausch, Dr. Candace O'Connor, and Ms. Cari Jacobs helped with the organization. Ms. Susan Isles is thanked for typing the manuscript.

REFERENCES

1. Blatteis CM: Functional anatomy of the hypothalamus from the point of view of temperature. In Szelényi Z, Székely M, editors: *Contributions to thermal physiology,* Budapest, 1980, Akademiai Kiado.
2. Boulant JA, Silva NL: Neuronal sensitivities in preoptic tissue slices: interactions among homeostatic systems, *Brain Res Bull* 20(6):871, 1988.
3. Boulant JA, Curras MC, Dean JB: Neurophysiological aspects of thermoregulation. In Wang LCH, editor: *Advances in comparative and environmental physiology,* vol 4, Berlin, 1989, Springer-Verlag.
4. Brengelmann G, Brown AC: Temperature regulation. In Ruch TC, Patton HD, editors: *Physiology and biophysics,* ed 19, Philadelphia, 1965, WB Saunders.
5. Brengelmann GL: Body temperature regulation. In Patton HD et al, editors: *Textbook of physiology: circulation, respiration, body fluids, metabolism, and endocrinology,* ed 21, Philadelphia, 1989, WB Saunders.

6. Brück K, Hinckel P: Thermoafferent networks and their adaptive modifications. In Schönbaum E, Lomax P, editors: *Thermoregulation: physiology and biochemistry,* New York, 1990, Pergamon Press.
7. Budd GM et al: Effects of fitness, fatness, and age on men's responses to whole body cooling in air, *J Appl Physiol* 71(6):2387, 1991.
8. Burke WEA, Mekjavić IB: Estimation of regional cutaneous cold sensitivity by analysis of the gasping response, *J Appl Physiol* 71(5):1933, 1991.
9. Cabanac M: Physiological role of pleasure, *Science* 173:1103, 1971.
10. Cagnacci A, Elliott JA, Yen SSC: Melatonin: a major regulator of the circadian rhythm of core temperature in humans, *J Clin Endocrinol Metab* 75:447, 1992.
11. Clapp JF III: The changing thermal response to endurance exercise during pregnancy, *Am J Obstet Gynecol* 165:1684, 1991.
12. Cossins AR, Bowler K: *Temperature biology of animals,* New York, 1987, Chapman & Hall.
13. Crawshaw LI: Temperature regulation in vertebrates, *Annu Rev Physiol* 42:473, 1980.
14. Crawshaw LI et al: Effect of local cooling on sweating rate and cold sensation, *Pflügers Arch* 354:19, 1975.
15. Crawshaw LI et al: Body temperature regulation in vertebrates: comparative aspects and neuronal elements. In Schönbaum E, Lomax P, editors: *Thermoregulation: physiology and biochemistry,* New York, 1990, Pergamon Press.
16. Crawshaw LI, O'Connor CS, Wollmuth LP: Ethanol and the neurobiology of temperature regulation. In Watson RR, editor: *Alcohol and neurobiology: brain development and hormone regulation,* Boca Raton, fla, 1992, CRC Press.
17. Dean JB, Boulant JA: Effects of synaptic blockade on thermosensitive neurons in rat diencephalon in vitro, *Am J Physiol* 257:R65, 1989.
18. Ducharme MB, Tikuisis P: In vivo thermal conductivity of the human forearm tissues, *J Appl Physiol* 70:2682, 1991.
19. Ekenvall L et al: α-Adrenoceptors and cold-induced vasoconstriction in human finger skin, *Am J Physiol* 255:H1000, 1988.
20. Falk B et al: Sweat gland response to exercise in the heat among pre-, mid-, and late-pubertal boys, *Med Sci Sports Exerc* 24(3):313, 1992.
21. Flavahan NA: The role of vascular α_2-adrenoreceptors as cutaneous thermosensors, *New Physiol Sci* 6:251, 1991.
22. Flavahan NA et al: Cooling and α_1- and α_2-adrenergic responses in cutaneous veins: role of receptor reserve, *Am J Physiol* 249:H950, 1970.
23. Freedman RR et al: Local temperature modulates $\propto_1$- and $\propto_2$-adrenergic vasoconstriction in men, *Am J Physiol* 32:H1197, 1992.
24. Fregly M: Activity of the hypothalamic-pituitary-thyroid axis during exposure to cold. In Schönbaum E, Lomax P, editors: *Thermoregulation: physiology and biochemistry,* New York, 1990, Pergamon Press.
25. Gautier H et al: Effects of hypoxia and cold acclimation on thermoregulation in the rat, *J Appl Physiol* 71(4):1355, 1991.
26. Giesbrecht GK et al: Treatment of immersion hypothermia by direct body-to-body contact, *FASEB J* 7:A441, 1993.
27. Grayson J: Responses of the microcirculation to hot and cold environments. In Schönbaum E, Lomax P, editors: *Thermoregulation: physiology and biochemistry,* New York, 1990, Pergamon Press.
28. Guyton AC: *Medical physiology,* Philadelphia, 1981, WB Saunders.
29. Hammel HT: Regulation of internal body temperature, *Annu Rev Physiol* 30:641, 1968.
30. Hardy JD: Physiology of temperature regulation, *Physiol Rev* 41:521, 1961.
31. Hardy JD: Body temperature regulation. In Mountcastle VB, editor: *Medical physiology,* vol 2, ed 2, St Louis, 1980, Mosby.
32. Hellstrom B, Hammel HT: Some characteristics of temperature regulation in the unanesthetized dog, *Am J Physiol* 213:547, 1967.
33. Hensel H: Cutaneous thermoreceptors. In Iggo A, editor: *Handbook of sensory physiology.* Vol 2. *Somatosensory system,* Berlin, 1973, Springer-Verlag.
34. Hensel H, Kenshalo DR: Warm receptors in the nasal region of cats, *J Physiol (Lond)* 204:99, 1969.
35. Hesslink RL Jr et al: Human cold air habituation is independent of thyroxine and thyrotropin, *J Appl Physiol* 72(6):2134, 1992.
36. Himms-Hagen S: Brown adipose tissue thermogenesis: role in thermoregulation, energy regulation and obesity. In Schönbaum E, Lomax P, editors: *Thermoregulation: physiology and biochemistry,* New York, 1990, Pergamon Press.
37. Hodgman CD, editor: *Handbook of chemistry and physics: a ready-reference book of chemical and physical data,* ed 43, Cleveland, 1962, Chemical Rubber.
38. Holy Bible (King James Version), I Kings 1:1-4, Boston, Whittemore Associates.
39. Hong S, Nadel ER: Thermogenic control during exercise in a cold environment, *J Appl Physiol* 47(5):1084, 1979.
40. Inoue Y et al: Regional differences in the sweating responses of older and younger men, *J Appl Physiol* 71(6):2453, 1991.
41. Jessen C: Thermal afferents in the control of body temperature. In Schönbaum E, Lomax P, editors: *Thermoregulation: physiology and biochemistry,* New York, 1990, Pergamon Press.
42. Khan F, Spence VA, and Belch JJF: Cutaneous vascular responses and thermoregulation in relation to age, *Clin Sci* 82:521, 1992.
43. Kleinebeckel D, Klussman FW: Shivering. In Schönbaum E, Lomax P, editors: *Thermoregulation: physiology and biochemistry,* New York, 1990, Pergamon Press.
44. Klement W, Arndt JO: The role of nociceptors of cutaneous veins in the mediation of cold pain in man, *J Physiol* 449:73, 1992.
45. Kluger MJ: Is fever beneficial?, *Yale J Biol Med* 59:89, 1986.
46. Malcolm RD, Alkana RL: Temperature dependence of ethanol depression in mice, *J Pharmacol Exp Ther* 35:306, 1983.
47. Mitchell JH et al: Acute response and chronic adaptation to exercise in women, *Med Sci Sports Exerc* 24(suppl 6):S258, 1992.
48. Mount LE: *The climatic physiology of the pig,* London, 1968, Edward Arnold.
49. Mount LE: *Adaptation to thermal environment: man and his productive animals,* Baltimore, 1979, University Park Press.
50. Mountcastle VB, editor: *Medical physiology,* vol 2, ed 14, St Louis, 1980, Mosby.
51. Nadel ER, Bullard RW, Stolwijk JAJ: Importance of skin temperature in the regulation of sweating, *J Appl Physiol* 31:80, 1971.
52. Nadel ER et al: Peripheral modifications to the central drive for sweating, *J Appl Physiol* 31:828, 1971.
53. Nadel ER, Stolwijk JAJ: Effect of skin wettedness on sweat gland response, *J Appl Physiol* 35(5):689, 1973.
54. Nadel ER et al: Mechanisms of thermal acclimation to exercise and heat, *J Appl Physiol* 37:515, 1974.
55. Newburgh LH: *Physiology of heat regulation and the science of clothing,* Philadelphia, 1949, WB Saunders.
56. Nishyasu T et al: Comparison of the forearm and calf blood flow response to thermal stress during dynamic exercise, *Med Sci Sports Exerc* 24:213, 1992.
57. Nobel PS: *Biophysical plant physiology and ecology,* New York, 1983, WH Freeman.
58. Pandolf KB et al: Human thermoregulatory responses during heat exposure after artificially induced sunburn, *Am J Physiol* 262:R610, 1992.
59. Pandolf KB et al: Human thermoregulatory responses during cold water immersion after artificially induced sunburn, *Am J Physiol* 262:R617, 1992.
60. Panksepp J: Hypothalamic integration of behavior: rewards, punishments, and related psychological processes. In Morgane PJ, Panksepp J, editors: *Handbook of the hypothalamus,* vol 3, part B, New York, 1980, Marcel Dekker.
61. Prezant DJ et al: Temperature dependence of rat diaphragm muscle contractility and fatigue, *J Appl Physiol* 69(5):1740, 1990.

62. Reinberg A, Smolensky M: Chronobiology and thermoregulation. In Schönbaum E, Lomax P, editors: *Thermoregulation: physiology and biochemistry,* New York, 1990, Pergamon Press.
63. Sawka MN: Physiological consequences of hypohydration: exercise performance and thermoregulation, *Med Sci Sports Exerc* 24(6):657, 1992.
64. Schmidt-Nielsen K: *Animal physiology: adaptation and environment,* ed 4, Cambridge, Eng, 1990, Cambridge University Press.
65. Segal SS, Faulkner JA, White TP: Skeletal muscle fatigue in vitro is temperature dependent, *J Appl Physiol* 61(2):660, 1986.
66. Sessler DI: Perianesthetic thermoregulation and heat balance in humans, *FASEB J* 7:638, 1993.
67. Shanahan TL, Czeisler CA: Light exposure induces equivalent phase shifts of the endogenous circadian rhythms of circulating plasma melatonin and core body temperature in men, *J Clin Endocrinol Metab* 73:227, 1991.
68. Simonsen L et al: Thermogenic response to epinephrine in the forearm and abdominal subcutaneous adipose tissue, *Am J Physiol* 263:E850, 1992.
69. Stitt JT: Prostaglandin E as the neural mediator of fever, *Yale J Biol Med* 59:137, 1986.
70. Stolwijk JAJ, Nadel ER: Thermoregulation during positive and negative work exercise, *Fed Proc* 32:1607, 1973.
71. Tamaki Y, Nakayama T: Effects of air constituents on thermosensitivities of preoptic neurons: hypoxia versus hypercapnia, *Pflugers Arch* 409:1, 1987.
72. Tankersley CG et al: Estrogen replacement in middle-aged women: thermoregulatory responses to exercise in the heat, *J Appl Physiol* 73(4):1238, 1992.
73. Wenger CB et al: Forearm blood flow during body temperature transients produced by leg exercise, *J Appl Physiol* 38(1):58, 1975.
74. Wenger CB et al: Nocturnal lowering of thresholds for sweating and vasodilation, *J Appl Physiol* 41:15, 1976.
75. Wood SC: Interactions between hypoxia and hypothermia, *Annu Rev Physiol* 53:71, 1991.

3 ACCIDENTAL HYPOTHERMIA

Daniel F. Danzl
Robert S. Pozos
Murray P. Hamlet

Cold modalities, although used for medical purposes for millennia, were not scientifically evaluated until the eighteenth century. The hemostatic, analgesic, and therapeutic effects of cold on a wide variety of conditions were well known. Although fever remained the most common disorder of thermoregulation, accidental hypothermia was also common and its treatment controversial. In addition to the biblical references to the truncal rewarming of King David by a damsel, various remedies were mentioned by Hippocrates, Aristotle, and Galen.[131,136,552]

The effects of cold on human performance are perhaps best documented in the annals of military history. A cold ambient temperature has turned the tide in many battles.[291,745] Xenophon's army experienced many cold casualties in Persia about 400 BC.[221] Alexander the Great was reputedly rendered comatose by hypothermia, as were many of the Roman legionnaires traversing the Alps. It was estimated that Hannibal lost approximately 20,000 of his 46,000 troops in 218 BC while crossing the Pyrenean Alps in northern Italy.[26,27]

Baron Larrey, Napoleon's chief surgeon, returned from Russia to France in 1812 with 350 healthy soldiers from the initial 12,000 in the 12th Division. His descriptions of the mental and physical effects of the cold during the approach to and retreat from the gates of Moscow included the insightful observation that victims of the cold placed closest to the campfire mysteriously died. Many of Napoleon's soldiers survived by crawling inside the warm carcasses of horses.[59,389]

Washington's troops were battered by the winter of 1777-1778, with nearly 10% "left to perish by winter's cold." In the Crimean War (1845-1855) more than 1000 French soldiers succumbed to the cold in the trenches. The lessons learned at Crimea had been forgotten by the time of World War I, in which the estimates of cold-related casualties included 115,000 British, 80,000 French, and 38,000 Italian troops. In World War II the Germans suffered at least 100,000 and the Americans 90,000 cold injuries. Of the American fatalities in Korea, 10% were cold related. At Goose Green in the Falklands (Malvinas) War of 1982 the temperature dropped at night to –4° C, resulting in many cases of hypothermia, frostbite, and trench foot.[13,221]

The majority of cold injuries encountered today affect the urban destitute and wilderness and sports enthusiasts.[174] Numerous cold-related tragedies have involved civilians, skiers, hunters, sailors, climbers, and swimmers.* Adolescents are psychologically prone to take risks and rarely employ wise measures to conserve heat and energy. The popularity of Arctic and mountain expeditions has led to an increase in persons at risk.[10,327,466] The toll on those challenging the environment has included climbers of Mt. McKinley, Mt. Everest, and Mt. Hood.[279]

Epidemiology

The wide scope of civilian hypothermia-related deaths continues to be a public health concern.[744] In most countries primary hypothermia deaths are considered violent and are classified as accidental, homicidal, or suicidal. Deaths from secondary hypothermia are usually considered natural complications of systemic disorders, including trauma, carcinoma, and sepsis.[799] The true incidence of secondary hy-

*References 79, 281, 348-350, 598, 656, 657.

pothermia throughout the world is unknown because hypothermic persons found indoors are likely to have other serious and diverting secondary medical illnesses[787] and because delays are common between hospital admission and death.[624] Thus secondary hypothermia is underreported. As expected, death certificate data more accurately quantify primary hypothermia.

Hypothermia occurs in a wide variety of locations and in all seasons.* In a multicenter North American survey of 428 cases of civilian accidental hypothermia, 69 occurred in Florida.[9,135] Urban settings account for the majority of cases in most of the industrialized countries.[140,332,717]

In the first epidemiologic survey of hypothermia in a North American population there was no evidence that low morning basal temperature is commonly found in a geriatric population sleeping at a normal ambient room temperature.[354] In another study in the United States a low morning body temperature was also uncommon in the elderly who remained indoors.[589,590] In contrast, 11.4% of the elderly were hypothermic in an early domestic survey in the United Kingdom in which the urine temperature was considered to be the core temperature.[219] The accuracy of those urine temperatures has since been questioned. Nevertheless, in one hospital-based study hypothermia was diagnosed in 3.6% of hospitalized patients who were over 65 years of age.[247] The incidence of chronic hypothermia in the elderly does not appear to be decreasing, and in some populations the fatality rates related to hypothermia have increased in persons over 75 years of age.[588,589]

Accidental hypothermia is best defined as the unintentional decrease of around 2° C in the "normal" core temperature of 37.2° to 37.7° C without disease in the preoptic and anterior hypothalamic nuclei (Table 3-1).[440] Hypothermia is both a symptom and a clinical disease entity.[156] When sufficient heat cannot be generated to maintain homeostasis and the core temperature drops below 30° C, the patient becomes poikilothermic and cools to the ambient temperature. Several clinical classifications have been proposed to facilitate discussion. The most practical division includes otherwise healthy patients with simple environmental exposure (primary), those with specific diseases producing hypothermia (secondary), and those with predisposing conditions. Other divisions reflect the etiology of hypothermia and include immersion versus nonimmersion and acute versus chronic heat loss.[441,495,599,690]

A variety of physiologic stressors and other factors can impair thermoregulation.[690] Age extremes, the state of health and nutrition, the type of exposure, and a multitude of intoxicants or medications can jeopardize thermostability by decreasing heat production or increasing heat loss. Physiologic stressors also include dehydration, sleep deprivation, and fatigue.[539] The compensatory responses to these challenges that increase heat loss via evaporation, radiation, conduction, and convection often fail.[441,599,777] Resultant mortality rates range from the ever-suspect none to well over 50% in many of the published clinical series, depending largely on the severity of risk factors and on patient selection criteria.[136,441,477,768,772]

For safety, experimental investigations of induced hypothermia in human volunteers terminate cooling at about 35° C. Naturally this precludes analysis of some of the more significant pathophysiologic features of moderate or severe hypothermia. Design limitations also occur in studies of anesthetized animals, since the results of these experiments require variable degrees of extrapolation to humans. For example, large differences exist both in the cardiovascular responses to interventions and in the amounts of peripheral musculature that are present, particularly in nonporcine animal models. As a result, clinical treatment recommendations must be predicated on the degree and duration of hypothermia and on the predisposing factors that are subsequently identified.[94,275,276,635,641]

Normal Physiology of Temperature Regulation

Warm-blooded animals precariously maintain a dynamic equilibrium between heat production and heat loss. The normal diurnal variation in humans is only 1° C.[226] Since physiologic changes occurring in humans are modified by predisposing or contributory factors, the normal responses to severe temperature depression require significant extrapolation.[48,67,346,512]

Basal heat production usually averages 40 to 60 kcal/m^2 body surface area per hour and increases with shivering thermogenesis.[470,574] Food ingestion, fever, activity, and cold stress increase heat production.[228] Normal thermoregulation in vertebrates involves the transmission of cold sensation to the hypothalamic neurons via the lateral spinothalamic tracts and the thalamus (Fig. 3-1). The physiologic characteristics of the three zones of hypothermia appear in Table 3-2. A complete discussion of the physiology of cold exposure and thermoregulation is presented in Chapter 2.

Pathophysiology

NERVOUS SYSTEM

Numbing cold is a well-known depressant of the central nervous system.[385,473,530,540] Clinical manifestations include impaired memory and judgment, slurred speech, and decreased consciousness. Although most patients are comatose below 30° C, some appear amazingly intact. Temperature-dependent enzyme systems in the brain do not function properly at cold temperatures that are well tolerated by the kidneys.[59]

*References 142, 166, 209, 400, 436, 477, 587, 589, 724, 768, 772.

Table 3-1 Fahrenheit to Centigrade Conversion Scales*

Fahrenheit	Centigrade	Fahrenheit	Centigrade
95	35	63	17.22
94	34.44	62	16.67
93	33.89	61	16.11
92	33.33	60	15.56
91	32.78	59	15
90	32.22	58	14.44
89	31.67	57	13.89
88	31.11	56	13.33
87	30.56	55	12.78
86	30	54	12.22
85	29.44	53	11.67
84	28.89	52	11.11
83	28.33	51	10.56
82	27.78	50	10
81	27.22	49	9.44
80	26.67	48	8.89
79	26.11	47	8.33
78	25.56	46	7.78
77	25	45	7.22
76	24.44	44	6.67
75	23.89	43	6.11
74	23.33	42	5.56
73	22.78	41	5
72	22.22	40	4.44
71	21.67	39	3.89
70	21.11	38	3.33
69	20.56	37	2.78
68	20	36	2.22
67	19.44	35	1.67
66	18.89	34	1.11
65	18.33	33	0.56
64	17.78	32	0

*C = (F − 32) × 5/9. Each 5° C = 9° F.

Neurons are initially stimulated by a 1° C drop in temperature.[556] However, the brain does not always cool uniformly during accidental hypothermia. After the initial increase a linear decrease occurs in cerebral metabolism by 6% to 10% per degree Centigrade from 35° to 25° C.[474] The electroencephalogram is abnormal below 33.5° C and becomes silent at 19° to 20° C.[180,210] The triphasic waves commonly noted in hypothermia have also been observed in various metabolic, toxic, and diffuse encephalopathies.[603] Visual evoked potentials, another objective measure of cerebral function, become smaller as the mercury drops.[617] After cerebral cortical function becomes impaired, lower brainstem functions are damaged.

Cerebrovascular autoregulation is surprisingly intact until the temperature drops below 25° C. Although vascular resistance is increased, a disproportionate redistribution of blood flow to the brain occurs. In one canine study, blood flow in the brain, muscle, kidney, and myocardium recovered quickly to control levels after rewarming. Flow deficits in the pulmonary, digestive, and endocrine systems persisted for up to 2 hours after rewarming.[17,767]

Chilling the peripheral nervous system increases muscle tension and preshivering tone and leads to shivering. Shivering, which is also centrally controlled, is a much more efficient heat producer than voluntary muscle contractions of the extremities.

CARDIOVASCULAR SYSTEM

Many of the cardiovascular responses that are caused by or associated with hypothermia have been well described but are not well understood.[393] Cold stress results in increased consumption of myocardial oxygen. Autonomic nervous system stimulation causes tachycardia and periph-

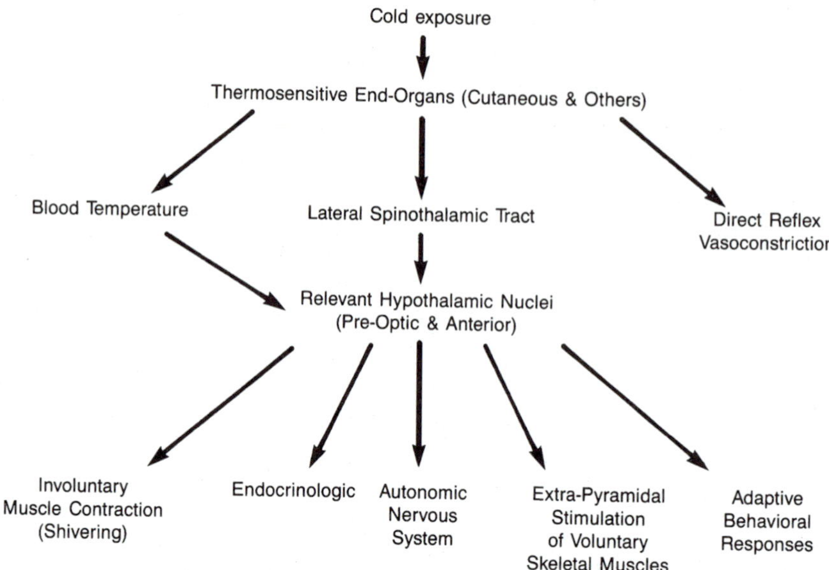

Fig. 3-1 Physiology of cold exposure.

eral vasoconstriction, both of which increase systemic blood pressure and cardiac afterload.[328] Following premonitory tachycardia, decremental bradycardia results in a 50% decrease in heart rate at 28° C.[50,661] Since this bradycardia is caused by decreased spontaneous depolarization of pacemaker cells, it is refractory to atropinization.[576]

During hypothermic bradycardia, unlike normothermia, systole is prolonged to a greater duration than diastole. In addition, the conduction system is much more sensitive to cold than is the myocardium, and thus the cardiac cycle is lengthened. Cold-induced changes in pH, oxygen, electrolytes, and nutrients also alter electrical conduction.[31]

Hypothermia progressively decreases mean arterial pressure and the cardiac index. Cardiac output drops to about 45% of normal at 25° C. Systemic arterial resistance was found by invasive hemodynamic monitoring to be increased in one group of patients.[273]

Even after rewarming, cardiovascular function may remain temporarily depressed. Impairment of myocardial contractility, metabolism, and peripheral vascular function can persist on rewarming.[737] Reduced myocardial contractility that resolves after warming has been documented with serial radionuclide ventriculography.[434]

Mild steady hypothermia in patients with poikilothermic thermoregulatory disorders causes electrocardiographic (ECG) alterations and conduction abnormalities.[439] First the PR, then the QRS, and most characteristically the QTC intervals are prolonged. Clinically invisible increased preshivering muscle tone can obscure the P waves; ST segment and T wave abnormalities are inconsistent.[458,675,734]

The J wave (Osborn wave or hypothermic hump; Fig. 3-2) was first described by Tomaszewski[731] in 1938. This wave is present at the junction of the QRS complex and ST segment. It is not prognostic but is potentially diagnostic.* J waves have been observed at any temperature below 32.2° C and are most frequently seen in leads II and V_6. When the core temperature falls below 25° C, J waves are commonly found in the precordial leads (especially V_3 or V_4). The size of the J waves also increases with temperature depression but is unrelated to arterial pH.[249,531] The J waves are usually upright in aVL, aVF, and the left precordial leads. The cause of these intriguing J deflections is not clear but may represent hypothermia-induced ion fluxes resulting in delayed depolarization or early repolarization of the left ventricle. Another remote possible explanation is the existence of an unidentified hypothalamic or neurogenic factor. J waves are not pathognomonic of hypothermia but are also associated with central nervous system lesions, focal cardiac ischemia, and sepsis. They may be present in young healthy persons.[155,726]

J waveform abnormalities, when pronounced, can simulate a myocardial infarction. In one case a hypothermic patient was mistakenly admitted to the coronary care unit.[243] The hypothermic ECG changes are not easily computer programmable for interpretation, so in this regard ECG computer programs are not infallible. We have been unable to find computer software that can successfully recognize and

*References 249, 314, 357, 542, 614, 636, 788.

Table 3-2 Characteristics of the Three Zones of Hypothermia

Stage	Core Temperature °C	Core Temperature °F	Characteristics
Mild	37.6	99.6 ± 1	Normal rectal temperature
	37.0	98.6 ± 1	Normal oral temperature
	36.0	96.8	Increase in metabolic rate and blood pressure and preshivering muscle tone
	35.0	95.0	Urine temperature 34.8° C; maximum shivering thermogenesis
	34.0	93.2	Amnesia, dysarthria, and poor judgment develop; maladaptive behavior; normal blood pressure; maximum respiratory stimulation; tachycardia, then progressive bradycardia
	33.0	91.4	Ataxia and apathy develop; linear depression of cerebral metabolism; tachypnea, then progressive decrease in respiratory minute volume; cold diuresis
Moderate	32.0	89.6	Stupor; 25% decrease in oxygen consumption
	31.0	87.8	Extinguished shivering thermogenesis
	30.0	86.0	Atrial fibrillation and other arrhythmias develop; poikilothermia; pupils and cardiac output two thirds of normal; insulin ineffective
	29.0	85.2	Progressive decrease in level of consciousness, pulse, and respiration; pupils dilated; paradoxical undressing
	28.0	82.4	Decreased ventricular fibrillation threshold; 50% decrease in oxygen consumption and pulse; hypoventilation
	27.0	80.6	Loss of reflexes and voluntary motion
Severe	26.0	78.8	Major acid-base disturbances; no reflexes or response to pain
	25.0	77.0	Cerebral blood flow one third of normal; loss of cerebrovascular autoregulation; cardiac output 45% of normal; pulmonary edema may develop
	24.0	75.2	Significant hypotension and bradycardia
	23.0	73.4	No corneal or oculocephalic reflexes; areflexia
	22.0	71.6	Maximum risk of ventricular fibrillation; 75% decrease in oxygen consumption
	20.0	68.0	Lowest resumption of cardiac electromechanical activity; pulse 20% of normal
	19.0	66.2	Electroencephalographic silencing
	18.0	64.4	Asystole
	16.0	60.8	Lowest adult accidental hypothermia survival[141]
	15.2	59.2	Lowest infant accidental hypothermia survival[524]
	10.0	50.0	92% decrease in oxygen consumption
	9.0	48.2	Lowest therapeutic hypothermia survival[512]

suggest the diagnosis of hypothermia. Such a capability can be important in rural and wilderness settings, since prehospital thrombolytic therapy will expand as the role of the field 12-lead ECG is refined.[134]

Below 32.2° C all types of atrial and ventricular dysrhythmias are commonly encountered.[104,168,188,726] Although atrial distention seems to cause the atrial arrhythmias, several mechanisms are postulated to cause ventricular irritability. The His-Purkinje system is more sensitive to cold than is the myocardium. As a result, conduction velocity decreases and electrical signals can disperse. Since the conduction time is prolonged more than the absolute refractory period, reentry currents can produce circus rhythms, which initiate ventricular fibrillation.

In addition to causing bradycardia, widening of the QRS complex, and prolongation of the QT interval, hypothermia increases the duration of action potentials (Fig. 3-3).[46,47] During rewarming, nonuniform myocardial temperatures can disperse conduction and further increase the action potential duration. This is yet another mechanism for the development of unidirectional blocks, which facilitate reentrant arrhythmias. In one study performed using temperatures between 25° and 20° C, myocardial conduction time was 400% of normal while the absolute refractory period rose only 228%. Another arrhythmogenic mechanism is the development of independent electrical foci that precipitate dysrhythmias.[121]

Selection of the class III antiarrhythmic drug *d*-sotalol may thus cause problems.[47] It has temperature-dependent effectiveness and lengthens prolonged action potentials more efficiently at long pacing cycle lengths. A more favorable drug would not further lengthen long action potentials in colder myocardial regions while lengthening short action potentials in warmer regions. This would reduce the dispersion of the action potential duration and the effective refractory period. A variety of electrolyte abnormalities can fur-

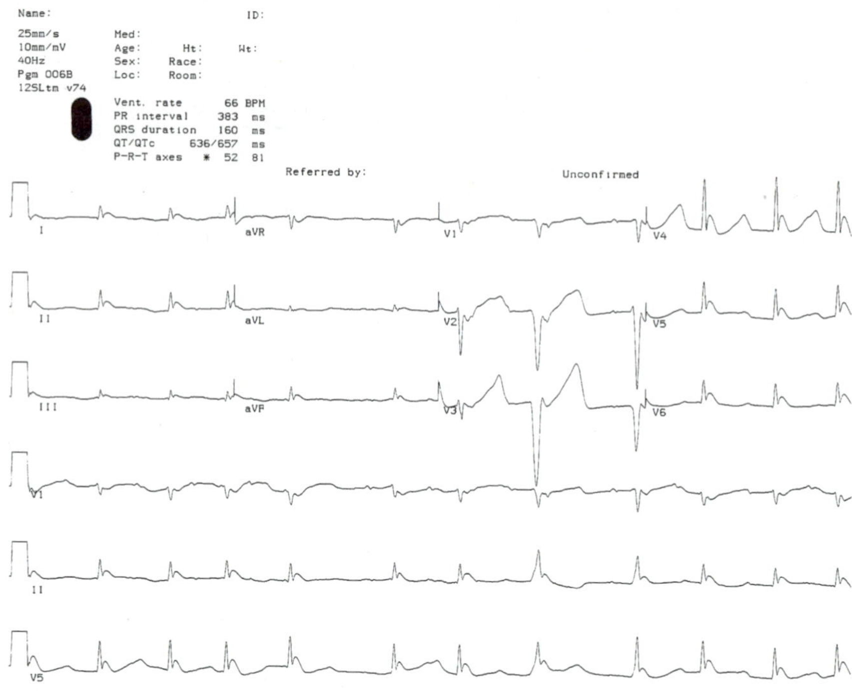

Fig. 3-2 The J or Osborn wave of hypothermia.

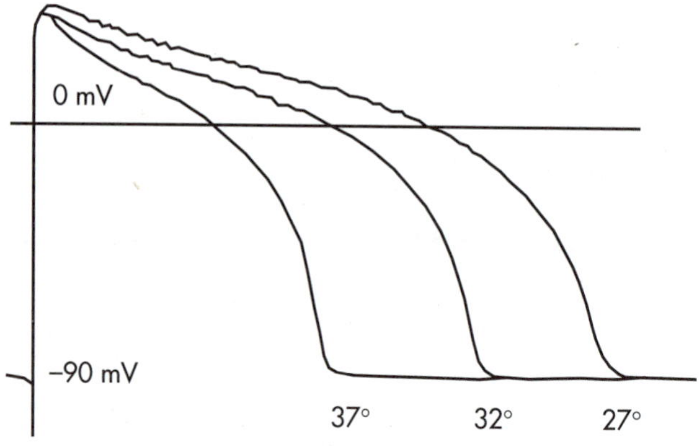

Fig. 3-3 Example of the effects of temperature on action potentials in cardiac cells.

ther complicate the situation during hypothermic conditions, since they exacerbate the effects of prolonged action potentials. Most conspicuously, hypothermia-induced cellular calcium loading mimics digitalis toxicity and may predispose to a forme fruste of torsades de pointes.[47,578]

Many explanations have been suggested for the development of hypothermia-induced ventricular fibrillation and asystole.[27,275] These rhythms often occur spontaneously below 25° C. The ventricular fibrillation threshold is decreased, as is the transmembrane resting potential. As previously mentioned, an independent focus or reentrant phenomenon develops. Since the heart is cold, the conduction delay is facilitated by the large dispersion of repolarization.[382] The action potential is also prolonged.[11] The increased temporal dispersion of the recovery of excitability is linked to ventricular fibrillation. In a way, nature's model of resistance to ventricular fibrillation is the heart of hibernating animals during rewarming.[326] Animals with this capacity seem to be protected by a shortened QT duration and a calcium channel handling system that prevents intracellular calcium overload.

Some reviews have implied that asystole is the more common rhythm seen on initial examination and that ventricular fibrillation is iatrogenic.[26,202,677] Possible causes of both of these rhythms include hypovolemia, tissue hypoxia, therapeutic manipulations, acid-base fluxes, autonomic dysfunction, and coronary vasoconstriction coupled with increased blood viscosity.*

The next major cardiovascular issue to consider is core temperature afterdrop, which refers to the continual decline in a hypothermic patient's temperature after removal from the cold. The pathophysiologic changes and clinical implications remain controversial.† A process that might contribute to afterdrop is the simple temperature equilibration between the warmer core and the cooler periphery. This would explain the afterdrop that has been demonstrated on isolated legs of beef and bags of gelatin.[758] Circulatory changes account for another set of observations. The coun-

*References 425, 498, 702, 705, 742, 767.

†References 143, 246, 274-276, 283, 323, 599, 686, 758, 775.

tercurrent cooling of blood that perfuses the cold extremities results in a core temperature decline until the existing temperature gradient is eliminated. This is particularly common during active external rewarming, when peripheral vasoconstriction and arteriovenous shunting are abruptly reversed.

The incidence and magnitude of core temperature afterdrop have varied widely in clinical experiments and in surgically induced hypothermia.* Hayward measured his own esophageal, rectal, tympanic, and cardiac temperatures (via flotation tip catheter) during rewarming after being cooled in 10° C water.[282] On 3 different days rewarming was achieved via shivering thermogenesis, heated humidified inhalation, and warm bath immersion. Coincident with a 0.3° C afterdrop during warm bath immersion, Hayward's mean arterial pressure fell 30% and his peripheral vascular resistance fell 50%. These results provide impressive support for the circulatory hypothesis.

Another study of peripheral blood flow during rewarming from mild hypothermia in humans suggests that only minimal skin blood flow changes can lead to afterdrop (Color Plate 7).[628] Harnett, Pruitt, and Sias[276] precipitated the largest core temperature afterdrops when their subjects were rewarmed with plumbed garments and heating pads. In summary, core temperature afterdrop appears to become most clinically relevant when a large temperature gradient exists between the periphery and the core, particularly in dehydrated, chronically cold patients. We have also observed major afterdrops when frostbitten extremities were thawed before thermal stabilization of the core temperature.

RESPIRATORY SYSTEM

Exposure to a big chill initially stimulates respiratory drive. Respiratory rate stimulation is followed by progressive depression of respiratory minute volume as cellular metabolism is depressed.[359,545] The respiratory rate often falls to 5 to 10 breaths/min below 30° C, and ultimately brainstem neurocontrol of ventilation fails.[395] Carbon dioxide production drops 50% for each 8° C fall in temperature.[441] When present in severe hypothermia, carbon dioxide retention and respiratory acidosis reflect the aberrant responses to normothermic respiratory stimuli. Some other pathophysiologic factors that contribute to a ventilation-perfusion mismatch include decreased ciliary motility, increased quantity and viscosity of secretions, respiratory distress syndrome, and noncardiogenic pulmonary edema.[93,534] The thorax loses elasticity while pulmonary compliance drops. The respiratory "bellows" stiffen and fail, since the contractile efficiency of the intercostal muscles and diaphragms declines.

A variety of other physiologic mysteries concerning hypoxia and hypothermia continue to be solved. For example, ectothermic vertebrates use an array of defense mechanisms in reaction to oxygen deprivation. They may reduce oxygen demand by behaviorally lowering their temperature or may favorably manipulate the oxyhemoglobin dissociation curve (see Fig. 3-4). Many of the pertinent potentially protective or detrimental factors that affect tissue oxygenation in endothermic humans are depicted in Box 3-1.

*References 116, 143, 246, 283, 323, 452.

RENAL SYSTEM

The kidneys respond briskly to hypothermia-induced changes in the capacitance of the vascular tree. Renal blood flow is depressed by 50% at 27° to 30° C, which decreases the glomerular filtration rate. Nevertheless, there is an initial large diuresis of this dilute glomerular filtrate, which does not clear nitrogenous wastes.[638,639]

The multifactorial etiology of the cold diuresis is still debated.[251,252] Some of the suggested mechanisms include inhibition of antidiuretic hormone (ADH) release and decrease in renal tubular function.[117,293,340,638] However, neither hydration nor ADH infusions seem to influence the diuretic response, which appears to be an attempt to compensate for an initial relative central hypervolemia caused by a vasoconstrictive overload of the capacitance vessels.

The diuresis is also possibly pressure related from impaired autoregulation in the kidney and may be caused by

BOX 3-1

OXYGENATION CONSIDERATIONS DURING HYPOTHERMIA

DETRIMENTAL FACTORS

Oxygen consumption increases with rise in temperature; caution if rapid rewarming; shivering also increases demand

Decreased temperature shifts oxyhemoglobin dissociation curve to the left

Ventilation-perfusion mismatch; atelectasis; decreased respiratory minute volume; bronchorrhea; decreased protective airway reflexes

Decreased tissue perfusion from vasoconstriction; increased viscosity

"Functional hemoglobin" concept: capability of hemoglobin to unload oxygen is lowered

Decreased thoracic elasticity and pulmonary compliance

PROTECTIVE FACTORS

Reduction of oxygen consumption: 50% at 28° C; 75% at 22° C; 92% at 10° C

Increased oxygen solubility in plasma

Decreased pH and increased Pa_{CO_2} shift oxyhemoglobin dissociation curve to right undiscovered effects on natriuretic polypeptide. Cold diuresis has circadian rhythmicity and correlates with periods of shivering. In experimental studies cold water immersion increases urinary output 3.5 times and the presence of ethanol impressively doubles that diuresis.[123] Regardless of the physiologic mechanism involved, progressive hemoconcentration occurs during the cold diuresis and absolute blood volume decreases. As the temperature continues to drop, kidney metabolism falls coincident with both chilling and the hypotensive hypoperfusion.[625]

COAGULATION

Significant advances in knowledge of the effects of temperature on coagulation continue to be reported.[553] One reason that coagulopathies often develop in hypothermic patients is that the enzymatic nature of the activated clotting factors is depressed by the cold.[157,204,594] In vivo the prolongation in clotting is proportional to the number of steps in the cascade. For example, at 29° C a 50% to 60% increase in the partial thromboplastin time (PTT) would be expected. However, kinetic tests of coagulation are normally performed in the laboratory at 37° C. It is essential to recognize that despite the potential multifactorial origin of a coagulopathy, the reversible hemostatic defect created by hypothermia may not be reflected by the "normal" prothrombin time (PT) or PTT.[609] Therefore the physician often observes a disparity between a clinically evident coagulopathy and "normal" clotting studies as reported by the laboratory. This coagulopathy is basically independent of clotting factor levels and cannot be confirmed by laboratory studies that are performed at 37° C. Treatment is rewarming, *not* simply administration of clotting factors.[595]

Thrombocytopenia is another cause of bleeding that becomes significant at 20° C.[83,665,746,747] Cold-induced thrombocytopenia was observed in 17 patients undergoing induced hypothermia. The average platelet count dropped from 184,000 to 37,000/ml^3 with maximal cooling.[653] Some mechanisms that have been proposed include direct bone marrow suppression and splenic or hepatic sequestration.[526,565,612] Thromboxane B_2 production by platelets is also temperature dependent, and therefore cooling the skin temperature in baboons produces a reversible platelet dysfunction.[98,741] Thrombocytopenia is a common but poorly recognized corollary of hypothermia in the elderly and in neonates.[63,110,172] During neonatal cold injury in one study, thrombocytopenia was present in six of seven infants.

Physiologic hypercoagulability develops during hypothermia, with appearance of a sequence similar to disseminated intravascular coagulation (DIC).[448,618] This results in a higher incidence of thromboembolism during hypothermia. Some of the postulated causes include thromboplastin release from cold tissue, simple circulatory collapse, and the release of catecholamines and steroids.[90] Since fibrin split product levels can be normal, bleeding is not always considered a hematologic manifestation of DIC. One distinctive hypothermic hematologic picture that has been reported includes thrombocytopenia, sideroblastic anemia, and erythroid hypoplasia.[526]

Whole blood viscosity increases with the hemoconcentration seen following diuresis and the shift of fluid out of the vascular compartments. Another cause of hyperviscosity unrelated to hematocrit is that red blood cells simply stiffen and have diminished cellular deformity when chilled.[572] The elevated viscosity of hypothermia is also exacerbated with cryoglobulinemia. Cryofibrinogen is a cold-precipitated fibrinogen occasionally seen in conjunction with carcinoma, sepsis, and collagen vascular diseases. The final mechanism that increases blood viscosity is the transient increase in platelet and red blood cell counts seen with mild surface cooling.[98] This could help to explain the epidemiologic observations of increased mortality from coronary and cerebral thromboses in winter.[352]

Predisposing Factors

For discussion purposes it is convenient and instructive to separate the factors that predispose to hypothermia into those that decrease heat production, increase heat loss, or impair thermoregulation.[136,441] Admittedly, there is significant overlap among these groups (Box 3-2).

DECREASED HEAT PRODUCTION

Thermogenesis is commonly decreased at both extremes of age.[418] In the elderly, neuromuscular inefficiency impairs shivering in conjunction with decreased physical activity.[70] The effects of aging on cold tolerance continue to be evaluated, since aging progressively diminishes homeostatic and cold adaptive capabilities.[39,793] Although most elderly persons have normal thermoregulation, they are prone to develop conditions that impair heat conservation.[23,95,231,446] For example, elderly surgical patients are at high risk for hypothermia.[485]

The elderly are physiologically less adept at increasing heat production and the respiratory quotient, which is the ratio of the volume of carbon dioxide produced to the volume of oxygen consumed per unit of time.[247,441,599] Impaired thermal perception, possibly caused by decreased resting peripheral blood flow, leads to poor adaptive behavior.* Metabolic studies also demonstrate that in severely hypothermic elderly persons lipolysis occurs in preference to glucose consumption.[692]

Neonates have a large surface area/mass ratio, a relatively deficient subcutaneous tissue layer, and virtually no behavioral defense mechanisms.[319] Newborn "unadapted" infants attempt to thermoregulate with an initial vasocon-

*References 114, 115, 220, 247, 446, 634, 751.

BOX 3-2

FACTORS PREDISPOSING TO HYPOTHERMIA

DECREASED HEAT PRODUCTION

- Endocrinologic failure
  - Hypopituitarism
  - Hypoadrenalism
  - Hypothyroidism
  - Lactic acidosis
  - Diabetic and alcoholic ketoacidosis
- Insufficient fuel
  - Hypoglycemia
  - Malnutrition
  - Marasmus
  - Kwashiorkor
  - Extreme physical exertion
- Neuromuscular physical exertion
  - Age extremes
  - Impaired shivering
  - Inactivity
  - Lack of adaptation

IMPAIRED THERMOREGULATION

- Peripheral failure
  - Neuropathies
  - Acute spinal cord transection
  - Diabetes
- Central failure/neurologic
  - Cardiovascular accident
  - Central nervous system trauma
  - Toxicologic
  - Metabolic
  - Subarachnoid hemorrhage
  - Pharmacologic
  - Hypothalamic dysfunction
  - Parkinson's disease
  - Anorexia nervosa
  - Cerebellar lesion
  - Neoplasm
  - Congenital intracranial anomalies
  - Multiple sclerosis
  - Hyperkalemic periodic paralysis

INCREASED HEAT LOSS

- Environmental
  - Immersion
  - Nonimmersion
- Induced vasodilation
  - Pharmacologic
  - Toxicologic
- Erythrodermas
  - Burns
  - Psoriasis
  - Ichthyosis
  - Exfoliative dermatitis
- Iatrogenic
  - Emergency childbirth
  - Cold infusions
  - Heatstroke treatment

MISCELLANEOUS ASSOCIATED CLINICAL STATES

- Multisystem trauma
- Recurrent hypothermia
- Episodic hypothermia
- Shapiro's syndrome
- Infections: bacterial, viral, parasitic
- Pancreatitis
- Carcinomatosis
- Cardiopulmonary disease
- Vascular insufficiency
- Uremia
- Paget's disease
- Giant cell arteritis
- Sarcoidosis
- Shaken baby syndrome
- Systemic lupus erythematosus
- Wernicke-Korsakoff syndrome
- Hodgkin's disease
- Shock
- Sickle-cell anemia
- Sudden infant death syndrome

striction and acceleration of metabolic rate. In contrast, "adapted" infants who are older than 5 days of age can increase lipolysis immediately and burn oxidative brown adipose tissue.[297,557,606]

The association between hypothermia and the mortality rate of premature infants has been well studied, and no cause-effect relationship has been found.[284] Although the smaller infants admitted to a neonatal intensive care unit are at the greatest risk of hypothermia, mortality was related to hypothermia only in the larger neonates.

Not surprisingly, emergency deliveries and resuscitations are responsible for most acute neonatal hypothermia. Some of the other common risk factors in early neonatal life are prematurity, low birth weight, inexperienced mother, perinatal morbidity, and low socioeconomic status.[794] In more chronically induced subacute hypothermia, lethargy, a weak cry, and failure to thrive are commonly observed.[386]

Many cold infants have paradoxical rosy cheeks and look surprisingly healthy. After the first few days of life, hypothermia frequently indicates septicemia and carries a high mortality rate.[126,184] Low weight and malnutrition were common findings in a series of 56 hypothermic infants who were 4 to 113 days of age.[674] Detection of hypothermia in a low birth weight neonate should suggest the possibility of intracranial hemorrhage; hypothermia has also been observed in the shaken baby syndrome.[158,430]

Endocrinologic failure, including hypopituitarism, hypoadrenalism, and myxedema, commonly decreases heat production.[237] Interestingly, congenital adrenal hyperplasia with mineralocorticoid insufficiency is more common in cold climates. This may be an adaptive response to prolonged exposure to cold temperatures, since the "normal" cold diuresis is reduced in these patients.[432] Hypothyroidism is often occult, with no history available regarding cold intolerance, dry skin, lassitude, or arthralgias. The physician should check for a thyroid scar or any history of thyroid hormone replacement. The degree of temperature depression correlates fairly directly with mortality.[214] Eighty percent of patients who are in myxedema coma, which is several times more common in females, are hypothermic.[2,173]

The body needs a continuous influx of fuel. The range of effects of insufficient nutrition extends from hypoglycemia to marasmus to kwashiorkor. Kwashiorkor is less often associated with hypothermia than is marasmus because of the insulating effect of the hypoproteinemic edema.[619] Central neuroglycopenia distorts hypothalamic function.[694] In one series of predominantly alcoholic patients with hypothermia, 41% were hypoglycemic.[208] Malnutrition decreases insulative subcutaneous fat and directly alters thermoregulation. In a series of 744 elderly women with femoral neck fractures, poor nutrition predisposed to hypothermia and its attendant clumsiness.[33] Partly because of fuel depletion, hypothermia is as great a threat as hyperthermia in marathon races run in cool climates. In a study of 62 runners, participants slowing from fatigue or injury late in a race were at serious risk of hypothermia.[462]

INCREASED HEAT LOSS

Poorly acclimated and insulated individuals often have high diaphoretic, convective, and evaporative heat losses during exposure to cold. Since the skin functions as a radiator, any dermatologic malfunction increases heat loss. Such erythrodermas include psoriasis, exfoliative dermatitis, and toxic epidermal necrolysis.[260,378,601,727] Hypothermia with hypernatremic dehydration is also seen in congenital lamellar ichthyosis.[229]

Burns and inappropriate burn treatment are additional causes of excessive heat loss.[413] Other iatrogenic causes include massive cold intravenous infusions and the overcooling of heatstroke victims.[363] When carbon dioxide is used for insufflation of the abdomen before laparoscopy, warming the gas[520] before administration helps prevent hypothermia.[546] Environmental immersion exposure is discussed in detail in Chapter 4.

Many pharmacologic and toxicologic agents both increase heat loss and impair thermoregulation. The most common of these is ethanol,[96,337,438] which interacts with every studied putative or proven thermoregulatory neurotransmitter, including serotonin and dopamine. Although ingestion of this cutaneous vasodilator leads to a feeling of warmth and perhaps visible flushing, it is the major cause of urban hypothermia.* In one series of 51 fatal cases of accidental hypothermia, two thirds of the victims were under the influence of alcohol and half were considered habitual drunkards.[4] In children with ethanol intoxication, hypothermia is a common effect.[447]

Ethanol is a poikilothermia-producing agent that directly impairs thermoregulation at high or low temperatures.[371,707] The body temperature is lowered both from cutaneous vasodilation with radiative heat loss and from impaired shivering thermogenesis. Chronic ethanol ingestion damages the mamillary bodies and posterior hypothalamus, which modulates shivering thermogenesis.[337,573-575] Ethanol also increases the risk of being exposed to the environment by modifying protective adaptive behavior.[372] The ultimate example is paradoxical undressing, which is the removal of clothing in response to a cold stress.[4] As an organic solvent, ethanol does confer a few theoretically redeeming qualities in the presence of freezing cold injuries by lowering the cellular freezing point.[251,252]

The neurophysiologic effects of ethanol are modified by the duration and intensity of exercise, by food consumption, and by applied cold stress.[224,227] Aging increases sensitivity to the hypothermic actions of ethanol in some primate experiments.[501] Chronic ingestion yields tolerance to its hypothermic effects, and at times rebound hyperthermia is seen during withdrawal. Conditions commonly associated with ethanol ingestion that adversely affect heat balance include immobility and hypoglycemia. Inhibition of hepatic gluconeogenesis coexists with malnutrition.[438,768,772] Hypothermic alcoholic ketoacidosis has been reported.[16,236] Intravenous thiamine is diagnostic and therapeutic for Wernicke's encephalopathy, which is another cause of reversible hypothermia.† The acute triad of global confusion, ophthalmoplegia, and truncal ataxia is often masked by hypothermia, and the temperature depression may persist for weeks.

IMPAIRED THERMOREGULATION

A variety of conditions that impair thermoregulation can be considered as having central, peripheral, metabolic, pharmacologic, or toxicologic effects.[150] Central conditions appear to directly affect hypothalamic function and frequently mediate vasodilation. Some common examples of traumatic

*References 4, 135, 203, 299, 309, 477, 730, 768.
†References 161, 347, 435, 450, 560, 600.

lesions include skull fractures, especially basilar, and intracerebral hemorrhages, most commonly chronic subdural hematomas. The pathologic lesions commonly associated with hypothermia include neoplasms, congenital anomalies, and Parkinson's disease.[97,217] Patients with Parkinson's disease or Alzheimer's disease, because of their global neurologic impairment, are behaviorally at particular risk. Finally, cerebellar lesions also impede heat production because of inefficient choreiform shivering.

Hypothermia can also occur in conjunction with Reye's syndrome.[713] In some patients with Hodgkin's disease, hypothermia is seen exclusively in previously febrile patients with advanced disease, independent of cell type.[77,335] This appears to be a disease-associated functional disorder of thermoregulation, similar to the hypothermia associated with anorexia nervosa.[468] Centrally induced hypothermia has been completely antagonized with thyrotropin-releasing hormone.[290]

Peripheral thermoregulation fails most characteristically following acute spinal cord transection.[8,20] Victims are functionally poikilothermic as soon as the peripheral vasoconstriction is extinguished.[469,567] Other peripheral impediments to thermostability include various neuropathies and diabetes mellitus. Hypothermia is more common in elderly diabetics than in the general population, even after exclusion of the subset of patients with diabetic metabolic emergencies.[508] The common denominator present in metabolic derangements may be the abnormal plasma osmolality that appears to interfere with hypothalamic function. Similar causes of hypothermia via this mechanism include hypoglycemia, diabetic ketoacidosis, and uremia.[262,322,706] Remarkably, the pH was 6.67 in one hypothermic survivor with lactic acidosis and 6.41 in another.[502]

Numerous medications and toxins in therapeutic or toxic doses impair centrally mediated thermoregulation and vasoconstriction.[411,460] In a single series of 103 critically ill patients with overdoses, 27 were hypothermic.[338] The usual offenders include barbiturates, benzodiazepines, phenothiazines, and the tricyclic antidepressants.[287] Reduction of the core temperature may also be a prodrome of lithium poisoning.[212] Organophosphates, narcotics, glutethimide, bromocriptine,[559] erythromycin, clonidine, fluphenazine, bethanechol, atropine, acetaminophen, and carbon monoxide have all been reported to cause hypothermia.* In experimental studies hypothermia following acute carbon monoxide poisoning was associated with increased mortality.[698]

Recurrent and episodic hypothermia are widely reported.[304,669] The recurrent variety is more common and is usually secondary to ethanol abuse, with one patient having survived 12 episodes.[476] Severe, recurrent presentations have also been caused by self-poisoning and anorexia nervosa.[164,671]

Patients with episodic hypothermia can be divided into two groups, with significant overlap.[725] In the first group, diaphoretic episodes precede the temperature decline, which lasts for several hours. Included in this group are patients with hypothalamic lesions and agenesis of the corpus callosum, which is termed Shapiro's syndrome.[566,626,650] The resultant hyperhidrosis and hypothermia have been successfully treated with clonidine, an α_2-adrenoceptor agonist.[752] The hypothermia seen with agenesis of the corpus callosum has also been associated with hypercalcemia and status epilepticus.[330] Since experimental sectioning of the corpus callosum does not induce hypothermia, associated lesions, including lipomas, probably cause this thermoinstability.[405,623,696]

This first group with brief episodic hypothermia also includes patients with spontaneous periodic hyperthermia.[167,218] This condition may reflect a diencephalic autonomic seizure disorder[487] and can be associated with paroxysmal hypertension. Both vasomotor and thermoregulatory mechanisms have been successfully treated with anticonvulsants.[151] Florid psychiatric symptoms often mask these intermittent hypothermic episodes. Idiopathic periodic hypothermia has also been noted in a patient with occult syringomyelia and bizarre behavior.[253]

The second category of patients with episodic hypothermia consists of persons who remain cold for days to weeks, rather than for hours. These patients have more seizure disorders, and the central hypothalamic thermostat is set abnormally low. Patients with intermittent hypothermia usually demonstrate some characteristics from both groups.[441,725] Circadian rhythm disturbances have also been observed in patients with neurologic disorders who have chronic hypothermia.[660]

Numerous infestations and infections can not only elevate but often depress core temperature. These include septicemia, pneumonia, peritonitis, meningitis, encephalitis, bacterial endocarditis, typhoid, miliary tuberculosis, syphilis, brucellosis, and trypanosomiasis.[76,404] Other diseases, in addition to cerebrovascular and cardiopulmonary disorders, that produce secondary hypothermia include lupus,[380] carcinomatosis, pancreatitis, and multiple sclerosis.[183,232] Hypothalamic demyelination has been one proposed mechanism to explain the episodic hypothermia observed in some patients with multiple sclerosis.[238,387]

Hypothermia can also result from the low cardiac output that follows a major myocardial infarction, which in one case was reversed by intraaortic balloon counterpulsation.[159,236] An additional hodgepodge of causes includes vascular insufficiency, giant cell arteritis, uremia, sickle cell anemia, Paget's disease, sarcoidosis, and sudden infant death syndrome.[19,171,441] Magnesium sulfate infusion during preterm labor has caused hypothermia with fetal and maternal bradycardia,[321,607] and hypothyroidism can be manifested as hypothermia following preeclampsia.[484]

---

*References 23, 51, 164, 254, 277, 384, 388, 407, 455, 523, 563.

TRAUMA

Of the variety of clinical entities that are associated with hypothermia, traumatic conditions causing hypotension and hypovolemia most dramatically jeopardize thermostability.* Mortality increases, but it is unclear whether that is because of the hypothermia or the injuries.[472] Recognition of hypothermia is often obscured by obvious hemorrhaging and injuries.[630] Conversely, traumatic neurologic deficits, including paresis and areflexia, can be misattributed to hypothermia.[8,20,567] In one study of trauma patients requiring operations, the mean temperature loss was greater in the emergency department than in the operating room.[257]

In one study that stratified the subjects for injury with the anatomic Injury Severity Scale (ISS), hypothermic patients had a higher mortality rate than similarly injured patients who remained normothermic.[336] Another study did not duplicate this finding.[684] However, those investigators stratified for injury using Trauma Revised Injury Severity Scale (TRISS) methodology, which is probably less valid during hypothermia because its physiologic components would overestimate injury severity. To illustrate this point, some component of hypotension might be normal for a given temperature.

A variety of adverse physiologic events accompany hypothermia with trauma.[464] A decrease in skin and core temperatures without compensatory shivering thermogenesis has been reported in a group of patients with major trauma as defined by the ISS.[412,431] Hypothermia directly causes coagulopathies in trauma patients through at least three avenues, which are discussed in the section on coagulation.[69] In review, the cascade of enzymatic reactions is impaired and plasma fibrinolytic activity is also enhanced. This produces a clinical presentation similar to DIC. In addition, platelets are poorly functional and become sequestered.

Hypothermia worsens the effects of endotoxins on clotting time in vitro and may synergistically exacerbate the coagulopathy seen in trauma patients.[205] The average temperature of 123 initially normothermic trauma patients in whom lethal coagulopathies developed was 31.2° C.[344] Hypothermia seems protective only when induced before shock occurs. This reduces adenosine triphosphate (ATP) utilization while ATP stores are still normal, as during elective surgery. Conversely, in trauma patients ATP stores are already depleted.

Presentation

When the patient's historical circumstances are available, they frequently suggest the presence of hypothermia.[69] The diagnosis of hypothermia becomes fairly simple when exposure is obvious, as with avalanche victims. However, subtle presentations predominate in urban settings, with patients often complaining only of vague symptoms including hunger, nausea, fatigue, and dizziness. Predisposing underlying illness or ethanol ingestion is also commonly present. Other clinical presentations include major trauma, immersion, overdose, and cerebrovascular accidents.[118,280,414,415,723]

With luck the overall constellation of physical findings will suggest the diagnosis (Box 3-3). During the head, eye, ear, nose, and throat examination, abnormal findings can include decreased corneal reflexes, mydriasis, strabismus, flushing, erythropsia, facial edema, rhinorrhea, and epistaxis. Mild hypothermia usually does *not* depress the human pupillary light reflex.[310,390] Cardiovascular findings following the initial tachycardia include bradydysrhythmias and hypotension. Heart sounds may be muffled and distant.

Tachypnea, an early respiratory finding, is usually followed by progressive hypoventilation accompanied by bronchorrhea and the presence of adventitious sounds. Since the gastrointestinal tract is depressed, abdominal distention or rigidity, ileus, obstipation, and poor rectal tone are frequently present. Gastric dilation is particularly common in neonates and in myxedematous adults. Genitourinary output ranges from initial polyuria because of cold diuresis to anuria. Interestingly, the incidence of testicular torsion reportedly increases because of cremasteric contractions.

Diffuse neurologic abnormalities vary widely. Some patients can still converse at 25° C and are normoreflexic. However, there is generally a progressive decrease in the level of consciousness proportionate to the degree of hypothermia. The presence of ataxia and dysarthria may mimic a cerebrovascular accident.[247] Speed of reasoning and memory registration are also impaired.[113] Amnesia, antinociception, anesthesia, or hypoesthesia can develop. Cranial nerve signs are present following bulbar damage from central pontine myelinolysis.[715] However, these extraocular muscle movement abnormalities, similar to extensor plantar responses, do not directly correlate with the degree of hypothermia.[206]

Hyperreflexia predominates from 35° to 32.2° C and is then followed by hyporeflexia. The plantar response remains flexor until 26° C, when areflexia develops. The knee jerk is usually the last reflex to disappear and is the first to reappear during rewarming. From 30° to 26° C, both the contraction and relaxation phases of the reflexes are prolonged equally. However, in myxedema the relaxation phase of the ankle reflex is more prolonged than is the contraction phase.[441] Spinal cord and other central nervous system lesions may be obscured by depressive neurologic changes that normally accompany hypothermia.[20,206]

Psychiatric presentations and suicide attempts associated with hypothermia are commonly misdiagnosed initially. Preexistent psychiatric disorders blossom again in the cold in some individuals who have become adjusted and stabilized in temperate climates.[506,507,721] Mental status alterations include anxiety, impaired judgment, perseveration,

*References 13, 33, 40, 431, 555, 615, 693.

BOX 3-3
SIGNS OF HYPOTHERMIA

HEAD, EYE, EAR, NOSE, THROAT
Mydriasis
Decreased corneal reflexes
Extraocular muscle abnormalities
Erythropsia
Flushing
Facial edema
Epistaxis
Rhinorrhea
Strabismus

CARDIOVASCULAR
Initial tachycardia
Subsequent bradycardia
Dysrhythmias
Decreased heart tones
Hepatojugular reflux
Jugular venous distention
Hypotension
Peripheral vasoconstriction

RESPIRATORY
Initial tachypnea
Adventitious sounds
Bronchorrhea
Progressive hypoventilation
Apnea

GASTROINTESTINAL
Ileus
Constipation
Abdominal distention or rigidity
Poor rectal tone
Gastric dilation in neonates or in adults with myxedema
Vomiting

GENITOURINARY
Anuria
Polyuria
Oliguria
Testicular torsion

NEUROLOGIC
Depressed level of consciousness
Ataxia
Dysarthria
Amnesia
Anesthesia
Areflexia
Poor suck reflex
Hypoesthesia
Antinociception
Initial hyperreflexia
Hyporeflexia
Central pontine myelinolysis

PSYCHIATRIC
Impaired judgment
Perseveration
Mood changes
Peculiar "flat" affect
Altered mental status
Paradoxical undressing
Neuroses
Psychoses
Suicide
Organic brain syndrome
Anorexia
Depression
Apathy
Irritability

MUSCULOSKELETAL
Increased muscle tone
Shivering
Rigidity or pseudo–rigor mortis
Paravertebral spasm
Opisthotonos
Compartment syndrome

DERMATOLOGIC
Erythema
Pallor
Cyanosis
Icterus
Scleral edema
Ecchymosis
Edema
Pernio
Frostnip
Frostbite
Panniculitis
Cold urticaria
Necrosis
Gangrene

neurosis, and psychosis.[620] Leaders of expeditions can become moody, apathetic, uncooperative, and risk taking.[580] Elderly patients often withdraw in confusion, become silent, and display lassitude and poor judgment. A peculiar flat affect is commonly observed, and the psychomotor impairment can resemble an organic brain syndrome.

Early in hypothermia, simply losing the effective use of the hands can be devastating. Appropriate behavior adapted to the cold, such as seeking a heat source, is often lacking.[115] An extreme example is paradoxical undressing.[360] The clothing is removed in a preterminal effort to address an impending thermoregulatory collapse, and many patients have been mistakenly described as sexual assault victims.[759] This phenomenon is also seen in hypothermic children.[666]

Musculoskeletal posturing can at its extreme extend to pseudo–rigor mortis. Preshivering muscle tone is increased before the core temperature drops to 35° C, and muscular rigidity, paravertebral spasm, and even opisthotonos may be present. Extremity compartment syndromes often develop because of associated conditions causing prolonged compression and immobility,[544,585] in addition to compartment hypertension seen during reperfusion of frostbitten extremities.

Dermatologic presentations of hypothermia include erythema, pallor, edema, and scleral edema. Cold urticaria, frostnip, frostbite, and gangrene should also cause the clinician to entertain this diagnosis.[331] Pernio has been observed in association with chronic myelomonocytic leukemia.[355]

Laboratory Evaluation

ACID-BASE BALANCE

The strategy for achieving and maintaining acid-base balance in hypothermia differs from that of normothermia in many regards.[107,149,169,315,703] After an initial respiratory alkalosis from hyperventilation when the person first becomes chilled, a common underlying disturbance is relative acidosis. The respiratory component of the acidosis is caused mainly by direct respiratory depression. In addition, as the temperature decreases, the solubility of carbon dioxide in the blood increases.[85] Some further contributors to the metabolic component of the acidosis include impaired hepatic metabolism and acid excretion, lactate generation from shivering, and decreased tissue perfusion. Nevertheless, reliable clinical prediction of the acid-base status in accidental hypothermia is not possible.[532] In one series of 135 cases 30% were acidotic and 25% alkalotic.[477]

Correction of arterial blood gases for temperature was initially suggested to aid in the clinician's interpretation of the pathophysiology involved in hypothermic arterial oxygenation and acid-base balance.[272,467,611,613,645] The controversy began in the 1950s when the protective effects of hypothermia during cardiac surgery led to the search for the most protective degree of ventilation.[780] The ideal strategy would minimize any potential cardiovascular and central nervous system complications during rewarming. If a pH electrode could be used at the patient's current core temperature, an uncorrected but exact pH value would be obtained. However, arterial blood samples are always warmed to 37° C before electrode measurements are obtained and are not measured at the patient's subnormal temperature. To correct for changes in temperature, Severinghaus's mathematical corrections have been subsequently applied.[644,645] In an airtight syringe with a constant bicarbonate content, the change in pH per °C of blood in vitro is –0.0147. Thus one could correct the pH by adding 0.0147 pH units per °C below 37° C. During correction the $Pa{O_2}$ also drops 7.2% and the $Pa{CO_2}$ drops 4.4% per °C in temperature.[85,356] The oxyhemoglobin dissociation curve (Fig. 3-4) shifts to the left because of the decreased partial pressure of dissolved gases. To interpret temperature-corrected values the clinician would need to compare results with the normal values at that temperature. For example, a $P{CO_2}$ of 40 mm Hg and a pH of 7.4 at 37° C are the equivalent of a $P{CO_2}$ of 30 mm Hg and a pH of 7.50 at 30° C. A $P{O_2}$ of 120 mm Hg at 37° C corresponds to a $P{O_2}$ of 59 mm Hg at 27° C and does not indicate arterial oxyhemoglobin desaturation.[683]

On the other hand, for accurate interpretation of uncorrected arterial blood gases as they are measured by electrodes at 37° C, the physician need only compare values with the well-known normal values at 37° C. This simplifies comparison of results from serial samples during rewarming. No matter what the temperature, if the uncorrected pH is 7.4 and the $P{CO_2}$ is 40 mm Hg, alveolar ventilation and acid-base balance are normal.[699,700]

Circulatory changes also prevent adequate mobilization and delivery of organic acids to the buffer systems. As in normothermia, mixed venous blood may best reflect acid-base status during resuscitation.[701,761] Despite flow changes in a moderately hypothermic canine model, a significant correlation persisted between arterial and mixed venous pH.[488] The arteriovenous change in pH was ±0.03 to 0.04

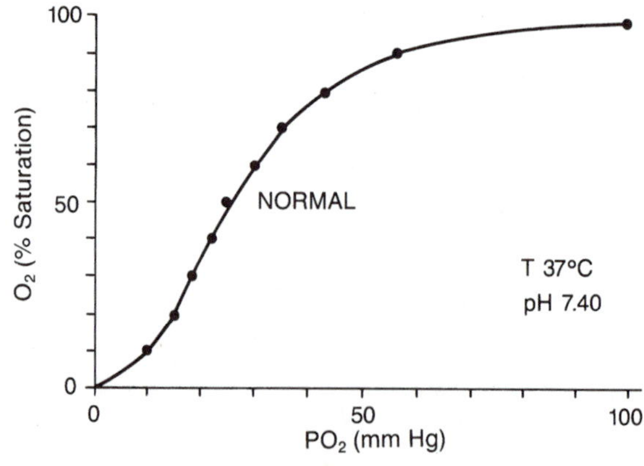

Fig. 3-4 Oxyhemoglobin dissociation curve at 37° C. At colder temperatures the curve shifts to the left.

pH unit. The buffering capacity of cold blood is also markedly impaired. In normothermia, when the PCO_2 increases 10 mm Hg, a decrease in pH of 0.08 unit occurs. At 28° C the decrease in pH doubles to 0.16.

Optimal strategy to maintain acid-base homeostasis during treatment of accidental hypothermia was challenged in the past. The accepted earlier assumption was that 7.42 was the ideal "corrected" patient pH at all temperatures and that therapy should be directed at maintenance of the corrected arterial pH at 7.42.[769,770] A better intracellular pH reference is electrochemical neutrality, at which pH equals pOH. Since the neutral point of water at 37° C is pH 6.8, Rahn has hypothesized that this normal 0.6 unit pH offset in body fluids should be maintained at all temperatures.[583,584,593] Since the neutral pH rises with cooling, so should blood pH (Fig. 3-5).

Rahn's hypothesis was motivated in part by his observation that Antarctic codfish survive far below the freezing point of water because of a glycoprotein antifreeze and are able to function in an extremely alkalotic state. This same blood pH variation, that is, a rise in pH with a decline in temperature, is seen in other cold-blooded vertebrates and invertebrates.[662,663] Relative alkalinity of tissues makes physiologic sense. Intracellular electrochemical neutrality ensures optimal function of the enzyme systems and transport proteins at all temperatures and allows excretion of the neutral intracellular waste product urea.[28,29]

Depressed metabolism and carbon dioxide generation are the physiologic responses to temperature depression, since each temperature has its associated metabolic rate. Ventilation is intrinsically adjusted to maintain a net charge on the defended parameter, the peptide-linked histidine imidazole buffering system.

One homeostatic approach to maintain a steady pH is to keep the bicarbonate content constant. This is achievable only if the total blood carbon dioxide content also does not change. Since carbon dioxide solubility increases with temperature depression, alveolar ventilation must increase to compensate by lowering the PCO_2. The active ectotherms exhibit this respiratory adaptation and do not depress their respiratory minute volume when cold. This response, termed the ectothermic or alpha-stat strategy, allows them to maintain the total bicarbonate and carbon dioxide content while increasing their pH. On the other hand, hibernating mammals are far more acidic and employ an acid-base strategy that suppresses metabolism.[503] This is termed the endothermic or pH stat strategy.

Several experimental and clinical studies have subsequently supported Rahn's breakthrough hypothesis. In one study a set of puppies with the corrected pH maintained at 7.4 had a 50% drop in cardiac performance after bypass.[36] The control group, left alkalotic, had normal cardiac indices and increased cerebral blood flow.[370,702,704] During systemic deep hypothermia in further canine studies, constraining the corrected pH to 7.4 caused myocardial damage, while relative alkalinity afforded myocardial protection.[36] Other advantages included improved electrical stability of the heart, since the fibrillation threshold of dogs markedly decreased when the corrected arterial pH was held at 7.4. In contrast, maintaining the pH at 7.4 during hypothermia in a rat model did not affect cardiac work response.[661] This suggests that the range of optimal extracellular pH is large in some species.[702]

During cardiopulmonary bypass, carbon dioxide is excreted and blood in the oxygenator does not reach equilibrium. To deal with this, supplemental ventilation with carbogen is one option. One ventilatory regimen including 5% carbon dioxide was optimal in a study of induced hypothermia.[271] Using 1% to 2% rather than 5% carbon dioxide in

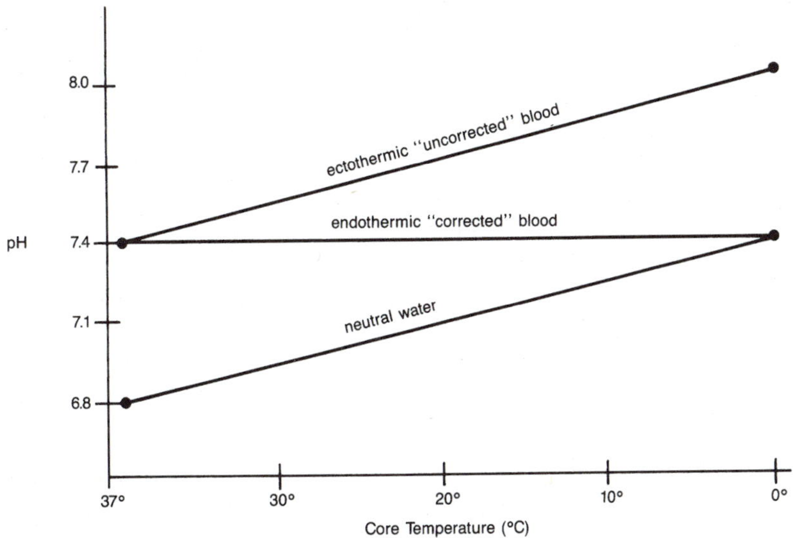

Fig. 3-5 Ectotherm's physiologic 0.6 pH unit offset from neutral water progressively diminishes if arterial blood gases are temperature corrected.

the oxygenator produced an uncorrected P_{CO_2} nearer 40 mm Hg and relative alkalosis in a study of 28 children on bypass with deep hypothermia.[461] Another advantage to adding a small fraction of carbon dioxide to the inspired mixture is the flattening and shifting of the oxyhemoglobin dissociation curve to the right (Fig. 3-4).[579]

In another study of 181 cardiac bypass patients, 121 consecutive patients were "endothermically" managed with "corrected" normal pH and P_{CO_2} values.[377] Ventricular fibrillation occurred in 49 (40%). Of the other 60 patients left "ectothermically" alkalotic, only 12 (20%) had spontaneous ventricular fibrillation.

These observations provide strong support for Rahn's hypothesis. The advantage that ectotherms obtain with a constant relative degree of alkalinity also applies to warm-blooded endotherms during hypothermic conditions when the 0.6 pH unit difference between the cell and blood is maintained. Potentially deleterious effects of this alkalosis on other organ systems have yet to be identified. However, it is clear that maintaining the corrected pH at 7.4 and P_{CO_2} at 40 mm Hg during hypothermia depresses cerebral and coronary blood flow and cardiac output and increases the incidence of lactic acidosis and ventricular fibrillation.[289]

HEMATOLOGIC EVALUATION

Hematologic evaluation is necessary except in the mildest exposure cases. The severity of any blood loss is easily underestimated, since the hematocrit value increases because of the decline in plasma volume and the 2% increase per 1° C fall in temperature.[342] In addition, total red blood cell mass might already be low because of a preexisting anemia, malnutrition, leukemia, uremia, or neoplasm.

The white blood cell count is frequently normal or low, even if sepsis is present. As a result, systemic leukopenia does not imply absence of infection, especially if the patient is at either age extreme, debilitated, intoxicated, or myxedematous or has secondary hypothermia.[50,404,653] The leukocyte count also drops during hypothermia because of the bone marrow depression and the hepatic, splenic, and splanchnic sequestration.

Serum electrolyte levels must be continuously monitored and rechecked during warming. Data from experimental and clinical settings demonstrate no reliable trends, and therefore no safe predictors of electrolyte values exist.[135,201,276] Serum electrolytes fluctuate with temperature, duration of exposure, and the rewarming technique selected. Both membrane permeability and sodium-potassium pump efficiency also change with temperature.[569,570] Isolated temperature depression per se has no consistent effect on the sodium and chloride levels until well below 25° C.[605] Plasma electrolyte levels are also affected by ongoing fluid shifts, prehydration, rehydration, and endocrine or gastrointestinal dysfunction.

Plasma potassium level is independent of temperature.[144,340,341] In experimental studies acute hypothermia causes a decline in serum potassium secondary to redistribution, which is reversible on rewarming.[680,681] However, empirical potassium supplementation during hypothermia often results in normothermic toxicity. From a clinical perspective, hypokalemia occurs as potassium moves into the musculature and not simply out of the body through kaliuresis.[52] The physiologically illogical discrepancy of a decreasing potassium level with a decreasing pH results from the greater intracellular than extracellular pH changes. Hypokalemia is much more common in prolonged or chronically induced hypothermia.[21,367,529]

Systemic potassium deficiencies can also be exacerbated by prior diuretic therapy, alcoholism, diabetic ketoacidosis, hypopituitarism, and inappropriate antidiuretic hormone secretion. The normal total body pool of potassium is about 3000 mEq, of which only 65 mEq is in circulation. Hypokalemic digitalis sensitivity can be masked by hypothermia, and gradual correction of persistent and severe hypokalemia during rewarming is necessary for optimal cardiac and gastrointestinal function.[599]

When hyperkalemia is identified, the physician should search for other causes of metabolic acidosis, crush injury or rhabdomyolysis, renal failure, postsubmersion hemolysis, or hypoaldosteronism. An important caveat is that temperature depression can increase hyperkalemic cardiac toxicity. Since the well-known diagnostic ECG changes are often obscured, and since ventricular fibrillation occurs with serum potassium levels below 7 mEq/L, serum potassium levels must be closely monitored. The cautious clinician should consider prophylactic administration of bicarbonate, insulin, or calcium in conservative doses.

Hypothermia also has no consistent effect on magnesium or calcium levels. Severe hypophosphatemia was reported in one patient during treatment of profound hypothermia.[403] In that case an intracellular phosphate shift was the postulated reason, since urinary excretion appeared minimal. Although increases in serum enzyme levels are not seen in mild experimental hypothermia, numerous serum enzymes are elevated when diffuse intracellular structural damage occurs in severe accidental hypothermia.[82,443,453] Creatine phosphokinase (CPK) levels over 200,000 IU have been observed, and rhabdomyolysis is often present in these instances.[585]

Inhibition of cellular membrane transport decreases glucose utilization. In addition, insulin release and activity are markedly reduced below 30° C. Since target cells are insulin resistant, hyperglycemia is commonly seen initially. Markedly elevated glucose levels often correlate with hyperamylasemia and increased cortisol secretion.*

Acute hypothermia initially elevates serum glucose levels through catecholamine-induced glycogenolysis. However, chronic exposure following exhaustion and

*References 124, 208, 442, 576, 672, 692, 772.

glycogen depletion leads to hypoglycemia, and the symptoms often resemble those of hypothermia. Cold-induced renal glycosuria is common and does not imply normoglycemia or hyperglycemia. When hypoglycemia and central neuroglycopenia are present, correction improves the level of consciousness only to that expected for the current core temperature.[223] Cholesterol and triglyceride levels are also often below normal.[692]

Hyperglycemia that persists during and after rewarming should suggest diabetic ketoacidosis or hemorrhagic pancreatitis. Insulin is ineffective until core temperature is well above 30° C and therefore should be withheld to avoid iatrogenic hypoglycemia after rewarming. While prior renal disease should be a consideration, blood urea nitrogen (BUN) and creatinine concentrations are often elevated because of decreased nitrogenous waste clearance by the cold diuresis. Because of ongoing fluid shifts, BUN is a poor reflector of circulatory volume status.

The relationship between primary accidental hypothermia and hyperamylasemia is poorly defined. While it appears to correlate with the severity of temperature depression,[86,592] preexisting or hypothermia-induced pancreatitis is present in up to 50% of the patients in some urban series.[443] Since the abdominal examination is frequently unreliable, the amylase level should be measured except in minor cases.[708] Ischemic pancreatitis is attributable to a microcirculatory collapse in hypothermia.[215] Decreased pancreatic blood flow activates many proteolytic enzymes. The extent of hyperamylasemia can correlate with mortality rates.[772] Hypothermia in the presence of hypothalamic astrocytomas and pancreatitis has also been reported.[86,278]

Treatment

PREHOSPITAL MANAGEMENT

Cold and exhaustion in combination are a common cause of hypothermia in the field.[268] The tolerance of the individual who is exposed depends on the temperature, the wind, and the clothing worn and its wetness. Mental and physical exhaustion with related depleted energy stores is the great unknown in many hypothermia episodes. It does not take extremely cold temperatures to produce hypothermia following energy depletion. As mental function decreases, the victim is unable to respond to the rising threat. Judgment is insidiously impaired, and the victim is not likely to take the necessary precautions to prevent further disaster.[480]

The presentation of patients who are awake covers a wide spectrum. Some patients are obtunded but conscious. The British term for this is the "stumbling slobbers" because of the obvious incoordination. Patients may or may not be shivering and often have a distant gaze and slurred speech.

Comatose patients must be handled carefully because their hearts are extremely sensitive to ventricular fibrillation and standstill. Rough handling during evacuation and transport is a common cause of ventricular fibrillation (Fig. 3-6). Gurneys should be carried or rolled *slowly* to avoid jostling, and "code 3 full lights and sirens" transport should be avoided if patients are perfusing adequately.

Field treatment of hypothermia is the art of the possible.[57,79] The initial rescuer and first responder often encounter considerable obstacles to the prime directive, which is the prevention of further heat loss.[479] Since cold, stiff, cyanotic patients with fixed and dilated pupils have been "reanimated," the treatment dictum for prehospital personnel remains, "No one is dead until warm and dead."[22,176,259] Unless patients are cold and dead, prehospital estimates of the reversibility of illness or injury should remain conservative pending transport. A succinct summary of prehospital care of the hypothermic patient is the dictum to rescue, examine, insulate, and transport.[1,686]

In certain imposing geographic settings, treatment protocols are helpful. They help standardize treatment while tacitly acknowledging that the available health care facilities may offer limited expertise and equipment.[621] Aeromedical transport is often ideal in these circumstances.[782] In difficult environments proper protocols with rehearsal and critique of mass casualty plans in the cold are far more important than similar adjuncts in flat and consistently sunny terrain.

The history obtained at the scene helps determine optimal treatment. A chronic course of hypothermia in an elderly indoor victim presents resuscitation challenges far different from an acute exposure or immersion episode. The pertinent past medical history regarding prior cardiopulmonary, endocrinologic, or neurologic conditions is particularly helpful.[91] The circumstances of discovery, duration of exposure, associated injuries or frostbite, and obvious pre-

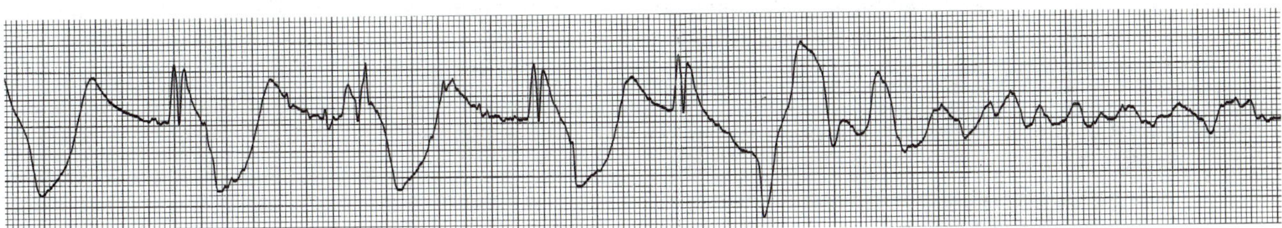

Fig. 3-6 In this patient ventricular fibrillation developed during a code 3 transport by emergency medical services to the emergency department. Note the pronounced J wave after the QRS complex.

disposing conditions should be recorded.[685] The Glasgow Coma Scale score, while not predictive, should be recorded. No prognostic neurologic scale during hypothermia has established validity, but trends are often useful.

Accurate field measurement of core temperature is generally impractical. Crude estimates based on the presence of shivering, level of consciousness, or behavior are often misleading. Electronic thermometers are generally unreliable, since they are calibrated for accuracy at room temperature. Indoors, truncal skin temperature may crudely suggest the severity of hypothermia. Low-reading glass oral thermometers that record down to 25° C give a rough estimate of the temperature in cooperative patients who are not tachypneic. These thermometers are often unreliable outdoors in cold ambient conditions.[596]

The failure to consider accidental hypothermia in the differential diagnosis can present unforeseen problems. For example, as discussed earlier, prehospital-initiated thrombolytic therapy is a growing feasibility. Current computer programs are unable to distinguish between myocardial injury and the pseudoinjury pattern that includes a J wave characteristic of hypothermia.[134] In rural and wilderness settings cellular transmission of computerized interpretations could result in unindicated thrombolytic therapy.

Prolonged field treatment should be avoided whenever possible, and the rescuer must attempt to prevent further heat loss (Box 3-4). The rescuer should consider and anticipate the presence of an irritable myocardium, hypovolemia, and a large temperature gradient between the periphery and the core.[481,482] Passive external rewarming with dry insulating materials minimizes conductive, convective, evaporative, and radiant heat losses.[189] Awake patients should have any wet clothing removed and should then be insulated with sleeping bags, insulated pads, bubble wrap, blankets, or even newspaper. If extrication will be delayed, it may be safe to give warm, sweet drinks, warm gelatin (Jello), Tang, juice, tea, or cocoa. Heavily caffeinated drinks should be avoided. Because a significant diuresis is usually associated with the cooling process, the victim's fluid balance must be assessed. Once mildly hypothermic patients are well hydrated, they can be walked out to safety.

Severely hypothermic patients should be handled gently and immobilized to prevent them from exerting themselves. Because of the autonomic dysfunction, patients should be kept in a horizontal position whenever possible to minimize orthostatic hypotension. Vigorously massaging cold extremities is also contraindicated, since skin rubbing, like ethanol, suppresses shivering thermogenesis and increases cutaneous vasodilation.

Field management of the comatose individual first involves ventilation to raise oxygen saturation. Mouth-to-mouth or mouth-to-nose rescue breathing is appropriate but may be difficult because of chest stiffness and the significant resistance to diaphragmatic motion. However, forced ventilation increases oxygenation, which helps to stabilize the heart electrically. Studies of hypothermic animals have shown that the single greatest factor in maintaining perfusion is oxygenation provided during severe hypothermia.

During storms prolonged field rewarming may be the only viable option until meteorologic conditions become more favorable for land or, preferably, aeromedical evacuation.[12,216] Hypothermia should be considered severe if a cold patient remains unresponsive following administration of 50% dextrose (25 g), naloxone (0.8 mg), and flumazenil (3 mg). Many prehospital medications freeze in solution. If this occurs, their pharmacologic activity after thawing is indeterminate.

An intravenous (IV) fluid challenge with 250 to 500 ml heated (37° to 41° C) 5% dextrose in normal saline solution should be given. If that is unavailable, any crystalloid infusion with dextrose can be used. Improvisation during transport is often helpful. For example, a plastic IV container can be placed under the patient's back, shoulders, or buttocks to add warmth and infusion pressure. Taping heat-producing packets to IV bags is another option. These heating agents come in the form of chemical packets or as phase change crystals, which produce heat for up to several hours. IV fluid compressors are bulb-inflating cuffs that surround IV pouches to maintain flow. The Israeli army has a spring steel

BOX 3-4

PREPARING HYPOTHERMIC PATIENTS FOR TRANSPORT

1. The patient must be dry. Gently remove or cut off wet clothing and replace it with dry clothing or a dry insulation system. Keep the patient horizontal, and do not allow exertion or massage of the extremities.
2. Stabilize injuries (i.e., the spine; place fractures in the correct anatomic position). Open wounds should be covered before packaging.
3. Initiate intravenous infusions (IVs) if feasible; bags can be placed under the patient's buttocks or in a compressor system. Administer a fluid challenge.
4. Active rewarming should be limited to heated inhalation and truncal heat. Insulate hot water bottles in stockings or mittens and then place them in the patient's axillae and groin.
5. The patient should be wrapped. The wrap starts with a large plastic sheet, on which is placed an insulated sleeping pad. A layer of blankets, a sleeping bag, or bubble wrap insulating material is laid over the sleeping bag; the patient is placed on the insulation; the heating bottles are put in place along with IVs, and the entire package is wrapped layer over layer. The plastic is the final closure. The face should be partially covered, but a tunnel should be created to allow access for breathing and monitoring of the patient.

compressor system for IV bags, but this is not yet commercially available.

Peripheral vessels may be difficult to locate, and IV lines are difficult to maintain during transport. Ideally, IV fluids should be warmed to body temperature or slightly higher, but total body warming is not accomplished with IV fluids in the field. The use of intraosseous infusions during hypothermia has not been reported, but this route may provide a reasonable pathway for fluid replacement in the field when peripheral vessels have collapsed and cannot be entered.

The methods selected to stabilize core temperature should be tailored to the severity of the hypothermia and the field circumstances.[240] Gently removing or cutting off wet clothing while the patient remains prone may be the best option to limit heat loss and prevent orthostasis. Passive external rewarming with waterproof insulation suffices for mild chronic hypothermia.[324]

"Field rewarming" is a misnomer, since adding much heat to a hypothermic patient in the field is extremely difficult.[190] Warmed IV solutions, heated sarongs, or heated humidified oxygen can provide only a small amount of heat input. Hot water bottles or heat packs can be placed in the axillae, in the groin, and around the neck. Casualty evacuation bags are available in many models and designs. Some have more insulation than others, and some have specialized zippers and openings that allow access to the patient during transport. Most bags are windproof and waterproof.

Based on rewarming experiments, Harnett and associates[274] contend that inhalation therapy is a safe technique for active rewarming of patients with profound hypothermia in the field. It helps to prevent respiratory heat loss, which represents an important percentage of heat production when the core temperature is below 32° C. Respiratory heat losses vary with humidity, ambient atmospheric temperature, and respiratory minute volume (RMV).[423] In another study the technical difficulties experienced while using inhalation rewarming devices in volunteers suggest the importance of proper instruction of the rescuer.[689]

Lloyd first recommended inhalation rewarming in 1971. His initial field device used a carbon dioxide and soda lime reaction to generate heat and moisture.[422,423] The original closed-circuit prototype with oxygen tank weighed 8 kg. The current version weighs 3 kg including the oxygen tank.[416] This unit consists of an oxygen cylinder, a demand valve, a 2 L reservoir bag, soda lime, and a pediatric water canister. An in-line thermometer measures the mean air temperature at the face mask. In the field, heat and moisture exchangers are practical, light, and inexpensive. However, they are less efficient than active humidifiers.[420]

The Douwens and Hayward Res-Q-Air (CF Electronics, Inc., Commack, N.Y.) is a lightweight, portable first aid device that delivers heated humidified air or oxygen at temperatures ranging from 42° to 44° C down to ambient conditions of −20° C. This system consists of a heating chamber connected via a corrugated hose to a one-way flow valve and an oronasal mask. The temperature is controlled by a transducer in the one-way flow valve that provides feedback to the electronic control circuits. Supplemental oxygen and bag adaptation are possible.

Although surface rewarming suppresses shivering, it may be the only option when the victim is isolated from medical care. Active external rewarming options include radiant heat, warmed objects placed on the patient, and body-to-body contact. Care must be exercised not to burn patients with hot objects, including commercially produced "hot packs." In experimental studies core temperature afterdrop was recorded with isolated upper truncal contact,[274,276] implying that total body contact rewarming may be hazardous. A hydraulic sarong or vest, in which heated water is circulated via hand pump, has been used in the past.[18] Although a dip in a hot spring would be nice for all parties concerned, immersion rewarming is dangerous in the field because monitoring and resuscitation capabilities are limited.

The Norwegian Personal Heater Heat Pac is a useful device for field transport of hypothermic patients. This device uses a single "D" battery and burns 30 hours on a single charcoal block. It is durable, lightweight (1 kg), efficient, and effective. It circulates hot air within a blanket or sleeping bag and provides a comfortable, warm and dry environment for transporting patients. It has gained the acceptance of most armies operating in northern climates, including those of Norway, Sweden, Finland, Canada, and the United States.

Prehospital life support for hypothermia differs from that for normothermia in many regards (Fig. 3-7). A patent airway and the presence of respirations must be established. The patient may appear apneic if the respiratory minute ventilation is significantly depressed. A common error is overzealous assistance of ventilation, which can induce hypocapnic ventricular irritability. The indications for prehospital endotracheal intubation are identical to those under normothermic conditions. Appropriate ventilation with 100% oxygen may protect the heart during the inevitable jostling of extrication and transport. Overinflation of the tracheal cuff with frigid ambient air should be avoided. As the patient warms, the air in the cuff can expand and kink the tube. Careful protection and fixation of the tubing of the cuff port during extremely cold conditions are necessary to prevent breakage and a cuff leak.[127]

Palpation of peripheral pulses is often difficult in vasoconstricted and bradycardic patients. An apparent cardiovascular collapse may actually reflect a depressed cardiac output that is nonetheless sufficient to meet minimal metabolic demands. Palpation and auscultation for at least 1 minute to establish spontaneous pulses would be wise. Iatrogenic ventricular fibrillation can easily result from unindicated chest compressions.

If a cardiac monitor is available and documents ventricular fibrillation or apparent asystole after maximal amplification of the QRS complex, the rescuer should defibrillate

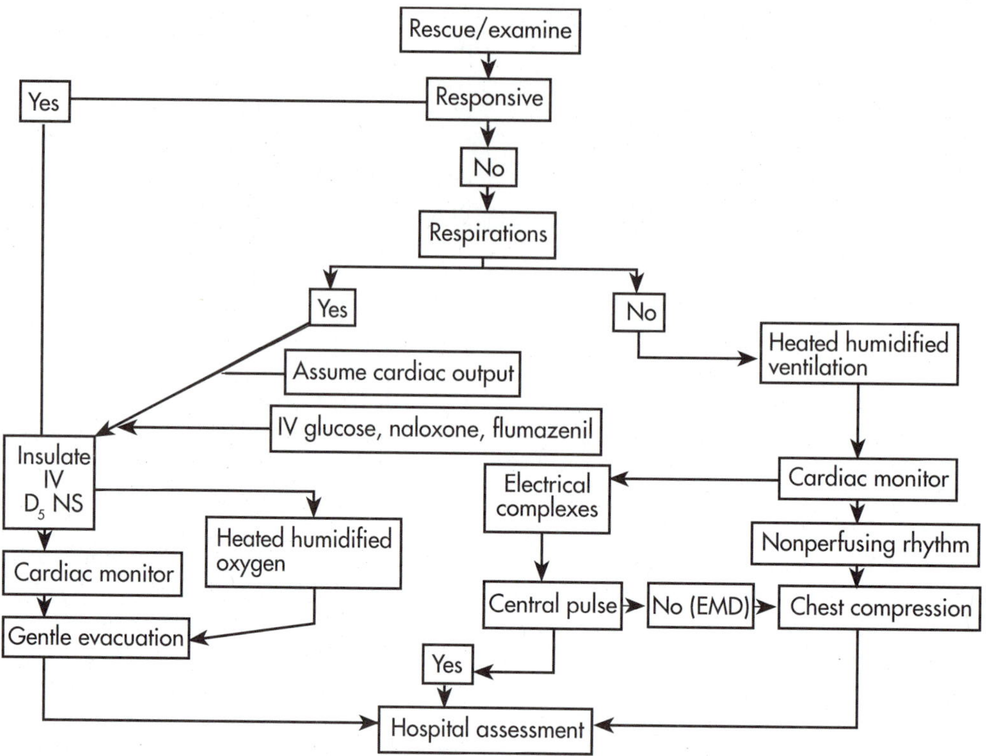

Fig. 3-7 Prehospital life support.

once with 2 watt sec/kg up to 200 watt sec.[465,710] Most monitors and defibrillators have not been tested for operation at temperatures below 15.5° C. Standard monitor leads do not always stick well to cold skin, so benzoin may be useful. If this fails, needle electrodes may be necessary. One author suggests puncturing the gel foam conventional monitor pad with a small-gauge injection needle.[762] Defibrillation should not be performed if electrical complexes are seen on the monitor. Unresponsive patients must be carefully assessed for a central pulse before they can be assumed to have electromechanical dissociation. The lowest temperature at which mechanical reestablishment of cardiac activity has been successful is 20° C,[141] and defibrillation attempts rarely succeed below 30° C.[425] If resuscitation in the field is unsuccessful, rewarming and cardiopulmonary resuscitation (CPR) should be continued during transport to the emergency department.

MANAGEMENT IN THE EMERGENCY DEPARTMENT

The history obtained from a hypothermic patient should be considered unreliable.[410] It is prudent to confirm hypothermia and monitor with continuous core temperature measurements. Diagnostic errors in the emergency department most commonly result from incomplete monitoring of the vital signs. Doppler ultrasound may be necessary to locate a pulse and should be supported by continuous ECG monitoring. The physician should address the requirements for resuscitation and initiate advanced life support when necessary (Box 3-5).

Some hospitals lack adequate equipment for accurate core temperature measurement.[655] Rectal measurements are most practical clinically but may not reflect cardiac or brain

BOX 3-5
RESUSCITATION REQUIREMENTS

Thermal stabilization
- Conduction
- Convection
- Radiation
- Evaporation
- Respiration

Maintenance of tissue oxygenation
- Adequate circulation
- Adequate ventilation

Identification of primary versus secondary hypothermia

Rewarming options
- Passive external rewarming
- Active external rewarming
- Active core rewarming

temperatures.[178] An indwelling thermistor probe placed to a depth of 15 cm is reliable unless adjacent to cold feces. Rectal temperature lags behind core temperature fluctuations and is also affected by lower extremity temperatures.[178,757,776]

Simultaneous esophageal temperature measurements may be helpful when airway protection is provided with endotracheal intubation. Since the upper third of the esophagus is near the trachea, probe reliability is often poor during heated inhalation therapy.[774-776] The correct selection, accuracy, and use of devices that measure urine temperature are debated.[179,219,354] Urine temperature has been of mixed value in screening for hypothermia in elderly patients.[408] Since intravascular hypothermia may cause arrhythmias in hypovolemic patients, monitoring of tympanic or bladder temperatures has also been suggested.[513]

Tympanic temperature closely approximates hypothalamic temperature.[757,781] Tympanic temperature can be accurately measured with thermometers designed to make contact with the tympanic membrane.[65] Since these are impractical except in anesthetized patients, external auditory canal thermometers that measure the infrared emission from the tympanic membrane were developed. These are not actually "tympanic" thermometers; however, most authors refer to them as tympanic thermometers.

Temperatures measured with external auditory canal thermometers were initially reported to correlate well with rectal and core temperatures.[255,659,720] However, investigators have found these thermometers to be poorly sensitive for fever when used in clinical settings.[353,792] No clinical studies of tympanic thermometers' ability to detect hypothermia have been reported.[499] Use of tympanic thermometers alone in patients with suspected hypothermia should await further study.

After temperature measurement, all clothing should be gently removed or cut off with minimal patient manipulation and the patient should be immediately insulated with dry blankets. A cardiac monitor is applied, and intravenous catheters are inserted as needed. Arterial catheter insertion has helped in the management of a few profoundly hypothermic patients. Pulmonary artery catheters have precipitated cardiac arrhythmias and should be reserved for complex cases.[490,491,550] Insertion of pulmonary artery catheters into cold vessels may lead to perforation of the pulmonary artery.[112] Central venous catheters should not be inserted into the right atrium, since this could precipitate arrhythmias.[658]

The accuracy of pulse oximetry during conditions of poor perfusion is unclear. In one study of hypothermic patients on cardiopulmonary bypass, the finger probes were inaccurate.[103] In another study the probes were fairly reliable if a vasodilating cream was applied first.[551] The value of end-tidal carbon dioxide measurements to assess adequacy of tissue perfusion and tracheal tube placement has been established at normal temperatures. However, most of these devices measure the carbon dioxide content only of dehumidified air and thus cannot be used during airway rewarming.

Laboratory evaluations to be considered, except in some cases of mild hypothermia, include blood sugar, arterial blood gases, complete blood cell count, electrolytes, BUN, creatinine, serum calcium, serum magnesium, serum amylase, prothrombin and partial thromboplastin times, platelet count, and fibrinogen level. A toxicologic screen should be considered if the level of consciousness does not correlate with the degree of hypothermia. Selective studies of thyroid function, cardiac isoenzyme levels, and serum cortisol levels are indicated.

Radiologic evaluation of poorly responsive patients must include cervical and other spine films to detect occult trauma. Chest radiographs may predict collapse during rewarming when cardiomegaly and redistribution of vascularity are already present. Abdominal films should be obtained when the physical examination is unreliable. Bowel sounds are usually diminished or absent in severe hypothermia, and rectus muscle rigidity is frequently present. Pneumoperitoneum, pancreatic calcifications, or hemoperitoneum may be noted. Small bowel dilation is associated with cold-induced mesenteric vascular occlusion, and colonic dilation is often present in conjunction with myxedema coma.

Nasogastric tube insertion should follow endotracheal intubation in moderate or severe hypothermia, since gastric dilation and poor gastrointestinal motility are common. Indwelling bladder catheters with urine meters are needed to monitor urine output and the cold diuresis.[286]

Fluid Resuscitation

Most fluid shifts are reversed by rewarming, and mild hypothermia usually requires only an IV lifeline. Although use of intraosseous infusions in hypothermia has not been studied, they may prove useful, particularly when vascular access is difficult as in children and vasoconstricted dehydrated patients. In more severe cases, volume shifts and elevated blood viscosity from hemoconcentration, lowered temperature, increased vascular permeability, and low flow state mandate aggressive fluid resuscitation.[269,522] The viscosity of blood increases 2% per °C drop in temperature; therefore hematocrit values over 50% are commonly seen. Low circulatory plasma volume is often coupled with elevated total plasma volume during rewarming.[276] Hemodilution is usually not a problem, and is seen only during massive crystalloid resuscitation of actively hemorrhaging patients.

The clinician should assume that patients will be significantly dehydrated, with free water depletion elevating the serum sodium concentration and osmolality. During the descent into a hypothermic state the normal physiologic cues for thirst become inactive and access to water is often difficult. Since hypothermia results in natriuresis, saline depletion may be present. Further causes of sodium losses include prior diuretic therapy and gastrointestinal losses. Preexisting total body sodium excess is seen with congestive heart failure, cirrhosis, and nephrosis. In these cases serum sodium and osmolality values are often normal. Rarely, serum sodium levels are low because of free water excess. Other causes include myxedema, panhypopituitarism, and inappropriate antidiuretic hormone secretion.[136,667]

Most patients with core temperature below 32.2° C should receive an initial fluid challenge with 250 to 500 ml of 5% dextrose in warmed normal saline solution. Theoretically, Ringer's lactate solution should be avoided, since a cold liver cannot metabolize lactate. Any potential advantages of colloids over crystalloids remain uncertain. In one experiment, normal saline solution had minimal lasting effects and did not hasten cardiovascular recovery from hypothermia.[605] In another, 10% low–molecular weight dextran solution increased plasma volume and decreased blood sludging.[163] A possibility is administering colloids to patients who are not responding to crystalloids.

It is important to monitor for the standard clinical signs of fluid overload, including rales, jugular venous distention, hepatojugular reflux, and S_3 cardiac gallop. Persistent cardiovascular instability often reflects *inadequate* intravascular volume.[195,273] In these cases properly placed central venous pressure catheters that do not irritate the right atrium have a role. Pulmonary wedge pressure measurements should generally be deferred until after rewarming.[181] The need for red blood cell transfusions is determined by the corrected hematocrit; blood dilution with warmed infusate does not cause significant hemolysis.[225]

In many cases rapid volume expansion is critical.[26,133] The circulatory volume is decreased, and peripheral vascular resistance is increased.[273] In neonates adequate fluid resuscitation markedly decreases mortality.[711] Adults receiving hemodynamic and pulmonary wedge pressure monitoring have shown improvement of cardiovascular efficiency during crystalloid administration.[273] Ventricular fibrillation that occurs immediately after rescue has been attributed not only to core temperature afterdrop, but also to vascular imbalance in patients who are moved from a horizontal supine position.[421] The fluxing relationship between the active vascular capacity and circulating fluid volume depends not only on the mechanism of cooling, but also on the method of rewarming.

The safety and efficacy of pneumatic antishock garments in hypothermia are unknown.[369] Their application presents several theoretic circulatory and limb hazards. Since the vasculature is already maximally vasoconstricted, provision of more peripheral vascular resistance by the garment should not be significant. Hypothermic patients, particularly those with frostbite, are at high risk for extremity compartment syndromes and rhabdomyolysis. Pneumatic trousers should be considered only for the temporary stabilization of coexistent exsanguinating major pelvic fractures.

Rewarming Options

PASSIVE EXTERNAL REWARMING

Since no controlled studies exist, rigid treatment protocols should not be suggested.[100,797] A versatile approach to rewarming can be developed after careful consideration of the results from animal experiments, human experiments on mild hypothermia, and various clinical reports (Box 3-6).[126,622,652,719]

The initial key treatment decision is whether to use active or passive rewarming (Box 3-7). Noninvasive passive external rewarming (PER) is ideal for the majority of previously healthy patients with mild hypothermia. The patient is covered with dry insulating materials in a warm environment to minimize the normal mechanisms of heat loss. When the wind is blocked, less heat escapes via radiation, convection, and conduction. Conditions with higher ambient humidities slightly limit respiratory heat loss.

Aluminized body covers significantly reduce heat loss.[191,298] Endogenous thermogenesis must generate an acceptable rate of rewarming for PER to be effective.[511,515] Humans are poikilothermic below 30° C, and metabolic heat production is less than 50% of normal below 28° C.[50] Shivering thermogenesis is also extinguished below 32° C. This thermoregulatory neuromuscular response to cold normally increases heat production from 250 to 1000 kcal/hr unless glycogen is depleted during cooling.[573]

BOX 3-6

REWARMING TECHNIQUES

PASSIVE EXTERNAL

Thermal stabilization
Insulation

ACTIVE

External
- Radiant heat
- Hot water bottles
- Plumbed garments
- Electric heating pads and blankets
- Forced circulated hot air
- Immersion in warm water

Core
- Inhalation rewarming
- Heated infusions
- Gastric and colonic lavage
- Mediastinal lavage
- Thoracic lavage
- Peritoneal lavage
- Extracorporeal blood rewarming
- Diathermy

Elderly patients in whom mild hypothermia develops gradually are acceptable candidates for PER. Peripheral vasoconstriction is maintained, which minimizes the circulatory component of core temperature afterdrop. When rewarming times are markedly prolonged (over 12 hours), complications increase.

The previous recommendations for rewarming rates with PER varied between 0.5° C and 2° C/hr.[128,131,135,441] Patients who are centrally hypovolemic, glycogen depleted, and without normal cardiovascular responses should be stabilized and rewarmed at a conservative rate.[117,177] However, in a recent multicenter survey the first (0.75° C ± 1.16), second (1.17° C ± 1.17), and third (1.26° C ± 1.28) hour rewarming rates for the elderly far exceeded 0.5° C per hour with no increase in mortality rate (Fig. 3-8).[135]

ACTIVE REWARMING

Active rewarming, which is the direct transfer of exogenous heat to a patient, is usually required with temperatures below 32° C. Rapid identification of any impediments to normal thermoregulation, such as cardiovascular instability or endocrinologic insufficiency, is essential.[201,397,417,477] Intrinsic thermogenesis may also be insufficient following traumatic spinal cord transection or pharmacologically induced peripheral vasodilation.[20] Some patient populations generally require active rewarming. For example, aggressive rewarming of infants minimizes energy expenditure and decreases mortality. In these circumstances vigorous monitoring for respiratory, hematologic, metabolic, and infectious complications is essential.[343,581,682,714,798]

Active External Rewarming

When active rewarming is needed, heat can be delivered externally or to the core. Active external rewarming (AER) techniques deliver heat directly to the skin.[203,471] Plumbed garments, hot water bottles, heating pads and blankets, and radiant heat sources have been used.[363,475,627] Forced air warming systems also efficiently transfer heat.[318,509] The Bair Hugger uses hot forced air circulated through a blanket.[399] In one study that rewarmed accidental hypothermia victims in the emergency department, rewarming shock and core temperature afterdrop were not noted.[795] Thermal injury to poorly perfused, vasoconstricted skin using some of the external heat application techniques is a hazard in both adults and children.[109,122,196]

Immersion in a 40° C circulating bath is another option. Monitoring, resuscitation, treatment of injuries, and maintenance of extremity vasoconstriction to prevent core temperature afterdrop are difficult. "Bobbing" CPR is impossible in the tub. In normothermic men with coronary artery disease the cardiovascular stress and arrhythmogenic response to immersion in a hot tub are mild and less than those induced by exercise.[6] In contrast, placing the hands and feet in warm water could theoretically open arteriovenous shunts and accelerate rewarming in acute hypothermia. The attraction to Scandinavian palmar heat packs may reflect this physiology.[642]

Initial concern with AER was expressed by Duguid, Simpson, and Stowers[168] in 1961, after 20 out of 23 of their patients died.[168] Retrospective analysis of numerous clinical series noted a disproportionately high mortality rate with AER.[258] In a small subset of one study the mortality rate was 64.3%.[477] Interpretation of the survival rates with AER is affected by various risk factors and patient selection criteria. In some reports "active" is an artificial description, since rewarming required more than 24 hours.[203] One author reported a 100% success rate with immersion rewarming.[222] DeRoubaix[153] successfully reanimated a 13-year-old boy in cardiopulmonary arrest at 25° C in a hut, turning him by the glow of a fire in a manner "similar to spit roasting."

Experimental and clinical reports have linked AER with peripheral vasodilation, hypotension, and core temperature afterdrop. In one canine model, three groups were treated with partial cardiac bypass, peritoneal dialysis, and AER with a circulating blanket.[495] The externally rewarmed group required more bicarbonate than did the other two groups, as well as two to three times the crystalloid volume to maintain cardiac filling pressures. Sudden periodic acidotic shifts in arterial pH were seen even when the temperature exceeded 30° C. These pH fluctuations were accompanied by a sudden conversion from sinus rhythm to ventricular fibrillation in some animals.

While previously healthy, young, acutely hypothermic victims are usually safe candidates for AER, it offers no major advantage.[130,245,246] Heat application that is confined to the thorax may mitigate many of the physiologic concerns pertaining to the depressed cardiovascular and metabolic systems, which are unable to meet accelerated peripheral demands.[274,275] Combining truncal AER with active core rewarming may further avert many potential side effects.[395,730]

BOX 3-7

INDICATIONS FOR ACTIVE REWARMING

Cardiovascular instability
Moderate or severe hypothermia (<32.2° C) (poikilothermia)
Inadequate rate or failure to rewarm
Endocrinologic insufficiency
Traumatic or toxicologic peripheral vasodilation
Secondary hypothermia impairing thermoregulation
Identification of predisposing factors (see Box 3-2)

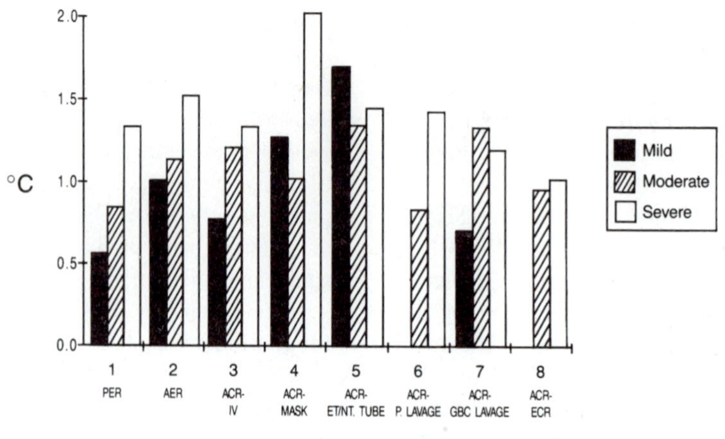

Fig. 3-8 First hour rewarming rates from a large multicenter survey. *PER,* Passive external rewarming; *AER,* active external rewarming; *ACR,* active core rewarming; *IV,* intravenous; *ET,* endotracheal tube; *NT,* nasotracheal tube; *P,* peritoneal lavage; *GBC,* gastric-bladder-colon lavage. (Data from Chang M, Gill T: *South Med J* 74:1509, 1981.)

Active Core Rewarming

A variety of techniques can effectively deliver heat to the core. Options include heated inhalation, IV fluids, gastrointestinal irrigation, peritoneal dialysis, extracorporeal rewarming, and diathermy. Average first hour rewarming rates reported with these techniques in one multicenter study are listed in Fig. 3-8.

Airway Rewarming. Heated, humidified oxygen inhalation has been studied extensively for both prehospital and emergency department rewarming.[420,610] The effectiveness of the respiratory tract as a heat exchanger varies with the technique and ambient conditions.[489,766] Since dry air has low thermal conductivity, complete humidification coupled with an inhalant temperature of 40° to 45° C is required. The main benefit of airway rewarming is the prevention of respiratory heat loss. Heat yield can represent 10% to 30% of the hypothermic patient's heat production when the respiratory minute volume is adequate.[263,283,586]

Rate of rewarming is greater through an endotracheal tube (ETT) than by mask.[477,478] In one series the reported rewarming rate with 40° C aerosol was 0.74° C per hour via mask and 1.22° C per hour via ETT.[477] In the multicenter survey the average first and second hour rewarming rates in severe cases were 1.5° to 2° C/hr. As expected because of the decremental efficiency at higher temperatures, the rate was slower in mild cases.[135]

The functional significance of a thermal countercurrent exchange in the cerebrovascular bed of humans continues to be explored.[148] This would affect the efficiency and influence of heated mask ventilation during hypothermia. Known as the rete mirabile, this system could preferentially rewarm the brainstem. Heated inhalation via face mask continuous positive airway pressure (CPAP) has been successfully used and offers a beneficial correction of the ventilation-perfusion mismatch.[87] Heated humidified oxygen via face mask may not be feasible in some patients with coexistent midfacial trauma.

The quantity of heat liberated during airway rewarming is produced mainly from the condensation of water vapor. The latent heat of vaporization of water in the lung is slightly lower than 540 kcal/g H_2O. This is multiplied by the liters per minute ventilation to calculate the quantity of heat transfer. When core temperature is 28° C, the rate of rewarming with heated ventilation at 42° C equals endogenous heat production.[504]

Heated humidified inhalation ensures adequate oxygenation, stimulates pulmonary cilia, and reduces the amount and viscosity of cold-induced bronchorrhea.[409,492,493] Although preexisting premature ventricular contractions (PVCs) may reappear during rewarming, there is no evidence that inhalation rewarming precipitates new, clinically significant ventricular arrhythmias.[135,138,139] Vapor absorption does not increase pulmonary congestion or wash out surfactant.[732] When the pulmonary vasculature is heated, warmed oxygenated blood that returns to the myocardium could attenuate intermittent temperature gradients.[37,493,494] The amplitude of shivering is also lowered, which is an advantage in more severe cases. In theory, this suppression could decrease heat production in mild hypothermia, although experimentally the core temperature continues to rise.[125,493]

There are numerous oxygenation considerations in hypothermia (Box 3-1).[38,358,493,786] The "functional" value of hemoglobin has been calculated at 28° C to be 4.2 g/10 g in patients on cardiopulmonary bypass.[207] The oxyhemoglobin dissociation curve also shifts to the left (Fig. 3-4). This impairs the release of oxygen from hemoglobin into the tissues. However, in canine experiments no evidence was found that this left shift impairs oxygen extraction by tissues during hypothermic conditions.[264]

Although some patients can self-adjust their RMV for current carbon dioxide production, this may not be the case in the presence of additional toxicologic or metabolic depressants.[646-648] A cascade nebulizer with an immersion heater is adequate equipment for patients with spontaneous respirations. Ideally, the inhalation hose has a surrounding warming wire. An in-line disposable temperature monitor is necessary.[670]

Without modification, many commercially available heated nebulizers do not allow the temperature to reach the desired 40° to 45° C. All modified equipment should be labeled to avoid routine use.[649] A volume ventilator with a heated cascade humidifier can also deliver CPAP or positive end-expiratory pressure (PEEP) if needed during rewarming. The airway rewarming rates clinically range from 1° to 2.5° C/hr.[135,477]

Heat and moisture exchangers function like artificial nares by trapping exhaled moisture and then returning it. They provide inadequate humidification for the treatment of accidental hypothermia. With prolonged use, endotracheal tube occlusion and atelectasis are both problems.[108,111,244] In the field, heat and moisture exchangers are practical, light, and cheap, although they are less efficient than active humidifiers.[420,424]

Airway rewarming is indicated in the field when equipment is available, and in virtually all cases when the core temperature is <32.2° C on arrival at the emergency department. Although airway rewarming provides less heat than some other forms of active core warming, it prevents normal respiratory heat and moisture loss. It is a safe, fairly noninvasive, practical technique in all settings.

Heated Infusions. Cold fluid resuscitation of hypovolemic patients can induce hypothermia.[383,651] In one series of previously normothermic patients with major abdominal vascular trauma the average postresuscitation temperature was 31.2° C in those with refractory coagulopathies.[344] IV fluids should be heated to 40° to 42° C, although some authors suggest that higher temperatures may be safe.[81] The amount of heat provided by solutions begins to become significant during massive volume resuscitations.[211] One liter of fluid at 42° C provides 14 kcal to a 70 kg patient at 28° C, elevating the core temperature almost ⅓° C.[504]

Microwave heating of IV fluids in flexible plastic bags is one widely available option.[5,15,637,765] The plasticizer in the polyvinyl chloride containers is stable to microwave heating. Thermal packs, jackets, or insulation on IV bags helps preserve heat.[56] Long lengths of IV tubing increase heat loss, especially at slow flow rates.[194] Heating times should be determined for each individual microwave oven and should average 2 minutes at high power for a 1 L bag of crystalloid. The fluid should be thoroughly mixed before administration, since "hot spots" are common in ovens. Fresh frozen plasma can also be thawed in under 5 minutes.

Blood preheated to 38° C in a standard warmer is useful, but clotting and shortened red blood cell life are hazards with blood warming packs.[49] Local microwave overheating hemolyzes blood. An alternative is to dilute packed red blood cells with warm calcium-free crystalloid.[394] The Level 1 Fluid Warmer (Life Systems, Inc., Southfield, Mich.) warms cold crystalloid and blood from 10° C to 35° C via a heat exchanger at flow rates of up to 500 ml/min.[71]

Rapid administration of fluid into the right atrium at a temperature significantly different from that of circulating blood may produce myocardial thermal gradients.[248,658,791] However, in one study heated IV fluid, up to 550 ml/min, was administered through the internal jugular vein without complication.[658]

We are investigating the use of amino acid infusions to accelerate energy metabolism. It has been observed that fever is common in patients receiving hyperalimentation. However, in patients recovering from elective surgery, amino acids have had no significant thermogenic effect.[292] We hope the results will differ in energy-depleted patients with chronically induced accidental hypothermia.

In summary, intravenous solutions and blood should routinely be heated during hypothermia resuscitations. Many varieties of blood warmers are available commercially, but in-line warmers are inadequate for rapid transfusions. Countercurrent in-line warmers and rapid warm saline admixture are the most efficient techniques.[316]

Heated Irrigation

Gastrointestinal irrigation. Heat transfer from irrigation fluids is usually limited by the available surface area, and therefore irrigation should not be used as the sole rewarming technique. Direct gastrointestinal irrigation is less desirable than irrigation via intragastric or intracolonic balloons because of the induced fluid and electrolyte fluxes. To avoid this, a double-lumen esophageal tube has been investigated, as have other modified Sengstaken tubes.[374,375] Patients should be tracheally intubated before gastric lavage. Because of the proximity of an irritable heart, overly vigorous placement of a large gastric tube seems ill advised. In the multicenter survey, gastric, bladder, and colon lavage rewarmed severely hypothermic patients at 1° to 1.5° C for the first hour and 1.5° to 2° C for the second hour.[135]

Commercially available kits designed for gastric decontamination are convenient (Fig. 3-9). The use of a Y connector and clamp simplifies the exchanges. The ideal dwell times for thermal exchange depend on the flow rates and may average several minutes. In direct gastric lavage, warmed electrolyte solutions such as normal saline or Ringer's lactate are administered via nasogastric tube.[402] After 15 minutes the solution is aspirated and replaced with warm fluids. Disadvantages include the small surface area

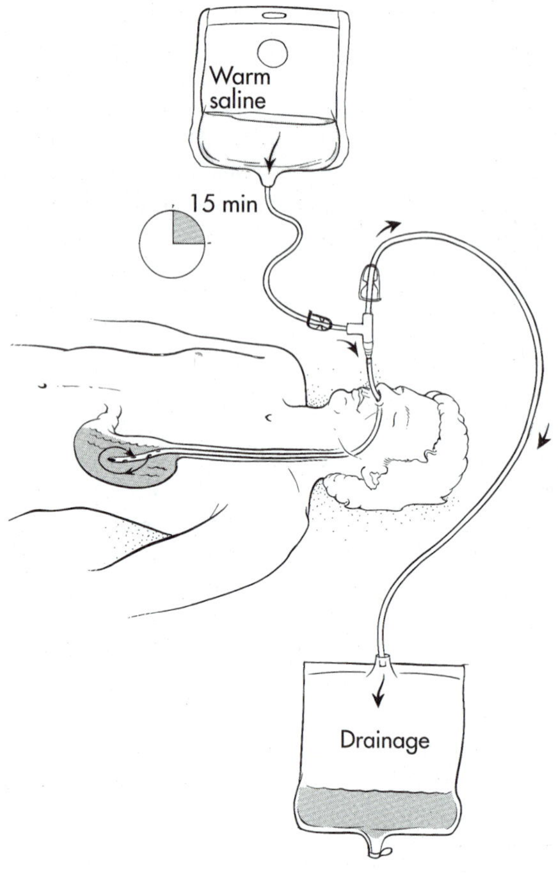

Fig. 3-9 Gastric lavage.

available for heat exchange and the large amount of fluid escaping into the duodenum.[74] Regurgitation is common, and the technique must be terminated during CPR. While some continue to support the concept of esophageal heat exchange, clinical success is limited.[762] In a well-designed study, esophageal heat exchange was ineffective in preventing perioperative hypothermia.[381]

Exceeding 200 to 300 ml aliquots may force fluid into the duodenum; therefore frequent fluid removal via gravity drainage minimizes "lost" fluid. A log of input and output is essential. This facilitates estimation of fluid balance during resuscitation and helps determine if irrigation should be abandoned in anticipation of dilutional electrolyte disturbances.

Bladder irrigation should also be limited to around 200 to 300 ml aliquots to prevent bladder distention. A number of esthetic obstacles must be overcome to maintain successful colonic irrigation.

Mediastinal irrigation. Mediastinal irrigation and direct myocardial lavage are alternatives in patients lacking spontaneous perfusion.[68,120,213] A standard left thoracotomy is performed while CPR is continued. Opening the pericardium is unnecessary unless an effusion or tamponade is present. The physician bathes the heart for several minutes in 1 to 2 L of an isotonic electrolyte solution heated to 40° C. This is followed by suctioning and replacement of warm fluids.[73]

The physician may attempt internal defibrillation at 1° to 2° C intervals after the myocardial temperature reaches 26° to 28° C. Unless a perfusing rhythm is achieved, lavage is continued until myocardial temperature exceeds 32° to 33° C. As suggested by O'Keeffe,[534] the standard postthoracotomy tube in the left side of the chest could provide an avenue for continued rewarming via thoracic irrigation.

A median sternotomy also allows ventricular decompression and direct defibrillation.[401] One potential disadvantage of both of these techniques is that open cardiac massage of a cold, rigid contracted heart may not generate flow.[7,132] Unless immediate cardiopulmonary bypass is an option, mediastinal irrigation and direct myocardial lavage are indicated only if cardiac arrest has occurred. In these circumstances personnel skilled in the technique should also initiate all other available rewarming modalities.

Closed thoracic lavage. Irrigation of the hemithoraces offers great promise as a rewarming adjunct.[30,74,75,547,754] Two large-bore thoracostomy tubes (36 to 40 Fr in adults; 14 to 24 Fr, ages 1 to 3; 20 to 32 Fr, ages 4 to 7) are inserted in one or both of the hemithoraces. One is placed anteriorly in the second to third intercostal space at the midclavicular line, and the other in the posterior axillary line at the fifth to sixth intercostal space. Normal saline heated to 40° to 42° C is then infused via a nonrecycled sterile system (Fig. 3-10, *A*). Hypothermic coagulopathies in extreme situations might necessitate the use of cautery at the incision sites.

A high-flow countercurrent fluid infuser (Level 1 Fluid Warmer)[72,496] heats (40° C) and delivers 1 L or preferably 3 L bags of normal saline into the afferent chest tube.[668] We prefer connecting into the Level 1 tubing with standard 3⁄16-inch-internal-diameter suction connection tubing and a sterilized plastic graduated two-way connector, since this facilitates adaptation to any size chest tube (Fig. 3-10, *A*). The effluent is then collected in a thoracostomy drainage set. The reservoir must be emptied frequently. Alternatively, when a single chest tube is used, 200 to 300 ml aliquots are used for irrigation and suctioning is through a Y connector. The Y connector is also useful for irrigating both hemithoraces with a single fluid warmer (Fig. 3-10, *B*).

Clinical experience with closed thoracic lavage is extremely limited. In some cases fluid has been infused into the anterior higher chest tube (afferent limb) and suctioned or gravity drained out the lower posterior tube (efferent limb) into a water seal chest drain.[266,267] Infusion inferoposteriorly with suction anteriorly can increase dwell times.[317] The efficiency of thermal transfer varies with flow rates and dwell times. If the patient has been successfully rewarmed, the upper tube should be removed and the lower one left in place to allow residual drainage.

Closed sterile thoracic lavage seems a natural choice in the emergency department during cardiac arrest resuscita-

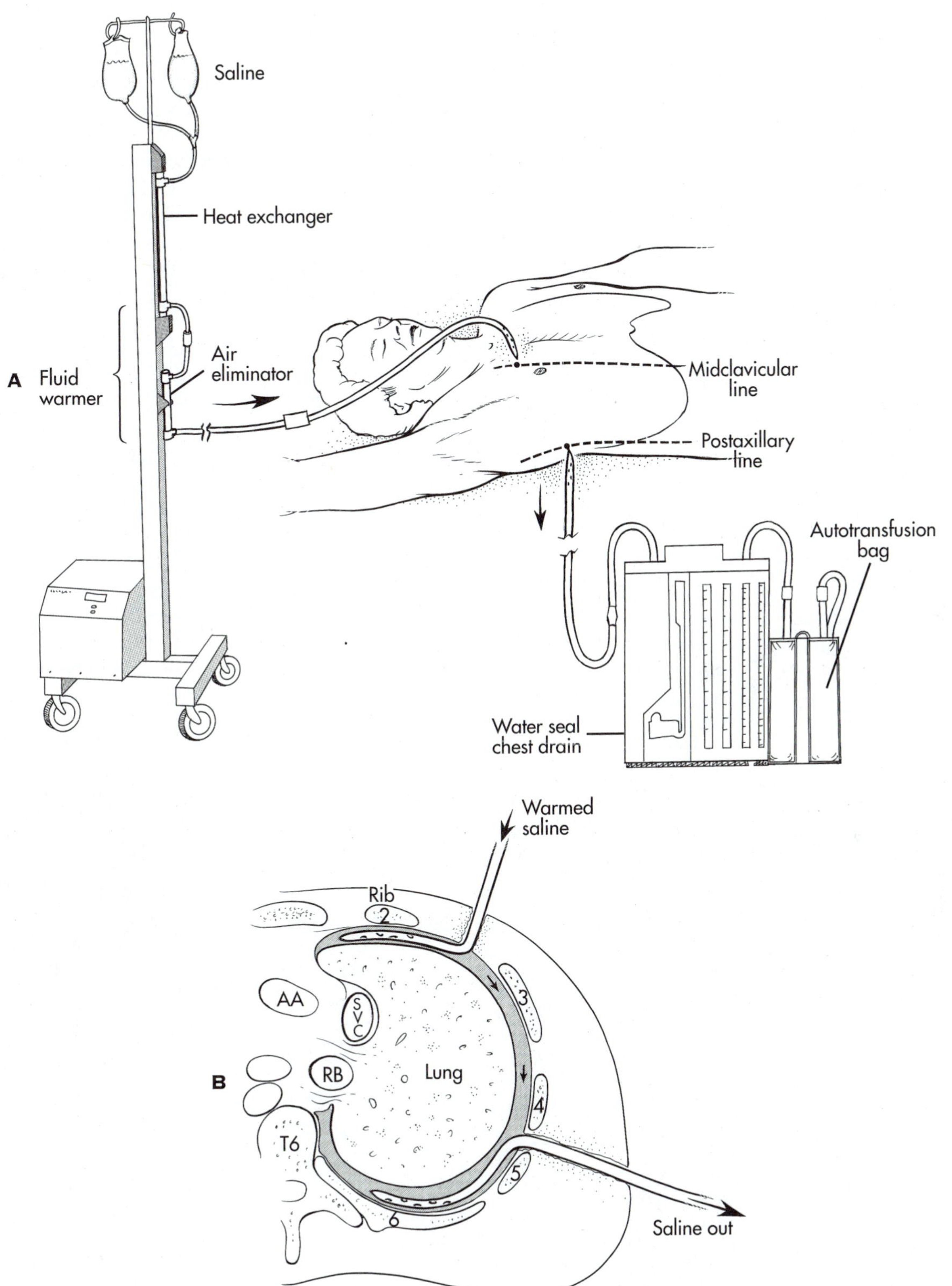

Fig. 3-10 Thoracic lavage. **A,** Cycle. **B,** Cross section.

tions. In patients who are perfusing, this technique should be considered hazardous unless extracorporeal rewarming capability is immediately available. Many hypothermic trauma patients receiving perfusion have been irrigated successfully in the operating room.[35]

The clinically reported rates range from 180 to 550 ml/min. The overall rate of rewarming should easily equal or exceed that achievable with peritoneal lavage, with the added benefit of preferential mediastinal rewarming. In addition, closed chest compressions during cardiac arrest can maintain perfusion. Open cardiac massage of a rigid, contracted heart may not be possible in severe cases before bypass, which was a problem with mediastinal irrigation.[7,132,429]

A variety of complications should be considered. Left-sided thoracostomy tube insertion into patients who are perfusing could easily induce ventricular fibrillation. Patients with pleural adhesions have poor infusion rates, and subcutaneous edema may develop. If the fluids are infused under pressure without adequate drainage, intrathoracic hypertension develops and causes the expected adverse cardiovascular effects. Insufficient data are available to assess the effects on pulmonary ventilation and perfusion.

Peritoneal lavage. Heated peritoneal lavage is a technique available in most facilities (Fig. 3-11).[391,599,602,676] Heat is conducted intraperitoneally via isotonic dialysate delivered at 40° to 45° C.[362,602] This technique is not a practical option in the field.

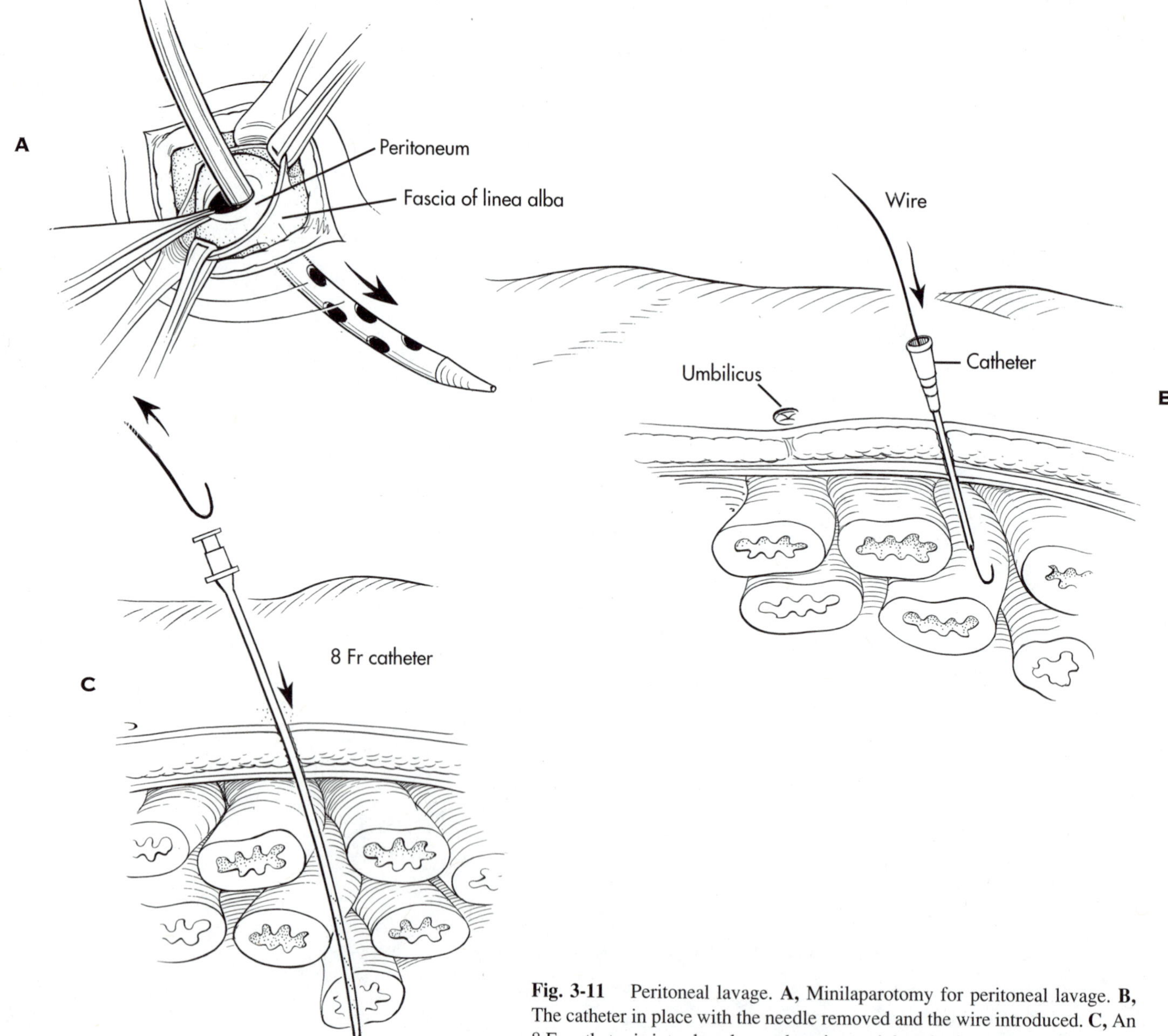

Fig. 3-11 Peritoneal lavage. **A,** Minilaparotomy for peritoneal lavage. **B,** The catheter in place with the needle removed and the wire introduced. **C,** An 8 Fr catheter is introduced over the wire, and the wire is then removed.

Before lavage is initiated, chest and abdominal radiographs should be obtained because subsequent films may reveal subdiaphragmatic air introduced during the procedure. The bladder and stomach must be emptied before insertion of the catheter. There are two popular variations of the technique for introducing fluid into the peritoneal cavity: the minilaparotomy and the percutaneous puncture.

The "minilap" requires an infraumbilical incision through the linea alba. A supraumbilical approach is necessary if previous surgical scars, a gravid uterus, or pelvic trauma is identified. The peritoneum is punctured under direct visualization and dialysis catheter(s) inserted. A much simpler and more rapid technique is the guidewire, or Seldinger, variation of the percutaneous puncture.[334] The site is infiltrated if necessary with lidocaine and a small stab incision is made. An 18- to 20-gauge needle penetrates the peritoneum, and a guidewire is introduced. Entry into the peritoneum is usually recognizable by a distinct "pop." A disposable kit is available (Arrow Peritoneal Lavage Kit [AK-0900], Arrow International Inc., Reading, Pa.). The 8 Fr lavage catheter is inserted over the wire and advanced into one of the pelvic gutters. Double-catheter systems with outflow suction speed rewarming.

Most authors have used normal saline or lactated Ringer's solution, but standard 1.5% dextrose dialysate solution with optional potassium supplementation can also be used.[668] Isotonic dialysate is heated to 40° to 45° C. Up to 2 L is then infused (10 to 20 ml/kg), retained for 20 to 30 minutes, and aspirated. The usual clinical exchange rate is 6 L/hr, which yields rewarming rates of 1° to 3° C/hr.* An alternative to consider in severe cases is a larger catheter, as found in cavity drainage kits (Arrow 14 Fr [AK-01601]) (Fig. 3-12). The catheter can be placed with the Seldinger technique. The higher drainage capability markedly increases exchange rates and minimizes dwell times necessary for maximal thermal transfer. The flow rate via gravity through regular tubing is approximately 500 ml/min, which can be tripled under infusion pressure.

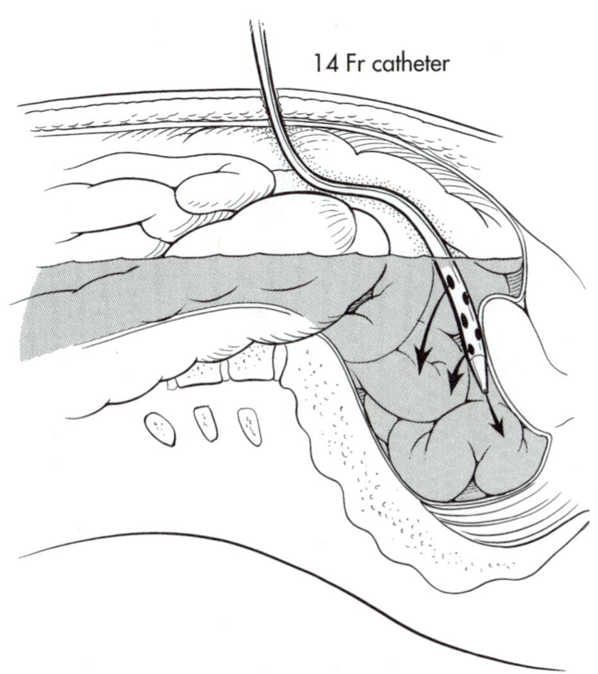

Fig. 3-12 Peritoneal lavage. A 14 Fr catheter is of greater caliber and can infuse fluids more rapidly.

A unique advantage of peritoneal dialysis is drug overdose and rhabdomyolysis detoxification when hemodialysis is unavailable. In addition, direct hepatic rewarming reactivates detoxification and conversion enzymes. Peritoneal dialysis worsens preexisting hypokalemia. However, vigilant electrolyte monitoring is essential before empirical modification of the dialysate. The presence of adhesions from previous abdominal surgery increases the complication rate and minimizes heat exchange. Only one third of the nonrenal dialyses were free of significant complications in one clinical report.[740] One of O'Connor's three stable and severely hypothermic patients developed ventricular fibrillation during the first exchange.[528,529]

Peritoneal dialysis during standard mechanical CPR was as effective as partial cardiac bypass in resuscitating severely hypothermic dogs.[496] Unlike the group of dogs receiving active external rewarming, peritoneal lavage rewarming did not require significantly greater quantities of crystalloids and bicarbonate. In another canine study, peritoneal dialysis at a rate of 12 L/hr rewarmed dogs more rapidly than did heated, humidified inhalation.[773] However, this exchange rate is rarely possible in humans. Bowel infarction may be a concern when using prolonged warm peritoneal dialysis in severe hypothermia with inadequate visceral perfusion during CPR.[34]

Peritoneal lavage should not be routinely used in treating stable, mildly hypothermic patients, because it is invasive. Extracorporeal rewarming should be available in the event of rare major complications, including ventricular fibrillation. In severe cases, the transfer of heat is lower than that achieved with cardiac bypass or hemodialysis.[144,554] This technique should be used in combination with all available rewarming techniques in cardiac arrest patients.

Extracorporeal Blood Rewarming

Cardiopulmonary bypass. A growing body of data suggests that partial or complete cardiopulmonary bypass (CPB) should be considered in severely hypothermic patients.† A major advantage of CPB is preservation of oxygenated flow if mechanical cardiac activity is lost during rewarming.‡ CPB is three to four times faster at rewarming than other active core rewarming (ACR) techniques and reduces the high blood viscosity associated with severe cases. CPB should also be considered when severe cases

*References 66, 154, 261, 325, 329, 562, 775.
†References 147, 296, 454, 459, 561, 728, 729, 739, 753.
‡References 84, 143, 162, 199, 311, 312, 379, 398, 729, 733, 778.

do not respond to less invasive rewarming techniques, in patients with completely frozen extremities, and when rhabdomyolysis is accompanied by major electrolyte disturbances.[333]

Various extracorporeal rewarming (ECR) techniques can be lifesaving modalities in selected profound cases of hypothermia.[279] Althaus describes complete recovery in three severely hypothermic tourists after prolonged periods of cardiac arrest and CPR.[7] In another review of 17 cases there were 13 survivors.[679]

The standard femoral-femoral circuit includes arterial and venous catheters, a mechanical pump, a membrane or bubble oxygenator, and a heat exchanger (Fig. 3-13).[54] A 16 to 30 Fr venous cannula is inserted via the femoral vein to the right atrium–inferior vena cava junction. The tip of the shorter 16 to 20 Fr arterial cannula resides at the aortic bifurcation. Closed chest compressions can be maintained during insertion and may help decompress the dilated nonbeating heart.[456]

Techniques are being developed to decrease the need for IV anticoagulation with heparin, which now limits clinical applicability.[755] Heparin-coated perfusion equipment has been used successfully without systemic heparinization in a patient with hypothermic cardiac arrest (23.3° C) and intracranial trauma.[748,749] The use of nonthrombogenic pumps, coupled with the enhanced physiologic fibrinolysis seen in the first hour of CPB, also has succeeded experimentally.[152]

Heated, oxygenated blood is returned via the femoral artery. Femoral flow rates of 2 to 3 L/min can elevate core temperature 1° to 2° C every 3 to 5 minutes. In Splittgerber's review the mean CPB temperature increase was 9.5° C/hr.[679] Most pumps are capable of generating full flow rates up to 7 L/min. Long[428] recommends considering the use of vasodilator therapy with IV nitroglycerin to facilitate perfusion. He initiates bypass flow rates at about 2 L/min and gradually increases to 4 to 5 L/min. Vasoactive agents may be needed to maintain the cardiac index at 30 or more and for a (low) systemic vascular resistance of 1000 or less.

The optimal temperature gradient and bypass rewarming rate are unknown. One study of rewarming via CPB in a swine model cooled to 23° C addresses this concern. An excessive temperature gradient between brain tissue and circulant adversely affected EEG regeneration.[597] The other theoretical concern is the possibility of increased bubbling if high perfusate temperature gradients are used. Most current investigators have used 5° C gradients[54,379] or 10° C gradients.[55] Eventually, neuromonitoring during rewarming will provide some answers. In severe cases evoked cerebral responses before EEG regeneration could help assess the recovering brain.

Complications with the standard technique include vessel damage, air embolism, hemolysis, disseminated intravascular coagulation, and pulmonary edema (Box 3-8). Endothelial leakage increases compartment pressures and exacerbates frostbite. If adequate flow rates of 3 to 4 L/min

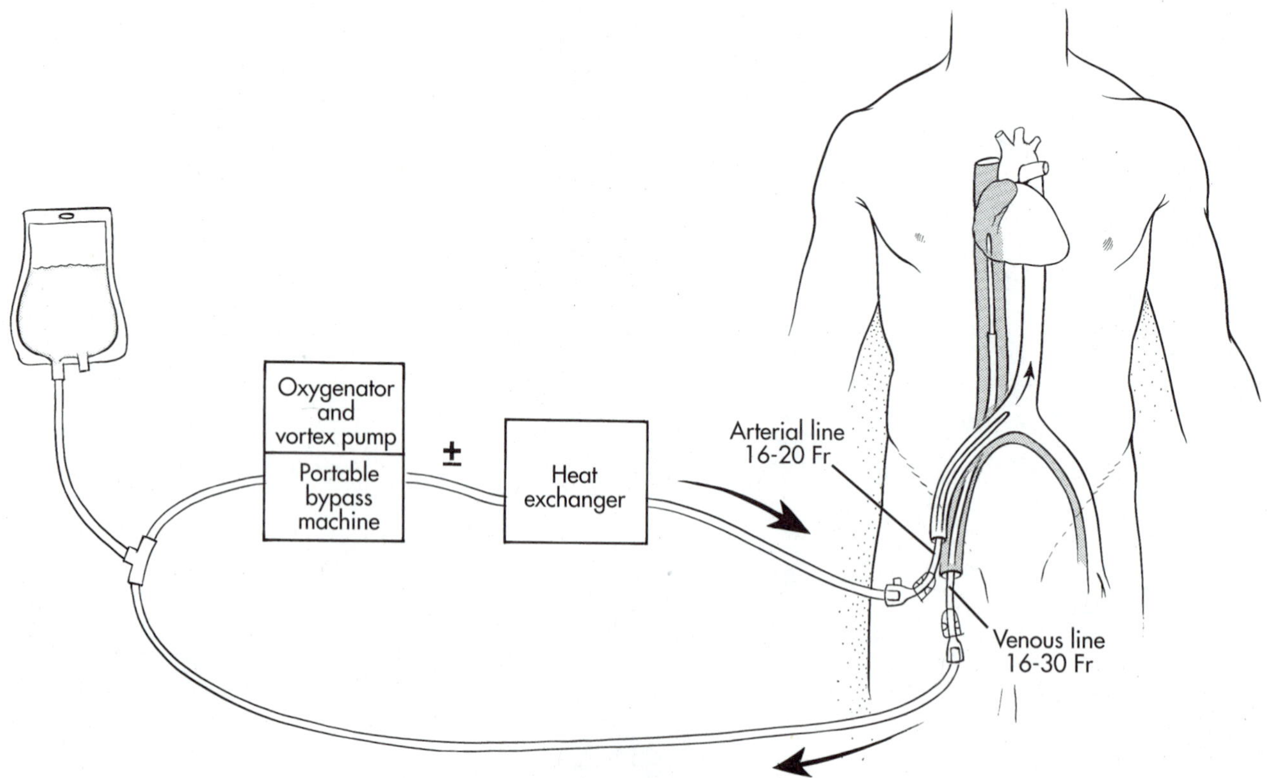

Fig. 3-13 Femoral-femoral bypass.

BOX 3-8

EXTRACORPOREAL REWARMING

COMPLICATIONS

Vascular injury
Air embolism
Pulmonary edema
Coagulopathies (hemolysis, disseminated intravascular coagulation)
Frostbite tissue damage
Extremity compartment syndromes

CONTRAINDICATIONS

CPR is contraindicated (see Box 3-9)
Lack of venous return
Intravascular clots or slush
Complete heparinization would be hazardous*

*Unless with athrombogenic tubing or adequate physiologic fibrinolysis.

(50 to 60 ml/kg/min) cannot be maintained, thoracotomy or a venous catheter with side holes, augmenting the intravascular volume, should be considered.

Arteriovenous rewarming. Another recently reported option is continuous arteriovenous rewarming through an artificial fistula.[233-235] Femoral arterial and venous catheters are percutaneously inserted and connected to the inflow and outflow ports of a countercurrent fluid warmer. In one study there was improved survival after moderately severe trauma. This technique requires a blood pressure of at least 60 mm Hg. One major advantage is that there is no need for a perfusionist, a pump, or systemic anticoagulation.

Venovenous rewarming. Extracorporeal venovenous rewarming is another option for warming and recirculating the blood. With this technique, blood is removed, usually from a central venous catheter, heated to 40° C, and returned via a second central or peripheral venous catheter. Flow rates of 150 to 400 ml/min have been achieved.[256]

The circuit is not complex and is more efficient than many other nonbypass modalities. However, there is no oxygenator, and since the method does not provide full circulatory support, volume infusion is the only option to augment inadequate cardiac output.

Another variation of the extracorporal venovenous circuit has been proposed.[527] Blood is removed from the femoral vein, heparinized, and sent through a blood rewarmer via an infusion pump accelerator. It is neutralized with protamine before reinjection into the subclavian or internal jugular vein, which would preferentially rewarm the heart.

Hemodialysis. Hemodialysis will become a more widely available and practical rewarming technique with the development of two-way flow catheters, which allow cannulation of a single vessel.[392,716] A Drake-Willock single-needle dialysis catheter can be used with a portable hemodialysis machine and external warmer. After central venous cannulation, exchange cycle volumes of 200 to 250 ml/min are possible. Although heat exchange is less than with standard two-vessel hemodialysis with CPB,[504] the ease of percutaneous subclavian vein placement is a major advantage. Inline hemodialysis also simplifies correction of electrolyte abnormalities. Local vascular complications, including thrombosis of vessels and hemorrhage secondary to anticoagulation, may occur.[643,736]

With all of these techniques there is no proof that rapid acceleration of the rate of rewarming improves survival rates. Potential complications of uncontrolled rapid rewarming in severe hypothermia include DIC, pulmonary edema, hemolysis, and acute tubular necrosis.[93]

In hypothermic cardiac arrest, rewarming should be attempted via CPB and hemodialysis when CPR is not contraindicated (Box 3-9), unless frozen intravascular contents are present that prevent flow. Clotted atrial blood or failure to obtain a venous return causes these techniques to fail. Because of this, and because the lowest temperature in a survivor of induced hypothermia was 9° C, we believe that ECR is unlikely ever to succeed below 5° C. If experienced personnel and necessary equipment are unavailable, all other rewarming techniques should be used in combination.[54,782]

Diathermy. Diathermy, the transmission of heat by conversion of energy, has been evaluated as a rewarming adjunct in accidental hypothermia.* Large amounts of heat can be delivered to deep tissues with ultrasonic (0.8 to 1 MHz) and low-frequency (915 to 2450 MHz) microwave radiation. Short-wave (13.56 to 40.68 MHz) modalities are high frequency and do not penetrate deeply.[276] Contraindications include frostbite, burns, significant edema, and all types of metallic implants and pacemakers.

*References 294, 426, 536, 537, 633, 695.

BOX 3-9

CONTRAINDICATIONS TO CARDIOPULMONARY RESUSCITATION IN ACCIDENTAL HYPOTHERMIA

Do-not-resuscitate status is documented and verified.
Obviously lethal injuries are present.
Chest wall depression is impossible.
Any signs of life are present.
Rescuers are endangered by evacuation delays or altered triage conditions.

From Danzl DF et al: *Ann Emerg Med* 16:1042, 1987. Developed in conjunction with the Wilderness Medical Society.

Under ideal conditions in a laboratory study, radiowave frequency (13.56 MHz) electromagnetic regional heating of hypothermic dogs after immersion did not damage tissue at 4 to 6 watts/kg and rapidly elevated the core temperature.[774] Zhong, Qinyi, and Mingjlang[798] successfully rewarmed 16 piglets with microwave irradiation "until they squealed and suckled." Subsequently, 20 of 28 human infants who were rewarmed with microwave irradiation at 90 to 100 watts survived. The temperature rose an average 1° C after 6 to 7 minutes, and the average infant required 45 minutes to achieve a rectal temperature of 36° C.

Both ultrasonic and low-frequency microwave diathermy have the potential to deliver large quantities of heat below the skin. As dosimetry guidelines are developed, potential complications and ideal application sites for this experimental technique deserve further study in the hospital. Someday this will be the ideal treatment. In the field setting, potential problems with power supply and electronic and navigational interference have compounded some of the physiologic problems.

Cardiopulmonary Resuscitation

Basic and advanced life support recommendations in hypothermia continue to evolve (Fig. 3-14).[139,187,687,688,760] Cardiac output generated with closed chest compressions maintains viability in selected patients with hypothermia.[543,691] The optimal rate and technique are unknown. Definitive prehospital determination of cardiac activity requires the aid of a cardiac monitor, since misdiagnosis of cardiac arrest is a hazard.[88,89] Peripheral pulses are difficult to palpate when extreme bradycardia is present with peripheral vasoconstriction.

Some authors contend that asystole is a more common presenting rhythm than is ventricular fibrillation (VF).[26] In the field, differentiating VF from asystole may be impractical.[510,677,771] Possible causes of VF include acid-base fluxes, hypoxia, and coronary vasoconstriction with increased blood viscosity.[376,498,702,742] Chest compressions and various therapeutic interventions have also been implicated. The role of acid-base fluxes is not clear. Mild alkalosis appears somewhat protective against VF during

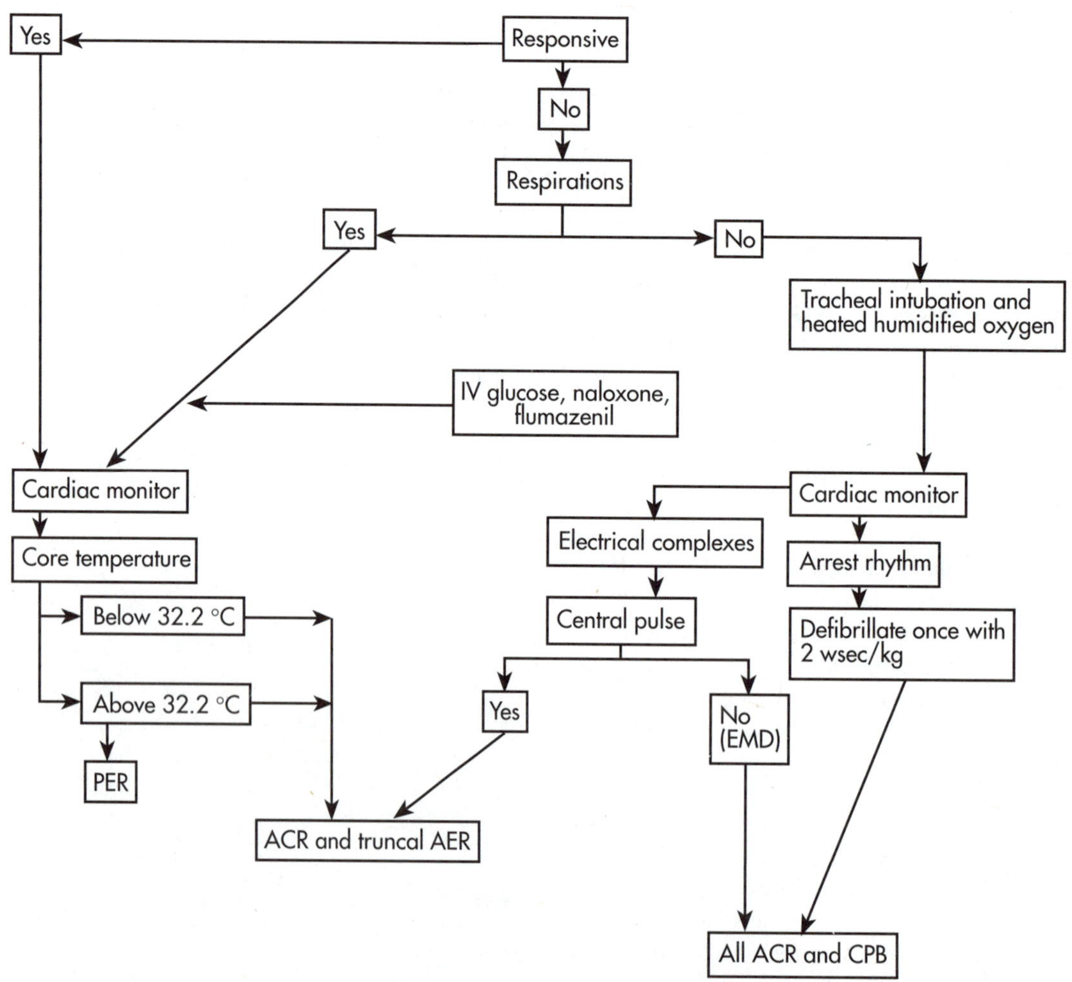

Fig. 3-14 Emergency department algorithm. *PER*, Passive external rewarming; *AER*, active external rewarming; *ACR*, active core rewarming; *CPB*, cardiopulmonary bypass.

controlled, induced hypothermia.[377] On the other hand, Southwick and Dalglish[677] have suggested that alkalosis correlates with VF versus mixed acidosis with asystole.

BLOOD FLOW DURING CHEST COMPRESSIONS

During normothermic conditions, blood flow partially results from phasic alterations in the intrathoracic pressure and not just from direct cardiac compression.[295,517,616] Niemann and associates[518] demonstrated that antegrade flow occurs without left ventricular compression in a normothermic canine model. Closed chest compressions increase intrathoracic pressure.[763] When thoracic inlet venous valves are competent, the resultant pressure gradient between arterial and venous compartments generates supradiaphragmatic antegrade flow.[750]

Some clinical observations have always challenged the supremacy of the "cardiac pump" model. For example, coughing asystolic patients temporarily remain conscious. Some tense, barrel-chested patients with chronic obstructive pulmonary disease survive after prolonged closed chest compressions. The cardiac pump model is predicated on closure of the mitral valve and opening of the aortic valve during chest compression. This allows forward stroke volume. During release of compression, transmitral flow can fill the left ventricle. Optimal cardiac output is thus generated by achieving the maximal compression rate, which allows maximal left ventricular end diastolic filling. Interestingly, transesophageal echocardiography in a canine model demonstrates mitral valve closure during chest compression except during low-impulse (downstroke momentum) compressions.[200] Compression of a cold, stiff chest wall may in fact be equivalent to low impulse.

In hypothermia the role of a "thoracic pump" with the heart as a passive conduit is an attractive hypothesis. The phasic alterations in intrathoracic pressure generated by compressions are equally applied to all of the cardiac chambers and thoracic vessels. The mitral valve remains open during compression, and blood continues to circulate through the left side of the heart.

Myocardial compliance can be severely reduced in hypothermia. Althaus[7] noted in one of three hypothermia survivors at thoracotomy that "the heart was found to be hard as stone and it is hardly conceivable how effective external cardiac massage could have been." Chest wall elasticity is also decreased with cold, as is pulmonary compliance.[146,173,743] Lastly, more force is needed to depress the chest wall sufficiently to generate intrathoracic vascular compartment pressure gradients. Despite the potential physiologic explanations, what cannot be refuted is that there are a large number of neurologically intact survivors after prolonged closed chest compressions. Once intrathoracic pressures have been measured during hypothermic closed chest compressions, we will have a better understanding.

Perfusion enhancement maneuvers remain largely unstudied in hypothermia. Ancillary abdominal binding, as with the abdominal compartment of antishock trousers, might favorably inhibit paradoxic diaphragmatic motion.[519] Simultaneous compression ventilation can increase flow in the left side of the heart.[517] Ventilation with the proper carbogen concentration would also allow high ventilatory rates while maintaining the uncorrected P_{CO_2} at 40 mm Hg. Placement of a counterpulsation intraaortic balloon is another option. Pneumatic-powered thoracic compression devices could be useful during prolonged resuscitations with limited availability of personnel and no bypass capabilities.

During hypothermic cardiac arrest in swine the cardiac output, cerebral blood flow, and myocardial blood flow averaged 50%, 55%, and 31%, respectively, of those achieved during normothermic closed chest compressions.[449] Blood flow to these areas did not decrease with time, unlike in the normothermic group. There was no significant difference in flow generated between normothermic and hypothermic swine at 20 minutes.

Hypothermic rheologic changes, including increased viscosity, also affect flow.[433] Peripheral vascular resistance would be expected to increase during vasoconstriction.[785,796] However, in the swine there was no difference in systemic and organ vascular resistance between normothermic and hypothermic CPR.[449]

In a multicenter survey of 428 cases, 9 of the 27 patients receiving CPR initiated in the field survived, as did 6 of 14 patients with emergency department–initiated CPR.[135] Based on these cases and a literature review, refinements of the American Heart Association's CPR standards in hypothermia have been proposed (Box 3-9).[135,187]

Since cardiac output is the product of heart rate and stroke volume, the optimal closed chest compression rate should be the fastest rate allowing optimal ventricular filling. Past recommendations have varied from "half" normothermic to normal rates. Many patients have recovered neurologically following slow compression rates. One recovered after 220 minutes at half the normal compression rate.[521] Probably the optimal rate has a direct linear relationship with the degree of hypothermia.[132]

Tissue decomposition, apparent rigor mortis, dependent lividity, and fixed, dilated pupils are not reliable criteria for withholding CPR.[101,187] Intermittent flow may provide adequate support during evacuation.[265,301,483,486] Therefore, CPR should not be withheld only because continuous chest compressions cannot be ensured.[32,92,529,558,570] The lowest temperature documented in an infant survivor of accidental hypothermia is 15.2° C, in an adult is 16° C, and in induced hypothermia is 9° C.[141,512,524] One patient recovered after 6½ hours of closed chest compressions.[406,632] In Saskatchewan in 1994 a 2-year-old child reportedly recovered from a core temperature of 57° F.

RESPIRATORY CONSIDERATIONS

When cardiopulmonary arrest develops during resuscitation, noncardiac causes are often pulmonary emboli or progressive respiratory insufficiency. Provision of an adequate oxygen supply is essential during rapid rewarming.[288] For each 10° C rise in temperature, oxygen consumption increases up to three times.[207]

Endotracheal intubation and ventilation decrease atelectasis and ventilation-perfusion mismatch. Complete airway protection averts aspiration, which is otherwise common in the setting of depressed airway reflexes, bronchorrhea, and ileus.[568] Carbon dioxide production also drops by half with an 8° C fall in the temperature. During induced hypothermia, carbogen (1% to 5% carbon dioxide added to oxygen) facilitates acid-base management by allowing adjustment of the fractional inspired CO_2 concentration ($FiCO_2$) while adjusting the ventilation.[461,756]

Past controversy regarding the hazards of endotracheal intubation reflected coincidental episodes and a miscitation by Fell of a series of hypothermic overdoses by Lee and Ames.[199,398] Fell stated that "endotracheal intubation was followed by cardiac arrest in a large proportion of cases," while Lee and Ames merely cautioned of that possibility. In a multicenter survey, endotracheal intubation was performed on 117 patients by multiple operators in various settings.[135] No induced arrhythmias were recognized, which is consistent with several reports.[730] Danzl and Miller[138,477] also nasotracheally intubated 40 hypothermic patients without incident, and Ledingham and Mone[396,397] did not note arrhythmias in their series of 44 cases. Potential arrhythmogenic factors include hypoxia, mechanical jostling, and acid-base or electrolyte fluctuations.

The indications for endotracheal intubation in hypothermia are identical to those in normothermia.[88,133,241] It is required unless the patient possesses intact protective airway reflexes. Ciliary activity is depressed in hypothermia, frothy sputum produces chest congestion, and the bronchorrhea resembles pulmonary edema. Fiberoptic or blind nasotracheal intubation is preferable to cricothyroidotomy when cold-induced trismus or potential cervical spine trauma is present. However, oral rather than nasal intubation may be advisable in significantly coagulopathic patients to avoid causing major epistaxis.

As expected, hypothermia prolongs the duration of neuromuscular blockade. With pancuronium the block is prolonged because metabolism into inactive metabolites is markedly decreased. Neuromuscular blockade is also prolonged with both vecuronium and atracurium.[463,608]

Resuscitation Pharmacology

The pharmacologic effects of medications are temperature dependent. The lower the temperature, the greater the degree of protein binding. Enterohepatic circulation and renal excretion are also altered, so abnormal physiologic drug responses should be anticipated. The usual clinical scenario is substandard therapeutic activity while the patient is severely hypothermic, progressing to toxicity after rewarming. For example, since hypothermia affects the metabolism of dilantin, toxicity may develop even after normothermic doses are given.[469] Medications should not be given orally because of decreased gastrointestinal function, and intramuscular medications should be avoided because they may be erratically absorbed from vasoconstricted sites.

Pharmacologic manipulation of respiratory drive, pulse, and blood pressure is generally not indicated. When relative tachycardia is not consistent with the temperature depression, the possibility of hypovolemia, hypoglycemia, or a toxicologic ingestion should be considered. Vasopressors are arrhythmogenic and cannot increase peripheral vascular resistance if the vasculature is already maximally constricted.[397] Vasodilators can precipitate core temperature afterdrop. If the intraarterial pressure is not consistent with the degree of hypothermia, judicious use of inotropic agents may be necessary.[549] In one clinical report dopamine was a successful adjunctive treatment.[582] Two patients with profound hypothermia following ethanol ingestion were resuscitated with low-dose dopamine support. In frostbite victims, however, the use of catecholamines may jeopardize the extremities.[428] Catecholamines also exacerbate preexistent occult hypokalemia.

The effect of temperature depression on the autonomic nervous system is still being investigated. In primates cooling produces a biphasic response in plasma catecholamine concentrations. After an initial increase the autonomic nervous system switches off at 29° C.[99] This suggests that catecholamine support might be useful below that temperature. The initial rise in catecholamine levels could also be caused by acute respiratory acidosis, which stimulates the sympathetic nervous system.[64,722]

Administration of dopamine alone or with lidocaine in another animal study improved cardiovascular function equivalent to a 5° C rise in temperature.[514] In one clinical series, endogenous catecholamine levels were elevated during bradycardia. As the levels dropped during rewarming, pulse rate increased.[270] Low-dose dopamine (1 to 5 µg/kg/min) or other catecholamine infusions should generally be reserved for severely hypotensive patients who do not respond to crystalloid resuscitation and rewarming.

THYROID

The most dramatic "Rip Van Winkle" rude awakening from hypothermic myxedema coma was Dr. Richard Asher's patient in the 1950s. He was successfully metabolically aroused from a 7-year 30° C slumber. Ironically, so was a quiescent oat cell carcinoma.

Cold induces stimulation of the hypothalamic-pituitary-thyroid axis. Unless myxedema is suspected, empirical therapy is not recommended.[145] A history of neck irradiation, radioactive iodine, Hashimoto's thyroiditis, or surgical treatment of hyperthyroidism should heighten the clinician's suspicion of myxedema. Failure to rewarm despite an appropriate course of therapy is a further clue.*

Myxedema coma is usually precipitated in elderly patients with chronic hypothyroidism who are stressed by trauma, infection, anesthesia, or medication ingestion.[445] Typical nonspecific laboratory abnormalities include hyponatremia, anemia, and liver enzyme and lipid elevations.[444] If myxedema coma is suspected, thyroid function studies, including serum thyroxine (T_4) by radioimmunoassay, triiodothyronine (T_3) resin uptake, and thyroid-stimulating hormone, should be obtained. It is also often interesting to measure the serum cortisol level.

Given the appropriate index of suspicion, the physician should administer 250 to 500 μg levothyroxine (T_4) intravenously over several minutes without waiting for confirmatory laboratory results. Daily injections of 100 μg are required for 5 to 7 days.[145] It is appropriate to consider adding at least 100 to 250 mg of hydrocortisone to the first 3 L of intravenous fluid. Absorption of T_4 is erratic if the drug is given orally or intramuscularly. The onset of action of T_3 is more rapid, which jeopardizes cardiovascular stability; therefore there is no current role for T_3 in acute replacement therapy.[2,145] The onset of action of T_4 is 6 to 12 hours, which is evidenced by continuous improvement of the vital signs during rewarming. Up to one half of the T_4 is eventually converted by the peripheral tissues into T_3.

STEROIDS

Acute cold stress and many coexisting disease processes stimulate cortisol secretion. The free active fraction of cortisol decreases as the temperature drops because of increased protein binding, and cortisol utilization is similarly decreased.[535] The increase in adrenocorticotropic hormone (ACTH) and adrenal steroid secretion may also be a neurogenic or emotional response in the conscious subject to an unpleasant environment. In rodents inhibition of ACTH secretion during hypothermia is mediated by decreased hypothalamic secretion of arginine vasopressin and oxytocin. This decreases pituitary responsiveness to corticotropin-releasing factor, inhibiting corticotropin release. Thus exogenous arginine vasopressin could prove helpful during rewarming.[239]

Canine experiments have demonstrated potential cerebral protective effects of 4 mg/kg dexamethasone IV in cold-injured cortical microcirculation.[678] However, in a clinical report, intracranial pressure remained normal without steroid supplementation during rewarming from 23° C.[21,525]

Cold exposure also induces adrenal unresponsiveness to ACTH. Therefore false diagnosis of decreased adrenal reserve is possible[197,198] and does not represent functional adrenal insufficiency, since ACTH levels return to normal after rewarming. Serum cortisol levels are commonly elevated. Secondary adrenal insufficiency resulting from panhypopituitarism may also coexist with myxedema. Empirical administration of steroids is not indicated unless hypoadrenocorticism is suspected based on a previous history of steroid dependence, suggestive physical findings, or an inexplicable failure to rewarm. The use of narcotic antagonists in hypothermia has been reported. Naloxone has been implicated in reducing the severity of hypothermia in drug overdoses and in spinal shock and appears to have activity at the mu receptor sites.[242,307]

Resuscitation Complications

ATRIAL ARRHYTHMIAS

All atrial arrhythmias, including atrial fibrillation, should have a slow ventricular response with the temperature depression. Atrial fibrillation was commonly noted below 32° C in one analysis of 60 ECGs from accidental hypothermia victims.[531] In half of these cases the rhythm was sinus, atrial, or junctional. In two other series atrial fibrillation was reported in 12 of 102 and in 12 of 33 cases.[533,772]

Atrial fibrillation usually converts spontaneously during rewarming, and digitalization is not warranted.[41,505,709] The AH interval prolongation present on His bundle electrocardiography is unresponsive to atropine.[320] Mesenteric embolization is a potential hazard when the rhythm converts back to sinus rhythm.

Hypothermia renders the negative inotropic effects of calcium channel blockers redundant.[285] Although verapamil has been used in the resuscitation of a profoundly hypothermic patient after near drowning,[368] any additional cerebral protective effects are still speculative. In summary, all new atrial arrhythmias usually convert spontaneously during rewarming and should be considered innocent. Attention should be directed toward correcting acid-base, fluid, and electrolyte imbalances while avoiding administration of atrial antiarrhythmics.

VENTRICULAR ARRHYTHMIAS

Prevention and ideal treatment of ventricular arrhythmias in hypothermia are complex issues. Since preexisting chronic ventricular ectopy may be suppressed in a cold heart, the physician noting these ectopic beats during rewarming is placed in a quandary. The history from the hypothermic patient may be unproductive, and the past cardiac history is often unavailable.[457]

Transient ventricular arrhythmias should generally be ignored. In one study of 22 continuously monitored patients with hypothermia, supraventricular arrhythmias were common (9 cases) and benign.[591] Ventricular extrasystoles developed in 10 patients, but none experienced ventricular

*References 24, 173, 214, 308, 604, 640, 738, 783.

tachycardia (VT) or VF during rewarming. The terminal rhythm in the 8 who died while being monitored was asystole, not VF. The energetics of the fibrillating hypothermic ventricle are under investigation, since asystole may consume less energy and be more protective.

Pharmacologic options are limited, since hypothermia induces complex physiologic changes that result in abnormal responses.[784] Drug metabolism and excretion are both progressively decreased. In normothermia, class IA ventricular antiarrhythmics have negative inotropic and indirect anticholinergic effects, and moderately decrease conduction velocity (Box 3-10).[742] Procainamide reportedly increases the incidence of VF during hypothermia. Quinidine has been useful during induced profound hypothermia,[170] preventing VF during cardiac manipulation at 25° to 30° C. There are no reports regarding the effects of disopyramide. In class IB, lidocaine is still waiting to be proved effective for prophylaxis and is ineffective in facilitating defibrillation.[14,516] In animal studies lidocaine and propranolol had minimal hemodynamic effects in hypothermia.[514] If normothermic effects persisted during hypothermia, the class IB agents would appear attractive because they minimally slow conduction while shortening the action potential duration (APD).

The class III agent bretylium tosylate, a unique bromobenzyl quaternary ammonium compound, has been extremely effective in several animal studies.[129,165,364,516] This class of agents seems most ideal pharmacologically, since it possesses direct antifibrillatory properties. However, the ability to prolong the action potential duration is temperature dependent. Ideally, a drug would lengthen the APD only in warmer regions to reduce dispersion.

Bretylium causes chemical sympathectomy and is both an antiarrhythmic and an antifibrillatory agent. Bretylium increases the VF threshold, APD, and effective refractory period. Interestingly, at least at normal temperatures, antifibrillatory effects occur more acutely than do antiarrhythmic effects. Nielson and Owman[516] found that bretylium beneficially increased the fibrillation threshold in cats, and Buckley, Bosch, and Bacaner[78] demonstrated efficacy in the prophylaxis and treatment of VF in a canine model. In that study, while 42% of the control dogs showed fibrillation, no dog given 15 mg/kg bretylium did. In the design of both of these studies, the drug was administered *before* hypothermia was induced. In a similarly designed canine study by Elenbaas and associates[182] bretylium failed to facilitate defibrillation at 22° C.

In the first study to evaluate the effects of bretylium administered *after* induction of hypothermia, Murphy, Nowak, and Tomlanovich[500] noted that only 1 of 11 dogs given bretylium (mean 40.5 mg/kg) before five invasive maneuvers developed VF. No dog, including control subjects, showed fibrillation during endotracheal intubation. Of note during discussions regarding prophylaxis, 3 of the 11 dogs converted to VF during the drug infusion. The effect of bretylium on plasma catecholamines and electrically induced arrhythmias has also been studied. Since catecholamine levels increase during cooling, the demonstrated protection appears to be due to alteration of the electrophysiologic properties of the cardiac tissues.[541] Amiodarone, another class III drug that possesses direct antifibrillatory activity, would be an interesting agent to study during hypothermic conditions. Also of note, magnesium sulfate at a dose of 100 mg/kg IV spontaneously defibrillated most patients on CPB at 30° C in one series of patients with induced hypothermia.[80] This occurred within minutes in two thirds of the cases.

Emergency transvenous intracardiac pacing of bradyrhythmias is extremely risky with cold hearts because it commonly precipitates ventricular fibrillation. New dysrhythmias that develop after rewarming may require pacing on rare occasions. External noninvasive pacing with low-resistance electrodes seems far preferable before stabilization.[192,193,497,550]

BOX 3-10

ANTIARRHYTHMIC AGENTS

Class I. Sodium channel blockers
- IA. Conduction and depolarization moderately slowed
  - Action potential duration (APD) and repolarization prolonged
    - Disopyramide
    - Procainamide
    - Quinidine
- IB. Conduction and depolarization minimally slowed
  - APD and repolarization shortened
    - Lidocaine
    - Mexiletine
    - Moricizine
    - Phenytoin
    - Tocainide
- IC. Conduction and depolarization markedly slowed
  - APD and repolarization prolonged
    - Encainide
    - Flecainide

Class II. β-Adrenergic blockers

Class III. Antifibrillatory properties
- APD prolonged
  - Amiodarone
  - Bretylium
  - *d*-Sotalol

Class IV. Calcium channel blockers
- Diltiazem
- Verapamil

Unclassified
- Adenosine
- Magnesium sulfate

In summary, although human data are sparse, bretylium is the only agent shown to have antiarrhythmic activity during hypothermic conditions.[365] Two cases of chemical ventricular defibrillation after infusion of bretylium 10 mg/kg in accidental hypothermia have been reported.[137,366] Bretylium appears to be the agent of choice for VF in hypothermia. Bretylium prophylaxis is investigational, since toxicity, optimal dosage, and particularly the ideal rate of infusion are unknown.

SEPSIS

The pathophysiology of sepsis in hypothermia continues to be unraveled.[42,43,105] Classic signs of infection, including erythema and fever, are absent. Rigors and shakes resemble shivering. Initial history, physical, and laboratory data are often unreliable, and therefore repeated evaluations and comprehensive culturing are mandatory in the emergency department.[571] The 10% subset of patients with sepsis syndrome who manifest a hypothermic response have a significantly increased frequency of shock and death,[105] and the hypothermia does not appear to be protective.

Hypothermia compromises host defenses and results in serious bacterial infections.[404] These significant infections can be accompanied by minimal inflammatory response. Some common etiologic organisms include gram-negative bacteria, gram-positive cocci, oral anaerobes, and Enterobacteriaceae.[491] Lewin, Brettman, and Holzman[404] cultured *Escherichia coli, Streptococcus pneumoniae,* two *Proteus* and *Klebsiella* species, *Staphylococcus aureus,* and *S. epidermidis.*

The core endotoxin components of gram-negative bacteria normally signal macrophages.[764] At normal or elevated temperature, active cytokine triggers include tumor necrosis factor, interleukin-1, and interleukin-6. The potential role of antiendotoxin monoclonal antibodies in patients with accidental but not cytokine-induced hypothermia is unresolved. Bone marrow release and circulation of neutrophils are compromised for up to 12 hours.[43] In addition, human and porcine neutrophils are susceptible to hypothermia.[697] In vitro, neutrophil migration and bacterial phagocytosis are reduced at 29° C.[3] Neutrophilic extermination of various bacteria, including *S. aureus* and *Streptococcus faecalis,* is also impaired.

Acquired neutrophil dysfunction has been identified.[102] In addition, hypothermia was associated with a decreased number of neutrophils in a series of 40 near-drowned children.[44,53] As a clinical demonstration of the importance of these factors, therapeutic maintenance of hypothermia to control cerebral edema in near drowning has been abandoned because of the substantial incidence of infectious complications.[53]

The reported incidence of infection varies dramatically with the patient's age and the clinical series reported.[160,404,772] In one group of 51 infants, 27 had sepsis.[126] While there were no reliable indicators of infection, some suggestive clues were present. Serum glucose and leukocyte abnormalities, anemia, uremia, and bradycardia were often identified. In addition to *Staphylococcus* and *Streptococcus,* the predominant organisms were *Haemophilus* and Enterobacteriaceae. Of Yagupsky's 57 hypothermic infants, 9 had sepsis.[789,790]

Lung infections, usually in the right upper lobe, were reported in 80 of 138 hypothermic infants by El-Radhi and coworkers.[184,185] Evaluation of the gastric aspirate was another diagnostic predictor of sepsis in 36 of 44 infected infants.[186] In five studies sepsis was found in 8% to 74% of hypothermic infants.[126,184-186,619] In this age group, empirical broad-spectrum antibiotics are warranted. Dagan and Gorodischer[126] recommend an intravenous aminoglycoside with ampicillin.

In adults the incidence of infection ranges from less than 1% to over 40%, depending on patient selection criteria.[135,404,490,772] In Lewin's series, serious soft tissue or pulmonary infections were present in 24 of 59 patients and in 9 the infection was undiagnosed at the time of hospital admission from the emergency department. Occult bacteremia was present in less than 1% of White's series of 102 patients, and results were negative in all of the 46 lumbar punctures. In other studies of hypothermic elderly patients admitted to hospitals, most have had evidence of probable or definite infections.[140]

Bacteremic infections were identified in 33 of 85 consecutive cases by Morris and co-workers.[490] In this series, 32 patients were hemodynamically monitored. Before patients were rewarmed, the combination of an elevated cardiac index and decreased systemic vascular resistance suggested bacteremia. This coincidental observation should prompt a search for infection with hemodynamic monitoring only when it is indicated for other reasons.[490,571] Surprisingly, no complications associated with right heart catheterization were reported in this series.

In summary, unlike children and the elderly, most previously healthy young adults do not need empirical antibiotic prophylaxis. However, treatment indications should be liberalized from normothermia. They should include failure to rewarm or any suspicion or evidence of aspiration, myositis, chest x-ray infiltrates, bacteriuria, or persistent altered mental status. In choosing broad-spectrum coverage, the physician should consider altered drug interactions, volumes of distribution, protein binding, hepatic metabolism, and renal excretion. The combination of an aminoglycoside with a broad-spectrum β-lactam antibiotic is often appropriate.

Forensic Pathology

Macromorphologic and micromorphologic lesions are variable and nonspecific in hypothermia, and there is no single pathognomonic finding at autopsy. Establishing hypothermia as the primary cause of death requires an adequate history of exposure and the absence of other lethal findings at necropsy. For example, unnatural deaths in nursing home patients may be significantly underreported for these reasons.[119]

Macroscopic skin changes can suggest the diagnosis. Hyperemia of the dorsum of the hands and knees is commonly found. Nonpathognomonic findings have been identified in the pancreas, lungs, and heart.[291,451] Pancreatic findings include fat necrosis, aseptic pancreatitis, and hemorrhage. Pulmonic changes consist of intraalveolar, interstitial, and intrabronchial hemorrhages. Hirvonen and Huttunen[299] also identified microscopic degeneration of the myocardium. In Coe's postmortem series an interesting anatomic observation in 45% of the hypothermic deaths was low lung weight.[106]

Bray, Luke, and Blackbourne[62] initially observed an increased vitreous glucose concentration in a group of plane crash victims who were immersed in icy water. This suggests that eye chilling might inhibit anaerobic glycolysis. A similar inhibition of glucose consumption and lactate production was also observed in experiments on decapitated sheep heads.[60,61]

An eye that has been directly exposed to the environment could be a chemical indicator of both the environmental and patient temperatures at the time of death. Vitreous humor chemistry profiles at autopsy on 133 patients revealed that glucose concentration and total carbon dioxide content varied inversely with temperature, with values significantly higher in the winter months.[61] An elevated vitreous glucose in a nondiabetic victim should suggest hypothermia.[106] The total urinary catecholamine content, particularly epinephrine, was high in one group of casualties known to be hypothermic.[300] Erosions of the gastric mucosa, termed Wischnewsky spots, are also frequently found.[45,712,735] In addition, exposure to extreme cold should be suspected when unusual intravascular hemolysis, which is seen after freezing of blood, is observed in a corpse.[361]

Prevention

To function optimally "as the water stiffens" requires an understanding of the principles of heat conservation and loss.[71,779] Well-trained and educated urban adults can participate in prolonged Arctic maneuvers safely.[654,718] To maintain core temperature in the narrow band necessary for peak functioning in cold environments, appropriate adaptive behavioral responses are essential.[302] Autonomic and endocrinologic mechanisms are only supplemental.[175,250,664]

Studies of human cold adaptation have reached highly variable conclusions. Explanations for these discrepancies include changes in core and shell temperatures and in metabolic rates before and after cold adaptation. Some observations are indicative of hypothermic insulative isometabolic cold adaptation associated with local cold adaptation of the extremities.[629]

Excellent physical conditioning with adequate rest and nutrition is paramount.[58,313] Hikers and skiers should always be accompanied by a partner and should wear effective thermal insulation. Wet inner garments must be changed promptly. Persons who exert themselves, including long-distance skiers, should switch garments depending on the current exertional heat production.[305,306,673] Since dehydration must be avoided, drinking from a cold stream is preferable to snow ingestion. Significant energy is needed to convert ice at 0° C into water at 0° C.[580]

All areas with a large surface area/volume ratio should be well insulated. The uncovered head can lose a large percentage of the body's total heat production. Adrenergic vasoconstriction does not occur effectively in the head and neck region.[252] That is why a nightcap, which was not originally Kentucky bourbon, is effective as a stocking cap worn to bed. Excellent synthetic insulating materials include Gore-Tex, Thinsulate, and taslanized nylon.

Flectalon, a web of aluminized polyvinyl chloride fibers, is a good insulating material.[303] In a comparison of its insulating efficacy with that of other materials, the "critical" temperature was determined. This is defined as the lowest environmental temperature at which the core temperature can be maintained without increased oxygen consumption. Flectalon lowers the critical temperature more than does Thinsulate and may prove useful as an insulator to prevent and treat hypothermia.

Under certain circumstances insidious hypothermia may develop during exposure to cold water because of the effects of increased insulation on compensatory physiologic events.[25,345] The army mnemonic "COLD," in reference to insulation with clothing, is *clean, open* during exercise to avoid sweating, *loose* layers to retain heat, and *dry* to limit conductive heat losses.[664] For a complete discussion of preventive measures, refer to Chapters 6 and 7.

Prevention of urban accidental hypothermia requires continual public education. For example, the optimal safe indoor temperature recommendation for the elderly has risen to 21.1° C.[115,419,548,577] Energy assistance and temporary sheltering are effective measures, and selective heating of sleeping quarters and the use of electric blankets are economical suggestions.[339] Prewarming the bed and bedroom at night may be the best overall advice to the elderly.[437]

Outcome

Even during normothermia there is often no consensus regarding the optimal duration of potentially unsuccessful resuscitative efforts.[538] Partially because of the dramatic reports of reanimations, the standard of care has been that "no one is dead until they are warm and dead." In reality, some victims are clearly dead when they are cold and dead, and it would be useful to safely identify them.[22]

Going to the medical literature to decide how to predict outcome is as scientific as when the ancients went to the oracle at Delphi, stirred some entrails, and predicted the outcome of the spring campaign. Survival is difficult to predict because of the variability of human physiologic responses to temperature depression.[564] The type and severity of the underlying or precipitating disease process are two determinants. Age extremes, while not statistically correlated with survival, are commonly associated with severe illnesses.[230,373] However, in a multicenter survey there were no significant age differences in mortality.[135]

Sex, trauma, infection, and toxin ingestions affected survival differently in multiple, uncontrolled clinical studies. There were no clinically significant differences in male versus female profiles in the multicenter survey.[135] From a large hypothermia data base a hypothermia outcome score has been developed that could enable multiple observers at differing sites to assess treatment modalities and outcome predictors. Prehospital cardiac arrest, low or absent blood pressure, elevated BUN, and the need for either endotracheal or nasogastric intubation in the emergency department were significant predictors of outcome after multivariant analysis.[133,351,631]

In a multiple regression analysis of 234 cases in Swiss clinics, prognostic factors were also assessed.[427] The biggest negative survival factors were asphyxia, slow rate of cooling, invasive rewarming, asystole, and development of pulmonary edema or adult respiratory distress syndrome. Positive predictors of survival included rapid cooling rate, presence of ventricular fibrillation during cardiac arrest, and narcotic or ethanol intoxication. In a study of 29 patients below 30° C, mode of cooling was the only independent risk factor.[564]

There is a need for some valid triage marker of death, since vital organ damage is difficult to predict. In one retrospective analysis of primarily avalanche burial victims, extreme hyperkalemia was noted on initial examination and resuscitation proved fruitless.[631] In the Mt. Hood tragedy the nonsurvivors also were hyperkalemic (serum potassium greater than 10 mmol/L).[279] However, in both of these reports asphyxia and compression injury may have been contributory.

SUMMARY

Accidental hypothermia continues to masquerade as a variety of disorders, challenging the clinician's diagnostic acumen and therapeutic versatility. Whereas birds can migrate and bears hibernate, humans still cannot acclimate to a three-dog night. While historical evidence of environmental exposure simplifies the diagnosis, subtle presentations are far more common, particularly in urban settings and in the elderly. The symptoms of hypothermia are often vague and reflect physiologic responses from all organ systems. The unwary urban clinician may misfocus on more obvious findings that suggest an alternative diagnosis: for example, medical, traumatic, toxicologic, neurologic, and psychiatric emergencies.

Several physical examination decoys complicate the clinical presentation of hypothermia. For example, a "relative" tachycardia disproportionate to the lowered temperature should trigger consideration of associated hypovolemia, hypoglycemia, or toxin ingestion. Initial hyperventilation seen in response to a cold stress normally wanes, since carbon dioxide production progressively declines. Persistent hyperventilation also reflects central nervous system disorder or underlying organic acidosis. A Glasgow Coma Scale score inconsistent with the temperature should not be dismissed as simple clinical variability. It may reflect toxicologic, traumatic, or infectious impairment of the central nervous system. Conversely, areflexia misattributed to hypothermia obscures the diagnosis of a spinal cord injury.

Field treatment is the art of the possible and should include gentle handling, insulation, and heated, humidified oxygen. Active external rewarming should be used only selectively and preferably should be limited to the trunk. The means of rewarming in the emergency department should be individualized and requires a versatile approach based on the pathophysiology, presentation, and available facilities. Active core rewarming with heated, humidified oxygen is a safe, practical option in all emergency departments and can be easily combined with other rewarming modalities.

Patients with mild primary accidental hypothermia can be rewarmed in the emergency department and discharged. Those with serious predisposing conditions require hospital admission and more intensive care. Moderately or severely hypothermic patients (below 32.2° C) require hospital admission if predisposing conditions, age extremes, or abnormal laboratory or toxicologic values are identified.

Transferring patients to specific centers specializing in a single rewarming technique is not generally warranted, since no survival advantage has been identified for any particular rewarming modality. Some severely hypothermic patients are best managed in facilities with cardiopulmonary bypass capabilities. Ultimately, the choice of specific rewarming techniques should reflect available expertise and resources.

REFERENCES

1. Adler AI: Arctic first aid (letter), *N Engl J Med* 326:351, 1992.
2. Ahmad S, Thaginsa A: Myxedema presenting as profound hypothermia-coma: a case report, *W Va Med J* 80:143, 1984.
3. Akriotis V, Biggar WD: The effects of hypothermia on neutrophil function in vitro, *J Leukocyte Biol* 37:51, 1985.
4. Albiin N, Eriksson A: Fatal accidental hypothermia and alcohol, *Alcohol Alcoholism* 19:13, 1984.
5. Aldrete JA: Preventing hypothermia in trauma patients by microwave warming of IV fluids, *J Emerg Med* 3:435, 1985.
6. Allison TG et al: Cardiovascular responses to immersion in a hot tub in comparison with exercise in male subjects with coronary artery disease, *Mayo Clin Proc* 68:19, 1993.

7. Althaus U et al: Management of profound accidental hypothermia with cardiorespiratory arrest, *Ann Surg* 195:492, 1982.
8. Altus P, Hickman JW, Nord HJ: Accidental hypothermia in a healthy quadriplegic patient, *Neurology* 35:427, 1985.
9. Altus P et al: Hypothermia in the sunny South, *South Med J* 73:1491, 1980.
10. Ambach E, Tributsch W, Henn R: Fatal accidents on glaciers: forensic, criminological, and glaciological conclusions, *J Forensic Sci* 36:1469, 1991.
11. Amlie JP et al: Effect of uniformly prolonged and increased basic dispersion of repolarization on premature dispersion on ventricular surface in dogs: role of action potential duration and activation time differences, *Eur Heart J* 6(D):15, 1985.
12. Andrew PJ, Parker RS: Treating accidental hypothermia, *Br J Med* 2:1641, 1978.
13. Andrews RP: Cold injury complicating trauma in the subfreezing environment, *Milit Med* 152:42, 1987.
14. Angelakos ET: Influence of pharmacologic agents on spontaneous and surgically-induced hypothermic ventricular fibrillation, *Ann NY Acad Sci* 80:351, 1959.
15. Anshus JS, Endahl GL, Mottley JL: Microwave heating of intravenous fluids, *Am J Emerg Med* 3:316, 1985.
16. Anwar A, Hamburger S: Alcoholic ketoacidosis, *Mo Med* 78:245, 1981.
17. Anzai T et al: Blood flow distribution in dogs during hypothermia and posthypothermia, *Am J Physiol* 234:H706, 1978.
18. Arnold JW, Eichenberger CH: The hydraulic sarong: emergency treatment device for accidental hypothermia, *JACEP* 4:438, 1975.
19. Ash SR: An explanation for uremic hypothermia, *Int J Artif Organs* 14:67, 1991.
20. Ashworth M et al: Missed injuries of the spinal cord, *Br Med J* 284:1334, 1982.
21. Astrup J et al: Increase in extracellular potassium in the brain during circulatory arrest: effects of hypothermia, lidocaine, and thiopental, *Anesthesiology* 55:256, 1981.
22. Auerbach PS: Some people are dead when they're cold and dead (editorial), *JAMA* 264:1856, 1990.
23. Avery WM: Accidental hypothermia, drugs and the elderly, *Am Pharm* 2:14, 1982.
24. Bacci V et al: Myxedema coma and cardiac arrest (letter), *JAMA* 245:920, 1981.
25. Bagian JP, Kaufman JW: Effectiveness of the space shuttle anti-exposure system in a cold water environment, *Aviat Space Environ Med* 61:563, 1990.
26. Bangs CC: Hypothermia and frostbite, *Emerg Med Clin North Am* 2:275, 1984.
27. Bangs CC, Hamlet MP: Hypothermia and cold injuries. In Auerbach P, Geehr E, editors: *Management of wilderness and environmental emergencies,* New York, 1983, Macmillan.
28. Baraka A: Hydrogen ion regulation during hypothermia: hibernators versus ectotherms, *Middle East J Anesth* 7:235, 1984.
29. Baraka AS et al: Effect of alpha-stat versus pH-stat strategy on oxyhemoglobin dissociation and whole-body oxygen consumption during hypothermic cardiopulmonary bypass, *Anesth Analg* 74:32, 1992.
30. Barr GL, Halvorsen LO, Donovan AJ: Correction of hypothermia by continuous pleural perfusion, *Surgery* 103:553, 1988.
31. Bashour TT, Gualberto A, Ryan C: Atrioventricular block in accidental hypothermia: a case report, *Angiology* 40:63, 1989.
32. Bass E: Cardiopulmonary arrest: pathophysiology and neurologic complications, *Ann Intern Med* 103:920, 1985.
33. Bastow MD, Rawlings J, Allison SP: Undernutrition, hypothermia, and injury in elderly women with fractured femur: an injury response to altered metabolism? *Lancet* 1:143, 1983.
34. Baumgartner FJ et al: Cardiopulmonary bypass for resuscitation of patients with accidental hypothermia and cardiac arrest, *Can J Surg* 35:184, 1992.
35. Baxter BT et al: Chest tube irrigation for postinjury hypothermia (letter), *Ann Emerg Med* 17:999, 1988.
36. Becker H et al: Myocardial damage caused by keeping pH 7.40 during systemic deep hypothermia, *J Thorac Cardiovasc Surg* 82:810, 1981.
37. Beran AV, Sperling DR: An improved method for inducing hypothermia and rewarming, *Aviat Space Environ Med* 50:884, 1979.
38. Bering EA Jr: Effects of profound hypothermia and circulatory arrest on cerebral oxygen metabolism and cerebrospinal fluid electrolyte composition in dogs, *J Neurosurg* 39:199, 1974.
39. Besdine RW: Hypothermia and accidental hypothermia. In Abrams WB, Berkow R, editors: *The Merck manual of geriatrics,* Rahway, NJ, 1990, Merck Sharp & Dohme Research Laboratories.
40. Best R, Syverud S, Nowak RM: Trauma and hypothermia, *Am J Emerg Med* 3:48, 1985.
41. Beyda EJ, Jung M, Bellet S: Effect of hypothermia on the tolerance of dogs to digitalis, *Circ Res* 9:129, 1961.
42. Biggar WD et al: Partial recovery of neutrophil functions during prolonged hypothermia in pigs, *J Appl Res* 60:1186, 1986.
43. Biggar WD, Bohn D, Kent G: Neutrophil circulation and release from bone marrow during hypothermia, *Infect Immun* 40:708, 1983.
44. Biggart MJ, Bohn DJ: Effect of hypothermia and cardiac arrest on outcome of near-drowning accidents in children, *J Pediatr* 117:179, 1990.
45. Birchmeyer MS, Mitchell EK: Wischnewski revisited: the diagnostic value of gastric mucosal ulcers in hypothermic deaths, *Am J Forensic Med Pathol* 10:28, 1989.
46. Bjornstad H, Tande PM, Refsum H: Cardiac electrophysiology during hypothermia: implications for medical treatment, *Arctic Med Res* 50:71, 1991.
47. Bjornstad H, Tande PM, Refsum H: Class III antiarrhythmic action of *d*-sotalol during hypothermia, *Am Heart J* 121:1429, 1991.
48. Black PR, van Devanter SV, Cohn LH: Effects of hypothermia on systemic and organ system metabolism and function, *J Surg Res* 20:49, 1976.
49. Blagdon J, Gibson T: Potential hazard of clotting during blood transfusion using a blood warming pack, *Br Med J* 290:1475, 1985.
50. Blair E: Physiology of hypothermia. In *Clinical hypothermia,* New York, 1964, McGraw-Hill.
51. Block R et al: Does hypothermia protect against the development of hepatitis in paracetamol overdose?, *Anaesthesia* 47:789, 1992.
52. Boelhouwder RU, Bruining HA, Ong GL: Corrections of serum potassium fluctuations with body temperature after major surgery, *Crit Care Med* 15:310, 1987.
53. Bohn DJ et al: Influence of hypothermia, barbiturate therapy and intracranial pressure monitoring on morbidity and mortality after near-drowning, *Crit Care Med* 14:529, 1986.
54. Bolgiano E et al: Accidental hypothermia with cardiac arrest: recovery following rewarming by cardiopulmonary bypass, *J Emerg Med* 10:427, 1992.
55. Bolte RG et al: The use of extracorporeal rewarming in a child submerged for 66 minutes, *JAMA* 260:377, 1988.
56. Bowen DR: Efficiency of the thermal jacket on the delivered temperature of prewarmed crystalloid intravenous fluid, *AANA J* 60:369, 1992.
57. Bowman W: *Outdoor emergency care: comprehensive first aid for non-urban settings,* Lakewood, Colo, 1988, National Ski Patrol System.
58. Bracker MD: Environmental and thermal injury, *Clin Sports Med* 11:419, 1992.
59. Brantigan CO, Paton B: Clinical hypothermia, accidental hypothermia and frostbite. In Goldsmith HS, editor: *Lewis practice of surgery,* New York, 1978, Harper & Row.
60. Bray M: The effect of chilling, freezing, and rewarming on the postmortem chemistry of vitreous humor, *J Forensic Sci* 29:404, 1984.
61. Bray M: The eye as a chemical indicator of environmental temperature at the time of death, *J Forensic Sci* 29:396, 1984.

62. Bray M, Luke JL, Blackbourne BD: Vitreous humor chemistry in deaths associated with rapid chilling and prolonged freshwater immersion, *J Forensic Sci* 28:588, 1983.
63. Breen EG et al: Impaired coagulation in accidental hypothermia of the elderly, *Age Ageing* 17:343, 1988.
64. Brimioulle S: Sympathetic nervous system activity during hypothermia, *Crit Care Med* 12:924, 1984.
65. Brinnel H, Cabanac M: Tympanic temperature is a core temperature in humans, *J Therm Biol* 14:47, 1989.
66. Bristow G: Treatment of accidental hypothermia with peritoneal dialysis, *Can Med Assoc J* 118:764, 1978.
67. Bristow G: Accidental hypothermia, *Can Anaesth Soc J* 31:S52, 1984.
68. Bristow G et al: Resuscitation from cardiopulmonary arrest during accidental hypothermia due to exhaustion and exposure, *Can Med Assoc J* 117:247, 1977.
69. Britt LD, Dascombe WH, Rodriguez A: New horizons in management of hypothermia and frostbite injury, *Surg Clin North Am* 71:345, 1991.
70. Brocklehurst JC, editor: *Textbook of geriatric medicine and gerontology,* New York, 1973, Churchill Livingstone.
71. Brooks CJ: Ship/rig personnel abandonment and helicopter crew/passenger immersion suits: the requirements in the North Atlantic, *Aviat Space Environ Med* 57:276, 1986.
72. Browne DA, deBoeck R, Morgan M: An evaluation of the Level 1 blood warmer series, *Anaesthesia* 45:960, 1990.
73. Brunette DD et al: Internal cardiac massage and mediastinal irrigation in hypothermic cardiac arrest, *Am J Emerg Med* 10:32, 1992.
74. Brunette DD et al: Comparison of gastric and closed thoracic cavity lavage in the treatment of severe hypothermia in dogs, *Ann Emerg Med* 16:1222, 1987.
75. Brunette DD, Sterner S, Ruiz E: Rewarming in severe hypothermia (letter), *Ann Emerg Med* 19:1076, 1990.
76. Bryant RE et al: Factors affecting mortality in gram-negative rod bacteremia, *Arch Intern Med* 127:120, 1971.
77. Buccini RV: Hypothermia in Hodgkin's disease, *N Engl J Med* 312:244, 1985.
78. Buckley JJ, Bosch CK, Bacaner MB: Prevention of ventricular fibrillation during hypothermia with bretylium tosylate, *Anesth Analg* 50:587, 1971.
79. Budd GM: Accidental hypothermia in skiers (editorial), *Med J Aust* 144:449, 1986.
80. Buky B: Effect of magnesium on ventricular fibrillation due to hypothermia, *Br J Anaesth* 42:886, 1970.
81. Burchman CA, Datta S, Ostheimer GW: Delivery temperature of heated intravenous solutions during rapid infusion, *J Clin Anesth* 1:259, 1989.
82. Buris L, Debreczeni L: The elevation of serum creatinine phosphokinase at induced hypothermia, *Forensic Sci Int* 20:35, 1982.
83. Burman LE: Hypothermia-induced thrombocytopenia (letter), *J R Soc Med* 81:619, 1988.
84. Caldwell C, Crawford R, Sinclair I: Hypothermia after cardiopulmonary bypass in man (letter), *Anesthesiology* 55:86, 1981.
85. Callaghan PB et al: Effect of varying CO_2 tensions on the O_2Hgb dissociation curve under hypothermic conditions, *Ann Surg* 154:903, 1961.
86. Camfield PR: Hypothalamic astrocytoma, hypothermia, and pancreatitis, *Arch Neurol* 41:1022, 1984.
87. Canivelt JL, Larbuisson R, Lamy M: Interest of face mask-CPAP in one case of severe accidental hypothermia, *Acta Anaesthesiol Belg* 40:281, 1989.
88. Carden DL: Intubating the hypothermic patient, *Ann Emerg Med* 12:124, 1983.
89. Carden DL et al: Hypothermia (clinical conference), *Ann Emerg Med* 11:497, 1982.
90. Carden DL, Nowak RM: Disseminated intravascular coagulation in hypothermia (letter), *JAMA* 247:2099, 1982.
91. Carden TS: Saving the hypothermic patient, *JAMA* 240:2761, 1978.
92. Carlsson C, Hagerdal M, Siesjo BK: Protective effect of hypothermia in cerebral oxygen deficiency caused by arterial hypoxia, *Anesthesiology* 44:27, 1976.
93. Carr ME, Wolfert AI: Rewarming by hemodialysis for hypothermia: failure of heparin to prevent DIC, *J Emerg Med* 6:277, 1988.
94. Casey LC et al: Development of a primate model of exposure hypothermia, *Adv Shock Res* 9:233, 1983.
95. Celestino FS, Van Noord GR, Miraglia CP: Accidental hypothermia in the elderly, *J Fam Pract* 26:259, 264, 1988.
96. Chan AW et al: Differential effects of R015-1788 in actions of chlordiazepoxide and ethanol, *Pharmacol Biochem Behav* 29:315, 1988.
97. Chang M, Gill T: Hypothermia, neurologic dysfunction, and sudden death in a man with carcinoma, *South Med J* 74:1509, 1981.
98. Chen RY, Chien S: Hemodynamic functions and blood viscosity in surface hypothermia, *Am J Physiol* 235:H136, 1978.
99. Chernow B et al: Sympathetic nervous system "switch-off" with severe hypothermia, *Crit Care Med* 11:677, 1983.
100. Chinard FP: Hypothermia treatment needs controlled studies, *Ann Intern Med* 90:990, 1979.
101. Chipman C et al: Criteria for cessation of CPR in the emergency department, *Ann Emerg Med* 10:11, 1981.
102. Clardy CW, Edwards KM, Gay JC: Increased susceptibility to infection in hypothermic children: possible role of acquired neutrophil dysfunction, *Pediatr Infect Dis* 4:379, 1985.
103. Clayton DG et al: A comparison of the performance of 20 pulse oximeters under conditions of poor perfusion, *Anaesthesia* 46:3, 1991.
104. Clements SD, Hurst JW: Diagnostic value of electrocardiographic abnormalities observed in subjects accidentally exposed to cold, *Am J Cardiol* 29:729, 1972.
105. Clemmer TP et al: Hypothermia in the sepsis syndrome and clinical outcome: the methylprednisolone severe sepsis study group, *Crit Care Med* 20:1395, 1992.
106. Coe JI: Hypothermia: autopsy findings and vitreous glucose, *J Forensic Sci* 29:389, 1984.
107. Coetzee A, Swanepoel C: The oxyhemoglobin dissociation curve before, during and after cardiac surgery, *Scand J Clin Lab Invest Suppl* 203:149, 1990.
108. Cohen DJ et al: Resuscitation of the hypothermic patient, *Am J Emerg Med* 6:475, 1988.
109. Cohen DN: Rewarming with hot packs (letter), *Am J Emerg Med* 3:371, 1985.
110. Cohen IJ et al: Thrombocytopenia of neonatal cold injury, *J Pediatr* 104:620, 1984.
111. Cohen IL et al: Endotracheal tube occlusion associated with the use of heat and moisture exchanges in the intensive care unit, *Crit Care Med* 16:277, 1988.
112. Cohen JA et al: Increased pulmonary artery perforating potential of pulmonary artery catheters during hypothermia, *J Cardiothorac Vasc Anesth* 5:235, 1991.
113. Coleshaw SR et al: Impaired memory registration and speed of reasoning caused by low body temperature, *J Appl Physiol* 55:27, 1983.
114. Collins KJ et al: Accidental hypothermia and impaired temperature homeostasis in the elderly, *Br J Med* 2:353, 1977.
115. Collins KJ, Exton-Smith AN, Dore C: Urban hypothermia: preferred temperature and thermal perception in old age, *Br Med J* 282:175, 1981.
116. Collis ML, Steinman AM, Chaney RD: Accidental hypothermia: an experimental study of practical rewarming methods, *Aviat Space Environ Med* 48:625, 1977.
117. Coniam SW: Accidental hypothermia, *Anaesthesia* 34:250, 1979.
118. Conroy JM et al: The big chill: intraoperative diagnosis and treatment of unsuspected preoperative hypothermia, *South Med J* 81:397, 1988.
119. Corey TS et al: Unnatural deaths in nursing home patients, *J Forensic Sci* 37:222, 1992.

120. Coughlin F: Heart-warming procedure, *N Engl J Med* 288:326, 1973.
121. Covino BG, Beavers WR: Changes in cardiac contractility during immersion hypothermia, *Am J Physiol* 195:433, 1958.
122. Crino MH, Nagel EL: Thermal burns caused by warming blankets in the operating room, *Anesthesiology* 29:149, 1968.
123. Cupples WA, Fox GR, Hayward JS: Effect of cold water immersion and its combination with alcohol intoxication on urine flow rate of man, *Can J Physiol Pharmacol* 58:319, 1980.
124. Curry DL, Curry KP: Hypothermia and insulin secretion, *Endocrinology* 87:750, 1970.
125. Daanen HA, Van De Linde FJ: Comparison of four noninvasive rewarming methods for mild hypothermia, *Aviat Space Environ Med* 63:1070, 1992.
126. Dagan R, Gorodischer R: Infections in hypothermic infants younger than 3 months old, *Am J Dis Child* 183:483, 1984.
127. Dahlgren BE, Nilsson HG, Viklund B: Tracheal tubes in cold stress, *Anaesthesia* 43:683, 1988.
128. Danzl DF: Accidental hypothermia. In Rosen P et al, editors: *Concepts and clinical practice,* New York, 1983, Mosby.
129. Danzl DF: Bretylium in hypothermia, *Wilderness Med* 4:5, 1987.
130. Danzl DF: Environmental thermal extremes, *Ann Emerg Med* 16:1029, 1987.
131. Danzl DF: Accidental hypothermia. In Rosen et al, editors: *Emergency medicine: concepts and clinical practice,* ed 2, St Louis, 1988, Mosby.
132. Danzl DF: Blood flow during closed chest compressions in hypothermic humans, *Wilderness Med* 7:12, 1991.
133. Danzl DF et al: Hypothermia outcome score: development and implications, *Crit Care Med* 17:227, 1989.
134. Danzl DF, O'Brien DJ: The ECG computer program: mort de froid, *J Wilderness Med* 3:328, 1992.
135. Danzl DF et al: Multicenter hypothermia survey, *Ann Emerg Med* 16:1042, 1987.
136. Danzl DF, Pozos RS, Hamlet MP: Accidental hypothermia. In Auerbach PS, Geehr EC, editors: *Management of wilderness and environmental emergencies,* ed 2, St. Louis, 1988, Mosby.
137. Danzl DF et al: Chemical ventricular defibrillation in severe accidental hypothermia, *Ann Emerg Med* 11:698, 1982.
138. Danzl DF, Thomas DM: Nasotracheal intubations in the emergency department, *Crit Care Med* 8:677, 1980.
139. Danzl DF, Vicario S, Thomas DM: Accidental hypothermia—advanced life support, *Ky Med Assoc J* 79:795, 1981.
140. Darowski A et al: Hypothermia and infection in elderly patients admitted to hospital, *Age Ageing* 20:100, 1991.
141. DaVee TS, Reineberg EJ: Extreme hypothermia and ventricular fibrillation, *Ann Emerg Med* 9:100, 1980.
142. Davidson M, Grant E: Accidental hypothermia: a community hospital perspective, *Postgrad Med* 70:42, 1981.
143. Davies DM, Millar EJ, Miller IA: Accidental hypothermia treated by extracorporeal blood-warming, *Lancet* 1:1036, 1967.
144. Davis FM, Judson JA: Warm peritoneal dialysis in the management of accidental hypothermia: report of five cases, *NZ Med J* 94:207, 1981.
145. Davis PJ, Davis FB: Hypothyroidism in the elderly, *Comp Ther* 10:17, 1984.
146. Deal CW, Warden JC, Monk I: Effects of hypothermia on lung compliance, *Thorax* 25:105, 1970.
147. Deimi R, Hess W: Successful therapy of a cardiac arrest during accidental hypothermia using extracorporeal circulation, *Anaesthesist* 41:93, 1992.
148. Deklunder G et al: Influence of ventilation of the face on thermoregulation in man during hyper- and hypothermia, *Eur J Appl Physiol* 62:342, 1991.
149. Delaney KA et al: Assessment of acid-base disturbances and their physiologic consequences, *Ann Emerg Med* 18:72, 1989.
150. DeLeeuw PW: Tale of the unexpected: hypothermia during vasodilation, *Nether J Med* 34:171, 1989.
151. DePlaen JL, Sepulchre D, Bidingija M: Paroxysmal hypertension and spontaneous periodic hypothermia, *Acta Clin Belg* 47:401, 1992.
152. DelRossi AJ et al: Heparinless extracorporeal bypass for treatment of hypothermia, *J Trauma* 30:79, 1990.
153. DeRoubaix JAM: Successful resuscitation in severe accidental hypothermia: a case report, *S Afr Med J* 57:374, 1980.
154. Desmeules H, Blais C: Hypothermie accidentelle: traitement d'un cas par irrigation peritoneale (Accidental hypothermia: treatment of a case using peritoneal irrigation), *Can Anaesth Soc J* 26:506, 1979.
155. DeSweit J: Changes simulating hypothermia in the electrocardiogram in subarachnoid hemorrhage, *J Electrocardiol* 5:193, 1972.
156. Dexter WW: Hypothermia: safe and efficient methods of rewarming the patient, *Postgrad Med* 88:55, 61, 1990.
157. Diaz JH, Cooper ES, Ochsner JL: Cold hemagglutination pathophysiology, *Arch Intern Med* 144:1639, 1984.
158. Dincsoy MY, Siddiq F, Kim YM: Intracranial hemorrhage in hypothermic low-birth-weight neonates, *Childs Nerve Syst* 6:245, 1984.
159. Doherty NE et al: Hypothermia with acute myocardial infarction, *Ann Intern Med* 101:797, 1984.
160. Doherty NE et al: Hypothermia and sepsis (letter), *Ann Intern Med* 103:308, 1985.
161. Donnan GA, Seeman E: Coma and hypothermia in Wernicke's encephalopathy, *Aust NZ J Med* 10:438, 1980.
162. Dorsey JS: Venoarterial bypass in hypothermia, *JAMA* 244:1900, 1980.
163. Drake CT, Lewis BJ: The plasma volume expanding effect of low molecular weight dextran in the hypothermic drug, *Surg Forum* 12:182, 1961.
164. Drenck NE, Staffeldt HV: Repeated deep accidental hypothermia, *Anaesthesia* 41:731, 1986.
165. Dronen S, Nowak RM, Tomlanovich MC: Bretylium tosylate and hypothermic ventricular fibrillation, *Ann Emerg Med* 9:335, 1980.
166. Duckworth WC, Cooper BC: Accidental hypothermia in the Bantu, *S Afr Med J* 38:295, 1964.
167. Duff RS et al: Spontaneous periodic hypothermia, *Q J Med* 30:329, 1961.
168. Duguid H, Simpson RG, Stowers JM: Accidental hypothermia, *Lancet* 2:1213, 1961.
169. Dula DJ: Use of IV bicarbonate in hypothermia, *JACEP* 8:48, 1979.
170. Dundee JW, Clarke RSJ: Pharmacology of hypothermia, *Int Anesth Clin* 2:857, 1964.
171. Dunne KP, Matthews TG: Hypothermia and sudden infant death syndrome, *Arch Dis Child* 63:438, 1988.
172. Easterbrook PJ, Davis HP: Thrombocytopenia in hypothermia: a common but poorly recognized complication, *Br Med J* 291:23, 1985.
173. Edelman IS: Thyroid thermogenesis, *N Engl J Med* 290:1303, 1974.
174. Edlich RF et al: Cold injuries, *Compt Ther* 15:13, 1989.
175. Edsall DW: Treatment of hypothermia (letter), *JAMA* 244:1902, 1980.
176. Edwards HA et al: Apparent death with accidental hypothermia, *Br J Anesth* 42:906, 1970.
177. Edwards RD Jr: Accidental hypothermia, *JACEP* 6:426, 1977.
178. Edwards RJ, Belyavin AJ, Harrison MH: Core temperature measurement in man, *Aviat Space Environ Med* 49:1289, 1978.
179. Ehrenkranz JRL: Urine temperature and core temperature, *JAMA* 255:1880, 1986.
180. Ehrmantraut WR, Ticktin HE, Fazekas JF: Cerebral hemodynamics and metabolism in accidental hypothermia, *Arch Intern Med* 99:57, 1957.
181. Eisenberg PR, Jaffe AS, Schuster DP: Clinical evaluation compared to pulmonary artery catheterization in the hemodynamic assessment of critically ill patients, *Crit Care Med* 12:549, 1984.
182. Elenbaas RM et al: Bretylium in hypothermia-induced ventricular fibrillation in dogs, *Ann Emerg Med* 13:994, 1984.

183. Ellis WW et al: Left ventricular dysfunction induced by cold exposure in patients with systemic sclerosis, *Am J Med* 80:385, 1986.
184. El-Radhi AS, Al-Kafaji N: Neonatal hypothermia in a developing country, *Clin Pediatr* 19:401, 1980.
185. El-Radhi AS et al: Infection in neonatal hypothermia, *Arch Dis Child* 58:143, 1983.
186. El-Radhi AS et al: Sepsis and hypothermia in the newborn infant: value of gastric aspirate examination, *J Pediatr* 103:300, 1983.
187. Emergency Cardiac Care Committee and Subcommittees: Guidelines for cardiopulmonary resuscitation and emergency cardiac care. IV. Special resuscitation situations: hypothermia, *JAMA* 268:224, 1992.
188. Emslie-Smith D: Accidental hypothermia: a common condition with a pathognomonic electrocardiogram, *Lancet* 2:492, 1958.
189. Ennemoser O, Ambach W, Flora G: Physical assessment of heat insulation rescue foils, *Int J Sports Med* 9:179, 1988.
190. Ereth MH, Lennon RL, Sessler DL: Limited heat transfer between thermal compartments during rewarming in vasoconstricted patients, *Aviat Space Environ Med* 63:1065, 1992.
191. Erickson RS, Yount ST: Effect of aluminized covers on body temperature in patients having abdominal surgery, *Heart Lung* 20:255, 1991.
192. Falk RH, Zoll PM, Zoll RH: Safety and efficacy of noninvasive cardiac pacing: a preliminary report, *N Engl J Med* 309:1166, 1983.
193. Faller JP, Rauscher M: Severe hypothermia: importance of temporary electrosystolic pacing until the end of the warming, *Nouv Presse Med* 7:3366, 1978.
194. Faries G et al: Temperature relationship to distance and flow rate of warmed IV fluids, *Ann Emerg Med* 20:1198, 1991.
195. Fedor EJ, Fischer B, Lee SH: Rewarming following hypothermia of two to twelve hours. I. Cardiovascular effects, *Ann Surg* 147:515, 1958.
196. Feldman KW, Morray JP, Schaller RT: Thermal injury caused by hot pack application in hypothermic children, *Am J Emerg Med* 3:38, 1985.
197. Felicetta JV, Green WL: Hypothermia and adrenocortical function, *Ann Intern Med* 90:855, 1979.
198. Felicetta JV, Green WL, Goodner CJ: Decreased adrenal responsiveness in hypothermic patients, *J Clin Endocrinol Metab* 50:93, 1980.
199. Fell RH et al: Severe hypothermia as a result of barbiturate overdose complicated by cardiac arrest, *Lancet* 1:392, 1968.
200. Feneley MP et al: Sequence of mitral valve motion and transmitral blood flow during manual cardiopulmonary resuscitation in dogs, *Circulation* 76:363, 1987.
201. Ferguson J, Epstein F, Van de Leuv J: Accidental hypothermia, *Emerg Med Clin N Am* 1:619, 1983.
202. Ferguson NV: Urban hypothermia, *Anaesthesia* 40:651, 1985.
203. Fernandez JP, O'Rourke RA, Ewy GA: Rapid active external rewarming in accidental hypothermia, *JAMA* 212:153, 1970.
204. Ferrara A et al: Hypothermia and acidosis worsen coagulopathy in the patient requiring massive transfusion, *Am J Surg* 160:515, 1990.
205. Ferraro FJ Jr et al: Cold-induced hypercoagulability in vitro: a trauma connection? *Am Surg* 58:355, 1992.
206. Fishbeck KH, Simon RP: Neurological manifestations of accidental hypothermia, *Ann Neurol* 10:384, 1981.
207. Fisher A et al: Oxygen availability during hypothermic cardiopulmonary bypass, *Crit Care Med* 5:154, 1977.
208. Fitzgerald FT: Hypoglycemia and accidental hypothermia in an alcoholic population, *West J Med* 133:105, 1980.
209. Fitzgerald FT, Jessop C: Accidental hypothermia: a report of 22 cases and review of the literature, *Adv Intern Med* 27:128, 1982.
210. Fitzgibbon FT, Hayward JS, Walker D: EEG and visual evoked potentials of conscious man during moderate hypothermia, *Electroencephalogr Clin Neurophysiol* 58:48, 1984.
211. Flancbaum L, Trooskin SZ, Pedersen H: Evaluation of bloodwarming devices with the apparent thermal clearance, *Ann Emerg Med* 18:355, 1989.
212. Follezou JY, Bleibel JM: Reduction of temperature and lithium poisoning, *N Engl J Med* 313:1609, 1985.
213. Foray J: Letter, *Ann Surg* 198:668, 1983.
214. Forester CF: Coma in myxedema: report of a case and review of the world literature, *Arch Intern Med* 111:734, 1963.
215. Foulis AK: Morphological study of the relation between accidental hypothermia and acute pancreatitis, *J Clin Pathol* 35:1244, 1982.
216. Fox JB et al: A retrospective analysis of air-evacuated hypothermia patients, *Aviat Space Environ Med* 59:1070, 1988.
217. Fox RH et al: Hypothermia in a young man with an anterior hypothalamic lesion, *Lancet* 2:185, 1970.
218. Fox RH et al: Spontaneous periodic hypothermia and diencephalic epilepsy, *Br Med J* 2:693, 1973.
219. Fox RH et al: Body temperatures in the elderly: a national study of physiological, social, and environmental conditions, *Br Med J* 1:200, 1973.
220. Fox RH et al: Diagnosis of hypothermia of the elderly, *Lancet* 1:424, 1971.
221. Francis TJR: Non-freezing cold injury: a historical review, *J R Nav Med Serv* 70:134, 1984.
222. Frank DH, Robson MC: Accidental hypothermia treated without mortality, *Surg Gynecol Obstet* 151:379, 1980.
223. Freinkel N et al: The hypothermia of hypoglycemia: studies with 2-deoxy-D-glucose in normal human subjects and mice, *N Engl J Med* 387:841, 1972.
224. Freinkel N et al: Alcohol hypoglycemia. I. Carbohydrate metabolism of patients with clinical alcohol hypoglycemia and the experimental reproduction of the syndrome with pure ethanol, *J Clin Invest* 42:1122, 1963.
225. Fried SJ, Satiani B, Zeeb P: Normothermic rapid volume replacement for hypovolemic shock: an in vivo and in vitro study utilizing a new technique, *J Trauma* 26:183, 1986.
226. Gale CC: Neuroendocrine aspects of thermoregulation, *Annu Rev Physiol* 35:391, 1973.
227. Gallaher MM et al: Pedestrian and hypothermia deaths among Native Americans in New Mexico: between bar and home, *JAMA* 267:1345, 1992.
228. Garry RC: Control of the temperature of the body, *Med Sci Law* 9:242, 1969.
229. Garty BZ et al: Hypernatremic dehydration and hypothermia in congenital lamellar ichthyosis, *Pediatr Derm* 3:65, 1985.
230. Gautam PC et al: Hypothermia in the elderly: sociomedical characteristics and outcome of 86 patients, *Public Health* 103:15, 1989.
231. Gautam PC et al: Hypothermia in the elderly: management in a purpose-built chamber, *Gerontology* 34:145, 1988.
232. Gayed NM: Hypothermia associated with terminal liver failure (letter), *Am J Med* 83:808, 1987.
233. Gentilello LM et al: Continuous arteriovenous rewarming: rapid reversal of hypothermia in critically ill patients, *J Trauma* 32:316, 1992.
234. Gentilello LM et al: Continuous arteriovenous rewarming: experimental results and thermodynamic model simulation of treatment for hypothermia, *J Trauma* 30:1436, 1990.
235. Gentilello LM, Rifley WJ: Continuous arteriovenous rewarming: report of a new technique for treating hypothermia, *J Trauma* 31:1151, 1991.
236. Geny C et al: Hypothermia, Wernicke's encephalopathy, and multiple sclerosis, *Acta Neurol Scand* 86:632, 1992.
237. Georgitis WJ, Hofeldt FD: Myxedema coma and cardiac arrest, *JAMA* 247:980, 1982.
238. Ghawche F, Destee A: Hypothermia and multiple sclerosis: a case with 3 episodes of transient hypothermia, *Rev Neurol (Paris)* 146:767, 1990.
239. Gibbs DM: Inhibition of corticotropin release during hypothermia: the role of corticotropin-releasing factor, vasopressin, and oxytocin, *Endocrinology* 116:723, 1985.
240. Giesbrecht GG et al: Effectiveness of three field treatments for induced mild (33.0° C) hypothermia, *J Appl Physiol* 63:2375, 1987.

241. Gillen JP et al: Ventricular fibrillation during orotracheal intubation of hypothermic dogs, *Ann Emerg Med* 15:412, 1986.
242. Glick SD, Guido RA: Naloxone antagonism of the thermoregulatory effects of phencyclidine, *Science* 217:1272, 1982.
243. Glusman A, Hasan K, Roguin N: Contraindication to thrombolytic therapy in accidental hypothermia, *Int J Cardiol* 28:269, 1990.
244. Goldberg ME et al: Do heated humidifiers and heat and moisture exchangers prevent temperature drop during lower abdominal surgery? *J Clin Anesth* 4:16, 1992.
245. Golden FStC: Recognition and treatment of immersion hypothermia, *Proc R Soc Med* 66:1058, 1973.
246. Golden FStC, Hervey GR: The mechanism of the after-drop following immersion hypothermia in pigs, *J Physiol* 272:26P, 1977.
247. Goldman A et al: A pilot study of low body temperature in old people admitted to hospital, *J R Coll Phys Lond* 11:291, 1977.
248. Gong V: Microwave warming of IV fluids in management of hypothermia, *Ann Emerg Med* 13:645, 1984.
249. Gould L et al: The Osborn wave in hypothermia, *Angiology* 36:125, 1985.
250. Graham T, Baulk K: Effect of alcohol ingestion on man's thermoregulatory responses during cold immersion, *Aviat Space Environ Med* 51:155, 1980.
251. Granberg PO: Alcohol and cold, *Arctic Med Res* 50:43, 1991.
252. Granberg PO: Human physiology under cold exposure, *Arctic Med Res* 50:23, 1991.
253. Gray HH, Smith LDR, Moore RH: Idiopathic periodic hypothermia and bizarre behaviour in the presence of occult syringomyelia, *Postgrad Med J* 62:289, 1986.
254. Greene JW, Craft L, Ghishan F: Acetaminophen poisoning in infancy, *Am J Dis Child* 137:386, 1983.
255. Green MM, Danzl DF, Praszkier H: Infrared tympanic thermography in the emergency department, *J Emerg Med* 7:437, 1989.
256. Gregory JS et al: Comparison of three methods of rewarming from hypothermia: advances of extracorporeal blood rewarming, *J Trauma* 31:1247, 1991.
257. Gregory JS et al: Incidence and timing of hypothermia in trauma patients undergoing operations, *J Trauma* 31:795, 1991.
258. Gregory RT, Doolittle WH: Accidental hypothermia. II. Clinical implications of experimental studies, *Alaska Med* 15:48, 1973.
259. Gregory RT et al: Treatment after exposure to cold, *Lancet* 1:377, 1972.
260. Grice KA, Bettley FR: Skin water loss and accidental hypothermia in psoriasis, ichthyosis, and erythroderma, *Br Med J* 4:195, 1957.
261. Grossheim RL: Hypothermia and frostbite treated with peritoneal dialysis, *Alaska Med* 15:53, 1973.
262. Guerin JM, Meyer P, Segrestaa JM: Hypothermia in diabetic ketoacidosis, *Diabetes Care* 10:801, 1987.
263. Guild WJ: Central body rewarming for hypothermia: possibilities, problems, and progress, *J R Naval Med Serv* 26:173, 1976.
264. Gutierrez G, Warley AR, Dantzker DR: Oxygen delivery and utilization in hypothermic dogs, *J Appl Physiol* 60:751, 1986.
265. Haavik PE, Dodgson M: Hypothermic circulatory arrest, *J Thorac Cardiovasc Surg* 88:1038, 1984.
266. Hall KN, Syverud SA: Closed thoracic cavity lavage in the treatment of severe hypothermia in human beings, *Ann Emerg Med* 19:204, 1990.
267. Hall KN, Syverud SA: Rewarming in severe hypothermia (letter), *Ann Emerg Med* 19:1076, 1990.
268. Hamlet MP: An overview of medically related problems in the cold environment, *Milit Med* 152:393, 1987.
269. Hamlet MP: The fluid shifts in hypothermia. In Pozos RS, Wittmers LE, editors: *The nature and treatment of hypothermia,* Minneapolis, 1983, University of Minnesota Press.
270. Hammerle AF et al: Plasma catecholamines in accidental hypothermia, *Klin Wochenschr* 92:654, 1980.
271. Haneda K et al: The importance of appropriate concentrations of inspired carbon dioxide on induced hypothermia under halothane-ether azetrope anesthesia, *J Cardiovasc Surg* 25:67, 1984.
272. Hansen JE, Sue DY: Should blood gas measurements be corrected for the patient's temperature? *N Engl J Med* 303:341, 1980.
273. Harari A et al: Haemodynamic study of prolonged deep accidental hypothermia, *Eur J Intensive Care Med* 1:65, 1975.
274. Harnett RM et al: Initial treatment of profound accidental hypothermia, *Aviat Space Environ Med* 51:680, 1980.
275. Harnett RM, Pruitt JR, Sias FR: A review of the literature concerning resuscitation from hypothermia. I. The problem and general approaches, *Aviat Space Environ Med* 54:425, 1983.
276. Harnett RM, Pruitt JR, Sias FR: A review of the literature concerning resuscitation from hypothermia. II. Selected rewarming protocols, *Aviat Space Environ Med* 54:487, 1983.
277. Hassel B: Hypothermia from erythromycin, *Ann Intern Med* 115:69, 1991.
278. Haugh RM, Markesbury WR: Hypothalamic astrocytoma: syndrome of hyperphagia, obesity, and disturbance of behavior and endocrine and autonomic function, *Arch Neurol* 40:560, 1983.
279. Hauty MG et al: Prognostic factors in severe accidental hypothermia: experience from the Mt. Hood tragedy, *J Trauma* 27:1107, 1987.
280. Hayes P: Diving and hypothermia, *Arctic Med Res* 50:37, 1991.
281. Hays RM, Jaffe KM, Ingman E: Accidental death associated with motorized wheelchair use: a case report, *Arch Phys Med Rehab* 66:709, 1985.
282. Hayward JS, Eckerson JD, Kemna D: Thermal and cardiovascular changes during three methods of resuscitation from mild hypothermia, *Resuscitation,* 11:21, 1984.
283. Hayward JS, Steinman AM: Accidental hypothermia: an experimental study of inhalation rewarming, *Aviat Space Environ Med* 46:1236, 1975.
284. Hazan J, Maag U, Chessex P: Association between hypothermia and mortality rate of premature infants—revisited, *Am J Obstet Gynecol* 164:111, 1991.
285. Hearse DJ, Yamamoto F, Shattaock MJ: Calcium antagonists and hypothermia: the temperature dependency of the negative inotropic and anti-ischemic properties of verapamil in the isolated rat heart, *Circulation* 70:I54, 1984.
286. Hector MG: Treatment of accidental hypothermia, *Am Fam Phys* 45:785, 1992.
287. Heh CW et al: Neuroleptic-induced hypothermia associated with amelioration of psychosis in schizophrenia, *Neuropsychopharmacology* 1:149, 1988.
288. Henneberg S et al: Effects of a thermal ceiling on postoperative hypothermia, *Acta Anaesth Scand* 29:602, 1985.
289. Hering JP et al: Influence of pH management on hemodynamics and metabolism in moderate hypothermia, *J Thorac Cardiovasc Surg* 104:1388, 1992.
290. Hernandez DE et al: Neurotensin-induced antinociception and hypothermia in mice: antagonism by TRH and structural analogs of TRH, *Regul Pept* 8:41, 1984.
291. Herr RD, White GL Jr: Hypothermia: threat to military operations, *Milit Med* 156:140, 1991.
292. Hersio K et al: Changes in whole body and tissue oxygen consumption during recovery from hypothermia: effect of amino acid infusion, *Crit Care Med* 19:503, 1991.
293. Hervey GR: Physiological changes encountered in hypothermia, *Proc R Soc Med* 66:1053, 1973.
294. Hesslink RL Jr et al: Radio frequency (13.56 MHz) energy enhances recovery from mild hypothermia, *J Appl Physiol* 67:1208, 1989.
295. Higano ST et al: The mechanism of blood flow during closed chest cardiac massage in humans: transesophageal echocardiographic observations, *Mayo Clin Proc* 65:1432, 1990.
296. Hill JG et al: Emergency applications of cardiopulmonary support: a multiinstitutional experience, *Ann Thorac Surg* 54:699, 1992.

297. Himms-Hagen J: Thermogenesis in brown adipose tissue as an energy buffer, *N Engl J Med* 311:1549, 1984.
298. Hindsholm KB et al: Reflective blankets used for reduction of heat loss during regional anesthesia, *Br J Anaesth* 68:531, 1992.
299. Hirvonen J, Huttunen P: Necropsy findings in fatal hypothermia cases, *Forensic Sci* 8:155, 1976.
300. Hirvonen J, Huttunen P: Increased urinary concentration of catecholamines in hypothermia deaths, *J Forensic Sci* 27:264, 1982.
301. Hochachka PW: Defense strategies against hypoxia and hypothermia, *Science* 231:234, 1986.
302. Hodgdon JA et al: Norwegian military field exercises in the Arctic: cognitive and physical performance, *Arctic Med Res* 50:123, 1991.
303. Holland BM et al: New insulating material in maintenance of body temperature, *Arch Dis Child* 60:47, 1985.
304. Holm IA et al: Recurrent hypothermia and thrombocytopenia after severe neonatal brain infection, *Clin Pediatr* 27:326, 1988.
305. Holmer I: Assessment of cold stress, *Arctic Med Res* 50:83, 1991.
306. Holmer I: Resultant clothing insulation during exercise in the cold, *Arctic Med Res* 50:94, 1991.
307. Holoday JW, Fadel AI: Naloxone acts at central opiate receptors to reverse hypotension, hypothermia, and hypoventilation in spinal shock, *Brain Res* 189:295, 1980.
308. Holvey DN et al: Treatment of myxedema coma with intravenous thyroxine, *Arch Intern Med* 113:89, 1964.
309. Hudson LD, Conn RD: Accidental hypothermia: associated diagnoses and prognosis in a common problem, *JAMA* 227:37, 1974.
310. Huet RCG, Harkliczek GF, Coad NR: Pupil size and light reactivity in hypothermic infants and adults (letter), *Intensive Care Med* 15:216, 1989.
311. Husby P et al: Accidental hypothermia with cardiac arrest: complete recovery after prolonged resuscitation and rewarming by extracorporeal circulation, *Intensive Care Med* 16:69, 1990.
312. Husby P et al: Deep accidental hypothermia with asystole: a successful treatment with heart-lung machine after prolonged cardiopulmonary resuscitation, *Tidsskr Nor Laegeforen* 111:183, 1991.
313. Hypothermia prevention, *MMWR* 37:780, 1988.
314. Ilia R et al: Atypical ventricular tachycardia and alternating Osborn waves induced by spontaneous mild hypothermia, *Pediatr Cardiol* 9:63, 1988.
315. Imon H et al: Optimal pH and $Pa{CO_2}$ during moderate hypothermia, *Jpn J Anesthesiol* 41:603, 1992.
316. Iserson KV, Huestis DW: Blood warming: current applications and techniques, *Transfusion* 31:558, 1991.
317. Iversen RJ et al: Successful CPR in a severely hypothermic patient using continuous thoracostomy lavage, *Ann Emerg Med* 19:1335, 1990.
318. Iwasaka H et al: Heat conservation during abdominal surgery, *Masui* 41:666, 1992.
319. Iyengar J, Bhakoo ON: Prevention of neonatal hypothermia in Himalayan villages: role of the domiciliary caretaker, *Trop Geogr Med* 43:293, 1991.
320. Jacob AI et al: A-V block in accidental hypothermia, *J Electrocardiol* 11:399, 1978.
321. Jadhon ME, Main EK: Fetal bradycardia associated with maternal hypothermia, *Obstet Gynecol* 72:496, 1988.
322. Jaffe N: Hypothermia: a diagnostic aid to hypoglycemia, *S Afr Med J* 40:569, 1966.
323. Jessen K: Immersion and accidental hypothermia, *Acta Med Port* 2:225, 1979.
324. Jessen K, Hagelsten JO: Search and rescue service in Denmark with special reference to accidental hypothermia, *Aerospace Med* 43:787, 1972.
325. Jessen K, Hagelsten JO: Peritoneal dialysis in the treatment of profound accidental hypothermia, *Aviat Space Environ Med* 49:426, 1978.
326. Johansson BW: The hibernator heart: nature's model of resistance to ventricular fibrillation, *Arctic Med Res* 50:58, 1991.
327. Johnson DE, Gamble WB: Trauma in the arctic: an incident report, *J Trauma* 31:1340, 1991.
328. Johnson DG et al: Plasma norepinephrine responses of man in cold water, *J Appl Physiol* 43:216, 1977.
329. Johnson LA: Accidental hypothermia: peritoneal dialysis, *JACEP* 6:556, 1977.
330. Johnson MH, Jones SN: Status epilepticus, hypothermia and metabolic chaos in a man with agenesis of the corpus callosum, *J Neurol Neurosurg Psychiatry* 48:480, 1985.
331. Johnston WE et al: Management of cold urticaria during hypothermic cardiopulmonary bypass, *N Engl J Med* 306:219, 1982.
332. Jolly BT, Ghezzi KT: Accidental hypothermia, *Emerg Med Clin North Am* 10:311, 1992.
333. Jones DR et al: The successful resuscitation of a hypothermic multitrauma patient, *W Va Med J* 87:298, 1991.
334. Jorge IC et al: A prospective randomized comparison between open and closed peritoneal lavage techniques, *J Trauma* 30:880, 1990.
335. Jung M et al: Hypothermia in Hodgkin's disease after exploratory laparotomy, *Klin Wochenschr* 66:552, 1988.
336. Jurkovich GJ et al: Hypothermia in trauma victims: an ominous predictor of survival, *J Trauma* 27:1019, 1987.
337. Kalant H, Le AD: Effects of ethanol on thermoregulation, *Pharmacol Ther* 23:313, 1984.
338. Kallenback J et al: Experience with acute poisoning in an intensive care unit: a review of 103 cases, *S Afr Med J* 59:587, 1981.
339. Kallman H: Protecting your elderly patient from winter's cold, *Geriatrics* 40:69, 1985.
340. Kanter GS: Renal clearance of sodium and potassium in hypothermia, *Can J Biochem Physiol* 40:113, 1962.
341. Kanter GS: Regulation of extracellular potassium in hypothermia, *Am J Physiol* 205:1285, 1963.
342. Kanter GS: Hypothermic hemoconcentration, *Am J Physiol* 214:856, 1968.
343. Kaplan M, Eidelman AI: Improved prognosis in severely hypothermic newborn infants treated by rapid rewarming, *J Pediatr* 105:470, 1984.
344. Kashuk JL et al: Major abdominal vascular trauma: a unified approach, *J Trauma* 22:672, 1982.
345. Kaufman JW, Bagian JP: Insidious hypothermia during raft use, *Aviat Space Environ* Med 61:569, 1990.
346. Kayser C: Physiological aspects of hypothermia, *Annu Rev Physiol* 19:83, 1957.
347. Kearsley JH, Musso AF: Hypothermia and coma in the Wernicke-Korsakoff syndrome, *Med J Aust* 2:504, 1980.
348. Keatinge WR: *Survival in cold water,* Oxford, Eng, 1969, Blackwell Scientific.
349. Keatinge WR: Accidental immersion hypothermia and drowning, *Practitioner* 219:183, 1977.
350. Keatinge WR: Hypothermia at sea, *Med Sci Law* 24:160, 1984.
351. Keatinge WR: Hypothermia: dead or alive? (editorial), *Br Med J* 302:3, 1991.
352. Keatinge WR et al: Increases in platelet and red cell counts, blood viscosity, and arterial pressure during mild surface cooling: factors in mortality from coronary and cerebral thrombosis in winter, *Br Med J* 289:1405, 1984.
353. Keeney RD et al: Evaluation of an infrared tympanic membrane thermometer in pediatric patients, *Pediatrics* 85:854, 1990.
354. Keilson L et al: Screening for hypothermia in the ambulatory elderly: the Maine experience, *JAMA* 254:1781, 1985.
355. Kelly JW, Dowling JP: Pernio: a possible association with chronic myelomonocytic leukemia, *Arch Dermatol* 121:1048, 1985.
356. Kelman GR, Nunn JF: Nomograms for correction of blood Po_2, Pco_2, pH and base excess for time and temperature, *J Appl Physiol* 21:1484, 1966.
357. Kennedy WL: Letter, *Ann Intern Med* 90:721, 1980.

358. Keykhah MM et al: Reduction of the cerebral protective effect of hypothermia by oligemic hypotension during hypoxia in the rat, *Stroke* 13:171, 1982.
359. Kiley JP, Eldridge FL, Millhorn DE: Respiration during hypothermia: effect of rewarming intermediate areas of ventral medulla, *J Appl Physiol* 59:1423, 1985.
360. Kinzinger R, Risse M, Puschel K: Irrational behavior in exposure to cold: paradoxical undressing in hypothermia, *Arch Kriminol* 187:47, 1991.
361. Kiuchi M, Kimura Y: unusual intravascular hemolysis in a case of fatal hypothermia, *Am J Forensic Med Pathol* 13:222, 1992.
362. Klarskov P, Amter F: Hypothermia after submersion: correction with peritoneal dialysis, *Ugeskr Laeger* 138:1937, 1976.
363. Klinge U et al: Hypothermia and polytrauma: a case report (28° C), *Anasth Intensivther Notfallmed* 25:436, 1990.
364. Kniffen FJ, Lomas TE, Cohnsell RE: The antiarrhythmic and antifibrillatory actions of bretylium and its o-iodobenzyl trimethylammonium analog, *J Pharmacol Exp Ther* 192:120, 1975.
365. Kobrin VI: Spontaneous ventricular defibrillation in hypothermia, *Kardiologiia* 31:19, 1991.
366. Kochar G, Kahn SE, Kotler MN: Bretylium tosylate and ventricular fibrillation in hypothermia (letter), *Ann Intern Med* 105:624, 1986.
367. Koht A, Cane R, Cerullo LJ: Serum potassium levels during prolonged hypothermia, *Intensive Care Med* 9:275, 1983.
368. Kollar DJ: Cerebral resuscitation by use of verapamil in a victim of near drowning, *Am J Emerg Med* 2:148, 1984.
369. Kolodzik PW et al: The effects of antishock trouser inflation during hypothermic cardiovascular depression in the canine model, *Am J Emerg Med* 6:584, 1988.
370. Kopf GS, Mirvis DM, Myers RE: Central nervous system tolerance to cardiac arrest during profound hypothermia, *J Surg Res* 18:29, 1975.
371. Koren G et al: Effect of hypothermia on the pharmacokinetics of ethanol in piglets, *Ann Emerg Med* 18:118, 1989.
372. Kortelainen ML: Drugs and alcohol in hypothermia and hyperthermia related deaths: a retrospective study, *J Forensic Sci* 32:1704, 1987.
373. Kramer MR, Vandijk J, Rosin AJ: Mortality in elderly patients with thermoregulatory failure, *Arch Intern Med* 149:1521, 1989.
374. Kristensen G, Drenck NE, Jordening H: A simple system for central rewarming of hypothermic patients, *Lancet* 2:1467, 1986.
375. Kristensen G et al: An oesophageal thermal tube for rewarming in hypothermia, *Acta Anaesthesiol Scand* 29:846, 1985.
376. Kristjanson MR, Bristow GK: Resuscitation from hypothermia-induced cardiac arrest, *Can Med Assoc J* 142:741, 1990.
377. Kroncke GM et al: Ectothermic philosophy of acid-base balance to prevent fibrillation during hypothermia, *Arch Surg* 121:303, 1986.
378. Krook G: Hypothermia in patients with exfoliative dermatitis, *Acta Derm Venereol* 40:142, 1960.
379. Kugelberg J et al: Treatment of accidental hypothermia, *Scand J Thorac Cardiovasc Surg* 1:142, 1967.
380. Kugler SL et al: Hypothermia and systemic lupus erythematosus, *J Rheumatol* 17:680, 1991.
381. Kulkarni P et al: Clinical evaluation of the oesophageal heat exchanger in the prevention of perioperative hypothermia, *Br J Anaesth* 70:216, 1993.
382. Kuo CS et al: Characteristics and possible mechanisms of ventricular arrhythmias dependent on the dispersion of action potential durations, *Circulation* 67:1356, 1983.
383. Kurskall MS et al: Evaluation of a blood warmer that utilizes a 40° C heat exchange, *Transfusion* 30:7, 1990.
384. Lacoutre PG, Lovejoy FH, Mitchell AA: Acute hypothermia associated with atropine, *Am J Dis Child* 137:291, 1983.
385. Lafferty JJ et al: Cerebral hypometabolism obtained with deep pentobarbital anesthesia and hypothermia (30° C), *Anesthesiology* 49:159, 1978.
386. Lamb FS, Rosner MS: Neonatal resuscitation, *Emerg Med Clin North Am* 5:541, 1987.
387. Lammens M, Lissoir F, Carton H: Hypothermia in three patients with multiple sclerosis, *Clin Neurol Neurosurg* 91:117, 1989.
388. Lanska D, Harsch HH: Hypothermic coma associated with thioridazine in a myxedematous patient (letter), *J Clin Psychiatry* 45:188, 1984.
389. Larrey DJ: Memoirs of Baron Larrey: surgeon. In *Chief of the grand armee,* London, 1961, Henry Renshaw (Translated by Lero-Dupre, La).
390. Larson MD et al: Isoflurane, but not mild hypothermia, depresses the human pupillary light reflex, *Anesthesiology* 75:62, 1991.
391. Lash RF, Burdete JA, Ozdil T: Accidental profound hypothermia and barbiturate intoxication: report of rapid "core" rewarming by peritoneal dialysis, *JAMA* 201:269, 1967.
392. Laub GW et al: Percutaneous cardiopulmonary bypass for the treatment of hypothermic circulatory collapse, *Ann Thorac Surg* 47:608, 1989.
393. Lauri T et al: Cardiac function in hypothermia, *Arctic Med Res* 50:63, 1991.
394. Leaman PL, Martyak GG: Microwave warming of resuscitation fluids, *Ann Emerg Med* 14:876, 1985.
395. Ledingham IM et al: Central rewarming system for treatment of hypothermia, *Lancet* 1:1168, 1980.
396. Ledingham IM, Mone JG: Treatment after exposure to cold, *Lancet* 1:534, 1972.
397. Ledingham IM, Mone JG: Treatment of accidental hypothermia: a prospective clinical study, *Br Med J* 280:1102, 1980.
398. Lee HA, Ames AC: Hemodialysis in severe barbiturate poisoning, *Br Med J* 1:1217, 1965.
399. Lennon RL et al: Evaluation of a forced-air system for warming hypothermic postoperative patients, *Anesth Analg* 70:424, 1990.
400. Leppaluoto J: Cold as a disabling factor in northern countries, *Arctic Med Res* 37:10, 1984.
401. Letsou GV et al: Is cardiopulmonary bypass effective for treatment of hypothermic arrest due to drowning or exposure?, *Arch Surg* 127:525, 1992.
402. Levitt MA et al: A comparative rewarming trial of gastric versus peritoneal lavage in a hypothermic model, *Am J Emerg Med* 8:285, 1990.
403. Levy LA: Severe hypophosphatemia as a complication of the treatment of hypothermia, *Arch Intern Med* 140:128-129, 1980.
404. Lewin S, Brettman LR, Holzman RS: Infections in hypothermic patients, *Arch Intern Med* 141:920, 1981.
405. Lewitt PA et al: Episodic hyperhidrosis, hypothermia, and agenesis of the corpus callosum, *Neurology* 33:1122, 1983.
406. Lexow K: Severe accidental hypothermia: survival after 6 hours 30 minutes of cardiopulmonary resuscitation, *Arctic Med Res* 50:112, 1991.
407. Lieh-Lai MW et al: Metabolism and pharmacokinetics of acetaminophen in a severely poisoned young child, *J Pediatr* 105:125, 1984.
408. Lilly JK, Boland JP, Zekan S: Urinary bladder temperature monitoring: a new index of body core temperature, *Crit Care Med* 8:742, 1980.
409. Linko K, Honkavaara P, Nieminen MT: Heated humidification in major abdominal surgery, *Eur J Anaesthesiol* 1:285, 1984.
410. Linning PE, Skulberg A, Abyholm F: Accidental hypothermia: review of the literature, *Acta Anaesthesiol Scand* 30:601, 1986.
411. Linton AL, Ledingham IM: Severe hypothermia with barbiturate intoxication, *Lancet* 1:24, 1966.
412. Little RA, Stoner HB: Body temperature after accidental injury, *Br J Surg* 68:221, 1981.
413. Livingston JH, Groggins RC: Clinical curio: hypothermia caused by treatment of a scald, *Br Med J* 228:771, 1984.
414. Lloyd EL: Hypothermia: the cause of death after rescue, *Alaska Med* 26:74, 1984.
415. Lloyd EL: Death in winter, *Lancet* 2:1434, 1985.

416. Lloyd EL: *Hypothermia and cold stress,* Rockville, Md, 1986, Aspen.
417. Lloyd EL: Treatment of accidental hypothermia with the Clinitron bed (letter), *Anaesthesia* 42:1121, 1987.
418. Lloyd EL: Hypothermia in the elderly, *Med Sci Law* 28:107, 1988.
419. Lloyd EL: Hypothesis: temperature recommendations for elderly people: are we wrong? *Age Ageing* 19:264, 1990.
420. Lloyd EL: Equipment for airway warming in the treatment of accidental hypothermia, *J Wilderness Med* 2:330, 1991.
421. Lloyd EL: The cause of death after rescue, *Int J Sports Med* Oct 13 Suppl 1:S196, 1992.
422. Lloyd EL et al: Accidental hypothermia: an apparatus for central rewarming as a first aid measure, *Scot Med J* 17:83, 1972.
423. Lloyd EL, Croxten D: Equipment for the provision of airway rewarming in the treatment of accidental hypothermia in patients, *Resuscitation* 9:61, 1981.
424. Lloyd EL, Frankland JC: Accidental hypothermia: central rewarming in the field, *Br Med J* 4:717, 1984.
425. Lloyd EL, Mitchell B: Factors affecting the onset of ventricular fibrillation in hypothermia, *Lancet* 2:1294, 1974.
426. Lloyd JR, Olsen RG: Radio frequency energy for rewarming of cold extremities, *Undersea Biomed Res* 19:199, 1992.
427. Locher T et al: Accidental hypothermia in Switzerland (1980-1987): case reports and prognostic factors, *Schweiz Med Wochenschr* 121:1020, 1991.
428. Long WB: Cardiopulmonary bypass for rewarming profound hypothermia patients: critical decisions in hypothermia, Annual International Forum, Portland, Ore, Feb 28, 1992.
429. Lucas SK, Schiff HV, Flaherty JT: The harmful effects of ventricular distention during postischemic reperfusion, *Ann Thorac Surg* 32:486, 1981.
430. Ludwig S, Warman M: Shaken baby syndrome: a review of 20 cases, *Ann Emerg Med* 13:104, 1984.
431. Luna GK et al: Incidence and effect of hypothermia in seriously injured patients, *J Trauma* 27:1014, 1987.
432. Lyen KR: Cold stress and congenital adrenal hyperplasia heterozygotes, *Med Hypoth* 12:77, 1983.
433. Lynch HF, Doph EF: Blood flow in small blood vessels during deep hypothermia, *J Appl Physiol* 11:192, 1957.
434. Maaravi AY, Weiss AT: The effect of prolonged hypothermia on cardiac function in a young patient with accidental hypothermia, *Chest* 98:1017, 1990.
435. Macaron C, Feero S, Goldflies M: Hypothermia in Wernicke's encephalopathy, *Post Med* 65(2):241, 1979.
436. MacDonell JE, Wrenn K: Hypothermia in the summer, *South Med J* 84:804, 1991.
437. Macey SM: Hypothermia and energy conservation: a trade off for elderly persons? *Int J Aging Hum Dev* 29:151, 1989.
438. MacGregor DC et al: The effects of ether, ethanol, propranolol, and butanol on tolerance to deep hypothermia, *Dis Chest* 50:523, 1966.
439. MacKenzie MA et al: Effects of steady hypothermia and normothermia on the electrocardiogram in human poikilothermia, *Arctic Med Res* 50:67, 1991.
440. Mackowiak PA, Wasserman SS, Levine MM: A critical appraisal of 98.6° F, the upper limit of the normal body temperature, and other legacies of Carl Reinhold August Wunderlich, *JAMA* 268:1578, 1992.
441. Maclean D, Emslie-Smith D: *Accidental hypothermia,* Philadelphia, 1977, JB Lippincott.
442. Maclean D, Murison J, Griffiths PD: Acute pancreatitis and diabetic ketoacidosis in hypothermia, *Br Med J* 2:59, 1974.
444. Maclean D, Murison J, Griffiths PD: Serum enzyme activities in accidental hypothermia and hypothermic myxoedema, *Clin Chim Acta* 52:197, 1974.
445. Maclean D, Taig DR, Emslie-Smith D: Achilles tendon reflex in accidental hypothermia and hypothermia myxoedema, *Br Med J* 2:87, 1973.
446. Macmillan AL et al: Temperature regulation in survivors of accidental hypothermia in the elderly, *Lancet* 2:165, 1967.
447. Madsen LP: Acute alcohol intoxication in children: diagnosis, treatment and complications, *Ugeskr Laeger* 152:2362, 1990.
448. Mahajan AL, Myers TJ, Baldini MG: Disseminated intravascular coagulation during rewarming following hypothermia, *JAMA* 245:2517, 1981.
449. Maningas PA et al: Regional blood flow during hypothermic arrest, *Ann Emerg Med* 15:390, 1986.
450. Mann MW, Degos JD: Hypothermia in Wernicke's encephalopathy, *Rev Neurol (Paris)* 143:684, 1987.
451. Mant AK: Autopsy diagnosis of accidental hypothermia, *J Forensic Med* 16:126, 1969.
452. Marcus P: Laboratory comparison of techniques for rewarming hypothermic casualties, *Aviat Space Environ Med* 49:692, 1978.
453. Marcus P, Edwards R: Serum enzyme levels during experimental hypothermia in man, *Q J Exp Physiol* 63:371, 1978.
454. Maresca L, Vasko JS: Treatment of hypothermia by extracorporeal circulation and internal rewarming, *J Trauma* 27:89, 1987.
455. Marruecos L et al: Clonidine overdose, *Crit Care Med* 11:959, 1983.
456. Martens P: Rewarming by extracorporeal circulation, *Intensive Care Med* 16:342, 1990.
457. Martin TG: Near drowning and cold water immersion, *Ann Emerg Med* 13:263, 1984.
458. Martinez-Lopez JI: Induced hypothermia: electrocardiographic abnormalities, *South Med J* 69:1548, 1976.
459. Martyn JW: Diagnosing and treating hypothermia, *Can Med Assoc J* 125:1089, 1981.
460. Matsuzaki M, Casella GA, Ratner M: Delta 9-tetrahydrocannabinol: EEG changes, bradycardia and hypothermia in the rhesus monkey, *Brain Res Bull* 19:223, 1987.
461. Matthews AJ, Stead AL, Abbott TR: Acid-base control during hypothermia, *Anaesthesia* 39:649, 1984.
462. Maughan RJ, Leiper JB, Thompson J: Rectal temperature after marathon running, *Br J Sports Med* 19:192, 1985.
463. Mazala M, Horrow JR, Storella RJ: Hypothermia and the action of neuromuscular blocking agents (letter), *Anaesthesia* 43:162, 1988.
464. McCallum AL: Update on trauma care in Canada: trauma and hypothermia, *Can J Surg* 33:457, 1990.
465. McDonald JL: Coarse ventricular fibrillation presenting as asystole or very low amplitude ventricular fibrillation, *Crit Care Med* 10:790, 1982.
466. McLennan JG, Ungersma J: Mountaineering accidents in the Sierra Nevada, *Am J Sports Med* 11:160, 1983.
467. McMillan IRK et al: Hypothermia: some observations on blood gas and electrolyte changes during surface cooling, *Ann R Coll Surg Engl* 16:186, 1955.
468. Mecklenburg RS et al: Hypothalamic dysfunction in patients with anorexia nervosa, *Medicine* 53:147, 1974.
469. Menard MR, Hahn G: Acute and chronic hypothermia in a man with spinal cord injury: environmental and pharmacologic causes, *Arch Phys Med Rehabil* 72:421, 1991.
470. Mercer JB: The shivering response in animal and man, *Arctic Med Res* 50:18, 1991.
471. Meriwether WD, Goodman RM: Severe accidental hypothermia with survival after rapid rewarming, *Am J Med* 53:505, 1972.
472. Meyer DM, Horton JW: Effect of moderate hypothermia in the treatment of canine hemorrhagic shock, *Ann Surg* 207:462, 1988.
473. Michenfelder JD, Milde JH: Failure of prolonged hypocapnia, hypothermia, or hypotension to favorably alter acute stroke in primates, *Stroke* 8:87, 1977.
474. Michenfelder JD, Milde JH: The relationship among canine brain temperature, metabolism, and function during hypothermia, *Anesthesiology* 75:130, 1991.
475. Miles JM, Thompson GR: Treatment of severe accidental hypothermia using the Clinitron bed, *Anesthesia* 42:415, 1987.

476. Miller JW, Danzl DF: Accidental hypothermia: a survivor of 12 episodes, *J Emerg Med* 1:407, 1984.
477. Miller JW, Danzl DF, Thomas DM: Urban accidental hypothermia: 135 cases, *Ann Emerg Med* 9:456, 1980.
478. Miller JW, Danzl DF, Thomas DM: Hypothermia treatment, *Ann Emerg Med* 10:396, 1981.
479. Mills WJ Jr: Field care of the hypothermic patient, *Int J Sports Med* Oct 13 Suppl 1:S199, 1992.
480. Mills WJ Jr: Summary of treatment of cold injury patient, *Alaska Med* 15:56, 1973.
481. Mills WJ Jr: Frostbite, *Alaska Med* 15:27, 1973.
482. Mills WJ Jr: Accidental hypothermia: management approach, *Alaska Med* 22:9, 1980.
483. Miyake T et al: Second report of an experimental study of cerebrocardiopulmonary resuscitation (CPR) in dogs with reference to a new continuous brain cooling method, using a Resusci Pump TM-1, *Resuscitation* 12:9, 1984.
484. Mizgala L, Lao TT, Hannah ME: Hypothyroidism presenting as hypothermia following pre-eclampsia at 23 weeks gestation: case report and review of the literature, *Br J Obstet Gynaecol* 98:221, 1991.
485. Moddeman G: The elderly surgical patient: a high risk for hypothermia, *AORN J* 53:1270, 1991.
486. Molina JE et al: Brain damage in profound hypothermia: Perfusion versus circulatory arrest, *J Thorac Cardiovasc Surg* 87:596, 1984.
487. Mooradian AD et al: Spontaneous periodic hypothermia, *Neurology* 34:79, 1984.
488. Moore EE, Good JT: Mixed venous and arterial pH: a comparison during hemorrhagic shock and hypothermia, *Ann Emerg Med* 11:300, 1982.
489. Moritz AR, Henriques FC, McLean R: The effects of inhaled heat on the air passages and lungs: an experimental investigation, *Am J Pathol* 21:311, 1945.
490. Morris DL et al: Hemodynamic characteristics of patients with hypothermia due to occult infection and other causes, *Ann Intern Med* 102:153, 1985.
491. Morris DL, Jande MA: Diagnosis of sepsis in the hypothermic patient, *J Clin Res* 30:519A, 1982.
492. Morrison JB, Conn ML, Hayward JS: Thermal increment provided by inhalation rewarming from hypothermia, *J Appl Physiol* 46:1061, 1979.
493. Morrison JB, Conn ML, Hayes PA: Influence of respiratory heat transfer on thermogenesis and heat storage after cold immersion, *Clin Sci* 63:127, 1982.
494. Morrison JB, Conn ML, Hayward JS: Accidental hypothermia: the effect of initial body temperatures and physique on the rate of rewarming, *Aviat Space Environ Med* 51:1095, 1980.
495. Moss J: Accidental severe hypothermia, *Surg Gynecol Obstet* 162:501, 1986.
496. Moss JF et al: A model for the treatment of accidental severe hypothermia, *J Trauma* 26:68, 1986.
497. Motin J et al: L'hypothermie accidentelle au cours des intoxications par less neuroleptiques et les tranquillis sants, *Lyon Med* 230:53, 1973.
498. Mouritzen CV, Anderson MN: Myocardial temperature gradients and ventricualr fibrillation during hypothermia, *J Thorac Cardiovasc Surg* 49:937, 1965.
499. Muma BK et al: Comparison of rectal, axillary and tympanic membrane temperatures in infants and young children, *Ann Emerg Med* 20:41, 1991.
500. Murphy K, Nowak RM, Tomlanovich MC: Use of bretylium tosylate as prophylaxis and treatment in hypothermic ventricular fibrillation in the canine model, *Ann Emerg Med* 15:1160, 1986.
501. Murphy MT, Lipton JM: Effects of alcohol on thermoregulation in aged monkeys, *Exp Gerontol* 18:19, 1983.
502. Murray BJ: Severe lactic acidosis and hypothermia, *West J Med* 134:162, 1981.
503. Musacchia XJ: Comparative physiological and biochemical aspects of hypothermia as a model for hibernation, *Cryobiology* 21:583, 1984.
504. Myers RA, Britten JS, Cowley RA: Hypothermia: quantitative aspects of therapy, *JACEP* 8:523, 1979.
505. Nahun LH, Phillips R: The effect of hypothermia on digitalis intoxication, *Conn Med* 23:568, 1959.
506. Nayha S: Autumn and suicide in northern Finland, *Arctic Med Res* 37:25, 1984.
507. Nayha S: The cold season and deaths in Finland, *Arctic Med Res* 37:20, 1984.
508. Neil HA, Dawson JA, Baker JE: Risk of hypothermia in elderly patients with diabetes, *Br Med J* 293:416, 1986.
509. Nelson MJ, Steele MT, Robinson WA: *Use of the Bair Hugger in the emergency department treatment of moderate to severe accidental hypothermia,* 8th Annual Scientific Meeting of the Wilderness Medical Society, Sept 20, 1992.
510. Nesemann ME et al: Asystolic cardiac arrest in hypothermia, *Wisc Med J* 82:19, 1983.
511. Neufer PD et al: Influence of skeletal muscle glycogen on passive rewarming after hypothermia, *J Appl Physiol* 65:805, 1988.
512. Niazi SA, Lewis FJ: Profound hypothermia in man: report of a case, *Ann Surg* 147:264, 1958.
513. Nicholson RW, Iserson KV: Core temperature measurement in hypovolemic resuscitation, *Ann Emerg Med* 20:262, 1991.
514. Nicodemus HF, Chaney RD, Herold R: Hemodynamic effects of inotropes during hypothermia and rapid rewarming, *Crit Care Med* 93:325, 1981.
515. Nielsen HK et al: Hypothermic patients admitted to an intensive care unit: a fifteen year survey, *Dan Med Bull* 39:190, 1992.
516. Nielson KC, Owman C: Control of ventricular fibrillation during induced hypothermia in cats after blocking the adrenergic neurons with bretylium, *Life Sci* 7:159, 1968.
517. Niemann JT et al: Blood flow without cardiac compression during closed chest CPR, *Crit Care Med* 9:380, 1981.
518. Niemann JT et al: Pressure synchronized cineangiography during experimental cardiopulmonary resuscitation, *Circulation* 64:985, 1981.
519. Niemann JT, Rosborough JP, Petikan P: Hemodynamic determinants of subdiaphragmatic venous return during closed-chest CPR in a canine cardiac arrest model, *Ann Emerg Med* 19:1232, 1990.
520. Nolan TE, Gallup DG: Massive transfusion: a recurrent review, *Obstet Gynecol Surv* 46:289, 1991.
521. Nordrehaug JE: Sustained ventricular fibrillation in deep accidental hypothermia, *Br Med J* 284:867, 1982.
522. Nose H: Transvascular fluid shift and redistribution of blood in hypothermia, *Jpn J Physiol* 32:831, 1982.
523. Noto T et al: Hypothermia caused by antipsychotic drugs in a schizophrenic patient, *J Clin Psychiatry* 48:77, 1987.
524. Nozaki R et al: Accidental profound hypothermia (letter), *N Engl J Med* 315:1680, 1986.
525. Nugent SK, Rogers MC: Resuscitation and intensive care monitoring following immersion hypothermia, *J Trauma* 20:814, 1980.
526. O'Brien H, Amess JA, Mollin DR: Recurrent thrombocytopenia, erythroid hypoplasia, and sideroblastic anemia associated with hypothermia, *Br J Haematol* 51:451, 1982.
527. O'Bryne P et al: Treatment of severe accidental hypothermia with a simple extracorporeal circuit, *Agressologie* 30:541, 1989.
528. O'Connor JP: The treatment of profound hypothermia with peritoneal dialysis, *Perit Dial Bull* 2:171, 1982.
529. O'Connor JP: Use of peritoneal dialysis in severely hypothermic patients, *Ann Emerg Med* 15:104, 1986.
530. O'Connor JV et al: The protective effect of profound hypothermia on the canine central nervous system during one hour of circulatory arrest, *Ann Thorac Surg* 41:255, 1986.
531. Okada M: The cardiac rhythm in accidental hypothermia, *J Electrocardiol* 17:123, 1984.

532. Okada M, Nishimura F: Respiratory function and acid-base status in accidental hypothermia assessed by arterial blood gas analysis, *Jpn J Med* 29:500, 1990.
533. O'Keeffe KM: Accidental hypothermia: a reviw of 62 cases, *JACEP* 6:491, 1977.
534. O'Keeffe KM: Treatment of accidental hypothermia and rewarming techniques. In Roberts JR, Hedges JR, editors: *Clinical procedures in emergency medicine*, Philadelphia, 1985, WB Saunders.
535. Oliver E, Miller JD, Norman JN: Steroids in secondary drowning (letter), *Lancet* 1:105, 1978.
536. Olsen RG: Reduced temperature afterdrop in rhesus monkeys with radio frequency rewarming, *Aviat Space Environ Med* 59:79, 1988.
537. Olsen RG, David TD: Hypothermia and electromagnetic rewarming in the rehesus monkey, *Aviat Space Environ Med* 55:1111, 1984.
538. O'Marcaigh AS et al: Cessation of unsuccessful pediatric resuscitation—how long is too long? *Mayo Clin Proc* 68:332, 1993.
539. Opstad PK, Bahr R: Reduced set point temperature in young men after prolonged strenuous exercise combined with sleep and energy deficiency, *Arctic Med Res* 6:122, 1991.
540. Orlowski JP et al: Hypothermia and barbiturate coma for refractory status epilepticus, *Crit Care Med* 12:367, 1984.
541. Orts A et al: Bretylium tosylate and electrically induced cardiac arrhythmias during hypothermia in dogs, *Am J Emerg Med* 10:311, 1992.
542. Osborn JJ: Experimental hypothermia respiratory and blood pH changes in relation to cardiac function, *Am J Physiol* 175:389, 1953.
543. Osborne L, Kamal El-Din AS, Smith JE: Survival after prolonged cardiac arrest and accidental hypothermia, *Br Med J* 289:881, 1984.
544. Osterman AL et al: Muscle ischemia and hypothermia: a bioenergetic study using "phosphorus nuclear magnetic resonance spectroscopy," *J Trauma* 24:811, 1984.
545. Otis AB, Jude J: Effects of body temperature on pulmonary gas exchange, *Am J Physiol* 188:355, 1957.
546. Ott DE: Correction of laparoscopic insufflation hypothermia, *J Laparoendosc Surg* 1:183, 1991.
547. Otto RJ, Metzler MH: Rewarming from experimental hypothermia: comparison of heated aerosol inhalation, peritoneal lavage and pleural lavage, *Crit Care Med* 16:869, 1988.
548. Otty CJ, Roland MO: Hypothermia in the elderly: scope for prevention, *Br Med J* 295:419, 1987.
549. Oung CM et al: Effects of hypothermia on hemodynamic responses to dopamine and dobutamine, *J Trauma* 33:671, 1992.
550. Pace NL: A critique of flow-directed pulmonary arterial catheterization, *Anesthesiology* 47:455, 1977.
551. Palve H: Pulse oximetry during low cardiac output and hypothermia states immediately after open heart surgery, *Crit Care Med* 17:66, 1989.
552. Paton BC: Accidental hypothermia, *Pharmacol Ther* 22:331, 1983.
553. Patt A, McCroskey BL, Moore EE: Hypothermia-induced coagulopathies in trauma, *Surg Clin North Am* 68:775, 1988.
554. Patton JF, Doolittle WH: Core rewarming by peritoneal dialysis following induced hypothermia in the dog, *J Appl Physiol* 33:800, 1972.
555. Pearn JH: Cold injury complicating trauma in subzero enviornments, *Med J Aust* 1:505, 1982.
556. Peran FK, Spaan G: Renshaw inhibition during local spinal cord cooling and warming, *Experientia* 26:978, 1970.
557. Perlstein PH et al: Adaptation to cold in the first three days of life, *Pediatrics* 54:411, 1974.
558. Perna AM et al: Cerebral metabolism and blood flow after circulatory arrest during deep hypothermia, *Ann Surg* 178:95, 1973.
559. Pfeiffer RF: Bromocriptine-induced hypothermia, *Neurology* 40:383, 1990.
560. Philip G, Smith JF: Hypothermia and Wernicke's encephalopathy, *J Pathol* 110:6, 1973.
561. Phillips SJ et al: Percutaneous cardiopulmonary bypass: application and indication for use, *Ann Thorac Surg* 47:121, 1989.
562. Pickering BG, Bristow GD, Craig DB: Case history number 97: core rewarming by peritoneal irrigation in accidental hypothermia with cardiac arrest, *Anesth Analg* 56:574, 1977.
563. Pierce EC: Treating acidemia in carbon monoxide poisoning may be dangerous, *J Hyperbaric Med* 1:87, 1986.
564. Pillgram-Larsen J et al: Accidental hypothermia: risk factors in 29 patients with body temperature of 30 degrees C and below, *Tidsskr Nor Laegeforen* 111:180, 1991.
565. Pina-Cabral JM, Ribeiro-da-Silva A, Almeida-Dias A: Platelet sequestration during hypothermia in dogs treated with sulphinpyrazone and ticlopidine: reversibility accelerated after intra-abdominal rewarming, *Thromb Haemost* 54:838, 1985.
566. Pineda M et al: Familial agenesis of the corpus callosum with hypothermia and apneic spells, *Neuropediatrics* 15:63, 1984.
567. Pledger HG: Disorders of temperature regulation in acute traumatic tetraplegia, *J Bone Joint Surg* 44:110, 1963.
568. Pontoppidan H, Beecher HK: Progressive loss of protective reflexes in the airway with advance of age, *JAMA* 174:2209, 1960.
569. Popovic V, Popovic P: *Hypothermia in biology and medicine*, New York, 1974, Grune & Stratton.
570. Popovic V, Popovic P: Survival of hypothermic dogs after 2-hour circulatory arrest, *Am J Physiol* 248:R308, 1985.
571. Potts DW, Sinopoli A: Infection, hypothermia, and hemodynamic monitoring, *Ann Intern Med* 102:869, 1985.
572. Poulos ND, Mollitt DL: The nature and reversibility of hypothermia-induced alterations of blood viscosity, *J Trauma* 31:996, 1991.
573. Pozos RS, Iaizzo PA: Shivering and pathological and physiological clonic oscillations of the human ankle, *J Appl Physiol* 71:1929, 1991.
574. Pozos RS et al: Human studies concerning thermal-induced shivering, postoperative "shivering" and cold-induced vasodilation, *Ann Emerg Med* 16:1037, 1987.
575. Pozos RS, Wittmers LE: *The nature and treatment of hypothermia*, Minneapolis, 1983, University of Minnesota Press.
576. Preston BR: Effect of hypothermia on systemic and organ system metabolism and function, *J Surg Res* 20:49, 1976.
577. Primrose WR, Smith LRN: Urban hypothermia, *Br Med J* 1:474, 1981.
578. Priori SG, Napolitano C, Schwartz PJ: Electrophysiologic mechanisms involved in the development of torsades de pointes, *Cardiovasc Drugs Ther* 5:203, 1991.
579. Prough DS et al: Response of cerebral blood flow to changes in carbon dioxide tension during hypothermic cardiopulmonary bypass, *Anesthesiology* 64:576, 1986.
580. Pugh LG: Accidental hypothermia in walkers, climbers, and campers: report to the medical commission on accident prevention, *Br Med J* 1:123, 1966.
581. Racine J, Jarjoui E: Severe hypothermia in infants, *Helv Paediatr Acta* 37:317, 1982.
582. Raheja R, Puri VK, Schaeffer RC: Shock due to profound hypothermia and alcohol ingestion: report of two cases, *Crit Care Med* 9:644, 1981.
583. Rahn H: Body temperature and acid-base regulation, *Pneumonologie* 151:87, 1974.
584. Rahn H, Reeves RB, Howell BJ: Hydrogen ion regulation, temperature, and evolution, *Am Rev Respir Dis* 112:165, 1975.
585. Raifman MA, Berant M, Lenarsky C: Cold weather and rhabdomyolysis, *J Pediatr* 93:970, 1978.
586. Ralley FE et al: Effect of heated humidified gases on temperature drop after cardiopulmonary bypass, *Anesth Analg* 63:1106, 1984.
587. Randall PE, Heath DF, Little RA: How common is accidental hypothermia? (letter), *Arch Emerg Med* 2:174, 1985.
588. Rango N: Old and cold: hypothermia in the elderly, *Geriatrics* 35:93, 1980.
589. Rango N: Exposure-related hypothermia in the United States, 1970-1979, *Am J Public Health* 74:1159, 1984.

590. Rango N: The social epidemiology of accidental hypothermia among the aged, *Gerontologist* 25:424, 1985.
591. Rankin AC, Rae AP: Cardiac arrhythmias during rewarming of patients with accidental hypothermia, *Br Med J* 289:784, 1984.
592. Read AE et al: Pancreatitis and accidental hypothermia, *Lancet* 2:1219, 1961.
593. Ream AK, Reitz BA, Silverberg G: Temperature correction of $Paco_2$ and pH in estimating acid-base status: an example of emperor's new clothes? *Anesthesiology* 56:41, 1982.
594. Reed RL et al: Hypothermia and blood coagulation: dissociation between enzyme activity and clotting factor levels, *Circ Shock* 32:141, 1990.
595. Reed RL et al: The disparity between hypothermic coagulopathy and clotting studies, *J Trauma* 33:465, 1992.
596. Reisinger KS, Kao J, Grant DM: Inaccuracy of the Clinitemp skin thermometer, *Pediatrics* 64:4, 1979.
597. Rekland T et al: Neuromonitoring in hypothermia and in hypothermic hypoxia, *Arctic Med Res* 50:32, 1991.
598. Renke W: Medical aspects of the survival of shipwrecked crewmen of the M/S "Kudowa Zdroj," *Bull Instit Maritime Trop Med Gdynia* 34:23, 1983.
599. Reuler JB: Hypothermia: pathophysiology, clinical settings, and management, *Ann Intern Med* 89:519, 1978.
600. Reuler JB, Girard DE, Cooney TG: Wernicke's encephalopathy, *N Engl J Med* 312:1035, 1985.
601. Reuler JB, Jones SR, Girard DE: Hypothermia in the erythroderma syndrome, *West J Med* 127:243, 1977.
602. Reuler JB, Parker RA: Peritoneal dialysis in the management of hypothermia, *JAMA* 240:2289, 1978.
603. Reutens DC, Dunne JW, Gubbay SS: Triphasic waves in accidental hypothermia, *Electroencephalogr Clin Neurophysiol* 76:370, 1990.
604. Ridgeway EC et al: Acute metabolic responses in myxedema to large doses of intravenous I-thyroxine, *Ann Intern Med* 77:549, 1972.
605. Roberts DE et al: Fluid replacement during hypothermia, *Aviat Space Environ Med* 56:333, 1985.
606. Robinson M, Seward PN: Environmental hypothermia in children, *Pediatr Emerg Care* 2:254, 1986.
607. Rodis JF et al: Maternal hypothermia: an unusual complication of magnesium sulfate therapy, *Am J Obstet Gynecol* 156:435, 1987.
608. Rodrigo N, Ranwala R: Delayed recovery following atracurium: a case report, *Eur J Anaesthesiol* 5:207, 1988.
609. Rohrer MJ, Natale AM: Effect of hypothermia on the coagulation cascade, *Crit Care Med* 20:1402, 1992.
610. Romet TT, Hoskin RW: Temperature and metabolic responses to inhalation and bath rewarming protocols, *Aviat Space Environ Med* 59:630, 1988.
611. Rosenfeld JB: Acid-base and electrolyte disturbances in hypothermia, *Am J Cardiol* 12:678, 1963.
612. Rosenkranz L: Bone marrow failure and pancytopenia in two patients with hypothermia, *South Med J* 78:358, 1985.
613. Rosenthal TB: The effect of temperature on the pH of blood and plasma in vitro, *J Biol Chem* 173:25, 1948.
614. Rothfield EL: Hypothermic hump, *JAMA* 213:626, 1970.
615. Rovito PF: Atrial caval shunting in blunt vascular injury, *Ann Surg* 205:318, 1987.
616. Rudikoff MT et al: Mechanisms of blood flow during cardiopulmonary resuscitation, *Circulation* 61:345, 1980.
617. Russ W et al: Effect of hypothermia on visual evoked potentials in humans, *Anesthesiology* 61:207, 1984.
618. Sabapathi R, Ridley C, Yen MC: Complete recovery from profound hypothermia associated with DIC, *Md Med J* 35:203, 1986.
619. Sadikali F, Owor R: Hypothermia in the tropics: a review of 24 cases, *Trop Geogr Med* 26:265, 1974.
620. Sampson JB: Anxiety as a factor in the incidence of combat cold injury: a review, *Milit Med* 149:89, 1984.
621. Samuelson T: Experience with standardized protocols in hypothermia, boom or bane? The Alaska experience, *Arctic Med Res* 50:28, 1991.
622. Samuelson T et al: Hypothermia and cold water near-drowning: treatment guidelines, *Alaska Med* 24:106, 1982.
623. Sander KB, Bommen M, Brook CG: Spontaneous hypothermia in a young boy, *Arch Dis Child* 58:230, 1983.
624. Sanderson L, Lybarger JA: Hypothermia-associated deaths—United States, 1968, 1980: leads from the MMWR, *JAMA* 255:307, 1986.
625. Sandhu JS et al: Acute renal failure in severe hypothermia, 14:591, 1992.
626. Sanfield JA et al: Altered norepinephrine metabolism in Shapiro's syndrome, *Arch Neurol* 46:53, 1989.
627. Sarman I, Can G, Tunell R: Rewarming preterm infants on a heated, water filled mattress, *Arch Dis Child* 64:687, 1989.
628. Savard GK et al: Peripheral blood flow during rewarming from mild hypothermia in humans, *J Appl Physiol* 58:4, 1985.
629. Savourey G, Vallerand AL, Bittel JH: General and local cold adaptation after a ski journey in a severe arctic environment, *Eur J Appl Physiol* 64:99, 1992.
630. Scalea TM et al: Injuries missed at operation: nemesis of the trauma surgeon, *J Trauma* 28:962, 1988.
631. Schaller MD, Fischer AP, Perret CH: Hyperkalemia: a prognostic factor during acute severe hypothermia, *JAMA* 264:1842, 1990.
632. Schissler P, Parker MA, Scott SJ Jr: Profound hypothermia: value of prolonged cardiopulmonary resuscitation, *South Med J* 74:474, 1981.
633. Schmicke P: Rewarming from accidental deep hypothermia by a short-wave therapy apparatus, *Anaesth Intensivther Notfallmed* 19:27, 1984.
634. Schneider J: Accidental hypothermia, *Gerontology* 13:156, 1983.
635. Schneider SM: Hypothermia: from recognition to rewarming, *Emerg Med Rep* 13:1, 1992.
636. Schwab RH et al: Electrocardiographic changes occurring in rapidly induced deep hypothermia, *Am J Med Sci* 248:290, 1964.
637. Schwaitzberg SD et al: Rapid in-line blood warming using microwave energy: preliminary studies, *J Invest Surg* 4:505, 1991.
638. Segar WE: Effect of hypothermia on tubular transport mechanisms, *Am J Physiol* 195:91, 1958.
639. Segar WE, Riley PA, Barila TG: Urinary composition during hypothermia, *Am J Physiol* 185:528, 1956.
640. Senior RM et al: The recognition and management of myxedema coma, *JAMA* 217:61, 1971.
641. Sereda WM: Treatment of hypothermia (letter), *CMAJ* 112:931, 1975.
642. Sessler DI, Moayeri A: Skin-surface warming: heat flux and central temperature, *Anesthesiology* 73:218, 1990.
643. Seuffert G: An Alaskan experience with cardiopulmonary bypass in resuscitating patients with profound hypothermia and cardiac arrest, *Alaska Med* 26:31, 1984.
644. Severinghaus JW: Blood gas calculator, *J Appl Physiol* 21:1108, 1966.
645. Severinghaus JW, Astrup PB: History of blood gas analysis. III. Carbon dioxide tension, *J Clin Monit* 2:60, 1986.
646. Severinghaus JW, Stupfel MA, Bradley AF: Alveolar dead space and arterial to end-tidal carbon dioxide differences during hypothermia in dog and man, *J Appl Physiol* 10:349, 1957.
647. Shanks CA: Heat gain in the treatment of accidental hypothermia, *Med J Aust* 2:346, 1975.
648. Shanks CA, Marsh HM: Simple core rewarming in accidental hypothermia, *Br J Anaesth* 45:522, 1973.
649. Shanks CA, Sara CA: Temperature monitoring of the humidifier during treatment of hypothermia, *Med J Aust* 2:1351, 1972.
650. Shapiro WR, Williams GH, Plum F: Spontaneous recurrent hypothermia accompanying agenesis of the corpus callosum, *Brain* 92:423, 1969.

651. Shaver J et al: Changes in epicardial and core temperature during resuscitation of hemorrhagic shock, *J Trauma* 24:957, 1984.
652. Sheehy TW, Navan RM: Hypothermia, *Ala J Med Sci* 21:374, 1984.
653. Shenaq SA et al: Effect of profound hypothermia on leukocytes and platelets, *Ann Clin Lab Sci* 16:130, 1986.
654. Shephard RJ: Some consequences of polar stress: data from a transpolar ski-trek, *Arctic Med Res* 50:25, 1991.
655. Sherman FT, Daum M: Hypothermia detection in emergency departments: how low does your thermometer go? *NY State J Med* 82:374, 1982.
656. Sherry E, Clout L: Deaths associated with skiing in Australia: a 32 year study of cases from the Snowy Mountains, *Med J Aust* 149:615, 1988.
657. Sherry E, Richards D: Hypothermia among resort skiers: 19 cases from the Snowy Mountains, *Med J Aust* 144:457, 1986.
658. Shields CP, Sixsmith DM: Treatment of moderate-to-severe hypothermia in an urban setting, *Ann Emerg Med* 19:1093, 1990.
659. Shinozaki T, Deane R, Perkins F: Infrared tympanic thermometer: evaluation of a new clinical thermometer, *Crit Care Med* 16:148, 1988.
660. Shinozaki M et al: Circadian rhythm disturbances in neurological patients with chronic hypothermia, *Prog Clin Biol Res* 341A:213, 1990.
661. Sinet M et al: Maintaining blood pH at 7.4 during hypothermia has no significant effect on work of the isolated rat heart, *Anesthesiology* 62:582, 1985.
662. Singer D, Bretschneider JH: Metabolic reduction in hypothermia: pathophysiological problems and natural examples. Part I, *Thorac Cardiovasc Surg* 38:205, 1990.
663. Singer D, Bretschneider JH: Metabolic reduction in hypothermia: pathophysiological problems and natural examples. Part II, *Thorac Cardiovasc Surg* 38:212, 1990.
664. Siple P: Clothing and climate. In Newburgh RW, editor: *Physiology of heat regulation and the science of clothing,* New York, 1968, LH Hafner.
665. Sircar P: Plasma volume bleeding and clotting time on hypothermic dogs, *Proc Soc Exp Biol Med* 87:194, 1954.
666. Sivaloganatham S: Paradoxical undressing due to hypothermia in a child, *Med Sci Law* 25:176, 1985.
667. Skandfer M et al: An experimental model for the study of transcapillary fluid balance in hypothermia, *Arctic Med Res* 50:127, 1991.
668. Sklar DP, Doezema D: Procedures pertaining to hypothermia. In Roberts JR, Hedges JR, editors: *Clinical procedures in emergency medicine,* 1991, Philadelphia, WB Saunders, pp 1100-1108.
669. Slotki IN, Oelbaum MH: Recurrent spontaneous hypothermia, *Postgrad Med J* 56:656, 1980.
670. Slovis CM, Bachvarov HL: Heated inhalation treatment of hypothermia, *Am J Emerg Med* 2:533, 1984.
671. Smith DK et al: Hypothermia in a patient with anorexia nervosa, *Metabolism* 32:1151, 1983.
672. Smith OKL: Insulin response in rats acutely exposed to cold, *Can J Physiol Pharmacol* 62:924, 1984.
673. Smolander J, Louhevaara V, Ahonen M: Clothing, hypothermia, *Lancet* 2:226, 1986.
674. Sofer S et al: Improved outcome of hypothermic infants, *Pediatr Emerg Care* 2:221, 1986.
675. Solomon A et al: The electrocardiographic features of hypothermia, *J Emerg Med* 7:169, 1989.
676. Soung LS et al: Treatment of accidental hypothermia with peritoneal dialysis, *Can Med Assoc J* 117:1415, 1977.
677. Southwick FS, Dalglish PH: Recovery after prolonged hypothermia, *JAMA* 243:1250, 1980.
678. Sowejimi T et al: Protective effects of steroids on the crotical microcirculation injured by cold, *J Neurosurg* 51:188, 1979.
679. Splittgerber FH et al: Partial cardiopulmonary bypass for core rewarming in profound accidental hypothermia, *Am Surg* 52:407, 1986.
680. Sprung J et al: Effects of acute hypothermia and beta-adrenergic receptor blockade on serum potassium concentration in rats, *Crit Care Med* 19:1545, 1991.
681. Sprung J et al: Potassium correction of hypothermic hypokalemia induces hyperkalemia after rewarming, *Can J Anaesth* 37:S69, 1990.
682. Stamm-Racine J, Ferrier PE: Management of neonatal hypothermia (letter), *J Pediatr* 106:532, 1985.
683. Stapczynski JS: Resuscitation from severe hypothermia, *Ann Emerg Med* 14:1126, 1985.
684. Steinemann S, Shackford SR, Davis JW: Implications of admission hypothermia in trauma patients, *J Trauma* 30:200, 1990.
685. Steinman A: Hypothermia, *Wilderness Med* 4:6, 1987.
686. Steinman A: Prehospital management of hypothermia, *Response* 6:18, 1987.
687. Steinman AM: The hypothermic code: CPR controversy revisited, *J Emerg Med Serv* 10:32, 1983.
688. Steinman AM: Cardiopulmonary resuscitation and hypothermia, *Circulation* 74(suppl IV):29, 1986.
689. Sterba JA: Efficacy and safety of prehospital rewarming techniques to treat accidental hypothermia, *Ann Emerg Med* 20:896, 1991.
690. Stewart CE: *Environmental emergencies,* Baltimore, 1990, Williams & Wilkins.
691. Stoneham MD, Squires SJ: Prolonged resuscitation in acute deep hypothermia, *Anaesthesia* 47:784, 1992.
692. Stoner HB, Little RA, Frayn KN: Fat metabolism in elderly patients with severe hypothermia, *Q J Exp Physiol* 68:701, 1983.
693. Strachan RD, Whittle IR, Miller JD: Hypothermia and severe head injury, *Brain Inj* 3:51, 1989.
694. Strauch BS et al: Hypothermia in hypoglycemia, *JAMA* 210:345, 1969.
695. Sturm JT, Logan MA: Microwave aids in external rewarming of hypothermia patients (letter), *Ann Emerg Med* 14:277, 1985.
696. Summers GD et al: Spontaneous periodic hypothermia with lipoma of the corpus callosum, *J Neurol Neurosurg Psychiatry* 944:1094, 1981.
697. Sung Y et al: Susceptibility of human and porcine neutrophils to hypothermia in vitro, *Pediatr Res* 19:1044, 1985.
698. Sutariya BB, Penny DG, Nallamothu BG: Hypothermia following acute carbon-monoxide increases mortality, *Toxicol Lett* 52:201, 1990.
699. Swain JA: Hypothermia and blood pH: a review, *Arch Intern Med* 148:1643, 1988.
700. Swain JA et al: Hemodynamics and metabolism during surface-induced hypothermia in the dog: a comparison of pH management strategies, *J Surg Res* 48:217, 1990.
701. Swain JA et al: Relationship of cerebral and myocardial intracellular pH to blood pH during hypothermia, *Am J Physiol* 260:1640, 1991.
702. Swain JA, White FN, Peters RM: The effect of pH on the hypothermic ventricular fibrillation threshold, *J Thorac Cardiovasc Surg* 87:445, 1984.
703. Swan H: The hydroxyl-hydrogen ion concentration ratio during hypothermia, *Surg Gynecol Obstet* 155:897, 1982.
704. Swan H: The importance of acid-base management for cardiac and cerebral preservation during open heart operations, *Surg Gynecol Obstet* 158:391, 1984.
705. Swan H et al: Cessation of circulation in general hypothermia. I. Physiologic changes and their control, *Ann Surg* 138:360, 1953.
706. Swartz RD et al: Hypothermia in the uremic patient, *Dialysis Transplant* 12:584, 1983.
707. Syapin PJ, Gee KW, Alkana RL: Ro 15-4513 differentially affects ethanol-induced hypnosis and hypothermia, *Brain Res Bull* 19:603, 1987.
708. Symbas PN et al: Influence of hypothermia on pancreatic function, *Ann Surg* 154:509, 1961.
709. Szekely P, Wynne NA: The effects of digitalis on the hypothermic heart, *Br Heart J* 22:647, 1960.

710. Tacker WA Jr et al: Transchest defibrillation under conditions of hypothermia, *Crit Care Med* 9:390, 1981.
711. Tafari N, Gentz J: Aspects of rewarming newborn infants with severe accidental hypothermia, *Acta Paediatr Scand* 63:595, 1974.
712. Takada M et al: Wischnevsky's gastric lesions in accidental hypothermia, *Am J Forensic Med Pathol* 12:300, 1991.
713. Taly AB et al: Hypothermia: an unusual manifestation of Reye's syndrome, *Ind J Med Sci* 44:237, 1990.
714. Tamarin FM, Conetta R, Brandstetter RD: Letter, *JAMA* 256:1723, 1986.
715. Tampi R, Alexander WS: Wernicke's encephalopathy with central pontine myelinolysis presenting with hypothermia, *NZ Med J* 95:342, 1982.
716. Tan S: Rewarming after cardiopulmonary bypass: a comparison of two methods, *Ann Acad Med Singapore* 19:350, 1990.
717. Tanaka M, Tokudome S: Accidental hypothermia and death from cold in urban areas, *Int J Biometeorol* 34:242, 1991.
718. Taylor MS: Cold weather injuries during peacetime military training, *Milit Med* 157:602, 1992.
719. Templin DW: Some historical aspects of the treatment of hypothermia, *Alaska Med* 26:13, 1984.
720. Terndrup T, Allegra JR, Kealy JA: A comparison of oral, rectal, and tympanic membrane-derived temperature changes after ingestion of liquids and smoking, *Am J Emerg Med* 7:150, 1989.
721. Theilade D: The danger of fatal misjudgment in hypothermia after immersion, *Anaesthesia* 32:889, 1977.
722. Therminarias A, Pellerei E: Plasma catecholamine and metabolic changes during cooling and rewarming in dogs, *Exp Biol* 47:117, 1987.
723. Thomandram SS et al: Survival after prolonged submersion in cold water without neurologic sequelae, *Arch Intern Med* 140:775, 1980.
724. Thomas DR: Accidental hypothermia in the sunbelt, *J Gen Intern Med* 3:552, 1988.
725. Thomas JD: Episodic hypothermia, *Lancet* 2:449, 1973.
726. Thompson R et al: Evolutionary changes in the electrocardiogram of severe progressive hypothermia, *J Electrocardiol* 10:67, 1977.
727. Timsit JF et al: Severe hypothermia occurring during the course of toxic epidermal necrolysis in patients treated with air-fluidized beds, *Arch Dermatol* 127:739, 1991.
728. Tisherman S et al: Resuscitation of dogs from cold-water submersion using cardiopulmonary bypass, *Ann Emerg Med* 14:389, 1985.
729. Tisherman SA et al: Profound hypothermia (less than 10° C) compared with deep hypothermia (15° C) improves neurologic outcome in dogs after two hours' circulatory arrest induced to enable resuscitative surgery, *J Trauma* 31:1051, 1991.
730. Tolman KG, Cohen A: Accidental hypothermia, *Can Med Assoc J* 103:1357, 1970.
731. Tomaszewski W: Changements electrocardiographiques observes chez un homme mort de froid, *Arch Mal Coeur* 31:525, 1938.
732. Toung JK et al: Alveolar surface activity following mechanical endotracheal ventilation with high-density water mist, *Anesth Analg* 49:851, 1970.
733. Towne WD, Geiss WP, Yanes HO: Intractable ventricular fibrillation associated with profound accidental hypothermia: successful treatment with partial cardiopulmonary bypass, *N Engl J Med* 287:1135, 1972.
734. Trevino A, Razi B, Beller BM: The characteristic electrocardiogram of accidental hypothermia, *Arch Intern Med* 127:470, 1971.
735. Tributsch W, Ambach E, Henn R: Forensic medicine aspects of death caused by hypothermia in high altitude, *Beitr Gerichte Med* 50:337, 1992.
736. Truscott DG, Firor WB, Clein LJ: Accidental profound hypothermia: successful resuscitation by core rewarming and assisted circulation, *Arch Surg* 106:216, 1973.
737. Tveita T et al: Hemodynamic and metabolic effects of hypothermia and rewarming, *Arctic Med Res* 50:48, 1991.
738. Urbanic RC, Mazzaferri EL: Thyrotoxic crisis and myxedema coma, *Heart Lung* 7:435, 1978.
739. Vaagenes P, Holme JA: Accidental deep hypothermia due to exposure, *Anaesthesia* 37:819, 1982.
740. Vaamonde CA et al: Complications of acute peritoneal dialysis, *J Chron Dis* 23:637, 1975.
741. Valeri CR et al: Hypothermia-induced reversible platelet dysfunction, *Ann Surg* 205:175, 1987.
742. Vandam LD, Brunap TK: Hypothermia, *N Engl J Med* 261:546, 1959.
743. Vapaaviori M: Changes in the static elastance and hysteresis of the chest wall and lung in normo-hypothermia, *Acta Physiol Scand* 5:49, 1962.
744. Varon J, Sadovnikoff N, Sternbach GL: Hypothermia: saving patients from the big chill, *Postgrad Med* 92:47, 1992.
745. Vaughn PB: Local cold injury—menace to military operations: a review, *Milit Med* 145:305, 1980.
746. Vella MA et al: Hypothermia-induced thrombocytopenia, *J R Soc Med* 81:228, 1988.
747. Villalobos TH et al: A cause of thrombocytopenia and leukopenia that occurs in dogs during deep hypothermia, *J Clin Invest* 37:1, 1958.
748. Von Segesser LK, Garcia E, Turina M: Perfusion without systemic heparinization for rewarming in accidental hypothermia, *Ann Thorac Surg* 52:560, 1991.
749. Von Segesser LK et al: Reduction and elimination of systemic heparinization during cardiopulmonary bypass, *J Thorac Cardiovasc Surg* 103:790, 1992.
750. Voorhees WD, Babbs CF, Tacker WA: Regional blood flow during cardiopulmonary resuscitation in dogs, *Crit Care Med* 8:134, 1980.
751. Wagner JA, Robinson S, Marino RP: Age and temperature regulation of humans in neutral and cold environments, *J Appl Physiol* 37:562, 1974.
752. Walker BR, Anderson JA, Edwards CR: Clonidine therapy for Shapiro's syndrome, *Q J Med* 82:235, 1992.
753. Walpoth BH et al: Accidental deep hypothermia with cardiopulmonary arrest: extracorporeal blood rewarming in 11 patients, *Eur J Cardiothorac Surg* 4:390, 1990.
754. Walters DT: Closed thoracic cavity lavage for hypothermia with cardiac arrest (letter), *Ann Emerg Med* 20:439, 1991.
755. Wang LS et al: A reevaluation of heparin requirements for cardiopulmonary bypass, *J Thorac Cardiovasc Surg* 101:153, 1991.
756. Ward M: *Mountain medicine,* London, 1975, Crosby Lockwood Staples.
757. Webb GE: Comparison of esophageal and tympanic temperature monitoring during cardiopulmonary bypass, *Anesth Analg (Cleve)* 52:729, 1973.
758. Webb P: Afterdrop of body temperature during rewarming: an alternative explanation, *J Appl Physiol* 60:385, 1986.
759. Wedin B, Vanggaard L, Hirvonen J: "Paradoxical undressing" in fatal hypothermia, *J Forensic Sci* 24:543, 1979.
760. Weil MH, Gazmuri RJ: Hypothermia after cardiac arrest, *Crit Care Med* 19:315, 1991.
761. Weil MH et al: Difference in acid-base state between venous and arterial blood during cardiopulmonary resuscitation, *N Engl J Med* 315:153, 1986.
762. Weinberg AD: Hypothermia, *Ann Emerg Med* 22:370, 1993.
763. Weisfeldt ML, Chandra N, Tsitlik J: Increased intrathoracic pressure—not direct heart compression—causes the rise in intrathoracic vascular pressures during CPR in dogs and pigs, *Crit Care Med* 9:377, 1981.
764. Wenzel RP: Anti-endotoxin monoclonal antibodies—a second look, *N Engl J Med* 326:1151, 1992.
765. Werwath DL et al: Microwave ovens: a safe new method of warming crystalloids, *Am Surg* 50:656, 1984.
766. Wessel HU, James GW, Paul MH: Effects of respiration and circulation on central blood temperature of the dog, *Am J Physiol* 211:1403, 1966.

767. Westin B, Sehgal N, Assali NS: Regional blood flow and vascular resistance during hypothermia in dogs, *Am J Physiol* 201:485, 1961.
768. Weyman AE, Greenbaum DM, Grace WJ: Accidental hypothermia in an alcoholic population, *Am J Med* 56:13, 1974.
769. White FN: A comparative physiological approach to hypothermia, *J Thorac Cardiovasc Surg* 82:821, 1981.
770. White FN: Reassuring acid-base balance in hypothermia: a comparative point of view, *West J Med* 138:255, 1983.
771. White JD: Cardiac arrest in hypothermia (letter), *JAMA* 244:2262, 1980.
772. White JD: Hypothermia: the Bellevue experience, *Ann Emerg Med* 11:417, 1982.
773. White JD et al: Controlled comparison of humidified inhalation and peritoneal lavage in rewarming immersion hypothermia, *Am J Emerg Med* 2:210, 1984.
774. White JD et al: Comparison of rewarming by radio wave regional hypothermia and warm humidified inhalation, *Aviat Space Environ Med* 55:1103, 1984.
775. White JD et al: Controlled comparison of radio wave regional hyperthermia and peritoneal lavage-rewarming after immersion hypothermia, *J Trauma* 25:989, 1985.
776. White JD et al: Rewarming in accidental hypothermia: radio wave versus inhalation therapy, *Ann Emerg Med* 16:50, 1987.
777. Whittle JL, Bates JH: Thermoregulatory failure secondary to acute illness, *Arch Intern Med* 139:418, 1979.
778. Wickstrom P et al: Accidental hypothermia: core rewarming with partial bypasss, *Am J Surg* 131:622, 1976.
779. Wilkerson JA: *Medicine for mountaineering,* ed 2, Seattle, 1975, The Mountaineers.
780. Willford DC et al: Importance of acid-base strategy in reducing myocardial and whole body oxygen consumption during perfusion hypothermia, *J Thorac Cardiovasc Surg* 100:699, 1990.
781. Wilson RD, Knapp C, Traver DL: Tympanic thermography: a clinical and research evaluation of a new technique, *South Med J* 64:1452, 1971.
782. Wisborg T, Husby P, Engedal H: Anesthesiologist-manned helicopters and regionalized extracorporeal circulation facilities: a unique chance in deep hypothermia, *Arctic Med Res* 50:108, 1991.
783. Wolf PD et al: Accidental hypothermia endocrine function during recovery, *J Clin Endocrinol Metab* 34:360, 1972.
784. Wong KC: Physiology and pharmacology of hypothermia, *West J Med* 138:227, 1983.
785. Wood JE, Bass DE, Iampietro PF: Responses of peripheral veins of man to prolonged and continuous cold exposure, *J Appl Physiol* 12:301, 1958.
786. Wood SC: Interactions between hypoxia and hypothermia, *Annu Rev Physiol* 53:71, 1991.
787. Woodhouse P, Keatinge WR, Colshaw SR: Factors associated with hypothermia in patients admitted to a group of inner city hospitals, *Lancet* 2:1201, 1989.
788. Wynne NA, Fuller JA, Szekely P: Electrocardiographic changes in hypothermia, *Br Heart J* 22:652, 1960.
789. Yagupsky P, Mares AJ, Gorodischer R: Pyloric stenosis associated with hypothermia (letter), *J Trop Pediatr* 32:270, 1986.
790. Yagupsky P, Sofer S: Infection in hypothermic infants (letter), *Pediatr Infect Dis* 5:112, 1986.
791. Yamada Y, Ysoshima A: Rapid warming of infusion solution, *Surg Gynecol Obstet* 160:400, 1985.
792. Yaron M et al: Inaccuracy of the infrared tympanic thermometer in the emergency department (abstract), *Ann Emerg Med* 21:654, 1992.
793. Young AJ: Effects of aging on human cold tolerance, *Exp Aging Res* 17:205, 1991.
794. Zabelle J et al: Risk factors for infantile hypothermia in early neonatal life, *Pediatr Emerg Care* 6:96, 1990.
795. Zachary L et al: Accidental hypothermia treated with rapid rewarming by immersion, *Ann Plast Surg* 9:238, 1982.
796. Zarins CK, Skinner DB: Circulation in profound hypothermia, *J Surg Res* 14:97, 1973.
797. Zell SC, Kurtz KJ: Severe exposure hypothermia: a resuscitation protocol, *Ann Emerg Med* 14:339, 1985.
798. Zhong H, Qinyi S, Mingjlang S: Rewarming with microwave irradiation in severe cold injury syndrome, *Chin Med J* 93:19, 1980.
799. Zumwalt RE, Kicklighter E: Deaths from hypothermia, *JAMA* 256:1136, 1986.

4 COLD WATER IMMERSION

Alan M. Steinman
John S. Hayward

Immersion in cold water is a hazard for anyone who participates in commercial or recreational activities in the oceans, lakes, and streams of all but the tropical regions of the world. Recreational water-related activities include swimming, hunting, fishing, sailing, power-boating, ocean kayaking, white-water rafting, canoeing, ocean-surfing, wind-surfing, and diving. Commercial activities involving water include fishing, shipping, offshore oil drilling, diving, and maritime military operations (for example, the Coast Guard and Navy) (Fig. 4-1).

The definition of cold water is variable. The temperature of thermally neutral water, in which heat loss balances heat production for a nude subject at rest, is approximately 33° C.[21] Hypothermia eventually results from immersion in water below this temperature. For practical purposes significant risk of immersion hypothermia usually begins in water colder than 25° C.[12,67,90] Table 4-1 shows the variation of water temperatures throughout the year at various sites.[185] Using 25° C as the definition of cold water, the risk of immersion hypothermia in North America is nearly universal during most of the year.

Cold water immersion is associated with two significant medical emergencies: near drowning and hypothermia. The risk of near drowning is discussed with respect to the physiologic consequences of sudden immersion in cold water and in the context of survival in rough seas. The management of submersion injuries is described in Chapter 48; diving injuries are discussed in Chapter 47.

Historical and Statistical Aspects

The history of humankind's association with the sea and with inland waters provides abundant examples of the effects of accidental cold water immersion. Case studies demonstrate the scope of the problem.

Perhaps the most famous occurrence was the sinking of the *Titanic* in 1912. After striking an iceberg at approximately 11:40 PM on April 14, the ship sank in calm seas. Water temperature was near 0° C. Of the 2201 people on board, only 712 were rescued, all from the ship's lifeboats. The remaining 1489 people died in the water, despite the arrival of a rescue vessel within 2 hours. Nearly all of these people were wearing "life preservers," yet the cause of death was officially listed as drowning.[121] More likely the cause of death was immersion hypothermia.[90,107]

In 1963 the cruise ship *Lakonia* caught fire and sank in approximately 18° C water off the coast of Madeira in fairly calm seas. Two hundred people abandoned ship into the sea; all wore self-righting life jackets, but 120 died. The cause of death for most victims was hypothermia. Since rescuers reported that small waves washed over the faces of unconscious people, drowning was probably the terminal event.[89] The extensive use of combat ships and aircraft in World War II, particularly in the north Pacific and north Atlantic oceans, provided many examples of accidental immersion in cold water. Molnar[127] reviewed several hundred of these cases. Among them was the following:

> A ship was rammed, and it sank in 3 minutes. Thirty survivors were picked up from rafts after exposure of 1½ to 4 hours. Some drowned and others died of exposure because the water was 39° F with high seas and a wind velocity of scale 7. Some of the survivors who held on to ropes couldn't let go and rescuers had to cut frozen rope to release them. It appears miraculous how the survivors could have endured such cold water. Most of those who were rescued were in an unconscious state and, when they became conscious complained of numbness of extremities and hands.

The Falklands War in 1982 provided further examples of immersion hypothermia related to naval combat. The Argentine cruiser *General Belgrano* sank in approximately 5° C water, resulting in the deaths of many sailors. Some of

Table 4-1 Mean Water Temperatures (°C)

Site	Jan.	Feb.	Mar.	Apr.	May	Jun.	Jul.	Aug.	Sep.	Oct.	Nov.	Dec.
Kodiak, Alaska	0	0	2	4	7	9	12	12	10	7	4	2
Victoria, B.C.	7	7	7	9	10	11	11	11	11	10	9	8
Astoria, Ore.	4	5	7	10	13	16	19	19	17	13	9	5
San Francisco, Calif.	11	11	12	12	12	12	13	13	12	12	11	11
San Diego, Calif.	14	14	15	16	17	18	20	20	20	18	16	15
Mobile, Ala.	10	10	14	21	23	28	29	29	27	23	19	14
Miami, Fla.	21	21	23	25	27	29	30	30	29	27	25	23
Norfolk, Va.	17	16	15	18	20	24	26	26	25	25	21	19
Cape May, N.J.	3	3	5	10	14	19	23	23	21	17	11	6
Traverse City, Mich.	2	1	1	1	1	3	5	10	10	6	5	4
Honolulu, Hawaii	24	24	24	24	25	25	26	26	27	26	25	25
Puerto Rico	26	26	26	26	26	27	27	27	28	27	27	26

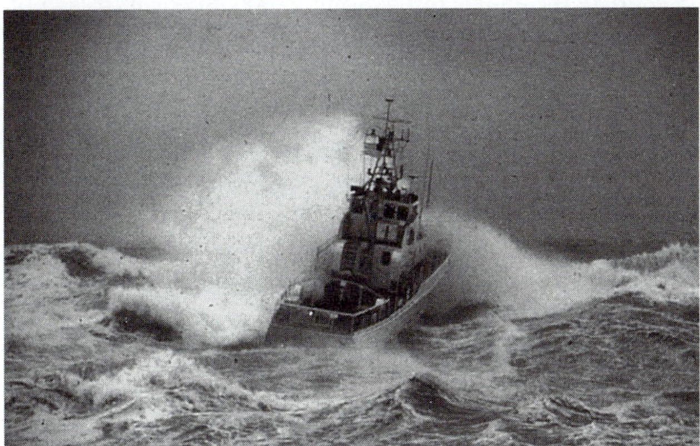

Fig. 4-1 Coast Guard rescue boat in rough seas.

the deaths from cold occurred even after the sailors had managed to emerge from the water into life rafts.

Numerous examples of maritime occupational accidents exist. In 1982 the offshore mobile oil-drilling platform *Ocean Ranger* collapsed in mountainous seas near Newfoundland, Canada. Water temperature was −1° C. Eighty-four workers were plunged into the water, and despite the presence of a rescue vessel, all died. Immersion hypothermia was a significant factor in these deaths, although the inability of the workers to combat the rough seas and maintain airway freeboard (the distance between the water surface and the mouth) was also a major problem.[115]

Fishing vessel mishaps are a common cause of immersion hypothermia. In 1983 the Alaskan fishing vessel *Saint Patrick* foundered in rough seas near Kodiak Island. The crew of 12, fearing the vessel would capsize, abandoned ship into 5° C water. Only 4 of them donned survival suits. Despite the excellent buoyancy and insulative properties of the suits, only 2 survivors ultimately made it to shore 24 hours later. Of the others, 9 succumbed to hypothermia or drowning. One was killed attempting landfall through the surf onto a rocky shore.[133]

Analysis of occupational accidents for fishermen from the United Kingdom between 1971 and 1980 showed that hypothermia and drowning were the most common causes of accidental death, with a death rate of approximately 1 per 1000 fisherman at risk from these causes.[144]

Recreational activities are a major source of immersion incidents. In 1983 Alaska had 253 deaths from accidental causes. Of these, 132 involved water-related deaths from either drowning or hypothermia.[34] For the entire United States, recreational boating fatalities for the years 1967 to 1976 averaged 1437 per year. A detailed analysis of the deaths for 1974 revealed that 15.7% were related to cold water immersion.[57] Of these, 43% occurred during fishing outings and 10% occurred during hunting activities.

A particularly poignant example of a recreational accident resulting in immersion hypothermia fatalities occurred in Lake Temiscamingue, Quebec, on June 12, 1978. A canoeing expedition of 27 schoolboys, aged 12 to 14, encountered a sudden change of weather on the lake. One of the four canoes tipped over when it turned broadside to the wind and 30 cm waves. The other three canoes capsized attempting to rescue the survivors. Four adults and all 27 boys were thrown into the 11° C water. All were wearing self-righting personal flotation devices (PFDs). Unfortunately, by the time the survivors could be rescued from shore the next day, 13 boys and 1 adult had died. The cause of death was officially listed as "asphyxiation, drowning and exhaustion."[27] The role of immersion hypothermia in these deaths was overlooked, either as a direct cause (the nonsurvivors were all found floating face up in their PFDs) or as a significant factor in drowning (for example, aspiration of water from wave action, secondary to unconsciousness, secondary to hypothermia).

The relatively high fatality rate from accidental immersion in cold water in various military, commercial, and recreational settings has stimulated technologic advances in protective clothing and rescue devices. The current availability of commonplace items of survival equipment (such as wet suits, dry suits, survival suits, and inflatable life rafts) is primarily a response to the needs of people who work in cold water environments. The value of various types of protective clothing is examined later in this chapter.

In summary, numerous case histories and statistical evidence document the significance of cold water immersion as a cause of the environmental emergencies of drowning and hypothermia. Although drowning is relatively easy to prevent (for example, through the use of personal flotation devices, water safety training, or restriction of alcohol use), hypothermia is not. Hypothermia is now more widely recognized than in the past, but prevention of immersion hypothermia is still a difficult and often expensive proposition. Therefore in regions of cold water the practice of safe boating and related procedures is essential.

Pathophysiology

Although the pathophysiology of immersion hypothermia is similar to that of hypothermia on land, a significant number of features distinguish immersion from nonimmersion cooling. Many clinically important characteristics of immersion hypothermia affect management of the cold patient in both prehospital and hospital settings. For a detailed examination of hypothermia pathophysiology, see Chapter 3.

RESPIRATORY SYSTEM CHANGES

Sudden immersion in cold water induces an initial reflex gasp, followed by hyperventilation.[26,118] Cold receptors deep in the skin provide a strong respiratory drive during the initial 1 or 2 minutes of immersion. Pulmonary ventilation increases up to fivefold as a result of elevation in both tidal volume and respiratory rate. After about 5 minutes tidal volume and respiratory rate decrease to levels consistent with metabolic requirements. Fig. 4-2 shows the typical response of lightly clothed subjects to sudden immersion in 0° C water.[65]

Respiratory responses to sudden immersion in cold water have significant practical consequences. The initial gasp potentiates aspiration of water and increases the risk of drowning. Hyperventilation, which can be prolonged in some individuals,[112] may potentiate reduced arterial Pco_2, with subsequent confusion and increased muscle tetany.[26] This is clearly detrimental for the survivor trying to remain afloat, particularly in rough water. Furthermore, the respiratory stimulation of cold water immersion significantly decreases underwater breath-holding duration. A recent study showed that mean breath-holding time of young, healthy volunteers decreased from 60 seconds in air to 15 to 25 seconds on sudden immersion in 0° to 15° C water.[70] This dramatic reduction has serious consequences for survivors attempting to escape from a submerged vehicle, capsized vessel, or ditched aircraft.[147,159] It also greatly increases the chance of drowning when white-water rafters and kayakers periodically submerge in very turbulent waters, even if they are wearing flotation devices.

CARDIOVASCULAR SYSTEM CHANGES

Immersion in cold water provokes substantial sympathetic output secondary to stimulation of cold receptors in the skin.[8,101] This results in marked peripheral vasoconstriction, which reduces muscle and cutaneous blood flow, shifts venous return to deep vessels, and potentiates countercurrent heat exchange in these deep vessels.[140,173] These effects increase total body insulation by restricting the flow of relatively warm blood through cold peripheral tissues. As a result the comparatively warm truncal "core" is surrounded by a "shell" of cold muscles (including truncal musculature) and other peripheral tissues. The metabolic consequences (such as lactic acidosis and electrolyte changes in peripheral tissues) may affect subsequent clinical management of the hypothermic patient.[139] Furthermore, the volume of relatively cold tissue that must be rewarmed during treatment may affect the choice of rewarming modality. This aspect of cardiovascular physiology is presented in the section on prehospital management strategies.

The extent of peripheral vasoconstriction may vary with water temperature. Immersion in water below 10° to 12° C is associated with vasodilation of cutaneous vessels, most likely caused by paralysis of vascular smooth muscle.[20] Whether this cold-induced vasodilation (CIVD) results in increased heat loss is controversial; some authors think that cooling rates accelerate when CIVD occurs,[91] while others have not seen changes in core temperature cooling rates secondary to the onset of observable skin CIVD.[65] The magnitude of CIVD varies with body heat content, so that after 1 hour, CIVD is not a significant contributor to heat loss.[172] Sympathetic discharge following cold water immersion has significant cardiac effects. Large increases in heart rate occur during the initial few minutes of immersion. As with respiratory changes, subsequent heart rates vary with metabolic requirements.[117] Fig. 4-3 shows typical heart rate responses of lightly clothed, nonexercising volunteers during immersion in 0° C water. Arterial pressure and cardiac output rose in response to the increase in both peripheral vasoconstriction and heart rate. One study on a human volunteer, in whom a Swan-Ganz catheter had been placed, showed that immersion in 10° C water induced a rise in systolic pressure from a preimmersion level of 130 mm Hg to between 180 and 190 mm Hg during most of a 2-hour immersion. Cardiac output increased from 5 to 6 L/min to 8 to 10 L/min.[69]

Electrocardiographic recordings during cold water immersion demonstrate occasional atrial and ventricular extrasystoles during the initial phase of increased sympathetic output.[94,139,140] Such cardiac dysrhythmias have been suspected as a cause of sudden death in cold water.[44,93,95] Although cold-induced ventricular fibrillation is rare above a core temperature of 32° C, it becomes increasingly likely at lower temperatures.[110,140] Proposed etiologic mechanisms for ventricular fibrillation in hypothermic patients include rapid changes in pH,[73,89] myocardial hypoxia,[90] hypercapnia or hypocapnia,[16,168] hypotension,[19] and myocar-

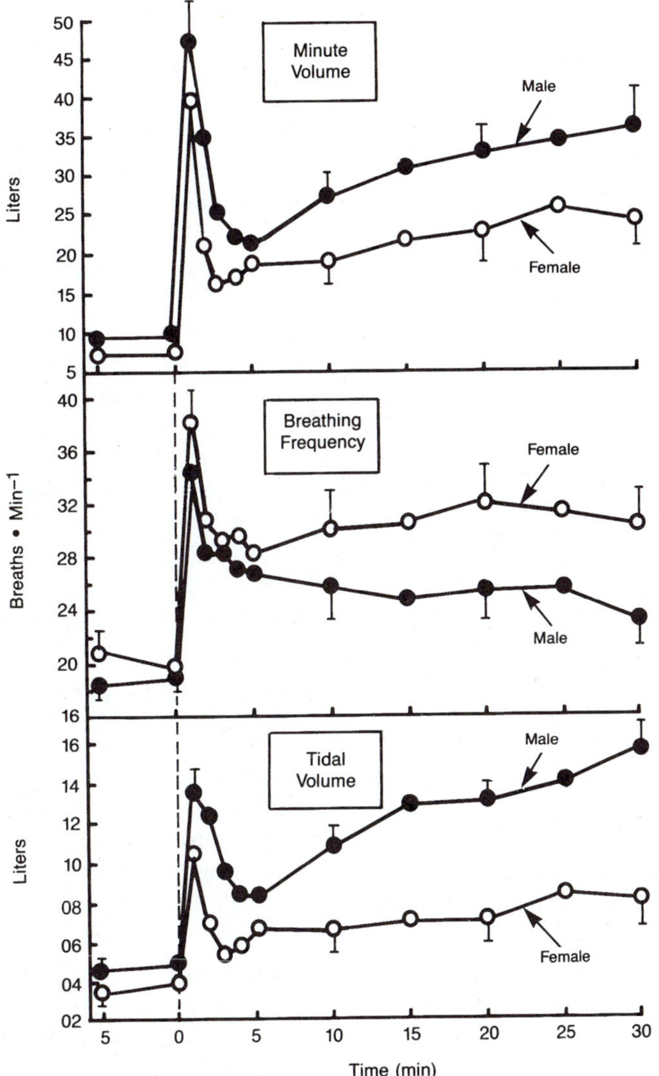

Fig. 4-2 Ventilatory changes in 21 lightly clothed, nonexercising humans during immersion in 0° C water. Representative standard errors are indicated. (From Hayward JS, Eckerson JD: *Aviat Space Environ Med* 55[3]:206, 1984.)

dial irritability with increased sensitivity to mechanical stimulation (such as chest wall compression or attempts to insert pacing wires).[110,140,155]

During cold water immersion, diuresis results from central hypervolemia, induced both by peripheral vasoconstriction with increased peripheral vascular resistance and by "hydrostatic squeeze" on tissues below the water's surface.[29,44] Hypervolemia, in turn, suppresses plasma renin activity and plasma aldosterone, which causes an increased urine flow rate.[29,39] Immersion in thermally neutral water doubles urine flow rate, whereas immersion in cold water can increase urine production by 350%.[29] Prolonged immersion can lead to significant hypovolemia, which has practical consequences during rescue and resuscitation of the hypothermic victim.

Other fluid changes occur during immersion hypothermia. Respiratory water losses follow inhalation of relatively dry air and exhalation of water-saturated air. In cold and dry climates respiratory water loss ranges from 300 to 500 ml/day.[55] Immersion hypothermia is associated with a fluid shift from intercellular to intracellular compartments.[11;30,55,146] Significant cerebral and pulmonary edema has been observed in survivors of severe hypothermia and as postmortem findings.[59]

CENTRAL NERVOUS SYSTEM CHANGES

Progressive depression of mental status occurs at core temperatures below 33° C, and loss of consciousness is common between 27° and 30° C.[110] In severe hypothermia

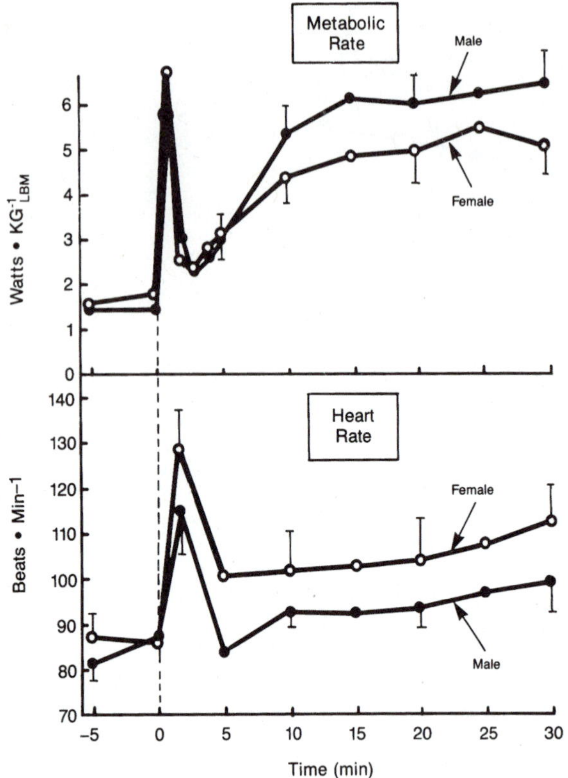

Fig. 4-3 Metabolic and heart rate change in 21 lightly clothed, nonexercising humans during immersion in 0° C water. Representative standard errors are indicated. *LBM,* Lean body mass. (From Hayward JS, Eckerson JD: *Aviat Space Environ Med* 55[3]:206, 1984.)

associated with unconsciousness, cerebral blood flow decreases in response to reduced cardiac output, increased blood viscosity, and decreased arterial pressure.[75,110] However, tolerance of the brain to hypoxia is increased in proportion to the decline in core temperature because of reduced tissue oxygen requirements. Studies in dogs showed that at a core temperature of 22° C, when oxygen consumption was only 25% of normal, the brain could tolerate 16 to 24 minutes of total circulatory and respiratory arrest.[51] At 10° C this tolerance increased to between 64 and 80 minutes. Before the widespread surgical use of cardiopulmonary bypass, deep levels of hypothermia were used to protect the brain and other tissues from anoxic damage during cardiac procedures.[50,51] Core temperatures of patients suffering accidental hypothermia are nearly always higher than 25° C,[122,125] with presumably shorter tolerance times for cerebral anoxia.

Electroencephalographic (EEG) changes in anesthetized, hypothermic humans show a progressive reduction of frequency and amplitude and an increased latency of evoked potentials.[39] However, in conscious, mildly to moderately hypothermic subjects cooled to 33° to 34° C in 10° C water, only minor changes in EEG frequency and amplitude and in visual-evoked responses occur.[39] Apparently an even lower brain temperature is required to cause significant impairment of conscious, integrative function. This does not mean that mild to moderate hypothermia has no consequences for mental performance. Even very minor impairment of brain physiology, when combined with prolonged, severe discomfort of cold stress and often fatigue, can result in irrational behavior. This is supported by the fact that marked behavioral changes have been observed to accompany mild to moderate levels of hypothermia.[10,77,107] Numerous case histories document the onset of hallucinations, impaired judgment, or other signs of disorganized mental activity in conscious hypothermic patients.[99,107,179] These have sometimes led hypothermic victims to remove their personal flotation devices, attempt to swim for shore, or abandon positions of relatively safety (such as atop an overturned boat or aboard a lifeboat), with tragic consequences.[62,106,159] Furthermore, intense discomfort of cold water immersion can produce panic, alarm, fear, or loss of the will to live, often associated with a fatal outcome.[107]

ENDOCRINE SYSTEM

Initial immersion in cold water produces a typical physiologic stress response. Catecholamine and adrenal steroid output is increased, leading to elevations in plasma and urinary levels of the hormones and their metabolites.[41] Plasma norepinephrine level can increase to approximately three times the preimmersion level and correlates well with metabolic rate.[85] Significant increases in blood lactate, free fatty acid, thyroxine, and triiodothyronine levels also occur.[84] Blood glucose level increases, and insulin level decreases. More severe levels of hypothermia are associated with a depressed metabolic rate. Glucose level may remain elevated even in deep hypothermia because of reduced output and effectiveness of insulin.[10]

MUSCULOSKELETAL SYSTEM CHANGES

The vasoconstriction that accompanies immersion in cold water is strong in all peripheral tissues (mainly muscle, fat, and skin), including those of the trunk region. Consequently, skeletal muscle and nerve temperatures decline rapidly. This is first noticeable in the limbs because of their faster cooling rate associated with their higher surface area/mass ratio. Limb strength, coordination, and response time deteriorate accordingly. A study of seminude subjects in 10° C water found that after the first 5 minutes of immersion, grip strength began to fall at a rate of approximately 1.8%/min.[26] Conduction velocity decreased in large fibers of the peripheral nerves; twitch time, in response to direct muscle stimulation, increased.

The decrease in strength and coordination has practical consequences. Impaired muscle performance may affect survivors' ability to swim, to stay afloat, or to pull themselves out of the water. Loss of fine motor skills may affect ability to use signaling devices (such as pyrotechnics, strobe lights, or a signaling mirror) or radios.[62,159]

METABOLIC HEAT PRODUCTION

Numerous studies have described the human response to cold water immersion.[20,68,120,167] During the first 15 minutes of immersion, initial effects are mainly a function of skin temperature as it rapidly cools to and stabilizes just above water temperature. For nonexercising and lightly clothed persons, metabolic heat production (H_m, in kilocalories per minute) and water temperature (T_w, in degrees Celsius) are related by the equation $H_m = 4.19 - 0.11\ T_w$.[67]

After approximately 15 minutes core temperature begins to decline, which induces further metabolic changes.[68] Fig. 4-4 shows the synergistic effects of skin and core temperature declines on metabolic rate. The thermoregulatory heat production of a human in cold water is highly correlated with shivering.[141,167] Maximum shivering thermogenesis in humans is approximately 4.5 times the resting rate of heat production.[68] Although shivering is affected by core temperature, it is driven primarily by skin temperature.[141] Fig. 4-4 shows that skin temperature rapidly increases during rewarming in a warm water bath. Above 33° or 34° C, this causes cessation of shivering and a sharp decline in metabolic rate, despite the presence of low core temperature.

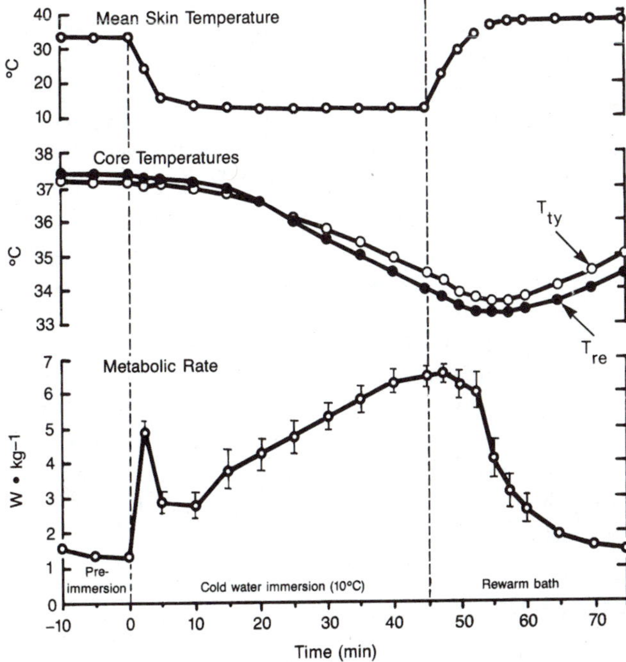

Fig. 4-4 The relationship among metabolic rate, skin temperature, and core temperature for lightly clothed, nonexercising males during cold water immersion and water bath rewarming. T_{ty}, Tympanic temperature; T_{re}, rectal temperature. (From Hayward JS, Eckerson JD: *Aviat Space Environ Med* 55[3]:206, 1984.)

HEAT LOSS AND COOLING RATE

The magnitude of heat loss to cold water is a function both of internal conductivity of heat from core to periphery and of heat loss from the surface of the body to the water.[130,167] Water has a specific heat 4000 times that of air and a thermal conductivity approximately 25 times greater.[130] Thus immersion in cold water is associated with a high rate of heat transfer from skin to water, at least 100 times greater than in air of the same temperature.[130] The resultant cooling or various body parts is a function of both regional blood flow and surface/volume relationships. Extremities and digits cool most rapidly, followed by the trunk.[62] The head also cools rapidly when exposed to cold water.[171]

During prolonged immersion, truncal heat losses are most crucial to survival.[62] Thermographic evidence shows that, despite marked peripheral vasoconstriction, heat losses are high in the groin, lateral and central thorax, and neck.[64] In the groin and neck, regions with a relatively thin layer of peripheral soft tissue, blood flow through the large, relatively superficial femoral vessels, carotid arteries, and jugular veins potentiates heat flow to the cold water. In the lateral and central thorax the relative absence of tissue insulation (muscle and subcutaneous fat), combined with high thermal conductivity of rib bone, potentiates heat loss from relatively warm lungs to the cold environment.

For a survivor immersed in cold water the rate of change of core temperature with time (cooling rate) is a function of the balance between metabolic heat production and heat loss to the water.[48,130] Heat production varies mainly with magnitude of shivering thermogenesis,[76,141] while heat loss varies with numerous factors (see later discussion). In general, for any given survivor, cooling rate in cold water is fairly linear once the core begins to cool.[58,67,165,166] This has been shown to be true for mildly hypothermic (core temperature 35° C) experimental subjects* and for moderately hypothermic experimental subjects (core temperature 33° C).[39,42] The only data that exist for severely hypothermic humans are those from the infamous Dachau concentration camp atrocities, in which conscious victims were cooled to death in ice water,[5] demonstrating the linearity of cooling rates.

Modifiers of Cooling Rate in Cold Water

INDIVIDUAL VARIATION

Heat production, heat loss, and cooling rates vary dramatically among subjects immersed in cold water. Individual morphologic differences account for a significant portion of the variation. The amount of subcutaneous body fat is the most important variable determining cooling rate

*References 58, 65, 67, 69, 165, 166.

through its effect on tissue insulation.[21,91] Cooling rate is inversely related to skinfold thickness. For example, subjects in the tenth percentile for skinfold thickness wearing light clothing in 5° C water have nine times the cooling rate of ninetieth percentile subjects.[136] Fig. 4-5 shows the linear relationship between change in core temperature and mean skinfold thickness. Body size and build (somatotype) are significant physiologic variables affecting cooling rates. Since body heat loss is proportional to surface area and body heat content is proportional to volume, somatotypes with large surface area/volume ratios (tall, skinny subjects) cool more quickly than do those with small ratios (short, fat, and well-muscled subjects).[154,169] Thus for any given body weight and level of body fat, mesomorphs cool more slowly than ectomorphs,[62,142] although this relationship may diminish with exercise in cold water.[155,170] Similarly, subjects with large body size have slower cooling rates than smaller subjects.[142] Children cool faster than adults.[154] The ability to shiver and thus produce metabolic heat is highly variable and affected by many factors: fatigue, hypoglycemia, state of health, muscle mass, alcohol and drug ingestion, age, and core temperature.[10] It is not known how long individuals can maintain an elevated shivering level or at what core temperature shivering fails. Various evidence suggests that shivering does not fail completely until unconsciousness occurs, at a brain temperature near 30° C or below.[64] Inability to shiver potentiates decline in core temperature. In one laboratory study approximately 10% of subjects failed to shiver on exposure to cold.[141]

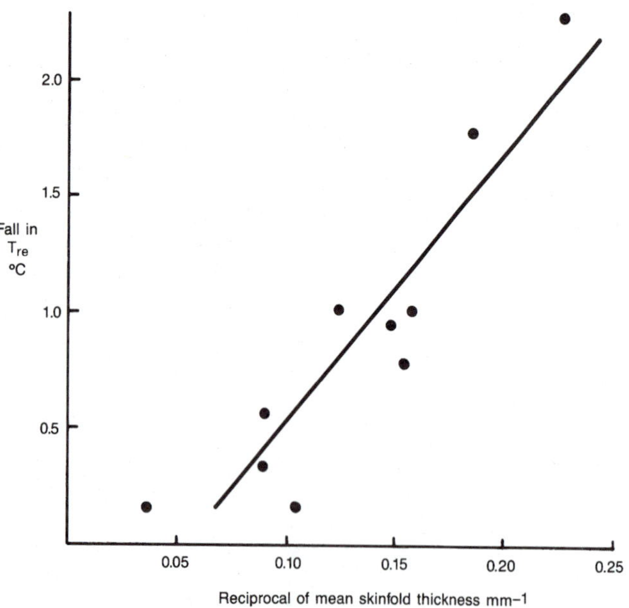

Fig. 4-5 The relationship between subcutaneous fat thickness in 10 men and the decline in rectal temperature during 30-minute immersions in stirred water at 15° C. Skinfold thickness is mean of readings at biceps, abdomen, subscapular, and subcostal sites. T_{re}, Rectal temperature. (From Keatinge WR: *Survival in cold water*, Oxford, 1969, Blackwell Press.)

Gender differences may also affect cooling rates. Because women generally have more subcutaneous fat than men, they have an advantage in terms of this component of tissue insulation. However, women tend to be smaller and to have less muscle mass than men and therefore have a larger surface/volume ratio, potentiating heat loss to the cold water.[19,130] These opposing factors may balance and result in similar cooling rates for women and men. Experimental evidence confirms this supposition.[67,175]

Individual differences in levels of aerobic fitness may affect cooling rates. Some studies have demonstrated increased tolerance to cold after physical training, although other studies have not confirmed this finding.[79] One experiment in 10° C water found that cooling rates varied inversely with endurance fitness level as determined by blood lactate levels.[84] Fitter subjects had a significantly longer immersion than did less fit subjects, independent of body fatness. However, caution should be applied to the idea that overall fitness is an advantage in cold water; the most powerful determinant of cooling rate is fatness, which itself is highly correlated with low fitness.

Numerous case histories support the variation in cooling rates. In July 1993 in the Strait of Georgia off the west coast of Canada, a man fell off a large ferry into water of 15° to 17° C. He drifted overnight for 8 hours before being rescued. He was only moderately hypothermic. Wide media coverage quoted professional rescuers (so-called experts) as saying that this was a "miracle." This erroneous and misleading assessment resulted from an inadequate understanding of the importance of individual variation in cooling rate associated with body physique. The survivor was 6'4" tall and weighed 220 pounds. His bulk of muscle and fat made him a very slow cooler and extended his survival time to nearly double the predicted value of about 5 hours. Therefore his survival was not a miracle but instead a predictable consequence of his body mass.

In summary, the cooling rate of each person in any one immersion situation is a result of multiple individual variables of physique and physiology. Accordingly, large differences in cooling rate are expected and account for a wide range of survival times around the average. This understanding is the basis of the general designations "slow coolers" and "fast coolers" used in Fig. 4-10.

WATER TEMPERATURE

Aside from individual physiologic differences, many exogenous variables affect the body's cooling rate. One of the most important is water temperature. The colder the water, the faster the cooling rate.[71,90] Fig. 4-6 graphically illustrates this relationship.

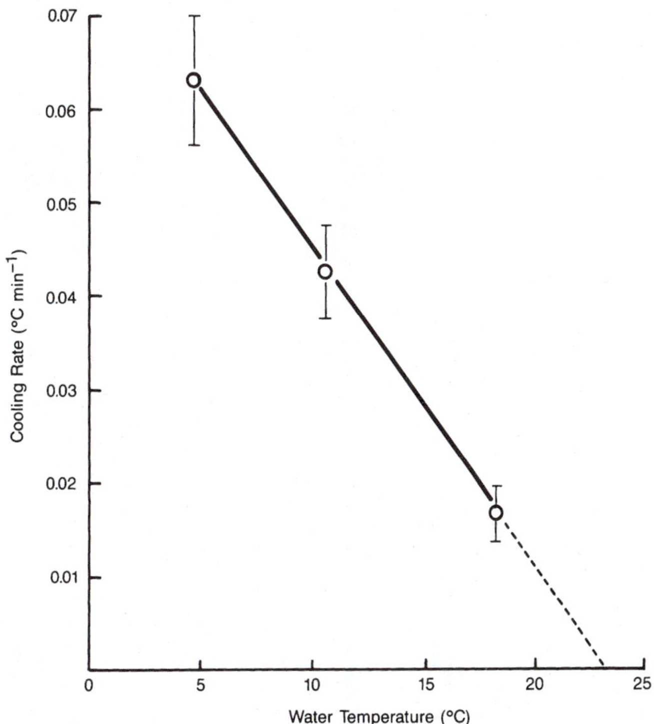

Fig. 4-6 The relationship between water temperature and the mean rectal temperature cooling rate in lightly clothed, nonexercising males and females during immersion in seawater. (From Hayward JS: The physiology of immersion hypothermia. In Pozos RS, Wittmers LE, editors: *The nature and treatment of hypothermia,* Minneapolis, 1983, University of Minnesota Press.)

CLOTHING

Protective clothing minimizes heat transfer to the environment. Most types of protective clothing take advantage of insulative properties of trapped air to limit heat loss. The thicker the layer of trapped air, the greater the insulation.[19] Insulative clothing developed for protection against hypothermia in air is generally inappropriate for immersion hypothermia. During immersion, trapped air is rapidly displaced by cold water.[165,183] Multiple layers of clothing, which in air would provide excellent insulation against extremely low temperatures, are rendered ineffective by immersion in water.

For adequate protection against immersion hypothermia, protective clothing must minimize conductive heat loss to the water. Most immersion protective garments take advantage of the insulative properties of air in a way that limits displacement of air by water. These garments are of either "wet" or "dry" design. "Wet" garments (such as wet suits, insulated coveralls, and thermal flotation jackets) do not exclude (but try to minimize) water between garment and wearer. "Dry" garments (survival suits or other watertight clothing) exclude water from access beneath clothing through the use of impermeable wrist, ankle, and neck seals and watertight zippers. In the case of "wet" garments, air is trapped within bubbles in closed-cell foam, which can either be tightly fitted, as in a standard "wet suit," or loosely fitted, as in specialized, foam-insulated coveralls. When the small amount of water underneath "wet," closed-cell foam garments is warmed and trapped, heat loss depends mainly on thickness of the foam insulation. In the case of "dry" garments, air may be trapped between the garment and the survivor's body. If the garment is also constructed of closed-cell foam, it traps additional air within the bubbles of the foam.

Different types of immersion protective clothing can have dramatic effects on a wearer's cooling rate. Table 4-2 shows a comparison of mean linear rectal temperature cooling rates for lean (12% body fat) male subjects immersed in 10° C calm water while wearing a variety of foam-insulated garments.[165] The relationship of protective clothing, cooling rates, and survival times in cold water is discussed in greater detail in the section on cold water survival.

ALCOHOL

Alcohol consumption is frequently associated with immersion hypothermia, since ethanol impairment of mental and motor performance is often the cause of accidental immersion.[36] Social drinking can result in carelessness.

Table 4-2 Mean Linear Cooling Rates for Lean Males Dressed in Various Types of Garments in 10° C Calm Water

Type of Protective Clothing	Cooling Rate (°C/hr ± SD)
Control (equivalent to ordinary street clothes)	3.2 ± 1.1
"WET DESIGN"	
Thermal "float coat" (loose-fitted, 5.4 mm closed-cell foam-insulated jacket)	1.6 ± 0.6
Short "wet suit" (custom-fitted, 3.2 mm closed-cell foam covering arms, trunk, and upper thighs)	1.2 ± 0.4
"Insulated coveralls" (loose-fitted, 3.2 mm closed-cell foam covering extremities and trunk)	1.0 ± 0.4
Full "wet suit" (custom-fitted, 4.8 mm closed-cell foam covering extremities and trunk	0.7 ± 0.3
"DRY DESIGN"	
"Immersion suit" (loose-fitted, 4.8 mm closed-cell foam with sealed openings)	0.5 ± 0.3

Intoxicated mariners or others near water often fall from a boat, ship, gangway, wharf, or bridge into the water. Drunken drivers capsize or collide. On the basis of frequency of occurrence alone, the consequences of alcohol ingestion warrant special consideration.

Studies on the effect of moderate doses of alcohol (blood alcohol levels of 50 to 100 mg/dl, the range associated with legal impairment) on cold stress have established the following:

1. Rate of heat loss is not significantly increased. Although alcohol normally causes increased peripheral blood flow ("flushing"), this response is abolished in cold water immersion.[40,81,126] Apparently the vasoconstrictive reflex to skin cooling is much stronger than the sedative effect of a moderate alcohol dose on the thermoregulatory system.
2. Rate of heat production is slightly decreased. A moderate ethanol dose inhibits the metabolic response to cold.[40,116] Shivering thermogenesis is reduced in cold water by approximately 10% to 20%.
3. Cooling rate is not significantly increased.[40,116] Because the body's cooling rate in cold water is influenced more by rate of heat loss than by rate of heat production, the slight reduction in shivering thermogenesis induced by moderate ethanol ingestion is outweighed by factors affecting heat loss (such as peripheral vasoconstriction and body fat). Since these do not vary with alcohol use when the person is cold stressed, cooling rate does not change.
4. Fatigue potentiates thermoregulatory impairment by alcohol. Exhaustive exercise leading to fatigue (characterized by hypoglycemia and depletion of glycogen reserves), combined with a moderate dose of ethanol, significantly reduces resistance to cold.[54,90] Alcohol inhibits gluconeogenesis,[52,86] so that the ability to provide glucose to maintain shivering is reduced. If a person enters cold water in this condition, cooling rate is likely to be greater than in the absence of ethanol.
5. Perception of cold is diminished. Experimental studies of humans in cold water show that moderate alcohol dosage to some extent relieves feelings of intense cold.[40,90] This cognitive alteration may be functionally related to reduced shivering response.
6. Cold-induced diuresis is increased. Alcohol inhibition of antidiuretic hormone augments immersion diuresis.[29] During the first hour of cold water immersion, urine flow rate can be more than six times normal (approximately 8 ml/min). For longer immersions, alcohol potentiates the development of dehydration and hypovolemia.

For most humans, high doses of alcohol (blood levels greater than 200 mg/dl) have an anesthetic effect. Major impairment of mental, motor, and involuntary function, such as thermoregulation, occurs. Such individuals cool faster. Alcoholics who "pass out" in cold locations ("urban hypothermia") rapidly and passively become hypothermic.[31,181] When highly intoxicated persons enter cold water (usually by falling in), hypothermia is seldom a problem because such persons usually drown quickly.

FOOD

For most situations of accidental immersion in cold water, type or quantity of food eaten before immersion has no important bearing on rate of body cooling. Hypothermic death is likely to occur before endogenous energy substrates are reduced to a point at which thermal defenses cannot be maintained. However, if the victim was deprived of food for a significant period before immersion (for example, spending several days in a lifeboat before it capsized), depletion of carbohydrate reserves would potentiate rapid cooling. Reduced availability of carbohydrates elicits a proportional decrement in heat production necessary for the response to cold.[111] Men who rested in a cold environment after an overnight fast showed reduced core cooling if they received substrate feeding high in carbohydrates.[176]

BEHAVIOR

Behavior in cold water has a pronounced effect on body cooling rate. The most obvious example is the difference between holding still and swimming. Several studies have shown that exercise in cold water increases cooling rate by

35% to 50%.[67,92] The major mechanism of this response is increased blood flow to skeletal muscles during activity. The resultant decrease in shell insulation[138,170,174] increases heat loss from the body more than can be compensated by increased heat production. Activity in cold water can also increase cooling rate by increasing the amount of water flow beneath any protective clothing (flushing effect).[3,4,165,183] Therefore holding still minimizes cooling rate in cold water.[7,82] Other beneficial behaviors for reducing cooling rate in cold water include minimizing the amount of body surface exposed to the water by adopting a fetal position (see Fig. 48-2), maximizing body-to-body contact with other survivors (see Fig. 48-3), and maximizing the amount of the body out of the water by the use of any buoyant object. Heat loss in cold air, even in wind, is significantly less than heat loss in water of a similar temperature.[87,166]

ACCLIMATIZATION

Although acclimatization of humans to heat is a well-established and quantitatively measurable phenomenon, acclimatization to cold is not as significant. Many studies have demonstrated that repeated exposure to cold air or water produces only minor changes in metabolic or insulative responses to subsequent whole body exposure to cold air.[13,17,101] No clear evidence exists for significant physiologic acclimatization to cold water immersion in terms of resistance to core cooling. The thermal challenge is of such magnitude that it overwhelms the limited capability of humans for physiologic cold acclimatization. Humans who spend prolonged periods in cold water, through either occupation or avocation (for example, channel swimmers), "acclimatize" by morphologic changes (they get fat), by technologic adaptation (they wear protective clothing), by physiologic conditioning (they get used to it), or by combinations of these.

Physiology of Afterdrop

Afterdrop is the phenomenon of continued core cooling immediately following removal of a hypothermia victim from cold stress. It can occur even if a victim is carefully insulated from heat loss to the environment and, seemingly paradoxically, during early stages of attempted rewarming. After cessation of immersion cooling, core regions of the body are still surrounded by a shell of colder tissues through which there is a declining gradient of temperature to the skin. Heat continues to be conducted from core to periphery until the magnitude of the gradient is reduced sufficiently for stabilization of core temperature.[47,178] The contribution of this conductive component to afterdrop varies with the site of measurement of core temperature. For example, the rectal region has a relatively large conductive afterdrop because it is surrounded by a large mass of cooler musculoskeletal and other soft tissue. The intrathoracic region (esophageal measurement site) has almost no conductive afterdrop because it is surrounded by a large mass of core tissues of similar temperature (heart and lungs) and a shell with relatively little musculoskeletal tissue (rib cage). A second, convective component to afterdrop derives from venous return of cooler blood from peripheral regions (for example, skeletal muscles of the trunk and extremities).[69,163] Exercise or significant external warming of skin (above 30° C) diminishes cold-induced vasoconstriction in this large mass of tissue and allows reperfusion of relatively cold tissue by relatively warm blood. Venous return of this blood results in further core cooling. This circulatory, convective component to afterdrop is especially evident in esophageal (or cardiac) temperature measurements[69] but can also be detected in rectal temperature.[149]

The circulatory (or convective) component of afterdrop was clearly demonstrated in a unique experiment on a human volunteer fitted with an indwelling Swan-Ganz catheter for measurement of cardiac temperature.[69] Rectal, esophageal, and tympanic temperatures were also recorded. Over 3 successive days three cold water immersions and three different types of rewarming were performed: shivering alone without exogenous heat; inhalation of heated, humidified air; and immersion in a warm water bath. No cardiac or esophageal afterdrop occurred with rewarming during shivering or during inhalation therapy, although an afterdrop was observed via the rectal and tympanic temperatures with these rewarming methods. Thus conductive afterdrop was observed, but circulatory afterdrop was not, since peripheral vasoconstriction was maintained. However, when the subject was immersed in the warm water bath and skin temperature was greater than 30° C, cardiac and esophageal temperatures demonstrated a conspicuous afterdrop. This is clearly evident for cardiac temperature in Fig. 4-7. Most significantly, this cardiac temperature afterdrop occurred precisely at the time when peripheral vascular resistance and mean arterial pressure fell 50% and 30%, respectively, most likely because of vasodilation in skeletal muscles of the trunk and proximal limbs (and less in the distal limbs).[149] Fig. 4-8 demonstrates these cardiovascular responses during bath rewarming in comparison with the other methods.

Afterdrop is thus a manifestation of two processes operating simultaneously: the conduction of heat down a thermal gradient from relatively warm core to relatively cold periphery and the venous return of blood cooled by flow through cold peripheral tissues. The relative importance of each varies with the site of measurement and with postimmersion treatment of the victim. The amount of afterdrop can vary from a small fraction of a degree Celsius to several degrees. In a strongly shivering victim with mild or moderate hypothermia, afterdrop of the vital thoracic and cranial core is inconsequential (about 0.5° C). In the absence of shivering thermogenesis and other thermoregulatory control associated with severe hypothermia (or with mild to moderate hypothermia when trauma or fatigue occur), afterdrop during

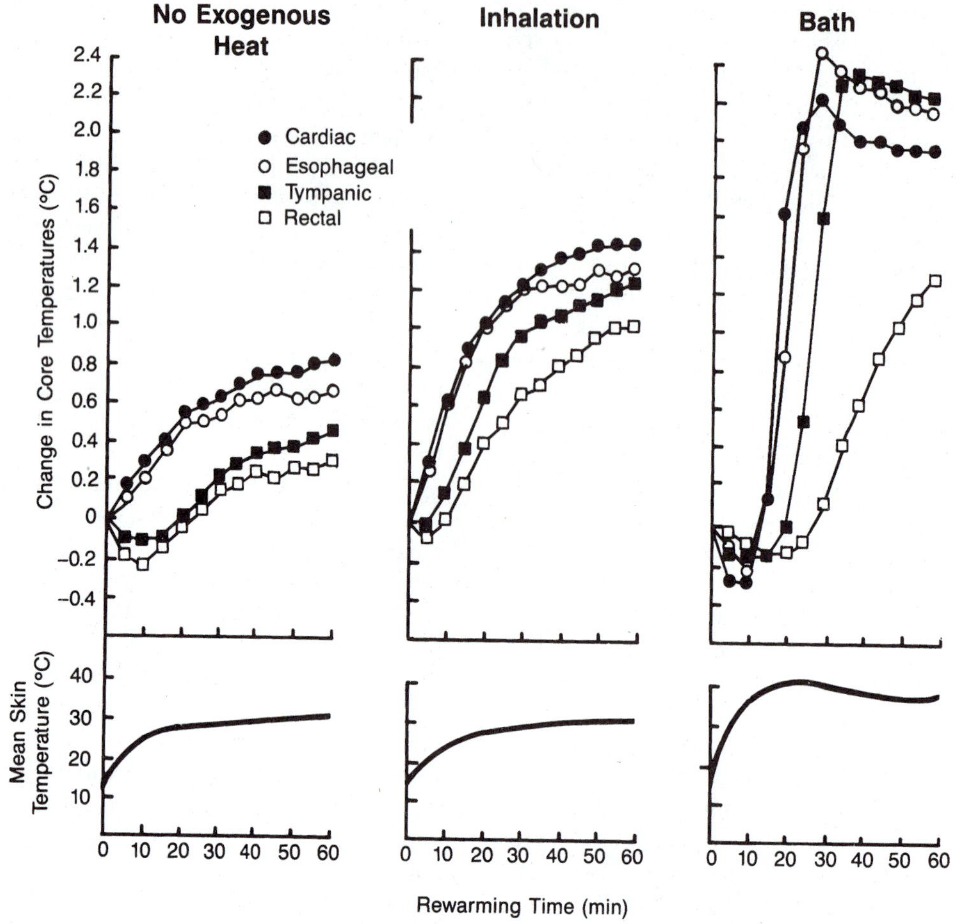

Fig. 4-7 Changes in core temperatures and mean skin temperatures during three methods of rewarming for a single subject: (1) no exogenous heat shivering inside a sleeping bag; (2) inhalation of heated, water-saturated air at 43° to 45° C; (3) immersion in a warm water bath at 41° to 42° C. (From Hayward JS, Eckerson JD, Kemma D: *Resuscitation* 11:21, 1984.)

the first half hour or more after rescue can be up to about 5° C, greatly increasing the probability of cardiac and central nervous system failure. Clearly, understanding of the afterdrop phenomenon is important for rescue and field management of patients with immersion hypothermia. The presence or absence of significant shivering is the most important, easy, and functionally relevant indicator of appropriate management.

Cold Water Survival

Cold water survival depends on avoidance of drowning and hypothermia and on the many factors related to these risks[159,160,166]:

1. Ability to swim
2. Ability to keep the head out of water (even without flotation aids)
3. Ability to avoid panic
4. Sea state
5. Availability and type of PFD
6. Availability of a life raft
7. Availability of other floating objects to increase buoyancy (such as a capsized boat)
8. Water temperature
9. Physical characteristics of the survivor
10. Type of protective clothing worn against immersion hypothermia
11. Behavior of the survivor in the water
12. Availability of signaling devices (whistles, flares, strobe lights, radios, and mirrors)
13. Proximity of rescue personnel

Drowning is the most immediate survival problem following water entry. To maintain airway freeboard and to avoid drowning, a survivor must possess the physical skills and psychologic aptitude to combat the effects of wave action.[28,159] Although a PFD assists in maintenance of airway freeboard, waves can still submerge a survivor's head, even in moderately calm seas.[43,103,160,184] To reduce the risk of drowning in rough seas, a survivor can increase effective airway freeboard by partially exiting the water (for example,

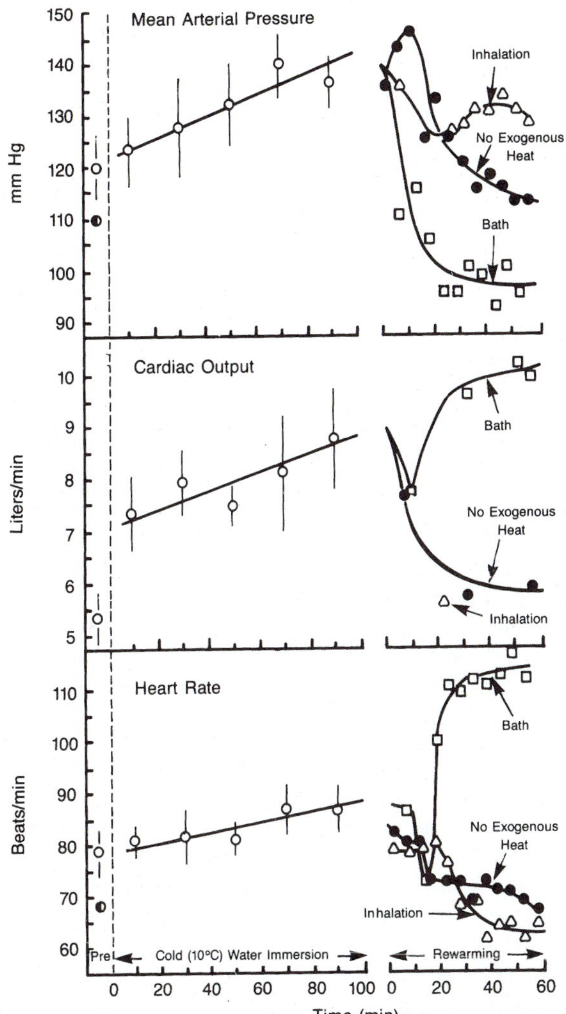

Fig. 4-8 Comparison of cardiovascular responses during cold water immersion and during rewarming by shivering (no exogenous heat), by inhalation of heated, water-saturated air at 43° to 45° C, or by immersion in a warm water bath at 41° to 42° C. (From Hayward JS, Eckerson JD, Kemma D: *Resuscitation* 11:21, 1984.)

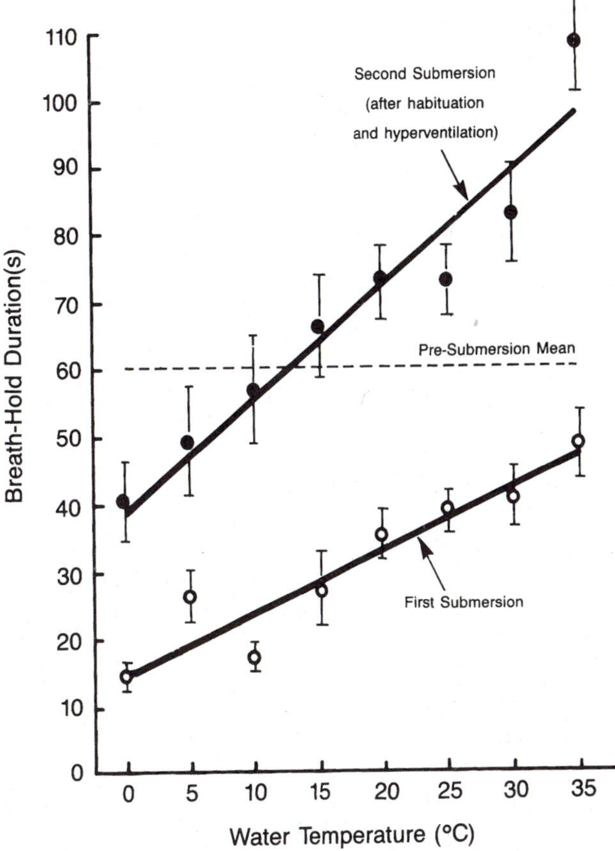

Fig. 4-9 Effect of water temperature on maximum breath-hold duration in young, physically fit human subjects (80 men and 80 women). First submersion was sudden after sitting comfortably in air at a mean temperature of 11.3° C. Second submersion followed 2 minutes of acclimatization to the water. The last 10 seconds of the acclimatization was accompanied by 10 seconds of hyperventilation. (From Hayward JS, Steinman AM: *Aviat Space Environ Med* 46:1236, 1975.)

clinging to an overturned vessel or other debris floating in the water) or by climbing totally out of the water into a life raft or onto a capsized vessel. In both these environments the survivor may still have to cope with the effects of cold wind, spray, and waves. Sudden immersion in cold water is accompanied by cardiorespiratory reflexes that can potentiate the risk of drowning. The abrupt release of sympathetic catecholamines potentiates the risk of incapacitating cardiac dysrhythmias in susceptible individuals or of myocardial infarction or cerebrovascular accident in persons with arterial disease or hypertension.[5,7] Sudden immersion in cold water initiates a reflex gasp and hyperventilation,[26,97,105] which significantly shorten breath-holding duration.[70,71] Fig. 4-9 illustrates this phenomenon. This reflex can have severe consequences for survivors attempting underwater egress from a submerged vehicle, capsized vessel, or aircraft or for survivors simply trying to maintain airway freeboard in a rough sea or white-water river.[147]

If a victim of cold water immersion can avoid drowning during the initial few minutes following water entry, prevention of hypothermia becomes an important problem. Survival time in cold water, based on the pathophysiologic effects of decreasing core temperature, is not a precise calculation. The large individual variations among survivors in morphology and state of health and fitness, combined with many exogenous variables affecting cooling rate (such as clothing, water temperature, sea state, flotation, and behavior), preclude exact predictions of survival time. However, sufficient experimental data and case history findings exist to allow generalizations. At a core temperature of 34° C, there is a significant deleterious effect on manual dexterity and "useful function" in cold water.[1,2,60,135] If a survivor is trying to combat rough seas, this level of dysfunction may potentiate drowning. At a core temperature of 30° C, unconsciousness is probable.[19,61,90,127] Even if a survivor is wearing a self-righting PFD designed to maintain airway freeboard in an unconscious person, drowning is probable at this core temperature in all but the calmest seas. At a core temperature of 25° C, cardiac arrest is probable.[5,90] Of these three core temperatures, 30° C is the most practical for defining the limits of survival in cold water.

For immersion hypothermia the most important variables affecting cooling rates in cold water are the following:

1. Water temperature
2. Survivor's physique
3. Type of protective clothing worn by the survivor
4. Sea state
5. Survivor's behavior in the water
6. Amount of the survivor's body immersed in the water

The advantage of body fat as an insulator against heat loss[21,91,98,169] and survivor behavior have been discussed previously in the section on pathophysiology and cooling rates. Using an extrapolation of linear cooling rate to 30° C, Fig. 4-10 shows predicted survival times of lightly clothed, nonexercising humans in cold water. The graph shows a line for the average expectancy and a broad zone that indicates the large amount of individual variability associated with different body size, build, and degree of fatness. The zone would include approximately 95% of the variation expected for adult and teenage humans under the conditions specified.[5,7] In the zone where death from hypothermia is highly improbable, cold water greatly facilitates death from drowning in the first 10 to 15 minutes, especially for those not wearing personal flotation devices.

A large number of studies over the past few decades have evaluated the relationship of different types of protective clothing to heat loss and cooling rates.* Nearly all of these have been conducted in calm water or in laboratory settings. As illustrated by the cooling rate data (Table 4-3), such studies have generally shown that in calm water, intact, "dry," and insulated garments (Fig. 4-11) provide better protection than do "wet" insulated garments and that well-insulated garments provide significantly better protection than do poorly insulated garments.

Although calm water studies have value in comparing the relative degree of protection afforded by different types of protective clothing, many immersion accidents occur in rough water.[2,15,58,90,127] In this environment a survivor's cooling rate may be affected by swimming to maintain airway freeboard,[7,82] passive body movements caused by waves,[131] flushing of cold water through "wet" suits,[165,183] and leakage of cold water into "dry" suits.[4,88,166] Two studies demonstrated significantly faster cooling rates for human volunteers wearing "wet" protective garments in rough water[165] or moving water[183] than for persons in calm water. Another recent study showed higher energy expenditure and faster cooling rates for subjects in a wave tank than for subjects in calm water.[60]

*References 3, 4, 22, 49, 56, 61, 63, 83, 88, 106, 119, 143, 165, 166, 182, 183.

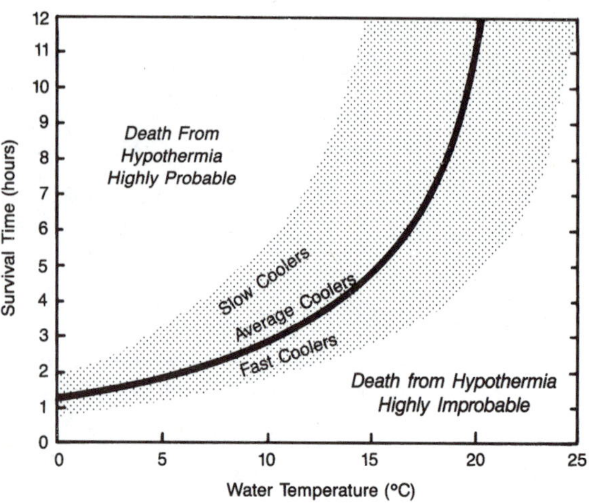

Fig. 4-10 Predicted calm water survival time (defined as the time required to cool to 30° C) in lightly clothed, nonexercising humans in cold water. The graph shows a line for the average expectancy and a broad zone that indicates the large amount of individual variability associated with different body size, build, fatness, physical fitness, and state of health. The zone would include approximately 95% of the variation expected for adult and teenage humans under the conditions specified. The zone would be shifted downward by physical activity (such as swimming) and upward slightly for heavy clothing or protective behaviors (such as huddling with other survivors or adopting a fetal position in the water). Specialized insulated protective clothing (for example, survival suits, wet suits) is capable of increasing survival time from 2 to 10 times (or more) the basic duration shown here. In the zone where death from hypothermia is highly improbable, cold water greatly facilitates death from drowning, often in the first 10 to 15 minutes, particularly for those not wearing flotation devices. (From Hayward JS: The physiology of immersion hypothermia. In Pozos RS, Wittmers LE, editors: *The nature and treatment of hypothermia,* Minneapolis, 1983, University of Minnesota Press.)

Fig. 4-12 shows a comparison of cooling rates for lean males dressed in different types of protective clothing in both calm and rough water at approximately 10° C.[165] The most dramatic differences occurred in the loose-fitted, "wet" protective clothing (such as the float coat and insulated coveralls), where cooling rates nearly doubled in rough seas over those in calm seas. This was primarily due to flushing of cold water through the garments. However, even the tight-fitted, full "wet" suit allowed a 30% faster cooling rate in rough water over that in calm water. The "dry" suit, which did not leak, showed no significant difference between calm and rough seas.

Estimated survival times in rough seas, based on experimental data, were published for thin males wearing different

Table 4-3 Comparison of Mean Cooling Rates for Thin Males* Wearing Various Types of Protective Clothing in 11.8° C Calm Water

Clothing Type	Mean Cooling Rate (°C/hr)†	Ratios to Control	
		Direct	Inverse
Dry, closed-cell foam insulation (4.8 mm thick)	0.31	0.14	7.35
Wet, closed-cell foam insulation (4.8 mm thick)	0.54	0.23	4.26
Dry, uninsulated (watertight shell over lightweight clothing)	1.07	0.47	2.15
Control (lightweight clothing alone)	2.30	1.00	1.00

*Mean body fat 9.1%.
†From Hayward JS et al: *Design concepts of survival suits for cold-water immersion and their thermal protection performance.* In Proceedings of the 17th Symposium of the SAFE Association, Van Nuys, Calif, 1980.

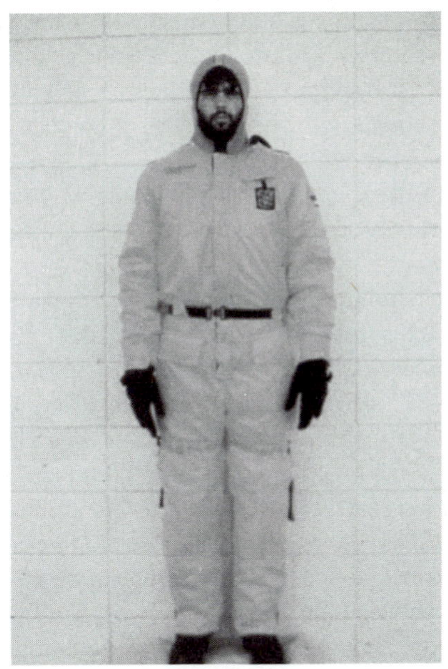

Fig. 4-11 Antiexposure coverall.

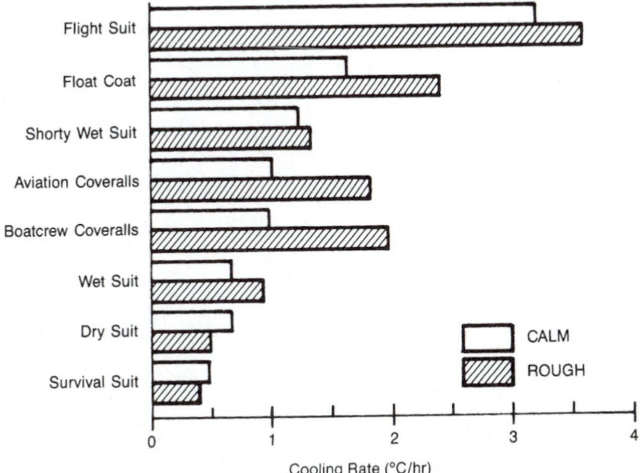

Fig. 4-12 A comparison of mean rectal temperature cooling rates in lean male subjects in calm versus rough seas at 10.7° C. *Flight suit,* Light clothing; *float coat,* loose-fitted, closed-cell foam insulated jacket; *shorty wet suit,* tight-fitted, closed-cell foam insulation covering trunk, arms, and upper thighs; *aviation and boatcrew coveralls,* loose-fitted, closed-cell foam insulated coveralls; *wet suit,* tight-fitted, closed-cell foam insulation covering entire trunk, arms, and legs; *dry suit and survival suit,* watertight ("dry"), closed-cell foam insulation covering trunk, extremities, hands, and feet. (From Steinman AM et al: *Aviat Space Environ Med* 58:550, 1987.)

types of protective clothing in 6° C water.[166] Table 4-4 shows these times for three different levels of survival. The following assumptions underlie these estimations:

1. Cooling rates are linear.*
2. Initial core temperature is 37.5° C.
3. Survivors are able to maintain airway freeboard until unconsciousness occurs at a rectal temperature of 30° C.
4. Self-righting flotation maintains airway freeboard when survivors are unconscious.

In comparing these estimated survival times with those of Fig. 4-10, the reader must recall that Fig. 4-10 concerns only survival to a core temperature of 30° C. Furthermore, the zone in the graph must be adjusted downward for rough seas and for survivors wearing only light clothing, and upward for survivors wearing insulated clothing. For 6° C water the survival times (to a core temperature of 30° C) correlate well between Fig. 4-10 and Table 4-4. We must emphasize that the estimates in Table 4-4 pertain to individuals with an average of only 11.1% body fat. Since many populations of adults (such as offshore oil workers) in the 30- to 50-year age range average 25% to 30% body fat, the estimates of "time to unconsciousness" and "time to cardiac arrest" must be considered conservative for a broader spectrum of adults.

Finally, survivor location has a significant effect on core temperature cooling rate and survival time. The U.S. Coast Guard and other rescue organizations recommend that a survivor of a maritime accident in cold seas get as much of the body out of the water as possible to minimize cooling rate and maximize survival time.[28,132,166,184] This recommendation derives from the higher thermal conductivity of water compared with air at the same temperature.[19] However, survivors exposed to cold air are still at risk from hypothermia secondary to convective, evaporative, and radiant heat losses.[7,19,87,152] In a rough sea environment, wind increases the magnitude of convective heat loss,[7,14] and spray and periodic wetting from breaking waves result in conductive heat loss. One study confirmed the above observations.[166] The cooling rates of thin male subjects, wearing different types of protective clothing, were compared for three survival situations:

1. Immersion in 6° C water with 5-foot breaking waves
2. Exposure to 7.7° C air, continuous water spray at 6°

*References 5, 58, 61, 65, 67, 165, 166.

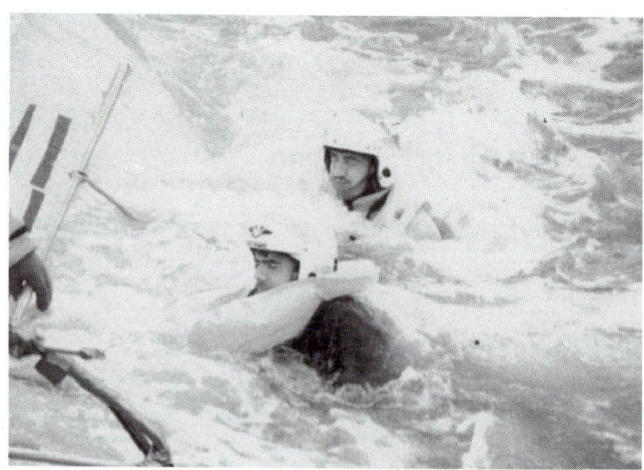

Fig. 4-13 Subjects testing cold water–protective clothing in simulated rough seas.

Table 4-4 Estimated Survival Times for Lean Subjects* Wearing Various Types of Protective Clothing in Rough Seas at 6.1° C

Clothing Type	Estimated Survival Time (hr) (95% Confidence Range)		
	Time to Incapacity (T = 34° C)	Time to Unconsciousness (T = 30° C)	Time to Cardiac Arrest (T = 25° C)
Control (lightweight clothing)	0.4-1.3	0.8-2.6	1.3-4.3
Torn, non-foam-insulated dry coverall (2″ tear in left shoulder)	0.9-2.7	1.6-5.2	2.5-8.4
Closed-cell foam–insulated, wet coverall (3.2 mm thick insulation in a loose-fitted coverall)	1.0-2.9	1.9-6.0	3.0-9.9
Closed-cell foam–insulated, custom-fitted wet suit (4.8 mm thick insulation; tight-fitted)	1.6-4.7	3.1-9.9	4.9-16.2
Intact, non-foam-insulated dry coverall (watertight shell over thick, fiberfill, insulated underwear)	2.9-8.8	5.7-18.2	9.1-30.0

Data from Steinman AM, Kubilis P: *Survival at sea: the effects of protective clothing and survivor location on core and skin temperature,* USCG Report CG-D-26-86, Springfield, Va, 1986, National Technical Information Service.
*Body fat 11.1%.

C, continuous 15 to 18 knots of wind, and occasional breaking waves while sitting atop an overturned boat (Fig. 4-13)

3. Exposure to 7.7° C air and occasional breaking waves while sitting in an open, one-man life raft (Fig. 4-14)

The results of the study are shown in Fig. 4-15. For each type of garment worn, cooling rates were considerably faster in the water than atop the boat (despite the effects of wind, spray, and breaking waves) or within the raft.

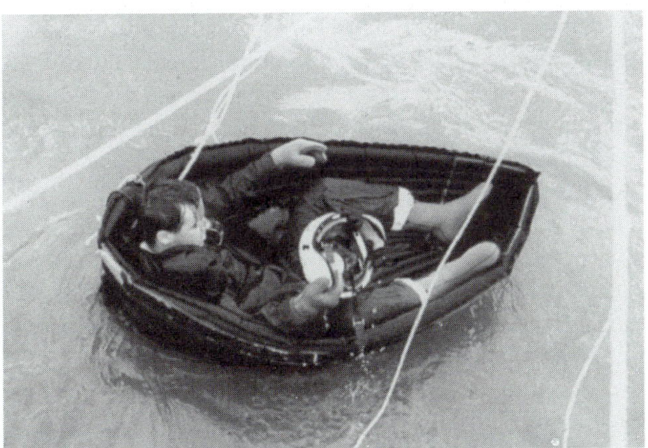

Fig. 4-14 Subject in experimental one-man life raft.

Survivors should therefore attempt to get as much of their bodies out of the water as possible, even if it means exposure to cold wind and spray. This recommendation is poorly understood, even by rescue and medical personnel who frequently work in wilderness environments. A widespread misunderstanding of the concept of "windchill" causes many to conclude that survivors have higher heat losses if they are exposed to wind, especially if they are wet, than if they are immersed in water.[166] Windchill (a term originally used by Siple and Passel[153] to describe the increase in heat loss from unprotected skin exposed to wind) is frequently used in the communication media without regard to the difference between exposed and unexposed skin. This misleads many to believe that the windchill temperature applies to both clothed and unclothed areas of the body. Furthermore, common experiences during recreational activities at the beach, lake, or swimming pool, where people subjectively feel colder after leaving the water (because of evaporative heat loss from the skin) than they do while swimming, reinforce the misunderstanding. This has occasionally led survivors to abandon a position of relative safety atop a capsized vessel and reenter the water, usually with tragic results. The sensation of coldness (which is skin dependent) does not reliably convey information about rate of heat loss when

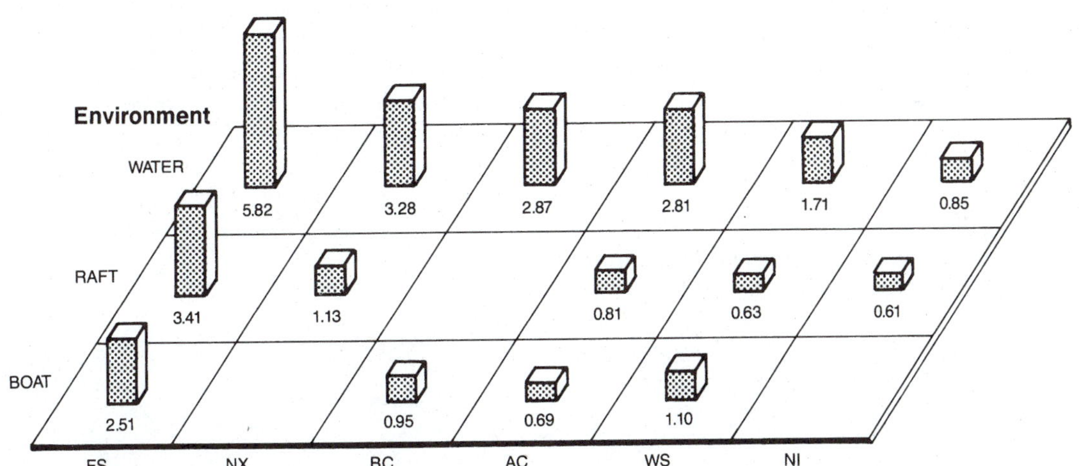

Fig. 4-15 Mean linear cooling rates (°C/hr) for lean males in three survival environments: *water,* immersion in 6.1° C breaking waves; *boat,* exposure to 7.7° C air with continuous 15 to 18 knots wind, water spray, and occasional breaking waves; these exposures followed an initial 5-minute immersion in 6.1° C water; *raft,* exposure to 7.7° C air in an open, one-man life raft, preceded by 5-minute immersion in 6.1° C water. *FS,* Flight suit; *BC,* boatcrew coveralls; *AC,* aircrew coveralls; *WS,* wet suit; *NI,* intact, non-foam-insulated, "dry" coveralls; *NX,* NI with a 2-inch tear in the left shoulder, thus permitting water to leak in and degrade the insulation. Blank squares indicate combinations of garment and environment that were not tested. (From Steinman AM, Kublis P: *Survival at sea: the effects of protective clothing and survivor location on core and skin temperature,* USCG Report CG-D-26-86, Springfield, Va, 1986, National Technical Information Service.)

two radically different environments such as air and water are compared.

Rescue and Management

Definitive hospital management of accidental hypothermia, whether it occurs in water or on land, is described in Chapter 3. This section describes prehospital management of moderate to severe hypothermia with specific reference to immersion pathophysiology. Patients who are only mildly hypothermic (exposed to cold water for a relatively short time, fully conscious, and vigorously shivering with a core temperature greater than 33° C) are usually capable of rewarming themselves without difficulty. These patients are generally not a medical emergency and usually do not require immediate transportation for definitive care. Medical personnel should exercise good clinical judgment in determining the severity of the problem and the need for urgent evacuation.

The primary goals in prehospital management of victims of accidental immersion hypothermia are prevention of cardiopulmonary arrest, stabilization of core temperature (as distinct from raising the core temperature), and transportation to a site of definitive medical care.[148,162] Definitive rewarming (that is, raising the core temperature) in the field is usually contraindicated, since the means to either diagnose or manage the many potential complications of severe hypothermia are unavailable in this setting. In unusual circumstances, when transportation to a site of definitive care is impossible, rewarming in the field, using the principles and techniques of management described in the following paragraphs, would be appropriate. Accordingly, prehospital management can be summarized simply as rescue, examine, stabilize, and transport.

RESCUE

Retrieval of a victim from cold water immersion must be performed with caution. Sudden reduction of the "hydrostatic squeeze" applied to tissues below the water's surface may potentiate hypotension, especially orthostatic hypotension.[29,44] Since a hypothermic patient's normal cardiovascular defenses are impaired,[139,145] the cold myocardium may be incapable of increasing cardiac output in response to a hypotensive stimulus. Hypovolemia, secondary to combined cold- and immersion-induced diuresis, potentiates these effects.[55,134] Peripheral vascular resistance may also be incapable of increasing, since vasoconstriction is already maximal because of cold stress. The net result is similar to suddenly deflating antishock trousers on a patient in hypovolemic shock: abrupt hypotension.[10,44] This has been demonstrated experimentally in mildly hypothermic human volunteers,[44] and it has been suspected as a cause of postrescue death in many immersion hypothermia victims.[46,164] Accordingly, rescuers should attempt to maintain hypothermic patients in a horizontal position during retrieval from the water and aboard the rescue vehicle (Fig. 4-16).[45,46,157,164] If the patient cannot be recovered horizontally, he or she should be placed in a supine posture as quickly as possible after removal from cold water.[164]

The patient's core temperature may continue to decline (depending on the site of measurement, the quality of insulation provided, and the patient's endogenous heat production) even after he or she has been rescued, because of the physiologic processes described earlier for "afterdrop." To diminish this effect, the patient's physical activity must be minimized. Conscious patients should not be required to assist in their own rescue (for example, by climbing up a scramble net or ship's ladder) or to ambulate once out of the water (as by walking to a waiting ambulance or helicopter)[9,10,125,148,164] Physical activity increases afterdrop, presumably by increasing perfusion of cold muscle tissue with relatively warm blood.[42] This blood is cooled; subsequent venous return (the circulatory component to afterdrop) contributes to a decline in myocardial temperature, increasing the risk of ventricular fibrillation.[69] Experiments on moderately hypothermic volunteers (esophageal temperature 33° C) demonstrated a threefold greater afterdrop during treadmill walking than while lying still.[42] Such an exercise-induced enhancement of afterdrop could precipitate postrescue collapse.

Throughout the rescue procedures and during subsequent management, hypothermic patients must be handled gently.[157] Excessive mechanical stimulation of the cold myocardium is another suspected cause of deaths after rescue.[107,110,125,140] Two cases from nonimmersion situations illustrate the problem. The Swiss Air Rescue Service recovered a 41-year-old man buried for over 2 hours by an avalanche.[6] He had barely detectable bradycardia and bradypnea and a core temperature near 22° C. During preparation for transport, he suffered cardiopulmonary arrest but was subsequently resuscitated successfully in the hospital following administration of CPR. In a similar case in the Sierra Nevada mountains of California, a 25-year-old

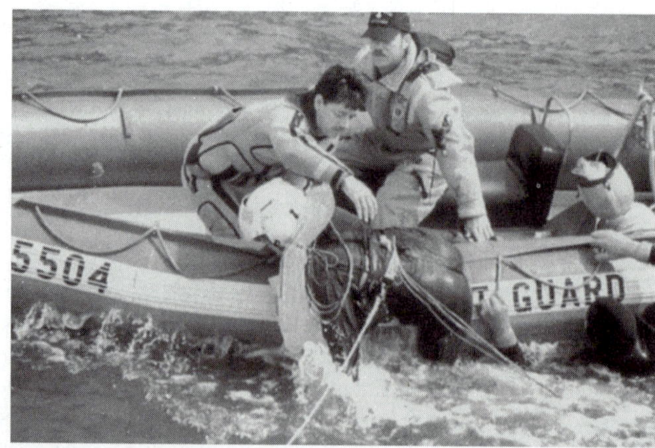

Fig. 4-16 Survivor being rescued from cold water into a Coast Guard boat.

woman became exhausted while cross-country skiing and was forced to remain overnight on the mountain. When discovered the next day, she was unconscious, with marked bradycardia, bradypnea, and a core temperature near 20° C. During rescue she suffered cardiopulmonary arrest but was successfully resuscitated following 3 hours of CPR during a difficult transport effort.[82]

EXAMINATION AND LIFE SUPPORT

Since hypothermia affects virtually every physiologic process, a severely hypothermic patient should be examined as would a victim of multiple trauma.[161] Rescuers should not focus solely on core temperature to the exclusion of other potentially life-threatening problems. In accordance with standard emergency medical procedures, the ABCs (airway, breathing, and circulation) of initial care must be practiced.[9,31,157,164] Rescuers should ensure an open airway and confirm the presence of adequate ventilation and circulation. If the patient is severely hypothermic, respirations and pulse may be slow, shallow, and difficult to detect.* Therefore rescuers should take 30 to 45 seconds to assess these vital signs.[157] If neither pulse nor breath is detectable, rescuers should commence CPR in accordance with normal basic life support protocols.[157,161] Cardiac rhythm should be carefully monitored, if possible. Percutaneous electrodes may be required to overcome interference from muscle fasciculations or shivering.[157] Endotracheal intubation and the administration of heated, humidified oxygen are useful in the management of apnea or hypoventilation.[157] Mouth-to-mouth or mouth-to-mask ventilations also provide heated, humidified ventilation (thus reducing further respiratory heat loss). If oxygen is available, it may supplement mouth-to-mouth or mouth-to-mask ventilation.

Hypothermic patients with *any* measurable pulses or respirations do not require the chest compressions of CPR, even though severe bradycardia and bradypnea may be present.[157,161] This differs from normothermic CPR protocols, where chest compressions may be indicated if bradycardia fails to provide sufficient cardiac output or systolic pressure.[157] Since the metabolic requirements of hypothermic patients are reduced, the observed bradycardia and bradypnea may still meet tissue oxygen requirements.[24,51,110] Inappropriate administration of chest compressions in an attempt to augment cardiac output may precipitate ventricular fibrillation from mechanical stimulation of the irritable myocardium.[110,125,186] If a victim of immersion in cold water is found floating face down, near drowning should be suspected and managed accordingly (see Chapter 48). In this case, correction of hypoxia is paramount, and consideration of hypothermia is of secondary importance.[148,157,164] Normal advanced cardiac life support (ACLS) protocols should not routinely be applied to severely hypothermic patients in cardiac arrest,[31,157,164] since management beyond basic life support differs from that used in normothermia.[157] Defibrillation and pharmacologic interventions are usually ineffective for myocardial temperatures below 30° C.[31,108,110,148,157] Furthermore, repeated defibrillatory shocks may damage the myocardium.[148,164] Although a successful defibrillation has been reported for a patient whose core temperature was 20° C, defibrillation should be limited to three shocks at 200 joules (J), 300 J, and 360 J, consecutively, in patients colder than 30° C.[157] Administered medications are not only ineffective but may accumulate to toxic levels, since drug metabolism by the hypothermic liver and kidneys is reduced.[9,140,145,164,180] For hypothermic patients with a core temperature >30° C, normal ACLS protocols may be used.[157] However, it may be necessary to extend the recommended interval for IV medications[157] because of the patient's reduced metabolic rate.

If the hypothermic patient is not in cardiopulmonary arrest, endotracheal or nasotracheal intubation should be performed gently. Insertion of pacemaker wires and central venous catheters has been suspected of precipitating ventricular fibrillation.[137,150] However, prior ventilation with 100% oxygen has been associated with decreased risk for this complication,[31,32,102,122] and none of these procedures should be withheld if specifically required.[157]

If the patient does not require immediate life support intervention, a thorough and systematic examination must be performed as quickly as possible before initiation of hypothermia therapy. Since severely hypothermic patients may have markedly depressed mental status, they may not respond normally to painful stimuli. Victims of immersion hypothermia may have suffered trauma before entering or while in the water. Skeletal and soft tissue injuries may be overlooked without careful examination.

Attention should be paid to the patient's mental status and other central nervous system signs. Rescuers should evaluate the level of consciousness, the presence or absence of shivering, and the pupillary size and light reflex. Pupils may appear fixed and dilated in an unconscious, severely hypothermic patient, simulating the appearance of death. The diagnosis of death should never be made in a hypothermic patient unless resuscitation efforts fail following adequate rewarming efforts.[9,31,104]

Vital signs should be carefully measured, with particular attention to core temperature. A low-reading thermometer (capable of recording down to 20° C) is required. Esophageal temperature (at the level of the atria) and tympanic membrane sensors measure the most accurate core temperature obtainable, since these measurements most closely parallel cardiac temperature.[25,69,139] Most rescue personnel are not equipped to measure esophageal temperature. Rectal temperature is the most easily obtained core temperature, yet rescuers often show reluctance to obtain a recording from this site in the field, and thermometer placement may cause an erroneous reading. If neither esophageal

*References 9, 31, 139, 151, 157, 161, 180.

nor rectal temperature is taken, oral or axillary temperature is often measured. Neither of these will be accurate in a victim of immersion hypothermia. Facial cooling affects oral temperature, and cold skin temperature affects axillary recordings.[113,117] However, the patient's true temperature will not be lower than indicated by an oral or axillary recording. Thus even superficial temperatures can be used in a limited way to monitor the patient's status, although this is not ideal. Hemorrhage should be controlled in the usual manner. Antishock trousers are normally contraindicated. Inflation of the trousers may force a sudden central bolus of cold, acidotic venous return from blood sequestered in the lower extremities.[10] Sudden temperature or pH changes may produce ventricular fibrillation in a cold myocardium already under 30° C.[16,107] This is particularly true for victims of immersion hypothermia, in which large temperature gradients exist between core and peripheral tissues.[49] Since hypothermia itself can cause hypotension without massive fluid losses, antishock trousers should be used only if the patient's hypotension is severe and secondary to hemorrhage.

INSULATION AND STABILIZATION

Following recovery of the patient from the water, and after management of immediate life-threatening emergencies, the next objective is prevention of further heat loss. Maximum insulation of the whole body from any further cooling by the environment is an obvious first requirement. The main goal for rescue personnel is to stabilize core temperature with a minimum of afterdrop from both conductive and convective components, which can depress cardiac temperature and potentiate ventricular fibrillation. All sources of heat loss (such as evaporation, conduction, convection, and radiation) should be controlled. If the patient cannot be totally insulated from evaporative cooling, wet clothing should be carefully removed. Movement of the patient must be kept to a minimum; clothing should be cut away if necessary. The patient's skin should be dried, and the patient should be protected by dry, insulative clothing and blankets, sleeping bag, or specialized rescue bag. This protection must include the head and neck. Incorporation of a windproof and waterproof layer is of obvious value. This is particularly important for patients requiring helicopter evacuation, since downwash from helicopter rotor blades can reach a wind speed of up to 100 mph.[148,164] Respiratory heat losses should be controlled. Hypothermic patients lose up to 13 kcal/hr through the inhalation of relatively cold, dry air and through the exhalation of water-saturated air at near core temperature.[52,80,114] The administration of heated, humidified air or oxygen at approximately 42° to 46° C can add up to 10 kcal/hr of heat to the patient, a net positive gain of 23 kcal/hr.[23,128,129,157] Although this is a relatively small amount of heat compared to the total kilocalories required to completely rewarm the hypothermic patient, heated and humidified ventilation is of value in insulating the airway from further evaporative heat loss.[23,31,72,107,164] Furthermore, heat is delivered to the core and may help to stabilize cardiac temperature,[72,107] minimizing the potential for afterdrop and ventricular fibrillation.

In an experimental study on mildly hypothermic human subjects, rectal and tympanic temperature afterdrops were smaller with inhalation warming than with shivering alone.[23] In another study, using a mildly hypothermic subject in whom a Swan-Ganz catheter had been placed in the right atrium, cardiac and esophageal temperatures showed no afterdrop with inhalation warming, compared with small afterdrops observed for rectal and tympanic membrane temperatures. All four temperature recording sites showed faster rates of rewarming with inhalation than with shivering alone.[69] Finally, animal studies have demonstrated stabilization of cardiac temperatures with the administration of heated and humidified oxygen.[78,109]

Administration of heated, humidified oxygen can be accomplished via endotracheal intubation or through a face mask. The former has the advantage of definitive airway control and direct delivery of heat to the lower respiratory tract.[31,107,124] The latter has the potential advantage of more efficient heat delivery to the brain through rewarming of oropharyngeal and nasopharyngeal tissues.[72] In either case, vigorous ventilation of the patient should be avoided to prevent relative hyperventilation and sudden extreme alkalosis and to minimize the risk of inducing ventricular fibrillation.[16] The patient should be allowed to breathe at his or her spontaneous ventilatory rate.

In a wilderness setting the ability to deliver heated, humidified air or oxygen can be accomplished with the use of commercial devices available for this purpose. Several systems have been devised[31] that are field compatible; one uses a portable stove to generate steam, which is cooled to a suitable temperature by a special valve, another uses the exothermic chemical reaction between soda-lime and carbon dioxide to generate both heat and water vapor,[107] and a third uses a battery-powered device that permits both spontaneous and forced ventilation. Homemade devices have also been used successfully. One easily assembled unit consists of nothing more than a Thermos bottle containing hot water. Oxygen or air is simply bubbled through the water, saturating the inhaled gas with warm water vapor.[133] Its disadvantage is that uniform temperature control is difficult to obtain. Treatment of the hypothermic patient in the field may also include the "conservative" application of moderate external heat to the neck, lateral and central thorax, and groin (areas with high potential for conductive heat transfer into the core). The intent is to add only a small amount of heat to the core to assist in temperature stabilization. This avoids heating too large an area of skin surface, which could stimulate central nervous system–mediated reflex relaxation of peripheral vasoconstriction. Moderate sources of heat include hot water bottles, chemical hot packs, heating pads, or other warmed objects. All must be separated from direct contact with the skin to prevent severe thermal burns.[161] Hypothermic skin is very sensitive to heat and is easily injured. Third-degree burns have resulted from application of a lukewarm hot water bottle.[133,164]

Body-to-body warming of the patient may be useful.[59] When wrapped together in a blanket or sleeping bag, a rescuer can donate body heat to a hypothermic patient. The rescuer should concentrate on thoracic contact (lateral chest to lateral chest). Lower extremity contact is unnecessary, so trousers need not be removed. As with the application of other warm objects, this strategy may retard afterdrop and potentiate slow rewarming. One advantage of body-to-body contact is its inability to warm the skin sufficiently to precipitate reflex vasodilation of peripheral tissues.[69] There are some early reports that body-to-body contact causes the hypothermic victim to stop shivering and perhaps to lose heat in certain situations. The variables remain to be quantified.

Administration of warmed intravenous fluids is beneficial in reversing hypothermia-induced dehydration and hypovolemia. Replacement of fluids before rewarming has been shown in dogs to augment cardiac output.[146] Dextrose 5% in water or normal saline, or normal saline alone, is preferable to lactated Ringer's solution, since a hypothermic liver may be unable to metabolize lactate normally.[164] Administration of 300 to 500 ml should be given fairly rapidly, with the remainder of the liter administered over the next hour.[9] In no case should cold intravenous fluids be administered. Plastic IV bottles can be easily carried inside a rescuer's clothing (preferably next to the skin) to keep the fluids warm.

The administration of oral fluid or food is contraindicated until the patient has recovered adequate cough and gag reflexes. Hot drinks are ineffective in warming a severely hypothermic victim (mainly because level of consciousness is incompatible with drinking) but may be useful in raising the morale of a mildly hypothermic survivor who is vigorously shivering and can manage his airway. Alcoholic beverages are contraindicated in all cases.

An algorithm summarizing the emergency management of the hypothermic patient is shown in Fig. 4-17. This protocol was recently published in the *Guidelines for Cardiopulmonary Resuscitation and Emergency Cardiac Care* of the American Heart Association and is reproduced with permission from the American Medical Association.[157] Additional techniques and explanations are provided in Chapter 3.

TRANSPORTATION

Once stabilization and insulation of the hypothermic patient have been accomplished, rescuers should transport the patient to an appropriate medical center for definitive rewarming. The receiving facility should be selected on the basis of knowledge and experience in managing hypothermic patients. In the same manner that victims of multiple trauma are most appropriately managed in trauma centers, severely hypothermic patients are best managed in hospitals equipped to handle potential complications and to provide core rewarming therapies. For example, a hospital with cardiac bypass rewarming capabilities may be a better choice for managing a severely hypothermic patient than a hospital without such qualifications, even though the former may require a longer transport time.

During transport to a site for definitive medical care, emergency medical personnel should frequently monitor the patient's core temperature and other vital signs. In addition, they should attach an electrocardiographic monitor, continue the administration of warmed IV fluids and heated, humidified air or oxygen, and continue the addition of mild external heat. Rescuers should maintain the hypothermic patient in a supine posture and should restrict the voluntary movements of conscious individuals. At the receiving facility, rescuers should ensure that the patient is carried, and not allowed to walk, to the treatment location.

In summary, prehospital rescue and management of immersion hypothermia require an understanding of the physiologic events occurring during both cooling and recovery. With such understanding, medical personnel can better prepare for and manage this potentially difficult environmental emergency. When prehospital care is performed safely and effectively, definitive hospital care is more likely to have a successful outcome.

Diving in Cold Water

Deliberate submersion in cold water, as with scuba diving, presents a challenge to thermoregulation. Since the development of insulative diving suits, cold stress for recreational divers has been limited to various amounts of peripheral cooling, with mild core hypothermia. Nevertheless, peripheral cooling can have important consequences for both mental and motor performance.[158,177] Impaired performance can potentiate life-threatening emergencies such as drowning (Chapter 48) and underwater diving emergencies (Chapter 47).

Diving carries a negligible risk of producing life-threatening levels of core hypothermia, except under special circumstances associated with military or commercial deep diving operations.[73,96] Dick[35] showed that for divers wearing 9 mm wet suits while performing routine tasks for 20 to 90 minutes beneath Antarctic sea ice (water temperature – 1.5° C), the mean fall in rectal temperature was only 0.3° C. Dunford and Hayward[37] showed that scuba divers wearing thin (3.2 mm) wet suits during 40 minutes of light activity at 24 m in 10° C water cooled an average of only 0.8° C by rectal temperature. Wolff and associates[183] showed that even thin people could stabilize body temperature while

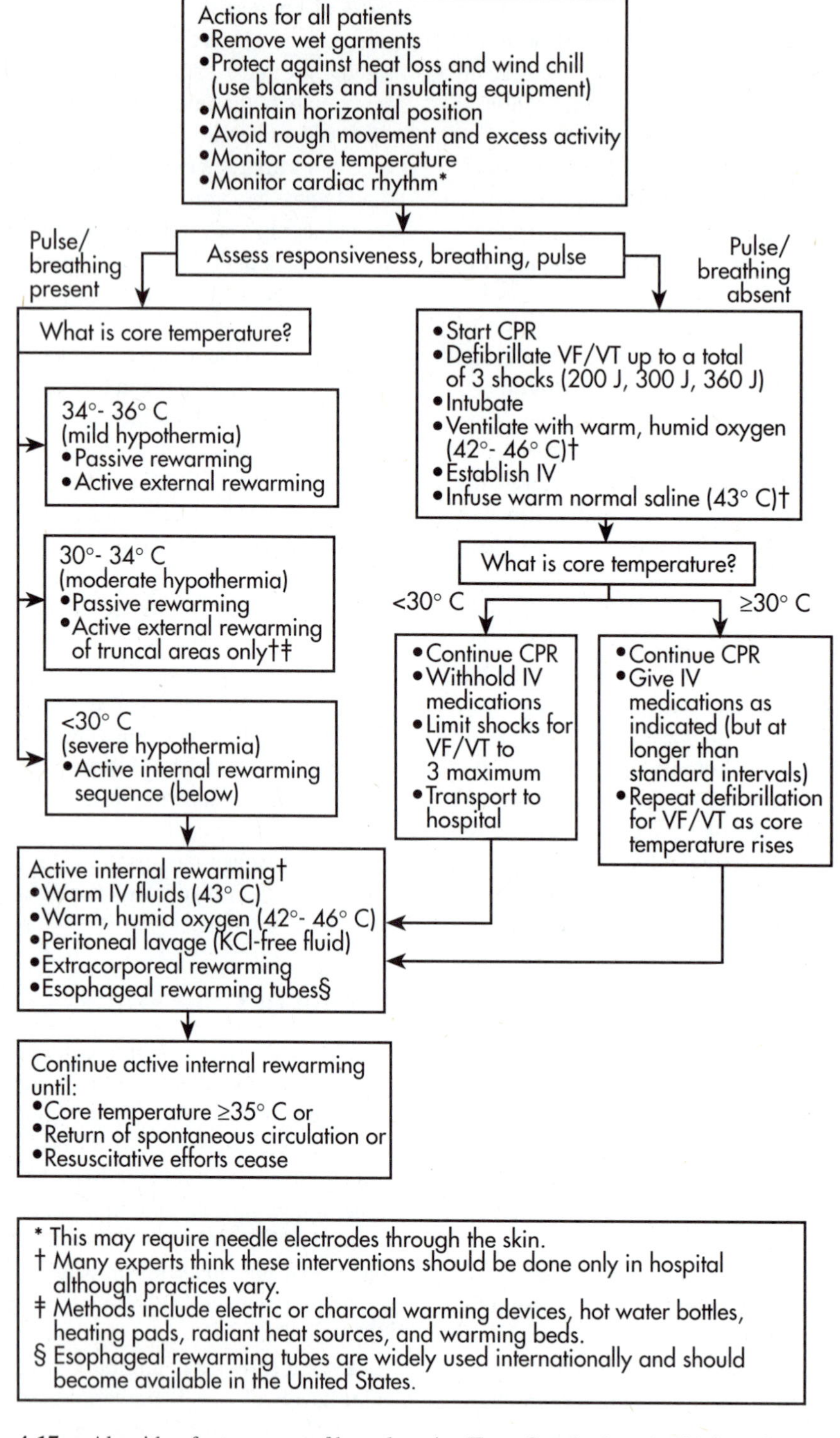

Fig. 4-17 Algorithm for treatment of hypothermia. (From Standards and guidelines for cardiopulmonary resuscitation [CPR] and emergency cardiac care [ECC], special resuscitation situations, *JAMA* 268[18]:2245, 1992.)

diving in water near 10° C and wearing 4 or 7 mm wet suits. Further study is required to ascertain whether repetitive dives in cold water, especially when accompanied by fatigue, can potentiate significant core hypothermia. Since dive duration is mainly determined by respiratory factors, the potential for developing severe levels of core hypothermia during normal scuba activity is similarly limited. Rescuers and divers should distinguish between peripheral cooling and core hypothermia; both are important problems, but the latter is rarely present to a significant degree.

REFERENCES

1. Air Standardization Coordinating Committee: *A technical basis for specifying the insulation of immersion protective clothing,* Air Standardization Coordinating Committee Air Standard 61/114C, 1984.
2. Allan JR: Survival after helicopter ditching: a technical guide for policy-makers, *Int J Aviat Safety* 1:291, 1983.
3. Allan JR, Elliot DH, Hayes PA: The thermal performance of partial coverage wet suits, *Aviat Space Environ Med* 57:1056, 1986.
4. Allan JR, Higenbottam C, Redman PJ: The effect of leakage on the insulation provided by immersion-protection clothing, *Aviat Space Environ Med* 56:1107, 1985.
5. Alexander L: *The treatment of shock from prolonged exposure to cold, especially in water,* Combined Intelligence Objectives Subcommittee Item No 24, Office of the Publication Board, Department of Commerce, Washington, DC, 1946.
6. Althaus U et al: Treatment of profound accidental hypothermia with circulatory arrest, *Schweiz Rundsch Med Prax* 67:1919, 1978.
7. American Society of Heating, Refrigerating and Air Conditioning Engineers (ASHRAE): Physiological principles, comfort and health. In *ASHRAE handbook of fundamentals,* New York, 1981, ASHRAE.
8. Arnett EL, Watts DT: Catecholamine excretion in men exposed to cold, *J Appl Physiol* 15:499, 1960.
9. Bangs CC: Treating hypothermia. In Wilkerson JA, Bangs CC, Hayward JS, editors: *Hypothermia, frostbite and other cold injuries,* Seattle, 1986, The Mountaineers.
10. Bangs CC, Hamlet MP: Hypothermia and cold injuries. In Auerbach P, Geehr E, editors: *Management of wilderness and environmental emergencies,* New York, 1983, Macmillan.
11. Barbour HG, McKay EA, Griffith WP: Water shifts in deep hypothermia, *Am J Physiol* 140:9, 1944.
12. Beckman EL, Reeves E: Physiological implications as to survival in water at 75° F, *Aerospace Med* 37:1135, 1966.
13. Bittel, JHM: Heat debt as an index for cold adaptation in men, *J Appl Physiol* 62(4):1627, 1987.
14. Breckenridge JR: Effects of body motion on convective and evaporative heat exchanges through various designs of clothing. In Hollies NRS, Goldman RF, editors: *Clothing comfort,* Ann Arbor, Mich, 1977, Ann Arbor Science.
15. Brooks CJ, Rowe KW: Water survival: 20 years of Canadian Forces aircrew experience, *J Aviat Space Environ Med* 55(1):41, 1984.
16. Brown EB, Miller F: Ventricular fibrillation following rapid fall in alveolar carbon dioxide concentration, *Am J Physiol* 169:56, 1952.
17. Bruck K, Baum E, Schwennicke HP: Cold-adaptive modifications in man induced by repeated short-term cold-exposures and during a 10-day and -night cold-exposure, *Pflugers Arch* 363:125, 1976.
18. Burton AC, Bazett HC: A study of the average temperature of the tissues, of the exchanges of heat and vasomotor responses in man by means of a bath calorimeter, *Am J Physiol* 117:36, 1936.
19. Burton AC, Edholm OG: *Man in a cold environment,* New York, 1969, Hafner.
20. Cannon P, Keatinge WR: The metabolic rate and heat loss of fat and thin men in heat balance in cold and warm water, *J Physiol* 154:329, 1960.
21. Carlson LD et al: Immersion in cold water and body tissue insulation, *Aerospace Med* 29:145, 1958.
22. Civil Aviation Authority (UK): *Report on hypothermia: evaluation of immersion suits carried out in a cold-water tank at Royal Naval Medical School,* Seafield Park, Civil Aviation Authority, Airworthiness Division, Barbazon House, Redhill, Surrey, 1975.
23. Collis KJ, Steinman AM, Chaney RD: Accidental hypothermia: an experimental study of practical rewarming methods, *Aviat Space Environ Med* 48:625, 1977.
24. Coniam SM: Accidental hypothermia, *Anesthesia* 34:250, 1979.
25. Cooper KE, Kenyon JR: A comparison of temperatures measured in the rectum, oesophagus, and on the surface of the aorta during hypothermia in man, *Br J Surg* 44:616, 1957.
26. Cooper KE, Martin S, Riben P: Respiratory and other responses of subjects immersed in cold water, *J Appl Physiol* 40:903, 1976.
27. *Coroner's report to the attorney-general following an inquest into the circumstances surrounding the death of 13 persons found drowned in Lake Temiscamingue on June 12, 1978,* Coroner's Report J/A.352: District of Temiscamingue, Province of Quebec.
28. Craighead FC, Craighead JJ: *How to survive on land and sea,* ed 4, Annapolis, MD, 1984, Naval Institute Press.
29. Cupples WA, Fox GR, Hayward JS: Effect of cold water immersion and its combination with alcohol intoxication on urine flow rate of man, *Can J Physiol Pharmacol* 58:319, 1980.
30. D'Amato HE, Hegnauer AH: Blood volume in the hypothermic dog, *Am J Physiol* 173:100, 1953.
31. Danzl DF: Accidental hypothermia. In Rosen et al, editors: *Emergency medicine: concepts and clinical practice,* St Louis, 1983, Mosby.
32. Danzl DF, Thomas DM: Nasotracheal intubations in the emergency department, *Crit Care Med* 8:677, 1980.
33. Danzl DF et al: Multicenter hypothermia survey, *Ann Emerg Med* 16:1042, 1987.
34. Department of Health and Social Services, Emergency Medical Services, 1983, State of Alaska.
35. Dick AF: Thermal loss in Antarctic divers, *Med J Aust* 140:351, 1984.
36. Drinking and drowning (editorial), *Br Med J* 1:70, 1979.
37. Dunford R, Hayward J: Venous gas bubble production following cold stress during a no-decompression dive, *Undersea Biomed Res* 8:41, 1981.
38. Epstein M: Water immersion and the kidney: implications for volume regulation, *Undersea Biomed Res* 11(2):113, 1984.
39. Fitzgibbon T, Hayward JS, Walker D: EEG and visual evoked potentials of conscious man during moderate hypothermia, *Electroencephalogr Clin Neurophysiol* 58:48, 1984.
40. Fox GR, Hayward JS, Hobson GN: Effect of alcohol on thermal balance of man in cold water, *Can J Physiol Pharmacol* 57:860, 1979.
41. Gale CC et al: Endocrine response to cold in man, *Fed Proc* 34:301, 1975.
42. Giesbrecht GG et al: Effectiveness of three field treatments for induced mild (33° C) hypothermia, *J Appl Physiol* 63:2375, 1987.
43. Girton TR, Wehr SE: *An evaluation of the rough-water performance characteristics of personal flotation devices (life-jackets),* USCG Rep USCG-M-84-1 (16714), Springfield, Va, 1984, National Technical Information Services.
44. Golden FStC: Problems of immersion, *Br J Hosp Med* 45:371, 1980.
45. Golden F: The present day state of hypothermia treatment. In Koch P, Kohfahl M, editors: *Unterkuhlung im Seenotfall,* 2nd Symposium, Cuxhaven FRG, Deutsche Gesellschaft zur Rettung Schiffbruchiger, 1982, p 43.
46. Golden F: Rewarming. In Pozos RS, Wittmers LE, editors: *The nature and treatment of hypothermia,* Minneapolis, 1983, University of Minnesota Press.
47. Golden FStC, Hervey GR: The mechanism of the after-drop following immersion hypothermia in pigs, *J Physiol* 272:26, 1977.
48. Goldman RF: *Immersion survival: the key factors,* Advisory Group for Aerospace Research and Development Conference Proceedings No 286, 1980.
49. Goldman RF et al: "Wet" versus "dry" suit approaches to water immersion protective clothing, *Aerospace Med* 37:485, 1966.
50. Gordon AS: Cerebral blood flow and temperature during deep hypothermia for cardiovascular surgery, *J Cardiovasc Surg* 3:299, 1962.
51. Gordon AS, Meyer BW, Jones JC: Open-heart surgery using deep hypothermia without an oxygenator, *J Thorac Cardiovas Surg* 40:787, 1960.
52. Graham T et al: Effect of alcohol ingestion on man's thermoregula-

tory responses during cold immersion, *Aviat Space Environ Med* 51:155, 1980.

53. Guild WJ: Central body rewarming for hypothermia: possibilities, problems and progress, *J R Nav Med Serv* 26:173, 1976.
54. Haight JSJ, Keatinge WR: Failure of thermoregulation in the cold during hypoglycemia induced by exercise and ethanol, *J Physiol* 229:87, 1973.
55. Hamlet MP: Fluid shifts in hypothermia. In Pozos RS, Wittmers LE, editors: *The nature and treatment of hypothermia,* Minneapolis, 1983, University of Minnesota Press.
56. Hampton IFG: *A report to UKOOA of a comparison of the thermal protection offered by a selection of survival suits,* Leeds, UK, 1976, University of Leeds Industrial Services Ltd.
57. Harnett RM, Bijlani MG: The involvement of cold water in recreational boating fatalities—I, *Accid Anal Prevent* 14:147, 1982.
58. Harnett RM et al: *Experimental evaluations of selected immersion hypothermia protection equipment,* USCG Report CG-D-79-79, Springfield, Va, 1979, National Technical Information Service.
59. Harnett RM, Pruitt JR, Sias FR: A review of the literature concerning resuscitation from hypothermia. I. The problem and general approaches, *Aviat Space Environ Med* 51:680, 1980.
60. Hayes PA, Sowood PJ, Cracknell R: *Energy expenditure and body cooling in man during immersion with and without waves: implications for thermal models,* Aircrew Equipment Group Report No. 519, RAF IAM, Farnborough, UK.
61. Hayward JS et al: *Design concepts of survival suits for cold-water immersion and their thermal protection performance.* In Proceedings of the 17th Symposium of the SAFE Association, Van Nuys, Calif, 1980.
62. Hayward JS: The physiology of immersion hypothermia. In Pozos RS, Wittmers LE, editors: *The nature and treatment of hypothermia,* Minneapolis, 1983, University of Minnesota Press.
63. Hayward JS: Thermal protection performance of survival suits in ice-water, *Aviat Space Environ Med* 55(3):212, 1984.
64. Hayward JS, Collis ML, Eckerson JD: Thermographic evaluation of relative heat loss areas of man during cold water immersion, *Aerospace Med* 44:708, 1983.
65. Hayward JS, Eckerson JD: Physiological responses and survival time prediction for humans in ice-water, *Aviat Space Environ Med* 55(3):206, 1984.
66. Hayward JS, Eckerson JD, Collis ML: Effect of behavioral variables on cooling rate of man in cold water, *J Appl Physiol* 38:1073, 1975.
67. Hayward JS, Eckerson JD, Collis ML: Thermal balance and survival time prediction of man in cold water, *Can J Physiol Pharmacol* 53:21, 1975.
68. Hayward JS, Eckerson JD, Collis ML: Thermoregulatory heat production in man: prediction equation based on skin and core temperatures, *J Appl Physiol* 42:377, 1977.
69. Hayward JS, Eckerson JD, Kemma D: Thermal and cardiovascular changes during three methods of resuscitation from mild hypothermia, *Resuscitation* 11:21, 1984.
70. Hayward JS et al: Temperature effect on the human dive response in relation to cold-water near-drowning, *J Appl Physiol* 56:202, 1984.
71. Hayward JS: Immersion hypothermia. In Wilkerson JA et al, editors: *Hypothermia, frostbite and other cold injuries,* Seattle, 1986, The Mountaineers.
72. Hayward JS, Steinman AM: Accidental hypothermia: an experimental study of inhalation rewarming, *Aviat Space Environ Med* 46:1236, 1975.
73. Hayward MG, Keatinge WR: Progressive symptomless hypothermia in water: possible cause of diving accidents, *Br Med J* 1182, 1979.
74. Hegnauer AH, Covino BG: Myocardial irritability in experimental immersion hypothermia. In Dripps Rd, editor: *Physiology of induced hypothermia,* Washington, DC, 1956, National Academy of Sciences.
75. Hernandez MJ: Cerebral circulation during hypothermia. In Pozos RS, Wittmers LE, editors: *The nature and treatment of hypothermia,* Minneapolis, 1983, University of Minnesota Press.
76. Hemingway A: Shivering, *Annu Rev Physiol* 4:397, 1963.
77. Hervey GR: Physiological changes encountered in hypothermia, *Proc R Soc Med* 66:1053, 1973.
78. Hornbein TF, Pavlin E, Chaney RD: Rewarming of hypothermic dogs with use of heated nebulized ventilation. In *Proceedings of the Scientific Assembly of the American Society of Anesthesiologists* (abstract), San Francisco, Calif, 1976.
79. Horvath, SM: Exercise in a cold environment. In Miller DI, editor: *Exercise and sport sciences reviews,* vol 9, Philadelphia, 1982, Franklin Institute Press.
80. Hudson MC, Robinson GJ: Treatment of accidental hypothermia, *Med J Aust* 1:410, 1973.
81. Hughes JH, Henry RE, Daly MJ: Influence of ethanol and ambient temperature on skin blood flow, *Ann Emerg Med* 13:597, 1984.
82. Hypothermia and survival, *Seagrant* 5:8, 1979.
83. Ilmarinen R: *Testing of immersion suits,* Helsinki, Finland, 1981, Finnish Board of Navigation.
84. Jacobs DA et al: Effects of endurance fitness on responses to cold water immersion, *Aviat Space Environ Med* 55:715, 1984.
85. Johnson DG et al: Plasma norepinephrine of man in cold water, *J Appl Physiol* 43:216, 1977.
86. Kalant H, Le AD: Effects of ethanol on thermoregulation, *Pharmacol Ther* 23:313, 1984.
87. Kaufman WC, Bothe DJ: Wind chill reconsidered, Siple revisited, *Aviat Space Environ Med* 57:23, 1986.
88. Kaufman J, Dejneka K: *Cold water evaluation of constant wear anti-exposure suit systems,* Rep No NADC-85092-60, Naval Air Development Center, Warminster, Pa, 1985.
89. Keatinge WR: Death after shipwreck, *Lancet* 2:1537, 1965.
90. Keatinge WR: *Survival in cold water,* Oxford, 1969, Blackwell Press.
91. Keatinge WR: The effects of subcutaneous fat and of previous exposure to cold on the body temperature, peripheral blood flow and metabolic rate of men in cold water, *J Physiol* 153:166, 1960.
92. Keatinge WR: The effect of work and clothing on the maintenance of the body temperature in water, *Q J Exp Physiol* 46:69, 1961.
93. Keatinge WR et al: Sudden failure of swimming in cold water, *Br Med J* 1:480, 1969.
94. Keatinge WR, Evans M: The respiratory and cardiovascular response to immersion in cold water, *Q J Exp Physiol* 46:83, 1961.
95. Keatinge WR, Hayward MG: Sudden death in cold water and ventricular arrhythmia, *J Forensic Sci* 26:459, 1981.
96. Keatinge WR, Hayward MG, McIver NKI: Hypothermia during saturation diving in the North Sea, *Br Med J* 1:291, 1980.
97. Keatinge WR, Nadel JA: Immediate respiratory responses to sudden cooling of the skin, *J Appl Physiol* 20:65, 1965.
98. Kollias J et al: Metabolic and thermal responses of women during cooling in water, *J Appl Physiol* 36:577, 1974.
99. Lathrop TG: *Hypothermia: killer of the unprepared,* ed 2, Portland, Ore, 1975, Mazamas Press.
100. LeBlanc J: Adaptation of man to cold. In Wang LCH, Hudson JW, editors: *Natural torpidity and thermogenesis,* New York, 1978, Academic Press.
101. Leblanc JA, Nadeau G: Urinary excretion of adrenaline and noradrenaline in normal and cold-adapted animals, *Can J Biochem Physiol* 39:215, 1961.
102. Ledingham IM, Mone JG: Treatment of accidental hypothermia: a prospective clinical study, *Br Med J* 280:1102, 1980.
103. Lifesaving jackets, *Geartest* No 13, Havant, Hampshire, UK, 1979, Geartest Ltd.
104. Lilja GP: Emergency treatment of hypothermia. In Pozos RS, Wittmers LE, editors: *The nature and treatment of hypothermia,* Minneapolis, 1983, University of Minnesota Press.
105. Lin YC: Circulatory functions during immersion and breath-hold dives in humans, *Undersea Biomed Res* 11(2):123, 1984.

106. Lippit MW, Sexton PG: *Thermal analysis of aircrew survival garments,* Naval Coastal Systems Center Tech Memo NCSC-TM-410-84, 1984.
107. Lloyd EL: *Hypothermia and cold stress,* Rockville, Md, 1986, Aspen Press.
108. Lloyd EL, Mitchell B: Factors affecting the onset of ventricular fibrillation in hypothermia, *Lancet* 2:1294, 1974.
109. Lloyd EL, Mitchell B, Williams JT: Rewarming from immersion hypothermia: a comparison of three methods, *Resuscitation* 5:5, 1976.
110. Maclean D: *Accidental hypothermia,* Oxford, 1977, Blackwell Press.
111. Mager M, Francesconi R: The relationship of glucose metabolism to hypothermia. In Pozos RS, Wittmers LE, editors: *The nature and treatment of hypothermia,* Minneapolis, 1983, University of Minnesota Press.
112. Malkinson TJ et al: Expired air volumes of males and females during cold water immersion, *Can J Physiol Pharmacol* 59:843, 1981.
113. Marcus P: Some effects of cooling and heating areas of the head and neck on body temperature measurement at the ear, *Aerospace Med* 44:397, 1973.
114. Marcus P: Laboratory comparison of techniques for rewarming hypothermic casualties, *Aviat Space Environ Med* 49:692, 1978.
115. Maritime Casualty Report, Mobile Offshore Drilling Unit (MODU) Ocean Ranger: *Capsizing and sinking in the Atlantic Ocean on 15 Feb 1982 with loss of life,* USCG 001 HQS 82, Springfield, Va, 1983, National Technical Information Service.
116. Martin S, Diewold RJ, Cooper DE: Alcohol, respiratory, skin and body temperature changes during cold water immersion, *J Appl Physiol* 43:322, 1977.
117. McKay WR: *Man in cold water: heart rate and electrocardiographic responses,* MSc thesis, Victoria, BC, 1977, University of Victoria.
118. Mekjavic IB, Bligh J: The pathophysiology of hypothermia, *Int Rev Ergonomics* 1:210, 1987.
119. Mekjavic IB, Gaul CA: Functional characteristics of helicopter pilot suits during cold water immersion and hot air exposure (abstract), *Ann Physiol Anthropol* 5(3):156, 1986.
120. Mekjavic IB, Morrison JB: Evaluation of predictive formulae for determining metabolic rate during cold-water immersion, *Aviat Space Environ Med* 57:671, 1986.
121. Mersey, Lord (Wreck Commissioner): *Report of a formal investigation into the circumstances attending the foundering on 15th April 1912 of the British Steamship 'Titanic' of Liverpool after striking ice in or near latitude 41° 46′N, longitude 50° 14′ north Atlantic Ocean, whereby loss of life ensued,* London, 1912, His Majesty's Stationery Office.
122. Miller JW, Danzl DF, Thomas DM: Urban accidental hypothermia: 135 cases, *Ann Emerg Med* 9:456, 1980.
123. Reference deleted in proofs.
124. Miller JW, Danzl DF, Thomas DM: Hypothermia treatment, *Ann Emerg Med* 10:396, 1981.
125. Mills WJ: Accidental hypothermia. In Pozos RS, Wittmers LE, editors: *The nature and treatment of hypothermia,* Minneapolis, 1983, University of Minnesota Press.
126. Mills WJ et al: The effect of ethanol on cold induced vasodilation. In Cooper KE et al, editors: *Homeostasis and thermal stress.* In Proceedings of the 6th International Symposium on Pharmacologic Thermoregulation, Basel, 1986, Karger.
127. Molnar GW: Survival of hypothermia by men immersed in the ocean, *JAMA* 131:1046, 1946.
128. Morrison JB, Conn ML, Hayes PA: Influence of respiratory heat transfer on thermogenesis and heat storage after cold immersion, *Clin Sci* 63:127, 1982.
129. Morrison JB, Conn ML, Hayward JS: Thermal increment provided by inhalation rewarming from hypothermia, *J Appl Physiol* 46(6):1061, 1979.
130. Nadel ER: Energy exchanges in water, *Undersea Biomed Res* 11(2):149, 1984.
131. Nadel ER et al: Energy exchanges of swimming man, *J Appl Physiol* 36(4):1073, 1975.
132. National Science Foundation: *Survival in Antarctica,* No 038-000-00549-9, Washington, DC, 1984, US Government Printing Office.
133. Nemiroff MJ: Personal communication, 1987.
134. Nose H: Transvascular fluid shift and redistribution of blood in hypothermia, *Jpn J Physiol* 32:831, 1982.
135. Nunneley SA, Wissler EH: *Prediction of immersion hypothermia in men wearing anti-exposure suits and/or life rafts,* AGARD Conf Proc No 286, 1980.
136. Nunneley SA, Wissler EH, Allan JR: Immersion cooling: effect of clothing and skinfold thickness, *Aviat Space Environ Med* 56:1177, 1985.
137. O'Keeffe KM: Outdoor health care: how not to be a babe in the woods or mountains, *Am J Nurs* 77:974, 1977.
138. Park YS, Pendergast DR, Rennie DW: Decrease in body insulation with exercise in cool water, *Undersea Biomed Res* 11:159, 1984.
139. Paton BC: Accidental hypothermia, *Pharmacol Ther* 22:331, 1983.
140. Paton BC: Cardiac function during accidental hypothermia. In Pozos RS, Wittmers LE, editors: *The nature and treatment of hypothermia,* Minneapolis, 1983, University of Minnesota Press.
141. Pozos RS, Wittmers LE. The relationship between shiver and respiratory parameters in humans. In Pozos RS, Wittmers LE, editors: *The nature and treatment of hypothermia,* Minneapolis, 1983, University of Minnesota Press.
142. Pugh LGCE et al: A physiological study of channel swimming, *Clin Sci* 19:257, 1960.
143. Reeps SM, Johanson DC, Santa Maria LJ: *Anti-exposure technology identification for mission specific operational requirements,* Rep No NADC-81081-60, Warminster, Pa, 1981, Naval Air Development Center.
144. Reilly MSJ: Mortality from occupational accidents to United Kingdom fishermen 1961-80, *Br J Ind Med* 42:806, 1985.
145. Reuler JB: Hypothermia: pathophysiology, clinical settings, and management, *Ann Intern Med* 89:519, 1978.
146. Roberts DE et al: Fluid replacement during hypothermia, *Aviat Space Environ Med* 56:333, 1985.
147. Ryack BL, Luria SM, Smith PF: Surviving helicopter crashes at sea: a review of studies of underwater egress from helicopters, *Aviat Space Environ Med* 57:603, 1986.
148. Samuelson T et al: Hypothermia and cold-water near-drowning: treatment guidelines, *Alaska Med* 24:106, 1983.
149. Savard GK et al: Peripheral blood flow during rewarming from mild hypothermia in humans, *J Appl Physiol* 58(1):4, 1985.
150. Schissler P, Parker MA, Scott, SJ: Profound hypothermia: value of prolonged cardiopulmonary resuscitation, *South Med J* 74:474, 1981.
151. Schneider SM: Hypothermia: from recognition to rewarming, *Emerg Med Rep* 13:1, 1992.
152. Shanks CA: Heat gain in the treatment of accidental hypothermia, *Med J Aust* 2:346, 1975.
153. Siple PA, Passel CF: Measurements of dry atmospheric cooling in subfreezing temperatures, *Proc Am Phil Soc* 89:177, 1945.
154. Sloan REG, Keatinge, WR: Cooling rates of young people swimming in cold water, *J Appl Physiol* 35:371, 1973.
155. Southwick FS, Dalglish PH Jr: Recovery after prolonged asystolic cardiac arrest in profound hypothermia: a case report and literature review, *JAMA* 243:1250, 1980.
156. Sowood PJ: Does intermittent exercise during cold water immersion affect the metabolic response to cold stress and the surface heat flux? (abstract), *Ann Physiol Anthropol* 5(3):157, 1986.
157. Standards and guidelines for cardiopulmonary resuscitation and emergency cardiac care, *JAMA* 268:2172, 1992.
158. Stang PR, Wiener EL: Diver performance in cold water, *Human Factors* 12:391, 1970.
159. Steinman AM: A few thoughts on water survival, *On-Scene Natl Maritime Search Rescue Rev* 2:12, 1984.

160. Steinman AM: A few more thoughts on water survival, *On-Scene Natl Maritime Search Rescue Rev* 3:14, 1984.
161. Steinman AM: Cardiopulmonary resuscitation and hypothermia, *Circulation* 74(suppl IV):IV-19, 1986.
162. Steinman AM: Prehospital management of hypothermia, *Response* 6:18, 1987.
163. Steinman AM: Hypothermia, *Wilderness Med* 4:6, 1987.
164. Steinman AM: Prehospital management of hypothermia: rescue, examine, insulate and transport, *J Emerg Med Serv* 1987.
165. Steinman AM et al: Immersion hypothermia: comparative protection of anti-exposure garments in calm versus rough seas, *Aviat Space Environ Med* 58:550, 1987.
166. Steinman AM, Kubilis P: *Survival at sea: the effects of protective clothing and survivor location on core and skin temperature,* USCG Rep No CG-D-26-86, Springfield, Va, 1986, National Technical Information Service.
167. Strong LH, Gee GK, Goldman RF: Metabolic and vasomotor insulative responses occurring on immersion in cold water, *J Appl Physiol* 58(3):964, 1985.
168. Swan H et al: Cessation of circulation in general hypothermia. I. Physiologic changes and their control, *Ann Surg* 138:360, 1953.
169. Timbal J, Loncle M, Boutelier C: Mathematical model of man's tolerance to cold using morphological factors, *Aviat Space Environ Med* 47:958, 1976.
170. Toner MM et al: Effects of body mass and morphology on thermal responses in water, *J Appl Physiol* 60(2):521, 1986.
171. Van de Linde FJG et al: Heat loss from the head in the cold (abstract), *Ann Physiol Anthropol* 5(3):130, 1986.
172. Van de Linde FJG, Romet TT: The effect of body heat content on finger temperature during and after hand immersion in cold water, *Ann Physiol Anthropol* 5(3):131, 1986.
173. Vanggaard L: Physiological reactions to wet-cold, *Aviat Space Environ Med* 46:33, 1975.
174. Wade CE, Veghte JH: Thermographic evaluation by relative heat loss by area in man after swimming, *Aviat Space Environ Med* 48:16, 1977.
175. Walsh CA, Graham TE: Male-female responses in various body temperatures during and following exercise in cold air, *Aviat Space Environ Med* 57:966, 1986.
176. Wang LCH, Man SFP, Belcastro AN: Improving cold tolerance in the exercising men: effects of substrates and theophylline. In Hiller HC, Musacchia GR, Wang LCH, editors: *Living in the cold: physiological and biochemical adaptations.* In Proceedings of the 7th International Symposium on Natural Mammalian Hibernation, New York, 1986, Elsevier Publications.
177. Webb P: Impaired performance from prolonged mild body cooling. In Bachrach AJ, Matzen MM, editors: *Underwater physiology VIII,* Bethesda, Md, 1984, Undersea Medical Society.
178. Webb P: Afterdrop of body temperature during rewarming: an alternative explanation, *J Appl Physiol* 60:385, 1986.
179. Wedin B, Vanggaard L, Hirven J: "Paradoxical undressing" in fatal hypothermia, *J Forensic Sci* 24(3):543, 1979.
180. Weinberg AD et al: *Cold weather emergencies: principles of patient management,* Branford, Conn, 1990, American.
181. Weyman AE, Greenbaum DM, Grace WJ: Accidental hypothermia in an alcoholic population, *Am J Med* 56:13, 1974.
182. White GR, Roth NJ: Cold-water survival suits for aircrew, *Aviat Space Environ Med* 50:1040, 1979.
183. Wolff AH et al: Heat exchanges in wet suits, *J Appl Physiol* 58(3):770, 1985.
184. US Coast Guard: *A pocket guide to cold-water survival,* Commandant Instruction M3131.6, Washington, DC, 1991, US Government Printing Office.
185. US Coast Guard: Commandant (G-OAV) data, 1986.
186. Zell SC, Kurtz KJ: Severe exposure hypothermia: a resuscitation protocol, *Ann Emerg Med* 14:339, 1985.

5 FROSTBITE AND OTHER COLD-INDUCED INJURIES

Robert L. McCauley
David J. Smith
Martin C. Robson
John P. Heggers

Cold-induced injuries are almost exclusively a result of humans' inability to properly protect themselves from the environment. Cold injuries may be either systemic or localized, depending on the temperature and length of exposure. Systemic injury is hypothermia, while localized injury is frostbite. Although much confusion exists in the literature regarding the myriad of clinical terms used to describe localized injury, the correct term is frostbite.

Historical Aspects

Numerous historical accounts discuss armies exposed to cold sustaining large numbers of cold-induced casualties. Although Hippocrates described some of the symptoms and sequelae of frostbite, cold injuries were probably not prevalent in ancient Greece. In 218 BC Hannibal lost nearly half of his army of 46,000 to cold injuries in only 15 days when they crossed the Pyrenean Alps. In 210 BC Xenophon described cold injuries suffered by Spartan soldiers during a retreat across the Carduchion mountains after leaving Alexander's armies. In 1778 Dr. James Thatcher wrote that 10% of George Washington's army had been left to perish in the winter cold during his campaign against the British soldiers.[73]

Despite these accounts, it was not until 1805 that the first official report was published on the effect of cold injury.[94] The first authoritative account of mass casualties was the description by Baron de Larrey, surgeon-in-chief of Napoleon's army during the invasion of Russia in the winter of 1812-1813.[36] Larrey wrote,

> When some external part of the body is caught by cold, instead of submitting it to heat, which provides gangrene, it is necessary to rub the affected part with substances containing very little calorick–for it is well known that the effect of calorick on an organized part that is almost deprived of life is marked by an acceleration of fermentation and putrefaction.[36]

Larrey introduced the concept of friction massage with ice or snow, the avoidance of heat in thawing, and the idea that cold injuries were similar to burn injuries. These concepts are better understood against the background as viewed by Larrey. Soldiers with cold injuries rapidly rewarmed their extremities over roaring fires (150° to 170° F) after long marches, only to renew the trek and refreeze their extremities the next day. Larrey recognized that warming was good, but cautioned against the use of excessive heat, and ultimately recognized the freeze-thaw-freeze cycle. Napoleon left France with 250,000 men and returned 6 months later with only 350 effective soldiers. The remainder were casualties to cold or starvation.

During the Crimean War (1854-1856) 300,000 French troops sustained 5000 cases of frostbite and 1000 deaths. During World War I (1917-1918), World War II (1941-1945), and the Korean conflict (1950-1953), at least 1 million cases of frostbite occurred. In November and December 1942 the Germans performed 15,000 amputations for cold injuries.[82] High-altitude frostbite, first described in 1943, was recognized from the treatment of aviators in World War II.[63] The most prevalent form of this injury was seen in B-17 and B-24 crews flying between 25,000 and 35,000 feet in temperatures of –32° to –43° C (–25° to –45° F). When attacked, the only way the waist gunners of the aircraft could operate their machine guns was to open the large waist pots through which the guns were fired. The gunners often took off their bulky mittens and jackets to improve the dexterity they felt was crucial to saving their lives.[84]

Until the 1950s treatment of cold injuries basically followed Larrey's guidelines. In 1956 experimental laboratory work by Merryman encouraged Hamill, the Public Health Service district medical officer in Tanana, Alaska, to try rapid rewarming at 100° F on a patient with frostbite and hypothermia.[10,52] This was the genesis and has become the cornerstone of the method currently used in Alaska and popularized by Mills.[52]

Factors Contributing to Frostbite

No comprehensive statistical data are available on the incidence of frostbite. The Royal College of Physicians in London estimated that 10% of elderly British home dwellers were hypothermic, but no comparable data were available for frostbite.[16] Frostbite is much more prevalent during military campaigns and is a known hazard for mountain climbers and explorers. In the nonadventurer civilian population, Mills collected 500 cases in Alaska by 1963; Cook County Hospital in Chicago recorded 843 cases from 1962-1972; Maria Hospital in Helsinki, Finland, reported 110 cases in 1968; and Detroit Receiving Hospital reported on 154 patients treated from 1982 to 1985.[4,23,34,51]

Physiologically, humans are tropical beings, better suited to losing heat than retaining it. When naked and at rest, a person's neutral environmental temperature is 28° C (82° F); with an environmental drop of only 8° C (14.5° F), the metabolic rate must double to avoid a lowering of body temperature. In comparison, the Arctic fox can maintain a steady thermal state within an external temperature of –40° C (–40° F) and by doubling its metabolic rate could cope with an outside temperature of –120° C (–184° F).

Putting on clothes in response to cold is not a reflex but requires a conscious decision. When the ability to decide or to act is impaired, there is a risk of cold-induced injury.[12] Alcohol has been implicated in many cases of frostbite.[29] Alcohol- or drug-intoxicated persons whose consciousness, judgment, or self-protective instincts are depressed often expose themselves to dangerous environmental hazards. Knize[29] noted that alcohol intake or mental instability led directly to cold injury in 50% of their patients. Once the injury had occurred, alcohol intake probably did not significantly alter the course of events. Barillo and associates[1] experimentally demonstrated increased mortality and a detrimental effect of ethanol on tissue perfusion associated with severe murine frostbite. Alcohol consumption promotes peripheral vascular dilation and increases heat loss. This may make an exposed part more susceptible to frostbite.

The type and duration of cold contact are the two most important factors in determining the extent of frostbite injury.[84] Touching cold wood or fabric is not nearly as dangerous as direct contact with metal, particularly by wet or even damp hands. Air alone is a poor thermal conductor. Cold alone is not nearly as dangerous a freezing factor as a combination of wind and cold.[90] Wind velocity in combination with temperature establishes the windchill index. For example, an ambient temperature of –6.7° C (20° F) with a 45 mph wind has the same cooling effect as –40° C (–40° F) temperature with a 2 mph breeze.[84] Thus it is important to think in terms of heat loss, not cold gain. Frostbite occurs when the body is unable to conserve heat or protect against heat loss.

Because many serious cases of frostbite originate at high altitude, it has been assumed that physiologic changes occurring with increased altitude make persons more prone to frostbite. However, present data suggest that reduction in atmospheric pressure has little or no effect on susceptibility to frostbite. Increased red blood cell concentration does not increase blood viscosity, impede capillary circulation, or have any other apparent bearing on cold injury.[84] On the other hand, deep, loose snow, which traditionally has been thought to insulate from the cold, may actually contribute to frostbite. Temperature measured beneath deep snow is frequently much lower than that on the surface. Washburn[84] recounts one expedition to Mt. McKinley, Alaska, when members of his party found it extremely difficult to keep their feet warm, despite a clear, sunny, –16° C (3° F) day with little wind. One member inadvertently dropped a thermometer in the snow and noted that it registered –25.6° C (–14° F). Feet must be dressed for the temperature at their level, not for surface temperature protection.

Development of frostbite does not depend simply on ambient temperature and duration of exposure. Along with wind chill, humidity and wetness also predispose to frostbite. Skin wetting adds an increment of heat transfer through evaporation and causes wet skin to cool faster than dry skin.[58] More important, water in the stratum corneum can terminate supercooling by triggering water crystallization not only in this layer, but also in the underlying tissue. Skin wetness is therefore conducive to frostbite because it allows crystallization to terminate supercooling after approximately half of the exposure time required by dry skin. This substantiates the clinical observation that "it has been found that supercooling displays itself in greater degree in skin that remains unwashed. Washing the skin encourages freezing, while rubbing the skin with spirit and anointing it with oil discourages it. The capacity to supercool greatly would seem to be connected with relative dryness of the horny layers of the skin. It is well known that Arctic explorers leave their skins unwashed."[39]

The degree of inadequacy of protective clothing varies with conditions and may contribute to insufficient conservation of body heat. Tight-fitting clothing may produce constriction, which hinders blood circulation and lessens the benefit of heat-retaining air insulation. Wet clothing transmits heat from the body into the environment because water is a thermal conductor superior to air by a factor of about 25.[29] Clothing that transmits moisture away from the body may be protective if an outer wind-resistant layer decreases heat loss. However, this wind-resistant layer must retain the same transmission capabilities; otherwise, clothing will still become moist. Clothes that decrease the amount of surface area may decrease frostbite risk. Mittens are more protective than gloves, since gloves have greater surface area and prevent air from circulating between fingers. Eighty percent of total body heat loss can occur through exposed head and neck areas. Poorly fitted boots notoriously generate frostbite injuries.

During World War II and the Korean conflict, clinical studies indicated that cold injuries occurred with higher frequency among soldiers in retreat.[62,88] Fatigue and apathy also increase the incidence of cold injury. When warfare is proceeding toward defeat or in conditions of starvation, soldiers often become indifferent to personal hygiene and clothing and the frequency of frostbite increases.[28] Overexertion increases heat loss. A large amount of body heat can be expended by panting, and perspiration further compounds the problem of chilling.[84] Both panting and sweating consume energy, which compounds the fatigue factor.

Impaired local circulation is a primary contributor to frostbite. Cigarette smoking causes vasoconstriction, decreased cutaneous blood flow, and tissue loss in random skin flaps.[37] Reus and colleagues[68] documented that smoking induced arteriolar vasoconstriction and decreased blood flow in a nude model. Although red blood cell velocity increased, the net effect was a decrease in blood flow in the cutaneous microcirculation during and immediately following smoking. Curiously, habitual heavy smokers do not appear to be more prone to frostbite. Other drugs known to have vasoactive properties may also predispose to or compound a frostbite injury. Disease states that alter tissue perfusion, such as atherosclerosis or arteritis, predispose to frostbite.

Based on clinical observations, an individual who has experienced prior cold injury is placed in a high risk category during subsequent cold exposure.[55,88] For undefined reasons, cold injury sensitizes an individual, so that subsequent cold exposure, even of a lesser degree, produces more rapid tissue damage.[29] Military studies emphasize that long periods of immobility contribute to the extent of cold injury.[29] Motion produces body heat and improves circulation, especially in endangered limbs.

Civilian clinical studies are inadequate for statistical evaluation of factors such as race and previous climatic environmental exposure.[29,47] Military studies suggest that dark-skinned soldiers are more susceptible than whites to cold injury under the same combat conditions.[62,90] Individuals from warmer climatic regions within the United States tend to be more susceptible.[88] There are no data to suggest influence of age or sex in the incidence of frostbite.

The Skin

The skin is an individual's interface with the environment, serving as an organ of protection. It controls the invasion of microorganisms, maintains fluid balance, regulates temperature, protects against injury from radiation and electricity, and provides immunologic surveillance. Each function is specifically related to a cell or area within the skin.[25]

The skin is a highly specialized bilaminate structure resting on a subcutaneous layer of padding. Generally the skin is about 1 to 2 mm in thickness, but it varies between 0.5 and 6 mm. The highly cellular epidermis and underlying dermis are in contact by multiple interpapillary ridges and grooves. The outermost layer of the epidermis, the stratum corneum, functions for protection. The innermost layer, the stratum germinativum or basal layer, contains the only proliferating cells within the epidermis. Between these two layers are keratinocytes in various stages of differentiation. Other cells derived from the neural crest (melanocytes) and mesenchyme (Langerhans' cells), as well as cells of unknown etiology (Merkel's cells), migrate into the epidermis and become organized in specific association with certain keratinocytes.

The dermal-epidermal junctions undulate in most areas of the body, increasing surface contact between the two layers to provide resistance to shearing. The dermal-epidermal junction is a complex of structures referred to as the basement membrane zone, which functions as a filter to inhibit or prevent passage of molecules greater than 40 kd.

The dermis, or deeper layer of skin, is 20 to 30 times thicker than the epidermis. It contains nervous, vascular, lymphatic, and supporting structures for the epidermis and harbors the epidermal appendages. Regions of the dermis differ in structural organization and biochemistry, and each responds uniquely to systemic disease, genetic disease, and environmental assault. The papillary dermis and reticular dermis compose the two main dermal zones. The dermis contains fibrous and nonfibrous matrix molecules. Fibrous proteins, primarily collagen, impart bulk, density, and tensile properties to skin, but also allow compliance and elasticity. Nonfibrous matrix molecules, glycosaminoglycans and glycoproteins, form ground substance that influences the osmotic properties of skin, permits cellular migration in a more fluid milieu, and serves as an integrative, continuous medium for all of the other structural elements.[25]

The papillary dermis is only slightly thicker than the overlying epidermis. Generally it is separated from the underlying reticular dermis by a horizontal plexus of vessels. This plexus provides the overlying papillary dermis with a rich blood supply. The papillary dermis is more commonly altered in environmentally induced skin lesions (such as actinic damage) than in systemic disease or inherited diseases of connective tissue metabolism.

The majority of dermis is reticular dermis. Epidermal appendages either terminate in the lower levels of the reticular dermis or penetrate even deeper into the subcutaneous tissue. Blood vessels pierce the dermis, yielding branches to hair follicles and sweat glands.

Thermoregulation is one body function in which the stratum corneum is not important. The rate at which heat is lost by radiation is a function of the temperature of the cutaneous surface, which in turn is a function primarily of the rate of blood flow through the skin. Heat is poorly conducted from warmer internal tissue to the cutaneous surface because adipose tissue is a good heat insulator.

Thus cutaneous circulation is key to the genesis of frostbite. Because of its role in thermoregulation, the normal blood flow of skin far exceeds its nutritional obligation. The skin holds a complex system of capillary loops that empty into a large subcapillary venous plexus containing the majority of the cutaneous blood volume. Under normothermic conditions, 80% of an extremity's blood volume is in the skin and muscle veins. Skin blood volume depends in part on the tone in the resistance and capacitance vessels, and tone in turn depends largely on ambient and body temperatures. Under basal conditions a 70 kg human has a total cutaneous blood flow of 200 to 500 ml/min. With external heating to maintain skin temperature at 41° C (105.8° F), this may increase to 7000 to 8000 ml/min, while cooling the skin to 14° C (57° F) may diminish it to 20 to 50 ml/min.

Blood flow through apical structures such as the nose, ears, hands, and feet varies most markedly because of richly innervated arteriovenous connections. Blood flow to hand skin can be increased from a basal rate of 3 to 10 ml/min/100 g of tissue to a maximum of 180 ml/min/100 g of tissue. This cutaneous vascular tone is controlled by both direct local and reflex effects. Indirect heating (warming a distant part of the body) results in reflex-mediated cutaneous vasodilation, whereas direct warming results in vasodilation dominated by local effects. When both types (central and peripheral) of heating or cooling are present, their effects are additive.

Cutaneous vessels are controlled by sympathetic adrenergic vasoconstrictor fibers. Vascular smooth muscles have both α- and β-receptors, although the significance of the β-receptors is yet to be defined. Vasodilation in the hands and feet is passive, so maximal reflex vasodilation occurs after sympathectomy. After sympathectomy, residual local control of vascular tone persists, so that direct heat or cold continues to alter blood flow.

When the hand or foot is cooled to 15° C (59° F), maximal vasoconstriction and minimal blood flow occur. If cooling continues to 10° C (50° F), vasoconstriction is interrupted by periods of vasodilation and an associated increase in blood and heat flow. This cold-induced vasodilation (CIVD), or "hunting response," recurs in 5- to 10-minute cycles to provide some protection from the cold. There is considerable individual variation in the amount of CIVD, which might explain some of the variation in susceptibility to frostbite. Prolonged repeated exposure to cold will increase CIVD and offer some degree of acclimatization. Eskimos, Lapps, and Nordic fishermen have a very strong CIVD response and very short intervals between dilations, which may contribute to maintenance of hand function in the cold environment.

There is little evidence that humans have any significant physiologic adaptation to cold. They remain homeothermic, warm weather, tropical animals who neither tolerate nor adapt well to the cold. They must find a well-defined microclimate to keep skin temperature close to 32.8° C (91° F). Normal skin maturation and tissue function rely on the maintenance of permeability and integrity of all tissue membranes. A steady rate relationship of prostaglandins, particularly PGE_2 (vasodilator) and $PGF_{2\alpha}$ (vasoconstrictor), is crucial for normal skin function. An imbalance may disrupt cell membrane equilibrium. This relationship is controlled through PGE_2-9-ketoreductase and nicotinamide adenine dinucleotide phosphate (NADPH). Low concentrations of PGE_2-9-ketoreductase found in normal skin emphasize an active biologic presence.

Frostbite Injury

The frostbite injury has classically been divided into four pathologic phases[32]:

1. Prefreeze phase. This is secondary to chilling and prior to ice crystal formation. Changes are caused by vasospasticity and transendothelial plasma leakage. Tissue temperature ranges from 3° to 10° C (37° to 50° F). Cutaneous sensation is generally abolished at 10° C (50° F).
2. Freeze-thaw phase. This is caused by actual ice crystal formation. Tissue temperature drops below the freezing point as the ambient environmental temperature dips below –15° to –6° C (5° to 21° F). Because of the underlying radiation of heat energy, skin must be supercooled to –4° C (24.8° F) to freeze. With no circulation, skin temperature may drop at a rate in excess of 0.5° C (1° F) per minute. After it is completely frozen, the tissue rapidly exhibits poikilothermy. The susceptibility of tissue to freezing varies, with endothelium, bone marrow, and nerve tissue more sensitive than muscle, bone, and cartilage.
3. Vascular stasis phase. This involves changes in blood vessels, including spasticity and dilation, and includes plasma leakage, stasis coagulation, and shunting.
4. Late ischemic phase. This is a result of thrombosis and arteriovenous shunting, ischemia, gangrene, and autonomic dysfunction.

Overlap occurs among these phases.[33] The changes during each phase vary with rapidity of freezing and duration and extent of injury. It is therefore conceptually clearer to divide pathologic changes occurring in frostbite into those resulting from direct cellular injury and those from indirect cellular effects. Changes caused by direct injury include the following[92]:

1. Extracellular ice formation
2. Intracellular ice formation
3. Cell dehydration and shrinkage
4. Abnormal intracellular electrolyte concentrations
5. Thermal shock
6. Denaturation of lipid-protein complexes

Cells subjected to a slow rate of cooling (hours) develop ice crystals extracellularly in the cellular interspaces. Rapid cooling (seconds to minutes) produces intracellular ice crystals, which are more lethal to the cell and less favorable for cell survival. In a clinical cold injury the slower rate of freezing does not produce intracellular crystals[49]; however, the extracellular ice formed is not innocuous. It draws water across the cell membrane, contributing to intracellular dehydration. The theory of cellular dehydration was originally proposed by Moran[59] in 1929 and subsequently supported by Merryman's study of "ice-crystal nucleation."[48] Cellular dehydration produces modification of protein structure by high electrolyte concentration, alteration of membrane lipids, alteration of cellular pH, and imbalance of chemical activity.[44,45] This phenomenon subsequently permits a marked and toxic increase of electrolytes within the cell, leading to partial shrinkage and collapse of its vital cell membrane. These events are incompatible with cell survival.

Not all the water within a cell is freezable. A small amount of unfrozen water, "bound water," constitutes up to 10% of the total water content and is held tightly in the protein complex within the cell. No matter how rapid or marked the cold injury, this bound water remains liquid. At temperatures below –20° C (–4° F), approximately 90% of available water is frozen.[92] Although the theory of ice crystal disruption of cell structure is attractive, it has yet to be conclusively proven.

Thermal shock defines the phenomenon of sudden and profound temperature change in a biologic system.[19] Precipitous chilling has been theorized to be incompatible with life, but the severity of this phenomenon is debatable. Another poorly understood concept is the manner in which subzero temperatures produce denaturation of lipid-protein complexes. One theory hypothesizes detachment of lipids and lipid protein from cell membranes as a consequence of the solvent action of a toxic electrolyte concentration within a cell.[40,41] There is no direct evidence supporting an alteration of enzyme activity during freezing, but DNA synthesis is inhibited.[27] On the other hand, there is indirect evidence of ox liver catalase inactivation caused by denaturation and structural alteration of lactic acid dehydrogenase after freezing and thawing.[42,78]

Indirect cellular damage secondary to progressive microvascular insults is more severe than the direct cellular effect. This is supported by the observation that skin tissue subjected to a standard freeze-thaw injury, which consistently produced necrosis in vivo, survived as a full-thickness skin graft when transplanted to an uninjured recipient site.[85] Conversely, uninjured full-thickness skin did not survive when transferred to a recipient area pretreated with the same freezing injury. Thus direct skin injury is reversible. The progressive nature of injury is probably secondary to microvascular changes.

Approximately 60% of skin capillary circulation ceases in the temperature range of 3° to 11° C, while 35% and 40% of blood flow ceases in arterioles and venules, respectively.[69] Capillary patency is initially restored in thawed tissue, but blood flow declines 3 to 5 minutes later. Three nearly simultaneous phenomena occur after thawing: momentary and initial vasoconstriction of arterioles and venules, resumption of capillary circulation and blood flow, and showers of emboli coursing through microvessels.[92] Ultimately there is progressive tissue loss caused by progressive thrombosis and hypoxia. This is similar to tissue loss seen in the distal dying random flap and the no reflow phenomenon. For both of these, in addition to the effect of arachidonic acid metabolites, oxygen free radicals have been shown to be detrimental and contribute to tissue loss. This may be the case in the frostbite injury.[9]

Considerable evidence points to the primary alteration of the cold injury being injury to vascular endothelium.[92] Seventy-two hours after a freeze-thaw injury there is loss of vascular endothelium in the capillary walls, accompanied by significant fibrin deposition. The endothelium may be totally destroyed, and fibrin may saturate the arteriole walls.[92] Ultrastructural derangement of endothelial cells following the thaw period has been observed by electron microscopy in capillaries of the hamster cheek pouch following subzero temperatures.[66] The endothelial injury was confirmed by demonstrating fluid extravasation from vessels almost immediately after thawing.[93] As in other forms of trauma, vascular endothelial cells swell and protrude inward into the lumen until they lyse.

Venules appear more sensitive to cold injury than are other vascular structures, partly because of lower flow rates. Arterioles, with a rate of flow almost twice that of venules, are less damaged by freezing and develop stasis later than venules. Capillaries manifest the fewest direct effects of cold injury, but their flow is quickly arrested as a result of their position between arterioles and venules. Generalized stasis and cessation of flow are noted at the point of injury within 20 minutes after freeze and thaw. "White thrombi" (blood cells and fibrin) follow platelet thrombi as blood flow progressively slows. Sludging and stasis result in ultimate thrombosis. Microangiography after cold injury shows that although spasm of the arterioles and venules exists, it is not marked enough to completely account for the decreased flow of progressive microvascular collapse.[2] It has been postulated that defects seen in angiograms are caused by local factors, possible thrombi. It has also been observed that vascular thrombosis following cold injury advances from the capillary level to that of the large vessels, and ultimately results in ischemic death of progressively larger areas.[31,32] Viable dermal cells may be observed histologically in cold-injured tissues for up to 8 days or until occlusion of local vessels occurs. This emphasizes that a major role is played by vascular insufficiency, and that direct injury to cellular structures and mechanisms may be reversible.

Because Cohnheim had shown changes in cold injury to be similar to changes seen in other inflammatory states, Robson and Heggers[70] postulated that progressive ischemia seen in frostbite might be due to the same inflammatory mediators responsible for progressive dermal ischemia in the burn wound. They evaluated blister fluid from patients with hand frostbite, measuring levels of PGE_2, $PGF_{2\alpha}$, and thromboxane B_2. Levels of the vasoconstricting, platelet-aggregating, and leukocyte-sticking prostanoids ($PGF_{2\alpha}$ and thromboxane A_2) were markedly elevated. The investigators postulated that massive edema following cold injury was due either to leakage of proteins caused by release of these prostanoids or to leukocyte sludging in the capillaries and increased hydrostatic pressure. Recent studies have confirmed the similarity between cold injury and the burn wound.[9]

Severe endothelial damage was observed by researchers studying a minimal cold injury model in the hairless mouse.[5] In addition, the sequence of endothelial damage, vascular dilation, vascular incompetence, and erythrocyte extravasation was confirmed. This led to speculation that arachidonic acid metabolites, which may originate from severely damaged endothelial cells, are important in progressive tissue loss. Significantly absent from in vivo and microscopic observations were vascular spasm, thrombosis, and fibrin deposition, all of which have previously been implicated as pathophysiologic mechanisms. A rabbit ear model demonstrated increased tissue survival following blockade of the arachidonic acid cascade at all levels.[67] The most marked tissue salvage resulted when specific thromboxane A_2 inhibitors were used. This has now been shown to be effective in clinical situations.[23]

SKIN CHANGES IN RESPONSE TO FROSTBITE

Reports in the 1940s documenting the histopathology of frostbite injury to the skin have been scarce and incomplete. Historically, studies by several investigators have been limited to skin biopsies without documentation of location, exposure time, temperature, or postinjury intervals.[75] More recently, experimental studies have been able to document the histopathology of skin changes under controlled conditions.

In 1988 Schoning and Hamlet[75] used a Hanford miniature swine model for frostbite injury (–75° C exposure for up to 20 minutes) to note progressive epithelial damage. Early changes included vacuolization of keratinocytes, with loss of intercellular attachments and pyknosis over a period of 1 week or more. This subsequently progressed to advanced cellular degeneration and the formation of microabscesses at the dermoepidermal junction. Later changes include epithelial necrosis and regeneration, both separately or together within the same tissue. Such histopathologic data favor the current standard of conservative management of frostbite injury.

However, Marzella and associates[43] used a New Zealand white rabbit ear model of frostbite injury and proposed that the skin necrosis induced by frostbite injury was merely a reflection of damage to the target cell: the endothelial cell. After submersion of a shaved rabbit ear in 60% ethyl alcohol at –21° C for 60 seconds, the entire microvasculature demonstrated endothelial damage within 1 hour; erythrocyte extravasation occurred within 6 hours. These early vascular changes in the rabbit ear model are in contradistinction to the timing of vascular changes in the Hanford miniature swine model reported by Schoning and colleagues. These authors performed biopsies on animals exposed to frostbite injury (–75° C for up to 20 minutes) and evaluated the specimens for vascular inflammation, medial degeneration, and thrombosis.[76] The earliest change documented both grossly and microscopically was hyperemia. Within 6 to 24 hours, leukocyte migration and vasculitis were noted. However, the most severe vascular changes of thrombosis and medial degeneration were not documented for 1 to 2 weeks following the injury.

Whether or not the changes in the epidermis are primary or secondary to damage to the underlying endothelial cells, it is clear that these tissues have a potential, although limited, capacity for regeneration. This further supports a conservative approach to the management of frostbite injury.

CLINICAL PRESENTATION

Classically frostbite has been described by its clinical presentation. Initially it is difficult to predict the extent of frostbite damage.[30,54] Mills[53] favors the use of two simple classifications: mild (without tissue loss) and severe (with tissue loss). Historically frostbite has been divided into "degrees of injury" based on acute physical findings after freezing and rewarming. First-degree injury shows numbness and erythema. There is a white or yellowish, firm plaque in the area of injury. There is no tissue loss, although edema is common. Second-degree injury results in superficial skin vesiculation (Fig. 5-1). A clear or milky fluid is present within the blisters, surrounded by erythema and edema. Third-degree injury shows deeper blisters, characterized by purple, blood-containing fluid (Color Plate 8). This indicates that the injury is into the reticular dermis and beneath the dermal vascular plexus. Fourth-degree injury is completely through the dermis and involves the relatively avascular subcuticular tissues (Color Plate 9). This tends to cause mummification, with muscle and bone involvement. Less severe bone injury in children may affect the growth plate and result in developmental digital deformities.[8,11]

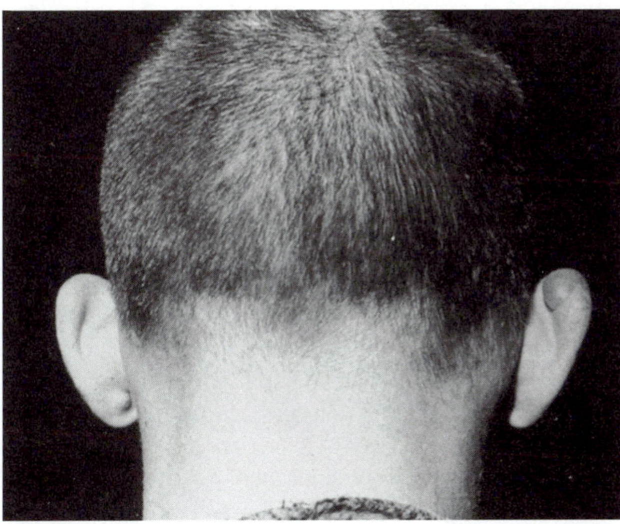

Fig. 5-1 Vesiculation of right ear with clear fluid characteristic of second-degree frostbite.

FROSTBITE SYMPTOMS

The severity of frostbite symptoms generally parallels the severity of the injury. In the civilian population, frostbite most frequently occurs on the extremities, with the lower extremity being far more common. It can also appear on the nose or ears and has been reported on the scrotum and penis in joggers.[84]

Mere numbness followed by tingling after rewarming does not constitute bona fide frostbite. Even in its mildest form, true frostbite damages the affected tissue. In most patients the initial clinical observation is coldness of the involved extremity, with numbness present in more than three fourths of patients. This ultimately causes the involved part to feel clumsy or absent and has been attributed to ischemia following intense vasoconstriction. When numbness is initially present, it frequently is followed by extreme pain (76% of patients) during rewarming. Throbbing pain begins 2 to 3 days after rewarming and continues for a variable period, even after the tissue becomes demarcated (22 to 45 days). After about a week the victim usually notices a residual tingling sensation, probably caused by ischemic neuritis. For this reason, this sensation tends to persist longer than do other symptoms. The severity of the injury usually defines the extent of neuropathologic damage. There may be a great deal of variation in symptoms, with some patients never noticing pain at the onset of the injury. In patients without tissue loss, symptoms usually subside within 1 month, while in those with tissue loss, disablement may exceed 6 months. In all cases symptoms are intensified by a warm environment. Other sensory deficits include spontaneous burning and electric current–like sensations. The burning sensation, which is frequently early in presentation, subsides within 2 to 3 weeks. This sensation is not present in victims with tissue loss. In victims without tissue loss it may resume on wearing shoes or increasing activity. The electric current–like shock is almost universal (97%) in patients with tissue loss. It usually begins 2 days after injury, lasts for about 6 weeks, and is particularly unpleasant at night. All frostbite victims experience some degree of sensory loss for at least 4 years after injury and perhaps indefinitely.

The clinical appearance of frostbite may be deceiving.[4,63] Only a few patients arrive with tissue still frozen. Originally the extremity appears yellowish white or mottled blue. It may be insensate and may appear frozen solid. Regardless of the depth of the injury, the extremity may have the appearance of being frozen. With rapid rewarming there is almost immediate hyperemia, even with the most severe injury. Sensation returns after thawing and persists until blebs appear. At this point, some effort may be made to assess the severity of the injury. Although "degrees" of injury have been defined, one usually differentiates between superficial (first- or second-degree) and deep (third- or fourth-degree) injuries. Even these distinctions are somewhat artificial, since the initial treatment of frostbite is identical. The degree system may have some importance in retrospective analysis of cases.

After the extremity is rewarmed, edema appears within 3 hours and lasts 5 days or longer, depending on the severity of the case.[63] Vesicles or bullae form 6 to 24 hours after rapid rewarming.[49,62] During the first 9 to 15 days, severely frostbitten skin forms a black, hard, and usually dry eschar whether vesicles are present or not (Color Plate 10).[62] Mummification forms an apparent line of demarcation in 22 to 45 days.[63]

Favorable prognostic signs include sensation to pinprick, normal color, warmth, and large, clear blebs that appear early and tend to extend to tips of the digits. Unfavorable signs include small, dark blebs that appear late and do not extend to the digit tips, the absence of edema, and the presence of cyanosis that does not blanch with pressure.[53]

Techniques that have been used to estimate the extent of injury and to predict ultimate tissue loss include intravenous radioisotope scanning (^{131}I RISA, ^{133}Xe, ^{99m}Tc MDP, ^{99m}Tc stannous pyrophosphate), angiography, routine roentgenography, and digital plethysmography. These modalities have also been recommended for estimating the vascular response to vasodilators and identifying tissue boundaries for surgical management. No prognostic technique is absolutely accurate in the immediate postthaw period; a delay of 2 to 3 weeks is necessary to exceed the period of transitory vascular instability.

OPHTHALMIC INJURIES

Ophthalmic injuries, particularly freezing of corneas, occur in individuals who try to force their eyes open in high-windchill situations. Snowmobilers and cross-country skiers are particularly susceptible. Blurred vision, photophobia, blepharospasm, tearing, and pain on rewarming suggest such an injury. Rapid rewarming and patching are the only effective treatments. Corticosteroids are contraindicated. Corneal transplantation may be required if keratitis and corneal opacification are irreversible and debilitating. Snowblindness caused by ultraviolet exposure is discussed in Chapter 1.

MANAGEMENT

In 1947 Hurley stated, "Tissue cells can be affected by freezing in three different ways: 1) a certain number of cells are killed; 2) a certain number remain unaffected; and 3) a large number are injured but may recover and survive under the right circumstances."[26] Obviously the major treatment effort must be to salvage as many cells in category 3 as possible.

Frostbite treatment is directed separately at the prethaw and postthaw intervals. If a patient is referred from a nearby location, no attempt at field rewarming may be indicated. Vigorous rubbing is ineffective and potentially harmful. The extremity should not be intentionally rewarmed during transport and should be protected against slow partial rewarming by keeping the patient away from intense campfires and car heaters. All constrictive and wet clothing should be replaced by dry, loose wraps or garments. The extremity is padded and splinted for protection, but no other treatment is initiated. Although there is a correlation between the length of time tissue is frozen and the amount of time required to thaw that tissue, there is no direct correlation between the length of time tissue is frozen and subsequent tissue damage. Therefore rapid transport of frostbite patients (within 2 hours) is appropriate. Otherwise, rapid rewarming should be instituted and the victim transported with protective dressings to prevent refreezing. Blisters should be left intact. Patients with long transport times are at greater risk for recurrent injury. All efforts should prevent subsequent refreezing, since this creates an infinitely worse result than does delayed thawing. A victim who must walk through snow should do so before thawing frostbitten feet. During transport the extremities should be elevated and tobacco smoking prohibited.[52] Alcohol ingestion is contraindicated.

Once in the emergency department, rapid rewarming should be started immediately. Associated traumatic injuries or medical conditions should be identified. Systemic hypothermia should be corrected to a core temperature of at least 34° C (93° F) before frostbite management is attempted. Fluid resuscitation is usually not a problem with frostbite injuries, although one case of rhabdomyolysis and acute renal failure has been reported.[73]

Treatment is directed at the specific pathophysiologic effects of the frostbite injury, either blocking direct cellular damage or preventing progressive microvascular thrombosis and tissue loss. Direct cellular damage is treated by rapid thawing of all degrees of frostbite with immersion in gently circulating water warmed to between 40° and 42° C (104° and 108° F) (Fig. 5-2).[29] Adherence to this narrow temperature range is important, since rewarming at lower temperatures is less beneficial for tissue survival,[17,23] and rewarming at higher temperatures may compound the injury by producing a burn wound.[56] Heated tap water (50° to 60° C or 122° to 140° F) is too hot and will cause profound discomfort and possible tissue damage. Frozen extremities should be rewarmed until the involved skin becomes pliable and erythematous at the most distal parts of the frostbite injury. This usually takes less than 30 minutes. Active motion during rewarming is helpful, but massage may compound the injury. Extreme pain may be experienced during thawing, and unless otherwise contraindicated, parenteral analgesics are administered. Rapid return of skin warmth and sensation with the presence of an erythematous color is a favorable sign, while the persistence of cold, anesthetic, and pale skin is unfavorable.

Rapid rewarming reverses the direct injury of ice crystal formation in the tissue. However, it does not prevent the progressive phase of the injury. McCauley and associates[46,47] have designed a protocol based on the pathophysiology of progressive dermal ischemia that has been quite successful in minimizing the production of local and systemic thromboxane by injured tissues (Box 5-1).

All but the most minor frostbite cases should be admitted to the hospital. Victims with minor injuries should be admitted if, after rapid rewarming, a warm environment cannot be ensured for the patient. No patient should ever be discharged into subfreezing weather. Even with a warm car waiting, the patient should be allowed to leave only with proper clothing (such as stocking cap, wool mittens, and wool socks).

Since the majority of frostbite injuries necessitate admission to the hospital, a discussion of the protocol is warranted. White or clear blisters, which represent more superficial injury, are debrided to prevent further contact of $PGF_{2\alpha}$ or TXA_2 with the damaged underlying tissues. Unlike the clear blisters, hemorrhagic blisters reflect structural damage to the subdermal plexus. It may be worthwhile to aspirate the thromboxane-containing fluid out of these blisters, but debridement may allow desiccation of the deep dermis and allow conversion of the injury to full thickness. Therefore hemorrhagic blisters are left intact. A specific thromboxane inhibitor is placed on the wounds to prevent further formation of this vasoconstricting mediator (Fig. 5-3). Aspirin was originally given systemically to block production of $PGF_{2\alpha}$ and TXA_2. Since the correct dose of aspirin is not known, aspirin has been replaced by ibuprofen.[86] Ibuprofen not only inhibits the arachidonic acid cascade, but also has the additional benefit of fibrinolysis. Elevation of the extremity minimizes dependent edema. Since edema inactivates the normal streptococcidioidal properties of the skin, parenteral penicillin is administered during the edema

BOX 5-1

PROTOCOL FOR RAPID REWARMING

1. Admit frostbite patients to a specialized unit if possible.
2. Do not discharge or transfer to another facility victims of acute frostbite requiring hospitalization unless it is necessary for specialized care. Transfer arrangements must protect the victim from cold exposure.
3. On admission, rapidly rewarm the affected areas in warm water at 40° to 42° C (104° to 108° F), usually for 15 to 30 minutes or until thawing is complete.
4. Upon completion of rewarming, treat the affected parts as follows:
   a. Debride white blisters and institute topical treatment with aloe vera (Dermaide aloe) every 6 hours.
   b. Leave hemorrhagic blisters intact and institute topical aloe vera (Dermaide aloe) every 6 hours.
   c. Elevate the affected part(s) with splinting as indicated.
   d. Administer antitetanus prophylaxis.
   e. For analgesia, administer morphine or meperidine (Demerol) intravenously or intramuscularly as indicated.
   f. Administer ibuprofen 400 mg orally ever 12 hours.
   g. Administer penicillin G 500,000 units intravenously every 6 hours for 48 to 72 hours.
   h. Perform hydrotherapy daily for 30 to 45 minutes at 40° C (104° F). The solution should meet the following specifications:
      (1) Large tank capacity—425 gallons
          Fill level estimate—285 gallons
          Sodium chloride—9.7 kg
          Calcium hypochlorite solution—95 ml
      (2) Medium tank capacity—270 gallons
          Fill level estimate—108 gallons
          Sodium chloride—3.7 kg
          Calcium hypochlorite solution—36 ml
      (3) Small tank capacity—95 gallons
          Fill level estimate—72 gallons
          Sodium chloride—2.5 kg
          Potassium chloride—71 g
          Calcium hypochlorite solution—24 ml
5. For documentation obtain photographs on admission, at 24 hours, and serially every 2 to 3 days until discharge.
6. Discharge patients with specific instructions for protection of the injured areas to avoid reinjury and follow up weekly until wounds are stable. If the patient is being discharged with no open lesions, instruct him or her to use wool socks, wear a hat, and use mittens instead of gloves to decrease the loss of heat between the fingers. Explain to patients that they are more susceptible to refreezing, so they should avoid exposure to cold and should wear warm clothing and shoes or boots if going outside is necessary. Give similar instructions to patients who are discharged with open lesions. Also instruct these patients to keep the affected extremity elevated and to take ibuprofen 400 mg orally every 12 hours. Aloe vera should be applied to the involved areas, or scarlet red ointment used if the open areas are small.

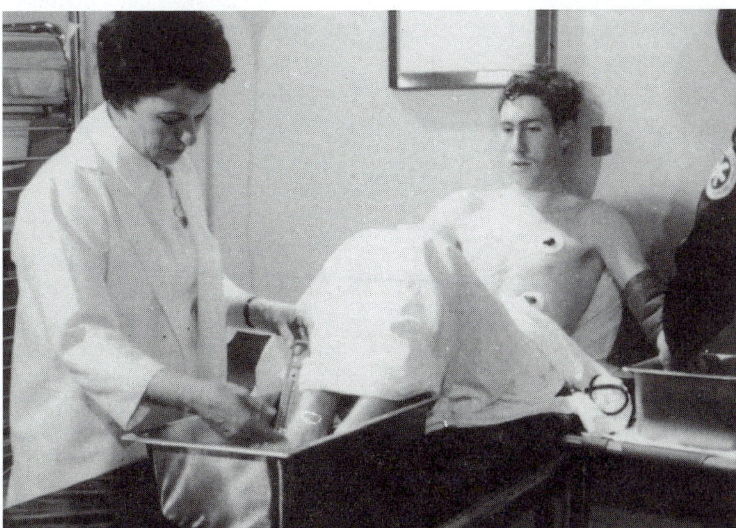

Fig. 5-2 Technique to rapidly warm all four extremities simultaneously. The water is 104° to 108° F (40° to 42° C), monitored by a thermometer, and circulated manually. Thawing is usually complete in 30 minutes, when the extremities are pliable and color and sensation have returned.

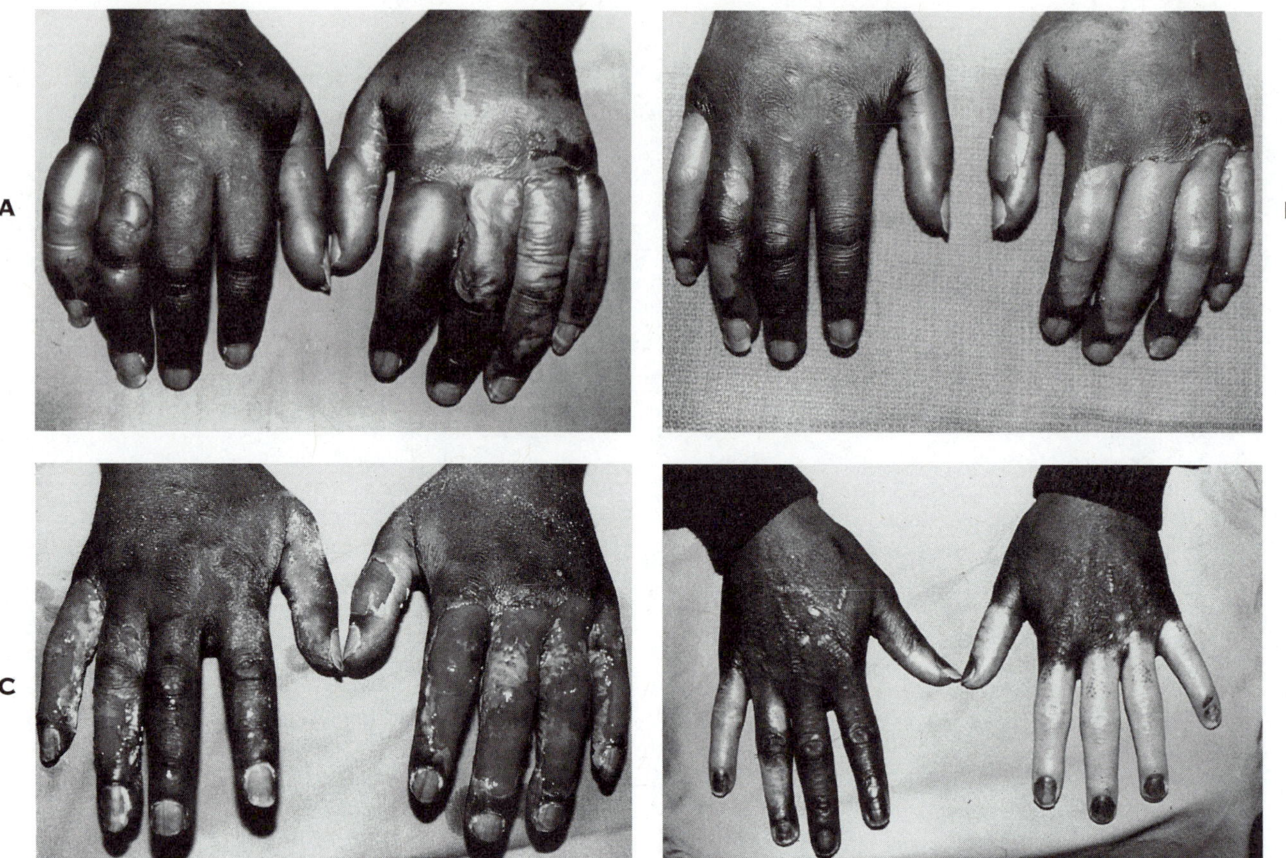

Fig. 5-3 **A,** Acute frostbite injury with clear fluid in superficial blisters. **B,** Blisters before treatment but after debridement. **C,** After 48 hours of therapy with topical aloe vera (Dermaide aloe). **D,** Sixteen days after injury.

phase of the injury.[12] Antitetanus prophylaxis is given if indicated by the patient's history. Tetanus killed thousands of Napoleon's soldiers in the Russian campaign. There was a report as recently as April 1985 documenting tetanus associated with a frostbite injury. Since frostbite generally involves injuries to the extremities, appropriate physical and occupational therapy should be initiated early. Daily hydrotherapy for active and passive range of motion is extremely valuable in the preservation of function.[15]

Between 1982 and 1985, 56 patients were treated with the previous frostbite protocol and 98 were treated by other "standard" methods. Of the 56 patients treated with the protocol, 18 were admitted with first-degree frostbite, 25 with second-degree frostbite, and 13 with third-degree frostbite. Thirty-two suffered acute frostbite, and 24 had subacute (presenting for treatment more than 24 hours after injury). The mean length of hospital stay for the acute protocol patients was 8.5 days and for the subacute group, 14.9 days. Overall, 67.9% of the protocol group healed without tissue loss, 25% healed with some tissue loss, and 7% required amputation. Of the nonprotocol patients, 11 were admitted with first-degree frostbite, 51 with second-degree frostbite, and 36 with third-degree frostbite. Fifty-six were acute cases, and 42 were subacute. The mean length of hospital stay was 17.5 days for the acute, nonprotocol patients and 19 days for the subacute group. Of this group, 32.7% healed without tissue loss, 34.6% healed with tissue loss, and 32.7% required amputation ($p < 0.001$, includes all groups of protocol-treated patients). These data indicate therapeutic efficacy of the protocol by virtue of less tissue loss, lower amputation rate, and significantly shorter hospital stay.

OTHER THERAPIES

A number of other therapeutic modalities have attempted to prevent progressive thrombosis and tissue loss. Most were proposed before the pathophysiology of the injury was found to be related to inflammatory mediators. These therapeutic attempts deserve comment. It has been observed that cold-injured vessels, shortly after thawing, became dilated and filled with clumps of erythrocytes. These clumps can be easily dislodged by gentle manipulation and do not represent true thrombosis. Although the mechanism that leads to erythrocyte clumping is not completely understood, it may reflect a cold-induced increase in blood viscosity. This suggests that the use of low–molecular weight dex-

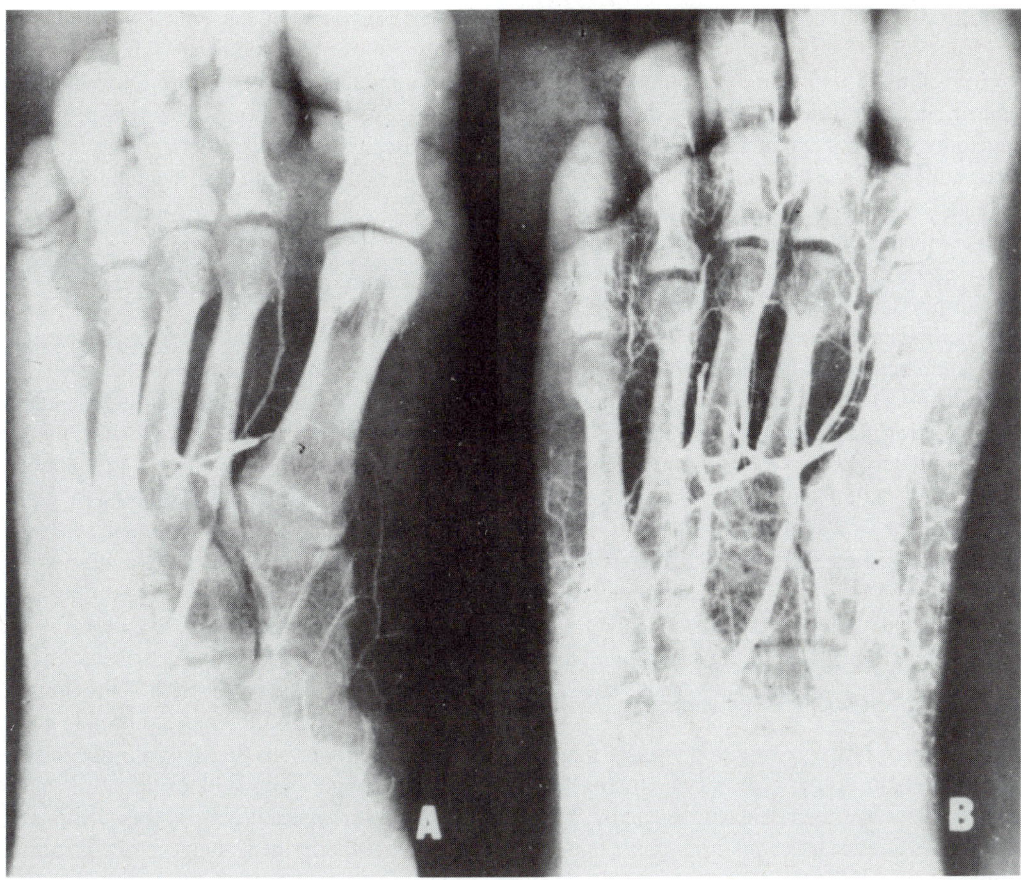

Fig. 5-4 Angiograms of the left foot of a 30-year-old man with cold injury. **A,** Initial angiogram. **B,** Angiogram taken 2 days after intraarterial injection of reserpine. (From Gralino BJ, Porter JM, Rosch J: *Radiology* 19:301, 1976.)

tran may be of benefit in the early treatment of frostbite. Although no controlled clinical trial of low–molecular weight dextran has been reported, there has been experimental evidence to support its use. Weatherly-White, Sjostrom, and Paton[85] demonstrated that the use of low–molecular weight dextran, 1 g/kg/day, protected against tissue loss in the rabbit ear model. This led to the suggestion that the use of 1 L of 6% dextran intravenously on the day of injury, followed by 500 ml on each of 5 successive days, might be of benefit.[71] With our present understanding of the etiology of frostbite, there appear to be few instances when it may be used and have demonstrable benefit.

Although true thrombi are not present in dilated, erythrocyte-filled vessels immediately after thawing, they form over the next few days. Thus heparin has been suggested as a possible treatment for frostbite. Lange and Loewe[35] demonstrated its usefulness in experimental frostbite. Subsequent investigations have been unable to substantiate these findings, and at the present time there is no evidence that heparin alters the natural history of the frostbite.[77]

Intraarterial reserpine has also been shown experimentally to be of use in frostbite. Porter and co-workers[64] reported its clinical use in five patients. Three of the patients were treated within 2 weeks of injury. Angiography of the involved extremities was performed before and after injection (Fig. 5-4). Reserpine appeared to be effective in relieving vasospasm. However, treatment did not retard progression of tissue loss. A multiarmed clinical study compared slow rewarming combined with intravenous dextran, intraarterial tolazoline, intraarterial reserpine, and various combinations of these drugs.[80] All of the drug treatments were superior to simple slow rewarming. However, rapid rewarming was as effective as any of the drug treatments. Therefore reserpine might be effective when patients are brought for treatment late and have not been rapidly rewarmed. To date, no anticoagulant or vasodilation treatment has proved useful in controlled clinical trials.

Several reports from Europe and the United States following World War II supported the use of sympathetic block and sympathectomy.[6] However, this remains controversial. If the sympathetic nervous system is involved, it seems reasonable that early sympathectomy would be beneficial. However, experimental evidence indicates that sympathectomy performed within the first few hours of injury increases edema formation and accelerates the pathologic process of tissue destruction.[18,85] On the other hand, sympathectomy performed 24 to 48 hours after thawing seems to hasten resolution of edema and decrease tissue loss.[18] The role of sympathectomy will not become clear until there is a verifiable clinical rating to evaluate results.[14] Similar problems exist in evaluation of the use of hyperbaric oxygen. Although some experimental data support its use, only occasional anecdotal cases are reported.[61] Furthermore, its use is predicated on the original theory of the frostbite injury, not the most recent experimental data.

Early surgical intervention has no role in the acute care of frostbite, unless there is ischemia from a constricting eschar or subeschar infection that cannot be controlled by topical antimicrobials. Decompressing escharotomy incisions are rarely necessary to increase the distal circulation. If such escharotomies are necessary to decompress digits and facilitate joint motion, incisions along the transaxial line are best. It is important that incisions avoid injury to the underlying structures. If uncontrolled infection is present early, escharotomy may be necessary. However, this is rare with the use of penetrating antibacterial agents such as mafenide acetate.

Surgical intervention is properly reserved for late treatment of frostbite. This is most often necessary if frostbite is very severe or if treatment has been delayed. Normally, aggressive therapeutic measures can prevent progressive injury and gangrene. If gangrene ensues, amputation or debridement with resurfacing may be necessary (Fig. 5-5). This should be accomplished only after the area is well demarcated, which generally requires 3 to 4 weeks. Historically, aggressive early debridement and attempted salvage have been thought to jeopardize recovering tissue and add to tissue loss. Gottlieb, Zachary, and Krizek[19] have taken a more aggressive approach to coverage of severe frostbite injury. Using technetium phosphate and bone scans, they identify nonperfused tissue by the tenth day following injury and surgically remove necrotic tissue. The remaining nonvascularized, nonviable, yet nonnecrotic and noninfected, tissue is salvaged by early coverage with well-vascularized tissue. Theoretically, if nonvascularized tissue has not undergone autolysis and is not infected, it should behave as a composite graft. Preliminary reports are promising.[19]

LATE SEQUELAE

Until 1957 little was recorded about the long-term sequelae of frostbite injuries. Blair, Schatzki, and Orr[3] studied 100 veterans of the Korean conflict 4 years after their injuries. In order of decreasing frequency, the victims reported excessive sweating, pain, coldness, numbness, abnormal skin color, and stiffness of the joints. In addition, the investigators noted frequent asymptomatic abnormalities of the nails, including ridges and inward curving of the edges. In general, the degree of long-term disability was related to the severity of the original injury. Symptoms were worse in cold than in warm weather. This is attributed to the fact that vessels do not react as well to stress.[79] Previously injured blood vessels do not constrict when exposed to cold as effectively as do normal vessels, and they do not dilate as effectively when vasoconstriction is blocked.

Probably hyperhidrosis is both a cause and a result of frostbite. Hyperhidrosis suggests the presence of an abnormal sympathetic nervous response induced by cold injury and is abolished by sympathetic denervation. Sensitivity to cold and predisposition to recurrent cold injury should suggest hyperhidrosis. Blanching and pain on subsequent cold exposure may be a nuisance or may be dramatic enough to suggest a diagnosis of Raynaud's phenomenon. Almost without exception a painful, shiny, cyanotic, and sweaty limb becomes warm, dry, and useful with sympathetic interruption. Schoning[74] examined the changes in the sweat

A
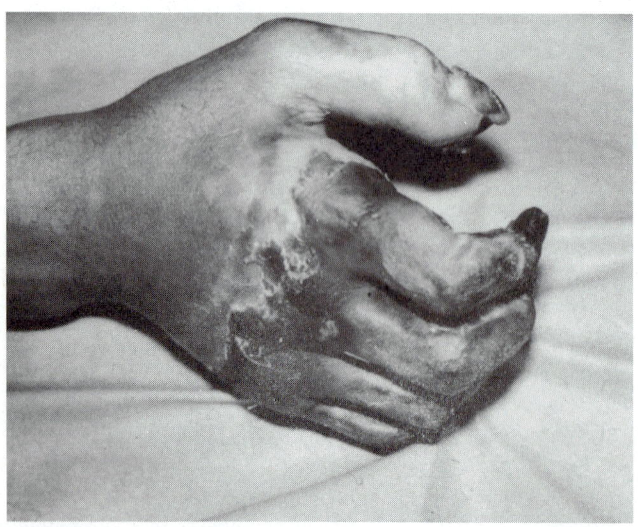

B
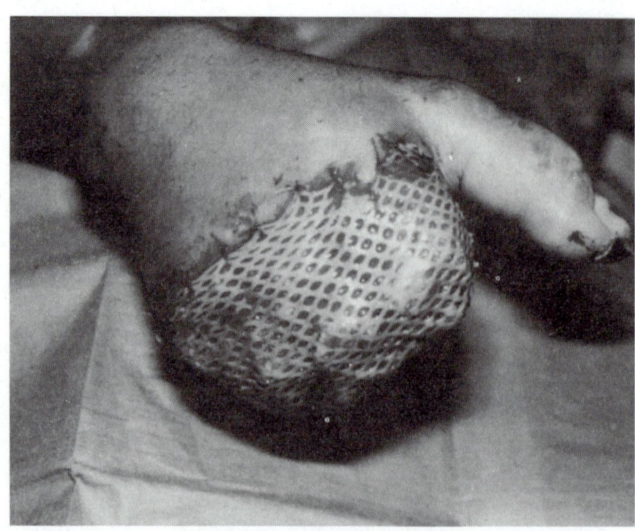

Fig. 5-5 **A,** Gangrene from third-degree frostbite. **B,** Treated with partial hand amputation in preparation for toe-to-hand transfer.

glands of the Hanford miniature swine after experimental frostbite injury to determine the etiology of hyperhidrosis. She noted that severe sweat gland changes were of two types: degeneration with necrosis and squamous metaplasia. Clearly, if hypohidrosis were a sequela of frostbite injury, morphologically normal and active sweat glands would be an expected finding. We may conclude that hyperhidrosis may lack histologic documentation.

The late abnormalities of change in skin color, including depigmentation of dark skin and appearance resembling erythrocyanosis in light skin, are most likely the result of ischemia.[3] Similarly, the nail abnormality is comparable to that seen with ischemia. Neither of these sequelae usually requires treatment.

Late symptoms of joint stiffness and pain on motion are relatively common and undoubtedly are related to the underlying scars and mechanical problems occasioned by the variety of amputations. "Punched-out" defects in subchondral bone of involved limbs have been noted. These localized areas of bone resorption generally appear within 5 to 10 months after injury and may heal spontaneously. Vascular occlusion is the probable cause of these lesions. Such bone involvement in close proximity to joint surfaces may help to explain joint symptoms.

The effects of frostbite on premature closure of epiphyses in the growing hand have recently been reemphasized.[87] The extent of premature closure has been correlated with the severity of the frostbite and noted in partial-thickness injuries. In the digits premature closure is more frequent from a distal to proximal direction (distal interphalangeal greater than proximal interphalangeal greater than metacarpophalangeal). The thumb has been less often involved. In only 2% of cases does partial epiphyseal closure cause angular deformity.

One of the characteristic features of frostbite is the surprising salvage possible in an apparently badly injured extremity. Amputation should therefore be performed with great conservatism and as late as possible. The line of demarcation may not be decided definitively for weeks or months after injury. As long as secondary sepsis does not intervene, patience often rewards both the patient and the surgeon with maximal length of the useful limb. This is particularly true in the upper extremities.

CONDITIONING AND PREVENTION

Frostbite can usually be prevented by experienced leadership, good physical condition, adequate food, and intelligently used equipment. Probably the two most important basic factors in prevention of frostbite are the heat-producing capacity of the body and the effectiveness of measures to conserve heat once it has been produced. The most fundamental defense against frostbite is a healthy body.

As previously noted, there are no data to support the belief that high altitude increases susceptibility based on changes in blood viscosity. On the other hand, living conditions at high altitude may contribute to increasing danger from frostbite. Cold becomes more intense, as do the violence and severity of storms. Shelter is less appealing and protective. Loss of sleep, inadequate diet, altered digestion, and nervous tension all contribute to a greater degree of fatigue than normally experienced at lower heights. Hypoxia reduces reasoning powers and leads to a tendency to laziness, carelessness, indecision, and lack of normal insight and judgment.[84]

The body requires the same amount of oxygen for various tasks regardless of the altitude. At higher altitudes, however, the body must process more air to gain that same amount of oxygen. Individuals must carefully regulate their activity; otherwise, they will not only exhaust the body, but will also cool it. Large quantities of heat can be lost through the lungs by panting and overexertion,[65] which also adds to fatigue.

At higher altitudes the natural protective mechanism of shivering is impaired and heat production during rest can be significantly reduced. If an individual becomes unable to exercise, the body cannot maintain adequate heat production. The body reduces blood flow to its surface and extremities in an effort to maintain core temperature. In such a situation no amount of insulation can prevent frostbite and nothing but vigorous warming and administration of oxygen can avert serious results. Since the use of auxiliary oxygen was introduced in mountaineering, frostbite has become less common.

Cold weather increases caloric needs, and variations in diet can have an effect on tolerance.[57] In the cold, cooking, dishwashing, thawing food, and melting water are arduous tasks. Fluid requirements far exceed what is empirically thought to be necessary.

Frostbite is rarely experienced by healthy individuals who are standing still and adequately clothed. It seems to be related almost always to factors such as fatigue, a sudden storm, an accident, or combinations of these. Alcohol intoxication is a frequent forerunner of frostbite. Injury to any part of the body, combined with fear or panic, can allow frostbite in a situation where climatic effects alone would not cause trouble to a seasoned, uninjured person.[84]

Because impaired local circulation is the primary cause of frostbite, anything with even a mildly adverse effect on normal peripheral circulation, such as tobacco or alcohol, should be avoided. Smoking results in varying degrees of diffuse vascular spasm, reducing normal peripheral circulation. Alcohol is not recommended at any time on the trail.[22]

Previous frostbite injury usually results in a prolonged reduction in tolerance to cold by the injured part. Conversely, the concept of physiologic adaptation to cold is extremely controversial. There can be no argument that Eskimos and Tibetans in cold, rugged climates "feel" cold much less than do nonnatives. They certainly seem to resist cold more than others and obviously tolerate cold better than those who live in temperate and tropical climates. However, many medical experts allege that this "resistance" is really no more than the result of experience in Arctic survival and day-to-day living. Furthermore, Eskimos, even though they do not feel cold as fast, freeze just as fast and badly as others, given the same actual contact situation. There is increasing evidence that tolerance exists, but even if it is proved, it may be of only academic interest. The basic reason most outdoorsmen are not frostbitten is that they tend to be in good physical condition and know how to act and dress properly.

Many physicians enjoy mountain climbing. Those involved in the Everest exploration wrote about the effects of cold and how to protect against it.[84] They suggested that overall physical well-being, good clothing, and intelligent operations in the field were by far the best insurance against frostbite. When a person is exhausted, hungry, ill, injured, or hypoxic, the chances for frostbite injury are increased.[22]

The following measures for frostbite protection are based on Washburn's recommendations[84]:

1. Dress to maintain general body warmth. In cold, windy weather the face, head, and neck must be protected, as enormous amounts of body heat can be lost through these parts.
2. Eat plenty of appetizing food to produce maximum output of body heat. Diet in cold weather at low altitude should tend toward fats, with carbohydrates intermediate and proteins least important. As altitude increases above 10,000 feet, carbohydrates become most important and proteins remain least.
3. Do not climb under extreme weather conditions, particularly at high altitudes on exposed terrain, or get too early a start in cold weather. The configuration of a mountain can help the climber find maximum shelter and solar warmth.
4. Avoid tight, snug-fitted clothing, particularly on the hands and feet. Socks and boots should fit closely, with no points of tightness or pressure. In putting on socks and boots, a person should carefully eliminate all wrinkles in socks. Old matted insoles are to be avoided.
5. Avoid perspiration under conditions of extreme cold; clothing that is adequately ventilated should be worn. If perspiring, remove some clothing or slow down.
6. Keep the feet and hands dry. Even with vapor-barrier boots, socks must not become too wet. All types of boots must be worn with great care during periods of inactivity, especially after exercise has resulted in damp socks or insoles. Wet socks in any type of boot soften the feet and make the skin more tender, greatly lowering resistance to cold and simultaneously increasing the danger of other foot injuries, such as blistering. Extra socks and insoles should always be carried. Light, smooth, dry, clean socks should be worn next to the skin, followed by one or two heavier outer pairs.
7. Wear mittens instead of gloves in extreme cold, except for specialized work like photography or surveying, in which great manual dexterity is required for short intervals. In these situations a mitten should be worn on one hand and a glove temporarily on the other. If bare finger dexterity is required, silk or rayon gloves should be worn, or all metal parts that must be touched frequently covered with adhesive tape. The thumbs should be removed and fists held in the palm of mittens occasionally to regain warmth of the entire hand.
8. Be careful while loading cameras, taking pictures, or handling stoves and fuel. The freezing point of gasoline (–57° C [–70° F]) and its rapid rate of evaporation make it very dangerous. Metal objects should never be touched with bare hands in extreme cold or in moderate cold when the hands are moist.
9. Mitten shells and gloves worn in extreme cold should be made of soft, flexible, dry-tanned deerskin, moose, elk, or caribou hide. Horsehide is less favorable because it dries stiffly after wetting. Removable mitten inserts or glove linings should be of soft wool.
10. Mittens should be tied together on a string hung around the neck or tied to the ends of parka sleeves. Oiled or greased leather gloves, boots, or clothing should never be used in cold weather operations.
11. Keep toenails and fingernails trimmed.
12. Hands, face, and feet should not be washed too thoroughly or too frequently under rough weather conditions. Tough, weatherbeaten face and hands resist frostbite most effectively.
13. Wind and high altitude should always be approached with respect. They can produce dramatic results when combined with cold. Exercise should not be too strenuous in extreme cold, particularly at high altitude, where undue exertion results in panting or very deep breathing. Cold inspired air will chill the whole body and under extreme conditions may damage lung tissue and cause internal hemorrhage.[84]
14. When a person becomes thoroughly chilled, it takes several hours of warmth and rest to return to normal, regardless of superficial feelings of comfort. A person recovering from an emergency cold situation should not venture out again into extreme cold too soon.
15. Avoid tobacco or alcohol at high altitudes and under conditions of frostbite danger.
16. A person who is frostbitten or otherwise injured in the field must remain calm. Panic or fear results in perspiration, which evaporates and causes further chilling.
17. Tetanus immunity should be current.

Other Cold-Induced Injuries

TRENCH FOOT (IMMERSION FOOT)

Another classification evaluates physical findings, but also adds the environmental conditions under which an injury occurred. In this scheme frostbite is viewed as the actual freezing of water in skin and subcutaneous tissues. It follows exposure at or below freezing, usually for more than 1 hour. In a series of 140 patients exposure to an ambient temperature of 20° F (–6.6° C) or less for 1 hour or more resulted in tissue loss.[29] Early symptoms are much like those of trench foot (immersion foot), with tingling and eventual numbness. Trench foot develops slowly over a period of hours to days without actual tissue freezing, because of exposure of wet feet to a temperature of 32° to 50° F (0° to 10° C).[28,88] This results in neurovascular damage without ice crystal formation. Immediately after exposure the skin appears erythematous, but it becomes pale and markedly swollen. Other early symptoms include numbness and painful paresthesias, followed by leg cramping. During the first few hours to days the limb is prehyperemic with swelling, diffuse discoloration, mottling, and hyposensitivity.

After 2 to 7 days the limb becomes hyperemic for a period of up to 6 weeks, during which the condition is marked by paresthesias, regional variation in superficial skin temperature, edema, vesiculation, ulceration, and occasionally gangrene. In the third, or hyperemic, phase the limb may return to normal temperature but remains exquisitely sensitive to cold. If the injury is severe, liquefaction gangrene may occur. Whether eventual tissue loss will occur is difficult to determine. Trench foot appears to have a better prognosis than frostbite, even when the extremities initially are clinically indistinguishable. This emphasizes a potential prognostic advantage of describing the environmental conditions.

FROSTNIP

Frostnip is superficial and reversible ice crystal formation associated with intense vasoconstriction. Chilblains result from chronic intermittent exposure to environmental conditions of high humidity and ambient temperature above freezing, without the development of tissue freezing. Frostnip is characterized by discomfort in the involved parts. The symptoms usually resolve spontaneously, and no tissue is lost. There is some question whether this qualifies as cold-induced injury, since neither frozen extracellular water nor progressive tissue loss is routinely demonstrated.

CHILBLAINS (PERNIO)

The chilblain ("cold sore") is a syndrome less severe than trench foot. It is seen most commonly in women and is characterized by localized erythema, cyanosis, plaques, nodules, and in rare severe cases hemorrhages, vesicles, bullae, and ulcerations on the exposed extremities, particularly the lower legs, toes, hands, and ears. The skin lesions appear 12 to 14 hours after exposure to cold and are characterized by intense pruritus and burning paresthesias. Tender, blue nodules follow rewarming and may persist for up to 14 days. Chronic pernio may occur in predisposed middle-aged women.

One histopathologic study of nine victims of pernio noted a unique lymphocytic vasculitis.[24] Edema of the papillary dermis was a variable feature, as was perivascular lymphocytic infiltration (characteristic of systemic lupus erythematosus, erythema multiforme, or drug eruption). In all likelihood trench foot and chilblains share a common pathophysiology that includes sympathetic instability and vascular hypersensitivity to cold, with microvascular stasis and thrombosis.

Management of the chilblain syndrome is supportive. The affected skin should be gently rewarmed as for frostbite, washed and dried, and dressed in dry, soft, sterile bandages. Elevation is essential to minimize swelling that predisposes to secondary bacterial infection. On occasion, healing is followed by hyperpigmentation. The victim is prone to recurrences on lesser exposure.

CRYOGLOBULINS

Cold-induced precipitation of serum proteins was first reported in a patient with multiple myeloma by Wintrobe and Buell.[91] Subsequently the term "cryoglobulin" was introduced to denote a group of serum proteins that have the common property of reversibly precipitating or gelling in the cold.[38] The vast majority of cryoglobulins are either intact monoclonal immunoglobulins (IgGs) or immunoglobulin complexes (that is, mixed cryoglobulins) in which one component, usually IgM, is directed against IgG.[21] Symptoms directly attributable to monoclonal cryoglobulins are quite variable and include cold intolerance with typical Raynaud's phenomenon, dependent purpura, cutaneous vasculitis with ulceration, retinal hemorrhages, coagulopathies, and cerebral thrombosis. In many cases, only inexact correlations exist among the concentration of the cryoglobulin, the temperature of cryoformation, and the presence of symptoms.[21] Of clinical relevance is the composition of the cryoprecipitate. Since acral temperatures of 30° C (86° F) are present in the hands and feet,[7] in vivo cryoprecipitation may directly contribute to impaired capillary blood flow in the extremities; this has been demonstrated by biomicroscopy of conjunctival and nailbed capillaries.[69] In patients with monoclonal cryo IgM the higher intrinsic viscosity of IgM compared with IgG is greatly amplified and attendant symptoms can often be directly related to hyperviscosity.[21]

In a large clinical series only two thirds of the patients had skin lesions or vasomotor attack at initial examination.[7] Cold sensitivity was apparent in less than half of these patients. Less common early symptoms were renal failure, mucosal bleeding, visual disturbance, or abdominal pain. In cryoglobulinemia without severe symptoms and in the absence of an underlying disease requiring active treatment, the decisions for treatment and type of treatment are difficult. Primary treatment should be directed toward minimizing cold exposure. Cyproheptadine (Periactin) 4 mg three or four times daily for approximately 1 to 2 weeks is useful when urticaria occurs.[83] This is probably due to its antihistamine and antikinin activity. Avoidance of prolonged standing is important in patients to prevent dependent purpura. With severe manifestations plasmapheresis may be required for emergency treatment.

COLD URTICARIA

Cold urticaria is a fairly common form of physical urticaria.[60] It is characterized by local or generalized wheals either on continuous cold exposure or on rewarming of sites previously exposed to cold. Local symptoms include redness, itching, wheals, and edema in cold-exposed skin. Systemic symptoms include fatigue, headache, dyspnea, tachycardia, and rare anaphylactic shock. Usually the diagnosis is made by an ice cube or ice water immersion test, in which a wheal reaction appears in the exposed skin within 20 minutes. Primary acquired cold urticaria is the most common form. It occurs at any age, has an equal male/female incidence, and tends to be self-limited, although it may become chronic. Secondary acquired cold urticaria is associated with an underlying disorder such as cold agglutinins or paroxysmal hemoglobinuria. Familial cold urticaria is rare.

The cause of cold urticaria is unknown. It has been reported to be mediated by IgE and IgM and to involve the release of histamine or other inflammatory mediators.[60,81] Avoidance of cold is not always effective in preventing cold urticaria, since the rate of cooling, not absolute temperature, appears to be the principal stimulus. Desensitization may achieve only short-term benefit. Cyproheptadine (Periactin) has been the most successful drug, but doxepin, hydroxyzine, and ketotifen have also been shown to be effective.[60,81]

REFERENCES

1. Barillo DJ et al: Detrimental effects of ethanol on murine frostbite, *Am Surg* 50:649, 1984.
2. Bellman S, Adams RJ: Vascular reactions after experimental cold injury, *Angiology* 7:339, 1956.
3. Blair JR, Schatzki R, Orr ND: Sequelae to cold injury in one hundred patients: follow-up study four years after occurrence of cold injury, *JAMA* 163:1203, 1957.
4. Boswick JA, Thompson JD, Jonas RA: The epidemiology of cold injuries, *Surg Gynecol Obstet* 149:326, 1979.
5. Bourne MH et al: Analysis of microvascular changes in frostbite injury, *J Surg Res* 40:26, 1986.
6. Bouwman DL et al: Early sympathetic blockade for frostbite: is it of value? *J Trauma* 20(9):744, 1980.
7. Brouet JC et al: Biologic and clinical significance of cryoglobulins: a report of 86 cases, *Am J Med* 57:775, 1974.
8. Brown FE, Spiegel PK, Boyle WE Jr: Digital deformity: an effect of frostbite in children, *Pediatrics* 71(6):955, 1983.
9. Bulkley GB: The role of oxygen free radicals in human disease processes, *Surgery* 94:407, 1983.
10. Campbell R: *General outcooling and local frostbite.* In Proceedings of the Symposium on Arctic Biology and Medicine. IV. Frostbite, Fort Wainwright, Alaska, 1964, Arctic Aeromedical Laboratory.
11. Carrera GF et al: Radiographic changes in the hands following childhood frostbite injury, *Skel Radiol* 6(1):33, 1981.
12. Cold hypersensitivity, *Br Med J* 1(5959):643, 1975.
13. Didlake RH, Kukora JS: Tetanus following frostbite injury, *Contemp Orthop* 10:69, 1985.
14. Ducuing J: Les troubles trophiques des produits par de froid sec en pathologic de guerre, *J Chir* 55:385, 1940.
15. Edstrom LE, Robson MC, Headley BJ: Evaluation of exercise techniques in the burn patient, *Burns* 4(2):113, 1977.
16. Fox RH et al: Body temperature in the elderly: a national study of physiological, social and environmental conditions, *Br Med J* 1:200, 1973.
17. Fuhrman FA, Crissman JM: Studies on gangrene following cold injury. VII. Treatment of cold injury by immediate rapid rewarming, *J Clin Invest* 26:476, 1947.
18. Golding MR et al: Protection from early and late sequelae of frostbite by regional sympathectomy: mechanism of "cold sensitivity" following frostbite, *Surgery* 53:303, 1963.
19. Gottlieb LJ, Zachary LS, Krizek TJ: *Aggressive surgical treatment of frostbite injuries.* Presented at Midwestern Association of Plastic Surgeons meeting, May 1987.
20. Greenfield ADM, Shepherd JT, Whelan RF: Cold vasoconstriction and vasodilatation, *Irish J Med Sci* 309:415, 1951.
21. Grey HM, Kohler PF: Cryoimmunoglobulins, *Semin Hematol* 10(2):87, 1973.
22. Headley BJ, Robson MC, Krizek TJ: Methods of reducing environmental stress for the acute burn patient, *Phys Ther* 55(1):5, 1975.
23. Heggers JP et al: Experimental and clinical observations on frostbite, *Ann Emerg Med* 16:1056, 1987.
24. Herman EW, Kezis JS, Silvers DN: A distinctive variant of pernio, *Arch Dermatol* 117:26, 1981.
25. Holbrook KA, Byers PH, Pinnell SR: The structure and function of dermal connective tissue in normal individuals and patients with inherited connective tissue disorders, *Scanning Electron Microscopy* 4:1731, 1982.
26. Hurley LA: Angioarchitectural changes associated with rapid rewarming subsequent to freezing injury, *Angiology* 8:19, 1957.
27. Johnson BE, Daniels F Jr: Enzymes studies in experimental cryosurgery of the skin, *Cryobiology* 11:22, 1974.
28. Kinmouth JB, Rob CG, Simeone FB: *The cryopathies in vascular surgery*, London, 1962, E Arnold.
29. Knize DM: *Cold injury in reconstructive plastic surgery: general principles,* vol 1, ed 2, Philadelphia, 1977, WB Saunders.
30. Knize DM et al: Prognostic factors in the management of frostbite, *J Trauma* 9(9):749, 1969.
31. Kulka JP: Histopathologic studies in frostbitten rabbits. In *Cold injury,* New York, 1956, Josiah Macy, Jr.
32. Kulka JP: Microcirculatory impairment as a factor in inflammatory tissue damage, *Ann NY Acad Sci* 116:1018, 1964.
33. Kulka JP: Vasomotor microcirculatory insufficiency: observations on non-freezing cold injury of the mouse ear, *Angiology* 12:491, 1961.
34. Kyosola K: clinical experiences in the management of cold injuries: a study of 110 cases, *J Trauma* 14(1):32, 1974.
35. Lange K, Loewe L: Subcutaneous heparin in the pitkin mastruum for the treatment of experimental human frostbite, *Surg Gynecol Obstet* 82:256, 1946.
36. Larrey DJ: *Memoirs of military surgery,* vol 2, Baltimore, 1814, Joseph Cushing.

37. Lawrence WT et al: The detrimental effect of cigarette smoking on flap survival: an experimental study in the rat, *Br J Plast Surg* 37:216, 1984.
38. Lerner AB, Barnum CP, Watson CJ: Studies of cryoglobulins. II. The spontaneous precipitation of protein from serum at 5° C in various disease states, *Am J Med Sci* 214:416, 1947.
39. Lewis T: Observations on some normal and injurious effects of cold upon the skin and underlying tissues: III. Frostbite, *Br Med J* 2:869, 1941.
40. Lovelock JE: Physical instability in thermal shock in red blood cells, *Nature* 173:659, 1954.
41. Lovelock JE: The denaturation of lipid-protein complexes as a cause of damage by freezing, *Proc R Soc Biol* 147:427, 1957.
42. Marhert CL: Lactate dehydrogenase isozymes: dissociation and recombination of subunits, *Science* 140:1629, 1963.
43. Marzella L et al: Morphologic characterization of acute injury to vascular endothelium of skin after frostbite, *Plast Reconstr Surg* 83(1):67, 1989.
44. Mazur P: Studies in rapidly frozen suspension of yeast cells by differential thermal analysis and conductometry, *Biophys J* 3:323, 1963.
45. Mazur P: Causes of injury in frozen and thawed cells, *Fed Proc* 24(suppl 14-15):5, 1965.
46. McCauley RL et al: Frostbite injuries: a rational approach based on the pathophysiology, *J Trauma* 23:143, 1983.
47. McCauley RL et al: Frostbite: methods to minimize tissue loss, *Postgrad Med* 88(8):67, 1990.
48. Merryman HT: Mechanisms of freezing in living cells and tissues, *Science* 124:515, 1956.
49. Merryman HT: The exceeding of a minimum tolerable cell volume in hypertonic suspension as a cause of freezing injury. In *The frozen cell,* London, 1970, Churchill.
50. Miller JW, Danzl DF, Thomas DM: Urban accidental hypothermia: 135 cases, *Ann Emerg Med* 9(9):456, 1980.
51. Mills WF Jr: Summary of treatment of the cold-injured patient, *Alaska Med* 15(2):56, 1973.
52. Mills WJ: Out in the cold, *Emerg Med,* Jan 1976, p 134.
53. Mills WJ Jr: *Clinical aspects of frostbite injury.* In Proceedings of the Symposium on Arctic Medicine and Biology. IV. Frostbite, Fort Wainwright, Alaska, 1964, Arctic Aeromedical Laboratory.
54. Mills WJ Jr: Frostbite, *Alaska Med* 15(2):27, 1973.
55. Mills WJ, Whaley R: *Frostbite: a method of management.* In Proceedings of the Symposium on Arctic Biology and Medicine. IV. Frostbite, Fort Wainwright, Alaska, 1964, Arctic Aeromedical Laboratory.
56. Mills WJ, Whaley R, Fish W: Frostbite: experience with rapid rewarming and ultrasonic therapy, *Alaska Med* 3:28, 1961.
57. Mitchell HH, Edman M: *Nutrition and climatic stress with particular reference to man,* Springfield, Ill, 1951, Charles C Thomas.
58. Molnar GW et al: Effect of skin wetting on fingercooling and freezing, *J Appl Physiol* 35(2):205, 1973.
59. Moran T: Critical temperature of freezing living muscle, *Proc R Soc Lond (Biol)* 105:177, 1929.
60. Neittaanmaki H: Cold urticaria: clinical findings in 200 patients, *J Am Acad Dermatol* 13:636, 1985.
61. Okuboye JA, Ferguson CC: The use of hyperbaric oxygen in the treatment of experimental frostbite, *Can J Surg* 11:78, 1968.
62. Orr KD, Fainer DC: Cold injuries in Korea clinic: the winter of 1950-1951, *Medicine* 31:177, 1952.
63. Orr KD, Fainer DC: *Cold injuries in Korea during winter of 1950-1951,* Fort Knox, Ky, 1951, Army Medical Research Laboratory.
64. Porter JM et al: Intra-arterial sympathetic blockage in the treatment of clinical frostbite, *Am J Surg* 132:625, 1976.
65. Pugh G: Expedition to Cho Oyo, *Geogr J (London)* 119:137, 1953.
66. Rabb JM et al: Effect of freezing and thawing on the microcirculation and capillary endothelium of the hamster cheek pouch, *Cryobiology* 11:508, 1974.
67. Raine TJ et al: Antiprostaglandins and antithromboxanes for treatment of frostbite, *Surg Forum* 31:557, 1980.
68. Reus WF et al: Acute effects of tobacco smoking on blood flow in the cutaneous micro-circulation, *Br J Plast Surg* 37:213, 1984.
69. Rinfret AP: *Cryobiology in cryogenic technology,* New York, 1962, Wiley.
70. Robson MC, Heggers JP: Evaluation of hand frostbite blister fluid as a clue to pathogenesis, *J Hand Surg* 6:43, 1981.
71. Robson MC, Krizek TJ, Wray RC: Care of the thermally injured patient. In *Management of trauma,* Philadelphia, 1979, WB Saunders.
72. Rosenthall L et al: Frostbite with rhabdomyolysis and renal failure: radionuclide study, *AJR* 137:387, 1981.
73. Schechter DS, Sarot 1A: Historical accounts of injuries due to cold, *Surgery* 63(3):527, 1968.
74. Schoning P: Experimental frostbite in the Hanford miniature swine. III. Sweat gland changes, *Int J Exp Pathol* 71:713, 1990.
75. Schoning P, Hamlet MP: Experimental frostbite in Hanford miniature swine. I. Epithelial changes, *Br J Exp Pathol* 70(1):41, 1989.
76. Schoning P, Hamlet MP: Experimental frostbite in Hanford miniature swine. II. Vascular changes, *Br J Exp Pathol* 70(1):51, 1989.
77. Schumaker HB et al: Studies in experimental frostbite: the effect of heparin in preventing gangrene, *Surgery* 22:900, 1947.
78. Shikama K, Yamazaki I: Denaturation of catalase by freezing and thawing, *Nature* 190:83, 1961.
79. Simeone FA: Surgical volumes of the history of the United States Army Medical Department in World War II: cold injury, *Arch Surg* 80:296, 1960.
80. Snider RL, Porter JM: Treatment of experimental frostbite with intra-arterial sympathetic blocking drugs, *Surgery* 77:557, 1975.
81. St.-Pierre JP, Kobric M, Rackham A: Effect of ketotifen treatment on cold-induced urticaria, *Ann Allergy* 55:840, 1985.
82. Vaughn PB: Local cold injury: menace to military operations; a review, *Milit Med* 145(5):305, 1980.
83. Wanderer AA, Ellis ES: Treatment of cold urticaria with cyproheptadine, *J Allergy Clin Immunol* 48:366, 1971.
84. Washburn B: Frostbite—what it is—how to prevent it—emergency treatment, *N Engl J Med* 266:974, 1962.
85. Weatherly-White RCA, Sjostrom B, Paton BC: Experimental studies in cold injury, *J Surg Res* 4:17, 1964.
86. Weissman G: Prostaglandins in acute inflammation. In *Current concepts,* Kalamazoo, Mich, 1980, Scope Publications.
87. Weuzl JE, Burke EC, Bianco AJ Jr: Epiphysical destruction from frostbite of the hands, *Am J Dis Child* 114:668, 1967.
88. Whayne TJ, DeBakey MF: *Cold injury, ground type,* Washington, DC, 1958, US Government Printing Office.
89. White JC, Scoville WB: Trench foot and immersion foot, *N Engl J Med* 232:425, 1945.
90. Wilson O, Goldman RF: Role of air temperature and wind in the time necessary for a finger to freeze, *J Appl Physiol* 29(5):658, 1970.
91. Wintrobe MM, Buell MV: Hyperproteinemia associated with multiple myeloma, *Bull Johns Hopkins Hosp* 52:156, 1933.
92. Zacarian SA: Cryogenics: the cryolesion and the pathogenesis of cryonecrosis. In *Cryosurgery for skin and cutaneous disorders,* St Louis, 1985, Mosby.
93. Zacarian SA, Stone D, Clater H: Effects of cryogenic temperatures in the microcirculation in the golden hamster cheek pouch, *Cryobiology* 7:27, 1970.
94. Zingg W: The management of accidental hypothermia, *Can Med Assoc J* 96:214, 1967.

6 DRESSING FOR THE COLD

Arthur L. Dickinson

Adaptation to cold environments
Management of thermoregulation
Selection of clothing

The term "hostile" is appropriate for a climate that is sufficiently cold, wet, or windy to require protective clothing. To have a safe and pleasurable experience, the sojourner into the wilderness must make correct decisions and take appropriate actions. The environment can be a harsh martinet that accepts no compromise from an uninformed wanderer and that allows no second chances because of poor judgment. As an example, the majority of hypothermia episodes in Colorado occur not in midwinter, but rather when the ambient temperature ranges between 30° and 50° F.

The purpose of this chapter is to present the facts necessary to minimize the risk of environmentally caused problems during recreation or work in cold, wet, or windy weather. Three statements summarize the concepts discussed in this chapter. First, humans have remarkably poor ability to make acute or chronic significant physiologic adaptations when exposed to a cold environment. Therefore knowledge about human physiology is of critical importance to the outdoorsman.

Second, persons physically active in a hostile environment must successfully manage their thermoregulatory system to be able to control the microclimate at the interface between skin and clothing.

Third, correct selection and use of clothing require appropriate balancing of the variables of intensity of activity, duration of activity, ambient temperature, wind, and precipitation.

Adaptation to Cold Environments

The human body can do little to adapt to a cold environment. This is in contrast to the body's robust ability to adapt and become more efficient when exercising in a hot, humid climate.

Cold, wetness, and wind challenge the body to maintain core temperatures above 35° C (94° F). Heat loss or inadequate heat production heightens the risk of physical discomfort, hypothermia, or surface cold injury such as frostnip or frostbite. Blood flow bears principal responsibility for maintaining peripheral temperature in cold weather and is the metabolic transport venue for oxygen, substrate fuel, and metabolic end products. Repeated exposure to cold seems to engender more efficient perfusion in the hands, but humans in the Western world have little other acclimatization capacity to cold exposure.

The one adaptable characteristic that can contribute to better tolerance of recreational activity in a cold environment is aerobic (physical work) capacity. When working muscles and the temperature regulation system must compete for the same limited blood supply, reduced demand for the same level of work in persons with higher aerobic capacity can mean an increased margin of safety when temperature regulation becomes critical. A second advantage is that at the same workload, aerobically fit individuals derive a greater percentage of energy from storage fat. This is in plentiful supply even in the slimmest individuals. Therefore, a lesser percent is required from the limited supply of carbohydrate foods, which need to be conserved in any wildland sojourn in cold weather.

It can therefore be concluded that the ability to exist safely in cold, wet, or windy environmental conditions does not depend (with the exception of aerobic capacity) on a robust, adaptable body, but on mastery and use of information that enables self-protection. Two major areas of information are critical: (1) knowledge of physiologic phenomena relative to exercise and temperature regulation and (2) knowledge of the insulation, ventilation, and protective properties of outdoor clothing and outfitting gear and how to employ clothing to best advantage in bad weather.

Management of Thermoregulation

As metabolic machines, humans produce heat profusely during recreational activity. Energy production escalates as the intensity of physical activity increases (Fig. 6-1). Somewhere between 82% and 90% of the energy produced is in the form of heat. Just sitting on a couch produces 60 to 70 kcal/hr, or a body temperature rise of 2° F if none of the heat is dissipated. A moderate hiking pace with a daypack or a steady cross-country ski stride could raise core temperature 8° F in an hour if the heat were not dissipated. Because

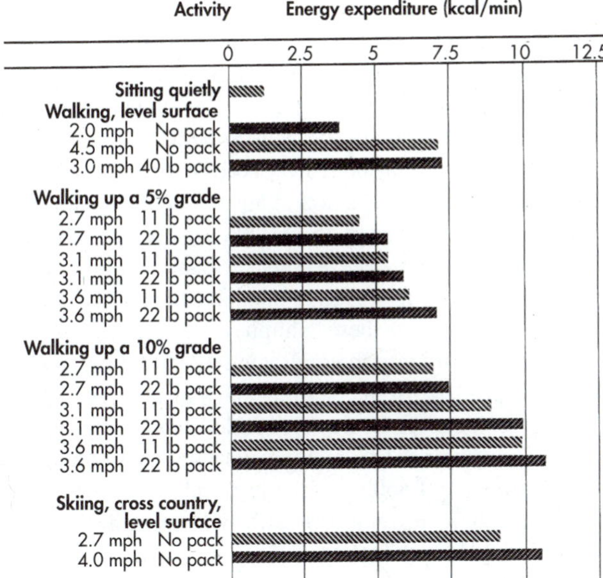

Fig. 6-1 Energy expenditures in kilocalories per minute for 160-pound men at rest and in selected recreational activity. Between 82% and 89% of energy expenditure is expected to be liberated as heat. (Data from Welsh D, Dickinson A, Byrnes WC, unpublished research, University of Colorado, 1982. Ski data from Wynder EL: *The book of health: the American health foundation,* New York, 1981, Franklin Watts.)

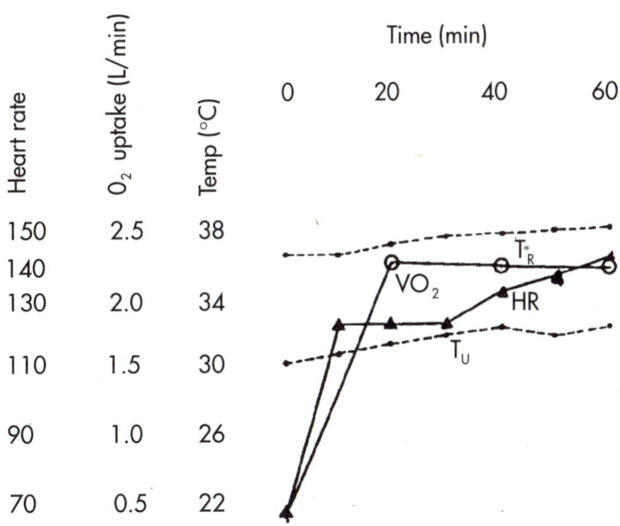

Fig. 6-2 Metabolic heat production during modest exercise with temperature at 21° C and relative humidity of 14%. (Data from Dickinson AL, Mood D: *The performance of Klimate recreational outerwear material in differing climatic conditions,* Technical report for Howe and Bainbridge, Boston, 1984.)

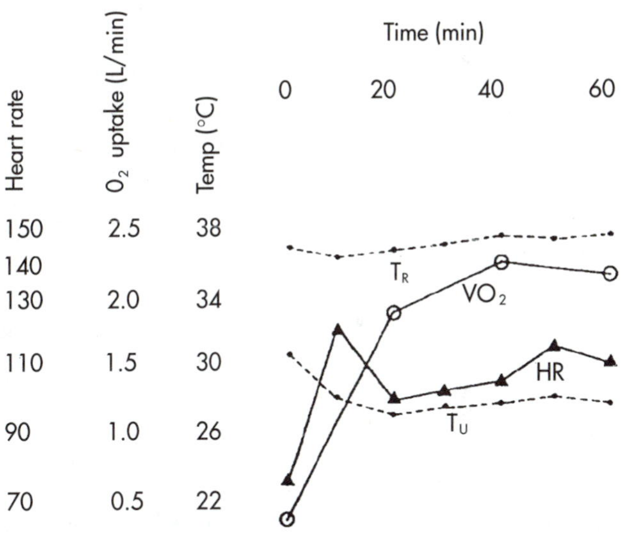

Fig. 6-3 Metabolic heat production during modest exercise with temperature at −19° C and 13.2 km/hr wind. (Data from Dickinson AL, Mood D: *The performance of Klimate recreational outerwear material in differing climatic conditions,* Technical report for Howe and Bainbridge, Boston, 1984.)

muscle can produce 100 times more heat at work than at rest, it would not take long with vigorous exercise to generate sufficient heat to melt a 5-pound block of ice and bring the water to a boil!

Thus generation of metabolic heat can be a threat to proper thermoregulation. It is remarkably easy to overdress for activity in cold weather, to sweat needlessly, and to thereby lose heat rapidly. The adverse effects of sweating in the cold are compounded by wearing clothing that sweat can permeate. This reduces garment temperatures to those of a refrigerator. The Eskimos have a saying that, while not based on the scientific process, has nevertheless survived the test of time: "If you sweat, you die."

Manufacturers of protective clothing have done a marvelous job of producing materials that preserve a warm microclimate for the body to maintain warmth at rest or at low levels of physical activity. However, most have not designed garments that can efficiently ventilate metabolic heat during more vigorous activity. The potential problem of metabolic heat production during modest exercise has been demonstrated (Figs. 6-2 and 6-3). Mean temperatures were recorded for five male subjects exercising at 50% of maximum oxygen uptake ($\dot{V}O_2max$), first in an ideal climate and dressed in T-shirt and shorts, and then dressed in three light layers of outdoor active wear. The subjects exercised at 0° F (−18° C) and faced an 8 mph breeze.

Although average upper body temperature (principally hand temperature) was lower in cold and windy conditions, core temperature did not change. Even when the workload was reduced to only half (now 25% of $\dot{V}O_2max$), mean skin temperature fell only 1° C (although hand temperature fell to 61° F), and core temperature remained the same as when exercising at 50% $\dot{V}O_2max$. Most important, when environmental temperature was raised from 0° F to 32° F (0° C) and the breeze was discontinued, even though the same light winter clothing was again worn, skin temperature increased dramatically *and sweating became profuse,* because heat production was significantly greater than heat loss. This experiment demonstrates the situation that occurs frequently and that puts active persons at risk of discomfort at best, and hypothermia at worst. Heat, lost at rates approximately 25 times greater through water than air, leaves the body in an accelerated fashion; clothing items that were comfortable when dry feel when wet as if they were just taken out of a cold attic. If core temperature is to be maintained, metabolism must be increased, accelerating depletion of carbohydrate energy stores that may already be in short supply.

To minimize the risk of this situation, a person venturing into a hostile environment must know what clothing is appropriate and how to use the garments correctly. The issue of clothing use is addressed later in the chapter.

Another fact to recall about human physiology is that humans have a limited supply of endogenous carbohydrate available as fuel for muscular activity, heat production, and brain metabolism. It has been calculated that most persons running at marathon pace have enough fat on board to fuel themselves for up to 600 miles. However, carbohydrate stores of glucose and glycogen in muscle and liver could propel a person for a distance of only about 15 miles! Therefore, during longer periods of outdoor activity, the combination of muscular activity and maintenance of body temperature can seriously deplete the limited fuel supply. Supplementation with carbohydrate snacks in cool, windy, or wet climatic conditions can be as important to the average person's safe and enjoyable completion of the day's activity as it would be to the long-distance runner or cyclist.

The energy cost of exercising in a cold environment compared with activities on a dry and sunny autumn day should be considered. The additional weight of clothing and other gear used to protect against the environment adds to the energy requirement, as can garment resistance at joints such as shoulders, knees, ankles, and feet. Pandolf, Haisman, and Goldman[11] calculated that these factors can increase the work cost of movement by 5% to 15%. If the surface being traversed is not firm, as it would be on a hiking path or groomed Nordic ski track, but instead is composed of soft or deep snow, sand, or water-soaked ground, the energy-efficient, hard surface–reactive force to lower extremity downward thrust is compromised. Force is attenuated and energy wasted until snow or earth underfoot packs with sufficient rigidity to counter the downward thrust of the body's mass through the foot, ski, or snowshoe. In addition, if the pattern of movement has to be modified, such as lifting the legs at hip and knee to walk through unpacked snow, additional energy is expended. It has been calculated that energy expenditure rises by one third for every 4-inch increase in snow depth.

At rest, such as when sitting in a canoe on an autumn day or ice fishing in the winter, body heat is lost principally (at least 60%) by radiation from 1.5 m^2 (average) of body surface area. Radiant heat forms a "Thermos bottle" of warmed air around a person, unless there is a breeze.

In the presence of moving air or when a person is moving, significant amounts of heat are lost by convection. Loose-fitting clothing pulled by body movement creates a bellowslike convective action of air between skin and clothing, purging body-heated air out, like smoke up a chimney. The neck, waistband, sleeves, pockets, and pant legs are the usual orifices. Using garments that have the ability to selectively loosen or close these "chimneys" to intentionally lose or conserve heat from the microclimate within the garment is always prudent. Some clothing, such as underwear, has a small percentage of Lycra fiber added for a snug fit. This maximizes its insulative and moisture wicking qualities by not allowing any flopping of the material, which would otherwise result in lessening of effectiveness when material loses contact with the skin.

Heat loss by conduction is the least frequent mode of transfer in a wildland hostile environment, although conductive heat loss (or heat gain, for that matter) occurs across the skin whenever it is in physical contact with matter 2° C cooler or warmer. Some common examples of heat conduction that occurs in outdoor recreational situations include sitting on rocks, lying on the ground, or being in contact with clothing that has been cooled by evaporation of sweat or by environmental moisture. An ineffective insulation system between foot and boot is a potentially serious example of convective heat loss. Absorbing heat by means of conduction is the method by which we reward a frostnipped cheek when we press an ungloved hand against it; conduction also occurs when a hypothermic body is rewarmed by being placed next to another body of normal temperature.

Unquestionably, the most important mode of heat loss is through evaporation of either sweat or environmental moisture in contact with the body surface. A body engaged in physical activity of sufficient vigor to produce sweating will lose 70% of body heat loss through evaporative cooling. Because cooling occurs at the site of evaporation and, of most consequence, when evaporation takes place on the surface of the skin, the value of garments that can transfer, or "wick," moisture away from the skin to be evaporated on outer layers of clothing is readily understood.

It helps to know the mechanisms of heat loss to critically evaluate the design and type of clothing material selected to be worn in a hostile environment. Being able to *selectively* control the amount of heat loss by evaporation and convection is the key to outfitting. Most important is the ability to regulate skin temperature in the trunk, where most sweat glands are located, the head and neck, and the areas of natural folds in the body—axillae, crotch, and backs of knees. Using buttons, zippers, and Velcro fasteners and simply adding or shedding layers of clothing are methods by which to regulate precisely the amount of heat loss. If one expects to be moderately to highly physically active, it is improper to rely solely on the clothing material to adequately ventilate to maintain the desired degree of body surface cooling. Despite manufacturer's claims about product ventilatory capability, exercise of greater intensity than walking a dog requires conscious temperature regulation. The challenge of outfitting is to maintain near normal body temperature, to conserve body energy stores, and to lose body heat to the extent that sweating is minimal. This requires balancing clothing to be worn against expected climatic conditions and assessing the intensity and duration of physical activity that will be required on the trip. Diagrammed, it is presented as:

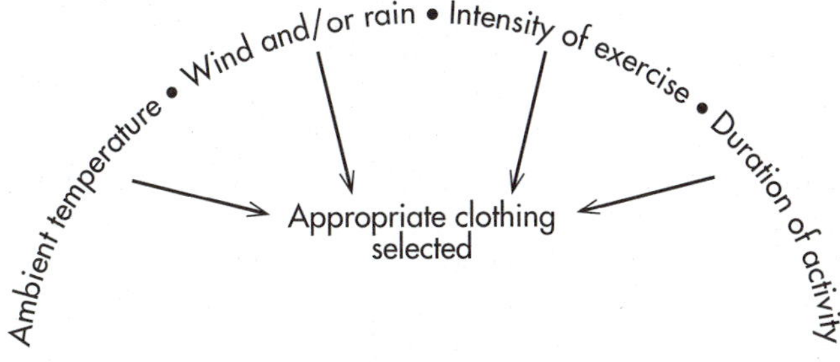

All of these factors influence thermoregulatory balance. *Selection of clothing is the single most important variable that the sojourner is usually empowered to manipulate toward achieving acceptable levels of thermoregulation.*

Selection of Clothing

The key aims of outfitting are abbreviated by the letters VIP—ventilation to selectively control heat storage and loss by adjusting clothing, insulation to control heat escape through convection and conduction, and protection against wind and rain, which greatly accelerate heat loss.

There is no material that is a fine insulator, yet protects superlatively from wind and rain. Product designers are milling and combining different forms of polyesters that result in much more versatile outer garments than those that were available a few years ago, but improvements in product design have made greater strides forward than have the types of basic materials worn in wildland excursions.

MATERIAL PROPERTIES IMPORTANT TO OUTDOOR ACTIVITIES

1. Thickness. The thicker the material, the greater the insulative value, so long as it stays dry. Thicknesses of an inch or more (except in sleeping bags) are rarely needed with the present materials available.
2. Fiber reaction to moisture. Four qualities are important:
   a. The ease of "wicking" action—of transferring moisture from body surface *to* material (hydrophilic) or transferring moisture from body surface *across* itself (hydrophobic) to other clothing
   b. Evaporative ability, or the rate of drying
   c. "Moisture regain," which is the amount of moisture a material can absorb before it feels cold
   d. The amount of insulative value a material loses when wet
3. Thermal conductance. The less the conductance, the better the insulation.
4. Resistance to wind. Fig. 6-4 helps to demonstrate the need for protection against wind. In this experiment, eight men and women wearing polypropylene underwear, cross-country ski uniforms with nylon turtleneck underneath, and hat and gloves, but no jacket or parka, exercised for 90 minutes in 0° F (−18° C) temperature at 50% to 60% $\dot{V}O_2max$ intensity, with no wind and when facing an 8 mph breeze.

The most commonly used clothing materials for outdoor activities are wool, cotton, nylon, polyester, and polypropylene. Natural down and synthetic fibers to replace down should be relegated to quiet times or activities such as alpine skiing where sitting on lifts, waiting in lift lines, and staying warm in the face of significant wind velocities and snow are the principal thermoregulatory challenges.

The four important material properties are different for each of the fibers cited.

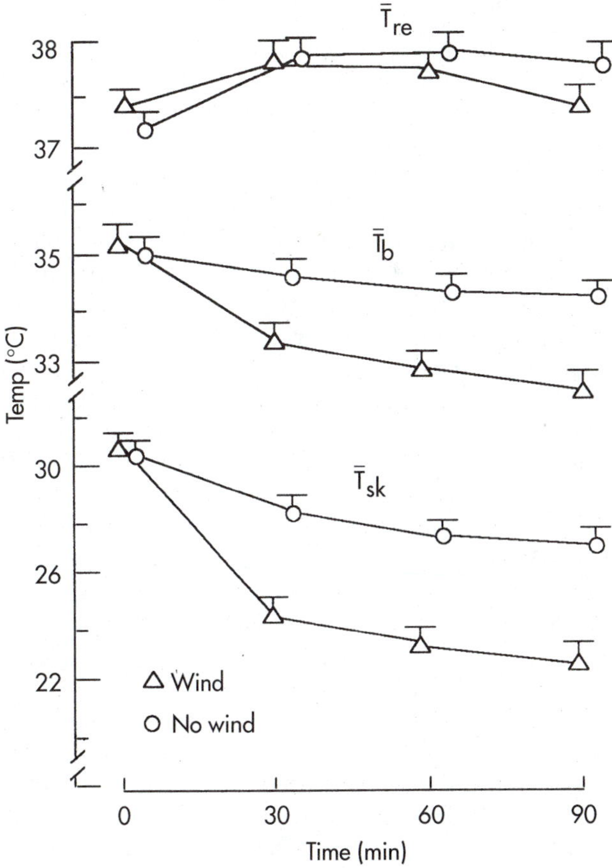

Fig. 6-4 T_{re}, T_{sk}, and T_b during exercise at −20° C. (Data from Haymes EM et al: *Med Sci Sports Exerc* 14[1]:41, 1982.)

Wool is a poor conductor of heat and therefore a good insulator. It has a moderate affinity to absorb moisture, but it can absorb a great deal—about 35% to 55% of saturation—before it feels wet. The evaporative ability (speed of drying) of wool is poor, but its fiber structure allows it to suspend water vapor without decreasing insulation.

Cotton feels great to a hiker in the summertime when, while he or she is struggling up a grade with a heavy pack, the lightest breeze hitting a sweaty shirt seems to have come straight from heaven. However, cotton has meager value in a harsh environment, where conservation of heat may be needed. Cotton loses up to 90% of its insulative value when wet, and it readily absorbs moisture (hence, it makes a great towel); its moisture regain is poor.

Polypropylene, like cotton, wicks moisture well, but unlike cotton it has a very low conductance index and high evaporative qualities. These properties are what make it so popular as an underlayer material for active outdoorsmen.

Nylon evaporates water quickly, is a good insulator, and has good quality of moisture regain. Because of its durability it is often the material preferred for outerwear. However, unless nylon is tightly knit, it does not screen wind and water well. It can be sprayed to provide more wind and water repellency, but this is at the expense of breathability. In any type of material, protection against moisture and ability to "breathe" are traded off. No material can do both in ideal fashion when intensities of activity are above 50% of $\dot{V}O_2max$, a level that a fit person can sustain for most of a day. W.L. Gore Company's high-profile Gore-Tex Teflon base was first laminated to nylon in outerwear garments that were breathable as well as water resistant.

Polyester is justifiably the most widely employed material in outdoor clothing today. The fibers can be formed into several sizes and configurations, thereby fashioning underlayer (underwear) garments, primarily insulative gear, such as the popular fleece jackets and even outer layer wind and moisture protective gear. Polyesters are poor conductors (good insulators), high in moisture regain, and (in some forms) good in wicking (moisture transfer). A greater versatility of form, smoother feel, and easier maintenance have elevated polypropylene to the favored underwear material. Polyester has replaced wool as the principal insulative layer material, usually as zippered or pullover jackets. The fibers can be fashioned to have some breathability, although in any but the lightest of breezes a wind-resistant shell over the fleece may be needed for comfort. Styles with a longer fleece pile, which have appeared since 1992, offer better protection against wind. When polyester is designed as an outer (protective) layer, fibers are woven more densely and a water- or wind-repellent sheath is sometimes laminated to it, possibly made of nylon and Lycra, or the outer surface can be sprayed with a water-repellent substance such as Ultrex. It is environmentally interesting that 80% of polyester fleece used in outdoorwear is processed from recycled plastic bottles.

Down and synthetic loft material are not often appropriate for clothing worn by the physically active, but they certainly have value when insulation is needed for quiet situations such as fishing, sitting around a campfire, using a sleeping bag, or other relatively inert functions. The greater the amount of "loft" possible in the material, the better the insulative value. Goose down has great loft ability. However, as with cotton, insulation capability plummets if down becomes wet. Down's moisture affinity is high and its drying rate is slow. Condensation that forms on the inner layer of down garments becomes a comfort problem.

There are synthetic hollow-core fibers such as Quallofil, Thinsulate (Thermaloft), or Polargard that approach the insulative value of down, are much less bulky, lose less insulative value when wet, and, being predominantly hydrophobic, dry more rapidly when wet. Alpine ski outerwear is a classic example of the use of nylon or polyester synthetic down. Most gloves designed for lower temperatures also use one of the synthetic loft products to achieve the insulative goal.

If a high level of warmth is an issue and a synthetic loft material is preferred in a sleeping bag or jacket, the buyer should look for a material that resists compression because reduced loft means reduced insulation. Many sleeping bags mix synthetic loft with a majority content of goose down to reduce moisture problems associated with 100% down.

In spite of continued improvements in the appropriateness of materials and the design of products, the *active* outdoorsman must still employ the principle of layering clothing to ensure the most comfortable, enjoyable, and *safe* experience in cold, wet, or windy conditions.

UNDERLAYER

Warmth and wicking ability are the principal requisites for layers next to the skin. Polyesters designed for moisture transfer and softness of feel and the older polypropylene best satisfy the needs of this layer. Three different weights (thicknesses) are usually available for purchase to give a selection relative to the amount of insulation desired.

Some manufacturers have added a small percentage of Lycra to the polyester to achieve a consistent snugness to the skin, able to withstand limb movement. This enables the garment to be somewhat more effective in both insulation and moisture transfer. On days when the temperature is above freezing and wind is not a worry, the underlayer may not be needed.

INSULATION LAYERS

Adequate insulation and ability to selectively ventilate are by far the most important characteristics of the insulative layers. With materials currently available, bulky and heavy clothing is easy to avoid. When protection from wind and moisture is not necessary, an insulation layer may also be the outermost layer.

Although appropriate material for insulation is readily available, finding products that are well designed for selective adjustment can be a challenge. Zippers or Velcro fasteners that vent areas around the trunk and the natural folds of axillae and neck are extremely important. Many jackets now use netting for the pockets, which is helpful, but more effective are zipper closure seams that extend from the inside of the upper arms down the side of the thorax. These can be opened to ventilate large areas. Also, ability to adjust tightness around waist, sleeves, and collar can augment the bellows actions of clothing movement by providing a chimney for air circulation.

PROTECTIVE LAYER

Wind and moisture can be serious challenges to thermoregulation, so protection against the elements and selective ventilation are the most important functions of the outer layer. If there is some ability of this layer and the insulative layer(s) to breathe and transfer moisture to the periphery, that is wonderful, but this is a secondary consideration.

Tightly knit, tough shells of nylon or wedded layers of nylon and polyesters are the most popular materials employed in the protective layer. Gore-Tex laminate remains the gold standard for qualities of both water resistance and breathability. In vigorous activity performed in rain or wet snow, however, *no* garment will satisfy the wearer because body heat production overwhelms the breathability of any material. On temperate days there may be no need for an insulative layer, so moisture transfer ability and ventilatory capacity can count heavily.

Special finishes sprayed or laminated to the polyester weave or microfiber construction have become increasingly popular for active outdoor wear. Somewhat less expensive and somewhat less moisture repellent, they have quite good breathability. Usually a polyester lining covers the inside of a protective garment of high nylon content to help compensate for its inability to transfer moisture.

Although the head is an area where a great deal of body heat can be lost, it is so easy to selectively control this loss with hats, hat liners of polyester or polypropylene, and face masks of polyester fleece that no real challenge exists here as long as the outdoorsman remembers to pack head protection. Knit bands to insulate forehead and ears and ordinary earmuffs are quite effective.

The wide variety of gloves and mittens made from polyester fleece, synthetic down, and wool, with a nylon outer cover where appropriate, ensures that hands are not injured by the cold. Glove liners are available when more insulation is needed. As with all cold weather apparel, gloves should not fit so snugly that peripheral blood flow is reduced.

Appropriate footwear remains a problem in cold environments. Boots are vulnerable to moisture and cold wherever they are stitched, although sealing compounds and waterproof tape can help. Instead of trying to keep moisture and cold out of the boot at the expense of sweaty feet, an alternative strategy now employed with the increased use of breathable and less waterproof boots is to use a Gore-Tex or comparable sock over the usual sock, with the intent of keeping the inner sock dry.

The following are general guidelines of outfitting for recreation and work in harsh environments:

1. For summer, early fall, and late spring, a cotton T-shirt is usually fine, but a weather-protective shell (top and bottom) and a long-sleeved top should be carried. A snack that is easily digested and has a high percentage of carbohydrate is needed. Large numbers of hypothermia cases occur when ambient temperatures range from 30° to 50° F. Perhaps rain, sleet, and wind are factors in the majority of these episodes.
2. For an ambient temperature of 32° F and above there is little need for underlayer bottoms, but a long-sleeved underlayer top is prudent. If wind is possible, or when the sun disappears behind the clouds, two layers of insulation should be available. Blue jeans or other cotton clothing should be left in the closet, but a hat should be brought. Garments for the trunk and arms should have selective ventilation capability.
3. For an ambient temperature of 20° to 30° F all three basic layers should be worn, but clothing should be ventilated or closed up as dictated by sun, wind, and intensity of exercise. A hat should be carried, although earmuffs or an earband is usually all that is needed. A dry, long-sleeved garment to change into or to add as an insulative layer is necessary.
4. For an ambient temperature of 0° to 19° F the ability to selectively ventilate is still necessary. Down should not be worn except in inactive periods. Old socks worn over boots add insulation, but booties for the same purpose can be purchased. A polypropylene or polyester hat liner is a judicious choice for the pack, as is a spare long-sleeved shirt. Glove liners are a good idea for the pack. For all temperatures, a high-carbohydrate snack should be packed.

REFERENCES

1. Askew EW: Nutrition for a cold environment, *Phys Sports Med* 17(12):77, 1989.
2. Dickinson AL, Mood D: *The performance of Klimate recreational outwear material in differing climatic conditions,* Technical report for Howe and Bainbridge, Boston, 1984.
3. Gavhed DCE, Nielson R, Holmer I: Thermoregulatory and subjective responses of clothed men in the cold during continuous and intermittent exercise, *Eur J Appl Physicol* 63:29, 1991.
4. Gonzales RR: Biophysical and physiological integration of proper clothing for exercise, *Exerc Sport Sci Rev* 15:261, 1977.
5. Graham TE: Thermal, metabolic and cardiovascular changes in men and women during cold stress, *Med Sci Sports Exerc* 20(5)(suppl): S185, 1988.
6. Haymes EM et al: Effects of wind on the thermal and metabolic responses to exercise in the cold, *Med Sci Sports Exerc* 14(1):41, 1982.

7. Holmer J, Elnas S: Physiological evaluation of resistance to evaporative heat transfer by clothing, *Ergonomics* 24:63, 1981.
8. Kaufman WC, Bothe D, Meyer SD: Thermal insulating capabilities of outdoor clothing materials, *Science* 215:690, 1982.
9. McCullough EA, Rohles FH Jr: Quantifying the thermal protection characteristics of outdoor clothing systems, *Human Factors* 25(2):191, 1983.
10. Nielson R, Endruski TL: Localized temperatures and water vapor pressures within clothing during alternate exercise/rest in the cold, *Ergonomics* 35(3):313, 1072.
11. Pandolf KB, Haisman MF, Goldman RF: Metabolic energy expenditure and terrain coefficients for walking on snow, *Ergonomics* 19(6):683, 1976.
12. Patton JF et al: Physiological responses to prolonged treadmill walking with external loads, *Eur J Appl Physiol* 63:89, 1991.
13. Teitlebaum A, Goldman RF: Increased energy cost with multiple clothing layers, *J Appl Physiol* 32:743, 1972.

7 POLAR MEDICINE

Bern Shen

Distinction between Arctic and Antarctic medicine
Importance of polar medicine
Brief history of human habitation in polar regions
Arctic medical problems
Antarctic medical problems
Overview and future developments

Like much of wilderness medicine, polar medicine's identity derives to a large extent from its setting. "Polar," however, can be defined in several different ways.[29] Geographically, the Arctic and Antarctic circles, at latitudes 66°33′ north and south, delimit areas in which the sun does not rise or set on at least 1 day of the year. A more functional definition is the 10° isotherm, which joins those areas in which the average temperature in the warmest month of the year is 10° C (50° F); this correlates roughly with the treeline. Still other definitions or subdivisions are based on the extent of permafrost, tundra, or sea ice.

For medical purposes the definition of "polar" is more complex. Although climate and geography are clearly important, the salient features of polar medicine are logistic and experiential. Unlike altitude medicine or hyperbaric medicine, for example, polar medicine is not unified by an underlying pathophysiology. Although fields such as the former are medicine *because of* their environment's effect on the human organism, polar medicine is largely medical practice *within* the setting.

Medical practice in spite of isolated settings is paradigmatic of wilderness medicine; the patient population is essentially if not literally a small demographic island. A provisional definition of polar medicine, then, could be formulated as "the practice of medicine in isolated settings"; to borrow an anthropologic term describing isolated "island" communities, it could be called Fourth World medicine.[53,113,157]

Distinction Between Arctic and Antarctic Medicine

Although the polar regions share the predominant attributes of cold and isolation, they display many important contrasts. The Arctic has been described as a sea nearly surrounded by land, while Antarctica is a land and ice mass circumscribed by ocean. The moderating effect of the North Polar waters compared with the elevation (2835 m) of the South Polar plateau accounts for the roughly 40° C (72° F) differences in wintertime low temperatures. On a plot of temperature versus humidity, the South Pole is more similar to Mars than to the rest of the earth.

Such environmental contrasts are reflected in population density and diversity of flora and fauna. In contrast to the Arctic's boreal forest, tundra, and growing population of over 2 million, Antarctica is a high, dry, icy desert continent with almost nonexistent flora and fauna, no indigenous population, and transient influxes of a few thousand people each summer and merely a few hundred in winter.

The differences in population patterns mark an important north-south disjunction in polar studies in general,[41] and in polar medicine in particular.[179] There are actually two overlapping but distinct spectra of medical problems—those of indigenous Arctic people and those of visitors to either polar region. As we shall see, many of the medical problems among the Inuit, Sami, Chukchi, Nenet, and other northern groups are those of populations making the often Faustian demographic and cultural transition to a Western industrialized society. Thus medical practice among these groups is similar to that among many other displaced aboriginal populations.

In contrast, medical problems among the usually young and fit scientific, commercial, tourist, or expedition personnel are often related to trauma and the environment and thus fall more appropriately under the purview of travel or expedition medicine. In a sense the current illnesses and health risks of the indigenous Arctic populations are the result of too much contact with other cultures, while those of the sojourners to either polar region are largely the result of too little connection with the culture and medical facilities of home.

The indigenous versus sojourner or essentially north-south disjunction in polar medicine poses a challenge to a meaningful synthesis. In the spirit of a trend in travel medicine,[69] I recognize that it makes sense to focus not only on the health of elite visitors to remote areas, but also on the health problems surrounding and sometimes even caused by them.

Rigorous discussions of health risks, practices, and outcomes ultimately depend on much finer resolution of local climate, culture, and occupational conditions. Even among the remarkably consistent linguistic cultures of the Arctic, there are clearly confounding variables in trying to metaanalyze, for example, health studies among reindeer herders in an isolated Sami village in northern Finland, Inuit apartment block dwellers in Nuuk, Greenland, and Alaskan pipeline workers on the North Slope. Likewise, in the Antarctic there are important differences among the living conditions and health determinants of a marine biologist on the Antarctic Peninsula, a geologist in the Dry Valleys, and a power plant mechanic at the South Pole Station.

Importance of Polar Medicine

INCREASE IN TOURISM AND EXPEDITIONS

The combined geographic polar regions cover about one sixth of the world's surface,[151] and their territory in the imagination has been enlarged by several remarkable expeditions and recent popular magazine articles and books.* Despite, or perhaps because of, the forbidding environment, tourism of various sorts to polar regions is increasing.[10,86,102,169] Junkets "to the North Pole" are popular despite being costly, and Antarctica has become a trendy destination for adventure seekers. Roughly 100,000 tourists a year visit Nordkapp on the tip of Norway,[100] even though no permanent settlement is there. At the other end of the globe, in 1980 it was estimated that 31,000 paying tourists, adventurers, or guests of national scientific expeditions had visited Antarctica.[126] More recently, roughly 3000 tourists a year have visited "the Ice" and commercial tourists have even been brought to the South Pole.

GEOPOLITICAL CONCERNS

The interest of governments in polar regions has not lagged behind that of tourists.[54,60,77,168,184] Political and territorial concerns have been important in both polar regions, and with increasing exploration of mineral and oil reserves[83] and fishing potential, migrating humans will bring medical problems with them. Although the Antarctic Treaty of 1959 prohibits territorial or commercial claims,[172] a number of nations have made sectoral claims on the continent, going so far as to ship pregnant women to Antarctica to give birth to Antarctic "citizens." Concern about the environmental impact of increasing human activity in polar regions† seems to be tempering the pace of development, but it appears likely that the pool of potential civilian and military[162] patients in polar regions will increase.

*References 31, 81, 87, 95, 102, 120, 123, 151.
†References 10, 57, 96, 106, 109, 169.

INCREASING RESEARCH ACTIVITIES

Scientific research has been a part of polar exploration throughout this century (Fig. 7-1).* There are scientific and medical journals devoted to the polar regions, and thousands of articles are indexed each year in the Antarctic Bibliography alone.[61] A new 45,000 square foot science facility has recently been completed at McMurdo,[52] and plans are being considered for replacement of the South Pole Station.[114] Here as well, some observers have discerned a north-south split, perceiving research in Antarctica as having more of a political motivation, and that in the Arctic as more practical in orientation.[38]

For both scientific and political reasons an important part of the scientific research in polar regions concerns environmental issues.[26,76] The remoteness of these regions enhances their value as a benchmark for studies of pollution, and studies have revealed several worrisome facts such as the prolonged effective half-life of radioactive fallout deposits[163] and increased chemical contamination of formerly pristine wilderness, particularly in animals high on the food chain.[26,58,163] As occupational and environmental health issues draw more attention in the next few years, this aspect of polar medicine will assume greater importance.

INTEREST IN ANALOGIES TO SPACE MISSIONS

Several articles and conferences have explored analogies between isolated polar research stations and space stations.[56,73,111,154,174] Data from polar (primarily Antarctic) stations tend to be more available and recent than

*References 4, 6, 7, 41, 147, 150, 170.

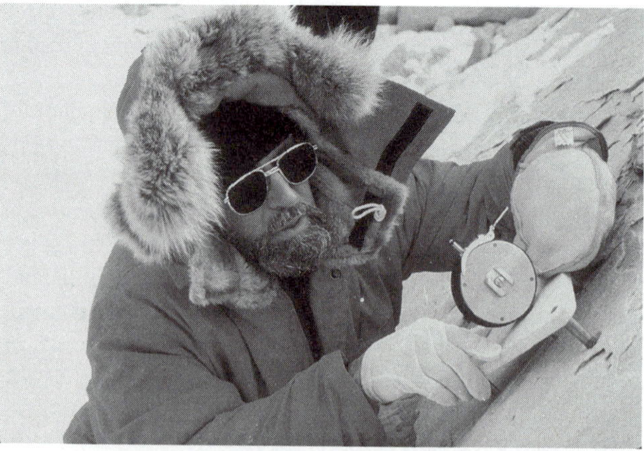

Fig. 7-1 Most human activity in Antarctica is related to scientific research in geology, glaciology, marine biology, upper atmosphere physics, and astronomy. (Courtesy National Science Foundation.)

from other space station analogs such as nuclear submarines.[173] Although the analogy is not perfect,[33] it seems useful. The immediate future of human spaceflight seems uncertain at this time, so polar studies may give planners more information of relevance to future space missions.[110]

Brief History of Human Habitation in Polar Regions

A perspective on the contrasts between Arctic and Antarctic medicine may be sharpened by review of an extremely brief summary of human habitation in the polar areas.

Humans are known to have inhabitated Arctic regions for at least 4500 years. Anthropologists have uncovered evidence for several waves of population migration from Siberia through northern Canada to Greenland. Each of these migrations was probably linked to climatic conditions, and each resulted in a distinct set of cultures. The general pattern was of a nomadic life with population densities of approximately 1 person per 400 km^2.[70,156] In more recent times this long-established and remarkable adaptation to a hostile environment has been disturbed. The pace of cultural change increased dramatically with sustained contact between Europeans and Inuit during the second half of the nineteenth century, when the whaling industry moved into Hudson Bay. In the early part of the twentieth century, religious missions, trading company posts, government stations, and eventually medical clinics and schools began to encourage permanent settlements,[70] roughly quadrupling the population density. This change in population distribution and the contact and sometimes conflict between the indigenous and European cultures had medical consequences.

In contrast to the Arctic, the known history of human exploration of the Antarctic is quite recent. Recorded sightings of the continent date only to around 1800, and "winter-over" sojourns did not occur for another century. One can also construct waves of settlement in Antarctica: sealing in the early nineteenth century, whaling in the early twentieth, and scientific since the mid-twentieth.[156] The heroic era of Antarctic exploration occupied the early years of the twentieth century, with exploits such as the highly publicized race for the South Pole between Roald Amundsen and Robert Scott in 1911, and the extraordinary survival of the crew of the 1914 *Endurance* expedition, led by Ernest Shackleton.[81] Perhaps because of these dramatic events, and perhaps because of the absence of an indigenous population and the scarcity of easily exploited resources, human activities in the Antarctic have retained a somewhat more expeditionary flavor than in the Arctic. This has helped to shape the contrasts in medical practice between North and South Polar regions.

Arctic Medical Problems

SOMATIC HEALTH PROBLEMS

Effects of Cultural and Demographic Transition

Medical problems among indigenous populations in the Arctic are characteristic of those of displaced aboriginal people elsewhere in the world. On the one hand, recent episodes such as the 1987 trichinosis outbreak in Salluit,[91,92] the 1980 rabies outbreak in the Svalbard Islands,[124] and continued problems with diphyllobothriasis[27] and toxoplasmosis[94] reflect diseases characteristic of nonindustrial life-styles. On the other hand, increased contact with industrialized cultures has brought problems as well as benefits. For many years health care has lagged behind national norms, with infant mortality in the Canadian Arctic greater than 10%, life expectancy in 1970 only 60% of the national average, and widely prevalent tuberculosis, alcoholism, and tobacco use.[98,99,156,177] Despite dedicated individual efforts, catastrophes such as the 1948 outbreaks of influenza originating at Cambridge Bay,[68] the 1949 polio epidemic among Hudson Bay Inuit,[68,101] and widespread tooth decay and even malnutrition with the introduction of new foods[68,70] have demonstrated negative medical consequences of cultural contact.

As indigenous Arctic populations and their environment make the cultural and demographic transition to a Western industrialized way of life, the spectrum of medical problems has shifted. Even isolated mining villages in Greenland no longer exhibit traditional patterns of illness.[48] Changing social patterns have resulted in disturbing trends; more than half the births in Greenland in the 1970s were to unwed mothers,[136] and the prevalence of gonorrhea and syphilis among Greenlanders is one in three,[53] raising concerns about transmissible diseases such as viral hepatitis and AIDS.[146]

Environmental and Occupational Health Problems

A consequence of the transition to industrialized life is a change in environmental health risks.[3] Popular attention has been focused by such recent catastrophes as the Severomorsk submarine base explosion in May 1984 and the *Exxon Valdez* accident in Prince William Sound. The nuclear accident at Chernobyl in May 1986 led to cesium 134 and 137 levels in reindeer meat 50 to 100 times those considered safe, forcing destruction of the Sami reindeer herds at the same time that lake fishing and berry picking were curtailed because of contamination.[53] Industrial emissions, including an estimated 100 million tons of sulfur dioxide annually from neighboring regions, have led to the phenomenon of the "Arctic haze," a gradual whitening of the historically deep blue Arctic sky.[53]

Environmental impacts have direct health consequences.[28,113,130] During the last 500 years, industrial pollution has led to a sevenfold increase in lead levels in human tissues in the Arctic.[53] Another recent survey found blood mercury levels above the normative limit in over 10% of Sami reindeer herders in northern Finland, an index of ocean contamination and concentration of heavy metals in fish.[90]

Nontoxicologic factors also make important contributions to Arctic morbidity and mortality. It is striking that Alaska's occupational death rate is five times that of the U.S. national average of 7.6 deaths per 100,000 workers.[135] This reflects in part inherently hazardous working conditions and occupations[14] and possible demographic biases of a young population.[82,139] Other factors, however, may play a role. Recently aircraft safety has attracted increasing attention.[25,139] Since aircraft are a predominant mode of transportation in polar regions, it is perhaps not surprising that Alaska accounted for almost one fourth of the fatal or serious commuter air crashes in the United States in a recent 5-year review.[135] Nonscheduled or commuter plane (less than 30 seats) flights commonly used in isolated areas may pose a sixfold risk of a fatal crash relative to scheduled airliner flights,[9,175] a figure not surprising given the often extremely challenging flying conditions.

PSYCHOSOCIAL HEALTH PROBLEMS

With social disruption and increased environmental and occupational health risks, it comes as no surprise that psychologic problems in the Arctic have achieved higher visibility in recent years. For a variety of reasons, stress seems to be higher in winter[55]; seasonal affective disorder, or SAD, is discussed below. One survey of over 7000 adults living north of the Arctic Circle found a prevalence of midwinter mental distress of 14% in men and 19% in women[55]; most other studies suggest that this figure may be low. Depression, suicidality, and domestic violence are prominent reasons for visits to the Baffin Consultation Service,[1,183] and conjugal violence has also been found to be a serious problem in communities near the Beaufort Sea.[35] Studies among scientific staff at research stations are relatively uncommon but show patterns of sleep disturbances, depression, and alcohol use reminiscent of those in Antarctic stations.[23]

The double apparent risk factors of high latitude and being a displaced aboriginal population have made alcohol abuse and concomitant violence a serious problem in the Arctic. In Greenland roughly 25,000 adults consume 28 million cans of beer a year, one of the highest per capita consumptions of alcohol in the world, and one in three Inuit dies a violent death.[53] Accidents are the leading cause of death in Greenland, and one third of these are estimated to be alcohol related, as are most of the crimes and domestic violence.[136] Similarly, in the Canadian Arctic, alcohol consumption is one and a half times the national average, and Inuit and Indians between 15 and 24 years have a suicide rate six times the national average.[53]

CURRENT AND FUTURE TRENDS

Fortunately, there are encouraging signs related to Arctic health care. The incidence of low birth weight (5.5% in the central Canadian Arctic) is low compared with many other populations.[40] Tuberculosis, which incapacitated up to 20% of the Canadian Inuit by 1950, has been largely brought under control.[70] Perhaps most surprisingly the age-standardized prevalence of diagnosed diabetes among circumpolar indigenous populations in Russia, Alaska, and Canada is low compared with the U.S. all-race prevalence of 23.5 per 1000 and quite low compared with the presumably genetically similar North American Indian groups.[185]

An important development in recent years has been the institution of trauma registries to track and target significant causes of morbidity and mortality.[44] A recent excerpt from Alaska's trauma registry reports that the leading category of death was firearms related (32%), while that of injury was falls (19%).[72] Recent research has increasingly emphasized that injury prevention is not solely a function of safer design of equipment, but a complex interplay of environment, activity, and people, notably including personal risk-taking behavior.[78] If current trends toward greater economic independence and education of Arctic peoples continue, such potentially modifiable health behaviors may recede in importance in coming years.

Antarctic Medical Problems

Medical practice, problems, and their study in the Antarctic are somewhat different from those in the Arctic. After a description of the U.S. medical stations in Antarctica, some highlights of health problems as a spectrum from primarily somatic to primarily psychologic are mentioned. As is increasingly appreciated, however, this dichotomy may be somewhat artificial; we have yet to develop taxonomically orthogonal, exhaustive, and mutually exclusive axes of polar medical problems.

MEDICAL STATIONS IN ANTARCTICA

The medical facilities in polar regions can be conveniently divided into permanent and expeditionary facilities, although a notable shift has occurred in the U.S. Antarctic Program "from an expeditionary to an operational attitude."[137] The United States maintains several small summer camps and three larger year-round stations: McMurdo (77°53′S, 166°40′E) on the Ross Ice Shelf, Palmer (64°46′S, 64°03′W) on the Antarctic Peninsula, and Amundsen-Scott (90°S) at the geographic South Pole. Roughly another 40 stations are maintained by a dozen other countries, mostly on the coast.

McMurdo on Ross Island is the largest settlement and major staging area for U.S. Antarctic activities. The summer population is about 1500 and the winter population is about

200. Monthly mean temperatures vary from –3° C in summer to –22° C in midwinter; cold weather limits aircraft operations and physically isolates McMurdo from late February to late August. The medical facilities consist of a well-equipped infirmary staffed during the summer by three physicians, three medical corpsmen, and several technicians; during the winter, staffing contracts to one physician and two medical corpsmen. The vast majority of patient visits are for routine minor medical problems. The rare patient requiring medical evacuation can be flown to Christchurch, New Zealand; fortunately, a logistically difficult winter evacuation has not been required since the 1960s.

Palmer Station on Anvers Island in the Antarctic Peninsula has summer and winter populations of about 40 and 10, respectively. With monthly mean temperatures between –10° C and 2° C, it is a popular Antarctic destination for cruise ships. Because of over a thousand visitors a year, there has been active debate regarding the proper role of station personnel in receiving commercial tourists.[137] This issue was highlighted during the 1992 season when a tourist suffered an apparent myocardial infarction and required evacuation. The infirmary has been recently reorganized to facilitate rapid access to emergency medications and equipment.[80]

In contrast to McMurdo and Palmer, Amundsen-Scott South Pole Station at 90°S is at an altitude of 2835 m on the polar plateau and has monthly mean temperatures of –28° C in December and –60° C in July. Its summer and winter populations are roughly 120 and 25, respectively. The biomed building, in an archway adjacent to the aluminum geodesic dome that shelters the main part of the station, has a fairly well-stocked pharmacy, dental equipment, x-ray darkroom, laboratory, and simple operating room. In recent years it has also been reorganized to include a "crash cart," more trauma supplies, and a more useful stock of medications; station personnel have undergone training in cardiopulmonary resuscitation and "trauma team" drills.[17,32,64,138] There have been recent cases of pulmonary edema and carbon monoxide poisoning, but fortunately no deaths since that following a cervical spine fracture in 1980.

SOMATIC HEALTH PROBLEMS

Many of the primarily somatic health problems in Antarctica have to do with cold, altitude, and trauma and are thoroughly covered in the chapters on those topics. In a midwinter setting where a tossed mug of coffee freezes before the liquid hits the ground, the dangers of frostbite are obvious. Anyone gasping for breath on "Heart Attack Hill" at the South Pole and losing 5 kg in the first 2 weeks from resting tachycardia and tachypnea can appreciate the physiologic stresses of rapid ascent to an equivalent of 3200 m. Likewise, the dangers of ultraviolet exposure at altitude with an ozone hole and reflection from a snow surface with an albedo of 80% to 90% can become painfully evident to the unwary visitor.[140] A few points, however, deserve further mention.

Cold-Related Problems

Cold, of course, is a dominant factor in polar medicine (Fig. 7-2). It can be a source of humor, such as in the infamous "300 Degree Club" at the South Pole, for which membership requires sprinting from a 200° F sauna to the Pole at –100° F while somewhat less than completely clothed. Similarly, the quintessential polar first aid story involves creative solutions to the problem of finding warm fluids,[2] but it would be reckless to forget the ever-present danger of such a hostile environment. Windchill commonly drops far below –72° C (–100° F), and it has been estimated that under the most severe winter conditions an inactive person in full polar clothing would undergo a life-threatening drop in core temperature to 27° C in only 20 minutes.[43] Airplane refueling crews and others working with liquids at ambient temperatures are constantly reminded that even a small splash can mean instant frostbite.

Rescue and treatment are complicated by the additional need for both victim and rescuer to avoid hypothermia and frostbite.[71] Disorientation and confusion from hypothermia,

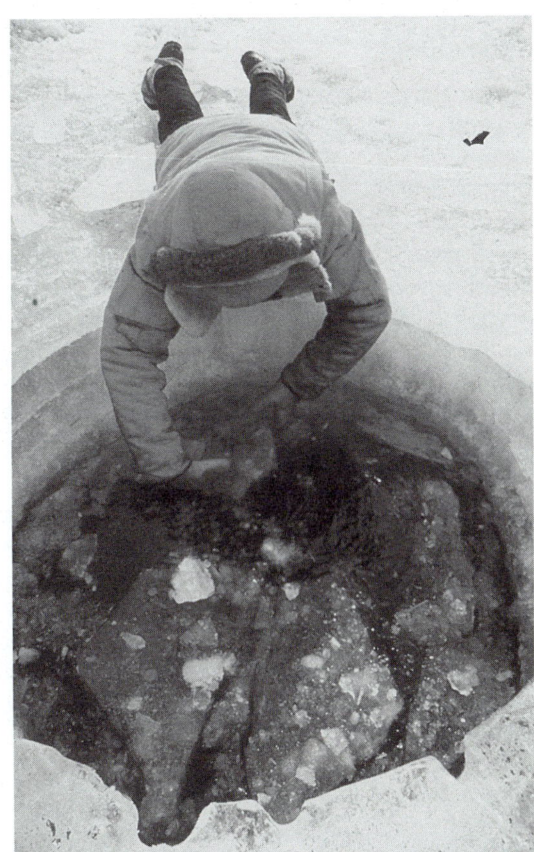

Fig. 7-2 Hypothermia is a constant threat in polar regions. (Courtesy National Science Foundation.)

clumsiness from bulky clothing, and degraded performance characteristics of equipment and intravenous (IV) fluids can complicate otherwise straightforward procedures. A recent case report describes almost immediate freezing of fluid in intravenous lines and shattering of the plastic IV tubing despite vigorous attempts to warm them.[71] Simple devices, such as air splints and pneumatic antishock garments, commonly used in warmer settings would be similarly unusable; in more sophisticated equipment, batteries would rapidly fail, unwinterized mechanical moving parts would seize, and metal objects would become dangerous sources of frostbite.

Clothing, not normally considered a medical topic, assumes special importance in the polar environment.[62,63,66] While the clothing used for many polar research programs in the summer seems adequate, a strong argument can be made for specialized winter gear, possibly adapted from the space program, that would allow relatively delicate manipulation of scientific equipment while offering protection from the cold. In fact, at temperatures below even that of most military specifications, material properties of equipment, including plastic electrical insulation, create unexpected and novel occupational hazards. Fortunately, the importance of ergonomic issues in the design of machinery as well as of clothing for polar conditions is receiving increased attention.[37,167]

Nutrition Studies

Nutrition has occupied a key niche throughout the history of polar expeditions.[39] Early expeditions in both polar regions provided several examples of nutritional illnesses, including scurvy and possible hypervitaminosis A and lead poisoning.[31,171] More sophisticated nutritional analyses have been possible in recent expeditions,[141,149] and advances continue to be made in development of lightweight but nutritionally dense rations.[36]

During the Canadian-Soviet transpolar ski trek, participants skiing some 20 km/day at a speed of about 3.5 km/hr while carrying 37 to 45 kg packs showed increased strength, decreased body fat, and increased HDL cholesterol, but a paradoxical drop in aerobic power, perhaps because of intensive pretrip conditioning and increased efficiency of skiing as the trip progressed.[140] Monika Christensen's expedition reported a daily expenditure of roughly 3000 kcal but noted that the men on the expedition consumed up to 6000 kcal/day by the end of the 2½-month trip, possibly related to the drop in temperature from –5° C to –40° C.[21] Although strenuous expedition activities can require caloric intake of up to 7000 kcal/day,[95,153] the applicability of these figures to more sedentary polar sojourners is probably limited.

Infection and Epidemiology

A number of studies have taken advantage of the physical isolation of Antarctic stations as a natural laboratory for infectious disease epidemiology, with particular reference to analogs in space colonies.[24] For example, transmission of *Escherichia coli* has been shown to correlate with population structure.[166] Since microorganisms are thought not to survive the cold long enough to be carried in by winds, midwinter respiratory tract infection outbreaks caused by parainfluenza viruses 1 and 3 and a rhinovirus in the absence of outside contacts have suggested that such organisms could persist in clothing or other fomites.[121] A similar study using swabs of 28 men isolated for a year demonstrated that *Staphylococcus aureus* could be temporarily suppressed but not permanently eradicated by antibacterial agents.[79]

Despite a widely reported leukopenia and decrease in cell-mediated immunity during the isolation of overwintering,[176] it is not clear whether persons emerging from Antarctic stations are more susceptible to infection. One study of 125 new and 75 winter-over crew at McMurdo during a 1977 outbreak of adenovirus type 21 showed that during a further 5-week isolation period 89% of the population were susceptible but only 15% were infected (much less than in usual outbreaks); no significant difference was found between winter-over crew and newcomers.[142]

Circadian Rhythms, Endocrine Studies, and Sleep Research

Pioneering studies of Natani and Shurley on sleep electroencephalograms at the old South Pole station demonstrated clear patterns of sleep disturbances and "free cycling" of the sleep-activity cycle.[104,144] Some of these findings have been extended in more recent studies. For example, among four subjects at a small winter-over camp, summer sleep cycles synchronized within the group and with clock time; during 126 days of sunless winter, rhythms free cycled in all four people but then resynchronized with reappearance of sun.[75] The degree of synchrony versus free cycling appears to depend on a number of factors, notably zeitgeber strength, although the number of subjects studied has not been large.[45]

A number of studies have examined the effect of prolonged polar residence on diurnal variations in the level of melatonin, whose role in free radical scavenging as well as sleep regulation is beginning to be elucidated.[115] Therapy with full-spectrum bright light (greater than 2500 lux) seems to facilitate daily resetting of the melatonin cycle.[97] Other endocrine fluctuations also appear to be correlated with the length of the day.[165]

Other endocrine studies have examined effects of prolonged residence in polar regions with a longer than diurnal time constant. Twenty-four-hour urinary excretion of catecholamines increases in the cold, but social stresses appear to overwhelm climatic determinants of catecholamine metabolism, correlating with increases in diastolic blood pressure and pulse during the year.[11] A more consistent pattern of decreased free thyroid hormones after several months has been demonstrated by several groups.[51,127] There has even been identified a pattern of increased pituitary release of thyroid-stimulating hormone in response to IV thyrotropin-releasing hormone and increased serum clearance of orally administered triiodothyronine (T_3), dubbed the "polar T_3 syndrome,"[128] but the clinical significance of these findings remains unclear.

Environmental Health Issues

Because of Antarctica's isolation, it seems a particularly disturbing site for litter and pollution. As in the Arctic, events such as the early problems with a nuclear reactor at McMurdo (since removed) and the 1989 oil spill from the *Bahia Paraiso* near Palmer Station,[108] and studies by groups such as Greenpeace have focused attention on environmental health risks in the Antarctic.[15a,106] Environmental inspections at a broad range of Antarctic stations have raised concern about toxic effluents and heavy metal residues,[122] as well as radioisotopes used for research.[137] In an attempt to address these issues, a number of countries have begun to implement more responsible waste management policies.

Occupational Health and Injury Prevention

Rigorous studies of risk are important for injury prevention (Fig. 7-3).[46] Unfortunately, they are complex and often bedeviled by challenges including unknown or controversial data, multiply determined effects, local variables, imprecise heuristics, and biases. For example, for purposes of occupational epidemiology, it may ultimately prove useful to stratify the Antarctic sojourner population into groups such as sport expeditions, military, commercial, and scientific, but the health behaviors of these groups overlap, and currently few studies have gone beyond aggregate descriptive statistics.

Even from these broad statistics, however, some figures emerge that may be useful cognitive anchors. Forty-five percent of medical cases in the Davis 1982 expedition were related to accidents.[30] A larger study of 1301 injuries among Australian expedition members found that 93% were minor, 3% were major, and 4% were environmental, working out to roughly one injury per person per year.[89] About 7% of the injuries were thought to be related to alcohol. There have been 52 deaths in the U.S. Antarctic Program since 1946, most related to aircraft accidents.[137] Other reports describe overuse and repetitive work syndromes and noise pollution[18,65]; often it is more difficult to adhere to standard occupational safety practices when in a remote location.[138] Environmentally related dermatologic problems may have an incidence of up to 40%.[88,129] A recent report highlights the use of cyanoacrylate glue to hasten healing of disabling fingertip fissures.[8]

Fire Safety

In the face of extreme cold, it is somewhat counterintuitive that fire has been labeled as "the major concern and principal danger at all Antarctic stations" (Fig. 7-4).[42,107] This initially surprising assessment rests on a number of factors. Cold temperatures severely limit the utility of water for fire suppression, and frequent high winds can fan fires. The extremely low absolute humidity in many polar regions results in an even lower relative humidity when outside air is warmed in station dwellings. This in turn leads to an increase in static electricity and dryness of combustibles, already at risk from frequent use of space heaters. Finally, alternative food and shelter are limited or nonexistent.

Elaborate predeployment training, frequent on-site drills, and a keen awareness of potential fire hazards have correlated with a satisfactory fire safety record to date, but this good fortune cannot be taken for granted. At least four major fires have occurred in Antarctica in the last 15 years[137]; fortunately, only one person died, but there were several injuries, and the Soviet Vostok winter crew had to endure 8 months without a power plant to supply heat.

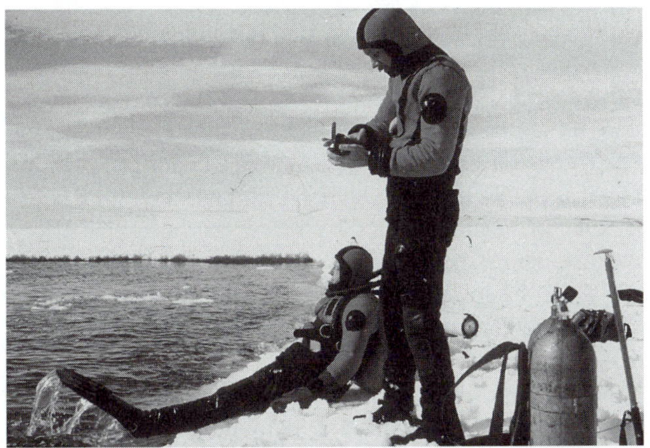

Fig. 7-3 Scientific research as well as support operations in polar regions often involve potential risks to health. (Courtesy National Science Foundation.)

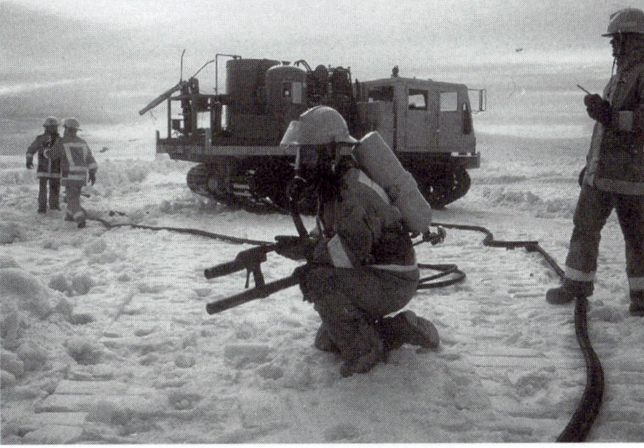

Fig. 7-4 Low temperatures complicate firefighting, making fire a major threat to polar stations. Here, crews train near McMurdo Base. (Courtesy National Science Foundation.)

Tourist Safety

Polar regions are imbued with a sense of the exotic, conjuring up "images of hardship, personal valor, danger, adventure, and of course, the hero."[137] As transportation increasingly opens up previously inaccessible areas, this image attracts growing tourist traffic and, with it, hot debate from both legal and environmental viewpoints.[15a]

The essential medicolegal issue is the extent of governmental organizations' responsibility for medical care of participants in nongovernmental activities, whether scientific, political, or commercial.[137] When a tourist group, particularly one including the older persons who can typically afford a $20,000 to $30,000 trip, requires aid beyond its own capabilities, whose responsibility is it? To what extent should a research station with limited medical supplies be required to divert some of those supplies to an individual who presumably bears responsibility for planning his or her own medical coverage? Should there be different policies for citizens of other countries?

Although the ethical course of action seems clear in the preceding scenarios, there is still uncertainty in our litigious society regarding the relative strengths of the Good Samaritan principle and the doctrine of assumed risk.[59] Perhaps eventually there will be a mandatory rescue insurance policy for tourists similar to the one currently being adopted in Mt. Rainier and Denali National Parks.[158]

Air Safety

As in the Arctic, reliance on aircraft for transportation has highlighted the critical importance of air safety. The worst air accident was the crash of an Air New Zealand tourist "flightseeing" DC-10 on Mt. Erebus in November 1979; this killed all 257 people aboard and effectively ended such flights, which had flown an estimated 11,000 tourists in the previous 2 years.[31] There have been 32 deaths in the U.S. Antarctic Program since 1946 from crashes related to either fixed-wing or rotor aircraft.[137] A ski-equipped LC-130 Hercules crashed at the remote D-59 camp in 1971. Fortunately, none of the 10 crew members aboard were injured, but during a salvage operation in 1987 another LC-130 bringing supplies to D-59 crashed nearby, killing 2 and injuring 9.

PSYCHOSOCIAL HEALTH PROBLEMS

For many polar living arrangements, psychosocial issues may be more important than strictly medical or environmental factors.* Psychiatric problems are mentioned even in reports of early expeditions,[31,160] and almost any participant in expeditions will recognize Thor Heyerdahl's observation:

> The most insidious danger on any expedition where men [sic] have to rub shoulders for weeks is a mental sickness which might be called "expedition fever"—a psychological condition which makes even the most peaceful person irritable, angry, furious, absolutely desperate because his perceptive capacity gradually shrinks until he sees only his companions' faults while their good qualities are no longer recorded by his grey matter.[160]

In fact, as Shurley notes, "minor mental troubles are both common and temporary."[143] This is particularly important since there is growing evidence that psychologic and somatic health issues are linked.[78,118] Stress can lead to increased risk of accidents, and conversely the fear of medical emergencies can lead to increased stress.[154] Confidence in the medical staff and facilities in isolated polar settings is a key factor in countering the concerns arising from isolation.

Alcohol Abuse

Adjustment to psychosocial stresses in polar communities depends on a complex array of sociocultural factors.[117,155] One coping mechanism is increased alcohol use. As in many isolated communities at high latitudes, alcohol abuse can disrupt rather than lubricate social interactions. At one station, annual per capita absolute alcohol consumption was calculated at 16.9 L.[176] At another a summer support staff member had to be terminated because of alcohol abuse and two winter-over staff had to be prohibited from purchasing alcohol from the station store; one of these actually required disulfiram to ensure abstinence.

At many Antarctic stations alcohol is easily available ("official" rations of two cases of beer plus either a bottle of liquor or two bottles of wine a week) and is actually subsidized. While relatively few serious incidents involving intoxicated staff have been reported, the potential for serious accidents remains real, particularly during winter when medical evacuation flights are impossible. Recommendations have called for routine monitoring of alcohol levels of anyone involved in an accident[137] or even prohibition of alcohol at Antarctic stations.[34]

Psychoneuroimmunology

The concept of psychologic or meteorologic modulation of immune function and other physiologic responses is gradually gaining some credence and remains largely unexplored. For example, perhaps an alternative explanation for leukopenia during winters is not absence of antigenic stimulation, as previously thought, but increased stress from interpersonal interactions.[13] In the last few years seasonal affective disorder has been largely accepted as a useful construct, and it will be intriguing to see if related findings, particularly by ex-Soviet station scientists, on weather-related pathophysiology are confirmed.

Psychologic stress at research stations may arise from several sources.[5,133] One is the environment itself; environmental severity has been found to be an independent predictor of hostility and anxiety after wintering over.[117] Perhaps more important is the perception of the environment. Newcomers to the South Pole station are usually observed

*References 23, 34, 49, 129, 140, 152.

wearing a full 12 kg polar outfit at –20° C for several weeks after arrival while the same individuals by midwinter may eventually think little of walking from the gym to their rooms at –60° C dressed only in running shorts and T-shirt.

Stress can also result from disjunction between a person's original motivation for joining the program and realities of life in the station. Studies suggest that people who go to Antarctic stations to seek thrills or to challenge themselves often have more difficulty sustaining their motivation and performance than those who go to accomplish a scientific mission or even those primarily motivated to earn money. In general, older individuals who are somewhat introverted, are able to set work goals and work toward them, and have broadly defined hobby interests seem to cope better with the social isolation and dynamics of wintering over.[34]

Small Group Dynamics

In addition to external climate and internal motivational factors, stress can arise from interpersonal interactions. Although there are many exceptions, participants in the Antarctic program often speak of a tendency for personnel to form cliques or microcultures. People may cluster according to ordinary personal chemistry, along lines of OAE (Old Antarctic Explorer) versus novice, winter-over versus summer status, or according to scientific, civilian, or military affiliation.[36] With time, such social clusters can be a source of support or of friction. Nuances of body language and proximity can take on heightened significance,[148] conferring a premium on social adaptability and compatibility.

Social isolation is of course an important factor in polar communities. Although this isolation has been lessened by modern communications and transportation, polar communities resemble in many ways the "asylums" studied by Goffman, "a place of residence and work where a large number of like-situated individuals, cut off from the wider society for an appreciable period of time, together lead an enclosed, formally administered round of life."[47]

A number of studies have drawn parallels between group processes in polar stations and those in other isolated and confined environments, such as submarines or in space.[74,105,111,173] Unfortunately, much of the submarine data is a decade or more old, raising questions of temporal drift and external validity, and the astronaut programs seem to have had little real interest in psychologic issues and so to have missed some opportunities for research in this field.[160]

Winter-Over Syndrome

Stressors such as those mentioned previously can result in what has been termed the winter-over syndrome. The historically oft-mentioned "Big Eye" or "20-foot stare in a 10-foot room" seems to be less common now, perhaps because the stations are increasingly comfortable and stimulating environments, but the constellation of depression, hostility, sleep disturbances, and impaired cognition seems to be both common and underreported.[154]

The winter-over syndrome is not a static condition, but a time- and individual-dependent process. At the South Pole research station, for example, winter-over staff characteristically report a recognizable pattern of fluctuating activity and mood. There is often a mixture of relief, pride, and fearful anticipation as the last LC-130 flight departs in mid-February, followed by a period of frenetic activity to beat inventory deadlines, file resupply orders, launch projects, and prepare the station for winter. As work and recreation routines develop, mood generally drops with the setting sun and increasing anticipation develops around the upcoming mid-winter airdrop of "freshies" (fruits and vegetables), mail, and supplies. There typically follows an August nadir, as the excitement surrounding the airdrop fades. Finally, a rise in mood generally occurs toward the end of the year, although studies at the Australian stations at Mawson and Macquarie Island suggest that the influx of new staff at station opening may actually be associated with increased depression.[176] As usual, the convenience of a descriptive label does not guarantee explanatory or predictive power or validity.

Seasonal Affective Disorder

A probable contributor to and confounder of the winter-over syndrome is the apparently fairly consistent exacerbation of stress and depression under conditions of winter or night. The term "seasonal affective disorder" (SAD) was first used in 1984 by Rosenthal and associates to describe the annual recurrence of bipolar affective disorder, hypersomnia, and overeating, which was alleviated by daily exposure to bright (2500 lux) light.[131,132] Although correlations with melatonin levels have been demonstrated, the detailed pathophysiology of SAD remains an active area of inquiry and may involve retinal signal transduction as well as timing of light intensity.* Sunlamps have been used informally in some Antarctic stations for years, and full-spectrum lighting has been installed in many public areas since 1987; given the current indoor lighting and self-selection of winter-overs, SAD may be no more prevalent in Antarctica than at lower latitudes.

Beneficial Effects of Isolation

An interesting point is that isolation may have positive as well as negative effects.[64] Isolation is not synonymous with loneliness and depression, as Amundsen reported from his sojourn at Framheim.[145] In one study it was found that, except for insomnia, the more severe the environment, the less severe the symptoms of depression, hostility, and anxiety.[119] In fact, a subset of "professional isolates" may actually prefer polar stations to "normal" society.[159]

---

*References 12, 84, 85, 97, 164, 182.

Reentry

An important issue familiar to many travelers and expedition members is that of reentry or social reintegration on return from a polar sojourn.[133] Although several studies suggest that personality traits are fairly stable during a polar stay, station personnel often require 6 months or more to normalize after returning from Antarctica.[160]

A question that has not been answered fully is whether subtle long-term disabilities might be induced by prolonged isolation at polar stations. Although there have been impressions of cognitive and sensory decrements after wintering over, these have not been confirmed in a number of studies.[160] As for somatic complaints a study of enlisted Navy personnel who wintered over between 1963 and 1973 found fewer hospitalizations for medical problems on follow-up than among a similar cohort who qualified for wintering over but did not actually go.[6]

Screening and Selection

Based on the preceding findings, several attempts have been made to refine the selection and screening process for successful polar sojourners.[180] These efforts have used a number of methods and instruments to cope with the methodologic constraints common to many studies of complex human systems.[19,50,129,160] Perhaps unsurprisingly, previous successful polar experience seems to be among the best predictors of subsequent high performance. In general, biographic data, peer ratings, psychometric testing, and interviews all seem helpful in selection, although each has weaknesses and inconsistencies.

Early studies led to the tripartite "ability, stability, compatibility" criteria for successful participation in the Antarctic programs.[50] This simple but useful scheme recognizes that technical skill, emotional equilibrium, and interpersonal skills all play important roles in an individual's performance and internal satisfaction. It would be desirable to improve measurement and predictive usefulness of these factors; such studies remain an active frontier for Antarctic research.

Overview and Future Developments

A point made early in this chapter was the challenge inherent in meaningfully synthesizing Arctic and Antarctic medicine. Reflection on some of the issues raised previously suggests several common areas of linkage and directions for future work.

ISSUES OF METHODOLOGY AND MEDICAL EPISTEMOLOGY

The state of knowledge about the Arctic and the Antarctic is still rudimentary. Studies in polar settings are often handicapped by extremely difficult research conditions and may never achieve the statistical power and validity expected of counterparts in more forgiving climes. Commonly encountered methodologic problems include most notably small sample sizes, unknown effect sizes, measurement of proxy variables, and multiple confounders.

In one study, cold tolerance of five Antarctic divers and five nondivers at the station were compared during a year using finger immersion tests with measurements of index finger pulp temperature, onset of cold-induced vasodilation, and pain scores.[15] No difference was found between the groups, perhaps, as the authors suggest, because of either whole body cooling or insufficient cold exposure during dives. In another review it was pointed out that simplifying assumptions of laboratory studies of cold adaptation may overlook the intermittent pattern of chilling and overheating under actual field conditions.[16] In yet another report, cardiac and respiratory functions were measured in Antarctic expedition members during a 3-month summer sojourn, and no persistent changes were noted; the authors suggest that the degree and duration of cold exposure may have been inadequate to produce notable changes.[181]

The preceding examples are offered not to level specific criticism; in fact, the studies were carefully performed and analyzed. As the authors themselves point out, however, inherent difficulties of research under polar conditions weaken the conclusions derived from it. Methodologic issues are perhaps even more complex in studies of social phenomena such as group dynamics, task performance, or depression. In these situations it may prove necessary to use multiple triangulating techniques of observational, qualitative, quasiexperimental, and experimental designs.[22,93,160] Given the high cost of supporting studies in a polar setting,[134] a major challenge is to design studies that can uncover meaningful results despite limited resources.

FOURTH WORLD MEDICAL DECISION MAKING

Given the relative paucity of rigorous studies on polar medical phenomena, a second challenge is to optimally design polar medical practice. Polar medical lore is replete with stories such as that of the physician of the 6th Soviet Antarctic Expedition who performed an appendectomy on himself[31] or those of retrospectively humorous cold-related injuries.[103] Although the basic principles of emergency medicine, epidemiology, occupational health, psychology, and other disciplines still apply in polar settings,[67] the spectrum of health problems and some important aspects of their management are undoubtedly skewed.[125] As with attempts to improve health care in the so-called developing countries, wholesale transplantation of the U.S. model of medicine may prove inappropriate. As polar medicine continues to evolve,[112] it will need to adapt the Western industrialized model to local conditions.

Fourth World medicine requires distillation of medical practice into a compact yet comprehensive package that will be robust enough to travel well. The usual, already tentative rules and thresholds of medical decision making are further stretched by novel constraints and the inherently unpredictable nature of a hostile environment.

Perhaps to a greater extent than in most settings, prevention and preparation are paramount in polar medicine. As might be imagined, the risks from even minor mishaps are exacerbated by cold and its effects on both humans and equipment, by altitude and impaired tissue oxygenation and wound healing, and by restricted dexterity and vision from bulky clothing. Isolation from medical facilities exerts a multiplier effect on these risks[139]; a victim extrication and resuscitation that would be routine in most urban or suburban U.S. settings presents an overwhelming challenge in polar settings.

With lives at stake, arguments have been made for planning for worst case scenarios rather than only for likely situations.[137,138] On the other hand, a realistic balance point on the cost/utility curve must be set for each situation based on estimated risks. As polar health workers have strived to build facilities and offer care of the highest quality, there have even been proposals for such luxuries as anesthesiologist-staffed helicopters and regionalized extracorporeal circulation equipment for rewarming hypothermic patients.[178] Such suggestions, while in line with the polar paradigm of projecting expertise into isolated regions, perhaps overemphasize therapeutic rather than preventive priorities. Given existing fiscal and logistic constraints, preventive measures should take priority over higher cost options.

A recurrent medical issue in polar stations involves contingency planning and the optimum level of inventory. This question applies equally to drugs, equipment, training, and personnel and is faced immediately by any incoming physician: given finite (even scarce) resources, space, and resupply, do I have enough X on station, have I completed enough training to handle Y, is there enough help available to take care of Z? "Just in time" principles of inventory management are not likely to be appropriate. This issue is well illustrated by the recurrent debate over whether to maintain a frozen blood bank at polar stations.[18,64,137,138]

A promising tool for both improved data gathering and medical diagnosis and treatment is informatics. When combined with improved communications systems, the computer offers a flexible and powerful solution to the problems of isolation.[20] Telemedicine embraces a broad range of possible activities, but the advantages of rapid access to organized data bases and remote consultations for radiology or via video are promising. Physiologic, psychologic,[161] and occupational health data[113] can be monitored or retrieved, ultimately unlinking geography and information flow.

Acknowledgments

I gratefully acknowledge the invaluable help and comments of Debbie Norris of Antarctic Support Associates, Dr. John Lynch of the National Science Foundation, and polar physicians Drs. Betty Carlisle, Danya Dilley, Matt Houseal, Michelle Raney, Joe Shields, and Bob Taber.

REFERENCES

1. Abbey S et al: Psychiatric consultation in the eastern Canadian Arctic. III. Mental health issues in Inuit women in the eastern Arctic, *Can J Psychiatry* 38(1):32, 1993.
2. Adler A: Arctic first aid, *N Engl J Med* 326(5):91, 1992.
3. Akerblom H: Human exposure to environmental hazards in the Arctic (editorial), *Arctic Med Res* 52(1):3, 1993.
4. Anderson P: Astrophysics goes south, *Science* 252(5012):1491, 1991.
5. Anderson C: Polar psychology: coping with it all, *Nature* 350(6316):290, 1991.
6. Anderson C et al: Research in Antarctica: exploring the still unexplored, *Nature* 350(6316):287, 1991.
7. Antarctic wilderness, *Nature* 348(6299):267, 1990.
8. Ayton J: Polar hands: spontaneous skin fissures closed with cyanoacrylate (Histoacryl Blue) tissue adhesive in antarctica, *Arctic Med Res* 52:127, 1993.
9. Baker S et al: Human factors in crashes of commuter airplanes, *Aviat Space Environ Med* 64:63, 1993.
10. Beck P: Regulating one of the last tourism frontiers: Antarctica, *Appl Geogr* 10(4):343, 1990.
11. Bodey A: *Human acclimatisation to cold in Antarctica, with special reference to the role of catecholamines,* Hobart, Australia, 1988, Australian National Antarctic Research Expedition (ANARE).
12. Bower B: Here comes the sun: scientists shed new light on winter depression, *Science News* 142:62, 1992.
13. Bower B: Marital tiffs spark immune swoon, *Science News* 144:153, 1993.
14. Brattebo G, Wisborg T, Fredriksen K: Crush injuries in Arctic offshore fisheries: initial treatment to prevent acute renal failure, *Arctic Med Res* 50(suppl 6):104, 1991.
15. Bridgman S: Peripheral cold acclimatization in Antarctic scuba divers, *Aviat Space Environ Med* 62(8):733, 1991.
15a. Broder IE, Keller LR: Fairness of distribution of risks with applications to Antarctica. In Mellers BA, Baron J, editors: *Psychological perspectives on justice,* New York, 1993, Cambridge University Press.
16. Budd G: Ergonomic aspects of cold stress and cold adaptation, *Scand J Work Environ Health* 15(suppl 1):15, 1989.
17. Carlisle E: *South Pole end of season report,* 1992, US Antarctic Program.
18. Carlisle E: *Palmer Station medical turnover report,* 1993, US Antarctic Program.
19. Cazes G et al: The quantitative and qualitative use of the Adaptability Questionnaire (ADQ), *Arctic Med Res* 48(4):185, 1989.
20. Chiang E, Wiesnet D, Merson R: Satellites: application to the United States Antarctic Program operations and the international potential. In Thomson R, editor: *Space and airborne technology applications to Antarctic operations,* Christchurch, NZ, 1989, Dept of Scientific and Industrial Research.
21. Christensen M: *90° south: final report,* London, 1988, Royal Geographical Society.
22. Cochran W: *Planning and analysis of observational studies,* New York, 1983, John Wiley.
23. Cochrane J, Freeman S: Working in Arctic and subarctic conditions: mental health issues, *Can J Psychiatry* 34(9):884, 1989.
24. Cosman B, Brandt-Rauf P: Infectious disease in Antarctica and its relation to aerospace medicine: a review, *Aviat Space Environ Med* 58(2):174, 1987.
25. Cottrell J et al: In-flight medical emergencies: one year of experience with the enhanced medical kit, *JAMA* 262:1653, 1989.

26. Cross M: Antarctica: exploration or exploitation? *New Scientist* 130(1774):29, 1991.
27. Curtis M, Bylund G: Diphyllobothriasis: fish tapeworm disease in the circumpolar north, *Arctic Med Res* 50(1):18, 1991.
28. Dahlstrom G: Work in the cold: an information and research program in occupational health, *Arctic Med Res* 51(suppl 7):92, 1992.
29. Dawson M: Arctic environments: the physical setting. In Jacobs M, Richardson J, editors: *Arctic life: challenge to survive,* Pittsburgh, 1983, Carnegie Institute.
30. Dick A: *Study of the health and physiological adaptation of an expedition in Antarctica, with special reference to occupational factors,* Hobart, Australia, 1987, Australian National Antarctic Research Expeditions.
31. *Antarctica: great stories from the frozen continent,* Sydney, Australia, 1985, Reader's Digest.
32. Dilley D: Personal communication, 1993.
33. Douglas W: Psychological and sociological aspects of manned spaceflight. In *The human experience in Antarctica: applications to life in space,* Sunnyvale, Calif, 1987, National Aeronautics and Space Administration.
34. Draggan S: *Performance in isolated environments,* 1987, Washington, DC, National Science Foundation.
35. Durst D: Conjugal violence: changing attitudes in two northern native communities, *Commun Mental Health J* 27(5):359, 1991.
36. Edwards J, Roberts D: The influence of a calorie supplement on the consumption of the meal, ready-to-eat in a cold environment, *Milit Med* 156(9):466, 1991.
37. Eisma T: Handling the cold with dexterity, *Occup Health Safety* 60(12):16, 1991.
38. Elzinga A, Bohlin I: Politics of science in polar regions, *Ambio* 18(1):71, 1989.
39. Feeney R: Food technology and polar exploration, *Arctic Med Res* 51:35, 1992.
40. Finnemore B: Low birth weight in the central Canadian Arctic, *Arctic Med Res* 51(3):117, 1992.
41. Fogg G: *A history of Antarctic science,* Cambridge, 1992, Cambridge University Press.
42. Fowler A: Antarctic logistics, *Oceanus* 31(2):80, 1988.
43. Freitas CD, Symon L: Bioclimatic index of human survival times in the antarctic, *Polar Rec* 23(147):651, 1987.
44. Frimodt-Moller B, Bay-Nielsen H: Classification of accidents in the Arctic: a suggestion for adaptation of the Nordic classification for accident monitoring, *Arctic Med Res* 51(suppl 7):15, 1992.
45. Gardner P et al: Adaptation of sleep and circadian rhythms to the Antarctic summer: a question of zeitgeber strength, *Aviat Space Environ Med* 62(11):1019, 1991.
46. Glickman T, Gough M, editors: *Readings in risk,* Washington, DC, 1990, Resources for the Future.
47. Goffman E: *Asylums: essays on the social situation of mental patients and other inmates,* Garden City, NY, 1961, Anchor Books.
48. Gottlieb J: Episodes of illness and medical service in a geographically isolated mine village in Greenland, *Arctic Med Res* 49(3):128, 1990.
49. Gunderson E: Psychological studies in Antarctica. In Gunderson E, editor: *Human adaptability to Antarctic conditions,* Washington, DC, 1974, American Geophysical Union.
50. Gunderson E, Palinkas L: *Review of psychological studies in the US Antarctic Program,* 1988, US Naval Health Research Center.
51. Hackney A, Hodgdon J: Thyroid hormone changes during military field operations: effects of cold exposure in the Arctic, *Aviat Space Environ Med* 63(7):606, 1992.
52. Haehnle R: Designing a new science facility for McMurdo Station, *Antarctic J US* 23(4):4, 1988.
53. Hall S: *The fourth world: the heritage of the Arctic and its destruction,* New York, 1988, Vintage Books.
54. Hamzah B, editor: *Antarctica in international affairs,* Kuala Lumpur, Malaysia, 1987, Institute of Strategic and International Studies.
55. Hansen V, Jacobsen B, Husby R: Mental distress during winter: an epidemiologic study of 7759 adults north of the Arctic Circle, *Acta Psychiatr Scand* 84(2):137, 1991.
56. Harrison A, Clearwater Y, McKay C: The human experience in Antarctica: applications to life in space, *Behav Sci* 34(4):253, 1989.
57. Hart P: Growth of Antarctic tourism, *Oceanus* 31(2):93, 1988.
58. Hemmings A, Hay J, Towle S: Environmental science: coming of age in Antarctica. In Hay J, Hemmings A, Thom N, editors: *Antarctica 150: scientific perspectives, policy futures,* Auckland, NZ, 1990, University of Auckland.
59. Herr R: The climb physician: an endangered species? (editorial), *J Wilderness Med* 1(3):144, 1990.
60. Herr R, Hall H, Haward M, editors: *Antarctica's future: continuity or change?* Hobart, Tasmania, 1990, Australian Institute of International Affairs.
61. Hibben S, editor: *Antarctic bibliography,* Superintendent of Documents No LC33.9, Washington, DC, 1992, Library of Congress.
62. Holmer I: Protective clothing against cold: performance standards as method for preventive measures, *Arctic Med Res* 51(suppl 7):94, 1992.
63. Holmer I, Gavhed D: Resultant clothing insulation during exercise in the cold, *Arctic Med Res* 50(suppl 6):94, 1991.
64. Houseal M: *Medical department of 1991 end-of-season report,* 1991, US Antarctic Program.
65. Houseal M: Lyme disease in the Antarctic, *N Engl J Med* 326(5):351, 1992.
66. Hubbs K: Antarctic Development Squadron Six (VXE 6) and its role in the test/evaluation of extreme cold weather clothing and equipment. In *US Navy Symposium on Arctic/Cold Weather Operations of Surface Ships,* Washington, DC, 1989, Department of the Navy.
67. Hughes E: Medical problems in the Antarctic, *Med J Aust* 143(3):95, 1985.
68. Illingworth F: *North of the Circle,* New York, 1951, Philosophical Library.
69. International Society of Travel Medicine: *2nd Conference on International Travel Medicine,* Atlanta, 1991.
70. Jacobs M, Richardson JI, editors: *Arctic life: challenge to survive,* Pittsburgh, 1983, Carnegie Institute.
71. Johnson D, Gamble W: Trauma in the Arctic: an incident report, *J Trauma* 31(10):1340, 1991.
72. Johnson M, Moore M, Kennedy R: Injuries in the Alaskan Arctic, *Arctic Med Res* 51(suppl 7):45, 1992.
73. Johnson R, Kingsley T: Antarctic research and lunar exploration: useful parallels. In *Space 88,* Albuquerque, 1988, American Society of Civil Engineers.
74. Kanas N: Psychological, psychiatric, and interpersonal aspects of long-duration space missions, *J Spacecraft Rockets* 27(5):457, 1990.
75. Kennaway D, Dorp CV: Free-running rhythms of melatonin, cortisol, elecrolytes and sleep in humans in Antarctica, *Am J Physiol* 260(6):R1137, 1991.
76. Kerr R: Ozone hole: not over the Arctic—for now (news), *Science* 256(5058):734, 1992.
77. Kimball L: *Southern exposure: deciding Antarctica's future,* Washington, DC, 1990, World Resources Institute.
78. Klen T: Accidents in the Arctic: a psychological point of view, *Arctic Med Res* 51(suppl 7):71, 1992.
79. Krikler S: *Staphylococcus aureus* in Antarctica: carriage and attempted eradication, *J Hyg* 97(3):427, 1986.
80. LaBarre R: *Palmer end-of-season report,* 1992, US Antarctic Program.
81. Lansing A: *Endurance: Shackleton's incredible voyage,* New York, 1986, Carroll & Graf.
82. Leigh J: Estimates of the probability of job-related death in 347 occupations, *J Occup Med* 29:510, 1987.
83. Lemonick M: Antarctica, *Time,* Jan 15, 1990.

84. Lewy A, Sack R: Light therapy and psychiatry, *Proc Soc Exp Biol Med* 183:11, 1986.
85. Lieberman H et al: Possible behavioral consequences of light-induced changes in melatonin availability, *Ann NY Acad Sci* 453:242, 1985.
86. Logan H: Tourism and other activities. In Hay J, Hemmings A, Thom N, editors: *Antarctica 150: scientific perspectives, policy futures,* Auckland, NZ, 1990, University of Auckland.
87. Lopéz B: *Arctic dreams: imagination and desire in a northern landscape,* New York, 1986, Scribner.
88. Lugg D: Antarctic epidemiology: a survey of ANARE stations 1947-72. In Edholm O, Gunderson E, editors: *Polar human biology,* London, 1973, Heinemann.
89. Lugg D, Gormely P, King H: Accidents on Australian Antarctic expeditions, *Polar Rec* 23(147):720, 1987.
90. Luoma P et al: Blood mercury and serum selenium concentration in reindeer herders in the Arctic area of northern Finland, *Arch Toxicol* 15(suppl):172, 1992.
91. MacLean J et al: Epidemiologic and serologic definition of primary and secondary trichinosis in the Arctic, *J Infect Dis* 165(5):908, 1992.
92. MacLean J et al: Trichinosis in the Canadian Arctic: report of five outbreaks and a new clinical syndrome, *J Infect Dis* 160(3):513, 1989.
93. Marshall C, Rossman G: *Designing qualitative research,* Newbury Park, Calif, 1989, Sage Publications.
94. McDonald J et al: An outbreak of toxoplasmosis in pregnant women in northern Quebec, *J Infect Dis* 161(4):769, 1990.
95. Mear R, Swan R: *A walk to the Pole: to the heart of Antarctica in the footsteps of Scott,* New York, 1987, Crown Publishers.
96. Meyer-Rochow V: Observations on an accidental case of raw sewage pollution in Antarctica, *Zentralb Hyg Umweltmed* 192(6):554, 1992.
97. Midwinter M, Arendt J: Adaptation of the melatonin rhythm in human subjects following night-shift work in Antarctica, *Neurosci Lett* 122(2):195, 1991.
98. Millar W: Smokeless tobacco use by youth in the Canadian Arctic, *Arctic Med Res* 49(suppl 2):39, 1990.
99. Millar W: Smoking prevalence in the Canadian Arctic, *Arctic Med Res* 49(suppl 2):23, 1990.
100. Modzelewski M: At the top of Europe, *New York Times,* Aug 29, 1993.
101. Moody J: *Arctic doctor,* New York, 1955, Dodd, Mead.
102. Murphy J: *South to the Pole by ski,* St Paul, Minn, 1990, Marlor Press.
103. Myhre U, Goode P, Miller I: Jogger's phimosis, *Br J Urol* 63(5):549, 1989.
104. Natani K et al: Long-term changes in sleep patterns in men on the South Polar plateau, *Arch Intern Med* 125:655, 1970.
105. National Aeronautics and Space Administration: *The human experience in Antarctica: applications to life in space,* Sunnyvale, Calif, 1987, National Aeronautics and Space Administration.
106. National Science Foundation: *US Antarctic Program final environmental impact statement,* Washington, DC, 1980, The Foundation.
107. National Science Foundation: *Survival in Antarctica,* Washington, DC, 1984, The Foundation.
108. National Science Foundation: *Antarctic J US* 24(2), 1989.
109. National Science Foundation: *Antarctic research: program announcement and proposal guide,* Washington, DC, 1993, The Foundation.
110. Nicholas J: Small groups in orbit: group interaction and crew performance on space station, *Aviat Space Environ Med* 58(10):1009, 1987.
111. Nicholas J, Foushee H: Organization, selection, and training of crews for extended spaceflight: findings from analogs and implications, *J Spacecraft Rockets* 27(5):451, 1990.
112. Norman J: Medical care and human biological research in the British Antarctic Survey Medical Unit, *Arctic Med Res* 48(3):103, 1989.
113. Norman J, Brebner J: Remote health: occupational health care in the Antarctic, *Occup Health (Lond)* 40:602, 1988.
114. Osgood S, Haehnle R: *Environment one: a master plan study for a new scientific research station at the geographic South Pole.* In International Cold Regions Engineering Specialty Conference, 6th (Feb 26-28), 1991, West Lebanon, NH, American Society of Civil Engineers.
115. Oxidation strongly linked to aging but quenched by ubiquitous hormone, *Science News* 144(7):109, 1993.
116. Palinkas L: Health and performance of Antarctic winter-over personnel: a follow-up study, *Aviat Space Environ Med* 57(10):954, 1986.
117. Palinkas L: Sociocultural influences on psychosocial adjustment in Antarctica, *Med Anthropol* 10(4):235, 1989.
118. Palinkas L: Going to extremes: the cultural context of stress, illness and coping in Antarctica, *Soc Sci Med* 35(5):651, 1992.
119. Palinkas L, Gunderson E, Burr, R: *Psychophysiological correlates of human adaptation in Antarctica.* In International Symposium on Antarctic Research, Tianjin, China, 1989, Ocean Press.
120. Parfit M: *South light: a journey to the last continent,* New York, 1985, Macmillan.
121. Parkinson A, Muchmore H, Scott E: Rhinovirus respiratory tract infections during isolation at South Pole Station, *Antarctic J US* 19(5):186, 1984.
122. Poorter MD, Schmidt S: Greenpeace environmental and scientific programme in Antarctica. In Hay J, Hemmings A, Thom N, editors: *Antarctica 150: scientific perspectives, policy futures,* Auckland, NZ, 1990, University of Auckland.
123. Porter E: *Antarctica,* New York, 1978, EP Dutton.
124. Prestrud P, Krogsrud J, Gjertz I: The occurrence of rabies in the Svalbard Islands of Norway, *J Wildl Dis* 28(1):57, 1992.
125. Priddy R: "Acute abdomen" in Antarctica, *Med J Aust* 143(3):108, 1985.
126. Pyne S: *The ice,* Iowa City, 1986, University of Iowa Press.
127. Reed H et al: Decreased free fraction of thyroid hormones after prolonged Antarctic residence, *J Appl Physiol* 69(4):1467, 1990.
128. Reed H et al: Changes in serum triiodothyronine (T_3) kinetics after prolonged Antarctic residence: the polar T_3 syndrome, *J Clin Endocrinol Metab* 70(4):965, 1990.
129. Rivolier J et al, editors: *Man in the Antarctic,* London, 1988, Taylor & Francis.
130. Rodahl K: Working in the cold, *Arctic Med Res* 50(suppl 6):80, 1991.
131. Rosenthal N et al: Antidepressant effects of light in seasonal affective disorder, *Am J Psychiatry* 142(2):163, 1985.
132. Rosenthal N et al: Seasonal affective disorder, *Arch Gen Psychiatry* 41:72, 1984.
133. Rothblum E: Psychological factors in the Antarctic (review), *J Psychol* 124(3):253, 1990.
134. Schneider C: Funding research in Antarctica: a look at NSF support to scientists, *Antarctic J US* 25(2):1990.
135. Schnitzer P, Bender T: Surveillance of traumatic occupational fatalities in Alaska: implications for prevention, *Public Health Rep* 107:70, 1992.
136. Schuurman H: *Canada's eastern neighbor: a view on change in Greenland,* Ottawa, Ontario, 1976, Ministry of Indian and Northern Affairs.
137. Schweickart R et al: *Safety in Antarctica,* Washington, DC, 1988, National Science Foundation.
138. Shen B: Report to Antarctic safety committee. In Schweickart R et al, editors: *Safety in Antarctica,* Washington, DC, 1988, National Science Foundation.
139. Shen B: Risks of travel in small aircraft: is commuter flying too dangerous? *Travel Med Advisor* 3(3):14, 1993.
140. Shephard R: Some consequences of polar stress: data from a transpolar ski-trek, *Arctic Med Res* 50(1):25, 1991.
141. Shephard R: Fat metabolism, exercise and the cold (review), *Can J Sport Sci* 17(2):83, 1992.

142. Shult P et al: Adenovirus 21 infection in an isolated Antarctic station: transmission of the virus and susceptibility of the population, *Am J Epidemiol* 133(6):599, 1991.
143. Shurley J: Physiological research at US stations in Antarctica. In Gunderson E, editor: *Human adaptability to Antarctic conditions,* Washington, DC, 1974, American Geophysical Union.
144. Shurley J et al: Sleep and activity patterns at South Pole Station, *Arch Gen Psychiatry* 22:385, 1970.
145. Simpson-Housley P: *Antarctica: exploration, perception and metaphor,* London, 1992, Routledge.
146. Skinhoj P: Epidemiology of viral hepatitis in circumpolar populations, *Arctic Med Res* 50(4):177, 1991.
147. Smith D: Stargazing at the South Pole, *New Scientist* 130(1774):33, 1991.
148. Sommer R: *Personal space: the behavioral basis of design,* Englewood Cliffs, NJ, 1969, Prentice-Hall.
149. Strivastava K, Kumar R: Human nutrition in cold and high terrestrial altitudes, *Int J Biometeorol* 36:10, 1992.
150. Stix G: Run silent, run (not so) cheap, *Sci Am* 269(4):26, 1993.
151. Stonehouse B: *North Pole, South Pole: a guide to the ecology and resources of the Arctic and Antarctic,* London, 1990, ION.
152. Strange R, Youngman S: Emotional aspects of wintering over, *Antarctic J US* 6:255, 1971.
153. Stroud M: Nutrition and energy balance on the "footsteps of Scott" expedition 1984-86, *Human Nutr Appl Nutr* 41A(6):426, 1987.
154. Stuster J: *Space station habitability recommendations based on a systematic comparative analysis of analogous conditions,* Mountain View, Calif, 1986, National Aeronautics and Space Administration.
155. Suedfeld R, Bernaldez J, Stossel D: The Plar Psychology Project (PPP): a cross-national investigation of polar adaptation, *Arctic Med Res* 48(2):91, 1989.
156. Sugden D: *Arctic and Antarctic,* Totowa, NJ, 1982, Barnes & Noble.
157. *Symposium on Medical Problems in Sparsely Populated Areas,* Oulu, Finland, 1978, Nordic Council for Arctic Medical Research.
158. Take a risk, pay the price, *New York Times,* Sept 19, 1993.
159. Taylor A: Professional isolates in New Zealand's Antarctic research programme, *Int Rev Appl Psychol* 18:135, 1969.
160. Taylor A: *Antarctic psychology,* Wellington, 1987, DSIR Science Information Publishing Centre.
161. Taylor A: *Collection and transmission of behavioural data by computer and satellite.* In International Symposium on Antarctic Research, Tianjin, China, 1989, Ocean Press.
162. Taylor M: Cold weather injuries during peacetime military training, *Milit Med* 157(11):602, 1992.
163. Thomas D et al: Arctic terrestrial ecosystem contamination (review), *Sci Total Environ* 122(1-2):135, 1992.
164. Thorington L: Spectral, irradiance, and temporal aspects of natural and artificial light, *Ann NY Acad Sci* 453:28, 1985.
165. Tkachev A, Ramenskaya E, Bojko J: Dynamics of hormone and metabolic state in polar inhabitants depend on daylight duration, *Arctic Med Res* 50(suppl 6):152, 1991.
166. Tzabar Y, Pennington T: The population structure and transmission of *Escherichia coli* in an isolated human community: studies on an Antarctic base, *Epidemiol Infect* 107(3):537, 1991.
167. Vayrynen S: Ergonomic design of machinery for use in the cold: a review based on the literature and original research, *Arctic Med Res* 51(suppl 7):87, 1992.
168. Vuori H: WHO and Nordic council for Arctic medical research: partners in health (editorial), *Arctic Med Res* 50(2):54, 1991.
169. Wace N: Antarctica: a new tourist destination, *Appl Geography* 10(4):327, 1990.
170. Walton D, editor: *Antarctic science,* Cambridge, 1987, Cambridge University Press.
171. Was the ill-fated Franklin expedition a victim of lead poisoning? *Nutr Rev* 47(10):322, 1989.
172. Watts A: *International law and the antarctic treaty system,* Hersch Lauterpacht Memorial Lectures, vol 11, Cambridge, 1992, Grotius Publications.
173. Weybrew B: Three decades of nuclear submarine research. In *The human experience in Antarctica: applications to life in space,* Sunnyvale, Calif, 1987, National Aeronautics and Space Administration.
174. Wharton R et al: *Use of analogs to support the Space Exploration Initiative,* Washington, DC, 1990, National Aeronautics and Space Administration and National Science Foundation.
175. Wiant C et al: Work-related aviation fatalities in Colorado 1982-1987, *Aviat Space Environ Med* 62:827, 1991.
176. Williams D: *Health, hormonal and stress-related studies on ANARE,* 1989, Hobart, Australia, Australian National Antarctic Research Expeditions.
177. Wilton P: "TB voyages" into high Arctic gave MDs a look at a culture in transition, *Can Med Assoc J* 148(9):1608, 1993.
178. Wisbory T, Husby P, Engedal H: Anesthesiologist-manned helicopters and regionalized extracorporeal circulation facilities: a unique chance in deep hypothermia, *Arctic Med Res* 50(suppl 6):108, 1991.
179. World Health Organization: *Health problems of local and migrant populations in Arctic regions,* 1979, The Organization.
180. World Health Organization: *Selection of personnel to work in circumpolar regions,* 1985, The Organization.
181. Xue Q et al: Changes in cardiac and respiratory function of Antarctic research expedition members, *Proc Chin Acad Med Sci* 4(2):112, 1989.
182. Yerevanian B et al: Effects of bright incandescent light on seasonal and nonseasonal major depressive disorder, *Psychiatry Res* 18:355, 1986.
183. Young L et al: Psychiatric consultation in the eastern Canadian Arctic. II. Referral patterns, diagnoses and treatment, *Can J Psychiatry* 38(1):28, 1993.
184. Young O: *Arctic in world affairs,* Seattle, 1989, University of Washington.
185. Young T et al: Prevalence of diagnosed diabetes in circumpolar indigenous populations, *Int J Epidemiol* 21(4):730, 1992.

8 HEAT-RELATED ILLNESSES

Roger W. Hubbard
Stephen L. Gaffin
Deborah L. Squire

Since the publication of the second edition of this text in 1989, rapid developments within the fields of immunology, molecular biology, and systemic and cell physiology have broadened the understanding of heat-related illnesses. A brief outline of a few advances that are opening new avenues of investigation serve as introduction to a more detailed discussion.

Systemic mechanisms underlying heatstroke based on recent studies of organ blood flow[181] and hemodynamics in heatstroke[231] are presented. New explanations of the causes and consequences of voluntary dehydration[211] are explored along with the expected impact of water and salt depletion on normal physiology and exercise performance.

The demonstration that strenuous exercise can produce systemic endotoxemia[51,61] and that endotoxins and the cytokine cascade have been implicated in acute heatstroke[55] and in other stressors such as fear and even depressed mood[236] may open new avenues of diagnosis and treatment. Thus we present an update to the classic systemic approach to understanding the physiologic dysfunction in heatstroke and, where possible, relate it to emerging shock models involving bacterial toxins and cytokines, such as tumor necrosis factor.

The views, opinions, and findings in this report are those of the authors and should not be construed as an official Department of the Army position, policy, or decision, unless so designated by other official documentation. Citations of commercial organizations and trade names in this report do not constitute an official Department of the Army endorsement or approval of the products or services of these organizations. We have adhered to the use of units and definitions described in *Aviation, Space and Environmental Medicine*[230] and the *Journal of Applied Physiology*.[46]

Overview of Heat Illness

It is convenient to classify the more familiar heat disorders such as heat syncope, heat exhaustion (including that induced by exertion, and water or salt depletion), heat cramps, and classic and exertional heatstroke into separate, well-defined categories. Even so, the symptoms often overlap. It is against this background of imperfect parity between the pure or ideal forms and the mixed bag reality that heat illnesses are discussed.

CLASSIC HEATSTROKE

Classic heatstroke occurs when environmental heat stress is maximal.[127,187,396] Populations at risk include the elderly, the poor (who lack adequate air conditioning), those who suffer from malnutrition, and those who have chronic diseases or substance addiction.[187] Because physical effort is *not* a primary determinant of excessive heat storage as it is of exertion-induced heatstroke, the onset of classic heatstroke is often slower. Predisposing factors commonly intervene over days rather than minutes or hours. As a result, there is often ample time for fluid and electrolyte imbalances to occur.

Under some circumstances passive hyperthermia can develop rapidly in extremely hot environments, such as when infants and small children are left in locked vehicles in the summer heat. This is also true for adults who are passengers in improperly ventilated or non-air-conditioned vehicles. For example, cabins and cargo spaces of military vehicles can reach 54° to 60° C within minutes under desert conditions, depending on environmental temperature and solar radiation.[207] Similar temperatures may occur in closed or confined spaces, such as enclosed attics, or in places, such as boiler rooms, where there is a high radiant load from machinery or power plants.[254] Individuals who depend on others for fluid intake because of age (the very young or the elderly) or illness are at risk of involuntary dehydration. Infants are more heat labile because of their immature thermoregulatory systems.[364] (See later discussion of thermoregulation in children.)

BOX 8-1

COMMONLY HELD FALLACIES REGARDING HEAT ILLNESS*

1. The sine qua non for diagnosis of heatstroke includes hot dry skin, temperature greater than 42° C, and coma.
2. Unlimited access to fluids allows the exercising individual to maintain adequate hydration despite heat stress.
3. Development of salt depletion–heat exhaustion requires 4 to 5 days of exposure to marked heat stress.
4. Consumption of commercially available electrolyte-containing beverages during exercise in the heat tends to return plasma potassium levels to resting values.
5. The primary underlying mechanisms for the development of heat cramps are hypokalemia and hypovolemia.
6. Consumption of excessive volumes of fluid to the point of development of nausea promotes the maximal clearance of free water by the kidneys.
7. When the patient is evaluated in the emergency department, a normal body temperature when combined with normal serum transaminases precludes the diagnosis of heatstroke.
8. The most physiologically appropriate method to achieve rapid reduction in body temperature from hyperthermia is the use of the warm air spray.
9. The risk of dilutional hyponatremia should preclude consumption of fluids in the absence of thirst.
10. Endotoxemia is a rare complication of ultramarathon running in the heat.
11. Review of the medical literature reveals that an individual sustaining a single episode of heatstroke remains at increased risk for future heat injury.
12. A high degree of aerobic conditioning, when combined with an appropriate period of heat acclimation, prevents the development of heat illness.
13. Adherence to published guidelines using wet bulb globe temperature to modify physical activity in the heat prevents the development of heat illness.
14. Carpopedal spasm is a relatively rare complication of exercise-induced heat exhaustion.
15. Violent shivering is a common complication in response to whole body cooling of patients with heat exhaustion.

*These fallacies are discussed in greater detail later in the chapter.

Heat Waves

When environmental heat stress is maximal, strenuous exercise is not required to produce heat illness.[127,174,187,396] Civilian populations are at increased risk for heat illness during heat waves. In Peking in 1743 a heat wave reportedly caused 11,000 deaths[379]; 411 cases of severe heatstroke in Nanjing were recently reported.[283] In a report by Ferris and colleagues,[138] 42 of 44 cases occurred within 8 consecutive days during which the maximum ambient temperature varied from 38.9° to 41.1° C (102° to 106° F). Temperatures within the patient's actual environment were probably much higher; this report predates the widespread availability of air conditioning. Only 7 of 44 persons were less than 50 years of age, and the greatest frequency of age distribution was in the range of 60 to 70 years.

Ellis[131,132] analyzed the General Mortality Tables of the Vital Statistics Reports of the United States for the period 1952-1967, during which there were five heat wave years (1952-1955 and 1966). During heat wave years the recorded average number of heatstroke or heat exhaustion deaths jumped from 179 to 820 deaths per year. The number of deaths classified as heat precipitated was more than 8000 during heat wave years.

The preceding figures suggest a reluctance to certify heatstroke or heat exhaustion as a cause of death or an underestimation in coding. Lack of recognition or too rigid reliance on the classic definitions of heatstroke can lead to underdiagnosis.[379] Thus epidemiologic estimates of the true incidence are probably conservative.

Host Factors

Hyperthermia commonly occurs in the presence of numerous and varied "host factors."[29,207] These include many that affect thermoregulation through heat loss mechanisms (for example, lack of acclimatization, fatigue, lack of sleep, dehydration, skin disorders), while others contribute to heat production (for example, obesity, lack of physical fitness, dehydration, febrile illness, sustained exercise).

Imbalances in fluids and electrolytes are common during hot spells, especially when salt losses in sweat are compounded by loss of appetite. Fluid and electrolyte losses resulting from illness (diarrhea or vomiting) often contribute to heat illness. In some cases dehydration is the primary cause of death.[379]

Combinations of factors that create a threat may be subtle. The presence of air conditioning in the home, workplace, and transportation may decrease the risk for the development of classic heatstroke. However, by diminishing the state of heat acclimatization and respect for the environment, air conditioning may increase a person's risk for developing exertional heatstroke. Intense and prolonged exposure during weekends and holidays accounts for many cases of sunburn and heat illness.

Although heatstroke may be due to accident, lack of knowledge, poor judgment, or neglect, it is a preventable illness. Therefore cases of fatal heatstroke should be investigated for criminal intent. In a most unusual incident an herbalist was convicted of manslaughter in Australia[289] because after he "treated" a young boy by "immersion in a heap of fermenting horse manure for forty minutes," the boy died of heatstroke. Educational efforts by both the media and the health care community aimed at parents of small children during heat waves should be made with the same enthusiasm as public service announcements of windchill factors during subzero temperatures. Coaches, organizers of races, and others responsible for the supervision or administration of sporting events or other activities in hot weather under conditions outside of heat stress guidelines should be held legally responsible for heat injuries among the participants. The military has long recognized the preventable nature of heat injuries that result from the intense physical activity in hot weather: "Commanding Officers of volunteers are very apt to err in this particular; and the spirit of their men is such that they shrink from complaint and persevere in efforts which may easily, under a burning sun, become dangerous to life."—*Lancet* (June 10, 1865).

EXERTIONAL HEATSTROKE

Exertional heatstroke often affects fit and highly motivated individuals participating in sporting events or undergoing performance tests such as those for firefighter and police candidates. With increased numbers of individuals participating in sports,[187,249,250] fitness activities such as jogging,[183] fun-running,[212,310,340,401] bicycling,[379] and long-distance sporting events,[443] the emergency physician can expect to see more exertional heat illness.[186] For example, an estimated 25 million Americans and 1 million Canadians participate in organized road races annually.[187] Furthermore, heat illnesses occur during such activities as participation in the Hadj[55] or in warfare during summer heat.[67]

During the period 1942-1944 there were at least 198 deaths from heat illness during military training in the United States.[362] Gardener and colleagues[155a] recently studied exertional heat illnesses in Marine recruits at Parris Island. The frequency of reported cases closely correlated with daily heat load (a combination of wet and dry bulb temperatures plus radiation) but did not correlate well with local dry bulb temperature. Most cases occurred between 7 and 9 AM, during training that would have been restricted at elevated heat loads later in the day. However, a fascinating observation was made that the frequency of heat illness depended on the temperature of the *previous day*. Regardless of the current temperature, if the day before was cool, the frequency of heat cases was low; if it was hot, the frequency was high. Gardener and associates thought that this could not have been related to an accumulated dehydration from the day before, since the recruits were forced to drink large amounts of water, enough to keep them urinating during the night. The presence of a high environmental temperature caused an unspecified physiologic *predisposition to heatstroke lasting for at least a day*.

Therefore even following widely published guidelines (based on wet bulb globe temperature, or WBGT) for physical activity does not preclude risks. Perhaps a better index should be developed. High rates of metabolic heat production (such as that produced when running) combined with conditions that limit evaporative heat loss (for example, high relative humidity, impermeable garments) appear to present a significant risk regardless of dry bulb temperature. Furthermore, prevention is complicated by the observation that conditions on the prior day contribute to the risk of heatstroke.

Heat Storage Rate

The increase in an individual's heat storage, as shown by a rise in core temperature (T_c), may be rapid (minutes to hours) and metabolic in origin because of overloaded heat loss mechanisms. For brief periods of intense effort, heat production may exceed 1000 kcal/hr.[327] For example, we previously reported[16] that an Olympic marathoner produced metabolic heat in excess of 1400 kcal/hr. Under conditions that limit heat dissipation, such as high humidity or the wearing of impermeable clothing, this rate of heat storage would approximate 0.5° C/min and produce heatstroke elevations in core temperature within 10 to 12 minutes. Even under a moderate workload (300 kcal/hr), a person who cannot sweat effectively and thereby dissipate heat can experience a rise in T_c of 5° C (9° F)/hr.[304,327]

Others at increased risk of heat illness because of occupation include miners,[442] heavy industry workers,[117,122] and individuals in the military.[67,279,280,293] The yearly pilgrimage to Mecca may result in hundreds of fatalities from heat illness.[238] Wearing impermeable garments during physical activity leads to rapid loss of sweat, overload of heat loss mechanisms, and hyperthermia. These events may occur voluntarily (dieters, wrestlers) or by occupation (firefighters, hazardous waste handlers). Some cases of exertional heatstroke have a genetic component.[324]

Failed thermoregulation can have its origin in the dysfunction of either central (hypothalamic) control or peripheral responses of heat loss mechanisms (sweating and vasodilation). A variety of drugs and toxins can produce hyperthermia and are implicated in some cases of severe heat illness.

Heat Stress and Thermoregulation

MECHANISMS OF HEAT TRANSFER

The human body obeys the laws of thermodynamics, as heat is transferred from a higher to a lower temperature.[134] The heat balance equation is derived from this law. Santee and Gonzalez[355] and Gonzalez[172] provide excellent discourse on characteristics of the thermal environment, the biophysics of heat transfer, the heat balance equation, and clothing considerations. When environmental temperature is higher than skin temperature, the body gains heat; when it is lower, the body loses heat. As a result, elevated environmental temperature adds to the heat burden of the body and interferes with heat dissipation. There are four mechanisms of heat transfer: conduction, convection, radiation, and evaporation. The environmental parameters that determine the potential for heat exchange constitute the thermal environment, which has been defined by Tracey and Christian[410] as "a biophysical aggregate of air temperature, wind speed, relative humidity, and radiation."

Conduction

Conduction is heat exchange between two surfaces in direct contact. It is generally the least important in quantitative terms, since behavioral thermoregulation generally intervenes (for example, we usually wear insulated boots while walking through snow). However, lying uninsulated while sleeping on either hot or cold ground can result in significant heat exchange, especially in a person under the influence of vasodilating drugs or alcohol. A person can usually hold a very hot cooking pot in a dry towel (containing a large number of tiny cells filled with air) without discomfort. However, if the towel is wet (the cells are filled with water), it rapidly heats up because of the much better conduction of heat through water than through air. Within a few seconds the pot becomes too hot to hold.

Convection

Convective heat exchange refers to heat transferred from a surface to a gas or fluid, usually air or water. It is a more complex process than conduction because the medium of heat transfer (air or water) is usually moving. The rate of heat exchange by convection depends on many variables, including the density of the fluid (for example, water versus the humidity of air), the temperature gradient, the surface area exposed, and the movement or flow rate of the fluid. Heat loss during cold water immersion is rapid because of the high thermal capacity of water, greater body surface exposed, and greater thermal conductivity of water (32 times that of air).[333,338] Convective heat exchange varies with the velocity of air movement. As ambient temperature (T_{amb}) approaches skin temperature (T_{sk}), the amount of heat loss becomes minimal. Once air temperature exceeds mean skin temperature, heat is gained by the body. Loose-fitting clothing maximizes convective and evaporative heat loss. By the same token, body motion alters heat exchange by convection both within and on the surface of clothing.

Radiation

Radiation refers to the transfer of heat between the body and its surroundings by electromagnetic waves. All matter absorbs and emits thermal radiation,[391] which is the "radiant energy emitted by a medium that is due solely to the temperature of the medium." Clothing reduces the radiant heat impinging on the skin from industrial sources (such as boilers and motors), as well as the solar load in broad daylight. Solar load is a major source of heat gain in hot climates—up to 250 kcal/hr in a seminude man[165] (approximately the same as walking; see later discussion) and 100 kcal/hr in a clothed man. The amount varies with the angle of the sun, season, clouds, and other factors. Concurrently, clothing affects the evaporative process.

Highly pigmented skin is protected from ultraviolet radiation, but it absorbs approximately 20% more heat than does nonpigmented or relatively nonpigmented skin.[233] Heat loss from the skin[190,349] by convection and radiation is maximized by increased skin blood flow (SkBF; at $T_{sk} > T_{amb}$). Although heat is carried by convection and conduction from the body core to the skin, the main role of elevated SkBF in a warm environment is to deliver the heat necessary to vaporize sweat.[167]

Evaporative Cooling

Evaporative, "wet," or insensible heat exchange is usually a one-way heat flow from a body surface to the environment. The heat exchange is insensible because the heat of vaporization (2.45 joules/kg) is "absorbed" without changing the measured temperature of the water as conversion from a liquid to a gaseous state occurs.

If the body is unable to maintain thermal equilibrium by radiation, convection, and conduction and core temperature rises, sweating must occur to permit heat loss by vaporization of water.[167] Evaporative heat loss is accompanied by the loss of 580 kcal/L of water evaporated or heat loss of approximately 1 kcal/1.7 ml of sweat evaporated (vaporized).

Since rates of gastric emptying can exceed 1 L/hr, a 1 L/hr sweat rate appears sustainable without significant dehydration if fluid is consumed. Higher sweat rates could theoretically achieve greater rates of heat loss (1500 ml/1.7 ml/kcal = 882 kcal) but are almost never achieved because of dripping sweat. Moreover, these high sweat rates are often at the expense of total body water, since drinking does not keep pace. Knochel[249] has estimated a more reasonable figure for an upper limit of heat dissipation as approximately 650 kcal/hr.

Certain parts of the body surface are more important than others in providing cooling through sweating. The scalp, face, and upper torso are most important. Only about 25% of total sweat is produced by the lower limbs.[427] Therefore, while wearing a shirt may be critical in the development of heat illness, wearing long or short pants is much less important. On the other hand, wearing protective head gear may be most important in the development of heat illness, as shown by a training exercise. In persons not wearing hats, the exercise was merely grueling, but of those with hats 33% suffered heat illness casualties,[195] as cited in Porter.[332]

The maximum rate of sweat vaporization depends on air dryness and movement. In a hot climate the limit to heat dissipation is a function of sweat rate and the "atmospheric cooling power" or maximal evaporative cooling capacity of the environment.[168,362] The environment's capacity to vaporize sweat varies primarily with humidity and also with wind velocity. As humidity approaches 100%, evaporative heat loss is minimized. The major effect of wind occurs in humid environments at a velocity between 0.5 and 5 m/sec.[134] Sweat that drips from the body provides no cooling, and sweat evaporated from clothing is considerably less efficient than sweat evaporated directly from skin.[134] Risk of hyperthermia increases with air temperature and humidity. As a result, military trainers and coaches tend to conduct early morning runs to avoid high ambient temperatures (elevated WBGT), and there has been an increased incidence of heat illness, despite the lower dry bulb temperatures, in humid climates. Sutton[400] pointed out that exertional heatstroke is reported more and more frequently during "fun runs" and marathons when the temperature is not particularly hot. This reinforces the simple definition that exertion-induced heatstroke occurs whenever the rate of heat production of an exercising individual exceeds the rate of heat loss, causing body temperature to rise to critical levels.

TEMPERATURE REGULATION

To prevent or appropriately manage heat illness, the clinician must understand thermal stress[147] and human thermoregulation.[167,185,398] Temperature regulation refers to both autonomic and behavioral thermoregulatory processes that modify the rates of heat production and heat loss by sweating, shivering, and variations in basal metabolism and peripheral vasomotor tone.[167] These processes act to maintain the temperature of the body within a restricted range under conditions of a variable internal or external heat load. The regulated temperature is generally considered that of the "body core," or T_c.

Behavioral Thermoregulation

To live, work, and reproduce successfully in arid or tropical climates, humans depend not only on physiologic mechanisms to acclimatize to heat but also on behavioral responses to assist temperature regulation. Thus they possess two control systems (behavioral and physiologic) to regulate body temperature.

Although behavioral responses augmenting shivering seem obvious in a cold environment (for example, seeking shelter, wearing clothes, and building fires), behavioral factors for thermoregulation in the heat (resting in the heat of the day, seeking shade or water when thirsty) are also important. Since behavioral responses represent conscious actions, sensations of thermal discomfort appear to anticipate actual changes in core temperature.[105]

Furthermore, simply because humanity has described thermoregulatory mechanisms for acclimatizing to heat, the reader should not infer that we originated as tropical animals.[145] As Hardy[185] has suggested, hyperthermia may simply represent a more serious problem than hypothermia so that humans have developed a greater capacity for heat elimination (vasodilation, sweating) than heat conservation (vasoconstriction).

On the other hand, the ability of organisms to tolerate high heat (thermophiles) has long fascinated biologists. It is thought that thermophilic organisms could be more primitive phylogenetically than temperature-sensitive organisms. This is based on the observation that all macromolecules of thermophiles are stable at high temperatures. The presence of thermophiles in many phylogenetic groups suggests a polyphyletic origin and the possibility that the common ancestral organism of all life was a thermophile.[60]

Heat Production

The basal metabolic rate of the average man (70 kg) in a sitting position amounts to approximately 50 to 60 kcal/hr/m^2 of body surface area or 100 kcal/hr.[254] With increased activity, metabolic heat production increases significantly (walking produces 250 to 300 kcal/hr; walking rapidly with a carried load, up to 400 to 450 kcal/hr) and may reach 20 times baseline level with strenuous exertion. Depending on the exercise task, 70% to 100% of the metabolic rate is released as heat, which needs to be dissipated to maintain thermal balance. If there were no means to dissipate heat, the addition of 70 kcal to a 70 kg person would theoretically be able to increase core temperature approximately 0.8° C (1.4° F), assuming the average specific heat of the human body is 0.8 (kcal/kg × °C).

Cellular metabolism increases 13% for each 1° C rise in temperature until the body approaches heatstroke temperature; at that point cellular metabolism may increase more rapidly. It is 50% above normal at 40.6° C.[70] The use of hyperthermia to treat cancer patients suggests that if blood pressure and pH are carefully controlled, temperatures in the 40° to 41° C range will often produce no systemic ill effects while killing cancerous cells.[66]

Body Temperature Ranges

Stolwijk[397] has estimated the range of normal internal temperatures (36° to 38° C) as well as the limits of body temperature for efficient thermoregulation (35° to 40° C). With heat stress or exercise during athletic events, body temperature increases to 40° to 42° C (104° to 107.6° F); this occurrence is well described.[114,304,443] Maron and colleagues[284] describe a marathoner who maintained a core temperature in excess of 41.5° C for at least 44 minutes during a race. Survival limits of body temperatures represent notable deviations from these ranges. For example, one case report[386] documents the survival of a heatstroke victim with a measured core temperature of 46.5° C (115.7° F).

Sensing, Relaying, and Central Integration Functions

Physiologic temperature regulation involves detecting changes in body temperature by sensory mechanisms and relaying thermal signals from central and peripheral locations to a central integrative area. This directs effector organs to increase or decrease heat storage appropriately.[167] These activities are mediated through the autonomic nervous system. Sensitive nerve endings within the hypothalamus and near the skin surface of most of the body act as thermoreceptors[195,306] to monitor core and skin temperature (T_c and T_{sk}).

The primary thermoregulatory responses are vasomotor alterations in blood flow and its distribution, shivering, and sweating. Sweating, skin blood flow, and forearm venous volume each have individual esophageal temperature thresholds that can be lowered by increasing the skin temperature.[360,431,432] An increase in skin temperature at any given core temperature increases the effector response. This type of temperature controller is called the proportional type, in engineering terms.

Mathematical modeling suggests that in the reflex control of skin blood flow, T_c is nine times as important as T_{sk}.[359] The importance of T_{sk} should not be minimized, however, because it varies over a much wider range than does T_c, which enables the system to accommodate to a wide range of environmental temperatures.

During exercise the increase in core temperature elicits an effector response (sweating) with minimal change in T_{sk}. This rise in body temperature is proportional to the increased metabolic rate and does not much depend on environmental temperature over a wide range.[311] However, as anyone who has experienced heat exhaustion knows, this relationship does not hold under extremely hot or humid conditions or conditions of maximum effort. This disparity between theory and common experience gave rise to the concept of prescriptive zone, or set of conditions in which the magnitude of the core temperature response for everyday work was independent of the environmental temperature.[270]

The preoptic area of the anterior hypothalamus of the brain is thought to be a primary site for integration and generation of a "thermal command signal." This area contains many neurons that alter their firing rate in response to warming or cooling.[56] The brain, which is well perfused relative to its mass, responds rapidly to only a few tenths of 1° C change in blood temperature.[39,40]

Although tympanic membrane temperature correlates less well with core temperature than does esophageal temperature, Benziger[39,40] was able to demonstrate that sweating and skin vasodilation increased linearly above a "set point" temperature of approximately 37° C (98.6° F). There is evidence that local heating accelerates sweating. Thus central and peripheral mechanisms cause sweating when skin temperature is elevated. Local heating may result in a greater release of neurotransmitter for a given sudomotor signal,[130] or the heating increases the gland sensitivity to a given dose of neurotransmitter.[321] Conversely, lower skin temperatures may inhibit sweating during exercise.[39] Since sweating is not completely abolished by cervical cord transection, spinal centers for temperature regulation appear to contribute.[408]

Set Point Hypothesis

The concept of the central nervous system as a functional interface between the thermosensors and thermoregulatory effectors that acts as a "central integrative area" is not accepted by all physiologists.[383] However, it provides a rationale for envisioning a thermostat, or "set point," that shifts all effector thresholds in the same direction.[167] This concept of a central thermostat or set point provides a conceptual framework that fits a variety of situations.

Heat-dissipating responses, such as venodilation, increased skin blood flow, and sweating, are the principal mechanisms involved in temperature regulation during exercise in the heat. Dilation of superficial veins increases the efficiency of heat convection from the core to skin and increases the time available for heat transfer between the blood and skin. The cutaneous vasculature is therefore an effector system in thermoregulation, because SkBF controls the rate of heat transfer between the body core and surface.[167,349] Unless the rate of heat storage exceeds the capacity of the thermoregulatory system (for example, a breakdown of thermolytic mechanisms), effector responses will increase until heat balance is restored.

Vasomotor System

The term "vasomotor system" refers only to the arterioles that control organ blood flow, vascular resistance, and arterial blood pressure.[349] Since arterioles and the heart together regulate blood pressure, a change in blood pressure is corrected by changes in vascular resistance or cardiac output.[167,186,349] Vasomotor adjustments optimize and regulate the distribution of cardiac output within and between different organ systems. Central thermal receptors alter vasomotor outflow to redirect blood flow to the skin.

Blood flow to the skin is under dual vasomotor control. In the cold, adrenergic vasoconstrictor fibers reduce skin blood flow.[146] However, during heat exposure, blood flow increases to the hands, lips, nose, and ears as a result of vasodilation, largely because of the withdrawal of vasoconstrictor tone.[146] Active sympathetic vasodilation[44] over most of the skin area[348] reduces vascular resistance below basal tone. Evidence[413] suggests a relationship between active sympathetic vasodilation and sweating, perhaps through the release of vasoactive intestinal polypeptide (VIP). The simultaneous release of both transmitters (VIP and acetylcholine) could help explain the apparent relationship between eccrine sweat secretion and cutaneous vasodilation.[275]

Venomotor System

The venomotor system controls the veins; it should be noted, however, that there is a dual venous drainage of the limbs. This consists of (1) deep veins that drain mainly from the muscles and have relatively poor sympathetic innervation[425] and (2) the richly innervated superficial veins draining the skin. Although venodilation and increased SkBF enhance heat transfer,[170] they act together to increase the amount of blood pooled in compliant peripheral vessels. As a consequence, filling of these veins reduces central blood volume; at some point the redistribution of blood could compromise venous return and cardiac filling.[348,349]

CARDIOVASCULAR STRAIN AND EXERCISE

Severe heat illness involves every system and affects the regulatory (cardiovascular), the integrative (neuroendocrine), and ultimately the basic cellular systems of the body. Probably no greater strain is put on the human body than heavy physical exertion in the heat. This impact of heat stress on the cardiovascular system represents the strain resulting from increased demand for cardiac output to transfer heat and water to the skin for evaporative cooling.

The hemodynamic displacement of blood to the periphery is aggravated by gravitational displacement of blood volume resulting from upright posture. In an upright human being about 70% of the blood volume is below heart level. Venous pooling of blood in the skin and in the great veins below the level of the heart leads to reduced venous return to the heart and consequent reduced cardiac filling.[348] If active skeletal muscle then vasodilates to supply the increased demands for blood flow in support of muscle metabolism, the competing demands for blood flow between vascular beds translate into a major regulatory problem.[349]

The potential conductance of the vasculature (skin 8 L/min^{-1}; viscera 3 L/min^{-1}; and muscle 65 to 70 L/min^{-1}) is enormous and far exceeds the pumping capacity of the normal human heart (about 22 L/min^{-1}).[222,350] Since the combined blood flow requirements of these vascular beds cannot be met, an inherent competition takes place between the mechanisms that maintain blood pressure and those that maintain blood flow to support metabolism and thermoregulation.[208]

The existence of a variety of heat illnesses as a phenomenon suggests five things: (1) the physiologic strain resulting in homeostatic failure produces heat illness; (2) a certain biologic variability is expressed in the response to heat and exercise; (3) hemodynamic stability often takes precedence over thermoregulation; (4) volitional behavior, expressed as exercise performance, is often maintained even as the risk of heat injury increases; and (5) the onset and increase in hyperthermia are not painful.[207]

Not surprisingly the physiologic threat to homeostasis is worsened when accompanied by fluid/electrolyte imbalance.[209,211] Treatment is then directed at the major sources of homeostatic failure: (1) cease the activity; (2) lie down; (3) cool down; and (4) rehydrate. Sometimes the cause of collapse or the other symptoms involved (such as headache, nausea, vomiting, and vertigo) is obvious; sometimes it is not readily appreciated.

Sweating

Although human eccrine sweat glands behave physiologically and pharmacologically as if under parasympathetic or cholinergic control, they also respond to adrenergic stimulation.[358] There are 2 to 3 million sweat glands distributed with decreasing frequency over the palms and soles, head, trunk, and extremities. The average density is about 100 to 200/cm^2; 1 g of sweat glands can secrete up to 250 g of sweat per day. Eccrine sweat is always hypotonic, contains variable concentrations of sodium, and is generally 99.5% water by weight.[134] It is important to remember, however, that a solution of 0.5% sodium chloride contains 5 g of salt per liter, a potential cause of serious salt depletion.

The process of sweat secretion and the sweat rate depend on activation of the sweat center in the hypothalamus, which discharges over the cholinergic fibers of the sympathetic nervous system. Rising blood temperatures increase both the number and the rate of sweat glands responding, until the body reaches a thermal equilibrium or the maximum sweat rate occurs.[167] Dehydration or hyperosmolality leads to reduced sweat rates,[361] with hyperosmolality the more effective (Fig. 8-1).

One of the highest sweat rates ever recorded in a human being was reported by our research group.[16] A world class distance runner produced sweat at 3.71 L/hr (after 19 days of heat acclimation training in Florida) during the 1984 Olympic marathon. Because the maximum rate of gastric emptying is much less than the maximum sweat rate (1.2 versus 3.7 L/hr), rehydration cannot keep pace with sweat losses under those conditions[17] and the athlete faces significant risk of dehydration.[18,19,208] Since rates of gastric emptying can exceed 1 L/hr, as a rule of thumb a 1 L/hr sweat rate appears sustainable without significant dehydration.

FLUID AND ELECTROLYTE IMBALANCE

Dehydration, as a dynamic change from euhydration to hypohydration, reduces or compromises the physiologic

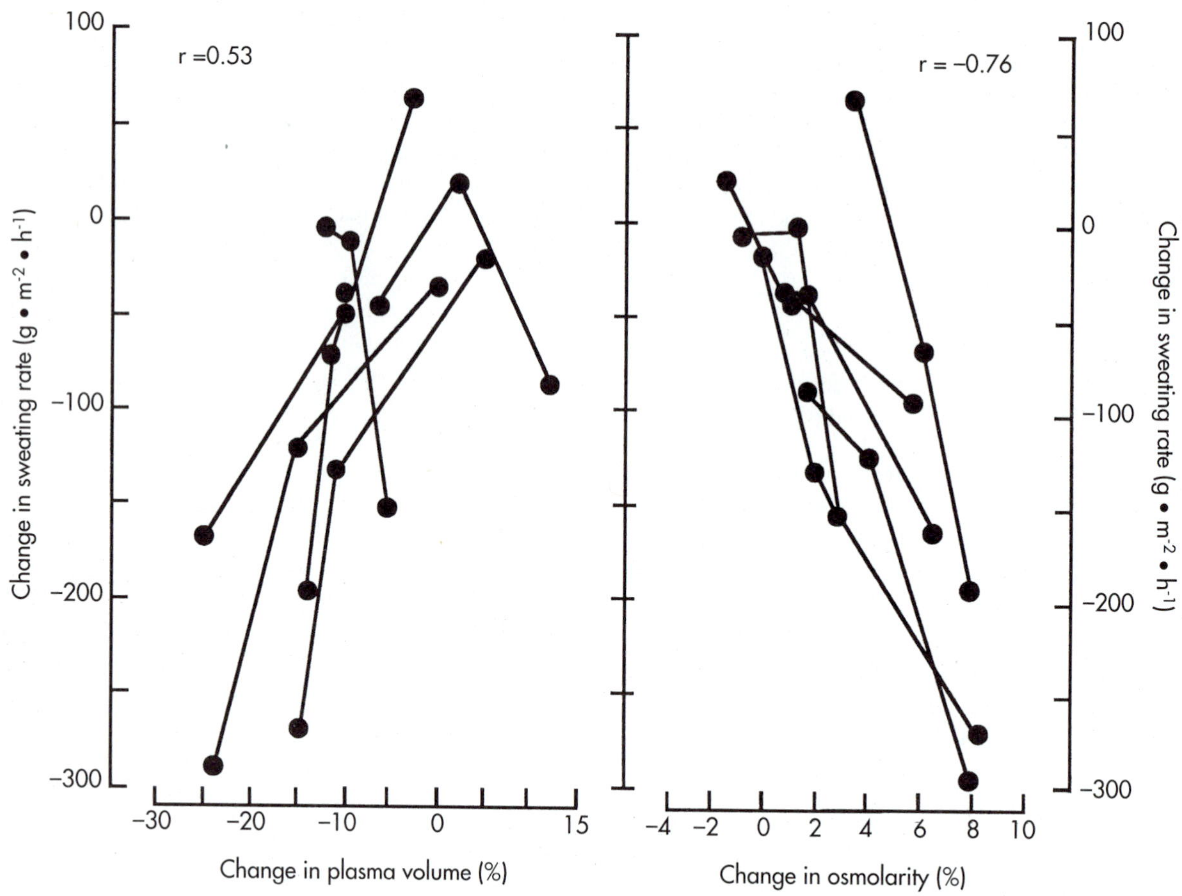

Fig. 8-1 Effect of reduced plasma volume or increased osmolarity on sweat rates in six individuals. (Redrawn from Sawka MN et al: *J Appl Physiol* 59:1394, 1985.)

advantages of physical training or heat acclimation. Involuntary dehydration can produce serious water deficits, such as found in persons cast adrift on tropical seas or stranded in the desert without water. Survival under these conditions requires knowledge of the trade-offs between physical activity and dehydration rate. Adolph and associates[1] described both the symptoms and the expected dehydration rates under these circumstances.

According to Marriott[285] the *minimum* unavoidable daily water loss approximates 1.5 L or about 2% of body weight as body water. Although hard work in the heat can elicit this magnitude of sweat loss in 1 hour (1.5 L/hr), rest in good shade can reduce sweat losses to minimum values (50 to 300 ml/hr at air temperatures from 80° to 100° F). If a 12% body weight loss as body water produces shock, survival time could vary between 1 and 5 days. *As a rule of thumb,[1] a person should carry 1 gallon of water for every 20 miles walked at night and 2 gallons for every 20 miles of desert walked during the day.*

Normal oxidation of carbohydrates produces a small amount of metabolic water that may have survival value. Approximately 500 ml may be produced per day, which represents 30% of the daily obligate water loss at rest. This represents only about 20 minutes of sweat-losing running time in the heat.

Voluntary Dehydration

Inadequate fluid intake also occurs where drinking *is* possible. Pitts and co-workers[330] emphasized that during work in the heat, *men never voluntarily drink as much water as they lose,* and they usually replace only two thirds of the net water loss. Adolph and co-workers[347] called this phenomenon voluntary dehydration and found that it increases with elevated sweat rate induced by higher ambient temperatures or work rate, inadequate time allowed for rehydration, and greater effort involved in acquiring water. Therefore as a general rule *all persons in the heat should be considered dehydrated* unless they have recently been forced to drink more water than they desired.

Thirst

The consumption of water depends on the palatability of beverages, which in turn depends on many factors such as water quality (turbidity, color, odor), temperature, and flavor. Our recent theoretical calculations and a review of the research involving thirst[211] suggest that thirst is delayed rather than inadequate.

The delay in thirst is a manifestation of the body's osmotic control because thirst does not become prominent until osmotic dehydration exceeds the renal capacity to deal with it physiologically. Although the osmoregulatory system appears to display large individual differences in both sensitivity and threshold,[343,345] the most potent stimulators of antidiuretic hormone (ADH) release and thirst are absolute and relative dehydration.[9]

Within any one individual the plasma vasopressin response (ADH release) is linearly related to plasma osmolality[345] and therefore to plasma sodium. Generally the range of body fluid osmolality in health is between 280 and 295 mOsm/kg H_2O.[135] For example, at an osmolality of 280 mOsm/kg H_2O, ADH release is almost completely inhibited and the urine osmolality is minimal (less than 100 mOsm/kg H_2O).

As dehydration occurs, the plasma ADH concentration rises (0.5 to 5 pg/ml) and conserves body water by increasing renal reabsorption of solute-free water.[344] This action of ADH increases urine concentration (a 1 mOsm plasma change increases urine osmolality by almost 100 mOsm/kg) and decreases flow. At the thirst threshold, urine flow is reduced 10 to 20 fold. Although there is wide variation in the individual thirst threshold, Vokes[421] estimates its average value at 295 mOsm/kg H_2O.

Chronic Hypohydration

The significant delay between the threshold for ADH release (greater than 280 mOsm) and the thirst threshold (greater than 295 mOsm) is important. It frees the individual from immediate drinking requirements in response to physiologic changes in osmolality. On the other hand, certain individuals and groups[211] maintain a chronic state of hypohydration just below the thirst threshold (294 mOsm/kg), which is equivalent to a total body water (TBW) deficit of some 2 L.

The following examples assume that the TBW in a 70 kg person is 42 L (about 60% of body weight), and that two thirds of this water (28 L) is intracellular and one third is extracellular (3.5 L of plasma and 10.5 L of interstitial fluid). By calculation,[135] the intravascular or plasma volume is equivalent to one twelfth of the total body water (42 L TBW/12 = 3.5 L plasma volume).

For example, assume:

$$(\text{Normal TBW}) \times (\text{Normal plasma}_{osm}) = (\text{Thirst TBW}) \times (\text{Thirst plasma}_{osm})$$

then

$$(42\text{ L}) \times (280\text{ mOsm/kg}) = (?\text{ L}) \times (295\text{ mOsm/kg});$$

$$(11{,}760\text{ mOsm}/295\text{ mOsm/kg}) = ?\text{ L} = 39.9\text{ L} = \text{TBW at the thirst threshold}$$

Then

$$(42\text{ L} - 39.9\text{ L}) = 2.1\text{ L} = \text{TBW deficit at the thirst threshold}$$

This degree of hypohydration at 295 mOsm/kg (2.1 L) represents nearly 3% of body weight ([2.1 kg/70 kg] × 100). Additional water loss through sweat of only 2.1 L (4.2 L total) now results in a water deficit equivalent to 6% of body mass. This 6% deficit causes performance decrements and increased risk of heat illness.

Primary Water Depletion

Hypohydration caused by primary water depletion and increased fluid losses is characterized by thirst and oliguria and is completely relieved by drinking pure water.[302] Sample calculations based on some commonly accepted estimates highlight the role of reduced water intake versus skipped meals and sweat (water and salt) losses in the dehydration process.

In the absence of sweating a pure water deficit caused by inadequate fluid intake occurs slowly but can lead eventually to symptoms of circulatory shock. Clinical shock from pure water deficit generally coincides with a sodium concentration above 170 mEq/L (normal range 135 to 145).[135] This water deficit can be estimated using the following formula:

$$\text{Water deficit (L)} = \text{TBW }(0.6 \times \text{wt in kg}) - (\text{TBW} \times \text{Desired plasma Na}^+/\text{Measured plasma Na}^+)$$

$$\text{Water deficit (L)} = 42\text{ L} - (42\text{L} \times 140\text{ mEq Na}^+/\text{L}/175\text{ mEq Na}^+/\text{L})$$

$$\text{Water deficit (L)} = 42\text{ L} - 33.6\text{ L} = 8.4\text{ L}$$

Thus in a pure water deficit sufficient to produce shock, an estimate of loss might be some 8.4 L of body water or 12% of body weight in a 70 kg person. At minimal rates of water loss (1.5 to 2.0 L/24 hr), this degree of dehydration could take 4 to 5 days to produce.

Therefore, by definition, if a pure water loss occurs (no salt loss), the loss would be apportioned over all the fluid spaces with two thirds of the loss from the intracellular water (8.4 L × 2/3 = 5.6 L), one third from the extracellular water (8.4 L/3 = 2.8 L), and one twelfth of this from the plasma space (8.4 L/12 = 700 ml). This loss represents approximately 20% of the plasma volume. In practice, usually less than one twelfth of the water loss comes from the plasma space because of its increased plasma protein oncotic pressure.

Sweat Salt Losses

In contrast to the case of primary water depletion is the situation in which an unacclimatized individual has skipped a prior meal and is producing hypotonic sweat (0.41% NaCl = 0.5 × normal plasma osmolality, taken to be 280 mOsm/kg H_2O) as the source of the body water deficit. This person begins exercise in the heat in a fully hydrated, normal state and over a 2- to 3-hour period loses 6% of body weight as sweat (4.2 L).

Assume that 0.5 isotonic saline is equivalent to an osmolality of 140 mOsm/kg (0.5 × 280 mOsm/kg). Then half of the fluid loss (4.2 L/2 = 2.1 L) is pure water and half (2.1 L) is normal saline (280 mOsm/kg). The extracellular space (3.5 L [plasma] + 10.5 L [interstitial] = 14 L; the sodium space) would lose 2.1 L of isotonic saline, of which the plasma contributes one fourth (3.5 L/14 L = 1/4). This is equivalent to 525 ml (2.1 L/4) of plasma volume.

In addition, the plasma would contribute one twelfth of the pure water deficit (2.1 L), or 175 ml (2.1 L/12). If these plasma volume losses are added (525 ml + 175 ml = 700 ml), the plasma could lose 20% of its volume ([100 ml/3500 ml] × 100), which is close to the shock threshold (Table 8-1).

Thus a 4.2 L sweat loss has theoretically as much impact on the plasma volume (20%) as twice the volume (8.4 L) of pure water loss (20%). In this example, however, inadequate salt and water intake (skipped meals, no drinking) has a role, as does the rapidity of sweat losses (hours versus days).

Rehydration With and Without Acclimatization

Sweating and normal thermoregulation have another impact on the predisposition to clinical states that is also widely unappreciated by trainers, coaches, and team physicians. Sweat salt losses by unacclimatized individuals can theoretically produce solute deficits having a profound impact on thirst and therefore on potential rehydration rates.

For example, if a non-heat-acclimatized person loses 6% of body weight (or 4.2 L) as hypotonic sweat (0.43% NaCl), there is a loss of 588 mOsm (34.4 g) of solute (140 mOsm/kg sweat × 4.2 kg). Upon this loss of 4.2 L of body water as sweat, the dehydrated plasma osmolality is only 295.6 mOsm/kg, compared with 311.1 mOsm/kg if only water had been lost. As a result, the person will consume theoretically only 80 ml of water (versus 1270 ml; see later discussion) before the thirst threshold (295 mOsm/kg H_2O) is reached. This represents only 1.9% of the water deficit (80 ml/4200 ml × 100). Consumption of a solute-rich meal or a fluid-replacement beverage about 2 hours before exercise potentially counteracts the sweat salt losses of a nonacclimatized individual. This probably also serves to explain, by and large, why water balance is not fully restored until mealtime in sweating, nonacclimatized individuals.

Another clinically and physiologically relevant aspect of this calculation should be emphasized. It is generally appreciated that with heat acclimation, subjects sweat sooner (at a lower T_c) and in larger volumes, increasing the requirement for replacement fluids.

Furthermore, late in the acclimatization process (7 to 10 days or more), persons generally produce a significantly more hypotonic sweat. If this sweat should contain a minimum sodium concentration (0.17% NaCl), the solute loss would be reduced to 235 (17 g) compared with 588 mOsm (see earlier discussion). The dehydrated plasma osmolality would be 305 mOsm/kg, and the subject would consume 1270 ml (a 16-fold increase) in returning to the thirst threshold (30.2% of the water deficit versus 1.9% above). Although this theoretically important aspect of acclimation on thirst and rehydration volumes has not been experimentally verified, it could significantly improve resistance to heat illness by maintaining more adequate body water stores.

Physiologic Consequences of Hypohydration

With these examples as a frame of reference, let us examine the impact of hypohydration on cardiovascular physiology and thermoregulation. Hyperosmolality, as in primary water depletion, increases the threshold temperatures for sweating and cutaneous vasodilation even without a fall in blood volume during exercise in the heat.[144] The effects of hypertonicity may be neurally mediated, since preoptic–anterior hypothalamic neurons are osmosensitive.[382] Moreover, hypovolemia secondary to increased hypohydration levels can mediate a systematic reduction of sweating rate during exercise in the heat.[143,361] Hypohydration of the plasma space as a result of lost salt and water combined with increased blood displacement to cutaneous vascular beds could compromise venous return and cardiac output.[303] Since decreased blood volume reduces central venous pressure[245] and cardiac filling pressure, hypohydration increases heart rate and decreases stroke volume.[5,354] In addition, it is likely that increases in plasma hematocrit and viscosity further reduce cardiac filling pressure as a result of increased resistance. In one series of patients with exertional heatstroke,[377] 35% were hypotensive with a systolic blood pressure below 90 torr. Similar findings have been reported in classic heatstroke.[174]

Sinus tachycardia is consistently present in heatstroke victims in response to excessive circulatory requirements.[375] Cardiac output and diastolic blood pressure are low, so pulse pressure is high.[379] Depending on the degree of hypoperfusion to vital organs, a person may experience shock.[249] Hypohydration compromises thermoregulation,[369] with linear increases in core temperature of about 0.15° C for each percent decrease in body weight during exercise in the heat.[361] Furthermore, by negating most of the thermoregulatory advantages conferred by high aerobic fitness and heat acclimatization,[65] hypohydration additionally increases the risk of heat illness.[379]

ACCLIMATIZATION

The process of human acclimatization to heat produces changes in thermoregulatory responses involving sweating, skin circulation, and thermoregulatory set point. Other changes that are equally impressive but not specifically thermoregulatory include important cardiovascular alterations (heart rate, stroke volume, and plasma volume) and endocrine adjustments. When these physiologic adjustments occur in response to heat exposure in a controlled laboratory setting, they are termed acclimation, and if induced by the natural environment, acclimatization.

Depending on a given individual's constitution, state of physical fitness, and thermal history, a given thermal stress and the intensity of exercise involved will likely produce some degree of thermal strain. However, each person acclimates to heat stress in his or her own way,[371] with considerable variation in indices of heat strain (weakness, rapid pulse, narrow pulse pressure, flushing of the face and neck, headache, shortness of breath, dizziness, cramps, nausea, and vomiting).

Physiologic Changes

In general, symptoms lessen as acclimation progresses. Nearly complete acclimation to a given level of daily exercise and heat stress can be achieved in 7 to 10 days (Fig. 8-2). Most authors agree that a program of physical training resulting in a high aerobic capacity improves physiologic responses at high ambient temperatures and hastens the acclimation process. In fact, with the exception that heat acclimation lowers metabolic rate, the physiologic changes produced by physical training are quite similar and include a lowered threshold temperature for the onset of skin blood flow, sweating (Fig. 8-3),[342] increased plasma volume, increased stroke volume, decreased heart rate, decreased skin temperature, decreased rectal temperature, and increased $\dot{V}O_2$max.[15] Practically this means that a fit but untrained person who runs a 500 m race and develops a rectal temperature of 40° to 43° C could, after acclimation, run the same race under the same environmental conditions and have a rectal temperature of only 37.5° C (Fig. 8-2).[249]

Although many controversial issues remain, a general rule is that either strenuous interval training or continuous exercise at an intensity greater than 50% $\dot{V}O_2$max accounts for about 50% of the improvements found with classic acclimation procedures.[166] This may be important to the individual who wants to prepare for an acute change in thermal climate but does not have the means to safely elevate his or her core temperature in the heat.

The primary mechanism of the heat acclimation process is to raise internal body temperature sufficiently to induce moderate sweating. This can be achieved with moderate exercise in the heat or by wearing more clothing in a cooler en-

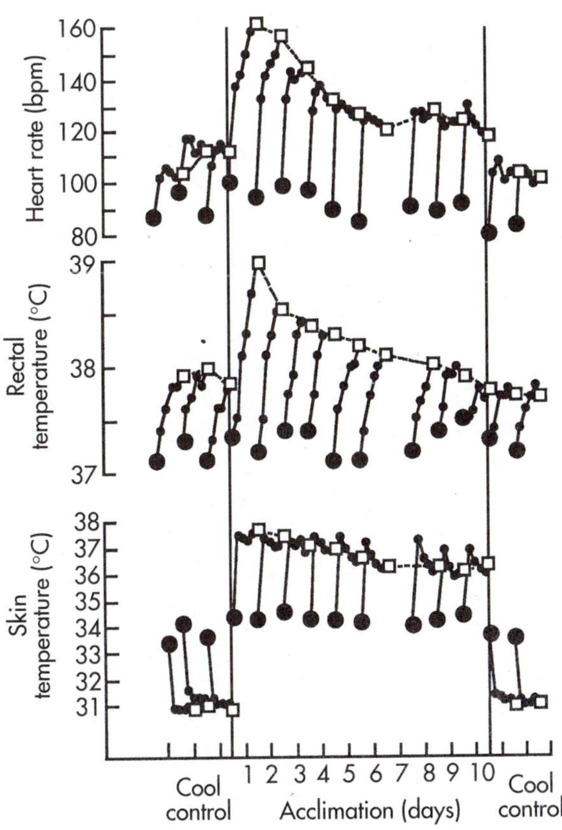

Fig. 8-2 Effect of 10 days' acclimation on heart rate and rectal and skin temperatures during a standard exercise (five 10-minute periods of treadmill, separated by 2-minute rests) in dry heat. Large circles show values before start of the first exercise period each day, with small circles showing successive values. Squares show the final values each day. Controls of exercise in cool environment before and after acclimation. (Redrawn from Eichna LW et al: *Am J Physiol* 163:585, 1950.)

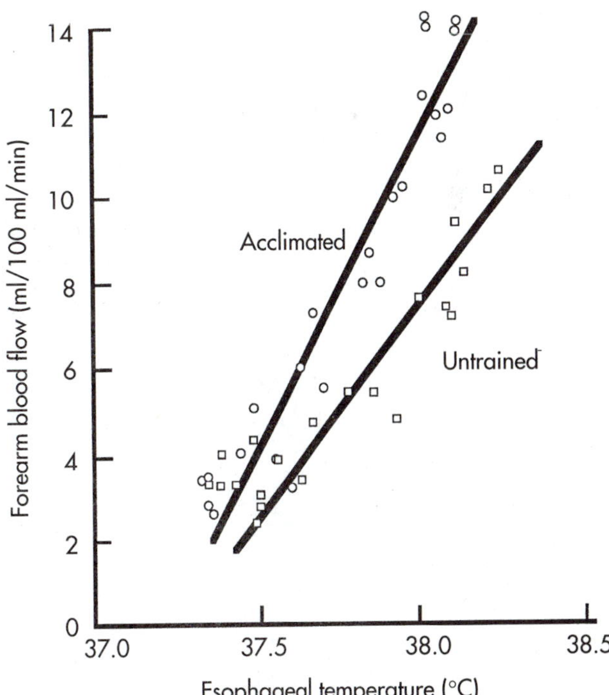

Fig. 8-3 Effect of acclimation on forearm blood flow versus esophageal temperature in one subject. (Redrawn from Roberts MF et al: *J Appl Physiol* 43:133, 1977.)

vironment. In the unacclimated individual, usually an hour per day of exercise in the heat is sufficient to produce an effect over days of exposure. As a rule 10 days of successive treadmill walks in dry heat lowers final exercise heart rates by about 40 beats/min, lowers rectal and skin temperatures by 1° and 1.5° C, respectively, and increases sweat production by about 10%.[128] Generally the degree of acclimation is related to the daily heat stress; that is, daily 100-minute bouts in the heat conferred more acclimation after 9 days than did 50-minute bouts.[271] Most of the improvement in heart rate occurs in 4 to 5 days, and the improvement is nearly complete after 7 days (Fig. 8-2). As heat acclimation progresses, the onset of thermal sweating occurs at lower core temperatures and the peak sweat rate is higher or even doubled (1.5 to 3 L/hr). Furthermore, the ability to sustain sweating for prolonged periods improves, along with more sweating in skin areas that sweated the least before acclimation. Acclimation tends to make the sweating response over different skin areas more uniform. These effects are not wholly central because changes in the glands themselves can be demonstrated pharmacologically.[91]

Heat acclimation increases the sweat glands' capacity to reabsorb sweat sodium at any given sweat rate.[4] Depending on the state of acclimation, the sodium concentration in sweat varies between approximately 5 and 60 mEq/L (10 to 20 mOsm/kg H_2O) (Table 8-1) and increases with sweat rate, but declines with the state of acclimation. The salt-sparing effect of acclimation seems to depend on the secretion of aldosterone, triggered by the combined effects of sodium depletion and heat stress.[256]

Skin vasodilation, especially in the forearm where it can be measured, occurs at a lower core temperature after acclimation (Fig. 8-3). Since these changes parallel the core temperature changes for sweating, they suggest that alterations are occurring in skin blood vessels at the same time as those in skin sweat glands.[147]

Changes in heart rate and plasma volume are both rapid and significantly correlated during the first week of acclimation.[371] The decrease in heart rate and increase in stroke volume may begin as early as the second day of work in the heat.[444] These changes are nearly complete by day 5, whereas final rectal temperatures are still declining with subsequent exposures. Although many authors have described the increases in plasma volume with days of exposure, conjecture surrounds the mechanisms involved, including salt retention, the addition of protein to the vascular space, and fluid shifts between compartments.[369] What is interesting, however, is a return of plasma volume to baseline levels after about 2 weeks without apparent thermoregulatory impairment.[30] Horowitz and colleagues[205] have shown that long-term acclimation in rats increased the compliance of the ventricle in isolated hearts, resulting in a greater diastolic volume at any end-diastolic pressure. This promising model has produced recent insights, detailed in the biochemical changes section that follows immediately.

Adaptation is clearly shown by the incidence of heat syncope among persons suddenly exposed to living in a hot environment (Fig. 8-4). Syncope, as described below, is caused by reduced cerebral blood flow resulting from a combination of peripheral blood pooling, reduced cardiac output, and orthostatic hypotension. Syncope peaks on the first day of heat exposure and falls to zero by day 5.

Although persons can acclimate to hot environments over a period of 1 to 2 weeks, they also deacclimate over the same period of time.

Biochemical Changes

Adaptations to high temperatures involve alterations in isoenzyme composition of metabolic enzymes in relation to their thermostability, that is, ability to resist thermal denaturation,[50,204,267] and having a higher proportion of "slow" myosin adenosine triphosphatase (ATPase).[205] Possibly as part of the same process, the metabolism of hearts isolated from heat-acclimated rats became more efficient in terms of amount of oxygen required per unit force time per gram of tissue.[203] Furthermore, evidence suggests that the induction of heat shock proteins may be involved, although this is not proved at present.

Table 8-1 Effect of Sweat Losses (Salt and Water) on Plasma Volume and Osmolality

Body Weight Loss		Hypotonic Sweat (Percent × 280 mOsm)															
		50%				25%				12.5%				As Pure Water			
		ΔPl Vol		ΔPl Osm		ΔPl Vol		ΔPl Osm		ΔPl Vol		ΔPl Osm		ΔPl Vol		ΔPl Osm	
%	L	ml	%	mOsm	Na	ml	%	mOsm	Na	ml	%	mOsm	Na	ml	%	mOsm	Na
0	0	0	0	280	140	0	0	280	140	0	0	280	140	0	0	280	140
2	1.4	−233	−6.7	285	142	−175	−5.0	287	144	−146	−4.2	288	142	−117	−3.3	290	145
4	2.8	−467	−13.3	290	145	−350	−10	295	148	−292	−8.3	298	149	−233	−6.7	300	150
6	4.2	−700	−20.0	296	148	−525	−15	303	152	−437	−12.5	307	154	−350	−10.0	311	156
8	5.6					−700	−20	312	156	−583	−16.7	318	159	−466	−13.3	323	162
10	7.0									−729	−20.8	329	164	−583	−16.7	336	168
12	8.4													−700	−20.0	350	175

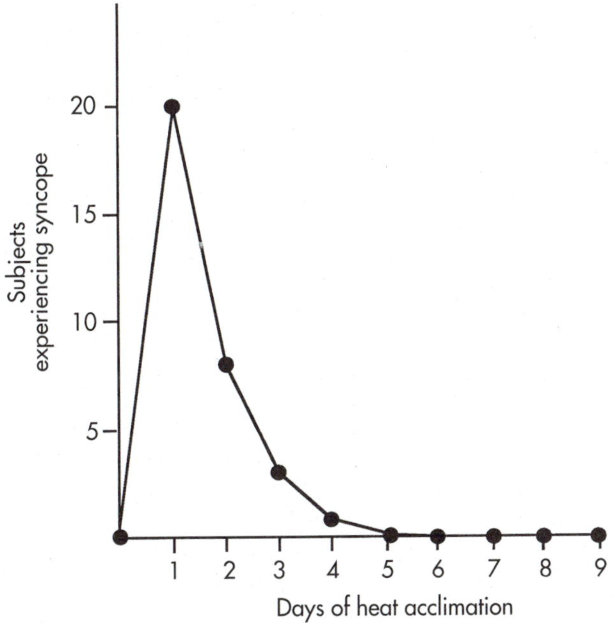

Fig. 8-4 Incidence of syncope among 45 subjects living in a hot environment for 24 hours each day and undergoing exercise trials. (Redrawn from Bean WB, Eichna LW: *Fed Proc* 2:144, 1943, by Hubbard RW, Armstrong LE. In Pandolf KB et al: *Human performance: physiology and environmental medicine at terrestrial extremes,* Indianapolis, 1988, Benchmark Press.)

An intriguing question is, "What is the fundamental event during heat-exercise stress that causes the biochemical and physiologic alterations in the body that ultimately result in heat tolerance?" At the moment this is unknown, but there is some reason to think that raising aldosterone concentrations could trigger an acclimation response by increasing the number of Na^+,K^+-ATPase membrane pumps. Aldosterone concentrations rise within a few minutes when humans are subjected to exercise in the heat.[150]

Green and co-workers[176] found that simply stimulating rabbit muscle by external low-frequency voltage over several days increased the number of Na^+,K^+ pumps in the sarcolemma by the fourth day, reaching a plateau on day 10. They also found that exercise training in humans caused a rise in the concentration of Na^+,K^+-ATPase pumps on sarcolemma within 1 week. They noted that at the same time the normal rise in plasma K^+ caused by severe exercise was reduced after acclimation; they suggested that it was the rise in the number of Na^+,K^+ pumps that attenuated the loss of K^+ from working muscle.[176]

The evidence of Horowitz and co-workers[205] strongly suggests that more than one state of acclimation exists: an initial short-term phase followed by a long-term phase. Subjected to a standard heat stress, unacclimated rats reached a target temperature of 41.5° to 42° C after 200 minutes, whereas after 5 to 7 days' acclimation at 34° C (short-term acclimation), it took 400 minutes (since they were much more efficient at dissipating heat), but after 28 days' acclimation (long-term), they required only 300 minutes (they became less efficient at losing heat). Furthermore, atria from short-term acclimated rats were less responsive to norepinephrine than were those from control animals while those from long-term acclimated rats recovered to preacclimation responsiveness.[267] With short-term acclimation there was an increase in one type of cardiac membrane receptor and a decrease in another, but on long-term acclimation both receptor types increased.[203] In the short-term phase, organ responsiveness to neurotransmitters decreased, but during the long-term phase it returned to control values. In summary, acclimation involves changes on a molecular level, including an increase in the number of Na^+,K^+-ATPase membrane pumps, which causes changes on a cellular level, leading to changes in organ function.

Heatstroke, Lipopolysaccharides, and Cytokines

BACTERIAL TOXINS

To absorb nutrients from ingested food, chyme remains in the small and large intestine for several hours to days. At body temperature, bacteria present in the gut also absorb nutrients from the chyme and reproduce rapidly, reaching concentrations of 10^9 to 10^{12} organisms/g.[158] Dead gram-negative bacteria slough off into their milieu large amounts of the highly toxic cell wall component lipopolysaccharide (LPS, endotoxin), which may reach concentrations of 1 mg/g in feces.

As long as LPS remains within the intestines, it shows no toxicity and any small amounts that "leak out" are rapidly inactivated by several mechanisms: some LPS is phagocytosed by bound Kupffer's cells within the liver reticuloendothelial system (RES), where it is partly detoxified and then bound by hepatocytes for further degrading[411]; some LPS binds to circulating antilipopolysaccharide antibodies[153]; some binds to high-density lipoprotein (HDL)[412]; and some binds to LPS-binding protein (LBP).[441]

Large amounts of LPS rapidly entering the circulation would overwhelm the protective systems, allowing LPS to express its toxic effects rapidly. At plasma concentrations below approximately 100 pg/ml, LPS initiates a cascade of molecular events that ultimately leads to nausea, vomiting, diarrhea, fever, and headache.[41] Higher concentrations can lead to conditions identical to those of gram-negative bacteremia, including vascular collapse, shock, and death.[76] In fact, at the time of death from gram-negative bacteremia in experimental animals, there may be no live bacteria in the plasma. High levels of circulating LPS appear to be the more immediate cause of septic shock.[434]

Intestinal Ischemia and Endotoxin Release

During exercise, blood flow to muscle may rise from a resting value of 1 to 2 ml/100 g/min to as high as 300 ml/100 g/min; blood flow also rises in the skin to provide cooling while maintaining blood flow to the heart, brain, and liver.[253] It is important that blood flow to the liver be maintained during heavy exercise to remove lactate and other metabolites from the blood and to provide glucose for energy. Although liver blood flow may decrease somewhat during exercise, glucose output may actually increase because of the influence of epinephrine and glucagon.[253]

In contrast, to maintain blood pressure during exercise and heat, blood flow to the intestines and kidney is probably greatly reduced, with regions of local ischemia and transitory gut wall damage—low enough to cause ischemic injury to the gut wall.[333,334] This reduced intestinal blood flow causes the diarrhea or water intoxication occasionally encountered during a marathon run as a consequence of the inability to resorb the water ingested during the race.[253] For example, in one extreme case, after winning a marathon in 1979, Derek Clayton stated that "two hours later . . . I was urinating quite large clots of blood, and I was vomiting black mucus and had a lot of black diarrhea."[142] The ultimate consequences of reduced gut blood flow may be severe.

Because of the high LPS gradient, almost any insult to the integrity of the gut wall leads to a rise in plasma LPS. Hemorrhage to 45 mm Hg reduced blood flow and therefore reduced oxygen transport to the walls of the stomach, small intestine, and sigmoid colon in swine.[296] This degree of hypoxemia in the cat has led to local elevations in the gut wall permeability barrier and caused endotoxemia.[154] In a swine model, blood flow through the superior mesenteric artery was progressively occluded.[140] Eventually the pH of the gut wall declined as a result of increasing tissue hypoxia and a local shift to aerobic or anaerobic metabolism with the production of lactate. At about the same time, LPS entered the circulation. Infusing LPS, itself, into swine caused marked hypotension, a reduction in superior mesenteric artery blood flow, an even larger increase in gut permeability,[140] and even the translocation of bacteria into the circulation.[430]

The size of putative "holes" in the gut wall accounting for the rise in LPS permeability depends on the duration of the ischemia. When the superior mesenteric artery of canines was occluded, LPS (molecular or micellar) leaked out into the circulation within 20 minutes, but the appearance in the circulation of whole live bacteria (several orders of magnitude larger) required 6 hours of occlusion.[325] Rats, however, required only 2 hours.[112]

In a different model, nonhuman primates first breathed a hypoxic gas mixture for an hour and then breathed oxygen.[155] A hypoxic reflex caused intestinal blood flow to fall, leading to ischemic injury to the gut wall and LPS translocation within only 5 to 10 minutes of the onset of hypoxia. On the other hand, when the gut flora had been reduced by administration of nonabsorbable antibiotics, both LPS and bacterial translocation were reduced to zero.[112,158]

Such studies together show that the permeability barrier in the gut wall is rapidly damaged by hypotension, reduced blood flow, and hypoxia, thus permitting LPS to enter the portal and systemic circulations at a high rate.

The development of secondary fever and infection with a high death rate is common following the cooling of patients with heatstroke.[380] The susceptibility of such patients to infections[380] may be due to a combination of changes in lymphocyte subpopulations together with the increase in gut wall permeability to LPS and bacteria caused by hyperthermia and its hypotension.[112]

CYTOKINES AND SHOCK

Cytokines are a wide class of protein cell regulators that control the timing, amplitude, and duration of the immune response. Originally they were called lymphokines and monokines because they were discovered in cells of the immune system. However, when it was established that they were also produced by a wide variety of cell types throughout the body, as well as by mechanisms unrelated to the immune response, they became known as cytokines.[88] They are relatively low–molecular weight (less than 80 kd) proteins, act at short range in a paracrine or autocrine manner rather than as circulating hormones,[116] and interact with high-affinity cell surface receptors regulating the transcription of several cellular genes, resulting in changes in cell behavior.[23] The various cytokines are extraordinarily active, have overlapping and important activities, and induce each other so that at present it is difficult to establish which cytokine has what critical function. Probably their local concentrations determine which regulatory influence a cytokine has at a particular time.

Endotoxin causes septic shock, but LPS itself does not appear to be a direct contact poison. Rather, LPS present in the blood is first bound by LPS-binding protein (LPB) to form a complex, which circulates until it encounters a specific high-affinity LPS receptor on macrophages. This receptor, CD-14, is attached to the surface membranes of macrophages through phosphoinositol.[367] Binding of CD-14 by the LPS-LBP complex initiates a cascade of reactions within the macrophage involving hypersecretion of immune mediators, the cytokines. Because of their inappropriate and excessive local concentrations, cytokines become highly toxic. Although the correlation between mortality and plasma concentration of any single cytokine is low in patients with sepsis, mortality correlates closely (p <.001) with a "score" consisting of a summation of the concentrations of individual cytokines.[79]

Most of the symptoms of gram-negative bacterial shock can be induced by injection of some of the purified cytokines alone. The first two (and most important) cytokines induced by LPS are tumor necrosis factor (TNF) and interleukin-1 (IL-1).[291] TNF causes hydrolysis of plasma membrane sphingomyelin and generation of ceramide, a second messenger.[255] Ceramide activates a serine-threonine protein phosphatase and is inhibited by okaic acid.[255] In humans,

TNF is usually detectable only at the onset of clinical responses.[291] TNF administration to humans causes fever, tachycardia, increase in stress hormones, and leukocytosis,[291] with the intensity of symptoms closely correlating with peak concentrations of TNF.

TNF rapidly induces IL-1, which causes fever, sleep, anorexia, and hypotension.[282] IL-1 acts directly on vascular endothelium (an organ the size of the liver if concentrated in one place) to increase local concentrations of nitric oxide and to raise circulating prostaglandin concentrations, ultimately resulting in vasodilation, hypotension, and possibly, shock.[116]

IL-1 may also have a more subtle effect. IL-1 changes the responses of arteries in different vascular beds to norepinephrine (NE),[331] and by so doing may cause abnormalities in regional blood flow. In one study IL-1 decreased NE-induced contraction by about 50% in the aorta, carotid, and pulmonary arteries, had no effect in hepatic and mesenteric arteries, and increased contraction in femoral arteries.[341] Elevations in circulating catecholamine concentration in persons with heatstroke have been reported.[3] The effects of TNF and IL-1 together are far greater than those of either alone.

Omega-6 Fatty Acids and Arachidonic Acid

At the biochemical level the binding of IL-1 to its specific membrane receptor activates G-protein, which increases intracellular cyclic adenosine monophosphate (cAMP) concentration, which in turn activates membrane phospholipases. It is activation of the phospholipases that ultimately leads to cell damage and organism pathophysiology.[80,169] The phospholipases break down phospholipid esters of fatty acids, including the omega-6 fatty acids, which predominate in cell membranes of an individual partaking of a normal Western diet.[217,264] Omega-6 fatty acids form arachidonic acid as their first major metabolite (Fig. 8-5).

Cells contain two major enzymes that can act on arachidonic acid: lipoxygenase and cyclooxygenase. Lipoxygenase causes arachidonic acid to enter a pathway leading to the formation of 5-HPETE and a series of toxic leukotrienes. Of them, LTB_4, LTC_4, and LTD_4 are the most important. LTB_4 induces inflammation, increases capillary leakage, and causes leukocytes to aggregate. LTC_4 and LTD_4 are the strong bronchoconstrictors involved in asthma.[93,182] Cyclooxygenase converts arachidonic acid into prostaglandin G_2, which is converted into PGH_2 with the formation of toxic free radicals. PGH_2 is a central metabolite on which a variety of enzymes act to form mainly toxic products such as thromboxane A_2 (TxA_2) and many different prostaglandins, including the toxic PGD_2. TxA_2 causes platelets to aggregate, is a strong vasoconstrictor, and increases capillary leakage. To a person in shock or with another circulatory disorder, such agents could convert a severe but treatable condition into a lethal one. In summary, eating a normal Western diet results in the presence of large amounts of omega-6 fatty acids in phospholipid cell membranes, predisposing to the formation of arachidonic acid and a large number of its toxic metabolites. For a review of prostaglandin and thromboxane biochemistry, see Oates and colleagues[319,320] and Bottoms and Adams.[52]

Fever

Fever, in contrast to exercise hyperthermia, represents a physiologic state in which the thermostat has been reset above 37° C by exogenous pyrogens released by bacteria or viruses[115] or from IL-1[131,223] and TNF.[301] It is now recognized that fever is also caused by IL-2 and interferons alpha and beta.[48]

Cytokines may be responsible in part for other clinical symptoms, including fatigue, malaise, and edema. α-Melanocyte stimulating hormone inhibits IL-1-induced fever and the acute phase response.[274] Interestingly, neutralizing antibodies to IL-1 and TNF have been found in the sera of both normal and sick individuals and may play a role in their regulation.[403]

Current evidence suggests that aspirin-like cyclooxygenase inhibitors interfere with IL-1-induced fever or shock responses by inhibiting prostaglandin synthesis.[323] Recently Jurivich and associates[224] described the effect of sodium salicylate on the human heat shock response and demonstrated that salicylate activation of DNA binding by the heat shock transcription factor (HSF) was comparable to activation attained during heat shock.

Defervation

Circulating pyrogens reach the thermoregulatory control center in the anterior hypothalamus and appear to act biochemically by inducing the synthesis of prostaglandins.[201,292] At the onset of a fever patients often feel "chilled" and shiver to elevate core temperature. A new, higher thermopreferendum, or preferred ambient temperature, is behaviorally established.[321] The physiologic change is even more important. Once this new set point temperature is established, the thermoregulatory center uses all available thermoregulatory mechanisms to maintain it. As a result, attempts at whole body cooling are met with sensations of extreme discomfort and violent shivering. Thus unsuccessful attempts to cool patients with suspected heat illness resulting in chills and violent shivering suggest coexistent infection or disease.

This prostaglandin-mediated pathway may be responsible for fever, for normal circadian temperature variation, for pathologic temperature elevations, and for temperature elevations related to stress.[38,248] Although there may be pyrogens that do not act via prostaglandins,[109,216] treatment if necessary should be directed at agents that block the action of the pyrogen at the hypothalamic receptor sites.

Since the external application of cold to reduce true fever is illogical[399] and often ineffective[26] even after an-

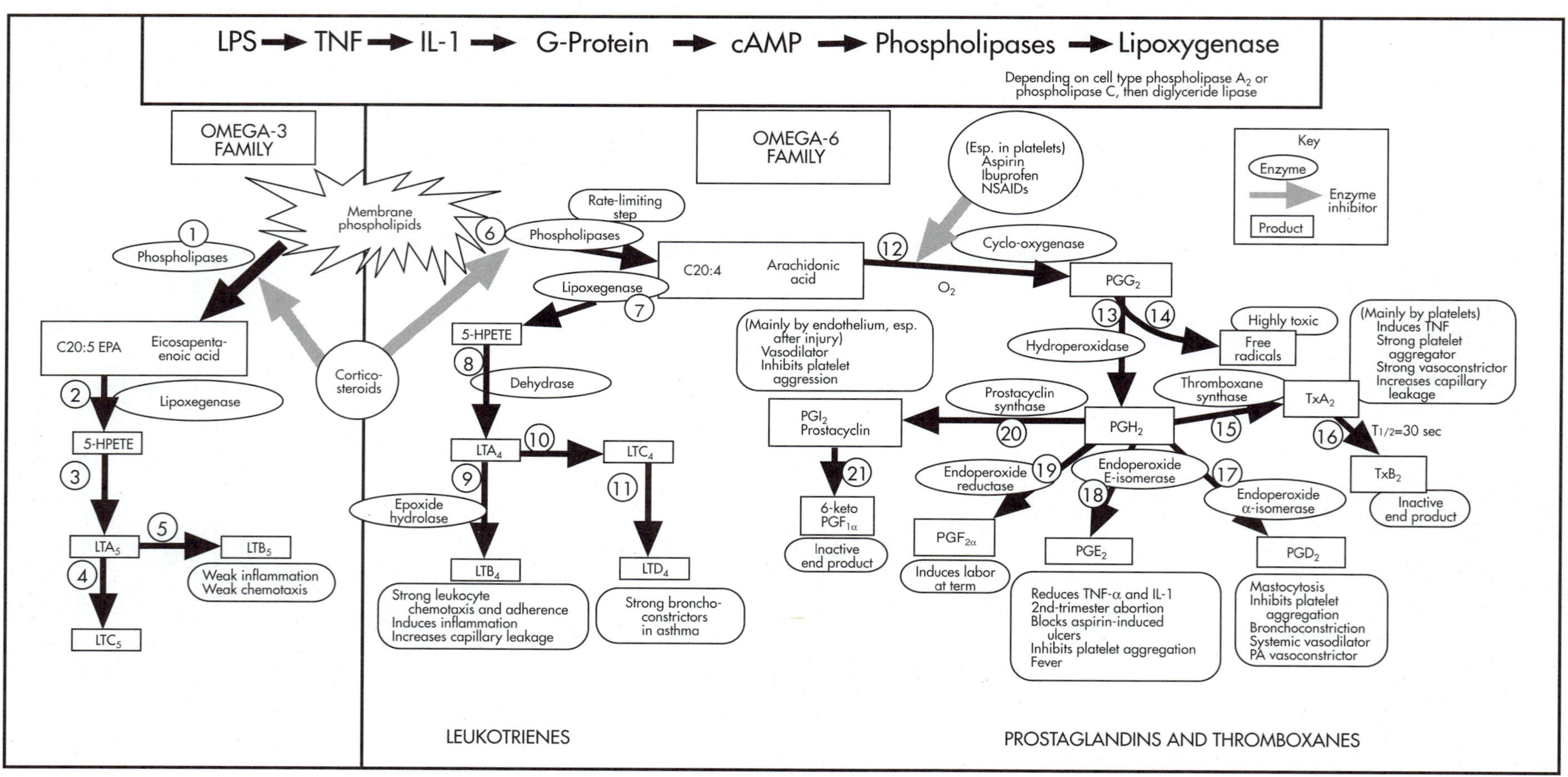

Fig. 8-5 Metabolism of omega-3 and omega-6 fatty acids induced by lipopolysaccharide or cytokines.

tipyretic therapy,[309] these results support the expectation that the elevated temperature set point is defended against environmental cooling. Therapy for fever that uses agents to block the causative molecular interaction is the most rational and clinically effective approach. Aspirin and other antipyretic agents, such as acetaminophen, indomethacin, ibuprofen, and other newer nonsteroidal antiinflammatory compounds, are effective and act either directly or indirectly through inhibition of the prostaglandin mechanism.[108] The release of pyrogens by exercise[72] and heatstroke has been noted.[254]

Should Antipyretic Therapy Be Routine?

In simple heat stress or mild hyperthermia produced by passive heat exposure or an exercise-induced increase in metabolism, body temperature will fall spontaneously toward normal levels.[301] The normal febrile response is generally self-limited in both magnitude and duration.[433] Vasopressin[417] and melanotropin[307] appear to act centrally to suppress temperature elevation and may be important in preventing extreme hyperthermia.

Although fever has long been recognized as a manifestation of disease[21] and may be identified as a debilitating problem even in the absence of other signs or symptoms,[429] antipyretic therapy should not be instituted routinely for every febrile episode.[141,175] Current opinion suggests that the febrile process has a role in host defense and that routine antipyretic therapy for fever is generally unnecessary and conceivably harmful,[399] especially with the link between aspirin and Reye's syndrome.[399] Instead, treatment should be based on evaluation of relative risks[45,121,247] in the individual case and reassessed if the anticipated benefits are not achieved.[399]

Fever and Resistance to Viral Infections

Resistance to murine,[35] porcine,[139] and canine[77] viral infections is reportedly enhanced by high temperatures. The eradication of viruses from different types of plants by long-term mild or moderate "whole body" hyperthermia followed by regeneration of virus-free plants by in vitro propagation of meristems is a generally applied technique of great economic significance.[422] Similarly, replication of DNA viruses appears to be inhibited by mild hyperthermia.[163,200,278] Measles virus membrane protein is selectively blocked at the level of mRNA translation by heating cultures to 39° C.[322]

Interestingly, viral infection can attenuate the production of heat shock proteins,[237,315,316,335] while on the other hand, heat stress might activate latent viruses.[161,314,449,450] Moreover, antipyresis increased viral shedding in ferrets.[213] Furthermore, activation of the reticuloendothelial system has been reported to improve heat tolerance in rats.[118] On the other hand, some host defense functions[351,416] that increase in vitro at 40° C level off or diminish at 42° or 43° C.[399]

EXPERIMENTAL BASIS FOR THE PARTICIPATION OF LIPOPOLYSACCHARIDE IN HEATSTROKE PATHOPHYSIOLOGY

Heatstroke temperatures greater than 43° C caused a large increase in permeability of isolated rat intestinal wall to LPS. This elevated permeability persisted even after the temperature was reduced to 37° C,[308] suggesting a temperature-induced injury to the gut wall. Gaffin and colleagues[157] investigated the time course of the movement of LPS through the intestinal wall into the circulation resulting from various insults (hypoxia, ischemia, and ionizing radiation) in nonhuman primates and evaluated the role of hyperthermia (T_{amb} = 41° C, RH = 100%, 3 to 4 hours) as a control. By directly measuring LPS with the *Limulus* amebocyte lysate method,[268] they found that as core temperature rose, the plasma LPS concentration was stable until 42° to 43° C (Fig. 8-6). At this temperature there was a sudden rise in LPS concentration, first in the portal vein, and 10 to 15 minutes later in the systemic circulation. This sequence appears to be the main route of LPS: out of the lumen of the intestines, through the portal vein and liver, and into the vena cava as a result of intestinal ischemia and heatstroke.[160]

In previous studies of infection, Gaffin and colleagues noted that when the concentration of live gram-negative bacteria or LPS rose, the detectable concentration of circulating antilipopolysaccharide antibodies fell because of consumption of LPS by its binding to specific antibodies.[434] It had been expected therefore that in the heatstroke experiments the concentration of natural antilipopolysaccharide antibodies would also immediately fall at 42° to 43° C. Contrary to expectations, natural anti-LPS began to decline at temperatures as low as 39° to 40° C (Fig. 8-6).[160] This suggests that as T_c rose to only 39° to 40° C, LPS actually commenced to leak into the circulation at a slow rate. As temperature continued to rise, at a certain point massive damage to the gut wall occurred, leading to rapid leakage of LPS into the portal vein. Currently it is not clear how much of this damage is caused by reduced oxygen delivery from reduced intestinal blood flow, how much by direct thermal damage of the gut wall, and how much by other causes.

Anti-LPS antibodies were protective against heatstroke in vervet monkeys up to a core temperature of 43.5° C but no higher.[159] This suggests that LPS-induced toxicity is important in the pathophysiology of heatstroke death only up to 43.5° C. Since anti-LPS provided no protection above this temperature, other mechanisms, such as direct thermal damage to nervous tissue, were more important.

LPS had previously been implicated as a factor in heatstroke death by indirect observations. Injection of very low doses of LPS leads to a rapid "tolerance" to ordinarily lethal doses of LPS.[177] DuBose and colleagues[119] found that administration of low doses of LPS protected rats against heatstroke and considered that LPS may be involved in heatstroke death, although they could not detect LPS in the circulation at the time. Consistent with a role for LPS they also

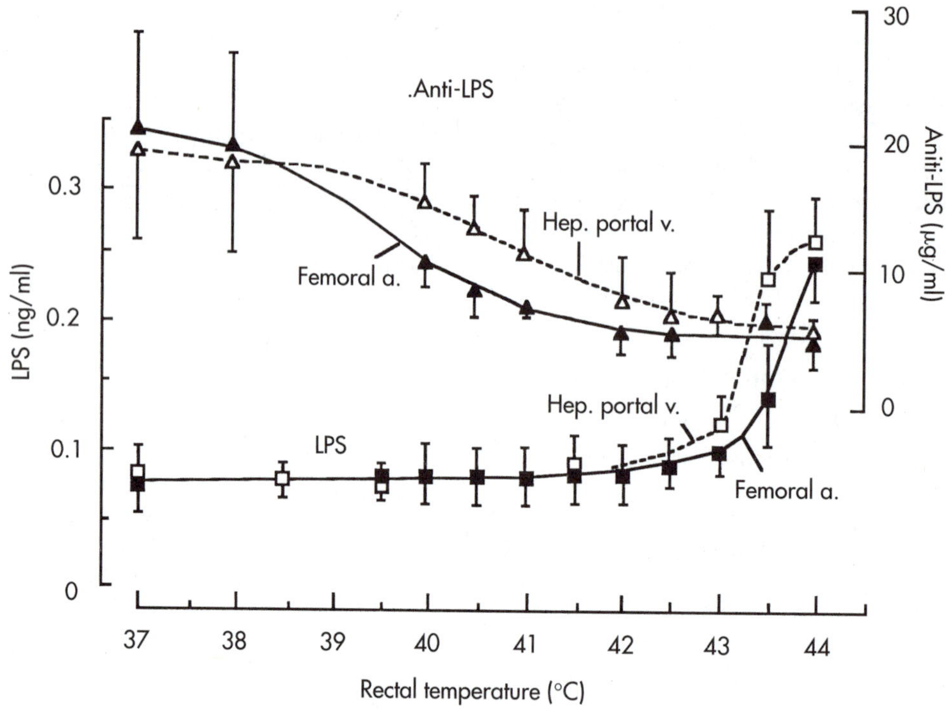

Fig. 8-6 Endotoxemia caused by heatstroke in anesthetized nonhuman primates. At T_{re} of 42° to 43° C, plasma lipopolysaccharide (LPS) concentration rose first in the hepatic portal vein and 10 to 15 minutes later in the systemic circulation. However, a decline in "consumed" anti-LPS antibodies occurred at temperatures as low as 39° to 40° C. (Redrawn from Gathiram P et al: *Circ Shock* 25:223, 1988.)

found[120] that when the activity of the reticuloendothelial system (the main mechanism for removal of LPS from the circulation) was reduced, the mortality of heatstroke increased. Gisolfi and co-workers[353] recently found the inverse effect. Rats were stressed with a T_{amb} of 47° to 50° C until their core temperatures reached 42.5° C and then were passively cooled. When they were injected with a high dose of LPS the next day, the mortality rate dropped from 71% in the control rats to zero in the heat-stressed rats.

The importance of LPS in heatstroke death was confirmed in an important study by Hayano[192] in a canine model of heatstroke. Hayano raised core temperature to 42.5° C, maintained this temperature for 3 hours, and then cooled the animals to 38° C, while taking serial blood samples through a catheter. He found that deaths occurred only in dogs that showed rises in plasma LPS concentrations. However, other pathophysiologic mechanisms were probably involved.

Exertional Heatstroke

Several recent studies support the idea that the immune system and LPS are involved in the pathophysiology of heatstroke. Leukocytosis is a general response to most forms of stress. It occurs following short-term and long-term muscular activity,[156] the administration of epinephrine or glucocorticoid, and excitement. Prolonged or severe exercise initiates mobilization and activation of neutrophils and causes proteolysis of skeletal muscle and production of acute phase proteins by the liver.[71] It has been suggested that exercise leads to local disruption of tissues and sloughing of tissue fragments that circulate and activate the complement system. This activation primes monocytes for further activation by LPS or by fragments of tissue subsequently damaged.[75]

Furthermore, severe exercise damaged renal function, causing a 100-fold increase in urinary excretion of proteins that was so profound that it led to an actual depletion of circulating antibodies.[331] Although it is well known that hyperthermia in humans results in a reduction in splanchnic blood flow,[333] only recently has sufficient evidence accumulated to provide a mechanism of how this may contribute to the pathophysiology of heatstroke. To consider the relationship of this evidence to heatstroke it is necessary to consider the contents of the intestinal lumen and the likely results of its leakage into the systemic circulation.

Fine and co-workers[173] noted in a heatstroke victim that the clinical signs, including blood clotting disturbances, were similar to those in septic shock cases. LPS activates a blood factor leading to disseminated intravascular coagulation,[288,451] a common complication of septic shock. The authors therefore suggested that LPS participates in the pathophysiology of heatstroke.

Since core temperatures of long-distance runners may rise above 40° C, we examined runners who collapsed during an ultramarathon (89.5 km) on a warm day[61] and those who managed to reach or who were carried into the medical tent at the finish line. Blood samples were taken from 98 patients before therapy. Eighteen of them had plasma LPS levels raised above normal values, including two in the 1 ng/ml lethal range! It should be noted that the body can tolerate short periods of much higher concentrations, and the conventional lethal concentration of 1 ng/ml refers to a long-term level even after all detoxifying mechanisms come into play.[434] While hypovolemia resulting from sweating may have caused a few "high normals" to cross into the elevated range, this could not have been the majority. Of those who finished the race, the smaller group with the low normal levels finished faster. Furthermore, this normal group had significantly higher levels of "natural" anti-LPS in their plasma; that is, the presence of high levels of anti-LPS antibodies correlated with low levels of LPS and better performance. This low LPS and high anti-LPS group also had reduced indices of nausea, vomiting, and headache and recovered faster (within 2 hours) than did the larger high LPS and low anti-LPS group (up to 2 days).

In triathlon participants the concentrations of anti-LPS antibodies fell and LPS rose at the end of the third race.[51] Some athletes had higher levels of "natural" anti-LPS antibodies than did others. When individuals were questioned about their training regimen, it became clear that those who trained the hardest in terms of miles swum, bicycled, and run the 3 weeks before the triathlon had the highest levels of anti-LPS. It may be that a part of the benefit of physical training is the increase in levels of natural anti-LPS antibodies. We proposed that as a result of severe training, temporary periods of intestinal ischemia occurred, leading to the entry of low to moderate levels of LPS into the circulation, which was enough to stimulate the immune system.

In a different study a marathon was run on a cold day.[311a] In this case no elevations in plasma LPS were seen. At present it is not clear what combinations of heat load and exertional factors are required for LPS increases.

Classic Heatstroke and Cytokines

The survival of hospitalized heatstroke patients is certainly related in part to the rapidity of cooling on entry to a hospital intensive care unit. This time factor may be important because of the time required for the production of cytokines, which is in the range of minutes to hours. Bouchama and colleagues[55] studied 17 Hadj patients with classic (nonexertional) heatstroke who were admitted to a hospital an average of 2 hours following the onset of heatstroke. They had core temperatures greater than 40.1° C and suffered from delirium, convulsions, and coma. Their plasma LPS concentrations ranged from 8 to 12 ng/ml, values that must be considered extremely high and in the potentially lethal range.[423] Furthermore, their TNF concentration was elevated by a factor of 8 to 247 pg/ml, and IL-1 was elevated to 480 pg/ml, a value 11 times that of healthy controls. The authors suggested that those cytokines exacerbated the hyperthermia of heatstroke, possibly through the induction of prostaglandins.

Bouchama and colleagues[54] further studied the immune systems of 11 patients with heatstroke. They compared the distribution of leukocyte subgroups and found in 9 of 11 patients a marked leukocytosis that increased with increasing core temperature. This resulted from a large increase in the number of T suppressor cytotoxic cells (CD8) and natural killer (NK) cells (CD16/CD56). There were also substantial decreases in T helper cells (CD4) and B cells (CD19) as a result of heatstroke. Rises in catecholamine levels also occurred during heatstroke.[3] Since the administration of epinephrine causes leukocytosis with an increase in NK and T suppressor cytotoxic cells, Bouchama suggested that the elevated catecholamine levels induced by heat stress caused the changes in lymphocyte subpopulations.

On the other hand, hyperthermia causes an increase in cortisol.[228,229] Cortisol administration is known to cause lymphocytopenia.[54] In the preceding study 2 of the 11 heatstroke patients had a decreased number of lymphocytes. To account for the reduction in lymphocytes, the authors suggested that in those two patients the effects of cortisol, rather than of catecholamines, were dominant. That is, changes in subpopulations of lymphocytes in heatstroke may depend (on an individual basis) on the relative rises in concentration of catecholamines and cortisol, as well as upon individual sensitivities to them. However, this is not yet clearly established.

Exertional Heatstroke and Cytokines

There are few recent studies of cytokines and exercise. Smith and colleagues[387] found little change in plasma cytokines after acute moderate exercise. However, this may have been due to faulty tissue taking, since when urine samples taken after a race were examined in a different study, large increases in interferon, TNF, IL-1, IL-6, and soluble IL-2r were found.[392] The authors further suggested that under conditions of stress the failure to detect changes in plasma cytokine concentrations may be due to rapid renal clearance from the circulation. Cannon and colleagues[73] found that "endogenous pyrogen" (now recognized as IL-1), which causes fever, was present in plasma taken after completion of severe exercise and that IL-1 was present in human skeletal muscle after eccentric exercise, conditions that damage skeletal muscle.[74] IL-1 causes muscle proteolysis by inducing branched chain keto acid dehydrogenase. This is a rate-limiting enzyme for the oxidation of amino acids in skeletal muscle. As this enzyme increases in concentration, amino acids are progressively oxidized, leading to muscle protein breakdown. Ingestion of vitamin E prevented a rise in IL-1 in vitro from leukocytes obtained from persons subjected to severe exercise.[75]

Haq and colleagues[184] examined blood samples taken from runners before and after a marathon race. Leukocyte levels rose from 7.8 to 22.9 × 10^9/L and cortisol concentration rose from 242 to 1004 nm/L. The concentrations of CD3, CD16 (NK T cells), and CD19 (B cells) lymphocytes fell, although no change in absolute lymphocyte count occurred.

Overtraining may be harmful. A combination of intense training and stress of competition makes some athletes immunosuppressed and more susceptible to infection. There may be a point at which laboratory techniques can quantitatively determine that the disadvantage of immunosuppression is greater than any benefit from exercise training and that exercise should be curtailed.[184]

Heat-Related Illnesses

VARIANTS OF HEATSTROKE

A number of clinical situations arise in which hyperthermia develops that is sufficiently severe (greater than 40° C) as to be considered for inclusion as a subgroup of exertional heatstroke. Malignant hyperthermia, neuroleptic seizures, and overdose of recreational drugs share the features of massive muscle contractions (with consequent overuse of high-energy compounds) and rhabdomyolysis—both features of exertional heatstroke.[252] Since the use of recreational drugs is not expected to decline significantly and the number of persons using neuroleptic drugs is probably on the increase, the involvement of heatstroke pathophysiology should be considered in treating those cases. Conversely, an apparent case of heatstroke in a summertime vacation area might be complicated by the preceding considerations.

Malignant Hyperthermia

Malignant hyperthermia is a rare and often fatal clinical syndrome involving hypermetabolism, triggered by halogenated anesthetics or depolarizing muscle relaxants.[94,426] It is believed that the anesthetic destabilizes membranes (such as the sarcoplasmic reticulum [SR]) associated with calcium pumping, leading to massive calcium entry into cells and activation of contractile apparatus, calmodulin, and a variety of calcium-sensitive enzymes. These in turn lead to muscle rigidity, hypercatabolism, fulminating hyperthermia, and metabolic acidosis.[94] In a strain of susceptible swine it is the calcium channel (ryanodine receptor) that is genetically defective and responsible for the effect.[426] In humans, malignant hyperthermia is due to a defect in a gene located on the short arm of chromosome 19 close to the calcium release channel of the SR.[24] Rhabdomyolysis, hyperkalemia, and myoglobinemia[366] are common, with plasma potassium levels rising as high as 10 mmol/L.[290] Dantrolene therapy appears critical for survival.

Neuroleptic Seizure

The treatment of psychiatric patients with neuroleptic drugs, as well as with antidepressants, antiemetics, and others,[125] may lead to the uncommon but often fatal neuroleptic malignant syndrome, characterized by hyperthermia as high as 42° C,[6] "lead pipe" skeletal muscle rigidity, dyspnea, coma, extrapyramidal syndrome, rhabdomyolysis, severe metabolic acidosis, leukocytosis, and elevated creatine phosphokinase.[193,223,406] A number of factors predispose to neuroleptic seizure, including dehydration, exhaustion, aggression, and restraints,[218] high environmental temperature, high doses of neuroleptics, abrupt discontinuation of antiparkinsonism agents, and administration of lithium.[125] Successful treatment includes immediate withdrawal of the drug, administration of dantrolene, and either oral bromocriptine or the combination of levodopa and carbidopa.[125]

Drug Overdose

While the toxicity of drug overdose is well recognized, it is not often appreciated that the hyperthermia attained can be in the range reported for heatstroke. Such hyperthermia has been induced with cocaine[114] and amphetamine derivatives such as MDMA ("ecstasy") and MDEA ("Eve").[407] Other components of this syndrome include hyperkalemia, rhabdomyolysis,[384] sympathetic hyperactivity, convulsions, rectorrhagia, psychosis, disseminated intravascular coagulation in the absence of positive blood cultures, and acute renal failure.[194]

Susceptibility to Heatstroke

There may be an inherited susceptibility to what appears to be exertional heatstroke. Muscle biopsy specimens taken from two men in military service who had recovered from exertional heatstroke had abnormal responses to halothane, a well-known cause of malignant hyperthermia.[426] Furthermore, muscles from members of their families had abnormal responses to halothane or ryanodine, a drug that binds to the Ca^{++} release channels of the sarcoplasmic reticulum.[202] A ryanodine contracture test has been proposed as an in vitro diagnostic test to screen for surgical patients who are susceptible to malignant hyperthermia.[202] This test might be useful in identifying, retrospectively, a possible subgroup of patients with exertional heatstroke.

CHANGES IN COGNITIVE FUNCTION

Changes in cognitive function appear to occur before the development of the physical symptoms associated with heat stress.[78] Time distortion,[33,34,107] memory impairment,[439] deterioration in attention, and decreased ability to calculate mathematical problems[81,178,438] are frequent cognitive characteristics associated with heat stress. Health care personnel should be trained to recognize that confusion, changes in affect, and impaired ability to function in the work environment can be early signs of heat injury under heat stress conditions.[78]

Vasovagal Syncope

Syncope is the cause of about 3% of emergency department visits and 6% of hospital admissions.[162] Syncope seen in emergency departments, outpatient departments, and long-term care settings is often of the vasovagal variety; clinical studies report it as the cause of syncope in 28% to 38% of patients aged 35 to 39 years.[111,227,287] Examples of benign presyncope or syncope resulting from diminished venous return to the heart because of blood pooling in the peripheral circulation include psychologic disturbances activating an autonomic vasodilation response; reflex syncope caused by heavy coughing, micturition, or pressure on an irritable carotid sinus; or reduced vasomotor tone caused by hypotensive drugs or alcohol.[126]

Interestingly, the same data bases suggest a decreased prevalence of vasovagal syncope in the old compared with the young.[273] Propranolol did not prevent the vasovagal reaction in response to head-up tilt.[273] Orthostatic hypotension is probably more common in older persons.[273] As a result, presyncope after the age of 40 may suggest a more serious condition (such as gastrointestinal bleeding, myocardial or valvular heat disease, or severe anemia). Cardiovascular syncope resulting from arrhythmia carries a 1-year mortality rate of about 30%.[226]

Hyperventilation Dizziness

Generalized cerebrovascular vasoconstriction with ischemia may occur as the result of a slight but prolonged increase in respiratory rate or tidal volume and may simply accompany an increase in anxiety.[126]

Heat-Induced Syncope

The clinical syndromes associated with exposure to heat vary in severity with cause and therefore so does the duration of central nervous system dysfunction. Transient or temporary loss of consciousness associated with a mild form of heat syncope has its origins primarily in the cardiovascular system. It is a problem of effective blood volume rather than an actual volume deficit.

The gravitational displacement of blood into dependent limbs of an upright and stationary person combined with hemodynamic displacement of blood into the peripheral circulation to support heat transfer at the body surface can temporarily compromise venous return, cardiac output, and cerebral perfusion. Patients are usually erect at the outset and sometimes report prodromal symptoms of restlessness, nausea, sighing, yawning, and dysphoria.[243] The hypotension results predominantly from vasodilation and bradycardia. This systemic disorder is considered self-limited because when the person faints, it is remedied by the assumption of a horizontal position.

Fainting is usually brief and responds to horizontal positioning and improved venous return. The patient should be allowed to rest in cooler, shadier surroundings and be offered replacement fluids, perhaps a commercial glucose-electrolyte product. The patient should be cautioned against protracted standing in hot environments, advised to flex leg muscles repeatedly while standing to enhance venous return, and warned to assume a sitting or horizontal position at the onset of warning signs or symptoms, such as vertigo, nausea, or weakness. Normally muscles in the legs act as a "second heart" and in concert with venous valves promote venous return, thereby counteracting orthostatic pooling and the predisposition to syncope. In fact, intramuscular pressure is higher in nonfainters.

The transient loss of consciousness in syncope must have a metabolic basis within ischemic cells of the brain. Despite this, the effects, although startling to onlookers and frightening to the patient, appear readily reversible. There is no risk of direct thermal injury to brain cells complicating the circulatory origin of this sudden decline in effective arterial volume.

The incidence of syncopal attacks falls rapidly with increasing days of work in the heat (Fig. 8-4), suggesting the importance of salt and water retention in preventing this disorder.[207] Thus individuals medicated with diuretics would be at increased risk. Knochel[254] has commented on the potential role that potassium depletion and hypokalemia could play by lowering blood pressure and blunting cardiovascular responsiveness. In stark contrast to simple syncope is the profound central nervous system dysfunction dominating the early course of heatstroke. Thus if a person faints in a setting where hyperthermia is possible and does *not* rapidly return to consciousness, heatstroke should be suspected and body temperature measured.

EXERTION-INDUCED SYNCOPE, CRAMPS, AND RESPIRATORY ALKALOSIS

Syncopal episodes associated with heat exhaustion in military personnel during basic training were described by Boyd and Beller.[36,37,58,59] In contrast to hypovolemic salt depletion, this heat exhaustion represents a rarely described nonclassic form of heat exhaustion characterized by hyperventilation, respiratory alkalosis, syncope, and tetany. A majority of these patients had experienced abdominal cramps, yet this type of heat exhaustion is independent of lactic acidosis and hyponatremia. Their observations were unique in several respects: the heat syncope episodes were not those classically described as the venous pooling or postural hypotension variety[31,311]; the patients with heat exhaustion exhibited a moderate to marked respiratory alkalosis, but only two appeared to be severely dehydrated; nearly all (16 of 17 patients) had severe abdominal or extremity muscle cramps; incapacitated trainees arrived at a heat ward within 10 to 30 minutes of the onset of symptoms; and brachial artery blood samples were drawn immediately on admission.

Clinical data recorded on admission are shown in Table 8-2. Almost all the casualties occurred in the afternoon during July 1971 at Fort Polk, Louisiana. All were diagnosed as heat exhaustion resulting from training in the field (12 of 17 while speed marching). Rectal temperatures on admission were elevated, even though the victims had been doused with water before evacuation (11 of 17) and a similar number had experienced syncope. Of 17 patients, 16 had abdominal or extremity muscle cramps as major symptoms. Serum electrolytes were in the normal range in the majority of the patients. However, hemoconcentration with elevated serum sodium level was observed in patients 4, 6, 11, and 15. Only 1 of 17 patients (patient 12) had a low serum sodium level and also experienced severe muscle cramps.

The majority of these patients were not water or salt depleted, and 15 of the 16 remaining patients with cramps had normal to elevated serum sodium and chloride levels (not shown). The mean arterial pH for this group of patients was 7.62 ± 0.03 (SEM), and 5 had a pH of 7.67 or greater. Arterial PCO_2 was reduced to a mean value of 23.5 ± 2 mm Hg. Thus all patients had moderate to marked respiratory alkalosis, and 9 had obvious tetany with carpopedal spasm.[59] The presence of carpopedal spasm and paresthesias in the distal extremities and perioral area helps distinguish this form of cramps from the classic variety.

These data associate exertion-induced heat exhaustion with a form of respiratory alkalosis characterized by syncope, tetany, and muscle cramps and may possibly be the result of "an exaggeration of the normal physiological ventilatory response to thermal extremes."[59] Hyperventilation with its resulting decrease in cerebral blood flow[234,378,424] could account for a significant number of cases of exercise-induced heat syncope. Recumbency, rest, and oral replacement of fluid and electrolyte deficits are usual recommendations. Rebreathing of expired air is directed at alleviating carpopedal spasms but should be done with extreme caution because of its hypoxemic effect.

Classic syncope is usually associated with postural hypotension, whereas heat exhaustion and heat cramps are usually associated with water and electrolyte imbalance.[263,266] Thus this series is a good example of the "mixed bag" reality of heat illness symptoms.

Anderson and associates[8] have suggested that heat-acclimated individuals are more prone to heat cramps based on increased exercise tolerance and greater maximum sweat rates combining to produce higher salt losses despite reduced sweat sodium concentrations. The basis for this assumption depends on significantly higher sweat rates (2.5 versus 1.5 L/hr) for the acclimated individuals and the notion that both groups would voluntarily work at maximum sweat rates for any given task. Most workers suggest that the opposite is true. Table 8-1 suggests higher salt losses for unacclimated individuals at any given sweat rate or volume of sweat lost. The differential diagnosis of heat cramps should also include exercise-induced peritonitis.[402]

Table 8-2 Clinical Data in 17 Patients with Heat Exhaustion

Case No.	Age	Activity	Syncope	Cramps	T_{re}	RR	Na^+	pH	PCO_2
1	19	Marching	Yes	Abd	99.6	24	142	—	—
2	20	Running mile	Yes	Legs/abd	98.4	30	145	—	—
3	20	Rifle range	No	No	99.4	24	143	—	—
4	21	Marching/running	Yes	Hands	100.4	22	162	7.47	34.0
5	21	Marching	No	Severe abd/legs	102.4	35	141	7.50	32.4
6	22	Marching	No	Legs	100.0	22	152	7.70	14.8
7	20	Rifle range	No	Mild	100.0	22	140	—	—
8	20	Marching	Yes	Abd/legs	100.8	30	145	7.52	28.8
9	20	Marching	No	Abd	101.4	24	—	7.69	19.8
10	18	Marching	Yes	Chest	100.8	18	140	7.56	29.4
11	19	Marching	Yes	Tetany	101.5	30	160	7.44	34.2
12	18	Marching	Yes	Severe	100.6	30	130	7.71	17.2
13	20	Marching	No	Mild	98.6	26	141	7.77	15.2
14	19	Marching	Yes	Abd/legs	100.7	30	145	7.76	16.3
15	23	Rifle range	Yes	Abd/legs	101.0	32	148	7.66	19.7
16	18	Marching	Yes	Chest/legs	101.2	28	148	7.78	14.7
17	17	Marching	Yes	Abd	101.6	22	146	7.53	28.4

RR, Respiratory rate; *Abd*, abdomen.

HEAT-INDUCED TETANY

Haldane[180] reported that men at rest hyperventilated in excessively hot environments. Adolph and Fulton[2] described dyspnea and tingling in the hands and feet of men being dehydrated in the heat. Wingfield[440] in 1941 presented the single case of a ship's engineer who experienced spontaneous hyperventilation and attacks of tetany during a voyage through the intense heat of the Persian Gulf. Since deliberate overbreathing by the subject would reproduce his symptoms, this appeared to be the first clinical description of heat-induced hyperventilation tetany.

Iampietro and co-workers[214,215] in our laboratory studied the physiologic changes and onset of symptoms (slight tingling of the feet and hands to more severe carpopedal spasms) during the exposure of male test subjects to hot, wet conditions. The frequency and severity of symptoms were apparently not related to the absolute change in measured parameters (P_{CO_2}, CO_2, pH, and T_{re}) but rather to the rate of change as depicted in Fig. 8-7.

As can be noted, there was no relationship between the absolute change and the incidence of symptoms, since the slopes of the lines were not significantly different from zero. In contrast, a direct relationship exists between the rate of change of the four parameters and the incidence of symptoms. When the subject's tolerance time was short, changes occurred rapidly and the incidence of symptoms was high; conversely, when the tolerance time was long, the same degree of change occurred but the incidence of symptoms was low. The authors speculated that "rapid changes lead to imbalance between intra- and extracellular compartments and that this imbalance may be one of the factors inducing symptoms." Again, treatment consists of rest, cooling, and rebreathing expired air.

The preceding information suggests that the cell membrane may be the locus of events (driving functions, activators, or inhibitors) affecting metabolic regulation and thereby driving homeostatic mechanisms to the limits of normal function. For example, Hochachka and Matheson[198,199] recently discussed ATPases and energy metabolism as proactive and reactive components in control of ATP turnover rates. In discussing the need for a new control paradigm for metabolic regulation, the authors came to the significant conclusion that "key control elements of energy-yielding pathways must lie essentially external to the pathways per se since the concentrations of none of the intermediates change by a factor large enough to directly cause the flux change."

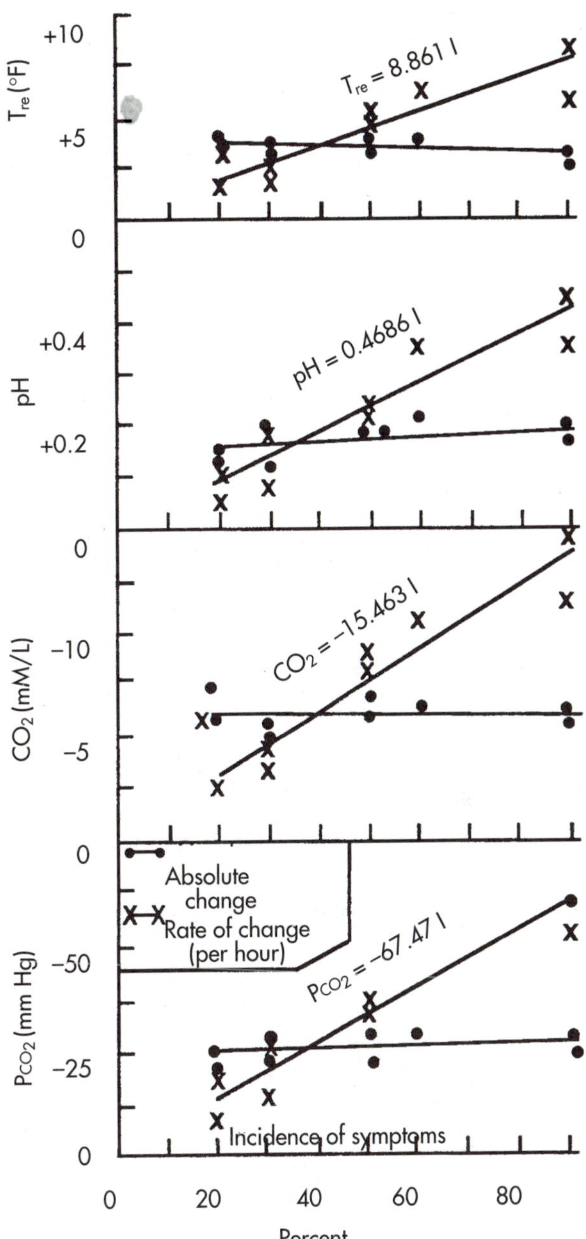

Fig. 8-7 Comparison of absolute change and rate of change of P_{CO_2}, CO_2, pH, and T_{re} with incidence of heat-induced tetany. Rate of change values were obtained by dividing the absolute change during exposure by the exposure time in minutes and multiplying by 60. (From Iampietro PF: *Fed Proc* 22:884, 1963.)

HEAT CRAMPS

Heat cramps are a frequent complication of heat exhaustion. For example, muscle cramps occurred in about 60% of 532 cases of heat exhaustion reviewed by Leithead and Lind[266,397] and in another 437 cases reported by Collings and associates.[90] However, the patient with salt depletion heat exhaustion is obviously ill and has numerous other symptoms. Cramps may not be either the earliest or the most prominent symptom, since fatigue, giddiness, nausea, and vomiting are common.

Heat cramps sometimes occur as the only complaint with minimal systemic symptoms. Talbott[404,405] published the classic description of heat cramps. During the 1930s, steel workers, coal miners, sugar cane cutters, and boiler operators were among the most common victims. Three factors common to most reports are that (1) cramps are preceded by several hours of sustained effort, combining (2) heavy sweating in hot surroundings with (3) the ingestion of large volumes of water. A fourth factor (see later discussion) may be cooling of the muscles. Talbott[405] recorded serum sodium levels ranging from 121 to 140 mEq/L. Thus the hyponatremia and hypochloremia diagnostic of heat cramps[254] might be due to a salt deficit or some degree of water intoxication. If overdrinking causes gastric distention, feelings of nausea[337] could trigger vasopressin release and contribute to renal water retention. Heat cramps are more common later in the day in an industrial setting; they sometimes occur while the person is showering and occasionally occur in the evening.[266] Since the brief, intermittent, or often excruciating contractions occur in muscles subjected to intensive activity and fatigue, and because exposure to heat in itself does not cause them, heat cramps is a misnomer.

Classic heat cramps are distinguished from hyperventilation-induced tetany because they generally involve voluntary skeletal muscle subjected to prior exertion. The cramps usually affect only a few muscle bundles at a time. As one bundle relaxes, an adjacent bundle contracts for 1 to 3 minutes. The cramp thus appears to wander over the affected muscle, but the pain can be excruciating in severe cases. Knochel and Reed[254] note that three precipitating conditions (exhaustive work, hemodilution, and cooling the muscle) can each account for depolarizing the muscle cell. This could explain the association of cramps with showering in cool water, since cooling slows sodium transport and depolarizes the cell.[385] The low incidence of heat cramps within the Indian Armed Forces[280] and the fact that Shibolet observed no cases within Israeli Defense Forces suggests that heat-acclimated individuals are less likely to experience them. This is consistent with Ladell's analysis[262] and Talbott's observation[405] that the incidence was greatest during the first few days of a heat wave. He also described the difficulty in distinguishing abdominal heat cramps from gastrointestinal upset.

Heat cramps generally respond quickly to salt solutions. Mild cases may be treated orally with 0.1% to 0.2% salt solutions (2 to 4 ten grain salt tablets [56 to 112 mEq] or ¼ to ½ teaspoon table salt dissolved in a quart of water). Cooling and flavoring enhance palatability. Oral salt tablets are gastric irritants and are not recommended. In severe cases intravenous isotonic saline (0.9% NaCl) or small amounts of hypertonic saline (3% NaCl) are administered by physicians for rapid relief.

HEAT EXHAUSTION

Classic heat exhaustion, like classic heatstroke, tends to develop over several days or longer and presents ample opportunity for electrolyte and water imbalance to occur. The hyponatremia and hypochloremia of patients with either heat cramps or salt depletion heat exhaustion often develop over 3 to 5 days[265] and usually manifest in the unacclimatized individual who has not fully developed his salt-conserving mechanisms.[388,389] Thirst is not as prominent in salt depletion heat exhaustion as are muscle cramps, nausea, and vomiting.[207,209] The major route of fluid and electrolyte imbalance (salt depletion, water depletion, water intoxication) involved in a particular heat exhaustion case[70,254,266,414] can be discovered from the events surrounding the collapse and a careful history.

Classic heat exhaustion is a manifestation of cardiovascular strain resulting from maintaining normothermia. The symptoms of heat exhaustion include various combinations of headache, dizziness, fatigue, hyperirritability, anxiety, piloerection, chills, nausea, vomiting, heat cramps, and heat sensations in the head and upper torso.[15,18,207] Clinical descriptions include tachycardia, hyperventilation, hypotension, and syncope. Although the boundary between heat exhaustion and heatstroke is usually defined as 39.4° to 40.0° C, the differential diagnosis is often tenuous[189] or even considered artificial.[379] The patient may collapse with either a normal or an elevated temperature (severe cases around 40° C), usually with profuse sweating. Spontaneous body cooling can occur, which is not prominent in severe heatstroke. The clinical determination of heat exhaustion is primarily a diagnosis of exclusion.[70]

The alternate forms of heat exhaustion are characterized by the type of fluid or electrolyte deficit (primarily pure water or salt deficiency), their underlying causes (prolonged heat exposure versus intense, short-term exertion), the intensity of the hyperthermia, and the absence or form of central nervous system disturbance. For example, Table 8-1 is a theoretical demonstration of the impact of body weight loss as either pure water or sweat of varying salt concentrations. If external cooling does not rapidly lower core temperature to normal or, conversely, precipitates severe shivering, intercurrent illness is suspected. It is our anecdotal experience that in the field approximately 20% of persons with suspected heat exhaustion have some form of viral or bacterial gastroenteritis. This is especially true if nonchlorinated water or ice is available.

At any percent body weight loss (Table 8-1) the decrement in plasma volume increases with the salt content of sweat. This would be the case for relatively unacclimated individuals. On the other hand, the more dilute the sweat (approaching a pure water deficit), the greater the increase in osmolality, plasma, sodium, and thirst. A more refined model such as this could be constructed from a basic hypothetical premise and, if it included derived values for hemoglobin or hematocrit concentrations, might provide a useful guide to diagnosis or therapy. Table 8-3 attempts to compare and contrast the various signs and symptoms of salt and wa-

Table 8-3 Signs and Symptoms of Salt and Water Depletion Heat Exhaustion

Signs and Symptoms	Salt Depletion Heat Exhaustion	Water Depletion Heat Exhaustion	Dilutional Hyponatremia[19,381a]
Recent weight gain	No	No	Yes
Thirst	Not prominent	Yes	Sometimes
Muscle cramps	In most cases	No	Sometimes
Nausea	Yes	Yes	Usually
Vomiting	In most cases	No	Usually
Muscle fatigue or weakness	Yes	Yes	No
Loss of skin turgor	Yes	Yes	No
Mental dullness, apathy	Yes	Yes	Yes
Orthostatic rise in pulse rate	Yes	Yes	No
Tachycardia	Yes	Yes	No
Dry mucous membranes	Yes	Yes	No
Increased rectal temperature	Yes	In most cases	No
Urine Na^+/Cl^-	Negligible	Normal	Low
Plasma Na^+/Cl^-	Below average	Above average	Below average

ter depletion heat exhaustion with dilutional hyponatremia. It is clear that at some point both syndromes share many symptoms. Vomiting and cramps appear to signal a significant sodium deficit in addition to some degree of water deficit.

HEAT ILLNESS AND COEXISTENT DISEASE

It has long been known that coexistent illness or infection predisposes an individual to heatstroke.[165] As emphasized by Wilcox,[437] a gastrointestinal (choleraic) type of heat illness occurred in 11.2% of his cases. The reverse is also true: heat waves produce excess deaths from all categories of disease. For example, Ellis[132] reported that in one heat wave week in New York in the late summer of 1948, deaths from diseases of the heart and arteries more than doubled (1364 versus 585), deaths from diabetes more than doubled, and pneumonia deaths tripled.

Despite data of this type, which suggest that infection predisposes to heat illness and that heat stress exacerbates illness,[269] little is known about the susceptibility to infection during heat exposure or the influence of infection on heat tolerance. In fact, a recent case report on temporary, acquired heat intolerance has called for further research into the effects of viral disease on thermoregulation.[232]

Clinical Observations in Heatstroke

The clinical manifestations of heatstroke vary, depending on whether the patient suffers from classic heatstroke or exertional heatstroke (Table 8-4). Some overlap in presentation may occur; treatment with a medication that places an elder at risk for classic heatstroke also places the exercising individual at risk for exertional heatstroke.

CHANGES IN BLOOD PARAMETERS

Hyperthermia in experimental animals or in humans results in temporary leukocytosis.[54,182] Disturbances in the blood coagulation system were present in all fatal cases of exertional heatstroke reported by Shibolet and co-workers.[378,380] Prothrombin levels were at 17% to 43%, depending on the severity of heatstroke, with thrombocyte values between 47 to $110 \times 10^3/mm^3$ and zero.[378,380] A similar disturbance in clotting proteins was found in a case of heatstroke by Graber,[173] who suggested that perhaps LPS participates in the pathophysiology of heatstroke.

Significant lay interest, scientific research, and commercial product development and marketing have focused on electrolyte abnormalities associated with physical exertion under a variety of conditions. The marked variability of electrolyte content in sweat and intensity of physical activity, along with ambient temperature and humidity and the preexisting state of hydration in the individual, all contribute to the degree of abnormalities observed.

Plasma Volume Changes

Physical exertion causes changes in plasma volume, which depends on a variety of factors: environmental conditions, intensity and duration of exercise, preexisting and coexisting state of hydration, and level of heat acclimatization. In a cool environment, plasma volume is maintained or even increased with exercise.[87] However, in the heat a few minutes' burst of supramaximal exercise causes a biphasic reduction in plasma volume.[27] Initially an increase in intracapillary hydrostatic pressure draws fluid from the intravascular to the extravascular space. The secondary reduction in plasma volume is believed to be caused by a transcapillary osmotic gradient created by the efflux of potassium and metabolites from the contracting muscle. Surprisingly, the

Table 8-4 Comparison of Classic and Exertional Heatstroke

	Classic	Exertional
Age group	Elderly	Men (15-45 yr)
Health status	Chronically ill	Healthy
Concurrent activity	Sedentary	Strenuous exercise
Drug use	Diuretics, antidepressants, antihypertensives, anticholinergics, antipsychotics	Usually none
Sweating	May be absent	Usually present
Lactic acidosis	Usually absent; poor prognosis if present	Common
Hyperkalemia	Usually absent	Often present
Hypocalcemia	Uncommon	Frequent
Hypoglycemia	Uncommon	Common
Creatine phosphokinase/aldolase	Mildly elevated	Markedly elevated
Rhabdomyolysis	Unusual	Frequently severe
Hyperuricemia	Mild	Severe
Acute renal failure	<5% of patients	25% to 30% of patients
Disseminated intravascular coagulation	Mild	Marked; poor prognosis
Mechanism	Poor dissipation of environmental heat	Excessive endogenous heat production and overwhelming of heat loss mechanisms

Modified from Knochel JP, Reed G: Disorders of heat regulation. In Kleeman CR, Maxwell MH, Narin RG, editors: *Clinical disorders of fluid and electrolyte metabolism,* New York, 1987, McGraw-Hill.

combined processes result in an overall reduction of plasma volume by 10% to 15% within 30 seconds.

The sweating associated with intense physical activity of 30 minutes or more causes a decrease in total body water; if these fluid losses are not replaced, a further reduction in plasma volume results.

Potassium

Normal concentration of potassium in sweat is 4 to 5 mmol/L. This concentration is not significantly affected by prolonged sweating, heat acclimation, or dietary intake of potassium.[98] Early studies reported development of potassium deficiency after repeated bouts of intense exercise under hot conditions.[251] This deficiency was believed to represent potassium loss in sweat. Later studies under similar conditions have documented normal plasma and muscle potassium levels associated with reduced urinary potassium excretion. The hyperkalemia that develops in heatstroke victims may represent failure of the sodium pump at the cell membrane level.

The literature is contradictory regarding the effect of heat stress on plasma potassium concentration. This may be expected if hypokalemia predisposes to heatstroke[150,229] and the resultant cellular damage returns plasma values to near normal or above. In some studies plasma K^+ levels in human subjects rose during heat and exercise.[149,329] During prolonged exercise, elevations in potassium concentrations are usually seen[370] and may cause vasodilation of terminal blood vessels within active skeletal muscles. Several days' training lowered this increase in extracellular K^+ for a given workload. It also improved cardiovascular stability and the ability to dissipate heat. Lundvall[277] thought that an increase in plasma potassium from exercise was caused by a large number of muscle membrane depolarizations. This elevated K^+ concentration could be reduced by insulin injection, but performance was not improved.

While classic heatstroke patients appear to have normal potassium levels, patients with exertional heatstroke often show hyperkalemia and rhabdomyolysis. However, Shibolet and co-workers[380] found variable potassium levels in their heatstroke patients ranging from hypokalemia to hyperkalemia. Anderson and co-workers[7] studied anesthetized and curarized cancer patients heated in a 50° C bath up to a core temperature of 42° C. They found that serum K^+ rose slowly to a plateau of 0.5 mEq/L above baseline, remained at this value for 3 hours, and then slowly declined, even though T_c remained at 42° C. The mechanism for this is not clear.

On the other hand, Shapiro and Cristal[373] stated that hyperthermia in humans leads first to hypokalemia, probably because of respiratory alkalosis, increased renal secretion, and loss in sweat. This is followed by metabolic acidosis and hyperkalemia when a potential combination of impaired renal function and general cellular damage develops. Khogali and colleagues[240] found that the majority of their patients suffering from heatstroke had hypovolemia but with normokalemia or hypokalemia, with concentrations as low as 2 mEq/L or less. Furthermore, once the hypovolemia had been corrected, their potassium levels fell still further. Morimoto[298] noted that during exercise and heating in humans there was a loss of potassium ion of 0.225 mEq/100 g body mass (70% into urine and 30% into saliva). The Na^+,K^+-ATPase pump appears stable up to 44° C, at which temperature the rate of ATPase is approximately double that at 37° C.[123,393,395]

Only about 2% of total body potassium is extracellular. Therefore the intracellular environment can act as a large potassium reservoir. K^+ passively diffuses outward, down the ion concentration gradient through potassium leak channels in the cell membrane, thus requiring a substantial proportion of metabolically derived ATP to pump them back inside the cell. Under conditions of hypoxemia the rate of ATP production falls, leading to a fall in the concentration of intracellular ATP. Eventually the Na^+,K^+-ATPase pumps fail to keep pace with the leak, leading to a net loss of K^+ from the cells[19] and a net gain into the blood.

The rate of activity of this pump increases with increasing temperature and with increases in serum Na^+ concentration. The Na^+,K^+-ATPase and K^+ leak channels are oppositely directed interfaces that regulate extracellular K^+ concentration. Agents that act on them can lead to rapid changes in plasma K^+ concentrations. Elevated plasma potassium concentrations not only depolarize excitable cell membranes according to the Nernst equation ($E_m \propto \log[\{K^+\}_{in}/\{K^+\}_{out}]$), but also decrease the rate of Na^+ entry during depolarization.[10] The net effect is to make the heart more refractory to excitation.

During hyperthermic stress of microswine, we found that plasma potassium concentration rose substantially (Fig. 8-8). In sheep exercising in heat, Khogali and coworkers[241] found a rise in potassium concentration. Francesconi and Mager[148] found in heat- and exercise-stressed rats that plasma potassium ion concentration rose during the heating period and that there was an inverse correlation between K^+ and survival time. Bowler[57] reported that in heat-stressed crayfish, hemolymph K^+ rose rapidly and nearly linearly with time of heat exposure. On the other hand, if the crayfish had been heat acclimated, there was a delay in K^+ rise and it rose at a much slower rate.

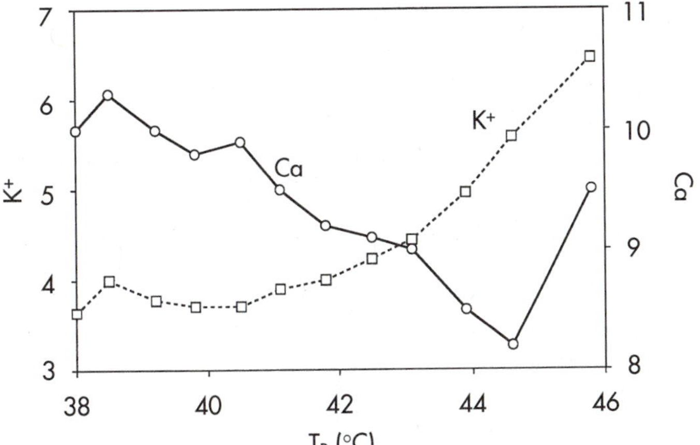

Fig. 8-8 Plasma potassium and calcium concentrations in an anesthetized miniature swine with induced heatstroke.

Sodium

Intracellular sodium content does not change significantly in response to heat treatment.[420,448] We, too, found no change in plasma Na^+ in heat-stressed microswine until a small rise occurred a few minutes before death.

Sweat concentration of sodium chloride may range from 10 to 60 mmol/L, depending on physical activity, heat exposure, the state of heat acclimation, and the amount of salt ingested.[62] Gender does not affect salt concentration in sweat, but studies have documented a lower salt content in the sweat of children as compared with adults.[12,113] Values rarely reach 40 mEq in prepubertal boys. The average American diet contains about 170 mEq of Na^+ per day, usually adequate to replace all Na^+ lost through sweating by the trained athlete. An athlete with an inadequate caloric intake, however, may also suffer from dietary mineral and salt deficiencies; supplementation may be required after moderate sweat losses. Failure to maintain normal salt intake may suppress triggering of the thirst mechanism by artificially lowering plasma osmolality, thereby reducing voluntary rehydration.

Effect of Physical Activity on Sodium Sweat Concentration

Rapid increase in exercise intensity rapidly produces increases in sweat electrolytes and a slower increase in serum electrolytes.[49,136,261] The concentration of electrolytes in sweat is highest just after beginning physical activity. Electrolyte concentrations then decrease with prolonged exercise.

Bohmer[49] measured the electrolyte concentration in sweat of elite athletes in a variety of sports (yachting, rowing, handball, and cycling). Initial values of sweat electrolytes were dependent on type of sport, duration of performance, and level of training. Cyclists and rowers, whose sports produce high-endurance capability, had significantly lower sodium content in sweat as compared with the yachtsmen. Furthermore, participation in an intensive training program led to a further reduction in sweat electrolyte concentration

Fukumoto and colleagues[151] investigated the differences in sweat composition between equal amounts of sweat induced by thermal stress alone and that induced by physical exercise. Both sodium and chloride concentrations were much lower in the sweat induced by thermal exposure than in that induced by running.

When large amounts of salt are lost through repeated sweating, sodium excretion in sweat is rapidly reduced, possibly as a passive result of falling body salt content. The sweat of a trained athlete may show a sodium content as low as 17 mmol/L (34 mOsm/kg), a level one-third that of a person who is untrained and unacclimated to the heat. Conversely, the untrained, unacclimatized "weekend warrior" or vacationer is at most risk for significant sodium losses when exercising in the heat (Table 8-1).

Effect of Heat Exposure on Renal Absorption of Sodium

After repeated days of exercise in the heat, active sodium conservation develops secondary to increased aldosterone production and enhanced renal absorption of sodium. Following a period of prolonged strenuous exercise and sweating, urinary excretion of sodium may almost cease temporarily.[100]

Sodium Deficiency

Exercise in temperate thermal environments is unlikely to result in a sodium deficiency requiring supplementation of the normal diet. Similarly, a brief (less than 2 hours) episode of moderate exercise in the heat rarely causes clinically significant hyponatremia. Hyponatremia may develop, however, when sweat loss exceeds 5 L/day. This may occur during the initial stage of acclimation to heat, during prolonged and repeated exercise in the heat (training camps), or during ultraendurance events, such as 50-mile runs or triathlons.[300]

Noakes, Goodwin, and Rayner[312] reported on four athletes who developed hyponatremia and water intoxication during endurance events lasting more than 7 hours. The cause was thought to be voluntary hyperhydration with hypotonic solutions, combined with moderate sweat sodium chloride losses. Athletes at risk were slower runners who competed at a lower intensity than did the top finishers. Armstrong and co-workers[19] reported an interesting case of symptomatic hyponatremia caused by voluntary intake of water with inappropriate ADH secretion and consequent renal shutdown. Such volume overload of the stomach is known to cause nausea, which is a strong stimulus for the production of ADH. New and interesting cases of hyponatremia from Grand Canyon National Park have recently been reported.[381a]

Calcium

Several studies suggest that hyperthermia leads to hypocalcemia as a result of deposition of calcium phosphates and calcium carbonates in injured skeletal muscles.[373] However, a rise in serum calcium concentration may occur at high temperatures because of acute renal failure or rhabdomyolysis.[250] On the other hand, we recently found a biphasic reduction in Ca^{++} concentration in microswine with heatstroke (Fig. 8-8). At approximately 41° C, Ca^{++} concentration declined, reaching a minimum at 44° C, and then rapidly rose to near baseline or baseline levels.

Indirect fluorescence methodology, as well as $^{45}Ca^{++}$ technique,[420] suggested that heating cells in culture to 45° to 45.5° C leads to a rise in cell membrane permeability[150] and an increase (0.1 micromolar) in intracellular calcium concentration. However, the rise in calcium observed by this method was probably too small to cause cell death.[124] Furthermore, when cells were loaded with Ca^{++} to a sixfold increase in total cell calcium content, they survived at 45° C, the same as did controls.[420]

Magnesium

Concentrations of magnesium in sweat vary from 0.02 to 5.0 mmol/L.[92,95,97-99,418] Magnesium losses in sweat during endurance exercise have been estimated to be about 1% of total body magnesium content.[99] Although conflicting studies exist as to the likelihood of hypomagnesemia secondary to losses in sweat, the consensus is that this is an unlikely phenomenon.[276] Assuming even the highest concentration of magnesium in sweat, significant depletion of magnesium is prevented by a concomitant rapid decrease in renal magnesium excretion.[98,418] The acute decrease in serum magnesium observed following prolonged intense exercise[36,346] may be caused by a temporary migration of Mg^{++} into erythrocytes[336] and actively contracting muscle,[95] as well as by losses in sweat.[97]

Phosphate

Hypophosphatemia is frequently seen in exertional heatstroke.[53] Heat stress caused a respiratory alkalosis that increased the rate of cellular uptake of phosphate and reduced phosphorus excretion.[299] Shapiro and Cristal,[373] however, suggested that this was due to increased renal clearance of phosphorus and decreased renal threshold, as well as to contributions from metabolic acidosis and increased uptake of phosphorus by the tissue cells. However, hypophosphatemia is not always reported and respiratory alkalosis does not always occur at the same time as hypophosphatemia.

Enzymes

At core temperatures of 41.8° to 42.2° C, aspartate aminotransferase (AST) and alanine aminotransferase (ALT) concentrations rose by factors of 25 and 8, respectively, and bilirubin concentration approximately doubled to 1.56 mg/dl.[329] Manjoo, Burger, and Kielblock[281] concluded that the rises in enzyme levels are a reliable index of tissue damage, which in turn is related to both the absolute body temperature elevation and the rate of rise in body temperature. They found that creatine kinase (indicates skeletal and cardiac muscle damage) was the most sensitive to increases in core temperature, followed by lactate dehydrogenase (indicates generalized tissue damage). In microswine with heatstroke, however, we found no changes in ALT, a rise in AST about an hour before death, and rises in CK and LDH only about 20 minutes before death.

Glucose

Heatstroke is known to lead to elevations in the stress hormones catecholamines and cortisol.[3] These hormones act in the liver to convert glycogen to glucose and lead to elevations in plasma glucose concentrations. Classic heatstroke patients were usually found to be hyperglycemic.[53,174] We also found rises in plasma glucose in approximately half of heat-stressed microswine with a sharp decline in highest temperatures at about 20 to 30 minutes after a rise in circulating insulin. In accordance with these observations, it has been reported that patients suffering from heat exhaustion were normoglycemic, but some patients with heatstroke were hypoglycemic.[102]

Clinical Management of Heat-Related Illness

As previously discussed, individuals exercising in the heat develop a spectrum of clinical illness ranging from syncope to heatstroke. Further discussion of the clinical management of heat illness will focus on heat exhaustion and heatstroke. The distinction between these two clinical diagnoses is somewhat artificial and may be difficult to establish in the field or at the medical facility.

HEAT EXHAUSTION

Heat exhaustion occurs in individuals who sweat profusely while participating in an endurance event or who engage in repeated bouts of exercise that result in significant sweat losses that remain unreplaced. Prolonged insensible sweat losses, such as occur while sitting in the sun in a moderate breeze, predispose to heat exhaustion if fluid and electrolyte losses are significant.

Problems with Recognition

The early symptoms of significant heat illness are often unrecognized or mistaken for malingering. Failure to attend to these symptoms puts the individual at great risk for thermal injury. Headache, confusion, drowsiness, and even euphoria may be important warning signals. Individuals who anticipate exposure to hot environmental conditions should be thoroughly versed in the manifestations of heat illness.

The patient with heat exhaustion may arrive at the medical facility with nausea and visual disturbances that mimic the prodrome of a migraine headache. Dizziness or syncope often leads to evaluation for arrhythmia or seizures. Chilling, piloerection, sweating, and moderately elevated temperature may lead a person to consider an infectious process. Development of altered mental status or ataxia raises the possibility of meningitis, encephalitis, or drug intoxication.

Treatment

Treatment is based on symptoms and focuses on reduction in both temperature and rehydration. The patient must stop exercising; although this appears to be intuitively obvious, persons who develop euphoria as an altered state of consciousness may resist this measure. Furthermore, later return to physical activity that day is contraindicated. When possible the victim should be removed from direct sunlight; restrictive clothing should be loosened. If the patient is unconscious or the rectal temperature is greater than 39° C, the patient should be treated as an incipient heatstroke victim and immediately evacuated to a medical facility following the guidelines below.

Body temperature may be lowered by a variety of means. When available, immersion in ice water facilitates the most rapid drop in body temperature.[101] Alternative measures in the field include sprinkling with water and fanning, or placing ice bags over the superficial great vessels (axillae and groin) and fanning.[242] Periodic toweling off of the skin renews the evaporative surface and facilitates evaporative cooling.

If the patient is alert, oral rehydration can be instituted with cold water or a fluid replacement beverage; the concentration of carbohydrate in such a beverage should not exceed 6% or intestinal absorption of fluid may be delayed. An initial target intake of 1 to 2 L over 2 to 4 hours is reasonable; greater intake results in an inappropriate diuresis. The victim should continue to rest and drink over the next 24 hours. As a general rule, for every pound of weight lost by sweating, 1 pint (2 cups or 500 ml) of fluid should be consumed. Total rehydration and replacement of electrolytes lost in sweat via oral intake may require 36 hours to complete.

After the acute episode the medical care provider should determine any possible host risk factors for heat illness and review with the patient signs of heat illness and preventive measures.

HEATSTROKE

Heatstroke is a true medical emergency; before 1950 the mortality rate was 40% to 75%.[11,82] Long-term survival is directly related to rapidity of institution of resuscitative measures.

Problems with Recognition

The traditional diagnosis of heatstroke required three signs: severe hyperthermia (T_c greater than 41° C), central nervous system disturbance, and cessation of sweating.[84] This symptom complex represents the extreme or full-blown heatstroke presentation; adherence to such strict criteria delays institution of critical interventional measures. We consider each of these criteria in turn.

Shibolet[377] reported changes in body temperature in heatstroke victims from the values documented in the field to the values obtained in the emergency department. The mean value in the field was 41.1° ± 0.8° C; the mean value on admission was 37.8° ± 1.2° C. Failure to obtain or record on-site rectal temperature may hinder prompt diagnosis; similarly, documentation of only mild elevation in body temperature should not preclude the diagnosis of heatstroke.

The patient's altered mental status may affect the ability of the emergency department personnel to obtain a detailed history regarding precipitating events. Lack of such information may also delay diagnosis. Emergency medical transport personnel should obtain this history before evacuating the patient and communicate the information to the appropriate medical staff.

Recent investigations have shown that cessation of sweating is only a late phenomenon of heatstroke.[188,339,380] At the time of collapse most heatstroke victims continue to sweat profusely. Failure to consider the diagnosis of heatstroke in the diaphoretic patient could be fatal.

Unless an alternative etiology is obvious, the previously healthy individual who collapses after physical exertion in hot weather should be considered to have exertional heatstroke.[82,379]

Diagnosis

Shibolet[377] noted that delay in temperature measurement or inaccurate methodology in obtaining initial temperature values often led to inappropriately low initial temperature determinations when compared with actual core temperature at the time of collapse. Loss of consciousness is a sine qua non to the diagnosis of heatstroke; with cessation of physical activity, heat production is markedly decreased. If the patient continues to sweat, body temperature will fall. Shapiro and Seidman[375] have proposed that the diagnosis of heatstroke should be considered in any "patient who has lost consciousness during exertion and demonstrates clinical and laboratory signs of heatstroke, even if body temperature was not found to be markedly elevated several hours after collapse." A history of prodromal symptoms as outlined in the section on heat exhaustion should markedly increase the index of suspicion for heatstroke.

Hyperthermia and central nervous system disturbance (coma, convulsions, confusion, or agitation) raise the possibility of a variety of central nervous system and systemic infections and disease processes (see Table 8-4). Evaluation for these disorders should proceed only after the diagnosis of heatstroke is ruled out. Markedly elevated levels of AST, ALT, and LDH may help in differential diagnosis[232]; the clinician should bear in mind that elevation of these enzymes may not occur for 24 to 48 hours after heat injury.[379]

Heatstroke Complications

The observed complications of heatstroke reflect the results of both direct thermal injury and cardiovascular collapse. Autopsy of persons with exertional heatstroke showed that they suffered from multiple hemorrhages, congestion, and cellular degeneration in most or all of the organs examined.[380] In exertional heatstroke in particular, rhabdomyolysis is usually present.[253] The chemical mediators of this damage have been previously discussed. A brief overview of the specific pathology found should provide a framework for discussion of the therapeutic and supportive management of heatstroke.

Central Nervous System. Marked sensitivity of the brain to thermal injury has been reviewed. The underlying pathology is brain edema and congestion, with petechial hemorrhage and neuronal degeneration noted on autopsy.[279] Cerebrospinal fluid pressure and hematologic features are normal.[379] Central nervous system dysfunction is directly related to the duration of hyperthermia and to circulatory failure.

In the previously cited series of heatstroke victims described by Shibolet,[377] coma occurred in 100% of patients, confusion or agitation or both in 100%, and convulsions in 72%. Pupillary constriction was present in 66% of cases.[239] Agitation, delirium, and hallucinations reflect central nervous system hyperirritability. Seizures occur in approximately 50% of cases.[239] Decerebrate rigidity, oculogyric crisis, and opisthotonos may develop; other findings may include loss of rectal sphincter tone, loss of skeletal muscle tone, and hemiplegia.[379] Cerebellar findings of dysarthria and ataxia are common.

Complete recovery occurs in most cases. However, chronic disability may develop in the form of mental deficiency, dysarthria, ataxia, aphasia, and hemiparesis.

Cardiovascular System. Hypotension does not always occur in heatstroke but is usually present in the fatal and severe cases.[380] This hypotension may persist, even following large volumes of fluid therapy with vasopressors. Thus hypotension is a late and ominous finding and may reflect failure of compensatory contraction of the mesenteric vessels. As vital organs are hypoperfused, shock develops. Left ventricular subendocardial hemorrhage and focal necrosis of cardiac muscle fibers are commonly found on autopsy.[279,379]

The extreme stress placed on the cardiovascular system of patients with heatstroke results in a universal finding of sinus tachycardia, often with rates exceeding 140 beats/min.[380] Pulse pressure is elevated in the face of low cardiac output and low diastolic blood pressure.[379] Electrocardiographic findings include ST segment and T wave abnormalities and conduction disturbances.[102] In microswine and monkeys, blood pressure was stable or rose until T_c reached 41° C and then declined until death.[157] In those studies, however, the heart rate rose to a plateau shortly after heating and commenced to rise at T_c of 41° C, peaking a few minutes before death.[157,160]

Pulmonary System. Hyperventilation is a common finding. Persistent hyperventilation may lead to respiratory alkalosis and tetany. Coma or seizures may predispose to pulmonary aspiration.[379] Pulmonary edema may become severe or fatal; disseminated intravascular coagulation may lead to adult respiratory distress syndrome.[129] Pulmonary infarctions have been found on autopsy.[279]

Renal System. Acute renal failure develops in 25% of heatstroke victims[249]; hypotension and resultant decreased renal blood flow constitute the primary underlying etiology. As in the central nervous system, thermal injury may cause direct cellular damage.[365] Disseminated intravascular coagulation and myoglobinuria offer further insult to renal tissue. Hematuria, pyuria, proteinuria, and hyaline and granular casts are seen on urinalysis. Eventually, oliguria and anuria may develop.

Hepatic System. Within 12 to 24 hours after heatstroke, elevated AST, ALT, and serum bilirubin levels can be detected.[235] Levels of AST greater than 1000 units are commonly seen in severe heatstroke.[32,419] Prothrombin level reaches its nadir 48 to 72 hours after heat injury.[361] Cholestasis and hepatocellular necrosis may develop.

Gastrointestinal System. Vomiting and diarrhea are common symptoms of heatstroke. Compensatory mesenteric vascular constriction may produce localized areas of mucosal injury. As previously discussed, the subsequent increase in serum LPS and its role as inducer of potentially damaging cytokines may play a critical part in both the morbidity and potential therapy of heatstroke. In the presence of disseminated intravascular coagulation, hematemesis and melena may develop.[379]

Hematologic System. White blood cell count may be as elevated as 20,000 to 30,000/ml. Platelet count is depressed, as are levels of clotting factors V and VIII. The commonly seen bleeding diathesis may be manifested as conjunctival hemorrhage, melena, purpura, hemoptysis, or hematuria.[379] The primary cause of this coagulopathy is thought to be release of thromboplastic substances secondary to endothelial damage, resulting in intravascular thrombosis and secondary fibrinolysis.[377] Other contributing factors may include direct inactivation of clotting factors by thermal injury, decreased hepatic production of clotting factors, and decreased production of platelets secondary to thermal injury to marrow megakaryocytes. Low levels of fibrinogen and elevated levels of fibrin split products, in the presence of thrombocytopenia, herald the onset of disseminated intravascular coagulation; clotting abnormalities most often peak 18 to 36 hours after the acute heat injury.[377]

Acid-Base and Electrolyte Abnormalities. Early in the course of heatstroke, respiratory alkalosis secondary to hyperventilation may be present. As anaerobic or aerobic glycolysis increases, serum lactate levels rise, creating a metabolic acidosis.

Hypernatremia reflects the associated dehydration common in heatstroke; sodium levels may, however, appear normal. In the face of dietary deficiency of sodium or profuse sweat losses, initial normonatremia may develop into hyponatremia upon rehydration. Potassium levels may be low or elevated, with hyperkalemia being associated with tissue damage and renal compromise. Hypocalcemia, hypomagnesemia, and hypophosphatemia may also occur. Although hypoglycemia may develop in cases of exertional heatstroke, hyperglycemia secondary to elevated catecholamine release may also be seen.

ON-SITE EMERGENCY MEDICAL TREATMENT

Heatstroke is a medical emergency. Rapid reduction of elevated body temperature is the keystone of management of heatstroke; the duration of hyperthermia may be the primary determinant of outcome.[249,380] Nevertheless, it is important to follow the ABCs of stabilization while cooling efforts are initiated.

In a comatose patient, control of the airway should be established by insertion of a cuffed endotracheal tube. When available, administration of supplemental oxygen may help meet the increased metabolic demands and treat the hypoxia commonly associated with aspiration, pulmonary hemorrhage, pulmonary infarction, pneumonitis, or pulmonary edema.[129,279] Positive-pressure ventilation is indicated if hypoxia persists despite supplemental oxygen administration.

As discussed previously, resuscitative measures may serve to lower body temperature rapidly. Monitoring and recording rectal temperature on site may be important to the accurate diagnosis of heatstroke. Vital signs should be monitored, with attention to blood pressure and pulse. Although normotension should not be taken as a reassuring sign, *hypotension should be recognized for the ominous sign it always represents.*

Circulatory access should be established by insertion of a large-gauge intravenous catheter. Administration of normal saline or Ringer's lactate should be begun. Recommendations regarding the rate of administration of fluids vary; whereas some authors advise a rate of 1200 ml over 4 hours,[318] others encourage a 2 L bolus over the first hour and an additional liter of fluid per hour for the next 3 hours.[375] Vigorous fluid resuscitation may precipitate development of pulmonary edema; careful monitoring is indicated.

Cooling measures should be initiated immediately. Cooling techniques are ineffective when the patient is having seizures; convulsions should be controlled by intravenous administration of 5 to 10 mg of diazepam as necessary. Rapid evacuation to an emergency medical facility is required.

Cooling Modalities

Much debate exists in the literature regarding the best approach to cooling heatstroke victims.[101,242,428] Since morbidity is directly related to duration of elevated core temperature, the efficiency of a given approach (how rapidly body temperature is lowered) assumes primary significance. Another consideration in choice of cooling modality is the need for access to the patient for continuous monitoring.

Khogali and associates[428] developed a body cooling unit designed to maximize evaporative cooling by maintaining cutaneous vasodilation and minimizing shivering. The patient is suspended on a net and sprayed from all sides with water at 15° C (59° F). Warm air (45° to 48° C) is blown over the victim. Cooling rates of 0.06° C/min have been obtained. Although this method is widely recommended as the treatment of choice, the rate of cooling is much less than that seen with ice water immersion.

Ice water immersion is an effective and easily available method of rapidly lowering core body temperature, although its use is one of the more hotly debated topics in the heatstroke literature. The increased thermal conductivity of water results in most cases in a reduction of core temperature to less than 39° C (102.2° F) in 10 to 40 minutes.[102] This reflects a mean rate of cooling of 0.13° C/min. Use of cold (but not iced) water resulted in a similar rate of cooling of 0.13° C/min.[318] Cold water immersion is less uncomfortable for the patient than immersion in iced water. In three series of exertional heatstroke victims in a military population (66 patients), *there were no fatalities* or permanent sequelae after treatment *with ice water immersion*.[36,102,317] Costrini[101] later reported 252 cases of heatstroke in Marines, all successfully treated with ice water immersion. Although other cooling methods reduce the rate of mortality, none has been so successful as ice water immersion.

In discussing an alternative cooling method, Khogali[237] summarizes the most commonly offered criticisms of ice water immersion:

1. Exposure to severely cold temperatures may cause peripheral vasoconstriction with shunting of the blood away from the skin, resulting in a paradoxical rise in core body temperature.
2. Induction of shivering (in response to the cold) may cause additional elevation in temperature.
3. Exposure to ice water causes marked patient discomfort.
4. Working in ice water is uncomfortable for medical attendants.
5. Access to the patient for monitoring of vital signs or administration of cardiopulmonary resuscitation is more difficult.
6. There is difficulty maintaining sanitary conditions should vomiting or diarrhea develop.

Although the first two criticisms may appear physiologically appropriate, review of the medical literature fails to provide documentation for a rise in body temperature following ice water immersion. In fact, decreased vascular resistance has been shown to persist during ice bath cooling to normothermia.[318] Other authors using ice water immersion for treatment of heatstroke did not find shivering problematic.[102] This is not an unexpected observation; since the hypothalamic set point for temperature regulation is not raised during heatstroke (unlike during febrile illness), the shivering response should only occur if the body temperature is allowed to fall below normal. When shivering has occurred, treatment with chlorpromazine (25 to 50 mg intravenously) has been effective.[219] Heatstroke victims rarely require cardiopulmonary resuscitation, so this concern should not preclude use of ice baths to treat heatstroke. The documented efficacy of ice water immersion in the rapid reduction of body temperature, and therefore morbidity and mortality, overrides any consideration of transient personal discomfort for the patient or medical attendants.

If other methods are used initially, any patient whose core body temperature does not reach 38.9° C within 30 minutes after beginning treatment should be placed in an ice water bath. A rapidly falling core temperature may not be accurately reflected by measured rectal temperature,[85] so with any cooling technique, active cooling should be discontinued when core body temperature falls to 39° C (102.2° F) to prevent inducing hypothermia.

A variety of ancillary modalities have been proposed to facilitate cooling, including administration of cold intravenous fluids, gastric lavage with cold fluids, and cooling inhaled air. While these therapies may cause lowering of body temperature, their effects are minimal compared with ice water immersion or effective evaporative cooling. Cooling blankets are ineffective in inducing the rapid lowering of body temperature required in treatment of heatstroke. Use of antipyretics is inappropriate and potentially harmful in heatstroke victims. Aspirin and acetaminophen lower temperature by normalizing the elevated hypothalamic set point caused by pyrogens; in heatstroke the set point is normal, with the temperature elevation reflecting failure of the normal cooling mechanisms. Furthermore, acetaminophen could induce additional hepatic damage; administration of aspirin could aggravate bleeding tendencies. Alcohol sponge baths are inappropriate under any circumstances, since absorption of alcohol may lead to poisoning and coma.

Hospital Emergency Medical Treatment. If control of the airway has not been previously established, insertion of a cuffed endotracheal tube provides protection from aspiration of oral secretions. As discussed previously, supplemental oxygen and, when necessary, positive-pressure ventilation should be provided.

Temperature should be continually monitored (at 5-minute intervals) by means of an esophageal or rectal probe. Cooling measures should be maintained for core body temperature greater than 38° C.

If not previously established, intravenous access should be obtained as quickly as possible. Administration of intravenous fluids (Ringer's lactate or normal saline) at a rate of 300 ml/hr will provide circulatory support without risking development of pulmonary or cerebral edema. Most heatstroke victims have a high cardiac index, low peripheral vascular resistance, and mild right-sided heart failure with elevated central venous pressure. Effective cooling results in vasoconstriction and increased blood pressure; therefore moderate fluid replacement is indicated in these cases. A Swan-Ganz pulmonary artery catheter may be necessary in the assessment of appropriate fluid supplementation. Some patients have a low cardiac index, hypotension, and elevated central venous pressure. These patients have been successfully treated with an isoproterenol drip (1 μg/min).[318] Patients with a low cardiac index, low central venous pressure, hypotension, and low pulmonary capillary wedge pressure should receive a fluid bolus.

Cardiac monitoring should be maintained during at least the first 24 hours of hospitalization. Use of norepinephrine and other α-adrenergic drugs should be avoided because they cause vasoconstriction, thereby decreasing cutaneous heat exchange. Anticholinergic drugs that inhibit sweating, such as atropine, should also be avoided.

As previously discussed, chlorpromazine may be used to treat uncontrollable shivering that might lead to rising body temperature. Chlorpromazine should be used advisedly, however, because it may cause hypotension or seizures and its anticholinergic effects may interfere with sweating. For these reasons some physicians prefer to use diazepam to control shivering.

A Foley catheter should be placed to monitor urinary output. Intravenous mannitol (0.25 mg/kg) or furosemide (1 mg/kg) may be used to promote renal blood flow and prevent damage from myoglobinuria and hyperuricemia.[375] Early dialysis should be considered if anuria, uremia, or hyperkalemia develops.

Cooling and hydration usually correct any acid-base abnormality; however, serum electrolytes, including glucose, should be monitored and appropriate modifications of intravenous fluids made.

Placement of a nasogastric tube connected to low continuous suction further controls oral and gastric secretions. Although antacids and histamine H_2 blockers have been used to prevent gastrointestinal bleeding, no studies to date demonstrate their efficacy in heatstroke patients.

As previously discussed, clotting disturbances peak 18 to 36 hours after onset of heat injury.[379] Coagulation tests (platelet count, prothombin time, fibrinogen levels, fibrin split products) should be obtained on admission and after 24 hours. Disseminated intravascular coagulation may develop 24 to 72 hours after admission and is marked by acute onset of bleeding from venipuncture sites, gingivae, nasal mucosae, lungs, or gastrointestinal tract. Disseminated intravascular coagulation is best prevented by rapid cooling of initial hyperthermia; treatment includes replacement of clotting factors and platelets by transfusion of fresh frozen plasma and platelets.

Prognosis

Rapid reduction of body temperature, control of seizures, proper rehydration, and prompt evacuation to an emergency medical facility now result in a 90% survival rate in heatstroke victims. As previously emphasized, the morbidity of heatstroke is directly related to the duration of hyperthermia.[374] A poor prognosis is associated with a core body temperature greater than 41° C, prolonged duration of hyperthermia, hyperkalemia, acute renal failure, and elevated serum levels of liver enzymes. Full recovery without evidence of neurologic impairment has been achieved even after coma of 24 hours' duration and subsequent seizures.[380] However, the persistence of coma after achievement of normothermia is a poor prognostic sign.[379]

Prevention

Prevention of heat illness rests on the awareness of host risk factors, adaptation of behavior and physical activity to these risk factors and the environmental conditions, and appropriate hydration during physical exercise in the heat. More aggressive media attention and education of the public as to heat illness and its prevention are indicated. Primary care physicians should incorporate this information in the anticipatory guidance of the routine health assessment. Despite a wealth of medical literature on heat injury, a few coaches continue to physically or psychologically force athletes to compete or run under conditions of heat stress. This practice should be viewed as irresponsible.

Awareness of Host Risk Factors

Any underlying condition that causes increased heat production, decreased heat dissipation, or dehydration will interfere with normal thermoregulatory mechanisms and predispose an individual to heat injury. The elderly may suffer from several of these conditions, which accounts for their risk for classic heatstroke. When healthy young adults exercise strenuously in the heat, exertional heatstroke may occur despite the absence of host risk factors.

Endocrine abnormalities, such as hyperthyroidism and pheochromocytoma, cause a marked increase in heat production. Acute febrile illness, by virtue of the elevated hypothalamic set point caused by pyrogens, also leads to increased body heat. The muscular activity associated with uncontrolled gross motor seizures or delirium tremens also releases significant metabolic heat.

The primary means of heat dissipation is the production and evaporation of sweat. Any condition that affects this process places the individual at risk for thermal injury. Poor physical conditioning, fatigue, cardiovascular disease, and lack of acclimation all limit the cardiovascular response to heat stress. Obesity places an individual at risk from reduced cardiac output, increased energy cost of moving extra mass, increased thermal insulation, and altered distribution of heat-activated sweat glands.[28] The elderly and the young show decreased efficiency of thermoregulatory function and increased risk of heat injury.

Several congenital or acquired abnormalities affect sweat production and evaporation. Ectodermal dysplasia is the most common form of congenital anhidrosis. Widespread psoriasis, scleroderma, miliaria rubra ("prickly heat" caused by plugging of the sweat ducts with keratin), or deep burns may also limit sweat production.

Dehydration affects both central thermoregulation and sweating. A mere 2% decrease in body weight through fluid loss produces an increase in heart rate, increase in body temperature, and decrease in plasma volume. In the otherwise healthy adult a gastrointestinal infection characterized by vomiting and diarrhea may cause sufficient dehydration to place the individual at risk for exertional heatstroke. More chronic conditions that may contribute to dehydration include diabetes mellitus, diabetes insipidus, eating disorders (especially bulimia), and mental retardation. Alcoholism and illicit drug use are among the 10 major risk factors for heatstroke in the general population.[244] Inhibition of ADH leading to a relative dehydration is a widely recognized effect of alcohol consumption.

Despite evidence that hypohydration limits physical performance,[13,68,69,409] voluntary dehydration continues to be routine in certain athletic arenas. Wrestlers, jockeys, boxers, and body builders commonly lose 3% to 5% of their body weight 1 to 2 days before competition. In addition to fluid and food restriction, other pathogenic weight control measures such as self-induced vomiting, laxatives and diuretics, and exposure to heat (saunas and hot tubs or "sauna suits") are often employed. Athletes undergoing rapid dehydration are at risk, not only of heat injury, but also of other serious medical conditions, such as pulmonary embolism.[104]

Box 8-2 highlights some of the medications that interfere with thermoregulation. Special attention should be given to the effect of antihistamines in reducing sweating. This class of medications is commonly obtained over the counter; the general population should be warned of the dangers of exercising in the heat when taking antihistamines.

BOX 8-2

DRUGS THAT INTERFERE WITH THERMOREGULATION

DRUGS THAT INCREASE HEAT PRODUCTION

Thyroid hormone
Amphetamines
Tricyclic antidepressants
Lysergic acid diethylamide (LSD)

DRUGS THAT DECREASE THIRST

Haloperidol

DRUGS THAT DECREASE SWEATING

Antihistamines (diphenhydramine)
Anticholinergics
Phenothiazines
Benztropine mesylate

Until recently the medical literature has commonly reported that sustaining an episode of heatstroke predisposes the individual to future heat injury. Whether this represented an inherent tendency to heat intolerance or an injury caused by the hyperthermia was not known. A recent study of heatstroke victims, however, refutes this belief.[14] Ten heatstroke patients were tested for their ability to acclimate to heat; by definition the ability to acclimate to heat indicates heat tolerance. Nine of these patients demonstrated heat tolerance within 3 months after the heatstroke episode; the remaining patient could acclimate to heat by a year after his heat injury. In no case was the heat intolerance permanent. Although individuals may show a transient heat intolerance following thermal injury, evidence for permanent susceptibility to thermal injury is lacking.

Adaptation to Environmental Conditions

Appropriate adaptation to hot environmental conditions encompasses many behaviors, including modification of clothing, degree of physical activity, anticipatory enhancement of physical conditioning, acclimation to heat stress, and attention to hydration.

Clothing. For the individual exercising under conditions of high heat, maximal skin exposure facilitates sweat evaporation. Clothing should be lightweight and of absorbent material. Different regions of the body are not equivalent in their sweat production[196]; the face and scalp account for 50% of total sweat production, while the lower extremities contribute only 25%. Toweling off the face to renew the evaporative surface and removing headgear whenever possible are important adjuncts to effective heat dissipation. While significant improvement in construction of athletic uniforms has been made, the uniforms and protective gear required by certain branches of the military and public safety officers continue to add to the risk of heat injury. Development of protective clothing that will also permit more effective heat dissipation is indicated.

Activity. Modification of physical activity should not be based only on the ambient temperature; humidity and, to a lesser degree, solar radiation contribute to heat stress. The wet bulb globe temperature (WBGT) is an index of heat stress that incorporates all three factors. This value may be calculated (Table 8-5) or obtained directly from portable heat stress monitors that measure all three parameters simultaneously and compute the WBGT. Alternatively, the heat index may be obtained from national weather stations. The current recommendations for the prevention of thermal injuries during distance running from the American College of Sports Medicine (ACSM) are based on the WBGT.[86] They state that "distance races (>16 km or 10 miles) should not be conducted when the WBGT exceeds 28° C (82.4° F). During periods of the year when the daylight dry bulb temperature often exceeds 27° C (80° F), distance races should be conducted before 9:00 AM or after 4:00 PM."

Table 8-6 presents a suggested modification of sports activity that is also based on the WBGT. Following ACSM guidelines, vigorous physical activity during the summer should be scheduled before 8 AM or after 6 PM to minimize exposure to solar radiation. *Early morning, however, is commonly the time of the highest humidity of the day.* It is important to note therefore that compliance with these recommendations does not remove all risk of heat injury. Development of another index of heat stress that provides a better basis for prevention of exertional heat stroke is indicated.

A qualitatively different modification of activity could effectively minimize the occurrence of classic heat stroke. Lack of residential air conditioning places the poor at risk during heat waves. By sitting in a cool or tepid bath periodically throughout the day, the individual can decrease the heat stress and thereby prevent heat injury.

Table 8-5 Wet Bulb Globe Temperature (WBGT) Heat Index

Temperature (°F)	Example
Wet bulb × 0.7 =	78 × 0.7 = 54.6
Dry bulb × 0.1 =	80 × 0.1 = 8.0
Black globe × 0.2 =	100 × 0.2 = 20.0
HEAT INDEX	82.6

Wet bulb reflects humidity. Dry bulb reflects ambient air temperature. Black globe reflects radiant heat load. Alternate equation: WBGT = (.567) Dry bulb temperature + (393) Environmental water vapor pressure + 3.94.

Table 8-6 Modification of Sports Activity Using Wet Bulb Globe Temperature

Index (°F)	Limitation
<50	Low risk for hyperthermia but possible risk for hypothermia
<65	Low risk for heat illness
65-73	Moderate risk toward end of workout
73-82	Those at high risk for heat injury should not continue to train; practice in shorts and T-shirts during the first week of training
82-84	Care should be taken by all athletes to maintain adequate hydration
85-87.9	Unacclimated persons should stop training; all outdoor drills in heavy uniforms should be cancelled
88-89.9	Acclimated athletes should exercise caution and continue workouts only at a reduced intensity; light clothing only
90 or above	Stop all training

Conditioning. The contribution of cardiovascular conditioning to thermoregulation has been discussed previously. Ideally, before exercising in the heat, an individual should train under temperate or thermoneutral conditions. For the previously sedentary individual an exercise regimen incorporating 20 to 30 minutes of aerobic activity 3 to 4 days a week will significantly improve cardiovascular function after 8 weeks.

It is important to remember that even physically active individuals may lack conditioning relative to a particularly stressful competition or activity. Heat illness in runners commonly occurs when novices exceed their training effort during races or when well-trained athletes increase their pace above normal during long-distance events.

Acclimation. On initial exposure to a hot environment, workouts should be moderate in intensity and duration. A gradual increase in the time and intensity of physical exertion over 8 to 10 days should allow optimal acclimation; children require 10 to 14 days to achieve a similar response. Acclimation can be begun in an anticipatory fashion by simulating hot environmental conditions indoors. If symptoms of heat illness develop during the acclimation period, all physical activity should be stopped and appropriate interventions begun. Acclimation is not facilitated by restricting fluid intake; in fact, conscious attention to fluid intake is required to prevent developing dehydration. As with physical conditioning, there are limits to the degree of protection that acclimation provides from heat stress. Given a sufficiently hot and humid environment, no one is immune to heat injury.

Hydration

Recommendations for fluid intake during physical activity are appropriate for a discussion on prevention of heat illness. The individual should be well hydrated before beginning physical activity in the heat; dehydration for any reason should preclude exertion while heat stressed. Eight ounces of water or appropriate fluid replacement beverage should be drunk 10 to 15 minutes before starting physical activity. Continued intake of 8 to 12 ounces of fluid every 20 to 30 minutes during exercise should be enforced or urine color should be monitored.[14a] Reliance on voluntary intake to maintain adequate fluid balance will result in development of significant dehydration. The traditional rules of some sports (such as field hockey, soccer, and rugby) unintentionally limit opportunities for hydration by failing to provide for timeouts and incorporating very brief half-times. During extremely hot and humid weather, team physicians, trainers, coaches, and officials should work together to incorporate additional breaks (quarters rather than halves) and provide unlimited access to fluids on the sidelines.

Preexercise and postexercise nude dry weights can guide additional fluid intake after exercise and before the next trial. For every pound of weight lost during activity, the individual should consume 1 pint (2 cups) of fluid over a period of several hours. Fluid loss should be replaced before return to activity in the heat; if a weight loss greater than 2% persists, the individual should be withheld from activity. Prehydration will forestall dehydration and enhance performance.

Rehydration

Once heat injury has progressed to the point of heatstroke, *intravenous replacement of fluid losses is required.* Ringer's lactate or normal saline is the initial intravenous fluid of choice, providing excellent expansion of intravascular volume without risking too rapid a correction of an unappreciated hyponatremia. The rate of administration of fluids should reflect preexisting or coexisting medical conditions. An initial rate of 1200 ml over 4 hours has been proposed.[318] *Supplemental potassium should be withheld until serum electrolyte levels are known.* This is important because some commercial beverages contain additional K^+. Future choice of fluids should reflect the individual's electrolyte status and cardiac and renal function.

Recommendations for maintaining oral hydration (or, more accurately, minimizing dehydration) are presented in the section on prevention of heat illness. The inability to rely on the thirst mechanism to prevent dehydration cannot be too strongly emphasized. Simple provision of fluids at the sideline during athletic practices and competitions or military training sessions is not sufficient. Scheduled breaks in activity (every 20 to 30 minutes depending on the degree of heat stress) for required consumption of fluids are now the standard of care.

Fluid Replacement Beverages. A more widely investigated and hotly debated topic is the appropriate fluid replacement during physical activity in the heat. Confusion has arisen over the need for replacement of electrolyte losses, as well as the advantages of carbohydrate supplementation.

White and Ford[436] studied the use of water versus an electrolyte-carbohydrate–containing beverage for fluid replacement of electrolyte losses equaling 1.9% and 3.5% in athletes. They found no significant difference in the maintenance of plasma volume between trials with water and the experimental formulations.

Early investigators promoted the consumption of sodium-containing fluid to prevent the development of hyponatremia during exercise. Johnson, Nelson, and Consolazio[221] used three commercial sports drinks, synthetic solutions containing the component individual minerals and glucose, and water as replacement fluids for men during 4 hours of physical activity. All solutions proved equally effective in maintaining water and mineral balance and moderate physical performance. The authors concluded that the major benefit of commercially available sports drinks was in their prevention of hypohydration resulting from voluntary increase in fluid intake on the basis of enhanced palatability; this conclusion has been drawn by other researchers in the field.[300,447]

The main characteristics of a solution that influence gastric emptying are osmolality and caloric content.[133] Which

Fig. 8-9 Model of the physiology and pathophysiology of heat stress and heatstroke. Core temperature has been divided into two regions to clarify physiologic mechanisms.

Normal Thermoregulation. Under a moderate heat load, as skin or core temperature (or both) rises, thermoreceptors (1) increase skin blood flow and (2) cause the secretion of sweat to (3) result in evaporative cooling. To prevent a drop in blood pressure (4), blood flow to the splanchnic regions and to muscle is reduced and (5) stroke volume and then (6) heart rate are increased. Then (7) catecholamines are secreted, followed by corticotropin-releasing factor (CRF), which leads to the secretion of adrenocorticotropic hormone followed by (8) cortisol. Catecholamines (9) cause leukocytosis, while cortisol (10) causes leukopenia leading to (11) changes in amounts of subsets of leukocytes. If the heat stress is prolonged and severe, the immunosuppression could (12) lead to subsequent increased susceptibility to infections. As temperature rises, (13) the respiratory rate increases. As a result of sweating, (14) plasma volume decreases and (15) hematocrit and (16) plasma osmolality rise, leading to (17,18) the sensation of thirst and ADH release. Reduced plasma volume (14), together with (4) reduced renal blood flow, leads to (19) rises in water-sparing hormones and reduced kidney function.

Impaired Homeostasis. As temperature continues to rise above approximately 40° C (104° F), direct hyperthermic damage (A1) to cells commences with increases in membrane fluidity and permeability, increases in metabolic rate including the activity of the Na^+,K^+-ATPase, increases in a variety of metabolites, and decreases in cellular ATP content. At about the same time the reduction in intestinal blood flow (4) becomes more severe, leading (A4) to ischemic injury of the gut wall. This in turn leads to rises in (A5) circulating lipopolysaccharide (LPS) and (A6) cytokines. By activating a blood factor (A7), LPS causes (A8) disseminated intravascular coagulation and its consequent rise in blood viscosity. Thermal injury of endothelia (A3), together with (A6) cytokines leads to (A9) enhanced metabolism of omega-6 fatty acids including (A10) the production of thromboxanes and leukotrienes, (A11) oxygen free radicals and further (A12) cellular injury, the probable production of the highly toxic nitric oxide, and (A13) increased vascular permeability. This leads to the loss of fluids into the tissues, and thus (A14) reduced venous return and (A15) consequent reduced central venous pressure. Through Starling's Law of the Heart (A16), cardiac output begins to fall. This is made more serious (A17) by electrolyte changes in the blood. Eventually (A18) blood pressure falls, leading (A19) to reduced tissue perfusion. In the case of the lung (A20), reduced perfusion leads to (A21) systemic hypoxemia and eventually (A22) ischemia of various tissues and organs and its consequent (A23) contribution to further cellular damage. (A24) Reduced blood flow to the brain (A25), as well as (A26) probable direct thermal denaturation, leads to damage of centrally mediated homeostatic mechanisms, (A27, A28) reduced skin blood flow and drop in cooling rate, and eventually (A29) a fall in respiration. In a separate pathway, cardiac output is also depressed as a result of (A30) a too rapid pulse rate causing (A31) incomplete cardiac filling. Electrolyte derangements are made more severe by (A32) an increased metabolic rate and (A33) reductions of renal blood flow in the kidney.

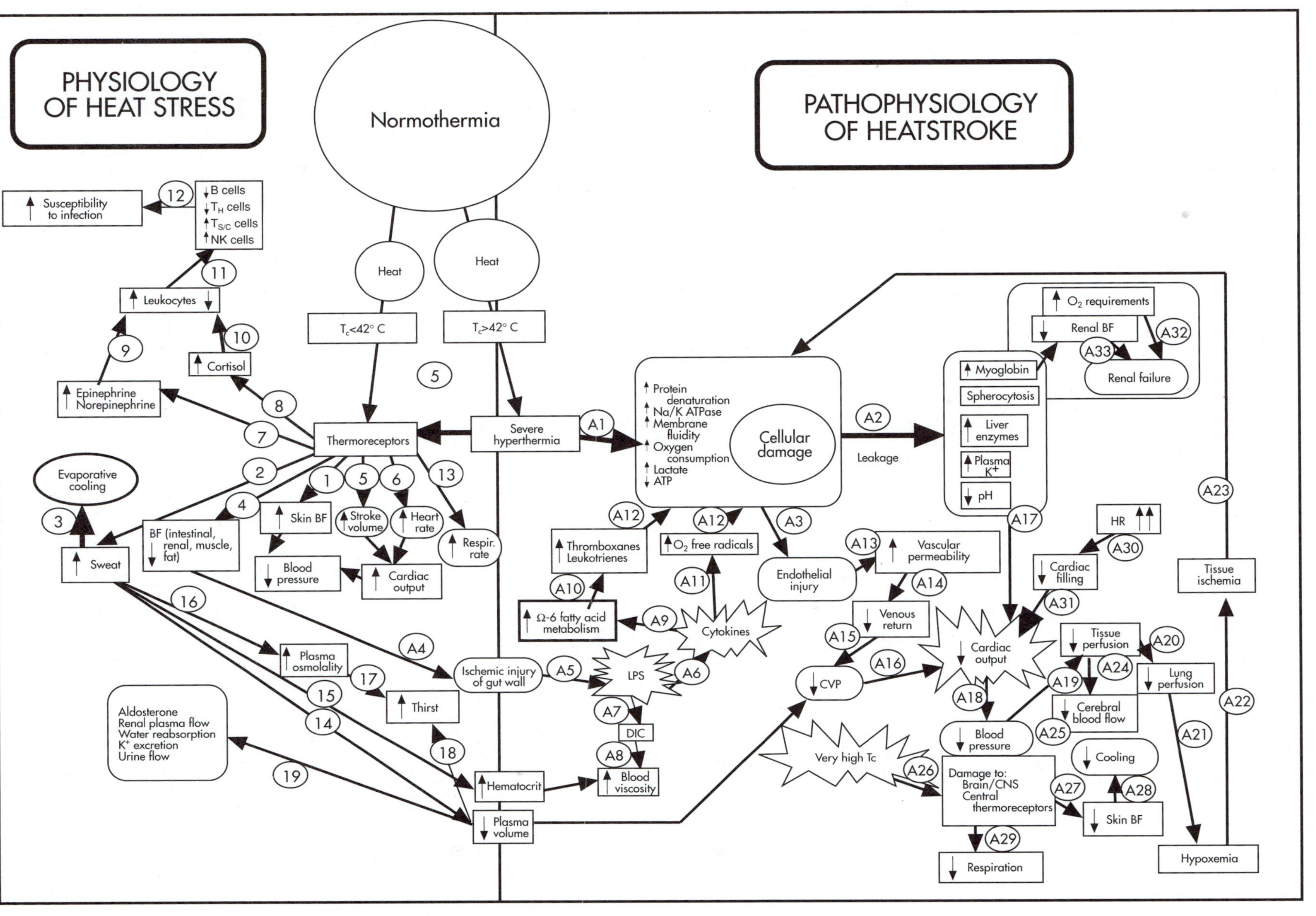

Fig. 8-9 For legend see opposite page.

factor predominates is influenced by physical activity and the temperature and volume of beverage. Early studies showed a delay in gastric emptying when the beverage contained more than 2.5% glucose, sucrose, or fructose. A more recent study by Davis and associates[110] found that a 6% sugar solution entered the blood as fast as a 2.5% solution or water. Seiple and co-workers[368] found no difference in gastric emptying time between water and beverages containing 5% and 7% carbohydrate (glucose polymers and fructose). Other investigators have confirmed that under exercise conditions 5% glucose polymer solutions show a gastric emptying rate similar to water.

Cold fluids empty from the stomach more rapidly than warm drinks. Drinking cold water increases the activity of the smooth muscle in the gastric wall, increasing motility. The commonly held belief that the consumption of cold water will result in stomach cramps has not been confirmed. Costill[96] has suggested that this phenomenon is more likely related to beverage volume than to its temperature.

Large volumes of liquid empty from the stomach more rapidly than do small quantities. Athletes, however, are uncomfortable exercising with a nearly full stomach. Indeed, while there may be a benefit to oral rehydration, if the nausea threshold is reached, a secondary increase in ADH secretion may impair the kidneys' ability to handle excess fluid and result in hyponatremia and water intoxication.[19,337] By drinking smaller amounts (150 to 250 ml) at 15- to 20-minute intervals, the athlete can maintain reasonable hydration while minimizing gastric filling.

A frequent argument for including sodium in fluid replacement beverages is to enhance intestinal absorption. Sodium transport is the major determinant of water absorption in the proximal small bowel. The active, coupled transport of sodium and glucose creates an osmotic gradient that pulls water from the lumen into the epithelial cells. Studies of carbohydrate-electrolyte solutions have shown their intestinal absorption to be equal to, but not better than, intestinal absorption of water.[300,435]

A sports drink needs to contain 5% to 10% carbohydrate in the form of glucose or sucrose to enhance endurance.[103] Many athletes, however, suffer cramps, nausea, and diarrhea after drinking a 10% glucose solution. An isocaloric glucose-polymer solution, however, has only one-fifth the osmotic pressure. This lower osmolality allows an increase in the carbohydrate content of a sports drink without risking the gastrointestinal side effects of a high osmolar drink. Several commercial polymer solutions are available.

Carbohydrate feeding during prolonged exercise enhances performance, whether assessed by exercise time to exhaustion or by time to complete a predetermined exercise task.[86,300] Glucose polymer solutions given before and during a soccer game resulted in sustained blood glucose and improved performance, although no difference in ratings of perceived exertion was found.[376] Whether use of these beverages spares muscle glycogen is a matter of current debate.

The use of carbohydrate solutions is not without disadvantages, however. These beverages are expensive, especially considering the limited athletic budgets of many school districts. In addition, the presence of such drinks may attract bees and yellowjackets into the vicinity of the athletes, placing them at risk for sting-induced allergic or anaphylactic reactions.

Under usual conditions the use of electrolyte-carbohydrate–containing beverages offers no advantage over water in maintaining plasma volume or electrolyte concentration or in improving intestinal absorption. Consumption of an electrolyte-containing beverage may be indicated under conditions of caloric restriction or repeated days of sustained sweat losses. Drinking carbohydrate solutions during prolonged exercise may enhance performance; athletes who might benefit are those involved in soccer, field hockey, rugby, and tennis. For these athletes use of glucose polymer solutions may be considered.

For the vast majority of individuals, however, the primary advantage of using electrolyte- or carbohydrate-containing drinks appears to enhance voluntary consumption. This factor should not be considered as insignificant if regulated intake is impossible.

Pathophysiology of Heat Stress and Heatstroke Model

A schematic model of normal thermoregulation and pathophysiology of heat stress and heatstroke (based on most of the preceding considerations) is shown in Fig. 8-9.

Acknowledgments

We gratefully acknowledge the dedicated assistance provided by SSG Donna Patterson, SGT Michael Koratich, SPC Michele Mayo, Ms. Kim Tartarini, and Ms. Diane Danielski.

REFERENCES

1. Adolph EF: *Physiology of man in the desert,* New York, 1947, Interscience.
2. Adolph EF, Fulton WB: The effects of exposure to high temperature upon the circulation in man, *Am J Physiol* 67:573, 1924.
3. Al-Hadramy MS, Ali F: Catecholamines in heat stroke, *Milit Med* 154:263, 1989.
4. Allan JR, Wilson CG: Influence of acclimatization on sweat sodium concentration, *J Appl Physiol* 38:708, 1971.
5. Allen TE, Smith DP, Miller DK: Hemodynamic response to submaximal exercise after dehydration and rehydration in high school wrestlers, *Med Sci Sports Exerc* 9:159, 1977.
6. Allsop P, Twigley AJ: The neuroleptic malignant syndrome: case report with a review of the literature, *Anaesthesia* 42:49, 1987.
7. Anderson RJ et al: Mechanism of effect of thoracic inferior vena cava constriction on renal water excretion, *J Clin Invest* 54:1473, 1974.
8. Anderson RJ et al: Heat injuries: early assessment and management. In Wolcott B, Rund DA, editors: *Emergency medicine annual,* vol 1, Norwalk, Conn, 1982, Appleton-Century-Crofts.

9. Andersson B: Regulation of water intake, *Physiol Rev* 58:582, 1978.
10. Andreoli TE et al: *Essentials of medicine*, ed 2, Philadelphia, 1990, WB Saunders.
11. Appenzeller O, Atkinson R: *Sports medicine: fitness training injuries*, Baltimore, 1981, Urban & Schwarzenberg.
12. Araki T, Toda Y, Matsushita K: Age differences in sweating during muscular exercise, *Jpn J Phys Fitness Sports Med* 28:239, 1979.
13. Armstrong LE, Costill DL, Fink WJ: Influence of diuretic-induced dehydration on competitive running performance, *Med Sci Sports Exerc* 17:456, 1985.
14. Armstrong LE, Deluca JP, Hubbard RW: Time course of recovery and heat acclimation ability of prior exertional heatstroke patients, *Med Sci Sports Exerc* 22:36, 1990.

14a. Armstrong LE, Hubbard RW: Application of a model of exertional heatstroke pathophysiology to cocaine intoxication, *Am J Emerg Med* 8:178, 1990.

15. Armstrong LE, Pandolf KB: Physical training, cardiorespiratory physical fitness and exercise heat tolerance. In Pandolf KB, Sawka MN, Gonzalez RR, editors: *Human performance physiology and environmental medicine at terrestrial extremes*, Indianapolis, 1988, Benchmark Press.
16. Armstrong LE et al: Heat acclimation during summer running in the northeastern United States, *Med Sci Sports Exerc* 19:131, 1986.
17. Armstrong LE et al: Preparing Alberto Salazar for the heat of the 1984 Olympic marathon, *Phys Sportsmed* 14:73, 1986.
18. Armstrong LE et al: Signs and symptoms of heat exhaustion during strenuous exercise, *Ann Sports Med* 3:182, 1987.
19. Armstrong LE et al: Symptomatic hyponatremia during prolonged exercise in heat, *Med Sci Sports Exerc* 25:543, 1993.

19a. Armstrong LE et al: Urinary indices of hydration status, *Int J Sports Nutr*, in press.

20. Astrup J, Blennow G, Nilsson B: Effects of reduced cerebral blood flow upon EEG pattern, cerebral extracellular potassium and energy metabolism in the rat cortex during bicuculline-induced seizures, *Brain Res* 177:115, 1979.
21. Atkins T: Fever: new perspective on an old phenomenon, *N Engl J Med* 308:958, 1983.
22. Ayala A et al: Hemorrhage induces an increase in serum TNF which is not associated with elevated levels of endotoxin, *Cytokine* 2:170, 1990.
23. Balkwill F: Cytokines: soluble factors in immune responses, *Curr Opin Immunol* 1:241, 1988.
24. Ball SP et al: Genetic linkage analysis of chromosome 19 markers in malignant hyperthermia, *Br J Anaesth* 70:70, 1993.
25. Ban E, Haour F, Lenstra R: Brain interleukin gene expression induced by peripheral dipolysaccharide administration, *Cytokine* 4:48, 1992.
26. Banet M: Mechanism of action of physical antipyresis in the rat, *J Appl Physiol* 64:1076, 1988.
27. Bar-Or O: Children and physical performance in warm and cold environments. In *Advances in pediatric sport sciences*, vol 1, Champaign, Ill, 1984, Human Kinetics.
28. Bar-Or O et al: Distribution of heat activated sweat glands in obese and lean men and women, *Hum Biol* 40:235, 1968.
29. Bartley JD: Heat stroke: is total prevention possible? *Milit Med* 142:528, 1977.
30. Bass DE, Henschel A: Responses of body fluid compartments to heat and cold, *Physiol Rev* 36:128, 1956.
31. Bean WB, Eichna LW: Performance in relation to environmental temperature, *Fed Proc* 2:144, 1943.
32. Beard MEJ et al: Jogger's heat stroke, *NZ Med J* 89:159, 1979.
33. Bell C, Provins K: Effects of high temperature environmental conditions on human performance, *J Occup Med* 4:202, 1962.
34. Bell C, Provins K: Relations between physiological responses to environmental heat and time judgement, *J Exp Psychol* 66:572, 1963.
35. Bell JF, Moore GJ: Effects of high ambient temperature on various stages of rabies virus infection in mice, *Infect Immun* 10:510, 1974.
36. Beller GA, Boyd AE: Heat stroke: a report of 13 consecutive cases without mortality despite severe hyperpyrexia and neurologic dysfunction, *Milit Med* 140:464, 1975.
37. Beller GA, Maher JT, Hartley LH: Changes in serum and sweat magnesium levels during work in the heat, *Aviat Space Environ Med* 46:709, 1975.
38. Benedek G et al: Indomethacin is effective against neurogenic hyperthermia following cranial trauma or brain surgery, *Can J Neurol Sci* 14:145, 1987.
39. Benziger TH: On physical heat regulation and the sense of temperature in man, *Proc Natl Acad Sci USA* 45:645, 1959.
40. Benziger TH: The diminution of thermoregulatory sweating during cold-reception at the skin, *Proc Natl Acad Sci USA* 47:740, 1961.
41. Berczi I, Bertok K, Bereznai T: Comparative studies on the toxicity of *E. coli* lipopolysaccharide endotoxin in various animal species, *Can J Microbiol* 12:1070, 1966.
42. Besedovsky H, Sorkin E: The immune response evokes changes in brain noradrenergic neurons, *Clin Exp Immunol* 27:1, 1977.
43. Biselli R et al: Influence of stress on lymphocyte subset distribution: a flow cytometric study in young student pilots, *Aviat Space Environ Med* 64:116, 1993.
44. Blair DA, Glover WE: Vasomotor fibers to the skin in the upper arm, calf and thigh, *J Physiol* 153:232, 1960.
45. Blatteis CM: Fever: is it beneficial? *Yale J Biol Med* 59:107, 1986.
46. Bligh J, Johnson KG: Glossary of terms for thermal physiology, *J Appl Physiol* 35:941, 1973.
47. Blood CG, Gauker ED: *The relationship between battle intensity and disease rates among Marine Corps infantry units. Final report no 92-1*, San Diego, 1992, Naval Health Research Center.
48. Bocci V: Central nervous system toxicity of interferons and other cytokines, *J Biol Regul Homeost Agents* 2:107, 1988.
49. Bohmer D: Loss of electrolytes by sweat in sports. In *Sport health and nutrition: the 1984 Olympic scientific congress proceedings*, vol 2, Champaign, Ill, 1986, Human Kinetics.
50. Borrelli MJ et al: Reduction of levels of nuclear-associated protein in heated cells by cycloheximide, D2O, and thermotolerance, *Radiat Res* 131:204, 1992.
51. Bosenberg AT et al: Strenuous exercise causes systemic endotoxemia, *J Appl Physiol* 65:106, 1988.
52. Bottoms G, Adams R: Involvement of prostaglandins and leukotrienes in the pathogenesis of endotoxemia and sepsis, *J Am Veterin Med Assoc* 200:1842, 1992.
53. Bouchama A et al: Mechanisms of hypophosphatemia in humans with heatstroke, *J Appl Physiol* 71:328, 1991.
54. Bouchama A et al: Distribution of peripheral blood leukocytes in acute heatstroke, *J Appl Physiol* 73:405, 1992.
55. Bouchama A et al: Elevated pyrogenic cytokines in heatstroke, *Chest* 104:1498, 1993.
56. Boulant JA: Hypothalamic control of thermoregulation. In Morgane PJ, Panksepp J, editors: *Handbook of the hypothalamus*, vol 3, Part A. *Behavioral studies of the hypothalamus*, New York, 1980, Marcel Dekker.
57. Bowler K: Heat death and cellular heat injury, *J Therm Biol* 6:171, 1981.
58. Boyd AE, Beller AG: Acid-base changes in heat exhaustion during basic training, *Proc Army Sci Conf* 1:114, 1972.
59. Boyd AE, Beller GA: Heat exhaustion and respiratory alkalosis, *Ann Intern Med* 83:835, 1975.
60. Brock TD: Life at high temperatures, *Science* 230:132, 1985.
61. Brock-Utne JG et al: Endotoxaemia in exhausted runners following a long distance race, *S Afr Med J* 73:533, 1988.
62. Brotherhood JR: Nutrition and sports performance, *Sports Med* 1:350, 1984.
63. Brown R, King MG, Husband AJ: Sleep deprivation-induced hyperthermia following antigen challenge due to opioid but not interleukin-1 involvement, *Physiol Behav* 51:767, 1992.

64. Burdon RH et al: Hyperthermia, Na^+K^+ATPase and lactic acid production in some human tumour cells, *Br J Cancer* 49:437, 1984.
65. Buskirk ER, Iampietro PF, Bass DE: Work performance after dehydration: effects of physical conditioning and heat acclimation, *J Appl Physiol* 12:189, 1958.
66. Bynum GD et al: Induced hyperthermia in sedated humans and the concept of critical thermal maximum, *Am J Physiol* 235:R228, 1978.
67. Caldwell JA Jr: A brief survey of chemical defense, crew rest and heat stress/physical training issues related to Operation Desert Storm, *Milit Med* 157:275, 1992.
68. Caldwell JE: Diuretic therapy and exercise performance, *Sports Med* 4:290, 1987.
69. Caldwell JE, Ahonen E, Nousiainen U: Differential effects of sauna-, diuretic-, and exercise-induced hypohydration, *J Appl Physiol* 57:1018, 1984.
70. Callaham ML: *Emergency management of heat illness: emergency physicians series,* North Chicago, Ill, 1979, Abbott Labs.
71. Campbell BG: Cocaine abuse with hyperthermia, seizures, and fatal complications, *Med J Aust* 149:387, 1988.
72. Cannon JG, Kluger MJ: Endogenous pyrogen activity in human plasma after exercise, *Science* 220:617, 1983.
73. Cannon JG et al: Physiological mechanisms contributing to increased interleukin-1 secretion, *J Appl Physiol* 61:1869, 1986.
74. Cannon JG et al: Increased interleukin 1 beta in human skeletal muscle after exercise, *Am J Physiol* 257:R451, 1989.
75. Cannon JG et al: Acute phase response in exercise. II. Associations between vitamin E, cytokines and muscle proteolysis, *Am J Physiol* 260:R1235, 1991.
76. Caridis DT et al: Endotoxaemia in man, *Lancet* 1:1381, 1972.
77. Carmichael LE, Barnes FD, Percy DH: Temperature as a factor in resistance of young puppies to canine herpesvirus, *J Infect Dis* 120:669, 1969.
78. Carter BJ, Cammermeyer M: Emergence of real casualties during simulated chemical warfare training under high heat conditions, *Milit Med* 150:657, 1985.
79. Casey LC, Balk RA, Bone RC: Plasma cytokine and endotoxin levels correlate with survival in patients with the sepsis syndrome, *Ann Intern Med* 119:771, 1993.
80. Chang J, Gilman SC, Lewis AE: Interleukin-1 activates phospholipase A2 in rabbit chondrocytes: a possible signal for IL-1 action, *J Immunol* 36:1283, 1986.
81. Chiles W: Effects of elevated temperatures on performance of a complex mental task, *Ergonomics* 2:89, 1958.
82. Choo MHHH: Clinical presentation of heat disorders. In Yeo PPB, Lin MK, editors: *Heat disorders,* Singapore, 1988, Headquarters Medical Services.
83. Clark BD et al: Detection of interleukin 1 alpha and 1 beta in rabbit tissues during endotoxemia using sensitive radioimmunoassays, *J Appl Physiol* 71:2412, 1991.
84. Clausen T: Regulation of active Na-K transport in skeletal muscle, *Physiol Rev* 66:542, 1986.
85. Clowes GHA, O'Donnell TF: Heatstroke, *N Engl J Med* 291:564, 1974.
86. Coggan AR, Coyle EF: Metabolism and performance following carbohydrate ingestion late in exercise, *Med Sci Sports Exerc* 21:59, 1989.
87. Cohen I, Mitchell D, Seider R: The effect of water deficit on body temperature during rugby, *S Afr Med J* 60:11, 1981.
88. Cohen S: Physiologic and pathologic manifestations of lymphokine action, *Hum Pathol* 17:112, 1986.
89. Cohen S, Tyrrell DA, Smith AP: Psychological stress and susceptibility to the common cold, *N Engl J Med* 325:606, 1991.
90. Collings GH, Shoudy LA, Shaffer FE: The clinical aspects of heat diseases, *Industr Med* 12:728, 1943.
91. Collins KJ, Crockford GW, Weiner JS: The local training effect of secretory activity on the response of eccrine sweat glands, *J Physiol* 184:203, 1966.
92. Consolazio CF, Matoush LO, Nelson RA: Excretion of sodium, potassium, magnesium and iron in human sweat and the relation of each to balance requirements, *J Nutr* 79:407, 1963.
93. Cook JA, Tempel GE, Ball HA: Eicosanoids in sepsis and its sequelae. In Halushka PV, Mais DE, editors: *Eicosanoids in the cardiovascular and renal systems,* Lancaster, UK, 1988, MTPP Press.
94. Cornet C, Moeller R, Laxenaoir MC: Clinical features of malignant hyperthermia crisis, *Ann Fr Anesth Reanim* 8:435, 1989.
95. Costill DL: Muscle water and electrolytes during acute and repeated bouts of dehydration. In Parizkova V, Rogozkin A, editors: *Nutrition, physical fitness and health,* Baltimore, 1978, University Park Press.
96. Costill DL: Water and electrolyte requirements during exercise, *Clin Sports Med* 3:639, 1984.
97. Costill DL, Branam G, Fink W: Changes in plasma renin and aldosterone, *Med Sci Sports Exerc* 8:209, 1976.
98. Costill DL, Cote R, Fink W: Muscle water and electrolytes following varied levels of dehydration in man, *J Appl Physiol* 40:6, 1976.
99. Costill DL, Miller JM: Nutrition for endurance sport: carbohydrate and fluid balance, *Int J Sports Med* 1:2, 1980.
100. Costill DL et al: Determination of human muscle pH in needle-biopsy specimens, *J Appl Physiol* 53:1310, 1982.
101. Costrini AM: Emergency treatment of exertional heatstroke and comparison of whole body cooling techniques, *Med Sci Sports Exerc* 22:15, 1990.
102. Costrini AM et al: Cardiovascualr and metabolic manifestations of heatstroke and severe heat exhaustion, *Am J Med* 66:296, 1979.
103. Coyle EF, Coggan AR: Effectiveness of carbohydrate feeding in delaying fatigue during prolonged exercise, *Sports Med* 1:446, 1984.
104. Croyle PH, Place RA, Hilgenberg AD: Massive pulmonary embolism in a high school wrestler, *JAMA* 241:827, 1979.
105. Cunningham DJ, Stolwijk JAJ, Wenger CB: Comparative thermoregulatory responses of resting men and women, *J Appl Physiol* 45:908, 1978.
106. Cunningham ET, DeSouza EB: Interleukin-1 receptors in the brain and endocrine tissues, *Immunol Today* 14:171, 1993.
107. Curley MD, Hawkins RN: Cognitive performance during a heat acclimation regimen, *Aviat Space Environ Med* 54:709, 1983.
108. Dascombe MJ: The pharmacology of fever, *Prog Neurobiol* 25:327, 1985.
109. Davatelis G et al: Macrophage inflammatory protein-1: a prostaglandin-independent endogenous pyrogen, *Science* 2432:1066, 1989.
110. Davis MM et al: Accumulation of deuterium oxide in body fluids after ingestion of D2O-labelled beverages, *J Appl Physiol* 63:2060, 1987.
111. Day SC et al: Evaluation and outcome of emergency room patients with transient loss of consciousness, *Am J Med* 73:15, 1982.
112. Deitch EA et al: Effect of hemorrhagic shock on bacterial translocation, intestinal morphology and intestinal permeability in conventional and antibiotic-decontaminated rats, *Crit Care Med* 18:529, 1990.
113. Dill DB, Hall FG, Van Beaumont W: Sweat chloride concentration: sweat rate, metabolic rate, skin temperature and age, *J Appl Physiol* 21:99, 1966.
114. Dill DB, Scholt L, MacLean D: Capacity of young males and females for running in desert heat, *Med Sci Sports* 9:137, 1977.
115. Dinarello CA, Cannon JG, Wolff SM: New concepts on the pathogenesis of fever, *Rev Infect Dis* 10:168, 1988.
116. Dinarello CA, Wolff SM: The role of interleukin-1 in disease, *N Engl J Med* 328:106, 1993.
117. Dinman BD, Horvath SM: Heat disorders in industry: a reevaluation of diagnostic criteria, *J Occup Med* 26:489, 1984.
118. DuBose DA, McCreary J, Sowders L: Correlation between plasma fibronectin level and experimental rat heat stress mortality, *J Appl Physiol* 59:706, 1985.
119. DuBose DA et al: Role of bacterial endotoxins of intestinal origin in rat heat stress mortality, *J Appl Physiol* 54:31, 1983.

120. DuBose DA et al: Relationship between rat heat stress mortality and alterations in reticuloendothelial carbon clearance function, *Aviat Space Environ Med* 54:1090, 1983.
121. Duff GW: Is fever beneficial to the host: a clinical perspective, *Yale J Biol Med,* 59:125, 1986.
122. Dukes-Dobos FN: Hazards of heat exposure: a review, *Scand J Work Environ Health* 7:73, 1981.
123. Dynlacht JR, Fox MH: Heat-induced changes in the membrane fluidity of Chinese hamster ovary cells measured by flow cytometry, *Radiat Res* 130:4, 1992.
124. Dynlacht JR, Hyun WC, Dewey WC: Changes in intracellular free calcium during hyperthermia: effects of local anesthetics and induction of thermotolerance, *Cytometry* 14:223, 1993.
125. Ebadi M, Pfeiffer RF, Murrin LC: Pathogenesis and treatment of neuroleptic malignant syndrome, *Gen Pharmacol* 21:367, 1990.
126. Edmeads J: Understanding dizziness: how to decipher this nonspecific symptom, *Postgraduate Med* 88:255, 1990.
127. Eichler A, McFee A, Root H: Heatstroke, *Am J Surg* 118:855, 1969.
128. Eichna LW et al: Thermal regulation during acclimatization in a hot, dry (desert type) environment, *Am J Physiol* 163:585, 1950.
129. El-Kassimi FA et al: Adult respiratory distress syndrome and disseminated intravascular coagulation complicating heat stroke, *Chest* 90:571, 1986.
130. Elizondo R: Local control of eccrine sweat gland function, *Fed Proc* 32:1583, 1973.
131. Ellis FP: Mortality from heat illness and heat-aggravated illness in the United States, *Environ Res* 5:1, 1972.
132. Ellis FP: Heat illness. I. Epidemiology. II. Pathogenesis. III. Acclimatization, *Trans R Soc Trop Med Hyg* 70:402, 1976.
133. Endres S et al: The effect of dietary supplementation with n-3 polyunsaturated fatty acids on the synthesis of interleukin-1 and tumor necrosis factor by mononuclear cells, *N Engl J Med* 320:265, 1989.
134. Epstein Y, Sohar E: Fluid balance in hot climates: sweating, water intake and prevention of dehydration, *Public Health Rev* 13:115, 1985.
135. Feig PU, McCurdy DK: The hypertonic state, *N Engl J Med* 297:1444, 1977.
136. Felig P, Johnson C, Levitt M: Hypernatremia induced by maximal exercise, *JAMA* 248:1209, 1982.
137. Felten DL et al: Noradrenergic sympathetic neural interactions with the immune system structure and function, *Immunol Rev* 100:225, 1987.
138. Ferris EB et al: Heat stroke: clinical and chemical observations on 44 cases, *J Clin Invest* 17:249, 1938.
139. Feruchi S, Shimizu Y: Effect of ambient temperatures on multiplication of attenuated transmissible gastroenteritis virus in the bodies of newborn piglets, *Infect Immun* 13:990, 1976.
140. Fink MP et al: Increased intestinal permeability in endotoxic pig, *Arch Surg* 126:211, 1991.
141. Fletcher JL Jr, Creten D: Perceptions of fever among adults in a family practice setting, *J Fam Pract* 22:427, 1986.
142. Fogoros RN: Runner's trots, *JAMA* 243:1743, 1980.
143. Fortney SM et al: Effect of blood volume on sweating rate and body fluids on exercising humans, *J Appl Physiol* 51:1594, 1981.
144. Fortney SM et al: Effect of hyperosmolality on control of blood flow and sweating, *J Appl Physiol* 57:1688, 1984.
145. Fox RH: Heat. In Edholm OG, Bacharach AL, editors: *The physiology of human survival,* London, 1965, Academic Press.
146. Fox RH, Edholm OG: Nervous control of the cutaneous circulation, *Br Med Bull* 19:110, 1963.
147. Fox RH et al: Acclimatization to heat in man by controlled elevation of body temperature, *J Physiol* 166:530, 1963.
148. Francesconi R, Mager M: Heat-injured rats: pathochemical indices and survival time, *J Appl Physiol* 45:1, 1978.
149. Francesconi R, Mager M: Hypo- and hyperglycemia in rats: effects on endurance and heat/exercise injury, *Aviat Space Environ Med* 54:1085, 1983.
150. Francesconi RP et al: Potassium deficiency in rats: effects on acute thermal tolerance, *J Thermal Biol* 16:77, 1991.
151. Fukumoto T, Tanaka T, Fujioka H: Differences in composition of sweat induced by thermal exposure and by running exercise, *Clin Cardiol* 11:707, 1988.
152. Furukawa M et al: Effects of hyperthermia on intracellular calcium concentration and responses of cancerous mammary cells in culture, *Cell Biochem Funct* 10:225, 1992.
153. Gaffin SL: Antibody therapy for shock. In Hardaway RM III, editor: *Shock: the reversible step toward death,* Littleton, Mass, 1988, PSG.
154. Gaffin SL et al: Protection against hemorrhagic shock in the cat by human plasma containing endotoxin-specific antibody, *J Surg Res* 31:18, 1981.
155. Gaffin SL et al: Hypoxia-induced endotoxemia in primates: role of the reticuloendothelial system function and anti-lipopolysaccharide plasma, *Aviat Space Environ Med* 57:1044, 1986.
156. Garrey W, Bryan W: Variations in white blood cell counts, *Physiol Rev* 15:597, 1935.
157. Gathiram P et al: Time course of endotoxemia and cardiovascular changes in heat-stressed primates, *Aviat Space Environ Med* 58:1071, 1987.
158. Gathiram P et al: Prevention of endotoxemia by non-absorbable antibiotics in heatstress, *J Clin Pathol* 40:1364, 1987.
159. Gathiram P et al: Anti-LPS improves survival in primates subjected to heat stroke, *Circ Shock* 23:157, 1987.
160. Gathiram P et al: Portal and systemic arterial plasma lipopolysaccharide concentrations in heat stressed primates, *Circ Shock* 25:223, 1988.
161. Geelen JMC et al: Heat-shock induction of human immunodeficiency virus, *J Gen Virol* 69:2913, 1988.
162. Gersh BJ, Hammill SC: Current recommendation for evaluating syncope, *Contemp Intern Med,* Oct 1990, p 80.
163. Gharpure M: A heat-sensitive cellular function required for the replication of DNA but not RNA viruses, *Virology* 27:308, 1965.
164. Gick CG, Ismail-Beigi F, Edelman IS: Hormonal regulation of Na K-ATPase. In Skou IC et al, editors: *The Na K pump, Part B, Cellular aspects,* New York, 1988, Alan R Liss.
165. Gilat R, Shibolet S, Sohar E: The mechanism of heatstroke, *J Trop Med Hyg* 66:204, 1963.
166. Gisolfi CV, Cohen JS: Relationships among training, heat acclimation and heat tolerance among men and women: the controversy revisited, *Med Sci Sports* 11:56, 1979.
167. Gisolfi CV, Wenger CB: Temperature regulation during exercise: old concepts, new ideas, *Exerc Sports Sci Rev* 12:339, 1984.
168. Givoni B, Goldman RF: Predicting rectal temperature response to work, environment and clothing, *J Appl Physiol* 32:812, 1973.
169. Godfrey RW, Johnson WJ, Hoffstein ST: Interleukin-1 stimulation of phospholipase in rat synovial fibroblasts: possible regulation by cyclooxygenase products, *Arthritis Rheum* 31:1421, 1988.
170. Goetz RH: Effect of changes in posture on peripheral circulation, with special reference to skin temperature readings and the plethysmogram, *Circulation* 1:56, 1950.
171. Golstein P et al: Cell death mechanisms and the immune system, *Immunol Rev* 121:29, 1991.
172. Gonzalez RR: Biophysics of heat transfer and clothing considerations. In Pandolf KB, Sawka MN, Gonzalez RR, editors: *Human performance physiology and environmental medicine at terrestrial extremes,* Indianapolis, 1988, Benchmark Press.
173. Graber CD et al: Fatal heat stroke: circulating endotoxin and gram-negative sepsis as complications, *JAMA* 216:1195, 1971.
174. Graham BS et al: Nonexertional heatstroke: physiologic management and cooling in 145 patients, *Arch Intern Med* 146:876, 1985.
175. Gray JD, Blaschke TF: Fever: to treat or not to treat, *Rational Drug Ther* 19:1, 1985.
176. Green HJ et al: Altitude acclimatization and energy metabolic adaptations in skeletal muscle during exercise, *J Appl Physiol* 73:2701, 1992.

177. Greisman SF, Hornick RB: Mechanisms of endotoxin tolerance with special reference to man, *J Infect Dis* 128(Suppl):S265, 1973.
178. Grether W: Human performance at elevated environmental temperatures, *Aerospace Med* 44:747, 1973.
179. Hahn GM: *Hyperthermia and cancer,* New York, 1982, Plenum.
180. Haldane JS: The influence of high air temperatures, *J Hyg* 55:495, 1905.
181. Hales JRS, Nielson B, Yanase M: Skin blood flow during severe heat stress regional variations and failure to maintain maximal level. In Milton AS, editor: Thermal physiology. In *Proceedings of the IUPS Thermal Commission Symposium,* Aberdeen, Scotland, Aug 1993, International Union of Physiological Science.
182. Hammarstrom S et al: Microcirculatory effects of leukotrienes C4 and D4 and E4 in guinea pig. In Lefer A, Gee MH, editors: *Progress in clinical and biological research: leukotrienes in cardiovascular and pulmonary function,* New York, 1985, Alan R Liss.
183. Hanson PG, Zimmerman SW: Exertional heatstroke in novice runners, *JAMA* 242:154, 1979.
184. Haq A et al: Changes in peripheral blood lymphocyte subsets associated with marathon running, *Med Sci Sports Exerc* 25:186, 1993.
185. Hardy JD: Physiology of temperature regulation, *Physiol Rev* 41:521, 1961.
186. Harrison MH: Effects of thermal stress and exercise on blood volume in humans, *Physiol Rev* 65:149, 1985.
187. Hart GR et al: Epidemic classical heat stroke: clinical characteristics and course of 28 patients, *Medicine* 61:189, 1982.
188. Hart LE, Egier BP, Shimizu AG: Exertional heatstroke: the runner's nemesis, *Can Med Assoc J* 122:1144, 1980.
189. Hart LE, Sutton JR: Environmental considerations for exercise, *Cardiol Clin* 5:245, 1987.
190. Havenith G, Middendrop HV: The relative influence of physical fitness, acclimatization state, anthropometric measures, and gender on individual reactions to stress, *Eur J Appl Physiol* 61:419, 1990.
191. Hayaishi O: Molecular mechanisms of sleep-wake regulation: role of prostaglandins D2 and E2, *FASEB J* 5:2575, 1991.
192. Hayano YH: Influence of induced hyperthermia on intestinal blood flow, translocation of endotoxin and other factors in mongrel dogs, *Masui* 40:769, 1991.
193. Heiman-Patterson TD: Neuroleptic malignant syndrome and malignant hyperthermia: important issues for the medical consultant, *Med Clin North Am* 77:477, 1993.
194. Henry JA, Jeffreys KJ, Dawling S: Toxicity and deaths from 3,4-methylenedioxymethamphetamine ("ecstacy"), *Lancet* 2:384, 1992.
195. Hensel H, Iggo A, Witt I: A quantitative study of sensitive cutaneous thermoreceptors with afferent fibers, *J Physiol* 153:113, 1960.
196. Herrman F, Prose PH, Sulzberger MB: Studies on sweating. V. Studies of quantity and distribution of thermogenic sweat delivery to the skin, *J Invest Dermatol* 18:71, 1952.
197. Hilton F: *The Paras,* London, 1983, British Broadcasting Corp.
198. Hochachka PW, Matheson GO: ATPases and energy metabolism as proactive and reactive components in control of ATP turnover rates. In Sutton JR, Coates G, Houston CS, editors: *Hypoxia and mountain medicine: advances in the biosciences,* vol 84, Oxford, 1992, Pergamon Press.
199. Hochachka PW, Matheson GO: Regulating ATP turnover rates over broad dynamic work ranges in skeletal muscles, *J Appl Physiol* 73:1697, 1992.
200. Hoggan MD, Roizman B: The effect of the temperature on inhibition of the formation and release of herpes simplex virus in infected FL cells, *Virology* 8:508, 1959.
201. Holmes SW, Horton EW: The identification of four prostaglandins in dog brain and their regional distribution in the central nervous system, *J Physiol* 195:731, 1968.
202. Hopkins PM, Ellis FR, Halsall PJ: Evidence for related myopathies in exertional heat stroke and malignant hyperthermia, *Lancet* 2:1491, 1991.
203. Horowitz M: Heat stress and heat acclimation: the cellular response-modifier of autonomic control. In Pleschka K, Gerstberger R, Pierau K, editors: *Integrative and cellular aspects of autonomic functions,* France, 1993, John Libbey Eurotext.
204. Horowitz M, Parnes S, Hasin Y: Mechanical and metabolic performance in the rat heart: effects of combined stress of heat acclimation and swimming training, *Basic Clin Physiol Pharmacol* 4(1-2):139, 1993.
205. Horowitz M et al: Heat acclimation: cardiac performance of isolated rat heart, *J Appl Physiol* 60:9, 1986.
206. Hubbard RW: Heatstroke pathophysiology: the energy depletion model, *Med Sci Sports Exerc* 22:19, 1990.
207. Hubbard RW, Armstrong LE: The heat illnesses: biochemical ultrastructural and fluid electrolyte considerations. In Pandolf KB, Sawka MN, Gonzalez RR, editors: *Human performance: physiology and environmental medicine at terrestrial extremes,* Indianapolis, 1988, Benchmark Press.
208. Hubbard RW, Armstrong LE: Hyperthermia: new thoughts on an old problem, *Phys Sports Med* 17:97, 1989.
209. Hubbard RW et al: Long term water and salt deficits: a military perspective. In *Military performance due to inadequate nutrition,* Washington, DC, 1986, National Academy Press.
210. Hubbard RW et al: Novel approaches to the pathophysiology of heat stroke: the energy depletion model, *Ann Emerg Med* 16:1066, 1987.
211. Hubbard RW: An introduction: the role of exercise in the etiology of exertional heatstroke, *Med Sci Sports Exerc* 22:2, 1990.
212. Hughson RL, Sutton JR: Heat stroke in a "run for fun," *Br Med J* 2:1158, 1978.
213. Husseini RH et al: Elevation of nasal viral levels by suppression of fever in ferrets infected with influenza viruses of differing virulence, *J Infect Dis* 145:520, 1982.
214. Iampietro PF: Heat-induced tetany, *Fed Proc* 22:884, 1963.
215. Iampietro PF, Mager M, Green EB: Some physiological changes accompanying tetany induced by exposure to hot wet conditions, *J Appl Physiol* 16:409, 1961.
216. Iriki M, Hashimoto M, Saigusa T: Threshold dissociation of thermoregulation effector responses in febrile rabbits, *Can J Physiol Pharmacol* 65:1304, 1987.
217. Irvine RF: How is the level of free arachidonic acid controlled in mammalian cells? *Biochem J* 4:3, 1982.
218. Jermain DM, Crismon ML: Psychotropic drug–related rhabdomyolysis, *Ann Pharmacother* 26:948, 1992.
219. Jesati RM: Management of severe hyperthermia with chlorpromazine and refrigeration, *N Engl J Med* 254:426, 1956.
220. Jiang CG et al: Immunosuppression in mice induced by cold water stress, *Brain Behav Immun* 4:278, 1990.
221. Johnson HL, Nelson RA, Consolazio CF: Effects of electrolyte and nutrient solutions on performance and metabolic balance, *Med Sci Sports Exerc* 20:26, 1988.
222. Johnson JM et al: Regulation of the cutaneous circulation, *Fed Proc* 445:2841, 1986.
223. Joshi PT, Capozzoli JA, Coyle JT: Neuroleptic malignant syndrome: life-threatening complication of neuroleptic treatment in adolescents with affective disorder, *Pediatrics* 87:235, 1991.
224. Jurivich DA et al: Effect of sodium salicylate on the human heat shock response, *Science* 255:1243, 1992.
225. Kampschmidt RF: The numerous postulated biological manifestations of interleukin-1, *J Leukoc Biol* 36:341, 1984.
226. Kapoor WN, Hammill SC, Gersh BJ: Diagnosis and natural history of syncope and the role of invasive electrophysiologic testing, *Am J Cardiol* 63:730, 1989.
227. Kapoor WN et al: Syncope in the elderly, *Am J Med* 80:419, 1986.
228. Kappel M et al: Effect of in vitro hyperthermia on the proliferative response of blood mononuclear cell subsets, and detection of interleukins 1 and 6, tumor necrosis factor-alpha and interferon-gamma, *Immunology* 73:304, 1991.

229. Kappel M et al: Effects of in vivo hyperthermia on natural killer cell activity, in vitro proliferative responses and blood mononuclear cell subpopulations, *Cell Exp Immunol* 84:175, 1991.
230. Kaufman WC et al: Standardization of units and symbols: revised, *Aviat Space Environ Med* 55:93, 1984.
231. Kaufmann SHE: Heat shock proteins and the immune response, *Immunol Today* 11:129, 1990.
232. Keren G, Epstein Y, Magazanik A: Temporary heat intolerance in a heatstroke patient, *Aviat Space Environ Med* 52:116, 1981.
233. Kerslake DM: *The stress of hot environments,* New York, 1972, Cambridge University Press.
234. Kety SS, Schmidt CF: The effects of active and passive hyperventilation on cerebral blood flow, oxygen consumption, cardiac output and blood pressure of normal men, *J Clin Invest* 25:107, 1961.
235. Kew MC, Bersohn I, Seftel H: The diagnostic and prognostic significance of the serum enzyme changes in heatstroke, *Trans R Soc Trop Med Hyg* 65:325, 1971.
236. Khansari DN, Murgo AJ, Faith RE: Effects of stress on the immune system, *Immunol Today* 11:170, 1990.
237. Khogali M: Epidemiology of heat illnesses during the Makkah pilgrimages in Saudi Arabia, *Int J Epidemiol* 12:267, 1983.
238. Khogali M: The Makkah body cooling unit. In Khogali M, Hales JRS, editors: *Heat stroke and temperature regulation,* Sydney, 1983, Academic Press.
239. Khogali M: Heatstroke and heat exhaustion, *Travel Traffic Med Int* 1:166, 1983.
240. Khogali M, Mustafa MKY: Clinical management of heat stroke patients. In Hales JRV, Richards DB, editors: *Heat stress: physical exertion and environment,* New York, 1987, Elsevier.
241. Khogali M et al: Induced heatstroke: a model in sheep. In Khogali M, editor: *Heatstroke and temperature regulation,* Sydney, Australia, 1983, Academic Press.
242. Kielblock AJ, VanRensberg JP, Franz RM: Body cooling as a method for reducing hyperthermia: an evaluation of techniques, *S Afr Med J* 69:378, 1986.
243. Kienzle MG: Syncope: mechanisms and manifestations, *Hosp Pract* 15:74, 1990.
244. Kilbourne EM et al: Risk factors in heatstroke, *JAMA* 247:3332, 1982.
245. Kirsch KA, Vonameln H, Wicke JH: Fluid control mechanisms after exercise dehydration, *Eur J Appl Physiol* 47:191, 1981.
246. Kluger MJ: Temperature regulation, fever and disease. In Robertshaw D, editor: *International review of physiology: environmental physiology III,* 20, Baltimore, 1979, University Park Press.
247. Kluger MJ: Is fever beneficial? *Yale J Biol Med* 59:89, 1986.
248. Kluger MJ: Further evidence that stress hyperthermia is a fever, *Physiol Behav* 39:763, 1987.
249. Knochel JP: Environmental heat illness, *Arch Intern Med* 133:841, 1974.
250. Knochel JP: Dog days and siriasis: how to kill a football player, *JAMA* 233:513, 1975.
251. Knochel JP: Role of glucoregulatory hormones in potassium homeostasis, *Kidney Int* 11:443, 1977.
252. Knochel JP: Heat stroke and related heat stress disorders, *Disease-a-Month* 35:301, 1989.
253. Knochel JP: Catastrophic medical events with exhaustive exercise: "white collar rhabdomyolysis," *Kidney Int* 38:709, 1990.
254. Knochel JP, Reed G: Disorders of heat regulation. In Kleeman CR, Maxwell MH, Narin RG, editors: *Clinical disorders of fluid and electrolyte metabolism,* New York, 1987, McGraw-Hill.
255. Kolesnick R: Ceramide: a novel second messenger, *Trends Cell Biol* 2:232, 1992.
256. Kosunen KJ et al: Plasma renin activity, angiotensin II and aldosterone during intense heat stress, *J Appl Physiol* 41:323, 1976.
257. Kreuger JM et al: Enhancement of slow-wave sleep by endotoxin and lipid A, *Am J Physiol* 251:R591, 1986.
258. Kronfol Z et al: Impaired lymphocyte function in depressive illness, *Life Sci* 33:2412, 1983.
259. Krueger JM et al: Putative sleep neuromodulators. In Montplaisir J, editor: *Sleep and biological rhythms,* Oxford, 1990, Oxford University Press.
260. Kreuger JM et al: Somnogenic cytokines and models concerning their effects on sleep, *Yale J Biol Med* 63:157, 1990.
261. Kunstlinger U, Ludwig HG, Stegemann J: Metabolic changes during volleyball matches, *Int J Sports Med* 8:315, 1987.
262. Ladell WSS: Heat cramps, *Lancet* 2:836, 1949.
263. Ladell WSS: Disorders due to heat, *Trans R Soc Trop Med Hyg* 51:189, 1957.
264. Lee JB, Katayama S: Prostaglandins, thromboxanes, and leukotrienes. In Wilson JD, Foster DW, editors: *Textbook of endocrinology,* Philadelphia, 1985, WB Saunders.
265. Leithead CS, Gunn ER: The aetiology of cane cutter's cramps in British Guiana. In *Environmental physiology and psychology in arid conditions,* Liege, Belgium, 1964, UNESCO.
266. Leithead CS, Lind AR: *Heat stress and heat disorders,* Philadelphia, 1964, Davis.
267. Levi E et al: Heat acclimation improves cardiac mechanics and metabolic performance during ischemia and reperfusion, *J Appl Physiol* 75:833, 1993.
268. Levin J, Bang F: Clottable protein in *Limulus:* its localization and kinetics of coagulation by endotoxin, *Thromb Haemost* 19:186, 1968.
269. Lewis GBH: Effect of altered environmental temperature on established infection, *Anaesth Intens Care* 16:338, 1988.
270. Lind AR: A physiological criterion for setting thermal environmental limits for everyday work, *J Appl Physiol* 18:51, 1963.
271. Lind AR, Bass DE: Optimal exposure time for development of acclimatization to heat, *Fed Proc* 22:704, 1963.
272. Lindquist S, Craig EA: The heatshock proteins, *Annu Rev Genet* 22:631, 1988.
273. Lipsitz LA et al: Reduced susceptibility to syncope during postural tilt in old age: is beta-blockage protective? *Arch Intern Med* 149:2709, 1989.
274. Lipton JM: Neuropeptide alpha-melanocyte-stimulating hormone in control of fever, the acute phase response and inflammation, neuroimmune networks, *Physiol Dis* 243, 1989.
275. Love AHG, Shanks RG: The relationship between the onset of sweating and vasodilation in the forearm during body heating, *J Physiol* 162:121, 1962.
276. Lukaski HC, Bolonchuk WW, Klevay LM: Maximal oxygen consumption as related to magnesium, copper and zinc nutriture, *Am J Clin Nutr* 37:407, 1983.
277. Lundvall J: Tissue hyperosmolality as mediator of vasodilation and transcapillary fluid flux in exercising skeletal muscle, *Acta Physiol Scand* 379(suppl):1, 1972.
278. Lwoff A: Factors influencing the evolution of viral diseases at the cellular level and in the organism, *Bacteriol Rev* 23:109, 1959.
279. Malamud N, Haymaker W, Custer RP: Heatstroke: a clinicopathological study of 125 fatal cases, *Milit Surg* 99:397, 1946.
280. Malhotra MS, Ventkataswamy Y: Heat casualties in the Indian Armed Forces, *Indian J Med Res* 62:1293, 1974.
281. Manjoo M, Burger FJ, Kielblock AJ: A relationship between heat load and plasma enzyme concentration, *J Therm Biol* 10:221, 1985.
282. Matnovani A, Bussolino F, Dejana E: Cytokine regulation of endothelial cell function, *FASEB J* 6:2591, 1992.
283. Mao ZC, Wang YT: Analysis of 411 cases of severe heat stroke in Nanjing, *Chin Med J* 104:256, 1991.
284. Maron MB, Wagner JA, Horvath SM: Thermoregulatory responses during competitive marathon running, *J Appl Physiol* 42:909, 1977.
285. Marriott HL: *Water and salt depletion,* Springfield, Ill, 1950, Charles C Thomas.
286. Martin AF et al: Identification and functional significance of troponin I isoforms in neonatal rat heart myofibrils, *Circ Res* 69:1244, 1991.

287. Martin GJ: Prospective evaluation of syncope, *Ann Emerg Med* 13:499, 1984.
288. McCabe WR: Endotoxin: microbiological, chemical, pathophysiological and clinical correlations. In Weinstein L, Fields BN, editors: *Seminars in infectious diseases,* vol 3, New York, 1980, Thieme-Stratton.
289. McCloskey BP: Manslaughter by heatstroke, *Med J Aust* 2:925, 1976.
290. Mehler J et al: Cardiac arrest during anesthesia induction with halothane and succinylcholine in an infant, *Anaesthetist* 40:497, 1991.
291. Michie HR et al: Detection of circulating tumor necrosis factor after endotoxin administration, *N Engl J Med* 319:1481, 1988.
292. Milton AS, Wendlandt S: Effects on body temperature of prostaglandins of the A, E, and F series of injection into the third ventricle of unanesthetized cats and rabbits, *J Physiol* 218:325, 1971.
293. Minard D, Belding HS, Kingston JR: Prevention of heat casualties, *JAMA* 165:1813, 1957.
294. Minton JE, Blecha F: Effect of acute stressors on endocrinological and immunological functions in lambs, *J Anim Sci* 68:3145, 1990.
295. Moldofsky H: Sleep disorders and chronic fatigue syndrome, *Ciba Found Symp* 173:262, 1993.
296. Montgomery A et al: Intramucosal pH measurement with tonometers for detecting gastrointestinal ischemia in porcine hemorrhagic shock, *Circ Shock* 29:319, 1989.
297. Moore NF, Pullin JSK, Reavy B: Inhibition of the induction of heat stock proteins in *Drosophila melanogaster* cells infected with insect picornavirus, *FEBS Lett* 128:93, 1981.
298. Morimoto T: Restitution of body fluid after thermal dehydration. In Hales JVS, Richards D, editors: *Heat stress: physical exertion and environment,* New York, 1987, Elsevier.
299. Mostellar ME, Tuttle EP: Effects of alkalosis on plasma concentration and urinary excretion of inorganic phosphate in man, *J Clin Invest* 43:138, 1964.
300. Murray R: The effects of consuming carbohydrate-electrolyte beverages on gastric emptying and fluid absorption during and following exercise, *Sports Med* 4:322, 1987.
301. Musacchia XJ: Fever and hyperthermia, *Fed Proc* 38:27, 1979.
302. Nadal JW, Pedersen S, Maddock WG: A comparison between dehydration from salt loss and from water deprivation, *Am J Physiol* 134:691, 1941.
303. Nadel ER: Circulatory and thermal regulations during exercise, *Fed Proc* 39:1491, 1980.
304. Nadel ER et al: Physiological defenses against hyperthermia of exercise, *Ann NY Acad Sci* 301:98, 1977.
305. Nakamura H et al: Recombinant human necrosis factor causes long-lasting and prostaglandin-mediated fever, with little tolerance, in rabbits, *J Pharmacol Exp Ther* 245:336, 1988.
306. Nakayama T et al: Thermal stimulation and electrical activity of single units of the preoptic region, *Am J Physiol* 204:1122, 1963.
307. Naylor AM, Cooper KE, Veale WL: Vasopressin and fever: evidence supporting the existence of an endogenous antipyretic system in the brain, *Can J Physiol Pharmacol* 65:1333, 1987.
308. Neuman F et al: Changes in membrane permeability to endotoxin in heat stroke, *Abstr Isr Soc Int Med Proc,* 1978, p 26.
309. Newman J: Evaluation of sponging to reduce body temperature in febrile children, *Can Med Assoc J* 132:641, 1985.
310. Nicholson RN, Somerville KW: Heat stroke in a "run for fun," *Br Med J* 1:1525, 1978.
311. Nielsen M: Die Regulation der Korpertemporature bei Muskelarbeit, *Skand Arch Physiol* 79:193, 1938.
311a. Noakes T, Gaffin S: Unpublished observations.
312. Noakes TD, Goodwin G, Rayner BL: Water intoxication: a possible complication during endurance exercise, *Med Sci Sports Exerc* 17:370, 1985.
313. Nover L: *Heat shock response,* Boca Raton, Fla, 1991, CRC Press.
314. Nover L: The glucose regulated proteins (GRP). In Nover L, editor: *Heat shock response,* Boca Raton, Fla, 1991, CRC Press.
315. Nover L: Inducers of HSP synthesis: heat shock and chemical stressors. In Nover L, editor: *Heat shock response,* Boca Raton, Fla, 1991, CRC Press.
316. Nover L, Scharf KD: Heat shock proteins. In Nover L, editor: *Heat shock response,* Boca Raton, Fla, 1991, CRC Press.
317. O'Donnell TF: Medical problems of recruit training: a research approach, *US Navy Med* 58:28, 1971.
318. O'Donnell TF, Clowes GHA: The circulatory abnormalities of heatstroke, *N Engl J Med* 287:734, 1972.
319. Oates JA et al: Clinical implications of prostaglandin and thromboxane A_2 formation, Part II, *N Engl J Med* 319:761, 1988.
320. Oates JA et al: Clinical implications of prostaglandin and thromboxane A_2 formation, Part I, *N Engl J Med* 319:689, 1988.
321. Ogawa T, Asayama M: Quantitative analysis of the local effect of skin temperature on sweating, *Jpn J Physiol* 36:417, 1986.
322. Ogura H et al: Selective inhibition of translation of the mRNA coding for measles virus membrane protein at elevated temperatures, *J Virol* 61:472, 1987.
323. Okusawa S et al: Interleukin-1 produces a shock-like state in rabbits: synergism with tumor necrosis factor and the effect of cyclooxygenase inhibition, *J Clin Invest* 81:1162, 1988.
324. Orimo S et al: Two familial cases with exertion-induced heatstroke: relationship to malignant hyperthermia, *Rinsho Shinkeigoku (Jpn)* 32:412, 1992.
325. Papa M et al: The effect of ischemia of the dog's colon on transmural migration of bacteria and endotoxin, *J Surg Res* 35:264, 1983.
326. Park YM et al: Stress-induced modulation of immune functions (abstract), *Aviat Space Environ Med* 64:449, 1993.
327. Passmore R, Durnin JVGA: Human energy expenditure, *Physiol Rev* 35:801, 1955.
328. Perotti MF et al: Calcium-dependent DNA fragmenation in human synovial cells exposed to cold shock, *FEBS Lett* 259:331, 1990.
329. Pettigrew RT et al: Circulatory and biochemical effects of whole body hyperthermia, *Br J Surg* 61:727, 1974.
330. Pitts GC, Johnson RE, Consolazio FC: Work in the heat as affected by intake of water, salt and glucose, *Am J Physiol* 142:253, 1944.
331. Poortmans JR, Jeanloz RW: Urinary excretion of immunoglobulins and their subunits in human subjects before and after exercise, *Med Sci Sports Exerc* 1:57, 1969.
332. Porter AM: Heat illness and soldiers, *Milit Med* 158:606, 1993.
333. Proppe DW: Alpha adrenergic control of intestinal circulation in heat-stressed baboons, *J Appl Physiol* R48:759, 1980.
334. Radigan LR, Robinbson S: Effects of environmental heat stress and exercise on renal blood flow and filtration rate, *J Appl Physiol* 2:185, 1949.
335. Reavy B, Pullin JSK, Moore NF: Transitional inhibition of heat-shock induced gene expression in picornavirus-infected *Drosophila melanogaster* cells, *Microbios* 38:91, 1983.
336. Refsum HE, Meen HD, Stromme SB: Changes in plasma amino acid distribution and urine amino acids excretion during prolonged heavy exercise, *Scan J Clin Lab Invest* 39:407, 1979.
337. Retchlin S: Neuroendocrinology. In Wilson JD, Foster DW, editors: *Textbook of endocrinology,* Philadelphia, 1985, WB Saunders.
338. Reuler JB: Hypothermia: pathophysiology, clinical settings, and management, *Ann Intern Med* 85:519, 1978.
339. Richards D, Richards R, Schofield J: Management of heat exhaustion in Sydney's *The Sun* City-to-Surf fun runners, *Med J Aust* 2:457, 1979.
340. Richards CRB, Richards DAB: Medical management of fun-runs. In Hales JRS, Richards DAB, editors: *Heat stress, physical exertion and environment,* Amsterdam, 1987, Elsevier.
341. Robert R, Chapelain B, Neliat G: Different effects of interleukin-1 on reactivity of arterial vessels isolated from various vascular beds in the rabbit, *Circ Shock* 40:139, 1993.
342. Roberts MF et al: Skin blood flow and sweating changes following exercise, training and heat acclimation, *J Appl Physiol* 43:133, 1977.

343. Robertson GL: The regulation of vasopressin function in health and disease, *Rec Prog Hormone Res* 33:333, 1977.
344. Robertson GL, Berl T: Water metabolism. In Brenner BM, Rector FC, editors: *The kidney,* Philadelphia, 1985, WB Saunders.
345. Robertson GL et al: The osmoregulation of vasopressin, *Kidney Int* 10:25, 1976.
346. Rose LI, Carroll DR, Lowe SL: Serum electrolyte changes after marathon running, *J Appl Physiol* 29:449, 1970.
347. Rothstein A, Adolph EF, Wills JH: Voluntary dehydration. In Adolph EF, editor: *Physiology of man in the desert,* New York, 1947, Interscience.
348. Rowell L: Cardiovascular aspects of human thermoregulation, *Circ Res* 52:367, 1983.
349. Rowell LB: Human cardiovascular adjustments to exercise and thermal stress, *Physiol Rev* 54:75, 1974.
350. Rowell LB: *Human circulation: regulation during physical stress,* New York, 1986, Oxford University Press.
351. Rozkowski W et al: Effect of hyperthermia on rabbit macrophages, *Immunobiology* 157:122, 1980.
352. Ruifrok ACC, Kanon B, Konings AWT: Correlation between survival and potassium loss in mouse fibroblasts after hyperthermia alone and after a combined treatment with X-rays, *Radiat Res* 101:326, 1985.
353. Ryan AJ et al: Acute heat stress protects rats against endotoxin shock, *J Appl Physiol* 73:1517, 1992.
354. Saltin B: Circulatory response to submaximal and maximal exercise after thermal dehydration, *J Appl Physiol* 19:1125, 1964.
355. Santee WR, Gonzalez RR: Characteristics of the thermal environment. In Pandolf KB, Sawka MN, Gonzalez RR, editors: *Human performance physiology and environmental medicine at terrestrial extremes,* Indianapolis, 1988, Benchmark Press.
356. Sapolsky RM: Stress in the wild, *Sci Am* 262:116, 1990.
357. Sapolsky RM: *Stress, the aging brain, and the mechanisms of neuron death,* Cambridge, Mass, 1992, MIT Press.
358. Sato K: The physiology, pharmacology and biochemistry of the eccrine sweat gland, *Rev Physiol Biochem Pharmacol* 79:51, 1977.
359. Sawka MN, Wenger CB: Physiological responses to acute exercise heat stress. In Pandolf KB, Sawka MN, Gonzalez RR, editors: *Human performance physiology and environmental medicine at terrestrial extremes,* Indianapolis, 1988, Benchmark Press.
360. Sawka MN et al: Heat exchange during upper- and lower-body exercise, *J Appl Physiol* 57:1050, 1984.
361. Sawka MN et al: Thermoregulatory and blood responses during exercise at graded hypohydration levels, *J Appl Physiol* 59:1394, 1985.
362. Schikele E: Environment and fatal heat stroke, *Milit Surg* 98:235, 1947.
363. Schlesinger MJ: Minireview: heat shock proteins, *J Biol Chem* 265:1211, 1990.
364. Schoenfeld Y, Udassin R: Age and sex differences in response to short exposure to extremely dry heat, *J Appl Physiol* 44:1, 1978.
365. Schrier RW et al: Renal metabolic and circulatory responses to heat and exercise, *Ann Intern Med* 73:213, 1970.
366. Schulte-Sasse U, Eberlein HJ: New findings and experiences in the field of malignant hyperthermia, *Anaesthetist* 35:1, 1986.
367. Scott RW: Therapeutic applications of neutrophil BPI, *Abstr Adv Diagnosis, Prevention & Treatment of Endotoxemia and Sepsis,* 3:1993.
368. Seiple RS et al: Gastric-emptying characteristics of two glucose polymer-electrolyte solutions, *Med Sci Sports Exerc* 15:366, 1983.
369. Senay LC: Temperature regulation and hypohydration: a singular view, *J Appl Physiol* 47:1, 1979.
370. Senay LC, Kok R: Effects of training and heat acclimatization on blood plasma contents of exercising man, *J Appl Physiol* 43:591, 1977.
371. Senay LC, Mitchell D, Wyndham CH: Acclimatization in a hot, humid environment: body fluid adjustments, *J Appl Physiol* 40:786, 1976.
372. Shapiro W, Wasserman AJ, Patterson JL: Mechanism and pattern of human cerebrovascular regulation after rapid changes in blood CO_2 tension, *J Clin Invest* 45:913, 1966.
373. Shapiro Y, Cristal N: Hyperthermia and heat stroke: effects on acid-base balance, blood electrolytes and hepato-renal function. In Hales JRS, Richards DAB, editors: *Heat stress: physical exertion and environment,* New York, 1987, Elsevier.
374. Shapiro Y, Rosenthal T, Sohar E: Experimental heatstroke, *Arch Intern Med* 131:688, 1973.
375. Shapiro Y, Seidman DS: Field and clinical observations of exertional heat stroke patients, *Med Sci Sports Exerc* 22:6, 1990.
376. Shephard JR, Leatt P: Carbohydrate and fluid of the soccer player, *Sports Med* 4:164, 1987.
377. Shibolet S: The clinical picture of heatstroke. In *Proceedings of the Tel HaShomer hospital,* Tel Aviv, 1962, Tel Aviv University.
378. Shibolet S, Fisher S, Gilat T: Fibrinolysis and hemorrhages in fatal heatstroke, *N Engl J Med* 266:169, 1962.
379. Shibolet S, Lancaster MC, Danon Y: Heatstroke: a review, *Aviat Space Environ Med* 47:280, 1976.
380. Shibolet S et al: Heatstroke: its clinical picture and mechanism in 36 cases, *Q J Med* New Series 36:525, 1967.
381. Shoham S et al: Recombinant tumor necrosis factor and interleukin 1 enhance slow-wave sleep in rabbits, *Am J Physiol* 253:R142, 1987.
381a. Shopes E: *Water intoxication: experience from the Grand Canyon (abstract).* Presented at 10th Annual Meeting of the Wilderness Medical Society, August 1994, Squaw Valley, Idaho, p 265.
382. Silva NL, Boulant JA: Effects of osmotic pressure, glucose and temperature on neurons in preoptic tissue slices, *Am J Physiol* 247:R335, 1984.
383. Simon E: Paradigms and concepts in thermal regulation of homeotherms, *NIPS* 2:89, 1987.
384. Singarajah C, Lavies NG: An overdose of ecstasy: a role of dantrolene, *Anaesthesia* 47:686, 1992.
385. Sjodin RA: *Transport in skeletal muscle,* New York, 1982, Wiley.
386. Slovis CM, Anderson GF: Survival in a heatstroke victim with a core temperature in excess of 46.5° C, *Ann Emerg Med* 11:269, 1982.
387. Smith JA et al: Cytokine immunoreactivity in plasma does not change after moderate endurance exercise, *Int J Sports Med* 11:179, 1990.
388. Sohar E, Adar R: Sodium requirements in Israel under conditions of work in hot climate. In *UNESCO/India Symposium on Environmental Physiology and Psychology, Lucknow, July 1962*, Paris, 1962, UNESCO.
389. Sohar E, Kaly J, and Adar R: The prevention of voluntary dehydration. In *UNESCO/India Symposium on Environmental Physiology and Psychology,* Lucknow, 1962, UNESCO.
390. Solomon GF et al: An intensive psychoimmunologic study of long-surviving persons with AIDS: pilot work, background studies, hypotheses, and methods, *Ann NY Acad Sci* 496:647, 1987.
391. Sparrow EM, Cess RD: *Radiation heat transfer,* Belmont, Calif, 1966, Wadsworth.
392. Sprenger H et al: Enhanced release of cytokines, interleukin-2 receptors and neopterin after long-distance running, *Clin Immunol Immunopathol* 63:188, 1992.
393. Stevenson AP, Galey WR, Tobey RA: Hyperthermia-induced increase in potassium transport in Chinese hamster cells, *J Cell Physiol* 115:75, 1983.
394. Stevenson AP et al: Appendix: application of compartmental analysis to the determination of ion fluxes in Chinese hamster cells, *J Cell Physiol* 115:75, 1983.
395. Reference deleted in proofs.
396. Stine RJ: Heat illness, *JACEP* 8:154, 1979.
397. Stolwijk JA: Responses to the thermal environment, *Fed Proc* 36:1655, 1977.
398. Stolwijk JAJ, Hardy JD: Control of body temperature. In Lee DHK, editor: *Handbook of physiology,* Bethesda, Md, 1977, American Physiological Society.

399. Styrt B: Antipyresis and fever, *Arch Intern Med* 150:1589, 1990.
400. Sutton JR: The medical problems of mass participation in athletic competition, *Med J Aust* 2:127, 1972.
401. Sutton JR, Hughson RL: Heatstroke in road races, *Lancet* 1:983, 1979.
402. Sutton JR, Sauder DN: Fever and abdominal pain following exercise, *Med Sci Sports Exerc* 21:S103, 1989.
403. Svenson M et al: IgG autoantibodies against interleukin-1 alpha in sera of normal individuals, *Scand J Immunol* 29:489, 1989.
404. Talbott JH: Heat cramps, In *Medicine,* Baltimore, 1935, Williams & Wilkins.
405. Talbott JH: Heat cramps, *N Engl J Med* 302:777, 1935.
406. Tamion F et al: Malignant neuroleptic syndrome during tiapride treatment, *Clin Exp* 10:461, 1990.
407. Tehan B, Hardern R, Bodenham A: Hyperthermia associated with 3,4-methylenedioxymethamphetamine ("Eve"), *Anaesthesia* 48:507, 1993.
408. Thauer R: Thermosensitivity of the spinal cord. In Hardy JD, Gagge AP, Stiwijk A, editors: *Physiological and behavioral temperature regulation,* Springfield, Ill, 1970, Charles C Thomas.
409. Torranin C, Smith DP, Byrd R: The effect of acute thermal dehydration and rapid rehydration on isometric and isotonic endurance, *J Sports Med Phys Fitness* 19:1, 1979.
410. Tracey CR, Christian KA: Ecological relations among space, time and thermal niche axes, *Ecology* 67:609, 1986.
411. Treon SP, Thomas P, Broitman SA: Lipopolysaccharide (LPS) processing by Kupffer's cells releases a modified LPS with increased hepatocyte binding and decreased tumor necrosis factor alpha stimulatory capacity, *Proc Soc Exp Biol Med* 202:153, 1992.
412. Ulevitch RJ, Tobias PS: Interactions of bacterial lipopolysaccharides with serum proteins. In Levin J et al, editors: *Bacterial endotoxins: pathophysiological effects, clinical significance, and pharmacological control,* New York, 1988, Alan R Liss.
413. Vaalasti A, Tainio H, Rechardt L: Vasoactive intestinal polypeptide (VIP)-like immunoreactivity in the nerves of human axillary sweat glands, *J Invest Dermatol* 85:246, 1985.
414. Vaamonde CA: In *Sodium: its biological significance,* Boca Raton, Fla, 1982, CRC Press.
415. Vaisman NA, Hahn TT: Tumor necrosis factor-alpha and anorexia: cause or effect, *Metabolism* 40:720, 1991.
416. VanOss CJ et al: Effect of temperature on the chemotaxis, phagocytic engulfment, digestion and O_2 consumption of human polymorphonuclear leukocytes, *J Reticuloendothel Soc* 27:561, 1980.
417. Veale WL, Kasting NW, Cooper KE: Arginine vasopressin and endogenous antipyresis: evidence and significance, *Fed Proc* 40:2750, 1981.
418. Vernon WB, Wacker WEB: Magnesium metabolism. In *Recent advances in clinical biochemistry,* New York, 1978, Churchill-Livingstone.
419. Vescia FG, Peck OC: Liver disease from heatstroke, *Gastroenterology* 43:340, 1962.
420. Vidair CA, Dewey WC: Evaluation of a role for intracellular Na^+, K^+, Ca^{2+}, and Mg^{2+} in hyperthermic cell killing, *Radiat Res* 105:187, 1986.
421. Vokes T: Water homeostasis, *Annu Rev Nutr* 7:383, 1987.
422. Wang PJ: Producing pathogen-free plants using tissue culture, *Plant Tissue Culture Newslett* 46:2, 1985.
423. Wardle N: Endotoxin and acute renal failure, *Nephron* 14:321, 1975.
424. Wasserman AJ, Patterson JL: The cerebral vascular response to reduction in arterial carbon dioxide tension, *J Clin Invest* 40:1297, 1961.
425. Webb-Peploe MM, Shepherd JT: Response of large hindlimb veins of the dog to sympathetic nerve stimulation, *Am J Physiol* 215:299, 1968.
426. Wedel DJ: Malignant hyperthermia and neuromuscular disease, *Neuromuscul Disord* 2:157, 1992.
427. Weiner JS: The regional distribution of sweating, *J Physiol (London)* 104:32, 1945.
428. Weiner JS, Khogali M: A physiological body-cooling unit for treatment of heatstroke, *Lancet* 1:507, 1980.
429. Weinstein L: Clinically benign fever of unknown origin: a personal retrospective, *Rev Infect Dis* 7:692, 1985.
430. Wells CL et al: Parenteral endotoxin and intestinal function. In Nowotny A, Spitzer JJ, Ziegler EJ, editors: *Cellular and molecular aspects of endotoxin reactions,* New York, 1990, Elsevier.
431. Wenger CB, Roberts MF: Control of forearm venous volume during exercise and body heating, *J Appl Physiol* 48:114, 1980.
432. Wenger CB et al: Interaction of local and reflex thermal effects in control of forearm blood flow, *J Appl Physiol* 58:251, 1985.
433. Werner J: Functional mechanisms of temperature regulation, adaptation, and fever: complementary system theoretical and experimental evidence, *Pharmacol Ther* 37:1, 1988.
434. Wessels BC et al: Plasma endotoxin concentration in healthy primates and during *E. coli* induced shock, *Crit Care Med* 16:601, 1988.
435. Wheeler KB, Banwell JG: Intestinal water and electrolyte flux of glucose-polymer electrolyte solutions, *Med Sci Sports Exerc* 18:436, 1986.
436. White J, Ford MA: The hydration and electrolyte maintenance properties of an experimental sports drink, *Br J Sports Med* 17:51, 1983.
437. Wilcox WH: The nature, prevention and treatment of heat hyperpyrexia, *Br Med J* 1:392, 1920.
438. Wing J: Upper thermal tolerance limits for unimpaired mental performance, *Aerospace Med* 36:960, 1965.
439. Wing JF, Touchstone RM: *The effects of high ambient temperature on short-term memory.* Technical Report AMRL-TR-65-103. Aerospace Medical Research Laboratories, Wright-Patterson Air Force Base, Ohio, 1965, Air Force Systems Command.
440. Wingfield A: Hyperventilation tetany in tropical climates, *Br Med J* 1:92, 1941.
441. Wright SD et al: Lipopolysaccharide (LPS) binding protein opsonizes LPS-bearing particles for recognition by a novel receptor on macrophages, *J Exp Med* 170:1231, 1989.
442. Wyndham CH: Survey of causal factors in heatstroke and their prevention in the gold mining industry, *J S Afr Inst Mining Metallurgy* 1:245, 1966.
443. Wyndham CH: Heatstroke and hyperthermia in marathon runners, *Ann NY Acad Sci* 128:1977.
444. Wyndham CH et al: Changes in central circulation and body fluid spaces during acclimatization to heat, *J Appl Physiol* 25:586, 1968.
445. Yamamoto K et al: Muramyl dipeptide–elicited production of PGD2 from astrocytes in culture, *Biochem Biophys Res Comm* 156:882, 1988.
446. Yamasu K et al: Activation of the systemic production of tumor necrosis factor after exposure to acute stress, *Eur Cytokine Netw* 3:391, 1992.
447. Yarrows SA: Weight loss through dehydration in amateur wrestling, *J Am Diet Assoc* 88:491, 1988.
448. Yi PN et al: Hyperthermia-induced intracellular ionic level changes in tumor cells, *Radiat Res* 93:534, 1983.
449. Zerbini M, Musiani M, La Placa M: Effect of heat shock on Epstein-Barr virus and cytomegalovirus expression, *J Cell Virol* 66:633, 1985.
450. Zerbini M, Musiani M, La Placa M: Stimulating effect of heat shock on the early stage of human cytomeglovirus replication cycle, *Virus Res* 6:211, 1986.
451. Zinner S, McCabe WR: Effects of IgM and IgG antibody in patients with bacteremia due to gram negative bacilli, *J Infect Dis* 133:37, 1976.

9 WILDLAND FIRES: DANGERS AND SURVIVAL

Kathleen Mary Davis
Robert W. Mutch

It is hard to know what to do with all the detail that rises out of fire. It rises out of a fire as thick as smoke and threatens to blot out everything. Some of it is true but doesn't make any difference. Some of it is just plain wrong. And some doesn't even exist, except in your mind, as you slowly discover long afterwards. Some of it, though, is true—and makes all the difference.

Norman Maclean: *Young Men and Fire*, 1992

Describing the 13 fatalities in the Mann Gulch fire near Helena, Montana, in 1949, Norman Maclean wrote, "They were still so young they hadn't learned to count the odds and to sense they might owe the universe a tragedy." The Mann Gulch fire has been called "the race that couldn't be won."[34] Although the crew increased their pace ahead of the fire, the fire accelerated faster than they until fire and people converged at the end of a race the firefighters could not win. Miraculously, three persons survived the fire. The foreman ignited an escape fire into which he tried to move the crew; two of the smokejumpers found a route to safety. Many improvements in a person's odds of surviving an encounter with a wildland fire have occurred since 1949. These advances include improved understanding of fire behavior, increased emphasis on fire safety and fire training, and development of personal protective equipment. But, as events such as the Colorado fires of 1994 show, tragedies continue to occur.

Whether the Mann Gulch fire, the 1871 Peshtigo fire in Wisconsin that killed 1150 people, the Great Idaho fire of 1910 that left 85 dead (Fig. 9-1), the 1947 Maine fires that produced 16 victims, or the 1991 Oakland fire that killed 25 people, wildland fires are as much a threat to human life, property, and natural resources on the North American continent as are hurricanes, tornadoes, floods, and earthquakes. This chapter describes the new look of this historical force and discusses current fire management policies, the nature and scope of wildland fire hazards, behavior of fires, typical injuries and fatalities, and survival techniques.

Wildland Fire Management and Technology

Programs for dealing with the overall spectrum of fire are collectively termed fire management.[2] They are based on the concept that fire and the complex interrelated factors that influence fire phenomena can and should be managed. In providing scientifically sound fire management programs that respond to the needs of people and natural environments, we must maintain full respect for the power of fire and the effects on both wildland environments and the people who live and work in them.[2]

Since the early 1900s, federal, state, and local fire protection agencies have routinely extinguished wildland fires to protect watershed, range, and timber values, as well as human lives and property. Lack of roads has not prevented application of an increasingly sophisticated technology of fire detection, fire danger rating systems, and fire suppression. Much progress has come from three fire science laboratories and two equipment development centers maintained by the U.S. Department of Agriculture (USDA) Forest Service. Lookout towers and foot trails of the 1930s have gradually been supplanted by patrol planes, some equipped with infrared heat scanners, and by other aircraft that can deliver firefighters, equipment, and fire-retarding chemicals to the most remote fire. These firefighting resources are organized under an Incident Command System that can easily manage simple to complex operational, logistical, planning, and fiscal functions associated with wildfire suppression actions.[4]

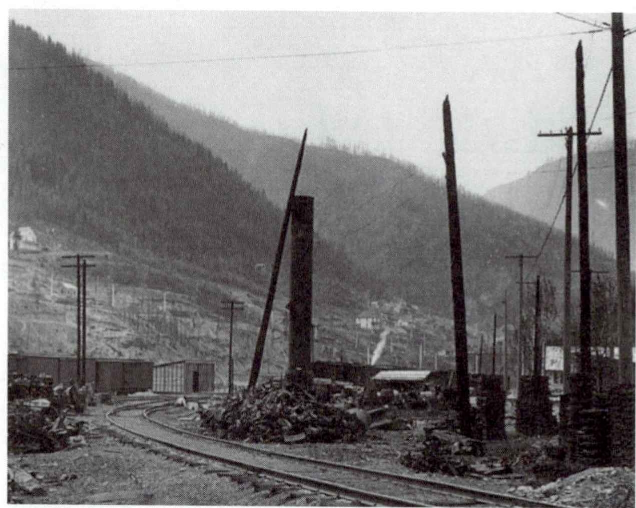

Fig. 9-1 Burned ruins of the foundry in Wallace, Idaho, furnish mute testimony to the destructive force of the 1910 fires. The cottage on the terrace was the only one left standing in that part of town. (Courtesy of the USDA Forest Service. Photo by R.H. McKay.)

Modern fire suppression technology, however, cannot indefinitely reduce the number of hectares burned, as demonstrated by several large fires in recent years: the Greater Yellowstone Area fires in 1988 (Fig. 9-2); Mack Lake fire in Michigan in 1980; Foothills fire near Boise, Idaho, in 1992; Silver Complex in Oregon in 1987; and Stanislaus Complex in California in 1989. The hard lesson learned from these fires and others is that wildfires are inevitable. Suppression may postpone large wildfires but will not prevent them. Effective fire exclusion in the past has caused wildland fuels to accumulate on an increasing amount of contiguous land, contributing to present-day fires of unnatural size and intensity in many plant communities (such as ponderosa pine, desert shrublands, and chaparral). Also, many areas in the United States have been struck by a forest health problem of unprecedented proportions.[24] Several factors have coincided to produce massive forest mortality, including drought, epidemic levels of insects and diseases, and unnatural accumulations of fuels as a result of fire exclusion. Beginning in the 1980s, large wildfires in the dead and dying forests have accelerated the rate of mortality, threatening people, property, and natural resources. Many agencies are now using prescribed fire more frequently, deliberately burning under predetermined conditions to reduce accumulations of fuels and to protect human life and property.

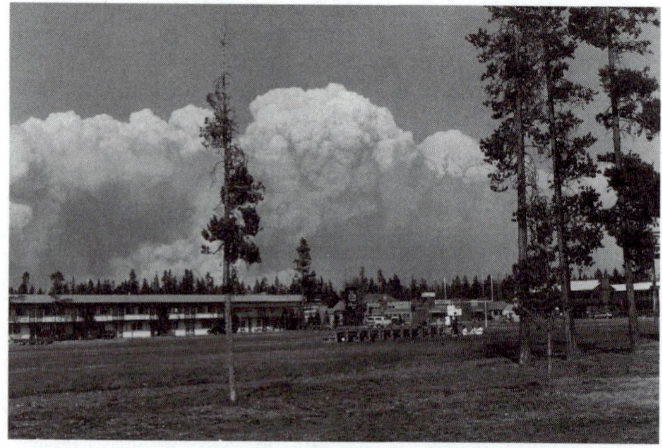

Fig. 9-2 The North Fork wildfire threatened the town of West Yellowstone, Montana, in 1988. (Photo courtesy of Linda Mutch.)

Research has indicated that fires are not categorically bad. Many plant communities in North America are highly flammable during certain periods in their life cycles. Annual grasses, ponderosa pine, and chaparral plant communities are flammable almost every dry season. Other communities, such as jack pine or lodgepole pine forests, may remain fire resistant during much of their life cycle, eventually becoming fire prone when killed by insects, diseases, and other natural causes. In contrast, the spread of nonnative grasses, such as cheatgrass and red brome, in the arid West has increased the frequency of fires in desert shrublands.

Evolutionary development in the presence of periodic wildland fires has produced plant species well adapted to recurrent fires. Wildland fires can benefit plant and animal communities. Disturbances such as fire tend to recycle ecosystems and maintain diversity.[17] Thus there is growing consensus that fire should be returned to wildland ecosystems where appropriate to perpetuate desirable fire-adapted plant and animal communities and to reduce fuel accumulations.

As a consequence of increasing awareness of the ecologic role and benefits of fire, several agencies are using fire as a resource management tool. A landmark report in 1963 to the National Park Service by the Advisory Board on

Wildlife Management[16] described how the western slope of the Sierra Nevada had been transformed by fire protection:

> When the forty-niners poured over the Sierra Nevada into California, those that kept diaries spoke almost to a man of the wide-spaced columns of mature trees that grew on the lower western slope in gigantic magnificence. Today much of the west slope is a dog-hair thicket of young pines, white fir, incense-cedar, and mature brush—a direct function of overprotection from natural ground fires. Not only is this accumulation of fuel dangerous to the giant sequoias and other mature trees, but the animal life is meager, wildflowers are sparse, and to some at least the vegetative tangle is depressing, not uplifting.

The board recommended that the Park Service recognize in management programs the importance of the natural role of fire in shaping plant communities. Many national parks and wildernesses now have approved fire management plans to allow prescribed fires.

PRESCRIBED FIRE

Prescribed fire, the intentional ignition of grass, shrub, or forest fuels for specific purposes according to predetermined conditions, is a recognized land management practice. Objectives of such burning vary: to reduce fire hazards after logging, expose mineral soil for seedbeds, regulate insects and diseases, perpetuate natural ecosystems, and improve range forage and wildlife habitat. In some areas managed by the National Park Service, USDA Forest Service, and Bureau of Land Management, naturally ignited fires may be allowed to burn according to approved prescriptions; fire management areas have been established in national parks and wildernesses from the florida Everglades to the Sierra Nevada in California (Fig. 9-3). Visitors are increasingly aware that prescribed natural fires provide an important environment for the enjoyment of park and wilderness experiences (Fig. 9-4).

Fires are not simply allowed to burn. Their spread is monitored to ensure that they remain in designated areas. Suppression measures, backed by modern fire control technology, are employed to protect human life and property and to contain fires within the management unit.

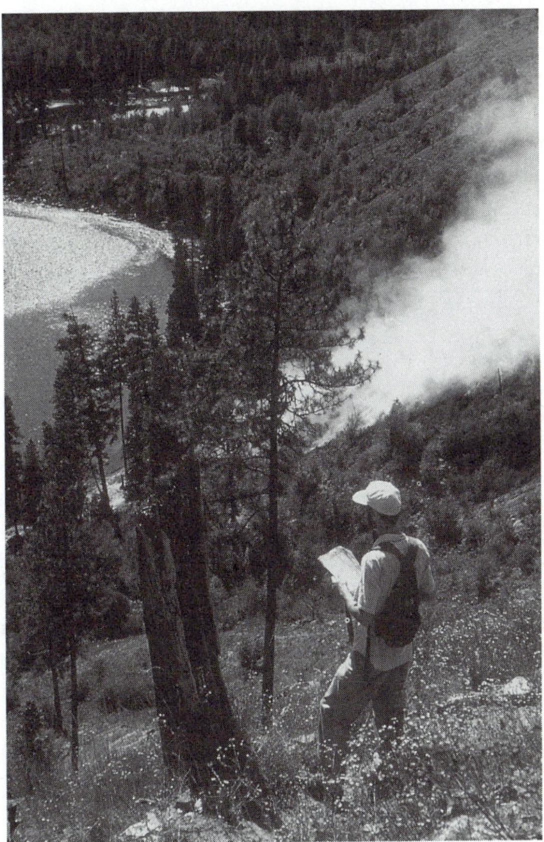

Fig. 9-3 Some lightning fires in wildernesses and national parks are now allowed to burn under observation to perpetuate natural ecosystems. (Courtesy of the USDA Forest Service.)

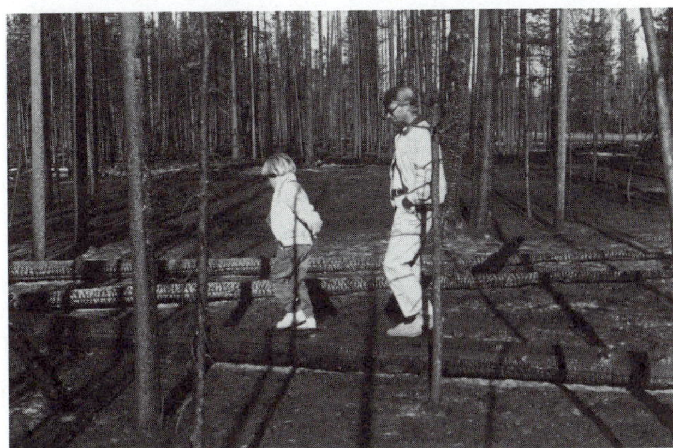

Fig. 9-4 Two visitors to Yellowstone National Park during the late summer of 1988 check out the recently burned forest. (Photo courtesy of Kathleen Davis.)

Wildland-Urban Interface: New Look of a Historical Problem

Today's wildland fire dilemma is compounded by several factors. Just as resource agencies are attempting to provide a more natural role for fire in wildland ecosystems, the general public is increasingly living and seeking recreation in many of these areas. Furthermore, past fire exclusion practices have contributed to the likelihood of larger fires burning at greater intensities as a result of abnormal fuel accumulations in some vegetation types. This combination of events can threaten the lives of the general public as well as emergency medical and firefighting personnel. Juxtaposition of people, property, and wildland fuel has resulted in the sacrifice of relatively safe perimeter fire suppression strategies in favor of directly protecting people and their possessions.[48] Direct suppression actions *within* the fire's perimeter place firefighters at a greater disadvantage from a safety standpoint.

Exposure to wildland fires is increasing for inexperienced people both in the backcountry and in the wildland-urban interface near apparently secure residences, recreational homes, and cabins. Thus what is known of fire behavior and fire survival principles must be readily available to emergency medical personnel, wildland dwellers, and recreationists. In fact, fire protection agencies have been making such information more available to the general public.

NATURE OF THE PROBLEM

Hot, dry, windy conditions annually produce high-intensity fires that threaten or burn homes where wildland and urban areas converge. The news media report startling losses of homes, watersheds, vegetation cover, wildlife habitat, and too often, human lives. The costs of property losses, resource losses, and suppression actions are staggering. Sadly, too few people learn from repeated lessons that they must understand wildland fire ecology and fire behavior. Residents of fire-prone environments need to understand that in some areas fires are inevitable, so that they can prepare to protect their lives and property better. Literature and personal consultation are available at no cost from many federal, state, county, and city firefighting agencies.

A question is whether the historical levels of destruction, injury, and fatality could be repeated today in the face of modern fire suppression technology. The answer requires an analysis of conditions that created high-intensity fire behavior in the forests of Idaho and Montana in 1910 (Fig. 9-5). Numerous conflagrations before and after the 1910 fires provide ample testimony to causative conditions. The Peshtigo, Michigan, Hinckley, Yacoult, and Maine fires burned hundreds of thousands of hectares and killed more than 2000 people between 1871 and 1947.

On the same day, October 8, 1871, that fire wiped out the town of Peshtigo, Wisconsin, the great Chicago fire devastated urban Chicago. Comparative statistics for those two fires highlight the destructive potential of wildland fires. The Peshtigo fire covered 518,016 hectares (1,280,000 acres) and killed 1150 people, whereas 860 hectares (2124 acres) burned and 300 lives were lost as a result of the Chicago fire.[47] The 1910 wildland fires had several common elements: many uncontrolled fires burning at one time; prolonged drought, high temperatures, and moderate to strong winds; and mixed conifer and hardwood fuels with slash from logging and land clearing. These large fires occurred primarily in conifer forests north of the 42nd meridian, or roughly across the northern quarter of the contiguous United States.[3] One critical element, which is not as likely to occur today as formerly, was the simultaneous presence of many uncontrolled fires. The effectiveness of modern fire suppression organizations has been greatly enhanced by their rapid growth and by the air deployment of firefighters and retardants to even the most remote wildland locations.

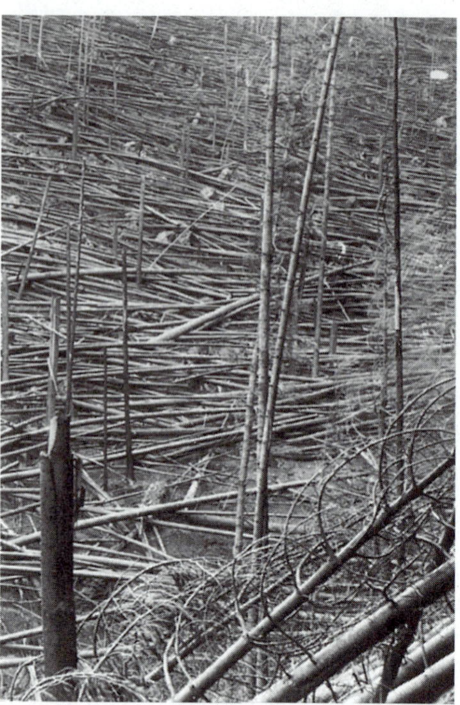

Fig. 9-5 These burned-over and wind-thrown trees resulted from the intense behavior of the 1910 forest fire near Falcon, Idaho. (Courtesy of the USDA Forest Service. Photo by J.B. Halm.)

High-velocity winds and more than 1600 individual fires contributed to the spread of the 1910 fires; it is unlikely that a multifire situation of that magnitude would occur today.

Prolonged drought, high winds, and flammable fuel types, however, are as significant to the behavior of high-intensity fires today as previously. In 1967 the Sundance fire in northern Idaho burned more than 22,627 hectares (55,910 acres) and killed two firefighters. In 1970 other fires burned approximately 40,470 hectares (100,000 acres) in the vicinity of Wenatchee, Washington. During the drought-stricken 1977 fire season in California, 21 major fires burned almost 150,000 hectares (370,000 acres). The largest of these fires, the remote Marble-Cone, spread through 70,418 hectares (174,000 acres) of flammable chaparral and mixed forest. The Sycamore fire near Santa Barbara, California, although only 324 hectares (800 acres) in size, destroyed more than 200 homes.

The benefits accrued by decreasing the number of uncontrolled fire starts have been offset by the tendency of people to live in fire-prone areas. For example, some of the fires most potentially damaging to human lives and property occur in areas rich in chaparral shrub fuel in California. Wilson[47] described the severe 1970 fire year in California, in which official estimates showed that 97% of 1260 fires occurring between September 15 and November 15 were held to less than 121 hectares (300 acres). The other 3% of the fires, fueled by a prolonged drought and fanned by strong Santa Ana winds, produced 14 deaths, destroyed 885 homes, and burned more than 242,820 hectares (600,000 acres). Ten years later the situation recurred over 28,330 hectares (70,000 acres) in southern California, resulting in the deaths of 5 persons and loss of more than 400 structures.

More recently, on October 20, 1992, a devastating fire occurred in the hills above Oakland and Berkeley, California (Color Plate 11). Burning embers carried by high winds from the perimeter of a small fire resulted in a major wildland-urban interface conflagration that killed 25 people, including a police officer and a firefighter, injured 150 others, destroyed nearly 2449 single-family dwellings and 437 apartment and condominium units, burned over 648 hectares (1600 acres), and did an estimated $1.5 billion in damage.[28] The scenario for disaster included a 5-year drought that had dried out overgrown grass, shrubs, and trees, making them readily ignitable. Other factors contributing to the disaster included untreated wood shingles, unprotected wooden decks that projected out over steep terrain, low relative humidity, high temperatures, and strong winds that averaged 32 km per hour (20 mph) and gusted up to 56 to 80 km per hour (35 to 50 mph). These severe conditions produced a voracious fire that consumed 790 homes in the first hour. Winds lessened to 8 km per hour (5 mph) by the first evening, and firefighters had the situation under control by the fourth day, but not before they had an awful glimpse of what future fires will be.

Wildland fires that threaten human lives and property are not exclusively located in southern California, since the exodus to wildland regions has become a national phenomenon. Fires burned more than 80,940 hectares (200,000 acres) in Maine in October 1947, killing 16 people; another 80,940 hectares (200,000 acres) burned in New Jersey in 1963. On July 16, 1977, the Pattee Canyon fire in Missoula, Montana, destroyed 6 homes (Fig. 9-6) and charred 486 hectares (1200 acres) of forests and grasslands in only a few hours.[9]

The 1985 wildland fire season was one of the most severe in this century; the national toll for that year paints a stark picture: 44 civilians and firefighters died, 1400 homes and structures were destroyed or damaged, and 1.2 million hectares (3 million acres) were burned.[43] On one day in Florida, May 17, a firefighter died, 40,470 hectares (100,000 acres) burned, 600 homes and other buildings were destroyed or damaged, and more than 1000 residents were safely evacuated. During 1986, in three states alone wildfires forced 13,500 people to evacuate their homes.

A human-caused fire starting on July 9, 1989, near Boulder, Colorado, raced through residential areas among the trees, destroying 44 homes and other structures and burning over 850 hectares (2100 acres). Losses for homes and natural resources were estimated at $10 million, and the cost to control the fire was another $1 million. This Black Tiger fire produced the worst fire losses in Colorado's history. The causes were familiar: lack of rainfall, high temperatures, strong winds, sloping topography, buildup of forest fuels, construction factors affecting the susceptibility of the homes to fire, combustible construction materials, poor access for emergency vehicles, and lack of home site main-

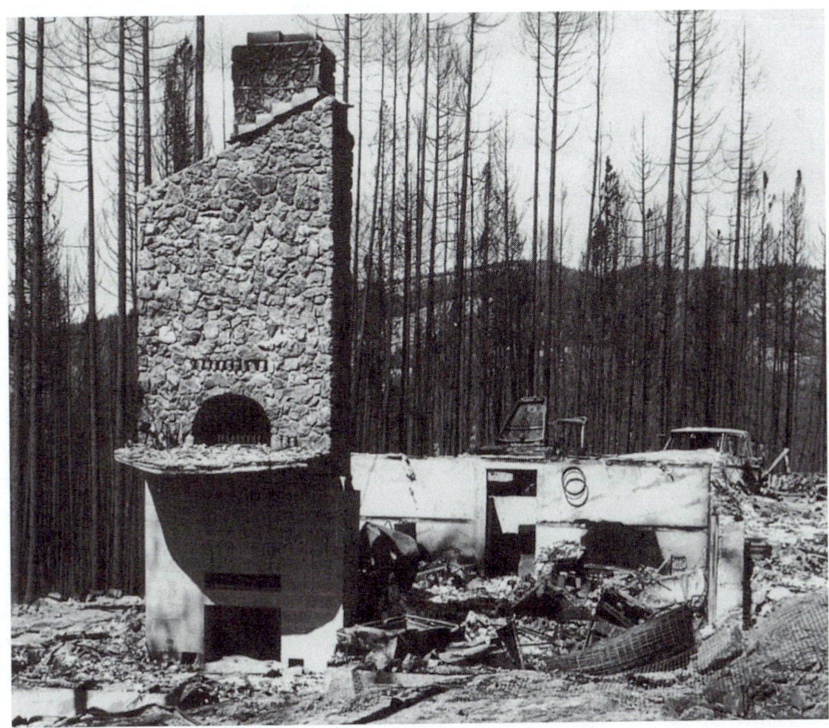

Fig. 9-6 A total of six homes in Missoula, Montana, were reduced to chimneys and foundations in the 1977 Pattee Canyon fire. (Photo courtesy of William C. Fischer.)

tenance for fire protection.[25] The conditions that led to the Black Tiger fire are still prevalent in many parts of Colorado as well as in other states. The Stephan Bridge Road fire in 1990, for example, spread across 2394 hectares (5916 acres) near Grayling, Michigan, destroying more than 76 homes and 125 other structures in approximately 5 hours.[26]

Fires at the wildland-urban interface also have increased internationally. For example, the Ash Wednesday fire disaster in 1983 burned more than 340,000 hectares (840,000 acres) of urban, forested, and pastoral lands in Victoria and South Australia, killing 77 and injuring 3500 persons and destroying 2528 homes.[43] A May 1987 wildfire in northern China added a new perspective regarding the devastating impact wildland fires may have on human lives, property, and natural resources. This fire reportedly burned over 404,700 hectares (1 million acres), killed almost 200 persons, seriously injured another 200, destroyed or damaged 12,000 houses, and forced nearly 60,000 people to evacuate their homes—clearly it was a disaster of major proportions. Protecting lives and property from wildfires at the wildland-urban interface presents one of the greatest challenges faced by wildfire protection agencies.

It is becoming increasingly rare to have a wildland fire situation that does not involve people. In spite of this, people are not fully aware of the fire risks and hazards of living and traveling in or near wildlands. *Risk,* in the jargon of the forest fire specialist, is the probability that a fire will occur. *Hazard* is the likelihood that a fire, once started, will cause unwanted results. Risk deals with causative agents; hazard deals with the fuel complex.[11] The results of two surveys indicated a general feeling of overconfidence by most residents toward the potential danger of forest fire. Eighty percent of Seeley Lake, Montana, forest residents who were interviewed thought that the forest fire hazard was low to moderate in their area.[10] Seventy-five percent of Colorado residents interviewed thought that the forest fire hazard was low or moderate in mountain subdivisions of their state.[15] Forest fire hazards in these two areas were much higher than the public estimates (Fig. 9-7).

Historical levels of fire-related injuries and fatalities probably will not occur again, since the numbers of uncontrolled fires burning at one time will be substantially fewer because of improved fire prevention, detection, and suppression techniques. Still, recent experiences in California, Colorado, Washington, and Michigan demonstrate that the exposure rate of people and property to fire risks and hazards will remain high because mobility facilitates living and recreating in wildlands. There is a growing need for the general public, emergency medical personnel, and fire suppression organizations to be well prepared to deal with wildland fire encounters.

WILDLAND LESSONS

The problems of living in a fire environment are no longer unique to southern California, as was thought when these urban interface fires gained national attention in the 1950s and 1960s. In recent years wildland-urban fire disasters have occurred from coast to coast. As more people move out of cities and into wildlands, these tragedies will recur. Following the recent disastrous fires in several states, recommendations for mitigating the impact of fires in the wildland-urban interface have been developed. The combined efforts of fire protection services, legislators, planners, developers, and the public and homeowners will be required to prevent the tragic loss of lives and homes in the wildlands (Box 9-1).[28]

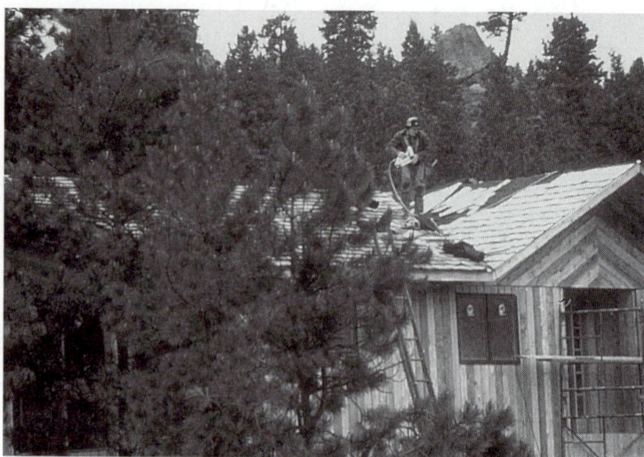

Fig. 9-7 Wildland fuels and flammable dwellings combine to pose significant threats to people and property. The wildland property owner must assume a major responsibility in designing and maintaining fire-safe buildings and surrounding land.

Recommendations to reduce the loss of life and property in the wildland-urban interface will be useless unless they are implemented at the grassroots level by all stakeholders. An excellent example of a community-based program is one implemented at Incline Village and Crystal Bay in the Lake Tahoe basin.[39] The objective of this program is to "reduce the potential for natural resource, property, and human life losses due to wildfire by empowering the communities' residents with the knowledge to address the hazard, providing the resources necessary to correct the problem, and encouraging the cooperative efforts of appropriate agencies." The three major components of this defensible-space program include neighborhood leader volunteers, a slash removal project, and agency coordination. The key to protecting life and property in the wildland-urban interface is property owners' realization that they have a serious problem and that their actions embody a significant part of the solution. In the Incline Village/Crystal Bay Plan, neighborhood leader volunteers are trained in defensible-space techniques and are expected to teach these techniques to their neighbors and to coordinate neighborhood efforts. Such concerted community action will greatly minimize the threats from Oakland-type "fires of the future."

It is also wise to have sensible land development practices, since tragedies arise not only from ignorance of fuels and fire behavior, but also from a greater concern for the esthetics of a homesite than for fire safety. Several aspects of

BOX 9-1

RECOMMENDATIONS TO REDUCE LOSS OF LIFE AND PROPERTY IN THE WILDLAND-URBAN INTERFACE

FIRE PROTECTION SERVICES

Ensure that all personnel receive regular cross-training in fighting wildfires and structural fires.

In urban departments, in particular, recognize the need to extinguish fires in wildland fuels by using thorough mop-up procedures.

Recognize the need for close coordination of response efforts among neighboring departments or agencies.

Develop specific mutual aid plans for coordinating resources to attack fires in the wildland-urban interface.

Schedule and conduct regular mutual aid training exercises.

Regularly schedule and conduct fire prevention and fire preparedness education programs for the general public and homeowners.

Conduct an assessment of fire risks and prepare a strategic plan to reduce these risks.

Work effectively with lawmakers and other government officials to help prevent unsafe residential and business development.

LEGISLATORS

Examine existing laws, regulations, and standards of other jurisdictions that are applicable for local use in mitigating hazards associated with wildland fires.

Adopt National Fire Protection Association Standard 299 for the Protection of Life and Property from Wildfire.[27] (The purpose of this standard is to provide criteria for fire agencies, land use planners, architects, developers, and local government for fire-safe development in areas that may be threatened by wildfire.)

Provide strong building regulations that restrict untreated wood shingle roofs and other practices known to decrease the fire safety of a structure in the wildlands.

PLANNERS AND DEVELOPERS

Create a map of potential problem areas based on fuel type and known fire behavior.

Evaluate all existing or planned housing developments to determine relative wildland fire protection ratings and advise property owners of conditions and responsibilities.

Ensure that all developments have more than one ingress-egress route.

Offer options for fire-safe buildings.

Provide appropriate fuel breaks or green belts in developments.

Ensure that adequate water supplies exist in developments.

Follow specifications in NFPA Standard 299 for the Protection of Life and Property from Wildfire.

PUBLIC AND HOMEOWNERS

Determine the wildfire hazard potential of the immediate area before buying or moving into any home.

Contact federal, state, and local fire services for educational programs and materials regarding fire protection.

Provide a defensible space around structures to help protect them.

Design and build nonflammable homes.

Urge lawmakers to respond with legislative assistance to require appropriate fire safety measures for communities.

development detract from fire safety in the wildland-urban interface[7,9]:

1. Lack of access to adequate water sources
2. Firewood stacked next to houses
3. Slash (that is, branches, stumps, logs, and other vegetative residues) piled on homesites or along access roads
4. Structures built on slopes with unenclosed stilt foundations.
5. Trees and shrubs growing next to structures, under eaves, and among stilt foundations.
6. Roads that are steep, narrow, winding, unmapped, unsigned, unnamed, and bordered by slash or dense vegetation that makes them impossible to drive on during a fire
7. Subdivisions on sites without two or more access roads for simultaneous ingress and egress
8. Roads and bridges without the grade, design, and width to permit simultaneous evacuation by residents and access by firefighters, emergency medical personnel, and equipment
9. Excessive slopes, heavy fuels, structures built in box canyons, and other hazardous situations
10. Lack of fuel breaks around homesites and in subdivisions
11. Living fuels that have not been modified by thinning, landscaping, or other methods to reduce vegetation and litter that contribute to fire intensity
12. Homes constructed with flammable building materials (wooden shakes, shingles)

Fire Behavior

URBAN AND WILDLAND FIRE THREATS

Safety precautions for wildland firefighting crew continually upgraded in light of new knowledge abo behavior. Information about hazards in the wildland-urban interface is now included in training programs and safety briefings. fire sites where people were injured or killed are visited afterward to assess fuel conditions, terrain features, probable wind movements at the time of the fire, and actions of firefighters (Fig. 9-8).

In reviewing such tragedies, a sobering observation is that crew members are almost always experienced and well-equipped firefighters, trained to anticipate "blowup" fire conditions. However, when visibility is lowered to 6 m (20 feet), noise levels preclude voice communication, eyes fill with tears, and wind blows debris in all directions, a person's judgment is badly impaired. Too often, previous training gives way to panic, which can lead to irrational decisions that result in serious injury or death.

This scenario is most evident in urban fires; the pattern of hysteria affecting persons trapped in burning buildings is familiar to fire chiefs. It is informative to review how fire kills in the urban setting and to compare this sequence of events with wildland fires. An adaptation from Owen describes what happens[30]:

> Heat rises rapidly to upper stories when a fire starts in the basement or on the ground floor. Toxic gases and smoke rise to the ceiling and work their way down to the victim—a vital lesson for families planning protective measures. Smoke poses the double problem of obscuring exit routes and contributing to pulmonary injury and oxygen deprivation.
>
> As the fire consumes oxygen, the ambient oxygen content drops, impairing neuromuscular activity. When the oxygen content drops below 16%, death by asphyxiation will ensue unless the victim is promptly evacuated. Asphyxiation, not fire itself, is the leading cause of fire deaths.
>
> Ambient temperatures may rise extremely rapidly from even small fires. Temperatures of 149° C (300° F) will cause rapid loss of consciousness and, along with toxic gases, will severely damage lung tissues. Warning devices may offer the only possibility for survival due to the rapid onset of debilitating symptoms.

Fire threats in urban and wildland situations have some obvious similarities and differences:

1. Smoke, heat, and gases are not as concentrated in wildland situations as in the confined quarters of urban fires.
2. Flames are not a leading killer in either the urban or wildland situation.
3. Although oxygen levels may be reduced near wildland fires, there is usually sufficient replenishment of oxygen in the outdoor environment to minimize deprivation. Asphyxiation, however, can also be an important cause of death in wildland fires.
4. Inhalation of superheated gases poses as serious a threat to life in wildland fires as in urban fires.
5. Wildland smoke does not contain toxic compounds produced by combustion of plastics and other house-

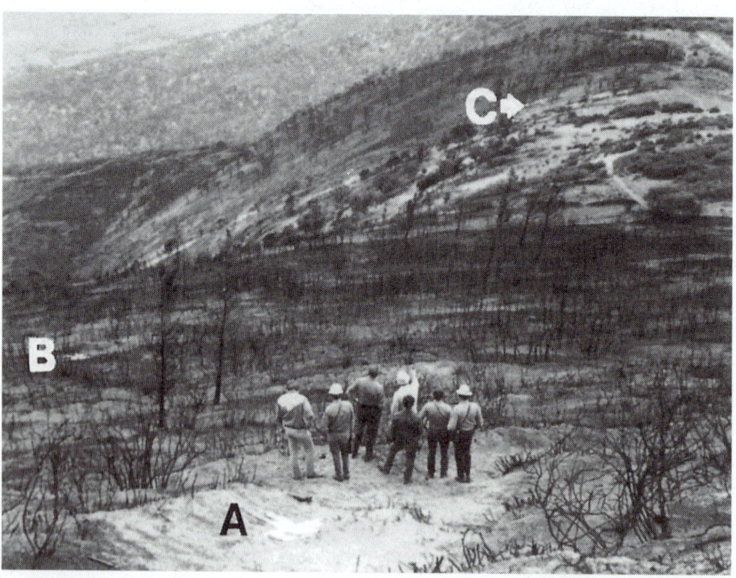

Fig. 9-8 In an attempt to avoid the intense heat of this brush fire in southwestern Colorado, four firefighters took refuge in the fireline, in the foreground at point *A*. Affected by intense convective and radiant heat and dense smoke, one individual ran into the fire and died at point *B*. Another individual ran approximately 1000 feet down the ridge, where his body was found at point *C*. The third fatality was a person who remained at point *A;* he died a short time after this position was overrun by fire. The only survivor also remained in a prone position at point *A* with his face pressed to the ground. At one point he reached back and threw dirt on his burning pants legs. The survivor sustained severe burns to the back of his legs, buttocks, and arms. The deaths of the other three individuals were attributed to asphyxiation. (Courtesy of the USDA Forest Service.)

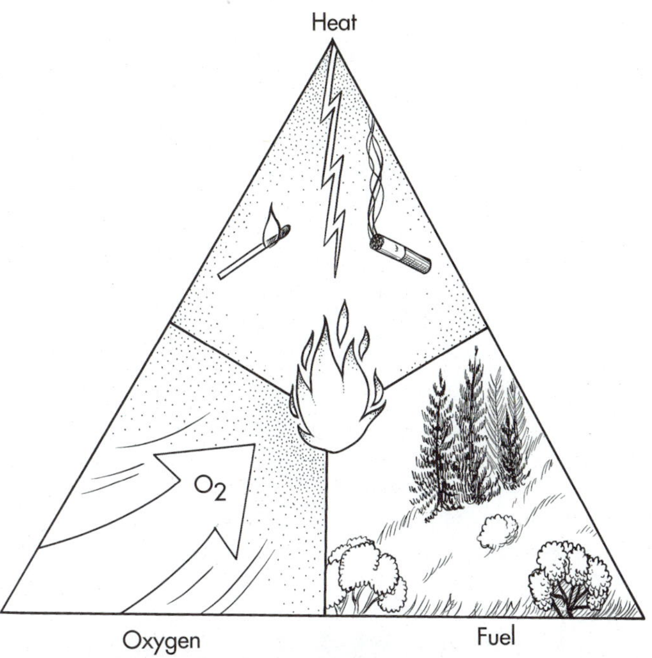

Fig. 9-9 Combustion is a process involving the combination of heat, oxygen, and fuel. An understanding of the variation of these three factors is fundamental to an understanding of fire behavior.

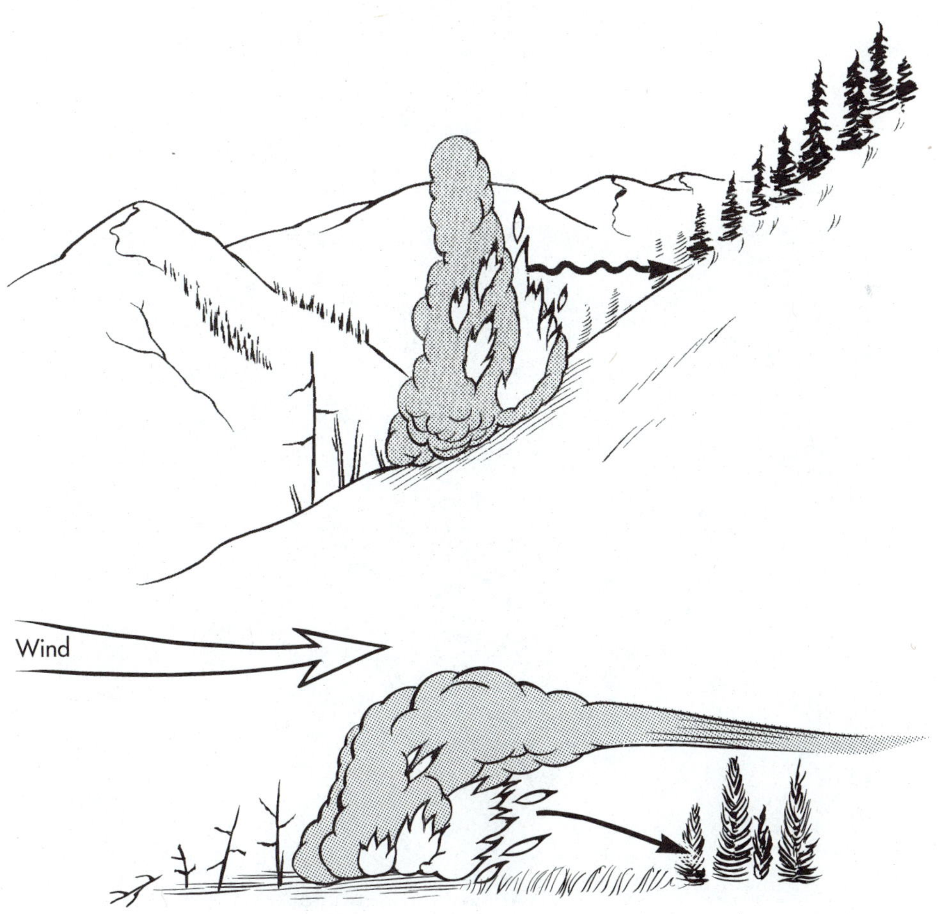

Fig. 9-10 Fuels and people upslope or downwind from a fire receive more radiant heat than on the downslope or upwind side.

hold materials, but it does impair visibility, contain carbon monoxide, and have suspended particulates that cause severe physical irritation of the lungs.

6. Automatic early-warning devices and sprinkler systems may protect people from serious injury or death in the urban environment, but in the wildland environment people must rely on their senses, knowledge, and skills to provide early warning of an impending threat to life.

FIRE BEHAVIOR KNOWLEDGE: A WILDLAND EARLY-WARNING SYSTEM

The science of fire behavior describes and predicts the performance of wildland fires in terms of rates of spread, intensity levels, ignition probabilities, spotting, and crowning potentials. *Spotting* is defined as a fire spread mechanism resulting from airborne firebrands or embers. *Crowning* is a fire spread mechanism that moves horizontally through the canopies of shrubs or trees. No two fires are exactly alike, since the possible combinations of fuel, weather, and topographic factors are almost infinite. Knowledge of current and predicted weather information and fire danger ratings can be obtained from local wildland fire protection agencies. Experienced firefighters routinely assess the probable behavior of fires using current and expected weather conditions in relation to local fuel and topographic conditions. It is equally important that the emergency medical person, backcountry recreationist, and wildland homeowner understand basic fire behavior principles to provide for adequate personal safety. A cardinal rule of fire safety is to base all actions on current and expected behavior of fires. Attention

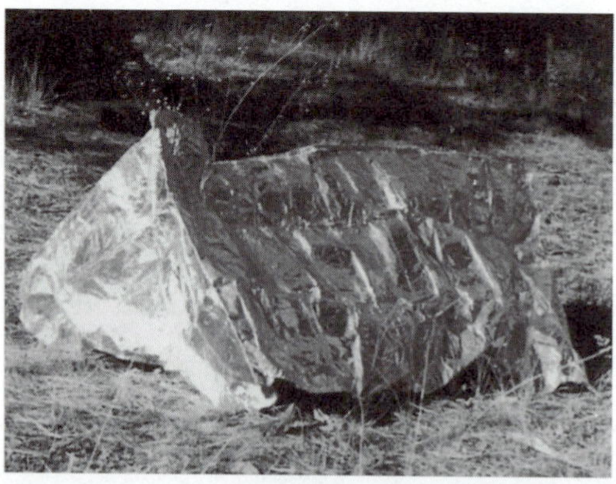

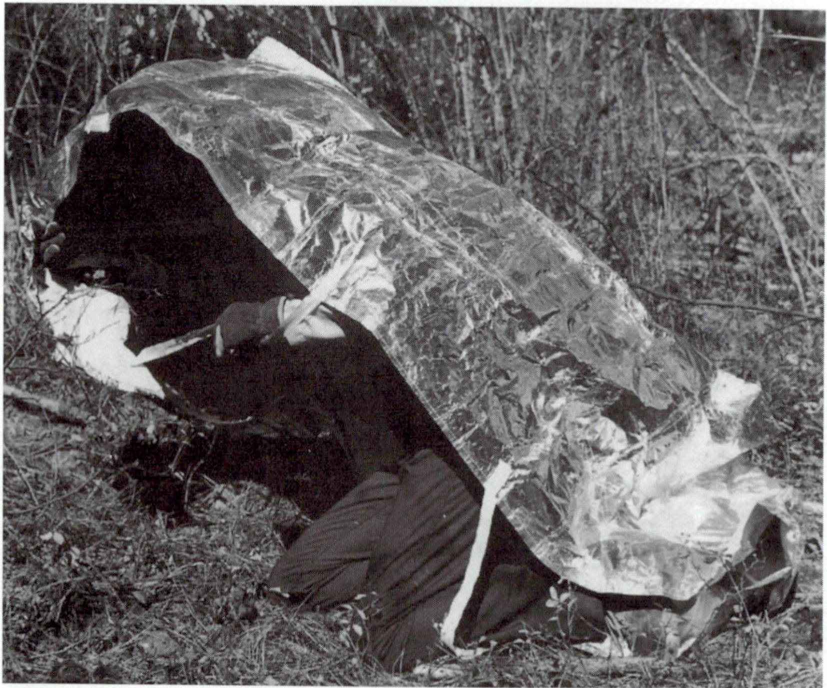

Fig. 9-11 An aluminized fire shelter, carried in a waist pouch, is deployed by firefighters as a last resort to provide protection from radiant heat and superheated air. (Photos courtesy of the USDA Forest Service.)

to simple principles, indicators, and rules should enable wildland users to anticipate and avoid fire threats.

Physical Principles of Heat Transfer

Heat, oxygen, and fuel are required in proper combination before ignition and combustion will occur (Fig. 9-9).[1] If any one of the three is absent, or if the three elements are not in proper balance, there will be no fire. Fire control actions are directed at disrupting one or more elements of this basic fire triangle. Because heat is critical in fire behavior, it is important to review different heat transfer methods.

With respect to a fire, heat energy is transferred by conduction, convection, radiation, and spotting; generally only the last three processes are significant in a wildland setting. Although conduction through solid objects is important in the burning of logs, this process does not transfer much heat outward from a flaming front.

Convection, or movement of hot masses of air, accounts for most heat transfer outward from the fire. Convective currents usually move vertically unless a wind or slope generates lateral movement. Convection is responsible for preheating fuels upslope and in shrub and tree canopies, which contributes further to a fire's spread and the onset of crown fires.

Radiation is the process by which heat energy is emitted in direct lines of rays; about 25% of combustion energy is transmitted in this manner. The amount of radiant heat transferred decreases inversely with the square of the distance from a point source. More radiant heat is emitted from a line of fire than from a point source. Radiant heat travels in straight lines, does not penetrate solid objects, and is easily reflected. It accounts for most of the preheating of surface fuel ahead of the fire front and poses a direct threat to people who are too close to the fire (Fig. 9-10). Many organized fire crew members carry aluminized fire shelters in belt pouches that can be deployed quickly when escape is not possible (Fig. 9-11). These shelters are used as a last resort to protect individuals from radiant heat.

Spotting is a mass transfer mechanism by which wind currents carry burning or glowing embers beyond the main fire to start new fires (Fig. 9-12). In this manner, fire spread may accelerate, unexpected fires will occur, and fire intensity and indraft winds may increase.

Factors in Wildland Fire Behavior

A wildland fire behaves according to variations in fuel, weather, and topography. Interactions among these factors and the fire are characterized in the following paragraphs. Early warning factors that signal the onset of hotter and faster burning conditions appear in Box 9-2.

Fuel. The more fuel that is burning, the hotter the fire will be. Certain types of fuel, such as chaparral, pine, and eucalyptus, burn more intensely because of their fine foliage that contains flammable oils. The size and arrangement of fuel also influence fire behavior. Small, loosely compacted fuel beds, such as dead grass, long pine needles, and shrubs, burn more rapidly than does tightly compacted fuel. Large fuels burn best when they are arranged so that they are closely spaced, such as logs in a fireplace. Scattered logs with no small or intermediate fuel nearby seldom burn unless they are old and rotten.

Weather. The greater the wind, the more rapid the spread of fire. Drier air and higher temperatures cause fuel to dry out more quickly; fire burns more intensely because drying creates more fuel. Prolonged drought makes more fuel available. Fires tend to burn more vigorously when atmospheric conditions are unstable.

The North American continent has been classified into 15 fire climate regions based on geographic and climatic factors (Fig. 9-13).[36] Major fire seasons, or periods of peak fire activity, can be used to warn emergency medical personnel and wildland users of the most probable times of year for life-threatening situations. Although the fire season for the southern Pacific coast is shown as June through September, critical fire weather can occur year round in the most southerly portion. Fire seasons are most active during spring

BOX 9-2

EARLY WARNING SIGNALS FOR HOTTER, FASTER BURNING CONDITIONS

FUEL

More fuel; drier fuel; dead fuel; flashy fuel (dead grass, pine needles, and shrubs); aerial fuel (combustible material suspended in crowns of high shrubs and trees, such as branches, needles, lichens, and mosses)

WEATHER

Faster winds; unstable atmosphere (indicators: gusty winds, dust devils, and good visibility); downdraft winds from dry thunderstorms and towering cumulus clouds (erratic and strong winds); higher temperatures, drought conditions, and lower humidities

TOPOGRAPHY

Steeper slopes; south- and southwest-facing slopes; gaps or saddles; chimneys and narrow canyons (Fig. 9-14)

FIRE BEHAVIOR

Rolling and burning pine cones, agaves, logs, hot rocks, and other debris igniting fuel downslope; spot fires that occur ahead of the main fire; individual trees that torch out, or areas of shrubs and trees that burn in a continuous crown fire; fires that smolder over a large area; many fires that start simultaneously; fire whirls that cause spot fires and erratic burning; intense burning with flame lengths greater than 1.2 m (4 feet); dark, massive smoke columns with rolling, boiling vertical development; lateral movement of fire near the base of a steep slope

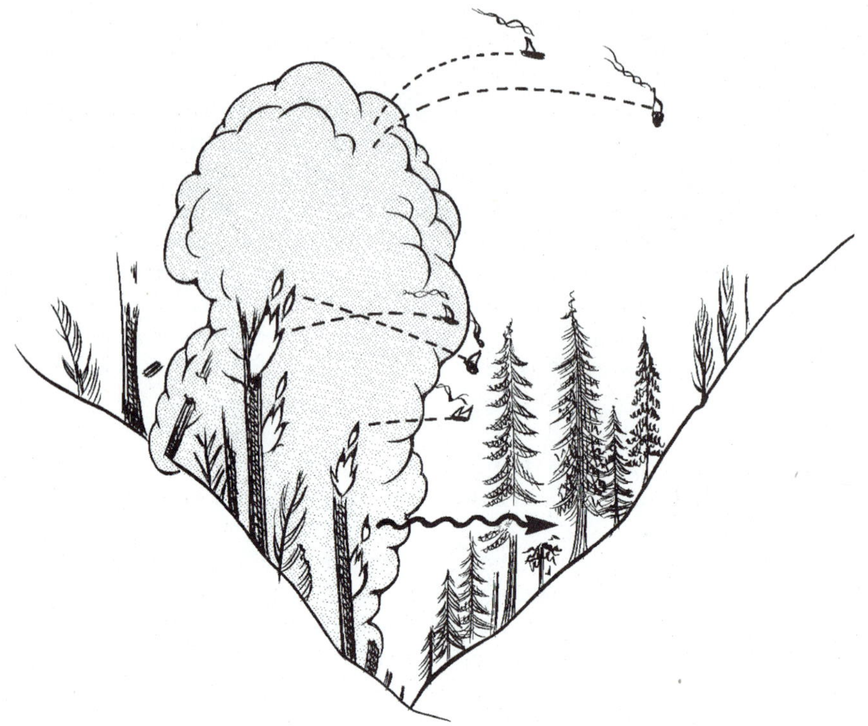

Fig. 9-12 Fuels and people on the slope opposite a fire in a narrow canyon are subject to intense heat and spot fires from airborne embers.

and fall in the Great Plains, Great Lakes, and North Atlantic regions.

Topography. The steeper the slope, the more rapid the spread of fire. Fire usually burns uphill, especially in daytime. Changes in topography cause changes in fire behavior. On steep terrain, rolling firebrands may cause a fire to spread *downhill*.

• • •

When a person encounters a wildland fire, the first step should be to review the principles and indicators of fire behavior, sizing up the situation in terms of fuel, weather, topographic factors, and observed fire behavior. After the fire's probable direction and rate of spread are estimated, travel routes that avoid life hazards can be planned (Fig. 9-15). The direction of the main body of smoke is often a good indicator of the direction the fire will take.

Extreme Fire Behavior

Several years of drought combined with a national forest health issue that has produced many dead and dying forests has set the stage for extreme fire behavior conditions that threaten people, property, and natural and cultural resources. Protection from these conditions requires an understanding of the crown fire process. As the name implies, a crown fire is a fire carried through the crowns, or foliage, of a forest or shrubland. Rothermel[33] described the conditions that produce a crown fire:

1. Dry fuels
2. Low humidity and high temperatures
3. Heavy accumulations of dead and downed fuels
4. Small trees in the understory, or "ladder fuels"
5. Steep slope
6. Strong winds
7. Unstable atmosphere
8. Continuous crown layer

The two most prominent behavior patterns of crown fires are wind-driven fires and plume-dominated fires. Each type of crown fire poses a distinct set of threats to people.

Wind-Driven Fire. A running crown fire can develop when winds increase with increasing elevation above the ground, driving flames from crown to crown (Fig. 9-16). Steep slopes can produce the same effect. Spread rates can vary from 1.6 to 11 km per hour (1 to 7 mph) and possibly faster in mountainous terrain.[33] A running crown fire is accompanied by showers of firebrands downwind, fire whirls, smoke, and the rapid development of a tilted convection column. As long as the wind remains fairly constant from one direction, the flanks of the fire can remain relatively safe. The greatest threat is to people who are at the head, or downwind, side of the fire. People also are at risk from long-distance spot fires that may ignite from flying embers as far as 1.6 km (1 mile) ahead of the main fire front.

Plume-Dominated Fire. An alternative form of crown

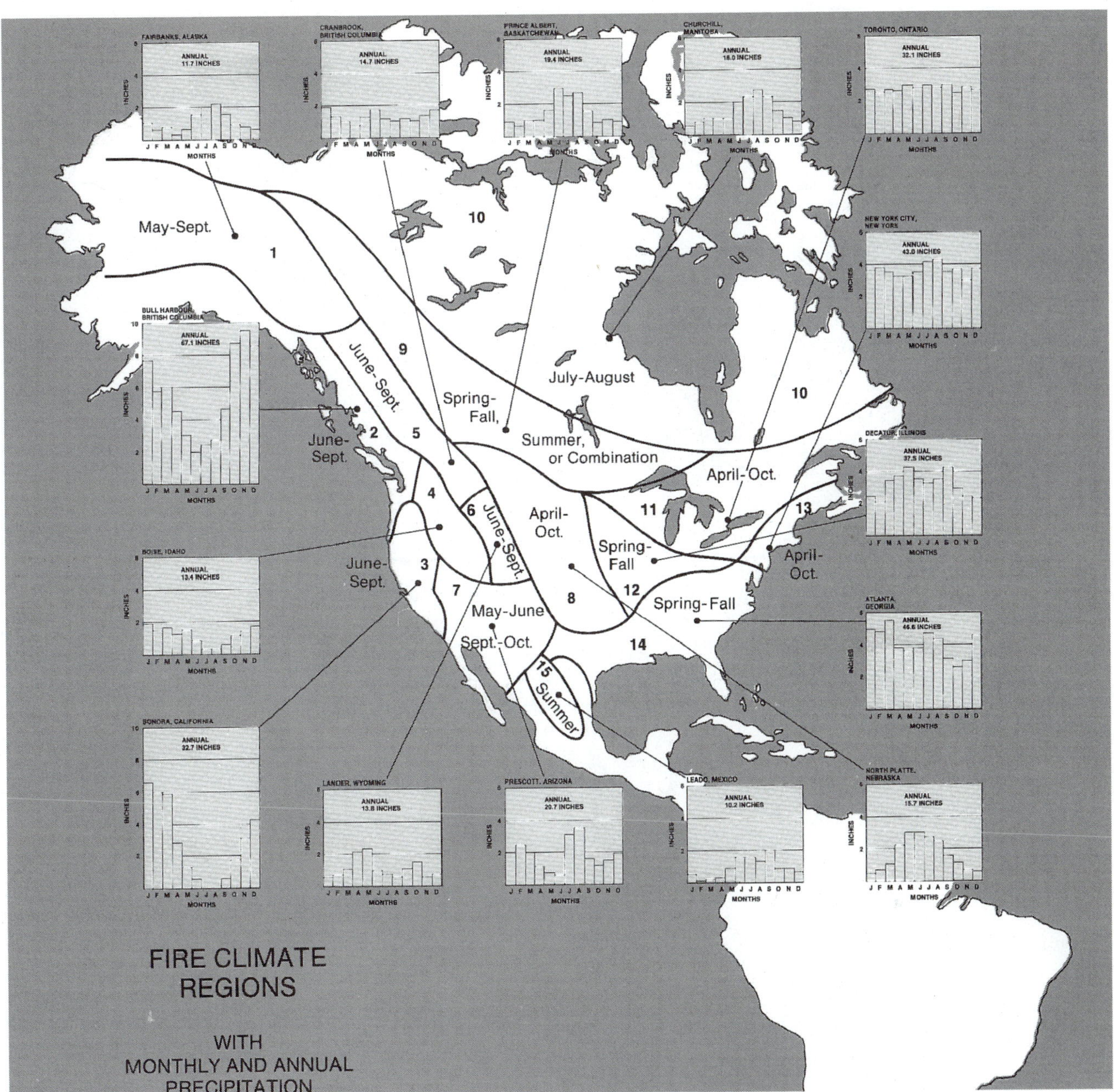

Fig. 9-13 Fire climate regions of North America, based on geographic and climatic factors, are as follows: (1) interior Alaska and the Yukon, (2) north Pacific Coast, (3) south Pacific Coast, (4) Great Basin, (5) northern Rocky Mountains, (6) southern Rocky Mountains, (7) Southwest (including adjacent Mexico), (8) Great Plains, (9) central and northwest Canada, (10) sub-Arctic and tundra, (11) Great Lakes, (12) Central States, (13) North Atlantic, (14) Southern States, and (15) Mexican central plateau. The bar graphs show the monthly and annual precipitation for a representative station in each of the fire climate regions. Months on the map indicate fire seasons. (From Schroeder MJ, Buck CC: *Fire weather*, Agricultural Handbook 360, 1970, USDA Forest Service.)

fire is one that develops with relatively low windspeeds or when windspeed decreases with elevation above the ground. This type of crown fire is called a plume-dominated fire because it is characterized by a towering convection column that stands vertically over the fire (Fig. 9-17). This type of fire poses a unique threat to people because it can produce spot fires in any direction around its perimeter. It can also spread rapidly as the combustion rate accelerates.

One form of a plume-dominated fire can be especially dangerous when a downburst of wind blows outward near

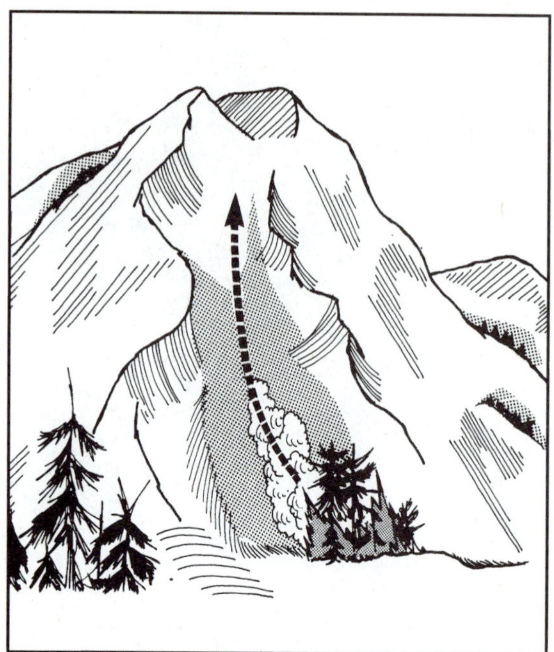

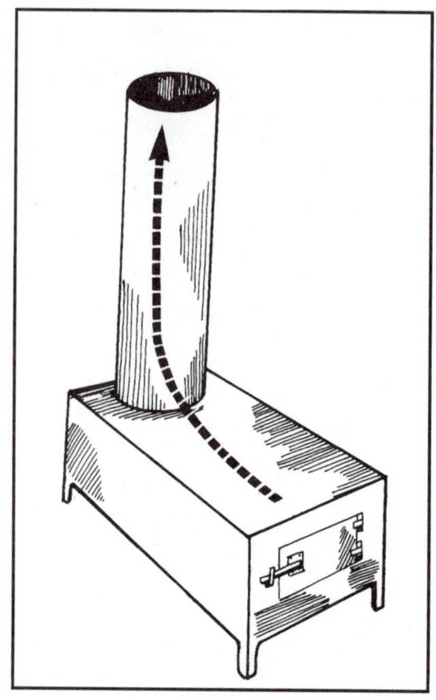

Fig. 9-14 Chutes, chimneys, and box canyons created by sharp ridges provide avenues for intense updrafts (like a fire in a stove) and rapid rates of spread. People should avoid being caught above a fire under these topographic conditions.

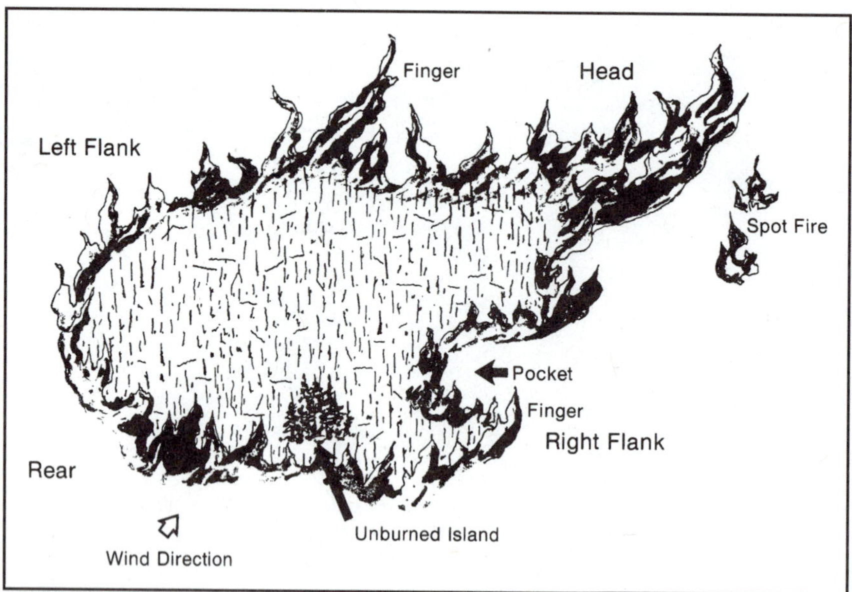

Fig. 9-15 The parts of a fire are described in terms of its left flank, right flank, head, and rear. There may also be unburned islands within the fire and spot fires ahead of the fire. The safest travel routes generally involve lateral movement on contours away from the fire's flank or movement toward the rear of the fire. Moving in front of a headfire should be avoided. The burned area inside the fire's perimeter can offer a safe haven, if the flaming perimeter can be safely penetrated by an individual.

the ground from the bottom of a convection cell. These winds can be extremely strong[14] and can greatly accelerate a fire. This type of wind occurred during the Dude fire north of Phoenix, Arizona, on June 26, 1990, when six firefighters were killed.

There are indicators that help to signal the onset of a downburst from a plume-dominated fire. The surest indicator is the occurrence of precipitation of any amount, even a light sprinkle, or the appearance of virga (evaporating rain) below a convective cell.[33] Another indicator is the rapid de-

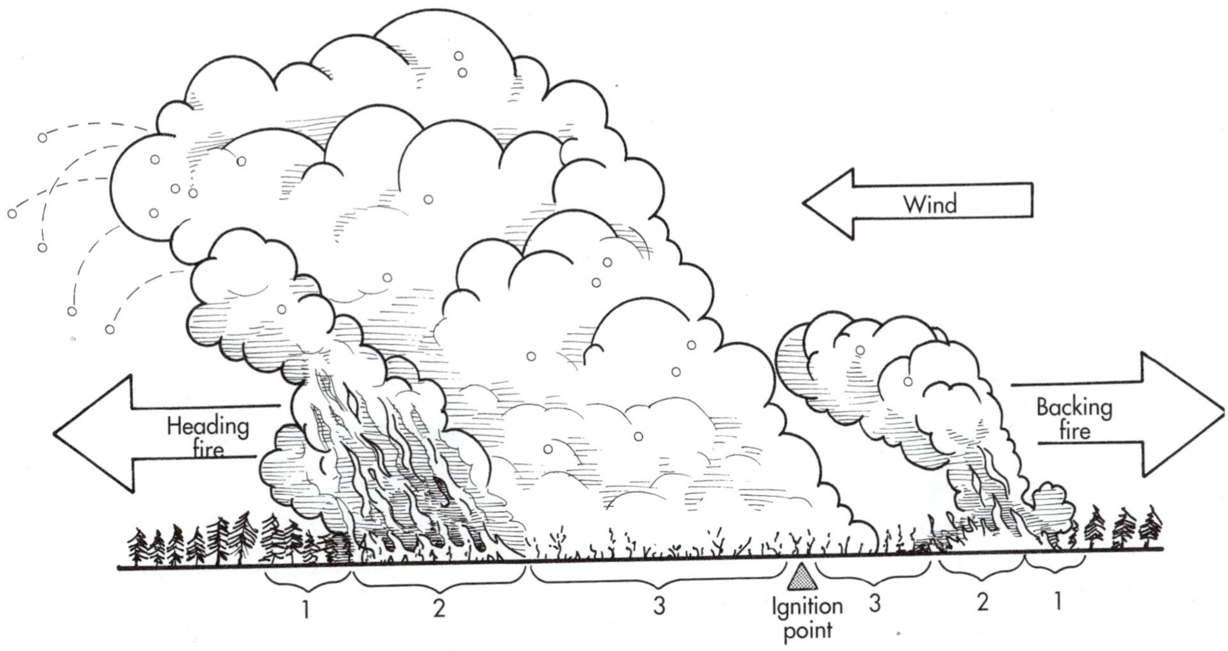

Fig. 9-16 Cross-sectional view of a wind-driven crown fire. People are most at risk on the downwind side of a wind-driven fire. This type of fire is caused by winds that increase in velocity with increasing elevation above the ground.

velopment of a strong convection column above the fire, or nearby thunder cells. A third and very short warning is the calm that develops when the indraft winds stop before the turnabout and outflow of wind from the cell. This brief period of calm may be accompanied by a humming sound just before the reversing wind flow arrives. If any of these indicators is present, the area should quickly be evacuated. The downburst may also break or uproot trees, creating an additional hazard for people.

Fires are seldom uniform and well behaved, so these descriptions of wind-driven and plume-dominated fire behavior may not be readily apparent. The behavior of these types of fires can be expected to change rapidly as environmental, fuel, and topographic conditions change.[33]

Table 9-1 Location of Bodies of 53 Persons Who Died in Tasmanian Fires, February 7, 1967

Location	No. of Deaths
Mustering stock	2
Firefighting	11
Traveling in a vehicle	2
Escaping from and found at some distance from houses	11
Within a few meters of houses	10
In houses	17

From McArthur AG, Cheney NP: *Report on southern Tasmania bushfires of 7 February 1967*, Hobart, Australia, 1967, Government Printer.

Fire-Related Injuries and Fatalities

Wildland fire disasters that result in injury and death occur worldwide. Most fatalities occur on days of extreme fire danger when people are exposed to abnormally high heat stress caused by weather or proximity to fires. Loss of life is dramatically highlighted under extreme burning conditions; however, many more people are injured than are killed by fires.

One of the worst fire disasters in Australia occurred on February 7, 1967, when 62 persons died in Tasmania.[19] Analysis of location and age of 53 individuals at the time of death is instructive (Tables 9-1 and 9-2). Most people whose bodies were found within or near houses were old, infirm, or physically disabled. More than one half of the houses vacated by the 11 people who traveled some distance before being killed were not burned. Most of these victims would probably have survived if they had remained in their homes. Most of the 11 firefighters who died were inexperienced. Many might have survived if they had observed fire behavior and safety rules.

A review of USDA Forest Service records between 1926 and 1976 showed that 145 men died in 41 fires from fire-induced injuries.[48] Large losses occurred in the Blackwater fire in Wyoming in 1937 and in the Rattlesnake fire in California in 1953, with 15 deaths each. Wilson's analysis of people lost to fires in areas protected by other federal, state, county, and private agencies indicated 77 fire-induced

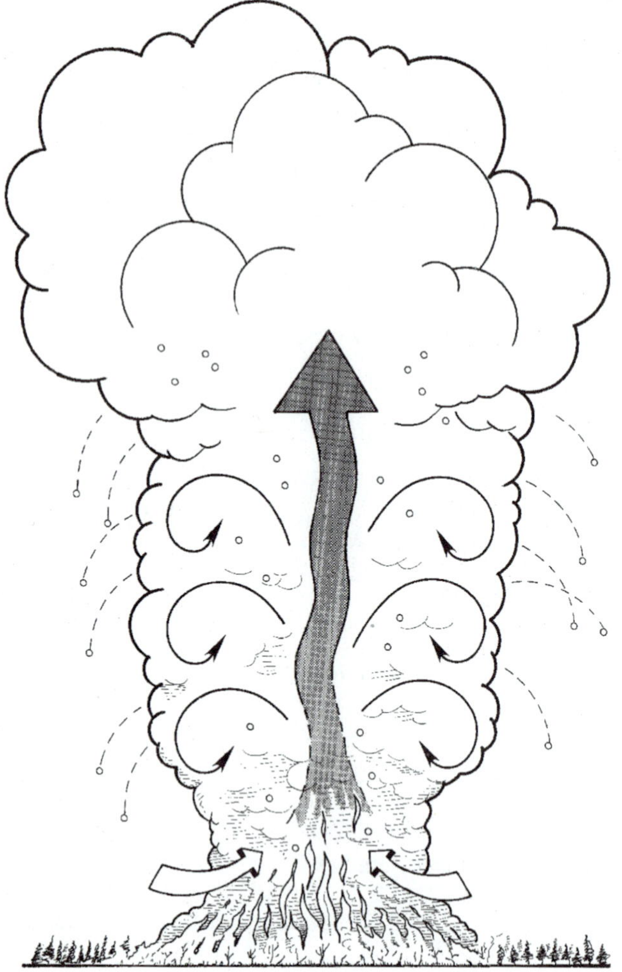

Fig. 9-17 Cross-sectional view of a plume-dominated crown fire. People are at risk around the complete perimeter of this type of fire because the fire can spread intensely or spot in any direction. This form of crown fire develops when wind velocities are relatively low or when velocities decrease with elevation above the ground. The convection plume above this type of fire may rise to 7600 to 9100 meters (25,000 to 30,000 feet) above the ground.

fatalities in 26 fires. The 1933 Griffith Park fire in southern California accounted for 25 fatalities and 128 injuries. Wilson[48] identified some common features connecting these fatal fires:

1. Relatively small fires or isolated sectors within larger fires seemed associated with most fatal incidents.
2. Flare-ups of presumed controlled fires seemed to be particularly hazardous. Fatalities occurred in the mop-up stage.
3. Unexpected shifts in wind direction or speed occasionally caused flare-ups in deceptively light fuels.
4. Gullies, chimneys, and steep slopes directed fires to run uphill.
5. The violent wind vortices left by helicopters and air tankers may have caused flare-ups in previously controlled areas.

Table 9-2 Age Distribution of 53 Persons Who Died in Tasmanian Fires, February 7, 1967

Age Group	Number in Group	Average Age
1-25	1	23
26-50	13	38
51-75	26	64
76-88	13	82

From McArthur AG, Cheney NP: *Report on southern Tasmania bushfires of 7 February 1967*, Hobart, Australia, 1967, Government Printer.

Wilson concluded that the hairline difference between fatal fires and near fatal fires was determined by the individual's reaction to a suddenly critical situation. Escapes were due to luck, circumstances, advance planning, a person's ability to avoid panic, or a combination of these factors. Frequently, poor visibility and absence of concise fire information threatened survival opportunities by creating confusion and panic.

Another analysis of 125 wildland fires, which included 236 fatalities and 66 near fatalities, revealed that the incidents were precipitated by the following basic situations[38]: fire running upslope 29.6%, sudden wind shift 20.8%, rapid rate of fire spread 13.6%, spot fires 9.6%, fire running downslope 6.4%, concentrated fuel flare-up 4.8%, downdrafts and gusts (overhead cumulus clouds) 4.0%, aircraft wake turbulence 0.8%, equipment failure 0.8%, and other (such as heart attack, electrocution) 9.6%.

NATIONAL FIRE PROTECTION ASSOCIATION FATALITY STUDY[29]

During the period from 1981 through 1990, 1221 firefighters died in the line of duty. Of these 1221 firefighters, 162 (or 13.3%) died as a result of wildland fires. The number of those deaths generally ranged between 15 and 22 per year with the exception of 6 deaths in 1982 and 12 deaths in 1983 (Fig. 9-18). Their distribution by region is shown in Fig. 9-19.

Almost three fourths of the deaths (117) occurred during fire suppression activities. The remaining 45 deaths occurred when firefighters were responding to or returning from such fires. The largest proportion of deaths during fire suppression activities was due to stress. These 35 deaths included 12 resulting from physical exertion at the fire scene.

The next major category involved firefighters who became caught or trapped—26 by fire progress and 1 by a falling object. Of the 26 firefighters overrun by fire, 17 died as a result of burns; the other 9 died of asphyxiation. The next category included 17 fatalities resulting from exposure to or contact with an object: 6 exposed to smoke, 6 exposed

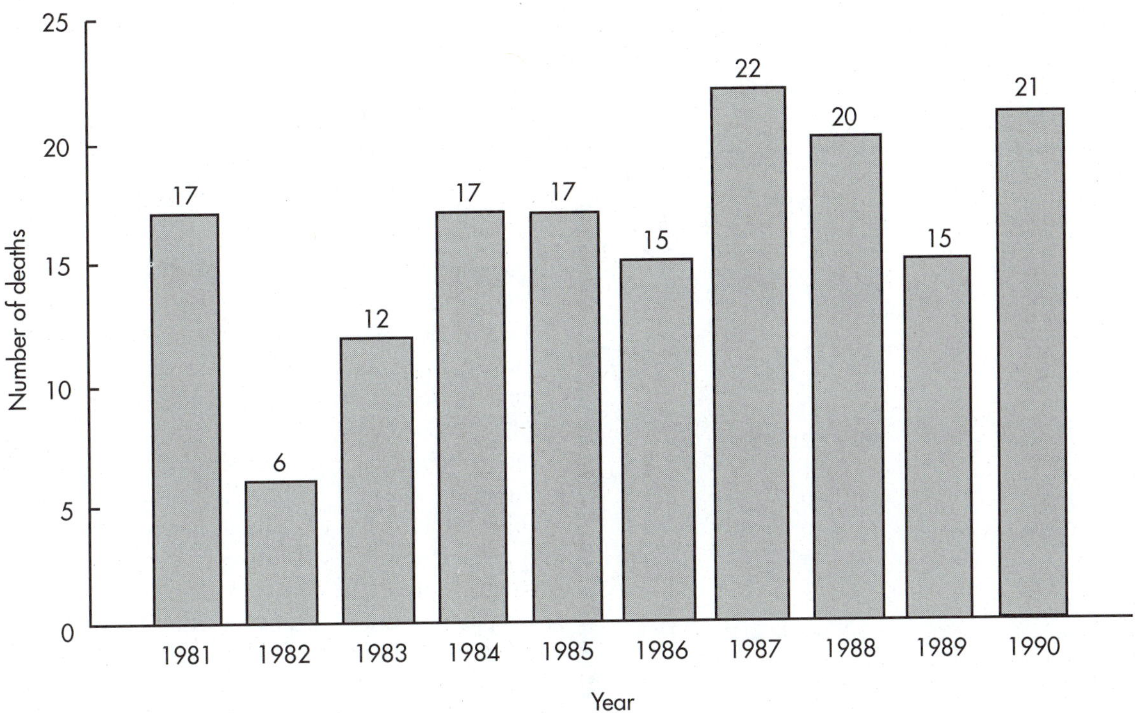

Fig. 9-18 Firefighter fatalities in the United States in wildland fires between 1981 and 1990.

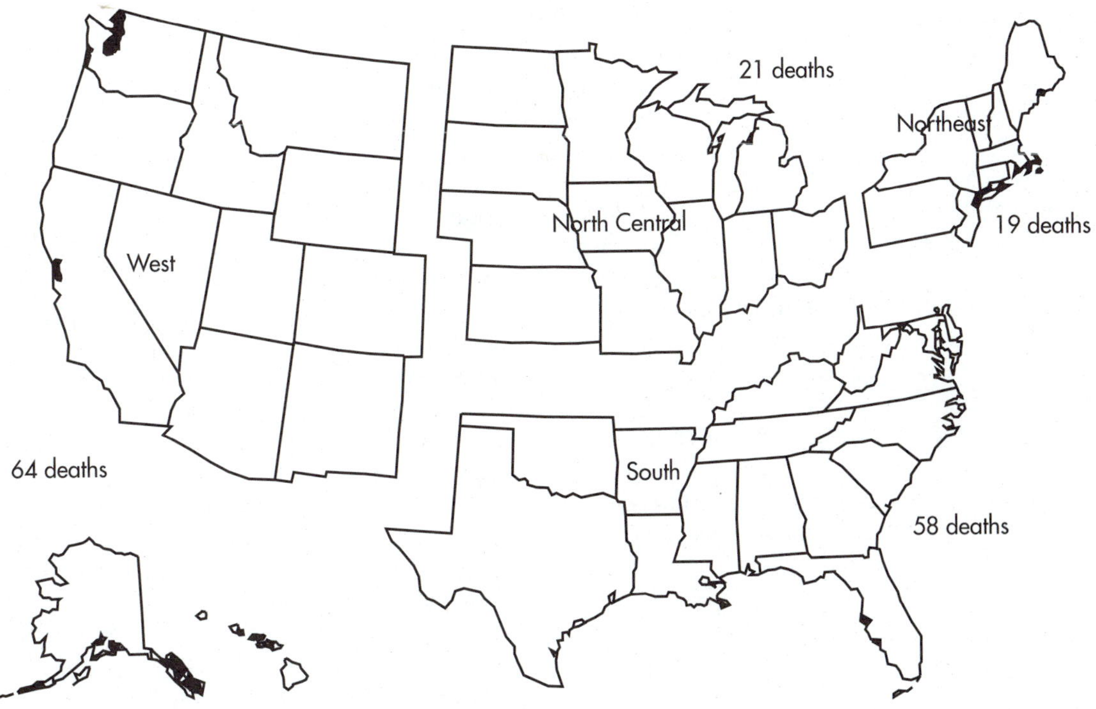

Fig. 9-19 Regional distribution of firefighter fatalities in wildland fires between 1981 and 1990.

to electricity, 3 overcome by hot weather, and 2 struck by lightning. Another 20 were killed in fire department apparatus accidents during fire suppression activities, including 16 in aircraft crashes.

The nature of fatal injuries is shown in Table 9-3. For this part of the National Fire Protection Association (NFPA) analysis, the deaths at the fire site were broken down by type of department—municipal departments (career or volunteer) or forestry agencies. A profile of the 117 victims at the wildland fire sites shows that 55 were members of municipal fire

Table 9-3 Wildland Firefighter Fatalities on the Fire Ground by Nature of Fatal Injury, 1981-1990

Cause of Death	Federal and State Wildland Agencies	Municipal		Total
		Volunteer	Career	
Heart attack	3	29	2	34
Internal trauma	21	5	0	26
Burns	13	1	1	15
Asphyxiation	9	1	1	11
Electric shock	3	5	0	8
Crushing	5	3	0	8
Heatstroke	0	1	2	3
Amputation	2	0	0	2
Stroke	2	0	0	2
Bleeding	0	2	0	2
Drowning	0	1	0	1
Fracture	1	0	0	1
Aneurysm	0	0	1	1
TOTAL	59	48	7	114

National Fire Protection Association: *Wildland fire fatalities 1981-1990*, Quincy, Mass, 1991, The Association.
Another three deaths involved members of fire brigades of paper companies: two died from burns and one suffered a heart attack.

departments (48 belonged to volunteer departments and 7 to career departments). The other 59 firefighters were career, seasonal, or contract employees of state and federal forestry agencies. The remaining 3 firefighters were employees of paper companies. As the table shows, heart attacks accounted for more than half of the deaths of municipal firefighters during fire suppression activities, while most of the deaths of state and federal employees were due to internal trauma and burns.

State and federal forestry officials believe that their rigid fitness requirements account for the low proportion of heart attack deaths. Of the 20 municipal heart attack victims for whom medical documentation was available, 12 had had prior heart attacks or bypass surgery, 4 had severe arteriosclerotic heart disease, 2 had diabetes, and 1 had hypertension; no medical documentation was available on the other victim. The lower proportion of heart attacks among wildland agency firefighters could also be a function of age. The median age of wildland firefighter victims was 35 years, while the median age for municipal firefighters was about 50 years.

NATURE OF INJURIES AND FATALITIES

Fire-related injuries and fatalities are a direct consequence of heat, flames, smoke, critical gas levels, or indirect injuries. Injuries and fatalities associated with wildland fires fall into categories of heat (direct thermal injury, inhalation, and heat stress disorders), flames (direct thermal injury and inhalation), smoke (inhalation and mucous membrane irritation), critical gas levels (oxygen, carbon monoxide, and carbon dioxide), and indirect effects (acute and chronic medical disability and trauma).

Although intense fires produce very high temperatures, they generally last for only a short time. The duration of intense heat increases with fuel load; thus intensity is greater in a forest fire where heavy fuels are burning than in a grass or shrub fire. Temperatures near the ground are lower because radiant heat is offset somewhat by inflow of fresh air and the fact that gases of combustion rise and are carried away by convection.[5] Measurements have demonstrated that close to the ground, within a few meters of flames reaching up to 11 m (36 feet), air temperatures may be less than 15° C (59° F) above ambient temperature. The breathing of heated air can be tolerated for 30 minutes at 93° C (199° F) and for 3 minutes at 250° C (482° F).[18] Death or severe pulmonary injury occurs when these limits are exceeded.

Thermal injuries of the respiratory tract frequently contribute to the clinical picture of smoke inhalation. Persons trapped in a fire may have no choice but to breathe flame or very hot gases. This usually results in a thermal injury to the tissues of the upper airway and respiratory tract, which is most commonly confined to the nose, nasopharynx, mouth, oropharynx, hypopharynx, larynx, and upper trachea. These injuries may result in edema accumulation that may obstruct the airway and produce asphyxia. Thermal injury to the respiratory tract can also cause tracheitis and mediastinitis.

Thermal injury to the airway should be suspected when thermal injuries to the head, face, and neck are noted. Suspicion is heightened by the presence of singed facial hair, burns of the nasal, oral, or pharyngeal mucosa, and stridor or dysphonia.[21,40,51] In association with a history of exposure to flame and hot gases in a closed space, these clinical findings strongly suggest the presence of a thermal injury to the airway. In view of the potential for acute airway obstruction, there is obvious urgency in establishing this diagnosis. Most experts who treat thermal injuries of the tracheobronchial tree advocate early visualization of the vocal cords by laryngoscopy and bronchoscopy.[22] Bronchoscopy is proving to be a useful predictor of the clinical course and urgency of intensive care unit intervention. In addition, there is one report of a significantly greater incidence of pneumonia and late mortality in persons with facial burns than in those without them.[49]

Burns of the lower trachea are rarely reported. In fact, injuries to and beyond the carina are difficult to produce when the trachea is cannulated and hot gases are delivered in the anesthetized dog.[20,50] Air has a very low specific heat and is therefore a poor conductor of thermal energy. In addition, the thermal exchange systems of the upper airway are quite efficient. The hot gas or flame is cooled sufficiently in the upper airway so that it does not burn the bronchi or more distal structures. It should be noted, however, that although water or steam in the hot gas mixture is probably rare, it is a far more efficient conductor of heat and permits significant thermal injury to the lower trachea and bronchi.

A delayed onset (2 to 24 hours after smoke inhalation) of pulmonary edema and adult respiratory distress syndrome is widely reported and should be anticipated. Whether this results from direct injury to alveoli, prolonged hypotension, or cerebral hypoxia and cerebral edema is unclear.

Heat stress is another fire-induced disorder.[37] This occurs when air temperature, humidity, radiant heat, and poor air movement combine with strenuous work and insulative clothing to raise body temperature beyond safe limits. Sweating cools the body as moisture evaporates. When water lost through sweating is not replaced, physiologic heat controls can deregulate and body temperature may rise, leading to heat exhaustion or heatstroke (see Chapter 8).

Direct contact with flames causes thermal injury, and death is inevitable when exposure is for long periods. Burns may be superficial, partial, or full thickness (see Chapter 10). Immediate death is the result of hypotension, hyperthermia, respiratory failure, and frank incineration.

The common cause of asphyxia in relation to wildland fire is smoke. Danger increases in locations where smoke accumulates because of poor ventilation, such as in caves, box canyons, narrow valleys, and gullies.

Dense, acrid smoke is particularly irritating to the respiratory system and eyes. Excessive coughing induces pharyngitis and vomiting. Keratitis, conjunctivitis, and chemosis may make it impossible to keep the eyes open.

There are concerns about the levels of oxygen, carbon monoxide, and carbon dioxide associated with fire. Critical levels may readily occur in a closed space and near burning or smoldering heavy fuels, but the open space of a wildland fire usually contributes to continual mixing of air. Misconceptions about lack of oxygen or excessive carbon monoxide and carbon dioxide in a wildland fire abound in the lay literature.

Flaming combustion can be maintained only at oxygen levels that exceed 12%, a level at which life can also be supported.[5,18] With continued indrafts of air that feed the flames, a fresh source of oxygen is usually present. Even mass fires, in which large tracts of land are burning, have rarely been found to reduce oxygen to hazardous levels. Low oxygen levels may occur, however, where there is little air movement, such as in caves (Fig. 9-20) or in burned-over land that continues to smoke from smoldering fuels.

Concentrations of carbon monoxide in excess of 800 parts per million (ppm) can cause death within hours. Most fires produce small quantities; however, atmospheric concentrations rarely reach lethal levels as a result of air movement. High concentrations appear to be associated with smoldering combustion of heavy fuels, such as fallen trees or slash piles, and carbon monoxide may also collect in low-lying areas or in underground shelters.[6] Outdoors, the danger lies in continual exposure to low concentrations that can result in increasing carboxyhemoglobin levels in blood. Prolonged exposure affects the central nervous system, resulting in headache, impaired judgment, progressive lethargy, decreased vision, and other psychomotor deficits.[48]

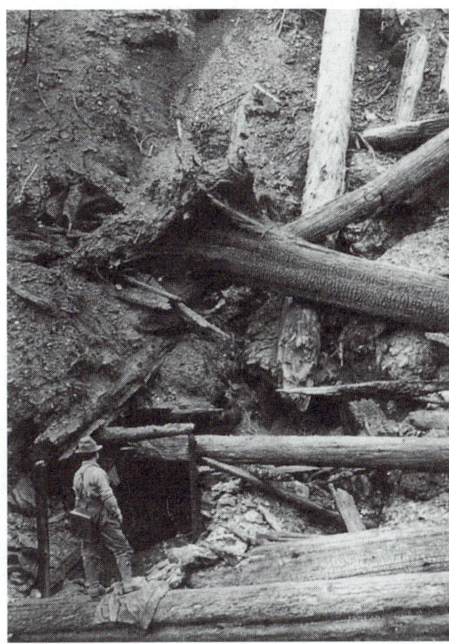

Fig. 9-20 Ranger Pulaski led 42 men and 2 horses to this mine tunnel near Placer Creek in northern Idaho to seek refuge from the 1910 fire. One man who failed to get into the tunnel was burned beyond recognition. All the men in the tunnel evidently were unconscious for a period of time. Five men died inside the tunnel, apparently from suffocation. The remainder of the crew was evacuated to the hospital in Wallace, where all recovered. (Courtesy of the USDA Forest Service. Photo by J.B. Halm.)

Studies have been conducted to measure levels of carbon monoxide around fires. Levels of 50 ppm were measured close to a prescribed burn in grass.[8] In another estimate, concentrations of 30 ppm were found roughly 61 m (200 feet) from the fire front. Studies on the 1974 Deadline and Outlaw forest fires in Idaho showed that firefighters were exposed to levels above the standards proposed by the National Institute of Occupational Safety and Health (35 ppm over an 8-hour period).[41]

It has been proposed that decreased ambient oxygen contributes to hypoxia and the overall picture of smoke inhalation (Table 9-4). This mechanism is at least variably operant. In studies in which standing gasoline was ignited in a closed bunker, the fire self-extinguished, while the ambient oxygen remained at 14%, a survivable level.[20] Subsequent work in which burning gasoline or napalm was injected into bunkers produced nearly complete and prolonged exhaustion of ambient oxygen. In light of the conflicting data it is difficult to classify definitively situations in which decreased ambient oxygen and subsequent hypoxia of exposed individuals contribute to the clinical picture of smoke inhalation. Studies in which ambient oxygen was measured by

Table 9-4 Human Response to Decreased Ambient Oxygen at Sea Level

Ambient Oxygen (%)	Human Response
20.9	Normal function
16-18	Decreased stamina and capacity for work
12-15	Dyspnea with walking; impaired coordination; variable impaired judgment
10-12	Dyspnea at rest; consciousness preserved; impaired judgment, coordination, and concentration
6-8	Loss of consciousness; death without prompt reversal
<6	Death in 6 to 10 minutes

scientists did not show significant depletion of the scene of the fire.[13]

Few data are available on levels of carbon dioxide around wildland fires. Although it may be produced in large quantities, it apparently never reaches hazardous concentrations, even in severe fire situations.[5,18]

The quantity of burning fuel and the type of topography affect levels of oxygen and toxic gases. Danger is greater in forest fires where heavy fuels burn over long periods of time than in quick-moving grass and shrub fires. Topography has a major influence; caves, box canyons, narrow canyons, gulches, and other terrain features can trap toxic gases or hinder ventilation, thereby preventing an inflow of fresh air. While most fatalities result from encounters with smoke, flames, and heat, critical gas levels can induce handicaps sufficient to render the victim more vulnerable to other hazards.

WILDLAND FIRES, AIR TOXINS, AND HUMAN HEALTH

In the United States about 80,000 firefighters are involved with suppression activities on 70,000 wildland fires that burn an average of over 0.8 million hectares (2 million acres) each year. In 1988 over 2 million hectares (5 million acres) of land were burned, with a total combined suppression cost in excess of $600 million. The firefighting effort has another cost that has not been quantified: the effect of smoke on firefighter health and productivity. Over the 4 months of the Greater Yellowstone Area fires, approximately 40% of the 30,000 medical visits made by wildland firefighters were for respiratory problems. More than 600 firefighters required subsequent medical care. In the Happy Camp area during the Klamath fire complex in California in 1987, ambient concentrations of carbon monoxide were measured as high as 54 ppm on a volume basis.[44] A better understanding of the effects of wildland fire smoke on people is clearly needed. The combustion products of concern include these classes of materials:

1. Particulate matter
2. Polynuclear aromatic hydrocarbons
3. Carbon monoxide
4. Aldehydes
5. Organic acids
6. Semivolatile and volatile organic compounds
7. Free radicals
8. Ozone
9. Inorganic fraction of particles

Large variances exist associated with the development of smoke combustion products and exposure to the materials of concern.[44] Ward and co-workers[45] indicated that the toxicity of the combination of combustion products depends on the relative concentrations of the individual compounds as well as the overall concentration and length of exposure. Individual toxicities are associated with many of the compounds found in smoke. The combined toxicity of these substances is not known. A detailed set of studies is being carried out to provide answers so that risk management options can be exercised. One of these studies suggested that wildland firefighters experience a small cross-seasonal decline in pulmonary function and an increase in several respiratory symptoms.[35] Eye irritation, nose irritation, and wheezing were associated with recent firefighting.

The strenuous work of fighting or escaping a fire magnifies chronic illnesses, age disabilities, exhaustion, and cardiovascular instability. Common trauma is induced by falling trees or limbs, rolling logs or rocks, vehicular accidents, poor visibility, panic, falling asleep in unburned fuels that later ignite, and leaving the safety of buildings and vehicles. Cuts, scrapes, scratches, lacerations, fractures, and eye injuries (foreign particles, smoke irritation, sharp objects) are other common afflictions. Poison oak, poison ivy, stinging insects, and poisonous snakes are additional sources of trauma during wildland fires. To avoid fire-related injuries and fatalities, a person must keep attuned to mental and physical stress levels and be aware of cumulative effects.[37] *Ignorance of this simple principle is disastrous.*

Wildland and Urban Interface Fire Survival Principles and Techniques

History has demonstrated repeatedly that individuals simply were not prepared to make correct judgments among survival alternatives under stress situations. Overconfidence, ignorance, bad habits, lack of preparation, and panic have quickly led to improper and unsafe actions during fire emergencies. The fact that fatal and near fatal accidents often have been associated with deceptively simple and easy fire situations reflects overconfidence and inappropriate human behavior patterns.[48] "Learning from mistakes" in these settings is not a reasonable education strategy for those in jeopardy; second chances are frequently unavailable.

To develop significant safety principles and rules, the USDA Forest Service organized a task force in 1957 to "study how we might strengthen our ways and means of preventing firefighting fatalities." One of the major recommendations of the task force was to adopt service-wide standard firefighting orders.

Ten standard firefighting orders were placed into operational practice during the 1957 fire season; later, 18 watchout situations were highlighted. Undoubtedly these preconditioned responses have been adopted by all wildland fire agencies and have saved lives and averted accidents. Almost without exception, when someone is injured or killed during fire suppression actions, it is not because something unexpected happened. Accidents generally result from violation of one or more fundamental principles. The growing opportunity for wildland fire encounters by emergency medical personnel and the public mandates that these people practice the same fire safety principles required of suppression agencies.

TEN STANDARD FIREFIGHTING ORDERS

Ten standard firefighting orders summarize fundamental principles of safety on the fireline (Box 9-3). While the orders were written for firefighters, they apply to all people working, living, or traveling near wildland fires. The orders are adapted below to remind emergency medical personnel, wildland homeowners, and recreationists of safety precautions:

BOX 9-3

TEN STANDARD FIREFIGHTING ORDERS

1. Keep informed of fire weather conditions, changes, and forecasts and how they may affect the area where you are located.
2. Know what the fire is doing at all times through personal observations, communication systems, or scouts.
3. Base all actions on current and expected behavior of the fire.
4. Determine escape routes and plans for everyone at risk and make certain that everyone understands routes and plans.
5. Post lookouts to watch the fire if you think there is any danger of being trapped, of increased fire activity, or of erratic fire behavior.
6. Be alert, keep calm, think clearly, and act decisively in order to avoid panic reactions.
7. Maintain prompt and clear communication with your group, firefighting forces, and command/communication centers.
8. Give clear, concise instructions and be sure that they are understood.
9. Maintain control of the people in your group at all times.
10. Fight fire aggressively, but provide for safety first. (Nonqualified and improperly equipped persons should fight fire only when it is necessary to assist injured persons.)

LCES: THE KEY TO SAFE PROCEDURES

LCES stands for lookouts, communications, escape routes, and safety zones. The following information is taken from Gleason's discussion[12] on applying LCES to safeguard people from the threats of wildland fires. In this context the LCES principles will be adapted to the safety and welfare of recreationists and emergency medical personnel who may be in the vicinity of a wildland fire.

The wildland fire environment has several basic hazards: lightning, volcanoes, fire-weakened trees, rolling rocks and logs, entrapment by running fires, respirable particulates, air toxins, and heat stress. When these hazards exist, there are two options:

1. Do not enter the environment.
2. Adhere to safe procedures. The key to these safe procedures is LCES.

These are the same items stressed in the standard firefighting orders. They should be viewed from a "systems" point of view, stressing the interdependence of the elements. For example, the best safety zone is of no value if the escape route does not offer timely access when needed. It is important that the LCES plan be identified to people well before it may be needed. The nature of wildland fires also dictates that LCES be redefined continuously to keep pace with changing conditions.

The LCES system is implemented in this manner:

1. Lookouts. Fixed lookouts or roving lookouts need to be in a position where both the hazard and the people can be seen. Lookouts must be trained to observe the wildland fire environment and to recognize and anticipate fire behavior changes. When the hazard becomes a danger, the lookout relays the information to the people so they can depart for the safety zone.
2. Communications. Communications is the vehicle that delivers the message to alert people to the approaching hazard. These communications must be prompt and clear.
3. Escape routes. These are the paths taken from a currently threatened position to an area free from danger. More than one escape route must be available. Escape routes are probably the most elusive component of LCES, since their effectiveness changes continuously. Escape routes must always provide access to safety zones in a timely manner.
4. Safety zones. These are locations where the threatened individual may find adequate refuge from the danger. The safety zones must be large enough to protect people from flames, radiant heat, convective

heat, and falling trees. The size of an effective safety zone will vary with changes in fuels, topography, wind conditions, and fire intensity.

EIGHTEEN WATCH-OUT SITUATIONS IN THE WILDLAND

Eighteen watch-out situations are stated below, with a short discussion of their relevance to emergency medical personnel and wildland users:

1. You are moving downhill toward a fire. Fire can move swiftly and suddenly uphill, so that constant observation must be made of fire behavior, fuels, and escape routes when walking downhill toward the fire. Assess the potential for fire to run uphill in every situation.
2. You are on a hillside where rolling, burning material can ignite fuel from below. When on a hillside below a fire, be watchful of burning materials, especially cones and logs, that can roll downhill and start a fire beneath you. Getting caught between two coalescing fires can be deadly.
3. Wind begins to blow, increase, or change direction. Wind has a strong influence on fire behavior, so be prepared to respond to any sudden changes.
4. The weather becomes hotter and drier. Fire activity increases, and its behavior changes more rapidly as ambient temperature rises and relative humidity decreases.
5. Dense vegetation with unburned fuel is between you and the fire. The danger in this situation is that unburned fuels can ignite. If the fire is moving away from you, be alert for wind changes or spot fires that may ignite fuels near you. Do not be overconfident if the area has burned once, because it could reignite if sufficient fuel remains.
6. You are in an unburned area near the fire where terrain and cover make travel difficult. The combination of fuel and difficult escape makes this a dangerous situation.
7. Travel or work is in an area that you have not seen in daylight. Darkness and unfamiliarity are a dangerous combination.
8. You are unfamiliar with local factors influencing fire behavior. When possible, seek information on what to expect from knowledgeable people, especially those from the area.
9. By necessity, you have to make a frontal assault on a fire with tankers. Any encounter with an active line of fire is dangerous because of proximity to intense heat, smoke, and flames, along with limited escape opportunities.
10. Spot fires occur frequently across the fireline. Generally, increased spotting indicates increased fire activity and intensity. Danger is that of entrapment between coalescing fires.
11. The main fire cannot be seen, and you are not in communication with anyone who can see it. The danger in this situation is in not knowing the location, size, and behavior of the main fire. Planning becomes guesswork, which is an unfavorable response.
12. An unclear assignment or confusing instructions have been received. Make sure that all assignments and instructions are fully understood.
13. You are drowsy and feel like resting or sleeping near the fireline in unburned fuel. This may lead to fire entrapment. *No one should sleep near a wildland fire.* If resting is absolutely necessary, choose a burned area that is safe from rolling material, smoke, reburn, and other dangers or seek a wide area of bare ground or rock.
14. Fire has not been scouted and sized up.
15. Safety zones and escape routes have not been identified.
16. You are uninformed on strategy, tactics, and hazards.
17. No communication link with crew members or supervisor has been established.
18. A line has been constructed without a safe anchor point.

FIFTEEN STRUCTURAL WATCH-OUT SITUATIONS FOR THE WILDLAND-URBAN INTERFACE

With the increasing necessity for crews to fight fires in the wildland-urban interface, these 15 structural watch-out situations were defined to increase awareness of structural fire dangers[42]:

1. Access is poor (for example, narrow roads, twisting, single lane with inadequate turning).
2. Load limits of local bridges are light or unknown; the bridges are narrow.
3. Winds are strong, and erratic fire behavior is occurring.
4. Area contains garages with closed, locked doors.
5. You have an inadequate water supply to attack the fire.
6. Structure windows are black or smoked over.
7. There are septic tanks and leach lines. (These are found in most rural situations.)
8. House or structure is burning with puffing rather than steady smoke.
9. Inside and outside construction of structures is wood with shake shingle roofs.
10. Natural fuels occur within 9 m (30 feet) of the structures.
11. Known or suspected panicked persons are in the vicinity.
12. Structure windows are bulging, and the roof has not been vented.

13. Additional fuels can be found in open crawl spaces beneath the structures.
14. Firefighting is taking place in or near chimney or canyon situations.
15. Elevated fuel or propane tanks are present.

REFUGE IN VEHICLES, BUILDINGS, AND FIRE SHELTERS

As stated previously, much of the heat from a fire is radiant energy. While its intensity at a given location may be high, it typically lasts for only a short time. Because radiant heat travels in straight lines, does not penetrate solid substances, and is easily reflected, seeking refuge in vehicles, buildings, or fire shelters is often lifesaving.

Vehicles

In the United States there have been several accounts of firefighters who have survived severe fire storms or the passage of fire fronts by taking refuge in vehicles. A few case histories follow, serving as examples of intense burning situations in which lives were saved because people stayed inside vehicles when the fire passed. These cases are from a chapter on survival techniques in an international report on fatal and near fatal wildland fire accidents[38]:

In 1958 a veteran Field Section Fire Warden and two young men were fighting forest fires that burned in heavy fuels near the Bass River State Forest in southern New Jersey. A 90 degree wind shift transformed the flank fire into a broad headfire, with advancing flames up to 12 m (40 feet). The men entered their vehicle, a Dodge W300 Power Wagon, which stood in the middle of a sand road 4 m (12 feet) wide. Simultaneously the engine and radio failed.

The Fire Warden repeatedly admonished the crewmen, who wished to flee, to stay in the truck. Subsequently the truck was rocked violently by convection currents and microclimatic changes generated by the flames. The men could neither see nor breathe because of smoke, and the cab began to fill with sparks that ignited the seat. The men stayed with the truck for only 3 or 4 minutes during the passage of the headfire, but they indicated later that the interval involved seemed more like 3 or 4 hours.

At the first opportunity all of them left the vehicle on the upwind side and crouched beside it to escape the searing heat and burning seats. The warden proceeded to burn his hand severely while disposing of a flaming gas can in the truck bed. While the young men escaped virtually unscathed, the older man suffered lung damage and remained on limited duty for 5 years. He has since recovered completely and retired.

In 1976 a firefighter died while fighting a grass fire near Buhler, Kansas, in Reno County. A flashover occurred from a buildup of gases on the lee side of a windbreak. A fire truck was caught in the flashover, and the firefighter working from the back of the vehicle ran and was killed. Although the truck burned, the driver was not seriously hurt.

In a 1962 California Division of Forestry fire in Fresno County, three men, followed by a flank fire that had turned into a headfire, raced back to their truck only a few feet ahead of the flames. The truck would not restart. After the main body of flames passed over the vehicle, the men jumped out in order to breathe, since the truck was burning. Almost completely blinded by smoke and heat, they stumbled headlong into matted fuels, and two received first- and second-degree burns. One man was not burned but had to be treated for smoke inhalation. The truck was a loss.

Sitting in a vehicle during a passing fire front is often perilous, but when a person is trapped, it is almost certain doom to attempt escape by running from the fire. The preceding case histories illustrate a few facts that, if remembered, may prevent panic:

1. The engine may stall and not restart.
2. The vehicle may be rocked by convection currents.
3. Smoke and sparks may enter the cab.
4. The interior, engine, or tires may ignite.
5. Temperatures increase inside the cab because the heat is radiated through the windows.
6. Metal gas tanks and containers rarely explode.
7. If it is necessary to leave the cab after the fire has passed, keep the vehicle between you and the fire.

The type of vehicle determines the amount of protection provided. Two travelers died in a fire in 1967 in Tasmania, Australia, when they were caught in a canvas-topped vehicle that afforded no protection.[18] A later fire in Australia led to further research on the protection provided by vehicles and the explosiveness of gasoline tanks. In 1969 at Lara, Victoria, Australia, a fast-moving grass fire crossed a four-lane expressway. Several cars stopped on the road in the confusion of smoke and flames. Seventeen people left the safety of their cars and perished. Six people stayed inside their vehicles and survived, even though one car ignited.

Over a period of several years investigations were carried out by the Forest Research Institute (now the Commonwealth Scientific and Industrial Research Organization [CSIRO], Division of Forest Research) in Canberra, Australia, in an attempt to collect accurate data and to dispel the misconceptions that cause persons to flee a safe refuge if trapped by fire.[5] Cars were placed between two burning piles of logging slash to study the ability of a car to shield against radiation. The test was a hotter, longer fire than would normally be encountered by passengers.

Car bodies halved the external radiation transmitted at the peak of the fire, but a person inside would have suffered severe burns to bare skin. Although air temperatures inside the car did not reach hazardous levels until well after the peak radiation had passed, smoke from smoldering plastic and rubber materials would have caused discomfort and made the car uninhabitable. In this study, metal gasoline tanks did not explode, whether intact on cars or separated and placed on a burning pile of slash. Apparently, when tanks are sealed, the space above the liquid contains a mixture too deficient in oxygen vapor for an explosion to occur.

Cheney[5,6] offered the following advice for survival when in a car and trapped by fire:

1. If smoke obstructs visibility, turn on the headlights and drive to the side of the road away from the leading edge of the fire. Try to select an area of sparse vegetation offering the least combustible material.
2. Attempt to shield your body from radiant heat energy by rolling up the windows and covering up with floor mats or hiding beneath the dashboard. Cover as much skin as possible.
3. Stay in the vehicle as long as possible. Unruptured gas tanks rarely explode, and vehicles usually take several minutes to ignite.
4. Grass fires create about 30 seconds of flame exposure, and chances for survival in a vehicle are good. Forest fires create higher intensity flames lasting for 3 to 4 minutes, lowering chances for survival. Staying in a vehicle improves chances for surviving a forest fire. Remain calm.
5. A strong, acrid smell usually results from burning paint and plastic materials, caused by small quantities of hydrogen chloride released from breakdown of polyvinyl chloride. Hydrogen chloride is water soluble, and discomfort can be relieved by breathing through a damp cloth. Urine is mostly water and can be used in emergencies.

Buildings

The decision to evacuate a house or remain and defend it is not easy to make. Fire services generally prefer that residents evacuate the threatened area so that agencies can concentrate on protecting structures (Fig. 9-21). Authorities also agree that evacuation of elderly, very young, infirm, and fearful people is usually a good idea. People should evacuate only if it can be accomplished safely, well in advance of any danger. Several principles should guide the evacuation decision[46]:

1. A fire within sight or smell is a fire that endangers you.
2. More unattended houses burn down.
3. Evacuation when fire is close is too late; evacuation must be done well before danger is apparent.
4. More people are injured and killed in the open than in houses.
5. Learn beforehand about community refuges.
6. Evacuate only to a known safe refuge.

Whether people can find refuge in buildings depends on the construction materials and the amount of preparation that has been made to reduce fuels around the structure. If a home is constructed amid a flammable vegetation type, plans and procedures to safeguard the home and its occupants are essential. A building usually offers protection during the passage of fire even if it ignites later, because it shields against radiant heat and smoke. After the fire passes, it may be necessary to exit if the building is burning.

Case histories from Australia demonstrate that homes provide safe havens.[18] In 1967 in Tasmania, 21 people left their houses as fire approached. All died, and some were within a few meters of the buildings. Many of the houses did not burn and therefore would have been refuges. Most people probably would have survived if they had remained in their dwellings.

When taking refuge in a building, people should be given useful jobs such as filling vessels with water, blocking cracks with wet blankets, and tightly closing windows and doors. If possible, lookouts should keep watch for spot fires on the outside of the building until the last minute. Staying in a house is usually safer than a hasty escape. Before fire

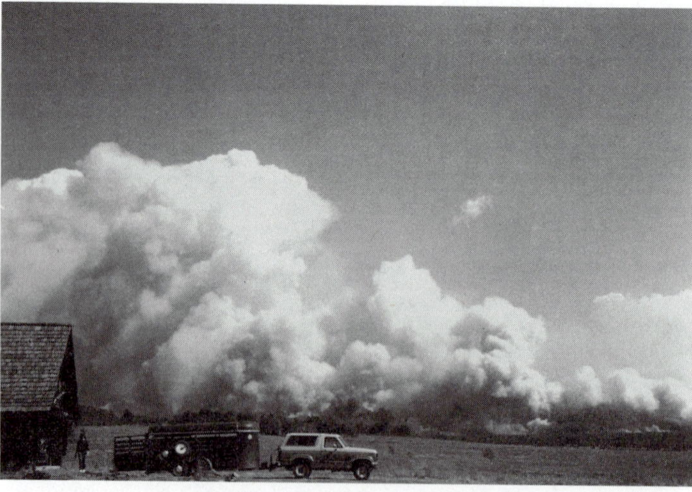

Fig. 9-21 Although the decision to evacuate a fire-threatened area is a difficult one, fire services generally prefer that residents evacuate so that agencies can concentrate on protecting structures. (Courtesy of Bob Mutch.)

approaches the house, the following precautions should be taken[39]:

1. If you plan to stay, evacuate your pets and all family members who are not essential to protecting the home.
2. Be properly dressed to survive the fire. Cotton fabrics are preferable to synthetics. Wear long pants and boots, and carry for protection a long-sleeved shirt or jacket, gloves, a handkerchief to shield the face, water to wet it, and goggles.
3. Remove combustible items from around the house. This includes lawn and poolside furniture, umbrellas, and tarp coverings. If they catch fire, the added heat could ignite the house.
4. Close outside attic, eave, and basement vents. This will eliminate the possibility of sparks blowing into hidden areas within the house. Close window shutters.
5. Place large plastic trash cans or buckets around the outside of the house and fill them with water. Soak burlap sacks, small rugs, and large rags. They can be helpful in beating out burning embers or small fires. Inside the house, fill bathtubs, sinks, and other containers with water. Toilet tanks and water heaters are an important water reservoir.
6. Place garden hoses so that they will reach any place on the house. Use the spray gun–type nozzle, adjusted to spray.
7. If you have portable gasoline-powered pumps to take water from a swimming pool or tank, make sure they are operating and in place.
8. Place a ladder against the roof of the house opposite the side of the approaching fire. If you have a combustible roof, wet it down or turn on any roof sprinklers. Turn on any special fire sprinklers installed to add protection. Do not waste water. Waste can drain the entire water system quickly.
9. Back your car into the garage and roll up the car windows. Disconnect the automatic garage door opener (in case of power failure, you cannot remove the car). Close all garage doors.
10. Place valuable papers and mementoes inside the car in the garage for quick departure, if necessary. All pets still with you should also be put in the car.
11. Close windows and doors to the house to prevent sparks from blowing inside. Close all doors inside the house to prevent drafts. Open the damper on your fireplace to help stabilize outside-inside pressure, but close the fireplace screen so that sparks will not ignite the room. Turn on a light in each room to make the house more visible in heavy smoke.
12. Turn off pilot lights.
13. If you have time, take down drapes and curtains. Close all venetian blinds or noncombustible window coverings to reduce the amount of heat radiating into the house. This provides added safety in case the windows give way because of heat or wind.
14. As the fire front approaches, go inside the house. Stay calm; you are in control of the situation.
15. After the fire passes, check the roof immediately. Extinguish any sparks or embers. Then, check the attic for hidden burning sparks. If you have a fire, get your neighbors to help fight it. For several hours after the fire, recheck for smoke and sparks throughout the house.

Fire Shelters

The fire shelter described earlier was developed by the Missoula Technology Development Center to reduce the number of serious burn injuries and fatalities among firefighters who become trapped while fighting wildland fires. Shelters, designed in the shape of a pup tent, protect the firefighter by reflecting radiant heat. Constructed of an aluminum foil–fiberglass cloth laminate, the shelter reflects approximately 95% of the radiant heat emanating from a fire. The shelter is credited with saving more than 220 lives since its introduction in the 1960s.[31] The main reason that fire shelters work well was demonstrated dramatically on August 29, 1985, when 73 firefighters were forced to take refuge in their shelters for approximately 1½ hours while a severe crown fire burned over them.[23] The incident took place during the Butte fire in the Salmon National Forest in Idaho. Observers described the crown fire that overran the firefighters as a standing wall of flame that reached 61 m (200 feet) above the treetops. Within the shelters firefighters experienced extreme heat for as long as 10 minutes. Shelters were so hot that they could be handled only with gloves. After leaving the shelters, some firefighters showed symptoms of possible carbon monoxide poisoning, including vomiting, disorientation, and difficulty in breathing. Emergency medical technicians administered oxygen to several individuals before evacuation. Five firefighters were hospitalized overnight for heat exhaustion, smoke inhalation, and dehydration. The consensus of those interviewed was that without the shelters, none would have survived.

ENTRAPMENT PROCEDURES

People must recognize that in some instances there may be no chance to escape a fire. When entrapment is imminent, injuries or death may be avoided by following entrapment procedures:

1. Do not panic. It is natural for most people to be afraid when trapped by fire. Accept this fear as natural. Once this has been done, clear thinking and intelligent decisions are possible. If fear becomes overwhelming, judgment is seriously impaired and survival becomes a matter of chance.

2. Do not run blindly or needlessly. Unless the path of escape is clearly indicated, do not run. Move downhill and away from the flank of the fire at a 45-degree angle where possible. Conserve your strength.
3. Enter the burned area. Particularly in grass, low shrubs, or other low fuels, do not delay if escape means passing through the flame front into the burned area. Move aggressively and parallel to the advancing fire front. Choose a place on the edge of the fire where flames are less than 1 m (3 feet) deep and can be seen through clearly, and where the fuel supply behind the fire edge has been mostly consumed. After covering exposed skin and taking several breaths, move through the flame front as quickly as possible. If necessary, get on the ground to move underneath smoke for improved visibility and to obtain fresh air for the move into the burned area.
4. Burn out. If you are in dead grass or low shrub fuels and the approaching flames are too high to run through, burn out as large an area as possible between you and the fire edge. Step into the burned area and cover as much of your exposed skin as possible. This action requires time for fuels to burn out, and as a last-ditch effort it may not be effective. It also does not work well in an intense forest fire.
5. Regulate breathing. Avoid inhaling dense smoke. Keep your face on the ground where there is usually less smoke. A dampened handkerchief held over the nose will help. Regulate breathing to coincide with the availability of relatively fresh air. If there is a possibility of breathing superheated air, a dry, not moist, cloth should be placed over the mouth. The lungs are better able to withstand dry heat than moist heat.
6. Protect against radiation. Many people who become victims of forest fires actually die before the flames reach them. Radiated heat quickly causes heatstroke, a state of complete exhaustion. Shielding that will reduce the heat rays must be found quickly in an area that will not burn. This may be provided by a shallow trench, crevice, large rock, running stream, large pond, vehicle, building, or the shore water of a lake. Do not seek refuge in an elevated water tank. Wells and caves generally should be avoided because oxygen may be quickly used up in these restricted places. Such refuges might be used as a last resort (Fig. 9-21). For protection against radiation, cover the head and other exposed skin with clothing or dirt.
7. Lie prone. In a critical emergency, lie face down in an area that will not burn. A person's chance of survival is greater in this position than if overtaken by fire when standing upright or kneeling.

Arnold "Smoke" Elser, an accomplished Montana outfitter, described how he helped his guests avoid entrapment by a forest fire in this personal communication:

> The fire began at the bottom of the canyon and proceeded up canyon as fires do. However, the wind currents carried the smoke to the east and not up the drainage to the north; therefore, we received no warning of the fire. The Monture Creek trail goes through some very old mature timber which was not burning as we approached. As my stock, the guests, and I arrived at the fire site and realized that we were in danger, we felt we should fall back and try to flank the fire to the east. Starting back toward this trail, we found a ground fire that made it very hazardous to travel in this direction. Because of my knowledge of the trail and terrain, I knew that our best bet would be to wet down the stock, guests, saddles and outer clothing and try to break through the head of the fire. We successfully did this, receiving only a few minor burns on the horses and the loss of some apparel tied to the backs of the saddles. Some lessons that I learned in this experience were that in handling livestock in a fire situation you must have a very close, firm hand on them. It is also very important that no one panics or shows any excitement, as this alarms the livestock and begins the panic run that is so well known. I found that by talking in very low monotone, keeping the pack stock and saddle stock very close together (head to tail), and moving on a good trail, we were able to come through this fire with virtually no harm.

Elser had these additional suggestions for wildland recreationists:

> Campers, whether they be livestock oriented, hikers, or boaters, should know where to camp to provide adequate fire barriers around campsites. All campers should consider at least one, and preferably two, safe escape routes and havens (such as rock piles, rivers, and large green meadows) away from heavy fuel areas. Campers should be alert to canyon air current conditions in critical fire seasons. The safety of many recreationists is threatened by nylon and other synthetic fabrics used in the manufacture of most backpacking equipment. These materials melt upon contact with heat. The very nature of good horse packing equipment is a deterrent to fire; canvas mantles that cover the gear and the canvas pack saddles are easily wet down. Leather items such as chaps, good saddle bags, and western hats [that] can shield against heat blasts all provide important protection for the horse user.

PROPER CLOTHING

Clothing provides protection against radiant heat, embers, and sparks, so it is sensible to dress appropriately (Fig. 9-22). Closely woven material is more resistant to radiation and less likely to ignite than is open-weave material. Natural fibers are best. Wool is more flame resistant than cotton, although cotton can be improved by chemical treatment to retard flammability. It must be emphasized that synthetic materials are a poor choice to wear near fire because they readily absorb heat, ignite, or melt.

Because closely woven materials that provide protection also restrict airflow, clothes should fit loosely to not interfere with dissipation of body heat. The advantage of cotton long johns or undergarments is that they absorb sweat, aid evaporation, and do not melt, unlike synthetics. Wearing excessive layers of clothing generally contributes to heat stress problems.

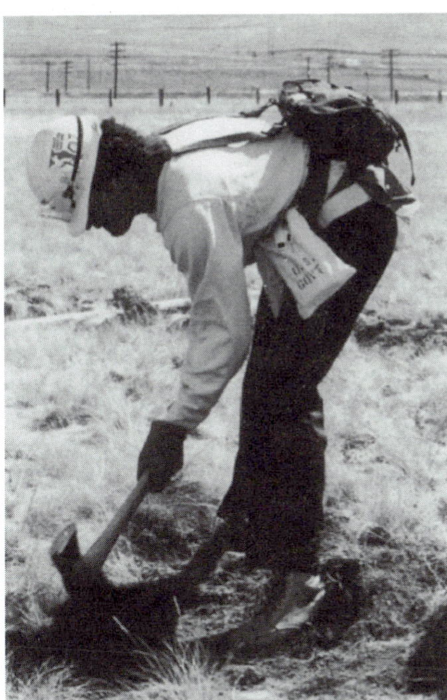

Fig. 9-22 Protective clothing for a firefighter includes hard hat and safety goggles, fire-resistant shirt and trousers, leather boots and gloves, and fire shelter carried in a waist pouch. Firefighters also carry canteens to ensure an adequate water supply in a heat-stressed environment. (Courtesy of the USDA Forest Service.)

As little skin as possible should be exposed to fire. Long trousers and a long-sleeved shirt should be worn. For maximum protection the shirt should be kept buttoned with sleeves rolled down.

Brightly colored (yellow or orange) coveralls or shirts are worn by organized firefighting crews. These colors improve safety and communications because they are visible in smoke, vegetation, and blackened landscapes.

Other essential apparel includes a safety helmet (hard hat), gloves (leather or natural fiber), leather work boots, woolen or cotton socks, a warm jacket for night wear, goggles, and a handkerchief. Clothing, backpacks, tents, and other camping equipment made of synthetics should be discarded when a person is close to a fire.

WATER INTAKE

Sweating, the primary method for body cooling, is an important physiologic function. Exhaling warm air and inhaling cooler air also helps to decrease body temperature. Because the cooling effect of sweat evaporation is essential for thermoregulation, it is important to replace fluids lost during strenuous work. In firefighting, water losses of 0.5 L/hr (1 pint/hr) are common, with losses of up to 2 L/hr (2 quarts/hr) under extreme conditions.[18] Unless water is restored regularly, dehydration may contribute to heat stress disorders, reluctance to work, irritability, poor judgment, and impatience.

The importance of dehydration cannot be overstressed. Thirst is not a good indicator of water requirements during strenuous work, so additional drinking of small quantities of water at regular intervals is recommended. A useful signal of dehydration is dark, scanty urine.

An excessive amount of electrolytes may be lost through sweating, which leads to nausea, vomiting, and muscle cramps. When meals are missed or unseasoned foods are eaten, electrolyte supplements may be necessary to replace lost salts. Sweetened drinks should be used as a source of energy if solid food is not available.

PERSONAL GEAR

Some rescue and medical missions take a few days. Therefore it is necessary to be prepared for extended periods and changing conditions in the backcountry (Box 9-4).

BOX 9-4

PERSONAL GEAR FOR RESCUE MISSIONS

1. Boots (leather, high-top, lace-up, nonslip soles, extra leather laces)
2. Socks (cotton or wool, at least two pairs)
3. Pants (natural fiber, flameproof, loose fitting, hems lower than boot tops)
4. Belt or suspenders
5. Shirt (natural fiber, flameproof, loose fitting, long sleeves)
6. Gloves (natural fiber or leather, extra pair)
7. Hat (hard hat and possibly a bandanna, stocking cap, or felt hat)
8. Jacket
9. Handkerchiefs or scarves
10. Goggles
11. Sleeping bag and ground cover
12. Map
13. Fire shelter
14. Food
15. Canteen
16. Radio (AM radio will receive better in rough terrain; FM is more line-of-sight; emergency personnel should have a two-way radio)
17. Bolt cutters (carried in vehicles to get through locked gates during escape from flare-ups or in the rescue of trapped people)
18. Miscellaneous items (mess kit, compass, flashlight, extra batteries, toilet paper, pencil, notepaper, flagging tape, flares, matches, can opener, wash cloth, toiletries, insect repellent, plastic bags, knife, first aid kit, and lip balm)

HOW TO REPORT A WILDLAND FIRE TO LOCAL FIRE PROTECTION AUTHORITIES

A caller should be prepared to provide the following information when reporting a fire:

1. Name of person giving the report
2. Where the person can be reached immediately
3. Where the person was at the time the fire was discovered
4. Location of the fire; is important to orient the fire to prominent landmarks such as roads, creeks, and mileposts on highways
5. Description of the fire: color and volume of the smoke, estimated size, and flame characteristics if visible
6. Whether anyone is fighting the fire at the time of the call

PORTABLE FIRE EXTINGUISHERS

People should know which extinguisher to select for a specific hazard in the home or recreational vehicle and be trained in its use. When a fire is discovered, the first step should be to evacuate occupants to safety and promptly report the fire to appropriate authorities. If the fire is small and poses no direct threat, an extinguisher should be used to fight it.

There are three major classes of fires. Class A fires are fueled by ordinary combustible materials such as wood, paper, cloth, upholstery, and many plastics. Class B fires are fueled by flammable liquids and gases such as kitchen greases, paints, oil, and gasoline. Class C fires are fueled by live electrical wires or equipment such as motors, power tools, and appliances. The right type of extinguisher must be used for each class of fire. Water extinguishers are used to control Class A fires by cooling and soaking burning materials. Carbon dioxide or dry chemical extinguishers are used to control Class B fires by smothering flames. Multipurpose dry chemical or liquefied gas extinguishers control Class A, B, or C fires by a smothering action. Liquefied gas extinguishers also produce a cooling effect. A dry chemical or liquefied gas extinguisher is recommended for recreational vehicles.

WILDFIRE FIGHTING TRAINING COURSE

"Wildfire Fighting," a self-contained 35 mm slide–audio cassette training program produced by the National Fire Protection Association, was designed to help paid and volunteer fire departments, forestry organizations, and individual volunteers prepare for such emergencies and carry out effective wildfire fighting operations. It includes useful information on prefire planning, mutual aid, logistical support, safety, fire ground organization, equipment and apparatus, and other topics essential for the safe and successful control of wildfires. The "Wildfire Fighting" program (NFPA Catalog Number SL-104; Harry Abraham, editor) can be ordered from the National Fire Protection Association, Batterymarch Park, Quincy, MA 02269.

Conclusions

Fire suppression efforts in the late 1800s and early 1900s were largely ineffective because of limited access, absence of trained firefighting organizations, and lack of a fire detection network. During these times many residents and numerous firefighters died in wildland fires in the United States and Canada. In the recent past, firefighters were more vulnerable to injuries and fatalities from wildland fires than was the general public. Today, with many people living and seeking recreation in wildlands, the odds for serious fire encounters are shifting toward an inexperienced populace. Large property losses and direct injuries are being reported in increasing numbers in the wildland-urban interface. Although wildland fires have not yet posed much of a threat to backcountry recreationists in the United States, the prospect for such confrontations is growing.

Experience with wildland fires allows us to conclude the following:

1. Residential shifts to the wildland-urban interface will increase exposures to life-threatening situations.
2. Prescribed fires in national parks and wildernesses will increase the likelihood that people will encounter fires.
3. The general public tends to underestimate existing fire hazards and is usually not experienced in avoiding fire threats.
4. In some instances, past fire exclusion practices have contributed to the development of more wildland fuel, setting the stage for greater rates of spread and higher intensity levels in some plant communities. The national ecosystem health issue has compounded this problem by producing vast expanses of dead and dying forests, increasing the threat to people from fast-moving, high-intensity fires.
5. Knowledge of fire behavior principles and survival rules will prepare people to take appropriate preventive measures in threatening situations.

The general public must share responsibility with suppression organizations to minimize fire hazards created by humans. Care with fire, proper cleanup of debris, and fuel reduction efforts on wildland property and the application of survival skills will minimize fire threats. Such precautions should become as commonplace in the wildland environment as smoke alarms and fire extinguishers have become in the home.

Wildland fire suppression agencies will continue to provide fast, safe, energetic initial attack responses to protect human life, property, and natural resources. Under conditions of prolonged drought, strong winds, low humidities, and high temperatures, some fires will escape even the best initial attack efforts, directly threatening human life and property. Emergency medical personnel will probably have increasing exposure to wildland fires and will need to know more about fire-related injuries, fire safety, and fire survival.

Acknowledgments

Line drawings on heat transfer and fire behavior are adapted from J.S. Barrows's *Fire Behavior in Northern Rocky Mountain Forests.* The booklet "Planning for Initial Attack" by the USDA Forest Service was a helpful reference on fire principles.

REFERENCES

1. Barrows JS: *Fire behavior in northern Rocky Mountain forests,* USDA Forest Service, Northern Rocky Mtn For and Range Exp Sta, Station 1951, Paper No 29.
2. Barrows JS: The challenges of forest fire management, *Western Wildlands* 1(3):3, 1974.
3. Brown AA, Davis P: *Forest fire: control and use,* ed 2, New York, 1973, McGraw-Hill.
4. California Department of Forestry: *Field operations guide (ICS-420-1),* Fire Protection Publications, Oklahoma State University, 1983.
5. Cheney NP: Don't panic—and live, *Nat Dev,* p 1, 1972.
6. Cheney NP: Personal communication, 1981.
7. Colorado State Forest Service: *Wildlife hazards: guidelines for their prevention in subdivisions and developments,* Ft Collins, 1977, Colorado State University.
8. Countryman CM: *Carbon monoxide: a firefighting problem,* USDA Forest Service, Pacific SW For and Range Exp Sta, 1971.
9. Fischer WC, Brooks DJ: Safeguarding Montana homes: lessons from the Pattee Canyon Fire, *Western Wildlands* 4(1):30, 1977.
10. Freedman JD: *A fire and fuel hazard analysis in the Seeley Lake area, Missoula County, Montana,* MA thesis, Missoula, 1980, University of Montana.
11. Freedman JD, Fischer WC: Forest home fire hazards, *Western Wildlands* 6(4):23, 1980.
12. Gleason P: LCES: the key to safe procedures, National Fire Protection Association, *Wildfire News and Notes* 5(2):1, 1991.
13. Gold A, Burgess WA, Clougherty EV: Exposure of firefighters to toxic air contaminants, *Am Ind Hyg Assoc J* 39:534, 1978.
14. Haines D: Downbursts and wildland fires: a dangerous combination, USDA Forest Service, *Fire Management Notes* 49(3):8, 1988.
15. Hulbert J: Fire problems in rural suburbs, *American Forests* 78(2):24, 1972.
16. Leopold AS et al: *Wildlife management in the national parks,* Trans American Wildlife and Natural Resources Conference 28:1, 1963.
17. Louks OL: Evolution of diversity, efficiency, and community stability, *Am Zool* 10:17, 1970.
18. Luke RH, McArthur AG: *Bushfires in Australia,* CSIRO Division of Forest Research, 1978, Australian Government Publishing Service.
19. McArthur AG, Cheney NP: *Report on Southern Tasmanian Bushfires of 7 February 1967,* Hobart, Australia, 1967, Government Printer.
20. Moritz AA et al: The effect of inhaled heat on the air passages and lungs, *Am J Pathol* 21:311, 1945.
21. Moylan JA: Smoke inhalation and burn injury, *Surg Clin North Am* 60:1533, 1980.
22. Moylan JA et al: Early diagnosis of inhalation injury using ^{133}xenon lung scan, *Ann Surg* 176:477, 1973.
23. Mutch RW, Rothermel RC: 73 fire fighters survive in shelters, *Fire Command* 53(3):30, 48, 1986.
24. Mutch RW: *Sustaining forest health to benefit people, property, and natural resources,* In Proceedings of the 1992 Society of American Foresters National Convention.
25. National Fire Protection Association: *Black Tiger fire case study,* Quincy, Mass, NFPA.
26. National Fire Protection Association: *Stephan Bridge Road fire case study,* Quincy, Mass, NFPA.
27. National Fire Protection Association: NFPA 299 *Protection of life and property from wildfire,* Quincy, Mass, 1991, NFPA.
28. National Fire Protection Association: The Oakland/Berkeley Hills fire, Quincy, Mass, NFPA.
29. National Fire Protection Association: *Wildland fire fatalities (1981-1990),* Quincy, Mass, 1991, NFPA.
30. Owen HR: *Fire and you,* Garden City, NY, 1977, Doubleday.
31. Putnam T: Your fire shelter: a facilitator discussion guide, Missoula Technology and Development Center, 1991, USDA Forest Service.
32. Radtke KWH: *A homeowner's guide to fire and watershed management at the chaparral-urban interface,* County of Los Angeles, Calif, 1982. (Available from Santa Monica Mountains Residents Association, 21656 Las Flores Hts Rd, Malibu, CA 90265; cost $0.50.)
33. Rothermel RC: *Predicting behavior and size of crown fires in the northern Rocky Mountains,* Research Paper INT-438, 1991, USDA Forest Service.
34. Rothermel RC: *Mann Gulch fire: a race that couldn't be won,* General Technical Report INT-299, 1993, USDA Forest Service.
35. Rothman N et al: Pulmonary function and respiratory symptoms in wildland firefighters, *Occup Med* 33(11):1163, 1991.
36. Schroeder JJ, Buck CC: Fire weather, Agr Handbook 360, 1970, USDA Forest Service.
37. Sharkey BJ: *Heat stress,* Missoula, Mont, 1979, USDA Forest Service, Missoula Equipment Development Center.
38. Smith A et al: Report of U.S.-Canadian task force study of fatal and near-fatal fire accidents, National Wildfire Coordinating Group, 1981 (unpublished report).
39. Smith E, Adams G: *Incline Village/Crystal Bay defensible space handbook,* Reno, Nev, 1991, University of Nevada Reno.
40. Stone JP et al: The transport of hydrogen chloride by soot from burning polyvinyl chloride, *J Fire Flammability* 4:42, 1973.
41. Tietz JG: *Firefighters' exposure to carbon monoxide on the Deadline and Outlaw fires,* Ed T 2424 (Smoke Inhalation Hazards), Missoula, Mont, 1975, USDA Forest Service, Equipment Development Center.
42. Tischendorf JW: Structural watch out situations for the wildland/urban interface. *Wildfire News and Notes* 5(3), National Fire Protection Association.
43. Tokle GO, Marker J: Wildfire strikes home! In Laughlin J, Page C, editors: *Report of the National Wildland/Urban Fire Protection Conference,* 1987.
44. Ward D: *Air toxics and fireline exposure,* Paper presented at 10th Conference on Fire and Forest Meteorology, Ottawa, Canada, 1989.
45. Ward D et al: The effects of forest fire smoke in firefighters: a comprehensive study plan. A special report for Congressional Committee of Appropriations for Title II—Related Agencies, USDA Forest Service and National Wildfire Coordinating Group, 1989.
46. Webster J: *The complete Australian bushfire book,* Melbourne, Australia, 1986, Thomas Nelson.
47. Wilson CC: Commingling of urban forest fires (a case study of the 1970 California near-disaster), *Fire Res Abs Rev* 13(1):35, 1971.
48. Wilson CC: Fatal and near-fatal forest fires, the common denominators, *Int Fire Chief* 43(9):9, 1977.
49. Wroblewski DA, Bower GC: The significance of facial burns in acute smoke inhalation, *Crit Care Med* 7:335, 1979.
50. Zapp JA: Fires, toxicity and plastics. In *Physiological and toxicological products,* 1976, Committee on Fire Research, National Research Council, National Academy of Sciences.
51. Zikria BA et al: Respiratory tract damage in burns: pathophysiology and treatment, *Ann NY Acad Sci* 150:618, 1968.

ADDITIONAL RECOMMENDED READINGS

Cohen S, Miller D: *The big burn,* Missoula, Mont, 1978, Pictorial Histories. (The Northwest's forest fire of 1910.)

Cottrell WH: *The book of fire,* Missoula, Mont, 1989, Mountain Press.

Gaylor HP: *Wildfires: prevention and control,* Bowie, Md, 1974, RJ Brady.

Pringle L: *Natural fire: its ecology in forests,* New York, 1979, William Morrow.

Radtke K: *Living more safely at the chaparral-urban interface.* USDA Forest Service and County of Los Angeles Dept of Forestry and Fire Warden, Pacific Southwest Forest and Range Exp Sta, 1981.

Webster J: *The complete Australian bushfire book,* 1986, Thomas Nelson.

10 EMERGENCY CARE OF THE BURNED PATIENT

Roberta Mann
David M. Heimbach

Epidemiology

Each year in the United States approximately 2 million individuals are burned seriously enough to seek the care of a physician, and about 70,000 of these require hospitalization. Fortunately, the number of deaths attributable to burns decreased from 12,000 in 1979 to 6000 in 1990. Although treatment facilities would like to take credit for this decrease, the most likely factor responsible is the widespread use of smoke detectors in both public and private dwellings. It has been estimated that more than 90% of burns are preventable and that most are caused by carelessness or ignorance. During the next few years the biggest contributions in decreasing burn mortality and morbidity may come not from medical scientists, but rather from improved engineering design and more successful programs in teaching burn prevention to the public.

Like other forms of trauma, burns frequently affect children and young adults. The hospital expenses and the social costs related to time away from work or school are staggering. Although most burns are limited in extent, a significant burn of the hand or foot may prevent a manual laborer from working for a year or more and in some cases may forever prevent a return to former activity. The eventual outcome for the burned patient is related to the severity of the injury, individual physical characteristics of the patient, motivation toward rehabilitation, and the quality of treatment of the acute burn.

Most persons with burns who are seen by physicians visit emergency departments, where judgment in triage, care plan for small burns, and initial management for major burns can influence survival of the patient and eventual cosmetic and functional results. Because most patients are young and about one third are children, they will live with the consequences of the acute treatment for an average of 50 years.

The decisions made at the initial contact with the patient require answers to the algorithm shown in Fig. 10-1. This chapter describes first responder care for major burns and is organized to guide assessment of burn severity and initial management of the serious burn, as well as to provide an initial treatment plan for minor burns.

Physiology

For burns other than chemical burns the primary events of injury occur during the time of heat contact. Coagulation necrosis takes place within cells and denaturation of collagen occurs in the dermis. Either blood vessels are completely destroyed or the endothelium is damaged severely enough to cause clotting, which leads to ischemic necrosis of remaining viable cells. The burn wound is not static. Surrounding the "zone of coagulation" is a zone of capillary and small vessel stasis. Red cells form into rouleaux, platelet and white cell aggregates form, and the circulation becomes stagnant. Over the next hours or even days the ultimate fate of the burn wound depends on the resolution or progression of this zone of stasis. Cells and tissue stroma release mediators to initiate the inflammatory response. Histamine, serotonin, prostaglandin derivatives, and the complement cascade all have roles. In patients with burns of less than 10% of the total body surface area (TBSA), the actions of these mediators are generally limited to the burn site itself. Capillary permeability increases, neutrophils marginate, and additional inflammatory cells (monocytes, macrophages) are attracted by chemotaxis to the site of injury, initiating the healing process.

As burns approach 20% TBSA, the local response becomes systemic. The capillary leak, permitting loss of fluid and protein from the intravascular compartment into the ex-

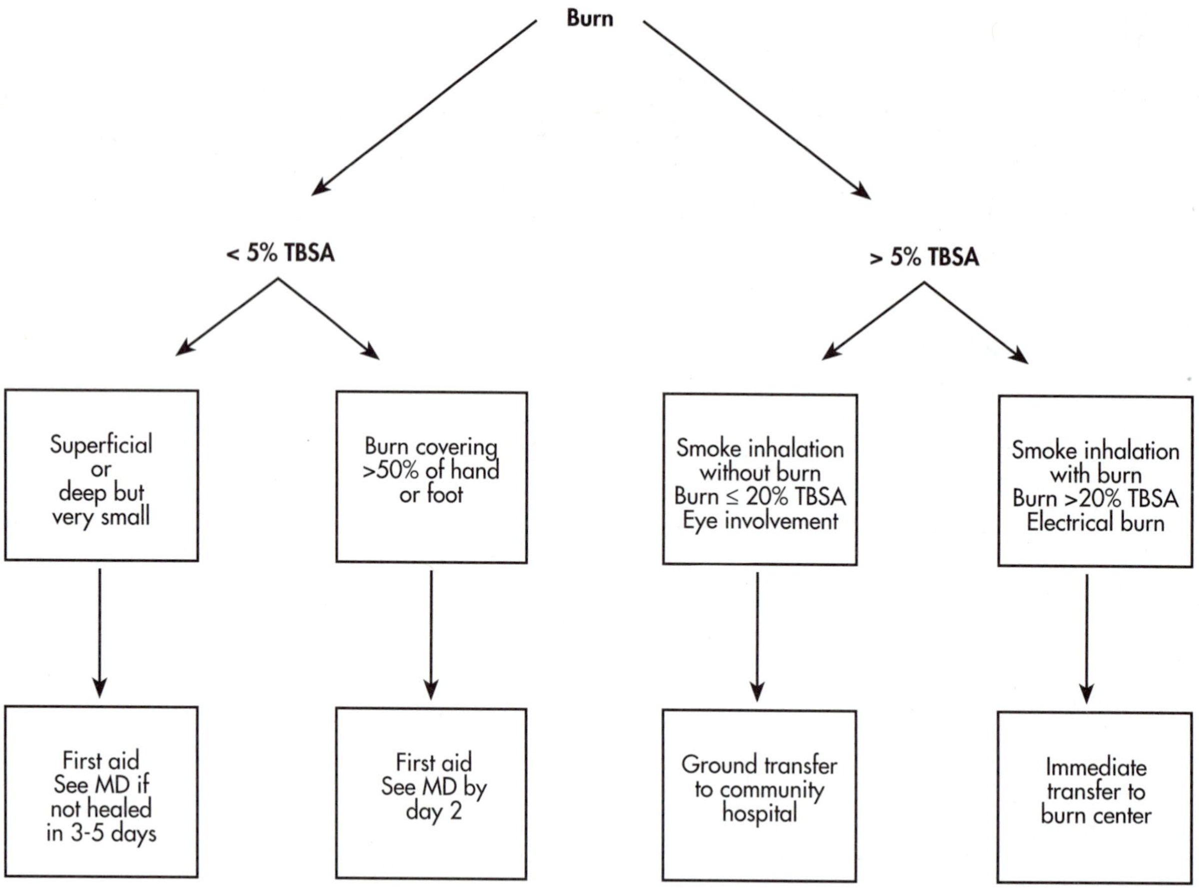

Fig. 10-1 Algorithm for decision making at the scene.

travascular compartment, becomes generalized. Cardiac output falls as a result of marked increased peripheral resistance, decreased intravascular fluid volume from the capillary leak, and the accompanying increase in blood viscosity. The decreased blood volume and cardiac output, accompanied by an intense sympathetic response, lead to decreased perfusion to the skin and viscera. Decreased flow to the skin can convert the zone of stasis to one of coagulation, increasing the depth of the burn. The capillary leak and depressed cardiac output lead to depressed central nervous system (CNS) function, and in extreme cases they result in severe cardiac depression with eventual cardiac failure in healthy patients or in myocardial infarction in patients with preexisting coronary artery disease. The first sign of CNS change is restlessness, followed by lethargy and finally coma. Without adequate resuscitation, burns of 30% TBSA frequently lead to acute renal failure, which in a patient with a severe burn almost invariably leads to a fatal outcome.

Cardiovascular changes begin immediately after a burn. The extent of these changes depends primarily on the size of the burn and to a lesser extent on the depth of burn. Most patients with uncomplicated burns of less than 15% TBSA can undergo oral fluid resuscitation with some salt-containing solution. As the burn extent passes 20% TBSA, massive shifts of fluid and electrolytes occur from the intravascular into the extravascular (extracellular) space. Reversal of the shifts begins during the second postburn day, but normal extracellular volume is not completely restored until 7 to 10 days after the burn. Unless the intravascular volume is repleted, classic hypovolemic shock occurs. An untreated person will die of cardiovascular collapse; if treatment is poor, irreversible acute tubular necrosis and renal failure will develop.

Types of Burns

SCALD BURNS

In civilian practice, scalds, usually resulting from hot water, are the most common cause of burns. Water at 140° F creates a deep partial-thickness or full-thickness burn in 3 seconds. At 156° F the same burn occurs in 1 second. Freshly brewed coffee from an automatic percolator is generally about 180° F. Boiling water always causes deep burns, and soups and sauces, which are thicker in consistency, remain in contact longer with the skin and often cause deep burns. In general, exposed areas tend to be burned less deeply than areas covered with thin clothing. Clothing retains the heat and keeps the liquid in contact with the skin for a longer time.

Immersion scalds are deep and severe burns.[21,31,97] Although the water may be cooler than with a spill scald, the duration of contact is longer and these burns frequently occur in small children or elderly patients with thin skin. Consequently, many states have passed legislation to set home and public hot water heaters to maximum temperatures well below 140° F.

Scald burns from grease or hot oil are generally deep partial thickness or full thickness. Cooking oil and grease, when hot enough to use for cooking, may be in the range of 400° F. Tar and asphalt burns are a special kind of scald. The "mother pot" at the back of the roofing truck maintains tar at a temperature of 400° to 500° F. Burns caused by tar directly from the mother pot are invariably full thickness. By the time the tar is spread on the roof, its temperature has decreased enough that most of the burns are deep partial thickness. Unfortunately, the initial evaluator cannot usually examine these burns because of the adherent tar. The tar should be removed by application of a petroleum-based ointment (such as Vaseline) under a dressing. The dressing may be removed and the ointment reapplied every 2 to 4 hours until the tar has dissolved. Only then can the extent of the injury and the depth of the burn be accurately estimated.[43,96]

FLAME BURNS

Flame burns are the next most common burn injuries. Although injuries in house fires have decreased with the advent of smoke detectors, a significant number of burn injuries still result from careless smoking, improper use of flammable liquids, automobile accidents, and clothing ignited from stoves or space heaters. Patients whose bedding or clothes have been on fire rarely escape without some full-thickness burns. Outdoor misadventures result from using cooking stoves fueled by white gasoline, taking lanterns into tents, smoking in a sleeping bag, and starting (or improving) charcoal fires with gasoline or kerosene.

FLASH BURNS

Flash burns are next in frequency. Explosions of natural gas, propane, gasoline, and other flammable liquids cause intense heat for a very brief time. For the most part, unignited clothing protects the skin in flash burns. Flash burns generally have a distribution over all exposed skin, with the deepest areas facing the source of ignition. Flash burns are partial thickness, with the depth dependent on the amount and kind of fuel that explodes. Although such burns generally heal without requiring extensive skin grafts, they may be very large and associated with significant thermal damage to the upper airway.

CONTACT BURNS

Contact burns result from hot metals, plastic, glass, or hot coals. Such burns are usually limited in extent but deep. Patients involved in industrial accidents commonly have both severe contact burns and crush injuries, since these accidents often occur from presses or from hot, heavy objects. With the increased use of wood-burning stoves, an increasing number of toddlers are burned each year. Their most common injuries are deep burns on the palms because the child falls with hands outstretched against the stove. Contact burns, especially in unconscious persons or those dealing with molten materials, are frequently fourth degree.[19,56,84] In the wilderness setting the most common contact burn is from hot coals. Intoxicated campers dance around and then into the campfire, architects of "river saunas" mishandle hot rocks, children fall into fires, and beach walkers may sustain deep burns when coals are buried in sand overnight. Even though the injured areas may be small, they can be deep and devastating when the hiker must walk a considerable distance on burned feet.[27]

ELECTRICAL BURNS

Electrical burns are actually thermal burns from very high-intensity heat. As electricity meets the resistance of body tissues, it is converted to heat in direct proportion to the amperage of the current and the electrical resistance of the body parts through which it passes. The smaller the body part through which the electricity passes, the more intense the heat and the less it is dissipated. Therefore fingers, hands, forearms, feet, and lower legs are frequently totally destroyed, whereas larger volume areas like the trunk usually dissipate the current enough to prevent extensive damage to the viscera, unless the contact point is on the abdomen or chest. Although cutaneous manifestations may appear limited, massive underlying tissue destruction may be present.[18,36,37,68]

Arc burns occur when current takes the most direct path rather than the one of least resistance. These deep and destructive wounds occur at joints that are in close apposition at the time of injury. Most common are burns of the forearm to the arm when the elbow is flexed and from the arm to the axilla if the shoulder is adducted when current passes from the upper extremity to the trunk.

Electrical burns cause a particular set of other injuries and complications that must be considered during the initial evaluation. As mentioned previously, injuries related to a fall are common. The intense associated muscle contractions may cause fractures of the lumbar vertebrae, humerus, or femur and may dislocate shoulders or hips.

Electrical cardiac damage may have symptoms like those of a myocardial contusion or infarction. Alternatively, the conduction system may be deranged. There can be actual rupture of the heart wall or of a papillary muscle leading to sudden valvular incompetence and refractory cardiac failure. Household current at 110 volts generally either does no damage or induces ventricular fibrillation. Alternating current is more likely to induce fibrillation than is direct current. If no cardiac abnormalities are present when a patient is first seen following shocks of 110 to 220 volts, the likelihood that they will appear later is small.

The nervous system is particularly sensitive to electricity. The most severe brain damage occurs when current passes through the head, but spinal cord damage is possible anytime current passes from one side of the body to the other.[47,51] Myelin-producing cells are susceptible. The devastating effects of transverse myelitis may develop days or weeks following injury. Conduction remains normal through existing myelin, but as the old myelin wears out, it is not replaced and conduction stops. Peripheral nerves are commonly damaged and may demonstrate severe permanent functional impairment.[23,33] Every patient with an electrical injury must have a thorough neurologic examination as part of the initial assessment. Myoglobinuria is a frequent accompaniment of severe electrical burns. Disruption of muscle cells releases cell fragments and myoglobin into the circulation to be filtered by the kidney. If untreated, this can lead to permanent renal failure.

Lightning strikes are discussed in Chapter 11. Several recent reviews are available.*

CHEMICAL BURNS

Chemical burns, usually caused by strong acids or alkalis are most often the result of industrial accidents, home use of drain cleaners, assaults, and other improper use of harsh solvents.† In contrast to thermal burns, chemical burns cause progressive damage until the chemicals are inactivated by reaction with the tissue or dilution by flushing with water. Although individual circumstances vary, acid burns may be more self-limiting than are alkali burns. Acid tends to "tan" the skin, creating an impermeable barrier that limits further penetration of the acid. Alkalis combine with cutaneous lipids and saponify the skin until they are neutralized. A full-thickness chemical burn may appear deceptively superficial, appearing as only a mild brownish surface discoloration. The skin may appear intact during the first few days after the burn, and then begin to slough spontaneously. Unless the observer can be absolutely certain, chemical burns should be considered deep partial thickness or full thickness until proven otherwise.

*References 24, 25, 28, 29, 57, 68.

†References 26, 38, 62, 64, 76, 79, 86.

Clinical Presentation

Cutaneous burns are caused by the application of heat or caustic chemicals to the skin. When heat is applied to the skin, the depth of injury is proportional to the temperature applied, the duration of contact, and the thickness of the skin.

The severity of the burn injury is related to the size of the burn, the depth of the burn, and the part of the body that is burned.

ESTIMATION OF BURN SIZE

Burns are the only quantifiable form of trauma. The single most important feature in predicting mortality, need for specialized care, and the complications expected from the burn is the overall burn size in proportion to the patient's total body surface. Treatment plans, including initial resuscitation and subsequent nutritional requirements, are derived directly from the size of the burn.

A general idea of burn size is provided by the "rule of nines." Each upper extremity accounts for 9% of TBSA; each lower extremity accounts for 18%; the anterior and posterior trunk each account for 18%; the head and neck account for 9%; and the perineum accounts for 1% (Fig. 10-2). While the "rule of nines" provides a reasonably accurate estimate of burn size, a number of more precise charts have been developed. A diagram of the burn can be drawn on a chart, so that a relatively precise calculation of burned area can be made from the accompanying total body surface area estimates given. Children under 4 years of age have much larger heads and smaller thighs in proportion to body size than do adults. In an infant the head accounts for nearly 20% of the TBSA; body proportions do not fully reach adult percentages until adolescence. To further increase accuracy in burn size estimation, especially when burns are in scattered body areas, the observer might calculate the unburned areas on a separate diagram. If the calculations of the unburned areas and the burned areas do not add up to 100%, the observer should begin again with a new diagram to calculate the burned areas. For smaller burns an accurate assessment of burn size can be made by using the patient's hand. The hand amounts to 2.5% TBSA. The dorsal surface accounts for 1%, the palmar surface for 1%, and the vertical surface for 0.5%.

DEPTH OF BURN

An understanding of burn depth requires an understanding of skin anatomy (Fig. 10-3). The epidermis, an intensely active layer of epithelial cells under layers of dead kera-

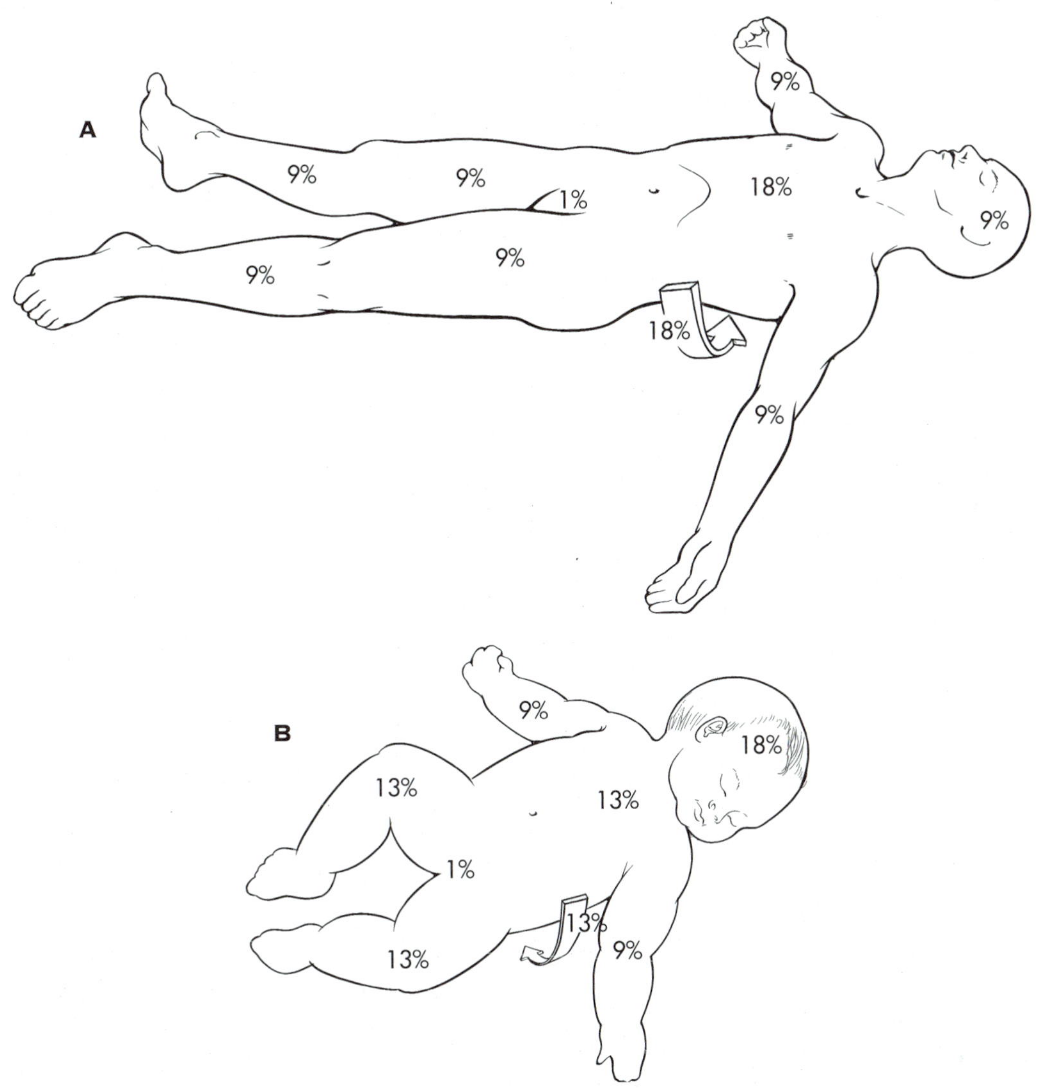

Fig. 10-2 Rule of nines used for estimating burned surface area. **A,** Adult. **B,** Infant.

tinized cells, is superficial to the active structural framework of the skin, the dermis. Although metabolically very active, the dermis has no regenerative capacity, and epithelial cells must eventually cover the surface of the dermis before the burn is healed. The skin appendages (hair follicles, sebaceous glands, and sweat glands) all contain an epithelial cell lining, so when the surface epidermis has been killed, epithelial covering must take place from overgrowth of the epithelial cells lining the skin appendages. As these cells reach the surface, they spread laterally to meet their neighbors, creating a new epithelial surface. As the burn extends deeper into the dermis, fewer and fewer appendages remain, and the epithelial remnants must travel farther to produce a new surface covering, sometimes taking many weeks to produce coverage. When the burn extends beyond the deepest layer of the skin appendages, the wound can heal only by epithelial ingrowth from the edges, by wound contraction, or by surgical transplantation of skin from a different site. The thickness of skin varies both with the age and sex of the individual and with the part of the body considered. While the thickness of the living epidermis is relatively constant, keratinized epidermal cells may reach a height of 5 mm on palms of hands and soles of feet. The thickness of the dermis, on the other hand, may vary from less than 1 mm on eyelids and genitalia to more than 5 mm on the posterior trunk. Although the proportional thickness of skin in each body area is similar in children, infant skin thickness in each specific area may be less than half that of adult skin; the skin does not reach adult thickness until adolescence. Similarly, in patients over 50 years of age, dermal atrophy causes all areas of skin to become quite thin.

Burns are classified by increasing depth as first degree, superficial partial thickness, deep partial thickness, full thickness, and fourth degree.

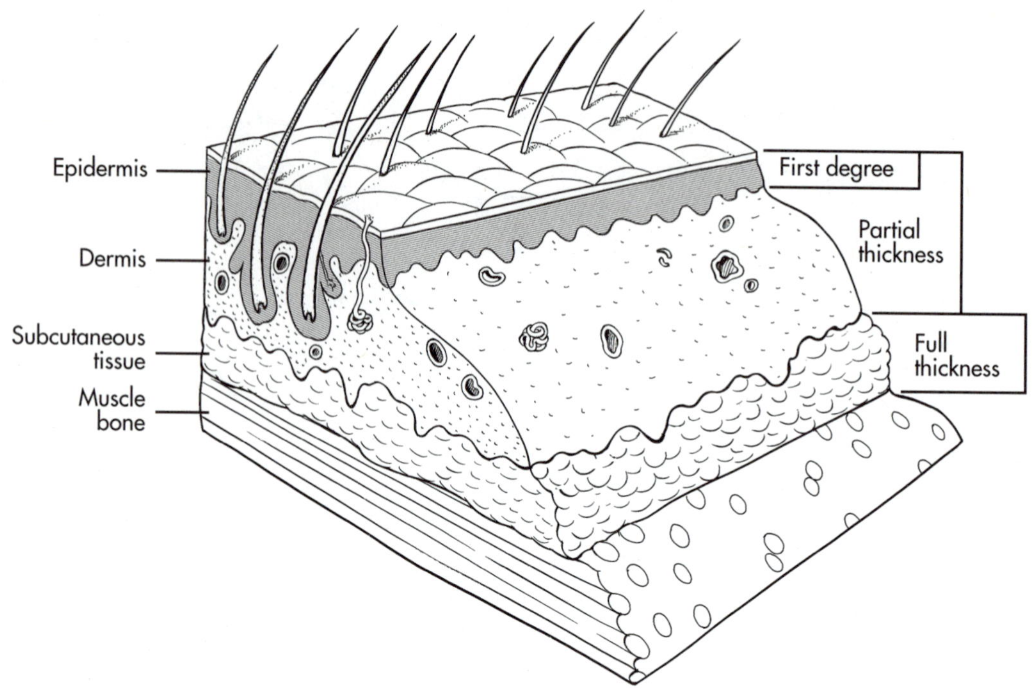

Fig. 10-3 Skin anatomy.

First-Degree Burns

First-degree burns involve only the epidermis. The prototype is mild sunburn. First-degree burns do not blister. They become erythematous because of dermal vasodilation and are quite painful, both spontaneously and when touched. Over 2 to 3 days the erythema and pain subside. By the fourth day the injured epithelium desquamates in the phenomenon of "peeling."

Superficial Partial-Thickness Burns

Superficial partial-thickness burns include the upper layers of dermis and characteristically form blisters with fluid collection at the interface of the epidermis and dermis. Blistering may not occur for some hours following injury. Burns initially thought to be first degree may therefore be diagnosed as superficial partial thickness by day 2. When blisters are removed, the wound is pink and wet and it is quite painful as currents of air contact it. The wound is hypersensitive to touch and blanches with pressure, and blood flow to the dermis is increased over that of normal skin. If infection is prevented, superficial partial-thickness burns heal spontaneously within 3 weeks without functional impairment. They rarely cause hypertrophic scarring, but in pigmented individuals the healed burns may never completely match the color of the surrounding normal skin.

Deep Partial-Thickness Burns

Deep partial-thickness burns also blister, but the wound surface is usually a mottled pink and white color immediately following the injury. The patient complains of discomfort rather than pain. When pressure is applied to the burn, capillary refill returns slowly or may be absent. The wound is often less sensitive to touch than is the surrounding normal skin. By the second day the wound may be white and is usually fairly dry. If infection is prevented, such burns heal in 3 to 9 weeks, but invariably do so with considerable scar formation. Unless active physical therapy is continued throughout the healing process, joint function may be impaired and hypertrophic scarring, particularly in pigmented individuals and children, becomes inevitable.

Full-Thickness Burns

Full-thickness burns involve all layers of the dermis and can heal only by wound contracture, epithelialization from the wound margin, or skin grafting. Full-thickness burns are classically described as leathery, firm, depressed when compared with adjoining normal skin, and insensitive to light touch or pinprick. Unfortunately, the difference in depth between a deep partial-thickness burn and a full-thickness burn may be less than 1 mm. Full-thickness burns are easily misdiagnosed as deep partial-thickness burns since the two types have many of the same clinical findings. For example, they may be mottled in appearance. They rarely blanch with pressure, and they may have a dry, white appearance. The burn may be translucent with clotted vessels visible in the depths. Some full-thickness burns, particularly immersion scalds, have a red appearance and can be confused with superficial partial-thickness burns by the uninitiated. However, these red, full-thickness burns do not blanch with pressure. Full-thickness burns develop a classic burn eschar. An eschar represents the structurally intact but dead and denatured dermis that, over days to weeks, separates spontaneously from the underlying viable tissue.

Fourth-Degree Burns

Fourth-degree burns involve not only all layers of the skin but also subcutaneous fat and deeper structures. These burns almost always have a charred appearance, and frequently only the cause of the burn gives a clue to the amount of underlying tissue destruction.

While these descriptions appear to separate burns into clearly defined categories, many burns have a mixture of characteristics that give the observer an imprecise diagnostic ability. Considerable research is under way to devise instruments that will more precisely measure the depth of injury. Much of current burn treatment depends on knowledge of the depth of the burn.

Treatment

CARE AT THE SCENE

Flame Burns

The first responder must remove the injured person from the source of heat. Because of the potential dangers of smoke inhalation in closed areas, the rescuer in a fire must take extreme caution not to become a victim. Persons with burning clothing should be prevented from running and should be made to lie down to keep flames and smoke away from the face. If water is not immediately available, the flames can be smothered with a coat or blanket. If nothing is available, the victim should be rolled slowly on the ground. Once the burning has stopped, the clothes should be removed. Unless all burned clothing is removed, some fabrics will continue to smolder and synthetic fabrics may melt, leaving a hot adherent residue on the victim that will continue the burning process.

Scalds and Grease Burns

The victim of a scald or grease burn must be removed from the source of heat. Any wet clothing or wrap should be removed, since fabric retains moist heat and may continue to burn skin that is in contact with the hot material. Accidents resulting from cooking indoors with grease are particularly hazardous. The startle response to a grease splatter may cause the victim to drop a pan of grease onto the fire, starting a kitchen fire that can rapidly become a dwelling fire.

Airway

Once flames are extinguished, primary attention must be directed to the airway. Any person rescued from a closed space or involved in a smoky fire should be considered at risk for smoke inhalation injury. If compressed oxygen is not available and the patient is coughing independently, he or she should be encouraged to continue to do so. If the victim is unconscious or the airway status is in question, the patient should be placed supine and the airway manipulated manually via the chin lift or jaw thrust maneuver. When possible, 100% oxygen should be administered by tight-fitting mask if smoke inhalation is suspected. If the patient is unconscious and if personnel are trained to insert an endotracheal tube, such a tube should be passed and attached to a source of 100% oxygen. If the airway has to be supported by a tight mask, the rescuers must be aware of the significant danger of aspiration of gastric contents. Air forced into the stomach distends it and causes vomiting. The mask prevents expulsion of the fluid, and the patient rapidly aspirates vomitus into the tracheobronchial tree. No unconscious supine patient should ever be left unattended.

Other Injuries and Transport

Once an airway is secured, the first responder should quickly assess the patient for other injuries and then transport him or her to the nearest hospital.[9,23,68] Patients should be kept flat and warm and should be given nothing by mouth. Aside from establishment of an airway, further resuscitation is unnecessary if the patient will arrive at a hospital within 30 minutes. For transport the patient should be wrapped in a clean, dry sheet and blanket. Sterility is not required.

Cold Application

Smaller burns, particularly scalds, may be treated with immediate application of cool water in hopes of limiting the extent of injury. The application of cold water is controversial, but immediate cooling does decrease the pain, possibly by a decrease in thromboxane production. By the time several minutes have passed, or after arrival in the emergency department, further cooling is not likely to alter the pathologic process. Ice water should not be used except on the smallest burns. Using ice on larger burns can easily induce systemic hypothermia and associated cutaneous vasoconstriction that can extend the thermal damage.

Swelling

During transport, constricting clothing and jewelry should be removed from burned and distal parts, since local swelling begins almost immediately. Constricting objects increase the swelling, and the removal of tight jewelry in the presence of distal edema is time consuming once swelling has occurred.

Electrical Burns

Electrical burns are particularly dangerous, both to the victim and to the rescuer. If the patient remains in contact with the source of electricity, the rescuer must avoid touching the victim until the current can be turned off or the wires cut with properly insulated wire cutters. Once the victim is removed from the source of current, airway, breathing, and circulation must be checked. Ventricular fibrillation or standstill is a common accompaniment to a major transthoracic current; cardiopulmonary resuscitation should be instituted if carotid or femoral pulses are not palpable. If pulses are present but the patient is apneic, mouth-to-mouth resuscitation alone may be lifesaving. Cardiopulmonary resuscitation should continue until a cardiac monitor can be obtained, which will direct treatment with epinephrine for cardiac standstill or defibrillation for ventricular fibrillation. Once an airway is established and pulses return, a careful search must be made for associated life-threatening injuries. Electrocuted patients frequently fall from heights and may have serious head or neck injuries. The intense tetanic muscle contractions associated with electrocution may fracture vertebrae or cause major joint dislocations. Patients with high-voltage electrical injuries should be treated with spinal precautions, and if necessary splints, until fractures can be ruled out.

Chemical Burns

Whenever possible, chemical burns should be thoroughly flushed with copious amounts of water at the scene of the accident. Chemicals will continue to burn until removed; washing for 5 to 10 minutes under a stream of running water may limit the overall severity of the burn. No thought should be given to searching for a specific neutralizing agent. Delay deepens the burn, and neutralizing agents may cause burns themselves; they frequently generate heat while neutralizing the offending agent, adding a thermal burn to the already potentially serious chemical burn.

First Aid at the Scene for Smaller Burns

Not all burns need immediate medical attention. Burns less than 5% TBSA (excluding deep burns of face, hands, feet, perineum, or circumferential extremity) can be treated successfully in a wilderness setting if adequate first aid supplies are available and wound care is performed diligently. Except for the very shallow burn that heals within a few days, most burns should be seen by a physician within 3 to 5 days after injury.

Burns should be washed thoroughly with plain soap and water and dried with a clean towel. Any obviously dead skin should be peeled off (which may be painful) or trimmed with sharp manicure scissors (usually painless). Large (greater than 2.5 cm), thin, fluid-filled blisters should be drained and the dead skin trimmed away. Small, thick blisters may be left intact. If any blister begins to leak fluid, it should be drained and trimmed to prevent a potential closed-space infection. Deep burns, as from a flame, are firm and leathery and do not require immediate debridement. A small tube of silver sulfadiazine cream and tubes of antibiotic (such as bacitracin) ointment should be available in the first aid kit. Either may be used and should be spread lightly over the wound. The wound may then be wrapped in dry, clean gauze, which does not have to be sterile. Simple dressings (one type of topical cream, plain gauze) are sufficient. Some patients prefer nonadherent dressings such as Telfa because they are less likely to stick to the wound during dressing changes. The same effect can be achieved by soaking (with water) a plain gauze dressing that appears stuck to the wound, waiting a few minutes, and then removing the dressing with additional water if necessary. Other dressings are available (antibiotic-impregnated silicone gel sheets, calcium alginate). Although patients may prefer one dressing over another for various reasons, no dressing has been shown conclusively to accelerate the healing of burn wounds. The first aid kit should be stocked with general use supplies; soaps and dressings designed specifically for burns are expensive and unnecessary.

Mobility of the wound area must be actively maintained, and concentrated efforts should be made to avoid dependent positioning, especially when the patient is resting or sleeping. Focal edema in a small burn wound can be painful and alarming and should be prevented with extremity elevation and active range-of-motion exercises several times a day. Wound care should be performed once a day if the dressing remains dry. A wet, sticky dressing needs more frequent wound care. If only the outer dressing is dirty, it may be changed as needed. For the quickest healing of superficial burns, daily wound care should remove all exudate and crust, both of which significantly retard wound healing. Items for the first aid kit include plain (not perfumed) soap, sharp scissors (large and small), small tube of silver sulfadiazine, tube(s) of bacitracin ointment, cotton gauze, Band-Aids, tape, and acetaminophen.

EMERGENCY DEPARTMENT CARE

The primary rule for the emergency physician is to "forget about the burn." Although a burn is usually readily apparent and often a dramatic injury, a careful search for other life-threatening injuries must take priority. Only after an overall assessment of the patient's condition should attention be directed to the specific problem of the burns. Assessment of the non–thermally injured patient is presented in Chapter 13; the following sections consider the specific problems encountered in the patient with burns.

RESUSCITATION

During the past 30 years more than a dozen resuscitation plans have been suggested. The goal of all resuscitation plans is to complete treatment with a living patient who has normally functioning kidneys and does not have cardiac failure or pulmonary edema. Nearly all of these plans use a combination of colloid and crystalloid solutions, but they vary considerably in the ratio of colloid to crystalloid, the timing of colloid administration, the sodium concentration of crystalloid solution, and to a much lesser extent in the total volume of fluid given.* Some require frequent changing of solutions, others require mixing of solutions, and some require careful monitoring of the patient's electrolytes. Intense controversy rages over the "best" resuscitation plan. The controversy, however, need not concern the physician without a special interest in burn physiology. There is general agreement on a few facts. A patient with very large burns will probably need both colloid and crystalloid. Initially, capillaries are permeable to both crystalloid and colloid solutions. The capillary leak to albumin and other large molecules repairs itself between the 6th and 24th hours.

The choice of formulas for initial resuscitation is probably of relatively little consequence as long as the rate of fluid administration is modified according to the patient's changing requirements as the hours pass. Because of its simplicity, ease of administration, and need for little blood chemistry monitoring, the formula developed by Baxter, known as the Baxter or Parkland formula, has been adopted by most hospitals and has been recommended officially by the American College of Surgeons Committee on Trauma.

According to the Baxter formula, crystalloid is given during the first 24 hours while the capillaries are still permeable to albumin and then colloid is given during the second 24 hours when the capillary leak has presumably sealed. Rapid administration of crystalloid solution results in early expansion of depleted plasma volume, which will return cardiac output toward normal. Once the capillary leak has sealed, colloid (usually in the form of albumin) remains the most effective solution to maintain plasma volume without further increasing edema. The Baxter formula was derived to provide specific replacement of known deficits measured by simultaneous determinations of red blood cell volume, plasma volume, extracellular fluid volume, and cardiac output during burn shock.

The first 24-hour and second 24-hour calculations are shown in Box 10-1. The formula calls for the administration of lactated Ringer's solution, 4 ml/kg body weight/percent body surface burned during the first 24 hours after the injury. Half of this fluid should be given in the first 8 hours and the second half during the next 16 hours. Fluid therapy during the second 24 hours consists of the administration of free water in quantity sufficient to maintain a normal serum sodium concentration, as well as plasma (or other colloid) to maintain a normal plasma volume.

The adequacy of resuscitation can best be judged by frequent measurements of vital signs, central venous pressure, and urine output and by observation of general mental and physical responses. Despite myriad new monitoring devices, urine output remains one of the most sensitive and reliable assessments of fluid resuscitation. In the absence of myoglobinuria a urine output of 0.5 ml/kg/hr in adults and 1.0 ml/kg/hr in children less than 10 kg ensures that renal perfusion is adequate. The patient's sensorium gives an indication of the state of cerebral perfusion and oxygenation. The patient should be alert and cooperative; confusion and combativeness are signs of inadequate resuscitation or warn of other causes of hypoxia.

BOX 10-1
BAXTER (PARKLAND) FORMULA

FIRST 24 HOURS—RINGER'S LACTATE

4 ml/kg/% burn in 24 hours
One half in first 8 hours
One half in second 16 hours

Example: 70 kg man with 50% burn

4 ml × 50% = 14,000 ml in 24 hours
7000 ml hours 1-8
3500 ml hours 8-16
3500 ml hours 17-24

SECOND 24 HOURS—ALBUMIN OR PLASMA AND MAINTENANCE

Maintain normal vital signs
Adequate urine output

Example: 70 kg man with 50% burn

250-500 ml plasma
2000-2500 ml D5W

Patients with burns of less than 50% TBSA can usually be resuscitated with a single large-bore peripheral intravenous (IV) line. Because of the high incidence of septic thrombophlebitis, lower extremities should be avoided as IV portals. Upper extremities are preferable, even if the IV line must pass through burned skin. Patients with burns larger than 50% TBSA or who have associated medical problems, are at the extremes of age, or have concomitant smoke inhalation should have additional central venous pressure monitoring. Because of the extremely unstable state of the circulation in patients with burns over 65%, such patients should be monitored in an intensive care setting where a Swan-Ganz catheter for measuring pulmonary wedge pressure and cardiac output is available.

The presence of myoglobinuria alters the resuscitation plan. Myoglobinuria results from the destruction of muscle cells with release of the red muscle pigment myoglobin. This is most often a problem in patients with associated crush injuries, electrical burns, or extremely deep thermal burns. Characteristic cola-colored urine is an indication to increase the amount of fluid given and to establish a diuresis of 70 to 100 ml urine per hour. An initial bolus of 12.5 g of

*References 4, 16, 32, 35, 41, 59, 63, 65.

mannitol with a repeat dose in 15 to 30 minutes should be considered.

ESCHAROTOMY

Careful monitoring of the peripheral circulation is required in patients with circumferential full-thickness burns of the extremities. The edema that forms beneath inelastic eschar increases tissue pressure to a point at which it exceeds lymphatic pressure, thereby further increasing edema. When the edema exceeds venous pressure and eventually approaches arterial pressure, it stops all circulation to the extremity distal to the constricted area.

The classic findings of a compartment syndrome, usually considered to be pain, paresthesias, pulselessness, and tense swelling, may or may not be present in the burned extremity. Therefore distal pulses should be carefully monitored with a Doppler ultrasound, and if any of the clinical signs mentioned above occur, or if Doppler signals disappear, an escharotomy should be performed immediately.

Escharotomy is performed as a ward procedure and does not require an anesthetic, since only insensate full-thickness burn is incised. An incision is made through the eschar into subcutaneous tissue, first along the lateral aspect of the extremity and, if symptoms or signs do not improve, along the medial aspect. The incisions need not be as deep as the investing muscle fascia, and bleeding can usually be easily controlled with an electrocautery and the use of topical clotting agents. If arrival to hospital will be within 6 hours, escharotomies should not be done in the field because the patient may bleed to death without proper equipment to control bleeding.

Circumferential full-thickness burns of the trunk in small children occasionally demand an escharotomy to improve pulmonary function. Chest wall escharotomies are made in the anterior axillary line bilaterally, extending from the clavicle to the costal margin. If the abdomen is involved with the burn, the inferior margins of the escharotomy may be connected transversely.

Fasciotomies are rarely needed in patients with thermal burns. However, if distal pulses do not return following medial and lateral escharotomies, fasciotomy should be considered. On the other hand, patients with electrical injuries frequently need fasciotomy. Careful monitoring of all patients with electrical burns and with burns associated with soft tissue trauma or fractures is mandatory. In these circumstances loss of pulses is a strong indication for urgent fasciotomy under general anesthesia in the operating room.

The need for escharotomy in the burned hand is somewhat controversial. Fingers burned badly enough to require escharotomy are frequently mummified, and the lack of muscles in the fingers puts less tissue at ischemic risk. Escharotomy done in fingers that may not require it runs the risk of exposing the interphalangeal joints, leading to subsequent infection that may ultimately require joint fusion or finger amputation. Both the palmar arch and digital vessels should be monitored with Doppler ultrasound in any significant hand burn. If the signals disappear over the palmar arch or in the digital vessels, consideration should be given to performance of a dorsal interosseous fasciotomy.

BURN WOUND MANAGEMENT

The burn wound should be cleansed initially with a surgical detergent. All loose, nonviable skin should be gently trimmed. Debridement should be done gently; small doses of intravenous narcotic are sufficient analgesia for this procedure. General anesthesia and operating room debridement should be avoided until resuscitation is complete, unless other surgical procedures are necessary.

Once the wound is cleansed, a topical chemotherapeutic agent should be applied. A detailed description of all the agents available is beyond the scope of this chapter, but those most commonly used in the United States and other industrialized countries contain silver sulfadiazine. It comes as a white cream, is soothing to the wound, has a good antimicrobial spectrum, and has almost no systemic absorption or toxicity.[7,40,81,90] The patient should be carefully questioned about allergy to sulfa drugs before their use, however, since allergic reactions are encountered in about 3% of patients. These reactions may be manifested clinically as pain after application rather than the soothing feeling that silver sulfadiazine usually provides. If an allergy is suspected (by history) a small (10 × 10 cm) patch of silver sulfadiazine should be applied as a test. The remainder of the wound can be dressed in bacitracin. If no local reaction occurs after 2 to 4 hours, an allergy is unlikely and silver sulfadiazine is the dressing of choice. If an allergy is confirmed, the patient should be referred to a burn center, where the next choice of topical antimicrobial would probably be silver nitrate solution.

OUTPATIENT BURNS

According to guidelines given above, the vast majority of patients with burns do not require hospitalization. In many cases the burn, if merely kept clean, heals spontaneously in less than 3 weeks with acceptable cosmetic results and no functional impairment. Unfortunately, good results in treating superficial minor burns may entice the unwary physician to treat more complex burns by the same methods. For the patient, the consequences of such a mistake can be the need for subsequent hospitalization, joint dysfunction, and hypertrophic scarring that may be difficult to correct, as well as considerable loss of time from work or school.

FIRST-DEGREE BURNS

Although first-degree burns are very painful, victims rarely seek medical attention unless the area burned is extensive. These patients do not require hospitalization, but control of the pain is extremely important. Aspirin or codeine may be adequate for small injuries, but for large burns, liberal use of a more potent narcotic for 2 to 3 days is indicated.

For topical medication we recommend one of the many proprietary compounds containing extracts of the aloe vera plant in concentrations of at least 60%. Aloe vera has antimicrobial properties and is an effective analgesic.[49,77] Anecdotal evidence suggests that it may decrease subsequent pruritus and peeling.

Burns from ultraviolet rays (sunlight, sunlamp) may initially appear to be only epidermal, but the injury may in fact be a superficial partial-thickness burn with blistering apparent only after 12 to 24 hours. Therefore the patient with such a burn should be cautioned about blisters and should be asked to return if they form, since wound management then becomes more important because of the potential for infection and subsequent scarring.

SUPERFICIAL PARTIAL-THICKNESS BURNS

Treatment of superficial partial-thickness burns presents little problem. If the wound is kept clean, the patient is kept comfortable, and the joints are kept active, these wounds heal in less than 3 weeks with minimal scarring and no joint impairment.

Initially the wound should be cleansed and debrided as described previously. Small blisters may be left intact. Biochemical analysis of the protein-banding pattern of burn blister fluid, obtained by polyacrylamide gel electrophoresis, has shown it to be similar to that of serum.[93] These authors suggest that the fluid is an exudate mainly from the vascular system, that it provides a good environment for the fibroblasts in the damaged site, and that it facilitates the healing process. Larger blisters are difficult to protect, however, and blister fluid is a rich culture medium for bacteria that live in the skin appendages. Therefore large blisters and small blisters in large burns should usually be totally removed with forceps and scissors. In some instances the blister fluid can be aspirated with a large-bore needle, allowing the blistered epidermis to remain on the wound as a biologic dressing. This dead epidermis, however, is fragile, tends to contract, and rarely stays in place except over small areas.

After debridement these wounds can sometimes be managed with a biologic dressing such as porcine xenograft.[5,95] Pigskin is available in frozen or lyophilized forms. After a biologic dressing is applied, the burn pain is markedly diminished, and if the xenograft "sticks," no further treatment is necessary except for a periodic wound check. When the burn reepithelializes, the xenograft desiccates and peels away from the new epidermis. Other synthetic dressings, such as those made from plastic film (Op-Site or Epigard) have achieved some popularity.[11,69,88] We find that these dressings adhere poorly (a leaking dressing is not an occlusive one) and provide no advantage. The most commonly used treatment is wound coverage with silver sulfadiazine and application of a light dressing to promote active range of motion. Some very small burns do not require topical agents. For small facial burns, bacitracin ointment may be a better choice than silver sulfadiazine cream because it is less drying.

Pain is managed as for first-degree burns, and the patient usually should return every 2 to 3 days until the wound heals or the patient has demonstrated the ability to manage the wound without supervision.

One home treatment regimen is to have the patient cleanse the wound once daily with tap water and reapply the topical agent and light dressing. During dressing changes, and as often as possible, all involved joints should be put through a full range of motion. The dressing may be unnecessary while the patient is at home, but the patient should dress the wound before leaving the house. This method is highly successful, but it is inconvenient and fairly painful and requires good patient cooperation.

Another treatment regimen advocated by some physicians is a single initial debridement and application of a bulky dressing to be left in place for several days without intermediate cleansing or dressing change. This method reduces pain, but the patient must be careful of the bandage. If the bandage is allowed to become saturated with fluid draining from the wound or to become dirty, it may promote infection.

The "exposure" method has little to recommend it. This method involves leaving the wound open, allowing the wound drainage to desiccate and form a scab. Controlled studies in animals have shown that desiccation and crust formation interfere with wound healing. Our experience has also shown that crusts crack over joints, cause considerable discomfort, and can hide infection.

DEEP PARTIAL-THICKNESS AND FULL-THICKNESS BURNS

Treatment of deep partial-thickness and full-thickness burns is a matter of grave concern. Full-thickness burns heal only by contraction and epithelialization from the periphery. Epithelium does not begin to migrate until the eschar is removed; the growth rate then is only about 1 mm/day. Thus healing of even a small full-thickness burn may involve many weeks of discomfort and disability.

Deep partial-thickness burns may take 4 to 8 weeks to heal and then leave an unacceptable scar. If a joint is involved, some loss of joint function is the rule. We have adopted a policy of early excision and grafting for such wounds.

Initial outpatient treatment can be followed by elective surgery as soon as it can be scheduled. Small wounds can be treated through day surgery; larger wounds located over dynamically important areas can be closed with only a day or two of hospitalization. The excision and grafting procedures should be done by a surgeon experienced in tangential wound excision.

The advantages of this aggressive approach—a pain-free patient with normal joint function, a better cosmetic result, and a rapid return to work or school—more than compensate for the brief hospitalization and the very small risk associated with minor operation.

Should the excision and grafting plan be unacceptable to the patient or the treating physician, the standard method of daily cleansing and application of silver sulfadiazine cream is used. Most full-thickness burns need grafting at about 3 to 4 weeks after the injury. Deep dermal burns should be seen by the physician frequently during the healing process; active physical therapy is crucial to ensuring a successful outcome.

Rehabilitation

Physicians who regularly care for people with burn injuries recognize that treatment goals extend far beyond healing of the wounds and survival of the patient. We aim to return patients at least to their preburn functional status physically and to ensure a smooth and timely reentry into family and social situations, including work or school. Awareness that recovery from burn injury often depends on a number of nonphysician health care workers is essential. Depending on the severity of the burn and the associated social situation, participation of nurses, nutritionists, occupational therapists, physical therapists, recreational therapists, social workers, vocational rehabilitation counselors, psychologists, pain management specialists, and clergy is commonly required.

Burn rehabilitation should be initiated by the first physician to see the patient. Once all systemic and wound issues have been addressed, proper positioning of wounded extremities or digits should be assessed by an occupational therapist who has been specially trained in burn management. Splints should be made immediately if deemed appropriate. Range-of-motion exercises should be started on the day of injury, and frequent follow-up by a physical therapist is essential. The best functional outcomes result from meticulous attention to early mobility. Patients almost universally choose not to move a burned body part, and an active ancillary burn staff is essential for satisfactory results. Burn scars require approximately a year to fade, soften, and mature. Physical therapy may be required throughout this time period or longer. Pressure garment therapy may be used in certain cases in an attempt to prevent the development of hypertrophic scars. The interested reader is referred to books dealing with acute burn care, reconstructive plastic surgery, and burn rehabilitation for further discussion.[1,8,14]

Inhalation Injury

EPIDEMIOLOGY

Of the nearly 50,000 fire victims admitted to hospitals each year, smoke or thermal damage to the respiratory tree may occur in as many as 30%.[71] Carbon monoxide poisoning, smoke poisoning, and thermal injury are three distinctly separate aspects of clinical inhalation injury and are discussed as such. Inhalation injury rarely occurs in an outdoor setting.

Carbon Monoxide Poisoning

Pathophysiology. Carbon monoxide (CO) is a colorless, odorless, tasteless gas that has an affinity for hemoglobin 200 times greater than that of oxygen. The most simply explained mechanism of action of CO is reversible displacement of oxygen on the hemoglobin molecule. Although worsening hypoxia is important, and the percentage of carboxyhemoglobin in the blood represents in large measure the degree of patient hypoxia, this simple mechanism cannot account for all of the experimental and clinical findings seen with exposure to CO. For example, an experimental group of dogs was exchange-transfused with blood containing 80% carboxyhemoglobin (COHb). They showed no symptoms. In a control group with COHb levels of 80% produced by inhalation of CO, all animals died. Furthermore, the degree of enzyme and muscle impairment may not correlate accurately with the levels of blood COHb.[15,20,30,50]

In vitro, CO combines reversibly with cardiac muscle myoglobin and heme-containing enzymes such as cytochrome oxidase a_3.[15] Despite its intense affinity, it readily dissociates according to the laws of mass action. The half-life of COHb in humans breathing room air is 4 to 5 hours. In humans breathing 100% oxygen, the half-life is reduced to 45 to 60 minutes.[54] In a hyperbaric oxygen chamber at 2 PSI, the half-life is 30 minutes, and at 3 atmospheres in a chamber it is reduced to 15 to 20 minutes.[92]

Clinical Presentation. Blood levels of COHb provide a laboratory measure to correlate with associated symptoms of CO poisoning. Levels less than 10% do not cause symptoms, although patients with exercise-induced angina may show decreased exercise tolerance. At levels of 20%, healthy persons complain of headache, nausea, vomiting, and loss of manual dexterity. At 30% they become confused and lethargic, and may show depressed ST segments on electrocardiogram. In a fire situation this level may lead to death as the victim loses both the interest and the ability to flee the smoke. At levels between 40% and 60% the patient lapses into coma, and levels much above 60% are usually fatal.

Therapy. Patients who have not been unconscious and who have a normal neurologic examination on admission almost always recover completely without treatment beyond administration of 100% oxygen. Patients who remain comatose once COHb levels have returned to normal have a poor prognosis, and in our experience they rarely awaken. While enthusiasts for hyperbaric oxygen treatment consider it a standard of care for CO poisoning,[2,3,52,61] many trauma physicians are skeptical.[78] The only controlled study done to date indicated that hyperbaric oxygen made no difference for moderate poisoning, and multiple treatments were no better than a single treatment for patients with severe poisoning.[72] Furthermore, when associated with a major burn, transport to a chamber delays definitive care and is associated with numerous complications, including emesis, seizures, eustachian tube occlusion, aspiration, hypocalcemia, agitation requiring restraints or sedation, arterial hypotension, tension pneumothorax, and cardiac dysrhythmia or arrest.[34,87]

Thermal Airway Injury

Pathophysiology. The term "pulmonary burn" is a misnomer. True thermal damage to the lower respiratory tract and lung parenchyma is extremely rare unless live steam or exploding gases are inhaled. The air temperature near the ceiling of a burning room may reach 540° C (1000° F) or more, but air has such poor heat-carrying capacity that most of the heat is dissipated in the nasopharynx and upper airway. The heat dissipation in the upper airway, however, may cause significant local thermal injury.

Clinical Presentation. Patients who have been in explosions (propane, natural gas, or gasoline) and have burns of the hands, face, and upper torso are particularly at risk for pharyngeal edema.

Therapy. Maintenance of the airway is the main concern with potential thermal airway injury. Patients injured in explosions should be examined for oropharyngeal erythema and edema. If these are present, the patient should be intubated for 24 to 72 hours until edema subsides. A simple test to determine if intubation should continue is to see if the patient can breathe around the endotracheal tube when the cuff is deflated. If so, the airway edema has probably resolved and extubation should be safe. If doubt exists, extubation should be performed over a fiberoptic bronchoscope or nasogastric tube, which allows easy replacement of the endotracheal tube if necessary. Since this is not a pulmonary parenchymal injury, the purpose of intubation is to protect the airway, not necessarily to assist with ventilation. Ventilator settings should be adjusted accordingly, and vigorous pulmonary toilet should be instituted to prevent the pulmonary problems (atelectasis and pneumonia) commonly seen in intubated patients.

Smoke Poisoning

Pathophysiology. Some 280 separate toxic products have been identified in wood smoke. Modern petrochemical science has now produced a wealth of plastic materials in homes and automobiles that when burned produce nearly all of these and many other products not yet even characterized.[45,66,85,99] Prominent by-products of incomplete combustion are oxides of sulfur, nitrogen, and many aldehydes. One such aldehyde, acrolein, causes severe pulmonary irritation and edema in concentrations as low as 10 ppm. Although the chemical mechanisms of injury may be different with different toxic products, the overall end organ response is reasonably well defined.* There is an immediate loss of bronchial epithelial cilia and decreased alveolar surfactant. Micro, and sometimes macro, atelectasis results and is compounded by mucosal edema in small airways. Wheezing and air hunger are common symptoms at this time. After a few hours, tracheal and bronchial epithelia begin to slough and hemorrhagic tracheobronchitis develops. In severe cases interstitial edema becomes prominent, resulting in a typical picture of the adult respiratory distress syndrome (ARDS). Pulmonary alveolar macrophages are poisoned, causing severe impairment of chemotaxis, which undoubtedly contributes to the high incidence of late pneumonia seen in patients with associated cutaneous burns. The activated neutrophils release superoxides and free radicals of oxygen, which together with other inflammatory mediators aggravate alveolar-capillary damage, leading to increased interstitial edema and impaired oxygenation.

Clinical Presentation. Any patient who has been indoors in a smoky fire and has a flame burn or was in an enclosed space should be assumed to have smoke poisoning until proven otherwise. The acrid smell of smoke on the victim's clothes should raise suspicion. Rescuers are often the most important historians and should be carefully questioned.

Careful inspection of the mouth and pharynx should be done early. Hoarseness and expiratory wheezes are signs of potentially serious airway edema or smoke poisoning. Copious mucus production and carbonaceous sputum are sure signs, but their absence should not raise false hopes that injury is absent. COHb levels should be obtained; elevated carboxyhemoglobin levels or any clinical symptoms of CO poisoning are presumptive evidence of associated smoke poisoning. In very smoky fires, COHb levels of 40% to 50% may be reached after only 2 to 3 minutes of exposure.[92]

Anyone with suspected smoke poisoning should have a set of arterial blood gases drawn. One of the earliest indicators is an improper ratio (P/F ratio) of the arterial PAO_2 to the percent of inspired oxygen (FIO_2). Normally the ratio is 400 to 500, whereas patients with impending pulmonary problems have a ratio of less than 300 (for example, PAO_2 of less than 120 with an FIO_2 of 0.40). A ratio of less than 250 is an indication for vigorous pulmonary therapy, not an indication for merely increasing the inspired oxygen concentration.

A number of authorities suggest the routine use of fiberoptic bronchoscopy.[12,55,74,81] It is inexpensive, quickly performed by an experienced clinician, and useful in accurately assessing edema of the upper airway. Aside from documenting the presence of tracheal erythema, however, it

*References 10, 17, 39, 42, 53, 54, 75, 83, 98, 99.

does not materially influence the treatment for smoke poisoning. Therefore it should be used only when the diagnosis is in doubt or for experimental studies.

We have correlated by multivariate analysis a constellation of historical items, signs, and symptoms with bronchoscopic findings in 100 consecutive patients with suspected smoke inhalation admitted to the University of Washington Burn Center in Seattle. If the patient had the combination of history of closed space fire, carbonaceous sputum, and a COHb level greater than 10%, there was 96% correlation with positive bronchoscopy. Presence of two of the above features dropped correlation to 70%, and if only one was present, the correlation dropped to 36%. As discussed previously, upper airway edema was best correlated with an explosion (flash burn) that involved both the face and the upper torso. Nearly 50% of such patients had significant upper airway edema and underwent prophylactic airway intubation.

Therapy. There is clear agreement that all patients burned in an enclosed space or having any suggestion of neurologic symptoms should be given 100% oxygen while awaiting measurement of COHb levels. This should be administered through a tight-fitting mask in the field. If the patient demonstrates labored breathing or if a prolonged transport time is anticipated, endotracheal intubation should be performed by trained personnel. One hundred percent oxygen can then be administered by ventilator.

Mucosal burns of the mouth, nasopharynx, and larynx respond with edema formation and may lead to upper airway obstruction at any time during the first 24 hours after the burn. Red or dry mucosa or small mucosal blisters should alert the observer to the possibility of subsequent airway obstruction; they also should raise suspicion that significant smoke inhalation may have occurred. Any patient with burns of the face should have a careful visual inspection of the mouth and pharynx; if abnormalities are found, the larynx should be examined immediately on arrival at the hospital. The presence of significant intraoral and pharyngeal burns is a clear indication for early endotracheal intubation, since the progressive edema may make later emergency intubation extremely hazardous, if not impossible.

The mucosal burns themselves are rarely full thickness and can be successfully managed with good oral hygiene. Once inserted, the endotracheal tube should remain in place for 2 to 5 days until the edema subsides.

Pulmonary functions early in the course of smoke poisoning are variably affected. Typically there are decreased lung volume (functional residual capacity) and vital capacity, evidence of obstructive disease with reduction in flow rates, increased dead space, and a rather rapid decrease in compliance. Surprisingly, much of the variability in pulmonary response appears to correlate with the severity of the associated cutaneous burn.[14] Without associated burns the mortality from smoke poisoning is low, the disease rarely progresses to ARDS, and symptomatic treatment usually leads to complete resolution of symptoms in a few days. In the presence of burns, smoke poisoning appears to approximately double the rate of mortality from burns of any size. Pulmonary symptoms (hypoxia, rales, rhonchi, wheezes) are seldom present on admission but may appear 12 to 48 hours following exposure. In general, the earlier the onset of symptoms, the more severe the disease.[91]

No standard treatment has evolved to ensure survival following smoke poisoning; each recommended treatment modality is tempered by opinion and the individual experience of the treating physician. In the presence of increasing laryngeal edema, nasotracheal or orotracheal intubation is indicated. A tracheostomy is never an emergency procedure and certainly should be avoided as initial airway management in patients with burns to the face and neck. A soft-cuffed endotracheal tube should be left in place for 3 to 5 days until the generalized oropharyngeal edema subsides.

Mild cases of smoke poisoning are treated with highly humidified air, vigorous pulmonary toilet, and bronchodilators as needed. Blood gases are drawn at least every 4 hours, and the P/F ratio is calculated. Worsening symptoms, difficulty in handling secretions, and a falling P/F ratio are all indications for intubation and respiratory assistance with a volume ventilator. If oxygenation is impaired (P/F ratio 250 or less), positive end-expiratory pressure (PEEP) or continuous positive airway pressure (CPAP) is initiated and increased by increments of 3 to 5 cm H_2O until no further improvement in the P/F ratio occurs or there is evidence of decreased cardiac output.

The physician must carefully search for other mechanical causes of poor ventilation (for example, restricted chest wall motion from full-thickness burns, pneumothorax from high ventilator pressures, or mechanical difficulties with the endotracheal tube).

Prophylactic antibiotics have no value in this chemical pneumonitis, and the subsequent burn management and treatment of eventual bacterial pneumonia can be made more difficult by the development of resistant organisms if antibiotics are used early.

Steroids are commonly used in patients with severe asthma. Clinicians dealing with smoke poisoning often use them for their spasmolytic and antiinflammatory actions. Several authors have studied the use of steroids, but a most convincing study comes from Moylan, who showed in a prospective blinded study of patients with smoke poisoning and associated major burns that the rates of mortality and infectious complications were higher in the steroid-treated patients. In patients without associated burns, Robinson and Seward[76] found that steroids did not alter the hospital course of patients admitted to the hospital following the MGM Grand and Hilton Hotel fires in Las Vegas in 1981.

The decision for hospital admission and the need for specialized care rest on the severity of symptoms from the smoke and the presence and magnitude of associated burns. Any patient who shows symptoms of smoke inhalation and has more than trivial burns should be admitted. If the burns are greater than 15% TBSA, the patient should probably be referred to a special care unit. In the absence of burns, admission depends on the severity of symptoms, presence of preexisting medical problems, and the social circumstances of the patient. Otherwise healthy patients with mild symptoms (only a few expiratory wheezes, minimal sputum production, COHb level less than 10%, and normal blood gas levels) can be watched for an hour or two and then discharged if they have a place to go and someone to stay with them. Patients with preexisting cardiovascular or pulmonary disease should be admitted for observation if they have any symptoms related to the smoke. Patients with moderate symptoms (generalized wheezing, mild hoarseness, moderate sputum production, COHb levels 5% to 10%, and normal blood gas levels) may be admitted for close observation and treated as for asthma. Severe symptoms (air hunger, severe wheezing, and copious [usually carbonaceous] sputum) require immediate intubation and ventilatory support in an intensive care unit setting.

Other Considerations

Burns are tetanus-prone wounds. The need for tetanus prophylaxis is determined by the patient's current immunization status. The treating physician should follow the recommendations of the American College of Surgeons.

All patients undergoing intravenous resuscitation should have an indwelling urinary catheter placed for hourly monitoring of urine output. Arterial lines are useful in patients who need frequent assessment of blood gases or who will need repeated blood sampling. Necessary laboratory work during the resuscitation phase is relatively minimal. Baseline blood chemistries should be drawn. If major operative procedures, such as fasciotomy or multiple escharotomies, are expected, blood should be sent for type and cross-matching for several units of whole blood. Blood gases are mandatory in any patient with a suspected inhalation injury, and arterial pH measurement is useful as an assessment of the overall treatment of shock. If the Baxter formula is used for resuscitation, frequent electrolyte determinations are not necessary because levels will remain in the normal range. By 48 hours, however, careful monitoring of serum sodium and potassium becomes important. High levels of circulating aldosterone result in an increase in renal potassium excretion, and varying degrees of evaporative water loss through eschar dramatically increase the free water requirements of burned patients. Hemoglobin and hematocrit levels are initially high and remain high or normal until the third or fourth postburn day. The blood glucose level commonly is elevated because of the glycogenolytic effect of elevated catecholamines, the gluconeogenic effect of elevated glucocorticoid and glucagon levels, and relative insulin resistance.[44,82,94,100] This well-described "stress diabetes" can become a problem in normal patients if glucose-containing solutions are given during resuscitation and frequently is a serious problem in patients with preexisting diabetes. All diabetic patients require careful monitoring of blood and urine glucose, and most require supplemental insulin during resuscitation.

All medications during the shock phase of burn care should be given intravenously. Subcutaneous and intramuscular injections are unreliably absorbed systemically, and their use should be avoided. Pain control is best managed with small intravenous doses of morphine given until pain control is adequate without affecting blood pressure.

Before the discovery of penicillin, 30% of burn patients died during the first week after the injury from overwhelming β-hemolytic streptococcal sepsis. The availability of penicillin decreased streptococcal infections but had no influence on mortality or the incidence of bacterial sepsis. Patients then survived the first postburn week only to die of gram-negative penicillin-resistant bacterial sepsis during the second or third week after the burn. The advent of effective topical chemotherapeutic agents applied directly to the burn wounds made possible the control of streptococcal infection, obviating the need for prophylactic penicillin. The use of prophylactic antibiotics in outpatient burns has not been carefully evaluated, so opinion is divided regarding its utility in patients not requiring hospitalization.

Stress ulceration of the stomach and duodenum was once a dread complication, occurring in nearly 30% of patients with burns. Protection of the gastric mucosa by immediate feeding through a small nasogastric tube or, failing that, with instillation of antacids or sucralfate has made stress ulcers rare.[48,61,70,73,89]

Psychosocial care should begin immediately. The patient and family must be comforted, and a realistic outlook regarding the prognosis of the burns should be given, at least to the patient's family. In house fires the patient's loved ones, pets, and many or all possessions may have been destroyed. If the family is not available, some member of the team, usually the social worker, should find out the extent of the damage in hopes of comforting the patient. If the patient is a child and the circumstances suggest that the burn may have been deliberately inflicted or resulted from negligence, physicians in most states are required by law to report their suspicion of child abuse to local authorities.

BURN SEVERITY AND CATEGORIZATION

Severity of injury is proportionate to the size of the total burn, the depth of the burn, the age of the patient, and associated medical problems or injuries. Burns have been classified by the American Burn Association and the American College of Surgeons Committee on Trauma into categories of minor, moderate, and severe.[6] Moderate burns are defined as partial-thickness burns of 15% to 25% of TBSA in adults (10% to 20% in children); full-thickness burns of less than 10% of TBSA; and burns that do not involve the eyes, ears, face, hands, feet, or perineum. Because of the significant cosmetic and functional risk, all but very superficial burns of the face, hands, feet, and perineum should be treated by a physician with a special interest in burn care in a facility that is accustomed to dealing with such problems. Major burns as described previously, most full-thickness burns in infants and elderly patients, and burns combined with diseases or injuries should also be treated in a specialized facility. Moderate burns can be treated in a community hospital by a knowledgeable physician as long as the other members of the health care team have the resources and knowledge to ensure a good result. Newer techniques of early wound closure have made burn care more complex, and an increasing number of patients with small but significant burns are being referred to specialized care facilities to take advantage of these concepts.

The criteria for admission to the hospital of patients with "minor" and "moderate" burns vary according to physician preference, the patient's social circumstances, and the ability to provide close follow-up. In some circumstances superficial burns as large as 15% can be successfully managed on an outpatient basis. In other circumstances burns as small as 1% may require admission because of the patient's inability or unwillingness to care for the wound. In general, the threshold for admission of elderly patients and infants should be low. Any patient (child or adult) who the physician suspects of having been abused must be admitted.

TRANSPORT AND TRANSFER PROTOCOLS

Once an airway is established and resuscitation is under way, burn patients are eminently suitable for transport.[9,22,46] Resuscitation can continue en route, since for the most part patients remain stable for several days. This was well proven during the Vietnam War, when burn victims were transported from Vietnam to Japan and then from Japan to the military burn center in San Antonio, Texas. The transport was generally accomplished during the first 2 weeks after the burn, with few complications occurring in about 1000 patients transferred.

Hospitals without specialized burn care facilities should decide where they will refer patients and work out transfer agreements and treatment protocols with the chosen burn center well in advance of need. If this is done, definitive care can begin at the initial hospital and continue without interruption during transport and at the burn center. In general, transfer should be from physician to physician, and contact should be established between them as soon as the patient arrives at the initial hospital.

The mode of transport depends on vehicle availability, local terrain, weather, and the distances involved. For distances of less than 50 miles, ground ambulance is usually satisfactory. For distances between 50 and 150 miles, many people prefer helicopter transport. It should be noted, however, that monitoring, airway management, and any changes in therapy are more difficult to achieve in a helicopter. All patients transported by air should have a nasogastric tube inserted and be placed on dependent drainage, since nausea and vomiting usually result during the flight. Two large-bore IV lines should be functional in case one stops working.

For distances over 150 miles, fixed-wing aircraft are usually satisfactory. Modern air ambulances are completely equipped flying intensive care units, and the personnel are usually well trained for both critical care and the peculiarities of patient care during flight (see Chapter 22).

The referring physicians must ensure that the patient's condition is suitable for a long transport and prepare the patient for the flight. The patient's airway must be secure. At 30,000 feet, planes can be pressurized to an altitude of about 5500 feet. Although supplemental oxygen can be given in flight, if the patient's oxygenation is marginal, performing intubation and starting mechanical ventilation before the transport may be preferable. Intubation is difficult en route, so if there is any question of upper airway edema, the patient should be intubated at the referring hospital. Burned patients have difficulty maintaining body temperature, and they should be wrapped warmly before transport. Bulky dressings, a blanket, and a Mylar sheet (usually available from the flight team) can help maintain body temperature. In case the patient has any cardiac irregularities, the plane must be equipped with electronic monitoring capability, since noise and vibrations in flight make clinical monitoring difficult.

Only after all other assessments are complete should attention be directed to the burn itself. If the patient is to be transferred from the initial hospital to a definitive care center during the first postburn day, personnel at the referring hospital can leave the burn wounds alone, merely calculating the size of burn for resuscitation and monitoring pulses distal to circumferential full-thickness burns. The patient can be wrapped in a clean sheet and kept warm until arrival at the definitive care center.

REFERENCES

1. Achauer, BM: *Burn reconstruction,* New York: 1991, Thieme Medical.
2. Adir Y, Bentur Y, Melamed Y: Hyperbaric oxygen for neuropsychiatric sequelae of carbon monoxide poisoning, *Harefuah* 122:562, 1992.
3. Adir Y et al: Hyperbaric oxygen treatment for carbon monoxide intoxication acquired in a sealed room during the Persian Gulf war, *Isr J Med Sci* 27:669, 1991.
4. Aharoni A et al: Burn resuscitation with a low-volume plasma regimen: analysis of mortality, *Burns* 15:230, 1989.
5. Alsbjorn BF: Biologic wound coverings in burn treatment, *World J Surg* 16:43, 1992.
6. American Burn Association: Hospital and prehospital resources for optimal care of patients with burn injury: guidelines for development and operation of burn centers, *J Burn Care Rehabil* 11:98, 1990.
7. Aoyama H, Yokoo K, Fujii K: Systemic absorption of sulphadiazine, silver sulphadiazine and sodium sulphadiazine through human burn wounds, *Burns* 16:163, 1990.
8. Artz CP, Moncrief JA, Pruitt BA Jr: *Burns: A team approach,* ed 2, Philadelphia, 1984, WB Saunders.
9. Baac BR et al: Helicopter transport of the patient with acute burns, *J Burn Care Rehabil* 12:229, 1991.

10. Barrow RE et al: Cellular sequence of tracheal repair in sheep after smoke inhalation injury, *Lung* 170:331, 1992.
11. Bauman LW et al: Bilaminate synthetic dressing for partial thickness burns: lack of cost reduction for inpatient care, *Am Surg* 57:131, 1991.
12. Bingham HG, Gallagher TJ, Powell MD: Early bronchoscopy as a predictor of ventilatory support for burned patients, *J Trauma* 27:1286, 1987.
13. Blinn DL, Slater H, Goldfarb LW: Inhalation injury with burns: a lethal combination, *J Emerg Med* 6:471, 1988.
14. Boswick JA JR: *The art and science of burn care,* Rockville, Md, 1987, Aspen.
15. Brown SD, Piantadosi CA: Reversal of carbon monoxide-cytochrome c oxidase binding by hyperbaric oxygen in vivo, *Adv Exp Med Biol* 248:747, 1989.
16. Carvajal HF, Parks DH: Optimal composition of burn resuscitation fluids, *Crit Care Med* 16:695, 1988.
17. Clark CJ et al: Role of pulmonary alveolar macrophage activation in acute lung injury after burns and smoke inhalation, *Lancet* 2:872, 1988.
18. Daniel RK et al: High-voltage electrical injury: acute pathophysiology, *J Hand Surg* 13:44, 1988.
19. Datubo-Brown DD, Gowar JP: Contact burns in children, *Burns* 15:285, 1989.
20. Della-Puppa T et al: Carbon monoxide poisoning and secondary neurologic syndrome: follow-up after hyperbaric oxygen therapy; preliminary results, *Minerva Anestesiol* 57:972, 1991.
21. Ding YL et al: Extensive scalds following accidental immersion in hot water pools, *Burns Incl Therm Inj* 13:305, 1987.
22. Ellis A, Rylah TA: Transfer of the thermally injured patient, *Br J Hosp Med* 44:206, 1990.
23. Engrav LH et al: Outcome and treatment of electrical injury with immediate median and ulnar nerve palsy at the wrist: a retrospective review and a survey of members of the American Burn Association, *Ann Plast Surg* 25:166, 1990.
24. Epperly TD, Steward JR: The physical effects of lightning injury, *J Fam Pract* 29:267, 1989.
25. Eriksson A, Ornehult L: Death by lightning, *Am J Forensic Med Pathol* 9:295, 1988.
26. Feldberg L, Regan PJ, Roberts AH: Cement burns and their treatment, *Burns* 18:51, 1992.
27. Field TO Jr, Dominic W, Hansbrough J: Beach-fire burns in San Diego County, *Burns Incl Therm Inj* 13:416, 1987.
28. Fontanarosa PB: Electrical shock and lightning strike, *Ann Emerg Med,* 1993, p 378.
29. Fulde GW, Marsden SJ: Lightning strikes, *Med J Aust* 153:496, 1990.
30. Gorman DF et al: A longitudinal study of 100 consecutive admissions for carbon monoxide poisoning to the Royal Adelaide Hospital, *Anaesth Intens Care* 20:311, 1992.
31. Graitcer PL, Sniezek JE: Hospitalizations due to tap water scalds, 1978-1985, *MMWR CDC Surveill Summ* 37:35, 1988.
32. Griswold JA et al: Hypertonic saline resuscitation: efficacy in a community-based burn unit, *South Med J* 84:692, 1991.
33. Grube BJ et al: Neurologic consequences of electrical burns, *J Trauma* 30:254, 1990.
34. Grube BJ, Marvin JA, Heimbach DM: Therapeutic hyperbaric oxygen: help or hindrance in burn patients with carbon monoxide poisoning? *J Burn Care Rehabil* 9:249, 1988.
35. Gunn ML et al: Prospective, randomized trial of hypertonic sodium lactate versus lactated Ringer's solution for burn shock resuscitation, *J Trauma* 29:1261, 1989.
36. Haberal M et al: Severe electrical injury, *Burns Incl Therm Inj* 15:60, 1989.
37. Hammond JS, Ward CG: High-voltage electrical injuries: management and outcome of 60 cases, *South Med J* 81:1351, 1988.
38. Herbert K, Lawrence JC: Chemical burns, *Burns* 15:381, 1989.
39. Herndon DN et al: Extravascular lung water changes following smoke inhalation and massive burn injury, *Surgery* 102:341, 1987.
40. Herruzo CR et al: Evaluation of the penetration strength, bactericidal efficacy and spectrum of action of several antimicrobial creams against isolated microorganisms in a burn centre, *Burns* 18:39, 1992.
41. Horton JW, White DJ: Hypertonic saline dextran resuscitation fails to improve cardiac function in neonatal and senescent burned guinea pigs, *J Trauma* 31:1459, 1991.
42. Hubbard GB et al: The morphology of smoke inhalation injury in sheep, *J Trauma* 31:1477, 1991.
43. James, NK, Moss AL: Review of burns caused by bitumen and the problems of its removal, *Burns* 16:214, 1990.
44. Jeffries MK, Vance ML: Growth hormone and cortisol secretion in patients with burn injury, *J Burn Care Rehabil* 13:391, 1992.
45. Jones J, McMullen MJ, Dougherty J: Toxic smoke inhalation: cyanide poisoning in fire victims, *Am J Emerg Med* 5:317, 1987.
46. Judkins KC: Aeromedical transfer of burned patients: a review with special reference to European civilian practice, *Burns Incl Therm Inj* 14:171, 1988.
47. Kanitkar S, Roberts AH: Paraplegia in an electrical burn: a case report, *Burns Incl Therm Inj* 14:49, 1988.
48. Kitajima MA et al: Gastric microcirculatory change and development of acute gastric mucosal lesions (stress ulcer), *Acta Physiol Hung* 73:137, 1989.
49. Klein AD, Penneys NS: Aloe vera, *J Am Acad Dermatol* 18(4 pt 1):714, 1988.
50. Kodama K et al: A case of "interval" form of acute carbon monoxide poisoning: brain MRI and therapeutic effect of hyperbaric oxygenation, *Rinsho Shinkeigaku* 30:420, 1990.
51. Koller J, Orsagh J: Delayed neurological sequelae of high-tension electrical burns, *Burns* 15:175, 1989.
52. Koren G et al: A multicenter, prospective study of fetal outcome following accidental carbon monoxide poisoning in pregnancy, *Reprod Toxicol* 5:397, 1991.
53. Leduc D et al: Acute and long-term respiratory damage following inhalation of ammonia, *Thorax* 47:755, 1992.
54. Linares HA, Herndon DN, Traber DL: Sequence of morphologic events in experimental smoke inhalation, *J Burn Care Rehabil* 10:27, 1989.
55. Lukånn J, Sånndor L, The importance of fiberbronchoscopy in respiratory burns, *Acta Chir Plast* 32:107, 1990.
56. Lyngdorf P: Occupational burn injuries, *Burns Incl Therm Inj* 13:294, 1987.
57. Massello W III: Lightning deaths, *Med Leg Bull* 37:1, 1988.
58. Mellins RB, Park S: Medical Progress: respiratory complications of smoke inhalation in victims of fires, *J Pediatr* 87:1, 1975.
59. Meuli M, Lochbuhler H: Current concepts in pediatric burn care: general management of severe burns, *Eur J Pediatr Surg* 2:195, 1992.
60. Meyer GW, Hart GB, Strauss MB: Hyperbaric oxygen therapy for acute smoke inhalation injuries, *Postgrad Med* 89:221, 1991.
61. Mittal PK et al: Sucralfate therapy for acid-induced upper gastrointestinal tract injury, *Am J Gastroenterol* 84:204, 1989.
62. Moran KD, O'Reilly T, Munster AM: Chemical burns: a ten-year experience, *Am Surg* 53:652, 1987.
63. Morehouse JD et al: Resuscitation of the thermally injured patient, *Crit Care Clin* 8:355, 1992.
64. Mozingo DW et al: Chemical burns, *J Trauma* 28:642, 1988.
65. Murison MS, Laitung JK, Pigott RW: Effectiveness of burns resuscitation using two different formulae, *Burns* 17:484, 1991.
66. Narita H et al: Smoke inhalation injury from newer synthetic building materials: a patient who survived 205 days, *Burns Incl Therm Inj* 13:147, 1987.
67. Palmer JH, Sutherland AB: Problems associated with transfer of patients to a regional burn unit, *Injury* 18:250, 1987.
68. Patten BM: Lightning and electrical injuries, *Neurol Clin* 10:1047, 1992.
69. Phillips LG et al: Uses and abuses of a biosynthetic dressing for partial skin thickness burns, *Burns* 15:254, 1989.

70. Prasad JK, Thomson PD, Feller I: Gastrointestinal haemorrhage in burn patients, *Burns Incl Therm Inj* 13:194, 1987.
71. Pruitt BA Jr et al: Evaluation and management of patients with inhalation injury, *J Trauma* 30:S63, 1990.
72. Raphael JC et al: Trial of normobaric and hyperbaric oxygen for acute carbon monoxide intoxication (see comments), *Lancet* 2:414, 1989.
73. Rath T, Walzer LR, Meissl G: Preventive measures for stress ulcers in burn patients, *Burns Incl Therm Inj* 14:504, 1988.
74. Richard P et al: Emergency tracheobronchoscopy in children with burns, *Ann Otolaryngol Chir Cervicofac* 107:195, 1990.
75. Riyami BM Changes in alveolar macrophage, monocyte, and neutrophil cell profiles after smoke inhalation injury, *J Clin Pathol* 43:43, 1990.
76. Robinson MD, Seward PN: Hazardous chemical exposure in children, *Pediatr Emerg Care* 3:179, 1987.
77. Rodriguez M, Cruz NI, Suarez A: Comparative evaluation of aloe vera in the management of burn wounds in guinea pigs, *Plast Reconstr Surg* 81:386, 1988.
78. Roy TM et al: Perceptions and utilization of hyperbaric oxygen therapy for carbon monoxide poisoning in an academic setting, *J Ky Med Assoc* 87:223, 1989.
79. Sawhney CP, Kaushish R: Acid and alkali burns: considerations in management, *Burns* 15:132, 1989.
80. Sawhney CP et al: Long-term experience with 1% topical silver sulphadiazine cream in the management of burn wounds, *Burns* 15:403, 1989.
81. Schneider W et al: Diagnostic and therapeutic possibilities for fibreoptic bronchoscopy in inhalation injury, *Burns Incl Therm Inj* 14:53, 1988.
82. Shangraw RE et al: Differentiation between septic and postburn insulin resistance, *Metabolism* 38:983, 1989.
83. Sharar SR et al: Cardiopulmonary responses after spontaneous inhalation of Douglas fir smoke in goats, *J Trauma* 28:164, 1988.
84. Shugerman R et al: Contact burns of the hand, *Pediatrics* 80:18, 1987.
85. Silverman SH et al: Cyanide toxicity in burned patients, *J Trauma* 28:171, 1988.
86. Singer A et al: Chemical burns: our 10-year experience, *Burns* 18:250, 1992.
87. Sloan EP et al: Complications and protocol considerations in carbon monoxide–poisoned patients who require hyperbaric oxygen therapy: report from a ten-year experience (see comments), *Ann Emerg Med* 18:629, 1989.
88. Smith DJ et al: Biosynthetic compound dressings: management of hand burns, *Burns Incl Therm Inj* 14:405, 1988.
89. Steen J et al: Antacid in the prevention of upper gastrointestinal bleeding in burns, *Acta Chir Scand Suppl* 547:93, 1988.
90. Stern HS: Silver sulphadiazine and the healing of partial thickness burns: a prospective clinical trial, *Br J Plast Surg* 42:581, 1989.
91. Stone HH, Martin JD Jr: Pulmonary injury associated with thermal burns, *Surg Gynecol Obstet* 129:1242, 1969.
92. Thom SR, Keim LW: Carbon monoxide poisoning: a review of epidemiology, pathophysiology, clinical findings, and treatment options including hyperbaric oxygen therapy, *J Toxicol Clin Toxicol* 27:141, 1989.
93. Uchinuma E et al: Biological evaluation of burn blister fluid, *Ann Plast Surg* 20:225, 1988.
94. van Gool JH et al: The relation among stress, adrenalin, interleukin 6 and acute-phase proteins in the rat, *Clin Immunol Immunopathol* 57:200, 1990.
95. Vanstraelen P: Comparison of calcium sodium alginate (Kaltostat) and porcine xenograft (E-Z Derm) in the healing of split-thickness skin graft donor sites, *Burns* 18:145, 1992.
96. Wachtel TL et al: Scalds from molten tar: an industrial hazard, *J Burn Care Rehabil* 9:218, 1988.
97. Walker AR: Fatal tapwater scald burns in the USA, 1979-86, *Burns* 16:49, 1990.
98. Wang CZ et al: Morphologic changes in basal cells during repair of tracheal epithelium, *Am J Pathol* 141:753, 1992.
99. Youn YK, Lalonde C, Demling R: Oxidants and the pathophysiology of burn and smoke inhalation injury, *Free Radic Biol Med* 12:409, 1992.
100. Ziegler MG, Morrissey EC, Marshall LF: Catecholamine and thyroid hormones in traumatic injury, *Crit Care Med* 18:253, 1990.

11 LIGHTNING INJURIES

Mary Ann Cooper
Christopher J. Andrews

Historical Overview

Humans have always viewed lightning with awe and trepidation.[173] Priests, the earliest astronomers and meteorologists, became proficient at weather prediction, interpreting changes in weather as omens of good or bad fortune, sometimes to the advantage of their political mentors. As a spectacular celestial event, lightning was often depicted in ancient cultures and religions.[79] A roll seal from Akkadian times (2200 BC) portrays a goddess holding sheaves of lightning bolts in each hand.[79] Next to her, a weather god drives a chariot and creates lightning bolts by flicking a whip at his horses, while priests offer libations. A relief found on a castle gate in northern Syria (900 BC) depicts the weather god Teshub holding a three-pronged thunderbolt.[142]

Beginning around 700 BC, Greek artists began to incorporate lightning symbols representing Zeus's tool of warning or favor. Aristotle noted that lightning resulted from the ignition of telluric fumes that made up storm clouds. Roman mythology saw lightning as more ominous than did the Greeks, with Thor using thunderbolts as tools of vengeance and condemnation so that Romans who were struck were denied burial rituals. Several Roman emperors wore laurel wreaths or sealskin to ward off lightning strikes. Important matters of state were often decided on observations of lightning and other natural phenomena. Both Seneca and Titus Lucretius discussed lightning in their treatises on natural events, and Plutarch noted that sleeping persons, having no spirit of life, were immune to lightning strikes.[79,113]

In Chinese mythology the goddess of lightning, Tien Mu, used mirrors to direct bolts of lightning.[142] She was one of five deities of the "Ministry of Thunderstorms" of ancient Chinese religion. Lightning also played a role in Buddhist symbolism and demonstrated Buddha's power and omniscience.

Although lightning is most frequently rendered as fire, it has also been represented as stone axes hurled from the heavens. French peasants carry a *pierre do tonnerre,* or lightning stone, to ward off lightning strikes. The Yakuts of eastern Asia regard rounded stones found in fields hit by lightning as thunder axes and often use the powdered stones in medicines and potions. In Africa the Basuto tribe views lightning as the great thunderbird Umpundulo, flashing its wings in the clouds as it descends to Earth.

Incidence of Injury

An estimated 2000 thunderstorms occur worldwide at any moment,[174] and lightning strikes the earth more than 100 times/sec. Although lightning strikes humans only in a fraction of these storms, a measurable number of deaths occur every year, with an estimated 1000 fatalities worldwide.[8] However, there is evidence that the incidence may be decreasing, at least in the United States. In a 34-year period ending in 1974 there were 6928 deaths from lightning in the United States,[178] whereas in a 17-year survey ending in 1986 there were only 1916.[58] *Storm Data,* a publication of the National Oceanic and Atmospheric Administration, reported 2566 deaths and 6270 injuries for approximately the same period.[163]

The apparent decrease in fatalities may be a result of several factors.[87,105,112] Increasing urbanization of the population leads to fewer deaths, since city people are seldom hit (lightning is more likely to strike a tall, metal-reinforced building than a person), although at least one study shows a disproportionate increase in urban lightning injuries compared to the population.[112]

Another reason for the overall decrease may be effective education in lightning safety. Although some have said that the decrease in fatal incidents may be a result of improved medical care, namely emergency medical services and advanced cardiac life support (ACLS), most emergency physicians will remember that widespread paramedic units and ACLS training were not available until the 1970s. The reason also may be that there are fewer thunderstorms. Reports of thunderstorm day frequencies during the period between 1951 and 1970 are 10% to 30% below the 70-year average for the central and eastern United States, Japan, South Africa, and parts of southern Europe.[36]

The final reason the fatality rate may seem to be decreasing is that fatalities are reported and collected in a different way. In 1953 the Public Health Service reclassified the injuries attributed to lightning. It now separately categorizes deaths that are secondarily related to lightning, such as those from forest fires or building fires kindled by lightning. Because of this reclassification, few reliable figures are obtainable for injuries and deaths directly caused by lightning. Lopez and Holle[111] studied hospital records, coroner's reports, and *Storm Data* reports.[111] On comparing the records to their own scanning of Colorado's major newspapers, they found that lightning injuries and fatalities were underreported by official records.

Estimates for lightning fatalities range between 50 and 300 annually in the United States.[167,173,174,178,187] Until Hurricane Andrew and the 1993 Mississippi River flooding, lightning was responsible for more fatalities annually in the United States than any other natural disaster, including earthquakes, blizzards, tornadoes, hurricanes, and volcanic eruptions, second only to flash floods.[178]

In the past, farmers, sailors, and other people who worked outdoors in isolated areas were the most frequently injured. Since the 1950s there has been a steady decrease in the number of farmers injured, in part because of the population shift to urban areas and also because of the mechanization of farming, which enables fewer farmers to cultivate much larger areas and provides enclosed, more lightning-proof farm vehicles.[112] Although the proportion of victims who are hikers, campers, golfers, and others in the outdoors for recreational purposes has grown, there is still a large work-related component.[78,87,112,140] A Colorado study showed that nearly 25% of deaths and 29% of injuries from lightning occurred during employment activities, with an alarming increase since the mid-1980s.[112] This information is consistent with the same group's study of Florida, in which 38% of lightning deaths were related to employment activities and only 32% to recreational activities.[87]

A significant proportion of deaths occur in multiples. In 1976 Weigel reported that 70% of deaths from lightning occurred as singlets, 15% in groups of two, and 15% in groups of three or more.[178] In a recent study, done in Colorado for the period 1950 through 1991, 89% of lightning fatalities occurred as singlets, 10% as doubles, and 1% as three or more.[112]

As might be expected, lightning deaths occur more frequently during the daytime when people are more active and outdoors. Seventy percent occur between noon and 6 PM, 20% between 6 PM and midnight, 10% between 6 AM and noon, and less than 1% between midnight and 6 AM. The majority of injuries occur in the summer, when thunderstorms are most frequent.[112,178]

Although lightning may occur without rain, it does not exist without thunder. Therefore the number of thunderstorm days, while not directly correlated with lightning injuries, is still an important indicator of where lightning incidents are likely to occur.[115,173] Belts drawn across the United States according to thunderstorm days (Fig. 11-1) indicate that Florida has more thunderstorm days than any other region.[115] Thunderstorms occur five times more frequently over high mountains and large plateaus than over coasts, and in low-altitude marsh districts more often than in low-altitude dry areas.[85]

Because lightning injuries are prevalent in mountainous areas and around large bodies of water such as river basins, the states with the largest number of lightning injuries tend to be those of the South, Gulf Coast, and Rocky Mountain area and along the Ohio, Mississippi, and Hudson rivers. For some reason, however, the greatest number of fatalities occur in the mid-Atlantic states, whereas the greatest proportionate mortality occurs in Wyoming, New Mexico, Arkansas, Missouri, and Florida.[59]

Buildings' susceptibility to lightning strikes is relative to their size, height, nature of construction, and insulation.[91] However, more thickly settled residential areas are five times less likely to be struck by lightning than are rural areas.[91] People are better protected in the city, where high buildings have metal frames and lightning protection devices, so that comparatively few injuries are reported in large cities.[178] A significant proportion of injuries occur to persons who are inside their homes or places of employment, although they are much less likely to be fatal.[112]

Since the space shuttle was hit by lightning, the National Aeronautics and Space Administration (NASA) has become interested in lightning injuries and methods of protecting against lightning damage. When the current density above a storm-prone area is measured and indicates that a discharge is likely, a small rocket carrying a wire attached to a ground or an object to be studied is launched. When the electric field is disturbed, a lightning discharge is catalyzed and usually travels down the wire. Both direct and indirect measurements can be made on the triggered lightning bolt. Using the results of some of these studies, NASA is able to examine the electric field at ground level under a cloud region and predict the likelihood of a lightning stroke before a launch. In the United States lightning detection grids have made it easier for meteorologists and cloud physicists to study light-

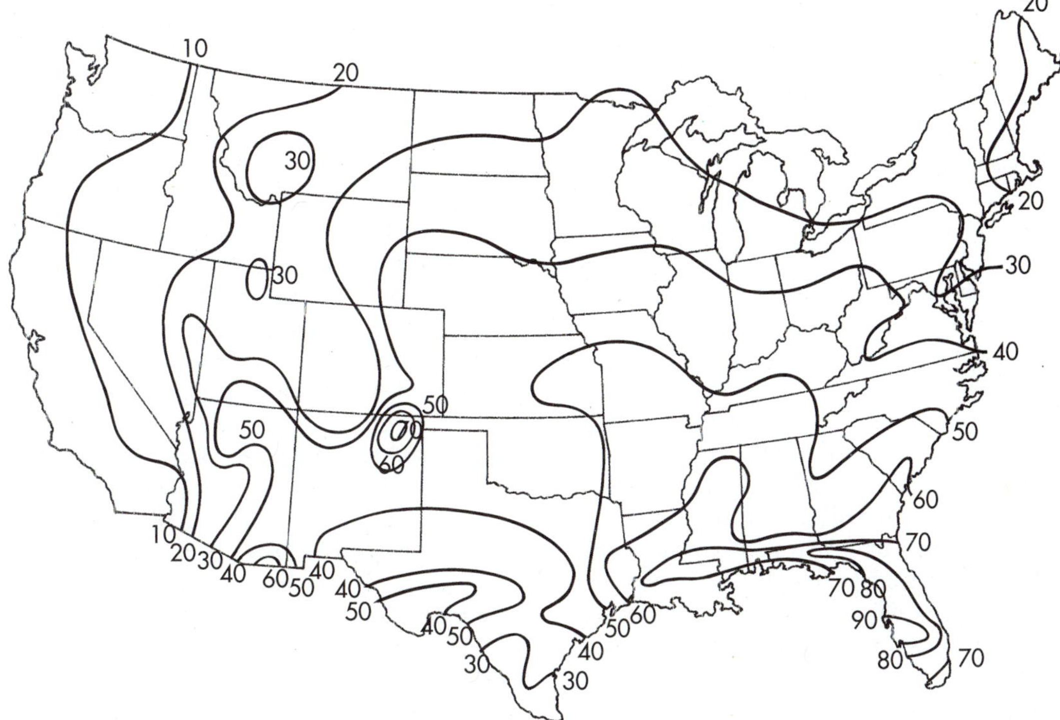

Fig. 11-1 Thunderstorm day map of the United States. (Modified from MacGorman DR, Rust WD: *Lightning strike density for the contiguous United States from thunderstorm duration records,* Pub No NUREG/CR03759, Washington, DC, 1984, Office of Nuclear Regulatory Research, U.S. Nuclear Regulatory Commission.)

ning and storms. Small hand-held lightning detection devices may soon be available at a reasonable cost and may decrease the incidence of lightning injuries at sporting and other recreational events.[170]

Myths and Superstitions

The Roman Pliny noted that a man who heard thunder was safe from the lightning stroke. In general this is true, since the light and strike precede the noise, depending on the distance from the lightning strike. However, some victims of direct hits report a sledgehammer-like effect of the force while seeing a bright light and occasionally hearing a loud noise.[161]

Many myths about lightning still persist today, including the notion that lightning strikes are invariable fatal. According to an American study of cases reported in the lightning literature since 1900, lightning strike carries a mortality of only 30%, and a morbidity of 70%.[44] A slightly different statistical interpretation of the same data yielded a mortality figure of 20%.[12-14] Since literature reports are usually biased toward the severe or interesting cases, a review of cases will tend to overestimate the mortality rate. In reality, mortality may be as low as 3% to 5%.

Generally only those who sustain immediate cardiopulmonary arrest die. Persons who are stunned or lose consciousness without cardiopulmonary arrest are highly unlikely to die, although they may still have serious sequelae.[44]

Most people know to seek shelter when storm clouds roll overhead. Few realize that one of the most dangerous times for a fatal strike is *before* the storm. Lightning may travel nearly horizontally as far as 10 km from the thunderhead and seem to occur "out of a clear blue sky," or at least when the day is still sunny. The faster the storm is traveling and the more violent it is, the more likely that a fatal strike will occur. Another time underestimated for the potential danger of lightning is the end of a thunderstorm, although injuries at this time are much more infrequent.

Most people believe that they are immune from lightning strikes if they are inside a building. Unfortunately, a significant proportion of injuries occur to persons who are in their homes or places of employment, especially if they are talking on the telephone.[6,11,112,148,184]

The "crispy critter" myth is the belief that the victim struck by lightning bursts into flames or is reduced to a pile of ashes. In reality, lightning often flashes over the outside of a victim, sometimes blowing off the clothes but leaving few external signs of injury and few if any burns.

Two other myths held by the public and many physicians are particularly harmful to lightning survivors: that "If you're not killed by lightning, you'll be OK," and "If there are no outward signs of lightning injury, the injury can't be serious." Medical literature, through lack of follow-up case reports, also implies that there are few permanent sequelae of lightning injury. However, in the last few years it has become apparent that permanent sequelae may occur. In addition, many lightning victims with significant sequelae had no evidence of burns acutely. Peripheral neuropathy and neuropsychologic symptoms, including severe memory difficulty, depression, and posttraumatic stress syndrome, may be debilitating.[47] Further study is needed to elucidate how malingerers may be distinguished from the many real victims of lightning injury.

Occasionally lighting victims show pathognomonic skin changes that are not true burns but have a fernlike pattern. At one time these patterns were thought to be imprints of the surrounding vegetation transferred onto the victim's skin by the lightning. Actually these fernlike patterns resemble fractals or the kind of pattern that can be obtained from placing a photographic plate in a strong electromagnetic field, which is what lightning produces for a short time around the victim.[86,169]

A myth still prevalent is that the lightning victim retains the charge and is dangerous to touch, since he or she is still "electrified." This myth has led to unnecessary deaths by delaying resuscitation efforts.

Medical literature and practice are plagued by myths that grew out of misread, misquoted, or misinterpreted data and continue to be propagated without further investigation. Not the least of these is the tenet that lightning victims who have resuscitation for several hours may still successfully recover. This belief seems to be grounded in the old idea of suspended animation—the concept that lightning is capable of shutting off systemic and cerebral metabolism, allowing rescuers a longer period in which to resuscitate the patient. This concept, credited to Taussig,[167] actually appeared some time before her article. In addition, the case recounted by Taussig that is the basis for this myth, when searched to its source, was a case report by Morikawa and Steichen.[127] The case does show a somewhat longer resuscitation period than usual, but not as miraculous as reported in Taussig's paper or as propagated in subsequent references to her paper.

In a study of lightning survivors, Andrews, Colquhoun, and Darveniza[7] have shown increasing prolongation of the QT interval, bringing up the theoretical possibility of torsades as a mechanism for the suspended animation reports. There is new evidence from animal experiments to support the teaching that respiratory arrest may persist longer than cardiac arrest.[5] This study, in which Australian sheep were hit with simulated lightning strokes, showed histologic evidence of greater damage to the respiratory centers than to the cardiac center in the fourth ventricle. Prolonged assisted ventilation *may* in some cases be successful after cardiac activity has returned.

Several booklets listing precautions for personal lightning protection appeared in the late 1700s and early 1800s.[123,131] One of the superstitions listed was that humans, by their presence, could attract lightning to a nearby object. A book of the times, *Catechism of Thunderstorms,* illustrated other myths.[101] Lightning was said to follow the draft of warm air behind a horse-drawn cart, so that coachmen were cautioned to walk their horses slowly through a storm.[161] Other precautions listed included seeking shelter away from tall trees and sheaves of corn if caught in the open and installing lightning rods for the protection of buildings and ships.

Historically, many remedies for resuscitation of lightning victims have been offered.[161] On July 15, 1889, Alfred West testified in a New York court that he was revived by "drawing out the electricity" when his feet were placed in warm water while his rescuer pulled on Mr. West's toes with one hand and milked a cow with the other.[23]

Other early attempts at resuscitation included friction to the bare skin, dousing the victim with a bucket of cold water, and chest compression.[161] An early attempt at cardiopulmonary resuscitation was given in 1807 when mouth-to-mouth ventilation was used for lightning victims and it was proposed that gentle electric shocks from galvanic batteries passed through the chest might be successful in resuscitating a victim of lightning.[31] Before that Benjamin Franklin had purposely electrocuted a chicken during a lightning experiment and reported successful resuscitation with mouth-to-beak ventilation.[74]

A myth in current treatment is that lightning injuries should be treated like other high-voltage electric injuries. Although lightning as an electric phenomenon follows the same laws of physics, the injuries seen with lightning are very different from high-voltage injuries and should be treated differently if iatrogenic morbidity and mortality are to be avoided.[45,46,48]

"Lightning never strikes the same place twice." In reality, the Empire State Building and the Sears Tower are hit thousands of times a year, as are mountaintops and radio-television antennas. If the circumstances facilitating the original lightning strike are still in effect in an area, the laws of nature will encourage further lightning strikes.

A common belief is that a person who is inside a building is safe from injury by lightning. Unfortunately, side flashes strike people through plumbing fixtures, telephones, and other appliances attached to the outside of the house by metal conductors.* Telephone companies include warnings in their directories against using telephones during thunderstorms. In addition, taking shelter in small sheds such as those on golf courses or hikers' lean-tos, especially above the tree level on a mountain, can be especially dangerous because lightning splashes onto the inhabitants.

*References 6, 49, 65, 91, 93, 103, 126, 139, 140, 152, 161.

Early Scientific Studies and Invention of the Lightning Rod

The study of electric phenomena is often traced to the publication of Gilbert's *De Magnete* in London in 1600. Experiments in France and Germany and by members of the Royal Society of London led to the invention of the Leyden jar in 1945.

Benjamin Franklin is generally regarded as the father of electric science and during his lifetime was known as the American Newton. Before his work it was thought that two distinct types of electric phenomena existed. Franklin's work unified these two forces, and he is responsible for renaming them as positive and negative charges.[74] He also proved with numerous experiments that lightning was an electric phenomenon and that thunderclouds are electrically charged, as demonstrated by the famous kite and key experiment.[73] He invented the lightning rod and announced its use in *Poor Richard's Almanack* in 1753:

> It has pleased God in his Goodness to Mankind, at length to discover to them the Means of securing their Habitation and other Buildings from Mischief by Thunder and Lightning. The Method is this: Provide a small Iron Rod (It may be made of the Rod-iron used by the Nailers) but of such a Length, that one End being three or four Feet in the moist Ground, the other may be six or eight Feet above the highest Part of the Building. To the upper End of the Rod fasten a Foot of brass Wire the Size of a common Knitting-needle, sharpened to a fine Point; the Rod may be secured to the House by a few small Staples. If the House or Barn be long, there may be a Rod and Point at each End, and a middling Wire along the Ridge from one to the other. A House thus furnished will not be damaged by Lightning, it being attracted to the Points, and passing thro the Metal into the Ground without hurting any Thing. Vessels also, having a sharp pointed rod fix'd on the Tops of their Masts, with a Wire from the Foot of the Rod reaching down, round one of the Shrouds, to the Water, will not be hurt by Lightning.

In the 1750s and 1760s the use of lightning rods became prevalent in the United States for the protection of both buildings and ships. Some scientists in Europe urged the installation of lightning rods on government buildings, churches, and other high buildings. However, religious advocates maintained that it would be blasphemy to install such devices on church steeples, since the churches received divine protection.[130] Because of this divine protection, some towns chose to store munitions in their churches, leading on more than one occasion to significant destruction and loss of life when the churches were hit by lightning.

Part of the delay in installing lightning rods in England may have been due to British distrust of the scientific theories of the upstart, newly independent United States. Years and numerous unsuccessful trials with English designs were required before the Franklin rod became accepted on Her Majesty's ships and buildings.[31]

At one time lightning rods were theorized to be diffusers of electric charges and could neutralize a storm cloud passing overhead, thus averting a lightning stroke.[161] This theory was in part an outgrowth of the observation of St. Elmo's fire, an aura appearing around the tip of lightning rods and ships' masts during a thunderstorm. This phenomenon is caused by the electron discharge that results from the strong electromagnetic field induced around the glowing object. Properly installed lightning rods have been shown to protect a building from damage by allowing the current to flow harmlessly to the ground, and to not attract lightning or diffuse the charge.[80]

The first Lightning Rod Conference was held in London in 1882. Recommendations from this conference were published that year and again in 1905. Further progress in the study of the properties of lightning came with the technical development of Sir Charles Vernon Boy's rotating camera and Dufour's high-speed cathode ray oscillograph, which helped to delineate physical properties of lightning, including the direction and speed of the strokes.

Various countries developed codes of practice for lightning protection (Germany 1924, United States 1929, Britain 1943, British colonies 1965). A variety of materials, including copper, aluminum, and iron, are recommended by these codes, which also specify the measurements and construction of the protective system, depending on the height, location, and construction of the structure to be protected.

Lightning strokes vary in power and frequency, depending on the terrain and geographic location. Complicated formulas have been devised to take into account the relative frequency of strikes in an area; the height, construction, and design of the building; and the degree of protection desirable, depending on whether it is a storage shed, house, school, hospital, or munitions factory.

A lightning protection system should be designed to take into account these factors plus the economic considerations of construction. Including a system in the initial design and construction is always easier and less expensive than modifying a completed building. In addition, except where prohibited by code, the owner may decide that a lightning protection system is not worth the expense, for example, for a mountain retreat that is seldom visited. For the design of a lightning protection system the reader is referred to five excellent references[29,79,80,116,175] and the Lightning Protection Institute, 3365 North Arlington Heights Road, Suite J, Arlington Heights, IL 60004, 800-488-6864.

Physics of Lightning Stroke

LIGHTNING DISCHARGE*

The study of lightning discharge and formation involves an entire branch of physics and meteorology and is extremely complex. We therefore illustrate here the simplified

*References 34, 78-80, 122, 173, 174, 178.

and most common mechanism of thundercloud formation and lightning strike.

Warm air can hold more moisture than cool air, so when a cold air front (high-pressure system) moves to a warm area (low-pressure system), the warm, moist, low-pressure air rises quickly through the cool, drier, high-pressure air (Fig. 11-2, *A*). As the warm air rises, the moisture condenses into water droplets and a cumulonimbus cloud is formed. As the water vapor condenses, the energy of condensation (or vaporization) is released and the cloud accumulates free energy. Sometimes the rising hot air overshoots the cloud and is picked up by the strong winds of the upper atmosphere, flattening out into the typical anvil-shaped thundercloud (Fig. 11-2, *B*).[79,147,173,174]

As the warm air rises, turbulence and induced friction cause complex redistribution of charges within the cloud (Fig. 11-2, *C*). Water droplets within the cloud acquire and increase their individual charges. A complex layering of charges, with large potential differences between the layers, results from the interaction between charged particles and internal and external electrical fields within the cloud .

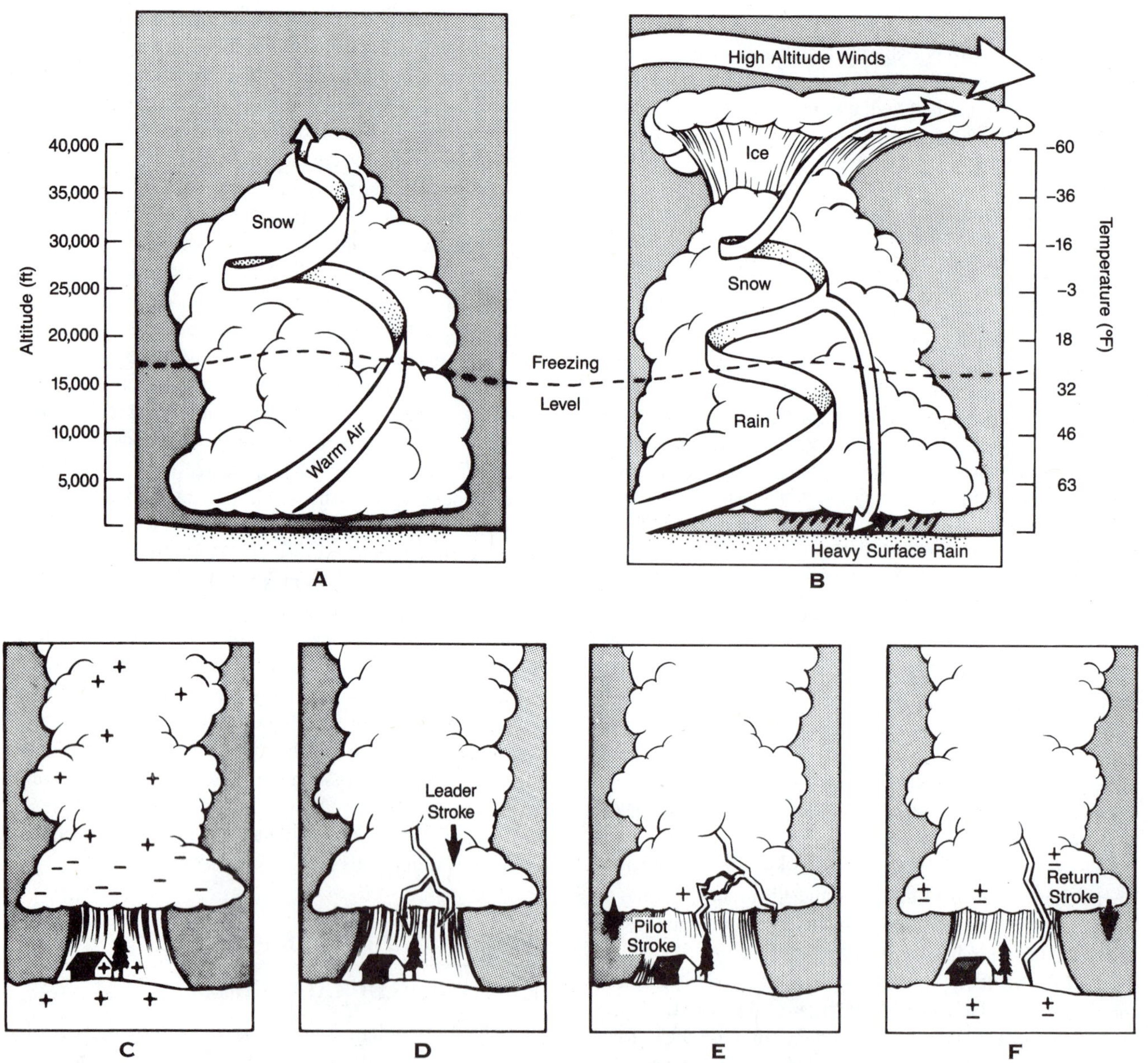

Fig. 11-2 **A,** Warm, low-pressure air rises and condenses into a cumulonimbus cloud. **B,** Typical anvil-shaped thundercloud. **C,** Water droplets within the cloud accumulate and layer charges. **D,** Relatively weak and slow stepped leader initiates the lightning strike. **E,** Positive pilot streamer rises from the ground to meet the stepped leader. **F,** Return stroke rushes from the ground to the cloud.

Generally lower layers of the thundercloud become negatively charged relative to the earth, particularly when the storm occurs over a flat plane. The earth, which normally is negatively charged relative to the atmosphere, has a strong positive charge induced as the negatively charged thunderhead passes overhead. The induced positive charge tends to flow as an upward current into trees, tall buildings, or people in the area of the thunderstorm cloud.

Normally, discharge of the potential difference is discouraged by the strong insulatory nature of air. However, when the potential difference between charges within the clouds or between the thundercloud and ground becomes sufficient, the charge may be dissipated as lightning.

A lightning stroke begins as a relatively weak and slow stepped leader from the cloud (Fig. 11-2, *D*). Although the tip of the leader may be luminous, the stepped leader itself is barely discernible with the unassisted eye. It travels with relatively short branched steps and forks ranging from 10 to 200 m in length. The leader travels at about one-third the speed of light (1×10^8 m/sec), and the potential difference between the tip and the earth ranges from 10 to 200 million volts. The leader ionizes a pathway that contains superheated ions, both positive and negative, thus forming a plasma column of very low resistance.

As the stepped leader progresses closer to earth with the large potential at its tip, more concentrated areas of induced charge build up on earth—particularly at the peaks of tall, relatively sharp objects. Several pilot streamers (Fig. 11-2, *E*) may rise vertically toward the stepped leader head. Ultimately one, or a small number, of the pilot streamers will contact the stepped leader head, thus completing a lightning channel of low resistance between cloud and ground. The stepped leader is said to "attach" to an object, and the process of joining is called attachment. As the low-resistance channel is formed by attachment, the potential difference between cloud and ground effectively disappears and the energy available is dissipated in an avalanche of charge between cloud and ground. This avalanche is referred to as the return stroke (Fig. 11-2, *F*) and is highly luminous. Subsequent to the discharge through the return stroke, the channel remains attached for a small amount of time, and with quick redistribution of charge from other regions of the cloud to the top of the channel (via J- and K- intracloud streamers), further return strokes may occur. Thus a lightning flash may be made up of multiple strokes (1 to 30, mean 4 to 5), and this causes a lightning flash to seem to flicker.

When a very tall building, such as the Empire State Building, is involved, or when high mountains rise into the clouds, the leader stroke may initiate from the building or mountain rather than from the cloud. In these cases a pilot stroke is rarely seen initiating from the cloud. The channel of ions that is formed by the leader stroke is maintained as a continuous stroke as the return stroke (misnamed in this instance) travels in the same direction from the ground or object to the cloud, dissipating the charge difference.

The tip of the stepped leader stroke is the most luminous of the sequence of strokes in each lightning discharge, since a huge amount of energy must be expended to overcome air resistance and ionize a channel. Because of the relative slowness and brilliance of the leader, lightning is perceived as traveling from the cloud to the earth, although the vast majority of energy is actually dissipated in the opposite direction with the return strokes. The direction of the return stroke is not visually perceived because of its tremendous speed and is recognized merely as an instantaneous brightening or flickering of the ionized pathway. Lightning may vary in color, either from the excitation of nitrogen atoms in the atmosphere (radiant light energy released as a bluish or reddish afterglow), or because the particles of dust through which the lightning passes are high in ion or mineral content (for example, smog, mining dust high in coal or iron content).[161]

DIAMETER AND TEMPERATURE OF LIGHTNING[79]

Many techniques could be used to measure the diameter or temperature of the lightning stroke. Unfortunately, all of the measurement techniques have artifact problems. Visual measurement of the stroke, using standard photography, usually shows the diameter of the main body of the stroke to be about 6 to 8 cm.

The diameter of the arc channel is sometimes measured indirectly, using measurements of holes and strips of damage that lightning produces when it hits aluminum airplane wings, buildings, or trees. Measurements vary from 0.003 to 8.0 cm, depending on the material destroyed, with hard metallic structures sustaining smaller punctures than relatively softer objects, such as trees. The ionized sheath around the tip of the bright leader stroke has never been measured but is estimated to be 3 to 20 m in diameter.

The temperature of the lightning stroke varies with the diameter of the stroke and has been calculated to be about 8000° C. Others estimate the temperature to be as high as 50,000° C. In a few milliseconds the temperature falls to 2000° to 3000° C, that of a normal high-voltage electric arc.

FORMS OF LIGHTNING[173]

Lightning occurs in many forms. As described previously, the most common is streak lightning (Fig. 11-3). Sheet lightning is a shapeless flash of light that represents lightning discharges within and between clouds. Sheet lightning may also be seen when lightning occurs over the horizon. Ribbon lightning is streak lightning driven by winds of the thunderstorm; the ionized air channel moves so rapidly across the earth that the successive secondary or return strokes seem to parallel one another. Bead lightning occurs

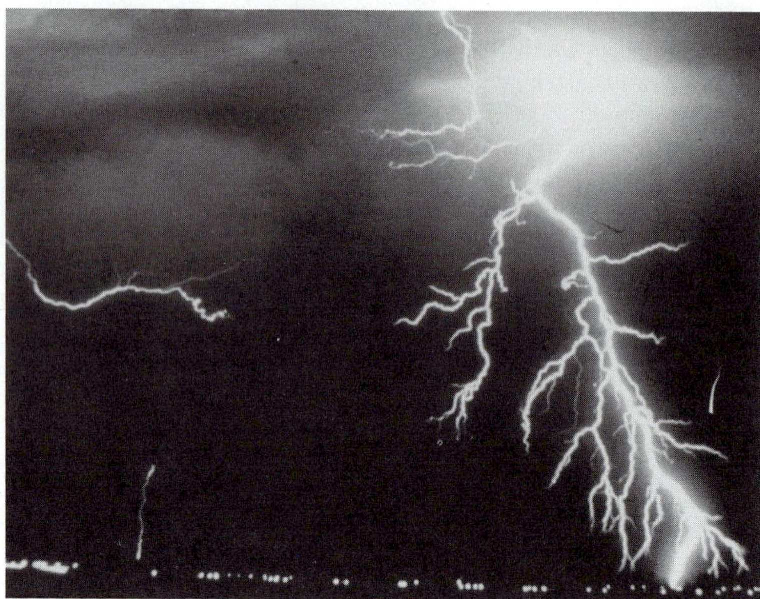

Fig. 11-3 Example of classic streak lightning.

when different areas of ionization and charge persist, lending a beadlike appearance to the afterstrokes. Another possible explanation of bead lightning may be perception of the bright end-on appearance of portions of a very jagged stroke.

The most unusual, least understood, and least predictable type of lightning is ball lightning. Taking the form of a softball-sized globe, ball lightning may enter a door of a house, travel down a hallway and out another door, or exhibit equally bizarre and inexplicable activity.[8,31,155]

Lightning may be either positive or negative in charge. Negative lightning is the more common. Positive lightning tends to occur during the winter, at the beginning of very violent thunderstorms, and with tornadoes and may have a very different injury profile from negative lightning. Unfortunately, not enough study has been made to develop any further medical characterizations.

THUNDER

There are two theories of thunder production. The first attributes thunder to shock waves resulting from the almost explosive expansion of air heated and ionized by the lightning stroke.[79,173,174] The second theory, less likely to be true, states that the superheated channel of ions cools rapidly and creates a vacuum. The thunderclap is produced when air rushes back into the vacuum.

A review of the facts and myths about thunder has led to several accepted statements[147]:

1. Cloud to ground lightning flashes produce the loudest thunder.
2. Thunder is seldom heard over distances greater than 10 miles.
3. The time interval between the perception of lightning and the first sound of thunder can be used to estimate the distance of the lightning stroke.
4. Atmospheric turbulence reduces the audibility of the thunder.
5. A heavy downpour of rain often immediately follows a strong clap of thunder.
6. The intensity of a pattern of thunder in one geographic location appears different from the pattern in another location.
7. The pitch of thunder deepens as the rumble persists.

The thunder clap from a lightning bolt that is close by is heard as a sharp crack. Distant thunder rumbles as the sound waves are refracted and modified by the thunderstorm's turbulence.[22] Using the difference in speeds between light and sound gives an estimate of the distance to the lightning stroke. To obtain the approximate distance to the flash in miles, a person can take the difference in seconds between the perception of the flash and the rumble and divide by five.

Mechanisms of Injury by Lightning[45]

Lightning is directly dangerous for four reasons: high voltage, secondary heat production, electromagnetic cellular effects, and explosive force. In addition, lightning may injure indirectly by kindling forest fires, house fires, and explosions or by dropping objects such as trees on occupied homes and automobiles.

Only injuries that are directly caused by lightning are discussed here. There are five primary mechanisms of injury: direct hit, splash, contact, step voltage, and blunt trauma.[46]

A direct strike is most likely to hit a person in the open who has been unable to find shelter. Any conductor that the victim carries, particularly if it is metal and carried above shoulder level, significantly increases the chances of a direct hit.[60,134,158]

A more frequent cause of injury is a splash. Splash injuries occur when lightning that has hit a tree or building splashes onto a victim who may have found shelter nearby.* The current, seeking the path of least resistance, may jump to a person whose body has less resistance than the tree or object that the lightning had initially contacted. There are multiple reports of side flashes indoors from metal objects, including plumbing and telephones.† Splashes may also occur from person to person when several people are standing close together.[16,27,98,114] On occasion, splashes occur from a fence or other long conductive object that was hit by lightning some distance away. Frequently groups of animals have been killed as they stood near a fence or sought shelter under trees.[78]

Contact injury occurs when the person is holding onto an object that is either directly hit or splashed by lightning.

Step voltage, also called stride voltage and ground current, is produced when lightning hits the ground or an object nearby.[21,23] The current spreads like a wave in a pond, diminishing as the radius from the strike increases. Contrary to the public's belief that the ground is a good "ground" (a good absorber of electrical energy), in reality electricity is difficult to pump into the ground. As a result, resistance to the flow of current is often greater in the ground than between the victim's feet, so if the victim's feet are at different distances from the origin of the strike, a large potential difference may exist between them. As a result, a current may preferentially pass up and through the lower resistance circuit made by the victim's legs and body rather than stay in the ground. Swimmers may also be affected by this mechanism as the current passes through them in the water.

Although ground current is less likely to produce fatalities than are direct hits or splashes, multiple victims and injuries are frequent. Large groups have been injured on baseball fields, at racetracks, while hiking, or during military maneuvers.‡

Persons who are not affected by the prior four mechanisms may nevertheless be injured by the explosive force of the shock wave produced as lightning hits nearby. It is not uncommon for a victim to be thrown by opisthotonic contractions initiated by the lightning strike. In addition, some have theorized that the person who is struck by lightning may suffer from explosive and implosive forces created by the thunderclap with resulting contusions and pressure injuries, including ruptured tympanic membranes.

*References 43, 53, 54, 60, 78, 157, 158, 161.
†References 49, 65, 91, 93, 103, 126, 139, 140, 152, 161.
‡References 19, 31, 56, 57, 98, 100, 129, 130.

Pathophysiology of Lightning Injury[45,46]

It is necessary to distinguish between lightning and generator-produced high-voltage electrical injuries, since there are significant differences between the mechanisms of injuries and their treatment. Although lightning is an electrical phenomenon and is governed by the laws of physics, it accounts for a unique spectrum of induced diseases that are best understood in light of specific physical properties of lightning.

Kouwenhoven determined six factors that affect the type and severity of injury encountered with electrical accidents (see Box 11-1): type of circuit, duration of exposure, voltage, amperage, resistance of the tissues, and pathway of the current.[89] The factor that seems most important in distinguishing lightning from high-voltage electric injuries is the duration of exposure to the current.

TYPE OF CIRCUIT

Lightning is neither a direct current nor an alternating current. At best, lightning is a unidirectional massive current impulse. The cloud to ground impulse results from the breakdown of a large electric field between cloud and ground, measured in millions of volts. Once connection is made with the ground, the voltage difference between cloud and ground disappears and a large current flows impulsively in a very short time. The study of such massive discharges of such short duration, particularly their effects on the human body, is not well advanced. Lightning is said to be a "current" phenomenon rather than a "voltage" phenomenon.

VOLTAGE, AMPERAGE, AND RESISTANCE

Lightning, being a current phenomenon, is not easily thought of in terms of classic Ohm's Law ($V = I \times R$) and

BOX 11-1

FACTORS AFFECTING SEVERITY OF ELECTRICAL BURNS

AC versus DC
Voltage
Amperage
Resistance
Pathway
Duration

power calculation (P = V × I) terms. This is because the voltage between cloud and ground disappears after lightning attachment occurs. The particular voltage being examined in these equations is unclear. Thus we must resort to alternative formulations of the equations.

The energy dissipated in a given tissue is determined by the current flowing through the tissue, and its resistance, by:

$$\text{Energy (heat)} = \text{Current}^2 \times \text{Resistance} \times \text{Time}$$

where a current flows through a resistance for time t.

As resistance goes up, so does the heat generated by passage of the current. In humans when low energy levels are encountered, much of the electric energy may be dissipated by the skin, so that superficial burns are often not accompanied by internal injuries.

Although lightning occasionally shows discrete entry and exit wounds, these are rare. Lightning more commonly causes only superficial streaking burns. The exception to this is when hot lightning occurs. Hot lightning is a prolonged stroke lasting up to 0.5 second and delivering a tremendous amount of energy, capable of exploding trees, setting fires, and acting like high-voltage electricity to produce injuries. Other factors not understood may contribute to the formation of deep burns, although deep burns similar to those of high-voltage electric injuries generally are rare with lightning.

PATHWAY, DURATION OF CURRENT, AND FLASHOVER EFFECT

The pathway of current through and over the body, the latter referred to as flashover, has been a matter of speculation.[88,132] Current has been thought to travel only in a sheet over the body surface. It has been found that in cranial lightning strike, flashover does indeed occur. However, a portion of the current may enter the cranial orifices—eyes, ears, nose, and mouth.[5,10] The entry of current would help to explain the myriad eye and ear symptoms that have been reported with lightning injury.

Andrews[5] further examined the functional consequences on cardiorespiratory function and concluded that the entry of current into the cranial orifices leads to the passage of current directly to the brainstem. In his study done on sheep, Andrews was able to demonstrate specific damage to neurons at the floor of the fourth ventricle in the location of the medullary cardiorespiratory control centers. From there it is

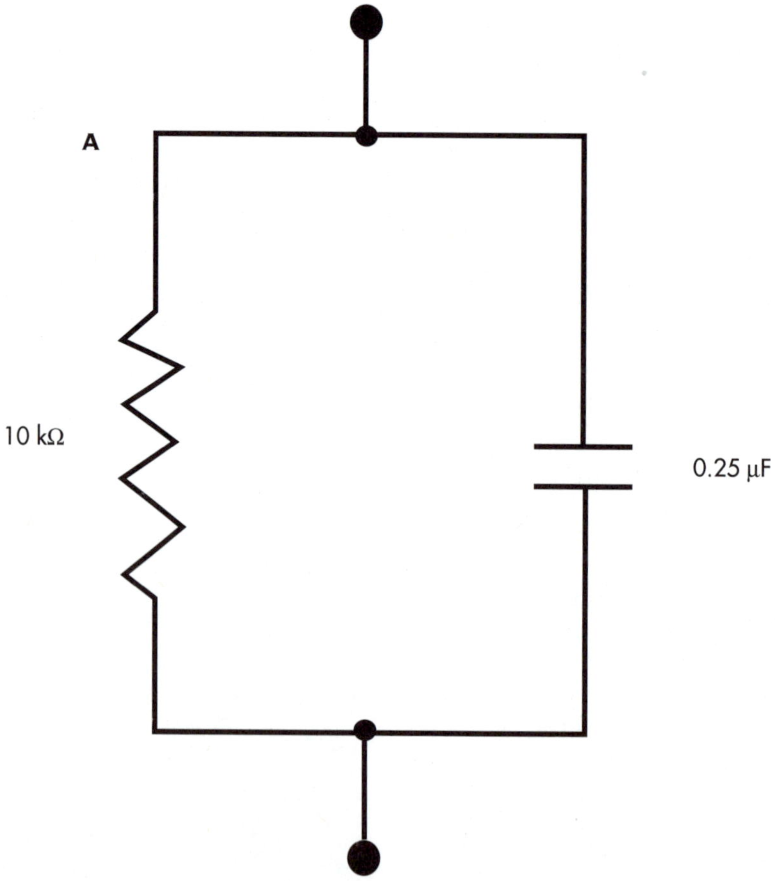

Fig. 11-4 **A,** Electrical model for human skin impedance.

postulated that current travels caudad via cerebrospinal fluid (CSF) and blood vessel pathways to impinge directly on the myocardium. Andrews[5] also showed histologic damage to the myocardium that is consistent with a number of autopsy reports of inferior myocardial necrosis.[102,114,118,129]

Mathematical modeling has been done of lightning strike to the human body.[5,8] Certain assumptions are made in any model, usually based on principles accepted in the literature.[24,26,107] Fig. 11-4, *A*, shows a model for skin resistance, and its connection to the internal body milieu is shown in Fig. 11-4, *B*. It will be noted that the internal body structures are regarded as purely resistive, whereas the skin contains significant elements of capacitance.[24,26,107]

The sequence of events during the strike started with the postulate that the stroke attached initially to the head of the victim. For a small fraction of time current flowed internally as the skin capacitance elements charged. At a voltage taken as 5 kV, the skin was assumed to break down. It is worth noting in the context of time scale that a lightning stroke is

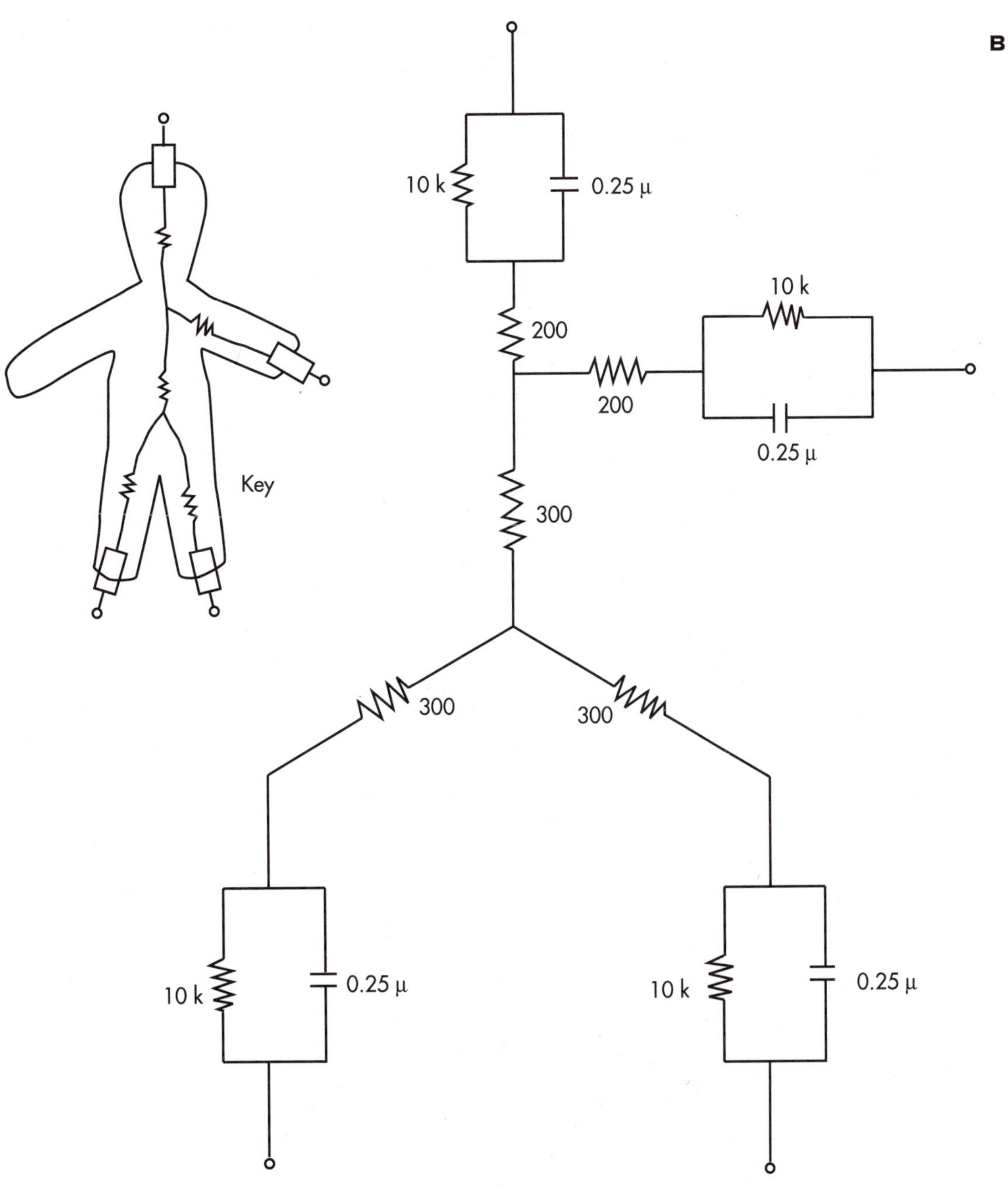

Fig. 11-4, cont'd. B, Model of human body for the purposes of examination of currents flowing during lightning strike.

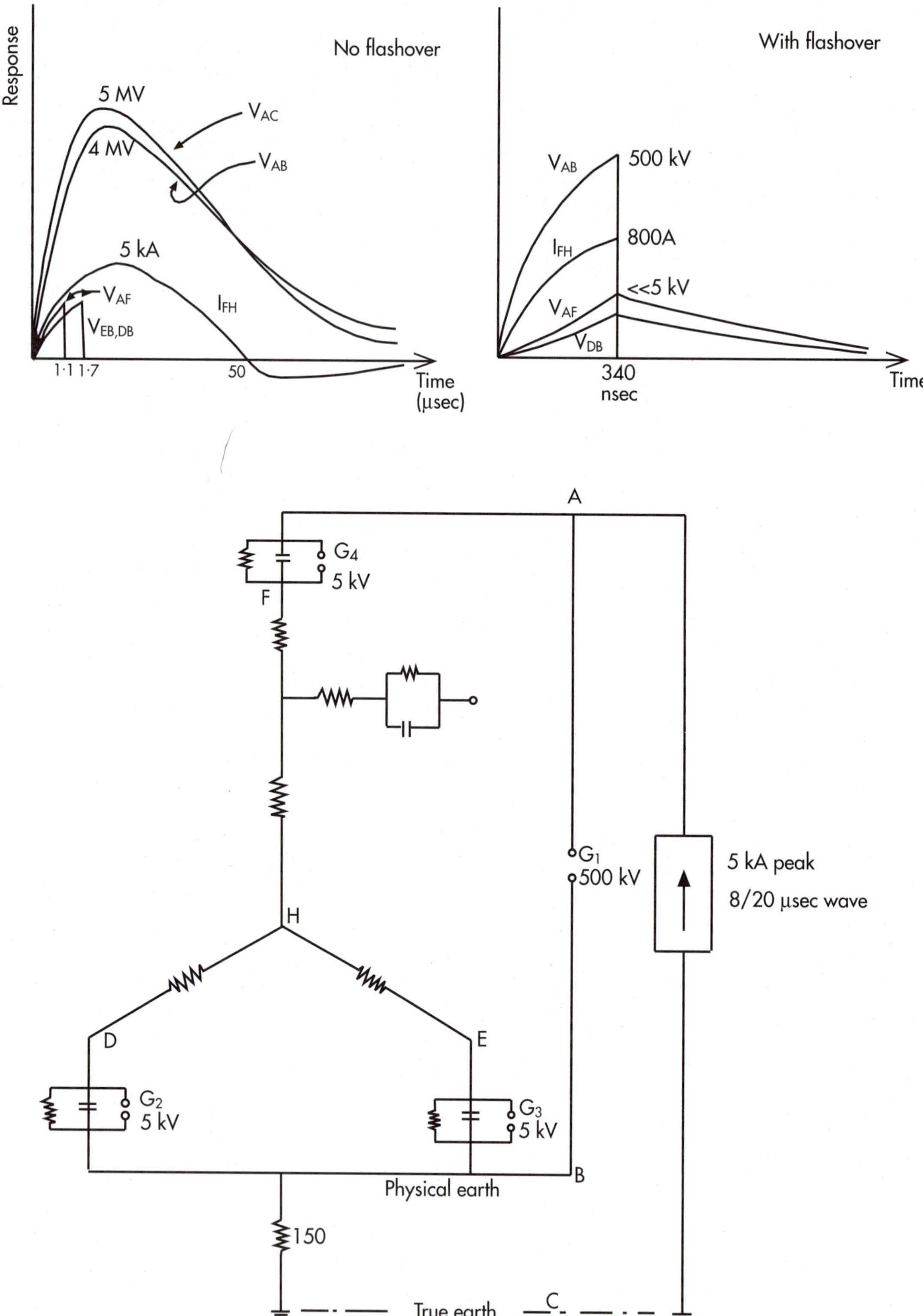

Fig. 11-5 Model of human body adapted for the circumstance of direct lightning strike. Responses of the body model are shown for cases of direct strike with and without subsequent flashover.

modeled as a current wave building to a maximum value in around 8 μsec. On the time scale found by others, this is the most likely course. Once the internal current increased, the voltage across the body to earth built up, and external flashover across the body occurred when the field reached the breakdown strength of air.

The results of mathematical modeling of these events are shown in Fig. 11-5, and the relative magnitudes of the various voltage components can be seen with their time scale. On this time scale the times to breakdown are short and most events occur early in the course of the stroke.

In summary, lightning applies a current to the human body. This current initially is transmitted internally, following which skin breaks down. Ultimately, external flashover occurs. Andrews[5] draws support for this model from measurements made in the experimental application of lightning impulses to Australian sheep. Further modeling of step voltage injury verified that for the erect human, this mechanism is less dangerous than is a direct strike.

Experimental evidence suggests that "a fast flashover appreciably diminishes the energy dissipation within the body and results in survival."[132] In addition, Ishikawa obtained experimental results with rabbits that are similar to the human data found by Cooper's study.[44,88,89]

As current flashes over the outside of the body, it may vaporize moisture on the skin and blast apart clothes and shoes, leaving the victim nearly naked, as noted by Hegner[85] in 1917:

> The clothing may not be affected in any way. It may be stripped or burned in part or entirely shredded to ribbons. Either warp or woof may be destroyed leaving the outer garments and the skin intact. . . . Metallic objects in or on the clothing are bent, broken, more or less fused or not affected. The shoes most constantly show the effects of the current. People are usually standing when struck, the current then enters or leaves the body through the feet [sic]. The shoes, especially when dry or only partially damp, interpose a substance of increased resistance. One or both shoes may be affected. They may be gently removed, or violently thrown many feet, be punctured or have a large hole torn in any part, shredded, split, reduced to lint or disappear entirely. The soles may disappear with or without the heels. Any of the foregoing may occur and the person not injured or only slightly shocked.

The amount of damage to the clothing or to the surface of the body is not an index to the severity of the injuries sustained within the body. Either may be disproportionately great or small.

BEHAVIOR OF CURRENT IN TISSUE

Electric current may be carried through tissue in a direct conduction fashion, obeying simple linear equations such as Ohm's Law. The result is heating of tissues under Joule's Law, with thermally induced cellular death and dysfunction. In addition, wherever there is an electric current, there is a magnetic field induced that may have as yet unexplained effects on body functions. The simple passage of current may interfere with neural and muscular function.[107]

Earlier in this century, electric injury was thought to occur not only because of thermal effects, but also because of some mysterious cellular effects.[21,23,92] Unfortunately, the technology was not available to investigate these effects and this idea was largely forgotten. In the last few years the theory of electroporation has been proposed. Cell wall integrity, enzyme reactions, protein shape and structure, and cell membrane "gates" and pumps operate by changes on the order of microvolts. It is not beyond the realm of imagination that passage of an electric current too small to produce significant thermal damage still may cause irreversible changes in these functions, leading to cell death or dysfunction.[107] Induction of electric charges by external electromagnetic fields also may be strong enough to produce noticeable effects in as yet unknown ways.

Injuries from Lightning

SEVERITY OF INJURY

Some of the most common signs and symptoms are listed in Box 11-2. Lightning is almost instantaneous in its action, difficult to report accurately, and seemingly unpredictable in its physical effects. Each case report of lightning injury has unique characteristics,[77] and symptoms may vary from trivial to fatal. For prognostic reasons victims generally can be placed in one of three groups.[45]

Minor Injury

These patients are awake and may report dysesthesia in the affected extremity from a lightning splash or in more serious strokes may report a feeling of having been hit on the

BOX 11-2

LIGHTNING INJURIES

IMMEDIATE

Ventricular asystole
Neurologic signs
- Seizures
- Deafness
- Confusion, amnesia
- Blindness

Contusion from shock wave
Chest pain, muscle aches
Tympanic membrane rupture

DELAYED

Dysesthesias, peripheral neuropathy
Neuropsychologic changes

head or having been in an explosion. They may or may not have perceived the lightning or thunder. They often suffer confusion, amnesia, temporary deafness or blindness, or temporary unconsciousness at the scene.[31] They seldom demonstrate any cutaneous burns or paralysis but may complain of paresthesias, muscular pain, confusion, and amnesia lasting from hours to days. Patients often have at least one tympanic membrane ruptured as a result of the explosive force of the lightning shock wave. Vital signs are usually stable, although occasional patients demonstrate transient mild hypertension.[82,167] Recovery is usually gradual and complete.

Moderate Injury

Moderately injured patients may be disoriented, combative, or comatose. They frequently exhibit motor paralysis, particularly of the lower extremities, with mottling of the skin and diminished or absent pulses.[52] Nonpalpable peripheral pulses may indicate arterial spasm[52] and sympathetic instability and should be differentiated from hypotension. However, if true hypotension occurs and persists, the patient should be scrutinized for fractures and other signs of blunt injury. Spinal shock from cervical or other spinal fractures, although rare with lightning, also may account for hypotension.

Occasionally these victims have suffered temporary cardiopulmonary standstill, although it is seldom documented.[161] Spontaneous recovery of the pulse is attributed to the heart's inherent automaticity. However, respiratory arrest that often occurs with lightning injury may be prolonged and lead to secondary cardiac arrest from hypoxia. Seizures may also occur.

First- and second-degree burns not prominent on admission may evolve over the first several hours. Rarely, third-degree burns may occur. Tympanic membrane rupture should be anticipated[44] and, along with hemotympanum, may indicate a basilar skull fracture.

Whereas the clinical condition often improves within the first few hours, patients are prone to have permanent sequelae such as sleep disorders, irritability, difficulty with fine psychomotor functions, paresthesias, generalized weakness, sympathetic nervous system dysfunction, and sometimes posttraumatic stress syndrome. A few cases of atrophic spinal paralysis have been reported.[27]

Severe Injury

Patients with severe injury may be in cardiac arrest with either ventricular standstill or fibrillation when first examined. Cardiac resuscitation may not be successful if the patient has suffered a prolonged period of cardiac and central nervous system (CNS) ischemia. Direct brain damage may occur from the lightning strike or blast effect. Tympanic membrane rupture with hemotympanum and cerebrospinal fluid (CSF) otorrhea is common in this group.

Patients with other signs of blunt trauma are likely to be victims of direct hits, although sometimes no burns are noted.

The prognosis is usually poor in the severely injured group because of direct lightning damage, often complicated by a delay in cardiopulmonary resuscitation.

DIFFERENCES BETWEEN INJURIES FROM HIGH-VOLTAGE ELECTRICITY AND LIGHTNING[8,45,46,48]

There are marked differences in injuries caused by high-voltage electric accidents and lightning (Table 11-1). Lightning contact with the body is almost instantaneous, often leading to flashover. Exposure to high-voltage electricity tends to be more prolonged because the victim freezes to the circuit. With skin breakdown, electric energy surges through the tissues with little resistance to flow, causing massive internal thermal injury that sometimes necessitates major amputations. Myoglobin release may be pronounced, and renal failure may occur. In addition, compartment syndromes requiring fasciotomy may occur. This is not the case with lightning injuries, in which fluid restriction and expectant care are usually the rule.

CARDIOPULMONARY ARREST

The most common cause of death in a lightning victim is cardiopulmonary arrest. In fact, a victim is highly unlikely

Table 11-1 Lightning Injuries

Factor	Lightning	High Voltage
Energy level	30 million volts, 50,000 amperes	Usually much lower
Time of exposure	Brief, instantaneous	Prolonged
Pathway	Flashover, orifice	Deep, internal
Burns	Superficial, minor	Deep, major injury
Cardiac	Primary and secondary arrest, asystole	Fibrillation
Renal	Rare myoglobinuria or hemoglobinuria	Myoglobinuric renal failure common
Fasciotomy	Rarely if ever necessary	Common, early, and extensive
Blunt injury	Explosive thunder effect	Falls, being thrown

(*p* <.0001) to die unless cardiopulmonary arrest is suffered as an immediate effect of the strike.[44] In the past, nearly 75% of those who suffered cardiopulmonary arrest from lightning injuries died, many because cardiopulmonary resuscitation was not attempted.

Cardiopulmonary arrest from lightning had previously been hypothesized and was recently confirmed to involve both a primary and a secondary arrest.[4,5,10,144,167] Injury first occurs with an immediate asystolic cardiac arrest and respiratory standstill. Because of the heart's automaticity, an organized series of contractions generally resumes within a short time.

Unfortunately, respiratory arrest caused by paralysis of the medullary respiratory center may last far longer than cardiac arrest. Unless the victim receives immediate ventilatory assistance, attendant hypoxia may induce arrhythmias and secondary cardiac arrest.

The course has been verified experimentally in sheep, with initial asystole, followed by resumption of a short run of bradycardia, then tachycardia, followed by an eventual blocks or bradycardia, and finally a second asystolic arrest.[5] Fig. 11-6 shows the result on respiratory rhythm of an impulse applied to the cranium of a sheep. An initial muscle spasm is seen, followed by cessation of natural rhythm. Fig. 11-7 shows the progress of myocardial activity of another sheep from impulse through asystole to secondary arrest.

Both asystole and ventricular fibrillation[102] have been reported with lightning strike. As noted in the animal work, asystole seems to be both the first and last response to the strike, as the secondary arrest rhythm of fibrillation deteriorates.[5] Premature ventricular contractions, ventricular tachycardia, and atrial fibrillation have been reported.[3,15,100,126,185]

It is not uncommon to find electrocardiographic (ECG) ST changes consistent with ischemia and damage in subepicardial, posterior, inferior, or anterior patterns.* Creatine phosphokinase MB isoenzyme elevation has been reported.[83,90,97,125,164] Elevation of serum glutamic oxaloacetic transaminase and lactic dehydrogenase has been

*References 3, 28, 61, 64, 66, 82, 90, 97, 98, 102, 110, 125, 129, 156, 164, 165, 167, 186.

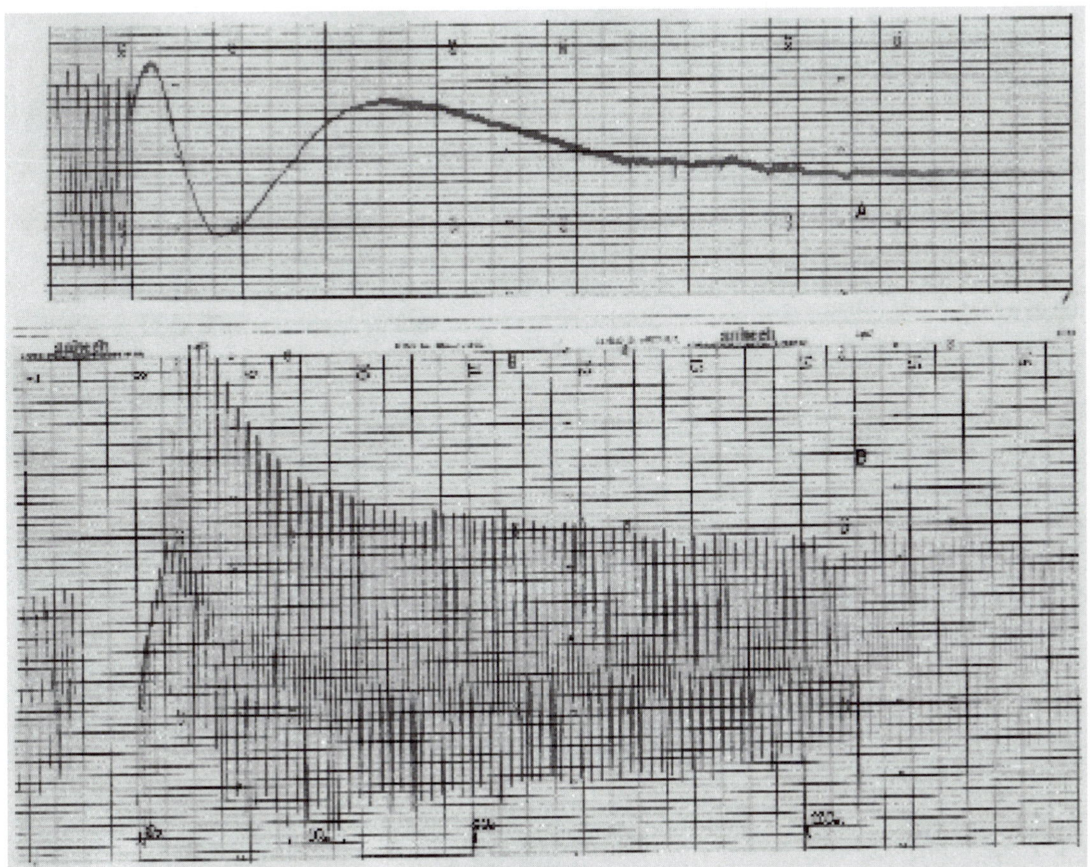

Fig. 11-6 Respiratory activity tracing in sheep struck by laboratory-generated lightning. *Top,* Where respiratory arrest did not occur. *Bottom,* Where respiratory muscle spasm occurred followed by respiratory arrest.

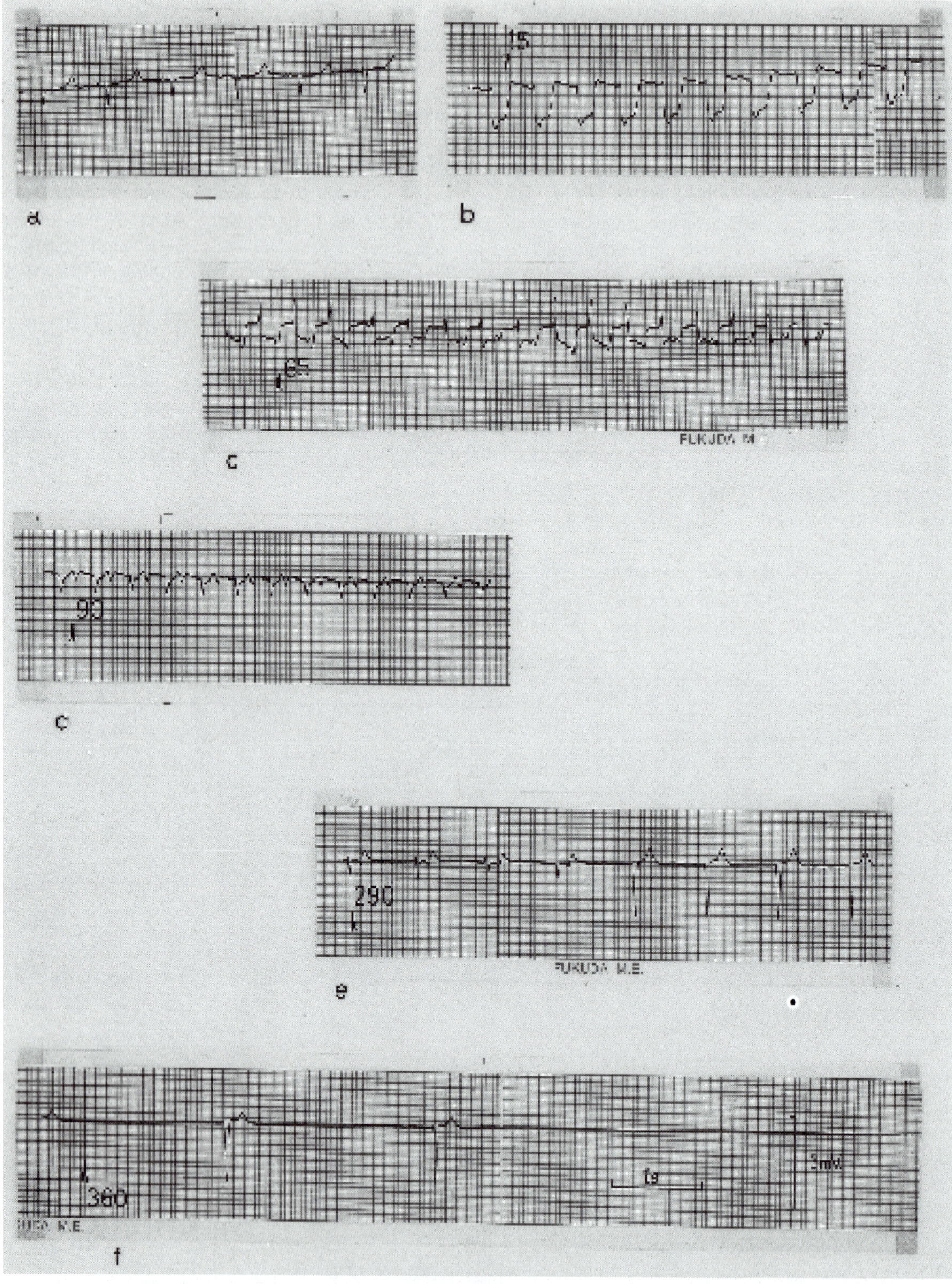

Fig. 11-7 Cardiac response in sheep (nonstandard leads) subjected to laboratory-generated lightning strike. **A,** Baseline. **B,** Initial morphology change, followed by, **C** to **E,** normalization of morphology, **C** and **D,** tachycardia, **E** and **F,** bradycardia, and, **F,** hypoxic secondary arrest. A short period of asystole was initially seen before tracing **B.**

reported but also may reflect concomitant trauma to other tissues.[83,102,185]

ECG changes may not occur until the second day, making the initial ECG a poor screening tool for ischemia. In addition, several authors stress that cardiac symptomatology may be inapparent on initial presentation.[98,164,166] Premature ventricular contractions were reported to begin in one patient nearly one week after presentation.[100] Whereas most ECG changes resolve within a few days, some may persist for months.[23,90,98]

A further phenomenon noted is the prolongation of QT interval following lightning strike.[7,55,97,133] This, too, has been verified in animal experiments (Fig. 11-8) in which the ischemic form of the ECG complexes gives way to normalization of morphology, followed by prolongation of the QT interval at 270 seconds after strike in sheep who did not suffer respiratory arrest. Another paper hypothesizes that the QT prolongation may have implications for the cessation of metabolism hypothesis if torsades is involved.[7]

Some reports have theorized that vascular spasm is a cause of cardiac damage.[161] However, ECG changes are not always consistent with vascular supply patterns in the heart.[82] Areas of focal cardiac necrosis have been reported in autopsies, and Andrews has shown histologic changes in sheep hearts.[5,102,114,118,129]

Pulmonary edema may accompany severe cardiac damage.[40,97,102,136] Pulmonary contusion, with severe hemoptysis and pulmonary hemorrhage,[160] has been reported and may be the result of blunt injury or direct lung damage.[27,40,136]

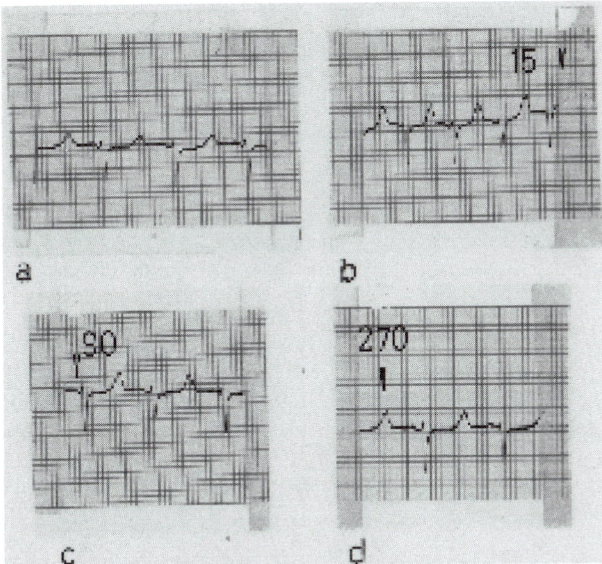

Fig. 11-8 Electrocardiogram (nonstandard leads) for sheep struck by laboratory-generated lightning. Asystolic arrest did not occur. QT was prolonged by 270 seconds after the strike.

NEUROLOGIC INJURIES

The second major cause of morbidity and mortality in lightning injuries is central nervous system damage.[75] When current traverses the brain, there can be coagulation of brain substance, formation of epidural and subdural hematomas, paralysis of the respiratory center, and intraventricular hemorrhage.[126,162,176] Autopsy findings include meningeal and parenchymal blood extravasation, petechiae, dural tears, scalp hematomas, and skull fractures.* Computed tomography (CT) of the head may show diffuse edema or intracranial hemorrhage.† Transient elevation of creatine phosphokinase BB has been reported.[83]

Direct cellular damage to the respiratory and cardiac centers in the fourth ventricle as well as the anterior surface of the brainstem has been shown in animal work.[5] If current enters through the orifices of the head, passes through the area of the pituitary and hypothalamus, and through the CSF into the retropharyngeal area, it is reasonable to expect signs and symptoms consistent with damage to these areas, including endocrine dysfunction and respiratory or cardiac arrest.

Seizures may accompany initial cardiorespiratory arrest as a result of hypoxia or intracranial damage.[120] They are usually transient but may continue for the first few days.

CT may show direct brain damage from blunt head injury in a limited number of victims, particularly those whose mental status deteriorates over time.[37,39,104,117,140] There have been reports of magnetic resonance imaging (MRI) findings in a few acutely injured patients.[38] Unfortunately, for patients with more chronic complaints, CT and MRI examinations are usually unremarkable.

Electroencephalographic (EEG) changes may isolate an epileptogenic focus in the acute phase in many lightning patients.[32,134,135] These patterns may be focal or diffuse, varying with the site and type of injury. Many of these patients do not experience seizures during hospitalization, and most usually have normalization of their EEG within a few months. Other victims, including children, have delayed seizures.[100] One severely injured patient was reported to have continued seizures after discharge to a nursing home.[127]

Obviously, if the victim has prolonged cardiopulmonary arrest, there may be anoxic brain injury that is not specific to lightning injury.

In Cooper's study of severely injured victims, nearly two thirds had some degree of lower extremity paralysis (keraunoparalysis), usually demarcating around the waist or the pelvis.[44] Almost one third of victims have upper extremity paralysis.[44] The affected extremities appear cold, clammy, mottled, insensate, and pulseless.[8,167-169] This is the result of sympathetic instability and intense vascular

*References 27, 41, 49-51, 60, 84, 99, 157, 182.
†References 37-39, 104, 117, 140, 159.

spasm, which has been likened to Raynaud's phenomenon in appearance and usually clears after several hours.[52,114] Fasciotomies are almost never indicated for lightning injuries, since any signs of compartment syndrome or distal ischemia usually clear with patient observation. Pulses can sometimes be elicited with a Doppler examination. Atrophic spinal paralysis has been reported, as have persistent paresis, paresthesias, incoordination, delayed and acute cerebellar ataxia, hemiplegia, and aphasia.* There is one report of quadriplegia developing 36 hours after injury and one of progressive muscle atrophy of the upper extremities.[18,27]

Nearly 72% of the victims in Cooper's study suffered loss of consciousness,[44] which may be an ominous sign, since nearly three fourths of these persons also suffered a cardiopulmonary arrest.[44] Those with cranial burns are two to three times more likely to suffer immediate cardiopulmonary arrest and have a three to four times greater probability of death.[44] Persons who are stunned or lose consciousness without cardiopulmonary arrest are highly unlikely to die,[44] although they may still have serious sequelae.

Whether or not victims have suffered loss of consciousness, they almost universally demonstrate anterograde amnesia and confusion, which may last for several days. Retrograde amnesia is less common. Often the patient appears to be well oriented and remembers his or her actions before the strike but may not be able to assimilate new experiences for several days, even when there is no external evidence of lightning burns on the head or neck. Patients often act like those who have experienced electroconvulsive therapy.[47]

Survivors may have persistent sleep disturbances, difficulty with fine mental and motor functions, dysesthesias, headaches, mood abnormalities, emotional lability, storm phobias, decreased exercise tolerance, and posttraumatic stress disorder.†

BURNS

Most people assume that because of the tremendous energy discharge involved, a lightning victim will be flash cooked.[31] Fortunately, the flashover effect saves most victims from more than minor burns. Although extensive third- and fourth-degree burns may occur in combination with skeletal disruption, they are rare.[3,41,67,157,177]

As shown in mathematical models, a portion of the lightning current may travel through the tissues.[5] If the electric field in the tissue becomes too large, electrons can be freed from their atoms. Referred to as dielectric breakdown,[107] this can cause a large increase in the flow of current and manifest as an electric arc. This may occur internal to the body or external to the body when the breakdown strength of air (2×10^6 V/m) is exceeded. Arclike burns can result. This happens more often with high-voltage electrical injury but may also occur with lightning.

Discrete entry and exit points are rare with lightning. The burns most commonly seen may be divided into five categories: linear burns; punctate, full-thickness burns; feathering or flowers; thermal burns from ignited clothing or heated metal; and combinations.

Linear burns (Fig. 11-9) often begin at the victim's head and progress down the chest, where they split and continue

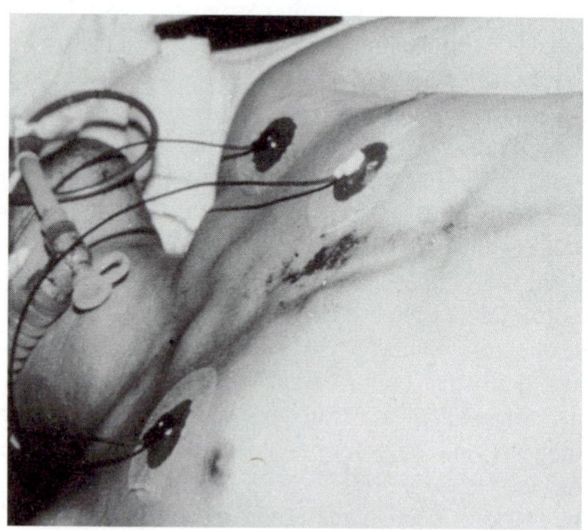

Fig. 11-9 Linear burns from lightning injury.

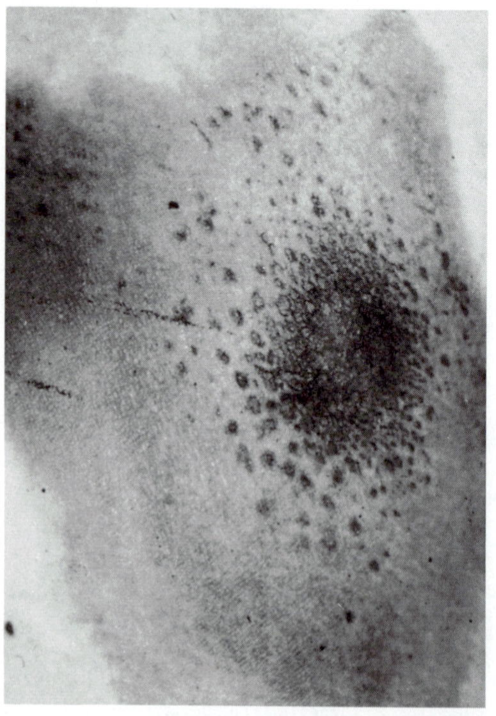

Fig. 11-10 Punctate burns from lightning injury. (Courtesy Art Kahn, M.D.)

*References 3, 15, 100, 109, 129, 150, 166, 183.

†References 47, 57, 67, 100, 129, 134, 148, 151.

down both legs. The burns generally are 1 to 4 cm wide and tend to follow areas of heavy sweat concentration, such as beneath breasts, down the midchest, and in the midaxillary line.[161] Linear burns are usually first- and second-degree burns that may be present initially or develop as late as several hours after the lightning strike. They may represent vaporization of the sweat into steam on the patient's body and are probably not true lightning burns.

Punctate burns (Fig. 11-10; Color Plate 12) are multiple, closely spaced, discrete circular burns that individually range from a few millimeters to a centimeter in diameter. They may be full thickness and resemble cigarette burns but are usually too small to require grafting.

Feathering burns (Fig. 11-11; Color Plate 13) are pathognomonic of lightning and are known by such names as Lichtenberg's flowers, filigree burns, arborescent burns, ferning, and keraunographic markings. These markings were once thought to represent photographic imprints of vegetation surrounding the victim.[114] The markings are now known not to be true burns, but cutaneous imprints from electron showers that track over the skin. The pattern found is similar to that on a photographic plate exposed to a strong electric field.[19,78,86,169]

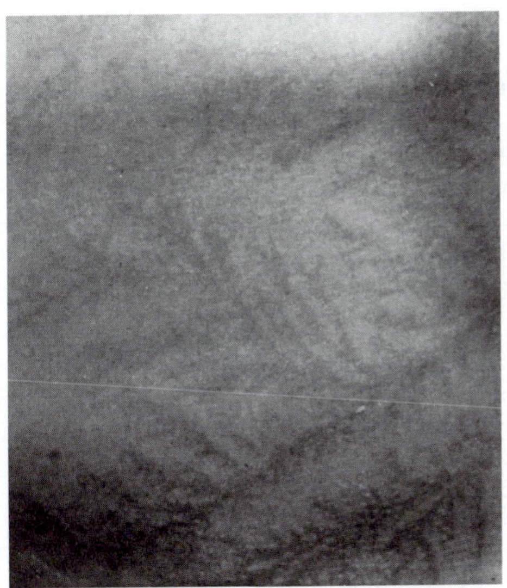

Fig. 11-11 Feathering burns.

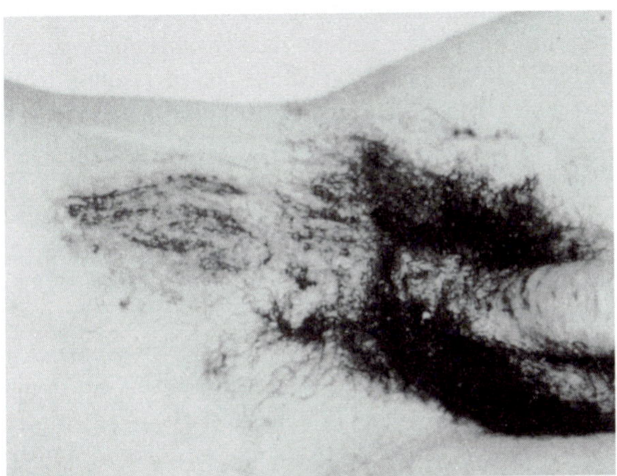

Fig. 11-12 Burn resulting from metal belt buckle or athletic supporter worn by a man struck by lightning.

On rare occasion clothing is ignited by lightning, causing severe thermal burns.[43,120] A victim wearing metal, such as a necklace or belt buckle, or carrying coins in his or her pocket may suffer second- and third-degree burns to adjacent skin as the objects become heated by the electric energy.[20,53,136] Fig. 11-12 shows the burn resulting from a metal belt buckle or athletic supporter worn by a young man who was struck while playing softball.

Victims of lightning may exhibit a combination of burns.

One author has related the prognosis of the patient to the location of the burns.[44] Patients who suffer cranial burns are four times more likely to die than those who do not have cranial burns ($p < .25$). Patients with cranial burns are two and a half times more likely to have a cardiopulmonary arrest than those who do not exhibit burns around the head and neck ($p < .025$).[44] Persons with leg burns are five times more likely to die than those who have no leg burns, perhaps because of a ground current etiology ($p < .05$).[44] The results of this study are consistent and further explained by animal work with entry of current through the cranial orifices and subsequent damage to the cardiac and respiratory centers.[5,10]

BLUNT AND EXPLOSIVE INJURIES

The victim of a lightning accident may be injured directly from the explosive force of lightning or from a fall (as from a horse or mountain ledge, out of a vehicle, or being hurled by endogenous opisthotonic force.)[17,20,134] Lightning victims incur a variety of fractures, including skull, ribs, extremities, and spine.* Rarely a burstlike injury of soft tissues occurs and discloses extensive underlying injuries, especially in the feet, where boots or socks may come apart (Fig. 11-13).[91]

Hemoglobinuria and myoglobinuria are seldom reported.[159,185] When they occur, they are usually transient. Myoglobinuric renal failure has not yet been reported, although one case has been verbally relayed to the first author (M.A.C.).

Persistent hypotension should alert the physician to blunt injuries to the chest, spine, lungs, heart, and intestines,[82,114,128] which may lead to complications of prolonged coma, pulmonary contusions,[160] heart failure, and ischemic bowel.

*References 18, 19, 41, 70, 143, 164.

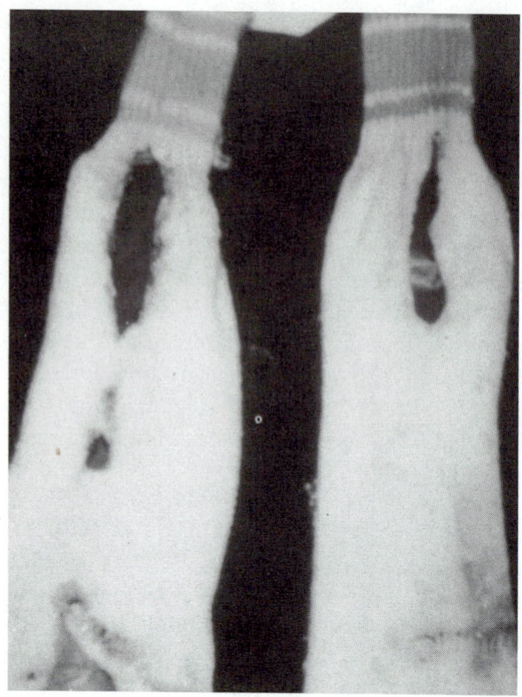

Fig. 11-13 Socks blown off during explosive lightning stroke.

Several patients have complained of jaw pain. At least one was found to have a styloid process fracture on the affected side. Many recovering victims believe that their premature arthritis may be a result of their injury, although no appropriately controlled studies have proven this.

EYE INJURIES

We have already drawn attention to the vulnerability of the cranial orifices as entry points for lightning current. It is therefore hardly surprising that significant ocular damage has been reported.[31,167] This observation applies equally to the auditory and olfactory apparatus.

Ocular injuries may occur in as many as 55% of persons struck by lightning and may be due to direct thermal or electrical damage, intense light, contusion from the shock wave, or combinations of these factors.[32]

Although cataracts most commonly develop within the first few days, they may occur as late as 2 years after the strike and are often bilateral.* Whereas the cataracts may be the typical anterior midperipheral type, posterior subcapsular opacities and vacuolization seem to occur more often with lightning injuries.[30] Corneal lesions, hyphema, uveitis, iridocyclitis, and vitreous hemorrhage occur with greater frequency than do choroidal rupture, chorioretinitis, retinal detachment, macular degeneration, and optic atrophy.† Diplopia, loss of accommodation, and decreased color sense have also been reported.[32,106]

Autonomic disturbances of the eye, including mydriasis, Horner's syndrome, anisocoria, and loss of light reflexes, may be transient or permanent.[32,114] Transient bilateral blindness of unknown etiology initially is not uncommon.[60,99] Intense photophobia may be present as the patient recovers.

Dilated or unreactive pupils should never be used as a prognostic sign or as a criterion for brain death in a lightning victim until all anatomic and functional lesions have been ruled out.[1]

*References 19, 30, 42, 62, 104, 130, 140, 171.

†References 30, 32, 104, 114, 125, 145.

EAR INJURIES

Temporary deafness is not uncommon.* It has been postulated that the intense noise and shock wave accompanying thunder may be responsible for sensorineural loss.[20] Newer work showing entry of lightning current through the cranial orifices could also account for some of the injuries seen.[5,10] Telephone-mediated lightning strikes may also account for otologic damage.[6,11,13,184]

Between 30% and 50% of lightning victims have rupture of one or both tympanic membranes, which may be from the shock wave effect, concomitant basilar skull fracture, or direct burn damage because of current flow into this orifice.[44] Cerebrospinal fluid otorrhea or hemotympanum may occur.[49] Disruption of the ossicles and mastoid has been reported.[20,49] Many cases of permanent deafness are noted in older literature.[154,167] Facial palsies, both acute and delayed, may occur from direct nerve damage by lightning.[20,125,141,180] Nystagmus, vertigo, and ataxia may result from otologic damage.[152,180,184]

FETAL SURVIVAL

The fetus of a pregnant woman who has been struck by lightning has an unpredictable prognosis.[35,44,72,138,146] Of 11 cases reported, nearly one half of the pregnancies ended in full-term live births, with no recognizable abnormality in the child.[41,167] Approximately one fourth resulted in live births with subsequent neonatal death; the remainder were stillbirths or deaths in utero.[81,138,179] There has been one report of a ruptured uterus after a lightning strike.[146]

HEMATOLOGIC ABNORMALITIES

Several unusual hematologic complications have been attributed to lightning injuries, including disseminated intravascular coagulation,[66] transiently positive Coombs' test,[119] and diGugliemo's syndrome, a type of erythroleukemia characterized by erythroblastosis, thrombocytopenia, and hepatosplenomegaly.[68] There have been some

*References 19, 76, 94, 98, 103, 167, 181, 184.

anecdotal reports of increased hypersensitivity, the development of allergies, and an increased risk of cancer in lightning victims, indicating perhaps an immunologic component to lightning injury, although this has not been studied in a controlled fashion.

ENDOCRINE AND SEXUAL DYSFUNCTION

One 32-year-old victim reported amenorrhea and premature menopause as a result of her injury. Others have reported menstrual irregularities, and there have been claimed cases of impotence. There also has been a report of hypersexuality in a male after a lightning strike that has not been authenticated by objective observers.

Recognition and Treatment of Lightning Injuries

DIAGNOSIS

The diagnosis of lightning injury may be difficult. A history of a thunderstorm, witnesses who can report having seen the strike, and typical physical findings in the victim make diagnosis easier.

However, lightning can strike on a relatively sunny day, or thunder may not be appreciated. If the victim is struck while working alone in a field, the diagnosis may be initially confused with other entities as listed in Box 11-3. In the past, persons have been suspected to have been the victims of assault because of the disarray of clothing and belongings.[161]

A diligent historical effort and careful physical examination at the earliest opportunity may help determine the true cause. Any person found with linear burns and clothes exploded off should be treated as a victim of lightning strike. Feathering burns are pathognomonic of lightning strike and occur in no other type of injury. Unfortunately, they are not always present. Another complex that is diagnostic of lightning strike includes linear or punctate burns, tympanic membrane rupture, confusion, and outdoor location, whether or not there is a history of a thunderstorm. Because there have been several cases of lightning sideflashes from indoor plumbing and telephone, the physician should suspect the cause in patients found confused and unconscious indoors after or during a thunderstorm.*

BOX 11-3

DIFFERENTIAL DIAGNOSIS OF LIGHTNING INJURY

Cerebrovascular accident
- Subarachnoid hemorrhage
- Intraventricular hemorrhage
- Stroke

Seizure disorder
Spinal cord injury
Closed head injury
Hypertensive encephalopathy
Cardiac arrhythmia
Myocardial infarction
Toxic ingestion (heavy metals)
Malingering, conversion reaction

INITIAL FIRST AID AND TRIAGE OF VICTIMS

As in any other emergency, the first steps are the ABCs: airway, breathing, and circulation. If the patient has had a cardiac arrest, cardiopulmonary resuscitation should be started immediately and a rescue vehicle called for transportation.

If the strike occurs far from civilization and evacuation is improbable, the victim will probably die unless pulse and respirations resume spontaneously in a short period of time. The heart may resume activity but may slip into secondary hypoxic arrest from refractory respiratory arrest. If the rescuer is successful in obtaining a pulse with cardiopulmonary resuscitation, ventilation should be continued until spontaneous adequate respirations resume, the patient is pronounced dead, continued resuscitation is deemed unfeasible owing to rescuers' exhaustion, or there is danger to their own survival.

When lightning strike involves multiple victims, resources and rescuers may not meet the demand and triage must be instituted.[16,28,167] Normally the rules of triage in multiple-casualty situations dictate bypassing dead persons for those who are moderately or severely injured and can benefit from resuscitation efforts. However, "resuscitate the dead" is the rule in lightning incidents, since victims who show some return of consciousness or who have spontaneous breathing are already on the way to recovery.[45,167] Survivors should be routinely stabilized and transported to the hospital for more thorough evaluation. In the field the most vigorous attempts at cardiopulmonary resuscitation should be directed to the victims who appear to be dead, since they may ultimately recover if properly resuscitated.[161]

The probability that lightning victims can recover after prolonged cardiopulmonary resuscitation (several hours) is not high. Other than for a few anecdotal reports,[63,104,124] there is no reason to believe that these patients will respond to prolonged efforts. Often in a remote setting the rescuer is emotionally tied to the victim by age as well as friendship and may tend to continue resuscitation past the point of fu-

*References 6, 9, 49, 65, 91, 93, 103, 126, 139, 140, 152, 161.

tility. In pronouncing a victim dead, the rescuer must be sure that other problems, such as hypothermia, are not clouding the victim's response to resuscitation efforts.

Other stabilization procedures, including splinting of fractures, intubation, spinal precautions, and institution of intravenous fluids and oxygen, should be accomplished, whenever indicated and feasible, before transport.

HISTORY AND PHYSICAL EXAMINATION

If witnesses are available, an eyewitness report is helpful, since victims are often confused and amnesic. The history should include a description of the event and the patient's behavior following the strike. Past medical history may be invaluable.

Like any other trauma victim, the patient must be totally undressed to facilitate a complete examination. Special note should be taken of the patient's vital signs, temperature, and level of consciousness. Since many victims are struck during a thunderstorm, they may be wet and cold. Hypothermia should be anticipated and treated appropriately (see Chapter 3).

The awake patient should be assessed for orientation and short-term memory. The lightning victim typically cannot assimilate information and may perseverate or ask repetitive questions during the examination. Continuing confusion or a deteriorating level of consciousness mandates CT of the head to rule out an intracranial event.

Examination of the patient's eyes is essential to establish reactivity and injury. Tympanic membrane rupture is an important indicator of lightning strike. Ossicular disruption may be one explanation for a patient's lack of appropriate response to verbal stimuli.

Although the pulmonary system may be affected by cardiac arrest, with complications of pulmonary edema or adult respiratory distress syndrome, it is uncommon to witness these initially. The cardiovascular examination should include distal pulses in all extremities, appreciation of arrhythmias, and evaluation of cardiac damage, including isoenzymatic and ECG changes.

The patient's abdominal examination occasionally demonstrates absent bowel sounds, which suggests ileus or indicates acute traumatic injury such as contusion of the liver, bowel, or spleen.

The examiner should document any skin changes. The patient's skin may show mottling, especially below the waist. Burns may be present initially but usually evolve and mature over a period of hours. Notation of pulses, color, and movement and sensory examination of the patient's extremities are essential.

The physical findings and mental state of minimally and moderately injured victims tend to change considerably over the first few hours; careful observation and documentation delineate the patient's course so that therapy can be appropriate. The minimally injured patient may sometimes be discharged to responsible persons or require only overnight observation, whereas the severely injured patient may require intensive care with mechanical ventilation, Swan-Ganz catheterization, antiarrhythmic medications, and other intensive interventions.

LABORATORY AND X-RAY TESTS

Minimum laboratory examinations include complete blood cell count and urinalysis (including a test for myoglobin). Blood tests indicated for the more severely injured patient include electrolyte screen, blood urea nitrogen (BUN), and creatinine. Serial cardiac enzyme and isoenzyme tests may be indicated in some cases. If the patient is to be placed on a ventilator, arterial blood gases will be necessary; if intracranial pressure monitoring is used, serum osmolality may be required.

An ECG is essential for all lightning victims and will frequently show QT prolongation even when otherwise normal.

A chest x-ray should usually be obtained. Cervical spine films should be taken if there is any evidence of cranial burns, contusions, loss of consciousness, or change in mentation that would make the physical examination unreliable, or if there are other historical considerations, such as a fall, that would recommend them. The patient who is unconscious, confused, or has a deteriorating level of consciousness requires a CT or MRI scan of the head to rule out blunt head trauma as well as ischemic injury. X-ray studies to rule out fractures, dislocations, and other injuries can be ordered as indicated by the physical examination and the physician's suspicions.

TREATMENT

Fluid Therapy

An intravenous lifeline is mandatory for the patient who shows unstable vital signs, unconsciousness, or disorientation. If the patient is hypotensive, fluid resuscitation with normal saline or Ringer's lactate solution is required, with the caution that significant cerebral edema may develop. Fluid restriction in normotensive or hypertensive patients is recommended because of this risk.

A Swan-Ganz catheter, arterial pressure, or central venous pressure monitoring system, as well as other critical care monitoring, may be indicated in the more severely injured patient. Careful intake and output measurement is necessary in the severely injured patient and requires the placement of an indwelling urinary catheter. Myoglobinuria is rare and usually transient when present, so that the mannitol diuresis, alkalinization, and aggressive fluid loading used with high-voltage electric injuries are rarely necessary. However, if burns are severe and extensive, resuscitation such as is necessary for high-voltage electrical injuries may be required.

Fasciotomy

Paralyzed and pulseless extremities seen with lightning injuries should not be treated like those caused by high-voltage injuries. Intense vascular spasm with lightning usually is a sequel to sympathetic instability. The victim's extremities should be treated expectantly. Steady improvement in the mottled, cool extremity, with return of pulses in a few hours, is the rule rather than the exception. Fasciotomies are rarely indicated unless the extremity shows no signs of recovery and raised intracompartmental tissue pressures are documented. Only one case necessitating fasciotomy has been reported.[3]

Antibiotics and Tetanus Prophylaxis

Prophylactic antibiotics are not indicated. Standard therapy should follow culture and identification of pathogens. Exceptions to this rule include open extremity or cranial fractures that violate the dura. In the latter case many neurosurgeons recommend antibiotic prophylaxis. Tetanus prophylaxis is mandatory if burns or lacerations are present.

Cardiovascular Therapy

Management of cardiac arrest is standard. In the patient who is not in a state of cardiac arrest, vasospasm may still make the peripheral pulses difficult to palpate. Usually femoral, brachial, or carotid pulses may be appreciated. A Doppler examination may be necessary to locate peripheral pulses and record blood pressure.

If a patient remains hypotensive on Doppler examination, fluid resuscitation may be necessary to establish adequate blood pressure and tissue perfusion. Causes of hypotension include major fractures, blood loss from abdominal or chest injuries, spinal shock, cardiogenic shock, and occasionally deep burns similar to high-voltage electric burns. As soon as an adequate central blood pressure is obtained, fluids should probably be restricted because of the high incidence of cranial injuries and cerebral edema.[102]

The patient who is without spontaneous or adequate respirations should be mechanically ventilated until brain death is declared, the patient resumes adequate ventilation, or the family decides to cease efforts.

All lightning victims, regardless of their condition, should have an ECG. Cardiac monitoring and serial isoenzyme measurements are indicated if there is any sign of ischemia or arrhythmia or if the patient complains of chest pain. Injury patterns, as well as arrhythmias, have been reported.[102] The indications for antiarrhythmic drugs and pressor agents are the same as for a suspected myocardial infarction.[102]

Prolongation of the QT interval has been reported by several authors in the past and has been proposed, when part of a torsades phenomenon, as a possible explanation for the reports of suspended animation with recovery.[7,55,97,133]

Transient hypertension may be so short lived as to require no acute therapy. However, several cases of hypertension have occurred 12 to 72 hours after lightning strike and seemed to respond well to β-blockers and other antihypertensive medications.[100,166] Use of newer antihypertensive agents with lightning injuries has not been reported but would probably be equally effective.

Treatment of Central Nervous System Injury

Every lightning victim should have a complete neurologic examination. If there is a history of loss of consciousness or if the patient exhibits confusion, hospital admission is necessary to observe the patient. The patient who has tympanic membrane rupture, cranial burns, or loss of consciousness or who shows a decreasing level of consciousness should have cervical spine radiologic examination, head CT, and possibly MRI. Serial CT scans may be useful in assessing ventricular hemorrhage and edema.

In the patient with persistent loss of consciousness, hyperventilation to maintain P_{CO_2} at 25 to 30 mm Hg may be useful to control cerebral edema.[104] If there are no other contraindications, the head should be elevated. Steroids probably are of as little benefit with lightning injuries as they are in other posttraumatic cerebral conditions.

Intracranial pressure monitoring may be a useful adjunct in patients with elevated intracranial pressure.[104,108] Cerebral edema may be managed with mannitol, furosemide, fluid restriction, and other standard therapies.[25,104,108,121,153] Although hypothermia was reported to contribute to complete recovery in one patient with prolonged cardiac arrest before resuscitation efforts, there is no firm evidence that this would benefit all patients.[144]

Early seizures are probably due to anoxia. If there is evidence of central nervous system damage or if seizures continue after adequate oxygenation and perfusion have been restored, standard pharmacologic intervention with diazepam, phenytoin, or phenobarbital should be considered.[102,120]

If paralysis does not improve, causes other than lightning, including blunt injury from a fall, may be responsible. In addition, spinal artery syndrome has been reported, perhaps caused by arterial spasm. A physical therapy program should be started before discharge. Unfortunately, in a number of patients peripheral neuropathies develop with continuing dysesthesias and weakness. These may respond to chronic pain management techniques, including combinations of nonsteroidal antiinflammatory drugs, carbamazepine, and tricyclic antidepressants.[8,9,47,69,148]

In recent years neuropsychologic deficits from lightning have become better appreciated.[46,47] Heightened anxiety states, hyperirritability, memory deficits, aphasia, sleep disturbance, posttraumatic stress disorder, and other evidence of brain damage should be assessed.[9,69,151] Some of these deficits are much like those suffered by victims of blunt head trauma. A rehabilitation program should be instituted early for these patients to return them to as functional a state as possible.

Often the victim's family and co-workers have difficulty understanding the change in personality that affects many of these victims. Neuropsychologic testing with appropriate therapy may be necessary. Certain personality types may predispose victims to more pronounced neuropsychologic symptoms.

The feeling of isolation and change that victims sometimes experience may lead to depression, substance abuse, and thoughts of suicide. Because of unfamiliarity with lightning injuries and their sequelae, many physicians are ill equipped to manage long-term care of lightning victims, leading the victim and the family to become angry.

Referral to Lightning Strike and Electric Shock Victims (LSESV) International, a support group founded in the late 1980s, can be of substantial help to victims and families. LSESV is located at 214 Canterbury Road, Jacksonville, NC 28540-5307, telephone 910-346-4708. Some local chapters have been formed in areas with a high incidence of lightning strikes.

Treatment of Burns

Lightning burns may be apparent at the time of admission but more commonly develop within the first few hours. They are generally superficial, unlike high-voltage electrical burns, and seldom cause massive muscle destruction. Vigorous fluid therapy and mannitol diuresis are not indicated. The patient's urine should be tested for myoglobin, although it is infrequently seen.[2,185] In the rare instance of myoglobinuria, intravenous mannitol and alkalinization of the urine with bicarbonate may be used. Overhydration with resultant cerebral edema probably has killed more lightning victims than has myoglobinuric renal failure.

Lightning burns are generally so superficial that they do not require treatment with topical agents. In the unusual instance of deep injury, topical therapy should be standard. Only in the rare instance of third-degree involvement is fasciotomy, amputation, or grafting necessary.

Treatment of Eye Injuries

Visual acuity should be measured and the patient's eyes thoroughly examined. Cataracts are not uncommon. Eye injuries should be treated in standard fashion and may require referral to an ophthalmologist.

Treatment of Ear Injuries

Simple tympanic membrane rupture is usually handled conservatively with observation until the patient's tissues return to normal.[20,152] Sensorineural damage to the auditory nerve and facial nerve palsies are not uncommon.[20,152] Loss of hearing mandates otologic evaluation.[181] Ossicular disruption or more severe damage may necessitate surgical repair. Otorrhea and hemotympanum are not uncommon and suggest basilar skull fracture. Complaints of pain around the angle of the patient's jaw should lead the physician to a search for occult fracture of the styloid process and other musculoskeletal damage.[52,125]

Treatment of Pregnant Victims

If a pregnant woman is struck, fetal viability must be assessed, including fetal heart tones and ultrasonography to observe fetal activity. Fetal death is treated with evacuation of the uterus.

Other Considerations

Gastric irritation is occasionally seen.[63,120] Histamine-2 antagonists or antacid therapy may be indicated. A nasogastric tube is appropriate if ileus or hematemesis occurs.[123] Peritoneal lavage or an abdominal CT scan may be indicated in comatose patients who remain hypotensive, since intestinal contusions and hemorrhage have been reported in other cases.[82,123]

Endocrine dysfunction, perhaps as a result of pituitary or hypothalamic damage, has occurred in some victims, including amenorrhea and impotence.

Pronouncing the Patient Dead

Dilated pupils should not be taken as a sign of brain death in the lightning victim.[1] EEGs may also show diffuse damage initially, only to clear with time. However, the patient who shows no response to resuscitative efforts, continues to become hypothermic, and meets current brain death criteria over a period of several hours to days may be pronounced dead with relative certainty.[82]

Precautions for Avoiding Lightning Injury*

Be aware of weather conditions and predictions before going on excursions or working in the open. Respect thunderstorms and their power. If you cannot avoid being outdoors, carry a small radio to monitor weather reports. Be prepared to seek shelter if a severe thunderstorm watch or warning is announced. Fatal lightning may strike as far as 10 km in front of the storm cloud, seeming to come out of the clear blue sky. Some victims have also underestimated the danger at the end of a storm.

If a storm strikes, seek shelter in a substantial building or in an all-metal vehicle, such as a car, but avoid convertibles. Small buildings, especially exposed metal sheds, offer variable protection, depending on the size and height of the building, since side flashes can occur to the occupants. Tents offer little protection because the metal support poles actually may act as lightning rods. Occupants of the tents should stay as far away from the poles and wet cloth as possible.

*References 71, 95, 96, 141, 167, 173, 174, 177.

If you are in an all-metal automobile (not a cloth-top convertible or Jeep), stay in it. The automobile will diffuse the current around you to the ground. It is a myth that rubber tires provide insulation, but it is true that the metal body generally affords protection.

If indoors during a thunderstorm, avoid open doors and windows, fireplaces, and metal objects such as pipes, sinks, radiators, and plug-in electrical appliances. Avoid using the telephone or a computer with a modem. A clothesline pole may act as a lightning rod and transmit lightning along the line.

Stay away from metal objects such as motorcycles, tractors, fences, and bicycles. Put down metal objects such as umbrellas or golf clubs. Metal cleats in shoes act as excellent grounding agents, and metal objects near the head make a person much more likely to be hit by lightning. Avoid areas near power lines, pipelines, fences, ski lifts, and other structural steel fabrications.[119]

If you are unable to find shelter, do not stand near tall isolated trees, on hilltops, or at a lookout or other exposed area. In the forest seek shelter in a low area under a thick growth of saplings or small trees. Seeking a clearing to avoid trees makes a person the tallest object in the clearing and more likely to be struck.

If you are totally in the open, stay far away from single trees to avoid lightning splashes. The position most likely to thwart lightning is still unclear. However, crouching down on both feet, kneeling, and rolling up in a ball all decrease the height of the person and minimize exposure to the ground current effects. Avoid seeking shelter in cornstalks, haystacks, or other objects that project above the ground. Caves, ditches, and valleys may provide some protection unless they are saturated with water, which may conduct the current.

If you are on the water, seek the shore. Avoid swimming, boating, or being the tallest object near the large open body of water. Lightning is attracted to metal masts and other objects projecting above the surface of the water and flows well through the water to injure swimmers, on the same principle as ground current injuries. Sheltering under a bridge or cliff while in the boat may provide some protection. Both sailboats and powerboats should be protected with lightning rods and grounding equipment attached to a metal keel or understructure of the boat.[116]

If a group of people is exposed, the persons should spread out and stay several yards apart, so that in the event of a strike, the fewest are injured seriously by ground current and by side flashes between persons.

Industrial Electrical Injuries[48]

Direct current (DC) causes only one third as much damage as alternating current (AC) of the same voltage and amperage. High-voltage commercial electricity usually alternates at about 60 cycles per second, just the right frequency to cause muscle tetany.[41] Because the victim is often working with the electrical source, the hands are the most frequently injured part of the body. The tetanic force triggered by the electricity causes the hand to freeze to the circuit, since the flexors of the forearm are stronger than the extensors. The current also arcs across flexed joints, producing kissing burns at each flexion point, including the wrist, elbow, and axilla.

The presence of water or sweat on the skin can lower resistance as much as 25 times. When the resistance of the dermis is lowered by moisture or diminished thickness, the applied energy preferentially courses through the inside of the body via lower resistance tissues. As a result, high-voltage electrical burns are characterized by deep muscle, nerve, and vascular damage, with variable overlying skin damage.

Both entry and exit wounds are usually seen with high-voltage electrical injuries, with diffuse, unpredictable damage occurring in between, similar to that of gunshot wounds.

Because the victim clasps the current source in his or her hand, the exposure is prolonged and the victim's skin breaks down, allowing the current to pass internally through the excellent electrolyte media of the blood and muscles. The external wound may appear fairly benign, hiding the extensive damage that may have occurred in deeper structures. For high-voltage injuries fasciotomies may be needed to maintain the circulation and viability of distal structures. Extensive amputations are not infrequent with high-voltage electrical injuries. Fluid loading, mannitol diuresis, and alkalinization may be necessary to prevent myoglobinuric renal failure.

Precautions for Avoiding Electrical Injury

Protection against the effects of electric current appears easy. Prevention is better than cure, and contact with any conductor should be avoided at all costs, on the assumption that the conductor is live. In the wilderness, high-voltage transmission lines are more likely to be encountered with attendant increased danger. Thus all intentional contact with conductors should be avoided. Persons should not climb pylons, swing from lines, or otherwise touch power lines.

Nonetheless, nonintentional contact with electrical conductors can occur. They may be hidden from view; insulation on normally touched apparatus may have been damaged or have aged; lines may have fallen; and any one of many other scenarios of accidental contact may occur. As a general principle, any item unidentifiable from a safe distance should be assumed harmful and not investigated until safety is ensured. This applies no less to electrical objects.

Persons working on electrical equipment should follow the procedures in Box 11-4.

BOX 11-4

PRECAUTIONS WHEN WORKING WITH ELECTRICAL EQUIPMENT

Do not work on live apparatus unless absolutely necessary.

If dealing with live equipment is unavoidable, work only in company, using appropriate safety dress (gloves, clothing, mats, etc.) and tools.

Wear clothing that leaves the minimum of bare flesh exposed. Do not wear metal components, such as belt buckles, or open footwear.

Near electrical fires, use fire extinguishers designed specifically for that task.

Do not use metal tools, such as metal tapes and poles, particularly if they are long and flexible.

BEFORE BEGINNING WORK

Determine which switch or circuit breaker controls the item to be worked on.

Open the switch or circuit breaker, or remove the fuse.

Firmly affix **Danger** signs to advise against reconnection by another party.

Test the apparatus to ensure that it is deenergized.

Test the testing device on a live circuit, after using it on the circuit to be worked on.

If possible, short to earth the active conductors after deenergization.

Once again, never work alone on electrical apparatus.

Residual current devices (RCDs), also known as ground fault circuit interrupters, sense any difference between current entering and leaving the line to which they are connected. Any difference must represent current conducted to the earth, and the circuit is immediately deenergized on the assumption the leak may be through a person. Since roughly 80% of accidents occur in this way, the RCD's importance is notable. RCDs are now required by code in new installations, particularly domestic ones, but they may be absent in older construction.

REFERENCES

1. Abt JL: The pupillary responses after being struck by lightning, *JAMA* 254:3312, 1985.
2. Akahane T, Okishio R: Lightning injury: report of two cases, *Burns* 10:45, 1983.
3. Amy BW et al: Lightning injury with survival in five patients, *JAMA* 253:243, 1985.
4. Andrews CJ: Comments on "Myocardial infarction after electrocution," *Med J Aust* 149:342, 1988.
5. Andrews CJ: *Studies in aspects of lightning injury,* doctoral dissertation, Brisbane, Australia, 1993, University of Queensland.
6. Andrews CJ: Telephone-related lightning injury, *Med J Aust* 157:823, 1992.
7. Andrews CJ, Colquhoun DM, Darveniza M: The QT interval in lightning injury with implications for the "cessation of metabolism" hypothesis, *J Wilderness Med* 4:155, 1993.
8. Andrews CJ et al: *Lightning injuries: electrical, medical, and legal aspects,* Boca Raton, Fla, 1992, CRC Press.
9. Andrews CJ, Darveniza M: Telephone mediated lightning injury: an australian survey, *J Trauma* 29:665, 1989.
10. Andrews CJ, Darveniza M: New models of the electrical insult in lightning strike. In Proceedings of the 9th International Conference on Atmospheric Physics, St Petersburg, Russia, 1992.
11. Andrews CJ, Darveniza M: *Determination of acoustic insult in telephone mediated lightning strike,* unpublished material, 1992.
12. Andrews CJ, Darveniza M, Mackerras D: A review of medical aspects of lightning injury. In Proceedings of the 1988 International Aerospace and Ground Conference on Lightning and Static Electricity, April 19-22, 1988, Oklahoma City, Okla, pp 231-250.
13. Andrews CJ, Darveniza M: Effects of lightning on mammalian tissue. In Proceedings of the 1989 International Conference on Lightning and Static Electricity, Sept 26-28, 1989, Bath, Eng, pp 4A.4.1-4A.4.4.
14. Andrews CJ, Darveniza M, Mackerras D: Lightning injury: a review of clinical aspects, pathophysiology and treatment, *Adv Trauma* 4:241, 1989.
15. Apfelberg D, Masters F, Robinson D: Pathophysiology and treatment of lightning injuries, *J Trauma* 14:453, 1974.
16. Arden GP et al: Lightning accident at Ascot, *Br Med J* 1:1453, 1956.
17. Auerbach P: Lightning strike, *Top Emerg Med* 2:129, 1980.
18. Baker R: Paraplegia as a result of lightning injury, *Br Med J* 4:1464, 1978.
19. Bartholome CW, Jacoby WD, Ranchand SC: Cutaneous manifestation of lightning injury, *Arch Dermatol* 111:1466, 1975.
20. Bergstrom L et al: The lightning damaged ear, *Arch Otolaryngol* 100:117, 1974.
21. Bernstein T: Effects of electricity and lightning on man and animals, *J Forensic Sci* 18:3, 1973.
22. Bernstein T: *Lightning death and injury in the United States, fourteen years (1968-1981),* Madison, 1982, University of Wisconsin.
23. Bernstein T: Theories of the causes of death from electricity in the late 19th century, *Med Instum* 9:267, 1975.
24. Biegelmeier G: New knowledge of the impedance of the human body. In Bridges J et al, editors: *Electric shock safety criteria,* New York, 1985, Pergamon Press.
25. Bruce DA: The pathophysiology of increased intracranial pressure. In *Upjohn current concepts,* Kalamazoo, Mich, 1978, Upjohn.
26. Bridges J et al, editors: *Electric shock safety criteria,* New York, 1985, Pergamon Press.
27. Buechner HA, Rothbaum JC: Lightning stroke injury: a report of multiple casualties from a single lightning bolt, *Milit Med* 126:775, 1961.
28. Burda CD: Electrocardiographic changes in lightning stroke, *Am Heart J* 72:521, 1966.
29. Burkhardt K: Protect your boat from lightning, *Sail,* Oct 1987, p 47.
30. Campo RV, Lewis RS: Lightning-induced macular hole, *Am J Otolaryngol* 97:792, 1984.
31. Cannel H: Struck by lightning: the effects upon the men and the ships of H M Navy, *J R Nav Med Serv* 65:165, 1979.
32. Castren JA, Kytila J: Eye symptoms caused by lightning, *Acta Ophthalmol* 41:139, 1983.
33. Chai JC: Human body responses to step voltages due to ground currents in lightning attachments. In Proceedings of the International Conference on Lightning and Static Electricity, October 6-8, 1992, Atlantic City, NJ, FAA Report No DOT/FAA/CT-92/20, pp P21–P2-10.
34. Chalmers JA: *Atmospheric electricity,* ed 2, London, 1967, Pergamon Press.
35. Chan YF, Sivasamboo R: Lightning accidents in pregnancy, *J Obstet Gynecol Br Common* 79:761, 1972.
36. Changnon SA: Secular trends in thunderstorm frequencies. In Dolesalek H, Reiter R, editors: *Electrical process in atmospheres,* Darmstadt, 1977, Steinkopff, p 482.

37. Cherington M, Vervalin C: Lightning injuries: who is at greatest risk? *Phys Sportsmed* 18:58, 1990.
38. Cherington M, Yarnell P, Hallmark D: MRI in lightning encephalopathy, *Neurology* 43:1437, 1993.
39. Cherington M, Yarnell P, Lammereste D: Lightning strikes: nature of neurological damage in patients evaluated in hospital emergency departments, *Ann Emerg Med* 21:575, 1992.
40. Chia BL: Electrocardiographic abnormalities and congestive cardiac failure due to lightning stroke, *Cardiology* 68:49, 1981.
41. Clark RO, Brighan JK: Death from lightning, *Lancet* 2:77, 1872.
42. Connole JV: Lightning and electric cataract, *Pa Med J* 38:939, 1935.
43. Cook AH, Boulting W: Two cases of injury by lightning, *Br Med J* 2:234, 1888.
44. Cooper MA: Lightning injuries: prognostic signs for death, *Ann Emerg Med* 9:134, 1980.
45. Cooper MA: Electrical and lightning injuries, *Emerg Med Clin North Am* 2:489, 1984.
46. Cooper MA: Medical aspects of lightning injury. In Proceedings of the 9th International Conference on Atmospheric Physics, St. Petersburg, Russia, 1992.
47. Cooper MA, Andrews CJ, ten Duis HJ: Neuropsychological aspects of lighting injury. In Proceedings of the 9th International Conference on Atmospheric Physics, St. Petersburg, Russia, 1992.
48. Cooper MA, Johnson K: Electrical Injuries. In Rosen P, Barkin RM, editors: *Emergency medicine, concepts and clinical practice,* ed 3, St Louis, 1992, Mosby, p 979.
49. Crawford AS, Hoopes BF: The surgical aspects of lightning stroke, *Surgery* 9:80, 1941.
50. Critchley M: The effects of lightning with especial reference to the nervous system, *Bristol Med Chir J* 49:285, 1932.
51. Critchley M: Neurological effects of lightning and of electricity, *Lancet* 1:68, 1934.
52. Currens JH: Arterial spasm and transient paralysis resulting from lightning striking an airplane, *J Aviat Med* 16:275, 1945.
53. Darling, Frier, Pedlow: Report of cases of lightning stroke, *Br Med J* 2:1522, 1905.
54. Dill AV: Notes on a case of death by lightning, *Br Med J,* Oct 10, 1942, p 426.
55. Dimikov GM: ECG changes in persons struck by lightning (title translated from Russian), *Klin Meditsima (Mosc),* 1966, p 95.
56. Dollinger S: Lightning-strike disaster among children, *Br J Med Psychiatry* 58:375, 1985.
57. Dollinger SJ, O'Donnell JP, Staley, AA: Lightning-induced disaster: effects on children's fears and worries, *J Counsel Clin Psychol* 52:1028, 1984.
58. Duclos PJ, Sanderson LM: An epidemiological description of lightning-related deaths in the United States, *Int J Epidemiol* 19:673, 1990.
59. Duclos PJ, Sanderson LM, Klontz KC: Lightning-related mortality and morbidity in Florida, *Pub Health Rep* 105:276, 1990.
60. Dunscombe-Haniball O: Accidents and injuries caused by lightning, *J Med Assoc S Afr* 1:1153, 1900.
61. Dupasquier C, Freeman J: Le foudroeiment, cardiac injury due to lightning, *Ann Fr Anesth Reanim* 5:601, 1986.
62. DuToit JS: Bilateral cataract caused by lightning, *J Med Assoc S Afr* 1:503, 1927.
63. Eaton RDP: Lightning injury, *Can Med Assoc J* 128:893, 1983.
64. Eber B et al: Myokardiale Schadigung nach Blitzschlag, *Z Kardiol* 78:402, 1989.
65. Edwards W: Injuries due to lightning striking a wireless aerial, *Br Med J* 2:294, 1925.
66. Ekoe JM et al: Disseminated intravascular coagulation and acute myocardial necrosis caused by lightning, *Int Care Med* 11:160, 1985.
67. Elwell EG: Non-fatal lightning burns, *Br Med J* 2:771, 1934.
68. Eng LIL, Sinnadurai C: Syndrome of erythremia di Gugliemo after lightning injury with autoimmune antibodies and terminating in acute monocytic leukemia, *Blood* 25:845, 1965.
69. Engelstatter GH: Psychological effects of lightning strike and electric shock injuries. In lecture notes, Third Annual International Meeting of Lightning Strike and Electric Shock Victims, Maggie Valley, NC, 1993.
70. Epperley TD, Stewart JR: The physical effects of lightning injury, *J Fam Pract* 29:267, 1989.
71. Ferstle J: The lowdown on lightning, *Backpacker,* July 22-23, 1986.
72. Flannery DB, Wiles H: Follow-up of a survivor of intrauterine lightning exposure, *Am J Obstet Gynecol* 142:238, 1982.
73. Franklin B: *Experiments and observations on electricity made at Philadelphia,* London, 1774, E Cave.
74. Franklin B: *The autobiography of Benjamin Franklin,* New Haven, Conn, 1973, Yale University Press.
75. Frayne JH, Gilligan BSL: Neurological sequelae of lightning stroke, *Clin Exp Neurol* 24:195, 1987.
76. Gabriell L: Unusual clinical picture of intermittent deafness in a subject struck by lightning, *Otorhinolaryngology* 31:79, 1965.
77. Gem W: Case of lightning stroke followed by recovery, *Lancet* 2:288, 1913.
78. Golde RH, Lee WR: Death by lightning, *Proc Inst Elec Eng* 123:1163, 1976.
79. Golde RH: *Lightning,* vols 1 and 2, London, 1977, Academic Press.
80. Golde RH: *Lightning protection,* New York, 1973, Chemical Publishing.
81. Guha-Ray DK: Fetal death at term due to lightning, *Am J Obstet Gynecol* 134:103, 1979.
82. Hanson GC, McIlzoraith GR: Lightning injury: two case histories and a review of management, *Br Med J* 4:271, 1973.
83. Harwood SJ, Catrov PG, Cole GW: Creatinine phosphokinase isoenzyme fraction in the serum of a patient struck by lightning, *Arch Intern Med* 138:645, 1978.
84. Heffernan D: Autopsy in a case of death by lightning, *Lancet* 2:266, 1877.
85. Hegner CF: Lightning—some of its effects, *Ann Surg* 65:401, 1917.
86. Hocking B, Andrews CJ: Fractals and lightning injury, *Med J Aust* 150:409, 1989.
87. Holle RL et al: Cloud-to-ground lightning related to deaths, injuries and property damage in central Florida. In Proceedings of the International Conference on Lightning and Static Electricity, Oct 6-8, 1992, Atlantic City, NJ, FAA Report No DOT/FAA/CT-92/20, pp 66-1–66-12.
88. Ishikawa T et al: Experimental study on the lethal threshold value of multiple successive voltage impulses to rabbits simulating multistroke lightning flash, *Int J Biometeor* 29:157, 1986.
89. Ishikawa T et al: Experimental studies on the effect of artificial respiration after lightning accidents, *Res Exp Med* 179:59, 1981.
90. Jackson SHD, Parry DJ: Lightning and the heart, *Br Heart J* 43:454, 1980.
91. Jaffe R: Electropathology—review of the pathological changes produced by electric current, *Arch Pathol* 5:839, 1928.
92. Jex-Blake AJ: Death by electric currents and by lightning, The Ghoulstonian Lectures, Lecture III, *Br Med J,* p 548.
93. Johnstone BR, Harding DL, Hocking B: Telephone-related lightning injury, *Med J Aust* 144:706, 1986.
94. Jones DT et al: Lightning and its effects on the auditory system, *Laryngoscope* 101:830, 1992.
95. Kitigawa N, Ohashi M, Ishikawa T: Safety guide against lightning hazards, *Res Lett Atmosph Electr* 10:37, 1990.
96. Kitigawa N et al: The nature of lightning discharges on human bodies and the basis for safety and protection. In Proceedings of the 18th International Congress on Lightning Protection, Munich, 1985, p 435.

97. Kliener JP, Wilkin JH: Cardiac effects of lightning stroke, *JAMA* 240:2757, 1978.
98. Kleinot S, Lkacko D, Keeley K: The cardiac effects of lightning injury, *S Afr Med J* 40:1141, 1966.
99. Knaggs RH: Unusual injuries caused by lightning stroke, *Lancet* 2:1216, 1894.
100. Kotagal S et al: Neurologic, psychiatric, and cardiovascular complications in children struck by lightning, *Pediatrics* 70:190, 1982.
101. Kraus J: *Gewittekatechismus, oder Unterricht uber Blitz und Donner, und wie man bey einem Gewitter sein Leben gegen den Blitz schutzen und die von Blitz getroggenen Menschen retten kann,* ed 5, Augsburg, 1914, Doll.
102. Kravitz H et al: Lightning injury, management of a case with ten-day survival, *Am J Dis Child* 131:413, 1977.
103. Kristensen S, Tveteras K: Lightning-induced acoustic rupture of the tympanic membrane (a report of two cases), *J Otolaryngol Otol* 99:711, 1985.
104. Krob MJ, Cram AE: Lightning injuries: a multisystem trauma, *J Iowa Med Soc,* June 1983, p 221.
105. Langley RL, Dunn KA, Esinhart JD: Lightning fatalities in North Carolina 1972-1988, *NC Med J* 52:281, 1991.
106. Lea JA: Paresis of accommodation following injury by lightning, *Br J Ophthalmol* 4:417, 1920.
107. Lee RC, Cravalho EG, Burke JF: *Electrical trauma: the pathophysiology, manifestations and clinical management,* Cambridge, Eng, 1992, Cambridge University Press.
108. Lehman LB: Successful management of an adult lightning victim using intracranial pressure monitoring, *Neurosurgery* 28:907, 1991.
109. Leys K: Spinal atrophic paralysis case following lightning stroke, *Edinburgh Med J* 49:657, 1942.
110. Lichtenberg R et al: Cardiovascular effects of lightning strikes, *J Am Coll Cardiol* 21:531, 1993.
111. Lopez RE et al: The underreporting of lightning injuries and deaths in Colorado, *Bull Am Meteorol Soc* (submitted 1993).
112. Lucretius CT: *De rerum natura,* Lugduni, 1534, Gryphium.
113. Lopez RE, Holle RL, Heitkamp TA: *Deaths, injuries, and material damage due to lightning in Colorado from 1950 to 1991 based on storm data,* unpublished material, 1993.
114. Lynch M, Shorthouse P: Injuries and death from lightning, *Lancet* 1:473, 1949.
115. MacGorman DR, Rust WD: Lightning strike density for the contiguous United States from thunderstorm duration records, Pub No NUREG/CR03759, Washington, DC, 1984, Office of Nuclear Regulatory Research, US Nuclear Regulatory Commission.
116. Maloney ES: *Chapman piloting, seamanship and small boat handling,* ed 57, New York, 1985, Hearst Marine Books.
117. Mann H, Kozic Z, Boulos MI: CT of lightning injury, *Am J Neuroradiol* 4:976, 1983.
118. Martyal GG, Ryan ME: Lightning "deaths" can be reversed, *Emerg Dept News,* 1979, p 26.
119. McCarthy LJ, Parker C: Positive antiglobulin tests in a boy struck by lightning, *J Lab Med* 305:283, 1982.
120. McCrady-Kahn UL, Kahn AM: Lightning burns, *West J Med* 134:215, 1981.
121. McGraw CP: Continuous intracranial pressure monitoring, review of techniques and presentation of method, *Surg Neurol* 6:149, 1976.
122. Meek JM, Craggs JD: *The lightning discharge, electrical breakdown of bases,* Oxford, 1953, Clarendon Press.
123. Milward T: Prolonged gastric dilatation as a complication of lightning injury, *Burns* 1:175, 1975.
124. Moran KT: Electric- and lightning-induced cardiac arrest reversed by prompt cardiopulmonary resuscitation, *JAMA* 255:2157, 1986.
125. Moran KT, Munster AM: Lightning injury: physics, pathophysiology and clinical features, *Irish Med J* 79:120, 1986.
126. Morgan Z et al: Atrial fibrillation and epidural hematoma associated with lightning stroke, *N Engl J Med* 259:956, 1954.
127. Morikawa S, Steichen F: Successful resuscitation after death from lightning, *Anesthesia* 21:222, 1960.
128. Moulson AM: Blast injury of the lungs due to lightning, *Br Med J* 289:1270, 1984.
129. Myers GJ, Colgan MT, Van Dyke DH: Lightning disaster among children, *JAMA* 238:1045, 1977.
130. Noel LP, Clarke WN, Addison D: Ocular complication of lightning, *J Pediatr Ophthalmol Strabismus* 17:245, 1985.
131. Nollet JA: *Lettres sur l'electricite,* Paris, 1753, Guerin & Delatour.
132. Ohashi M, Kitagawa N, Ishikawa T: Lightning injury caused by discharges accompanying flashover—a clinical and experimental study of death and survival, *Burns* 12:496, 1986.
133. Palmer ABD: Lightning injury causing prolongation of the QT interval, *Post Med J* 63:891, 1987.
134. Panse F: Electrical trauma. In *Handbook of neurology,* vol 23, p 683.
135. Patterson JH, Turner JWA: Lightning and the central nervous system, *J R Army Med Corps* 82:73, 1944.
136. Peters WJ: Lightning injury, *Can Med Assoc J* 128:148, 1983.
137. Pethebridge K, Williams W: *Australian electrical wiring: theory and practice,* New York, 1985, McGraw-Hill.
138. Pierce MR, Henderson RA, Mitchell JM: Cardiopulmonary arrest secondary to lightning injury in a pregnant woman, *Ann Emerg Med* 15:597, 1986.
139. Plueckhahn VD: Injury and death caused by lightning, *Med J Aust* 144:673, 1986.
140. Poulson P, Knudstrup P: Lightning causing inner ear damage and intracranial haematoma, *J Laryngol Otol* 100:1067, 1986.
141. Prentice SA: Death by lightning, *Med J Aust* 2:252, 1973.
142. Prinz H: *Feur, Blitz and Funke,* Munich, 1965, Bruckman.
143. Pritchard EAB: Changes in the central nervous system due to electrocution, *Lancet* 1:1163, 1934.
144. Ravitch MM et al: Lightning stroke, *N Engl J Med* 264:36, 1961.
145. Raymond LF: Specific treatment of uveitis, lightning induced: an auto-immune disease, *Am J Allergy* 27:242, 1969.
146. Rees W: Pregnant woman struck by lightning, *Br Med J* 1:103, 1965.
147. Remillard WJ: *The acoustics of thunder,* Technical Memo No 44 (unpublished), Cambridge, Mass, 1960, Acoustic Research Laboratory, Harvard University.
148. Shantha TR: Causalgia induced by telephone-mediated lightning electrical injury and treated by interpleural block, *Anesth Analg* 73:507, 1991.
149. Shapiro MB: Lightning cataracts, *Wisc Med J* 83:23, 1984.
150. Sharma M, Smith A: Paraplegia as a result of lightning injury, *Br Med J* 2:1464, 1978.
151. Shaw D, York-Moore ME: Neuropsychiatric sequelae of lightning stroke, *Br Med J* 1957, p 1152.
152. Shaw GP, Atkinson LS: Hearing loss secondary to lightning strike, *Otolaryngology* 2:233, 1981.
153. Shulman K, Marmarou A, Miller JD: *Intracranial pressure IV,* Berlin, 1980, Springer-Verlag.
154. Silverman N: Unilateral deafness as a sequel to nonfatal lightning trauma, *J Ind State Med Assoc* 29:530, 1936.
155. Singer S: *The nature of ball lightning,* New York, 1971, Plenum Press.
156. Sinha AK: Lightning-induced myocardial injury, a case report with management, *Angiology* 36:327, 1985.
157. Skan DA: Death from lightning-stroke, with multiple injuries, *Br Med J* 1:666, 1949.
158. Slingerland I: Lightning stroke, *NY State Med J* 14:466, 1914.
159. Smith J: Lightning injuries, *J Emerg Nurs* 9:248, 1983.
160. Solterman B, Frutiger A, Kuhn M: Lightning injury with lung bleeding in a tracheotomized patient, *Chest* 99:240, 1991.
161. Spencer HA: *Lighting, lightning stroke and its treatment,* London, 1932, Bailliere, Tindal & Cox.
162. Stanley LD, Suss RA: Intracerebral hematoma secondary to lightning strike: case report and review of the literature, *Neurosurgery* 16:686, 1985.

163. Storm data, *NOAA* 27:12, 1985.
164. Strasser EJ, Davis RM, Menshey JJ: Lightning injuries, *J Trauma* 17:315, 1977.
165. Subramanian N, Somasundaram B, Periasamy JK: Cardiac injury due to lightning—report of a survivor, *Ind Heart J* 37:72, 1985.
166. Suri ML, Vijayan GP: Neurological sequelae of lightning, *J Assoc Phys Ind* 26:209, 1978.
167. Taussig H: "Death" from lightning and the possibility of living again, *Ann Intern Med* 68:1345, 1968.
168. ten Duis HJ, Klasen HJ: Keraunoparalysis, a 'specific' lightning injury, *Burns* 12:54, 1985.
169. ten Duis HJ et al: Superficial lightning injuries—their "fractal" shape and origin, *Burns* 13:141, 1987.
170. Thunderstorm Sensor, Lightning Location and Protection, Inc., 2705 E. Medina Road, Suite 111, Tucson, AZ 85706, 602-741-2838.
171. Tiscornia A: Bilateral cataract from lightning stroke, *JAMA* 77:1930, 1921.
172. Uman MA: *Understanding lightning,* Carnegie, Pa, 1971, Bek Technical Publications (reissued as *All about lightning,* New York, 1986, Dover).
173. US Department of Commerce: *Lightning,* Pub No API 70005, Washington, DC, 1970, US Government Printing Office.
174. US Department of Commerce: *Thunderstorms,* Pub No AA-PI 75009, Washington DC, 1976, US Government Printing Office.
175. Viemeister RE: *The lightning book,* Boston, 1972, MIT Press.
176. Wakasugi C, Masui M: Secondary brain hemorrhages associated with lighting stroke: report of a case, *Jpn J Legal Med* 40:42, 1986.
177. Wehe WA: Report of a case of burns from lightning, *Int J Surg,* 1918, p 191.
178. Weigel E: Lightning, the underrated killer, *NOAA* 6:2, 1976.
179. Weinstein L: Lightning: a rare cause of intrauterine death with maternal survival, *South Med J* 72:632, 1979.
180. Weiss KS: Otologic lightning bolts, *Am J Otolaryngol* 1:334, 1980.
181. West G: Lightning as a cause of hearing loss, *Md State Med J* 4:35, 1955.
182. Wilks G: Case of lightning stroke, *Lancet* 2:655, 1879.
183. Woods J: Spinal atrophic paralysis following lightning stroke, *S Afr Med J* 26:92, 1952.
184. Wright JW, Silk KL: Acoustic and vestibular defects in lightning survivors, *Laryngscope,* 1974, p 1378.
185. Yost JW, Holmes FF: Myoglobinuria following lightning stroke, *JAMA* 228:1147, 1974.
186. Zeana CD: Acute transient myocardial ischemia after lightning injury, *Int J Cardiol* 5:207, 1984.
187. Zegel FH: Lightning deaths in the United States: a seven-year survey from 1959 to 1965, *Weatherwise* 20:169, 1967.

12 EXPOSURE TO RADIATION FROM THE SUN

Josiah Friedlander
Nicholas J. Lowe

Solar Radiation

SOLAR SPECTRUM

Solar radiation encompasses the electromagnetic spectrum from short, high-energy cosmic rays, gamma rays, and x-rays to the longer, lower energy ultraviolet (UV), visible, infrared (IR), microwaves, and radiowaves (Fig. 12-1). Between 30% and 40% of solar radiation, including most of the harmful portions, is absorbed in the atmosphere by the ozone layer at 15 to 35 km above sea level.[22] High-energy radiation (wavelength less than 10 nm) displaces electrons from incident tissue to form ions. Therefore radiation in this category, including gamma rays and x-rays, is termed ionizing radiation. Since UV, visible, and shorter IR waves lack the energy to do this, they are categorized as nonionizing radiation.

The radiation striking the earth is approximately 50% visible (wavelength 400 to 800 nm), 40% IR (1300 to 1700 nm), and 10% UV (10 to 400 nm). The ultraviolet spectrum is divided for convenience into UVA, accorded 320 to 400 nm; UVB, from 290 to 320 nm; UVC, from 100 to 290 nm; and vacuum UV, from 10 to 100 nm.[9] The human eye cannot detect wavelengths other than those in the visible range. Vacuum UV, UVC, and the shortest UVB are screened by the ozone layer, which eliminates essentially all UVR under 290 nm. Little UVA is filtered in the atmosphere. The remaining UV that reaches the ground is about 10% UVB and 90% UVA at midday. UVB intensity declines from the noontime apex, but UVA intensity remains relatively constant throughout the day.[32]

FACTORS GOVERNING RADIATION INTENSITY

Radiation intensity varies substantially according to many factors, including time of day, altitude, latitude, and season. Eighty percent of UVR delivered to the earth's surface reaches the ground between 9 AM and 3 PM, with 65% between 10 AM and 2 PM. This is the time of day when the path that UVR travels is the most direct and therefore the shortest. As the day goes on, the distance that the energy must travel through the atmosphere (where incident UVR is most effectively absorbed) is longer and thus the energy is attenuated. UVR intensity increases 4% to 5% for every 1000 feet ascended, primarily as a function of lessening fog, dust, and smoke.

During summer the sun's path is more directly overhead so the path solar energy must travel is shorter. Hence, summer sun is stronger than winter sun. Closer to the equator the path the energy travels is also shorter, leading to more intense flux on the ground.

Radiation is reflected efficiently by snow and ice (80% to 85%) but can also be reflected by many other light-colored or reflective substances, including sand (20%), grass (2.5%), and bright metal, white, and water surfaces (10% to 100%) depending on angle of incidence and other factors. Interestingly, choppy water reflects more effectively than smooth. As the afternoon progresses, the sun's incident angle increases and therefore a larger percentage of UVR is reflected, although the UVR intensity itself decreases.[32]

Solar radiation that strikes humans on the earth's surface is a combination of sunlight and skylight. Sunlight is the unreflected component of solar radiation, while skylight is solar radiation reflected by clouds, air pollutants, and moisture. Usually skylight provides more of the UVR that reaches the surface. Peak sunlight at noontime provides as much UVR as does skylight. In areas with little air pollution and low humidity such as the desert, a higher proportion of the UVR comes from sunlight.[32]

Other important factors to consider in terms of UVR exposure are elements such as wind, humidity, and water ex-

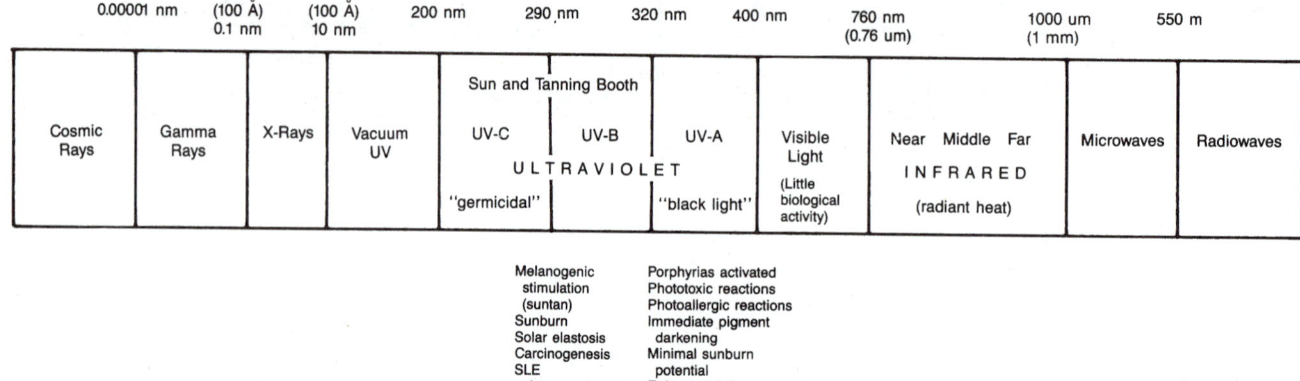

Fig. 12-1 Electromagnetic (solar) spectrum.

posure. An individual's perception of total UVR exposure is lessened when the skin is cooled by a brisk breeze. UVR penetrates well-hydrated skin up to four times as effectively as it does dry skin because of changes induced in the refractive index of the skin. Moist skin does not reflect or scatter incident UVR as effectively. Subjects who keep the skin well hydrated by frequent water immersion (as in swimming) or sunning in a humid environment have increased UV absorption.[32]

Finally, ozone (O_3), which is continuously generated and degraded in the stratosphere, provides an effective screen against virtually all radiation below 290 nm. The ozone eliminates essentially all vacuum UV and UVC. A large part of UVB is also filtered by the stratospheric ozone, but UVA arrives at the earth's surface virtually undiminished. The primary dermatologic concern about chlorofluorocarbon-enhanced degradation of the ozone layer is that more UVB will reach the surface of the earth, causing a dramatic rise in the deleterious effects of excessive solar exposure.[32]

Acute Effects of Radiation on the Skin

Depending on its physical properties, each wavelength produces different effects: energy carried, depth of penetration, and absorption by tissue. UVC has not been demonstrated to cause human health problems, even at relatively high dosages. Artificially generated UVC from germicidal lamps and arc welders appears to be safe. Although UVC is more energetic than UVB and UVA, it has little potential to induce melanogenesis ("tanning") or other radiation-induced effects because of its limited penetration beyond the outermost stratum corneum.[32]

UVB exposure leads to melanogenesis, sunburn, nonmelanoma skin cancer, premature aging, reactivation of herpes labialis,[36] and the nonenzymatic production of vitamin D. About 95% of the UVB presented to human skin is absorbed in the epidermis. Only 10% to 20% of UVB penetrates the dermis.

By contrast, UVA wavelengths effectively penetrate the dermis. UVA is responsible for most photoallergic and a few phototoxic reactions, as well as for the loss of elastosis seen in photoaged skin. A common artificial source of UVA is a Wood's lamp.

SUNBURN

Erythema, the most familiar manifestation of UVR exposure, occurs in a biphasic manner. The early portion of this reaction, known as immediate pigment darkening (IPD), is mediated by UVA and lasts 15 to 30 minutes. UVA-induced erythema is marked in some individuals, but undetectable in others. Delayed erythema, a function primarily of UVB dosage, begins 2 to 8 hours after exposure and reaches a maximum in 24 to 36 hours with erythema, pruritus, and pain in the sun-exposed areas. This reaction resolves over a 3- to 5-day period and initiates increased melanogenesis, which reaches an apex at 2 to 3 weeks.[32]

The minimal erythema dose (MED) is defined as the amount of UVB exposure after which minimally perceptible erythema can be detected. UVB at 307 nm is the most efficient wavelength for erythema. The dosage of UVA required to elicit erythema, 20 to 70 J/cm^2, is 600 to 1000 times that required for UVB, which ranges from 220 to 100 mJ/cm^2.[20] Although the intensity of UVA at noon is typically 10 times that of UVB, UVB radiation is responsible for 98% to 99% of delayed erythema development.

A typical MED value for an individual who burns easily and tans slightly is 20 minutes at midday in midsummer. An exposure of 5 MED produces a painful sunburn. At 10 MED, edema, vesiculation, and bulla formation often occur. Skin necrosis leading to scarring and uneven pigmentation may result. Depending on the area involved, severe sunburn can cause the systemic symptoms of "sun poisoning," including fever, nausea, vomiting, severe headache, prostration, and even shock.[32]

Microscopically, changes are detectable as early as 30 minutes after UVR exposure. Epidermal changes include intracellular edema, vacuolization, and swelling of melanocytes and the development of characteristic "sunburn cells." In the dermis, UVR initially leads to interstitial edema and endothelial cell swelling. Later, perivenular edema, degranulation and loss of mast cells, decrease in numbers of Langerhans' cells, neutrophil infiltration, and erythrocyte extravasation develop. This reaction reaches its apex at 24 hours and resolves over 3 to 5 days.[32]

Sunburn cells are dyskeratotic keratinocytes with pyknotic nuclei and homogeneous eosinophilic cytoplasm. Sunburn cell formation is maximal at 18 to 24 hours after exposure and resolves in 3 to 7 days.[32] These cells occur in proportion to the amount of skin's UVB exposure. UVA is less effective in the development of sunburn cells.[17]

Later changes include hyperkeratosis (increased scale), acanthosis (epidermal thickening), disorganization and misalignment of keratinocytes, dermal vascular ectasia, and mononuclear perivascular infiltration.[20]

Treatment of Acute Sunburn

No truly effective therapies for the acute symptoms of a sunburn have been developed. Fortunately, the symptoms resolve over 2 to 3 days, usually without sequelae. Simple and safe therapies are usually the best to recommend.

Cool compresses, frequent cool showers or baths, and lotions containing menthol may provide significant symptomatic relief. The use of teabags, oatmeal, calamine, aloe, baking soda, cornstarch, or talcum powder has not been demonstrated to provide any additional benefits. Topical agents with benzocaine may provide symptomatic relief, but benzocaine is known to be sensitizing.

Oral analgesics may be necessary for some individuals. Although acetaminophen, aspirin, or ibuprofen is usually sufficient, occasionally narcotics such as acetaminophen with codeine are necessary.

When administered early in the course of a sunburn, antiprostaglandins such as nonsteroidal antiinflammatory drugs (NSAIDs) are helpful in reducing erythema. Although NSAIDs do not reverse the damage incurred by the skin, they are touted enthusiastically by some as a useful therapy. Topical indomethacin cream has been demonstrated to diminish or delay UVB-induced erythema when applied prophylactically 1 hour before exposure. Interestingly, the indomethacin appears to work both by inhibiting prostaglandin synthesis and by acting as a UVB blocker. Indomethacin cream has an SPF of 4 to 5. Unfortunately, topical indomethacin has no effect on UVA-induced erythema or sun damage and the cream is not available in the United States.[32]

Corticosteroids, both topical and systemic, are also relatively ineffective in reducing sunburn erythema. Topical corticosteroids blanch a low-intensity sunburn, but not as effectively as indomethacin. Systemic steroids are also ineffective in ameliorating the symptoms of most sunburns. However, persons with systemic symptoms of sun poisoning may benefit from a few days of systemic corticosteroid therapy.[32]

SOLAR RADIATION AND THE IMMUNE SYSTEM

UVR is known to suppress the mixed lymphocyte reaction in the skin, a measure of immune function. There is some question as to whether sunscreens can prevent this UVR-induced dysfunction.[28,45] Two other measurements of immune function, contact hypersensitivity to 2,3-dinitrofluorobenzene and inhibition of transplanted UVR-induced tumor cell growth, are suppressed in chronically UVR-exposed mice. No protection is provided by an SPF 15 sunscreen containing padimate O as the active ingredient, although a similarly rated sunscreen containing 2-ethylhexyl-*p*-methoxy cinnamate prevents this immunosuppression.[31]

SOLAR RADIATION AND OCULAR INJURY

The eyes are extremely sensitive to UVR overexposure. Ocular injuries may be categorized anatomically from anterior to posterior. A sunburnlike reaction of the cornea and conjunctivae from mild excessive UVR is termed "snow blindness." This occurs more commonly at altitudes where UVR intensity is higher. Because of snow's excellent optical reflective properties, this condition is frequently seen in skiers and hikers in snowy areas. A variant occurs in those who frequent tanning salons. The UVA generated by the tanning machines can actually penetrate the lid of an otherwise unprotected but closed eye and induce a corneal injury.

Brief exposure to high-intensity UVR, such as from a welder's torch, may also cause photokeratitis.

Symptoms of photokeratitis begin 2 to 12 hours after exposure and include erythema, increased lacrimation, and a gritty sensation. Depending on the severity of the injury, other manifestations may include photophobia, chemosis, overwhelming pain, and blepharospasm. This condition is usually self-limited, resolving over a couple of days.

The examining physician notes intense conjunctival injection, along with corneal pitting on staining with fluorescein. Visual acuity is generally unaffected, although it may be difficult to assess because of patient discomfort.

UVA can induce ocular injuries, but UVB is the more common etiologic agent for photokeratitis. Unfortunately, no protective phenomenon analogous to tanning occurs in the eye. Skiers and mountain climbers should be advised to wear protective sunglasses with attached side panels to reduce peripheral reflected radiation. When these are unavailable, sunglasses may be improvised using cardboard with a narrow slit for viewing. Sunscreen applied to eyelids may provide additional protection.

Treatment for acute photokeratitis must be directed at pain control. The use of topical anesthetics during the initial examination often provides significant relief, but ongoing use of these substances is discouraged because of their negative effect on healing. If iritis is associated with the keratitis, topical mydriatic-cycloplegic therapy (such as tropicamide 1%–cyclopentolate 0.5 to 1% or homatropine 5%) may be beneficial in relieving pain. Subsequently, short-term narcotic analgesics and sedatives may be necessary. Corticosteroids are of no proven use and should be avoided because they predispose to infection. When there appears to be breakdown of corneal integrity, judicious bilateral use of topical antibiotic ointments and patching may be useful as prophylaxis against infection.

More serious and permanent anterior ophthalmic injuries may occur via exposure to intense sources of UVR. Examples include UVR lasers, which can induce cataracts within 24 hours after exposure to radiation in the 295 to 325 nm range. Even more dramatically, cataracts can develop nearly instantaneously after exposure to an intense source near 365 nm.

Cumulative industrial exposure has been implicated in the development of glassblower's and furnaceman's cataracts. This relationship has been demonstrated epidemiologically, although the pathophysiologic mechanism is unclear.

For persons at risk, it is important to emphasize the damage that can occur and to counsel on prevention through the use of protective eyewear. Currently the only therapy for fully formed cataracts is surgical extraction.

Retinal injury most often results from prolonged direct viewing of the sun. Usually the discomfort and even severe pain that result from staring at the sun are enough to discourage individuals from continuing. However, prolonged sungazing does occur during a solar eclipse when the observed intensity of the sun's rays is lessened. Even when the general guidelines of viewing an eclipse only through photographic film are followed, observers sometimes develop "eclipse retinopathy" or solar retinitis. Other circumstances such as drug abuse (for example, LSD), religious rituals (a Brahman ritual in India involves sungazing), and viewing the sun through binoculars can lead to solar retinitis.

The optical characteristics of the eye actually increase the risk for severe injuries to the retina. The lens focuses incident radiation onto the foveal portion of the macular retina, the area of highest visual acuity. The intensity of the solar radiation at the lens is thus increased substantially by the time it strikes the fovea.

Clinical findings of mild solar retinitis may be limited to local edema. Extensive changes including retinal atrophy, foveal cysts, or even permanent holes in the fovea (accompanied by development of a central scotoma) can occur with more intense cumulative exposure.

Detection of the extent of often subtle changes requires the skills of an expert ophthalmologist and sophisticated examination techniques such as fluorescein angiography. Systemic corticosteroids are useful in ameliorating the edema and inflammation.[32]

Chronic Effects of Solar Radiation on the Skin

The two major adaptive responses in the skin initiated by UVR exposure are melanogenesis (tanning) and thickening of the stratum corneum. Tanning occurs as a result of de novo production of melanin in melanocytes. UVB enhances the binding of circulating melanocyte-stimulating hormone (MSH) to melanocytes, leading to melanocyte proliferation, dendritic arborization, and pigment production. Interestingly, UVB actually induces melanocyte proliferation in both exposed and covered areas of the body.[20]

Melanin is produced from tyrosine through several enzymatically controlled reactions. The initial, rate-limiting step is the conversion of tyrosine into dihydroxyphenyalanine (DOPA). The melanin, incorporated into organelles called melanosomes, is then distributed to surrounding keratinocytes (Fig. 12-2). Some melanosomes remain intact in the keratinocytes as they keratinize and migrate to become the stratum corneum. However, others are degraded enzymatically into an amorphous form that is deposited in the interstitium. This amorphous melanin undergoes oxidation in the "immediate pigment darkening" reaction when exposed to UVA radiation.[32]

Melanin absorbs, reflects, and scatters UVR and also acts as a free radical trap. Although persons of all skin types have approximately the same number of melanocytes, black-skinned persons have approximately 400 melanosomes per basal epidermal cell, four times as many as the

A

Tyrosine

Tyrosinase

Dopa

Melanin

5,6,-Dihydroxyindole

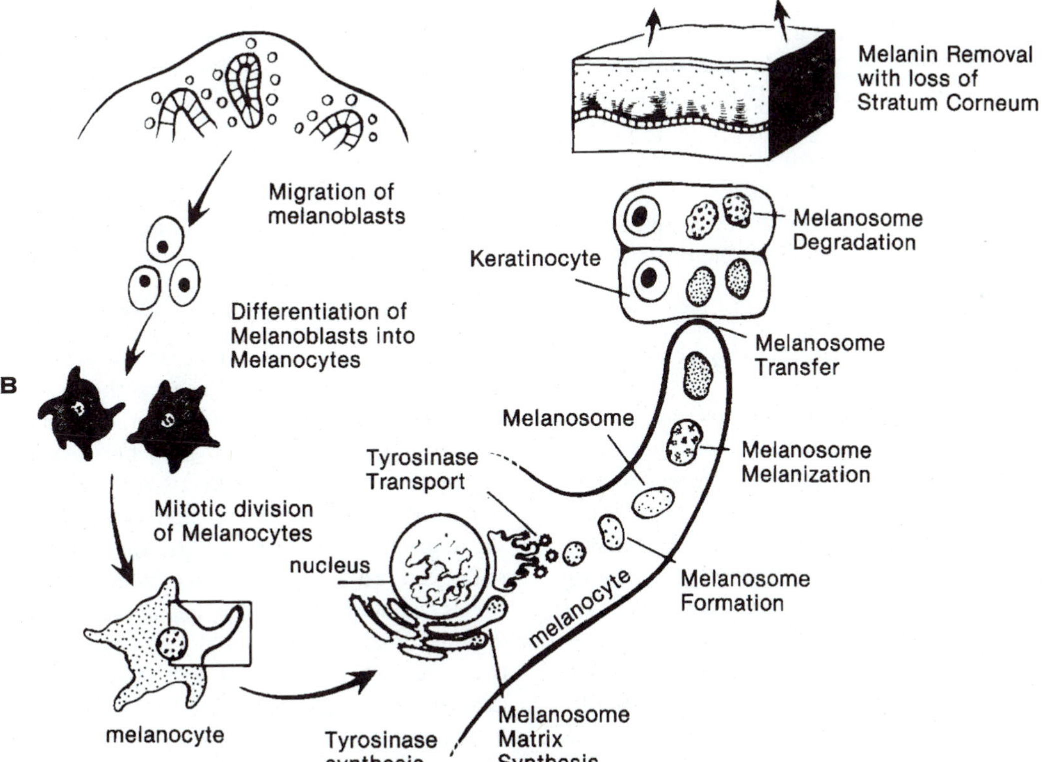

Fig. 12-2 **A,** Biosynthesis of tyrosine-based melanin. **B,** Morphologic and metabolic pathway of epidermal melanin pigmentation. (From Isselbacher KJ et al, editors: *Harrison's principles of internal medicine,* ed 9, New York, 1980, McGraw-Hill.)

typical pale white person.[32] This difference reduces the UVA and UVB penetration into the dermis by a factor of five in blacks as compared with whites and is responsible for the 30-fold increase in the typical MED value for blacks.[20]

Tanning induces a maximal SPF increase of 2 to 4 against further UVR exposure. Even with a "protective tanning base," whites are susceptible to a significant amount of UVR-induced damage.[32]

The skin surface is composed of a layer of densely keratinized cells called the stratum corneum. In response to chronic UVB exposure the stratum corneum can hypertrophy to six times its original thickness via increased synthesis of keratin by basal keratinocytes. This response is independent of pigmentary changes, as evidenced by its occurrence in albinoes. The stratum corneum is particularly hypertrophied on the palms and soles, which explains why these areas are so resistant to sun damage.[32] Thickened stratum corneum absorbs or reflects 90% to 95% of incident UVB, so that just 5% to 10% reaches the basal keratinocytes, melanocytes, and superficial dermal vascular system.[15] Interestingly, chronic UVA exposure does not induce a similar proliferation of the stratum corneum.[20]

Although UVA exposure at high dosage (such as in a tanning salon) can produce erythema and melanogenesis, it does not provide the same degree of protection as a naturally acquired UVB suntan. This is due to at least two factors. UVA does not induce thickening of the stratum corneum, an important protective factor induced by UVB. Also, the pigmentary changes induced by UVA exposure occur primarily in the basal layer while those initiated by UVB are distributed throughout the epidermis. Although these differences are not detectable by the casual observer, they can be distinguished histologically and in terms of their protective effect.[32]

SOLAR RADIATION AND PHOTOAGING

Human skin changes in grossly and microscopically detectable ways over the lifetime of an individual. However, exposure to excessive amounts of solar radiation greatly increases the rate at which skin ages. Dermatoheliosis ("photoaging") is the wrinkled, leathery skin seen prematurely in persons chronically exposed to the sun. Photoaging is induced by chronic exposure to all portions of the solar spectrum, including UVA, UVB, and infrared.[21] In fact, the only other clinically significant cause of photoaging that has been documented is cigarette smoking. A person who smokes more than 10 cigarettes a day is statistically more likely to have older-appearing skin than that of an age-matched and sun exposure–matched control subject.

Grossly, photoaged skin appears wrinkled and atrophic with mottled pigmentation. Superimposed are hypopigmented macules as well as hyperpigmented lentigines ("liver spots" or "sun spots"), telangiectasia, and raised, roughened, precancerous actinic keratoses.

Microscopically, as skin ages normally, the epidermis atrophies, the dermis becomes hypocellular, the vasculature remains intact, and collagen forms a stable, increasingly cross-linked matrix. By contrast the epidermis of photoaged skin becomes acanthotic (thickened), the dermis becomes hypercellular (because of fibroblast and mast cell proliferation), and the vessels become tortuous and dilated. Elastic fibers degenerate into a thickened, amorphous mass, displacing the normal collagen in a process termed elastosis. These changes are detectable in most whites before 30 years of age.[20] Shorter UVA, in the 320 to 340 nm range, is probably responsible for the bulk of UVA-induced photodamage.[21]

Chronic exposure to solar radiation also has dramatic effects on the life span of fibroblasts and keratinocytes. It is well documented that human fibroblasts in vitro divide only a limited number of times before they die. Although the mechanism remains unclear, the number of times they replicate correlates with the age of the subject from whom the fibroblasts are obtained. More recent studies have demonstrated that fibroblasts and keratinocytes from a given individual replicate more times if obtained from an unexposed area of the body than if derived from more chronically sun-exposed tissue.[44] This implies that solar radiation exposure increases the turnover or decreases the regenerative capacity of human skin and thus hastens skin aging.

Some good news is on the horizon. Scientific studies have documented histologic and physical improvement in photodamaged skin after treatment with topical tretinoin (0.1% retinoic acid) cream. Although work continues, these results are welcomed by dermatologists and patients.[46]

SOLAR RADIATION AND CANCER

Solar radiation–induced local immune suppression may induce or promote nonmelanoma skin cancer (NMSC). UVR definitely induces NMSC in mice. Transformation of normal cells into malignant probably results from UVR-initiated DNA mutation. Patients with xeroderma pigmentosum, who lack the usual reparative enzymes for damaged DNA, are at greatly increased risk for NMSC. Although cumulative UVB appears to be more closely linked to NMSC development, UVA also plays a role. Both can induce thymine dimer formation, which may be an initiating step in cell transformation. Also, UVA has been demonstrated to augment the development of UVB-induced NMSC in hairless mice.[20]

Epidemiologic studies of cumulative sun exposure and the incidence of NMSC in normal humans are also extremely strong. The risk of basal cell carcinoma in Atlanta, Georgia, is 50% greater than that in Minneapolis, Minnesota. The age-adjusted risk for squamous cell carcinoma in Atlanta is four times that in Minneapolis. The mutagenicity of a joule of UVB at 300 nm is 1000 times that of a joule of UVA at 330 nm. The carcinogenic effects probably correlate with the mutagenicity, and thus UVB can be assumed to be many times more carcinogenic than UVA.[42]

The data on malignant melanoma (MM) are not as clear. Nevertheless, MM is probably induced or promoted in some way by UV exposure. Recent trends have shown an alarming rise in development of MM. Risk factors for the development of MM are complex and do not correlate with cumulative UVB exposure. However, intermittent intense sunlight exposure may correlate with the development of melanoma.[12] As mentioned earlier, UVB actually induces melanocyte proliferation in both exposed and covered areas of the body. This may explain why MM sometimes occurs in areas without significant prior sun exposure.[20]

Garland, Garland, and Gorham[12] postulate that broader use of sunscreens that primarily protect against UVB wavelengths encourages susceptible individuals to spend more time in the sun. These persons receive a larger cumulative dose of solar radiation outside the UVB range. Increased exposure to non-UVB solar radiation may initiate or promote the development of skin cancers of both the basal cell and melanoma types.

SUN EXPOSURE IN ANIMALS

Animals are generally much more resistant than humans to the effects of UVR exposure. Small areas of certain animals, such as a collie's nose and the eyelids of collies and sheep dogs are both hairless and poorly pigmented. A solar radiation–induced dermatitis can develop in these areas under conditions of high solar flux. With severe and repeated episodes, even squamous cell carcinoma has been described.[32]

Sunscreens

HISTORY AND DEVELOPMENT

In 1928 the world's first commercial use of a sunscreen, an emulsion of benzyl salicylate and benzyl cinnamate, was reported in the United States. In the 1930s a 10% solution of phenyl salicylate (Solol) appeared on the Australian market. In 1935 lotions of quinine oleate and quinine bisulfate were available in the United States. In 1943 PABA was patented, introducing this popular agent and subsequently its derivatives. The U.S. military used red petrolatum, a physical blocking agent, as a sunblock during World War II. Their efforts also led to the popularization of other UV-filtering agents, including glyceryl PABA, 2-ethylhexyl salicylate, digalloyl trioleate, homomenthyl salicylate, and dipropylene glycol salicylate.[39] Most early agents were directed toward UVB, the portion of the sun's spectrum responsible for the most palpable and distressing effect, the familiar sunburn.

Parsol 1789 (abobenzone or 4-t-butyl-4′-methoxydibenzoylmethane), an agent broadly effective in the UVA spectrum, is now marketed in combination with UVB blocking agents. These formulations provide broad-spectrum chemical sun protection to the U.S. consumer.

A new subclass of physical blockers, micronized reflecting powders, have recently been made available from a variety of manufacturers. Unlike traditional physical blockers, micronized reflecting powders are invisible. They provide broad-spectrum protection against UVR similar to that of the traditional products. The powders should prove useful to UVR-sensitive patients resistant to physical blockers for cosmetic reasons. An additional benefit is that they do not cause photosensitization.

Future trends in the development of sunscreens include products with efficacy against UVC (which may become more important with further erosion of the ozone layer) and agents directed against infrared (because of concerns about IR-induced photoaging).

EVALUATION OF SUNSCREENING AGENTS

Agents Against UVB

The U.S. Food and Drug Administration (FDA)-approved technique to assess the efficacy of a sunscreen in the UVB portion of the spectrum is determination of the sunscreen protection factor (SPF). SPF is defined as the ratio of the time of UVR exposure necessary to produce minimally detectable erythema in sunscreen-protected skin to the time for unprotected skin.

A typical testing protocol is as follows. Skin, ideally in a non-sun-exposed area such as the buttocks or lower back, is covered with lightproof adhesive foil. Areas of foil 1 cm^2 are removed sequentially so that each area receives a defined dose of UVB. The following day the patient returns and the areas are assessed for erythema. The amount of exposure necessary to generate barely detectable erythema is determined.

One day later, sunscreen is applied uniformly with a pipette at 2 mg/cm^2 or 2 $\mu l/cm^2$. The sunscreen is allowed to dry for 15 minutes, and then the subject is irradiated for incrementally increasing times based on the estimated SPF, which is usually determined spectrophotometrically. The volunteer is asked to return 24 hours later, at which time the skin is reexamined. The minimal erythema dose of UVB for the protected skin is determined. The SPF is then calculated from the ratio of the protected MED to the unprotected MED.[23]

There is some controversy about whether SPF thus defined accurately reflects the action spectra for induction of skin cancer in humans. Also, application of 2 mg/cm^2 correlates to using at least 1 ounce over the body's surface. Since studies have revealed that most individuals apply about 0.75 ounce (1.5 mg/cm^2 or 1.5 $\mu l/cm^2$), the in vivo SPF is sometimes significantly less than the listed SPF.[14]

Agents Against UVA

Currently no consensus has been reached on a technique to assess a protection factor in the UVA portion of the spectrum. In part, the confusion is due to limited knowledge about the harmful effects of UVA radiation. It is obvious that UVB causes sunburn and that this is undesirable, if for no other reason than the associated discomfort. UVA can cause erythema, but only after a much larger dose. However, the action spectra for other UVA-induced phenomena (such as photosensitivity dermatitis, photoaging, and possible effects in the development of MM and NMSC) are not specifically defined. In addition, the various techniques used by the different investigators do not correlate well with one another.[35]

The UVA protection factor (APF) is defined analogously to SPF and simply assesses the time until erythema develops in UVA-exposed skin. The reliability of such testing is questionable because of the inadequacy of current filters used on the light sources to generate pure UVA beams, as well as the long exposure times required.[35] Recently, however, Cole and VanFossen[5] described a high-intensity UVA source that they contend is a more effective method to assess UVA protection based on either erythema or tanning in an unsensitized individual.

Phototoxic protection factor (PPF) was developed to decrease the UVA dose necessary to achieve a detectable difference in erythema. This involves sensitizing the subject's skin with 8-methoxypsoralen (8-MOP), either topically or orally, and then comparing the MED, as is done for UVB sunscreen testing.[26]

Immediate pigment darkening (IPD), a UVA- and visible spectrum–mediated transient oxidation of preexisting melanin, has also been used to evaluate UVA sunscreen efficacy.[19] IPD has been criticized because it does not reflect any UVA-induced damage to the skin, either acutely or chronically.[1] In addition, IPD testing must be performed on individuals with darker skin because pale-skinned individuals who are most in need of protection do not demonstrate easily measurable IPD.[1]

The monochromatic protection factor (MPF) is defined as the ratio of the photocurrent (measured by a spectroradiometer) measured through plain Transpore tape (3M Company, St. Paul, Minn.) to the photocurrent measured through sunscreen-coated tape at a given wavelength. According to Diffey and Robson,[6] this in vitro method provides close agreement with in vivo recorded SPF data. Other techniques include spectrophotometrically comparing sunscreeen applied to either quartz crystal[35] or excised, treated epidermis,[37] with the untreated surface as a control.

Finally, the inhibition of sunburn cell formation by sunscreen in 8-MOP-sensitized skin in both mice[35] and humans[40] has been used to assess UVA sun protection. The inciting wavelength for sunburn cells is in the UVB range, but this is shifted into UVA by sensitization with 8-MOP.[13] The limitations of these final two techniques are obvious in light of the difficulty in ensuring a correlation between these in vitro tests and the human response.

Substantivity

Substantivity is the characteristic of a sunscreen that reflects how effectively the advertised degree of protection is maintained under adverse conditions, including repeated water exposure or sweating. According to the FDA, a sunscreen is declared water resistant if it can maintain its original SPF after two 20-minute immersions. A sunscreen is considered waterproof if it retains its protective integrity after four 20-minute immersions.[18] Substantivity is enormously important, since sunscreens are used outdoors in settings where abundant sweating and repeated immersion in water are common.

ACTIVE SUNSCREEN INGREDIENTS (TABLE 12-1)

Protectants Against UVB

PABA. PABA (paraaminobenzoic acid) has been available since 1943 and was popular in the 1950s and

Table 12-1 FDA-Approved Sunscreen Ingredients (1993)

Product	Approved Percent of Product
CHEMICAL BLOCKERS	
UVA Absorbers	
Oxybenzone	2-6
Sulisobenzone	5-10
Dioxybenzone	3
Methyl anthralinate	3.5-5
Avobenzone	3*
UVB Absorbers	
Aminobenzoic acid (PABA)	5-15
Amyl dimethyl PABA (padimate A)	1-5
2-Ethoxyethyl-1 *p*-methoxy cinnamate	1-3
Diethanolamine *p*-methoxy cinnamate	8-10
Digalloyl trioleate	2-5
Ethyl 4-bis (hydroxypropyl) aminobenzoate	1-5
2-Ethylhexyl-2-cyano-3,3 diphenylacrylate	7-10
Ethylhexyl-*p*-methoxy cinnamate	2-7.5
2-Ethylhexyl salicylate	3-5
Glyceryl aminobenzoate (glyceryl PABA)	2-3
Homomenthyl salicylate	4-25
Lawsone with dihydroxyacetate	0.25% with 3%
Octyl dimethyl PABA (padimate O)	1.4-8
2-Phenylbenzimidazole-5-sulfonic acid	1.4
Thethanolamine salicylate	5-12
PHYSICAL BLOCKERS	
Red petrolatum	30-100
Titanium dioxide	2-25

*Available in the United States (1993) in Photoplex, Filteray, and Shade UVA Guard.

1960s. For a variety of reasons, PABA is now used infrequently as a sunscreen. Its absorption peak at 296 nm[39] is relatively far from the UVB-induced erythema peak at 307 nm. It is poorly soluble in water and must be used as a 5% to 15% solution in alcohol. After application, PABA effectively penetrates the stratum corneum, where it is trapped and remains bonded via hydrogen bonding to epidermal proteins. This greatly enhances its substantivity[10] but also increases the risk for contact or photocontact dermatitis. Sensitivity of this sort is seen in up to 4% of the population.[8] PABA can cause a stinging sensation when applied and stains both cotton and synthetic fabrics. After photooxidation this can leave a permanent yellow discoloration.[30]

PABA Derivatives. PABA esters are created by addition of hydrocarbon groups to the PABA molecule. Many of these molecules are an improvement over PABA in that they are water soluble and do not penetrate the stratum corneum. The most widely used of the PABA derivatives is padimate O, or octyl dimethyl PABA. Its absorption peak is around 300 nm in nonpolar solvents, ranging to 316 nm in polar solvents.[39] Padimate O is relatively stable chemically, making it less likely to stain clothing.[41] Padimate A (amyldimethyl PABA) is similar to padimate O and is also used in combination with other agents. Neither ester stains clothing, although both can cause stinging when applied.

Another derivative, glyceryl PABA, has frequently been implicated as the etiologic agent in both contact and photocontact dermatitis. However, after careful testing it appears that contaminating impurities, including benzocaine, may actually have been responsible.[7]

Salicylates. These agents are ortho-disubstituted aromatic compounds with a peak absorption around 300 nm. Two compounds of this type, octyl salicylate and homomenthyl salicylate (homosalate), are currently approved in the United States. Although not very effective as sunscreens, they have the benefit of being exceptionally stable, essentially nonsensitizing, and water insoluble, leading to high substantivity. They are also useful as solubilizers of other poorly soluble sunscreen ingredients such as the benzophenones.[39] They are used commonly in "PABA-free" products.[41]

Cinnamates. 2-Ethylhexyl-1 *p*-methoxy cinnamate (Par-sol MCX) (absorption maximum 310 to 311 nm),[8] 2-ethoxyethyl-*p*-methoxy cinnamate (Cinoxate) (UV absorption maximum 310 nm),[8] diethanolamine-methoxy cinnamate, and octyl methoxy cinnamate are available in the United States. These are effective in blocking UVB but have poor substantivity; they are generally found in combination with other agents.[27] Cinoxate is the cinnamate most often noted to cause contact and photocontact dermatitis. Cross-sensitization is seen with other cinnamates, found in balsam of Peru, balsam of Tolu, coca leaves, and cinnamon oil.[7]

Protectants Against UVA

Benzophenones. Benzophenones are aromatic ketones that absorb predominantly in the UVA portion of the spectrum between 320 and 350 nm. For example, oxybenzone has an absorption maximum of 326 nm in polar solvents compared with 352 nm in nonpolar solvents. Benzophenone-3 (sulisobenzone) and dioxybenzone are also approved for the U.S. market.[39] Oxybenzone is frequently implicated as the etiologic agent in photocontact allergy, although reactions have also been reported with dioxybenzone.[7]

Dibenzoylmethanes. Dibenzoylmethanes are substituted diketones that undergo keto-enol tautomerism on absorption of UVR. The keto form of the dibenzoylmethanes has a UV absorption maximum of 260 nm while the enol form absorbs above 345 nm. Parsol 1789 (avobenzone or 4-t-butyl-4′-methoxy-dibenzoylmethane), with an absorption maximum at 355 nm, is the only agent of this class available in the United States. Although these compounds are capable of a high degree of UV absorption, they are unstable and can undergo photoisomerization to compounds that are not protective. Parsol 1789 has been shown to have a loss of protective power as high as 36% because of photodegradation.[39] Even Parsol 1789 does not provide significant protection against UVA radiation close to 400 nm.[33]

Physical Blockers

Physical blocking agents such as zinc oxide, titanium dioxide, iron oxide, kaolin, icthammol (ichthyol),[30] red veterinary petrolatum, talc ($MgSiO_2$), and calamine (FeO_2) are composed of particles of a size that scatter, reflect, or absorb solar radiation in the UV, visible, and even infrared ranges. Twenty percent zinc oxide, 20% titanium dioxide, and 1% iron oxide have been spectrophotometrically demonstrated to reduce transmittance in the UVA and visible ranges to a maximum of approximately 20%. However, a combination of the zinc and iron oxides is synergistic, effectively reducing transmittance in the UVA and visible ranges to as low as 1.5%. These data were confirmed in vivo in a hematoporphyrin derivative–sensitized guinea pig model.[33]

Older physical blockers have the disadvantage that they are comedogenic, must be applied in a relatively thick layer, and melt in the sun, staining clothing. They are opaque and therefore visible, making them cosmetically undesirable for many individuals. These formulations have found a market in young people who apply brightly pigmented products in limited areas. However, this does not provide protection for untreated areas. Because of the efficacy and broad-spectrum coverage of physical blockers, they are potentially important for persons with certain photosensitivity disorders.

Recently developed micronized preparations now available in the United States provide an excellent option within this class of sunscreens. Micronized physical blockers are suspensions of finely ground material such as titanium dioxide that reflect at wavelengths shorter than the visible spectrum. Since they do not reflect in the visible spectrum, they are invisible and thus more cosmetically acceptable. Micronized titanium dioxide is chemically stable and does not cause any photoallergic or contact dermatitis.

Micronized sunscreens are more effective at the shorter UV wavelengths. A major difficulty in formulating micronized sunscreens is in preventing agglomeration of the particles. If this occurs, the portion of the spectrum reflected will shift into the visible range and the product will have characteristics of traditional opaque physical blockers.

In the field a variety of physical blockers can be concocted that, although somewhat messy, provide good photoprotection. Ashes from charcoal or wood, clay paste, axle grease, and covering the head with tree branches or clothing are all possible options.[32]

Vehicle

The choice of vehicle for a sunscreen is important for several reasons. First, the proper vehicle can enhance a sunscreen's substantivity or ability to remain on the skin and be effective. Second, the wrong vehicle may act as a skin irritant, induce a phototoxic or photoallergic reaction, or be comedogenic. Finally, a solvent may modify the sunscreening agent because of its polarity and thereby dramatically shift the absorption spectrum of the agent toward or away from the desired range.[25]

Systemic Photoprotection

Over the years a variety of systemic agents have been investigated as oral agents for sunscreening purposes. The appeal is threefold. First, oral agents are convenient. Second, they provide coverage for the entire body. Third, they are likely to eliminate the concern over substantivity so critical for topically applied products. Included in the list of these products are PABA, antihistamines, aspirin, indomethacin, retinol, ascorbic acid, α-tocopherols (such as vitamins A, C, and E), corticosteroids, psoralens, β-carotene, and antimalarials. The last three are used in some individuals with certain photosensitivity dermatoses (see later discussion). Otherwise, these agents have been disappointing for persons with normal skin.[44]

Sun Protective Clothing

Although UVB is partially reflected by clothing, lightweight fabrics typically worn in summertime do not even provide an SPF of 15. Once these fabrics are damp from sweat or water, their SPF falls. The weave of a fabric does not appear to have a dramatic effect on the flux of solar radiation through garments. In fact, it has been shown that a tightly woven cotton fabric provides less protection against UV exposure than a shirt of white knitted fabric. Solumbra, a maker of sun protective wear, manufactures clothing that has been demonstrated in vivo to provide an SPF greater than 30 regardless of color or moisture content.[38] Such special fabrics are useful for some photosensitivity sufferers. Practitioners should be aware that some fabrics provide protection via an applied coating that may lose efficacy over time.

Other Barriers

Window glass effectively blocks UVR below 320 nm, thus providing solid protection against UVB. Tinted windows and the plastic interleaf found in auto windshields effectively block nearly all UVA.[16] However, front and side window tinting sufficient to protect individuals with UVA-sensitive skin is illegal in many areas because of concerns about reduced driver visibility and limited ability for law enforcement officers to see what is happening inside an auto with closed windows.

Sun Protection

SUN PROTECTION FOR NORMAL SKIN

Chronic exposure to UVB leads to deleterious effects on human skin, including photoaging and NMSC. Application of a UVB blocking sunscreen decreases the risk for development of NMSC.[32] Therefore we recommend that patients use sunscreens as described in Table 12-2.

In addition, all individuals should be encouraged to stay indoors or seek shade during the peak hours of solar radiation flux from 10 AM to 2 PM. A hat or a sun visor is a useful addition. Patients with pale complexions should be reassured that fair skin is attractive. Those who insist on darker skin should use a self-tanning lotion containing dihydroxyacetone (DHA). Tanning salons should be avoided because intense UVA exposure provides limited protection and induces photoaging and photoallergic reactions.

Individuals who spend a significant amount of time outdoors, particularly in areas of high solar flux, should be cautioned about the acute and chronic risks of UV exposure and should be advised as to how to properly protect themselves. Included in this list of individuals are naturalists, skiers, hikers, bicyclists, fishermen, mountain climbers, and gardeners as well as members of certain professions (such as farmers and farm workers, lifeguards, meter readers, postal delivery persons, and police officers walking a beat).

Finally, information about sun protection should be disseminated to children at an early age. Childhood is typically the time of life when maximal sun exposure occurs. Childhood sunburns are implicated in increasing risk for malignant melanoma[20] and NMSC and thus should assiduously be avoided. It has been calculated biostatistically that if children consistently used an SPF 15 sunscreen through the age of 18, the occurrence of NMSC could be reduced by 78%. If an SPF 7.5 product were used throughout life, the risk of NMSC would decrease 97%.[42,43]

Tables 12-3 and 12-4 list many of the suncreening formulations currently available in the United States.

Table 12-2 Skin Types and Recommended Sunscreen Protection Factors

Type	Characteristic	Examples	Suggested SPF: Routine Day	Suggested SPF: Outdoor Activity
I	Always burns easily, never tans	Celtic or Irish extraction; often blue eyes, red hair, freckles	15	25-30 (waterproof)
II	Burns easily, tans slightly	"Fair-skinned" individuals; often have blond hair	12-15	25-30 (waterproof)
III	Sometimes burns, then tans gradually and moderately	Most whites	8-10	15 (waterproof)
IV	Burns minimally, always tans well	Hispanics and Asians	6-8	15 (waterproof)
V	Burns rarely, tans deeply	Middle Easterners, Indians	6-8	15 (waterproof)
VI	Almost never burns, deeply pigmented	Blacks	6-8	15 (waterproof)

SUN PROTECTION FOR PHOTOSENSITIVE SKIN

A variety of skin disorders occur as a result of, or can be exacerbated by, exposure to solar radiation. Photosensitivity disorders are conveniently divided into phototoxic, photoallergic, and nontoxic, nonallergic disorders. Phototoxic disorders generally can be described as an exaggerated but otherwise normal response to light. Photoallergies are an abnormal or atypical dermal reaction to a chemical substance to which the sufferer has previously been photosensitized. The final category encompasses innate or acquired disorders that can worsen after exposure to solar radiation.

A general precaution must be noted when suggesting a strategy to protect a patient with photosensitivity dermatitis. These persons also tend to be supersensitive to chemicals. Many manufacturers are developing superpotent sunscreens with high SPF values that rely on high concentrations of several sunscreening agents used together. At these higher concentrations all persons are at increased risk of chemical irritation and sensitization. However, individuals with a preexisting photosensitivity dermatitis are at particularly high risk.[23]

Phototoxicity

Phototoxicity can occur in any individual exposed to photosensitive agents and radiant energy of sufficient intensity. It should be suspected in anyone seeking treatment for a sunburn out of proportion to the extent of UVR exposure. Although the etiology is unknown, phototoxicity does not involve the immune system. One postulated mechanism is that the offending agent is incorporated into cells. The incident UVR at a specific wavelength is absorbed by this chemical as a chromophore. This initiates development of an exaggerated sunburn.

Phototoxic reactions occur most frequently in persons with type I and II skin and least frequently in children and black-skinned persons. The onset is typically minutes to hours after UV exposure; dermatologic manifestations are those of an exaggerated sunburn, sometimes with formation of blisters or bullae. When the sensitizing substance is ingested, the dermatitis occurs only in the areas of sun exposure demarcated by clothing lines. If the etiologic agent is applied topically, the areas affected are those to which the agent was applied where sun exposure also occurred. The reaction resolves without sequelae. Although UVB is usually involved, it is wise to use a broad-spectrum sunscreen and to withdraw the offending agent.[32]

External agents commonly implicated in phototoxic reactions are listed in Box 12-1.[30]

A large number of plants elaborate photoactive substances, such as furocoumarins (particularly psoralens), which can induce phototoxic reactions (Table 12-5).[30] This category of phototoxic reaction is termed phytophotodermatitis. It has been noted in vegetable pickers and other food handlers, as well as in naturalists. Flower leis given to visitors in Hawaii have also been implicated.

Phytophotodermatitis is commonly exploited by dermatologists as part of a therapeutic regimen to control psoriasis and to repigment the skin of persons with vitiligo. Patients are administered psoralens either topically or orally and then are exposed to controlled doses of UVA. This is called PUVA (psoralen UVA).

Psoralens are also incorporated into sunscreens as a suntan-enhancing agent in Europe. Unfortunately, this can lead to severe and possibly lethal sunburns in some individuals and also increases the risk of skin cancer, since it is documented that psoralens in combination with UVA increase the risk for development of NMSC.[30]

Table 12-3 Sunscreen Formulations Available in the United States (1993)

Product	SPF	Ingredients
Solbar PF (Person and Covey)	50 (waterproof)	Cream: oxybenzone, octyl methoxy cinnamate, octocrylene
PreSun 46 (Westwood)	46 (waterproof)	Lotion: padimate O, oxybenzone
Coppertone Moisturizing Sunblock 45 (Plough)	45 (waterproof)	Lotion: ethylhexyl-*p*-methoxy cinnamate, 2-ethylhexyl salicylate, octocrylene, oxybenzone, vitamin E, aloe
Water Babies Sunblock (Plough)	45 (waterproof)	Lotion: ethylhexyl-*p*-methoxy cinnamate, 2-ethylhexyl salicylate, octocrylene, benzyl alcohol
Shade Sunblock (Plough)	45 (waterproof)	Lotion: ethylhexyl-*p*-methoxy cinnamate, octocrylene, oxybenzone, 2-ethylhexyl salicylate, benzyl alcohol
Vaseline Intensive Care Block Out (Chesebrough-Ponds)	40 (waterproof)	Lotion: padimate O, ethylhexyl-*p*-methoxy cinnamate, oxybenzone, 2-ethylhexyl salicylate, titanium dioxide
PreSun 39 Creamy Sunscreen (Westwood)	39 (waterproof)	Cream: padimate O, oxybenzone, cetyl alcohol
Bullfrog (Chattem)	36 (waterproof)	Gel: benzophenone-3, octocrylene, octyl methoxy cinnamate, isostearyl alcohol
Aloe Up (Aloe Up)	30 (waterproof)	Lotion: homosalate, octyl methoxy cinnamate, oxybenzone, octyl salicylate
Aloe Up Water Sports (Aloe Up)	30 (waterproof)	Lotion: octyl methoxy cinnamate, benzophenone-3, octyl salicylate, homosalate
Coppertone Moisturizing Sunblock 30 (Plough)	30 (waterproof)	Lotion: ethylhexyl-*p*-methoxy cinnamate, 2-ethylhexyl salicylate, homosalate, oxybenzone, vitamin E, aloe
Coppertone Kids (Plough)	30 (waterproof)	Lotion: octocrylene, ethylhexyl-*p*-methoxy cinnamate, oxybenzone, 2-ethylhexyl salicylate
Neutrogena Sunblock (Neutrogena)	30 (waterproof)	Lotion: ethylhexyl-*p*-methoxy cinnamate, octocrylene, methyl anthralinate
Sundown Sunblock Ultra (Johnson & Johnson)	30 (waterproof)	Lotion: ethylhexyl-*p*-methoxy cinnamate, 2-ethylhexyl salicylate, octocrylene, oxybenzone, benzyl alcohol, 2-ethylhexyl salicylate, benzophenone-3
PreSun Active Clear Gel (Westwood)	30 (waterproof)	Gel: octyl methoxy cinnamate, oxybenzone, octyl salicylate
Johnson's Baby Sunblock (Johnson & Johnson)	30 (waterproof)	Lotion: benzophenone-3, octyl methoxy cinnamate, octyl salicylate, titanium dioxide
Shade Sunblock (Plough)	30 (waterproof)	Stick: ethylhexyl-*p*-methoxy cinnamate, oxybenzone, 2-ethylhexyl salicylate, homosalate Lotion: ethylhexyl-*p*-methoxy cinnamate, oxybenzone, 2-ethylhexyl salicylate, homosalate, benzyl alcohol, phenethyl alcohol
Sea & Ski Block Out for Kids (Carter)	30 (waterproof)	Lotion: padimate O, octyl methoxy cinnamate, oxybenzone
Solbar PF (Person and Covey)	30	Lotion: octocrylene, octyl methoxy cinnamate, oxybenzone, SD alcohol 40
Water Babies Sunblock (Plough)	30 (waterproof)	Lotion: ethylhexyl-*p*-methoxy cinnamate, oxybenzone, 2-ethylhexyl salicylate, homosalate, benzyl alcohol
Bain de Soleil Protecteur Gentil Under Eye Protecteur (Richardson-Vicks)	30	Stick: ethylhexyl-*p*-methoxy cinnamate, oxybenzone, 2-ethylhexyl salicylate
T1-Screen (Fischer)	30 (waterproof)	Lotion: ethylhexyl-*p*-methoxy cinnamate, oxybenzone, 2-ethylhexyl salicylate, 2-ethylhexyl 2-cyano-3,3-diphenacrylate
Vaseline Intensive Care Block Out (Chesebrough-Ponds)	30 (waterproof)	Lotion: ethylhexyl-*p*-methoxy cinnamate, oxybenzone, 2-ethylhexyl salicylate, titanium dioxide
PreSun 29 Sensitive Skin Sunscreen (Westwood)	29 (waterproof)	Cream: octyl methoxy cinnamate, oxybenzone, octyl salicylate, cetyl alcohol
PreSun for Kids (Westwood)	29 (waterproof)	Cream: octyl methoxy cinnamate, oxybenzone, octyl salicylate, cetyl alcohol
Aloe Up (Aloe Up)	25	Lotion: homosalate, octyl methoxy cinnamate, benzophenone-3
Body Glove (Promenity)	25 (waterproof)	Lotion: octyl methoxy cinnamate, oxybenzone, titanium dioxide
Water Babies Sunblock (Plough)	25 (waterproof)	Cream: ethylhexyl-*p*-methoxy cinnamate, 2-ethylhexyl salicylate, homosalate, oxybenzone, benzyl alcohol
Coppertone Moisturizing Sunblock (Plough)	25 (waterproof)	Lotion: ethylhexyl-*p*-methoxy cinnamate, 2-ethylhexyl salicylate, homosalate, oxybenzone, benzyl alcohol, vitamin E, aloe

Table 12-3 Sunscreen Formulations Available in the United States (1993)—cont'd

Product	SPE	Ingredients
Shade Sunblock (Plough)	25	Gel: ethylhexyl-*p*-methoxy cinnamate, octyl salicylate, homosalate, oxybenzone, SD alcohol 40
Bain de Soleil Protecteur Gentil Body Silkening Creme (Richardson-Vicks)	25 (waterproof)	Cream: padimate O, ethylhexyl-*p*-methoxy cinnamate, oxybenzone, benzyl alcohol
Bain de Soleil Protecteur Gentil Facial Creme (Richardson-Vicks)	25 (waterproof)	Cream: padimate O, ethylhexyl-*p*-methoxy cinnamate, oxybenzone
Bain de Soleil Protecteur Gentil Body Silkening (Richardson-Vicks)	25	Stick: padimate O, ethylhexyl-*p*-methoxy cinnamate, oxybenzone, dioxybenzone
Eclipse 25 (Eclipse)	25 (water resistant)	Lotion: octyl methoxy cinnamate, titanium dioxide, oxybenzone, octyl salicylate
Hawaiian Tropic Baby Faces Sunblock (Tanning Research)	25 (waterproof)	Lotion: 2-ethylhexyl-*p*-methoxy cinnamate, oxybenzone, octyl salicylate, methyl anthralinate
Neutrogena Sunblock Stick (Neutrogena)	25	Stick: octyl methoxy cinnamate, benzophenone-3, octyl salicylate
Sundown Sunblock Ultra (Johnson & Johnson)	25	Lotion: octyl methoxy cinnamate, oxybenzone, octyl salicylate, titanium dioxide, cetyl alcohol
PreSun 23 (Westwood)	23 (waterproof)	Lotion: ethylhexyl-*p*-methoxy cinnamate, oxybenzone, 2-ethylhexyl salicylate
PreSun for Kids (Westwood)	23 (waterproof)	Cream: padimate O, oxybenzone
Aloe Up (Aloe Up)	20 (waterproof)	Spray mist: padimate O, octyl methoxy cinnamate, oxybenzone, octyl salicylate, SD alcohol 40
Child Garde (Eclipse)	20 (waterproof)	As above
Sundown Sunblock Ultra (Johnson & Johnson)	20 (waterproof)	Lotion: octyl methoxy cinnamate, octyl salicylate, oxybenzone, titanium dioxide, cetyl alcohol
Bain de Soleil Protecteur Gentil Body Silkening Spray (Richardson-Vicks)	20 (waterproof)	Lotion: padimate O, oxybenzone, ethylhexyl-*p*-methoxy cinnamate, octyl salicylate, titanium dioxide, cetyl alcohol
TI-Screen (Fischer)	20	Lotion: ethylhexyl-*p*-methoxy cinnamate, oxybenzone, 2-ethylhexyl salicylate, SD alcohol 40
Bullfrog (Chattem)	18 (waterproof)	Gel: octocrylene, benzophenone-3, octyl methoxy cinnamate, isostearyl alcohol Stick: benzophenone-3, octyl methoxy cinnamate, isostearyl alcohol
Bullfrog for Kids (Chattem)	18 (waterproof)	Gel: octocrylene, octyl methoxy cinnamate, octyl salicylate
Neutrogena Chemical Free* (Neutrogena)	17	Lotion: micronized titanium dioxide
TI-Screen Natural* (Fischer)	16 (waterproof)	Cream: micronized titanium dioxide
Body Glove Everyday (Promenity)	15	Lotion: octyl methoxy cinnamate, oxybenzone
Body Glove Bug and Sun (Promenity)	15	Lotion: octyl methoxy cinnamate, oxybenzone
Block Out by Sea & Ski (Carter)	15 (waterproof)	Cream: padimate O, octyl methoxy cinnamate, oxybenzone
Block Out Clear by Sea & Ski (Carter)	15	Lotion: padimate O, octyl methoxy cinnamate, SD alcohol 40
Caribe Sports Screen (Caribe)	15	Lotion: ethyl dihydroxypropyl PABA
Coppertone Moisturizing Sunblock (Plough)	15 (waterproof)	Lotion: ethylhexyl-*p*-methoxy cinnamate, oxybenzone, benzyl alcohol, vitamin E, aloe
Coppertone Kids 15 (Plough)	15 (waterproof)	Lotion: ethylhexyl-*p*-methoxy cinnamate, oxybenzone, 2-ethylhexyl salicylate, homosalate
DuraScreen (Penederm)	15	Lotion: octyl methoxy cinnamate, benzophenone-3, octyl salicylate, titanium dioxide
Filteray (Borroughs-Wellcome)	15 (water resistant)	Lotion: avobenzone, padimate O, benzyl alcohol
Hawaiian Tropic 15 Plus Sunblock (Tanning Research)	15 (waterproof)	Lotion: ethylhexyl-*p*-methoxy cinnamate, oxybenzone, methyl anthralinate
Johnson's Baby Sunblock (Johnson & Johnson)	15	Cream and lotion: octyl methoxy cinnamate, octyl salicylate, oxybenzone, titanium dioxide, stearyl alcohol, cetyl alcohol
Neutrogena Sunblock (Sunblock)	15 (waterproof)	Lotion: octyl methoxy cinnamate, octyl salicylate, methyl anthralinate

Continued.

Table 12-3 Sunscreen Formulations Available in the United States (1993)—cont'd

Product	SPE	Ingredients
No More Tears* (Johnson & Johnson)	15	Lotion: micronized titanium dioxide and zinc oxide
Noskote Sunblock Creme (Plough)	15 (waterproof)	Cream: ethylhexyl-*p*-methoxy cinnamate, 2-ethylhexyl salicylate, oxybenzone, benzyl alcohol
Oil of Olay Lotion (Procter & Gamble)	15	Lotion: ethylhexyl-*p*-methoxy cinnamate, 2-phenylbenzimidazole-5-sulfonic acid
Photoplex Broad Spectrum Sunscreen (Herbert Labs)	15 (water resistant)	Lotion: padimate O, avobenzone, benzyl alcohol
PreSun 15 Facial (Westwood)	15	Cream: padimate O, oxybenzone, benzyl alcohol, cetyl alcohol Stick: padimate O, oxybenzone, petrolatum
PreSun 15 Creamy (Westwood)	15 (waterproof)	Cream: padimate O, oxybenzone, cetyl alcohol
PreSun 15 Sensitive Skin Sunscreen (Westwood)	15 (waterproof)	Cream: octyl methoxy cinnamate, oxybenzone, octyl salicylate, cetyl alcohol
Purpose Lotion (Johnson & Johnson)	15	Lotion: methyl anthralinate, octyl methoxy cinnamate, titanium dioxide
Ray Block (Del Ray)	15	Lotion: padimate O, benzophenone-3, SD alcohol
Shade Sunblock (Plough)	15 (waterproof)	Gel: 2-ethylhexyl-*p*-methoxy cinnamate, octyl salicylate, oxybenzone, SD alcohol 40 Lotion: 2-ethylhexyl-*p*-methoxy cinnamate, oxybenzone, benzyl alcohol, phenethyl alcohol
Shade UVA Guard (Plough)	15 (water resistant)	Lotion: octyl methoxy cinnamate, avobenzone, oxybenzone
Solbar Plus 15 (Person & Covey)	15 (waterproof)	Cream: padimate O, oxybenzone, dioxybenzone
Solbar PF (Person & Covey)	15 (water resistant)	Cream: Octyl methoxy cinnamate, oxybenzone
Solbar PF Sunscreen (Person & Covey)	15	Liquid: octyl methoxy cinnamate, oxybenzone, SD alcohol 40
Sundown Sunblock Ultra (Johnson & Johnson)	15 (waterproof)	Cream: octyl methoxy cinnamate, octyl salicylate, oxybenzone, titanium dioxide, stearyl alcohol, cetyl alcohol
Sundown Sunblock Ultra (Johnson & Johnson)	15 (waterproof)	Lotion: padimate O, octyl methoxy cinnamate, oxybenzone, benzyl alcohol, stearyl alcohol
Total Eclipse Oily and Acne Prone Skin Sunscreen (Eclipse)	15	Lotion: padimate O, oxybenzone, glyceryl PABA, alcohol
Total Eclipse Sunscreen Moisturizing (Eclipse)	15 (waterproof)	Lotion: padimate O, oxybenzone, octyl salicylate in moisturizing base
TI-Screen (Fischer)	15 (water resistant)	Lotion: ethylhexyl-*p*-methoxy cinnamate, oxybenzone
TI-Baby (Fischer)	15 (water resistant)	Lotion: ethylhexyl-*p*-methoxy cinnamate, oxybenzone
Vaseline Intensive Care Moisturizing Sunblock (Chesebrough-Ponds)	15 (waterproof)	Lotion: ethylhexyl-*p*-methoxy cinnamate, oxybenzone
Vaseline Intensive Care Baby Moisturizing Sunblock (Chesebrough-Ponds)	15 (waterproof)	Lotion: ethylhexyl-*p*-methoxy cinnamate, oxybenzone
Vaseline Intensive Care UV Lotion (Chesebrough-Ponds)	15	Lotion: ethylhexyl-*p*-methoxy cinnamate, oxybenzone
Water Babies Sunblock by Coppertone (Plough)	15 (waterproof)	Lotion: ethylhexyl-*p*-methoxy cinnamate, oxybenzone, benzyl alcohol
Aloe Up (Aloe Up)	12 (waterproof)	Lotion: octyl methoxy cinnamate, benzophenone-3
Purpose Lotion (Johnson & Johnson)	12	Lotion: octyl methoxy cinnamate, oxybenzone
Banana Boat (Sun)	10 (waterproof)	Lotion: ethylhexyl-*p*-methoxy cinnamate, oxybenzone, aloe, vitamin E
Caribe Clear Face Screen (Caribe)	10	Lotion: benzophenone-3, homosalate
Hawaiian Tropic Sunscreen (Tanning Research)	10 (waterproof)	Lotion: padimate O, oxybenzone
Original Eclipse Sunscreen (Eclipse)	10	Lotion: padimate O, glyceryl PABA
Snootie by Sea & Ski (Carter)	10	Lotion: padimate O
Bullfrog (Chattem)	9 (waterproof)	Gel: benzophenone-3, octyl methoxy cinnamate, isostearyl alcohol
Aloe Up (Aloe Up)	8 (waterproof)	Lotion: octyl methoxy cinnamate, benzophenone-3
Banana Boat (Sun)	8 (waterproof)	Lotion: padimate O, oxybenzone, aloe, vitamin E
Body Glove (Promenity)	8 (waterproof)	Lotion: octyl methoxy cinnamate, oxybenzone

Table 12-3 Sunscreen Formulations Available in the United States (1993)—cont'd

Product	SPE	Ingredients
Neutrogena Sunless Tanning (Neutrogena)	8	Lotion: octyl methoxy cinnamate
Neutrogena Sunblock (Neutrogena)	8 (waterproof)	Lotion: octyl methoxy cinnamate, methyl anthralinate
PreSun 8 Creamy (Westwood)	8 (waterproof)	Cream: padimate O, oxybenzone, cetyl alcohol
Hawaiian Tropic Aloe PABA Sunscreen (Tanning Research)	8 (waterproof)	Lotion: padimate O, oxybenzone, aloe
TI-Screen (Fischer)	8 (water resistant)	Lotion: ethylhexyl-*p*-methoxy cinnamate, oxybenzone
Coppertone Moisturizing Sunscreen (Plough)	8 (waterproof)	Lotion: ethylhexyl-*p*-methoxy cinnamate, oxybenzone, benzyl alcohol, vitamin E, aloe
Sundown (J&J)	8 (waterproof)	Cream: octyl methoxy cinnamate, octyl salicylate, oxybenzone, titanium dioxide
Sundown Maximal (J&J)	8 (waterproof)	Lotion: padimate O, oxybenzone, benzyl alcohol, stearyl alcohol
Almay Moisturizing Lotion (Almay)	6 (water resistant)	Lotion: ethylhexyl-*p*-methoxy cinnamate, 2-ethylhexyl salicylate, oxybenzone
Almay Sunless Tanning Lotion (Almay)	6	Lotion: ethylhexyl-*p*-methoxy cinnamate, oxybenzone
Aloe Up Suntan Oil (Aloe Up)	6	Oil: octyl methoxy cinnamate
Banana Boat (Sun)	6 (waterproof)	Lotion: padimate O, aloe, vitamin E
Hawaiian Tropic Sunscreen (Tanning Research)	6 (waterproof)	Lotion: padimate O, oxybenzone
Coppertone Moisturizing Sunblock (Plough)	6 (waterproof)	Lotion: ethylhexyl-*p*-methoxy cinnamate, oxybenzone, benzyl alcohol, vitamin E, aloe
Sundown Extra (Johnson & Johnson)	6 (waterproof)	Lotion: padimate O, oxybenzone, benzyl alcohol, stearyl alcohol
Almay Protective Tanning Gel (Almay)	4	Gel: 2-phenylbenzimidazole-5-sulfonic acid
Aloe Up (Aloe Up)	4 (waterproof)	Lotion: octyl methoxy cinnamate, benzophenone-3
Sea & Ski Golden Tan (Carter)	4	Lotion: padimate O
Sundown Moderate (Johnson & Johnson)	4 (waterproof)	Lotion: padimate O, oxybenzone, benzyl alcohol, stearyl alcohol
Hawaiian Tropic Dark Tanning with Sunscreen (Tanning Research)	4 (waterproof)	Lotion: octyl methoxy cinnamate, methyl anthralinate
Tan Magnifier by Coppertone (Plough)	4	Lotion: ethylhexyl-*p*-methoxy cinnamate
Coppertone Lite Tanning (Plough)	4 (waterproof)	Lotion: ethylhexyl-*p*-methoxy cinnamate
Coppertone Moisturizing Suntan (Plough)	4 (waterproof)	Lotion: ethylhexyl-*p*-methoxy cinnamate, oxybenzone, benzyl alcohol, vitamin E, aloe
Coppertone Moisturizing Suntan (Plough)	2 (waterproof)	Oil: homosalate, vitamin E, aloe
Coppertone Lite Tanning (Plough)	2	Oil: 2-ethylhexyl salicylate
QT by Coppertone (Plough)	2	Lotion: ethylhexyl-*p*-methoxy cinnamate
Sea & Ski Baby Lotion Formula (Carter)	2	Lotion: padimate O
Coppertone Dark Tanning Spray (Plough)	2 (waterproof)	Oil: ethylhexyl-*p*-methoxy cinnamate, vitamin E, aloe
Maxafil (Gen Derm)	NA	Oil: cinoxate, methyl anthralinate
A-FII (Gen Derm)	NA	Cream: methyl anthralinate, titanium dioxide (dark or neutral tint)
Ray-Nox (Torch)	NA	Cream: PABA, stearyl alcohol, cetyl alcohol
RV Paque (Elder)	NA	Cream: red petrolatum, zinc oxide, and cinoxate in a water-resistant base

*Micronized physical blockers ("chemical free").

Table 12-4 Lip Sunscreen Formulations Available in the United States (1993)

Product	SPF	Ingredients
Water Babies Little Licks by Coppertone (Plough)	30	Lip balm: ethylhexyl-*p*-methoxy cinnamate, oxybenzone, 2-ethylhexyl salicylate
Bain de Soleil Lip Protecteur (Richardson Vicks)	30	Lip balm: ethylhexyl-*p*-methoxy cinnamate, oxybenzone, 2-ethylhexyl salicylate, oleyl alcohol, petrolatum
Aloe Kote (Aloe Up)	25	Lip balm: homosalate, octyl methoxy cinnamate, oxybenzone, aloe
PreSun 15 Lip Protector (Westwood)	15	Lipstick: padimate O, oxybenzone, petrolatum
ChapStick Sunblock 15 (Robins Consumer)	15	Lip balm: padimate O, oxybenzone, cetyl alcohol, tartrazine
Eclipse Lip and Face Protectant (Eclipse)	15	Stick: padimate O, oxybenzone
Hawaiian Tropic 15 Sunblock Lip Balm (Tanning Research)	15	Lip balm: padimate O, oxybenzone
Lipkote by Coppertone (Plough)	15	Lip balm: ethylhexyl-*p*-methoxy cinnamate, oxybenzone, vitamin E, aloe
Daily Conditioning Treatment for Lips (Blistex)	15	Lip balm: padimate O, oxybenzone, petrolatum, cetyl alcohol
Blistek (Blistex)	10	Lip balm: padimate O, oxybenzone, dimethicone, cetyl alcohol; regular, mint, and berry flavors
RV PABA (Elder)	NA	Lipstick: PABA

Photoallergy

Photoallergy involves interaction of the immune system and solar radiation. Photoallergic reactions are rare and usually require UVA exposure. Individuals with this disorder have previously been exposed to the responsible agent and, after reexposure to it and UVR, develop the dermatitis within 24 to 48 hours later. The reaction resembles a contact dermatitis and primarily involves sun-exposed areas, although it may spread to adjacent unexposed skin. Photoallergy can be seen with minimal substance and UVR exposure and resolves fully after elimination of the allergen except for occasional postinflammatory hypopigmentation. Both ingested and applied substances can be responsible. Common offenders include some of the agents added to soaps, cosmetics, and perfumes. Because of the length of time between contact with the inciting agent and development of the dermatologic manifestation, neither patient nor doctor may be able to relate the two. Photopatch testing is often necessary to identify the etiologic agent. Since the UVA portion of the spectrum is most often responsible, it is important to use an effective UVA sunscreen product.[32]

Other Photosensitivity Disorders

The third category of photodermatoses, those responses that are neither phototoxic nor photoallergic, include several disorders discussed in the following paragraphs. Since affected persons are extremely sensitive to the sun, they need a highly efficacious sunscreen or properly tested sun protective clothing.

Polymorphous Light Eruption. Polymorphous light eruption (PMLE) is a common, idiopathic skin eruption that occurs in susceptible individuals on exposure to more intense than usual solar irradiation (290 to 365 nm).[24] PMLE affects 10% to 14% of the white population, a majority of them female, with onset usually in the first three decades of life. Typically, PMLE manifests as some combination of pruritic papules, macules, vesicles, plaques, or confluent erythema 1 to 2 days (2 hours to 5 days) after sun exposure on areas of unprotected skin. PMLE is seen most commonly at the beginning of summer or during a visit to a geographic clime with a higher solar flux. The reaction resolves over 7 to 10 days if additional sun exposure is avoided. As the name suggests, the reaction is polymorphic; in a given individual it usually has a single morphology that remains constant.

Investigators have variously implicated UVA, UVB, UVC, visible radiation, x-rays, and even α-particles in the action spectrum. Often, PMLE flares can be prevented by use of newer broad-spectrum sunscreens. A recent study of an Inuit Indian population demonstrated that at least 18 of 30 were sensitive to UVA. According to the physician evaluators in this study, 86% of the 21 patients who completed the study obtained good to excellent results using a sunscreen containing padimate O and avobenzone.[11]

It must be kept in mind that sunscreens providing modest UVA protection (such as benzophenones) are poorly effective for persons with PMLE. Many patients benefit from prophylactic PUVA photochemotherapy, while others respond to oral agents, including antimalarials or β-carotene.[44] Some may have to avoid the sun entirely and to wear effective sun protective clothing.

Porphyria. Porphyrias are caused by an inherited or acquired abnormality in the heme metabolic pathway. Substrate for the affected enzyme accumulates, leading to

BOX 12-1
AGENTS THAT MAY CAUSE PHOTOSENSITIVITY*

ANTICANCER DRUGS
Dacarbazine* (DTIC-Dome)
Fluorouracil (Fluoroplex; others)
Methotrexate (Mexate; others)
Procarbazine (Matulane)
Vinblastine (Velban)

ANTIDEPRESSANTS
Amitriptyline (Elavil; others)
Amoxapine (Asendin)
Desipramine (Norpramin; Pertofrane)
Doxepin (Adapin; Sinequan)
Imipramine (Tofranil; others)
Isocarboxazid (Marplan)
Maprotiline (Ludiomil)
Nortriptyline (Aventyl; Pamelor)
Protriptyline (Vivactil)
Trimipramine (Surmontil)

ANTIHISTAMINES
Cyproheptadine (Periactin)
Diphenhydramine (Benadryl; others)

ANTIMICROBIALS
Antifungals (Fentichlor; Multifungin; Jadit)
Demeclocycline* (Declomycin; others)
Doxycycline (Vibramycin; others)
Griseofulvin (Fulvicin-U/F; others)
Methacycline (Rondomycin)
Minocycline (Minocin)
Nalidixic acid* (NegGram)
Oxytetracycline (Terramycin; others)
Sulfacytine (Renoquid)
Sulfadoxine-pyrimethamine (Fansidar)
Sulfaguanidine
Sulfamethazine (Neotrizine; others)
Sulfamethizole (Thiosulfil; others)
Sulfamethoxazole (Gantanol; others)
Sulfamethoxazole-trimethoprim (Bactrim, Septra; others)
Sulfanilamide
Sulfapyridine
Sulfasalazine
Sulfathiazole
Sulfisoxazole (Gantrisin; others)
Tetracycline (Achromycin; others)

ANTIPARASITIC DRUGS
Bithionol* (Bitin)
Chloroquine (Aralen)
Hydroxychloroquine
Pyrvinium pamoate (Povan)
Quinine

ANTIPSYCHOTIC DRUGS
Chlorpromazine (Thorazine; others)
Chlorprothixine (Taractan)
Fluphenazine (Permitil; Prolixin)
Haloperidol (Haldol)
Perphenazine (Trilafon)
Piperacetazine (Quide)
Prochlorperazine (Compazine; others)
Promethazine (Phenergan; others)
Thioridazine (Mellaril)
Thiothixene (Navane)
Trifluoperazine (Stelazine; others)
Triflupromazine (Vesprin)
Trimeprazine (Temaril)

DIURETICS
Acetazolamide (Diamox)
Amiloride (Midamor)
Bendroflumethiazide (Naturetin; others)
Benzthiazide (Exna; others)
Chlorothiazide (Diuril; others)
Cyclothiazide (Anhydron)
Furosemide (Lasix)
Hydrochlorothiazide (HydroDIURIL; others)
Hydroflumethiazide (Diucardin; others)
Methyclothiazide (Aquatensen; Enduron)
Metolazone (Diulo; Zaroxolyn)
Polythiazide (Renese)
Quinethazone (Hydromox)
Trichlormethiazide (Methahydrin; others)

HYPOGLYCEMICS
Acetohexamide (Dymelor)
Chlorpropamide (Diabinese; Insulase)
Glipizide (Glucotrol)
Glyburide (DiaBeta; Micronase)
Tolazamide (Tolinase)
Tolbutamide (Orinase; others)

NONSTEROIDAL ANTIINFLAMMATORY DRUGS
Benoxaprofen (Oraflex)
Ketoprofen (Orudis)
Naproxen (Naprosyn)
Phenylbutazone (Butazolidin; others)
Piroxicam (Feldene)
Sulindac (Clinoril)

SUNSCREENS
6-Acetoxy-2,4,-dimethyl-*m*-dioxane (preservative in sunscreens)
Benzophenones (Aramis; Clinique; others)
Cinnamates (Aramis; Estee Lauder; others)

Continued.

*Common.

BOX 12-1
AGENTS THAT MAY CAUSE PHOTOSENSITIVITY*—cont'd

SUNSCREENS—cont'd

Oxybenzone (Eclipse; PreSun; others)
PABA esters (Eclipse; Block Out; Sea & Ski; others)
Para-aminobenzoic acid (PABA—Pabagel; Pabanol; PreSun; others)

OTHERS

Amiodarone* (Cordarone)
Bergamot oil, oils of citron, lavender, lime, sandalwood, cedar* (used in many perfumes and cosmetics; also topical exposure to citrus rind oils)
Benzocaine
Captopril (Capoten)
Carbamazepine (Tegretol)
Chlordiazepoxide (Librium)
Coal tar and derivatives (containing acridine, anthracene, naphthalene, phenanthrene phenols, thiophene)
Contraceptives, oral (Norethynodrel)
Cyclamates (calcium cyclamate, sodium cyclohexylsulfamate)
Diethystilbestrol
Disopyramide (Norpace)
Dyes (acridine, acriflavine, anthraquinone, eosin, erythrocine, fluorescein, methylene blue, methyl violet, orange red, rose bengal, toluidine blue, trypaflavine, trypan blue)
Furocoumarins: psoralens (trioxsalen, methoxsalen, psoralen)
Gold salts (Myochrysine; Solganal)
Hexachlorophene (pHisoHex; others)
Isotretinoin (Accutane)
6-Methylcoumarin (used in perfumes, shaving lotions, and sunscreens)
Mestranol
Musk ambrette (used in perfumes)
Quinidine sulfate and gluconate
Saccharine
Tattoo dye (red or yellow cadmium sulfide)

the clinical manifestations. There are a wide variety of porphyrias because of the complexity of heme biosynthesis.

Photosensitivity begins in childhood on sun-exposed areas with the acute development of vesicles, bullae, and hyperpigmentation or hypopigmentation. The skin is also more sensitive than normal to trauma. With chronic exposure the skin scars atrophically with mutilating deformities of exposed areas, including cicatrizing alopecia. Other manifestations are highly variable, depending on the type of porphyria.[3] The action spectrum is in the visible range from 400 to 410 nm (Soret band), and thus these unfortunate individuals must be protected by a physical blocking agent or by adequate clothing. Some sufferers respond to oral β-carotene.[44]

Solar Urticaria. Solar urticaria is a rare, rapidly developing reaction to sun or UV exposure (290 to 515 nm).[24] Minutes after exposure, sensitive individuals develop pruritus followed by the urticaria and erythema. The reaction rarely lasts longer than 24 hours.

This syndrome encompasses different subsets. Some individuals produce a serum factor, which after inoculation into a normal subject transiently permits induction of solar urticaria in the recipient. This group appears to generate an immunoglobulin of the IgE class, which causes the reaction. These subjects can rightfully be classified among those with photoallergies. Others cannot transfer the reaction passively, and the mechanism for the development of solar urticaria is unknown.

Antihistamines are effective at high doses in a minority of patients. Maintenance solar exposure and PUVA therapy have also been used successfully in some. Patients should be phototested to determine the wavelengths that promote their reaction and then provided with a protective sunscreen. Alternatively or in addition, they may be instructed to avoid the sun whenever possible.[2]

Chronic Actinic Dermatitis. Chronic actinic dermatitis encompasses the gamut of disease previously described as chronic photosensitivity dermatitis or actinic reticuloid.[24] Seen in older, predominantly male patients, this dermatosis manifests initially as erythematous macules and plaques in sun-exposed areas, including the face, exposed areas of scalp, rim of the ears, back of the neck, forearms, and back of the hands. These lesions have been called chronic photosensitivity dermatitis. With time this disorder can evolve into the lichenified, infiltrated lesions of actinic reticuloid with superimposed areas of edema and vesiculation during acute flare-ups. A clinical diagnosis in these patients should be confirmed by demonstrating a low threshold for reaction across a broad portion of the UV and short visible (blue) spectrum (290 to 360 nm).

On histologic examination the skin condition initially resembles a contact dermatitis but can progress with actinic reticuloid to the pattern of a cutaneous T cell lymphoma. The portion of the spectrum causing the reaction varies from one individual to another. Thus phototesting and careful selection of sunscreens or avoidance of the sun are mandated in the management of these individuals. Treatment options

Table 12-5 Common Plants and Lichens Causing Photodermatitis

Common Name	Botanical Name	Family
Lime	*Citrus aurantifolia*	Rutaceae
Citron	*Citrus medica (C. acida)*	
Bitter orange	*Citrus aurantium*	Rutaceae
Lemon	*Citrus limon*	Rutaceae
Bergamot	*Citrus bergamia*	Rutaceae
Gas plant, burning bush	*Dictamnus albus (D. fraxinella)*	Rutaceae
Common rue	*Ruta graveolens*	Rutaceae
Persian lime (Tahitian)	*Citrus aurantifolia,* "Persian" *Phebalium argenteum*	Rutaceae
Cow parsley, wild chervil	*Anthriscus sylvestris*	Umbelliferae
Celery	*Apium graveolens*	Umbelliferae
Giant hogweed	*Heracleum mantegazzianum*	Umbelliferae
	Heracleum maximum (H. dulce)	Umbelliferae
Parsnip (garden variety)	*Pastinaca sative (P. urens)*	Umbelliferae
Cow parsley	*Heracleum sphondylium*	Umbelliferae
Parsnip (wild parsnip)	*Heracleum giganteum*	Umbelliferae
Fennel	*Foeniculum vulgare*	Umbelliferae
Dill	*Anethum graveolens*	Umbelliferae
	Peucedanum ostruthium	Umbelliferae
Wild carrot, garden carrot	*Daucus carota*	Umbelliferae
Masterwort	*Peucedanum ostruthium*	Umbelliferae
	Ammin majus	Umbelliferae
Angelica	*Angelica archangelica*	Umbelliferae
Figs	*Ficus carica*	Moraceae
Milfoil, yarrow	*Achillea millefolium*	Compositae
Stinking mayweed	*Anthemis cotula*	Compositae
Buttercup	*Ranunculus* spp.	Ranunculaceae
Mustard	*Brassica* spp.	Cruciferae
Bind weed	*Convolvulus arvensis*	Convolvulaceae
Agrimony	*Agrimonia eupatoria*	Rosaceae
Goose foot	*Chenopodium* spp.	Chenopodiaceae
Scurfy pea, bavchi	*Psoralea corylifolia*	Leguminosae
St. John's wort	*Hypericum perforatum*	Hypericaceae
	Hypericum crispum	Hypericaceae
	Schinopsis quebracho-colorado	
Red quebracho	*Schinopsia lorentzii*	Anacardiaceae
Lichens	*Parmelia* spp.	Lichen (symbiotic association between fungi and algae) commonly grouped with fungi
	Hypogymnia spp.	
	Pseudovernia spp.	
	Cladonia spp.	
	Platismatia spp.	
	Physcia spp.	
	Umbilicaria spp.	
	Cetraria spp.	

include oral azathioprine, PUVA with or without prednisone, etretinate, and cyclosporine.[34]

Persistent Light Reaction. In most patients a chemical photosensitivity dermatitis resolves within a week or two if the offending agent is eliminated.[24] A subset of individuals (usually older men) continue to overreact to the sun in spite of careful avoidance of the putative photosensitizer. This condition is called persistent light reaction and sometimes resolves in months, although it may persist indefinitely. For some persons the reaction is so severe that it results in a generalized exfoliative dermatitis. On histologic study the tissue shows a dense, perivascular, round cell infiltrate.

In some cases the mechanism for persistent light reaction is ongoing exposure to some chemical that is not correctly identified and eliminated. In other instances the offending agent has bonded to dermal proteins in such a way that it cannot be eliminated. Often the reaction is idiopathic. The action spectrum (290 to 400 nm) is usually in the UVB range, although overlap into UVA is common. Phototesting to determine appropriate protective sunscreens and avoidance of the sun are usually effective in minimizing flare-ups.[2]

Lupus Erythematosus. Cutaneous lupus erythematosus (LE) occurs in two broad forms, discoid LE and subacute cutaneous LE.[24] The lesions of discoid LE are typically found on the head and neck and are well defined, variably sized scaly patches that heal leaving atrophy, scarring, and pigmentary changes. Subacute cutaneous LE manifests as papulosquamous or polycyclic lesions around the neck, on the outer aspects of the arms, and on the trunk. These lesions are milder than those of discoid LE and heal without scarring or atrophy.[4] Although UVB appears to be more prominent in LE, UVA also plays a role in some individuals.[16] The spectrum of action is 290 to 330 nm.

Interestingly, exacerbations of noncutaneous lupus (such as nephritis) are sometimes seen after sun exposure.[44] Thus it is necessary to provide these patients with a broad-spectrum sunblock and encourage them to avoid the sun. Oral antimalarials such as chloroquine have been used with limited success.[44] Recently an open label trial of a broad-spectrum sunscreen containing padimate O and avobenzone reduced clinical severity of cutaneous LE over a 4-week period.[4]

Xeroderma Pigmentosum. Xeroderma pigmentosum is an autosomal recessive disorder that stems from a genetic defect in the ability to repair UVB-induced dimers.[24] This leads to a high frequency of mutations and premature development of skin neoplasms, including malignant melanoma and basal cell and squamous cell carcinoma. One study noted that the median age at which skin cancer develops in patients with xeroderma pigmentosum was 8 years, compared with 60 in the general population. Other clinical manifestations include sun sensitivity, skin atrophy, and increased freckling. Photophobia and other ocular manifestations, including severe UV-induced conjunctivitis and keratitis, are common. Progressive neurologic deterioration occurs in about 40% of victims. The spectrum of action is 290 to 340 nm.

After diagnosis, treating physicians should aim for careful protection against the sun and vigilant detection of skin cancer. Eye protection should also be emphasized.[22,44]

Vitiligo. Vitiligo is an idiopathic, acquired patchy depigmentation syndrome. Although harmless, it is cosmetically problematic. UVR exposure in depigmented skin does induce hypertrophy of the stratum corneum, but the chronically amelanotic nature of the skin makes it susceptible to premature actinic damage and skin cancer. Individuals with this disorder should be cautioned to avoid sun exposure and to use adequate sun protection to prevent painful burns in depigmented areas. PUVA has been demonstrated to be an effective treatment for vitiligo, resulting in a cosmetically acceptable degree of repigmentation in 50% to 70% of patients, although certain body areas notoriously respond poorly.[29]

Albinism. Oculocutaneous albinism is an autosomal recessive defect in the formation of melanosomes. Although melanocytes are present, these individuals are either hypomelanotic or amelanotic in the skin and hair. Patients living in areas of high solar flux uniformly develop premalignant (actinic keratoses) or malignant (NMSC) skin lesions by early adulthood if they are not careful to apply sunscreens and avoid unnecessary sun exposure. Melanoma is rare, although the reason for this is unclear.[29]

SUMMARY

Understanding the effects of sun on the skin continues to evolve. A relationship between UVB exposure and the development of basal cell and squamous cell carcinoma has been documented. It appears likely that high-dose exposure to UVR increases the risk for malignant melanoma. Chronic exposure to either UVA or UVB increases the rate of skin aging.

Development of new, highly effective sunscreens of both the traditional chemical kind and newer micronized physical blockers ("chemical-free") continues. More effective UVB-blocking formulations may lead to increased cumulative sun exposure and thus UVA exposure. However, only time will delineate the impact of such exposure on the rates of skin cancer and skin aging. Meanwhile, physicians may benefit their patients most by discouraging sun exposure and encouraging prudent and frequent use of sunscreens.

Children, as well as adults with a likelihood of increased sun exposure, should be warned of the short- and long-term consequences of UVR on the skin and should be instructed regarding sun protection. Any person who has one of the many photosensitivity dermatoses must receive counseling about the special requirements to protect his or her skin.

REFERENCES

1. Agin PP, Stanfield JW: Letter, *J Am Acad Dermatol* 27:136, 1992.
2. Bernhard JD et al: Abnormal reactions to ultraviolet radiation. In Fitzpatrick TB et al, editors: *Dermatology in general medicine*, ed 3, New York, 1987, McGraw-Hill.
3. Bickers DB, Pathak MA; The porphyrias. In Fitzpatric TB et al, editors: *Dermatology in general medicine*, ed 3, New York, 1987, McGraw-Hill.
4. Callen JP et al: Safety and efficacy of a broad spectrum sunscreen in patients with discoid or subacute cutaneous lupus erythematosus, *Cutis* 47:130, 1991.
5. Cole C, VanFossen R: Measurement of sunscreen UVA protection: an unsensitized human model, *J Am Acad Dermatol* 26:178, 1992.
6. Diffey BL, Robson JJ: A new substrate to measure suncreen protection factors throughout the ulraviolet spectrum, *Soc Cosmet Chem* 40:127, 1989.
7. Dromgoole SH, Maibach HI: Suncreening agent intolerance: contact and photocontact sensitization and contact urticaria, *J Am Acad Dermatol* 22:1068, 1990.
8. Dromgoole SH, Maibach HI: Contact sensitization and photocontact sensitization of sunscreening agents. In Lowe NJ, editor: *Physician's guide to sunscreens*, New York, 1991, Marcel Dekker.

9. Epstein JH: Biologic effect of sunlight. In Lowe NJ, editor: *Physician's guide to sunscreens,* New York, 1991, Marcel Dekker.
10. Fisher AA: Sunscreen dermatitis: para-aminobenzoic acid and its derivatives, *Cutis* 50:190, 1992.
11. Fusaro RM, Johnson JA: Topical photoprotection for hereditary polymorphic light eruption of American Indians, *J Am Acad Dermatol* 24:744, 1991.
12. Garland CF, Garland FC, Gorham ED: Rising trends in melanoma: an hypothesis concerning sunscreen effectiveness, *Ann Epidemiol* 3:103, 1993.
13. Garmyn M, Sohrabvand N, Roelandts R: Modification of sunburn cell in 8-MOP-sensitized mouse epidermis: method of assessing UVA sunscreen efficacy, *J Invest Dermatol* 93:642, 1989.
14. Gottlieb A, Bourget T, Lowe NJ: Sunscreens: effects of amounts of application of sun protection factors. In Lowe NJ, editor: *Physician's guide to sunscreens,* New York, 1991, Marcel Dekker.
15. Harber LC, DeLeo VA, Prystowsky JH: Intrinsic and extrinsic photoprotection against UVB and UVA radiation. In Lowe NJ, editor: *Physician's guide to sunscreens,* New York, 1991, Marcel Dekker.
16. Johnson JA, Fusaro RM: Broad spectrum photoprotection: the role of tinted auto windows, sunscreens and browning agents in the diagnosis and treatment of photosensitivity, *Dermatology* 185:237, 1992.
17. Kaidbey KH: The photoprotective potential of the new superpotent sunscreens, *J Am Acad Dermatol* 22:449, 1990.
18. Kaidbey KH: Substantivity and water resistance of sunscreens. In Lowe NJ, editor: *Physician's guide to sunscreens,* New York, 1991, Marcel Dekker.
19. Kaidbey KH, Barnes A: Determination of UVA protection factors by means of immediate pigment darkening in normal skin, *J Am Acad Dermatol* 25:262, 1991.
20. Kaplan LA: Suntan, sunburn and sun protection, *J Wilderness Med* 3:173, 1992.
21. Kligman LH, Kligman AM: Ultraviolet radiation-induced skin aging. In Lowe NJ, editor: *Physician's guide to sunscreens,* New York, 1991, Marcel Dekker.
22. Kraemer KH: Heritable diseases with increased sensitivity to cellular injury. In Fitzpatrick TB et al, editors: *Dermatology in general medicine,* ed 3, New York, 1987, McGraw-Hill.
23. Lowe NJ: SPF: comparative techniques and selection of UV sources. In Lowe NJ, editor: *Physician's guide to sunscreens,* New York, 1991, Marcel Dekker.
24. Lowe NJ: UVA photoprotection. In Lowe NJ, editor: *Physician's guide to sunscreens,* New York, 1991, Marcel Dekker.
25. Lowe NJ, Weingarten D, Wortzman M: Sunscreens and phototesting, *Clin Dermatol* 6:40, 1988.
26. Lowe NJ et al: Indoor and outdoor efficacy testing of a broad spectrum sunscreen against ultraviolet A radiation in psoralen-sensitized subjects, *J Am Acad Dermatol* 17:224, 1987.
27. Luftman DB, Lowe NJ, Moy RL: Sunscreens: update and review, *J Dermatol Surg Oncol* 17:744, 1991.
28. Mommaas AM et al: Analysis of the protective effect of topical sunscreens on the UVB-induced suppression of the mixed lymphocyte reaction, *J Invest Dermatol* 95:313, 1990.
29. Mosher DB et al: Disorders of the melanocytes. In Fitzpatrick TB et al, editors: *Dermatology in general medicine,* ed 3, New York, 1987, McGraw-Hill.
30. Patel NH, Highton A, Moy RL: Properties of topical sunscreen formulations, *J Dermatol Surg Oncol* 18:316, 1992.
31. Reeve VE et al: Differential protection by two sunscreens from UV radiation-induced immunosuppression, *J Invest Dermatol* 97:624, 1991.
32. Roberts J: Exposure to the sun. In Auerbach P, editor: *Management of wilderness and environmental emergencies,* ed 2, St Louis, 1989, Mosby.
33. Roelandts RJ: Which components in broad spectrum sunscreens are most necessary for adequate UVA protection? *Am Acad Dermatol* 25:999, 1991.
34. Roelandts RJ: Chronic actinic dermatitis, *J Am Acad Dermatol* 28:240, 1993.
35. Roelandts RJ, Sohrabvand N, Garmyn M: Evaluating the UVA protection of sunscreens, *J Am Acad Dermatol* 21:56, 1989.
36. Rooney JF et al: Prevention of ultraviolet-light-induced herpes labialis by sunscreen, *Lancet* 338:1419, 1991.
37. Sayre RM, Agin PP: A method for the determination of UVA protection for normal skin, *J Am Acad Dermatol* 23:429, 1990.
38. Sayre RM, Lowe NJ: Personal communication, 1943.
39. Shaath NA: Evolution of modern sunscreen chemicals. In Lowe NJ, Shaath NA, editors: *Sunscreens: development, evaluation and regulatory aspects,* New York, 1990, Marcel Dekker.
40. Stanfield JW et al: Ultraviolet A sunscreen evaluations in normal subjects, *J Am Acad Dermatol* 20:744, 1989.
41. Sterling GB: Sunscreens: a review, *Cutis* 50:221, 1992.
42. Stern RS: Sunscreen use and non-melanoma skin cancer. In Lowe NJ, editor: *Physician's guide to sunscreens,* New York, 1991, Marcel Dekker.
43. Stern RS, Weinstein MC, Baker SG: Risk reduction for non-melanoma skin cancer with childhood sunscreen use, *Arch Dermatol* 122:537, 1986.
44. Taylor CR et al: Photoaging/photodamage and photoprotection, *J Am Acad Dermatol* 22:1, 1990.
45. Van Praag MCG et al: Effect of topical sunscreens on the UV-radiation induced suppression of the alloactivating capacity in human skin in vivo, *J Invest Dermatol* 97:629, 1991.
46. Weiss JS et al: Topical tretinoin improves photoaged skin: a double-blind vehicle controlled trial, *JAMA* 259:527, 1988.

13 WILDERNESS TRAUMA EMERGENCIES

John A. Morris, Jr.
Marc F. Swiontkowski
Henry J. Herrmann

The management of wilderness trauma is based on military and civilian prehospital principles, which include rapid assessment, treatment, and, if necessary, evacuation. These principles and those promulgated by the Committee on Trauma of the American College of Surgeons (ACS) are formally taught in the ACS Advanced Trauma Life Support (ATLS) program. Any physician planning to be a medical officer on a wilderness expedition should be familiar with the material taught in the ATLS program.

Establishing Priorities

There are three immediate priorities in managing wilderness trauma:

1. Control yourself. It is normal to feel anxious when confronted with an injured victim. However, anxiety must not be transmitted to the victim or other members of the expedition team. One must be in control of oneself to take control of the situation.
2. Control the situation. The first priority in controlling the situation is ensuring the safety of the noninjured members of the party. Expeditious evacuation of a victim requires that all expedition members function at maximum efficiency; even minor injuries to other members in the group can jeopardize physical strength and functional manpower.

   While the physician member of the team may not be the expedition leader, his or her position is automatically elevated during a medical crisis. However, this does not mean that the physician should dominate the evacuation planning process. While the expedition leader must rely on the medical assessment provided by the physician, the leader is best prepared to plan the evacuation.
3. Overview. The victim's general condition should be evaluated. Is the victim in immediate distress from a condition that requires relatively simple management, such as airway control? Is the victim in such a precarious environmental situation that he or she needs to be moved before resuscitation? Is the victim properly protected from the elements, including sun, wind, cold, and water?

After the victim has been placed in a stable, relatively safe environment, the examining physician is ready to implement the five steps of wilderness trauma management: primary survey, resuscitation, secondary survey, plan, and packaging.

The purpose of the primary survey is to identify and begin initial management of life-threatening conditions by assessing the following:

1. Airway maintenance and cervical spine stabilization
2. Breathing
3. Circulation, with control of significant external hemorrhage
4. Mental status
5. Exposure

After the primary survey is performed, resuscitation efforts are begun. The level of resuscitation depends on the equipment and expertise available. At a minimum, resuscitation consists of control of external hemorrhage. In the emergency department, resuscitation would also include the administration of oxygen and intravenous fluids.

The third step is the secondary survey, a head-to-toe evaluation of the trauma victim that uses inspection, percussion, and palpation techniques to evaluate each of the body's five regions: head and face, thorax, abdomen, skeleton, and skin. Following this survey the examining physician should formulate a plan. It is useful to record all observations on paper if circumstances permit.

The first step in determining a plan is to compile a list of injuries. The next step is to determine if any injury warrants evacuation. Should an evacuation be by air, ground, or water? Aeromedical evacuation is expensive and, depending on the environment, could be a risk to both the victim and the medical evacuation team. Aeromedical evacuation should be considered only for victims with potentially life- or limb-threatening injuries or where the environment requires such a modality.

Packaging the patient for evacuation is the final step. The evacuation effort requires organization, coordination, and great effort on the part of the entire expedition team.

Primary Survey

The first step in management of wilderness trauma is the primary survey, including assessing the airway, cervical spine, breathing, circulation, mental status, and exposure.

AIRWAY AND CERVICAL SPINE

The upper airway should be assessed for patency. Chin lift (Fig. 13-1) or jaw thrust (Fig. 13-2) may be helpful in establishing an airway. Specific attention should be directed toward the possibility of cervical spine fracture. The victim's head and neck should never be hyperextended or hyperflexed to establish or maintain an airway. Approximately 10% of victims with head injuries or facial fractures have a concomitant cervical spine fracture. Such a fracture should be assumed to exist in any person with a significant injury above the clavicle. The integrity of the cervical spine can be accurately assessed only by radiography.

BREATHING

The victim's chest should be exposed and chest wall movement observed. Conditions that lead to asymmetric

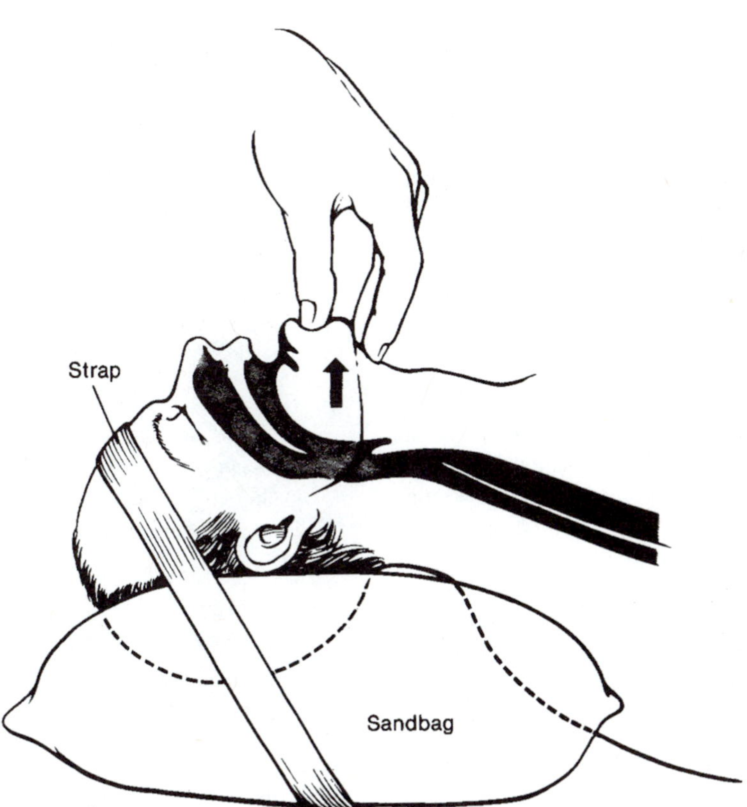

Fig. 13-1 Chin lift. This procedure requires two people. One person stabilizes the neck. The other opens the airway using his or her thumb to grasp the chin just below the lower lip, while the fingers of the same hand are placed underneath the anterior mandible and the chin is gently lifted.

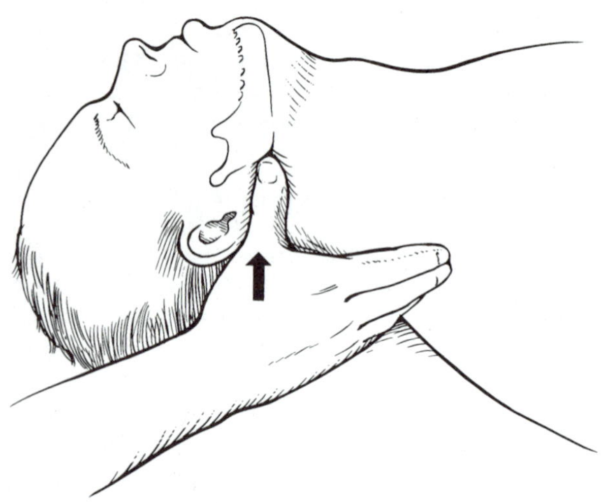

Fig. 13-2 Modified jaw thrust. This procedure requires only one person to perform the dual tasks of stabilizing the neck and establishing an airway. The hands are placed on either side of the neck to hold traction, and the thumbs are used to push up on the angles of the mandible. In this position the index finger can also be used to check for a carotid pulse.

movement include tension pneumothorax, open pneumothorax, and flail chest. These conditions are discussed in detail in the section on thoracic trauma.

CIRCULATION

Evaluation of circulation is divided into assessment of cardiac output and control of major external hemorrhage. Manometric blood pressure measurement is not easily performed in the field. However, important information regarding perfusion and oxygenation can be obtained rapidly by taking the victim's pulse, looking at skin color, and checking capillary refill time.

The victim's pulse should be assessed first. Although these are only general estimates and carry some inaccuracy, if a radial artery pulse is palpable, the systolic blood pressure is over 80 mm Hg; if the femoral artery pulse is palpable, the blood pressure is above 70 mm Hg; and if the carotid artery pulse is palpable, the blood pressure is above 60 mm Hg.

Skin color and capillary refill allow a rapid initial estimation of peripheral perfusion. Pressure applied to the thumbnail or hypothenar eminence causes underlying tissue to blanch. In a normovolemic person, color returns to the nailbed within 2 seconds. In a hypovolemic, poorly oxygenated person, capillary refill requires more than 2 seconds. If hypovolemia is suspected, on the basis of either absent pulses or a prolonged capillary refill time, the examiner should immediately look at the neck veins. Distended neck veins in the presence of hypotension suggest either tension pneumothorax or pericardial tamponade. Flat neck veins suggest hypovolemia.

CONTROL OF HEMORRHAGE

Major hemorrhage can occur in only four areas: into the chest, abdomen and retroperitoneum, or thigh or onto the ground. Exsanguinating external hemorrhage should be identified and controlled during the primary survey. Blood loss is managed in the field by direct pressure on the wound. Tourniquets should not be used unless bleeding cannot be controlled with direct pressure and the rescuer accepts the responsibility for potential limb loss. In the field little can be done about significant intrathoracic or intraabdominal hemorrhage; proper stabilization of a femoral fracture minimizes blood loss into the thigh.

MENTAL STATUS

A mental status evaluation using the Glasgow Coma Scale (Box 13-1) establishes the victim's level of consciousness using eye opening, verbal response, and motor response. For instance, the victim may be described as opening eyes to pain, talking in a confused fashion, or localizing only to deep pain. The neurologic assessment should be repeated often if it is at any time abnormal. Deterioration in mental status evaluation may portend a poor prognosis. A variety of conditions other than intracra-

BOX 13-1

GLASGOW COMA SCALE

This scale evaluates the degree of coma by determining the best motor, verbal, and eye opening response to standardized stimuli.

EYE OPENING	
Spontaneous	4
To voice	3
To pain	2
None	1
VERBAL RESPONSE	
Oriented	5
Confused	4
Inappropriate words	3
Incomprehensible words	2
None	1
MOTOR RESPONSE	
Obeys command	6
Localizes pain	5
Withdraw (pain)	4
Flexion (pain)	3
Extension (pain)	2
None	1
TOTAL	

nial injury, such as hypothermia, can affect mental status.

Pupil size and reaction are also part of the mental status evaluation. If the pupils are not equal and reactive to light, a mass lesion or direct ocular injury should be suspected.

EXPOSURE

Full physical evaluation requires removal of all clothing in an appropriately protected environment. After the examination, the victim should be kept in a warm and dry environment.

Resuscitation

Resuscitation follows the primary survey. The extent to which resuscitation can be performed depends on the skill and experience of the rescuer, equipment, and environmental conditions. Under optimal circumstances, resuscitation allows oxygenation, fluid administration, monitoring of vital signs, and placement of a cardiac monitor and nasogastric and urinary catheters. Obviously, this type of resuscitation cannot be performed in the wilderness environment. Here, resuscitation may be limited to oral administration of warm, high-calorie fluids and maintenance of victim comfort and temperature. Because of the potential for pulmonary aspiration, no fluids should be given orally to any victim with a significant closed head injury.

Secondary Survey

The secondary survey begins with physical examination of the head and moves in a systematic fashion through a more detailed physical examination of the face, neck, chest, abdomen, pelvis, extremities, and skin. The neck is examined independently of the thoracolumbar spinal cord. The entire spinal examination is discussed in the section on orthopedic injuries. Examination of the pelvis, which follows abdominal examination, is also discussed in the section on orthopedic injuries.

INJURIES TO THE HEAD AND FACE

Secondary survey of the head and face builds on information gathered in the mental status evaluation performed during the primary survey. Elements of the Glasgow Coma Scale are repeated, and a more detailed search for focal neurologic signs is initiated. The scalp is thoroughly palpated for tenderness, depressions, and lacerations. Finally, the bones of the face, including the zygomatic arch, maxilla, and mandible, are palpated for fractures.

HEAD AND FACE ANATOMY

The skull is composed of two groups of bones that construct the face and cranium. Cranial bones are divided into the calvarium and base. The calvarium is composed of frontal, ethmoid, sphenoid, parietal, and occipital bones. The calvarium is especially thin in the temporal regions, while the base of the skull is irregular with outcroppings, such as the anterior temporal fossa.

The skull is covered by the scalp. The two most clinically important scalp layers are the dermis and galea aponeurotica. The galea is a thick fibrous tissue layer overlying the calvarium. Located between the dermis and the galea is a rich vascular network characteristic of the scalp. When lacerated, these vessels can be a significant source of hemorrhage.

Inside the skull the brain is covered by three membranous layers: (1) a thick and fibrous dura, (2) a thinner arachnoid layer, and (3) the innermost pia. In the urban setting, defining the precise layer of injury has therapeutic and prognostic significance; in the wilderness environment this distinction is meaningless because all major head injuries are managed similarly with respect to evacuation.

PHYSICAL EXAMINATION

The hallmark of brain injury is an altered level of consciousness. Physical examination begins with reestimation of the Glasgow Coma Scale. Evaluation of the eye-opening response begins with the victim's response to conversation and proceeds through a response to a painful stimulus (which should not be applied to an injured face).

If the victim's eyes are swollen shut because of facial trauma, the examination should proceed to the verbal response. The victim's orientation to time, place, and person should be assessed. Next the victim's speech is assessed for confused conversation or inappropriate words or concepts. The examiner should note whether the victim can verbalize or make incomprehensible sounds or whether he or she is silent.

The best motor response is perhaps the most useful index of brain injury. If a victim does not follow commands, a painful stimulus should be applied either over the sternum or to the supraorbital rim. If the victim does not follow commands but localizes to pain, this may indicate a significant injury and the rescuer should be concerned about airway maintenance. If the victim simply withdraws in a generalized fashion in response to a painful stimulus, this is an indication for definitive airway control via endotracheal intubation, if the equipment and expertise are available. Absence of motor response or abnormal decorticate posturing to the administration of a painful stimulus immediately following an injury is a poor prognostic sign.

Although a direct blow to the globe can cause traumatic mydriasis, and although 5% to 10% of the population has a congenital anisocoria, neither of these diagnoses should be assumed in a victim in the wilderness environment who manifests mental status changes.

FOCAL SIGNS

Following the estimation of the Glasgow Coma Scale and the pupillary examination, the victim should be examined for the presence of neurologic focal findings, which can be either motor or sensory deficits. Sensory deficits follow general dermatome patterns described in Fig. 13-3. Reflex changes in the absence of altered mental status do not mandate evacuation unless associated with a spinal cord injury.

With the exception of the performance of gag and corneal reflex evaluations, the brainstem cannot be satisfactorily evaluated in the wilderness environment. The doll's eyes maneuver should never be performed without complete radiologic evaluation of the cervical spine. Icewater caloric tests add nothing to an evacuation decision and should not be performed outdoors.

SPECIAL SITUATIONS

Several situations that occur in the outdoor environment mandate rapid evacuation. These include depressed skull

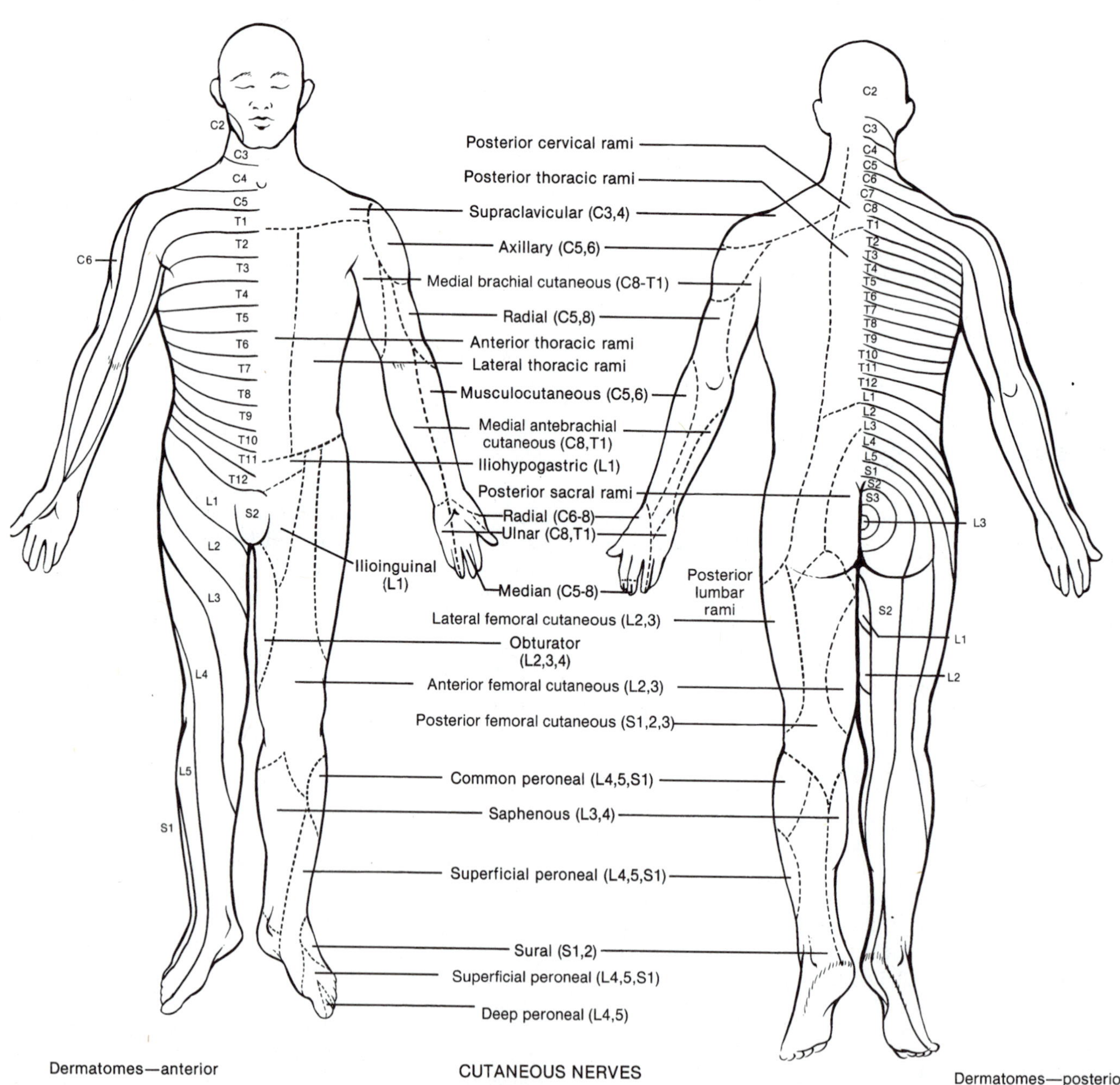

Fig. 13-3 Dermatome pattern, the skin area stimulated by spinal cord elements. Sensory deficits follow general dermatome patterns.

fracture, basilar skull fracture, and penetrating trauma. A depressed skull fracture is either open or closed. The diagnosis is often made by palpation of the head and scalp. If a depression is suspected on physical examination, the wound should not be probed, nor should any bony fragment be removed or elevated. The victim should receive broad-spectrum intravenous antibiotics chosen for penetration of the blood-brain barrier (cefuroxime, adult dose 1.5 g intramuscularly) and be immediately evacuated.

A person with a basilar skull fracture often appears confused, agitated, or combative. Battle's sign, or ecchymosis in the mastoid region, is often associated with hemotympanum and basilar skull fracture. Raccoon eyes, or periorbital ecchymoses, are also frequently associated with basilar skull fracture.

A person with penetrating trauma to the head requires immediate evacuation even if at the time of the initial presentation he or she does not demonstrate mental status changes. Foreign bodies piercing the head or neck should be removed only in the operating room by a qualified surgeon.

HISTORY

With a suspected head injury, a history of the accident is helpful. The elapsed time of unresponsiveness affects the evacuation decision. A description of the accident includes whether the patient fell and struck his or her head, the distance of the fall, and the landing surface. If the victim was struck on the head by a falling object, a depressing or axial loading force is suggested. If the victim was struck on the head while wearing protection such as a climbing helmet, the force may have been dissipated. The victim's status immediately following a suspected head injury should be considered. Descriptions of nausea, vomiting, seizure activity, fecal or urinary incontinence, and drug or alcohol ingestion are important.

EVACUATION

Deciding whether to evacuate a patient with a closed head injury requires considerable judgment and expertise. The decision can be simplified by dividing patients with closed head injuries into three groups based on the risk of having either an intracranial mass lesion or a brain contusion. The high-risk group includes patients with depressed levels of consciousness, indicated by a Glasgow Coma Scale score of 13 or less. Focal neurologic signs or decreasing level of consciousness requires evacuation. All persons with penetrating skull injuries or those who have evidence of a depressed or basilar skull fracture require immediate evacuation.

The low-risk group includes persons who have suffered a blow to the head but are asymptomatic or complain only of mild headache and dizziness. They may also have a small scalp hematoma, laceration, contusion, or abrasion but remain alert without focal neurologic signs. Victims with low-risk criteria have less than 1:1000 chance of having a significant brain injury.[31]

The group for which the evacuation decision is most difficult is the moderate-risk group. These victims have a history of a brief loss of consciousness or change in consciousness at the time of injury or a history of progressive headache, vomiting, or posttraumatic amnesia. If any of these signs is present in the face of other system injury, the victim must be evacuated immediately. If these signs are present in isolation and evacuation can be performed in less than 12 hours, the evacuation should proceed. If a victim has moderate risk criteria associated with an isolated head injury, and if evacuation will take longer than 12 hours, it is probably reasonable to observe the victim for 4 to 6 hours while evacuation plans are being made. If the victim improves to normalcy during the observation period, it is reasonable to continue the observation period. However, if at any time the victim's mental status deteriorates or symptoms worsen, evacuation must be immediate.

Major Maxillofacial Trauma

PRIMARY SURVEY

A victim suffering major head and neck injuries requires appropriate emergency care and timely transport to a properly equipped trauma center. As with any major injury, management consists of the primary survey, resuscitation, secondary survey, planning, and evacuation. The person conducting the primary survey should remember the factors characteristic of head and neck injuries. The airway may be compromised because of aspiration of blood, avulsed teeth or dental appliances, direct trauma and swelling, or a retrusive tongue secondary to mobile mandibular fracture. The consequences of mishandling a cervical spine fracture while opening the airway could be disastrous. Therefore the neck should not be hyperextended. The spine is supported, manually at first and then with rigid immobilization. The mouth should be cleared of blood, vomitus, avulsed teeth, and dentures. (Dentures should be kept with the patient, since they are helpful for definitive fixation.) The airway can be maintained by chin lift, jaw thrust, traction on the tongue with gauze or a safety pin (Fig. 13-4), an oropharyngeal airway, endotracheal intubation, or cricothyroidotomy.

The next feature of the primary survey is the circulation, which includes severe bleeding. Techniques to control bleeding in the maxillofacial region include direct pressure over a sterile dressing and judicious use of digital pressure on the external carotid artery.[12] Intraoral bleeding may be controlled by having the patient bite firmly on a gauze pad. The primary survey and resuscitation phases of management are completed as for any other injury.

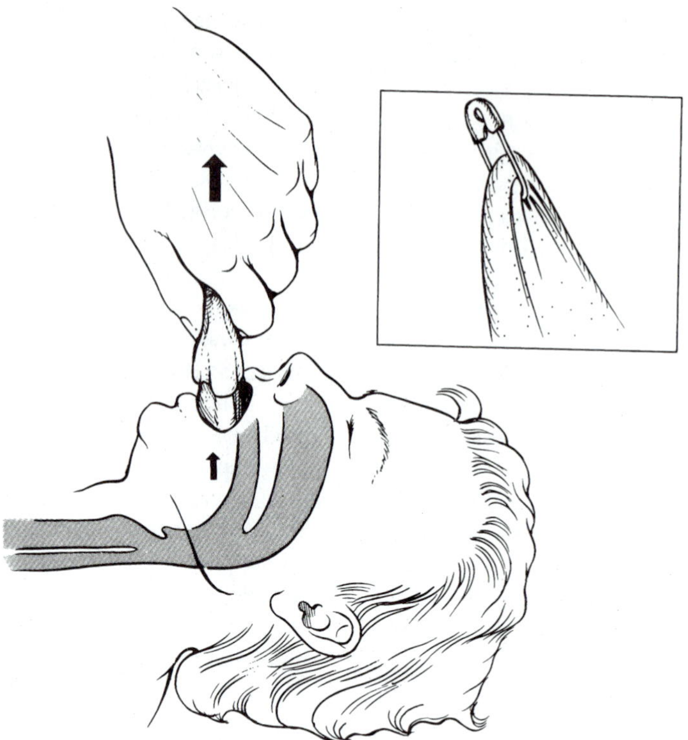

Fig. 13-4 A safety pin may be used to apply tongue traction if the tongue cannot be held using a dry cloth or gauze bandage.

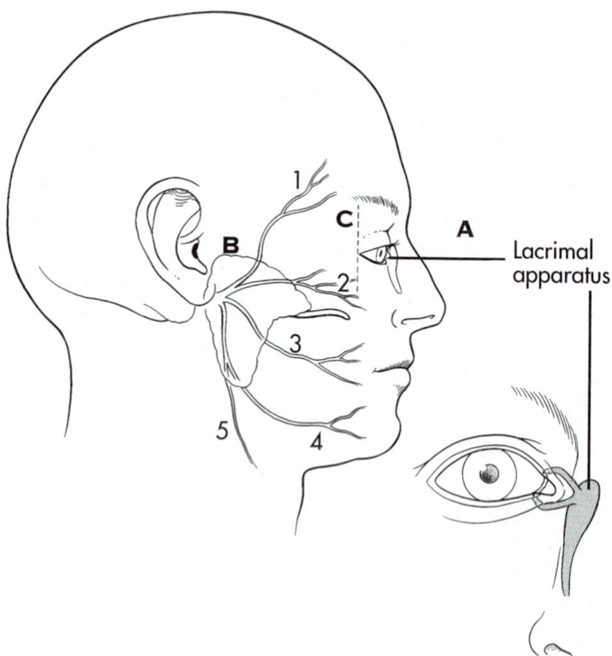

Fig. 13-5 Structures that may be injured by facial lacerations. *A,* Lacrimal drainage system. *B,* Parotid duct. *C,* Line drawn through the lateral canthus of the eye. Facial nerve injuries posterior to this line should be repaired as soon as possible. *1-5,* Branches of cranial nerve VII. (Redrawn from *Oral and maxillofacial surgery services in the emergency department,* Rosemont, Ill, 1992, American Association of Oral and Maxillofacial Surgeons.)

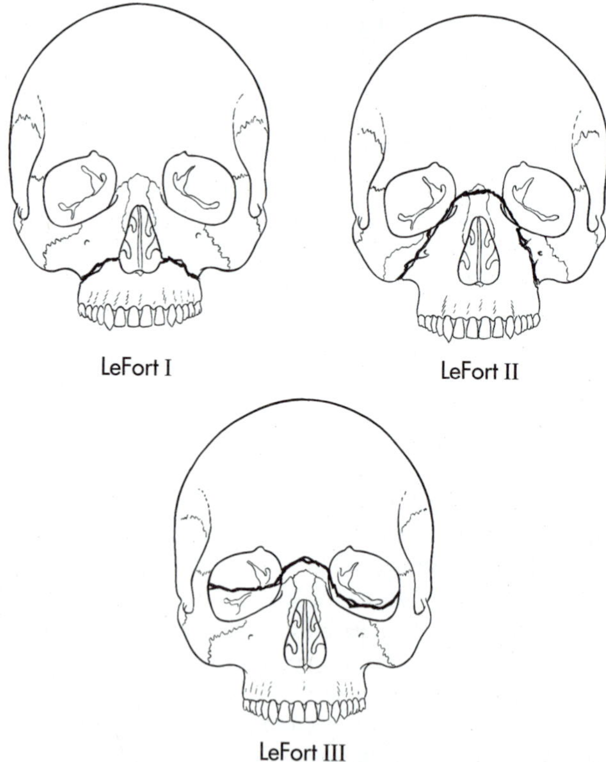

Fig. 13-6 Classification of midface fracture. (Redrawn from *Oral and maxillofacial surgery services in the emergency department,* Rosemont, Ill, 1992, American Association of Oral and Maxillofacial Surgeons.)

SECONDARY SURVEY

The secondary survey of the head and neck area includes examination of soft tissues and palpation of the scalp and facial bones. Facial lacerations may be complicated by damage to associated structures (Fig. 13-5). Injury to the lacrimal drainage system is present if a probe inserted into the punctum at the medial corner of the lid emerges into the laceration. Damage to the parotid duct is suspected if there is a buccal nerve paralysis or leakage from the wound when Stensen's duct is irrigated with saline solution. Facial nerve damage is sought by observing the patient move the eyebrows, eyelids, and mouth. If nerve injury occurs behind a vertical line through the lateral canthus of the eye, evacuation for immediate repair is recommended.[37]

Deformity, crepitus, and mobility are signs of fracture but may be masked by swelling. Inability to occlude the teeth properly and sublingual hematoma are also evidence of mandibular fracture. Restricted opening or deviation of the jaw when opening, preauricular tenderness, and premature occlusion on the injured side, especially when coupled with trauma to the chin, suggest condylar fracture. Another sign of mandibular fracture is pain elicited by placing one hand over each angle of the jaw and pressing inward.[27]

Midface fractures are classified as LeFort I, II, or III (Fig. 13-6). Tenderness and ecchymosis over the fracture site and malocclusion are signs of midface fracture. LeFort III fractures are often associated with airway compromise, visual disturbances, and cerebrospinal fluid rhinorrhea. Other fracture sites include the nasal bone, the zygomatic complex, the orbit, and the frontal sinus.

Maxillofacial trauma is often associated with intracranial injury. The secondary survey is continued to the rest of the body, since 17% of patients with mandibular fractures have other facial fractures and 10% have injuries outside the head and neck.[10]

Field treatment of facial fractures includes elevation of the patient's head to reduce bleeding and swelling and temporary stabilization with bandages. Narcotics should be used only if absolutely necessary, and then judiciously. Narcotic analgesics may cause respiratory depression, which can aggravate trauma-impaired breathing, or may mask changes in mental status. After the preceding steps have been taken, the victim is ready for evacuation.[22,29,37]

EMERGENCY DEPARTMENT TREATMENT

Early care of a patient with maxillofacial trauma builds on emergency field treatment and prepares the victim for definitive care, usually performed in the operating room by a maxillofacial surgeon. Emergency department treatment includes a more comprehensive head and neck examination, radiographs, laboratory tests, intravenous fluids, and early care of soft tissue injuries.

Complete diagnosis of maxillofacial injuries requires careful examination and adequate radiographs. Cervical spine fractures should also be sought by radiograph. Computed tomography adds valuable information about the location and severity of facial fractures.[11,12,30]

Another objective of emergency department treatment in head and neck trauma is to control bleeding not adequately treated in the field. Blind clamping of blood vessels should be avoided because of the proximity of facial nerve branches. Ligation of the external carotid artery at the angle of the mandible is favored over ligation of the maxillary artery via a Caldwell-Luc approach.[22] Hemostasis of torn vessels in the maxillary sinuses may be accomplished with fracture reduction or nasal tamponade or both. Lacerations should not be sutured until fractures are reduced and repaired. Hemostasis, debridement of foreign material, irrigation, dressing, and initiation of antibiotic therapy are appropriate procedures for the emergency department physician.[22,37]

Injuries to the Thorax

In the wilderness environment, blunt thoracic injuries usually result from falls or direct blows to the chest. Immediate, life-threatening thoracic injuries include airway obstruction, tension pneumothorax, sucking chest wound, massive hemothorax, flail chest, and cardiac tamponade. The hallmark of significant thoracic injury is tissue hypoxia. Fortunately, less than 15% of patients with major thoracic trauma require a chest operation. Most thoracic trauma can be temporarily managed with simple procedures readily available in the field.

PHYSICAL EXAMINATION

Inspection

Inspection of the victim with thoracic trauma begins by exposing the patient's chest. The airway is assessed for patency and air exchange, and the pattern of breathing is noted. In the immediate postinjury period most trauma victims are tachypneic, partly from pain and partly from anxiety. Dyspnea, cyanosis, the use of accessory muscles of respiration, or intercostal muscular retraction is abnormal.

Chest wall movement during respiration should be symmetric. Paradoxic chest wall movement is associated with flail chest. The chest wall should be inspected for contusions and abrasions, which may herald underlying bony or visceral injury.

Distention of the external jugular veins in a person who has just suffered thoracic trauma and is hypotensive or tachycardic (heart rate greater than 130 beats/min) suggests impairment of venous return. This finding is associated with tension pneumothorax or pericardial tamponade. In tension pneumothorax, deviation of the trachea is opposite the lesion.

Palpation

The thorax should be palpated systematically for bony tenderness, starting at the distal clavicles and working medially toward the sternum. The sternum is divided into the manubrium, gladiolus (body), and xiphoid cartilage. The manubrium is joined to the gladiolus by fibrocartilage, but mobility at this junction is minimal.

Each rib should be palpated individually. Ribs 1 to 7 are vertebrosternal; their costal cartilages join the sternum. Ribs 8, 9, and 10 are vertebrochondral, with each costal cartilage commonly joining the cartilage of the rib above. Ribs 11 and 12, vertebral ribs, have no attachment to the sternum. Point tenderness over a rib can be associated with contusion or fracture. Displaced fractures can be palpated; occasionally, bone grating can be felt during respiration.

Subcutaneous emphysema may extend up into the neck and down to the level of the inguinal ligaments. In the trauma situation, subcutaneous emphysema is invariably associated with a pneumothorax.

Vocal Fremitus

Vocal fremitus is a form of vibratory palpation.[8] During speech the victim's vocal cords emit vibrations in the bronchial air column that are conducted to the chest wall. Diminished vocal fremitus is associated with pneumothorax or hemothorax. To test for vocal fremitus, the examiner applies the palmar arch of the examining hand against the person's anterior chest wall. The person is asked to repeat "1, 2, 3," using the same pitch and intensity of voice with each repetition. If the vibrations are not well perceived, the patient is asked to lower the pitch of the voice. The chest should be symmetric, left to right.

Percussion

Percussion is used to detect changes in the normal density of an organ. Percussion of the chest is performed by placing the examining fingertip on the chest wall and sequentially striking the fingertip with the tip of the finger of the other hand. In the trauma victim, dullness replacing resonance in the lower lung suggests hemothorax. Hyperresonance or tympany replacing resonance occurs only with a large pneumothorax or tension pneumothorax.

Auscultation

If a stethoscope is not available, primitive chest auscultation can be performed using a rolled piece of cardboard or paper. The absence of sounds normally produced by the tracheobronchial air column indicates blockage in the airways or abnormal filtering of sound by fluid within the pleural cavity. In the trauma victim, this is invariably associated with pneumothorax or hemothorax.

BLUNT CHEST TRAUMA

Blunt chest trauma in the wilderness is most often associated with either a direct blow or a deceleration injury.

Rib Fractures

Rib fractures range in severity from an isolated nondisplaced single fracture, which causes only minor discomfort, to a major flail segment, which can be associated with an underlying hemopneumothorax and pulmonary contusion. Rib fractures are characterized by painful respiration, most severe on inspiration. Victims often breathe in a characteristically rapid, shallow pattern. Point tenderness is palpated over the fracture, and displacement can occasionally be detected. Rib fractures are detected with a compression test in which pressure is exerted on the sternum while the patient lies supine. This elicits pain over the fracture site.

Isolated rib fractures are managed with oral analgesics and rest. Thoracic taping and splinting are not necessary or helpful. Multiple rib fractures are significant because of the potential seriousness of associated injuries and increased pain. However, this pain responds well to an intercostal nerve block. Victims with multiple rib fractures need to be evacuated as conditions permit. Following the administration of an intercostal block, a person may regain the ability to hike out of the wilderness.

Costochondral Separation

It is difficult to distinguish between a rib fracture and costochondral separation. Pain is invariably anterior over the costochondral junction. Pain increases with inspiration and worsens with direct palpation. Costochondral separation also responds to intercostal nerve block and oral analgesics.

Sternal Fracture

A sternal fracture is usually associated with a direct blow to the anterior chest wall. The injury is characterized by severe, constant chest pain that worsens with direct palpation. Sternal instability is unusual and can be associated with a significant underlying visceral injury, including pulmonary and myocardial contusions. The victim should be immediately evacuated by litter or helicopter.

Pneumothorax

Simple pneumothorax can occur from an injury that allows air to enter through the thoracic wall or, more commonly, from an injury to the lung, which permits air to exit into the pleural space. Symptoms include tachypnea, a resonant hemithorax, absence of breath sounds, and tactile fremitus.

In the wilderness environment, tube thoracostomy is rarely possible. Fortunately, although victims with isolated pneumothorax complain of chest pain, they are not completely disabled. With a nerve block to control pain, ambulation facilitates evacuation. It may be easier to set a slow pace with frequent rest periods than to perform an unnecessary litter evacuation.

Hemothorax

Hemothorax is invariably associated with multiple rib fractures resulting from a direct blow to the chest. The primary cause of a hemothorax is laceration of the lung, intercostal vessel, or internal mammary artery. The victim complains of chest pain, tenderness associated with the rib fractures, inspiratory pain, and dyspnea. Vocal fremitus is absent, percussion may be flat or dull, and breath sounds are diminished or absent.

In the wilderness environment a chest tube should not be placed unless proper equipment is available and evacuation will be delayed. Needle aspiration of a hemothorax is unnecessary in the immediate postinjury period. Isolated hemothorax from blunt trauma leading to shock is unusual and commonly associated with other massive injuries.

Tension Pneumothorax

A tension pneumothorax develops when a one-way air leak follows lung rupture or chest wall penetration. Air is forced into the thoracic cavity with no means of escape, and pressure mounts within the hemithorax. The mediastinum is shifted to the contralateral side, which impedes venous return from both the superior and the inferior venae cavae. Cardiac output is diminished and the patient soon exhibits signs and symptoms of shock. Victims with tension pneumothorax manifest distended neck veins and tracheal deviation away from the side of the lesion. There is unilateral absence of breath sounds, and the hemithorax is hyperresonant or tympanitic. Respiratory distress, cyanosis, and frank cardiovascular collapse may occur.

Tension pneumothorax mandates rapid chest decompression. This procedure is performed by inserting a needle or catheter into the chest and converting the tension into an open pneumothorax. Ideally, a 14-gauge catheter is inserted percutaneously over the second rib in the midclavicular or anterior axillary line (Fig. 13-7). Once the rib is identified with the tip of the needle, the needle is marched over the anterior superior surface of the rib and inserted through the intercostal muscles and pleura into the hemithorax. As the pressure within the hemithorax is released, a distinct release of air is heard. The plastic catheter is advanced over the tip of the needle, the needle withdrawn, and the catheter left in place to ensure continued decompression. Because tension pneumothorax is commonly associated with severe injury, the victim should be evacuated to a medical facility as rapidly as possible. A rubber glove or finger cot can be attached to the external catheter opening to create a unidirec-

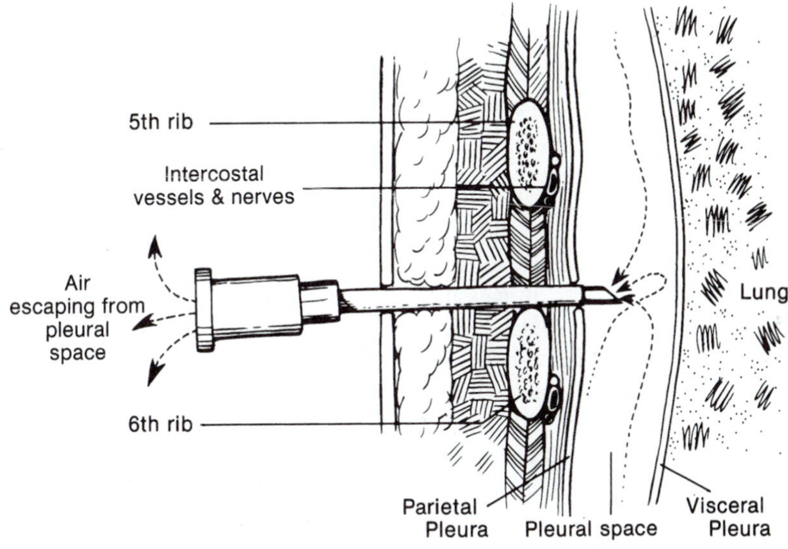

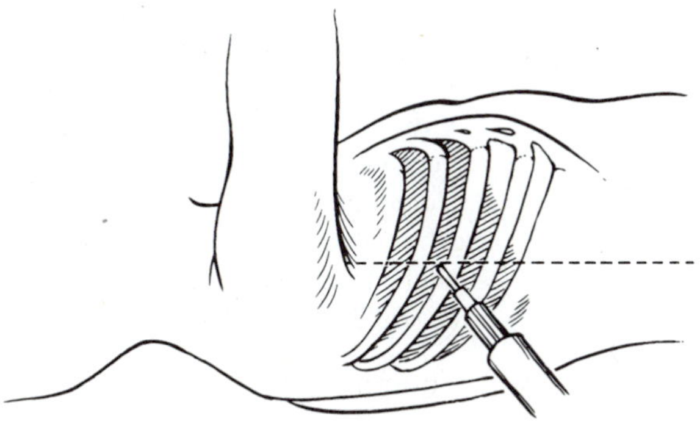

Fig. 13-7 Needle decompression of tension pneumothorax. This procedure is performed only for tension pneumothorax in patients with hemodynamic instability.

tional flutter valve that allows continuous egress of air from the pleural space.

Flail Chest

When a series of three or more ribs is fractured in both the anterior and posterior plane, a portion of the chest wall may be mechanically unstable. As negative intrathoracic pressure develops during inspiration, the unstable segment paradoxically moves inward and inhibits ventilation. A flail segment indicates a severe direct blow to the chest wall with associated multiple rib fractures and decreased tidal volume, often with associated underlying pulmonary contusion. The contusion can be expected to progressively impair ventilation and oxygenation over the succeeding 48 hours. Victims will often tolerate a flail segment for the first 24 to 48 hours, after which they require mechanical ventilation.

Any victim with a flail segment should be rapidly evacuated. Because the victim is usually incapable of participating in evacuation, a litter should be prepared or aeromedical evacuation considered. Intercostal nerve block may assist in short-term management of pain and pulmonary toilet. External chest wall supports, including taping or stabilization with sandbags, are contraindicated. These measures hinder chest wall movement, decrease vital capacity, and are less effective than intercostal nerve block in pain control.

Injuries to the trachea, bronchi, great vessels, esophagus, and diaphragm are rare and not amenable to diagnosis or treatment in the wilderness environment.

PENETRATING CHEST TRAUMA

At a minimum, penetrating chest trauma above the nipple line is associated with hemopneumothorax. It may also be associated with significant visceral injury. A victim with penetrating chest trauma below the nipple line often has intraabdominal penetration in addition to possible thoracic injury. Such a victim requires immediate rapid evacuation.

The open ("sucking") chest would produces profound intrathoracic physiologic alterations. Normal chest expansion creates negative intrathoracic pressure, which pulls air into the trachea and allows the lungs to expand. When the diaphragm and chest relax, positive pressure creates expiration. If the chest wall sustains an injury approximately two-thirds the tracheal diameter, negative intrathoracic pressure required for inspiration is lost, the ipsilateral lung collapses, and the loss of negative intrathoracic pressure affects the good lung. Consequently, it is important to rapidly reconstruct chest wall integrity. Initially, this is most easily done by placing a hand over the sucking chest wound. Field treatment includes placing a petrolatum gauze on top of the wound, covering it with a 4 × 4 gauze pad, and taping it on three sides (Fig. 13-8). The untaped fourth side serves as a relief mechanism to prevent tension pneumothorax. Persons with sucking chest wounds should be rapidly evacuated to sophisticated medical care.

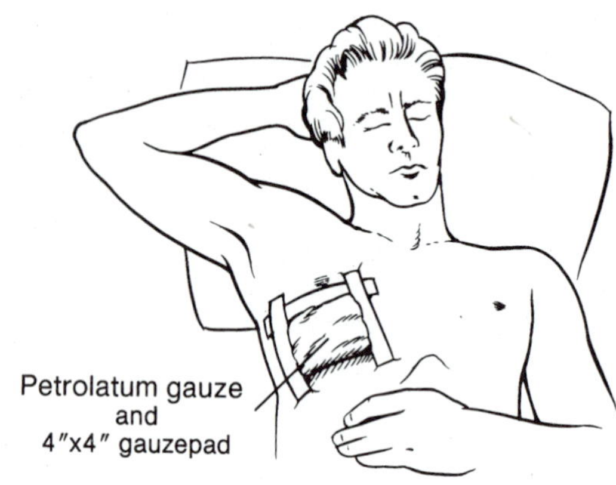

Fig. 13-8 Treatment of a sucking chest wound. Sealing the wound with a gel defibrillator pad works best because this pad adheres to wet or dry skin. Petrolatum gauze or Saran Wrap also works well.

Injuries to the Abdomen

Intraabdominal injuries in the wilderness setting are unique because they are often difficult to recognize. *However, once recognized or suspected, all intraabdominal injuries require immediate evacuation.*

PENETRATING INJURIES

Penetrating injuries may result from gunshot or stab wounds. The social context in which these injuries occur (accidental, intentional, or self-inflicted) makes little difference in the wilderness setting. Recrimination, guilt, and blame only interfere with the paramount goal of immediate evacuation.

Gunshot Wounds

Low-caliber gunshot injuries often present with small entrance and no exit wounds. High-caliber, high-velocity gunshot injuries may have relatively innocuous entrance wounds but be associated with large, disfiguring exit wounds and extensive internal injuries. No matter what the caliber or trajectory and no matter where the entrance and exit, all gunshot wounds from the nipple line to the inguinal ligament should be presumed to have penetrated the abdominal cavity and created an intraabdominal injury. These injuries mandate immediate surgical intervention. A victim of gunshot wounds to the head, chest, abdomen, or groin should undergo immediate evacuation accompanied by the administration of broad-spectrum antibiotics (cefoxitin, adult dose 2 g intramuscularly). Gunshot wounds are discussed in Chapter 14.

Shotgun Injuries

Shotgun injuries to the torso are managed in the same manner as gunshot wounds. Shotgun injuries have a potentially lower incidence of underlying visceral injury than gunshot wounds, but there is often extensive soft tissue damage requiring surgical debridement. The potential exists for delayed development of peritonitis from a single penetrating pellet to the viscera. Consequently, shotgun injuries should also be treated with emergency evacuation and broad-spectrum antibiotics (cefoxitin, adult dose 2 g intramuscularly).

Occasionally a close-range shotgun blast results in a soft tissue defect large enough for injured bowel to extrude through the wound. The injured bowel should not be placed back into the abdomen. Injured bowel displaced from the abdominal cavity conceptually should be treated as though it were an enterocutaneous fistula. Since evacuation is often delayed in the wilderness, it is better to have fecal contents outside, rather than inside, the peritoneal cavity. The exteriorized bowel should be kept moist and covered at all times. Uncovered bowel outside the peritoneal cavity rapidly desiccates and becomes nonviable, mandating later surgical resection. Exposed bowel should be covered with an abdominal pad or cloth moistened with sterile saline, at best, or with drinking water, at worst. The dressing should be checked and remoistened at least every 2 hours.

Stab Wounds

The penetrating object is usually a knife but may be as varied as a piton, ski pole, or tree limb. Any deep skin laceration from the nipple line to the groin should be considered to have damaged an intraabdominal organ. While the odds of an abdominal gunshot wound injuring a visceral organ exceed 95%, the odds of a stab wound causing the same injury are between 50% and 60%.

In certain urban hospitals the high incidence of negative surgical explorations for stab wounds has led to a more selective approach toward the patient with an abdominal stab wound.[35] This approach uses local wound exploration, diagnostic peritoneal lavage, and frequent physical examination.

Although no data exist addressing the management of stab wounds in the wilderness environment, the following approach is reasonable. If the wound extends into subcutaneous tissue, the evacuation decision depends on the results of local wound exploration. This procedure is simple to perform, even in the wilderness environment. The skin and subcutaneous tissue are infiltrated with local anesthetic, and the laceration is extended several centimeters to clearly identify the anterior fascia. It is helpful to use lidocaine (Xylocaine) 1% with epinephrine to minimize the slight but annoying bleeding that can impair visualization. The wound should never be probed with any instruments.

If thorough exploration of the wound shows no evidence of anterior fascial penetration, and if the patient demonstrates no evidence of peritoneal irritation, the wound can be closed with Steri-Strips, dressed, and the evacuation process delayed. Wound exploration is confined to the area from the costal margin to the inguinal ligament. Local wound exploration is contraindicated in wounds that extend above the costal margin. It is possible for such exploration to communicate with a small pneumothorax, exacerbating respiratory distress. If local wound exploration does not demonstrate fascial penetration, physical examination should be performed every few hours for the succeeding 24 hours. If no peritoneal signs develop and the patient feels constitutionally strong, a remote expedition may resume with caution and an eye to evacuation should the victim become ill. In the wilderness environment it is prudent to have a low threshold for evacuation because of the technical difficulties in performing wound exploration, such as insufficient light and inadequate instruments.

BLUNT INJURIES

Blunt intraabdominal injury is commonly associated with falls. Abdominal injuries are often associated with fractures or closed head injuries. Often the decision for evacuation is made on the basis of other injuries; however, the wilderness physician must be attuned to the potential for intraabdominal hemorrhage as an occult isolated injury.

For descriptive purposes the abdomen may be divided into the thoracic, true, and retroperitoneal compartments. The thoracic abdomen contains the liver, spleen, stomach, and diaphragm. The liver, spleen, and more rarely, stomach may be injured by direct blows to the ribs or sternum. Twenty percent of persons with multiple left lower rib fractures have ruptured spleens.[34] A direct blow to the epigastrium may result in increased intraabdominal pressure with subsequent rupture of liver or diaphragm. The true abdomen contains the small bowel, large bowel, and bladder. Isolated bowel injuries are rare in the wilderness setting. Blunt bladder or rectal injury usually occurs in conjunction with a severe pelvic fracture and carries high mortality. The retroperitoneal abdomen contains the kidneys, ureters, pancreas, and great vessels. It is notoriously difficult to evaluate by physical examination.

Although much progress has been made in the last decade to evaluate the presence of blunt intraabdominal injury, modalities such as computed tomography, ultrasound, and diagnostic peritoneal lavage are irrelevant in a wilderness setting. The wilderness physician must have a high index of suspicion and perform a superlative physical examination.

Physical Examination

The physician looks for signs of early shock: tachypnea, tachycardia, delayed capillary refill, weak or thready pulse, and cool or clammy skin. Physical examination of the abdomen begins with inspection. Contusions and abrasions may be the only harbingers of occult visceral injury. Periumbilical ecchymosis associated with abdominal hemorrhage (Cullen's sign) is virtually never present in a victim with acute abdominal trauma. Abdominal distention secondary to hemorrhage is a very late sign and never present before shock and cardiovascular collapse. Abdominal inspection should survey the flanks, lower chest, and back. Inspection of the back should follow palpation of the spine while the patient is supine. The patient should be carefully log-rolled if there is any suspicion of spinal injury.

Looking for muscle guarding, the examiner gently palpates the abdomen in all four quadrants. *Any* persistent guarding following wilderness trauma mandates rapid evacuation. Percussion tenderness is an indicator of peritoneal irritation, also mandating evacuation. The presence or absence of bowel sounds has little prognostic significance. Bowel sounds may be present in the face of significant intraabdominal hemorrhage or, conversely, be absent in victims when extraabdominal injuries induce ileus.

Referred Pain

Pain referred to the left shoulder (Kehr's sign) strongly suggests the presence of a ruptured spleen. This pain is often exaggerated by placing the victim in Trendelenburg position, increasing the amount of left upper quadrant blood irritating the diaphragm. Pain from the retroperitoneal abdomen associated with injuries to the kidney or pancreas may be referred to the back. However, referred pain is usually a late finding and not helpful in the evaluation of acute trauma.

Gross hematuria that does not clear immediately or is coupled with an associated injury, such as pelvic fracture or abdominal or back pain, requires immediate evacuation. To minimize blood loss, the victim should be kept stationary and the evacuation team brought as close to the victim as possible.

In a wilderness setting, rectal and vaginal examination adds little to the evacuation decision. The unstable pelvic fracture associated with rectal and vaginal injuries is usually the determinant for evacuation.

SHOCK

The best way to manage shock is to prevent it with rapid diagnosis, aggressive resuscitation, and rapid transport to an operating room for definitive care. The wilderness setting provides distinct limitations to aggressive resuscitation and rapid transport.

If intravenous fluids are available, a large-bore (14- or 16-gauge) catheter should be placed in the antecubital fossa. Ideally, lactated Ringer's or normal saline solution should be administered in sufficient volume to maintain urine output at 30 to 50 ml/hr, systolic blood pressure greater than 90 mm Hg, and pulse rate below 110 beats/min.

In certain areas blood may be available before the victim reaches a trained surgeon and operating room. Human immunodeficiency virus is now endemic in the blood supply of some Third World countries, especially in central Africa. Most trauma victims in the expedition environment are young and have superb underlying vigor. With proper titration of crystalloid to maintain tissue perfusion, such persons can tolerate red blood cell volumes in the 10% to 12% range without significant long-term sequelae. Consequently, the administration of blood products may be delayed until an operating room and safe blood supply are available. Before traveling overseas, the physician should investigate potential problems in the local blood supply.

In the absence of intravenous therapy, little can be done for treatment of shock in the wilderness beyond general supportive measures, such as maintaining the victim in a warm sheltered environment, minimizing movement (to the extent compatible with the rapid evacuation), and attempting oral administration of warmed fluids if the victim's airway is stable and the victim is capable of purposeful swallowing. Trendelenburg positioning (head down, feet up) provides a transient shift in peripheral intravascular volume to the central circulation. Military antishock trousers (MAST) are rarely used in the wilderness because they are bulky, are difficult to transport, and should not be inflated for longer than 2 hours.

Injuries to the Skeletal System

In the wilderness environment, the individual who initially manages the patient with a musculoskeletal injury should be alert to a number of factors. First, the caregiver should know the cause of the injury. He or she should also determine the direction of the injury's force in relation to the individual or limb so that the victim can later be examined for injuries to adjacent bones and joints. The time of the injury should be noted; for many injuries the length of time to treatment determines prognosis. The environment in which the accident has occurred is another important consideration. Cold, wind, or heat exposure may negatively affect the victim's condition and should be reported to the physicians at the definitive care center. Open wounds, especially those that communicate with fractures, may have variable outcomes depending on environmental conditions. A covered, clean puncture wound with associated tibia fracture occurring in a cold environment has a much lower risk of infection and chronic osteomyelitis than does an uncovered ragged laceration with associated comminuted tibia fracture occurring in a tropical environment.

Once the patient has been stabilized, the skeletal system should be examined in detail. This examination is an orderly process that begins with the spine, moves to the pelvis, and ends with the extremities.

Injuries to the Spine

CERVICAL SPINE

In the wilderness setting, fractures or dislocations of the cervical spine are a result of falls from significant heights or of high-velocity ski or vehicular injuries. Because of the high degree of association between head and cervical spine injury, an individual with a significant head injury should also be considered to have a cervical spine injury. This is especially true when an individual has lost consciousness. Ideally, a person with a suspected cervical spine injury should be placed on a backboard with rolls on either side of the head and then evacuated.

Fractures of the cervical spine frequently result in neurologic deficit. Fractures of the C1-2 complex generally result from axial loading (a C1 ring fracture—Jefferson's fracture) or an acute flexion injury (a C2 posterior element fracture—hangman's fracture). Generally a complete neurologic injury at this level is unsurvivable owing to paralysis of respiratory muscle function. Therefore surviving patients generally have a partial deficit or are neurologically intact. Fractures of the axial cervical spine may be a result of flexion, extension, rotational forces, or combinations of these. The most common mechanism of injury is flexion, and the most common level of injury at C5-6.[5]

Fractures and dislocations may result in partial or complete neurologic injury distal to the fracture or in no neurologic injury at all. Partial injuries to the spinal cord result from typical patterns of injury. Because flexion injuries are the most common type of injury to the cervical spine, the anterior cord syndrome is the most commonly seen serious neurologic picture. A careful neurologic examination in the field to grade motor strength and to document sensory response to light touch and pinprick yields important information that should be reported to the treating physician at the definitive care facility. The presence or absence of the Babinski reflex should be noted as well.

When appropriate supplies are available, a rectal examination should be performed. Complete lack of tone and failure of the sphincter muscles to contract when pulling on the penis or clitoris (the bulbocavernosus reflex) indicate the presence of spinal injury.

When individuals with cervical spine fractures or dislocations are transported, the neck must be stabilized to prevent further injury to the spinal cord or nerve roots at the level of the fracture or dislocation. Since approximately 28% of patients with cervical spine fractures have fractures elsewhere in the spine, the entire spine must be protected during transport.[5]

Occasionally, pure flexion injuries can result in dislocation of one or both of the posterior facets without fracture or neurologic injury. The patient may complain only of neck pain and limitation of motion. If so, the same precautions should be taken as for cervical injuries; that is, the patient should be transported with the neck rigidly immobilized. With this injury, great posterior instability is present (since the interspinous ligament is ruptured), and any further flexion stress could produce a cord injury.

THORACOLUMBAR SPINE

Fractures of the thoracolumbar spine occur most frequently at the thoracolumbar junction. Because the thoracic spine is well splinted by the thoracic cage, when axial or flexion loads are applied, the ribs prevent loading of the thoracic vertebral bodies and transmit the forces to the upper lumbar levels. In the wilderness setting these fractures are generally produced by falls from significant heights or by high-velocity sporting vehicular trauma. With rapid deceleration in the seated position (which happens in a snowmobile), a significant flexion moment is produced with the fulcrum at the thoracolumbar junction (Figure 13-9). Similarly, when an individual jumps or falls and reaches the ground in the upright position, a flexion moment at the thoracolumbar junction is produced as the weight of the upper torso falls anterior to the center of gravity. For this reason, thoracolumbar spine fractures are frequently associated with major fractures of the hindfoot (particularly calcaneus fractures). With this mechanism of injury and single or bilateral calcaneus fractures, a spine fracture should be assumed and the patient should be transported with spine precautions.

With the above injury, careful neurologic examination must be performed as a part of the secondary survey. Particular attention must be paid to the dermatomal response to light touch and pinprick, motor function, and the presence or absence of the cord level reflexes. If the patient has sustained a significant head injury, it should also be assumed that he or she has a spinal injury. The

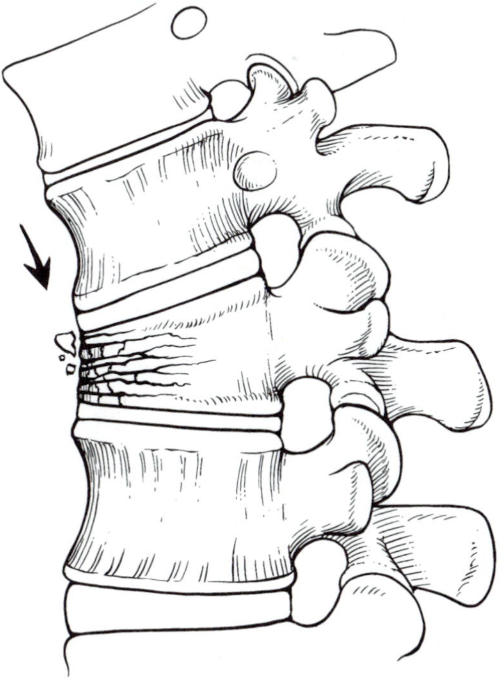

Fig. 13-9 Wedge compression fracture from axial or flexion loading at the thoracolumbar junction.

victim should be log-rolled, maintaining perfect spinal alignment, and a backboard should be placed beneath the victim. The scoop stretcher is an excellent alternative that does not require rolling the individual. Following a spine fracture with cord level injury, significant fluctuations in sympathetic tone may occur. Therefore, if equipment is available, blood pressure should be monitored frequently during transportation. Since fluctuations in sympathetic tone may also prohibit the normal response to environmental heat or cold, body temperature should be monitored frequently and appropriate steps taken to cool or warm the patient.

Injuries to the Pelvis

In the wilderness setting, fractures of the pelvis are generally associated with falls from significant heights, high-velocity ski accidents, or vehicular trauma. The direction of the force is directly related to the fracture and has important implications for definitive management.[45,47] Pennal and Tile[38,47] divide pelvic fractures into anteroposterior compression injuries, lateral compression injuries, and vertical shear injuries. Not included in this classification are simple, nondisplaced inferior or superior ramus fractures or avulsion fractures. On clinical examination these simple fractures are generally identifiable by an area of tenderness not associated with detectable instability.

The key factor in initial management of pelvic fractures is identification of posterior injury to the pelvic ring. Posterior ring fractures or dislocations are associated with a greater incidence of significant hemorrhage, neurologic injury, and mortality than are other pelvic fractures. The diagnosis of a posterior ring fracture is based on instability of the pelvis associated with posterior pain, swelling, ecchymosis, and motion. Patients with posterior ring fractures must be immediately evacuated on backboards, with care taken to minimize leg and torso motion.

In general, lateral compression injuries are stable injuries with impaction of the posterior structures. These fractures are less frequently associated with the above complications. AP compression injuries demonstrate anterior instability along with palpable ramus fractures or gapping of the public symphyses. Fractures of this type are generally associated with an appreciable incidence of bladder, prostatic, or urethral injury. Definitive care is directed toward providing posterior stability for vertical shear fractures and those few lateral compression injuries with unstable posterior fractures. AP compression injuries, when anterior symphyseal gapping is significant, are managed by stabilization with internal or external fixation. When the symphysis is widened more than 2.5 cm, injury to the anterior capsular structures of the sacroiliac joint is present and stabilization is mandated.

Injuries to the Extremities

PHYSICAL EXAMINATION

Physical examination of the extremities is divided into circulatory function, nerve function, skeletal function, and joint function.

Circulatory Function

Injury to the major vessels supplying the limbs can occur with penetrating or blunt trauma. Fractures can produce injury to the vessels by direct laceration (rarely) or by stretching, which produces intimal flaps. These flaps can immediately occlude the distal flow or can expose critical intimal cells. This exposure leads to platelet aggregation and delayed occlusion. For this reason, repeated examination of the circulatory function of the limb is mandatory before and after the patient's arrival at the definitive care center. The color and warmth of the skin of the distal extremity must be assessed. Distal pallor and asymmetric regional hypothermia could mean a vascular injury. Pulses palpated in the upper extremity should include the brachial, radial, and ulnar. Hand-held battery-powered sound Doppler units may be available at fully equipped treatment centers and are useful in assessing these pulses. Blood loss and hypothermia may make these pulses difficult to assess. In the field the pulses of obese individuals can also be difficult to evaluate; therefore temperature and color become the keys to the diagnosis. Any suspected major arterial injury mandates immediate evacuation after appropriate splinting of the limb.

Nerve Function

Nerve function may be impossible to assess in an unconscious or uncooperative patient. Whenever possible, however, it is important to establish the status of nerve function to the distal extremity after the patient is stabilized. The initial findings can then be periodically compared with additional examinations during transportation of the patient. A deteriorating neurologic status has important implications for definitive care of the patient.

Sensory examination should be carefully documented with regard to light touch and pinprick. The unique area of supply for the peripheral nerves is important to assess for extremity injuries. For spinal and pelvic injuries the dermatomal distribution of the spinal nerve should be addressed. This distinction between peripheral nerve and nerve root level should be maintained. Muscle function should be assessed by observing active function and grading the strength of each group against resistance. In the case of potential spinal cord injury the presence or absence of the Babinski and bulbocavernosus reflexes should be noted.

Skeletal Function

The long bones of the lower extremity serve as the major structural supports for locomotion. Those of the upper extremity stabilize the soft tissues, enabling positioning of the hand in space. A visible angulated deformity should alert the examiner to the existence of a fracture; appropriate splinting should be performed after the limb is aligned with axial traction. Palpable crepitus confirms the diagnosis. Radiographic confirmation follows at the definitive treatment center.

Other than noting the degree and orientation of the limb's position when the victim is found, there is no reason to delay in aligning and splinting fractures. Making the distinction between joint injuries and intraarticular or very proximal or distal fractures is difficult for even the experienced practitioner and must wait until the patient arrives at a definitive care facility. Similarly, distinguishing a ligamentous injury from a fracture is difficult at the level of the wrist and ankle. Since the initial care of these classes of injuries is identical, this differentiation is not required for initial treatment in the field.

Joint Function

Muscle forces act across the joints to improve the position of the lower limbs for ambulation and of the hand for handling objects. Each joint has a certain minimum function to allow for stability and a normal range of motion. Making the diagnosis of a joint injury in the field allows appropriate splinting and prevents further damage during transport.

Palpation of the long bones should begin distally and proceed across all joints. Palpable crepitus at the joint level mandates application of an appropriate splint. If the patient is able to cooperate, the examiner should request that the patient move every joint through an active range of motion. This exercise quickly focuses the examination on the location of the injury. When this is not possible, passive motion of each joint should be evaluated after palpation of the joint for crepitus and swelling. Crepitus, swelling, deformity, or a block to motion should prompt the application of a splint.

If the joint is dislocated, it should be promptly reduced following completion of the neurocirculatory examination. Reduction of the joint generally relieves the patient's discomfort considerably. After reduction, stability of the involved joint should be assessed by careful, controlled motion.

Joints that have associated fractures or interposed soft tissues are frequently unstable after reduction. In these circumstances more care must be taken in applying splints to prevent redislocation during splinting. The details of the reduction maneuver, including orientation of the pull, amount of force involved, degree of patient sedation, and residual instability of the joint, should be reported to the definitive care physician.

SPLINTING TECHNIQUES

In cases of suspected cervical or thoracolumbar spine trauma, the patient should be transported on a hard surface. Backboards or scoop stretchers are most effective for this purpose; however, in remote settings improvisation with any hard piece of wood, fiberglass, or straight tree limbs lashed together may be necessary. If injury of the cervical spine is suspected, a roll of clothes or water bottle should be placed on either side of the head to prevent rotational movement. These objects should be as high as the patient's midface on either side. Tape applied from the supporting stretcher across the objects and the patient's forehead will add further stability. Any patient with a suspected major pelvic injury should be transported with similar techniques, and the lower extremities should be stabilized to prevent motion.

For fractures or dislocations about the shoulder, a commercially available sling or improvised triangular bandage will suffice and will provide considerable relief by taking the weight of the arm off the injured structure(s). Whenever possible, splinting of the upper extremity should be done in the position of function. Occasionally, it may be difficult to place the elbow with a joint injury in 90 degrees of flexion and neutral pronation-supination.

The limb should be securely fixed to the splint with tape or elastic bandages. Air splints are available that when inflated can adequately splint the upper extremity in this position. The advantages of these splints are that they are lightweight and compact. Splints may also be made from plaster or fiberglass, which can be cut to shape and length and applied over cotton softroll. Wooden or metal splints, custom-made or improvised, can serve the same function if these other materials are not available.

The primary aim in splinting is to immobilize the limb securely in the functional position until definitive care can be reached. Hand splints should be applied with the metacarpophalangeal joints flexed 90 degrees and the interphalangeal joints extended. This position places the collateral ligaments at maximum length and prevents later joint contracture. The lower extremity should be positioned for transport with the hip and knee extended and the ankle in neutral. In cases of hip or femur fractures or dislocations, traction should be applied whenever possible, improvising when necessary (Fig. 13-10). Most commonly a Thomas splint with a Spanish windlass is available. The ring of the splint rests against the patient's ischium and pubis, and traction is applied through the windlass, stabilizing the joint or fracture fragments. More recently the Kendrick traction device has become available. This splint is light and packaged for easy transportation. If commercial splints are unavailable, the injured leg can be strapped to the noninjured leg, with a tree limb or walking stick placed between them. If possible, the patient should be transported on a backboard.

With the lower leg, air splints provide adequate immobilization of the tibia-fibula fractures or ankle fractures and dislocations. Splints made from plaster or fiberglass may be applied with Ace wraps over cotton padding. Custom-made or improvised metal splints can be held in place with elastic bandages or tape. The ankle should be held in neutral and the splint firmly applied. Patients with unstable lower ex-

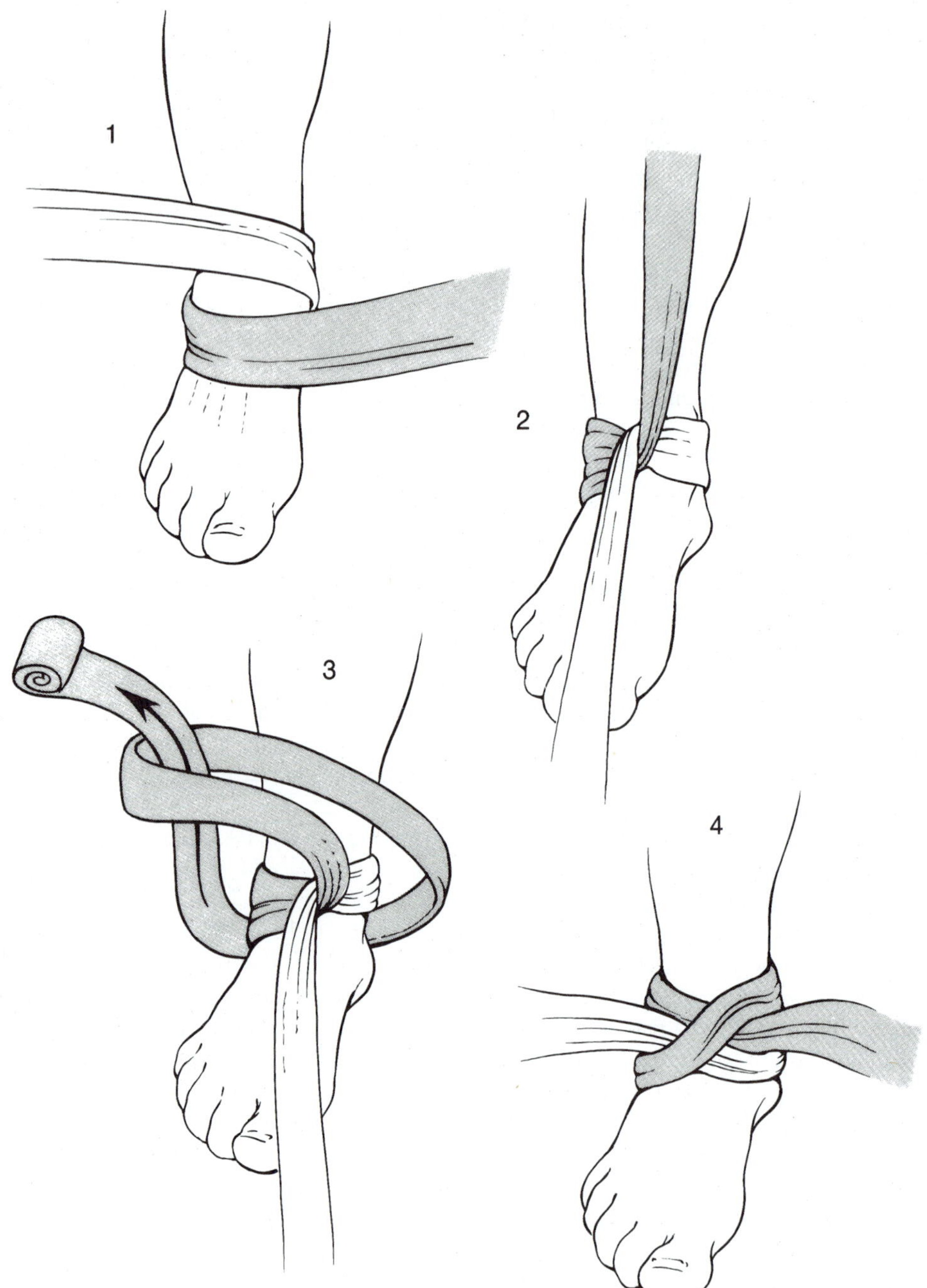

Fig. 13-10 Improvisation of an ankle wrap to be used for traction.

tremity fractures or dislocations should be transported recumbent with the limb elevated.

OPEN FRACTURES

General care of open fractures in the outdoor environment depends on evacuation time. If evacuation can be completed within 8 hours, the fracture should be realigned, broad-spectrum antibiotics given (cefoxitin, adult dose 2 g intramuscularly), and the extremity splinted. These fractures require immediate operative irrigation, debridement, and stabilization. If evacuation time exceeds 8 hours, irrigation, limited debridement, and stabilization should be attempted in the field. Unfortunately, the incidence of osteomyelitis is high.

AMPUTATIONS

In the wilderness environment, amputation victims require immediate evacuation. Treatment includes hemorrhage control by direct pressure, as described in the primary survey. Tourniquets are virtually never indicated. Without cooling, an amputated part remains viable for only 4 to 6 hours; with cooling, viability may be extended to 18 hours. The amputated part should be cleaned with water, wrapped in a moistened sterile gauze or towel, placed in a plastic bag, and transported on ice. The amputated part should accompany the victim throughout the evacuation process.

COMPARTMENT SYNDROMES

A compartment syndrome exists when locally increased tissue pressure compromises local circulation and neuromuscular function. In the wilderness setting, compartment syndromes most frequently occur in association with fractures or severe contusions. This syndrome can occur when the victim has been lying for some time across a limb with body weight occluding the arterial supply. Elevated local tissue pressure (greater than 30 mm Hg) accompanies acute hemorrhage and microvascular leakage or revascularization following ischemia.

The lower leg and forearm are the most common sites for a compartment syndrome, because tight fasciae encase the muscle compartments in these regions and because these areas are frequently involved with fractures or severe contusions. Compartment syndromes have also been described in the thigh, hand, foot, and gluteal regions.

The conscious patient complains of severe pain, which seems out of proportion to the injury. The muscle compartments feel extremely tight, and applied pressure increases the pain. The cooperative patient notes decreased sensation to light touch and pinprick stimuli in the areas supplied by the nerve(s) traversing the compartment. Most commonly this is noted on the dorsum of the foot in the first webspace, caused by pressure affecting the deep peroneal nerve in the anterior compartment of the leg. Stretching muscles within the compartment produces severe pain. The most reliable signs of a compartment syndrome are pain, tight compartments, hypoesthesia, and pain on passive stretch. Pulselessness, pallor, and slow capillary refill may never be seen, even with the most severe compartment syndrome.

When a compartment syndrome is recognized, emergency evacuation must be expedited. The victim must be definitively treated in the first 6 to 8 hours after onset of this condition to optimize return of function to the involved limb. Measurement of compartmental pressures is a useful adjunct to clinical diagnosis performed at most definitive care facilities. Emergency fasciotomy, the treatment of choice, is performed to relieve the pressure, which untreated can produce nerve and muscle cell death within 12 hours. Limited fasciotomies can be performed in the field by an experienced surgeon if evacuation will require more than 8 hours.

UPPER EXTREMITY FRACTURES

Clavicle

Fractures of the clavicle generally occur in the middle and lateral thirds of the bone and are typically associated with direct blows or with falls onto the lateral shoulder. These fractures frequently occur with snow skiing. The patient complains of shoulder pain, which may be poorly localized. Motion of the arm or shoulder exacerbates the pain. The examiner can localize the problem by gentle palpation to identify the area of maximum tenderness. The presence of crepitus at the clavicle confirms the diagnosis. Although rare, clavicle fractures can be associated with a pneumothorax as the cupula of the lung is punctured; therefore the chest should be auscultated for equal breath sounds when a stethoscope is available. The presence of shortness of breath and deep pain on inspiration should increase the suspicion of clavicle fracture. Clavicle fractures may also be associated with injuries to the brachial plexus and axillary artery or subclavian vessels. A thorough neurocirculatory examination of the affected extremity must be performed. The skin should be examined carefully, since 3% to 5% of clavicle fractures may be open because of the subcutaneous location of the bone. The presence of a significant open wound, a suspected pneumothorax, or nerve or vascular injury should prompt evacuation. The field treatment for a clavicle fracture consists of a figure-8 bandage or sling, along with judicious use of analgesics.

Humerus

A fracture of the humeral shaft may be produced by a direct blow or torsional force on the arm. These fractures frequently occur with falls, rope accidents, and skiing accidents. Fractures of the midshaft and junction of the middle and distal one third of the humeral shaft violate the spiral groove path of the radial nerve. When the injured individual complains of arm pain with associated deformity and crepitus, the sensory and motor function of the radial nerve must be carefully checked as a part of the overall neurocirculatory examination. When a fracture of the humeral shaft is suspected, an appropriate coaptation splint of plaster, fiberglass, or wood should be firmly applied with an elastic bandage on the medial and lateral sides of the humerus (Fig. 13-11). A sling should be used for comfort.

Fractures of the proximal humerus are frequently difficult to differentiate from a shoulder dislocation in the acute phase. The mechanism is frequently a high-velocity fall onto an abducted, externally rotated arm or a direct blow to the anterior shoulder. These situations frequently occur in skiing accidents. The patient complains of severe pain around the shoulder and with any motion of the arm. Palpable crepitus with arm motion confirms the diagnosis of a proximal humerus fracture. To determine the presence of anterior fullness, which would imply associated anterior humeral head dislocation, the examiner should use the uninjured side as a

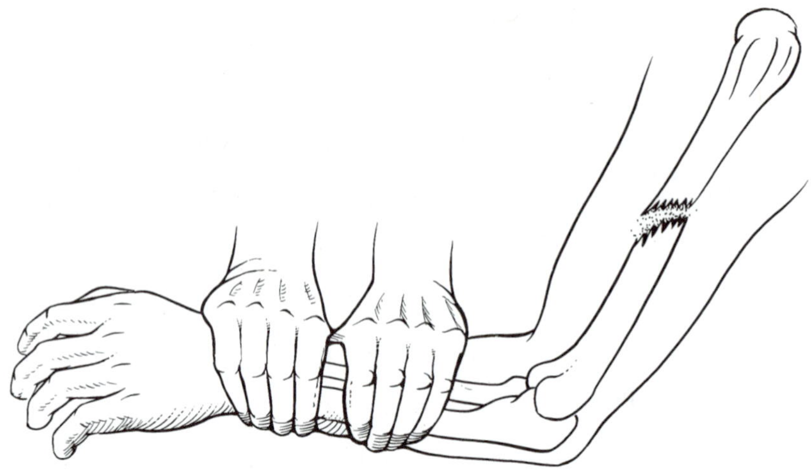

Fig. 13-11 To control pain, a fractured humerus should be stabilized manually until a splint can be applied.

reference and palpate the anterior aspect of the injured shoulder firmly while rotating the arm. If this injury is identified and definitive care is more than an hour or two away, reduction should be attempted. Using available sedation, the trunk must be stabilized while the treating individual applies firm longitudinal traction in line with the arm. A second individual should then apply anterior pressure to the humeral head to ease it back into the glenoid joint space. The application of an arm sling is the appropriate field management for a proximal humeral fracture. Associated significant distal nerve or vascular injury should prompt evacuation.

Fractures of the distal humerus are more frequently extraarticular in children and intraarticular in adults. Children generally sustain supracondylar fractures with an extension moment across the elbow in falls from heights. The peak age of incidence is 4 to 8 years, although these fractures can also occur in adults. Deformity, swelling, pain, and crepitus are present, and the diagnosis is fairly obvious. Careful neurocirculatory examinations must be performed. If the radial pulse is absent, an attempt at flexing or extending the elbow should be made while the radial pulse is palpated. If the pulse improves, the limb should be splinted in that position for transportation. The motor examination should focus on flexion of the thumb and distal interphalangeal joint of the index finger, since injury to the anterior interosseous nerve is frequently associated with these fractures.

The adult with pain, crepitus, deformity, and swelling after a fall should have a splint applied after the neurocirculatory examination. The splint should be applied with the elbow at 45 or 90 degrees of flexion, depending on the comfort of the patient. Because crepitus is more often associated with fractures than with dislocations, radiographs should be made before any attempt at reduction. Evacuation should be performed promptly in the presence of an open fracture or neurocirculatory deficit.

Radius

Radial shaft fractures are more commonly associated with motor vehicle or industrial accidents but may occur in the wilderness setting in the case of a fall with angular or axial loading of the forearm. A radial shaft fracture may be associated with a dislocation of the distal radioulnar joint (Galeazzi fracture); therefore the wrist must be examined for tenderness, swelling, and deformity when a fracture of the radial shaft is suspected. The patient generally complains of pain, and deformity and crepitus are identified over the radial shaft after a fall or direct blow. Any motion of the arm exacerbates the pain. When a fracture of the ulna is also present, the both-bone forearm fracture, forearm instability is marked. The joint above (elbow) and the joint below (wrist) should always be clinically examined for tenderness, crepitus, and deformity. Once a fracture of the radius or both bones of the forearm is identified, the wrist, forearm, and elbow should be splinted in the position of function.

Fractures of the radial head generally occur in young to middle-aged adults who fall onto outstretched hands. The patient complains of pain about the elbow with loss of full extension. There is pain at the radial head on the lateral side of the elbow with gentle pressure and rotation of the forearm. Fractures of the radial head frequently produce hemarthrosis of the elbow. This is identifiable by fullness posterior to the radial head and anterior to the tip of the olecranon. A fluid wave is ballottable. If the equipment is available and the examiner is confident about the diagnosis, the hemarthrosis may be aspirated and 5 ml of lidocaine instilled. The elbow should be moved through a gentle range of motion and then placed in a posterior splint in 90 degrees of flexion with neutral pronation and supination. On prolonged expeditions when definitive care cannot be reached, these splints should be removed at 5 days and intermittent active range of motion exercises performed with reapplication of the splint for comfort. With more comminuted radial head fractures, attempts at motion produce pain and crepitus and little progress in motion is seen. With nondisplaced or minimally displaced radial head fractures, early motion prevents permanent loss of elbow motion.

Fractures of the distal metaphyseal radius are generally associated with falls onto outstretched hands in older osteoporotic individuals. In the wilderness setting these fractures occur in younger adults with falls from significant heights onto outstretched hands. Intraarticular distal radius fractures are often associated with fractures of the ulnar styloid. Pain, deformity, and crepitus are obvious. A distal neurocirculatory examination should be carefully performed, focusing on the sensory function of the median nerve. With significant deformity at the wrist, longitudinal traction should be applied following appropriate sedation and a splint that immobilizes the wrist and elbow should also be applied. In cases of open fractures, significant neurologic deficits distally, or abnormal circulatory examination, splinting should be prompt. The limb should be kept elevated above the heart during transportation.

Ulna

Ulnar shaft fractures are most often associated with fractures of the radial shaft at the same level. When isolated, they most often occur as a result of direct blows, the so-called nightstick fracture. A fracture of the ulnar shaft can be associated with dislocation of the radial head (Monteggia lesion), and elbow function should be carefully assessed. In the wilderness setting the most frequent mechanism of injury is bracing a fall or collision with the forearm. Pain, localized swelling, and crepitus are present. A long-arm splint should be applied in the position of function. An open fracture is indication for prompt evacuation.

Fractures of the proximal ulna (olecranon) occur as a result of a fall onto the posterior elbow or with an avulsion mechanism with a violent asymmetric contraction of the triceps. The patient may be unable to extend the elbow actively against gravity if the triceps is dissociated from the forearm with a complete fracture of the olecranon. On initial examination the patient has pain, significant swelling, and ecchymosis. There may be a palpable gap in the olecranon, and the fracture may be open. In cases of severe trauma the olecranon fracture may be associated with an intraarticular fracture of the distal humerus. This diagnosis can be made only radiographically. After the distal neurocirculatory examination is complete and examination of the shoulder and wrist has been performed, the splint should be applied in the position of function. An open fracture, absent pulse, severe swelling, or neurologic deficit should prompt immediate evacuation.

Wrist

Wrist fractures occur because of significant rotational forces or high axial loading forces, such as those occurring with falls onto the hand. The patient first complains of pain and later of swelling about the wrist. Any use of the hand or rotation of the forearm produces significant pain. Many fractures of the carpal bones are associated with wrist dislocations. When such an injury is suspected, reduction of the fracture should be performed by grasping the hand in a handshake fashion and pulling with axial traction.

Precise diagnosis of fractures of the carpus is not possible in the absence of radiographs. The most common fracture is that of the scaphoid. This diagnosis is suspected because the patient's area of maximum tenderness is in the anatomic snuffbox (Fig. 13-12). When the examiner notes this and appropriate splinting materials are available, a thumb spica splint should be applied, immobilizing both the radius and the thumb metacarpal. Another common fracture is that of the hook of the hamate bone. The patient complains of pain at the base of the hypothenar eminence, which is the point of maximum tenderness. This injury frequently occurs when the hand is used to apply great force to an object with a handle on it, such as an ax or hammer, and great resistance is met. A short-arm splint suffices for this injury, as well as for other suspected carpal injuries, until definitive treatment can be obtained. Open fractures or those accompanied by median nerve dysfunction should be managed by evacuation.

Metacarpals

Fractures of the metacarpal base or shaft occur with crushing injuries or with axial loads when rocks or other immovable objects are struck. Fractures at the base of the digit metacarpals are suspected when tenderness, crepitus, and occasionally deformity are present. These should be managed with a short-arm splint. The same findings are generally present with shaft fractures.

Fractures of the metacarpal necks also occur by the same mechanism. The 5th and 4th metacarpals are most frequently involved. These fractures occur at the base of the knuckles and can be associated with significant rotational deformities. Rotation of the metacarpal should be checked by observing the orientation of the fingernails as the metacarpophalangeal and the interphalangeal joints are flexed 90 degrees. The fingernails should be parallel to one another and perpendicular to the orientation of the palm. The terminal portions of the digit should point to the scaphoid tubercle.

When malalignment or significant shortening is noted, rotation and reduction with traction on the involved digit should be attempted. Immobilization of a fractured metacarpal shaft or neck is accomplished by applying an aluminum splint (or stick) to the volar surface and taping the involved digit to the next digit with the metacarpophalangeal joint at 90 degrees. This is the point of maximum length of the collateral ligaments, and immobilizing the joint in this position prevents contracture of these ligaments with subsequent loss of motion.

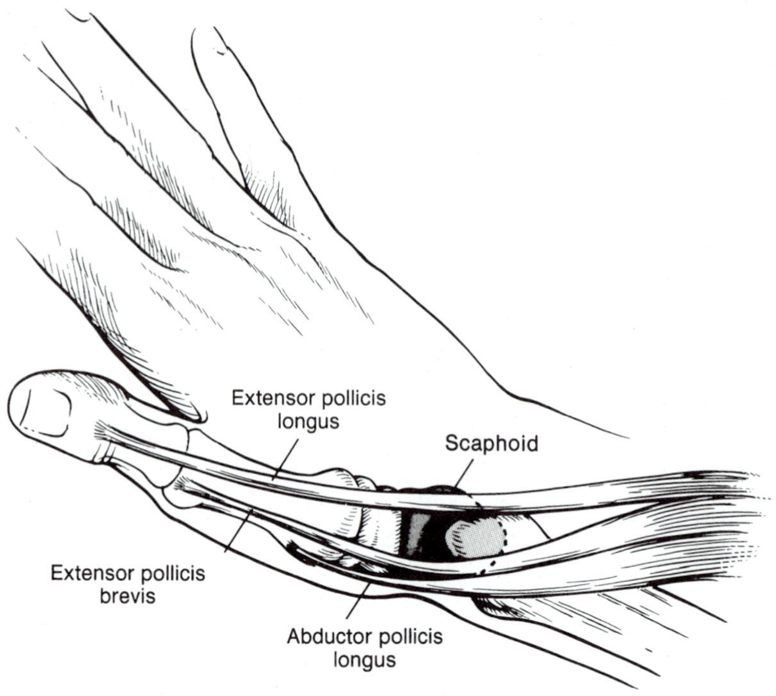

Fig. 13-12 The scaphoid (navicular) bone sits in the "anatomic snuffbox" of the radial aspect of the wrist.

Fractures of the base of the thumb metacarpal often occur when an individual falls with objects grasped between the index finger and thumb. This position is common when ski poles are grasped. Fractures of the base of the thumb metacarpal are difficult to differentiate from ulnar collateral ligament injuries to the thumb. When this fracture is suspected, the thumb and wrist should be immobilized in a thumb spica splint. Open metacarpal fractures need cleansing, debridement, and presumptive antibiotic therapy for 48 hours or until definitive care can be obtained.

Phalanges

Fractures of the digital phalanges occur as a result of crush injuries, or when the digits are caught in ropes or within equipment being used to pull up objects. Angular or rotational deformity and crepitus make these fractures obvious. Without radiographs, intraarticular fractures with subluxations or dislocations are difficult to differentiate from interphalangeal joint dislocations. These fractures should be reduced by grasping the digit and applying traction. Fractures of the shaft of the phalanges should be reduced by applying traction and correcting the deformity. Both types of fractures should be immobilized by taping the injured digit to the neighboring uninjured digit or by taping the digit to a volar splint. Nailbed fractures or crushes should be cleansed with soap, a sterile dressing applied, and a protective volar splint applied to prevent further injury.

UPPER EXTREMITY DISLOCATIONS AND SPRAINS

Sternoclavicular Joint

The sternoclavicular joint is generally injured by a fall onto an abducted shoulder. The usual direction of the dislocation is with the medial head of the clavicle going anterior to the manubrium of the sternum. A direct blow to the sternum may also produce this injury as well as associated rib fractures. The patient complains of pain in the region of the sternum and frequently has difficulty taking a deep breath. When the dislocation is posterior, significant pressure may be placed on the esophagus and superior vena cava. The patient may complain of difficulty swallowing and have engorgement of all of the veins of the face and upper extremities—superior vena cava obstruction syndrome. A step-off between the sternum and medial head of the clavicle (compared with the uninjured side) confirms this diagnosis.

Reduction should be attempted as soon as possible. A large roll of clothing or other firm object should be placed between the scapulae, and the patient should be placed on a firm surface. Sharp, firm pressure, directed posteriorly, should be applied to both shoulders. This maneuver should be repeated several times with a larger object placed between the scapulae if reduction attempts are initially unsuccessful. If the patient remains in extremis, the midshaft clavicle may be grasped with a towel clip or pliers and forcefully pulled out of the thoracic cavity. This type of dislocation requires evacuation. Anterior dislocations should be managed with a sling.

Acromioclavicular Joint

The acromioclavicular joint is injured by a blow on top of the shoulder (Fig. 13-13). First-degree acromioclavicular joint injury is an injury to the capsule between the acromion and the clavicle; no superior migration of the clavicle is seen. Second-degree acromioclavicular joint injury is a complete capsular disruption with the coracoclavicular ligaments remaining intact. Superior migration of the clavicle relative to the acromion of one-half the diameter of the clavicle is noted. Third-degree acromioclavicular joint injury is

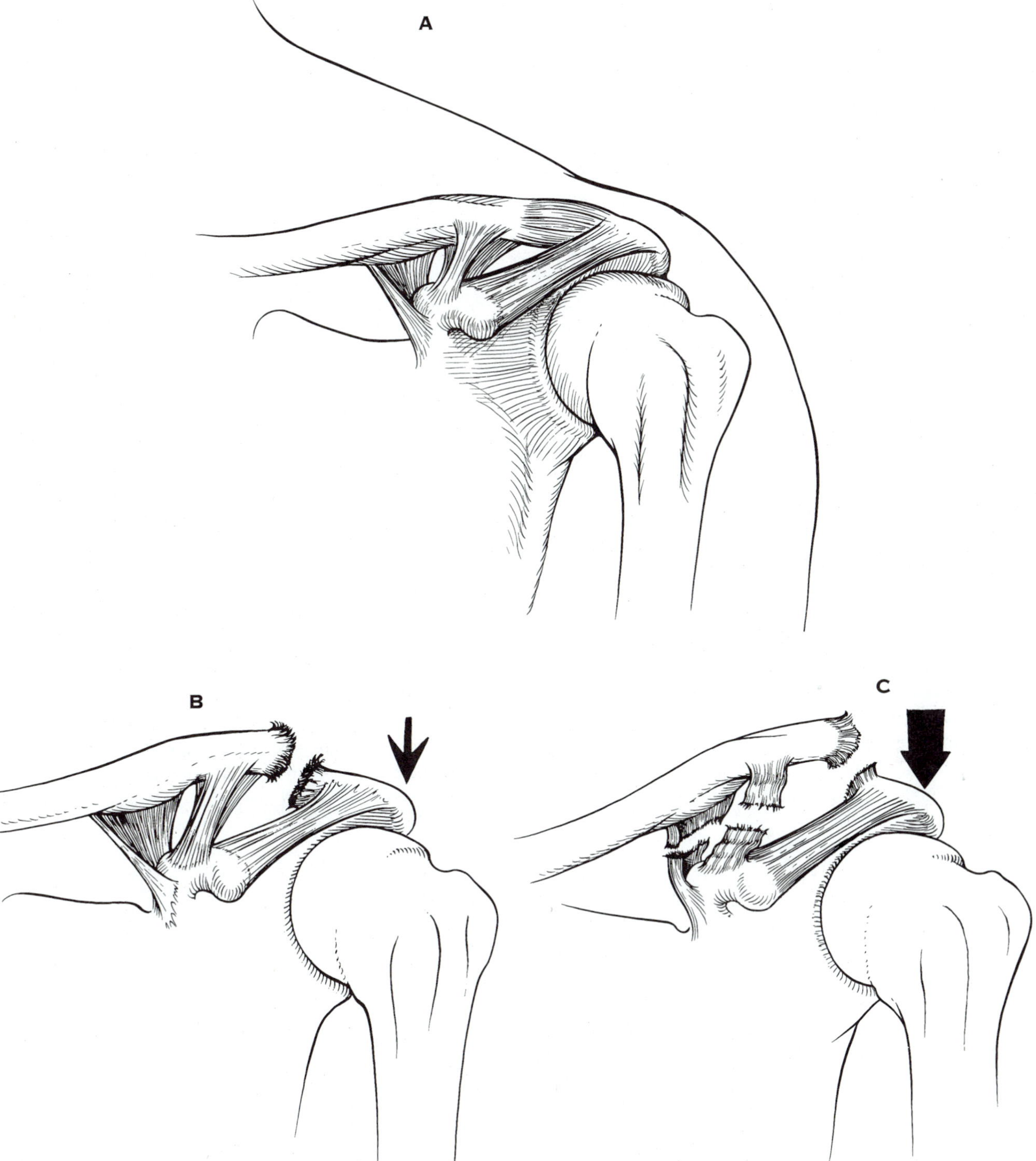

Fig. 13-13 Acromioclavicular joint injury. **A,** Normal anatomy. **B,** Second-degree injury. **C,** Third-degree injury.

total disruption of the joint capsule and the coracoclavicular ligaments, which allows superior migration of the clavicle of up to 2 cm. Because using the hand increases pain, the arm on the affected side should be placed in a sling. As long as the individual can tolerate the discomfort associated with such an injury, evacuation is not mandatory.

Glenohumeral Joint

The shoulder joint is generally dislocated anteriorly or anteriorly and inferiorly. The usual mechanism of injury is a blow to the arm in the abducted and externally rotated position. This frequently occurs in skiing as the individual crosses his or her ski tips or goes forward on a mogul and lands face first with the arm(s) in this position. Anterior shoulder instability can be recurrent in 30% to 50% of individuals.[17]

Recurrent dislocations and dislocations in younger patients may be easier to reduce than first-time dislocations in older patients. The examiner should do a thorough motor, sensory, and circulatory examination of the involved extremity. Axillary and musculocutaneous nerves should be carefully assessed, since they are the nerves most commonly injured with anterior dislocation. Anterior dislocations are more common in older individuals; therefore serial examinations of distal pulses, capillary refill, and forearm compartments should be made in these individuals.

The preferred method for reduction is linear traction along the line of the extremity while the torso is stabilized with a blanket or rope (Fig. 13-14). Narcotic or benzodiazepine premedication can be extremely helpful but should be avoided in the multiply injured patient. If the shoulder cannot be reduced after three attempts, evacuation is indicated. The Hippocratic maneuver of placing a foot in the axilla of the injured limb should be avoided because of increased pressure on the structures within the axillary sheath. If the reduction maneuver is successful, the arm should be placed in a sling until definitive care is reached. Because there is a significant incidence of fractures of the tuberosities with these injuries, x-ray examination is required to make the diagnosis and evacuation is mandated. An alternative method of relocation is to have the victim lie prone over a log or makeshift platform and to apply downward traction on the affected arm. This may be accomplished with or without attached weight (5 to 10 pounds) to the limb in conjunction with the scapula rotation technique.

Posterior dislocations of the glenohumeral joint make up less than 5% of shoulder dislocations. They result from a direct blow to the anterior shoulder; they also occur as a result of marked internal rotation that occurs with grand mal seizures. The patient complains of significant pain and loss of shoulder motion. Generally, external rotation is completely lost. Using palpation, the examiner can usually detect posterior fullness not found on the uninjured side. The reduction maneuver, aftercare, and indications for evacuation are similar to those for anterior dislocation.

Elbow

Dislocations of the elbow occur with hyperextension or axial loads from falls onto the outstretched hand. They are generally posterior and lateral. The diagnosis is obvious, with posterior deformity at the elbow and foreshortening of the forearm. Following a careful examination of the distal sensory, motor, and circulatory status, reduction should be performed. With countertraction on the upper arm, linear traction should be applied with the elbow slightly flexed and the forearm in the original degree of pronation or supination. Premedication with opiates or benzodiazepines can be extremely helpful. Reduction provides nearly complete relief of pain and restoration of normal surface anatomy. Following reduction a posterior splint should be applied with the elbow in 90 degrees of flexion and the forearm in neutral position. A sling should be used for comfort. If reduction is not successful after

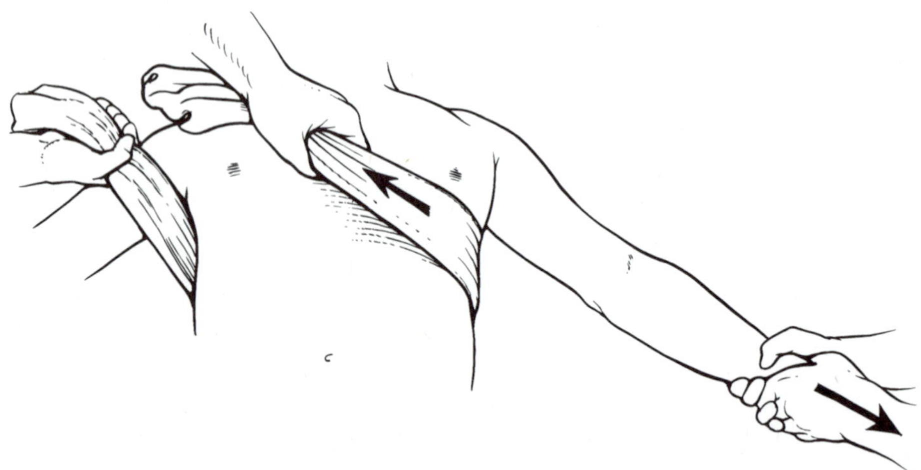

Fig. 13-14 Traction and countertraction for dislocated shoulder reduction.

three attempts or if a nerve or vascular injury is suspected, a splint should be applied to the arm as it lies and evacuation initiated.

Wrist

As noted in the previous section, wrist dislocations are frequently associated with carpal fractures. These injuries are generally produced by falls onto the outstretched hand. A wrist dislocation may be difficult to differentiate from a fracture of the distal radius on clinical grounds alone. However, in either case a reduction maneuver in the field is indicated. This should be performed after careful assessment of distal neurocirculatory function, emphasizing median nerve function. The hand is grasped in the handshake fashion, countertraction is placed on the upper arm, and linear traction is applied. Significant force is required, and premedication, if available and indicated, may be extremely helpful. If reduction is unsuccessful after three attempts or if there is median nerve dysfunction, evacuation is indicated. A short-arm splint should be applied if reduction is successful, and the arm should be elevated above the heart as much as possible until the definitive care center can be reached. Pain and tenderness about the wrist with no significant deformity should be considered an intercarpal ligamentous disruption or a carpal fracture, and a short-arm splint should be applied.

Metacarpophalangeal Joint

Metacarpophalangeal joint dislocations are rare and may be produced by crush injuries or injuries occurring when the hand is caught in a rope. These dislocations may be dorsal or volar. Generally, dorsal dislocations are easily reduced by linear traction along the finger. Volar palmar dislocations may be irreducible, since the head of the metacarpal becomes entrapped between the volar ligaments. These dislocations frequently require open reduction. If reduction of a digital metacarpophalangeal joint dislocation is successful, a volar splint should be applied with the joint held at 90 degrees of flexion. If reduction is unsuccessful, the joint should be splinted in the position of comfort and definitive treatment should be obtained as soon as possible.

The thumb metacarpophalangeal joint is the one most commonly injured. Injury to the ulnar collateral ligament of this joint results from a valgus stress, generally from a ski pole. This can occur when an individual falls holding an object in the first webspace. Detectable clinical instability documented by lateral stress x-ray studies is an indication for surgical repair. A thumb spica splint should be applied and definitive care sought within 10 days of the injury.

Proximal Interphalangeal Joint

Proximal interphalangeal joint dislocations are common. These injuries occur with axial loading of a finger when an individual attempts to catch an object. These dislocations can also result when a finger becomes entangled in a rope or another piece of equipment. They are generally volar (middle phalanx in relationship to the proximal) and are easily reduced with longitudinal traction. A volar splint should be applied and the finger taped to the splint in 10 degrees of flexion. Early motion of the joint should be initiated to regain full extension. When the dislocation is dorsal, the central slip of the extensor mechanism may be ruptured. For this reason the joint should be slightly hyperextended as the splint is applied after reduction. With either a volar or distal dislocation, definitive care must be sought as soon as possible.

Distal Interphalangeal Joint

The distal interphalangeal joint is less frequently injured than the proximal interphalangeal joint. Volar dislocation or subluxation may result in disruption of the terminal extensor mechanism. After reduction with traction, the joint should be examined for full active extension. If an extension lag is noted, the joint should be splinted in 15 degrees of hyperextension for 3 weeks. Ultimately an x-ray examination must be performed to rule out an intraarticular fracture.

Occasionally, when an object is firmly grasped and then pulled away, rupture of the flexor profundus tendon occurs. On examination, active flexion of the distal interphalangeal joint is absent. The digit should be splinted in flexion and the patient seen by an upper extremity surgeon within 10 days.

LOWER EXTREMITY FRACTURES

Femur and Patella

In general, healthy, active individuals sustain fractures of the proximal femur only in falls from significant heights or from high-velocity injuries sustained during water or snow skiing. These fractures occur in the femoral neck or intertrochanteric region. When there is no injury to the head or spinal cord, the patient complains of pain about the proximal thigh. In all but the thinnest individuals there is little local reaction in terms of swelling or deformity around the hip region to aid in diagnosis. Any movement of the affected limb produces significant pain. In many cases the affected limb is noticeably shortened and externally rotated. Following a careful sensory, motor, and circulatory examination, the limb should be realigned and a Kendrick, Thomas, or REEL splint applied, if available. If none is available, the victim should be transported on a backboard, with the limbs strapped together or to a board with a tree limb placed between them. Fracture of the femoral neck is associated with a significant risk of posttraumatic femoral head necrosis. Without a radiograph these fractures are impossible to distinguish from intertrochanteric fractures. Because there is evidence that emergency treatment of a fracture of the femoral neck decreases the risk of posttraumatic necrosis,[46] patients in whom this injury is suspected should be evacuated rapidly.

Fractures of the femoral shaft occur with similar mechanisms; however, crepitus and maximum deformity are noted at midthigh. After neurocirculatory examination the limb should be placed in traction or protected as noted previously. These fractures may be open injuries; therefore the victim's pants should be split open to complete the examination. Discovery of an open wound should prompt rapid evacuation.

Fractures of the distal end of the femur are frequently intraarticular and occur with high-velocity loading when the knee is flexed. With axial loading of the femur the patella becomes the driving wedge and the femoral condyles are impacted. A patella fracture may result, or the condyles of the distal femur may be split. With a patella fracture the injury may be obvious on deep palpation. These injuries are often open, since there is very little soft tissue overlying this sesamoid bone. The definitive diagnosis is made radiographically. After initial examination of nerve and vessel function the limb should be realigned. At this point crepitus may be noted, as well as significant instability in the case of a distal femur fracture, which will not be seen with a patella fracture. A posterior splint should be applied to the realigned limb for transportation. As with all fractures, open wounds in the region of the fracture or an abnormal nerve or vascular examination should prompt immediate evacuation.

Tibia and Fibula

The tibial plateau is the broad intraarticular surface of the upper tibia that articulates with the distal femur. This area can be fractured with falls or jumps from heights. Frequently, angulatory moments across the knee are associated. A valgus moment produces a fracture of the lateral tibial plateau, whereas a varus moment produces a medial plateau fracture. Pain, swelling, and deformity are obvious on initial examination. With a tibial plateau fracture, hemarthrosis quickly becomes evident, with significant swelling about the knee. Because of anatomic tethering of the popliteal artery by the fascia of the soleus complex, arterial injuries may result from these fractures, especially when they are associated with knee dislocations. Distal pulses and capillary refill must be serially examined at 1-hour intervals. The possibility of a compartment syndrome must be kept in mind. After initial examination the limb should be carefully realigned and a posterior splint applied for transportation.

Tibial shaft fractures are associated with fibular shaft fractures in 90% of cases. These fractures result from high-impact trauma. Before the development of higher, anatomically conforming ski boots, this fracture was the most common skiing injury because the body rotated around a fixed foot (that is, a ski caught against a rock or tree stump), which produced a torsional, spiral fracture of the tibia and fibula.

The tibial shaft fracture is the most common type of open fracture in the wilderness setting. When this injury is suspected, the entire limb must be inspected for distal sensory, motor, and circulatory function before realignment of the limb. A posterior splint should be applied for transportation. Great care must be taken in serially examining the limb for the possibility of a compartment syndrome, since this is the most common location for this problem.

Ankle

The intraarticular distal tibia, medial malleolus, distal fibula, or any combination of these may be involved in an ankle fracture, generally produced by large torsional moments about a fixed foot. With the distal tibia, axial loading from a fall or jump may also be involved. The examiner notices significant pain and swelling as the shoe is removed. Palpation along the medial and lateral malleoli confirms the clinical suspicion. After the shoe is removed to inspect the skin for open wounds, neurocirculatory examination should be performed.

If there is a rotational deformity in the ankle, the ankle should be realigned with gentle traction before a posterior splint is applied with the ankle in neutral. During transportation the limb should be elevated above the level of the heart with the victim supine on a backboard, if possible.

Tarsal Bone

The calcaneus and talus are most often fractured during falls or jumps from significant heights when the victim lands on his or her feet. With a calcaneus fracture, significant heel pain, deformity, and crepitus are immediately evident after the boot is removed. A talus fracture may be impossible to differentiate on clinical grounds from an ankle fracture. With an ankle fracture, tenderness and deformity are at the level of the malleoli, while with the talus fracture. tenderness and swelling are distal to the malleoli. Fortunately, talus fractures are generally not associated with ankle fractures but may be associated with dislocations of the subtalar joint. With the latter the deformity is more significant. Talus fractures occur when the foot is forced into maximum dorsiflexion. Knowing the point of the foot's impact with the ground is helpful in differentiating the two fractures. Fractures of the other tarsal bones are exceedingly rare but would be defined by localizing the tenderness to a specific site. A short-leg splint with extra padding should be applied for all these fractures, and the limb should be elevated during transportation. If a talus fracture is suspected, evacuation of the victim should be expedited, since posttraumatic necrosis of the talar body is a common complication.

Metatarsal

Fractures at the bases of the metatarsals often occur in combination with midfoot dislocation. These injuries frequently occur across the entire midfoot joint and are commonly associated with fractures at the bases of the 2nd and 5th metatarsals. These injuries usually occur with axial loading of the foot while it is in maximum plantar flexion. This mechanism is most commonly produced with vehicular trauma and in the wilderness most frequently occurs with snowmobiling. The victim complains of midfoot pain and swelling; once the shoe is removed, crepitus and tenderness are noted at the base of the metatarsals. Generally, overall alignment of the foot is maintained, but stressing the midfoot by stabilizing the heel and placing stress across the forefoot in the varus and valgus directions reveals any instability present. The foot should be placed in a well-padded posterior splint and elevated whenever possible. Under no circumstances should a victim with a suspected midfoot fracture-dislocation be allowed to ambulate, since swelling would intensify and further injury to the midfoot might result.

Metatarsal shaft fractures occur with crush injuries and with falls or jumps from moderate heights. Midshaft metatarsal fractures also occur as stress, or so-called march, fractures. These injuries are often the result of prolonged hiking or running with poor preconditioning. Dull pain at the midshaft of a metatarsal (often the 2nd or 5th) may be converted to more severe pain with associated crepitus by a jump from a log or rock. Pain and localized tenderness are the hallmarks of this diagnosis. These fractures may be temporarily managed with a stiff-soled boot or orthotic insert. In cases of fracture instability or extreme pain a short-leg splint should be applied and no further weight bearing allowed.

Phalanx

Toe phalanges are fractured by crush injuries or when heavy objects are dropped on the foot. These injuries can be prevented by the use of steel-toed or hard-toed boots. The great toe phalanx fracture can be a significant problem as force is placed on the great toe during the toe-off phase of weight bearing. Phalanx fractures are managed by taping the toe to an adjacent uninjured toe with cotton placed between. Stiff-soled boots minimize discomfort with weight bearing.

LOWER EXTREMITY DISLOCATIONS AND SPRAINS

Hip

Posterior hip dislocations are produced by axial loading of the femur with the limb relatively adducted.[40] They generally occur as a result of vehicular trauma but can occur following a fall or sledding or skiing accident. With posterior dislocation the victim complains of severe pain about the hip. The affected limb appears shortened and adducted, and any hip motion increases the pain. It is not clinically possible to determine if there is an associated acetabular fracture. In the case of the rare anterior dislocation the limb is abducted and flexed. This type of dislocation is generally produced by wide abduction of the hip as a result of a significant force.

The victim should be placed supine for a complete survey of all organ systems. The distal limb should be carefully examined for associated fractures, and a careful sensory and motor examination performed. If it will be more than 6 hours before the victim can be evacuated to a definitive care center, closed reduction should be attempted. The victim should remain on a flat, hard surface, and analgesia should be provided with narcotic or benzodiazepine or both if available. An assistant should stabilize the pelvis by placing both palms on the anterior iliac crests. The treating individual should bend the knee and apply linear traction in line with the thigh in the case of an anterior dislocation and with the hip flexed 30 degrees in the case of a posterior dislocation. If this maneuver fails to reduce the hip, evacuation must be expedited because there is a direct relationship between the time to reduction and the incidence of osteonecrosis of the femoral head. This complication can be devastating in young individuals.

Knee

Knee dislocations are obvious because of the amount of deformity involved. The tibia may be dislocated in any of four directions relative to the distal femur. The most common direction is anterior (tibia anterior to the femur). This injury represents a true emergency because of the high incidence of associated vascular injury, which occurs because of tethering of the popliteal vessels along the posterior border of the tibia by the soleus fascia. A knee dislocation is a high-velocity injury most commonly produced by vehicular trauma or falls. When this injury is suspected, a careful screening neurocirculatory examination must be performed. Intact distal pulses do not definitively rule out an arterial injury. Intimal flap tears can produce delayed thromboses of the artery.

After the initial examination, linear traction should be applied to the limb in order to reduce the knee. This is generally successful regardless of direction of the dislocation. For transportation a posterior splint should be applied to the limb and the victim moved on a backboard. The examiner must be vigilant to the possibility of an arterial lesion or emerging compartment syndrome. Evacuation must be carried out on an emergency basis because of the risk of loss of the limb.

Frequently the patellofemoral joint is dislocated. Because of the increased femorotibial angle in females, this injury is far more common in women. Generalized ligamentous laxity may predispose to this problem. Dislocation of the kneecap may result from a twisting injury or asymmetric quadriceps contraction during a fall. These mechanisms routinely occur with hiking, climbing, or skiing accidents. The patella lies lateral to the articular distal femur. Although neurovascular injuries rarely occur in association with this injury, the screening examination should be conducted.

The patella can often be reduced by straightening the knee. If this is not successful, gentle pressure should be applied to the patella to push it back up onto the distal femoral articular groove. A knee splint should be applied with the joint in extension. Weight bearing should be avoided, but if this is not possible, further damage is unlikely. The knee should be kept in extension until definitive care can be obtained. A radiograph is ultimately required to rule out osteochondral fractures, which are frequently associated with this injury.

Ankle

Ankle dislocations are almost always accompanied by fractures of both malleoli. These dislocations generally occur with falls onto uneven surfaces or with twisting injuries of moderate velocity. The area about the ankle should be carefully observed for open injuries. A neurocirculatory examination is conducted to obtain a baseline status. The ankle joint should then be aligned by grasping the posterior heel, applying traction with the knee bent (to relax the gastrocsoleus complex), and bringing the foot into alignment with the distal tibia. Following this maneuver the foot should be reexamined, wounds dressed, and a posterior splint applied. During transport the limb should be elevated above the level of the heart.

The most common musculoskeletal injury occurring in the wilderness or sport setting is an ankle sprain. Ligament sprain, or tearing of the fibers, is separated into three grades. Grade 1 injury is partial disruption of some of the ligament fibers represented grossly by mild intersubstance hemorrhage. Grade 2 injury is complete disruption of a portion of the ligament fibers. The main substance of the ligament remains intact, and the injury is characterized by moderate hemorrhage with grossly visible torn ligament fibers. Grade 3 injury is complete disruption of the ligament fibers, which in the correct setting results in instability of the related joint.

The medial ligament complex consists of the deltoid ligament, which runs from the medial malleolus to the talus (Fig. 13-15). The ligament complex on the lateral side is much more complex and consists of three separate liga-

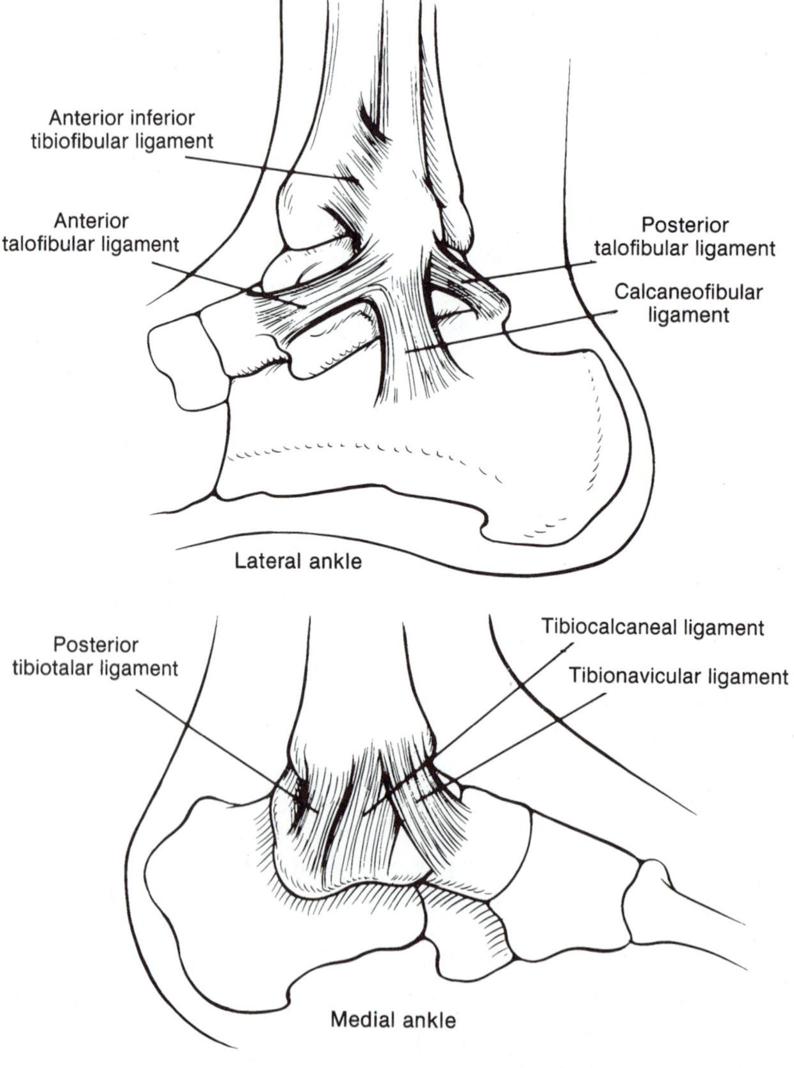

Fig. 13-15 Ligament complexes of the ankle.

ments named for their origins and insertions: the calcaneofibular ligament, the anterior talofibular ligament, and the posterior talofibular ligament (Fig. 13-15). The lateral ligament complex is the most frequent site of an inversion injury. When such an injury occurs, the shoe and sock should be removed and the screening neurocirculatory examination conducted. Each ligament should be individually palpated for tenderness, and the ankle should then be evaluated for instability with the anterior drawer test. This test is performed by stabilizing the tibia with one hand and grasping the posterior heel to pull the foot forward with the other hand. If the talus slides forward within the ankle mortise (using the uninjured side as a comparison), the injury is representative of a grade 3 ligament disruption. The foot and ankle should be placed into a posterior splint or air splint. If possible the victim should not bear weight on the limb. If this examination does not reveal instability, indicative of a grade 1 or 2 ankle sprain, the victim may be treated by application of an elastic bandage or taping of the ankle. Commercially available stirrup air splints also aid in ambulatory management of these injuries.

Radiographs are required to definitively rule out small talar avulsion fractures. This type of inversion injury is also infrequently associated with fractures at the insertion of the peroneus brevis tendon. The examiner may identify the presence of this injury with point tenderness at the base of the 5th metatarsal, but a radiograph is required for definitive diagnosis. Early management is the same as for a sprain.

Hindfoot

The subtalar joint may infrequently be dislocated in a significant fall or jump when an individual lands off balance or on an uneven surface. The calcaneus may be dislocated medially or laterally relative to the talus, the latter being slightly more common. The position of the heel relative to the ankle should be assessed. With either dislocation a reduction should be attempted if it will be more than 3 hours until the victim can be transported to a definitive care center. If no other injuries are apparent, a sedative may be used.

Medial dislocations are reduced more easily than lateral dislocations, in which the posterior tibial tendon frequently becomes displaced onto the lateral neck of the talus, blocking the reduction. The maneuver is the same: the heel is grasped with the knee flexed (relaxing the gastroc-soleus complex), linear traction is applied, and the heel is brought over to the ankle joint. This maneuver is generally successful for medial dislocation, but lateral dislocation, especially when associated with open wounds, often requires open treatment. After reduction is attempted, a posterior splint is applied and the limb elevated above the heart. Even if the reduction is successful, the victim should not be allowed to bear weight until definitive care is obtained.

Midfoot

Midfoot (Lisfranc's) dislocations are generally associated with one or more fractures at the base of the metatarsals, most commonly the 2nd and 5th metatarsals. Midfoot dislocations occur with axial loading of the foot in maximum plantar flexion. The forefoot is generally displaced laterally relative to the midfoot when the injury is initially unstable. More commonly the foot is normally aligned. There is significant swelling in association with tenderness at the base of the 1st, 2nd, and 5th metatarsals. With dorsal-plantar-oriented force, instability and crepitus are frequently noted. After the neurocirculatory examination is complete, the physician should stress the forefoot by stabilizing the heel and applying a varus and valgus directed force. If the forefoot is unstable and associated with significant swelling, pain, or crepitus, a midfoot dislocation should be considered to be present. A short-leg splint is applied, and the foot elevated above the heart during transportation. The individual should not be allowed to bear weight.

Metatarsophalangeal and Interphalangeal Joints

Metatarsophalangeal joint dislocations of the toes are relatively uncommon but can occur in the great toe with moderate axial force. Crush injuries and rock climbing accidents while the victim is wearing flexible-soled shoes can produce this injury; wearing boots with reinforced toe boxes of adequate depth generally prevents it. Injuries of this type at the great toe may be associated with fractures of the metatarsal or phalanx; the dislocation is generally distal. Because these may be open fractures, the foot must be inspected.

The lesser metatarsophalangeal joints are generally dislocated laterally or medially. The most common mechanism for this injury is striking unshod toes on immovable objects. The toes should be relocated by applying linear traction with the victim supine and the weight of the foot used as countertraction. Similar mechanisms produce dislocations of the interphalangeal joints, which are also reduced by applying linear traction with gentle manipulation. Once reduced, the injured toe should be taped to the adjacent toe for 1 to 3 weeks, and a protective boot with stiff sole and deep toe box should be worn.

EVACUATION DECISION

The issues surrounding the decision to evacuate an orthopedically injured individual vary depending on the goals and support of the expedition. A group of 25 climbers in the Himalayas with physician support and a field hospital at base camp will have very different criteria for evacuating an injured person than will a family of four spending a week hiking in the Rockies. In all cases party leaders should have a plan for contacting evacuation support teams if a serious injury occurs.

Musculoskeletal injuries that warrant immediate evacuation to a definitive care center include any suspected cervical, thoracic, or lumbar spine injuries. A victim who has a suspected pelvic injury with posterior instability, significant suspected blood loss, or injury to the sacral plexus should receive emergency evacuation on a backboard. Any open fracture requires definitive debridement and care within 18 hours to prevent development of deep infection, and should prompt emergency evacuation. Broad-spectrum antibiotics (cefoxitin, adult dose 2 g intramuscularly) should be administered early in the postinjury course.

Victims with suspected compartment syndromes must be evacuated on an emergency basis. Joint dislocations involving the hip or knee warrant immediate evacuation because of the associated risk of vascular injury or posttraumatic osteonecrosis of the femoral head. Lacerations involving a tendon or nerve warrant urgent evacuation to a center where an upper extremity surgeon is available. In all but the most serious wilderness expeditions, arrangements should be made to evacuate the victim when the treating individuals are not reasonably sure of the injury with which they are dealing or its appropriate management.

Injuries of the Skin

Major lacerations are often the most obvious sign of trauma; however, injuries to the integument are rarely life threatening. Contusions, abrasions, and lacerations should cause the examiner to focus on areas of potential occult injury. Contusions often overlie extremity fractures or, when present on the torso, suggest the potential for underlying visceral injury. Extremity lacerations may be associated with fractures or may extend into the joint space.

The four basic types of skin injuries are lacerations, crush injuries, stretch injuries, and puncture wounds. Lacerations rarely require closure in the wilderness environment. Crush injuries are often associated with significant tissue necrosis, impaired healing, and increased rate of infection; fortunately, they are rare in the wilderness. Stretch injuries produce a split in the skin but, more important, may be associated with underlying nerve or tendon damage. Puncture wounds often appear innocuous but have a high propensity for infection.

WOUND MANAGEMENT

To minimize infection, promote healing, and decrease the need for evacuation, wilderness wound management incorporates four steps: examination, anesthesia, cleaning and debridement, and definitive wound care.

Examination

The first step in wound management is examination, which must be performed in good light conditions after hemostasis has been achieved. Extremity injuries require detailed evaluation of distal neurovascular function before administration of local anesthesia.

Anesthesia

Administration of anesthesia occurs before mechanical wound cleansing and definitive care. Three methods of anesthetic administration applicable in the wilderness setting are topical anesthesia, local anesthesia, and regional anesthesia.

Topical Anesthesia. Topical anesthesia was originally introduced for mucosal lacerations but has been shown to be effective for skin lacerations. TAC (sterile tetracaine 0.5%, adrenalin 1:2000, and cocaine 11.8% in saline) is the topical anesthetic of choice. The solution is soaked into a sterile gauze and placed directly over the wound for 7 to 10 minutes. This may provide good analgesia and simultaneously assist in achieving hemostasis by a combination of direct pressure on the wound and vasoconstriction. Disadvantages include the potential for a slightly increased rate of infection and the fact that TAC solution is not as versatile an analgesic as lidocaine, which can be used for both local and regional infiltration.

Local Anesthesia. Local anesthesia using an injection of 1% lidocaine (without epinephrine) is the standard method for achieving soft tissue analgesia. In adults the maximum injectable dose of lidocaine subcutaneously is 300 to 400 mg. (For children, the maximum dose is 4 mg/kg.) The area of soft tissue to be anesthetized is injected circumferentially. Lidocaine should not be injected directly from within the wound to the periphery because this increases the chance of introducing bacteria and foreign material deeper into soft tissue.[34] The injection should proceed from the periphery of the wound, with each successive needle stick entering the skin through an area anesthetized by the previous injection.

Local anesthesia can be administered with relatively little discomfort using a small 25-gauge needle and a 1 cc tuberculin syringe. While using a small syringe may increase the time required to anesthetize a large wound, this method minimizes both the anesthetic dose and the distortion of soft tissue planes, facilitating soft tissue repair. Pain associated with the administration of local anesthesia is due to acidity and stretching of nerve endings within the dermis and subcutaneous tissue. Burning sensation associated with the administration of lidocaine is directly proportional to the rate of administration. Buffered (addition of bicarbonate) lidocaine invokes less pain. Administration of local anesthesia in small concentrated dosages under low pressure minimizes irritation of the sensitive nerve endings.

Regional Anesthesia. Regional anesthesia, defined as sensory nerve blockage proximal to the wound, is an excellent mode of anesthesia administration for wounds of the upper and lower extremity. The two types of blocks are regional nerve blocks and the Bier block. Regional nerve blocks require skill, practice, and a detailed knowledge of regional anatomy; they are not suitable for the first-time user in the wilderness environment. The Bier block uses the venous system to administer the anesthetic agent. It is useful for large lacerations or reduction of fractures in the distal extremity. The Bier block is convenient in the wilderness environment in that it does not require the skill level of regional nerve blocks.

A Bier block is administered by cannulating a vein on

the dorsum of the hand or foot, preferably using a 20-gauge butterfly needle. The butterfly is secured using tape, after which the arm or lower leg is elevated for several minutes to decrease intravascular volume. The extremity is then padded with rolled gauze at a site proximal to the injury. The gauze wrap serves as a protective layer between the skin and a tourniquet, which is applied subsequently.

The ideal tourniquet is a blood pressure cuff; however, a piece of rubber tubing, bandanna, or rope may be used if a cuff is not available. The purpose of the tourniquet is to obliterate vascular inflow to the extremity by maintaining a pressure gradient of approximately 50 mm Hg above systolic pressure. One percent lidocaine is administered in a 25 ml bolus in the upper extremity or a 35 ml bolus in the lower extremity. The anesthetic agent diffuses from the intravascular space into the soft tissue. The tourniquet may remain inflated for up to 90 minutes. The Bier block requires 10 to 15 minutes for complete analgesia of the distal extremity to develop. Care must be taken not to release the tourniquet for 20 minutes after the bolus of lidocaine, since this may release a potentially toxic dose into the vascular system. After 20 minutes the risk diminishes because much of the lidocaine has moved into the soft tissues where it becomes bound to protein.

Cleaning and Debridement

Hair Removal. In the wilderness a battery-operated electric razor is rarely available. A safety razor works well on the scalp where hair removal is mandatory for wound evaluation, cleaning, and debridement. In other areas of the body, hair removal is rarely required except when micropore tape is used for definitive wound closure. The eyebrows should never be shaved.

Mechanical Cleaning. Mechanical cleaning of the wound is a vital component of wilderness wound management. These wounds are often contaminated with mud, dirt, and foreign bodies. Much has been written about wound irrigants, but in the wilderness setting, drinking water may be the only irrigation solution available. Caustic disinfectants kill normal cells at the same rate they kill bacteria and should not be added to irrigation fluid. Simple soaking does not clean the wound, and scrubbing with an abrasive material only increases tissue damage.

The most effective mode of mechanical cleaning is moderate- to high-pressure irrigation, accomplished by attaching an 18-gauge needle to a 35 to 50 cc syringe and forcibly injecting the irrigant into the wound. This procedure provides an irrigation pressure of approximately 7 to 8 PSI and significantly reduces wound bacterial counts while it flushes small particulate matter from the wound. Depending on the wound size, up to 1 L of irrigant may be required for the initial phase of mechanical cleaning.

Debridement. The next step is debridement, defined as the surgical removal of wound debris and devitalized tissue. The simplest method of debridement is wound excision, wherein all wound edges are sharply debrided using a scalpel. Following excision the wound is carefully explored to remove additional debris and foreign material. Debridement is followed by another round of high-pressure irrigation. When inspection of the wound reveals no evidence of debris or necrotic tissue, the wound is ready for definitive wound care.

Definitive Wound Care

In the wilderness the risk of infection precludes suture closure. Here, definitive wound management should be accomplished by open wound management with delayed primary closure or primary closure using micropore tape. The use of surgical staples is as yet unproven in a wilderness setting. This apparently nonsurgical approach to definitive wound care in the wilderness represents an approach based on sound surgical principles and minimizes the risk of long-term morbidity associated with infection, while preserving function and cosmesis. Delayed repair and cosmetic revision are facilitated if tissue and underlying structures have not been compromised by infection.

LACERATIONS

Treatment of lacerations in the wilderness follows the wound management procedures outlined previously. However, the treatment varies depending on the body region in which the laceration occurs.

Scalp Lacerations

The extent and severity of scalp lacerations are often initially obscured by surrounding hair that is matted with blood. Hydrogen peroxide and water effectively remove this material. Hair surrounding the laceration is removed using a safety razor. Hair removal should be limited to the immediate area of the laceration, since the surrounding hair can later be twisted into strands and used to approximate the wound edges if necessary. Once the margins of the scalp laceration have been defined, local or topical anesthetics may be applied.

Physical examination of a scalp laceration should determine the integrity of the galea. Significant galeal laceration or the presence of a degloving injury may mandate evacuation. This is especially true in victims with mental status changes. An extensive scalp laceration bleeds freely, and if it follows a fall or direct blow to the head, it may be associated with an underlying skull fracture. Superficial scalp lacerations often bleed freely and may require pressure dressings to achieve hemostasis.

Minor scalp lacerations can be effectively treated in the wilderness setting. After the application of analgesia and wound exploration, mechanical high-pressure irrigation should be employed. Surgical debridement of scalp wounds should be kept to an absolute minimum because it may be difficult to mobilize wound edges to cover the resulting soft tissue defect. In addition, cosmesis is not a significant concern on the hair-covered scalp. Acceptable closure of a minor scalp laceration can be performed using strands of hair to approximate wound edges. This method minimizes the degree of shaving necessary if micropore tape closure were used.

Facial Lacerations

Lacerations to the face are relatively simply to manage in the wilderness, because they rarely damage significant underlying structures. However, if injuries to the facial nerve or parotid or lacrimal ducts occur, they can always be repaired secondarily.

Analgesia for lacerations to the face can be achieved by either local or topical methods. High-pressure irrigation is the method of choice for mechanical cleaning, and surgical debridement should be limited to obvious areas of necrotic tissue. The face has an excellent blood supply; consequently, wound closure using micropore tape is effective and often produces satisfying cosmetic results.

Torso Lacerations

Torso lacerations require evaluation for fascial penetration. If the anterior fascial layer is penetrated, the injury should be considered not as a skin injury, but rather as an injury to the underlying region, that is, the chest or abdomen.

Analgesia for torso lacerations can be either local or topical. Mechanical cleaning consists of irrigation and surgical debridement, which can be liberal because the soft tissue planes are readily mobilized to cover the defect. Wound management can be a wet-to-dry dressing with either delayed primary closure or a primary closure using micropore tape. The dirty wound should *never* be closed. If any wound shows signs of infection 3 to 5 days after the injury, it should be opened and wet-to-dry dressings initiated.

Extremity Injuries

Management of extremity lacerations in the wilderness environment requires careful judgment because of the potential involvement of underlying structures. This is especially true with the hand, where critical structures lie perilously close to the surface. Therefore a detailed neurovascular evaluation of all extremity lacerations should be performed. Mechanical cleaning should include high-pressure irrigation, removal of foreign bodies, and minimal surgical debridement on the hands and feet. Analgesia can be either local or regional, and wound closure tends toward delayed primary closure rather than micropore tape approximation. Any evidence of neurovascular functional compromise with a hand wound mandates evacuation.

Hand Injuries

Severe contusions to the hand commonly occur with crush or rope injuries. The hand should be carefully protected if marked swelling and pain with motion are present. If no joint instability or fracture is identified, a bulky hand dressing should be applied with the wrist dorsiflexed 10 degrees, the thumb abducted, and the metacarpophalangeal joints flexed 90 degrees, the position of function. Cotton wadding or bandages can be placed in the palm and between the fingers, and an elastic bandage used as an overwrap. A volar splint allows this position to be maintained until definitive care is reached.

Lacerations of the finger flexor or extensor tendons occur with accidents involving knives or other sharp objects. A flexor tendon laceration, partial or complete, can be a serious problem if not repaired early. The open wound should be cleansed and loosely taped closed (if the wound is clean), and the finger splinted in slight flexion at the interphalangeal joints and in 90 degrees of flexion at the metacarpophalangeal joint. To achieve optimal results, this injury should be managed by a hand surgeon within the first 3 to 5 days. For extensor tendons the open wound should be cleansed, taped closed, and a splint applied with the metacarpophalangeal joints in slight flexion and the interphalangeal joints extended. The victim should be seen by an orthopedic surgeon within 7 days.

The nerves most commonly injured by laceration include the superficial radial nerve at the wrist, ulnar nerve at the elbow or wrist, and median nerve at the wrist. Digital nerves are commonly lacerated in accidents with knives. In general, the wound should be cleansed and taped loosely and a splint applied to the wrist and hand. The victim should be seen by a hand surgeon experienced in microsurgery within 7 days.

PUNCTURE WOUNDS

Puncture wounds carry significant infection risk where organic contamination is frequent. Significant puncture wounds to the torso should be treated according to the guidelines outlined in the section on penetrating trauma to the chest and abdomen. Puncture wounds to the extremities should be unroofed if they are proximal to the wrist or ankle. The unroofed wound should be irrigated using high-pressure irrigation and then packed open with sterile gauze. Delayed primary closure with tape can occur at 48 to 96 hours. Puncture wounds to the hands and feet should not be explored in the absence of detailed knowledge of anatomy. If this expertise is not available, the wound should be cleaned and the patient started on antibiotics.

If the skin is punctured with a fishhook, the skin surrounding the entry point should be gently scrubbed with soap and water. After the skin is clean, gentle pressure should be applied along the curve toward the point while pulling on the hook. If the hook is not easily removed, the barb is caught in the tissue. In this case the hook must be removed by firmly pushing it through the skin so that the barb appears. The shaft or barb should be cut off and the remainder of the hook pulled back out of the skin. The two holes should be washed and left open with a simple dry dressing. An alternative method of removal advocated by some is to yank the hook from the skin while applying pressure into the curve of the hook to disengage the barb. If a hook enters the skin anywhere near the eye, removal should not be attempted; the victim should be immediately taken to a medical facility.

BURNS

Major burns are unusual in the wilderness setting and require urgent evacuation. Simple first aid principles in the treatment of major burns include immediately controlling the fire, removing smoldering clothing, and keeping the burned area clean and dry. The victim's temperature and hydration should be maintained throughout the evacuation process. A first-degree burn is characterized by pain and erythema without blister formation and is managed conservatively by immobilization and dry dressing coverage. Second-degree burns are characterized by pain, erythema, and blister formation. The blisters should remain intact unless grossly infected, and the burned area should be immobilized and covered with a bulky dry sterile dressing. Third-degree burns are characterized as full-thickness burns, with loss of all skin elements, both dermal and epidermal. The skin has a gray leathery appearance, and the burn does not blanch to pressure, indicating thrombosis of dermal and subdermal blood vessels. The burned area is anesthetic to touch, although deep pressure sensation may be preserved.

Treatment of major burns should follow the principles outlined in the primary survey. Burns to the respiratory tract insidiously compromise the airway. They are characterized by carbonaceous sputum, singed nasal vibrissae, and oropharyngeal inflammation. Stridor is a late sign of oropharyngeal burns and mandates immediate intubation or tracheostomy.

Fluid resuscitation of burn victims depends on the body surface area (BSA) burned and the depth of the burn. In the first 24 hours after the burn, victims with major burns require 2 to 4 ml of balanced salt solution per kilogram body weight per percent BSA burned. Half of this solution is administered in the first 8 hours, and the remainder over the next 16 hours. Adequate fluid resuscitation provides a urine output of 50 ml/hr in an adult or 1 ml/hr/kg in a child. Topical antibiotics are not necessary for initial field management of major burns.

Criteria for immediate evacuation of burn victims include second-degree burns involving 10% or more of BSA, third-degree burns of 5% BSA, all but extremely minor burns involving the face, eyes, ears, hands, feet, or perineum, or any burn associated with a fracture. Because a circumferential third-degree burn to the distal extremity or a digit may result in compromise of vascular inflow, this burn may require escharotomy.

Burns are discussed in greater detail in Chapter 10.

Dental Emergencies

Acute conditions involving the mouth and related structures can disrupt recreational activities in the outdoors. A simple toothache, although not life threatening, can cause disabling pain. At the other end of the spectrum, odontogenic infection or major facial trauma is associated with high morbidity and mortality. Diagnosis and treatment of dental emergencies falling into the broad categories of pain, infection, and trauma are discussed. Sections on local anesthesia, the dental first aid kit, and prevention follow.

SUBACUTE BACTERIAL ENDOCARDITIS

Medical personnel are reminded to seek a history of heart murmur before intraoral manipulations that are likely to cause bacteremia. Patients with most types of heart murmurs should be premedicated to prevent subacute bacterial endocarditis. Some of the regimens recommended by the American Heart Association are given in Box 13-2.

MAXILLOFACIAL PAIN

The causes of maxillofacial pain are myriad, and diagnosis of head and neck syndromes can be exceedingly difficult. Box 13-3 lists some pain-producing conditions. Fortunately, most of these syndromes are relatively rare. Only the most commonly encountered are discussed here.

PULPITIS

The common toothache is caused by inflammation of the dental pulp. The patient may have difficulty identifying the

BOX 13-2

ANTIBIOTIC PROPHYLAXIS FOR PREVENTION OF SUBACUTE BACTERIAL ENDOCARDITIS

The following are dosages for adults undergoing oral procedures:

STANDARD REGIMEN

Amoxicillin 3.0 g po 1 hour before procedure
1.5 g po 6 hours after initial dose

REGIMEN FOR ALLERGIC PATIENTS

Erythromycin stearate 1.0 g po 2 hours before procedure
0.5 g po 6 hours after initial dose

PARENTERAL REGIMENS

Ampicillin 2.0 g IV or IM 30 minutes before procedure
1.0 g IV or IM 6 hours after initial dose

or

Vancomycin 1.0 g IV administered over 1 hour, beginning 1 hour before procedure; no repeat dose

From Dhaani AS et al: *JAMA* 264(22):2919, 1990.

BOX 13-3
CONDITIONS THAT CAUSE FACIAL PAIN

Pulpalgia (acute, chronic, hyperplastic)
Periapical periodontitis (acute, chronic, suppurative, cystic)
Periodontal infections
- Periodontal abscess
- Acute necrotizing ulcerative gingivitis
- Primary herpetic gingivostomatitis
- Pericoronitis

Myofascial pain-dysfunction syndrome
Neurologic pain
- Trigeminal neuralgia
- Trigeminal neuritis
- Herpes zoster neuritis

Atypical facial pain
Psychogenic facial pain
Dental causalgia
Vascular pain
- Migraine headache
- Temporal arteritis
- Cluster headache

Referred pain
- Referred pulpalgia
- Referred pain of subacute thyroiditis
- Referred pain of myocardial infarction or angina pectoris

Sinus and paranasal pain

offending tooth, since the pain often radiates or is referred from one dental arch to the other or to the eye or ear region. The painful tooth is rarely sensitive to percussion or palpation. An obvious cause, such as a large carious lesion, is sometimes found on examination of the mouth, but often all of the teeth appear intact. If the pulpitis is mild, the condition is characterized by pain that is elicited only by hot, cold, or sweets and disappears within seconds when the stimulus is removed. A moderate pulpitis is characterized by increasing severity of pain and an increasing interval between the removal of the stimulus and the resolution of pain. In its most severe form, pulpitis causes severe, continuous, and debilitating pain.

Emergency treatment recommendations are as follows:

1. Mild pulpitis (characterized by transient thermal sensitivity). Examine the mouth visually. Structures will likely appear within normal limits. However, if a defect is found, it should be temporarily filled. Reassure the patient. While this condition is annoying, rapid progression is unlikely.
2. Moderate pulpitis (longer episodes of pain). Proceed as for mild pulpitis. Treat with nonnarcotic analgesics.
3. Severe pulpitis (severe, continuous pain). The preferred approach is pain relief through local anesthesia followed by evacuation of the patient. A nerve block with bupivicaine 2% with 1:200,000 epinephrine (Marcaine) provides about 8 hours of pain relief without central nervous system depression. Narcotics, even in large doses, might not provide adequate analgesia and might compromise the victim's ability to participate in evacuation. In extraordinary circumstances an experienced rescuer could locate the offending tooth, expose the pulp, remove the inflamed pulpal tissue with a barbed broach, and cover the opening with temporary filling material.

PERIAPICAL PERIODONTITIS

Inflammation of the supporting structures of a tooth is characterized by constant, often throbbing pain. Unlike in pulpitis the affected tooth is easily located. The patient can usually point to the exact source of the pain, or the examiner may gently percuss individual teeth, observing for tenderness. The area over the apex of the tooth is usually tender to palpation, but there is no frank swelling, which differentiates this condition from infectious processes. Trauma to a tooth can result in periapical inflammation, but the most common cause is egress of breakdown products from necrotic pulp. Minor swelling around the apex extrudes the tooth slightly, causing increased forces on the tooth during occlusion and thus intensified pain. Emergency treatment includes a soft diet in addition to the analgesics or anesthetics or both. Ideally the opposing tooth is shortened to relieve occlusal forces. Because this is often impractical in the field, the sufferer should be given a strip of leather or something similar to place between the teeth on the nonpainful side. This will keep the offending tooth out of occlusion and reduce pain.

MYOFASCIAL PAIN-DYSFUNCTION SYNDROME

In myofascial pain-dysfunction (MPD) syndrome, pain originates in muscles (usually the posterior cervical musculature or the muscles of mastication) and in their highly innervated fascial attachments to bone. The pathophysiology, in part, consists of a cycle of muscular hyperactivity and spasm, causing ischemia, pain, and psychologic stress, all of which increase muscular hyperactivity in a positive feedback loop. Dysfunction refers to findings such as deviation of the jaw on opening or inability to open the mouth wide. MPD syndrome may be associated with internal derangements of the temporomandibular joint.

Participants in outdoor activities are exposed to certain risk factors for MPD syndrome. Stress and the resulting parafunctional activity (grinding and clenching the teeth) are probably the leading initiators of MPD. Increased function, such as that required to chew granola, jerky, and other foods common on wilderness expeditions, is another factor that may precipitate an acute episode of MPD syndrome.

MPD syndrome is characterized by unilateral facial pain, tenderness in the affected muscles, possible unilateral headache, and associated dysfunction (pain on chewing, inability to occlude the teeth normally, trismus, joint sounds, lateral deviation of the mandible on opening). Emergency treatment consists of resting the muscles (soft diet and decrease in parafunctional activity) and applying moist heat. Analgesics should be given on a consistent schedule, rather than as needed, to break the cycle of pain and spasm. Muscle relaxants or sedatives, such as diazepam, are used only if primary treatment is ineffective.[13]

APHTHOUS ULCERS

The etiology of aphthous ulcers is unclear. They may represent an autoimmune attack on the oral mucosa followed by secondary infection.[42] They appear as round, superficial lesions with a red halo, occur on movable mucosa, and can be quite painful. Patients usually give a history of similar ulcerations. The lesions typically last 10 to 14 days. Many treatments have been proposed, and none has been found predictably effective. The best approach to management appears to be topical steroids, which reduce pain and hasten healing by 3 to 4 days. A mixture of fluocinonide 0.05% ointment (Lidex) and Orabase can be laid gently over ulcer 6 to 8 times per day, especially after meals and before bedtime. The medications should not be mixed until just before application, and the mixture should not be rubbed into the lesion. Other options include premixed preparations (Kenalog in Orabase), which are more convenient but deliver approximately 10% of the antiinflammatory effect; Decadron elixir 0.5 mg/5 ml four times a day (rinse with 5 ml for 2 minutes and expectorate), or for very severe cases systemic steroids.

ORAL INFECTIONS

Viral Infections

Use of sunblocking preparations on the lips helps prevent outbreaks of herpes labialis, which may be treated with oral acyclovir (Zovirax) 200 mg five times a day for 5 days. It is important to begin treatment as soon as the patient becomes aware of a prodromal paresthesia or "tingle." Primary herpetic gingivostomatitis is characterized by a thin zone of very red, painful gingiva next to the teeth. Other areas of mucosa, such as the tongue, may also be involved, and close inspection may reveal tiny vesicles or ulcers. Sore throat, lymphadenopathy, and low-grade fever are also present. Like other viral infections of the oral cavity, herpes labialis is self-limited. The patient should be reassured that the condition will resolve in about 10 days. Treatment is symptomatic and includes analgesics and soothing mouth rinses such as warm saline solution or a mixture of equal amounts of Benadryl elixir 12.5 mg/5 ml, Kaopectate, and Xylocaine Viscous 2% (rinse and expectorate 5 ml every 2 hours).

Yeast Infections

Oral yeast infections are found most commonly in individuals who are debilitated, immunocompromised, or taking antibiotics. Classic oral candidiasis is characterized by white patches on the mucosa that can be rubbed off, leaving a red, raw surface. Candidiasis can also be manifest as erythematous mucosa, without any sign of white patches, or as chronic angular cheilitis. Treatment is antimycotic mouth rinses (Nystatin oral suspension 100,000 units/ml, rinse with 5 ml for 2 minutes and swallow four times a day for 10 days) or lozenges (clotrimazole troche [Mycelex] 1 four times a day, leave in mouth 5 minutes and expectorate remains). In the field Nystatin preparations meant for vaginal use suffice (Mycostatin vaginal suppository, used as an oral lozenge three times a day for 10 days).

Bacterial Infections

Bacterial infections in the maxillofacial region are a serious health threat. In a wilderness setting they should be treated aggressively. The majority of odontogenic infections are caused by mixed populations of aerobes and anaerobes. Table 13-1 lists the most common bacteria associated with oral infections. These organisms are almost always present in normal oral flora, but because of a change in the relative amounts of various bacteria or in the oral environment, these mixed populations become virulent.

The behavior of various organisms, such as the production of collagenase or hyaluronidase, determines the clinical

Table 13-1 Average Reported Incidence of Microorganisms Isolated from Pulpal and Periapical Infections

Microorganism	Percent
Streptococcus (α-hemolytic and nonhemolytic)	50
Veillonella spp.	29
Propionibacterium	20
Anaerobic *Streptococcus*	18
Staphylococcus	16
Bacteroides spp.	15
Streptococcus faecalis	13
Candida albicans	7
Fusobacterium	5
Neisseria spp.	5
Lactobacillus spp.	5
Proteus spp.	4
Escherichia coli	4
Diphtheroids	4
Actinomyces spp.	4

From Topazian TG, Goldberg MH: *Oral and maxillofacial infections*, Philadelphia, 1987, WB Saunders.

presentation. Thus an infection may localize as an abscess or be present as a diffuse cellulitis. Oral infections generally spread slowly, but rapid spread to deep facial spaces may occur. Regional lymphadenopathy is common, whereas severe systemic symptoms are rare. Although bone is often involved, osteomyelitis is uncommon.[39,48]

Acute Apical Abscess and Cellulitis

Acute apical infection begins with bacterial infusion of the dental pulp. The organisms spread to surrounding bone through the apical foramen. Bacteria erode the cortical plate along the path of least resistance. Since the apices of most teeth are located to the facial aspect of the jaw, swelling is much more common in the facial soft tissues than in those on the lingual side.

The patient has pain and swelling, often fluctuant and usually in the buccal vestibule. The patient often gives a history of prior toothache, but early in this infection tooth pain is often absent. The offending tooth can be localized by percussion, consideration of the site of swelling and condition of individual teeth, and use of radiographs if available. The affected tooth does not respond to hot or cold. The primary treatment for an apical abscess is drainage. This can be accomplished with extraction, incision, or endodontic therapy. The treatment chosen depends on the equipment and personnel available, the advisability of retaining the offending tooth, and ultimately, clinical judgment. Antibiotics are necessary only if complicating factors exist (see Box 13-4).

Incision and drainage is often the treatment of choice in an emergency situation. This procedure can be performed by a nondentist using commonly available supplies.[3,19] It is indicated for fluctuant swellings caused by apical abscess and may also be effective for nonfluctuant swelling associated with infection. Infiltration of local anesthetic is unlikely to be successful because of a decreased local pH. Adequate anesthesia can often be obtained by applying cold to the area to be incised. Ethyl chloride, ice, or snow may be used. An incision is made from the point of maximum fluctuance down to bone in one swift movement, and the beaks of a hemostat or a knife handle is used to spread the incision. A T-shaped drain may be improvised from a piece of latex glove (Fig. 13-16); it may be retained without sutures, or a cotton wick can be placed. Hydration, a soft diet, analgesics, and warm saline rinses are helpful adjunct measures.

Dental extractions are considered definitive treatment and should be attempted in the field only under extraordinary circumstances. Extraction requires trained personnel, specialized instruments, and profound anesthesia, which may be difficult to obtain in the wilderness. Premedication with a sedative, a narcotic, or both may be necessary, as may dental radiographs. Intraoperative and postoperative complications are common. Providers of emergency care should focus on treating pain and infection with local anesthetics, analgesics, incision and drainage, and antibiotics as appropriate for each case. Extraction or other definitive care can be rendered after evacuation.

BOX 13-4

INDICATIONS FOR ANTIBIOTIC USE FOR ORAL INFECTIONS

- Prophylaxis for subacute bacterial endocarditis
- Local infections
  - Immunocompromise
  - Inadequate drainage
  - Delay to definitive care
- Disseminated infections
  - Lymphadenopathy
  - Fascial plane involvement
  - Systemic symptoms
- Compound maxillofacial fractures involving tooth-supporting bone
- Exarticulation of teeth
- Soft tissue wounds open for 6 hours or more before definitive care

From Topazian RG, Goldberg MH, editors: *Oral and maxillofacial infections*, ed 2, Philadelphia, 1987, WB Saunders.

Chronic Apical Abscess

The hallmark of chronic apical infection is a draining fistula or "gum boil." Because the bacteria have a route of escape, they do not cause pressure or pain, although the tooth may be mildly sensitive during eating. A gum abscess is not truly an emergency, but if the patient is overly concerned that it may worsen before definitive care is provided, it can be treated with antibiotics.

Periodontal Abscess

A periodontal abscess is a proliferation of bacteria between gingiva and tooth. Swelling is near the gingival margin, rather than in the vestibule. The tooth is sensitive to percussion but responds appropriately to hot and cold. There is always communication between the abscess and the mouth. The passage can be found by probing with a small, blunt instrument. This anaerobic infection is not aggressive and can be treated simply. Under local anesthesia the infection is drained through the gingival sulcus using a blunt instrument; no incision is necessary. Hot saline rinses are prescribed. Quick recovery is almost invariable.

Pericoronitis

Pericoronitis is an infection of the gingival flap around a partially erupted tooth. The most common site is the mandibular third molar. The infection is usually caused by streptococci and seldom produces purulence. The condition may mimic streptococcal pharyngitis or tonsillitis.

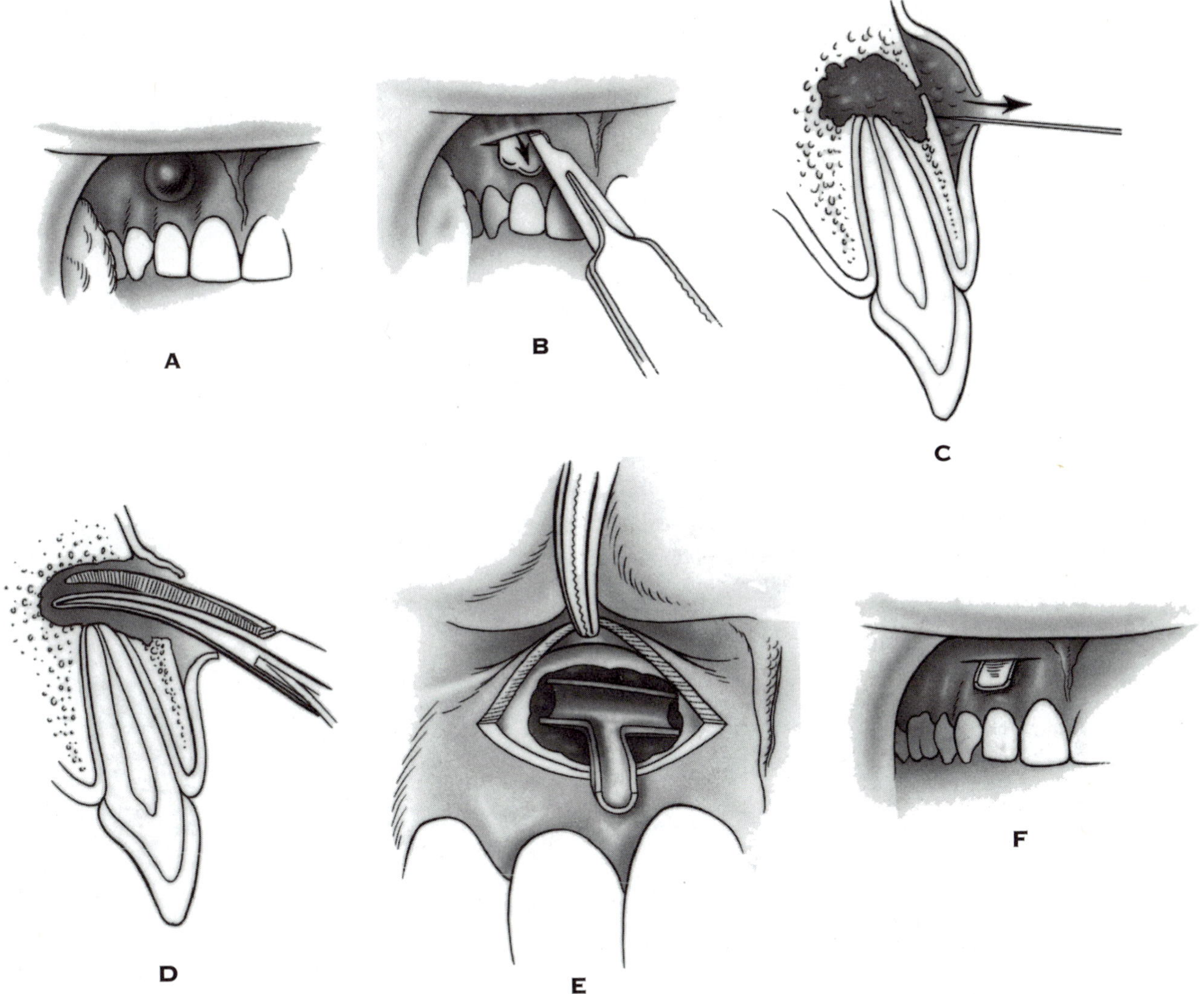

Fig. 13-16 Incision and drainage technique. **A,** Fluctuant abscess. **B,** Abscess incised with scalpel. Purulent drainage removed by suction or caught in gauze sponges. **C,** Cross section showing incision carried to the bone. **D,** The incision is spread with a hemostat. **E,** A T drain will often stay in place without sutures. **F,** Drain in place. (Redrawn from Ingle JI, Beveridge EE: *Endodontics,* ed 2, Philadelphia, 1976, Lea & Febiger.)

The primary site of infection is tender, and trismus is a common sign. Field treatment consists of curettage of the area around the tooth and under the flap. In the absence of proper dental instruments a small, curved hemostat suffices. The space under the flap is irrigated with a syringe, and the patient receives hot saline rinses every 2 hours and antibiotic therapy.

Deep Fascial Space Infections

Acute apical infections occasionally spread beyond the local area. The most commonly involved spaces are the canine, buccal, and masticator spaces and the floor of the mouth.

The canine space is defined by the levator anguli oris muscle, levator labii superioris muscle, and the maxilla. Infection originates in a maxillary canine tooth. Swelling causes the eye to close on the affected side. The infection is drained through an intraoral approach.

The buccal space is bounded by the buccinator muscle, skin of the cheek, zygomatic arch, and angle of the mandible. The offending tooth is a maxillary or mandibular posterior. Drainage is obtained extraorally.

The masticator spaces are divided into the masseteric, pterygoid, superficial temporal, and deep temporal, all of which communicate. The hallmark of involvement is trismus. Swelling may be minimal because of the overlying muscle mass. The masseteric and pterygoid spaces are drained at the angle of the mandible, while the temporal space may be drained from an intraoral approach or through an incision just superior to the zygomatic arch.

The floor of the mouth is bounded by the mentalis muscle, oral mucosa, mandible, hyoid bone, and platysma muscle. The mylohyoid muscle subdivides the space into sublingual and submandibular spaces. These communicate posteriorly and with their counterparts across the midline. Infection originates in a mandibular tooth. If the sublingual space alone is infected, an intraoral approach is used to avoid damage to Wharton's duct. If the submandibular space is involved, an extraoral approach is used. All incisions in the facial area are made parallel to branches of the facial nerve.[23,44]

Fascial space infections are potentially life threatening because they increase the likelihood of sepsis, may cause cavernous sinus venous thrombosis or mediastinitis, and may compromise the airway. The most feared infection is Ludwig's angina, or bilateral submandibular space infection, which elevates the tongue, obstructs breathing, and is associated with a high mortality rate.

Evaluation of severe infection includes serial recording of systemic parameters, a cranial nerve examination, and radiography if available. Trismus denotes involvement of the masticator spaces. Primary or secondary salivary gland involvement is excluded by expression of clear saliva. Treatment includes airway management, fluid and electrolyte management, aggressive incision and drainage, and intravenous antibiotics. Any person with a suspected fascial space infection should be evacuated immediately.

Use of Antibiotics

The indications for antibiotic use in dental conditions are given in Box 13-4. For uncomplicated local infections, drainage is the only treatment needed. Penicillin and erythromycin are the most commonly used antibiotics in dental practice, but broad-spectrum drugs typically carried on wilderness expeditions are acceptable.[18,48] Combination antibiotic therapy is not indicated except for life-threatening sepsis or when organisms particularly sensitive to combination therapy have been identified.[48]

BOX 13-5

CLASSIFICATION OF DENTAL TRAUMA

INJURIES TO THE HARD DENTAL TISSUES AND PULP

Crown infraction
Uncomplicated crown fracture
Complicated crown fracture
Uncomplicated crown-root fracture
Complicated crown-root fracture
Root fracture

INJURIES TO THE PERIODONTAL TISSUES

Concussion
Subluxation
Intrusive luxation
Extrusive luxation
Lateral luxation
Exarticulation

INJURIES TO THE SUPPORTING BONE

Comminution of alveolar socket
Fracture of alveolar socket wall
Fracture of alveolar process
Fracture of jaw

INJURIES TO SOFT TISSUES

Laceration of gingiva or oral mucosa
Contusion of gingiva or oral mucosa

From *International classification of diseases and stomatology,* ed 2, Geneva, 1978, World Health Organization.

DENTAL TRAUMA

A classification of traumatic injuries to the teeth and supporting structures is given in Box 13-5. These injuries often occur in combination, with one tooth exhibiting two or more injuries or with several teeth exhibiting various sequelae of trauma. All traumatic dental injuries require definitive treatment, but proper emergency treatment improves the prognosis and makes the patient more comfortable. Treatment of most injuries requires, or is at least facilitated by, the infiltration of local anesthetic.

History and Examination

In addition to gathering standard historical data, the treatment provider should ask about loss of consciousness, nausea, vomiting, or dizziness. Information about how and when the injury occurred should be elicited, and the patient should be asked about any abnormal cold sensitivity, malocclusion, or previous injury to the area. The region should be cleansed of blood and debris to unmask soft tissue injuries and facilitate diagnosis. Any lacerations should be carefully examined to determine if they penetrate through the lip or contain foreign material.

All the teeth should be examined for fractures. A blow to the chin or whiplash injury may produce fractures of the posterior teeth as the mandible is forcibly closed. Fractured teeth should be examined for pulp exposure. This requires drying the tooth with gauze and observing carefully. Each tooth is percussed with an instrument handle. Tenderness denotes injury to the periodontal ligament. A high, metallic sound indicates ankylosis. Each tooth is tested for abnormal mobility. Electrical pulp vitality testing, dental radiographs, and soft tissue radiographs are obtained if possible.[1,2]

Treatment

Crown Infraction. Blows to the teeth sometimes produce small craze lines in the enamel. These superficial fractures look like tiny surface cracks on an old porcelain dish. The patient should be assured that damage is minimal.

Uncomplicated Crown Fracture. The tooth has been fractured, but no pulp tissue is visible. The tooth may be sensitive to cold, but otherwise all test results are within normal limits. Usually no treatment is necessary. Irritating sharp edges may be smoothed with a fingernail file. If thermal sensitivity is moderate to severe, a soothing topical anti-inflammatory dressing (Intermediate Restorative Material [IRM], L.D. Caulk Co., Milford, Del.) can be held in place with aluminum foil or adhesive tape.[4]

Uncomplicated Crown-Root Fracture. Diagnosis and treatment of an uncomplicated crown-root fracture are identical to those of an uncomplicated crown fracture, except that the fracture is nearly vertical, leaving a small, chisel-shaped fragment attached only by the palatal gingiva (Fig. 13-17). Removal of this mobile fragment makes the patient much more comfortable.

Complicated Crown Fracture. In a complicated crown fracture the pulp has been exposed. A small exposure that has not been grossly contaminated is capped with calcium hydroxide (Dycal, L.D. Caulk Co., Milford, Del.) or IRM. If the exposure is large, or if the pulp tissue has been exposed for more than 24 hours, about 2 mm of tissue should be amputated with a sharp, sterile instrument. If bleeding continues for more than a few minutes, a cotton pellet soaked in anesthetic solution, hydrogen peroxide, or Dycal can be used to obtain hemostasis. The top of the canal is filled with Dycal or IRM, and the tooth is protected as in crown fracture.

Complicated Crown-Root Fracture. The tooth has been fractured obliquely, resulting in a mobile fragment attached to the palatal gingiva as well as a pulp exposure. First the mobile fragment is removed as in crown-root fracture. Then the pulp exposure is treated as in complicated crown fracture.

Root Fracture. Root fracture may be difficult to diagnose without radiographs. There is slight to severe malposition of the crown, but this could be caused by luxation of the entire tooth or root fracture with luxation of the coronal fragment. The tooth should be repositioned as precisely as possible and splinted rigidly. Hard tissue union of the fragments usually occurs within 3 months. If the coronal fragment proves impossible to stabilize and definitive treatment is days away, the mobile fragment should be removed. No attempt should be made to extract the apical fragment.

Concussion and Subluxation. Concussion and subluxation are injuries to the tooth's supporting structures (periodontal ligament, bone, and gingiva) that cause sensitivity to percussion. The tooth remains in its proper position. In subluxation the tooth is abnormally mobile, while in concussion mobility is normal. Emergency treatment consists of shortening the opposing tooth so that the patient may occlude comfortably.

Intrusion. A tooth that has been driven into the bone by

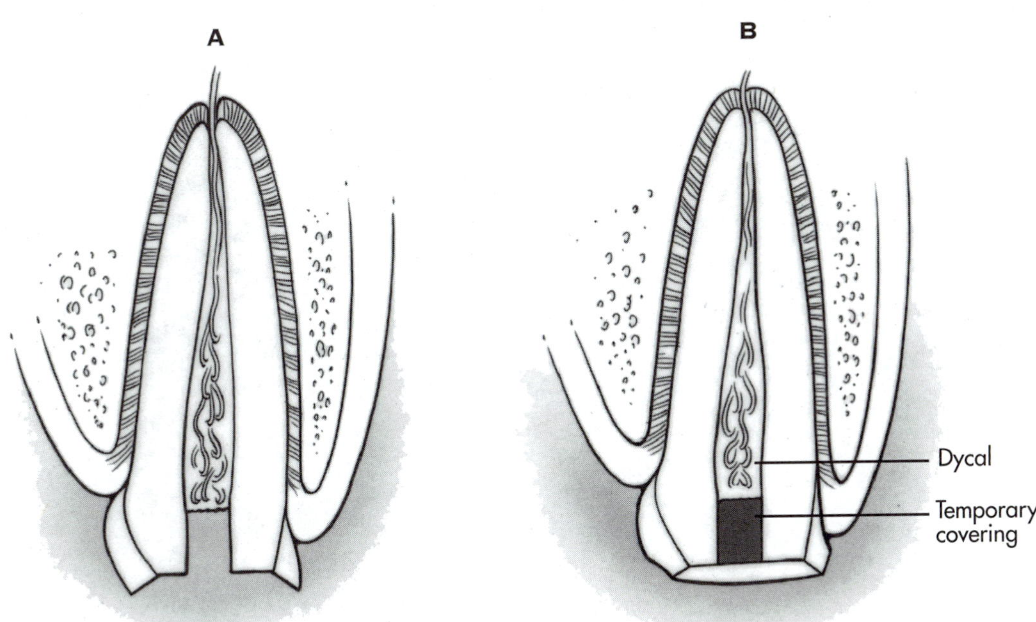

Fig. 13-17 **A,** Uncomplicated crown root fracture. **B,** Treatment for complicated crown root fracture. (Redrawn from Andreasen JO, Andreason FM: *Essentials of traumatic injuries to the teeth,* Copenhagen, 1990, Munksgaard.)

a vertical force demonstrates little mobility and a high, metallic tone on percussion. Emergency treatment is palliative only. Endodontic treatment (to prevent inflammatory root resorption) and orthodontic extrusion should begin within 2 weeks of injury. Intrusion is associated with a poor long-term prognosis.

Extrusion. The extruded tooth is partially displaced from its socket and extremely mobile. Gentle, steady pressure is used to reposition the tooth, allowing time to displace the blood that has collected in the apical region of the socket. In this and other injuries requiring teeth to be reduced, the patient's occlusion is the best guide to proper position. If the patient bites and contacts only the injured tooth, further positioning is necessary. After reduction the tooth is nonrigidly splinted for 2 to 3 weeks.

Lateral Luxation. In lateral luxation the tooth is often displaced by a horizontal blow, yet not mobile because the apex is locked into its new position in the alveolar bone. A high, metallic tone on percussion is another clue that this has occurred. Fig. 13-18 shows how two fingers are used to reduce the tooth. One finger gently guides the apex down and back while the other repositions the crown. The tooth may snap back into position and be quite stable. Splinting is necessary if mobility is present after reduction.

Exarticulation. When a tooth is totally avulsed from bone, the prognosis after replantation depends on the health of the periodontal ligament cells, some of which are still attached to the root surface and some of which line the socket wall. To preserve the vitality of these cells, the time before replantation should be kept to a minimum. If the tooth must be stored, it should be placed in tissue culture medium, physiologic saline, milk, or saliva, in that order of preference. The tooth should be handled only by the crown. The root surface should never be scrubbed, curetted, or treated with disinfectants. It should be gently rinsed with saline solution to remove debris. Clotted blood should be removed from the socket by the use of gentle irrigation and suction; the socket walls should not be scraped. The tooth should be eased back into place with slow, steady pressure. After replantation the tooth is nonrigidly splinted for 1 week, and antibiotic therapy and antitetanus prophylaxis are begun. Endodontic therapy should be instituted within 2 weeks.[1,2,37]

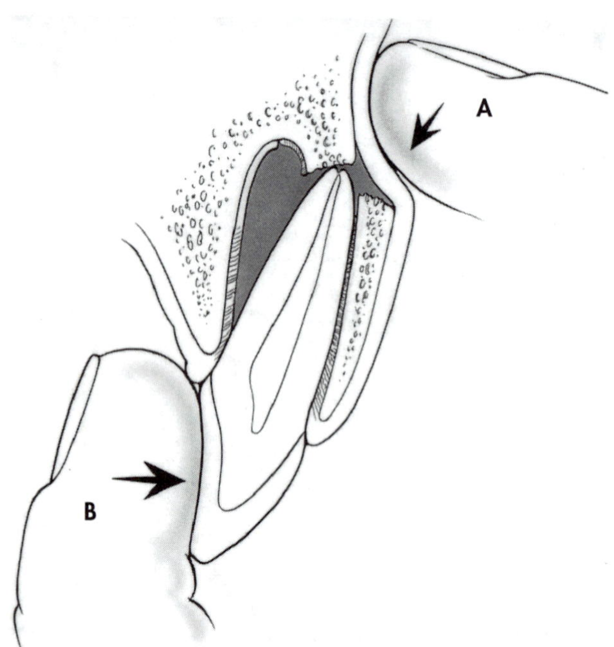

Fig. 13-18 Reduction of lateral luxation. (Redrawn from Andreasen JO, Andreason FM: *Essentials of traumatic injuries to the teeth,* Copenhagen, 1990, Munksgaard.)

The preferred approach to avulsion or severe luxation is immediate reduction in the field, followed by evacuation for definitive treatment. The next most desirable option is to store the tooth properly and to transport patient and tooth for replantation within a few hours of injury. If field conditions prevent either course of action, a delayed replantation procedure is indicated. The tooth should be stored dry. Three weeks after the injury the necrotic pulp tissue is removed and the tooth is disinfected, fluoridated, and surgically replanted. Delayed replantation aims to produce ankylosis between tooth and bone.[2]

Alveolar Segment Fracture. Alveolar segment fracture is characterized by displacement of two or more teeth as a unit. The teeth are not mobile with respect to one another. The apices may be locked into their abnormal position as in lateral luxation. The segment is repositioned (this may be painful even with local anesthesia). Rigid splinting is placed for 4 to 6 weeks.

Splinting. When the goal of splinting is a normal, fibrous union between tooth and bone, a short-term, nonrigid technique is used. When hard tissue union is desired (for example, root fracture or alveolar segment fracture), longer term rigid splinting is used. For fractures of the jaws or alveolar segments, arch bar and wire splints are often used. This technique is contraindicated for stabilizing individual teeth because as the wires are tightened, the mobile tooth is extruded. Bonding to adjacent teeth using acid-etched composite is the treatment of choice.[2,36]

The rescuer lacking adequate materials must use ingenuity and improvisation in splinting teeth. Fig. 13-19 shows how a suture can be used to hold a tooth in place. A crude

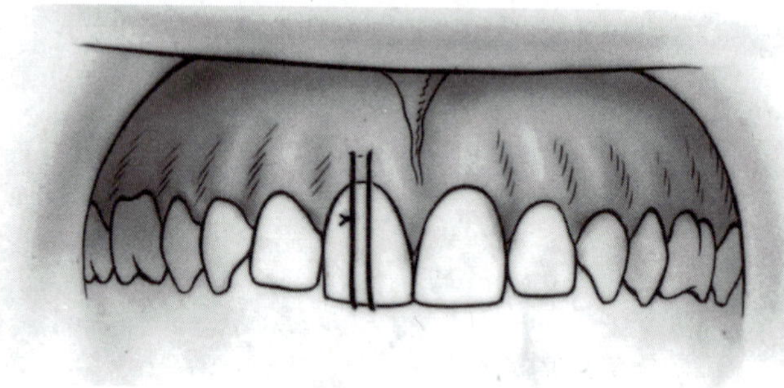

Fig. 13-19 Suture used to stabilize a loosened or avulsed tooth.

arch bar can be cut from a SAM splint and dead-soft wire obtained from copper wiring or twist ties.

Injuries to Primary Teeth. Injuries to the deciduous teeth offer unique challenges, not the least of which is behavior management of a young child. Splinting is very difficult because of the small amount of tooth structure available. In general, heroic efforts should not be made to save primary teeth. Exarticulated deciduous teeth should not be replanted. Severely extruded teeth, infected teeth, or those intruded into the developing permanent tooth should be extracted. Because the permanent tooth follicle lies to the lingual side of the primary root, the typical frontal impact displaces the crown palatally but levers the root apex away from the permanent tooth (Fig. 13-20). Most minor subluxations and luxations require only symptomatic treatment. As long as the displaced tooth does not interfere with occlusion, reduction is contraindicated. Spontaneous repositioning often occurs over a period of weeks. Fragments of primary roots need not be extracted because normal resorption will occur.[1,2]

SOFT TISSUE INJURIES

Wounds of the oral mucosa and face should be treated after repair of hard tissue injuries. Lacerations are likely to be reopened if closed before intraoral manipulations. Soft tissue injuries should be thoroughly irrigated and cleansed of foreign debris. The excellent blood supply to this region means that wounds may be closed with sutures or wound closures with little fear of infection, as long as treatment can be accomplished within 6 hours of injury.

Through and through lacerations, which are common in the lower lip, are treated as follows: the mucosa is closed from an intraoral approach, the surgeon rescrubs and obtains sterile instruments, and the wound is irrigated and is closed in layers from an extraoral approach. Lacerations crossing the vermilion border of the lip require careful alignment to avoid future disfigurement.

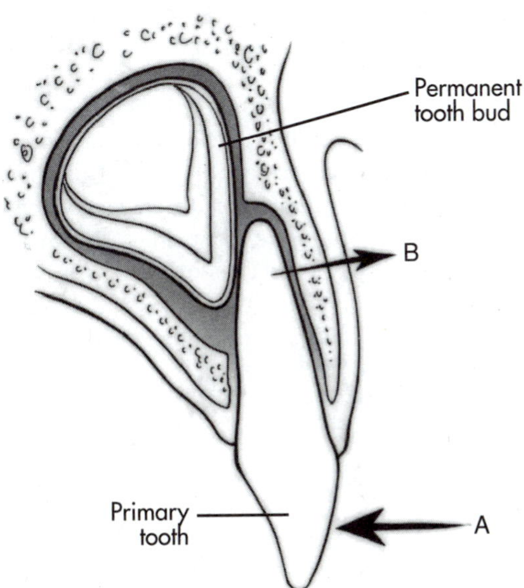

Fig. 13-20 Trauma to a deciduous tooth. *A,* Direction of typical force as the child falls forward. *B,* Apex of deciduous tooth is levered away from the developing permanent tooth.

LOCAL ANESTHESIA

Local anesthesia is a prerequisite to many emergency dental procedures. A knowledge of nerve block techniques is often needed for fracture reduction, pain relief in areas of infection, and many procedures involving mandibular teeth. However, anesthesia in many less complicated cases can be obtained by infiltration. About 2 ml of local anesthetic solution is placed as close to the apex of the tooth as possible, just above the periosteum of the buccal cortical plate. Holding the syringe parallel to the long axis of the tooth ensures that the needle tip is guided in the proper direction (Fig. 13-21). Lidocaine 2% with 1:100,000 epinephrine is commonly used, although 2% bupivicaine with 1:200,000 epinephrine is useful for long-term pain relief. Other local anesthetics could be substituted.[28]

DENTAL FIRST AID KIT

Items necessary to manage dental emergencies can be added to a wilderness first aid kit without a large sacrifice of space or weight.

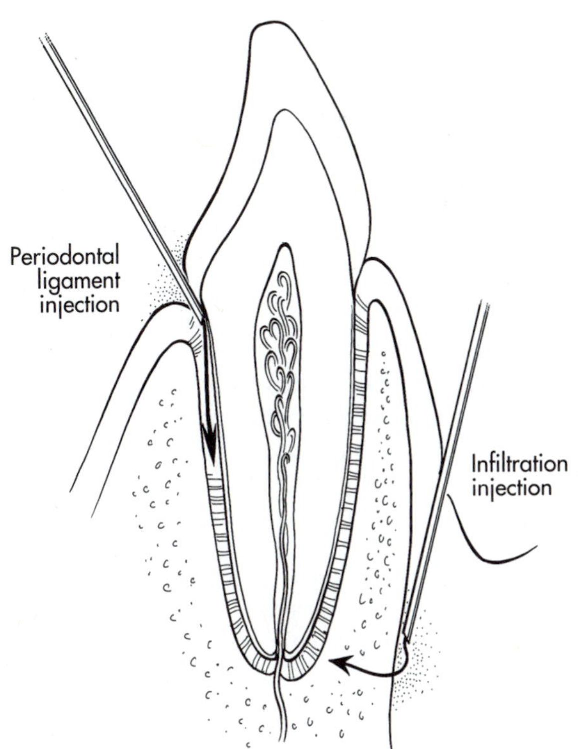

Fig. 13-21 Position of the needle for infiltration of local anesthetic.

Cavit (Premier Co., Norristown, Penn.) is temporary filling material that requires no mixing and is easy to use. The treatment provider squeezes a small amount of material from the tube and places it in the tooth. A dental packing instrument (or cotton tip applicator or toothpick) is wetted to prevent sticking. The Cavit is packed well, and any excess is removed. The patient bites down to displace material that would interfere with occlusion. The filling sets a few minutes after contact with saliva.

Zinc oxide–eugenol cements (Intermediate Restorative Material [IRM], L.D. Caulk Co., Milford, Del.) consist of a liquid and a powder. Mixing begins with the addition of powder to a few drops of the liquid component. Keep adding powder to make a dough that is as dry as possible. More powder is used on instruments to keep the mixture from sticking. The material is inserted and shaped as explained previously. Zinz oxide–eugenol cements have several advantages over Cavit. Most important is the soothing effect of eugenol on teeth with pulpitis. Zinc oxide–eugenol mixtures are significantly stronger than Cavit and can be mixed to a doughy stage for filling or less thickly for use as a cement. However, the liquid tends to leak from its container and lend a pervasive odor to backpack and tent, and the cements are difficult to mix and a sticky mess to insert into the tooth.

Barbed broaches are tiny instruments used to remove vital pulp tissue. Profound anesthesia is necessary. Anesthetic solution may be injected directly into the pulp as a last resort. A broach is inserted into the canal as far as possible without binding against the canal walls. The broach is turned clockwise 10 turns and then removed with the attached pulpal tissue.

A more complete kit for extended expeditions would include a 151 Universal extraction forceps and straight elevator for extracting teeth. Bite registration putty (Express, 3M Co., St. Paul, Minn.) can be used to fabricate temporary crowns and semirigid splints. With clean, dry hands (not letting powder from latex gloves contaminate the putty) the treatment provider kneads together equal amounts of components A and B. The material is molded into the desired shape, and any excess is trimmed with a sharp knife or scissors after 4 minutes' setting time. A mouth mirror, syringe, 30-gauge needles, and anesthetic carpules complete the kit. These items fit in a small case that weighs 14 ounces. A custom dental first aid kit is preferred over commercial dental "travel kits," which contain unnecessary items and lack essentials.

In an outdoor situation, techniques must often be adapted or improvised depending on the items available. For example, Fig. 13-19 shows how a suture can be used to splint an avulsed or extruded tooth. A temporary filling can be fashioned from softened candle wax, a hickory twig can be chewed to form a makeshift toothbrush, and a Swiss Army knife can be used to perform a drainage procedure.

PREVENTION

The vast majority of dental emergencies can be prevented. Lip balm with sunscreen can inhibit herpes labialis outbreaks. Routine professional care and good personal oral hygiene prevent many odontogenic infections and painful, inflammatory conditions. Before any extended travel in remote areas, thorough examination, radiographs, periodontal care, and treatment of troublesome teeth are advised.

In the wilderness, daily oral hygiene not only helps prevent dental emergencies but also contributes to an overall sense of well-being and buoys morale in difficult circumstances, as when an expedition is tent bound by bad weather. Toothpaste is not essential, since mechanical removal of plaque and stimulation of the gingiva are the most important aspects of oral care.

Acute Abdomen

In the wilderness environment the critical distinction between the surgical and nonsurgical abdomen determines whether the patient should be evacuated. Pain, anorexia, nausea, vomiting, and fever are characteristic manifestations of an acute abdominal disorder. Tenderness and guarding suggest that surgery is needed.

The approach to the patient with abdominal pain begins with a detailed history, which includes the person's age, sex, systemic symptoms, and past medical history. This information provides a framework for more detailed questioning about the character of the pain, including mode of onset, severity, and precipitating and palliating factors.

In persons 15 to 40 years of age, females are more likely to have abdominal pain, but males have a higher incidence of surgical disease. Common genitourinary causes for abdominal pain in men include epididymitis and testicular torsion. Common causes in women include pelvic inflammatory disease, urinary tract infection, dysmenorrhea, and ectopic pregnancy.

Pain is the hallmark of the surgical abdomen (Table 13-2). It can be characterized by mode of onset, severity, localization, and precipitating factors. The onset of abdominal pain can be explosive, rapid, or gradual. The patient who is suddenly seized with explosive, agonizing pain is most likely to have rupture of a hollow viscus into the free peritoneal cavity. Colic of renal or biliary origin may also be sudden in onset but seldom causes pain severe enough to prostrate the patient. If the patient has rapid onset of pain that quickly worsens, acute pancreatitis, mesenteric thrombosis, or small bowel strangulation should be suspected. The patient with gradual onset of pain is likely to have peritoneal inflammation, such as that accompanying appendicitis or diverticulitis.

The severity of the pain may be characterized as excruciating, severe, dull, or colicky. Excruciating pain unresponsive to narcotics suggests an acute vascular lesion, such as rupture of an abdominal aneurysm or intestinal infarction. Both conditions are unusual in the wilderness environment.

Table 13-2 Differential Diagnostic Features of Abdominal Pain

Disease	Location of Pain and Prior Attacks	Mode of Onset and Type of Pain	Associated Gastrointestinal Symptoms	Physical Examination
Acute appendicitis	Periumbical or localized generally to right lower abdominal quadrant	Insidious to acute and persistent	Anorexia common; nausea and vomiting in some	Low-grade fever; epigastric tenderness initially; later, right lower quadrant
Intestinal obstruction	Diffuse	Sudden onset; crampy	Vomiting common	Abdominal distention; high-pitched rushes
Perforated duodenal ulcer	Epigastric; history of ulcer in many	Abrupt onset; steady	Anorexia; nausea and vomiting	Epigastric tenderness; involuntary guarding
Diverticulitis	Left lower quadrant; history of previous attacks	Gradual onset; steady or crampy	Diarrhea common	Fever common; mass and tenderness in left lower quadrant
Acute cholecystitis	Epigastric or right upper quadrant; may be referred to right shoulder	Insidious to acute	Anorexia; nausea and vomiting	Right upper quadrant pain
Renal colic	Costovertebral or along course of ureter	Sudden; severe and sharp	Frequently nausea and vomiting	Flank tenderness
Acute pancreatitis	Epigastric penetrating to back	Acute; persistent, dull, severe	Anorexia; nausea and vomiting common	Epigastric tenderness
Acute salpingitis	Bilateral adnexal; later, may be generalized	Gradually becomes worse	Nausea and vomiting may be present	Cervical motion elicits tenderness; mass if tuboovarian abscess is present
Ectopic pregnancy	Unilateral early; may have shoulder pain after rupture	Sudden or intermittently vague to sharp	Frequently none	Adnexal mass; tenderness

Severe pain readily controlled by medication is characteristic of peritonitis from a ruptured viscus or acute pancreatitis. Dull, vague, poorly localized pain suggests an inflammatory process and is a common initial presentation of appendicitis. Colicky pain characterized as cramps and rushes is suggestive of gastroenteritis. The pain from mechanical small bowel obstruction is also colicky but has a rhythmic pattern, with pain-free intervals alternating with severe colic. Peristaltic rushes may be heard during the severe colic. The peristaltic rushes associated with gastroenteritis are not necessarily coordinated with the colicky pain.

APPENDICITIS

Acute appendicitis is the most common cause of a surgical abdomen in patients under the age of 30 years. Acute appendicitis is really more than one single disease entity. In terms of physical signs and symptoms, appendicitis proceeds from inflammation to obstruction to ischemia to perforation, all within approximately 36 hours. The patient's symptoms reflect the stage of the disease. Unfortunately, the time frame for the progression of these clinical events is highly variable.

Differential diagnosis of appendicitis includes gastroenteritis and mesenteric adenitis, the most common inflammatory disorders in adults. The first symptom of gastroenteritis is typically vomiting, which precedes the onset of pain and is often associated with diarrhea; it is rarely associated with localizing signs or muscular spasm. Bowel sounds are usually hyperactive. A rectal examination rarely shows abnormalities in gastroenteritis but frequently does so in adults with appendicitis. Mesenteric adenitis is often preceded by an upper respiratory tract infection and is associated with vague abdominal discomfort that often begins in the right lower quadrant. Abdominal examination reveals only mild right lower quadrant tenderness that is often not well localized.

The incidence of pelvic inflammatory disease in young women with abdominal pain confounds the diagnosis of appendicitis. Lewis and associates[24] found that if the onset of abdominal pain occurred within 7 days of menses, the incidence of pelvic inflammatory disease was twice that of appendicitis. However, if the menstrual period began 8 or more days before the onset of abdominal pain, appendicitis was twice as likely as pelvic inflammatory disease. This one piece of history coupled with a careful pelvic examination can help delineate the diagnosis in female patients.

Once the diagnosis of a surgical abdomen is made, evacuation is mandated. If appendicitis is suspected, the patient may be able to participate in the evacuation. If the evacuation time is over 12 hours, broad-spectrum antibiotics (cefoxitin, adult dose 2 g intramuscularly) should be administered. Hydration should be maintained and pain medication administered as needed.

REFERENCES

1. Andreasen JO: *Traumatic injuries to the teeth,* ed 2, Philadelphia, 1981, WB Saunders.
3. Antrium DD: Dental emergency: incision and drainage technique for non-dental personnel, *US Navy Med* 75(1):20, 1984.
4. Antrium DD: Treatment of traumatic dental injuries by non-dental personnel, *US Navy Med* 74(3):18, 1983.
5. Bohlman HH, Ducker TB, Lucas JT: *Spine and spinal cord injuries in the spine,* Philadelphia, 1982, WB Saunders.
6. Christiansen G: Kit for temporary treatment of dental emergencies by laymen found useful, *Clin Res Assoc Newslett* 11(2):4, 1987.
7. Committee on Rheumatic Fever and Infective Carditis of the Council on Cardiovascular Disease in the Young: Prevention of bacterial endocarditis: a statement for health professionals, *Circulation* 70:1123a, 1987.
8. DeGowin EL, DeGowin RL: *Bedside diagnostic examination,* ed 4, New York, 1981, Macmillan.
9. Dhaani AS et al: Prevention of bacterial endocarditis: recommendations of the American Heart Association, *JAMA* 264(22):2919, 1990.
10. Ellis E, Moos KF, El-Attar AS: Ten years of mandibular fractures: an analysis of 2,137 cases, *Oral Surg* 59:129, 1985.
11. Finkle DR et al: Comparison of diagnostic methods used in maxillofacial trauma, *Plast Reconstruct Surg* 75:32, 1985.
12. Frame JW, Wake MJS: Evaluation of maxillofacial injuries by use of computerized tomography, *J Oral Maxillofac Surg* 40:482, 1982.
13. Fricton JR et al: Myofascial pain syndrome of the head and neck: a review of clinical characteristics of 164 patients, *Oral Surg* 60:623, 1985.
14. Griffee MB et al: *Bacteroides melaninogenicus* and dental infections: some questions and answers, *Oral Surg* 54(4):486, 1982.
15. Hall HD et al: Effect of time of extraction on resolution of odontogenic cellulitis, *J Am Dent Assoc* 77:626, 1968.
16. Heintz WD: The case for mandatory mouth protectors, *Sports Med* 3:61, 1975.
17. Hovelius L et al: Recurrences after initial dislocation of the shoulder: results of a prospective study of treatment, *J Bone Joint Surg* 65A:343, 1983.
18. Hurt DE, King TJ, Fuler GE: Antibiotic susceptibility of bacteria isolated from oral infections, *J Oral Surg* 36:527, 1978.
19. Ingle JI, Beveridge EE: *Endodontics,* Philadelphia, 1976, Lea & Febiger.
20. Kennedy JC: Complete dislocation of the knee joint, *J Bone Joint Surg* 45A:889, 1963.
21. Kerr DA, Ash MM, Millard HD: *Oral diagnosis,* ed 6, St Louis, 1983, Mosby.
22. Kruger E, Schilli W: *Oral and maxillofacial traumatology,* Chicago, 1982, Quintessence.
23. Laskin D: Anatomic considerations in diagnosis and treatment of odontogenic infections, *J Am Dent Assoc* 69:308, 1964.
24. Lewis FR et al: Appendicitis: a critical review of diagnosis and treatment in 1,000 cases, *Arch Surg* 110:677, 1975.
25. Lewis VL et al: Facial injuries associated with cervical fractures: recognition of patterns and management, *J Trauma* 25:90, 1985.
26. Lister G: *The hand: diagnosis and indications,* Edinburgh, 1984, Churchill Livingstone.
27. Luyk NH, Ferguson JW: The diagnosis and initial management of the fractured mandible, *Am J Emerg Med* 9:352, 1991.
28. Malamed SF: *Handbook of local anesthesia,* ed 2, St Louis, 1986, Mosby.
29. Manson PN: Maxillofacial injuries, *Emerg Med Clin North Am* 2:761, 1984.
30. Manson PN et al: Toward CT-based facial fracture treatment, *Plast Reconstruct Surg* 85:202, 1990.
31. Masters SL et al: Skull x-ray examinations after head trauma: recommendations by a multidisciplinary panel and validation study, *N Engl J Med* 316(2):84, 1987.
32. Matsen FA III: *Compartmental syndromes,* New York, 1980, Grune & Stratton.
33. Matsen FA, Winquist RA, Krugmire RB: Diagnosis and management of compartment syndromes, *J Bone Joint Surg* 62A:286, 1980.
34. Mills J, Ho MT, Trunkey DD: *Current emergency diagnosis and treatment,* Los Altos, Calif, 1983, Lange.
35. Nance FC et al: Surgical judgment in the management of penetrating wounds of the abdomen: experience with 2,212 patients, *Ann Surg* 193:639, 1931.
36. Oikarinen K: Tooth splinting: a review of the literature and consideration of the versatility of a wire composite splint, *Endodont Dent Traumatol* 6:237, 1990.
37. *Oral and maxillofacial surgery services in the emergency department,* Rosemont, Ill, 1992, American Association of Oral and Maxillofacial Surgeons.
38. Pennal GF et al: Pelvic disruption: assessment and classification, *Clin Orthop* 157:12, 1980.
39. Sabiston CB, Grigsby WR, Seggerstrom N: Bacterial study of pyogenic infections of dental origin, *Oral Surg* 41:430, 1976.
40. Schatzker J, Barrington TW: Fractures of the femoral neck associated with fractures of the same femoral shaft, *Can J Surg* 11:297, 1968.
41. Schneider RC, Kahn EA: Chronic neurologic sequelae of acute trauma of the spine and spinal cord. I. The significance of the acute flexion or "teardrop" fracture—dislocation of the cervical spine, *J Bone Joint Surg* 38A:985, 1956.
42. Scully C, Porter SR: Recurrent aphthous stomatitis: current concepts of etiology, pathogenesis and management, *J Oral Pathol Med* 18:21, 1989.
43. Shafer WG, Hine MK, Levy BM: *A textbook of oral pathology,* ed 4, Philadelphia, 1983, WB Saunders.
44. Shapiro AH, Sleeper E, Turalnick W: Spread of infection of dental origin: anatomical and surgical considerations, *Oral Surg* 3:1407, 1950.
45. Slatis P, Huittinen VM: Double vertical fractures of the pelvis: a report on 163 patients, *Acta Chir Scand* 138:799, 1972.
46. Swiontkowski MF, Winquist RA, Hansen ST: Fractures of the femoral neck in patients between the ages of twelve and forty-nine years, *J Bone Joint Surg* 66A:837, 1984.
47. Tile M: *Fractures of the pelvis and acetabulum,* Baltimore, 1984, Williams & Wilkins.
48. Topazian RG, Goldberg MH: *Oral and maxillofacial infections,* Philadelphia, 1987, WB Saunders.

14 HUNTING INJURIES

Edward J. Otten

Even as Nimrod the mighty hunter before the Lord.

Genesis 10:9

Anthropologists have many theories concerning the origins and importance of hunting in the evolution of the human species. The physical attributes of bipedal locomotion, binocular vision, and an opposable thumb all make humans more efficient hunters. Whether these exist because humans have an innate compulsion to hunt or whether humans are hunters because of these traits is debatable. There is no debate, however, that human social evolution, language, the use of tools, and domestication of animals are directly related to more efficient hunting. In a survival situation, and in some ways with regard to evolution, hunter-gatherer animals have a distinct advantage over strictly vegetarian animals because of the relative food value of meat over plants. Hunters tend to be males. Approximately three fourths of all calories in modern hunter-gatherer groups are derived from plants, and this portion of the food is usually supplied by the women in the group. Even in Eskimo tribes where plants make up little of the diet, the women do most of the fishing while the men hunt.

Hominids were at a disadvantage, even in groups, when hunting large animals or driving off other predators from their kills until they began using stones, long bones, and sticks to enhance their relatively weak teeth and claws. Implements for hunting and skinning animals were the earliest tools found by anthropologists. Human cultural evolution followed closely the technologic changes in weapons, although sports, business, and war had replaced the need for hunting in most cultures even by the time Nimrod walked the earth. Bows and arrows, slings, spear throwers, nets, harpoons, traps, and firearms were designed to extend the reach and increase the lethality of the human hand. Unfortunately, humans discovered that they could kill each other with these weapons. Since the discovery of gunpowder, the development of weapons technology has surpassed all other forms of human endeavor, including medicine and transportation.[4,5]

Hunting in the United States

Only a few cultures still depend on hunting as their primary food-gathering method. Examples are the Mbuti tribe, Andaman Islanders, and Eskimos. Many cultures, however, use hunting to supplement agriculture, plant gathering, or raising livestock. Most hunting in the United States is done for sport or pleasure, although in some areas of the country hunting and trapping are still the primary source of income for a few people. The total number of hunters and trappers is unknown. Many participate illegally and are not licensed. Throughout the United States 30 million hunting licenses were sold in 1988. Although hunting seasons are regulated and relatively short, hunters spent 16 million visitor-days in the national forests.

The North American Association of Hunter Safety Coordinators, a division of the New York State Office of Wildlife Management, reported 860 fatal hunting injuries during the 4-year period 1983-1986, with a total of 6992 injuries from firearms. Interestingly, 34% of the total injuries and 89% of the handgun injuries were self-inflicted. Shotguns accounted for 106 of the fatalities and 906 of the total injuries, while rifles accounted for 79 fatalities and 465 injuries. Hunting injuries are only a small portion of the total number of unintentional firearm deaths in the United States. Of 131 firearm deaths in California from 1977 to 1983, only eight were the result of hunting accidents.[6,7,14,18,24,28] Hunting injury data may be inaccurate for a number of reasons. Many minor nonfatal injuries may go unreported, and most states do not differentiate accidental firearm hunting deaths from deaths that occur during any other activity. Also, automobile and all terrain vehicle accidents that occur while hunting, or gunshot wounds inflicted while "cleaning a gun" at home, could be considered nonhunting injuries.

TYPES OF INJURY ENCOUNTERED

Most injuries to hunters are the same types of injury seen in backpackers, fishermen, and climbers. Frostbite, sprains,

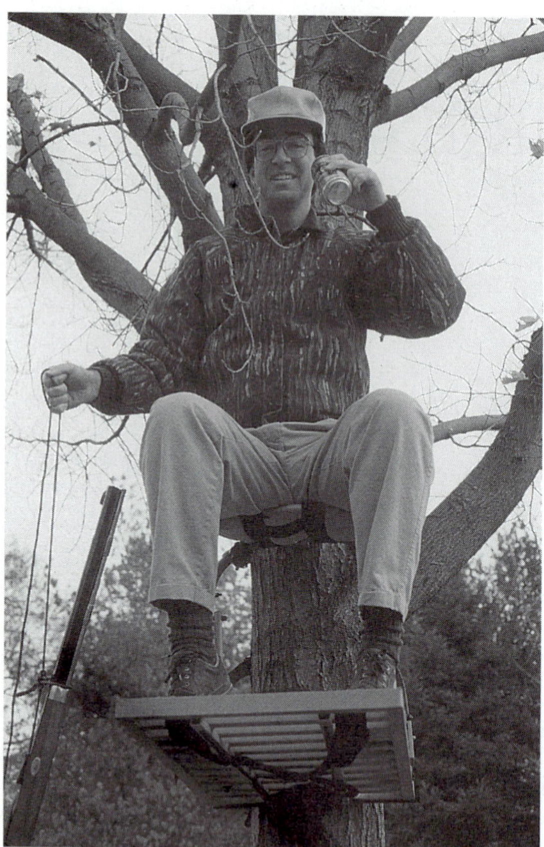

Fig. 14-1 The wrong way to use a tree stand. This hunter is not wearing a safety harness, is drinking alcohol, and is pulling his firearm into the tree stand with the muzzle pointing upward.

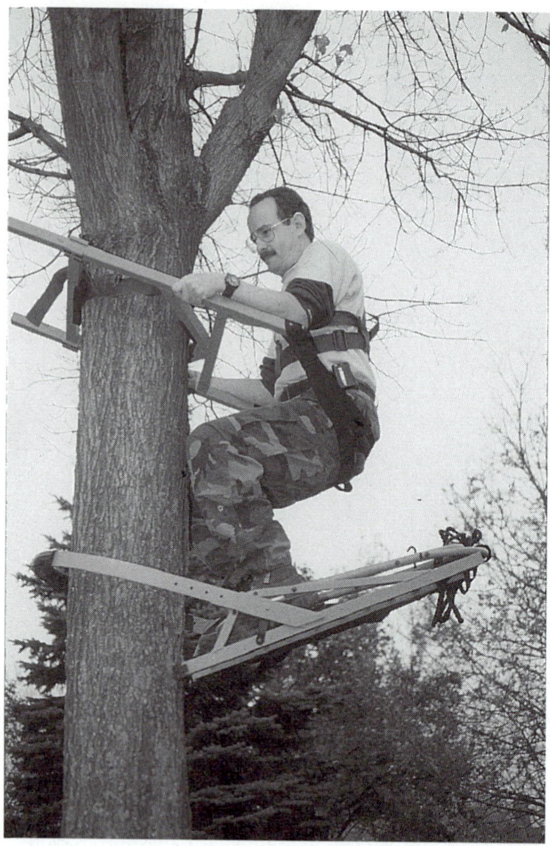

Fig. 14-2 A commercially produced tree stand that can be used to climb the tree and that obviates the need for a ladder or steps, which are the cause of many falls.

burns, and fractures occur with the same frequency in hunters as in others who visit wilderness areas.

A common type of injury in hunters that is not associated with weapons is the tree stand injury. Tree stands are platforms designed to hold hunters several feet off the ground so they can more easily kill large game. Whether homemade or of commercial design, the platforms generally are small and attached to the trunks of trees, with some method, usually a ladder or steps, for climbing the tree (Figs. 14-1 and 14-2). Hunters often fall asleep in the platforms and fall off, or fall while climbing up or down trees. At least half of these injuries could be prevented if all hunters wore tree stand safety harnesses. While most of the injuries are similar to those seen with any type of fall, occasionally a hunter drops a firearm, which discharges, or falls on an arrow or rifle, causing an additional weapons injury (Fig. 14-3). Over 10 years, injuries of this type in Georgia accounted for 36% of reported hunting injuries and 20% of hunting fatalities.[23,25]

Injuries that are unique to hunters are those caused by their weapons. Most hunting is done with firearms. Shotguns and rifles are more commonly used, although handguns are increasing in popularity. Other types of weapon include the bow or crossbow and arrow. These are popular because an extended hunting season is allowed in several states if this type of "primitive" weapon is used. The rationale is that these weapons are less dangerous to innocent bystanders at long range compared with rifles and shotguns and that more skill is needed to hunt with this type of weapon.

Other weapons are used for hunting but are less likely to be encountered. For example, spears, harpoons, and nets are used by some hunters in the Arctic, Australia, and Africa. Trap injuries may be included in the definition of hunting injuries. Most traps are designed to catch and hold small game. Injuries usually occur when a trapper triggers a spring-loaded trap prematurely. Crush injuries and puncture wounds to the hands are most common. Hikers occasionally tread on unmarked traps, and domestic animals such as dogs are accidentally caught in poachers' traps. Another problem with traps occurs when an animal (wild or domestic) is caught in a trap and attacks the trapper while being released. Many knife lacerations occur when hunters clean game. Lack of familiarity with the process or techniques for field dressing and cleaning game is the likely cause. Failing to wear protective gloves, using the wrong type of knife, working with bloody, slippery material, and having cold hands all contribute to accidents.

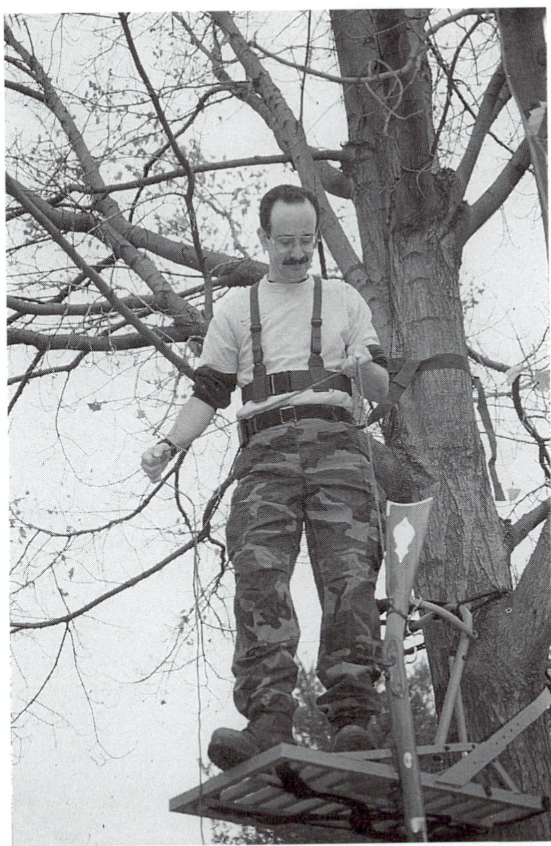

Fig. 14-3 The correct way to bring a firearm into the tree stand, with the muzzle pointing down and the hunter wearing a safety harness at all times.

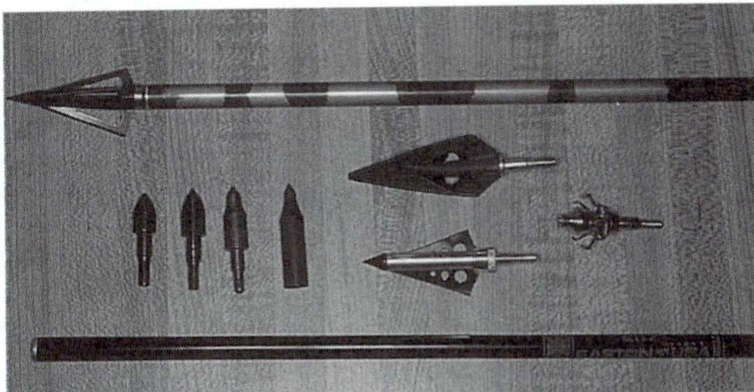

Fig. 14-4 Types of arrows. *Top,* Aluminum shaft arrow with hunting broadhead. *Middle (left to right),* Four field points of various weights: two types of broadheads and small game blunt hunting head with spring claws to prevent arrow loss from burrowing to ground. *Bottom,* Fiberglass shaft for interchangeable heads.

Arrow Injuries

Modern arrows are usually made from aluminum, graphite, or fiberglass, although many beginners still use inexpensive wooden arrows. A number of types of arrowhead are in use, such as field points and target points, but most injuries are due to broadheads. These come in a variety of sizes and shapes and are designed to inflict injury by lacerating tissue and blood vessels, thereby causing bleeding and shock. Unlike firearms, which are designed to kill quickly by tearing tissue and transferring large amounts of energy, arrows usually kill more slowly with less tissue damage (Fig. 14-4).[3,13] Arrows are propelled by a conventional bow, which may be straight, recurve, or compound, or by a crossbow. The force used to propel the arrow is usually measured in "draw weight," which is the number of foot-pounds necessary to draw a 28-inch arrow to its full length. The higher the pound draw, the more powerful the bow and the deeper the penetration the same type of arrow will have. Arrows have a much shorter range than bullets and must be more accurately placed to kill the animal quickly; therefore most shots are taken under 50 m. Because brush and tree branches can easily deflect an arrow, most shots are taken with a clear field of view. For these reasons target identification is usually not a problem and a bow hunter is less likely to shoot another hunter. Most arrow injuries occur when hunters fire illegally at night in heavy brush and are not sure of their target. Another common injury occurs when a hunter runs after a wounded animal and falls on an arrow that was to be used for a second shot or falls out of a tree stand onto an arrow. A loaded crossbow is similar to a loaded gun. Hunters have been accidentally shot when dropping the weapon or snagging the trigger on a branch or fence. Hunting arrowheads are quite sharp; injuries commonly occur when a hunter is sharpening the blade of the arrow or returning an arrow to the quiver.

Injuries from Firearms

Firearms discharge a projectile by using air, modern fast-burning powders, or old-fashioned black powder. Air guns use a spring or carbon dioxide cartridge to push the projectile from the barrel. While air guns are quite accurate at short distances, the projectiles cannot usually penetrate skin from distances greater than 100 m. Air guns are commonly used by children, who cannot legally obtain or use other types of firearms. Well-meaning parents buy them as toys, erroneously believing them to be safe. The wounds they cause can be lethal, especially from the spring-propelled guns, which can send out lead pellets at sufficiently high velocities to penetrate bone. Black powder weapons use a solid propellant that is ignited with a spark from flint striking steel or a percussion cap. When ignited, the propellant is rapidly converted to a gas that expands and pushes a lead ball out of the barrel of the weapon. These weapons are quite accurate and are used to hunt large game such as deer and elk. The injuries from black powder weapons are similar to those from modern weapons and are discussed below. The same precautions should be used when hunting with or shooting any type of firearm, whether the propellant is air or gunpowder.[15,17,27]

The powder (propellant) in weapons that use modern gunpowder is encased in a brass or aluminum shell for rifles and handguns and in a plastic or paper shell for shotguns.

Shells are open on one end for the actual projectiles to be inserted, and in the case of shotgun shells, plastic or cotton wadding is used to keep the projectiles from moving around inside the shells. The powder is detonated from the opposite end by an explosive primer that is in either the rim of the shell, as with the .22 caliber long rifle cartridge, or the middle of the shell, as with the 12-gauge shotgun shell or 30/30 rifle cartridge. Detonation occurs when the firing pin on the weapon strikes the primer, igniting the powder. Upon detonation the powder produces a rapidly expanding gas that pushes the projectile (and wadding) out of the barrel of the weapon. Not all of the powder is burned, so that in case of close proximity wounds, powder stippling may appear on clothing or skin. With contact wounds the escaping gases may cause bursting of the skin and a stellate laceration near the point of entrance. The projectile may vary in size and shape from 1 mm in circumference and a few milligrams in weight to 2 cm in circumference and 100 g in weight. The projectiles are usually made of lead or steel and may be covered with a copper jacket. They are usually single when shot from a rifle or pistol and multiple when fired from a shotgun, although some hunters prefer large single (deer slug) rounds fired from shotguns.

Hundreds of types of bullets or rounds are available for firearms. They may be factory loaded or hand loaded, which adds the variables of propellant amount and type. Small arms are classified according to caliber, which is expressed in fractions of an inch; for example, .22 caliber means the diameter of the bullet is 0.22 inch; .45 caliber is 0.45 inch; and so forth. The caliber may be expressed in metric measurement; for example a 9 mm bullet is 9 mm in diameter, which also happens to be 0.357 inch. This system can be made more complicated when considering the amount of powder used, the year the bullet was adopted, or the name of the person who first introduced the round. Examples of these types are .45/70 (70 grains of powder), .30-06 (adopted in 1906), and .35 Whelen (the man who developed the round). Shotgun terminology is a little less complicated, based on the number of lead balls, the diameter of the barrel, and how many lead balls it takes to make a pound. For example, a 12-gauge shotgun has a barrel that is the same diameter as a lead ball that weighs 1⁄12 pound, a 20-gauge, 1⁄20 pound. The higher the gauge, the smaller the barrel and the smaller the round. The only exception is the .410 shotgun, which is caliber .410 or 0.410 inch in diameter. The recent introduction of the term "magnum" refers more to the type and amount of powder than to the size of the bullet used (Figs. 14-5 and 14-6).

The type and severity of wounds inflicted by a firearm depend on several factors. The most often quoted factor, but the least important, is the amount of energy the bullet (projectile) has when leaving the firearm. The kinetic energy formula, $KE = \frac{1}{2} MV^2$, can be applied to any moving object or to calculate the muzzle energy for a particular type of firearm. Energy increases much more as a function of the velocity of the bullet than as a function of the mass. For this reason most firearms are classified according to muzzle velocity. The higher the velocity of the bullet, the greater the energy and the greater the potential for injury. Firearms with muzzle velocities greater than 2500 feet/sec are considered high velocity, 1500 to 2500 feet/sec medium velocity, and less than 1500 feet/sec low velocity (Table 14-1). Bullets cause damage to tissue by crushing. The energy of a bullet may be transmitted to the tissue in part or in total depending on the surface area the bullet presents to the tissue. Bullets that strike at an angle, yaw, mushroom, or fragment present more surface area than do bullets that stay in one axis and maintain one shape. Hunting bullets are designed to manipulate shape and composition in order to maximize surface area. By the Geneva Convention, military bullets must have a full metal jacket and be less than .50 caliber. This is designed to minimize surface area. However, most military

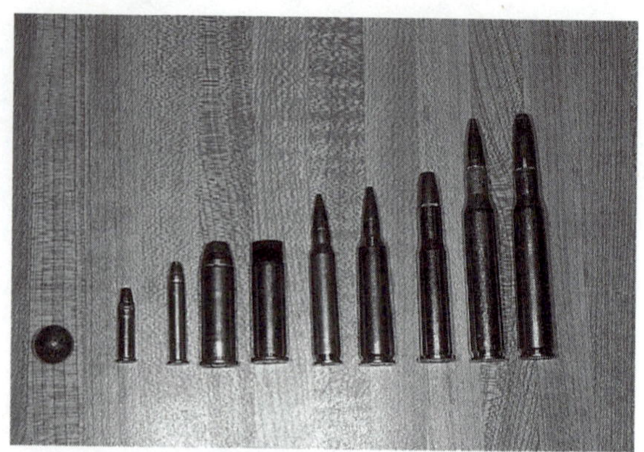

Fig. 14-5 Examples of hunting bullets. *Left to right,* .50 caliber black powder lead bullet, .22 caliber long rifle lead bullet, .44 magnum semijacketed hollowpoint bullet, .44 magnum shotshell, .223 caliber (5.56 mm) full metal jacket bullet, .22/250 caliber semijacketed soft point bullet, .30/30 caliber soft point flat nose bullet, .270 caliber pointed soft point bullet, and .30-06 caliber round nose soft point bullet.

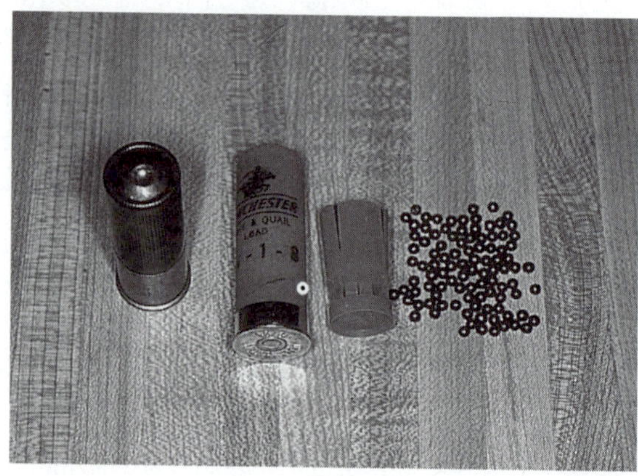

Fig. 14-6 Examples of shotgun rounds. *Left to right,* 12-gauge slug round, empty 12-gauge plastic round, plastic 12-gauge wadding, and number six shotgun pellets.

Table 14-1 Comparison of Bullet Caliber, Weight, Velocity, and Muzzle Energy

Caliber	Weight (Grains)	Muzzle Velocity (Feet/Sec)	Muzzle Energy (Foot-pounds)
.22	40	1080	90
.223	55	3250	1280
.44 magnum	180	1600	1045
.30/60	150	2750	2500

rounds travel at such high velocities (greater than 2700 feet/sec) that fragmentation reliably occurs even with full metal jackets. Fragmentation may also occur when a bullet strikes bone and sends splinters in several directions. The bone fragments cause injuries within the body similar to those from bullet fragments and may even exit the body to injure bystanders. Another phenomenon that occurs is temporary cavitation, which occurs at all velocities to some degree but becomes a factor only at high velocities. A permanent cavity occurs when a bullet or fragment crushes tissue. The bullet also creates a radial dispersion wave as a result of acceleration of tissue away from its path, which creates a temporary cavity. This wave is well tolerated by most elastic tissue such as muscle, bowel, and lung; however, inelastic tissues such as liver or brain do not tolerate it and may be severely damaged by the temporary cavity. In high-velocity bullet wounds the temporary cavity may be several times larger than the permanent cavity. The total effect of high energy, fragmentation, mushrooming, yaw, and temporary cavity formation injures tissue. While the kinetic energy formula cannot be denied, the other factors are probably more important to injury production. The type of tissue struck is the most important factor. As can be seen from Table 14-1, the .22 caliber long rifle bullet has a low mass and velocity and thus a low muzzle energy, yet more fatalities have occurred from this round than from any other. It is very inexpensive, can be fired from a number of rifles and handguns, is commonly used to hunt game, and is not thought of as particularly dangerous by inexperienced hunters. For these reasons most people are shot by this round. The bullet is highly lethal when striking the brain, the heart, or a major blood vessel.*

Other rare problems associated with firearms are explosions that occur within the firearm itself. These can cause burns or fragment-type injuries. When firearms are loaded with excessive amounts of powder or the wrong powder is used in reloading bullets, the resultant detonation may cause the frame or cylinder of the firearm to explode. The burning powder or fragments of metal can cause injuries to the shooter. These injuries usually occur to the face and hands; penetrating eye injuries are also common. Obstruction of the barrel of the firearm by snow, mud, or other foreign material may cause a similar explosion.

*References 1, 2, 8-12, 16, 22, 26.

TREATMENT OF HUNTING INJURIES

The treatment of hunting injuries involves standard principles and priorities of trauma care. Airway, breathing, circulation, bleeding control, immobilization of the spine and fractured extremities, wound care, and stabilization of the patient for transport should be performed in an expedient manner. The patient should always be disarmed to prevent accidental injury to the rescuer or further injury to the victim. Removing the firearm or arrow from the vicinity of patient care is usually sufficient, but ideally the firearm should be made safe by removal of the ammunition and opening of the firing chamber. Arrows should be placed in a quiver, or the points may be wrapped in cloth to prevent injury.

The management of common traumatic injuries and illnesses, such as hypothermia and mountain sickness, is no different except for one important point: *always disarm the patient.* A patient with a charged weapon and a head injury or change in mental status for any reason presents an immediate danger to a well-meaning rescuer. If the person attempting to offer aid to an injured hunter is not familiar with weapons, it is usually best to move the weapon several feet from the victim and point it in a direction where an accidental discharge will do the least harm.

Arrow Injuries

Lacerations from razor-sharp hunting points are not unusual and can be treated like any similar laceration. The wound should be irrigated, any foreign material removed, and the laceration closed primarily. Victims pierced by an arrow should be stabilized, and the arrow should be left in place during transport if possible. Attempts to remove the arrow by pulling it out or pushing it through the wound may cause significantly more injury and should be avoided. It is acceptable to cut off the shaft of the arrow and leave 3 or 4 inches protruding from the wound to make transport easier if this can be accomplished with a minimum of arrow movement. A large pair of paramedic-type shears can usually cut through an arrow shaft if it is stabilized during cutting. The portion of the arrow that remains in the wound should then be fixed with gauze pads or cloth and tape. A similar approach should be used for spears and knives. The patient should be transferred as quickly as possible to an operating room where the arrow can be removed under controlled conditions. Radiographs are helpful to identify associated anatomic structures before removal is attempted in the operating room (Fig. 14-7).

Gunshot Wounds

Emergency department care of the gunshot wound includes securing the airway, placing two intravenous lines in

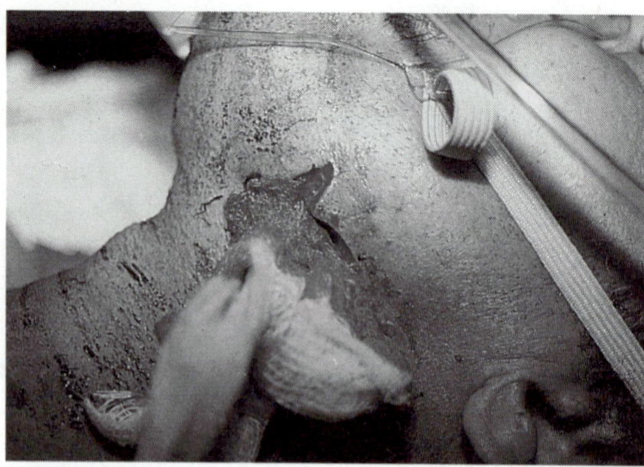

Fig. 14-7 Arrow wound to the left side of the neck near the mandible. The shape of the wound resembles the blades of the broadhead as shown in Fig. 14-4.

unaffected extremities, performing cardiac monitoring, and providing oxygen therapy. The patient with a neck wound and expanding hematoma should be endotracheally intubated as soon as possible. If endotracheal intubation is not possible, a needle cricothyrotomy followed by a tube cricothyrotomy should be performed. Relief of tension pneumothorax with a needle or tube thoracostomy or occlusion of a sucking chest wound should be done immediately. Any external bleeding should be controlled by direct pressure. A radiograph should be obtained of the involved area, and where there is a presumed entrance wound without an exit wound, multiple x-ray studies may be needed to find the location of the bullet. On rare occasion, bullets have been observed to embolize from the chest area via the aorta to the lower extremity arteries or to the heart via the vena cava. A type and cross-match and basic trauma laboratory tests should be performed. Tetanus toxoid and immunoglobulin should be administered as indicated by the patient's history. Broad-spectrum antibiotics should be administered to cover the wide range of pathogens associated with gunshot wounds, especially with complex wounds to the abdomen and extremities. Patients in shock should be taken to the operating room immediately. If this is not possible, type O-negative or type-specific blood should be transfused. Autotransfusion, when available, can be an ideal way to replace lost blood in the patient in shock. Military antishock trousers or pneumatic antishock garments have not been shown to be beneficial in the treatment of shock secondary to penetrating trauma. Emergency thoracotomy is indicated for patients who have lost vital signs shortly before reaching the emergency department or while in the emergency department. Injuries to the heart or great vessels can be occluded with Foley catheter balloons, pericardial tamponade can be relieved, and the aorta can be cross-clamped. Hypothermia is commonly unrecognized in the trauma victim and may lead to coagulopathy, cardiac arrhythmias, or electrolyte disturbances. Rectal temperatures should be obtained, and only warmed fluids and blood given to the patient.

Many myths associated with the management of gunshot wounds should be repudiated. The size or caliber of a bullet cannot easily be determined from the size of the wound; skin is quite elastic and stretches before being torn by a blunt bullet. The path of the bullet cannot be determined by connecting the entrance and exit wounds, since bullets may bounce and only a fragment may exit. The exit wound may be larger or smaller than the entrance wound, and the point of entrance or exit is not easily determined by looking at the wound. Wounds from high-velocity bullets are similar to other types of wounds, and standard rules of debridement should be followed. Wide debridement of normal-appearing tissue is unnecessary and should not be done. In general, victims of gunshot wounds should be evacuated quickly and stabilized if possible. Most victims (80%) of gunshot wounds to the chest who survive the first 30 minutes can be treated with a thoracostomy tube and observation. All gunshot wounds to the abdomen should be explored in the operating room. Radiographs should be used to identify bullets, bullet fragments, and bony injuries. Extremity wounds can be treated conservatively unless signs of vascular injury are present. Experience in combat has shown that vascular injuries do best when identified and treated immediately. Obviously, major bony injuries and nerve injuries eventually need operative therapy, but immediate intervention is rarely necessary. Most important, the underlying injury cannot be determined by examination of the external wound.

Vascular injuries may not be identified during the initial examination; therefore noninvasive, portable, Doppler ultrasound studies can be extremely valuable in the emergency department. Contrast angiography should be performed on any patient with a suspected vascular injury. The removal of the bullet or bullet fragment is not necessary unless the bullet is intravascular, intraarticular, or in contact with nervous tissue such as the spinal cord or a peripheral nerve. Bullets found during exploratory laparotomy or wound debridement should be removed, but it is unnecessary to explore soft tissue such as muscle or fat solely to remove a bullet. Shotgun pellets that have minimal penetration can be removed from the skin with a forceps. Often the plastic or cloth wadding is found in superficial shotgun wounds and should be removed. Shotgun blasts may produce large soft tissue defects that need extensive debridement and either skin grafting or surgical flap rotation to maximize coverage. Patients with powder burns should have as much of the powder residue removed as possible with a brush under local anesthesia. The powder will tattoo the skin if it is not removed, and the deep burns may need dermabrasion or surgical debridement (Fig. 14-8).[1,8,16,26]

Retained lead bullets and shotgun pellets for the most part are not hazardous; however, when they are within joint spaces or the gastrointestinal tract, significant amounts of lead can be absorbed and toxicity can occur.[21]

A

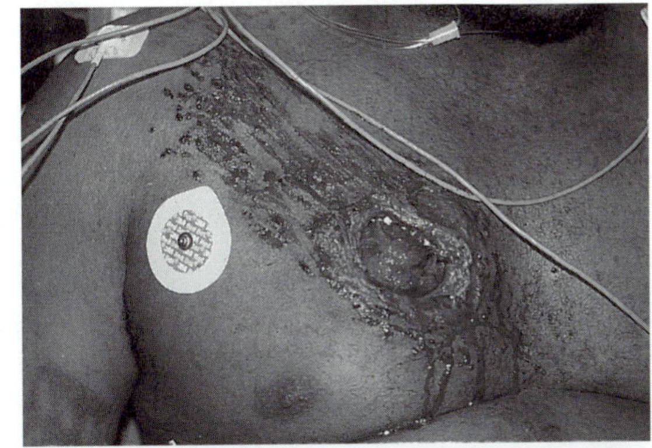

B

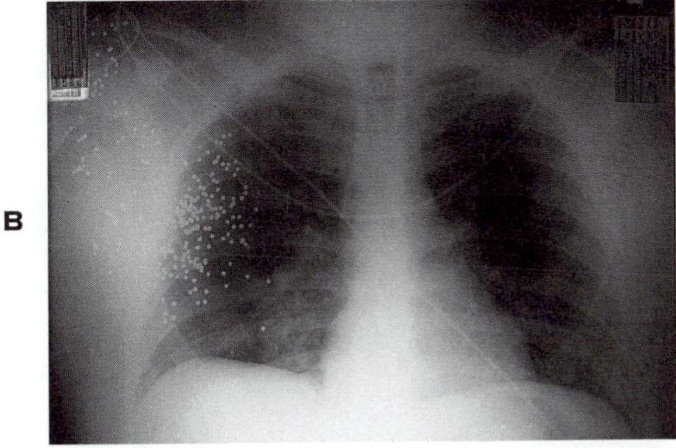

Fig. 14-8 **A,** Close-range 12-gauge shotgun wound to the right side of the upper chest. The large central wound was caused by the plastic wadding, and the pellets have struck at an angle toward the shoulder. The patient was turning to the right when shot. The external appearance of the wound indicates a massive injury to the chest. **B,** Chest radiograph of the patient in **A.** No pellets have penetrated the chest, and there was no pneumothorax, pulmonary contusion, or vascular injury. The injury was totally superficial, and the patient was admitted for observation and local wound care.

PREVENTION OF HUNTING INJURIES

Most state fish and wildlife agencies have recognized that hunters are at risk for injuries and have tried to develop programs to minimize morbidity and mortality. National organizations such as the Boy Scouts of America and the National Rifle Association have been teaching firearm and hunting safety for decades. The Hunter Education Association and the North American Association of Hunter Safety Coordinators (NAAHSC) have attempted to identify high-risk groups and situations by collecting data on both fatal and nonfatal hunting-related injuries. NAAHSC-approved Hunter Safety Programs are available in every state, and all states except Alaska, Massachusetts, and South Carolina require the course before issuing a license to hunt. These courses are roughly 12 hours long and cover hunter responsibility, firearms and ammunition, bow hunting, personal safety, game care, and wildlife identification. They stress respect for the wilderness and a rational approach to game management. All hunters, potential hunters, and persons going into hunting areas should take one of these courses. Approximately 650,000 hunters complete a hunter safety course annually. Since the first course given in Kentucky in 1946, more than 18 million hunters have been certified.

Most injuries could probably be prevented by following a few simple rules. Nonhunters should be aware of hunting seasons and designated hunting areas and wear international orange clothing articles while in hunting areas. Hunters should always be sure of their target before shooting, use safety harnesses in tree stands, and use appropriate technique and tools for cleaning game. Tree stands should be well constructed. Hunters should never consume alcohol or mind-altering drugs that might interfere with their judgment. Eye protection in the form of safety glasses should be worn while hunting or target shooting to prevent injuries from ricocheting fragments and shotgun pellets. High-frequency hearing loss is common in hunters because of the loud report of the firearm. While earplugs and headsets can protect the hunter, they are impractical for most hunting and are used mainly for target shooting. Some hunters use a single ear plug for the ear closest to the muzzle of the firearm. This protects the ear most likely to be injured but still allows the hunter to hear approaching game and other hunters. Bow hunters should always use wrist and finger protection to prevent injuries from the arrow fletching and the bowstring. All arrows should be carried in a quiver until ready for use. The arrow broadhead should always be pointed away from the hunter. These few steps would probably eliminate most hunting injuries.[19,20]

Fishing Injuries

Sport fishing is associated with a large number of relatively minor injuries compared with hunting. The usual problems associated with outdoor recreation are common among fishermen: sunburn, frostbite, hypothermia, near drowning, sprains, fractures, motion sickness, and heat illness. Lacerations are relatively more common because of the use of knives to cut bait and fishing lines and to clean fish. These lacerations are often contaminated with a variety of marine and freshwater pathogens that may increase the incidence of wound infection. Thorough debridement of the wound and copious irrigation with sterile saline solution are the best initial methods to prevent infection (see Chapters 51 and 52).

FISHHOOK INJURIES

Fishhooks are designed to penetrate the skin of fish easily and to hold fast while the fish is played and landed. To perform this dual role, they are extremely sharp at the tip, have a barb just proximal to the tip, and are curved so that the more force applied to the hook, the deeper it penetrates. Fishhooks may be single or in clusters of two, three, or four to increase the chance of catching the fish. Some state fishing laws limit the number of hooks allowed on a single line when fishing for certain game fish to make it more sporting. Unfortunately, the increased number of hooks on a lure or line also increases the chance of catching a fisherman. The most common fishhook punctures occur when fish are removed from hooks. The combination of sharp hooks, slippery fish, and an inexperienced fisherman leads to puncture wounds or embedded fishhooks. Many fishermen use commercial fishhook removers or large Kelly forceps to remove hooks. Some fishing guides simply cut the hook with a side-cutting pliers; they believe the remaining segment of hook will eventually oxidize in the victim and disintegrate. Often, fishhooks are stepped on with a bare foot or fishermen catch themselves or another person on the backcast.

Fishhooks can penetrate skin, muscle, and bone. They may pierce the eye or the penis. Care must be taken in removing a fishhook so that further damage to underlying structures is avoided. The first step is to remove the portion of the hook that is embedded from any attached lines, fish, bait, or lure. This is best done with a sharp side-cutting pliers. A bolt cutter may be needed for large, hardened hooks. A number of techniques are used for removing embedded fishhooks, but all involve a certain amount of movement of the hook, which causes increased pain. A local anesthetic should be infiltrated around the puncture site to minimize pain and movement of the patient. The first method can be used if the hook is not deeply embedded. Pressure is applied along the curve of the hook while the hook is pulled away from the point. Because the barb is on the inside of the curve of the hook, this enlarges the entrance hole enough to allow the barb and point to pass through. Sometimes a string looped through the curve of the hook facilitates the process. If the hook is deeply embedded, pressure can be applied along the curve of the hook until the point and barb penetrate the skin at another place, and then the barb can be cut off and the remainder of the hook backed out (Fig. 14-9). Fishhooks embedded in the eye should be left in place, the eye covered with a metal patch or cup, and the patient referred to an ophthalmologist for further care. Rarely, hooks become embedded in bone or cartilage; this patient must be taken to the operating room to have the hook removed via a surgical incision.

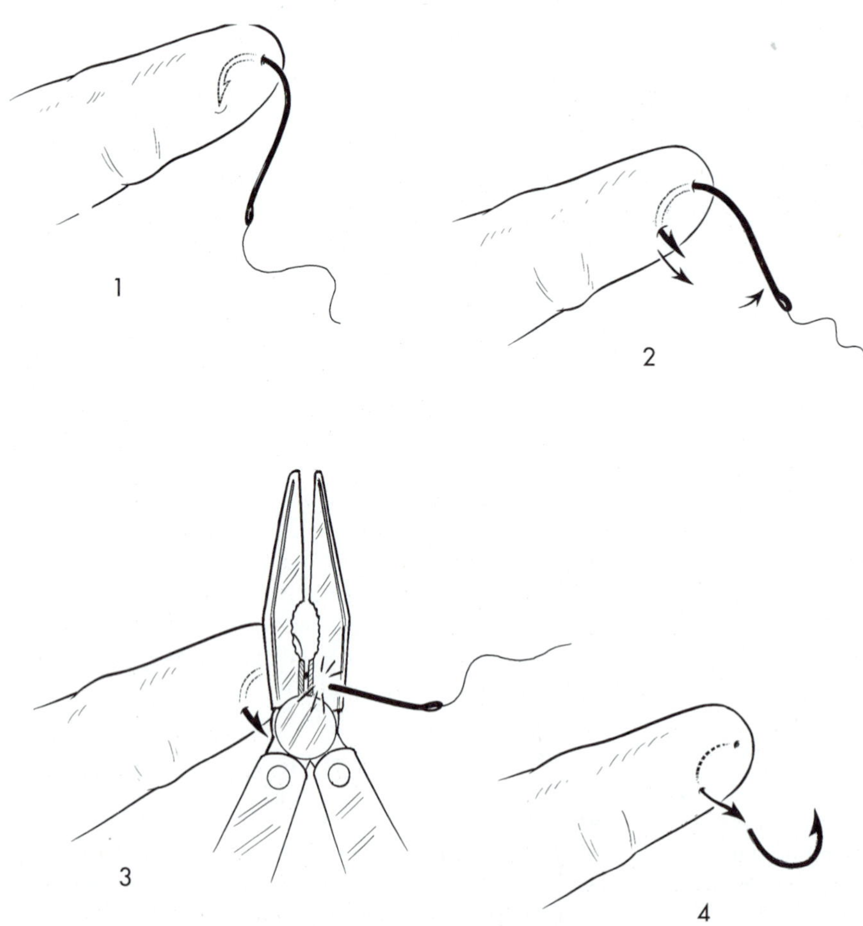

Fig. 14-9 Removal of a fishhook that has penetrated a fingertip.

FISHING SPEAR INJURIES

Fishing spears, like fishhooks, are designed to penetrate and hold fish. They may be jabbed or thrown or propelled by rubber straps or carbon dioxide cartridges. The more force used to propel the spear, the deeper penetration into tissue. While arrows are designed to cause bleeding and bullets to cause crushing, fishing spears are designed to hold the fish until it drowns or is otherwise dispatched. Spears may penetrate the human chest or abdominal cavity, skull, or any other anatomic area. Some bleeding may occur, especially if major blood vessels are struck. The victim should be removed from the water as soon as possible and immediate attention given to airway, breathing, and bleeding control. The spear should be stabilized in place, and the patient immediately transported to a medical facility. Penetrating neck and chest injuries may require endotracheal intubation and tube thoracostomy. If a spear is embedded in the cheek and interfering with the patient's airway, cutting it off with a bolt cutter and removing it through the mouth is permitted. Spears in all other locations should be left in place, although they may be cut off to facilitate transportation or improve the patient's comfort (Fig. 14-10).

A

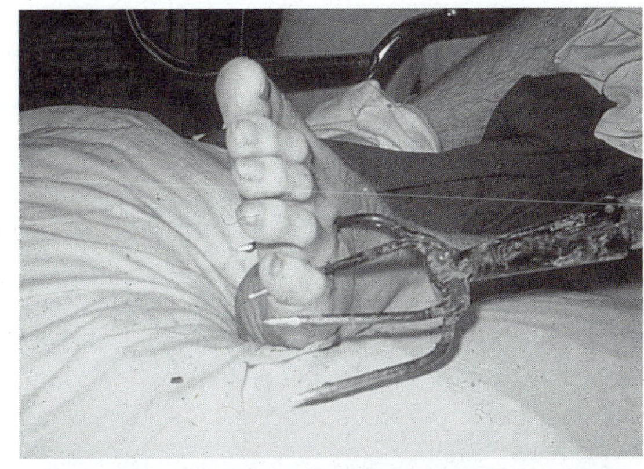

B

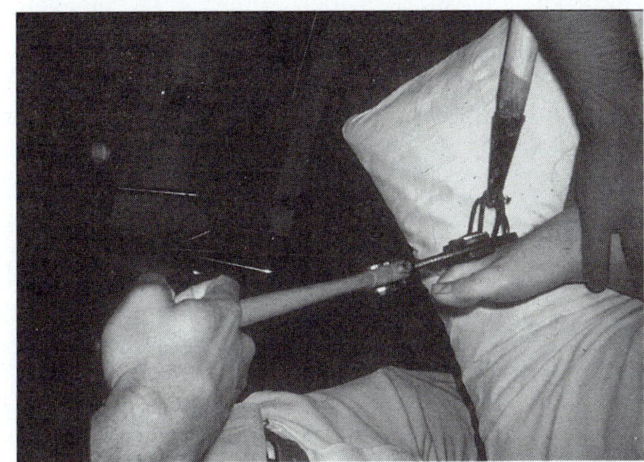

Fig. 14-10 **A,** Male patient with a multipronged fishing spear through the foot. He said he saw something move and he speared it. **B,** Same patient with the spear being cut off in the emergency department with a bolt cutter. The patient was taken to the operating room to have the remainder of the spear removed.

REFERENCES

1. Adams DB: Wound ballistics: a review, *Milit Med* 147:831, 1982.
2. Amato JJ et al: Bone as a secondary missile: an experimental study in the fragmentation of bone by high-velocity missiles, *J Trauma* 29:609, 1989.
3. Bear F: *Fred Bear's world of archery,* Garden City, NY, 1979, Doubleday.
4. Blumenschine RJ, Cavallo JA: Scavening and human evolution, *Sci Am* 267:90, 1992.
5. Campbell BG: Hunting and the evolution of society. In *Humankind emerging,* Boston, 1979, Little, Brown.
6. Carter GL: Accidental firearm fatalities and injuries among recreational hunters, *Ann Emerg Med* 18:406, 1989.
7. Cole TB, Patetta MJ: Hunting firearm injuries, North Carolina, *Am J Public Health* 78:1585, 1988.
8. Fackler ML: Wound ballistics: a review of common misconceptions, *JAMA* 259:2730, 1988.
9. Fackler ML, Ballamy RF, Malinowski JA: The wound profile: Illustration of the missile-tissue interaction, *J Trauma* 28:S21, 1988.
10. Fackler ML, Bellamy RF, Malinowski JA: Wounding mechanism of projectiles striking at more than 1.5 km/sec, *J Trauma* 26:250, 1986.
11. Fackler ML, Malinowski JA: The wound profile: a visual method for quantifying gunshot wound components, *J Trauma* 25:522, 1985.
12. Fackler ML et al: Bullet fragmentation: a major cause of tissue disruption, *J Trauma* 24:35, 1984.
13. Hain WH: Fatal arrow wounds, *J Forensic Sci* 34:691, 1988.
14. Lambrecht CB, Hargarten SW: Hunting-related injuries and deaths in Montana: the scope of the problem and a framework for prevention, *J Wilderness Med* 4:175, 1993.
15. Lawrence HS: Fatal nonpowder firearm wounds: case report and review of the literature, *Pediatrics* 85:177, 1990.
16. Lindsey D: The idolatry of velocity, or lies, damn lies and ballistics, *J Trauma* 20:1068, 1980.
17. Lucas RM, Mitterer D: Pneumatic firearm injuries: trivial trauma or perilous pitfalls? *J Emerg Med* 8:433, 1990.
18. National Safety Council: *Accident facts 1987,* Washington, DC, 1987, The Council.
19. *Ohio hunter safety education student handbook,* Ohio Division of Wildlife, Seattle, 1981, Outdoor Empire.
20. Pryce D: *Safe hunting,* New York, 1974, David McKay.
21. Stromberg BV: Symptomatic lead toxicity secondary to retained shotgun pellets, *J Trauma* 30:356, 1990.
22. Sykes LN, Champion HR, Fouty WJ: Dum-dums, hollow-points, and devastators: techniques designed to increase wounding potential of bullets, *J Trauma* 28:618, 1988.
23. Tree stand–related injuries among deer hunters—Georgia, 1979-89, *MMWR* 38:697, 1989.
24. US Department of the Interior, Fish and Wildlife Service: *1985 national survey of fishing, hunting and wildlife associated recreation,* Washington, DC, 1988, US Government Printing Office.
25. Urquhart CK et al: Deer stands: a significant cause of injury and mortality, *South Med J* 84:686, 1991.
26. Walker ML, Poindexter JM, Stovall I: Principles of management of shotgun wounds, *Surg Gynecol Obstet* 170:97, 1990.
27. Walsh IR et al: Pediatric gunshot wounds—powder and non-powder weapons, *Pediatr Emerg Care* 4:279, 1988.
28. Wintemute GJ et al: Unintentional firearm deaths in California, *J Trauma* 29:457, 1989.

15 WILDERNESS SURVIVAL

Warren D. Bowman

This chapter examines the human body's requirements for homeostasis and the way they can be satisfied in a wilderness environment where little oxygen, food, or water may be available and where extremes of heat or cold may exist. Although improvisation and living off the land are mentioned, *anticipation, prevention,* and especially *preplanning* are much more important and form the core of this discussion. As an example taken from Antarctic exploration, Roald Amundson's style of thorough preparation should be emulated, rather than Robert Scott's amateurish muddling.[8]

The outcome of an encounter with severe environmental stress varies with the type, magnitude, and duration of the stress and with the stressed subject's resources. These resources include the state of acclimatization and physical integrity, particularly conditioning and the presence of illness or injury; experience; equipment and the ability to improvise intelligently; and such intangibles as "backcountry common sense" and the will to survive. The recommendations in this chapter are based on personal experience, the opinion of survival experts, and analysis of actual survival situations. General principles are emphasized, but "tricks of the trade" may at times hold the key to life or death. Unfortunately, most of the lay literature emphasizes tales of misfortune, hazardous adventures, and mindless bravado in the face of unnecessary hardships (often incurred by the errors of the participants), while great deeds go unrecorded or forgotten because the experience and competence of the adventures kept catastrophic, "newsworthy" experiences to a minimum. In the words of Corneille, "To vanquish without risk is to triumph without glory."[5]

Increased leisure time and growing interest in outdoor activities put more people into settings where survival situations can develop. The cross-country skier, winter mountaineer, and winter camper may be exposed to extremes of cold and storm. The expeditionary mountaineer may explore regions where winter exists the year round and where it is difficult to supply the body's requirements for oxygen. The desert or tropical traveler may be exposed to extremes of heat and humidity. Passengers in aircraft, seacraft, or land vehicles may be stranded in almost any type of environment. A common thread in the development of life- or limb-threatening emergencies seems to be the unexpected occurrence of severe environmental conditions, such as winter storms, for which wilderness travelers were unprepared, accompanied by the traveler's insistence on traveling in extreme conditions rather than staying put in a snug bivouac. Physicians who participate in wilderness recreation or treat adventurers need to be aware of the physiologic and psychologic impacts of environmental stress and how related deleterious effects can be prevented and treated.

The knowledgeable traveler should give considerable forethought to the unexpected and approach the preventive aspects of survival in an orderly fashion. This includes being familiar with weather forecasts, strategizing worst-case scenarios, including emergency items in the backpack, avoiding solo travel in the wilderness, and leaving notice of the projected route and expected time of return. With good planning, deteriorating weather or an injury-forced bivouac becomes more of an inconvenience than a life-threatening ordeal.

For survival the body requires a constant supply of oxygen, a core temperature regulated within relatively narrow limits (perhaps 75° to 107° F [24° to 42° C]), water, food, and a generous amount of self-confidence, faith, and the will to live. For comfort and optimum performance, body temperature must be close to normal and the body must be rested, well nourished, in top physical condition, and free from disease and injury. Although these requirements are discussed separately, they are interrelated. The most immediate are maintenance of body integrity (through accident prevention) and regulation of body temperature. However, dehydration, starvation, and exhaustion make temperature maintenance more difficult and interfere with the rational thought and agility required to prevent accidents. Insufficient oxygen becomes a contributing factor at extreme altitude or in the case of suffocation caused by avalanche burial or carbon monoxide poisoning from cooking in an unventilated shelter. Abundant food and water are of little value to a hypothermic person dying of insufficient clothing and shelter or to the victim of heatstroke, even though lack of food and water eventually weaken and kill an otherwise healthy individual. Lack of self-confidence, faith, and the will to live may cause an attitude of panic and defeatism that prevents a person from taking timely survival actions such as conserving energy, preparing shelter, or lighting a fire. Poor physical conditioning or the presence of illness or injury may interfere with the body's ability to produce heat by shivering or lose heat by sweating and increasing skin perfusion, and can hamper wood gathering, shelter building, and other actions necessary for survival.[4]

The most important organ for survival is the human brain, since voluntary actions such as preparedness, regulation of energy expenditure, adjustment of clothing, and seeking shelter are more important than involuntary mechanisms of adaptation to heat or cold.

Oxygen

As a human ascends from sea level, the body is subjected to increasing cold, decreasing oxygen, increasing solar radiation, and decreasing atmospheric pressure. For every 1000 feet (305 m) of altitude gain, the ambient temperature drops by about 4° F (2.2° C), the barometric pressure drops by about 20 mm Hg (0.1 mb/m), and the amount of ultraviolet radiation increases by about 5%. The percentage of oxygen in the atmosphere remains constant, but the partial pressure of oxygen diminishes with altitude so that at 10,000 feet (3077 m) it is only two-thirds that at sea level and at 18,000 feet (5488 m) only half.[3]

In acute exposure to high altitude the effects of hypoxia can lead initially to symptoms of fatigue, weakness, headache, loss of appetite, nausea, vomiting, shortness of breath on exertion, insomnia, and Cheyne-Stokes respirations (see Chapter 1).

These symptoms are probably present to some degree in everyone who goes suddenly from sea level to 8000 feet (2462 m) or above. The clinical effects of hypoxia are often difficult to separate from those of cold, high winds, dehydration, and exhaustion. Serious degrees of acute mountain sickness are unusual below 12,000 to 14,000 feet (3692 to 4308 m) but have been reported in trekkers as low as 7500 feet (2308 m). Anyone who intends to attain these altitudes should be familiar with disorders related to altitude. At any height, oxygen in ambient air may be prevented from reaching the cellular level because of interruption of normal transport pathways, generally by illness or injury. Possible examples of this in the wilderness include the following[4]:

1. Insufficient oxygen in inspired air from suffocation in avalanche burial, near drowning, or living in a poorly ventilated snow cave
2. Upper airway obstruction caused by a facial injury, blockage by the tongue in a comatose patient, or aspiration of foreign material
3. Interference with proper lung function caused by pneumonia, pulmonary edema, pulmonary hemorrhage, atelectasis, hemothorax, pneumothorax, or chest wall injury
4. Circulatory insufficiency caused by myocardial infarction, pericardial tamponade, hemorrhagic shock, or pulmonary embolism
5. Interference with respiratory control after injury to the respiratory center or hyperviscosity-induced brainstem infarction
6. Interference with the oxygen-carrying capacity of the blood caused by anemia or carbon monoxide poisoning

The emergency and definitive treatment of each of these conditions follows standard techniques and includes administration of oxygen. Carbon monoxide poisoning is probably a greater hazard than is generally appreciated. Many famous polar explorers, including Byrd, Andree, and Stefansson, were killed by or had narrow escapes from the effects of stoves operated in tightly enclosed living areas.[12]

Regulation of Body Temperature

Humans are called homeotherms because as warm-blooded creatures they maintain a body temperature that varies within very narrow limits despite changes in environmental temperature. In poikilotherms, or cold-blooded animals, body temperature varies with that of the environment. Homeothermy is necessary to support the enzyme systems of the human body, which function best at 98.6° to 100° F (37° to 37.5° C). In vitro the speed of enzymatic reactions tends to double for each 10° C rise in temperature, until the enzyme starts to denature. The human body can be thought of as a heat-generating and heat-dissipating machine whose internal temperature is the net result of opposing mechanisms that tend to increase or decrease body heat production, increase or decrease body heat loss, and increase or decrease addition of heat from the outside. Through these mechanisms the internal body temperature can usually be regulated successfully despite ambient temperatures that in temperate climates vary well over 100° F (52° C) from the coldest to the hottest seasons of the year.

Basal body heat production occurs at a rate of about 50 kcal/m^2/hr. This can be increased by muscular activity (involuntary [shivering] and voluntary), eating, inflammation and infection (fever), and in response to cold exposure. Shivering can increase heat production by up to five times the basal rate; vigorous exercise can increase heat production by up to 10 times. Cold exposure increases hunger, the secretion of epinephrine, norepinephrine, and thyroxine, and semiconscious activity such as foot stamping and dancing in place. Eating provides not only needed calories but also the specific dynamic action (SDA) of food, which is the temporary increase in basal metabolic rate that occurs during digestion alone. The SDA of protein is five to seven times higher than that of fat and carbohydrate. However, the onset of the SDA is much faster with carbohydrate than with protein or fat. In hot weather, body heat production can be decreased by decreasing muscular activity and avoiding foods with a high SDA.

In cold weather, heat can be added to the body by close approximation to a fire or other heat source, by sunlight exposure, and by ingesting hot food and drink. In hot weather, external heat addition can be decreased by staying in the shade, wearing clothing that provides shelter from the sun, and avoiding hot objects and hot food and drink.

The body loses heat to the environment by conduction, convection, evaporation, radiation, and respiration. It may gain heat from the environment by the same mechanisms (except for evaporation). The relative importance of these mechanisms depends on such variables as temperature, humidity, wind velocity, cloud cover, insulation, contact with hot or cold objects, sweating, and muscular exercise. For the purpose of illustration, in still air at a temperature of 70° F (21° C), radiation, conduction, and convection together account for 70% of total heat loss, evaporation accounts for 27%, and urination, defecation, and respiration for only 3%. During work, however, evaporation may account for up to 85% of heat loss.[4]

It is useful to think of the body as composed of a core (heart, lungs, liver, adrenal glands, central nervous system, and other vital organs) and a shell (skin, muscles, and extremities). Most of the adjustments in response to cold or heat exposure occur in the shell. They are designed to maintain a relatively constant core temperature; in cold weather the body is prepared to sacrifice parts of the shell to frostbite in order to preserve the core temperature.

The importance of avoiding travel and seeking shelter during storms and extreme cold cannot be overemphasized. The additive chilling effect of wind when added to cold is impressive. Windchill charts (Fig. 15-1) show the relationship between actual temperature, wind velocity, and "effective" temperature at the body surface. "Windchill" refers only to the *rate* of cooling; the actual temperature reached is no lower than it would be if wind were absent (unless evaporation of liquid is occurring from the body surface). The increase in heat loss as the wind rises is not linear; rather, it is roughly proportional to the *square root* of the wind speed.

At moderate ambient temperatures the body's core temperature is kept stable by constant small adjustments in metabolic rate, muscular activity, sweating, and skin circulation. When the body is chilled, automatic and semiautomatic mechanisms increase internal heat production through a slight increase in the metabolic rate, by shivering, and by semiconscious activities such as foot stamping, and reduce heat loss by diminishing sweat production and shell circulation. The body's surface area is reduced by a strong compulsion to curl up into a ball. At the same time the brain tells the body to decrease heat loss by adding insulation and wind protection, to seek shelter, and to increase heat gain by such things as increasing muscular activity, building a fire, seeking sunlight, and eating.[4]

When the body overheats, these actions are reversed. The body increases heat loss by increasing circulation to the skin and extremities and increasing sweating. These mechanisms require more water, which stimulates the thirst response. Heat production is decreased because of a feeling of sluggishness and languor, leading to a reduction in physical activity and in the amount of heat produced by muscles. The brain tells the body to decrease heat gain and increase heat loss by providing shelter from the sun, removing clothing, and fanning oneself.

Cold Weather Survival

Body temperature in a cold environment is maintained by decreasing body heat loss, increasing body heat production, and adding external heat. The most efficient of these methods is conservation of body heat by decreasing heat loss, generally by using clothing and shelter.

To obtain maximal heat production, the body should be kept in the best possible physical condition. This is particularly important for persons with sedentary jobs who participate in vigorous outdoor sports and for rescue personnel who may be subject to severe, unplanned, prolonged physical stress. A suitable physical conditioning program should develop both aerobic and motor fitness. The goal of aerobic exercise is efficient extraction of oxygen from alveolar air. This skill is best developed by rhythmic endurance exercises such as running, cross-country skiing, cycling, swimming, and using exercise bicycles and Nordic skiing simulators. The most effective activities are those that exercise lower and upper extremities simultaneously. Exercise should be vigorous enough to produce a heart rate of 75% of the age-related maximum (0.75 × [220 − the participant's age]) for at least 15 minutes 4 days a week. Motor fitness, which includes strength, power, balance, agility, and flexibility, is developed by vigorous competitive team sports, selected calisthenics, and weight-lifting exercises.

Heat loss from conduction and convection can be prevented by interposing substances of low thermal conductivity between the body and outside air. Clothing creates a microclimate of warmed, still air next to the skin surface. Clothing's value depends on how well it traps air and prevents its motion, the thickness of the air layer, and whether

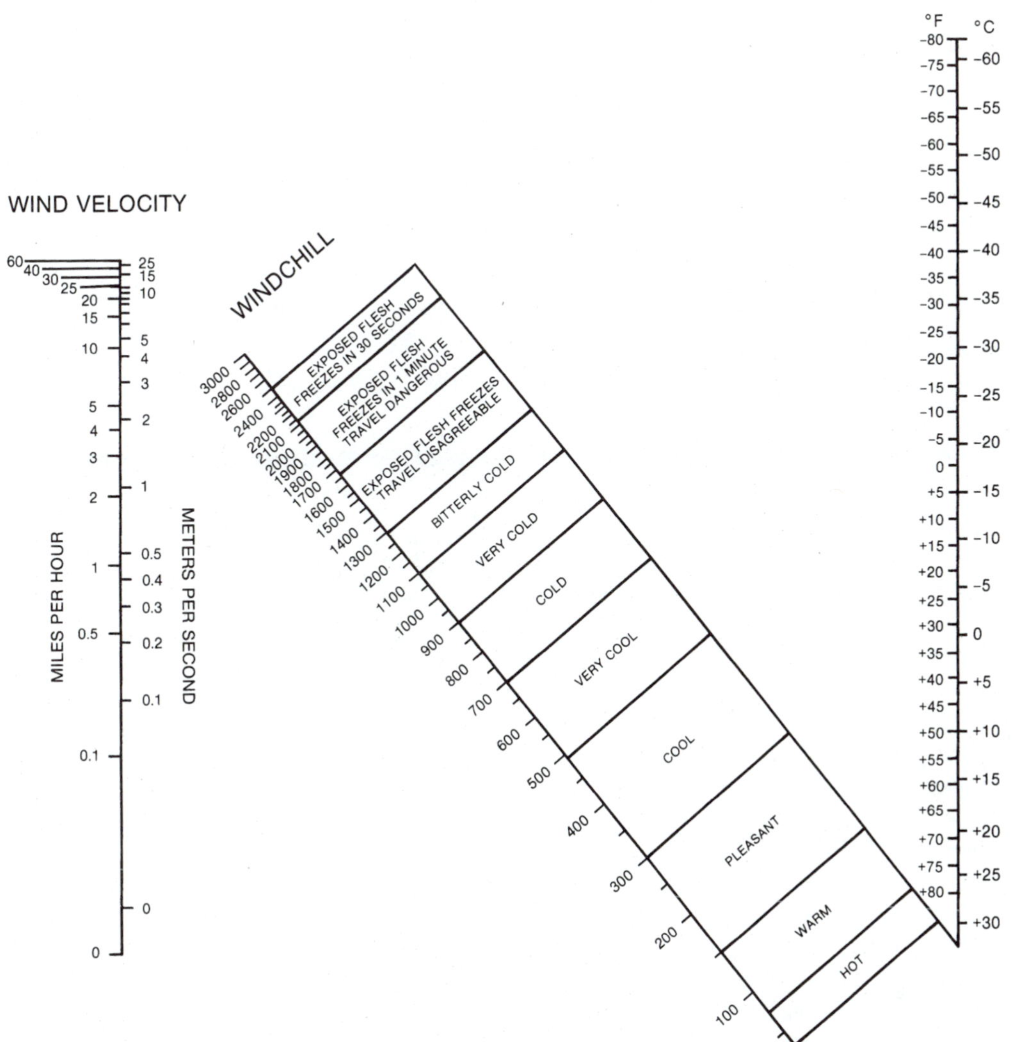

Fig. 15-1 Line chart showing windchill and state of comfort under varying conditions of temperature and wind velocity. The numbers along the left margin of the diagonal center block refer to the windchill factor, that is, the rate of cooling in kilocalories per square meter per hour of an unclad, inactive body exposed to specific temperatures and wind velocities. Windchill factors above 1400 are most hazardous.

effectiveness is reduced by wetting (Table 15-1). Traditional insulating materials are wool, down, foam, and older synthetics such as Orlon, Dacron, and polyester. Wool retains warmth when wet because of a moderately low wicking action and a unique ability to suspend water vapor within its fibers without affecting its low thermal conductance. It can absorb a considerable amount of water without feeling wet but is heavier than synthetics and harder to dry. Cotton, particularly denim and corduroy, is a poor insulator. It dries slowly because of the lower evaporative ability; high thermal conductance is further increased by wetting. Cotton has no place in the backcountry in cold weather. Orlon, acrylic, and polyester were developed in an attempt to duplicate the properties of wool without wool's higher cost. They are used in hats, sweaters, and long underwear. They are almost as warm and not as itchy as wool, and they evaporate moisture better. There are a number of new fabrics woven from fibers that have lower thermal conductance, high insulating ability, and better wicking action than do conventional fibers. Examples include polypropylene, treated polyester such as Capilene, and hollow polyester such as Thermax. Other new insulating materials include Thermolactyl, a combination of acrylic and polyester; Hollofil II and Quallofil, hollow synthetic fibers designed on the principle of reindeer hair; polyester pile, which is light, dries easily, and stays warm when wet because its fibers do not absorb water; and Thinsulate and Thermolite, which are microfibers that provide good insulating ability with less bulk.

Table 15-1 Fiber Characteristics

Fabric	Specific Gravity* (Ratio to Water)	Thermal Conductance† (cal/m²)	Evaporative Ability‡	Wicking Ability	Moisture Regain§
Wool	1.32	2.10	Low	Moderate	17
Cotton	1.54	6.10	Low	High	7.9
Nylon	1.14	2.40	High	Low	4
Polyester	1.38	2.40	High	Low	1
Acrylic	1.15	2.40	High	High	1
Olefin (polypropylene)	0.91	1.20	High	High	5

Modified from Davis AK: *Nordic skiing—a scientific approach,* 1980, University of Minnesota, Minneapolis.
*The lower the specific gravity, the better the insulating ability.
†The lower the thermal conductance, the slower the flow of heat from the body.
‡The higher the evaporative ability, the shorter the amount of time a fiber will be wet, that is, in a reduced insulative state.
§Moisture regain is the amount of moisture a fiber can absorb before feeling wet.

Persons in the outdoors should use the "layer principle" of clothing, which is effective in preventing overheating as well as chilling. Multiple layers of clothing provide multiple layers of microclimate. Layers are added or subtracted as necessary, avoiding excessive perspiration that saturates clothing with moisture and causes increased heat loss from conduction and evaporation. Since water conducts heat 25 to 32 times faster than does air at the same temperature, exertion leading to sweating and wetting of clothing should be avoided. Clothing should be easily adjustable, sweaters should be of the zipper or cardigan type, and outer layers should be cut full enough to allow expansion of inner layers to their full thicknesses. Zippers in the axillary and lateral thigh areas are useful for ventilation.

Loss of heat from convection can be prevented by wearing windproof outer garments of nylon, tightly woven cotton-nylon blends, or water-resistant laminates such as Gore-Tex. Typical examples include a parka with hood and a pair of windproof pants (regular or bib style) or ski warm-up pants.

The loss of heat from infrared radiation also can be prevented by insulation, emphasizing proper covering for body parts with a large surface area/volume ratio. A source of considerable heat loss is the uncovered head, which can dissipate up to 70% of total body heat production at ambient temperatures of 5° F (−16° C), partly because the body does not reduce blood supply to the head and neck as it does to the extremities in cold weather. High heat loss by radiation during cold nights can be decreased by sleeping in a tent or under a tarp instead of in the open. Coverage for the head, ears, hands, and feet should not restrict circulation. A useful new item of clothing developed for the skiing public is the "neck warmer."

Heat loss from the respiratory tract can be diminished by avoiding overexertion and overheating with excessively heavy breathing. When it is extremely cold, inspired air can be warmed by pulling the parka hood out in front of the face to form a "frost tunnel."

Heat loss from conduction occurs by direct contact with a colder object. Sitting down on a pack, foam pad, log, or other object of lower heat conductivity is preferable to sitting in the snow or on a cold rock. At low temperatures bare skin freezes to metal. This can be avoided by wearing light gloves when handling metal objects. Gasoline or other liquids with freezing points lower than that of water can cause frostbite if accidentally poured on the skin at low temperatures. During bivouacs in snow shelters, contact with the snow can be avoided by using a foam pad or improvising a mattress of evergreen boughs, grass, or dry leaves. A cold and injured person needs insulating material between the body and the snow or cold ground, as well as over and around him or her.

Heat loss from conduction and evaporation can be lessened by avoiding wetting and by changing to dry clothes or drying out quickly when wet. Ideally, outer clothing should be windproof, should not collect snow, and should shed water but not be waterproof, since waterproof garments prevent evaporation of sweat. A number of new fabrics, of which Gore-Tex is the most popular, accomplish this reasonably well and are desirable for maritime climates and summer storms.

DRESSING FOR COLD WEATHER

Anyone who ventures outdoors in cold weather should carry clothing for the most extreme environmental conditions that are likely to be experienced.

First Layer

Long Underwear. Long underwear can be made of 85% to 100% wool. If considerable exertion and sweating are anticipated, polypropylene, Capilene, or Thermax blends may be preferable because of their superior ability to wick moisture away from the skin. Duofold and other fabrics containing cotton should be avoided for reasons mentioned previously. Net underwear is preferred by some, but it should be made of wool. Other synthetics such as polyester, Orlon, and acrylic are satisfactory.

Socks. One or two pairs of wool socks of the ragg variety are excellent, preferably with an additional pair of light polypropylene socks worn underneath next to the skin. At least one spare pair of wool socks should be carried.

Second Layer

Shirt. Shirts should be made of light, soft wool or a suitable synthetic and should have long sleeves. Large breast pockets with buttons or Velcro are handy to carry items such as sunglasses and a compass. Shirts should open completely in front or at least have a half-zipper. A turtleneck feature protects the neck, as do neck gaiters and mufflers. Either of the latter can be pulled up to protect the lower face.

Pants. Wool pants are best, as knickers or long pants. Army surplus wool pants are inexpensive and durable.

Foot Gear. The type of boot chosen depends on the type of activity and the expected environmental temperatures. For moderate temperatures, sturdy leather climbing boots made of full-thickness leather, 6 to 8 inches in height with rubber lug soles and roomy enough to accommodate the desired numbers of socks, are ideal. They must be long enough that the toes do not strike the front of the boot when walking downhill. Boots should be laced firmly enough that the heel does not move, but not so tightly that circulation is restricted and the toes cannot be wiggled easily.

For colder temperatures double boots are preferable. These can be all leather or have outer shells of plastic or nylon with inner boots of felt or foam. The Canadian type of shoe-pak (such as the Sorel) with a removable inner felt liner is a good choice for snowshoeing and other nontechnical outdoor activities in the cold. Special double ski boots are available for ski touring, Telemark skiing, and ski mountaineering, depending on whether three-pin or mountaineering ski bindings are used. Gaiters should be used in snow country to keep snow out of the tops of the boots. These should be high enough to reach to the knee and should open in front.

Hat. Hats should be of the stocking variety, made of wool, Orlon, polypropylene, or wool-polypropylene, and large enough to cover the ears. Bomber caps with bills and pull-down earflaps are popular. Some arrangement should be provided to protect the face from cold wind. This can be a balaclava feature or a separate face mask. A useful combination is a ski hat with a "neck warmer" that can be pulled up to cover most of the lower face.

Glove Liners. Light polypropylene gloves are useful for moderately cold conditions or when fine finger movements are required, as in adjusting ski bindings.

Third Layer

Parka. The parka can be a standard ski or mountain parka filled with down, Dacron, Quallofil, Thinsulate, or other lofting material. A more versatile combination is two separate garments: a pile jacket plus a Gore-Tex shell. The shell should have a hood with a drawstring, a two-way zipper with an overlying weather flap closed with snaps, hand warmer pockets, a cloth flap to protect the chin from the metal zipper pull, and zippered openings under the armpits. Cargo pockets should have zippers and be located where they can be reached by the person wearing a pack with a fastened waist belt. The shell should be finger-tip length unless bibs are worn.

Wind Pants. Wind pants should be light and water repellent; Gore-Tex is a good choice. Long, zippered side openings are useful to permit donning them without removing boots, as well as for ventilation and access to inner pants pockets.

Hand Gear. Mittens are warmer than gloves. Excellent three-layer mitten sets are available that include windproof shells with leather palms and two sets of removable pile mittens, at least one of which is kept in place by Velcro. Another good system is a thin, polypropylene glove liner inside a heavy wool (Dachstein, ragg, or wool-polypropylene) mitten inside a Gore-Tex shell. An option that gives more finger dexterity in moderately cold conditions is a polypropylene glove liner inside a fingerless wool glove inside a shell. Shells should have easily accessible "nose-warmers," be long enough to cover the wrists, and have palms of soft leather or sticky fabric for holding ice axes and ski poles securely.

Fourth Layer

The above three layers are usually worn on the body. A fourth layer should be easily available in the pack. This should include a vest or jacket filled with down or synthetic lofting material and a pair of pile or quilted pants. For high-altitude mountaineering, special insulated overboots or lined gaiters should be available.

Rain Gear. In moderate climates or in spring conditions when rain or wet snow may be encountered, outer garments of Gore-Tex or similar material should be used. For maritime climates and during seasons of heavy rain it is probably best to have separate sets of outer garments: a light, thin, windproof nylon jacket and pants and a waterproof (coated nylon) jacket and pants.

Vapor Barrier Principle

The theory behind the use of waterproof garments close to the skin is that saturation of outer garments with sweat (with resulting reduction in insulating value) is prevented and sweating is reduced. This seems to work better in very cold weather than at moderate temperatures. A light garment of polypropylene or similar material should be worn next to the skin, with the waterproof garment over this. Persons with hyperhidrosis and those who object to a clammy feeling next to the skin may not like a vapor barrier system.

METHODS FOR INCREASING HEAT PRODUCTION

Heat production can be increased by raising the level of muscular activity. A cold person should loosen boots, walk around, stamp the feet, jump in place, swing the arms, and wiggle fingers and toes. Shivering is involuntary and generates considerable heat.

The ingestion of food provides calories and the SDA of the food. It is preferable to eat often in cold weather, at least every 2 hours on the trail. Snacks should be high in carbohydrate. Because alcohol may lower blood sugar, impair judgment, and increase peripheral vasodilation, it should be avoided outdoors in cold weather. Nicotine-induced peripheral vasoconstriction may predispose to frostbite.

SHELTER

Everyone who spends time in the wilderness should practice the construction of several types of emergency survival shelters. The function of a shelter is to provide an extension of the microclimate of still, warm air furnished by clothing and to contain heat generated by the body, a fire, or other heat source. A properly designed shelter should be constructed easily and rapidly with simple tools and should give good protection from wind, rain, and snowfall. The type and size of shelter depend on the presence or absence of snow cover and its depth, on natural features of the landscape, and on whether firewood or a stove and fuel are available. If external heat cannot be provided, a shelter must be small and windtight to preserve body heat.

Advantage can be taken of small trees, branches, thick grass, leaf piles, small caves, and snow holes under downed trees or dense evergreens. If possible, a shelter should be constructed in the timber. Generally, shelters partway up the side of a ridge are warmer than those in a valley, since cold air tends to collect in valleys and basins during the night. Exposed, windy ridges above timberline are quite cold. Areas exposed to rockfalls and avalanches or under dead trees or large, dead limbs should be avoided. If open water is available, one may wish to camp close by, although in nonsurvival conditions camps should be at least 100 feet from bodies of water. To avoid drifting snow, tents and shelters should be located with the entrance at right angles to the prevailing winds. Snow is a good insulator (Table 15-2), with heat conductivity ⅒,₀₀₀ that of copper and about the same as wool felt, so that snow shelters may be warmer than other types of constructed shelters so long as the inhabitants remain dry. Contact with the snow or cold ground is avoided by using a foam pad, dry leaves, or grass or (in survival conditions only) by constructing a bed of evergreen boughs.

Table 15-2 Thermal Conductivity of Various Substances

Substance	Conductivity*	Temperature Measured (°C)
Air	0.006	0
Down	0.01	20
Polyester (hollow)	0.016	
Polyester (solid)	0.019	
Snow (old)	0.115	0
Cork	0.128	30
Sawdust	0.14	30
Wool felt	0.149	40
Cardboard	0.5	20
Wood	0.8	20
Dry sand	0.93	20
Water	1.4	12
Brick	1.5	20
Concrete	2.2	20
Ice	5.7	0

*Conductivity is the quantity of heat in gram calories transmitted per second through a plate of material 1 cm thick and 1 cm^2 in area when the temperature difference between the sides of the plate is 1° C.

Natural Shelters

Caves and alcoves under overhangs are good shelters and can be improved by building wind walls with rocks, snow blocks, or brush. A fire should be built so that heat reflects onto the occupant. This can be accomplished by positioning the fire 5 to 6 feet from the back of the shelter, with a reflector wall of logs or stones on the opposite side of the fire; the occupant should sit between the fire and the back of the shelter (Fig. 15-2).

In deep snow, large fallen logs and bent-over evergreens frequently have hollows under them that can be used as small caves. Cone-shaped depressions in the snow around the trunks of evergreens ("tree wells") can be improved by digging them out and roofing them over with evergreen branches or a tarp. If building a fire is not possible, the shelter should be small to retain body heat. A fire can be built to one side of such a shelter, and the heat will reflect off the snow toward the occupant. There must be a ventilation hole directly above the fire, and the fire should not be at risk from falling snow by being located under snow-laden branches.

Artificial Shelters

When no snow is available, shelters can be constructed of small trees, branches, brush, and boughs. A tarp can be rigged into a lean-to type of shelter. In cold weather the most satisfactory form is a lean-to with two sides closed with brush, a fire at the open front, and a wall of logs or stones to reflect heat into its interior (Fig. 15-3).

Snow Shelters

Although a small snow cave large enough for one person can be dug with a ski or cooking pot as a shovel, larger ones (Fig. 15-4) take several hours to dig with good shovels and

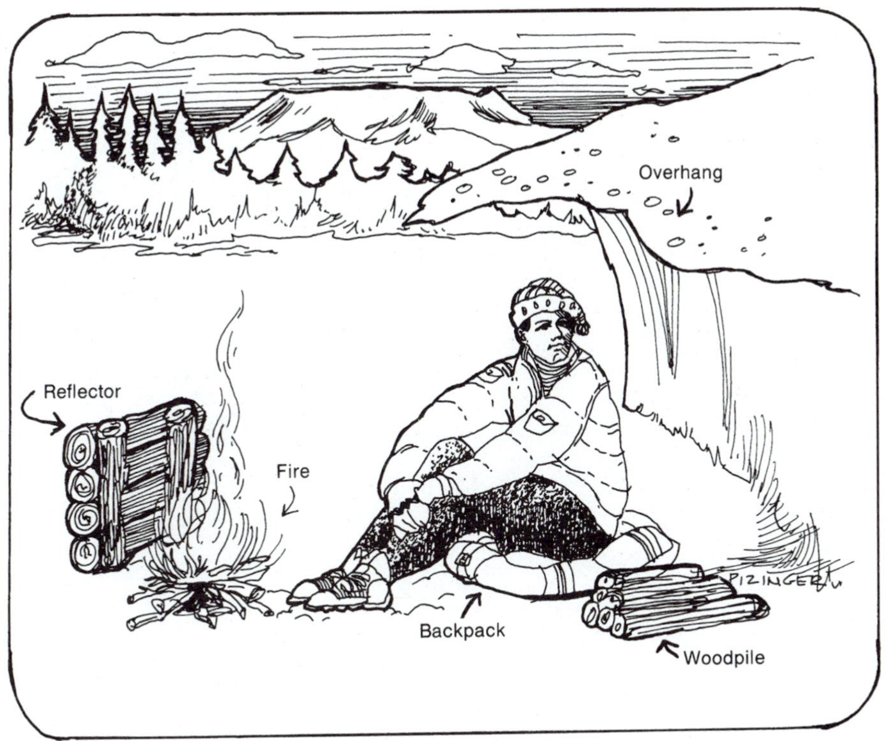

Fig. 15-2 Natural shelter.

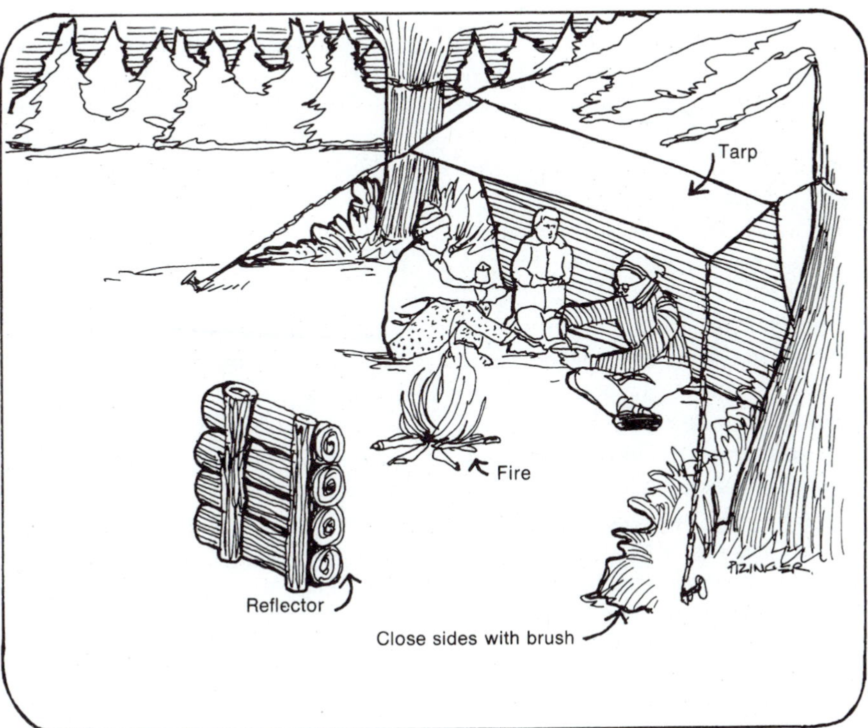

Fig. 15-3 Lean-to-shelter. Sides should be closed with brush or snow.

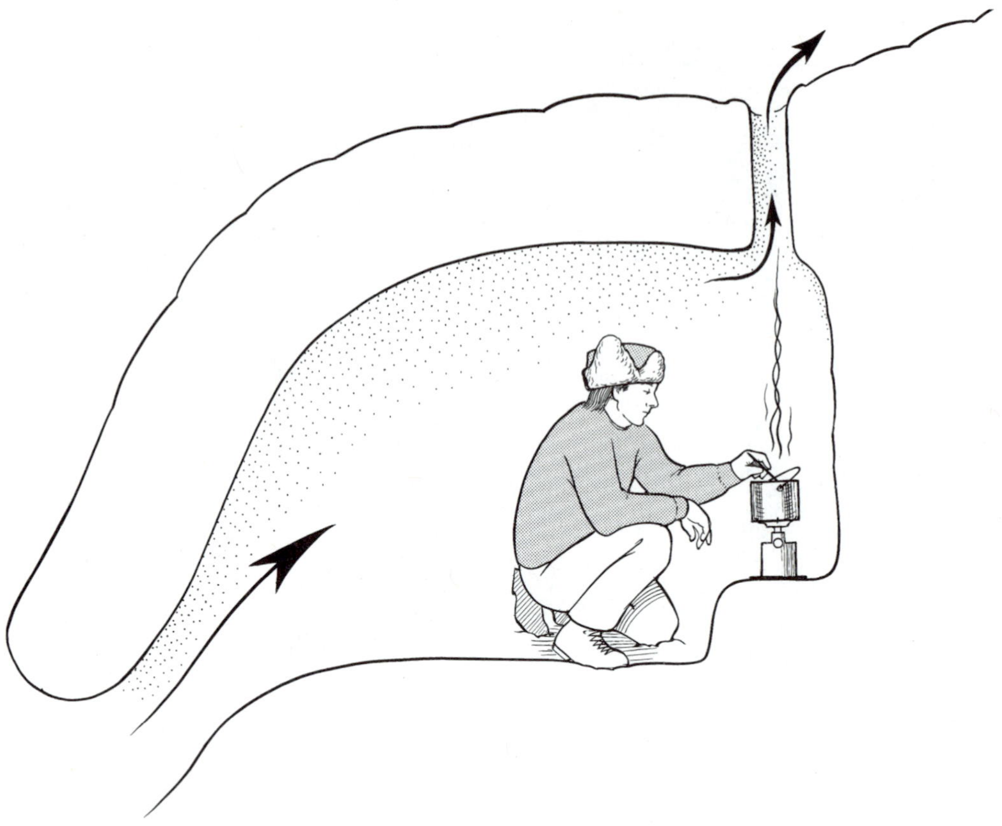

Fig. 15-4 Snow cave.

usually cause the digger to become quite wet. Igloos are comfortable but require time, experience, and a certain amount of engineering skill. They are not recommended to the novice.

A snow trench is the easiest and quickest shelter. It can be dug wherever the snow is 3 feet or deeper or can be piled to that depth. A 4 × 6 foot trench can be dug in 20 minutes, one end roofed over with a tarp or boughs, and a fire built at the opposite end (Fig. 15-5).

If a large tarp and a stove are available, a trench can be dug that is as comfortable as a snow cave and will hold three people. The object is to keep the maximal amount of snow around and over the trench. The trench is dug so that it is as narrow as possible at the surface while still permitting the digger room enough to shovel; a suitable size is 4 feet wide and 8 feet long. It is undercut at the back and sides so that the bottom is 6 to 7 feet wide and 9 to 10 feet long (Fig. 15-6). The entrance is made narrow so that it will contain heat and can be closed with a small plastic sheet or a pack. Four or more skis or small tree trunks are laid from side to side over the top of the trench, with ski poles or branches interwoven at right angles. A tarp is then laid on top of these and snow piled around its edges to hold it down. When the entrance is closed, a small stove plus the body heat of the occupants will raise the interior temperature to 25° to 30° F (−4° to −1° C). Higher temperatures should be avoided, so that clothing and bedding will not become wet from melting snow.

Above the timberline in deep, wind-packed snow, a similar trench can be roofed with snow blocks that are laid horizontally, set as an A-frame, or laid on skis (Fig. 15-7). Chinks between the blocks are caulked with snow.

Tents and Bivouac Sacs

Tents are generally comfortable and dry, but in very cold weather they are not as warm as snow shelters. They are preferable to snow shelters at mild temperatures, with damp snow conditions at temperatures above freezing, or when the snow cover is minimal. Bivouac sacs are carried by climbers on long alpine-style climbs or for emergencies. They are usually made of Gore-Tex or waterproof fabric and hold one or two persons. Many modern packs have extensions so that when used with a cagoule or anorak (roomy, knee-length, hooded pullover garments) they form an acceptable bivouac sac.

VEHICLES

Persons stranded in automobiles or downed airplanes can survive using the equipment in the vehicles. Survivors should *stay with the vehicle* rather than try to go for help, since a vehicle is much more visible to rescuers than is a

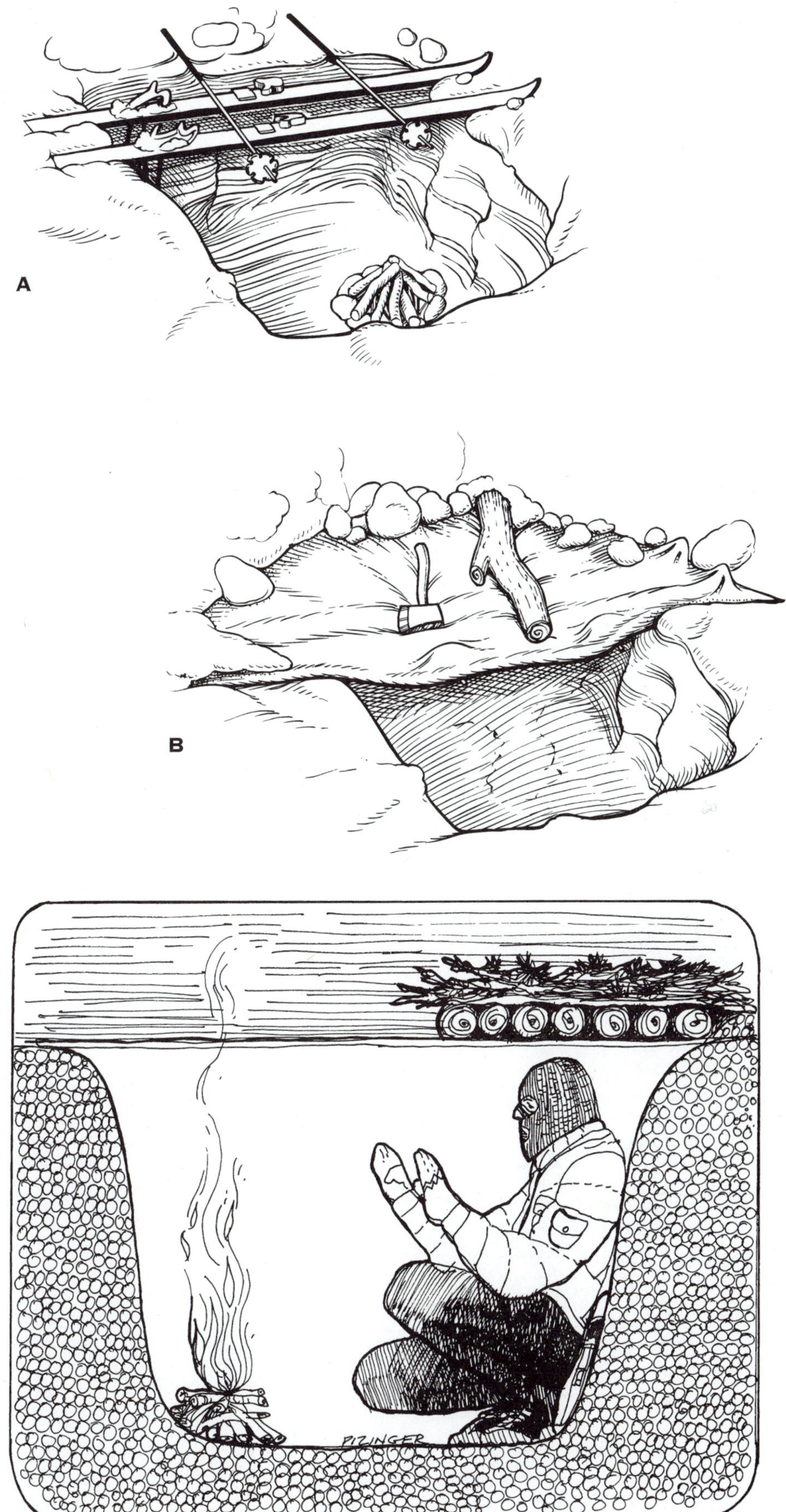

Fig. 15-5 Snow trench. **A,** A pit is dug and overlaid with skis. **B,** A tarp is secured with snow and heavy objects. **C,** A fire is built at the opposite end.

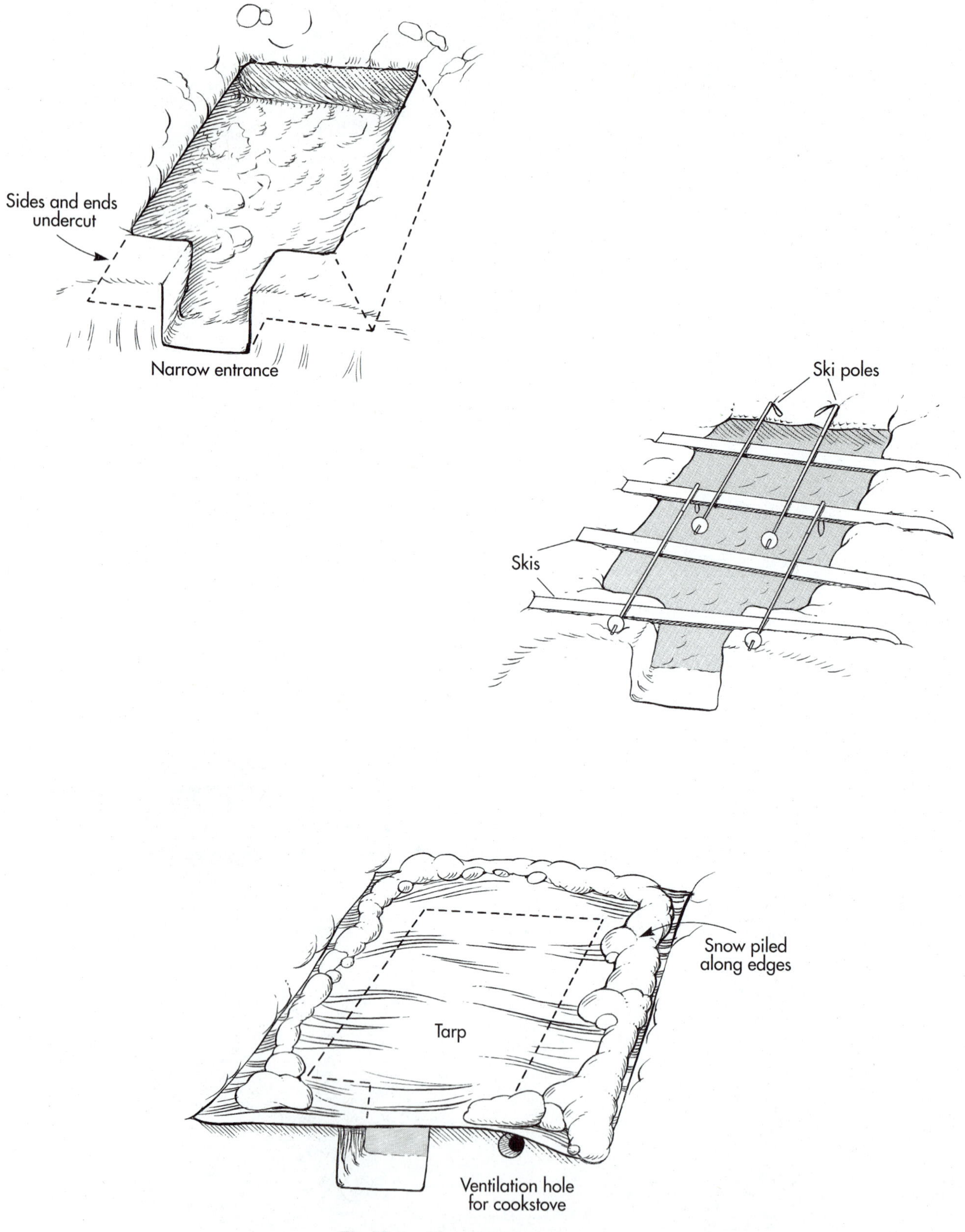

Sides and ends undercut
Narrow entrance
Ski poles
Skis
Snow piled along edges
Tarp
Ventilation hole for cookstove

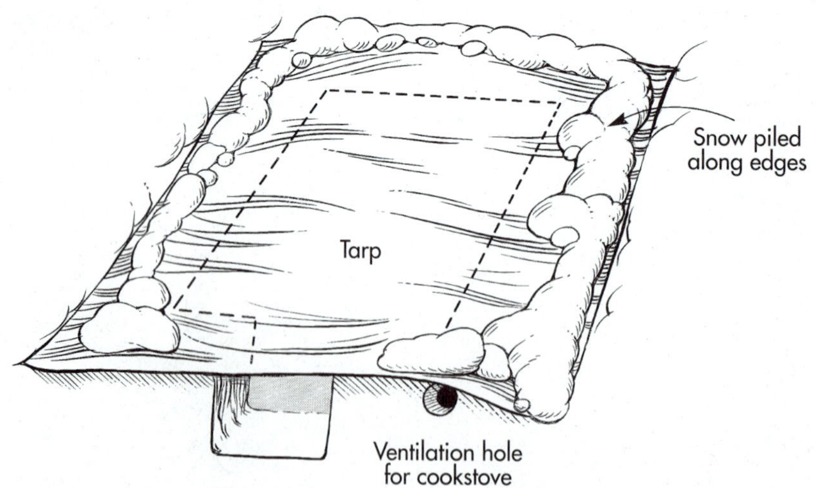

Fig. 15-6 Three-person snow trench.

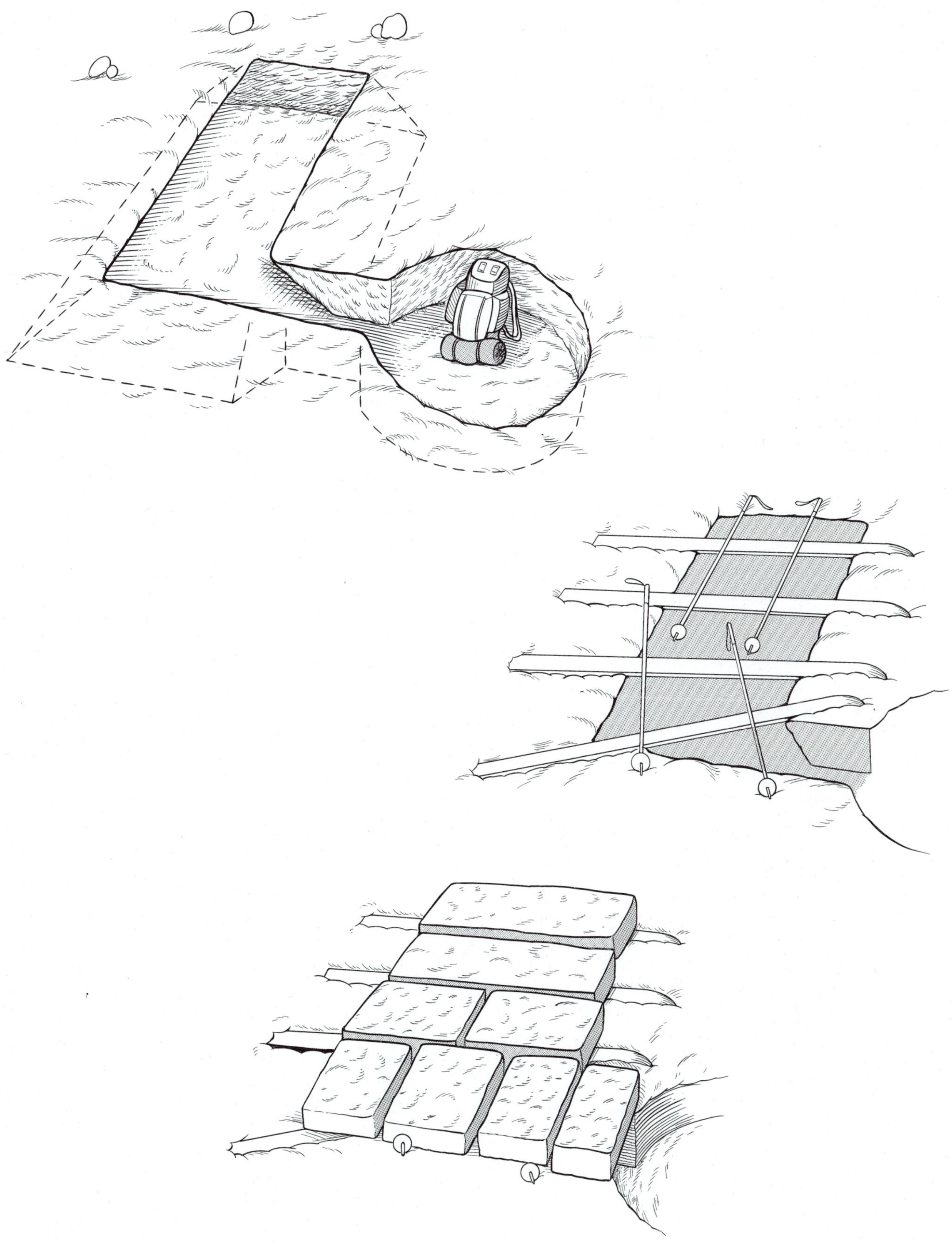

Fig. 15-7 Above-timberline snow trench.

person. Floor mats and upholstery can be used for insulation, but it is much better to have a vehicle survival kit containing extra clothing and blankets (see Appendix D).

Automobiles[18]

In cold weather, drivers should keep their vehicles in the best possible mechanical condition, using winter-grade or 10/40 grade oil, the proper amount of radiator antifreeze, and deicer fluid for the fuel tank. Snow tires, preferably studded (illegal in some states), are desirable, but chains should be carried as well. Four-wheel drive is optimal, and front-wheel drive superior to rear-wheel drive. The battery should be kept charged, the exhaust system free of leaks, and the gas tank full. A citizen's band radio is useful. The marooned driver should tie a brightly colored piece of cloth to the antenna and at night should leave the inside dome light on to be seen by snowplows and rescuers (headlights use too much current). If necessary for heat, the motor and heater can be run for 20 minutes of each hour (after checking to see if the exhaust pipe is free of snow). To avoid carbon monoxide poisoning, a downwind window should be kept cracked 1 to 2 inches. Reusable carbon monoxide detectors are available and can be carried in the survival kit. One or two large candles should be carried to provide heat and light if the gasoline supply runs out. Two candles can raise the interior temperature well above freezing.

Airplanes

Airplane fuselages are poorly insulated. Unless a stove or other heating device is available, survivors are usually better off constructing a shelter that can be more easily heated, outside but near the aircraft. Batteries and cigarette lighters can be used as fire starters, with oil and gasoline as fuel (see below).

ADDITION OF HEAT FROM THE OUTSIDE

Fire Building

The ability to build a fire under adverse conditions is an essential skill that should be practiced by persons who engage in outdoors activities (Fig. 15-8). Necessary equipment includes a sturdy knife, a candle, and waterproof matches. In addition, a tube of chemical fire starter (available in most outdoor stores) is highly recommended, especially for wet climates.

To burn, a fire needs air, but not too much air. The fire site should be out of the wind behind a rock or log, or in a snow pit. If the fire is built on bare ground, all burnable material such as moss and grass should be cleaned off by scraping the ground surface down to mineral soil over an area at least 3 feet in diameter. If snow is too deep to be removed down to bare ground, the fire should be built on a platform of green logs.

Building a fire requires three types of combustible material: tinder, kindling, and fuel. Tinder is any type of finely divided, highly flammable material. It must be dry. Examples include grass and leaves, inner bark of birch trees, shavings from dry sticks, cotton balls, small sticks, and fine grades of steel wool. The easiest available natural material is "squaw wood"—small dry twigs on the lower, dead branches of evergreens. The wet, outer wood of small branches can be shaved off or they can be split lengthwise into several thinner lengths with a knife to expose the dry core. The tinder is arranged in lean-to form by placing it against a larger branch, smallest sticks on the bottom and larger ones on top, separated just enough so that air can reach each piece. To conserve matches, one match should be used to light a candle or segment of fire starter, which in turn lights the tinder. The flame should be placed under the middle of the lean-to of tinder so that lower pieces will set fire to higher pieces.

Kindling is larger material, usually larger pieces of squaw wood or larger branches that have been split lengthwise with a knife. Once the tinder is burning well, these larger pieces of dry wood are added.

Fuel is the largest material, usually branches and trunks of dead trees several inches or more in diameter. These should be split if an ax is available. Standing dead wood is preferable to wood lying on the ground, and wood that has lost its bark to wood with bark, because both will be drier and less rotten than their alternatives. Fuel is added after the kindling is burning well.

Several times as much fuel should be collected as will be needed. When dead branches are gathered, only those that snap loudly when broken off should be selected. If no ax or saw is available, the fire can be built next to a large, downed log, which may catch and burn for several days. Long, dead sections of trees can be shortened by laying them across a fire so that when they burn through, two shorter sections result. Fires generally should be kept small, both to conserve wood and to allow them to be approached closely.

A fire can be started without matches by using an automobile cigarette lighter, or batteries and steel wool. A "wire" can be made by twisting and pulling out a fine-grade (such as 4-0) steel wool. This will catch fire if the ends are touched to the positive and negative terminals of two fresh C or D batteries in tandem. A fire starter can be made by stripping the insulation from the middle of a wire and wrapping the bare portion 7 to 10 times around a dry stick. If the two ends of the wire are touched to the terminals of an automobile battery, the wire will become red hot and the stick will ignite (the wire should be long enough that the flame is not close to the battery, where it could ignite hydrogen gas produced by the battery).

When scraped hard with a file or knife blade, commercial "metal matches" made of magnesium will produce showers of sparks that will ignite tinder such as fine steel wool, cotton, or very small dry shavings. Oil or gasoline can be used as fuel if poured over a container full of dirt or sand.

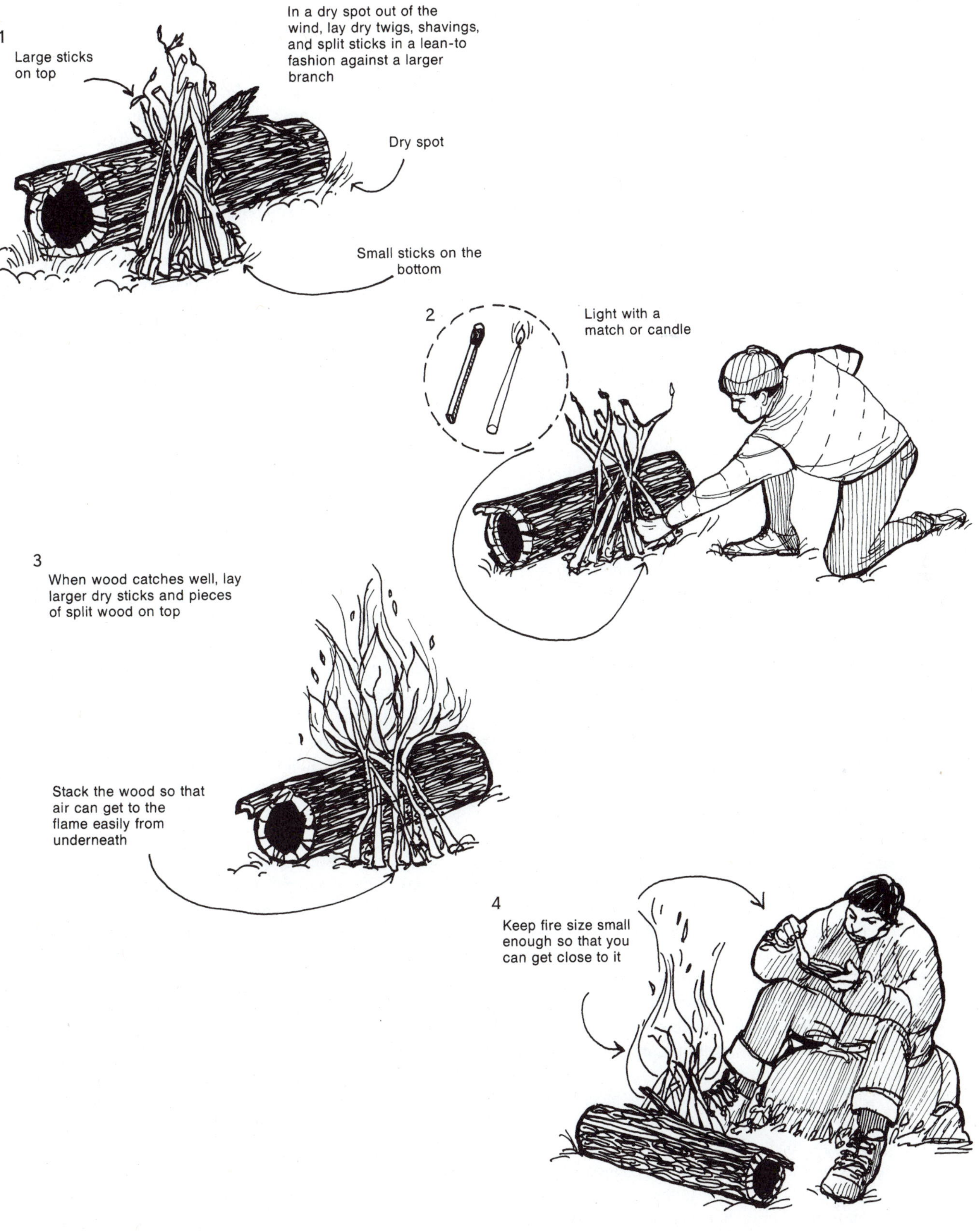
1
Large sticks on top
In a dry spot out of the wind, lay dry twigs, shavings, and split sticks in a lean-to fashion against a larger branch
Dry spot
Small sticks on the bottom
2
Light with a match or candle
3
When wood catches well, lay larger dry sticks and pieces of split wood on top
Stack the wood so that air can get to the flame easily from underneath
4
Keep fire size small enough so that you can get close to it
PIZINGER

Fig. 15-8 Building a fire.

FOOD

The human body requires a daily supply of calories, carbohydrate, protein, fat, minerals, and vitamins. Carbohydrates supply calories and are essential for replacement of muscle glycogen. If diet is inadequate, body stores of fat and protein will be depleted to provide calories. A moderately active 70 kg male normally requires the food equivalent of 2800 kcal/day, but if exercising in cold weather he may require more than twice this amount. Protein intake should be at least 65 g/day and carbohydrates should make up 60% to 70% of the diet.

Although most persons in a survival situation worry more about food than anything else, food is usually less important than shelter or water because a person can survive for weeks without food, even in cold weather. However, there must be enough water and energy expenditure must be kept to a minimum. Most ski mountaineering or climbing parties carry adequate supplies of food; problems arise if food is exhausted, lost, or contaminated. Bare ridges, high mountains above timberline, and dense evergreen forests are difficult places to find wild food, even in summer. Success is more likely on river and stream banks, on lake shores, in margins of forests, and in natural clearings. Since in most cases the amount of wild food found by an untrained individual will not provide enough calories to replenish the energy expended in searching for it, it is important *always to carry extra food for emergencies.*

Here are a few general rules about wilderness edibles. However, there are many exceptions to them; no unfamiliar wild food should be eaten except in extreme circumstances.[6,9,15] For detailed discussions of poisonous plants and mushrooms, see Chapters 37 and 38.

1. All wild foods except fruits and berries should be cooked. This will make them more palatable, more digestible, and safer to eat.
2. Persons in the outdoors should know the edible plants and animals of their own familiar areas. Similar lifeforms are often found in other similar areas.
3. Plants to avoid include mushrooms, buttercups, bulbs, plants with umbrella-shaped flowers, wild beans and peas, all unknown berries except blue and black ones, and all plants with milky or colored sap or shiny leaves. Compound berries (such as raspberries and blackberries) are safe to eat.
4. No one should eat large quantities of a strange plant food without first testing it.[15]
   a. Touch the plant's sap or juice to the inner forearm or tip of the tongue.
   b. If there are no ill effects, boil plant parts in two changes of water, 5 minutes per change. Place 1 teaspoonful of the product in the mouth for 5 minutes and chew but do not swallow it. If a burning, nauseating, or bitter taste results, immediately spit it out. If no unpleasant effect occurs, swallow it and wait 8 hours.
   c. If after 8 hours there are no ill effects, such as nausea, cramps, or diarrhea, eat 2 tablespoonfuls and wait an additional 8 hours.
   d. If no ill effects occur at the end of this period, consider the plant edible.
5. All land mammals, birds, and birds' eggs can be eaten. The entire carcass, both fat and lean, should be eaten, except for seal and polar bear livers. Crustaceans, mollusks, insects, some amphibians (except for toads), and reptiles can be eaten. Salamanders and frogs should be skinned. Fish, crustaceans, and mollusks should be eaten promptly because they spoil quickly. Fish and meat can be preserved by drying. Black mussels, Pacific reef fish, "puffers," and any fish that looks "ugly" should be avoided (see Chapter 53).
6. Edible parts of wild plants may include roots, leaves (especially young leaves), stems (usually require peeling), shoots, buds, grass seeds, inner bark (aspen, cottonwood, birch, willow, lodgepole pine, and Scotch pine), nuts, and berries (except as noted in 3 above).

Animal Food[6,9-11,14,15]

Mammals and birds can be trapped, snared, or shot. Some, such as spruce hens and porcupines, can be clubbed. Fish can be hooked, speared, or trapped. However, to secure this type of food, the hunter must locate the animal. On land this can be done by searching for signs such as trails, droppings, burrows, dens, and bedding areas. Carnivore dung usually contains hair and bone; herbivore dung has indigestible plant parts. Trails lead to feeding and watering places. Successful hunting requires patience, skill at stalking, and knowledge of animal behavior. The best times to hunt are at dawn and dusk as animals are moving to or from their bedding areas.

Small animals can be snared or trapped, which may be more efficient than physically hunting them on foot. Snares should be baited or located on a game trail at a place where the animal has no choice but to enter the snare. This can be a naturally narrow area or one that is prepared. Snare loops can be made from any type of bare wire or improvised from strips of green bark, cord, shoelaces, or clothing strips, but light, strong wire such as 28-gauge piano wire is best. A small loop is tied at one end of the wire, and the main loop is made by feeding the other end through the small loop (Fig. 15-9, *A*). The main loop is adjusted to catch the animal around the neck and to fit the expected size of the prey. Snares using loops are effective because the animal almost always lunges forward, tightening the loop around its neck. Some type of locking device[15] should be included to prevent a wire loop from loosening after the animal is in it (Fig. 15-9, *B*). Snares should be set at midday when animals are bedded down. The person should approach the area at a 90-degree angle to the trail, set the snare, and back away. He or

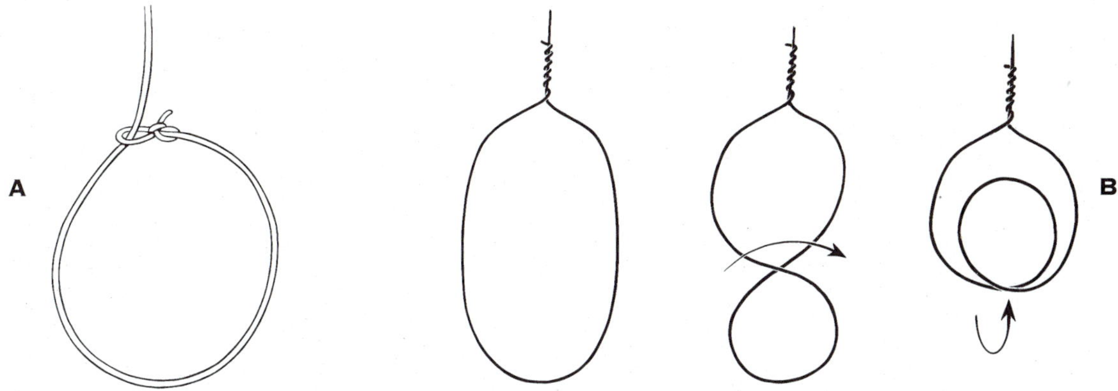

Fig. 15-9 Snare loop. **A,** Simple snare loop. **B,** Locking device for a wire snare loop.

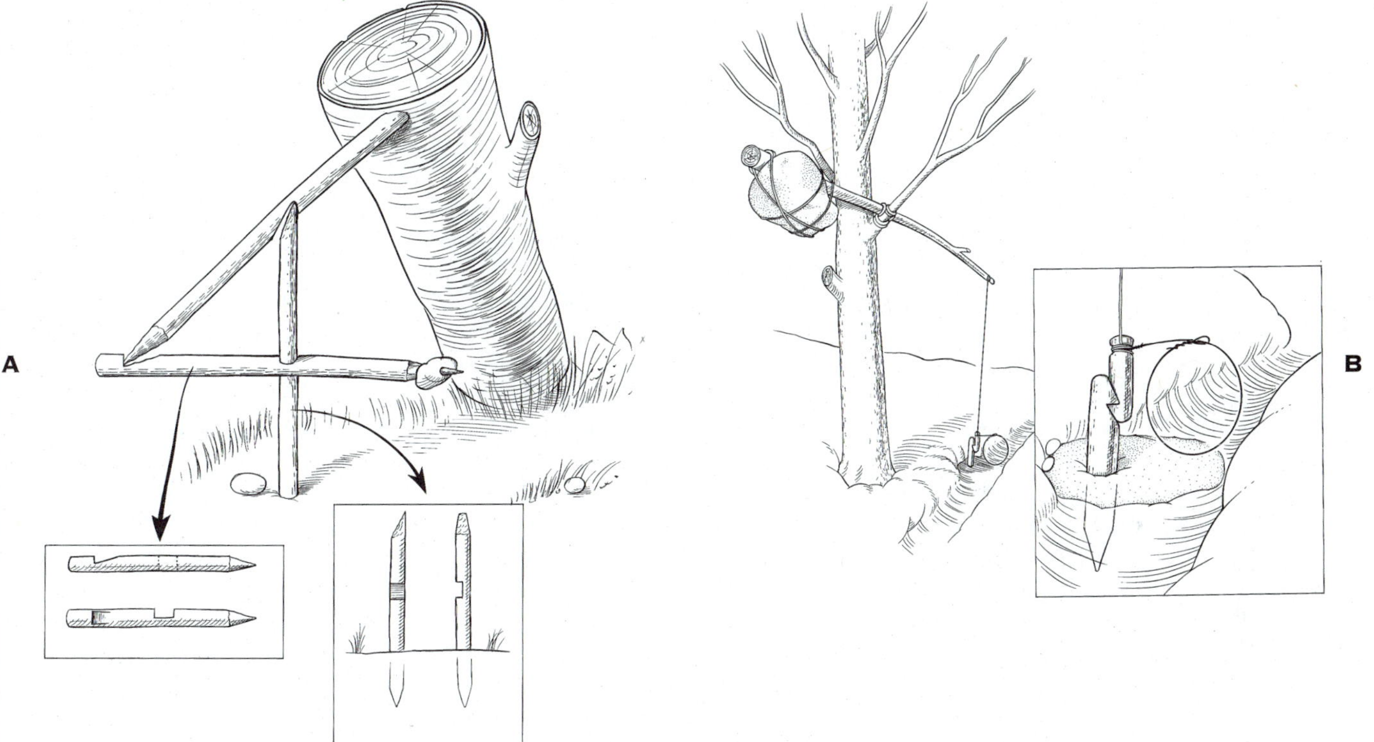

Fig. 15-10 **A,** Figure-4 deadfall. **B,** Twitch-up snare.

she should keep downwind from the expected location of the animal and not walk on the game trail. Natural surroundings should be disturbed as little as possible. Snares and traps should be checked twice daily.

Many different types of snares have been invented; some are simple loops, but most include a trigger arrangement that releases when disturbed by the animal's movement and allows a counterweight to pin the animal or a bent sapling to straighten and hoist it off the ground (Fig. 15-10). Snares can also be set at the mouths of dens and burrows. In general, one animal is caught for every 15 snares set.

Birds can be caught with baited fishhooks or snares.

Fish can be secured with hook and line, traps, and spears. Emergency survival kits should contain several hooks and a long length of line. Insects, smaller fish, worms, shellfish, or meat can be used as bait, or lures can be improvised from pieces of brightly colored cloth, feathers, or bits of shiny metal. In open streams the best places to fish are pools below falls and behind rocks. Locating fish is more difficult in the winter when they retreat into the deep part of lakes. However, holes can be cut in the ice of frozen lakes. The best time to fish is early morning or late evening. An effective fish spear is the split-shaft type (Fig. 15-11, *A*). A

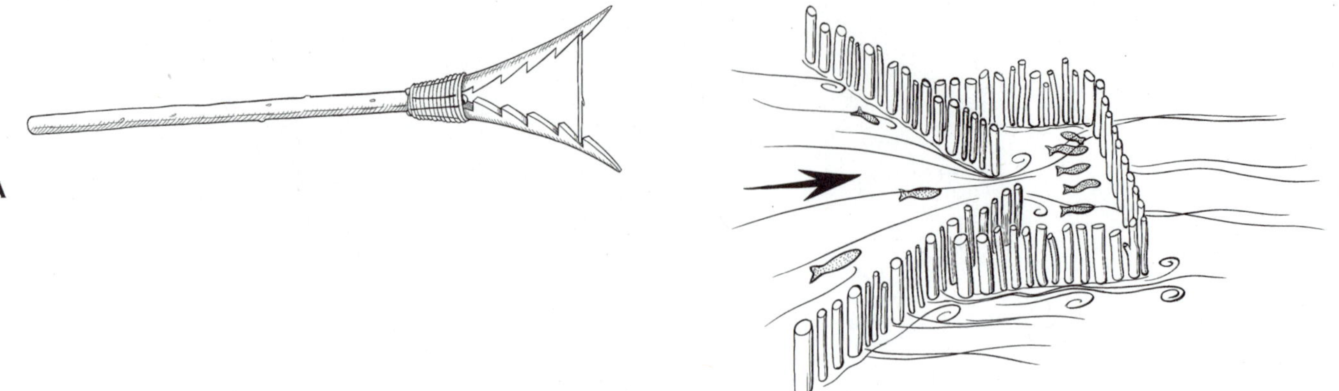

Fig. 15-11 **A,** Split-shaft fish spear. **B,** Fish trap.

spear works best if it is used to pin a fish against the bottom or bank so the fish can be grasped with the hands before it works loose.

In streams, fish traps can be made by using rocks or vertical willow branches to build an enclosure with a funnel-shaped opening whose narrow end extends well into the enclosure (Fig. 15-11, *B*). It should be located so that the current drives fish into the wide end of the funnel. Another type of trap can be made by tying the neck and sleeves of a T-shirt closed, placing the shirt with the tail propped open in the water at the downstream end of a pool where fish have been seen, and chasing the fish into the shirt.

Another way to catch large fish (at least 10 inches long) is by "tickling." This involves crawling slowly upstream along a stream bank, feeling underneath the bank and under nearby logs for fish. They usually lie still with their heads upstream. If a fish is felt, the hand can slowly move forward, grasp the fish at the gills, and flip it onto the bank.[10] "Tickling" fish and constructing and using fish traps are obviously difficult in winter when streams are snow covered and the ability to work in water or on snowy stream banks is limited because of the cold and the consequences of becoming wet.

Plant Food[6,9-11,14,15]

Edible plants (Fig. 15-12) are common in mountain meadows and even in forests, although considerable energy may be needed to dig up or gather plant material. This is especially true during the winter months, when gathering roots and berries may require removing snow from large areas and digging in frozen ground. Pine cones can be picked from trees. Single leaf, sugar, limber, whitebark, pinon, and Coulter pine cones contain edible nuts. The plant gatherer should look for unopened cones, scorch them over a fire to partially burn off the pitch, and split them by pounding with a rock. The nuts are removed and roasted. Acorns are another good source of food; they should be boiled for an hour with three changes of water to remove the bitter tannic acid. Cattails and arrowheads can be found in low-lying, marshy areas and lakeshores. In spring the sheathed top spike of the cattail can be boiled and eaten and the sprouts can be eaten raw. Pollen from the blooming flower spike can be used like flour. The roots are fibrous but contain much starchy material and can be boiled or roasted. Arrowhead tubers can be boiled or roasted for 30 minutes and eaten after peeling.

Dandelions, wooly louseworts, wild onions, elk thistle, and bistort can sometimes be found under the snow in mountain meadows. The roots of all these plants are edible and nourishing but should be boiled. However, since many bulbs are poisonous, only those that have an onion odor should be eaten. The young leaves and shoots of ferns can be boiled and eaten, and the leaves of mountain sorrel can be eaten raw. Wild rose hips are edible. Elk thistle stems are edible if peeled and boiled. Dandelion leaves can be eaten after boiling in several changes of water to remove the bitter taste. The inner bark of aspen, cottonwood, birch, willow, lodgepole pine, and Scotch pine is edible.

Berries such as huckleberries, raspberries, crowberries, cranberries, bearberries (kinickinnick), salmonberries, and thimbleberries can sometimes be found under or over the snow and are edible (Fig. 15-13).

Certain types of lichen can be eaten. Iceland moss should be boiled for an hour, reindeer moss boiled or roasted, and rock tripe dried and then boiled.

WATER

Water comprises about 60% of the body weight of an average young adult male; the value for a female is slightly lower. The percentage of water tends to decrease with age. Daily water loss includes about 1200 ml of urine, 1000 ml through the skin and lungs, and 300 ml in the stool. Since about 700 ml of water is produced daily by metabolism of food, a minimum daily intake of 1800 ml is necessary in a temperate climate at sea level to avoid dehydration. In a hot, dry climate, at high altitude, or with exertion, insensible losses and sweating increase considerably. Up to 2 L/hr can

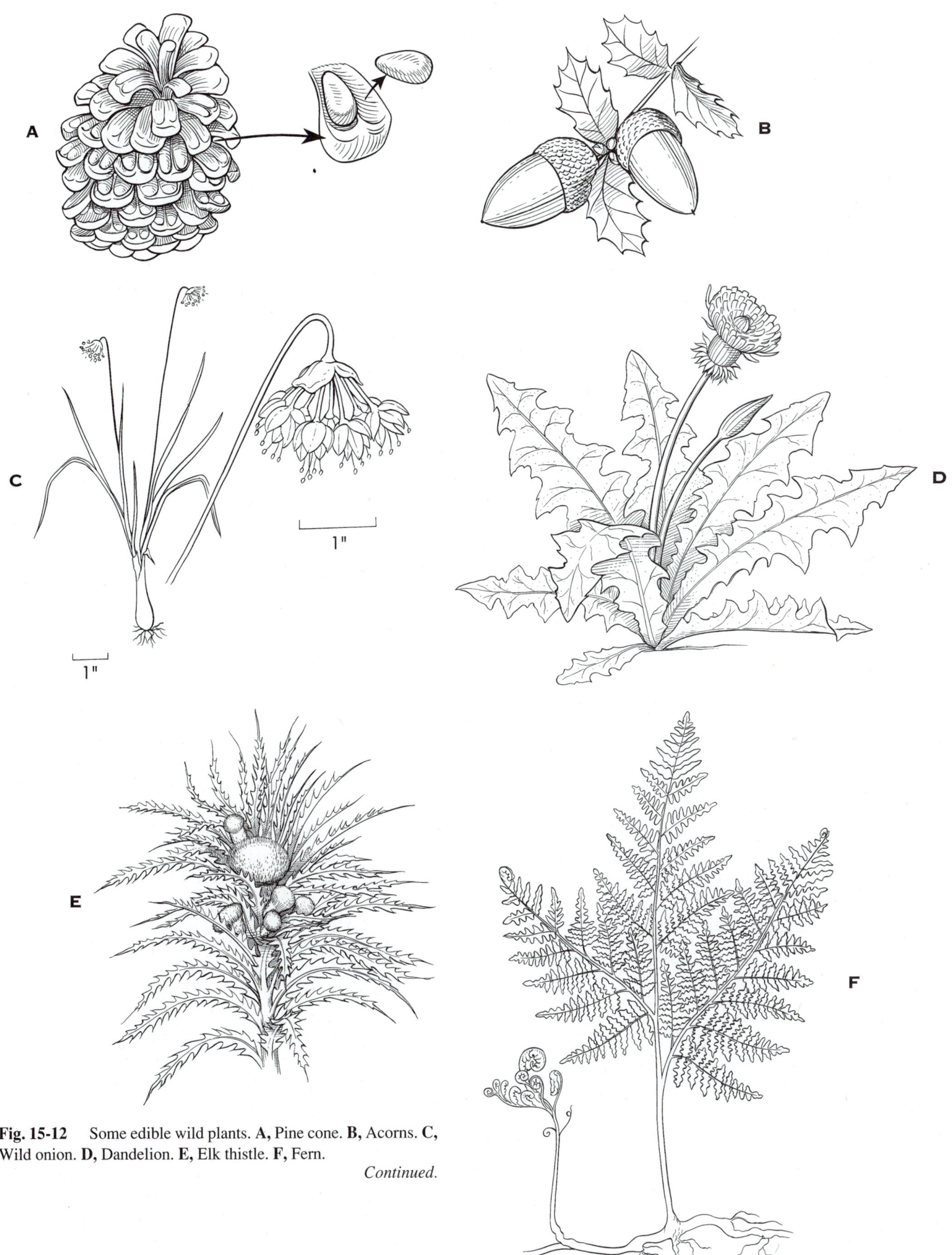

Fig. 15-12 Some edible wild plants. **A,** Pine cone. **B,** Acorns. **C,** Wild onion. **D,** Dandelion. **E,** Elk thistle. **F,** Fern.

Continued.

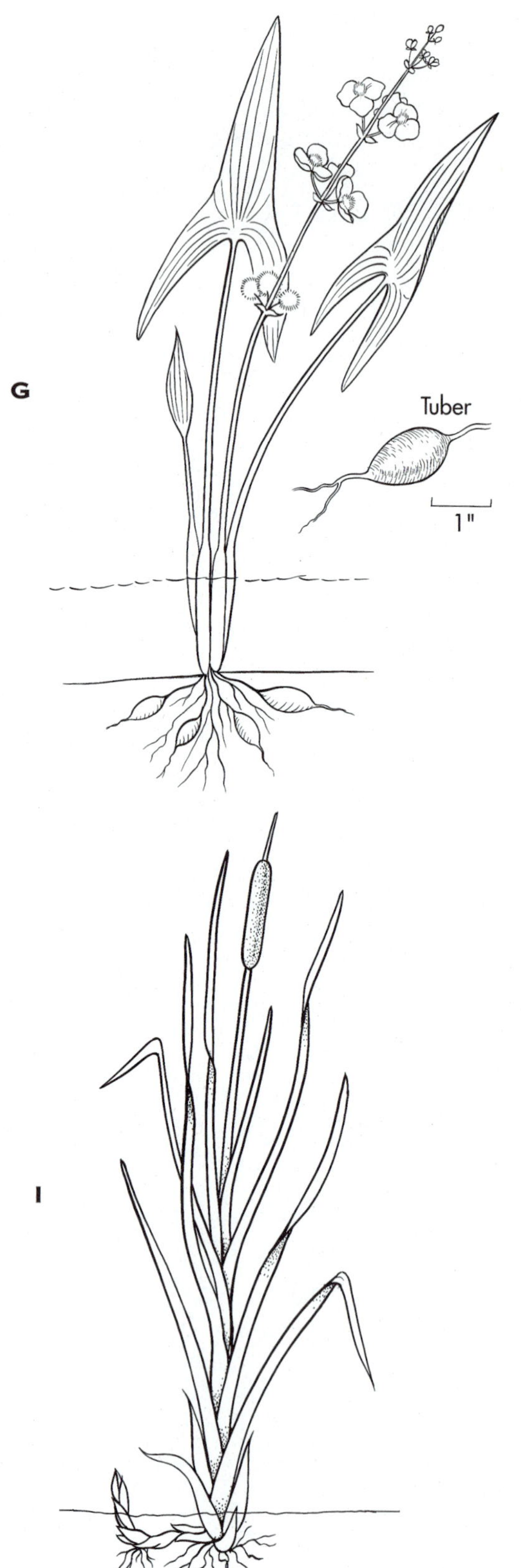

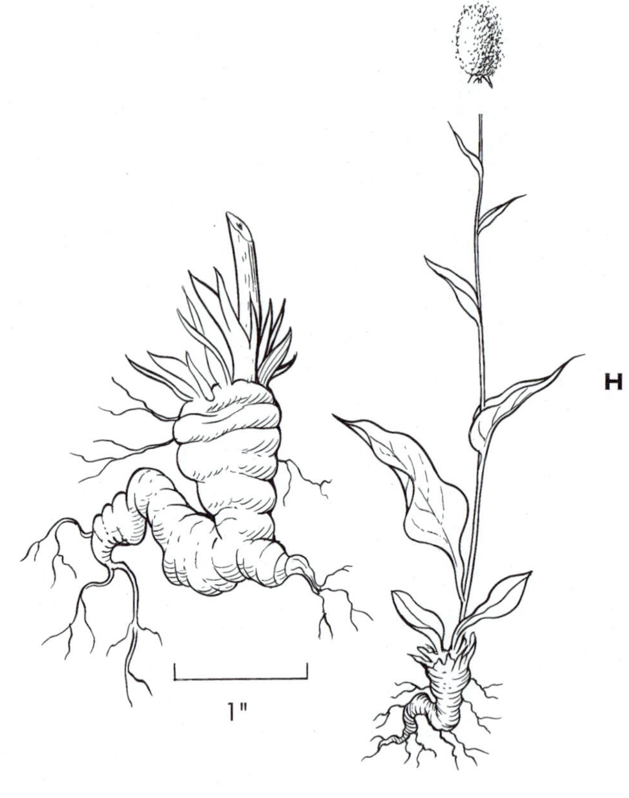

Fig. 15-12, cont'd. G, Arrowhead. **H,** Bistort. **I,** Cattail.

be lost during very hard exercise such as Nordic ski racing. In cold weather thirst is decreased, so that an individual may not replace fluids adequately. At subfreezing temperatures and in locations above the snow line the lack of liquid water and the effort and fuel required to melt snow compound the problem. Almost all surface water should be considered contaminated by animal or human wastes, with the possible exception of small streams descending from untracked snowfields or high, uninhabited areas. At altitudes below 18,000 feet (5488 m), simply bringing water to a boil will kill *Giardia* cysts and most harmful bacteria and viruses. Water can also be disinfected by filtration or addition of chemicals (see Chapter 43).

Active efforts must be made to prevent fluid deficit. Whenever open water is encountered, individuals should drink heartily and fill all empty canteens. Each morning enough snow should be melted to provide everyone with at least a canteenful for the day. At night, no one should go to bed thirsty. Melting ice or hard snow is more efficient than melting light, powdery snow. On warm, sunny days, snow can be spread on a dark plastic sheet to melt.

At high altitudes at least 3 L of water a day should be provided for each person. If intake is adequate, 1 to 1.5 L of light-colored urine is excreted per day. Adding fruit flavors or making hot drinks improves the palatability of water. Electrolyte drinks and salt tablets are generally unnecessary in cold weather, since the electrolytes lost in sweat are easily replaced by a normal diet. When fuel is exhausted and

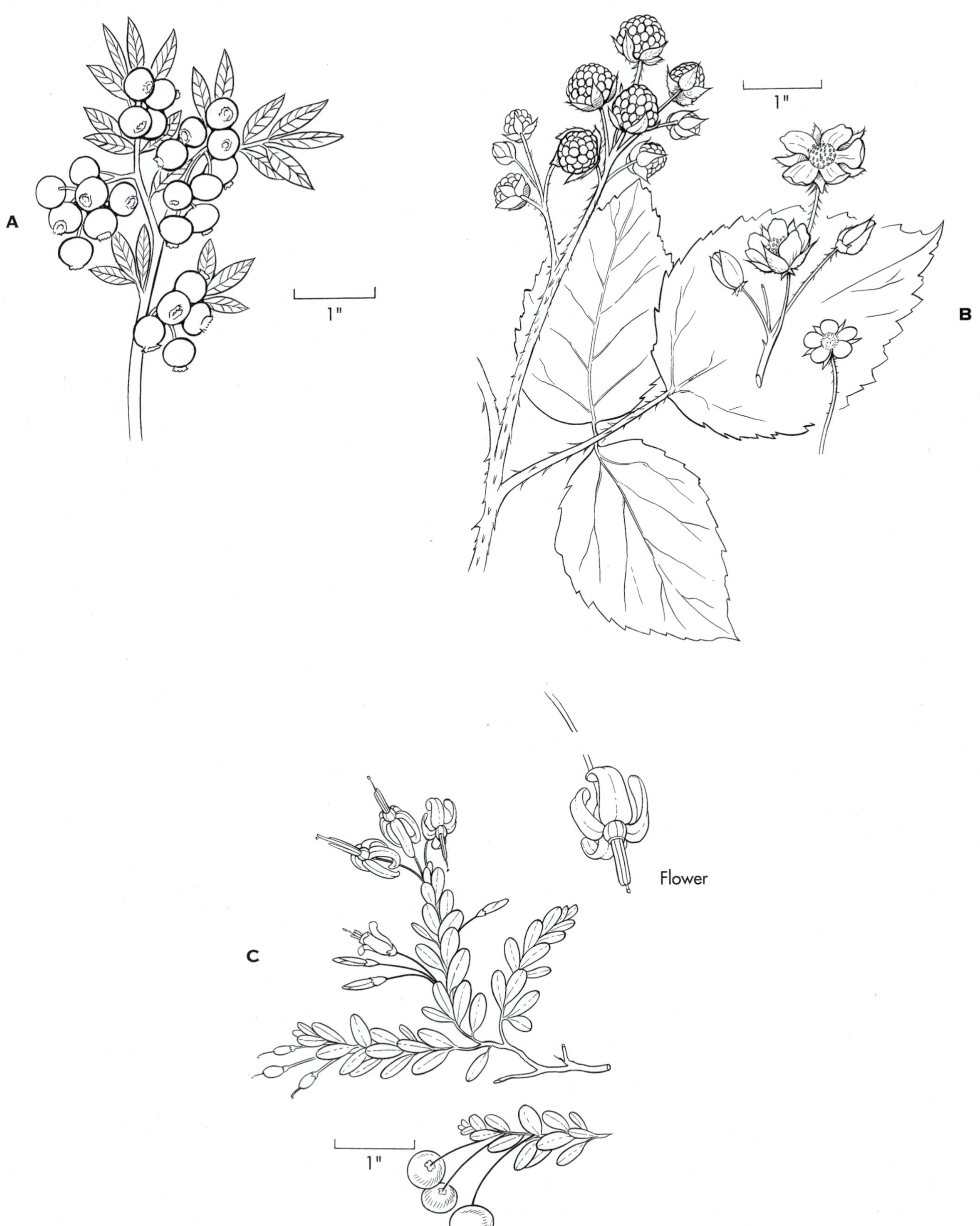

Fig. 15-13 Some edible berries. **A,** Blueberry. **B,** Blackberry. **C,** Cranberry.
Continued.

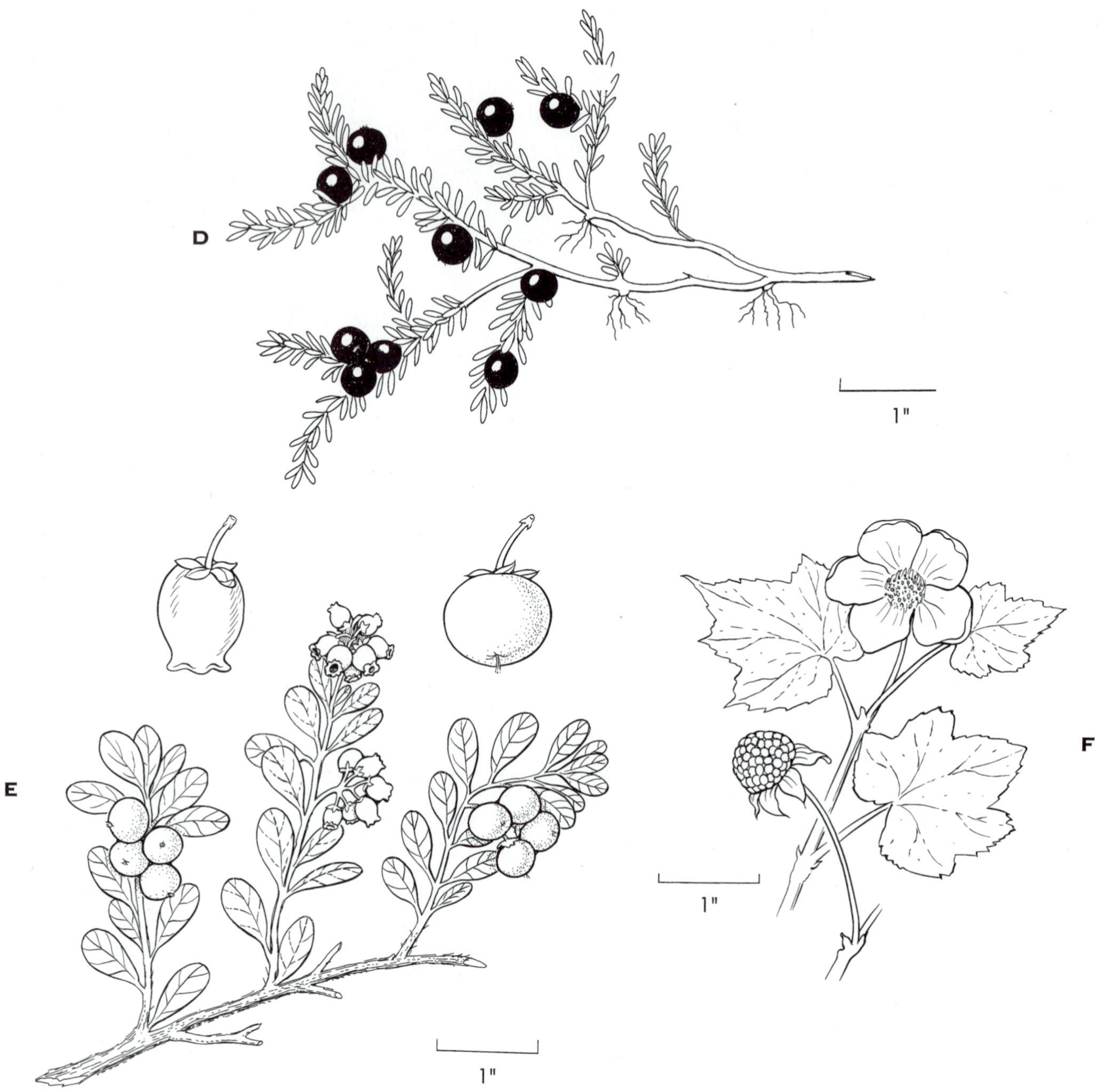

Fig. 15-13, cont'd. **D,** Crowberry. **E,** Bearberry. **F,** Salmonberry.

snow must be melted, trekkers must descend below the timberline to find open water or wood for fuel. When water supplies are limited, overexertion should be avoided ("ration your sweat").

EMERGENCY OVERSNOW TRAVEL

Oversnow travel in deep snow is almost impossible without skis or snowshoes. Even though travel per se may be unwise, wilderness foot travelers should know how to improvise snowshoes from natural materials if they are stranded by a late or early season snowstorm. Emergency snowshoes (Fig. 15-14, *A*) can be made from poles that are 6 feet long, ¾ to 1 inch thick at the base, and ¼ inch thick at the tip and sticks that are ¾ to 1 inch thick and 10 inches long.[2] Twelve long poles and 12 short sticks are needed. For each snowshoe, the six long poles are placed side by side on the ground and the middle point of the poles is marked. One short stick is lashed crosswise to the tail (base) of the poles, and three short sticks are lashed side by side just forward of the center of the poles where the toe of the boot will rest. Two sticks are lashed where the heel of the boot will strike the snowshoe. The tips of the six poles are tied together. Each binding (Fig.

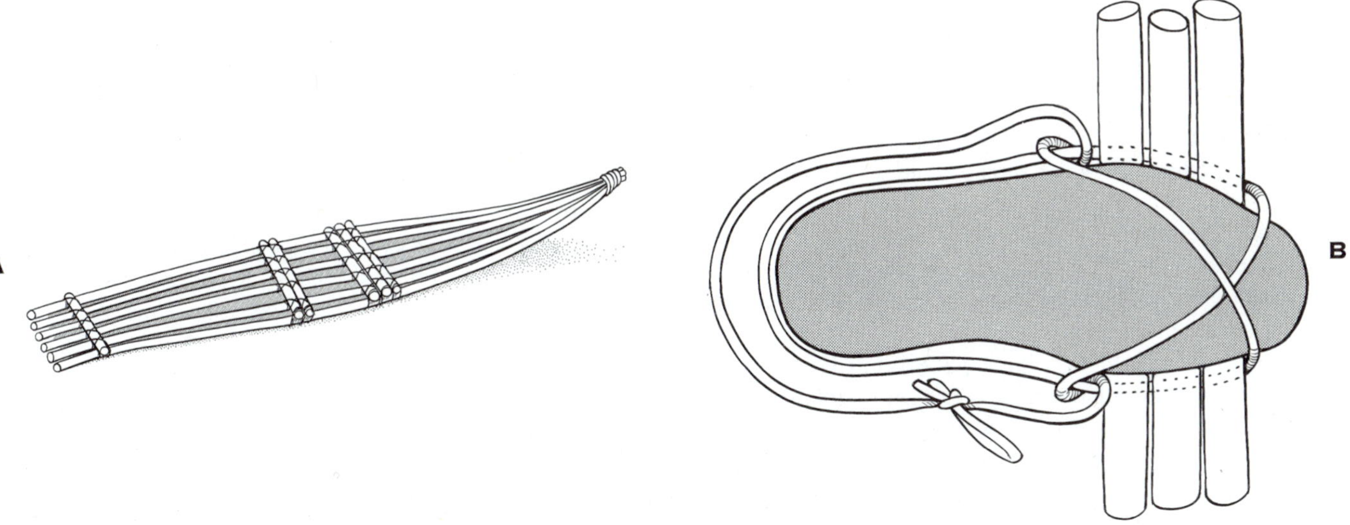

Fig. 15-14 **A,** Emergency snowshoe. **B,** Detail of snowshoe binding.

15-14, *B*) is made of a continuous length (about 6 feet) of nylon cord, preferably braided, since it will eventually fray. The midpoint of the cord is positioned at the back of the boot above the bulge of the heel. Each end of the cord is run under the three side-by-side short sticks at the side of the boot, then up and across the boot toe so that it crosses the other end on top of the toe, forming an X. Then each end is looped around the cord running along the opposite side of the boot and the ends are brought around the back of the boot heel. The cord is pulled tight around the boot and the ends are tied together at the lateral side of the heel.

On walking, the tip of the snowshoe should rise, the boot heel should rise, and the boot sole should remain on the snowshoe.

Hot Weather Survival

Environmental conditions predisposing to serious heat stress can be found in most temperate zone regions during the summer months and in the tropics the year round. The amount of heat stress is proportional to both temperature and relative humidity, so that a tropical jungle environment with a relatively lower temperature and higher humidity can be just as dangerous as a drier desert environment with a relatively higher temperature. Serious heat illness occurs when endogenous heat production plus exogenous heat gain forces the core temperature to dangerous levels (more than 104° to 105° F [40° to 46° C]) despite the body's cooling mechanisms. These mechanisms include involuntary cutaneous vasodilation and sweating, plus voluntary mechanisms such as seeking shelter from the sun, avoiding excess insulation and heat-producing physical activity, and replacing lost fluids and electrolytes. For a detailed discussion of heat illness, refer to Chapter 8.

The body adapts better to heat and altitude than to cold. It acclimatizes to heat by increasing the blood volume, dilating skin blood vessels, and improving cardiac efficiency so as to carry more heat from the body core to the shell. The process of acclimatization takes about 10 days, during which the subject starts to perspire at a lower temperature, the volume of perspiration increases, and the perspiration contains fewer electrolytes.

The following discussion emphasizes survival in a desert environment; for jungle survival suggestions, see Chapter 16.

PRACTICAL METHODS FOR ADJUSTING TO HOT WEATHER[3]

Heat loss by conduction, convection, and radiation can be increased by exposing the maximum amount of skin to the circulating air. This should be done only when in the shade; when in the sun, skin should be completely protected by clothing. Because heat loss and sweating may be impaired by sunscreens, a good compromise is to cover the face and hands with a sunscreen with a high sun protection factor (SPF) number (see Chapter 12) and wear a long-sleeved shirt and long trousers of tightly woven, loose-fitting, light-colored (preferably white) cotton. If desired, ventilation holes can be cut at the axillae and groin. Hydration is maintained by drinking adequate fluids, some of which can contain electrolyte supplements. Optimal hydration maintains blood volume and shell circulation and supports the sweating mechanism. Enough water *must* be carried or be available in the field. Water bottles should be wrapped with clothing to insulate them and buried in the backpack.

The layer principle of clothing is recommended, especially in the desert. Layers can be taken off during the heat of the day and added at night when the dry desert air cools rapidly. Since high winds and sandstorms occur frequently in desert areas, a wind-resistant parka and pants are necessary; since rainstorms occasionally occur as well, the garments should also be water repellent.

Because of its high thermal conductivity, poor insulating ability, and good wicking ability, cotton—which is avoided in cold weather—is probably the fabric of choice for hot weather clothing. Clothing should be loose to improve air circulation.

Before exposure to prolonged or strenuous hot weather exertion, individuals should allow time for acclimatization.

Heat gain from the environment can be minimized by using clothing to protect the head and body from the direct rays of the sun. A hat with a wide brim or a Foreign Legion–style cap with a neck protector and ventilation holes in the crown is recommended. A neck protector can be improvised from a T-shirt or bandanna.

Travelers should seek shelter during the hottest part of the day. Caves and overhangs can be used, but gulleys and other dry watercourses should be avoided because of the danger of flash floods. A sun shelter can be made by suspending a tarp from brush or cacti or by laying the tarp on a framework of poles. Travelers who become stranded in a vehicle should lie *under* it. Because desert air is much cooler a foot above or a few inches below the ground surface, the desert traveler should lie on a platform or in a scooped-out depression rather than directly on the ground.

Direct contact with the hot ground and other hot objects, particularly hot metal, should be avoided. Sturdy hiking or climbing boots should be worn to protect the feet, not only from the hot ground but also from sharp rocks, the spines of cacti, and snakes. Gaiters should be worn or improvised from strips of cloth to keep sand and insects out of boots and socks. The hands should be protected with leather gloves. Rest periods should be taken in the shade rather than in the direct sun. High-quality sunglasses should be used to protect the eyes; sunglasses can be improvised from a piece of cardboard or wood with a slit cut for each eye.

Body heat production can be minimized by avoiding muscular exertion during periods of high heat and humidity. Traveling should be done only early in the morning, late in the evening, or at night.

DESERT SURVIVAL[6,9,11,14,15]

About 20% of the earth's land surface is made up of desert. Desert areas average less than 10 inches (25.4 cm) of rainfall annually. Deserts range from barren sand or gravel plains without a living plant for a hundred miles to areas of grass and thorny bushes that can support camels and goats. Despite lack of moisture, many kinds of plants and animals have adapted to the hot, arid environment and are able to thrive in many deserts.

Deserts heat up rapidly during the day, but because of low humidity and the low specific heat of the ground they cool rapidly at night. Daily temperature extremes may range as widely as 45° F (21° C). These temperature changes produce alternate expansion and contraction of rocks, causing them to break up into smaller and smaller fragments and eventually to form gravel or sand. Lack of rainfall reduces the eroding effect of water, so that wind and windborne sand are the most important agents of erosion. When the rare rains occur, water tends to run off rather than sink into the ground. Thus flash floods may occur and dry water courses (arroyos, wadis, or dry washes) are familiar landscape features. Sudden weather changes are common; desert travelers in the fall, winter, and spring should be prepared for cold as well as hot weather. Dust storms and strong solar glare can be hazardous.

Southerly deserts may be hot all year round, whereas northern ones may have four recognizable seasons. The hottest recorded desert temperatures have been 134.4° F in the Sahara at Azizia and 134° F in Death Valley, California.[9] The ground can become so hot that feet may be burned through shoes, and serious burns can result from touching exposed metal. Desert plants have developed special characteristics that enable them to conserve water and survive long periods of drought. Some have extensive root systems that quickly absorb rainfall moisture, while others have exceptionally long roots that reach down to the water table. Many plants are dormant during the hottest season; others have thick external coverings that resist evaporative losses. Still others are able to store water during wet seasons to allow survival through dry periods. Desert animals forage and hunt during the cool of the evening and night, and rest in cool places during the day.

Food

Food is difficult to obtain in true deserts but is less important than water. A survivor can live several weeks without food if water is available. There is more natural food available in the deserts of the American southwest than in Old World deserts such as the Sahara and Gobi (Fig. 15-15). No plant with milky juice should be eaten. All cactus fruits are edible, and the leaves of flat-leaved cacti (such as the prickly pear) can be peeled and eaten, preferably after boiling. Wild cherries, wild celery, wild currants, wild onions, acacia beans, and pinon nuts are found in some areas. Grass seeds and the soft part of grass stalks are edible. Kangaroo rats, jeroboas, rabbits, prairie dogs, lizards, tortoises, snakes, and insects, particularly locusts, are all edible. Small mammals and birds can be trapped or snared as described previously. If firearms are available, larger animals such as antelope, deer, foxes, and badgers can be procured and leftover meat dried in the sun.[9,14,15] If water is limited, however, it is wise to base the diet on carbohydrate rather than protein, since more water is required to excrete the waste products of protein in the urine.

Water

There is no substitute for water in the desert, although a person can prolong life in a survival situation by decreasing water loss. Waterholes and oases are rare in deserts. They

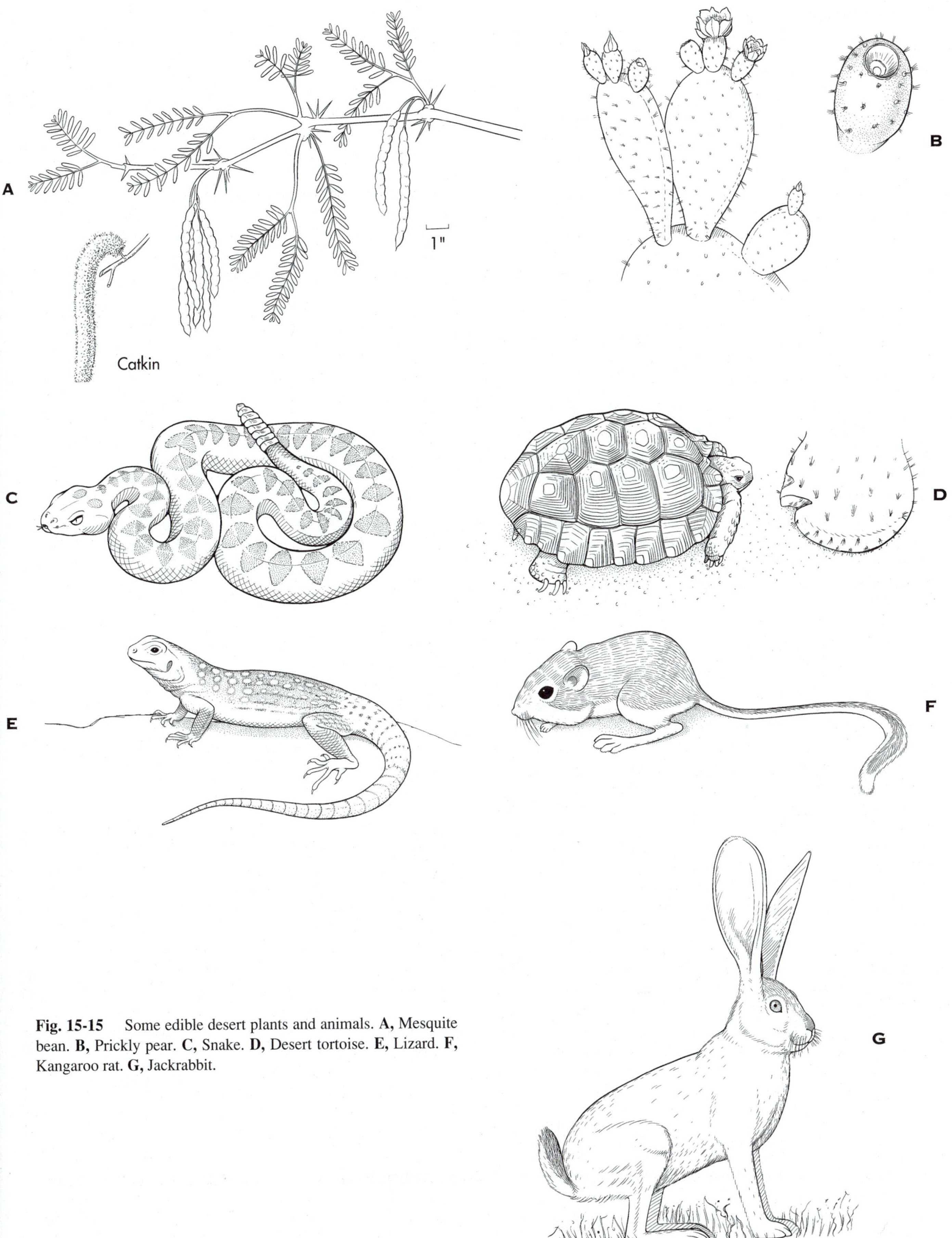

Fig. 15-15 Some edible desert plants and animals. **A,** Mesquite bean. **B,** Prickly pear. **C,** Snake. **D,** Desert tortoise. **E,** Lizard. **F,** Kangaroo rat. **G,** Jackrabbit.

occasionally may be located by watching the behavior of animals and birds, which travel toward water at dawn and dusk. Animal trails tend to lead to water and may be joined by other trails and become wider as they approach it. Birds may circle before landing at a waterhole, especially in the morning. A pool of water that has no animal tracks and droppings around it should be avoided because it may be poisonous. Muddy and dirty water should be filtered through cloth, and all water should be treated chemically or by filtration (see Chapter 43) or boiling before drinking. Persons should not drink urine or water from a vehicle radiator (which contains glycols). Table 15-3 shows the expected days of survival in the desert in relation to the amount of water available.

A useful device for producing potable water in the desert is a solar still (Fig. 15-16). The materials needed include a 6 × 6 foot piece of sturdy, clear plastic sheeting (preferably reinforced with duct tape in the center), a shovel, a 6- to 8-foot piece of surgical tubing, a 1-quart plastic bowl of the Tupperware type, duct tape, and a knife. A cone-shaped hole is dug about 3½ feet in diameter and 18 to 20 inches deep. This should be dug in a low area where water would stand the longest after a rain. The bowl, with the surgical tubing taped securely to its bottom, is placed in the center of the hole. The plastic sheet is placed loosely on top of the hole and weighted by a fist-sized rock in the center so that it sags into a cone whose apex is just above the bowl. Crushed desert vegetation, especially barrel and saguaro cactus, is placed inside the hole to provide additional moisture. The edges of the hole are sealed with dirt and rocks piled around the rim on top of the plastic sheet. Urine is placed inside the hole in an open container. Water from a vehicle radiator should not be used, since the glycols will distill along with the water.

The still should not be opened once it starts operating. It will produce 1 pint to 1 quart of water per 24 hours without added urine or vegetation, and up to 4 quarts with it. The surgical tubing is used to suck water from the bowl periodically as it collects.

If vegetation is plentiful, another type of solar still can be made from a large, clear plastic bag.[13] On a slope, a hole several feet in diameter is dug with a craterlike rim surrounded by a moat that drains downhill into a small hole. The bag is centered on the large hole with its edges over the moat and its mouth downhill at the small hole. An upright stick is placed inside the bag in the middle, and clean rocks are put along the "crater rim" to keep the bag anchored and ballooned out. The bag is reinforced with duct tape where the stick tents it. After the bag is filled with vegetation, its mouth is tied shut. The vegetation should not touch the sides of the bag or spill onto the part of the bag that is over the moat. The warmth of the sun causes water to evaporate from the vegetation and condense on the inside of the bag, run down into the part of the bag that is over the moat, run

Table 15-3 Expected Days of Survival at Various Environmental Temperatures and with Varying Amounts of Available Water

	Maximum Daily Temperature in Shade (°F)	Available Water per Man (U.S. Quarts)					
		0	1	2	4	10	20
No walking	120	2.0	2.0	2.0	2.5	3.0	4.5
	110	3.0	3.0	3.5	4.0	5.0	7.0
	100	5.0	5.5	6.0	7.0	9.5	13.5
	90	7.0	8.0	9.0	10.5	15.0	23.0
	80	9.0	10.0	11.0	13.0	19.0	29.0
	70	10.0	11.0	12.0	14.0	20.5	32.0
	60	10.0	11.0	12.0	14.0	21.0	32.0
	50	10.0	11.0	12.0	14.5	21.0	32.0
Walking at night and resting thereafter	120	1.0	2.0	2.0	2.5	3.0	
	110	2.0	2.0	2.5	3.0	3.5	
	100	3.0	3.5	3.5	4.5	5.5	
	90	5.0	5.5	5.5	6.5	8.0	
	80	7.0	7.5	8.0	9.5	11.5	
	70	7.5	8.0	9.0	10.5	13.5	
	60	8.0	8.5	9.0	11.0	14.0	
	50	8.0	8.5	9.0	11.0	14.0	

From Adolph et al: *Physiology of man,* New York, 1947, Interscience.

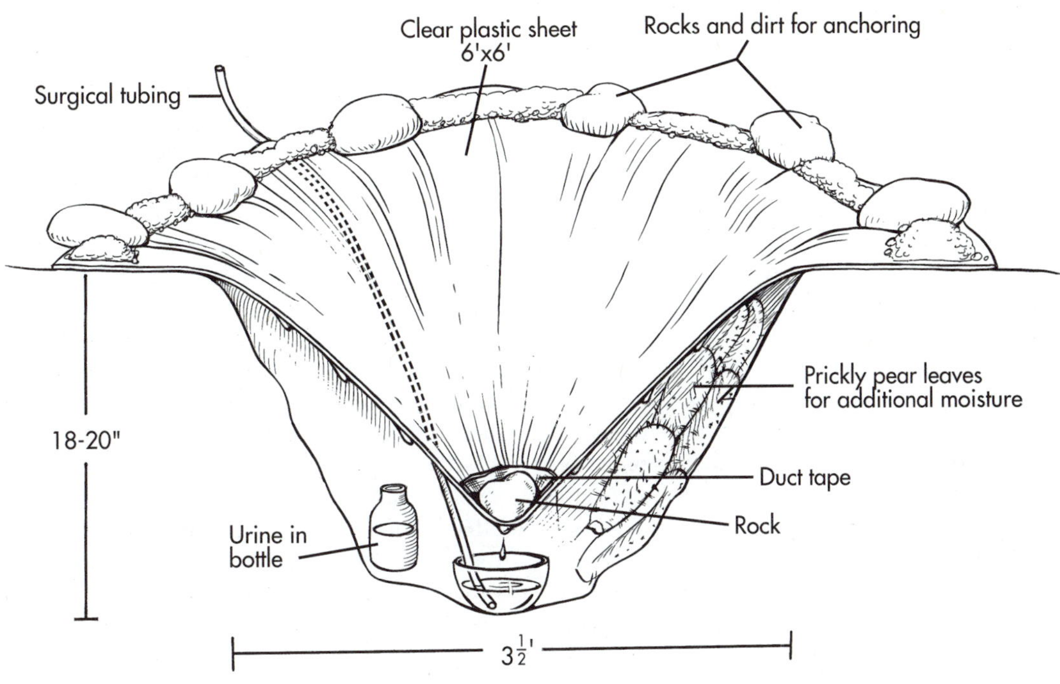

Fig. 15-16 Solar still.

downhill toward the mouth of the bag, and collect in the part of the bag's neck that is in the small hole. The mouth of the bag can be opened and the water poured out as needed.

Preparing for a Possible Survival Situation

Basic survival equipment and skills for anyone interested in wilderness travel should include the following:

1. Physical conditioning and healthful habits
2. Ability to swim well
3. Expertise in the use of a map and compass and in finding directions without a compass. A person should be able to identify the Big Dipper (Northern Hemisphere only) and follow the "pointers" (farthest stars on the bowl of the Dipper) to the North Star (Polaris). On a sunny day a nondigital watch set to standard time can be used to find direction. When the hour hand is pointed toward the sun, south will be one half of the shorter of the two distances between the hour hand and 12 o'clock.
4. Ability to build a fire under adverse conditions
5. A working knowledge of local weather patterns. The backcountry should be avoided during times of high hazard. In the United States the best source of weather information is the National Weather Service, which broadcasts on a 24-hour basis at frequencies of 162.40 or 162.55 MHz VHF-FM. Many multichannel radios receive this frequency; there are also inexpensive, lightweight radios that receive only this frequency. In evaluating avalanche conditions, the traveler needs to know what the weather conditions have been over the *previous few days* as well. The U.S. Forest Service provides warnings of dangerous avalanche conditions in many mountainous areas, especially in the western states.
6. Familiarity with the special medical problems of the type of wilderness involved. For example, for cold weather and high-altitude travel, familiarity with the prevention, diagnosis, and treatment of hypothermia, frostbite, and acute mountain sickness is needed. Travel in the desert and tropics requires familiarity with tropical infections, snakebite, tropical skin diseases, and heat illness. Basic principles of prehospital emergency care and the improvisation of splints and bandages must be understood. A person who has not had special training in prehospital field care should not assume that standard medical school or other professional training confers expertise in this area.
7. A survival kit containing equipment appropriate for the topography, climate, and season (see appendixes to chapter)
8. Ability to construct appropriate types of survival shelters
9. A working knowledge of the characteristics of natural hazards and of how to predict and avoid them. These include forest fire, lightning strike, avalanche, rockfall, cornice fall, flash flood, white

water, deadfall, storms of various kinds, and hazardous animals and plants.

10. Reading and analyzing accounts of survival experiences. The American Alpine Club's "Accidents in North American Mountaineering"[1] and the U.S. Forest Service's accounts of avalanche accidents[17] contain good examples from the standpoint of mountain and winter environments. There are many accounts in the popular literature of the experiences of travelers stranded by shipwreck or plane crash.
11. Awareness of the psychologic aspects of a survival situation and of errors in judgment that can lead to a survival emergency. A common error is to continue on a predecided course such as reaching a distant hut despite conditions that would make a more prudent person bivouac or turn back.[7] Many anxieties that paralyze action may appear in a survival situation. These include fear (of the unknown, being alone, wild animals, darkness, weakness, personal failure, discomfort, suffering, and death); surrender, which results in chaotic thought, inactivity, and loss of the will to live; and panic, the uncontrolled urge to run from the situation. Panic interferes with good judgment, resulting in inappropriate actions such as abandoning weaker companions or otherwise dividing the party, and discarding vital survival equipment. Useless flight saps available energy, leading to exhaustion and hastening death. The person must have faith in his or her abilities and equipment and in the likelihood that rescuers will arrive.
12. Knowledge of edible plants and animals of the area of projected travel. Basic hunting, trapping, and fishing skills are very valuable.
13. Awareness that a person should never travel into the wilderness alone and should always let others know the destination and expected time of return

Faith and the Will to Survive

In a survival emergency a person who has adequate oxygen, a stable body temperature, shelter, water, and food may still die if unable to withstand the psychologic stress. Conversely, persons have survived amazing hardships with little more than a strong determination to live. If a person possesses the necessary skills and has a minimum of survival equipment (see appendixes to the chapter), the odds are strongly in his or her favor. Medical personnel have the advantage of being trained to suppress panic. Fear and surrender are normal reactions that must be opposed by whatever psychologic tools are available. In some cases religious faith and the desire to rejoin loved ones have been credited with survival. No one can predict what his or her own reaction will be. Groups faced with emergencies testify that courage and leadership appear in unexpected places.

One of the hardest decisions is whether to stay put and wait for rescue or try to "walk out." In general it is better to use the time to prepare a snug shelter and conserve strength as long as there is any chance of rescue. Travel should never be attempted in severe weather, in desert daytime heat, or in deep snow without snowshoes or skis. If there is no chance of rescue, the proper course is to prepare as best possible, wait for good weather, and then travel in the most logical direction.

Signaling

Aside from the use of radios and other electronic equipment, signaling devices are either auditory or visual. Three of anything is a universally recognized distress signal: three whistle blasts, three shots, three fires, three columns of smoke. The most effective auditory device is a whistle. An effective ground-to-air signaling device is a glass signal mirror, which can be seen up to 10 miles away, but this requires sunlight. A traveler stranded in a vehicle should remain with the vehicle, since an automobile or airplane is much more visible than a person. Smoke is easily seen by day, and a fire or flashlight by night. On a cloudy day, black smoke is more visible than white; the reverse is true on a sunny day.

Black smoke can be produced by burning parts of a vehicle, such as rubber or oil, and white smoke by adding green leaves or a small amount of water to the fire. Ground signals should be as large as possible—at least 3 feet wide and 18 feet long—and should contain straight lines and square corners, which are not found in nature. They can be tramped out in dirt or on grass or can be made from brush or logs. In snow the depressions can be filled with vegetation to increase contrast. Many pilots do not know the traditional 18 International Ground-to-Air Emergency Signals. They have recently been replaced with five easily memorized signals adopted by the International Convention on Civil Aviation[15,16]:

- V I require assistance
- X I require medical assistance
- N No
- Y Yes
- → Proceeding in this direction

Air-to-ground signals:

- Message received and understood: rock plane side to side
- Message received but not understood: make a complete righthand circle

APPENDIX A

Sample Basic Wilderness Survival Kit

Shelter building equipment:

- Plastic or nylon tarp
- ⅛-inch nylon cord, braided, 50 feet
- Folding saw

Fire building equipment:
- Waterproof matches
- Candle
- Firestarter
- Sharp, sturdy hunting knife

Signaling equipment:
- Whistle
- Card with ground-to-air signals
- Two quarters for pay phone
- Signal mirror
- Flashlight

Other:
- Compass
- Map
- Metal pot with bale
- Cup and spoon
- Toilet paper
- Sunburn cream
- Lip salve
- Spare mittens and socks
- Emergency food
- Water disinfection equipment: chemicals or filter
- First aid kit
- Sunglasses
- Canteen (full)

Additional considerations:
- Fishhooks and line
- No. 28 piano wire for snares

APPENDIX B

Sample Winter Survival Kit

Basic survival items from Appendix A

Spare clothing for severe weather, enough for at least four layers total

Snow shovel: the best choice is the collapsible type resembling a small grain scoop, available in most mountaineering and Nordic ski shops

Optional items: piece of Ensolite or Therm-a-Rest mattress, sleeping bag, Gore-Tex bivouac sac, stove and fuel, light ax, snow saw

APPENDIX C

Sample Desert Survival Kit

Basic survival items from Appendix A

Foldup GI shovel, short handle type

Items for construction of four solar stills:
- Four sheets of clear plastic, 6 × 6 feet, reinforced in the center by a cross of duct tape
- Four pieces of surgical tubing, 6 to 8 feet long
- Four 1-quart Tupperware-type bowls

5-Gallon water jug, *full*

1 L wide-mouth bottle for use as urinal

Spare sunglasses

Heavy gloves

Citizen's band radio

Optional: Light rifle or target pistol with ammunition

APPENDIX D

Vehicle Survival Kit[18]

Sleeping bag or two blankets for each occupant

Extra winter clothing, including boots, for each occupant

Emergency food

Waterproof matches

Long-burning candles, at least 2

First aid kit

Pocket knife

Pot or coffee can

Toilet paper

Citizen's band radio

Flashlight with extra batteries

Extra quart of oil

Chains

Snow shovel

Tow chain

Small sack of sand

Two jugs of water

Tool kit

Gas line deicer

Flagging

Flares

Ax

Folding saw

APPENDIX E

Sample Survival First Aid Kit

Cravats, at least 2

Roll of 3-inch Kling gauze

Roll of 2-inch adhesive tape

2-inch rubberized (Ace) bandage

Band-Aids

Nonadhering sterile gauze pads

Sterile compresses

Steel sewing needle

Single-edged razor blade

Thermometer (low-reading for cold conditions)

Aspirin or acetaminophen, 325 mg tablets

Acetaminophen, 325 mg, with codeine, 30 mg, or propoxyphene, 100 mg, with acetaminophen, 650 mg

Diphenhydramine, 25 or 50 mg capsules

Small bottle of povidone-iodine solution

Splinting materials can usually be improvised using ski poles, ice axes, hammers, branches, poles, and parts of backpacks or vehicles

Physicians may wish to take an injectable narcotic, such as meperidine or morphine

REFERENCES

1. *Accidents in North American mountaineering,* New York, the American Alpine Club, Inc., and Banff, the Alpine Club of Canada (published yearly).
2. *Aircrew survival,* Department of the Air Force, Washington, DC, 1985, U.S. Government Printing Office.
3. Bowman WD: *Winter first aid manual,* ed 4, Denver, 1984, National Ski Patrol System.
4. Bowman WD: *Outdoor emergency care,* ed 2, Denver, 1993, National Ski Patrol System.
5. Corneille P: *Le Cid,* Act II, Scene 2, 1636.
6. Craighead FC Jr, Craighead JJ: *How to survive on land and sea,* ed 3, Annapolis, Md, 1956, US Naval Institute; ed 4, revised by Smith RE, Jarvis DS, 1984.
7. Fear G: *Surviving the unexpected wilderness emergency,* Tacoma, Wash, 1979, Survival Education Association.
8. Huntford R: *The last place on earth,* New York, 1986, Atheneum.
9. Nesbitt PH, Pond AW, Allen WH: *The survival book,* New York, 1959, Funk & Wagnalls.
10. Patterson CE: *Surviving in the wilds,* Toronto, 1979, Personal Library Publishers.
11. Shanks B: *Wilderness survival,* New York, 1987, Universe Books.
12. Stefansson V: *Unsolved mysteries of the Arctic,* New York, 1938, Macmillan.
13. Stoffel R, Lavalla R: *Survival sense for pilots and passengers,* Olympia, Wash, 1980, Emergency Response Institute.
14. *Survival,* Field Manual 21-76, Washington, DC, 1986, Department of the Army, US Government Printing Office.
15. *Survival training,* Washington, DC, 1985, Department of the Air Force, US Government Printing Office.
16. Whitmore PB, Bunstock J: *The W.I.S.E. man's guide to wilderness survival,* Lincoln, Neb, 1985, Astonisher Press.
17. Williams K, Armstrong B: *The snowy torrents: avalanche accidents in the United States 1972-1979,* Jackson, Wyo, Teton Bookshop Publishing.
18. *Winter driving booklet,* Cheyenne, Wyo, 1984, Wyoming Disaster and Civil Defense.

ADDITIONAL RECOMMENDED READINGS

Auerbach PS: *Medicine for the outdoors,* Boston, 1991, Little, Brown.

Lansing A: *Endurance,* New York, 1976, Avon.

The NSPS ski mountaineering manual, Denver, 1980, National Ski Patrol.

Olsen LD: *Outdoor survival skills,* Chicago, 1990, Chicago Review Press.

Randall G: *Cold comfort: keeping warm in the outdoors,* New York, 1987, Nick Lyons Books.

Riley MJ: *Don't get snowed: a guide to mountain travel,* Matteson, Ill, 1977, Greatlakes Living Press.

Rutstrum C: *Paradise below zero,* New York, 1974, Collier Books.

Simer P, Sullivan J: *The National Outdoor Leadership School's wilderness guide,* New York, 1983, Simon & Schuster.

Slonim NB, editor: *Environmental physiology,* St Louis, 1974, Mosby.

Survival in Antartica, Washington, DC, 1984, National Science Foundation.

Tejada-Flores L: *Backcountry skiing,* San Francisco, 1981, Sierra Club Books.

Troebst CC: *The art of survival,* Garden City, NY, 1965, Doubleday.

Waterman J: *Surviving Denali,* New York, 1983, American Alpine Club.

Wilkerson J, editor: *Medicine for mountaineering,* ed 4, Seattle, 1992, The Mountaineers.

Wilkinson E: *Snow caves for fun and survival,* Denver, 1986, Windsong Press.

16 JUNGLE TRAVEL AND SURVIVAL

John B. Walden

Persons who venture into the tropical rainforest step into an exotic and mysterious environment. However, it can also be unforgiving. Preparedness makes the difference between misery and pleasure.

Tropical Environment

In these forests lies a virtually limitless supply of excitement, joy and wonder to be encountered in new illuminations on the constructs and workings of life on earth.

T.E. Lovejoy[17]

Tropical rainforests, located between the Tropic of Cancer (23°27′ N latitude) and the Tropic of Capricorn (23° 27′ S latitude), are regions with at least 4 inches of precipitation per month and a mean annual monthly temperature exceeding 75° F with no frost occurring.[8] Facts and figures fail to capture the essence of the tropical rainforests and their extraordinary biologic diversity. Seen from the air, the forest stretches from horizon to horizon in an incredibly green carpet. In season the crowns of trees in full blossom dot the landscape with vivid splashes of red, orange, and yellow. Even sizable streams may be hidden beneath the emerald canopy. Rivers, usually muddy yellow or black, snake through the forest; early morning or late afternoon sun transforms these braided rivers into glistening, mirrorlike strands of liquid silver.

Observed from the forest floor, the jungle is entrancing. In virgin, deep forest, all is muted and shadowy save for random shafts of light that stream down to spotlight labyrinths of oddly shaped branches and spectacularly colored flowers. Shrubs and herbaceous plants are scarce in forest away from the flood plain, so it is relatively easy to walk undisturbed. The dimness is broken occasionally by areas bathed in bright light from larger holes in the canopy caused by a recently fallen tree, a sandy beach, or cutting and burning by humans. It is in these sunlit areas that the traveler encounters the lush and nearly impenetrable wall of foliage portrayed in adventure films. The tidy textbook division of vegetation into distinct tiers is somewhat arbitrary and not easily confirmed, even by the experts.[23]

In addition to the upland *terra firme* forests, there are lowland forests that remain submerged for several months each year. Such forests, or *várzeas,* make up only a small percentage of forested land, but they are infinitely more fertile than their nonflooding and nutrient-poor counterparts.

Despite environmental differences within the jungle, the basics of travel remain the same.

Trip Preparation

READING

Back issues of *National Geographic* provide an excellent introduction to the people and places the traveler plans to visit. *The Emerald Realm,*[8] a National Geographic Society special publication, is a superb overview of the world's tropical forests. The references cited at the end of this chapter offer insights into the complex inner workings of the moist tropical forest.[18,21,23,31,32] The books by Kritcher[15] and Forsyth and Miyata[11] are especially helpful.

Trips into the rainforest should be scheduled for the dry season because trails are more serviceable for trekking at that time. Information on weather patterns may be obtained from missionaries, anthropologists, agencies of national governments, and the excellent series *World Survey of Climatology,* edited by Werner Schwerdtfeger.[27]

ATTITUDE

The main attribute for which experienced expedition leaders look in selecting participants is a sense of humor; the ability to see the bright side when times get rough may be an asset more valuable than physical conditioning. Houston[13] and others have discussed the role of humor as a predictor of success. Erb[9] noted that successful or failed participation in wilderness ventures also is a significant predictor. Experienced group leaders rely on their intuition during the interview process to recognize when a potential expedition member may not work out.

A number of expedition leaders privately note that two individuals who have a sexual relationship often form a team within a team, to the detriment of the expedition as a whole.

CONDITIONING

Indigenous peoples in jungle regions are almost always slender. After trekking with large numbers of nonindigenous men and women in equatorial regions, I have observed that overweight or powerfully built individuals, particularly men, seem to fare the worst, especially with heat-related illness. Getting down to an ideal weight pays off on the trail.

Although being in reasonably good shape helps, a person need not be an elite athlete to trek through the jungle and enjoy the experience. Good leg strength, acquired by training with stair-climbing exercise machines, offers appropriate preparation.

To keep up with native porters and guides, the prospective expedition member should practice hiking at a fast pace. Once in the jungle, travelers should try to imitate the energy-saving, fluid rhythm of the locals.

Because trekkers frequently encounter single-log bridges, a well-developed sense of balance is desirable. Walking in the rails of train tracks or on curbs may help in preparation. An even better activity is to go to the woodlands and practice walking on logs. Head stability is important. Equilibrium can be enhanced by avoiding brisk head movements and by employing the "gaze-anchoring" technique of tightrope walkers: fix the gaze on a spot at the end of the log and do not stare down at the spot just ahead of the feet.[1,4,22]

IMMUNIZATIONS

Travelers to rainforest regions should protect against the following diseases through vaccination or prophylactic medications:

1. Diphtheria, tetanus
2. Hepatitis A, hepatitis B
3. Measles, mumps, rubella
4. Polio
5. Typhoid
6. Yellow fever (in certain regions of tropical Africa and South America)
7. Malaria

Malaria is prevalent throughout the tropics. Before travel to malarious areas the appropriate prophylaxis is needed. Updated information on the risk of malaria in various regions may be obtained through the International Travelers' Hot Line service of the Centers for Disease Control and Prevention (404-332-4559). *The Medical Letter on Drugs and Therapeutics* issue on parasitic diseases, published every 2 years, is an excellent source for current recommendations on preventing and treating malaria (see Chapter 45).

Persons traveling into remote regions of Amazonia where Indian groups live in isolation should receive yearly influenza vaccinations to reduce the likelihood of inadvertently transmitting disease to these high-risk native inhabitants. Protection against meningococcal disease and rabies should be considered where circumstances warrant. Cholera vaccine is not very effective and is generally administered to satisfy the entry requirements of the few countries that continue to require vaccination.

MEDICAL KIT

The Wilderness Medical Society points out that it is inappropriate to pack medications and equipment when no team member has the knowledge or experience to use them safely.[14] The following basic medical kit (Box 16-1) is adequate for personal use in the rainforest setting (see Chapter 17 for additional recommendations regarding wilderness medical kits):

BOX 16-1

MEDICAL KIT FOR JUNGLE TRAVEL

Bactroban ointment (30 g)
Benadryl 50 mg tablets (15)
Cipro 500 mg tablets (20)
Elimite 5% cream (60 g)
EpiPen auto-injector (2)
Flagyl 250 mg tablets (21)
Lotrisone cream (15 g)
Motrin 600 mg tablets (30)
Nix 1% shampoo (2 oz)
Pepto-Bismol tablets (48)
SAM splint (1)
Sodium Sulamyd ophthalmic solution 10% (15 ml)
Sunscreen 4 oz tubes (2)
Toradol 30 mg single-dose syringe (2) plus 10 mg tablets (12)
Xylocaine 2 ml single-dose vials (3) plus disposable syringes and needles

1. Bismuth subsalicylate tablets (Pepto-Bismol). Pepto-Bismol is an effective over-the-counter preparation for preventing and treating common traveler's diarrhea. It also is useful for heartburn and indigestion. Pepto-Bismol tends to turn the tongue and stool black.
2. Diphenhydramine hydrochloride 50 mg capsules (Benadryl). Benadryl is safe and effective as an antihistamine, for motion sickness, and as a nighttime sleep aid.
3. Ciprofloxacin hydrochloride 500 mg tablets (Cipro). Cipro is highly active against the important bacterial causes of enteritis, including *Escherichia coli, Vibrio cholerae, Salmonella, Shigella, Campylobacter jejuni, Aeromonas,* and *Yersinia entercolitica.*
4. Clotrimazole and betamethasone dipropionate cream (Lotrisone). Lotrisone has the dual advantage of having antifungal properties and a sufficiently potent steroid for steroid-sensitive rashes.
5. Epinephrine auto-injector (EpiPen/EpiPen Jr. Auto-Injector). For emergency treatment of severe allergic reactions to insect stings, foods, or drugs, EpiPen/EpiPen Jr. provides a virtually foolproof delivery system for speeding a single dose of epinephrine into the victim's bloodstream.
6. Ibuprofen 600 mg tablets. Ibuprofen is a good choice for mild to moderate pain from such problems as menstrual cramps, rheumatoid arthritis, and osteoarthritis. It also lowers elevated body temperature caused by common infectious diseases.
7. Ketorolac (Toradol) 60 mg for injection. Ketorolac provides good short-term relief for moderate to severe pain. It is preferred over narcotics only because it is less likely to cause problems with customs officers and police.
8. Lidocaine hydrochloride. This local anesthetic agent may be required for relief of the excruciating pain resulting from stingray envenomation and conga ant or caterpillar stings. It should be infiltrated around the wound area.
9. Metronidazole 250 mg tablets. Metronidazole is excellent for treating giardiasis, acute amebic dysentery, or *Trichomonas* vaginitis.
10. Mupirocin ointment 2% (Bactroban). The ointment should be immediately applied to burns, abrasions, lacerations, and ruptured blisters, which can rapidly become infected in the tropics.
11. Permethrin 5% cream and 1% shampoo. Many natives, especially in the tropics of Central and South American, are infested with scabies and head lice. Travelers who have been in close contact with heavily infested tribal peoples should apply permethrin cream and shampoo before returning home.
12. SAM splint. This remarkable splint is lightweight, waterproof, reusable, and not affected by temperature extremes.
13. Sulfacetamide sodium ophthalmic solution 10% (Sodium Sulamyd). This is excellent for treating conjunctivitis, corneal ulcers, or other superficial ocular infections.
14. Sunscreen. Sunscreen is essential in open areas such as rivers or jungle clearings. Sunscreens designated "waterproof" retain their full sun protection factor rating for longer periods during sweating or water immersion than do products designated water resistant. Opaque formulations are excellent for the nose, lips, and ears. Visitors to the tropics should wear lightweight, long-sleeved shirts and a wide-brimmed hat when exposed to the sun for prolonged periods (see Chapter 12).

Common sense dictates supplementary items. Women on long trips might wish to add miconazole vaginal suppositories to treat yeast infections; older men might take a 16 Fr Foley catheter and sterile lubricating jelly for dealing with problems arising from prostatic hypertrophy.

GEAR

The idea is to travel as light as possible. The more stuff that is packed, the greater the likelihood of breakdowns, complications, and misery. "Equipment freaks"[29] who go in for lots of unnecessarily expensive, colorful gear will be disappointed by the following discussion of basic equipment. These items have, however, withstood the test of time over years of long-distance tropical trekking.

Gear must hold up under difficult jungle travel conditions that include heat, wetness, and mud. At this writing there is no line of advertised gear ideally suited for the traveler who plans to spend time off the beaten path in the tropics. In the United States, L.L. Bean, Inc. (Freeport, ME 04033) and Recreational Equipment, Inc. (REI) (1700 45th Street East, Sumner, WA 98352-0001) are good sources for reasonably priced and reliable equipment, which, while not always ideal for the tropics, is usually satisfactory (see Chapter 17).

Footwear

Since feet absorb more punishment than any other part of the body, suitable footwear is the single most important item of gear. This is the one place where a person absolutely must not carry inferior equipment. If the feet cannot go, nothing can go.

Military-style "jungle boots" are unsuitable for serious, long-distance trekking. After an hour of hard walking through streams and muddy trails, blisters will form on every surface of the foot and the skin will peel off in sheets, bringing a jungle trip to a premature end. Furthermore, safely crossing log bridges and mossy,

BOX 16-2

GEAR FOR JUNGLE TRAVEL

Trail shoes (1 pair)
Camp boots (1 pair)
Socks (3 pairs)
Hat (1)
Pullover (1)
Shirts
  Long-sleeved (2)
  Short-sleeved (2)
Pants (2 pairs)
Undergarments
  Underpants (3)
  Sports bra (2)
Poncho (1)
Flannel sheet
Hammock or Therm-a-Rest
Mosquito net
Backpack for porter
Personal backpack
Antifogging solution for eyeglasses
Batteries
Binoculars
Camera equipment and film
Campsuds
Candles
Cup/plate
Ear plugs
Fishing supplies
Garbage bags
  30-gallon size (4)
  13-gallon size (4)
Headlamp
Inflatable cushion
Insect repellent
Laminated map(s)
Machete
Waterproof matches/cigarette lighter
Pen
Toilet paper
Pocket tool
Poly bottles (2)
Razor/battery-operated shaver
Sensi sport sponge
Spoon
Sunglasses
Umbrella
Whistle
Zipper bags
  Gallon size (5)
  Quart size (5)
  Pint size (5)

slime-covered river rocks is almost impossible in these boots.

Two pair of shoes are needed: one suitable for the wet, slippery conditions imposed by the trail and another that meets the need for dryness and comfort in camp.

Trail Shoes. The following features are desirable in trail shoes:

1. Uppers that hit just above or just below the ankles. Some people choose a high-cut design, reasoning that the extra height gives some added snake protection.
2. Extra protection over the big toe. Protective rubber or leather toecaps help keep the big toe from being severely battered and bruised.
3. Moderately deep-tread outsoles. Traction on rugged and muddy terrain is important. Running shoes with hard, "high-impact" soles should not be worn because they become slippery on wet logs or river rocks.
4. Quick drying time. Uppers of Cordura nylon and split leather, in addition to resisting abrasion and being somewhat breathable, dry out surprisingly fast when placed in the sun. Even though hiking shoes usually become soaked within minutes on the trail, it is a psychologic boost to start off each new day with dry (or less than soggy!) shoes. Since jungle travelers can be in waist-high water many times each day while on the trail, waterproof shoes with Gore-Tex liners are not essential.
5. Snagproof design. Shoes or boots with "quick-lace" steel hooks should be avoided: vines and weeds become tangled around the metal hooks, causing the wearer to stumble and pulling the laces untied. Shoelaces should always be double knotted.
6. Light weight

Camp Boots. Footwear needs are very different in camp. Being wet on the trail is one thing, but the trekker wants dry feet in camp. Here are the key features:

1. A boot. Shoes, although excellent for the trail, do not work out well in camp. A boot that comes to midcalf keeps mud off the feet and pants.
2. Rubber construction. Rubber remains an excellent material for keeping water away from the feet.
3. Rubber lug soles for traction. When rubber-soled boots are worn, however, extreme caution is needed when crossing wet or dry log bridges and walking on

slippery moss or slime-covered rocks by the river's edge.

4. Light weight. On the trail, camp boots must be carried in a pack, so the lighter the better.

The Nokia Piha Boot (stock number 791) sold by Hitchcock Shoes, Inc., 225 Beal Street, Hingham, MA 02043 (617-749-3260) is the perfect boot for camp. Its features include all-rubber construction, lug soles, light weight, and durability. It is absolutely waterproof. The boot is 10 inches high and rolls up to consume minimal space in a pack. (The North American distributor of the Piha Boot is Nordic Footwear, Ltd., 4981 Highway 7 East, Unit 12-A, Suite 154, Merkham, Ontario, Canada L3R1N1.)

Other Options. The lightweight, comfortable, mesh/neoprene fabric "water" shoes that have become popular in recent years for beach and sailboarding activities may have a place on river trips in which substantial time will be spent in dugout canoes or rubber rafts.

Thongs and open-toe sandals are fine for most towns and cities in the tropics, but in certain jungle regions such as the Amazon Basin, exposed feet invite hordes of biting insects, including burrowing jigger fleas.

The jungle traveler must never go barefoot. Plant spines and glass can puncture the feet, and larvae of ubiquitous parasitic diseases such as hookworm and strongyloidiasis can enter through the skin.

Socks. Cotton socks should be worn in the jungle to decrease the risk of blisters from wet trail shoes, to reduce insect bites (particularly from no-see-ums), and to lessen the risk of lacerations from sawgrass.

Clothing

In many countries military green or camouflage-style clothing is strictly contraindicated. This is particularly true in military dictatorships or in remote border regions. To be mistaken for a guerilla or foreign infiltrator by the military, police, or security (undercover) forces can lead to harassment, detention, or worse.

Hat. For protection from radiant heat and things that tend to land on a person's head in the forest, the traveler should wear a lightweight, light-colored hat that has a medium or wide brim. It need not be waterproof, but it should be made of material that can be wadded up. A useful feature is a fastener on each side to snap the brim up for traveling on the trail. A pith helmet is fine for open savanna and river trips, but on the trail, branches would knock it off a person's head every few minutes.

Pullover. A drenching rain may leave a person feeling chilled and uncomfortable, particularly when traveling mainly by canoe or raft. (Chilling generally is not a problem when hiking on the trail so long as the person keeps moving.) A Dacron polyester fleece pullover such as L.L. Bean's Polarlite Pullover, REI's Polarlite Sweater, or one of the excellent pullovers made by Patagonia will keep a person warm. When these garments get wet, they should be wrung out so that they continue to offer thermal protection. Professional white-water boatmen working in tropical regions generally pack a polyester outerwear garment.

Shirts. Two light-colored, ultralightweight, long-sleeved cotton shirts should be taken. One of these shirts will be the trail shirt. At the end of the day, it should be washed and rinsed so that it will be ready, although perhaps still damp, the next morning. The second shirt can be used in camp or as a spare for the trail.

In camp, if there are not many no-see-ums and mosquitoes, a lightweight, short-sleeved cotton shirt comes in handy. Two should be packed. A four-pocket style called the *guayabera,* favored by men throughout Latin America and the Caribbean, is ideal.

Pants. Two pairs of lightweight, light-colored cotton pants are needed. One pair is worn on the trail during the entire trip. Trail pants should be washed often. The other pair is worn around camp and in towns along the way. Jeans become waterlogged as soon as they become wet and are totally unsuitable for tropical trekking.

Undergarments. Underpants and sports bras should be made of cotton.

Poncho. An ultrathin waterproof poncho is useful on rafting or canoe trips and in villages but is worthless on the trail.

Bedding

Flannel Sheet. First-time visitors to tropical rainforests are surprised to discover how uncomfortably cold it gets between midnight and sunrise. A cotton sheet does not provide enough warmth, a blanket is too heavy, and a summer-weight sleeping bag retains too much body heat. A flannel sheet, sewn together like a mummy bag (40 × 90 inches), but without a taper, provides suitable warmth either in a hammock or on a pad.

Many inhabitants of the tropical forests sleep with their feet near a fire that is tended throughout the night. They have learned that the chill of damp, cool jungle nights can be lessened as long as the feet stay warm. Using disposable "warm packs" wrapped within a sock accomplishes essentially the same thing.

Hammock. Soft, cloth hammocks are exquisitely comfortable and lovely to look at, but they are too bulky and too heavy for trips. After a few days they begin to smell. Fishnet cotton hammocks are comfortable and lightweight but tend to fall apart within hours or days. The so-called camping tent-hammocks or military tent-hammocks seem adequate, but they are usually bulky, heavy, impossible to sling properly, extremely uncomfortable, hot (one trekker described his as a "jungle sweat-lodge"), unstable, and *never* able to keep the rain out in a heavy tropical downpour.

The nylon SuperHammock has proved nearly ideal for jungle travel (Model EZ-190 sold by E-Z Sales Manufacturing, 1432 West 166 St., Gardena, CA 90247). It is compact, lightweight, durable, and reasonably comfortable. It cannot rot or absorb odors. For easier handling, the ski rope tie-end lines that are sold with the SuperHammock should be replaced with ⅜-inch double-braided rope.

Therm-a-Rest. The Term-a-Rest foam pad is the choice of expedition organizers throughout the world. It combines the insulating qualities of foam and the cushioning of an air mattress, rolls up to a compact size, and inflates on its own when the valve is opened.

The traveler who will be sleeping on a pad should pack a good-quality 1½ × 2½ yard plastic ground sheet. The ground sheet should not be placed directly on the jungle floor, where stinging insects and snakes abound. It should be used only in a hut or on an elevated platform. The ground sheet may also come in handy for temporary rain protection and for keeping bow spray off a person or gear during water travel.

Mosquito Netting. A mosquito net designed for use with a hammock is basically a rectangular box that is open at the bottom with sleeves at each end panel for the passage of the ropes by which the hammock is slung. Such nets are hard to find outside the tropics. Fortunately, a serviceable mosquito net can easily be made from "no-see-um netting," which is available from REI. Instructions for sewing the netting are given in Fig. 16-1.

Backpacks

A sturdy, well-designed backpack should be used to carry gear. On serious jungle treks porters are present. This frees expedition members to carry much lighter loads.

Backpack for Porter. An internal-frame backpack of 3000 to 4000 cubic inch capacity is a good size. It should have external pockets for quick access to liter-sized water bottles.

Indigenous peoples the world over are accustomed to carrying packs and hauling loads with a strap known as a tumpline slung over the forehead or chest. Many natives, including Amazonian Indians, dislike using the shoulder straps that come as standard equipment on backpacks. Given enough straps, almost any native porter can quickly rig a satisfactory tumpline on a backpack.

Personal Pack. A daypack of 1200 to 2000 cubic inch capacity is useful for carrying a camera, snack food, and other gear that must be kept handy. A waterproof liner will keep perspiration from wicking into the bag and wetting everything inside. The pack should have two outside pockets for quick access to liter-sized water bottles.

Pack for River Trips. A durable, waterproof "dry" bag, used by river runners, is worth considering, especially if the trip will involve spending days or weeks at a time in dugout canoes or rubber rafts. Most of these packs, however, cannot stand up to the demands of long-distance overland trekking. The straps tend to be uncomfortable and frequently rip out on the trail.

Other Useful Items

Antifogging Solution for Eyeglasses. Antifog solution, available from dive shops, reduces humidity-induced fogging of glasses.

Batteries. Alkaline batteries should be brought from home. Batteries sold in Third World nations do not last long and often leak.

Binoculars. The traveler who is an avid bird watcher or enjoys watching butterflies or seeking out orchids high on distant limbs will want to pack a pair of binoculars that are lightweight, compact, shockproof, and waterproof or water resistant.

Camera Equipment and Film. Older-style cameras with mechanical shutters are reliable in regions of high humidity; professionals often choose the totally waterproof Nikonos. Many professional photographers use two lenses in the tropics: a wide-angle to normal zoom and an 80 to 200 mm telephoto zoom. A fast fixed-focal-length lens (*f*1.4) works effectively in the low-light conditions under the jungle canopy. (My preferences are a 24 mm wide-angle *f*/2.8, a 50 mm "normal" *f*/1.4, and a 105 mm macro *f*/2.8.)

Water-resistant or waterproof point-and-shoot cameras are worthy of consideration. Although they are less versatile and overall less reliable than mechanical cameras, their convenience offsets these drawbacks.

In the low-light conditions of the tropical forest, moderately "fast" film is essential unless a tripod is brought. Kodachrome 200 Professional (PKL) or Ektachrome 400 Professional (EPL) is an excellent choice. Both films produce sharp images and very saturated colors.

Camera Case or Bag. Hard-bodied Pelican cases are waterproof and virtually indestructible. The silver gray color cuts down on heat absorption and is preferred by professional photographers working in hot climates. The cases are ideal for rafting or canoe trips, but bulky for trekking. On the trail, waterproof "dry" bags protect equipment.

Camp Soap. A biodegradable soap should be used. The soap Campsuds works in hot, cold, fresh, or salt water and cleans just about anything: dishes, clothing, hair, and skin.

Candles. Electricity tends to fail at unpredictable times in small towns and even in cities in Third World countries. Travelers should carry dripless candles, but spring-loaded candle lanterns should be avoided. They give off an anemic glow, gum up, get crushed or broken, and basically waste space in the pack.

Cup and Plate. A large Lexan polycarbonate cup is unbreakable, does not retain taste or odor, and serves the role of cup, bowl, and plate. Travelers who feel the need for an actual plate should buy one made of indestructible Melamine.

Ear Plugs. Travel in the tropics often involves flying in incredibly loud helicopters, cargo planes, or short take-off and landing (STOL) aircraft. Sponge ear plugs that roll up and fit in the ear canal offer inexpensive, effective protection against hearing damage.

Fishing Supplies. For additional "food insurance" the jungle traveler should carry 75 feet of 20-pound-test fishing line, a 12-inch steel leader with swivel, and a few hooks. Breakdown travel rods and spincast reels should be considered for sport fishing or adding fresh meat to the daily provisions. Throughout the tropics most species of fish find Rat-L-Trap lures, particularly the chrome and blue combination, irresistible.

Garbage Bags. Four 30-gallon capacity and four 13-gallon capacity large plastic garbage bags come in handy for holding clothes, bedding, and other items that must stay absolutely dry and for keeping dirty boots isolated from clean items in the backpack.

Headlamp. Battery-operated headlamps offer hands-free convenience and are perfect for reading at night in the hammock or making a stumble-free, late night dash to the latrine. The REI Cordless Headlamp is lightweight, durable, and inexpensive. It shines up to 14 hours on four AA batteries.

Inflatable Cushion or Pillow. If a lot of time will be spent sitting in a dugout canoe or aluminum boat, a small, durable, cloth-covered inflatable cushion is recommended.

Insect Repellent. To repel mosquitoes, flies, ticks, chiggers, fleas, and gnats (but not no-see-ums), buy any spray insect repellent containing 15% to 30% *N,N*-diethyl-meta-toluamide (DEET). Avoid formulations containing higher than 30% DEET, often called "jungle juice." They may pose health hazards (see Chapter 34).

Technique is critical when applying insect repellent. Before dressing, the person should spray the ankles, lower legs, and waist. After the socks are put on, a band should be sprayed around the top; a band should also be sprayed around both pant legs to midcalf. A light spray to the shirt, front and back, may also help. The hands should be sprayed, rubbed vigorously, and run through the hair. Some repellent should be dabbed on the face, neck, and ears, carefully avoiding the eyes.

No-see-ums, which are tiny gnats that abound throughout the tropics of the Americas, are in many regions the single most common source of insect annoyance. They tend to be especially active near sunset and love to feast on the flesh of humans emerging from a cleansing bath in a jungle stream. No-see-ums cannot bite through even the thinnest cloth and are repelled by Skin So Soft (SSS), sold by Avon. (SSS is not effective against ticks, fleas, flies, and chiggers and offers little protection against mosquitoes.) SSS should be applied liberally and often to the wrists, knuckles, bare ankles, face, ears, and scalp. Men with full beards seem to be especially troubled by tiny gnats and may benefit by applying small amounts of SSS to the beard area.

Laminated Map. Accurate maps exist for most regions on earth. It pays to search out the best map available and laminate photocopied portions that are relevant to a particular itinerary.

Machete. A machete is the single essential tool for jungle survival and for the many tasks in camp and on the trail that require steel with a sharp edge. A proper machete (long, heavy, and well made) in experienced hands is worth its weight in gold. Also, machetes make excellent gifts and are often more desirable than cash for payment of services.

The machete is not used to hack at the foliage in a frenzy. In the hands of an expert the finely honed machete is swung with rhythm and grace; cuts are made sparingly and selectively with near surgical precision.

Machetes are dangerous tools. It is especially hazardous to use a machete in the rain or when cutting wet grass; the weapon may fly right out of the hand. Also, when cutting brush, the worker often encounters sawgrass. The resulting skin lacerations, which are not noticed at the first because sawgrass is razor sharp, may take a week or two to heal. Because of the risks involved, an experienced individual should be in charge of transporting and using the machete.

Matches or Cigarette Lighter. Waterproof, windproof Hurricane Matches light when damp and stay lit for several seconds even in the strongest wind. Many jungle travelers prefer a butane cigarette lighter.

Pen. The Fisher Space Pen (Fisher Pen Company, Forest Park, IL 60130) writes upside down without pumping, under water and over grease, and in hot and cold temperature extremes. It has an estimated shelf life of over 100 years.

Pocket Tool. The favorite pocket tool for the outdoors enthusiast is the Swiss Army knife. The essential options are a main blade, can opener, bottle opener, flathead screwdriver, and Phillips screwdriver.

The Leatherman Pocket Survival Tool deserves consideration. It is compact and easy to carry in its belt sheath and has 12 useful implements, including needle-nosed pliers.

The Gerber Sportsman's Tool provides 10 useful implements, including pliers (unfortunately not needle nosed). It comes with a rotproof nylon belt sheath. The knife blades and screwdrivers do not lock in place.

Poly Bottles. High on the list of essential gear are two quart or liter size wide-mouth water bottles made of high-density polyethylene or Lexan polycarbonate.

A 2-ounce, heavy-duty poly bottle comes in handy for carrying a salt and pepper mixture to add flavor to boiled plantains and yucca.

Razor or Battery-Operated Shaver. Both men and women should carry lightweight disposable razors. Most men find that lightweight, AA battery–operated shavers give two shaves a day for up to 2 weeks before requiring a change of batteries. However, men need a razor shave every few days because the battery-operated models cannot maintain a uniformly close shave indefinitely.

Sport Sponge. The sport sponge, made of microporous material, is lightweight, compact, and mysteriously superabsorbent. It replaces the bulky, hard-to-dry, rot- and odor-prone cotton towel. With the Sensi or any similar brand the body and even hair can be dried in a fraction of the time it takes with a traditional towel.

Spoon. The knife-spoon-fork sets that nestle together are unnecessary. Humans do not need a fork to eat. With a knife blade, all that is necessary is a good table spoon made of either Lexan polycarbonate or stainless steel.

Sunglasses. Sunglasses should be polarized with full UV protection. Many travelers prefer sunglasses with red-tinted lenses. Because red is the complement of green, these lenses make the jungle foliage stand out intensely and sharply, giving the illusion of enhanced contrast and depth of field. Eyeglass retainers, such as Chums or Croakies, hold eyeglasses securely during vigorous activity. L.L. Bean sells a rugged, hard-shell sport glasses case made of impact-resistant Lexan polycarbonate.

Toilet Paper. American toilet paper is much softer than toilet paper purchased in Third World countries. The traveler should never wipe with jungle leaves. An alternative is to adopt the habit of native people: wipe with the left hand and then rinse the hand with water.

Umbrella. A collapsible umbrella comes in handy in tropical cities and in remote villages when walking from hut to hut. It also offers excellent protection from the sun on canoe or raft trips.

Whistle. A high-quality plastic or metal whistle attached by a lanyard to a belt loop can be used to signal someone in case the trekker strays off the path.

Zipper Bags. Heavy-duty zipper freezer bags are excellent for organizing medicines, toiletries, and other small objects. Five each of the gallon, quart, and pint sizes should be brought.

Coping With the Jungle Environment

A visit to the rainforests of the New World tropics can be either a sublime experience or a hellish ordeal.

Adrian Forsyth and Ken Miyata[11]

WETNESS

The superhumid lowland rainforest gets up to 400 inches of rain a year; by contrast, Indiana averages about 40 inches a year. In the higher elevation cloud forest there is a continuous, dense cloud cover throughout the year accompanied by a constant mist or drizzle. In such a setting of heat and high humidity, people become mentally fatigued as a result of being constantly wet. At some point it occurs to most people who spend a lot of time in the jungle, particularly during the rainy season, that they will never be dry again . . . ever.

Fortunately, travelers can be perfectly content during even long stays in the tropics if they employ basic strategies for coping with the physical and psychologic burden of wetness. There are three fundamentals of living with wetness:

Revelation No. 1. Wetness is as much a state of mind as it is a physical condition.

Revelation No. 2. It's OK to be wet!

Revelation No. 3. Your body, particularly your feet, must be dry in camp and at night.

Newcomers to the tropics commonly waste inordinate energy in behaviors designed to avoid getting wet. Experienced travelers, on the other hand, stride right on through streams and puddles without skipping a beat.

Dryness while trekking or working during the daylight hours is not a requisite for physical or mental health. Wetness does not equate with illness, significant discomfort, or dampened spirits. People can tolerate being wet throughout much of the day if they know for certain that they have a dry change of clothes to wear in camp and that they will be dry at night. In addition to the psychologic benefits, being dry at night means that maceration is less likely to develop in intertriginous areas.

Bedding and clothing can be protected from moisture by careful wrapping in plastic garbage bags. Despite all efforts, however, eventually certain "dry" items become damp or accidentally soaked. In such instances the wet articles should be spread out on shrubs and bushes. They will dry within 2 hours in full sun. Cloth dried over a wood fire tends to pick up unpleasant odors that repeated washing will not remove.

HEALTH ISSUES

Health Risks

The subject of the tropics causes many people to think about tropical diseases and conjure up visions of textbook cases of filariasis in Polynesian Islanders whose scrotal sacs are distended to the size of watermelons and must be carried around in wheelbarrows. Their imagination may dwell on such animals as the candirú, a matchstick-sized parasitic catfish that can penetrate the urethra of a bather who carelessly voids into Amazon Basin waters. The piranha has received such bad press that it comes as a surprise to most travelers that there is not a single documented case of human fatality resulting from attack by a school of crazed piranha.

Malaria, hepatitis, and motor vehicle accidents are the three leading health problems in most tropical regions. From a practical standpoint, tropical travelers who venture off the beaten path can expect to be exposed to situations with an inherent risk of bodily harm and a number of potentially serious diseases such as leishmaniasis, onchocerciasis, and Chagas' disease. Bouts of diarrhea or other annoyances are a near certainty, regardless of the extent of precautions taken. However, death is an unlikely consequence of venturing into the leafy realm of the topics.

Duration of Jungle Travel

After 2 to 3 weeks of travel in remote areas, the general health of expedition participants almost inevitably deteriorates as a result of a steady accumulation of insect bites and injuries sustained in falls and close encounters with noxious plants. Trekkers with minimal previous jungle experience may quickly tire of a diet of unfamiliar food and understandably miss the comforts of home. For these reasons, experienced leaders prefer to limit expeditions to 3 weeks.

Preventing Heat-Related Illness

The following guidelines should be considered to prevent heat-related illness.

1. Before undertaking long-distance trekking in the tropics, acclimatize by spending at least 5 days in a hot, humid environment and engaging in moderate daily exercise there. This acclimatization will be lost within a week if not maintained.[12]
2. Avoid alcohol and certain drugs. Medications such as β-blockers, anticholinergics, and diuretics increase the likelihood of heat-related illness and should be avoided if possible.
3. Wear lightweight, light-colored, and loose-fitting cotton clothing and a wide-brimmed hat.
4. Whenever possible, have a native porter carry all gear.
5. Maintain adequate hydration. The following schedule has proved satisfactory for the strenuous exercise of trekking: Before setting off on the trail, drink a liter of disinfected water. A half hour later drink a second liter. One hour after the second liter, drink a third, then consume approximately 1 L every 2 to 4 hours throughout the day while on the trail.

Heat cramps, often severe, tend to occur when large amounts of water are ingested without adequate salt replacement. Oral rehydration salts (ORS) come in premeasured packets that, when added to a liter of disinfected water, provide an ideal balance for replacing lost electrolytes. It is a good idea to drink at least 1 L of water containing rehydration salts before setting out on the trail and a second liter with them after especially strenuous days. ORS packets are distributed throughout the developing world by the World Health Organization and UNICEF, but they are hard to come by in the commercial market overseas. In the United States, ORS packets may be obtained from Jianas Brothers, 2533 Southwest Boulevard, Kansas City, MO 64108, 816-421-2880.

Sport mixtures such as Gatorade are tasty and will to some degree maintain adequate electrolyte balance, but not nearly as well as ORS. Salt tablets are not recommended because they are gastric irritants and may actually delay acclimatization because of aldosterone suppression.[12]

Heat-related illness is discussed in greater detail in Chapter 8.

COPING WITH UNEXPECTED ISOLATION IN THE JUNGLE

Sometimes travelers face unexpected isolation in the jungle. Various factors contribute to this state of affairs, such as inclement weather, mechanical problems, or political turmoil that shuts down public transportation.

Many people stuck in a remote locale respond with anger and irritability. This attitude certainly does not improve the situation and can be devastating in the context of group dynamics. It is far better to accept the situation and use the additional time to appreciate the esthetic qualities of the tropical forest. Unhurried strolls along a jungle path reveal small and captivating discoveries. Photography can help keep the spirits high and foster creativity. Paperback books are an invaluable ally in overcoming the blahs.

It helps to shift out of gear mentally and allow the intellectual machinery to idle. Nearly everyone has had the experience of driving for hours and arriving at a destination with virtually no recollection of anything. The same thing can be accomplished in the village setting by just lying around in a hammock. The hours and the days pass surprisingly fast. This experience is akin to cruising in a sailboat with no engine . . . the person learns patience and develops an appreciation that the rhythms of nature are not governed by the ticking of a clock. For many visitors to the jungle, unexpected isolation opens up a new world as they come to experience the biospheric cadence.

CAMP LIFE

Shelter

Natives rarely spend the night in makeshift shelters, and even then only because of absolute necessity. With few exceptions it is best to use existing dwellings for slinging a hammock or putting down a sleeping pad.

Common courtesy governs the placement of a hammock or sleeping pad inside the hut of a native. Certain spots are used throughout the day or night for domestic duties. Also, there are often places in huts where no one ever sits or sleeps or where only men or women are permitted out of custom. Since travelers will not know where such taboo spots are, they should ask before bedding down.

Under circumstances where huts are not available for use, a properly used tarpaulin provides satisfactory shelter from the rain. Waterproof, rip-stop polyethylene tarps (7 × 9 feet), although bulky, are acceptable. If pack space is a concern, REI's compact, lightweight Coated Nylon Tarp in the 7 × 9 foot size is a good choice. Tarps of this type must be well sealed before use. Seam Grip is an excellent sealer.

Fig. 16-1 illustrates a typical method of erecting a tarp. First a fairly stout line is run between two trees at a height of 7 to 8 feet off the ground and is cinched tight. Next the long axis of the tarp is centered over the rope and a rope attached to the middle grommet on each end is tied to the tree. Then the corner grommets are tied to whatever trees, bushes, or strong clumps of grass are handy. In addition to the corner tie-downs, a tie-down in the middle on each side is helpful. The sides of the roof should be made high enough to enter

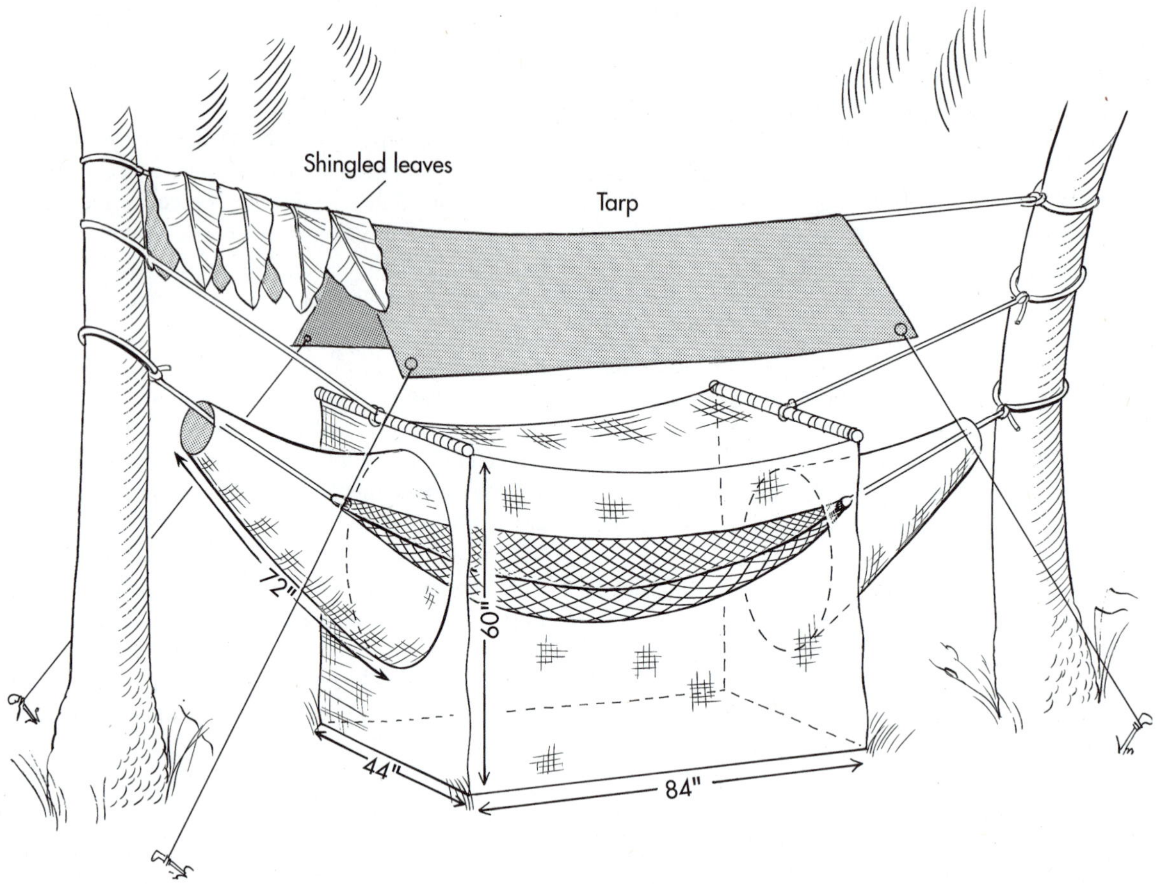

Fig. 16-1 Construction of mosquito netting for use with a hammock: sleeve hole = 88 inches in circumference; small hole = 18 inches in circumference; smallest holes (for supporting sticks) = 4 inches in circumference.

and exit conveniently, yet not so high that driving rain can come in at an angle.

Once the tarp is up, the hammock ropes are run through the sleeves of the mosquito net. Then the hammock is slung. It should be suspended high enough that it will not sag to the ground during the night as it naturally gives under an adult's weight. Next the mosquito net is suspended. The ropes running from tree to tarp, from tree to mosquito net, and from tree to hammock should be sprayed with Deet insect repellent to keep ants and other pests from using the ropes as trails. Finally, a few broad leaves (banana leaves or heliconia is perfect) are folded down at the spine and one or two are draped over the bare rope extending from the tree to the tarp, allowing the leaf nearest the tarp to "shingle" onto the tarp. This keeps rain from running down the tarp and hammock ropes.

Knowledge of two knots is needed for slinging a hammock. These knots always hold and always come undone quickly without jamming.

The *half hitch* is used to tie the hammock to a horizontal beam (Fig. 16-2):

1. Pass the working end of the rope around the object to which it is to be secured.
2. Pass the working end of the rope around again without crossing over itself.
3. Bring the end over and around the standing part and through the loop that has just been created. You have just made a half hitch.
4. Make a second half hitch below the first half hitch.
5. Pull tight.

The *camel hitch* is used to tie the hammock to a vertical post so securely that the user can sleep soundly knowing the knot will stay exactly where it was tied (Fig. 16-3):

1. Make three turns around the vertical pole.
2. Bring the working end up and over the turns.
3. Make a turn at the top and pass the end back under itself.
4. Make a second turn at the top and pass the end back under itself.

Never assume that just because the stars are twinkling brightly in a clear sky, the conditions will stay that way for long. In minutes, clouds can move in and shed rain that falls

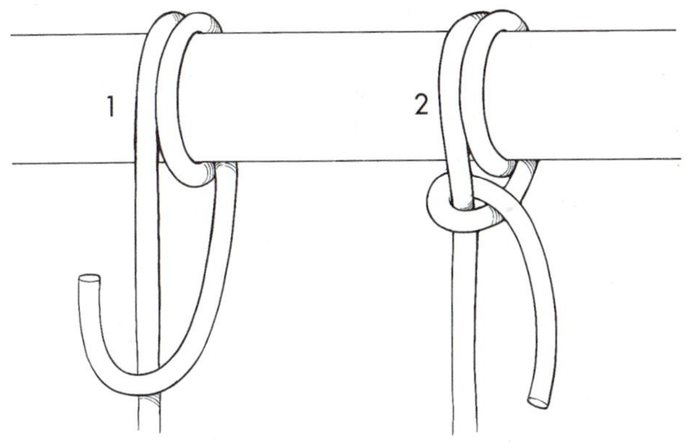

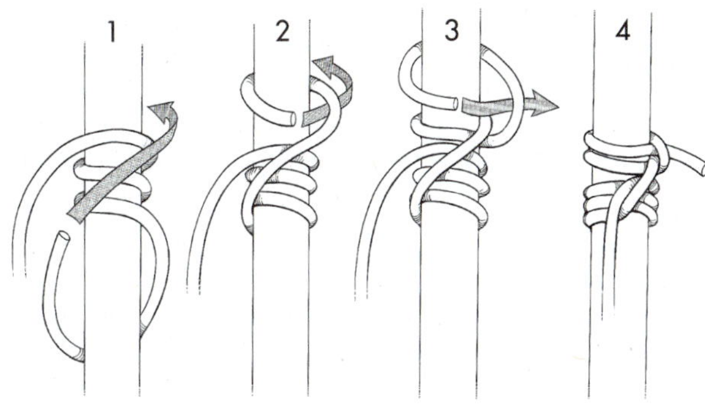

Fig. 16-3 Camel hitch.

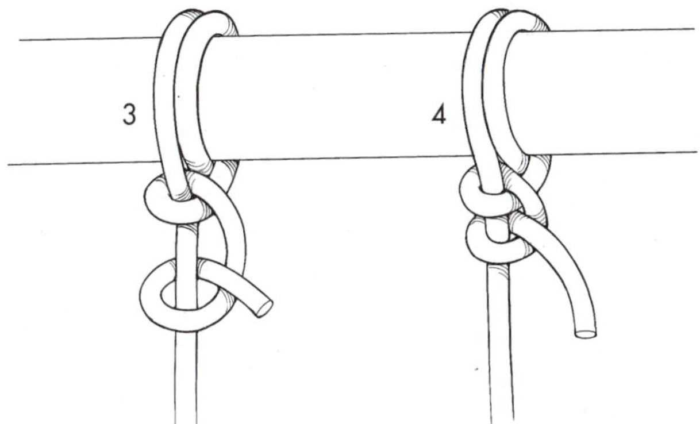

Fig. 16-2 Half hitch knot.

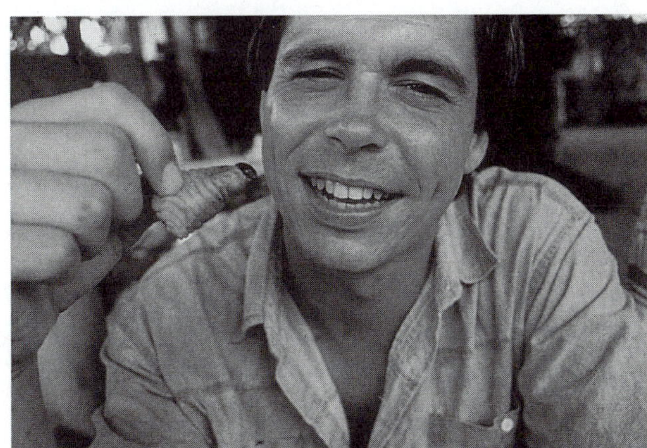

Fig. 16-4 The palm grub is a favorite of Amazonian Indians.

hard enough to shake the earth. A person who has not prepared shelter thoughtfully and well will pay the consequences.

The use of a tent as shelter in the tropical rainforest is not recommended. Clearing a tent space is time consuming, and the stumps remaining from cutting saplings and bushes invariably perforate the floor. Air does not circulate; after a restless night sweltering in the tent the traveler emerges tired, sticky, and irritable.

Food

Solitary travelers or small groups usually do not need to pack in large amounts of food. Edibles are always available in areas inhabited by friendly natives; the locals must be eating something. As a general rule, food is safe to eat if it is peeled, cooked, or boiled.

Travelers in the tropics must open the mind to eating the food that is available locally. Most creatures, whether they walk, crawl, slither, hop, scuttle, swim, or fly, are good to eat. So, persons confronted with boiled caiman (alligator), cooked capybara (a 50 kg rodent), or a plate of roasted palm grubs (larvae of *Rhynchophorus* spp.) should eat and be glad for food on the table. Raw palm grubs, up to 5 inches long, are quite tasty and are a great favorite of Amazonian Indians. They are eaten by slashing open the thin integument with the thumbnail, extracting and discarding the intestinal tract, placing the opened skin to the mouth, and sucking out the turgid contents. Like so many unpleasant-looking edible things (the oyster comes to mind), the palm grub is a great delicacy (Fig. 16-4).

In addition to palm grubs, more than 20 species of edible insects, including ants and termites, are collected year round by the people of Amazonia.[7] Large (10-inch diameter!) hairy spiders, *Theraphosa leblondi,* are often captured and roasted on an open fire. After the barbed hairs are singed off, the spider is placed in the embers away from the hottest part of the fire. Prepared in this manner spiders have a pleasant, shrimplike taste.

Indians of the Americans have perfected the art of smoking fish and meat so that they remain safe to eat for long periods. It is common to see huge hunks of tapir meat or monstrous slabs of 100-pound catfish resting on racks, coal black from the smoking process.

The tropics have an abundance of flora as food. The yard-long heart of palm is cool and delicious when eaten in its raw state or may be included in a soup spiced with tropical herbs. Several tropical fruits that make their way to grocers in North America and Europe should be familiar to the traveler: the papaya, excellent with a layering of lime juice; the mango, pungent but superb; and the juicy, sweet pineapple. In recent years consumers outside the tropics have experienced the delights of the passionfruit (*Passiflora* spp.) in fruit-based drinks. There are numerous New World fruits that often have no name in English and generally have not found their way into the world market: chirimoya, guanabana, pitahayas, naranjilla, uchuva, tamarillo, zapote, sapotilla, and badea, to name a few.[16,20,30] The boiled fruit of the peach palm, *Guillielma gasipaes,* is nutritious and flavorful.

The banana and its cousin, the plantain, provide a large percentage of the total caloric intake of natives in the American and African tropics. Curiously, in many native villages it is difficult to find the sweet, finger-length bananas and the common yellow bananas that are exported by the billions from tropical countries. It is, alas, the green plantain that features prominently in the daily fare of inhabitants of the tropics. The plantain cannot be faulted because of any disagreeable taste, since it has little taste at all. It is the fruit's exceptional dryness that makes it so unpalatable. Indeed, the most hardened tropical traveler may emit an audible groan when served a plate of dry, roasted plantains.

Yucca (manioc or cassava), *Manihot esculenta,* is a staple source of carbohydrate nutrition throughout the Americans and much of tropical Africa. There are two kinds of yucca, the "sweet" and the "bitter." They are both the same species but differ in the distribution and amount of a poisonous constituent, a cyanogenic glycoside, in the root.[26] To the eye, sweet and bitter yucca cannot be easily distinguished; one must know which variety was planted. Sweet yucca, commonly encountered in the eastern lowlands of the Andean countries of Colombia, Ecuador, and Peru, is eaten after the bark containing the toxic substance is peeled off and the root is boiled. In bitter yucca, the poison is more concentrated and distributed throughout the root, so it must be extracted before consumption. Amerindians have devised an ingenious apparatus, the *tipití,* that expresses the poisonous juice from the peeled and grated flour of the manioc roots.

Travelers in a large group should carry dried, packaged foods, since the host village might not be able to provide sufficient foodstuffs or they might pass through truly isolated or unexplored regions that are uninhabited. Packaged foods should be carried by travelers in regions where the locals are known to be unfriendly.

Dried instant food simply needs the addition of water to make a good and hearty meal. A few selections should be tried before a large supply for field use is ordered. It is not necessary to add hot water to all packaged foods; adding purified, ambient-temperature water produces acceptable results for most foods. Drawbacks to prepackaged foods include the expense, the space they take up, and the matter of dealing with the empty foil packages.

I carry the following supplemental food items for 2- to 3-week treks into remote but inhabited jungle regions: one 2-ounce heavy-duty poly bottle filled with salt and pepper mixed half and half, a few pounds of rice, a tin of long-keeping butter (or oil) for cooking the rice, a few tins of tuna, and a couple of pounds of hard caramels for trail snack treats.

Potable Water

Potable Aqua (tetraglycine hydroperiodide 16.7%) tablets are recommended for treating water because they are easy to use and have proved effective in killing bacteria, viruses, and most parasite cysts (see Chapter 45).

Water filters have gained popularity in recent years and are standard equipment on high-altitude expeditions. Filters are not recommended for purifying jungle water; they clog up with silt every few minutes and must be cleaned frequently.

HAZARDS (REAL AND IMAGINED)

The following hazards were chosen for discussion because they are commonly encountered in the wilderness jungle setting—or because people think they are. Additional insights and viewpoints, particularly with respect to treatment, are given by other authors throughout this book.

Arthropods

Ants. The conga ant, *Paraponera clavata,* 1 to 1½ inches long, is the terror of the American tropics. The bite of these large black ants can produce intense pain and fever for up to 24 hours, hence the Spanish name *veinte-cuatro* (twenty-four). Fortunately, they are conspicuous because their large, shiny black bodies tend to stand out against foliage. Special caution is needed when ducking under or climbing over trees that have fallen over the trail; ants are often found in these fallen trees. A conga bite requires strong pain medication and perhaps the injection of lidocaine at the bite site.

Travelers should avoid touching trees and bushes. Many plants in the tropics harbor colonies of ant "protectors" in a relationship in which the plants provide a home and food for the ants and the ants provide aggressive defense of the plants.

Fire ants are common throughout the tropics and subtropics. Their bite causes discomfort, but not excruciating pain.

Chiggers. Chiggers, a form of mite, are a problem throughout the equatorial regions. Whereas temperate-climate chiggers may cause mild discomfort for a few days, the tropical chigger sets up an inflammatory and allergic reaction that often persists for weeks.

In the South American tropics, chiggers are found in grassy fields such as jungle airstrips and yards around mission compounds. Walking through chigger-infested areas without protection could leave a person covered with chigger bites. After a few days the victim begins to itch mildly.

As the days pass, the itching intensifies and seems to come in waves. A curious feature of chigger infestation is that at times the itching seems to be centered in one area, such as the legs, and a few hours later another area may feel on fire.

Prevention is the best treatment. Areas known to be infested with chiggers should be avoided when possible. Spraying shoes or boots and lower pant legs with repellent containing DEET is highly effective.

Pretreatment of clothing with permethrin has been recommended. Travelers in the tropics should *never* walk through grassy areas in shorts. A number of remedies have been proposed, none of which is universally successful in eliminating or shortening the course of the infuriating itch.

Jigger Flea. *Tunga penetrans,* the jigger flea or chigoe, originally was found in South and Central America but now has spread to East and West Africa and India. The fertilized female flea enters the feet through cracks in the soles, between the toes, and around the toenails. At about the time the flea eggs are ripe for release, intense itching sets in and the ensuing scratching helps release large numbers of flea eggs.

Natives are familiar with the appearance and symptoms of jigger flea infestation and have developed expertise in plucking them out so that the jigger does not burst during extraction, an occurrence that generally leads to impressive complications. A sterile needle should be supplied for the extraction.

Myiasis. Myiasis (skin infestation by fly larvae) is common in many regions of sub-Saharan Africa (the tumbu fly, *Cordylobia anthropophaga*) or Central and South America (the human botfly, *Dermatobia hominis*). The victim finds an itchy swelling that slowly enlarges into a lesion with a single breathing pore from which bubbles a clear or slightly bloody drainage. Later, movement is felt under the skin as the developing larva wriggles around.

Removing the larvae before they emerge on their own is generally advised, if only for esthetic reasons: there is something inherently unpleasant about harboring a moving, growing maggot under the skin. Surgical excision, however, should be undertaken with caution because accidental rupture of the larval tegument can lead to secondary infections. Various methods have been employed to close off the breathing pore so the larva will emerge on its own; such methods include the application of bacon fat, meat, chewing gum, or petroleum jelly.

Scorpions and Spiders. Stinging scorpions and venomous spiders are common throughout the tropics and provide yet another reason to exercise caution before sitting down or placing a hand on logs, bushes, or the ground.

Venomous Moths, Butterflies, and Caterpillars. The larvae and adults of a number of moths (genus *Hylesia*) and butterflies bear venomous hairs that may cause skin eruptions. The rash may result from direct contact with the adults or larvae or by windblown hairs. The pain resulting from direct contact with certain Amazonian caterpillars can be excruciating and disabling.

In the Amazon tropics, noxious smoke from the burning of garbage (such as the plastic wrappers of freeze-dried food) may cause tree-dwelling caterpillars to loosen their hold on overhead branches and rain down on unwary campers below.

Treatment of lepidoptera envenomation, discussed in Chapter 31, may require injection of lidocaine at the site of intense pain and the administration of analgesics, antihistamines, and corticosteroids. Moth hairs may be removed with the sticky rolling lint removers used for clothing.

Wasp and Bee Stings. The sudden, intense pain from the sting of certain species of tropical wasps and bees can be so severe that it knocks the victim to the ground as though hit with an electric shock. Wearing of perfumes and brightly colored or flower-patterned clothing should be avoided.[14] Bird watchers should not venture too close to the hanging nests of yellow-rumped caciques and oropendolas because wasps are invariably associated with these nests.

Fish

Stingray. The stingray, a flattened, cartilaginous cousin of the shark, may be encountered buried just beneath the surface of the bottom ooze in tropical rivers and streams throughout the Amazon Basin, Africa, and Indochina. Rays inflict injury by lashing upward with the tail, driving a barbed venomous spine deep into the victim's foot, ankle, or lower leg. This produces agonizing pain often accompanied by headache, vomiting, and shortness of breath. After the initial phase of envenomation passes, tissue death may set in. Wearing shoes or boots when wading in water does not always prevent the stingray from jabbing its barb into the foot or leg. Prevention lies in shuffling the feet along the bottom so that the ray will have enough warning to glide away safely (see Chapter 51).

Electric Eel. The so-called electric eel (actually an eel-shaped fish) is encountered from Guatemala to the La Plata River in South America and is especially common in the Amazon region. A person can drown after being stunned by the jolt this fish delivers.

Electric eels are said to prefer deep water. Inhabitants of regions heavily infested with eels report that a slight tingling sensation of the skin may be felt when one is close at hand. No practical way of preventing these shocks is known, although legends tell of explorers in years past driving horses through infested waters so that the eels discharged their "batteries" and were rendered harmless to humans wading in the river.

Candirú. The candirú is a toothpick-sized parasitic catfish that inhabits Amazonian waters and may invade the urethra of humans who are voiding. Orifice penetration by the wily candirú can be prevented by wearing a tight bathing suit and not urinating underwater. The British author Redmond O'Hanlon feared this fish so much that he invented an anti-candirú device using a tea-strainer to fit over his penis![19] There are various native methods of dislodging these fish from the urethra, including drinking a tea made from the green fruit of the jugua tree, *Genipa americana L.* Two to five grams of vitamin C taken by mouth may serve the same purpose (see Chapter 52).[3]

Piranha. As previously noted, there are no confirmed human deaths resulting from piranha attack. These fish have, however, nipped off the fingertips of canoeists who carelessly dangled their hands in the water in a sort of trolling mode.

Mammals

Bats. Vampire bats are found throughout Mexico, Central America, and South America, especially in areas that have large cattle ranches. Sleeping humans are unaware of the presence of a feeding bat; the phlebotomy is painless. Both vampire and fruit bats carry rabies. Sleeping under mosquito netting prevents bat bites. The risk of rabies can be reduced by prophylactic human diploid cell vaccine.

Dogs. Most native groups keep dogs around for hunting. Populations with a history of recent tribal warfare often keep packs of dogs close by as an early warning system. These semiwild dogs should be treated with caution; threatening them may cause immediate attack, since they are not easily intimidated. When approaching huts or villages, the traveler should allow porters to go first so they can deal with the dogs.

Dogs that are intent on biting often adopt particular behavior patterns. The traveler should be hypervigilant of the dog that, when protecting its territory, crouches low, straightens its back and tail, emits a deep guttural growl, and stares fixedly at a specific part of the person's anatomy. When such behavior is observed, an attack is imminent. At this point a sharp blow to the nose with the foot or a stick may be the only way to deflect the attack. Some dog experts recommend freezing in place as a way of avoiding attack by a dog whose space has been invaded. It is best to avoid making direct eye contact with a dog that exhibits aggressive behavior.

Jaguars. Jaguar attacks are exceedingly rare. The following recommendations for deterring a jaguar attack are based on advice for avoiding a cougar attack. Increase your apparent size by raising your arms above the head and waving an object such as a backpack or stick or opening a jacket. Yell, shout, whistle, or speak loudly and forcefully in a low, deep tone of voice. Back away slowly; do not turn your back and run.[6]

Reptiles

Snakes. Snakebites are rare; 450,000 person-hours of field work at sites in Costa Rican rainforests were documented without a single snakebite.[5]

Most poisonous snakes tend to blend into their surroundings, and nonnatives rarely see them. This fact is the basis for the most effective protection: putting a jungle-reared guide in front on the trail. Natives almost always spot a poisonous snake and can quickly dispatch it.

Snakes are often encountered along the shoreline of rivers and small streams. Particular caution is needed when hiking in such areas or when disembarking from a canoe or rubber raft. In the forest the hiker should always step up onto a log and then step away from the log: it should *not* be straddled (snakes often are encountered where the log makes contact with the jungle floor). Since many venomous snakes in the tropics are heat seeking and hunt at night, caution is needed when walking around in camp at night. Trips to the toilet after dark should be kept to a minimum.

Anacondas (water boas) feature in the folklore of all native cultures in the regions of Amazonia where these enormous snakes (up to 30 feet long) live. These nonpoisonous snakes kill by looping coils around prey and then tightening the coils, suffocating the victim. There are anecdotal reports of anacondas attacking and swallowing humans, particularly children and women bathing at the edge of jungle streams, but such stories are unconfirmed.

Alligators and Crocodiles. Alligators and crocodiles appear torpid as they lie sunning themselves. Such creatures can move amazingly fast when they want to; humans cannot outswim or outrun a charging crocodile.

Bites should be treated with thorough cleaning of the wound, surgical debridement if necessary, tetanus prophylaxis, and an appropriate antibiotic. A study of the oral flora of 10 alligators captured in Louisiana revealed various aerobic and anaerobic organisms responsive to trimethoprim-sulfamethoxaole.[10]

Plants

Armed or Spine-Bearing Plants. Spine-bearing trees abound in forested areas of the tropics. The peach palm *(Bactris gasipaes),* a tall, slender palm whose fruit mesocarp is much prized by natives, is found from Nicaragua to Bolivia. The trunk of this tree is ringed with needle-sharp spines (Fig. 16-5). Peach palms often grow alongside trails. Contact with this palm can result in penetration of spines deep into the flesh. Spines that enter a joint space may re-

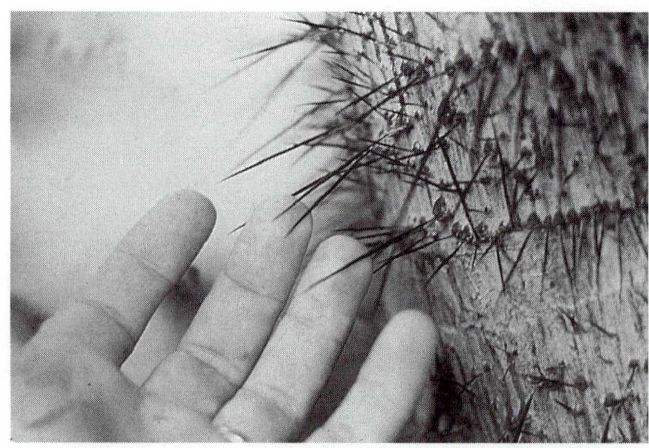

Fig. 16-5 Needle-sharp spines ring the "peach palm."

quire surgical extraction. Secondary infection and an inflammatory response often occur.

Hallucinogenic Plants. Jungle-dwelling tribes throughout Central and South America use hallucinogenic plants. To ignore the ubiquity of psychoactive drugs among Amerindians is to deny a key element in understanding the rich and complex weave of Indian life. Powerful drugs such as ayahuasca (*Banisteriopsis* spp.), *Brugmansia* spp., the virola snuffs, and yopo *(A. peregrina)* are used within an indigenous sacred context allowing, for example, a shaman to "see" and to know the truth.[24-26]

Should the traveler partake of hallucinogens? Some argue, with a certain validity, that outsiders cannot acquire insight into Indians' drug-induced sense of the cosmos without ingesting their mind-altering drugs. However, given the very real risks of emerging with a damaged sense of identity in the home culture—a virtual blurring of the sense of reality—and lingering unpleasant aftereffects, it is wise to avoid these powerful intoxicants.

Sawgrass. In many regions of the tropics, sawgrass is an ever-present nuisance. Blades of this grass can slice into exposed skin like a surgical scalpel. Even when treated with antibiotic ointment, the lacerations often take 1 to 2 weeks to heal. Hikers should carefully avoid touching sawgrass; special care is needed when working with a machete.

Miscellaneous Hazards

Falling Trees. Tropical trees do not have deep roots and often fall in relatively modest winds. In many regions of the world the risk of snakebite is significantly lower than the risk of injury or death from falling trees.

Little can be done to anticipate or avoid trees that fall in a windstorm or simply because they are old and rotted. In the forest, hammocks should be slung away from large trees. Travelers setting up camp should always look up at the branches of any trees near camp; although the base of the tree may appear sound, areas high up may be rotted.

Fording Rivers. The hiker should never attempt to cross a fast-flowing or deep river with a pack on the back. Regaining footing in a rapidly moving current can be difficult. Unless experienced in crossing such streams, the traveler should take the hand of a native guide or porter.

Log Bridges. On frequently used trails, natives generally place a single log across creeks, ravines, and swampy areas. These log "bridges" may be up to 20 feet high and 75 feet long. Since there is generally nothing to hold onto, good balance is essential. Because a backpack seems to significantly impair balance, a porter should carry it across. (See the discussion of balance in this chapter under "Trip Preparation.")

Mercury Contamination. Travelers to the Amazon Basin should be aware of the serious, widespread contamination of waterways by mercury that gold miners *(garimpeiros)* use to process their ore. Of the commonly available portable water treatment and filtration systems, none claims to remove dissolved heavy metal compounds such as mercury. Travelers should exercise caution in choosing rivulets as a source of potable water in areas where mercury contamination is known or suspected.

Rising Rivers. Streams, particularly narrow ones bounded by vertical banks, can rise 20 feet in a few hours as a result of intense rains. Camp should not be set up on an island or beach in a small canyon during the rainy season. A cloudburst in the headwaters can send a wall of water rushing downstream even though it may be a clear, moonlit night at the campsite.

Traveling with Children in the Tropics

The following guidelines should be considered when trekking with children in the tropical forest:

1. Do not attempt a daylong hike. Indigenous children can hike all day in the humid tropical forest; a nonnative child cannot. A hike of 1 to 2 hours is plenty for preadolescents, or 2 to 3 hours for children aged 12 to 16. Do not subject a child to jungle trail conditions unless the child has had extensive experience hiking in temperate climates.
2. Do not attempt difficult or dangerous trails.
3. Avoid trekking during the rainy season.
4. Keep the child well hydrated.
5. Provide proper footwear (running or hiking sneaker-type shoes or boots with an adequate tread). Avoid leather boots.
6. Keep the child ahead of you and behind a native guide. Children should not be out of sight on the trail.
7. When wading across rivers, have an adult native guide hold the child's hand.
8. *Always* have children wear a properly sized life vest while rafting, taking canoe trips, or crossing deep, swift, or wide rivers.
9. Do not allow a child to carry any equipment in a daypack other than 2 L bottles of drinking water.
10. Ensure that routine vaccinations are up to date. Special vaccinations such as yellow fever and typhoid should be considered for certain jungle areas. Hepatitis A protection using immune globulin (IG) is recommended. Antimalarials are indicated.

A special word of caution regarding swimming: any child who plans to visit the tropics should be a strong swimmer. Many natives begin swimming in infancy and are accustomed to bathing and playing in deep or rapidly flowing water that would be extremely hazardous to visiting children. Swimming holes are often located in the swift-flowing outer loop of jungle rivers where depths may reach 6 feet or more within a yard of the shoreline.

Survival

Every year, inexperienced people enter the jungle and get lost. After a person ventures but a few yards into the forest, especially jungle that has been cleared and is now a tangle of secondary growth, everything begins to look the same. *To avoid getting lost, travelers should always have an experienced guide when traversing unfamiliar territory.*

Occasionally travelers are left behind on the trail by indigenous guides. Unintentional desertion happens when trekkers hire natives who have had no experience with neophytes. Realizing almost at once that their charges cannot keep up on the trail, the guides run ahead and sit down to rest, not knowing that others cannot navigate the trail alone. Travelers who want to avoid being left behind on the trail should hire a guide who is experienced in traveling with nonnatives.

RESCUE STRATEGIES

The focus of survival in the jungle should be geared toward efforts that will get the traveler out—fast.

Lightweight, hand-held aircraft VHF band transceivers are excellent for emergency communications. Visitors to remote areas should ascertain beforehand the radio frequencies that potential rescue aircraft might use. VHF transceivers are line-of-sight instruments, so they are most useful when aircraft are overhead without objects such as trees or mountains between the hand-held unit and the aircraft. When weight is not a major issue, single sideband (SSB) transceivers should be considered. Within the next few years, portable satellite transceivers will become the system of choice for worldwide emergency communications.

Lightweight global positioning system (GPS) units are the size of a paperback novel and display precise latitude, longitude, and altitude. Such information is extremely useful when communicating with rescue aircraft.

Canoeists, rafters, or trekkers contemplating an expedition into largely uninhabited and unexplored regions should consider buying a compact emergency position-indicating radio beacon (EPIRB). The new 406 MHz EPIRB units offer a reliable method of alerting various rescue services via a global satellite system. These units should be activated only in a true emergency when lives are at risk.

In many regions of the world the Missionary Aviation Fellowship (MAF) provides air service into remote airstrips in small villages. If assistance is needed, a hand-held ratio transmitter can be used to call an MAF short take-off and landing (STOL) aircraft.

Bush pilots appreciate having information on the condition of seldom used airstrips. A crude but acceptable device for measuring airstrip hardness is constructed and used as follows: Cut a pole exactly 2 inches in diameter and approximately 6 feet long. Starting exactly 6 inches from one end, taper that end to a point. Lash a cross-member on the pole and have a person weighing approximately 170 pounds stand with assistance on the cross-member. Make a map of the strip, noting the depth to which the pointed end of the pole sinks into the earth at several dozen sites. Communicate this information to the pilot by radio. If the pole goes in only 2 inches in most areas, the strip is considered ideal; 2 to 4 inches is marginal; penetration beyond 4 inches indicates that the airstrip is unsuitable for landing and take-off.

If rescue is not feasible, the traveler should continually move downstream at a fast pace. In inhabited areas there is usually a trail running alongside a stream. From time to time the trail may veer away from the stream where natives have cut a path to connect two villages by the shortest distance rather than following the meandering course of the river. Marking the trail every 10 yards with a machete makes it easier to return to the starting point. To avoid confusion, the traveler should mark trees only on one side of the trail. In the jungle setting, navigation with a compass for a distance of more than 200 yards is fraught with hazard. Travelers should not attempt to cut overland if lost, inexperienced, or on their own unless a significant landmark is visible or sounds of humans or domesticated animals, indicating a settlement, are clearly heard.

A raft may be constructed by lashing logs together with rope or tough, pliable jungle vines. Balsa trees *(Ochroma pyramidale),* encountered throughout much of Amazonia,

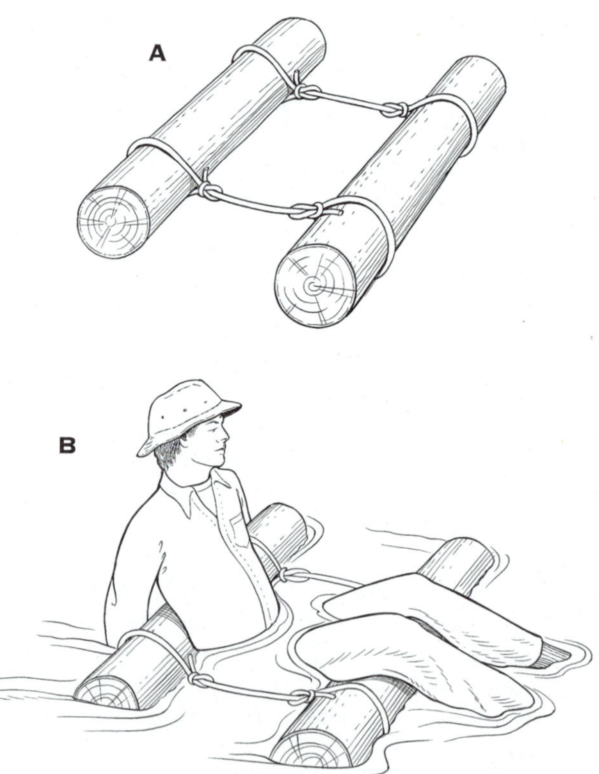

Fig. 16-6 Log flotation device. **A,** Two lightweight logs are tied together to create the log flotation device. **B,** Log flotation device in action.

make the best rafts. Balsa is often found growing alongside rivers and has the following characteristics: tall, columnar trunk with branches and leaves bunched at the top, which gives the tree a "skinny" look; beige or gray-beige trunk; bark that is smooth but tends to flake, giving it a mottled appearance; and broadly heart-shaped, more or less three-lobed leaves. The key feature of balsa wood is its remarkably light weight.

A log flotation device may be fashioned by using two balsa logs or other lightweight wood placed 2 feet apart and tied together (Fig. 16-6).[28]

A "brush" raft may be constructed by placing buoyant vegetation within clothing or a poncho. Dry leaf litter ("duff") or plants such as water hyacinth may be used.[28]

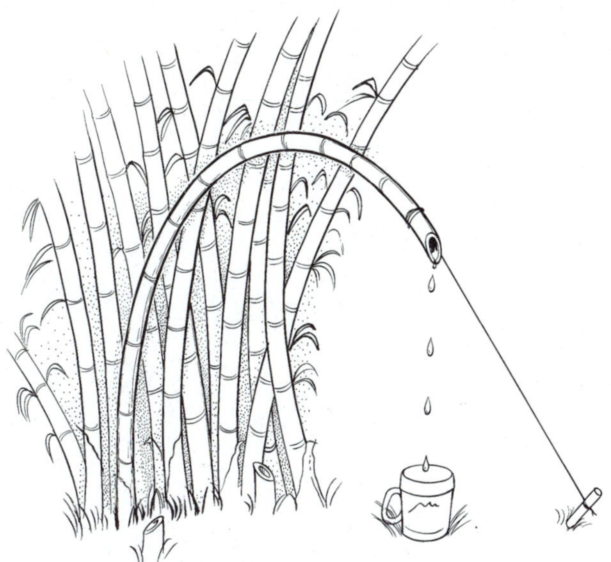

Fig. 16-7 Bamboo can be source of water.

FOOD

Food is readily available. Even abandoned villages yield enough fruit and vegetables on which to survive. Root crops such as taro, yams, and yucca should be sought. Yucca roots should be shredded or pounded and then boiled to release the toxic compounds they contain. As an extra precaution, the wet pulp should be flattened into a "pancake" and cooked on a grate to drive off any remaining volatile hydrogen cyanide gas.

All land crabs, mammals, birds, freshwater fish, turtles, snakes, and lizards are edible but should be cooked first to eliminate parasites.[2] It is virtually impossible to kill game without firearms. In inexperienced hands, traps and snares are not effective. Much better results are obtained from fishing.

For additional general rules regarding wilderness edibles, see Chapter 15.

WATER

Water may be made safe by boiling or using chemical disinfectants such as Potable Aqua tablets. Drinkable water may be found in lianas, often called "water vines," throughout jungle regions. Vines that contain water are fairly easy to identify because they tend to resemble the "grapevines" of North American forests and have rough, scaly bark. These vines may be several inches thick and contain surprising amounts of crystal-clear water. Vines that do not contain drinkable water tend to have a smoother bark and when cut exude a sticky, milky liquid. Travelers should *not* drink from vines that contain milky, latexlike sap; these vines are poisonous. Maximal amounts of water are collected from water-bearing vines if the first cut is high on the vine and the second cut is lower on the vine near the ground.

Water may be trapped within sections of certain types of green bamboo. Bamboo that contains water makes a sloshing sound when shaken. Water also may be obtained from green bamboo stalks by bending a stalk over, tying it down,

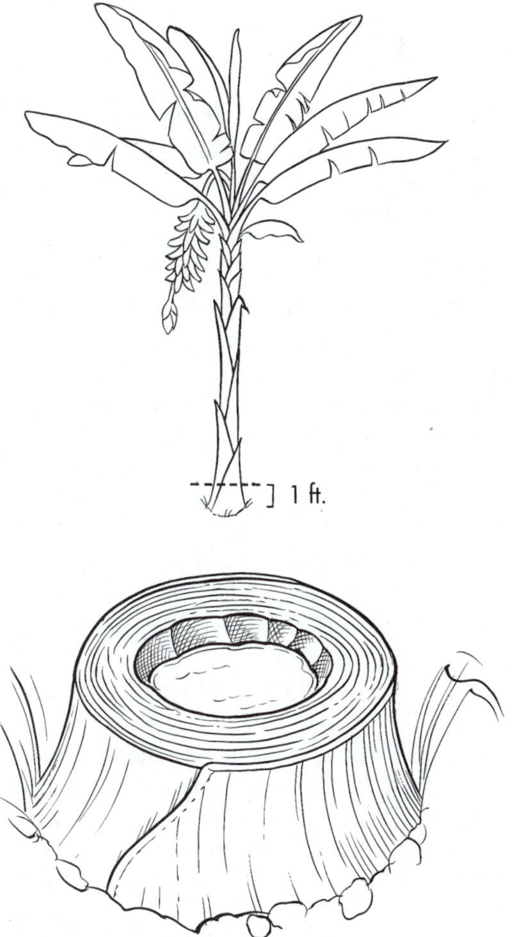

Fig. 16-8 Water collected from banana plant.

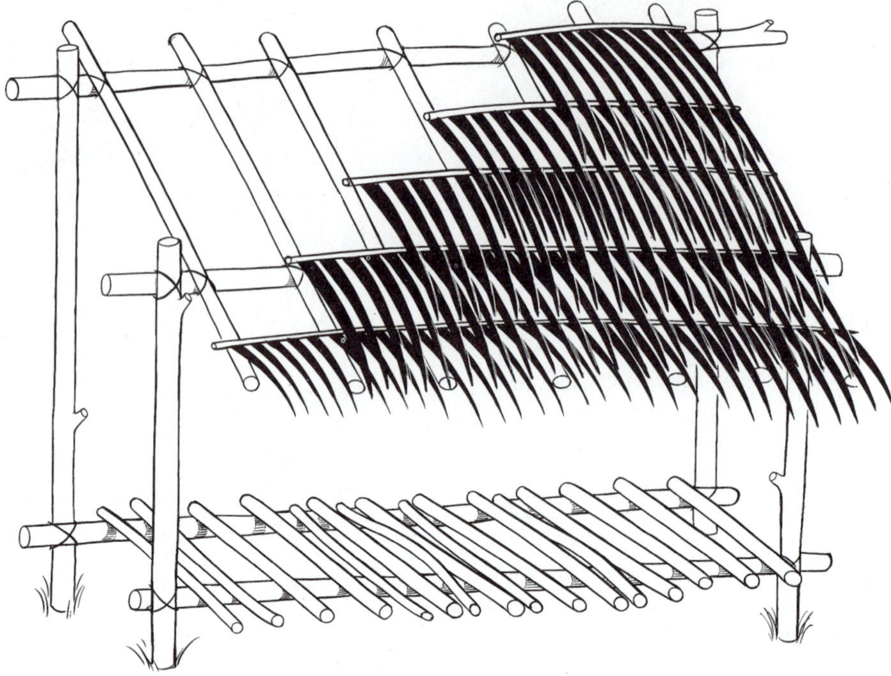

Fig. 16-9 Sleeping platform.

and cutting off the top. Water dripping from the severed tip can be collected in a container during the night (Fig. 16-7).[28]

Large amounts of water can be found in the voluminous natural cisterns formed by the cuplike interiors of epiphytes (air plants) such as bromeliads. The water should be strained through a cloth.[28]

Water may be collected from a banana or plantain plant by cutting the plant approximately 1 foot above the ground and scooping out the center of the stump into a bowl shape. The hollow thus formed fills immediately with water. The first two fillings have a bitter taste and should be dipped out. The third and subsequent fillings are drinkable. A banana plant can furnish water in this fashion for several days (Fig. 16-8).[28]

In coastal regions unripe (green) coconuts provide adequate supplies of refreshing milk. The milk of mature coconuts has a laxative effect and should be avoided.

SHELTER

In an emergency it is possible to construct a proper shelter using only plant materials. Fig. 16-9 illustrates the basics of constructing a sleeping platform and lean-to.

A covering can be made from tropical palms by selecting a suitable ground-hugging species or chopping down a slender tall palm (palm trees with spines often provide the best fronds) and separating each frond into halves. This is accomplished by grasping the frond at the distal end, separating the leaves as though parting hair down the middle,

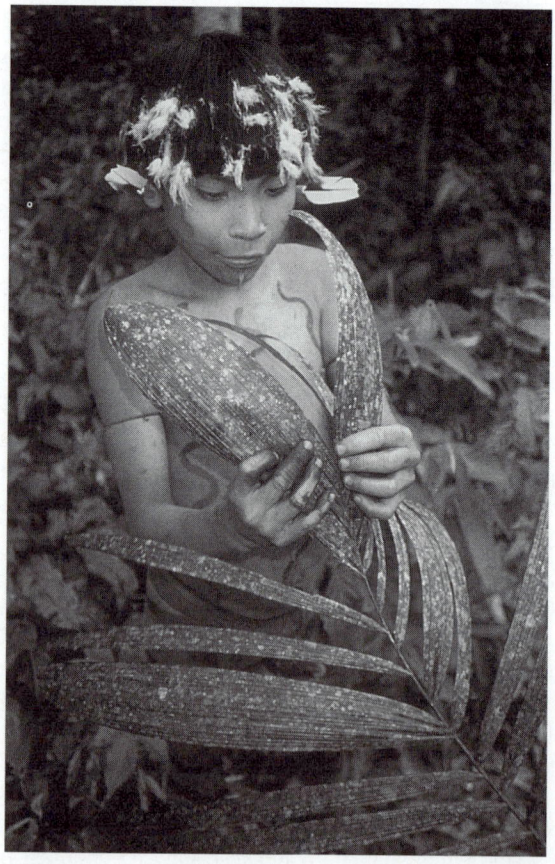

Fig. 16-10 Indian splitting a frond to make a covering for a lean-to.

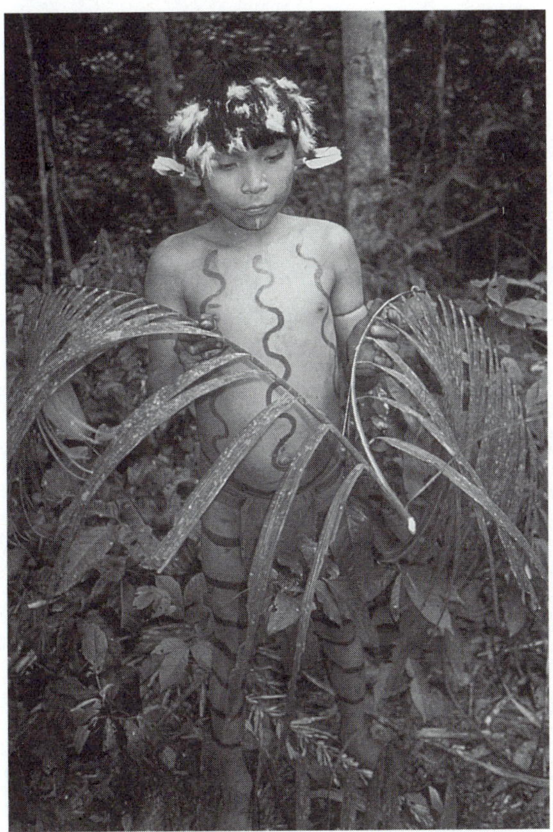

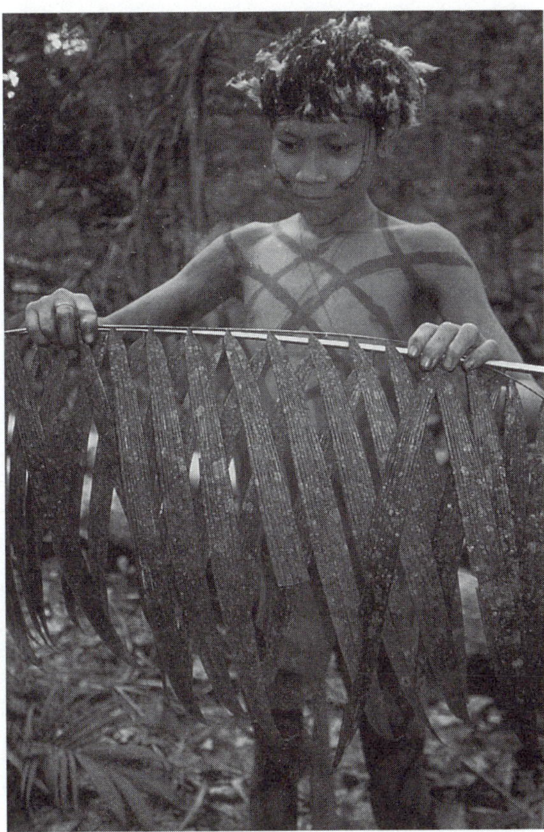

Fig. 16-10, cont'd. For legend see opposite page.

and with a quick jerk splitting the frond in two (Fig. 16-10). The halves should be overlapped like shingles and secured to the roof framework.

It is much easier to construct an adequate shelter using a tarpaulin (see "Camp Life" in this chapter).

REFERENCES

1. Berthoz A, Pozzo T: Intermittent head stabilization during postural and locomotory tasks in humans. In Amblard B, Berthoz A, Clarac F, editors: *Development, adaptation and modulation of posture and gait,* Amsterdam, 1988, Elsevier.
2. Bowman WD: Wilderness survival. In Auerbach PS, Geehr EC, editors: *Management of wilderness and environmental emergencies,* ed 2, St Louis, 1989, Mosby.
3. Breault JL: Candiru: Amazonian parasitic catfish, *J Wilderness Med* 2(4):312, 1991.
4. Clement G, Pozzo T, Berthoz A: Contribution of eye position to control of the upside-down standing posture, *Exp Brain Res* 73(3):569, 1988.
5. Colwell RK: A bite to remember, *Natural History* 94(4):2, 1985.
6. Conrad L: Cougar attack: case report of a fatality, *J Wilderness Med* 3(4):387, 1992.
7. Dufour DL: Insects as food, *Am Anthropologist* 89(2):383, 1987.
8. *The emerald realm: earth's precious rainforests,* Washington, DC, 1990, National Geographic Society.
9. Erb BD: Predicting success in wilderness ventures, *Wilderness Med Lett* 7(3):8, 1990.
10. Flandry F et al: Initial antibiotic therapy for alligator bites, *South Med J* 82(2):262, 1989.
11. Forsyth A, Miyata K: *Tropical nature,* New York, 1984, Scribner's.
12. Goodman P, Kurtz KJ, Carmichael J: Medical recommendations for wilderness travel, *Postgrad Med* 77(8):173, 1985.
13. Houston CS: Who will you take on a high mountain expedition? *Wilderness Med Lett* 7(3):11, 1990.
14. Iserson KV, editor: *Position statements,* Point Reyes Station, Calif, 1989, Wilderness Medical Society.
15. Kritcher JC: *A neotropical companion,* Princeton, NJ, 1989, Princeton University Press.
16. *Lost crops of the Incas,* Washington, DC, 1989, National Academy Press.
17. Lovejoy TE: Foreword. In Forsyth A, Miyata K: *Tropical nature,* New York, 1984, Scribner's.
18. Myers N: *The primary source,* New York, 1984, WW Norton.
19. O'Hanlon R: *In trouble again,* New York, 1990, Vintage Books.
20. Olaya Cl: *Frutas de America,* Bogota, Colombia, 1991, Editorial Norma.
21. Perry DR: The canopy of the tropical rainforest, *Sci Am* 251(5):138, 1984.
22. Pozzo T, Berthoz A, Lefort L: Head stabilization during various locomotor tasks in humans, *Exp Brain Res* 82(1):97, 1990.
23. Richards P: The tropical rainforests, *Sci Am* 229(6):58, 1973.
24. Schultes RE: *Where the gods reign,* Oracle, Ariz, 1988, Synergetic Press.

25. Schultes RE, Hofmann A: *Plants of the gods,* New York, 1979, McGraw-Hill.
26. Schultes RE, Raffauf RF: *The healing forest,* Portland, 1990, Dioscorides Press.
27. Schwerdtfeger W, editor: *World survey of climatology,* 16 vols, New York, 1969-1986, Elsevier Scientific.
28. *Survival: AF Regulation 64-4,* vol 1, Washington, DC, 1985, Department of the Air Force.
29. Theroux P: *The happy isles of Oceania,* New York, 1992, Putnam's.
30. Weatherford J: *Indian givers,* New York, 1988, Crown.
31. Wilson EO: Threats to biodiversity, *Sci Am* 261(3):108, 1989.
32. Wilson EO, editor: *Biodiversity,* Washington, DC, 1988, National Academy Press.

17 WILDERNESS EQUIPMENT AND MEDICAL SUPPLIES

Steven C. Zell
Philip H. Goodman

The foremost challenges of wilderness recreation are the prevention and management of injury and illness. Medical care may be greatly delayed for the person who becomes disabled many hours from civilization. Unnecessary suffering can be minimized by educating the traveler, planning each trip carefully, and carrying appropriate medical, first aid, and emergency supplies.

Large expeditions usually enlist experienced medical professionals in logistic planning. Unfortunately, most smaller groups trekking into the wilds do not have access to this professional expertise. Even when a physician is a party member, he or she is usually not specifically trained in wilderness medicine. This text details medical management in the wilderness setting. This chapter is intended to complement that material by summarizing recommendations for selecting medical provisions for a variety of wilderness experiences. The first part of the chapter is an overview of important preventive measures and risk factors for wilderness travel. The second part highlights assembly of the medical kit and provides quick references intended for persons engaging in low-risk wilderness travel. The indexes for contingency and medical supplies (see Figs. 17-2 and 17-3) are intended primarily for persons with medical experience and allow a more sophisticated selection of supplies based on duration of travel and distance from medical care. The final section of the chapter updates the use of equipment and medical supplies, describing specific high-technology items that are not standard to the basic wilderness medical kit.

Before any travel in the wilderness, it is important to understand the epidemiology of wilderness injuries because such information helps in the selection of components of the first aid kit. Incidents can be broadly categorized into traumatic injuries associated with wilderness travel and medical illness related to specific recreational or environmental hazards. Data from the National Outdoor Leadership School emphasize that injuries account for most of the incidents requiring medical attention; sprains and strains are the most common, followed by soft tissue injuries. Fractures and dislocations account for less than 5% of traumatic injuries. In addition, medical illness is uncommon (1.5 per 1000 person days of travel) and is most often due to a nonspecific viral syndrome. Less common illnesses described include dermatologic problems from sun exposure, rashes, diarrhea, headache, and pain from dental caries. Environmental issues predominantly relate to high-altitude illness and hypothermia, with their importance increasing as a function of altitude and duration of cold exposure. Both can occur regardless of the level of prior physical conditioning.

Preparing for Travel

GENERAL PREPAREDNESS

It is the responsibility of the trip coordinator to assess the health limitations of the group. A questionnaire for this purpose is provided in Appendix A at the end of the chapter. The coordinator should confidentially but frankly discuss medical problems with each candidate and require a medical evaluation if uncertainty exists. The safety of the individual and the group is the coordinator's first priority. Boxes 17-1 and 17-2 give checklists for preparedness.

BOX 17-1

CHECKLIST FOR GENERAL PREPAREDNESS

Physical conditioning
Immunizations (especially tetanus)
Planning of potential rescue and evacuation routes and leaving an itinerary with person to initiate rescue if group does not return on time
Proper clothing and equipment
Medical-alert medallion or card (illness, allergy, medication)
Water disinfection (chemicals or devices)
Sunglasses, sunscreen, and adhesive blister pads
Historical appraisal of weather conditions:
National Climatic Data Center (704-259-0682) (United States and global cities; small fee)
State climatologists
National and state park services

Fitness

Healthy Participants. Active, healthy individuals should begin a graduated exercise program at least 2 months before departure to minimize the deleterious effects of muscular, metabolic, and mental fatigue. This is especially important for persons going to high altitude; aerobic capacity in a sedentary person drops about 4% for each 1000 feet (300 m) above the 4000-foot (1200 m) level, but the loss is only half as great in an aerobically fit individual (see Chapter 1). Careful stretching of muscle groups may increase efficiency and lessen the likelihood of soft tissue injury during exertion and minor accidents.

If excessive environmental heat is anticipated, preparatory exercise in a hot, humid environment (simulated with sweat clothing) for 1 hour daily for at least 7 days before departure will increase plasma volume (aldosterone effect) and sweat rate, while lowering myocardial oxygen demand and sweat sodium content. This acclimatization will be lost within a week if not maintained (see Chapter 2).

Persons with Preexisting Medical Problems. Participants with preexisting cardiovascular or pulmonary disease should have a medical evaluation.

Cardiovascular contraindications to travel, especially at higher elevations, include evidence of recent or unstable myocardial ischemia, serious dysrhythmias, active heart failure, recurrent deep venous thrombosis, severe anemia, and sickle cell disease.[6] Chronic pulmonary disease precludes travel at elevations above 5000 feet (1500 m) if hypoxemia (Po_2 less than 60 mm Hg or less than 90% hemoglobin saturation) is present at sea level. In those with questionably compromising disease, or in those traveling to extreme elevations, ear oximetry or actual oxygen consumption measurements may be performed during the course of treadmill testing to better define work capacity and detect desaturation with exercise. Patients with moderate sea level hypoxia (Po_2 60 to 70 mm Hg) can probably travel safely by air and to high-altitude destinations, provided they are not anemic and the arterial Po_2 is above 50 mm Hg while breathing an O_2 mixture corresponding to the elevation of the destination.[3]

Many prescription drugs predispose to heat-, cold-, and altitude-related illness. Diuretics contract intravascular volume and may thus impair heat transfer to the skin. The anticholinergic action of antihistamines, phenothiazines, and tricyclic antidepressants may result in hypothalamic dysfunction and diminished sweating. Whenever possible, alternate preparations should be considered for use during wilderness travel.

Alcohol should generally be avoided. Alcohol induces

BOX 17-2

CHECKLIST OF PRETRAVEL MEASURES FOR DEVELOPING COUNTRIES

Predetermine local sources of medical help
Important phone numbers for obtaining up-to-date travel warnings
Centers for Disease Control and Prevention:*
International Traveler's Hotline 404-332-4559
Department of State Citizens Emergency Center 202-647-5225
Immunization information and advice
Local health department
USPHS booklet: *Health Information for International Travel,* U.S. Government Printing Office, Washington, DC 20402. HHS Pub. No. (CDC) 85-8280
Required immunizations as defined by the World Health Organization
Yellow fever: listing of countries requiring this vaccine found in HHS publication above
Immunizations requiring an update
Tetanus-diphtheria
Measles (if born after 1956 and unvaccinated), mumps, and rubella
Polio
Influenza
Immunizations for special circumstances
Hepatitis A immune globulin
Hepatitis B
Rabies
Meningococcal vaccine
Typhoid fever
Japanese encephalitis

BOX 17-3

GUIDELINES DURING TRAVEL PERIODS IN UNDERDEVELOPED COUNTRIES

General recommendations
- Contact U.S. embassy on arrival.
- Avoid ice, unboiled or unbottled water, and uncooked food.
- Avoid wading or swimming in lakes and canals of populous regions.
- Avoid blood transfusions and use of needles. Practice safe sex guidelines, especially in Africa and Southeast Asia.
- Take necessary precautions against insects, especially mosquitoes.
  - Avoid nocturnal travel.
  - Use a repellent containing DEET.
  - Sleep in a well-screened area.

Initiate recommended chemoprophylaxis based on travel itinerary.
- Malaria: On return, continue medications for another 4 weeks.
- Traveler's diarrhea

peripheral vasodilation and may lead to net heat *gain* in hot environments and excessive heat *losses* in cool, windy, or wet conditions. In addition, alcohol's effects on judgment and sensory perception may result in failure to acknowledge early symptoms of environmental illness.

Patients with serious medical allergies or active illnesses should have an appropriate medical identification bracelet, anklet, medallion, or wallet card, and they should store their personal medications in a protected but accessible location in their pack.

Oral Hygiene and Health

Mild sore throat and a foul taste are common when traveling in the mountains and in cool weather, probably because of mouth breathing and enhanced loss of moisture from the upper respiratory tract. Carrying a supply of hard candies or medicated lozenges (such as Cepacol or Chloraseptic) is recommended. Saline spray may be used to keep nasal passages hydrated.

Toothache is common at high altitude. Since treatment of early caries and loose fillings (which may trap expanding air) can prevent this misery, the trip coordinator should insist that all party members have dental examinations before the trip. On the trail, frequent brushing may be impractical; flossing after meals, rinsing well with water, and chewing sugar-free gum will help maintain oral hygiene en route.

Urine containers may be appropriate to carry if prolonged adverse weather is a possibility. Funnel-like devices that connect to urine containers are helpful for women (such as Lady-J, available from Campmor; see Appendix C at the end of the chapter). Groups camping in a delicate ecology or when close to a lake or river should use a lightweight, portable commode with disposable plastic holding bags.

Hikers whose feet sweat excessively may benefit from talc or a medicated powder (for example, tolnaftate; see Table 17-2). Keeping feet and socks dry minimizes the tendency to blister formation and reduces heat loss in the cold.

Travelers to cold and aquatic environments are especially prone to overdrying of the skin. Regular application of a lubricating lotion such as Eucerin, Lubriderm, or Keri lotion may help to forestall microtrauma and cracking of the epidermis.

Education in First Aid and Wilderness Safety

Participants should be encouraged to take general courses in first aid and wilderness safety. Agencies that offer general and specialized training in skiing, mountaineering, river-rafting, and other types of wilderness medicine are listed in Appendix D at the end of the chapter. Locally organized programs may be found through the American Red Cross, sporting goods stores, and continuing education departments of local colleges.

Before departure the trip coordinator should review the emergency supplies with the rest of the group. The proper use of mechanical devices should be demonstrated, and indications for the use of medications should be discussed. Groups planning an extended or high-risk outing may wish to conduct a day of mock injury evaluation and management.

FACTORS IN TRIP PLANNING

The five major considerations in planning a trip are (1) the maximum anticipated delay in obtaining medical assistance, (2) total duration of the outing, (3) level of risk associated with a particular activity and environment, (4) group-related factors, and (5) requirements for special equipment and supplies for high-risk expeditions.

Availability of Medical Care

The longer the maximum anticipated delay in obtaining advanced medical assistance, the more likely the irreversible loss of neurologic function, limb, or life. The anticipated delay must take into account that in very rural areas the nearest physician or hospital may not be equipped to handle a major wilderness injury or illness. An extreme case example is the planning of emergency access to a recompression chamber for members of a deep-sea diving expedition. A more typical example is a deeply penetrating arm laceration. As the hours pass, the likelihood of infection grows. If the victim can reach advanced medical help within an hour, it will suffice to control bleeding and apply a few sterile gauze squares held in place by improvised cravats or tape. If definitive care is several hours away, irrigation with water containing a topical disinfectant is desirable. If the delay in care will be over 6 hours, a decision will have to be made whether to close the wound in the field or to evacuate the victim to medical care. (Trauma issues are discussed in Chapter 13.)

The estimate of the anticipated delay depends on the type of rescue services available, the method of contacting them, the terrain and weather, and the number of able persons. Party members should agree in advance on simple emergency distress signals, such as whistle or flashlight bursts in groups of three. Usually, uninjured party members have to make contact with outside agencies.

Manually evacuating the victim is another option, but this requires a relatively mobile victim or at least six carriers if the victim is immobilized. In this regard it is important to know whether other groups might be trekking in the same vicinity. If access is controlled by permit, the administering agency should be asked about the itinerary of neighboring parties. The decision to carry a victim out must be based on a realistic appraisal of the hours it would take messengers to reach aid versus a manual evacuation effort to traverse the greatest distance or worst weather and terrain foreseeable. The use of radio communications is discussed later in the chapter.

Trip Duration

The likelihood of mishap rises as the trip duration increases. This is partly attributable to unpredictable weather and the cumulative effects of fatigue and overuse syndromes. In addition, long trips usually involve extensive planning, significant financial investment, and time away from work. Party members are therefore reluctant to cut the trip short and are more willing to continue in the face of mild medical disability and equipment failure. Groups planning to be away from civilization for more than a week should have a maximally diversified list of medical and contingency items.

Environment and Risk of Activities

Weather, terrain, and activity interact and increase the risk of illness or injury. Particularly hazardous combinations include winter climbing, mountaineering, skiing, and primitive white-water kayaking. The anticipated ranges of weather and terrain must therefore be figured into estimates of the maximum delay to medical assistance (see earlier discussion). A very readable text that offers a general explanation of weather and a specific discussion of the climatology of major domestic recreation areas is the Sierra Club's *Weathering the Wilderness.*[9] U.S. and global historical summary data indicating temperature ranges, winds, and duration, type, and amount of precipitation can be obtained from the National Climatic Data Center (see Box 17-1 and Appendix D at the end of the chapter). State and national park services and state climatology offices are also sources of such information about their territories. The National Weather Service office nearest the travel site can provide short-term forecasts and in many regions broadcasts weather information between 162.40 and 162.55 MHz VHF (see Appendix D).

Group Size

The size of the group indirectly influences the selection of emergency gear. A victim should almost never be left unattended while help is sought; a party of two or three will find it difficult to evacuate an injured member. For this reason a minimum party of four is recommended for all but short, low-risk trips. At the other extreme, a very large party entails more careful planning because it will probably encounter a greater variety of injuries and illnesses. Extremes of group size may justify classification of the trip as high risk for planning purposes.

Medically trained individuals traveling with a group at high risk of trauma or illness may wish to carry supplies requiring special expertise for proper use (Boxes 17-4 and 17-5). Some of the necessary skills may be acquired in advanced first aid, paramedic, or nursing classes. Intramuscular and intravenous medications should be administered

BOX 17-4

CHECKLIST FOR HIGH-RISK OUTINGS: DEVICES REQUIRING SPECIAL MEDICAL TRAINING

Airway, nasopharyngeal (impaired mental status; resuscitation)
Cricothyrotomy cannula or catheter (e.g., Abelson cannula—see Appendix C at the end of the chapter)
Chest tube set (chest trauma; empyema—practical only on major expeditions)
Glucose testing strips and buccally absorbed glucose preparation (if diabetic on trip; strips must be protected from freezing)
Ophthalmoscope with blue filter and fluorescein strips to stain corneal lesions (retinal hemorrhages; anterior eye examination—practical only on expeditions)
Oxygen (hypoxemia, shock, cerebral-pulmonary edema, impaired mental status)
Sphygmomanometer (anaeroid, plastic housing—practical only on expeditions)
Stethoscope (lightweight, noise-reducing; e.g., Lifescope—see Appendix C)
Suction device (mechanical) (clearing oral cavity; chest tube drainage—practical only on expeditions)
Surgical tools (practical only on remote expeditions)

BOX 17-5

CHECKLIST FOR HIGH-RISK OUTINGS: MEDICATION REQUIRING SPECIAL MEDICAL TRAINING*

GENERAL USE

Intravenous (IV) solutions (isotonic) and tubing (for hydration, route for IV medications)†
Needles and syringes (for intramuscular [IM] and IV medications)
Antibiotic, IM (practical only for expeditions) (e.g., ceftriaxone)
Beta agonist metered-dose inhaler (for asthma, anaphylactic reaction)
Dextrose 50% injection (hypoglycemia, nontraumatic coma, hyperthermia)
Nitroglycerin tablets (angina pectoris)
Ophthalmic anesthetic (e.g., proparacaine or tetracaine‡ 0.5%) (to facilitate eye examination and to provide short-term analgesia only)

HIGH RISK OF INSECT BITES

Epinephrine‡ 1:1000 injection (for severe allergic reaction, cardiac arrest)
Diphenhydramine injection§ (for allergic reaction, nausea, mild sedation)

HIGH RISK OF TRAUMA

Nalbuphine†‡ (Nubain) or butorphanol†‡ (Stadol) injectable (for pain, pulmonary edema) and include naloxone (Narcan)†‡ to antagonize narcotic-induced respiratory depression or hypotension
Diazepam‡ (or lorazepam [Ativan‡]) injectable (for major sedation; seizures)

HIGH RISK OF ALTITUDE ILLNESS

Corticosteroid injection (e.g., dexamethasone†) (cerebral-pulmonary edema, severe allergic reaction, asthma)
Furosemide injection§ (cerebral-pulmonary edema)
Nifedipine for pulmonary edema

HIGH RISK OF SNOWBLINDNESS

Ophthalmic cycloplegic (e.g., cyclopentolate 1%) (for pain due to snowblindness)
Ophthalmic corticosteroid-antibiotic combination (e.g., Maxitrol) (recommended for short-term use in snowblindness *only* if blue filter ophthalmoscopic exam using fluorescein stain rules out herpetic keratitis)

*See text for comments on considerations of dispensing medication.
†Do not use after freezing.
‡Protect from prolonged exposure to high temperatures and bright light.
§Stable after freezing provided that no cracking or leakage has occurred.

only by those with formal training in the indications, dosing, and risks of those drugs. Inclusion of medical supplies such as oxygen and intravenous fluids would be reasonable only for search and rescue (see Chapter 21), high-risk expeditions, or research studies. Items such as surgical tools, chest tubes, and mechanical suction devices would be appropriate only for extremely high-risk expeditions[7] and military excursions.

Special Equipment and Supplies for High-Risk Expeditions

A host of recreational activities have inherent risks that may dictate specialized equipment beyond a basic medical kit. Mountain climbing not only poses a risk from traumatic injury but also subjects the climber to high-altitude illness and may require portable oxygen or a pressurized bag for treatment of victims suffering the ill effects of extreme altitude. Extreme cold exposure might dictate the need for technical devices to provide warmed intravenous fluids and humidified oxygen for expeditions at high risk and distant from emergency services. Adventurous white-water sports place the participants at risk from freshwater drowning, and such expeditions might consider carrying an oral airway for cardiopulmonary resuscitation. Cycling poses soft tissue injuries from abrasions that require occlusive water-based gels for proper wound care. Travel to underdeveloped nations in which mosquitoes transmit deadly infectious diseases requires specialized equipment such as protective netting for sleeping, chemical repellents to treat clothing, and medications to manage traveler's diarrhea. Table 17-1 lists common recreational activities and identifies specialized equipment purchases that may be considered for high-risk expeditions.

Assembling the Medical Kit

The emergency kit may be broken down into five components (see Boxes 17-6 through 17-9): (1) survival items carried on the person, (2) personal first aid equipment and drugs carried in the pack, (3) a share of community supplies carried in the pack, (4) specialized equipment and supplies to deal with environmental and recreational haz-

Table 17-1 Recreational Activities Requiring Specialized Equipment

	Specialized Equipment					
Recreational Activity	**High Altitude**	**Cold Exposure**	**Water Sports**	**Bicycling**	**Climbing and Hiking**	**Third World Travel**
Backpacking		X	X		X	
Mountain climbing and expeditions	X	X	X		X	X
Rock climbing					X	
Winter backcountry camping and skiing		X			X	
Cycling				X		
Water sports			X			X
Fishing			X		X	
Hunting		X	X		X	
Search and rescue		X	X		X	
International travel and trekking			X		X	X

Recommended specialized equipment for each recreational activity is denoted by an X in the appropriate column and itemized in Box 17-8. Lists are comprehensive and intended for groups at a distance from medical help or involved in a high-risk adventure; not all items may be needed for low-risk travel. Purchase of specialized equipment should be based on the foundation of a comprehensive medical kit as highlighted in Box 17-10.

BOX 17-6

CONTENTS OF A PERSONAL MEDICAL KIT

ON-PERSON ITEMS

Identification
Swiss Army knife or razor blade
Nylon cord
Whistle
Lighter or waterproof matches
Poncho
Adhesive compress and tape
Bandanna

IN-PACK ITEMS

Personal first aid material
Prescription medications, labeled (in plastic or waterproof aluminum box)
Over-the-counter medications noted in the comprehensive first aid kit (see Box 17-10)

BOX 17-7

CONTENTS OF A MEDICAL KIT FOR EXPEDITIONS AND THE MEDICALLY TRAINED

Comprehensive first aid kit for the management of trauma (see Box 17-10)
Repair materials (see Table 17-5)
Appropriate prescription medications (see Box 17-5 and Tables 17-2 and 17-3)
Indicated equipment based upon recreational and environmental hazards (see Box 17-8)
Medical devices requiring specialized training (see Box 17-4)

ards (see p. 424), and (5) items stored in the vehicle. The components of a well-equipped first aid medical kit designed for the management of trauma and common medical problems are itemized in Box 17-10. However, for the medically inexperienced, consideration can be given to a host of commercially packaged wilderness first aid kits (see Fig. 17-1 and Appendix C at the end of the chapter). Experienced persons who want to tailor a medical kit for expeditions involved in high-risk travel may wish to move on to the discussion of selecting contingency supplies (Figs. 17-2 and 17-3).

Survival Items Carried on the Person

A sudden fall, avalanche, or swamping can quickly separate victim and gear. In anticipation of this, many experienced wilderness travelers carry a bare minimum of survival items on their person at all times (see Box 17-6). These typically include assorted adhesive compress strips, knife or razor blade, butane lighter or matches (preferably the waterproof, strike-anywhere type), plastic whistle, length of thin nylon cord, and bandanna (which can double as a cravat or sling). These items can be compactly stored inside a plastic bag or small stuff sack and may be carried in either a pocket

BOX 17-8

SPECIALIZED EQUIPMENT FOR RECREATIONAL AND ENVIRONMENTAL ACTIVITIES

HIGH ALTITUDE

Gamow Bag and accessories
- Gamow Tent
- Breathing Bladder
- Portable air compressor

EPAP mask with headstrap
Portable pulse oximeter

COLD EXPOSURE

External thermal stabilizer bag
Res-Q-Air
Hot-Sack IV Warmer
Grabber Warmers
Hotronic Foot Warmers
Space Thermal Reflective Survival Bag
Low-reading thermometer

WATER SPORTS

CPR Microshield
Katadyn or MSR WaterWorks filter

BICYCLING

All-Terrain Cyclist Kit
Hydrogel occlusive dressing

MOUNTAIN CLIMBING AND HIKING

SAM splint
Air-Stirrup ankle brace

TROPICAL AND THIRD WORLD TRAVEL

Sawyer Extractor
Permethin repellent
TropicScreen mosquito net
Oral Rehydration Salts packets

or a small fannypack (the zippered, passport-size waist belts sold at luggage stores are comfortable and inexpensive). As noted previously, all travelers should carry some form of identification on their persons, and those with serious medical allergies or active illnesses should have an appropriate medical alert bracelet, anklet, medallion, or wallet card. Those with a history of bee, wasp, or ant anaphylactic allergy should carry at least two preloaded syringes of 1:1000 epinephrine solution (EpiPen; Ana-Kit) in a cool dark compartment and should inform others in the party of the medicine's location and proper usage.

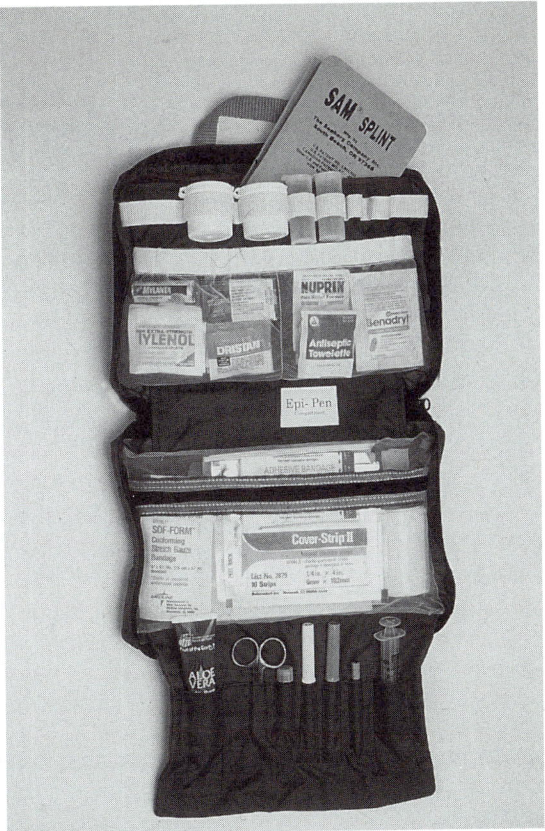

Fig. 17-1 Prepackaged wilderness first aid kits are available from many manufacturers. Kits are neatly organized and rugged, with detachable inner pouches that are useful for day trips. Bags are water resistant to allow for white-water use. A surprisingly large amount of first aid material can be carried, as shown in the illustration.

Personal Items Carried in the Pack

Certain basic contingency "essentials" should be carried on virtually every venture. These include map, compass, knife, flashlight, fire source, pencil and paper, coins for telephone calls, and sunglasses. In addition, extra clothing, food, and water should be carried in proportion to the risk associated with the trip. At least one extra pair of dark sunglasses should be carried in the group. Improvised or "Eskimo" sunglasses, made by cutting small slits in a piece of cardboard, plastic, or cloth, can be tied or taped over the eyes to block most incoming ultraviolet light yet permit adequate vision for travel.

A host of over-the-counter medications may be useful for wilderness travel, especially for low-risk outings of short duration. Some commonly required nonprescription items that may be of value are listed in Box 17-10. Of prime importance is the control of pain associated with trauma. For mild to moderate pain, aspirin, acetaminophen, or a non-

BOX 17-9

CHECKLIST: RECOMMENDED IN-VEHICLE EMERGENCY SUPPLIES

FIRST AID KIT

As for trail, but include large burn dressings
Boards for splint construction
Backboard, short or folding long (e.g., Junkin—see Appendix C at end of chapter)

RESCUE AND SURVIVAL

Avalanche probe poles, collapsing*
Bags, large plastic
Blankets, wool and space-blankets
Climbing rope and hardware†
Candles, long-burning
Flashlight
Food and water (in canteen)
Ice ax†
Matches (waterproof) or lighter
Radio, citizens band
Rope
Saw with metal-cutting blade
Small stove, pot or coffee can, and utensils
Ski climbing skins, snowshoes*
Tarp, plastic
Toilet paper

AUTOMOTIVE

Aluminum foil to cover windows (minimizes heat loss or gain)
Cables to jump battery
Chains with tighteners (with repair links and special pliers)*
Fire extinguisher
Flares, 10-minute (at least six) (can also serve as fire starter)
Gloves
Oil, extra can
Shovel, metal or Lexan with short or collapsing handle
Tool kit (consider inclusion of a small ax)
Tow chain or cable
Wheel chock or wedgeblocks

*Winter weather supplies.
†Mountain terrain supplies (special training needed).

BOX 17-10

CONTENTS OF A COMPREHENSIVE MEDICAL KIT

WOUND MANAGEMENT

Irrigation syringe with 18-gauge needle
Povidone-iodine solution USP 10%
Wound closure strips
Butterfly closures
Tincture of benzoin
Alcohol pads
Moleskin
Antiseptic towelettes
Scalpel with no. 11 or 15 blade
Latex surgical gloves

BANDAGING MATERIALS

Lamino Trauma Dressing
4 × 4 sterile dressing pads
Eye pad
Nonadherent sterile dressing
3-inch sterile gauze bandage
Elastic bandage wrap with Velcro closure
Adhesive cloth tape
Band-Aids
Cotton-tipped applicators

OVER-THE-COUNTER MEDICATIONS

Extra Strength Tylenol
Nuprin (Ibuprofen 200 mg)
Benadryl
Actifed
Mylanta II antacid
Imodium AD
Rectal glycerine suppositories
Saline eye wash
Glutose paste
Hydrocortisone cream 1%
Neosporin antibiotic ointment
Tinactin antifungal cream
Aloe vera gel

MISCELLANEOUS EQUIPMENT

Folding scissors
Forceps for removal of splinters and ticks
Thermometer
SAM splint
Triangular bandage and safety pins
Plastic resealable (Zip-Lock) bags

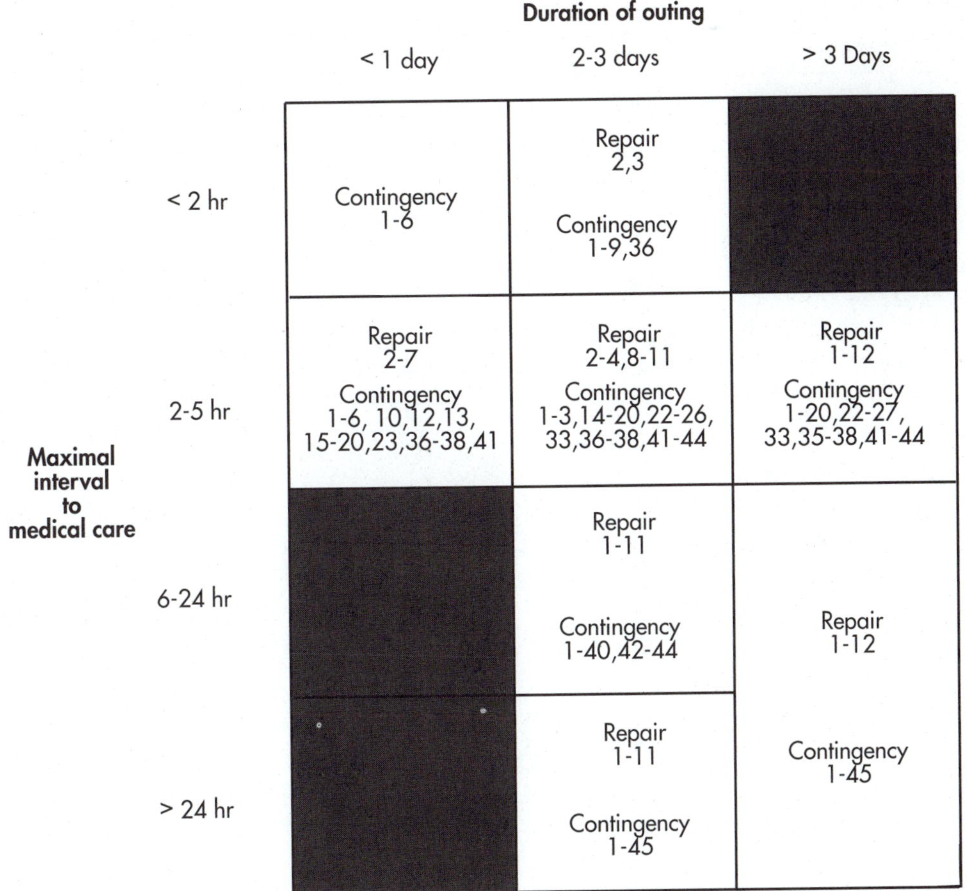

Fig. 17-2 Recommendations for contingency and repair items needed for wilderness travel, grouped based on the duration of outing (vertical columns) and the maximum interval to medical care (horizontal columns). Numbers refer to the descriptions of contingency and repair items found in Tables 17-4 and 17-5. For each list, only the items relevant to the actual type of outing should be considered.

steroidal antiinflammatory drug is effective. Decongestants are helpful to treat symptoms associated with upper respiratory infections, and their antihistaminic effects are useful for the treatment of allergies and insomnia. Gastrointestinal complaints are common, necessitating antacids and an antidiarrheal agent.

Saline eye wash is helpful for irritated eyes and to remove foreign objects. A host of topical creams are needed to treat superficial infections of the skin, and a steroid ointment is of value for treatment of rashes or contact dermatitis. Aloe vera gel is useful for treatment of frostbite and injuries from burns or excessive sun exposure.

Frequently needed first aid material and personal medications are carried in stuff sacks or plastic box containers. Medication containers should be stored in an accessible but thermally and physically protected location in each individual's pack because capsules and suppositories may melt if exposed to extreme heat. Many injectable medications are unstable after exposure to extremes of heat, cold, or light (see Box 17-5 and Appendix A, Chapter 21). Dressings, bandages, and adhesive materials should be kept in a plastic bag within their container to protect them from moisture.

Medications should be stored in unit dose sheets or screw-top plastic bottles labeled with the patient's and physician's names, generic and trade drug names, dispensing information, and expiration date. Medications requiring a prescription with directions for their use (Tables 17-2 and 17-3) should be secured in a watertight plastic or aluminum box. The trip coordinator should ask each member of the party to check that any expired medications are replaced and that capsules and suppositories are intact.

Community Supplies Carried in the Pack

As mentioned at the beginning of the chapter, traumatic injuries represent the greatest concern during wilderness travel. A comprehensive medical kit is the most important community item (see Box 17-10). Emphasis is placed on the management of wounds and stabilization of injuries through appropriate bandaging. Suture material is not recommended

Table 17-2 Topical Medications for Wilderness Travel

Classification	Recommended	Examples	Indications	Contraindications	Side Effects
1. Antibiotic irrigation, topical	Povidone-iodine 10% solution (diluted to 1%)	Betadine	Wounds; burns; blisters	Iodine sensitivity	Local skin reaction **(R)**
2. Antibiotic ointment, topical	Povidone-iodine; bacitracin-polymixin B	Betadine ointment, Polysporin	Burns; abrasions; contaminated lacerations; blisters	Known local sensitivity to ingredients	Local burning **(O)**, skin reactions **(R)**
3. Antibiotic, ophthalmic	Sulfonamide-containing preparation	Sodium sulamyd 10% ointment	Conjunctivitis; snow-blindness; corneal abrasions	Known allergy to sulfonamides	Transient stinging **(C)**; allergic reaction **(R)**
4. Antibiotic/ antiinflammatory, otic	Antimicrobial plus hydrocortisone 1%	Acetic acid 2% plus hydrocortisone 1% (VoSol HC)	Ear pain (worsened by pulling, itching, discharge)	Allergy to ingredients **(R)**; suspected perforation of eardrum (**R** in adults)	Local irritation; allergic reaction **(R)**
5. Antifungal, topical	Miconazole 2%; or ketoconazole 2% cream	Monistat, Micatin, or Nizoral	Athlete's foot, and fungus or yeast infection in groin, under breasts, under arms	None	Local skin irritation **(R)**
6. Corticosteroid cream, topical	High-potency fluorinated compounds (e.g., betamethasone, fluocinolone, halcinonide)	Synalar-HP 0.2%, Diprosone 0.05%, Lidex 0.05%	Rash, swelling due to plant contact and insect bites	Minimize application to skin of face and groin	(Short-term) worsening of some infections
7. Decongestant spray, nasal	Xylometazoline or oxymetazoline; phenylephrine 0.5%	Otrivin, Afrin, Duration, Dristan	Nasal congestion; sinusitis; nasal bleeding	None	Dizziness **(R)**, tremor **(R)**, dysrhythmia **(R)**

Numbers refer to the classification scheme in Fig. 17-3.

C, Common, >10%; **O,** occasional, 1%-10%; **R,** rare, 1%; **D,** dose-related; **Rx,** requires an individual prescription for use in the United States; **OTC,** available over the counter at general pharmacies in the United States; **Ind,** recommended to be dispensed to each party member; **Group,** recommended to be acquired for the group size indicated.

Dosage (Adult)	Quantity	Alternative Drugs	Comments
Irrigate wounds (dilute 10:1 with sterile water); paint burn, abrasion, and blister. For emergency water disinfection, add 16 drops 10% povidone-iodine to each quart of water, allowing 30 min contact before drinking	Per wk: small squeeze-bottle per 4-6 people **(OTC; Group)**	Chlorhexidine (Hibiclens) (do not use to disinfect water)	Plain soap useful for superficial wounds. For deep wounds, use high-pressure irrigation from 35 cc syringe with 18-gauge needle. Chlorhexidine more stable than povidone-iodine at prolonged high temperature (and for storage in vehicle).
After irrigation, apply thin layer twice daily	Per trip: several individual packets per person **(OTC; Ind)**	Silver sulfadiazine 1% (Silvadene)—best choice for burns and possibly frostbite, but relatively expensive and potential sulfa allergy; neomycin not recommended because of occasional sensitivity	Povidone-iodine is active against yeast, fungi, protozoa as well as bacteria.
Deposit inside lower lid every 4 hr and at bedtime	Per trip: smallest tube **(Rx; Ind)**	Polymixin B-bacitracin (Polysporin)	Avoid topical preparation of systemic drugs (e.g., penicillins, tetracycline, gentamicin) and neomycin because sensitization could lead to future reaction.
Four drops into ear (keep upward for 5 min) four times/day for 7 days	Per wk: 10 ml bottle **(Rx; Ind)**	Antibacterial (usually neosporin-HC combinations) (Corticosporin; otic Neo-Cort-Dome; Coly-Mycin)	Neosporin may sensitize to some systemic antibiotics.
Rub in 2-3 times per day until eruption clears	Per trip: One 30 g tube per 4-5 persons **(Rx; Group)**	Clotrimazole (Lotrimin) cream, tolnaftate (Tinactin), and Desenex powders are useful to prevent foot and groin fungus, but Tinactin cream and Desenex ointment are not optimum agents for treatment; nystatin (Mycostatin) is relatively unstable to heat	May use cool soaks to soothe; dry skin well before applying cream.
Rub in thoroughly 2-3 times daily while skin is still moist after washing, as needed for itching	Per trip: 15 g per 4-6 people **(Rx; Group)**	Also use cold compress or soaks; oral antihistamines	Not helpful for sunburn; if rash worsens, discontinue corticosteroid and consider fungus (see no. 5). Consider oral steroid for contact dermatitis involving face, groin, or more than 25% body surface.
2 sprays (5-10 sec apart) to each nostril every 8-12 min	Per wk: 15 ml spray bottle **(OTC; Ind)**	See Oral decongestant in Table 17-3	Use only for several days continuously to prevent reactive congestion and tolerance. Phenylephrine can also be used in an emergency as inhaled bronchodilator.

Continued.

Table 17-2 Topical Medications for Wilderness Travel—cont'd

Classification	Recommended	Examples	Indications	Contraindications	Side Effects
8. Dental filling, temporary	Premixed filling paste	Cavit	Pain from chipped tooth or lost filling	None	None
9. Sunscreen	Methoxy cinnamate/ oxybenzone combinations	Tiscreen, Piz Buin, Solbar PF	Minimize sunburn, windburn	Known local sensitivity to ingredients (esp. PABA)	Local skin irritation (**R**)
10. Sunscreen, lip balm	See Sunscreen above	Chap Stick Sunblock 15	Minimize sunburn, chafing; prevent herpes labialis	See Sunscreen above	See Sunscreen above

Numbers refer to the classification scheme in Fig. 17-3.
C, Common, >10%; **O,** occasional, 1%-10%; **R,** rare, 1%; **D,** dose-related; **Rx,** requires an individual prescription for use in the United States; **OTC,** available over the counter at general pharmacies in the United States; **Ind,** recommended to be dispensed to each party member; **Group,** recommended to be acquired for the group size indicated.

on the list of items because of the likelihood of subsequent infection. Large wounds are best treated with sterile pressure dressings.

Bulky and heavy items, including most stock first aid and contingency supplies, should be labeled and distributed among the members of the group for storage and transport. A cross made from strips of tape or cloth should be placed on the pack overlying the compartment containing the first aid items. This allows ready access by any member of the party in an emergency situation. Repair materials are best kept in clearly labeled stuff sacks, or aluminum or plastic boxes independent of the first aid and medical supplies.

Items Stored in the Vehicle

A complete emergency kit in the vehicle (see Box 17-9) is highly recommended. It will facilitate further stabilization of an injured person evacuated to a trailhead. The vehicle kit should also provide material necessary to deal with accidents encountered along the highway and to cope with the environment if the occupants are stranded by automotive trouble or natural disaster. Several large burn dressings and a neckboard with strapping will fit in a standard trunk or other recess. Although only large vehicles can accommodate the usual full-length backboard, a folding backboard is now available from Junkin Safety Appliance Co. (see Appendix C at the end of the chapter). The remaining contents of an emergency kit will fit in a medium (6W × 12L × 9H) or large (8W × 18L × 14H) war surplus ammunition box, or a toolbox of similar size.

SELECTING CONTINGENCY SUPPLIES: ADVANCED EXPEDITION PLANNING

Individuals with medical training involved with risky wilderness travel may opt to design their own medical kit. Adventurous expeditions may wish to include a host of prescription medications that require advanced knowledge (see Box 17-5) and carry special devices requiring medical training (see Box 17-4). In addition, specialized equipment to handle expected environmental and recreational hazards can create a heavy burden (see Box 17-8). An appropriate emergency kit would be one that is just adequate in content, but not too heavy or bulky. A commonly used approach is to prepare a separate list for every anticipated combination of trip factors; this is practical only when considering a limited scope of wilderness activities (see references 2, 7, and 10 and Appendix B at the end of the chapter). Presented here is an alternative approach: assess each of the trip planning factors discussed previously, then refer to a cross-tabulation of these factor levels to obtain the recommended contents of a tailored kit. This makes the risks explicit and the listing general. It does, of course, require the user to filter the final kit contents so that they are appropriate for the specific wilderness terrain anticipated. The cross-tabulations in the indexes in Figs. 17-2 and 17-3 provide suggestions for contingency/repair equipment and medications, respectively.

Using a Wilderness Index

The wilderness indexes were developed to assist persons with advanced first aid[4] or medical training,[5] and to advise lay travelers on the appropriate contents of medical

Dosage (Adult)	Quantity	Alternative Drugs	Comments
Dry tooth, insert paste, allow to set 15 min	Per trip: small (7 g) tube (obtain from dentist) **(Group)**	Small amounts of zinc oxide powder and eugenol	Very short shelf life once unsealed (hardens). Temporary filling must be replaced by permanent dental work upon return.
SPF (sun protection factor) of 15 or more; apply more frequently for sweating or water immersion	As anticipated for trip conditions **(OTC; Group)**	Opaque sunblock cream; esp. useful on nose, lip, ear	Ointments > creams > lotions for sweat and water resistance and for protection against frostbite.
As needed	Per wk: 1 tube **(OTC; Ind)**	Opaque sunblock containing titanium or zinc oxide	May be helpful in preventing recurrent labial herpes.

kits. In Figs. 17-2 and 17-3 a unique "square" of recommendations is found at the intersection of the horizontal column "Duration of Outing," and the vertical column "Maximum Interval to Medical Care." Numbers refer to the descriptions of contingency and repair equipment (Tables 17-4 and 17-5) and medications (Tables 17-2 and 17-3). The drug doses listed in Table 17-3 are intended for nonpregnant, young or middle-aged adults in good health. Reduced doses are often necessary for children, the elderly, and those with end-organ disease (especially renal, hepatic, and cardiac). The personal physician should modify the doses appropriately.

For each listing, only those items relevant to the actual type of outing should be considered. For example, equipment needed *only* for snow travel would be inappropriate for kayaking.

A Sample Journey

The month is April, and the goal is a 21-mile round trip cross-country ski tour to the top of Mt. Whitney (elevation 14,495 feet; 4418 m) in the Sierra Nevada mountains. The team consists of four cross-country skiers who have completed an American Red Cross advanced first aid course, as well as an avalanche seminar offered to the public by the National Ski Patrol System. The trip duration will be 2 to 3 days, depending on weather and snow conditions. The base camp will be at 12,500 feet (3810 m). Were a skier to become disabled en route, one of the others would remain with the victim while the remaining two would ski out to the nearest telephone or source of help (no longer than an 8-hour ski from any point along the route). Helicopter evacuation to the nearest hospital would usually be accomplished within the next 6 hours; even foul weather should not extend the maximum interval to medical care beyond 24 hours. The trip is high risk in terms of trauma, cold injury, and equipment failure and could result in high-altitude illness. The following steps refer to the indexes in Figs. 17-2 and 17-3.

1. Determine maximum interval to medical care. In the example given, "6-24 hr" would be the appropriate horizontal column.
2. Determine trip duration. In the example given, "2-3 days" would be the appropriate vertical column.
3. Find the "square" of recommended items. On each index the intersection of the horizontal and vertical columns defines a square of items. Note the reference item numbers listed and find the suggested items in the tables recommended in each figure legend.
4. Eliminate items that are clearly inappropriate for this trek. In the example given, a prolonged rescue effort or evacuation effort would be unlikely, considering the need for oral item 2 (Fig. 17-2) (amphetamine stimulant). There will be no foreign travel, eliminating the need for item 7 (traveler's diarrhea antibiotic).

In the example given, the items remaining are *contingency supplies:* 1-40, 42-44; *repair items:* 1-11; *topical medications:* 1, 2, 7, 9, 10; and *oral medications:* 1, 3, 4, 10-12, 14.

Finally, emphasis must be placed on the recreational

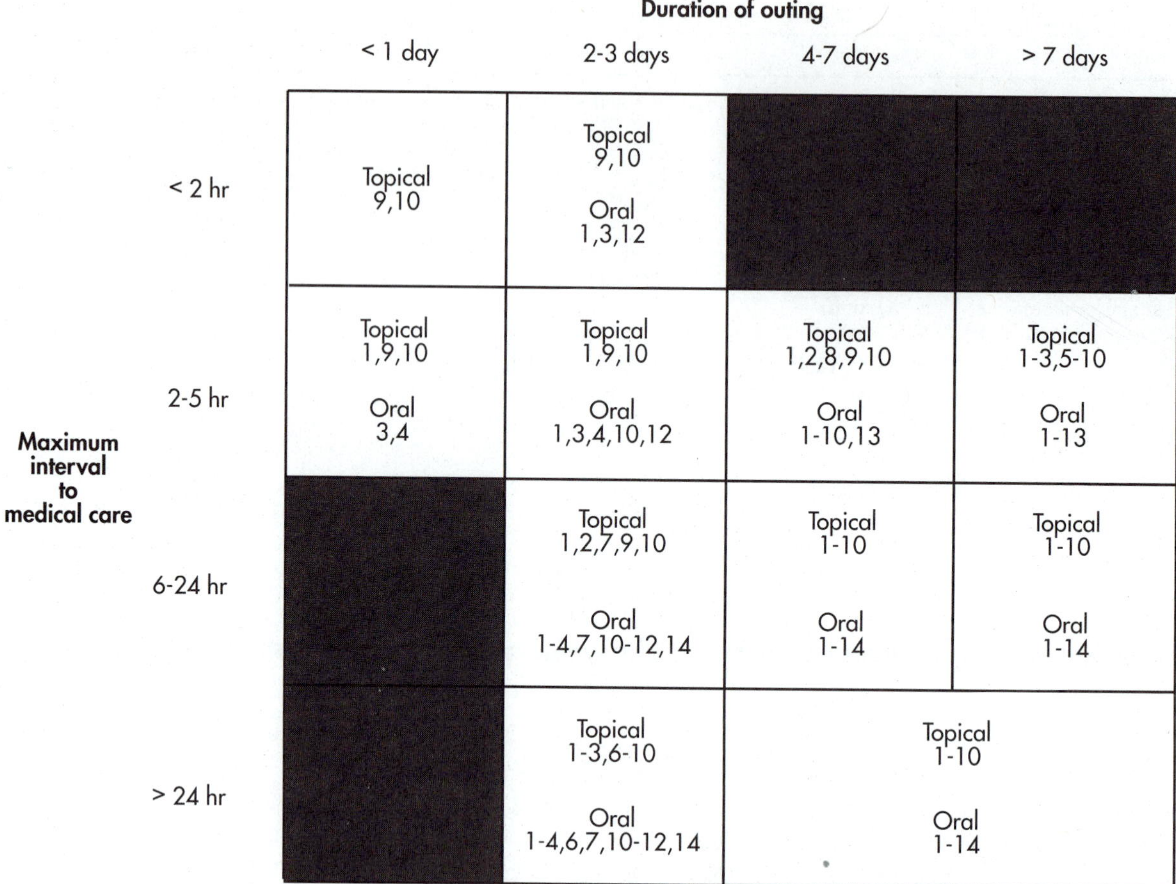

Fig. 17-3 Recommendations for both topical and oral medications needed for wilderness travel, grouped based on the duration of outing (vertical columns) and the maximum interval to medical care (horizontal columns). Numbers refer to the descriptions of topical and oral medications found in Tables 17-2 and 17-3, respectively. For each list, only the items relevant to the actual type of outing should be considered. Physicians traveling with groups at high risk should also consider the inclusion of devices and drugs listed in Boxes 17-4 and 17-5. The doses recommended Tables 17-2 and 17-3 are intended for nonpregnant, young, or middle-aged adults in good health. Reduced doses may be required for children, the elderly, and those with medical disorders. In all situations, the traveler's personal physician should recommend the appropriate doses.

and environmental hazards likely to be encountered during travel. In this example the dangers relate mainly to high altitude and cold exposure. Specialized equipment that may be of value under the conditions described is listed in Box 17-8. Because of proximity to a medical center able to provide prompt helicopter evacuation, a Gamow Bag would not be mandated for the treatment of high-altitude illness. In addition, the need to carry technical equipment to provide warmed intraveneous solutions or humidified oxygen is offset by a prompt helicopter rescue. However, frostbite can occur rapidly, and an individual might wish to carry a Grabber Warmer because of its low weight and easy packability (see section for product descriptions).

MULTIFUNCTIONALITY AND IMPROVISATION IN SELECTION OF TRIP SUPPLIES

Most wilderness travel places severe limitations on the weight and bulk of personal gear. Multifunctionality and improvisation (see Chapter 18) therefore are recurrent themes in the selection of travel items. Examples of multifunctionality include using spare socks as extra mittens, extra clothing as splint padding, foam sleeping pad cut into squares as a seat or knee pad or as a base for a stove, tape as a butterfly wound closure or as a moleskin substitute, a tongue depressor as a finger splint or emergency fire-starting tinder, a small road flare as an emergency fire starter, and a metal canteen as a cooking pot. A *sturdy* straight or lock-back folding knife may find separate utility as a hammer, digging instrument, ax, lever, or stake. The addition of a Swiss Army type of multiple-tool knife provides backup blades, scissors, saw, awl, screwdrivers, and tweezers. Imaginative uses of plastic bags include a cold compress (filled with ice or snow), a sandbag to stabilize a neck or fracture (filled with dirt, sand, or snow), an emergency poncho (a hole made for the head), a vapor-barrier sleeping garment for a cold-weather bivouac (one large bag as poncho plus another over the lower body), an evaporative still to collect and purify water, a surface to absorb solar heat and melt snow, a container for avulsed tissue or excretions, a map case, and of course a trash bag!

Improvisation is easiest in wooded environments. Branches or roots may provide the material for splints, emergency bedding and shelter, emergency snowshoes, or a makeshift litter or toboggan. In other terrains a pack frame or rigid material may facilitate splinting. In mountaineering skiing, splints and toboggans may be partially improvised from skis and poles with the help of lightweight adapter kits (see National Ski Patrol in Appendix C at the end of the chapter).

RADIO COMMUNICATIONS

A radio system for communication is usually warranted only for split groups or on extremely hazardous trips. A party that will be split into subgroups could use hand-held radios operating either on the citizens band or the low-band VHF frequencies (*Rescue* magazine, Appendix D). Both types of radio permit local communications between transceivers; furthermore, a party member situated atop a local peak or ridge can use a third transceiver to relay information between otherwise isolated party subgroups below. Citizens band radios are the least expensive (about $100 for a 5-watt transceiver) and may be used to call for help by contacting citizens or officials monitoring emergency channel 9. Unfortunately, citizens band channels are characterized by a high level of background noise that greatly limits the effective range of communication (often to less than 1 mile in line of sight). Low-band VHF radios are quieter and moderately more expensive (about $200 for a 2-watt transceiver with a range of 2 to 3 miles in line of sight) but cannot be used to directly contact emergency services. High-band VHF and UHF units, less noisy and more expensive, usually are used to communicate across rugged terrain indirectly via networks of radio repeaters situated atop local peaks. Repeaters are necessary because the direct signal of hand-held radios cannot wrap around local hills or ridges (that is, they are primarily useful for line-of-sight communications). Repeater networks are operated by local authorities (sheriffs, search and rescue organizations, park and forest services) and use special electronic access codes not generally accessible to the public. However, if a party is traveling in some quasiofficial capacity (such as for ski patrol, disaster, search and rescue, military training, or authorized wilderness research), the official agencies may authorize use of their frequencies.

CLOTHING

Technologic advances in clothing include materials such as Gore-Tex that are resistant to penetration by water droplets (rain) but relatively permeable to vapor (sweat). Gore-Tex has become a popular outer cloth for jackets, pants, gloves, boots, and tents. However, water resistance may be lost if the material is soiled, and high sweat rates may exceed its capacity to ventilate adequately. Thus individuals who perspire excessively may be better served by a combination of a removable waterproof shell over a more "breathable" primary garment.

For cold weather travel, jacket or parka selection is important. Traditional parkas consist of down or polyester fiber-filled nylon shells. Down garments are extremely warm, lightweight, and compressible, but they lose almost all insulating value when wet and are difficult to dry. Polyester fiberfill (such as Polargard; Dacron Hollofill) is heavier and less compressible than down but retains significant insulation value when wet and is much easier to dry. Polyolefin fiberfill (Thinsulate) jackets are less compressible but lighter, less bulky, and more wind resistant than other fiberfills. Newer lightweight polyester "fiberpile" knits are warm, lightweight, very breathable, and quick to dry. Unfortunately, they lose their insulating properties in the wind, and cannot be compressed for packing.

Polypropylene has been widely accepted as a thin, soft, innermost layer for use in undergarments, glove liners, face masks, and caps. Polypropylene wicks away moisture without absorbing it. Thermax, a new hollow core polyester fiber, and Capilene, a treated polypropylene material, perform similar functions.

In general, loose layering of garments offers the least bulky and most versatile protection from cold and wind. In warm weather, clothing should be lightweight, loose fitting, and light colored. Cotton is comfortable and usually adequate, but when wet it may transmit a large amount of ultraviolet light.

Boots for hiking and mountaineering should be coated with a water repellent and thoroughly broken in (worn for 10 to 20 miles of walking) before the trip. Foot surfaces that feel warm or become reddened during this process should be noted, and adhesive pads (moleskin or Spenco 2nd Skin; see below) should be applied prophylactically over these spots for the first few days on the trail. A bulky wool sock worn over a thin, tightly woven inner sock (nylon, polypropylene, cotton, or wool) is a good way to minimize friction blistering. Applying foot powder helps to keep the skin dry and diminishes friction.

Table 17-3 Oral Medication for Wilderness Travel

Classification	Recommended	Examples	Indications	Contraindications	Side Effects
1. Acute mountain sickness (AMS)	Acetazolamide	Diamox	Prevention and treatment of AMS (headache, sleep disturbance, lassitude, nausea, incoordination)	Concurrent diuretic medications; sulfa allergy	Tingling **(C)**; fatigue, drowsiness, nausea **(O)** *Caution:* Toxicity (confusion, lethargy, incontinence) may develop with the concomitant use of aspirin or Pepto-Bismol
2. Amphetamine stimulant	Dextroamphetamine 5 mg tablets	Dexedrine	Life-threatening mental fatigue	None in indicated setting	Stimulation **(D)**; anorexia **(C)**; GI disturbance **(C)**; tremor and headache **(O)**
3. Analgesic/ antiinflammatory, oral nonnarcotic	Aspirin, enteric-coated preferred	Generic, Ecotrin, Cosprin, Easprin	Moderate pain; high-grade fever (T >102° F, 39° C)	Aspirin sensitivity **(O)**; bleeding tendency **(R)**; ringing in ears **(D)**; chronic kidney disease	GI upset **(C)**; easy bruising or bleeding **(R)**
4. Analgesic, oral narcotic	Aspirin (or acetaminophen) with 30 mg codeine	Empirin or Empracet No. 3; Tylenol No. 3	Moderate to severe pain; disabling cough	Respiratory difficulty, head injury; other sedative drugs or alcohol; narcotic allergy; possible surgical abdomen (rigid and tender with fever, weakness, vomiting) *Caution:* Toxicity may develop from concomitant use of aspirin and acetazolamide (see Acute mountain sickness)	Respiratory depression and hypotension **(D)**; drowsiness, vomiting, constipation **(C)**; rash **(R)**

Numbers refer to the classification scheme in Fig. 17-3. Doses listed in Table 17-3 are intended for nonpregnant, young, or middle-aged adults in good health. Reduced doses may be required for children, the extreme elderly, and those with medical disorders. In all situations the traveler's personal physician should recommend appropriate doses.

C, Common, >10%; **O,** occasional, 1%-10%; **R,** rare, <1%; **D,** dose-related; **Rx,** requires an individual prescription for use in the United States; **OTC,** available over the counter at general pharmacies in the United States; **Ind,** recommended to be dispensed to each party member; **Group,** recommended to be acquired for the group size indicated.

Dosage (Adult)	Quantity (Per Trip)	Alternative Drugs	Comments
Prevention: 150-250 mg every 12 hr, or 500 mg sustained action capsule, for 1 day before and 1-2 days into ascent Treatment: 250 mg every 8-12 hr as needed for up to 48 hr	10-12 tablets **(Rx; Ind)**	Oxygen is helpful but not curative; potent diuretics not recommended for AMS: oral dexamethasone for treatment of severe AMS only	Prevent AMS by slow ascent and sleeping at lowest altitude possible. Best treatment for severe or prolonged (>24-48 hr) AMS is descent by at least 2000 ft. Avoid alcohol and sedatives. Observe for symptoms of pulmonary and cerebral edema (see also Corticosteroid below and in Box 17-5).
5-10 mg every 4-6 hr as needed	6 tablets **(Rx; Ind)**	Methylphenidate (Ritalin) 5 mg tablets	Only for high-risk conditions in remote regions, e.g., search and rescue work, mountain or ice climbing, exploratory kayaking. Be aware of local restrictions on drugs with abuse potential.
Two 325 mg tablets every 6 hours as needed	12-15 per person **(OTC; Group)**	Ibuprofen (Rufen, Advil) 400-600 mg every 6 hours	Other antiinflammatory drugs useful but require Rx (e.g., Indocin, Naprosyn, Clinoril, Tolectin, Trilisate, Dolobid) and have similar side effects—recommend trial for patient tolerance before outing. Acetaminophen good for mild pain and fever, but products above more useful for outdoor-related pain (esp. sunburn and musculoskeletal injury).
1-2 tablets every 4-8 hr as needed	12-24 tablets **(Rx; Ind)**	Aspirin (or acetaminophen) with oxycodone 5 mg; acetaminophen with hydrocodone 5 mg; the following have higher abuse potential and may require special prescriptions and authorization to carry: codeine 30 mg; oxycodone 5 mg; meperidine 50 mg; levorphanol 2 mg; hydromorphone 2 mg. Buccal morphine tablets (containing either 6 or 10 mg base) may provide analgesia.	Individuals vary in type and degree of side effect experienced—trial or brief regimen under controlled circumstances may be appropriate.

Continued.

Table 17-3 Oral Medication for Wilderness Travel—cont'd

Classification	Recommended	Examples	Indications	Contraindications	Side Effects
5. Antacid	High-potency antacid tablets with simethicone	Mylanta II; Riopan II	Epigastric or "gas" discomfort; heartburn	Chronic kidney disease. Aluminum-containing antacids should not be taken within 4 hr of chloroquine.	Diarrhea **(C)**; constipation **(O)**
6. Antibiotic, oral, general	Two or three of the following broad-spectrum oral agents: cefadroxil (Ultracef, Duricef) 1 g; ciprofloxacin (Cipro) 500 or 750 mg; doxycycline (Vibramycin) 100 mg; erythromycin (E-Mycin, Eryc) 333 mg; trimethoprim-sulfamethoxazole (Bactrim DS, Septra DS) 160/800 mg; amoxicillin 500 mg-clavulanate 125 mg (Augmentin 500)		Infection: GI, GU, lung, oral, sinus, skin	Known allergy (avoid doxycycline in pregnancy)	Cefadroxil, ciprofloxacin, erythromycin, amoxicillin-clavulanate: abdominal pain, nausea, diarrhea **(O)** Doxycycline: abdominal pain, nausea, diarrhea **(C)**; photosensitivity **(O)**; rash **(R)** Trimethoprim-sulfamethoxazole: see Antibiotic for traveler's diarrhea below
7. Antibiotic, oral, for traveler's diarrhea	Trimethoprim 160 mg, sulfamethoxazole 800 mg	Bactrim DS; Septra DS	Prevention on crucial trip or in those with underlying illness; treatment for prolonged loose stooling and cramps, fever and weakness	Sulfa allergy (sulfamethoxazole component)	Rash **(O)**; GI and neurologic symptoms **(R)**; photosensitivity **(R)**

Numbers refer to the classification scheme in Fig. 17-3. Doses listed in Table 17-3 are intended for nonpregnant, young, or middle-aged adults in good health. Reduced doses may be required for children, the extreme elderly, and those with medical disorders. In all situations the traveler's personal physician should recommend appropriate doses.

C, Common, >10%; **O,** occasional, 1%-10%; **R,** rare, <1%; **D,** dose-related; **Rx,** requires an individual prescription for use in the United States; **OTC,** available over the counter at general pharmacies in the United States; **Ind,** recommended to be dispensed to each party member; **Group,** recommended to be acquired for the group size indicated.

Dosage (Adult)	Quantity (Per Trip)	Alternative Drugs	Comments
1-2 tablets as needed (to maximum of 12/day)	12 tablets per person **(OTC; Group)**	Other antacids	Drink a full glass of water with each dose.
Cefadroxil, ciprofloxacin, doxycycline: one dose every 12 hr for at least 5 days Erythromycin, amoxicillin-clavulanate: one dose every 8 hr for at least 5 days *Preferred sites:* Cefadroxil: skin, oral, sinus > lung >> GU (500 mg q12h) Ciprofloxacin: GU, GI, lung > skin, sinus (750 mg q12h) Doxycycline: lung, GU > skin (includes aquatic) (100 mg q12h) Erythromycin: lung, skin, oral > sinus, GU >> GI (333 mg q8h) Trimethoprim-sulfamethoxazole: GU, lung, sinus > skin (includes aquatic) >> oral (one DS q12h) Amoxicillin: lung, GU, sinus, skin > GI (500 mg q8h)	14-20 **(Rx; Ind)**	Also acceptable, but more cumbersome, are rational combinations of more site-specific agents, e.g., dicloxacillin (skin), metronidazole (giardiasis), norfloxacin (GI, urinary)	See also Antibiotic, oral, for traveler's diarrhea. Individuals vary in type and degree of side effects experienced—a brief trial of the regimen under controlled circumstances may be appropriate.
Prevention: 1 dose daily through 2 days after return *Treatment:* 1 dose every 12 hr for 3 days	At least 6 (see General oral antibiotic)	*Prevention:* doxycycline 100 mg daily or norfloxacin 200 mg daily *Treatment:* trimethoprim 250 mg every 12 hr or ciprofloxacin 500 or 750 mg every 12 hr	*See footnote.

*Traveler's diarrhea is usually mild and subsides spontaneously within 4 days—reserve antibiotics for indications above and for treatment of dysentery (blood and mucus). During diarrhea, avoid milk products and solids, but maintain fluid intake and electrolytes—the U.S. Public Health Service recommends drinking alternately from each glass: (1) 8 oz fruit juice with ½ tsp honey, corn syrup, or sugar with a pinch of table salt, and (2) 8 oz carbonated or boiled water with ¼ tsp baking soda. Alternatively, packets of electrolyte powder (to mix with water) may be useful for isolated, high-risk travel. Bismuth subsalicylate (Pepto-Bismol) liquid and tablets are reported to be about 60% effective in preventing *E. coli* diarrhea, but the large quantity necessary may be impractical to carry; also, toxicity may develop from concomitant use of salicylates or acetazolamide.

Giardiasis onset is usually delayed by at least 2 weeks after exposure—for prolonged trip consider metronidazole (250 mg every 8 hr for 5 days) or quinacrine (100 mg after meals three times a day for 5 days).

For severe diarrhea in *E. histolytica* amebiasis risk areas, medical evaluation advised, but consider carrying metronidazole (750 mg every 8 hr for 5 days) plus iodoquinol (650 mg every 8 hr for 3 weeks).

For prolonged stay in areas of intestinal worms, carry: for ascariasis, hookworm, and trichuriasis—mebendazole (100 mg twice daily for 3 days); for strongyloidiasis—thiabendazole (25 mg per kg twice daily for 3 days); for common tapeworms—niclosamide (1 g, repeat in 1 hr).

Continued.

Table 17-3 Oral Medication for Wilderness Travel—cont'd

Classification	Recommended	Examples	Indications	Contraindications	Side Effects
8. Antidiarrheal agent	Loperamide 2 mg capsule	Imodium	Persistent frequent, watery stools causing cramps or compromised activities	Blood or pus in stool; suspected *Shigella* or *Campylobacter* infection; possible surgical abdomen (rigid and tender, with fever, weakness, vomiting); known bacterial cause, inflammatory bowel disorder; diarrhea following antibiotics	Dry mouth, drowsiness, **(O); ** abdominal pain **(R)**
9. Antiemetic/ antinausea, rectal suppository	Promethazine 25 mg suppository	Phenergan	Severe nausea, vomiting when oral agent not tolerated (see Antihistamine, oral)	Risk of hypothermia; heavy sedation from injury, illness, or other drugs; high fever, known phenothiazine reaction	Sedation **(D)**; dry mouth, blurred vision **(O)**
10. Antihistamine, oral	Diphenhydramine 25 mg capsules	Benadryl; generic	Mild nausea or motion sickness; itching; allergy; mild sleeplessness	Active asthma (drug dries secretions); sedation from illness or other drugs	Drowsiness **(C, D)**; thickened respiratory secretions **(O)**; abdominal pain **(R)**
11. Corticosteroid, oral	6-14 day tapering doses of methylprednisolone or prednisone tablets	Medrol Dosepak (prepackaged—6-day tapering of methylprednisolone)	Severe contact dermatitis (poison oak, ivy, sumac); severe sunburn; anaphylaxis; treatment of cerebral edema (incoordination, stupor—in coma, oral medications cannot be given, see Box 17-5)	Active peptic ulcer disease; diabetes; concurrent infection	Fluid retention **(O)**; others **(R)** during very short-term use

Numbers refer to the classification scheme in Fig. 17-3. Doses listed in Table 17-3 are intended for nonpregnant, young, or middle-aged adults in good health. Reduced doses may be required for children, the extreme elderly, and those with medical disorders. In all situations the traveler's personal physician should recommend appropriate doses.

C, Common, >10%; **O,** occasional, 1%-10%; **R,** rare, <1%; **D,** dose-related; **Rx,** requires an individual prescription for use in the United States; **OTC,** available over the counter at general pharmacies in the United States; **Ind,** recommended to be dispensed to each party member; **Group,** recommended to be acquired for the group size indicated.

Dosage (Adult)	Quantity (Per Trip)	Alternative Drugs	Comments
1-2 capsules after each unformed stool (maximum 8/day, 3 days)	12-16 **(Rx; Ind)**	Diphenoxylate with atropine (Lomotil) tablets	Before using antidiarrheal, try clear liquid diet to decrease diarrhea; maintain fluid intake.
25 mg per rectum every 12 hr as needed	4 suppositories **(Rx; Ind)**	Prochlorperazine (Compazine) 25 mg suppository	(See also Antihistamine, oral.) Promethazine has prominent phenothiazine and antihistamine action; keep suppositories protected from heat and pressure; for motion sickness (adults only), consider scopolamine disk (Transderm Scop) 0.5 mg, whole or half patch every 3 days to skin behind ear (scopolamine may cause toxic psychosis).
25-75 mg every 6-8 hr as needed	6-8 tablets **(OTC** or **Rx; Ind)**	Hydroxyzine (Atarax) 25 mg tablets; chlorpheniramine (Chlor-Trimeton) 4 mg tablets; terfenadine (Seldane) 60 mg tablets	Chlorpheniramine or terfenadine is the least sedating, but nausea and itching relief may depend on sedation. At high altitude, antihistamines may worsen sleep patterns; benzodiazepines are preferable for sleep if acetazolamide is effective.
30-60 mg/day of methylprednisolone or 50-100 mg prednisone for 1-3 days, decreased gradually over the subsequent 4-14 days; may be given in split daily doses for cerebral edema	1 Medrol Dosepak **(Rx; Ind)** for concern of dermatitis only, or up to 100 tablets of methylprednisolone (4 mg) or prednisone (5 mg) for concern of cerebral edema	Dexamethasone 0.5 mg tablets (starting dose 4-12 mg/day)	Drug treatment for cerebral edema does *not* substitute for prompt descent of at least 2000 ft. (See also Corticosteroid, topical in Table 17-2 and Corticosteroid, injectable in Box 17-5.)

Continued.

Table 17-3 Oral Medication for Wilderness Travel—cont'd

Classification	Recommended	Examples	Indications	Contraindications	Side Effects
12. Decongestant, oral	Pseudoephedrine 30 mg tabs	Sudafed	Nasal congestion; sinus discomfort	Uncontrolled high blood pressure	Dry mouth, fast pulse, sleep difficulty **(O)**
13. Laxative	Senna derivative	Senokot	Symptomatic constipation	Fever, weakness, vomiting, rigid or tender abdomen	—
14. Sedative, oral	Triazolam 0.125 mg tablets	Halcion	Sleeplessness, including jet lag; anxiety; muscle spasm	Coexisting sedation from alcohol, drugs, illness	Drowsiness, dizziness **(D);** loss of coordination **(O);** anterograde amnesia **(R)**

Numbers refer to the classification scheme in Fig. 17-3. Doses listed in Table 17-3 are intended for nonpregnant, young, or middle-aged adults in good health. Reduced doses may be required for children, the extreme elderly, and those with medical disorders. In all situations the traveler's personal physician should recommend appropriate doses.

C, Common, >10%; **O,** occasional, 1%-10%; **R,** rare, <1%; **D,** dose-related; **Rx,** requires an individual prescription for use in the United States; **OTC,** available over the counter at general pharmacies in the United States; **Ind,** recommended to be dispensed to each party member; **Group,** recommended to be acquired for the group size indicated.

EYEWEAR

The appropriate use of sunglasses and goggles will protect eyes from sunlight, wind, and dust. Sunglasses that will be used extensively in the wilderness should be made of either glass or polycarbonate. Most outdoor equipment retailers offer a wide selection of nonprescription lenses made of these materials. In addition, many name-brand and custom varieties can be obtained from an eye specialist in prescription configuration. The major variables to consider when buying sunglasses are light transmission, lens construction, coloration, and polarization. Lenses for aquatic, desert, snow, and high-altitude use should absorb 85% to 95% of visible light and essentially all (greater than 99%) ultraviolet (UV) radiation. This degree of visible light absorption can be easily achieved with glass, plastic, or polycarbonate lenses. (The serious wilderness trekker will have to obtain another, less dark pair for use while driving a vehicle.) Soft contact lenses that absorb UV are also available.

Plastic lenses scratch easily and generally are not recommended for extensive wilderness trekking. Lenses that darken with increasing sun intensity (photochromic) are currently available only in glass. Only one type of photochromic lens, Photosun II, blocks enough visible light when fully darkened (about 90%) to be seriously considered for extremely bright or reflective conditions. Although many glass lenses block only 90% to 97% of UV light, some manufacturers use a new coating that absorbs over 98% of UV. Complete UV light absorption can readily be achieved with polycarbonate. Polycarbonate lenses are lightweight, scratch resistant, and shatterproof (a major advantage over glass lenses for wilderness sports, in which impact is a major consideration). Polycarbonate models that absorb at least 99% UV are manufactured under such brand names as All Weather, Bolle, Gargoyles, Gentex, Learjet, Ski-Optics, Suncloud, and Wings.

The choice of lens color is based largely on personal preference. Although yellow or rose lenses may appear to enhance contrast or hazy (flat) light conditions, research studies have found no consistent benefit. Polarization decreases reflected solar glare from horizontal water, snow, and ice surfaces and is highly desirable for winter mountaineering, skiing, and aquatic wilderness sports. Glass, but not polycarbonate, lenses are available with polarization, although an external clip-on flip-up plastic polarizer (about $12) can be added to the polycarbonate lenses. These clip-on polarizers absorb an additional 50% of the remaining transmitted light (increasing visible light absorption from, say, 90% to 95%) and may be of additional benefit in bright conditions. Recreational Equipment Incorporated (REI) (see Appendix C at the end of the chapter) offers a polarizer sandwiched between two glass lenses.

Other considerations include price, optical gradient and mirroring, frame construction, and peripheral features. A pair of high-quality nonprescription sunglasses generally costs between $20 and $100. More expensive models are

Dosage (Adult)	Quantity (Per Trip)	Alternative Drugs	Comments
60-90 mg every 6-8 hr as needed	12-24 tablets **(OTC; Group)**	Ephedrine, phenylpropanolamine, or isopropamide (with or without an antihistamine)	Use nasal decongestant spray concurrently (see Table 17-2).
2-4 tablets at bedtime or twice daily	6-8 tablets per person **(OTC; Group)**	Other stimulants not recommended. Bulk agents (e.g., psyllium preparations) may be useful prophylactically.	Infrequent stooling is common during travel—encourage fluids and bulk in diet; senna products are helpful for narcotic-induced constipation, and unlike with other agents, the bowel will not habituate.
0.125-0.375 mg 1 hr before retiring	4-6 tablets **(Rx; Ind)**	Oxazepam (Serax) 15 mg tablets	At high altitude, first try acetazolamide (see Acute mountain sickness) for sleeplessness.

often priced for their fashionable appearance rather than optical merit. "Gradient" lenses may be darker (or mirrored) at the top or bottom to preferentially block direct or reflected sunlight, respectively. This feature is desirable for aquatic, desert, and high-altitude travel but probably unnecessary for most backpacking activity. Sunglass frames should be composed of nylon, Lexan, silicone-graphite, or metal rather than brittle plastic. Frame hinges preferably use a bolt and nut rather than a pin. It is recommended that for extended wilderness use, nuts be specially sealed (such as with Locktite) and pins be sealed with cyanoacrylate Super Glue. Sunglass models with side shields and nose protectors are recommended for snow, desert, and aquatic terrain. Retention (neck) straps are recommended for any activity involving climbing or skiing. For water sports a lanyard may be attached from the frame over the back to a belt loop. High-impact frames (such as RecSpecs) with polycarbonate lenses are available for hazardous sports such as climbing, white-water venturing, and hang-gliding.

MEDICAL SUPPLIES

Wound Care Material

Needles and other surgical tools may be crudely "sterilized" by being rubbed vigorously with a prepackaged towelette containing alcohol, chlorhexidine (Hibistat), povidone-iodine (Betadine), or benzalkonium chloride. After the instruments are rubbed with alcohol or Hibistat towelettes, the residual alcohol can be ignited for additional effect. Flame sterilization to red hot may also be acceptable. A less efficient method is to immerse the tool in boiling water for about the same duration recommended to disinfect water for drinking.

Forcefully ejecting irrigant solution from a 20 or 35 cc syringe through an 18- or 19-gauge needle generates pressures adequate to dislodge bacteria and microscopic particles from contaminated wound surfaces. Unfortunately, the literature does not specify how "clean" an irrigant solution must be. Since the primary goal of irrigation is the removal of debris, it seems reasonable that water pure enough to drink should be adequate for irrigation, especially if povidone-iodine solution is added.

Significant advances in wound care include Tegaderm adhesive dressings and Spenco 2nd Skin. Tegaderm is a transparent 3 × 3 adhesive covering for clean wounds that provides a barrier to water, dust, and dirt, while allowing oxygen to penetrate. It can be left in place for several days, provided no wound complications arise. Spenco 2nd Skin is a polyethylene oxide gel laminate for placement over blistering skin and burns. Like moleskin products, 2nd Skin reduces friction damage to the underlying skin. 2nd Skin may offer additional protection by redistributing pressure and absorbing exudate. It is an excellent product to carry, especially for bicycling, in which abrasion injuries are common.

Table 17-4 Contingency Supplies for Wilderness Travel

Item	Description, Quantity (No.), (Weight)*	Comment
1. Whistle	Nonmetal, shrill (1 oz)	Emergency signal (bursts of three)
2. Knives	A sturdy folding or straight knife plus a multi-tool knife	e.g., Swiss Army type
3. Maps	Trail and topographic (1 oz) (some per group)	Plastic coated or with cover
4. Compass, fluid-filled	≤2° gradations (1-2 oz)	Know area declination
5. Flashlight	Two C cell most efficient; lithium or alkaline No. 1 (6-8 oz)	Headlamp attachment desirable
6. Sunglasses	With side and nose blocks; polycarbonate or glass lens (1-3 oz)	>98% UVB filtering; >85% light absorption
7. Rescue and survival guide	Condensed (3-6 oz) (per group)	Learn basic air-to-ground signals (see Appendix B)
8. Pencil and paper	Waterproof paper preferred (2 oz)	
9. Quarters	Two (1 oz)	Phone calls; wrap in plastic and tape inside kit
10. Accident report forms	Waterproof preferred, two (1 oz) (per group)	
11. Spare sunglasses	(1-3 oz) (per group)	May improvise—make slits in cardboard, cloth
12. Toilet paper, small roll	One (1 oz)	Store in plastic bag
13. Matches, waterproof	"Strike-anywhere" type, 12	Store in plastic bag
14. Spare bulb, batteries	(1-3 oz)	Store in plastic bag
15. Closed-cell foam pads	1 × 1 ft sections, one to three (3 oz)	e.g., Ensolite; to insulate stove, seats, use as cervical collar or splint pads
16. Avalanche cord	Red; metal arrows (2 oz)	Attach to body
17. "Space" blanket	56 × 84 inches, two or three (1 oz)	Emergency insulation (replace every 3 yr)
18. Surveyor's trail tape	Bright color 50 ft (1 oz) (per group)	Trail, avalanche site markers
19. Utility cord	Nylon 25-50 ft (2 oz)	Shelter; utility
20. Heat source	Candle; fuel tabs, one or two (2 oz)	
21. Emergency toboggan kit	Variable (per 2-3 persons)	Convert skis and poles; e.g., NSP (see Appendix C)
22. Goggles	Rose or amber (4 oz)	Double lens, polarized preferred
23. Radio beacon	(8 oz); e.g., Pieps, Skadi, Ortovox	Use in avalanche terrain
24. Scraper	Metal edged (1 oz)	Ice and wax removal
25. Shovel	Lexan or aluminum (16-32 oz) (per 1-3 persons)	e.g., REI (see Appendix C)
26. Face mask	Leather, silk, or synthetic (1 oz)	
27. Aerial flares; ground smoke bombs	Red smoke, two to four (1 oz) (per group)	Rescue signal
28. "Bungie" elastic cords with hooks	6-12 inch #1-2 (1 oz)	Pack compression; lash equipment to pack
29. Swami belt	1-inch webbing 10-20 ft (4-8 oz)	Waist, seat harness
30. Carabiner, locking type	Aluminum, two or three (3 oz)	Climbing or rappel harness; rope brake; Prusik handle
31. Rescue pulley	Small, one or two (2 oz)	Cliff, crevasse rescue
32. Rope, Perlon or Goldline	5.5-9 mm 50-75 ft (8-16 oz) (per group)	Rescue, evacuation
33. Magnifying lens	8-15 × (1 oz) (per group)	Snow crystal exam; map reading; splinter removal; fire starter
34. Altimeter	≤20-ft accuracy (2 oz) (per group)	Altitude orienteering; barometric changes
35. Saw	Wire or blade (2-15 oz) (per 1-4 persons)	Fuel or shelter (cuts wood, snow, ice)
36. Extra food and candy	1-day supply (8-16 oz)	Prevent hypothermia
37. Extra clothing	Wool preferred	Sock doubles as mitten
38. Signal mirror	Unbreakable preferred (1 oz)	
39. Road flare	5-minute, one or two (3 oz)	Rescue signal; emergency fire starter
40. Extra ski wax	Klister or two-wax system (3 oz)	
41. Emergency shelter	"Tube" tent, tarp, or bivvy sack (3-16 oz)	May improvise with large plastic bags
42. Extra water	1 pint, metal preferred (18 oz)	Metal canteen can be heated directly
43. Thermometer, outdoor	In protective case (0.5 oz) (per group)	Snow, water, air temp
44. Lens antifogger	Liquid or stick (1 oz)	For glasses, goggles
45. Climbing skins, adhesive	"Skinny" type (11-16 oz)	Urgent snow climbing, or slowing descent

Numbers refer to the classification scheme in Fig. 17-2.

*Quantity is per person per trip, unless otherwise specified; weight given is per individual item, in ounces (35 oz = 1 kg = 2.2 lb).

Table 17-5 Repair Supplies for Wilderness Travel

Item	Description, Quantity, Weight*	Comment
1. Needle or sewing awl	With heavy thread (1 oz)	Clothing, pack repair
2. Screwdrivers	Flat and Phillips No. 2 (3-6 oz)	For skis, No. 3 "posidrive" (or filed down No. 2 Phillips)
3. Tape, duct or reinforced strapping	1-2 inches wide, 5 yards (2 oz) (per person per trip)	
4. Wire	Braided steel, 3-6 ft (2 oz)	Repair of binding, boot, snowshoe, and pack
5. Awl	On multifunction knife (2 oz) (per person per trip)	Repair of clothing, pack, shelter
6. Visegrip pliers	5-inch (5-8 oz)	
7. Glue	Two-component epoxy, or meltable nylon glue stick (1 oz)	
8. Spare bale and screws	Two	Repair of ski binding
9. "P-tex" ski base stick	Meltable No. 1 (1 oz)	Repair of plastic ski base
10. Spare ski tip	Plastic or aluminum (3-5 oz)	
11. Spare crampon wrench	No. 1 (one)	
12. Knife sharpener	Diamond-bar, ceramic, or stone (2-3 oz)	

Numbers refer to the classification scheme in Fig. 17-2.
*Quantity is per group unless specified; weight given is per individual item, in ounces (35 oz = 1 kg = 2.2 lb).

Topical Medications

Sweat, water, wind, dirt, and friction inherent in wilderness travel diminish the efficacy of topical sunscreens and corticosteroids. For this reason sunscreen products containing methoxy cinnamates in combination with oxybenzones (Table 17-2) are recommended to provide high substantivity,[8] or "staying power" (see Chapter 12). A sunscreen sun protection factor (SPF) of at least 15 is recommended for wilderness travel by anyone even mildly susceptible to sunburn, since the goal is to prevent the burn entirely.

Topical corticosteroids are especially useful for contact dermatitis and insect bites. They may alleviate suffering and obviate the need for systemic drugs. Maximally potent fluorinated corticosteroid preparations (such as betamethasone, flucinolone, flucinonide, and halcinonide) are recommended (Table 17-2) for use under the harsh circumstances of wilderness travel; it is extremely unlikely that any complications would result from short-term use.

Intravenous and Classified Drugs

Although injectable medications could be prescribed for individual laypersons, a medically trained member of the party would have to administer the drugs. Such injectable drugs would rarely be needed, and since they are often temperature sensitive, are fragile, and expire quickly, it is not recommended that these drugs (with the exception of epinephrine) be carried routinely on wilderness outings (see Appendix A, Chapter 21). A trip portending an extremely high risk of illness or injury should include a certified health professional controlling a customized drug kit (selected from Boxes 17-4 and 17-5). Party members should be made aware of, and consent to, the extraordinary hazards of such a trip. In addition, they should be familiar with local sources of health services.

Narcotic analgesics should be used to treat pain only if mild analgesics such as aspirin and acetaminophen are inadequate, mental status is not clouded (as might occur with head trauma), and respiratory difficulty is not present (unless it is due solely to discomfort) (see Box 17-5 and Table 17-3). Oral narcotic-containing products are appropriate for moderately severe pain. If indicated by the circumstances, appropriately trained personnel may carry injectable narcotic preparations. Although products with agonist-antagonist activity such as nalbuphine (Nubain) or butorphanol (Stadol) are recommended to limit respiratory depression at higher doses, the narcotic antagonist naloxone (Narcan) should still be included for use in the event of oversedation. A promising new development is buccal morphine (13.3 mg, equivalent to 10 mg of base). Placed between the upper lip and gum above the front teeth, buccal morphine has analgesic effect and duration comparable to the same dose given intramuscularly[1] and can be removed in the event of oversedation, respiratory depression, or hypotension. Information on the marketing status of this drug is available from Forest Laboratories (see Appendix D at the end of the chapter).

A short-acting central nervous system amphetamine stimulant (Table 17-3) may be justifiably carried during extremely high-risk activity, such as winter mountaineering, in which the participant might have to overcome fatigue in order to assist in a rescue effort or to reach aid. The small quantity prescribed on a one-time basis is unlikely to be associated with misuse.

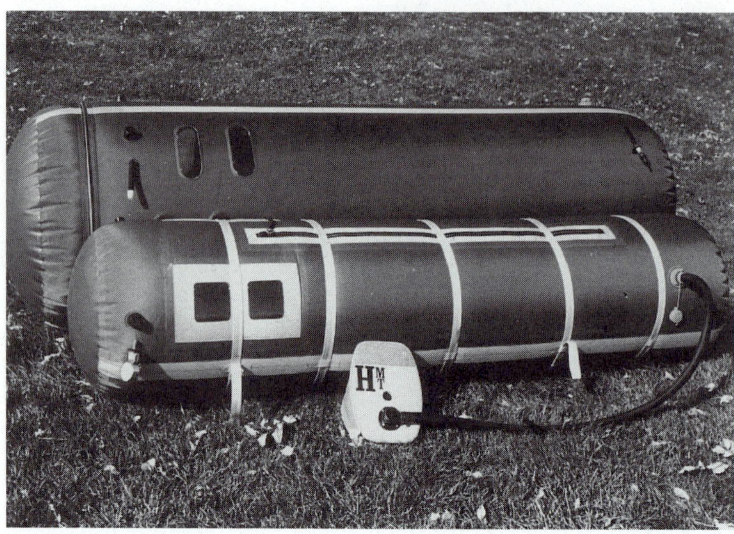

Fig. 17-4 Gamow Bag *(foreground)* and Tent. Attached is the foot pump required to pressurize the compartment to 2 pounds per square inch. The tent is roughly 50% larger, and its extra height allows the person to sit upright, an important feature in someone suffering from pulmonary edema. Four windows are strategically located to permit observation. Entry is via a lengthwise zipper.

SPECIFIC EQUIPMENT PURCHASES

This section reviews specialized items that are not basic to the comprehensive medical kit but may be needed for certain high-risk recreational activities. Box 17-8 itemizes such equipment, and descriptions of products, their usage, and indicated circumstances are given here. Suppliers and their unique products are listed in Appendix C.

High-Altitude Exposure

The Gamow Bag (Fig. 17-4) is a portable hyperbaric chamber resembling a large sleeping bag with a window. It has been shown to be effective for the treatment of high-altitude pulmonary and cerebral edema. Constructed of nylon, the bag is foldable and has a packing weight of 14.5 pounds. It is 7 feet long and has a diameter of 21 inches. The bag is pressurized with a foot pump at a rate of 10 to 20 strokes per minute and has relief valves pressurized to 2 pounds per square inch, allowing the venting of expired air. In situations such as a remote clinic that has electricity, a mechanical compressor can be used to avoid the fatiguing task of foot pumping.

A Breathing Bladder has been introduced. One end of this large nylon bag connects to a face mask, and the other to one of the pressure relief valves of the Gamow Bag. The patient inhales uncontaminated air from the Gamow Bag, and the exhaled air flows down a plastic tube into the bladder. This obviates the need for manual foot pumping of the bag for a 15- to 30-minute period until the bladder becomes full. It is then necessary to operate the foot pump again to repressurize the bag. The bladder is an excellent alternative for expeditions at very high altitude that are far from medical evacuation and when a prolonged period of resuscitation is anticipated.

The recently developed Gamow Tent operates on the same principles as the Gamow Bag. It is nearly 50% larger, and the added height allows a victim to sit upright.

The aforementioned devices are expensive and intended for expeditions going to extremes of altitude (greater than 14,000 feet) or in dangerous situations that prevent an easy, rapid descent (for example, ice climbing on a steep glacial crevasse).

Cold Exposure

Equipment purchases for cold exposure relate to the stabilization and resuscitation of victims with accidental exposure hypothermia. For most travel, removal of an individual from exposure and prevention of further heat loss are sufficient measures when medical assistance is nearby. Persons engaging in low-risk travel can use a sleeping bag wrapped with a Space Emergency Blanket to provide a capsule that preserves heat and allows thermal recovery. The latter product is made of a lightweight material capable of reflecting and retaining over 80% of radiated body heat. Another helpful product is the Grabber Warmer. Useful in the prevention of frostbite, these small pads undergo a chemical reaction on exposure to the air, producing heat. Grabber Warmers can maintain a temperature of 150° F for 7 hours or more. They can be placed in gloves, shoes, and pockets for the prevention of frostbite.

For more serious expeditions involving high-risk travel or distant from medical rescue or assistance, several highly sophisticated products may be of value. For victims of severe exposure hypothermia, elevation of the core temperature in addition to prevention of further body heat loss may be critical in life-threatening cases. Inhalation of warm, hu-

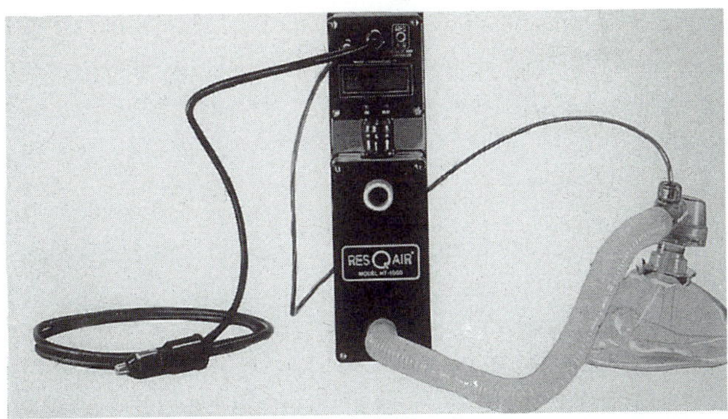

Fig. 17-5 The Res-Q-Air system for delivery of warm, saturated air. The unit is portable and battery run for use in the field. Its use requires minimal training. Temperature is adjusted by a single control dial.

midified air provides an excellent method of heat exchange and is now possible with portable field units. The Res-Q-Air (Fig. 17-5) provides warm, saturated air by using a battery-operated device that requires a small amount of water and delivers heat for inhalation via an attached hose and face mask. The unit is simple to operate, has a temperature control valve, and runs for an hour on battery power. It is small (9 × 3 × 2 inches), weighs 4½ pounds, and is portable. In the event that emergency intravenous fluids may be required, an intravenous bag warmer, the Hot-Sack, can be used. This product comes in a soft, rugged portable case and has its own battery power source. Temperature within the bag remains at 98° F, so that intravenous fluids are kept warm. The bag has a protective sleeve to place over intravenous tubing to maintain warmth.

Advanced expeditioners and persons involved in cold water search and rescue should consider the purchase of a Hypothermic Stabilizer Bag. This product consists of an internal, high-pile fabric that wicks water to allow quick drying of hypothermic victims. The thermal properties far exceed those of an equivalent-thickness conventional down sleeping bag, and the product requires no additional insulation underneath for support and comfort. A key feature involves the ability to perform complete cardiopulmonary resuscitation through an access window over the chest. The stabilizer's outer cover is made of water-resistant material and has carrying handles to allow for safe transport of victims (Fig. 17-6).

Water Sports

The principles of water disinfection are covered in Chapter 43, but the design features of a filtration system that produce acceptable water for consumption need to be highlighted. Key design features are (1) an adequate pore size of the filter to remove bacteria and protozoan cysts (0.2 μm or less), (2) a filter element that either has activated charcoal or is impregnated with silver or iodine for local antibacterial action, (3) a pump-feed mechanism that forces water

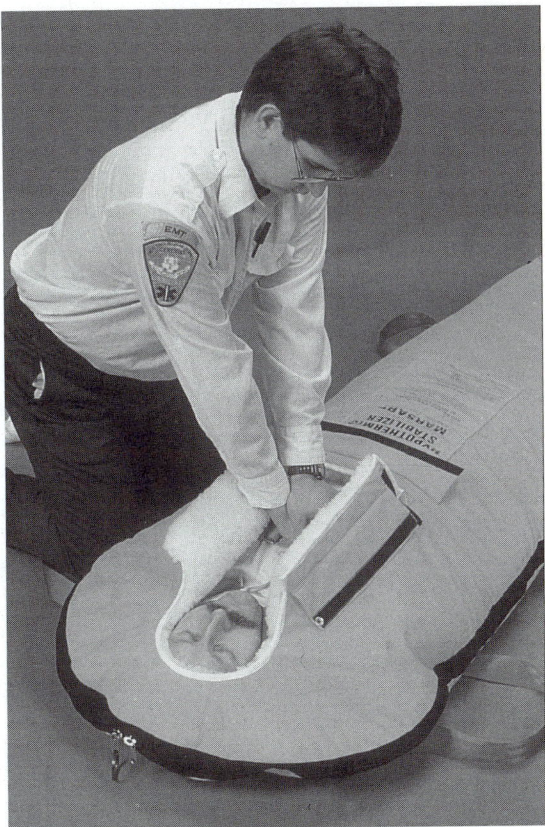

Fig. 17-6 Hypothermic Stabilizer bag. This excellent prehospital transport device allows the passive rewarming of victims suffering from cold exposure and is especially useful in cold water immersion because of the drying ability of its high-pile fabric. The unit weighs only 12 pounds and measures 12 × 13 inches when packaged in a portable case.

through the filter housing, (4) a device that can be easily disassembled and cleaned for proper maintenance, and (5) a product having durability and simplicity of use. Noteworthy filters that have most of the desirable features include the Katadyn water filter, PUR filter, and MSR WaterWorks.

Bicycling

Several prepackaged kits for the cyclist can be purchased. Persons who want to upgrade the basic first aid kit to treat injuries unique to cycling should consider the abrasions and minor burns likely to be encountered. Proper wound management requires a protective pad that is nonadherent, cools the skin and absorbs exuded fluids. A number of breathable water-based gels, such as Spenco 2nd Skin, exist for this purpose.

Mountain Climbing and Hiking

In wilderness travel above the treeline or on shipboard, the inclusion of more advanced splinting products should be considered. The SAM splint weighs only 4 ounces. Its coated aluminum strips unfold to provide rigid longitudinal support. It could also function as a cervical collar, although the neck would still have to be immobilized. (At least two SAM splints are needed to stabilize an entire extremity). More elaborate devices, including an air-stirrup ankle brace having an inner liner of adjustable air cells blown up through a valve, exist. If activity will predispose to high risk of femoral fracture and a traction splint is desirable, the Kendrick traction device should be considered.

Third World Travel

Travelers to underdeveloped countries are at risk of infection from a host of diseases transmitted by insect bites. For travel outside of urban areas, the risks are especially great when sleeping unprotected in the outdoors. A lightweight bed net that can enclose two persons should be carried (see Fig. 34-8). Further protection against mosquitoes can be achieved by spraying the nets with permethrin. For bites from insects, spiders, and snakes, the Sawyer Extractor may be of value. Several topical medications that combine an anesthetic (benzocaine) along with a cooling agent (menthol), such as Sawyer's Sting Aid or Itch Balm Plus, may be helpful in dealing with troublesome bites or allergic reactions. Because of the high risk of a bout of traveler's diarrhea, consideration should be given to carrying oral rehydration packets. Commercially prepackaged units contain essential elements that allow oral rehydration when combined with 1 L of sterilized water.

LEGAL CONSIDERATIONS

Chapter 55 presents general legal issues concerning wilderness and environmental emergencies, including the dispensation of prescription drugs. It is advisable, from both a medical and legal perspective, that travelers have their personal physician explain and prescribe in advance any medications indicated in Tables 17-2 and 17-3. It is *not* acceptable for prescription medications to be shared among travelers.

Physicians traveling as equal members of the party may render emergency treatment to others under the protection of Good Samaritan laws, but physicians sponsored in any way by the travel organization may be held to the standard of care of a professional physician-patient relationship.

➠ SUMMARY

Provided that an individual is moderately active and without life-threatening illnesses, travel into the outdoors may be encouraged. The trip coordinator should review the health status and experience of potential participants, emphasize preventive measures, and carefully weigh important risk factors. An array of supplies to deal with potential medical problems can be appropriately selected. Specific prescription medication may be authorized for responsible individuals to forestall serious disability or discomfort resulting from injury or illness en route. Physicians traveling with a wilderness party may wish to carry additional medications and devices.

REFERENCES

1. Bell MD et al: Buccal morphine—a new route for analgesia? *Lancet* 1:71, 1985.
2. Bowman W: Data-based first aid, *Response!* 6:12, 1987.
3. Goodman PH: Medical emergencies during air travel: aircraft resources and guidelines for Good Samaritan physicians, *Postgrad Med* 80(8):54, 1986.
4. Goodman PH: Guidelines for the selection of medical and emergency equipment for wilderness travel, *Ski Patrol,* Spring 1985, p 32.
5. Goodman PH, Kurtz KJ, Carmichael J: Primary care in the wilderness, three-part series, *Postgrad Med* 77:173, 1985; 77:253, 1985; 77:202, 1985.
6. Houston CS: Altitude illness, *Postgrad Med* 74:231, 1983.
7. Illingsworth R: Medical equipment for expeditions, *Br Med J* 282:202, 1981.
8. Kaidbey KH, Kligman AM: An appraisal of the efficacy and substantivity of the new high-potency sunscreens, *J Am Acad Dermatol* 4:566, 1981.
9. Reifsnyder WF: *Weathering the wilderness,* San Francisco, 1980, Sierra Club Books.
10. Wehbring J: The rescue pack, *Response!* 6:34, 1987.

APPENDIX A

Health Questionnaire for Wilderness Travel (Page 1 of 2)

TRIP COORDINATOR: ______________________ Dates of trip: __________-__________

Trip Location: ______________________ Major type of activity: ______________________

Please provide the following information (use another sheet of paper if necessary): (All information will be used *confidentially* by the coordinator to promote the safety of the party)

Name ______________________ Age _____ Height _____ Weight _____

Address ______________________ What is your overall HEALTH? (circle one)

______________________ Poor Fair Good Excellent

Phone ( ) ______________________

Person to contact in EMERGENCY:

Contact's Name ______________________

Contact's Phone ( ) ______________________

What is your overall PHYSICAL condition?

Poor Fair Good Excellent

MEDICAL DATA

1. Allergies (drug, pollen, food, etc.—be specific) .... (YES) (NO)
2. Allergies (insect bites—be specific) .... (YES) (NO)
3. Diabetes .... (YES) (NO)
4. Epilepsy, Seizures, or Convulsions .... (YES) (NO)
5. Heart Problems .... (YES) (NO)
6. Kidney Problems .... (YES) (NO)
7. Injuries or Problems with Joints: (Specify which side, EXPLAIN problem)
   A. Ankle .... (YES) (NO)
   B. Knee .... (YES) (NO)
   C. Hip .... (YES) (NO)
   D. Fingers/Toes .... (YES) (NO)
   E. Wrist .... (YES) (NO)
   F. Elbow .... (YES) (NO)
   G. Shoulder .... (YES) (NO)
   H. Back/Spine .... (YES) (NO)
   I. Other .... (YES) (NO)

Modified from Green P: *The outdoor leadership handbook,* Tacoma, Wash, 1982, Emergency Response Institute.

Health Questionnaire for Wilderness Travel (Page 2 of 2)

8. Have you ever had: (EXPLAIN problem)

   A. Mountain sickness .... (YES) (NO)

   B. Cerebral edema .... (YES) (NO)

   C. Pulmonary edema .... (YES) (NO)

   D. Heatstroke .... (YES) (NO)

   E. Sun/snow blindness .... (YES) (NO)

   F. Frostbite .... (YES) (NO)

   G. Hypothermia/exposure .... (YES) (NO)

   H. Immersion foot .... (YES) (NO)

   I. Excessive nosebleeds .... (YES) (NO)

   J. Asthma .... (YES) (NO)

   K. Ulcers .... (YES) (NO)

   L. Bowel problems .... (YES) (NO)

   M. Broken bones .... (YES) (NO)

9. List any medical problems, illnesses, injuries, or chronic conditions that you have presently or have had in the last 3 years (be as specific as possible):

10. List any MEDICATIONS that you are currently taking (include the dosing, if possible):

APPENDIX B

Annotated Bibliography of First Aid and Medical Planning

1. American Alpine Club: *Accidents in North American mountaineering,* New York, American Alpine Club. (113 E. 90th Street; 10128). Annually published review of the important findings of accident investigations.
2. American Red Cross: *Advanced first aid and emergency care,* ed 2, Garden City, NY, 1979, Doubleday. 320 pp. 16 oz. (available from local offices of the ARC). Accepted guidelines for advanced first aid, best reviewed in a classroom format before travel.
3. Auerbach P: *Medicine for the outdoors,* Boston, 1991, Little, Brown. 412 pp. 16 oz. (34 Beacon Street; 02106; 800-343-9204) Comprehensive guide for lay persons who travel in all environments. Includes general information, major medical-surgical problems, minor disorders, environment-related problems, drugs and doses. Especially welcome are sections covering diving illness, hazardous marine life, wild plant poisoning, and wildland fires. **Highly recommended that a copy be carried by a lay person responsible for medical care for any type of extended wilderness travel.**
4. Bowman W: *Outdoor emergency care: comprehensive first aid for non-urban settings,* ed 2, Lakewood, Colo, 1993, NSPS. (133 S. Van Gordon; 80228; 303-988-1111.) Developed for ski patrollers, provides an up-to-date, comprehensive guide to the prevention, recognition, and management of injuries and illness encountered in nonurban settings. **Highly recommended reading for participants in all varieties of skiing.**
5. Brown R: *Emergency/survival handbook,* ed 4, Bellevue, Wash, 1987, American Outdoor Safety League. 45 pp. 3 oz. (P.O. Box 3301; 98009). A lightweight, pocket-size guide to first aid that follows ARC standards. Includes wax-impregnated cover for emergency fire starting and Mylar centerfold for signalling.
6. Darvill F: *Mountaineering medicine,* ed 13, Berkeley, Calif, 1992, Wilderness Press. 101 pp. 3 oz. (2440 Bancroft Way; 94704; 415-843-8080). Lightweight, easily carried reminder of the principles of first aid and basic medical care for the mountain environment.
7. Hackett P: *Mountain sickness: prevention, recognition and treatment.* New York, American Alpine Club. (113 E. 90th Street; 10028). Thorough review of the current understanding of this problem. **Recommended reading for all travelers to high altitude.**
8. Lentz M et al: *Mountaineering first aid,* ed 3, Seattle, 1985, The Mountaineers. 104 pp. (306 Second Ave West; 98119; 800-553-4453). Good review of mountaineering first aid, most appropriate for classroom or individual reading in advance of departure.
9. *Medical Letter on Drugs and Therapeutics.* (56 Harrison Street, New Rochelle, NY 10801.) A four-page newsletter published every 2 weeks. Provides regular updates and expert opinion on the use of sunscreens, antibiotics, drugs for parasitic diseases, high-altitude illness, corticosteroids, rehydration solutions, and use of drugs in pregnancy. Requires familiarity with medical terminology and concepts. **Recommended reading for physicians serving as advisors to wilderness travelers.**
10. *Wilderness Medicine Letter.* (P.O. Box 2463 Indianapolis, IN 46206.) The newsletter of the Wilderness Medical Society. Reviews of recent publications, notification of events and meetings, official position statements, and commentary by experts in the field. **Highly recommended reading for physicians serving as advisors to travelers.**
11. Wilkerson J, ed: *Medicine for mountaineering and other wilderness activities,* ed 4, Seattle, 1992, The Mountaineers. 414 pp. 16 oz. (1011 SW Klickitat Way; 98134). Comprehensive coverage of the prevention, recognition, and advanced field management of mountaineering injuries and illnesses. Many sections are easily understood by general reader, but chapters on medical illness require familiarity with medical terminology and concepts, and a working knowledge of basic first aid is assumed. **Recommended that a single copy be carried by the person responsible for medical care of a large group on an extended or high-risk mountaineering outing.**
12. Wilkerson J, Bangs C, Hayward J: *Hypothermia, frostbite and other cold injuries,* Seattle, 1986, The Mountaineers. 105 pp. (306 Second Ave. West; 98119; 800-553-4453). Excellent overview that explains, in lay terms, the metabolic disturbances underlying cold injury, as well as practical methods of preventing and treating these disorders. Especially welcome is the chapter on immersion injuries containing valuable information for those involved in aquatic sports. **Highly recommended reading for all travelers to cold weather, mountain, and aquatic wilderness environments.**

APPENDIX C

Suppliers Listed in Text and Tables

Many of the products cited in this chapter can be found in outdoor equipment retail stores or pharmacies. The sources listed below provide specialized products referred to in the text.

1. **Adventure Medical Kits,** P.O. Box 2586, Berkeley, CA 94602; 510-632-1442 (supplier of well-designed

medical kits that are prepackaged for a range of specific recreational activities, such as bicycling, whitewater rafting, and backcountry travel)

2. **Campmor,** Paramus, NJ; 800-226-7667 (Lady-J urinal guide)
3. **C.F. Electronics, Inc.,** 5 Brayton Court, Commack, NY 11725; 516-499-8085 (RES-Q-AIR and IV HOT-SACK plus accessories; sophisticated equipment for the serious expedition traveler to areas of extreme cold)
4. **Chinook Medical Gear, Inc.,** 2805 Wilderness Place, Suite 700, Boulder, CO 94520; 800-766-1365 (the most complete catalog retailer for wilderness medical supplies; carrier of the Gamow Bag; good beginning source for the person in need of a wide variety of medical supplies)
5. **Gilbert Surgical Instruments, Inc.,** P.O. Box 458, Bellmawr, NJ 08031; 609-933-2770 (Abelson Emergency Cricothyrotomy Cannula)
6. **Grabber International West,** 205 Mason Circle, Concord, CA 94520; 510-680-0777 (manufacturer of a variety of packaged miniheaters with accessories useful for preventing cold-related injuries of the hands, feet, and face)
7. **Junkin Safety Appliance Co.,** 3121 Millers Ln., Louisville, KY 40216; 502-775-8303 (folding aluminum full-length backboard, 15 lb)
8. **MARSARS/Great Eastern Marine, Inc.,** 205 Myrtle St., Shelton, CT 06484-4015; 900-545-2071 (manufacturer of water and ice rescue equipment; a hypothermic stabilizer bag and additional accessory heat packs are available)
9. **Medixchoice,** 1750 Joe Crosson Dr., Suite D2, El Cajon, CA 92020; 619-258-0105 (Kendrick traction device, 16 oz)
10. **Mountain Safety Research,** P.O. Box 24547, Seattle, WA 98124; 206-624-7048 (manufacturer of high-performance and lightweight stoves, as well as the WaterWorks filtration system)
11. **National Ski Patrol System, Inc.** (NSP), 133 S. Van Gordon, Ste. 100, Lakewood, CO 80228; 303-988-1111 (various first aid supplies and equipment for winter skiing and mountaineering sold by catalogue to NSP members)
12. **Outdoor Research,** 1000 1st Ave. So., Seattle, WA 98134; 800-421-2421 (diverse array of tote bags, medical travel kits, and stuff sacks useful for international travel)
13. **Patagonia, Inc.,** P.O. Box 86, Ventura, CA 93002; 805-643-8616 (Capilene underclothing; variety of outdoor clothing)
14. **Recreational Equipment, Inc.** (REI), P.O. Box 88126, Seattle, WA 98138-0126; 206-323-8333 (Thermax underclothing; variety of sunglasses, outdoor gear and clothing)
15. **Seaberg Co.,** P.O. Box 734, South Beach, OR 97366; 503-867-4726 (SAM folding splint, 4 oz)
16. **Travel Medicine Inc.,** 351 Pleasant St., Suite 312, Northampton, MA 01060; 800-872-8633 (specializing in educational books and handy supplies for international travel; source of insect repellents, clothing, and nets for mosquito protection)

APPENDIX D
Sources of Information About Wilderness Emergencies

1. **American River Touring Association,** 24000 Casa Loma Rd., Groveland, CA 95321; 800-323-2782 (Nonprofit organization that sponsors basic and leadership courses for river-rafting and kayaking).
2. **Emergency Response Institute,** 1819 Mark Street N.E., Olympia, WA 98506; 206-491-7785 (Publishes books and sponsors symposia on search and rescue, emergency preparedness, survival, and outdoor leadership).
3. **Forest Laboratories Inc.,** NY; attention: Dr. J.M. Schor; 150 E. 58th St., NY, NY 10155; 212-421-7850 (Information on the availability of buccal morphine sulfate preparation).
4. **National Association for Search and Rescue (NASAR),** P.O. Box 3709, Fairfax, VA 22038; 703-352-1349 (Educational association that provides conferences, symposia, and training in search and rescue and emergency response, including communications; sponsors *Rescue* magazine [JEMS Communications, 1947 Camino-Vida Roble, Suite 200, Carlsbad, CA 92008; 619-431-9797]).
5. **National Climatic Data Center,** Federal Building, Asheville, NC 28801-2696; 704-271-4800 (Provides historical weather summaries for US and many foreign cities; small fee for materials. Telephone first to determine availability of relevant data).
6. **National Ski Patrol System, Inc.** (NSP), 133 S. Van Gordon, Ste. 100, Lakewood, CO 80228; 303-988-1111 (Sponsors training programs in winter emergency care, avalanche, and ski mountaineering, some that are open to the public; sells equipment and first aid supplies through catalogue to NSP members).
7. **National Weather Service** in city near region of travel; for further information, write: Attn. W/OM 15 × 2, Silver Spring, MD 20910 (The NWS nearest the travel site can provide forecasts, and in many regions, provides broadcasts over NOAA Weather Radio on frequencies between 162.40 and 162.55 mHz, including 3- to 5-day forecasts and avalanche warnings).

8. **Outward Bound Training Institute/Kurt Hahn Leadership Center,** 121 N. Sterling St., Morganton, NC 28655-3443; 704-437-6112 (Nonprofit educational organization that uses the mountain, river, and ocean wilderness settings to provide stimuli for personal development; separate leadership training courses available).
9. **Undersea and Hyperbaric Medical Society,** 9650 Rockville Pike, Bethesda, MD 20814; 301-942-2980 (Nonprofit organization that sponsors workshops and meetings on the prevention and treatment of diving injuries and illnesses treatable with hyperbaric oxygen. Publishes bimonthly newsletter, *Pressure,* and two research publications, *Undersea Biomedical Research* and *Journal of Hyperbaric Medicine*).
10. **Wilderness Education Association,** Department of Recreation Resources, Colorado State University, Fort Collins, CO 80523; 303-223-6252 (Nonprofit educational organization that sponsors, in conjunction with colleges, a 5-week National Standards Program for Outdoor Leadership Certification).
11. **Wilderness Medical Society,** P.O. Box 2463, Indianapolis, IN 46206-2463; 317-631-1745 (Nonprofit organization of medical and related professionals interested in the prevention and treatment of wilderness injuries and illnesses. Publishes quarterly newsletter, *Wilderness Medicine Letter,* covering wilderness medicine meetings, literature review, field management, and position statements. Publishes *Wilderness and Environmental Medicine* [formerly *Journal of Wilderness Medicine*], the official academic publication of the society.)

18 WILDERNESS IMPROVISATION

Eric A. Weiss
Howard J. Donner

At the heart of wilderness medicine is improvisation, an amazing amalgam of formal medical science integrated with an adventurous twist of creative and commonsense problem solving.

Defined as "to fabricate out of what is conveniently at hand," improvisation encompasses infinite variations, with few absolute rights and wrongs. Wilderness improvisation occurs within a creative environment, limited more often by imagination than by personnel or equipment.

General Guidelines

A person working with complex improvised systems should always test his or her creation on a noninjured person ("work out the bugs") before applying it to a patient. Materials that lend themselves to improvisation should be included in the wilderness survival kit. This will greatly enhance the efficiency of any improvised system. Creativity is needed when searching for improvisational materials. The victim's gear can be harvested to provide needed items (for example, backpacks can be dismantled to obtain foam pads and straps). When possible, construction of improvised systems should be practiced at home before they are required in an actual rescue.

Improvised Airway Management

The most common cause of airway obstruction in the semiconscious or unconscious victim is relaxation of the oropharyngeal muscles, which allows the tongue to slide back and obstruct the airway. If only one rescuer is present, maintaining a patent airway with the jaw thrust or chin lift technique precludes further first aid management. A nasal trumpet type of airway can be improvised from a Foley catheter, a radiator hose, a solar shower hose, siphon tubing, or an inflation hose from a kayak flotation bag or sport pouch.

A temporary airway can be established by attaching the anterior aspect of the victim's tongue to the lower lip with two safety pins. An alternative to puncturing the lower lip is to pass a string through the safety pins and hold traction on the tongue by securing the other end to the victim's shirt button or jacket zipper.

If neither an oral nor a nasal airway can be established, cricothyroidotomy is indicated. The barrel of a 3 cc or 1 cc syringe with the plunger removed can be cut at a 45-degree angle at its midpoint to create an improvised cricothyroid airway device. After a vertical 1 cm incision is made through the skin over the cricothyroid membrane, the larynx is stabilized between the fingers and the pointed end of the syringe is inserted through the membrane and aimed caudad (toward the buttocks).

The proximal flange of the syringe barrel helps secure the device to the neck and prevents it from completely entering the trachea and being aspirated. Other potential cricothyroid airways include small flashlight casings, pen casings, small pill bottles, and large-bore needles and catheters.

Ear, Nose, and Throat Emergencies

Epistaxis is a common problem in travelers. The reduced humidity in airplanes, cold climates, and high-altitude environments can produce drying and erosion of the nasal mucosa. Other etiologic factors include facial trauma, infections, and inflammatory rhinitis. Although most cases of epistaxis are minor, some present life-threatening emergencies.[25]

Anterior epistaxis from one side of the nasal cavity occurs in 90% of cases.[5] If pinching the nostrils together for a full 10 minutes does not control the bleeding, nasal packing may be needed. A piece of cotton or gauze soaked with a vasoconstrictor such as Afrin or Neo-Synephrine Nasal

Spray can be inserted into the nose and left in place for 5 to 10 minutes. Vaseline-impregnated gauze or strips of a nonadherent dressing can then be packed into the nose so that both ends of the gauze remain outside the nasal cavity. This prevents the patient from inadvertently aspirating the nasal packing.[25]

To completely pack the nasal cavity of an adult patient, a minimum of 3 feet of packing is required to fill the nasal cavity and tamponade the bleeding site.[5] Expandable packing material such as Weimert Epistaxis Packing or the Rhino Rocket is available commercially. A tampon or balloon tip from a Foley catheter can also be used as improvised packing.[25]

Anterior nasal packing blocks sinus drainage and predisposes the patient to sinusitis. Prophylactic antibiotics are usually recommended until the pack is removed in 48 hours.[25]

If the bleeding site is located posteriorly, a 14 to 16 Fr Foley catheter with a 30 ml balloon can be used to tamponade the site.[7] The catheter should be prelubricated with either Vaseline or a water-based lubricant. The catheter is inserted through the nasal cavity into the posterior pharynx. The balloon is then inflated with 10 to 15 ml of water and gently withdrawn back into the posterior nasopharynx until resistance is met. The catheter is secured firmly to the patient's forehead with several strips of tape. The anterior nose is then packed in front of the catheter balloon as described earlier.

Esophageal foreign bodies may cause significant morbidity. Respiratory compromise caused by tracheal compression or by aspiration of secretions can occur. Mediastinitis, pleural effusions, pneumothorax, and abscess may be seen with perforations of the esophagus from sharp objects or pressure necrosis caused by large objects.[15]

The use of a Foley balloon-tipped catheter has been reported to be a safe method for removing blunt esophageal foreign bodies.[3,4,9] Success rates of 98% have been cited.[4] Complications associated with this method include laryngospasm, epistaxis, pain, esophageal perforation, and tracheal aspiration of the dislodged foreign body.[15] Sharp, ragged foreign bodies or an uncooperative patient precludes use of this technique.[22]

A 12 to 16 Fr Foley catheter is lubricated and placed orally into the esophagus with the patient in a sitting position. After the patient is placed in a Trendelenburg position, the catheter is passed beyond the foreign body and the balloon is inflated with water. The catheter is withdrawn with steady traction until the foreign body can be removed from the hypopharynx or expelled by coughing. Care must be taken to avoid lodging the foreign body in the nasopharynx. Any significant impedance to withdrawal should terminate the attempt.[22] Use of this technique is recommended only in extreme wilderness settings or when endoscopy is not available.

Improvised Splinting and Traction*

CERVICAL SPINE INJURIES

Because of its mobility, the cervical spine is the region of the spinal column most commonly injured in trauma. Any obvious or suspected cervical spine injury demands full spinal immobilization with use of both a rigid or semirigid cervical collar and long board immobilization. Historically, dogma about cervical spine injuries has specified a "splint 'em as they lie" approach. Transporting a patient who is not in anatomic position is arduous in the backcountry. It is uncomfortable for the patient, is difficult for the rescuers, and most important, increases the risk of further injury. In general, gentle axial traction back to anatomic position is indicated unless (1) return to anatomic position causes a significant increase in pain or focal neurologic deficit or (2) movement of the head and neck results in any noticeable mechanical resistance.[13a]

All cervical spine injuries (or suspected injuries) deserve full long board immobilization. Movement of the pelvis and hips in a lateral direction is potentially more dangerous than anterior-posterior movement; therefore it is appropriate during extended transport to allow gentle flexion at the hip with immobilization in that position if it is more comfortable for the patient. Soft pads behind the knees and the small of the back also add to the patient's comfort during a long transport.[6a]

Cervical Collars

Cervical collars should always be viewed as an adjunct to full spinal immobilization and never used alone. The improvised cervical collar should be used in conjunction with manual cervical spine stabilization followed by complete immobilization of the patient on a spine board. A properly applied and fitted collar is a primary defense against axial loading of the cervical spine, particularly in an evacuation that involves tilting of the patient's body uphill or downhill. Improvised cervical collars have in the past had a bad reputation, and textbooks continue to depict them made from a simple cravat wrapped around the neck. This type of system is of course no more effective than the soft cervical collars often used by urban plaintiffs trying to impress a jury.

An improvised cervical collar can work effectively *only* if it has the following features:

1. It is rigid or semirigid.
2. It fits properly (many improvised designs are too small).
3. It does not choke the patient.
4. It allows the patient's mouth to open if vomiting occurs.

*Specific aspects of fracture care are covered in detail in other chapters. This chapter focuses on improvised *systems*, not on definitive orthopedic *management*. Improvised systems rarely provide the same degree of protection as commercial systems. Good judgment is needed.

The following are improvisational approaches to cervical collars.

SAM Splint Cervical Collar. A cervical collar can be made from a SAM splint in the following way: Create a bend in the splint approximately 6 inches from the end of the splint. This bend will form the anterior post. Then, create flares for the mandible. Apply the anterior post underneath the chin and bring the remainder of the splint around the neck and apply the splint to the chest, ensuring the appropriate chin-to-chest distance by angling the end of the splint somewhat inferiorly. Take up circumferential slack by creating lateral posts. Finally, squeeze the back to create a posterior post and secure with tape (Fig. 18-1).

Closed-Cell Foam System. The best closed-cell foam systems incorporate a full-size or three-quarter-length pad folded longitudinally into thirds and applied by being centered over the back of the patient's neck and wrapped forward. The pad is crossed under the chin, contoured underneath opposite axillae, and secured. If the pad is not long enough, extensions can be taped or tied on. This system also works well with blankets, beach towels, or even a rolled plastic tarp. Small flexible cervical collars that do not optimally extend the chin-to-chest distance should be avoided.

Padded Hip Belt. A padded hip belt removed from a large internal or external frame backpack can sometimes be modified to work perfectly. Wider is usually better. Excess circumference can be taken up by overlapping the belt and securing the excess material with duct tape.

Clothing. Bulky clothing, such as a fiberpile jacket, can be used to make a cervical collar. Often, prewrapping a wide Ace wrap around the jacket compresses the material to make it more rigid and supportive.

Improvised Spinal Immobilization

As noted, the improvised cervical collar is only an adjunct to full spinal immobilization. Two immobilization systems are (1) short board immobilization, which is useful for short-duration transport (that is, getting the patient out of immediate danger) or when used in conjunction with a long board; and (2) long board immobilization, used for definitive immobilization during extensive transport.

All systems should be used in conjunction with a rigid or semirigid cervical collar, as described previously. Improvised lateral "towel rolls" are often added to these systems for additional head and neck support. These rolls can be improvised from small sections of Ensolite. Alternatively, a U-shaped head support or "horse collar" can be made from any rolled garment, blanket, tarp, or tent fly; this is placed over the patient's head in an inverted U and used in conjunction with the improvised cervical collar and spine board. Hiking socks or stuff bags filled with dirt, sand, or gravel also work well for this purpose. Stuff bags filled with snow for support should *never* be used because the snow can melt during transport and allow excessive head and neck motion. However, snow-filled stuff bags can act as temporary support while more definitive systems are being constructed. Another excellent system uses a folded SAM splint to create a "head bed" style of cradle for the head. When properly constructed, this device eliminates the need for blanket rolls or a cradle.

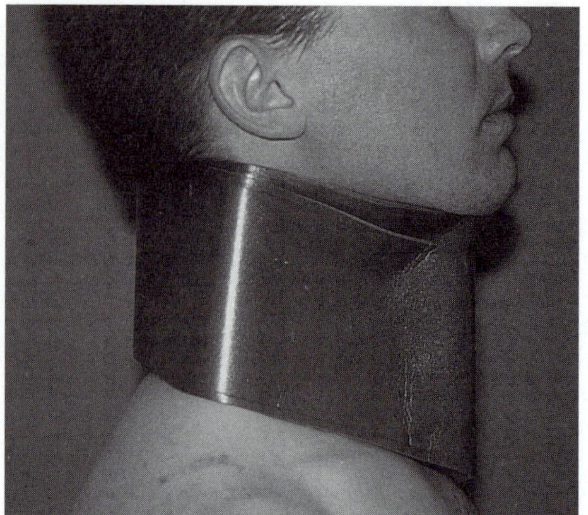

A

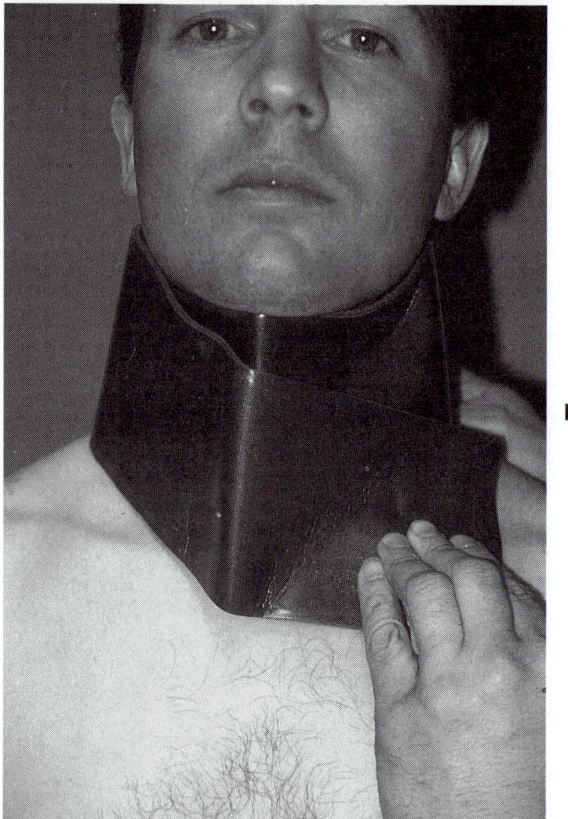

B

Fig. 18-1 **A,** Side view of cervical collar fashioned from SAM splint. **B,** Frontal view. The end is angled inferiorly to provide an adequate chin-to-chest distance.

Improvised Short Board Immobilization

Internal frame pack and snow shovel system. Some internal frame backpacks can be easily modified by inserting a snow shovel through the centerline attachment points (the shovel handgrip may need to be removed first). The patient's head is taped to the lightly padded shovel (Fig. 18-2); in this context the shovel blade serves as a head bed for the patient. The beauty of this system is that it incorporates the remainder of the pack suspension as designed (that is, shoulder and sternum straps with hip belt). It works well in conjunction with other long board designs, such as the continuous loop system (see section on continuous loop system below).

Inverted pack system. An efficient short board can be made with use of an inverted internal or external frame backpack. The padded hip belt is used as a head bed, and the frame is used as a short board in conjunction with a rigid or semirigid cervical collar (Fig. 18-3).

The pack is turned upside down, and the patient's shoulders and torso are lashed to the pack. The waist belt is fastened around the patient's head, in similar fashion to the top section of a Kendrick extrication device. The hip belt is typically too large, but excess circumference can be taken up with bilateral Ensolite rolls. Unlike the snow shovel system, this system requires that a way be devised to lash the patient to the splint.

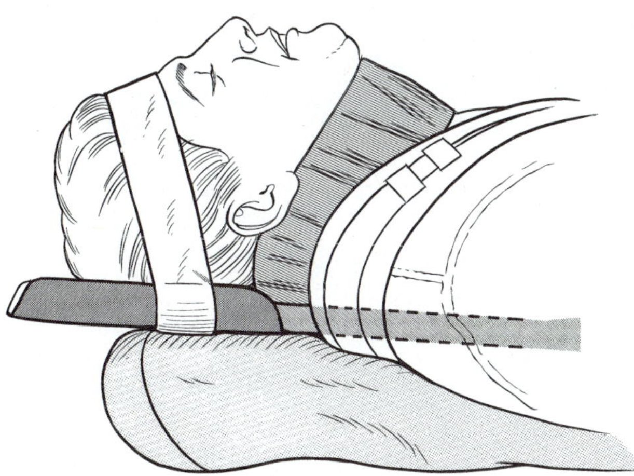

Fig. 18-2 Head immobilized on a padded shovel.

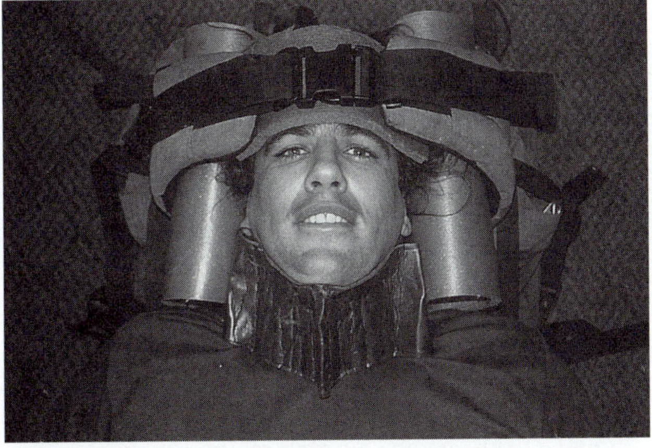

Fig. 18-3 Short board using an inverted pack system. The backpack waistbelt can be seen encircling the head.

Snowshoe system. A snowshoe can be made into a fairly reliable short board (Fig. 18-4). The snowshoe is padded and then rigged for attachment to the patient as shown.[14a]

Improvised Long Board Immobilization

Continuous loop system. For the continuous loop system (also known as the daisy chain, cocoon wrap, or mummy litter), the following items are needed:

1. A long climbing or rescue rope
2. A large tarp
3. Sleeping pads (Ensolite or Therm-a-Rest)
4. Stiffeners (such as skis, poles, snowshoes, canoe paddles, tree branches)

The rope is laid out with even U-shaped loops as shown in Fig. 18-5. The midsection should be slightly wider to conform to the patient's width. A small loop is tied at the foot end of the rope. A tarp is placed on the laid rope. On top of the tarp, foam pads are laid the full length of the system (the pads can be overlapped to add length). Then stiffeners are laid on top of the pads in the same axis as the patient. Multiple foam pads are added on top of the stiffeners. The patient is placed on the pads. The daisy chain is formed by bringing a single loop through the pretied loop, pulling loops toward the center, and feeding through the loops brought up from the opposite side. It is important to take up rope slack continuously. When the patient's armpits are reached, a loop is brought over each shoulder and tied off (or clipped off with a carabiner) (Fig. 18-5).

One excellent modification involves the addition of an inverted internal frame backpack. This can be incorporated with the padding and secured with the head end of the rope. The pack adds rigidity and padding, and the padded hip belt serves as a very efficient head and neck immobilizer.

Backpack frame litters. Functional litters can be constructed from external frame backpacks. Traditionally two frames are used, but three or four frames (as illustrated in Fig. 18-6) make for a larger, more stable litter. Cable ties or fiberglass strapping tape simplifies this fabrication. These litters can be reinforced with ice axes or ski poles.

Kayak system. Properly modified, the kayak makes an ideal rigid long board improvised litter. The seat must first be removed, along with sections of the upper deck if necessary. A serrated river knife (or camp saw) makes this improvisation much easier. Open deck canoes can be used almost as is, once the flotation has been removed.

Canoe system. Many rivers have railroad tracks that run parallel to the river canyon. The tracks can be used to slide a canoe by placing the boat perpendicular to the tracks and pulling on both bow and stern lines.

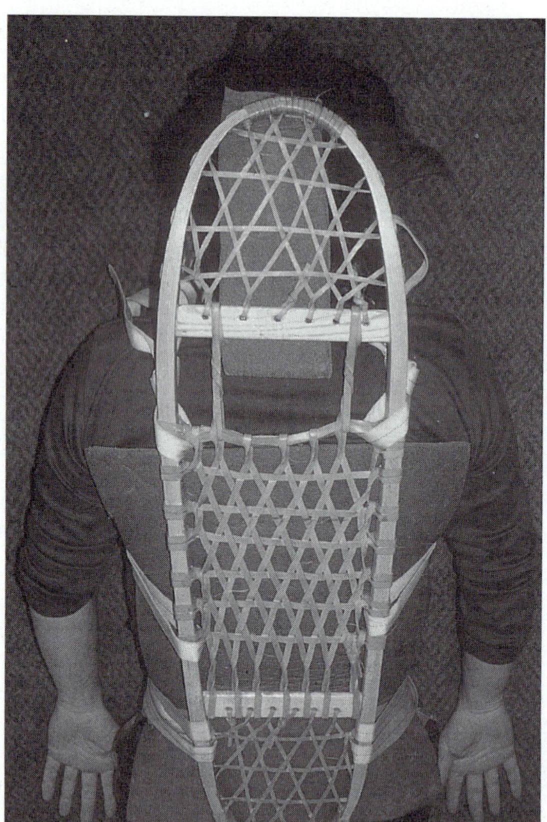

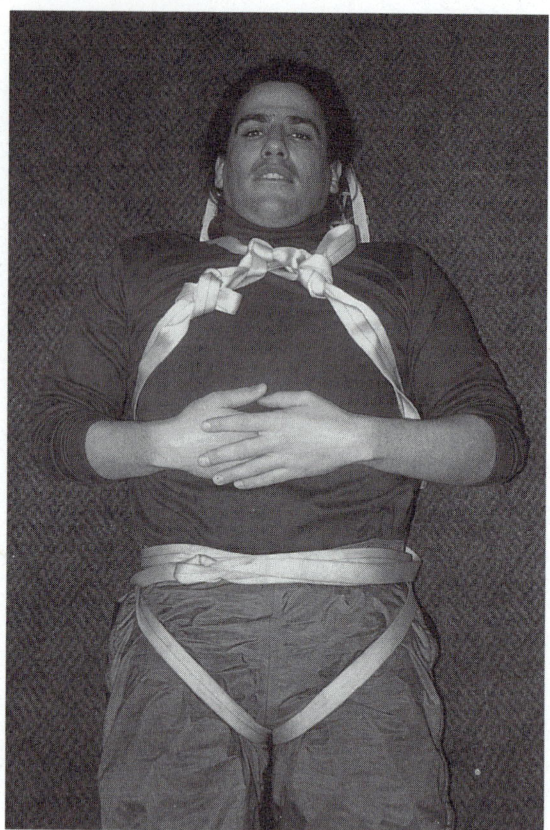

Fig. 18-4 Improvised snowshoe short board. A well-padded snowshoe is prerigged with webbing and attached to the patient as shown. This system can also be used in conjunction with long board systems such as the continuous loop system.

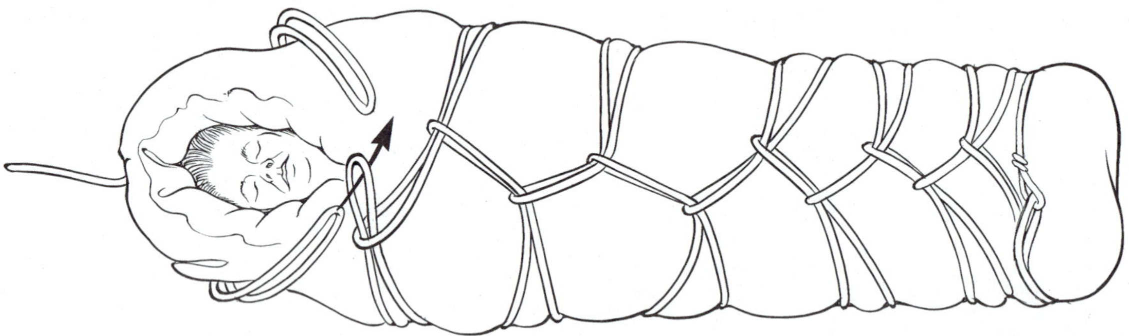

Fig. 18-5 Continuous loop or "mummy" litter made with a climbing rope. Not visible are stiffeners such as skis and poles placed underneath the patient to add structural rigidity. It is important to pad between the stiffeners and the patient (see text).

TRACTION

Why are improvised traction systems so crucial? Traction can be lifesaving in certain situations.[4a] The importance of femoral traction in urban emergency medicine is generally accepted. In the backcountry environment, traction is essential for two fundamental reasons: (1) the general inability to provide intravenous volume expansion and (2) prolonged transport time to definitive care.

The primary purpose of backcountry femoral traction is to *limit blood loss into the thigh.* For a constant surface area, the volume of a sphere is greater than the volume of a cylinder. Pulling (via traction) the thigh compartment back into its natural cylindrical shape limits blood loss into the soft tissue. Although the main objective is to control hemorrhage and prevent shock, enhanced patient comfort and decreased potential for neurovascular damage are important

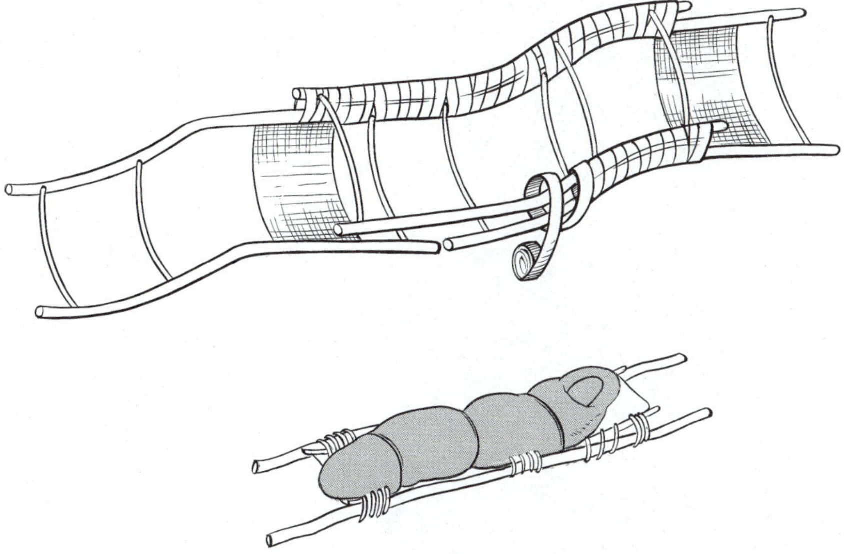

Fig. 18-6 Backpack frame litter.

secondary benefits. Properly applied, improvised femoral traction can save lives in the backcountry, particularly on extended transports where intravenous fluids are not available.

General Principles of Traction

The potential variety of traction designs is unlimited, but five key design principles should be considered when evaluating any femoral traction system:

1. Does the splint provide inline traction? Or, does the splint incorrectly pull the patient's leg off to the side or needlessly plantar flex the patient's ankle?
2. Is the splint comfortable? This one is easy: ask the patient.
3. Does the splint compromise neurologic or vascular function? Constantly check the patient's distal neurovascular function.
4. Is the splint durable, or will it break when subjected to backcountry stresses? As stated earlier, it might help to try the traction design on an uninjured patient and then knock the device around a bit to determine its strength.
5. Is the splint cumbersome? Many reasonable splint designs become so bulky and awkward that litter transport, technical rescue, or helicopter evacuation is impossible. For example, a full-length ski splint is not compatible with evacuation in a small helicopter.

Femoral Traction Systems

Every femoral traction system has six components:

1. Ankle hitch
2. Rigid support
3. Traction mechanism
4. Proximal anchor
5. Method for securing the splint to the leg
6. Additional padding

Ankle Hitch. A variety of techniques are used for anchoring the distal extremity to the splint. Many of these techniques work well, but some are impossible to recall in an emergency. The reader should choose an easy-to-remember technique and practice it.

Single runner system. A long piece of webbing, shoelace, belt, or rope can be looped over itself and one end brought through the middle to create a stirrup. After being rotated away from the person by 180 degrees, the hitch is slipped over the shoe and ankle.

Double runner system. This is a very straightforward technique. Two short webbing loops ("runners") are laid over and under the ankle as shown (Fig. 18-7, *A*). The long loop sides are passed through the short loop on both sides (Fig. 18-7, *B*) and adjusted as needed (Fig. 18-7, *C*). One advantage of this system is that it is infinitely adjustable, which enables the rescuer to center the pull from any direction. As always, proper padding is essential, especially for long transports. The patient's boot can distribute the pressure over the foot and ankle but will obscure visualization and palpation of the foot. A reasonable compromise is to leave the boot on and cut out the toe section for observation.

Patient's boot system. Another efficient system uses the patient's own boot as the hitch. Two holes are cut into the side walls of the boot just above the midsole and in line with the ankle joint. A piece of nylon webbing or a cravat is threaded through and the ankle hitch is complete (Fig. 18-8). Cutting away the toe may be necessary for neurovascular assessment.

Buck's traction. For extended transport, Buck's traction can be improvised using a closed-cell foam pad (Fig. 18-9). The pad is wrapped around the lower leg as shown; a stirrup

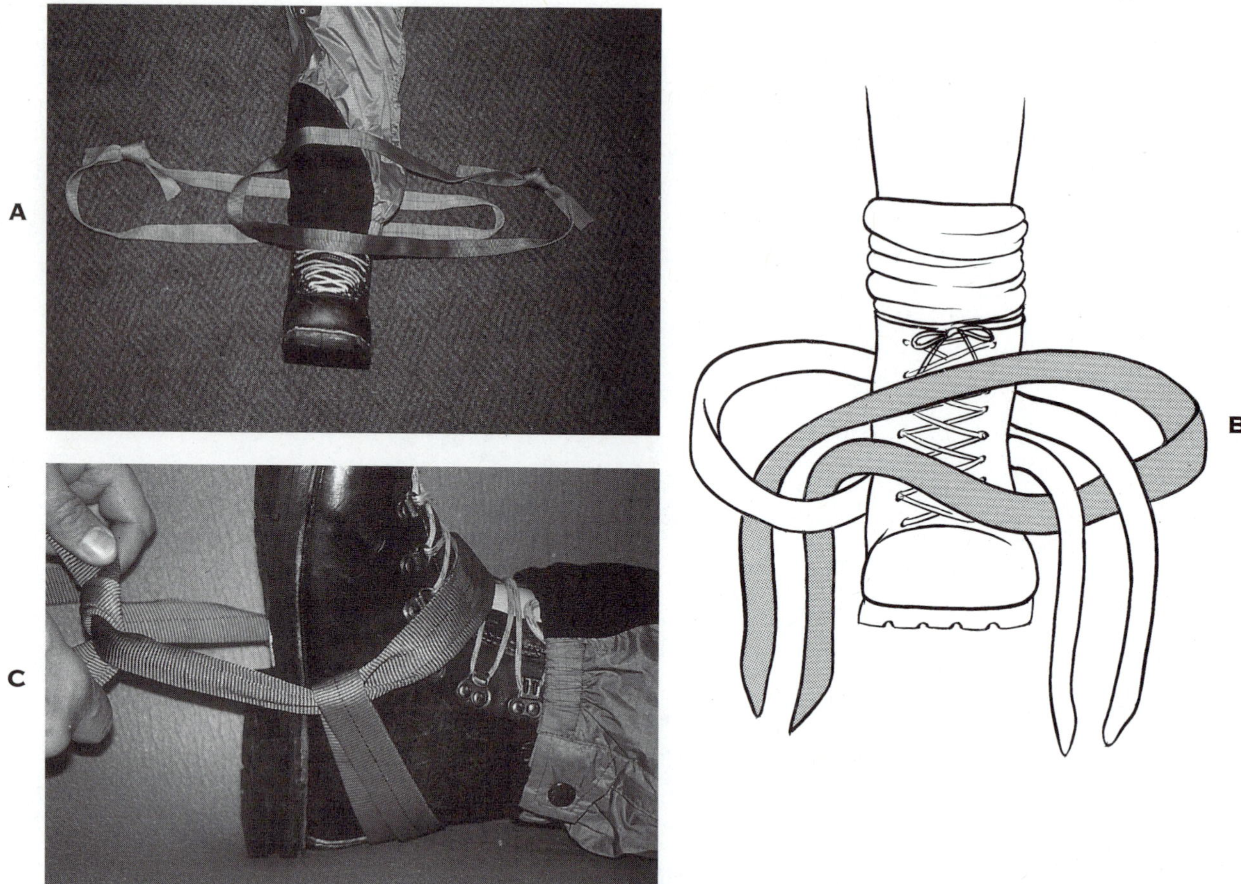

Fig. 18-7 Double runner ankle hitch. **A** and **B,** Two webbing loops (runners) are laid over and under the ankle. **C,** Completed double runner ankle hitch. The beauty of this system is its infinite adjustability. The traction can be easily centered from any angle, ensuring in-line traction.

is then looped below the foot from medial calf to lateral calf. This assembly is then fastened with a second cravat wrapped circumferentially around the calf over the closed-cell foam (duct tape or nylon webbing can be used instead of cravats). This system greatly increases the surface area over which the stirrup is applied and decreases the potential for neurovascular complications and dermal ischemia. In addition, improvised Buck's traction can be used to manage backcountry hip fractures. However, recent literature indicates that this technique has little benefit.[1] If Buck's traction is used for a hip injury, smaller amounts of traction (roughly 5 pounds or less) should be used.

Rigid Support. The rigid support can be fabricated as a unilateral support (similar to the Sager traction splint or Kendrick traction device) or as a bilateral support, such as the Thomas half ring or Hare traction splint. Unilateral supports tend to be easier to apply than bilateral supports. The following are some ideas for rigid support.

Double ski pole or canoe paddle system. This is fashioned like a Thomas half ring, with the interlocked pole straps slipped under the proximal thigh to form the ischial support. Some mountain guides carry a prefabricated drilled ski pole section or aluminum bar that can be used to stabilize the distal end of this system (Figs. 18-10 and 18-11).

Single ski pole or canoe-kayak paddle. In this system a single ski pole or paddle is used either between the legs, which is ideal for bilateral femur fractures, or lateral to the injured leg. The ultimate rigid support is an adjustable telescoping ski pole used laterally. The pole can be adjusted to the appropriate length for each patient, making the splint compact for litter work or helicopter evacuation (Fig. 18-12).

Tent poles. This system employs conventional sectioned tent poles. The poles can be fitted together to create the ideal length rigid support. Because of their flexibility, tent poles must be well secured to the leg to prevent them from flexing out of position. A blanket pin or bent tent stake (Fig. 18-13) can be placed in the end of the pole to provide an anchor for the traction system. Alternately, a Prusik knot (Fig. 18-14) can be used to secure the system to the end of the tent pole (Fig. 18-15).

Miscellaneous. Any suitable object, such as a canoe or kayak paddle (Fig. 18-15), two ice axes taped together at the handles, or a straight branch, can be used to make a rigid support. Although skis immediately come to mind as suitable rigid components, they are too cumbersome to work ef-

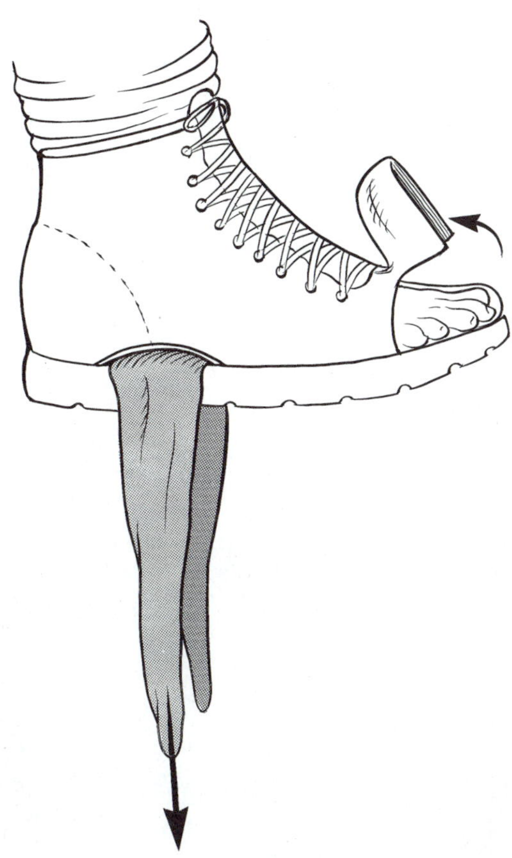

Fig. 18-8 Traction using cut boot and cravat.

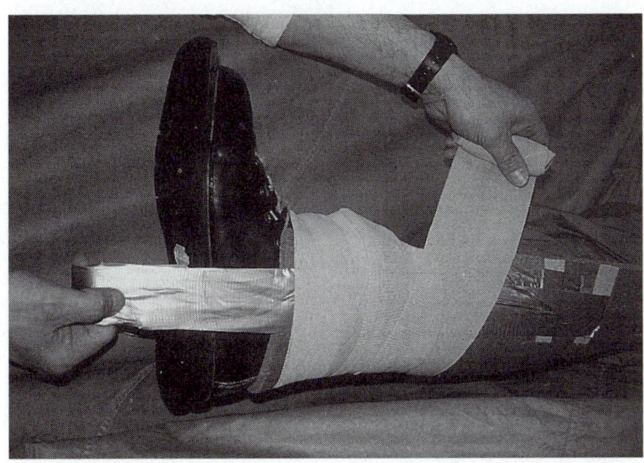

Fig. 18-9 Buck's traction. Duct tape stirrups are added to a small foam pad that is wrapped around the leg. The entire unit is wrapped with an Ace bandage. This system helps distribute the force of the traction over a large surface area.

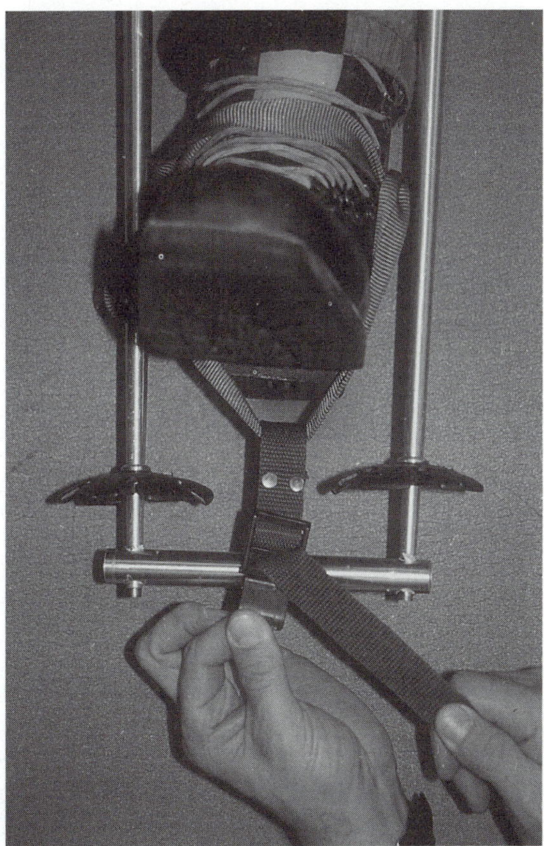

Fig. 18-10 Double ski pole system with prefabricated cross-bar and webbing belt traction. A prefabricated drilled ski section is used to attach the ends of two ski poles. Traction is applied with a webbing belt and sliding buckle.

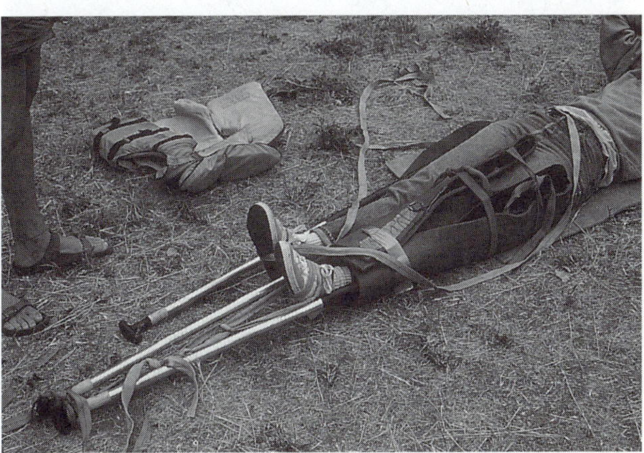

Fig. 18-11 Two canoe paddles with Ensolite padding and ankle stirrup fashioned for traction splinting of a femur fracture.

fectively. Because of their length, skis may extend far beyond the patient's feet or require placement into the axillae, which is unnecessary and inhibits the patient's mobility (for example, sitting up during transport). Premanufactured canvas pockets, available from the National Ski Patrol System, provide a ski tip and tail attachment grommet for use with the ski system.

Traction Mechanism. The first modern popularized improvised traction mechanism was the Boy Scout–style Spanish windlass. Although these systems work and look good in the movies, they can be awkward to apply and are often not durable. The windlass can unspin if it is inadvertently jarred and can apply rotational forces to the leg.

The amount of traction required is primarily a function

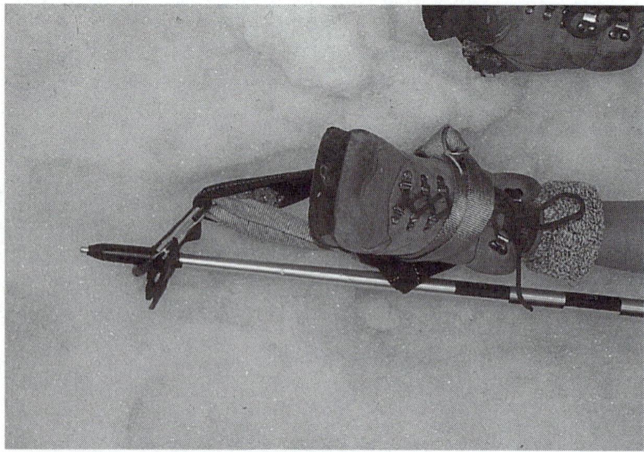

Fig. 18-12 Single ski pole system. An adjustable telescoping ski pole is used as the rigid support. A stirrup is attached to a carabiner placed over the end of the pole. Traction is applied by elongating the ski pole while another rescuer provides manual traction on the patient's leg. Additional padding and securing follow (not shown).

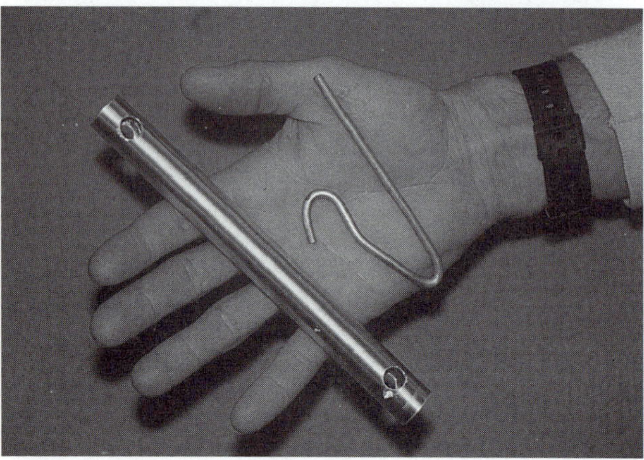

Fig. 18-13 Prefabricated drilled tent pole section and bent tent stake. The ski pole section is used to stabilize the end of a double ski pole traction system. This can be improvised on site if necessary. The bent tent stake serves as a distal traction anchor if a tent pole is used as the rigid support.

of patient comfort. A general rule is to use 10% of body weight or about 10 to 15 pounds for the average patient. After the traction is applied, rescuers should always recheck distal neurovascular function (circulation, sensation, movement).

Cam lock or Fastex-like slider. This simple, effective system uses straps that have a Fastex-like slider. Such straps are often used as waist belts or to hold items to packs. Alternately, a cam lock with nylon webbing can be used. The belt is attached to the distal portion of the rigid support and then to the ankle hitch. Traction is easily applied by cinching the nylon webbing.

Trucker's hitch. A windlass can be easily fashioned using small diameter line (parachute cord) and a standard

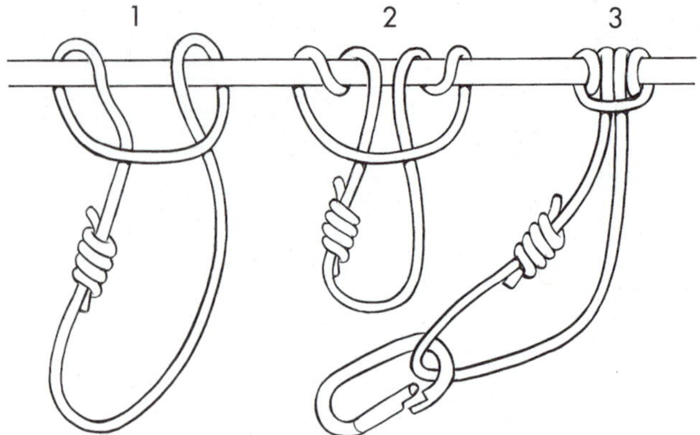

Fig. 18-14 A Prusik knot made from a small diameter cord is used as an adjustable distal traction anchor.

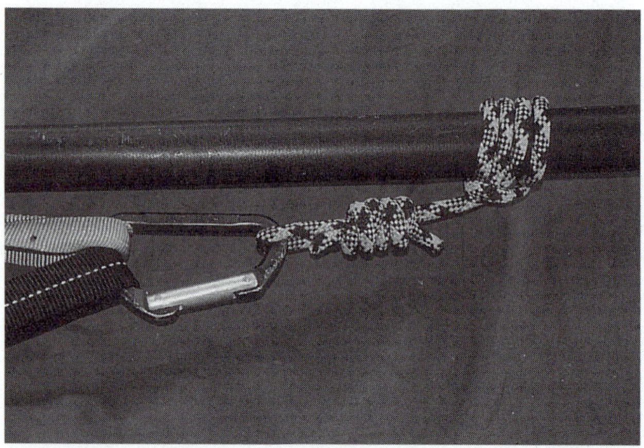

Fig. 18-15 Two Prusik wraps are shown. Three or four wraps provide additional friction and security. If the Prusik knot slips, it can be easily taped in place.

trucker's hitch for additional mechanical advantage (Fig. 18-16).

Prusik knot. Almost any system can be rigged with a Prusik knot (see Fig. 18-14). Prusiks are ideal for providing traction from rigid supports with few tie-on points (such as a canoe paddle shaft or a tent pole). The Prusik knot can be used to apply the traction (by sliding the knot distally) or simply as an attachment point for one of the traction mechanisms already mentioned.

Litter traction. If no rigid support is available and a rigid litter such as a Stokes is being used, traction can be applied from the rigid bar at the foot end of the litter. If this system is used, the patient must be immobilized on the litter with adequate countertraction, such as inguinal straps.

Proximal Anchor. The simplest proximal anchor uses a single ischial strap, which can be made from a piece of climbing webbing or a prefabricated strap, belt, or cam lock (Fig. 18-17). A cloth cravat can be used in a pinch. On the river a life jacket can be used (Fig. 18-18). When climbing, a climbing harness is ideal. The preferred system is a proxi-

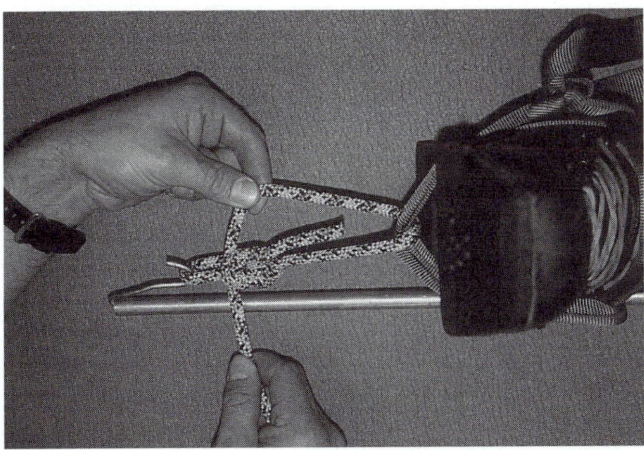

Fig. 18-16 Tent pole traction with trucker's hitch. A bent tent stake is placed into the end of the tent pole as the distal traction anchor. A simple trucker's hitch is used to provide traction.

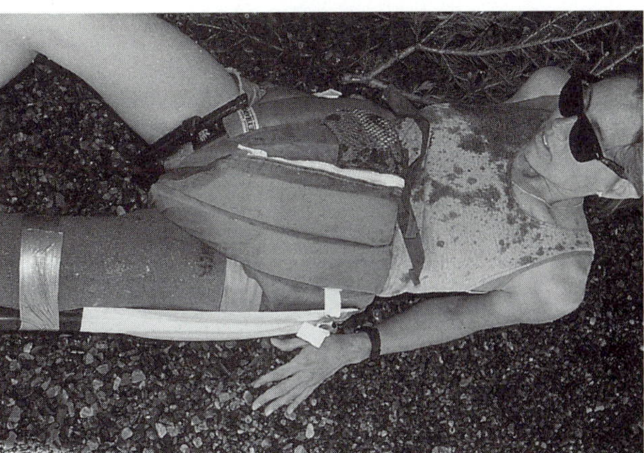

Fig. 18-18 Life jacket proximal anchor. An inverted life jacket worn like a diaper forms a well-padded proximal anchor. A kayak paddle is rigged to the life jacket's side adjustment strap.

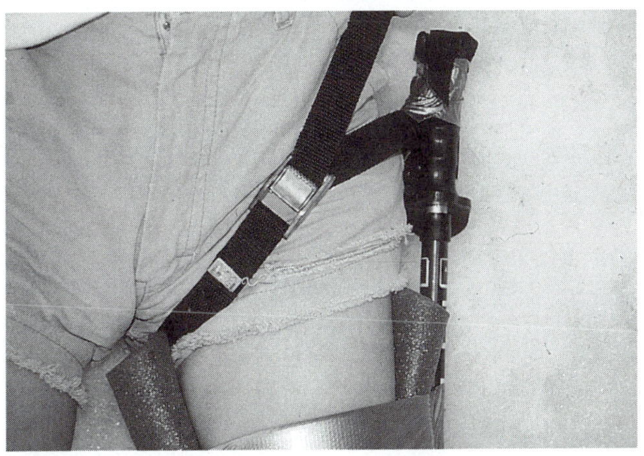

Fig. 18-17 Proximal anchor using cam lock belt. The belt is applied as shown. A ski pole is used laterally as the rigid support. Duct tape is useful for securing components. Padding is helpful but is not always necessary if the patient is wearing pants.

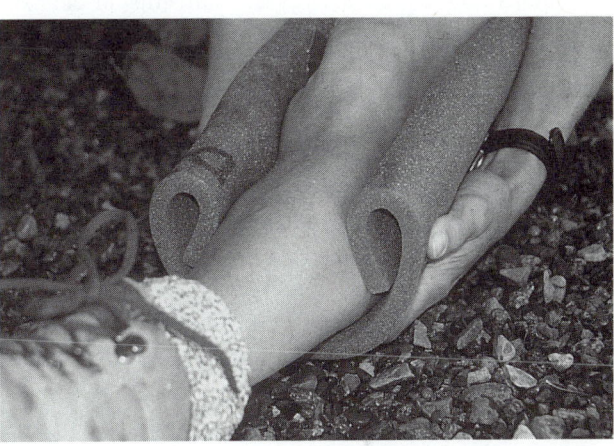

Fig. 18-19 Folding Ensolite padding often provides better visualization of the extremity than does a circumferential wrap.

mal ischial strap, but a padded medial support (analogous to a Sager splint) can also be used. When a medial traction system (Sager analog) is used, the inguinal area should be generously padded. A folded SAM splint attached to the proximal end of the rigid support works well.

Securing and Padding. All potential pressure points should be checked to ensure they are adequately padded. An excellent padding system can be made by first covering the upper and lower leg with a folded length of Ensolite (Fig. 18-19). This is preferred over a circumferential wrap because the folded system allows for visualization of the extremity. The patient will be more comfortable if femoral traction is applied with the knee in slight flexion (padding placed beneath the knee during transport). The splint must be secured firmly to the leg. Almost any straplike object will work, but a 4- to 6-inch Ace bandage wrapped circumferentially will provide a comfortable and secure union. Finally, the ankles or feet should be strapped or tied together to give the system additional stability. Tying the ankles together also prevents the injured leg from excess external rotation and jarring during transport.

EXTREMITY SPLINTS

All fractures should be splinted before the patient is moved unless the patient's life is in immediate danger. In general, the splint should incorporate the joints above and below the fracture. If possible, the splint should be fashioned on the uninjured extremity and then transferred to the injured one.

On ski trips, skis and poles can be used as improvised splints. On white-water trips, canoe and kayak paddles can be used in a similar manner. Airbags used as flotation for kayaks and canoes can be converted into pneumatic splints for arm and ankle injuries. The minicell or ethafoam pillars found in most kayaks can be removed and carved into pieces to provide upper and lower extremity splints. A life jacket can be molded into a cylinder splint for knee immobilization or into a pillow splint for the ankle.

The flexible aluminum stays found in internal frame packs can be molded into upper extremity splints. Other improvised splinting material includes sticks or tree limbs, rolled-up magazines, books or newspapers, ice axes, tent poles, and dirt-filled garbage bags or fanny packs.

Ideally a splint should immobilize the fractured bone in a functional position. In general, "functional position" means that the legs should be straight or slightly bent at the knee, the ankle and elbow bent at 90 degrees, the wrists straight, and the fingers flexed in a curve as if the person were attempting to hold a can of soda or a baseball.

Splints can be secured in place with strips of clothing, belts, pieces of rope or webbing, pack straps, Ace wraps, or gauze bandages.

TRIANGULAR BANDAGE MYTH

One of the most ubiquitous components of first aid kits and one of the easiest to replace through improvisation is the triangular bandage. The need to carry this bulky item, which is commonly used to construct a sling and swath bandage for shoulder and arm immobilization, can be eliminated by carrying two or three safety pins. Pinning the shirt sleeve of the injured arm to the chest portion of the shirt effectively immobilizes the extremity against the body (Fig. 18-20, *B*).

If the patient is wearing a short-sleeved shirt, the bottom of the shirt can be folded up and over the arm to create a pouch. This can be pinned to the sleeve and chest section of the shirt to secure the arm (Fig. 18-20, *A*).

Triangular bandages are also used for securing splints and constructing pressure wraps. Common items such as socks, shirts, belts, pack straps, webbing, shoe laces, fanny packs, and underwear can easily be substituted.

Improvised Wound Management

The same principles that govern wound management in the emergency department also apply in the wilderness. The main problem faced in the wilderness is access to adequate supplies. The decision to close a wound primarily or pack it open should take into account the mechanism of injury, the age of the wound, the site of the wound, the degree of contamination, and the ability to effectively clean the wound.

WOUND IRRIGATION

The primary determinants of infection are bacterial counts and amount of devitalized tissue remaining in the wound.[12] Ridding a wound of bacteria and other particulate matter requires more than soaking and gentle washing with a disinfectant.[14] Irrigating the wound with a forceful stream is the most effective method of reducing bacterial counts and removing debris and contaminants.[16,21] The cleansing capacity of the stream depends on the hydraulic pressure

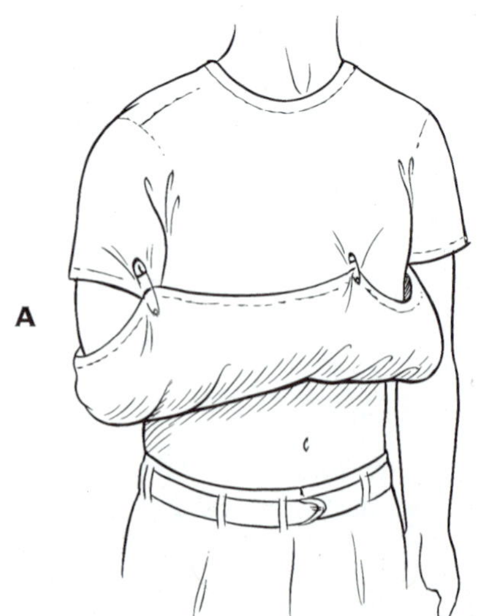

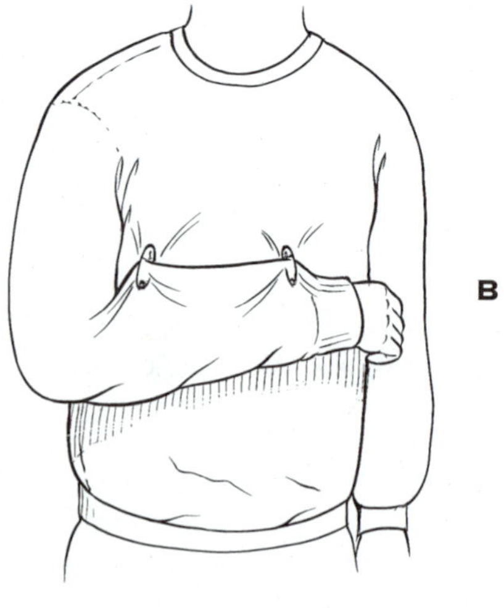

Fig. 18-20 Techniques for pinning the arm to the shirt as an improvised sling. **A,** With a short-sleeved shirt the bottom of the shirt is folded up over the injured arm and secured to the sleeve and upper shirt. **B,** With a long-sleeved shirt or jacket the sleeved arm is simply pinned to the chest portion of the garment.

under which the fluid is delivered.[11,20] Irrigation is best accomplished by attaching an 18- or 19-gauge catheter to a 35 cc syringe or a 22-gauge needle to a 12 cc syringe. This creates hydraulic pressure in the range of 7 to 8 lb/in^2 and 13 lb/in^2, respectively.[11,18,20] The solution is directed into the wound from a distance of 1 to 2 inches at an angle perpendicular to the wound surface and as close to the wound as possible. The amount of irrigation fluid will vary with the size and contamination of the wound, but should average no less than 250 ml.[11] Remember: "The solution to pollution is dilution."

There is a lack of consensus on which irrigation solution is the best for open wounds. Those who subscribe to the dogma that nothing should enter a wound that could not be instilled safely into the eye believe that normal saline is the best solution.[6,13] In a study of 531 patients with traumatic wounds, there was no significant variation in infection rates among sutured wounds irrigated with normal saline, 1% povidone-iodine, or pluronic F-68 (Shur-Clens).[8]

Tap water was recently found to be as effective for irrigating wounds as sterile saline. In fact, the infection rate was significantly lower after irrigation with tap water, and no infections resulted from the bacteria cultured from the tap water.[1]

Improvised wound irrigation requires only a puncturable container to hold the water, such as a sandwich or garbage bag, and a safety pin or 18-gauge needle (see Box 18-1).

WOUND CLOSURE

Before a wound is closed, all foreign material and grossly devitalized tissue should be removed. Debridement can be done with scissors, a knife, or any other sharp object. Wounds can be closed with sutures, staples, tape, pins, or glue. Although suturing is still the most widely used technique, stapling and gluing are ideal methods for closing wounds in the wilderness.

Clinical studies of the use of staples to close traumatic lacerations have found various advantages of stapling over suturing: wound tensile strength is greater, there is less inflammation, the time required for closure is shorter, and fewer instruments are needed.[19] Most important, the cosmetic outcome is not compromised.[10] Staplers are lightweight, presterilized, and easy to use.

WOUND TAPING

Skin tapes are useful for shallow, nongaping wounds and have several advantages over suturing, including reduced need for anesthesia, ease of application, decreased incidence of wound infection, and availability. Any strong tape can be used to improvise skin tape strips, but duct tape works especially well (see Box 18-2). Puncturing holes in the tape before application helps to prevent exudate from building up under the tape.

Although benzoin is usually applied to the skin before the tape to augment adhesion, cyanoacrylate glue (Crazy Glue) works better. If benzoin is available, the two can be used in combination.

Wound taping does not work well over joints or on hairy skin surfaces unless the hair is first removed. Scalp lacerations can sometimes be closed by tying opposing strands of hair to approximate the wound edges.

BOX 18-1
RECOMMENDED TECHNIQUE FOR WOUND IRRIGATION

1. Fill a sandwich or garbage bag with water.
2. Disinfect the water with iodine tablets, iodine solution, or povidone-iodine or by boiling it.
3. Normal saline can be made by adding 2 teaspoons of salt (9 g) per liter of water.
4. Seal the bag.
5. Puncture the bottom of the bag with an 18-gauge needle, safety pin, fork prong, or knife tip.
6. Squeeze the top of the bag forcefully while holding it just above the wound, directing the stream into the wound.
7. Use caution to ensure that none of the irrigation fluid splashes into your eyes.

BOX 18-2
WOUND TAPING TECHNIQUE

1. Obtain hemostasis and dry the wound edges.
2. Apply benzoin or cyanoacrylate glue to the skin adjacent to the wound. Benzoin should be left to dry until it becomes tacky, but the tape should be applied to the glue while the glue is still wet.
3. Tape should be cut to quarter-inch or half-inch widths, depending on the size of the laceration, and to a length that allows for 2 to 3 cm of overlap on each side of the wound.
4. Secure one half of the tape to one side of the wound. Oppose the opposite wound edge with a finger while the tape is secured to the other side.
5. Wound tapes should have gaps of 2 to 3 mm between them to allow for serous drainage.
6. Cross-stays of tape can be placed perpendicular over the tape ends to prevent them from peeling off.
7. Additional glue can be applied to the tape edges every 24 hours to reinforce adhesion.

GLUING

Although Histoacryl (butyl-2-cyanoacrylate) tissue adhesive is frequently used in Europe and Canada for sutureless skin closure,[24] it has not yet been approved by the Food and Drug Administration for use in the United States. When applied to the skin surface, Histoacryl provides strong tissue support and peels off in 4 to 5 days without leaving evidence of its presence.[23] It provides a faster and less painful method for closing lacerations than does suturing and has yielded similar cosmetic results in children with facial lacerations.[17] Histoacryl evokes a mild acute inflammatory reaction with no tissue necrosis.[23]

Histoacryl has also been used successfully to treat superficial painful fissures of the fingertips ("polar hands"), which commonly occur in cold climates and at high elevations.[2]

Crazy Glue or Super Glue (ethyl-2-cyanoacrylate) is a shorter chain cyanoacrylate derivative that is readily available in the United States. Compared with Histoacryl, it releases more heat during polymerization and produces a severe acute inflammatory reaction, with tissue necrosis and a chronic foreign body giant cell response.[23] Its use for routine wound closure cannot be recommended at this time.

RING REMOVAL

Rings should be removed quickly from injured fingers and after any trauma to the hands. Progressive swelling may cause rings to act as tourniquets. If a ring cannot be removed with soap or lubricating jelly, the string wrap technique can be employed. A 20-inch length of fine string, dental floss, umbilical tape, or thick suture is passed between the ring and the finger. The string is pulled so that most of it is on the distal side of the digit and then is wrapped around the swollen finger from proximal to distal. The wrapping should begin next to the ring and continue past the proximal interphalangeal joint. Successive loops of the wrap should be placed close enough together to prevent any swollen skin from bulging between the strands. The ring is removed by unwinding the proximal end of the string and forcing the ring over the distal string. If the string is not long enough, the technique may require repeated wraps (Fig. 18-21).

BOX 18-3
TECHNIQUE FOR GLUING LACERATIONS

1. Oppose the wound edges manually to a desirable position.
2. Apply a thin film of tissue adhesive to the opposed skin edges.
3. Hold the wound edges together for 60 seconds, until full polymerization has taken place.
4. Wounds under tension should be reinforced with Steri-Strips or improvised tape strips glued to the skin.

Improvisational Toolkit

Some people, convinced they could whittle a Swan-Ganz catheter from a tree branch if they had to, enter the wilderness with nothing more than a Swiss Army knife. However, a little foresight and preparation make improvisation much easier. Efficiency translates into speedy preparation and assembly, which ultimately results in better patient care. The following section lists items that will make improvisation easier in the field.

KNIFE

The knife can be a fairly simple model, but it should have an awl for drilling holes into skis, poles, sticks, and so

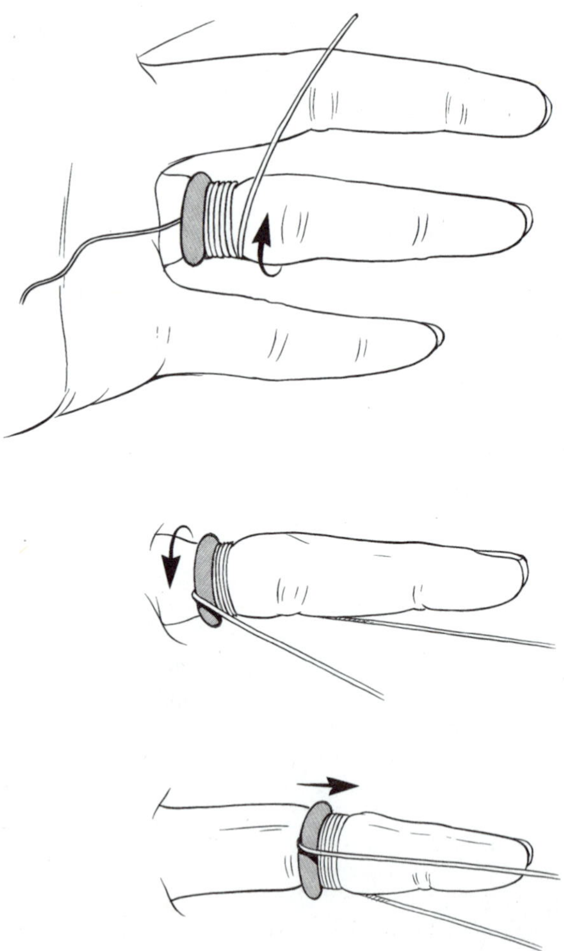

Fig. 18-21 String technique for removing a ring from a swollen finger.

on. The awl on a Swiss Army knife works quite well for this purpose. This allows the rescuer to create well-fitted components during improvisation (for example, a drilled cross-bar attached to drilled ski tips for an improvised rescue toboggan).

TAPE

Some form of strong, sticky, waterproof tape should be carried. (This is one item that *cannot* be improvised.) Either cloth adhesive tape (already in the medical kit) or duct tape should be used. Duct tape is ideal for almost all tasks. It can even be used on skin when needed (for example, to close wounds, treat blisters, or tape an ankle). Some persons may be sensitive to the adhesive. Fiberglass strapping tape has greater tensile strength and is ideal for joining rigid components, such as taping two ice axes together. However, it is less sticky than duct tape and not as useful for patching torn items. Extra tape can be carried by wrapping lengths of it around pieces of gear.

PLASTIC CABLE TIES

Lightweight cable ties can be used to bind almost anything together instantaneously (for example, binding pack frames together for improvised litters or ski poles together for improvised carriers). They are also perfect for repairing many items in the backcountry.

PARACHUTE CORD

Parachute cord has hundreds of uses in the backcountry. It can be used for trucker's hitch traction and for tying complex splints together. Parachute cord is light, and a good supply should be carried.

SAFETY PINS

Safety pins have a variety of uses (see Box 18-4).

WIRE

Braided picture-hanging wire works well because it is supple and ties like line. Its strength makes it superior for repairing and improvising components under an extreme load, such as fabricating improvised rescue sleds or repairing broken or detached ski bindings.

BOLTS AND WING NUTS

Bolts and wing nuts make the job of constructing an improvised rescue sled much easier (see section on rescue sleds). Bolts will be useful only if holes can be created to put them through. Therefore a knife with an awl is needed for drilling holes through skis, poles, and so on.

PREFABRICATED CROSS-BAR

The prefab cross-bar can be used for double ski pole traction splint systems. A cross-bar can be easily fabricated in the field from a branch or short section of the patient's ski pole, but carrying a prefabricated device such as a 6-inch predrilled ski pole section saves time (Fig. 18-10).

ENSOLITE (CLOSED-CELL FOAM) PADS

Since the introduction of Therm-a-Rest-type inflatable pads, closed-cell foam has become increasingly scarce; however, closed-cell foam (Ensolite) is still the ultimate padding for almost any improvised splint or rescue device. The uses for closed-cell foam are virtually unlimited. Even die-hard Therm-a-Rest fans should carry a small amount of closed-cell foam, which doubles as a comfortable seat

BOX 18-4

USES OF A SAFETY PIN

- Using two safety pins to pin the anterior aspect of the tongue to the lower lip in order to establish an airway in an unconscious patient whose airway is obstructed
- Replacing the lost screw in a pair of eyeglasses to prevent the lens from falling out
- Improvising glasses: Draw two circles in a piece of duct tape where your eyes would fit. Use the pin to make holes in the circles, then tape this to your face. The pinholes will partially correct myopic vision and protect the eyes from ultraviolet radiation. Slits can also be used for improvised sunglasses.
- Neurosensory skin testing
- Puncturing plastic bags for irrigation of wounds
- Removing embedded foreign bodies from the skin
- Draining an abscess or blister
- Relieving a subungual hematoma
- As a fishhook
- As a finger splint (mallet finger)
- As a sewing needle, using dental floss as thread
- Holding gaping wounds together
- Replacing a broken clothing zipper
- Holding gloves or mittens to a coat sleeve
- Unclogging jets in a camping stove
- Pinning triage notes to multiple victims
- Removing a corneal foreign body (with ophthalmic anesthetic)
- In a sling and swath for shoulder or arm injuries
- To fix a ski binding
- To extract the clot from a thrombosed hemorrhoid
- To pin a strap or shirt tightly around the chest for rib fracture support
- Tick removal

cushion and is lightweight. Furthermore, unlike inflatable pads, Ensolite will not puncture and deflate.

Therm-a-Rest pads also have their place. They can be used as padding for many long bone splints and immobilizers (one example is an improvised universal knee immobilizer). An inflatable pad can also be used to cushion pelvic fractures. First the deflated pad should be wrapped around the pelvis. Then the pad is secured with tape and inflated, creating an improvised substitute for military antishock trousers (MAST device).

FLUORESCENT SURVEYOR'S TAPE

Surveyor's tape can be used much like Hansel and Gretel's bread crumbs to help relocate a route into or out of a rescue scene. It is also ideal for marking shelters in deep snow and can serve as a wind sock during helicopter operations on improvised landing zones. Surveyor's tape is not biodegradable, so it should always be removed from the site after the rescue is completed.

SPACE BLANKET OR LIGHTWEIGHT TARP

For improvising hasty shelters in times of emergency, some form of tarp is essential. In the snow a slit trench shelter can be built in a matter of minutes using a tarp. Otherwise, the complex and time-consuming construction of improvised structures such as snow caves, igloos, or tree branch shelters might be necessary. Typically, little time or help is available for this task during emergencies. In addition, tarps are essential for "hypothermia wraps" when managing injured patients in cold or wet conditions. The only advantage of a space blanket over other tarps is its small size, which means there is a good chance it was packed for the trip.

SAM SPLINT

Introduced in 1985, the SAM splint (Fig. 18-22) has largely filled the niche formerly occupied by military-style ladder splints and wire mesh splints. The SAM splint is exceptionally versatile. It weighs approximately 4½ ounces and rolls up into a space approximately the size of a Kerlix bandage. It is made of a thin sheet of malleable aluminum sandwiched between two thin layers of closed cell foam. The splint initially has no rigidity, but after structural U-shaped bends are placed along the axis of the splint, it becomes quite rigid.

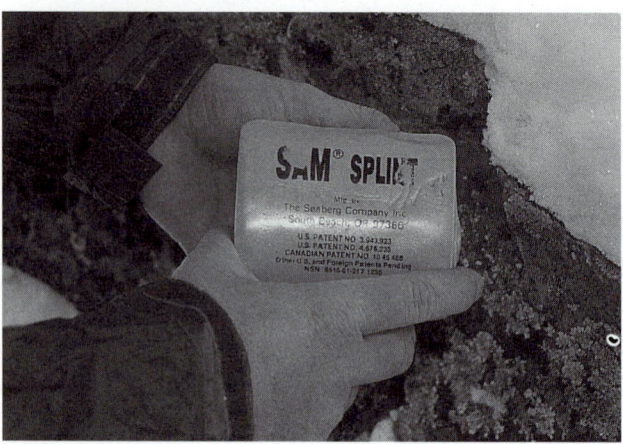

Fig. 18-22 The SAM splint consists of a thin sheet of malleable aluminum sandwiched between two thin layers of foam. It can be easily molded to injured extremities and becomes rigid after U-shaped bends are placed into the aluminum.

Improvised Eyeglasses

Exposure of unprotected eyes to ultraviolet radiation at high altitudes may result in photokeratitis (snow blindness). Symptoms are delayed, and the victim is often unaware that an eye injury is developing. When sunglasses are lost at 14,000 feet in the snow, photokeratitis can develop in a mere 20 minutes. Improvised sunglasses can be fashioned from duct tape, cardboard, or other light-impermeable material that can be cut. Cardboard glasses with narrow eye slits can be taped over the eyes for protection.

Slits can also be cut into a piece of duct tape that has been folded over on itself with the sticky sides opposing. After a triangular wedge is removed for the nose, another piece of tape can be applied to secure the glasses to the head.

Pinhole tape glasses can improve vision in a myopic person whose corrective lenses have been lost. With myopia, parallel light rays from distant objects focus in front of the retina. The pinhole directs entering light to the center of the cornea, where refraction (bending of the light) is unnecessary. Light remains in focus regardless of the refractive error of the eye (Fig. 18-23). Pinhole glasses decrease both illumination and the field of vision. Therefore a piece of duct tape or cardboard should be punctured repeatedly with a safety pin, needle, fork, or other sharp object until enough light can enter to focus on distant objects, and the device should be secured to the face.

Improvised Transport

CARRIERS

Two-Hand Seat*

Two carriers stand side by side. Each carrier grasps the other carrier's wrists with opposite hands (for example, right to left). The victim sits on the rescuers' joined forearms. The carriers each maintain one free hand to place behind the

*Both the two-hand seat and the four-hand seat are useful only for very short carries over gentle terrain.

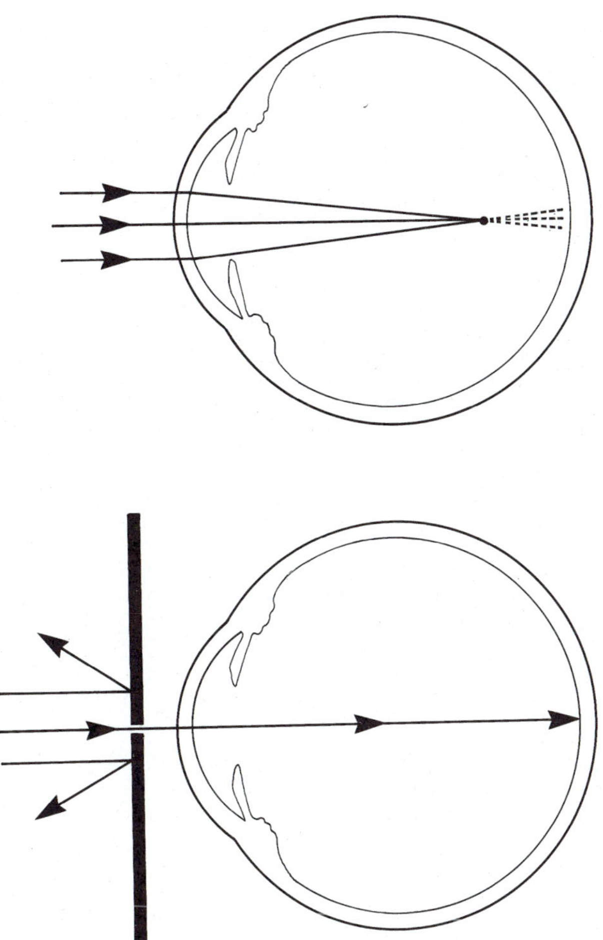

Fig. 18-23 Pinhole in cardboard to improve vision in person with myopia.

back of the victim for support (support hands can be joined). This system places great stress on the carriers' forearms and wrists.

Four-Hand Seat

Two carriers stand side by side. Each carrier grasps his own right forearm with his left hand, palms facing down. Each carrier then grasps the forearm of the other with his free hand to form a square "forearm" seat. With the forearm seat, the patient must support himself with a hand around the rescuers' backs.

Ski Pole or Ice Ax Carry

Two carriers with backpacks stand side by side with four ski poles or joined ice ax shafts resting between them and the base of the pack straps (Fig. 18-24). The ski poles or ice ax shafts can be joined with cable ties, adhesive tape, duct tape, wire, or cord. Because the rescuers must walk side by side, this technique requires wide open, gentle terrain. The victim sits on the padded poles or shaft with his arms over the carriers' shoulders.

Split-Coil Seat ("Tragsitz")

The split-coil seat transport uses a coiled climbing rope to join the rescuer and victim together in a piggy-back fashion (Fig. 18-25). The patient must be able to support himself to avoid falling back, or must be tied in.

Two-Rescuer Split-Coil Seat

The two-rescuer split-coil seat is essentially the same as the split-coil Tragsitz transport, except that two rescuers split the coil over their shoulders. The patient sits on the low point of the rope between the rescuers (Fig. 18-26). Each rescuer maintains a free hand to help support the patient.

Backpack Carry

A large backpack is modified by cutting leg holes at the base. The victim sits in it like a baby carrier.

Nylon Webbing Carry

Nylon webbing can be used to attach the victim to the rescuer like a backpack (Fig. 18-27). At least 15 to 20 feet of nylon webbing is needed to construct this transport. The center of the webbing is placed behind the patient and brought forward under his armpits. The webbing is then crossed and brought over the rescuer's shoulders, then down around the patient's thighs. The webbing is finally brought forward and tied around the rescuer's waist. Additional padding is needed for this system, especially around the posterior thighs of the patient.

LITTERS (NONRIGID)

Many nonrigid litter systems have been developed over the years. These systems are best suited for transporting noncritically injured patients over moderate terrain. They should *never* be used for trauma patients with potential spinal injuries.

Blanket Litter

A simple nonrigid litter can be fabricated from two rigid poles, branches, or skis and a large blanket or tarp. The blanket or tarp is wrapped around the skis or poles as many times as possible and the poles are carried. The blanket or tarp should not be simply draped over the poles. For easier carrying, the poles can be rigged to the base of backpacks. Large external frame packs work best, but internal frame packs can be rigged to do the job. Alternatively, a padded harness to support the litter can be made from a single piece of webbing, in a design similar to a nylon webbing carry.

Tree Pole Litter

The tree pole litter is similar to the blanket litter described previously. In the tree pole litter, instead of a blanket or a tarp, the side poles are laced together with webbing or rope and then padded. Again, the poles may be fitted through pack frames to aid carrying. To give this litter more

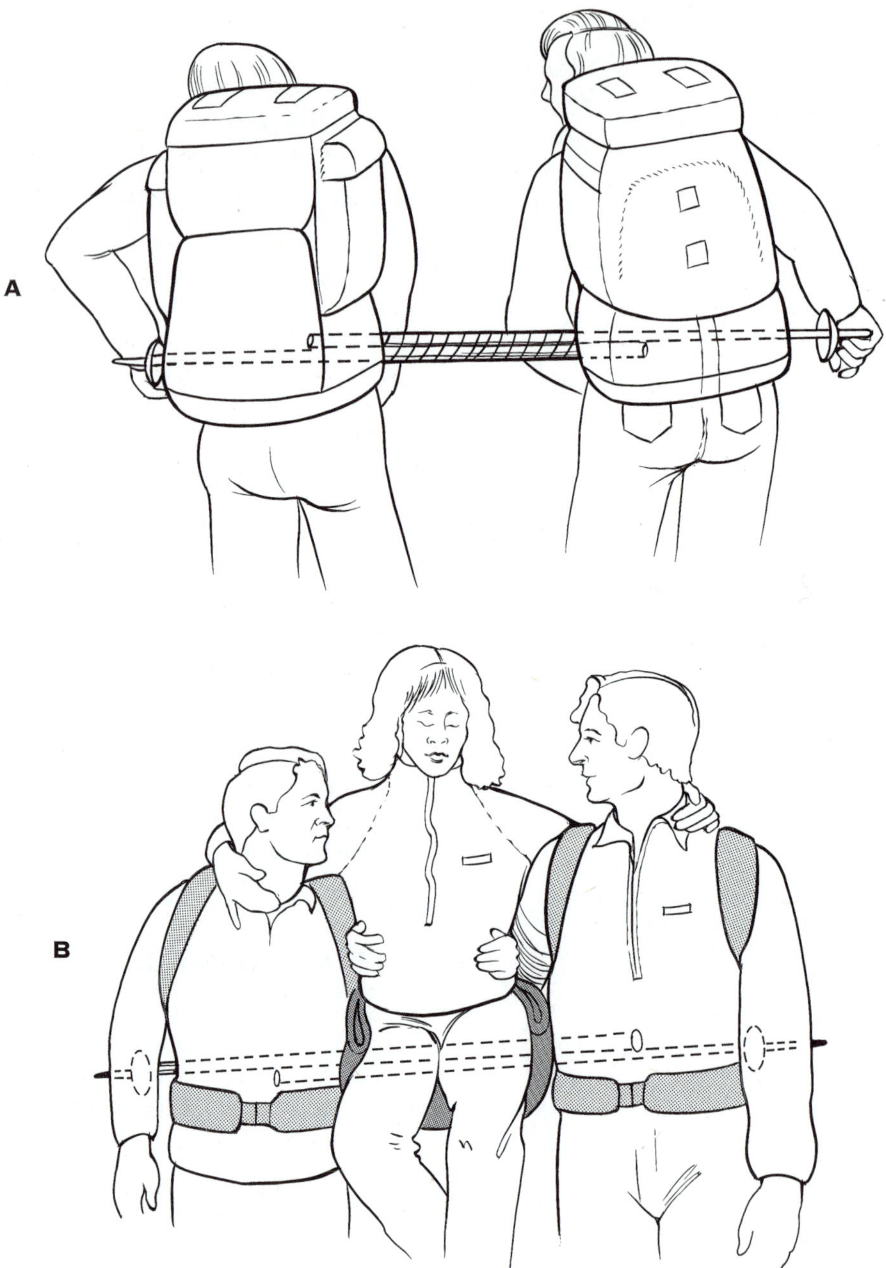

Fig. 18-24 Ski pole seat. **A,** Ski poles are anchored by the packs. **B,** The victim is supported by the rescuers.

stability and to add tension to the lacing, the rescuer should fabricate a rectangle with rigid cross-bars at both ends before lacing.

Parka Litter

Two or more parkas can be used to form a litter (Fig. 18-28). Skis or branches are slipped through the sleeves of heavy parkas, and the parkas are zipped shut with the sleeves inside. (Ski edges should be taped first to prevent them from tearing through the parkas.)

Internal Frame Pack Litter

The internal frame pack litter is constructed from two to three full-size internal frame backpacks, which must have lateral compression straps (day packs are suboptimal). Slide poles or skis through the compression straps; the packs then act as a support surface for the victim.

Life Jacket Litter

Life jackets can be placed over paddles or oars to create a makeshift nonrigid litter.

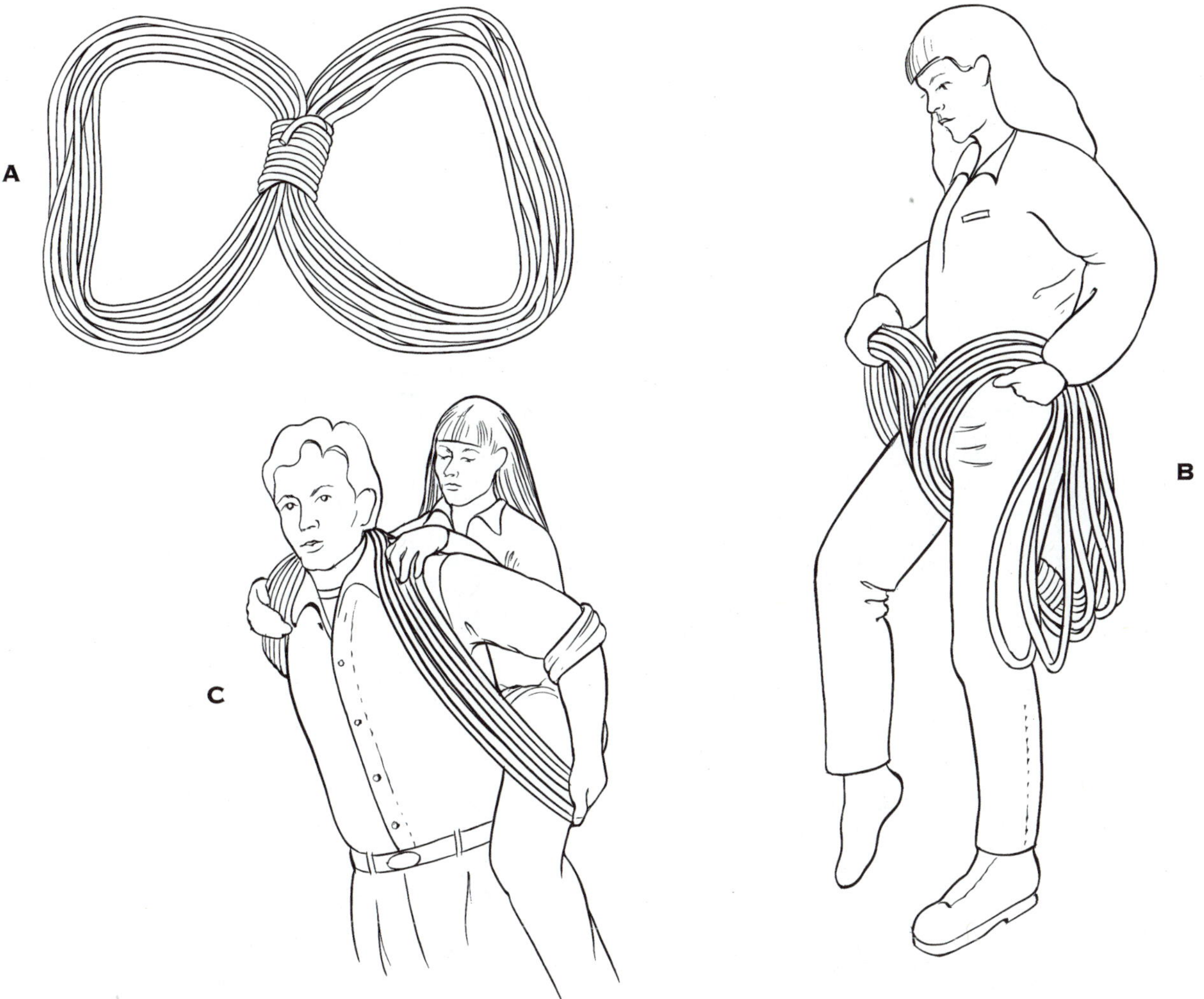

Fig. 18-25 Split-coil seat. **A,** Rope coil is split. **B,** Victim climbs through rope. **C,** Rescuer hoists the sitting victim.

Rope Litter

On mountaineering trips the classic rope litter can be used, but this system offers little back support and should never be used for victims with suspected spine injuries. The rope is uncoiled and flaked onto the ground with 16 180-degree bends (eight on each side of the rope center). The rope bends should approximate the size of the finished litter. The free rope ends are then used to clove hitch off each bend (leaving 2 inches of bend to the outside of each clove hitch). The leftover rope is threaded through the loops at the outside of each clove hitch. This gives the rescuers a continuous handhold and protects the bends from slipping through the clove hitches. The rope ends are then tied off (Fig. 18-29). The litter is padded with packs, Therm-a-Rest pads, or foam pads. This improvised litter is somewhat ungainly and requires six or more rescuers for an evacuation of any distance. A rope litter can be tied to poles or skis to add lateral stability if needed.

Improvised Rescue Sled or Toboggan

A sled or toboggan can be constructed from one or more pairs of skis and poles that are lashed, wired, or screwed together. Many designs are possible. Improvised rescue sleds may be flimsy and often bog down hopelessly in deep snow. Nonetheless, they can be useful for transporting a patient over short distances (to a more sheltered camp or to a more appropriate landing zone). They have sometimes been used for more extensive transports, but they do not perform as well as commercial rescue sleds.

To build an improvised rescue sled-toboggan, the rescuer needs a pair of skis (preferably the patient's) and two pairs of ski poles; three 2-foot-long sticks (or ski pole sections); 80 feet of nylon cord; and extra lengths of rope for sled hauling.

The skis are placed 2 feet apart. The first stick is used as the front cross-bar and is lashed to the ski tips. Alternately, holes can be drilled into the stick and ski tips with an awl, and

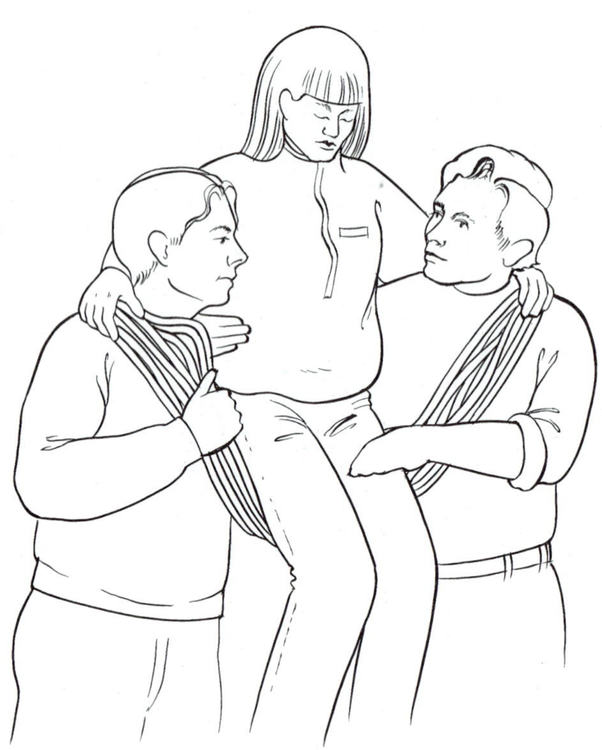

Fig. 18-26 Two-rescuer split-coil seat. Balance could be improved by using a longer coil to carry the victim lower.

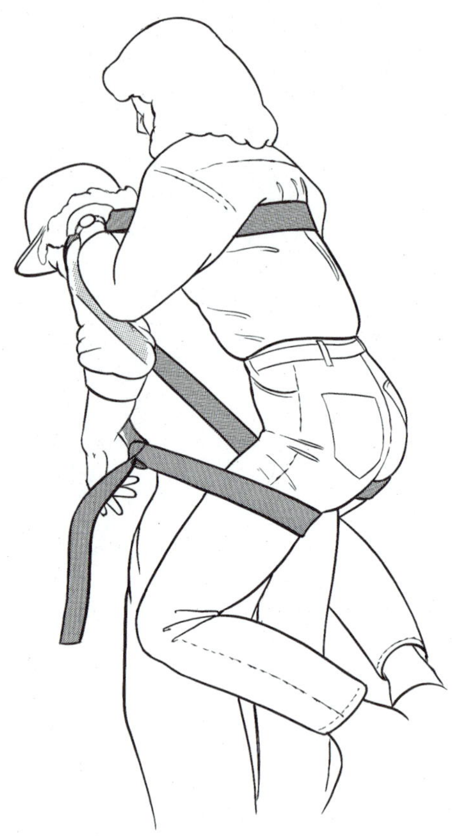

Fig. 18-27 Webbing carry. Webbing crisscrosses in front of the victim's chest before passing over the shoulders of the rescuer.

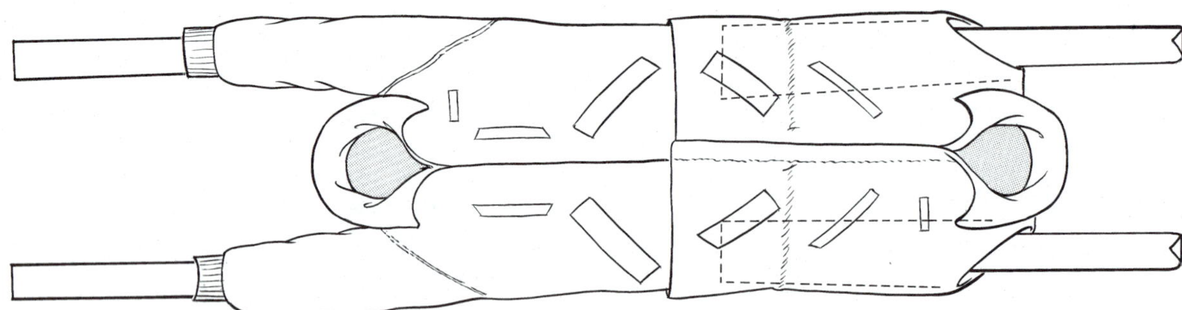

Fig. 18-28 Parka litter. On the right the sleeves are zipped inside to reinforce the litter.

bolts can be used to fasten them together. The middle stick is lashed to the bindings. One pair of ski poles is placed over the cross-bars (baskets over the ski tips) and lashed down. The second set of poles is lashed to the middle stick with baskets facing back toward the tails. A third rear stick is placed on the tails of the skis and lashed to the poles. The lashings are not wrapped around the skis; the cross-bar simply sits on the tails of the skis under the weight of the patient. Nylon cord is then woven back and forth across the horizontal ski poles. The hauling ropes are passed through the baskets on the front of the sled. The ropes are then brought around the middle cross-bar and back to the front cross-bar. This rigging system reverses the direction of pull on the front cross-bar, making it less likely to slip off the ski tips.[22a]

Another sled design incorporates a predrilled snow shovel incorporated into the front of the sled. A rigid backpack frame can also be used to reinforce the sled. This requires drilling holes into the ski tips and carrying a predrilled shovel. This system holds the skis in a wedge position and may offer slightly greater durability.[19a]

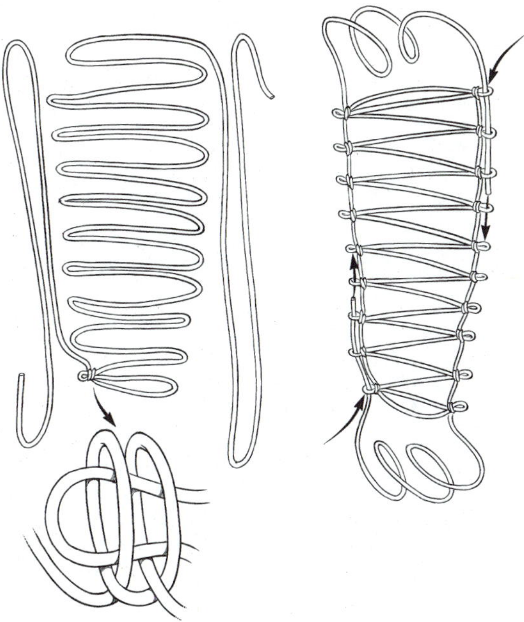

Fig. 18-29 Rope litter.

A Final Note

Under certain conditions, improvised systems are entirely *suboptimal* and may not meet standard of care criteria. It would, for example, be ill advised to fabricate a litter for transporting a patient with a suspected spine injury when professional rescue is only a few miles away. An improvised litter system might be entirely appropriate, however, if the injured person is 40 miles out in Alaska's Brooks Range and needs transport to a sheltered camp or potential helicopter landing zone. The context of the situation should be considered. At times, persons are obligated to do whatever they can, and a resourceful approach to problem solving combined with a little ingenuity could save a victim's life.

REFERENCES

1. Anderson GH et al: Preoperative skin traction for fractures of the proximal femur, *J Bone Joint Surg* 75B(5):794, 1993.

1a. Angeras MH, Brandberg A: Comparison between sterile saline and tap water for the cleansing of acute traumatic soft tissue wounds, *Eur J Surg* 158:347, 1992.

2. Ayton JM: Polar hands: spontaneous skin fissures closed with histoacryl blue tissue adhesive in Antarctica, *Arctic Med Res* 52:127, 1993.

3. Bancewicz J: Oesophageal bolus extraction by balloon catheter, *Br Med J* 1:1142, 1978.

4. Bigler FC: The use of a Foley catheter for removal of blunt foreign objects from the esophagus, *J Thorac Cardiovasc Surg* 51:759, 1966.

4a. Borschneck AG: Why traction? *J Emerg Med Serv* 10:44, 1985.

5. Bratton JR: Epistaxis management: conservative and surgical, *J S Carolina Med Assoc* 80:395, 1984.

6. Bryant CA et al: Search for a non-toxic surgical scrub solution for periorbital lacerations, *Ann Emerg Med* 5:317, 1984.

6a. Chan D et al: The effect of spinal immobilization on healthy volunteers, *Ann Emerg Med* 23(1):48, 1994.

7. Cook PR, Renner G, Williams F: A comparison of nasal balloons and posterior gauze packs for posterior epistaxis, *Ear Nose Throat J* 64:446, 1985.

8. Dire D: A comparison of wound irrigation solutions used in the emergency department, *Ann Emerg Med* 19:704, 1990.

9. Dunlap LB: Removal of an esophageal foreign body using a Foley catheter, *Ann Emerg Med* 10:101, 1981.

10. Dunmire SM et al: Staples versus sutures for wounds closure in the pediatric population, *Ann Emerg Med* 18:448, 1989.

11. Edlich RF: Current concepts of emergency wound management, *Emerg Med Rep* 5:22, 1984.

12. Edlich RF et al: Principles of emergency wound management, *Ann Emerg Med* 17:1284, 1988.

13. Edlich RF, Sinkinson CA: Current concepts of emergency wound management. Part II, *Emerg Med Rep* 5:173, 1984.

13a. Isaac J, Goth P: *The Outward Bound wilderness first aid handbook,* New York, 1991, Lyons & Burford.

14. Lammers RL et al: Effect of povidone-iodine and saline soaking on bacterial counts in acute, traumatic, contaminated wounds, *Ann Emerg Med* 19:709, 1990.

14a. Lyons S, Wilderness Professional Training, Crested Butte, Colo: Personal correspondence, 1994.

15. Nandi P, Ong GB: Foreign body in the esophagus: review of 2394 cases, *Br J Surg* 65:5, 1978.

16. Peterson L: Prophylaxis of wound infections, *Arch Surg* 50:177, 1945.

17. Quinn JV et al: A randomized, controlled trial comparing a tissue adhesive with suturing in the repair of pediatric facial lacerations, *Ann Emerg Med* 22:1130, 1993.

18. Rodeheaver GT et al: Wound cleansing by high pressure irrigation, *Surg Gynecol Obstet* 141:357, 1975.

19. Roth JH, Windle BH: Staple versus suture closure of skin incisions in a pig model, *Can J Surg* 31:19, 1988.

19a. Schimelpfenig T, Lindsey L: *NOLS wilderness first aid,* Wyoming, 1991, NOLS Publications.

20. Sinkinson CA: Maximizing a wound's potential for healing, *Emerg Med Rep* 10:11, 1989.

21. Stevenson T et al: Cleansing the traumatic wound by high-pressure syringe irrigation, *J Am Coll Emerg Phys* 5:17, 1976.

22. Taylor RB: Esophageal foreign bodies, *Emerg Med Clin North Am* 5:2, 1987.

22a. Tilton B: *The basic essentials of rescue from the backcountry,* Indiana, 1990, ICS Books.

23. Toriumi DM et al: Histotoxicity of histoacryl when used in a subcutaneous site, *Laryngoscope,* April 1991.

24. Watson DP: Use of cyanoacrylate tissue adhesive for closing facial lacerations in children, *Br Med J* 299:1014, 1989.

25. Yonkers AJ et al: Etiology and management of epistaxis, *Ear Nose Throat J* 60:453, 1981.

19 CHILDREN IN THE WILDERNESS

Barbara C. Kennedy
Douglas A. Gentile

Once the territory of a few adventurous or unique individuals, the wilderness today attracts an ever broader range of explorers. This includes the pediatric age group, as parents seek to share the joys and lessons of wilderness travel with their children. In 1990, of the estimated 11 million people participating in backpacking and wilderness camping, nearly 25% were under 17 years of age.[69] Millions of other children annually visit national parks and recreation areas or travel to developing countries.

Wilderness travel with children requires special preparation and places extra demands on parents. However, it also affords unique opportunities. Parents and children interact in a setting distant from the stresses of work and school. Isolated from the distractions of television and modern life, children experience new environments and participate in activities that enrich their lives and provide valuable lessons. These activities bring families together as they learn to rely on one another for support, entertainment, and camaraderie.

Physicians and other health care professionals can encourage and facilitate such undertakings by providing medical guidelines and recommendations for wilderness travel with children. This chapter focuses on how children differ from adults and how to prevent, recognize, and treat the medical problems children are likely to encounter in a wilderness setting. Because wilderness travel may encompass travel to foreign countries, pediatric travel immunizations and malaria prophylaxis, along with common pediatric medical problems seen during travel to and within developing countries, are also reviewed.

What Makes Children Different

SIZE AND SHAPE

Children differ from adults in a number of physical, physiologic, and psychologic aspects. The most obvious difference is size. Children may vary over 20-fold in size, from the average 7-pound baby to the 140-pound adolescent. Accordingly, medications and fluids must be calculated on an individual basis, based on the weight of the child. Table 19-1 lists average weights for age. This variation in size also influences a child's risk for the development of serious complications from envenomations.

Many snakes, spiders, scorpions, and poisonous marine animals deliver the same unit dose of venom regardless of the size of the victim; children often experience greater toxicity because of the increased dose of venom per kilogram of weight.

Children are not only smaller than adults; they also have a larger surface area to mass ratio. For example, a 7-pound infant has 2.5 times more body surface area per unit weight than a 140-pound adult. In addition to the larger body surface area, the part of the body most often left exposed, the

Table 19-1 Average Weights for Age

Age (years)	Weight	
	kg	lb
1	10	22
3	15	33
6	20	44
8	25	55
9.5	30	66
11	35	77

Modified from National Center for Health Statistics percentiles, *Am J Clin Nutr* 32:607, 1979.

head, takes up a larger proportion of the body in a young child (Fig. 19-1). As a result, children experience greater exposure to environmental factors, such as cold, heat, and solar radiation. They are also more likely to suffer toxic effects from topical agents, such as insect repellents and medications.

MUSCULOSKELETAL SYSTEM

The musculoskeletal system in children differs from that in adults in several important ways. A child nearly doubles in height between birth and 2 years, and again between 2 and 18 years. In some respects this rapid growth makes a child's bones much more forgiving; the remodeling potential is much greater than in adults. Nonunion or a permanent angulation deformity of a metaphysis is unusual in children owing to the active osteogenic potential of the periosteum. Because of the active periosteum, fractures in the pediatric population heal rapidly. For example, a fractured femur typically heals in 3 weeks in a newborn compared with 20 weeks in a 20-year-old.[11] The strong, pliable periosteum also permits the development of greenstick and buckle fractures, which are not seen in the adult population. These fractures with their intact periosteum are quite stable with little swelling or crepitus. If nondisplaced, they are often incorrectly dismissed as sprains.

Another key difference between the musculoskeletal systems of children and adults is that children have an open growth plate, or physis, at the ends of long bones that connects the metaphysis to the epiphysis (Fig. 19-2). The growth plates consist of soft cartilaginous cells that have the consistency of rubber and act as shock absorbers. They protect the joint surfaces from suffering the grossly comminuted fractures seen in adults. However, because the growth plate is more vulnerable to injury than the strong ligaments or capsular tissues that attach to the epiphysis, a true sprain in a child is rare. Any significant juxtaarticular tenderness in a child should be assumed to be a growth plate injury. Such an injury is most common at the ankle (lateral malleolus), the knee (distal femur), and the wrist (distal radius). Physeal fractures have been classified into five Salter-Harris groups (Fig. 19-2). Salter-Harris I and II fractures generally heal without complications. However, Salter-Harris III and IV fractures often require open reduction of displaced fractures to realign the joint and growth plates and to permit normal growth. A Salter-Harris V fracture has a poor prognosis; the impaction and crushing of some or all of the growth plate may result in a bony bridge that prevents future growth, or it may produce unequal, angulated growth. Consequently, any significant injury, especially if it involves the growth plate, requires a full evaluation in a medical facility.

CARDIOVASCULAR AND RESPIRATORY SYSTEMS

The basic physiologic parameters change greatly from infancy to childhood to adulthood. These differences are important to recognize in order to avoid unnecessary and potentially harmful interventions in healthy children, and yet recognize and intervene when abnormal vital signs are truly present. For example, a blood pressure of 65/35 mm Hg, pulse rate of 160 beats/min, and respiratory rate of 40 breaths/min are considered ominous vital signs for an adult. However, these vital signs are normal in a 2-month-old infant.[27] Although blood pressure readings may not be available in a wilderness setting, it is possible to assess the strength of the pulse and determine the pulse and respiratory rate of an ill child. In general, infants and children have

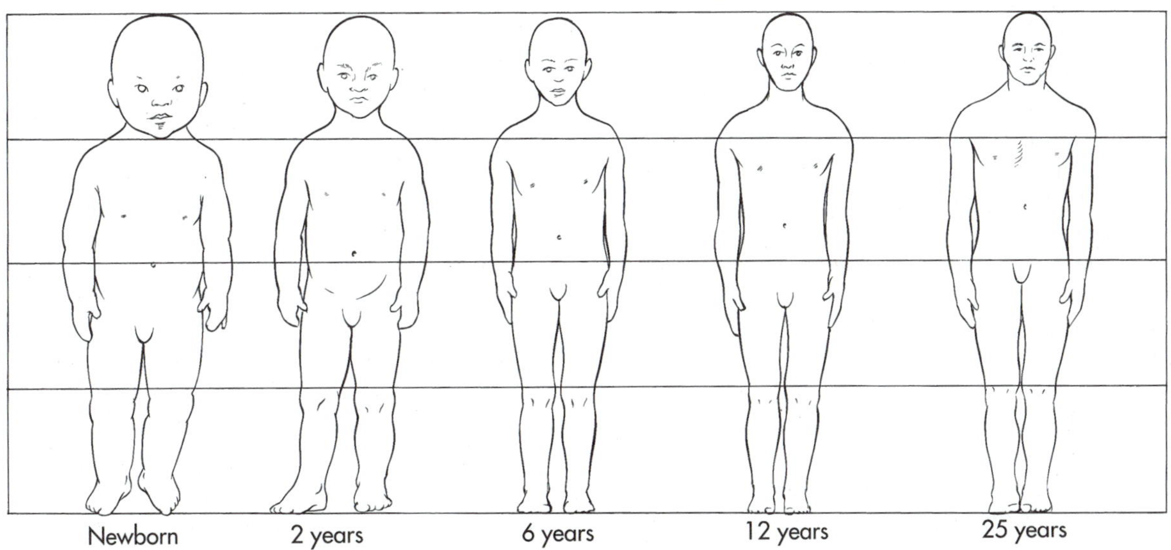

Fig. 19-1 Body proportions.

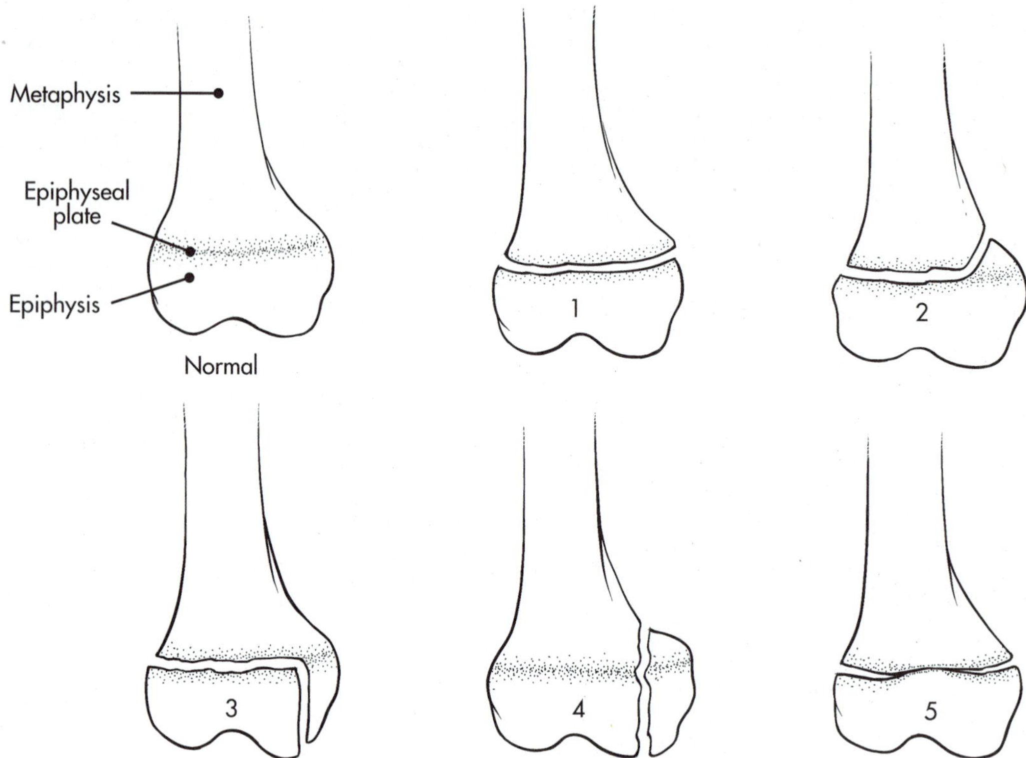

Fig. 19-2 Salter-Harris classification of physeal fractures.

greater respiratory and heart rates and a lower blood pressure than adults. The normal values for various age groups are presented in Table 19-2.

Table 19-2 Age-Specific Resting Heart Rate and Respiratory Rate*

Age	Heart Rate (Beats/Min)	Respiratory Rate (Breaths/Min)
2-5 mo	140 ± 40	40 ± 12
6-11 mo	135 ± 30	30 ± 10
1-2 yr	120 ± 30	25 ± 8
3-4 yr	110 ± 30	24 ± 6
5-7 yr	100 ± 30	21 ± 5
8-11 yr	90 ± 30	20 ± 4
12-15 yr	85 ± 30	18 ± 3

*Mean rate ± 2 SD.

THERMOREGULATION

Because environmental extremes are often encountered when traveling in wilderness areas, it is important to recognize that thermoregulation is less efficient in children than in adults. A number of physiologic and morphologic differences make children more susceptible than adults to heat illness.[70] During exercise, children generate more metabolic heat per unit mass than do adults. Children also have lower cardiac output at a given metabolic rate, resulting in a lower capacity to convey heat from the body core to the periphery.[18] Because of their larger surface area to mass ratio, children also gain heat more rapidly from the environment than do adults when ambient temperature exceeds skin temperature. Under these same conditions, cooling from conduction, convection, and radiation ceases to be effective, leaving evaporation (sweating) as the only effective means of heat dissipation.[59] Unfortunately, children have a lower capacity for evaporative cooling, possibly because of decreased sweat volume, regional differences in sweat patterns, and a higher sweat point (the rectal temperature when sweating starts).[18,29] Finally, children acclimatize to hot environments at a slower rate than adults.[81]

Children are also at greater risk for hypothermia. Their larger surface area to mass ratio causes them to cool more rapidly than adults in cold environments. Children have less subcutaneous fat and thus less "natural" insulation. Infants in particular have an inefficient shivering mechanism.[15] Humans are poorly adapted to a cold environment and must rely on adaptive behavioral responses such as seeking shelter and dressing appropriately to maintain body heat. Infants and young children are not capable of these responses and must rely on their caregivers to provide shelter and appropriate clothing.

IMMUNOLOGY AND INFECTIONS

Children experience a greater number of infections than adults. The average 1-year-old has six to eight infections per year, while the average adult has only three to four infections per year.[46] Infections in children tend to be more severe. The younger the child, the more likely that a given infection represents a first exposure. A first-exposure infection is more likely to cause fever and produce severe symptoms than a reexposure, in which the infection is modified by the antibodies produced from the first exposure. Young children are also less likely to have cross-reacting antibodies from a previous infection with an antigenically related organism.[46]

Many common respiratory or viral infections produce more severe symptoms in children because of anatomic differences. Children have narrower respiratory passages, such as the bronchioles, eustachian tubes, and larynx, that are easily obstructed by edema and mucus. This obstruction worsens the symptoms, prolongs clearance of infection, and increases the risk of secondary infection. Pertussis or "whooping cough" is a classic example of the differences in severity of infection between children and adults. Nearly 20% of infants with pertussis have severe complications such as pneumonia, seizures, or encephalopathy, while this illness develops as a simple cold in most adults.[51]

General Considerations and Expectations

Children of different ages have different needs and abilities. Expectations regarding distances to travel, pace, and safety issues vary depending on age (Table 19-3). This section explores the key issues regarding wilderness travel with children of various ages and provides general expectations for each age group. A number of helpful books that discuss different aspects of wilderness activities with children are listed under "Additional Recommended Readings" at the end of the chapter.

FIRST 2 YEARS

Travel Expectations

Children in their first 2 years can travel almost anywhere, although they place extra demands on their caretakers and require attention and care nearly all of their waking hours. The distances these children are able to travel depend mainly on the adult's hiking abilities, since the children are usually carried. Most children are content in front carriers (infants) or back carriers (older infants and toddlers) and can easily travel for hours at a time. However, because of their increased risk of illness and limited communication skills, infants must be watched closely for signs of infection, hypothermia, hyperthermia, and altitude illness. Parents must be prepared to give prompt treatment or evacuate to seek medical attention should any signs of illness develop. Evacuation plans should be formulated before departure.

Entertainment in this age group is simple. A few small toys, which can be attached to the carrier on a short string, the natural surroundings, and a little parental attention provide ample amusement. A toddler can spend hours examining rocks, leaves, and sticks and rarely tires of a parent's undivided attention. If a child is comforted by a pacifier, it can be attached to the child's shirt or carrier, with extras packed for emergencies.

Safety

As babies becomes more active with rolling, crawling, and then walking, they require constant attention. Bells attached to their shoes may function as an alerting device, ringing when they are on the move. These children are often considered "grazing creatures," putting everything they come across into their mouths. When they are not being car-

Table 19-3 Age-Specific Expectations for Wilderness Travel

Age	Expectation	Safety Issues
0-2 yr	Distance traveled depends on the adults; child carriers used	Provide "safe play area," e.g., tent floor, extra tarp laid out; bells on shoes; ipecac syrup
2-4 yr	Difficult age; stop every 10-15 min; hike ½ to 2 miles on own	Dress in bright colors; teach how to use whistle; ipecac syrup
5-7 yr	Hike 1-3 hr/day; cover 3-4 miles over easy terrain; rest every 30-45 min	Carry whistle: three blows = "I'm lost," 2 blows = "We are coming"; carry own pack with mini first aid kit and water
8-9 yr	Hike a full day with easy pace; cover 6-7 miles over variable terrain; if taller than 4 feet, can use framed pack	As for 5-7 yr, plus: teach map use and route finding; precondition by increasing maximum distances by ≤10%/week; watch for overuse injuries; keep weight of pack ≤20% of body weight
10-12 yr	Hike a full day at moderate pace; cover 8-10 miles over variable terrain	As for 8-9 yr
Teenagers	Hike 8-12 miles at adult pace; may see a decrease in pace or distance with growth spurt	As for 8-9 yr

ried, it is best to have a child-proofed area for them to play in, such as a tent floor or an extra tarp laid out. Toxic ingestions are a possibility in this age group, and parents should be prepared. Syrup of ipecac to induce emesis after certain toxic ingestions should be included in the first aid kit.

Food and Drink

Nourishment in the first 2 years is fairly simple. Infants in their first 4 to 6 months require only breast milk or formula. As long as the mother remains healthy, breast feeding is the safest and most convenient way to feed an infant. However, if the mother is not nursing or not available, formula may be used. Formula is most conveniently carried in a powdered form and mixed as needed. The water for formula may be boiled once a day and stored in individual bottles with airtight lids. The powder for the formula is added just before feeding. Any unused, reconstituted formula should be discarded after 2 to 3 hours at room temperature.

Baby cereals can be carried conveniently in a dry form to be mixed with formula or breast milk. Dry cereals mixed with breast milk or formula have a higher nutritional value than ready-to-feed cereals in jars. Jars of commercial pureed foods may be carried, but the empty jars must be packed out. Once a jar of baby food has been opened, it should be used for only that meal. Without refrigeration, opened jars of baby food spoil quickly. Some families prefer to bring a hand grinder and make their own pureed foods. Some helpful resources on preparing homemade baby food are included in the recommended readings at the end of the chapter.

By 9 to 12 months many babies are eating finger foods. Parents should be cautioned to avoid any hard round foods, such as peanuts or candies, that a baby may choke on. Up to 1 year of age, honey should be avoided because of an increased risk of botulism, a potentially fatal illness. Parents may also want to also avoid citrus foods, which may cause rashes around the mouth and in the diaper area. Any new foods should be tested at home first to be certain the baby will accept it when away from home.

All water for drinking must be disinfected by boiling, iodination, or the use of small-pore filters. Chronic iodide poisoning and neonatal goiter have been associated with prolonged ingestion of large amounts of iodine,[83] although small amounts ingested for water disinfection appear safe.[77] Nonetheless, if both boiled water and iodinated water are available, it is prudent to use the boiled water for the infants and small children. In addition, infants and small children often reject the taste of iodinated water. Iodine must be kept out of reach of small children; severe acute toxicity can occur with an ingestion of just 2 to 4 g.

Diapers

Most children under the age of 2 years are in diapers, either disposable or cloth. Soiled diapers in a wilderness environment require special care. Thin paper diaper liners may be purchased to help collect the stool. The stool and liner should be buried in a trench at least 6 inches deep and 200 feet from any water source. If disposable diapers are used, they should be packed out after the stool has been removed and buried. The used disposable diaper should be wrapped and placed in a double bag for packing out. To reduce weight, urine-soaked diapers may be set out in the sun to dry before repacking. The new superabsorbent diapers may be left on babies much longer and still keep their bottoms dry. However, superabsorbent diapers cannot be dried out as easily and the urine cannot be wrung out of them. Consequently they add significant weight for the rest of the trip. Some families, especially on longer trips, prefer to use cloth diapers, which may be washed out and reused. Cloth diapers must be changed more frequently, since they are not as absorbent; extras should be packed. Washing cloth diapers is labor intensive and time consuming and requires an abundant supply of water. A washbasin will be needed, and the diapers will have to be washed in hot soapy water. The diapers should be rinsed at least twice to remove irritating soap residue, and the waste water dumped where it will not pollute, at least 200 feet from a water source. Families should avoid prefolded cloth diapers because they take too long to dry.

Equipment

Infants and young children are not capable of extended hikes, and their parents may wish to transport them in carriers. Excellent front and back carriers are now available. Most front carriers work well from infancy until an age when babies can sit fairly well, typically 6 to 9 months. It is important that a front carrier extend up high enough in the back to completely support the baby's head. Once a child is sitting well, back carriers are preferred. Back carriers function on the same principle as framed backpacks, redistributing the weight off the shoulders and onto the hips. Many back carriers are able to stand alone and can double as a highchair. Children must be strapped into back carriers, since it is easy for a child to be catapulted out of a carrier if the adult bends over or falls.

Sleeping bags are available for infants and toddlers. However, in a warm climate a few blankets may be sufficient, and in a colder climate a snowsuit works quite well. Children, including young infants, need their own sleeping pads. The sleeping pads protect them from hard, rough ground under the tent and insulate them from the cold ground at night.

Shoes for young children should protect their feet and allow for full range of movement. The best shoes for toddlers are lightweight and flexible. They need shoes that stay on well, since children often flip their shoes off while in a carrier. Velcro-strapped shoes stay on well and are easy to put on and take off. Since children often lose shoes, an extra pair should be included.

2 TO 4 YEARS

Travel Expectations

Children 2 to 4 years old are the most challenging to take into the wilderness. Two-year-olds become easily frustrated and throw temper tantrums, often as a result of the collision between adult restrictions and rules and their desires for independence and control. By 2 years of age, children are becoming too heavy to carry for prolonged periods, but they are still incapable of hiking long distances on their own. They are just gaining bladder and bowel control, and accidents are frequent. Despite these difficulties wilderness trips with this age group can be successful with appropriate planning, preparation, and readjustment of expectations.

A key ingredient to successful wilderness trips with small children is to keep things slow, simple, and flexible. This is the age of independence and assertion. The children need to be given some control and allowed to set a pace. Adults should also encourage young children to express their natural curiosity and enthusiasm for the outdoors by letting them stop to explore their surroundings. Parents can enjoy rediscovering nature through the eyes of their children by getting down and exploring rocks and tide pools and observing a caterpillar's crawl with their children. Parents should expect to stop at least every 15 minutes while hiking. If a diversion or a stimulus is needed to get the children hiking again, parents can begin a story or favorite song and continue it while hiking. With patience and plenty of time, parents can expect children in this age group to travel ½ to 2 miles over easy terrain.

Safety

Unfortunately, 2- to 4-year-olds are notorious for exploring their environment by either wandering off or putting whatever they come across into their mouths. These young children must be watched closely and cautioned to keep wild mushrooms, plants, stones, and any nonfood item out of their mouths. Parents should continue to carry syrup of ipecac in the first aid kit for potential toxic ingestions. The campsites selected should be away from dangers such as steep drop-offs and fast or deep water. Children are easier to locate if dressed in brightly colored clothing. As children get older, they may carry a whistle to call for help when they are lost. The standard distress signal is three blows to indicate "I'm lost" or "I need help"; the response is two blows to indicate "help is coming." Parents should teach children to "stay put" once they discover they are lost and wait to let help come to them. If children panic and start running when they realize they are lost, they increase the chance not only of getting injured, but also of getting farther from the family.

Food

The diet of 2- to 4-year-olds is usually quite simple, but very individual. They tend to have strong preferences and dislikes. Unfortunately, most children this age do not like the convenient "all-in-one-pot" cooking common around campfires. Foods should be tested at home first to be sure they are acceptable. Nutritious snacks such as raisins, granola bars, bagels, crackers, string cheese, and fruit leathers can be packed; these snacks sometimes become a child's meal. Small children should not be given items that they may choke on, such as peanuts and hard, round candies. Hot dogs are one of the most common foods that children choke on. Cutting hot dogs into bite-size pieces decreases the risk. At least one adult member should be trained in basic cardiopulmonary resuscitation and know how to assist a choking child.

Toileting

Most children are becoming toilet trained by the end of their third year. However, accidents are common and parents need to be prepared with extra dry clothing that is readily accessible. Children should be taught correct toileting procedure for a wilderness environment. Stools should be deposited at least 200 feet from a water source, buried in a hole approximately 6 inches deep, and completely covered. Many families carry a special trowel for this purpose. Some groups staying in one location for more than a day dig a specific toileting trench, 12 to 18 inches deep, to be used multiple times. They then add enough dirt after each use to cover all waste. Children need help learning to squat over the trench and to bury their stools.

It may be years before children gain reliable nighttime bladder control, so parents should be prepared for accidents. Cotton and down sleeping bags should be avoided because they lose their insulating abilities and take a long time to dry when wet. Fortunately, there are many synthetic bags available with fills such as Polarguard, Quallofil, and Hollofil, which maintain warmth and loft when wet.

SCHOOL AGE (5 YEARS AND UP)

Travel Expectations

Once children enter the school years, their abilities and attention span increase dramatically. This enables them to participate more actively in many outdoor activities. Children are hungry for knowledge and readily absorb information about nature and outdoor activities. They enjoy being included in the initial planning, as well as in the field activities such as setting up camp, cooking, and cleaning up. School-age children can understand maps and often enjoy following their progress from one point to another. This is an ideal age to explain to them the rules of living in and traveling through wilderness areas. The examples and rules parents set for appropriate behavior in a wilderness at this age may become lessons engraved for a lifetime.

When parents are planning for hiking trips, it is important that they have appropriate expectations for children's differing abilities (Table 19-3). An individual child's hiking ability can be estimated by hikes around the neighborhood or in a local park. If this becomes a routine, the children become preconditioned, increase their endurance, and learn to pace themselves. More important, parents can get a good estimate of what to expect and test methods for motivating their children. It is better to underestimate than to overestimate a child's ability. Parents should also remember that children, like adults, have good and bad days, so allowances should be made.

Safety

School-age children can learn to become more self-sufficient and in tune with their surroundings. They can be taught to recognize their surroundings, so they are less likely to get lost. Landmarks can be pointed out; children should learn how different landmarks can look from different perspectives. They should periodically turn around so they can see where they came from as well as where they are going. As children advance in the school years, they can learn survival skills, such as how to build a shelter, secure food, maintain warmth, use a signal mirror, and use a map and compass. As with the previous age group, they should carry a whistle and know how to use it appropriately.

Equipment

Children like to feel important, capable, and self-sufficient. These feelings are enhanced if they are allowed to carry some of their own gear. Even 5-year-olds like to carry their own soft backpacks. Items they can carry in the packs include snacks, a favorite small toy, tissues or a handkerchief, lip balm, a small ziplock trash bag, and a whistle. As the children grow, the contents of their backpacks should reflect their increasing independence with more self-care and survival items. In addition to the preceding items, they may wish to carry their own water bottle, a mini first aid kit (adhesive bandages, wipes, personal medication), sunscreen, insect repellent, and other survival items as they learn to use them. The maximum weight of these packs should be 20% of the child's body weight until he or she has had significant backcountry experience and has proved that more can be carried comfortably. Once children reach 4 feet in height, they can be fitted for a framed backpack. When a backpack is properly fitted, the waistband should be just over the hipbones and the shoulder strap anchor points should be 1 to 2 inches below each shoulder crest. With a framed pack children can carry even more of their gear. However, the total weight should be gradually increased to allow the child to become comfortable with the heavier loads.

Environmental Illnesses

HIGH-ALTITUDE ILLNESS

High-altitude illness (see Chapter 1) can be viewed as a continuum that includes acute mountain sickness (AMS) through the life-threatening conditions high-altitude pulmonary edema (HAPE) and high-altitude cerebral edema (HACE). AMS usually develops within 24 hours of ascent. The incidence and severity depend on individual susceptibility as well as the rate of ascent and the altitude attained, particularly the sleeping altitude. The true incidence is unknown but probably falls between 10% and 20% at 2500 m (8200 feet) in adults.[31] The incidence in children is reported at 28% at similar altitudes.[76]

Symptoms

The cardinal symptoms of AMS are a bitemporal, throbbing headache, anorexia, and malaise. Children appear particularly prone to nausea and vomiting. Other symptoms include lassitude, dizziness, dyspnea on exertion, and fragmented sleep. Infants may display nonspecific findings including irritability, poor feeding, and sleep disturbance. Manifestations of severe AMS include dyspnea at rest and ataxia, which presage HAPE and HACE, respectively.

Treatment

Acetazolamide has been convincingly shown to reduce the incidence of AMS in adults.[34] Pretreatment with this agent mimics the acclimated state by inducing a hyperchloremic metabolic acidosis and a compensatory increase in respiration. There are no published studies of its efficacy in children, but clinical experience suggests that it is beneficial. The primary indication for acetazolamide prophylaxis in children is a history of recurrent AMS despite graded ascent.[76] Acetazolamide is given at 5 to 10 mg/kg/day, in two divided doses, up to a maximum daily dose of 500 mg. It should be started 24 hours before ascent and continued for 48 hours at altitude. Side effects include nausea and somnolence; paresthesias may be particularly bothersome in children. Dexamethasone also prevents or reduces symptoms of AMS in adults, but there is little experience with its use for this purpose in children.

Treatment of mild AMS requires halting the ascent and allowing time for acclimatization to occur. *Proceeding to higher altitude in the presence of symptoms is contraindicated* and may lead to the life-threatening conditions HAPE and HACE. Symptomatic therapy includes rest and acetaminophen for headache. In children older than 2 years of age or greater than 10 kg, prochlorperazine (Compazine) relieves nausea and vomiting and has the advantage of increasing the hypoxic ventilatory response.[49] However, children are more susceptible to the extrapyramidal symptoms from phenothiazines, and the medication should be stopped if such symptoms develop. Prochlorperazine is given at 0.4 mg/kg/day, orally or rectally, in 3 or 4 divided doses. Descent is unequivocally the most successful treatment for AMS and is mandatory if symptoms progress or fail to improve. While descent should proceed as far as necessary for improvement, 500 to 1000 m is often sufficient. If immediate descent is not possible, oxygen (1 to 2 L/min) should be administered if available. Limited studies examining dexamethasone and acetazolamide for the treatment of AMS suggest that both are effective.[26,43] Dexamethasone should probably be reserved for patients with deterioration of consciousness or truncal ataxia.

Prevention

The safest and surest method of preventing high-altitude illness is to allow for acclimatization via a graded ascent. No exact guidelines exist, especially considering the variable susceptibility to altitude illness. However, general recommendations for children (and adults) without altitude experience are listed in Box 19-1. Day trips to higher altitude should feature return to lower altitude to sleep in order to aid acclimatization.[28]

Reentry pulmonary edema refers to the development of HAPE in long-term residents of high-altitude areas on reascent from a trip to low altitude. Children and adolescents are particularly susceptible. Symptoms usually begin within a day of reascent and include cough, shortness of breath, vomiting, and chest pain. Rales are characteristic on examination. Treatment with bed rest and oxygen usually suffices.[66,68]

COLD INJURY

As previously noted in the section on thermoregulation, children cool more rapidly than adults and often lack the knowledge and judgment to initiate responses that will maintain warmth in a cold environment. As a result, parents participating in cold weather recreation with children should be able to recognize, treat, and preferably prevent hypothermia and frostbite.

BOX 19-1

RECOMMENDATIONS FOR PREVENTING HIGH-ALTITUDE ILLNESS

Avoid abrupt ascent to a sleeping altitude higher than 3000 m (9843 feet).

Spend 2 or 3 nights at 2500 to 3000 m before going higher.

Avoid abrupt increases of greater than 500 m in sleeping altitude.

Modified from Hackett PH, Roach RC: *Ann Emerg Med* 16:980, 1987.

HYPOTHERMIA

Hypothermia (see Chapter 3) is defined as a core body temperature below 35° C (95° F). At this temperature the body no longer generates enough heat to maintain body functions. The condition is considered moderate or mild when the core temperature is above 32° C (89.6° F) and severe when it is below 32° C.[15] The signs and symptoms of hypothermia are listed in Table 19-4, although these are not invariable. The most important clue to significant hypothermia is altered mental status. The child who begins to undress or to stumble and make inappropriate remarks should be evaluated for hypothermia. Physicians should caution parents that hypothermia can develop at moderate temperatures if adverse climatic conditions are compounded by illness, fatigue, dehydration, inadequate nutrition, or wet clothing.

Treatment

For the hypothermic child, field rewarming begins with limiting further exposure to the cold environment. Wet clothing should be removed, and the child's head and neck protected from further heat loss. Placing the child, together with a normothermic person, in a sleeping bag insulated from the ground provides external warming. Hot water bottles, insulated to prevent burns, may also be placed in the axillae and groin and around the neck. If the child is alert, oral hydration with warm fluids containing glucose repletes glycogen and corrects dehydration, which frequently accompanies hypothermia. Signs of severe hypothermia dictate immediate evacuation if conditions permit; rescuers should handle the victim gently to prevent precipitating arrhythmias.

Table 19-4 Signs and Symptoms of Hypothermia

Temperature	Signs and Symptoms
35°-37° C (95°-98.6° F)	Sensation of cold, shivering, increased heart rate, slight incoordination in hand movements
32.2°-35° C (90°-95° F)	Increased muscular incoordination, stumbling gait, decrease or loss of shivering, weakness, apathy, drowsiness, confusion, slurred speech
29.4°-32.2° C (85°-90° F)	Loss of shivering, confusion progressing to coma, inability to walk or follow commands, paradoxical undressing, loss of vision
<29.4° C (<85° F)	Rigid muscles; decreased blood pressure, heart rate, and respiratory rate; dilated pupils; appearance of death

Modified from Auerbach PS: *Medicine for the outdoors,* Boston, 1991, Little, Brown.

Prevention

When preparing for cold weather activities, children should dress in layers to allow clothing to be added or subtracted as necessary, thus avoiding excessive perspiration yet maintaining warmth. Since children generally avail themselves of any opportunity to get wet, clothing that maintains low thermal conductance when wet is particularly important; conductive heat loss may increase 25 times in wet clothing.[13] Wool retains warmth when wet because of its unique ability to suspend water vapor within the fibers; however, it is heavier than synthetics and takes much longer to dry. Cotton has a high thermal conductance that increases greatly when wet; it is a poor choice for wilderness activities in cold weather. New synthetic materials (polypropylene, Capilene, Thermax) wick moisture away from the skin and dry quickly, making them ideal for an inner layer. An insulating layer may incorporate wool, polyester pile, Thinsulate, or similar materials. Windproof and water-resistant outer garments decrease heat loss from convection and keep children dry. Hats and mittens are essential; the uncovered head of a child dissipates up to 70% of total body heat production at ambient temperatures of 5° C.[7]

FROSTBITE

Localized cold injury results in frostbite (see Chapter 5). Predisposing factors include wet skin, constricting garments that hinder blood circulation, fatigue, contact with cold metal, and windchill. If skin temperature drops below 10° C, cutaneous sensation is generally abolished and injury may go unnoticed. Skin cooled to –4° C freezes.[40]

Frostbite has traditionally been divided into degrees of injury, much like burns. First-degree injury manifests with numbness, erythema, and edema without tissue loss. Second-degree frostbite results in superficial blistering, while third-degree injury produces deeper blisters containing bloody fluid. Fourth-degree injury extends through the dermis to subcuticular tissues. In children, frostbite that extends into bone may affect the growth plate and result in skeletal deformities.[8,37]

Treatment

Rapid rewarming constitutes the primary treatment of frostbite and is best accomplished by immersion in water warmed to 40° to 42° C.[30] This narrow temperature range maximizes rewarming speed, while preventing compounded injury from a burn wound. Thawing usually takes 30 to 45 minutes and is complete when the skin is soft and pliable. Although field rewarming is indicated unless evacuation can be effected quickly, great care should be taken to avoid refreezing; refreezing causes far more damage than delayed thawing. Vigorous rubbing should also be avoided because it is ineffective and potentially harmful. After thawing, blister fluid should be aspirated to prevent further contact with tissue-damaging prostaglandins and thromboxanes, and a sterile dressing applied.[30]

HEAT ILLNESS

Families participating in wilderness activities in hot climates must take special precautions to avoid heat illness (see Chapter 8); children do not tolerate the demands of exercise in the heat as well as adults. Parents planning wilderness ventures with children in hot climates can follow some simple guidelines for avoiding heat illness. The most obvious entails reducing the duration and intensity of activities under conditions of high climatic heat stress, keeping in mind that the risk of heat illness depends on relative humidity, wind velocity, and radiant heat, as well as standard dry bulb thermometer temperature. Fig. 19-3 gives a rough guide for activity levels based on temperature and relative humidity.

Children should be fully hydrated before prolonged exercise and actively encouraged to drink fluids at regular intervals. Provision of pleasantly flavored drinks may aid fluid intake. When not actively encouraged to drink, exercising children will progressively dehydrate, even when water is freely available.[4] As little as a 2% decrease in body weight through fluid loss results in increased heart rate and body temperature and decreased plasma volume. Water losses of 4% to 5% of body weight reduce muscular work capacity by 20% to 30%.[70]

A child eating a normal diet does not require electrolyte replacement unless sweating is prolonged or excessive.[21] Children have a lower concentration of salt in their sweat compared with adults. This, along with the overall decrease in the amount of sweat a child generates, decreases the need for salt supplemention.[29] Salt tablets can cause gastric irritation and hypernatremic dehydration and should be avoided. Since sweat evaporated from clothing contributes less to cooling than sweat evaporated from skin,[14] children should change out of sweat-soaked clothing and wear dry, lightweight, loose-fitting clothing. Finally, children acclimatize to the heat slower than do adults, often taking 10 to 14 days to fully acclimate. The intensity and duration of exercise should be gradually increased over this period.[10]

Infants and neonates are most vulnerable to heat illness. Under high climatic heat stress, infants fed undiluted cow's milk or formula may develop marked salt retention and dehydration. They should be given extra water or dilute feedings.[12,73] The lower osmolar load of breast milk appears to protect against heat illness and hypernatremia.[73]

Early signs and symptoms of heat illness include flushing, tachycardia, weakness, mild confusion, headache, and nausea. Vomiting often occurs in children. Sweating may be present or absent. If heat illness develops, children should be removed from obvious sources of heat, including direct sunlight, and have their clothing removed. Evaporative cooling

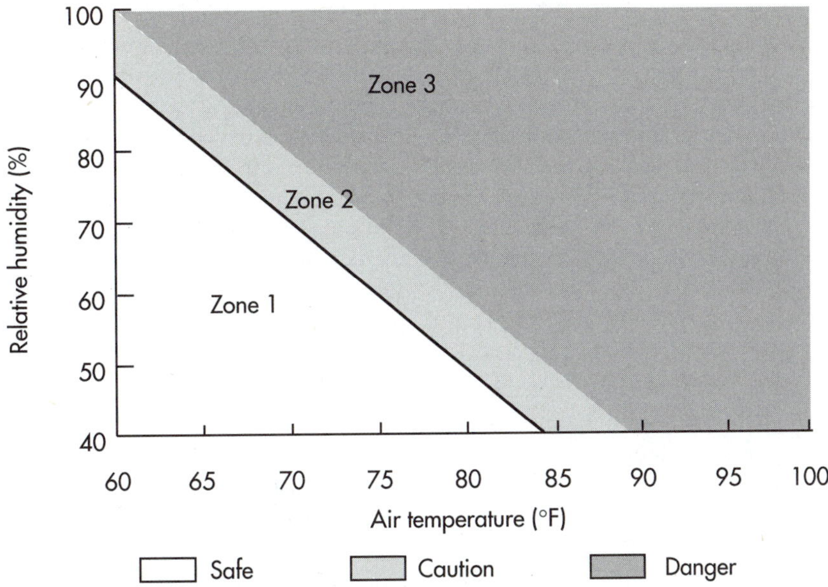

Fig. 19-3 Activity levels based on temperature and relative humidity.

can be increased in the field by vigorous fanning after spraying or sprinkling the victim with water. If available, ice packs or cold compresses placed in the groin and axilla and on the scalp also aid cooling. If the child is alert, dehydration may be corrected with oral fluids. Progression of symptoms or failure to respond mandates immediate evacuation.

SUN DAMAGE

The hazards of overexposure to sunlight include sunburn, photoaging, skin cancer, and phototoxic and photoallergic reactions (see Chapter 12). Preventing ultraviolet damage to the skin should start in childhood, since 80% of a person's lifetime sun exposure occurs before 21 years of age.[3] Recent evidence suggests that the risk of developing malignant melanoma is at least double if a person has had one or more severe sunburns in childhood. This risk is even higher if a child is light skinned with a propensity to burn rather than tan.[23,54,85]

The ultraviolet wavelengths UVA and UVB are principally responsible for the harmful effects of solar radiation. UVB is primarily responsible for suntan and sunburn. However, it also promotes the development of skin cancer and aging of the skin. UVB increases 4% for every 1000-foot gain in elevation over sea level. Therefore a backpacker at 10,000 feet will have a 40% increase in UVB exposure. UVA, which is 10 to 100 times more abundant than UVB, is only 0.001 as potent at inducing sunburn. It is also less affected than UVB by changes in season or solar zenith angle. UVA is primarily responsible for photosensitivity reactions and solar urticaria. It also contributes to skin cancer and skin aging. A number of drugs often used in adolescence, such as tetracycline, vitamin A derivatives (Retin A, Accutane), and nonsteroidal antiinflammatory drugs (NSAIDs), increase the risk of photosensitivity reactions and the need for UVA protection. Consequently, it is important to use sunscreens that protect against both UVA and UVB.

The harmful effects of ultraviolet radiation from the sun can be reduced if parents are educated to the dangers of sun exposure and encouraged to use sun protective clothing and sunscreens early in their children's lives. Studies indicate that the regular use of a sunscreen with a sun protection factor (SPF) of at least 15 for the first 18 years of life reduces a person's lifetime risk of developing nonmelanoma skin cancer by 78%.[71] The use of sunscreen in teenagers—a population adults often have little influence over—is positively associated with having parents who insisted on sunscreen use when the teenagers were younger children.[3]

Sunscreens

Most sunscreens have ingredients such as PABA, PABA-esters, cinnamates, salicylates, and anthranilates that protect the skin from sun damage by absorbing primarily UVB. Dibenzoylmethane absorbs only UVA. Benzophenones block UVB and to a lesser degree UVA.[36] Sunscreens that combine ingredients that protect the skin from both UVB and UVA are the most effective. A recently developed product, micronized titanium dioxide, which reflects ultraviolet light in a fashion similar to the sun block zinc oxide, is nearly colorless yet retains the ability to scatter sunlight.

The SPF is a measure of a sunscreen's effectiveness. It is measured in terms of the minimal dose (in length of time) of UV radiation required to cause skin erythema. Sunscreens with SPF of 30 or higher provide a superior degree of photoprotection and almost completely prevent the cellular changes seen with sunburn.[35]

Water-resistant sunscreens maintain their effectiveness for up to 40 minutes of water immersion, whereas waterproof sunscreens maintain their effectiveness for up to 80 minutes of water immersion.[36] Either should be reapplied if longer times are spent in the water, or sooner if the water is turbulent. Excessive sweating and rubbing of the skin are also indications for reapplication.

Sun Protective Clothing

Appropriate clothing is important in minimizing sun damage. Hats with brims help to protect the face from sun exposure. Clothing made from tightly woven fabrics is more protective than clothing made from loosely woven fabric. For example, loosely woven fabrics such as that in most T-shirts have an SPF of only 5. Most clothing loses even more of its protective effect when wet. However, a few manufacturers (Frogskin, Inc., 800-845-9531; Sun Precautions, Inc., 800-882-7860) are now marketing high-SPF (25 to 30) protective clothing. This specialized sun protective clothing is cool and lightweight, dries quickly, and can maintain its full SPF capabilities even when wet.

Treatment

When sunburn occurs, the mainstay of treatment is cool compresses, topical antipruritics, and NSAIDs.[36] Recent studies indicate that a high-potency topical steroid, betamethasone dipropionate, may work synergistically with NSAIDs to reduce the UVB-induced erythema by as much as 42% to 58% if used early in the burning process.[32] Strong topical steroids should be used judiciously, since just a 7-day course may suppress the hypothalamic-pituitary-adrenal axis. As always, the best cure is prevention.

Bites and Stings

Bites and stings occur commonly in the pediatric age group. In 1992, the American Association of Poison Control Centers recorded 70,272 calls regarding bites and envenomations; 44% involved patients 17 years of age or younger. Remarkably, major morbidity occurred in less than 0.1% of cases, and there were no deaths in patients less than 17 years of age.[45] This emphasizes the need for appropriate triage to determine which children require aggressive therapy and to avoid potentially harmful field interventions.

SNAKES

Most snakebites can be prevented. Children up to 10 years of age are particularly likely to handle snakes and have a higher rate of bites than any other age group.[17] They also suffer more severe envenomation syndromes than do adults.[82] Children should be instructed not to handle snakes, reach blindly into crevices, or turn over rocks and fallen limbs. A useful adage is that hands and feet should never go where the eyes cannot see. When walking through endemic areas, hikers should stay on trails and wear long, loose pants and boots that extend above the ankle. Campsites should be on open ground, away from woodpiles or rockpiles. A recently developed negative-pressure suction device (The Extractor, Sawyer Products, Safety Harbor, Fla.) removed up to 30% of injected venom (in an animal model) if used within 3 minutes of the bite.[72] No incision over the bite is necessary. Parents traveling to snake-infested areas should consider adding this product to their medical kit. For a detailed discussion of snakebites see Chapter 28.

HYMENOPTERA

Hymenoptera stings (bees, wasps, hornets, and ants) are the most common cause of envenomation in children. Although Hymenoptera venom possesses intrinsic toxicity, the amount delivered is small and multiple stings are necessary for significant human morbidity.[25] However, the venoms are potent antigens capable of producing IgE-mediated anaphylaxis in sensitized individuals. Although children appear less susceptible to systemic sting reactions than adults,[79] physicians should educate parents in the management of Hymenoptera stings, particularly if a child has had a previous severe reaction.

Hymenoptera stings usually produce local pain, swelling, and erythema. If a stinger is present, it should be flicked or scraped out, taking care to avoid squeezing an attached venom sac. Applying ice or cool compresses when available reduces pain and swelling. Elevation and immobilization are indicated for large local reactions on extremities. In older children, oral antihistamines may provide additional symptomatic relief.

Early signs of a systemic reaction include generalized pruritus, urticaria, angioedema, bronchospasm, and laryngeal edema; their presence mandates medical evaluation. Epinephrine is the drug of choice for systemic sting reactions and should be administered in the field if available (0.01 mg/kg subcutaneously).[80] Parents without a medical background may prefer the EpiPen Jr. or EpiPen. Both contain a spring-loaded automatic injector that delivers 0.3 mg (EpiPen) or 0.15 mg (EpiPen Jr.) of epinephrine subcutaneously when triggered by pressing the device against the thigh. The EpiPen Jr. is appropriate for children up to 15 kg, while the regular EpiPen is appropriate for larger children and adults. Since up to half of all patients with anaphylactic reactions have no forewarning,[56] epinephrine belongs in all wilderness medical kits. For a detailed discussion of Hymenoptera stings see Chapter 31.

MOSQUITOES

Mosquitoes not only present a high nuisance potential but serve as vectors for disease (see Chapter 34). A number of steps can be taken to avoid mosquitoes (see Box 19-2). A proper wardrobe provides an excellent physical barrier to

BOX 19-2

MOSQUITO AVOIDANCE

Wear long-sleeved shirt and pants.
Minimize outdoor activities at dusk.
Use mosquito netting to cover the heads of infants and children, and in sleeping area.
Spray clothing, netting, and screens with permethrin repellents (Permanone or Duranon).
Use insect repellents with no more than 35% DEET, on exposed skin only, avoiding hands of young children (they often end up in the mouth). Apply DEET products over any other creams such as sunscreen to minimize absorption and maximize the repellent effect.
Keep DEET out of reach of small children; it is toxic.

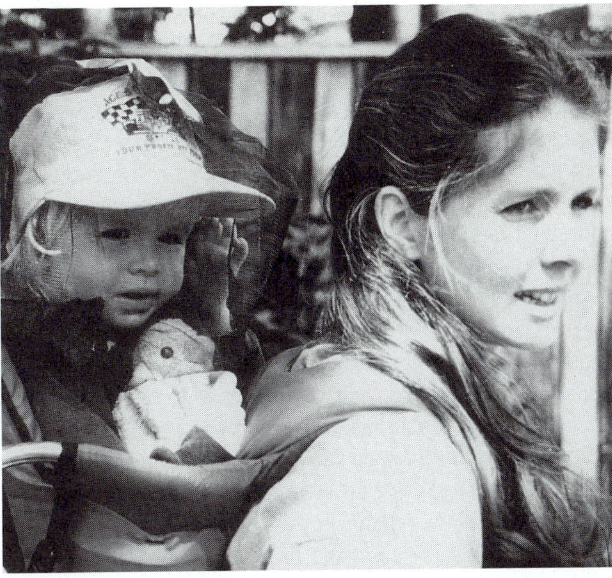

Fig. 19-4 Mosquito netting draped over a child's hat. (Courtesy Scott Kehl.)

mosquitoes; this should include ankle-high footwear, pants cinched at the ankles or tucked into socks, long-sleeved shirt, and a full-brimmed hat. Mosquito netting draped over a child's hat will protect the face and neck without the toxic side effects occasionally seen with repellents (Fig. 19-4). Mosquito netting, especially in the sleeping area, has been found to reduce the mosquito attack rate by 97%.[84]

Repellents containing DEET (*N,N*-diethyl-meta-toluamide) are effective against mosquitoes, ticks, blackflies, and many other arthropods. Although generally of low toxicity,[78] DEET is absorbed cutaneously and toxic encephalopathy associated with its use has been reported.[58] Children appear at particular risk, perhaps because of their greater surface area to mass ratio.[74] High concentrations of DEET may also cause dermatitis with erythema, bullae, skin necrosis, and residual scarring.[41] While products containing 100% DEET are commercially available, long-acting formulations of 35% DEET appear equally effective in protecting against mosquitoes, with much less potential for toxicity.[64] Although available data do not permit precise safety guidelines, it seems prudent to avoid using products containing higher than 35% DEET in children. DEET products can be applied over other creams such as sunscreen to minimize absorption and maximize repellent effect. Parents should also be cautioned to keep DEET out of the reach of small children, since ingestions may be fatal.[84]

The pesticide permethrin, available as a 0.5% spray (Permanone, Duranon Tick Repellent), is safe and effective against arthropods, especially ticks.[65] Unlike DEET repellents, these permethrin products are applied to fabric or netting and should not be applied to the skin. Permethrins as a class have low toxicity in mammals. The combination of DEET applied to exposed skin and permethrin treatment of clothing is particularly effective in protecting against mosquito bites and ticks.[44,67] The protective effect of mosquito netting is greatly enhanced when the netting is impregnated with permethrin.[84] Permethrin repels mosquitoes even when holes or tears are present in the netting.

Foreign Travel with Children

Traveling with children to wilderness areas within developing countries entails the risks not only of wilderness travel, but also of encountering poor sanitation conditions with consequent exposure to bacteria, viruses, protozoa, and helminths not usually seen in the developed world. Preparation for foreign travel with children includes appropriate immunizations, malaria prophylaxis when indicated, and guidance regarding prevention and treatment of medical problems common to foreign travel.

GENERAL RECOMMENDATIONS

General advice to parents should include a discussion of precautions for daily activities. The most common travel-related health problems occur through the ingestion of contaminated foods and water. Advice for preventing the ingestion of harmful organisms via food and drink is given in Box 19-3. Scabies and lice infestations can become a significant problem if the family is staying in teahouses or if there is close contact with the local children. Permethrin cream (Elimite) is safe and effective for the treatment of infestations with both lice and scabies in children as young as 2 months old. One application is curative. Parents should be advised about the hazards of mosquitoes as vectors of diseases and about the safest and most effective means of avoiding these vectors (Box 19-2). Consultation should also include the health hazards of swimming in fresh water (schistosomiasis, noncholera *Vibrio* infection, and leptospirosis). When outside in rural areas with limited sanitation, children should wear shoes (not sandals) and be discouraged from playing in the dirt, to avoid infection with skin-penetrating parasites (*Strongyloides stercoralis* and hookworm). Children's impulsive behaviors, smaller size, and lack of prior immunity place them at greater risk for complications from the preceding hazards.

Parents of children with special medical conditions should carry a pertinent medical summary with them and be given resources for specialty physicians in the destination countries. Foreign specialty physicians may be found in international medical specialty directories. A generous supply of necessary medications with instructions on what to do should symptoms worsen must be included in the medical kit. An extra supply of all essential medications should be kept with either the parents or the patient in case the medical kit gets lost or separated from the patient when the medication is needed. Some travelers in endemic areas for hepatitis B and AIDS carry their own needles and syringes for emergency use. The International Association for Medical Assistance to Travelers (417 Center St., Lewiston, NY 14692; phone: 716-754-4883) has a directory of qualified physicians worldwide who speak English.

RECOMMENDATIONS FOR PROBLEMS ENCOUNTERED WHILE TRAVELING

Parents may also need advice regarding common problems encountered with travel itself. They should be aware of methods to help children cope with the boredom and restlessness that comes from being confined while traveling. Telling stories, reading, and playing simple games can help pass the time. Parents may wish to prepare small activity packs or bags with paper, pencils, crayons, cards, travel puzzles, or small toys. A few special treats can be held out to be presented at particularly taxing times.

Motion Sickness

Children are commonly afflicted by motion sickness, which can turn a wonderful adventure into a nightmare. Bumpy rides, especially during air and ocean travel, are the most common settings. Emotional upset, noxious odors, and ear infections can make the symptoms worse. Children experiencing motion sickness are often pale and sweaty and feel nauseated and weak. They may vomit, but unfortunately this does not provide prolonged relief. Children known to be susceptible to motion sickness should be seated in the middle or near the front of the boat, plane, or car where the motion is minimized. They should be encouraged to look at objects far away and avoid focusing on close objects such as books. Some children get significant relief from using headphones to listen to tapes of music or stories. Dimenhydrinate (Dramamine) started 1 hour before departure and repeated every 6 hours can help those known to be prone to motion sickness. If dimenhydrinate is not available, diphenhydramine (Benadryl) may also be effective. Both medications may cause drowsiness, and diphenhydramine occasionally causes a paradoxic hyperexcitability in children. Scopolamine patches, commonly used in adults, should not be used in children because children are particularly susceptible to the side effects of belladonna alkaloids, including scopolamine. Whether this particular administration system might release too much scopolamine and consequently produce serious side effects in children is not known.[52]

Eustachian Tube Dysfunction

Eustachian tube dysfunction causes discomfort that results from a pressure disequilibrium between the eustachian tube and the surrounding atmospheric pressure.[42] It may be particularly bothersome when flying. Swallowing often helps relieve the pressure disequilibrium and may be facilitated by drinking, or for the breast-fed infant, nursing. Older children may wish to chew gum or practice yawning. When eustachian tube dysfunction is a recurrent problem, an oral antihistamine and long-acting decongestant nasal spray may be given 1 hour before the flight.

IMMUNIZATIONS

Foreign travel with children requires obtaining the immunizations required specifically for travel and may require modification of the routine childhood immunization schedule. Table 19-5 lists a number of sources for up-to-date information about the travel immunizations and malaria prophylaxis recommended for different geographic areas. Information that will be necessary to evaluate which immunizations and malaria prophylaxis are needed includes the following:

1. Countries of travel
2. Length of time in each country
3. Location of destinations (rural versus urban)
4. Time of year
5. Type of lodging and eating facilities
6. Previous immunizations
7. Age and weight of the child

Special immunizations required for travel may need to be adapted for children (Table 19-6). The risk of acquiring diseases covered by many routine childhood immunizations (diphtheria, pertussis, tetanus, measles, polio, and hepatitis B) is greater when traveling to developing countries. Consequently, children who have not completed their primary series of immunizations may require a shortening of the intervals between vaccinations or extra doses to maximize protection before travel (Table 19-7).

Ideally a visit to discuss travel plans and start immunizations should be made at least 6 weeks before travel. Not all immunobiologic agents recommended for travel are compatible, and some require multiple doses. Therefore the selection of immunizations to be given at any one time and the

Table 19-5 Resources for Up-to-Date Travel Immunizations and Malaria Prophylaxis Recommendations

Resource		Comments
Centers for Disease Control and Prevention (CDC): 404-332-4555		Updated recorded message, with fax available, via a touch tone phone menu
CDC Meningitis and Special Pathogen Branch: 404-639-3087		The most recent update on meningococcal activity
CDC Division of Vector-borne Viral Diseases: 303-221-6400		The latest information on yellow fever and other arboviral infections
Regional US. Public Health Service Quarantine Stations		
Chicago	312-686-2150	12 Noon–8 PM (Central Time)
Honolulu	808-541-2552	6 AM–3 PM (Hawaii time)
Los Angeles	213-215-2365	8 AM–5 PM (Pacific Time)
Miami	305-526-2910	8 AM–5 PM (Eastern time)
New York	718-917-1685	8 AM–10 PM (Eastern Time)
San Francisco	415-876-2872	8 AM–4 PM (Pacific Time)
Seattle	206-442-4519	8 AM–5 PM (Pacific Time)

interval between immunizations are important. Table 19-7 presents recommendations for the timing and sequence of both specific travel immunizations and the routine childhood immunizations that may be needed in preparation for foreign travel. In general, all toxoids, inactivated vaccines, and live-attenuated vaccines may be given simultaneously. Exceptions are those against yellow fever and cholera, which should not be given simultaneously or within 3 weeks of each other. Live attenuated vaccines should be given either simultaneously or at least 30 days apart because theoretically the immune responses could be impaired if the live vaccines were given within 30 days of each other. Immune globulin interferes with antibody production of the live attenuated virus vaccines against measles, mumps, and rubella (MMR). Thus it should not be given with MMR vaccine. If immune globulin is given first, the MMR vaccination should be delayed by at least 6 weeks and preferably 3 months to obtain an adequate immunogenic response. When both are needed for travel, it is best to give the MMR vaccine first. The immune globulin can be given closer to the time of travel, at least 2 weeks and preferably 4 weeks after the MMR vaccine. Immune globulin does not interfere with antibody production of the live viral vaccines against polio (oral vaccine) and yellow fever and may be given at the same visit.[57] Vaccines that require multiple doses or early administration include hepatitis B, typhoid, Japanese encephalitis, rabies, yellow fever, and MMR (if immune globulin is to be given near departure).

MALARIA

In visits to developing countries in the tropics, the risk for acquiring malaria from mosquito bites is significant. Even areas where the overall risk is relatively low may have foci of intense transmission. In addition to personal protective measures (Box 19-2), chemoprophylaxis is recommended for travelers to countries where malaria is endemic. *Plasmodium vivax* and *P. falciparum* are the two most abundant species responsible for malaria. The most lethal plasmodium, *P. falciparum,* has developed widespread resistance to chloroquine, the old standard for chemoprophylaxis, and in some areas has developed multidrug resistance. Therefore chemoprophylaxis varies depending on the area of travel.

Chloroquine (Aralen) is still the drug of choice for travelers to the few areas where chloroquine-resistant strains of *P. falciparum* are not a problem (Central America north of Panama, Haiti and the Dominican Republic, and the Middle East), or areas where falciparum malaria does not occur (Egypt and the Middle East). Chloroquine prophylaxis should be given weekly, starting 1 week before travel into a malarial area, and continued for 4 weeks after leaving a malarious region. Chloroquine is passed through the breast milk, although not in sufficient quantities to protect the infant. Therefore a breast-fed infant should receive chloroquine prophylaxis in the standard recommended doses (Table 19-8). Chloroquine is not readily available in a liquid form in the United States. The powder, which is extremely bitter, may be suspended in a syrup or mixed with food. Instant pudding effectively masks the bitter taste and makes the medicine more palatable. An acceptable-tasting syrup is available in most developing countries under the name Nivaquine. Chloroquine should be kept out of the reach of children; as little as 1 g may be fatal in small children.[52] If a toxic chloroquine ingestion occurs, immediate evacuation of the stomach with syrup of ipecac or lavage is indicated, with prompt transport of the child to a medical facility.

In most areas with chloroquine-resistant malaria, pregnant women and children less that 15 kg in weight should take chloroquine weekly and add *proguanil (Paludrine)* daily. Proguanil is not available in the United States but may be purchased in most tropical countries. Nonpregnant woman and children over 15 kg in weight should take *mefloquine (Lariam)* when in most chloroquine-resistant areas. Mefloquine, like chloroquine, is given weekly, starting 1 week before entering a malarious area and continuing for 4

Table 19-6 Travel Vaccines for Children

Vaccine	Give if Recommended for Area of Travel* and:	Dose	Booster	Comments
Typhoid	Age >6 mo Stay >2 wk Eating at nontourist facilities	2 doses, 4 wk apart 6 mo–10 yr: 0.25 ml SC >10 yr: 0.5 ml SC *or* Oral typhoid (if >5 yr) 4 capsules (1 po qod × 4)	Injection booster q 3 yr Oral booster q 5 yr	Injection may cause fever; give acetaminophen prophylactically Oral has less side effects 70%-90% effective
Hepatitis B	Not previously immunized	Recombivax HB 3 doses at 0, 1, 6 mo <11 yr: 0.25 ml IM 11-19 yr: 0.5 ml IM >19 yr: 1 ml IM *or* Engerix-B 3 doses at interval of 0, 1, 6 mo <11 yr: 0.5 ml IM >11 yr: 1 ml IM	?	Some protection after just one or two doses
Immune globulin (IG) for hepatitis A	Stay >2 wk Eating at nontourist facilities	<3 mo stay: 0.02 ml/kg IM (maximum 2 ml) >3 mo stay: 0.06 ml/kg IM (maximum 5 ml)	Booster q 5 mo	Give as close to departure as possible Give IG at least 2 wk (preferably 4 wk) after MMR; MMR should not be given within 6 wk (preferably 3 mo) of IG Hepatitis A vaccine (HAV) may soon be available
Yellow fever	Age >9 mo Not allergic to eggs, pregnant, or immunocompromised	0.5 ml SC at least 10 days before departure	Booster q 10 yr	Available in state-approved travel clinics Do not give within 3 wk of cholera vaccine
Japanese encephalitis	Age >1 yr Stay >3 mo during epidemic season	3 doses at interval of 0, 7, 30 days; 1-3 yr: 0.5 ml SC >3 yr: 1 ml SC	Booster q 2 yr	Children at greatest risk Available in special travel clinics in U.S. and through U.S. consulate of endemic countries 95% effective
Meningococcal	During epidemic season	0.5 ml SC	Booster in 2 yr if first dose was given when <4 yr old	Required for travel to certain parts of Saudi Arabia
Rabies	Stay >3 mo High risk of contact with wild animals Spelunkers	3 doses at interval of 0, 7, 28 days 1 ml IM	None unless post exposure	Children at greater risk If exposed and previously immunized, give vaccine 1 ml IM at 0 and 3 days If exposed and *un*immunized give: Rabies IG 20 IU/kg, half at site and half IM Rabies vaccine, 5 doses, 1 ml at 0, 3, 7, 14, 28 days
Cholera	Age >6 mo Required for entry into some countries, but not routinely recommended by Centers for Disease Control and Prevention or World Health Organization	0.2 ml SC	None	Only 50% effective for only 3-6 mo Do not give within 3 wk of yellow fever vaccine

*See Table 19-5 for up-to-date sources regarding specific travel immunizations recommended for area of travel.

Table 19-7 Recommended Timing and Sequence of Immunizations for Foreign Travel*

4-6 Wk Before Departure	1 Wk After Initial Visit	Week of Departure
Typhoid-inactivated injection† (minimum of 28 days between doses)		Typhoid-inactivated injection† *or* Oral Typhoid (Ty2la)‡ (may be given at first visit)
Japanese encephalitis† (day 0)	Japanese encephalitis† (day 7)	Japanese encephalitis† (day 30)
Rabies† (day 0)	Rabies†(day 7)	Rabies† (day 28)
Yellow fever‡ (more than 10 days before departure and 3 wk before cholera)		Cholera† (may be given at first visit if yellow fever not given)
Meningococcal vaccine† (may be given wk of departure)		Meningococcal vaccine† if indicated and not given at earlier visit
		Immune globulin (IG) for hepatitis A prevention
ROUTINE IMMUNIZATIONS (IF PRIMARY SERIES NOT ALREADY COMPLETED)		
DPT (DT§, P†) at least three doses (primary series) before travel is desired, earliest at 4 wk of age, then every 4 wk until three given; fourth dose may be given 6 mo after third		DPT: additional dose if primary series not yet completed Td if >6 yr old and 10 yr lapse from previous DPT
Hepatitis B† (day 0)		Hepatitis B† (day 28); third dose due in 5 mo
MMR‡ if >6 mo old should have at least one dose (if available, give just measles when between 6 and 12 mo), if school age second dose is desired before travel; if first dose was before 12 mo old then repeated at 15 mo; if IG is also to be administered, give MMR 2 wk (preferably 4 wk) before IG		MMR‡ (if not given at first visit)
OPV‡ at least three doses (primary series) before travel is desired, given every 4 wk until three doses received; if travel starts before 6 wk of age, give an additional dose but do not count as part of primary series		OPV‡: give if primary series not completed or if <7 yr old and more than 6 wk has lapsed since third dose and fourth dose not yet received
Haemophilus b vaccine† given per standard recommendations, no adaptations made for foreign travel		

*Give only immunizations indicated for area of travel, length of stay, type of accommodations, high-risk activities, and beyond a minimum age.
†Inactivated vaccine.
‡Live attenuated virus vaccine.
§Toxoid.

weeks after leaving a malarious area. In Southeast Asia, West Africa, and Papua New Guinea, where multidrug-resistant *P. falciparum* exists, the combination of *proguanil and sulfisoxazole* has been shown to be effective as prophylaxis.[5] This regimen is taken daily and continued for 4 weeks after leaving malarious areas. Sulfisoxazole should not be given to children under 2 months of age or to anyone allergic to sulfa drugs.

Primaquine is an antimalarial drug used to prevent emergence of *P. vivax* and *P. ovale* after heavy exposure or prolonged (many months) exposure to mosquitoes, since routine chemoprophylaxis does not kill the exoerythrocytic stages of these *Plasmodium* species. Primaquine is taken daily for 2 weeks after leaving a malarious area. Primaquine should not be given to anyone with glucose-6-phosphate dehydrogenase (G-6-PD) deficiency.

Pyrimethamine-sulfadoxine (Fansidar) is recommended as a standby for treatment if symptoms of malaria develop.[5] Pyrimethamine-sulfadoxine is given as a one-time dose. Prophylaxis with this drug is not recommended because of the risk of Stevens-Johnson syndrome. Pyrimethamine-sulfadoxine should not be given to an infant less than 2 months old or to anyone allergic to sulfa drugs.

TRAVELER'S DIARRHEA

Traveling to wilderness areas or developing countries requires leaving behind modern sanitation and reliably disinfected tap water. Unfortunately, this places travelers at increased risk for diarrheal illness. Traveler's diarrhea has been reported to affect 25% to 50% of travelers from low-risk to high-risk countries.[48] Traveler's diarrhea has been

Table 19-8 Malaria Chemoprophylaxis

Medication	Indications	Dose
Chloroquine (Aralen)	Travel to chloroquine-sensitive areas (Caribbean, Central America north of Panama, Middle East, Egypt, Iraq, Turkey) Safe for children <15 kg and pregnant women	Given weekly* 5 mg/kg base (8.3 mg/kg salt) up to 300 mg base Liquid form not available in United States; children unable to swallow capsules may mix premeasured powder from capsules with foods such as instant pudding to mask bitter taste
Proguanil (Paludrine)	Add to chloroquine in most chloroquine-resistant area for child <15 kg and pregnant women Not available in United States; may be purchased overseas	Given daily with chloroquine weekly* <2 yr 50 mg 2-6 yr 100 mg 7-10 yr 150 mg >10 yr 200 mg
Mefloquine (Lariam)	Child ≥15 kg in most chloroquine-resistant areas	Given weekly* 15-19 kg ¼ tablet 20-30 kg ½ tablet 31-45 kg ¾ tablet >45 kg 1 tablet
Proguanil plus sulfisoxazole	Multidrug-resistant area, i.e., Southeast Asia, West Africa, Papua New Guinea Avoid in child <2 mo	Proguanil as above, with sulfisoxazole 75 mg/kg/day, daily and continued for 4 weeks after leaving malarious area
Primaquine	After prolonged stay (many months) in malarious area or heavy exposure to mosquitoes in endemic area Avoid if G-6-PD deficient	Given daily 0.3 mg/kg base for 14 days after leaving malarious area
Pyrimethamine-sulfadoxine (Fansidar)	Standby for *treatment* if symptoms of malaria develop Avoid in child <2 mo	Given as a one-time dose 5-10 kg ½ tablet 11-20 kg 1 tablet 21-30 kg 1½ tablets 31-45 kg 2 tablets >45 kg 3 tablets

*Weekly malaria chemoprophylaxis is administered beginning 1 to 2 weeks before entering an endemic area, throughout travel in the area, and for 4 weeks after leaving the endemic area.

defined as greater than three unformed stools in a day, or any number of such stools when accompanied by additional symptoms, such as fever greater than 38° C, abdominal cramping, vomiting, or blood or mucus in the stools.[53] In small children the course tends to be more severe and prolonged, lasting from 3 days to 3 weeks.[53] Traveler's diarrhea can be caused by bacteria, viruses, protozoa, or parasitic worms. Enterotoxigenic *Escherichia coli* organisms are responsible for 50% of traveler's diarrhea. Rotavirus and Norwalk-like viruses account for another 30%.[48] Children's hygiene habits provide increased exposure to these pathogens and place them at higher risk. Preventing diarrhea and other illnesses in remote or foreign areas requires a combination of proper disposal of human waste products, hand washing, dietary precautions, and water disinfection.[2]

Prevention

Standard recommendations for prevention of traveler's diarrhea are based primarily on known potential vehicles for transmission of the illness (see Box 19-3). Transmission is

BOX 19-3

PREVENTION OF TRAVELER'S DIARRHEA

1. Eat only well-cooked vegetables, meats, and seafood.
2. Eat only fruit that you can peel.
3. Drink only disinfected water, carbonated beverages, or hot teas or coffee.
4. Drink or eat only pasteurized dairy products.
5. Use only ice cubes made from disinfected water.
6. Breast feed infants.
7. If using formula prepare with disinfected water or use ready-to-feed.
8. Wash hands before eating or preparing food.
9. Brush teeth with disinfected water.
10. Avoid food from street vendors.

through fecal-oral contamination, with water and food the most common vehicles. Data suggest that careful selection and preparation of food and beverages can decrease the risk of acquiring traveler's diarrhea.[2] Washing hands thoroughly before eating decreases bacterial carriage and also serves as a reminder to children of the need for precautions. The "boil it, cook it, peel it, or forget it" rule implies that all raw vegetables and salads should be avoided, meats and seafood should be well cooked, and fruits need to be properly peeled.[39] Unpasteurized dairly products should be avoided. In developing countries, tap water and ice made from untreated water are not considered safe. Even bottled water is suspect.[6] Bottled and carbonated soft drinks, beer, and wine appear safe. Boiled or otherwise disinfected water should be used for drinking or preparation of formula. Breast feeding is safest for young infants. See Chapter 43 for a complete discussion of water disinfection.

Treatment

The major cause of morbidity and mortality in infants and small children with diarrhea is dehydration. Signs of dehydration in children are listed in Box 19-4. Children young enough to be wearing diapers should be wetting them at least every 8 hours. If not, they should be considered dehydrated. The cornerstone of therapy is oral rehydration, which can be used alone in 90% of cases, especially if instituted early.[62] Parents traveling to developing countries or wilderness areas with children should carry a powdered oral rehydration solution (ORS) or a recipe for a homemade solution (see Box 19-5). Powdered ORS is readily available in most developing countries through the World Health Organization (WHO) and may be obtained in the United States from Jianas Brothers, Kansas City, Missouri (816-421-2880). Rice-based ORS, similar to the one in Box 19-5, has been shown to be more effective than the standard glucose-based ORS and may decrease the stool output by up to 36% in the first 24 hours.[47,55] However, because of hydrolysis of its starches, the rice-based ORS is stable only for 12 hours, after which time it should be discarded and a new solution made.[61]

For rapid rehydration of mild to moderate dehydration, 60 to 90 ml/kg should be administered over the first 4-hour period and repeated until signs of dehydration resolve.[61] The solution should contain 75 to 90 mEq/L sodium and 2% to 2.5% carbohydrate (Table 19-9). If a solution with more than 3% glucose is used, the osmotic pressure exerted by the glucose in the intestinal lumen produces fluid losses greater than absorption, and diarrhea may be exacerbated. Most colas and juices contain nearly 10% to 15% glucose or carbohydrate and consequently are not appropriate rehydration solutions.[24,75] The high sodium concentration in the rehydration solution poses a risk for hypernatremia if the solu-

BOX 19-4

SIGNS OF DEHYDRATION

MILD

Slightly dry mucous membranes
Increased thirst
Decreased urine output

MODERATE

Sunken eyes
Sunken fontanelle
Poor skin turgor
Dry mucous membranes

SEVERE

Signs of moderate dehydration plus one or more of the following:
- Rapid thready pulse
- Cyanosis
- Rapid breathing
- Delayed capillary refill
- Lethargy
- Coma

Modified from Goepp JG, Santosham M: *Prin Pract Pediatr Updates* 1:1, 1993.

BOX 19-5

HOMEMADE ORS*

Mix:
1 tsp (5 g) of salt
1 cup (50 g) of rice cereal
to 1 quart (1 L) of drinking water

Modified from *Med Lett* 33:107, 1991.
*This solution is stable for only 12 hours, after which time it should be discarded and a new solution made.

Table 19-9 Field Treatment of Dehydration

	Rehydration Solution	Maintenance Solution
Volume	60-90 ml/kg/4 hr* (1-1.5 oz/lb/4 hr)	75-150 ml/kg/day* (1-2.5 oz/lb/day)
Electrolytes		
Na^+ (mEq/L)	75-90	50-60
Glucose (%)	2-2.5	2-2.5
K^+ (mEq/L)	20	20
Base (mEq/L)	30	30

Modified from Goepp JG, Santosham M: *Prin Pract Pediatr Updates* 1:1, 1993.
*Add 10 ml/kg or about 4 ounces for each diarrheal stool and 5 ml/kg or about 2 ounces for each bout of emesis.

tion is used for maintenance fluids or to prevent dehydration. For maintaining hydration an ORS given alternately with a low-sodium fluid (water or human milk) will avert hypernatremia. Alternately, a separate solution containing 50 to 60 mEq/L sodium can be used. Maintenance fluid volumes are 75 to 150 ml/kg/day. An additional 10 ml/kg or 4 ounces can be given for each diarrheal stool and 5 ml/kg or 2 ounces for each episode of emesis.[38] If vomiting develops, most children will still tolerate ORS if given in small volumes (5 to 10 ml) every 5 minutes. Feeding of solid food should be continued during and after diarrhea.[9,60] Severe dehydration requires prompt medical attention.

While oral hydration should be the cornerstone of therapy for diarrhea and dehydration, a few medications appear to be helpful. Antibiotic chemoprophylaxis remains controversial for adults and cannot be recommended for children.[33] Treatment at the onset of symptoms of traveler's diarrhea with the combination antibiotic trimethoprim-sulfamethoxazole or with trimethoprim alone reduces the number of unformed stools, duration of illness, and abdominal symptoms in adults.[19] Extrapolating to children, administration of trimethoprim (4 mg/kg/dose) and sulfamethoxazole (20 mg/kg/dose) twice a day for 3 days for acute traveler's diarrhea appears reasonable, and anecdotal evidence suggests that it is efficacious.[48]

Loperamide is an opioid analogue without central effects that has antimotility properties and that appears safe and effective in children. When studied in a group of children 3 months to 3 years at four times the recommended dose (0.8 mg/kg/day compared with standard of 0.2 mg/kg/day), it decreased the duration of diarrhea by approximately 24 hours without adverse side affects.[16] When loperamide was used concomitantly with trimethoprim-sulfamethoxazole in adults with traveler's diarrhea, the duration of diarrhea was decreased from 59 hours to 1 hour.[20] However, any antimotility agent should be stopped if signs of dysentery (blood in the stools or fever higher than 38.4° C) develop.

Bismuth subsalicylate (Pepto-Bismol) has been shown to decrease stool output by 30% when given in a dose of 100 mg/kg/day.[22] This treatment appears safe and effective, giving a peak mean salicylate level of 11.5 mg/dl, well below levels considered toxic (greater than 40 mg/dl). However, this treatment may not be practical because of the large volumes required (1 ml/kg every 4 hours), which could be 6 ounces daily for the average 9-year-old.

Pediatric Wilderness Medical Kits

When a family will be traveling in remote areas, the medical kit must be adapted to meet the special needs of the children. Actual items carried vary depending on the ages of the children and any preexisting medical conditions, length of travel, specific environmental conditions encountered, and medical sophistication of the adults. Although there is considerable room for individual preference in assembling a medical kit, the following discussion focuses on medical problems commonly encountered during wilderness travel with children and on the basic medical supplies (Box 19-6) and medications (Table 19-10) for managing those situations.

To reduce weight and bulk, medications selected for a wilderness medical kit should have multiple uses. For example, diphenhydramine is effective for allergic symptoms, pruritus, and motion sickness and as a sleep aid. Desitin, best known for its use in preventing diaper rash, is also an

BOX 19-6

PEDIATRIC WILDERNESS MEDICAL KIT: BASIC SUPPLIES

- Assorted adhesive bandages
- Butterfly bandages or Steri-Strips
- Gauze pads
- Cotton-tipped applicators
- Gauze roll
- Nonadherent dressings
- Tape
- Moleskin or Spenco 2nd Skin
- Eye patches
- Triangular bandage or sling
- Elastic bandage
- Povidone-iodine solution 10% (use to cleanse wounds and disinfect water)
- Antiseptic wipes (benzalkonium chloride)
- Antibacterial soap
- Tincture of benzoin
- Alcohol wipes
- Lightweight malleable splint (SAM splint)
- Needles
- Safety pins
- Syringe, 20 to 35 cc (for wound irrigation)
- 18-Gauge plastic catheter or irrigation tip (for wound irrigation)
- Bulb syringe
- Digital thermometer
- Scissors
- Tweezers
- Sunscreen waterproof cream, SPF of at least 15
- Insect repellent (no more than 35% DEET)
- First aid book

Table 19-10 Pediatric Wilderness Medical Kit: Medications

Medication	Indications	Dose
TOPICAL MEDICATION		
Antibiotic ointment, i.e., Bacitracin-polymyxin B (Polysporin)	Superficial skin infections	Apply as directed 1-3 times/day
Anesthetic-antipruritic ointment, i.e., pramoxine	Contact dermatitis; bug bites; sunburn	Apply to affected areas 3-4 times/day
Topical corticosteroid, i.e., 1% hydrocortisone	Contact dermatitis; atopic dermatitis; insect bites; sunburn	Apply to affected areas 2-3 times/day (avoid >1% hydrocortisone on face and groin)
Antifungal cream, i.e., miconazole (Micatin)	Yeast diaper dermatitis; athlete's foot; ringworm; jock itch	Apply as directed twice per day
Desitin cream	Irritation diaper rash; sun block	Apply a thin coat as needed for diaper rash; apply a thick coat for sun block
Anesthetic eye drops, i.e., proparacaine ophthalmic*	Removal of superficial ocular foreign body	1 drop in affected eye for removal of foreign body (must protect eye with patch for at least 1 hr after use)
Eyewash	Removal of superficial ocular foreign body	Flush as directed (may improvise with sterile water and flush with syringe)
Antibiotic eye drops, i.e., tobramycin (Tobrex)*	Purulent conjunctivitis; corneal abrasion; otitis externa	Use as directed every 2-4 hr; apply once per day and cover with eye patch for corneal abrasion
ORAL MEDICATION		
Diphenhydramine (Benadryl) 12.5 mg/5 ml elixir 25 mg capsules 50 mg capsules	Allergic symptoms; itching; insomnia; nausea; motion sickness	1.25 mg/kg/dose every 4-6 hr (usually causes drowsiness, may cause hyperactivity and restlessness in children)
Acetaminophen 80 and 160 mg chewable tabs 80 mg/0.8 ml drops 160 mg/5 ml elixir	Fever control; minor aches and pain	10-15 mg/kg/dose every 4-6 hr
Acetaminophen with codeine* 120 mg acetaminophen and 12 mg codeine/5 ml	Severe pain; severe cough	As per acetaminophen or 0.5-1.0 mg/kg/dose codeine every 4-6 hr
Ibuprofen 100 mg/5 ml elixir* 200 mg caplets	Fever control; pain relief	5-10 mg/kg/dose every 6 hr, maximum 40 mg/kg/day
Dimenhydrinate (Dramamine) 12.5 mg/5 ml elixir 50 mg chewable tab	Motion sickness	1-1.5 mg/kg/dose 1 hr before departure and then every 6 hr (may cause drowsiness)
ORAL ANTIBIOTICS (CHOOSE ONE OR TWO)		
Amoxicillin* 125 mg chewable tab 250 mg chewable tab 250 mg capsule	Otitis media; sinusitis; pharyngitis; pneumonia/bronchitis; urinary tract infections	10-15 mg/kg/dose 3 times/day (chewable with pleasant "bubble gum" taste)
Amoxicillin-clavulanate (Augmentin)* 125 mg chewable tab 250 mg chewable tab 250 mg coated tab	As per amoxicillin; animal bites; skin infections; for resistant organisms	10 mg/kg/dose 3 times/day (may cause GI upset and diarrhea; chewable with slightly bitter taste)
Trimethoprim-sulfamethoxazole (TMP/SMX) (Bactrim, Septra)* 40 mg TMP and 200 mg SMX per 5 ml 80 mg TMP and 400 mg SMX scored tab	Otitis media; urinary tract infections; traveler's diarrhea; wounds acquired in an aquatic environment	4 mg/kg/dose TMP and 20 mg/kg/dose SMX twice per day (avoid in infant <2 mo)

*Prescription medication.

Continued.

Table 19-10 Pediatric Wilderness Medical Kit: Medications—cont'd

Medication	Indications	Dose
ORAL ANTIBIOTICS (CHOOSE ONE OR TWO)—cont'd		
Cefixime (Suprax)* 100 mg/5 ml suspension 200 mg coated tab 400 mg coated tab	Otitis media; pharyngitis; bronchitis; urinary tract infections	8 mg/kg/dose once per day (pleasant-tasting liquid; no refrigeration needed; comes as a powder to be mixed with water for oral suspension when needed; discard 14 days after reconstituted)
OTHER PREPARATIONS		
Epinephrine* (premeasured syringe) 0.15 mg EpiPen Jr. 0.3 mg EpiPen	Anaphylaxis; asthma	0.15 mg up to 15 kg; 0.3 mg over 15 kg
Syrup of ipecac	Induce vomiting for certain toxic ingestions	15 ml followed by 1-2 glasses of water, repeated in 20 min if no emesis
Oral rehydration (ORS) packets 1 packet per liter (quart)	Dehydration	60-90 ml/kg over 4 hr, repeat until signs of dehydration resolve
FOREIGN TRAVEL ADD:		
Loperamide (Imodium) 1 mg/5 ml 1 mg caps	Significant diarrhea	0.2-0.8 mg/kg/dose every 6 hr (discontinue if any signs of dysentery develop)
Trimethoprim-sulfamethoxazole*	Traveler's diarrhea; see above	See above
Oral rehydration packets	Dehydration	See above
Permethrin 5% cream (Elimite)*	Lice; scabies	Apply to skin from head to feet, wash off after 8-12 hr
TRAVEL TO HIGH ALTITUDE ADD:		
Acetazolamide (Diamox)*	Recurrent AMS despite graded ascent	5-10 mg/kg/day, up to 500 mg, in 2 doses, start 24 hr before ascent and continue for 48 hr at altitude
Prochlorperazine (Compazine)*	Nausea and vomiting seen with AMS	0.4 mg/kg/day, orally or rectally, in 3-4 divided doses, not recommended for children <2 yr or <10 kg
SNAKE-INFESTED AREAS ADD:		
The Extractor† (a negative-pressure suction device)	Poisonous snakebites	Apply within 3 min of bite

*Prescription medication.
†Sawyer Products, Safety Harbor, Fla.

excellent sun block, since it contains 40% zinc oxide. A broad-spectrum antifungal cream such as miconazole covers not only tineal infections (ringworm, jock itch, and athlete's foot), but also *Candida* infections (diaper rash and vaginitis).

Since most children under 5 cannot swallow pills, liquid or chewable medications are preferred. Most children can chew tablets once their first molars are present (about 15 months). Before that time, chewable medications can be crushed between two spoons and mixed with food. Liquid medications add excess weight and the potential for leaks. If used, they should be stable at room temperature and have a reasonable shelf life. If a child dislikes the taste of medication, it may be camouflaged in a food such as instant pudding, which is easily carried in a powdered form and is often effective at masking bitter tastes.

Painful musculoskeletal injuries are a potential complication of wilderness activities, and pain medication for children should be included in the medical kit.

Acetaminophen not only relieves minor aches and pains but also is effective for fever control. It is well tolerated by most children and available in many pleasant-tasting forms for children unable to swallow pills: chewable 80 mg or 160 mg tabs, an elixir, and concentrated drops.

Ibuprofen appears to be more effective than acetaminophen for pain and fever control. Its duration of action is

6 to 8 hours, compared with 4 to 6 hours for acetaminophen. Ibuprofen is available as 200 mg pills and an elixir (100 mg/5 ml). Currently a prescription is required to obtain the elixir form.

Tylenol with codeine combines the analgesic effects of a centrally acting agent, codeine, with a peripherally acting analgesic, acetaminophen. It is indicated for the treatment of moderate to severe pain. Acetaminophen has the added effect of fever control, while codeine has antitussive properties. Codeine can cause respiratory depression and elevate intracranial pressure, especially in the presence of head injury, and its use should be avoided in situations where this may be a concern.

Two or three antibiotics will cover most bacterial infections encountered in children. All of the following antibiotics provide coverage for otitis media, sinusitis, pneumonia, and urinary tract infections. Some have added indications as noted. Age, allergies, intolerance, and past experience must be taken into account when antibiotics are selected. All oral antibiotics require a prescription.

Amoxicillin-clavulanate (Augmentin) provides excellent coverage for recurrent pharyngitis, soft tissue infections, animal bites, and infections when a resistant organism is anticipated. The most common side effect is diarrhea, with a frequency of 9%. The diarrhea may be lessened with a decrease in the dose. A secondary superinfection, candidal diaper dermatitis, can occur and may be treated with an antifungal cream. Amoxicillin-clavulanate is available in chewable tablets (125 mg and 250 mg) and is given three times per day.

Trimethoprim-sulfamethoxazole (Septra, Bactrim) is recommended for traveler's diarrhea and wounds sustained in an aquatic environment.[1] It is available in a liquid form that does not require refrigeration and is given only twice per day.

Amoxicillin is available in pleasant-tasting chewable tablets (125 mg and 250 mg) and is given three times per day. Amoxicillin is familiar to and well tolerated by most children.

Cefixime (Suprax) is particularly effective for resistant organisms that produce β-lactamase enzymes, as are often seen in otitis and sinusitis. It is available in a powdered form that can be reconstituted with water when needed and does not require refrigeration. However, it starts to lose efficacy 14 days after reconstitution and should be discarded at that time. Cefixime may be given just once per day, and a 10-day course for the average 1-year-old totals less than 2 ounces.

Ciprofloxacin (Cipro), a new quinolone, has a broad spectrum of coverage and is often recommended as an antibiotic of choice for adults. Its use has been discouraged in children because of a potential problem with arthropathic effects on weight-bearing joints; however, a recent study involving more than 600 children has found only a 1.3% rate of reversible arthralgia and no evidence of arthropathy.[63] Ciprofloxacin should not be routinely recommended for children; however, in special situations the benefits of its use may outweigh the risks.

INFANTS AND SMALL CHILDREN

A family traveling with an infant must be particularly vigilant in monitoring their child's state of health. Infants become hypothermic, hyperthermic, septic, and dehydrated more rapidly than adults or older children. A thermometer and appropriate lubricant should be included in the medical kit for monitoring rectal temperature. A temperature over 38° C in a child less than 4 months of age requires evacuation for medical evaluation. Digital oral thermometers are recommended, since they are less likely to break, are easy to read, and are three to four times faster than a glass thermometer. Some emit an audio alarm when the reading is ready.

Infants are less tolerant of problems with excess mucus; a bulb syringe is handy for suctioning mucus from the oropharynx and nasal passages. A few drops of saline solution (¼ tsp of salt in 1 cup of water) instilled into the nares a few minutes before aspiration helps to loosen the mucus. Nasal aspiration should be reserved for times of most need, such as before feeding and sleep, since the procedure can be irritating to the nose and child. Other uses for a clean bulb syringe include flushing foreign bodies from ears and administering enemas.

Away from the conveniences of home, diapers tend to be changed less frequently; consequently, diaper rash may become a problem. A good barrier cream, such as Desitin, may be helpful and should be started at the first signs of irritation. If the rash progresses despite appropriate treatment, an antifungal cream such as miconazole may be used.

Children under 5 years are notorious for putting everything into their mouths, including wild mushrooms, medicines not intended for them from the medical kit, and other toxic substances. Consequently, they need to be watched closely. The medical kit should be kept in a safe place, and syrup of ipecac should be included to treat potential toxic ingestions.

REFERENCES

1. Auerbach PS et al: Bacteriology of the freshwater environment: implications for clinical therapy, *Ann Emerg Med* 9:1016, 1987.
2. Backer HD: Infectious diarrhea from wilderness and foreign travel. In Auerbach PS, Geehr EC, editors: *Management of wilderness and environmental emergencies,* St Louis, 1989, Mosby.
3. Banks B et al: Attitudes of teenagers toward sun exposure and sunscreen use, *Pediatrics* 89:40, 1992.
4. Bar-or O et al: Voluntary hypohydration in 10- to 12-year-old boys, *J Appl Physiol* 48:104, 1980.
5. Barry M: Medical considerations for international travel with infants and older children, *Infect Dis Clin North Am* 6:389, 1992.
6. Blaser MJ: Environmental interventions for the prevention of travelers' diarrhea, *Rev Infect Dis* 8(suppl 2):S142, 1986.
7. Bowman W: Wilderness survival. In Auerbach PS, Geehr EC, editors: *Management of wilderness and environmental emergencies,* St Louis, 1989, Mosby.

8. Brown FE, Spiegel PK, Boyle WE: Digital deformity: an effect of frostbite in children, *Pediatrics* 71:955, 1983.
9. Claeson M, Merson MH: Global progress in the control of diarrheal diseases, *Pediatr Infect Dis J* 9:345, 1990.
10. Committee on Sports Medicine, American Academy of Pediatrics: Climatic heat stress and the exercising child, *Pediatrics* 69:808, 1982.
11. Conrad EU, Rang MC: Fractures and sprains, *Pediatr Clin North Am* 33:1523, 1986.
12. Danks DM, Wevv DW, Allen J: Heat illness in infants and young children, *Br Med J* 2:287, 1962.
13. Danzl DF, Pozos RS, Hamlet MP: Accidental hypothermia. In Auerbach PS, Geehr EC, editors: *Management of wilderness and environmental emergencies,* St Louis, 1989, Mosby.
14. Derslake D: *The stress of hot environments,* Cambridge, Eng, 1972, Cambridge University Press.
15. Dexter W: Hypothermia, *Postgrad Med* 88:55, 1990.
16. Diarrhoeal Disease Study Group: Loperamide in acute diarrhea in childhood: results of a double blind, placebo controlled multicentre clinical trial, *Br Med J* 289:1263, 1984.
17. Downey D, Omer G, Moheb M: New Mexico rattlesnake bites: demographic review and guidelines for treatment, *J Trauma* 31:1380, 1991.
18. Drinkwater BL et al: Response of prepubertal girls and college women to work in the heat, *J Appl Physiol* 43:1046, 1977.
19. Dupont HL et al: Treatment of travelers' diarrhea with trimethoprim/sulfamethoxazole or trimethoprim alone, *N Engl J Med* 307:841, 1982.
20. Ericsson CD et al: Treatment of travelers' diarrhea with sulfamethoxazole and trimethoprim and loperamide, *JAMA* 263:257, 1990.
21. Exertional heat injury, *Med Lett* 23:63, 1981.
22. Figueroa-Quintaanilla D: A controlled trial of bismuth subsalicylate in infants with acute watery diarrheal disease, *N Engl J Med* 328:1653, 1993.
23. Gallagher R: Suntan, sunburn, and pigmentation factors and the frequency of acquired melanocytic nevi in children, *Arch Dermatol* 126:770, 1990.
24. Goepp J, Santosham M: Oral rehydration therapy, *Princ Pract Pediatr Updates* 1:1, 1993.
25. Gonzalo M et al: Acute renal failure due to multiple stings by Africanized bees, *Ann Intern Med* 104:210, 1986.
26. Grissom CK et al: *Acetazolamide in the treatment of acute mountain sickness: clinical efficacy and effect on gas exchange.* Abstract from Sixth Annual Scientific Meeting of the Wilderness Medical Society, July 14-20, 1990, Snowbird, Utah, Wilderness Medical Society.
27. Guidelines for cardiopulmonary resuscitation and emergency cardiac care, *JAMA* 268:2199, 1992.
28. Hackett PH, Roach RC, Sutton JR: High altitude medicine. In Auerbach PS, Geehr EC, editors: *Management of wilderness and environmental emergencies,* St Louis, 1989, Mosby.
29. Haymes EM, McCormick RJ, Buskirk ER: Heat tolerance of exercising lean and obese prepubertal boys, *J Appl Physiol* 39:457, 1975.
30. Heggars JP et al: Experimental and clinical observations on frostbite, *Ann Emerg Med* 16:1056, 1987.
31. Houston CS: Incidence of acute mountain sickness at intermediate altitudes (letter), *JAMA* 261:3551, 1989.
32. Hughes G: Synergistic effects of oral nonsteroidal drugs and topical corticosteroids in the therapy of sunburn in humans, *Dermatology* 184:54, 1992.
33. Johnson PC, Dupont HL, Ericsson CD: Chemoprophylaxis and chemotherapy of travelers' diarrhea in children, *Pediatr Infect Dis* 4:620, 1985.
34. Johnson TS, Rock PB: Acute mountain sickness, *N Engl J Med* 319:841, 1988.
35. Kaidbey K: The photoprotective potential of the new superpotent sunscreens, *J Am Acad Dermatol* 22:449, 1990.
36. Kaplan LA: *Wilderness dermatology: an overview.* Abstract, Third Annual Winter Wilderness Medicine, March 24, 1993, Sun Valley, Idaho.
37. Kelly K et al: Profound accidental hypothermia and freeze injury of the extremities in a child, *Crit Care Med* 18:679, 1990.
38. Kleinman R: We have the solution: now what's the problem? *Pediatrics* 90:113, 1992.
39. Kozicki M, Steffen R, Shar M: "Boil it, cook it, or forget it": does this rule prevent travelers diarrhea? *Int J Epidemiol* 14:169, 1985.
40. Kulka JP: Observations on non-freezing cold injury of the mouse ear, *Angiology* 12:491, 1961.
41. Lamberg SE, Mulrennan JA: Bullous reaction to diethyl toluamide (DEET), *Arch Dermatol* 100:582, 1969.
42. Levin EB: Middle ear disease. In Hoekelman RA, editor: *Principles of pediatrics: health care of the young,* New York, 1978, McGraw-Hill.
43. Levine BD et al: Dexamethasone in the treatment of acute mountain sickness, *N Engl J Med* 321:1707, 1989.
44. Lillie TH, Schreck CE, Rahe AJ: Effectiveness of personal protection against mosquitoes in Alaska, *J Med Entomol* 25:475, 1988.
45. Litovitz TL, Holm KC, Clancy C: 1992 annual report of the American Association of Poison Control Centers toxic exposure surveillance systems, *Am J Emerg Med* 11:494, 1993.
46. Moffet HI: General concepts. In *Pediatric infectious diseases,* Philadelphia, 1975, JB Lippincott.
47. Mota-Hernandez F: Rice solution and World Health Organization solution by gastric infusion for high stool output diarrhea, *Am J Dis Child* 145:937, 1991.
48. Nahlen BL et al: International travel and the child younger than two years. II. Recommendation for prevention of traveler's diarrhea and malaria chemoprophylaxis, *Pediatr Infect Dis J* 8:735, 1989.
49. Olson LG, Hensley MJ, Saunders NA: Augmentation of ventilatory response to asphyxia by prochlorperazine in humans, *J Appl Physiol* 53:637, 1982.
50. Reference deleted in proofs.
51. *Pertussis: report of the Committee on Infectious Diseases,* Elk Grove Village, Ill, 1991, American Academy of Pediatrics.
52. *Physicians' desk reference,* ed 46, Montvale, NJ, 1992, Medical Economics Data.
53. Pitzinger B: Incidence and clinical features of traveler's diarrhea in infants and children, *Pediatr Infect Dis J* 10:719, 1991.
54. Pope D et al: Benign pigmented nevi in children, *Arch Dermatol* 128:1201, 1992.
55. Rahnan A: Rice-ORS shortens the duration of watery diarrhoeas, *Trop Geogr Med,* 1990, p 230.
56. Reisman RE: Stinging insect allergy, *J Allergy Clin Immunol* 64:3, 1979.
57. *Report of the Committee on Infectious Disease,* Elk Grove Village, Ill, 1991, American Academy of Pediatrics.
58. Robbins PJ, Cherniack MG: Review of the biodistribution and toxicity of the insect repellent *N,N*-diethyl-m-toluamide (DEET), *J Toxicol Environ Health* 18:503, 1986.
59. Robinson MD, Seward PN: Heat injury in children, *Pediatr Emerg Care* 3:114, 1987.
60. Salahuddin S: A traditional diet as part of oral rehydration therapy in severe acute diarrhoea in young children, *J Diarrh Dis Res* 9(3):258, 1991.
61. Santosham M: A comparison of rice-based oral rehydration solution and "early feeding" for the treatment of acute diarrhea in infants, *J Pediatr* 166:868, 1990.
62. Santosham M, Brown KH, Sack RB: Oral rehydration therapy and dietary therapy for acute childhood diarrhea, *Pediatr Rev* 8:273, 1987.
63. Schaad U: Role of the new quinolones in pediatric practice, *Pediatr Infect Dis J* 11:1043, 1992.
64. Schreck CE, Kline DL: Personal protection afforded by controlled-release topical repellents and permethrin-treated clothing against natural populations of *Aedes taeniorhynchus, J Am Mosq Control Assoc* 5:77, 1989.
65. Schreck CE, Snoddy EL, Spielman A: Pressurized sprays of perme-

thrin or DEET on military clothing for personal protection against *Ixodes dammini, J Med Entomol* 28:396, 1986.

66. Scoggin CH et al: High-altitude pulmonary edema in the children and young adults of Leadville, Colorado, *N Engl J Med* 297:1269, 1977.
67. Sholdt LL et al: Field bioassays of permethrin-treated uniforms and a new extended duration repellant against mosquitoes in Pakistan, *J Am Mosq Control Assoc* 4:233, 1988.
68. Sophocles AM, Bachman J: High-altitude pulmonary edema among visitors to Summit County, Colorado, *J Fam Pract* 17:1015, 1983.
69. *Sports participation in 1990: series 1,* Mt Prospect, Ill, 1990, National Sporting Goods Association.
70. Squire DL: Heat illness: fluid and electrolyte issues for pediatric and adolescent athletes, *Pediatr Clin North Am* 37:1085, 1990.
71. Stern RS, Weinstein MC, Baker SG: Risk reduction for nonmelanoma skin cancer with childhood sunscreen use, *Arch Dermatol* 122:537, 1986.
72. Sullivan JB: Snakebite. In Callaham ML, editor: *Current therapy in emergency medicine,* Philadelphia, 1987, BC Decker.
73. Taj-Eldin S, Falaki N: Heat illness in infants and small children in desert climates, *J Trop Med Hyg* 71:100, 1968.
74. Tenenbein M: Severe toxic reactions and death following the ingestion of diethyltoluamide-containing insect repellents, *JAMA* 258:1509, 1987.
75. The management of acute diarrhea in children: oral rehydration, maintenance, and nutritional therapy, *MMWR* 41:1992.
76. Theis MK et al: Acute mountain sickness in children at 2835 meters, *Am J Dis Child* 147:143, 1993.
77. Thomas WC et al: Iodine disinfection of water, *Arch Environ Health* 19:124, 1969.
78. US Environmental Protection Agency: *N,N*-Diethyl-m-toluamide (DEET), Pesticide Registration Standard, Washington, DC, 1980, Office of Pesticide and Toxic Substances.
79. Valentine MD: Insect venom allergy: diagnosis and treatment, *J Allergy Clin Immunol* 73:299, 1984.
80. Valentine MD, Lichtenstein LM: Anaphylaxis and stinging insect hypersensitivity, *JAMA* 258:2881, 1987.
81. Wagner JA et al: Heat tolerance and acclimatization to work in the heat in relation to age, *J Appl Physiol* 33:616, 1972.
82. White R, Weber R: Poisonous snakebite in Central Texas, *Ann Surg* 213:466, 1991.
83. Wolff J: Iodide goiter and the pharmacologic effects of excess iodide, *Am J Med* 47:101, 1969.
84. Wyler D: Malaria chemoprophylaxis for the traveler, *N Eng J Med* 329:31, 1993.
85. Zanetti R: Cutaneous melanoma and sunburns in childhood in a southern European population, *Eur J Cancer* 28A:1172, 1992.

ADDITIONAL RECOMMENDED READINGS

Brody J: *Jane Brody's good food book,* New York, 1987, Bantam.

Castle S: *The complete new guide to preparing baby foods,* New York, 1992, Bantam.

Cornell J: *Sharing nature with children,* Nevada City, Calif, 1979, Dawn Publications.

Doan M: *Starting small in the wilderness,* San Francisco, 1979, Sierra Club.

Euser B: *Take 'em along,* Evergreen, Colo, 1987, Cordillera Press.

Foster L: *Take a hike!* San Francisco, 1991, Sierra Club.

Hodgson M: *Wilderness with children,* Harrisburg, Pa, 1992, Stackpole Books.

Silverman G: *Backpacking with babies and small children,* Berkeley, Calif, 1986, Wilderness Press.

Sisson E: *Nature with children of all ages,* New York, 1982, Prentice-Hall.

20 WOMEN IN THE WILDERNESS

Joseph F. Mortola
Gunhilde M. Buchsbaum

Increasing numbers of women have become participants in both vocational and recreational expeditions to remote areas for extended intervals of time. Experience from these excursions has indicated that women and men exhibit far more similarities than differences in their ability to withstand novel environments. However, significant disparities in cardiovascular, pulmonary, and metabolic physiology between men and women mandate that different adaptations occur during acclimation. Moreover, women bring an exquisitely sensitive neuroendocrine system and more complex reproductive anatomy to the wilderness environment.

In the context of their neuroendocrine system, women demonstrate more dramatic adaptation to physically and psychologically stressful situations. The most obvious of these adaptations is induction of a cascade of endocrine events that serve as endogenous contraception[124] and result in complete amenorrhea in up to 20% of elite athletes.[31] This neuroendocrine response protects women from the dangers of pregnancy and the demands of neonates, which may constitute a significant threat to survival during extreme environmental contingencies. Many of the unique challenges encountered by women in the wilderness are the result of incomplete expressions of this adaptive endogenous contraceptive response. The manifestations include a variety of menstrual cycle abnormalities that may be encountered during strenuous physical activity. Other challenges result from physiologic differences between men and women.

Preparation for Women on Wilderness Expeditions

CARDIOVASCULAR ACCLIMATION

On average, women have smaller bodies than men. Mean differences in acclimation to wilderness environments between women and men result more from disparity in overall size and body surface area than from intrinsic sexual dimorphism. With respect to cardiovascular function, women have lower mean stroke volume, cardiac index, and end-diastolic and end-systolic left venticular volume. Although the *efficiency* of cardiac activity, as measured by indexes that correct for heart size, is similar between sexes,[119] women at rest maintain total oxygen delivery and blood flow at levels similar to men by compensating for the lower stroke volume with increased heart rate. After a number of variables are controlled for, women have heart rates that average 6 to 14 beats/min higher than age-matched men.[47] This relationship is least consistent in young adults, however, where several studies have shown that young men may actually have higher heart rates than women.[59] With advancing age, stroke volume, cardiac index, and end-diastolic and end-systolic volumes decline in both sexes. However, the rate of decline is more rapid in men,[59] so that older men and women show fewer differences than do their younger counterparts.

The disparity between younger men and women in cardiovascular parameters is highly dependent on exercise training. In sedentary individuals, for instance, the stroke index (which is a measure of stroke volume corrected for body size) increases significantly more in men than in women who go from supine rest to maximal upright exercise. This difference is less pronounced when women and men who have undergone endurance training are compared.[140] A similar phenomenon occurs when the primary measure of aerobic power, $\dot{V}O_2max$, is compared between sedentary and trained men and women. The lower $\dot{V}O_2max$ in sedentary women, however, may account for this more rapid adaptation to acute hypoxia.[103] Taken together, current evidence indicates that women undergoing vigorous physical activity can increase their performance dramatically by endurance training. On average, because of their smaller size, more endurance training is likely to be necessary than for men to achieve maximal aerobic capacity.

THERMAL ACCLIMATION

Women adapt more easily to hot, wet environments than do men. This results from a lower sweat rate than in men of equal fitness and size, which decreases the risk of dehydration.[64] In contrast, the higher sweat rate in men is more advantageous in hot, dry environments where perspiration decreases the risk of hyperthermia, provided ample fluid replacement is available. Once acclimated to dry heat, women substantially increase their sudorific response and have sweat and body weight losses equal to those of men.[130] Evidence suggests that once acclimated to such an environment, women actually perform better. For women planning wilderness expeditions to hot dry environments, acclimation is of paramount importance. This can occur with a 2-week training interval in a hot environment. A similar acclimation to heat may occur if the training is done in temperate environments (21° C), but requires 8 to 11 weeks.[48]

On average, women in cold environments adapt better than do men. This may be due to part to thicker subcutaneous fat. Decreased insulation that results from the lower muscle mass of women may be disadvantageous only at extremes of temperature. Although adaptation to cold environments is more dependent on body size, physical fitness, and degree of acclimation than on sex itself,[50] exercise performed during cold exposure has been shown to be more effective in maintaining body heat in women than in men.[88]

ADAPTATION TO WILDERNESS ENVIRONMENTS DURING PREGNANCY

Pregnancy constitutes a state in which multiple physiologic adaptations occur to accommodate the needs of a growing fetus. Cardiac output and oxygen consumption are increased at rest. During exercise, manifestations of decreased respiratory reserves, including lower carbon dioxide production and a decreased respiratory exchange rate,[97] may become apparent. This predisposes to a decreased tolerance for anaerobic exercise in untrained women during the second and third trimesters.[6] However, steady maintenance of an exercise program during pregnancy actually decreases the amount of oxygen required to perform a similar task in the nonpregnant state.[25] Therefore pregnant women in wilderness environments may perform as well as or better than in the nonpregnant state, provided that endurance training is steadily maintained throughout the pregnancy.

Because pregnancy sometimes has unpredictable complications, appropriate evacuation contingencies are particularly important. Prenatal care should be continued during wilderness expeditions. During the second and third trimesters, weekly blood pressure monitoring should be performed. A blood pressure greater than 140/90 mm Hg recorded after 15 minutes of rest indicates that evacuation is required because of developing preeclampsia. Auscultation of the fetal heart is performed monthly, with an expected rate between 120 and 160 beats/min. In the absence of a complication such as preeclampsia, there is no evidence that exercise in pregnancy is detrimental to the developing fetus.[29,78]

ANEMIA PROPHYLAXIS

Several aspects of female reproductive function predispose to anemia. Normal cyclic vaginal bleeding results in mean hemoglobin ranges that are significantly lower in women (12 to 16 g/dl) than in men (14 to 18 g/dl). Not infrequently, women with dysfunctional uterine bleeding or anatomic uterine defects, such as uterine myomas, are significantly more anemic. Because of the demands of wilderness expeditions, anemia can constitute a serious health risk, particularly at high altitudes.[51] There is some evidence that women are more susceptible to acute mountain sickness (AMS) than are men.[52,53] AMS in mild form includes headaches, anorexia, nausea, and malaise. More severe forms include altered consciousness, ataxia, pulmonary edema, and coma. The specific manifestation of pulmonary edema as a feature of severe AMS appears to be less common in women.[117] Women living at high altitudes have a lower incidence of chronic mountain polycythemia than do men,[72] perhaps as a result of lower hematocrit. During pregnancy, however, a fourfold higher incidence of toxemia is noted at high altitudes.[96] For this reason prolonged high-altitude exposure is not recommended for pregnant women. Regardless of altitude, women embarking on wilderness expeditions should have a hematocrit test to determine red blood cell volume at least 1 month before departure. In the event that anemia is recognized and iron deficiency is determined to be the cause, supplementation should be prescribed at a dose of 300 mg of ferrous sulfate three times a day. The predominant side effect is constipation, so the dose must be titrated to minimize this uncomfortable symptom.

In addition to lower hematocrit values in most women, iron deficiency is more common in women during periods of sustained strenuous exercise and physical activity. Iron supplementation has been shown not only to increase iron stores in elite athletes, but also to improve their exercise capacity as measured by oxygen consumption ($\dot{V}O_2max$). Three hundred milligrams a day is more than sufficient to achieve these beneficial effects in women who are not anemic.[85]

GYNECOLOGIC PREPARATION

Gynecologic examination of a woman preparing for a strenuous wilderness experience is directed at detecting preventable difficulties. Particular attention is directed to examination of the uterus to detect the presence of fibroids that may result in irregular, profuse, and hormonally unresponsive bleeding. In addition, careful adnexal examination should be performed to detect ovarian masses that may rupture acutely during strenuous exercise. For the most part these masses are physiologic cysts that respond to gonadotropin suppression by oral contraceptive agents.

All women who are sexually active should have a test for early pregnancy detection before a wilderness expedition. Pregnancy is not a contraindication to involvement in an expedition, provided the fetus is at least 8 weeks' gestational age and clearly demonstrated by ultrasonographic examination to be intrauterine. Ruptured ectopic pregnancies are a clearly preventable potential cause of mortality in women remote from medical care.[36,37] Moreover, pregnancies earlier than 8 weeks carry a 25% chance of miscarriage[126] and may pose an unacceptably high risk of serious hemorrhage if travel is remote from an area where dilatation and curettage to control hemorrhage are available.

Contraception is recommended in women undertaking wilderness expeditions because it serves two important purposes. The first is the prevention of early pregnancy occurring just before or during the trip. The risks of early pregnancy remote from medical care have been discussed. For this indication, any effective method of contraception is suitable. The second advantage is the prevention of irregular, dangerous, and sometimes difficult to diagnose uterine bleeding. This latter prophylaxis is available only through the use of hormonal contraceptive agents. Three methods of hormonal contraception are available: the oral contraceptive pill, indwelling slow release progestin formulation (Norplant), and injectable progestin (Depo-Provera). The last compound was approved in the United States for contraception only in 1993.[110]

For a woman planning an expedition who is not currently using a hormonal contraceptive, the oral contraceptive pill is the agent of choice. These agents are associated with less uterine bleeding than the progestational agents Norplant and Depo-Provera. The large variety of oral contraceptive formulations available can be divided into three categories: monophasic pills, multiphasic pills, and progestin-only pills (the "mini-pill"). Of these the progestin-only pills are associated with the highest incidence of unpredictable and irregular vaginal bleeding and are therefore the least desirable. The selection of either a monophasic or biphasic formulation depends primarily on patient and physician preference.

In the event that a patient cannot tolerate the oral contraceptive pill, either because of a medical contraindication or because of undesirable side effects, barrier methods are recommended. There appears to be little justification for attempting either Norplant or Depo-Provera unless a 6-month trial before the expedition is possible. The trial is recommended to identify subjects susceptible to abnormal uterine bleeding.

BOX 20-1

BASIC SUPPLIES FOR WOMEN'S HYGIENE

Sanitary napkins or tampons
Plastic bags for tampon storage
Toilet paper (store in plastic bag)
Cotton underwear
Lady-J Urinal Guide (available from Campmor, Paramus, N.J.) if long periods of poor weather are anticipated
Vaginal speculum (if trained medical professional accompanies expedition)

Concern exists regarding increased thrombotic potential of estrogen compounds* contained in both monophasic and multiphasic oral contraceptives. Extensive study has demonstrated that serious thrombotic events are not significantly increased before the age of 35[105] and lethal events have no greater incidence in women between the age of 35 and menopause who do not smoke.[107] However, the interactive effects of the thrombogenic potential of oral contraceptive agents and the higher incidence of thrombosis that may accompany high-altitude exposure[34,113,114] have not been studied. In women undergoing high-altitude exposure the unknown risk of increased thromboembolism may not be justified based on the rationale of eliminating gynecologic emergencies. At present the birth control pill should not be routinely recommended for such expeditions.

MEDICAL AND HYGIENE SUPPLIES FOR WILDERNESS EXPEDITIONS INVOLVING WOMEN

Because women have more complex reproductive systems than men, appropriate supplies make wilderness expeditions more comfortable. The supplies recommended during wilderness travel are given in Box 20-1.

Table 20-1 provides a list of medications that are particularly important on expeditions when women are involved. These are used to treat the most common problems, including dysmenorrhea, urinary tract infections, vaginitis, and irregular uterine bleeding. Also included is a pregnancy test kit.

Physiologic Adaptations to Physically Stressful Environments

BONE STRENGTH

Increasing attention has been devoted to the study of bone strength in women. Normative data indicate that at all

*References 3, 13, 21, 100, 125, 139.

Table 20-1 Medicines Specific to Women's Health

Medication	Indication	Dose	Length of Trip (hr)
Acetaminophen 325 mg	Dysmenorrhea	1-2 every 3-4 hr	>24
Trimethoprim-sulfamethoxazole* double strength	Urinary infection	1 twice a day for 3 days	>72
Ampicillin* 250 mg	Urinary infection	1 four times a day for 7 days	>72
Metronidazole† 250 mg	Nonyeast vaginitis	1 three times a day for 7 days	>72
Miconazole cream	Yeast vaginitis	Nightly for 3 nights	>24
Estrogen 2.5 mg	Nonpregnant irregular vaginal bleeding	1 twice a day	>48
Pregnancy test kit	Irregular vaginal bleeding	As needed	>48

*Trimethoprim-sulfamethoxazole is contraindicated in individuals with sulfa allergy, and ampicillin is contraindicated in individuals allergic to penicillin.
†Metronidazole (Flagyl) has not been shown to be safe in pregnancy. The other medications suggested may be used in both pregnant and nonpregnant patients.

ages of adult life women have lower bone density than men.[69] In younger years these differences are of little clinical consequence under most circumstances. However, after menopause, women undergo greatly accelerated bone loss.[58,61,76,95] To some degree this loss of bone can be retarded by weight-bearing exercise[116] and calcium supplementation.[54,106] With respect to fracture risk, vigorous physical activity is a double-edged sword. On the one hand, exercise promotes bone strength.[4,71] On the other hand, it increases the risk of fracture by increasing exposure of bones to trauma. The extent to which exercise and calcium protect against bone loss depends on nonenvironmental factors.[60] Family history of osteoporosis and race are risk factors for osteoporosis; white and Asian women are more susceptible than blacks.

Estrogen administration has been definitively shown to maintain bone strength in postmenopausal women[75,99] and therefore presumably to decrease fracture risk.[46] In this regard, estrogen is more effective than either calcium or exercise.[115] Even active postmenopausal women should be prescribed estrogen supplementation, provided no contraindications exist. These include previous breast or uterine cancer or previous thromboembolic events. Menopausal women who have not had a hysterectomy also require progestin supplementation as prophylaxis against the endometrial hyperplasia and carcinoma that may result from unopposed estrogen. The most extensively studied estrogen-progestin regimen includes 0.625 mg of conjugated equine estrogen (Premarin) on days 1 through 25 of each month and 10 mg of medroxyprogesterone acetate (Provera) on days 16 through 25. With this schedule, menses reliably occurs during the last few days of each calendar month. In the case of wilderness or remote travel involving menopausal women, this is optimal treatment. A variety of other schedules have been proposed for maintenance of bone strength. These include continuous daily administration of conjugated equine estrogens and medroxyprogesterone acetate. When this regimen is used, the dose of medroxyprogesterone acetate can be reduced to 2.5 mg/day. This is particularly suited to women who experience mood changes and breast tenderness when taking higher doses of progestin. On this schedule, women eventually cease menstruation. However, in some women up to 1 year of therapy may be required to achieve sufficient endometrial atrophy to result in complete amenorrhea. During this time, bleeding may occur at irregular and unpredictable times. It is therefore less well suited to women on vigorous journeys remote from medical care.

In younger women, particularly distance runners, the absence of menstrual periods signals a state of estrogen deprivation. After 1 to 3 years of this condition, dramatic declines in bone density have been observed.[17] This places young women at a greatly increased risk for stress fractures.[87] To minimize these risks, a strong recommendation for oral contraceptives is made. To be maximally effective in preventing osteoporosis, estrogen therapy (such as with the birth control pill) should be instituted as early as possible after the onset of a 6-month period of amenorrhea. Alternatively, a combined cyclic combination of conjugated equine estrogens and medroxyprogesterone acetate may be prescribed, as advocated for postmenopausal women. The latter is preferable for women who show poor tolerance to oral contraceptive agents because of either physical or mood-related side effects.

NORMAL MENSTRUAL CYCLICITY

Menstrual cycle disturbances are more common during wilderness expeditions. These result from the physical and psychologic stresses that attend such demanding experiences. An understanding of normal menstrual cycle physiology is therefore relevant.

The normal menstrual cycle is the result of a complex series of integrated events that involve the hypothalamus, pituitary gland, ovary, and uterus (Fig. 20-1). The pivotal

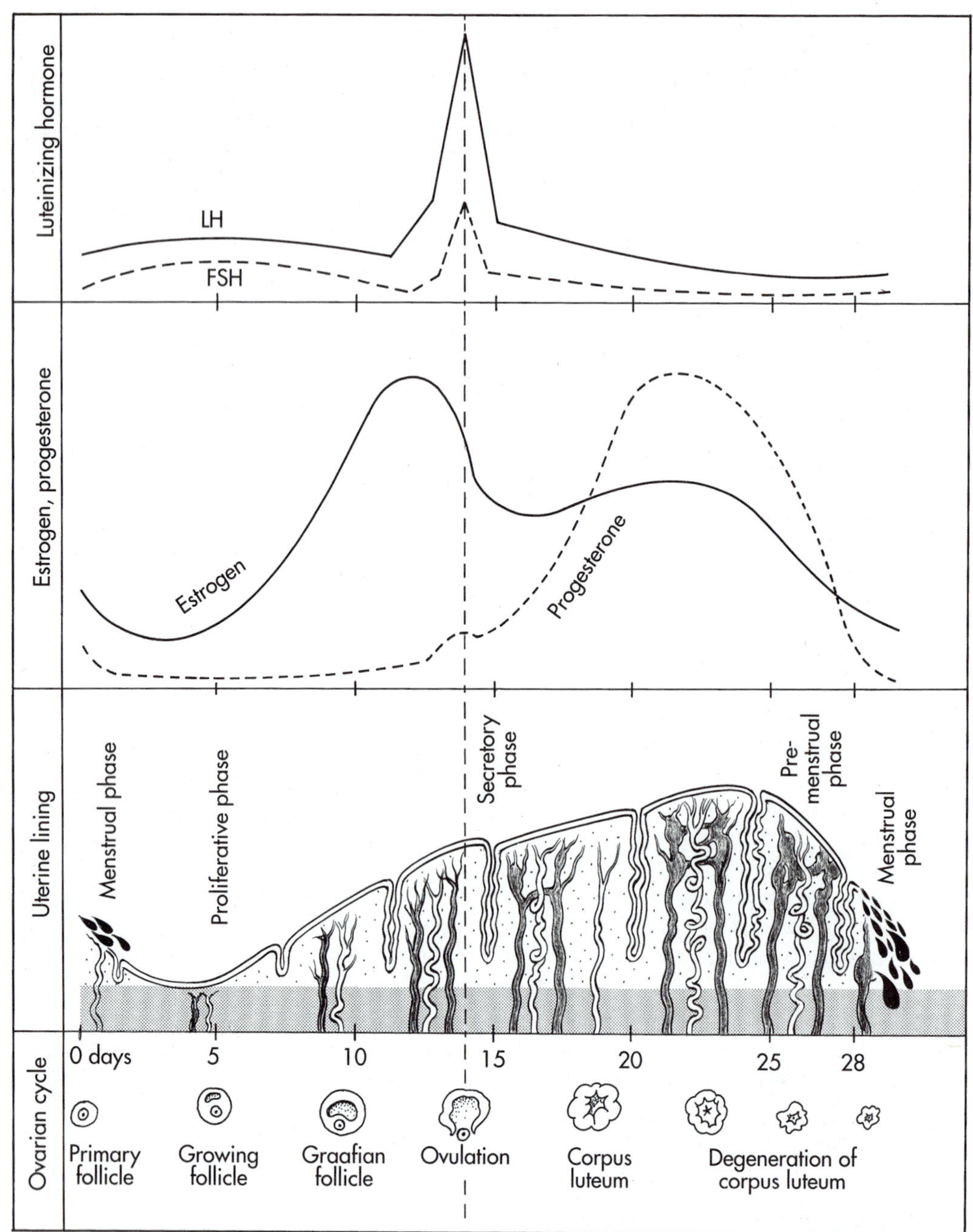

Fig. 20-1 Diagrammatic representation of normal human ovarian and endometrial cycle. (Redrawn from Shaw ST Jr, Roche PC: Menstruation. In Finn CA, editor: *Oxford reviews of reproduction and endocrinology,* vol 2, Oxford, Eng, 1980, Oxford University Press.)

event in the normal menstrual cycle is generation of the midcycle luteinizing hormone (LH) surge. This surge is generated when a critical level of estradiol is produced by the ovary.[136] Estradiol levels in this critical range exert positive feedback on the LH-producing gonadotrophs in the pituitary. At lower levels and at supraphysiologic levels the feedback of estradiol on LH secretion is inhibitory.[135] It is only within the critical midrange that feedback of estradiol facilitates pituitary release of LH. This triphasic effect of estrogen, although well documented empirically, is poorly understood.[22]

Ovarian production of estrogen essential to normal menstrual cyclicity is the result of an interaction between two cell types.[56] The thecal cell, which is located in the ovarian stroma, is LH responsive and produces androgens.[94] The granulosa cell is primarily follicle-stimulating hormone

(FSH) responsive. Under the influence of this gonadotropin the granulosa cell converts androgens to estrogen by aromatization of the first ring of the androgen molecule.[121] Thus, for menstrual cyclicity to occur, trophic stimuli from the pituitary (LH and FSH) must be supplied to the ovary.[93] The essential trigger for release of pituitary LH and FSH is pulsatile delivery of gonadotropin-releasing hormone (GnRH) from the hypothalamus.[67] In most human experiments the frequency of pulsatile release of hypothalamic GnRH is inferred from circulating concentrations of LH. GnRH itself has an extremely short half-life and appears in the peripheral circulation in essentially unmeasurable amounts.[9] In contrast, circulating serum levels of LH show distinct oscillations over the course of the day. Such oscillations are referred to as pulses. Extensive animal data have demonstrated that a peripherally detected pulse of LH bears a one-to-one temporal relationship with a hypothalamic burst of GnRH.[27,74] Although GnRH is also a potent releaser of FSH, the long half-life of FSH[28] in the peripheral circulation does not permit precise identification of discrete bursts of the hormone. For this reason the frequency of GnRH bursts from the hypothalamus is better inferred from the measurement of circulating LH.[70] If the hypothalamic frequency of GnRH is sufficiently reduced, inadequate pituitary release of LH and, probably more important, FSH will ensue.[68] Under these circumstances insufficient estradiol production by the ovary is observed and normal menstrual cyclicity cannot occur.

Within the ovary during the first half of the menstrual cycle, FSH acts not only to induce aromatase, which converts androgens to estrogens, but also to induce granulosa cell proliferation. The proliferation results in more FSH receptor[83] in the dominant follicle[92] and thereby stimulates further growth.[57] Each follicle contains an oocyte. The development of the oocyte is arrested during meiosis until follicular growth occurs.[91,120] Thus, during the first half of the menstrual cycle (follicular phase), both oocyte maturation and estradiol production occur. At the end of the follicular phase the granulosa cell acquires LH receptors,[138] which earlier in the cycle were present only on the theca cell. The acquisition of these receptors permits ovulation in response to the LH surge.[123]

During the second half of the cycle (luteal phase), the steroidogenesis of the ovary changes so that large amounts of progesterone, as well as estradiol, are produced.[84] The majority of this progesterone production is from the remaining cells of the structure, which constituted the dominant follicle in the earlier part of the cycle.[90] The steroidogenic structure in the second half of the cycle is termed the corpus luteum.[2] Although progesterone has a variety of physiologic functions, the most important is adequate preparation of the endometrium to accept implantation of a fertilized embryo. Continued production of progesterone depends on LH from the pituitary gland.[49] The pulsatile pattern of this LH is markedly different from that seen during the follicular phase. The luteal phase LH secretion is characterized by infrequent but robust LH pulses. The mean pulse frequency during the middle of the luteal phase is once every 216 minutes, as compared with once every 72 minutes in the middle of the follicular phase.[39] Despite continued LH secretion, the corpus luteum has a finite life span.[63] If pregnancy occurs, the 2-week life span of the corpus luteum is extended for several additional weeks by human chorionic gonadotropin (hCG),[30] a hormone produced by the developing placenta.[102] In the absence of hCG the corpus luteum begins to decline 7 days after ovulation and estrogen and progesterone production decline.

It is the decline in the levels of estrogen and progesterone that results in menstrual bleeding when pregnancy does not occur.[55] The effect of estrogen on the endometrium is to induce proliferation.[66] During the follicular phase of the cycle the estrogen-dominant environment results in endometrial growth. During the luteal phase, progesterone decreases estrogen receptors and proliferation is markedly reduced. The effect of progesterone, however, is to transform the endometrium into a structure with increasing glandular complexity[134] and increasing secretory activity.[101] This secretory activity is optimal for implantation. At the end of the cycle, when production of both estrogen and progesterone by the corpus luteum is decreasing, the endometrium undergoes degeneration and menstrual bleeding ensues.

MENSTRUAL CYCLE ABNORMALITIES IN THE ATHLETE

Highly trained athletes, such as those who often participate in demanding wilderness experiences, have a high incidence of menstrual cycle abnormalities.[80] In 1976 more than half of the women athletes competing in the Olympic Games reported menstrual cycle irregularity,[137] as compared with only 10% in the Tokyo Olympics in 1964.[128] Whether this represented an increase in the true incidence of abnormalities or greater reporting is uncertain. The highest rates of abnormal menstrual cycles have been reported in distance runners, among whom the incidence of amenorrhea reaches 50% (Fig. 20-2).[111] Increased menstrual abnormalities have also been reported in swimmers,[86] ballet dancers,[65] and field athletes. The incidence of amenorrhea appears to depend on the type of sport undertaken.[132] In runners and ballet dancers the incidence of amenorrhea correlates with the degree of physical exertion.[109] In swimmers, however, the incidence of amenorrhea is lower and remains at approximately 12% regardless of the intensity of exercise. It appears that exercise, even at more moderate levels, is associated with increased menstrual dysfunction.[38] Joggers who completed 5 to 30 miles per week had fewer menses per year than did their sedentary counterparts.[33] In 1985 Bullen and co-workers[15] demonstrated that women exposed to a graded rigorous exercise program had incidences of anovulation that reached 42% when unaccompanied by weight loss, and as high as 63% in the presence of weight loss. These figures compared with a 10.6% incidence in the general population.

In a classic study by Frisch and associates,[43] menarche was delayed an average of 3 years in ballet dancers who began exercising before menarche (Fig. 20-3). Similar findings are observed in young female gymnasts.[127] In a study of college-age athletes engaged in running and swimming, a delay of menarche was also reported.[43] Earlier, Frisch and McArthur[42] proposed that the loss of body fat might be responsible for the change in menstrual cyclicity. In anorexia nervosa the incidence of amenorrhea is so high as to be required for the diagnosis by the *Diagnostic and Statistical Manual* of the American Psychiatric Association.[5] More recently, several investigators have postulated that psychogenic stress is sufficient to cause amenorrhea.[11,41] Thus it is uncertain in highly trained athletes whether psychogenic stress factors play a role in the amenorrhea. While a preliminary report suggested that amenorrheic athletes may exhibit more stress than do their cyclic counterparts,[45] the overall conclusions of the limited studies available have

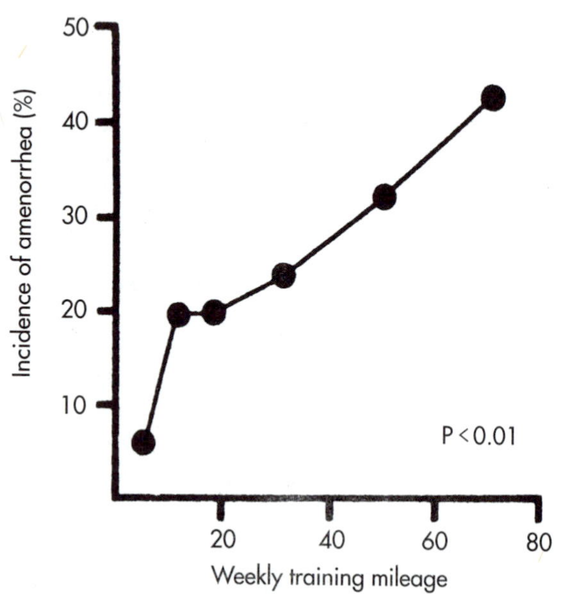

Fig. 20-2 Incidence of amenorrhea in women runners based on weekly training distance. (From Feicht CB, Johnson TS, Martin BJ: *Lancet* 2:1145, 1978.)

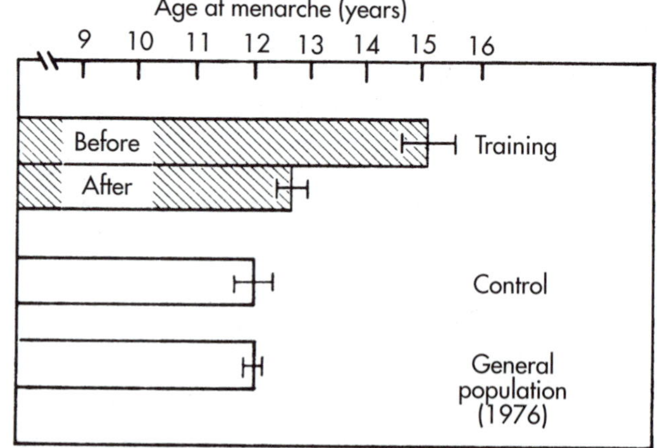

Fig. 20-3 Timing of menstruation in girls who begin exercise training before puberty versus after puberty. (From Frisch RE et al: *JAMA* 246:1559, 1981.)

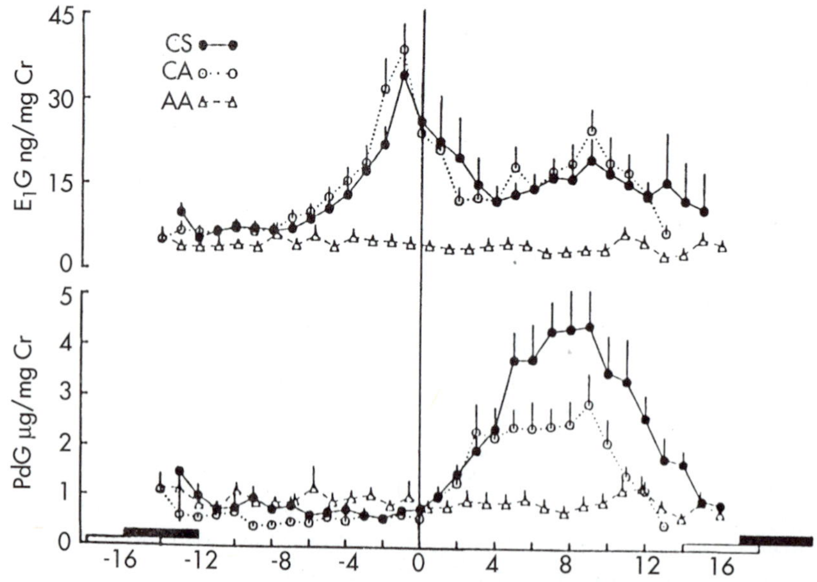

Fig. 20-4 Urinary metabolites of estradiol (E_1G) and progesterone *(PdG)* in amenorrheic athletes *(AA)*, cycling athletes *(CA)*, and sedentary control women *(CS)* with timing of menses in CS *(dark box)* and CA *(open box)*. (From Loucks AB et al: *J Clin Endocrinol Metab* 68:402, 1989.)

not supported a role of psychogenic stress in exercise-induced amenorrhea.[79,89] Although the combination of severe psychogenic stress and acute weight loss in anorexia nervosa consistently produces amenorrhea, the applicability of this model to exercise-induced amenorrhea is doubtful. Several studies have shown that when exercise is interrupted in ballet dancers, menses return without a change in body fat or the ratio of body fat to lean mass.[1,10] Methodologic flaws in measuring the proportion of body fat to lean mass in vivo characterized many early correlational studies.[62] More recently, underwater weighing techniques for determination of body fat were used to determine that no statistical differences exist between cycling and amenorrheic athletes.[81]

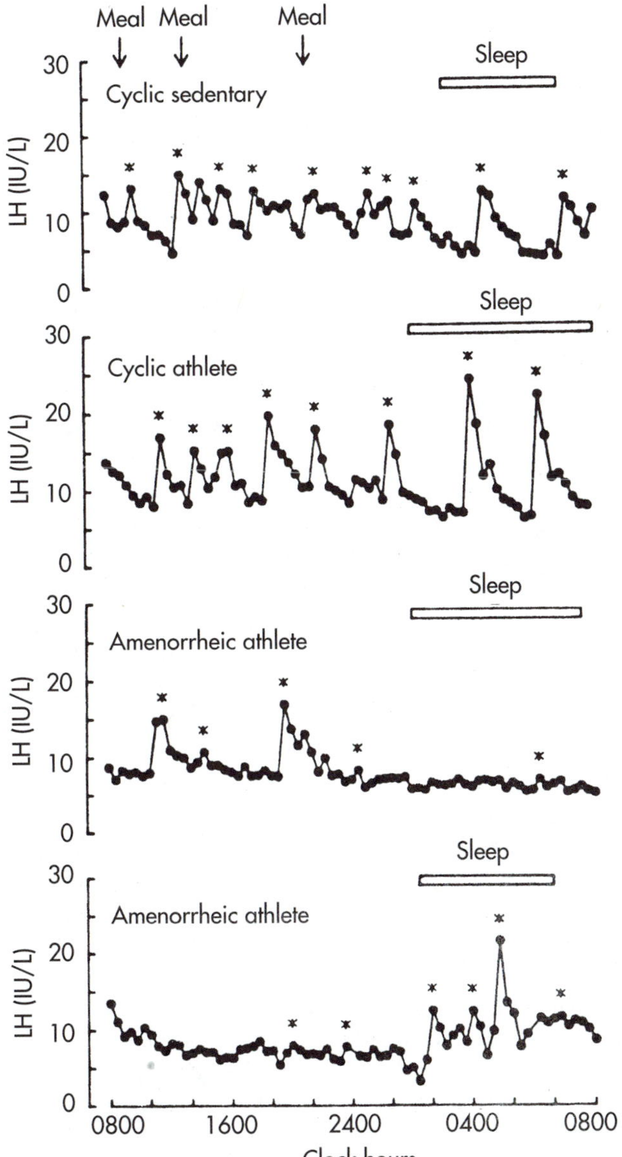

Fig. 20-5 Serum LH levels drawn at 20-minute intervals in cycling controls, cycling athletes, and amenorrheic athletes. The asterisks indicate statistically significant pulses. (From Loucks AB et al: *J Clin Endocrinol Metab* 68:402, 1989.)

Amenorrhea is the most dramatic and worrisome form of menstrual disturbance in women athletes. Anovulatory cycles also occur in this population. In addition, in women who do ovulate, an extremely high incidence of inadequate luteal phase progesterone production is observed (Fig. 20-4). This was first reported by Shangold and colleagues[112] and has subsequently been replicated by several other investigators.[12,14,104] Similar results were reported in an experiment in which sedentary women were exposed to graded exercise. In this population the incidence of luteal phase deficiency reached 63%.[15]

The mechanism underlying anovulation and amenorrhea is alteration in the normal pulse frequency of GnRH. Loucks and co-workers[81] have demonstrated decreased early follicular phase LH pulse frequency in cycling athletes as compared with normal controls, and an even further decrease in LH pulse frequency in amenorrheic athletes (Fig. 20-5). Of interest, the decreased pulse frequency was accompanied by an increased pulse amplitude in the athletes who retained normal menstrual cycles. This may have reflected an increased pituitary reserve of LH in this population as a result of fewer LH pulses as compared with control subjects (Fig. 20-6). In amenorrheic athletes, pulse amplitude was similar to that of controls. The decreased pituitary reserve of LH in this population as compared with cycling athletes may reflect a decline in LH synthesis, as well as decreased number of LH pulses. LH pulse frequency bears a one-to-one correspondence with GnRH pulse frequency.[26] It has previously been demonstrated that at very low frequencies of GnRH stimulation, FSH is produced in excess of LH.[27] This was confirmed in the study by Loucks and colleagues, when in response to a fixed bolus of exogenous GnRH, pituitary FSH release was found to be maximal in the amenorrheic athletes.

The mechanism of decreased GnRH pulsatile activity remains to be discerned. To be sure, it is only one of myriad acute and chronic physiologic changes observed in athletes. In response to maximal exercise challenge, acute changes occur in the form of increases in prolactin, cortisol, adrenocorticotropic hormone, β-endorphin, norepinephrine, growth hormone, melatonin, and prolactin.[7,18,19,32,40] Of these, alterations in the cortisol axis persist at rest. Elevated 24-hour cortisol levels in amenorrheic athletes have been well documented. There has been some evidence that increased cortisol levels may result in decreased GnRH-LH release. The extent to which these cortisol axis alterations may be responsible for the decreased LH in amenorrheic athletes remains to be determined. Another axis that exhibits chronic changes in highly trained athletes is the thyroid axis.[82] Although thyroid-stimulating hormone (TSH) levels appear to be unchanged, decreased circulating thyroid hormone levels are observed. These decreased circulating levels of thyroid hormone may in some degree reflect estro-

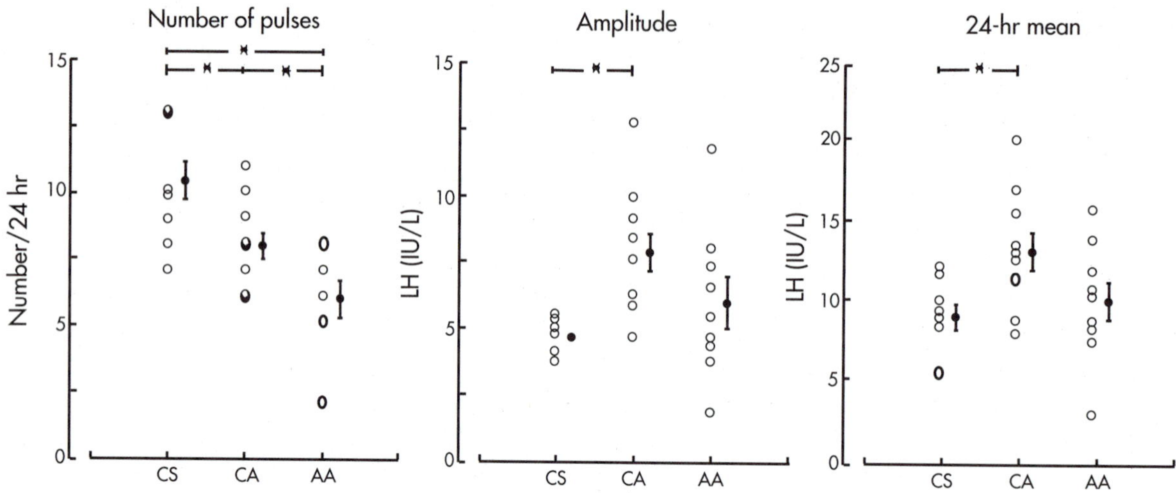

Fig. 20-6 Individual values and group means (±SE) for luteinizing hormone *(LH)* pulse frequency, pulse amplitude, and transverse mean LH concentrations in cycling sedentary women *(CS)*, cycling athletes *(CA)*, and amenorrheic athletes *(AA)*. (From Loucks AB et al: *J Clin Endocrinol Metab* 68:402, 1989.)

gen deficiency. In addition, decreased levels of thyroid hormone reduce sex hormone binding globulin (SHBG) and through this mechanism may influence menstrual cyclicity as well.

The clinical significance of amenorrhea in highly trained athletes undergoing strenuous expeditions is the influence that hypoestrogenism has on bone density. Although amenorrhea occurs most commonly in runners, high degrees of physical exertion from any source, including wilderness expeditions, may produce amenorrhea. All women with amenorrhea are at significant risk for loss of bone strength. In 1971 Drinkwater and co-workers[36] first found the association between decreased bone density and amenorrhea in female athletes. Since that time, these results have been replicated by several investigators.[17,87] The decline in bone density seen in amenorrheic athletes can be impressive, 13% within the first 3 years. This may advance the bone age by as much as 20 years in the athlete in her midtwenties. Because of this the importance of estrogen and progestin supplementation in this population is paramount.

DYSFUNCTIONAL UTERINE BLEEDING

Dysfunctional uterine bleeding refers to unexpected menstrual bleeding in the absence of an anatomic cause. Although the term is rather vague in that it does not imply a distinct etiology, it is useful in the context of wilderness medicine in that emergency treatment can be instituted that will prevent further blood loss before more definitive diagnosis. Before the diagnosis of dysfunctional uterine bleeding, anatomic causes should be excluded. The most common anatomic cause of bleeding in reproductive women is uterine fibroids (myomas). These are usually readily diagnosed by pelvic examination. Findings on examination consistent with uterine fibroids include an enlarged, irregularly shaped uterus.[16] Other causes more difficult to diagnose include endometrial polyps and cervical disease.[122] Fortunately, cervical disease rarely develops acutely and is easily diagnosed by visual inspection during the preexpedition physical examination. Even in the presence of uterine fibroids or endometrial polyps, hormonal therapy may be an effective temporizing step before definitive therapy.

Dysfunctional uterine bleeding may result from a variety of hormonal imbalances. In a woman taking oral contraceptive pills the bleeding most commonly results from a relative deficiency of estrogen as compared with progesterone at the level of the endometrium.[133] This occurs despite the supraphysiologic doses of estrogen contained in birth control pills. Early in the course of oral contraceptive use the endometrial tissue gradually thins. This initially causes shedding of endometrium with accompanying bleeding. Later the uterus may be relatively denuded of endometrium, which, if it does not result in amenorrhea, often causes prolonged and irregular bleeding patterns. The optimal therapy for dysfunctional uterine bleeding in a woman taking birth control pills is to supply estrogen. This may be done by administration of conjugated equine estrogen (Premarin) in doses of 10 mg/day, usually given as 2.5 mg four times a day. Should this not be available, high doses of birth control pills are usually efficacious. In this case,[100] four pills a day should be prescribed for up to 1 week. In general, the latter therapy is less acceptable because of side effects and changes in lipid levels and coagulation times. Moreover, bothersome side effects can occur, including headaches, fluid retention, and depression.

In adult women not using oral contraceptives, dysfunctional uterine bleeding may be the result of either estrogen deficiency or estrogen excess. Estrogen deficiency states typically are seen in women with a history of stress, exercise, or restricted diet. In this case, estrogen supplementation in the form of Premarin in the doses discussed previously is the most effective initial treatment. Estrogen excess states usually accompany a polycystic ovary–like syndrome. On physical examination these women tend to be somewhat obese and have evidence of hirsutism. Generally they have a history of intervals of several months of amenorrhea separated by heavy and often prolonged periods. These women are usually best treated with a progestational agent. Medroxyprogesterone acetate (Provera) 10 to 20 mg/day is adequate.

In either estrogen-deficient or estrogen-excess dysfunctional uterine bleeding, if more specific therapy is not available, four oral contraceptive pills a day may be prescribed acutely. In the case of estrogen deficiency, with this regimen sufficient estrogen is available to decrease or stop the bleeding. In the case of estrogen excess, advantage is taken of the progestin component of the pill.[118]

Ectopic Pregnancy

Ectopic pregnancy is a medical emergency and requires prompt evacuation of the patient to a facility with surgical capability. In the last stages the woman with an ectopic pregnancy has an acute abdomen with peritoneal signs, the absence of high-grade fever, and orthostatic hypotension.[129] Shoulder pain is due to diaphragmatic irritation from intraperitoneal blood. At this stage, management is straightforward and evacuation measures should be instituted. Shock is likely to develop rapidly, and the patient's blood pressure requires close monitoring until the time of evacuation. Vigorous fluid resuscitation should be instituted.

Ectopic pregnancies occur in approximately 1 in 100 pregnancies.[35] Risk factors include previous abdominal surgery, particularly pelvic surgery, previous use of an intrauterine device for birth control, previous history of pelvic inflammatory disease, and previous ectopic pregnancy.[23,24,73,131]

Ectopic pregnancies most commonly rupture after 7 weeks of gestation (5 weeks after conception), although ruptured ectopic pregnancies as early as 5 weeks of gestation occur.[20] Usually, abnormal vaginal bleeding and abdominal pain precede the rupture. For this reason, all episodes of abnormal vaginal bleeding in wilderness environments must be evaluated early. *Early diagnosis and evacuation are lifesaving in ectopic pregnancy.*

A previous, apparently normal menstrual period is sometimes observed in ectopic pregnancy. In retrospect, this will have occurred because of inadequate hCG production by the ectopic pregnancy to maintain the corpus luteum. As a result, progesterone production is decreased and endometrial shedding accompanied by menstrual flow occurs. Recently, simple and highly accurate 2-minute urine pregnancy testing kits have become available. These may be stored for periods of time at room temperature.[8] The most reliable is the ICON from Hybridtech, Inc., San Diego, Calif. Such kits should be included in the medical supplies of an expedition in which women are involved, and in which evacuation will require more than a few hours. They should be used liberally in all cases of abnormal vaginal bleeding. Because of the remarkable sensitivity and specificity of properly selected kits, false-positive and false-negative results are exceedingly rare. A negative test virtually excludes the diagnosis of ectopic pregnancy. To ensure adequate performance of the test and viability of the reagents, only tests with an internal positive reference should be used.

Vaginitis

Vaginitis generally is easily managed in wilderness settings, provided the medical kit includes an antifungal agent and metronidazole. Vaginitis need not be treated except for the comfort of the patient. If a trained individual is available, a speculum should be part of the medical supply kit and a vaginal examination should be performed to determine if the organism is *Candida, Trichomonas,* or *Gardnerella.* Other vaginitides are rare. Vaginal yeast is a thick curdy discharge with the predominant symptom of itching. The treatment is an antifungal agent such as miconazole vaginally for 3 successive nights. With *Gardnerella* and *Trichomonas* infections the discharge is usually thin and often malodorous. *Trichomonas* and *Gardnerella* are treated with metronidazole. A thorough course includes 250 mg of metronidazole four times a day for 1 week. An alternative therapy suggested for *Trichomonas* is 2 g orally as a single dose[98] or 1 g orally twice a day.

Shark and Bear Attacks

The association of menstrual blood with attacks by bears and sharks has been suggested. Evidence indicates that bear attacks are much more likely to occur because the animal is provoked, startled, or hungry. The association with menstrual bleeding, although suggested, has not been established. Nonetheless, the odor of menstrual blood may attract a variety of animals. Appropriate hygiene is enhanced by placing used tampons or sanitary napkins in sealed plastic bags and storing or disposing of them away from the campsite.

Sharks are considerably more dangerous than bears. The species most commonly associated with human attack include the great white, tiger, blue hammerhead, and great reef. Of these, the great white shark is considered the most dangerous. Swimming in shark-infested waters should always be considered dangerous (see Chapter 51). In particular, any open wound should be considered a risk factor for shark attack. Sharks can detect blood in water when concentrations are as low as one part per million. Although there is no definitive evidence that menstrual bleeding attracts sharks, all bloody fluids, including menstrual flow, should be considered contraindicated in shark-infested waters.

Psychologic Adaptations to Wilderness

No evidence has shown one sex is psychologically better equipped for strenuous expeditions than the other. Expeditions that include both men and women have the difficulty of making appropriate provisions for privacy. This is required not only for bowel and bladder elimination, but also for changes of tampons or napkins. Appropriate consideration for privacy should be adapted to the particular expedition. As has been previously addressed, women have more disruption of reproductive physiology in psychologically stressful situations than do men. Stress reduction is therefore particularly important for women in wilderness expeditions to prevent menstrual dysfunction. There is no clearly superior technique of stress reduction, and different techniques work better for different individuals. These may include meditation, yoga, or open communication and expression of concern about interpersonal matters during the expedition.

Emergency Childbirth

Although childbirth should never be planned for a wilderness expedition, unexpected childbirth may be encountered. Should this occur, the following guide is offered.

ASSESSMENT OF CERVICAL DILATATION

In emergency situations, labor should be allowed to progress without intervention until the mother experiences the desire for involuntary expulsive efforts (the desire to push). At this point, a vaginal examination should be performed (with a clean glove if available) to determine the extent of cervical dilatation. Often the mother involuntarily expresses expulsive efforts before full dilatation. Full dilatation is ensured on vaginal examination by feeling the head of the baby for 360 degrees with no cervical tissue palpable. Most often, cervical tissue is palpated anteriorly (toward the mother's symphysis) before full dilatation. The mother should be encouraged to refrain from voluntary pushing until full cervical dilatation is determined. Because of the risk of infection, repeated vaginal examinations to determine full dilatation should not be performed more frequently than every 30 minutes.

PREPARATION

To the extent possible, clean surroundings should be provided at the site of the expected birth. The mother should be appropriately positioned so that the *buttocks are elevated*. This is important because the most difficult part of birth is delivery of the infant's anterior shoulder. Anterior shoulder delivery is eventually assisted by posterior traction on the infant toward the sacrum of the mother. Sufficient room should be available to allow this to occur. If this is impossible to achieve, consideration should be given to allowing the mother to deliver in the lateral position with a second assistant elevating the top leg. Delivery in the squatting position is also acceptable, although a less controlled delivery usually results. If two clamps and scissors are available, these should be readied in the event of a tight umbilical cord around the infant's neck.

DELIVERY

Once full dilatation is reached and the delivery area readied, labor should be allowed to progress spontaneously. The mother is encouraged to push during contractions and to rest between contractions. When the infant's head is visible at the vaginal introitus, the perineum should be permitted to stretch slowly.

Delivery should be accomplished during a uterine contraction. At the start of the contraction the mother should be encouraged to push. During this effort, gentle *countertraction* is applied against the baby's head while the perineum is supported between the vagina and rectum using pressure with the other hand. The purpose of this maneuver is to promote gentle stretching of the perineum and avoid tearing. When the baby has appeared up to the level of the eyebrows, the mother should be instructed to push very gently or not at all, while the assistant to the delivery extends the chin, which is palpated through the maternal perineum (Fig. 20-7). Countertraction against the oncoming head is maintained during this maneuver. Once the baby's head is delivered, the operator should allow the infant to begin a 90-degree turn so that the head faces laterally. The infant's neck should then be palpated to ascertain the presence of an umbilical cord. If a nuchal cord is present, and attempt should be made to slip the cord over the baby's head. If this is not possible, the cord should be occluded with two clamps and cut in between. Alternatively, string may be used to *tightly* tie the cord in two places, and a cut made between them. Tight occlusion of the cord is essential to prevent profuse bleeding by the baby. If a suction apparatus is available, the nose and mouth should be cleaned of fluid before the delivery proceeds. If this is not available, a finger or tissue should be used to remove as much amniotic fluid as possible. The infant's head should then be gently pushed posteriorly and the mother instructed to push forcefully until the anterior shoulder is delivered (Fig. 20-8). Once this has occurred, the remainder of the birth will proceed smoothly. The mother should be instructed to push very gently until the posterior shoulder is delivered. As she does so, upward traction should be applied. Further suctioning of the

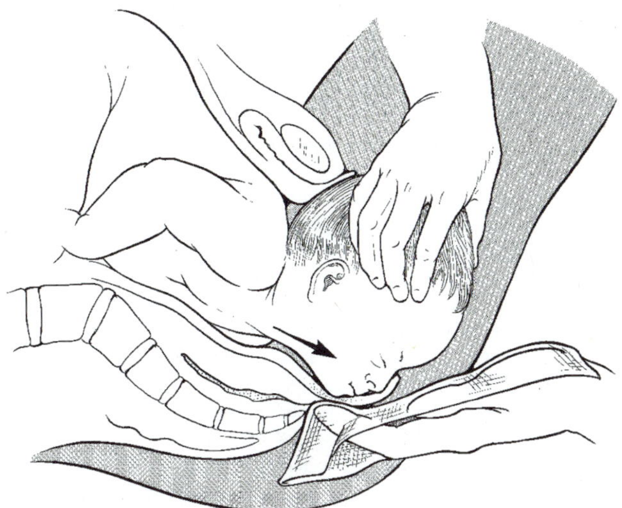

Fig. 20-7 Technique of controlled delivery of the head demonstrating upward pressure on the fetal chin and countertraction on the oncoming occiput. (Redrawn from Pritchard JA, MacDonald PC: *Williams obstetrics,* ed 16, New York, Appleton-Century-Crofts.)

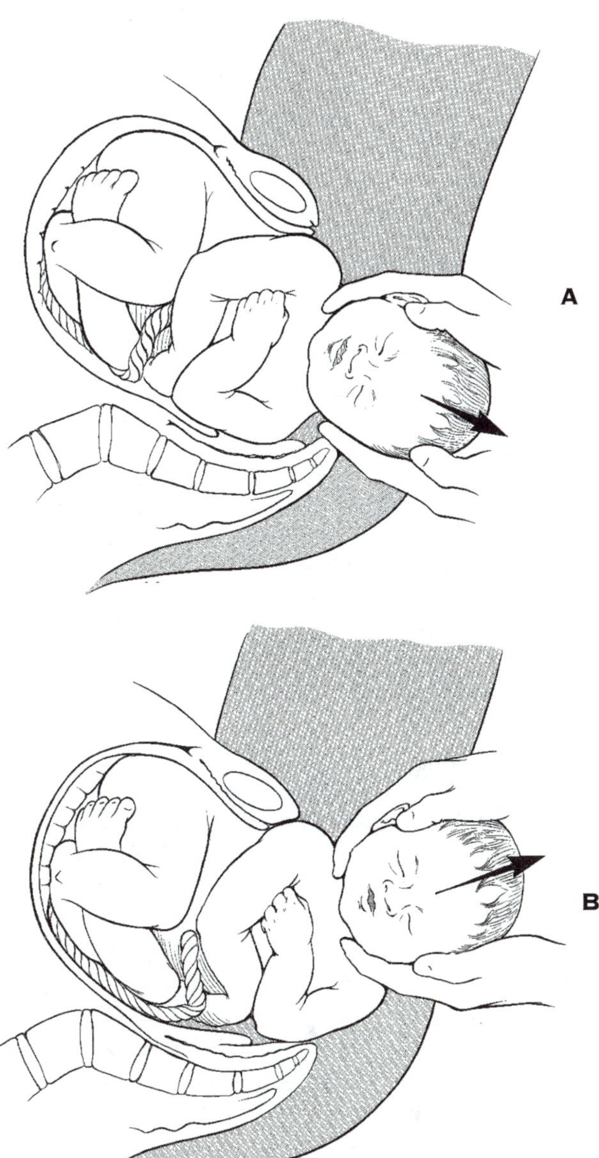

Fig. 20-8 **A,** Gentle downward traction to facilitate descent of the anterior shoulder. **B,** Delivery of anterior shoulder complete: gentle downward traction to deliver the posterior shoulder. (Redrawn from Pritchard JA, MacDonald PC: *Williams obstetrics,* New York, Appleton-Century-Crofts.)

airway should be undertaken, and the baby should be gently stimulated to cry. This may be done by flicking the foot with a finger or vigorous massage of the body and extremities. Should the baby fail to cry or have airway difficulty, the umbilical cord should be immediately ligated and cut and resuscitative efforts begun. If respiratory efforts are normal, the umbilical cord can be ligated and cut leisurely. In any case, attention should turn to the infant.

RESUSCITATION OF THE INFANT

The infant should be immediately dried vigorously and placed in the warmest spot possible. The mother's abdomen may be used to provide warmth. The infant should then be gently stimulated. This is best effected by vigorous rubbing with a dry towel. If no breathing efforts are observed, the pulse should be taken at the umbilical cord or over the precordium. If the pulse is less than 60 beats/min or respirations are absent, the airway should be cleared and infant cardiopulmonary resuscitation (CPR) should be started. Infant CPR is performed by placing two fingers over the precordium and supplying 100 compressions per minute. Two breaths after each 15 compressions are recommended. These are delivered as short puffs, with the resuscitator's mouth placed over both the infant's nose and mouth.

ATTENTION TO THE MOTHER

After the infant is stabilized, the mother's perineum should be inspected for lacerations and direct pressure and packs applied to minimize bleeding. Separation of the placenta should be determined. Signs of placental separation include lengthening of the umbilical cord and often an increase in bleeding. The placenta should be delivered primarily by maternal pushing, with only very gentle traction on the umbilical cord by the assistant.

Since emergency births rarely are accomplished in clean environments, antibiotic therapy for the mother should be instituted if available. Cephalosporins are the treatment of choice and should be administered for 48 hours.

POSTPARTUM BLEEDING

Postpartum bleeding is a common event. The most effective measure to control bleeding is vigorous uterine massage. This should initially be attempted abdominally. If it fails to control hemorrhage, bimanual massage should be undertaken with one hand in the vagina and the other on the uterine fundus, palpated through the abdomen. This may have to be repeated frequently during the first few hours after birth. It will be uncomfortable for the mother but is essential to minimize hemorrhage.

BREECH DELIVERIES

Breech deliveries are potentially dangerous in suboptimal settings. To the extent possible, a breech delivery should be allowed to proceed spontaneously until the sacrum of the infant is visible through the vagina. The assistant should then deliver the legs by flexing each knee and pulling gently to deliver each leg. (In some breech presentations the legs are already flexed.) The assistant should then place a towel over the infant's back and place his or her hands over the sacrum (not higher because of the large infant adrenal glands). In this position the assistant should help guide the infant out, but traction should not be applied. Once the scapulae are visible, the infant should be rotated in such a way that the shoulders are oriented into the anterior and posterior direction. The assistant's fingers are then used to deliver each of the infant's arms. The most difficult part is delivery of the head. To assist in this, the assistant's hand should be placed into the vagina and the infant's head maximally flexed. This is done by placing the second and fourth fingers over the infant's cheekbones and the third finger either on the chin or in the mouth. Firm flexion of the chin should then be applied as the mother is instructed to push. The remainder of the care of the mother and infant should proceed as described previously.

➠ SUMMARY

Safe participation by women in wilderness expeditions requires careful evaluation of gynecologic health before departure. Because of physiologic differences, specific conditioning programs are highly advantageous to women. In both women of reproductive age and postmenopausal women, particular attention should be directed toward preventing dangerous uterine bleeding and bone fractures. In women of reproductive age, steps should be taken to avoid the dangers of pregnancy and childbirth in wilderness situations. With the use of these precautions, women will be at no greater risk than men in wilderness settings.

REFERENCES

1. Abraham SF et al: Body weight, exercise and menstrual status among ballet dancers in training, *Br J Obstet Gynecol* 89:507, 1982.
2. Aedo A-R et al: Ovarian steroid secretion in normally menstruating women. II. Contribution of the corpus luteum, *Acta Endocrinol* 95:212, 1980.
3. Ambrus CM et al: Effect of contraceptive drugs on the coagulation system, *Hematol Rev* 2:163, 1970.
4. Aloia JF et al: Prevention of involutional bone loss by exercise, *Ann Intern Med* 89:356, 1978.
5. American Psychiatric Association Committee on Nomenclature: *Diagnostic and statistical manual of mental disorders, Edition III-Revised,* Washington, DC, 1987, The Association.
6. Artal R et al: Pulmonary responses to exercise in pregnancy, *Am J Obstet Gynecol* 154(2):378, 1986.
7. Baker ER et al: Plasma gonadotropins, prolactin, and steroid concentrations in female runners after a long-distance run, *Fertil Steril* 38:38, 1982.
8. Barnes RB, Roy S, Yee B: Reliability of urine pregnancy tests in the diagnosis of ectopic pregnancy, *J Reprod Med* 30:827, 1985.
9. Barron JL, Miller RP, Searle DI: Metabolic clearance and plasma half-disappearance time of D-TRP[6] and exogenous luteinizing hormone-releasing hormone, *J Clin Endocrinol Metab* 54:1169, 1982.
10. Beillewicz WZ, Fellows HM, Hytten EA: Comments on the critical metabolic mass and the age of menarche, *Ann Hum Biol* 3:51, 1976.
11. Berga S et al: Neuroendocrine aberrations in women with functional hypothalamic amenorrhea, *J Clin Endocrinol Metab* 68:242, 1989.
12. Bonen A et al: Profile of selected hormones during menstrual cycles of teenage athletes, *J Appl Physiol* 5:545, 1981.
13. Bottinger LE et al: Oral contraceptives and thromboembolic disease: effects of lowering oestrogen content, *Lancet* 1:1097, 1980.
14. Boyden T et al: Sex steroids and endurance running in women, *Fertil Steril* 39:629, 1983.
15. Bullen BA et al: Induction of menstrual disorders in untrained women by strenuous exercise, *N Engl J Med* 312:1349, 1985.
16. Buttram VC, Reiter RC: Uterine leiomyomata: etiology, symptomatology, management, *Fertil Steril* 36:433, 1981.
17. Cann CE et al: Decreased spinal mineral content in amenorrheic women, *JAMA* 251:626, 1974.
18. Carr DB et al: Plasma melatonin increases during exercise in women, *J Clin Endocrinol Metab* 53:224, 1981.
19. Carr DB et al: Physical conditioning facilitates the exercise-induced secretion of beta-endorphin and beta-lipotropin in women, *N Engl J Med* 305:560, 1981.
20. Cartwright PS, Vaughn B, Tuttle D: Culdocentesis and ectopic pregnancy, *J Reprod Med* 28:88, 1984.
21. Carvalho A et al: Coagulation abnormalities in women taking oral contraceptives, *JAMA* 237:857, 1977.
22. Chappel SC et al: Studies in rhesus monkeys on the site where estrogen inhibits gonadotropins: delivery of 17-estradiol to the hypothalamus and pituitary gland, *J Clin Endocrinol Metab* 52:1, 1981.
23. Chavin W: The rise in ectopic pregnancies—exploration of possible reasons, *Int J Gynecol* 20:341, 1982.
24. Chow W-H, Daling JR, Weiss NS: IUD use and subsequent tubal ectopic pregnancy, *Am J Public Health* 76:536, 1986.
25. Clapp JF III: Oxygen consumption during treadmill exercise before, during, and after pregnancy, *Am J Obstet Gynecol* 161(6 Pt 1):1458, 1989.
26. Clark IJ, Cumming JT: The temporal relationship between gonadotropin releasing hormone (GnRH) and luteninizing hormone (LH) secretion in ovariectomized ewes, *Endocrinology* 111:1737, 1982.
27. Clark IJ et al: Effects on plasma luteinizing hormone and follicle stimulating hormone of varying frequency and amplitude of gonadotropin releasing hormone pulses in ovariectomized ewes with hypothalamic-pituitary disconnection, *Neuroendocrinology* 39:214, 1984.
28. Coble YD Jr et al: Production rates and metabolic clearance rates of human follicle stimulating hormone in premenopausal and postmenopausal women, *J Clin Invest* 48:359, 1969.

29. Collings CA, Curet LB, Mullin JP: Maternal and aerobic exercise program, *Am J Obstet Gynecol* 145(6):702, 1983.
30. Csapo AL, Pulkkinen MO, Wiest WG: Effects of lutectomy and progesterone replacement in early pregnant patients, *Am J Obstet Gynecol* 115:579, 1973.
31. Cumming DC, Rebar RW: Exercise and reproductive function in women, *Am J Ind Med* 4:113, 1983.
32. Cumming DC et al: Acute exercise related changes in women runners and non-runners, *Fertil Steril* 36:421, 1981.
33. Dale E, Gerlach DH, Wilhite AL: Menstrual dysfunction in distance runners, *Obstet Gynecol* 54:47, 1979.
34. Dickinson JG et al: Altitude related deaths in seven trekkers in the Himalayas, *Thorax* 38:646, 1983.
35. Dorfman SF: Deaths from ectopic pregnancy, United States, 1979-1980: clinical aspects, *Obstet Gynecol* 64:386, 1984.
36. Drinkwater BL et al: Bone mineral content of amenorrheic and eumenorrheic athletes, *N Engl J Med* 311:277, 1984.
37. Edmonds DK, Lindsay KS, Miller JF, et al: Early embroyonic mortality in women, *Fertil Steril* 38:447, 1982.
38. Feicht CB, Johnson TS, Martin BJ: Secondary amenorrhea in athletes, *Lancet* 2:1145, 1978.
39. Filicori M et al: Characterization of the physiologic pattern of epidosic gonadotropin secretion throughout the human menstrual cycle, *J Clin Endocrinol Metab* 62:1136, 1986.
40. Fraioli F et al: Physical exercise stimulates marked concommitant increase of beta-endorphin and adrenocorticotropic hormone (ACTH) in peripheral blood in man, *Experientia* 36:987, 1980.
41. Fries H, Nillius SJ, Petterson F: Epidemiology of secondary amenorrhea. II. A retrospective evaluation of etiology with special regard to psychogenic factors, *Am J Obstet Gynecol* 118:473, 1974.
42. Frisch RE, McArthur JW: Menstrual cycles: fatness as a determinant of minimum weight for height necessary for their maintenance or onset, *Science* 185:949s, 1974.
43. Frisch RE, Wyschak G, Vincent LE: Delayed menarche and amenorrhea in ballet dancers, *N Engl J Med* 303:17, 1980.
44. Frisch RE et al: Delayed menarche and amenorrhea of college athletes in relation to the onset of training, *JAMA* 246:1559, 1981.
45. Galle PC et al: Physiologic and psychologic profiles in a survey of women runners, *Fertil Steril* 39:363, 1983.
46. Genant HK et al: *Quantitative computed tomography for spinal and mineral assessment in osteoporosis.* Proceedings of the Copenhagen International Symposium on Osteoporosis, 1984, Aalborg Stiftsbogtrykkeri.
47. Gillum RF: The epidemiology of resting heart rate in a national sample of men and women: associations with hypertension, coronary heart disease, blood pressure, and other cardiovascular risk factors, *Am Heart J* 116(1 Pt 1):163, 1988.
48. Gisolfi CV, Cohen JS: Relationships among training, heat acclimation, and heat tolerance in men and women: the controversy revisited, *Med Sci Sports* 11(1):56, 1979.
49. Goodman AL, Hodgen GD: The ovarian triad of the primate menstrual cycle, *Recent Prog Horm Res* 39:1, 1983.
50. Graham TE: Thermal, metabolic, and cardiovascular changes in men and women during cold stress, *Med Sci Sports Exerc* 20(5 Suppl):S185, 1988.
51. Hachett PH, Rennie D, Levine HD: The incidence, importance and prophylaxis of acute mountain sickness, *Lancet* 2:1149, 1979.
52. Hannon JP: Comparative altitude adaptability in young men and women. In Follinsbee LJ et al, editors: *Environmental stress,* New York, 1978, Academic Press.
53. Harris CW, Shields JL, Hannon JP: Acute altitude sickness in females, *Aerospace Med* 37:1163, 1966.
54. Heaney RP, Recker RR, Saville PD: Menopausal changes in calcium balance performance, *Lab Clin Med* 92:953, 1978.
55. Henzl MR et al: Lysosomal concept of menstrual bleeding in humans, *J Clin Endocrinol Metab* 34:860, 1972.
56. Hillier SG, Reichart LE, Van Hall EV: Control of preovulatory follicular estrogen biosythesis in the human ovary, *J Clin Endocrinol Metab* 52:847, 1981.
57. Hillier SG et al: Intraovarian sex steroid hormone interactions and regulation of follicular maturation: aromatization of androgens by human granulosa cells in vitro, *J Clin Endocrinol Metab* 50:640, 1980.
58. Horseman A, Nordin BEC, Crilley RG: Effect on bone of withdrawal of oestrogen therapy, *Lancet* 2:33, 1979.
59. Hossack KF, Bruce RA: Maximal cardiac function in sedentary normal men and women: comparison of age-related changes, *J Appl Physiol* 53(4):799, 1982.
60. Jaszmann LJB: Epidemiology of the climacteric syndrome. In Campbell S, editor: *Management of the menopause and postmenopausal years,* Lancaster, Eng, 1976, MTP Press.
61. Johansson BW et al: On some late effects of bilateral oophorectomy in the age range of 15-30 years, *Acta Obstet Gynecol Scand* 54:449, 1975.
62. Johnston FE: Systematic errors in the mellitis cheek equation to predict body fat in lean females, *N Engl J Med* 312:588, 1985.
63. Karsch JF et al: Functional luteolysis in the rhesus monkey: the role of estrogen, *Endocrinology* 98:553, 1986.
64. Kenney WL: A review of comparative responses of men and women to heat stress, *Environ Res* 37(1):1, 1985.
65. Kirkendahl DR, Calebrese LH: Physiologic aspects of dance, *Clin Sports Med* 2:525, 1983.
66. Kistner RW: Endometrial alterations associated with estrogen and estrogen-progestin combinations. In Norris HJ, Hertig AT, Abel MR, editors: *The uterus,* Baltimore, 1973, Williams & Wilkins.
67. Knobil E: The neuroendocrine control of the menstrual cycle, *Curr Prog Horm Res* 36:42, 1980.
68. Knobil E: Patterns of hypophysiotropic signals and gonadotropin secretion in the rhesus monkey, *Biol Reprod* 24:44, 1981.
69. Knoweldon J, Buhr AJ, Dunbar O: Incidence of fractures in persons over 35 years of age, *Br J Prev Soc Med* 18:130, 1964.
70. Kohler PO, Ross GT, O'Dell WE: Metabolic clearance and production rates of human luteinizing hormone in pre- and postmenopausal women, *J Clin Invest* 47:38, 1968.
71. Krolner B et al: Physical exercise as prophylaxis against involutional bone loss: a controlled trial, *Clin Sci* 64:541, 1983.
72. Kryger M et al: Excessive polycythemia at high altitude: role of ventilatory drive and lung disease, *Am Rev Respir Dis* 118:659, 1978.
73. Levin AA, Shoenbaum SC, Stubblefield PG: Ectopic pregnancy and prior induced abortion, *Am J Public Health* 72:253, 1982.
74. Levine J et al: Simultaneous measurement of luteinizing releasing hormone and luteinizing hormone release in unanesthetized, ovariectomized sheep, *Endocrinology* 111:1149, 1982.
75. Lindsay R et al: Long term prevention of post-menopausal osteoporosis by oestrogen, *Lancet* 1:1038, 1976.
76. Lindsay R et al: Bone response to termination of oestrogen therapy, *Lancet* 1:1325, 1978.
77. Lostroh AJ, Johnson RE: Amount of interstitial cell stimulating hormone and follicle stimulating hormone required for follicular development, uterine growth and ovulation in the hypophysectomized rat, *Endocrinology* 79:991, 1966.
78. Lotgering FK, Gilbert RD, Longo LD: The interactions of exercise and pregnancy: a review, *Am J Obstet Gynecol* 149(5):560, 1984.
79. Loucks AB, Horvath SM: Exercise induced stress responses of amenorrheic and eumenorrheic runners, *J Clin Endocrinol Metab* 59:1109, 1984.
80. Loucks AB, Horvath SM: Athletic amenorrhea: a review, *Med Sci Sports Exerc* 17:56, 1985.
81. Loucks AB et al: Alterations in the hypothalamic-pituitary ovarian and hypothalamic-pituitary-adrenal axes in athletic women, *J Clin Endocrinol Metab* 68:402, 1989.
82. Loucks AB et al: Hypothalamic-pituitary-thyroidal function in eumenorrheic and amenorrheic athletes, *J Clin Endocrinol Metab* 75:514, 1992.

83. Louvet JP, Vaitukaitis JL: Induction of follicle-stimulating hormone (FSH) receptors in rat ovaries by estrogen priming, *Endocrinology* 99:758, 1976.
84. Macdonald GJ, Greep RO: Ability of luteinizing hormone (LH) to acutely increase serum progesterone during the secretory phase of the rhesus menstrual cycle, *Fertil Steril* 23:466, 1972.
85. Magazanik A et al: Effect of an iron supplement on body iron status and aerobic capacity of young training women, *Eur J Appl Physiol* 62(5):317, 1991.
86. Malina RM et al: Age at menarche and selected menstrual characteristics in athletes at different competitive levels and in different sports, *Med Sci Sports Exerc* 10:18, 1978.
87. Marcus RC et al: Menstrual function and bone mass in elite women distance runners, *Ann Intern Med* 102:158, 1985.
88. McArdle WD et al: Thermal adjustment to cold-water exposure in resting men and women, *J Appl Physiol* 56(6):1565, 1984.
89. McArthur JW et al: Hypothalamic amenorrhea in runners of normal body composition, *Endocrinol Res Commun* 7:13, 1980.
90. McNatty KP, Sawyers RS: Relationship between the endocrine environment within the graafian follicle and the subsequent rate of progesterone secretion by human granulosa cells in vitro, *J Endocrinol* 66:391, 1975.
91. McNatty KP et al: The microenvironment of the human antral follicle: inter-relationships among the steroid levels in antral fluid, the population of granulosa cells and the status of the oocyte in vivo and in vitro, *J Clin Endocrinol Metab* 49:851, 1979.
92. McNatty KP et al: Metabolism of androstenedione by human ovarian tissues in vitro with particular reference to reductase and aromatase activity, *Steroids* 34:429, 1979.
93. McNatty KP et al: Steroidogenesis by recombined follicular cells from the human ovary in vitro, *J Clin Endocrinol Metab* 51:1286, 1980.
94. McNatty KP et al: Thecal tissue from human ovarian follicular cells in vitro, *Steroids* 36:53, 1980.
95. Meema S, Meema H: Menopausal bone loss and osteoporosis, *Isr J Med Sci* 12:601, 1976.
96. Moore LG: Altitude-aggravated illnesses: examples from pregnancy and prenatal life, *Ann Emerg Med* 16(9):965, 1987.
97. Morton MJ et al: Exercise dynamics in late gestation: effects of physical training, *Am J Obstet Gynecol* 152(1):91, 1985.
98. Morton RS: Metronidazole in the single dose treatment of trichomoniasis in men and women, *Br J Venereal Dis* 48:525, 1972.
99. Nachtigall LE et al: Estrogen replacement therapy. I. A 10-year prospective study of the relationship to osteoporosis, *Obstet Gynecol* 53:227, 1979.
100. Nelson L, Rybo G: Treatment of menorrhagia, *Am J Obstet Gynecol* 110:713, 1971.
101. Noyes RW, Hertig AG, Rock J: Dating the endometrial biopsy, *Fertil Steril* 1:3, 1950.
102. Owens OM, Ryan KJ, Tulchinsky D: Episodic secretion of human chorionic gonadotropin during early pregnancy, *J Clin Endocrinol Metab* 53:1307, 1981.
103. Paterson DJ et al: Maximal exercise cardiorespiratory responses of men and women during acute exposure to hypoxia, *Aviat Space Environ Med* 58(3):243, 1987.
104. Prior JC et al: Reversible luteal phase defects and infertility associated with marathon training, *Lancet* 2:269, 1982.
105. Ramcharan S et al: The Walnut Creek contraceptive drug study. III. An interim report: a comparison of disease occurrence leading to hospitalization or death in users of oral contraceptives, *J Reprod Med* 25:346, 1980.
106. Riggs BL et al: Effect of fluoride/calcium regimen on vertebral fracture occurrence in postmenopausal osteoporosis, *N Engl J Med* 306:446, 1982.
107. Rosenberg L et al: Oral contraceptives use in relationship to nonfatal myocardial infarction, *Am J Epidemiol* 11:59, 1980.
108. Royal College of General Practioners: Oral contraceptive study: oral contraceptives, venous thrombosis and varicose veins, *J R Coll Gen Pract* 28:393, 1978.
109. Sanborn CF, Martin BJ, Wagner WW: Is athletic amenorrhea specific to runners? *Am J Obstet Gynecol* 143:859, 1982.
110. Schwallie PC, Assenzo JR: Contraceptive use—efficacy study utilizing medroxyprogesterone acetate administered as an intramuscular injection once every 90 days, *Fertil Steril* 24:331, 1973.
111. Schwartz B et al: Exercise induced amenorrhea: a distinct entity? *Am J Obstet Gynecol* 141:662, 1981.
112. Shangold M et al: The relationship between long-distance running, plasma progesterone and luteal phase length, *Fertil Steril* 31:131, 1979.
113. Singh I, Chohan IS, Mathew NT: Fibrinolytic activity in high altitude pulmonary edema, *Ind J Med Res* 57(2):210, 1969.
114. Singh I et al: High altitude pulmonary edema, *Lancet* 1:229, 1965.
115. Smith EL: Exercise for the prevention of osteoporosis, a review, *Phys Sports Med* 10:72, 1982.
116. Smith EL, Redden W, Smith PE: Physical activity and calcium modalities for bone mineral increase in aged women, *Med Sci Sports Exerc* 13:60, 1981.
117. Sophocles AM, Bachman J: HAPE in Vail, Colorado, 1975-1982, *West J Med* 144:569, 1986.
118. Speroff L, Glass RH, Kase N: *Clinical gynecologic endocrinology and infertility,* ed 3, Baltimore, 1986, Williams & Wilkins.
119. Sullivan MJ, Cobb FR, Higginbotham MB: Stroke volume increases by similar mechanisms during upright exercise in normal men and women, *Am J Cardiol* 67(16):1405, 1991.
120. Tsafriri A, Pomerantz SH, Channing CP: Inhibition of oocyte maturation by porcine follicular fluid: partial characterization of the inhibitor, *Biol Reprod* 14:511, 1976.
121. Tsang BK, Armstrong DT, Whitfield JF: Steroid biosynthesis by isolated human ovarian follicular cells in vitro, *J Clin Endocrinol Metab* 51:1407, 1980.
122. Valle RF: Hysteroscopic examination of patients with abnormal uterine bleeding, *Surg Gynecol Obstet* 153:521, 1981.
123. Van de Weile RL et al: Mechanisms regulating the human menstrual cycle, *Rec Prog Horm Res* 26:63, 1970.
124. Van der Walt LA, Wilmsen EN, Jenkins T: Unusual sex hormone patterns among desert dwelling hunter-gatherers, *J Clin Endocrinol Metab* 46:658, 1978.
125. Vessey MP, McPherson K, Yeates D: Mortality in oral contraceptive users, *Lancet* 1:549, 1981.
126. Warburton D, Fraser FC: Spontaneous abortion risks in man: data from reproductive histories collected in a medical genetics unit, *Am J Hum Genet* 16:1, 1964.
127. Warren MP: The effects of exercise on pubertal progression and reproductive function in girls, *J Clin Endocrinol Metab* 51:1150, 1980.
128. Webb JL, Millan DL, Stoltz CJ: Gynecologic survey of American female athletes competing at the Montreal Olympic games, *J Sports Med Phys Fitness* 19:409, 1975.
129. Weckstein LN: Current perspective on ectopic pregnancy, *Obstet Gynecol Surv* 40:259, 1985.
130. Wells CL: Responses of physically active and acclimated men and women to exercise in a desert environment, *Med Sci Sports Exerc* 12(1):9, 1980.
131. Westrol L, Bengtsson LPH, Mardh P-A: Incidence, trends and risks of ectopic pregnancy in a population of women, *Br Med J* 282:583, 1981.
132. Wilmore JH, Brown CH, Davis AJ: Body physique and composition of the female distance runner, *Ann NY Acad Sci* 301:764, 1977.
133. Wilson EW: Lysosome function in normal endometrium and endometrium exposed to contraceptive steroids. In Diczfalusy E, Fraser IS, Webb FTG, editors: *WHO Symposium on Steroid Contraception and Endometrial Bleeding,* 1980.

134. Wynn RM, Wooley RS: Ultrastructural changes in the human endometrium. II. Normal post-ovulatory changes, *Fertil Steril* 18:721, 1967.
135. Yen SSC, Lein A: The apparent paradox of the negative and positive feedback control system on gonadotropin secretion, *Am J Obstet Gynecol* 126:942, 1976.
136. Young JR, Jaffe RB: Strength-duration characteristics of estrogen effects on gonadotropin response to gonadotropin releasing hormone in women. II. Effects of varying concentrations of estradiol, *J Clin Endocrinol Metab* 42:432, 1976.
137. Zaharieva EL: Survey of sportswomen at the Tokyo Olympics, *J Sport Med Phys Fitness* 5:215, 1965.
138. Zaleznik AJ, Midgely AR, Reichert LE Jr: Granulosa cell maturation in the rat: increased binding of human chorionic gonadotropin following treatment with follicle-stimulating hormone in vivo, *Endocrinology* 95:818, 1974.
139. Zuck TF et al: Implications of depressed antithrombin-III activity associated with oral contraceptives, *Surg Gynecol Obstet* 133:609, 1971.
140. Zwiren LD, Cureton KJ, Hutchinson P: Comparison of circulatory responses to submaximal exercise in equally trained men and women, *Int J Sports Med* 4(4):255, 1983.

21 SEARCH AND RESCUE

Donald C. Cooper
Patrick H. LaValla
Robert C. Stoffel

As ever-increasing numbers of hikers, campers, climbers, and general outdoor users turn to our wildlands for recreation, the medical community and search and rescue (SAR) organizations will contend with a growing number of lost, sick, and injured persons. Wilderness search, rescue, and medical intervention are unique in several ways. All aspects of SAR are enormously time consuming. Simply getting the message concerning a lost or injured person out of a wilderness area may take several days. Organizing a team, equipment, and transportation requires a variable amount of time depending on the level of preparedness of the rescue organization. To find, gain access to, and transport the victim to definitive care completes a lengthy process. Because a large number of people are involved in a wilderness rescue (six or eight people are required to carry a litter 1 mile), logistic considerations such as food, shelter, and transport quickly create their own problems. Searchers and rescuers are subjected to the same risks and environmental stresses that compromise victims. To obviate further tragedy, rescue personnel must have a heightened awareness of potential danger and adverse conditions. In addition to basic and advanced life support training, rescuers must have extensive wilderness experience, combining practicality with creativity and resourcefulness, as well as training in such areas as survival, improvisation, communications, leadership, navigation (for example, map and compass, loran, global positioning system), first aid (at least), and specific search and rescue techniques. Many interventions, such as cardiopulmonary resuscitation, tube thoracostomy, tracheal intubation, and intravenous therapy, are difficult if not impossible in the wilderness setting. Examinations may be hampered by the bulky clothing necessary to keep the victim warm and dry. Medications and equipment are subject to rough handling and extremes of temperature, which may render them ineffective, unsterile, or inoperative (Appendix A at the end of the chapter provides some information on drug stability). Finally, decision making that optimizes patient care while not unduly risking the well-being of SAR workers requires experienced leadership grounded in both common sense and technical skill. Perhaps the demands of SAR were best summarized by the wise rescuer who said that climbers, divers, hikers, and other outdoor enthusiasts get to choose where they practice their skills, but search and rescue personnel have no such choice. The situation, usually urgent, dictates where and when rescuers practice their art. The same situation that already compromised at least one person's health or well-being subsequently endangers the search and rescue participants.

This chapter is intended as a primer to introduce medical professionals to the unique search, rescue, and medical problems encountered in wilderness and backcountry situations. We discuss the rudiments of SAR coordination, resources, and specialized problems. This information will help medical personnel understand the SAR community and provide an educational foundation that might help to prevent situations requiring rescue.

Search and Rescue—An Overview

Search and rescue systems provide the response for overdue, lost, injured, or stranded people, usually in connection with outdoor activities and environments. In the context of SAR, "wilderness" can take on several meanings. For instance, most consider wilderness to be regions that are uninhabited and uncultivated. Personnel may be called out to search a natural area such as a large park or desert, but it is equally likely that a search will be urban, in an area devastated by a natural disaster such as an earthquake or hurricane. Since the majority of the U.S. population resides in urban areas, emergency responders and SAR personnel are far more likely to encounter an urban wilderness than a natural one. However, this chapter focuses on the nonurban setting.

SAR emergencies vary nationally, as do the responders. Programs, equipment, and personnel differ geographically in accordance with local needs and available resources.

SAR can probably be best defined as "finding and aiding people in distress—relieving pain and suffering."[9] SAR involves a great many volunteers and entails a multitude of skills. For example, the eruption of Mt. St. Helens, one of the nation's most catastrophic disasters, resulted in the largest peacetime search and rescue operation in the history of the United States.

SAR operations can benefit comprehensive emergency management, providing a training ground and experience builder for disaster response capability at the most elementary level. The management concepts used in SAR operations establish foundation principles for providing response capability to large-scale emergencies and disasters. Nearly every type of hazard mentioned in comprehensive emergency management plans (local and state disaster coordination plans developed in all states) requires search and rescue.[10] Management of these SAR operations can range from directing the actions of a few responders in a small community hit by a minor earthquake to managing an effort involving thousands of searchers in a large urban calamity. Often, large situations involve several political subdivisions and coordination of air and ground resources. Local governments and other agencies that participate in SAR response must coordinate diverse multiskilled responders. In addition, many agencies that collectively support multiorganizational SAR responses operate under their own specific statutory authority.

SAR operations entail a motivating time factor that focuses on a successful conclusion: finding or rescuing a lost subject before he or she succumbs to the effects of the environment, injuries, or a specific hazard. To be effective, extremely diverse organizations must be drawn together in a life-threatening situation with a commonality of purpose; this is even more true during a community-wide disaster.

SEARCH AND RESCUE IN THE UNITED STATES

National Search and Rescue Plan[13]

Very few people are familiar with the national SAR systems that provide response and assistance for overdue, missing, or stranded persons. Although SAR involves many agencies and volunteers, the federal government assumes some responsibilities for overall coordination, especially coordination of federal or military resources requested by local or state agencies. The *National Search and Rescue Plan,* a document that identifies federal responsibilities, is the basis for the *National Search and Rescue Manual,* which discusses search and rescue organization, resources, methods, and techniques. Although the federal government provides guidance, local and state government agencies are expected to assume responsibility for initial SAR response commensurate with their capabilities and within their geographic boundaries. In general, the federal role is to coordinate local, state, and federal agencies in order to create a cooperative national SAR network. According to the *National Search and Rescue Plan,* all maritime or navigable water SAR is the responsibility of the U.S. Coast Guard, and all inland SAR is the responsibility of the U.S. Air Force. These two military organizations are the federal coordinating agencies for federal resources used in responding to SAR incidents within their respective areas of responsibility (Fig. 21-1).

Air Force Rescue Coordination Center

The Aerospace Rescue and Recovery Service operates the Air Force Rescue Coordination Center (AFRCC), which is the federal agency responsible for coordinating SAR activities in the 48 contiguous states. The AFRCC's prime mission is to coordinate SAR for both military and civilian personnel. The AFRCC is centrally located at Scott Air Force Base, Illinois, 20 miles east of St. Louis, Missouri. It is operated 24 hours a day by personnel trained and experienced in SAR operations. The center is equipped with telephone, teletype, and hot-line communications. A resource file lists all federal, state, local, and volunteer organizations capable of conducting or assisting in SAR operations. However, the AFRCC is not authorized to commit federal funds to hire SAR resources. A list of Mexican and Canadian SAR coordinating agencies is available. The center is administratively divided into three sections: an operations section to conduct individual SAR missions; a directorship to provide overall management and formulate SAR plans, agreements, and policy; and a reports section to maintain data and records.

Federal Aviation Administration

Through its Air Route Traffic Control Centers and Flight Service Stations, the Federal Aviation Administration (FAA) monitors and flight-follows aircraft that file flight plans in the inland region. In some cases, individual citizens contact an FAA facility when they know of a probable SAR situation involving aircraft. Therefore the FAA is usually the first agency to alert the AFRCC about an emergency involving an overdue aircraft. The AFRCC is tied directly into the FAA's teletype network, and agency facilities use the teletype to initially alert the AFRCC.

Once the AFRCC is alerted, it works with the FAA to determine the urgency of the situation. Initially all radio communications are reviewed to ascertain as closely as possible the last location of the aircraft in distress. Concurrently, other FAA facilities begin to check all possible recovery airports for the missing aircraft. The AFRCC contacts relatives and friends of the pilot or passengers aboard the missing aircraft, in the hope of establishing the

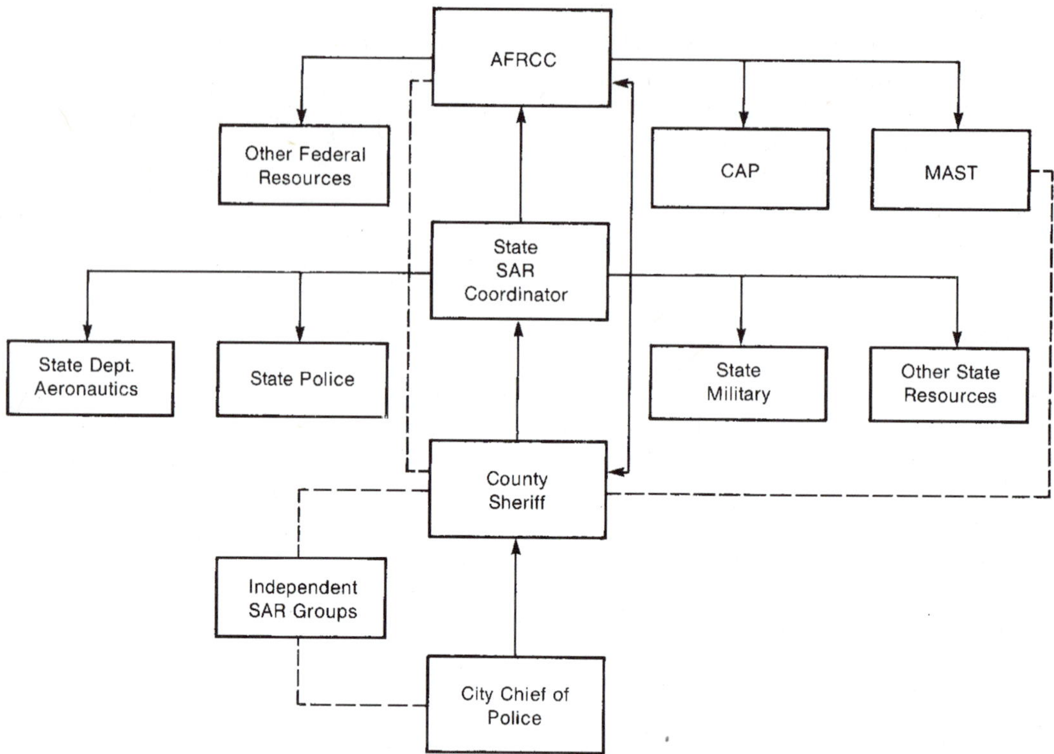

Fig. 21-1 Search and rescue (SAR) request and communication channels. The dotted lines show the channel for communication and information; the solid lines show the channel for requesting SAR mutual aid and assistance. *AFRCC,* Air Force Rescue Coordination Center; *CAP,* Civil Air Patrol; *MAST,* Military Assistance to Safety and Transportation.

whereabouts of the aircraft and gathering information about the persons aboard. The AFRCC attempts to get a description of the aircraft's capabilities and nuances and data on the emergency equipment aboard and the pilot's intentions. The FAA and AFRCC have learned that the majority of alerts for missing aircraft are generated by failure of the pilot either to finish the flight plan or to inform some person or agency of his or her intentions. For this reason only a small percentage of alerts issued by the FAA result in an actual airborne search for a missing aircraft.

Since the enactment of federal law requiring most aircraft to be equipped with an emergency locator transmitter (ELT), the AFRCC has worked closely with the FAA to locate the source of ELT signals. All ELT signals reported to FAA facilities are immediately forwarded to the AFRCC and investigated by both organizations as probable distress signals.

Civil Air Patrol

Throughout the United States the Civil Air Patrol provides most responses to downed or missing aircraft. The patrol is a private, nonprofit corporation of volunteers who provide emergency response and aviation safety education. On request, the Civil Air Patrol will provide to the authority in charge of the air search or rescue effort the following: mission coordinators; aircraft, pilots, and observers; ground search teams; base camp support; and communications networks. When officially given a task and involved in a search or rescue mission, patrol members are reimbursed by the U.S. Air Force for communication expenses and fuel and oil expenses incurred by aircraft or ground vehicles. In addition, because members constitute an official auxiliary of the Air Force, all Civil Air Patrol members are covered by the Federal Worker's Compensation Act in the event of injury. Current statistics show that Civil Air Patrol members respond to three fourths of all air SAR missions.

State's Role: Coordination and Support

All states have passed legislation that provides for direct support to local government entities during emergencies or life-threatening situations. Approximately 22 of the 50 states have a state agency responsible for overall coordination and support for local SAR problems. This support can take many forms, but most often it is in the area of coordination and "one-stop shopping" for resources. Each state must establish an agency or central location that is familiar with all aspects of emergency management and the resources available to aid in life-threatening situations. Many of the resources available belong to the state and can be used to aid local jurisdictions.

A number of states, especially in the Northwest, have designated a state agency to be responsible for directing and coordinating air SAR activities. These state departments or divisions of aeronautics develop and maintain aviation search and rescue response programs with cooperation and support from local and federal agencies. It has been our experience that this system works far better than those in other areas of the country that rely on the federal government to initiate and carry out aircraft SAR activities.

If a local emergency manager, sheriff, or fire chief requests outside assistance in the form of specialized teams, search dogs, air support, or enhanced communications, the state agency for civil defense, emergency services, or emergency management can in most cases locate the nearest resources available and coordinate the response. If any federal resources are needed, such as air support or military personnel, the state agency provides a direct link to that resource. For instance, the AFRCC at Scott Air Force Base in Illinois has working agreements with the majority of states that are updated annually. Technically, the resources of local and state governments must have been exhausted or be unequal to a task before federal support can be rendered. However, policy provides for immediate aid when time is critical and in life-or-death situations. Much discretion is given to military installation commanders regarding aid to civilian authorities as long as the primary (military) mission of the resource is not impaired. In fact, most commanders appreciate the opportunity to fly actual missions. Access to these resources must be gained through the state and the AFRCC.

A good example of this coordination and relationship took place recently in a state that was undertaking a major search effort for a missing child. The local sheriff's deputy coordinating the search effort needed air support desperately to transport searchers into higher areas and to search some difficult terrain. Access to the area was limited and time considerations were critical. The child was inadequately clothed for the weather conditions and several severe weather fronts were expected within 48 hours. The deputy also thought that a few good search dog teams would pay high dividends within some of the designated search areas. A request for helicopter support was made to the state department of emergency management. No private or commercial helicopter resources were available in the surrounding area. (Military aircraft cannot fly a mission of this type if civilian resources are available in the area, especially if it takes business away from private enterprise.) The state agency made a call to the AFRCC and requested support from a base located over a hundred miles north of the county where the search was being conducted. They also asked if the aircraft could detour slightly and pick up two search dogs and handlers. Less than 45 minutes after the original request, Air Force helicopters were airborne. The dogs and their handlers were transported to the search scene and participated in the search. The dog teams were ultimately successful.

Every state's emergency management agency is responsible for providing support, guidance, training, and coordination to local political subdivisions within that state. As such, it produces a vital behind-the-scenes effort to help local jurisdictions prepare for emergencies, including SAR. The state also initiates the laws necessary to enhance effective actions for SAR response. Such legislation often indemnifies volunteer SAR teams, provides their medical coverage and insurance, and in some cases replaces personal property lost during SAR work. Although most volunteers work willingly until the job is done, this recognition and coverage by the state often provide additional incentives for volunteer participation.

Local Response

The official response to the call for a wilderness SAR situation is usually delegated to a political subdivision within the state. The legal responsibility for SAR is generally vested with the county sheriff or chief law enforcement officer at the local level, but this varies by region and state. In some cases it is the responsibility of state police agencies, in others, of land management agencies. The SAR response for one jurisdiction may differ greatly from that for another. For instance, many national parks in some areas of the country handle all of their own SAR incidents. Others jointly manage the function, while some rely entirely on outside resources. National forest land is managed solely by forest service personnel, but in SAR this federal agency only supports the functions of the local sheriff's department.

In urban areas, police officers, firefighters, emergency medical technicians, and civil defense emergency organizations maintain some degree of disaster and emergency readiness through daily missions that involve SAR work. Fire departments have historically been responsible for rescue and response to emergencies within certain geographic or political areas. Many are augmented by volunteers. Law enforcement agencies also maintain full-time, efficient response systems designed for their particular SAR requirements. Ambulance and rescue vehicles operated by a variety of private enterprises and volunteer organizations augment existing local government services. Through local emergency response planning and coordination, these services respond to a spectrum of everyday emergencies, including fires, collapsed buildings, hazardous material spills, vehicle extrications, and home medical emergencies.

County sheriffs, reserve law enforcement, volunteer fire departments, and a variety of volunteer and rescue units have been established to address local SAR problems. Delivery of search and rescue aid to rural and wilderness areas often presents many special logistic problems, which may be compounded by distance, terrain, and weather. The demand for wilderness SAR is often seasonal and unpredictable. Volunteer mountain rescue units, Explorer search and rescue groups, search and rescue dog teams, Civil Air Patrol squadrons, motorized units, and many types of volunteer composite teams (teams having a variety of capabilities) are usually formed locally in response to the type and nature of recurring SAR problems. Regardless of who does it or what type of SAR emergencies occur, local resources and effort must be developed because they are closest to the problem. State and federal resources are subject to problems with time lag, distance, weather, and logistics. The same storm or disaster that incapacitates a local area may also prohibit outside (and sometimes inside) emergency response and resupply.

Although official agency responses differ greatly around the country, one major factor remains constant: the dedicated and unfailing willingness of volunteers to respond and work until the job is done. The volunteer effort in SAR nationwide is the backbone of aid to people in distress, as is stated in the rescue service motto: "These Things We Do That Others May Live." The volunteer response has proved crucial to wilderness-type situations. Volunteer organizations, communications, and special skills cannot be replaced by any "official agency" resources.

Organization of a Search and Rescue Event

Search and rescue requires people who take action and meet objectives to achieve a common goal, often with one or more lives in the balance. For any combination of actions to be effective in a particular situation, the enterprise must be systematically coordinated and organized. All participants must know their responsibilities, what is expected of them, who is in charge, and to whom they should answer. If this knowledge is lacking, the effort can quickly become chaotic, ineffective, and very probably, dangerous. Nowhere are these issues more important than in an emergency situation where time is of the essence.

Emergency response research is clear and specific. The four operational problems that continue to arise during emergency responses in the United States are ambiguity of authority, inability to communicate between agencies, poor use (or no use) of specialized resources, and unplanned negative interactions with the news media.[9,10] Accordingly, the key elements for success in SAR operations continue to be good coordination of resources (the right people and equipment in the right place at the right time), effective communications, and good management practices with trained leaders.[10]

INCIDENT COMMAND SYSTEM

The system designed to address the challenges of managing emergency incidents, including SAR, is called the Incident Command System (ICS). It has been in use in the United States for many years.[3] This function-based system was designed to be adaptable to various types and sizes of incidents in a proactive, rather than a reactive, manner. The system groups similar tasks into five functional areas: command, operations, planning, logistics, and finance. Each of these functions is performed at every incident to one degree or another, and all can easily be expanded as the size and complexity of the situation dictate. This expansion, however, is based in the premise that the span of control—the ratio of the subordinates to each supervisor—should never exceed seven to one and should more commonly be five to one. When this is exceeded, another level is added to the hierarchy to maintain an acceptable span of control (Fig. 21-2).

Command

The command section is led by the incident commander and provides overall management for the incident. Within ICS the command section is responsible for dealing with other agencies (liaison officer), for dealing with the news media and other external influences (information officer), and for the overall safety of the operation and its participants (safety officer). If the incident is too small for these functions to be performed by separate individuals, the incident commander performs them.

As mentioned earlier, unplanned negative interactions with the news media are one of the four operational problems that continue to plague SAR efforts. It is crucially important to properly address the functions of the information officer (sometimes called the public information officer [PIO]). Proper interaction with the news media and other external influences (family members, political officials, and so on) can dramatically affect the success of an SAR event, at least in the public's eye. SAR managers are correct to presume that how they deal with these influences may well dictate their future, professionally and otherwise. A skilled SAR manager sees interaction with these influences as an opportunity to gain assistance from the general public and from powerful individuals, not as a challenge to be overcome.

Operations

The operations section is led by the operations section chief, who is responsible for coordinating and performing all tactical operations. This role is commonly performed by the incident commander until the incident becomes large and complex enough that the function must be performed by another individual. Examples of functional groups that might fall under the operations section are emergency medical services, hazardous materials, firefighting, law enforcement, search, rescue, and recovery. Depending on the situation, additional operational functions may be required. For instance, traffic control might be required at a vehicle accident, ventilation might be required at a fire scene, and so on. The system permits "operations" to mean any tactics required to meet the goals of the incident action plan.

When multiple casualties are involved in an incident, their triage, treatment, and transport fall under the purview of the operations section. In such an incident the operations

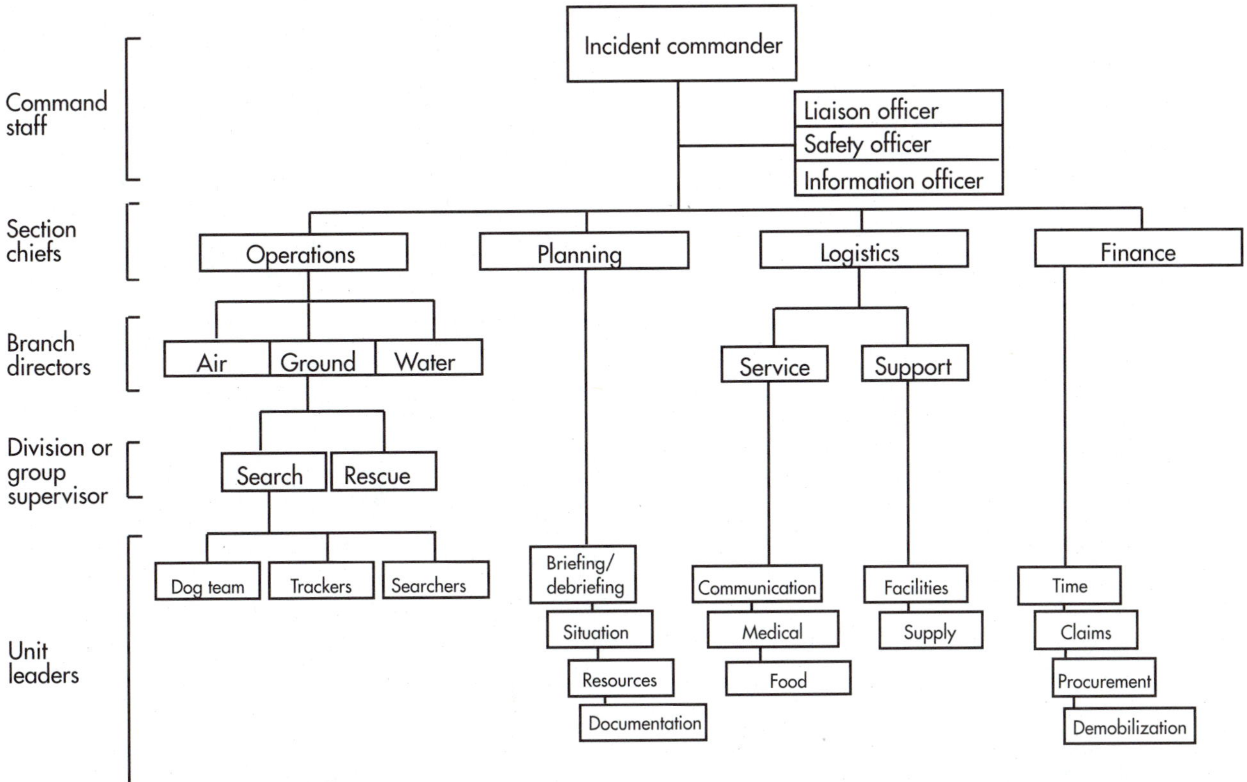

Fig. 21-2 Functional hierarchy of the Incident Command System commonly used in search and rescue in the United States. (From Cooper DC, LaValla PH, Stoffel RC: *Search and rescue fundamentals: basic skills and knowledge to perform search and rescue,* ed 3, Olympia, Wash, 1993, Emergency Response Institute.)

section is divided into functional groups, often including at least triage, treatment, and transport groups. The person in charge of managing and coordinating the efforts of each group is called the group supervisor.

If the operations section is better divided using geography than function, a "division" rather than a "group" is formed. For instance, injured persons at an auto accident might be found on two sides of a road. An east division and a west division might be established to deal with the geographic separation of the resources. The supervisor of each division would answer to the operations chief.

To respond to specific challenges within an incident, a task force or strike team might be formed. A task force uses similar units to meet an objective. For instance, a number of three-person tracking teams could be assembled into a task force, then assigned a leader and communications to meet a common objective. A strike team, on the other hand, is a collection of dissimilar resources assembled for a specific mission. For instance, two three-person tracking teams and three dog teams could be combined, assigned a leader and common communications, and charged with accomplishing a particular mission. These two combinations of resources permit the necessary flexibility in resource allocation.

Planning

The planning section is led by the planning section chief, who is responsible for collecting, evaluating, and distributing all incident information. As with the other sections, the incident commander performs this function unless the size and complexity of the incident dictate otherwise.

In SAR the planning section is particularly important because it evaluates evidence and determines, based on what has been learned, what future actions should be taken or how current actions should be modified. Because such interpretation and evaluation often require great technical knowledge, personnel such as hazardous materials specialists, physicians, structural engineers, and others with specialized training help the planning section develop and revise the incident action plan.

Examples of the planning section tasks include the following:

1. Developing, revising, and distributing the incident action plan

2. Developing, procuring, and maintaining any written documents such as maps and sketches
3. Predicting future events and establishing contingencies based on predictions
4. Tracking the status of all resources
5. Documenting all incident activities

Logistics

The logistics section is led by the logistics section chief, who is responsible for providing personnel, equipment, and supplies for the entire incident. This awesome task involves ensuring that personnel are available, rested, and fed; that all equipment, including communications equipment, is available and operable; that vehicles are fueled and repaired; and that medical care is provided for all incident personnel. Basically, logistics is charged with seeing that the physical tools required to meet the overall objectives are available, operable, and maintained.

Finance

If the size and complexity of the incident prevent the incident commander from monitoring finances, the finance section is led by the finance section chief. This section is responsible for tracking all financial data for the incident, such as personnel hours, resource costs, costs for damage survey, and injury claims and compensation.

Since most agencies involved in SAR can handle financial issues on their own, and since most incidents are small and of short duration, the incident commander usually performs the functions of this section. Only in the largest or most complex incidents is it necessary for the incident commander to assign an individual or staff to perform finance section duties.

Four Phases of a Search and Rescue Event: The Incident Cycle

Every search and rescue event goes through four consecutive phases: locate, access, stabilize, and transport.[4] This sequence, however, could more accurately be described as a continuum that begins with planning or preplanning for the incident. Since planning for the next incident should be affected by what happened during the last, the incident cycle is actually continuous and only pauses between incidents. Once first notice of an incident has been received and the locate phase begins, the goal is to progress through the access, stabilize, and transport phases as quickly, safely, and efficiently as possible. Planning between incidents allows decisions to be made in a calm environment without the urgency that often accompanies an SAR operation. Such plans identify who will be in charge, the organization of the operation, specific procedures, viable alternatives, and other decisions that are best made before an incident occurs (Fig. 21-3).

LOCATE PHASE

The first step in addressing any emergency situation is locating the subject or subjects in need of assistance. This may be as simple as asking for an address or as complex as conducting an extended search (one lasting more than 2 hours[14]) for a lost person or persons. If the subject is easily found, rescuers can quickly move into the access phase. However, if locating the subject is difficult, this phase may turn into the crux of the SAR problem.

First Notice

The first notice of an incident is often conveyed by relatives who report an injury or missing person, by a witness to an incident, by a government agency reporting distress signals (such as Emergency Locator Transmitter), by bystanders who perceive a problem, or by a 911 call. Once the initial notice is received, the individual taking the information must know what to do and whom to call next.

Planning Data and Its Uses

Information gathered at the onset of an incident begins an ongoing investigation. It is used to determine the appropriate response and to help predict how the subject or subjects might react to the situation. This information is called "planning data" and includes any information that might affect what should be done to resolve the situation. Examples of planning data include the name of the subject, the situation that caused the problem, the last known location of the subject, the subject's physical and mental condition, the subject's plans (where was he or she going?), what resources are available, weather information (present and predicted), geographic information, and the history of similar incidents in the area. The purpose of collecting all this information is to help decide what to do next while predicting what the subject might do to help or hinder the situation.

The investigation and gathering of information continue throughout the incident and are used to modify initial plans. As new information is acquired, an action plan is developed and revised until the end of the incident cycle, when planning for the next incident commences.

Once information is gathered, the urgency of the situation is assessed by someone in charge. This assessment ultimately determines the speed, level, and nature of any response and may indicate whether a nonurgent or an emergency response is needed. The specific information used in urgency determination includes the age and condition of the subject, current and predicted weather, and relevant hazards. Box 21-1 is an Urgency Determination Form, which can be used by SAR managers to determine how urgent their response should be. Urgency contributes to allowable risks and thus influences searcher safety—a primary consideration for search managers.

Search Tactics

During the initial "locate" phase of the incident, emphasis is on searching for the subject. Exactly how to accomplish

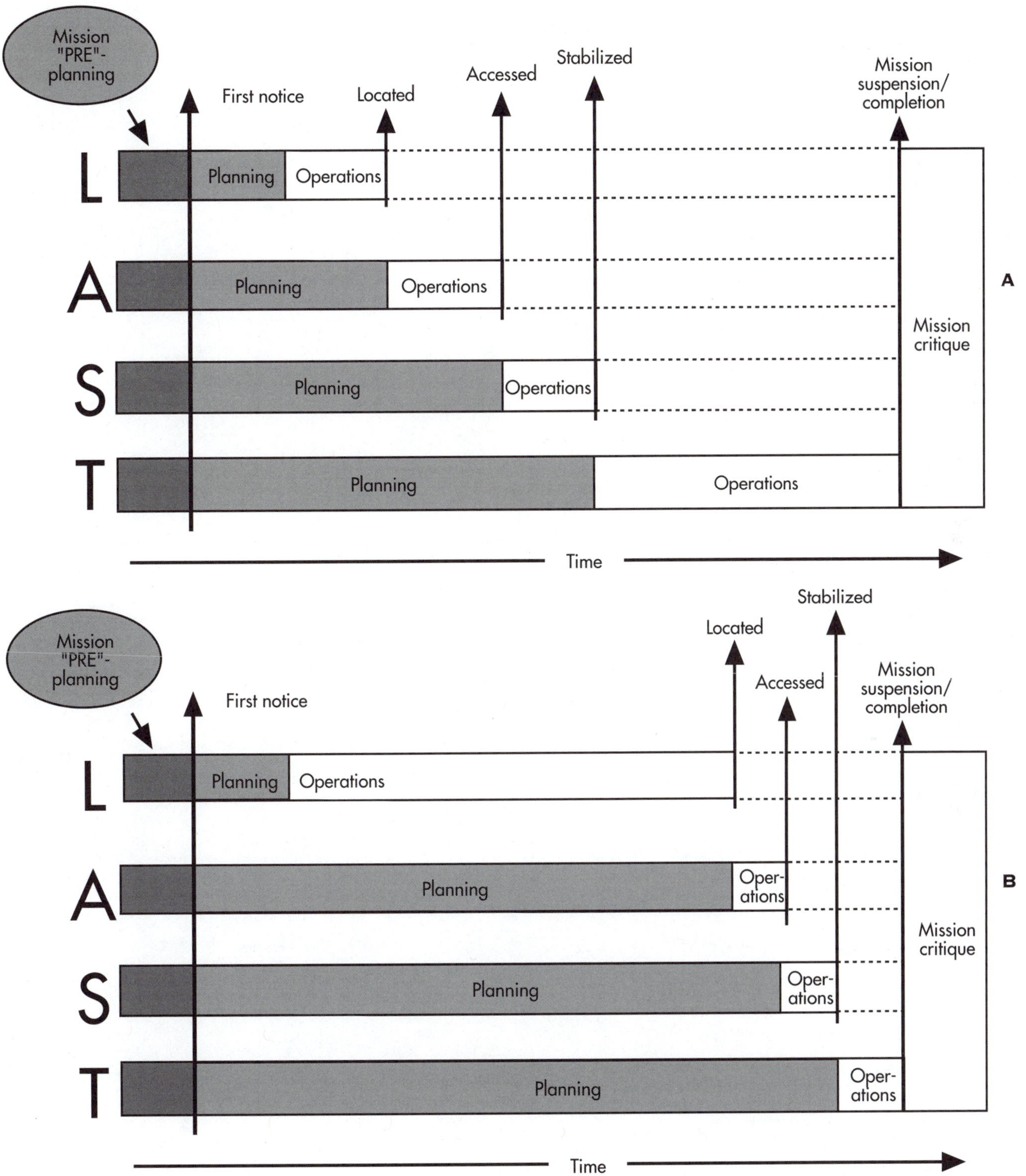

Fig. 21-3 The time-specific components of an SAR event vary with the type of incident. Note that all components take place in both incidents, but simply take different amounts of time. **A,** Typical rescue operation. **B,** Typical search operation.

BOX 21-1

URGENCY DETERMINATION FORM

On the following chart, the lower the numerical rating of the factor, the higher the relative urgency, and the higher the rating, the lower the urgency. Range = 7 to 21. Add up the score and assess the urgency using the graph.

7	9	11	13	15	17	19	21
Highest Urgency			Intermediate Urgency				Lowest Urgency

SUBJECT PROFILE	Rating
Age	
Very young	1
Very old	1
Other	2-3
Medical Condition	
Known or suspected injured or ill or mental problem	1-2
Healthy	3
Known fatality	3
Number of Subjects	
One alone	1
More than one (unless separation is suspected)	2-3
SUBJECT EXPERIENCE PROFILE	
Not experienced, does not know area	1
Not experienced, knows area	1-2
Experienced, not familiar with area	2
Experienced, knows area	3
WEATHER PROFILE	
Past or present hazardous weather	1
Predicted hazardous weather (8 hr or less)	1-2
Predicted hazardous weather (more than 8 hr)	2
No hazardous weather predicted	3
EQUIPMENT PROFILE	
Inadequate for environment and weather	1
Questionable for environment and weather	1-2
Adequate for environment and weather	3
TERRAIN AND HAZARDS PROFILE	
Known hazardous terrain or other hazards	1
Few or no hazards	2-3

Date Completed: ____________ Time: ____________ Total Score: ____________

From Cooper DC, LaValla PH, Stoffel RC: *Search and rescue fundamentals: basic skills and knowledge to perform search and rescue,* ed 3, Olympia, Wash, 1990, Emergency Response Institute.

this is a priority, especially if this part of the incident cycle is expected to be a problem. SAR managers first initiate techniques that increase the chances of locating the subject in the shortest time. These techniques are generally termed "tactics" and involve some action performed to find the subject. These actions can be passive, not requiring actual field searching, or active, requiring deployment of searchers in the field. Examples of passive tactics include confining the search area to limit movement of the subject and people into and out of the area, identifying and protecting the point last seen (PLS) or the last known position (LKP), and attracting the subject, if he or she is expected to be responsive.

Generally, passive techniques are quicker and easier to apply, so they are started first. As the incident progresses, active tactics are initiated. In SAR management, efforts are almost universally made to apply quick response resources in areas likely to offer early success. The best resources are put in the best areas as early as possible. In addition, identifying and protecting the PLS or LKP are crucial passive techniques that can mean the difference between success and failure of the entire effort.[9]

Active techniques include sending teams of searchers into an area to search for clues or the subject. They are categorized by level of thoroughness. For instance, a fast, relatively nonthorough search of high-probability areas is called a type I search (see Table 21-1). Type II techniques can be applied when relatively rapid searches of large areas are desired. Thoroughness may increase, but more important, efficiency improves because larger areas can be searched with the same or fewer resources. Thus success is achieved sooner. Type III techniques are applied only when the absolute highest level of thoroughness is required. Unfortunately, this is almost always at the expense of time and efficiency. Basically, the greater the thoroughness, the less efficient the technique.

Clues and Their Value

Clues are discovered during the investigative and tactical phases of a search. Their importance cannot be overemphasized. They may take the form of physical evidence such as a footprint or discarded item, or an account by a witness, or information gleaned from the investigation. Clues serve as the rudder that steers the overall search operation. Relevant clues are the basis for all search strategy and can determine or modify all actions. Their powerful influence should be obvious; this is why searchers are taught to be "clue conscious" and to seek clues, not just subjects. There are many more clues than there are subjects.

People generate clues. A person exudes scent, takes up space, and, when traveling, leaves evidence of passing. This evidence is often discoverable if the appropriate resource is applied in a coordinated, organized search effort. Searchers must be sophisticated enough to discover this evidence and interpret its meaning before it is destroyed or decays. Since

Table 21-1 Summary of Active Search Tactics

	Type I	Type II	Type III
Criterion	Speed	Efficiency	Thoroughness
Objective	Quickly search high-probability areas and gain information on search area	Rapid search of large areas	Search with absolute highest probability of detection
Definition	Fast initial response of well-trained, self-sufficient, and very mobile searchers, who check areas most likely to produce clues or the subject the soonest	Relatively fast, systematic search of high-probability segments of the search area that produce high results per searcher hour of effort	Slow, highly systematic search using the most thorough techniques to provide the highest possible probability of detection
Considerations	Works best with responsive subject; offers immediate show of effort; helps define search area; clue consciousness is critical; planning is crucial for effective use; often determines where not to search	Often employed after hasty searches, especially if clues were found; best suited to responsive subjects; often effective at finding clues; between-searcher spacing depends on terrain and visibility	Marking search segment is very important; should be used only as a last resort; very destructive of clues; used when other methods of searching are unsuccessful
Techniques	Investigation (personal physical effort); check last known position for clues; follow known route; run trails and ridges; check area perimeter, confine area; check hazards and attractions	Open grid line search with wide between-searcher spacing; compass bearings or specific guides are often used to control search; often applied in a defined area to follow up a discovered clue; no overlap in area coverage; critical separation; sound sweeps	Closed grid or sweep search with small between-searcher spacing; searched areas often overlap adjacent teams for better coverage
Usual team makeup	Two or three very mobile, well-trained, self-sufficient searchers	May include three to seven skilled searchers, but usually just three	Four to seven searchers, including both trained and untrained personnel
Most effective resource	Investigators; trained hasty teams; human trackers; dogs; aircraft; any mobile trained resource	Clue-conscious search teams; human trackers and sign-cutters; dogs; aircraft; trained grid search teams	Trained grid search teams

discoverable evidence important to a search effort is often easily destroyed, it is important to protect it from damage until it is completely analyzed.

Search Resources

"Resources" are defined as all personnel and equipment available, or potentially available, for assignment to incident tasks; information on the status of resources should be maintained.[14] Specific types of active tactics are categorized by the resource that performs them, such as dog teams, human trackers, ground search teams, and aircraft. Other common resources include management teams (for example, overhead teams, public information officers), water-trained responders (for example, river rescue, divers), cold weather responders (for example, ice climbers, avalanche experts, ski patrollers), specialized vehicle responders (for example, snowmobiles, four-wheel-drive trucks, all-terrain vehicles, mountain bikes, horses), and technical experts (for example, communications experts, interviewers, chemists, rock climbers, physicians, cavers). In addition to these, other less common resources might also be available. These could include attraction devices (such as horns, flags, lights, sirens), mine detectors (military), noise-sensitive equipment (super microphones), infrared devices (forward-looking infrared [FLIR] on aircraft, night vision equipment), thermistors, and even witches, seers, prophets, and diviners.

Just about anything imaginable may be available for use in a SAR incident. Their use is limited only by the creativity of those in charge. Here we discuss a few of the most common.

Dogs. Dog teams are a common type of active search resource in the wilderness and are composed of a dog (occasionally more than one) and a human handler. The dog uses scent to search for and follow a subject while the handler interprets signals from the dog and searches visually for evidence. Three common types are tracking dogs, trailing dogs, and air-scenting dogs.

Tracking dogs follow scent on the ground from a person's footsteps and usually very closely follow the trail where a person traveled, regardless of the wind. Trailing dogs follow scent that has fallen onto the ground from the subject along the route of travel. Unlike the tracking dog, the trailing dog may follow the scent at some distance from the actual tracks of the subject, and may therefore be more affected by wind. Tracking and trailing dogs are most effective when used in areas that have not been contaminated by humans other than the subject. Also, weather and time tend to work to destroy scent available to these types of dogs, so the earlier they are used in a search, the better their chances of finding something.

Air-scenting dogs work off-lead to follow a subject's scent to its source. Specifically bred and trained air-scenting dogs can even discriminate between individual humans. They may detect scent from articles of clothing and can often follow it to discover a person buried in rubble or snow or even submerged under water. Wind is very important to this type of dog, as are other environmental forces such as sun and rain. But as long as the source exists, an air-scenting dog can usually detect the scent carried in air currents and follow it to the source.

Human Trackers. Human trackers use their visual senses to search for evidence left by a person's passing. Human trackers "cut" or look for "sign" or discoverable evidence by examining the area where the subject probably would have passed. This process of looking for the first piece of evidence from which to track is called "sign cutting." Following the subsequent chain or chronology of sign is called "tracking."[5]

In SAR, most trackers use a stride-based approach called the step-by-step method. This simple, methodical method emphasizes finding every piece of possible evidence left by a subject. However, its most important role is undoubtedly its ability to determine quickly the direction of travel of the subject and thus limit the search area.

Ground Search Teams

Hasty teams. A hasty team is an initial response team of well-trained, self-sufficient, highly mobile searchers whose primary responsibility is to check out the areas most likely to first produce the subject or clues (trails, roads, roadheads, campsites, lakes, clearings, and so on). Their efficiency and usefulness are based on how quickly they can respond and the accuracy of initial information.

Ideally, hasty teams should include two or three individuals who are knowledgeable about track and signs. They should be clue and subject oriented, familiar with the local terrain and dangers in the area, and completely self-sufficient. Also necessary are the ability to skillfully interview witnesses and to use navigational skills with pinpoint accuracy. Team members should be trained at least in advanced first aid. Hasty teams usually operate under standard operating procedures, so they do not have to wait for specific instructions. They carry all the equipment they might need to help themselves and the lost subject for at least 24 hours.

Grid teams. Grid searchers use a more systematic approach to searching. They usually examine a well-defined, usually small, segment to discover evidence. The classic approach to grid searching involves several individuals (almost always too many) standing in a line, shoulder to shoulder, walking through an area in search of either evidence or subjects. The distance between searchers can be varied to change thoroughness and efficiency (wide spacing is less thorough and more efficient). However, such resource-intensive approaches to searching are generally preferred less than those that use fewer personnel in a more efficient manner (such as tracking, dogs, or aircraft). In addition, close-spaced grid searching tends to damage evidence and is generally difficult to coordinate.

While grid searching may be an acceptable approach in certain limited circumstances, experience has shown that when the subject of a search is a person, searching in this thorough manner should be used only as a last resort. Experiments involving grid searching have suggested that it is better to place searchers farther apart. This improves efficiency and use of resources.

Aircraft. Aircraft serve the same purpose as grid searchers, only from a greater distance, at a greater speed, over a larger area, and usually with a lower level of thoroughness.

Within a search effort, aircraft can serve both as a tactical tool to look for clues and as transportation for personnel and equipment. Both fixed- and rotor-wing aircraft have their place in SAR and, like other resources, have their advantages and limitations. Among the most obvious limitations are the expense and complex use requirements of aircraft. Aircraft not only require specialized personnel and cost a great deal to operate, they also have very strict weather and environmental restrictions. For instance, it would be difficult to search from an aircraft in a snowstorm, and terrain may prevent searching certain areas from the air. However, most of these difficulties can be adequately addressed and minimized in a well-developed preplan.

Search Management Considerations[9]

State-of-the-art searching for lost persons has come a long way from the familiar lining-up of volunteers shoulder to shoulder and walking in a straight line to search an area. Many new lifesaving concepts have been developed by the national SAR community. By borrowing from psychology, mathematics, and business and analyzing research on past incidents, search management has evolved into a sophisticated science. By studying human behavior, statistics, probabilities, leadership, and management, search managers have been able to improve search effectiveness and efficiency.

Search management is determined by two general considerations: where am I going to look for the lost person? (strategy) and how am I going to find the lost person? (tactics). To be effective, modern searchers follow several basic principles and techniques:

1. Respond urgently—*a search is an emergency.*
2. Confine the search area.
3. Search for clues.
4. Search at night.
5. Search with a plan in an organized manner.
6. Grid search (type III) as a last resort.

Every day, firefighters, paramedics, police officers, and other emergency responders receive calls to perform their duties, and often they can only guess what they will find once they arrive. In searching, too, the concept of the "firehouse" response has evolved. This concept calls for emergency responders, much like emergency physicians, to assume the worst and hope for the best. Thus they respond with "lights and siren" to most calls just in case the situation is serious. Furthermore, they often respond in this way even when the reporting party specifies that the situation is minor, claiming that a certain percentage of individuals reporting incidents are wrong in their assessment. Essentially, the situation is considered an emergency until proven otherwise.

For years, searching has been considered less urgent than other emergencies. While emergency responders were running with lights and sirens to situations reported as "women not feeling well" or "dumpster on fire," reports of a lost child or an overdue hiker were relegated to the "let's wait and see" category. Through years of experience, search managers now know that a search is as much an emergency as any other call for help. Furthermore, if an urgent response is mustered, the situation can be resolved faster, more successfully, and usually with less effort. Thus a search should be considered an emergency that justifies an urgent response, a high priority, a thorough assessment, and immediate action.

Data analysis from thousands of SAR missions has made it possible to predict where the subject might be and to assess the relative probability that the subject is or is not within the search area. This quantification of the chances that the lost person or clue is in the search area is called probability of area (POA). Research on various types and methods of ground search patterns and the ability of a resource (such as dogs, ground searchers, or helicopters) to detect a lost person or clue has produced a similar concept, called "probability of detection" or POD. POD is a quantification of the probability that a search resource will find the lost person or clue if it indeed is in the area being searched. Further application of this "probability" theory allows the development of an overall probability of success (POS), the product of POA and POD (POD × POA = POS). Such a POS can be used by a skilled search manager in the planning stages of a search to predict the outcomes of specific resource field applications.

Modern search management is also based on the use of what is called a complete "subject profile." Such a profile identifies as much as is known about the missing subject, including general state of health, past experiences, and state of mind, through the use of a form called the Lost Person Questionnaire. This information is collected and used by search managers to predict how an individual would react in various situations.

Analysis of past incidents and how the involved individuals behaved in given circumstances has offered great insight for search managers. Several studies of lost person behavior have been conducted over the years, including the ground-breaking work of the late William G. Syrotuck.[12] Mr. Syrotuck's work produced the concept of geographic probability zones around the point last seen and defined categories of lost persons based on the fact that individuals with similar characteristics behave in similar ways. Such efforts have taught search managers the importance of collecting behavioral data on lost persons, as well as the predictive value of such data.

ACCESS PHASE

After the subject is located, the search is over. Rescuers must now gain access to the subject to assess and treat injuries, evaluate the situation, and mitigate the problem. Accomplishing these objectives may be as simple as walking into a room with the subject or as complex as reaching an astronaut in space. Regardless, planning for this eventuality should be complete and ready to be carried out at the conclusion of the locate phase.

Once rescuers reach a subject, the situation and scene must be assessed. In emergency services terminology this is called the size-up. The size-up consists of identifying hazards to the subject and rescuers, then developing a strategy to deal with the problems. For instance, a subject might be trapped by a winter storm in a high alpine environment. Safety considerations for rescuers entering such a hostile and dangerous environment would certainly influence further actions and may well take precedence over the entire rescue effort (Fig. 21-4).

Specialized skills may be required for rescuers to safely gain access to the scene. For instance, rescuers may need to rappel to a patient who has fallen onto a ledge in terrain like the Grand Canyon. Or rescuers may need to climb sheer rock faces to reach an injured mountaineer on Half Dome in Yosemite National Park. These are examples of how complex the access phase of a rescue may be and point to the importance of thorough and proper planning (Fig. 21-5).

If the size-up indicates that the situation or environment is so hazardous that remaining on scene poses an immediate threat to the subject, accelerated rescue techniques may be required. Accelerated rescue techniques are immediate actions required to remove a subject from a dangerous environment without stabilization. They often entail deviations from local standard operating procedures and protocols. Examples of such situations include poisonous gas environments (for example, in caves), fires, unstable terrain (such as avalanches and rock slides), adverse weather (hurricanes, thunderstorms, severe snowstorms), or any hostile environment that threatens the subject, rescuers, or both.

STABILIZE PHASE

Once the rescuers have access to the subject, medical management commences. This process usually follows accepted procedures, starting with primary and secondary physical examinations and basic and advanced life support. The goal of medical stabilization is usually to prepare the

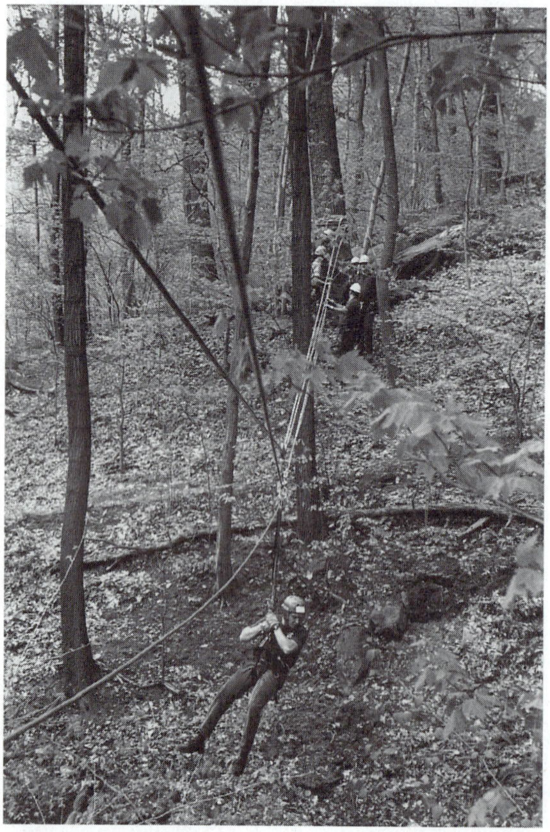

Fig. 21-4 Specialized, and often complex, skills may be required to gain access to a patient. Here a rescuer is lowered to a victim of a fall in a deep ravine.

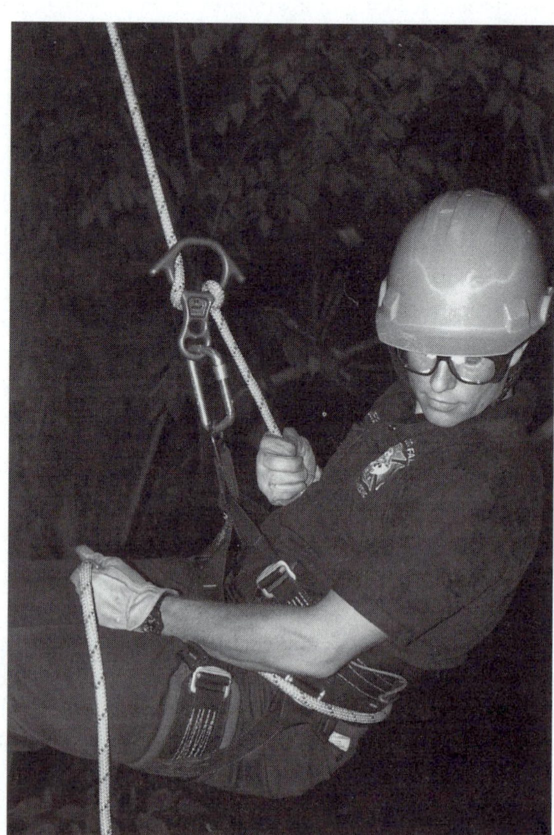

Fig. 21-5 Rappeling is a skill commonly used in the access phase of SAR. Note the use of head, hand, and eye protection.

subject for transportation to a definitive care facility. If medical care is not required, confirming this fact may be all that is required at this stage before moving into the transport phase.

Stabilization, like assessment, should continue throughout the transport phase. It should include full body immobilization, usually in a litter; specific site immobilization of fractures and related injuries; treatment of shock and other hemodynamic compromise; and protection from the environment. The overall objective is to prepare the patient for transport to definitive care while maintaining his or her comfort and safety.

TRANSPORT PHASE

In the fourth phase of SAR the subject is moved to definitive care. For this to occur, the stabilized subject must be "packaged" so that he or she can be moved safely and efficiently while stabilization and assessment continue. Transportation types range from foot travel, with the subject walking on his or her own, to evacuation by aircraft. The appropriate mode of transportation is determined by weather, type and severity of injuries, overall urgency, terrain, available resources, and other related factors.

Equipment

Today's rescues occur in many remote and unusual environments and often require extremely technical rescue equipment and skills. Responders trained in the appropriate techniques and technologies should be the only personnel to apply them. Much of the gear and many of the techniques have been derived from those first developed by mountaineers, climbers, cavers, and more recently, white-water enthusiasts.

Rescue equipment is generally broken down into three broad categories: personal gear, rescue software, and rescue hardware. Personal equipment includes such items as footwear, gloves, helmets, articles of clothing, eye protection, and other protective apparel. Software is such equipment as rope, webbing, slings, and harnesses that are made of soft, strong synthetic materials specifically designed and manufactured for rescue. Hardware is such equipment as carabiners, cams, friction devices, pulleys, and litters made of steel and alloys specifically designed and manufactured to endure the rigors of rescue.

Personal Equipment. Rescuers must often wear special equipment to protect them from accidents and hazards. Head, eye, and hand protection is considered mandatory in virtually all rescue environments. Additional personal equipment requirements are dictated by the rescue environment and the specific needs of the situation (Fig. 21-6).

Special gear. In addition to the usual challenges of the rescue environment, certain hazards require specialized equipment. Examples of such equipment include fire-resistant clothing worn by structural and wildland firefighters, personal flotation devices (PFDs) used by rescuers in and around water (Fig. 21-7), netting used in outdoor settings when insects become a problem, bulletproof garments used by law enforcement and military rescue personnel, and chemical protective suits worn when exposure to hazardous materials is possible.

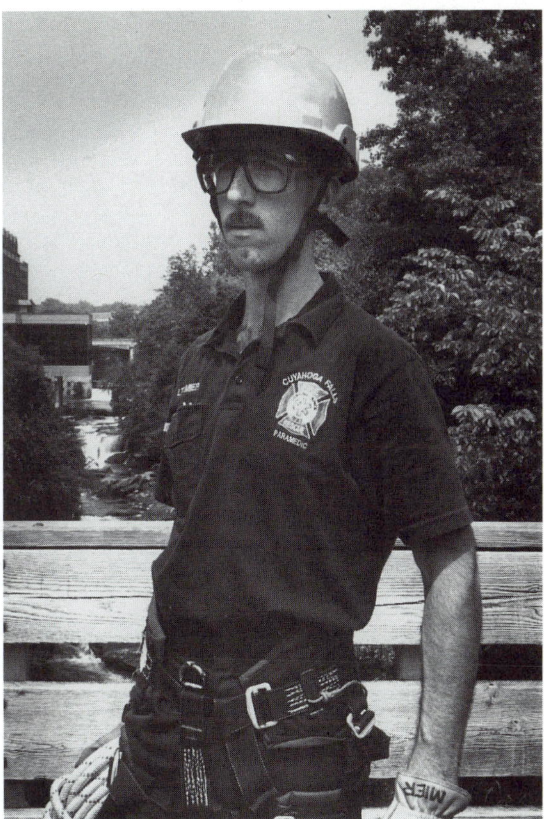

Fig. 21-6 Even though the personal equipment necessary is dictated by both the rescue environment and the needs of the specific situation, it includes head, hand, and eye protection as a minimum.

No clothing or protective gear meets all the requirements for involvement in or around a rescue scene. Rescuers study situations so that they understand all hazards before anyone becomes involved. Their conclusions help them identify protective equipment requirements. Gear that may be necessary for one environment can be dangerous in another. Firefighter's turnout gear may be required in a structure fire but can be deadly in a river rescue situation. Every rescuer is responsible for understanding the rescue environment and how to best prepare for it.

Software

Rope. Rope is by far the most versatile piece of rescue equipment and serves as the universal link in most rescue environments. The material from which the rope is made (such as nylon, polyester, or polyolefins) and the design (laid, kernmantle, flat) are important in the consideration of the use for which a rope is intended.

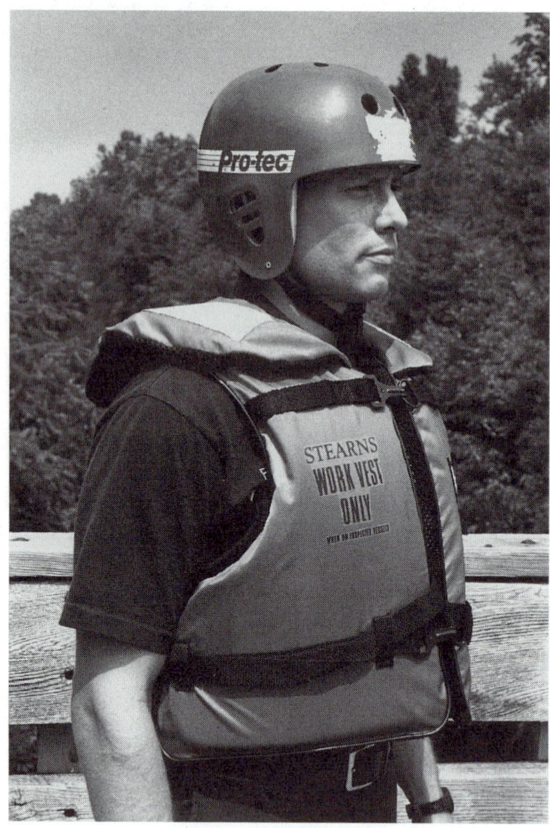

Fig. 21-7 Rescuer wearing a personal flotation device (PFD) and helmet often used for rescue in and around moving water.

In most rescue environments, nylon is preferred because of its overall strength, resistance to abrasion, and ability to stretch and absorb energy. Natural fiber ropes such as hemp are not even considered for use in rescue—synthetic materials are far better. Although design and amount of materials used influence strength, new one-half-inch-diameter nylon rescue rope usually has a tensile strength in excess of 9000 pounds (Fig. 21-8).

The most common design of rescue rope is "kernmantle," a term derived from the German meaning "core in sheath." With this design a core of material (often parallel fibers) is surrounded by a braided sheath. The sheath protects the inner core, which supplies much of the strength of the overall rope. Other designs such as laid (twisted) and braided are also used in rescue rope.

Kernmantle rope is either "dynamic" or "static." Dynamic kernmantle stretches more than 4% of its length to absorb the impact of a fall and is used primarily in lead climbing. Static kernmantle stretches less (no more than 4% of its length); it is used in rescues where a great deal of stretch would be a nuisance or even dangerous.

Because of the importance of rope in the rescue chain, frequent inspection, care, and maintenance are important. Rope used in rescue is kept clean, inspected often, and protected from sharp edges, high temperatures, sunlight, chemicals, and abrasion. In addition, a detailed history of rescue ropes is kept so that an educated decision can eventually be made regarding each rope's removal from rescue service.

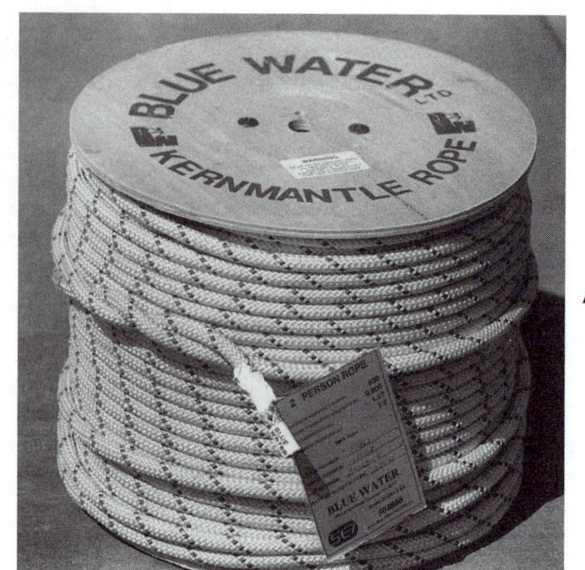

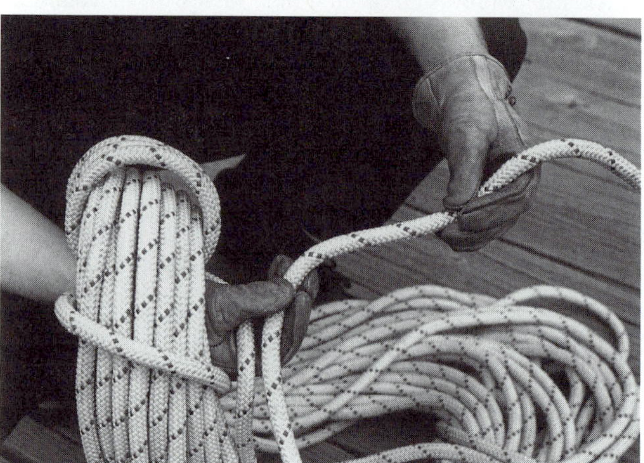

Fig. 21-8 **A,** Spool (600 feet) of half-inch, nylon, static, kernmantle rope of the type commonly used in rescue. Note the attached label, which shows that the product meets NFPA 1983, the National Fire Protection Association's Standard on Fire Service Life Safety Rope, Harnesses, and Hardware. This standard is one of very few in existence regarding rescue software. Its application to nonfire service rescue remains controversial. **B,** Rescue rope being checked for damage before use.

Webbing. Flat rope or webbing is another common link in rescue systems. It comes in two common configurations: flat and tubular. Tubular webbing is manufactured as a tube is such a way as to seem flat when in use. In cross section, however, it is obviously tubular and a bit less stiff than true flat webbing. One-inch-diameter tubular webbing can be used in rescues to tie anchor slings and harnesses. It has a tensile strength of approximately 4000 pounds when new (Fig. 21-9).

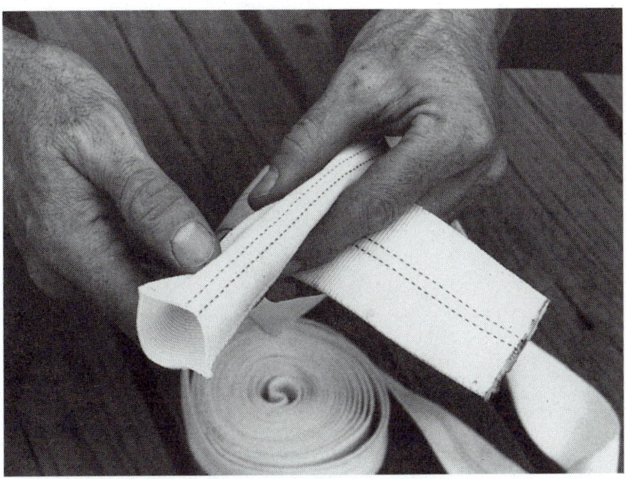

Fig. 21-9 Tubular webbing with cross section visible on the left.

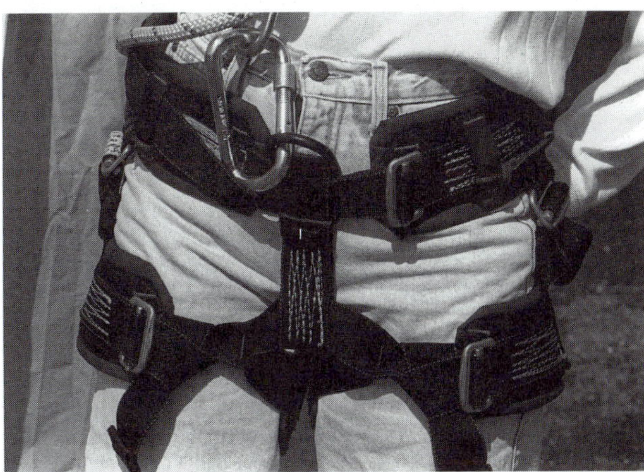

Fig. 21-10 Common type of rescue seat harness. Note attachment ring in front.

Flat webbing is flat in cross section. Its strength is directly proportional to the amount of material used in its manufacture. Automobile seat belts are an example of the material used in rescue harnesses, anchor slings, and anywhere strong, flat software is beneficial.

Harnesses. Harnesses come in many sizes and shapes; they are used to attach something (usually a rope) to a person's body. They may be "full-body," encompassing the thorax and the pelvis; "seat," encompassing only the pelvis (Fig. 21-10); or "chest," encompassing only the thorax. Each type of harness has its use and associated advantages and disadvantages. Classically, the most common harness for climbing has been the seat harness. However, rescue practitioners have been trying to standardize the full-body harness for rescuer use, the separate seat and chest harnesses having only limited special use by trained individuals.

Webbing can be tied into a large loop (runner) and applied to a person in such a way as to serve as an improvised harness. Although this is not a preferred method of attachment to a rope, it can work if other harnesses are not available.

Hardware

Carabiners. Carabiners are large, safety-pin-type mechanisms used to connect various elements of a rescue system such as a rope and anchor. They are occasionally called biners, snap links, or crabs, and consist of a spring-loaded gate that pivots open, a spine that supports most of the load and lies opposite the gate, a latch, and depending on the specific style, a locking mechanism (Fig. 21-11).

Steel and aluminum are the two materials from which carabiners are most commonly made. Size for size, steel is stronger and heavier, but aluminum is lighter and stronger pound for pound. In rescue, steel is almost always preferred unless weight is a factor, as in remote alpine situations.

Common shapes of carabiners include oval, D, offset D, pear, and large offset D. The design best suited for any situation is dictated by the specific use. No matter what the shape, carabiners used in rescue usually have a mechanism for locking the gate closed so that opening it takes a special effort. This design feature not only improves the strength of the device, but also reduces the chances that a carabiner will open accidentally at a bad time.

Descending devices. Many different descending devices exist today, but all do primarily the same thing: apply friction to the rope to allow controlled lowering of a person or load. The most common descending devices in rescue are the figure-8 plate and the brake bar rack.

The figure-8 plate gets the name from its general shape. It has two rings of different sizes. The larger ring produces friction on the rope, while the smaller ring is used primarily as an attachment for the load (the rescuer during rappel). Friction is produced by passing a bight of rope through the large ring and passing it around the small ring, then attaching the small ring to either an anchor (for a lowering system) or a rescuer's harness (for a rappel or abseil) with a locking carabiner (Fig. 21-12).

The brake bar rack, or simply "the rack," uses either steel or aluminum bars on a steel rack to produce friction on a rope. When the rope is threaded alternately around the bars and the load or rescuer is attached to the "eye" in the rack, friction is applied. The number of bars applied to the rope and the distance between them can be varied to change the friction. This variable friction allows versatility not available with the figure-8 plate; however, the rack takes a bit more training to use safely (Fig. 21-13).

Cam ascenders. Ascenders are devices that grip or hold the rope. They have been adapted from climbing and caving equipment, where they are used to ascend or climb a fixed rope. In rescue, they are used to climb fixed lines when necessary, but they can also be used in hauling systems to grip the rope. In this way they hold fast when the rope is pulled in one direction while allowing the rope to slide easily when it is pulled in the other direction (Fig. 21-14).

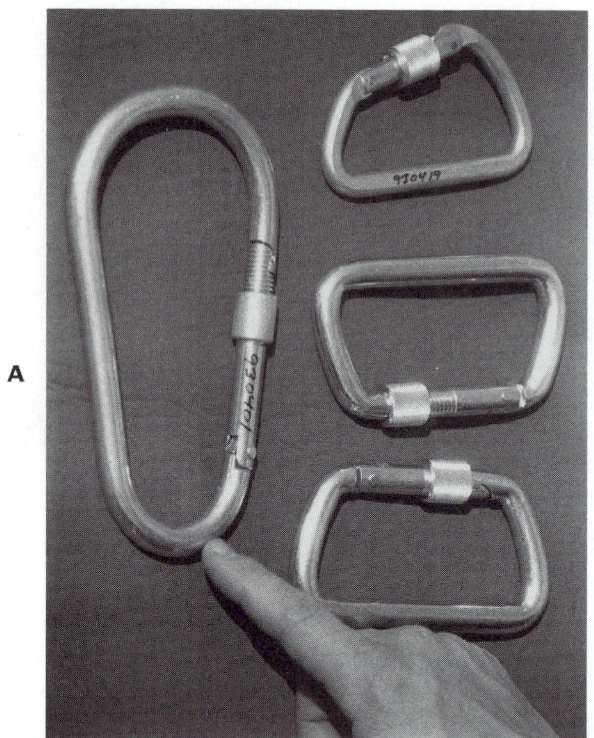

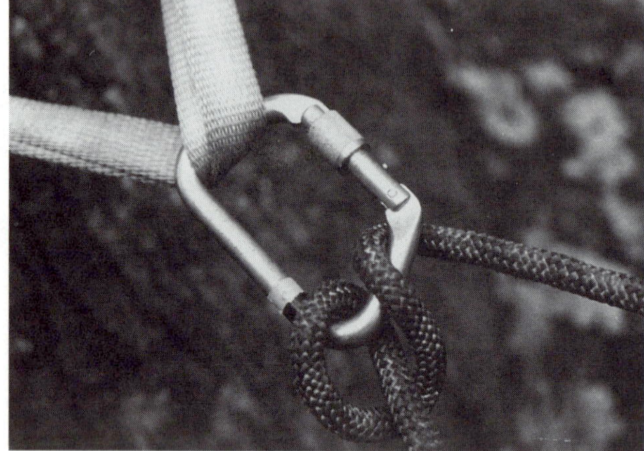

Fig. 21-11 **A,** Various types of carabiners. *Upper right,* Offset D locking steel. *Middle and lower right,* Large D locking steel. *Left,* Large, pear-shaped locking steel. **B,** Large D steel locking carabiner in use with a Münter hitch as a belay. Note that locking carabiners should always be locked when in use.

When cams are used to climb a rope, one is fixed to the rope and supports the load while the other is moved into position ahead. When this action is alternately repeated, a skilled climber can move up a rope with relative speed and ease.

Pulleys. Pulleys are simple machines that apply a turning wheel to reduce friction on a rope as it rounds a turn. In rescue, these metal devices serve primarily to change the direction of a rope, such as within a mechanical advantage system. The "sheave" is the wheel or pulley, and there may

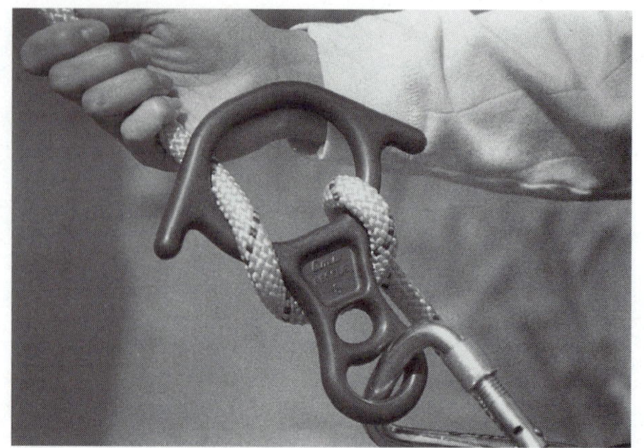

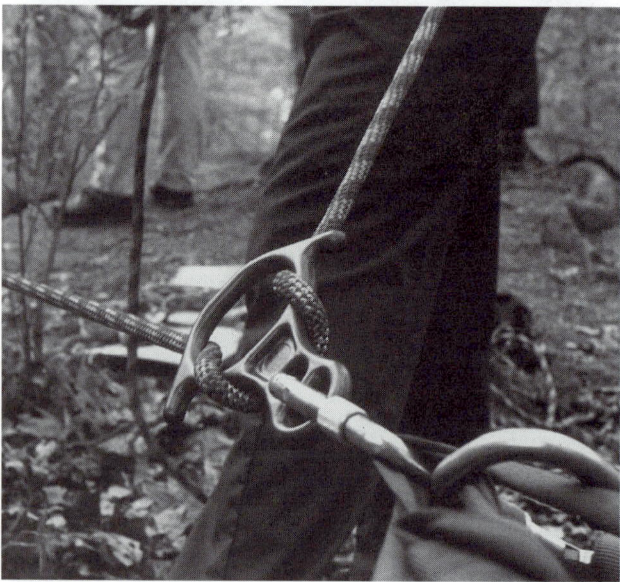

Fig. 21-12 **A,** Example of figure-8 plate descending device commonly used in rescue. **B,** Figure-8 plate in use as a belay.

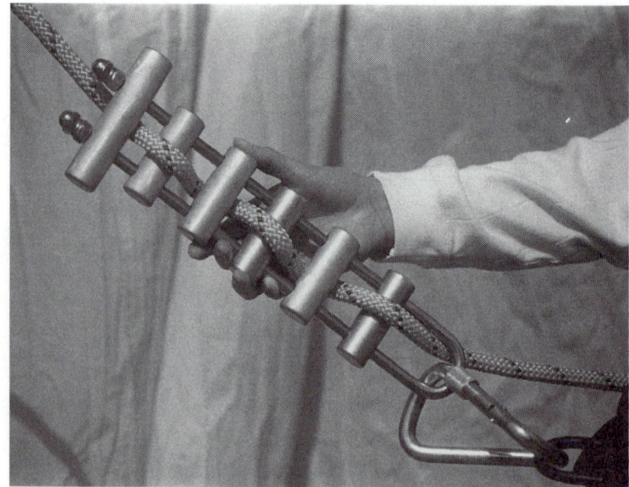

Fig. 21-13 One type of brake bar rack with rope attached.

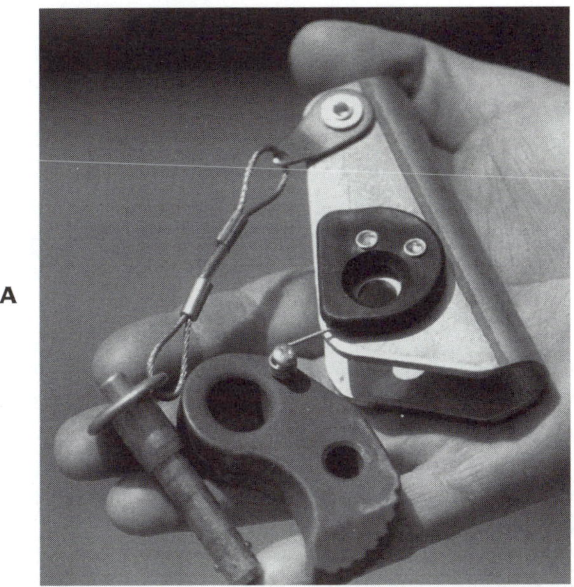

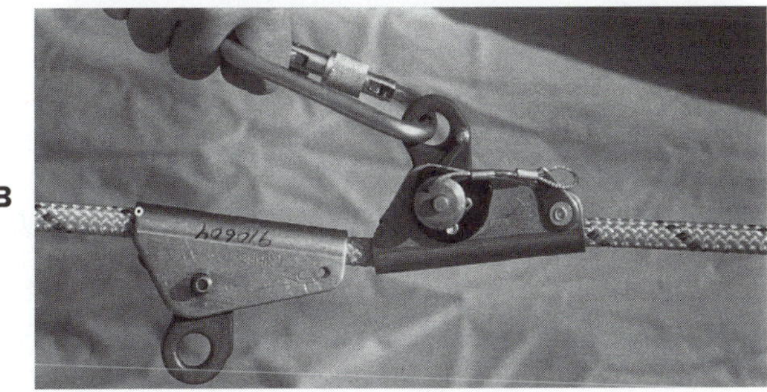

Fig. 21-14 **A,** Gibbs cam ascender dismantled and ready to be applied to the rope. Shell on right, cam in middle, pin on left. **B,** Two Gibbs cam ascenders applied to the rope. When the eye of the cam is pulled, the cam squeezes the rope and holds fast. When the cam is released, the device can be moved on the rope.

be more than one. The "side plate" or "cheek" is the side of the device that makes contact with the anchor at the "hook," which is usually the weakest part. The axle or "sheave pin" is what the wheel turns on; it is supported by the side plates. In rescue pulleys the side plates are movable so that the pulley can be attached to a rope anywhere along its length (Fig. 21-15).

The larger the diameter of the pulley, the more efficient the device. That is, the bigger the pulley, the more friction (theoretically) is reduced. A rule of thumb often used by rescuers is that a pulley with the largest diameter possible should be used, but never less than four times the diameter of the rope. Therefore, since half-inch (11 mm) rope is commonly used in rescue, a pulley diameter of at least 2 inches should be used.

A variation of the pulley is the edge roller. This device uses 4- to 6-inch open-face pulleys to both reduce the friction of a rope passing over an edge and reduce damage to the rope by protecting it from excess abrasion. Single units can protect the rope from 90-degree angles, while multiple units tied together can provide protection for complex projections.

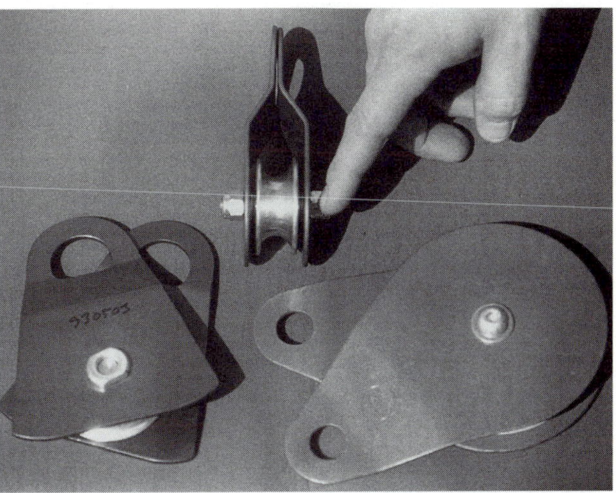

Fig. 21-15 Various types and sizes of pulleys commonly used for rescue. *Top,* 2-inch. *Left,* 2-inch, Prusik-minding. *Right,* 4-inch.

Litters. Litters or stretchers are the conveyances in which patients are transported when they cannot travel under their own power. New high-technology materials and designs have greatly improved the choices available. In past years, rescuers were forced to settle for either wooden backboards, old military stretchers, the wire Navy Stokes basket, or the "scoop" stretcher. Today, strong, lightweight synthetic materials and inventive designs have improved the strength, weight, durability, and comfort of litters (Fig. 21-16).

The goals have not changed during the continuing evolution of the perfect wilderness transportation device. Rescuers still want a device that is comfortable for a patient in pain, serves well as a platform for assessment and medical care during transport, allows for full-body immobilization while offering complete security, and protects its occupants from the rescue environment (Fig. 21-17).

Techniques

Patient Packaging. Stabilizing a patient for transport is termed packaging. When either injuries or travel distance indicates that the patient must be carried, a litter is usually used. The litter serves both as a convenient vehicle for transport and as a full-body splint.

Physically strapping a patient into a litter is relatively easy, but making it comfortable and effective in terms of splinting can be a challenge. Generally, the following goals must be considered.

1. Package the patient to avoid causing additional injury.
2. Ensure the patient's comfort and warmth.
3. Immobilize the patient's entire body in such a way as to allow continued assessment during transport.

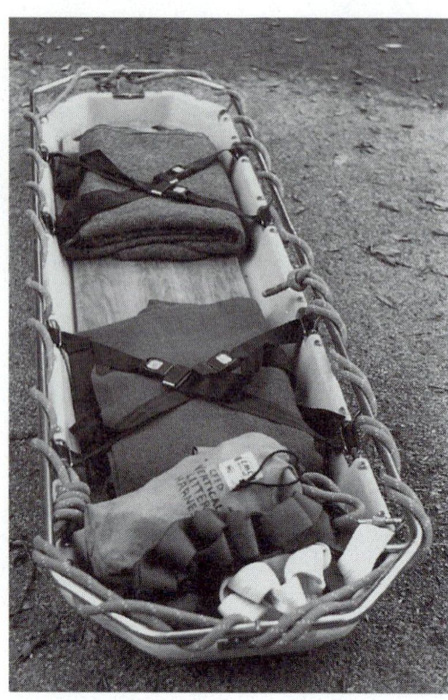

Fig. 21-16 One type of basket litter with equipment for raising and patient packaging strapped inside. Note long backboard and wool blankets.

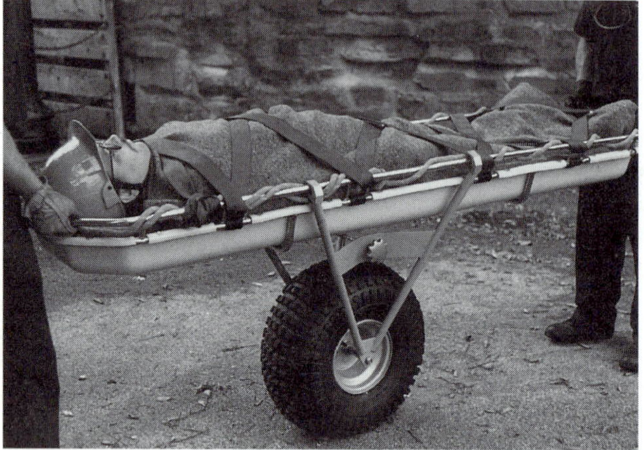

Fig. 21-17 Attachments such as this wheel allow fewer rescuers to carry the litter and patient with ease, even over rough terrain.

4. Package the patient neatly so that the litter can be moved easily and safely.
5. Ensure that the patient is safe during transport by securing him or her within the litter and belaying the litter as necessary.

A common approach to packaging a patient entails using a long or short backboard for immobilization, then placing the patient on the board into the litter. Insulation and padding can be added above and below the patient as needed, but a cover of some type should always be used to protect the patient from falling material. A helmet and face shield (or goggles) are also recommended to protect the head and face from projectiles. Tape or webbing serves well to immobilize the helmeted head, and a cervical collar is applied if possible. Once a seat harness is applied to the patient's pelvis and a cover is put in place, a 30-foot piece of webbing laced back and forth through the sides of the litter secures the patient. Because it might become necessary to log-roll the patient in the litter to prevent aspiration of emesis, attachment of the patient within the litter should allow very little sliding or other movement in any direction. Tying the harness the patient is wearing tightly to the siderails of the litter can help (Fig. 21-18).

Litter Carry. Carrying a litter in the wilderness is difficult and requires many resources. It takes at least six rescuers to carry a patient in a litter a short distance (¼ mile or less) over relatively flat terrain. With six rescuers, four can carry the litter while the other two clear the area in the direction of travel and assist in any difficult spots. However, depending on terrain and the weight of the patient, all six rescuers may be needed to safely carry the litter any distance. If the travel distance is longer, many more rescuers are needed (Fig. 21-19).

Technical Evacuation. In steeper terrain when there is a chance that the litter might slide downhill, ropes are used to enhance the safety of transport. When the terrain is gently sloping and litter bearers will carry most of the weight of the litter, a belay rope is tied to the litter and used to help bearers maintain control. In such situations one end of a rope is tied to the litter while a person belays the other end using a belay device and a good anchor. This type of rescue is called a low-angle or scree evacuation.

A high-angle evacuation is one in which the litter's weight is borne primarily by one or more ropes. In these situations, such as when the litter is to be lowered or raised over an edge, much more care must be taken to ensure that

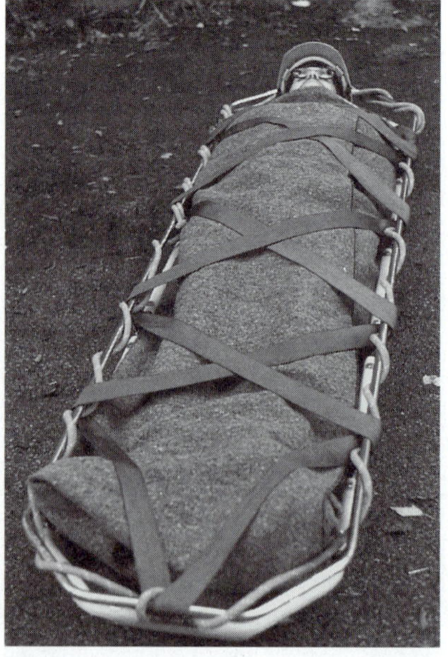

Fig. 21-18 Patient in litter packaged for carrying.

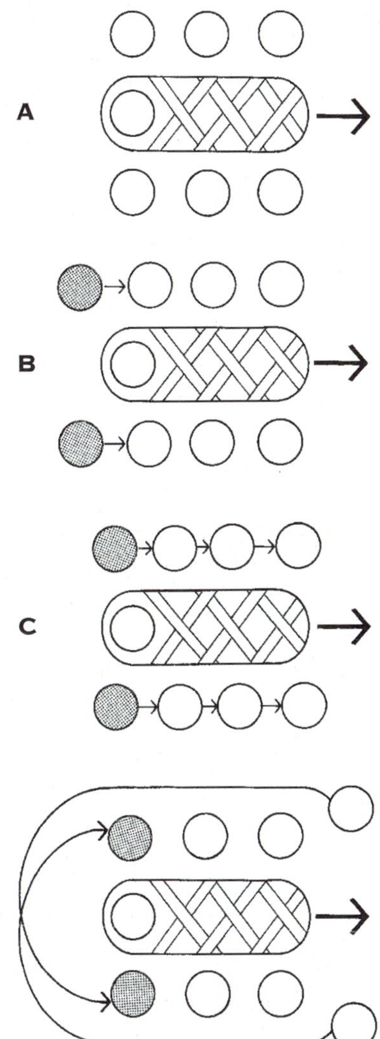

Fig. 21-19 Litter-carrying sequence. **A,** Six rescuers are usually required to carry a litter but may need relief over long distances (greater than ¼ mile). **B,** Relief rescuers can rotate into position while the litter is in motion by approaching from the rear. As relief rescuers move forward, others progressively move forward **(C)** until the forwardmost rescuers can release the litter (peel out) and move to the rear **(D).** Rescuers in the rear can rotate sides so that they can alternate carrying arms. Carrying straps (webbing) can also be used to distribute the load over the rescuers' shoulders. In most cases the litter is carried feet first with a medical attendant at the head monitoring airway, breathing, level of consciousness, and so on.

the equipment and personnel are prepared to endure the extreme stresses of such situations. The nature of these types of rescue is such that only the best-trained and best-equipped rescuers should attempt them.

When the litter must be lowered from a height, a lowering system is set up. Good anchors are selected and a belay device is used to lower the load under control. This type of rescue uses gravity and is therefore preferred over a system that pulls the load up.

When a litter must be raised from below, a raising or hauling system is used. In a raising system, anchors are placed and mechanical advantage is applied to raise the load. Since mechanical advantage systems can cause more severe stresses to equipment than the load alone, great care must be taken to ensure the quality of the equipment and the plan before proceedings.

Anatomy of a Search and Rescue Incident

To summarize how all of the previously discussed information fits together, it is convenient to dissect a SAR incident into its component parts and then analyze how all the parts fit together.

From the SAR operative's perspective, an actual callout is merely an interruption of planning for an incident. That is, people involved in SAR are constantly in a state of readiness, prepared to respond. When a situation occurs, this planning stage is suddenly interrupted by the report of an incident or first notice. The individual taking the information is charged with conveying it to the appropriate authority. The authority determines the urgency, continues the investigation process, begins to develop an operational strategy, and generates an incident action plan. At the same time, those in charge begin to muster appropriate resources to carry out the action plan. In SAR this is termed resource callout, or just callout.

Once notified of an incident, individual resources are gathered at a collection point and signed in. The sign-in process enhances safety and allows tracking of resources, which helps those in charge determine the quantity and type of resources available. Once signed in, resources are allocated to assignments designed to meet the goals of the action plan within a reasonable time. This physical implementation of plans in the field is called tactics and is a direct outgrowth of the incident action plan.

Allocation of resources in the field continues until there is reason to suspend a phase of the operation. If the subject is found, the search is suspended and the access phase can commence. Once rescuers have access to the subject, the focus turns to stabilization and transportation. If at any point the operation cannot be continued (for example, the subject was never found, access cannot be gained, transportation is impossible), suspension and demobilization may occur without completion of the entire cycle. The decision to discontinue active search efforts is difficult and involves complex management issues, almost always of the no-win variety.

When a situation is resolved, mission suspension and demobilization begin. In larger incidents this may involve structured deactivation of multiple resources, pulling teams out of the field, dismantling facilities, completing documentation, and returning resources to service. Basically, everyone finishes what he or she was doing and gets ready to do it again. All of this takes planning and preparation and should be addressed in the overall preplan long before it is required.

After every incident, participants realize that if they had it all to do again, they would do some things differently. If these thoughts and ideas are not documented, they can be lost and future responses will repeat past mistakes. This is one reason that every incident should contain some type of evaluation of the entire mission, known as the critique. The critique can be formal, involving every participant at a sit-down meeting, or informal, involving just a brief discussion of recent events. The critique documents lessons learned and provides a basis for revising the preplan. Thus the cycle continues and lessons learned from one mission influence the next.

Search and Rescue Environments Within the Wilderness Setting[4]

Search and rescue teams throughout the world are frequently called on to solve complex problems in a wide spectrum of environments. Even within the wilderness environment addressed in this text, widely diversified subenvironments exist that present unique sets of problems and hazards to SAR personnel. When confronted with the numerous and dangerous environmental conditions found in the wilderness setting, SAR personnel must be prepared to work where others have been unable to cope. A military motto becomes the SAR credo: "Adapt, improvise, overcome."

Some of the specialized subenvironments and their associated conditions within which SAR team members may have to work are listed in Box 21-2.

It is beyond the scope of this text to discuss in detail how SAR personnel adapt to each of these environments, but it is important to note that adaptation and improvisation are required in nearly all wilderness situations. The particular improvisation depends on the situation, as well as the skill and experience of the individuals involved.

Regardless of the type of rescue environment encountered by rescuers, the following general rules should be followed:

1. Use technical personnel for technical rescue.
2. If the subject is dead, evacuate only when there is no risk to fellow team members, or at least when the hazard has been assessed and the risk justified.
3. Stabilize the subject before evacuating; continue stabilization during transport.
4. Find, plan, and use the easiest route for evacuation.
5. If a litter must be carried, appoint someone to serve as route finder, with a radio and markers, to report potential hazards and problems.
6. Litter teams of six to eight persons per team should be used, with three teams minimum. Normally, there should be no more than 20 minutes per shift. Additional personnel may also be required to carry equipment.
7. Use accepted procedures to care for and protect the victim.
8. A radio carrier brings up the rear.
9. If using a helicopter for evacuation, make sure:
   a. That the subject is briefed.
   b. That the subject is protected.
   c. That someone goes with the subject who knows what has been done medically.

Special Environments in Search and Rescue

Specialized SAR environments produce diverse problems and potential complications. Each environment presents its own obstacles to increase the complexity and difficulty of particular rescues.

Technical Rock. Mountaineering, rock climbing, and casual scrambling have created a need for specialized SAR expertise. Individuals and groups involved in rock rescue have refined and developed techniques for most situations. The hallmark of a technical rock rescuer is the ability to improvise and modify tools or techniques to meet any crisis. He or she must be comfortable using climbing gear and being exposed to heights.

Once an individual has been located in a rock environment and the situation surveyed, it is necessary to gain access. Local groups familiar with particular well-known areas will have already solved this problem. The solution will involve either climbing up or dropping down to the victim. Safety for all persons involved is paramount, because an accident during a rescue is almost always catastrophic. Climbing up to the victim requires a knowledge of rock-climbing techniques, and proper equipment and familiarity with its use are critical. Local outing clubs or mountaineering stores can be contacted for more detailed assistance. Specialized technical rock rescue teams, such as those sanc-

BOX 21-2

SEARCH AND RESCUE CONDITIONS

Mountainous terrain	Air shafts
Vertical rock	Fast water and white-water streams
Vertical ice	Coastal white-water surf
Flat ice and ice holes	Flash floods
Snow fields and avalanches	Slow-rising floods
Crevasses	High winds and storms
Caves	Seas and lakes
Mines	Snow and blizzard conditions
Wells	Hazardous material dump sites
Booby-trapped stills and gardens	

tioned by the Mountain Rescue Association, routinely practice climbing techniques and solving vertical rescue problems.

Caves and Mines. Standard obstacles in the environment include poor communications, extreme darkness, difficulty in lighting, small and wet spaces, and questionable atmosphere. The various environments included here are collectively termed "confined spaces" in the urban setting.

The levels of moisture in a water, or "live," cave can vary over a considerable range. Some are merely muddy; others have flowing rivers. Caves in the western United States are generally drier than eastern caves; however, humidity, wetness, and cold temperatures create potential for hypothermia in both areas, a fact that is greatly underestimated. Flooding is often a great problem, and many cavers have died because of inattention to the weather on the outside. During heavy rains, the caves become natural drains for streams. Wind and temperature are other underestimated problems associated with cave and mine emergencies. It is not unusual for strong winds to develop along subterranean passages, which intensifies convective air chilling.

Confined passages, low crawls, and squeezes pose unique problems for the rescue of injured cavers. The use of standard items such as litters, backboards, and splints may be impossible in such places. Confined passages with varying, often toxic, constituent gases can lead to difficulties for victims and rescuers alike. Occasionally, self-contained breathing apparatus, surface-supplied air, or self-contained underwater breathing apparatus is required. The potential for toxic gases justifies extensive atmospheric monitoring while operating in the underground environment.

An essential part of any cave or mine rescue operation is thorough orientation to the hazards associated with a particular underground area. This involves pinpointing the locations of pits, waterfalls, siphons, canyons, and other difficult formations that may pose problems in extrication, search, or safety. Many caves have been mapped by the National Speleological Society and the National Park Service.

The real difficulties may begin only after a victim is located. The goal is to move the person rapidly, safely, and comfortably to the surface. Without practice underground, that task will be virtually impossible. Neoprene exposure bags similar to body bags have been used for this purpose and keep the individual dry and protected during what may be a very long and slow evacuation.

Medical care procedures must be performed under dark, cold, and muddy conditions. Experienced cave rescuers agree that repackaging supplies and equipment for underground use is essential. Streamlining kits, packs, and containers is imperative for unobstructed passage through tight spaces in the cold, damp conditions.

Team members must carry a minimum of 24 hours of light in a helmet-mounted lamp, two additional sources of light with spare bulbs and batteries, and waterproof matches and candles. Other equipment needed might include the following:

1. A high-quality helmet with chin strap and headlamp attachment
2. Sturdy, warm clothes and gloves for damp, dirty conditions for up to 24 hours; the material should be wool and the fit should allow good mobility
3. Lug-soled boots that are light and drain water
4. Nonstretch, specialized caving rope that is highly resistant to abrasion
5. Wrap-around-style litter (or even an old conveyor belt) that can aid in dragging an injured person through small passages: a common Stokes litter may work well
6. Wet suits for longer missions in extremely wet caves
7. Harnesses and slings resistant to chemicals and water
8. Plastic sheeting to divert water around a victim during evacuation
9. Small portable pumps, a siphon hose, and plastic to divert, dam, or pump water around areas during operations
10. Warm food and drink carried in thermally insulated containers

Essential caving skills include all of the capabilities for rock climbing, including vertical rope technique, ascending, rappeling, belaying, and being comfortable working at the end of a rope. All of these skills must be practiced until they can be done in the cold and wet without the benefit of light. Team practices are conducted both on the surface and underground with participants being forced to work in mud, suffocatingly tight squeezes, soaking waterfalls, and complete darkness. This may be a difficult evolution for even the most experienced rescuer to endure, but just another "hang in the hole" for a seasoned caver.

White-Water—River. There are dozens of potentially dangerous problems in the river SAR (white-water) situation (see Chapter 49). Log and debris piles at various bends in the river can function as "strainers" for the recreational victim, but they may be death traps for the would-be rescuer. The banks of the stream may be deeply undercut with treacherous overhanging debris and snags that can catch on clothing, equipment, and skin. Combined with muddy and rapidly rising water, these factors render river rescue difficult and unpredictable.

In fast-moving water the single greatest problem is that responders underestimate the power and threat of moving water. Foolhardy heroics and overenthusiasm frequently lead to further tragedy. Cold water immersion coupled with wind and cold temperatures predisposes everyone to hypothermia. Wet clothing, darkness, and injury add to the insult. The noise of moving water may obviate clear communications, and poor contact between the victim and rescuers or among the rescuers leads to confusion and danger.

All potential responders in this environment must know how to read the water for capsize points and other dangerous phenomena. The hydraulics of low-head dams, collapsed bridges, and other submerged structures can produce a drowning machine for unsuspecting individuals. Rescue team members must know how to protect themselves in fast-moving water at all times. Mandatory in this environment are good judgment, strong swimming ability, knowledge of all types of technical systems and equipment used in climbing, and a thorough understanding of river dynamics and hydraulic influences.

White-water and river rescue equipment needs. In addition to standard rescue equipment, the following items should be considered when establishing rescue capability in the white-water and river environment:

1. Inflatable rafts or boats (Hard boats may not be as stable and are usually less preferred. Inflatables should be at least 14 to 16 feet long and 6 feet wide with separate air chambers. The "spider boat" with two pontoons joined together in a catamaran-style craft makes an excellent, stable rescue platform for moving water.)
2. A line gun or crossbow adaptation that will shoot a line at least 200 feet
3. Power winch or simple "come-along" that can be carried to remote sites
4. Lengthy (150 to 300 feet) durable floating ropes in rope bags
5. Floating throw-rope bags with approximately 60 feet of line
6. A lightweight litter with enough flotation to keep a packaged patient's head out of the water; standard rescue litters often have adaptations for this purpose
7. Fire-hose end caps with air-hose adapters, which allow the fire hose to be inflated with air and used in a shore-based rescue
8. PFDs for every rescuer who will be exposed to the water environment; wet suits and helmets for rescuers who will be directly involved in moving water
9. Dry extra clothing for victims and rescuers
10. Portable "loudhailer" or public address system
11. Portable lighting systems
12. Detailed maps, aerial photographs, or both, of the area as well as information regarding river hazards during high, medium, and low water levels
13. Dry, buoyant storage bags for sensitive gear
14. Reliable, watertight communications capability for white-water noise and moisture conditions
15. Small surfboardlike styrofoam boards for swimming in moving water

White-Water—Surf. Like river white water, ocean surf can present some very different problems in rescue, since there is no "average" beach. There are recurring rescue situations that pose unique problems in the white-water surf environment.

Along with the potential for immersion hypothermia, lacerations and contusions can result from being dashed against barnacle-encrusted rocks in the wild and unpredictable ocean surf. Contact with venomous sea life is always a possibility. However, the greatest threat to ocean beach users is the action of the water itself and the possibility of drowning through inattention or unfamiliarity with ocean surf hazards in the form of runouts, undertows, and rips.

Runout. A runout occurs when an offshore sandbar or ledge is built up over a long period. Millions of tons of water flow over the bar during daily tidal changes. Eventually the water may equal or exceed the level outside the bar. Any weak spot in the bar usually gives way, causing a funnel effect (Fig. 21-20). Water rushes toward the bar at a terrific rate, sweeping everything with it. This common phenomenon can be easily spotted from the beach. Usually 15 to 50 yards wide, it is characterized by choppy, jumbled-up little waves. The water often has a dirty, foamy, or debris-laden surface moving seaward. If a bar is visible offshore, definite breaks can be seen where the water pours through. Surfers often seek runout currents for fast transportation out beyond shoreline waves.

Swimmers caught in a runout have two options. They may swim parallel to the shoreline out of the strip of current,

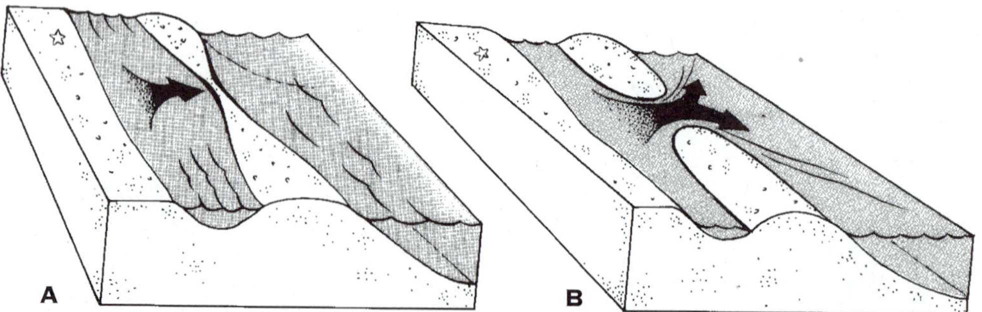

Fig. 21-20 Runout. **A,** This phenomenon begins with an offshore sandbar. As waves roll in, the water level builds up behind the bar until a section gives way. **B,** As the sandbar "dam" gives way, the water develops a very rapid current running seaward. The recommended action is to swim across the current until out of the pull.

or if the bar is visible (usually characterized by breaking waves), they may relax and let the current complete its runout. About 25 yards beyond the bar the current dissipates. This is an offshore phenomenon—current force increases near the bar but is often negligible near shore.

Rip. A far worse problem close to the beach is a rip, which can knock children and even adults off their feet and carry them to deep water in seconds. Rips are caused by a slight depression on the beach where wave water rushes after breaking on shore. Water rushing to the depression soon becomes an irresistible seaward flow (Fig. 21-21). It may be as narrow as 15 yards at its source and usually does not travel as far as a runout. Rips generally dissipate a few yards beyond the breakers. A rip looks like a runout, with a streak of turbulent discolored water or a line of foam leading directly out from shore. A swimmer has the same options as in a runout, either to swim parallel to the beach or to relax and ride the current until it ebbs. A person who swims straight toward the beach will never make it. A beach with several rips moving up and down in unpredictable patterns is very dangerous. An unwary swimmer could panic and drown.

Undertow. On narrow, steep beaches a type of current known as undertow can be found. It is caused by gravity acting on water thrown up on the beach by wave action. Water retreating back down the steep shore continues under oncoming waves (Fig. 21-22). Undertow is usually of very short duration and is ended by the next breaking wave. Wading near shore on a steep beach, an individual could be pulled under in this current and find himself or herself quickly in deep water. If the person resists the current, the next wave may break directly on the person's back. In some circumstances this could cause traumatic injury, especially to the neck and back. A person caught in an undertow should let the current pull until it ceases, then swim to the surface and ride the next wave into shore.

Cold, Snow, and Ice. Perhaps no other type of SAR environment requires a more broadly based foundation of personal and team skills than winter snow and ice. These skills include downhill and cross-country skiing, snowshoeing, technical climbing, winter survival, and a good understanding of snow and ice physics. Unlike rock, snow and ice conditions change on a daily and even minute-to-minute basis. The effects of gravity, wind, temperature, slope, heat exchange, load factors, and avalanche (see Chapter 25) continually impose problems for missions under these conditions. Technical and nontechnical SAR problems in snow and ice environments take longer to address and are more taxing, technical, and complex. Combined with shorter days, extremes of weather, and the ever-present threat of hypothermia and localized cold injuries, technical missions of this type are unacceptable for all but the most experienced SAR personnel.

Versatility and improvisation are essential components of the overall strategy that must be used in snow and ice. Transportation of the victim is often one of the most difficult problems, but it can usually be resolved through detailed preplanning. Innovations such as covering a litter with a canvas cover or improvising an attachment to cross-country skis are clever solutions to common winter problems. Commercial products such as the Hegg Sled and the Sked Litter have streamlined the laborious task of transporting injured people through snow and ice.

Magnitude and Causes of Problems in Wilderness Search and Rescue

It is impossible to report the exact number of backcountry search and rescue missions that occur each year in the United States. Some estimates are in excess of 100,000. In the United States, no federal agency is charged with gathering these data. With rare exception, only in the last few years have some states and local jurisdictions begun to collect and analyze SAR mission numbers and related information. Through the efforts of organizations such as the National Association for Search and Rescue, this vital information is now being used as a data base to predict victim behavior and to improve the efficiency of SAR management.

Most wilderness accidents are the result of inexperience or lack of preparation, often aggravated by fatigue, lowered

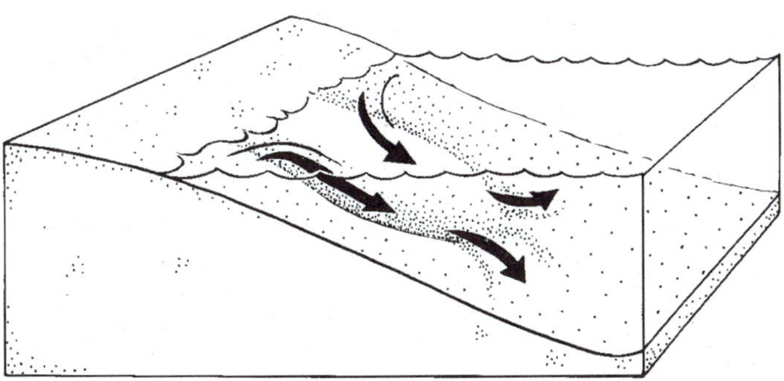

Fig. 21-21 Riptide. A depression in the beach floor concentrates returning water into a strong current. To escape, a person should ride with the current or swim to the side and out of the pull.

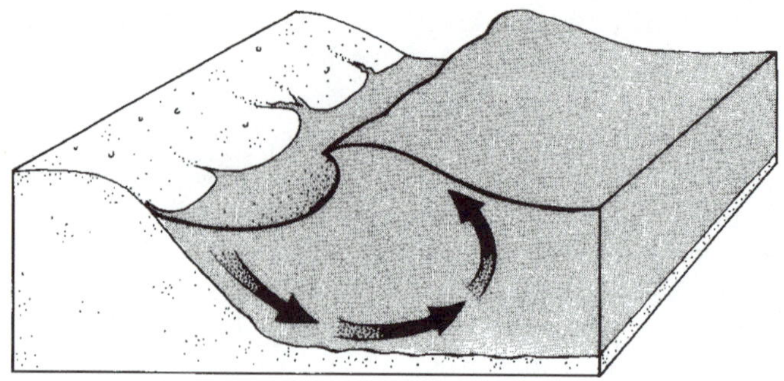

Fig. 21-22 Undertow. This hazard usually develops on a steep beach where the water returns rapidly seaward after being tossed up by wave action. A person should never fight this action but should relax and rise on the next wave.

body temperature, and other medical management problems, rather than the direct result of natural phenomena such as avalanche or rock fall.

In an effort to save lives through education, the Washington State Department of Emergency Management Search and Rescue Division has been recording statistics on search and rescue missions for over 20 years. The goal of this effort has been to find out what factors in each search and rescue mission may have caused a problem for the subject. Box 21-3 is an overview of that data, compiled in an attempt to create a preventive SAR subject profile.

In addition to the factors listed in Box 21-3, the data pointed out some extremely interesting characteristics. Using broad-based generalizations, the analysts were able to further describe a potential SAR victim. While the data were gathered only from the State of Washington, they have application in nearly every state and have to some degree been substantiated by other statistics.

The average SAR victim is a composite outdoorsman (for example, hunter, fisherman, skier, hiker, climber, boater, photographer). Most do not do any of these activities well and are not members of organized groups that specialize in these pursuits. Most reside in densely populated areas and travel some distance for recreation and outdoor pursuits. They usually travel too fast and too far to acclimatize well to the terrain, altitude, and environmental conditions encountered. Interviews show that they also generally ignore signs of weather change, environmental hazards, body indicators, and written warnings concerning danger or safety. Most wilderness or backcountry emergencies are solved by either the victim or outside help within 72 hours. The decisions and actions taken by the victims during the first 6 hours of the situation (such as emergency shelter, improving clothing, firecraft, signaling) are the most critical and influence the outcome most heavily. Of all the precipitating factors, weather contributes the most to misery, carelessness, and the ultimate SAR mission.

Not long ago, Dr. Warren Bowman compiled data from three independent sources in an effort to identify training and equipment for more efficient responses to remote-area SAR problems. Dr. Bowman examined the data from three studies[1]:

1. *Accidents in North American mountaineering,* published by the American Alpine Club and the Alpine Club of Canada, for the 6-year period 1980-1985. There were 353 accidents, not including 32 miscellaneous fractures. There were 183 deaths, victims who either were found dead or died shortly after being reached, for a total of 536 incidents.
2. McLennan JG, Ungersma J: Mountaineering accidents in the Sierra Nevada, *Am J Sports Med* 11(3):160, 1983. There were 215 accidents and 17 deaths, all on class V climbs. The authors estimated that more than 60% of injuries were associated with acute mountain sickness and over 10% with hypothermia.
3. Schussman LC, Lutz LJ: Mountaineering and rock climbing accidents, *Physician Sports Med* 10(6):53, 1982. There were 144 accidents and 30 deaths in Grand Teton National Park from 1970 to 1980.

BOX 21-3

FACTORS THAT CONTRIBUTED TO SURVIVAL SITUATIONS AND SEARCH AND RESCUE MISSIONS

Improper clothing, footgear, or both
Lack of rest (fatigue)
Lack of adequate water (dehydration)
Hypothermia or hyperthermia
Too ambitious an undertaking for skills or proficiency
Poor physical condition, lack of motivation, or both
Inadequate or improper food
Little or no planning
Inadequate party for the goal, and lack of leadership
Itinerary confusing or not known to others
Individuals could not recognize a physical, mental, or environmental threat
No preparation for adverse weather
Unfamiliarity with terrain and lack of map or compass
"It can't happen to me" philosophy

Although the data are limited to mountaineering accidents and do not accurately describe the full spectrum of injuries and the equipment needed for problems that might be encountered in other wilderness environments, Bowman's study clearly revealed the need for more accurate and thorough analysis of localized mission data (see Table 21-2 and Box 21-4, which summarize data).

Disaster and Urban Search and Rescue: The Next Important Step in Search and Rescue

While some will insist that urban SAR is a fire service responsibility, in many parts of the country it is done exclusively by law enforcement and in other locations by emergency medical services (EMS) or other volunteers.

Urban search and rescue operations include locating people incapacitated and in need of assistance, stabilizing them, and relocating them to a safe place by means of light or heavy rescue techniques. The place of safety may be an evacuation or relocation center, a field first aid station, triage center, casualty collection point, or hospital; the morgue is another possible destination.

Within rescue circles it is known that mountaineering and the industry that supplies mountaineering equipment have changed the science of light rescue over the past decade. New technologies have enhanced the cutting edge, but dissemination of the information needed to those who need to know it has been extremely poor. Only recently have urban rescue squads, firefighters, EMS responders, and law enforcement officers begun to use and modify the techniques and equipment of mountain rescue and recreational climbing to fit urban rescue needs.

Until the mid-1980s, familiarity with heavy rescue was a hit-or-miss affair left to public and private construction firms, utilities, and engineering agencies. If the need arose, officials grabbed whatever equipment and expertise were available and hoped they were sufficient.

With the major earthquakes in Mexico City (1985), Armenia (1989), and California (1989), and the associated urban SAR problems, the federal government began a significant effort to develop an urban SAR capability throughout the United States. The Federal Response Plan

Table 21-2 Analysis of Injuries by First Aid Equipment Required

Category	Percentage of Total	First Aid Equipment/Action Required
Death on arrival or shortly thereafter	34.0	None
Leg or ankle fracture	11.4	Splint (long or short leg), pain medications. If open, see "Laceration."
Multiple injuries (various combinations of head, chest, abdominal, and extremity injuries)	10.0	Dressings, bandages, airways, suction, bag mask, splints, cravats, IVs or MAST, oxygen, Kendrick Extrication Device (KED), pain medications, cricothyrotomy set, chest tube, Foley catheter, urinal, petrolatum gauze
Head injury	7.0	Dressings and bandages, extrication collar, airways, suction, KED, oxygen, Foley catheter, urinal, IVs
Frostbite	6.7	Stove, pot, thermometer, dressings
Arm, wrist fracture	3.4	Short arm splint, sling, pain medications. If open, see "Laceration"
Hypothermia	3.2	Rewarming device, stove, shelter-building equipment or tent, sleeping bag, IVs
Pulmonary edema	3.0	Descent to lower altitude, oxygen, furosemide
Vertebral fracture	3.0	Extrication collar, KED, pain medications
Laceration	2.4	Dressings, bandages, sterile saline for irrigation, antiseptic soap
Hand fracture	1.3	Splint, wad of gauze, sling, pain medications. If open, see "Laceration"
Knee sprain, dislocation	2.0	Cravat, elastic bandage, long leg splint, plastic bag for snow
Femur fracture	1.5	Traction splint, pain medications, MAST or IVs. If open, see "Laceration"
Foot fracture or crush injury	1.3	Splint (long or short leg), pain medications. If open, see "Laceration"
Contusion	1.0	Plastic bag for snow, splint (if extremity)
Ankle sprain	1.0	Adhesive tape or elastic bandage, plastic bag for snow
Cerebral edema	0.7	Oxygen, descent to lower altitude, dexamethasone, airways, suction
Shoulder dislocation	0.7	Cravats for sling, pain medications
Hip, pelvis fracture	0.5	Backboard (Thompson or Stokes litter), pain medications, Foley catheter, urinal
Heat injury	0.5	Poncho for shade, cold water
Lightning injury	0.5	Dressings and bandages, antiseptic soap, pocket mask, airways, oxygen, monitor-defibrillator, IVs
Facial injuries	0.5	Airways, oxygen, dressings, bandages
Bites, stings (including anaphylaxis)	0.4	Epinephrine, diphenhydramine (see "Laceration")
Pneumonia	0.1	Antibiotics, oxygen
Chest, rib bruises	0.05	Adhesive tape, elastic bandage

BOX 21-4

PRIORITY FIRST AID EQUIPMENT

MOST USEFUL

Airways
Alcohol sponges
Arm or hand splint (wire, SAM splint)
Dressings, bandages, Kling, tape, cravats, Ace wrap
Extrication collar (can use SAM splint)
Flashlight
Germicidal soap
Heat-generating device (heat pads, Heatpak, Heat Treat)
Light traction splint (Sager or Kendrick Traction Device)
Litter
Long leg air splint
Lubricant for thermometer
Notebook and pencil, tags
Pain medications
Plastic bags (for snow, sprain and contusion treatment)
Pocket mask
Portable, short backboard (KED, Oregon Spine Splint)
Safety pins
Scissors
Seam ripper
Sterile irrigation solution (IV bag of 0.9% saline)
Suction device (bulb or syringe)
Syringe (20 cc) for irrigating
Thermometer (low-reading for cold weather and high altitude; regular for hot weather)
Urinal or pee bottle
Vasoline gauze

USEFUL BUT HEAVY, EXPENSIVE, OR NEEDING SPECIAL EXPERTISE

Bag-mask
Chest tube set (Heimlich valve, McSwain dart)
Cricothyrotomy set
Foley catheter, gloves, lubricant, clamp, and plug
For allergic reactions and anaphylaxis: bee sting kit, EpiPen, Benadryl
For high altitude: Diamox, Decadron, Lasix
For pneumonia and other infections: antibiotics
IV solutions, sets, needles
Military antishock trousers (MAST)
Oxygen
Suction device (mechanical)

LESS USEFUL

Defibrillator
Instant glucose
Cardiac monitor
Short leg air splint

RESCUER'S PERSONAL GEAR

Extra clothing
Food and hot drinks
Ice ax, ice hammer, ski poles, Ensolite, Therm-a-Rest (use for splint improvisation)
Poncho
Stove, gas, cooking pot
Tent, bivouac sac

outlines the concepts on which the U.S. Urban Search and Rescue (US&R) Operations System is based. This system uses the Department of Defense as the lead agency but eventually involves nearly every federal agency, including the Federal Emergency Management Agency (FEMA). From these efforts 25 US&R response teams have been established around the country, based on standardized equipment, organizational structure, personnel qualifications, and operating procedures. Their mission is to work as part of a federal effort to locate, extricate, and provide initial medical treatment to victims trapped in structures that have collapsed during a disaster.[6]

APPENDIX A
Drug Stability Information

Stability data on drug products are nearly always based on studies done in controlled environmental conditions. It is often difficult to ascertain whether a drug product can be safely used after storage under conditions other than those specified by the manufacturer.

The question of stability of drug products pertains not only to the drug itself, but to the container in which it is packaged. If, for example, a parenteral drug packaged in a syringe for ready use is frozen, the drug itself may be fully potent, but the sterility of the product may be lost. Hairline cracks in the syringe may have resulted from freezing.

Thus, for most of the drug products listed, stability and sterility cannot be guaranteed if stored under conditions other than those recommended by the manufacturers.

Mannitol Injection 5%-25%. Stable at higher air temperatures. Solutions of 15% or higher crystallize out at lower temperatures, but will resolubilize when warmed to 80° C. Sterility cannot be guaranteed if frozen.

Lidocaine 1% Injection. Lidocaine is a relatively stable drug, but excessive heat or cold decreases shelf life. It should be stored between 15° and 40° C. It may be used after thawing, provided the container is completely intact and the solution remains clear. Lidocaine with epinephrine exposed to temperatures over 40° C for a long period should not be used (loss of epinephrine effect).

Sodium Bicarbonate Injection, 50 ml. The manufacturer specifically states "Do not freeze." If frozen, this product should not be used.

Naloxone Hydrochloride, 0.4 mg/ml. Protect from light during storage. Should not be used after being frozen. Store between 15° and 30° C.

Diphenhydramine Injection, 10 mg/ml. Drug (injection, elixir, tablets) is stable after freezing. Container should be checked for cracks or leakage. Store in light-resistant container, preferably at 15°-30° C.

Dexamethasone Injection, 4 mg/ml. Sensitive to light and extremes of temperature. Do not store at high temperature for long periods (maintains full potency for 6 months up to 40° C and up to 3 months at 50° C). Do not use after freezing.

Tetanus Toxoid, 0.5 ml. Do not use after freezing. Should be refrigerated; however, remains stable for months when stored at room temperature.

Meperidine Hydrochloride, 100 mg/ml. May be used after thawing if the solution shows no signs of precipitation or cloudiness and if the ampules or vials show no signs of cracking or leaking. Should be stored at 15°-30° C, protected from light. Retains full potency at 20° C for 1 month; at 35° C for 6 months; and at 45° C for 3 months.

Calcium Chloride 10% Solution. Drug pH is altered significantly if frozen or exposed to temperatures over 40° C. The product should not be used if either occurs.

Penicillin GK Injection. Stable in powder form for 2-3 years if stored at no greater than 30° C; higher temperatures cause potency to decrease.

Procaine Penicillin G Injection. Should be refrigerated; however, is stable at room temperatures for 6 months. Higher temperatures would increase hydrolysis and decrease potency. May be frozen and retain potency.

Furosemide Injection. May be used after freezing, barring evidence of cracking, leaking, or other damage to glass. All intact ampules or syringes, when returned to room temperature, should be vigorously shaken to redissolve any constituents that may have crystallized out of solution. Discoloration may occur when exposed to light, but potency is retained.

Gamma Benzene Hexachloride Lotions. The lotion and shampoo become thick when frozen, but do not lose effect. Effect of high temperatures unknown. Protect from light. Spray should not be exposed to temperatures below –2° C or above 54° C.

Glucagon Injection. In powder form, should be refrigerated, but is stable at room temperature for several weeks. When diluent is added to powder, resulting solution may be used for up to 3 months, if refrigerated. Thawing will not affect activity. Cloudy or thick diluent should not be used. Do not use if stored at temperatures greater than 35° C for an extended period.

Intravenous Solutions (D5W, D5NS, etc.). Effects of freezing these solutions are unknown. Incomplete resolubilization, especially with electrolyte solutions, seems a real danger.

Morphine Sulfate Injection, Solution, and Soluble Tablets. Exposed to air, morphine sulfate loses its water of hydration; it may darken on prolonged exposure to light. Store at 15°-30° C; avoid freezing. Freezing does not affect potency but may create insoluble particles.

Prochlorperazine Injection, Solution, Tablets, and Capsules. Store in tight, light-resistant containers. Store at 15°-30° C; avoid freezing. Discard discolored (impotent) solution.

Promethazine Injection, Tablets, Solution, and Suppositories. Protect from light. Store oral and parenteral products at 15°-30° C; store suppositories at 2°-8° C. Avoid freezing.

Antacids. Aluminum hydroxide gel suspension should not be frozen. Avoid freezing milk of magnesia. Upon freezing, many antacids separate into water and gel layers, which will probably not affect therapeutic value of the product, but will probably affect taste and prevent reformation of the emulsion, even with shaking.

Epinephrine Injection (Salts and Solutions). Epinephrine darkens upon exposure to light and air. Oxidation causes a color change to pink, then brown. Epinephrine should be stored at 25° C; avoid freezing. Heat above 40° C may inactive the product.

Diazepam Injection, Capsules, and Tablets. Protect from light and store at a temperature less than 40° C, preferably at 15°-30° C; avoid freezing. When frozen, diazepam tends to flocculate and precipitate. Rewarm with warm water; if no precipitate is visible, the product may be used.

Acetaminophen Elixir and Drops. Store at temperatures between 15° and 30° C, not above 40° C. Avoid freezing. Stability after freezing is unknown.

Acknowledgments

Thanks to Robert J. Matutat, Pharm. D. (UCLA), and Philip E. Johnston, Pharm. D. (Vanderbilt), for their help in preparing Appendix A.

REFERENCES

1. Bowman WD Jr: *Winter first aid manual,* ed 2, Denver, 1976, National Ski Patrol System, Inc.
2. Bowman W: Search and rescue: data-based first aid, *Wilderness Med,* April 1987.
3. Carlson GP, editor: *Incident Command System, National Interagency Incident Management System,* Stillwater, 1983, Fire Protection Publications, Oklahoma State University.
4. Cooper DC, LaValla PH, Stoffel RC: *Search and rescue fundamentals: basic skills and knowledge to perform search and rescue,* ed 3, Olympia, Wash, 1990 (revised 1993), Emergency Response Institute.
5. Cooper DC, Taylor A: *Fundamentals of mantracking: the step-by-step method,* ed 2, Olympia, Wash, 1992, Emergency Response Institute.
6. Federal Emergency Management Agency: *The Federal Response Plan,* PL 93-288, as amended, Washington, DC, 1991, Superintendent of Documents.

7. Ganong WF: Respiratory adjustment in health and disease. In *Review of medical physiology,* ed 7, Los Altos, Calif, 1975, Lange Medical Publications.
8. Geehr EC: Mountain rescue and preparation: environmental medical emergencies, *Topics Emerg Med* 2(3), 1980.
9. LaValla PH, Stoffel RC: *Search is an emergency: a text for managing search operations,* Olympia, Wash, 1987 (revised 1993), Emergency Response Institute.
10. LaValla PH, Stoffel RC: *Blueprint for community emergency management: a text for managing emergency operations,* Olympia, Wash, 1983 (revised 1991), Emergency Response Institute.
11. Miller AT Jr: Altitude. In Slonin NB, editor: *Environmental physiology,* St Louis, 1974, Mosby.
12. Syrotuck WG: *Analysis of lost person behavior,* Westmoreland, NY, 1977, Arner Publications.
13. United States Air Force: *National search and rescue manual,* volume 1, *National search and rescue system,* AFM 64-2, Washington, DC, 1986, Superintendent of Documents.
14. Worsing RA Jr, editor: *Basic rescue and emergency care,* Park Ridge, Ill, 1990, American Academy of Orthopaedic Surgeons.

22 AEROMEDICAL TRANSPORT

S. Marshal Isaacs
Charles E. Saunders
Bruno Dürrer

Rapid provision of appropriate definitive care to the acutely ill and injured is a major goal of all emergency medical services (EMS) systems throughout the world. The ability to rapidly transport and initiate treatment of severely ill or traumatized patients is important in decreasing morbidity and mortality. This is particularly germane to wilderness and environmental emergencies, where medical resources are scarce, transport times to definitive care facilities are often prolonged, and terrain and weather conditions are inherently difficult. Aeromedical transport crews can deliver emergency medical care at the scene while the time to definitive care can be markedly decreased. This maximizes the patient's chance for a successful recovery.

Aeromedical Evolution

Rapid evacuation of trauma victims from an injury scene to the location of definitive care is a modern concept with roots in antiquity. In the New Testament, an early instance of prehospital care and transport was documented: "a certain Samaritan . . . went to him and bound up his wounds, pouring oil and wine, and set him on his own beast and brought him to an inn, and took care of him."[79]

It has been said that the greatest impetuses to the advancement of emergency care and transportation have been epidemics and wars.[62] Before the classical Greco-Roman period, injured soldiers were often left on the battlefield to die. However, Homer described the use of chariots to evacuate fallen warriors during the Trojan War.[49] Napoleon's forces devised horse-drawn carriages, or *ambulance volantes,* for the same purpose.[53] The North American Indians devised the travois, a litter that could be pulled by a person or animal to transport the ill or injured.[60] The U.S. Army began a similar practice during the Seminole War of 1835-1842 and used it again in the Civil War. Major Jonathan Letterman established the process of rapidly clearing wounded soldiers to a point behind the battle line where they could be further triaged to an expectant area for persons with mortal wounds, a local treatment area for the walking wounded, or a hospital if definitive care was feasible. The central concept was efficient access to surgery for the victim of trauma.

These developments were soon followed by the invention of flying machines. In France, Richet had prophesied the potentials of air transport in 1869.[62] This was before the first balloon airlift. The prophesy was validated the following year during the Franco-Prussian War when the first documented aeromedical evacuations took place. During the Prussian siege of Paris, 160 wounded soldiers were evacuated and transported by hot air balloon over enemy lines.[83]

In the United States air evacuation took place soon after the Wright brothers flew in 1903.[40] Grossman and Rhoades presented their idea of air transport of patients to the War Department in 1910, but the government refused to fund them. It was not until World War I that the U.S. military began to employ aircraft to carry injured soldiers, and this occurred only rarely. However, the French transported patients as early as 1912 aboard Dorland ARII fighters converted to carry litters, despite the government's objection to the concept of aeromedical transport: "Are there not enough dead in France today without killing the wounded in airplanes?"[40]

The United States began employing its first dedicated air ambulances in 1920, using the deHavilland DH-4A, followed by the Cox-Klemin XA-1. World War II saw the widespread application of fixed-wing aircraft for evacuation. More than 1.4 million were transported from front-line hospitals to tertiary care facilities, with only 46 deaths en route.[88] During this time the concept of medical care during transport was implemented. In November 1942 the War Department began to train flight surgeons, flight nurses, and enlisted medical personnel for aeromedical transport.[40] It was also during this year that Igor Sikorsky produced a rotor-wing aircraft, called a "helicopter," which the army configured with external litters. It was used in an air evacuation for the first time in 1944 in Burma.[37]

Helicopters did not enjoy widespread use until more reliable machines became available. The Sikorsky S-51 and later the Bell 47-B were deployed over the rugged terrain and uncertain roads of Korea with great success to provide wide-scale evacuation of wounded soldiers to Mobile Army Surgical Hospital (MASH) units. Although only 11 dedicated "Medevac" helicopters were employed, more than 17,700 casualties were evacuated. For the first time, injury victims could travel directly from the point of injury to definitive surgical care.

This set the stage for the Army helicopter evacuation ("Dust Off") operations in Vietnam in 1962. With the Bell UH-1A Iroquois ("Huey") under the leadership of Major Charles Kelly, the Army's 57th Medical Detachment became known for the courage and hard work of flight crews that flew despite darkness, adverse weather, and enemy fire. Later, the turbine-powered Bell model UH-1H was used to evacuate up to nine patients at a time by hoist from above a dense jungle canopy. By 1967, 94,000 injured men had been evacuated.[70]

As air evacuation matured, the time from wound to definitive care declined from 18 hours in World War I to between 1 and 2 hours in Vietnam.[91] Although medical advances have contributed to improved survival, battlefield mortality has steadily declined from 18% in World War I to 1.8% in Vietnam, perhaps more because of rapid aeromedical transport to definitive care (Table 22-1).

Unfortunately, emergency medical care for civilians greatly lagged behind the developments in the military. In the late 1960s rescue efforts were more organized, skilled, and rapidly performed for a man shot in the Vietnam conflict than for a civilian injured on U.S. highways.[62] Civilian ambulances were said to be no faster than taxis.[78]

Civilian transport began to change dramatically in the United States in 1966 when the National Academy of Sciences–National Research Council put forth the white paper *Accidental Death and Disability: The Neglected Disease of Modern Society* (U.S. Department of Health, Education and Welfare). This document was the impetus for improving EMS systems through the country. It was not long before the civilian sector began to emulate the military model.

Outside the United States, Germany and Switzerland had developed a network of helicopter and fixed-wing air evacuation and transport services that continue to provide rapid access to care from even the most remote areas.[39] The first U.S. civilian aeromedical program was begun in 1969 as a joint effort between the Maryland State Police and the University of Maryland Center for the Study of Trauma (now the Maryland Institute for Emergency Medical Service Systems). There, certain hospitals were designated as trauma centers, to which victims of highway and other trauma were flown by police pilot-paramedic teams in a primary response role at the accident scene. Since 1970 the service has flown more than 199,000 missions (G. Shields: Personal communication, Maryland State Police, 1993).

With the development of faster and more powerful helicopters, reconfiguration of fixed-wing aircraft for aeromedical needs, enhanced knowledge of aeromedical physiology, and experience accumulated through more than 50 years of transport experience, the acceptance, utilization, and success of aeromedical transport are universal. The role of aeromedical transport in the wilderness setting continues to evolve as its importance in providing rapid emergency medical care to the sick and injured is recognized.

Table 22-1 Mortality Rates and Evacuation Times During Major Wars

Conflict	Evacuation Time (hr)	Mortality Rate (%)
World War I	18	18.0
World War II	4-6	3.3
Korea	2-4	2.4
Vietnam	1-2	1.8

From Stewart RD: *Trauma Q*, May 1985, pp 1-13.

Types of Aeromedical Transport Programs

HOSPITAL-BASED PROGRAMS

The most ubiquitous type of program is hospital based. Helicopter service is often provided in primary (to the accident scene) and secondary (to the community hospital emergency department) response roles. In addition, many hospitals provide fixed-wing transport in a secondary response role for long-distance transports or for instances when weather conditions preclude flying under visual flight rules (VFR).

According to the Association of Air Medical Services, in early 1994 there were more than 175 hospital- or health care provider–affiliated and 20 freestanding rotor-wing transport programs in the United States. These services transported more than 172,000 patients in 1993. Nationally, approximately 70% of all flights are interfacility transports and 30% are flights from the scene.[64]

In a hospital-based transport program the hospital frequently leases the helicopter from a vendor, who also supplies the pilots, maintenance, and fuel. The hospital has the responsibility for providing the medical crew and determining the configuration of the crew. In addition, the program directors are responsible for medical control and quality improvement.

The hospital may choose to own the aircraft and contract with a vendor for operations or employ its own pilots and mechanics. In most cases the helicopter resides on a helipad atop or near the hospital, while the crew, which may consist of a specially trained flight nurse, flight paramedic, and a physician, is quartered in the hospital ready for immediate launch (see "Medical Team Configuration").

NON-HOSPITAL-BASED PROGRAMS

Non-hospital-based service is provided by an entity that may be supported by a consortium of hospitals or it may be an independent corporation, an ambulance service, or an aviation fixed-base operator (FBO). The aircraft may be owned or leased by the entity or by an aviation contractor. Although this is not a common model for helicopter services in the United States, many fixed-wing services operate in this fashion. A corporate airplane may be provided on demand for use in an air ambulance mode with its interior reconfigured, or a dedicated airplane may be provided with a custom air-ambulance interior configuration (usually under a Supplemental Type Certificate).

PUBLIC SAFETY, POLICE, OR STATE SERVICES

The aircraft (usually a helicopter) may be owned and operated by a governmental agency such as the state highway patrol and operated under part 135 of the Federal Aviation Regulations (FAR). As in the Maryland model, flight personnel typically include police pilots and emergency medical technician-paramedics.

MILITARY ASSISTANCE TO SAFETY AND TRAFFIC PROGRAM

The Military Assistance to Safety and Traffic (MAST) program was established to supplement the civilian EMS systems. Under this program, air medical evacuation services are supplied by active-duty military medical units to the extent that their training budgets allow, provided they can use actual patient transports in lieu of training exercises. The MAST mission is "secondary"; it is available only when its personnel and equipment are not being used in support of the unit's primary mission. MAST may be requested by the local EMS or disaster management agency. Typical aircraft include the Bell UH-1 and Sikorsky UH-60 (Blackhawk). The medical crew usually consists of medical corpsmen.

OTHER MILITARY RESOURCES

The U.S. Air Force provides aeromedical transport in support of U.S. military disaster conditions. This service can be requested through the Airlift Command at Scott Air Force Base in Illinois. Other available resources include the Air National Guard, which operates C-130 transports for air evacuation, and the U.S. Coast Guard, which operates Aerospatiale Dauphins and Sikorsky H-3 helicopters for search and rescue. In addition, many states have organizations, such as the California Department of Forestry, that may be called on to assist in search and rescue operations in preparation for aeromedical transport.

Patient Mission Types

PRIMARY RESPONSE

In a primary response role the aeromedical transport service responds to an accident scene or field location, usually at the request of police, fire, or local EMS personnel, and serves as the initial and sole mechanism of transport to the hospital. In this instance the aeromedical crew may function as "first responders." Helicopters are most suited to a primary response role. The required response times must be short (less than 10 minutes from call to lift-off); thus the flight crew must be stationed at or near the launch site 24 hours a day. The service radius ("stage length") is short (typically less than 50 miles), and crews need to be experienced in techniques for landing in proximity to obstacles, under poor conditions, and on uncertain surfaces. In prehospital situations, patients' conditions vary widely and often little or no assessment or stabilization is performed before arrival of the flight crew. Medical personnel must possess a high degree of training and experience and should possess at a minimum emergency medical technician (EMT) skills required for patient extrication and stabilization at the scene.

SECONDARY RESPONSE

In the secondary response role a patient has already been transported by other means to a hospital where some degree of stabilization may have occurred. The aeromedical service transports the patient in the early stages of care from the emergency department of a hospital to a facility better equipped to offer definitive care. Response times required for this type of mission must be competitive with one-way ground transport times. Stage lengths are short to intermediate (150 miles). The transport vehicle is commonly a helicopter, although in some remote and wilderness areas, fixed-wing services are also suited to this role. Flight crews used in a secondary response vary depending on the needs of the patient (see "Medical Mission Types"). The responding aeromedical service typically consists of flight nurses, paramedics, and in some cases flight physicians.

TERTIARY RESPONSE

A tertiary response is one in which a hospital inpatient who requires specialized services unavailable at the current facility or who requests relocation is transported to a new facility. Tertiary transports may involve helicopters or fixed-wing aircraft, depending on the level of urgency, stage length, and the cost of transport.

Medical Mission Types

The needs of different patient types may be categorized by medical problem; this in turn dictates the requirements of the aeromedical transport service. In most hospital-based helicopter programs the majority of patients transported are categorized as adult trauma, cardiac, or medical noncardiac. A number of programs offer or specialize in pediatric, neonatal, perinatal, and organ transplant services, for which specialized crews and equipment may be required. In addition, aeromedical transport programs that provide search and rescue operations require specialized equipment and training.

TRAUMA PATIENTS

Trauma patients transported in the primary or secondary response modes may account for 20% to 60% of a hospital-based helicopter service's transport activity, depending on the hospital's function and capability as a trauma center and the relationship between the aeromedical service and the community EMS and public safety network. In a study of one urban setting it was noted that 20% of helicopter missions were to injury scenes, which were located at a mean distance of 14.4 miles from the hospital. Nineteen percent of transports involved patients with penetrating trauma, while 81% suffered blunt trauma (66% from motor vehicle accidents). The most common organ system injuries involved the head (65%), extremities (39%), chest (31%), and abdomen (27%). The overall mortality of transported patients was 24%. The most common procedures required at the scene were endotracheal intubation (41%) and cardiopulmonary resuscitation (CPR) (18.7%). The most common life-threatening conditions were cardiac arrest (18.7%), airway obstruction (5.1%), cardiac tamponade (3.2%), and tension pneumothorax (1.7%).[34]

A multicenter study of blunt trauma victims transported by helicopter aeromedical services from both urban and rural environments found a mean trauma score of 13 (of 16), mean age of 29 years, and overall mortality rate of 15%.[8]

These and other studies indicate the need for skilled crews in the transport of trauma patients.[93] Medical personnel must have the ability to assess the patient adequately to detect frequent in-flight complications and to intervene with appropriate procedures, including intravenous cannulation, endotracheal intubation, CPR, chest decompression, and at times a surgical airway (see Box 22-1).

In wilderness areas the flight crew must be skilled at victim extrication and operating in rugged terrain. They must be familiar with standard trauma care and the range of clinical entities most frequently seen in the wilderness setting. In addition, because resources may be limited and backup unavailable, they may be required to function semiautonomously. For this reason, protocols and standing orders are valuable. Most important are training, skill, and judgment.

BOX 22-1

TRAUMA CARE ABOARD EMERGENCY MEDICAL SERVICES HELICOPTERS

MECHANISM OF INJURY

Motor vehicle accident
Fall
Industrial or agricultural accident
Gunshot or stab wound
Burn
Sporting accident
Drowning
Hypothermia

PROCEDURES PERFORMED BY FLIGHT CREW

Endotracheal intubation
Cardiopulmonary resuscitation
Intravenous lines
Central venous access
Extrication and splinting
Bladder catheterization
Nasogastric tube insertion
Venous cutdown
Tube thoracostomy
Cricothyrotomy
Pericardiocentesis
MAST garment application

CARDIAC DISEASE

Patients with most cardiac disease most often are transported in a secondary or tertiary response role, by either helicopter or fixed-wing aircraft. They typically account for 20% to 50% of an aeromedical service's transport activity. The conditions of these patients are often medically complex. Technologically sophisticated treatment modalities may include antiarrhythmics, vasopressors, inotropes, vasodilators, thrombolytic agents, cardiac monitoring, arterial and central venous pressure monitoring, pacemakers, implantable defibrillators, and intraaortic balloon counterpulsation devices.[24,31,38,51] The flight crew must have sophisticated knowledge, expertise, and experience and sometimes includes a cardiac critical care nurse and a physician.

PATIENTS WITH MEDICAL, NONCARDIAC CONDITIONS

Patients with medical, noncardiac conditions, like those with cardiac disease, are most commonly transported in the secondary or tertiary response mode by either helicopter or fixed-wing aircraft. This group consists largely of patients with acute neurologic disease or shock, or who require assisted ventilation.[42] The spectrum of potential in-flight challenges includes cardiovascular problems, arrhythmias, hypotension, respiratory difficulties requiring acute airway management, seizures, and alterations in level of consciousness. The flight team must possess the ability to manage an airway and operate a ventilator. Additional considerations relate to the cabin environment and need for pressurization if hypoxemia is present, if barotrauma is likely, or if trapped gas exists, as well as the need to predict the requirement for and manage finite oxygen resources in flight.

PEDIATRIC PATIENTS

Pediatric patients may have traumatic or medical conditions.[9,45] In a study of 636 pediatric patients transported by air in the Salt Lake City area, 57.5% were transported by helicopter and 37.5% by fixed-wing aircraft, with a mean stage length of 207 miles (helicopter, 82 miles; fixed-wing, 452 miles). Less than 1% of flights were from the scene. The patient age ranged from 3 weeks to 16 years with 45% less than 1 year old. Trauma was the most common diagnosis (15.3% head injury, 9.3% multiple injuries), followed by neurologic illness (24.2%), respiratory failure or infection (20.1%), gastrointestinal or genitourinary problems (10.2%), metabolic disease (9.2%), cardiovascular disease (6%), and general pediatric surgical problems (5.7%). The overall mortality was 7%.[61] Many of the considerations for pediatric transport are similar to those for adults, especially with older children. However, infants may require an incubator, and in all cases flight crews must be experienced in caring for infants and children. Specifically, knowledge of pediatric advanced cardiac life support skills, including pediatric drug dosages, airway sizes, and fluid management, is essential.

PERINATAL PATIENTS

The need for expedient evaluation, preparation, and transport of the obstetric-gynecologic patient is increasing. Types of problems include ectopic pregnancy, pelvic inflammatory disease, toxic shock syndrome, abnormal fetal presentation, multiple gestation, diabetes in pregnancy, placenta previa, abruptio placentae, disseminated intravascular coagulation, preeclampsia-eclampsia, and preterm labor. The decision to transport patients in advanced preterm labor should be based on such factors as distance between hospitals, time required to cover the distance, personnel available for the transport, gestational age, and speed with which labor has progressed. The flight crew must be knowledgeable about these problems and comfortable with their treatment, so as to ensure a favorable outcome for both mother and child.

NEONATES

Neonates have unique anatomy and physiology, and the diseases that affect them require specific knowledge and skills by those involved in their transport. Specific issues include newborn assessment, including assignment of an Apgar score, airway clearance, temperature, homeostasis, and familiarity with neonatal resuscitation.[3] Access to references concerning neonatal emergency drug dosages should be available.[2,73]

The ability to perform umbilical vein catheterization is an important skill for any member of the transport team involved in neonatal care. In addition, knowledge of fluid, electrolyte, and glucose requirements is essential.[54] The flight crew involved in the transport of a neonate often includes a neonatal nurse and a neonatologist.

SEARCH AND RESCUE

Wilderness search and rescue is a unique aspect of aeromedical care and transport that requires a significant amount of training and expertise. Most aeromedical aircraft in the United States are not suited for search and rescue operations (see "Aircraft for Search and Rescue"). Most standard crews are not trained in search and rescue techniques. However, many aeromedical helicopters and some fixed-wing aircraft become involved in search and rescue activities, so it is important to be familiar with certain medical aspects of search and rescue. In addition, outside the United States, persons providing aeromedical transport are frequently involved in search and rescue activities. For a full discussion of search and rescue, see Chapter 21.

The keys to a successful search and rescue operation include proper communications, transport, evacuation, and medical treatment, all performed in the setting of favorable weather conditions and topography. The helicopter, equipped with a winch and preferably twin engines, is the most efficient means of providing search and rescue in the wilderness setting; it is essential for this role in mountainous regions. As a prognostic factor, a long delay between the time of the accident and the call for assistance, combined with a serious injury, has a deleterious effect on the outcome of the patient.

Helicopters are helpful in a number of search and rescue activities, including low-altitude search activity, search area evaluation, and movement of supplies and equipment. In some instances they may be the only means of extrication and rescue from the scene. Fixed-wing aircraft, on the other hand, are useful only for search area evaluation and secondary transport.

In the United Kingdom the Royal Air Force operates a helicopter search and rescue service that flew 1490 missions from 1980 to 1989, almost all of which involved vacationers along the coasts or in the mountains.[56] The Danish helicopter rescue service was founded in 1966 and uses a Sikorsky (S-61) helicopter. Since 1973 its crew has included a physician trained in aerospace medicine and helicopter transport. From 1973 to 1989 it flew 5733 missions, in 2075 of which direct medical intervention occurred. The most frequently encountered problems were abdominal trauma and cardiopulmonary diseases.[97]

In the high Alps more than 90% of all rescues are performed using helicopters (3000 per year).[4] Of these, 5% are combined rescues; that is, the helicopter carries the rescuers below cloud level, near the site of the accident. Only 5% of mountain rescues are purely ground rescues, mainly necessitated by visibility.[77] Currently a network of search and rescue systems extends throughout the Alps. In some countries (France, Italy, Germany, Austria, and Spain), air rescues are managed partially or totally by the army or the state. The aircraft most commonly used for this purpose are the Alouette III, Lama, Ecureil (French), Bolkow 105, 117 (German), Augusta AK 117 (Italian), and Bell (United States). In Switzerland the rescue system in remote terrain is managed by the Swiss Alpine Club and three air rescue companies, Swiss Air Rescue (REGA), Air Glaciers, and Air Zermatt. Switzerland may be unique in that its 18 strategically placed helicopter rescue bases allow an aircraft to reach any accident scene within 15 minutes of take-off. Since the foundation of REGA in 1952, more than 150,000 patients have been transported by either fixed-wing aircraft or helicopter.

Today up to 8000 patients (5500 from accident scenes) are transported by helicopter every year. Twenty percent of these rescues require a winch, with one third of all winch operations occurring in accident sites that are difficult to reach.[29] More than 75% of all persons rescued by winch were thought to have injuries requiring physician assistance at the scene. Eight percent of all Swiss air rescue missions are physician assisted, while the other 20% have a paramedic in charge. All the physicians and rescue crews are physically fit and trained in alpine techniques, since two thirds of all rescue missions performed from 1990 to 1993 were in topographically remote and difficult terrain (Color Plate 14).

Difficult helicopter search and rescue operations are those that involve low visibility, strong winds, night missions, high-angle rescues, and long-line winch operations (extension of the winch cable up to 120 m). In addition, in mountainous regions, power cables and transport cables present a considerable risk. In all cases the rescue risks to the flight crew (as well as to the patient) must be weighed against the degree of injury and risk of further morbidity. During the last 15 years Switzerland has lost three ambulance helicopters to accidents.

Despite the increasing number of people who participate in alpine sports, including mountain climbing, downhill skiing, mountain biking, and paragliding[30] (Table 22-2), the number of casualties during the last 5 years has remained constant at about 150 deaths a year in the Swiss Alps. This is thought to be due largely to the efficient medical-assisted helicopter rescue service in Switzerland.

In addition to search and rescue in mountainous regions, aeromedical rescue presents great challenges to the medical and flight crews involved in rescues from sea and white water, floods, vertical rocks, and avalanches.

Optimal medical treatment of any patient who is rescued begins immediately at the site of the accident unless weather conditions are deteriorating or the scene is inherently unstable. The patient with potential multiple system trauma should be evacuated with the use of a rescue net or sac with spine immobilization. Those with minimal or isolated injuries may be evacuated by use of climbing harnesses or rescue belts.[28] The decision to evacuate (hoist) before or after medical treatment is delicate, and whether to provide intravenous medication before the hoist and complete injury evaluation is a difficult decision even in the best of settings.

For the diagnosis and treatment of hypothermia, special core temperature thermometers and equipment for delivering warmed humidified oxygen and intravenous fluids are available. A thorough understanding of the pathophysiology and treatment of hypothermia (Chapter 3), acute mountain sickness (Chapter 1), and frostbite (Chapter 5) is essential for all those involved in search and rescue activities.

Aeromedical Aircraft

Many aircraft can be adapted to the air ambulance role. Each has its strengths and limitations. On the other hand, not

Table 22-2 Mountaineering Accidents in the Swiss Alps, 1992 (N = 1845 Persons)

Activity	Number of Patients Rescued
Delta gliding	18
Paragliding	196
Off-slope skiing	35
Ski touring	238
Mixed climbing	456
Rock climbing	178
Hiking	723

From Dürrer B, Hassler R, Mosimann U: *Mountaineering accidents in the Swiss Alps & rescue activities of the Swiss Alpine Club, 1992.*

all aircraft are suited for aeromedical transport in the wilderness environment or for search and rescue. Because these craft must support a critically ill individual in a hostile environment, certain flight limitations take on physiologic significance. Matching the physical characteristics of the aircraft to the needs of the mission and the demands of the environment in which it will function is vitally important.

CABIN SPACE

Cabin space should be considered not only in terms of total interior volume in cubic feet, but also with regard to floor space, headroom, and the ergonomics of cabin layout. Ample headroom should be available for the patient to lie comfortably on a secured stretcher and for access by two crew members to all parts of the body, specifically the head for intubation, the chest for CPR, and the extremities for monitoring perfusion. Some helicopters, such as the Aerospatiale AStar/TwinStar or the MBB BO-105, provide ample upper body access but only limited lower body access while in flight. The relationship of flight crew members when seated (and secured by the belt) in proximity to the patient is important. The ideal configuration places one medical crew member at the patient's head for airway management and verbal interaction and one at the patient's side to monitor vital signs and perform necessary non-airway-related procedures. This arrangement is typified by the MBB BK-117 helicopter (Fig. 22-1).

While some rotor-wing aircraft, such as the BK, are theoretically capable of transporting two patients, this greatly increases demands on the flight crew and the aircraft and diminishes access to both patients. Policies and procedures regarding two-patient transport in these aircraft should be carefully considered.

Cabin space is more generous in fixed-wing aircraft. Cabin-class airplanes, such as the Beech King Air and Piper Cheyenne III, provide an aisle and capability to carry more than one patient and additional crew or family members.

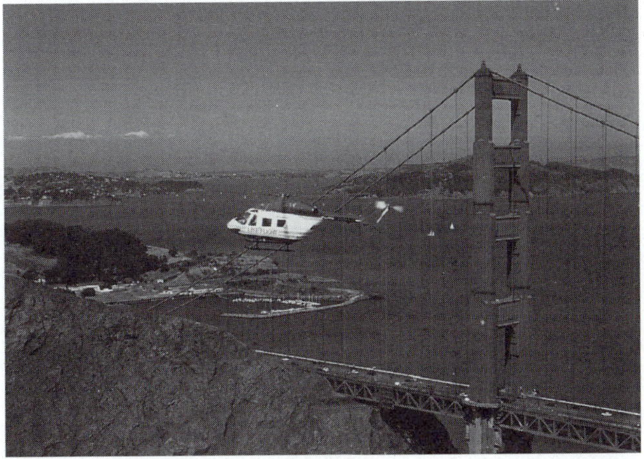

Fig. 22-1 Stanford LifeFlight MBB BK-117. (Courtesy Geralyn Martinez.)

ACCESS FOR PATIENT LOADING

The cargo door should be wide enough that the patient's stretcher can be maneuvered into the aircraft without undue tilting, and it should be positioned comfortably near stretcher height to obviate the need for strenuous lifting during ground loading. Standard door configurations on many aircraft do not meet these needs. The "clamshell" doors on an MBB BK-117 helicopter and the oversized cargo door on a Gulfstream Commander 1000 work well for patient loading (Fig. 22-2).

USEFUL LOAD

One of the most important considerations for a given patient transport is the aircraft's useful load. This difference between the maximum take-off weight and the basic empty weight is a reflection of the load-carrying capability. In most EMS helicopters the useful load ranges between 1500 and 2800 pounds. On-board avionics, medical equipment, fuel,

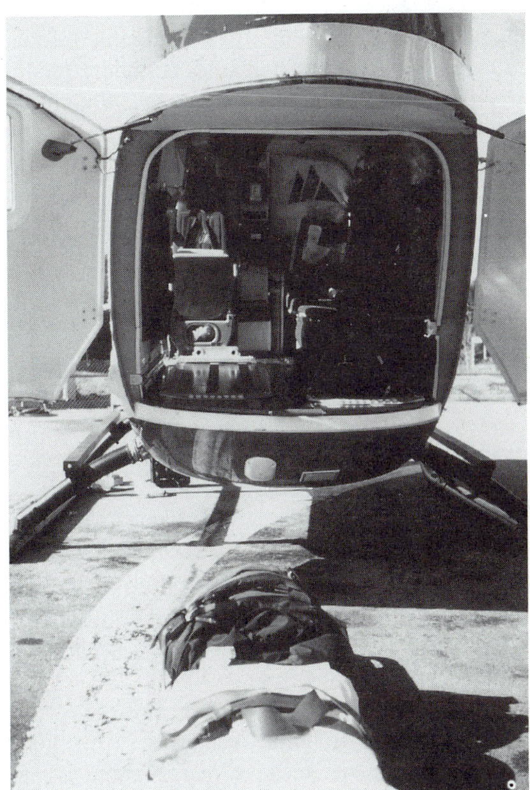

Fig. 22-2 MBB BK-117 with rear clamshell doors open. (Courtesy Susan Lockman, Stanford LifeFlight.)

Maximum takeoff weight[a]		________
Less basic empty weight[b]	–	________
Less fuel on board[c]	–	________
Less pilot and crew	–	________
Less medical gear[d]	–	________
Maximum "patient payload"	=	________

[a]Maximum takeoff weight is certificated for each aircraft type and can be found in the operating manual.

[b]Basic empty weight includes added avionics, permanent equipment, fluids, and unusable fuel. It is different for each aircraft, and is recorded in the aircraft's operating manual.

[c]The quantity of fuel on board depends on the mission needs. Divide round trip distance by cruise speed to yield time en route. Add time for warm-up, climb, approach, and a 30 minute reserve (VFR), to yield total engine time. Multiply total engine time by rate of fuel consumption, to yield total fuel consumed. Fuel weighs 6 lbs/gal.

[d]Medical gear includes carry-on and nonpermanent items.

Fig. 22-3 Weight calculation aboard aircraft.

and crew weights must be subtracted from this value to yield the maximum allowable patient weight (Fig. 22-3). Fuel weighs 6 pounds per gallon; a twin-engine helicopter may burn 70 gallons per hour (420 pounds per hour), requiring it to carry 600 pounds or more fuel for a 30-minute-radius flight (with 30-minute reserve). Thus it becomes evident that a flight crew of three weighing a total of 500 pounds with a full load of fuel, oxygen, and medical gear may not have the capability to carry even a small patient, especially on a hot day when the helicopter's performance (lift) is reduced. This consideration can become critical on flights from the accident scene, where terrain obstacles may require vertical take-off and climb-out, demanding maximum helicopter performance.

WEIGHT AND BALANCE

Not only must the weight of the loaded aircraft remain at or below the maximum certificated take-off weight for that aircraft, but the center of gravity (CG) must lie within fore and aft limits established by the manufacturer. Each loading configuration places the CG in a unique position, which must be calculated by the pilot before flight, or the flight characteristics may be adversely affected, compromising safety. This consideration may dictate where certain pieces of medical equipment, such as oxygen bottles, may be placed or where heavier crew members must sit.

On flights from the accident scene the patient's weight is approximated only just before departure. With pressure to hasten departure, accurate weight and balance calculations are difficult. For that reason the aircraft employed must have enough margin in the CG envelope that CG limits are not easily exceeded for the given mission profile.

CRUISE SPEED

One of the most basic reasons for transporting a patient by air is to take advantage of the greater speed of aircraft compared with ground vehicles. This allows the patient earlier arrival at the destination and minimizes time spent out of the hospital. Not only do aircraft have a speed advantage, but they can travel in a straight line from origin to destination without the curves and deviations present in surface travel. For an aircraft to compete with a ground vehicle in speed in a primary or secondary response mode, it must be at least twice as fast as an ambulance, since the helicopter must fly round trip (outbound to destination and inbound with patient) in the time that the ambulance would travel one way. This is possible with most EMS helicopters, unless the referral location has no suitable landing area (necessitating a time-consuming transit of crew and stretcher to and from the location), ground "packaging" times for the flight crew with the patient are excessive, or an ambulance has a clear, straight highway as a means of alternative transport.

Most EMS helicopters are capable of cruise speeds in the 120 to 150 mph range, although a headwind or tailwind may hinder or improve these figures (Table 22-3). Piston-twin aircraft have a cruise speed range of 220 to 275 mph, turboprop aircraft of 300 to 385 mph, and jets of 400 to 535 mph or more.[22,71]

Table 22-3 Helicopters Frequently Used for Aeromedical Transport

Helicopter	Cruise Speed (mph)	Engine(s)	SHP	Useful Load (lb)	Service Ceiling (ft)	Range (Miles)*
Bell 206L-3	130	SE-T	650	1950	20000	325
AStar 350D	140	SE-T	615	1868	15000	379
TwinStar 355F1	147	TE-T	420 each	2391	13120	368
MBB BO-105 CBS	145	TE-T	420 each	2732	17000	334
Agusata 109A II	163	TE-T	420 each	2605	15000	359
Bell 222UT	152	TE-T	684 each	3376	15800	380
MBB BK-117	160	TE-T	650 each	2645	17000	368
Sikorsky S-76	167	TE-T	650 each	4700	15000	550
Dauphin 2	161	TE-T	700 each	4118	15000	564

Data from Collins RL et al: *Flying 1985 annual & buyer's guide,* New York, 1985, Ziff-Davis; and 1987 hospital aviation directory, *Hosp Aviat* 6(4):8, 1987.
SE-T, Single engine, turbine; *TE-T,* twin engine, turbine; *SHP,* shaft horse power.
*Range includes fuel for warmup, taxi, climb, and 30-minute reserve.

RANGE

Aircraft range is limited by the amount of fuel, which is a function of fuel tank capacity and useful load. In most cases, a trade-off is made between payload and fuel; the more weight in fuel, the less weight in passengers (or patients). The maximum time aloft can be calculated by dividing usable fuel on board by rate of fuel burn per hour at cruise speed. Multiplying maximum time aloft by cruise speed yields the maximum range. The Federal Aviation Administration (FAA), under FAR part 91.23, requires that a 45-minute fuel reserve remain at the conclusion of all flights conducted under instrument flight rules (IFR), and a 30-minute reserve under visual flight rules (VFR). Most EMS helicopters operate under VFR, while most fixed-wing operations are IFR. Because helicopters typically fly to and from a point at which refueling is not available, round-trip fuel must be carried; this effectively limits the customary radius of operation to approximately half the range (less VFR reserves). Although it is possible to refuel en route to an airport, this adds to the flight time. Thus helicopters typically operate within a radius of 150 miles or less, unless the transport is one-way outbound or unless refueling at the destination is feasible. Fixed-wing aircraft operate from airport to airport; hence the radius of operation is closer to the maximum range with reserves. Most fixed-wing aircraft are capable of ranges in excess of 1000 miles, with some jets able to travel up to 2000 miles.

PRESSURIZATION

The partial pressure of oxygen in the atmosphere declines with increasing altitude so that at 18,000 feet it is one-half that at sea level. Part 91.32 of FAR requires the use of supplemental oxygen for the pilot at flight altitudes above 12,500 feet for longer than 30 minutes.[32] Above 14,000 feet, supplemental oxygen must be used by the pilot and all *minimum required* flight crew at all times. Technically a medical flight crew member is not a *required* minimum crew member for the operation of the aircraft; neither is the copilot of an aircraft operated under FAR part 135 and certified for single-pilot operations (as is the case with most aeromedical aircraft). Thus the medical crew member is not required to wear supplemental oxygen, although doing so would be prudent, especially for smokers. In addition, oxygen use is recommended for all above 14,000 feet at night, since night vision deteriorates rapidly at altitude without oxygen. At altitudes greater than 15,000 feet, in addition to the above requirements, each occupant must be provided with supplemental oxygen (although there is no legal requirement to use it). The effects of hypoxia with increases in altitude are more pronounced in patients with lung disease and preexisting hypoxia; this necessitates supplemental oxygen at much lower altitudes.

To eliminate the need to provide supplemental oxygen, pressurization is available in many larger, fixed-wing aircraft (Table 22-4). A pressurized aircraft is able to pump air into the cabin to maintain a pressure differential between the cabin and outside air, generally 4 to 8 pounds per square inch (PSI). This allows the cabin atmosphere to be maintained at or below the equivalent of an 8000-foot altitude, despite actual altitudes of 30,000 feet or higher.[63] Pressurization obviates the need for supplemental oxygen for crew members and nonpatient passengers, but passengers with lung disease may still require it. Also, by limiting the drop in cabin pressure that occurs with altitude, changes in trapped gas volumes, such as in endotracheal (ET) tube cuffs, air splints, and the gastrointestinal tract, can be decreased or eliminated.

On the other hand, helicopters are nonpressurized and generally fly at lower altitudes where altitude-related hy-

Table 22-4 Fixed-Wing Aircraft Used for Aeromedical Transport

Aircraft	Cruise Speed (mph)	Cabin	Engines	Useful Load (lb)*	Service Ceiling (ft)	Range (Miles)†	Take-Off (ft)‡
Seneca III	221	NP	TE-P	1921	25000	721	1250
Baron 58TC	277	NP	TE-P	2447	25000	1150	2700
Cessna 402C	245	NP	TE-P	2774	26900	1164	2200
Navaho 350	250	NP	TE-P	2533	24000	1200	2200
Cessna 414	258	P	TE-P	2386	30800	1300	2600
Cessna 421	277	P	TE-P	2807	30200	1522	—
Cessna 441	330	P	TE-T	4124	35000	2195	—
Cheyenne II	293	P	TE-T	4053	31000	1275	2500
Cheyenne III	347	P	TE-T	4448	35000	1789	3200
MU-2	317	P	TE-T	3975	27300	1412	—
King Air F90	309	P	TE-T	4383	31000	1315	2900
Commader 1000	323	P	TE-T	3965	30750	2149	
Citation I	410	P	TE-J	5222	41000	1500	3000
Lear 25D	509	P	TE-J	7150	51000	1600	4000

Data from Collins RL et al: *Flying 1985 annual & buyers guide,* New York, 1985, Ziff-Davis; 1987 hospital aviation directory, *Hosp Aviat* 6(4):8, 1987; and McNeil EL: *Airborne care of the ill and injured,* New York, 1983, Springer-Verlag.

NP, Nonpressurized; *P,* pressurized; *TE-P,* twin-engine, piston; *TE-T,* twin-engine, turboprop; *TE-J,* twin-engine, turbojet/turbofan.

*Useful load excluding avionics, fuel, passengers.

†Range estimated at cruise speed, less 45-minute reserve.

‡Approximate nonbalance-field take-off length.

poxia is unlikely. One exception occurs in mountainous regions where altitudes required to rescue victims or cross mountain passes may exceed 12,000 feet. Reasons for transporting patients at higher altitudes include terrain avoidance, the need to surmount adverse weather (which usually occurs within 20,000 feet above ground), and the fact that greater speed and fuel efficiency can be obtained at higher altitudes.

SERVICE CEILING

The service ceiling is the maximum altitude at which an aircraft can still maintain a 100 foot per minute rate of climb. It is important in predicting an aircraft's ability to climb above adverse terrain and weather, and to take advantage of favorable winds aloft in order to maximize ground speed. In the western United States, mountainous areas require flight at least 2000 feet above the highest terrain along the route of flight, which means a 12,000- to 16,000-foot service ceiling. These altitudes restrict most helicopters and require use of supplemental oxygen in nonpressurized airplanes. Flight operations that typically require flight at these altitudes should have access to aircraft with sufficiently high service ceilings and pressurization.

RUNWAY LENGTH

Although not a factor in helicopter operations, runway length restricts certain fixed-wing aircraft from landing. Most airports in rural areas have runway lengths between 2000 and 4000 feet. Higher performance airplanes usually have progressively longer runway requirements and may be unable to land and take off safely on these strips. Thus, when transport from a rural location with a short runway is requested, it is important to determine the capability of the aircraft being used. Piston twin aircraft can usually operate safely from a 2500- to 3000-foot strip but may have difficulty with 2000 feet; turboprop airplanes require 2500 to 3500 feet; and jets usually require runway lengths of 4000 feet or more.[63] The take-off roll for airplanes increases with increasing temperature and airport altitude; on a hot day, many airplanes may be incapable of taking off from a short runway if heavily loaded.

In winter conditions, operating on icy runways may pose a safety hazard for braking. Turboprop airplanes and jets have a reverse thrust mode that can slow the aircraft on rollout without braking.

WEATHER OPERATIONS

Adverse weather conditions that may affect a given flight include restrictions in visibility resulting from precipitation, fog, haze, or clouds, as well as airframe icing, turbulence, and wind shear. Flight during instrument meteorologic conditions (IMC) requires adherence to instrument flight rules (IFR), while visual meteorologic conditions (VMC) allow alternative use of visual flight rules (VFR).

VMC conditions for airplanes are defined as visibility of at least 3 miles and ceiling of at least 1000 feet (departing from an airport in controlled airspace).[32] The ability to fly IFR not only improves the likelihood that the mission can be undertaken and completed safely should clouds or adverse weather be present, but also permits the air traffic control center to follow the flight and properly separate aircraft.

IFR capability has drawbacks. Sophisticated and expensive equipment and training are required. Virtually all fixed-wing aircraft are capable of IFR operations, but most EMS helicopters are not. IFR operations are conducted from airport to airport (where an instrument approach is available), yet most helicopters travel to and from nonairport points without an instrument approach. The percentage of actual missions canceled or aborted because of IMC conditions is small in most rotor-wing programs. In a recent study it was determined that inadvertent excursions into IMC conditions occurred about 1.3 times per pilot per year, and the anticipated percentage of operations that would be conducted IFR, if it were available, was 9.4%.[69] For most hospital-based programs the cost of upgrading to a more expensive IFR-equipped helicopter (especially if a copilot is necessary for IFR certification), plus the added expense of maintaining pilot IFR proficiency, would be prohibitive.

PERFORMANCE

Closely related to aircraft speed is its ability to climb, expressed in feet per minute (fpm). Known as performance, this ability dictates the type of aircraft used for a given aeromedical transport mission (Table 22-2). The greater the performance (a complex function of power, weight, wing, propeller, and air density characteristics), the better the aircraft's ability to outclimb adverse weather or to avoid rising terrain or obstacles. Helicopters are unique in their ability to hover above the ground effect, that is, to climb vertically out of the supporting cushion of air produced by the rotor wash. Helicopters perform better when they can get a running start, building up forward speed while still in the cushion of ground effect until translational lift is developed. Translational lift results from the forward to backward flow of air over the rotor blades. A helicopter's ability to climb vertically out of ground effect is limited by horsepower and weight. On a hot day at high altitude, performance may be insufficient to take off vertically.[47] This must be considered when selecting a landing site away from an airport. If a confined space surrounded by obstacles is selected, a vertical take-off may be required. For this reason, twin-engine helicopters are becoming more common in EMS operations, especially when calls to accident scenes are frequent.[18]

Fixed-wing aircraft are virtually all twin-engine, not only for enhanced speed, performance, and cabin space, but also for the necessary redundancy of systems required for IFR operations under FAR part 135. If one engine fails, a second is available to allow flight to be maintained; however, if failure occurs during take-off, single-engine climb performance may not be adequate to provide lift. This fact may be critical if insufficient altitude has been gained to allow a return to the airport before obstructions are encountered. Therefore single-engine climb performance for various types of aircraft must be considered, especially if operating out of high-altitude airports, in hot weather, or in mountainous regions (Table 22-4). In general, single-engine climb performance is about 200 to 290 fpm in piston twins, 600 to 900 fpm for turboprops, and 1000 to 2000 fpm for jets.[63] The airplane with the best single-engine climb performance will provide the greatest margin of safety, but the cost of equipment, pilot training, and adequate runways will be high.

AIRCRAFT FOR SEARCH AND RESCUE

Search and rescue is a special type of aeromedical transport that demands aircraft uniquely suited to this role. The aircraft should have good visibility to the sides and below, the ability to fly slowly and to hover, the ability to land away from an airport, and adequate performance in high-density altitude conditions. In addition, certain extrication situations require the capability to hoist victims from rugged or hostile terrain.

Helicopters are the vehicle of choice for search and rescue. Twin-engine, turbine-powered helicopters are the most advantageous. Examples are the Aerospatiale Allouette, MBB BO-105, and BK-117 (Fig. 22-4). The MBB helicopters are used by REGA (Swiss Air Rescue), which specializes in alpine wilderness rescue. Civilian helicopters in common use in search and rescue operations have cruise speeds between 125 and 160 mph and can lift between 2000 and 3000 pounds (less weight of crew and fuel).[63] Few hospital-based EMS helicopters are configured for winch operations, and hospital flight crews are typically not trained in search and rescue techniques. The search and rescue mission differs from other types of medical missions in its requirement for low-level flight over potentially hostile terrain, its use of flight crews for visual surveillance for survivors or wreckage, the need for a prolonged hover if winch operations occur, and the need for flight crew training in wilderness survival principles if a mishap occurs. Experience and training in these activities are essential for safety.

Military helicopters, such as the Sikorsky UH-60 operated by the Army under the MAST program, are better suited to search and rescue than are civilian EMS helicopters. The UH-60 has a maximum gross weight of 20,250 pounds, with an approximate payload of 5800 pounds. It typically cruises at 138 mph, with a maximum airspeed of 222 mph. It is capable of hoist operations, with a 250-foot cable and a 600-pound gross lifting weight. With the use of a jungle penetrator apparatus, up to three individuals may be hoisted simultaneously from above a forest canopy. Crew members on board a typical medical evacuation mission in-

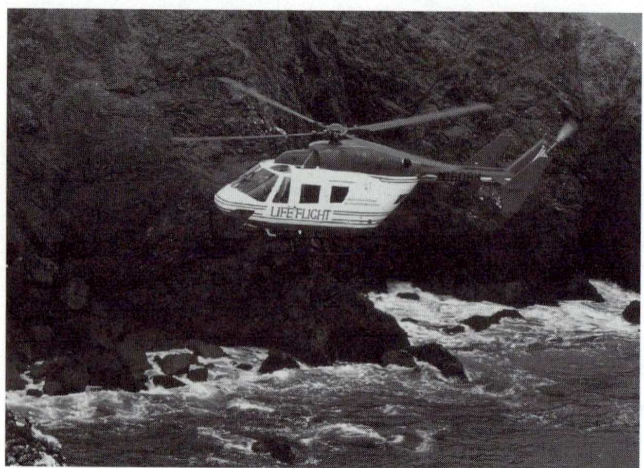

Fig. 22-4 Stanford LifeFlight MBB BK-117 used for search and rescue mission. (Courtesy Geralyn Martinez.)

clude the pilot, copilot, crew chief, and a flight "medic" (medical corpsman). Without the hoist the UH-60 is capable of carrying four litters or seven ambulatory patients (or various combinations of litter and ambulatory patients); with the hoist, three litter and two ambulatory patients, or six ambulatory patients, may be carried. The flight crews are trained for search and rescue, particularly in hostile terrain, and in using the winch. However, specialized medical equipment (such as a ventilator or pacemaker) and medications may not be available. In addition, the crew may not be skilled at certain advanced clinical procedures, such as venous cutdown, chest tube insertion, and cricothyrotomy.

Search and rescue over water requires special technique. The pilot must hover in a position to keep the victim in visual contact (that is, at the pilot's 2 o'clock position) if possible, without causing excessive rotor wash. A floating smoke marker helps as a point of visual reference. A flight crew member enters the water or descends onto the deck of the boat to stabilize and secure the patient, who is then hoisted aboard the helicopter.

In mountainous areas special hazards exist. Not only are high-density altitudes encountered, which may limit an aircraft's performance, but local weather patterns may be erratic. On the leeward side of mountains or ridges, severe downdrafts could prevent a helicopter from hovering out of ground effect. The landing site selected should be free of terrain obstacles and should allow for a long shallow approach and departure. Open areas away from the leeward side of mountains or ridges are preferable. For additional information on helicopters in search and rescue, see Chapter 21.

PILOT REQUIREMENTS

Helicopter EMS operations are usually conducted VFR, and the FAA has established minimum requirements for pilot experience. FAR part 135.243 specifies that the pilot in command of a helicopter carrying passengers for hire must have at least 500 hours of flight time, including at least 100 hours of cross-country time with 25 hours at night. Fixed-wing operations are typically IFR, and under these circumstances pilots must have at least 1200 hours of flight time, including 500 cross-country, 100 night, and 75 hours of actual or simulated instrument time. They must also be instrument rated and possess a commercial certificate.

Most EMS helicopter pilots have a great deal more experience than the minimum requirements; in one survey 59% had more than 4000 hours and none had fewer than 2000 hours.[33] The pilot in command is solely responsible for the safety of all persons aboard the aircraft and must decide whether to accept or decline a mission. For this reason the pilot is often not told the nature of the medical mission until a decision to go is made. This decision should be based solely on the destination, weather conditions, environmental circumstances, and estimated time at the scene, airport, or destination facility. No mention of patient type or severity should be made to the pilot before the launch decision is made so that this decision is objective.

COMMUNICATIONS

Helicopter EMS units must have the capability to communicate on VHF frequencies assigned for air traffic control, flight service, and local airport Unicom. In addition, the ability to communicate with ground EMS and public safety via VHF and UHF frequencies is essential. Air use frequencies are accessible through standard aircraft communications transceivers, but EMS communications require additional radio equipment designed for this purpose. Additional needs include communication with the helicopter's base station, either on a locally assigned public use frequency or a Federal Communications Commission (FCC)-assigned discrete frequency in the VHF airband. Another means of communication is aircraft 800 MHz radiotelephones that can access the surface telephone network. Communication over airband frequencies requires strict adherence to FAA communications guidelines and the possession of a radiotelephone operator permit from the FCC.[27]

MEDICAL EQUIPMENT AND IN-FLIGHT MONITORING

On-board medical supplies and equipment are typically tailored to the needs of a specific transport program and include medications, airway and ventilation supplies, dressings and bandages, intravenous fluids, immobilization devices, military antishock trousers (MAST), stretchers, and so forth.[74] The Department of Transportation, in conjunction with the American Medical Association, has published guidelines for on-board equipment for air ambulance operation (see Box 22-2).[94]

BOX 22-2

DEPARTMENT OF TRANSPORTATION–AMERICAN MEDICAL ASSOCIATION GUIDELINES FOR ON-BOARD MEDICAL EQUIPMENT FOR AEROMEDICAL TRANSPORT

BASIC MEDICAL EQUIPMENT RECOMMENDED FOR EACH FLIGHT

1/patient	Litter or stretcher with approved restraints
2/patient	Sheets
2/patient	Blankets
1/patient	Pillow with cover impervious to moisture
1/patient	Pillowcase
1 set	Spare sheets and pillowcase (if weight and space allow)
1 unit	Medical oxygen with manual control; adjustable flowmeter with gauge (0 to 15 L/min); attachment for humidification (**Note:** The oxygen unit must be attached to the aircraft in an approved manner. The amount of oxygen to be carried is determined by multiplying the prescribed flow rate times the length of time the patient must be on oxygen and adding a 45-minute reserve. The minimum amount of oxygen carried should be enough to supply one patient for 1 hour at 10 L/min. It may be necessary to carry a portable oxygen unit if oxygen is not available for patient transfer at some point in the flight.)
2 each	Oxygen masks in adult, child, and infant sizes
6	Connecting tubes
1	Oxygen key
1 unit	Portable suction with connecting tubes
2 each	Suction catheters (various sizes)
2	Tonsil suction tips
1 unit	Squeeze bag-valve-mask unit capable of receiving oxygen through an inlet, and delivering 80% to 100% oxygen through the mask; with masks in adult, child, and infant sizes (bags in adult and small child/infant sizes)
1 unit	Oxygen-powered, manually triggered breathing device (100 L/min flow rate)
1	Blood pressure cuff, sphygmomanometer
1	Stethoscope (**Note:** To record blood pressure readings, a Doppler or electronic stethoscope may be required if noise or vibration levels are high. An electronic unit must not cause electromagnetic interference on aircraft equipment.)
2 each	Oropharyngeal airways in adult, child, and infant sizes
1	Emesis basin
1	Urinal or bedpan or both
1/patient	Sound suppressors
1	Pneumatic antishock trousers with pressure relief valve
2	Cervical collars
2	20-gallon trash bags
1 box	Ziplock plastic bags or similar product
1	Flashlight, 2 D batteries or equivalent with spare batteries and bulb
2	Locking hooks (or other positive locking device for intravenous fluid containers)
1 qt.	Drinking water
12	Paper cups

DRESSINGS AND SUPPLIES KIT, DESIGNED TO BE CARRIED ON EACH FLIGHT

4	Cardboard or air splints or equivalent in arm and leg sizes
12	Tongue depressors
2	Mouth gags or padded tongue depressors
1	Bandage scissors
4	Tourniquets
1 each	Rolls of adhesive tape, ½, 1, 2, 3 inch
1 each	Rolls of paper tape, various sizes
4	Kling bandages or equivalent
1	3-inch elastic bandage
1	4-inch elastic bandage
4	Kerlix rolls or equivalent
2 pairs	Sterile gloves
3	Petrolatum gauze
1 box	Adhesive bandages
6	Disposable surgical face masks
2 each	Syringes, 3, 5, and 10 cc (TB and insulin)
3 each	Needles, 18, 20, and 22 gauge
3 each	Needles, 19, 21 gauge, scalp/vein
2	Surgical dressings
24	Sterile gauze pads
6	Nonsterile gauze pads
2	Triangle bandages
2	Wrist restraints
2	Eye covers
1 roll	Aluminum foil, sterilized and wrapped
1	Large safety pin
2	Clinical thermometers
4	Airsick bags
12	Waterless towelettes
1 box	Tissues

MEDICATION AND INTRAVENOUS KIT, DESIGNED TO BE CARRIED ON EACH FLIGHT

2	Epinephrine HCl, 1:1000, 1 ml, prefilled syringe
2	Epinephrine HCl, 1:10,000, 10 ml, prefilled syringe with intracardiac needle
2	Aminophylline inj. IM, 500 mg in 2 ml ampules
4	Atropine sulfate, 0.5 mg in 5 ml prefilled syringe
2	Diphenhydramine HCl, 50 mg/ml, 1 ml prefilled syringe
2	Dextrose, 25 g/50 ml, prefilled syringe

Continued.

BOX 22-2

DEPARTMENT OF TRANSPORTATION–AMERICAN MEDICAL ASSOCIATION GUIDELINES FOR ON-BOARD MEDICAL EQUIPMENT FOR AEROMEDICAL TRANSPORT—cont'd

2	Intravenous injection sets with micro dripper
2	Lidocaine HCl, 2g/10 ml, prefilled syringe
3	Lidocaine HCl, 20 mg/ml, 5 ml prefilled syringe
6	Naloxone HCl, 0.4 mg/ml, 1 ml ampules
1	Nitroglycerin, 0.4 mg, sublingual tablets, 100
2	Digoxin inj., 0.5 mg/2 ml ampules
4	Furosemide, 10 mg/ml, 2 ml ampules
2	Chlorpromazine HCl, 25 mg/ml, 1 ml ampules
6	Sodium bicarbonate inj., 3.75 mg/50 ml, prefilled syringe
2	Morphine sulfate, 15 mg/ml, prefilled syringe
1	Hydrocortisone sodium succinate, 100 mg/vial
1	Methylprednisolone sodium succinate, 1000 mg/vial
1	Plasma protein fraction, 250 ml with infusion set
2	Sterile water for injection 20 ml
3	Diazepam, 5 mg/ml, 2 ml prefilled syringe
6	Alcohol swabs
1	Phenylephrine HCl, 0.25%, nasal spray
2	Ammonia inhalant solution, 0.5 ml ampule
2	Isoproterenol HCl, 1:5000, 1 ml ampules
1	Tourniquet
1	0.9% sodium chloride inj., 500 ml bag
1	0.9% sodium chloride inj., 250 ml bag
1	Lactated Ringer's inj., 250 ml bag
1	Lactated Ringer's inj., 500 ml bag
2	Lactated Ringer's inj., 1000 ml bag
3	Needles, 15 gauge, 1½ inch
1	Dextrose, 5% in water, 250 ml
1	Dextrose, 5% in water, 500 ml
1	Dextrose, 5% in normal saline, 250 ml
1	Dextrose, 5% in normal saline, 500 ml
1	Pressure pack or infusion pump
1 each	Drip tubing, regular and pediatric
2	Armboards
6	Alcohol wipes
1	Clean hemostat
1 each	Sterile hemostat, curved and straight
1	Nasogastric tube, 14 gauge
2	Sterile normal saline for injection, 20 ml
2 pair	Sterile gloves
1	Knife handle
1	Subclavian set
1	No. 15 blade
1	Intravenous infusion cuff
1 each	Rolls of tape, 1 and 2 inch

AIRWAY MANAGEMENT KIT, DESIGNED TO BE CARRIED ON EACH FLIGHT

1	Laryngoscope with curved and straight blades in various sizes; spare batteries and bulb
As required	Adapters for attaching endotracheal tubes to oxygen etc.
1	Rubber-shod forceps
1	Magill forceps
1	Esophageal obturator airway with gastric suction capability
1	McSwain dart or Heimlich valve
1	Syringe, 60 cc
1	Needle, 14 gauge
1	Syringe, 10 cc
1 each	Rolls of adhesive tape, 1 and 2 inch
1	Viscous lidocaine HCl, 2%
1 tube	Surgical lubricant

BURN KIT, TO BE CARRIED WHEN REQUIRED

3	Normal saline, 1 cc in plastic container
1	57 × 80 inch sterile burn sheet
5 packs	Xeroform gauze, 5 × 9 inch
1	Irrigating syringe, 50 cc
2 pairs	Sterile gloves
4	Kerlix rolls
2 packs	Fluffy gauze

POISON DRUG OVERDOSE KIT, TO BE CARRIED WHEN REQUIRED

1	Irrigation tray
1	Surgical stomach tube for lavage
1 each	Specimen bottles for urine, gastric, and miscellaneous
2 each	Stomach tubes, 14, 16, 18 Fr
1	Rubber stomach tube No. 20
1 tube	Lubricant
1 box	Glucagon, 1 unit
2	Ipecac syrup, 30 ml
1	Physostigmine salicylate, 1 mg/ml, 2 ml ampules
1	Pralidoxime chloride, 1 g kit
1	Activated charcoal, 10 g

OBSTETRIC KIT, TO BE CARRIED WHEN REQUIRED

1	Disposable obstetric pack with sheets, cord clamps, DeLee suction, plastic bag, silver swaddler, sterile gloves
2	Oxytocin, 10 units/ml, 1 ml ampule
1	Episiotomy scissors
1	Ring forceps

PEDIATRIC KIT, TO BE CARRIED WHEN REQUIRED AND ALWAYS WITH OBSTETRIC KIT

1	Pediatric laryngoscope handle with blades
1 each	Pediatric endotracheal tubes with stylette, 2.5, 3, 3.5, 4 Fr
1	Pediatric Magill forceps
2	Bulb syringes
2	DeLee suction

BOX 22-2

DEPARTMENT OF TRANSPORTATION–AMERICAN MEDICAL ASSOCIATION GUIDELINES FOR ON-BOARD MEDICAL EQUIPMENT FOR AEROMEDICAL TRANSPORT—cont'd

2	Pediatric drip IV tubing
1 each	Feeding tubes, 3.5, 5, 8 Fr
1	Pediatric blood pressure cuff, sphygmomanometer

ADDITIONAL EQUIPMENT FOR TRAUMA PATIENTS, TO BE CARRIED WHEN REQUIRED

1	Scoop stretcher
1	Long backboard
1	Foley catheter set
1	Femur traction splint
1	Suture kit

ADDITIONAL EQUIPMENT FOR CARDIAC PATIENT, TO BE CARRIED WHEN REQUIRED

1 unit	Cardiac monitor with strip chart recorder
1 each	Spare ECG electrode for each lead
1	Spare roll of ECG recording paper
1 unit	Defibrillator with four pads and conductive gel (defibrillator may come as a unit with the cardiac monitor)
1	Rubber mat or other means of electrically isolating the patient from the aircraft
1	Cardiac board

ADDITIONAL EQUIPMENT FOR SPECIFIC PATIENTS, TO BE CARRIED WHEN REQUIRED

1 unit	Respirator capable of continuous venilation, with ventilator, tubing, exhaled volume measuring device, set of tracheostomy endotracheal adaptors
1 unit	Incubator, with all equipment suitable for neonatal care

Modified from Department of Transportation, National Highway Traffic Safety Administration, American Medical Association Commission on Emergency Medical Services: *Air ambulance guidelines,* Washington, DC, 1981.

POWER

Most aircraft systems operate from 14 or 28 volts DC power supplied by an engine-driven alternator or generator. This is not adequate to operate most medical devices, which require 110 to 120 volts AC. Such devices cannot be used without an internal battery of sufficient charge to provide power for the duration of the mission, or unless a 110 to 120 volt AC power source is available from a power invertor, which must be installed under a Supplemental Type Certificate. Power invertors are common components of EMS helicopters and dedicated fixed-wing aircraft that have been retrofit with a custom air-ambulance cabin configuration, but they may not be a standard component in fixed-wing aircraft that support a dual role and use an interchangeable corporate configuration.

STRETCHER

The patient stretcher must be secured to the aircraft according to the requirements of FAR part 23.561 or 25.561 for seats, which are: 3.0 g's upward (2.0 g's part 25), 9.0 g's forward, and 1.5 g's sideways. For helicopters the requirements are: 1.5 g's upward, 4.0 g's forward, and 2.0 g's sideways. Special configurations, especially those incorporating oxygen bottles and metal framework, may require an STC. Other guidelines (recommendations only) for stretcher configurations are for clear view and access to the patients with at least 30 inches of headroom and at least 12 inches of aisle beside the head. The stretcher should be at least 19 inches wide by 73 inches long.[94] If the patient is positioned with head forward, the acceleration that occurs during take-off of a fixed-wing aircraft may cause venous pooling in the lower extremities and transient hypotension. To prevent this, the patient can be positioned with feet forward.

CLIMATE CONTROL

The aircraft must be capable of maintaining a comfortable interior environment (recommended 75° F). During summer months the extensive glass area on a helicopter can produce a greenhouse effect, which may necessitate air conditioning for the comfort of both crew and patient.

LIGHTING

Lighting should be available to enable the crew to attend to the patient's needs, yet not interfere with cockpit operations. Curtains or other physical barriers may satisfy this need.

SUCTION

Suction is a requirement for ambulance operations in most states and should be available at all times during aeromedical transport. Integral suction as a custom retrofit system or a portable battery-powered device can be employed.

OXYGEN

In general, enough oxygen should be provided for the flight, plus a 45-minute reserve (IFR; 30 minutes VFR). In addition, oxygen should be carried to allow for ground handling time at either end. The amount of oxygen required can be obtained by multiplying the desired flow rate in liters per minute by the total duration of transport and patient loading and unloading. The capacities of various types of oxygen tanks and their respective weights are shown in Table 22-5. Some portable ventilators have a gas-driven logic circuit that requires additional air or oxygen. Electrically powered ventilators have a lower requirement for oxygen but carry the additional need for a power invertor. In most cases patients are transported with oxygen supplied by nasal cannulae (1 to 6 L/m). A single E-sized oxygen cylinder is adequate for short flights, although backup cylinders are usually carried. Patients intubated and maintained on 100% oxygen, as well as those ventilated on long flights, will exceed the capacity of an E cylinder quickly. In such cases several E cylinders or an H cylinder will be required.

VENTILATORS

On short flights, most patients can be bag ventilated manually, with the addition of a positive end-expiratory pressure (PEEP) valve as needed. Manual ventilation has drawbacks. Minute ventilation can rarely be precisely controlled, leading either to respiratory acidosis or more commonly to alkalosis. The patient's tidal volume limits may be exceeded with resultant pulmonary barotrauma. More important, the medical attendant will be completely occupied with ventilation and is thus unavailable to perform other tasks. This takes on added importance if complex infusions are being administered or in-flight complications occur. The likelihood that manual ventilation will be unsatisfactory increases with the duration of transport, the medical complexity of the patient, and the severity of underlying lung disease.

Compact ventilators are available for use in the aeromedical transport environment.[12] The simplest are pressure ventilators with a timing valve mechanism that will deliver a predicted minute ventilation at a given rate and tidal volume adjustable to patient size. These require that the patient have normal airway compliance. If airway resistance increases, smaller tidal volumes will result and tidal volumes usually cannot be varied independently from rate. Volume-cycled ventilators are superior and available in configurations in which tidal volume and rate can be varied independently. Oxygen bottles, a 50 PSI regulator, high-pressure gas lines, a patient breathing circuit, and source of humidification need to be present.

Table 22-5 Oxygen Tank Specifications

Cylinder Size	Weight (lb)	Capacity* (L)	Endurance† (hr) At 2 L/min	Endurance† (hr) At 10 L/min
D	11	356	2.0	1.0
G	32	1200	10.0	2.0
Q	70	2320	19.3	3.8
H and Q	150	6900	57.5	11.5

From National EMS Pilot's Association: *Hosp Aviat* 5(6):17, 1986.
*At 70° F, 14.7 PSI. Capacity varies with ambient conditions.
†Estimated endurance; actual values may vary.

INFUSION DEVICES

Several methods of intravenous (IV) infusion delivery are available in the aeromedical setting: gravity-feed microdrip or macrodrip tubing with the drip rate manually adjusted, gravity-fed automatic infusion regulators with a closed-loop drip monitoring feedback mechanism controlling drip rate, and infusion pumps. If a pump is employed over moderate or long transport distances, the internal battery power will be inadequate, necessitating an external source of power, usually an AC power invertor. With infusions that must be carefully maintained, an infusion pump is preferable. With frequent patient movement and manipulation, tubing can bend and kink, altering resistance to fluid flow. Air trapped in tubing (or in glass IV bottles) can expand with changes in altitude and increase or decrease the infusion pressure. Thus a reliable servocontrolled infusion system provides a margin of safety.

MONITOR-DEFIBRILLATOR

Combination monitor-defibrillators operate from internal batteries when 110 to 120 volts AC is not available. Other monitors capable of pressure monitoring from arterial lines or pulmonary artery catheters may be used, but these may have limited usefulness on flights of short duration in which vibration and motion (turbulence) can introduce artifact and erroneous readings, as may occur aboard a helicopter. Dedicated fixed-wing aircraft that frequently transport critically ill patients over long distances may find a greater role for these devices. Recently, noninvasive blood pressure measuring devices have been found to have reasonable accuracy in most patients, although sensitivity of the device may be insufficient.[58]

Concern has been expressed over the potential hazards of defibrillation while airborne. Recent reports from actual trials support its safety.[24,44] Caution is still advised, and care should be taken to ensure that crew and aircraft systems are isolated from potential electrical contact. (See "Problems in Aeromedical Transport.")

OXIMETRY

A fairly recent technologic innovation of potential great use in the prehospital environment is the noninvasive oximetry method of monitoring hemoglobin saturation. Pulse oximeters, as these devices are known, use a colorimetric method and function by placement of a soft probe over a fingertip, in a thin skinfold such as an earlobe, or against the conjunctiva.[1,86] They may be extremely useful in aeromedical transport where other methods to detect changes in respiratory status are difficult.

END-TIDAL CARBON DIOXIDE

End-tidal carbon dioxide monitoring involves the use of a sensor placed in the path of exhaled gas from the endotracheal tube of an intubated patient. These devices indicate systemic PCO_2 and are useful in assessing adequacy of ventilation.

TRANSCUTANEOUS PO_2 AND PCO_2

Oxygen and carbon dioxide sensors noninvasively monitor PO_2 and PCO_2 after placement over a hyperemic cutaneous surface. Hyperemia is enhanced by heating the skin with a thermocouple, which may be uncomfortable, and hence is usually reserved for use in neonates.

NONINVASIVE CARDIAC OUTPUT

Cardiac output, stroke volume, and other hemodynamic variables can be monitored noninvasively by measuring transthoracic electrical bioimpedance through standard electrocardiographic electrodes and processing the signal with devices available for this purpose.[81] First used by the National Aeronautics and Space Administration for monitoring astronauts, the technique has been adapted for civilian aeromedical environments. Baseline impedance values can serve as a guide to intrathoracic fluid status.[80]

MECHANICAL RESUSCITATORS

Cardiac arrest resuscitation while airborne in a small cabin is difficult and physically demanding. In most instances a standard medical crew of two will be completely occupied in performing chest compressions and ensuring ventilation. Additional tasks may be impossible. For this reason a mechanical resuscitator may be employed to prevent fatigue and to free crew members for other tasks.[68] Mechanical resuscitators are gas-powered devices capable of providing ventilation and chest compressions automatically. Some models provide only chest compressions.

Flight Crew

CREW CONFIGURATION

One of the continuing controversies in aeromedical transport involves crew composition (Table 22-6). The ideal crew composition is a matter of debate and varies considerably with the mission profile. When the aircraft is involved in a primary response to the accident scene, there may be a benefit from the inclusion of an EMT. The transport of patients whose illness or injuries are complex, or whose clinical conditions are markedly unstable, may benefit from the presence of a physician. All aeromedical transport programs include one or more of the following providers in the transport medical crew.

EMERGENCY MEDICAL TECHNICIAN–PARAMEDIC

EMTs are increasingly a part of the aeromedical flight team. In 1993, 71% of rotor-wing transport programs reported using an EMT-Paramedic (EMT-P) as a member of the flight team, as opposed to 44% in 1988.[15] Paramedics vary in their level of training depending on the state in which they work but commonly follow Department of Transportation guidelines, which include three levels of certification. EMT-Basic provides basic ambulance, rescue, and first aid skills. EMT-Intermediate may include IV and intubation skills. The EMT-Paramedic level allows such skills as intubation, IV techniques, medication administration, defibrillation, and dysrhythmia recognition and treatment. For an aeromedical flight team member, additional training relating to the aeromedical environment is desirable.[84,94]

EMTs can be of particular value in operations where frequent interaction with ground EMS is necessary. In some regions helicopter EMS service is integrated into the regional primary response network so that they arrive at the accident scene before ground units. In such an event, flight team members experienced in scene assessment and victim extrication are essential.

FLIGHT NURSE

At least one flight nurse is a component of almost all aeromedical transport programs; in 1993, 21% of rotor-wing programs reported using two flight nurses as the sole team members.[15] Critical care or emergency nursing experience is usually a prerequisite, with additional training that includes patient assessment, ACLS, a trauma life support course, prehospital care skills, certain procedures such as endotracheal intubation, advanced intravenous cannulation techniques, and in some cases needle thoracotomy, venous cutdown, cricothyrotomy, and other specialized patient care activities (Table 22-6). In many cases the flight nurse is also a certified EMT.

Table 22-6 Medical Attendants in Aeromedical Transport, 1988-1993

	Percentages				
	1988	**1990**	**1991**	**1992**	**1993**
HELICOPTER					
Medical crew					
One attendant	8	3	3	2	2
Two attendants	92	97	97	98	98
Crew configuration					
RN/paramedic	44	54	53	57	71
RN/RN	15	11	11	19	21
RN/physician	10	12	11	10	3
RN/other	17	15	20	7	2
Other	14	8	5	7	3
Regular-duty shift length					
8 hours	2	2	4	6	3
12 hours	62	68	70	82	63
24 hours	18	16	15	11	10
12 and 24 hours	9	9	5	0	19
Other	9	5	6	1	5
FIXED-WING AIRCRAFT					
Medical crew					
One attendant	17	17	10	4	5
Two attendants	83	83	90	96	95
Crew configuration					
RN/paramedic	41	38	36	54	59
RN/RN	17	15	25	18	24
RN/physician	5	3	2	0	6
RN/other	22	35	32	18	9
Other	15	9	5	10	2
Regular-duty shift length					
8 hours	—	3	2	2	8
12 hours	46	43	50	47	46
24 hours	14	14	14	19	8
Other	40	40	34	32	38

From Cady G: *Air Med J* 12(9):308, 1993.

FLIGHT PHYSICIAN

The experience and training of a physician involved in aeromedical transport depend on his or her role. If functioning as the on-line medical control physician, he or she communicates via radio or 800 MHz radio telephone with the flight crew, monitors care, and gives necessary orders. In the United States physicians fly as a component of the flight team in a minority of aeromedical transport programs. In fact, in 1993 only 3% of all rotor-wing transport programs reported the routine use of a physician, as compared with 10% in 1988.[15] In helicopter EMS operations an emergency physician or trauma surgeon may be appropriate, whereas with fixed-wing transport of ICU patients an intensivist may be of value.

Physicians functioning in this role must have a current level of skill and expertise sufficient to address a wide range of clinical problems. They must also possess additional training relative to the airborne environment, including flight physiology, aircraft operations, and prehospital care (see Box 22-3). Most important, they must function in this role with sufficient frequency so as to maintain their skills and remain safe and comfortable within the aeromedical setting. In doing so, they may be an asset to the flight team, rather than a distraction or a liability.

A number of studies performed during the late 1980s and early 1990s attempted to answer the question of whether a physician crew member has an effect on the outcome of patients transported by helicopter.* Without question each study was performed by investigators who had markedly different backgrounds and biases and whose methods used to answer this question varied greatly. Not surprisingly, some studies concluded that a physician crew member had a positive impact on patient outcome, while others found no difference in outcome between similar cohorts of patients transported by flight crews with two nurses or a nurse and a paramedic. What is without question is that the cost of using a physician crew member is substantially higher than the cost of a nurse-nurse or nurse-paramedic crew configuration. Some argue that this higher cost would be offset by the decrease in hospital stay or lost person-years that would occur if a physician were a standard member of the flight crew. In our opinion, with advanced training in critical procedures and treatment protocols combined with on-line medical direction, a nonphysician flight crew functions in most cases as well as a crew that includes a physician. There is no objective evidence to support the benefit of a physician as a standard flight crew member.

CREW MEMBER STRESS

By its nature, aeromedical transport involves moving a gravely ill patient into an adverse environment with limited resources. Under these conditions a medical crew of only two or three persons must perform complex tasks, solve difficult problems, and make life or death decisions. They must perform in a physically confining space that may be uncomfortable, and they must do so under time pressure and with little or no physical assistance. In some cases, rescuers' lives may be at risk. In few other arenas of civilian medical care does this scenario occur.

"Stress" describes an array of adverse physiologic and psychologic reactions that occur when a person perceives a threat to existence. Although stress is not proven to diminish performance, it may be responsible for errors, faulty judg-

*References 5, 6, 14, 41, 43, 76, 85, 87.

BOX 22-3

SPECIALIZED TRAINING FOR AEROMEDICAL TRANSPORT

- Aviation physiology
  - Atmospheric pressure changes with altitude
  - Gas expansion with altitude
  - Changes in partial pressure of oxygen with altitude
  - Effects of motion and acceleration
  - Effects of noise and vibration
  - Changes in temperature and humidity
- Aircraft safety
- Aircraft systems and equipment operations
- In-flight emergency procedures
- Survival techniques
- Patient extrication and immobilization
- Patient loading and handling aboard an aircraft
- Patient care techniques in the aeromedical environment
- Respiratory support and ventilation aboard the aircraft
- Pertinent Federal Aviation Administration regulations and procedures
- Familiarity with the local EMS system
- Radio communications skills and techniques
- Hazardous materials response procedures
- Record keeping and documentation in aeromedical transport
- Preflight, in-flight, and postflight procedures
- Clinical procedures
  - Cardiopulmonary resuscitation aboard the aircraft
  - Defibrillation aboard the aircraft
  - Intravenous cannulation
  - Endotracheal intubation
  - Tube thoracostomy
  - Needle thoracotomy
  - Cricothyrotomy
  - Central vein catheterization
  - Pericardiocentesis
  - Nasogastric tube insertion
  - Bladder catheterization
  - Antishock trouser application
  - Interosseous line placement
  - Umbilical vein catheterization

ment, and uneven manual skill performance. It may also have an effect on the physical and psychologic health and satisfaction of the flight crew member.[16]

Not surprisingly, when anxiety among aeromedical crew members was measured during patient flights, its level was found to be significantly higher than during a baseline period on the ground.[89] Factors that correlate with high in-flight anxiety levels include adverse weather conditions (such as low ceilings and high winds), severity of the patient's medical condition, complexity of illness or injuries, and the crew member's fatigue.

Efforts should be made to minimize stress among crew members. This includes frequent and adequate training, continuing education and feedback, adequate medical backup, including on-line medical direction, written protocols, and treatment guidelines that can aid in difficult judgment decisions, a supportive rather than an intimidating or critical quality assurance program, adequate rest, and safe weather minimums. Both routine mission debriefing and critical incident stress debriefing (CISD) should be an integral part of all transport programs.[65,66]

Flight Physiology

Aeromedical care is different from ground-based care not only because of special equipment and the space-limited environment, but also because of the hostile physical milieu.

HYPOXIA AND ALTITUDE

The earth is blanketed by a sea of air. The troposphere lies in the first 30,000 to 60,000 feet and contains atmospheric moisture. This allows vertical convection currents, as well as a temperature decline with increasing altitude at a lapse rate of 2° C per 1000 feet. Virtually all atmospheric weather occurs in this layer. Above this level lies the stratosphere, extending from 60,000 to 100,000 feet, where temperature remains relatively constant and no moisture or vertical convection currents exist.

Air exerts pressure on everything it touches in an amount equal to the weight of the column of air above the point of reference. At sea level the atmospheric pressure is 14.7 PSI or 760 mm Hg. As the person ascends, there is a progressively smaller air mass remaining to exert weight and the pressure diminishes. At 18,000 feet the atmospheric pressure is one half that at sea level, and at 28,000 feet it is one third as great (Fig. 22-5). Similarly, under the weight of air, individual molecules tend to compact, so that the density of air is also greatest at the surface and diminishes with increasing altitude.

These phenomena underlie most of the important physiologic consequences of flight. Air is composed of several gases, of which oxygen makes up approximately 21%, an amount that is relatively constant despite increasing altitude (Table 22-7).[74] Henry's Law states that the quantity of gas that goes into solution depends on the partial pressure of that gas (and its solubility characteristics) as exerted at the air-water interface. The partial pressure of oxygen in alveolar air (P_{AO_2}) is determined by multiplying the fractional composition of oxygen in inspired air (F_{IO_2}) by the atmospheric pressure (barometric pressure, P_B) after the opposing vapor pressure of water (P_W, 47 mm Hg) has been subtracted. This is the basis of the alveolar air equation

$$P_{AO_2} = F_{IO_2} \times (P_B - P_W) - P_{CO_2}/R$$

where P_{CO_2} is the arterial P_{CO_2} and R is the respiratory quotient (approximately 0.8). Arterial P_{O_2} (P_{aO_2}) in normal individuals is within 10 to 15 mm Hg of the P_{AO_2}. With lung

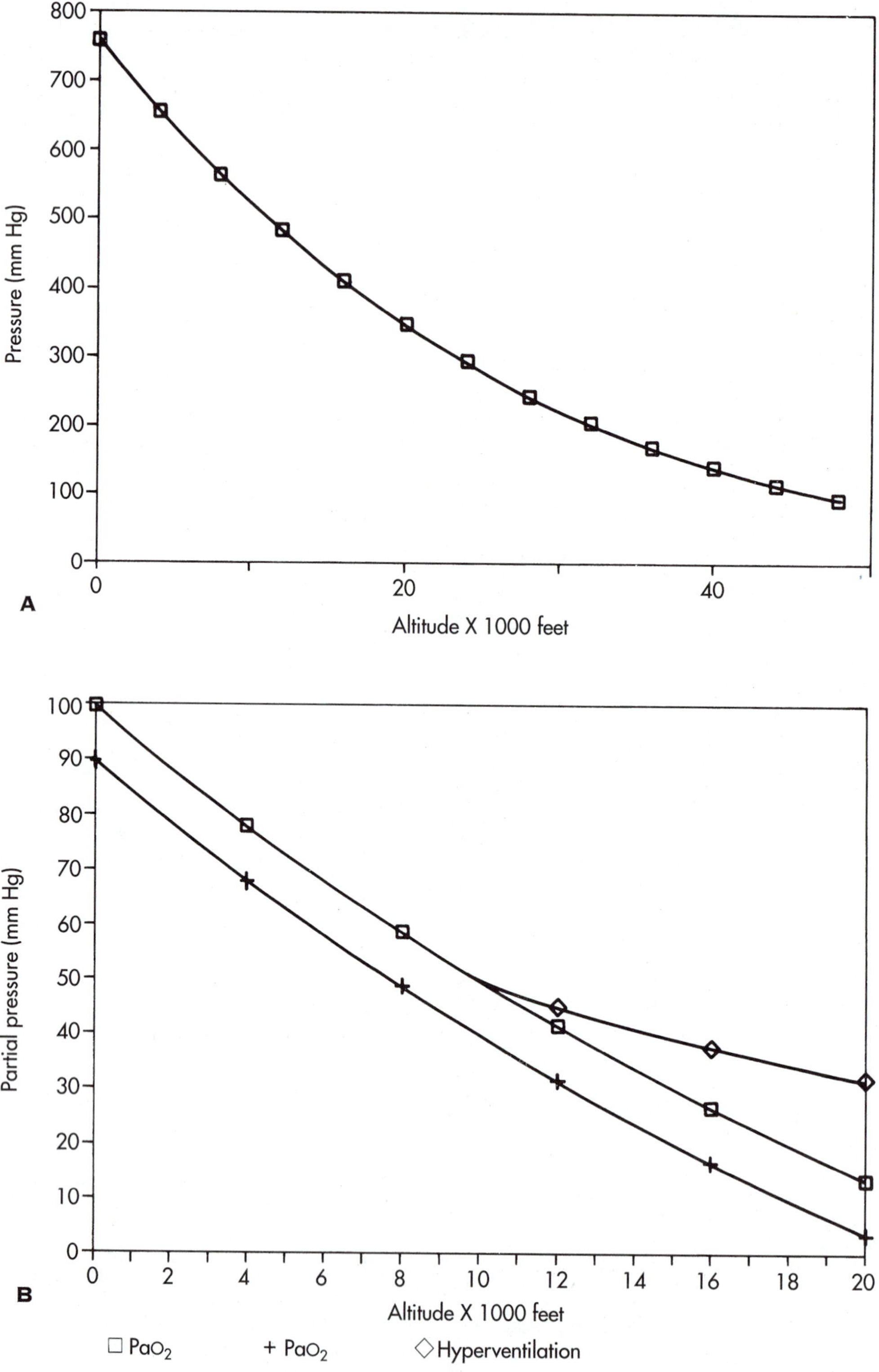

Fig. 22-5 **A,** Atmospheric pressure versus altitude. **B,** Alveolar and arterial oxygen tensions versus altitude.

Table 22-7 Composition of Air

Gas	Percent
Nitrogen	78.09
Oxygen	20.95
Carbon dioxide	0.03
Other gases	0.07
Water vapor	1-5 at sea level

From Del Vecchio RJ: *Physiologic aspects of flight,* Oakdale, NY, 1977, Dowling College Press.

disease characterized by ventilation-perfusion mismatch, intrapulmonic shunting, or severe diffusion defects, the alveolar-arterial oxygen gradient is much larger and higher amounts of inspired oxygen are required to produce sufficient oxygenation of arterial blood. The atmospheric Po_2, PAO_2, and the Pao_2 all decline with altitude (Fig. 22-5). To some extent arterial Po_2 can be maintained slightly through hyperventilation as Pco_2 is reduced, but eventually Pao_2 will decline below 60% and hemoglobin will begin to desaturate markedly.

It is important during aeromedical transport to maintain hemoglobin saturation at or above 90%. Knowledge of the patient's preflight Pao_2 will enable a calculation of the patient's alveolar/arterial oxygen gradient, which can then be subtracted from the PAO_2 calculated for the anticipated en route altitude (or cabin altitude in a pressurized craft) to yield the expected en route Pao_2. Nomograms can be devised for this purpose (Fig. 22-6). If the en route expected Pao_2 is unacceptably low, supplemental oxygen is required. The Fio_2 required to maintain the alveolar Po_2 at a given level can be calculated from the alveolar air equation as follows:

$$Fio_2 = (PAO_2 + Pco_2/R)/(P_B - P_W)$$

Or, if $Pco_2 = 40$, $R = 0.8$, and $P_W = 47$ mm Hg, then:

$$Fio_2 = (PAO_2 + 50)/(P_B - 47)$$

This allows PAO_2 to be determined by adding the Pao_2 desired (the minimum acceptable is 60 mm Hg) to the known alveolar/arterial oxygen gradient (calculated from the preflight blood gas). P_B can be estimated over the first 15,000 feet of ambient or cabin altitude as follows:

$$P_B = 760 - (23 \times \text{Alt})$$

where Alt is the altitude above sea level in thousands of feet. In most cases transport cabin environments rarely exceed these altitudes, since pressurized craft are usually capable of maintaining cabin pressure equal to that at altitudes at or below 8000 feet and nonpressurized craft must provide supplemental oxygen above 15,000 feet. Even a modest increase in Fio_2 is usually enough to maintain oxygenation under these circumstances, unless a severe alveolar/arterial oxygen gradient exists, in which case the addition of positive end-expiratory pressure (PEEP) may be necessary. The above equation would predict that a Pao_2 of 80 mm Hg at sea level on 40% oxygen would require an Fio_2 of 50% at 8000 feet to be maintained. The use of an oximeter can make the monitoring of oxygenation much easier. Simply put, as altitude increases, a fall in oxygen saturation can be treated with increases in Fio_2.

EFFECTS OF PRESSURE CHANGES

Trapped Gas

Boyle's Law states that the volume of a gas varies inversely with pressure. This means that trapped gases expand as an aircraft ascends to higher altitude (and lower pressure) and contract as it descends. The volume change can be determined from the equation

$$P_1 \times V_1 = P_2 \times V_2$$

Clinically, this is manifested by such alterations as expansion or contraction of air splints or MAST pants, changes in endotracheal tube cuff size, expansion of bowel gas in cases of intestinal obstruction or ileus, expansion of pneumothorax airspace, and expansion of air trapped in IV lines (or glass IV bottles) (Table 22-8). Certain precautions must be taken, such as the use of plastic IV bags and frequent monitoring of pressure cuffs.

Dysbarism

Decompression sickness occurs mainly in scuba divers who ascend too soon after a dive. Lower ambient pressure allows nitrogen bubbles to form in the microcirculation, causing ischemia and tissue damage (see Chapter 47). Care must be taken in the transport of an ill or injured diver to allow a surface interval of at least 12 hours before transport. An alternative is to attain at least a level D (PADI) dive stage, with a cabin altitude not to exceed 8000 feet. If an individual must be transported abruptly after submersion, the transport must be conducted at the lowest possible safe altitude in a pressurized aircraft, to reduce the risk of decompression sickness or air embolism.

MOTION AND ACCELERATION

Aircraft not only move through space in a rectilinear fashion, which cannot be detected by human senses in the absence of visual cues, but also rotate about three axes: longitudinal (roll), vertical (yaw), and horizontal (pitch) (Fig. 22-7). Motions about these axes are sensed by the semicircular canals located in the inner ear. Sensations from these organs are useful as an adjunct to visual cues. However, they may quickly lead to spatial disorientation, a phenomenon experienced commonly by individuals traveling in a turbulent environment without a visual frame of

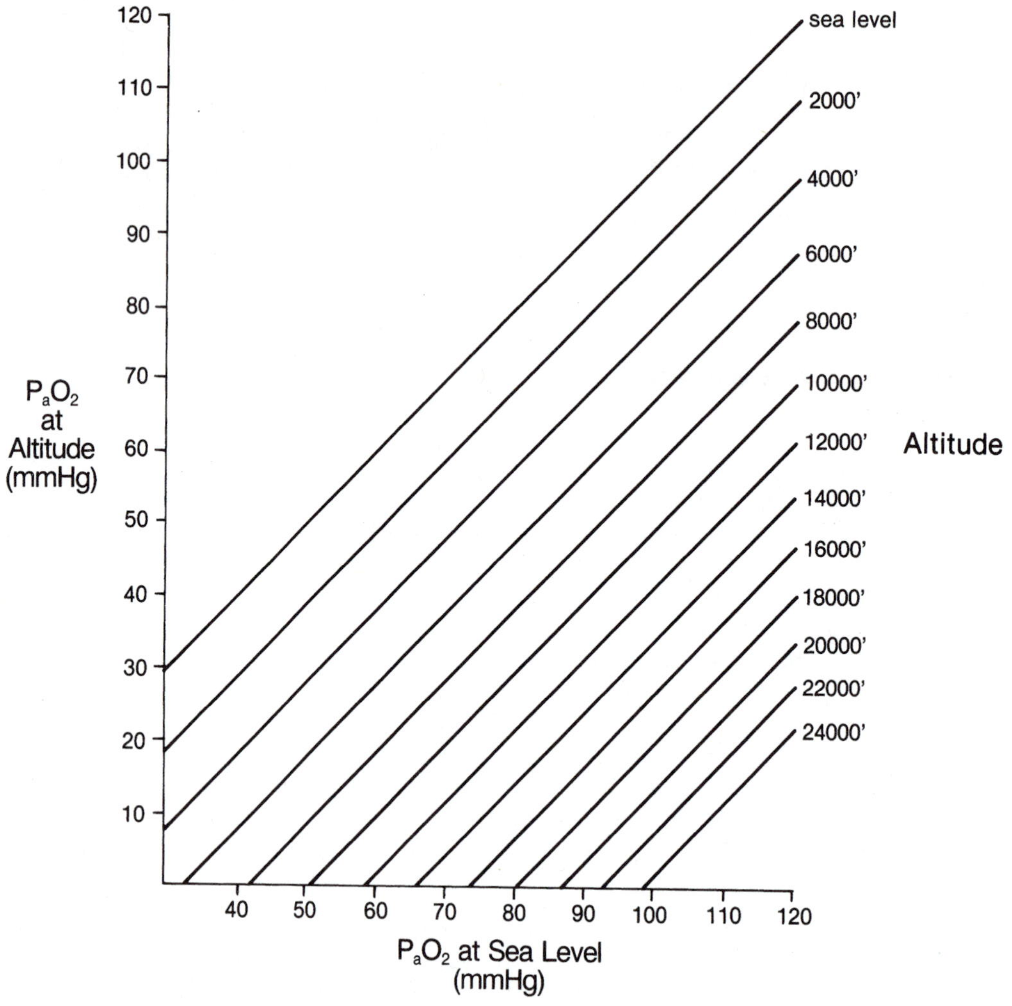

Fig. 22-6 PaO_2 at altitude versus PaO_2 at sea level. Locate the sea level PaO_2 on the x axis and intersect with the cruise altitude (on the diagonal). Read across to find the PaO_2 at altitude (y axis).

reference. For example, when an aircraft enters a bank to the right, the sensation may be initially correctly interpreted. However, after roll-out of the stationary bank to a neutral position, a sensation of rolling into a left bank may be sensed. If uncorrected, apprehension may follow. The best remedy for this effect is to maintain a visual reference to the correct position.

Vestibular stimuli, especially in turbulence with limited or no visual frame of reference, may result in motion sickness, manifested most commonly as nausea or vomiting. This occurs with both patients and flight crews. It can be counteracted with antiemetics such as antihistamines (such as dimenhydrinate 50 mg orally) or phenothiazines (such as prochlorperazine 10 mg orally); however, these may produce sedation and are potentially hazardous in flight. Recently, transdermal scopolamine patches applied behind the ear have been used as an effective prophylactic agent for nausea and vomiting during flight.

Table 22-8 Clinical Manifestations of Trapped Gas Expansion

Trapped Gas Location	Clinical Manifestations
Intestinal lumen	Abdominal pain, distension
Pleural space	Pneumothorax, tension pneumothorax
Subcutaneous	Subcutaneous emphysema
Paranasal sinuses	Facial pain
Middle ear	Ear pain
Dental root	Tooth pain
Blood	Air embolism, decompression sickness
Air splints, antishock trousers	Compartment syndrome, ischemia
IV bottle and tubing	Flow rate increase
Blood pressure cuff	Tourniquet effect
Endotracheal tube cuff	Air leak, hypoventilation

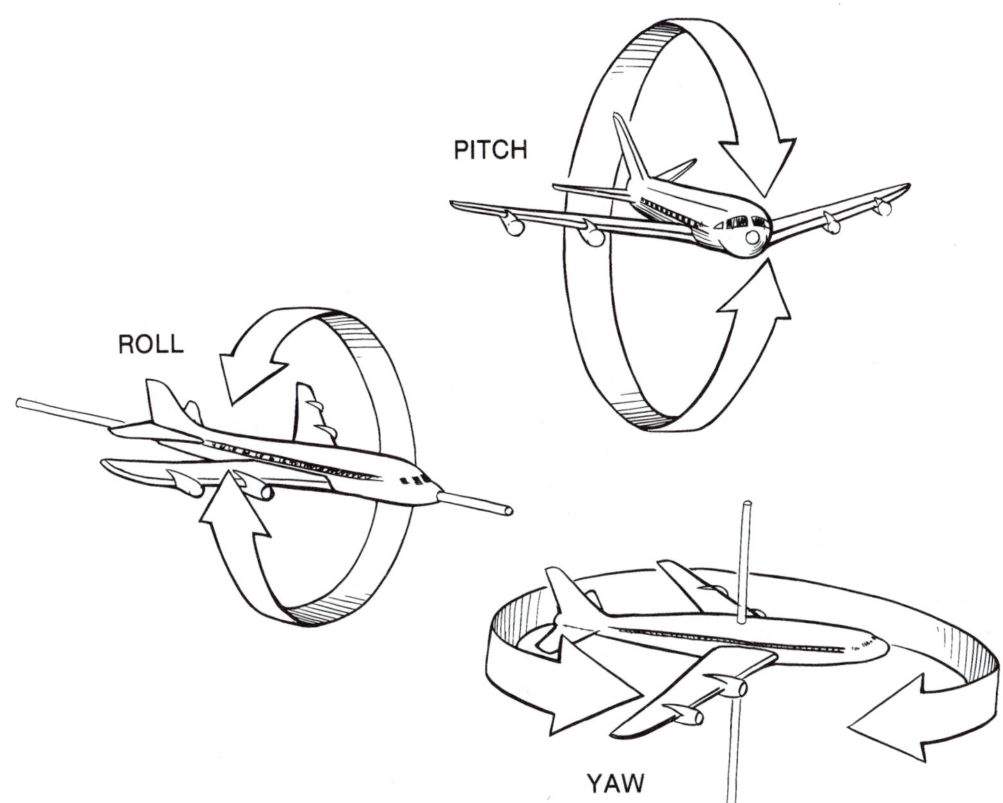

Fig. 22-7 Axes of movement in aviation.

NOISE AND VIBRATION

Noise and vibration are components of all aircraft environments, especially helicopters. The most obvious impact of noise is on communications within the cabin, particularly with the patient, since he or she is least likely to have a headset and access to the aircraft's intercom. In addition, the patient's breath sounds are difficult if not impossible to hear, and thus other means to identify changes in respiratory status, such as pulse oximetry, must be employed.

Headsets are essential for effective communication among flight crew members aboard a helicopter, although they are usually unnecessary aboard larger fixed-wing aircraft. Noise may lead to permanent defects in auditory acuity if exposure is prolonged or recurrent. Veteran pilots commonly demonstrate 10 to 20 dB reductions in high-frequency auditory acuity. Noise and vibration may also lead to stress and fatigue.

Common Aeromedical Transport Problems

PRETRANSPORT PREPARATION

Once the decision to transport a patient by air is made and the appropriate aeromedical service is contacted, preparations must be made to ensure patient safety and comfort and to aid the flight crew in patient care. In a study of the causes of ground delays in a rural interhospital helicopter transport program, it was found that at the time of arrival of the flight team, 31% of patients required minor interventions (insertion of intravenous lines or a nasogastric tube, blood transfusion, bladder catheterization, antishock trouser application) before liftoff, and 33% required major interventions (endotracheal intubation, tube thoracostomy, or central venous access).[55] When no intervention was required, the mean ground time was 31.2 minutes, compared with 57.4 minutes when one or more major interventions was required.

To minimize delays, pretransport preparations should be made for victims of acute trauma. These are listed in Box 22-4.

PATIENT COMFORT

Motion, vibration, noise, temperature variations, dry air, changes in atmospheric pressure, confinement to a limited position or backboard, and fear of flying may all contribute to patient discomfort.

PATIENT MOVEMENT

Patient handling and movement can contribute to morbidity and mortality in unstable patients.[95] All transported

BOX 22-4
PRETRANSPORT PREPARATIONS

SCENE RESPONSE

Secure airway
Stabilization on a rigid spine board with cervical immobilization device, neck rolls, and tape
Two large-bore intravenous lines
Antishock garment applied
Landing zone selected and secured

INTERHOSPITAL TRANSPORT

Secure airway
Stabilization on a rigid spine board with cervical immobilization device, neck rolls, and tape
Two large-bore intravenous lines
Tube thoracostomy for pneumo/hemothorax
Bladder catheterization (if not contraindicated)
Nasogastric catheterization (if not contraindicated)
Lactated Ringer's solution hanging
Typed and cross-matched blood if available
Extremity fractures splinted (traction splinting for femur fractures)
Copies of all available emergency department records and laboratory results, including a description of the mechanism of injury

patients should be adequately secured to the stretcher with safety straps to prevent sudden shifting of position or movement of a secured fracture. During transport from the ground to the aircraft cabin, attempts should be made to limit sudden pitching of the stretcher. Department of Transportation guidelines recommend design of cabin access such that no more than 30 degrees of roll and 45 degrees of pitch may occur to the patient-occupied stretcher during loading.[63] The stretcher, in turn, should be adequately attached to the floor.

Motion sickness in the patient may be treated with an antiemetic such as promethazine (25 mg orally, intravenously, or intramuscularly) or prochlorperazine (5 to 10 mg orally, intravenously, or intramuscularly). Scopolamine disks are useful for prolonged flight and do not require parenteral or oral administration, although their antiemetic effects are not always uniform and may not occur until 4 to 6 hours after application. They may be best used to decrease motion sickness in members of the flight crew.

NOISE

Noise can be avoided with hearing protectors, which are devices similar to headphones but without internal speakers. Inexpensive hearing protectors are available as deformable foam ear plugs. In some cases headphones may be used in an awake patient if the crew desires the patient to be able to communicate on the intercom system.

RESPIRATORY DISTRESS

Patients with respiratory disease or distress should have immediately treatable conditions addressed before lift-off. Endotracheal intubation is essential if airway patency is threatened or if adequate oxygenation cannot be maintained with supplemental oxygen. It is better to err on the side of caution when making a decision about a patient's airway. During flight it is easier to treat restlessness in an intubated patient than airway obstruction or apnea in a nonintubated patient.

Nearly all patients should receive supplemental oxygen. FIO_2 should be increased with increasing cabin altitude (Fig. 22-8) to maintain a stable PO_2. When oxygen saturation monitoring is unavailable and pretransport arterial oxygen content unknown, 100% oxygen may be administered throughout the flight to ensure adequate oxygenation. Patients with chronic lung disease who are prone to hypercapnia may have a deterioration in condition if the hypoxic drive is eliminated. In these patients the least oxygen necessary to maintain saturation above 90% is advisable; this amount may be estimated in advance or calculated from the alveolar air equation. Close in-flight monitoring is essential. Finally, altitude changes may affect endotracheal cuff volume, so cuff pressure must be checked frequently.

CARDIOPULMONARY RESUSCITATION AND CARDIAC DEFIBRILLATION

CPR in an aircraft is difficult. The rescuers must perform several tasks simultaneously while ventilating the lungs or compressing the chest, all in a physically confining space. The crew must be familiar with modifications in technique.[46] As previously mentioned, there should be no concern with airborne defibrillation if all electronic navigational equipment on the aircraft has a common ground, as mandated by the FAA standards. Despite cramped quarters and sensitive electrical equipment, defibrillation can be safely performed in all types of aircraft currently used for emergency transport utilizing standard precautions routinely used during defibrillation on the ground.[25,96]

COMBATIVENESS

Patients may be combative to the point that they pose a threat to the safety of the flight and crew. An uncontrollable patient may cause sudden shifts in aircraft balance or may strike a crew member or important flight instruments or equipment. Such patients should be properly restrained in advance, and there should be no hesitation in sedating them temporarily. If sedation is necessary, a careful neurologic examination documented beforehand is essential. Useful

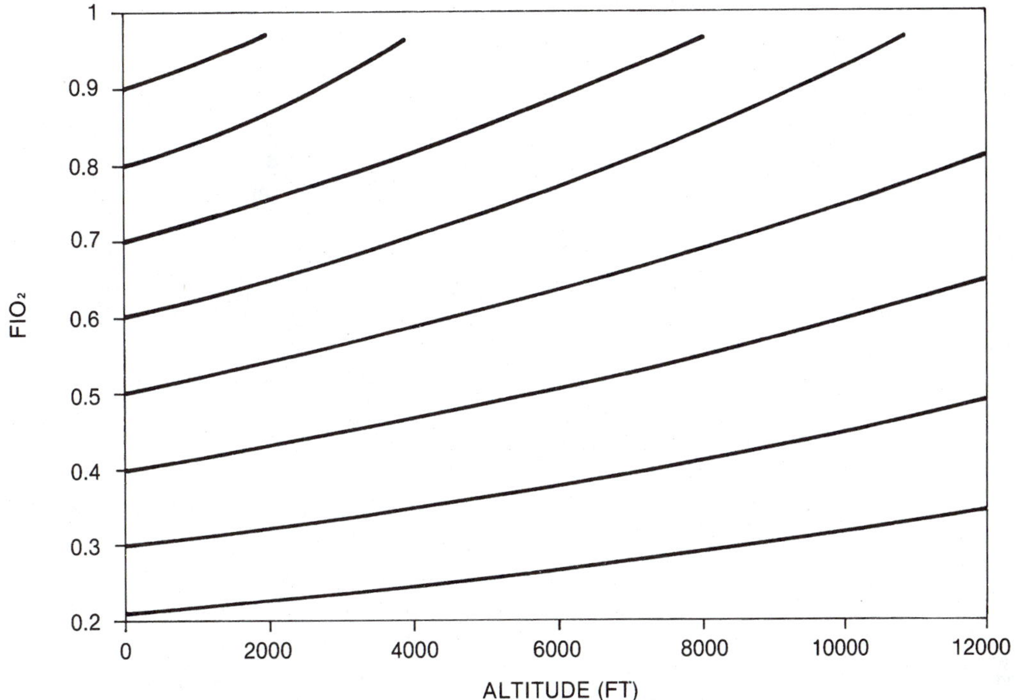

PB	ALT					FIO_2				
760	0	0.21	0.30	0.40	0.50	0.60	0.70	0.80	0.90	1.00
707	2000	0.23	0.32	0.43	0.54	0.65	0.76	0.86	0.97	PP
656	4000	0.25	0.35	0.47	0.59	0.70	0.82	0.94	PP	PP
609	6000	0.27	0.38	0.51	0.63	0.76	0.89	PP	PP	PP
564	8000	0.29	0.41	0.55	0.69	0.83	0.97	PP	PP	PP
523	10000	0.31	0.45	0.60	0.75	0.90	PP	PP	PP	PP
483	12000	0.34	0.49	0.65	0.82	0.98	PP	PP	PP	PP
	A-a:	15	79	150	222	293	364	435	507	578

Calculated from the alveolar air equation under standard temperature and pressure conditions. PP = Positive pressure required, PB = Barometric pressure (mmHg), ALT = altitude (feet), A-a = Alveolar–arterial oxygen gradient (mmHg).
X axis: enroute altitude
Y axis: FIO_2 required to maintain PO_2 = 90 mmHg
To calculate the FIO_2 necessary to maintain PO_2 = 90 mmHg at a specific altitude, choose the value on the Y axis closest to that necessary to maintain PO_2 = 90 mmHg at sea level (altitude = 0 ft) and follow the corresponding line across to the new altitude (X axis). The proper FIO_2 is the Y value corresponding to the new X value.

Fig. 22-8 Fio_2 required to maintain Po_2 at 90 mm Hg (varying with altitude).

agents include diazepam (5 to 20 mg intravenously) or shorter acting agents such as midazolam (2 to 10 mg intravenously or intramuscularly.) Paralyzing agents, such as pancuronium, vecuronium, and succinylcholine, have the advantage of not actually altering the sensorium, but they require airway control with endotracheal intubation.[92] In addition, it is necessary to sedate a patient who is paralyzed to facilitate intubation and transport.

ENDOTRACHEAL INTUBATION

Endotracheal intubation may be difficult to perform while airborne, especially in a confining cabin, and therefore should take place before departure if possible. This is especially true in trauma victims with head injuries and in burn victims who have carbonaceous sputum or hoarseness. Special techniques are available to supplement standard methods of intubation, including a lighted stylet, endotracheal tubes with controllable tips, and digital intubation. Sedation or pharmacologic paralysis may be necessary. As of 1992, 106 aeromedical transport programs in the United States reported using neuromuscular blocking agents; 39 use them to facilitate intubations, and 67 use them once a patient is intubated in order to manage the patient's combativeness and ensure airway patency.[82] Induction of paralysis before intubation in the aeromedical setting is controversial. One study reported a 96.6% success rate using succinylcholine to facilitate intubation, with 3.4% of patients requiring an emergency surgical airway.[67] Besides the need for surgical airway if intubation is unsuccessful, concerns exist about cervical spine manipulation during intubation in the paralyzed patient, unrecognized esophageal intubation in a nonbreathing patient, and the relative contraindications to the use of succinylcholine in certain patients. As shorter acting nondepolarizing paralytic agents (such as mivacurium) are developed, further study of this adjunct to airway and combativeness control in the aeromedical setting will be forthcoming.[52]

In some flight programs, nonphysician flight crew members are taught to perform emergency cricothyrotomies. While occasionally lifesaving, this procedure is often difficult to perform and should be undertaken only as a final method to secure an emergency airway.

THROMBOLYSIS

The air transport of patients with acute myocardial infarction often involves the use of thrombolytic therapy. Because bleeding is a major adverse effect of thrombolytic agents, a recent study was undertaken to determine if air transport resulted in a higher incidence of bleeding complications compared with a similar cohort of patients given thrombolytic drugs who were transported by ground ambulance. The study concluded that helicopter transport of patients with acute myocardial infarction after initiation of thrombolysis is safe acutely and without a clinically significant increase in bleeding complications.[35]

FLIGHT SAFETY

Because aeromedical transport involves medical care delivered in a hostile environment, the patient and crew are at risk of injury or death in the event of a mishap. For that reason, flight crew training and program emphasis must be directed toward safety.

The pilot is ultimately responsible for the safety of the aircraft's occupants and is trained not only to operate the aircraft skillfully and safely, but also to provide necessary safety instructions and guidance to crew members and passengers. Safety practices vary depending on the type of aircraft, but common practices include the following.

Approaching the Aircraft

Helicopters with turning rotor blades must be approached only from the front and sides and only while under pilot observation (Fig. 22-9). The tail rotor must be given wide berth, especially on helicopters with rear doors. It is advisable in such cases to station a crew member in a safe position to direct approaching individuals away from the tail rotor. Shutting down the helicopter's engines completely, when the situation allows, is prudent before patient loading and unloading. Approaching in a crouched position minimizes the risk of contact with the rotor blades should a sudden gust of wind or movement of the aircraft cause them to dip. Loose clothing and debris should be secured (Box 22-5).

Fixed-wing aircraft should be approached with similar precautions regarding propellers. This is especially important in aircraft with access doors in front of the wing and engine nacelles. Engine shutdown on the side of entry enhances safety of loading and unloading.

Safety Belt Use

The use of safety belts (preferably with shoulder harnesses, especially in helicopters) is an important safety measure. However, certain patient care activities, such as endotracheal intubation and CPR, may be impossible to perform with safety belts secured. The design and selection of aircraft and interior configurations should allow maximal access to the patient with the crew members properly restrained. Throughout the flight the crew members and patient should remain restrained as much as possible in smooth air and at all times in rough air. Movement inside the cabin affects aircraft balance. An aircraft loaded near its aft center of gravity limit may be unsafely balanced if a crew member moves to a new position within the cabin. Changes in position should be preceded by consultation with the pilot. A light aircraft is sensitive to turbulent air, and appropriate precautions must be taken to avoid being injured from sudden motion.

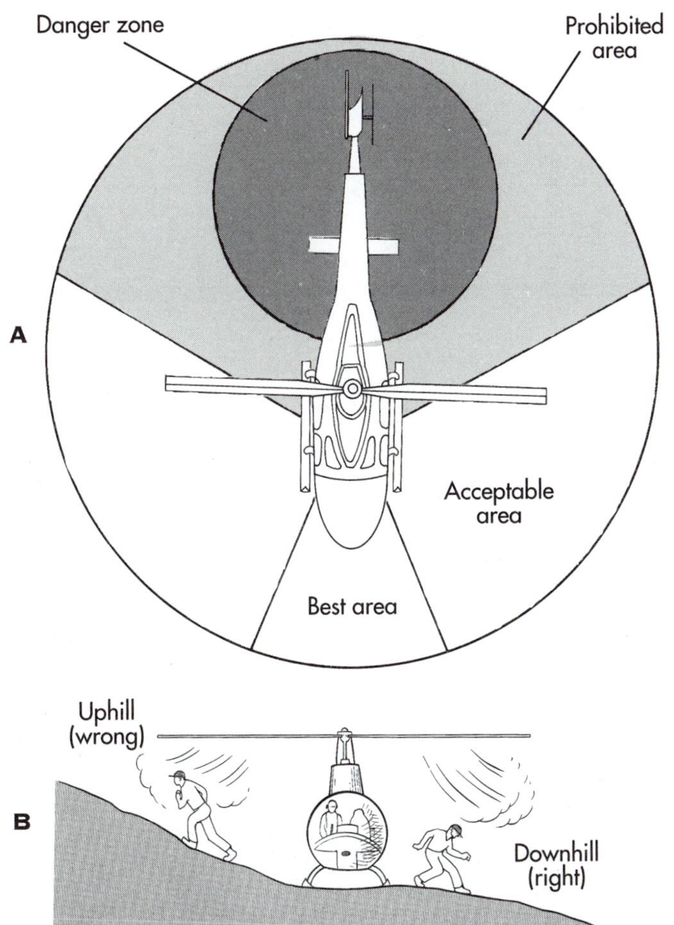

Fig. 22-9 Helicopter safety. **A,** Safe approach zones. **B,** The proper way to approach or depart a helicopter.

Proper Use of Aircraft Equipment

Crew members must be familiar with all aircraft equipment they may be required to operate in flight or in an emergency. This includes all aircraft doors, the fire extinguisher, communications equipment, oxygen equipment, electrical outlets, and so forth. In addition, crew members must be familiar with emergency shutdown procedures. Finally, before take-off, door security must be confirmed by a crew member familiar with the operation of the door.

In-Flight Obstacle Reporting

An extra pair of eyes can be invaluable to a pilot in a busy airspace or on a scene approach complicated by trees and electrical or phone wires. Primarily important in VFR conditions, assistance with obstacle identification can enhance the safety of the mission; however, flight should not occur under conditions in which obstacle reporting by a crew member is essential to safety, since the crew member must then divide attention between patient care and obstacle reporting.

BOX 22-5

HELICOPTER SAFETY

DO:

Approach and depart downhill.
Use crouched position.
Approach after visual contact and approval from pilot.
Await direction of flight crew.
Approach from the front or the sides.
Secure area first of people and then of loose debris.

DON'T:

Approach or depart uphill.
Use tall intravenous poles or other objects.
Use loose sheets or clothing.
Smoke tobacco within 50 feet.
Run near the aircraft.
Drive a vehicle within 30 feet.
Shine headlights or flashlights toward the aircraft.

Ground Coordination and Control

Enthusiastic rescue personnel or curious onlookers may approach the aircraft in a hazardous manner. Flight crew members must be able to communicate with ground units during the landing phase to ensure adequate scene preparation; they may be required to perform crowd control while on the ground. This requires directing individuals away from the rotor blades, propellers, or other hazardous equipment at the scene. If loading or unloading the patient while the rotors or propellers are still turning ("hot loading" or "hot off-loading") is believed to be necessary, special precautions for ground crews, flight crew, and the patient must be undertaken.

Emergency Procedures

Well-rehearsed emergency procedures should be standard operating procedure. These procedures should address in-flight fires, electrical failures, loss of pressurization, engine failure, emergency landing with and without power, precautionary landing away from an airport, and other in-flight emergencies.

Survival

Emergency or precautionary landings away from an airport are followed by a period of time before rescue occurs. Under adverse environmental conditions and with injured victims, survival may depend on specific actions by the crew. Techniques such as communicating distress signals and locator information, providing emergency shelter, using aircraft fuel for fires or signals, tending to the emergency medical needs of victims, and obtaining emergency food

Table 22-9 Major and Primary Causes and Severity of Aeromedical Accidents, 1972 to 1989

	Percentages		
	1972-1985	1987-1988	1989
MAJOR CAUSES			
Weather	30	30	17
Engine failure	18	9	0
Obstacle strike	18	10	33
Control loss	9	20	17
Other	25	40	33
PRIMARY CAUSE			
Pilot error	64	60	83
Mechanical failure	30	30	0
Unknown	6	10	17
ACCIDENT SEVERITY			
Fatal	36	50	67
Injury	28	30	17
Damage only	36	20	17

From Collett HM: *J Air Med Transport* 9(2):12, 1990.

Table 22-10 Effect of Weather on Accident Seriousness

Severity of Accident	Weather-Related	Percentage
Fatal	14/21	67
Injury	3/17	18
Damage only	1/32	3

From Collett HM: *Hosp Aviat* 5(11):15, 1986.

Table 22-11 Environment of Fatal Accidents

Visibility	Accidents	Percent
Day visual meteorologic conditions	3	14
Night visual meteorologic conditions	4	19
Day marginal	4	19
Night marginal	10	48
TOTAL	21	100

From Collett HM: *Hosp Aviat* 5(11):15, 1986.

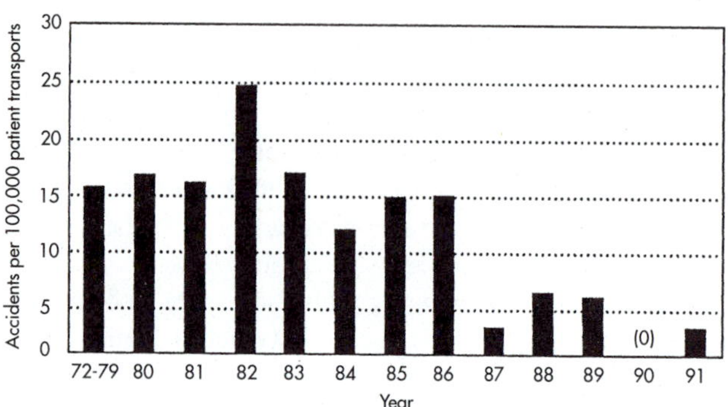

Fig. 22-10 Aeromedical helicopter accident rate, 1972 to 1991. (From Preston N: *J Air Med Transport* 11[2]:14, 1992.)

and water should be addressed in prescribed survival procedures and training.

Aeromedical Accidents

Recent attention has been focused on EMS helicopter accidents. Statistics from 1986 indicate a rotor-wing accident rate estimated to be 17.65 per 100,000 transports with 5.88 fatalities per 100,000 transports.[36] Aviation accident rates are typically reported in relation to flight hours. EMS fatalities therefore amounted to 6.0 per 100,000 flight hours, compared with 3.3 for the helicopter industry in general. However, the EMS rate has been on the decline, with 3.0 accidents per 100,000 transports reported in 1991 (Fig. 22-10).[75,90]

Examining the causes of EMS accidents reveals that 64% to 84% are due to pilot error, approximately 23% to mechanical causes, and 3% to unknown causes.[19] Of accidents caused by pilot error, 67% had adverse weather as a contributing factor (Table 22-9).[17] In all, 67% of fatal weather-related accidents occur at night and 86% of all fatal accidents occur at night or in marginal weather conditions (Table 22-10).[20] This is despite the fact that only 35% to 40% of all EMS helicopter flights occur at night. The most common phase of flight for weather-related accidents was en route (86%), with 14% occurring on departure and none on approach (Table 22-11).

Only 5% of fatal EMS helicopter accidents occur in flights to or from the scene, although such flights account for 24% of EMS helicopter missions.[21] When scene-related accidents occur, they result in fatalities 9% of the time and injuries 35% of the time, suggesting a low-energy impact as compared to an en route crash. Causal factors related to scene accidents include wire and obstacle strikes (70%), loss of control (18%), and mechanical failure (12%). The landing phase is involved in scene-related accidents in 41% of cases, whereas the take-off phase is involved in 59%. Because 40% of scene-related accidents occur at night and approximately 40% of helicopter EMS flights occur at night, scene accidents do not appear more hazardous at night than in the day. Single-engine helicopters have more often been involved in engine failure accidents (77%) than have twin-engine craft (the two types are approximately equal in number in the EMS industry).

Recommendations for enhancing safety include instituting stringent guidelines to limit flights at night or in adverse weather, increasing pilot proficiency training, and reducing pilot fatigue and workload factors. Decisions concerning the appropriateness of air transport regarding utilization and weather should be based on general protocols that are not subject to the emotional turmoil of a medical crisis.[10] The trend in the industry has been toward twin-engine helicopters for increased margin of safety from engine failure accidents. Interestingly an article published in 1989 in the *British Medical Journal* discussed the possibility of using blimps and hot air balloons, which offer some of the advantages of the conventional aeromedical transport with an appreciable improvement in safety.[23]

In addition, for dedicated EMS helicopter flights there is a statistically strong relationship between the ability to fly under IFR and a lower accident rate.[57] In 1992, however, the Association of Air Medical Services published its new voluntary standards for rotor- and fixed-wing aircraft and considered the question of whether all helicopters should be required to have IFR capability. This was not mandated because of the tremendous expense and likely infrequency of use by many programs.[59]

Landing Zones

A suitable landing site for a helicopter should be flat, open, and free of loose objects, with clear landing and take-off routes. The National EMS Pilots Association recommends a landing zone of 60 × 60 square feet for a small helicopter such as a Jet Ranger to 120 × 120 feet for a large helicopter such as a Bell 412.[98]

Dispatch and Communications

The dispatch center is the focal point for communications during aeromedical transport operations. Dispatchers receive incoming requests for service, obtain necessary information relative to the launch decision, coordinate the interaction between essential parties, "scramble" the flight crew, assemble and maintain necessary information regarding destination, weather, local telephone numbers, and frequencies, follow the progress of the flight, input data into the system data base, and communicate with ground EMS units and hospitals. Communication may occur through a combination of methods: land telephone lines into a dispatch switchboard, hospital-EMS net transceiver, discrete frequency transceiver (communications with aircraft), or walkie-talkie radios. Familiarity with the EMS system and EMS communications is essential for successful dispatch.

Flight following is an important part of aeromedical safety and involves tracking the position of the aircraft during a mission by plotting the location according to position reports from the pilot at 10- to 15-minute intervals. If an accident or in-flight emergency occurs, the dispatcher is soon aware and can initiate search and rescue to a precise location, which enhances the chances of survival.

Appropriate Use of Aeromedical Services

Aeromedical transport combines skilled treatment and stabilization capability with rapid access to definitive care, but not without risk, and at high cost ($1 to $2 million per year for a program, or about $2000 per transported patient, which is approximately 400% higher than ground transport).[13] However, the comparative risk of aeromedical transport must be placed in perspective against the risk of patient death from nonreferral or from less timely ground transport with limited medical capability en route.

Although not proven, advanced provider skill levels during prehospital care are considered beneficial, especially in severely ill or injured patients.[50] In rural and wilderness environments, advanced life support (ALS) services may be made more readily available by EMS helicopters. This is especially true in areas that are difficult or impossible to reach by ground.

The speed of access to definitive care is another consideration in choosing the mode of transport. In isolated rural or wilderness locations the helicopter may be the only means of expedient access. Prolonged victim extrication allows time for a helicopter to arrive at the scene, decreasing total transport time and thereby increasing the advantage of helicopter transport.

Another factor to be considered is patient comfort. This is especially evident on long transports and over rough roads. Although a helicopter moves in three dimensions, fore and aft acceleration is usually steady, without the starting and stopping motions present during ground transport. However, helicopters typically travel within 3000 feet of the ground's surface and are more subject to turbulence than are high-flying fixed-wing aircraft, the most comfortable method of long-distance transport.

Whether aeromedical transport reduces mortality when compared with ground transport has not been determined definitively. An uncontrolled national multicenter study of trauma patients transported by helicopter showed a 21% reduction in mortality from that expected based on predictions from the Trauma Score–Injury Severity Score (TRISS) methodology and national normative trauma outcome data.[8]

A similar study using the TRISS methodology comparing actual mortality with helicopter versus ground transport showed a 52% reduction from expected mortality when patients were transported by air, versus no reduction in expected mortality when transport occurred by ground.[7]

Another study using TRISS methodology found a benefit of aeromedical transport only in patients with severe trauma (a probability of survival less than 90%).[11]

In September 1990 the Association of Air Medical Services (AAMS) issued a position paper on the appropriate use of emergency air medical services. In January 1992 these recommendations were accepted by the California Medicaid provider as reasonable criteria for the use of air medical transport. In a study period during 1992 and 1993, 558 consecutive patient transports were reviewed and 98% had met at least one of the AAMS appropriate use criteria.[72]

The risk of aeromedical transport can be placed in perspective if the overall risk of death using ground transport, estimated from the trauma score, is compared with the risk when patients are transported by air. Assuming a reduction in risk of between 21% and 52% when transport is by air, the additional risk of death from crashes (6 per 100,000 transports, or 0.006 per transport) is negligible in comparison to the benefits. This is probably true, however, only for patients with moderate to severe, but nonmortal, injuries (that is, trauma scores between 5 and 14). Those having minor injuries, with near 100% likelihood of survival, are unlikely to gain additional benefit; those having mortal injuries, with little hope of survival, are unlikely to be saved by any means attempted or employed.

The decision to transport a patient by air requires judgment and a realistic appraisal of the risks. A patient should be transported by air only if he or she is so ill that transport is necessary; if ground transport is unavailable, delayed, or unable to reach the patient; or if aeromedical transport would reduce the risk of death by permitting more rapid access to definitive care, providing greater medical skill en route, or both.

SUMMARY

It has been estimated that since aircraft took to the sky to assist in the emergency transport of the sick and injured, more than 1 million patients have been transported over 100 million miles. With a conservative estimate of mortality reduction of even 10%, close to 100,000 patients may owe their lives to the speed and skill provided by aeromedical transport teams.[48]

REFERENCES

1. Abraham E, Lee G, Morgan MT: Conjunctival oxygen tension monitoring during helicopter transport of critically ill patients, *Ann Emerg Med* 15:782, 1986.
2. American Academy of Pediatrics: Emergency drug dosages for infants and children and naloxone use in newborns: clarification, *Pediatrics* 83(5):803, 1989.
3. Apgar V: A proposal for new method of evaluation of the newborn infant, *Anesth Analg* 32:260, 1953.
4. Bagnoud B et al: *Mountain rescue today, colour atlas of mountain medicine,* London, 1991, Wolfe.
5. Baxt WG: Is there a role for flight physicians on EMS rotorcraft? *Trauma Quarterly* 39, May 1985.
6. Baxt WG, Moody P: The impact of a rotocraft aeromedical emergency care service on trauma mortality, *JAMA* 249:3047, 1983.
7. Baxt WG, Moody P: The impact of a physician as part of the aeromedical prehospital team in patients with blunt trauma, *JAMA* 257:3246, 1987.
8. Baxt WG et al: Hospital-based rotocraft aeromedical emergency care services and trauma mortality: a multicenter study, *Ann Emerg Med* 14:859, 1985.
9. Black RE et al: Air transport of pediatric emergency cases, *N Engl J Med* 207:1465, 1982.
10. Blue B: Aeromedical transport, *J Fam Pract* 36(3):269, 1993.
11. Boyd CR, Corse KM, Campbell RC: Emergency interhospital transport of the major trauma patient: air versus ground, *J Trauma* 29(6):789, 1989.
12. Branson RD et al: Utilization of mechanical ventilators in hospital based air ambulance programs, *Hosp Aviat* 5(1):6, 1986.
13. Burney RE, Fischer RP: Ground versus air transport of trauma victims: medical and logistical considerations, *Ann Emerg Med* 15:1491, 1986.
14. Burney RE et al: Comparison of aeromedical crew performance by patient severity and outcome, *Ann Emerg Med* 21(4):375, 1992.
15. Cady G: 1993 program survey, *Air Med J* September, 1993.
16. Cauthorne CV, Fedorowicz RJ: Sociological impacts of work/rest schedules on pilots, and their perceptions of performance, *Hosp Aviat* 5(1):14, 1986.
17. Collett HM: Scene-related accidents, *Hosp Aviat* 5(12):17, 1986.
18. Collett HM: Weather related accidents, *Hosp Aviat* 5(11):15, 1986.
19. Collett HM: Mechanical failure accidents, *Hosp Aviat* 6(1):11, 1987.
20. Collett, HM: Year in review, *Hosp Aviat* (6)1:3, 1987.
21. Collett HM: 1989 accident review, *J Air Med Transport* 9(2):12, 1990.
22. Collins RL et al: *Flying 1985 annual & buyers guide,* New York, 1985, Ziff-Davis.
23. Cottrell JJ, Garrard C: Emergency transport by aeromedical blimp, *Br Med J* 298(6677):869, 1989.
24. Dedrick D et al: *Airborne defibrillation study* (abstract), Washington, DC, 1986, Seventh Annual ASHBEAMS Scientific Assembly.
25. Defibrillation safety in emergency helicopter transport, *Ann Emerg Med* 18(1):69, 1989.
26. Del Vecchio RJ: *Physiologic aspects of flight,* Oakdale, NY, 1977, Dowling College Press.
27. Dispatch and communications, *Hosp Aviat* 6(1):5, 1987.
28. Dürrer B: Practical problems of fixation and evacuation in mountain rescue. Proceedings of the International Congress of Mountain Medicine, Crans, Montana, 1991.
29. Dürrer B: REGA winch rescues 1983 and 1984. Proceedings of the International Aeromedical Evacuation Congress, 1985, Zurich, p 108.
30. Dürrer B, Hassler R, Mosimann U: *Mountaineering accidents in the Swiss Alps and rescue activities of the Swiss Alpine Club, 1992.*
31. Ehrenwerth J, Sonja S, Hackel A: Transport of critically ill adults, *Crit Care Med* 14:543, 1986.
32. Federal Aviation Administration, Department of Transportation: *Federal aviation regulations.* In FAR-AIM 1986, Seattle, 1986, ASA.
33. Fifth annual aircrew survey, *Hosp Aviat* 5(10):19, 1986.
34. Fischer RP et al: Urban helicopter response to the scene of injury, *J Trauma* 24:946, 1984.
35. Fromom RE et al: Bleeding complications following initiation of thrombolytic therapy for acute myocardial infarction: a comparison of helicopter-transported and nontransported patients, *Ann Emerg Med* 20(8):1991.
36. Golby SB: Critical care, *AOPA Pilot* 30:39, 1987.
37. Golby SB: Dust off, *AOPA Pilot* 30:46, 1987.
38. Gore JM et al: Evaluation of an emergency cardiac transport system, *Ann Emerg Med* 12:675, 1983.
39. Green B: The aeromedical programs of West Germany, *Hosp Aviat* 6(3):6, 1987.
40. Guiford FR, Soboroff BJ: Air evacuation, *J Aviat Med* 18(6):601, 1947.

41. Hamman BL et al: Helicopter transport of trauma victims: does a physician make a difference? *J Trauma* 31(4):490, 1991.
42. Harless KW et al: Civilian ground and air transport of adults with acute respiratory failure, *JAMA* 240:361, 1978.
43. Harris BH: Performance of aeromedical crew members: training or experience? *Am J Emerg Med* 4:409, 1986.
44. Harris BH: Defibrillation in helicopters, *Ann Emerg Med* 12:517, 1983.
45. Harris BH, Orr RE, Boles ET: Aeromedical transportation for infants and children, *J Pediatr Surg* 10:719, 1975.
46. Hensleigh C, Yelser F: Helicopter megacode, *J Aeromed Health Care* 18:1984.
47. High altitude operations, *Hosp Aviat* June 1984, p 4.
48. Hoffman L: Worth their weight in gold, *EMN,* Jan 1992.
49. Homer: *The Iliad,* Middlesex, Eng, 1982, Penguin Books (translated by EV Rieu).
50. Jacobs LM et al: Prehospital advanced life support: benefits in trauma, *J Trauma* 24:8, 1984.
51. Kaplan L, Walsh D, Burney RE: Emergency aeromedical transport of patients with acute myocardial infarction, *Ann Emerg Med* 16:55, 1987.
52. Kern L, Komon H: An evaluation of Mivacurium chloride: can it be effective in the prehospital setting? (abstract), *Air Med J* 12(9):1993.
53. Larrey JD: *Memorires de chirurgie militaire et campagnes,* Paris, 1812, J Smith.
54. Lee G: *Flight nursing: principles and practice*, St Louis, 1991, Mosby.
55. Leicht MJ et al: Rural interhospital helicopter transport of motor vehicle trauma victims: causes for delays and recommendations, *Ann Emerg Med* 15:450, 1986.
56. Liskiewicz WJ: An evaluation of the Royal Air Force helicopter search and rescue services in Britain with reference to Royal Air Force Valley 1980-1989, *J R Soc Med* 85f(12):727, 1992.
57. Low R et al: Factors associated with accidents involving EMS helicopters, *Air Med J* 9:35, 1993.
58. Low RB, Martin D: Accuracy of blood pressure measurements made aboard helicopters, *Ann Emerg Med* 16:510, 1987.
59. Lumpe D: Association of air medical services publishes new voluntary standards, *JEMS* 10:28, 1992.
60. MacDonald RC, Banks JG, Ledingham I: Transportation of the injured, *Injury* 12(3):225, 1979.
61. Mayer TA, Walker ML: Severity of illness and injury in pediatric air transport, *Ann Emerg Med* 13:108, 1984.
62. Mckenny S: Aeromedical evolution, *AMJ*, May-June 1986, p 22.
63. McNeil EL: *Airborne care of the ill and injured,* New York, 1983, Springer-Verlag.
64. Merrill N, Executive Director, Association of Air Medical Services: Personal communication, Dec 1993.
65. Mitchell JT: Stress: the history, status and future of critical incident stress debriefings, *JEMS* 11:47, 1988.
66. Mitchell JT: Stress: development and functions of a critical incident stress debriefing team, *JEMS* 12:43, 1988.
67. Murphy-Macabobby M et al: Neuromuscular blockade in aeromedical airway management, *Ann Emerg Med* 21(6):1992.
68. National Conference on Cardiopulmonary Resuscitation and Emergency Cardiac Care: Standards and guidelines for cardiopulmonary resuscitation (CPR) and emergency cardiac care (ECC), *JAMA* 255:2905, 1986.
69. National EMS Pilot's Association: Single pilot IFR survey, *Hosp Aviat* 5(6):17, 1986.
70. Neel S: Army aeromedical evacuation procedures in Vietnam, *JAMA* 204(4):309, 1968.
71. 1987 hospital aviation directory, *Hosp Aviat* 6(4):8, 1987.
72. O'Malley R, Watson-Hopkins M: Monitoring the appropriateness of air medical transports, *Air Med J* 9:332, 1993.
73. *Pediatric drug chart,* ed 3, Oregon, 1993, InforMed.
74. Poulton TJ, Kisicki PA: Physiologic monitoring during civilian air medical transport, *Aviat Space Environ Med* 58:367, 1987.
75. Preston N: 1991 air medical accident rates, *J Air Med Transport* 11(2):14, 1992.
76. Rhee KJ et al: Is the flight physician needed for helicopter emergency medical services? *Ann Emerg Med* 15:174, 1986.
77. Rohrer W et al: *Swiss air rescue medical statistics 1990/1991.*
78. Rosen P et al: Prehospital care: an integrated concept of emergency medicine, *Top Emerg Med* 1(4):19, 1980.
79. Sandmel S, editor: *The new English Bible,* Luke 10:33-35.
80. Saunders CE: Use of transthoracic electrical bioimpedance in assessing thoracic fluid status in emergency department patients, *JAMA* 257:1899, 1987.
81. Saunders CE, Glass E: Noninvasive cardiac output measurement during airborne critical care transport using impedance cardiography (abstract), Washington, DC, 1986, Seventh Annual ASHBEAMS Scientific Assembly.
82. Sayre MR, Weisgerber I: The use of neuromuscular blocking agents by air medical services, *J Air Med Transport,* Jan 1992.
83. Secretary of the Air Force: *Aeromedical evacuation,* Background Information Rep No 68-3, US Air Force Office of Information, 1968.
84. Shea D: The role of nurses and paramedics on EMS rotorcraft, *Trauma Q,* May 1985, p 33.
85. Shufflebarger C, Townsend R: Letter to the editor, *JAMA* 258:2378, 1987.
86. Shufflebarger C et al: Transconjunctival oxygen monitoring as a predictor of hypoxemia during helicopter transport, *Am J Emerg Med* 4:501, 1986.
87. Snow N, Hull C, Severns, J: Physican presence on a helicopter emergency medical service: necessary or desirable? *Aviat Space Environ Med,* 57:1176, 1986.
88. Sredl DM: *Airborne patient care management: a multidisciplinary approach,* St Louis, Mo, 1983, Medical Research Associates.
89. Stanley L, Saunders CE: Stress in aeromedical transport crews: objective measurement in-flight and associated factors (abstract), Milwaukee, Wis, 1987 Eighth Annual ASHBEAMS/NFNA Conference.
90. Steinbrunn RN: Preventing and controlling inadvertent IFR, *Air Med J* 9:315, 1993.
91. Stewart RD: Prehospital care of trauma, *Trauma Q,* May 1985, p 1.
92. Syverud SA et al: Prehospital use of neuromuscular blocking agents in a helicopter ambulance program, *Ann Emerg Med* 16:500, 1987.
93. Thomas F, Clemmer TP, Orme JF: A survey of advanced life support procedures being performed by physicians and nurses used on hospital aeromedical evacuation services, *Aviat Space Environ Med* 56:1213, 1985.
94. US Department of Transportation, National Highway Traffic Safety Administration; American Medical Association Commission on Emergency Medical Services: *Air ambulance guidelines, 1981.*
95. Waddell G et al: Effects of ambulance transport in critically ill patients, *Br Med J* 1:386, 1975.
96. Waggoner RR et al: Airborne defibrillation . . . the sequel, *J Air Med Transport,* Feb 1991.
97. Wegman F et al: Sixteen years with the Danish search and rescue helicopter service, *Aviat Space Environ Med* 61(5):436, 1990.
98. Whitman J: *Preparing a landing zone,* NEMSPA, Sept 1991.

23 WILDERNESS EMERGENCY MEDICAL SERVICES AND RESPONSE SYSTEMS

Franklin R. Hubbell

Sequence of events in backcountry rescue
Team organization and function
Training of wilderness emergency medical technicians

When an accident or medical crisis of any kind occurs in the wilderness or backcountry, away from access to immediate assistance, a chain of events begins to occur that will hopefully lead to a successful rescue. The chain of events and how it unfolds vary tremendously depending on the part of the world in which the critical events occur. At the current time a national or international standard for wilderness emergency medical services and response does not exist. Instead, the configurations of personnel and policies reflect local and national influences (Box 23-1).

The American Alpine Club's Safety Committee gathers, reviews, and analyzes mountaineering accidents that have occurred throughout North America and publishes the annual report *Accidents in North American Mountaineering*. The data collected for that report illustrate not only the necessary diversity of wilderness and mountain rescues, but also some of the current limitations. The following is a summary of data from *Accidents in North American Mountaineering*.

It should be noted that many of the recommendations in Box 23-2 still need considerable development and may be considered controversial. In particular, specialized wilderness medical training with standardized protocols has yet to be developed. This issue is currently being addressed specifically by a Wilderness Medicine Task Group organized through the American Society for Testing and Materials (ASTM), an international consensus standard-setting body.

Wilderness emergency medicine is a combination of emergency medical training and outdoor-wilderness skills. Blending of these elements is essential but is not necessarily natural or easy. The art and science of prehospital emergency medicine began over 20 years ago, and it has evolved into a highly regimented and well-defined subspecialty of emergency medicine. Thousands of individuals have been trained as first responders, EMTs, and paramedics, and a well-organized emergency medical services (EMS) system exists nationwide. This statement is somewhat misleading because each state has its own EMS system and standards. A truly national uniform standard does not exist. However, each state has a well-organized EMS system designed to respond rapidly to crises and provide appropriate emergency care.

Training programs that focus on rapid response, rapid intervention, and rapid transport to advanced care facilities exist nationwide. Prehospital personnel are trained to work within the framework of the "golden hour," when time is precious and critical actions save lives. This is the nationally accepted urban standard to which all EMS personnel are currently trained. While this standard is appropriate for evaluating and training urban EMS personnel and response systems, it is not appropriate for rural, wilderness, mountain, or "extended" EMS personnel and response systems. In these situations patient care is measured in hours and days rather than minutes.

Traditional EMS recognizes rapid notification (the 911 system), dispatch, response, assessment, thorough prehospital care, transport, evaluation, and critical care in a hospital emergency department. Rapidity is the most critical factor that distinguishes urban emergency medical care from wilderness emergency medical care. But time is not the only difference. Wilderness emergency medicine is governed by a complex set of medical skills and protocols, equipment requirements, and other specialized skills, including different attitudes or psychologic requirements, which call for premeditated action. A productive mental attitude comes from the individual's training, expertise, and experience in the outdoors.

In mountain and wilderness outdoor activities, including mountain and wilderness rescue, haste makes waste. Ill-applied haste may in certain circumstances cost lives. As a re-

BOX 23-1

MOUNTAIN SEARCH AND RESCUE FACTORS IN THE UNITED STATES

1. Search and rescue is the responsibility of national parks, state parks, county sheriffs, or state conservation officers, depending upon the state or park.
2. The vast majority of backcountry and technical rescues are carried out by volunteer rescue groups.
3. Ninety percent of all rescues are carryouts on foot rather than airlifts by helicopter or fixed-wing aircraft.
4. At least 95% of rescues are performed without physicians present, instead using the skills of first responders, emergency medical technicians (EMTs), and paramedics, who may or may not be trained in wilderness medicine and rescue techniques.
5. Only two of the major climbing areas, Yosemite and Grand Teton National Parks, use helicopters extensively.
6. Only Denali National Park uses fixed-wing aircraft extensively and helicopters occasionally.
7. Only three national parks have rangers who are trained specifically for technical rescue, advanced medical support, and helicopter operations. These are Yosemite, Grand Teton, and Mt. Rainier National Parks.
8. National and state parks are not mandated with a "duty to rescue." However, virtually all parks provide rescue service. Most parks have a budget for these activities.
9. Many roadside climbing areas and popular backcountry areas are not within the jurisdictions of parks. Technical and backcountry rescues carried out at these locations are often performed by local rescue squads, fire departments, and ambulance units, usually without the benefit of specialized training or technical backcountry skills.

sult, wilderness and mountain rescue teams must achieve a balance between the urgency of the situation and the necessity to be fully prepared and aware of the incident. This is not an easy or natural blend of emotions and skills. On one hand, there are trained EMS professionals who are always primed and ready to go and who feel comfortable moving rapidly, acting quickly, and thinking on their feet. On the other hand, there are the skilled outdoorspersons who are always eager and willing to get into the backcountry but who understand the necessity of thorough preparedness. This philosophy involves making sure that each individual is prepared. The team must be organized and know where it is going, what injuries to anticipate, and how weather will affect the rescue. This is a difficult task that requires recognition of the differences between short-term and long-term care during a rescue, so that a safe and successful extended care rescue can be achieved.

Mountain rescue, wilderness rescue, rural rescue, whitewater rescue, expedition medicine, disaster medicine, air-sea rescue, search and rescue, cave rescue, and avalanche rescue are all likely to be extended rescues. Once rescue personnel reach a victim, they will most likely be with the person for hours, providing extended emergency care. The terms "extended rescue" and "extended emergency care" refer to rescue efforts that are outside the first hour.

Sequence of Events in Backcountry Rescue

The principles and standards of a wilderness or mountain rescue (extended care rescue), including organization, specialized skills and knowledge, and essential components

BOX 23-2

RESCUE PERSONNEL AND TRAINING IN THE UNITED STATES

1. Most technical rescue personnel in the United States are climbers or skiers who have added rescue techniques and medical training to their skills.
2. There are about 600,000 emergency medical technicians (EMTs) in the United States.
3. There are a growing number of wilderness EMTs trained in the skills of extended patient care in the backcountry environment.
4. Key skill elements of medical training for wilderness medical and rescue training include the following.
   a. Thorough patient assessment skills and monitoring
   b. Technical skills and the authority to perform the following:
      (1) Airway management, to include endotracheal intubation.
      (2) Shock management to include IV therapy
      (3) Use of the military antishock trousers (MAST) garment
      (4) Oxygen administration
      (5) Use of appropriate medications
         (a) Epinephrine for anaphylactic reactions
         (b) Antibiotics for compound fractures
         (c) Acetazolamide, nifedipine, and furosemide for acute high-altitude problems
         (d) Pain medications for musculoskeletal trauma
      (6) Field rewarming techniques
      (7) Field reduction of fracture-dislocations
   c. Patient packaging and transportation skills
5. Key skill elements of technical training for rescue personnel in the United States include the following:
   a. Appropriate climbing skills for terrain (rock, ice, snow, glacier)
   b. Radio communications skills and protocols
   c. Helicopter and fixed-wing protocols

of the team, can best be illustrated by reviewing the sequence of events during a typical backcountry rescue in North America (Box 23-3).

OCCURRENCE OF THE CRITICAL EVENT

The critical event occurs when an individual participating in an activity away from immediate help is suddenly stricken by injury or illness. The key factor is immobilization. The fact that the injured or ill person cannot self-evacuate or move to seek shelter or stay warm results in the need for a rescue. Once the victim or others in the party realize this, the need to seek help becomes obvious.

MAKING THE DECISION TO GET HELP

Before anyone leaves to seek assistance, the victim's companions should assess the victim by performing a physical examination, record vital signs, determine the level of consciousness, provide appropriate emergency care, and move the victim into protective shelter. Patient information should be summarized in a note that accompanies the individual(s) going for help. A map depicting the exact location and a list of the other members in the party, with information on how well prepared they are to endure the environmental conditions, should be included. The individual(s) going for help should carry appropriate provisions. To prepare adequately generally takes 30 minutes to 1 hour. However, thorough preparation rarely occurs. Often, someone suddenly yells "I'll get help" and disappears, running down the trail with sparse vital knowledge.

With the improvements and availability of communications technology, such as cellular phones and global positioning systems, backcountry adventurers may have more rapid access to the EMS system from the mountains. Whether this will increase the number of inappropriate callouts remains to be determined.

BOX 23-3

SEQUENCE OF EVENTS IN BACKCOUNTRY RESCUE

1. The critical event occurs: an injury or illness that requires assistance and evacuation.
2. A decision is made to "get help" and someone goes for help.
3. The emergency medical system is notified of the emergency.
4. The emergency medical system is activated, or "dispatched."
5. Eventually the "extended rescue team" is notified and mobilized.
6. The rescue team assembles and organizes, then leaves the trailhead (may be preceded by a "hasty team").
7. The team locates the victim.
8. The team provides appropriate "extended emergency care."
9. The team organizes and evacuates the patient to the appropriate facility.
10. The team returns to base, is debriefed, and prepares for the next rescue.

NOTIFYING THE EMERGENCY MEDICAL SYSTEM

Eventually the messenger notifies someone in authority that an emergency has occurred and that help is needed. Usually, the request is made to a central 911 system. If no central service is available, a local dispatch agency is notified. The agency notifies the closest emergency medical service, which can be a rescue squad, ambulance corps, fire department, or first response team.

ACTIVATING THE EMERGENCY MEDICAL SYSTEM

Notification of an emergency usually occurs via pagers that are worn by individual members. An alert tone is followed by an oral message describing the emergency, its location, and the type of response required.

At this point a wide variety of events can occur, involving agencies within and outside the EMS system. Even in areas of the United States with well-organized extended care rescue teams, the team may be notified last. Ideally they should be notified immediately, but all too often this is not the case. Instead, local agency responders are notified and rush around trying to determine how quickly they can reach the patient.

The first and foremost principle in extended care rescues is that *haste makes waste and costs lives.* As was mentioned earlier, this is the point where the worlds of EMS and extended rescue or care meet and often clash. Eventually the authorities realize that the situation demands the specialized skills of the extended care or technical rescue team.

NOTIFYING AND MOBILIZING THE EXTENDED RESCUE TEAM

The first step is to notify team members. In many parts of the United States, organized and coordinated extended rescue teams do not exist, so a "team" is created of relatively untrained volunteers willing to hike in and assist in the rescue effort. The task of further organizing and coordinating the rescue effort generally falls onto the shoulders of a local rescue squad, fire service, or police department, which may or may not be willing and prepared to manage and execute an extended or technical rescue.

In the parts of the United States where backcountry use is common and backcountry accidents occur with regularity, extended care rescue teams have generally evolved from local EMS teams with skilled outdoor enthusiasts. Some teams offering local search and rescue capabilities may be coordinated locally (such as the Appalachian Mountain Club, SOLO, and Mountain Rescue Service in the White Mountains of New Hampshire); other teams may be part of a nationwide system responding to incidents throughout the country and be coordinated on a regional or national level (such as the National Cave Rescue Commission). Coordination of extended care rescue teams may also come under the jurisdiction of a law enforcement body, such as state conservation officers (for example, New Hampshire Fish & Game), sheriff's department (for example, the Los Angeles County Sheriff in California), or a statewide coordinating system (for example, the Pennsylvania Search and Rescue Council or the Virginia Search and Rescue Council). Organized teams can be quite sophisticated in their dispatching function so that all members can be notified simultaneously, or they may use a more "low-tech" telephone tree to notify members.

ASSEMBLING AND ORGANIZING THE RESCUE TEAM

Once members are notified, they assemble at a common location (rescue station) to organize the rescue effort. The first task is to define the type of rescue in order to establish equipment needs. Estimating the time it will take to effect the rescue and assessing the need for other agency involvement and assistance are also primary tasks. The questions to be answered and the variables may include the following:

1. Time of day: will this be a night rescue?
2. Weather: what are the current weather conditions at the rescue location and what is the forecast?
3. When did the accident occur?
4. What are the supposed injuries?
5. How many victims are there?
6. How many people are in the victim's party?
7. How well prepared are they?
8. Does anyone in the party have medical expertise?
9. Do we know the exact location, or is this a search and rescue?
10. Is a "hasty team" needed? Has it left for the scene yet?
11. Is each of the team members prepared? Does each have personal equipment, a bivouac kit, head lamp, food, and water?
12. Is each member trained and skilled in this particular type of rescue?
13. Who is on the medical team?
14. Who is on the evacuation team?
15. Is the team equipment organized and divided up?
16. How urgent is the situation? Is a helicopter required? Is one available?
17. Are the weather conditions appropriate for an air rescue?
18. Will multiple agencies be involved? If so, are radio frequencies coordinated?

Once the team is assembled and all pertinent issues have been addressed satisfactorily, the team is transported to the trailhead (launch point) to begin the search.

It is common practice for a hasty team to start out ahead of the main team. Once the hasty team has enough information to locate the patient, they travel as light as possible, with only enough gear to ensure their own safety and the capacity to manage the victim's primary injuries. The point is to get a small team to the patient as quickly as is reasonably possible in order to deliver primary care and apprise the rest of the team of the victim's condition, equipment needs, and environmental concerns.

LOCATING THE VICTIM

How much time it takes to locate the victim varies tremendously. This depends on distance, terrain, weather conditions, mode of transportation, and whether the exact location of the victim is known. A general rule of thumb for a team responding on foot is that it will take 1 hour for each mile through the backcountry. If a search is involved, all bets are off. A search and rescue effort can involve many agencies, individuals, and days (see Chapter 21).

PROVIDING APPROPRIATE "EXTENDED EMERGENCY CARE"

Once the patient is located, appropriate medical care can be provided. The rescue team should ensure its own safety; wet clothes should be replaced with warm dry clothing and members should check for emerging problems within their group. While the medical team cares for the patient, the evacuation team should concern itself with securing shelter, preparing warm drinks, establishing and maintaining communications, and planning and organizing the evacuation.

Expedition members with the patient should be attended to. Often they have been affected by the environment while waiting for the rescue team to arrive. They may need to be assessed and treated for hypothermia, frostbite, heatstroke, heat exhaustion, and dehydration.

Regardless of what has transpired before the medical team has arrived, a complete patient assessment is essential. It cannot be assumed that all the injuries have been uncovered or that the medical condition(s) has been managed properly (Box 23-4).

In the extended care environment it is necessary to monitor the patient for any *changing* conditions that would indicate an underlying problem requiring attention. Awareness of environmental emergencies is particularly important, with constant care to prevent hypothermia, frostbite, heatstroke, heat exhaustion, and dehydration. To do this, it is necessary to monitor and the patient and write a new SOAP note at least every 15 minutes:

BOX 23-4

PATIENT ASSESSMENT

PRIMARY SURVEY: LOCATING AND TREATING LIFE-THREATENING PROBLEMS

A—Airway Management

Is the airway open?
Is the airway going to *stay* open?

B—Breathing

Is air moving in and out?
Is the airway quiet or silent?
Is breathing effortless?
Is the respiratory system intact?
Is breathing adequate to support life?

C—Circulation

Is there a pulse?
Is bleeding well controlled?
Is capillary refill normal (less than 2 sec)?
Is circulation adequate to support life?

D—Disability

Conscious versus unconscious
Level of consciousness—
  Awake/Verbal/Painful/Unconscious (AVPU) or Glasgow Coma Scale
Cervical spine stabilization

E—Environment

Internal versus external
Is the patient warm and dry?
Protected from the cold ground
Protected from the elements

SECONDARY SURVEY: WHAT'S WRONG AND HOW SERIOUS IS IT?

Vital signs: Indicate the condition of the patient
  RR—respiratory rate and effort
  PR—pulse rate and character
  BP—blood pressure (systolic/diastolic)
  LOC—level of consciousness (AVPU or Glasgow Coma Scale)
  TP—tissue perfusion: skin color, temperature, and moisture
  Capillary refill (less than 2 sec)
Patient examination: Head-to-toe examination to locate injuries
AMPLE history: **A**llergies
  Medicines
  Past medical history
  Last food/drink
  Events leading up
SOAP NOTE: To record and organize patient data
  Subjective: Age, sex, mechanism of injury, chief complaint
  Objective: Vital signs, patient examination, AMPLE history
  Assessment: Problem list
  Plan: Plan for each problem

Subjective: Is the patient comfortable, too hot, too cold, hungry, thirsty, or in need of urination or defecation?
Objective: Vital signs—are they stable? Record these. Patient examination—recheck all dressings, bandages, and splints; are they still controlling bleeding? Are they too tight or too loose? (Swelling limbs can cause bandages or splints to impede circulation, resulting in ischemic injuries or worsening frostbite or snakebite.)
Assessment: Has the initial assessment changed?
Plan: Is the rate of evacuation still the same?

EVACUATING THE PATIENT TO THE APPROPRIATE FACILITY

During the process of providing emergency care, part of the team was designated as the evacuation team. This group has taken the time to evaluate the various options for evacuation. The first information they need is provided by the medical team leader, since they need to know the status of the patient in order to establish the pace. If the patient's condition is stable, time is less important; if the patient's condition is critical, time is at a premium.

The evacuation team must explore different options. If speed is a consideration, weather conditions are reviewed and the availability of a helicopter-assisted rescue is determined. If a helicopter is not an option, the fastest route out is established. If time or speed is not a critical issue, the safest means of evacuation that will be easiest on the patient and rescuers is defined. A general rule for the duration of an evacuation is that it will take 1 to 2 hours for every mile to be covered, requiring six well-rested litter bearers for every mile. Thus a 4-mile carryout will most likely require a 24-member litter team and can take from 4 to 8 hours to complete. Eventually the team reaches a trailhead and the victim is transferred to an ambulance for transport to a hospital emergency facility.

RETURNING TO BASE

The team returns to base to reorganize equipment in preparation for the next extended rescue, and to debrief. Because people are exhausted and hungry, the debriefing session is often cancelled. However, establishing a mechanism to debrief the rescue effort is imperative so that they can learn from the shared experience, discuss patient care, and air problems. Whenever several different emergency organizations with disparate rescue and emergency personnel combine to perform a complex rescue, there may be tension, bruised egos, and concerns about the medical care provided or the evacuation plan used. These problems deserve to be discussed and managed in real time as expediently as possible so the teams will cooperate successfully, improve their performance, and provide the best possible patient care on the next rescue. This process minimizes the burnout syndrome that can occur with volunteer teams.

Team Organization and Function

The organization of an extended care rescue team is based on both the training of individuals and the type of rescue. The structures of teams can vary from loosely knit groups of friends with no hierarchy to paramilitary organizations with rigid leadership roles.

Team members require personal knowledge, experience, and expertise in the particular aspect of extended care and rescue in which they will participate, as well as knowledge and expertise in the principles of extended emergency care, extended rescue techniques, and technical rescue skills.

PERSONAL KNOWLEDGE, EXPERIENCE, AND EXPERTISE

Individuals who want to be part of an extended rescue team need to acquire outdoor skills *before* they become part of a rescue team. Every member must have extensive knowledge of likely environmental emergencies: hypothermia, frostbite, heat syndromes, snakebite, dehydration, lightning strike, and so forth. Each must understand general principles of weather behavior. Rescuers need to be comfortable with route finding, map and compass, personal preparedness, and bivouac and survival skills. The knowledge, skills, and equipment that a skilled outdoorsperson will always have are often referred to as "the ten essentials" (see Box 23-5). The same skills, knowledge, and equipment commonly used by the outdoor enthusiast are essential on a mountain rescue.

EXTENDED RESCUE TECHNIQUES AND SKILLS

Specific skills and techniques applicable to a particular situation include those of search and rescue, vertical and technical rock climbing, and white-water navigation. Snow

BOX 23-5

THE TEN ESSENTIALS

1. *Attitude*
   Positive belief that you can make things better
   Will to survive
2. *Fuel to burn: food*
   High-carbohydrate foods that require no preparation
   High-carbohydrate foods that can be made into a drink
3. *Quench your thirst: water*
   A minimum of 2 L/day if not active
   Up to 3 L/hr if active
   Ability to make more pure disinfected water
4. *Stay warm and dry: clothing*
   Warm clothing that retains heat even if wet
   Waterproof raingear, top and bottom
5. *Get dry: shelter*
   Ability to improvise shelter or bivouac
   A bivouac ("bivy") kit (see Box 23-6)
6. *Get warm: fire*
   Ability to warm water (stove, candle, fire)
   Ability to build a fire (waterproof matches and tinder)
   Ability to make kindling or tinder (folding knife)
7. *Know where you're going: navigation*
   Map and compass skills and route-finding skills
   Ability to move about at night (headlamp)
8. *Know the environment: weather*
   Basic understanding of weather patterns
   Knowledge of how to react to severe weather, lightning
9. *Getting help: signaling*
   Whistle, preferably plastic
10. *Providing help: first aid kit*
    Basic small personal trauma kit

BOX 23-6

BIVOUAC KIT

Two large garbage bags (emergency shelter or raingear)
10 × 10 foot sheet of plastic and 100 feet of parachute cord (shelter)
Emergency space blanket (shelter, ground cloth)
Stocking cap (warmth)
Spare socks (warmth and can act as spare mittens)
Metal cup (to warm liquids)
Gelatin (to make a drink)
Two plumber's candles (to warm water or start fire)
Waterproof matches or lighter
Knife
Compass
Whistle

All of these items fit neatly into a small stuff sack that is 6 × 6 inches and weighs less than 1 pound when filled.

BOX 23-7

KNOWLEDGE, SKILLS, AND EQUIPMENT FOR EXTENDED RESCUE TEAMS

MOUNTAINEERING SKILLS

Understanding fabrics and clothing systems and their seasonal variations (see Chapter 6)
- Fabrics and fibers
- Layering techniques
- Vapor barrier systems
- Waterproof fabrics, raingear systems
- Footgear

Personal protection equipment
- Helmets
- Harnesses
- Gloves
- Goggles, sunglasses
- Hearing protection

Backcountry equipment
- Internal or external frame packs and soft packs
- Shelter (natural and human-made)
- Specialty equipment: snow shoes, crampons, ice axes, stoves, skis

Backcountry travel
- Route finding
- Map and compass: map reading, dead reckoning, types of maps, compass reading, bearings, magnetic versus true bearing, triangulation, global positioning systems

Survival skills: the ten essentials
- Shelter and warmth; emergency bivouac ("bivy") kits
- Food, water

Understanding how backcountry travel and rescue vary with the seasons

Understanding how backcountry travel and rescue vary with different environments
- Alpine
- Desert
- Forest
- Water (swamp, river, lake, ocean)
- Tropics
- High altitude

Low-impact camping and rescue work

Basics of weather and weather forecasting
- Principles of barometric pressure
- Clouds and their significance in weather forecasting
- Prevailing weather patterns in the rescue area

Personal fitness
- Physical conditioning
- Nutrition and hydration requirements for different activities

MOUNTAIN AND EXTENDED EMERGENCY MEDICAL SKILLS

Emergency medical training should be at a minimal level of first responder or higher (emergency medical technician, paramedic, registered nurse, nurse practitioner, physician's assistant, or physician). Regardless of the level, training must include specific information on wilderness and extended emergency care procedures. Topics of extended care training and principles should include the following:

Patient assessment system

Cardiopulmonary resuscitation

Airway management, including endotracheal intubation and needle decompression for tension pneumothorax

Shock and control of bleeding, including the use of intravenous (IV) therapy for fluid resuscitation

Long-term wound care and prevention of infection

Musculoskeletal injury management, including specific information on diagnosis and long-term management of the following:
- Sprains and strains
- Fractures, including how to reduce or realign angulated fractures
- Diagnosis and reduction of dislocations
- Management of compound fractures
- Management of chest injuries, including decompression of a tension pneumothorax with a needle thoracostomy
- Spinal cord injury diagnosis and management
- Head injury, including recognition and management of increasing intracranial pressure

Management of environmental emergencies
- Hypothermia and frostbite, including the use of IV fluids
- Heatstroke and heat exhaustion, including the use of IV fluids
- Dehydration and nutrition, acute and during evacuation
- Lightning injuries
- Animal attacks, insect bites, and reptile and marine envenomations, including anaphylactic reactions and the use of epinephrine and antihistamines
- Contact dermatitis, such as poison ivy, oak, and sumac
- Sunburn and snow blindness
- High-altitude injuries, including acute mountain sickness, high-altitude pulmonary edema, high-altitude cerebral edema
- Near drowning

Diagnosis and management of acute medical emergencies
- Chest pain (myocardial infarction, angina, costochondritis)
- Shortness of breath (asthma, anaphylaxis, pneumothorax)
- Seizures and cerebrovascular accidents
- Acute abdomen (peritonitis, constipation, diarrhea)
- Pyelonephritis and septic shock

Patient lifting and handling techniques (body elevation and movement [BEAM] and free of any movement [FOAM])

Improvising techniques: "emergency medicine barehanded" (see Chapter 18)

BOX 23-7

KNOWLEDGE, SKILLS, AND EQUIPMENT FOR EXTENDED RESCUE TEAMS—cont'd

- Bloodborne pathogens and infectious disease prevention
- Monitoring of bodily functions (hunger, thirst, and need to excrete)
- General understanding and appreciation for the difference between urban (short-term) and wilderness (long-term) emergency care

MOUNTAIN AND EXTENDED RESCUE SKILLS

- Understanding equipment used in wilderness search and rescue operations, including maintenance and care
  - Ropes, slings, carabiners, harnesses, helmets
  - Litters, litter harnesses, haul systems
  - Litter patient packaging equipment
- Basic radio communications
  - Care and maintenance of communications equipment
  - Procedures and protocols
- Basic helicopter operations and procedures
  - Approach to a helicopter
  - Safety considerations
  - Landing zones
  - Haul techniques
  - Interagency relations
- Basic understanding of search procedures
- Basic understanding of rescue procedures
- Basic understanding of Incident Command System and its use in search and rescue management
- Basic rope handling and knot tying skills
  - How to care for and handle ropes
  - Rappeling, belaying, and braking techniques
  - Knots
    - Figure-8
    - Figure-8 follow through
    - Figure-8 on a bite
    - Double figure-8
    - Double fisherman
    - Prusik
    - Tensionless hitch (round turn and two half hitches)
    - Water
    - Half hitch and full hitch
    - Bowline
    - Alpine butterfly
- Specific rescue training
  - Water search
  - White-water
  - Avalanche
  - Technical or vertical (rock)
  - Cave

LEADERSHIP

- Leadership and followship training

or winter camping or avalanche rescue may be required, depending on the environment. Formulating a list of the knowledge and skills required for members of extended rescue and mountain rescue teams is a current task of an ASTM F32 subcommittee. Extended rescue teams should require their members to have at a minimum the working knowledge and equipment in Box 23-7.

Knowledge is acquired over time. Specific medical, rescue, and technical skills are obtained and retained through courses, continuous training, and refresher programs. Appendix A at the conclusion of this chapter provides a list of schools, institutes, and organizations that are involved in mountaineering research, standards development, and training programs.

WILDERNESS AND MOUNTAIN RESCUE TEAM ORGANIZATION

Organization of wilderness and mountain rescue teams is where the greatest diversity exists, since no universal standard has been established. Teams vary from local mountain rescue teams with extreme skills and qualifications for providing mountain rescue care to informal collections of friends without leadership. Other, more "professional" teams are operated under the jurisdiction of law enforcement agencies with paramilitary hierarchy and leadership. This diversity is particularly noticeable in the United States because the vast majority of teams are composed of volunteers who are not reimbursed for their rescue efforts.

In Europe, mountain rescue teams are professional and employ full-time personnel. They charge for rescue efforts, with the fees providing money for personnel, equipment, helicopters, technical gear, and ongoing training. As with any "profession," standards have evolved. As a result, there are more standards in Europe than in North America. Still, there is variation from European country to country, especially in leadership and organization.

It cannot be overemphasized that in many parts of the world, especially remote and wild areas, organized and available rescue teams do not exist. If someone is in need of help, the expedition team necessarily becomes the rescue team.

Training of Wilderness Emergency Medical Technicians

The best way to develop an appreciation for the vast difference between what is required of the traditional (urban) emergency medical technician (EMT) and the extended care or wilderness emergency medical technician (WEMT) is to compare their respective course curriculums.

The Department of Transportation (DOT) is responsible for developing and updating the EMT curriculum. This curriculum is considered to be the minimum national standard for EMT students to qualify for the National Registry or an individual state practical and written examination. Passage of such an examination enables a student to become certified as a National Registry or state EMT.

A national standard for WEMT curricula does not yet exist. ASTM has a task force dedicated to developing such a standard. Despite the lack of a DOT-like standard, there are several similar curricula for wilderness emergency care at the EMT level. Based on the recommendations of the Wilderness Medical Society and other groups that address the issues of wilderness prehospital emergency medicine, these curricula adhere to the same principles of long-term patient care, which can be used for comparison with the standard DOT curriculum.

A WEMT course typically contains all of the material in the DOT EMT course curriculum plus what is necessary to acquire the skills attendant to long-term wilderness emergency care. Typical EMT courses are approximately 100 hours with 10 additional hours of emergency department observation time. The WEMT module carries an additional 48 to 80 hours of training.

A typical WEMT course outline appears in Box 23-8. The topics in boldface are peculiar to a WEMT program, while the other topics are the required topics covered in a DOT EMT course. Hours per topic illustrate the time required for both EMT and WEMT training. This outline is arranged in the current DOT EMT recommended format, with the WEMT material added on a per topic basis; topics are not necessarily listed in the order that they would be taught for a particular course. An explanation of the extended emergency medical care material that WEMTs must learn follows.

INTRODUCTION TO EMERGENCY CARE

"Wilderness versus urban emergency care" is an introductory presentation to illustrate the differences between urban ("golden hour") emergency care and extended, or "wilderness," emergency care. For WEMTs it will in certain instances be necessary to learn two different modalities of therapy, one for short-term (less than 1 hour) care and one for long-term or extended (several hours to days) care.

"Backcountry rescue gear inspection" is a hands-on review of gear for the outdoor practice sessions and backcountry mock rescues. It is essential that the course staff inspect the participants' boots, clothing, raingear, and rescue equipment to determine their adequacy for the particular environment in which they will be deployed. Inspecting equipment not only ensures the safety of each individual in the course, but also teaches a standard for preparedness, awareness, and attention to details that is critical for wilderness travel and emergency care.

"Medical legal issues" is usually offered early in a course, so that the participants are aware of the legal concerns surrounding practicing medicine as EMTs and WEMTs. WEMTs need to be aware of protocols that may exist in the state where they will become licensed.

"The human animal—our natural physiologic limits" is an overview lecture of how humans fit into the natural environment and of their daily nutritional requirements and natural limitations. The WEMT must understand physiologic limits such as those of endurance, temperature, and altitude, and the consequences when they are exceeded.

PATIENT ASSESSMENT SYSTEMS

"Patient assessment in the wilderness and practice" takes the newly learned skills of patient assessment and adapts them to the backcountry. The WEMT needs to be knowledgeable and skillful in wilderness patient assessment, a step-by-step approach to the first 5 minutes of scene safety and patient care. The WEMT will develop an awareness of potential life-threatening dangers in the environment, how to ensure personal safety and the safety of others, how to approach a victim safely, how to perform primary and secondary surveys to determine the extent and severity of injuries, and what impact the environment might have on the patient.

AIRWAYS, OXYGEN, AND MECHANICAL AIDS TO BREATHING

"Airways, oxygen, cardiopulmonary resuscitation, and mechanical aids to breathing in the wilderness environment—uses and limitations" addresses one of the most important lifesaving and life-maintaining skills in emergency medicine, the ability to establish and maintain a patent airway. Unfortunately, most EMTs are not provided with the training and tools they need to properly maintain an open airway in an unconscious patient. Failure to perform endotracheal intubation can be disastrous for a patient.

Endotracheal intubation is commonly used by paramedics and advanced life support (ALS) personnel in cardiac arrest settings and for unconscious, unresponsive patients. In the extended care environment the use of intubation in a cardiac arrest situation is not nearly as common as it is for the normothermic, unconscious, and unresponsive patient, who has probably suffered head trauma. In this situation, without intubation, the only way to maintain a patent

BOX 23-8
EMT AND WEMT COURSE CURRICULA AND HOURS PER TOPIC*

1. Introduction to emergency care
   Wilderness versus urban emergency care (1 hour)
   Backcountry rescue gear inspection (1 hour)
   Medical legal issues (1 hour)
   Bloodborne pathogens
   Overview of human systems—anatomy and physiology (2 hours)
   The human animal—our natural physiologic limits (2 hours)
2. Patient assessment systems
   Primary survey—ABCs (1 hour)
   Secondary survey (1 hour)
   Patient assessment practice (2 hours)
   Patient assessment in the wilderness and practice (3 hours)
3. Cardiopulmonary resuscitation (8 hours)
   Mannequin practice and certification (8 hours)
      Cardiopulmonary resuscitation (CPR) teaching, practice, and testing to American Heart Association standards
4. Airways, oxygen, and mechanical aids to breathing (3 hours)
   Airways, oxygen, CPR, and mechanical aids to breathing in the wilderness environment—uses and limitations (6 hours)
      Airways: oropharyngeal, nasopharyngeal, esophageal obturator airway, endotracheal intubation
      Oxygen administration
      Suction techniques
5. Bleeding and shock (3 hours)
   Shock, intravenous (IV) fluids, and long-term patient care (4 hours)
   Practice starting IV infusions and fluid administration (4 hours)
   Use of pneumatic antishock garments (PASG) (3 hours)
   Use of PSAG in the wilderness (1 hour)
6. Soft tissue injuries (3 hours)
   Long-term wound care (1 hour)
7. Principles of musculoskeletal care
   Fractures of the upper extremities (3 hours)
   Fractures of the pelvis, hip, and lower extremities (3 hours)
   Fracture laboratory—practice in assessment and management (3 hours)
   Musculoskeletal trauma management in the wilderness (3 hours)
8. Injuries of the head, face, eye, neck, and spine (3 hours)
   Practical laboratory: spinal cord injury management (SCIM) (3 hours)
   Head trauma, increasing intracranial pressure (1 hour)
   SCIM: Long-term care and improvising (1 hour)
9. Injuries to the chest, abdomen, and genitalia (3 hours)
   Chest trauma in the wilderness (3 hours)
10. Medical emergencies I (3 hours)
      Poisoning, bites and strings, heart attack, stroke, dyspnea
    Medical emergencies II (3 hours)
      Diabetes, acute abdomen, communicable disease, seizure, substance abuse, and pediatric emergencies
    Medical emergencies in the wilderness (3 hours)
11. Emergency childbirth (3 hours)
12. Burns and hazardous materials (3 hours)
    Long-term care of burns (1 hour)
13. Environmental emergencies (3 hours)
    Hypothermia, frostbite, immersion foot (4 hours)
    Heatstroke, heat exhaustion, dehydration (4 hours)
    Drowning (2 hours)
    High-altitude emergencies (2 hours)
    Barotrauma (2 hours)
    Animals that bite and sting (2 hours)
    Plants —contact dermatitis (2 hours)
    Marine animals that bite and sting (2 hours)
14. Psychologic aspects of emergency care (3 hours)
15. Lifting and moving patients (3 hours)
    Use of Stokes litters and improvising litters (3 hours)
16. Principles of vehicle extrication (4 hours)
    Practice laboratory (3-8 hours)
    Principles of backcountry evacuation (4 hours)
    Search and rescue organization and execution (4 hours)
    Wilderness mock rescue with or without overnight (8-12 hours)
17. Ambulance operations I (3 hours)
    Ambulance operations II (3 hours)
    Helicopter-assisted rescues (3 hours)
18. Review (3-6 hours)
    Testing—written and practical examinations (16-20 hours)
19. Emergency department observation time (10 hours)

*Topics in boldface are peculiar to WEMT programs, while the other topics are required topics covered in a DOT EMT course.

airway while lifting, moving, and transporting a patient in a litter is to place the patient on his or her side. Gravity pulls the tongue forward and allows secretions to drain from the mouth. Oropharyngeal, nasopharyngeal, and esophageal obturator airways and tongue pin-pull techniques may temporarily keep the tongue from occluding the airway, but they are ineffective in preventing vomitus, blood, or saliva from entering the airway. Also, during an evacuation in a Stokes litter, constant monitoring of a patient's airway is virtually impossible, which makes endotracheal intubation of paramount importance. The WEMT needs to know how to establish and maintain a patent airway, including endotracheal intubation.

"Oxygen administration" presents the use of supplemental oxygen, for which both EMTs and WEMTs follow the same general guidelines. Even though oxygen is important to prehospital care, its use has significant logistic limitations in the backcountry.

The WEMT needs to realize that carrying large quantities of oxygen into the backcountry is impossible. Small D and E cylinders can be carried, but each provides high-flow oxygen for only 20 to 30 minutes. Oxygen is a compressed gas in a tank, so as it expands, it cools dramatically and may contribute to hypothermia. To prevent this, the gas should be preheated by wrapping the oxygen tubing around a chemical heat pack during administration.

"Suction techniques" presents the use of suction devices to clear the airway, which is similar for EMTs and WEMTs. Hand-operated, as distinct from battery-operated, suction devices are usually used.

BLEEDING AND SHOCK

"Shock, intravenous fluids, and long-term patient care" and "practice starting IV infusions and fluid administration" provide information about the care of patients in shock.

In the urban management of shock the essential component is recognition. Once shock is recognized, the patient can be rapidly transported to an emergency department or intercepted by paramedics for definitive care, namely fluid resuscitation.

In the extended care environment, WEMTs have to be able to manage the shock syndrome by providing appropriate definitive care. During extended evacuations, WEMTs need to know how to administer intravenous fluids to stabilize hypovolemia. This includes starting a peripheral intravenous line, maintaining the catheter placement, using proper fluids, and prewarming the solutions before and during administration.

"Use of pneumatic antishock garments (PASG) in the wilderness" discusses the use of these garments for patients in shock. The value of treating shock using PASG versus intravenous therapy is argued. As long as an intravenous line can be established and maintained, fluid administration is the definitive method for managing shock. The WEMT must be aware that the PASG has other uses. In the extended care situation, it may be invaluable to stabilize a fractured pelvis to control internal blood loss and prevent shock. It may be useful in conjunction with a traction splint for a fractured femur. An added benefit is that the PASG provides a comfortable and well-padded ride for the patient in a Stokes litter.

It is equally important that WEMTs recognize the limitations of a PASG. The primary drawback in the backcountry is the potential for cold injury. Once the apparatus is inflated, the decrease in peripheral circulation greatly increases the risk for cold injuries or frostbite to the lower extremities. This can be prevented by properly packing the feet with chemical heat packs and properly insulating the lower extremities in the litter. Careful monitoring of the lower extremities every 15 minutes is essential.

SOFT TISSUE INJURIES

"Long-term wound care" covers proper wound management once bleeding has been controlled, and further care if it will require more that 12 hours to bring the victim to definitive care. The principles of long-term wound care are to stabilize the wound and prevent and control infection.

To prevent infection, the WEMT has to know how to sterilize or disinfect fluid and how to use it to properly debride and rinse out a contaminated wound. Once the wound is cleaned and debrided, the edges can be approximated but not tightly closed, since this may increase the risk of abscess formation and a life-threatening infection. Training in suturing techniques to close wounds is not currently recommended.

Even the most fastidiously cleaned wound can still become infected, particularly in a remote setting, because of the constant exposure to microbes. Recognition of wound infections and appropriate management are important. The WEMT must learn to use specific antibiotics in extended care settings of greater than 3 days and for prophylaxis with grossly contaminated wounds and compound fractures. Antibiotic therapy is not controversial, since there are a variety of safe broad-spectrum antibiotics that can cover most wound infections with minimal risk of a severe allergic reaction. Antibiotics are not to be used cavalierly, but in certain circumstances the benefits clearly outweigh the risks.

PRINCIPLES OF MUSCULOSKELETAL CARE

"Musculoskeletal trauma management in the wilderness" presents the treatment of injuries. In an urban setting the primary concern with fracture and dislocation care is that the injury site be splinted properly to prevent further injury. In the extended care environment the primary concern is to maintain proper circulation distal to the site of the injury. This may require straightening an angulated fracture or reducing a dislocation.

When an angulated fracture occurs, distal circulation can be impaired partially or totally. This puts the soft tissues at considerable risk for ischemic injury or frostbite. Under normal circumstances it would take hours for moderate ischemia to cause an irreparable soft tissue injury, but in the backcountry, extended time under hostile weather conditions frequently occurs, which decreases the amount of heat and oxygen being transferred to the extremity.

Knowing how to properly straighten out angulated fractures significantly decreases the risk of secondary ischemic injury and frostbite, controls bleeding at the fracture site, and diminishes pain. It is much easier to splint and stabilize a fracture in proper position if it is straight than if it is angulated.

Approximately 3 additional hours of training is needed to teach a WEMT how to straighten an angulated fracture and reduce dislocations. Without an x-ray study it is impossible to see the exact positioning of bone fragments or disarticulated joints, making it difficult to know exactly how to manipulate the bone. The concern here is that if a jagged bone end is moved improperly, a secondary injury might occur. Part of a neurovascular bundle could be severed, a fascial sheath surrounding a muscle could be cut, or the ends could erupt through the skin. Fortunately, all of these structures are richly endowed with pain receptors. If the sharp end of a bone fragment begins to impinge, it causes a dramatic increase in pain at the site. A commonly used technique is to straighten out the angulated site slowly while under constant gentle traction. With each 1 to 2 cm of movement the patient is asked if the new position is better or worse (causes less or more pain). If the pain diminishes with movement, the reduction is proceeding properly; if pain increases, all movement is stopped and the extremity is returned to the previous position of improvement. While still under gentle traction, the extremity is repositioned and another attempt at reduction is made.

As long as nothing is forced and movement is achieved slowly under gentle traction, angulated fractures can be easily realigned and dislocations reduced without the need for pain medication or any risk of further injury.

Musculoskeletal injuries in the long-term care setting must be carefully monitored. It is essential to reinspect the injury site at reasonable intervals for circulation, sensation, and motion. Fracture sites swell; as a result, even the best splint can act as an inadvertent tourniquet. Immobilized extremities cool because of lack of activity and impaired circulation, also increasing the risk of ischemic injury or frostbite.

INJURIES OF THE HEAD, FACE, EYE, NECK, AND SPINE

"Head trauma, increasing intracranial pressure" addresses one of the leading causes of death from backcountry accidents. Many who die of head trauma in the wilderness would have survived in an urban setting because of rapid access to definitive care. The WEMT must be able to recognize a potentially serious head injury long before the victim is at risk of brainstem herniation.

In the extended care environment there are few situations when the team should hurry. One such situation is the presence of significant head trauma, for which the only appropriate care may be rapid evacuation to a facility where the patient can be put into the hands of a neurosurgeon.

It is important not only to establish the level of consciousness, but also to have a method of monitoring it. To evaluate and monitor the level of consciousness, the AVPU (**A**wake, **V**erbal, **P**ain, **U**nresponsive) scale is used. Within the primary survey an initial evaluation of disability or neurologic status is made using the AVPU scale. After that, level of consciousness is reevaluated every 15 minutes to observe for any evidence of increasing intracranial pressure.

INJURIES TO THE CHEST, ABDOMEN, AND GENITALIA

Chest trauma is significant for the WEMT because it can result in a pneumothorax that can evolve into a tension pneumothorax. WEMTs need to be taught how to inspect, palpate, percuss, and auscultate the chest for significant injuries to the respiratory system. Training an individual how to detect breath sounds, determine the presence of a pneumothorax, and monitor a pneumothorax for its development into a tension pneumothorax is not difficult. Unlike increasing increasing pressure, for which there is little to do but evacuate, a tension pneumothorax can be relieved, increasing the chance of survival. The easiest and most effective technique for a WEMT to learn is needle thoracostomy in the fifth intercostal space, midaxillary line.

MEDICAL EMERGENCIES

Medical emergencies in the wilderness are usually diagnosed easily if EMTs are aware of the essential signs and symptoms.

ENVIRONMENTAL EMERGENCIES

The typical EMT course includes 3 to 6 hours of training in the management of environmental emergencies. A WEMT course will have a minimum of 22 hours of additional training in environmental emergencies.

"Hypothermia, frostbite, and immersion foot" covers cold injuries, which are among the most common environmental injuries seen in the backcountry. The WEMT has to understand principles of thermoregulation; heat production and heat loss; recognition of hypothermia, frostbite, and immersion foot; and appropriate care.

"Heatstroke, heat exhaustion, and dehydration" provides necessary information about the balance of heat production and heat loss in a hot environment and the fluid requirements necessary to support physiologic cooling. WEMTs need to know how to recognize and provide long-term care for victims of heatstroke, heat exhaustion, and dehydration.

LIFTING AND MOVING PATIENTS

"Use of Stokes litters and improvising litters" discusses the primary device for evacuation from the backcountry. Even when a helicopter is used, the patient is usually "packaged" in a litter before being loaded. WEMTs need to know the specific techniques for patient packaging in a litter to protect and support injuries. Use of the proper carrying techniques and methods of belaying a litter up or down a steep slope is critical to the safety of everyone involved.

AMBULANCE OPERATIONS

"Helicopter-assisted rescues" describes the use of helicopters in backcountry rescue efforts and evacuation. WEMT training should address the dangers, hazards, and limitations of helicopters.

APPENDIX A

Research, Standards, and Program Resources

The following is a list of organizations and committees dedicated to some aspect of extended medical, rescue, and technical training. Many are also active in mountain, wilderness, marine, or disaster rescue and management efforts.

American Alpine Club
710 Tenth Street, Suite 100
Golden, CO 80401
303-384-0110
Resource: Publishes *Accidents in North American Mountaineering* and *The American Alpine Journal* annually. Has committees dedicated to establishing and promoting standards in safety and education in mountaineering.

American Mountain Guides Association
P.O. Box 2128
Estes Park, CO 80517
303-586-0571
Resource: Dedicated to establishing and maintaining standards for mountaineering and professional mountain guides. Publishes quarterly *Mountain Bulletin.*

Appalachian Mountain Club
P.O. Box 298
Gorham, NH 03581
603-466-2727
Resource: Active mountain rescue team which offers a variety of workshops on outdoor skills, environmental issues, and wilderness medical and rescue skills. Publishes quarterly *Appalachia.*

Appalachian Search and Rescue Conference
P.O. Box 440, Newcomb Station
Charlottesville, VA 22904
804-674-2400 (emergencies only)
Resource: Wilderness EMS agency, search and rescue, course and materials development.

American Society for Testing and Materials
1916 Race Street
Philadelphia, PA 19103
215-299-5400 for Committees F-30 on EMS and F-32 on search and rescue
Resource: National and international standards-setting organization, currently with committees dedicated to developing standards to extended care, rescue, and search and rescue.

Center for Emergency Medicine of Western Pennsylvania
230 McKee Place, Suite 500
Pittsburgh, PA 15213-4904
Resource: Offers various wilderness EMT and wilderness command physician training courses.

International Society for Mountain Medicine
Clinique Generale de Sion
1950 Sion, Switzerland
Resource: An international organization dedicated to research and education in mountaineering. Publishes quarterly *The Newsletter of the ISMM.*

Mountain Rescue Association
2144 South 1100 East, Suite 150-375
Salt Lake City, UT 84106
303-567-9584
Resource: National wilderness rescue organization dedicated to the development of standards and certification of mountain rescue teams.

Nantahala Outdoor Center
US 19 West, Box 41
Bryson City, NC 28713
704-488-2175
Resource: Offers a variety of courses on white-water rescue and wilderness medical and rescue training.

National Association for Search and Rescue
P.O. Box 3709
Fairfax, VA 22038
703-352-1349
Resource: National information resource for search and rescue as well as certifications in various search functions and wilderness emergency medicine. Publishes quarterly journal *Response.*

National Cave Rescue Commission
c/o National Speleological Society
Cave Ave.
Huntsville, AL 35810
205-852-1300
EMERGENCY: *National Rescue Coordination 1-800-851-3051*
Resource: Active national cave rescue team.

National Ski Patrol System, Inc.
Ski Patrol Building, Suite 100
133 South Van Gordon
Lakewood, CO 80228
303-988-1111
Resource: Active rescue teams and ski patrols. Offers a winter emergency care (WEC) course, various ski patrol certifications, avalanche training, and introductory mountaineering training.

Stonehearth Open Learning Opportunities (SOLO)
RFD #1 Box 163
Conway, NH 03818
603-447-6711
Resource: An international organization dedicated to developing and offering a variety of courses and certifications in wilderness and marine medicine, rescue, leadership, and outdoor skills. An active mountain rescue team.

Union Internationale des Associations d'Alpinisme (UIAA)
(International Union of Alpine Associations)
President of the UIAA Medical Commission
University of Salzburg, Institute of Sports Science
Salzburger Platz 130,
A-5710 Kaprun Austria
Resource: An international organization dedicated to the promotion of standards, safety, awareness, and education in mountaineering worldwide. Produces multiple publications on mountain safety and medicine.

United States Coast Guard Headquarters
2100 Second Street, SW
Washington, DC 20593-0001
202-267-1012 (Boating Operations)
Resource: Active national marine rescue military organization. Source of information and various boating-related certifications.

Wilderness Medical Associates
RFD 2, Box 890
Bryant Pond, ME 04219
207-665-2701, 800-742-2931
Resource: Offers a variety of courses and cerifications in wilderness medical and rescue courses.

Wilderness Medical Society
P.O. Box 2463
Indianapolis, IN 46206
317-631-1745
Resource: A physician-based national wilderness medical organization with various committees dedicated to education in wilderness emergency medicine. Particular attention to education for physicians. Publishes quarterly newsletter and *Wilderness and Environmental Medicine* (formerly *Journal of Wilderness Medicine).*

Wilderness Medicine Institute
300 Tenth Street
P.O. Box 9
Pitkin, CO 81254
303-641-3572
Resource: Offers a variety of courses and certifications in wilderness medicine and rescue. Publishes bimonthly *Wilderness Medicine Newsletter.*

Wilderness Professional Training
P.O. Box 759
Crested Butte, CO 81224
303-349-5939
Resource: Offers a variety of courses and certifications in wilderness medicine and rescue.

RECOMMENDED READINGS

American Academy of Orthopedic Surgeons: *Emergency care and transportation of the sick and injured,* ed 5, Menasha, Wis, 1971, George Banta.

Auerbach P: *Medicine for the outdoors,* Boston, 1991, Little, Brown.

Bowman W: *Outdoor emergency care,* ed 2, Denver, 1993, National Ski Patrol.

Caroline N: *Emergency medical treatment,* ed 3, Boston, 1982, Little, Brown.

Grant H, Murray R: *Emergency care,* ed 6, Washington, DC, RJ Brady.

Hafen B, Karren K: *Prehospital emergency care and crisis intervention,* ed 4, Englewood, Colo, 1992, Morton.

Henry M, Stapleton E: *EMT prehospital care,* Philadelphia, 1992, Saunders.

Houston C: *Going higher: the story of man and altitude, 1990.*

Iverson KV, editor: *Position statements of the Wilderness Medical Society,* Point Reyes Station, Calif, 1989, Wilderness Medical Society.

Schimelpfenig T, Lindsey L: *NOLS wilderness first aid,* Lander, Wyo, 1991, National Outdoor Leadership School.

Setnicka T: *Wilderness search and rescue,* Boston, 1980, Appalachian Mountain Club.

Stewart C: *Environmental emergencies,* Baltimore, 1990, Williams & Wilkins.

US Department of Transportation, National Highway Traffic Safety Administration: *Emergency medical technician-ambulance: national standard curriculum,* ed 3, Washington, DC, 1984, US Government Printing Office.

Wilkerson J, editor: *Medicine for mountaineering,* ed 4, Seattle, 1993, The Mountaineers.

Williamson J, editor: *Accidents in North American mountaineering,* Golden, Colo, American Alpine Club, published yearly.

24 NATURAL AND HUMAN-MADE HAZARDS: MITIGATION AND MANAGEMENT ISSUES

Sheila B. Reed

The term "hazard" is usually applied to rare or extreme events in the natural or human-made environment. Hazards can adversely affect human life or property to the extent of causing a disaster, or major disruptive situation. "Natural" hazards are caused by biologic, geologic, seismic, hydrologic, or meteorologic processes in the natural environment and include drought, flood, earthquake, volcanic eruption, and severe storms. When natural hazards occur close to vulnerable human settlements, structures, and economic assets, the normal functioning of a society may be disrupted and extraordinary emergency interventions may be necessary to save lives and the environment.

Human-made hazards are derived from human interactions with the environment, human relationships and attitudes, and the use of technology. For example, transportation accidents, petrochemical explosions, mine fires, building collapses, oil spills, hazardous waste leaks, and nuclear power plant failures are disasters where the principal and direct causes are human actions. Many hazards have both natural and human components; for example, desertification results from arid conditions, erosion, and overgrazing, landslides may occur from poorly planned construction on unstable hillsides, and flooding is sometimes caused by dam failures.

The distinction between many natural causes of hazards and contributions of humans to disastrous situations is becoming increasingly blurred. As populations grow and expand, pressure on land resources may force settlement in vulnerable areas, where hazards such as volcanic eruptions, earthquakes, or floods can become major disasters. Pest infestations may lead to famine in food-deficient areas, incidences of disease might become an epidemic because of overcrowding, and drought may become famine where food shortages result from combinations of lack of rainfall and displacement of people. The recent focus on global warming emanates from studies of the effects of climatic conditions and environmental pollution. Variables in these studies form such complex interactions that even computerized models have difficulty predicting the outcomes. Hazards with combination causes result in complex disasters and often in complex emergencies. Whatever their causes, disasters have serious political, economic, social, and environmental implications. In less developed areas, disasters can severely set back or reverse development efforts.

Disaster Management

This chapter focuses on hazards with a significant geophysical component, from a disaster management perspective. Disaster management encompasses all aspects of planning for and responding to disasters, including predisaster and postdisaster activities. It refers to the management of both the risks and the consequences of disasters. Components of disaster management include vulnerability and risk assessment, disaster mitigation and preparedness, and disaster assessment. Selection of management options depends on the type of hazard and whether the onset is likely to be slow or rapid.

SLOW- VERSUS RAPID-ONSET HAZARDS

Hazards may develop gradually and persist for a long time or may arise suddenly and be resolved rapidly. Rapid-onset hazards often occur with violent intensity and have profound effects on the surrounding environment, resulting in measurable numbers of casualties and damage. Slow-onset climatic changes brought on by deforestation, drought, desertification, or environmental pollution change the suitability of different parts of the world to agriculture and also affect the flora and fauna. The effects of slow-onset disasters are often insidious, and their impact can be measured only through environmental studies and in terms of reduction in quality of life and productivity for the affected population. The study of disaster management, formerly focused mainly on natural hazards, now encompasses a range of slow- and rapid-onset disasters and their natural and human causes.

It is conservatively estimated that between 1.5 and 2 million people have been killed in rapid-onset disasters since 1946, or an average annual death toll of 35,000 to 50,000. The biggest killers are earthquakes, tropical cyclones, and floods. Most deaths are concentrated in a relatively small number of communities, predominantly in poorer nations of Asia, Latin America, and Oceania. In comparison, North America, Europe, Japan, and Australia have average annual death tolls that rarely exceed a few hundred persons.

Although no comprehensive data are available for economic losses from rapid-onset hazards, a few examples illustrate the scale of the problem. Annual worldwide losses from tropical cyclones are estimated at between $6 and $7 billion. For landslides the comparable figure exceeds $1 billion. These figures only hint at the human impact of destruction. The eruption of Colombia's Nevado del Ruiz volcano in 1985 killed approximately 22,000 people and left 10,000 more homeless. Hurricane Andrew's impact on Florida in 1992 destroyed 30,000 homes, damaged 60,000, and left 350,000 people homeless, with damage estimates of $16 billion. An earthquake in south central India in October 1993 claimed at least 30,000 lives.

The relative human, economic, and social impacts of rapid-onset disasters are usually greatest in small, poor nations. The 1985 earthquake in Mexico City caused economic losses equivalent to roughly 3.5% of Mexico's gross national product (GNP). Hurricane Fifi in 1974 caused losses in Honduras that exceeded 35% of the country's GNP. Hurricane Allen in 1980 caused losses in St. Lucia equivalent to 89% of the nation's GNP and destroyed 90% of the nation's banana crop, which normally accounts for 80% of the country's agricultural output.

Economic losses from rapid-onset hazards are increasing at a rapid pace. In the United States, damage to buildings from earthquakes, tropical cyclones, and floods is expected to increase from approximately $6 billion in 1978 to more than $11 billion in the year 2000 if no additional loss reduction measures are undertaken. A major earthquake in Tokyo would probably kill more than 30,000 people, cause the collapse of 60,000 houses, and set fire to more than 400,000 homes.

Slow-onset disasters take an even greater toll, but precise figures are difficult to find. Drought currently affects more people than any other disaster; worldwide, droughts have been estimated to affect more than 18 million people each year during the 1960s, more than 24 million people during the 1970s, and 101 million from 1980 to 1989. During the early 1980s, drought affected up to 30 million people in Africa alone. Droughts have led to famines, resulting in large numbers of deaths and displacements. Increasing desertification in arid areas may be contributing to droughts. Desertification, or decline in biologic productivity, extends to 70% of total productive arid lands or 3.6 billion acres worldwide and may adversely affect the quality of life for 10% of the world population, including urban dwellers.

Possible global warming is predicted in the next century from increased atmospheric carbon dioxide caused by burning of fossil fuels, deforestation, and generation of methane. If this occurs, sea levels will rise and coastal cities worldwide will be inundated. A rise of 1 m in sea level could flood 15% of arable land in Egypt's Nile Delta and completely submerge the tiny island of the Maldives, inhabited by 200,000. Hundreds of millions of people will also be affected if increased ultraviolet radiation is delivered to the earth's surface as a result of stratospheric ozone depletion caused by continued release of chlorofluorocarbons.

Although global warming and ozone depletion are threats to the future, other forms of environmental pollution, such as water and air pollution, affect life today. Massive oil spills make headlines, and adverse health effects are seen from contamination and smog. Deforestation, particularly in the tropical rainforests, is highly significant. In addition to its contribution to possible global warming, it increases vulnerability to droughts, landslides, and floods.

ASSESSING VULNERABILITY AND RISK

Not all hazards become disasters. Whether or not a disaster occurs depends on the magnitude, intensity, and duration of the event and the vulnerability of the community. For example, a severe earthquake is not a disaster unless it significantly disrupts a community by creating large numbers of casualties and substantial destruction. Effective disaster management requires information about the magnitude of the risk faced and how much importance society places on the reduction of that risk. Risks are often quantified in aggregated ways (for example, a probability of 1 in 23,000 per year of an individual's dying in an earthquake in Iran). The importance placed on risk of a hazard is likely to be influenced by the nature of the risks faced on a daily basis. In Pakistan, where communities are regularly afflicted by floods, earthquakes, and landslides, people use their meager resources to protect against what they perceive to be greater risks, such as disease and irrigation failure. In California, where risk of disease is low, communities choose to initiate programs against natural disasters.

Differences in vulnerability are often defined as the susceptibility of buildings, infrastructure, economy, and natural resources to damage from hazards. Many aspects of vulnerability, however, cannot be described in monetary terms and should not be overlooked, such as personal loss of family, home, and income and related human suffering and psychosocial problems. While communities in developed nations may be just as prone to hazards as are communities in poor nations, the wealthier communities are often less vulnerable to damage. Although southern California and Managua, Nicaragua, are both prone to earthquakes, California is less vulnerable to damage because of strictly enforced building codes, zoning regulations, earthquake preparedness training, and sophisticated communications systems. In 1971 the San Fernando earthquake in California measured 6.4 on the Richter scale but caused minor damage and 58 deaths, while an earthquake of similar magnitude struck Managua 2 years later and reduced the center of the city to rubble, killing approximately 6000. Similarly, in wealthy countries, drought and resulting loss of food production and groundwater are managed by use of food surpluses and treated water, but drought in poor nations often leads to deaths from famine and to sickness and death from contaminated water supplies.

DISASTER MITIGATION STRATEGIES

Mitigation involves not only saving lives and reducing injury and property losses, but also reducing the adverse consequences of hazards to economic activities and social institutions. Where resources are limited, they should be directed toward protecting the most vulnerable elements. Vulnerability also implies a lack of resources for rapid recovery.

For most risks associated with natural geophysical hazards, such as volcanic eruptions, tsunamis, and tropical cyclones, little or no opportunity is available to reduce the hazard itself. In these cases the emphasis must be placed on reducing the vulnerability of the elements at risk. However, for technologic and human-made hazards or slow-onset hazards such as environmental pollution and desertification, reducing the hazard is likely to be the most effective mitigation strategy.

Actions by planning authorities to reduce vulnerability can be "active," where desired actions are promoted through incentives, or "passive," where undesired actions are prevented by use of controls and penalties. The range of mitigation options can include the following.

Engineering and Construction

Engineering measures range from large-scale engineering works to strengthening individual buildings and to small-scale community based projects, such as training to incorporate better protection into traditional structures like buildings, roads, and embankments.

Physical Planning Measures

Careful location of new facilities, particularly community facilities such as schools, hospitals, and infrastructure, plays an important role in reducing settlement vulnerability. In urban areas, deconcentration of elements especially at risk is an important principle. Specific procedures include hazard mapping and development of a master plan containing land use control guidelines. Hazard occurrence probabilities can be extrapolated from historical data and used to create hazard maps to show regional variation. Hazard mapping can be detailed by an inventory of people or things that are exposed or vulnerable to the hazard. In France, the Zones Exposed to Risks of Movements of the Soil and Subsoil (ZERMOS) plan produces landslide hazard maps at scales of 1:25,000 or larger that are used as tools for mitigation planning. The maps portray degrees of risk of various types of landslides, including activity, rate, and potential consequences.

Economic Measures

The linkages among different sectors of the economy may suffer more disruption from disaster than may the physical infrastructure. Diversifying and strengthening the economy are important ways to reduce risk. Within a strong economy, governments can use economic incentives to encourage individuals or institutions to take disaster mitigation actions.

Management and Institutional Measures

Building disaster protection takes time and needs support from programs of education, training, and institution building to provide the professional knowledge and competence required. Development of forecasting and warning systems are important protective measures.

Societal Measures

Mitigation planning should aim to develop a "safety culture" in which all members of society are aware of the hazards they face, know how to protect themselves, and support the protection efforts of others and communities as a whole. Specifically, these include conducting community education programs and planning and practicing evacuation procedures.

DISASTER PREPAREDNESS

A disaster preparedness plan for sudden-onset hazards such as earthquakes, volcanic eruptions, tropical cyclones, and floods usually contains the following elements:

1. Identification and mapping of the hazard zones; registration of valuable and movable property
2. Identification of safe refuge zones to which the population will be evacuated in case of danger
3. Identification and maintenance of evacuation routes
4. Identification of assembly points for persons awaiting transport for evacuation
5. Means of transport and traffic control
6. Shelter and accommodation in the refuge zone
7. Inventory of personnel and equipment for search and rescue
8. Hospital and medical services for treatment of injured persons
9. Security in evacuated areas
10. Formulation and communication of public warnings and procedures for communication in emergencies
11. Provisions for revising and updating the plan

Preparedness measures for slow-onset disasters such as drought include early warning systems that alert authorities to precursory conditions and allow preparations to avert famine and displacement.

DISASTER ASSESSMENT AND POSTDISASTER NEEDS

Assessments regularly conducted during the recovery process help to identify needs that lead to appropriate types of assistance. In the cases of slow-onset hazard types such as desertification, deforestation, and environmental pollution, a distinct postdisaster period usually does not exist; thus ongoing impact assessment is vital. The initial response to a rapid-onset hazardous event includes the following steps by local authorities:

1. Evacuation
2. Emergency shelter
3. Search and rescue
4. Medical assistance
5. Provision of short-term food and water
6. Water disinfection and purification
7. Epidemiologic surveillance
8. Provision of temporary lodging
9. Reopening of roads
10. Reestablishment of communications networks and contact with remote areas
11. Brush and debris clearance
12. Disaster assessment
13. Provision of inputs for recovery and rehabilitation

Nature of Hazards

Many kinds of natural hazards and hazards partially rooted in natural systems exist. Many of these occur infrequently or affect only small populations. One example is the eruption of toxic gases from several volcanic lakes in Cameroon that killed 2000 people in 1984 and 1986. Other rare events such as meteor impacts may occur only once every few centuries. Other widespread but minor phenomena that damage property but do not generally cause loss of life include land subsidence and sinkholes. Some hazards, such as snowstorms, often occur in areas that are prepared to deal with them so that they rarely become disasters.

Eleven hazards that affect large populations are discussed here and can be categorized as follows:

Geologic hazards—earthquakes, tsunamis, volcanic eruptions, landslides

Climatic hazards—tropical cyclones, tornadoes, floods, drought

Environmental hazards—environmental pollution, deforestation, desertification

To plan appropriate responses to implement emergency medical care and other measures to save or restore physical and mental health of affected populations, officials first need to understand the causal phenomena, characteristics, and predictability of the hazards and the factors that contribute to vulnerability. Further, examination of the effects the hazard has had on humans, property, and the environment can promote measures that may prevent or lessen casualties and destruction.

EARTHQUAKES

Earthquakes are among the most destructive and feared of natural hazards. They may occur at any time of year, day or night, with sudden impact and little warning. They can destroy buildings in seconds, killing or injuring the inhabitants. Earthquakes not only destroy entire cities but may destabilize the government, economy, and social structure of a country.

Causal Phenomena

The earth's crust is a rock layer of varying thickness from a depth of about 10 km under the oceans to 65 km under the continents. The theory of plate tectonics holds that the crustal plates ride on the mobile mantle and give rise to stresses in the crust when they contact each other. Stresses occur along the plate boundaries by pulling away from, sliding alongside, and pushing against one another. All of these movements are associated with earthquakes.

The areas of stress at plate boundaries that release accumulated energy by slipping or rupturing are known as faults. Elastic rebound occurs when the maximum point of supportable strain is reached and a rupture occurs, allowing the rock to rebound until the strain is relieved (Fig. 24-1). Usually the rock rebounds on both sides of the fault. The point of rupture is called the focus and may be located near the surface or deep below it. The point on the surface directly above the focus is termed the epicenter (Fig. 24-2).

The energy generated by an earthquake is not always released violently but can be small or gradual. Minor earth tremors are recorded daily in the United States, but whether

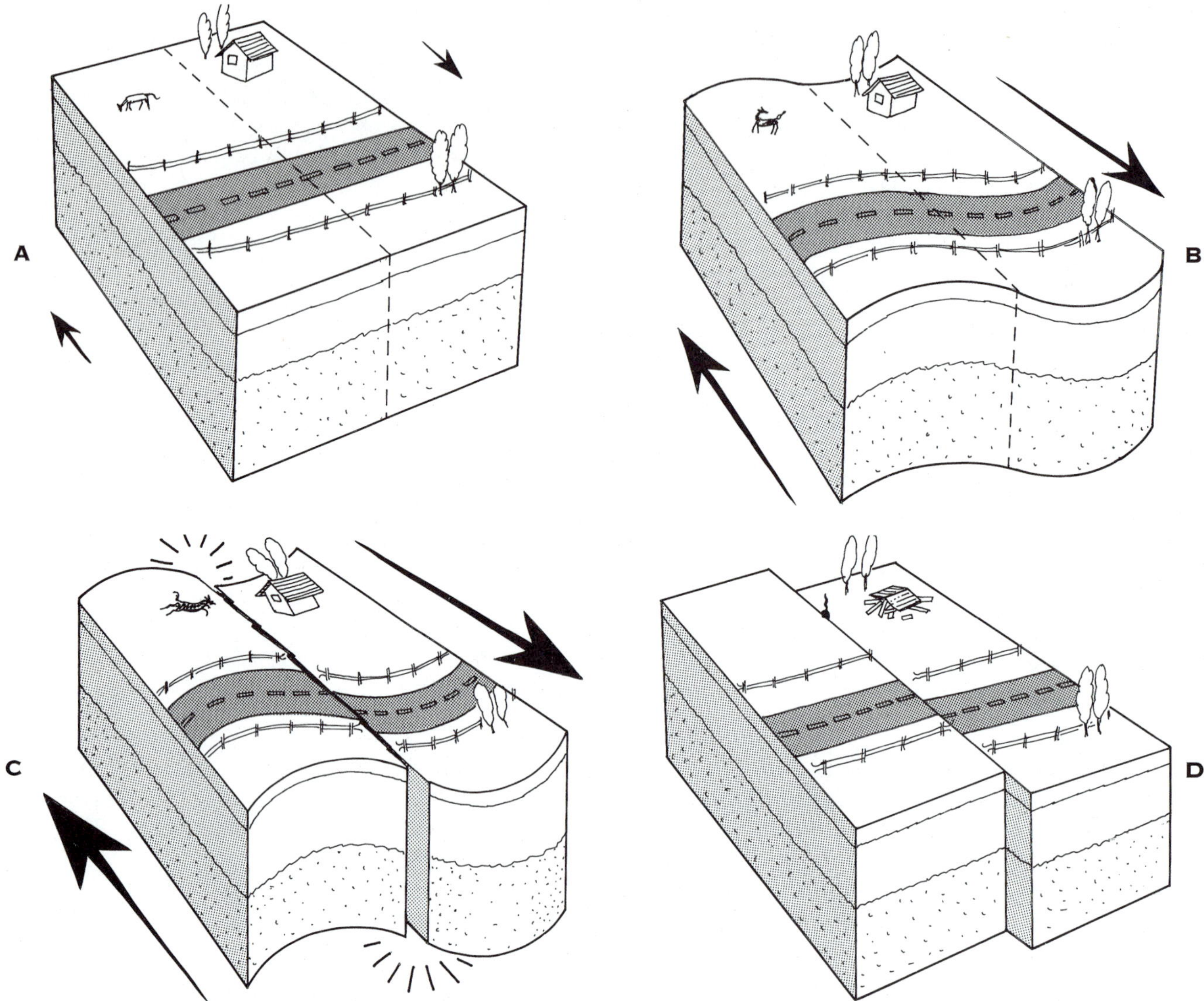

Fig. 24-1 Elastic rebound in earthquake. **A,** Forces build up over time. **B,** Crust deforms. **C,** Crust snaps. **D,** Plates slide.

they are caused by the same processes that relatively infrequently level a city is not known. Most damaging earthquakes seem to be associated with sudden ruptures of the crust.

Characteristics

The actual rupture process may last from a fraction of a second to a few minutes for a major earthquake. Seismic (from the Greek *seismos,* meaning shock or earthquake) waves are generated that last from less than a tenth of a second to nearly a minute and cause ground shaking. The seismic waves propagate in all directions, causing vibrations that damage vulnerable structures and infrastructure.

There are three types of seismic waves. The body waves (P, or primary, and S, or secondary) penetrate the body of the earth, vibrating fast (Fig. 24-3). P waves travel at about 24,000 kph and provide the initial jolt that causes buildings to vibrate in an up and down motion. S waves travel about 16,000 kph in a movement similar to the snap of a whip, causing a sharper jolt that vibrates structures from side to side and usually resulting in the most destruction. The third type of waves, surface waves, vibrate the ground horizontally and vertically and cause swaying of tall buildings, even at great distances from the epicenter.

Earthquake focus depth is an important factor in determining the characteristics of the waves. Shallow focus earthquakes are extremely damaging because of their proximity to the surface. The earthquake may be preceded by preliminary tremors and followed by aftershocks of decreasing intensity.

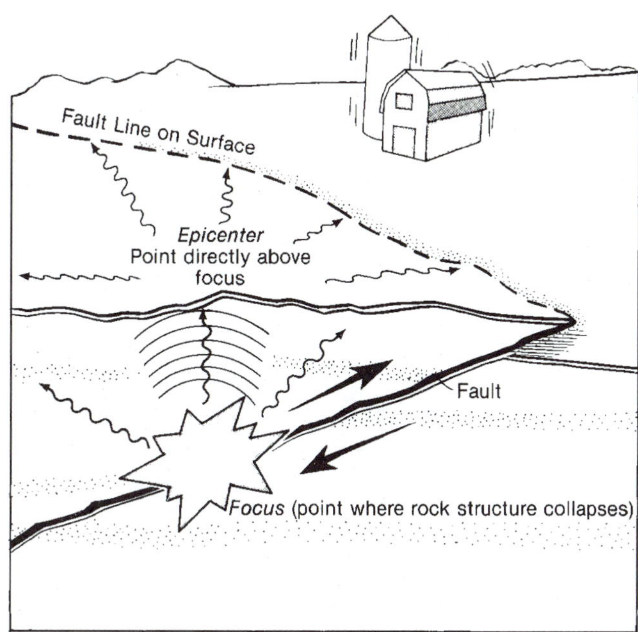

Fig. 24-2 Motion of the earth's plates causes increased pressure at faults where the plates meet. Eventually the rock structure collapses and movement occurs along the fault. Energy is propagated to the surface above and radiates outward. Waves of motion in the earth's crust shake landforms and buildings, causing damage. (Courtesy Disaster Management Center, University of Wisconsin.)

Measurement of Magnitude and Intensity

Earthquake magnitude, or amount of energy released, is determined by use of a seismograph, which records ground vibrations. The Richter scale mathematically adjusts the readings for the distance of the instrument from the epicenter. The Richter scale is logarithmic; an increase of one magnitude signifies a 10-fold increase in ground motion, or roughly 30 times the energy. Thus an earthquake with a magnitude of 7.5 releases 30 times more energy than one with 6.5 magnitude. The smallest quake to be felt by humans is of magnitude 3, while the largest quakes recorded under this system are from 8.8 to 8.9 in magnitude.

The earthquake intensity scale measures the effects of the earthquake where it occurs. The most widely used scale of this type is the modified Mercalli scale, which expresses the intensity of earthquake effects on people, structures, and the earth's surface in values from I to XII (see Box 24-1). Another, more explicit scale used in Europe is the Medvedev-Sponheuer-Karnik (MSK) scale.

Locations and Predictability

Most earthquakes (95%) occur in well-defined zones near the boundaries of the tectonic plates. These areas bordering the Pacific Ocean are called the circum-Pacific belt. Areas traversing the East Indies, the Himalayas, Iran, Turkey, and the Balkans are called the Alpide belt. Earthquakes also occur along the ocean trenches such as around the Aleutians, Tonga, Japan, and Chile and within the eastern Caribbean. Some earthquakes occur in the middle of the plates, possibly indicating where earlier plate boundaries might have been. These include the New Madrid earthquake in 1811 and the Charleston earthquake in 1816 in the United States, the Agadir earthquake in 1960 in Morocco, and the Koyna earthquake in 1967 in India.

Earthquake prediction was a constant preoccupation for early astrologers and prophets. Some signs noted by observers were buildings gently trembling, animals and birds becoming excited, and well water turning cloudy and smelling bad. These signs are still valid, although the behavior of animals might be ruled out as difficult to interpret. Reasonable risk assessments of potential earthquake activity can be made with confidence based on the following:

1. Knowledge of seismic zones or areas most at risk, gained through study of historical incidence and plate tectonics
2. Monitoring of seismic activity by use of seismographs and other instruments (the U.S. Geological Survey monitors 80 countries)
3. Use of community-based scientifically sound observations such as elevation and turbidity of water in wells and radon gas escape into well water

Earthquake Hazards

Earthquakes produce many direct and sometimes indirect effects. Landslides, flooding, and tsunamis are considered secondary hazards and are also discussed separately in this chapter.

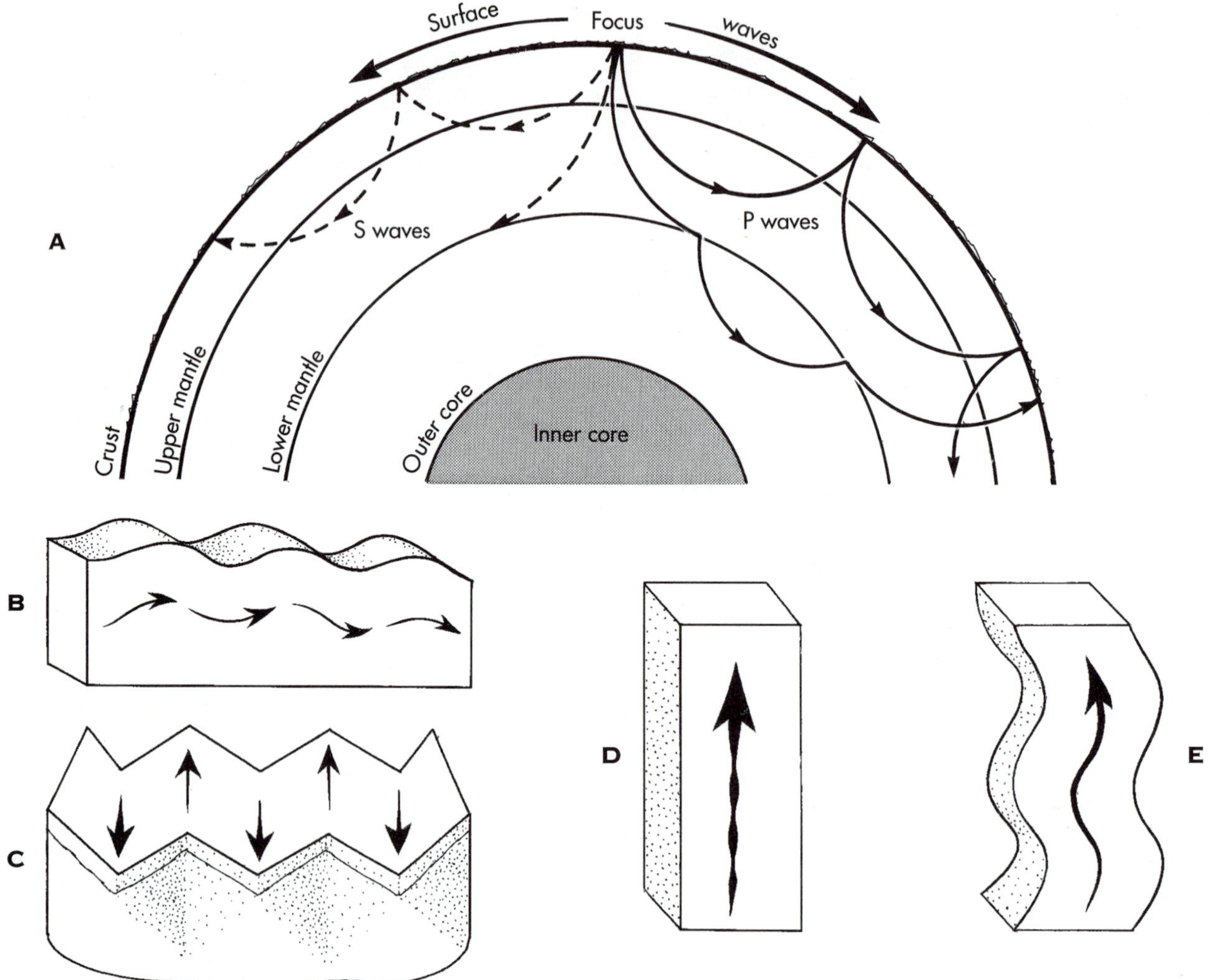

Fig. 24-3 **A,** Propagation of seismic waves in an earthquake. Surface waves vibrate the ground, **B** and **C,** horizontally and, **D** and **E,** vertically.

Fault Displacement and Ground Shaking. Fault displacement, either rapid or gradual, may damage foundations of buildings on or near the fault area or may displace the land, creating troughs and ridges. Ground shaking causes more widespread damage, particularly to the built environment. The extent of the damage is related to the size of the earthquake, the closeness of the focus to the surface, the buffering power of the area's rocks and soil, and the type of buildings being shaken. Aftershocks may cause further damage and may recur for weeks or even years after the initial event.

Ground Failure and Liquefaction. Seismic vibrations may cause settlement beneath buildings when soils consolidate or compact. Certain types of soil, such as alluvial or sandy soils, are more vulnerable to failure. Liquefaction is a type of ground failure that occurs when saturated soils lose strength and collapse or become liquefied. During the 1964 earthquake in Nigata, Japan, the ground beneath earthquake-resistant buildings became liquefied, causing the buildings to lean up to 45 degrees from the vertical. Most of these buildings were later jacked back into an upright position and reoccupied.

Lateral Spreads and Flow Failure. Lateral spreads involve the lateral movement of large blocks of soil as a result of liquefaction in a subsurface layer. Lateral spreads generally develop on gentle slopes with horizontal movement of 10 to 15 feet. However, where conditions are favorable and duration of ground shaking is extended, movements can be 100 to 150 feet. During the 1964 Alaska earthquake, more than 200 bridges were damaged or destroyed by lateral spreading of flood plain deposits toward river channels. In the 1906 San Francisco earthquake, a number of major pipelines were broken by lateral spreading, hampering efforts to fight fires that caused most of the damage to the city. In 1989, the Marina District in San Francisco, built on soft landfill, suffered damage from lateral spreading.

BOX 24-1

MODIFIED MERCALLI INTENSITY SCALE OF 1931

I Not felt except by a very few under especially favorable circumstances.

II Felt only by a few persons at rest, especially on upper floors of buildings. Delicately suspended objects may swing.

III Felt quite noticeably indoors, especially on upper floors of buildings, but many people do not recognize it as an earthquake. Standing motorcars may rock slightly. Vibration like passing of truck. Duration estimated.

IV During the day felt indoors by many. Outdoors by few. At night some awakened. Dishes, windows, doors disturbed; walls make creaking sound. Sensation like heavy truck striking building. Standing motor cars rocked noticeably.

V Felt by nearly everyone; many awakened. Some dishes, windows, etc., broken. A few instances of cracked plaster. Unstable objects overturned. Disturbances of trees, poles, and other tall objects sometimes noticed. Pendulum clocks may stop.

VI Felt by all; many frightened and run outdoors. Some heavy furniture moved; a few instances of fallen plaster or damaged chimneys. Damage slight.

VII Everybody runs outdoors. Damage negligible in buildings of good design and construction, slight to moderate in well-built ordinary structures, considerable in poorly built or badly designed structures. Some chimneys broken. Noticed by persons driving motor cars.

VIII Damage slight in specially designed structures, considerable in ordinary substantial buildings with partial collapse, great in poorly built structures. Panel walls thrown out of frame structures. Fall of chimneys, factory stacks, columns, monuments, and walls. Heavy furniture overturned. Sand and mud ejected in small amounts. Changes in well water. Persons driving motor cars disturbed.

IX Damage considerable in specially designed structures. Well-designed structures thrown out of plumb, greatly in substantial buildings with partial collapse. Buildings shifted off foundations. Ground cracked conspicuously. Underground pipes broken.

X Some well-built wooden structures destroyed. Most masonry and frame structures with foundations destroyed; ground badly cracked. Rails bent. Landslides considerable from river banks and steep slopes. Shifted sand and mud. Water splashed (slopped) over banks.

XI Few, if any, (masonry) structures remain standing. Bridges destroyed. Broad fissures in ground. Underground pipelines completely out of service. Earth slumps and land slips in soft ground. Rails bent greatly.

XII Damage total. Practically all works of construction are damaged greatly or destroyed. Waves seen on ground surface. Lines of sight and level are distorted. Objects are thrown upward into the air.

Flow failure, in which either a layer of liquefied soil rides on top of another or blocks of intact material ride on top of liquefied soil, can be catastrophic. Flow failures usually form in loose, saturated sands or silts on slopes greater than 3 degrees. They can originate either on land or underwater. Some of the most damaging flow failures have occurred underwater in coastal areas, carrying away large sections of port facilities and generating large sea waves. Some flow failures on land have been as much as a mile in length and breadth, such as those induced by the 1920 earthquake in Kansu, China, which killed 200,000 people.

Landslides. Slope instability may cause landslides during an earthquake. Steepness, weak soils, and presence of water may contribute to vulnerability from landslides. Liquefaction of soils on slopes may lead to disastrous slides. The most abundant types of earthquake-induced landslides are rock falls and rock slides, usually originating on steep slopes.

Flooding. Tsunamis may be generated by undersea or near-shore earthquakes and may break over the coastline with great destructive force. Other flooding may be caused by *seiches* (back and forth wave action in bays), or by failures in dams and levees.

Typical Adverse Effects of Earthquakes

Ground shaking can damage human settlements, buildings and infrastructure (particularly bridges), elevated railways, railways, water towers, water treatment facilities, utility lines, pipelines, electrical generating facilities, and transformer stations. Aftershocks can do a great deal of damage to already weakened structures. Significant secondary effects include fires, dam failures, and landslides, which may block waterways and cause flooding. Damage may occur to facilities using or manufacturing dangerous materials, resulting in chemical spills. Communications facilities may break down. Destruction of property may have a serious impact on shelter needs, economic production, and living standards of the affected community. Depending on their level of vulnerability, many people may be homeless in the aftermath of an earthquake.

The casualty rate is often high, especially when earthquakes occur in areas of high population density, particularly when streets between buildings are narrow, buildings are not earthquake resistant, or the ground is sloping and unstable; or where adobe or dry stone construction with heavy upper floors and roofs is common.

Casualty rates may be high when quakes occur at night because the preliminary tremors are not felt in sleep and people are not tuned in to receive media warning. In daytime, people are particularly vulnerable if in large unsafe structures such as schools and offices. Casualties generally decrease with distance from the epicenter. As a rule of thumb, quakes result in three times as many injured survivors as persons killed. The proportion of dead may be higher with major landslides and other secondary hazards. In areas where houses are of lightweight construction, especially with wood frames, casualties are generally much lower and earthquakes may occur regularly with no serious, direct effects on human populations.

The most widespread medical problems are fracture injuries. Other health threats may occur with secondary flooding (see "Floods"), when water supplies are disrupted (earthquakes can change levels in the water table) and contaminated water is used or water shortages exist, and where people are living in high-density relief camps, where epidemics may develop or food shortages exist.

TSUNAMIS

Tsunami is a Japanese word meaning harbor wave. Although tsunamis are sometimes called tidal waves, they actually have nothing to do with the tides. The waves originate from undersea or coastal seismic activity, landslides, and volcanic eruptions. They ultimately break over land with great destructive power, often affecting distant shores.

Causes and Characteristics

The geologic movements that cause a tsunami are produced in three major ways (Fig. 24-4). The foremost cause is fault movement on the sea floor, accompanied by an earthquake. The second most common cause is a landslide occurring underwater or originating above the sea and then plunging into the water. The highest tsunamis ever reported were produced by a landslide at Lituya Bay, Alaska, in 1958. A massive rock slide produced a wave that reached a high water mark of 1740 feet above the shoreline. A third cause of a tsunami is a submarine explosion from volcanic eruption.

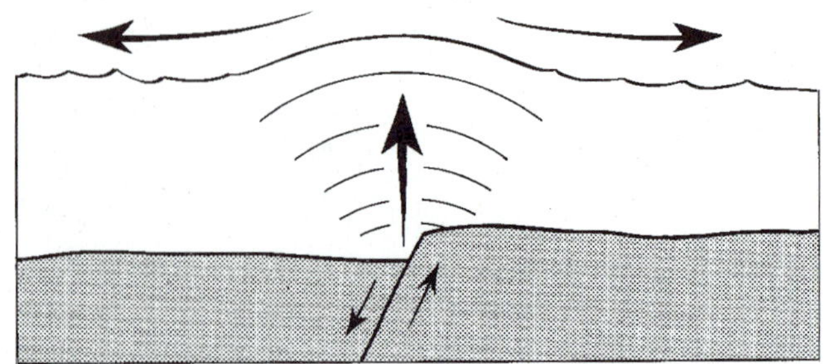

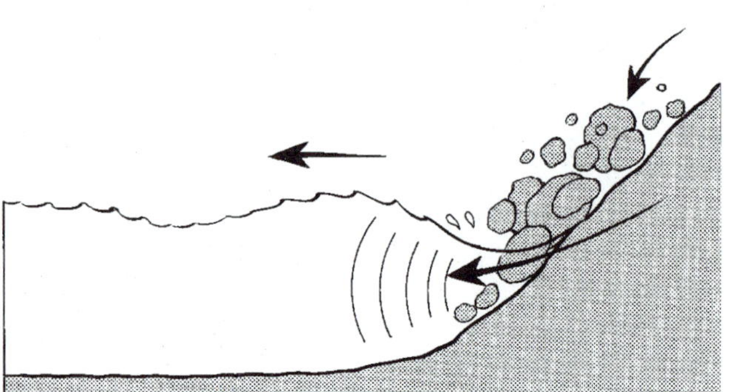

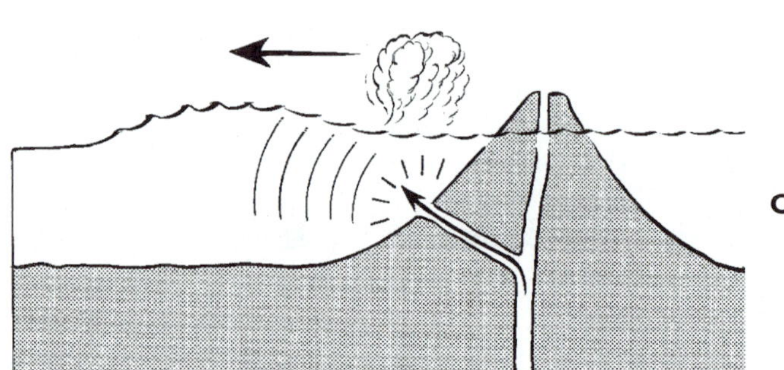

Fig. 24-4 Tsunamis are produced in three ways. **A,** Fault movement on the sea floor. **B,** Landslide. **C,** Submarine explosion from volcanic eruption.

Tsunami waves differ from ordinary deep ocean waves, which are produced by wind blowing over water. Normal waves are rarely longer than 300 m from crest to crest. Tsunami waves, however, may measure 150 km between successive wave crests. Tsunamis travel much faster than ordinary waves. Compared with normal wave speed of around 100 kph, tsunamis in the deep water of the ocean may travel at the speed of a jet airplane—800 kph! In spite of their speed, tsunamis increase the water height only 30 to 45 cm and often pass unnoticed by ships at sea. In 1946 a ship's captain on a vessel lying offshore near Hilo, Hawaii, claimed he could feel no unusual waves beneath him, although he saw them crashing on the shore.

Contrary to popular belief, the tsunami is not a single giant wave. It is possible for a tsunami to consist of 10 or more waves, termed a tsunami wave train. The waves follow each other in 5- to 90-minute intervals.

As tsunami waves approach the shore, they begin to change. The shape of the near-shore sea floor influences how tsunami waves will behave. Where the shore drops off quickly into deep water, the waves are smaller. Areas with long shallow shelves, such as the major Hawaiian islands, allow formation of very high waves. In the bays and estuaries, seiches where the water sloshes back and forth can amplify waves to some of the greatest heights ever observed.

As the waves approach shore, they travel progressively slower, finally decreasing to about 48 kph.

On shore, the initial sign of a tsunami depends on what part of the wave first reaches land; a wave crest causes a rise in the water level and a wave trough causes a recession. The rise may not be significant enough to be noticed by the general public. Observers are more likely to notice the withdrawal of water, which may leave fish floundering on the sea floor. A tsunami does not always appear as a vertical wall of water, known as a bore, as typically portrayed in drawings. More often, the effect is that of an incoming tide that floods the land. Normal waves and swells may ride on top of the tsunami wave, or the tsunami may roll across relatively calm inland waters.

The flooding produced by a tsunami may vary greatly from place to place over a short distance owing to a number of variables. These include submarine topography, shape of the shoreline, reflected waves, and modification of waves by seiches and tides. The Hilo tsunami of 1946, originating in the Aleutian Trench, produced 30-foot waves in one location and only half that height a few miles away. The sequence of the largest wave in the tsunami wave train also varies, and the destructiveness is not always predictable. In 1960 in Hilo, many people returned to their homes after two waves had passed, only to be swallowed up in a giant bore that in this case was the third wave.

Predictability. Tsunamis have occurred in all oceans and in the Mediterranean Sea, but the great majority of them occur in the Pacific Ocean, simply because the rim of the Pacific Ocean basin is the most geologically active region in the world. The zones stretching from New Zealand through East Asia, the Aleutians, and the western coasts of the Americas all the way to the South Shetland Islands are characterized by deep ocean trenches, explosive volcanic islands, and dynamic mountain ranges.

About 180 tsunamis were recorded between 1900 and 1970 in the Pacific. Of these, 35 caused casualties and damage only locally, while nine struck areas throughout the Pacific. A Tsunami Warning System (TWS) was developed in Hawaii shortly after the 1946 Hilo tsunami and is headquartered in the Pacific Warning Center in Honolulu, Hawaii. It has been improved and expanded and now consists of 62 tide stations, 77 seismic stations, and hundreds of points for dissemination of information. There are 24 member countries in the Pacific basin.

The TWS works by monitoring seismic activity from a network of seismic stations. A tsunami is almost always generated by an undersea earthquake of magnitude 7 or greater. Therefore special warning alarms sound when a quake measuring 6.5 or over occurs anywhere near the Pacific. A tsunami watch is declared if the epicenter is close enough to the ocean to be of concern. Government and voluntary agencies are then alerted and local media are activated to broadcast information. The five nearest tide stations monitor their gauges, and trained observers watch the waves. With positive indicators a tsunami warning is issued.

The TWS met with general success in saving lives during the tsunamis of 1952 and 1957 in Hawaii. In 1960, however, two major earthquakes occurring a day apart rocked the coast of Chile in South America. The first registered 7.5 on the Richter scale and produced a small but noticeable wave in Hilo Bay. The second registered a stunning 8.5, more than 30 times the energy of the first, and authorities predicted generation of a large, destructive tsunami. When the waves hit Hilo, 15 hours after the earthquake, not all of the public had taken the warnings seriously and 61 people were killed. About 7 hours later the tsunami struck Japan, killing 180. When information of conditions in Chile reached TWS, it was learned that three giant waves had destroyed villages along a 500-mile stretch of coastal South America, arriving only 15 minutes after the earthquake.

The Chilean government in recent years has experimented with use of satellite technology to provide nearly immediate warnings of potentially tsunamigenic earthquakes. Project THRUST (Tsunami Hazards Reduction Utilizing Systems Technology) can provide lifesaving tsunami hazard information in an average elapsed time of 2 minutes within its communication radius. In conjunction with this satellite communications network, historical data, model simulations, and emergency operations plans are used.

Factors Contributing to Vulnerability

The following major factors contribute to vulnerability to tsunamis:

1. Growing world population, increasing urban concentration, and larger investments in infrastructure, particularly on the coastal regions; some of these settlements and economic assets sit on low-lying coastal areas likely to be affected by tsunamis
2. Lack of tsunami-resistant buildings and site planning
3. Lack of a warning system or lack of sufficient education for the public to create awareness of the effects of a tsunami and unpredictable intensity; for example, having observed relatively moderate tsunamis in 1952 and 1957, citizens at Hilo in 1960 actually converged on the coast to watch the waves come in, with catastrophic results

Typical Adverse Effects

The force of water in a bore can raze everything in its path with pressures of up to 10,000 kg/m^2. The flooding effect of a tsunami, however, most greatly affects human settlements by water damage to homes and businesses, roads, and infrastructure.

Withdrawal of tsunami waves also causes significant damage. As the waves are dragged back toward the sea, bottom sediments are scoured out, collapsing piers and port facilities and sweeping out foundations of buildings. Entire beaches have disappeared and houses have been carried out to sea. Water levels and currents may change unpredictably, and boats of all sizes may be swamped, sunk, or battered.

Casualties and Public Health. Deaths occur principally from drowning, as water inundates homes or neighborhoods. Many people may be washed out to sea or crushed by the giant waves. Some injuries occur from battering by debris. Little evidence exists of tsunami flooding directly causing large-scale health problems. In some cases malaria mosquitoes may increase breeding owing to collection of water in trapped pools. Open wells and other groundwater may be contaminated by saltwater and debris or sewage. Normal water supplies may be inaccessible for days because of broken water mains.

Crops and Food Supplies. Flooding and damage by tsunami waves may result in the following:

1. The harvest may be lost, depending on time of year.
2. Land may be rendered infertile from saltwater incursion from the sea.
3. Food stocks not moved to high ground are damaged.
4. Animals not moved to high ground may perish.
5. Farm implements may be lost, hindering tillage.
6. Boats and fishing nets may be lost.

VOLCANIC ERUPTIONS

A volcano is a vent or chimney to the earth's surface from a reservoir of molten rock, called magma, deep in the crust of the earth. Approximately 600 volcanoes are active (have erupted in recorded history) in the world today, and many thousands are dormant (could become active again) or extinct (are not expected to erupt again). On average, about 50 volcanoes erupt every year. Since AD 1000 more than 300,000 people have been killed directly or indirectly by volcanic eruptions, and at present about 10% of the world's population lives on or near potentially dangerous volcanoes.

Volcanology, the study of volcanoes, has experienced a period of intensified interest following five major eruptions in the 1980s and early 1990s: Mt. St. Helens in the United States (1980); El Chichon in Mexico (1982); Galunggung in Indonesia (1982), Nevado del Ruiz in Colombia (1985), and Mt. Pinatubo in the Philippines (1991). Although the Mt. St. Helens eruptions were predicted with remarkable accuracy, predictive capability on a worldwide basis for more explosive eruptions has not been achieved. No recognized immediate precursors to the eruption of El Chichon were known. It caused the worst volcanic disaster in Mexico's history. Ineffective implementation and evacuation measures in spite of sufficient warnings resulted in more than 22,000 deaths from the eruption of Nevado del Ruiz. Galunggung erupted for 9 months, disrupting the lives of 600,000 people. Despite a major evacuation effort from Mt. Pinatubo, 320 people died mainly from collapse of ash-covered roofs. A study of these eruptions underscores the importance of predisaster geoscience studies, volcanic hazard assessments, volcano monitoring, contingency planning, and enhanced communications between scientists and authorities. The world's most dangerous volcanoes are in densely populated countries where only limited resources exist to monitor them.

Causal Phenomena

The basic ingredients for a volcanic eruption are magma and an accumulation of gases beneath an active volcanic vent, which may be either on land or below the sea. Magma is composed of silicates containing dissolved gases and sometimes crystallized minerals in a liquidlike suspension. Driven by buoyancy and gas pressure, the magma, which is lighter than surrounding rock, forces its way upward. As it reaches the surface, the pressures decrease, enabling the dissolved gases to effervesce, pushing the magma through the volcanic vent as they are released.

The chemical and physical composition of magma determines the amount of force with which a volcano erupts. Magmas that are less viscous allow gas to be released more easily. More viscous magma, perhaps containing a greater concentration of solid particles, may confine these gases longer, allowing greater pressures to build up. This greater pressure may lead to more violent eruptions.

Types of Volcanoes

Four types of volcanoes are illustrated in Fig. 24-5.

Cinder Cones. Cinder cones are built up from explosive eruptions that accumulate layers of pumice, ash, and other volcanic debris. They are relatively short (about 300 m from the base), have steep slopes, and usually have a crater at the top. The Paracutin volcano in Mexico came to life in 1943 after emitting steam from cracks in the soil of a farmer's cornfield. A violent earthquake followed. Sand and rocks piled up around the newly formed opening. After a series of explosions a crater formed and eventually lava flowed down the slopes. After the first day the cone was 37 m high. In 1 week it was 170 m high, and within 10 weeks it was 338 m and spread over hundreds of hectares. During 9 years of activity, about 260 square km were covered with ash, which destroyed a nearby town.

Composite Volcanoes. Composite volcanoes, or stratovolcanoes, are steep-sided, symmetric cones built of alternating layers of lava, ash, and cinders that may reach a height of about 2400 m. A conduit system within the volcano allows magma to rise to the surface. Some of the most scenic mountains in the world are composite volcanoes, such as Mt. Fujiyama in Japan, Mt. St. Helens in the United States, and Mt. Vesuvius in Italy. When the hardened plug at the volcano's throat is blasted out by the built-up pressure, it can be the most devastating type of volcanic eruption.

Shield Volcanoes. A shield volcano forms from consecutive deposits of lava spreading out in all directions over great distances from the central vent and creating a domelike shape resembling a warrior's shield. The slope on the flanks of the volcano is only a few degrees. Mauna Loa on the island of Hawaii is a magnificent shield volcano, rising 4207 m above

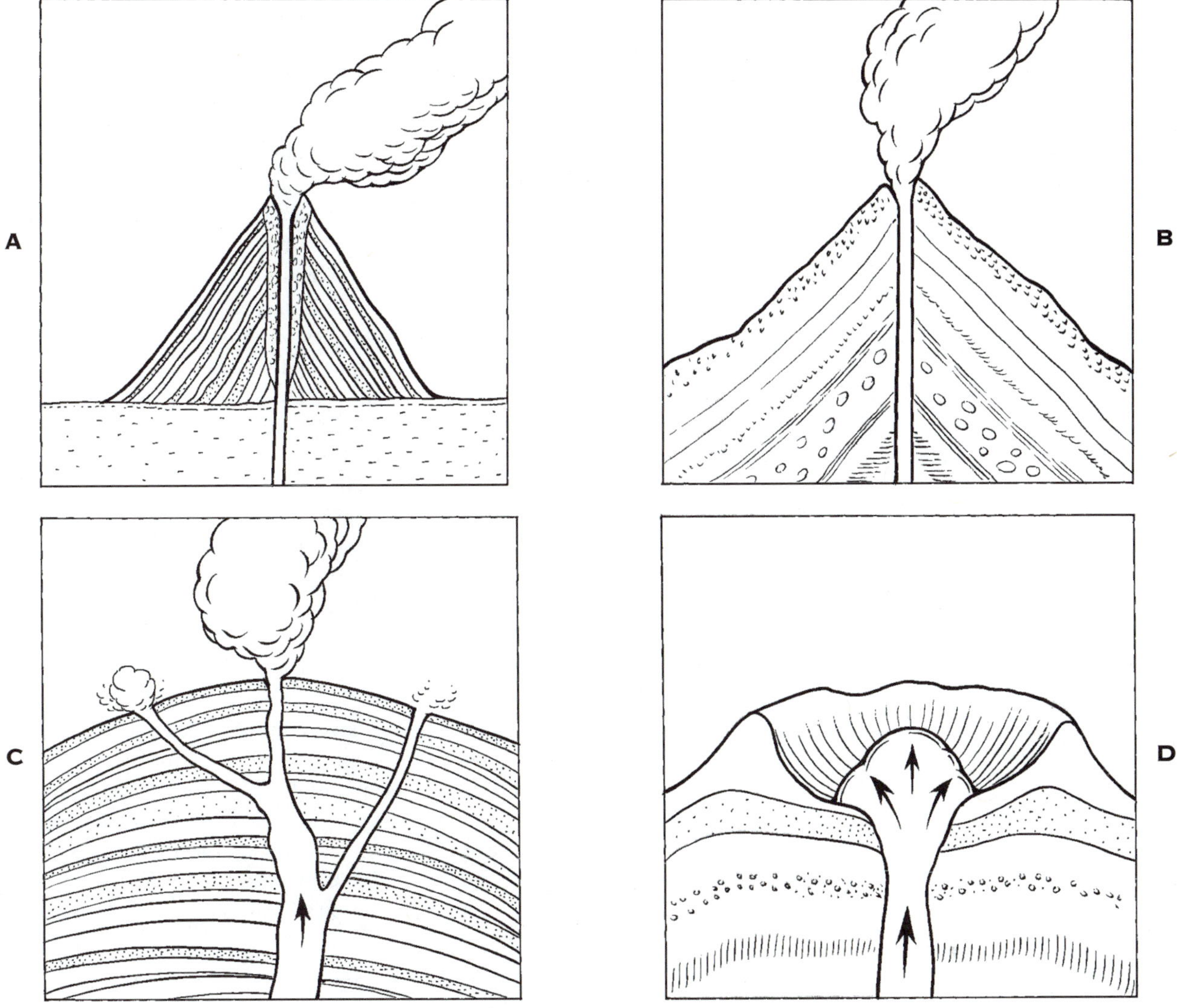

Fig. 24-5 Types of volcanoes. **A,** Cinder cone. **B,** Composite volcano. **C,** Shield volcano. **D,** Lava dome.

sea level. It is one of six volcanoes, including the submarine volcano Loihi, that are still in the process of building the Hawaiian Islands.

Lava Domes. Lava domes usually occur within the craters or on the flanks of large composite volcanoes. The lava is viscous and, instead of flowing, piles up and hardens around the vent, growing from within and ultimately exploding and fragmenting. Mt. Pelee in Martinique, West Indies, is an example of a lava dome.

General Characteristics of Volcanic Eruptions

The effects of volcanic eruptions on life and property vary with the type of material ejected and the extent of the deposits.

Ash Falls. Almost all volcanoes emit ash, but emissions vary widely in volume and intensity. Heavy ash falls can cause complete darkness or drastically reduce visibility. Fine material from great eruptions may travel around the world and affect world climate. Clouds of dust and ash can remain in the air for days or weeks and spread over large distances. Ash falls may occur with other eruptive phenomena, particularly pyroclastic flows, described in the next section. The majority of deaths from the Mt. Pinatubo eruption occurred when rains from a typhoon wetted the ash on rooftops, causing their collapse.

Pyroclastic Flows. Pyroclastic (meaning fire-broken in Greek) flows are the most dangerous of all volcanic phenomena because there is virtually no defense against them. They are horizontally directed explosions or blasts of gas containing ash and larger fragments in suspension. They travel at great speed and burn everything in their path. The flows move like a snow or rock avalanche because they contain a heavy load of dust and lava fragments that are denser than the surrounding air. Gas continues to be released as they travel, creating a continuously expanding cloud.

Various types of pyroclastic flows exist, but all are characterized by their high speed, mainly in a horizontal direction and at very high temperatures. The pyroclastic flows from the Mt. St. Helens eruption in 1980 moved at rates up to 870 kph, and pyroclastic deposits found 2 days after the blast at the foot of the mountain registered temperatures of more than 700° C. The greatest distance recorded by such flows in historical times is 35 km.

Volcanic Mudflows and Debris Flows (Lahars). Enormous quantities of ash and larger fragments, called tephra, accumulate after an eruption on the steep slopes of a volcano, sometimes to a depth of several meters. When mixed with water, the volcanic debris is transformed into a material that flows easily downhill, like wet concrete. *Lahar* is an Indonesian word for debris flows or mudflows. A primary debris flow is caused by eruptive activity such as melting of snow and ice by hot volcanic materials, and a secondary debris flow results when heavy rainfall saturates the deposits.

The rate of flow is affected by the volume of mud and debris, the viscosity, and the slope and character of the terrain. Velocity may reach 100 kph, and distance traveled may exceed 100 km. Mudflows and debris flows can be very destructive. They have buried entire towns, such as Armero, Colombia. They can silt up waterways, causing floods and changing river courses.

Lava Flows. Lava flows are formed by hot, molten lava flowing from a volcano and spreading over the surrounding countryside. Depending on the viscosity, a flow may move a few meters per hour. It is usually slow enough that living creatures can move to safety. Sometimes the edges break off, causing small hot avalanches.

Volcanic Gases. Gas is a product of every eruption and may also be emitted by the volcano during periods of inactivity, either intermittently or continually. Volcanic gas is composed mostly of steam, although often present are large amounts of toxic sulfur dioxide, hydrogen sulfide, and smaller but measurable amounts of toxic hydrochloric and hydrofluoric acid gases. Carbon dioxide is often a major component of volcanic gas and is an asphyxiant because it is much denser than air and tends to travel to and through low-lying areas and valleys. Several mountain climbers and skiers in Japan were overcome by hydrogen sulfide fumes in a valley near the Kusatsushirane volcano, and eventually an alarm system was installed. In 1986 nearly 1800 people were asphyxiated by gas bursts from crater lakes in Cameroon.

Tsunamis. Tsunamis, described previously, are generated by movement of the ocean floor possibly caused by a volcano. In a study of volcanic eruptions in the past 1000 years, human fatalities resulting from indirect tsunami wave hazards were as significant as those from pyroclastic flows and primary mudflows.

Location of Volcanoes

Volcanoes that have erupted in historical times are in clearly defined volcanic belts (Fig. 24-6). Like earthquakes, volcanoes are essentially plate boundary phenomena, indicating enormous geologic forces where tectonic or crustal plates exert forces on one another. Most volcanoes are in the Pacific Ocean, and half of these are in the western Pacific area. A large proportion of volcanoes occur in island arcs,

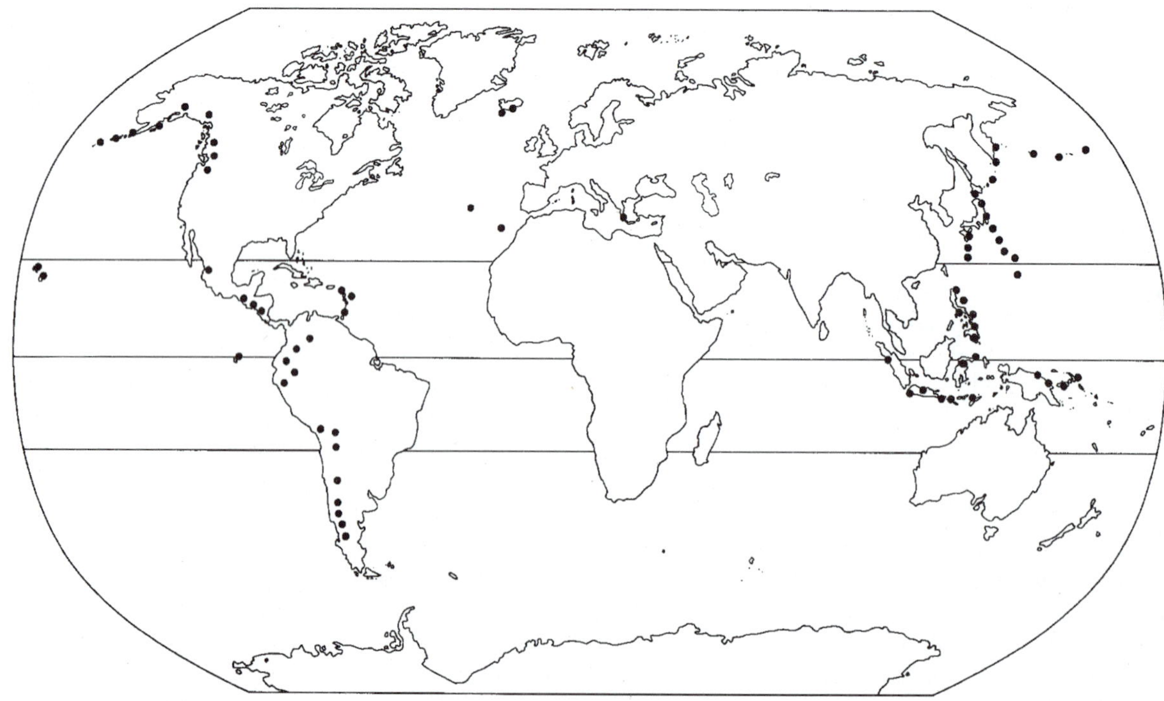

Fig. 24-6 Map of volcanic eruptions shows clearly defined volcanic belts.

the longest of which is the Aleutian Islands, extending more than 4762 km from Alaska to Asia. Other examples are Japan, the Philippines, Indonesia, New Hebrides, and Tonga. Each arc is associated with a deep ocean trench. The east coast of the Pacific is also the site of many volcanoes, ranging from the United States to Central and South America. Submarine volcanoes account for two thirds of the earth's volcanism, and while they cause few primary effects, they can be responsible for tsunamis and other earthquake-related phenomena.

In the Atlantic Ocean, volcanic activity is far less extensive and generally occurs in two locations: the midoceanic ridges and the West Indies. Rift volcanoes, such as those in Iceland and East Africa, account for about 15% of the known active volcanoes. Isolated regions of volcanic activity exist in about 100 places in the world. These mysterious hot spots lie deep within the interior and cause volcanoes in the plates moving above them, not necessarily on the plate boundary. Apparently the Hawaiian Islands were formed in sequence as the Pacific plate passed over a single hot spot.

Predictability

Systematic surveillance of volcanoes, begun early in this century at the Hawaiian Volcano Observatory, indicates that most eruptions are preceded by measurable geophysical and geochemical changes. Short-term forecasts within hours or months may be made through volcano monitoring techniques that include seismic monitoring, ground deformation studies, and observations and recordings of hydrothermal, geochemical, and geoelectrical changes. By carefully monitoring these factors, scientists were able to predict within hours 13 eruptions of Mt. St. Helens, which took place between June 1980 and December 1982.

The best basis for long-term forecasting (within a year or longer) of a possible eruption is through geologic studies of the past history of each volcano. Each past eruption has left records in the form of lava beds. These are deposits and layers of ash and tephra that can be studied to determine the extent of the flows and length of time between eruptions.

Problems in Eruption Forecasting and Prediction. While significant progress has been made in long-term forecasting of volcanic eruptions, monitoring techniques have not progressed to the point of yielding precise predictions. For the purposes of warning the public and avoiding false alarms that create distrust and chaos, ideal predictions should provide precise information concerning the place, time, type, and magnitude of the eruption. The remarkable monitoring of events at Mt. St. Helens and Mt. Pinatubo lends hope to future improvements in technique. However, these methods need to be tested at other volcanoes and for more explosive eruptions.

The greatest constraint to predictability is lack of baseline monitoring studies, which depict the full range of characteristics of the volcano. Interpretation of baseline data enables differentiation of the precursory pattern of an actual eruption from other volcanic activity, such as intrusion of magma under the surface, which is sometimes termed aborted eruption. Before the 1982 eruption of El Chichon, virtually nothing was known of its history of frequent and violent eruptions. No monitoring was conducted before or during the brief eruption.

Developing countries suffer the greatest economic losses from volcanic eruptions. More than 99% of eruption-caused deaths since 1900 have been in developing countries. Because of shortages of funds and trained personnel, monitoring is also poorest in these countries.

Factors Contributing to Vulnerability

Rich volcanic soils and scenic terrains attract people to settle on the flanks of volcanoes. These people are more vulnerable if they live downwind from the volcano, in the path of historical channels for mud or lava flows, or close to waterways likely to flood because of silting. Structures with roof designs that do not resist ash accumulation are vulnerable even miles from a volcano. All combustible materials are at risk.

Typical Adverse Effects

Casualties and Health. Deaths can be expected from pyroclastic and mud flows and to a much lesser extent from lava flows and toxic gases. Injuries may occur from impact of falling rock fragments and from being buried in mud. Burns to the skin, breathing passages, and lungs may result from exposure to steam and hot dust clouds. Ash fall and toxic gases may cause respiratory difficulties for people and animals. Nontoxic gases of densities greater than air, such as carbon dioxide, can be dangerous when they collect in low-lying areas. Water supplies contaminated with ash may contain toxic chemicals and cause illness. Deaths have also occurred indirectly from starvation and from tsunami waves.

Settlements, Infrastructure, and Agriculture. Complete destruction of everything in the path of pyroclastic, mud, or lava flows should be expected, including vegetation, agricultural land, human settlements, structures, bridges, roads, and other infrastructure. Structures may collapse under the weight of ash, particularly if the ash is wet. Falling ash may be hot enough to cause fires. Flooding may result from waterways filling up with volcanic deposits or from melting of large amounts of snow or glacial ice. Rivers may change course because of oversilting. Ashfall can destroy mechanical systems by clogging openings such as those in irrigation systems and airplane and other engines. Communication systems could be disrupted by electrical storms developing in the ash clouds. Transportation by air, land, and sea may be affected. Disruption in air traffic from large ash eruptions can have serious effects on emergency response.

Crops in the path of mud, pyroclastic, or lava flows are destroyed, and ashfall may render agricultural land temporarily unusable. Heavy ash loads may break the branches of fruit or nut trees. Livestock may suffer from inhaling toxic gases or ash. Ash containing toxic chemicals, such as fluorine, may contaminate the grazing lands.

LANDSLIDES

Landslides are a major threat each year to human settlements and infrastructure. "Landslide" is a general term covering a wide variety of landforms and processes involving the movement of soil and rock downslope under the influence of gravity. Although landslides may take place in conjunction with earthquakes, floods, and volcanoes, they are much more widespread and over time cause more property loss than any other geologic event.

Causal Phenomena

Landslides occur as a result of changes, either sudden or gradual, in the composition, structure, hydrology, or vegetation of a slope. These changes can be caused by the following:

1. Vibrations from earthquakes, blasting, machinery, traffic, and thunder; some of the most disastrous landslides have been triggered by earthquakes
2. Changes in water content caused by heavy rainfall and rises in groundwater levels
3. Removal of lateral support by erosion, previous slope failure, construction, excavation, deforestation, or loss of stabilizing vegetation
4. Loading with weight of rain, hail, snow, accumulation of loose rock or volcanic material, stockpiles of rock, waste piles, and weight of buildings and vegetation
5. Weathering and other physical or chemical actions that decrease strength of rocks and soils over time

Landslides in urban areas are often induced by human actions, such as interruption of water courses and a change in the water table or new construction involving "cut and fill" methods that disrupt slope stability.

General Characteristics

Landslides usually occur as secondary effects of heavy storms, earthquakes, and volcanic eruptions. The materials that compose landslides are divided into two classes: bedrock and soil (earth and organic matter debris). A landslide may be classified by its type of movement (Fig. 24-7).

Falls. A fall is a mass of rock or other material that moves downward by falling or bouncing through the air. These are most common along steep road or railroad embankments, steep escarpments, or steeply undercut cliffs, especially in coastal areas. Large individual boulders can cause significant damage.

Slides. Resulting from shear failure (slippage) along one or several surfaces, the slide material may remain intact or break up.

Topple. A topple is caused by overturning forces that rotate a rock out of its original position. The rock section may have settled at a precarious angle, balancing itself on a pivotal point from which it tilts or rotates forward. A topple may not involve much movement, and it does not necessarily trigger a rockfall or rock slide.

Lateral Spread. Large blocks of soil spread out horizontally by fracturing off the original base. Lateral spreads occur generally on gentle slopes, usually less than 6%, and typically spread 3 to 5 m but may move from 30 to 50 m where conditions are favorable. Lateral spreads usually break up internally and form numerous fissures and scarps. The process can be caused by liquefaction whereby saturated, loose sands or silts assume a liquefied state. A lateral spread is usually triggered by ground shaking (as with an earthquake). During the 1964 Alaskan earthquake, more than 200 bridges were damaged or destroyed by lateral spreading of floodplain deposits near river channels.

Flows. Flows move like a viscous fluid, sometimes very rapidly, and can cover several miles. Water is not essential for flows to occur; however, most flows form after periods of heavy rainfall. A mudflow contains at least 50% sand, silt, and clay particles. A lahar is a mudflow that originates on the slope of a volcano and may be triggered by rainfall, sudden melting of snow or glaciers, or water flowing from crater lakes. A debris flow is a slurry of soils, rocks, and organic matter combined with air and water. Debris flows usually occur on steep gullies. Very slow, almost imperceptible flows of soil and bedrock are called creeps. Over long periods of time, creeps may cause telephone poles or other objects to tilt downhill.

Landslide Predictability

The velocity of landslides varies from extremely slow (less than 0.06 m/year) to extremely fast (greater than 3 m/sec), which might imply a similar variation in predictability. In absolute terms, however, predicting the actual occurrence of a landslide is extremely difficult, although situations of high risk, such as forecasted heavy rainfall or seismic activity combined with landslide susceptibility, may lead to estimation of a time frame and possible consequences.

Estimation of landslide hazard potential includes historical information on the geology, geomorphology (study of landforms), hydrology, and vegetation of a specific area. Structural features that may affect stability include sequence and type of layering, lithologic changes, planes, joints, faults, and folds. The most important geomorphologic consideration in the prediction of landslides is the history of landslides in a given area.

The source, movement, amount of water, and water pressure must be studied. Climatic patterns combined with soil type may cause different types of landslides. For example, when monsoons occur in tropical regions, large debris slides of soils, rocks, and organic matter may occur. Plant cover on slopes may have either a positive or negative stabilizing effect. Roots may decrease water runoff and increase soil cohesion, or conversely may widen fractures in rock surfaces and promote infiltration.

Factors Contributing to Vulnerability

Settlements built on steep slopes, weak soils, or cliff tops, at the base of steep slopes, on alluvial outwash fans, or

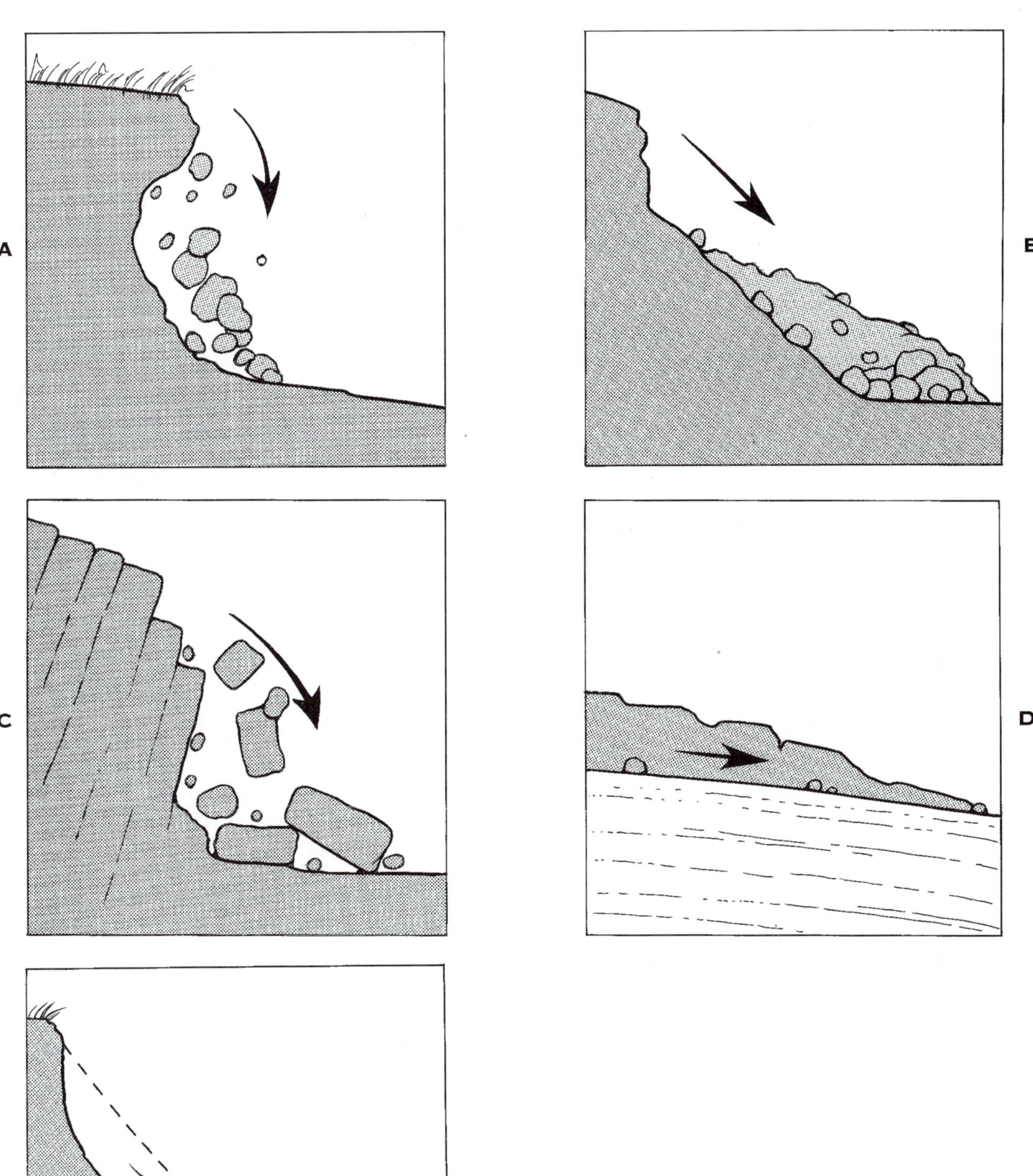

Fig. 24-7 Landslides classified by their type of movement. **A,** Fall. **B,** Slide. **C,** Topple. **D,** Lateral spread. **E,** Flow.

at the mouth of streams emerging from mountain valleys are all vulnerable. Roads and communication lines through mountainous areas are in danger. In most types of landslides, damage may occur to buildings even if foundations have been strengthened. Infrastructural elements, such as buried utility lines or brittle pipes, are vulnerable.

Typical Adverse Effects

Anything on top of or in the path of a landslide will be severely damaged or destroyed. In addition, rubble may damage lines of communication or block roadways. Waterways may be blocked, creating a flood risk. Casualties may not be widespread, except in the case of massive movements caused by major hazards such as earthquakes and volcanoes.

In addition to direct damage from a landslide, many indirect adverse effects occur. These include loss of productivity of agricultural or forest lands (if buried), reduced real estate values in high-risk areas and lost tax revenues from these devaluations, adverse effects on water quality in streams and irrigation facilities, and secondary physical effects, such as flooding.

Casualties. Fatalities have resulted from slope failure where population pressure has prompted settlement in areas vulnerable to landslides. Casualties may be caused by collapse of buildings or burial by landslide debris. Worldwide, approximately 600 deaths occur per year, mainly in the circum-Pacific region. The estimate for loss of life in the United States is 25 lives per year, greater than the average loss from earthquakes. Catastrophic landslides have killed many thousands of persons, such as the debris slide on the slopes of Huascaran in Peru triggered by an earthquake in 1970, which killed over 18,000 people. In January 1989, barely 6 weeks after an earthquake killed 25,000 people in Armenia, another quake struck the republic of Tadjikistan, 50 km southwest of the capital city of Dushanbe. This quake registered 5.8 on the Richter scale. The earthquake triggered a landslide of hillside soils that had become wet with melted snow. The liquefied soil spilled downhill and eventually covered an area about 8 km long and 1 km wide. The total volume of mud was more than 10 million m^3. The epicenter of the earthquake was located in the village of Sharora. This village and several others were engulfed with mud that killed 200 and left 30,000 homeless. Mud deposits reached a height of 25 m in Sharora, causing rescue efforts to be abandoned. Later the area was declared a national monument.

TROPICAL CYCLONES

The World Meteorological Organization (WMO) uses the generic term "tropical cyclone" to cover weather systems in which winds exceed "gale force" (minimum of 34 knots or 63 kph). Tropical cyclones are rotating, intense low-pressure systems of tropical oceanic origin. "Hurricane-force" (63 knots or 117 kph) winds mark the most severe type of tropical storm. They are called hurricanes in the Caribbean, the United States, Central America, and parts of the Pacific; typhoons in the northwest Pacific and east Asia; severe cyclonic storms in the Bay of Bengal; and severe tropical cyclones in south Indian, South Pacific, and Australian waters. For easy identification and tracking, the storms are generally given alternating masculine and feminine names, or numbers that identify the year and annual sequence.

Tropical cyclones are the most devastating of seasonally recurring rapid-onset natural hazards. Between 80 and 100 tropical cyclones occur around the world each year. Devastation by violent winds, torrential rainfall, and accompanying phenomena, including storm surges and floods, can lead to massive community disruption. In the last decade the official death toll in individual tropical cyclones reached 140,000 (Bangladesh, 1991), and damages approached $10 billion in Hurricane Gilbert (1988) and Hurricane Hugo (1989). The damages from Hurricane Andrew in Florida and Louisiana in 1992 totaled $16 billion.

Causal Phenomena

The development cycle of tropical cyclones may be divided into three stages: formation and initial development, full maturity, and modification or decay. Depending on their tracks over the warm tropical seas and proximity to land, they may last from less than 24 hours to more than 3 weeks (the average duration is about 6 days). Their tracks are naturally erratic but initially move generally westward, then progressively poleward into higher latitudes where they may make landfall, or into an easterly direction as they lose their cyclonic structure.

Formation and Initial Development Stage. Four atmospheric and oceanic conditions are necessary for development of a cyclonic storm (Fig. 24-8):

1. A warm sea temperature (greater than 26° C to a depth of 60 m) provides abundant water vapor in the air by evaporation.
2. High relative humidity (degree to which the air is saturated by water vapor) of the atmosphere to a height of about 7000 m facilitates condensation of water vapor into water droplets and clouds, releases heat energy, and induces a drop in barometric pressure.
3. Atmospheric instability (an above average decrease of temperature with altitude) encourages considerable vertical cumulus cloud convection when condensation of rising air occurs.
4. A location of at least 4 to 5 latitude degrees from the equator allows the influence of the forces as the earth's rotation (Coriolis force) takes effect and induces cyclonic wind circulation around a low-pressure center.

The atmosphere can usually organize itself into a tropical cyclone in 2 to 4 days. This process is characterized by increasing thunderstorms and rain squalls at sea. Meteorologists can monitor these processes with weather satellites and radar from as far as 400 miles away from the storm. The

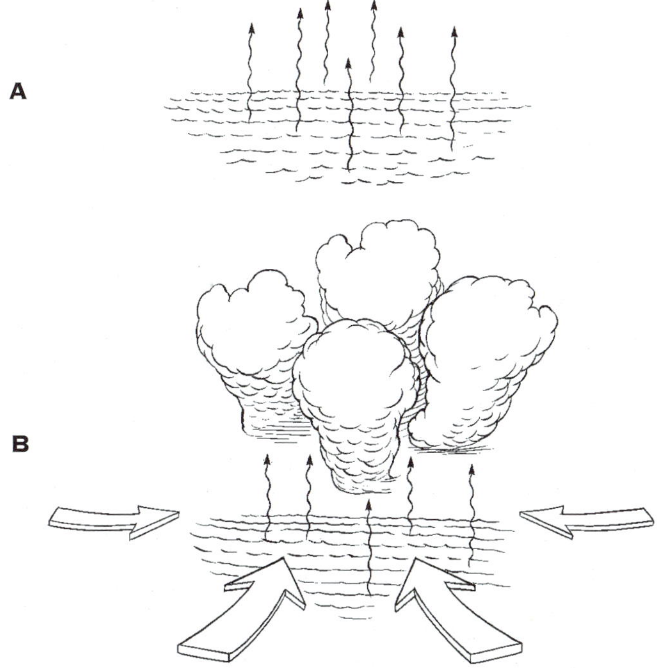

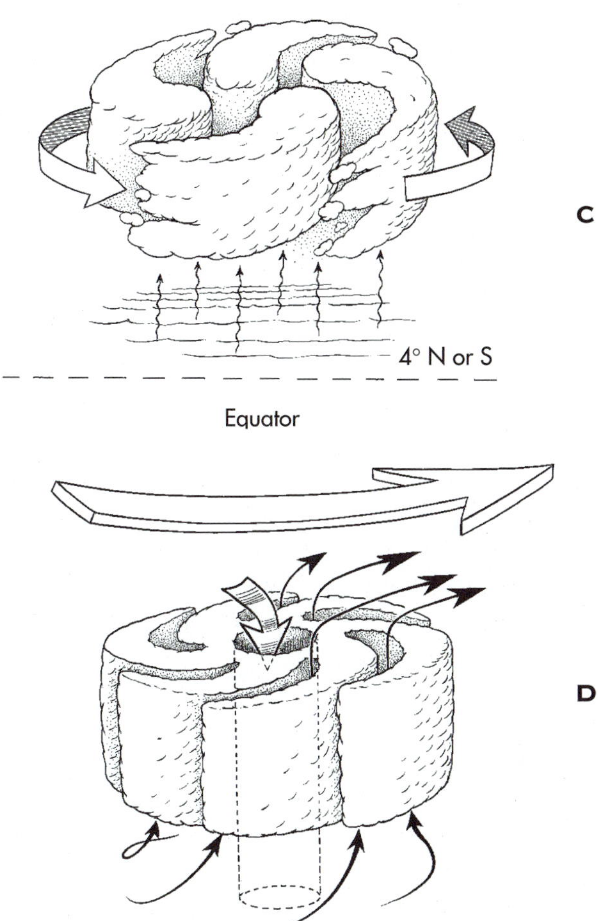

Fig. 24-8 Cyclone formation. **A,** Warm seas (greater than 26° C) cause rising humid air. **B,** Cooler high-altitude temperatures cause formation of cumulonimbus clouds. The surrounding air moves toward the central low-pressure area. **C,** Cumulonimbus clouds form into spiraling bands. The Coriolis effect causes winds to swirl around the central low-pressure area. **D,** High altitude dispels the top of the cyclonic air system. Dry high-altitude air flows down the "eye." Hurricane force winds circle around the eye.

existence of favorable conditions for cyclone development determines the cyclone season for each monitoring center. In the Indian and south Asian region the season is divided into two periods, from April to early June and from October to early December. In the Caribbean and United States, tropical storms and hurricanes reach their peak strengths in middle to late summer. In the Southern Hemisphere, the cyclone season extends from November to April or May, but occasionally cyclones occur in other months in lower latitudes.

Mature Tropical Cyclones. As viewed by weather satellites and radar imagery, the main physical feature of a mature tropical cyclone is a spiral pattern of highly turbulent giant cumulus thundercloud bands. These bands spiral inward and form a dense, highly active central cloud core that wraps around a relatively calm and cloud-free "eye." The eye typically has a diameter of 20 to 60 km in which light winds occur and looks like a black hole or dot surrounded by white clouds.

In contrast to the light wind conditions in the eye, the turbulent cloud formations extending outward from the eye accompany winds of up to 250 kph, sufficient to destroy or severely damage most nonengineered structures in the affected communities. These strong winds are caused by a horizontal temperature gradient that exists between the warm core of the cyclone (up to 10° C higher than the external environment) and the surrounding areas, and results in a correspondingly high pressure gradient.

Weakening Stage of a Tropical Cyclone. A tropical cyclone begins to weaken in terms of its central low pressure, internal warm core, and extremely high winds as soon as its sources of warm moist air begin to ebb or are abruptly cut off. This would occur during landfall, by movement into higher latitudes, or through influence of another low-pressure system. The weakening of a cyclone does not mean that danger to life and property is over. When the cyclone hits land, especially over mountainous or hilly terrain, widespread riverine and flash flooding may last for weeks. The energy from a weakening tropical cyclone may be reorganized into a less concentrated but more extensive storm system causing widespread violent weather.

General Characteristics

Tropical cyclones are characterized by their destructive winds, storm surges, and exceptional level of rainfall, which may cause flooding.

Destructive Winds. The strong winds generated by a tropical cyclone circulate clockwise in the Southern Hemisphere and counterclockwise in the Northern Hemisphere, while spiraling inward and increasing toward the cyclone center. Wind speeds progressively increase toward the core as follows:

1. 150 to 300 km from the center of a typical mature cyclone, winds of 63 to 88 kph
2. 100 to 150 km from the center, storm force winds of 89 to 117 kph
3. 50 to 100 km from the center, winds in excess of hurricane force, 117 kph or greater
4. 20 to 50 km from the center, the edge of the inner core contains winds 250 kph or greater

As the eye arrives, winds fall off to become almost calm, but rise again just as quickly as the eye passes and are replaced by hurricane force winds from a direction nearly the reverse of those previously blowing.

The Beaufort scale is used to classify the intensity of the storms. It estimates the wind velocity by observations of the effects of winds on the ocean surface and familiar objects. Both the United States (Saffir-Simpson Potential Hurricane Damage Scale) (see Box 24-2) and Australia (Cyclone Severity Categories) use country-specific scales that estimate potential property damage in five categories. The Philippines recently increased its typhoon warning signal numbers from three ranges of wind speeds to four in order to take into account the lower standards of building structures and regional variations.

BOX 24-2

SAFFIR-SIMPSON HURRICANE SCALE

SCALE NO. 1

Winds of 74 to 95 mph. Damage primarily to shrubbery, trees, foliage, and unanchored mobile homes. No real damage to other structures. Some damage to poorly constructed signs. And/or storm surge 4 to 5 feet above normal. Low-lying coastal roads inundated, minor pier damage, some small craft in exposed anchorage torn from moorings.

SCALE NO. 2

Winds of 96 to 100 mph. Considerable damage to shrubbery and tree foliage; some trees blown down. Major damage to exposed mobile homes. Extensive damage to poorly constructed signs. Some damage to roofing materials of buildings; some window and door damage. No major damage to buildings. And/or storm surge 6 to 8 feet above normal. Coastal roads and low-lying escape routes inland cut by rising water 2 to 4 hours before arrival of hurricane center. Considerable damage to piers. Marinas flooded. Small craft in unprotected anchorages torn from moorings. Evacuation of some shoreline residences and low-lying island areas required.

SCALE NO. 3

Winds of 111 to 130 mph. Foliage torn from trees; large trees blown down. Practically all poorly constructed signs blown down. Some damage to roofing materials of buildings; some window and door damage. Some structural damage to small buildings. Mobile homes destroyed. And/or storm surge of 9 to 12 feet above normal. Serious flooding at coast and many smaller structures near coast destroyed; larger structures near coast damaged by battering waves and floating debris. Low-lying escape routes inland cut by rising water 3 to 5 hours before hurricane center arrives. Flat terrain 5 feet or less above sea level flooded inland 8 miles or more. Evacuation of low-lying residences within several blocks of shoreline possibly required.

SCALE NO. 4

Winds of 131 to 155 mph. Shrubs and trees blown down; all signs down. Extensive damage to roofing materials, windows, and doors. Complete failure of roofs on many small residences. Complete destruction of mobile homes. And/or storm surge 13 to 18 feet above normal. Flat terrain 10 feet or less above sea level flooded inland as far as 6 miles. Major damage to lower floors of structures near shore due to flooding and battering by waves and floating debris. Low-lying escape routes inland cut by rising water 3 to 5 hours before hurricane center arrives. Major erosion of beaches. Massive evacuation of all residences within 500 yards of shore possibly required, and of single-story residences on low ground within 2 miles of shore.

SCALE NO. 5

Winds greater than 155 mph. Shrubs and trees blown down; considerable damage to roofs of buildings; all signs down. Very severe and extensive damage to windows and doors. Complete failure of roofs on many residences and industrial buildings. Extensive shattering of glass in windows and doors. Some complete building failures. Small buildings overturned or blown away. Complete destruction of mobile homes. And/or storm surge greater than 18 feet above normal. Major damage to lower floors of all structures less than 15 feet above sea level within 500 yards of shore. Low-lying escape routes inland cut by rising water 3 to 5 hours before hurricane center arrives. Massive evacuation of all residential areas on low ground within 5 to 10 miles of shore possibly required.

From National Oceanic and Atmospheric Administration: *Tropical cyclones of the North Atlantic Ocean, 1871-1977,* Asheville, NC, 1978, National Climatic Center, p 25.

Storm Surges. The storm surge, defined as the rise in sea level above the normally predicted astronomic tide, is frequently a key or overriding factor in a tropical storm disaster. As the cyclone approaches the coast, the friction of strong on-shore winds on the sea surface, in combination with the "suction effect" of reduced atmospheric pressure, can pile up the seawater along a coastline near a cyclone's landfall well above the predicted tide level for that time. In cyclones of moderate intensity, the effect is generally limited to several meters, but in the case of exceptionally intense cyclones, storm surges of up to 8 m can result.

Of the countries experiencing cyclonic storms, those most vulnerable to storm surges are those with low-lying land along the closed and semienclosed bays facing the ocean. These countries include Bangladesh, China, India, Japan, Mexico, the United States, and Australia. Prevailing on-shore winds and low pressures from winter depressions in nontropical latitudes, as in countries bordering the North Sea, are also subject to storm surges that require substantial mitigation measures, such as dykes.

Exceptional Rainfall Occurrences. The world's highest rainfall totals over 1 to 2 days have occurred during tropical cyclones. The highest 12- and 24-hour totals, 135 cm and 188 cm, respectively, have both occurred during cyclones at La Reunion Island in the southwestern Indian Ocean. The very high specific humidity condenses into exceptionally large raindrops and giant cumulus clouds, resulting in high precipitation rates. When a cyclone makes landfall, the rain rapidly saturates even dry catchment areas and rapid runoff may explosively flood the usual water courses as it creates new ones.

The relationship between rainfall and wind speed is not always proportional. For instance, if the atmosphere over land is already saturated with moisture, rainfall will be strongly enhanced and the cyclone will weaken slowly. If the atmosphere is dry, the rainfall will be greatly reduced and the cyclone will decay faster. Thus landfall of even a relatively weak tropical cyclone may result in extensive flooding.

Predictability

Tropical cyclones form in all oceans of the world except the South Atlantic and South Pacific east of 140° W longitude. Nearly one quarter form between 5° and 10° latitude of the equator and two thirds between 10° and 20° latitude. It is rare for a tropical cyclone to form south of 20° to 22° latitude in the Southern Hemisphere; however, they occasionally form as far north as 30° to 32° in the more extensive warmer water of the Northern Hemisphere. They are mainly confined to the warmer 6 months of the year but have occurred in every month in the western North Pacific.

The locations, frequencies, and intensities of tropical cyclones are well known from historical observations and, more recently, from routine satellite monitoring. Tropical cyclones do not follow the same track except coincidentally over short distances. Some follow linear paths, others recurve in a symmetric manner, and still others accelerate or slow down and seem stationary for a time. For this reason, predicting when, where, and if a storm will hit land is often difficult, especially with islands. In general, the difficulty in forecasting increases from lower to higher latitudes, while the margin of error in determining the cyclone center decreases as landfall approaches.

Special warning and preparedness strategies for evacuation from offshore facilities or closure of industrial plants must be worked out relating the costs and benefits of those strategies against the uncertainties of precision in the forecasts. For general community purposes that require a minimum 12 hours of preparedness time, the imprecision in forecasting the location of landfall within 24 hours should be generally tolerable, bearing in mind that highly adverse cyclonic weather usually commences about 6 hours before landfall of the cyclone.

Regrettably, progress in reducing forecasting errors has remained slow in the last two decades despite huge investments in monitoring systems. However, substantial progress has been made in the organization of warning and dissemination systems, particularly through regional cooperation. The activities of national meteorologic services are coordinated at the international level by the World Meteorological Organization (WMO). Forecasts and warnings are prepared within the framework of the WMO's World Weather Watch (WWW) program. Under this program, meteorologic observational data are provided nationally, and data from satellites and information provided by the regional centers are exchanged around the world.

The WWW system includes 8500 land stations, 5500 merchant ships, aircraft, special ocean weather ships, automatic weather stations, and meteorologic satellites. A tropical cyclone is first identified and then followed from satellite pictures. A complex Global Telecommunications System relays the observations. Ultimately, however, the responsibility for providing forecasts and warnings to the local population regarding tropical cyclones and the associated winds, rains, and storm surges falls upon the national services. Unfortunately, many of the less developed countries, where most deaths from tropical cyclones occur, do not possess state-of-the-art warning systems.

Factors Contributing to Vulnerability

Human settlements located in exposed, low-lying coastal areas are vulnerable to the direct effects of a cyclone, such as wind, rain, and storm surges. Settlements in adjacent areas are vulnerable to floods and mudslides or landslides from the resultant heavy rains. The death rate is higher where communications systems are poor and warning systems are inadequate.

The quality of structures determines resistance to the effects of the cyclone. Those most vulnerable are lightweight structures with wood frames, older buildings with weakened walls, and houses made of unreinforced concrete block (Fig. 24-9). Infrastructural elements particularly at risk are telephone and telegraph poles, fishing boats, and other maritime industries.

Typical Adverse Effects

Structures are damaged and destroyed by wind force, through collapse from pressure differentials, and by flooding, storm surge, and landslides. Standing crops may be lost to floods, storm surges, and seawater salinity. Salt from storm surges may also be deposited on agricultural lands and increase groundwater salinity. Fruit, nut, or lumber trees may be damaged or destroyed by winds, flood, or storm surges. Plantation-type crops such as bananas are extremely vulnerable. Erosion can occur from flooding and storm surges.

Casualties and Public Health. Relatively few casualties occur because of the high winds in cyclonic storms. Storm surges may cause many deaths, but usually few injuries among survivors. Because of flooding and possible contamination of water supplies, malaria and other viruses may be prevalent several weeks after the flooding.

Water Supplies. Open wells and other groundwater supplies may be temporarily contaminated by flood waters and storm surges. They are considered contaminated by pathogenic organisms only if dead bodies of people or animals are lying in the sources or if sewage is swept in. Normal water sources may be unavailable for several days.

Crops and Food Supplies. The combination of high winds and heavy rains, even without flooding, can ruin standing crops and tree plantations. Food stocks may be lost or contaminated if the structures in which they were held have been destroyed or inundated. Food shortages may occur until the next harvest. Tree and food crops may be blown down or damaged and must be harvested prematurely.

Communications and Logistics. Communications may be severely disrupted as telephone lines, radio antennas, and satellite disks are brought down, usually by wind. Roads and railroad lines may be blocked by fallen trees or debris, and aircraft movements may be curtailed for at least 12 to 24 hours after the storm. Modes of transportation such as trucks, carts, and small boats may be damaged by wind or flooding. The cumulative effect of all damage is to impede information gathering and transport networks.

Preparedness Measures in India

Tropical cyclones struck the same coastal areas of the Indian state of Andhra Pradesh in 1978 and 1990. On the

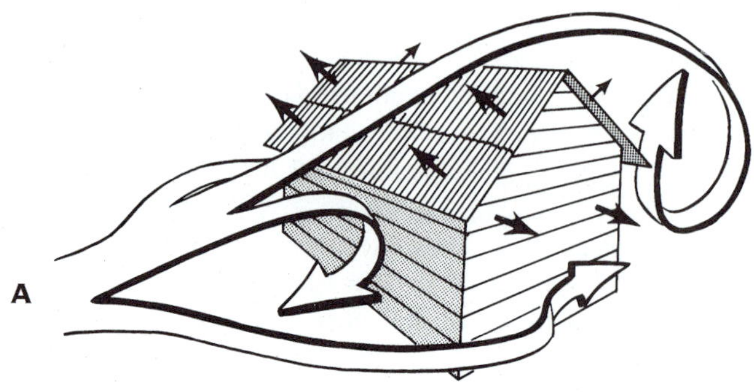

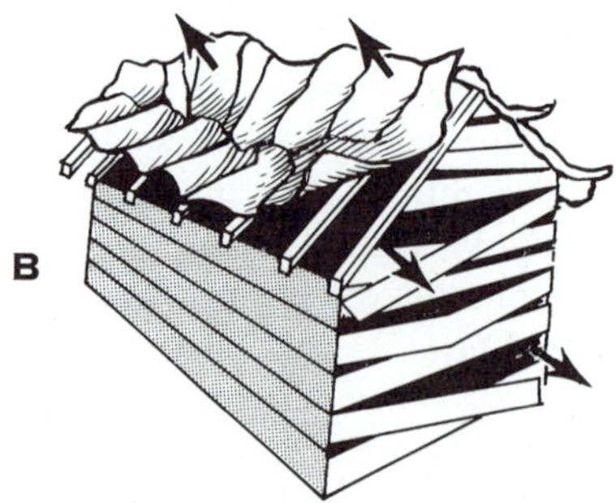

Fig. 24-9 How high winds damage buildings. **A,** Wind blowing into a building is slowed at the windward face, creating high pressure. The airflow separates as it spills around the building, creating low pressure or suction at the end walls, roof, and leeward walls. **B,** The roof may lift off and the walls blow out if there is not special reinforcement to the structure. (Courtesy Disaster Management Center, University of Wisconsin.)

first occasion about 10,000 perished. In 1990, despite significant increases in population, fewer than 1000 died. What factors made the critical difference?

A program of improved monitoring and warning dissemination had been developed by the Indian government. This included use of a domestic satellite, an upgraded cyclone contingency preparedness plan, and enhanced community awareness. Widespread evacuation procedures were initiated by the state counter-disaster committee 48 hours ahead of forecasted landfall. A total of 651,865 people were evacuated from 546 villages to 1098 emergency relief camps by 2019 evacuation teams using 745 transport vehicles. People had also been instructed by the media to go to the camps before the commencement of the cyclonic weather.

TORNADOES

Tornadoes are the most dramatic example of a class of storms, often called severe local storms, which includes thunderstorms and hailstorms. Severe local storms a few miles to a few tens of miles in diameter are often accompanied by unusually strong, gusty winds that can cause severe damage, by heavy local rain that can cause flash floods, and by lightning, hail, and sometimes tornadoes. These intense vortices may be only a few hundred feet in diameter but can contain winds in excess of 300 mph, capable of tearing roofs off houses and lifting houses, trees, and vehicles hundreds of feet through the air. Tornadoes have been known to occur in swarms, with as many as several dozen affecting an area of hundreds of thousands of square miles in a single day.

Causal Phenomena

Tornadoes and other severe local storms result from intense, local atmospheric instability, usually caused by solar heating of the earth's surface, which causes intense convective columns. A tornado is an intense vortex in which air spirals inward and upward. It is frequently, but not always, visible as a funnel cloud hanging part or all of the way from the generating storm to the ground. The upper portion of the funnel consists of water droplets, while the lower portion usually consists of dust and soil being sucked up from the ground. The funnel size may range from a few meters to a few hundred meters in diameter and from 10 m to several kilometers high. The funnel may undergo changes in appearance during the tornado's lifetime. There may be a single well-defined funnel, multiple funnels, or funnels that appear to consist of several ropelike strands. Tornadoes may be as loud as the roar of a freight train.

Tornadoes are the most violent event associated with thunderstorms. They occur in many parts of the world but are most frequent and fierce in the United States. As many as 1000 may strike the United States each year, mostly in the central plains and southeastern states, although they have occurred in every state, mostly in the spring and summer. Of all the natural hazards in the United States, thunderstorms with associated winds, rain, hail, lightning, and tornadoes rank first in number of deaths, second in number of injuries, and third in property damage.

The most common type of tornado is small and lasts only a minute or two, causing minor damage over a track often less than 300 feet wide and 1 to 2 miles long. Most tornado-related deaths, injuries, and property damage are caused by relatively infrequent, large, and long-lasting tornadoes whose paths may be more than 1 mile wide and more than 100 miles long over a period of several hours.

Predictability

Although conditions favorable to tornado formation can often be predicted a number of hours in advance, the areas in which these conditions are found may cover hundreds of thousands of square miles. It is impossible to predict where individual tornadoes will occur. When a warning is issued, a tornado has already formed and the threatened population may have only a few minutes to take cover. In the United States, when tornadoes are considered likely within a well-defined region, a tornado watch is issued. When a tornado is actually detected, either visually or on radar, a tornado warning is issued.

Factors Contributing to Vulnerability

Most injuries from tornadoes are caused by flying or falling debris, usually from destroyed structures. The quality of structures will determine resistance to the effects of the cyclone. Those most vulnerable are lightweight structures with wood frames, older buildings with weakened walls, mobile homes, and houses made of unreinforced concrete blocks. Thorough education regarding taking shelter from flying debris is essential to reduce deaths and injuries.

Examples of Tornado Outbreaks

In March 1925 a tornado struck Missouri, Illinois, and Indiana, killing 689 people. On April 11, 1965, an outbreak of at least 37 tornadoes struck Iowa, Wisconsin, Illinois, Indiana, Michigan, and Ohio, killing 271 people, injuring more than 3000, and causing $300 million in damage. On April 3 and 4, 1974, an outbreak of 147 tornadoes struck Illinois, Indiana, Michigan, Ohio, West Virginia, Virginia, Kentucky, Tennessee, North Carolina, South Carolina, Georgia, and Alabama, killing 335 people, injuring more than 5500, affecting more than 27,000 households, and causing more than $600 million in damage. More than half the deaths were caused by less than 5% of the tornadoes. The worst of these struck Xenia, Ohio. It cut a swath of destruction half a mile wide and 16 miles long, killed 34 people, injured 1150, and damaged or destroyed 2400 homes. On May 31, 1985, 43 tornadoes struck Ohio, Pennsylvania, New York, and southern Ontario, killing 87 people.

FLOODS

Throughout history, people have been attracted to the fertile lands of the floodplains, where their lives have been made easier by virtue of proximity to sources of food and water. Ironically, the same river or stream that provides sustenance to the surrounding population also renders humans vulnerable to disaster by periodic flooding. Floods can arise from abnormally heavy precipitation, dam failures, rapid snow melts, river blockages, or even burst water mains. Flood disasters are second only to droughts in the total number of people affected worldwide. Flood disasters, however, are more numerous than droughts, and their number is increasing. While flooding is considered a natural process, it is greatly exacerbated today by farming, deforestation, urbanization, and poor management of watershed areas.

Every year in Bangladesh, large tracts of land are submerged during the monsoon season, a normally beneficial process that deposits a rich layer of alluvial soil. The floods originate from three great river systems in the Himalayan mountains: the Ganges, the Brahmaputra, and the Meghna. In the summer of 1988 the rivers reached their highest levels in history, and 60% of the land was flooded. At least 1500 people died in the floods, and 49 million were affected by crop loss and damaged homes.

In the aftermath of the flooding, cases of diarrheal diseases reached epidemic proportions, with 50,000 cases reported daily. The risk of other diseases such as hepatitis, typhoid fever, and measles was elevated because of contaminated water supplies. Destruction of almost 4 million hectares of crops and partial damage to 3 million hectares left a shortfall in annual grain requirements of 1 million tons and placed the population at risk of famine. In the flood of 1974 in Bangladesh, affecting 50% of the land, 27,500 perished from subsequent disease and starvation. Fortunately, timely arrival of food aid in 1988 averted a famine crisis.

Types of Floods

Flash Floods. These are usually defined as floods that occur within 6 hours of the beginning of heavy rainfall. This type of flooding requires rapid localized warnings and immediate response by affected communities if damage is to be mitigated. Flash floods are normally a result of runoff from a torrential downpour, particularly if the catchment slope is unable to absorb and hold a significant part of the water. Other causes of flash floods include dam failure or sudden breakup of ice jams or other river obstructions. Flash floods are potential threats particularly where the terrain is steep, surface runoff is high, water flows through narrow canyons, and severe rainstorms are likely.

River Floods. River floods are usually caused by precipitation over large catchment areas, by melting of the winter accumulation of snow, or sometimes by both. The floods take place in river systems with tributaries that may drain large geographic areas and encompass many independent river basins. In contrast to flash floods, river floods normally build up slowly, are often seasonal, and may continue for days or weeks. Factors governing the amount of flooding include ground conditions (the amount of moisture in the soil, vegetation cover, depth of snow, cover by impervious urban surfaces such as concrete) and size of the catchment basin (Fig. 24-10).

Coastal Floods. Some flooding is associated with tropical cyclones (also called hurricanes and typhoons). Catastrophic flooding from rainwater is often aggravated by wind-induced storm surges along the coast. Saltwater may flood the land by one or a combination of effects from high tides, storm surges, or tsunamis. As in river floods, intense rain falling over a large geographic area will produce extreme flooding in coastal river basins.

Contribution by Humans to Flooding

Floods are naturally occurring hazards but can become disasters when human settlements occupy the floodplain. Population pressure is now so great that people have accepted the risk associated with floods because of the greater need for a place to live. In the United States, for example, billions of dollars have been spent on flood protection programs since 1936. In spite of this, the annual flood hazard has become greater because people have moved to and built on floodplains faster than engineers can design better flood protection.

Increase in population combined with poor resource management have resulted in new types of flooding. Conversion of forests in the catchment area to pasture and arable land means that less water is held in the upper reaches of the catchment basin, and the increased runoff water flows rapidly to the plains, with the effect of more frequent, unexpected, and severe flooding.

Another type of flood becoming more common is urban flash flooding. Buildings and roads cover the land, preventing infiltration, so that rainwater runs over the impervious surfaces and forms artificial streams. Inattention to maintenance of drainage systems, especially after long dry spells when dust, debris, and overgrown vegetation have blocked natural water flow, can accentuate the degree of flash flooding.

Predictability

Riverine flood forecasting estimates river level stage, discharge, time of occurrence, and duration of flooding, especially of peak discharge at specific points along river systems. Flooding resulting from precipitation, snow melt in the catchment system, or upstream flooding, is predictable from 12 hours to as much as several weeks ahead. Forecasts issued to the public result from regular monitoring of the river heights and rainfall observations. Flash flood warnings, however, depend solely on meteorologic forecasts and knowledge of local geographic conditions. The very short lead time for the development of flash floods does not permit useful monitoring of actual river levels for warning purposes.

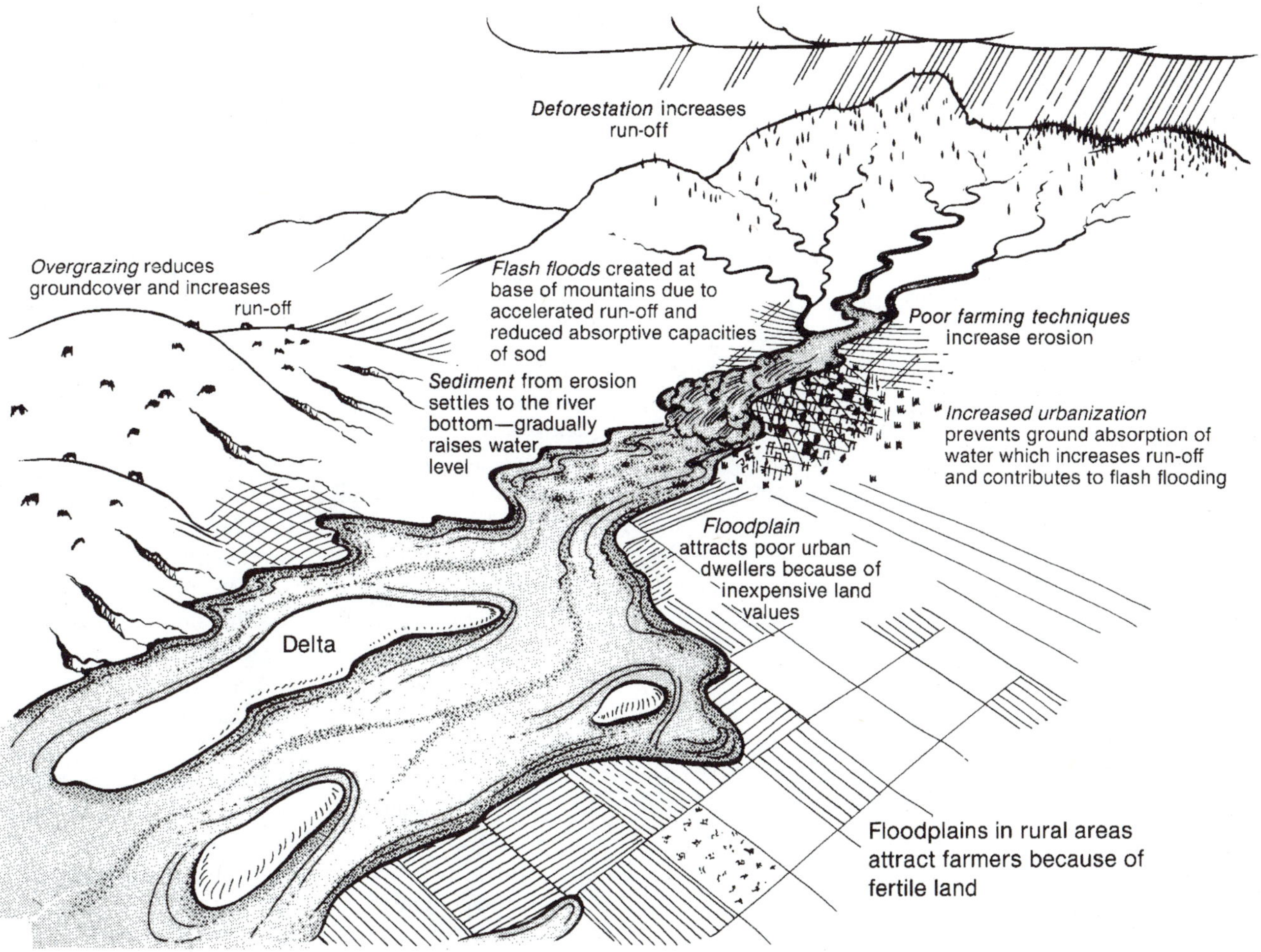
Deforestation increases run-off
Overgrazing reduces groundcover and increases run-off
Flash floods created at base of mountains due to accelerated run-off and reduced absorptive capacities of sod
Poor farming techniques increase erosion
Sediment from erosion settles to the river bottom—gradually raises water level
Increased urbanization prevents ground absorption of water which increases run-off and contributes to flash flooding
Floodplain attracts poor urban dwellers because of inexpensive land values
Delta
Floodplains in rural areas attract farmers because of fertile land

Fig. 24-10 Flooding and its causes. (Courtesy Disaster Management Center, University of Wisconsin.)

For comparison with previous flood events and conversion to warning information, assessment of the following elements should be included: flood frequency analysis, topographic mapping and height contouring around river systems with estimates of water-holding capacity of the catchment area, precipitation and snow melt records, soil filtration capacity, and (if in a coastal area) tidal records, storm frequency, topography, coastal geography, and breakwater characteristics.

An effective means of monitoring floodplains is through remote sensing techniques. The images produced by satellites can be interpreted to map flooded and flood-prone areas. Other efforts to improve forecasting are being implemented by United Nations organizations such as the WMO using WWW and the Global Data Processing System. These systems are strategic when flood conditions exist across international boundaries. The great majority of river and flash flood forecasts, however, depend on observations made by national weather services for activation of flood alert warnings.

Vulnerability

At notable risk in floodplain settlements are buildings made of earth or with soluble mortar, buildings with shallow foundations, or buildings that are nonresistant to water force and inundation. Infrastructural elements at particular risk include utilities such as sewer systems, power and water supplies, and machinery and electronics belonging to industry and communications. Of great concern are food stocks and standing crops, confined livestock, irreplaceable cultural artifacts, and fishing boats and other maritime industries.

Other factors affecting vulnerability are lack of adequate refuge sites above flood levels and accessible routes for reaching those sites. Also, lack of public information about escape routes and other appropriate response activities renders communities more vulnerable.

Typical Adverse Effects

Structures are damaged by receiving the force of impact of flood waters, floating away on rising waters, becoming inundated, collapsing because of undercutting by scouring or erosion, and being struck by water-borne debris.

Damage is likely to be much greater in valleys than in open, low-lying areas. Flash floods often sweep away everything in their path. In coastal areas, storm surges are destructive both on inward travel and on outward return to the sea. Mud, oil, and other pollutants carried by water are deposited and ruin crops and building contents. Saturation of soils may cause landslides or ground failure.

Casualties and Public Health. Currents of moving or turbulent water can knock down and drown people and animals in relatively shallow depths. Major floods may result in large numbers of deaths from drowning, particularly among the young and weak, but generally inflict few serious but nonfatal injuries requiring hospital treatment. Slow flooding causes relatively few direct deaths or injuries but often increases the occurrence of snakebites.

Endemic disease will continue in flooded areas, but little evidence exists of floods directly causing any large-scale additional health problems apart from diarrhea, malaria, and other viral outbreaks 8 to 10 weeks following the flood.

Water, Crops, and Food Supplies. Open wells and other groundwater supplies may be contaminated temporarily by debris carried by flood waters or by saltwater brought in by storm surges. They are contaminated by pathogenic organisms, however, only if dead bodies of people or animals are caught in the sources or if sewage is swept in. Normal sources of water may not be available for several days.

An entire harvest may be lost along with animal fodder, resulting in long-term food shortages. Food stocks may be lost by submersion of crop storage facilities, resulting in immediate food shortages. Grains quickly spoil if saturated with water, even for a short time. Most agricultural losses result from the inundation of crops or stagnation by standing water, as in the 1988 Bangladesh flood.

Large numbers of animals, including draught animals, may be lost if they are not moved to safety. This may reduce the availability of milk and other animal products and services, such as preparation of the land for planting. These losses, in addition to possible loss of farm implements and seed stocks, may hinder future planting efforts.

Floods bring mixed results in terms of their effects on the soil. In some cases land may be rendered infertile for several years following a flood because of erosion of the topsoil or salt permeation, as in the case of a coastal flood. Heavy silting may have adverse effects or may significantly increase fertility of the soil.

In coastal areas, where fish provide a source of protein, boats and fishing equipment may be lost or damaged.

On the positive side, floods may flush out pollutants in the waterways. Other positive effects include preserving wetlands, recharging groundwater, and maintaining the river ecosystems by providing breeding, nesting, and feeding areas for fish, birds, and wildlife.

DROUGHT

Of all natural disasters, droughts potentially have the greatest economic impact and affect the greatest number of people. Earthquakes and cyclones can have enormous physical intensity but are invariably of short duration and geographically limited. The death toll from such disasters can be very high if urban or densely populated rural areas are affected. By contrast, droughts affect large geographic areas, often covering whole countries or parts of continents. Droughts may last for months and in some cases several years. They have a direct and significant impact on food production and the overall economy.

A general working definition of drought might be a "temporary reduction in water or moisture availability significantly below the normal or expected amount for a specified period." How the normal amount is measured is of critical importance and may be defined in two ways:

1. A reduction of water availability might qualify for the use of the term "drought" when it falls below 80% of the average availability over the preceding 20 years. However, within naturally fluctuating climate and weather systems, the period selected as the basis for estimating the average may be significantly misleading.
2. All societies tend to stabilize their socioeconomic systems around what is perceived to be the normal rainfall. This perception is heavily weighted toward recent experience. Thus, after 10 years with above average rainfall, a society may have become used to the wetter state and perceive the first year of average rainfall as a drought.

Drought Types

There are three types of drought: meteorologic, hydrologic, and agricultural (Fig. 24-11). The first two describe a physical event, whereas the third describes the particular impact of the first two on an area of human activity, namely agricultural production. Meteorologic drought involves a reduction in rainfall for a specified period (day, month, season, year) below a specified amount, usually defined as some proportion of the long-term average for the specified time period. Its definition involves only precipitation statistics. Hydrologic drought involves a reduction in water resources (streamflows, lake levels, groundwater, underground aquifers) below a specified level for a given period. Its definition involves data on availability and offtake rates in relation to the normal operations of the system (domestic, industrial, irrigated agricultural) being supplied.

Agricultural drought is the result of meterologic and hydrologic droughts on this particular area of human activity. To achieve optimum growth, crops must have particular temperature, moisture, and nutrient requirements met during their growth cycle. If moisture availability falls below the optimum amount during the growth cycle, crop growth will be impaired and yields reduced. Because of the complexity

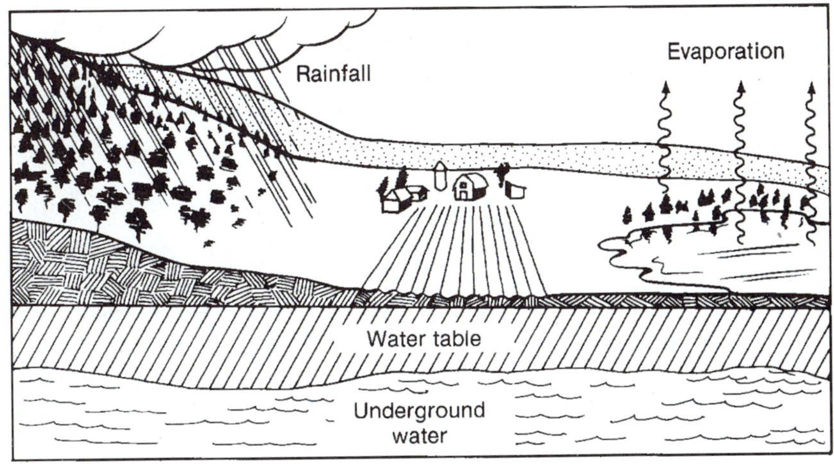

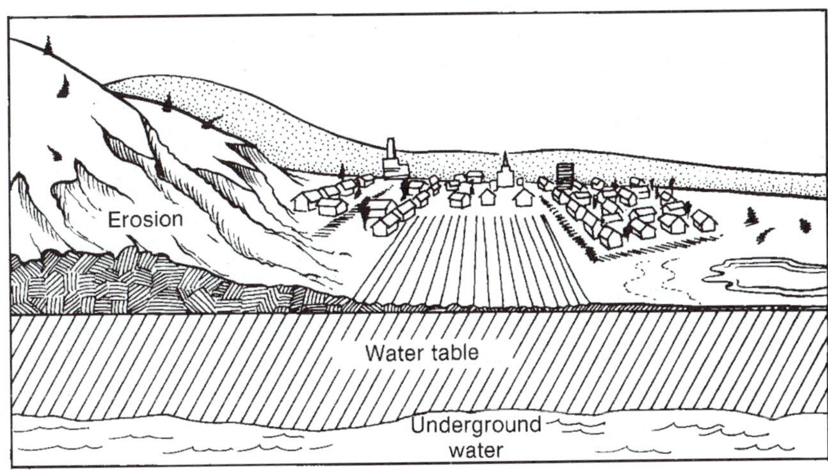

Fig. 24-11 The drought cycle. Meteorologic changes reduce rainfall, while urbanization, overgrazing, deforestation, and farming reduce soil water retention. As normal hydrologic balance is disrupted, topsoil erodes and the water table is lowered, making recovery difficult. Food and drinking water reductions induce human migration from the area. (From *Natural hazards: causes and effects,* Madison, Disaster Management Center, University of Wisconsin.)

of the relationships involved, agricultural drought is difficult to measure. A fall in yields may be due to insufficient moisture, but it may also stem from many factors, including unavailability of fertilizers, lack of weeding, presence of pests and crop diseases, lack of labor at critical periods in the growth cycle, and unattractive crop prices. Because of all the factors capable of affecting yields, meteorologic drought and agricultural drought are not always synonymous.

Causal Phenomena

Rainfall deficit may be due to one or more factors, such as an absence of available moisture in the atmosphere, large-scale subsidence (downward movement of air within the atmosphere) that suppresses convective activity, and the absence of rain-producing systems. Changes in such factors involve changes in weather systems ranging from local to regional to global. While it may be possible to indicate the immediate cause of a meteorologic drought in a particular location, it is often not possible to pinpoint the underlying cause.

Short-term drought episodes (1 to 3 years) can often be linked to global-scale fluctuations in the atmosphere and oceans elsewhere in the world. Thus, the El Niño/Southern Oscillation (ENSO) phenomenon, which involves the periodic invasion of warm surface water into the normally colder waters off the Pacific coast of South America, affects the levels of rainfall in many different parts of the world, including southeastern Africa. However, the process that causes the invasion by the warmer currents is incompletely understood.

Many causes of long (a decade or more) dry regimes have been postulated. Among the local causes are human-induced changes in albedo (reflectivity) of the ground surface or in soil moisture or both. Such changes are hypothesized to be caused by vegetation loss from overgrazing and deforestation either in the general vicinity or upwind of the area along the line of the prevailing, moisture-carrying winds. Such changes may involve biogeophysical feedback mechanisms, so that once started, the changes perpetuate the drought conditions.

On a larger scale, the link between sea surface temperatures and rainfall is a possible cause of the long, dry regimen. The fact that the southern Atlantic has been consistently and anomalously warmer than the northern Atlantic since 1970 may be related to the predominantly dry period in the Sahel since the mid-1960s.

One of the main problems with the postulations involving human-induced change is that of distinguishing human-induced change from natural long-term fluctuations. For example, rainfall in the western Sahel fluctuates periodically on a time scale of around 50 years, with the predominantly dry period since the mid-1960s being part of such a cycle. However, reliable rainfall data series for the Sahel and many other parts of the world are available only for the last 80 to 90 years. This is too short a period to support the assertion of such a rainfall cycle, since five or six cycles are needed for predictive purposes.

Predictability

Of the major natural disasters, a drought is unique in terms of the length of time between the first indications that it is developing and the point at which it begins to have a significant impact on the population of the affected area. The length of such "warning time" varies significantly among societies. In many countries the warning time is on the order of several months, but it may be much less, perhaps a matter of a few weeks. Whatever the period, the warning time is sufficient for a response by a government to mitigate the impact of the drought before it becomes significant.

Through modern meteorologic monitoring and telecommunication systems, preventing excess mortality resulting from food shortages caused by drought alone has become possible. However, droughts may continue to contribute to famines because other factors such as conflict and international politics are now responsible for propelling economic hardships caused by drought into a famine, as in Ethiopia in 1984 and 1987 and in Somalia in 1992.

During the last two decades, systems for reporting on meteorologic, agricultural, crop marketing, and other indicators, such as nutritional status, have been improved to provide early warning information. In most countries such systems have involved the creation of early warning units located in an appropriate department of the central government into which the meterologic department and agricultural extension and statistics department feed information. Regional groupings such as CILSS (Comit Permanent Inter-Etats de Lutte Contre la Secheresse dans la Sahel, or Permanent Inter-State Committee for Drought Control in the Sahel) in West Africa and SADCC (Southern African Development Coordinating Conference) have established regional early warning systems that combine the output of the national systems with information from other sources, such as remote sensing information from satellites.

Factors Contributing to Vulnerability

Agricultural production is more vulnerable to drought in irrigated areas to the degree that water needs are met by the irrigation supply. Another factor that influences vulnerability is moisture retention of soil. In many arid and semiarid areas of the tropics, sandy soils can promote crop growth only with frequent and evenly spaced rains. Deficiencies in moisture supply at critical growth stages can significantly reduce yields.

The adaptive behavior of farmers can affect vulnerability. Farmers may respond to intermittent rains with repeated replantings of the same crop variety, while others may replant using other varieties. Some farmers may not have seed reserves or be in a position to purchase replacement seeds and may experience a crop failure while other farmers in the same area may produce a satisfactory harvest. Households dependent on animal products for survival may be vulnerable if grazing and watering supplies diminish.

Typical Adverse Effects

The effects of drought on agriculture and concomitant socioeconomic costs can lead to intense human suffering and famine. Initial reduction in income for farmers results in reduced agriculture-related employment, increased defaulting on loans, reduced government earnings and foreign exchange, and increased prices of staple foods. Increasing inflation rates then render certain population groups—notably the poorest or subsistence groups—unable to purchase food. They may switch to cheaper foods, reduce their intake, sell their assets to raise funds, or migrate to areas where food is available or employment opportunities exist.

The act of migration produces stress and increased morbidity. Reduced food intake leads to deterioration of nutritional status and reduced ability to resist infection. Morbidity is also increased because of drying up of water sources and reduction in water quality. The social costs include breakup of communities and families. Competition for water may lead to local conflicts.

ENVIRONMENTAL POLLUTION

The population of the earth doubled to 5.2 billion people in the period spanning from 1950 to 1991. Global economic activity has quadrupled. Despite the rate at which natural resources are being consumed in the world, many poor countries still desperately need the benefits accompanying industrialization and economic growth. In general, people in developing countries are much more vulnerable to the effects of environmental degradation because they are poorer and depend more directly on the land.

Causes of Air and Water Pollution

Various parts of the environment are subjected to the effects of toxic (poisonous) chemicals produced in manufacturing, such as paint and metal production, and the burning of fossil fuels such as gasoline, coal, and oil. Some of these chemicals are heavy metals, such as lead, that are essentially nondegradable. Other toxic compounds, such as pesticides, are purposely introduced into the environment. Toxic chemicals may accumulate and affect the quality of air and water. Other pollutants of importance are from biologic sources such as human wastes, soil sediments, and decaying organic matter.

Air Pollution. Much of the world's urban population breathes polluted air at least part of the time. Sulfur dioxide, a major pollutant, is a corrosive gas harmful to humans and the environment. Electricity generation using fossil fuels is the key source of this compound in industrialized countries. In developed countries the burning of fossil fuels also contributes. Other air pollutants include nitrogen oxides, carbon dioxide, and lead, mainly from vehicle exhaust.

Marine Pollution. Sewage is the major cause of ocean pollution. Raw sewage containing human excreta and domestic wastes is disposed of in large quantities directly into the ocean. In the summer of 1993, thousands of ocean beaches were closed in the United States because of high levels of pathogens from human and animal wastes. Industrial effluents are also piped into the ocean. Other pollutants include marine litter, spills of petroleum, and other chemical compounds such as those containing mercury and dumped radioactive substances.

Freshwater Pollution. Human waste and other domestic wastewaters are often discharged directly into nearby bodies of water, particularly in urban areas. In developing countries this waste may be completely untreated. Industrial effluents from papermaking, chemical, metalworking, textile, and food processing industries reach bodies of water by direct discharge or by leaching from dumps.

Clearing the land for agricultural uses and following such agricultural practices as irrigation and use of fertilizers and pesticides have seriously affected water quality in many countries. Deforestation on an unprecedented scale has led to soil erosion, causing accelerated runoff and sediment deposits in riverbeds. The sediment level in rivers may increase 100-fold in deforested areas during rainy seasons.

Runoff of nitrogen from fertilizers, particularly in industrialized nations, renders some water unfit to drink without treatment. Use of irrigation systems may lead to increased salinity of water sources and saltwater intrusion on coastal areas where water is withdrawn. Approximately 25% of the world's pesticide production is used in developing countries, mainly on cash crops. Accumulations of pesticide toxins are found in food, soil, and water. Although data on Africa are lacking, studies in Asia indicate that rivers and lakes in Indonesia and Malaysia have very high levels of polychlorinated biphenyls (PCBs) and some pesticides.

Ozone Depletion

Ozone is a form of oxygen composed of three atoms of oxygen. Most atmospheric ozone is concentrated in the upper atmosphere, or stratosphere. The ozonosphere, or the ozone layer, is 11 to 24 km above the earth. Ozone screens out harmful wavelengths of ultraviolet radiation from the sun, protecting life on earth. Ultraviolet light is associated with increased skin cancer and cataracts and reduced phytoplankton in the oceans. Thinning of the ozone layer is caused by chlorofluorocarbons (CFCs), chemicals used in refrigeration, foam products, and aerosol propellants.

The CFCs that damage the ozone layer may also contribute to global warming. Although they compose a fraction of greenhouse gases, they account for 20% of the warming trend caused by radiative trapping potential (10,000 times greater than that of carbon dioxide).

Global Warming

Global temperatures appear to be higher today than they have been since 1862, when temperatures were first recorded by instrumentation. The last 10 years include the six hottest temperatures ever recorded. One explanation for this increase is perhaps a global warming caused by the "greenhouse effect."

The term "greenhouse effect" is used to describe the role of certain atmospheric gases such as carbon dioxide, methane, and water vapor in trapping radiation that would otherwise leave the atmosphere. Without this canopy of gases and clouds, the temperature of the earth would be extremely cold. The atmospheric gases therefore behave similarly to a greenhouse.

Since the beginning of the Industrial Revolution in the late eighteenth century, carbon dioxide in the atmosphere has increased by nearly 25%, mostly owing to combustion of coal, oil, natural gas, and gasoline. Currently a strong scientific consensus is evolving that buildup of greenhouse gases should lead to a warming of global atmosphere. Computer models used to examine the climatic effects of increasing carbon dioxide suggest that if it doubles, global temperatures would increase on average by 3° to 5° C.

Trees play a vital role in recycling carbon dioxide by taking it in, transforming it chemically, storing the carbon, and releasing oxygen into the air. When trees are cut down, left to decay, or burned, they release stored carbon to the air as carbon dioxide. Recently in Central Africa the virgin rainforests were found to have air pollution levels comparable to those in industrial areas. A major cause of this pollution is the fires that rage for months across huge stretches of land to clear shrubs and trees for the production of crops and grasses. Deforestation has been estimated to account for 20% of total atmospheric content of carbon dioxide. The effects of acid rain (pollutants that are held in the clouds and fall back to earth in rainwater) and air pollution in Europe, Canada, and the United States also contribute to the increase of carbon dioxide.

Another greenhouse gas is methane. Methane is generated by bacteria as they break down organic matter. It is emitted largely by landfills, cattle, and fermenting rice paddies. The concentration of methane gas in the atmosphere has doubled in the past 200 years, mainly with the expansion of animal husbandry and rice cultivation, an increased number of landfills, and leaking natural gas pipelines.

The greenhouse effect is still a subject of controversy in the scientific community. Both the magnitude and the timing of the warming and future climatic changes are uncertain. The status can be summarized as follows:

Fact: Greenhouse gases are responsible for keeping the planet warmer than it would be otherwise.

Fact: Concentrations of greenhouse gases are increasing at unprecedented rates.

Theory: Continued greenhouse gas emissions will lead to global warming.

General Characteristics and Adverse Effects

Air Pollution. Pollution of the troposphere (lower atmosphere) is damaging to agricultural crops, forests, aquatic systems, buildings, and human health. Primary pollutants often react to form secondary pollutants (acidic compounds), a frequent cause of environmental damage. The following effects are possible:

1. Crop and vegetation damage by injury to plant tissue, increasing susceptibility to disease and drought
2. Decline in forests caused by leaf damage by acidic compounds, acidic soils, and stresses of multiple pollutants
3. Damage to aquatic ecosystems so that they no longer support life
4. Degradation of building materials, such as metal, stone, and brick
5. Adverse impact on human health by damage to respiratory tracts

Marine Pollution. Marine pollution has the following major effects:

1. Spread of pathogens from human wastes; these include viruses and protozoa that cause hepatitis, cholera, typhoid, and other contagious diseases
2. Release of undegradable materials such as plastics and netting that may injure marine mammals
3. Oil pollution from oil spills
4. Spread of hazardous chemicals and radioactive substances into the marine ecosystem where they may accumulate in seafood

Freshwater Pollution. Freshwater pollution results in the following adverse effects:

1. Untreated wastewater carries viruses and bacteria from human feces into human drinking water, which can result in illness or even in infant mortality
2. Eutrophication, or decay of organic matter, which decreases oxygen levels in water, upsetting the balance of the aquatic ecosystem
3. Adverse health of persons drinking untreated water from tainted sources; water acidification reduces its capacity to support aquatic life
4. Runoff sediment from eroded soil deposits in drainage basins, reducing the basins' capacity and exacerbating flooding
5. Salinization from irrigation with harmful effects on downstream agriculture
6. Pesticides and fertilizer chemicals that accumulate in water and affect tissues in living organisms

Ozone Depletion. As the ozone layer thins, more medium wave ultraviolet light (UV-B) will reach the earth. Nonmelanoma skin cancer will certainly increase in light-skinned individuals and people living near the equator. UV-B also reduces the ability of the body's immune system to fight foreign substances entering through the skin. Diseases of the eye, such as cataracts and deterioration of the cornea and retina, are also associated with ultraviolet light.

Effects on marine life. UV-B radiation can penetrate the ocean's surface, damaging fish larvae and juveniles and the phytoplankton base of the food chain, affecting growth and reproduction. Since fish provide 14% of the animal protein consumed worldwide (60% of that in Japan), the impact could be significant.

Global Warming. The impacts of global warming are still uncertain. Computer models are unable to make reliable predictions of regional changes. The following changes *may* occur.

Sea level rise. Melting of the Arctic ice sheets and alpine glaciers could cause the seas to expand and sea levels to rise. Depending on the degree of global warming, the seas will rise 30 cm to 2 m by 2075, jeopardizing coastal settlements and marine ecosystems. A rise of 1 m in sea level could flood 15% of arable land in Egypt's Nile Delta and would flood 12% of Bangladesh, displacing 11 million people. The tiny island of the Maldives, inhabited by 200,000, would be submerged.

Climate change. Natural disasters such as superhurricanes could become common. A temperature increase of a few degrees in tropical seas can intensify hurricane production. The warmer oceans may bring an increase in occurrence of the El Niño phenomenon near the coast of Peru. El Niño is the incursion of warm surface water to the coast and occurs every 3 to 7 years with disastrous effects. This phenomenon inhibits phytoplankton growth, causes fish and shellfish to migrate or die, and forces higher forms of life, such as birds and human beings, dependent on the sealife to migrate or die.

Other climatic changes could lead to warmer and drier conditions in middle latitudes, higher temperatures in semitropical and tropical areas, and higher rates of evaporation. Rainfall patterns may also change. The combined effects of increased carbon dioxide and climate changes may alter plant and animal productivity. Plants may actually grow faster and larger but may have reduced nutritive value.

Changes in ecosystems. In warmer climates, grasslands, savannas, and deserts may be expected to expand, rendering them vulnerable to increased degradation through erosion and fire. Animal species that could not adapt to the temperature increases would have to relocate to survive, a difficult task, given population pressures on land. Plant species unable to adapt would perish.

Public health impact. Global warming might affect mortality because of heat stress and increase the incidence of respiratory diseases, allergies, and reproductive illnesses. Geographic ranges of vector-induced diseases, such as mosquito-borne malaria and yellow fever, and parasitic diseases might increase.

Prediction and Measurement

Air and Water Pollution. Pollutants are measured all over the world, but to a much lesser degree in developing countries. The most comprehensive data collection system is the Global Environment Monitoring System (GEMS), of the United Nations Environmental Programme (UNEP), which provides data on sulfur dioxide and particulate matter in urban air and contaminants in water resources. Pollution production is related to per capita consumption, so that as countries develop, pollution also tends to increase.

Ozone Depletion. Ozone levels are regularly monitored each year, especially in the Southern Hemisphere, where a seasonal ozone hole opens over Antarctica every year. Twenty million tons of CFC were manufactured and have either escaped or will escape to the atmosphere.

Greenhouse Effect. Greenhouse gas emissions are regularly measured all over the world. But even if the exact levels of future greenhouse emissions were available, difficulties would arise in predicting the effects on global climate. Climatic models are used to study climate change, but the models differ in their interpretation of all the various interactions in the earth's systems. This is partly because information being put into the system for analysis is not complete or is poorly understood.

Possible Risk Reduction Measures

Air and Water Pollution. Most nations are acting individually to control air pollution. Basic requirements are to set ambient air quality standards that measure pollutants at a distance from the source and set controls on acceptable levels, and to require that every source of an air pollutant meet certain emission limits. In some cases, humans may have to develop the technologies to make the latter possible.

Pollution control of coastal areas in the past has proved that recovery is possible to some extent. The banned pesticide DDT, which was present in many forms of marine life, is now decreasing in concentration. Most strategies for protecting the oceans must address broader ranges of pollutants from sewage to industrial effluents. More effort should be focused on establishing policy for protection of coastal areas on national and international levels.

Improvement of soils can decrease the possibility of water contamination by toxic chemicals and decrease runoff, thereby lessening silting and sedimentation of waterways. Establishing terraces and contour bounds, stabilizing sand dunes, building check dams, and planting trees and shrubs can help to stabilize soil. Watershed mapping, management, and protection are also of vital importance in ensuring a safe and plentiful drinking water supply. Proper systems to dispose of human waste should be promoted.

Regulations must be established and enforced by government agencies to protect citizens against the toxic effects of pesticides and other chemicals. Improvement of soils will also help to absorb and degrade toxins. Further studies must be made on the effects of pesticide residues. Farmers may use crop types resistant to pests or use an integrated approach to pest management, requiring less pesticide.

Ozone Depletion. International cooperation to limit CFC emissions intends to reduce production and use of CFCs in industrialized nations by 50% from 1986 levels before the year 2000, but developing countries are allowed to increase their use slightly. Meanwhile, research is attempting to address the need for CFC substitutes, for minimizing loss to the atmosphere, and for recycling. Countries can regulate import and use of aerosols and disposal of refrigeration units.

Global Warming. Since burning of fossil fuels (at least in theory) is the primary cause of global warming, it appears that developed countries are mainly at fault and that poorer countries are more likely to be the victims. Scientists, however, estimate that 20% of greenhouse gases (mainly carbon dioxide) results from deforestation, a trend occurring at a devastating rate in developing countries, particularly in tropical rainforests. In any case, global warming could affect the entire planet and steps can be taken to prepare for its effects and to prevent its acceleration. Successful strategies would include the following:

1. Reduce the rate of deforestation. Plant trees to solve community needs for wood, such as fuel wood, or to provide profits for individual farmers with agroforestry.
2. Increase the efficiency of energy production and use. Promote energy efficiency in urban areas and support renewable energy sources such as wind, water, geothermal, and solar power. These may be of great use in areas where no electricity sources exist.
3. Develop regulations to curb pollution from traffic emissions and industry in urban areas.

Education is a vital tool for environmental awareness. Only through understanding the relationships of ecosystems and long-term effects of degradation will people be motivated to act. Women's groups in India have established a tree protection lobby. Their motto is "trees are not wood," a concept that promotes trees as a vital part of the ecosystem involving carbon dioxide exchange to the air and a root system to hold down the soil. Education regarding the environment should begin in the early grades. Education for adults may take place in farmers' cooperatives, women's cooperatives, and village settings or may accompany programs to distribute seeds and tools. Use of the media, such as television, radio, and posters or newspapers, is an effective method to reach many people in a short time.

Trying to Save the Black Sea

The Black Sea, named for the dark clouds and fierce storms that affect its shores each autumn, faces an even darker future. The residues of modern agriculture and industry now threaten its marine life and the air quality of its bordering countries of Bulgaria, Romania, Turkey, and parts of the new Commonwealth of Independent States. The Black Sea is particularly vulnerable to pollution, as it collects 10 times more water per square meter of surface area than any other sea or ocean. It is fed by several major rivers, which carry in a large portion of the pollutants. The most important is the Danube, which flows through eight highly industrialized countries, all using chemically intensive agricultural practices.

In addition, the Black Sea has natural pollutants—organic matter collected over thousands of years, now decaying and diminishing the supply of oxygen in the water vital to life. In the unique two-stratum structure of the sea, where saltwater from the Mediterranean forms a bottom layer and fresh water a top layer, toxic hydrogen sulfide produced from the decomposing matter remains on the bottom layer, where oxygen is not present. Construction of irrigation works and dams has reduced the flow of fresh water into the Black Sea, so that the toxic layer that was previously 200 m below the surface has now risen to a depth of only 80 to 100 m.

Further deterioration of the Black Sea and air pollution from industries around it could be economically disastrous to the surrounding countries that depend on it to draw tourists. The resource-poor country of Bulgaria has developed a 20-year plan to save the sea and to bolster tourism. The plan calls for the following:

1. A total ban on discharge of any pollutants into the sea
2. Regulation of development of concentrated industrialization in the coastal zone
3. Environmental monitoring by 20 different institutions in coordination with UNEP
4. Restricting the inflow of fertilizers and the building of dams
5. Proliferation of blue mollusks to eat plankton, which use up the precious oxygen; shellfish cultivation is also a possibility
6. Holding a convention to assess the sea's environmental problems and draw up a blueprint to attack them; this plan would be closely linked to the international effort to address the pollution problems of Europe's major rivers

DEFORESTATION

Approximately 34% of the earth, or 4.5 billion hectares, is covered by forests and woodlands that supply fuel wood, wood products, food, and medicinal sources. Trees protect the land by controlling water runoff and by preventing erosion, soil infertility, and desertification. Absorption of carbon dioxide and water by trees and release of oxygen to the air help to moderate local and global climates. In addition, forests and woodlands promote and protect diversification of species.

Deforestation is the removal or damage of vegetation in a region that is predominantly tree covered. Deforestation is a slow-onset hazard that may contribute to disasters caused by flooding, landslides, and drought. Deforestation reaches critical proportions when large areas of vegetation are removed or damaged, harming the land's protective and regenerative properties. The rapid rate of deforestation in some parts of the world is a driving force in the yearly increase of flood disasters in these areas.

More than 11.1 million hectares of tropical forests and woodlands are converted into agriculture, pasture lands, or other uses every year. This includes 7.3 million hectares of tropical forest (6.1 million hectares of moist forest) and 3.8 million hectares of open and savanna woodland. Less than 10% of the land being deforested is replanted every year. Although the amount of forest land coming under protection or conservation is growing, the future still poses problems because of rapidly increasing pressures of development and exploitation.

Causal Phenomena

The increase in agriculture, firewood collection, and unregulated timber harvesting is the principal and immediate reason for deforestation. Beneath the obvious causes are fundamental problems in development, such as the use of inefficient agricultural practices, insecure land tenure, rising unemployment, rapid population growth, and failure to regulate and preserve forest lands.

Farming. The major cause of forest loss is the spread of farming. Land may be cleared for commercial ventures such as sugarcane, coffee, or rubber plantations, a principal cause of deforestation in Central America. In tropical rainforests, both legal and illegal colonists are trying to farm the former jungle lands, where soil conditions are fragile. Up to 90% of the nutrients are in vegetation rather than in the soil. When the forest is cut and burned, a nutrient surge occurs in the soil, lending initial fertility. After cropping and exposure to sun and rain, however, soil fertility rapidly declines, and the area becomes unproductive, perhaps prompting the farmer to slash and burn new forest areas.

Many traditional people in the Amazon Basin, Central Africa, and Southeast Asia still practice shifting cultivation techniques, allowing fallow periods between cropping for soils to regenerate. This practice becomes unsustainable if populations increase to the extent of forcing people into smaller areas. Insecure land tenure or fixed land titles may also force overuse of the land.

Because of crowded conditions in cities and farm areas, many people migrate to areas of marginal fertility, where they must keep moving their fields to produce sufficient food. Where this occurs, the migrant farmer may damage timber, wildlife, and human resources. In Venezuela, which has a high rate of unemployment and rising numbers of landless peasants, 30,000 families live and farm in national parks, forest reserves, and other legally protected areas. An influx of shifting cultivators who settled on the watershed above the Panama Canal has caused increased silting of a major reservoir that supplies Panama City.

Grazing. In Central and South America, large areas of tropical forest have been cleared to create grazing lands. A major portion of this can be attributed to economic enterprises designed for meat production. The Brazilian government has granted large land concessions to both domestic and foreign corporations wanting to raise cattle in the Amazon area. In Central America, virgin forest is being destroyed by ranchers who intend to export beef to the United States.

Firewood Collection. Firewood collection can contribute to the depletion of tree cover, particularly in lightly wooded areas. Because of a lack of alternative fuels and fuel-efficient stoves, this is especially a problem in Africa and in Asian highland countries such as Nepal. In areas of dense woods, dead material may fill local requirements for fuel. The outright destruction of trees for fuel occurs most commonly around cities and towns, where commercial markets for firewood and charcoal exist. Well-organized groups and individuals bring fuel wood by vehicle, pack animal, and cart into many cities, hastening local deforestation.

Fuel wood crisis. One hundred million people in developing countries cannot meet their minimum needs for energy, and close to 1.3 billion consume fuel wood resources faster than they are being replenished. In parts of West Africa today, some urban families spend one fourth of their income on wood or charcoal for cooking. In India, firewood is subsidized for the poor to prevent starvation.

Logging. Extensive logging in humid tropical forests, particularly in Asia and in temperate and mountainous forests, is conducted by large multinational corporations for export or to fill building needs in cities. The procedure usually involves either "clear cutting" or "creaming," or selective logging, of the forest's small proportion of valued species. Creaming (even though a less radical alternative to clear cutting) still causes significant damage to vegetation and wildlife, facts that are not apparent from the statistics. A study in Indonesia revealed that logging operations damaged or destroyed about 40% of trees left behind. The roads created by logging operations may encourage settlers to enter the forest and begin slash and burn agriculture, so that eventually even more of the forest is lost.

General Characteristics

Trees play a vital role in regulating our atmosphere, ecosystems, and weather systems. They recycle carbon dioxide, a gas now increasing in the atmosphere and thought to contribute to global warming. They release moisture to the air, thus contributing to rainfall and moderating local and global climate. Their roots trap nutrients, improve soil fertility, and also trap pollutants, keeping them from the water supply. They provide habitats for species, engendering diversity. They nurture traditional cultures by giving shelter, wood, food, and medicinal products. These benefits are lost as trees are destroyed.

The root systems of vegetation help retain water in the soil, anchor the soil particles, and provide aeration to keep soil from compacting. When vegetation dies, the nutrients go back to the soil. When root systems are removed, soil becomes destabilized. Water tends to flow off the top of the soil instead of percolating in, and it carries valuable topsoil along with it. This soil eventually forms sediment in the drainage basins.

Deforestation poses the most immediate danger by its contribution to these other hazards:

1. Destabilized soils are more susceptible to landslides and may increase the landslide risk in areas vulnerable to earthquakes and volcanoes.
2. Loss of moisture from deforestation may contribute to drought conditions, which in turn may trigger famines. Soil nutrients may also be lost through erosion of topsoil, resulting in decreased food production and possible chronic food shortages.
3. Erosion and dry conditions, combined with loss of vegetation and soil compaction, result in desertification and unproductive lands.
4. Dryness may accelerate the spread of fires.
5. Loss of carbon dioxide from dying trees and fires may add to global warming.
6. Research has proved conclusively that deforestation of watersheds, especially around smaller rivers and streams, can increase the severity of flooding, reduce streamflows, dry up springs in dry seasons, and increase the amount of sediment entering waterways.

Of all the hazards associated with deforestation, flooding is perhaps the most serious. Usually, curative measures, rather than preventive, such as dredging and dam building, are taken to solve flooding problems. As flooding worsens in developing countries, more attention is given to protection of watersheds. In India, flood damages between 1953 and 1978 averaged $250 million per year. Today, even more people live in flood-prone areas. Possibly flood problems will not be lessened without reforestation of the increasingly denuded hills of northern India and Nepal.

Predictability

Measurement and monitoring of forested areas may be conducted through ground level sampling and aerial or satellite surveys. Each method has drawbacks. Ground sampling is tedious and hard to extrapolate, aerial surveys are expensive, and satellite imagery poses difficulty in distinguishing forest from other vegetation. Combinations of methods usually produce the best results. Vague definitions in the study of deforestation still make exact determinations and forecast difficult. For instance, at what point does selective logging become deforestation? Or, if farmland has been left to regrow, did deforestation occur?

Three different prediction methods follow:

1. One type of study predicts future deforestation rates by extrapolating present rates of deforestation into the future. If the present rate of deforestation at 6.1 million hectares per year were to continue, the tropical moist forests would be completely cleared in 177 years. Where deforestation is more acute, the losses will be more serious. Cote d'Ivoire and Nigeria annually lose about 5.2% of their forests, while Costa Rica, Sri Lanka, and El Salvador lose between 3.2% and 3.6%. Each of these countries could lose all forests between the years 2007 and 2017.
2. Another forecast for 43 tropical countries was made using a mathematical model, which assumed that when forests in a country fell to a critical level, governments would take action to prevent further deforestation. Considerably more optimistic, the results predicted deforestation rates to decrease to between 0.9 and 3.7 million hectares per year in 2030.
3. Perhaps the bleakest theoretical forecast incorporates the effects of population growth and increasing consumption, which might be assumed to increase the rate of deforestation worldwide. However, growth of economies and technologies at the same time may assist to cur:ail the deforestation process if governments take appropriate action.

Typical Adverse Effects

The specific impacts of deforestation include the following:

1. Loss of soil fertility in the tropics and loss of productive capacity
2. Soil erosion and deposition of sediment
3. Increased runoff
4. Reduction in rainfall and increase in temperature
5. Destruction of biodiversity and traditional cultures
6. Loss of "free" goods such as fuels, food, and medicines
7. Exacerbation of other disasters

Impact on Economy. Most developing countries are already importers of forest products, especially paper. The fact that the amount of wood and wood products available per person in the world is falling (thus, increasing in price) combined with shortages of foreign currencies suggests that import of forest products will be increasingly prohibitive for these countries. Commercially marketed firewood is becoming more scarce, and prices are growing higher. Wood for construction is also scarce in many countries, which adversely affects the availability of housing.

Possible Risk Reduction Measures. These include various types of forest management, reforestation, and community participation in those activities. Most governments now recognize the vital importance of national forestry programs. Foresters help people meet their basic needs for forest products, and not always from the traditional forest or concentrated woodlot. For instance, forestry practiced by many farmers on their own land has been shown in some cases to be more environmentally effective. Reforestation has become intrinsically interwoven with other government policies that affect the population. Forestry therefore should be considered an integral part of land use and natural resource planning sectors of government.

Forests should be viewed by governments as capital resources to be managed. Management of the system should discourage concessionaires or other land users from practices that are not sustainable. Good management encourages highly selective harvesting without undue waste of remaining trees, especially in tropical forests. For any country to address its loss of forests and ensure that forests will yield economic benefits well into the future, certain steps must be taken:

1. Forest law or basic forest policy must be written that clearly states the objective of long-term sustainable management of the forest.
2. Forest regulations or management guidelines must be written and followed.
3. Sufficient financial and human resources must be allocated to do the job.

Forest management must be considered in the broadest sense of land use planning to include solutions for people as well as for trees. Compromises between complete destruction of the forests and complete conservation might entail regulated clearing of forests for shifting cultivation, habitation, or hunting; voluntary and intentional protection of forests or individual species by designating areas for reserves or national parks; and enrichment of the forest with species from other places. The last option may be considered risky, since pests and other species-specific problems may accompany the species.

Many unresolved scientific issues in forest management remain. How can the ever-expanding areas of secondary vegetation and degraded soils be managed to be more productive to the local people? Since most primary forests have disappeared, what sort of forest can we establish that would be stable and productive, and which would ensure the conservation of biologic diversity? What types of further basic ecologic research do we need in order to manage natural forests?

Social Forestry in Thailand

A project was begun in 1980 by Thailand's Royal Forestry Department (RFD) aimed at restoring the depleted forests. In just one generation since 1960, Thailand's forests had been reduced by half as its population doubled. The challenge facing the government was to restore the forests while permitting the expanding population to earn a living through farming.

The 8000 Thais living on 10,000 hectares near Nakhon Ratchasima on the Khorat Plateau had used slash and burn agriculture for years, destroying the forest. To develop the project, a survey was conducted for an entire year to determine the cropping patterns of the settlers and their expectations for the future. The RFD discovered that most wished to remain on the land and farm. Sixty percent of the land was suitable for farming, and that part would be used as incentive to encourage permanent settlement. The remaining 40% would be reforested by the RFD to prevent erosion of the hillsides and destruction of watersheds. The plan called for village councils to be formed and infrastructural inputs provided, such as roads, schools, and health centers.

The results of the project have been heartening. The trees planted by RFD grew rapidly and prompted villagers to plant 3.5 million seedlings. Complementary projects were initiated, including beekeeping, cottage industries, and crop diversification. The RFD provided training to its own staff, including experience with successful social forestry programs in other countries.

Many problems remain in Thailand. During the past 30 years the total amount of forest replanted is equivalent to only 1 year of cutting. Much timber is being harvested for profit without a permit. The relentless population growth and poverty place constant pressure on forest resources. However, the government is committed to future projects of this kind. Today it is national policy in Thailand to return 40% of the country to forest. This is crucial for Thailand if it is to become a major exporter of timber again.

DESERTIFICATION

Desertification may be simply described as the spread of desertlike conditions but is more broadly defined as the decline in biologic productivity or production potential resulting from a long-term process of degradation or change in climate. It occurs throughout dry areas (not only on the edges of natural deserts), affecting both developed and developing regions such as Africa, the Middle East, India, Pakistan, China, Australia, the Commonwealth of Independent States, the southwestern United States, and Greece. The most significant factor contributing to desertification is poor land use practices by human populations. A slow-onset disaster, desertification worsens conditions of poverty, brings malnutrition and disease, and destabilizes the social and economic bases of affected countries.

Causal Phenomena

Role of Climate. Vulnerability to desertification and the severity of its impact are partially governed by climatic conditions of an area. The lower and more uncertain the rainfall, the greater the potential for desertification. Other influencing factors are seasonal patterns of rainfall and high temperatures that increase evaporation.

The world's drylands are found in two belts centered approximately on the Tropic of Cancer and the Tropic of Capricorn (23.5° north and south of the equator, respectively) and cover one third of the earth's surface. More than 80% of the total area of drylands is found on just three continents: Africa (37%), Asia (33%), and Australia (14%). The drylands can be further classified into hyperarid, arid, and semiarid zones, depending on the average amount of rainfall received per year. Other factors, such as temperature and soil conditions, must be considered when determining the dryness ratio.

Both natural and human-derived climatic changes may contribute to desertification. Natural effects, such as long-term climatic cycles and the basic earth-sun geometry, have resulted in drier conditions in the Sahara. Human influence is associated with the predicted global warming trend and local climatic changes where deforestation has reduced the moisture-holding capacity of soil and has decreased cloud formation. The result is less rainfall and higher temperatures.

Despite the common misperception that desertification is caused by the desert advancing itself, land degradation can occur at great distances from deserts. Desertification usually begins as a spot on the land where land abuse has been excessive; from that spot, land degradation can spread outward with continued abuse. Many believe that droughts are responsible for desertification, but the reverse is more likely: desertification may actually contribute to droughts. Droughts increase the likelihood that the rate of degradation will increase. However, when the rains return, well-managed lands recover from droughts with minimal adverse effects.

Role of Land Use Management. Desertification can be brought about through any use of drylands that does not take into account their limitations and the contrasts in productivity and vulnerability that characterize them. Overcultivation occurs when farmers crop land more intensively than permitted by natural fertility and fail to compensate by adding fertilizer or by letting the land lie fallow for soil fertility to regenerate. Overcultivation reduces fertility of the soil, damages its structure, and leaves it vulnerable to erosion. Farmers may quit traditional methods of ensuring long-term soil fertility for many reasons, including drought, increasing need to produce because of population growth, cropping on marginal rangelands unsuitable for long-term production, land tenure restrictions confining sectors of the population to marginal lands, mechanized farming, and expansion of cash cropping.

While a large part of agricultural production in developing countries fills subsistence needs, some cash crops are grown to add to foreign exchange. A feature of most cash crops, however, is their extreme demand for nutrients and optimum site conditions. Degradation of land occurs directly through improper management of such crops, and indirectly by displacing subsistence crops and pastoralism to marginal lands. These conditions occurred in the 1950s and 1960s when cultivation of groundnuts expanded in West Africa and Sudan, taking over grazing lands. One reason was the attempt by France to combat the U.S. domination of the vegetable oils market. Incentives were provided by use of artificially high prices and may have contributed to the 1970 Sahelian drought disaster.

Overgrazing is a major cause of desertification (rangelands account for 90% of desertified lands) and occurs when too many animals are pastured. The number of cattle in Niger, for example, increased an estimated 450% between 1938 and 1961 and an additional 29% by 1970, when the majority were killed by starvation. Livestock density increases when herd sizes grow too large in wet years and cannot be sustained in dry years. Lucrative markets for meat in places like Nigeria and the Middle East have caused the establishment of cattle ranches where concentrated activity threatens land with poor returns for the investment. The introduction of better veterinary care has also decreased mortality rates. The introduction of deep wells increases availability of water, allowing larger, less mobile herds that congregate in the well area and degrade the vegetation and soil.

Poor irrigation management. The concept of using irrigation to ward off the threat of crop failure during drought seems a logical one and has thus been promoted by many development agencies. Ironically, poor management of irrigation projects has been a cause of desertification. In some cases productivity falls and soils become salinized, alkalized, or waterlogged. The major problem is usually inadequate drainage, and damage may be irreversible. A key example is the Greater Mussayeb irrigation project in Iraq, begun in 1953. By 1969 waterlogging was widespread and two thirds of the soil was saline. In 1970 a project to reclaim the salinized land was begun, but by 1976, because of technical and organizational limitations, the project still had not been successful. Egypt, Iraq, and Pakistan have lost more than 25% of their irrigated areas to salinization and waterlogging.

Deforestation. Land is cleared for agriculture, livestock, and fuel wood production, among other purposes. Deforestation is the first step toward desertification, removing vegetative barriers and exposing land to sun, wind, and rain. In Africa, demands for fuel wood and charcoal exert considerable stress on wood resources.

Role of Policy in Desertification. Population growth and economic expansion also contribute to desertification. When government and multilateral policies do not keep pace with population growth by using appropriate agricultural technologies to increase food production, desertification can be induced as increasing amounts of land are used and soil nutrients are not replenished. If government policy does not alleviate poverty, the poor are driven by expansion of urban populations or cash cropping enterprises to occupy marginal lands, which become more densely populated. This places more stress on the land. Governments often choose to expand cash crop cultivation to improve foreign currency holdings, rather than promote food security for the poor.

General Characteristics

The two main characteristics of desertification, the degradation of soil and degradation of vegetation, have the same result: reduction of productivity.

Degradation of Soil. Vegetation normally protects soil from being washed away by rain and also from splash erosion by impact of raindrops. The raindrops move the soil particles and pack them together on the surface, sealing the pores and thereby decreasing infiltration and increasing runoff. Sheet erosion is a more serious form of erosion in which fine layers of topsoil carrying soil nutrients are washed away. Unless the nutrients are replenished artificially, crop yields decline. Gullies are created by the runoff and, unless reclaimed by conservation measures, render the land unusable.

Wind erosion. Wind erosion occurs when finer components of the soil, such as silt, clay, and organic matter that contain most of the nutrients, are blown away, leaving behind the less fertile sand and coarse particles. Sand itself may start to drift, forming dunes, but this accounts for a minor proportion of the effects of wind erosion. Strong winds may form dust storms that damage crops by shredding leaves.

Soil compaction. Nearly complete compaction can occur when soil of poor structure is compressed by heavy machinery or by hooves of large herds of animals. A less serious form of compaction, called surface crusting, results when high-speed mechanical cultivation or dry season cultivation turns particles into thin powder, which then forms a crust when pelted with raindrops. Crusting and compaction make the soil less permeable for germination of new plants.

Waterlogging (salinization and alkalinization). These effects result from poor management of irrigation and water supplies in general. When the soil is waterlogged, the upward movement of saline in groundwater leaves salt on the surface when the water evaporates.

Degradation of Vegetation. Vegetation in arid lands adapts to the cycle of water availability by adjusting its growth. The drier the area, the farther apart plants grow. Some plants grow only during the rainy seasons. Degradation of vegetation occurs initially in the early stages of desertification with deforestation, but later it continues after soil fertility declines.

There are two main forms of vegetation degradation. The first is overall reduction of density of the vegetation cover, or biomass. The second is a more subtle change in types of vegetation to less productive forms. For instance, rangeland perennial grasses may be replaced by less palatable annual varieties, or more saline-tolerant crops such as barley would have to be substituted for traditional crops because of low yields from waterlogging and salinization.

Predictability

Insufficient progress has been made to quantify the extent of desertification and its progression. Data bases are incomplete or do not exist for many countries and governments. They often fail to address the problem, since the payoffs seem long term. To improve predictability, identify problem areas, and initiate investigation of causes, constant monitoring of dryland ecosystems must be carried out. Socioeconomic indicators showing trends in human health, income, and welfare must be collected. Scientists on a national level may conduct aerial photographic surveys of vegetation and aerial and ground animal counts. Meteorologic predictions of rainfall levels may be useful to predict drought.

Global surveillance of drylands can be achieved through use of remote sensing. However, not enough detail is always present in the satellite photos to distinguish preconditions for desertification. Comparison of imagery over years should help distinguish desertification from short-term fluctuations in the environment caused by climatic changes. In the future, data on the extent of degraded soils should be enhanced by the Global Assessment of Soil Degradation, sponsored by the United Nations Erosion Project and the International Soil Reference and Information Centre in the Netherlands.

Rate and Scope of Desertification

Desertification affects drylands in more than 100 countries but is concentrated in Asia and Africa, which account for 70% of all desertified land. Scientists have tried to quantify the areas desertified on a worldwide basis. The physical damage, in reduction of productivity of soils and loss of vegetation, is described previously. The number of casualties cannot be scientifically extrapolated, but certainly deaths do occur, perhaps directly as a result of famine or indirectly because of a reduction in standards of living.

In terms of social impact, an estimated 280 million rural people are affected at least by moderate desertification, and the number rises to 470 million (10% of the world population) when urban dwellers are included. Eighty-five percent of the rural population is farm based but occupies only 15% of the drylands, making the impact of desertification very serious. The population affected by desertification is also vulnerable to the effects of droughts and famines.

Estimates of the rate of desertification vary. One estimate claims that over 202,000 km^2 of land, or an area the size of Senegal, is desertified each year.

Acknowledgments

This chapter draws on several publications. The structure and much of the content come from *Introduction to Hazards,* a teaching module prepared for the Disaster Management Training Programme of the United Nations Development Program (UNDP). I also used excerpts from the chapter on this subject by Abram B. Bernstein and Paul Thompson, which appeared in the previous edition of this text. Information in the drought section came from *Drought and Famine,* another UNDP training module, written by John Borton and Nigel Nicholds. Another background document was *Natural Hazards: Causes and Effects,* published by the Disaster Management Center of the University of Wisconsin. I would like to thank Paul Thompson and Jim Good of InterWorks for their collaboration on this project and Robert L. Southern of Weather Associates for his input on the tropical cyclone section.

RECOMMENDED READINGS

Dudley WC, Lee M: *Tsunami!* Honolulu, 1988, University of Hawaii Press.

El-Baz F, Hassan MHA, editors: *Physics of desertification,* Amsterdam, 1986, Martinus Nijhoff.

Erikson J: *Volcanoes and earthquakes,* Blue Ridge Summit, Pa, 1988, Tab Books.

Gere JM, Shah HC: *Terra non firma,* New York, 1984, WH Freeman.

Grainger A: *The threatening desert: controlling desertification,* London, 1990, Earthscan.

Hanley ML: Can the Black Sea be saved? *World Development* 3(2):6, 1990.

Hays WW, editor: *Facing geologic and hydrologic hazards,* Washington, DC, 1981, US Government Printing Office.

Lorca E: Integration of the THRUST project into the Chile Tsunami Warning System, *Nat Hazards 4:293,* 1991.

Mitigating natural disasters, phenomena, effects and options, New York, 1991, United Nations Disaster Relief Organization.

Natural hazards primer, Washington, DC, 1990, Organization of American States.

Tilling RI: Volcanic hazards and their mitigation: progress and problems, *Rev Geophys* 27(2):237, 1989.

United States Geological Survey: *Earthquakes and volcanoes,* 1989, p 21.

Vickers DO: Tropical cyclones, *Nature and Resources* 27(1):31, 1991.

Volcanic emergency management, New York, 1985, United Nations Disaster Relief Organization.

Wilhite DA, Glantz MH: Understanding the drought phenomenon: the role of definitions, *Water International* 10:111, 1985.

World Resources Institute: *World resources 1988-89,* New York, 1988, Basic Books.

World Resources Institute: *World resources 1990-91,* Oxford, Eng, 1990, Oxford University Press.

25 AVALANCHES

Knox Williams
Betsy R. Armstrong
Richard L. Armstrong

An avalanche is a mass of snow that slides down a mountainside. In the United States, approximately 100,000 avalanches occur annually, of which about 100 cause injury, death, or destruction of property. Based on reported incidents, about 150 people a year are caught in avalanches (that is, they are bodily involved in the moving snow or its effects). Sixty are partly or wholly buried, 13 sustain injury, and 15 are killed. Average annual property damage is approximately $440,000.[2] This chapter describes the properties of the mountain snowpack that contribute to avalanche formation and describes avalanche safety techniques.[1]

Properties of Snow

PHYSICAL PROPERTIES

Although snow cover appears to be nothing more than a thick, homogeneous blanket covering the ground, it is in fact one of the most complex materials found in nature. It is highly variable and goes through significant changes in relatively short periods of time.

In nature, snow cover is variable on both the broad geographic scale (Antarctic snow is quite different from snow found in the Cascade Mountains of North America) and on the microscale (where snow conditions may vary greatly from one side of a rock or tree to the other). All snow crystals are made of the same substance, the water molecule, but local environmental conditions control the type and character of snow found at a given location. At a single site the snow cover varies from top to bottom, resulting in a complex layered structure.

Individual layers may be quite thick or very thin. In general, thicker layers represent consistent conditions during one storm, when new snow crystals falling are of the same type, wind speed and direction vary little, and temperature and precipitation are fairly constant. Thinner layers, perhaps only millimeters in thickness, often reflect conditions between storms, such as the formation during fair weather of a melt-freeze crust, a period of strong winds creating a wind crust, or the occurrence of surface hoar, the winter equivalent of dew. Delicate feather-shaped crystals of surface hoar deposited from the moist atmosphere onto the cold snow surface overnight offer a beautiful glistening sight as they reflect the sun of the following day. However, they are very fragile and weak, and once buried by subsequent snowfalls, may be major contributors to avalanche formation.

One property of snow is strength or hardness, which is of great importance in terms of avalanche formation. Snow can vary from light and fluffy, easy to shovel, and especially delightful to ski through, to heavy and dense, impossible to penetrate with a shovel, and hard enough to make it very difficult for a skier to carve a turn, even with sharp metal edges. The arrangement of the ice skeleton and the changing density (or the mass per unit volume) produce this wide range of conditions. In the case of snow, density is determined by the volume mixture of ice crystals and air. The denser the snow layer, the harder and stronger it becomes, as long as it is not melting.

The density of new snow can have a wide range of values. This depends on how closely the new snow crystals pack together, which is controlled by the shape of the crystals. The initial crystals have a variety of shapes, and some pack more closely together than others (Fig. 25-1). For example, needles pack more closely than stellars and as a consequence may possess a density three to four times that of stellars.

Wind can alter the shape of new snow crystals, breaking them into much smaller pieces that pack very closely together to form wind slabs. These in turn may possess a density 5 to 10 times that of new stellars falling in the absence of wind. Because these processes occur at different times and locations at the surface of the snow cover and are buried by subsequent snowfalls, a varied, nonhomogeneous layered structure results. Therefore what may seem to the casual

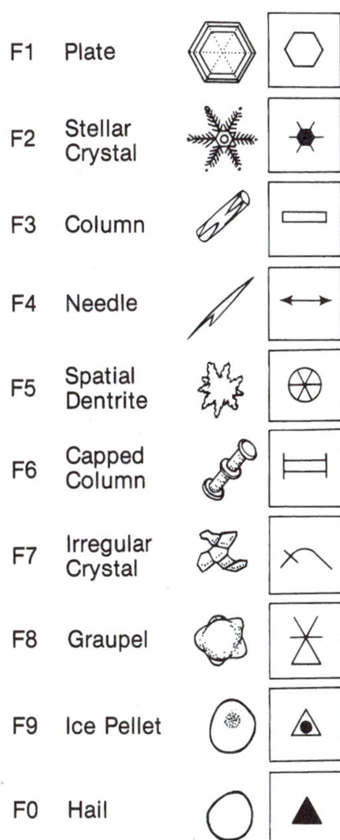

Fig. 25-1 International classification of solid precipitation. (From the International Association of Scientific Hydrology.)

observer to be minor variations in atmospheric conditions can have an important influence on the properties of snow.

After snow has been deposited on the ground, the density increases as the snow layer settles vertically or shrinks in thickness. Because an increase in density equals an increase in strength, the rate at which this change occurs is important with respect to avalanche potential. Snow can settle simply because of its own weight. It is highly compressible because it is composed mostly of empty airspace within an ice skeleton of snow crystals. In a typical layer of new snow, 85% to 95% of the volume is empty airspace. Individual ice crystals can move and slide past each other, and because the force of gravity causes them to move slowly downward, the layer shrinks. The heavier the snow above and the warmer the temperature, the faster this settlement proceeds.

At the same time the complex, intricate shapes that characterize the new snow crystals begin to change. They become rounded and suitable for closer packing. Intricate crystals change because they possess a shape that is naturally unstable. New snow crystals have a large surface area/volume ratio and are composed of crystalline solid close to its melting point. In this aspect, snow crystals are almost unique among materials found in nature. Surface energy physics dictates that this unstable condition will change; the warmer the temperature, the faster the change. Under very cold conditions the original shapes of the snow crystals are recognizable after they have been in the snow cover for several days or even a week or two. As temperatures warm and approach the melting point, such shapes disappear within a few hours to a day. Changes in the shape or texture of snow crystals are examples of initial metamorphism. The geologic term "metamorphism" defines changes that result from the effects of temperature and pressure. As the crystal shapes simplify, they can pack more closely together, enhancing further settlement (Fig. 25-2).

The changes generally occur within hours to a few days. The structure of snow cover changes over a period of weeks to months via other processes. Settlement, which may initially have been rapid, continues at a much slower rate. Other factors begin to exert dominant influences on metamorphism. These factors include the difference in temperature measured upward or downward in the snow layer, called the temperature gradient.

Averaged over 24 hours, snow temperatures generally are coldest near the surface and warmest near the ground at the base of the snow cover, creating a temperature gradient across a snow layer sandwiched between cold winter air and relatively warm ground (Fig. 25-3). The temperature gradient crosses both ice and large void spaces filled with air. Within the ice skeleton the temperature adjacent to the ground is warmer than that of the snow layer just above, and this pattern continues through the snow cover in the direction of the colder surface.

Warm air contains more water vapor than does cold air; this holds true for the air trapped within the snow cover. The greater the amount of water vapor, the greater the pressure. Therefore both a pressure gradient and a temperature gradient exist through the snow cover. When a pressure difference exists, the difference naturally tends to equalize, just as adjacent high and low atmospheric pressure centers cause movement of air masses. Pressure differences within snow cause vapor to move upward through the snow layers. The air within the layers of the snow cover is saturated with water vapor, with a relative humidity of 100%. When air moves upward to a colder layer, the amount of water vapor that can be supported in the airspace diminishes. Some vapor changes to solid water and is deposited on the surrounding ice grains. We witness a similar process when warm, moist air in a heated room comes in contact with a cold windowpane. The invisible water vapor is cooled to its ice point, and some of the vapor changes state and is deposited as frost on the window.

Fig. 25-4 shows how the texture of the snow layer changes during this temperature-gradient process. Water molecules sublimate from the upper surfaces of a grain. The vapor moves upward along the temperature (and vapor) gradient and is deposited as a solid ice molecule on the underside of a colder grain above. If this process continues long enough (it continues as long as a strong temperature gradient exists), all grains in the snow layer are trans-

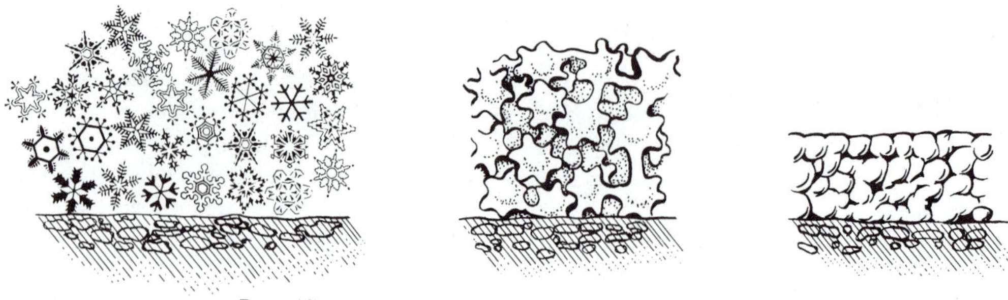

Fig. 25-2 Settlement. As the crystal shapes become more rounded, they can pack more closely together and the layer settles or shrinks in thickness.

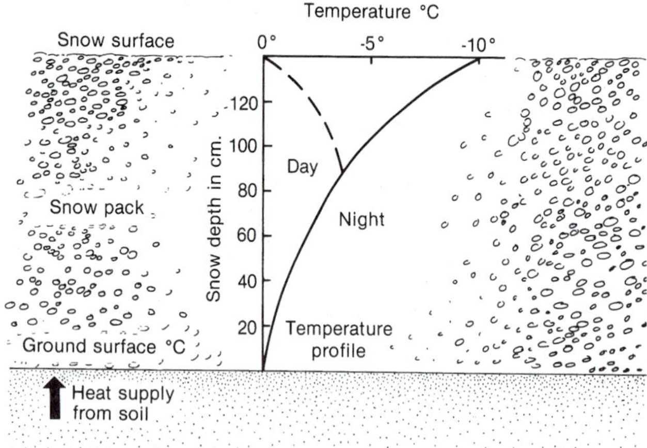

Fig. 25-3 When an insulating layer of snow separates the warm ground from the cold air, a temperature gradient develops across the snow layer.

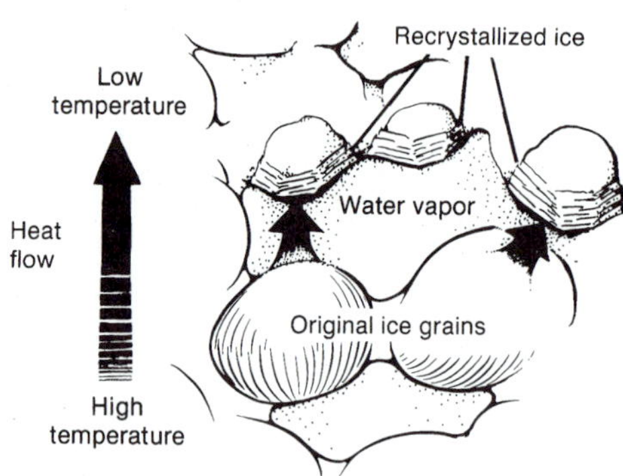

Fig. 25-4 In the temperature-gradient process, ice sublimates from the top of one grain, moves upward as water vapor, and then is deposited on the bottom surface of the grain above. If conditions allow this process to continue long enough, all of the original grains are lost as the recrystallization produces a layer of totally new crystals.

formed from solid to vapor and back to solid again; that is, they totally recrystallize. New crystals are completely different in texture from their initial form. They become large, coarse grains with facets and sharp angles and may eventually evolve into a hollow cup form. Examples of these crystals are shown in Figs. 25-5 through 25-7. The process is called temperature-gradient metamorphism, or kinetic metamorphism, and well-developed crystals are commonly known as depth hoar.

Depth hoar is of particular importance to avalanche formation. It is very weak because there is little or no cohesion or bonding at the grain contacts. Depth hoar or temperature-gradient snow layers can be compared to dry sand. Each grain may possess significant strength, but a layer composed of grains is very weak and friable because they lack connections. Thus depth hoar is commonly called sugar snow. Depth hoar usually develops whenever the temperature gradient is equal to or greater than about 10° C per meter. In the cold, shallow snow covers of a continental climate, such as that of the Rocky Mountains, a gradient of this magnitude is common within the first snow layers of the season. Therefore a layer of depth hoar is frequently found at the bottom of the snow cover, and the resulting low strength becomes a significant factor for future avalanches.

In the absence of a strong temperature gradient, a totally different type of snow texture develops. When the gradient is less than about 10° C per meter, there is still a vapor pressure difference and upward movement of vapor through the snow layers, but at a much slower rate. As a result, water vapor deposited on a colder grain tends to cover the total grain in a more homogeneous manner, rather than showing the preferential deposition characteristic of depth hoar. This process produces a grain with a smooth surface of more rounded or oblong shape. Over time, vapor is deposited at the grain contacts (concavities), as well as over the remaining surface of the grain (convexity). Connecting bonds formed at the grain contacts give the snow layer strength over time (Fig. 25-8). Bond growth, called sintering, yields a cohesive texture, in complete contrast to the cohesionless texture of depth hoar. This type of grain has been referred to by various terms (destructive metamorphism, equitemperature metamorphism, and equilibrium metamorphism), but can generally be described as fine-grained or well-sintered (bonded) snow. Rounded and interconnected grains are shown in Fig. 25-9.

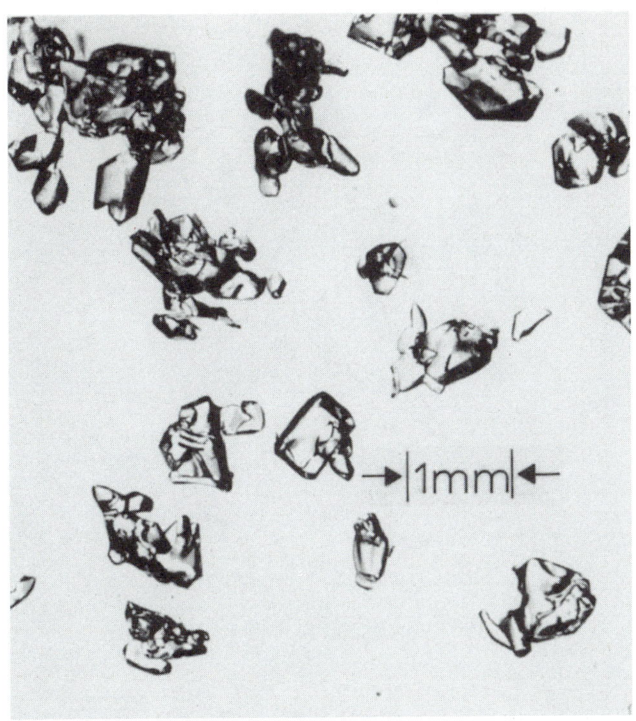

Fig. 25-5 Beginning temperature-gradient process: facets and angles are visible. (R. Armstrong photo.)

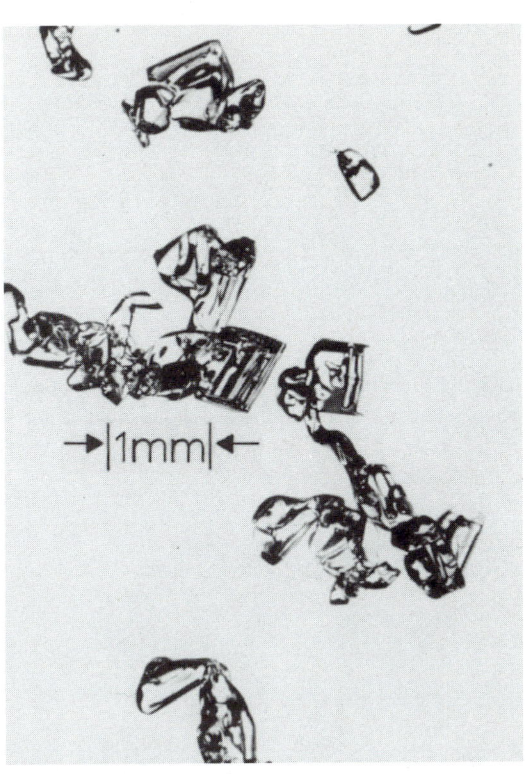

Fig. 25-6 As the temperature-gradient process continues, the crystals grow in size and stepped features are visible. (R. Armstrong photo.)

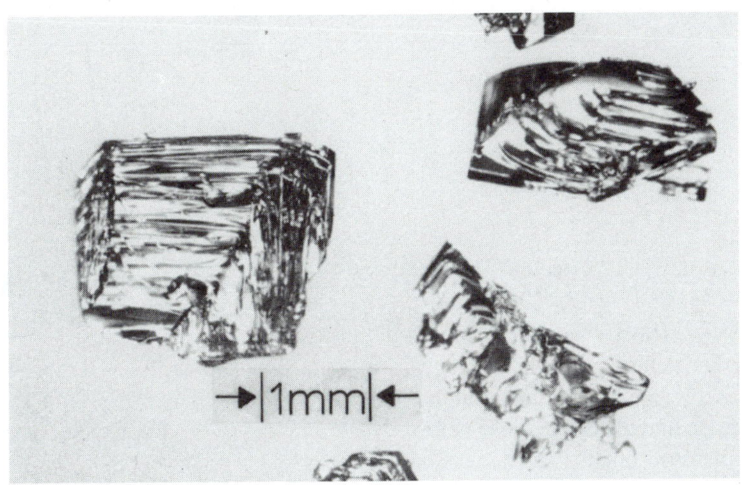

Fig. 25-7 Advanced temperature-gradient crystals attain a hollow cup-shaped form. (R. Armstrong photo.)

The preceding paragraphs describe the "big picture" in terms of what happens to snow layers after they have been buried by subsequent snowfalls. If the layer is subfreezing (that is, if no melt is taking place), one of the two processes described previously is occurring, or perhaps a transition exists between the two. Within the total snow cover these processes may occur simultaneously, but only one can take place within a given layer at a given time. Both processes accelerate with warmer snow temperature because water vapor is involved. The temperature gradient across the layer determines whether the process involves the growth of weak depth hoar crystals or the development of a stronger snow layer with a sintered, interconnected texture.

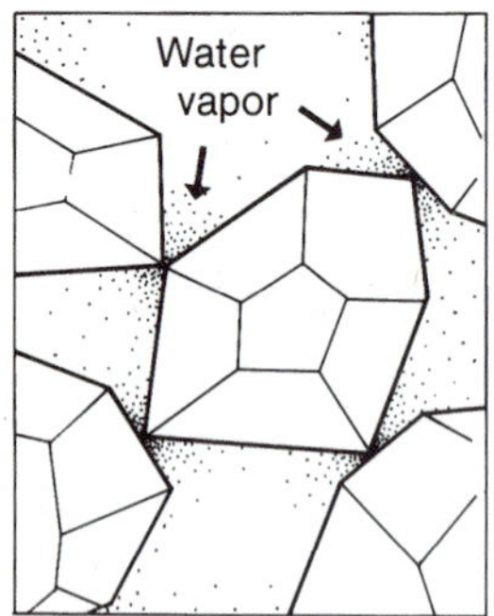

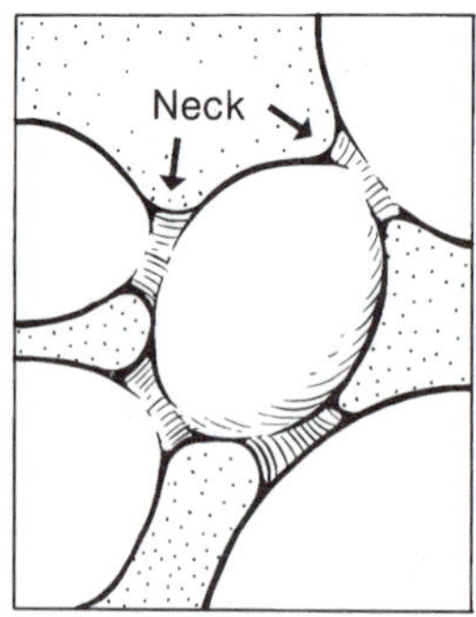

Fig. 25-8 Equitemperature grain growth. In the presence of weak temperature gradients, bonds grow at the grain contacts.

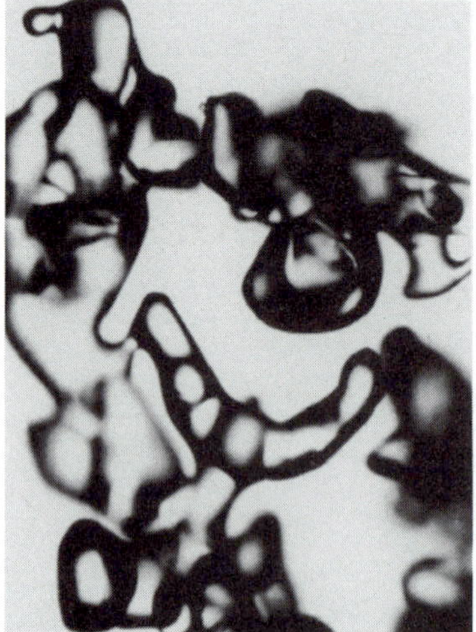

Fig. 25-9 Bonded or sintered grains resulting from equitemperature metamorphism. (S. Colbeck photo.)

SLAB AVALANCHE FORMATION

There are two basic types of avalanche release. The first is point, or loose snow, avalanche (Fig. 25-10). A loose snow avalanche involves cohesionless snow and is initiated at a point, spreading out laterally as it moves down the slope to form a characteristic inverted V shape. A single grain or a clump of grains slips out of place and dislodges those below on the slope, which in turn dislodge others. The avalanche continues as long as the snow is cohesionless and the slope is steep enough. This type of avalanche usually involves only small amounts of near-surface snow.

The second type of avalanche, the slab avalanche, requires a cohesive snow layer poorly anchored to the snow below because of the presence of a weak layer. The cohesive blanket of snow breaks away simultaneously over a broad area (Fig. 25-11). A slab release can involve a range of snow thicknesses, from the near-surface layers to the entire snow cover down to the ground. In contrast to a loose snow avalanche, a slab avalanche has the potential to involve very large amounts of snow.

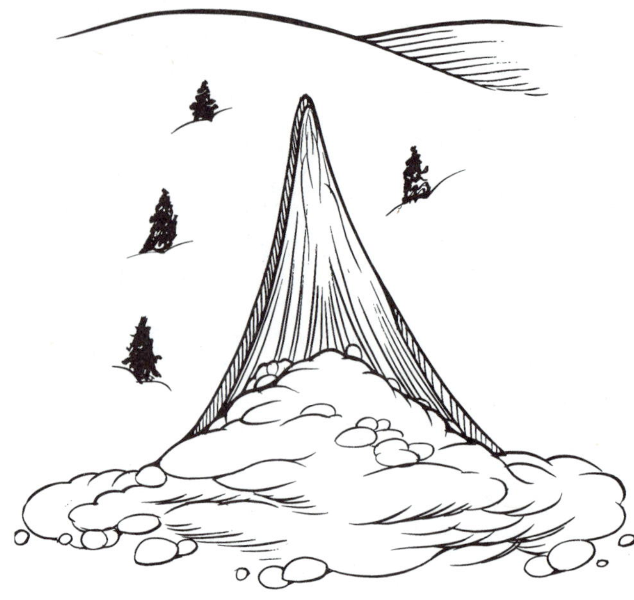

Fig. 25-10 Loose snow or point-release avalanche.

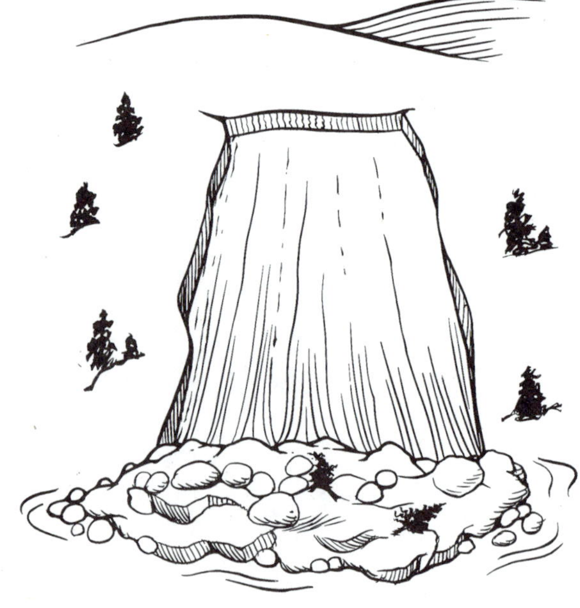

Fig. 25-11 Slab avalanche.

To understand the conditions in snow cover that contribute to slab avalanche formation, it is essential to reemphasize that snow cover develops layer by layer. Although a layered structure can develop by metamorphic processes, distinct layers develop in numerous other ways, most of which have some influence on avalanche formation. The layered structure is directly tied to the two ingredients essential to the formation of slab avalanches: the cohesive layer of snow and the weak layer beneath. If the snow cover is homogeneous from the ground to the surface, there is no danger of slab avalanches, regardless of the snow type. If the entire snow layer is sintered, dense, and strong, stability is very high. Even if the entire snow cover is composed of a very weak layer of depth hoar, there is still no hazard from slab avalanches because the cohesionless character does not allow propagation of the cracks necessary for slab avalanches to form. However, the combination of a basal layer of depth hoar with a cohesive layer above, for example, does provide exactly the ingredients for slab avalanche danger. For successful evaluation of slab avalanche potential, information is needed about the entire snowpack, not just the surface. A hard wind slab at the surface may seem strong and safe to the uninitiated, but when it rests on a weaker layer, which may be well below the surface, it may fail under the weight of a skier and be released as a slab avalanche.

Many snow structure combinations can contribute to slab formation. One scenario involves thick layers of weak snow, which result from development of depth hoar early in the season. The typical combination of climatic factors that produce these layers is early winter snowfalls followed by several weeks of clear, cold weather. Even at higher elevations in the mountains, snow cover on the slopes with a southerly aspect may melt off during a period of fair weather. However, in October and early November the sun angle is low enough that steep slopes with a northerly aspect receive little or no direct heating from the sun. Snow remains on the ground, but not without change. Snow on north-facing slopes experiences optimal conditions for depth hoar formation; a thin, low-density snow cover (maximum opportunity for vapor flow) is sandwiched between the warm ground, still retaining much of its summer heat, and the cold air above. This snow layer recrystallizes over a period of weeks. When the first large storm of winter arrives in November, cohesive layers of wind-deposited snow accumulate on a very weak base, setting the scene for a widespread avalanche cycle. Fig. 25-12 describes other combinations that result in brittle or cohesive layers of snow upon a weak layer.

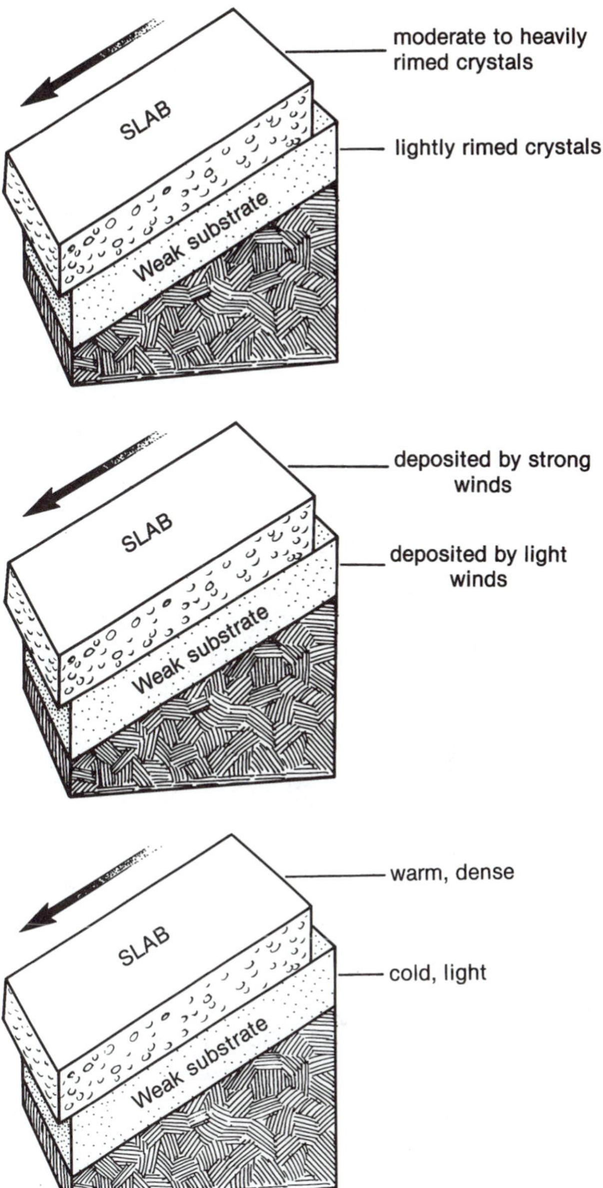

Fig. 25-12 Snow layer combinations that often contribute to avalanche formation.

MECHANICAL PROPERTIES

How Snow Deforms on a Slope

Almost all physical properties of snow can be easily seen or measured. A snowpit provides a wealth of information regarding these properties, layer by layer, throughout the thickness of the snow cover. However, even detailed knowledge of these properties does not provide all the information necessary to evaluate avalanche potential. The current mechanical state of the snow cover must be considered. Unfortunately, for the average person these properties are virtually impossible to measure directly.

Mechanical deformation occurs within the snow cover just before its failure and the start of a slab avalanche. Snow cover has a tendency to settle simply from its own weight. When this occurs on level ground, the settlement is perpendicular to the ground and the snow layer densifies and gains in strength. The situation is not so simple when snow rests on a slope. The force of gravity is divided into two components, one tending to cause the snow layer to shrink in thickness, and a new component acting parallel to the slope, which tends to pull the snow down the slope. Downslope movement within the snow cover occurs at all times, even on gentle slopes. The speed of movement is slow, generally on the order of a few millimeters per day up to millimeters per hour within new snow on steep slopes. The evidence of these forces is often clearly visible in the bending of trees and damage to structures built on snow-covered slopes. Although the movement is slow, when deep snow pushes against a rigid structure, the forces are significant and even large buildings can be pushed off their foundations.

Snow deforms in a highly variable fashion. It is generally described as a viscoelastic material. Sometimes it deforms as if it were a liquid (viscous) and at other times it responds more like a solid (elastic). Viscous deformation implies continuous and irreversible flow. Elastic deformation implies that once the force causing the deformation is removed, some small part of the initial deformation is recovered. The elasticity of snow is not so obvious, primarily because the amount of rebound is very small compared with that of more familiar materials.

In regard to avalanche formation, it is important to know when snow acts primarily as an elastic material and when it responds more like a viscous substance. These conditions are shown in Fig. 25-13. Laboratory experiments have shown that conditions of warm temperatures and slow application of force favor viscous deformation. We see examples of this as snow slowly deforms and bends over the edge of a roof or sags from a tree branch. In such cases the snow deforms but does not crack or break. In contrast, when temperatures are very cold or when force is applied rapidly, snow reacts like an elastic material. If enough force is applied, it fractures. We think of such a substance as brittle; the release of stored elastic energy causes fractures to move through the material. In the case of snow cover on a steep slope, forces associated with accumulating snow or the weight of a skier may increase until the snow fails. At that point, stored elastic energy is released and is available to drive brittle fractures over great distances through the snow slab.

The slab avalanche provides the best example of elastic deformation in snow cover. While the deformation cannot actually be seen, evidence of the resultant brittle failure is clearly present in the form of the sharp, linear fracture line and crown face of the slab release (Fig. 25-14). The crown face is almost always perpendicular to the bed surface, evidence that snow has failed in a brittle manner.

To fully understand the slab avalanche condition or the stability of the snow cover, its mechanical state must be considered. Snow is always deforming downslope, but throughout most of the winter the strength of the snow is sufficient to prevent an avalanche. The snow cover is layered, and some layers are weaker than others. During periods of snowfall, blowing snow, or both, an additional load, or weight, is being applied to the snow in the starting zone, the snow is creeping faster, and these new stresses are beginning to approach the strength of the weakest layers. The weakest layer has a weakest point somewhere within its continuous structure. If the stresses caused by the load of the new snow or the weight of a skier reach the level at which they equal the strength of the weakest point, the snow fails completely at that point (Fig. 25-15). This means that the strength at that point immediately goes to zero. This is analogous to what would happen if someone on a tug-of-war team were to let go of the rope. If the remainder of the team were strong enough to make up for the lost member, not much would change immediately. The same situation exists with the snow cover. If the surrounding snow has sufficient strength to make up for the fact that the strength at the weakest point has now gone to zero, nothing happens beyond perhaps a local movement or settlement in the snow. If, however, the surrounding snow is not capable of doing this, the area of snow next to the initial weak point fails, and then the area next to it, and the chain reaction begins.

As the initial crack forms in the now unstable snow, the elastic energy is released, which in turn drives the crack further, releasing more elastic energy, and so forth. The ability of snow to store elastic energy is essentially what allows large slab avalanches to occur. As long as the snow properties are similar across the avalanche starting zone, the crack will continue to propagate, allowing entire basins, many acres in area, to be set in motion within a few seconds.

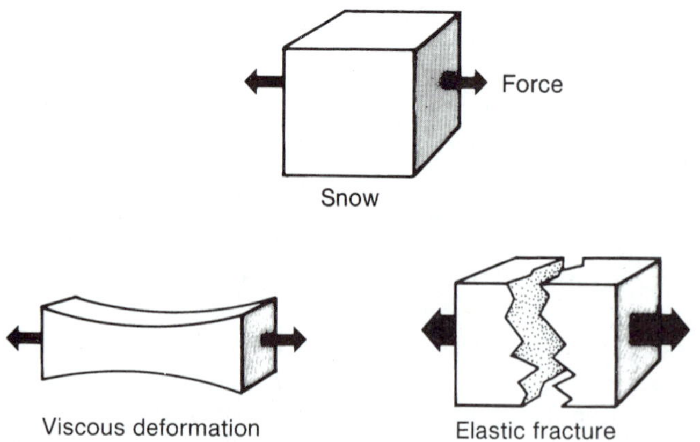

Fig. 25-13 Depending on prevailing conditions, snow may deform and stretch in a viscous or flowing manner, or it may respond more like a solid and fracture.

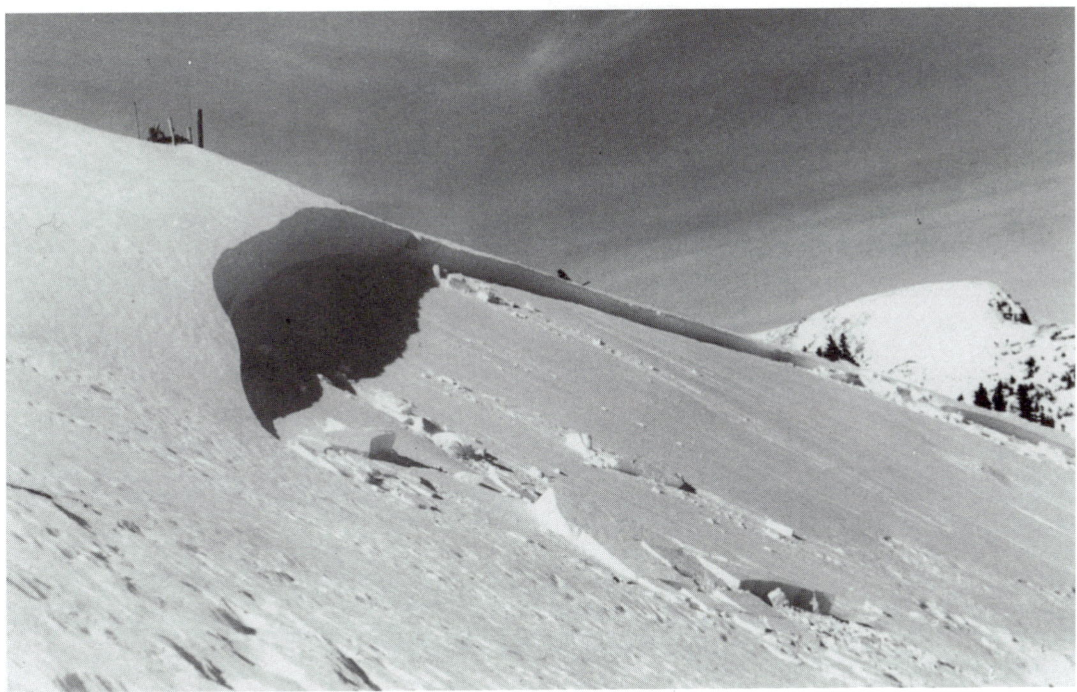

Fig. 25-14 The consistent 90-degree angle between crown face and bed surface of the avalanche shows that slab avalanches result from an elastic fracture. (A. Judson photo.)

Avalanche Dynamics

The topic of avalanche dynamics includes how avalanches move, how fast they move, and how far and with how much destructive power they travel. The science of avalanche dynamics is not well advanced, although much has been learned in the past few decades. Measured data for avalanche velocity and impact pressure are still lacking. While any environmental measurement presents its own set of problems, it is obvious that opportunities for making measurements inside a moving avalanche are extremely limited. Although avalanche paths exist in a variety of sizes and shapes, they all have three distinct parts with respect to dynamics (Fig. 25-16). In the starting zone, usually the steepest part of the path, the avalanche breaks away, accelerates down the slope, and picks up additional snow. From the starting zone the avalanche proceeds to the track, where it remains essentially constant and picks up little or no additional snow as it moves; the average slope angle has become less steep and frequently the snow cover is more stable than in the starting zone. Small avalanches often stop in the track. After traveling down the track, the avalanche reaches the runout zone. Here the avalanche motion ends, either slowly as it decelerates across a gradual slope such as an alluvial fan, or abruptly as it crashes into the bottom of a gorge or ravine. As a general rule, the slope angle of starting zones is 30 to 45 degrees, of the track is 20 to 30 degrees, and of the runout zone is less than 20 degrees.

Few actual measurements of avalanche velocities have been made, but enough data have been obtained to provide some typical values for the various avalanche types. For the highly turbulent dry-powder avalanches, the velocities are commonly in the range of 75 to 100 mph, with rare examples in the range of 150 to 200 mph. Such speeds are possible for powder avalanches because large amounts of air in the moving snow greatly reduce the forces resulting from internal friction. As snow in the starting zone becomes dense, wetter, or both, movement becomes less turbulent and a more flowing type of motion reduces typical velocities to the range of 50 to 75 mph. During spring conditions when the snow contains large amounts of liquid water, speeds may reach only about 25 mph (Fig. 25-17).

In most cases the avalanche simply follows a path down the steepest route on the slope while being guided or channeled by terrain features. However, the higher speed avalanche may deviate from this path. Terrain features, such as the side walls of a gully, which would normally direct the flow of the avalanche around a bend, may be overridden by a high-velocity powder avalanche (Fig. 25-18). The slower moving avalanches, which travel near the ground, tend to follow terrain features, giving them somewhat predictable courses.

Because avalanches can travel at very high speeds, the resultant impact pressures can be significant. Smaller and medium-sized events (impact pressures of 1 to 15 PSI) have the potential to heavily damage wood frame structures.

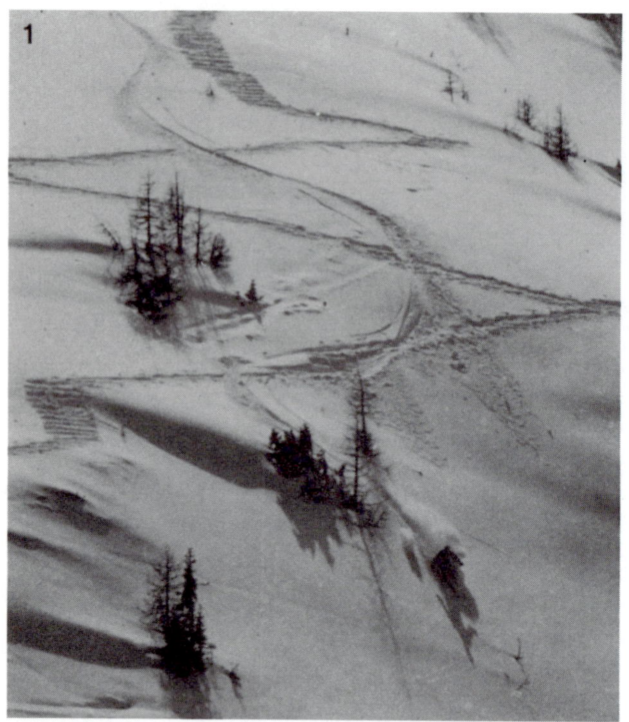

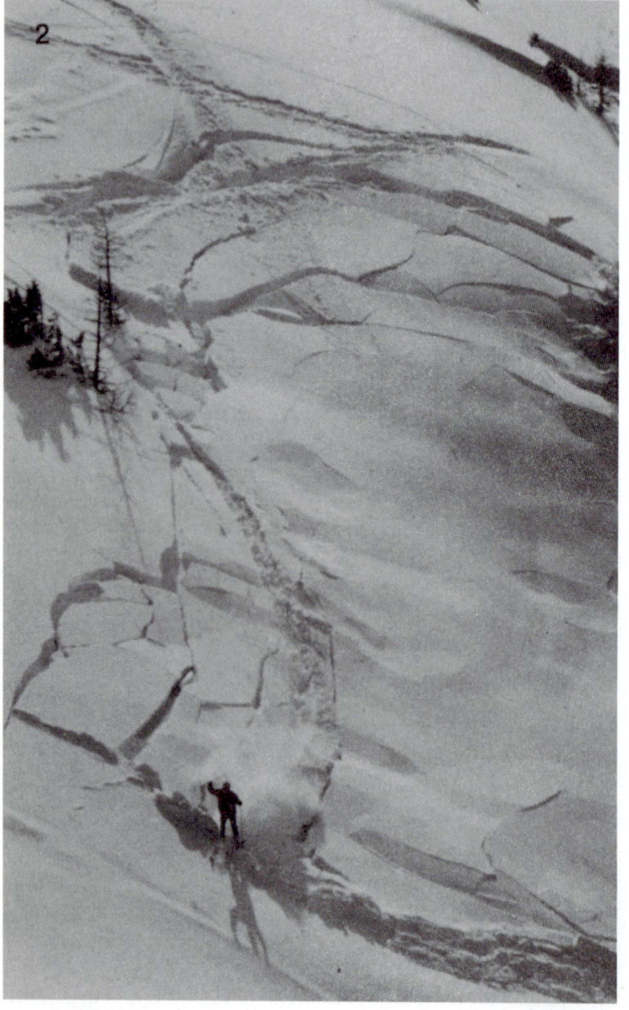

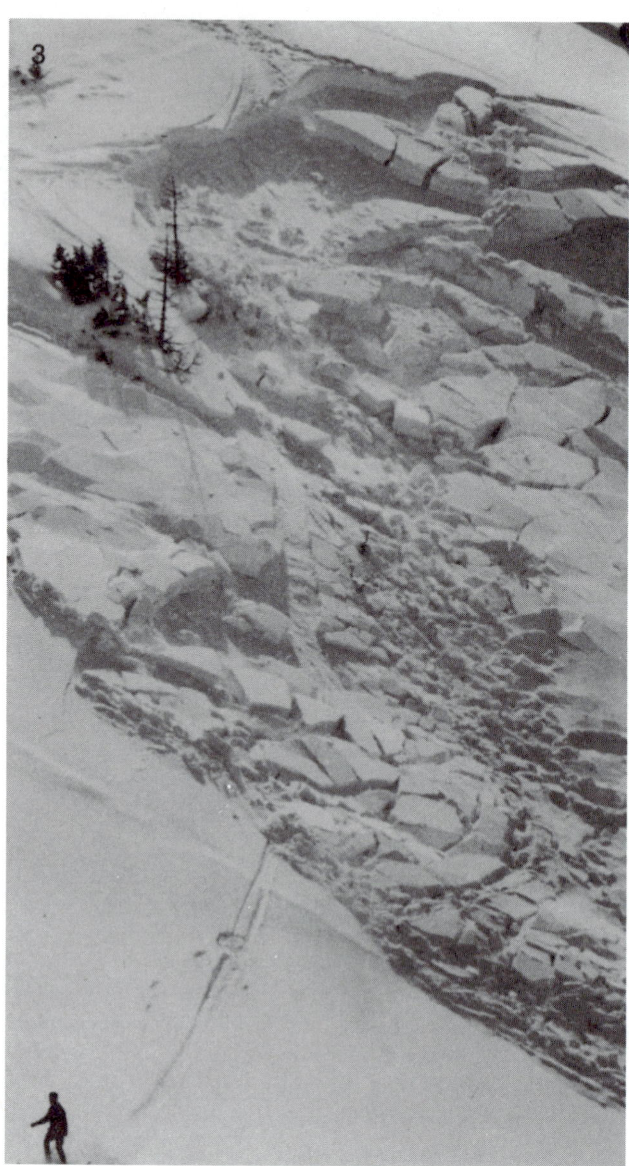

Fig. 25-15 Slab avalanche released by a skier. (R. Ludwig photo.)

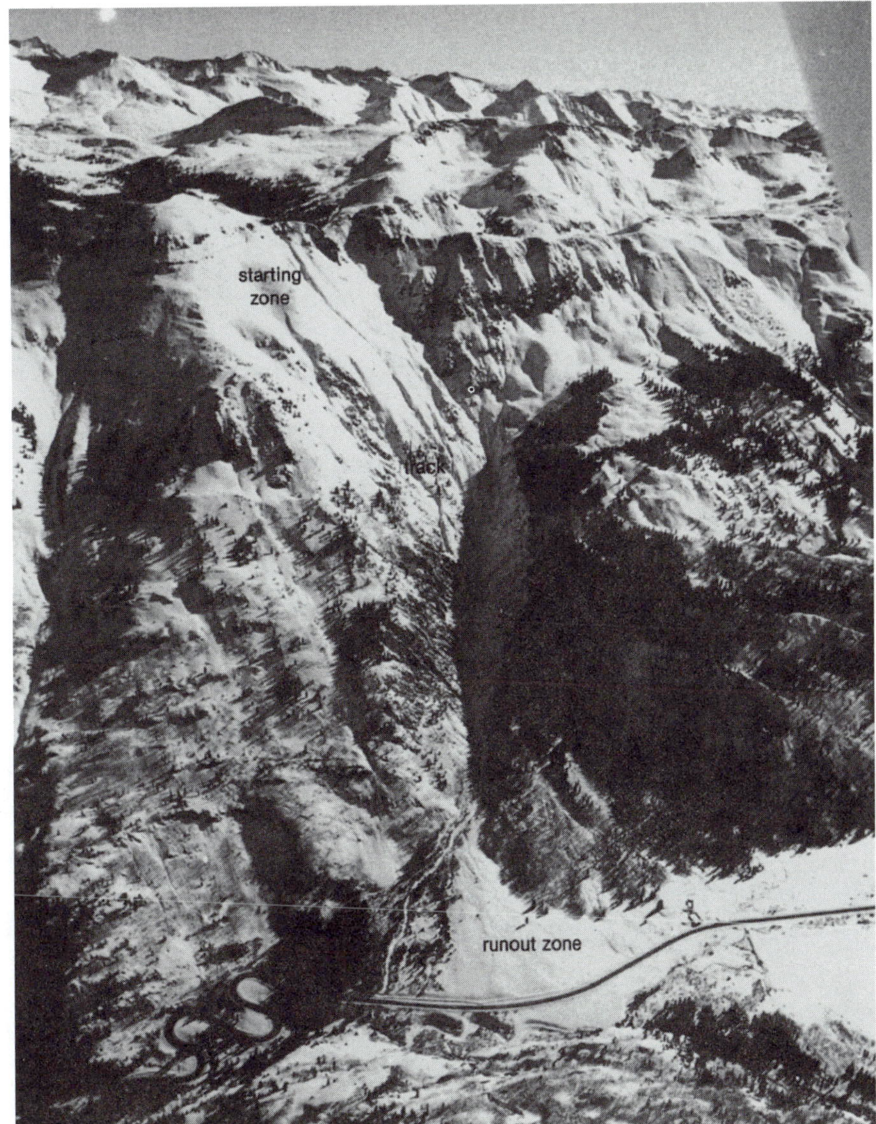

Fig. 25-16 The three parts of an avalanche path: starting zone, track, and runout zone. (B. Armstrong photo.)

Extremely large avalanches (impact pressures of more than 150 PSI) possess the force to uproot mature forests and even destroy structures built of concrete.

Some reports of avalanche damage describe circumstances that cannot be easily explained simply by the impact of large amounts of fast-moving dense snow. Some observers have noted that as an avalanche passed, some buildings actually exploded, perhaps from some form of vacuum created by the fast-moving snow. Other reports indicate that a structure was destroyed by the "air blast" preceding the avalanche, because there was no evidence of large amounts of avalanche debris in the area. However, this is more likely to be damage resulting from the powder cloud, which may only comprise a few inches of settled snow, yet contributes significantly to the total impact force. The presence of the snow crystals can increase the air density by a factor of three or more. A powder cloud traveling at a moderate dry avalanche speed of 60 mph could have the impact force of a 180 mph wind, well beyond the destructive capacity of a hurricane.

Identifying Avalanche Path Characteristics

Characteristics such as elevation, slope profiles, and weather determine whether a mountain can produce avalanches. The ingredients of an avalanche, snow and a steep enough slope, are such that any mountain can produce an avalanche if conditions are exactly right. To be a consis-

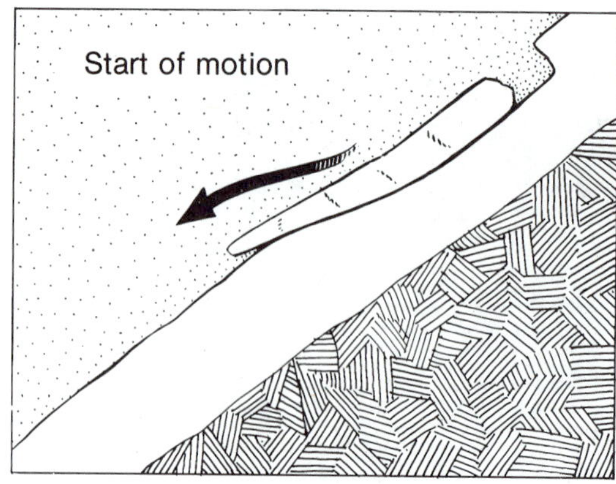

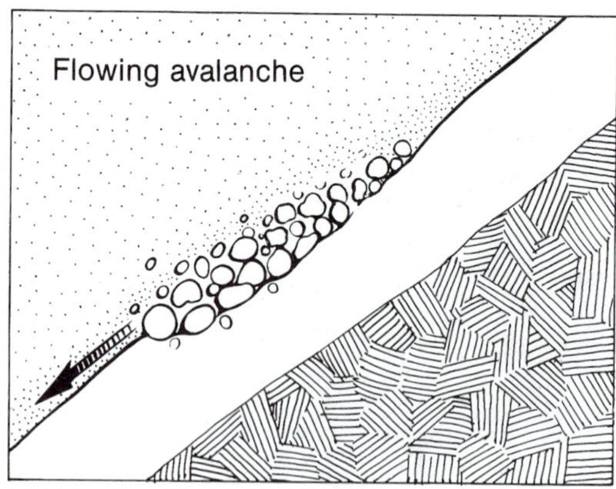

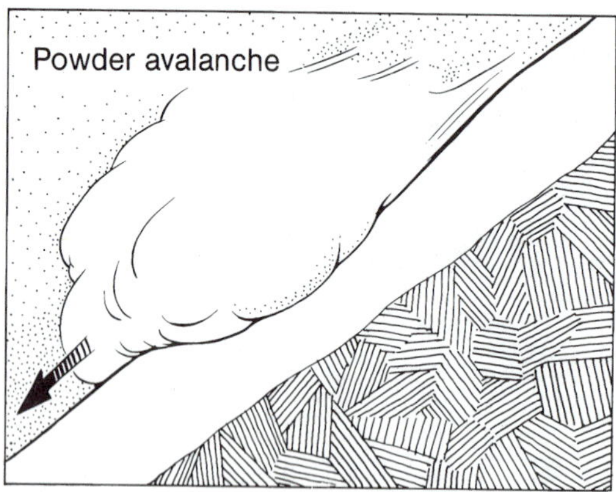

Fig. 25-17 A dry-snow avalanche may have a slowing motion and travel near the surface or, with lower density snow and higher velocities, the turbulent dust cloud of the powder avalanche develops.

tent producer of avalanches, a mountain and its weather must work in harmony.

ELEVATION

Mountains must be at high enough latitudes or high enough in elevation to build and sustain a winter snow cover before their slopes can become avalanche threats. Temperature drops steadily with elevation. This has the obvious effect of allowing snow to build up deeper and remain longer at higher elevations before melting depletes the snow cover. A less obvious effect of the temperature and elevation relationship on avalanche formation is the demarcation called treeline. This is the level above which the combined effects of low temperature, strong winds, and heavy snowfall prevent tree growth.

The treeline can be quite variable in any mountain range, depending on the microclimates. On a single mountain, treeline is generally higher on south slopes than on north slopes (in the Northern Hemisphere), because more sunshine leads to warmer average temperatures on southern exposures. Latitudinal variation in the elevation of treeline ranges from sea level in northern Alaska to almost 12,000 feet in the Sierras of southern California and the Rockies of New Mexico.

Mountains that rise above treeline are more likely to produce avalanches. Dense timber anchors the snowpack so avalanches can seldom start. Below treeline, avalanches can start on slopes having no trees or only scattered trees, a circumstance arising either from natural causes, such as a streambed or rockslide area, or from human-made causes such as a clearcut. Above treeline, avalanches are free to start, and once set in motion, they can easily cut a swath through the trees below. The classic avalanche path is one having a steep bowl above treeline to catch the snow and a track extending below treeline. Avalanches run repeatedly down the track and ravage whatever vegetation grows there, leaving a scar of small or stunted trees that cuts through larger trees on either side.

STEEPNESS

In snow that is thoroughly saturated with water, so that a slush mixture is formed, the slope needs only to have a slight tilt to produce an avalanche. For example, a wet-snow avalanche in Japan occurred on a beginners' slope at a ski area. The slope was only 10 degrees, but the avalanche was big enough to kill seven skiers. This extreme applies only to a water-saturated snowpack, which behaves more like a liquid than a solid.

A more realistic slope is 22 degrees, the "angle of repose" for granular substances such as sand and dry, unbonded snow. Round grains will not stack up in a pile having sides much steeper than 22 degrees before gravity rearranges the pile. Dry-snow avalanches have occurred on slopes of 22 to 25 degrees; these are rare, for snow grains are seldom round and seldom touch without forming bonds. A useful minimum steepness for producing avalanches is 30 degrees. Avalanches occur with the greatest frequency on slopes of 30 to 45 degrees. These are the angles in which the balance between strength (the bonding of the snow trying to hold it in place) and stress (the force of gravity trying to pull it loose) is most critical. On even steeper slopes the force of gravity wins; snow continually rolls or sloughs off, preventing buildup of deep snowpacks.

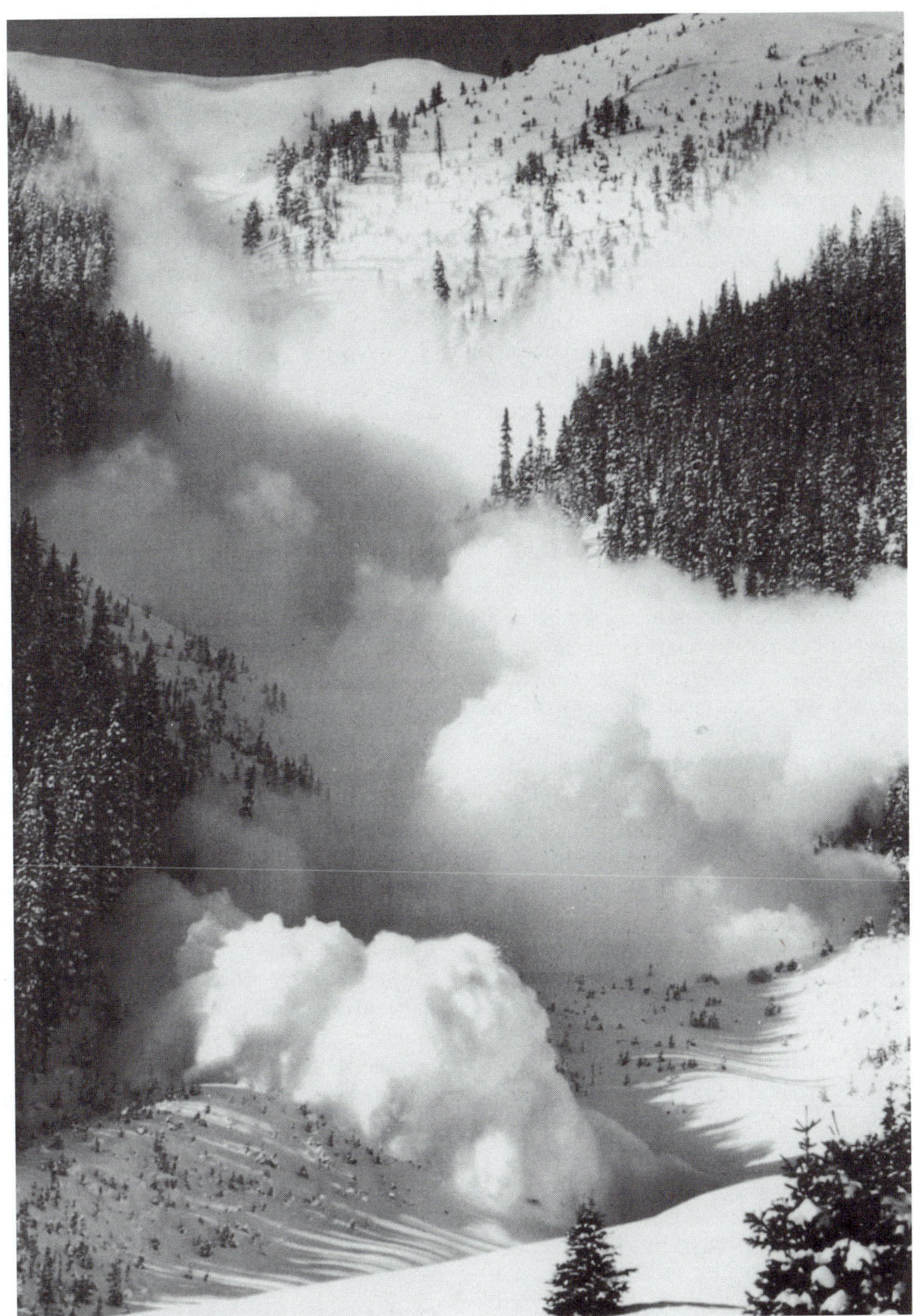

Fig. 25-18 The large powder cloud associated with a fast-moving dry-snow avalanche. (R. Armstrong photo.)

Exceptions exist, such as damp snow plastered to a steep slope by strong winds.

ORIENTATION

Avalanches occur on slopes facing every point of the compass. Steep slopes are equally likely to face east or west, north or south. There are factors, however, that cause more avalanches to fall on slopes facing north, northeast, and east than those facing south through west. These relate to slope orientation with respect to sun and wind. The sun angle in Northern Hemisphere winters causes south slopes to get much more sunshine and heating than do north slopes, which frequently leads to radically different snow covers. North slopes have deeper and colder snow covers, often with a substantial layer of depth hoar near the ground. South slopes usually carry a shallower and warmer snow cover, laced with multiple ice layers formed on warm days between storms. Most ski areas are built on predominantly north-facing slopes to take advantage of deeper and longer lasting snow cover. At high latitudes, such as in Alaska, the winter sun is so low on the horizon and heat input to south slopes is so small that there are few differences in the snow covers of north and south slopes. The effect of the prevailing west wind at midlatitudes is important. Storms most often move west to east, and storm winds are most frequently from the western quadrant: southwest, west, or northwest. The effect is to pick up fallen snow and redeposit it on slopes facing away from the wind, that is, onto northeast, east, and southeast slopes. These are the slopes most often overburdened with wind-drifted snow. The net effect of sun and wind is to cause more avalanches on north- through east-facing slopes.

AVALANCHE TERRAIN

The frequency with which a path produces avalanches depends on a number of factors, with slope steepness a major factor. The easiest way to create high stress is to increase the slope angle; gravity works that much harder to stretch the snow out and rip it from its underpinnings. A slope of 45 degrees produces many more avalanches than one of 30 degrees. However, specific terrain features are also important.

Broad slopes that are curved into a bowl shape and narrow slopes that are confined to a gully efficiently collect snow. Those having a curved horizontal profile, such as a bowl or gully, trap blowing snow coming from several directions; the snow drifts over the top and settles as a deep pillow. On the other hand, the plane-surfaced slope collects snow efficiently only if it is being blown directly from behind. A side wind scours the slope more than loads it.

The surface conditions of a starting zone often dictate the size and type of avalanche. A particularly rough ground surface, such as a boulder field, will not usually produce avalanches early in the winter, since it takes considerable snowfall to cover the ground anchors. Once most of the rocks are covered, avalanches will pull out in sections, the area between two exposed rocks running one time, and the area between two other rocks running another. A smooth rock face or grassy slope provides a surface that is too slick for snow to grip. Therefore full-depth avalanches are distinctly possible; if the avalanche does not run during the winter, it is likely to run to ground in the spring, once melt water percolates through the snow and lubricates the ground surface.

Vegetation has a mixed effect on avalanche releases. Bushes provide anchoring support until they become totally covered; at that point they may provide weak points in the snow cover, since air circulates well around the bush, providing an ideal habitat for the growth of depth hoar. It is common to see that the fracture line of an avalanche has run from a rock to a tree to a bush, all places of healthy depth hoar growth.

A dense stand of trees can easily provide enough anchors to prevent avalanches. Reforestation of slopes devoid of trees because of logging, fire, or avalanche is an effective means of avalanche control. Scattered trees on a gladed slope offer little if any support to hold snow in place. Isolated trees may do more harm than good by providing concentrated weak points on the slope.

Factors Contributing to Avalanche Formation

The factors that contribute to avalanche release are terrain, weather, and snowpack. Terrain factors are fixed; however, the state of the weather and snowpack changes daily, even hourly. Precipitation, wind, temperature, snow depth, snow surface, weak layers, and settlement are all factors determining whether an avalanche will occur.

SNOWFALL

New snowfall is the event that leads to most avalanches; more than 80% of all avalanches fall during or just after a storm. Fresh snowfall adds weight to existing snow cover. If the snow cover is not strong enough to absorb this extra weight, avalanche releases occur. The size of the avalanche is usually related to the amount of new snow. Snowfalls of less than 6 inches seldom produce avalanches. Snows of 6 to 12 inches usually produce a few small slides, and some of these harm skiers who release them. Snows of 1 to 2 feet produce avalanches of larger size that present a considerable threat to skiers and pose closure problems for highways and railways. Snows of 2 to 4 feet are much more dangerous, and snowfalls greater than 4 feet produce major avalanches capable of large-scale destruction. These figures are guidelines based on data and experience and must be considered with other factors to arrive at the true hazard. For example, a snowfall of 10 inches whipped by strong winds may be serious; a fall of 2 feet of feather-light snow in the absence of wind may produce no avalanches.

SNOWFALL INTENSITY

The rate at which snowfall accumulates is almost as important as the amount of snow. A snowfall of 3 feet in one day is far more hazardous than 3 feet in 3 days. As a viscoelastic material, snow can absorb slow loading by deforming or compressing. Under a rapid load the snow cannot deform quickly enough and is more likely to crack, which is how slab avalanches begin. A snowfall rate of 1 inch per hour or greater sustained for 10 hours or more is generally a red flag indicating danger. The danger worsens if snowfall is accompanied by wind.

RAIN

Light rain falling on a cold snowpack invariably freezes into an ice crust, which adds strength to the snow cover. At a later time the smooth crust could become a sliding layer beneath the new fall of snow. Heavy rain (usually an inch or more) greatly weakens the snow cover. First, it adds weight. An inch of rain is the equivalent in weight to 10 to 12 inches of snow. Second, it adds no internal strength of its own (in the form of a skeleton of ice, as new snow would), while it dissolves bonds between snow grains as it percolates through the top snow layers, reducing strength even further.

NEW SNOW DENSITY AND CRYSTAL TYPE

A layer of fresh snow contains only a small amount of solid material (ice); the large majority of the volume is occupied by air. It is convenient to refer to snow density as a percentage of the volume occupied by ice. New snow densities usually range from 7% to 12%. In the high elevations of Colorado, 7% is an average value; in the more maritime climates of the Sierras and Cascades, 12% is a typical value. Density becomes an important factor in avalanche formation when it varies from average values.

Wet snowfalls or falls of heavily rimed crystals, such as graupel, may have densities of 20% or greater. A layer of heavier than normal snow presents a danger because of excess weight. Snowfall that is much lighter than normal, 2% to 4% for example, can also present a dangerous situation. If the low-density layer quickly becomes buried by snowfall of normal or high density, a weak layer has been introduced into the snowpack. By virtue of low density, the weak layer has marginal ability to withstand the weight of layers above, making it susceptible to collapse. Storms that begin with low temperatures but then warm up produce a layer of weak snow beneath a stronger, heavier layer.

Density is closely linked to crystal type. Snowfalls consisting of graupel, fine needles, and columns can accumulate at high densities. Snowfalls of plates, stellars, and dendritic forms account for most of the lower densities.

WIND SPEED AND DIRECTION

Wind drives fallen snow into drifts and cornices from which avalanches begin. Winds pick up snow from exposed, windward slopes and drive it onto adjacent, leeward slopes, where it is deposited into sheltered hollows and gullies.

A speed of 15 mph is sufficient to pick up freshly fallen snow. Higher speeds are required to dislodge older snow. Speeds of 20 to 50 mph are the most efficient in transporting snow into avalanche starting zones. Speeds greater than 50 mph can create spectacular banners of snow streaming from high peaks, but much of this snow is lost to evaporation in the air or is deposited far down the slope away from the avalanche starting zone.

Winds play a dual role in increasing avalanche potential. First, wind scours snow from a large area (of a windward slope) and deposits it in a smaller area (of a starting zone). Wind can thus turn a 1-foot snowfall into a 3-foot drift in a starting zone. The rate at which blowing snow collects in bowls and gullies can be impressive. In one test at Berthoud Pass, Colorado, the wind deposited snow in a gully at a rate of 18 inches per hour. Another wind effect is that blowing snow is denser after deposit than before. This is because snow grains are subjected to harsh treatment in their travels; each collision with another grain knocks off arms and sharp angles, reducing size and allowing the pieces to settle into a denser layer. The net result of wind is to fill avalanche starting zones with more and heavier snow than if the wind had not blown.

TEMPERATURE

The role of temperature in snow metamorphism is played over a period of days, weeks, and even months. The influence of temperature on the mechanical state of the snow cover is more acute, with changes occurring in minutes to hours. The actual effect of temperature is not always easy to interpret; while an increase in temperature may contribute to stabilization of the snow cover in one situation, it might at another time lead to avalanche activity.

In several situations an increase in temperature clearly produces an increase in avalanche potential. In general, these include a rise in temperature during a storm or immediately after a storm, or a prolonged period of warm, fair weather such as occurs with spring conditions. In the first example the temperature at the beginning of snowfall may be well below freezing, but as the storm progresses, the temperature increases. As a result the initial layers of new snow are light, fluffy, low density, and relatively low in strength, while the later layers are warmer, denser, and stiffer. Thus the essential ingredients for a slab avalanche are provided within the new snow layers of the storm: a cohesive slab resting on a weak layer. If the temperature continues to rise, the falling snow turns to rain, a situation not uncommon in lower elevation coastal mountain ranges. Once this happens, avalanches are almost certain, because as the rain falls, additional weight is added to the avalanche slope, but no additional strength is provided as it is whenever a layer of snow accumulates.

The second example may occur following an overnight snowstorm that does not produce an avalanche on the slope of interest. By morning the precipitation stops and clear skies allow the morning sun to shine directly on the slopes. The sun rapidly warms the cold, low-density new snow, which begins to deform and creep downslope. The new snow layer settles, densifies, and gains strength. At the same time, it is stretched downhill and some of the bonds between the grains are pulled apart; thus the snow layer becomes weaker. If more bonds are broken by stretching than are formed by settlement, there is not enough strength to hold the snow on the slope and an avalanche occurs.

In these first two examples the complete snow cover generally remained at temperatures below freezing. A third example occurs when a substantial amount of the winter's snow cover is warmed to the melting point. During winter, sun angles are low, days are short, and air temperatures are cold enough that the small amount of heat gained by the snow cover during the day is lost during the long cold night. As spring approaches, this pattern changes, and eventually enough heat is available at the snow surface during the day to cause some melt. This melt layer refreezes again that night, but the next day more heat may be available, so that eventually a substantial amount of melting occurs and melt water begins to move down through the snow cover. As melt water percolates slowly downward, it melts the bonds that attach the snow grains and the strength of the layers decreases. At first the near-surface layers are affected, with the midday melt reaching only as far as the uppermost few inches, with little or no increase in avalanche hazard. If warm weather continues, the melt layer becomes thicker and the potential for wet snow avalanches increases. The conditions most favorable for wet slab avalanches occur when the snow structure provides the necessary layering. When melt water encounters an ice layer or impermeable crust, or in some cases a layer of weak depth hoar, wet slab avalanches are likely to occur.

DEPTH OF SNOW COVER

Of the snowpack factors contributing to avalanche formation, this is the most basic. When the early-winter snowpack covers natural anchors such as rocks and bushes, the start of the avalanche season is at hand. North-facing slopes are usually covered before other slopes. A scan of the terrain usually suffices to weigh this clue, but another method can be used to determine the time of the first significant avalanches. Long-term studies show a relationship between snow depth at a study site and avalanche activity. For example, along Red Mountain Pass, Colorado, it is unlikely that an avalanche large enough to reach the highway will run until close to 3 feet of snow covers the ground at the University of Colorado's snow study site. At Alta, Utah, once 52 inches of snowpack have built up, the first avalanche to cover the road leading from Salt Lake City can be expected.

NATURE OF THE SNOW SURFACE

How well new snow bonds to the old snow surface is a key factor in determining whether an avalanche will release within the layer of new snow or deeper in the snowpack. A poor bond, usually new snow resting on a smooth, cold surface with snowfalls of 1 foot or more, almost always produces a new-snow avalanche. A strong bond, usually onto a warm, soft, or rough surface, may produce nothing at all, or if weaknesses lie at deeper layers of the snow cover, a large snowfall will cause avalanches to pull out older layers of snow in addition to the new snow layer. These avalanches have more potential for destruction. A cold, hard snow surface offers little grip to fresh, cold snow. Ice crusts are commonly observed to be avalanche-sliding surfaces. The crust could be a sun crust, rain crust, or a hardened layer of firm snow that has survived the summer. Firm layers are especially dangerous in early winter when first snows fall.

WEAK LAYERS

Any layer susceptible to collapse or failure because of the weight of the overburden is a weak link. Of the snowpack contributory factors, this is the most important, for a weak layer is essential to every avalanche. The weak layer releases along what is called the failure plane, sliding surface, or bed surface.

One common weak layer is an old snow surface that offers a poor bond for new snow. Another weak layer that forms on the snow surface is hoar frost, or surface hoar. This is the solid equivalent of dew. On clear, calm nights, it forms a layer of feathery, sparkling flakes that grow on the snow surface. The layer can be a major contributor to avalanche formation when buried by a snowfall. Many avalanches have been known to release on a buried layer of surface hoar, sometimes a layer more than 1 month old and 6 feet or more below the surface.

A weak layer that is almost always found in the snowpacks that blanket the Rocky Mountains and occasionally the Cascades and Sierra Nevadas is temperature-gradient snow, or depth hoar. The way to decide whether a temperature-gradient layer is near its collapse point is to test the strength of the overlying layers and the support provided around the edges of the slope. This is no easy task. One method is to try jumping on your skis while standing on a shallow slope. Collapse is a good indication that similar snow cover on a steeper slope will produce an avalanche. Often skiers and climbers cause inadvertent collapses while skiing or walking on a depth hoar–riddled snowpack. The resulting "whoomf" sound is a warning of weak snow below.

Finally, a weak layer can be created within the snow cover when surface melting or rain causes water to percolate into the snow and then fan out on an impermeable layer, thereby lubricating that layer and destroying its shear strength. Combining the contributory factors on a day-by-day basis is the avalanche forecaster's art. Every avalanche must have a weak layer to release on, so knowledge of snow stratigraphy, or layering, and what sort of applied load will cause a layer to fail is the essence of forecasting.

Safe Travel in Avalanche Terrain

The first major decision often faced in backcountry situations is whether to avoid or to confront a potential avalanche hazard. A group touring with no particular goal in mind will probably not challenge avalanches. For this group, being able to recognize and avoid avalanche terrain is sufficient education. In the other extreme, mountaineering expeditions that have specific goals and are willing to wait out dangerous periods or take severe risks to succeed need considerably more information.

The ability to travel safely in avalanche terrain requires special preparations, including education and possession of safety and rescue equipment. The group should have the skills required to anticipate and react to an avalanche.

IDENTIFYING AVALANCHE TERRAIN

Because most avalanches release on slopes of 30 to 45 degrees of pitch, judging steepness is a prime skill in recognizing potential avalanche areas. An inclinometer is an instrument used to measure slope angles. Some compasses are also equipped for this purpose; a second needle and a graduated scale in degrees can be used to measure slope angles. A ski pole may be used to judge approximate slope steepness. When dangled by its strap, the pole becomes a plumb line from which the slope angle can be "eyeballed."

Evidence of fresh avalanche activity identifies avalanche slopes: the presence of fracture lines and the rubble of avalanche snow on the slope or at the bottom. Other clues are swaths of missing trees or trees that are bent downhill or damaged, especially with the uphill branches removed. Above treeline, steep bowls and gullies are almost always capable of producing avalanches.

ROUTE FINDING

Good route-finding techniques are necessary for safe travel in avalanche terrain (Fig. 25-19). The object of a good route in avalanche country is more than avoiding avalanches. It should also be efficient and take into account the abilities and desires of the group when choosing a route that is not overly technical, tiresome, or time consuming. The safest way to avoid avalanches is to travel above or below and well away from them. When taking the high route, the traveler should choose a ridgeline that is above the avalanche starting zones. It is safest to travel the windward side of the ridge. The snow cover is usually thinner and windpacked, with rocks sticking through: not the most pleasant skiing, but safe. Cornice collapses present a very real hazard; they should be avoided by staying on the roughened snow more to windward.

Skiers taking the low route in the valley should not linger in the runouts of avalanche paths. Even though it is unlikely that a skier traveling along the valley could trigger an avalanche high up on the slope, the skier should not boost the odds of getting caught in an avalanche released by natural forces far above. Slopes of 30 degrees or more should be avoided. By climbing, descending, and traversing only in gentle terrain, avalanche terrain can be avoided.

STABILITY EVALUATION TESTS

Skiers can perform several tests of stability. On a small slope that is not too steep (and therefore will not avalanche), the skier can try a ski test by skiing along a shallow traverse and then setting the ski edges in a hard check. Any cracks or settlement noises indicate that the same slope, if steeper, would have probably avalanched, and on the steeper slope it would have taken less weight or jolt to cause the avalanche.

Another test is to push a ski pole into the snow, handle end first. This helps to feel the major layering of the snowpack. For example, the skier may feel the layer of new snow, midpack stronger layers, and depth hoar layers, if the pole is long enough. Hard-snow layers and ice lenses resist penetration altogether. This test reveals only the gross layers; thin weak layers, such as buried surface hoar or a poor bond between any two layers, cannot be detected. Thus the ski pole test has limited value.

A much better way to directly observe and test snowpack layers is to dig a hasty snowpit. (This is an excellent use of the shovel that, in the next section, we recommend that the skier carry.) In a spot as near as possible to a suspected avalanche slope without putting the traveler at risk, a pit 4 to 5 feet deep and 3 feet wide should be dug. With the shovel, the uphill wall is shaved until it is smooth and vertical. Now the layers of snow can be observed and felt. The tester can see where the new snow touches the layer beneath, poke the pit wall with a finger to test hardness, and brush the pit wall with a paintbrush to see which layers are soft and fall away and which are hard and stay in place after being brushed. By grabbing a handful of depth hoar the skier can see how large the grains are and how poorly they stick together.

The shovel shear test gauges the shear strength between layers and thus locates weak layers. First a column of snow is isolated from the vertical pit wall. Both sides and the back of the column are cut with the shovel or a ski, so that the column is free standing. The dimensions are a shovel's width on all sides. The tester inserts the shovel blade at the back of the column and gently pulls forward on the handle. An unstable slab will shear loose on the weak layer, making a clean break; the poorer the bond, the easier the shear. A five-point scale is used to rate the shear: "very easy" if it breaks as the column is being cut or the shovel is being inserted; "easy" if a gentle pull on the shovel does the job; "moderate" if a slightly stronger shovel-pry is required; "hard" if a solid tug is required; "very hard" if a major effort is needed to break the snow. Generally, "very easy" and "easy" shears indicate unconditionally unstable snow, "moderate" means conditionally unstable, and "hard" and "very hard" mean stable.

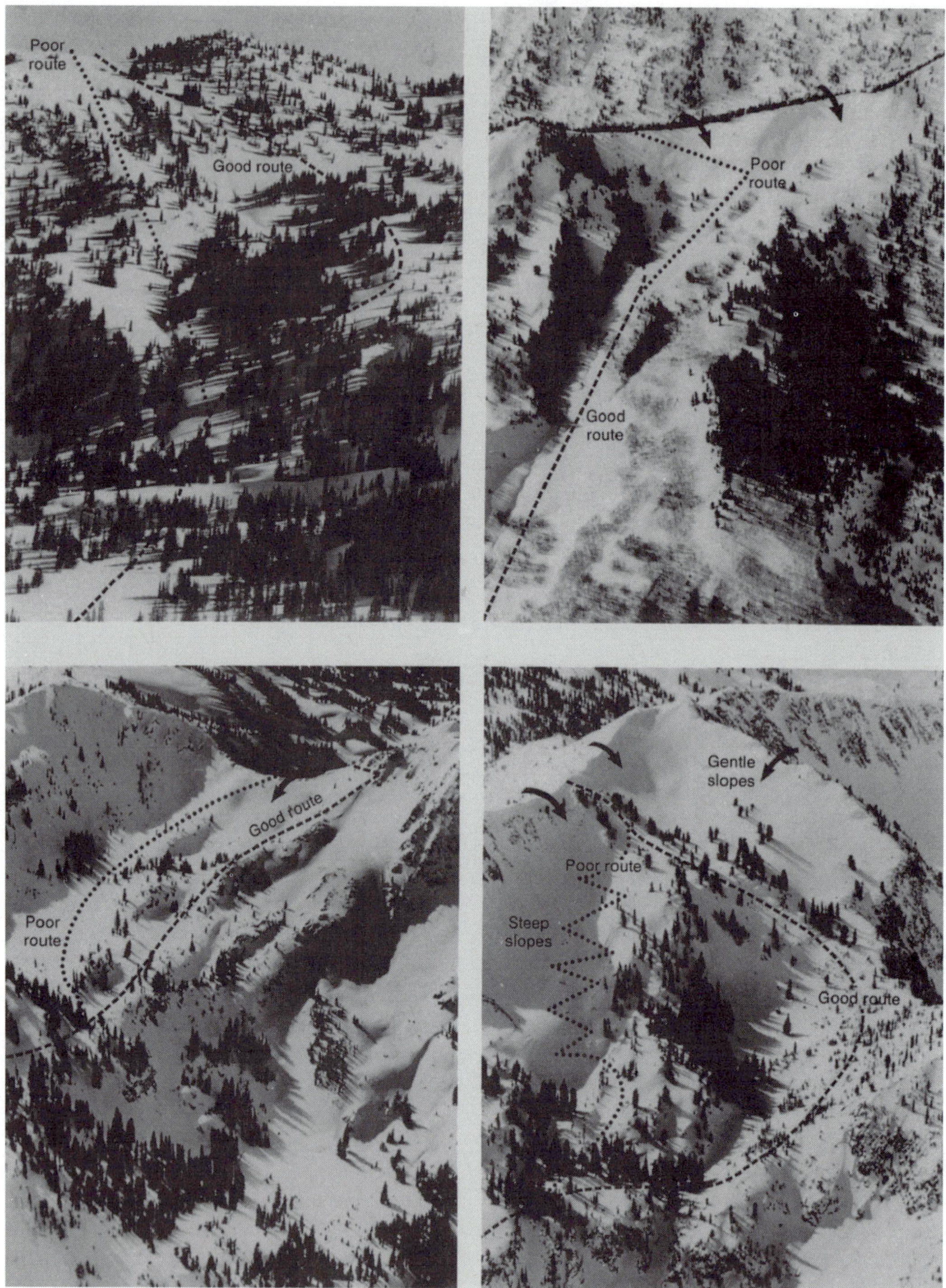

Fig. 25-19 Four ski-touring areas showing the safer routes *(dashed lines)* and the more hazardous routes *(dotted lines)*. Arrows indicate areas of wind loading. (From USDA Forest Service: *Avalanche handbook,* Agricultural Handbook 489, USDA. Alexis Kelmer photo.)

The value of the shovel shear test is that it can find thin weak layers undetectable by any other method. Its shortcoming is that it is not a true test of stability, since it does not indicate the amount of weight required to cause shear failure.

A test that does a better job of indicating actual stability is the Rutschblock or shear block test. This test is calibrated to the skier's weight and the stress he or she would put on the snow. Again, a snowpit is dug with a vertical uphill wall, but the pit must be about 8 feet wide. By cutting into the pit wall, the skier isolates a block of snow that is about 7 feet wide (a ski length) and goes back 4 feet (a ski pole length) into the pit wall. Both sides and the back are cut with a shovel or ski, so that the block is free standing. Wearing skis, the skier climbs around and well uphill from the isolated block and carefully approaches it from above. With skis across the fall line, the skier gently steps onto the block, first with the downhill ski and then the uphill ski, so that he or she is standing on the isolated block of snow. If the slab of snow has not yet failed, gently flexing the knees applies a little more pressure. Next some gentle jumps are tried. The stress should be by jumping harder until the block eventually shears loose or crumbles apart.

The interpretation of the results is: "extremely unstable" if the block fails while the skier is cutting it, approaching it from above, or merely standing on it; "unstable" if it fails with a knee flex or one gentle jump; "moderately stable" if it fails after repeated jumps; "very stable" if it never fails but merely crumbles. These are objective results that help answer the bigger question—Will it slide?—and help the mountain traveler decide how much risk to take.

AVALANCHE SAFETY EQUIPMENT

The first piece of safety equipment the skier or climber should own is a shovel. It can be used to dig snowpits for stability evaluation and snow caves for overnight shelter. A shovel is also needed for digging in avalanche debris, since such snow is far too hard for digging with the hands or skis.

The shovel should be sturdy and strong enough to dig in avalanche debris, yet light and small enough to fit into a pack. There is no excuse for not carrying a shovel. Shovels are made of aluminum or high-strength plastic and can be collapsible. Many good types are available in mountaineering stores. Some ski patrollers carry grain scoops to ensure that they can dig quickly and efficiently in avalanche debris.

Several pieces of equipment are designed specifically for finding buried avalanche victims. The first is a collapsible probe pole. Organized rescue teams keep rigid poles in 10- or 12-foot lengths as part of their rescue caches. The recreationist can buy probe poles of tubular steel that come in 2-foot sections that fit together to make a full-length probe. Ski poles with removable grips and baskets can be screwed together to make an avalanche probe. Survivors of an accident use probes to search for buried victims.

An avalanche cord is orange or red rope, approximately 50 feet long, that can be coiled and attached to a belt. When traveling in avalanche terrain, a skier or climber strings the cord out behind. The idea is that if an avalanche releases and the victim is buried, the cord will float and some portion of it will come to rest on the surface. Rescuers follow the cord, or probe in the immediate area, to locate the victim.

Avalanche cords have saved lives. However, tests done in the early 1970s by the International Vanni Eigenmann Foundation of Milan, Italy, showed that avalanche cords were only marginally effective. In tests performed by attaching an avalanche cord to a sandbag dummy tossed onto an avalanche path, a portion of the avalanche cord was visible on the surface only 40% of the time.

Avalanche rescue beacons, or transceivers, have become the most-used personal rescue devices worldwide. When used properly, they are a fast and effective way to locate buried avalanche victims. In the United States these have become standard issue for ski area patrollers involved in avalanche work and for helicopter-skiing guides and clients. They are also commonly used by highway departments, search and rescue teams, and an increasing number of winter recreationists. Since beacons were introduced in the United States, they have saved at least 30 lives. In recent years about two or three lives per winter have been saved by beacons.

Transceivers act as transmitters that emit a signal on a frequency of 2275 Hz or 457 kHz. A buried victim's unit emits this signal, while the rescuers' units receive the signal. The signal carries about 100 feet and, once picked up, guides searchers specifically to the buried unit.

Two types of beacons are sold in the United States: 2275 Hz frequency and dual frequency (2275 Hz and 457 kHz). All are compatible with one another. In other countries there have been instances in which incompatible units operating on different frequencies were used in rescues, with fatal results. To avoid such catastrophes in the future, the International Commission for Alpine Rescue (ICAR) in 1986 decided to recommend standardization of beacons on the 457 kHz frequency after 1990.[4] The 457 kHz frequency is thought to be superior to 2275 Hz because a greater range leads to faster recovery times. Following the recommendation of ICAR, Canada dropped 2275 Hz beacons on January 1, 1993. The sale and use of 2275 Hz beacons will cease in the United States as of December 31, 1995. After that date, all beacons sold worldwide will be on the 457 kHz frequency. Dual-frequency beacons will, of course, always be compatible with the new single-frequency standard of 457 kHz. However, dual-frequency units suffer from slightly reduced range and shorter battery life.

Merely possessing a beacon does not ensure its lifesaving capability. Frequent practice is required to master a beacon-guided search, which is not straightforward. Skilled practitioners can find a buried unit in less than 5 minutes once they pick up the signal. Since speed is of the essence in avalanche rescue, beacons are obvious lifesavers. The best safety equipment is a beacon for a quick find and a shovel for a quick recovery.

CROSSING AVALANCHE SLOPES

Travel through avalanche country always involves risk, but certain travel techniques can minimize that risk. Proper travel techniques might not prevent an avalanche release but can improve the odds of surviving. The timing of a trip has a lot to do with safety. Most avalanches occur during and just after storms. Waiting a full day after a storm has ended can allow the snowpack to react to the new snow load and gain strength.

Before crossing a potential avalanche slope, the skier or hiker should get personal gear in order by tightening up clothing, zipping up zippers, and putting on hat, gloves and goggles. A person should be padded and insulated if trapped. If a heavy mountaineering pack is carried, the straps should be loosened or slung over one shoulder only, so that the pack can be easily discarded if the person is knocked down. A heavy pack makes a person top-heavy, making it difficult to swim with the avalanche. The skier should remove pole wrist straps and ski runaway straps, because poles and skis attached to a victim hinder swimming motions and only serve to drag the victim under. Finally, a person wearing a rescue beacon should be certain it is transmitting.

If possible, the person should cross low on the slope, near the bottom or in the runout zone. Crossing rarely causes a release in the starting zone far above. The greater risk is getting hit by an untimely natural release from above. If crossing high without reaching the safety of the ridge is necessary, the starting zone should be traversed as high as possible and close to rocks, cliff, or cornice. Should the slope fracture, most of the sliding snow will be below and the chance of staying on the surface of the moving avalanche will be better. Invariably, the person highest on the slope runs the least risk of being buried.

A person who must climb or descend an avalanche path should keep far to the sides. Should the slope fracture, escaping to the side improves the chance of surviving. Only one person at a time should cross, climb, or descend an avalanche slope; all other members should watch from a safe location. Two commonsense principles lie behind this advice. First, only one group member is exposed to the hazard, leaving the others available as rescuers. Second, less weight is put on the snow. All persons should traverse in the same track. This not only reduces the amount of work required, but also disturbs less snow, which lowers the chance of avalanche release.

Skiers and climbers should never drop their guard on an avalanche slope. They should not stop in the middle of a slope, but only at the edge or beneath a point of protection, such as a rock outcropping. It is possible for the second, third, or even tenth person traversing or skiing down a slope to trigger the avalanche. Trouble should always be anticipated, and an escape route such as getting out to the side or grabbing a tree should be kept in mind.

SURVIVAL OF VICTIMS

Escaping to the Side

The moment the snow begins to move below the person, he or she has a split second to make a decision or make a move. Whether on foot, skis, or snowmobile, the person should first try to escape to the side of the avalanche or try to grab onto a tree. Staying on one's feet or snow machine gives some control and keeps the head up. Escaping to the side gets the person out altogether or to a place where the forces and speeds are less. Turning skis or the snow machine downhill in an effort to outrun the avalanche is a bad move, for the avalanche invariably overtakes its victims.

The person should shout and then close the mouth. Shouting alerts companions to what is happening. Clamping the mouth shut and breathing through the nose prevents inhalation of a mouthful of snow.

Swimming

A person knocked off his or her feet should attempt to swim with the avalanche. Cumbersome or heavy gear should be discarded. Ski poles should be tossed away; with luck the avalanche will strip away the skis. The victim should get away from the snow machine. Swimming motions with the arms and legs increase the freedom to maneuver the body. The purpose is to maintain a position near the surface. Any swimming motions will do, but if the person has been thrown forward and is being carried head first downhill, the breast stroke with the arms (similar to body surfing) should be used; if being carried down feet first, the person should try to roll onto his or her back and attempt to "tread water" with the arms and legs.

Reaching the Surface

Avalanches come to a stop when they flow out onto more gentle terrain. A victim may have a second or two when he or she feels the sensation of slowing down. This is a crucial point in the ordeal, the best chance to reach the surface. The person should thrust upward with swimming motions and try to burst through to the surface. Unless very deeply buried at this time, the person will probably know which way is up. All possible strength should be exerted to get the head, an arm, or even a hand above the surface. Even if the person cannot get his or her head out, being near the surface greatly improves the odds for survival. If any clue is on the surface, it gives the rescuers something to see. A hand should be used to clear a breathing space over the mouth.

RESCUE BY SURVIVORS

Marking the Last-Seen Point

A survivor or eyewitness to an accident needs to act quickly and positively. The rescuer's actions over the next several minutes may mean the difference between life and death for the victim. First, the victim's last-seen point should be fixed and marked with a piece of equipment, clothing, a tree branch, or anything that can be seen from a distance downslope. It is most often safe to move out onto the bed surface of the avalanche that has recently run. It is dangerous when the fracture line has broken at midslope, leaving a large mass of snow still hanging above the fracture.

Searching for Clues

The fall line should be searched below the last-seen point for any clues of the victim. The snow should be scuffed by kicking and turning over loose chunks to look for anything that might be attached to the victim or that will give the victim's trajectory and narrow the search area. Shallow probes should be made into likely burial spots with an avalanche probe, ski, ski pole, or tree limb. Likely spots are the uphill sides of trees and rocks, and benches or bends in the slope where snow avalanche debris is concentrated. The toe of the debris should be searched thoroughly; many victims are found in this area.

Rescue Beacons

If the group was using beacons, all survivors must immediately switch their units to receive mode. While making the fast scuff-search for visual clues, survivors should at the same time search the debris, listening for the beeping sound coming from the buried beacon. When they pick up the signal, they will be able to narrow the search area quickly. If skilled in this kind of search, they will pinpoint the burial site in a few minutes.

Probing

Probing avalanche debris is a simple but slow method for searching for buried victims. A probe line is composed of up to a dozen rescuers with avalanche probes, or sounding rods, who stand elbow to elbow on the avalanche debris. Ideally, probes should be 3 to 4 m long. Once the whole area is probed without a find, the proper decision is to do it again. In rescues with enough manpower, shovelers stand nearby to check out any possible strike. The line does not stop in such an event but continues to march forward with its methodical "down, up, step" cadence.

Coarse probing is four to five times faster than the more thorough technique called fine probing. For a coarse probe, probers straddle a distance of 50 cm and are spaced 75 cm apart (Fig. 25-20). This leaves 25 cm between the toes of adjacent probers. Probes are pushed into the center of the straddled span. Upon command from the leader, the line advances one step, about 70 cm. (Where terrain is steep or probers are few, an alternative is to stand "fingertip-to-fingertip." Probers probe first on one side of their body, then on the other.) This method gives about a 70% chance of finding the victim.

After several passes of coarse probing with no results, a fine probe is done, usually when the objective is body recovery. For this method the line is arranged as for coarse probing. Each searcher probes in front of the left foot, in the center of the straddled position, and in front of the right foot. On signal the line advances 30 cm and repeats the three probes. This method gives a 100% probability of finding a victim. The probe holes are spaced 25 by 30 cm, or 13 probes per square meter. On average, 20 searchers can fine probe an area 100 by 100 m in 16 to 20 hours.[5]

Avalanche Guard

If the threat of a second avalanche exists, one person should stand in a safe location to shout out a warning. This gives the searchers a few seconds to flee to safety. Rescues are often carried out in dangerous conditions, and self-preservation should be a major consideration.

Going for Help

A difficult question in rescues is when to seek outside help. If the accident occurs in or near a ski area and there are several rescuers, one person can be sent to notify the ski patrol immediately. If only one rescuer is present, the correct choice becomes harder. The best advice is to search the surface hastily but thoroughly for clues before leaving to notify the patrol. If a patrol phone is close, the rescuer should notify the patrol and then return immediately to resume the search.

If the avalanche occurs in the backcountry far from any organized body of rescuers, all party members should remain at the site. The guiding principle in backcountry rescues is that survivors search until they cannot or should not continue. When deciding when to stop searching, the safety of the search party must be weighed against the decreasing survival chances of the buried victim.

One exception exists to the rule of all party members staying to search. When there are a large number of survivors, two people can go out to secure help and the search party will still have a sizable rescue force on hand.

Three-Stage Rescue

A full-scale operation is divided into three stages. The first stage is the hasty search column. This group, composed of as many people as are on hand, heads swiftly to the site carrying probes, shovels, and first aid equipment. They scuff the avalanche for clues and probe likely areas in hopes of making a quick find. The person reporting the avalanche often accompanies this column back to the site.

The second stage brings the main body of rescuers to the site. They carry bulkier equipment needed for search, resuscitation, and evacuation: more probes and shovels, toboggans, sleeping bags, resuscitation equipment, medical supplies, and a trained avalanche dog and handler, if available. Ideally, stage two should begin 10 to 15 minutes after stage one.

The third stage brings in support for stages one and two, in the case of a prolonged rescue. Included are fresh rescuers to take over for cold and tired searchers, hot food and drink, tents, warm clothing, and lighting equipment. Avalanche dogs and handlers can provide additional searching power.

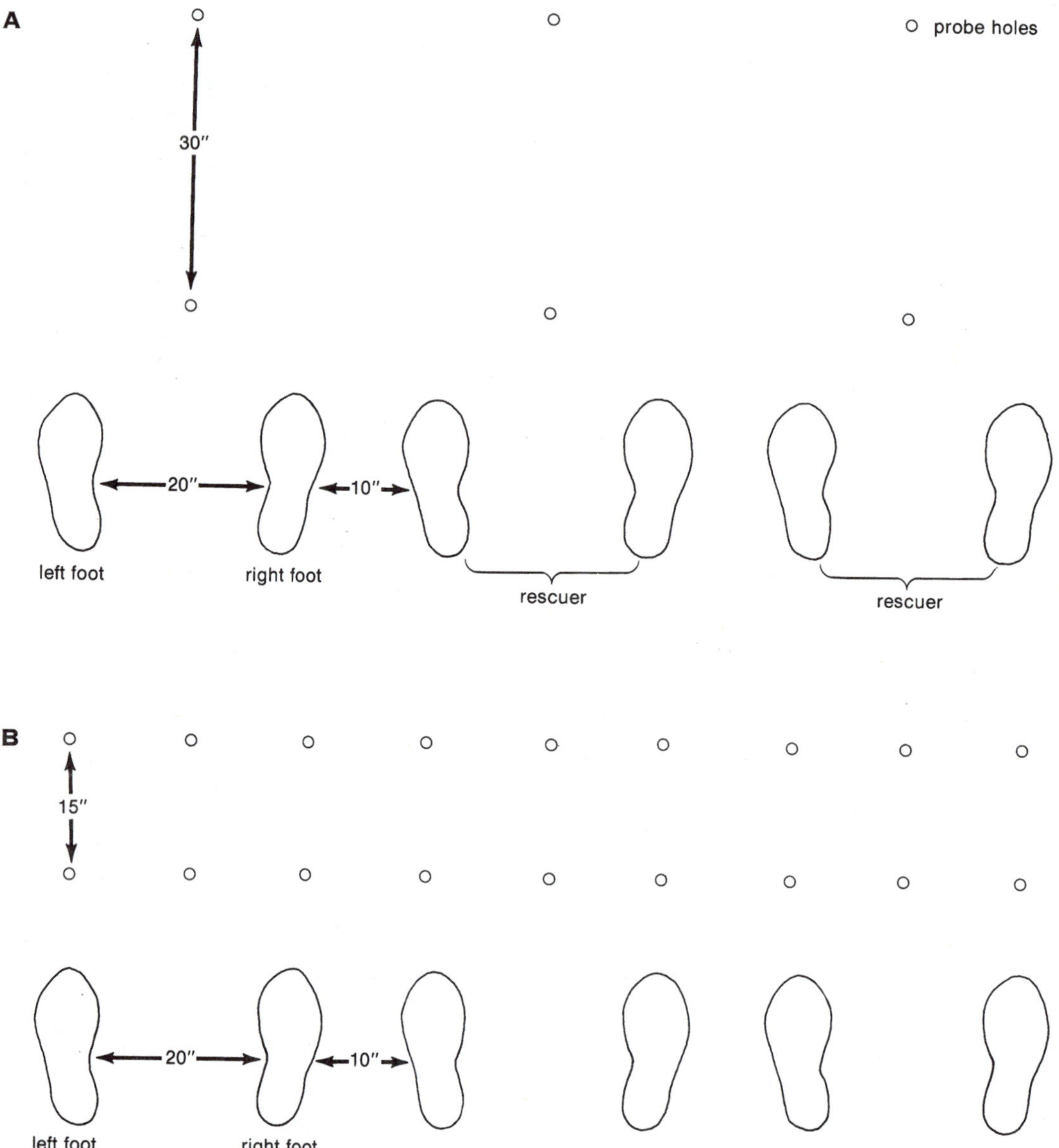

Fig. 25-20 **A,** Coarse and, **B,** fine avalanche probing.

The Modern Avalanche Victim

Avalanche deaths have increased in the United States each decade since 1950. Fig. 25-21 shows annual deaths; Fig. 25-22 shows these numbers averaged over 5-year periods. From 1950 to 1993, 417 people died in avalanches. Of these, 369 (88%) were men and 48 (12%) were women. The average age of all victims is 31 years. The youngest was 6; the oldest, 66.

Fig. 25-23 shows the activity groups for the victims. Most victims (76%) were pursuing some form of recreation at the time of their accident, with climbers, ski tourers, and lift skiers heading the list. The distinction between ski tourers and lift skiers is that lift skiers pursue their sport in and around developed ski areas and rely on lifts to get them up the hill. This category includes skiers who leave the area boundary or ski into "closed" areas within the ski area boundary. The ski tourers category includes ski mountaineers, backcountry skiers, helicopter and snowcat skiers, and snowshoers. Among nonrecreation groups, the persons at work category includes ski patrollers, highway personnel, and others who were on the job when avalanches struck. Since 1950, 14 states have registered avalanche fatalities (Fig. 25-24).

STATISTICS OF AVALANCHE BURIALS

Numerous factors affect a buried victim's chances for survival: time buried, depth buried, clues on the surface,

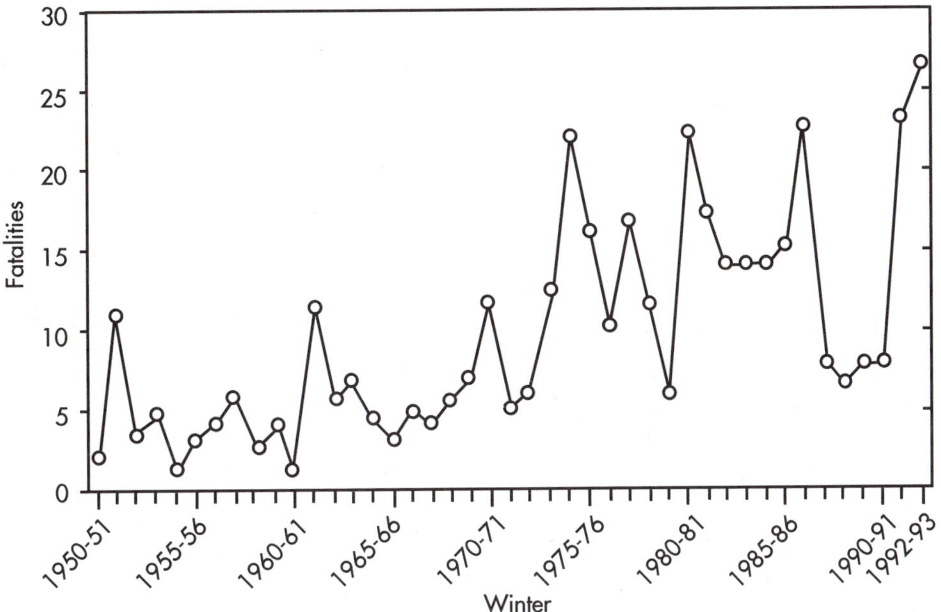

Fig. 25-21 Avalanche fatalities in the United States from the winters of 1950-51 to 1992-93.

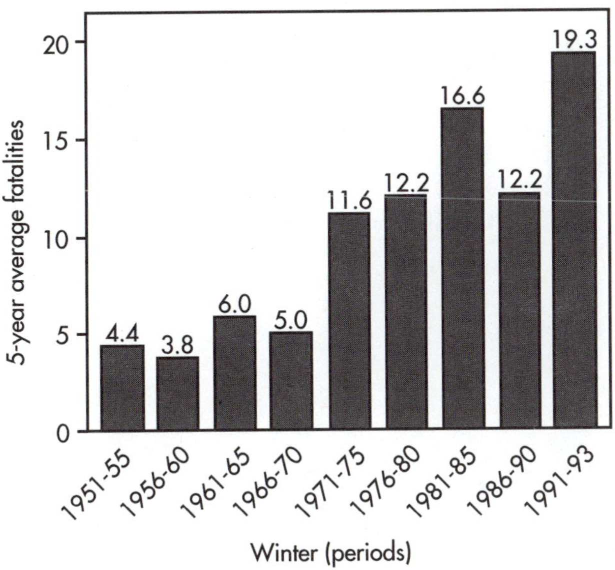

Fig. 25-22 Avalanche fatalities in the United States averaged by five-winter periods, 1950-51 to 1992-93.

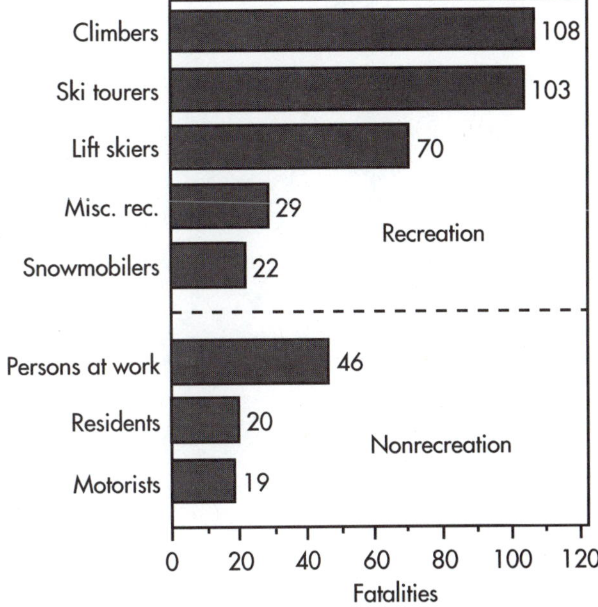

Fig. 25-23 Avalanche fatalities in the United States from 1950-51 to 1992-93 by activity categories.

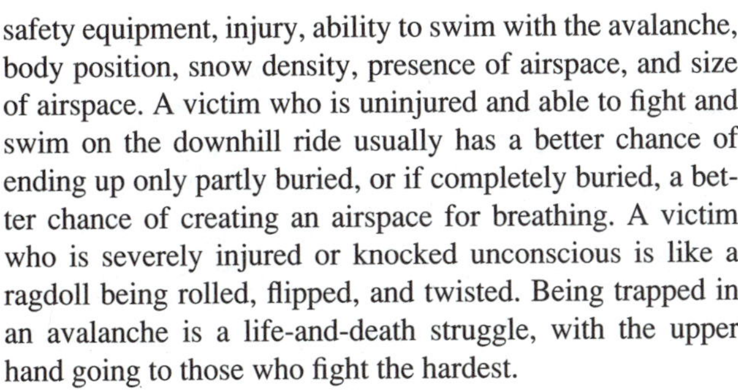

safety equipment, injury, ability to swim with the avalanche, body position, snow density, presence of airspace, and size of airspace. A victim who is uninjured and able to fight and swim on the downhill ride usually has a better chance of ending up only partly buried, or if completely buried, a better chance of creating an airspace for breathing. A victim who is severely injured or knocked unconscious is like a ragdoll being rolled, flipped, and twisted. Being trapped in an avalanche is a life-and-death struggle, with the upper hand going to those who fight the hardest.

Avalanches kill in two ways. First, serious injury is always possible in a tumble down an avalanche path. Trees, rocks, cliffs, and the wrenching action of snow in motion can do horrible things to the human body. About one third of all avalanche deaths are caused by trauma, especially to the head and neck. Second, snow burial causes suffocation in two thirds of avalanche deaths. The problem of breathing in an avalanche does not start with being buried. A victim being carried down in the churning maelstrom of snow has an

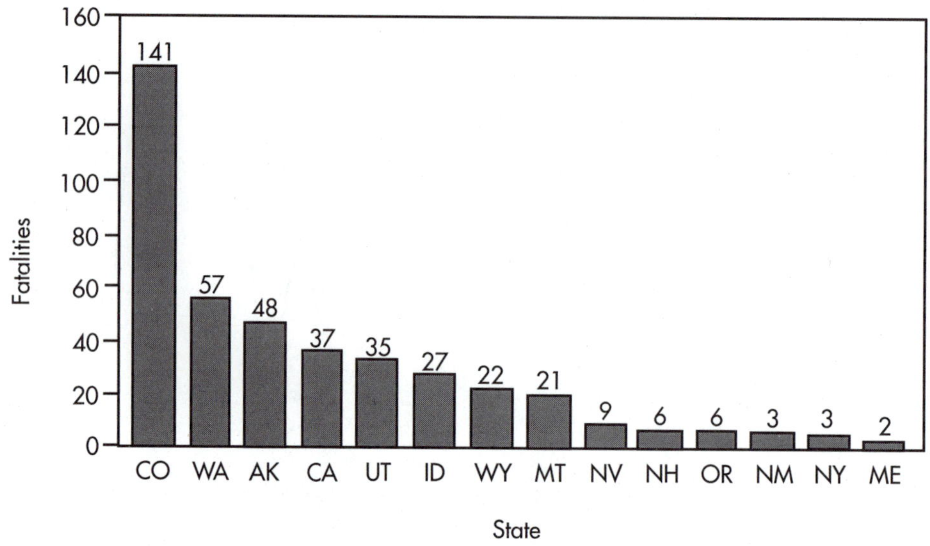

Fig. 25-24 Avalanche fatalities in the United States from 1950-51 to 1992-93 by state.

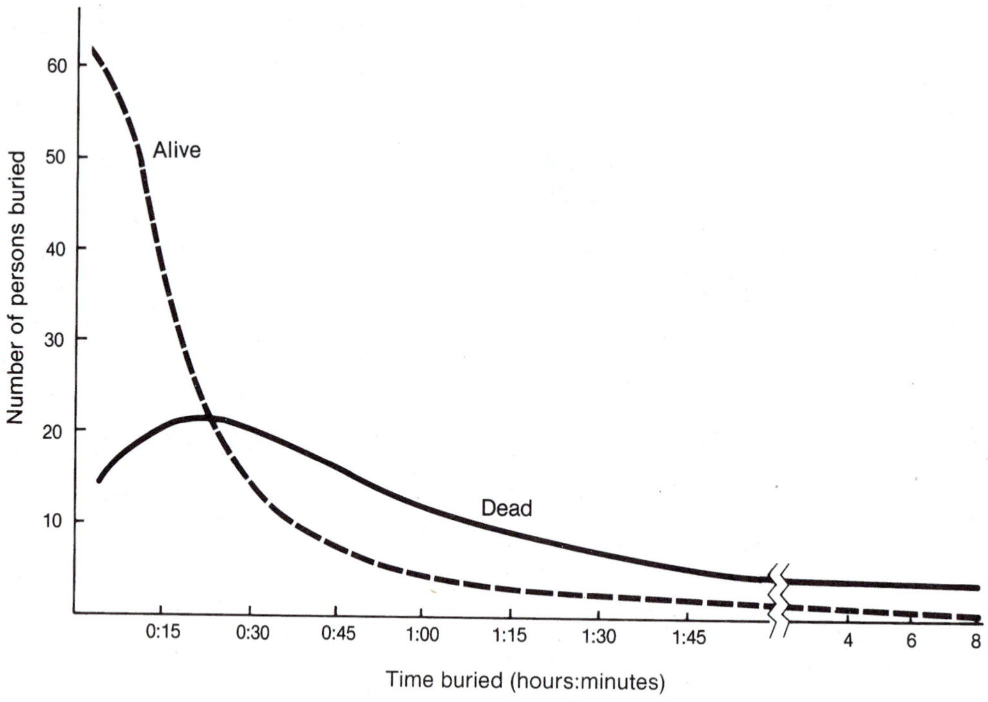

Fig. 25-25 Length of time buried for U.S. avalanche fatalities and survivors in direct contact with the snow (not in a structure or vehicle), 1950-51 through 1986-87.

extraordinarily hard time breathing. Inhaled snow clogs the mouth and nose; suffocation occurs quickly if the victim is buried with the airway already blocked. Snow that was light and airy when a skier carved turns in it becomes viselike in its new form. Where the snow might have been 80% air to begin with, it might be less than 50% air after an avalanche. The snow is much less permeable to airflow, making it harder for the victim to breathe.

Snow sets up hard and solid after an avalanche. It is almost impossible for victims to dig themselves out, even if buried less than a foot deep. Hard debris also makes recovery very difficult in the absence of a sturdy shovel. The pressure of the snow in a burial of several feet sometimes is so great that the victim is unable to expand his or her chest to draw a breath. Warm exhaled breath freezes on the snow around the face, eventually forming an ice mask that cuts off

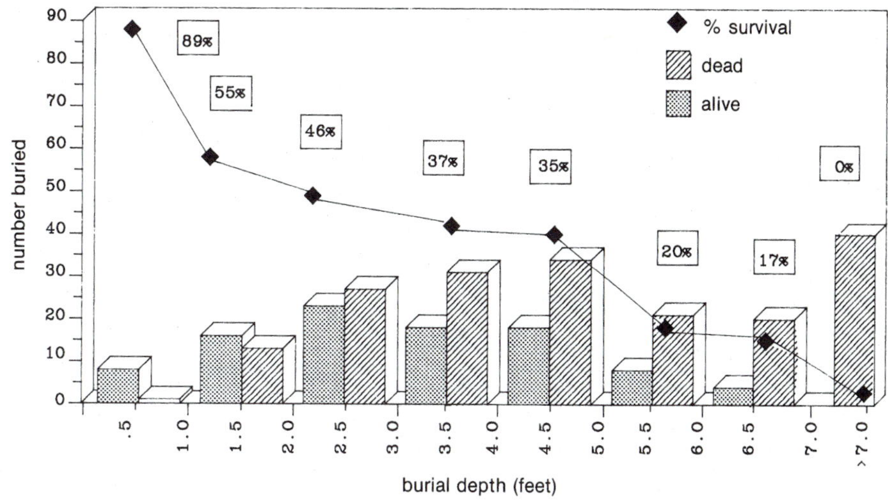

Fig. 25-26 Depth of burial for U.S. avalanche fatalities and survivors and percentage survival for victims in direct contact with the snow (not in a structure or vehicle) 1950-51 through 1986-87.

all airflow. It takes longer than snow-clogged airways, but the result is still death by suffocation.

The statistics on survival are derived from a large number of avalanche burials. In compiling these figures, we have included only persons who were totally buried in direct contact with the snow. We have not included victims buried in the wreckage of buildings or vehicles, for such victims can be shielded from the snow to allow sizable airspaces. Under favorable circumstances such as this, some victims have been able to live for days. In 1982, Anna Conrad lived for 5 days at Alpine Meadows, California, in the rubble of a demolished building, the longest survival on record in the United States.

A completely buried victim has a poor chance of survival. Fig. 25-25 shows decreasing survival with increasing burial time. In the first 15 minutes, more persons are found alive than dead. Between 16 to 30 minutes, an equal number are found dead and alive. After 30 minutes, more are found dead than alive and the survival rate continues to diminish. The important point is that speed is essential in the search. In favorable circumstances, buried victims can live for several hours beneath the snow; therefore rescuers should never abandon a search prematurely. A miner in Colorado who was buried by an avalanche near a mine portal was able to dig himself out after being buried for approximately 22 hours and nearly 6 feet deep. However, after several hours the diminishing probability of finding a live victim should be weighed against the safety of the search party.

Survival is interrelated with both time and depth of burial, as shown in Fig. 25-26. Survival probabilities diminish with increasing burial depth. To date, no one in the United States who has been buried deeper than 7 feet has been recovered alive.

STATISTICS OF RESCUE

A buried victim's chance of survival directly relates not only to depth and length of time of burial, but also to type of rescue. Table 25-1 compiles the statistics on survival as a function of type of rescue. Buried victims rescued by party members or groups at the accident site have a much better chance of survival than those rescued by organized rescue groups, time being the major influencing factor. Of those found alive, 59% were rescued by party members and 25% by an organized rescue party.

Table 25-2 describes methods of rescue for buried avalanche victims. Seventy-seven percent of victims (63/82) who were buried with a body part (such as a hand) or an attached object (such as a ski tip) protruding from the snow were found alive. In some cases this was simply good luck, but in many cases it was the result of actively fighting or swimming with the avalanche or of thrusting a hand upward when the avalanche began to slow down. Either way, this statistic shows the advantages of a shallow burial: less time required to search, shorter digging time, and the possibility of attached objects or body parts being visible on the debris. Of the fatalities in this category, many were skiing alone, with no one to spot the hand or ski tip and provide rescue.

Organized probe lines have found more victims than any other method, but because of the time required, most victims (88%) are recovered dead. Only 14 people were found alive by this method, with 102 recovered dead.

Rescue transceivers are an efficient method to locate victims. Since the first transceiver rescue in 1974, 19 of 39 buried victims (49%) have been recovered alive. Although some transceiver rescues have been textbook examples, where the victim's transceiver signal is located in minutes, everyone in the party has shovels, and the victim is dug out in a short time, 59% of victims are found dead. The more

Table 25-1 Type of Rescue for Buried Avalanche Victims in Direct Contact with Snow, Based on a Sample of 421 Burials in the United States from 1950-51 to 1986-87

	Self-Rescue	Rescue by Party Members	Rescue by Organized Team	Total
Found alive	27 (16%)	96 (59%)	41 (25%)	164
Found dead	—	45 (18%)	212 (82%)	257

Table 25-2 Method of Rescue (First Contact) for Buried Avalanche Victims, Based on a Sample of 490 Avalanche Burials in the United States from 1950-51 to 1986-87

Method	Found Alive	Found Dead	Total
Attached object or body part	63	19	82
Hasty search or random probe	14	23	37
Coarse or fine probe	14	102	116
Rescue transceiver	19	20	39
Avalanche cord	1	0	1
Acoustic contact	11	1	12
Avalanche dog	2	14	16
Other (digging, bulldozer)	13	13	26
Found after long time span	0	26	26
Not found, not recovered	0	24*	24
Not known	16	26	42
Inside vehicle	20	10	30
Inside structure	16	27	43
TOTAL	188	305	493

*Eleven persons died in an ice avalanche, bodies not recovered.

practice and experience with transceivers on the part of the rescuers, the faster the find and recovery.

Despite the insulating properties of snow, 12 victims who were shallowly buried were able to yell and be heard by rescuers (acoustic contact). An unfortunate case was the man whose moans were heard, but who was dead when uncovered 20 minutes later.

Trained search dogs are capable of locating buried victims very quickly, but because they are often brought to the scene only after extended periods of burial, there have been few live rescues. In the March 1982 avalanche disaster at Alpine Meadows, California, a dog made the first live recovery of an avalanche victim in the United States. Since then, dogs have effected two additional live recoveries: a highway worker on Wolf Creek Pass, Colorado, in February 1989 and a skier at Kirkwood Meadows, California, in January 1993.

A trained dog can search more effectively than can 30 searchers. Search dogs move rapidly over avalanche debris, using their sensitive noses to scan for human scent diffusing up through the snowpack. Dogs have found bodies buried 10 m deep, but have also passed over some buried only 2 m deep.[3] They are not 100% effective. Search and rescue teams and law enforcement agencies work closely with search dog handlers, and trained search dogs are becoming common fixtures at several ski areas in the western United States.

These statistics point out the extreme importance of rescue skills. Organized rescue teams, such as ski patrollers, must be highly practiced. They must have adequate training, manpower, and equipment to perform a hasty search and probe of likely burial spots within a minimum time span. For backcountry rescues the message is clear that a buried victim's best hope for survival is to be found by his or her companions. The need to seek outside rescue units practically ensures a body recovery mission.

APPENDIX A
Public Information

Twenty-four-hour regional avalanche information is available, generally from November through April, by calling recorded messages. Additional information can often be found through local forest service ranger districts, parks, or ski areas.

CALIFORNIA

Lake Tahoe/Donner Summit (Truckee)
916-587-2158
Central-Eastern Sierra (Mammoth Lakes)
619-934-6611

COLORADO

Colorado Rockies (Denver/Boulder)
303-275-5360
Colorado Rockies (Fort Collins)
303-482-0457
Colorado Rockies (Colorado Springs)
719-520-0020
Northern Colorado Rockies (Summit County)
303-668-0600
Northern Colorado Rockies (Vail)
303-827-5687
Central Colorado Rockies (Aspen)
303-920-1664
Southern Colorado Rockies (Durango)
303-247-8187

IDAHO

Smokey, Sawtooth, and Pioneer Mountains (Ketchum)
206-622-8027

MONTANA

Northwest Mountains (Whitefish)
406-257-8606
South Central Mountains (Bozeman)
406-587-6981
Southern Mountains (Cooke City)
406-838-2259
Southern Mountains (West Yellowstone)
406-646-7912

OREGON

Southern Washington Cascades and Mt. Hood area (Portland)
503-326-2400

UTAH

Sundance/Mt. Timpanogos area (Provo)
801-374-9770
Tri-Canyon area (Salt Lake City)
801-364-1581
Mt. Ogden south to the Tri-Canyons (Ogden)
801-621-2362
East of Tri-Canyons (Park City)
801-649-2250
North Wasatch (Logan)
801-752-4146
La Sal Mountains (Moab)
801-259-7669

WASHINGTON

Washington Cascades and Olympics (Seattle)
206-526-6677

WYOMING

Teton, Wyoming, and Wind River Mountains (Teton Village)
307-733-2664

CANADA

Banff National Park (Banff)
403-762-1460
Canadian Rockies (Calgary and Edmonton)
403-243-7253
Canadian Rockies (Vancouver)
604-290-9333

APPENDIX B
Avalanche Education

Several organizations teach basic and advanced avalanche awareness and training courses. Beyond those listed here, many local colleges and universities, ski patrols, and recreation departments offer courses.

Alaska Avalanche School
Alaska Mountain Safety Center
9140 Brewster's Drive
Anchorage, AL 99516
907-345-3566 (day), 907-345-7736 (evening)

American Avalanche Institute
c/o Rod Newcomb
Box 308
Wilson, WY 83014
307-733-3315

Blue Lake Centre
Box 850
Hinton, Alta, Canada TOE 1B0
403-865-4741

Brighton Ski Touring Center
P.O. Box 17848
Salt Lake City, UT 84117
801-531-9171

Canadian Avalanche Association Training Schools
Box 2759
Revelstoke, B.C., Canada V0E 2S0
604-837-2435

Canadian Ski Patrol System
National Avalanche Training Officer
RR2 Okotoks, Box 1117
Okotoks, Alta, Canada T0L 1T0
403-938-2131 or 403-938-2101

Federation of Mountain Clubs of British Columbia
336-1367 West Broadway
Vancouver, B.C., Canada V6H 4A9
604-737-3053

The Mountain School, Inc.
P.O. Box 728
Renton, WA 98057
206-266-2613

National Avalanche School
National Avalanche Foundation
133 South Van Gordon St., Suite 100
Lakewood, CO 80228
303-988-1111

National Ski Patrol
c/o Lin Ballard
170 Misty Vale
Boulder, CO 80302
303-449-8619

Nordic Ski Institute
Box 1050
Canmore, Alta., Canada T0L 0M0
403-678-4102

Paragon Guides
P.O. Box 130
Vail, CO 81658
303-926-5299

Sierra Ski Touring
c/o Dave Beck
Box 176
Gardnerville, NV 89410
702-782-3047

Sierra Wilderness Seminars
P.O. Box 707
Arcata, CA 95521
707-822-8066

Silverton Avalanche School
c/o San Juan Mountain Search and Rescue
Box 4
Silverton, CO 81433

Summit County Avalanche Seminar
Summit County Rescue Group
P.O. Box 1794
Breckenridge, CO 80424

Colleges and universities that offer avalanche and snow related courses:

Montana State University
Department of Engineering and Engineering Mechanics
Bozeman, MT 59715

Sierra College
Forestry Department
5000 Rocklin Road
Rocklin, CA 95677

University of British Columbia
Department of Geophysics
Vancouver, B.C.
Canada V6T 2A4

University of Utah
Department of Geography
Salt Lake City, UT 84102

Utah State University
Forestry Department
UMC 52
Logan, UT 84322

Utah Technical College at Provo
P.O. Box 1609
Provo, UT 84603
Attn: Wayne Kearny

Wenatchee Valley College
c/o Lee Rowe
5th Street
Wenatchee, WA 98801

APPENDIX C
Avalanche Safety Equipment Manufacturers and Suppliers

Alpine Research, Inc.
1803 South Foothills Highway
Boulder, CO 80303
303-642-7844
Backcountry ski equipment, survival gear, rescue beacons

Black Diamond Equipment, Ltd.
2084 East 3900 South
Salt Lake City, UT 84124
801-278-5533
Backcountry ski equipment, clothing, survival gear, rescue beacons

Cascade Toboggan
25802 West Valley Highway
Kent, WA 98032
206-852-0182
Shovels, probes, rescue beacons, other rescue equipment

Climb High
1861 Shelburne Road
Shelburne, VT 05482
802-985-5055
Backcountry ski and expedition equipment, rescue beacons, shovels, probes, and clothing

Eastern Mountain Sports
1 Vose Farm Road
Peterborough, NH 03458
603-924-9571
(or local retail store)
Backcountry ski equipment, clothing, survival gear, rescue beacons

Exploration Products
North 3005 Industrial Lane, Bldg S21
Spokane, WA 99216
509-927-8101
Rescue beacons, survival gear

Hydro-Tech
4658 N.E. 178th St.
Seattle, WA 98155
206-362-1074
Snowpit instruments

Lawtronics
326 Walton
Buffalo, NY 14226
716-839-0630
Skadi rescue beacons

Life Link
P.O. Box 2913
Jackson Hole, WY 83001
800-443-8620
Snowpit instruments, shovels, probes, rescue beacons, other rescue equipment

Mountain Safety Research
4225 2nd Avenue South
Seattle, WA 98134
206-624-857
Survival gear, probes, other rescue equipment

Mt. Tam Sports
Box 111
Kentfield, CA 94914
415-461-8111
Snowpit instruments, rescue equipment, first aid equipment

The North Face
999 Harrison St.
Berkeley, CA 94710
800-323-8333
(or local retail store)
Backcountry ski equipment, clothing, survival gear, rescue beacons

Recreational Equipment, Inc.
P.O. Box 88125
Seattle, WA 98138-2125
206-323-8333
(or local retail store)
Backcountry ski equipment, clothing, survival gear, rescue beacons

Wasatch Touring
702 East 100 South
Salt Lake City, UT 84102
801-359-9361
Snowpit instruments, probes, shovels, rescue beacons

REFERENCES

1. Armstrong BR, Williams K: *The avalanche book,* Golden, Colo, 1992, Fulcrum.
2. *Avalanche notes,* Fort Collins, Colo, Westwide Data Network, US Forest Service.
3. Bryson S: *Search dog training,* Pacific Grove, Calif, 1984, Boxwood Press.
4. Meier F: *A standard frequency for avalanche beacons: what's going on in Europe?* Proceedings of International Snow Science Workshop, Lake Tahoe, Calif, Oct 22-25, 1986.
5. Perla R, Martinelli M Jr: *The avalanche handbook,* Agriculture Handbook 489, Washington, DC, 1976, USDA Forest Service.

ADDITIONAL RECOMMENDED READINGS

The Avalanche Review, P.O. Box 510904, Salt Lake City, UT 84151 (official publication of the American Association of Avalanche Professionals).

Colbeck SC, editor: *Dynamics of snow and ice masses,* New York, 1980, Academic Press.

Daffern T: *Avalanche safety for skiers and climbers,* ed 2, Seattle, Wash, 1992, Cloudcap.

Fraser C: *Avalanches and snow safety,* New York, 1978, Charles Scribner.

Fredston J, Fesler D: *Snow sense: a guide to evaluating avalanche hazard,* ed 3, Anchorage, 1988, Alaska Avalanche School, Alaska Mountain Safety Center.

Gallagher D, editor: *The snowy torrents: avalanche accidents in the United States 1910-1966,* 1967, Alta Avalanche Study Center, USDA Forest Service.

LaChapelle ER: *The ABC's of avalanche safety,* ed 2, Seattle, Wash, 1985, The Mountaineers Books.

Nakaya U: *Snow crystals: natural and artificial,* Cambridge, Mass, 1954, Harvard University Press.

Williams K: *The snowy torrents: avalanche accidents in the United States 1967-71,* USDA Forest Service General Technical Report RM-8, Fort Collins, Colo, 1975.

Williams K, Armstrong B: *The snowy torrents: avalanche accidents in the United States 1972-79,* Jackson, Wyo, 1975, Teton Bookshop Publishing Co.

26 NATURAL DISASTER MANAGEMENT

Eric K. Noji

- Nature of disaster
- Past problems in natural disaster management
- Information management systems for disaster response
- Health care needs in specific natural disasters
- Practical issues in natural disaster response
- Some public health problems associated with natural disasters

Throughout history, natural disasters have exacted a heavy toll of death and suffering (Tables 26-1 and 26-2). During the past 20 years they have claimed about 3 million lives worldwide, have adversely affected the lives of at least 800 million more people, and have resulted in property damage exceeding $23 billion.[70,95,103] Recent natural catastrophes have included the Armenia earthquake in 1988, Hurricane Hugo and the California earthquake in 1989, the Bangladesh cyclone in 1991, and Hurricane Andrew in 1992. The future appears to be even more frightening. Increasing population density in floodplains and in earthquake- and hurricane-prone areas points to the probability of future catastrophic natural disasters with millions of casual-

Table 26-1 Crude Disaster Mortality by Type, 1960-1969, 1970-1979, and 1980-1989

	Deaths		
Disaster Type	**1960-69**	**1970-79**	**1980-89**
Floods	28,700	46,800	38,598
Cyclones	107,500	343,600	14,482
Earthquakes	52,500	389,700	53,740
Hurricanes			1,263
Other disasters			1,011,777
TOTAL			1,119,860

From Office of US Foreign Disaster Assistance: *Disaster history: significant data on major disasters worldwide, 1900-present,* Washington, DC, 1990, Agency for International Development.

Table 26-2 Selected Natural Disasters of the Twentieth Century*

Year	Event	Location	Approximate Death Toll
1900	Hurricane	USA	6,000
1902	Volcanic eruption	Martinique	29,000
1902	Volcanic eruption	Guatemala	6,000
1906	Typhoon	Hong Kong	10,000
1906	Earthquake	Taiwan	6,000
1906	Earthquake/fire	USA	1,500
1908	Earthquake	Italy	75,000
1911	Volcanic eruption	Philippines	1,300
1915	Earthquake	Italy	30,000
1916	Landslide	Italy, Austria	10,000
1919	Volcanic eruption	Indonesia	5,200
1920	Earthquake/landslide	China	200,000
1923	Earthquake/fire	Japan	143,000
1928	Hurricane/flood	USA	2,000
1930	Volcanic eruption	Indonesia	1,400
1932	Earthquake	China	70,000
1933	Tsunami	Japan	3,000
1935	Earthquake	India	60,000
1938	Hurricane	USA	600
1939	Earthquake/tsunami	Chile	30,000
1945	Flood/landslide	Japan	1,200
1946	Tsunami	Japan	1,400
1948	Earthquake	USSR	100,000
1949	Flood	China	57,000
1949	Earthquake/landslide	USSR	20,000
1951	Volcanic eruption	Papua New Guinea	2,900
1953	Flood	North Sea coast	1,800
1954	Landslide	Austria	200
1954	Flood	China	40,000
1959	Typhoon	Japan	4,600
1960	Earthquake	Morocco	12,000
1961	Typhoon	Hong Kong	400
1962	Landslide	Peru	5,000

*Disasters selected to represent global vulnerability to rapid-onset disasters.

Table 26-2 Selected Natural Disasters of the Twentieth Century—cont'd

Year	Event	Location	Approximate Death Toll
1962	Earthquake	Iran	12,000
1963	Tropical cyclone	Bangladesh	22,000
1963	Volcanic eruption	Indonesia	1,200
1963	Landslide	Italy	2,000
1965	Tropical cyclone	Bangladesh	17,000
1965	Tropical cyclone	Bangladesh	30,000
1965	Tropical cyclone	Bangladesh	10,000
1968	Earthquake	Iran	12,000
1970	Earthquake/landslide	Peru	70,000
1970	Tropical cyclone	Bangladesh	300,000
1971	Tropical cyclone	India	25,000
1972	Earthquake	Nicaragua	6,000
1976	Earthquake	China	250,000
1976	Earthquake	Guatemala	24,000
1976	Earthquake	Italy	900
1977	Tropical cyclone	India	20,000
1978	Earthquake	Iran	25,000
1980	Earthquake	Italy	1,300
1982	Volcanic eruption	Mexico	1,700
1985	Tropical cyclone	Bangladesh	10,000
1985	Earthquake	Mexico	10,000
1985	Volcanic eruption	Columbia	22,000
1988	Hurricane Gilbert	Caribbean	343
1988	Earthquake	Armenia SSR	25,000
1989	Hurricane Hugo	Caribbean	56
1990	Earthquake	Iran	40,000
1990	Earthquake	Philippines	2,000
1991	Tropical cyclone	Bangladesh	140,000
1991	Volcanic eruption	Philippines	800
1991	Typhoon/flood	Philippines	6,000
1991	Flood	China	1,500
1992	Hurricane Andrew	USA	52
1993	Earthquake	India	10,000

Data from Office of US Foreign Disaster Assistance: *Disaster history: significant data on major disasters worldwide, 1900-Present,* Washington, DC, 1990, Agency for International Development; and National Geographic Society: *Nature on the rampage, our violent earth,* Washington, DC, 1987, National Geographic Society.

ties.[72,145] Because of the massive impact of disasters on human health, the United Nations General Assembly has declared the 1990s to be the International Decade of Natural Disaster Reduction and has called for a global effort to reduce the impact of these untoward events.[138]

Many natural disasters of large magnitude occur in remote areas, far from towns and hospitals. The roads frequently become impassable, bridges collapse, and inclement weather adds to the difficulties. The more remote the area, the longer it takes for external assistance to arrive, and the more the community will have to rely on its own resources, at least for the first several hours, if not days. Friends, neighbors, and relatives conduct the initial search and rescue of victims, provide basic first aid, and transport the injured to the nearest health care facilities.

Good disaster management must link data collection and analysis to an immediate decision-making process.[15] The overall objective of disaster management from a public health perspective is to assess the needs of disaster-affected populations, match available resources to those needs, prevent further adverse health effects, implement disease control strategies for well-defined problems, evaluate the effectiveness of disaster relief programs, and improve contingency plans for various types of future disasters.[54]

Clearly the effects of disasters on the health of populations are quantifiable. Common patterns of morbidity and mortality following certain disasters can be identified.[144] Better epidemiologic knowledge of the causes of death and types of injuries and illnesses caused by natural disasters is clearly essential to determine the relief supplies, equipment, and personnel needed to respond effectively to such situations.[2,15,69] In addition, results of disaster research serve as the basis for providing informed advice about the probable health effects of future disasters, for establishing priorities for action by emergency medical services, and for emphasizing the need for accurate information as the basis for relief management decisions.[15,60]

Proper planning and execution of disaster medical aid programs require knowledge of the types of disasters that might occur, the morbidity and mortality that might result, and the consequent medical care needs. Therefore emergency responders should be expert on how to handle the type of disaster most prevalent in their own community, since each type of disaster is characterized by different morbidity and mortality patterns and has different health care requirements.[15,101] For example, hospitals along the Gulf Coast of the United States should plan for hurricanes, while those in California should plan for earthquakes.[38,69,80]

In addition, specific types of medical and health problems tend to occur at different times following a natural disaster's impact. With earthquakes, for example, the problem of severe injuries that require immediate trauma care must be handled mainly at the time and place of impact. The problem of increased risk of disease transmission can be handled later, however, since it takes longer to develop and the greatest danger occurs with crowding and poor sanitation. Effective emergency medical response depends on anticipating the different medical and health problems before they arise and on delivering the appropriate interventions at the precise times and places where they are needed most.[126]

This chapter discusses the nature of disasters, medical and health needs associated with natural disasters, practical issues of disaster response, and how medical and public health relief efforts should be organized in advance of a disaster and managed at the time of an emergency.

Nature of Disaster

Before a discussion of disaster management, the term "disaster" must be defined. According to the World Health Organization, a disaster is a sudden ecologic phenomenon of sufficient magnitude to require external assistance.[110,147] At the community level this can be defined operationally as any community emergency that seriously affects people's lives and property and that exceeds the capacity of the community to effectively respond to that emergency.[78]

The essence of a disaster is substantial environmental damage, which may or may not be accompanied by large numbers of casualties. For semantic clarity, this chapter refers to limited incidents creating relatively small numbers of casualties and slight environmental disturbance as "multiple casualty incidents." The term "disaster" is reserved for incidents that cause great disruption of the physical and social environments and require extraordinary resources and special medical care, even in the absence of mass casualties.

True disasters affect a community in numerous ways. Roads, telephone lines, and other transportation and communication links are often destroyed. Public utilities and energy supplies may be disrupted. Substantial numbers of victims may be rendered homeless. Portions of the community's industrial or economic base may be destroyed or damaged. Casualties may require medical care, and damage to food sources and utilities may create public health threats.

Past Problems in Natural Disaster Management

In ancient times, little mitigation was possible against the effects of disaster. Today, in contrast, communications inform us rapidly of disasters and allow us to quickly and efficiently initiate medical aid to victims. This requires adequate planning and brisk execution. Medical aid in many previous disasters has been well intentioned but poorly organized, with limited benefits.[53,110]

Health decisions made during emergencies are often based on insufficient, nonexistent, or even false information, which results in inappropriate, insufficient, or unnecessary health aid, waste of health resources, or countereffective measures.[126] For example, large amounts of useless drugs and other consumable supplies are frequently sent to a disaster site. After the 1976 earthquake in Guatemala, 100 tons of unsorted medicines were airlifted to the country from foreign donors.[43,45] Of these supplies, 90% were of no value, since they consisted of medications that had expired, were already opened, or carried labels written in foreign languages. A similar situation occurred after the 1988 Armenian earthquake, when international relief operations sent at least 5000 tons of drugs and consumable medical supplies. Because of the difficulties with identification and sorting, only 30% of the drugs were immediately usable by the health workers in Armenia; 11% were useless, and 8% had expired. Ultimately, 20% of all the drugs provided by international aid had to be destroyed.[4] Other examples of inappropriate aid include sending mobile hospitals and teams of specialized trauma or emergency medicine specialists that arrive much too late and sending unprepared medical volunteers when nonmedical relief workers (such as sanitary engineers) would probably be more appropriate. The arrival of unprepared and inexperienced foreign personnel may damage the relief effort by tying up communication, transportation, and housing. These problems are all compounded in the vacuum created by the disaster, including the lack of communication, transportation, local supplies and support, and a decision-making structure. Since these relief operations are often conducted under the watchful eye of the media, medical relief efforts are often pejoratively called "the second disaster."[83]

Information Management Systems for Disaster Response

Over the past several years, efforts have been made to develop rapid and valid disaster damage assessment techniques.[136,148] These techniques must be able to define quickly the overall effects of the disaster impact, the nature and extent of the health problems, groups in the population at particular risk for adverse health events, specific health care needs of the survivors, local resources to cope with the event, and the extent and effectiveness of the response to the disaster by local authorities.[78,130] Guha-Sapir and Lechat have developed useful attributes for indicators for needs assessment in earthquakes ("quick and dirty" surveys). These have highlighted simplicity, speed of use, and operational feasibility.[68] The techniques employed, which are the use of sample and systematic surveys and the establishment of simple reporting systems, are methodologically straightforward. Given suitable personnel and transport, reasonably accurate estimates of relief needs could be obtained quickly.[32] Problems may arise, however, with the interpretation of data, particularly incomplete data, and in developing countries where predisaster health and nutritional levels are unknown.

The ultimate goal of the surveillance is to prevent or reduce the adverse health consequences of the disaster itself, as well as to optimize the decision-making process associated with management of the relief effort. These epidemiologic objectives can be simply defined as the surveillance cycle: the collection of data, analysis of data, and response to data.[54] The surveillance cycle must be repeated many times: immediately; with rapid, "quick and dirty" assessments of problems using the most rudimentary data collection techniques; then with short-term assessments involving the establishment of simple but reliable sources of data; and subsequently, with ongoing surveillance to identify continuing problems and monitor the response to the interventions chosen.

Field surveillance methods vary greatly by disaster setting and by the personnel and time available. Early field surveys must be simple and address the essential basic questions requiring immediate answers that will directly prevent loss of life or injury. Subsequently, surveys can address issues such as the availability of medical care, assessment of the need for specific interventions, and epidemic control (a rumor clearinghouse), each of which demands more careful investigation. Surveillance must be sensitive to monitor the impact of relief on the health problems of the population and to determine whether the effort is having a tangible impact on the population or if new strategies are needed.[133] Surveillance becomes an iterative, cycling process in which simple health outcomes are constantly monitored and interventions assessed for efficacy.

Finally, linking the information gathered after disasters to a management decision process is important.[69] The information is clearly an essential requirement for determining appropriate relief supplies, equipment, and personnel needed to respond effectively to a catastrophic event. In the rapid evolution of a disaster relief program, major decisions regarding relief are made early, hastily and often irreversibly, so the need for reliable early data to assist in making these decisions is vital. An organized approach to data collection in disaster situations can greatly improve decision making and can predict a variety of options that disaster managers need to face. The availability of questionnaires that were prepared before the disaster and can be adapted and modified quickly assists in an efficient data collection operation. Therefore standardized procedures for collecting data during disasters need to be developed so that the information is available for operational decisions and action.

Operational decisions vary depending on the phase of the disaster. In the early phase of relief, basic needs of water, food, clothing, shelter, and medical care must be met, after which the longer term process of rebuilding proceeds. Relief aid can often be squandered by overreacting to minor problems when excitement is great, needs are extensive, and scrutiny by the media is omnipresent.[126] Since everyone in the disaster area feels needs and experiences loss, the challenge of the early assessment is to decide where early intervention will prevent the greatest loss of life or severe morbidity. The postimpact phase requires information on long-term rehabilitation and restoration of health services. Epidemiologic assessment, prioritization of needs, and ordering an appropriate response can have a major impact on the community's ability to return to normalcy in both the short and longer term.

Health Care Needs in Specific Natural Disasters

Natural hazards that can cause substantial property damage, economic dislocation, and medical problems include earthquakes and associated phenomena, volcanic eruptions, and extreme weather incidents (see Chapter 24). Accounts of morbidity and mortality recorded after previous disasters can predict the medical care needs of future disasters and provide a foundation for disaster response planning.

FLOODS

Floods are the most common natural disasters. They affect more people worldwide and cause greater mortality than any other type of natural disaster.[70,104,145] They occur in almost every country, but 70% of all flood deaths occur in India and Bangladesh (Fig. 26-1).[95] In the United States, floods cause more deaths than any other natural disaster, with most fatalities resulting from flash floods.[58]

Fast-flowing water carrying debris such as boulders and fallen trees accounts for the primary flood-related injuries and deaths. Not surprisingly, the main cause of death from floods is drowning, followed by various combinations of trauma, drowning, and hypothermia with or without submersion.[11] Persons submerged in cold water for up to about 40 minutes have been successfully resuscitated with 100% recovery of neurologic function.[104] Unfortunately, such resuscitations from clinical death require technologically advanced measures, which may not be available for days following a flood even in a highly developed country such as the United States.

Among flood survivors, the proportion requiring emergency medical care is reported to vary between 0.2% and 2%.[127,131] Most injuries requiring urgent medical attention are minor and include lacerations, skin rashes, and ulcers.[110] However, flood-associated lacerations are frequently contaminated, so primary wound closure should be done with

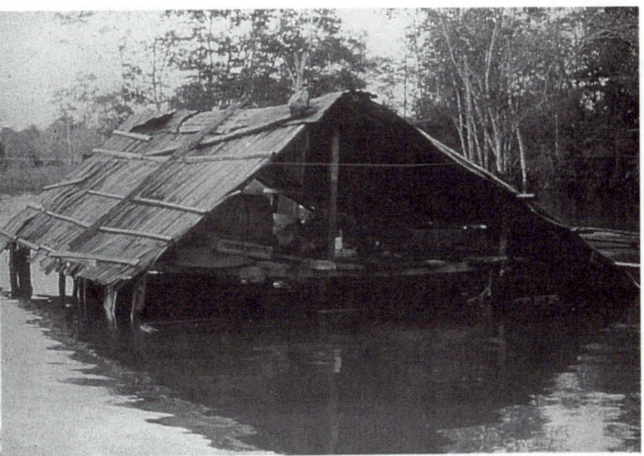

Fig. 26-1 During the summer of 1988, monsoon rains resulted in the most severe flooding ever recorded in Bangladesh. Water covered three fourths of the land area of Bangladesh and caused up to 40 million persons to be displaced from their homes. (Courtesy Centers for Disease Control and Prevention, U.S. Public Health Service.)

caution. Primary closure without careful evaluation of the wound almost always requires reopening and additional treatment within 24 to 48 hours.[11]

Increased incidence of snakebites was reported following floods in India and the Philippines.[141] In India, most snakebites were by cobras that had been driven by rising floodwaters to seek higher ground near towns and villages.

For some floods, substantial numbers of casualties caused by fire have been documented.[104] Fast-flowing water can break oil or gasoline storage tanks. If the film of oil is ignited, the fire may spread to buildings on land.

From a public health viewpoint, floods may disrupt water purification and sewage disposal systems, cause toxic waste sites to overflow, or dislodge chemicals stored above ground.[46] In addition, makeshift evacuation centers with insufficient sanitary facilities may become substantially overcrowded.[111] The combination of these events may contribute to increased exposure to highly toxic biologic and chemical agents. Examples include the potential for waterborne disease transmission of such agents as enterotoxigenic *Escherichia coli, Shigella, Salmonella,* and hepatitis A virus.[127] The risk of transmission of malaria and yellow fever may be increased because of enhanced vector-breeding conditions.[110] In 1973, Ussher reported that the most serious problems encountered after a Philippine flood were viral upper respiratory tract infections, which were probably caused by crowded conditions in temporary shelters.[110,141]

Despite the potential for communicable diseases to follow floods, mass vaccination programs are counterproductive for a variety of reasons. They not only divert limited personnel and resources from other critical relief tasks, but also may create a false sense of security and cause persons who have been vaccinated to neglect basic hygiene.[44] Unfortunately, after floods the public often demands typhoid vaccine and tetanus toxoid, although no epidemics of typhoid after floods have ever been documented in the United States.[57] In addition, antibodies to typhoid following immunization take several weeks to develop, and even then, vaccination protects only moderately. Likewise, mass tetanus vaccination programs are not indicated. Management of flood-associated wounds should include appropriate evaluation of the injured person's tetanus immunization history, and the person should be vaccinated only if indicated.

The proper approach to the problem of communicable diseases is to set up an epidemiologic surveillance system so that an increase in cases of communicable diseases in the flood-stricken area can be identified quickly. Particular attention should be given to diseases endemic to the area. For example, when floods occur in areas with endemic arthropod-borne encephalitides, arthropods known to transmit the disease should be monitored and areas should be sprayed if the vector population increases significantly after the flood.

TROPICAL CYCLONES (HURRICANES OR TYPHOONS)

Cyclones, hurricanes, and typhoons have killed hundreds of thousands and injured millions of people during the last 20 years (Fig. 26-2).[72,103] From 1900 to 1989 more than 13,000 people lost their lives in hurricanes in the United States (Table 26-3).[52] The greatest natural disaster in U.S. history occurred on September 8, 1900, when a hurricane struck Galveston, Texas, and killed more than 6000 people.[56,95] The most financially costly natural disaster in U.S. history resulted from the impact of Hurricane Andrew in Florida and Louisiana in 1992, with insured losses exceeding $20 billion. In 1970, deaths resulting from a single trop-

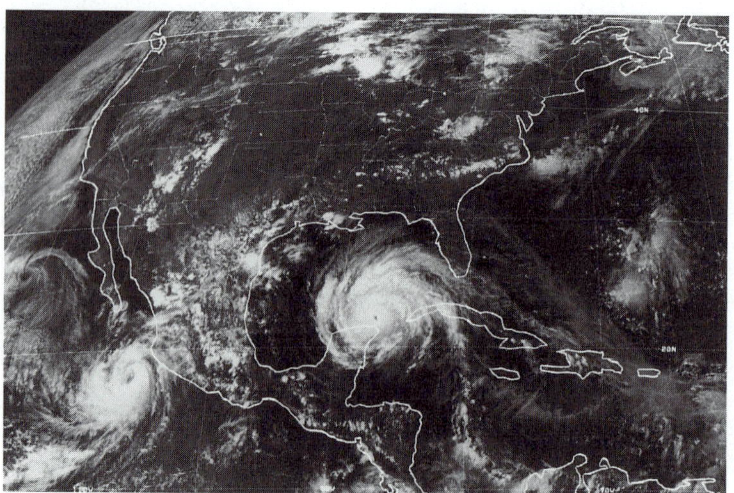

Fig. 26-2 Satellite image of a hurricane and a cyclone striking Mexico simultaneously. (Courtesy World Health Organization and Office of the UN Disaster Relief Coordinator.)

Table 26-3 Hurricanes Causing More Than 100 Deaths in the United States, 1900-1982

Storm/Area	Year	Deaths
Texas (Galveston)	1900	6000
Florida (Lake Okeechobee)	1928	1836
South Texas, Florida (Keys)	1919	600-900*
New England	1938	600
Florida (Keys)	1935	408
Audrey/Louisiana, Texas	1957	390
Northeast United States	1944	390†
Louisiana (Grand Isle)	1909	350
Louisiana (New Orleans)	1915	275
Texas (Galveston)	1915	275
Camille/Mississippi, Louisiana	1969	256
Florida (Miami)	1926	243
Diane/Northeast US	1955	184
Florida (Southeast)	1906	164
Mississippi, Alabama, Florida (Pensacola)	1906	134
Agnes/Northeast US	1972	122

From French JG: Hurricanes. In *The public health consequences of disasters,* Atlanta, 1986, Centers for Disease Control, US Public Health Service.
*Includes over 500 lost on ships at sea.
†Includes 344 lost on ships at sea.

ical cyclone striking Bangladesh were estimated to exceed 250,000. As population growth continues along vulnerable coastal areas, deaths and injuries resulting from tropical cyclones will increase.[67]

Although hurricane winds do great damage, wind is not the biggest killer in a hurricane. Hurricanes are classic examples of disasters that trigger secondary effects such as tornadoes and flooding that, together with storm surges, can cause extraordinarily high rates of morbidity and mortality. This was seen following the 1991 cyclone and sea surge in Bangladesh in which 140,000 people drowned.[63] Nine of 10 hurricane fatalities are drownings associated with storm surges.[55,56,109] The major rescue problem is locating persons stranded by rising waters and evacuating them to higher land. Other causes of deaths and injuries include burial beneath houses collapsed by wind or water, penetrating trauma from broken glass or wood, blunt trauma from floating objects or debris, or entrapment by mud slides that may accompany hurricane-associated floods.[31,71] Many of the most severe injuries occur to persons who are in mobile homes during the storm or who are injured or electrocuted during the postdisaster cleanup.[28,29,113]

Most persons who seek medical care after hurricanes do not require sophisticated surgical or intensive care services and can be treated as outpatients.[118] The great majority suffer from lacerations caused by flying glass or other debris[71]; a few have closed fractures and other, mostly penetrating injuries.[37] Longmire and associates studied injuries associated with Hurricane Frederic (1984) and Hurricane Elena (1985).[84,85] They found a statistically significant increase in lacerations, puncture wounds, chain saw injuries, burns, gasoline aspiration, gastrointestinal complaints, insect stings, and spouse abuse in the 2 weeks after the hurricane. The authors concluded that minor trauma being treated in the outpatient setting created an urgent demand for primary care physicians and nurses skilled in managing minor surgical emergencies. In addition, although the number of chain saw injuries was small, the time-consuming nature of treating such wounds increased significantly the demands placed on remaining emergency department personnel to treat people with other injuries. As with flood-related wounds, emergency medical care providers should be aware that such wounds may contain highly contaminated material such as soil or fecal matter.[108,112] Because of this danger, primary wound closure should be done with caution.

People are often severely crowded in storm shelters.[30] As with flood disasters, this crowding increases the probability of disease communication via aerosol or fecal-oral routes, particularly when sanitary facilities are insufficient.[16]

In summary, trauma after a cyclone is not usually a major public health problem when compared with the need for water, food, clothing, sanitation, and other hygienic measures.[131] Studies demonstrate that sending fully equipped mobile hospitals and specialized surgical teams that arrive much too late at the disaster site is an ineffective response to a cyclone disaster, and that nonmedical relief (such as epidemiologists, sanitary engineers, shelter, food, and agricultural supplies) is probably more effective in reducing mortality and morbidity. On the other hand, field hospitals and emergency medical teams from outside the disaster-affected area may indeed be useful in providing ongoing primary health care services to the community when all other health care facilities have been destroyed or severely damaged. This was the case in St. Croix after Hurricane Hugo[118] and in south Florida after Hurricane Andrew.[140] These situations reemphasize the importance of conducting rapid assessments of public health needs before sending relief personnel and materials to a disaster.[111]

TORNADOES

Tornadoes are among the most most violent of all natural atmospheric phenomena (Fig. 26-3).[95] Although almost 700 tornadoes occur in the United States each year, only about 3% result in severe injuries requiring hospitalization.[125] Of 14,600 tornadoes studied between 1952 and 1973, only 497 caused fatalities, and 26 of these events accounted for almost half of the fatalities.[59] The Centers for Disease Control and Prevention has reviewed the public health impact of tornadoes in great detail.[125]

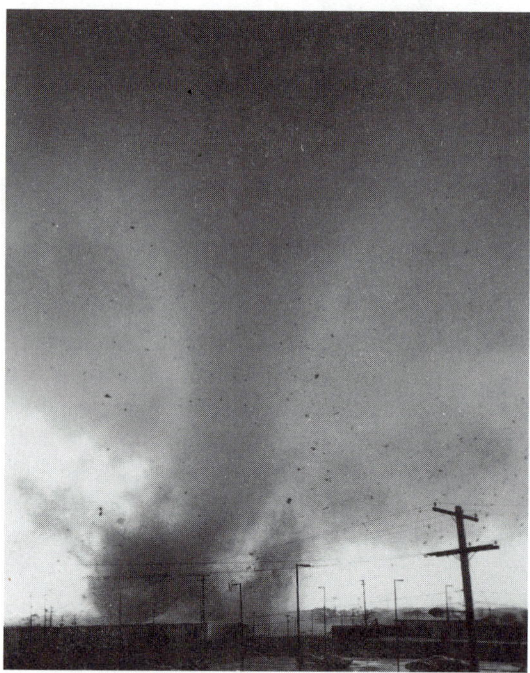

Fig. 26-3 Tornado striking McConnell Air Force Base, Kansas, April 26, 1991. (Courtesy U.S. Air Force.)

The destruction caused by tornadoes results from the combined action of their strong rotary winds and the partial vacuum in the center of the vortex.[94] For example, when a tornado passes over a building, the winds twist and rip at the outside. Simultaneously, the abrupt pressure reduction in the tornado's eye causes explosive pressures inside the building. Walls collapse or topple outward, windows explode, and the debris from this destruction can be driven as high-velocity missiles through the air. Buildings of unreinforced masonry, wood frame buildings, and those with large window areas are likely to suffer the most extensive damage.[82] Thus building practices may be largely responsible for the severity of injury resulting from tornadoes.[20]

In the last 50 years tornadoes have been responsible for more than 9000 deaths.[62] About 4% of all injuries sustained were fatal. For every person seriously injured or killed, approximately 44 others required some emergency medical attention.[65]

A review of the published literature shows characteristic patterns of injuries (fatal and nonfatal) sustained by victims of tornado disasters. The leading cause of death is craniocerebral trauma,[18,88] followed by crushing wounds of the chest and trunk.[6,127] Fractures are the most frequent nonfatal injury. Also frequent are lacerations, penetrating trauma with retained foreign bodies, and other soft tissue injuries. A high percentage wounds among tornado casualties are heavily contaminated.[19,73] In many instances foreign materials such as glass, wood splinters, tar, dirt, grass, and manure are deeply embedded in areas of soft tissue injury.[88] Wound contamination appears to be a major factor contributing to the high rate of postoperative sepsis for tornado victims who require surgery, even under conditions in which patients receive highly skilled and prompt surgical debridement. Sepsis is common in both minor and major injuries; sepsis affects one half to two thirds of patients with minor wounds.[6] Hight and co-workers examined the postoperative course of patients after the Worcester tornado in the 1950s and found sepsis in 12.5% to 23.0% of orthopedic and neurosurgical patients with lacerations.[73] In addition, they noted three cases of gas gangrene; however, they reported no cases of tetanus.

Three studies have looked specifically at the species of bacteria that contaminate wounds sustained during tornadoes.[19,60,76] These revealed frequent infection with aerobic gram-negative bacilli, presumably derived from soil.

VOLCANIC ERUPTIONS

Volcanic eruptions have claimed more than 266,000 lives in the past 400 years, with fatalities occurring in about 5% of all eruptions.[17,128] Some of the more catastrophic eruptions in history include the eruption of Krakatoa (Indonesia), which caused the deaths of 36,000 people; that of Mt. Pelee in 1902, which caused the destruction of St. Pierre in Martinique and the deaths of 28,000 people; that of Nevado del Ruiz, in Colombia, which claimed 25,000 lives; and that of Mt. Pinatubo in the Philippines, with effects still ongoing because of persistent mudflows. The U.S. Geological Survey has identified about 35 volcanoes in the western United States and Alaska that are likely to erupt in the future. Most of these are in remote rural areas and are not likely to result in disaster. A few, like Mt. Hood, Mt. Shasta, Mt. Rainier, and the volcano underlying Mammoth Lakes in California, are near population centers.[5,12] Because of the increasing population density in areas of volcanic activity, volcanic hazards are of growing concern.[39,72,95]

Eruptions have immediate life-threatening health effects through suffocation from inhalation of massive quantities of airborne ash, scalding from blasts of superheated steam, and surges of lethal gas (Table 26-4).[10,13] Pyroclastic flows and surges are particularly lethal.[8] These are currents of extremely hot gases and particles that flow down the slopes of a volcano at tens to hundreds of meters per second and cover hundreds of square kilometers. Because of their suddenness and speed, pyroclastic flows and surges are difficult to escape.

Mudflows or lahars account for at least 10% of volcano-related deaths.[143] These are flowing masses of volcanic debris mixed with water. The mud is sometimes scalding hot, and entrapped persons may sustain severe burns. A relatively minor eruption of snow-capped Nevado del Ruiz in 1985 triggered lahars from the volcano's icecap that buried more than 22,000 persons in Colombia, South America.[128]

An indirect effect of volcanic activity is the accumulation of toxic volcanic gases in deep crater lakes.[105,129]

Table 26-4 Principal Health Effects of Eruptions in the Vicinity of the Volcano

Eruptive Event	Consequence	Health Impact
Explosions	Lateral blast, rock fragments	Trauma, skin burns
	Air shock waves	Lacerations from broken windows
Hot ash release	Glowing avalanches	Skin and lung burns
	Ash flows and falls	Asphyxiation
	Lightning	Electrocution
	Forest fires	Burns
Melting ice, snow, and rain accompanying eruption	Mudflows, floods	Engulfing, drowning
Lava	Forest fires	Burns
Gas emissions: sulfur dioxide, carbon monoxide, carbon dioxide, hydrogen sulfide, hydrogen fluoride	Pooling in low-lying areas and inhalation	Asphyxiation, airway constriction
Radon	Radiation exposure	Lung cancer
Earthquakes	Building damage	Trauma

From Baxter PJ, Bernstein RS, Buist AS: *Am J Public Health* 76:84, 1986.

Sudden release of these gases can be catastrophic; carbon dioxide released from Lake Monoun and Lake Nyos in Cameroun in 1984 and 1986, respectively, claimed 1800 lives. Other toxic effects of these gas releases include pulmonary edema, irritant conjunctivitis, joint pain, muscle weakness, and cutaneous bullae. In the rare event of a ground-level release of toxic gases or aerosols (for example, from a vent opening to the atmosphere from the side of the volcano), equipment for monitoring atmospheric concentrations of sulfur dioxide, hydrogen sulfide, hydrofluoric acid, carbon dioxide, and other gases should be available.[10,13]

A volcanic eruption may also generate tremendous quantities of ashfall.[93,119] Buildings have been reported to collapse from the weight of ash accumulating on roofs, resulting in severe trauma to the occupants.[89] The ash can also be irritating to the eyes (causing corneal abrasions), mucous membranes, and respiratory system.[87] Upper airway irritation, cough, and bronchospasm, as well as exacerbation of chronic lung diseases, are common findings in symptomatic patients.[8] In extremely high concentrations (for example, in the path of a pyroclastic flow or near the volcanic vent during an ashfall), volcanic ash may cause severe tracheal injury, pulmonary edema, and bronchial obstruction leading to death from acute pulmonary injury or from suffocation.[89] After the eruption of Mt. St. Helens in 1980, 23 immediate deaths were reported (Fig. 26-4). Postmortem examinations revealed that 18 of these resulted from asphyxia.[49] In the majority of the asphyxiated victims the ash mixed with mucus and formed plugs that obstructed the principal airways (trachea and main bronchi). Finally, a delayed onset of ash-induced mucus hypersecretion or obstructive airway disease may occur.[9]

Victims recovered from volcano-generated mudflows may suffer from severe dehydration, burns, and eye infections.[50,51] Reports of surgical care following the volcanic eruption in Colombia in 1985 showed that primary closure of wounds contaminated by mud and other volcanic material resulted in major complications.[106] These complications included gangrene necessitating amputation, osteomyelitis, compartment syndrome, and sepsis.

In summary, most volcanic deaths are caused by immediate suffocation and, to a lesser extent, by burns or blunt trauma. Advanced cardiac and trauma life support capabilities, even if immediately available, would probably arrive too late to save asphyxiated victims. Patients with acute respiratory distress have a great potential to develop severe respiratory distress syndrome. For these patients it is advisable to arrange admission to an intensive care unit where appropriate respiratory supportive measures are available, ranging from continuous positive airway pressure to mechanical ventilation with positive end-expiratory pressure.[89] In conclusion, hospitals in the vicinity of both active and dormant volcanoes should be prepared to deal with a sudden influx of victims with severe burns and lung damage from inhalation of hot ash, as well as multiple varieties of trauma.[8,13]

EARTHQUAKES

An earthquake of great magnitude is one of the most destructive events in nature. During the past 20 years, earthquakes have caused more than a million deaths and injuries worldwide.[103] In the United States, approximately 1600 deaths attributed to earthquakes have been recorded since colonial times, of which more than 1000 have occurred in California (Fig. 26-5).[132] Hospitals and other health care facilities are particularly vulnerable to the damaging effects of an earthquake. Because of loss of power and water supply,

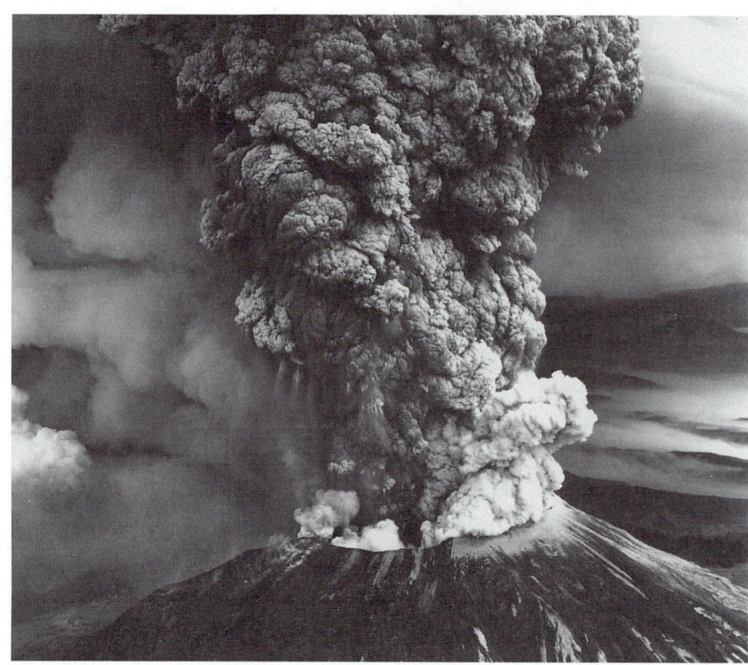

Fig. 26-4 Eruption of Mt. St. Helens, Washington State, May 18, 1980. (Photograph courtesy of the U.S. Geological Survey.)

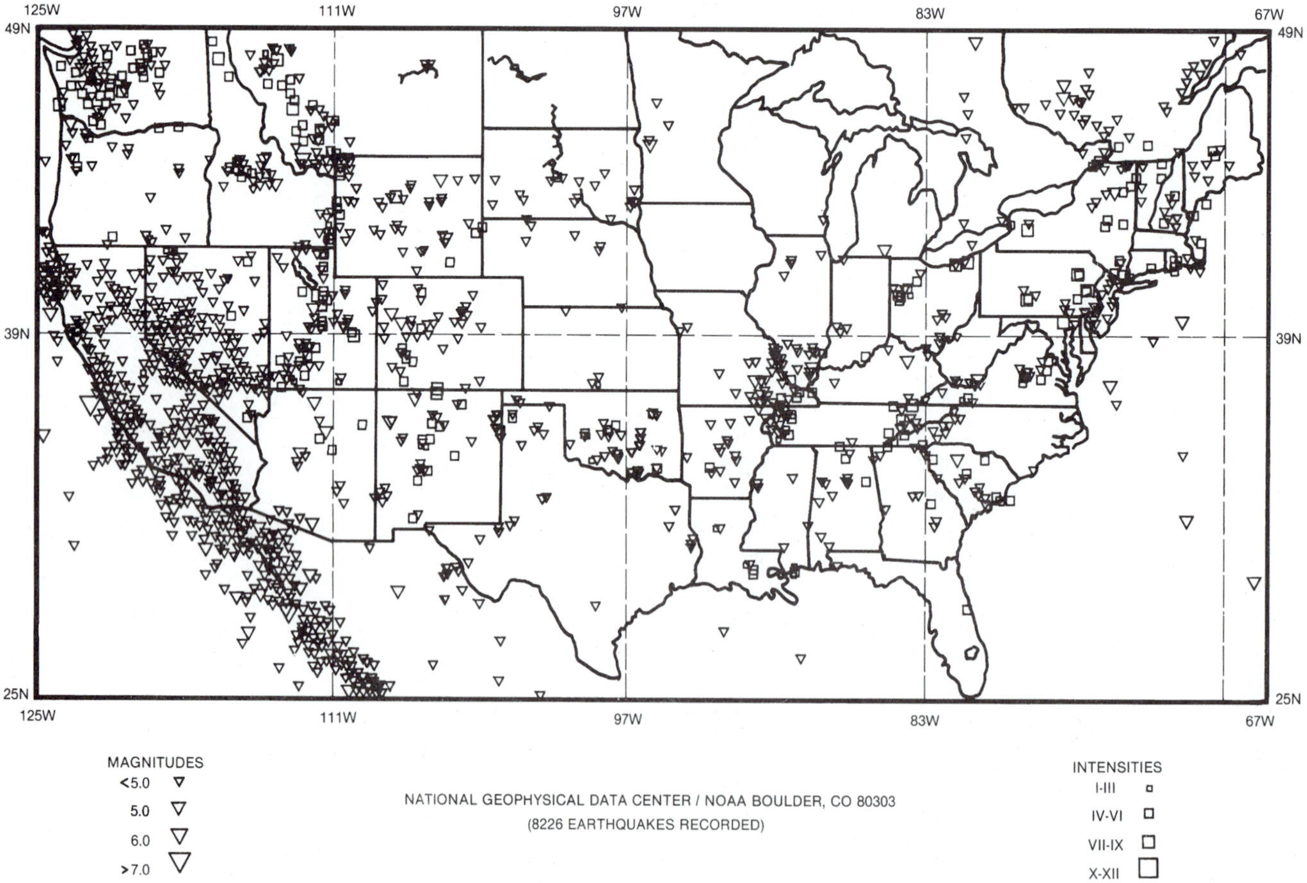

125W 111W 97W 83W 67W

49N 39N 25N

MAGNITUDES
<5.0
5.0
6.0
>7.0

NATIONAL GEOPHYSICAL DATA CENTER / NOAA BOULDER, CO 80303
(8226 EARTHQUAKES RECORDED)

INTENSITIES
I-III
IV-VI
VII-IX
X-XII

Fig. 26-5 Earthquake risk in the continental United States. Triangles represent active seismic areas from January 1937 to May 1987.

equipment, such as x-ray machines, kidney dialysis machines, ventilators, and blood analyzers, and hospital facilities such as intensive care units and surgical theaters cannot function normally when they are most needed.[3,100,116]

In reviewing historical accounts of earthquakes, disaster medical planners should note injury type or diagnostic classification among survivors, which determines the medical care needed after the event. The primary cause of death and injury from earthquakes is the collapse of buildings that are not adequately designed for earthquake resistance, are built with inadequate materials, or are poorly constructed (Fig. 26-6).[61,86] Studies have shown that factors determining the number of people killed when a building collapses include how badly they are trapped, how severely they are injured, how long they must wait for rescue, and how long they can survive without medical attention.[35,36,102]

Deaths resulting from major earthquakes can be instantaneous, rapid, or delayed. Instantaneous death can be caused by severe crushing injuries to the head or chest, external or internal hemorrhage, or drowning from earthquake-induced tidal waves (tsunamis). Rapid death occurs within minutes or hours and can be caused by asphyxia from dust inhalation or chest compression, hypovolemic shock, or exposure (for example, hypothermia). Delayed death occurs within days and can be caused by dehydration, hypothermia, hyperthermia, crush syndrome, or postoperative sepsis.[124]

As with most natural disasters, the majority of those requiring medical assistance have minor injuries such as superficial lacerations, sprains, and bruises.[114] The next most frequent reason for seeking medical attention is simple fractures not requiring operative intervention.[127] For example, after the 1968 earthquake south of Khorasan, Iran, only 368 (3.3%) of 11,254 persons injured required inpatient care.

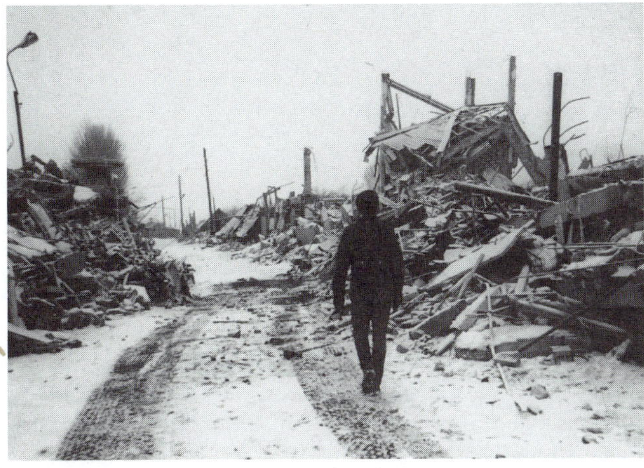

Fig. 26-6 Main street in devastated Armenian village showing complete collapse of all buildings following December 7, 1988, earthquake. (Eric K. Noji photo.)

Hospitalized patients included those with serious multiple fractures or internal injuries, hypothermia, sepsis from wound infections, or multiple organ failure requiring surgery or other intensive care services.[91]

More detailed inpatient information is available from data collected on 4832 patients admitted to hospitals following the 1988 earthquake in Armenia.[102] Consistent with findings from other major earthquakes, combination injuries constituted 39.7% of the cases. Superficial trauma such as lacerations and contusions was the most frequently observed (24.9%), followed by head injuries (22%), lower extremity injuries (19%), crush syndrome (11%), and upper extremity trauma (10%).

Infected wounds and gangrene were major problems following the Armenian earthquake.[98] Persons who have been trapped by rubble for several hours or days may also develop compartment syndromes requiring fasciotomy or amputation. These persons may have significant rhabdomyolysis and must be watched closely for signs and symptoms of crush syndrome such as hypovolemic shock, hyperkalemia, renal failure, or fatal cardiac arrhythmias.[14,96,99] Following the 1988 earthquake in Armenia, more than 1000 victims trapped in collapsed buildings developed crush syndrome as a result of limb compression; 323 developed secondary acute renal failure requiring renal dialysis.[96]

Heavy dust is produced by crumbling buildings immediately following earthquakes. For trapped victims, this dust is a life-threatening hazard that may cause asphyxiation or upper airway obstruction.[74] Fulminant pulmonary edema from dust inhalation may also be a delayed cause of death.[124] Asbestos and other particulate matter in the dust are both subacute and chronic respiratory hazards for trapped victims, as well as for rescue and cleanup personnel. The degree of hazard depends on the characteristics and toxicity of the dust.[132]

Burns and smoke inhalation from fires used to be major hazards after an earthquake. For example, following the 1923 earthquake in Tokyo, more than 140,000 people perished, principally because of fires that broke out in a city where most buildings were constructed from highly flammable paper (shoji) and wood material. Since 1950, however, the incidence of burns has decreased considerably.[36]

To maximize saving trapped victims and increase their chances of survival, search and rescue teams must respond rapidly after a building collapses.[97] Studies of the 1980 Campania-Irpinia, Italy, earthquake[41,42] and the 1976 Tangshan, China, earthquake[149] show that the proportion of trapped people found alive declined as delay in extrication increased. In the Italian study a survey of 3619 survivors showed that 93% of those who were trapped and survived were extricated within the first 24 hours and that 95% of the deaths recorded occurred while the victims were still trapped in rubble.[42] Estimates of the survivability of victims buried under collapsed earthen buildings in Turkey and China indicate that within 2 to 6 hours less than 50% of those buried are still alive.[41,42]

Although we cannot determine whether a trapped person dies immediately or survives for some time under the debris, we can safely assume that more people would be saved if they were extricated sooner. Safar,[123] studying the 1980 earthquake in Italy, concluded that 25% to 50% of victims who were injured and died slowly could have been saved if lifesaving first aid had been rendered immediately. As suggested by these data, if any significant reduction in earthquake mortality is to be achieved, appropriate search and rescue action must be provided within the first 2 days after the impact.

Paralleling the speed required for effective search and extrication is the speed with which emergency medical services must be provided. The greatest demand occurs within the first 24 hours.[134] In fact, injured people usually seek medical attention at emergency departments only during the first 3 to 5 days, after which time hospital case mix patterns return almost to normal. A good example of the crucial importance of early demand for emergency care is seen in the number of admissions to a field hospital after the 1976 earthquake in Guatemala.[43,45] From day 6 on, admissions fell dramatically despite intensive efforts to find injured people in remote rural areas of the impact zone, indicating that specialized field hospitals that arrived a week or more after an earthquake are generally too late to help during the emergency phase. After the Armenian earthquake, only 22 (2.4%) of the 902 patients requiring hospitalization at a large hospital were admitted 7 or more days after the impact.[102]

With most earthquakes, trauma caused by the collapse of buildings is the cause of most deaths and injuries. However, a surprisingly large number of patients require acute care for nonsurgical problems such as acute myocardial infarction, exacerbation of chronic diseases such as diabetes or hypertension, anxiety and other mental health problems, respiratory disease from exposure to dust and asbestos fibers from rubble, and near drowning because of flooding from broken dams. An example of the adverse effects of an earthquake on medical conditions was observed after a magnitude 6.7 earthquake in Athens, Greece. A 50% increase in deaths from myocardial infarction was documented during the first 3 days after the earthquake, peaking on the third day.[79,137] Finally, an earthquake may precipitate a major technologic disaster by damaging or destroying nuclear power stations, hospitals with dangerous biologic products, hydrocarbon storage areas, and hazardous chemical plants.

As with most natural disasters, the risk of secondary epidemics is minimal, and only mass vaccination campaigns based on results of epidemiologic surveillance are appropriate following earthquakes.[135]

Practical Issues in Natural Disaster Response

MASS CASUALTY CARE

A disaster may create casualties in excess of the capacity of the local health care system. The approach to patient evaluation and treatment is quite different under disaster situations resulting in large numbers of casualties.[23,24,47] Disaster medical care under these circumstances is of a different style and quality from that usually practiced. While some principles of medical care are unchanged in a mass casualty incident, others must be altered to achieve the best overall result.[117] The health care system must adapt to this situation with four measures: simplifying care (austerity); rationing care (adopting a triage ethic); calling for outside help; and in circumstances of catastrophe, instituting mass care measures typical of battlefield medicine. Many compromises in work methods eliminate attention to details that would be required in less urgent situations. Physicians and nurses often perform procedures beyond the scope of their usual practices. Professional functions and roles are widely shared among physicians, nurses, and paramedics. These adaptations allow available resources to serve more victims.

AUSTERITY

To be effective, disaster medical care must be confined to basic measures, adequate to preserve life and function. Examinations, techniques, appliances, and drugs that are not essential to patient survival or preservation of function are luxuries. It may be necessary to perform fracture reductions and other minor surgical procedures with oral narcotic analgesia only. Orthopedic devices are often improvised. Use of outdated drugs is sometimes acceptable, rather than using no drugs. The level of austerity is determined by the health care personnel, supplies, and equipment available at the disaster treatment site.

TRIAGE AND RATIONING

Initial management of mass casualties includes triage, basic field stabilization, and transportation. In general, triage can be defined as the prioritization of patient care based on severity of injury or illness, prognosis, and availability of resources.[120,121] The goal of triage therefore is to select those patients in greatest need of immediate medical attention and to arrange for that treatment. It is a concept born on the world's battlefields, by which victims are classified and treated based on the seriousness of their injuries. Military surgeons long ago recognized that the number of victims produced in battle could overwhelm medical resources. Some persons suffer injuries that would be fatal even under ideal circumstances where resources are unlimited. In mass casualty situations, one no longer can concentrate all resources on the management of a single critically ill patient. Attempts at salvaging mortally wounded individuals with heroic measures under conditions of limited personnel and supplies may deprive other victims of care for life-threatening, but readily correctable, conditions. The "walking wounded" sustain injuries that are survivable even if the provision of definitive medical care is significantly delayed. Thus, in the humanitarian interest of providing the greatest good for the greatest number of persons, methods of classification have been developed that facilitate treatment prioritization. The first victims treated are those with life-threatening injuries that can be readily stabilized without the expenditure of massive amounts of limited resources. The next priority is persons who have sustained injuries likely to have significant morbidity, which would be appreciably lessened by early intervention. Catastrophically injured patients (for example, those with burns involving 95% body surface area) who have a minimal chance for survival despite optimal medical care are provided comfort measures and may need to be left to die (see Box 26-1). Spending time on patients who are not likely to live leaves other patients who might be saved awaiting care. If too much time intervenes, these patients also may become nonsalvageable. In addition to the nature and urgency of the patient's systemic condition,

BOX 26-1

DESCRIPTION OF IMMEDIATE AND DELAYED CASES IN SIMPLE TRIAGE DURING MULTIPLE CASUALTY INCIDENTS, AND IN MILITARY TRIAGE DURING MASS CASUALTY INCIDENTS

SIMPLE TRIAGE

Immediate (Priority I)

Asphyxia
Respiratory obstruction from mechanical causes
Sucking chest wounds
Tension pneumothorax
Maxillofacial wounds in which asphyxia exists or is likely to develop
Shock caused by major external hemorrhage
Major internal hemorrhage
Visceral injuries or evisceration
Cardiopericardial injuries
Massive muscle damage
Severe burns *over* 25% body surface area
Dislocations
Major fractures
Major medical problems readily correctable
Closed cerebral injuries with increasing loss of consciousness

Delayed (Priority II)

Vascular injuries requiring repair
Wounds of the genitourinary tract
Thoracic wounds without asphyxia
Severe burns *under* 25% body surface area
Spinal cord injuries requiring decompression
Suspected spinal cord injuries without neurologic signs
Lesser fractures
Injuries of the eye
Maxillofacial injuries without asphyxia
Minor medical problems
Victims with little hope of survival under the best circumstances of medical care

MASS CASUALTY TRIAGE WITH AN OVERWHELMING NUMBER OF INJURIES

Immediate (Priority I)

Asphyxia
Respiratory obstruction from mechanical causes
Sucking chest wounds
Tension pneumothorax
Maxillofacial wounds in which asphyxia exists or is likely to develop
Shock caused by major external hemorrhage
Dislocations
Severe burns *under* 25% body surface area*
Lesser fractures*
Major medical problems that can be handled readily

Delayed (Priority II)

Major fractures (if able to stabilize)*
Visceral injuries or evisceration*
Cardiopericardial injuries*
Massive muscle damage*
Severe burns *over* 25% body surface area*
Vascular injuries requiring repair
Wounds of the genitourinary tract
Thoracic wounds without asphyxia
Closed cerebral injuries with increasing loss of consciousness*
Spinal cord injuries requiring decompression*
Suspected spinal cord injuries without neurologic signs
Injuries of the eye
Maxillofacial injuries without asphyxia
Complicated major medical problems*
Minor medical problems
Victims with little hope of survival under the best of circumstances of medical care

Courtesy Office of Emergency Services, State of California.
*Conditions that have changed categories.

triage decisions must be sensitive to factors affecting prognosis, such as age, general health, physical condition of the patient, the qualifications of the responders, and availability of key supplies and equipment.[117]

Triage procedures are routinely used in civilian multiple or mass casualty incidents and are essential in disaster incidents. Prioritization of victims may be needed with smaller numbers of casualties when environmental conditions, remote settings, or unusual circumstances limit availability of medical care or ease of evacuation. The decision to evacuate persons who stand a reasonable chance of survival before others who are mortally injured may be necessary in settings of high-angle technical mountain rescue, complicated cave rescue, or extended overland transport from isolated wilderness regions, particularly when air evacuation is unavailable or infeasible. Effective triage is critical to the success of any disaster care operation and should be performed by a senior and knowledgeable provider. The essential differentiation to be made is "now" versus "not now." In disaster triage the moribund patient unlikely to survive is classified as "not now," when in ordinary circumstances he or she would be "immediate."

Numerous triage methods have been discussed in the medical literature.[77,90,139] Methods fall into two classes: qualitative and quantitative. Qualitative methods classify patients into subjective categories (immediate, delayed, minor, expectant, and so on). Two-tier, three-tier, four-tier, and five-tier systems have been described (see Box 26-2). Any qualitative triage method can be used successfully in a disaster. Each ranks patients relative to others and to the available care, and each requires periodic reconsideration for treatment.

Quantitative methods assign an objective score to each patient based on initial clinical status. Various schemes based on anatomic indicators of injury severity, physiologic measurements, and mechanisms of injury have been developed to predict certain types of outcomes such as survival. The Trauma Score is one such system used in trauma research as a predictor of outcome.[33,34] Many emergency medical systems use the revised Trauma Score for field triage and as a guide for patient routing in tiered trauma treatment systems.[33] While experienced physicians frequently rely on their best medical judgment to triage patients, medically inexperienced personnel may benefit from such an algorithmic approach to assessment and triage. Suppose that several members of an isolated mountain village were injured during an earthquake, that the village had only one health care worker, and that evacuation and treatment resources were limited. Decisions would have to be made regarding who would be evacuated first and who would be treated first. A trauma assessment based on physiologic variables could provide a relatively objective evaluation of the patient's condition and a rational basis for the allocation of scarce resources. The use of such standardized scoring systems for triage decisions, however, remains to be studied in the disaster setting. Triage methods founded on scoring systems require familiarity with the scoring systems. They cannot be used by disaster medical personnel unfamiliar with their application or modification.

BOX 26-2

TRIAGE RATING SYSTEMS

FIVE-TIER SYSTEM (USED IN MILITARY TRIAGE)

Dead or will die
Life threatening—readily correctable
Urgent—must be treated within 1 to 2 hours
Delayed—noncritical or ambulatory
No injury—no treatment necessary

FOUR-TIER SYSTEM

Immediate—seriously injured, reasonable chance of survival
Delayed—can wait for care after simple first aid
Expectant—extremely critical, moribund
Minimal—no impairment of function, can either treat self or be treated by a nonprofessional

THREE-TIER SYSTEM

Life threatening—readily correctable
Urgent—must be treated within 1 to 2 hours
Delayed—no injury, noncritical, or ambulatory

TWO-TIER SYSTEM

Immediate versus delayed
- Immediate—life-threatening injuries that are readily correctable on scene, and those that are urgent
- Delayed—no injury, noncritical injuries, ambulatory victims, moribund, and dead

MECHANICS OF THE TRIAGE PROCESS

Triage should begin as soon as trained medical personnel arrive on the scene. A rapid survey is performed, noting the number of victims, hazards to victims and rescuers, and the need for additional help. This information should be relayed rapidly to the communication centers responsible for the dispatch of emergency services, so that additional help can be mobilized as early as possible. The most qualified medical person present should be designated the provisional triage officer. The triage officer should not be assigned other duties and should not become extensively involved in patient care. During the initial survey, each victim is rapidly assessed for immediately correctable life-threatening problems such as airway obstruction, vigorous hemorrhage, or nonfatal penetrating chest injuries. Initial care should be limited to correction of these problems. In other words, resuscitation and definitive care clearly have no role at this stage. Care should be limited to manually opening airways and controlling external hemorrhage.[122] Physical hazards may influence the decision to provide further care on site or delay additional therapy until victims are transported a safe distance away to a casualty collection point. As additional experienced emergency medical personnel arrive, the role of triage officer should be assumed by the most experienced and knowledgeable person(s) present. Advanced medical knowledge is an asset in minimizing triage errors. However, field-experienced physicians are relatively rare. Successful disaster triage under mock conditions can be performed by appropriately trained advanced emergency medical technicians or by experienced nurses. Triage is a dynamic process. Continued clinical deterioration or improvement may change the initial decision to evacuate or treat a victim. Triage should be performed each time the responsibility for the care of a victim is transferred.[142]

ADJUNCTS TO TRIAGE

A triage tag is a paper tag intended to show the triage category in which a patient has been classified. Most bear color codes designating triage category. All enforce the use of the particular scheme of categorization for which they were designed, such as "immediate," "delayed," "minor," and "expectant," depending on injury severity and prognosis. Most are deliberately simple, like the METTAG (Fig. 26-7, *A*), and bear only minimal information to identify the patient and indicate triage class and site of injury. Others carry more information and serve as an abbreviated medical record (Fig. 26-7, *B*). Vayer, Ten Eyck, and Cowan[142] reviewed the use of triage tags in disasters and reported that the tags had been used effectively in only a few multiple casualty incidents. These authors recommend that triage tags be abandoned and replaced by a system of "geographic triage" that sorts casualties into areas reserved for patients of similar priority for treatment. Simultaneously, some disaster medical systems are recasting their "triage tags" as "victim tracking tags" used to track victims in an elaborate evacuation system.

ON-SITE MEDICAL CARE

Determining how much and what type of care to administer at the disaster site depends on several factors.[107] If the number of patients is small and sufficient prehospital per-

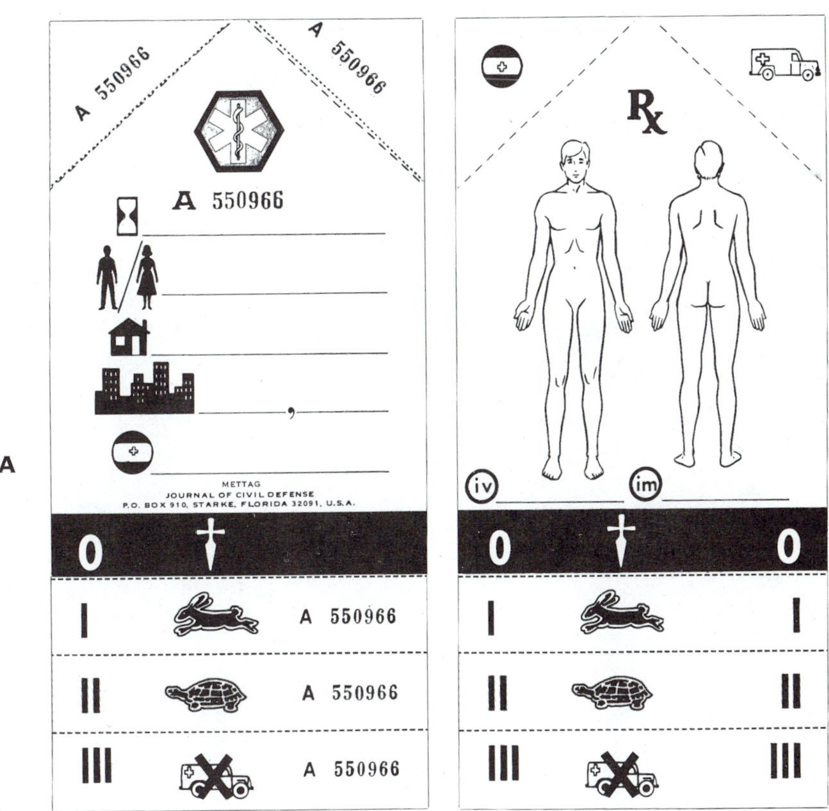

Fig. 26-7 Examples of disaster tags. **A,** METTAG. (Courtesy of Journal of Civil Defense, Starke, Fla.)

Continued.

PRINT ALL INFORMATION

ATTACH TAG SECURELY TO PATIENT

DISASTER TAG

PINK COPY FOR: Administration
WHITE COPY FOR: Admitting
HARD COPY FOR: Patient Record

№ 317363

HOSPITAL

ADMITTING

NAME (Last) (First) (Initial)

LOCATION WHEN INJURED

ADDRESS | PHONE

DESCRIPTION (Height, Weight, Hair, Eyes, Complexion, Build, Race, Marks, Clothing, Articles)

DATE / / | TIME A.M. P.M. | AGE | SEX | RELIGION

NOTIFY IN CASE OF EMERGENCY | RELATIONSHIP

ADDRESS | PHONE

MEDICAL

ALLERGIC TO

TENTATIVE DIAGNOSIS

INITIAL TREATMENTS (See Details on Reverse Side)

☐ AIRWAY ☐ TOURNIQUET
☐ SPLINT ☐ INJECTION

INITIAL ROUTING DIRECTIONS

☐ MAJOR SURGERY ☐ MINOR SURGERY ☐ FIRST AID
☐ X-RAY ☐ ICU ☐ CCU ☐ OBSERVATION
☐ MORGUE ☐ OTHER ______

TRIAGE

CARE CLASSIFICATION

☐ IMMEDIATE (Life Support)
☐ DELAYED
☐ DEAD

If Immediate Care Affix Red Label

If Delayed Care Affix Black Label

DO NOT DETACH TAG FROM PATIENT UNTIL INCORPORATED IN PATIENT'S RECORDS.

SEE REVERSE SIDE FOR TREATMENT RECORD, DISPOSITION AND INSTRUCTIONS

MEDICATIONS	Medications	Dose	Time	By
	Tetanus Toxoid		AM PM	
	Antitetanic Serum		AM PM	
	T.A.T. With Gas Gangrene		AM PM	
			AM PM	
			AM PM	
			AM PM	

TOURNIQUETS	Limb	Time On	Time Off
		AM PM	AM PM
		AM PM	AM PM

CONDITION AND DISPOSITION

ADMITTED TO (Room, Surgery, ICU, CCU, Other)

TRANSFERRED TO	DATE	TIME
	/ /	A.M. P.M.
☐ DISCHARGED ☐ DIED	/ /	A.M. P.M.

SIGNATURE OF DOCTORS

INSTRUCTIONS

1. Complete as many items as possible without delaying necessary care.
2. Be sure to attach label under "Care Classification" to indicate the level of care required.
   a. Immediate Care indicates a patient in need of life supporting medical service.
   b. Delayed Care indicates a patient where medical service needs are postponable without further endangering life.
3. Indicate time whenever tourniquet is released and reapplied.
4. Use the labels attached to identify patient's belongings or other records with this disaster tag.
5. Forward the top, pink copy to Administration, and the white copy to Admitting. Keep the hard copy with the Patient.

APPROVED BY HOSPITAL COUNCIL OF SOUTHERN CALIFORNIA 4/72

SECURLINE' DISASTER TAG
Reorder Number 2100
PRECISION GRAPHICS DIVISION
Precision Dynamics Corp. 3031 Thornton Ave., Burbank, Calif 91504 · USA · (213) 849-6111

№ 317363

№ 317363

№ 317363

№ 317363

DELAYED

B

Fig. 26-7, cont'd. B, More detailed disaster tag. (Courtesy Precision Graphics Division, Precision Dynamics Corp., Burbank, Calif.)

sonnel and transportation resources are available, on-site medical care can proceed in a fairly normal manner, with rapid stabilization and transportation to nearby hospitals. When extrication is prolonged, potentially lifesaving interventions, such as intravenous fluids for hypovolemic shock, should be instituted.[122] On the other hand, early rapid transportation with a minimum of treatment should be practiced in such circumstances as danger to rescuers and casualties from fire, explosion, falling buildings, hazardous materials, and extreme weather conditions.[40]

With an overwhelming number of casualties that exceed transportation capacities, advanced field medical treatment may be beneficial, since hours may pass before seriously injured patients can be evacuated.[7] This may necessitate the establishment of field hospitals with operating theater capabilities.[92] Such a field hospital may be set up in a large building such as a school or church. Casualties are brought to the field hospital from the disaster site for further assessment and initial treatment of injuries. After a period of observation and stabilization, they are either sent home or transported to a hospital.

Evacuation of the minor injured and ambulatory may rapidly overwhelm local hospitals before the arrival of the more severely injured.[115] Under these conditions it may be better not to evacuate the severely injured, but to treat them locally.

COMMUNICATION FROM DISASTER SITE TO HOSPITAL

Local emergency communications or the disaster operations center should alert hospitals in the affected area of a possible mass or multiple casualty situation. This report should include number of injured and, specifically, number of seriously injured and number for whom ambulatory treatment is sufficient.[22] Hospitals should report to the local emergency communications center the following information:

1. Bed availability
2. Number of casualties received thus far
3. Number of additional casualties that the hospital is prepared to accept.
4. Specific items in short supply

SPECIFIC CLINICAL ISSUES IN FIELD CARE OF DISASTER PATIENTS

The purpose of this section is not to review all aspects of mass casualty care, but to address some concepts of care that are not found in the routine management of emergency patients.

For example, wound infections may occur in virtually all types of disasters. Infected wounds and gangrene were major problems following the Armenian earthquake.[98] In hurricanes or tornadoes, persons may be cut by flying glass and other potentially highly contaminated material.[110,147] Because of this, all wounds should be copiously flushed with saline. Primary closure of heavily contaminated wounds may result in major complications, as was the case following the Armero volcanic eruption in Colombia. If lacerations are old (more than 6 to 12 hours) or appear contaminated, they should be treated by debridement and left open for primary delayed closure for a 3-day period.[21] This allows an opportunity to observe the wound for the development of infection. For tetanus prophylaxis all patients should receive a tetanus booster, and if the wound is highly contaminated, tetanus immune globulin (Hypertet) should be administered.

Patients with blunt trauma—for example, victims of earthquakes who have been trapped by rubble for several hours or days—should be watched closely for signs and symptoms of crush syndrome, such as cardiac arrhythmias and renal failure. Fulminant pulmonary edema from dust inhalation may also be a delayed cause of mortality for victims of building collapse.[98]

Austerity, rationing, and expediency may cause disaster medical care to be of lesser absolute quality than medical care delivered in the community under normal circumstances. However, disaster circumstances that exceed the capacity of available medical care resources establish a different community standard of care aimed at directing scarce resources selectively to victims who can receive the most benefit.

Some Public Health Problems Associated with Natural Disasters

EPIDEMICS

Natural disasters are often followed by rampant rumors of epidemics (such as typhoid, cholera, or rabies) or unusual conditions such as increased snakebites and dog bites. Such unsubstantiated reports gain great public credibility when printed as facts in newspapers or reported on television or radio. For example, following disasters in developing countries, any disruption of the water supply or sewage treatment facilities has usually been accompanied by rumors of outbreaks of cholera or typhoid. Such rumors may well have reflected psychologic fears and anxieties about a disastrous event rather than the true perception of an imminent problem. Although natural disasters do not usually result in outbreaks of infectious disease, under certain circumstances disasters may increase disease transmission.[1,126] In addition, information on disease incidence in most developing countries is poor, and some outbreaks may have been missed by public health authorities.[13,44] The most frequently observed increases in communicable disease are caused by fecal contamination of water and by respiratory spread (for example, measles in refugee camps).[26,27]

During the past 40 years, outbreaks of communicable disease following natural disasters have been unusual; however, disasters do have elements that can contribute to transmission of disease, and persons responsible for managing disaster relief operations should establish a surveillance system and institute appropriate sanitary and medical measures to prevent outbreaks.[15,60a,66,126,146] Mass vaccination programs, however, are rarely necessary.[25] Finally, a clearinghouse for rumors should be established to investigate those that have merit in a timely fashion, dispel those that are obviously false, and inform the public of hazards where a response is required. This concept has been helpful not only in developing countries, but also in disasters occurring in urban settings of industrialized countries.

DISPOSITION OF DEAD BODIES

The public and government authorities are usually greatly concerned about the danger of disease transmission from decaying corpses (Fig. 26-8). Responsible health authorities should recognize, however, that the health hazards associated with unburied bodies are minimal, particularly if death resulted from trauma.[75] Such bodies are unlikely to cause outbreaks of diseases such as typhoid, cholera, or plague, although they may transmit agents of gastroenteritis or food poisoning to survivors if the bodies contaminate streams, wells, or other water sources.[110] Despite the negligible health risk, dead bodies represent a delicate social problem. Demands for mass burial or cremation are certainly not justified on public health grounds, and mass cremations require tremendous quantities of fuel.

➠ SUMMARY

This chapter discusses health effects of some of the more important sudden-impact natural disasters (Table 26-5) and outlines the requirements for effective emergency medical and public health response to these events. Sound epidemiologic knowledge of the causes of death and of the types of injuries and illnesses caused by disasters is clearly essential when determining what relief supplies, equipment, and personnel are needed to respond effectively in emergency situations.[110] The overall objective of disaster management is to

A

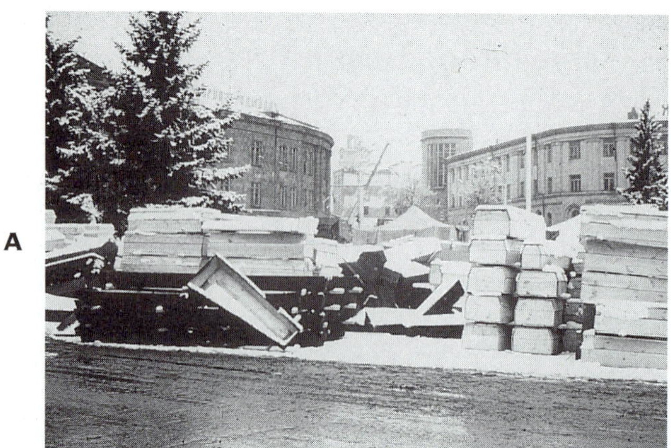

B

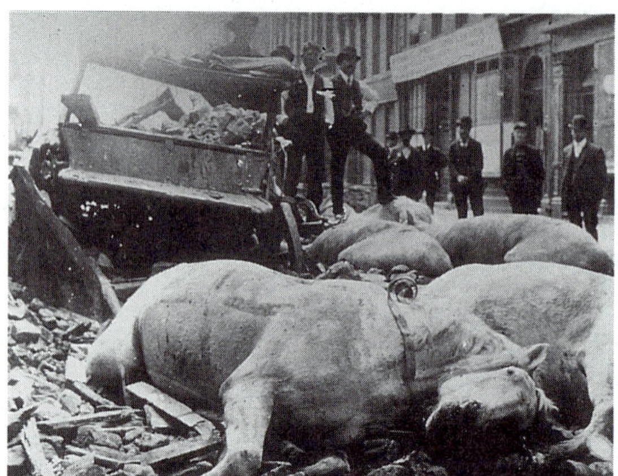

Fig. 26-8 **A,** Coffins lining the street in the city of Leninakan following the 1988 earthquake in Armenia. (Eric K. Noji photo.) **B,** Three horses were killed as a result of falling debris during the 1906 San Francisco earthquake. (Photo courtesy Eric Swenson, U.S. Geological Survey.)

Table 26-5 Short-Term Effects of Major Natural Disasters

Effects	Earthquakes	High Winds (Without Flooding)	Tsunamis	Floods/Flash Floods
Deaths	Many	Few	Many	Few
Severe injuries requiring extensive care	Overwhelming	Moderate	Few	Few
Increased risk of communicable diseases	Potential (but small) risk following all major disasters (probability rises as overcrowding increases and sanitation deteriorates)			
Food scarcity	Rare (may occur because of factors other than food shortage)	Rare	Common	Common
Major population movements	Rare (may occur in heavily damaged urban areas)	Rare	Common	Common

Modified from *Emergency health management after natural disaster,* Office of Emergency Preparedness and Disaster Relief Coordination, Scientific Publication No 407, Washington, DC, 1981, Pan American Health Organization.

assess the needs of disaster-affected populations, to match resources to needs efficiently, to prevent further adverse health effects, to evaluate relief program effectiveness, and to plan for future disasters.

All natural disasters are unique in that each affected region of the world has different social, economic, and health backgrounds. Some similarities exist, however, among the health effects of different natural disasters, which if recognized can ensure that health and emergency medical relief and limited resources are well managed.[69]

REFERENCES

1. Aghababian RV, Teuscher J: Infectious diseases following major disasters, *Ann Emerg Med* 21:362, 1992.
2. Armenian HK: *Methodologic issues in the epidemiologic studies of disasters.* In Proceedings of the International Workshop on Earthquake Injury Epidemiology: implications for mitigation and response, Baltimore, 1989, Johns Hopkins University, p 95.
3. Arnold C, Durkin M: *Hospitals and the San Fernando earthquake of 1971: the operational experience,* San Mateo, Calif, 1983, Building Systems Development, Inc, p 1.
4. Autier P et al: Drug supply in the aftermath of the 1988 Armenian earthquake, *Lancet* 335:1388, 1990.
5. Bailey RA et al: The Volcano Hazards Program: objectives and long-range plans, US Geological Survey Open-File Report 83-400, 1983.
6. Bakst HJ et al: *The Worcester County tornado: medical study of the disaster,* Washington, DC, 1954, National Research Council, Committee on Disaster Studies.
7. Baskett P, Weller R: *Medicine for disasters,* London, 1988, Wright.
8. Baxter PJ: Volcanoes. In Gregg MB, editor: *The public health consequences of disasters,* Atlanta, 1989, Centers for Disease Control.
9. Baxter PJ, Bernstein RS, Buist AS: Preventive health measures in volcanic eruptions, *Am J Public Health* 76(suppl):84, 1986.
10. Baxter PJ et al: Medical aspects of volcanic disasters: an outline of the hazards and emergency response measures, *Disasters* 6:268, 1982.
11. Beinin L: *Medical consequences of natural disasters,* Berlin, 1985, Springer-Verlag.
12. Bernstein RS, Baxter PJ, Buist AS: Introduction to the epidemiological aspects of explosive volcanism, *Am J Public Health* 76(suppl):3, 1986.
13. Bernstein RS et al: Immediate public health concerns and actions in volcanic eruptions: lessons from the Mt. St. Helens eruptions, May 18-October 18, 1980, *Am J Public Health* 76(suppl):25, 1986.
14. Better OS, Stein JH: Early management of shock and prophylaxis of acute renal failure in traumatic rhabdomyolysis, *N Engl J Med* 322:825, 1990.
15. Binder S, Sanderson LM: The role of the epidemiologist in natural disasters, *Ann Emerg Med* 16:1081, 1987.
16. Bissell R: Delayed-impact infectious disease after a natural disaster, *J Emerg Med* 1:59, 1983.
17. Blong RJ: *Volcanic hazards: a sourcebook on the effects of eruptions,* North Ryde, Australia, 1984, Academic Press.
18. Brenner SA, Noji EK: Head injuries and mortality in tornado disasters (letter), *Am J Public Health* 82:1296, 1992.
19. Brenner SA, Noji EK: Wound infections after tornadoes (letter), *J Trauma* 33:643, 1992.
20. Brenner SA, Noji EK: Risk factors for death and injury in tornadoes: an epidemiologic approach. In Church C et al, editors: *The tornado: its structure, dynamics, prediction, and hazards,* Washington, DC, 1993, American Geophysical Union.
21. Burkle FM, Sanner PH, Wolcott BW, editors: *Disaster medicine,* New York, 1984, Medical Examination Publishing.
22. Butman AM: *Emergency training: responding to the mass casualty incident: a guide for EMS personnel,* Westport, Conn, 1982, Educational Direction.
23. Butman A: The challenge of casualties en masse, *Emerg Med* 15(7):110, 1983.
24. Byrd TR: Disaster medicine: toward a more rational approach, *Milit Med* 145:270, 1980.
25. Centers for Disease Control: Current trends in flood disasters and immunization—California, *MMWR* 32:171, 1983.
26. Centers for Disease Control: Outbreak of diarrheal illness associated with a natural disaster—Utah, *MMWR* 35:662, 1986.
27. Centers for Disease Control: Health assessment of the population affected by flood conditions—Khartoum, Sudan, *MMWR* 38:785, 1989.
28. Centers for Disease Control: Medical examiner/coroner reports of deaths associated with Hurricane Hugo—S. Carolina, *MMWR* 38:754, 1989.
29. Centers for Disease Control: Update: work-related electrocutions associated with Hurricane Hugo, *MMWR* 38:718, 1989.
30. Centers for Disease Control: Surveillance of shelters after Hurricane Hugo—Puerto Rico, *MMWR* 39:41, 1990.
31. Centers for Disease Control: Medical examiner reports of deaths associated with Hurricane Andrew—Florida: preliminary report, *MMWR* 41:641, 1992.
32. Centers for Disease Control: Rapid health needs assessment following Hurricane Andrew—Florida and Louisiana, *MMWR* 41:696, 1992.
33. Champion HR: Trauma triage, *J World Assoc Emerg Disaster Med* 3(2):1, 1987.
34. Champion HR et al: The Trauma Score, *Crit Care Med* 9:672, 1981.
35. Coburn AW, Hughes RE: Fatalities, injury and rescue in earthquakes. In *2nd Conference of the Development Studies Association,* Manchester, Eng, 1987, University of Manchester.
36. Coburn AW, Murakami HO, Ohta Y: *Factors affecting fatalities and injury in earthquakes: engineering seismology and earthquake; disaster prevention planning internal report,* Hokkaido, Japan, 1987, Hokkaido University.
37. Cohen SP, Raghavulu CV: *The Andhra Pradesh cyclone of 1977,* New Delhi, India, 1979, Vikas.
38. Contzen H: Preparations in hospital for the treatment of mass casualties, *J World Assoc Emerg Disaster Med* 1:118, 1985.
39. Cuny F: *Disasters and development,* Oxford, Eng, 1983, Oxford University Press.
40. Currance PL, Bronstein AC: *Emergency care for hazardous materials exposure,* St Louis, 1988, Mosby.
41. de Bruycker M, Greco D, Lechat MF: The 1980 earthquake in southern Italy: morbidity and mortality, *Int J Epidemiol* 14:113, 1985.
42. de Bruycker M et al: The 1980 earthquake in southern Italy: rescue of trapped victims and mortality, *Bull WHO* 61:1021, 1983.
43. de Ville de Goyet C, Jeannee E: Epidemiological data on morbidity and mortality following the Guatemala earthquake, *IRCS Med Sci Soc Med* 4:212, 1976.
44. de Ville de Goyet C, Zeballos JL: Communicable diseases and epidemiological surveillance after sudden natural disasters. In Baskett P, Weller R, editors: *Medicine for disasters,* London, 1988, Wright.
45. de Ville de Goyet C et al: Earthquake in Guatemala: epidemiologic evaluation of the relief effort, *Pan Am Health Organ Bull* 10:95, 1976.
46. Dietz VJ et al: Health assessment of the 1985 flood disaster in Puerto Rico, *Disasters* 14:164, 1990.
47. Dubouloz M: An introduction to disaster medicine, *Bull Int Civil Defence,* August 1983, p 25.
48. Editorial: Disaster epidemiology, *Lancet* 336:845, 1990.
49. Eisele JW et al: Death during the May 18, 1980, eruption of Mount St. Helens, *N Engl J Med* 305:931, 1981.

50. Falk H et al: *Mount St. Helens volcano health report No 18,* Atlanta, 1980, Centers for Disease Control.
51. Falk H et al: *Mount St. Helens volcano health report No 19,* Atlanta, 1980, Centers for Disease Control.
52. Federal Emergency Management Agency: *Principal threats facing communities and local emergency management coordinators: a report to the US Senate Committee on Appropriations,* Washington, DC, 1992, FEMA Office of Emergency Management.
53. Foege WH: Public health aspects of disaster management. In Last JM, editor: *Public health and preventive medicine,* ed 11, New York, 1980, Appleton-Century-Crofts.
54. Foege WH: Public health aspects of disaster management. In Last JM, editor: *Public health and preventive medicine,* Norwalk, Conn, 1986, Appleton-Century-Crofts.
55. Frazier K: *The violent face of nature: severe phenomena and natural disasters,* New York, 1979, William Morrow.
56. French JG: Hurricanes. In Gregg MB, editor: *The public health consequences of disasters,* Atlanta, 1989, Centers for Disease Control.
57. French JG, Holt KW: Floods. In Gregg MB, editor: *The public health consequences of disasters,* Atlanta, 1989, Centers for Disease Control.
58. French JG et al: Mortality from flash flood: a review of National Weather Service Reports, *Public Health Rep* 98:584, 1983.
59. Galway G: Relationship of tornado deaths to severe weather watch areas, *Monogr Weather Rev* 103:737, 1975.
60. Gilbert DN et al: Microbiologic study of wound infections in tornado casualties, *Arch Environ Health* 26:125, 1973.
60a. Glass RI, Noji EK: Epidemiologic surveillance following disasters. In Halperin WE, Baker EL, Monson RR, editors: *Public health surveillance,* New York, 1992, Van Nostrand Reinhold.
61. Glass RI et al: Earthquake injuries related to housing in a Guatemalan village, *Science* 197:638, 1977.
62. Glass RI et al: Injuries from the Wichita Falls tornado: implications for prevention, *Science* 207:734, 1980.
63. Glass RI et al: Health effects of the 1991 Bangladesh cyclone: report of a UNICEF evaluation team, New York, 1992, UNICEF.
65. Gordon PD: *Special statistical summary—deaths, injuries and property loss by type of disaster, 1970-1980,* Washington, DC, 1982, Federal Emergency Management Agency.
66. Gregg M: *Management of surveillance operations following a disaster,* Atlanta, 1979, Centers for Disease Control.
67. Gross EM: The hurricane dilemma in the United States, *Episodes: International Geoscience Newsmagazine* 14:36, 1991.
68. Guha-Sapir D: Rapid needs assessment in mass emergencies: review of current concepts and methods, *World Health Stat Q* 44:17, 1991.
69. Guha-Sapir D, Lechat MF: Information systems and needs assessment in natural disasters: an approach for better disaster relief management, *Disasters* 10:232, 1986.
70. Guha-Sapir D, Lechat MF: Reducing the impact of natural disasters: why aren't we better prepared? *Health Policy and Planning* 1:118, 1986.
71. Gurd CH, Bromwich A, Quinn JV: The health management of Cyclone Tracy, *Med J Aust* 1:641, 1975.
72. Hagman G: *Prevention better than cure,* Stockholm, 1984, Swedish Red Cross.
73. Hight D et al: Medical aspects of the Worcester tornado disaster, *N Engl J Med* 254:267, 1956.
74. Hingston RA, Hingston L: Respiratory injuries in earthquakes in Latin America in the 1970s: a personal experience in Peru (1970); Nicaragua (1972-3); and Guatemala (1976), *Disaster Med* 1:425, 1983.
75. Hooft PJ, Noji EK, Van de Voorde HP: Fatality management in mass-casualty incidents, *Forensic Sci Int* 40:3, 1989.
76. Ivy JH: Infections encountered in tornado and automobile accident victims, *J Ind Med Assoc* 61:1657, 1968.
77. Jacobs L et al: An emergency medical system approach to disaster planning, *J Trauma* 19:157, 1979.
78. Jenkins AL, van de Leuv JH,: *Disaster planning in emergency department organization and management,* ed 2, St Louis, 1978, Mosby.
79. Katsouyanni K, Kogevinas M, Trichopoulos D: Earthquake-related stress and cardiac mortality, *Int J Epidemiol* 15:326, 1986.
80. Katz LB, Pascarelli EF: Planning and developing a community hospital disaster program, *Emerg Med Serv,* Sept/Oct 1978, p 70.
81. Kerr RA: Volcanoes to keep an eye on, *Science* 221:634, 1983.
82. Kindel S: Penny-wise, pound-foolish, *Forbes* 17:170, 1985.
83. Lechat MF: Updates: the epidemiology of health effects of disasters, *Epidemiol Rev* 12:192, 1990.
84. Longmire AW, Burch J, Broom LA: Morbidity of Hurricane Elena, *South Med J* 81:1343, 1988.
85. Longmire AW, Ten Eyck RP: Morbidity of Hurricane Frederic, *Ann Emerg Med* 13:334, 1984.
86. Malilay J: Medical and healthcare aspects of the 1992 earthquake in Egypt. In *Report of the Earthquake Engineering Research Institute Reconnaissance Team,* Oakland, 1992, Earthquake Engineering Research Institute.
87. Malilay J: *Volcanic eruption of Cerro Negro, Nicaruagua, April, 1992.* Report to the Pan American Health Organization (PAHO), Washington, DC, 1992, PAHO Emergency Preparedness and Disaster Relief Coordination Unit.
88. Mandelbaum I, Nahrwold D, Boyer DW: Management of tornado casualties, *J Trauma* 6:353, 1966.
89. Manni C, Magalini S, Proietti R: Volcanoes. In Baskett P, Weller R, editors: *Medicine for disasters,* London, 1988, Wright.
90. Marian JF, Bougarte W: Disaster preparedness. In Schwartz GR et al, editors: *Principles and practice of emergency medicine,* Philadelphia, 1978, WB Saunders.
91. Memarzadeh P: *The earthquake of August 31, 1968, in the south of Khorasan, Iran.* In Proceedings of the joint IHF/IUA/UNDRO/WHO Seminar, Manila, 1978, World Health Organization Regional Office.
92. Nancekievill D, Finch P: The role of hospital mobile medical teams at a major accident. In Cowley RA, editor: *Proceedings of mass casualties: a lessons learned approach,* June 1982.
93. Nania J, Bruya TE: In the wake of Mount St. Helens, *Ann Emerg Med* 11:184, 1982.
94. National Oceanic and Atmospheric Administration, US Department of Commerce: *Tornado,* Washington, DC, 1973, US Government Printing Office.
95. National Research Council: *Confronting natural disasters: an international decade for natural disaster reduction,* Washington, DC, 1987, National Academy Press.
96. Noji EK: Acute renal failure in natural disasters, *Renal Failure* 14:245, 1992.
97. Noji EK: Medical consequences of earthquakes: coordinating medical and rescue response, *Disaster Management* 4:32, 1991.
98. Noji EK: Medical and healthcare aspects of the 1988 earthquake in Soviet Armenia, *Earthquake Spectra* (suppl):101, 1989.
99. Noji EK: Prophylaxis of acute renal failure in traumatic rhabdomyolysis (letter), *N Engl J Med* 323:550, 1990.
100. Noji EK, Jones NP: Hospital preparedness for earthquakes. In Tomasik KM, editor: *Emergency preparedness: when disaster strikes,* Plant, Technology & Safety Management Series, Oakbrook Terrace, Ill, 1990, Joint Commission on the Accreditation of Healthcare Organizations.
101. Noji EK, Sivertson KT: Injury prevention in natural disasters: a theoretical framework, *Disasters* 11:290, 1987.
102. Noji EK et al: The 1988 earthquake in Soviet Armenia: a case study, *Ann Emerg Med* 19:891, 1990.
103. Office of US Foreign Disaster Assistance: *Disaster history: significant data on major disasters worldwide, 1900-present,* Washington, DC, 1992, Agency for International Development.

104. Orlowski J: Floods, hurricanes, and tsunamis. In Baskett P, Weller R, editors: *Medicine for disasters,* London, 1988, Wright.
105. Othman-Chande M: The Cameroon volcanic gas disaster: an analysis of a makeshift response, *Disasters* 2:96, 1987.
106. Oxtoby MJ, Broome CV, Pinzon MR: Late mortality in Nevado del Ruiz victims. In *Disaster chronicles No. 4, the volcanic eruption in Colombia, November 13, 1985,* Washington, DC, 1986, Pan American Health Organization.
107. Oyen O: The on-scene medical organization, *J World Assoc Emerg Disaster Med* 1(2):115, 1985.
108. Pan American Health Organization: *The effects of Hurricane David, 1979, on the population of Dominica,* Disaster report no. 1, Washington, DC, 1979, The Organization.
109. Pan American Health Organization: *Report on disasters and emergency preparedness for Jamaica, St. Vincent and Dominica,* Disaster report no. 2. Washington, DC, 1980, The Organization.
110. Pan American Health Organization: *Emergency health management after natural disaster,* Scientific publication no. 407, Washington, DC, 1981, PAHO Office of Emergency Preparedness and Disaster Relief Coordination.
111. Pan American Health Organization: *Assessing needs in the health sector after floods and hurricanes,* Technical paper no. 11, Washington, DC, 1987, The Organization.
112. Pan American Health Organization: *Hurricane Gilbert in Jamaica, September, 1988,* Disaster report no. 5, Washington, DC, 1989, The Organization.
113. Philen RM et al: Hurricane Hugo—1989, *Disasters* 15:177, 1992.
114. Pointer JE et al: The 1989 Loma Prieta earthquake: impact on hospital care, *Ann Emerg Med* 21:1228, 1992.
115. Quarantelli EL: *Delivery of emergency medical services in disasters: assumptions and realities,* New York, 1983, Irvington.
116. Reitherman R: How to prepare a hospital for an earthquake, *J Emerg Med* 4:119, 1986.
117. Roding H: Triage and its ethical problems, *J World Assoc Emerg Disaster Med* 3(3):10, 1987.
118. Roth PB et al: The St. Croix disaster and the National Disaster Medical System, *Ann Emerg Med* 20:391, 1991.
119. Rubin CH, Noji EK: Impact of the eruption of Mt. Hudson on livestock in Argentina, *Bull Global Volcanism Network* 16:5, 1991.
120. Rund D, Rausch T: *Triage,* St Louis, 1981, Mosby.
121. Rutherford WH: Sorting patients, sometimes called triage, *Disaster Med* 1(1):121, 1983.
122. Safar P: Resuscitation potentials in mass disasters, *J World Assoc Emerg Disaster Med* 2:34, 1986.
123. Safar P: Resuscitation potentials in mass disasters, *Prehosp Disaster Med* 2:34, 1986.
124. Safar P, Pretto EA, Bircher NG: Resuscitation medicine including the management of severe trauma. In Baskett P, Weller R, editors: *Medicine for disasters,* London, 1988, Wright.
125. Sanderson LM: Tornadoes. In Gregg MB, editor: *The public health consequences of disasters,* Atlanta, 1989, Centers for Disease Control.
126. Seaman J: Disaster epidemiology: or why most international disaster relief is ineffective, *Injury* 21:5, 1990.
127. Seaman J: Epidemiology of natural disasters, *Contrib Epidemiol Biostat* 5:1, 1984.
128. Sigurdsson H, Carey S: Volcanic disasters in Latin America and the 13th November 1985 eruption of Nevado del Ruiz volcano in Colombia, *Disasters* 10:205, 1986.
129. Sigurdsson H: Gas bursts from Cameroon crater lakes: a new natural hazard, *Disasters* 12:131, 1988.
130. Smith GS: Development of rapid epidemiologic assessment methods to evaluate health status and delivery of health services, *Int J Epidemiol* 18(suppl):S2, 1989.
131. Sommer A, Mosley WH: East Bengal cyclone of November, 1970, *Lancet* 1:1029, 1972.
132. Stratton JW: Earthquakes. In Gregg MB, editor: *The public health consequences of disasters,* Atlanta, 1989, Centers for Disease Control.
133. Surmieda RS et al: Surveillance in evacuation camps after the eruption of Mt. Pinatubo. In *Public health surveillance and international health,* Atlanta, 1992, Centers for Disease Control.
134. Thiel CC et al: 911 EMS process in the Loma Prieta earthquake, *Prehosp Disaster Med* 7:348, 1992.
135. Toole MJ: Communicable disease epidemiology following disasters, *Ann Emerg Med* 21:418, 1992.
136. Toole MJ, Tailhades M: Disasters: what are the needs? How can they be assessed? *Trop Doct* 219(suppl):18, 1991.
137. Trichopoulos D, Katsouyanni K, Zavitsanos X: Psychological stress and fatal heart attack: the Athens 1981 earthquake natural experiment, *Lancet* 1:441, 1983.
138. UN General Assembly: *International decade for natural disaster reduction: report of the Secretary-General. 43rd session, agenda item 86. A/43/723. 18 October 1988,* New York, 1988, United Nations.
139. US Air Force: *Medical planning for disaster and casualty control,* Washington, DC, 1967, US Air Force Medical Service.
140. US Public Health Service: *Hurricane Andrew,* Situation report no. 6, Rockville, Md, 1992, US Public Health Service.
141. Ussher JH: Philippine flood disaster, *J Res Naval Med Serv* 59:81, 1973.
142. Vayer JS, Ten Eyck RP, Cowan ML: New concepts in triage, *Ann Emerg Med* 15:927, 1986.
143. Walker GPL: Volcanic hazards, *Interdisc Sci Rev* 7:148, 1982.
144. Western K: *The epidemiology of natural and man-made disasters: the present state of the art. Dissertation for the academic diploma in tropical public health London School of Hygiene and Tropical Medicine,* London, 1972, University of London.
145. Wijkman A, Timberlake L: *Natural disasters: acts of God or acts of man,* New York, 1984, Earthscan.
146. Woodruff B et al: Disease surveillance and control after a flood—Khartoum, Sudan, 1988, *Disasters* 14:151, 1990.
147. World Health Organization: Emergency care in natural disasters: views of an international seminar, *WHO Chron* 34:96, 1980.
148. World Health Organization: *Rapid health assessment protocols,* Geneva, 1990, Emergency Preparedness and Response Office, The Organization.
149. Yong S: Medical support in the Tangshan earthquake: a review of the management of mass casualties and certain major injuries, *J Trauma* 27:1130, 1987.

27 THE CHANGING ENVIRONMENT

James K. Mitchell
Keith Harrington

- Issues of environmental change
- Impacts of environmental change on wilderness areas
- Consequences of environmental change
- What might be done about limiting environmental change?

Three miles southwest of the Kremlin, not far from Moscow's Olympic Stadium, lies the Novodevichiy Cemetery, one of the most celebrated burying places in Russia. Amid ornate memorials to former leaders now out of favor, like Gromyko and Khrushchev, and to giants of the arts, such as Chekhov and Shostakovich, stands a white marble pedestal carrying the sculpted head of Vladimir Illich Vernadsky (1863-1945). Little known in the West, Vernadsky was a prescient observer of the emerging role of humans as makers of the global environment. It was he who first announced that we are living at a time when the power of mankind to change the earth now rivals that of geologic processes.[4] In the past, students of natural history could regard the human life span as a mere blink of a cosmic eye that witnessed little environmental change. Today we are faced with the prospect that the planet may be fundamentally transformed by humans, perhaps within a few decades, but more probably over the space of one or two generations.

This situation has not come about all at once, or equally everywhere. On a global scale, it has gradually built up over centuries, although the local manifestations of increased human agency have been sometimes masked by other processes. For example, conversion of "natural" ecosystems to "managed" ecosystems is a dominant feature on the global scale, but in some parts of the world (such as the United States and Western Europe) managed ecosystems are also being abandoned.[46]

The complications of environmental change might best be appreciated with the aid of a time machine such as the one envisioned by H.G. Wells in 1935. Imagine, for a moment, being in a mature pine forest in southern New England. What might be observed as the machine slips into the past at this location?

The surrounding landscape comes clearly into view. The pine trees shrink slowly down into youth as the years wind back, for most of today's pines trace their origin to the abandonment of farm lands at or near the turn of the century. The pines disappear entirely in the late nineteenth century and are replaced by shrubs and eventually by grasses. By the mid-1800s the local vicinity is completely open and appears as a shifting mosaic of agricultural crops and pasture, rotated in time and space. This is the high tide of farming in New England. Thereafter, the sequence goes into reverse. By the eighteenth century, trees begin to return, connecting the remnant patches of presettlement vegetation. Gradually the forest closes in and traces of human presence fade. Little breaks the monotony, apart from occasional fires started by lightning or native Americans clearing seasonal cultivation patches, or major windstorms that topple weaker trees. As the sixteenth century approaches, clearly the landscape is essentially similar from decade to decade.

The time traveler's dominant impression is one of change. The preceding sequence of changes has been documented by many analysts of the New England landscape.[43] The sequence might be different elsewhere but is no less dynamic. Sometimes the changes are sudden and dramatic, and sometimes they are slow and imperceptible.* Sometimes

*Arguments between uniformitarians (who give primacy to continuous, small-scale changes) and catastrophists (who favor change as a function of intermittent large-scale events) have continued for more than a century. Although the uniformitarian position has dominated among earth scientists, recent evidence in support of catastrophic explanations is compelling. For example, the fossil record indicates that mass extinctions have occurred throughout the globe at many times in the past. (See Martin PS, Klein RG, editors: *Quaternary extinctions: a prehistoric revolution,* Tucson, 1984, University of Arizona Press.) Some analysts argue that the age of dinosaurs ended 65 million years ago when a massive meteor collided with the earth, perhaps striking the Gulf of Mexico near the Yucatan Peninsula. (See Alvarez W, Asaro F: What caused mass extinction? *Sci Am* 263[4]:78, 1990.) The impact may have thrown sufficient dust into the atmosphere that solar radiation was reflected back into space, causing global temperatures to plummet. A similar although smaller effect was noted in 1992 when volcanic Mt. Pinatubo in the Philippines spewed ash, dust, and gases into the atmosphere and lowered mean global temperature by an estimated 2° C. (See Dutton EC, Christy JR: Solar radiative forcing at selected locations and evidence of global lower troposphere cooling following eruptions of El Chichon and Pinatubo, *Geophys Res Lett* 19[23]:2313, 1992.)

they are "natural" (for example, storms) and sometimes they are caused by humans (for example, forest clearance). For the bulk of human history, natural changes have seemed to dominate, although in fact people have been major shapers of the environment for millennia.[26] A casual observer of the New England landscape might conclude that the well-wooded 1990s scene is more "natural" than the cleared fields of the 1850s. However, today's scene is just as much a product of human choices as that of the nineteenth century, albeit different in composition and appearance.

In any event, deciding whether human or natural factors are responsible for a given environmental change is often difficult; both factors tend to operate interdependently (Fig. 27-1). It is widely believed that people have reached a critical threshold as environmental modifiers; they are able to equal or surpass the effects of nature. Portentous changes are becoming manifest in the entire biosphere. We can at last begin to speak of a human "transformation" of the global environment.[22]

This chapter addresses environmental change and its human dimensions, with special attention to implications for environmental and wilderness medicine. What types of changes are likely to occur? How will they affect the natural environment, especially wilderness areas? What will be the consequences for society in general and for medical practitioners in particular? Can anything be done to improve our

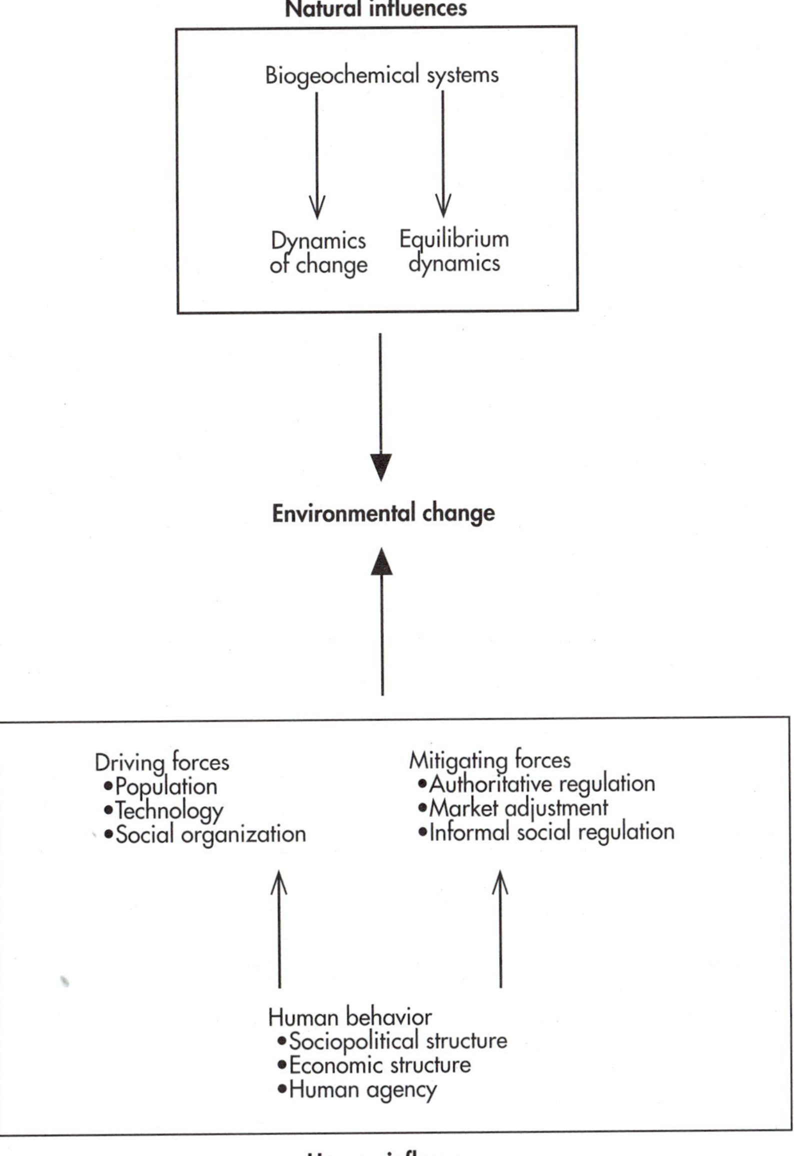

Fig. 27-1 Human and natural forces for environmental change. (Modified from Kates RW, Turner BL II, Clark WC: The great transformation. In Turner BL II, editor: *The earth as transformed by human action,* Cambridge, Eng, 1990, Cambridge University Press.)

chances of successfully negotiating this impending time of dislocation and discontinuity?

Issues of Environmental Change

In recent years a number of environmental change issues have come to prominence. They include climate change, stratospheric ozone depletion, erosion of biodiversity, population growth, and burgeoning pollution. These issues affect all environments, from urban centers to remote wilderness areas. In the discussion that follows, they are examined on a variety of scales. Although each scale is characterized by different expressions of change, all are interconnected. Local changes can aggregate to produce global effects, and global changes have many different disaggregated local effects.[53]

CLIMATE CHANGE

Weather is the state of the atmosphere at any specific time. Climate is the average weather pattern at a particular location. Weather and climate are usually described by such measures as temperature, precipitation, pressure, humidity, and wind speed and direction. In most parts of the world these measures have been recorded for less than a century, so the actual historical record of direct observations is relatively brief compared with the human tenure of the earth. However, scientists are often able to extend the historical record by constructing synthetic climate data from other evidence such as tree rings, fossils, concentrations of plankton in ocean sediments, pollen in sedimentary rocks, and isotopes of carbon and oxygen in rocks and glacial ice. For example, narrow intervals between annual growth rings in trees and thin layers of organic material in lake sediments usually indicate cold dry conditions. Clues like these permit investigators to open a window on past climates.

Fig. 27-2 illustrates trends in average global temperature during the past 10,000 years. Note that the global temperature has been in flux throughout this period. Not only has weather varied about long-term average conditions, but the averages themselves have changed over time. For example, during the most recent ice age (about 10,000 years ago), average global temperatures were approximately 6° C cooler than at present.[15] In other words, a massive environmental change (the Wisconsin ice age) was connected with a relatively small climatic change. Fortunately, the climate has remained within a range that sustains life for most of the earth's history, and the changes have occurred at very slow rates over thousands to millions of years.

Currently a broad consensus exists among atmospheric scientists that global temperatures may rise significantly in coming decades.[27] Although the global climate system is

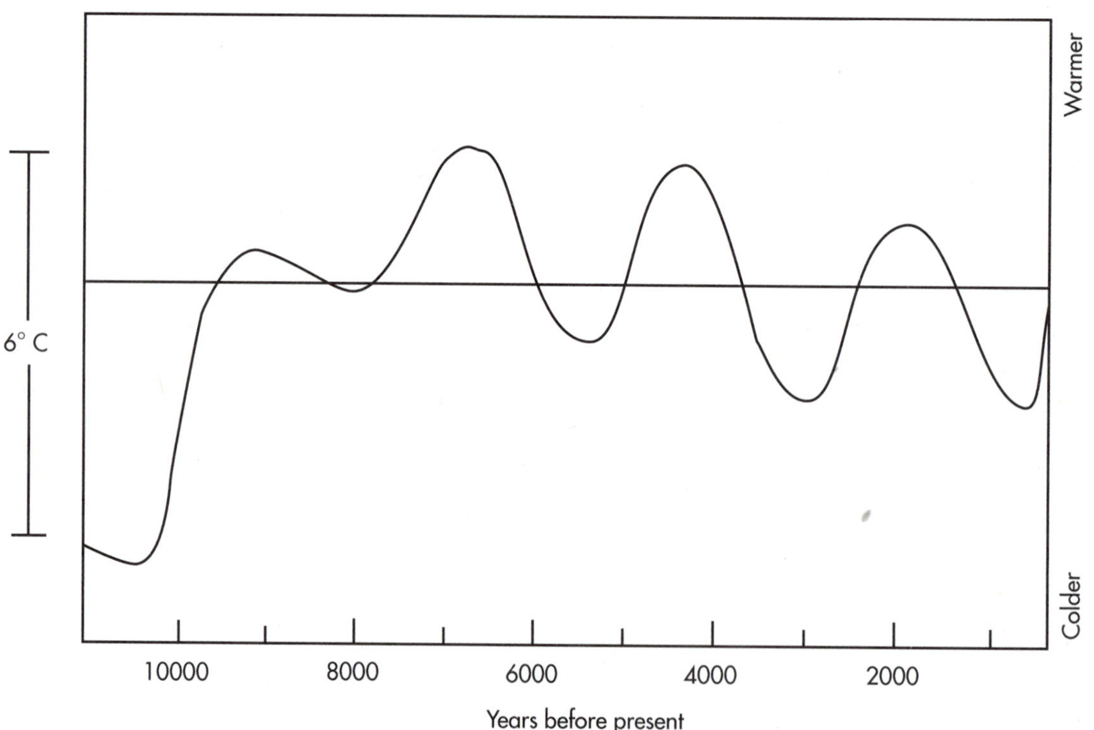

Fig. 27-2 Variations of mean global temperature during the past 10,000 years. Horizontal line represents present global average temperature. (Modified from Henderson-Sellers A, Robinson PJ: *Contemporary climatology,* New York, 1991, Wiley.)

enormously complex, two factors point toward warming. First, it is known that certain greenhouse gases warm the atmosphere by trapping short-wave radiation reflected from the earth's surface when it is heated by solar radiation. Second, atmospheric concentrations of these gases, which include carbon dioxide, methane, and nitrous oxide, are steadily increasing. Normally the materials in greenhouse gases pass through long biogeochemical cycles between natural sources and natural sinks. For example, sulfur enters the atmosphere as sulfur dioxide from volcanic eruptions and washes back to the oceans in the form of mildly acid rainfall whose constituents are later incorporated into bottom sediments. Human activities can increase source loads (for example, emissions) and reduce the absorptive capacities of natural sinks. In the case of carbon dioxide, the greenhouse gas about which there is most concern, both processes are at work simultaneously. Emissions of carbon dioxide have been increasing as energy-hungry societies burn petroleum hydrocarbons, coal, and wood. At the same time, forests that usually absorb huge amounts of atmospheric carbon dioxide are being systematically cleared.[56]

Atmospheric scientists are currently struggling to estimate how climate might change as greenhouse gases accumulate. For this purpose they rely heavily on general circulation models (GCMs) that mathematically simulate the global climate system. The chemistry and physics of climate are complex and the models, although increasingly sophisticated, are still in their infancy. Their accuracy is constrained both by the limits of current knowledge about the dynamics of the atmosphere and by the computational power of the most advanced supercomputers. They are also hedged with other limitations. For example, the present generation of GCMs is too coarse to provide more than a broad-gauge portrayal of atmospheric conditions in a lattice of regions over the earth's surface. They do not reveal storm systems that bring most of the weather to mid and high latitudes. They also do not incorporate the role of clouds as reflectors and absorbers of energy. They do not satisfactorily account for all of the carbon dioxide that is believed to have been liberated into the atmosphere through human activities. Nonetheless, many have considerable confidence in the accuracy of GCMs because of their relative success in replicating present and past climates.

The Intergovernmental Panel on Climate Change (IPCC), a joint United Nations–World Meteorological Organization committee of leading earth scientists, has synthesized existing research on climate change. Their conclusions are sobering. If nothing is done to alter present patterns of energy use and land use, there will be twice the preindustrial age (mid-eighteenth century) concentration of greenhouse gases in the atmosphere by 2030. This will probably raise mean global temperature about 0.3° C per decade to 1° C above the present value by 2025 and to 3° C above the present value by 2100.[16]

While the IPCC estimates embody a consensus about global warming, the level of agreement declines as researchers attempt to forecast the resulting impacts, especially at regional and local levels. An enhanced greenhouse effect would have a greater effect on the global climate than temperature alone. Solar radiation provides the energy that drives the climate system. The effects of a warmer atmosphere could produce a cascade of changes in many climate variables. For example, precipitation patterns might change in ways that do not mirror temperature fluctuations.

GCMs generally indicate that lower latitudes and lower elevations will be less affected by anticipated climate changes than upper latitudes and higher elevations. Probably a mosaic of regional and local changes will occur along a spectrum from strongly positive to strongly negative depending on how, when, and where they occur. For example, tropical islands might experience heavier precipitation combined with more frequent severe storms and rising sea levels. The net impacts of such changes are difficult to assess. For Malé and other heavily populated low-lying islands of the Indo-Pacific Ocean, the results could be disastrous, while other places, such as high-standing islands of the Caribbean, could see offsetting agricultural benefits.[39]

More than any other factor, the rate of climate change is of concern to humans. General circulation models indicate that absolute changes in temperature will be smaller than those that have occurred at other times during the earth's history. However, the anticipated climate changes would still occur at a rate and magnitude that are unprecedented in human experience. Whereas past changes usually occurred slowly enough for plants and animals to adapt or migrate, examples of mass extinctions following rapid change exist. Many scientists fear that today and in the future insufficient time and undeveloped areas will be available for plants and animals to make similar adjustments.

While changes of average climate would have important long-term consequences, variations in extreme weather might produce the most immediate and significant impacts.[28] Droughts, floods, and tropical cyclones are unusual events in today's climate. If mean climates change, changes in the frequency and severity of these extremes would probably also occur and become manifest well before the permanent shifts could be confirmed. The geographic distribution of such events would also be affected. As a result, natural hazards would be likely to pose increased risks to society. Moreover, exposure and vulnerability to extreme events would probably be exacerbated because populations at risk might respond to the new conditions on the basis of outdated information and assumptions.[11] We might find that our previous experience prepared us to "fight the last war" rather than the new one.

STRATOSPHERIC OZONE DEPLETION

The stratosphere is a distinct layer of the upper atmosphere that occurs between 9 and 35 miles above the ground. It contains significant concentrations of ozone (O_3), a gas that is formed when solar radiation splits ordinary oxygen atoms.* The stratospheric ozone layer absorbs most of the ultraviolet (UV) radiation from space that would otherwise damage plant and animal species.

During the 1970s and 1980s, researchers discovered that stratospheric ozone was being lost and that the ozone layer was thinning to the point of disappearance, particularly in polar regions.[30] Chlorofluorocarbons (CFCs) were held to be at fault. For decades, these synthetic compounds had been manufactured in large quantities, mainly for use as aerosol propellants and refrigerants. Once CFCs escape into the atmosphere, they remain stable until reaching the stratosphere, where they decompose under the action of UV radiation. Chlorine atoms are released and bond with ozone atoms, breaking them down into oxygen and other products. As a result, the ozone shield is weakened or removed.

If the ozone layer is sufficiently depleted, intensity of UV radiation that reaches the earth's surface could be significantly increased. This could have deleterious consequences for human populations and for plant and animal species. For humans, increased incidence of skin cancer, cataracts, and immune system suppression are three recognized effects of high UV exposure. While humans might take precautions to protect themselves against UV radiation, such as reducing time spent outdoors, or adding sun blocks, glasses, and clothes, nonhuman species may not be able to make the necessary adaptations. Serious disruption of human and agricultural systems is possible.

During their winter seasons, the Antarctic[40] and to a lesser extent the Arctic[25] have been experiencing elevated levels of UV radiation. "Ozone holes" have been clearly traced to CFCs. Depletion of stratospheric ozone is not completely understood but is occurring so rapidly and has such grave potential effects that governments have felt compelled to act. An international agreement, the Montreal Protocol, has been reached to phase out CFC usage by 1996. However, chlorine atoms are extremely long lived in the stratosphere, perhaps persisting for 100 to 200 years. Even if all CFC usage ceases by 1996 (an ambitious assumption), the prospect of additional ozone depletion will continue for many decades.

EROSION OF BIODIVERSITY

Loss of species is a serious global problem that comes under the heading "erosion of biodiversity." Biodiversity is not an agent of change like greenhouse gas buildup or ozone depletion. It is an index or conceptual framework against which all environmental changes can be considered.[51] Like climate change and ozone depletion, biodiversity has a range of dimensions from global to local. The two aspects of biodiversity of greatest importance are numbers and interconnections of species.

It is estimated that the earth is home to 3 to 8 million species. About 1.7 million of these have been cataloged.[44] The estimate's wide range shows how little is known about the planet's biologic resources. Ecosystems in temperate and high latitudes have relatively few species in comparison with those of the tropics. For example, tropical forests may have 2 to 10 times as many species as temperate forests.[12]

Paleobiologic research indicates that the number and type of species have varied greatly over time. New species evolve through adaptive genetic mutations, while others perish because of competitive pressures of natural selection. Emergence and disappearance rates depend on the speed and direction of environmental change and the ability of species to adjust. What is most troubling about the recent record is the disappearance of so many species. Over 115 species of mammals and 171 species of birds are known to have become extinct since 1600 (Table 27-1). On some oceanic islands, such as Hawaii, the disappearance of native animal species is almost total. The rate of human alteration

Table 27-1 Species and Subspecies of Mammals and Birds Considered To Have Become Extinct Since 1700

Location	Mammals	Birds
Continents		
Africa	11	0
Asia	11	6
Australia	22	0
Europe	7	0
North America	22	8
South America	0	2
Total	73	16
Pelagic	1	0
Islands		
Continental		
Africa	0	2
Asia	4	0
Australia	0	2
North America	4	3
Oceanic		
Pacific Ocean	4	109
Indian Ocean	4	18
Atlantic Ocean	23	20
Mediterranean Sea	2	1
Total (all islands)	41	155
TOTAL (all locations)	115	171

Data from Diamond JM: Historic extinctions: a rosetta stone for understanding prehistoric extinctions. In Martin PS, Klein RG, editors: *Quaternary extinctions: a prehistoric revolution,* Tucson, 1984, University of Arizona Press.

*Ozone also accumulates near ground level as a by-product of the photochemical modification of exhaust gases from automobiles and other sources of pollution. Concentrations of this type of ozone are sometimes reported in local news media, but the ground-level "ozone problem" should not be confused with the stratospheric one.

of habitats and ecosystems has so accelerated in recent decades that 20% of all species may be lost by the year 2000.[31] Commercial forestry and fishing have proved particularly injurious to biodiversity because they harvest desirable species and destroy undesirable species at the same time. Agriculture and animal husbandry also contribute to species extinctions.

For many people the protection of threatened species is a moral imperative. For others it is a luxury. Quite apart from moral issues, the rising rate of species extinction has practical implications.[45] For example, loss of the planet's genetic stock hampers the search for wild strains of domestic crops that are resistant to pests and diseases that plague high-yield domestic varieties. The so-called Green Revolution was built on this principle, and prospects for relieving global hunger are closely connected to it.

Biodiversity is also important in the stability of global ecosystems. For example, the extent to which entire species can be eliminated from an ecosystem before it collapses is unknown. Most ecologists believe that ecosystems containing a wide diversity of organisms are more resilient to change than those with few species. Regardless of the degree of resilience, biodiversity and environmental change may be connected by negative feedback relationships. Thus environmental change may lead to a loss of biodiversity that in turn produces lowered resistance to pressures for further change.

The importance of preserving biodiversity is illustrated by the worldwide decline of shark populations. In the early 1980s the U.S. National Marine Fishery Service encouraged increased shark fishing for human consumption as a means of reducing pressure on other species such as tuna. Along the east coast of the United States the result has been a rapid increase in commercial shark landings, from 135 in 1979 to 5729 in 1991.[33] Recreational landings of sharks may have risen proportionately. Demand for shark meat is rising, driven partly by Asian partiality to shark fin soup, which fetches up to $60 a serving, and by a growing U.S. market for shark steaks, which retail at $3 to $4 per pound.[33] As a result, numbers of sharks are falling in U.S. waters, and the effects are rippling through marine ecosystems. Florida's Atlantic stone crab fishery has collapsed; sharks eat octopuses, which are important stone crab predators. As shark numbers have fallen, numbers of octopuses have exploded. This example illustrates what can happen when the top of the food chain in an ecosystem is disrupted. Similar effects can occur lower down the food chain but are often less obvious. The loss of biodiverse marine plankton has recently emerged as an important global environmental concern.

POPULATION GROWTH

Human population is one of the primary driving forces behind contemporary environmental change. Beginning with the Reverend Thomas Malthus (1766-1834), many people have argued that rising populations must eventually deplete resources and degrade environments because the earth is, for all intents and purposes, a closed system.[21] In the absence of interplanetary space travel on a scale impossible at present, to destinations that are now unknown and perhaps nonexistent, the earth is our only home. Leaving aside the counterargument that human ingenuity can make possible the support for larger populations indefinitely, clearly from the perspective of burdens on the physical environment, how people live is more important than the number of people. All other things being equal, richer societies place heavier burdens on the physical environment than poorer ones.

The global population has undergone unprecedented growth in the last several centuries (Fig. 27-3). By 1800 the earth's population was approximately 1 billion. By 1920 it had doubled. Three billion was reached in 1960, and the present estimate is over 5 billion. The United Nations estimates that more than 8 billion people will be on earth by the year 2025.[54] Numbers may level out to between 12 and 15 billion by 2100. Most of the new growth is likely to occur in developing countries of Asia, Africa, and Latin America (Table 27-2). The recent experience of China suggests that the process of development can itself perpetuate or increase historical rates of population growth, at least until economic conditions improve significantly.

POLLUTION

Unwanted by-products of production and consumption that exceed the absorptive capacity of the environment are known as pollution. Pollution comes in many forms, including solid physical materials, liquid chemical compounds, and energy (for example, thermal pollution). Some pollutants (such as certain isotopes of plutonium) are highly toxic even in small amounts. Many materials that are beneficial in small amounts can be deleterious in large quantities. For example, phosphorus is a nutrient that limits biologic productivity in coastal and marine ecosystems. Small amounts of phosphorus can increase algal growth at the bottom of marine food chains. But when larger amounts of phosphorus-rich runoff from fertilizers or septic systems enter these environments, the entire population of algae can begin a period of explosive growth ("bloom"). Extensive blooms can produce "red tides" or "brown tides."[8] This occurs when algae prevent light from penetrating coastal waters and the decomposition of dead algae consumes dissolved oxygen. Large fish kills are a frequent result.

The preferences of people for quick and convenient disposal of pollutants into available environmental sinks (such as soil, streams, groundwater, oceans, and atmosphere) have sometimes been validated by incomplete science. For decades in the United States and elsewhere, scientists advised policymakers that "the solution to pollution is dilution." As a result, physical and chemical wastes have been

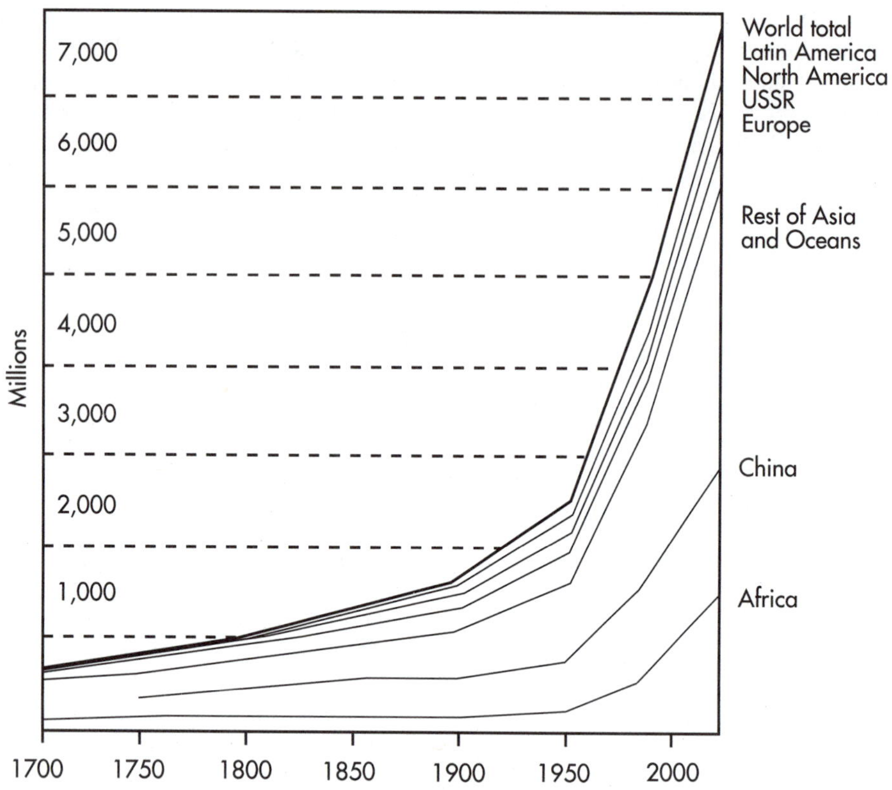

Fig. 27-3 Global population (1700-2020). (Modified from Demeny P: Population. In Turner BL II, editor: *The earth as transformed by human action,* Cambridge, Eng, 1990, Cambridge University Press.)

Table 27-2 Average Annual Percentage Rates of Population Increase

	1700-1750	1750-1800	1800-1850	1850-1900	1900-1950	1950-1985	1985-2020
Africa	0.0	0.0	0.1	0.4	1.0	2.6	2.7
Asia	0.3	0.5	0.5	0.3	0.8	2.1	1.4
Europe	0.3	0.6	0.7	0.7	0.6	0.6	0.1
Russia	0.3	0.7	1.0	1.0	0.7	1.2	0.6
North America	0.8	1.0	3.2	2.6	1.2	1.3	0.6
Latin America	0.8	0.5	1.2	1.6	1.6	2.6	1.6
Oceania	—	—	—	—	1.6	1.9	1.2
WORLD TOTAL	0.25	0.44	0.55	0.54	0.84	1.88	1.45

From Demeny P: Population. In Turner BL II, editor: *The earth as transformed by human action,* Cambridge, Eng, 1990, Cambridge University Press.

released into environments that had finite capacities for absorbing them. Once the absorptive capacities were reached, a variety of serious problems occurred. These included biologically "dead" rivers (such as Cleveland's Cuyahoga River), "dead" lakes (such as Lake Erie), and "dead" seas (such as the sewage sludge dumping ground in the New York Bight off the coasts of New Jersey and Long Island). Although some of these conditions can be reversed, the processes are slow, costly, contentious, and often incomplete. Also, a growing body of evidence suggests that the aggregate effect of pollution may be jeopardizing the functioning of fundamental earth systems. The buildup of atmospheric carbon dioxide is an excellent example of this process.

Despite a large volume of evidence, the effects of pollutants on receiving environments are not fully known. This is partly because of a lack of scientific knowledge about the normal (unpolluted) functioning of some environments, such as deep oceans and tropical forests. The sheer volume and variety of materials released into the environment and their interactions complicate the study of effects of any single pollutant. Sometimes the effects of pollutants are subtle, long delayed, and far removed from the point of origin, making it difficult to connect causes and consequences. Sometimes experts disagree about evidence of pollution impacts collected in the field and evidence acquired from laboratory experiments. Even the impacts of well-studied events like the *Exxon Valdez* tanker grounding are in dispute.[38] Nonetheless, there is a broad consensus that the absorptive capacity of receiving media is not inexhaustible and that pollution is a growing world problem that is pushing society against the limits of environmental resilience.

Impacts of Environmental Change on Wilderness Areas

Clearly wilderness areas are likely to be affected significantly by global environmental change. Before taking up that subject we will clarify terms and usage of the word "wilderness."

Western cultures frequently portray "natural" and "human" as mutually exclusive concepts. As far as the earth's environments are concerned, however, the reality is more complex. Our environments are arranged on a continuum from intensely human-constructed places, such as cities, to places where the human presence is small, intermittent, or nonexistent, such as wilderness areas. Most places show evidence of both human and natural influences.

No consensus exists about the meaning of "wilderness," and no comprehensive maps of wilderness areas are available. However, most analysts recognize that the term refers to places that have some or all of the following three characteristics: few or no permanent resident human populations, unmanaged biogeochemical systems, and no significant modification by modern technology. Places that meet these criteria might include deep oceans, high mountains, deserts, circumpolar lands, certain oceanic islands, coastal fringes, most areas of active vulcanicity, and some of the world's great forests (such as taiga and tropical rainforests).*

The three criteria are best regarded as necessary but not sufficient to identify an area as wilderness. Spatial dimensions must also be taken into account. An acre of wetland that is surrounded by shopping malls would not be considered wilderness even if it is in biologically pristine condition. As a rule of thumb, a wilderness should encompass at least several square miles.

If the foregoing criteria were to be applied to the United States, they would include a great diversity of environments. Most would be marginal lands and waters, that is, beyond the boundaries of areas that are permanently settled at present and perhaps without prospects for human occupancy or use in the long term. Some protected areas within the ecumene (inhabited lands) might also qualify as wilderness because they are administered as such. But most protected areas, such as national parks, national forests, and national recreational areas, would probably not meet all three major wilderness criteria because they are often subject to intensive management of residual plant and animal populations as well as to human visitors.[24]

CONVERSION OF WILDERNESS

In many parts of the world the frontiers of wilderness areas are being pushed back as land is converted to managed uses. Economic growth and population increases are the ultimate driving forces of this conversion at the global scale. At local and regional levels a variety of conversion processes are apparent. These include resource extraction industries, such as mining and forestry; agriculture; animal husbandry; tourism; and commercial and residential uses.[32] These processes are not confined to land. They also affect freshwater and shallow water marine environments. Tourism is exerting pressure on coral reefs in Belize, Kenya, and many other countries.

Most land conversion is driven by demands for additional cropland. The highest levels of land conversion are found in developing countries with rapidly growing populations (Table 27-3). Most of the world's prime agricultural lands have been brought under cultivation, so attention has turned to other terrains that are spatially and agriculturally marginal.[2] Often these are wilderness areas. For example, during the last four decades many formerly unpopulated parts of Sumatra and Borneo have been settled by government-sponsored "transmigrants" from the heavily populated Indonesian island of Java.

Land conversion may fragment existing wilderness areas by dividing them into smaller blocks. This process is well advanced in the Amazon rainforest of Brazil where new long-distance, government-built roads bring settlers.[49] As a result, ecologic "islands" that may not be sustainable are created. Forest edge environments replace deep forest ones. The islands may be too small to retain the previous diversity of species. Governments often attempt to protect such islands by designating them as parks or wilderness areas, but this may be insufficient to prevent further

*How should formerly developed areas that have reverted to unmanaged states be classified? Many such areas can be found in Western Europe and North America (for example, the Adirondack Mountains of New York). Often, radical differences exist between predevelopment conditions and reverted conditions. For the purposes of this discussion, such areas are considered wilderness.

Table 27-3 Global Land Use Changes (1700-1980)

Region	Vegetation Types	Percentage Changes				
		1700-1850	1850-1920	1920-1950	1950-1980	1700-1980
Tropical Africa	Forests and woodlands	−1.6	−4.6	−6.8	−9.6	−20.9
	Grassland and pasture	0.9	2.8	3.6	2.5	10.1
	Croplands	29.5	54.4	54.5	63.2	404.5
North Africa/ Middle East	Forests and woodlands	−10.5	−20.6	−33.3	−22.2	−63.2
	Grassland and pasture	−0.4	−0.6	−1.3	−3.4	−5.6
	Croplands	35.0	59.3	53.5	62.1	435.0
North America	Forests and woodlands	−4.4	−2.8	−0.5	0.3	−7.3
	Grassland and pasture	−0.1	−11.3	−2.7	0.1	−13.7
	Croplands	1566.7	258.0	15.1	−1.5	6666.7
Latin America	Forests and woodlands	−1.7	−3.6	−7.0	−9.6	−20.3
	Grassland and pasture	2.1	4.0	8.4	9.6	26.2
	Croplands	157.1	150.0	93.3	63.2	1928.6
China	Forests and woodlands	−28.9	−17.7	−12.7	−15.9	−57.0
	Grassland and pasture	−0.7	−0.3	−0.3	−1.6	−2.9
	Croplands	158.6	26.7	13.7	24.1	362.1
South Asia	Forests and woodlands	−5.4	−8.8	−13.1	−28.3	−46.3
	Grassland and pasture	0.0	0.5	0.0	−1.6	−1.1
	Croplands	34.0	38.0	38.8	54.4	296.2
Southeast Asia	Forests and woodlands	−0.4	−2.0	−2.0	−2.9	−7.1
	Grassland and pasture	−1.6	−7.3	−7.9	−12.4	−26.4
	Croplands	75.0	200.0	66.7	57.1	1275.0
Europe	Forests and woodlands	−10.9	−2.4	−0.5	6.5	−7.8
	Grassland and pasture	−21.1	−7.3	−2.2	1.5	−27.4
	Croplands	97.0	11.4	3.4	−9.9	104.5
Russia	Forests and woodlands	−6.2	−7.5	−3.5	−1.2	−17.3
	Grassland and pasture	0.9	−0.4	−0.4	−0.5	−0.3
	Croplands	184.8	89.4	21.3	7.9	606.1
Pacific developed countries	Forests and woodlands	0.0	−2.2	−1.1	−4.7	−7.9
	Grassland and pasture	−0.2	−1.3	−0.8	−2.7	−4.9
	Croplands	20.0	216.7	47.4	107.1	1060.0
TOTAL	Forests and woodlands	−4.0	−4.8	−5.1	−6.2	−18.7
	Grassland and pasture	−0.3	−1.3	0.5	0.1	−1.0
	Croplands	102.6	70.0	28.1	28.3	466.4

From Richards JF: Land transformation. In Turner BL II, editor: *The earth as transformed by human action*, Cambridge, Eng, 1990, Cambridge University Press.

changes. In any case, to be effective, such places often require intensive management of ecosystems and visitors, which defeats the objective of designating them as wilderness in the first instance. Moreover, the management actions may ripple through the ecosystems in unforeseen ways, perhaps contributing to the long-term conversion process.

HUMAN PENETRATION OF WILDERNESS AREAS

Wilderness areas may be degraded without being converted to other uses. This usually occurs in one of three ways: direct impacts from increasing human presence; indirect effects of conventional industrial technologies in adjacent areas; and global effects of innovative, powerful, and often high-risk technologies.

Direct Impacts

Few parts of the planet have not been explored by humans at ground level. Formerly remote areas are being penetrated for a variety of reasons. Canada's James Bay is slowly being altered by a huge hydropower scheme; gold prospecting has intruded into the innermost recesses of Amazonia and Angola; and Philippine coral reefs are subject to cyanide poisoning in pursuit of aquarium fish.[10]

The penetration of wilderness is facilitated by modern industrial technologies, especially transportation technologies. For example, road building encourages invasion of wilderness areas for recreation, resource extraction, or other purposes. The roads themselves have environmental impacts ranging from vegetation clearance to drainage impedance, but their roles as conduits of change are even more significant. They bring new people, exotic materials, and different life-styles to remote places. Similar inroads are made by boats and aircraft and their support facilities.

As economic gain is an important incentive for wilderness penetration, recreational and esthetic needs are also increasing visitation. Hunting and fishing have long attracted visitors to wilderness areas like the Boundary Waters Canoe Area of northern Minnesota. Such pursuits are being reinforced by "ecotourism." An increasing number of people want to visit remote areas to appreciate pristine beauty. For many people who formerly might have sought out Yellowstone National Park and the Grand Canyon, the destinations of choice include places like Antarctica, the high Himalaya, Amazonia, and even Siberia. The more remote the destination, the more attractive. Since most ecotourists want to visit the wilderness for only brief periods, they are whisked in and out by the most modern transportation technologies.

Visits from ecotourists can change wilderness environments. Seemingly insignificant impacts that are repeated can eventually become major problems. In the Masai Mara Reserve of Kenya's Serengeti Plains, the savanna ecosystem has been altered by successive photographic safaris. Safari camps require open campfires; fuel wood is scavenged from fallen trees that would otherwise provide important ecologic niches for local plants and animals. Climbing expeditions on Mt. Everest have reported large volumes of garbage left by earlier expeditions. Decomposition is slow in the dry mountain air. The scarring of scientific sites in Antarctica by discarded refuse and vehicle tracks is well known. Even the Galapagos Islands, the one-time archetypical wilderness of Charles Darwin, are succumbing to the effects of their popularity with ecotourists. Geographers from the United States are assisting the government of Ecuador in carrying capacity studies that will be the basis for land use regulations and other development controls to limit further degradation of these internationally valued sites.

Indirect Impacts

One of the most potent indirect impacts on wilderness areas follows the introduction (inadvertent or intentional) of nonnative species. Negative impacts have been demonstrated in the United States countless times, such as after the introduction of English sparrows, Asian gypsy moths, and Africanized "killer" bees. One recent example occurred in Glacier National Park. Pack trips within the park were curtailed because horses were introducing exotic species of grasses picked up from stable feed and passed through the digestive tract within the feces.

The problems of small islands and introduced species are legendary. Guam's experience with the brown tree snake is a good example.[34] These snakes are native to New Guinea, but several managed to travel to Guam on airplanes in 1962. They thrived in the absence of native snakes or predators. Now Guam has as many as 30,000 brown tree snakes per square mile, and they have devastated native bird species. These snakes are beginning to show up in the Hawaiian Islands, where conditions are also favorable for colonization. The potential outcome is discouraging, although efforts to intercept the snakes are being increased.

High-Risk Technologies

Technologic risks are an increasingly familiar threat to modern industrial society. Such risks are usually perceived as limited to accidents in urban industrial zones like Bhopal, India, where over 3000 people died following the accidental release of methylisocyanate gas in 1984. However, some technologies have the potential to affect very large areas at great distances from the point of origin, up to and including the entire global environment.

Biotechnology exemplifies the powerful, high-risk technologies. Through genetic engineering, new organisms are being created, primarily for agricultural purposes. Nuclear technologies are another example. Like biotechnologies, they are characterized by considerable uncertainty about potential impacts. For decades after World War II, a massive nuclear war between the United States and the Soviet Union was a serious possibility that would have brought catastrophic changes to the earth as a whole.[41] Many military nuclear facilities were located in remote areas throughout the United States and the Soviet Union. With the end of the Cold War this threat has diminished, although regional nuclear conflicts among lesser powers are still possible. The risks for nuclear weapons accidents also remain. Nuclear bombs have been lost at sea, improperly managed nuclear wastes have exploded in the Ural Mountains and elsewhere, and military nuclear wastes are buried on small Pacific islands, often within reach of rising sea levels. Environmental contamination around nuclear weapons manufacturing plants in the United States has been reported, and nuclear submarine propulsion systems have been discarded into the Arctic Ocean north of Russia.

Civilian uses of nuclear technologies pose risks to wilderness areas. Accidents like the explosion and fire at the Chernobyl nuclear power station have had global repercussions. Deposition of highly radioactive fallout in Arctic areas of Scandinavia demonstrates that no wilderness is immune from the effects of major nuclear accidents.[3] The proposed placement of a repository for high-level nuclear waste in Yucca Mountain in the middle of semiarid Nevada provides another example of the connection between high-risk technologies and wilderness areas.[7]

Consequences of Environmental Change

Research on global environmental change continues to reveal an ever greater number of connections between human and natural systems. Linkages among species in a given ecosystem, among different ecosystems, and among global biogeochemical systems have been described. Providing details about all vulnerable systems is not possible, but the range of interconnections can be illustrated by the example of coral reefs. Such reefs are among the most prized of wilderness ecosystems. Major reefs, like the Great Barrier Reef of Australia and the reefs off Belize, are national and international treasures.

Coral reefs cover only 0.17% of the ocean floor—an area about the size of Texas.[13] However, the importance of such reefs far exceeds their physical extent. Their biologic diversity is second only to that of tropical forests; their productivity is among the highest in the world; they protect adjacent lands from wave action, nourish valuable fish populations, and generate millions of dollars in tourist revenues.

When subject to physical or chemical stress, coral "bleaches," losing color as a consequence of biochemical changes. Such stresses may be caused by fluctuations in sea level, temperature, or salinity and by pollution. Although reefs sometimes recover, bleaching often leads to death of the coral organisms and decomposition or disintegration of the reefs. In 1987, marine scientists began to notice high levels of coral bleaching and mortality off Puerto Rico. A worldwide pattern of severe coral bleaching began to emerge.[5] Some scientists interpreted the problem as a harbinger of global warming, but it is unclear that this is the case. Nonetheless, coral reefs are vulnerable to temperature changes and sea level increases, so that the threat of future damage is considerable. The best estimate now available is that sea level may rise an average of 1 m by 2100. Healthy reefs can grow upward by as much as 10 cm per decade, which may allow some reefs to adjust to rising sea level. But if reefs are unhealthy—the evidence of bleaching suggests that many are—the rate of inundation may well exceed the coral's ability to keep pace.[50]

Among the stresses that afflict coral reefs are coral mining for cement, dredging for navigation, coral collection for aquariums, and disruption by divers and commercial fishing. Many places also experience significant biochemical effects from coastal pollution and sediment or pollution runoff from land.

The loss of coral reefs is already significant. Estimates suggest that 5% to 10% of the world's living reefs have been destroyed by human activities. An additional 60% are thought to be at risk over the next 20 to 40 years.[55] The consequences for society are potentially enormous. The physical protection of coastlines could be drastically reduced. The locally rich fisheries of coral islands could be diminished to the impoverished levels that typify deep oceans. Prized tourist attractions would disappear together with the revenues they generate. Opportunities for the recovery of medicinal products from reef organisms could well be lost.* Finally, the genetic resources of the planet could be further eroded. These are just some of the consequences of environmental change for one type of wilderness area. Similar, perhaps larger, effects may occur elsewhere.

ENVIRONMENTAL CHANGE AND MEDICAL EMERGENCIES

The causes and characteristics of many medical emergencies, and perhaps also the appropriate responses, are directly and indirectly connected with the environment in which they occur. This text contains many examples of emergency medicine challenges that are posed by environments in general and wilderness environments in particular. In some cases an environmental agent causes a medical emergency (for example, reptile bites, altitude sickness, wild animal attacks). In others the environment affects the treatment of problems that are not environmentally created (for example, wilderness trauma and surgical emergencies, hunting injuries, wilderness medical liability). In many cases the environment serves as both agent and context. Inasmuch as the process of environmental change is global in scope, it probably will also affect emergency medicine. A number of examples follow.

Increasing human penetration of wilderness areas is steadily driving up the number of wilderness emergencies. In 367 U.S. national parks, the number of search and rescue missions per million visits has climbed from 12.0 (1987) to 19.4 (1991). More than 5000 rescues occurred in 1991—a 78% increase over a 5-year period.[37] The costs of a single rescue can exceed $100,000; the National Park Service spent over $3 million on search and rescue operations in 1991. Park service personnel may be exposed to high risk when called on to retrieve inexperienced and underequipped parties. Given the rising cost of such operations, it has been proposed that individuals who participate in risky adventures should post rescue bonds before departing into the wilderness. The combination of increasing populations and projected changes in environmental conditions can only add to the costs and difficulties of search and rescue in wilderness areas in the future.

As settlement advances into wilderness areas, new patterns of disease are likely to form. For example, African land conversion from unmanaged wetlands to irrigated agriculture may spread the range of schistosomiasis and other water-borne diseases that are associated with drainage canals.[47] Likewise, more people may be exposed to virulent diseases of wilderness ecosystems. Conversion of tropical

*Kainic acid, used in the diagnosis of Huntington's chorea, has already been developed from coral reef organisms. (See *The Economist,* June 13, 1992.)

forest in Africa may increase exposure to malaria carried by mosquitoes, onchocerciasis (river blindness) carried by simulium flies, and trypanosomiasis (sleeping sickness) carried by tsetse flies.

Pollutants often migrate into wilderness areas ahead of people. Air pollution is particularly mobile. Higher smokestacks have been a common means of diluting airborne pollutants, but they also allow these materials to disperse more widely. Trees and lakes in New York State's Adirondack Mountains have been affected by acid rains transported from the Ohio Valley, and once clear vistas in the Grand Canyon have been obscured by smoke from a distant coal-fired power plant. The growing severity of winter haze in the Arctic is a further problem.[52] Although the Arctic is a remote area, increasing haze has been observed there for almost a century. This smog consists of many different industrial pollutants that originate far to the south in industrial areas, especially the heavy manufacturing industries of Russia. Intense cold is perhaps the most obvious environmental health hazard in the Arctic, but the buildup of industrial air pollutants may also have significant health effects both directly on the body and indirectly through uptake by food sources in the Arctic environment.

The effect of weather on human mortality has long been a focus of biometeorologic research.[18] A range of medical conditions that are weather related are listed in Box 27-1. To take but one, well-established linkages exist between high summer temperatures and human mortality, especially among the elderly.[20] Although "global warming" need not mean that all parts of the earth will experience significantly elevated temperatures, some researchers are convinced that summer heat waves are likely to become more extreme, leading to increased mortality from this cause.[19]

BOX 27-1

CAUSES OF DEATH CONSIDERED TO BE WEATHER RELATED

Active rheumatic fever
Adverse effect of medicinal agents
Cerebrovascular disease
Complications of medical care
Complications of pregnancy and childbirth
Contusion and crushing of intact skin surface
Diseases of the arteries, arterioles, and capillaries
Diseases of the blood and blood-forming organs
Diseases of the digestive system
Disease of the musculoskeletal system and connective tissue
Diseases of the nervous system and sense organs
Diseases of the skin and subcutaneous tissue
Diseases of the veins and lymphatics
Effects of foreign body entering through orifice
Endocrine, nutritional, and metabolic diseases
Fractures of the skull, spine, trunk, and limbs
Hypertensive disease
Influenza
Injury to nerves and spinal cord
Intracranial injury
Ischemic heart disease
Neoplasms: benign and malignant
Superficial injury
Toxic effects of substances of chiefly nonmedical sources

Modified from Kalkstein LS, Davis RE: *Ann Assoc Am Geographers* 79(1):44, 1989.

The medical effects of UV radiation have already been noted. Further erosion of the stratospheric ozone layer will undoubtedly increase the likelihood of cataracts, skin cancers, and immune system diseases. Reduction of biodiversity threatens to reduce the availability of natural materials that have medicinal value. Ethnobotanists are currently working with traditional shamans in Amazonia to catalog the medicinal properties of plants in tropical forests. Marine species are also an important source of new medicines. Scientists have recently extracted from sharks a powerful agent against bacteria, fungi, and parasites that may spur research into naturally occurring antibiotics.

The "ozone hole" is a dramatic example of the expanding capacity of humans to modify the biosphere. Usually the process is inadvertent, and wilderness areas are not singled out for attention. Sometimes, however, the very remoteness and isolation of wilderness areas encourages dramatic environmental changes. Such was the case in northwest Alaska in 1962 when the U.S. government buried 15,000 pounds of radioactive soil at Point Hope.[35] The project was conducted by the U.S. Geological Survey acting in conjunction with the Atomic Energy Commission. The intent was to study effects of Arctic environments on radioactive isotopes. However, the burial was illegal; no public hearings were held, no markers were erected, and high-level wastes instead of low-level wastes were included. When the land was returned to the Inupiat (Eskimos) in 1971, they were not informed about the buried soils. They now attribute current elevated cancer rates to living and hunting for many years in a contaminated area. Government officials reject this view. The Point Hope case is not an isolated example. There is significant evidence that metropolitan governments have often tended to regard wilderness peripheries and their populations as dispensable when issues of national security and the welfare of metropolitan residents are at stake.[9]

COMPLEXITY AND UNCERTAINTY

Although we have ample reason to be concerned about the environmental changes that lie ahead for wilderness areas, the subject is hedged with complexity and uncertainty. The potential for change exists, but it is difficult to be certain how fast and how far such changes will proceed. The following two cases illustrate some of the dimensions of complexity and uncertainty.

The north (Na Pali) coast of the Hawaiian island of Kauai is representative of wilderness areas that are particularly vulnerable to climate change. It is one of the most remote and beautiful places in Hawaii, accessible only on foot, from the ocean, or by air, weather permitting. The potential for increased rainfall, storminess, and sea level rise could radically alter this wilderness. For example, increased rainfall on Kauai's massive central peak, Mount Waialeale ("the wettest place on earth"), would make hiking on steep Na Pali access trails that are already subject to erosion and landslides difficult. The few available campsites near beaches may be eliminated by rising sea level. Sea caves that can be entered only by inflatable small powerboats during calm conditions may become inaccessible. Flash floods in Na Pali streams may erode archeologic sites, and increased moisture in the air would add to the mistiness that is now only an occasional feature of the area. Offshore waters host migrating whales that can be seen from the coast, but increased soil erosion might add to sediment loads and discourage these highly valued mammals.

As the Na Pali coast becomes increasingly hazardous to visitors on foot, larger numbers may try to enter by helicopter, with more high technology–dependent visitors and fewer low technology–dependent ones. Health and safety emergencies may increase, or the mix of emergencies may change. Already the skies over Na Pali are crowded with noisy aircraft. Several crashes and deaths occur every year. Leptospirosis from Na Pali streams is now a health hazard and may become worse. The bacteria were introduced from Southeast Asia in imported rats and pigs. In 1989 the Hawaiian Islands reported 66 cases of leptospirosis with two resulting deaths.[36] Despite the potential for problems, no one can yet say with certainty which, if any, of these changes will come about. Nonetheless, we see strong indications that the Na Pali coast will not remain in its present state.

A second case that illustrates the complex interplay of environmental linkages and the potential for problems is provided by the highlands of Papua New Guinea.[1] Since the sweet potato was introduced to this area in the 1500s, it has become a staple crop for residents of remote mountain valleys. Sweet potatoes are susceptible to frost damage and tend to deplete mountain soils. In response to these constraints, villagers have developed specialized social and agricultural adjustments including the practice of "mounding" and a complex system of resource exchanges between residents of higher elevations and lower elevations. Global warming might reduce the frost hazard, but increased precipitation or increased UV radiation could also threaten crop survival. At present we have no way of confirming the extent and severity of possible changes. But clearly a delicately worked out system of human ecology like this one would not remain unaffected by climate changes of the type that are anticipated in the next several decades.

What Might Be Done About Limiting Environmental Change?

At the beginning of this chapter we suggested that change is a dominant, perhaps "normal," feature of the world's landscapes and environments. What is different about the present era of environmental change is the extent to which it is directly attributable to human decisions and actions. It seems unlikely that people will stand by and do nothing if the anticipated changes are perceived as threatening, especially if they are also perceived as caused by humans. However, also likely are responses to environmental change that will not be motivated solely by concern about environmental hazards, such as medical emergencies in wilderness areas. Recognition is growing throughout the world that improved environmental quality is an appropriate goal for all countries, not just developed ones. Therefore public policies toward the environment will seek both to mitigate risks such as those connected with environmental emergencies and to secure rewards by safeguarding and enhancing valued resources such as wilderness areas. Let us briefly examine some recent activities that provide clues to future public policies at the global, national, and local levels.

INTERNATIONAL ACTIONS

The first Earth Day (April 22, 1970) ushered in an important era of environmental politics in the United States.[6] The immediate result was a striking increase in public awareness of environmental issues. The United Nations Conference on the Human Environment (Stockholm, 1972) played a similar role on the international stage. In June 1992 the United Nations Conference on Environment and Development (UNCED) marked the twentieth anniversary of the Stockholm meeting and focused attention squarely on the global environment and emerging issues of environmental change. Several significant international agreements that addressed the task of slowing environmental change were signed[14]:

1. The Rio Declaration, a broad agreement on principles of environmental management and development
2. The Convention on Climate Change, a nonbinding treaty for industrialized and developing countries that is intended to stabilize and eventually reduce greenhouse gas emissions
3. The Convention on Biodiversity, a nonbinding treaty that establishes a framework to preserve the planet's biologic diversity and to share products derived from genetic stocks

These agreements are unusual because they broadly and directly link issues of environmental management to issues of economic development and because they took place under the glare of international publicity in a global forum. Many other international agreements are more narrowly targeted and have been signed without such fanfare. They include, for example, the Montreal Protocol on CFCs, the Convention on International Trade in Endangered Species of Wild Fauna and Flora (CITES), the London Dumping Convention, the World Heritage List, and various agreements about the protection of Antarctica. (CITES aims to limit trafficking in endangered species, and the Dumping Convention bans ocean disposal of wastes.)

Important as agreements among governments are, they do not constitute the only kind of international action to limit environmental change. Increasingly, nongovernmental organizations have become significant international policy actors. Such organizations can serve as catalysts for responsible environmental management by marshaling public support for governmental agreements. They can also take action themselves, as in the case of so-called debt-for-nature swaps.

Debt-for-nature swaps were first begun in 1987 as an innovative way to accomplish three goals: to ease the debt burdens of developing countries, to relieve the international banking community of risky development loans, and to protect important environmental resources in debt-ridden developing countries. The mechanism operates as follows. An environmental organization purchases some of the debt of a developing country from a lien-holding institution. Since no one expects the loans to be paid back in the near future, they have lost their luster as financial instruments and can be purchased well below face value. The organization then forgives the debt in return for the debtor country's agreement to undertake environmental protection measures. These may include establishing preservation areas or deferring environmentally destructive development proposals. Debt-for-nature swaps offer one means for private organizations in the developed world to make a direct commitment to limiting unwanted environmental changes in developing countries. However, at present they fall short of being an adequate solution because the amount of debt greatly exceeds the funds that are available for buy-backs.

NATIONAL ACTIONS

Because national states retain sovereignty over most of the resources within their borders, they are still the most powerful institutions for managing the global environment. For example, the U.S. government has authority to regulate pollution, manage federal lands, and control waste disposal.[42] It also has important supervisory and review powers over the actions of state governments. Finally, it has strong indirect influence on economic factors that are deeply implicated in environmental issues.

Together with business and industry, environmental interest groups are important nongovernmental participants in shaping U.S. environmental policy. Although direct action groups like Greenpeace often receive publicity in the mass media, most U.S. environmental groups are political lobbying organizations. As shown in Table 27-4, membership in the major environmental organizations has increased greatly in the last two decades, especially during the Reagan presidency when environmental issues were widely perceived to have been ignored by the U.S. government.[29]

New environmental interest groups are also joining the fray. For example, the American Medical Association has recently formed an Environmental Health Task Force that is charged with studying harmful environmental issues such as waste disposal and ozone depletion. In addition, the

Table 27-4 National Environmental Lobbying Organizations

	Membership (in Thousands)					
Organization (Year Founded)	**1960**	**1969**	**1972**	**1979**	**1983**	**1990**
Sierra Club (1892)	15	83	136	181	346	560
National Audubon Society (1905)	32	120	232	300	498	600
National Parks and Conservation Association (1919)	15	43	50	31	38	100
Izaak Walton League (1922)	51	52	56	52	47	50
The Wilderness Society (1935)	10	44	51	48	100	370
National Wildlife Federation (1936)	—	465	525	784	758	975
Defenders of Wildlife (1947)	—	12	15	48	63	80
Environmental Defense Fund (1967)	—	—	30	45	50	150
Friends of the Earth (1969)	—	—	8	23	29	30
Natural Resources Defense Council (1970)	—	—	6	42	45	168
Environmental Action (1970)	—	—	8	22	20	20
TOTAL	123	819	1117	1576	1994	3103

Modified from Mitchell RC, Mertig AG, Dunlap RE: *Soc Nat Resources* 4:219, 1991.

National Association of Physicians for the Environment was established in April 1992 to educate physicians about environmental hazards to human health and to develop recommendations for policymakers.[17]

LOCAL ACTIONS

One of the most popular environmental slogans of recent years is "Think Globally, Act Locally." This advice recognizes that most environmental issues need to be addressed at the grassroots level if they are to be resolved successfully. In local communities the effects of environmental problems are most forcefully felt by individuals, and the "not in my back yard" (NIMBY) syndrome is a powerful deterrent to projects with perceived negative impacts on environment and health.[48] For example, opposition to creating sites for sanitary landfills has raised garbage disposal costs to the point that recycling has become an accepted part of daily activities for many Americans. In other words, the political pressure of the NIMBY syndrome has yielded significant environmental benefits.

Nontraditional leaders are an emerging facet of local environmental activism. In the United States, women play key leadership roles in many local environmental groups. The same is true in developing countries such as India (the Chipko Movement) and Kenya (the Greenbelt Movement).[23] Chico Mendes, a Brazilian rubber-tapper who urged a slowdown in clearance of Amazonian forests, is another widely heralded example.

Looking across the range of environmental change issues and responses, new institutions and new philosophies of human-nature relations are emerging and are being linked to a broad range of public concerns. Issues of environmental change are now seen as intertwined with issues of economics and security. In other words, the principle of diversity in natural systems, which imparts resilience in the face of stress, is now being replicated in social systems. This is a hopeful sign at a time when environmental changes are unprecedented in rate and magnitude.

➠ SUMMARY

Environmental change has been a characteristic feature of the earth's history, but today the changes are unprecedented in human experience. Nonetheless, people are capable of taking positive steps to confront and manage anticipated changes, despite the complexity and uncertainty. During the next several decades, wilderness areas will be particularly affected by environmental transformations that occur within and around them—perhaps more so that at any comparable period in the past. Like other sectors of society, emergency medicine and emergency medical systems will face new challenges as a result. Wilderness medical systems may need to be redesigned with particular attention to improving their flexibility.

REFERENCES

1. Allen BJ: Adaptation to frost and recent political change in highland Papua New Guinea. In Allan NJR, Knapp GW, Stadel C, editors: *Human impacts on mountains,* Totowa, NJ, Rowman & Littlefield.
2. Allen JC, Barnes DF: The causes of deforestation in developing countries, *Ann Assoc Amer Geographers* 75:163, 1985.
3. Anspaugh LR, Catlin RJ, Goldman M: The global impact of the Chernobyl reactor accident, *Science* 242(4885):1513, 1988.
4. Bailes KE: *Science and Russian culture in an age of revolution: V.I. Vernadsky and his scientific school (1863-1945),* Bloomington, 1990, Indiana University Press.
5. Bunkley-Williams L, Williams EH: Global assault on coral reefs, *Nat Hist,* April 1990, p 46.
6. Cahn R, Cahn P: Did Earth Day change the world? *Environment* 32(7):16, 1990.
7. Carter LJ: *Nuclear imperatives and public trust: dealing with radioactive waste,* Washington, DC, 1987, Resources for the Future.
8. Cherfas J: The ocean fringe—under siege from the land, *Science* 248:163, 1990.
9. Dalby S: Ecopolitical discourse: "environmental security" and political geography, *Prog Human Geogr* 16(4):503, 1992.
10. Derr M: Raiders of the reef, *Audubon* 92:48, 1992.
11. Dracup JA, Kendall DR: Floods and droughts. In Waggoner PE, editor: *Climate change and U.S. water resources,* New York, 1990, Wiley, p 243.
12. Erwin TL: Beetles and other insects of tropical forest canopies at Manaus, Brazil, sampled by insecticidal fogging. In Whitmore TC, Chadwick AC, editors: *Tropical rain forest ecology and management,* Oxford, 1993, Blackwell Scientific, p 59.
13. Goreau TJ: Control of atmospheric carbon dioxide, *Global Environ Change* 2(1), March 1992, p 5; Salvat B: Coral reefs—a challenging ecosystem for human societies, *Global Environ Change* 2(1):12, 1992; Weber R: Reviving coral reefs, *State of the world 1993,* Worldwatch Institute, New York, 1993, WW Norton, p 42.
14. Haas PM, Levy MA, Parson EA: How should we judge UNCED's success? *Environment* 34(8):6, 1992.
15. Henderson-Sellers A, Robinson PJ: *Contemporary climatology,* New York, 1991, Wiley.
16. Houghton JT, Jenkins GJ, Ephraums JJ, editors: *Climate change: the IPCC scientific assessment,* New York, 1990, Cambridge University Press.
17. *The Internist,* May 1992 (referenced in *Environment* 34[6]:21, 1992).
18. Jones TS: Morbidity and mortality associated with the July 1980 heat wave in St. Louis and Kansas City, Missouri, *JAMA* 247:3327, 1982.
19. Kalkstein LS: *The impacts of predicted climate changes upon human mortality,* Publications in Climatology Series XLI (1), Newark, 1988, University of Delaware.
20. Kalkstein LS, Davis RE: Weather and human mortality: an evaluation of demographic and interregional responses in the United States, *Ann Assoc Amer Geographers* 79(1):44, 1989.
21. Kates RW: The human environment: the road not taken, the road still beckoning, *Ann Assoc Amer Geographers* 77(4):525, 1987.
22. Kates RW, Turner BL II, Clark WC: The great transformation. In Turner BL II et al, editors: *The earth as transformed by human action: global and regional changes in the biosphere over the past 300 years,* Cambridge, Eng, 1990, Cambridge University Press, p 1.
23. Lake RW: Rethinking NIMBY, *J Am Planning Assoc* 87:97, 1993.
24. Machlis GA, Ticknell TL: *The state of the world's parks: an international assessment of resource management, policy, and research,* Boulder, Colo, 1985, Westview Press.
25. Mahlman JD: Global change: a looming Arctic ozone hole, *Nature* 360(6401):209, 1992.
26. Marsh GP: *Man and nature; or the earth as modified by human action.* (orig. 1864), Cambridge, 1965, Belknap Press of Harvard University

Press. Thomas Jr WL: *Man's role in changing the face of the earth,* Chicago, 1956, University of Chicago Press.

27. Mintzer IM, editor: *Confronting climate change,* New York, 1991, Cambridge University Press.
28. Mitchell JK, Ericksen NJ: Effects of climate change on weather-related disasters. In Mintzer IM, editor: *Confronting climate change,* New York, 1991, Cambridge University Press, p 141.
29. Mitchell RC, Mertig AG, Dunlap RE: Twenty years of environmental mobilization: trends among national environmental organizations, *Society Nat Resources* 4:219, 1991.
30. Morrisette PM et al: Prospects for a global greenhouse accord: lessons from other agreements, *Glob Environ Change* 1(3):209, 1991; Haas PM: Policy responses to stratospheric ozone depletion, *Glob Environ Change* 1(3):224, 1991.
31. Myers N: *The shrinking ark,* Oxford, Eng, 1980, Pergamon Press.
32. National Academy of Sciences: *Conversion of tropical moist forests,* Washington, DC, 1980, National Academy Press.
33. *New York Times,* July 7, 1991.
34. *New York Times,* July 14, 1992.
35. *New York Times,* December 12, 1992.
36. *New York Times,* December 29, 1992.
37. *New York Times,* March 28, 1993.
38. *New York Times,* April 30, 1993.
39. Pernetta JC: Impacts of climate change and sea level rise on small island states: national and international responses, *Glob Environ Change* 2(1):19, 1992.
40. Pitari G, Viscunti G, Verdecchia M: Global ozone depletion and the Antarctic ozone hole, *J Geophys Res* 97(8):8075, 1992.
41. Pittock AB et al: *Environmental consequences of nuclear war,* SCOPE 28, New York, 1986, Wiley.
42. Platt RH: *Land use control: geography, law, and public policy,* Englewood Cliffs, NJ, 1991, Prentice-Hall.
43. Raup H: View from John Saunderson's farm: a perspective for the use of the land, *Forest History* 10(1):1, 1966; Merchant C: *Ecological revolutions: nature, gender, and science in New England,* Chapel Hill, 1989, University of North Carolina Press.
44. Raven PH: We're killing our world, Keynote address, Feb 14, 1986, Chicago, American Association for the Advancement of Science.
45. Reid WV, Miller KR: *Keeping options alive: the scientific basis for conserving biodiversity,* Washington, DC 1989, World Resources Institute.
46. Richards JF: Land transformation. In Turner BL II et al, editors: *The earth as transformed by human action: global and regional changes in the biosphere over the last 300 years,* Cambridge, Eng, 1990, Cambridge University Press, p 163.
47. Rosenfield PL, Bower B: Management strategies for mitigating adverse impacts of water development projects, *Prog Water Technol* 11(1-2):285, 1979.
48. Shiva V: *Staying alive: women, ecology, and development,* Atlantic Highlands, NJ, 1988, Zed Books.
49. Smith NJH et al: Environmental impacts of resource exploitation in Amazonia, *Glob Environ Change* 1(4):313, 1991.
50. Smith SV, Buddemeier RW: Global change and coral reef ecosystems, *Annu Rev Ecol Systemetics* 23:89, 1992.
51. Solbrig OT: The origin and function of biodiversity, *Environment* 33(5):16-20, 1991.
52. Stonehouse B, editor: *Arctic air pollution,* New York, 1986, Cambridge University Press; Soroos MS: The odyssey of Arctic haze: toward a global atmospheric regime, *Environment* 34(10):6, 1992.
53. Turner BL II et al, editors: *The earth as transformed by human action: global and regional changes in the biosphere over the past 300 years,* Cambridge, Eng, 1990, Cambridge University Press.
54. United Nations: *World demographic estimates and projections,* New York, 1988.
55. Wilkinson CR: Coral reefs are facing widespread extinctions: can we prevent these through sustainable management practices? Address at International Symposium on Coral Reefs, Guam, 1992.
56. Wood WB: Tropical deforestation: balancing regional development demands and global environmental concerns, *Glob Environ Change* 1(1):23, 1990.

28 NORTH AMERICAN VENOMOUS REPTILE BITES

John B. Sullivan, Jr.
Willis A. Wingert
Robert L. Norris, Jr.

Animal venom poisoning differs from chemical poisoning because of the complex nature and activity of proteins in venom. An industrial chemical may exert a pharmacologic action on only one or two organ systems, but venom contains many enzymes and proteins that can simultaneously damage local tissues, blood vessels, cellular blood elements, and myoneural junctions. The multiple components in venom may act independently or synergistically. Pathophysiologic sequelae may range from simple local edema and pain to massive tissue edema, hypotension, coagulopathy, and shock. The physician confronted with an envenomed patient must be prepared not only to administer antivenin but also to counter many physiologic dysfunctions involving circulation, respiration, and coagulation.

Snakes inhabit terrain from elevations below sea level to above timberline. Most snakes prefer the ground, but some climb trees or swim. Although the natural habitat of all venomous reptiles is in sparsely inhabited areas such as deserts and swamps, no clinician dealing with emergencies is exempt from treating envenomation, even in a large urban emergency department. City dwellers in increasing numbers venture into the reptiles' habitats for recreation or to collect these animals for display in their homes or as pets. Furthermore, foreign or exotic snakes are brought into the United States in relatively large numbers, either legally or by smuggling, and are maintained by private individuals in "underground" zoos. Collectors of these often brightly colored and attractive reptiles sometimes mistake venomous for nonvenomous species and may handle the animals carelessly. The venomous coral snake, for example, has many mimics.

Complicating the problem of envenomation is the application of ill-advised, empirical, and sometimes mutilating therapy, much of which has no pharmacologic or scientific basis and, indeed, may be based on folklore. Examples are traditional internal use of alcohol ("snakebite medicine"), wide surgical incisions of bitten extremities, injudicious and wrong application of tourniquets, and use of cryotherapy, which imposes frostbite on already damaged tissues. Envenomation should be approached as scientifically as other poisonings:

1. Make the diagnosis.
2. Determine the severity of poisoning.
3. Monitor vital signs and support blood pressure and respirations as necessary.
4. Neutralize the poison as completely as possible with specific antivenin when appropriate.
5. Monitor the patient for worsening of envenomation and need for further antivenin.
6. Restore functional joint patterns with appropriate wound care and physiotherapy.

Epidemiologic Aspects of Snake Venom Poisoning

Statistics reported by the American Association of Poison Control Centers (AAPCC) listed 3425 bites from all indigenous U.S. snakes, (venomous and nonvenomous) in 1990, 4033 bites in 1991, and 4675 in 1992.[41-43] Of a total of 12,133 bites reported by the participating centers, there were no deaths in 1990, one death in 1991, and one in 1992. These statistics reflect the low mortality associated with snake venom poisoning in the United States. The incidence of morbidity following bites in this country is unknown but probably quite high.[22] There is a reported incidence of 3.74 bites per 100,000 population.[74] Nineteen species of poisonous snakes account for these bites (Table 28-1).

The two main families of venomous snakes indigenous to the United States are Crotalidae (pit vipers) and Elapidae (coral snakes). Of the Crotalidae, three genera inhabit the United States: *Crotalus* and *Sistrurus,* or rattlesnakes, which include 15 species (Color Plates 15, 16, and 17), and *Agkistrodon,* which includes the cottonmouth (water) moccasin *(A. piscivorus)* and the copperhead *(A. contortrix)* (Color Plates 18 and 19). The Elapidae, or coral snakes (genera *Micrurus* and *Micruroides*), are limited geographically to the southern and southwestern states and account for only 20 to 25 human bites each year, less than 0.5% of all envenomations (Color Plates 20 and 21).[67]

The highest bite rates are found in southern states: North Carolina (18.79:100,000 population per year), Arkansas (17.23), Texas (14.70), Mississippi (10.83), and Louisiana (10.25). The southwestern desert states also have a respectable incidence: Arizona (7.83) and New Mexico (7.54).[66]

About 90% of envenomations occur between April and October, as may be expected, since snakes are poikilothermic and more active in warm months of the year.[58] One half of bites occur from 2 to 9 PM.[66,99] The incidence is much higher in males (9:1).[99] Young adults (especially males) have a higher incidence of envenomation, and 50% of all bites occur in the age group 18 to 28 years.[67,99] Almost all bites are on the extremities, with 80% on the finger and hand and 15% on the foot and ankle.[99] At least 40% of bites are not accidental; that is, they occur when a poisonous snake is purposely handled. Many bites are associated with alcohol ingestion by the victim.[99]

Crotalidae (Pit Vipers)

ANATOMY, PHYSIOLOGY, AND HABITS OF CROTALIDAE

The majority of snakebites are caused by the Crotalidae family, or pit vipers, so called because of a depression or pit in the maxillary bone. This pit is located midway between and below the level of the eye and the nostril on each side of the head. This organ is believed to be a sensory infrared heat–detecting organ, which enables the snake to locate warm-blooded prey or enemies even in absolute darkness.[66] The pit guides the direction of the strike and possibly determines the amount of venom to be released from the venom gland, according to the size or heat emission of the prey.[7] These thermal receptors are exquisitely sensitive to infrared radiation and can detect changes in temperature of as little as 0.003° C.[52] However, the maximal range of this organ is believed to be only 14 inches.[37] Snakes are deaf to most airborne sounds, since they lack an external ear, and their vision is indistinct with no fovea in the retina.[37] However, their sense of smell is keen. The major stimuli in the form of volatile chemical substances are brought to the smell detection organs by the protruding forked tongue. Snakes are very sensitive to ground-conducted vibrations, probably by conduction through the stapes of the middle ear.[37]

Rattlesnakes, like most reptiles, are relatively inactive animals compared with mammals. Snakes generally do not travel long distances in search of prey and cannot sustain maximal physical activity for a prolonged period. Muscular energy is limited by a single functional lung and a three-chambered heart with a pulmonary shunt resulting from an incomplete ventricular septum. Therefore blood in the dorsal aorta has a reduced oxygen content; oxygenation of peripheral tissue and augmentation of blood pressure are limited.[37] In addition, snake skin lacks integumentary glands with which to eliminate excess body heat produced by excessive muscular activity. The rattlesnake's top speed of travel is 3 mph, equivalent to a human's moderate walking pace.

Snakes lack internal means of regulating body temperature. Thus environmental temperature variations influence their activity. Snakes become immobile at temperatures below 8° C and cannot survive for more than 12 minutes at temperatures above 42° C. Their optimal temperature range is 27° to 32° C, which occurs in evenings and at night in southern states and southwestern deserts.[37] Therefore snakes are nocturnal feeders and winter hibernators, the latter usually in rocky dens. Snakes mate in the spring, and in most cases the young are born between August and October. Influenced by temperature and food supply, their maximal growth rate occurs in the first 2 years of life. The life span of some captive snakes has exceeded 30 years.

Venomous snakes are strict carnivores and capable of inflicting a fatal bite at birth. Their food consists largely of small nocturnal mammals, especially rodents, birds and bird eggs, frogs, lizards, and other snakes. The copperhead's diet includes a high proportion of insects.[77] Snakes secure prey by lying coiled and immobile beside animal trails or burrows. Aided by a keen sense of smell and heat receptors, the snake detects and locates a passing mammal. When the prey comes within striking range, which is usually a distance half the length of the snake, the snake opens its mouth wide, erects its fangs, and lunges forward, briefly burying its fangs into the prey to inject a lethal dose of venom. The amount of venom released is based on the snake's estimate of the victim's size.[37] The speed of the strike is extremely rapid, approximately 8 feet per second.[96] The strike is usually directed slightly downward, but rattlesnakes may strike hori-

Table 28-1 Major Venomous Snakes of North America

Area	Common Name	Scientific Name	Usual Habitat and Characteristics
Northeastern states	Cottonmouth	*Agkistrodon piscivoris*	Average adult male length 30-45 inches (maximum 6 feet); semiaquatic: swamps, lakes, sluggish streams; swims and crawls with head raised at an angle of 45 degrees; pugnacious
	Copperhead	*A. contortrix*	Average adult length 24-36 inches (maximum 4 feet); wooded mountains, damp meadows, along old stone walls, near abandoned buildings; may climb bushes and low trees in search of food; usually docile
	Timber rattlesnake	*Crotalus horridus horridus*	Average adult length 36-48 inches (maximum 6 feet); wooded, mountainous areas, usually in second-growth timber; may stray into farmlands in harvest season; basks and hibernates in rocky bluffs and ledges; usually retreats if disturbed
Southeastern states	Cottonmouth	*A. piscivoris*	Lagoons, sluggish waterways; basks by day on logs, stones, or branches near water; when disturbed, vibrates tail and opens mouth wide to reveal white lining
	Copperhead	*A. contortrix*	Frequents both lowland swamps and uplands
	Eastern diamondback rattlesnake	*C. adamanteus*	Average adult length 42-66 inches (maximum 8 feet); low coastal areas, scrub palmetto, low brush, and dry pine woods, often close to water; sometimes found in farmlands; largest and most dangerous rattlesnake in U.S.; usually does not retreat when disturbed
	Canebrake rattlesnake	*C. horridus atricaudatus*	Average adult length 36-48 inches (maximum 6 feet); lowlands, swamps, and cane thickets; related to northern timber rattlesnake; mild mannered
	Pigmy rattlesnake	*Sistrurus miliarius*	Average adult length 15-22 inches (maximum 31 inches); usually found near water: lakes, rivers, floodplains, swamps, and marshes; alert and bad tempered, but rarely inflicts serious bites
	Eastern coral snake	*Micrurus fulvius fulvius*	Average adult length 23-32 inches (maximum 4 feet); grasslands and dry open woods, sometimes along streams or in piles of garden compost; usually docile and seldom bites unless handled; diurnal
Central states	Cottonmouth	*A. piscivoris*	See *A. piscivoris* above
	Copperhead	*A. contortrix*	See *A. contortrix* above
	Massasauga rattlesnake	*S. catenatus*	Average adult length 18-28 inches (maximum 3 feet); prairie regions, dry wooded land, grasslands, in woodpiles and cellars under steps, in hay fields; bogs and marshes in northeastern region; secretive, not usually aggressive, but bites readily if cornered
	Timber rattlesnake	*C. horridus horridus*	Wooded rocky hills, basking on ledges
	Prairie rattlesnake	*C. viridis viridis*	Average adult length 36-48 inches (maximum 5 feet); dry grasslands, rocky hills, on open mountain slopes to 9000 feet; diurnal, but avoids intense light and heat; irritable
	Great Basin rattlesnake	*C. viridis lutosus*	Average adult length 24-35 inches (maximum 4 feet); arid to semiarid rocky areas
Southwestern states	Cottonmouth	*A. piscivoris*	Near water in central and eastern Texas
	Copperhead	*A. contortrix*	Wooded hills in central and eastern Texas
	Pigmy rattlesnake (Color Plate 15)	*S. miliarius*	Grasslands in southeast Arizona; New Mexico to southern Texas
	Massasauga rattlesnake	*S. catenatus*	Prairie lands in Texas and Arizona
	Northern black-tailed rattlesnake	*C. molossus*	Average adult length 36-48 inches (maximum 5 feet); southern regions of southwestern states, extending into Mexico; characteristic solid black tail
	Prairie rattlesnake	*C. viridis viridis*	Dry hills and grasslands
	Sidewinder	*C. cerastes*	Average adult length 18-25 inches (maximum 30 inches); desert areas, sandy flats, sand dunes, arid rocky hillsides; rests with body buried in the sand; has elevated hornlike scale above the eye; not highly irritable
	Mojave rattlesnake	*C. scutulatus scutulatus*	Average adult length 30-40 inches (maximum 4 feet); lowlands, in southeastern Arizona and northern Mexico (desert and arid areas); moderately irritable; highly toxic venom

Table 28-1 Major Venomous Snakes of North America—cont'd

Area	Common Name	Scientific Name	Usual Habitat and Characteristics
	Western diamondback rattlesnake	*C. atrox*	Average adult length 36-66 inches (maximum 7 feet); lowlands and rocky hillsides; diurnal; large, bold, aggressive snake often found in open and cultivated areas and near farm buildings; raises head and loop of neck high above coils in striking
	Red diamondback rattlesnake	*C. ruber ruber*	Average adult length 40-50 inches (maximum 5 feet); similar to western diamondback; hisses loudly when disturbed; less irritable than western diamondback
	Texas coral snake	*Micrurus fulvius tenere*	Average adult length 23-32 inches (maximum 4 feet); see eastern coral snake
	Sonoran coral snake (Color Plate 20)	*Micruroides euryxanthus*	Average adult length 12-16 inches (maximum 20 inches); limited to Arizona and New Mexico; smaller than *M. fulvius;* antivenin not available for this species; no fatalities reported
Pacific	Northern Pacific rattlesnake	*C. viridis oreganus*	Average adult length 36-48 inches (maximum 5 feet); semiarid areas from sea level to 11,000 feet; avoids extremes of heat and moisture; may be found in suburban areas and farmlands; northern California, Washington, and Oregon; highly toxic venom
	Southern Pacific rattlesnake	*C. viridis helleri*	Same as above, except found in southern California
	Great Basin rattlesnake	*C. viridis lutosus*	Arid and semiarid areas in eastern Oregon
	Western diamondback rattlesnake	*C. atrox*	Confined to narrow zone of dry, rocky hills and sandy desert in southwestern California and Baja California; active during the day in cool weather
	Red diamondback rattlesnake	*C. ruber ruber*	See *C. ruber ruber* above
	Sidewinder	*C. cerastes*	See *C. cerastes* above
	Mojave rattlesnake	*C. s. scutulatus*	Mojave Desert area in southern California

zontally or even upward at a 45-degree angle. Although the strike is usually single and from a coiled position, rattlesnakes may strike from almost any position and may strike several times. The strike is more an injection than a bite, so the fragile fangs and jaw articulation are less at risk. The potent venom is designed to immobilize the prey rapidly so that it cannot escape beyond the snake's area of sensory detection (about 20 feet), to prevent a retaliatory struggle that would injure the snake, and to begin digestion of the prey. After the victim is subdued, the snake swallows it head first. This is facilitated by a loose muscular (rather than connective tissue) articulation between the upper and lower jaws, which permits the ingestion of amazingly large prey. However, these articulations have a disadvantageous lack of rigidity and strength, so a large struggling rodent can readily break a rattlesnake's jaw.

IDENTIFYING CHARACTERISTICS OF CROTALIDAE

Four distinguishing characteristics of the Crotalidae are facial pits, vertical elliptical pupils ("cat's eye"), a triangular head distinct from the remainder of the body, and a single row of subcaudal scutes or scales (Fig. 28-1). The genera *Crotalus* and *Sistrurus* are further characterized by rattles, which are interlocking horny segments formed on the tail as the snake periodically sheds its skin during growth (Fig. 28-2). The snake's age in years is not determined by the number of rattles, since molting occurs from one to four times annually, depending on temperature, food, moisture, age, health, and possibly other factors. Rattles are commonly missing as a result of injury. The characteristic buzz occurs when the tail vibrates from 20 to 85 cycles per second, in direct relation to the environmental temperature.[37] *Strikes may occur without a preliminary warning buzz.*

Venom Apparatus

The venom apparatus consists of a gland, duct, and one or more fangs on each side of the head (Fig. 28-3). The venom glands are located at the outer edge of the upper jaw, immediately below the eye, and are analogous to the human parotid glands. Each secretory cell synthesizes all components, both toxic peptides and digestive enzymes.[79] The gland is contracted by an external jaw muscle to discharge the venom. Since these muscles have an innervation separate from that of the biting mechanism, the snake can control the amount of venom to be discharged and injected. This is quantitated by the weight and size of the victim. Therefore discharge is not an all-or-none phenomenon, and pit vipers rarely discharge the full contents at a single bite. High-speed

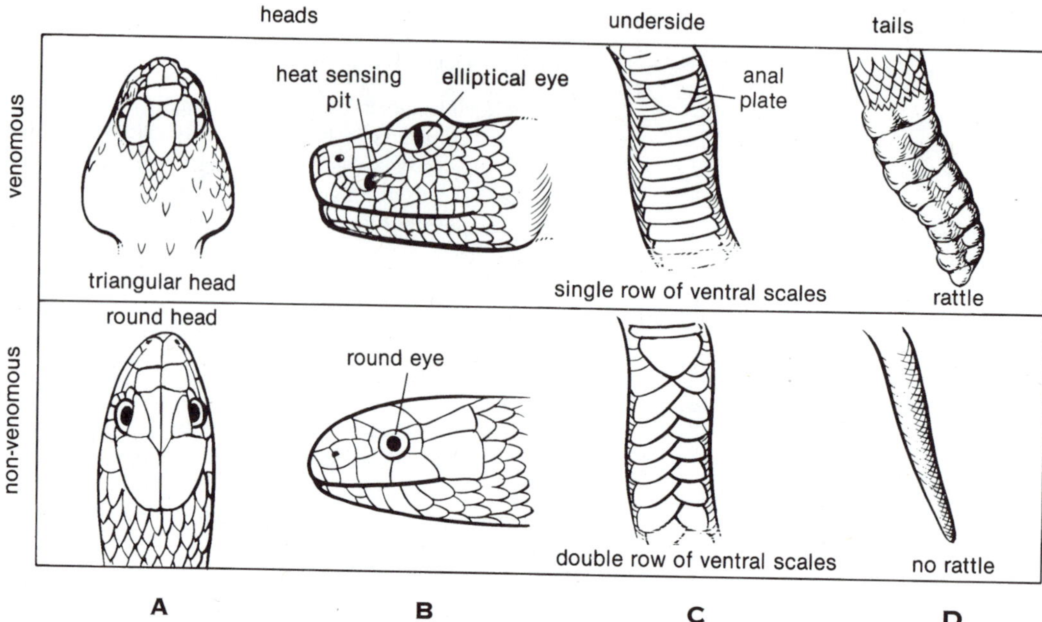

Fig. 28-1 Identification of venomous pit vipers. **A,** Triangular head. **B,** Elliptical eye; heat-sensing facial pits on sides of head near nostrils. **C,** Single row of ventral scales leading up to anal plate. **D,** Rattles on tail (baby rattlesnakes have only "buttons" but are still quite venomous).

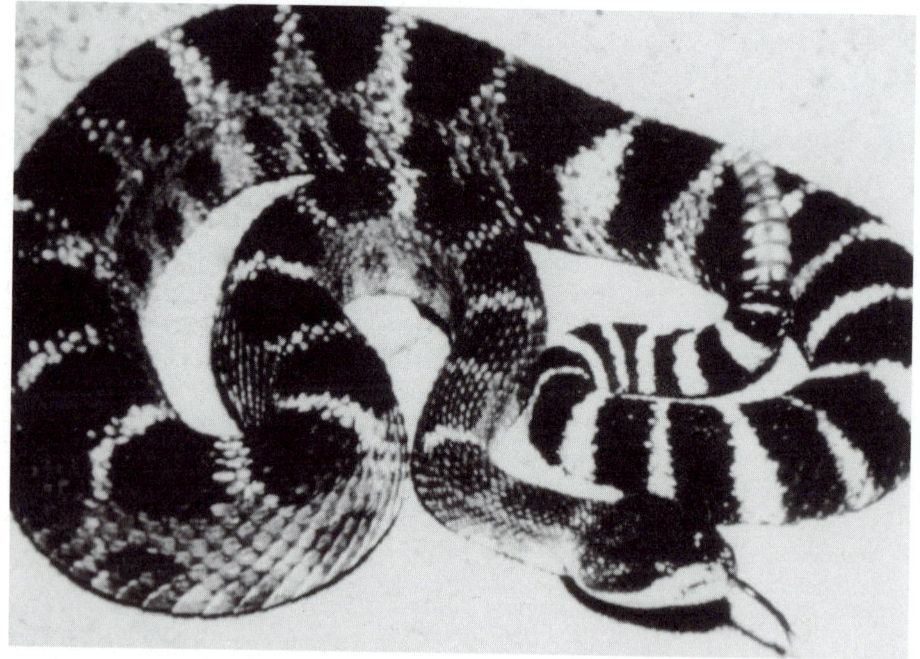

Fig. 28-2 Northern Pacific rattlesnake *Crotalus viridis oreganus.*

sensory feedback in the heat-detecting pit enables the snake to make split-second adjustments in the force and direction of the strike and in the quantity of venom injected. Most rattlesnakes discharge between 25% and 75% of their venom when they bite a human.[77] After discharge, venom is completely replenished in as little as 21 days. Lethal peptides are replenished first, probably as a defense mechanism.[18]

The venom glands are connected by ducts to two elongated hollow upper maxillary teeth or fangs, which have a slitlike opening near the tip. The ducts empty into the fang sheath, which itself contains venom in a small pocket. When not in use, the fangs are folded against the upper jaw, along the roof of the mouth. During the strike the fangs rotate down and forward so that their base is at a right angle to the

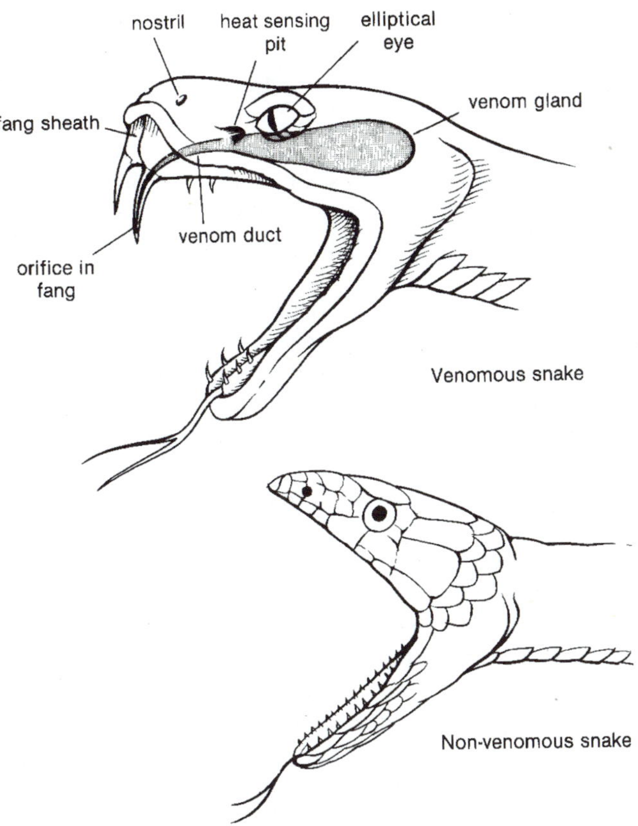

Fig. 28-3 Venom apparatus of a pit viper, consisting of a gland, duct, and one or more fangs on each side of the head.

jaw. In adult snakes the fangs vary from 8 to more than 20 mm in length. Fangs of large snakes may penetrate to the muscles of humans and may perforate rubber or even leather boots.[52] Reserve fangs may move into position before the functional fang is shed. Therefore a victim may demonstrate from one to four fang marks at the site of a single bite.

Venom

Crotalus venom is a complex substance having three functions: immobilization, killing, and digestion of prey. Venom of older snakes appears to be less lethal than that of younger snakes, although the former is present in greater quantity. Venom is a multiple-component poison consisting of proteins and peptides and affects many tissues primarily or secondarily.

Chemically, venom consists of 90% water, 5 to 15 enzymes, 3 to 12 nonenzymatic proteins and peptides, and at least 6 as-yet-unidentified substances. Isoelectric focusing of *Crotalus* venom demonstrates that many different proteins are isolated as stainable protein bands.

The lethal venom components responsible for immediate death of prey are low–molecular weight peptides and polypeptides (20– to 28–amino acid chains, molecular weight 4800 to 100,000).[69] These components have been shown by electron microscopy to damage endothelial cells of vascular walls, to dilate the perinuclear space, to create endothelial blebs, and to lyse the plasma membrane of cells. These insults cause transient microangiopathic vascular permeability to both plasma proteins and erythrocytes,[60] manifested by fluid loss into tissue spaces. This ultimately results in hemoconcentration, lactic acidosis, and hypovolemic shock, followed by death of the prey.

Tissue destruction is both local and diffuse, caused by various enzymes designed by nature to aid in and hasten digestion of prey. The more important enzymes and their actions follow:

1. Proteolytic enzymes or proteases. Trypsinlike action damages muscle and subcutaneous tissues, leading to necrosis.[76]
2. Hyaluronidase. Cleavage of internal glycoside bonds to various acid mucopolysaccharides decreases the viscosity of connective tissue and allows other fractions of venom to spread through involved tissues.
3. Phospholipase A_2. This is an esterolytic enzyme, common to all pit viper venoms, that specifically catalyzes hydrolysis of the ester bond at the C-2 position of lecithin. This action releases a molecule of fatty acid and lysolecithin. The latter substance damages mast cell membranes and provokes histamine release from mast cells. Since red blood cell membranes contain lecithin, the normal permeability of the cell wall may be altered, allowing water to enter the cell without regulation. This may lead to hemolysis. Phospholipase A_2 also causes necrosis of muscle fibers; the enzyme damages the plasma membrane of muscle cells within minutes, disrupts intracellular organelles, and causes an influx of calcium and an efflux of creatine and creatine kinase.[24]
4. L-Amino acid oxidase. This enzyme causes tissue destruction by catalyzing oxidation of amino acids and gives venom its characteristic yellow color.[53]
5. Thrombinlike enzymes and amino acid esterases. These enzymes act as defibrinating anticoagulants, promoting fibrin clot formation by incompletely splitting fibrinopeptide A or B from the fibrinogen molecule. Factor XIII is not activated. The result is formation of an unstable fibrin clot, readily lysed by plasmin and by proteolytic enzymes in the venom. Afibrinogenemia, thrombocytopenia, and an increase in fibrin split products follow.
6. Other enzymes. Other enzymes whose pharmacologic actions have not been fully determined include collagenase, RNAse, DNAse, and arginine ester hydrolase.

Pathophysiologic Effects of Crotalid Venom

The components of venom differ in relative amounts among species of pit vipers. Therefore the pathophysiology and human symptoms from the effects of venom may vary among offending species. For example, subcutaneous hemorrhage is common in bites by eastern diamondback *(Crotalus adamanteus)* and Pacific rattlesnakes *(C. viridis oreganus* and *C. viridis helleri);* edema may be less severe following bites by the Mojave *(C. scutulatus scutulatus),* pigmy *(Sistrurus miliarius),* massasauga *(S. catenatus),* and sidewinder rattlesnakes *(C. cerastes)* in some cases, and far less severe in the copperhead *(Agkistrodon contortrix).*[77]

Because of the multiple protein and peptide biotoxins in crotalid venom, human pathophysiology is diverse and can involve multiple organ systems. Primarily, venom produces local tissue and microvascular damage leading to local tissue necrosis, hemorrhage, and extravasation of intravascular volume. As venom is spread via lymphatics and blood, the damage spreads. The major toxic effects occur within local tissue, blood vessels, and blood components. However, virtually every other organ system is vulnerable, including the central nervous system.

Local Tissue and Microvasculature: Pathophysiology

Pathologic examination of venom-injected muscle reveals hemorrhage, myoedema, interstitial edema, and myonecrosis.[61] Electron microscopy studies of tissues injected with *Crotalus* venom reveal that endothelial cells of the microvasculature swell and rupture, leaving large gaps in these vessels for fluid extravasation.[61] The earliest pathophysiologic changes in the vessel endothelium are dilation of the endoplasmic reticulum and perinuclear space, followed by intracellular bleb formation and cytolysis. As endothelial cells rupture, platelets eventually fill areas left by cytolysis.[61]

Damage to microvascular endothelial cells leads to the interstitial edema so frequently seen in crotalid envenomation syndromes. The proteases, hyaluronidases, and phospholipase A_2 all damage cell membranes. It is of interest to note that this type of endothelial cell damage is seen microscopically in a variety of tissue injury states such as ischemia, and may be a general injury response of endothelial cells.[61]

Intravascular hemolysis is seen after crotalid venom injection and is thought to be the result of phospholipase A_2 actions on erythrocyte membranes, releasing lysolecithin, the causative agent of hemolysis.[61]

Pathophysiologic Effects on the Clotting System

Platelet aggregation occurs at sites of endothelial cell damage in the microvasculature. It has been demonstrated that venom from crotalid species produces platelet aggregation and that this aggregation can be blocked using IgG purified from Wyeth antivenin.[5] The release of adenosine-5-diphosphate (ADP) from platelets may also play a role in local platelet aggregation, since ADP has been shown to induce platelet aggregation.[5]

Pathophysiologic effects on the clotting system can be manifested as true disseminated intravascular coagulation (DIC), a DIC-like syndrome, hypofibrinogenemia with or without thrombocytopenia, or hypofibrinogenemia with or without fibrinolysis.[26] Coagulopathies are commonly seen after crotalid envenomation (Color Plate 22).

Coagulation changes result from the presence of a thrombinlike enzyme in crotalid venom that clots fibrinogen.[3] *Crotalus adamanteus* (eastern diamondback rattlesnake) venom possesses significant thrombinlike enzyme activity. Physiochemical studies on *C. adamanteus* venom confirmed that this procoagulant enzyme, crotalase, is a glycoprotein with a molecular weight of 32,700.[45] This enzyme acts directly on fibrinogen without affecting other blood proteins. Venom from adult *Crotalus atrox* (western diamondback rattlesnake) has strong fibrinolytic activity.[3] Research has shown that adult *C. atrox* venom contains two fibrinolytic enzymes having molecular weights of 60,000 and 21,500.[3] Of clinical interest, the coagulopathy produced by younger *C. atrox* may differ from that caused by the adult snake. Juvenile snakes up to 8 months of age appear to have more fibrinogen clotting activity than do adult snakes.[72]

Venom from adult *C. atrox* can render human plasma and purified fibrinogen incoagulable.[63] Fibrinogen is a dimeric molecule composed of two sets of three different polypeptide chains. The attack on fibrinogen by the fibrinolytic enzymes in *C. atrox* venom appears to preferentially degrade the A_2 chain first and then the Bb chain of purified fibrinogen. However, fibrinogen in human plasma demonstrated only Bb chain cleavage.[63]

Cardiovascular Pathophysiology

Hemostatic changes following crotalid envenomation result from a combination of venom-induced increased vascular permeability and hemorrhage. Venom-induced shock is manifested by a combination of hypotension, lactic acidemia, hemoconcentration, and hypoproteinemia.[84] Low–molecular weight venom peptides infused into animal models produce hypotension, lactic acidosis, and rise in hematocrit.[84] Rattlesnake venom–induced shock is essentially hypovolemia complicated by coagulopathy.[84] Release of histamine, bradykinin, and other vascular amines may also contribute to hypotension and extravascular fluid extravasation.[84]

Muscle and Neuromuscular Pathophysiology

Venom-induced myonecrosis has been studied extensively with *Crotalus viridis viridis* (prairie rattlesnake) venom.[61] Vacuole formation within muscle cells occurs before necrosis. Clinically, myonecrosis is not commonly seen, since venom is usually deposited subcutaneously and not intramuscularly. Studies of the neuromuscular effects of crotalid venom have been confined to venom of *Crotalus scutulatus scutulatus* (Mojave rattlesnake). There is a geographic variation in Mojave rattlesnake venom properties. Envenomation by the Mojave rattlesnake has been depicted as producing predominantly neurotoxic effects with a paucity of local tissue effects. However, this is certainly not the case in clinical envenomation syndromes in Arizona.

Mojave venoms A and B, so named for geographic locations of the snakes, result in different pathophysiologic pictures in humans.[20] Mojave venom A is found in snakes inhabiting California, Utah, and southwestern Arizona. Venom B is localized around the Phoenix region.[20] Venom A appears to be more toxic. Data indicate that venom B produces more local tissue destruction and edema than does venom A.[20] Venom B appears to be higher than venom A in proteolytic activity and in hemorrhagic activity. Venom patterns by gel electrophoresis showed differences in protein between venom A and venom B.[20] Venom A contains Mojave toxin, the neurotoxic protein characteristically producing neuromuscular weakness and paralysis after envenomation. This geographic variation in Mojave rattlesnake venom may explain divergent clinical pictures of envenomation caused by the same snake. Mojave toxin is an acidic protein that consists of a basic phospholipase A_2 and an acidic peptide subunit.[28] This protein has been demonstrated to be neurotoxic, acting at the presynaptic site in the neuromuscular junction.[28] The mode of action of Mojave toxin appears to be similar to that of other presynaptically acting toxins. Mojave toxin has multiple binding and activity sites and multiple pathophysiologic effects, in addition to causing neuromuscular blockade. This is reasonable, since the effects of phospholipases are seen at multiple tissue sites. The pathophysiologic effects of crotalid venom vary from snake to snake even within a single species. In general, the vascular endothelium and the clotting system are the two main targets that when damaged produce the majority of clinical features seen after envenomation. Loss of vascular volume, hemorrhage, and coagulopathy are the major consequences of venom injection into humans, which can result in massive tissue edema, shock, bleeding, and coagulation defects.

BOX 28-1

SIGNS AND SYMPTOMS OF ENVENOMATION IN 227 PATIENTS*

SYMPTOMS	
Weakness	80%
Nausea, vomiting	70%
Paresthesias	73%
Pain	60%
SIGNS	
Fang marks	100%
Swelling	98%
Ecchymoses	27%
Fasciculations	19%
Hypotension	11%
Bullae	6%
Necrosis	4%
LABORATORY ABNORMALITIES	
Fibrinogen	35%
Fibrin split products	39%
Prothrombin time	15%
Proteinuria	9%
Hematuria	8%

*Treated at the Los Angeles County–University of Southern California Medical Center, 1975-1985.

CROTALIDAE CLINICAL ENVENOMATION SYNDROMES

Clinical envenomation syndromes vary with the amount of venom deposited and the protein content of venom. Estimates are that nonenvenomed bites occur in 22% of victims.[77]

Signs and symptoms (Box 28-1) depend on a number of factors. As previously noted, pit vipers rarely discharge the full contents of their venom glands at a single bite. Although the heat-detecting pit organ is believed to regulate the amount of venom discharged according to the size of the prey, these heat receptors seem to be confused by the large amount of heat radiated by a human. Consequently, on any given strike, the amount of venom released may vary from little or none to almost the entire content of the glands. Of 225 patients referred to the University of Southern California, 2% were not envenomed, 26% were mildly envenomed with minimal signs and symptoms, 61% received moderate envenomations, and 11% had severe symptoms.[99] However, nonenvenomed patients are unlikely to require referral, which may have skewed the data.

Other important factors determining the amount of venom released include the age, size, and species of snake (Table 28-2). As noted in Table 28-2, the venom glands of the eastern diamondback *(Crotalus adamanteus)* contain a large amount of very potent venom, compared with that contained in the sidewinder *(C. cerastes)* or the copperhead *(Agkistrodon contortrix)*. Pit vipers are venomous at birth, but their glands do not contain as much venom as the glands of the adult. The age, size, and health of the victim, along with the nature, location, depth, and number of bites and the length of time the snake attaches, determine the severity of envenomation and must be considered in the management of poisoning. Finally, clothing and shoes may decrease fang penetration or totally deflect the strike.

Crotalid envenomation is characterized by the presence of one or more fang marks, pain, and some edema at the bite site. Pain and edema are initially localized to the area immediately surrounding the bite site and occur within minutes after envenomation. If venom is injected near a blood vessel or intravenously, moderate to severe symptoms can begin rapidly. Hypotension and shock have occurred quickly after intravenous deposition of venom.[84] The distance between

Table 28-2 Comparative Toxicity of Snake Venoms

Species	Average Length of Adult (Inches)	Approximate Yield, Dry Venom (mg)	Intraperitoneal LD_{50} Mice (mg/kg)	Intravenous LD_{50} Mice (mg/kg)
RATTLESNAKES (CROTALUS)				
Eastern diamondback *(C. adamanteus)*	32-65	300-700	1.89	1.68
Western diamondback *(C. atrox)*	30-65	175-320	3.71	4.20
Prairie *(C. viridis viridis)*	32-46	35-100	2.25	1.61
Southern Pacific *(C. viridis helleri)*	32-48	75-150	1.60	1.29
Mojave *(C. s. scutulatus)*	22-40	50-90	0.23	0.21
Sidewinder *(C. cerastes)*	18-30	18-40	4.00	—
MOCCASINS (AGKISTRODON)				
Cottonmouth *(A. piscivorus)*	30-50	90-145	5.11	4.00
Copperhead *(A. contortrix)*	24-36	40-70	10.50	10.92
CORAL SNAKES (MICRURUS)				
Eastern coral *(M. fulvius)*	16-28	2-6	0.97	—

Modified from Russell FE, Puffer HW: *Clin Toxicol* 3:433, 1970.

fang marks varies from 0.5 to 4.0 cm, and the depth of the puncture wounds can be from 1 to 8 mm.[77] Because of the superficial nature of most bites, venom is deposited into subcutaneous tissues, and rarely subfascially or into muscles.

Almost immediately after the bite, most victims experience local burning pain, which usually is not severe. Progressive local swelling appears within 5 minutes. Without treatment, edema may progress rapidly and involve an entire injured extremity within 1 hour if envenomation is severe. Generally, however, edema spreads more slowly over a period of 6 to 12 hours. This edema is soft, pitting, and limited to subcutaneous tissues (Fig. 28-4). The envenomation syndrome is a spectrum ranging from mild edema with localized pain to edema and ecchymosis involving an entire extremity, accompanied by coagulopathy. In addition, severe envenomation can involve hypotension, shock, and coma along with coagulopathy (see Box 28-1). Ecchymosis caused by destruction of blood vessels and red blood cells may occur within several hours (Fig. 28-5) (Color Plate 23). Hemorrhagic blebs and bullae develop at the site of the bite within 6 to 36 hours and may progress proximally along the involved extremity (Figs. 28-6 and 28-7).

Paresthesias of the scalp, face, and lips, along with periorbital muscle fasciculations, indicate that a significant envenomation has occurred. Some patients complain of a metallic taste in the mouth. General symptoms include weakness, sweating, nausea, and faintness.

Venom proteins are carried by the lymphatics; therefore lymphangitis and lymphadenopathy are common. Hemorrhage may occur throughout the body as soon as 6 hours after envenomation. Hemorrhage can be manifested as skin petechiae, epistaxis, hematemesis, melena, hemoptysis, and blindness. If no treatment is administered, hypovolemic shock and pulmonary edema may develop. The bites of some Mojave rattlesnakes may produce neuromuscular blockade leading to respiratory paralysis. Paralysis initially appears as cranial nerve deficits (hoarseness, difficulty swallowing, and ptosis) and progresses to the diaphragm. Bites

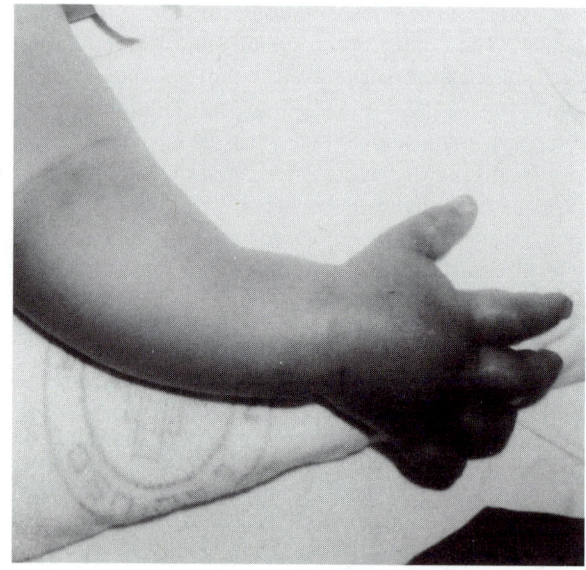

Fig. 28-4 Moderate rattlesnake envenomation in an 18-month-old boy 12 hours after bite, showing fang mark and fang scratch on wrist with ecchymosis and edema of extremity to axilla. The patient required 25 vials of antivenin.

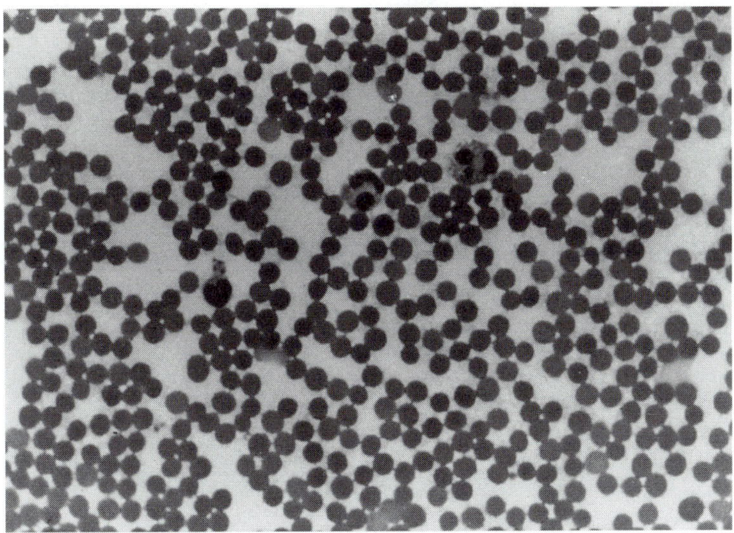

Fig. 28-5 Red blood cell destruction caused by pit viper venom. Swelling and pyknocytosis can be seen 12 hours after the bite.

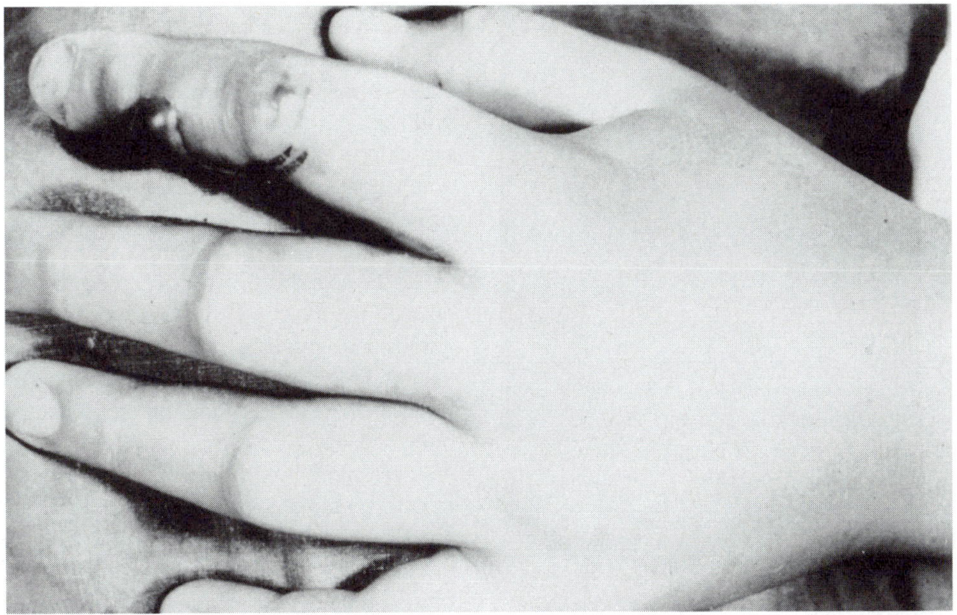

Fig. 28-6 Mild rattlesnake envenomation, left index finger, 4 hours after bite. Note hemorrhagic bleb at the site of the bite, subcutaneous hemorrhage, and swelling of the hand. All laboratory values were within normal range.

from the southern Pacific rattlesnake *(Crotalus viridis helleri)* have been known to produce intense muscle fasciculations leading to difficulty breathing. This can be corrected with antivenin administration.

MANAGEMENT OF CROTALID ENVENOMATION

Snake venom poisoning is a medical emergency. Treatment should reduce venom effects, minimize tissue damage, prevent complicated sequelae, and maintain vital signs.

Management is guided by the severity of envenomation. Envenomation grading systems are of value in deciding how much antivenin to administer. The easiest and most clinically applicable system indicates grades of mild, moderate, or severe (see Box 28-2).

It is of great importance to remember that the envenomation grade can change over time. Initially diagnosed mild envenomation can become severe in a few hours. Venom,

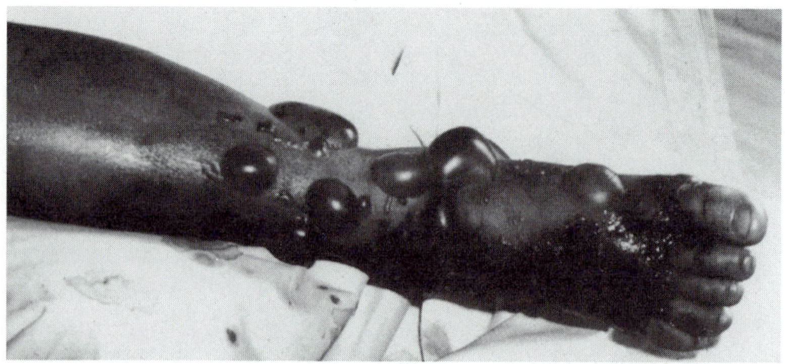

Fig. 28-7 Hemorrhagic blebs and edema 24 hours after rattlesnake bite in dorsum of right foot. The patient recovered with tissue loss at the site of the bite, requiring a small graft. Platelet count, prothrombin time, and hematocrit were abnormal.

BOX 28-2

DEGREES OF CROTALID ENVENOMATION

No envenomation: fang marks, but no local or systemic reactions

Minimal envenomation: fang marks, local swelling and pain, but no systemic reactions

Moderate envenomation: fang marks and swelling progress beyond the site of the bite; systemic signs and symptoms, such as nausea, vomiting, paresthesias, or orthostatic changes; laboratory abnormalities such as hemoconcentration, and mild coagulation parameter changes

Severe envenomation: fang marks present with marked swelling of the extremity, subcutaneous ecchymosis, severe symptoms, and marked coagulopathy with thrombocytopenia, hypofibrinogenemia, prolonged prothrombin and partial thromboplastin times, increased fibrin split products, increased creatine phosphokinase, proteinuria, and hematuria.

like any drug or toxin, has pharmacokinetic parameters of absorption from sites of deposition, distribution into tissues, and elimination from the body.

Pitfalls and errors in diagnosis and management of clinical envenomation syndromes can be avoided (see Box 28-3).

Prehospital Management

Many historically recommended first aid measures for snakebite have never been proved valuable in controlled studies. Such procedures as incision and suction or application of tourniquets and tight constriction bands complicate management by creating devitalized tissue or secondarily infected wounds. Only the following prehospital procedures are necessary.

1. Avoid panic. Excitement and hysteria result in nausea, faintness, dizziness, hyperventilation, and other stress reactions that obscure differentiation of bites between poisonous and nonpoisonous snakes.

The victim should retreat out of the snake's striking range, which is approximately the length of the snake. Since snakes are defensive animals and rarely actually attack, they will remain immobile or attempt to retreat if given the opportunity. Second bites occur primarily in small children who are paralyzed with fright within 2 or 3 feet of the snake or in individuals who persist in harassing the snake in spite of the first bite.

If the snake is killed, it can be transported to the hospital with the patient. However, killing the snake can be dangerous and produce another bitten victim. It is not absolutely necessary to identify the snake to treat the bite appropriately. Identification of the snake species is helpful only because of the variation in venom toxicity among species; more toxic venom increases the amount of antivenin required to treat a bite. If it is known that only a single species of snake inhabits a given geographic area, procuring the snake is not necessary. Most snakes have a limited range of activity and can be found within 20 feet of the site of the accident, even after several hours. If the snake is killed, it should not be directly handled, but should be transported in a closed container to the hospital where a herpetologist or other trained person can identify it. The dead snake can be collected using a stick that is longer than the snake. Decapitated head reactions persist for 20 to 60 minutes, and the severed head of a snake can envenom a person.[33]

2. Immobilize the bitten extremity. This is performed by splinting as if for a fracture. Experiments with crotalid venom in rabbits and with elapid venom in monkeys indicate that local tissue necrosis is diminished by immobilization and that systemic absorption of elapid venom is delayed.[80,92] For the same reason, the victim should reduce physical activity to a minimum.

BOX 28-3

ERRORS IN DIAGNOSIS AND TREATMENT OF CROTALID ENVENOMATION

Not considering snake venom poisoning in the case of an edematous, ecchymotic extremity in a child who was playing in an area where snakes may be found
Not looking for fang marks at the site of pain
Not considering that envenomation grade can change with time and thus that the clinical status of the patient may worsen over a period of time
Attempting to support the blood pressure with vasopressor drugs without adequate volume resuscitation
Not checking initial coagulation studies and repeating these at a later time (within 12 hours)
Not considering the diagnosis of envenomation because a snake was not seen
Delaying antivenin administration to perform a skin test in a severely envenomed patient
Not administering antivenin early in the envenomation course with the presence of progressive signs and symptoms
Not administering adequate amounts of antivenin
Not having epinephrine immediately available at the bedside during antivenin administration
Failing to premedicate patients with antihistamines and expanding intravascular volume (when safe to do so) before beginning antivenin
Not considering administration of broad-spectrum prophylactic antibiotics
Not realizing that antivenin can successfully reverse coagulopathy more than 24 hours after envenomation
Leaving a constriction band or tourniquet on an extremity for a prolonged period
Not skin testing appropriately; that is, not administering the proper dose of horse serum intradermally
Skin testing with horse serum when there is no intention to administer antivenin
Performing a fasciotomy without measured substantial elevation in intracompartmental pressure

3. Obtain medical assistance. The victim should be transported to the nearest medical facility, either on an improvised stretcher or by ambulance if circumstances permit (many bites occur in urban areas, often in the patient's home or garage). If the victim is alone, he or she should walk slowly, resting periodically and using a makeshift crutch if the lower extremity is involved, until help is reached. Again, activity should be kept to a minimum.

Evacuation of a victim depends on the number of rescuers available, the ruggedness of the terrain, and transportation facilities available in the area. If the evacuation involves many hours of hiking over rugged terrain, good judgment may dictate that the victim remain in an area easily identifiable from the air while a companion hikes out of the wilderness to obtain helicopter evacuation. If the victim is many hours from medical care, such as backpacking in a wilderness area, or if severe symptoms develop rapidly, the victim should be placed at rest and activity kept to a minimum. The bitten extremity should be immobilized by splinting. To maintain renal flow and to attempt to control intravascular volume, the victim should drink as much of any available fluid as possible, preferably at least 2 L in 24 hours, in frequent small amounts unless vomiting is a problem.

Other First Aid Measures

In 1979, a technique involving an elastic bandage pressure wrap was approved for use in Australia as an effective first aid measure for elapid bites. This pressure-immobilization technique has been studied using the venoms of Australian snakes, cobras, and one North American pit viper.[91-93] The technique involves applying a broad elastic bandage over the bite site as soon as possible after a bite (see Fig. 29-2). The bitten extremity is kept still and clothes are left on while the bandage is applied. The bandage is started over the bite site and wrapped proximally until the entire extremity is wrapped as tightly as one would strap a sprained ankle. The extremity is then immobilized with a splint. The efficacy of pressure-immobilization depends on collapsing small, superficial lymphatic and venous vessels to retard venom uptake and distribution. The technique has been demonstrated to significantly delay the onset of symptoms in humans bitten by Australian elapids.[4,9,57,71] Possible disadvantages of this method include increased local tissue damage in crotalid bites because of the necrotizing effect of crotalid venom if it remains localized to certain sites over time. Australian snake venom has little or no necrotizing effect.

In animal studies using *Crotalus adamanteus* (eastern diamondback rattlesnake) venom, the systemic absorption of venom was minimized by the pressure-immobilization method as compared with controls.[91] However, when the pressure wrap was removed, massive edema, discoloration, and ecchymosis rapidly developed in the envenomed extremity and sudden abnormal elevations in prothrombin time and partial thromboplastin time occurred.[91] Further research is necessary before this technique can be recommended routinely for pit viper envenomations.

Electric shock therapy can be dangerous to patients and has no proven value in managing bites by pit vipers.[1,91] The use of electric shock therapy arose from a report in the United States of a farmer who used high-voltage, low-amperage, direct current to treat bee stings. Soon afterward, this technique was used to manage snake venom poisonings in Ecuador. In the 34 cases reported, humans bitten by Ecuadorian venomous snakes responded favorably to electric shock applied to the wound.[23] Up to five shocks by a direct current of 20 to 25 kV, 1 mA, applied to the bite site within 30 to 120 minutes after 36 individual bites, resulted either in no development of expected symptoms or in cessation of progression of symptoms already present.[19] The biologic basis of this treatment is unknown, the species of snakes (with two exceptions) were not stated, and there is a high incidence (78%) of protective antibodies to snake venoms in Ecuadorian tribesmen.[45] The technique is being challenged by animal experimentation. In animal studies, there appears to be no increase in survival or improvement in morbidity with the use of electroshock therapy.[13,29,34,88]

The classic recommendations to apply a tourniquet, to incise and suck the wound, or both have become highly controversial. Tourniquets and constricting bands can interfere with estimation of severity of envenomation and lead to underestimation of the quantity of antivenin required.[99] No valid evidence has shown that constriction bands influence the outcome of envenomation in humans, although animal research suggests a beneficial effect of a lymphoocclusive constriction band.[8] Incision and suction appear to have originated in the Hindu system of medicine, *Ayurveda,* between 1000 and 600 BC. The procedure, including placement of a tourniquet above the wound and local cautery, was described by the Hindu physician Sushruta,[44] and except for cautery, differs little from traditional twentieth-century recommendations. McCullough and Gennaro[48] found that suction removed over 50% of radioisotope-labeled venom injected into canine subcutaneous tissue if the suction was instituted within 3 minutes of injection. These data have never been verified in humans, nor has a clear improvement been demonstrated in survival of experimental animals after this technique.[87] Data from Los Angeles County–University of Southern California Medical Center (LAC-USCMC) compared 147 victims who received first aid with 78 who received none, and found no significant difference in severity of the bite; the grade of envenomation was not related to the use of first aid.[99] Animal studies using a negative-pressure suction device called "The Extractor" (Sawyer Products, Safety Harbor, Fla.), have demonstrated removal of up to 30% of crotalid venom proteins if used within 3 minutes after a bite.[6] The device comes with four different-size suction cups, which attach to the barrel of the supplied syringe. After the appropriate-size cup is attached to cover the entire bite site, the plunger of the syringe is pulled out to its full length. The cup and syringe unit is then applied over the bite site and the plunger pushed all the way down. This creates negative pressure over the bite site. Serosanguineous fluid and venom may be seen extruding from fang marks. The suction device should be applied within 3 minutes of the bite and should be left in place for 30 minutes for maximum effectiveness. Because of the high negative pressure (nearly 1 atm) obtained with this device, an incision over the bite site is not required. Currently The Extractor is undergoing clinical trials in human envenomation cases. Since no incision is necessary, the device may be superior to incision and suction because it does not introduce bacteria into the wound.

Cryotherapy is not recommended, since it may be significantly detrimental to envenomed tissues. Experimental evidence has failed to demonstrate any beneficial effects on morbidity or mortality. Freezing or vasoconstricting already compromised tissues may contribute to necrosis. No well-controlled in vitro data or prospective human observations support the contention that low temperatures induced by cooling diminish envenomation. Although the hypothesis that snake venom enzyme activity diminishes with tissue cooling is attractive, it remains to be confirmed.

The use of antivenin in the field is unwise. Backpacking the extensive equipment and drugs necessary to administer intravenous antivenin, especially when the *minimum* recommended dose is five vials,[99] would be cumbersome. The risk of a severe anaphylactic reaction to horse serum without adequate available treatment, such as endotracheal intubation, oxygen, and epinephrine or dopamine, outweighs the potential benefits of field administration of antivenin. This critical treatment should be applied by a knowledgeable professional in a setting suitable for intensive monitoring and resuscitation. Most bites are not severe, the victim rarely dies in the first 24 hours, and medical evacuation systems have improved greatly to decrease transport times.

Emergency Department and Hospital Management

The majority of pit viper envenomations result in morbidity related to tissue edema and coagulopathy. Rarely does death occur from envenomation, and when it does, it usually results from an intravenous bolus of venom, delayed diagnosis and treatment, or mismanagement of the envenomation syndrome. Treatment of envenomation in a medical facility involves the following sequence of events, which depend on the presenting condition of the patient.[100]

Establishing a Physiologic Baseline

1. Perform a rapid evaluation of presenting signs and symptoms. Inquire about the time of the envenomation, the first aid applied, a previous history of snakebite treatment, and any known allergies, especially sensitivity to horse serum and antibiotics. Ask the patient about tingling or numbness around the mouth and scalp. Record vital signs carefully. Establish at least one intravenous line in the unbitten extremity if evidence of envenomation is present. If volume replacement is necessary, the initial fluid of choice is a crystalloid such as normal saline or Ringer's lactate. If the patient is hypotensive and fails to respond to the infusion of 1 to 2 L of saline (20 to 40 ml/kg in a child), the resuscitation fluid should be changed to albumin. Animal research suggests that this compound stays inside the leaky vasculature longer and results in improved survival when used as an adjunct to crystalloids.[83]

2. Inquire about current medications. Note if the patient is taking β-adrenergic receptor blocking agents, because these can potentiate some effects of anaphylaxis and diminish its recognition.[32]
3. Attempt to identify the species of the offending snake, if possible with the aid of a herpetologist.[69] Time usually permits at least venomous and nonvenomous species to be differentiated. If expert consultation is not available, observe the size of the snake; large snakes potentially cause more serious bites because they have a larger quantity of toxic venom in the venom glands.
4. Draw blood for complete blood count and differential, peripheral blood smear (note erythrocyte spherocytosis or pyknocytosis), platelet count, fibrinogen, prothrombin time, partial thromboplastin time, and fibrin split products. Obtain a sample as soon as possible for initial blood typing and screening, and if envenomation is estimated to be moderate or severe, have several units of blood set aside for the patient. Circulating venom and antivenin may interfere with the proper type and cross-match of blood products. Obtain electrolytes, blood urea nitrogen, creatinine, creatine phosphokinase (a marker for muscle necrosis), and urinalysis (note hematuria or proteinuria).
5. Measure and record the circumference of the injured extremity at the level of edema and approximately 4 inches proximal to this level. Recheck every 15 minutes until progression has ceased, and then monitor hourly for 24 hours.
6. Determine the severity of envenomation and need for antivenin. Grading the severity of envenomation helps determine the amount of antivenin to be administered or if antivenin is required at all. Severity of poisoning depends on a number of variables: genus, species, and size of the snake; size of the patient; amount of venom injected; consequent activity of the patient; and type of first aid rendered. Larger snakes generally have more venom in their venom glands. However, the venom of a small *C. atrox* (western diamondback rattlesnake) can carry extremely potent fibrinogen clotting activity. At this time, there is no widely available clinically applicable test to determine toxic concentrations of venom either in tissue or in serum. An enzyme-linked immunosorbent assay (ELISA) for detecting North American pit viper venom in concentrations of 10 to 100 ng/ml has been developed.[55] ELISA provides a sensitive method for detecting snake venom in tissues and biologic fluids within 60 minutes.[55] The reagents for ELISA are inexpensive, and testing can be carried out by a clinical laboratory. However, current use of ELISA for detecting venom is limited to forensic cases and to validate diagnosis of crotalid venom poisoning after treatment. For now, clinical signs and symptoms must be used to estimate severity of poisoning.
7. If the treating physician is unfamiliar with managing snake venom poisoning, consultation with a regional poison center is strongly recommended. Regional poison centers approved by the AAPCC provide physician clinical toxicology consultation 24 hours a day. All AAPCC-approved regional centers follow similar medical standards in managing envenomations and can provide the expertise necessary to manage the patient appropriately.

At LAC-USCMC, the University of Arizona Health Sciences Center, and Stanford University Medical Center, a simple grading system is used based on local and systemic effects of venom (see Box 28-2).

If signs and symptoms of envenomation do not develop within 6 hours of observation, all vital signs remain within normal limits, and laboratory coagulation profiles remain normal, the patient can be discharged from the emergency department and rechecked within 12 to 24 hours. Signs and symptoms may rarely develop later than 6 hours after a bite that was originally asymptomatic.[30] All wounds should be cleaned and the patient instructed to observe for wound infection (see "Antibiotics and Wound Care in Snakebite"). Tetanus immunization should be made current with tetanus toxoid if 5 years has elapsed since the last immunization.

If any signs of venom poisoning exist, the patient should be admitted to the hospital and the need for antivenin assessed.

Determining the Need for Antivenin. Antivenin is the mainstay of therapy for snake venom poisoning. Antivenin efficacy resides in high-affinity antibody, which binds to venom proteins with the objective of enhancing venom elimination.

Commercial antivenin has been available for crotalid envenomation syndromes in the United States since 1947. It has been established that venoms of four pit viper species *(Crotalus atrox, Crotalus adamanteus, Bothrops atrox,* and *Crotalus durissus terrificus)* contain antigens that are sufficiently cross reactive to provide a reliable common immunogen source for hyperimmunizing horses.[77] Horses were chosen for production of hyperimmune serum because of their size and the ease of obtaining a large volume of antiserum. Hyperimmune serum is produced by gradually immunizing horses with mixtures of the four venoms plus an adjuvant to stimulate the immune system. Currently 28 laboratories in 23 countries produce antivenin commercially, and all of these antivenins are of equine source.[7] Wyeth Laboratories' production of polyvalent Crotalidae antivenin involves ammonium sulfate fractionation of hyperimmune serum. This procedure concentrates antibodies as well as other proteins. The final product is a sterile vial of equine polyvalent antivenin, containing approximately 1 g of lyophilized protein.

The Wyeth polyvalent antivenin is standardized by its ability to neutralize the toxicity of a specific quantity of venom injected intravenously into mice and is effective in envenomation by any North, Central, or South American pit viper. Wyeth also manufactures a commercial antiserum against venom of the eastern coral snake *(Micrurus fulvius).* This antivenin is *not* effective for bites of the Arizona coral snake *(Micruroides euryxanthus),* whose venom is less toxic than that of its eastern relative.

The poor quality of most antivenins has been recognized since 1969.[12] Multiple production and manufacturing processes and the differing efficacies of testing procedures have caused purity and antibody concentration of antivenin products to vary. Antivenins from all producers still contain a variety of heterologous proteins that produce adverse effects in human beings. These proteins include equine albumin, β_1 and β_2 globulins, α_1 and α_2 globulins, and IgG_1 and IgM (Box 28-4 and Fig. 28-8).

In 1967 the Expert Committee on Biological Standardization of the World Health Organization called for development of new and better methods to produce purified antivenin devoid of adverse human effects. Potency assays were changed and have since been based in terms of lethal dose (LD), the equivalent weight in milligrams of reference venom neutralized by a specified quantity of antivenin, and protection of a stated proportion of animals. Antivenin lots prepared by individual manufacturers must be tested by this standard. Efficacy in human beings had been virtually ignored until enough field anecdotal clinical data could be collected. The clinical efficacy of antivenin is now established, but adverse reactions of serum sickness and occasional anaphylaxis continue to be serious problems in managing envenomations.

BOX 28-4

WYETH ANTIVENIN PROTEIN QUANTITATION

IgG	2900.0 mg/ml
IgM	75.0 mg/ml
Total protein	9.4 g/dl
Albumin	0.28 g/dl
$Alpha_1$	0.74 g/dl
$Alpha_2$	3.50 g/dl
Beta	2.76 g/dl
Gamma	2.12 g/dl

Progress achieved in terms of immunotherapy of drug-induced toxicity has not been paralleled with respect to immunotherapy of venom poisoning. Despite the heterologous nature of Wyeth antivenins, they remain the current standard of therapy in managing indigenous Crotalidae and Elapidae envenomations in the United States. A new product, composed of sheep-derived, purified Fab fragments, has been recently tested in humans in the United States and shows great promise.

Like any equine serum source product, antivenin contains many nonimmunoglobulin proteins in addition to venom-specific IgG. Quantitative protein electrophoresis of Wyeth antivenin and horse serum from six separate lots demonstrated the wide variety of proteins present (Fig. 28-8).[89] As shown by these data, the process of ammonium sulfate precipitation of hyperimmune serum does not adequately purify the final product. Each vial of antivenin from these six lots contained between 1 and 2 g of equine protein.[89] Ammonium sulfate processing causes denaturation and loss of variable amounts of specific neutralizing IgG. Since this process is

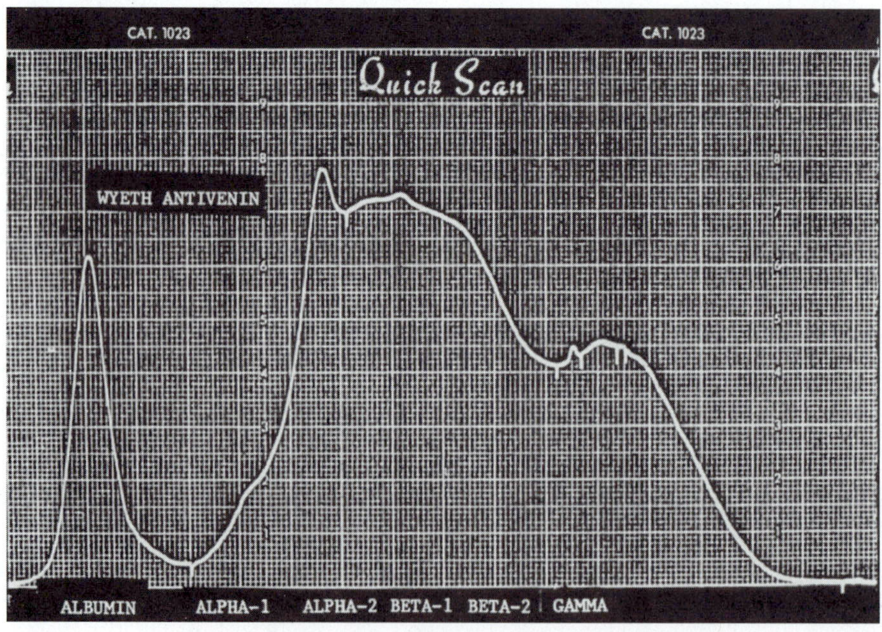

Fig. 28-8 Protein electrophoresis of Wyeth antivenin, demonstrating presence of multiple proteins.

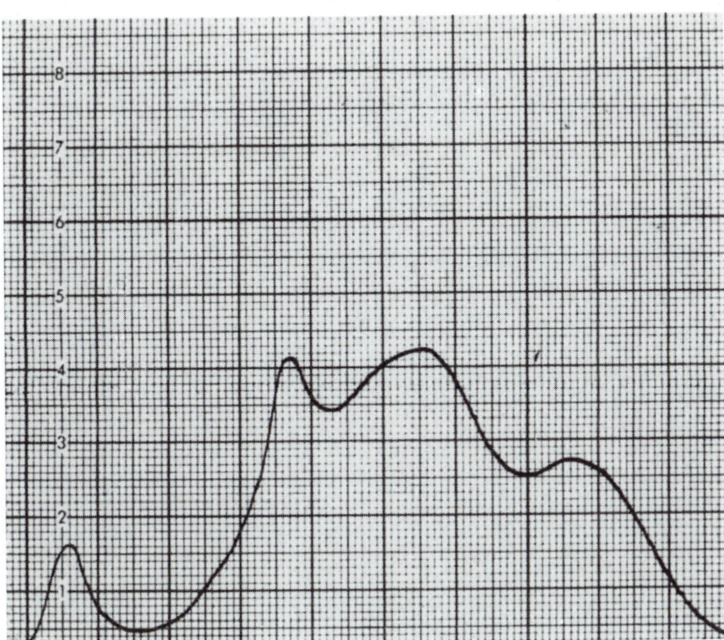

Fig. 28-9 Quantitative protein electrophoresis of Wyeth antivenin. Note reduced albumin peak with concentration of β- and gamma globulins (reading left to right). After ammonium sulfate precipitation.

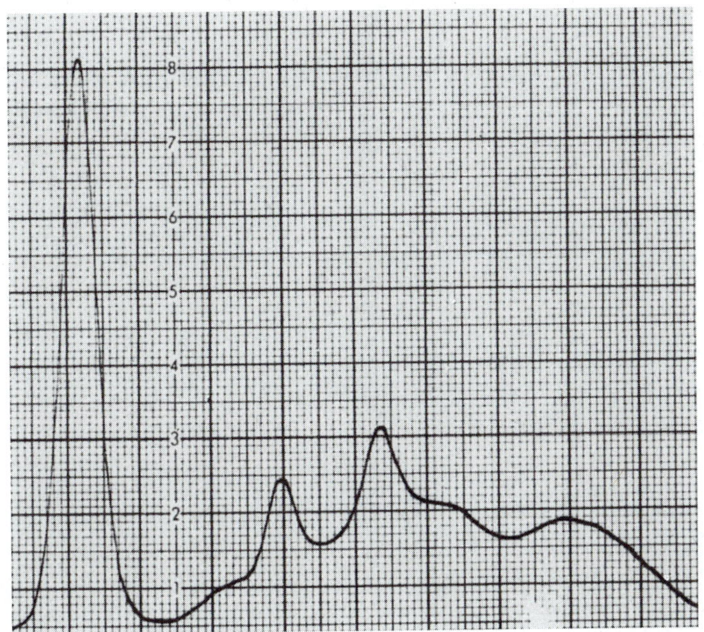

Fig. 28-10 Quantitative protein electrophoresis of Wyeth hyperimmune horse serum. Before ammonium sulfate precipitation.

currently used to produce commercial antivenin, the drug not only contains many extraneous proteins, but also is so dilute that large quantities are required to treat clinical envenomations. Considering that a person with a moderate to severe envenomation will receive 20 to 30 vials of antivenin, it is easy to understand why the incidence of serum sickness is so high.

The multiple protein content of commercial antivenin is further demonstrated in studies comparing antivenin, hyperimmune horse serum, and normal horse serum (Figs. 28-9, 28-10, and 28-11; Boxes 28-4, 28-5, and 28-6).[89] These

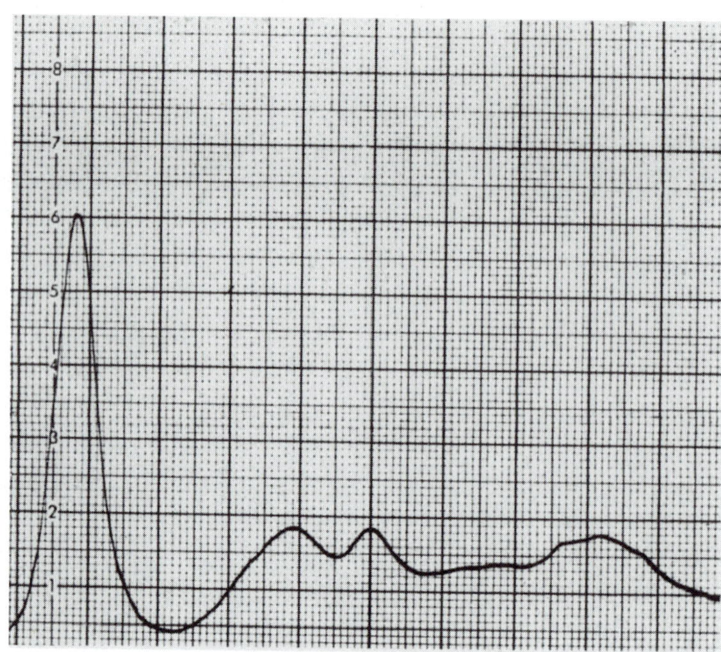

Fig. 28-11 Quantitative protein electrophoresis of normal horse serum.

BOX 28-5

HYPERIMMUNE HORSE SERUM PROTEIN QUANTITATION

IgG	2500.00 mg/ml
IgM	48.00 mg/ml
Total protein	5.50 g/dl
Albumin	1.88 g/dl
$Alpha_1$	0.26 g/dl
$Alpha_2$	1.55 g/dl
Beta	0.78 g/dl
Gamma	1.04 g/dl

BOX 28-6

NORMAL HORSE SERUM PROTEIN QUANTITATION

IgG	240.00 mg/ml
IgM	19.00 mg/ml
Total protein	0.90 g/dl
Albumin	0.30 g/dl
$Alpha_1$	0.06 g/dl
$Alpha_2$	0.20 g/dl
Beta	0.15 g/dl
Gamma	0.20 g/dl

comparisons demonstrate that antivenin contains the same protein pattern found in hyperimmune serum and horse serum. In fact, total IgG concentration in antivenin generally does not differ appreciably from hyperimmune serum (Boxes 28-4 and 28-5).[89] Total IgG in the six lots of Wyeth antivenin studied varied between 16% and 25% of total protein, substantiating the dilute nature of the product with respect to neutralizing antibody.[89]

Clinical Use of Antivenin. Snake venom poisoning is a clinical spectrum ranging from mild to severe (see Box 28-2). The amount of antivenin administered in cases of envenomation varies as a function of severity of the syndrome. Guidelines exist to aid the clinician in management and in determining the need for antivenin (Box 28-7). Also, the package insert accompanying the product is a useful guide to determining the need for and the starting doses of antivenin to be used in clinical cases.

Not every envenomed patient requires antivenin. A patient with a mild envenomation can be managed without antivenin. In this instance, observation alone is warranted and the patient can be monitored for worsening of the syndrome. A point of caution: a mild syndrome can become moderate or severe over a period of hours. If antivenin is not initially administered, close observation is still mandatory.

Before antivenin administration in a relatively stable patient, skin testing can be done with the dilute horse serum test material supplied in the Wyeth kit in an effort to predict the risk of anaphylaxis. Skin testing should be performed

BOX 28-7

ANTIVENIN DETERMINATION GUIDELINES

No envenomation	No antivenin
Minimal	0 or 5 vials
Moderate	10-20 vials
Severe	20 or more vials

only if the physician intends to use antivenin. Routine skin testing with horse serum is not appropriate if the decision to administer antivenin has not been made. A proper skin test can be predictive of hypersensitivity to horse serum.

Skin testing is accomplished by intradermal administration of 0.01 to 0.03 ml of horse serum, which is supplied in a dilution of 1:10 in the kit. A positive reaction to skin testing is erythema or pseudopodia at the site within 30 minutes of skin test application. Proper intradermal administration of the skin test is important in determining hypersensitivity to horse serum. A skin test administered subcutaneously may not show a positive reaction in an allergic individual. Skin testing with antivenin is not recommended unless it is diluted at least 1:100. Antivenin has been shown to contain approximately seven times the concentration of protein as the horse serum supplied in the Wyeth kit.[89] Also, there is a 70.8% coefficient of variation in the amount of albumin in antivenin, compared with a 15.5% coefficient of variation in albumin concentration in the skin test material.[89] Because albumin is a major allergen, using antivenin for skin testing exposes the patient to a highly variable and concentrated mixture, unless it is adequately diluted. During both skin testing and antivenin administration, anaphylaxis should be anticipated; appropriate drugs and equipment should be available to manage this crisis.

A negative skin test does not guarantee that acute hypersensitivity reactions or anaphylaxis will not occur during antivenin infusion. Early clinical symptoms of anaphylaxis include a hot, flushed feeling, nausea, and dyspnea. Patients with a history of allergy to horse serum, asthma, or history of general allergic manifestations should be considered at risk for acute hypersensitivity reactions to antivenin administration. A high index of suspicion for anaphylaxis must be maintained regardless of skin test results. Furthermore, in a severely envenomed patient, a positive skin test does not contraindicate the administration of antivenin. On many occasions, severely poisoned patients with positive skin tests have received adequate doses of antivenin without allergic sequelae after pretreatment with diphenhydramine and cimetidine. Considering these points, it is reasonable, when faced with a patient exhibiting severe symptoms, to proceed with antivenin administration without delaying to perform a skin test, while remaining highly vigilant for any sign of reaction.

Route and Dosage of Antivenin. The most effective and rapid route of antivenin administration is intravenous. Gennaro[18] reported that antivenin labeled with radioactive iodine accumulated at the site of the bite significantly faster after intravenous than after intramuscular or subcutaneous injection. Furthermore, in severe envenomations the systemic circulation may already be compromised and antivenin will be distributed slowly from intramuscular or intracutaneous sites. Antivenin should never be injected into a finger or toe. Because of the dilute nature of antivenin, the volume required in most envenomations is too large to give by any route but intravenous. Furthermore, if a reaction to the antivenin develops, it is advantageous to be able to shut off the infusion—a luxury not available after intramuscular or intracutaneous administration.

Antivenin dose is based on severity of envenomation. Adequate dosage, particularly in children, cannot be overemphasized. Children receive more milligrams of venom per kilogram of body weight than do adults, have less body water with which to dilute venom, and have less inherent resistance to its effects. Therefore children may require *larger* doses per unit of body weight than do adults. The recommended starting amounts of crotalid antivenin listed in Box 28-7 should be administered over a period of 1 to 2 hours in either adults or children using the clinical status of the patient, as well as the envenomation grading, as guides.

The Wyeth antivenin kit contains the following items:

1. One vial of antivenin containing approximately 1 g of lyophilized, sterile, heterologous, equine antiserum with preservatives (phenol 0.25% and thimerosal 0.005%) (In a freeze-dried state the antivenin remains stable and there is no need to keep it refrigerated.)
2. One 10 ml vial of bacteriostatic injection water with preservative (0.001% phenylmercuric nitrate) (any sterile diluent may be substituted)
3. One vial of normal horse serum diluted 1:10 for skin testing
4. Package insert

Each vial of antivenin must be separately prepared by dissolving the lyophilized antiserum with 10 ml of warmed saline or bacteriostatic water. Using warm diluent (approximately 37° C) will significantly speed the rate of dissolution of this relatively insoluble product. Excessive vigorous shaking of the reconstituted vials will result in more denatured protein, which appears as foam. Gentle shaking or swirling will ensure slow but proper dissolution of the product. This initial preparation is further diluted before administration. Final dilution depends on both the amount of antivenin required and the size of the patient. For adults, an initial dilution of 1:2 or 1:4 of reconstituted antivenin (for example, five vials diluted equals 50 ml in 200 ml 0.5 normal saline) is recommended.

The initial dilute antivenin infusion should be started slowly at a rate of 1 ml/min while the patient is observed for either an anaphylactic (IgE-mediated) or anaphylactoid (mast cell degranulating or complement activating) reaction. If no reaction occurs after 10 minutes, the speed of the infusion may be increased until the total amount is infused in 1 to 2 hours.

In children the rate and amount of intravenous fluid are based on body weight. Ten ml/kg/hr is a safe infusion rate. Close observation of urine output is required if more than 150 ml/kg/24 hr is administered.

Patients bitten by the Mojave rattlesnake *(Crotalus scutulatus)* require careful evaluation because the venom, while very lethal, may cause only moderate swelling and the symptoms of poisoning are frequently delayed.[96] If the offending snake is identified as *C. s. scutulatus,* the initial dose of antivenin should be 10 vials.

Copperhead *(A. contortrix)* venom is the least toxic of pit viper venoms and usually does not require antivenin therapy.[77]

To be most effective, antivenin should be given within the first 4 to 6 hours after the bite. The antivenin has less value as time passes, but exactly how long after envenomation antivenin can still be effective is unknown. Our experiments with the injection of radioisotope-labeled venom in rabbits indicate the presence of some circulating venom component at least 96 hours after the injection. Russell and Sullivan have observed the efficacious administration of antivenin 24 hours after bites of an eastern diamondback *(Crotalus adamanteus)* and a prairie rattlesnake *(C. viridis viridis)* bite.[77] It is possible that a symptomatic patient, such as one having coagulation defects with active hemorrhage, would benefit from antivenin administered up to 72 hours after envenomation.

Clinical Reactions to Antivenin. Equine source antivenin is highly allergenic, and adverse reactions occur in three clinical forms: acute anaphylaxis of type I IgE–mediated hypersensitivity; anticomplement reactions that clinically resemble anaphylaxis; and serum sickness.

Acute anaphylaxis and anticomplement reactions are uncommon, but do occur with the current equine antivenin. Type I hypersensitivity reactions are mediated by IgE and occur in response to antigenic challenge by the equine proteins in antivenin. Since antivenin contains a wide variety of equine serum proteins, it is difficult to implicate one single class of molecules as the cause.[89] Both careful questioning about a patient's allergic history and readiness to manage anaphylaxis are important in the treatment of snake venom–poisoned patients.

Anticomplement reactions are thought to be responsible for some of the acute reactions following antivenin administration. Anticomplement reactions are usually manifested as urticarial rashes and hypotension on the initial infusion of antivenin.[90,97] The anticomplement reaction is thought to result from immunoglobulin aggregates and other protein aggregates in antivenin.[90,97] These aggregates may initiate complement activity via activation of the C5a component of complement.[90,97] Overall, the anticomplementary activity of antivenin constitutes a low risk. This reaction is thought to occur most often when concentrated antivenin is given rapidly. The severity of the reaction may be limited by cautious expansion of the victim's intravascular volume with crystalloids before the administration of antivenin.

The syndromes produced by anaphylaxis and anticomplement reactions are similar in clinical features: nausea, warm flushed feeling, urticarial rash, hypotension, and bronchospasm. Immediate administration of 0.3 to 0.5 ml of 1:1000 concentration of aqueous epinephrine subcutaneously can prevent further progression of anaphylaxis. A single dose of epinephrine given at the onset of the syndrome may be all that is required. If administration of epinephrine is delayed and anaphylaxis is allowed to progress, it becomes more difficult to reverse. In this situation and in severe episodes of anaphylaxis, intravascular volume may be depleted. Rapid restoration of intravascular volume with normal saline is critical in reversing hypotension. Since the release of histamine by basophils and mast cells is the pharmacologic lesion of anaphylaxis, administration of intravenous histamine antagonists (diphenhydramine and cimetidine) is an important second-line therapy. Corticosteroids are not first-line pharmacotherapy for anaphylaxis; however, steroids can be beneficial in helping moderate the course of anaphylaxis and should be given early, since pharmacologic activity does not take place for 4 to 6 hours after administration.[35]

All patients with anaphylaxis should be closely observed for recurrence of the syndrome. Oxygen, equipment for endotracheal intubation, and suction equipment should be readily available.

Patients taking β-adrenergic–blocking drugs who have anaphylaxis can be difficult to manage and may have higher morbidity.[32] β-Receptor–blocking drugs can competitively block adenyl cyclase receptors on efferent cells and increase airway resistance in both asthmatic and nonasthamatic individuals.[32] β-Blockers inhibit adenyl cyclase, resulting in lowered intracellular cyclic adenosine monophosphate and a lowered threshold of mediator release.[32] Clinical cases of severe anaphylaxis with unresponsive bradycardia in patients taking β-blockers have been associated with much more difficult clinical resuscitation courses as well as higher morbidity and mortality.[2] Aggressive management of these patients with epinephrine and intravenous fluids is essential.

Serum sickness, a type IV hypersensitivity reaction, occurs 1 to 4 weeks after antivenin treatment and is manifest as urticarial rashes, arthralgias, and occasionally fever. McCullough and Gennaro[48] reported a 75% incidence of serum sickness to some degree after the administration of snake antivenin. Wainschel has observed that some degree of serum sickness usually develops in patients who receive more than 70 ml (seven vials) of antivenin.[99,101]

Serum sickness is caused by production of circulating immune complexes as a result of excess antivenin proteins.

Deposition of antigen-antibody complexes in vascular beds increases vascular permeability through local release of vasoactive amines. The complexes also activate complement and chemotactic factors, attracting neutrophils; these release proteolytic enzymes and basic proteins, which in turn cause local tissue destruction. Finally, the complexes induce histamine release from mast cells, which further increases capillary permeability.

Serum sickness usually is first manifested by urticaria, often generalized, and pruritus. Symptoms then progress to edema, arthralgias, fever, swollen joints, lymphadenopathy, and occasionally peripheral neuritis with pain and weakness in the extremities.

Corticosteroids are the drugs of choice for treatment of serum sickness and should be administered at the onset of urticaria. Adults should receive up to 60 mg of prednisone daily in two to four divided doses, depending on the progression of symptoms. If the presenting symptoms are not severe, the equivalent of 10 mg of prednisone orally every 6 hours may be preferred. For children, prednisone, 0.14 to 2 mg/kg/day in four doses by any route, may be administered according to the severity of symptoms. The corticosteroids should be given regularly until all signs and symptoms have subsided for 24 hours and then gradually tapered over 72 hours while the patient is observed closely for recurrence of symptoms. Longer tapering may be necessary to avoid transient adrenal insufficiency.

Antihistamines are of value in providing sedative and antipruritic effects.[74,99] Treatment with antihistamines and corticosteroids usually resolves the problem without sequelae.

Serum-Sensitive or Skin Test–Positive Individuals. Unfortunately, in severe envenomations, when time is a critical factor in neutralization of toxins, only a small quantity of antivenin can be administered by the desensitization method recommended in the antivenin package insert. A useful procedure in patients at risk for death or loss of limb is to begin therapy with administration of 50 to 100 mg (2 mg/kg in children) of diphenhydramine (Benadryl) and 300 mg (5 to 10 mg/kg in children) of cimetidine intravenously. Large doses of intravenous steroids can also be given in an effort to mitigate delayed effects. This is followed by slow intravenous administration of one vial (10 ml) of antivenin diluted 1:20 in 0.45 normal saline over a period of 60 minutes. The patient must be observed closely for signs and symptoms of anaphylaxis, usually heralded by the appearance of urticaria. If anaphylaxis does not occur, four vials of antivenin diluted 1:10 (360 ml 0.45 normal saline) may be added at a rate tolerated by the patient, while still closely observing pulse and blood pressure. Diphenhydramine may be repeated if urticaria appears. Diluted antivenin is then administered at a slow rate until the symptoms of envenomation are controlled.

Many patients with a positive skin test have been administered antivenin without adverse effects after pretreatment with intravenous antihistamines. The use of corticosteroids in envenomation syndromes remains controversial. The true role of corticosteroids in venom poisoning is to help prevent or lessen hypersensitivity reactions. The onset of corticosteroid pharmacologic activity, however, is 4 to 6 hours after administration. Administering steroids early in high-risk cases may mitigate a later reaction, especially if further antivenin administration becomes necessary.

Therapeutic dilemmas occur in severely envenomed patients allergic to antivenin. Pretreatment with intravenous H_1 and H_2 antihistamines followed by cautious infusion of dilute antivenin and administration of corticosteroids has been recommended.[12,15] Still, serious acute reactions develop in some patients. For patients with true IgE-mediated hypersensitivity, simultaneous infusion of epinephrine and antivenin has been advocated.[12] Although this method can successfully deliver small amounts of antivenin over several hours, its clinical efficacy may not be fully realized, since antivenin is very dilute with respect to its high-affinity IgG content.[89] The incidence of anaphylaxis will be significantly reduced when the new Fab antivenin becomes available.

Patients who require antivenin, but in whom signs of anaphylaxis develop despite this procedure, present a problem in clinical judgment and in the design of therapy. A method used successfully by Wainschel at LAC-USCMC, which requires considerable clinical acumen by an experienced observer, is intravenous injection of antivenin concomitantly with epinephrine.[101] A solution of 1:10,000 epinephrine is attached "piggyback" to an intravenous crystalloid solution in another extremity; 0.3 to 1.0 ml of the epinephrine infusion is started first, followed by 0.1 to 0.2 ml of antivenin solution through the second intravenous line. The physician observes the patient closely for signs of anaphylaxis and continues to alternate epinephrine with the serum as slowly as necessary. An alternative infusion technique for epinephrine, 1 mg in 250 ml normal saline, is described in Chapter 30. Eventually the patient may not require epinephrine with each dose of antivenin. However, in these patients serum sickness frequently develops within a week.

The Arizona Poison and Drug Center has been consulted in many cases involving clinical reactions to antivenin. These cases have been complicated by acute anaphylaxis and serum sickness reactions. Concern over the safety of simultaneous epinephrine and antivenin infusion in highly allergic patients prompted reevaluation of this method of treatment in selected patients. Our clinical experience in managing such patients who refused or could not safely receive antivenin therapy showed little morbidity and no mortality when antivenin was withheld.

Five patients with severe crotalid envenomations were managed by this method. One patient refused antivenin, two suffered anaphylactic reactions after skin testing, and two developed anaphylaxis after initiation of the antivenin infusion. These patients were hospitalized and managed symptomatically. Envenomed limbs were immobilized and elevated, and physical therapy was started when results of coagulation studies returned to normal. Only one patient, who was bitten on the index finger and refused antivenin, sustained any tissue loss; however, this was minimal and his finger regained completely normal function within 1 year of the bite.

Use of this unconventional approach is limited. In many subsequent cases, patients allergic to equine antivenin have been safely managed by pretreatment with diphenhydramine, cimetidine, and steroids, followed by very slow administration of dilute antivenin. Withholding antivenin in significant envenomations leads to the potential for bleeding complications and worsening coagulopathy, although these were not found in this series. Treatment of coagulopathy with cryoprecipitate or fresh-frozen plasma can be attempted should this occur. In a patient in our series who received several doses of fresh-frozen plasma over a period of days, no immediate reversal of coagulopathy occurred. The prothrombin-like venom proteins must be neutralized with antivenin administration, concurrent with the administration of fresh-frozen plasma, to successfully reverse a coagulopathy. Along with abnormal increases in the prothrombin time (PT) and partial thromboplastin time (PTT), severe thrombocytopenia and hypofibrinogenemia may be present. Levels of fibrinogen degradation products may or may not be increased. The effect of venom on circulating platelets is probably a combination of increased platelet adhesiveness to damaged blood vessels and tissues local to the site of the bite, as well as direct action of venom on platelets to cause platelet aggregation.[5] In vitro experiments have demonstrated that the venoms of *Crotalus atrox* (western diamondback rattlesnake), *Crotalus adamanteus* (eastern diamondback rattlesnake), *Crotalus viridis helleri* (southern Pacific rattlesnake), and *Crotalus scutulatus scutulatus* (Mojave rattlesnake) all produce direct human platelet aggregation, which is prevented by affinity-purified IgG from commercial antivenin.[5] Clinical experience has shown that marked thrombocytopenia with platelet counts as low as 2000/mm^3 occurs after crotalid bites.[94] Also, the platelet count may not return to normal for 4 to 7 days and may not be influenced by antivenin administration.[38] Platelet infusions have been administered in some cases without significant improvement in platelet counts.[94] In other clinical cases the only coagulation defect may be moderate to profound thrombocytopenia, which reverses over a period of 4 to 7 days. The clinician should be aware that bleeding can occur during a coagulopathy phase and the patient should be closely watched for signs of hypovolemia and bleeding. Should bleeding occur, rapid administration of fresh-frozen plasma or cryoprecipitate is necessary and can temporarily help terminate the bleeding. However, it has been our clinical observation that antivenin is always required for rapid reversal of hypofibrinogenemia, as well as the prolonged PT and PTT, even if cryoprecipitate or fresh-frozen plasma is administered. Thus withholding antivenin in allergic patients necessitates close observation, prolongs hospital stay, and increases cost. Finally, the potential for worsening morbidity is not excluded.

The nonantivenin approach is recommended only for selected cases. Current management of patients who have a positive skin test or who manifest urticarial reactions to horse serum skin testing requires readministration of more dilute antivenin after administration of intravenous antihistamines (H_1 and H_2) and corticosteroids. Similarly, reactions to antivenin administration after a negative skin test should be treated with readministration of more dilute antivenin after pretreatment with antihistamine. Patients refusing antivenin are not coerced into accepting antivenin therapy.

Antibiotics and Wound Care in Snakebite. Secondary wound site infection can be prevented by administering a broad-spectrum antibiotic, such as a second-generation cephalosporin. Pathogenic bacteria, predominantly gram-negative and anaerobic organisms, are present in snakes' mouths.[32] Wound cultures can be obtained to determine specific antibiotic need after infection appears. Antibiotics need not be used for trivial bites, which rarely become secondarily infected. Antibiotics are indicated if the bite has been contaminated by an incision, and particularly by oral suction. The flora of the human mouth includes at least 42 species of pathogenic organisms. Antibiotics of choice in wounds contaminated with human mouth bacteria are either broad-spectrum cephalosporins such as cefadroxil (Duricef) 500 mg twice daily for 5 days, or dicloxacillin 250 to 500 mg four times daily for 7 to 10 days. Aerobic and anaerobic cultures of rattlesnake venom have demonstrated the presence of 58 strains of aerobic bacteria and 28 strains of anaerobes.[21] These include *Clostridium, Pseudomonas, Proteus, Micrococcus, Enterobacter, Staphylococcus, Streptococcus, Corynebacterium,* and *Citrobacter*.[21] *Clostridium tetani* was not present in these cultures, but the organism is carried into the fang puncture wound by contamination with soil, dirt on the skin, or nonsterile first aid procedures. If the patient has been immunized adequately in the past, 0.5 ml of tetanus toxoid is sufficient. If the status of immunity is questionable, 250 to 500 units of tetanus hyperimmune globulin should also be administered.

The extremity should be well immobilized in a position of function on a splint padded to prevent pressure necrosis. The extremity should be maintained at or slightly below heart level until after antivenin has been administered; elevation is employed after that time. Between the third and fifth day, the hemorrhagic blebs, vesicles, and superficial necrotic tissue should be debrided surgically. Most tissue necrosis occurs during the first 3 days, and premature disruption of vesicles or damaged tissue during this initial period results in further tissue injury or bleeding. Debridement should not be delayed beyond the seventh day. After debridement the envenomed area should be cleansed daily with diluted antiseptics such as povidone-iodine or hydrogen peroxide. Early skin grafting should be considered if extensive tissue destruction has occurred. Early active physiotherapy is essential to allow restoration of joint function.

Surgical Intervention and Fasciotomy

Massive edema resulting from extremity injury can potentially result in a compartmental syndrome. Since most snakebites occur on the extremities and hands, knowledge of the various muscle compartments is beneficial in monitoring a patient should massive edema occur after a bite. There are well-defined fascial compartments in the hand, forearm, arm, and lower leg.[27] There are two fascial compartments in the upper arm (anterior-flexor and posterior-extensor). The forearm has two compartments, flexor and extensor (Color Plate 24). The flexor compartment of the forearm contains the median and ulnar nerves, along with the radial and ulnar arteries. The extensor compartment contains the radial nerve. The hand compartments are the thenar compartment, midpalmar compartment, hypothenar compartment, and deep palmar compartment. The leg has four fascial compartments: anterior, lateral, superior posterior, and deep posterior (Color Plate 25).

Compartmental syndromes result from increased tissue pressure in a closed fascial space. This directly compromises circulation and neurologic function of the injured extremity. Most snakebites result in venom's being injected subcutaneously and not subfascially into muscle. Thus edema contained in envenomed extremities is mainly subcutaneous and not intracompartmental. The diagnosis of a compartmental syndrome in snakebites can be difficult unless there is obvious neurologic dysfunction. An envenomed extremity can be extremely painful, both at rest and on movement. The extremity may appear cyanotic because of subcutaneous bleeding, and pulses may be difficult to palpate because of massive edema. Capillary fill can be normal and arterial pulses palpable even in the presence of a fully developed compartmental syndrome. In these situations, compartmental pressure monitoring and creatine kinase measurements are necessary to guide management. Currently available invasive methods for measuring compartmental pressure include the wick catheter technique, direct needle insertion, and the slit catheter technique. Compartmental measurements may be intermittent or continuous. To achieve a continuous compartmental reading, the monitoring system uses an infusion pump connected to a three-way stopcock and polyethylene tubing that will deliver 0.5 to 0.7 ml of normal saline per day into the compartment of interest. To ensure accuracy, the pressure transducer should be at the same level as the extremity being monitored.[46]

Direct needle insertion uses fluid-filled (normal saline) tubing connecting an 18- to 21-gauge needle to a pressure transducer. Sterile normal saline is introduced into the monitoring tubing continuously to allow constant monitoring of intracompartmental pressure.[27,46]

The wick catheter technique is similar in that a slow pump infusion system is combined with a pressure transducer to allow continuous low-flow fluid infusion into the compartment using a catheter with a small wick of suture at the terminal end.[56] The catheter is introduced into the compartment by a 14-gauge needle and the needle withdrawn.

The slit catheter method employs PE60 polyethylene tubing, 20 cm in length, with multiple 2 mm slits in the end of the catheter. A blunt-tipped 20-gauge needle is attached to the end of the catheter and a pressure line connects the catheter to a low-pressure transducer. The catheter unit is introduced into the compartment with a 14-gauge needle.[73]

The level of intracompartmental pressure that indicates the need for surgical intervention in a snakebitten extremity is generally accepted to be 30 mm Hg or greater, as accurately measured by one of the three techniques described.[17,56] Capillary blood pressure is approximately 20 to 25 mm Hg, so when tissue fluid pressure exceeds 30 mm Hg, capillary pressure cannot maintain blood flow.[56] It should be remembered that a patient who is hypotensive will be more susceptible to tissue ischemia at lower compartmental pressures. Other authorities have shown that compartmental pressures greater than 55 mm Hg are associated with significant loss of neuromuscular function.[46] Thus using a compartmental pressure of 30 mm Hg or greater will help avoid unnecessary tissue damage from compartmental syndromes. In a clinical series of envenomed patients using the wick catheter technique, measurements of compartment pressures never exceeded 20 mm Hg, even in grossly edematous extremities.[16,56]

Continuous monitoring of intracompartmental muscle pressures is the most accurate way to follow pressure elevations in an envenomed extremity. However, this may not always be possible because of patient and mechanical factors. Occasionally, only a one-time measurement is available. Also, continuous monitoring of one compartment ignores rising pressures in other compartments. Once a pressure of 30 mm Hg or greater is verified, surgical decompression of the muscle compartment is indicated.

As a primary mode of therapy in snakebite management, prophylactic fasciotomy cannot be recommended.[87] Garfin and associates[17] injected rattlesnake venom into both intact and fasciotomized muscle compartments of experimental animals. While intracompartmental pressures increased in both groups, the amount of muscle necrosis was not different. Decompression before envenomation did not prevent necrosis. It appears that necrosis is the direct result of venom enzymes, proteases, and phospholipase, rather than of an increase in intracompartmental pressures.

Noninvasive vascular studies of swollen envenomed extremities by pulse volume recorder and Doppler flowmeter have demonstrated no decrease in pulsatile arterial flow during maximal swelling, even when the skin temperature was decreased.[12] Increased tissue pressure, either subcutaneous or compartmental, was not severe enough to cause ischemia in the limb.[12]

Massive limb edema with ecchymosis is commonly seen in moderate to severe crotalid envenomations. Before surgical decompression is conducted, a compartmental syndrome should be demonstrated using appropriate monitoring techniques.[17] At the University of Arizona Health Sciences Center, we have successfully avoided the need for fasciotomy even in grossly swollen, ecchymotic limbs by compartmental monitoring demonstrating normal compartmental pressures. In addition, we successfully lowered intracompartmental pressure of one patient by the administration of mannitol along with antivenin, thus avoiding fasciotomy.

PROGNOSIS OF CROTALID ENVENOMATION

Death is uncommon if antivenin is given without delay and in adequate amounts. The fatality rate in treated cases is less than 1%. Permanent disability and amputation are less frequent since cryotherapy has fallen into disuse. Of the more than 860 patients who have been treated at LAC-USCMC, no deaths or amputations have occurred that can be attributed to venom poisoning.[79,99] However, several amputations were necessitated by frostbite induced by cryotherapy. Radical first aid procedures such as wide and deep incisions, followed by secondary infection, have required tendon repair and plastic surgery. It is now quite evident that the vast majority of crotalid envenomations do not result in tissue loss, loss of an extremity or digit, or loss of life when properly managed. Even when antivenin is withheld from severely allergic individuals, few permanent tissue sequelae occur.

RESEARCH AND DEVELOPMENT OF A NEWER ANTIVENIN

Purification of IgG(T) by Immunosorbent Affinity Chromatography

Investigations since 1980 using immunosorbent polyacrylamide affinity chromatography developed by Sullivan and Russell have yielded highly purified, equine antibody IgG(T) with high affinity for crotalid venoms.[80,89] Quantitative protein electrophoresis, along with immunoelectrophoresis of the affinity-isolated antibody versus Wyeth antivenin, has revealed the purity of the isolated antibody compared with the heterologous nature of Wyeth antivenin.[80,89] Antivenin contains multiple proteins besides IgG, including albumin, α- and β-globulins, and gamma globulins, including IgM (Figs. 28-8 and 28-9; Box 28-4). Protein electrophoresis of the affinity-purified antibody reveals a single peak of immunoglobulin (Fig. 28-12). Immunoelectrophoresis of the affinity-purified antibody versus Wyeth antivenin developed with anti–horse serum reveals a single precipitin band for the purified product and multiple bands for the commercial antivenin (Fig. 28-13), indicating the heterologous protein content of Wyeth antivenin and the purity of the affinity-isolated antibody. This purified antibody belongs to a subclass of equine IgG called IgG(T) (Fig. 28-14) and has unique features that set it apart from other horse immunoglobulins.[49] IgG(T) is an acidic antibody with high carbohydrate content, in contrast to the alkaline nature of other animal and human IgG antibodies; it does not fix complement by the classical pathway, and it has limited precipitability with antigens, favoring the formation of intramolecular bonds by bivalently binding to repeating antigenic determinants.[49]

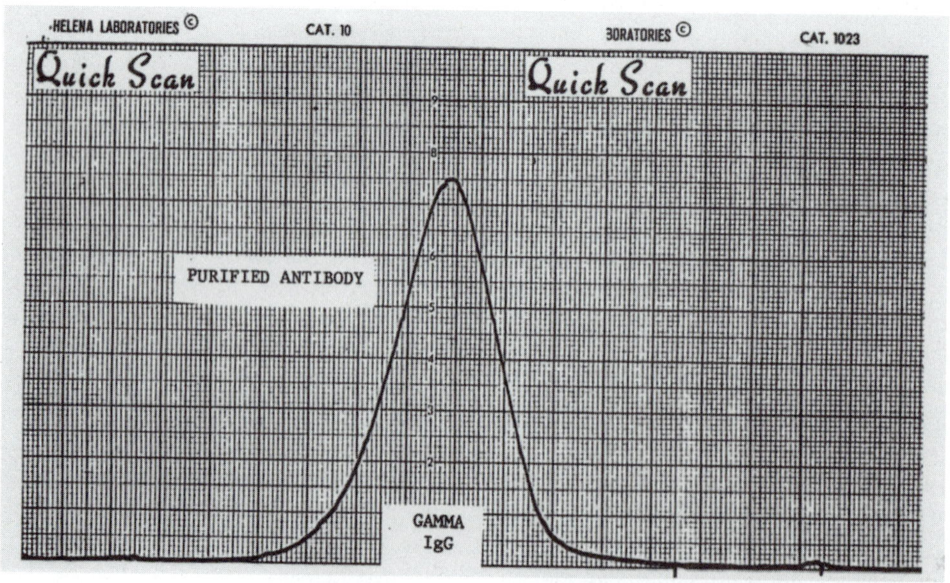

Fig. 28-12 Protein electrophoresis demonstrating single peak of immunoglobulin IgG(T).

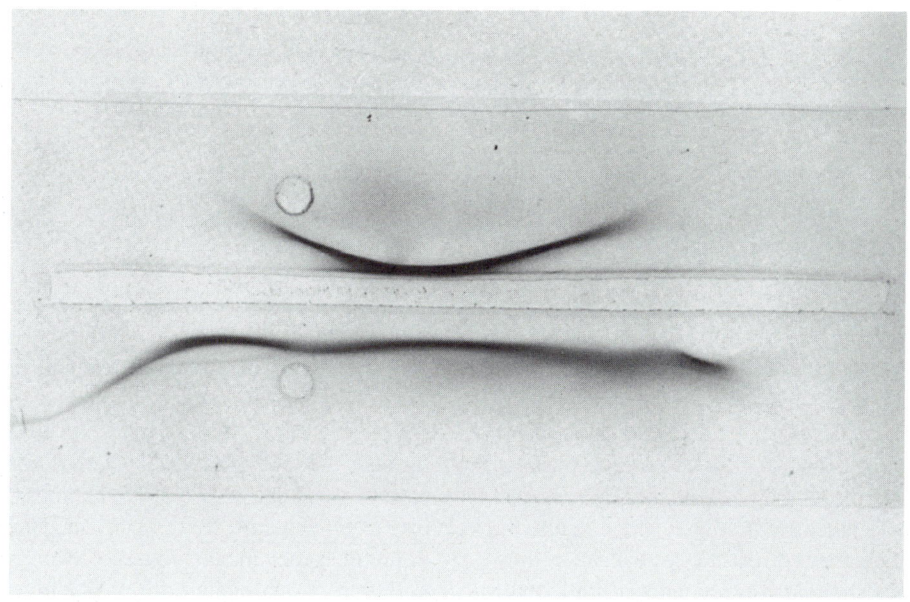

Fig. 28-13 Purified antibody on top; anti–horse serum in the middle trough; Wyeth antivenin on bottom. Note presence of multiple precipitin bands with Wyeth antivenin, indicating the presence of multiple extraneous proteins.

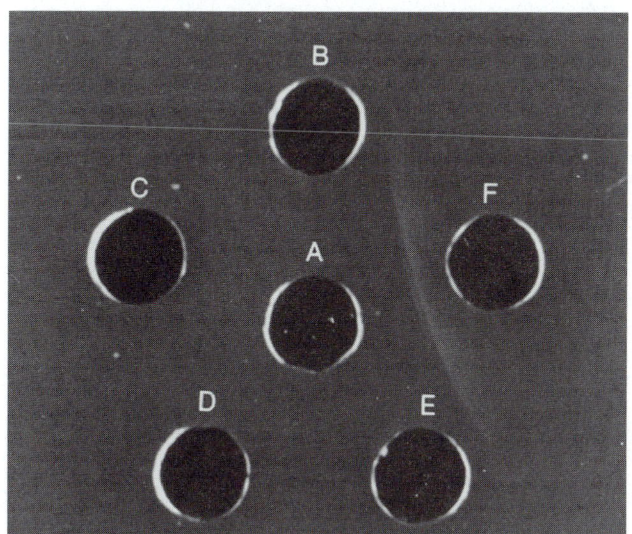

Fig. 28-14 Precipitin band to anti-IgG(T), showing that the purified IgG is mainly IgG(T). **A,** Purified antibody. **B,** Anti-IgG. **C,** Anti-IgG(T). **D,** Anti-IgM. **E,** Anti-IgA. **F,** Blank.

Studies, both in vivo and in vitro, have demonstrated the superior efficacy of purified IgG(T) over classic antivenin in neutralizing venom pathophysiology of *Crotalus atrox, Crotalus admanteus, Crotalus s. scutulatus,* and *Crotalus viridis helleri.* Further studies with leukocyte histamine release assays, using leukocytes from humans sensitized to antivenin, as well as guinea pig anaphylaxis models, demonstrated that purified IgG(T) did not provoke histamine release in these sensitized cells or produce anaphylaxis in horse serum–sensitive animals.[80] Previous studies comparing affinity isolated IgG(T) with whole antivenin further demonstrated the superior efficacy of the purified antibody in lethality protection, and prevention of muscle necrosis, subcutaneous hemorrhage, direct cytotoxicity, platelet aggregation, and fibrinogen clotting.[80]

Conclusions from these investigations are that affinity-isolated polyvalent IgG(T) yields a superior immunotherapeutic agent compared with present antivenin.[80] This research opened the way for further development of a new antivenin.

Whole Antibody Versus Fab Fragments

To be effective, immunotherapy for venom poisoning must drastically alter the pharmacokinetics of the venom proteins and increase venom elimination. The success of antibody reversal of poisons depends on establishing a concentration gradient from tissue receptor sites into the plasma. Unless there is a large effect on this redistribution of the toxin, the immunoglobulin will not successfully alter the clinical course of the poisoning. To be maximally effective, immunotherapy should provide enhanced elimination of the drug or toxin. The antibody-toxin interaction is dynamic in that toxin can be released to rebind to receptor sites.

Because of the large molecular weight of IgG (150,000 daltons), its elimination requires immune cell clearance. Many venom proteins are in the molecular weight range of 20,000 to 90,000. The molecular weight cutoff for renal clearance is in the upper range of 50,000. This poses the hypothetical problem of IgG actually delaying venom clearance because of its large size. Clinical pharmacokinetic studies of crotalid venom and antivenin have not yet been performed. One pharmacokinetic study using radiolabeled scorpion venom and partially purified IgG demonstrated very contrasting distributions and eliminations.[31] The intravenous administration of labeled IgG in an animal model produced a triexponential equation consistent with a three-compartment model. A rapid distribution half-life of 1.1 hours was followed by a slower phase half-life of 9.6 hours. The actual elimination half-life for the IgG was 43.3 hours. In contrast, the whole venom had a distribution half-life of 5.6 minutes and an elimination half-life of 6.4 hours.

Purified Fab fragments have been produced from IgG(T) using papain digestion and molecular size exclusion of active fragments.

Comparing the pharmacokinetics of animal IgG and Fab fragments described in other studies has yielded solid evidence of the superior clearance properties of the active fragments. [89] The smaller Fab fragments retain the affinity of the much larger IgG but are renally eliminated rather than requiring clearance by cells of the immune system. Thus the use of Fab(T) fragments could enhance clearance of venom proteins because many of these proteins are under the 50,000 molecular weight cutoff for renal elimination. In addition to enhanced clearance of venom, Fab fragments would be much less immunogenic than would whole antibody. Fab fragment antivenins are promising new modes of therapy for envenomation (Box 28-8).

The concept of producing monoclonal antibodies against venom antigens is not new. However, the practicality of monoclonal antibodies is uncertain because snake venom is composed of hundreds of toxic proteins, each protein having multiple antigenic sites. Because of this, multiple monoclonal antibodies would have to be produced. Instead, it appears that the future treatment of snake venom poisoning may be with polyclonal, polyvalent Fab fragments. Preliminary clinical trials with sheep Fab fragments directed against crotalid venom have been concluded. Sheep Fab fragments have historically been shown to be safe for human use and are easy to produce.

BOX 28-8

CHARACTERISTICS OF Fab FRAGMENTS AS COMPARED WITH IgG

- Distribution t½ of Fab is much shorter than that of IgG (0.3 versus 4 hours)
- Fab elimination t½ is shorter than that of IgG (9 to 13 versus 61 hours)
- Fab volume of distribution is greater than that of IgG (8.7 times)
- Fab is renally excreted versus immune system elimination of IgG
- Fab affinity for antigen is same as that of IgG
- Fab is much less immunogenic than is IgG

Elapidae (Coral Snakes)

EPIDEMIOLOGY

Two members of the coral snake family, Elapidae, occur in the United States: the western coral snake *(Micruroides euryxanthus)* (Color Plate 20), found in Arizona and New Mexico, and the eastern coral snake *(Micrurus fulvius)* (Color Plate 21), distributed from coastal North Carolina through the Gulf states to western Texas (Fig. 28-15). The eastern coral snake is more dangerous. Coral snakes favor dry, open, brushy, or sandy ground near rivers or lakes. Sometimes they may be found in loamy soil under leaf accumulations.[95] The elapids differ from pit vipers in having very short fangs fixed at the anterior part of the maxilla, round pupils, and subcaudal scales in a double row. The color pattern is characteristic, with red, black, and yellow or white bands completely encircling the body. The snout is completely black. Since many nonpoisonous mimics occur in coral snake territory, the rule of thumb for identifying a coral snake is by the sequence of colors: red bands bordered by yellow (or white) indicate a venomous animal: thus "red on yellow, kill a fellow; red on black, venom lack." This rule applies to all coral snakes native to the United States, but does not apply to species found south of Mexico City, Mexico.

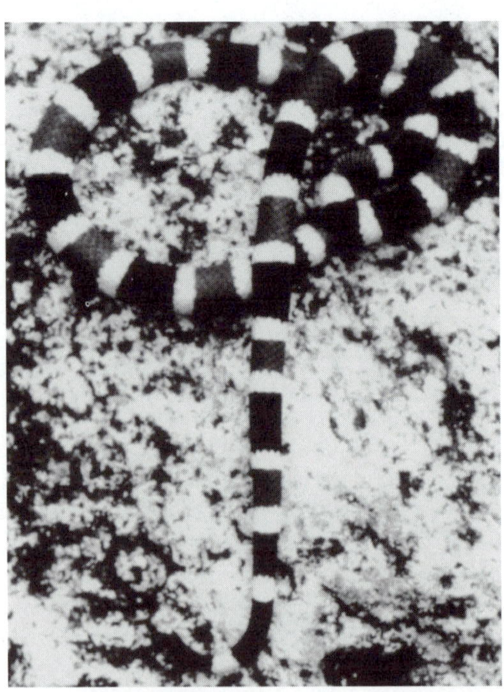

Fig. 28-15 Coral snake *(Micrurus fulvius)*.

The coral snake is slender, ranges in length from 50 to 110 cm (20 to 44 inches), feeds chiefly on small lizards and other snakes, and is diurnal. Most coral snakes are shy, docile animals and do not bite unless handled or deliberately provoked. The small mouth and fangs make it difficult for the snake to bite anything larger than a finger, toe, or fold of skin. The coral snake tends to hang on and chew, rather than to strike and release like the rattlesnake.

ELAPIDAE CLINICAL ENVENOMATION SYNDROMES

The bite of the eastern coral snake *(Micrurus fulvius)* produces little or no pain and no local edema or necrosis. The venom is primarily neurotoxic. Paresthesias and muscle fasciculations are common at the site of the bite. Flaccid paralysis and respiratory failure can develop over the course of several hours. The incidence of envenomation is lower than that with rattlesnakes because only about 40% of coral snake bites result in significant envenomation.[77] Signs and symptoms of envenomation range from local swelling, nausea, and vomiting to weakness, dizziness, paresthesias, and respiratory paralysis. Thirty-nine victims of eastern coral snake envenomation over a 12-year period revealed the following clinical manifestations after bites: local edema (40%), paresthesias (35%), nausea (30%), vomiting (25%), weakness (15%), diplopia (10%), dyspnea (10%), diaphoresis (10%), myalgia (10%), fasciculations (5%), and confusion (5%).[36] No deaths have been reported from coral snake bites in Florida since 1959.[79]

Diagnosis of coral snake bite can be difficult. Fang marks are hard to see but may be identified by expressing blood from the small puncture sites.[59]

Within 90 minutes of envenomation the bitten extremity may feel weak or numb. Several hours later, systemic symptoms appear, which include tremors, drowsiness or euphoria, and marked salivation. After 5 to 10 hours, slurred speech and diplopia herald the onset of cranial nerve palsies. Bulbar paralysis is manifested as dysphagia and dyspnea.[47] The curare-like effect of the venom may cause total flaccid paralysis. Death is associated with respiratory and cardiac failure. Onset of bulbar paralysis, dysphagia, and respiratory paralysis may be delayed by up to 13 hours after the bite.[36]

MANAGEMENT OF ELAPIDAE ENVENOMATION

Antivenin against eastern coral snake *(Micrurus fulvius)* venom was developed in 1967 (Antivenin, *Micrurus fulvius*). It is equine in source and produced by Wyeth Laboratories. The same precautions for acute reactions must be undertaken in the administration of eastern coral snake antivenin as for crotalid antivenin.

Since it is difficult to ascertain early whether envenomation by the coral snake has occurred, treatment and observation are mandatory. Early treatment with antivenin is advised in any suspected bite with envenomation, since signs and symptoms can be delayed for up to 12 hours. Also, the symptoms are difficult to reverse once the onset occurs because the venom binds to nerve sites and is not easily displaced, even with antivenin. Thus, early administration of four to six vials of antivenin is warranted in patients definitely bitten by an eastern coral snake even if no signs or symptoms are present.[36] One vial of antivenin is estimated to neutralize 2 mg of this snake's venom. Large coral snakes can inject 20 mg of venom, four to five times the human lethal dose.[15] Delay in administering antivenin can result in progression of symptoms to the point that intubation and mechanical respiratory support may be necessary. Once respiratory paralysis occurs, ventilatory support may be required for up to 7 days.[36] Bulbar paralysis may signal imminent respiratory failure, which carries a significant risk of aspiration.[36] It is therefore important to proceed with prompt endotracheal intubation in any patient with signs of bulbar dysfunction.

Management of a victim of envenomation by the Arizona coral snake *(Micruroides euryxanthus)* is purely supportive as there is no commercially available antiserum against its venom. However, no fatal bites have been reported with this species.

NATURAL COURSE OF ELAPIDAE ENVENOMATION

Persons who go untreated after envenomation by coral snakes can experience a serious life-threatening course of respiratory distress, muscle fasciculations leading to highly elevated serum creatine kinase, and other neurologic manifestations. One report of the course of a 36-year-old bitten man who was allergic to antivenin described respiratory muscle paralysis, myoglobinemia, difficulty in swallowing and handling secretions, and intubation and ventilatory support for 6 days, as well as other supportive care in the intensive care unit.[36]

Envenomation by Exotic Snakes

Many species of exotic snakes are housed in scientific collections, zoos, and private collections of amateur herpetologists and nonprofessional snake fanciers. Annually, about 75,000 snakes, including more than 6800 belonging to venomous species, are legally imported into the United States and an additional number are smuggled and may fall into the collections of individuals who are unskilled snake handlers.[92] Of all snake envenomations in the United States, the proportion resulting from exotic snake bites is reported to be 4% to 13%.[65,77,99] Consequently, a physician occasionally may be confronted with the management of a bite by a king cobra *(Ophiophagus hannah)*, mamba (*Dendroaspis* spp.), or fer-de-lance (*Bothrops* spp.). The most common exotic snakes involved in bites in the United States are the species and subspecies of cobras *(Naja naja)*. The major species identified in private possession are cobras, gaboon vipers *(Bitis gabonica)*, African puff adders *(Bitis arietans)*, kraits (*Bungarus* spp.), European vipers (*Vipera* spp.), European asp *(Vipera aspis)*, and mambas (*Dendroaspis* spp.)[77]

The approach to evaluation and management of victims bitten by foreign snakes imported into the U.S. is detailed in Chapter 29.

Venomous Lizards

The only two species of venomous lizards in the world are found in North America. The Gila monster *(Heloderma suspectum)* (Color Plate 26) and the Mexican beaded lizard *(H. horridum)* (Color Plate 27) are closely related. Both possess venom glands and grooved teeth capable of envenoming humans.

The Gila monster and the Mexican beaded lizard are found only in the Great Sonoran Desert area in southern Arizona and northwestern Mexico. However, human envenomations are not restricted to these geographic areas, since bites are occasionally incurred during careless handling of captive specimens by amateur collectors.[78]

Both lizards are large (300 to 400 cm) reptiles with large flat heads, bulging mandibular muscles, and relatively long, round, thick tails. The limbs are short and stubby. Although these lizards appear sluggish and lumbering when relaxed, they are capable of remarkably quick lunges and bites when feeding or engaged in defense. The color of the Gila monster's thick skin ranges from pink to orange on black. The beaded lizard is a darker purple on black.

VENOM AND VENOM APPARATUS

The venom apparatus consists in part of paired inferior labial glands located on either side of the lower jaw. Each gland contains several lobes with separate ducts that carry the venom to the mucous membranes between the lower lip and jaw, close to the base of the teeth. The teeth are solid, lance-shaped, sharp, recurved, and grooved on the anterior and posterior surfaces. Each half of the jaw has 9 or 10 teeth, the largest and most deeply grooved located nearest the discharge orifice of the venom glands.

Human envenomation occurs when venom is drawn into puncture wounds through capillary action along the grooved surfaces of the teeth, especially when the lizard retains its grasp and chews for an extended period. Not all bites result in envenomation, since the lizard may only nip the victim, may bite without chewing, or may not expel venom from the glands to the infralabial area during a bite. Russell has noted that of 15 cases observed, only 9 involved envenomation.[74]

The venom is a complex mixture of enzymes, including amine oxidase, phospholipase A, protease, hyaluronidase, kallikrein, and serotonin.[50,51,102] The lethal dose for humans is estimated at 5 to 8 mg; Russell[77] estimates that an animal's venom glands contain approximately 17 mg of venom. The major pathophysiologic actions in experimental animals are systemic hypotension and respiratory arrest.[70,77,79]

MEDICAL ASPECTS

Heloderm wounds usually are simple punctures, although teeth may break off or be shed during the bite and remain in the wound. Pain, often severe and burning, appears at the wound site within 5 minutes and may radiate up the extremity.[75,79,86] Intense pain may last from 3 to 5 hours and then subside after 8 hours. Edema occurs at the wound, usually within 15 minutes, and progresses slowly in variable degrees up the extremity.[79,86] Cyanosis or blue discoloration may appear around the wound. The victim may feel weak and faint and become diaphoretic. The wound site may remain tender for 3 to 4 weeks after the bite.[77,79] Usually, little tissue necrosis occurs. In humans, severe hypotension is rarely observed and no coagulation defects have been noted.[77,79]

Gila monsters may hang on tenaciously during a bite, and mechanical means may be required to loosen the grip of the jaws; rescuers have used pliers, chisels, crowbars, or incision of the jaw muscles with a sharp knife.[86]

TREATMENT

The wound should be cleansed thoroughly with a soap or iodophor solution. Infiltration of the puncture wounds with 1% lidocaine using a 25-gauge needle and then probing the wounds to detect the presence of shed or broken teeth can help prevent future infection from a foreign body.[77] Soft tissue radiographs may be useful. Intense pain may require analgesics in doses appropriate for the patient's age and weight. The vital signs, especially blood pressure, should be monitored closely. The extremity should be immobilized in a functional position and elevated to help decrease extremity pain and edema. Intravenous crystalloid solutions such as normal saline should be administered if massive limb edema occurs. Hypotension can also be successfully managed using intravenous normal saline. Tetanus prophylaxis is standard. The wound should be observed for secondary infection, although antibiotics usually are not required.[77] Follow-up care is the same as for any penetrating reptilian wound: dry sterile dressings, along with daily cleansing with an antiseptic solution. Physical therapy may be necessary to prevent contractures and restore function.

Snakebite in Pregnancy

The management of snake venom poisoning in a pregnant woman is no different from that of anyone else, with the following exceptions:

1. No studies have demonstrated the effect of venom on the developing fetus, but it can be presumed to be detrimental, since venom proteins probably cross the placental barrier. Therefore early aggressive management with antivenin is recommended, along with fetal monitoring.
2. If anaphylaxis from antivenin develops in a pregnant woman, administration of epinephrine should be avoided if possible because it may drastically reduce uterine blood flow.[14] Ephedrine, a noncatecholamine adrenergic agent, does not affect uterine blood flow at normal doses of 25 to 50 mg intravenously and should be used as a first-line agent. At these doses, ephedrine is primarily a β-receptor agonist and raises blood pressure by increasing heart rate. Also, the β-receptor agonism of ephedrine acts to prevent further histamine release from basophils and mast cells in anaphylaxis. Further therapy includes intravenous diphenhydramine, cimetidine, and crystalloid or colloid fluids to replace lost intravascular volume.

The pregnant snakebitten woman is a medical dilemma, and no additional guidelines have been established to date. The pathophysiologic effects of snake venom on human pregnancy and the fetus are unknown. One case report of a pregnant woman envenomed by *Bothrops jararaca* reported abruptio placentae as an outcome of the envenomation syndrome.[103] It should be assumed that the effects of the venom on the fetus and the placental-uterine unit are detrimental. Early obstetric consultation and ultrasonographic evaluation of the fetus and placenta are recommended.

Prevention of Venom Poisoning

The best method of avoiding snakebite is to avoid poisonous snakes.[81] Snakes generally are afraid of humans and retreat to safety if given an opportunity. Unless accidentally and suddenly confronted at very close range, a snake is unlikely to strike a comparatively huge human.

These rules should be followed when in snake-infested territory:

1. Avoid the known habitats of snakes, which are generally areas in which the snake seeks protection: swamps; rocky ledges; wood, stone, and rubbish piles; caves and deserted mines; and deserted buildings, especially in rural areas.
2. Do not put any part of your body, especially hands and feet, into places you cannot first inspect. Snakes often lie next to a fallen tree or under a rock. Do not sit on or step over a log if the other side is not visible. Walk on clear paths as much as possible. Carry a walking stick to prod logs and rocks before stepping over them. Do not reach blindly into bushes or under rocks.
3. Wear adequate protective clothing. The majority of bites are on the hands (80%) (from handling) and the lower legs and feet (15%)[99]; this speaks for the value of wearing leather boots that rise just below the knee and sturdy trousers (for men and women) when walking in snake-infested areas.
4. Avoid hiking alone in snake-infested areas unless you are experienced and knowledgeable about the area.
5. Avoid walking at night in snake-infested areas, especially in southwestern deserts and mountains. If you must walk, wear boots and carry a flashlight and walking stick. Most venomous snakes avoid direct sunlight and are most active during the moderate temperatures of the night.
6. Do not handle snakes unless you are an experienced herpetologist or very familiar with the identification and habits of snakes. Every year many victims are bitten because they handle a snake carelessly, especially while intoxicated; attempt to pick up a freshly killed rattlesnake; or go out of their way to kill snakes, without knowledge of their habits and habitats.

REFERENCES

1. Anker RL, Straffon WG, Loiselle DS: Retarding the uptake of "mock venom" in humans—comparisons of three first-aid treatments, *Med J Aust* 1:212, 1982.
2. Awai LE, Ekori YA: Insect sting anaphylaxis and beta-adrenergic blockade—a relative contraindication, *Ann Allergy* 53:48, 1984.
3. Bajwa S, Markland F, Russell F: Fibrinolytic enzyme(s) in western diamondback rattlesnake *(Crotalus atrox)* venom, *Toxicon* 18:285, 1980.
4. Balmain R, McClelland KL: Pantyhose compression bandage: first-aid measure for snake bite, *Med J Aust* 2(5):240, 1982.
5. Bar-Or D, Sullivan J, Black E: Neutralization of Crotalidae venom induced platelet aggregation by affinity chromatography-isolated IgG to *Crotalus viridis helleri* venom, *Clin Toxicol* 22(1):1, 1984.
6. Bronstein AC et al: Negative pressure suction in field treatment of rattlesnake bite, AACT, Kansas City, 1985 (abstract).
7. Bullock TH, Diecke FPJ: Properties of an infrared receptor, *J Physiol* 134:47, 1956.
8. Burgess JL et al: Effects of constriction bands on rattlesnake venom absorption: a pharmacokinetic study, *Ann Emerg Med* 21(9):1086, 1992.
9. Busack SD: Amphibians and reptiles imported into the U.S., Wildlife Leaflet 506, 1974, US Fish and Wildlife Service.
10. Cable DM et al: Prolonged defibrination after a bite from a "nonvenomous" snake, *JAMA* 251(7):925, 1984.
11. Carlson RW, Schaeffer RC, Whigham H: Rattlesnake venom shock in the rat: development of a method, *Am J Physiol* 229(6):1668, 1975.
12. Curry SC et al: Non-invasive vascular studies in management of rattlesnake envenomations to extremities, *Ann Emerg Med* 14:1081, 1985.
13. Dart RC, Lindsey D: Snakebites and shocks, *Ann Emerg Med* 17(11):1262, 1988.
14. Entman SS, Moise KJ: Anaphylaxis in pregnancy, *South Med J* 77(3):402, 1984.
15. Fix JD: Venom yield of the North American coral snake and its clinical significance, *South Med J* 73:737, 1980.

16. Garfin SR, Mubarak SJ, Davidson TM: Rattlesnake bites—current concepts, *Clin Orthop* 140:50, 1979.
17. Garfin SR et al: Rattlesnake bites and surgical decompression: results using a laboratory model, *Toxicon* 22:177, 1984.
18. Gennaro JF: Observations on the treatment of snakebite in North America. In Keegan HL, MacFarlane WV, editors: *Venomous and poisonous animals and noxious plants of the Pacific region,* New York, 1963, Pergamon.
19. Glass TG: Treatment of rattlesnake bites (letter), *JAMA* 247:461, 1982.
20. Glenn JL et al: Geographical variation in *Crotulus scutulatus scutulatus* (Mojave rattlesnake) venom properties, *Toxicon* 21(1):119, 1983.
21. Goldstein EJ et al: Bacteriology of rattlesnake venom and implications for therapy, *J Infect Dis* 140:818, 1979.
22. Grace TG, Omer GE: The management of upper-extremity pit viper wounds, *J Hand Surg* 5(2):168, 1980.
23. Guderian RH, MacKenzie CD, Williams JF: High-voltage shock treatment for snakebite (letter), *Lancet* 2(8500):229, 1986.
24. Gutierrez JM: Myonecrosis induced by *Bothrops asper* venom: pathogenesis and treatment, Second American Symposium on Animal, Plant and Microbial Toxins, May 1, 1986.
25. Hardy DL: Envenomation by the Mojave rattlesnake *(Crotalus scutulatus scutulatus)* in southern Arizona, USA, *Toxicon* 21(1):111, 1983.
26. Hasiba U, Rosenbach L, Rockwell D: DIC-like syndrome after envenomation by the snake, *Crotalus horridus horridus, N Engl J Med* 292:505, 1975.
27. Haynes J, Berg E: Compartment syndrome of the upper extremity, *Curr Concepts Trauma Care,* 10, 1985.
28. Ho CL, Lee CY: Presynaptic actions of Mojave toxin isolated from Mojave rattlesnake *(Crotalus scutulatus)* venom, *Toxicon* 19:889, 1981.
29. Howe NR, Meisenheimer JL: Electric shock does not save snakebitten rats, *Ann Emerg Med* 17(3):245, 1988.
30. Hurlbut KM et al: Reliability of clinical presentation for predicting significant pit viper envenomation, *Ann Emerg Med* 17(4):438, 1988.
31. Ismail M, Shibl A, Morad A: Pharmacokinetics of I^{125} labeled antivenin to the venom from the scorpion, *Androctonus amoreuxi, Toxicon* 21:47, 1983.
32. Jacobs RL et al: Potential anaphylaxis in patients with drug-induced beta-adrenergic blockade, *J Allergy Clin Immunol* 68:125, 1981.
33. Jenkins MS, Russell FE: Physician therapy for injuries produced by rattlesnakes. In Kaiser E, editor: *Animal and plant toxins,* 1973, Nilheim Goldman Verlag.
34. Johnson EK, Kardong KV, Mackessy SP: Electric shocks are ineffective in treatment of lethal effects of rattlesnake envenomation in mice, *Toxicon* 25(12):1347, 1987.
35. Kelly JF, Patterson R: Anaphylaxis—course, mechanisms, and treatment, *JAMA* 227:1431, 1974.
36. Kitchens CS, VanMierop LH: Envenomation by the eastern coral snake *(Micrurus fulvius fulvius), JAMA* 258:1615, 1987.
37. Klauber IM: *Rattlesnakes: their habitats, life histories and influence on mankind,* vol 1, ed 2, Berkeley, 1972, University of California Press.
38. LaGrange RG, Russell FE: Blood platelet studies in man and rabbits following *Crotalus* envenomation, *Proc West Pharmacol Soc* 13:99, 1970.
39. Ledbetter EO, Kutcher AT: The aerobic and anerobic flora of rattlesnake fangs and venom, *Arch Environ Health* 19:770, 1969.
40. Lee BY et al: Management of compartment syndrome, *Am J Surg* 148:383, 1984.
41. Litovitz TL et al: 1990 annual report of the American Association of Poison Control Centers National Data Collection System, *Am J Emerg Med* 9(5):461, 1991.
42. Litovitz TL et al: 1991 annual report of the American Association of Poison Control Centers National Data Collection System, *Am J Emerg Med* 10(5):452, 1992.
43. Litovitz TL et al: 1992 annual report of the American Association of Poison Control Centers Toxic Exposure Surveillance System, *Am J Emerg Med* 11(5):494, 1993.
44. Majno G: *The healing hand,* Cambridge, Mass, 1975, Harvard University Press.
45. Markland F, Damus P: Purification and properties of a thrombin-like enzyme from the venom of *Crotalus adamanteus* (eastern diamondback rattlesnake), *J Biol Chem* 246:6460, 1971.
46. Matsen FA, Winquist RA, Krugmire RB: Diagnosis and management of compartmental syndromes, *J Bone Joint Surg* 62A(2):286, 1980.
47. McCullough NC, Gennaro JF: Evaluation of venomous snake-bite in the southern United States, *J Fla Med Assoc* 49:959, 1963.
48. McCullough NC, Gennaro JF: Treatment of venomous snake-bites. In *Snake venoms and envenomations,* New York, 1971, Marcel Dekker.
49. McGuire TC, Archer BG, Crawford TB: Equine IgG and IgG(T) antibodies—dependency of precipitability on both antigen and antibody structure, *Mol Immunol* 16:787, 1979.
50. Mebs D: Biochemistry of kinin-releasing enzymes in the venom of the viper *Bitis gabonica* and of the lizard *Heloderma suspectum.* In Sicuteri F, editor: *Bradykinin and related kinins: cardiovascular biochemical and neural actions,* New York, 1970, Plenum Press.
51. Mebs D, Raudonat HW: Biochemical investigations on *Heloderma* venom, *Inst Butantan Simp Int* 33:907, 1960.
52. Minton SA: Snakebite in the Midwestern region, *Indiana University Medical Center Bull* 14:28, 1952.
53. Minton SA: Snakes and snake venoms. In *Venom diseases,* Springfield, Ill, 1974, Charles C Thomas.
54. Minton SA: Electric shock treatment of snakebites, *Wilderness Med* 4(2):4, 1987.
55. Minton SA: Present tests for detection of snake venom: clinical applications, *Ann Emerg Med* 16:932, 1987.
56. Mubarak SJ, Owen CA, Hargens AR: Acute compartment syndromes: diagnosis and treatment with the aid of the wick catheter, *J Bone Joint Surg* 60A(8):1091, 1978.
57. Murrell G: The effectiveness of the pressure/immobilization first aid technique in the case of a tiger snake bite, *Med J Aust* 2(6):295, 1981.
58. Nobel GK, Schmidt A: The structure and function of facial and labial pits of snakes, *Proc Am Phil Soc* 77:263, 1937.
59. Norris RL, Dart RC: Apparent coral snake envenomation in a patient without fang marks, *Am J Emerg Med* 7:402, 1989.
60. Ownby CL: Pathology of rattlesnake envenomation. In Tu AT, editor: *Rattlesnake venoms,* New York, 1982, Marcel Dekker.
61. Ownby CL, Kainer RA, Tu AT: Pathogenesis of hemorrhage induced by rattlesnake venom, *Am J Pathol* 76(2):401, 1974.
62. Ownby CL et al: Ability of anti-venin to myotoxin A from prairie rattlesnake *(Crotalus viridis viridis)* venom to neutralize local myotoxicity and lethal effects of myotoxin A and homologous crude venom, *Toxicon* 21(1):35, 1983.
63. Pandya B, Rubin R, Olexa S: Unique degradation of human fibrinogen by proteases from western diamondback rattlesnake *(Crotalus atrox)* venom, *Toxicon* 21(4):515, 1983.
64. Parrish HM: Ophidiasis: an unusual occupational hazard, *Ind Med Surg* 27:63, 1958.
65. Parrish HM: Analysis of 450 fatalities from venomous animals in the United States, *Am J Med Sci* 245:129, 1963.
66. Parrish HM: Incidence of treated snakebites, *US Public Health Rep* 81:269, 1966.
67. Parrish HM, Goldner JC, Silverberg SL: Comparison between snakebites in children and adults, *Pediatrics* 36:251, 1965.
68. Parrish HM, Khan MS: Bites by coral snakes: report of 11 representative cases, *Am J Med Sci* 253:561, 1967.
69. Pattabhiraman TR, Bufkin DC, Russell FE: Some chemical and pharmacological properties of toxic fractions from the venom of the southern Pacific rattlesnake, II, *Proc West Pharmacol Soc* 17:227, 1974.
70. Patterson RA: Smooth muscle stimulating action of venom from the Gila monster *Heloderma suspectum, Toxicon* 7:321, 1969.

71. Pearn J et al: First-aid for snake-bite: efficacy of a constrictive bandage with limb immobilization in the management of human envenomation, *Med J Aust* 2(6):293, 1981.
72. Reid HA, Theakston DG: Changes in coagulation effects by venoms of *Crotalus atrox* as snakes age, *Am J Trop Med Hyg* 27:1053, 1978.
73. Rorabeck CH, Castle GSP, Logan J: The slit catheter: a new device for measuring intracompartmental pressures, *Orthop Surg,* p 515.
74. Russell FE: Snakebite. In Conn HF, editor: *Current therapy,* Philadelphia, 1958, WB Saunders.
75. Russell FE: First aid for snake venom poisoning, *Toxicon* 4:285, 1967.
76. Russell FE: Snake venom poisoning in the United States, *Med Arts Sci* 23:3, 1969.
77. Russell FE: *Snake venom poisoning.* Philadelphia, 1980, JB Lippincott.
78. Russell FE: Snake venom poisoning in the United States, *Annu Rev Med* 31:247, 1980.
79. Russell FE, Bogert C: Gila monster—its biology, venom and bite—a review, *Toxicon* 19(3):341, 1981.
80. Russell FE, Sullivan JB, Egen NB: Preparation of a new antivenin by affinity chromatography, *Am J Trop Med Hyg* 34:141, 1985.
81. Russell FE, Wingert WA: Unpublished data.
82. Schaeffer RC et al: The histochemistry of the venom glands of the rattlesnake *Crotalus viridis helleri, Toxicon* 10:295, 1972.
83. Schaeffer RC et al: The effects of colloidal and crystalloid fluids on rattlesnake venom shock in the rat, *J Pharmacol Exp Ther* 206:687, 1978.
84. Schaeffer RC et al: Cardiovascular failure produced by a peptide from the venom of the southern Pacific rattlesnake, *Crotalus viridis helleri, Toxicon* 17:447, 1979.
85. Simon TL, Grace TG: Envenomation coagulopathy in wounds from pit vipers, *N Engl J Med* 305:443, 1981.
86. Stahnke HL, Heffron WA, Lewis DL: Bite of the Gila monster, *Rocky Mt Med J* 67:25, 1970.
87. Stewart ME, Greenland S, Hoffman JB: First-aid treatment of poisonous snakebite: are currently recommended procedures justified? *Ann Emerg Med* 10:331, 1981.
88. Stoud C et al: Effect of electric shock therapy on local tissue reaction to poisonous snake venom injection in rabbits, *Ann Emerg Med* 18(4):447, 1989.
89. Sullivan JB: Past, present, and future immunotherapy of snake venom poisoning, *Ann Emerg Med* 16:938, 1987.
90. Sutherland SK: Serum reactions—an analysis of commercial antivenoms and the possible role of anticomplimentary activity in de-novo reactions to anti-venins and antitoxins, *Med J Aust* 1:613, 1977.
91. Sutherland SK, Coulter AR: Early management of bites by the eastern diamondback rattlesnake *(Crotalus adamanteus):* studies in monkeys *(Macaca faxciularis), Am J Trop Med Hyg* 30(2):497, 1981.
92. Sutherland SK, Coulter AR, Harris RD: Rationalization of first-aid measures for elapid snakebite, *Lancet* 183, 1979.
93. Sutherland SK et al: First aid for cobra *(Naja naja)* bites, *Ind J Med Res* 73:266, 1981.
94. Tallon RN et al: Letter to the editor, *N Engl J Med* 305:1347, 1981.
95. US Navy, Bureau of Medicine and Surgery: *Poisonous snakes of the world,* rev ed, Washington, DC, 1968, US Government Printing Office.
96. Van Riper W: Measuring the speed of a rattlesnake's strike, *Anim Kingdom* 57:50, 1954.
97. Waldesbuhl M, Renata A, Meylan A: Anticomplementary activity of gamma-immunoglobulins and their subunits, *Immunochemistry* 7:185, 1970.
98. Watt CJ, Gennaro JF: Pit viper bites in south Georgia and north Florida, *Trans South SA* 77:378, 1966.
99. Wingert WA, Chan LS: A review of rattlesnake bites and rationale for recommended treatment, *West J Med,* in press.
100. Wingert WA, Pattabirhaman T, Russell FE: Unpublished data.
101. Wingert WA, Wainschel J: Envenomation by poisonous snakes, *South Med J* 68:1015, 1975.
102. Zarafonetis CJD, Kalas JP: Serotonin degradation by homogenates of tissues from *Heloderma horridum,* the Mexican beaded lizard, *Nature* 195:701, 1962.
103. Zugaib M et al: Abruptio placentae following snakebite, *Am J Obstet Gynecol* 151:754, 1985.

29 NON–NORTH AMERICAN VENOMOUS REPTILE BITES

Sherman A. Minton
Robert L. Norris, Jr.

Snake envenomation is a significant cause of morbidity and mortality in some parts of the world. The only attempt to evaluate snakebite as a global problem was undertaken in 1954 under the auspices of the World Health Organization.[71] The estimate was an annual incidence of 300,000 bites with 30,000 to 40,000 deaths. Because the methodology was faulty, the estimate of incidence was probably much too low. Although reporting from many parts of the world is inadequate, there is general agreement that the highest incidence of snakebite occurs in regions where dense human populations coexist with a dense population of venomous snakes, people are engaged in agriculture by nonmechanized methods, and most people reside in small villages. Geographically, these regions include Southeast Asia, sub-Saharan Africa, and tropical America.

The epidemiologic patterns of snakebite in the United States and Europe have changed since 1950. Before that time the pattern largely involved persons engaged in agriculture or living in rural environments, although the number of snakebites was far fewer than those reported from tropical regions. Over the past 40 years the number of bites from handling captive snakes in a hazardous fashion has increased. In the experience of one of us, 50 of 97 bites by identified or presumed venomous snakes were inflicted by captive snakes; 33 bites were by snakes in private collections, rather than zoos or research institutions. Also increasing are venomous snake hunting and live capture by private individuals at community-sponsored events such as "rattlesnake roundups." The popularity of snake keeping as a hobby has increased greatly. While most species kept in captivity are not dangerous, some people regularly acquire venomous species and others do so occasionally. In a few cases venomous snakes are incorrectly identified and sold as innocuous species. Many of the snakes in the pet trade are not native to the nations where they are sold. Boa constrictors and ball pythons are harmless exotics popular in the United States, while the nonvenomous North American king snakes *(Lampropeltis)* and rat snakes *(Elaphe)* are popular in Europe. Venomous species also appear in the international trade. Cobras, large African vipers of the genus *Bitis,* and green arboreal vipers (*Trimeresurus* spp.) from Southeast Asia are among the species commonly sold in the United States, while rattlesnakes are prized by collectors in Europe. An informal survey in southern California indicated that nearly 2000 venomous snakes were kept by herpetologists and snake collectors in that area in the early 1960s.[61] Before 1960, bites by nonnative venomous snakes in the United States made up approximately 4% of total bites, largely confined to workers in research laboratories, zoos, and other public displays. However, in 1972, 15% of 410 hospital-treated snakebites were inflicted by nonnative species.[33] In the experience of one of us since 1981, 36 of 50 bites by captive venomous snakes were inflicted by nonnative species, with roughly a third by cobras. An emergency department physician in an urban hospital in the eastern or midwestern United States is almost as likely to be confronted with a bite of an exotic venomous snake as with that of a species native to North America.

Snakebite is a negligible hazard for tourists engaged in sight-seeing or recreation unless they deliberately capture or handle local reptiles. The risk for those involved in engineering projects, exploration, military operations, scientific fieldwork, and humanitarian activities in regions where venomous snakes are common is somewhat higher, but nevertheless small. Hardy[29] reported three bites by the large pit viper *Bothrops asper* during 1.5 million person-hours in the field at four operations in Belize, Costa Rica, and Guatemala.

Snakes of Medical Importance

Snakes are a distinctive and specialized group of reptiles represented by about 2700 species. However, their classification at the family level and beyond has always presented problems to taxonomists. Recent taxonomic changes involving medically important species include redivision of the pit viper genera *Agkistrodon* (North America and Asia), *Bothrops* (tropical America), and *Trimeresurus* (southern Asia) and the recognition that some wide-ranging species, such as the Asian cobra *(Naja naja)* and saw-scaled viper *(Echis carinatus),* are actually groups of several similar species. A summary of the major snake families is given in Table 29-1. All species in the families Viperidae, Elapidae, Hydrophiidae, and Atractaspididae, plus an unknown but significant number in the family Colubridae, are venomous. Box 29-1 lists the most medically important venomous species for certain areas of the world.

COBRAS

Strictly speaking, these are snakes of the genus *Naja,* but the term is often applied to other snakes of cobralike habitus, particularly the king cobra *(Ophiophagus hannah),* ringhals *(Hemachatus),* water cobras *(Boulengerina),* and tree cobras *(Pseudohaje).* Spreading the neck to form a hood is common to all, although this behavior is seen in numerous other snakes of several families, including some nonvenomous species. Nearly all cobras are large snakes, 1.2 to 2.5 m in total length, with the king cobra occasionally reaching 5 m. Cobras of the genus *Naja* occur throughout Africa and tropical and subtropical Asia, except in deserts. They live in a wide variety of habitats and adapt well to agricultural and suburban situations. The king cobra is restricted to forest areas in southeastern Asia; the ringhals, water cobras, and tree cobras inhabit sub-Saharan Africa. The African *Naja nigricollis, N. mossambica,* and *Hemachatus* have fangs modified for ejecting jets of venom anteriorly and somewhat upward for distances up to 3 m with remarkable accuracy; these are the "spitting cobras." This habit is rarely seen in Southeast Asian cobras.

MAMBAS

Mambas are slender elapid snakes constituting the genus *Dendroaspis.* They are usually 1.5 to 2.2 m long, although the black mamba *(D. polylepis)* may reach 4 m. There are four species, which inhabit most of tropical Africa. Mambas are at least partially arboreal, very alert and active, and aggressive under some circumstances.

KRAITS

There are about a dozen species of south Asian elapids of the genus *Bungarus.* Their average lengths are 1 to 1.2 m,

Table 29-1 Major Snake Families

Group	Distribution	Remarks
Blind snakes Families: Typhlopidae and Leptotyphlopidae	Tropical and warm temperate zones	Very small, wormlike snakes; none venomous
Boas and pythons Family: Boidae	Mostly tropical and warm temperate zones; pythons in Old World only	Includes both large and small species; none venomous
"Typical" snakes Family: Colubridae	Almost worldwide except for Arctic, Antarctic, southern Australia, and certain islands	Large and extremely varied family; many species with venom glands and posterior maxillary fangs, but few capable of causing clinically significant envenomation
Burrowing asps Family: Atractaspididae	Africa, limited areas of Middle East	About 15 species, all venomous; rather small burrowers; large maxillary fangs used singly with backward stabbing motion
Cobras, mambas, coral snakes, kraits, and others Family: Elapidae	Tropical and warm temperate zones	About 180 species, all venomous; fangs at anterior end of maxillae
Sea snakes Family: Hydrophiidae	Mostly Southeast Asian and Australian coastal waters	About 50 species, all venomous; fangs similar to those of Elapidae
Pit vipers Family: Viperidae Subfamily: Crotalinae	The Americas and much of Asia	About 120 species, all venomous; highly movable fangs on much reduced maxillae; heat-sensing pits between eyes and nostrils
Old World vipers Family: Viperidae Subfamily: Viperinae	Africa, Europe, and Asia	About 40 species, all venomous; fangs like those of pit vipers; no heat-sensing pits

BOX 29-1
THE MOST IMPORTANT SPECIES OF VENOMOUS SNAKES IN VARIOUS REGIONS OF THE WORLD

UNITED STATES AND CANADA

Diamondback rattlesnakes *(Crotalus adamanteus* [Color Plate 16] and *C. atrox)*
Timber rattlesnake *(C. horridus)* (Color Plate 17)
Prairie rattlesnake *(C. viridis viridis)*
Pacific rattlesnake *(C. viridis helleri* and *C. v. oreganus)*
Pigmy rattlesnake *(Sistrurus miliarius)* (Color Plate 15)
Copperhead *(Agkistrodon contortrix)* (Color Plate 19)
Cottonmouth *(Agkistrodon piscivorus)* (Color Plate 18)

MEXICO, CENTRAL AMERICA, WEST INDIES

Western diamondback rattlesnake *(Crotalus atrox)*
Mexican west-coast rattlesnake *(C. basiliscus)*
Tropical rattlesnake *(C. durissus),* several subspecies
Cantil *(Agkistrodon bilineatus)*
Terciopelo, barba amarilla *(Bothrops asper)*
Fer-de-lance *(Bothrops lanceolatus, B. caribbaeus)*
Lora, green palm viper *(Bothriechis lateralis)*
Eyelash viper *(Bothriechis schlegelii)*
Hognose viper *(Porthidium nasutum)*
Central American coral snake *(Micrurus nigrocinctus)*

NORTHERN SOUTH AMERICA (TO ABOUT 15° S)

Tropical rattlesnake *(Crotalus durissus),* several subspecies
Terciopelo, mapana, vibora equis *(Bothrops asper* and *B. atrox)*
Neuwied's lancehead *(Bothrops neuwiedi)*
Amazonian tree viper *(Bothriopsis bilineata)*
Hognose vipers *(Porthidium nasutum, P. lansbergii)*
Bushmaster *(Lachesis muta)* (Color Plate 28)
Amazonian coral snake *(Micrurus spixii)*
Red-tail coral snake *(M. mipartitus)*

SOUTHERN SOUTH AMERICA

Brazilian rattlesnake *(Crotalus durissus terrificus)*
Jararaca *(Bothrops jararaca)*
Jararacussu *(B. jararacussu)*
Neuwied's lancehead *(B. neuwiedi)*
Urutu *(B. alternatus)*
Southern coral snake *(Micrurus frontalis)*

EUROPE

European viper *(Vipera berus)*
Asp viper *(V. aspis)*
Nose-horned viper *(V. ammodytes)*

NEAR AND MIDDLE EAST

Levantine viper *(Vipera lebetina)*
Palestine viper *(V. palaestinae)*
Saw-scaled vipers *(Echis carinatus* and *E. coloratus)*
Desert horned viper *(Cerastes cerastes)*

INDIAN SUBCONTINENT AND SRI LANKA

Russell's viper *(Vipera russellii)*
Saw-scale viper *(Echis carinatus)*
Hump-nose viper *(Hypnale hypnale)*
Indian krait *(Bungarus caeruleus)*
Asian cobras *(Naja naja* and *N. kaouthia)*
Sea snakes, especially the beaked sea snake *(Enhydrina schistosa),* important in some coastal areas.

SOUTHEAST ASIA INCLUDING PHILIPPINES AND MOST OF INDONESIA

Russell's viper *(Vipera russellii)* (Color Plate 29)
Malayan pit viper *(Calloselasma rhodostoma)*
White-lipped tree viper *(Trimeresurus albolabris)*
Wagler's pit viper, temple viper *(T. wagleri)*
Mangrove viper *(T. purpureomaculatus)*
Malayan krait *(Bungarus candidus)*
Asian cobras (chiefly *Naja atra, N. kaouthia, N. philippiensis, N. sputatrix,* and *N. sumatrana*)
King cobra *(Ophiophagus hannah)*
Beaked sea snake *(Enhydrina schistosa)*
Annulated sea snake *(Hydrophis cyanocinctus)*
Hardwicke's sea snake *(Lapemis curtus hardwickii)*

FAR EAST (EASTERN CHINA, TAIWAN, KOREA, JAPAN)

Mamushis *(Agkistrodon blomhoffii, A. halys, A. intermedius)*
Hundred-pace snake *(Deinagkistrodon acutus)*
Okinawa habu *(Trimeresurus flavoviridis)*
Chinese habu *(T. mucrosquamatus)*
Chinese green tree viper *(T. stejnegeri)*
Many-banded krait *(Bungarus multicinctus)* (Color Plate 30)
Chinese cobra *(Naja atra)* (Color Plate 31)
Annulated sea snake *(Hydrophis cyanocinctus)*

NORTHERN AUSTRALIA, NEW GUINEA AND ASSOCIATED ISLANDS

Death adders *(Acanthophis antarcticus* and *A. praelongus)*
Taipan *(Oxyuranus scutellatus)* (Color Plate 32)
Mulga snake, king brown snake *(Pseudechis australis)*
Papuan black snake *(Pseudechis papuanus)*
Brown snakes *(Pseudonaja textilis, P. nuchalis)*
Ikaheka snake *(Micropechis ikaheka)*
Sea snakes, particularly *Astrotia stokesi, Aipysurus laevis, Lapemis curtus*

SOUTHERN AUSTRALIA AND TASMANIA

Tiger snakes *(Notechis scutatus* [Color Plate 33] and *N. ater)*
Copperhead *(Austrelaps superbus)*
Death adder *(Acanthophis antarcticus)*
Mulga snake, king brown snake *(Pseudechis australis)*

BOX 29-1

THE MOST IMPORTANT SPECIES OF VENOMOUS SNAKES IN VARIOUS REGIONS OF THE WORLD—cont'd

Red-bellied black snake *(Pseudechis porphyriacus)*
Brown snakes *(Pseudonaja)*, several species

NORTH AFRICA TO SOUTHERN EDGE OF SAHARA

Desert horned viper *(Cerastes cerastes)*
Saw-scale vipers *(Echis pyramidum, E. ocellatus)*
North African rock viper *(Vipera mauritanica)*
Puff adder *(Bitis arietans)*
Egyptian cobra *(Naja haje)*
Spitting cobra *(Naja pallida)*
Burrowing asp *(Atractaspis microlepidota)*

CENTRAL AND SOUTHERN AFRICA

Saw-scale vipers *(Echis pyramidum, E. ocellatus)*
Puff adder *(Bitis arietans)*
Rhinocerus viper *(B. nasicornis)*
Gaboon viper *(B. gabonica)*
Green tree viper *(Atheris squamiger)*
Night adders *(Causus rhombeatus, C. maculatus)*
Spitting cobras *(Naja mossambica, N. nigricollis)*
Egyptian cobra *(N. haje)*
Cape cobra *(N. nivea)*
Ringhals *(Hemachatus haemachatus)*
Black mamba *(Dendroaspis polylepis)*
Green mambas *(D. angusticeps* [Color Plate 34], *D. viridis)*
Burrowing asps *(Atractaspis)*, several species
Boomslang *(Dispholidus typus)* (Color Plate 35)

with two species reaching 2 m. They have short fangs and highly toxic venom, are nocturnal, and are often found close to human dwellings. Bites are uncommon, but the case fatality rate is high.

CORAL SNAKES

All medically important species of coral snakes are in the genus *Micrurus*, which includes about 50 species distributed from the southern United States to central Argentina. Nearly all are in the 0.6 to 1.2 m size range. Most have tricolor patterns of red, yellow, and black. A few species are bicolor. It must be emphasized that the rules and mnemonics for distinguishing coral snakes from their mimics become progressively less reliable from central Mexico southward, something a few herpetologists have learned to their sorrow. Coral snakes are secretive and not often encountered. The dozen or so species of oriental coral snakes *(Calliophis, Maticora)* are widely distributed, but uncommon and little known.

AUSTRALIAN ELAPIDS

Elapids are the dominant snakes of Australia, New Guinea, and islands north to the Solomons; there are about 85 species. All are fairly closely related and seem to be part of one evolutionary radiation, which also includes the sea snakes. In appearance, the diverse lot ranges from small (40 to 60 cm) and essentially innocuous burrowers to the coastal taipan *(Oxyuranus scutellatus)*, which may reach a length of 3.3 m and is occasionally aggressive. The death adders *(Acanthophis)* are viperlike in appearance with wide heads and thick bodies. Other dangerous species are the tiger snakes *(Notechis)*, which may be plentiful in the well-populated eastern coastal districts of Australia, the brown snakes *(Pseudonaja)*, which are quick and may be dangerous if cornered, and large snakes of the genus *Pseudechis*, which includes the red-bellied black snake *(P. porphyriacus)* and king brown snake *(P. australis)*. The venoms of most of these snakes are highly toxic.

SEA SNAKES

The 50 or so species of sea snakes inhabit tropical and subtropical sections of the western Pacific and Indian Oceans over the continental shelves, but the pelagic sea snake *(Pelamis platurus)* also occurs on the western coasts of America from Baja California to Ecuador and is occasionally found in Hawaiian waters. Similarity in plasma and venom proteins indicates that sea snakes are closely related to Australian terrestrial elapids. (See Chapter 52 for additional information.)

EURASIAN VIPERS

The genus *Vipera* includes approximately a dozen species. Russell's viper *(V. russelli)* is found from Pakistan to Taiwan and is one of the world's most dangerous snakes, having a highly lethal venom. It adapts well to agricultural environments. Other dangerous large species are the Levantine viper *(V. lebetina)*, found from North Africa to Pakistan, and the Palestine viper *(V. palaestinae)*, which is native to the Middle East. The European viper *(V. berus)* has one of the most extensive ranges of any land snake and is found from the British Isles to Korea and the eastern limits of the former USSR. It is relatively small (60 to 75 cm). Other species important in Europe are the asp viper *(V. aspis)*, Iberian viper *(V. latasti)*, and nose-horned viper *(V. ammodytes)*. These cause numerous bites, but the case fatality rate is low.

DESERT VIPERS

The saw-scaled vipers *(Echis)* may cause more fatalities than any other snakes in the world.[84] These snakes live in arid and semiarid regions from India through the Middle East to west Africa; however, they often thrive on cultivated land. Their name comes from the sawtooth ridges on the lateral scales that are rubbed together to produce a warning sound. These small snakes are rarely more than 60 cm in length but are highly irritable and quick to strike. The venoms cause severe coagulopathy. *Cerastes* has two species in North Africa and the Middle East, including the horned viper of Egypt. These snakes are highly adapted to desert conditions. They are relatively small, and their bites are rarely fatal. Two other species in this group are the Persian horned viper *(Pseudocerastes persicus)* and the leaf-nosed viper *(Eristicophis macmahoni)*, both occurring in the Middle East and Pakistan. They are uncommon and of little medical importance.

AFRICAN VIPERS

The genus *Bitis* has 12 species and occurs throughout Africa exclusive of the northern deserts. The wide-ranging puff adder *(B. arietans)* also occurs in western Saudi Arabia. All are stout, wide-headed snakes. They vary in size from *B. peringueyi* (rarely exceeds 30 cm) to the Gaboon viper *(B. gabonica)*, which may reach a length of 2 m and a weight of about 10 kg. Habitat ranges from desert to rainforest. The puff adder is a major cause of snakebites in most parts of Africa where it is found. It prefers grassland and often lives near villages. *Atheris* is an arboreal African viper genus with eight species. The snakes are usually 50 to 65 cm long, and some have a bizarre appearance that makes them popular with zoos and hobbyists; bites are infrequent. Night adders of the genus *Causus* are widespread in Africa south of the Sahara. They are usually 50 to 70 cm long and may be plentiful around fields and villages. Bites are numerous, but fatalities are almost unknown.

AGKISTRODON COMPLEX PIT VIPERS

The 15 species in this pit viper group are found from the eastern United States to Central America and throughout much of Asia. They are characterized by large shields on the crown of the head—a presumably primitive condition in viperid snakes. American copperheads *(A. contortrix)* and cottonmouths *(A. piscivorus)* are discussed in Chapter 28. The closely related cantil *(A. bilineatus)* is native to Mexico and Central America. The mamushi *(A. blomhoffii)* of Japan, Korea, and eastern China, Siberian pit viper *(A. halys)* of Asian Russia and Mongolia, and the Central Asian pit viper *(A. intermedius)*, found from Iran to Korea, are all common snakes, usually 60 to 80 cm long and of moderate build. They are the only venomous snakes in much of central and northeastern Asia and cause many snakebites. The case fatality rate is low. The Malayan pit viper *(Calloselasma rhodostoma)* is a distinctive species of Southeast Asia that inhabits forests at low elevation and is particularly common on rubber plantations. It is a major cause of snakebites. The hundred-pace snake *(Deinagkistrodon acutus)* is a large (1.2 to 1.5 m) snake with a strongly upturned snout. It is native to forests in south China and Taiwan and is dangerous, but uncommon.

ASIAN LANCE-HEAD PIT VIPERS

In older terminology, this is the genus *Trimeresurus*, now subdivided by many herpetologists. It includes approximately 40 species. They are distributed from southern India to Indonesia, the Philippines, and the southern islands of Japan. The most dangerous species are large (to 2.3 m), slender snakes with very wide heads. They are often called *habus*, a Japanese name, are mostly terrestrial, and may have large populations in sugarcane fields and other areas of cultivation. The Okinawa habu *(T. flavoviridis)* accounts for a high incidence of snakebites on the southern Ryukyu Islands.[63] The Chinese habu *(T. mucrosquamatus)* has a wide range in Southeast Asia and is another plentiful and dangerous species. Arboreal species are often predominantly green, are 60 to 100 cm long, and are found throughout the range of the group. *T. albolabris*, the white-lipped bamboo viper, is the most widely distributed member of this group. These vipers cause many snakebites, but fatalities are rare. A third group (*Ovophis* to some) includes five species of stout, short vipers found in mountainous terrain. They seem to be of little medical importance. Wagler's pit viper is a widely distributed arboreal species usually assigned to the genus *Tropidolaemus*. Its venom contains a peculiar heat-stable toxin; however, bites do not seem to differ from those of arboreal *Trimeresurus*.

NEOTROPICAL PIT VIPERS

Most of these snakes were formerly assigned to the genus *Bothrops*, which ranges from eastern Mexico to southern Argentina and on a few islands of the West Indies. The genus contains approximately 30 species, most of which are of medical importance. These are medium to long snakes (0.7 to 2.5 m) of moderate to heavy build with distinct triangular heads. Habitat ranges from semiarid grasslands to rainforests; several species adapt well to banana and sugarcane plantations. Among the more dangerous species are *B. atrox, B. asper, B. jararaca,* and *B. lanceolatus.* While they have many Spanish and Portuguese names, the name "fer-de-lance" is often used for these snakes in English language publications. Species of *Bothrops* account for most of the serious snakebites in Latin America. Fifteen arboreal species formerly in *Bothrops* are now in the genera *Bothriopsis* and *Bothriechis.* They are slender snakes with large heads and are 50 to 100 cm in length. Most have the color green in their pattern. The eyelash viper *(Bothriechis schlegelii)* is a well-known example that accounts for about 20% of venomous snakebites in Costa Rica. Fatalities are rare. Fourteen other former *Bothrops* species constitute the genus *Porthidium,* which has been further subdivided by some authorities. These are small to moderate-sized (45 to 100 cm) snakes with heavy bodies and wide heads. They are found from eastern Mexico to northern South America, usually in forests and often in highlands. They are terrestrial. Bites are fairly common, but fatalities very rare. The bushmaster *(Lachesis muta)* is the largest pit viper, usually 1.5 to 2.5 m, but occasionally reaching 3.6 m. It has extraordinarily rough scales in the middorsal region and a distinct tail spine. It is found in lowland forests from southern Nicaragua to eastern Brazil and is uncommon. Bushmaster bites are rare, but the case fatality rate is high.

RATTLESNAKES

The 31 species of rattlesnakes occur from southern Canada to Uruguay and eastern Argentina, although only two species occur south of the isthmus of Tehuantepec in Mexico. All except one insular species in Baja California can be identified by the presence of a rattle. Rattlesnakes are discussed in detail in Chapter 28.

BURROWING ASPS

The 15 species of the genus *Atractaspis* were formerly considered vipers because they have viperlike fangs; however, they have several unique features that justify their recognition as a separate family. They are small (50 to 80 cm), moderately slender with small heads, and uniformly black or brown. They are found throughout most of sub-Saharan Africa and in small areas of the Middle East. They frequent habitats ranging from forest to semidesert and are burrowers that may emerge at night and after rains. Bites are fairly common in some parts of Africa, but fatalities are infrequent.

COLUBRID SNAKES

The colubrids are an enormous and taxonomically untidy family of snakes that lack anterior fangs and the primitive features associated with boas and a few other groups of snakes (labial heat-sensing pits, pelvic spurs, and so on). Some herpetologists partition this family, but there is little agreement on what divisions should be recognized. In most parts of the world they make up the majority of snake species and are absent only from the Arctic and Antarctic, southern Australia, and some islands. Many species have grooved fangs in the rear of the upper jaw and others have enlarged but ungrooved rear teeth. While the vast majority of these species are harmless, more than 50 species of colubrid snakes in 30 genera have caused human envenoming. The great majority of cases are mild because the venom-injecting apparatus is inefficient and the quantity of venom small. There have, however, been serious and fatal envenomations.[45] Most colubrid bites involve the handling of snakes believed to be harmless. Among the more important species are the boomslang *(Dispholidus),* twig snakes (*Thelotornis* spp.), Japanese garter snake *(Rhabdophis tigrinus),* and brown treesnake *(Boiga irregularis).*

Venom Apparatus

The venom apparatus of snakes functions mainly to immobilize and kill prey, although it may also be an important means of defense. Some modification of dentition is seen in all venomous snakes, although in some colubrids it may be no more than enlargement of a pair of posterior maxillary teeth. The most highly modified dentition is that of vipers, in which a single large tubular or deeply grooved fang is attached to a greatly reduced maxillary bone. These fangs have a wide range of rocking movement. Burrowing asps (*Atractaspis* spp.) have large viperlike fangs used one at a time with a backward stabbing motion as the lower jaw is shifted to the opposite side. They can bite with the mouth virtually closed. Fangs of elapid snakes are short, tubular or grooved, and attached to a longer maxillary bone that may bear additional teeth and has a limited degree of rocking movement. Fangs of sea snakes are even shorter; the maxillary bone is long and usually bears additional teeth. Fangs of colubrids are at the rear of the maxillary bone and nearly always preceded by additional teeth. The fangs often are grooved.

Snake venoms are produced in a pair of glands usually located between the eye and the angle of the mouth, although in one genus of oriental elapids *(Maticora),* two species of burrowing asps *(Atractaspis),* and two species of night adders *(Causus)* the glands are tubular and extend well back into the body. Histologic and histochemical studies show secretory cells of various types in all snake venom glands.[5,36] Space for venom storage in the lumen of the gland is greatest in viperids and some elapids (such as cobras), less in other elapids and sea snakes, and very small in colubrids. Musculature for emptying the glands is best developed in viperids, moderately effective in elapids and sea snakes, and relatively ineffective in colubrids. This is reflected in quantities of venom injected in natural bites and amounts that can be obtained by extraction.

Snake Venoms

There is an immense volume of literature on the biochemistry and pharmacology of snake venoms. The venoms themselves are colorless to amber liquids whose solid content is mostly protein. Pharmacologically active substances include enzymes, polypeptide toxins, glycoproteins, and substances such as nucleotides, small peptides, and biogenic amines. Many of the enzymes and toxins are very stable. Dried snake venoms can retain lethality and some enzyme activity after three decades of storage.

The postsynaptic neurotoxins are probably the best understood snake venom toxins. These are found in most elapid and sea snake venoms. They bind to the nicotinic acetylcholine receptors competitively with acetylcholine and produce a nondepolarizing neuromuscular blockade. The short toxins have 60 to 62 amino acids and four disulfide bridges; the long toxins have 71 to 74 amino acids and five disulfide bridges.

Presynaptic neurotoxins inhibit release of acetylcholine at the neuromuscular junction. Toxins in this group have phospholipase A_2 activity, occur in a variety of elapid and viper venoms, and are similar to myotoxins in some sea snake venoms. The phospholipases of this group have 110 to 125 amino acids and six or seven disulfide bonds. Their neurotoxicity and myotoxicity are not related to hydrolytic activity.

With the exception of sea snake venom, nearly all snake venoms affect blood coagulation, although not always to a clinically significant degree. Thrombinlike activity that converts fibrinogen to fibrin is characteristic of pit viper venoms. The fibrin so formed is abnormal and easily lysed. Enzymes responsible for this activity have been isolated from venoms of the Malayan pit viper *(Calloselasma)*, eastern diamondback rattlesnake *(Crotalus adamanteus)*, hundred-pace snake *(Deinagkistrodon)*, and jararaca *(Bothrops jararaca)*. These enzymes in sublethal doses produce nonclotting blood and do not cause platelet aggregation. Prothrombin activation with formation of thrombin is seen particularly with venoms of the Russell's viper *(Vipera russelli)* and saw-scaled vipers (*Echis* spp.). It is also seen with venoms of several Australian elapid snakes, some pit vipers, and the dangerous colubrid snakes. Enzymes responsible have been isolated from Russell's viper and saw-scaled viper venoms. Some venoms have more than one type of anticoagulant activity.

Hemorrhage and necrosis are commonly seen with snakebites, particularly those inflicted by vipers. Although commonly attributed to proteolytic enzymes, several hemorrhagic factors that have been isolated have little or no proteolytic activity.[53] Disruption of the vascular basement membrane is their main mode of action.

Extensive myonecrosis is often seen with bites by sea snakes, some Australian elapids, and some rattlesnakes. Myotoxins have been isolated from several venoms. Most myotoxins show phospholipase A_2 activity, which is more pronounced in those derived from elapids.

The so-called cardiotoxin first described from cobra venom and subsequently found in venoms of some other related snakes is a strongly basic polypeptide whose basic action is to produce irreversible depolarization of cell membranes. A specific cardiotoxin with quite different structure and action is found in venoms of some burrowing asps. Its action is directly on the heart, producing atrioventricular block.[89]

Hyaluronidase has been reported from nearly all reptilian venoms studied. It facilitates spread and absorption of other venom components. A number of other enzymes, such as phosphodiesterase, L-amino acid oxidase, 5′ nucleotidase, and acetylcholinesterase, are present in many snake venoms, but their roles in clinical snake envenomation are poorly understood. Most of the clinical effects of envenomation result from several venom components acting in concert, so venom effects may be compounded by endogenous release of autopharmacologic compounds such as histamine and bradykinin.

Signs and Symptoms of Snake Venom Poisoning

The complexity and diversity of snake venoms are reflected in the wide array of signs and symptoms that can occur after envenomation. The precise clinical picture and degree of severity of any specific venomous snakebite depend on many factors, including the species of snake and its age, size, health, and geographic origin, the anatomic location of the bite, the size and health of the victim, what therapeutic interventions are employed, and so forth. The treating physician must anticipate multisystem dysfunction in any victim of snake venom poisoning. The patient is best served by the doctor who remains vigilant for any constellation of signs, symptoms, and laboratory findings regardless of the species of snake implicated. A general description of presenting signs and symptoms for the various families of venomous snakes is found in Box 29-2.

ELAPIDS

Local findings after most elapid envenomations are unimpressive compared to those seen after typical viperid venom poisoning (see below) (Color Plate 36). In many cases it may be difficult to find distinct fang marks.[69,92] The degree of pain varies depending on the species involved. Often local pain is a minor complaint, but it may be significant after bites by certain cobra species such as the king cobra *(Ophiophagus hannah)*.[24] Regional lymphadenopathy may be present. While significant local soft tissue swelling is uncommon after most elapid envenomations,[12] some

BOX 29-2

SIGNS AND SYMPTOMS AFTER SNAKE VENOM POISONING

ELAPIDS (COBRAS, MAMBAS, KRAITS, AUSTRALIAN VENOMOUS SNAKES, CORAL SNAKES)

Local

Findings may be absent or minimal
Significant pain occurs with some species
Regional lymphadenopathy
Necrosis occurs with some species

Systemic

Neurotoxicity (cranial nerve dysfunction, altered mental status, peripheral weakness and paralysis, respiratory failure)
Cardiovascular failure
Coagulopathy
Myonecrosis
Renal failure

SEA SNAKES

Local

Trivial
Fang marks may be difficult to identify

Systemic

Neurotoxicity (cranial nerve dysfunction, peripheral weakness and paralysis, respiratory failure)
Myotoxicity with resulting muscle pain and tenderness, myoglobinemia, myoglobinuria, and hyperkalemia (may precipitate cardiac dysrhythmias and renal failure)

VIPERS AND PIT VIPERS

Local

Pain
Soft tissue swelling
Regional lymphadenopathy
Ecchymosis, bloody exudate from fang marks
Early absence of local findings does not rule out significant envenomation
Local necrosis may be significant

Systemic

Essentially any organ system may be involved
Cardiovascular toxicity (hypotension, pulmonary edema)
Neurotoxicity (cranial nerve dysfunction, peripheral weakness) with some species
Hemorrhagic diathesis (bleeding from any system is possible)
Renal failure

BURROWING ASPS

Local

Single fang puncture mark common
Pain
Some swelling
Occasional local necrosis

Systemic

Nausea, vomiting
Diaphoresis
Fever
Occasional respiratory distress, cardiac dysrhythmias (A-V block)
Rare fatalities

COLUBRIDS (REAR-FANGED)

Local

Mild to moderate local swelling, pain, and ecchymosis
Bloody exudate from fang marks

Systemic

Nausea, vomiting
Coagulopathy with its attendant complications
Renal dysfunction

species, such as the African spitting cobras *(Naja mossambica* and *N. nigricollis)*[76,77] and some of the Asiatic cobras (*Naja naja* spp.),[59,67,75] may produce early edema as an indication of envenomation.

The swelling can progress with time to involve the entire bitten extremity. With some of these species, local tissue necrosis may be profound (Color Plate 37).[58,60,75,76,86] Some Australian elapids, such as the taipan (*Oxyuranus* spp.) and tiger snake (*Notechis* spp.), are capable of inducing significant myonecrosis and coagulopathy as well.[18,22,58,60,92] Renal failure has been reported as a complication of envenomation by some elapids.[13,30,60]

Neurotoxicity is a major component of the clinical picture seen after most elapid envenomations. The time of onset of neuropathic signs and symptoms after envenomation is quite variable. It appears to be most rapid after serious cobra and mamba bites, and most delayed after some coral snake envenomations. In certain situations the onset may be delayed for 10 hours or more.[60] The earliest systemic manifestations of envenomation by most elapids are signs of cranial nerve dysfunction (especially ptosis, but also difficulty swallowing, dysphonia, and blurred vision).[75] Paresthesias, muscle fasciculations, peripheral weakness, and paralysis, including paralysis of respiratory muscles, may soon follow.[94] Alteration of mental status (drowsiness, hallucinations) is not uncommon.[75] Other associated systemic symptoms include hypersalivation and diaphoresis.[12,54] In cases of severe envenomation, cardiovascular depression may result in hypotension and pulmonary edema.[60,90]

Eye exposure to venom from any of the spitting cobras or ringhals results in immediate burning pain and tearing. Significant systemic absorption does not occur after such exposure, but corneal ulceration, uveitis, and permanent blindness can follow untreated incidents.[60,85] Bites by spitting cobras often manifest violent local reactions with hemorrhages and necrosis, but rarely neurotoxicity.

SEA SNAKES

Local findings at the bite site after sea snake envenomation are usually trivial. In serious cases, systemic symptoms usually appear within 2 hours.[79] The bite site may show several tiny puncture wounds from the fangs and other teeth, but local pain and soft tissue swelling are negligible (Color Plate 38). The fang marks may be difficult to see if not diligently sought.[80]

Sea snake venoms demonstrate significant neurotoxicity in animal studies and in human envenomations.[13,60,80] Neurologic dysfunction is manifested by hypersalivation, dysphagia, dysarthria, muscle spasm, and paralysis.* Patients remain conscious if hypoxia is prevented.[80] Envenomation is also characterized by trismus[54] and significant, diffuse myopathic findings.[58,60] The myotoxic components of sea snake venoms may cause a tremendous outpouring of potassium and myoglobin from injured muscle. Hyperkalemia may precipitate cardiac dysrhythmias; myoglobinuria can lead to acute renal failure.[7] Untreated sea snake envenomation may cause significant muscle pain and weakness for months.[58,60] Death after sea snake envenomation may result from respiratory failure caused by paralysis of the diaphragm, hyperkalemic cardiac arrest, or acute renal failure.[80] More information regarding sea snakes can be found in Chapter 52.

VIPERS AND PIT VIPERS (VIPERIDS)

The effects of envenomation by Eurasian and African vipers and Asian and neotropical pit vipers are very similar to those seen after bites by the pit vipers of North America, as discussed in Chapter 28. Severe pain, local soft tissue swelling, subcutaneous ecchymosis, and bloody exudation from the fang marks begin within minutes. Regional lymphadenopathy may be present within 30 to 60 minutes, and soft tissue swelling may progress to impressive proportions over several hours. The trunk and even the contralateral extremity may become edematous. Lack of soft tissue swelling does not rule out the possibility of significant envenomation.[51] After 12 to 24 hours, serum-filled vesicles and hemorrhagic bullae may appear and ecchymoses may spread throughout the involved extremity.[13]

Systemic envenomation may result in a vast array of signs and symptoms such as blurred vision, alteration in taste sensation, weakness, dizziness, diaphoresis, nausea, vomiting, diarrhea, fever, headache, abdominal pain, and bleeding at any of a number of anatomic sites.[2,44,54,60] Hypotension and shock may occur over a variable time course. Early on, hypotension is caused primarily by pooling of blood in the pulmonary and splanchnic vasculatures. After several hours, transudation of fluid into the bitten extremity and peritoneal cavity, hemolysis, and systemic bleeding may play a role.

Coagulopathy is a characteristic finding after systemic venom poisoning by saw-scaled vipers (*Echis* spp.)[15,32,44,56,60] and is also seen after bites by individuals of some populations of *Vipera russelli* and many neotropical and Asian pit vipers.[51] Victims can bleed at any of a number of sites, including the bite wound, soft tissues, gastrointestinal tract, respiratory tract, brain, and kidneys. The venoms of some populations of *V. russelli* are also capable of producing massive intravascular coagulation and hemolysis.[34,51]

While neurologic findings after pit viper venom poisoning in North America are uncommon, they have been reported after bites by the South American rattlesnake (*Crotalus durissus*) and by a number of vipers in the Eastern hemisphere, including the Berg adder (*Bitis atropos*),[85] Palestine viper (*Vipera palaestinae*)[15,81] and some populations of Russell's viper (*V. russelli*).[83] Such signs and symptoms may include cranial nerve dysfunction, muscle paralysis, and respiratory failure.[31,49]

Patients may have an altered sensorium (from lethargy to coma) as a result of hypotension, hypoxia, intracranial bleeding, and possibly direct venom effects. While seizures have been reported, they are uncommon and probably secondary to cerebral hypoxia.

Multifactorial renal failure may occur as a complication of viperid envenomation, much as it does with North American pit vipers or Australian elapids. Etiologic factors include myoglobinuria, hemoglobinuria, hypotension, and possibly direct venom nephrotoxicity. This is especially common after bites of the Russell's viper and saw-scaled viper (*Echis carinatus*).[13,56,60] Onset may be delayed for several days, and any complaints of costovertebral angle pain should arouse suspicion of impending renal failure.[51]

Local bite site necrosis and myonecrosis may be severe after viperid envenomation and may necessitate surgical intervention (grafting procedures or amputations).[44] While the vast majority of effective bites by viperids result in venom deposition into subcutaneous tissues, the possibility of subfascial injection exists. In these rare cases, direct myotoxic-

*References 23, 57, 59, 66, 79, 80.

ity can produce muscle necrosis. If muscle swelling is significant, a compartment syndrome may develop. The signs and symptoms of a compartment syndrome are closely mimicked by the findings after a typical subcutaneous envenomation (swelling, discoloration or cyanosis, pain on palpation, paresthesias). The diagnosis of a compartment syndrome can be confirmed by documenting elevated intracompartmental pressures. This has significant treatment implications, as discussed below.

BURROWING ASPS

Envenomation by any of the burrowing asps (*Atractaspis* spp.) may result in severe symptoms, although fatalities have thus far been reported from only *A. microlepidota* and *A. irregularis*.[15-17] Patients bitten by these snakes may have severe local pain followed by numbness, soft tissue swelling, lymphadenopathy, vomiting, diaphoresis, and fever.[15,17,85] Systemic coagulopathies may occur.[15,17,26] Local vesicles can be seen at the bite site, and local tissue necrosis occurs rarely.[10,17,85] The cause of death after experimental *Atractaspis* envenomation has been attributed to venom-induced coronary vasospasm.[39]

COLUBRIDS (DISPHOLIDUS, THELOTORNIS, RHABDOPHIS)

Envenomation by some of the rear-fanged colubrids may have severe consequences. Fatalities have been reported after bites by the boomslang *(Dispholidus typus),* the bird or twig snake *(Thelotornis kirtlandii),* and the Japanese garter snake or yamakagashi *(Rhabdophis tigrinus)*.[38,46,48] Severe, life-threatening envenomation has also occurred after bites by the red-necked keelback *(R. subminiatus)*.[8,20,41] Signs and symptoms of envenomation by these snakes include mild soft tissue swelling and, in severe cases, coagulopathy not unlike that seen with viperid venom poisoning.* Other associated findings may include variable local pain, headache, nausea, vomiting, ecchymoses, jaundice, and abdominal pain.† Renal dysfunction has been reported after *D. typus, T. kirtlandii,* and *R. tigrinus* envenomations.[38,42,48,65] A worrisome aspect of bites by these snakes is that the onset of signs of serious envenomation may be delayed by many hours and possibly even days.[12,21]

Management

FIRST AID MEASURES

Prehospital management of a bite by any potentially venomous snake involves placing the victim at rest, offering reassurance, and providing expeditious transport to the nearest facility equipped to handle such an emergency (Fig. 29-1). Above this, any first aid measure employed should at least do no further harm and should in no way delay arriving at medical care.

A proven technique of limiting systemic distribution of venom after elapid and sea snake bites involves immediately wrapping the entire bitten extremity with a crepe or elastic bandage followed by splinting with any available object (compression and immobilization; Fig. 29-2).* The wrap is applied at approximately the tension that would be used to strap a sprained ankle. The splinted extremity should then be maintained at approximately heart level.

The use of this technique in cases of viperid envenomation is controversial. In a single, small laboratory study, compression and immobilization have been demonstrated to limit pit viper venom dispersal from the bite site without worsening necrosis[68]; it is possible that localizing a potentially necrotizing venom in the region of the bite site may exacerbate tissue loss.[28] Clinical experience with the use of compression and immobilization in human victims of viperid envenomation is lacking. In making the decision to use compression and immobilization for a victim envenomed by a viperid snake, the rescuer must weigh the risks against potential benefits. If it appears that the bite should have only local implications (for example, the offending reptile is a small, relatively nontoxic viper), it may be best to avoid compression and immobilization. If, on the other hand, the bite is potentially life threatening, use of the technique may be wise. Such a scenario might involve a large or virulent snake, multiple bites, or a prolonged evacuation time. If the victim is several hours from medical care and antivenin availability and has suffered what appears to be a severe viperid bite, the compression and immobilization technique may buy valuable time.

Respiratory and cardiovascular status should be supported to the extent possible under field conditions. If the time to reach medical care is prolonged and nausea and vomiting are not significant problems, the victim should be encouraged to drink frequent, small volumes of clear, nonalcoholic liquids to support his or her intravascular volume.

Other first aid measures occasionally recommended for snake bites lack sufficient laboratory or clinical evidence to prove their effectiveness. Using a sharp instrument to open the fang marks in the field probably does more harm than good by exacerbating local bleeding (especially in cases with a coagulopathy), introducing bacteria into the wound under nonsterile conditions, and further devascularizing the wound in circumstances where perfusion may already be impaired.

Applying suction to the wound using a mechanical device such as "The Extractor" (Sawyer Products, Long Beach, Calif.; Fig. 29-3) without incising the bite probably does no harm, and there is some evidence that this may re-

*References 20, 38, 42, 45, 48, 62.

†References 12, 20, 38, 45, 48, 62, 65.

*References 3, 23, 28, 50, 55, 79.

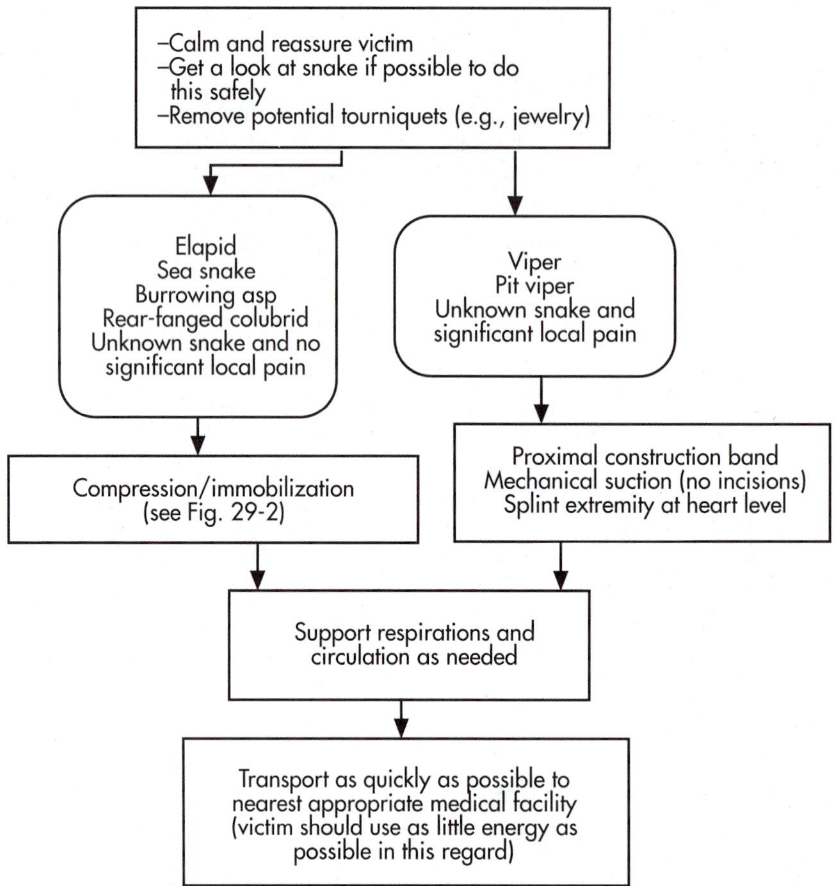

Fig. 29-1 First aid measures for venomous snakebite.

move a small percentage of venom load from the site.[6,7] Further description of "The Extractor" is found in Chapter 28.

The use of measures such as local cooling, electric shock, and the application of topical agents is to be condemned; these lack efficacy and may actually worsen local tissue damage or the overall clinical outcome. Preliminary work, for example, suggests that cold application actually drives some deleterious venom components deeper into tissues.[61] Further discussion of cryotherapy and electric shock is found in Chapter 28.

There is no easy answer to the question of how best to evacuate a victim of significant snakebite from a remote field situation. The key principles are getting the victim to medical care as soon as possible and limiting the victim's physical activity to minimize cardiac output and systemic circulation of venom. If the victim is alone and unlikely to be found for several hours, he or she should apply first aid measures and then attempt to hike out, pausing for frequent rest stops. If a lower extremity is involved, a makeshift crutch can be fashioned to assist ambulation. If one companion is present and prompt transportation to medical care is unavailable, first aid measures should be applied and the victim placed at rest. If unconscious, the victim should be placed in a "recovery position" (left lateral decubitus position with his or her head downhill and the left knee bent) to keep the airway open and decrease the risk of aspiration. The companion can then hike out in search of help. Any plan to carry the victim out must take into account the local terrain, weather conditions, and overall distance.

HOSPITAL MANAGEMENT

The initial hospital management of a victim of snake venom poisoning should involve an assessment of respiratory and cardiovascular status (Fig. 29-4). A patient who is demonstrating significant respiratory distress or is otherwise in extremis should be promptly intubated to support ventilation and prevent aspiration. Oxygen should be administered to all victims initially while rapid assessment takes place. Cardiac and pulse oximetry monitoring should be started.

Hypotension is treated initially with intravenous fluid. Crystalloids such as Ringer's lactate or normal saline should be started through at least two large-bore intravenous lines. Having two lines also allows for the simultaneous administration of fluids, drugs, and antivenin when indicated. If hypotension persists after the rapid infusion of approximately

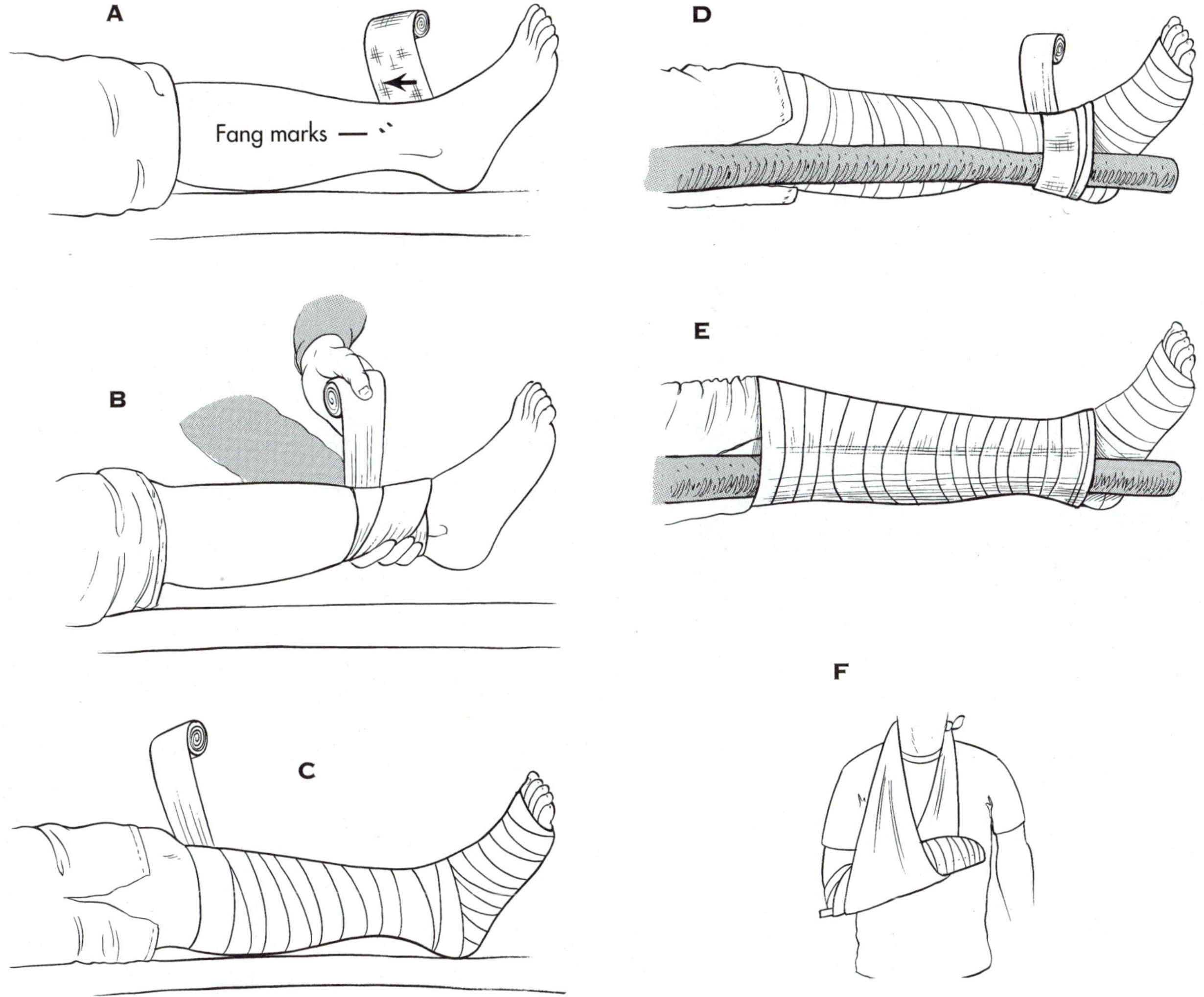

Fig. 29-2 The Australian compression and immobilization technique. This technique has proven effective in the management of elapid and sea snake envenomations. Its efficacy in viperid bites has yet to be evaluated clinically.

2 L of crystalloid in an adult or 20 to 40 ml/kg in a child, the treating physician should change to a colloid such as albumin. Animal research has demonstrated an improvement in physiologic parameters and survival with the use of albumin.[64] Vasopressors should be used only after intravascular volume has been restored. The inappropriate use of vasopressors where volume was required led to prolonged hypotension, multiple organ failure, and deaths that were probably preventable.[29]

In the case of victims who report being bitten by a snake but appear well, several questions must be addressed. First, was the snake venomous? Being able to identify the venomous species indigenous to an area is important. Hospital emergency wards should maintain color photographs of the local snake species to aid in identification.

If the snake has been identified as venomous and the patient remains asymptomatic, was he or she actually bitten? A careful search for puncture wounds should be made. In some cases of sea snake bites and with bites by some of the smaller venomous snakes, such as coral snakes, identifying fang marks can be difficult.[52,80]

If bitten, was the victim envenomed? A relatively high number of bites by venomous snakes occur without injection of venom; these are "dry bites." Absence of envenomation is seen in approximately 20% to 30% of viper bites.[37] Most elapid species produce dry bites in approximately 50% of cases; in Australia the rate approaches 70%.[70] The incidence of dry bites reaches approximately 75% with sea snakes[37,58] and is even higher with rear-fanged colubrids.[45] A careful history regarding current symptoms and a rapid physical examination looking for abnormalities should be performed. Careful evaluation and monitoring of the victim's vital signs are important. If a compression and immobilization device has been applied in the field and the patient

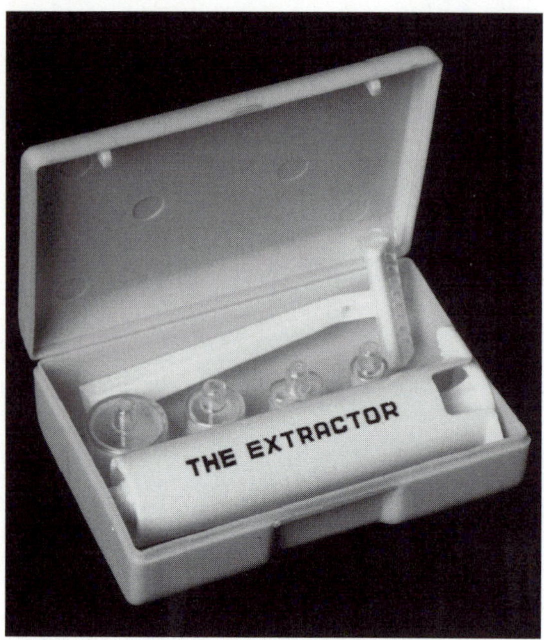

Fig. 29-3 "The Extractor." A device for applying mechanical suction to snakebites in the field.

is asymptomatic, it should be removed (after intravenous access has been secured and appropriate antivenin has been located) to assess the bitten extremity. If obvious signs of envenomation develop, the device should be immediately reapplied and left in place until antivenin administration has begun. If a totally occlusive vascular tourniquet has been applied in the field, a looser constriction band (to diminish only superficial venous and lymphatic return) should be applied proximally and intravenous access should be secured. The arterial tourniquet can then be removed while closely observing the victim for sudden deterioration when stagnant, acidic blood (with or without venom) is released to the central circulation. If signs of significant envenomation are present on arrival, appropriate antivenin administration should begin before removal of any compression and immobilization device or constriction band (although tourniquets are best replaced by constriction bands as soon as possible to avoid adding ischemic insult to venom-induced tissue damage).

Snake venom detection kits are available in Australian hospitals to help detect the presence of venom in a bitten individual and identify the offending indigenous species.[60,72] This technique, which is both sensitive and specific, employs an enzyme-linked immunosorbent assay (ELISA) to identify venom in tissue fluid taken from the bite site or in the victim's urine.[72,73] The test is less reliable using blood samples.[92]

If envenomation has occurred, what is the apparent severity of the poisoning? If the victim is in extremis, this question is already answered. If the patient appears relatively stable, however, the answer is not so simple. It must be remembered that in some cases of snake venom poisoning, there may be a delay of many hours before significant signs or symptoms appear. Likewise, it is critical to understand that snake venom poisoning is a dynamic process, so a patient who looks well one minute may be in respiratory distress and hypotensive the next. The wise physician expects multisystem involvement after snake venom poisoning and anticipates deterioration in the victim's clinical status.

The history and physical examination help determine the severity of each case. The bitten extremity should be marked at two proximal locations and the circumferences at these sites monitored every 15 minutes for progressive swelling until it is clear that such swelling has ceased. Rapidly progressive swelling indicates a worsening clinical situation. Lack of swelling, however, does not rule out significant envenomation.

Laboratory evaluations are also helpful in determining severity. Initial studies that might be obtained are outlined in Box 29-3. A complete blood cell count can detect a drop in red blood cell mass if bleeding or hemolysis is occurring. Alternatively, early hemoconcentration may be found as a result of intravascular fluid transudation. Leukocytosis is not uncommon, and the platelet count is an index of consumptive coagulopathy. The peripheral blood smear may reveal microangiopathic hemolysis. A sample for blood typing and screening should be obtained as soon as possible, since venom toxins or antivenin may later interfere with this procedure. Blood coagulation studies (prothrombin time, partial thromboplastin time, fibrinogen level, and fibrin degradation products) can aid in gauging severity. Urine samples should be checked at the bedside with reagent strips for the presence of blood. If positive, formal urinalysis and measurement of urine myoglobin should be performed. Stool should also be tested for gross or occult blood. Baseline electrolyte and renal function studies are important in cases where hyperkalemia or renal failure are potential complications. Liver function parameters help assess hepatic toxicity. In some cases creatinine kinase levels may help determine the presence of envenomation by documenting myotoxicity. If elevated, isoenzymes should be checked. If envenomation appears to have been significant, an electrocardiogram and chest radiograph should also be obtained to help evaluate cardiopulmonary effects. Arterial blood gases should be measured and followed if there is evidence of respiratory involvement or circulatory embarrassment. Signs or symptoms of intracranial bleeding should be evaluated by a computed tomographic scan.

The key principles of treating any significant snake envenomation are sound supportive care of the victim's physiologic status and the use of appropriate antivenin when available. Antivenins are available for the vast majority of the world's medically important venomous snakes. A list of the manufacturers producing antivenins around the world can be found in a 1991 review by Theakston and Warrell.[74]

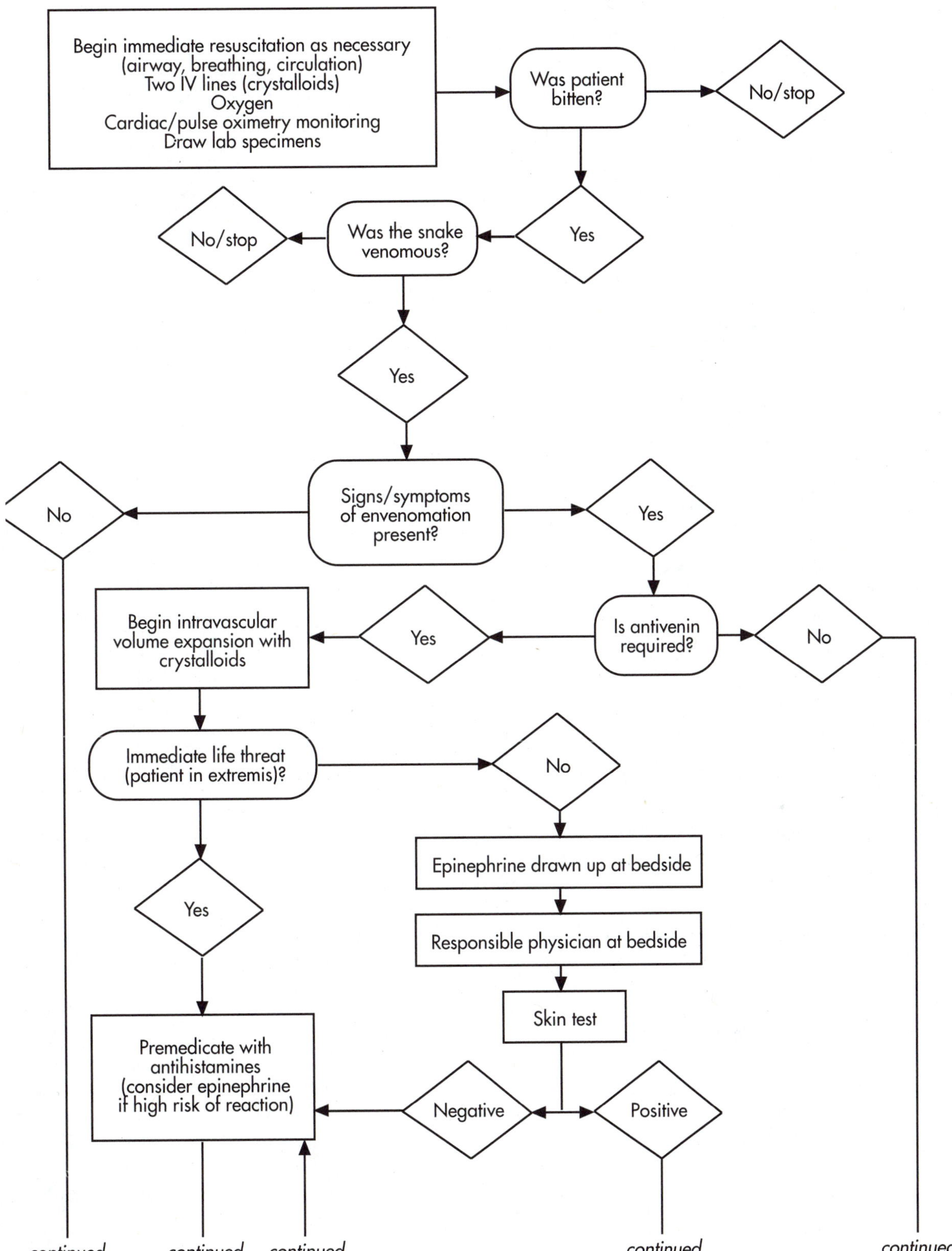

Fig. 29-4 Guidelines for the hospital management of venomous snakebite.
Continued.

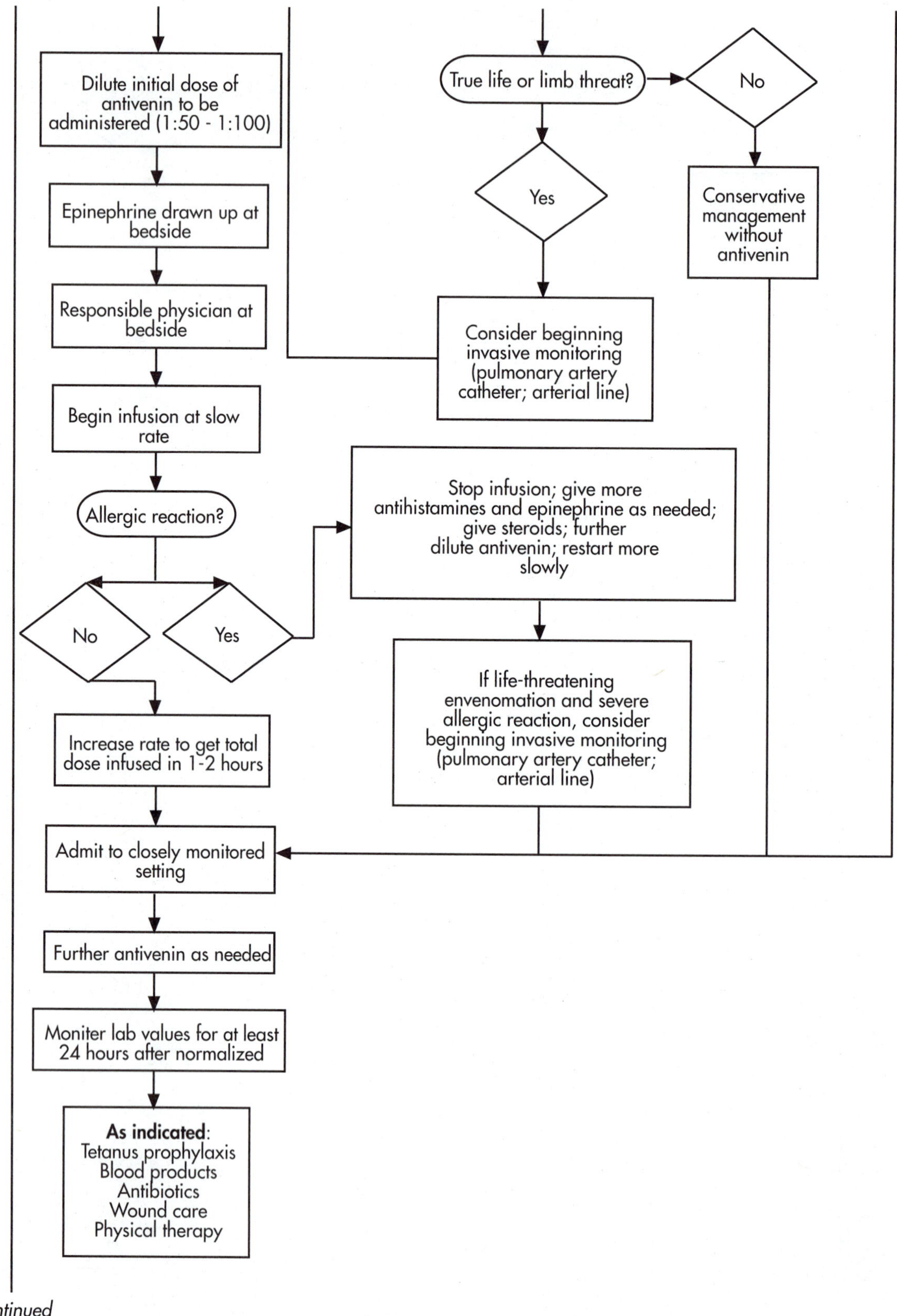
Dilute initial dose of antivenin to be administered (1:50 - 1:100)
Epinephrine drawn up at bedside
Responsible physician at bedside
Begin infusion at slow rate
Allergic reaction?
No
Yes
Increase rate to get total dose infused in 1-2 hours
Stop infusion; give more antihistamines and epinephrine as needed; give steroids; further dilute antivenin; restart more slowly
If life-threatening envenomation and severe allergic reaction, consider beginning invasive monitoring (pulmonary artery catheter; arterial line)
True life or limb threat?
Yes
No
Consider beginning invasive monitoring (pulmonary artery catheter; arterial line)
Conservative management without antivenin
Admit to closely monitored setting
Further antivenin as needed
Moniter lab values for at least 24 hours after normalized
As indicated:
Tetanus prophylaxis
Blood products
Antibiotics
Wound care
Physical therapy
continued

Fig. 29-4, cont'd. For legend see preceding page.

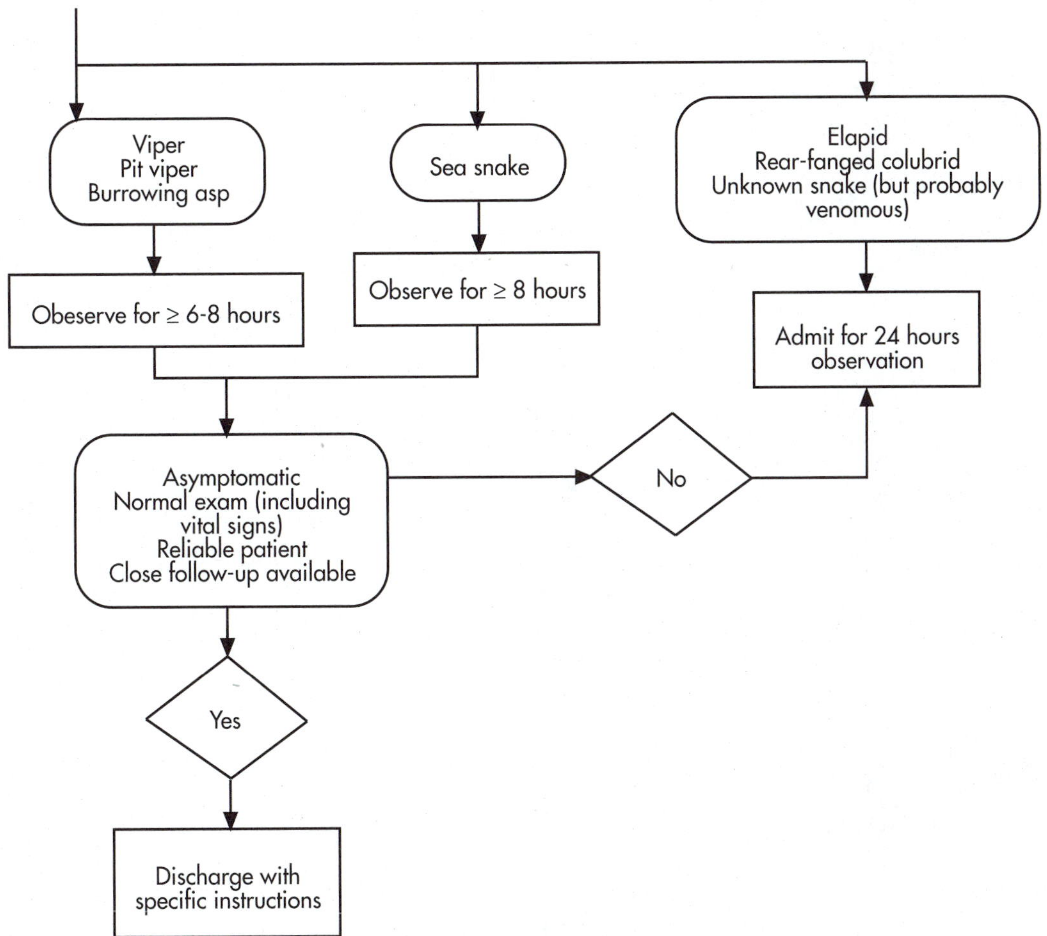

Fig. 29-4, cont'd. For legend see p. 723.

Currently there is no specific antivenin for *Atractaspis* species, and the majority of these bites follow a benign clinical course.[77] Likewise, no antivenins for colubrid envenomations are widely available, although antivenins against *Dispholidus typus* and *Rhabdophis tigrinus* venoms are produced in South Africa and Japan, respectively, for use in these regions. Management of envenomation by burrowing asps and colubrids relies almost entirely on sound supportive care. The bitten extremity should be splinted and elevated. Mild analgesics may be required in some cases, and antibiotics are indicated if secondary infection occurs. If a coagulopathy develops, careful assessment of the coagulation status of the patient is vital. Fresh-frozen plasma may replace depleted coagulation factors,[48,62] and blood products may be needed to counter a declining hematocrit, but there is a danger of adding fuel to an ongoing consumptive coagulopathy with resulting exacerbation of intravascular clot deposition.[42] Use of intravenous steroids (hydrocortisone, 15 mg/kg/day) and ε-aminocaproic acid (70 mg/kg initially, then 15 mg/kg/day) has been reported beneficial in some cases.[40] The use of heparin to combat ongoing intravascular coagulation has also been recommended but is controversial.[38,65] These modalities have no effect on any direct venom toxicity to the vasculature and internal organs.[48]

For an antivenin to be effective in snake venom poisoning, it must contain antibodies to the specific deleterious antigens present in the offending snake's venom. In regions where more than one antivenin is available to treat bites by various indigenous snakes, identifying the specific snake takes on added importance. In Australia, where multiple monospecific antivenins are available, this task is aided by the ELISA kits mentioned previously. In regions where the only antivenin available is a polyvalent product, identifying the specific snake is less critical as long as all medically important indigenous species are covered by the antivenin.

Using an antivenin developed for unrelated species is generally of no benefit unless cross-protection has been previously demonstrated. There is, however, significant risk in attempting to use a heterologous antivenin, since all commercially available products are of equine origin, and therefore carry the risks of allergic phenomena, as described in Chapter 28. In some instances, however, heterologous antivenins have demonstrated significant cross-protection.[43]

BOX 29-3

DIAGNOSTIC STUDIES IN EVALUATION OF VENOMOUS SNAKEBITE VICTIMS

BLOOD AND SERUM

Type and cross-match
Complete blood cell count
Peripheral smear
Coagulation studies (fibrinogen, fibrin degradation products, partial thromboplastin time, prothrombin time)
Electrolytes; glucose; creatinine; blood urea nitrogen; liver enzymes; bilirubin
Arterial blood gases
Myoglobin; creatinine kinase

URINE

Bedside tests (glucose, blood, myoglobin [on each voided specimen])
Urinalysis

STOOL

Test for blood

RADIOGRAPHS

Chest (if over 40 years old, history of underlying cardiopulmonary disease, or severe envenomation)
Bite site soft tissue films (if retained fangs possible)
Computed tomography of the brain (if presentation suggests intracranial hemorrhage)

ELECTROCARDIOGRAM

If patient is over 40 years old, has a history of underlying cardiopulmonary disease, or has a severe envenomation

An excellent example of this is the efficacy of Commonwealth Serum Laboratory's tiger snake *(Notechis)* antivenin against sea snake venoms.[4,23,66,79] This should be considered the second-line agent to be used if specific sea snake antivenin is not available.[80] As research continues and clinical experience is gained, our understanding of the antigenic relationships between venoms of seemingly unrelated snake taxa will expand and the list of cross-protective antivenins will grow.

If there is a choice between a polyvalent antivenin developed to counter the effects of venom poisoning by several snake species found in a geographic area and a monovalent serum specific for one species of snake, the monovalent product should be used if the snake has been definitively identified. It will provide more specific protection with a smaller burden of extraneous, allergenic proteins ineffective against the offending snake's venom. Recommendations regarding antivenin choices can be obtained from experts in snake envenomation or from the *Antivenin Index,* which is produced and periodically updated by the American Association of Zoological Parks and Aquariums.[1] This resource contains a list of medically important snakes of the world (scientific and common names), recommended antivenins for these species, a list of antivenin inventories maintained by participating institutions in the United States, and a list of manufacturers of antivenins around the world. It can be purchased by writing to The American Zoo and Aquarium Association, Oglebay Park, Wheeling, WV 26003-1698. Assistance in locating stocks of antivenin within the United States can be obtained by using the *Antivenin Index* or consulting the University of Arizona Poison Control Center (telephone number 602-626-6016).

Once the decision has been made to administer antivenin and an appropriate agent has been located, preparations for administration should begin promptly. The patient's intravascular volume should be expanded with crystalloid infusion unless there is a contraindication (such as a history of congestive heart failure). Volume expansion may blunt a hypotensive response that could occur as a result of direct complement activation by antivenin proteins. An appropriate dose of 1:1000 aqueous epinephrine (0.01 ml/kg up to 0.5 ml total) should be drawn up in a syringe and placed at the patient's bedside before any antivenin is administered. If the patient appears stable, time might be taken to perform a skin test as outlined in the product package insert in an attempt to predict an anaphylactic response to the equine serum. The test is, however, neither sensitive nor specific—a significant number of false positives and false negatives occur. Furthermore, a positive skin test does not contraindicate the use of antivenin if a significant life or limb threat exists. A conjunctival test for hypersensitivity is occasionally recommended, but this technique is extremely unreliable and uncomfortable and should be abandoned.[61]

If a snakebite victim is obviously unstable and in need of immediate antivenin, it is reasonable to forgo allergy testing and commence with administration of the antiserum at an initial slow rate with the treating physician at the bedside, ready to intervene at the earliest sign of reaction. A more complete discussion of the potential complications associated with any commercially available snake antivenin is found in Chapter 28.

If the skin test is negative or the decision is made to proceed without skin testing, the patient should be premedicated with intravenous antihistamines. In an adult, 50 to 100 mg of diphenhydramine (child, 1 to 2 mg/kg) and 300 mg of cimetidine (child, 5 to 10 mg/kg) or equivalent agents can be given. In cases where antivenin is clearly needed and an increased risk of anaphylaxis is a concern (for example, because of a history of allergy to horses or prior reaction to antivenin), premedicating the patient with a small dose of subcutaneous 1:1000 epinephrine (0.3 to 0.5 ml in adults; 0.01 ml/kg in children) should be considered if there are no contraindications (such as coronary artery disease or severe hypertension).

The total antivenin dose to be administered should be added to a bag of diluent (5% dextrose in water or crystalloid) at a dilution of 1:50 to 1:100. The infusion should be begun intravenously at a very slow rate (a few milliliters per minute) with the physician in immediate attendance. If no reaction occurs after a few minutes, the rate can be progressively increased so that the total dose is administered in approximately 1 to 2 hours. If the patient is in extremis, however, the infusion should be hastened accordingly. Antivenin should not be administered by local or intramuscular injection because it is less effective by these routes, and if a reaction occurs, there is no way to discontinue the drug.[12]

If an early reaction occurs, the antivenin should be temporarily halted and the reaction treated as suggested in Chapter 28. The infusion can then usually be restarted at a slower rate. Further diluting the antivenin may also be helpful. Managing a victim with life-threatening envenomation who has a serious allergic reaction to antivenin is difficult.

Choosing the appropriate initial dose of antivenin can be guided by the package insert for the chosen product. Antivenin can generally be withheld in an apparently dry bite or minor envenomation while the patient is closely observed for any development or progression of signs or symptoms. For a few species of snakes, antivenin should be administered after *any* bite by an identified specimen regardless of whether symptoms or signs are present. An example would be any bite inflicted by a krait (*Bungarus* spp.) or large (greater than 50 cm in length) coral snake (*Micrurus* spp.). This is to prevent the onset of problems that can be rapidly progressive and difficult to halt.

Currently the potency of different antivenins is variable, and it is difficult to make general recommendations regarding dosages. For a moderate envenomation, 20 to 50 ml of reconstituted (if lyophilized) antivenin is a reasonable dose for many products, to be further diluted before initial administration.[60] In a severe envenomation, especially with evidence of neurotoxicity, 100 to 150 ml is more appropriate.[60] If signs and symptoms or laboratory abnormalities continue to progress after the initial dose is given, more antivenin should be administered. Children should receive the same doses as adults, or even higher, since they often incur larger envenomations in proportion to their body surface area and intravascular volume.[47,60] It may be possible in the future to guide antivenin dosing by ELISA techniques that quantitate circulating venom.[11]

Victims who have been obviously envenomed, particularly those requiring antivenin, should be admitted to a unit where they can receive close cardiopulmonary monitoring until overall stability is achieved. Any abnormal laboratory values should be remeasured frequently in these patients for at least 24 to 48 hours or until normalized. Cases of delayed coagulopathy after antivenin treatment have been reported and may result from delayed release of venom from depot sites such as skin blisters.[60]

Patients bitten by venomous snakes who are totally without signs or symptoms create challenging disposition decisions. If a viperid snake is implicated in such a bite, it is usually safe to discharge the victim after 4 to 6 hours of close observation, provided the clinical picture remains completely normal. For sea snakes, 8 hours is reasonable; for elapids, 24 hours is safer.[12,80] Suspected boomslang *(Dispholidus typus)* or bird or twig snake (*Thelotornis* spp.) bites should be observed in the hospital for 24 hours, and if coagulation studies remain normal at that time, the patient can be discharged. It is wise to admit a patient for 24 to 48 hours of observation if there is any indication that envenomation has occurred (such as mildly abnormal vital signs) or if patient reliability is in doubt. If the decision is made to send a patient home, he or she should receive explicit discharge instructions concerning bed rest for 24 hours, increased fluid intake, and symptoms for which he or she should watch (increased pain, swelling, dizziness, shortness of breath, numbness, weakness). Follow-up within 24 hours should be arranged for reevaluation.

If a coagulopathy is present and associated with clinically significant bleeding, administration of appropriate blood products should be considered. It is important that antivenin administration begin if possible before such products are given. It is not infrequent after some viperid bites to obtain laboratory parameters indicating severe coagulopathy *without* evidence of significant, clinical hemorrhage.[44,56] Such cases can be treated with antivenin and close observation with the patient on strict bed rest while blood products are withheld.

While other treatment modalities in snake venom poisoning have demonstrated variable anecdotal benefit, the use of such techniques does not replace proper conservative care and appropriate antivenin use. Edrophonium and neostigmine have been reported to reverse neuromuscular blockade temporarily after cobra envenomation.[60,75,88] The combination of edrophonium and atropine might be tried in a situation of impending respiratory failure in a victim of cobra or krait bite when antivenin is not immediately available. Care should be exercised in the use of these agents because either may stimulate a cholinergic crisis. Attempts to temporize in a patient with impending respiratory failure are likely to result in aspiration with complications.[35] It is wiser to proceed with prompt endotracheal intubation before frank respiratory failure occurs.

Ethylenediamine tetraacetic acid (EDTA) has been touted as an inhibitor of snake venom proteases,[44,61] but its clinical efficacy has not been demonstrated. In fact, an increase in mortality has been demonstrated in animal models when EDTA was given intravenously to treat pit viper venom poisoning.[61]

Other modalities recommended in the past that lack evidence to support routine use include the application of topical agents (such as potassium permanganate) to "deactivate" venom; routine fasciotomy of the bitten extremity (see later discussion); immediate exploration, debridement, or excision of the bite site; administration of heparin to counter disseminated intravascular coagulopathic abnormalities; and high-dose steroids. Renal failure can best be prevented by aggressively treating hypotension, maintaining adequate urinary output, and using antivenin appropriately. Myoglobinuria should be treated in standard fashion with sodium bicarbonate, mannitol, or loop diuretics. If renal failure develops, care should be directed at maintaining proper electrolyte balance. Peritoneal dialysis or hemodialysis is often required in such cases. Hemodialysis has been anecdotally reported to improve peripheral muscle weakness in victims of severe sea snake envenomation with acute renal failure, probably by reversing hyperkalemic and uremic effects on venom-damaged muscle fibers.[66] It should be understood, however, that dialysis cannot remove circulating venom components, and the indications for dialysis are the same as for any other cause of acute renal failure.

Wound care of the bitten extremity should be managed as described in Chapter 28. Antibiotics (first-generation cephalosporins, ampicillin, erythromycin, tetracycline, and others) may be given prophylactically in cases of envenomation with significant local soft tissue changes in an attempt to limit secondary infection, although the actual incidence of infection is low.[14] Antibiotics may be particularly important if any misdirected attempt was made to incise the bite site under unsterile field conditions.[93] Early physical therapy aimed at returning the bitten extremity to its maximal level of function is important, especially in patients with significant soft tissue swelling or necrosis.

If concern exists about the possibility of a compartmental syndrome, intracompartmental pressures can be rapidly and easily checked using any of a number of devices designed for this purpose, such as the wick catheter. If the pressure in an involved compartment is greater than 30 to 40 mm Hg in a normotensive patient, this may exceed the capillary perfusion pressure in the muscles. Ischemia may result if the situation is not addressed, usually by means of a fasciotomy. The pressure at which ischemia ensues is even lower in hypotensive snakebite victims, so the threshold for performing a fasciotomy may need to be lowered in this setting. It must be emphasized that the overall incidence of compartment syndromes after venomous snakebite is quite low,[19,25,87] and "prophylactic" fasciotomies in patients without objectively documented elevated intracompartmental pressures are inappropriate.

The management of a victim with ocular exposure to spitting cobra venom must begin with immediate and copious irrigation of the eyes with any readily available, suitable fluid.[60,85] Prompt treatment may help prevent the local complications of such exposure. Close ophthalmologic follow-up is important to rule out corneal ulceration or uveitis.

Victims who receive equine antivenin are at risk for immune complex–mediated delayed serum sickness, usually 1 to 2 weeks after administration. This risk increases in direct proportion to the total dose of antivenin administered. The signs, symptoms, and management of this complication are discussed in Chapter 28.

Active Immunization

Rituals and techniques for immunization against snake venom have been practiced for centuries in various parts of the world.[46] More recently, modern immunologic methods have been used. Beginning in 1965, 43,446 individuals in the Ryukyu Islands of Japan, an area of very high snakebite incidence, were immunized with habu *(Trimeresurus flavoviridis)* venom toxoid. Follow-up after about 5 years indicated equivocal results, and no further large-scale trials were undertaken, but experimental work continues. Immunization of individuals against other snake venoms has been carried out.[63,78]

Mortality

While mortality rates are extremely variable throughout the world, more than 95% of deaths from snakebites occur in underdeveloped countries with inadequate or remote medical resources.[11] The causes of death in fatal cases of elapid envenomation are respiratory paralysis, coagulopathy, renal failure, and cardiac failure.[12,61,91] In viperid-related fatalities, the cause of death is usually protracted hypovolemic shock.[12] This is often related to inadequate fluid resuscitation, inappropriate use of vasopressors, or inadequate or delayed use of antivenin. Sea snake fatalities are related to respiratory failure, cardiac dysrhythmias, or renal failure.[9,60,80] The average time to death after envenomation is 5 hours in elapid bites, 2 to 3 days in viperid bites, and 12 to 24 hours in sea snake bites.[59]

SUMMARY

While mortality rates for bites by venomous snakes remain high in some parts of the world, this is primarily because of the scarcity of appropriate medical resources. Bites by these same species to keepers of exotic snakes in the United States and Europe are rarely fatal when care is sought early and appropriate antivenin is readily available.

People traveling in the field in foreign countries should educate themselves concerning the dangerous fauna they may encounter. Field guides or textbooks illustrating the indigenous venomous snakes should be studied, and any available medical care in the area should be researched before it is needed. Resources such as the Arizona Poison Control Center (telephone number 602-626-6016) are available for consultation in cases of snake venom poisoning. This center maintains a consultant on call who can offer assistance to physicians dealing with cases of snake envenomation. It can also help locate sources of foreign antivenins stocked in institutions within the United States.

Once in the field, avoidance measures should be observed to prevent exposure to venomous snakes. Hands and feet should never be placed where one cannot see; walking barefoot at night should be strictly avoided; sufficient commotion should be made when trekking through thick undergrowth to give snakes ample warning to move out of the way; and no attempt should be made to kill or capture a snake unless the traveler is an experienced herpetologist. As with any aspect of wilderness travel, a little forethought and caution can help ensure that a "once-in-a-lifetime" adventure does not result in an "end-of-a-lifetime" disaster.

REFERENCES

1. *Antivenom index,* Wheeling, WV, 1989, American Association of Zoological Parks and Aquariums, American Association of Poison Control Centers.
2. Audebert F, Sorkine M, Bon C: Clinical gradation and ELISA quantification of envenomations following viper bites in France, *Toxicon* 30:488, 1992.
3. Balmain R, McClelland KL: Pantyhose compression bandage: first-aid measure for snake bite, *Med J Aust* 2(5):240, 1982.
4. Baxter EH, Gallichio HA: Cross-neutralization by tiger snake *(Notechis scutatus)* antivenine and sea snake *(Enhydrina schistosa)* antivenine against several sea snake venoms, *Toxicon* 12(3):273, 1974.
5. Bdolah A: The venom glands of snakes and venom secretion. In Lee CY, editor: *Snake venoms,* Berlin, 1979, Springer-Verlag.
6. Bronstein AC, Russell FE, Sullivan JB: Negative pressure suction in the field treatment of rattlesnake bite victims, *Vet Hum Toxicol* 28:485, 1986.
7. Bronstein AC et al: Negative pressure suction in field treatment of rattlesnake bite, *Vet Hum Toxicol* 28:297, 1985.
8. Cable D et al: Prolonged defibrination after a bite from a "nonvenomous" snake, *JAMA* 251:925, 1984.
9. Carey JE, Wright EA: The site of action of the venom of the sea snake *Enhydrina schistosa, Trans R Soc Trop Med Hyg* 55(1):153, 1961.
10. Chajek T et al: Anaphylactoid reaction and tissue damage following bite by *Atractaspis engaddensis, Trans R Soc Trop Med Hyg* 68:333, 1974.
11. Chippaux JP: Production and use of snake antivenin. Vol 5 in Tu AT, editor: *Handbook of natural toxins: reptile venoms and toxins,* New York, 1991, Marcel Dekker.
12. Christensen PA: The treatment of snakebite, *S Afr Med J* 43:1253, 1969.
13. Chugh KS, Sakhuja V: Renal disease caused by snake venom. Vol 5 in Tu AT, editor: *Handbook of natural toxins: reptile venoms and toxins,* New York, 1991, Marcel Dekker.
14. Clark RF, Selden BS, Furbee B: The incidence of wound infection following crotalid envenomation, *J Emerg Med* 11:583, 1993.
15. Coppola M, Hogan DE: Venomous snakes of Southwest Asia, *Am J Emerg Med* 10:230, 1992.
16. Corkill NL, Ionides CJP, Pitman CRS: Biting and poisoning by the mole vipers of the genus *Atractaspis, Trans R Soc Trop Med Hyg* 53:95, 1959.
17. Corkill NL, Kirk R: Poisoning by the Sudan mole viper *Atractaspis microlepidota* Gunther, *Trans R Soc Trop Med Hyg* 48:376, 1954.
18. Currie B, Theakston D, Warrell D: Envenoming from the Papuan taipan *(Oxyuranus scutellatus canni), Toxicon* 30:501, 1992.
19. Curry SC et al: Noninvasive vascular studies in management of rattlesnake envenomations to extremities, *Ann Emerg Med* 14(11):1081, 1985.
20. Ferlan I et al: Preliminary studies on the venom of the colubrid snake *Rhabdophis subminiatus* (red-necked keelback), *Toxicon* 21:570, 1983.
21. Fitzsimons DC, Smith HM: Another rear-fanged South African snake lethal to humans, *Herpetologica* 14:198, 1958.
22. Frost J: Tiger snake envenomation, *Med J Aust* 1:440, 1980.
23. Fulde GWO, Smith F: Sea snake envenomation at Bondi, *Med J Aust* 141:44, 1984.
24. Ganthavorn S: A case of king cobra bite, *Toxicon* 9:293, 1971.
25. Garfin SR: Rattlesnake bites: current hospital therapy, *West J Med* 137(5):411, 1982.
26. Gunders AE, Walter HJ, Etzel E: Case of snake-bite by *Atractaspis corpulenta, Trans R Soc Trop Med Hyg* 54:279, 1960.
27. Hardy DL: *Bothrops asper* (Viperidae) snakebite and field researchers in Middle America, *Biotropica* 26(2):198, 1994.
28. Hardy DL: Snakebite update: *Crotalus* envenomation in Tucson, 1973-1980 and comments on the new Australian method of first aid for elapid snakebites. Presented September 22, 1982, at the Annual Conference of the American Association of Zoos, Parks and Aquariums, Scottsdale, Arizona.
29. Hardy DL: Fatal rattlesnake envenomation in Arizona: 1969-1984, *Clin Toxicol* 24(1):1, 1986.
30. Hood VL, Johnson JR: Acute failure with myoglobinuria following tiger snake bite, *Aust NZ J Med* 4:415, 1974.
31. Hurwitz BJ, Hull PR: Berg adder bite, *S Afr Med J* 45:969, 1971.
32. Iddon D, Hommel M, Theakston RDG: Characterisation of a monoclonal antibody capable of neutralising the haemorrhagic activity of west African *Echis carinatus* (carpet viper) venom, *Toxicon* 26:167, 1988.
33. Jenkins M, Russell FE: Physical therapy for snake venom poisoning, *Phys Ther* 54:1298, 1974.
34. Jeyarajah R: Russell's viper bite in Sri Lanka: a study of 22 cases, *Am J Trop Med Hyg* 33(3):506, 1984.
35. Kitchens CS, Van Mierop LHS: Envenomation by the eastern coral snake *(Micrurus fulvius fulvius):* a study of 39 victims, *JAMA* 258(12):1615, 1987.
36. Kochva E: The origin of snakes and evolution of the venom apparatus, *Toxicon* 25:65, 1987.
37. Kunkel DB et al: Reptile envenomations, *J Toxicol Clin Toxicol* 21(4&5):503, 1983-84.
38. Lakier JB, Fritz VU: Consumptive coagulopathy caused by a boomslang bite, *S Afr Med J* 43:1052, 1969.
39. Lee S et al: Coronary vasospasm as the primary cause of death due to the venom of the burrowing asp, *Atractaspis engaddensis, Toxicon* 24:285, 1986.
40. Mandell F et al: Major coagulopathy and "nonpoisonous" snake bites, *Pediatrics* 65(2):314, 1980.
41. Mather HM, Mayne S, McMonagle TM: Severe envenomation from "harmless" pet snake, *Br Med J* 1(6123):1324, 1978.
42. Mebs D et al: A fatal case of snake bite due to *Thelotornis kirtlandii.* In Rosenberg P, editor: *Toxins: animal, plant and microbial,* Oxford, 1978, Pergamon Press.
43. Minton SA: Paraspecific protection by elapid and sea snake antivenins, *Toxicon* 5(1):47, 1967.
44. Minton SA: *Venom diseases,* Springfield, Ill, 1974, Charles C Thomas.
45. Minton SA: Venomous bites by nonvenomous snakes: an annotated bibliography of colubrid envenomation, *J Wilderness Med* 1:119, 1990.
46. Minton SA, Minton MR: *Venomous reptiles,* New York, 1980, Scribners.
47. Mitrakul C et al: Clinical features of neurotoxic snake bite and response to antivenom in 47 children, *Am J Trop Med Hyg* 33:1258, 1984.
48. Mittleman MB, Goris RC: Death caused by the bite of the Japanese colubrid snake *Rhabdophis tigrinus* (Boie) (Reptilia, Serpentes, Colubridae), *J Herpetol* 12(1):109, 1978.
49. Montgomery J: Two cases of ophthalmoplegia due to Berg adder bite, *Cent Afr J Med* 5(4):173, 1959.

50. Murrell G: The effectiveness of the pressure/immobilization first aid technique in the case of a tiger snake bite, *Med J Aust* 2(6):295, 1981.
51. Myint-Lwin et al: Bites by Russell's viper *(Vipera russelli siamensis)* in Burma: haemostatic, vascular, and renal disturbances and response to treatment, *Lancet* 2:1259, 1985.
52. Norris RL, Dart RC: Apparent coral snake envenomation in a patient without fang marks, *Am J Emerg Med* 7:402, 1989.
53. Ohsaka A: Hemorrhagic, necrotizing, and edema-forming effects of snake venoms. In Lee CY, editor: *Snake venoms,* Berlin, 1979, Springer-Verlag.
54. Parrish HM: *Poisonous snakebites in the United States,* New York, 1980, Vantage Press.
55. Pearn J et al: First-aid for snake-bite: efficacy of a constrictive bandage with limb immobilization in the management of human envenomation, *Med J Aust* 2(6):293, 1981.
56. Prentice CRM: Acquired coagulation disorders, *Clin Haematol* 14:413, 1985.
57. Reid HA: Myoglobinuria and sea-snakebite poisoning, *Br Med J* 1:1284, 1961.
58. Reid HA: Snakebite in the tropics, *Br Med J* 3:359, 1968.
59. Reid HA, Lim KJ: Sea-snake bite: a survey of fishing villages in northwest Malaya, *Br Med J* 2:1266, 1957.
60. Reid HA, Theakston RDG: The management of snake bite, *Bull WHO* 61:885, 1983.
61. Russell FE: *Snake venom poisoning,* New York, 1983, Scholium International.
62. Saddler M, Paul B: Vine snake envenomation, *Cent Afr J Med* 34(2):31, 1988.
63. Sawai Y: Vaccination against snake bite poisoning. In Lee CY, editor: *Snake venoms,* Berlin, 1979, Springer-Verlag.
64. Schaeffer RC et al: The effects of colloidal and crystalloidal fluids on rattlesnake venom shock in the rat, *J Pharmacol Exp Ther* 206(3):687, 1978.
65. Spies SK, Malherbe LF: Boomslangbyt met afibriongnemie, *S Afr Med J* 36:834, 1962.
66. Sitprija V, Sribhibhadh R, Benyajati C: Haemodialysis in poisoning by sea-snake venom, *Br Med J* 3:218, 1971.
67. Stueven H et al: Cobra envenomation: an uncommon emergency, *Ann Emerg Med* 12(10):636, 1983.
68. Sutherland SK, Coulter AR: Early management of bites by the eastern diamondback rattlesnake *(Crotalus adamanteus):* studies in monkeys *(Macaca fascicularis), Am J Trop Med Hyg* 30(2):497, 1981.
69. Sutherland SK, King K: *Management of snake-bite injuries,* Hurstville, 1991, Royal Flying Doctor Service of Australia.
70. Sutherland SK: Mr Ram Chandra and snakebite, *Med J Aust* 1:457, 1979.
71. Swaroop S, Grab B: Snakebite mortality in the world, *Bull WHO* 10:35, 1954.
72. Theakston RDG: The application of immunoassay techniques, including enzyme-linked immunosorbent assay (ELISA), to snake venom research, *Toxicon* 21:341, 1983.
73. Theakston RDG, Pugh RNH, Reid HA: Enzyme-linked immunosorbent assay of venom-antibodies in human victims of snake bite, *J Trop Med Hyg* 84:109, 1981.
74. Theakston RDG, Warrell DA: Antivenoms: a list of hyperimmune sera currently available for the treatment of envenoming by bites and stings, *Toxicon* 29(12):1419, 1991.
75. Tiger ME, Brecher E, Bevan D: Cobra bite in Philadelphia, *Penn Med* 87:53, 1975.
76. Tilbury CR: Observations on the bite of the Mozambique spitting cobra *(Naja mossambica mossambica), S Afr Med J* 61:308, 1982.
77. Tilbury CR, Branch WR: Observations on the bite of the southern burrowing asp *(Atractaspis bibronii)* in Natal, *S Afr Med J* 75:327, 1989.
78. Toriba M, Sawai Y: Venomous snakes of medical importance in Japan. In Gopalakrishnakone P, Chou LM, editors: *Snakes of medical importance Asia-Pacific Region,* Singapore, 1990, Venom and Toxin Research Group, University of Singapore.
79. Tu A, Fulde G: Sea snake bites, *Clin Dermatol* 5:118, 1987.
80. Tu AT: Biotoxicology of sea snake venoms, *Ann Emerg Med* 16(9):1023, 1987.
81. Van Mierop LHS: Poisonous snakebite: a review—snakes and their venom, *J Fla Med Assoc* 63(3):191, 1976.
82. Warrell DA: Snakes and snake bite, *Br Med J* 2(6133):352, 1978.
83. Warrell DA: Tropical snake bite: clinical studies in Southeast Asia, vol 1. In Harris JB, editor: *Natural toxins animal, plant, microbial,* Oxford, Eng, 1986, Clarendon Press.
84. Warrell DA, Arnett C: The importance of bites by saw-scaled or carpet vipers *(Echis carinatus):* epidemiological studies in Nigeria and a review of world literature, *Acta Trop* 33:307, 1976.
85. Warrell DA, Ormerod LD, Davidson NM: Bites by the night adder *(Causus maculatus)* and burrowing vipers (genus *Atractaspis*) in Nigeria, *Am J Trop Med Hyg* 25:517, 1976.
86. Warrell DA et al: Necrosis, haemorrhage and complement depletion following bites by the spitting cobra *(Naja nigricollis), Q J Med* 45(177):1, 1976.
87. Watt CH: Treatment of poisonous snakebite with emphasis on digit dermotomy, *South Med J* 78(6):694, 1985.
88. Watt G et al: Positive response to edrophonium in patients with neurotoxic envenoming by cobras *(Naja naja philippinensis):* a placebo-controlled study, *N Engl J Med* 315:1444, 1986.
89. Weiser E et al: Cardiotoxic effects of the venom of the burrowing asp, *Atractaspis engaddensis* (Atractaspididae, Ophidia), *Toxicon* 22:767, 1984.
90. Wetzel WW, Christy NP: A king cobra bite in New York City, *Toxicon* 27:393, 1989.
91. White J: Elapid snakes: venom toxicity and actions; aspects of envenomation; management of bites. In Covacevish J, Davis P, Pearn J, editors: *Toxic plants and animals: a guide for Australia,* Brisbane, 1987, Queensland Museum.
92. White J: Snakebite: an Australian perspective, *J Wilderness Med* 2:219, 1991.
93. Wingert WA, Chan L: Rattlesnake bites in southern California and rationale for recommended treatment, *West J Med* 148:37, 1988.
94. Wingert WA, Wainschel J: Diagnosis and management of envenomation by poisonous snakes, *South Med J* 68(8):1015, 1975.

30 ANTIVENINS AND IMMUNOBIOLOGICALS: IMMUNOTHERAPEUTICS OF ENVENOMATION

Rivka S. Horowitz
Richard C. Dart

Principles of antivenin therapy
Adverse effects of antivenin
Use of specific antivenins
Experimental approaches to immunotherapeutics

The ideal therapeutic agent effectively treats or prevents a designated medical condition and is free of adverse effects. Commercially available antivenins clearly fall short of the mark. The vast majority of antivenins are equine derived and thus possess the potential adverse immunologic effects inherent in the administration of foreign proteins. Although antivenin lowers the morbidity and mortality associated with envenomation, it may produce its own untoward and potentially life-threatening effects. As a result, many physicians are reluctant to administer antivenin even to patients who have a clear indication for its use.

Worldwide, over 60 commercial laboratories produce almost 200 different antivenin preparations for the treatment of snake, arachnid, fish, and coelenterate envenomations. Theakston and Warrell[53] have compiled a list of hyperimmune sera available for the treatment of venom poisoning.

A detailed account of all internationally available antivenins is beyond the scope of this chapter, which focuses on the immunotherapeutics of North American envenomation, particularly antivenins directed against North American pit vipers.

One caveat to this approach must be stressed. Zoos and amateur snake enthusiasts are likely to house nonindigenous, exotic snakes. Physicians must expeditiously exploit all available resources to identify and acquire the appropriate antivenins for unusual envenomations. One such resource, the *Antivenin Index,* is compiled by the American Association of Zoological Parks and Aquariums and the American Association of Poison Control Centers (AAPCC). The *Index* lists the location of foreign antivenins stocked by zoos in the United States. Guidance for use of these antivenins and general snakebite management may be obtained through an AAPCC-certified poison center.

Principles of Antivenin Therapy

HISTORICAL PERSPECTIVE

Immunotherapy against snake venom dates to 1887 with the first report of successful immunization in birds. Sewall[42] reported that pigeons injected with increasing but sublethal doses of *Sistrurus catenatus catenatus* (Eastern massasauga) venom became resistant to venom doses seven times the lethal dose. Seven years later, Calmette reported that serum from animals inoculated with venom from the cobra, *Naja naja,* protected against injection of that venom.[9] Simultaneously, Phisalix and Bertrand[35] reported the same phenomenon with the European viper, *Vipera berus.*

Within a decade of Sewall's landmark experiment, Calmette produced the first therapeutic antivenin derived from hyperimmunizing horses with cobra venom.[10] In addition to its efficacy against cobra envenomation, Calmette claimed it was effective against snake venoms from a variety of diverse genuses. Although Calmette overestimated the effectiveness of his antivenin, stating that it was effective against all neurotoxic venoms,[9] he and others recognized another important principle of immunotherapy still operative today, that of interspecies cross-reactivity.

Another pioneer in the study and production of antivenin, Vital Brazil, further demonstrated both specificity and cross-reactivity through the production of numerous monospecific and polyspecific antivenins. A monospecific antivenin is derived from hyperimmunizing animals with the venom of a single species, whereas polyspecific antivenin is produced either by inoculating animals with the venom of more than one species or by pooling different monospecific antivenins into a final product. Brazil recognized the need for polyspecific antivenins, since snakebite victims were often unable to differentiate among the variety of poisonous snakes indigenous to an area.[15]

To ensure an adequate supply of venom for his research, Brazil organized a unique exchange network throughout the countryside of São Paulo, Brazil. He convinced government and railroad officials to allow free passage for snakes shipped to his institute and sent devices for snake capture and crates for transport to anyone requesting them. He offered one vial of serum (antivenin) for every snake shipped to him. A further incentive for trapping and transporting additional snakes was obvious: any farmer sending six snakes would receive a syringe and needle for administering the serum.[15] After more than a decade of operating his exchange program, Brazil claimed a significant decrease in mortality from snakebites.[6,15]

NEUTRALIZING ANTIBODY

The foundation of antivenin therapy is the antigen-antibody interaction. The component of antivenin responsible for its therapeutic activity is the IgG molecule. This neutralizing antibody inactivates the antigen by specific, noncovalent, antigen-antibody binding. Thus a neutralizing antibody to phospholipase A, a common constituent of snake venoms, prevents or attenuates the neurotoxic or myotoxic activity associated with this venom component.

Understanding the structure of IgG helps to explain both the mechanism of action and the adverse reactions of antivenins. An IgG molecule weighs approximately 150,000 daltons and is composed of two functional parts: the antigen binding site, consisting of two Fab portions, and the effector site, or Fc region (Fig. 30-1). Specific binding of the antigen to the Fab binding sites neutralizes further activity of the antigen. The Fc region of IgG is responsible for binding and activating immune system cells (phagocytes, macrophages, mast cells, and so on) and triggering a host of immunologic responses. These reactions, which include degranulation of mast cells and activation of the complement cascade, are partly responsible for the immediate, life-threatening allergic reactions to antivenin.

The large size of the IgG antibody (150,000 daltons) has important implications for the immunogenicity, distribution, and elimination of these neutralizing antibodies. Large–molecular weight entities in general (IgG and other large antivenin components) are more likely to trigger immunologic reactions than are smaller ones.[54] In addition, the large size of IgG may limit more extensive distribution into tissue compartments. The ideal neutralizing antibody would be expected to have a large volume of distribution, implying more extensive tissue penetration and access to venom components. Under normal physiologic conditions, however, protein molecules like IgG remain in the in-

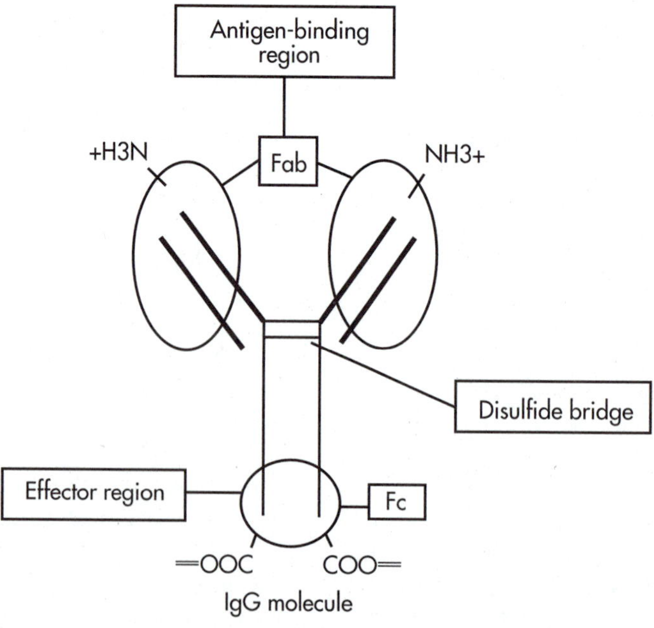

Fig. 30-1 Schematic diagram of an IgG molecule. The antigen-binding region (Fab portion) is present at the amino-terminal end. The effector region (Fc portion) interacts with the immune system cells and resides at the carboxyl end of IgG. Note the disulfide bridge.

travascular space and therefore have small volumes of distribution. Theoretically, this may limit the effectiveness of IgG in binding antigen within tissue compartments.

Finally, large molecules like IgG may have long elimination half-lives, which may predispose them to further immunologic complications. Theoretically, the more rapid the clearance of foreign proteins, the less time they will be available to form immune complexes with endogenous antibodies. These complexes may precipitate in tissues, resulting in clinical disease, that is, serum sickness. Molecules with molecular weights greater than 50,000 exceed the threshold for filtration and excretion by the kidneys. Elimination of neutralizing antibodies and antibody-antigen complexes therefore occurs via the reticuloendothelial system. This process prolongs the elimination half-life compared to simple renal excretion and may predispose patients to serum sickness.

In an attempt to resolve the problems associated with the large size of the antibody molecule, methods for enzymatic cleavage of IgG with pepsin and papain have been developed. The resultant fragments, Fab_2 and Fab (Figs. 30-2 and 30-3), are effective in neutralizing venom components while avoiding the above-mentioned problems associated with the large IgG molecule (see "Advent of Fab Immunotherapy").

MODERN PRODUCTION OF ANTIVENIN

It is clear that currently available antivenins have numerous disadvantages despite their general efficacy against venom poisoning. Efforts to maximize the neutralizing potential of antivenin while minimizing its immunogenicity have become the principal goal of modern antivenin production.

Advances in the understanding of the physiology of antivenin production have occurred since the late 1800s. Nevertheless, commercial manufacture of antivenin relies on the same principles of equine hyperimmunization with snake venom described over a hundred years ago.

All antivenins follow a two-step production process. First, a neutralizing antibody is produced by immunization of a host animal with sublethal doses of venom. This antibody is but one of many proteins present in the resulting immune serum preparation. Step two involves purification of antivenin with reduction in the fraction of nonneutralizing proteins. The preparation is then concentrated and packaged in its final lyophilized or liquid form.

The only commercially available antivenin in the United States against pit viper envenomation is Antivenin (Crotalidae) Polyvalent Wyeth. Manufacture of this antivenin has changed little since its introduction in 1954. In this process, horses are immunized with increasing doses of venom from four crotalid species: *C. adamanteus* (eastern diamondback), *C. atrox* (western diamondback), *C. durissus terrificus* (South American or tropical rattlesnake), and *Bothrops atrox* (fer-de-lance), plus adjuvant for immune system stimulation.[36] The resultant hyperimmune serum is subjected to an ammonium sulfate precipitation, which removes a variety of plasma proteins. Unfortunately, a fraction of neutralizing antibody is also lost in this process, resulting in diminished potency. The product is then precipitated, filtered, resuspended, and lyophilized. The final concentrated antivenin contains 1.5 to 2 g of horse protein, only 15% to 25% of which is IgG.[47]

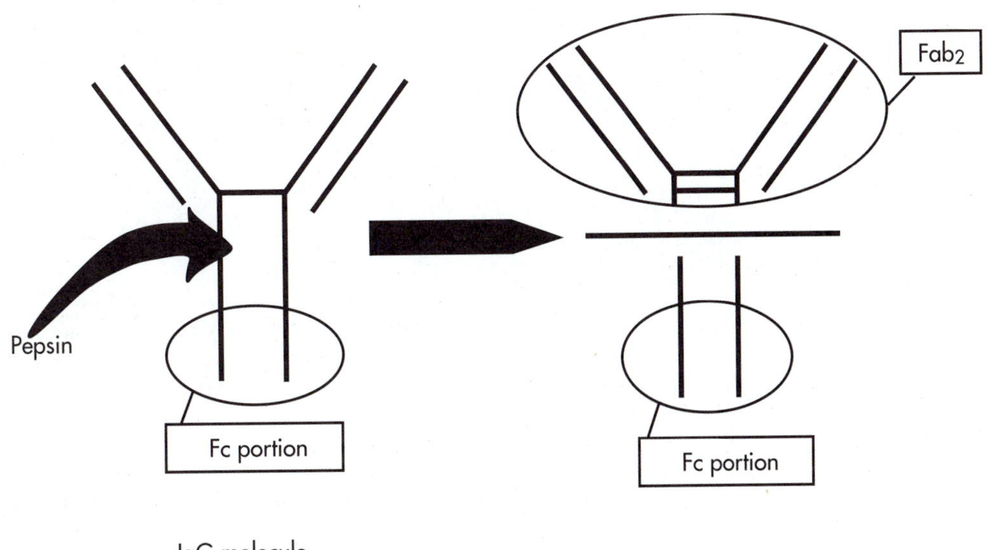

Fig. 30-2 Proteolytic cleavage of IgG results in predictable substituent fractions. Pepsin digestion produces an Fc and a Fab_2 fraction. Fab_2 consists of two Fab portions connected by a disulfide bridge. Molecular weight of Fab_2 is 100,000 daltons.

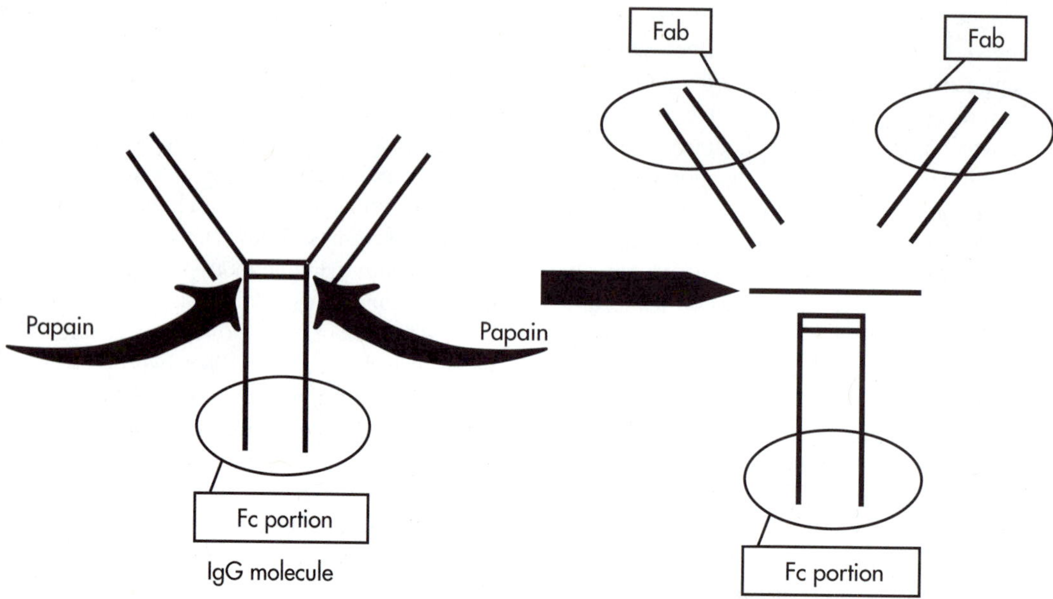

Fig. 30-3 Proteolytic cleavage of IgG results in predictable substituent fractions. Papain digestion of IgG yields the Fc and two Fab segments for each IgG molecule. Molecular weight of Fab is 50,000 daltons.

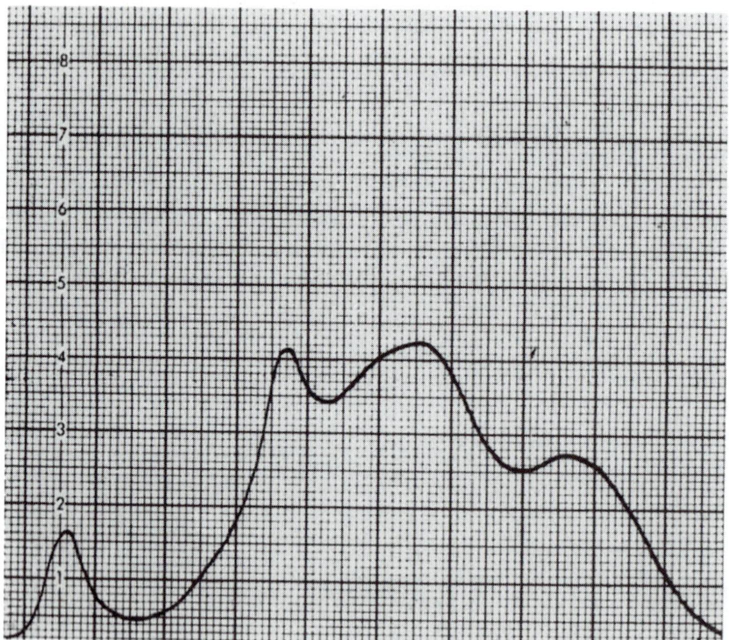

Fig. 30-4 Serum protein electrophoresis of Wyeth antivenin. The chromatogram demonstrates the presence of nonneutralizing protein in the antivenin. The four peaks noted above, from left to right, are albumin, α_2, β, and γ.

Because of the incomplete purification, the Wyeth polyvalent crotalid antivenin contains significant amounts of other equine serum proteins, such as albumin, α- and β-globulins, and IgM, which contribute to its immunogenicity. Sullivan has quantified the relative contributions of nonneutralizing proteins to the final antivenin product (Fig. 30-4; Box 30-1).[47]

These impurities notwithstanding, the Wyeth antivenin preparation is effective against all crotalids native to North, Central, and South America despite the fact that it is prepared from only four species. This cross-reactivity enables a single preparation of antivenin to be effective against any clinically significant pit viper envenomation.

BOX 30-1

QUANTITATION OF PROTEINS IN SAMPLES OF WYETH ANTIVENIN

IgG	2900 mg/ml
IgM	75 mg/ml
Total protein	9.4 g/dl
Albumin	0.28 g/dl
$Alpha_1$	0.74 g/dl
$Alpha_2$	3.50 g/dl
Beta	2.76 g/dl
Gamma	2.12 g/dl

Adverse Effects of Antivenin

Although equine-derived antivenin is clinically effective, its heterologous nature presents several problems. These include life-threatening anaphylactic and anaphylactoid reactions and the more common, but self-limiting, serum sickness (described later in the chapter). As mentioned previously, the purification process results in denaturation of a portion of the protective IgG fraction.[47] Thus, to provide adequate reversal of venom poisoning in clinical practice, multiple vials of antivenin must be administered, further potentiating possible adverse effects.

ANAPHYLACTIC AND ANAPHYLACTOID REACTIONS

The spectrum of human immunologic responses to antivenin is well documented. Introduction of heterologous protein may precipitate type I hypersensitivity reactions. This syndrome results from IgE-mediated degranulation of mast cells and release of vasoactive mediators, including histamine, leukotriene, platelet activating factor, adenosine, and neutrophilic and eosinophilic chemotactic factors.[27] These substances induce vasodilation and increased capillary permeability and result in hemodynamic instability. The resultant hypotension is often accompanied by bronchospasm, laryngospasm, and ultimately death, in the absence of pharmacologic intervention.

A second syndrome, clinically indistinguishable from anaphylaxis but not IgE mediated, is referred to as "anaphylactoid." In this syndrome, mast cell degranulation is postulated to occur as a result of direct interaction of nonneutralizing antivenin protein or the Fc segment of the IgG molecule itself with mast cell membranes. This often occurs in association with activation of the complement cascade.[50] In addition, large nonneutralizing proteins present in antivenin, as well as aggregates of IgG itself,[4,14,20] may directly activate the complement system, resulting in release of vasoactive mediators with subsequent hypotension, bronchospasm, and airway compromise.

TREATMENT OF ACUTE SERUM REACTIONS

The most feared complications of antivenin administration are anaphylactic and anaphylactoid reactions. The resultant hypotension, bronchospasm, and airway compromise require rapid, appropriate management on the part of the treating physician. These life-threatening sequelae may occur whether antivenin is administered as the skin test or in the full antivenin dose.

Management of allergic reactions should include epinephrine (as intravenous bolus or infusion), antihistamines (both H_1 and H_2 blockers) (Table 30-1), and aggressive airway support if necessary.

MANAGEMENT OF THE ANTIVENIN-ALLERGIC PATIENT

Patients with significant envenomation and a history of allergy to equine-derived antivenin or to horse serum present a difficult challenge. The decision to treat with standard antivenin (Antivenin [Crotalidae] Polyvalent Wyeth) must be based on strong clinical and laboratory indications and requires careful risk-benefit analysis. A patient with a history of allergy to antivenin who requires antivenin because of life- or limb-threatening symptoms may be successfully supported with epinephrine, antihistamines (both H_1 and H_2 blockers) (Table 30-1), and careful attention to airway management. Patients who have experienced life-threatening allergic reactions to antivenin may not necessarily have recurrent reactions when rechallenged. Nevertheless, it is prudent to pretreat such patients with epinephrine and antihistamines (diphenhydramine and cimetidine) before antivenin administration.

SERUM SICKNESS

In addition to the acute effects associated with antivenin administration, a delayed type III hypersensitivity reaction is well described. This entity, known as serum sickness, has a significant incidence,[13,51] particularly in patients receiving more than seven or eight vials of antivenin.[19,55]

The syndrome of serum sickness was originally described in 1905 by two pediatricians, von Pirquet and Schick, who noted that children receiving equine-derived streptococcal antitoxin sometimes developed fever, lymphadenopathy, and rash.[30] They coined the term "serum sickness" to describe this constellation of symptoms resulting from the administration of heterologous serum.

Modern definitions of this syndrome have varied little from the original description. Serum sickness is a spectrum of disease, typically characterized by fever, malaise, urticaria, lymphadenopathy, arthralgias, and less commonly,

Table 30-1 Recommendations for the Treatment of Antivenin-Induced Anaphylaxis or Anaphylactoid Reaction

	Epinephrine		Antihistamines	
	Infusion	**Bolus**	**Diphenhydramine**	**Cimetidine**
Adult	1-4 μg/min IV	0.5-1.0 ml of 1:10,000 solution IV	50 mg IV stat, then 50 mg IV q6h, prn	300 mg IV stat, then 300 mg IV q6h, prn
Child	0.01-1.0 μg/kg/min IV	0.01 mg/kg of 1:10,000 solution IV	1 mg/kg IV stat, then 1 mg/kg IV q6h prn	5-10 mg/kg IV stat, then 5-10 mg/kg IV q6h, prn

glomerulonephritis and neuritis. The onset of symptoms usually occurs within 1 to 2 weeks after exposure to foreign antigens, in this case, heterologous protein in antivenin.

The pathophysiology of this disorder results from nonspecific deposition of immune complexes (antigen-IgG) in susceptible tissue. Under nonpathologic conditions, these complexes are cleared by the reticuloendothelial system without sequelae. However, in the presence of abnormal vascular permeability and slight antigen excess, precipitation of immune complexes occurs. In addition, there is a predilection for immune complex deposition in tissues whose vasculature has a filtering function.[7] These complexes diffuse between endothelial cells and deposit along the basement membrane.[28] The interaction of immune complexes trapped in the vascular wall with vasoactive mediators results in complement activation, further release of vasoactive mediators, and exacerbation of the inflammatory process. This process characteristically occurs in skin, synovial joints, and the glomerular apparatus, resulting in the clinical manifestations of serum sickness.[12,27,57]

Treatment of Serum Sickness

A large percentage of patients receiving more than seven or eight vials of the standard, equine-derived anticrotalid antivenin develop serum sickness.[19,55] The spectrum of illness in this syndrome is highly variable and may range from mild urticaria, malaise, and low-grade fever to debilitating arthralgias and myalgias. Fortunately, although well described, glomerulonephritis and neuritis are rare complications. The variability of the syndrome requires that treatment be tailored to individual clinical needs.

Patients with serum sickness should receive antihistamines such as diphenhydramine or hydroxyzine and, except in the mildest cases, a 7- to 10-day course of high-dose steroids. Clinical illness typically resolves within 1 to 2 weeks.

In summary, although effective, Antivenin (Crotalidae) Polyvalent Wyeth is replete with potential problems. These include the presence of significant amounts of nonneutralizing but immunogenic equine proteins and the precipitation and inactivation of neutralizing antibodies in the process of manufacturing, thus necessitating the administration of multiple vials of antivenin.

Use of Specific Antivenins

This section covers general aspects of antivenin use for envenomation by the black widow spider, coral snake, and pit vipers. Specific indications for each antivenin are covered in their respective chapters (see Chapters 28, 29, and 32), as are specialized or experimental antivenins directed against the venoms of such creatures as scorpions (see Chapter 35) and stonefish, box-jellyfish, and sea snakes (see Chapter 52).

ARACHNID ANTIVENIN

Black Widow Spider

The only nonsnake antivenin approved by the Food and Drug Administration (FDA) for use in the United States is indicated for envenomation by the black widow spider, *Latrodectus mactans* (see Chapter 32). Antivenin *(Latrodectus mactans)* MSD is derived from hyperimmunizing horses with *Latrodectus* venom and is effective in counteracting the pain typically associated with severe envenomations. It is used frequently in Australia and not unexpectedly is associated with a low but measurable incidence of anaphylaxis and serum sickness.[52]

Fortunately, the venom from the black widow spider rarely results in life-threatening manifestations. Patients can usually be managed effectively with adequate doses of narcotic analgesics and benzodiazepines. There are conditions, however, in which *Latrodectus* antivenin may be indicated. In general, patients with underlying medical problems such as coronary artery disease or chronic obstructive pulmonary disease, whose pain may trigger secondary ischemic events, or who may not be able to tolerate large doses of narcotics or benzodiazepines may be appropriate candidates for antivenin. Pregnancy and extremes of age have often been cited as indications for antivenin.[29,40] Overall, the consensus in the United States is that little justification exists for using a product that may induce life-threatening allergic reactions when effective alternative therapy is available.[29]

SNAKE ENVENOMATION

In contrast to black widow spider bites, venomous snakebites (see Chapters 28 and 29) do not afford the luxury of withholding antivenin when signs of envenomation are present. There is no effective alternative therapy for clinically significant snake envenomations other than commercially available antivenin. In the setting of venomous snakebites, early intervention with adequate doses of antivenin reduces the morbidity and mortality associated with envenomation.[39]

The currently available antivenins in North America for indigenous snakebites are the equine-derived Antivenin (Crotalidae) Polyvalent Wyeth, and eastern coral snake antivenin, Antivenin *(Micrurus fulvius)*.

CORAL SNAKES (ELAPIDAE)

The American Association of Poison Control Centers reported 27 coral snake bites (family Elapidae) in 1991.[23] An effective antivenin is available only for the Eastern *(Micrurus fulvius fulvius)* and Texas *(M. fulvius tenere)* coral snakes. Envenomation by these two species is associated with more serious systemic findings than typically occurs with their Arizona (Sonoran, *Micruroides euryxanthus*) counterpart.[21,38] Signs of local envenomation are minimal, with neurotoxicity in the form of bulbar and respiratory paralysis developing up to 12 hours after the bite.

Immunotherapy for *Micrurus fulvius* envenomation requires intravenous administration of four to six vials of Antivenin *(Micrurus fulvius)* (Equine Origin).[37] Additional vials may be necessary as clinically warranted.[21] Antivenin should be given to patients who have been bitten by an Eastern coral snake that has "chewed" on the affected part and who have evidence of fang penetration through the skin.[21]

Early antivenin treatment is recommended, since cranial nerve dysfunction and respiratory paralysis from Eastern coral snake envenomation may be easier to prevent than to reverse once established.[21] It is possible that once venom components are bound to neuronal target tissue, either they are not readily removed by antivenin, or the end-organ toxicity they induce is not readily reversible. Thus early administration of antivenin, preferably within 8 hours of the bite, has been advocated.[21] As with any equine-derived product, skin testing is mandatory and preparations for treatment of anaphylaxis must be in place. (Skin testing may be omitted if the patient is hemodynamically unstable as a result of envenomation.)

PIT VIPERS (CROTALIDAE)

The only FDA-approved antivenin for the treatment of pit viper envenomation in the United States is Antivenin (Crotalidae) Polyvalent Wyeth. Indications for its use include signs and symptoms of progressive envenomation, as manifested by increasing local or systemic effects, or laboratory abnormalities consistent with envenomation (see Chapter 28).

A careful history must be elicited from all envenomed patients. This should include allergy to horse dander, history of atopic reactions, and previous allergy or exposure to horse serum. Patients with positive histories may be at greater risk for allergic reactions to antivenin.

Once the decision to administer antivenin has been made, a skin test should be placed to determine horse serum sensitivity. Skin testing may be omitted for patients in extremis from snake envenomation, since immediate treatment may be lifesaving.

Skin testing should never be done unless a decision to administer antivenin has been made, since life-threatening allergic reactions may occur from skin testing alone. Finally, the patient must be in an intensive care setting, with adequate intravenous access and resuscitation equipment at hand. The attendant staff must be prepared to treat acute anaphylaxis whenever skin testing is performed or antivenin is infused.

Protocol for Skin Test

The manufacturer recommends the following protocol for skin testing[36]:

1. 0.02 to 0.03 ml of a 1:10 dilution of antivenin or 0.02 to 0.03 ml of horse serum (provided in the kit as prediluted 1:10 solution) is injected intradermally.
2. A similar control dose of normal saline is injected at a distant site for comparison.
3. Patients with a history of sensitivity to horse serum, who nevertheless require antivenin therapy, should be skin tested using a dilution of 1:100 of antivenin or normal horse serum.
4. A positive skin test is usually manifest within 5 to 30 minutes and is characterized by a wheal with or without erythema.[36]

That a significant percentage of both false-positive and false-negative skin tests occurs is well documented in the literature. Therefore a negative skin test does not rule out the potential for anaphylaxis associated with the administration of antivenin. Equally important, a positive skin test does not contraindicate the use of antivenin if the patient's life or limb is threatened.[26,36,39] The purpose of a skin test is to identify a patient with obvious severe hypersensitivity so that the health care team can be prepared to manage an allergic reaction.

Administration of Antivenin (Crotalidae) Polyvalent Wyeth

In general, 10 vials of antivenin are administered initially, although the clinical severity of the bite may necessitate higher initial doses. Eastern diamondback rattlesnake *(C. adamanteus)* envenomations, for example, are typically more severe and may require an initial dose of 10 to 20 vials of antivenin.

Although seemingly a minor detail, dissolving the lyophilized antivenin is yet another challenge in managing the snakebite patient. Ten milliliters of diluent (bacteriostatic water for injection, USP) provided with each antivenin kit is added to the lyophilized antivenin. Gentle swirling and rotating of the vials are mandatory to avoid inactivating the neutralizing component, IgG. Vigorous handling or shaking while solubilizing the antivenin may result in partial denaturation of IgG. This process takes 20 to 30 minutes per vial, so enlisting the help of staff results in more rapid completion of the solubilizing process.

Once in solution, the vials of antivenin are diluted in 250 to 500 ml D_5W or normal saline. The initial rate of infusion should be slow, coupled with frequent clinical assessment for evidence of an allergic reaction. If well tolerated, the remainder of the infusion should be administered over 1 hour.

The initial rate of antivenin infusion in patients with positive skin tests should be even slower than for the skin test–negative patients. Pretreatment of these patients with epinephrine and antihistamines is advocated by some[32] but is not universally recommended. We support their use. If no allergic reaction occurs, the residual infusion may proceed over the next 1 to 2 hours.

If anaphylaxis develops during administration of antivenin, the infusion is stopped and aggressive airway management and pharmacologic intervention are initiated. Patients should receive epinephrine and antihistamines (both H_1 and H_2 blockers) (Table 30-1). Persistent life-threatening, systemic signs of venom poisoning may necessitate restarting the antivenin infusion. Under these conditions the antivenin should be further diluted and given at a slower rate than the initial infusion. The patient should be pretreated with antihistamines and epinephrine, and when required, epinephrine should be simultaneously infused at a second intravenous site (see Chapter 28).

Experimental Approaches to Immunotherapeutics

PURIFICATION OF EQUINE-DERIVED ANTICROTALID IgG(T)

In an effort to eliminate the deleterious effects of Antivenin (Crotalidae) Polyvalent Wyeth, several novel approaches have been explored. These include purification of Wyeth antivenin, affinity purification of Fab fragments, use of avian-derived antibodies, and production of monoclonal antibodies.

Sullivan and Russell successfully purified a neutralizing class of IgG antibody (subclass IgG[T]) from the Wyeth antivenin preparation using affinity purification techniques.[41,47,48] Numerous assays, both in vitro and in vivo, have demonstrated the superiority of this IgG(T) fraction over commercial antivenin. Purified IgG attenuated or prevented venom-induced lethality in mice, human fibrinogen clot formation, human embryonic lung cell culture cytotoxicity, human platelet aggregation, and tissue hemorrhage and necrosis in mice.[3,41,48]

The purified IgG is also less antigenic than the Wyeth preparation.[41,47,48] Guinea pigs previously sensitized with horse serum did not develop anaphylaxis when challenged with IgG(T). In contrast, sensitized animals challenged with the commercially available antivenin developed a syndrome consistent with anaphylaxis.[18,41,47,48] Furthermore, human leukocytes from patients known to be sensitized to horse serum released increased amounts of histamine in vitro when challenged with either commercially available antivenin or horse serum. In contrast, leukocytes from the same sensitized patients challenged with the affinity-purified IgG fraction produced no increase in histamine release.[48]

The advantages of affinity-purified antibody are that large amounts of neutralizing IgG(T) can be isolated with relatively simple methodology[47] and that the final product contains less nonneutralizing heterologous protein[47] and is therefore less immunogenic and more concentrated in neutralizing antibodies.[41,47,48]

Like the standard antivenin, these pooled, affinity-purified IgG fractions derived from four species of pit viper demonstrate effective neutralization of toxicity from other pit viper species.[3,41,47,48]

AVIAN-DERIVED ANTICROTALID IgG

In another approach to this problem, Carroll and associates[11] have developed a purified, avian-derived crotalid antivenin. In this experimental model, laying hens are repeatedly injected with inactivated venom from three crotalid species: *C. atrox* (western diamondback), *Trimeresurus flavoviridis* (habu), and *C. durissus terrificus* (South American or tropical rattlesnake). Affinity purification of IgG from egg yolk yields neutralizing antivenin, which is significantly more potent, on a protein weight basis, than the Wyeth preparation in neutralizing the three crotalid venoms tested.

In addition to the relatively low estimated production cost, avian-derived antivenin has an important advantage over mammalian antivenin in that it does not fix complement.[11] Although the untoward effects attributed to complement activation (such as anaphylactoid reactions and cytotoxicity) are avoided, serious adverse reactions may still occur, especially in patients with allergies to egg products.

ADVENT OF Fab IMMUNOTHERAPY

A further advance in immunotherapy for envenomation involves the use of specific Fab to neutralize venom (Fig. 30-3). There are theoretical advantages for the use of these smaller antibody fragments. The "perfect" immunotherapeutic agent should have the following characteristics: (1) high specificity and affinity for the antigen, (2) rapid and extensive tissue distribution so that it will reach and bind the antigen in a timely fashion, (3) low antigenicity, and (4) rapid clearance from the body.[47] Based on clinical and experimental data, Fab appears to satisfy these criteria.

ADVANTAGES OF Fab VERSUS IgG

Digoxin Antidote Experience

A large body of evidence from both animal and human experiments supports the efficacy and superiority of purified Fab compared to whole IgG. Much of the evidence comes from animal and human experience with digoxin intoxication. Extensive experience with the digoxin antidote, Digibind, demonstrates that ovine-derived digoxin-specific Fab fulfills the criteria for an effective immunotherapeutic agent, and is superior in some respects to whole IgG antibodies.[8,24,45]

Kinetic Advantages and Immunologic Efficacy of Fab Versus IgG

In the baboon and rabbit models, distribution and elimination half-lives for digoxin-specific Fab were significantly shorter (0.28 to 0.32 and 9 to 13 hours, respectively) than those of the digoxin-specific IgG molecules (4 and 61 hours, respectively).[45] In addition, the volume of distribution of digoxin-specific Fab is significantly greater than that of the whole IgG antibody, reflecting its more extensive tissue distribution. In this model, therefore, Fab was more rapidly and extensively distributed to tissue sites than was IgG.[45]

Similar kinetic analysis in the dog model of digoxin poisoning revealed significantly shorter distribution half-lives with Fab than with the whole IgG antibody (0.54 hour versus 2.28 hours, respectively). This correlated with shorter mean time to reversal of digoxin-induced cardiotoxicity in the Fab-treated group (36 minutes versus 85 minutes in the IgG group).[24]

As important as the proven efficacy of ovine-derived Fab[1,44,58] is the absence of anaphylaxis or serum sickness despite its extensive use in clinical practice. Digoxin-specific Fab (Digibind) is a safe and effective therapy for the rapid reversal of digoxin-induced cardiotoxicity. The antidote has also been used to manage intoxication from wild oleander.

OVINE-DERIVED Fab ANTIVENIN

Affinity-Purified Fab Anti–Vipera Berus Antivenin

In an attempt to reduce the incidence of untoward immunologic reactions, an affinity-purified Fab antivenin effective against *Vipera berus* (European viper) has been developed.[43] Preliminary data from clinical trials in Sweden demonstrate decreased morbidity after treatment with Fab.[34] Equally important, neither anaphylaxis nor serum sickness has occurred.

Polyvalent Crotalid Antivenin, Ovine Fab (Lyophilized)

An important advance in the immunotherapeutics of crotalid envenomation has recently been achieved with the production of a purified Fab crotalid antivenin, Polyvalent Crotalid Antivenin (Ovine Fab Lyophilized). This product is derived from sheep immunized with venom from four species of pit viper (*C. atrox* [western diamondback], *C. adamanteus* [eastern diamondback], *C. scutulatus scutulatus* [Mojave rattlesnake], and *Agkistrodon piscovorus piscovorus* [eastern cottonmouth]) and is in clinical trial in the United States.

Successful reversal of the clinical manifestations of crotalid envenomation using polyspecific anticrotalid Fab can be anticipated based on (1) the effectiveness of digoxin-specific Fab immunotherapy, (2) the promising clinical trials using Fab antivenin directed against *V. berus*,[34] and (3) the protection against venom-induced lethality in mice after the administration of specific Fab.[49]

Although analogies can be made between the successful treatment of digoxin toxicity with Digibind and the use of purified Fab fragment antivenin for snake envenomation, there are some important differences. (1) Unlike digoxin, snake venom is a heterogeneous mixture of antigens varying greatly in size and structure. The antigenicity of each venom component may vary greatly depending on its physical characteristics. (2) Unlike snake venom, digoxin does not cause permanent cellular damage to target cells. Thus, once digoxin is bound to Digibind, the cellular toxicity is reversed. The same may not be true of toxic effects of venom. (3) The relatively small size of digoxin (781 daltons) and the Fab portion (50,000 daltons) permits the complex to be renally excreted. In addition, there is evidence to support endogenous renal catabolism of such small complexes.[2,22,46,56] This will probably not be true of much larger Fab-venom immune complexes.

Venom is a complex mixture of proteins, glycoproteins, and peptides, with molecular weights ranging from several thousand to greater than 100,000.[39] Fab complexed to small-molecular-weight venom components may be cleared renally. The majority of venom proteins, however, have molecular weights greater than 20,000 daltons and would be too large to be filtered and excreted by the kidney when complexed to Fab. This may result in significantly longer elimination half-lives of venom-Fab complexes. Theoretically, this may allow sufficient time for dissociation of the venom-Fab complex, resulting in the release of active venom components.

IS THERE A ROLE FOR MONOCLONAL ANTIBODIES?

In the ongoing search for the "perfect" antivenin, we have evolved in sophistication from the earliest recorded production of antivenin in 1896 by Calmette[10] to the present development of Fab immunotherapy.

Advances in molecular biology have made the use of monoclonal antibodies commonplace in research.[16] A monoclonal antibody is a single, unique molecule produced in large quantity by a clone of cultured B cells. The role of monoclonal antibodies in venom research and experimental immunotherapeutics is currently being explored.

Reports describing the production of monoclonal antibodies directed against specific venom components and activities are appearing in the literature with great frequency. Monoclonal antibody–based ELISA immunoassays can be used to measure the concentration of venom components and may be more accurate and sensitive than other currently available bioassays.[5] Furthermore, this technique has diagnostic potential, since it can be used to detect unique venom components after envenomation.[31]

In addition, successful isolation of monoclonal antibodies directed against specific venom activities suggests promising new therapeutic potential. For example, monoclonal antibodies directed against venom components with antithrombin-like,[31] antihemorrhagic,[17,33] antimyotoxic,[25] and other activities have been purified. Preincubation of several classes of antiphospholipase A_2-monoclonal antibodies neutralized the myotoxic activity in mice typically seen with *Bothrops asper* (fer-de-lance) envenomation.[25]

Despite these advances, there are significant theoretical problems with the use of monoclonal antibodies for the therapy of venom poisoning. Traditionally, we have defined an effective antivenin as having a broad spectrum of activity capable of counteracting a wide array of clinical sequelae. Because of the complex and heterogeneous nature of venoms with their innumerable antigenic sites, such antivenin would require pooling of many different monoclonal antibodies.

In addition, a major advantage of a polyclonal antivenin is its ability to neutralize the effects of venoms of related species within the same genus or family. The very specificity that enables monoclonal antibodies to target unique antigenic determinants might render it impractical as an isolated therapeutic modality against envenomation.[25,47]

Nevertheless, with continued isolation of monoclonal antibodies capable of neutralizing specific clinical effects of envenomation such as myotoxic effects[25] and thrombinlike activity,[31] we may eventually develop "libraries" of monoclonal antibodies capable of targeting and counteracting predominant signs and symptoms of envenomation. Thus adjunctive immunotherapy with monoclonal antibodies in conjunction with a broad-spectrum antivenin may provide the exquisite sensitivity against specific adverse reactions typically absent in standard antivenin.

After a slow start, advances in molecular biology are finally being applied to envenomation therapeutics. We can anticipate a multitude of novel immunotherapeutic modalities in the future.

REFERENCES

1. Antman EM et al: Treatment of 150 cases of life-threatening digitalis intoxication with digoxin-specific Fab antibody fragments: final report of a multicenter study, *Circulation* 81:1744, 1990.
2. Arend WP, Silverblatt JF: Serum disappearance and catabolism of homologous immunoglobulin fragments in rats, *Clin Exp Immunol* 22:502, 1975.
3. Bar-Or D et al: Neutralization of Crotalidae venom induced platelet aggregation by affinity chromatography isolated IgG to *Crotalus viridis helleri* venom, *Clin Toxicol* 22:1, 1984.
4. Barandun S et al: *Clinical applications of immunoglobulin (gamma globulin): a review of current findings,* Basel, Switzerland, 1982, Sandoz Products.
5. Bignami GS et al: Monoclonal antibody–based enzyme-linked immunoassays for the measurement of palytoxin in biological samples, *Toxicon* 30:687, 1992.
6. Brazil V: *Le defense contre l'ophidisme,* ed 2, São Paulo, 1914, Pocai & Weiss.
7. Buhner D, Grant JA: Serum sickness, *Dermatol Clin* 3:107, 1985.
8. Butler VP Jr et al: Effects of sheep digoxin-specific antibodies and their Fab fragments on digoxin pharmacokinetics in dogs, *J Clin Invest* 59:35, 1977.
9. Calmette A: L'immunisation artificielle des animaux contre le venin des serpents et al therapeutic experimentale de morsures venimeuses, *CR Soc Biol* 46:120, 1894.
10. Calmette A: *Le venin de serpants: physiologie de l'envenomation; traitment des morsures venimeuses par le serum des animaux vaccines,* Paris, 1896, Societe de Editions Scientifiques.
11. Carroll SB, et al: Comparison of the purity and efficacy of affinity purified avian antivenoms with commercial equine crotalid antivenoms, *Toxicon* 30:1017, 1992.
12. Cochrane CG, Koffler D: Immune complex disease in experimental animals and man, *Adv Immunol* 16:185, 1973.
13. Corrigan P, Russell FE, Wainschel J: Clinical reactions to antivenin, *Toxicon* 1(suppl):457, 1978.
14. Day NK, Good RA, Wahn V: Adverse reactions in selected patients following intravenous infusions of gamma globulin, *Am J Med* 76(suppl 3A):25, 1984.
15. Hawgood BJ: Review article: pioneers of anti-venomous serotherapy: Dr. Vital Brazil (1865-1950), *Toxicon* 30:573, 1992.
16. Henry R, Begent J, Pedley RB: Monoclonal antibody administration: current clinical pharmacokinetic status and future trends, *Clin Pharmacokinet* 23:85, 1992.
17. Iddon D, Hommel M, Theakston RDG: Characterization of a monoclonal antibody capable of neutralizing the haemorrhagic activity of the West African *Echis carinatus* (carpet viper) venom, *Toxicon* 26:169, 1988.
18. Jeter WS, Russell FE, Sullivan JB: Short communication: anaphylaxis in guinea pigs challenged with antivenin preparations, *Toxicon* 21:729, 1983.
19. Jurkovich GJ et al: Complications of Crotalidae antivenin therapy, *J Trauma* 28:1032, 1988.
20. Kirkpatrick CH: Allergic histories and reaction of patients treated with digoxin immune Fab (ovine) antibody, *Am J Emerg Med* 9 (suppl 1):7, 1991.
21. Kitchens C, Van Mierop L: Envenomation by the eastern coral snake *(Micrurus fulvius fulvius):* a study of 39 victims, *JAMA* 258:1615, 1987.
22. Lathem W et al: The demonstration and localization of renal tubular reabsorption of hemoglobin by stop flow analysis, *J Clin Invest* 39:840, 1960.
23. Litovitz TL et al: 1991 annual report of the American Association of Poison Control Centers, *Am J Emerg Med* 10:452, 1992.
24. Lloyd BL, Smith TW: Contrasting rates of reversal of digoxin toxicity by digoxin-specific IgG and Fab fragments, *Circulation* 58:280, 1978.

25. Lomonte B et al: Neutralization of myotoxic phospholipases A2 from the venom of the snake *Bothrops asper* by monoclonal antibodies, *Toxicon* 30:239, 1992.
26. Malasit P et al: Prediction, prevention and mechanism of early (anaphylactic) antivenom reactions in victims of snake bites, *Br Med J* 292:17, 1986.
27. Melvold R: Review of immunology. In Patterson R et al, editors: *Allergic diseases: diagnosis and management,* ed 4, Philadelphia, 1993, JB Lippincott.
28. Michael AF Jr et al: Acute poststreptococcal glomerulonephritis, *J Clin Invest* 45:237, 1966.
29. Moss H, Binder L: A retrospective review of black widow spider envenomation, *Ann Emerg Med* 16:188, 1987.
30. Mygind N: *Essential allergy,* Oxford, Eng, 1986, Blackwell Scientific Publications.
31. Nakamura M, Kinjoh K, Kosugi T: Production of a monoclonal antibody against the thrombin-like enzyme, habutobin, from *Trimeresurus flavoviridis* venom, *Toxicon* 30:1177, 1992.
32. Otten EJ, McKimm D: Venomous snakebite in a patient allergic to horse serum, *Ann Emerg Med* 12:624, 1983.
33. Perez JC, Garcia VE, Huang SY: Production of a monoclonal antibody against hemorrhagic activity of *Crotalus atrox* (Western diamondback rattlesnake) venom, *Toxicon* 22:967, 1984.
34. Persson H, for the *V. berus* Fab antivenom study group: initial experience with *Vipera berus* specific Fab antivenom, abstract, *European Association Poison Centers and Clinical Toxicologists,* Istanbul, Turkey, 1992, p 3.
35. Phisalix C, Bertrand G: Sur le proriete antitoxique du sang des animaux vaccines contre le venin des vipere, *CR Soc Biol* 46:111, 1894.
36. Product information, Antivenin (Crotalidae) Polyvalent, Wyeth.
37. Product information, Antivenin *(Micrurus fulvius)* Equine Origin, Wyeth.
38. Russell FE: Bites by the Sonoran coral snake, *Micruroides euryxanthus, Toxicon* 5:39, 1967.
39. Russell FE: *Snake venom poisoning,* ed 2, New York, 1983, Scholium International.
40. Russell FE, Marcus P, Streng JA: Black widow spider envenomation during pregnancy, *Toxicon* 17:188, 1979.
41. Russell FE et al: Preparation of a new antivenin by affinity chromatography, *Am J Trop Med Hyg* 34:141, 1985.
42. Sewall H: Experiments on the preventive inoculation of rattlesnake venom, *J Physiol Lond* 8:203, 1887.
43. Smith DC et al: An affinity purified ovine antivenom for the treatment of *Vipera berus* envenoming, *Toxicon* 30:865, 1992.
44. Smith TW: Review of clinical experience with digoxin immune Fab (ovine), *Am J Emerg Med* 9(suppl 1):1, 1991.
45. Smith TW et al: Immunogenicity and kinetics of distribution and elimination of sheep digoxin-specific IgG and Fab fragments in the rabbit and baboon, *Clin Exp Immunol* 36:384, 1979.
46. Spiegelberg HL, Weigle WO: The catabolism of homologous and heterologous 7S gamma globulin fragments, *J Exp Med* 121:323, 1965.
47. Sullivan JB: Past, present, and future immunotherapy of snake venom poisoning, *Ann Emerg Med* 16:938, 1987.
48. Sullivan JB, Russell FE: Isolation and purification of antibodies to rattlesnake venom by affinity chromatography, *Proc West Pharmacol Soc* 25:185, 1982.
49. Sullivan JB et al: Protection against *Crotalus* venom lethality by monovalent, polyclonal F(ab) fragments: in search of a better snake trap (abstract), *Vet Hum Toxicol* 26:400, 1984.
50. Sutherland SK: Serum reactions: an analysis of commercial antivenoms and the possible role of anticomplementary activity in de-novo reactions to antivenoms and antitoxins, *Med J Aust* 1:613, 1977.
51. Sutherland SK, Lovering KE: Antivenoms: use and adverse reactions over a 12-month period in Australia and Papua New Guinea, *Med J Aust* 2:671, 1979.
52. Sutherland SK, Trinca JC: Survey of 2144 cases of red-back spider bites, *Med J Aust* 2:620, 1978.
53. Theakston RDG, Warrell DA: Antivenoms: a list of hyperimmune sera currently available for the treatment of envenoming by bites and stings, *Toxicon* 29:1419, 1991.
54. Wingert WA: Editorial: treatment of Crotalid envenomation: conservative vs. anticipatory, *J Wilderness Med* 3:113, 1992.
55. Wingert WA, Chan L: Rattlesnake bites in southern California and rationale for recommended treatment, *West J Med* 148:37, 1988.
56. Wochner RD, Strober W, Waldmann TA: The role of the kidney in the catabolism of Bence Jones proteins and immunoglobulin fragments, *J Exp Med* 126:207, 1967.
57. Wolff SM: The vasculitic syndromes. In Wyngaarden JB, Smith LH Jr, Bennett JC, editors: *Cecil textbook of medicine,* ed 19, Philadelphia, 1992, WB Saunders.
58. Woolf AD et al: Results of multicenter studies of digoxin-specific antibody fragments in managing digitalis intoxication in the pediatric population, *Am J Emerg Med* 9:16, 1991.

31 ARTHROPOD ENVENOMATION AND PARASITISM

Sherman A. Minton
H. Bernard Bechtel

The phylum Arthropoda contains about four fifths of the known animals of the world, and insects are the largest group of arthropods. Insects are an important part of the biota of all terrestrial and freshwater environments that support life; only in marine environments are they relatively unimportant. More species of insects exist than of any other form of multicellular life, and they may well exceed all other land animals in biomass. There are very few substances of plant or animal origin that some insects cannot use as food, and in their feeding they play a vital role in recycling organic compounds. They compete with other organisms for the world's food supplies but are themselves a major food source for many forms of life. They are essential for the pollination of many plants.

Insect life cycles are diverse and often complex, involving developmental and sexual stages that are widely different in morphology and ways of life. Although sexual reproduction is the rule, parthenogenesis and pedogenesis occur. Some groups, such as ants, bees, and termites, have developed a high degree of social organization. During at least part of its life cycle, an insect's body is divided into three distinct regions (head, thorax, and abdomen), with three pairs of legs attached to the thorax. Except for a few primitive or parasitic groups, most adult insects have wings.

The greatest direct medical importance of insects is associated with their feeding on human blood and tissue fluids. In doing so, they often inject salivary secretions. This is a highly effective method of transmitting pathogenic microorganisms; moreover, the secretions are often allergenic and sometimes toxic. Other insects may carry human pathogens passively on their feet or mouthparts or in their digestive tracts.

Venoms have evolved in several insect groups, and venomous insects may attack humans, sometimes with lethal results. Skin, hair, and secretions of insects may be irritant or allergenic, producing cutaneous and respiratory syndromes. Finally, insects can be highly annoying.

Venomous Insects

HYMENOPTERA (BEES, WASPS, AND ANTS)

By far the most important venomous insects are members of the order Hymenoptera, including bees, wasps, and ants (Fig. 31-1). They vary in size from minute to large (up to 60 mm in body length). The abdomen and thorax are connected by a slender pedicle that may be quite long in certain wasps and ants. Bees and most wasps are winged as adults; ants are wingless, except for sexually mature adults during part of the life cycle. Mouthparts are adapted for chewing but in some species are modified for sucking. The life cycle includes egg, larva, and pupa stages before emergence of adults. Immature stages may be protected and provided with food by the adult. Both animal and plant foods are used. Many species are parasitic on other arthropods. All ants and many species of bees and wasps are social insects. Colonies range in size from a few dozen individuals to many thousands. In cold climates, most individuals die in autumn, leaving the fertilized females to winter over and found new colonies in the spring.

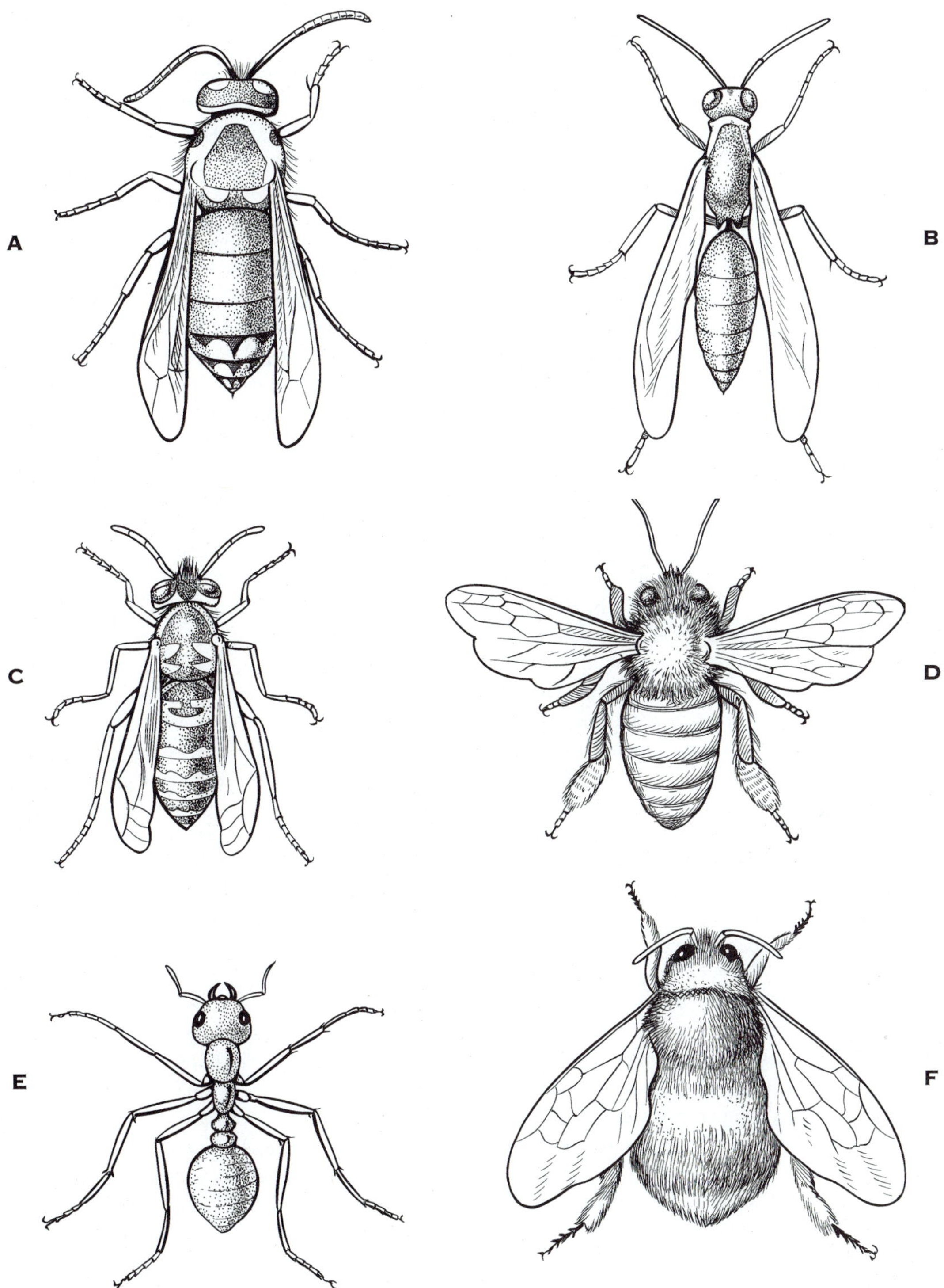

Fig. 31-1 Representative venomous Hymenoptera: **A,** hornet *(Vespula maculata);* **B,** wasp *(Chlorion ichneumerea);* **C,** yellowjacket *(Vespula maculiforma);* **D,** honey bee *(Apis mellifera);* **E,** fire ant *(Solenopsis invicta);* **F,** bumblebee (*Bombus* species).

Bees

The honey bee *(Apis mellifera)* is one of the few domesticated insects and is maintained in hives in many countries. Numerous geographic races of the honey bee exist; the Italian bee *(A. m. ligustica)*, a common domestic strain of Europe, is also widely distributed in the United States. Feral honey bee colonies usually nest in hollow trees or crevices in rocks but may nest in the walls of occupied buildings.

An event of considerable health and economic significance in the Americas has been the spread of an African race of the honey bee *(A. m. scutellata,* also referred to as *A. m. adansoni)*. This race was introduced from Africa into Brazil because it was thought to be a more efficient honey producer in the tropics. It is characterized by large populations (one queen may lay tens of thousands of eggs), frequent swarming, nonstop flights of at least 20 km, and a tendency toward mass attacks following minimal provocation.

The first escapes from hives occurred in the state of São Paulo in 1957, and the "Brazilian killer bees," or "Africanized bees," have spread widely. Cold climate seems to have stopped their southern spread in Argentina, but they have moved steadily northward 200 to 300 miles per year and in October 1990 reached the southern border of the United States. Unless they acquire greater resistance to winter conditions, their range in the United States will be confined to Florida, the Gulf Coast, southern Texas, and parts of southern California and Arizona.[182] The greatest impact of Africanized bees in the United States will probably be economic, related to decreased honey production and less effective pollination of crops. They also present a threat to human health. Africanized bee colonies are extremely sensitive to disturbance, respond faster in greater numbers, and are up to 10 times more active in stinging than are European bees. However, the quantity of venom per sting is slightly less in African bees, with no significant biochemical or allergenic difference between the venoms.[123,165]

About 350 fatal attacks have been documented, of which at least 70 have occurred in Venezuela during 1977 and 1978.[113,183] From newspaper accounts we have learned of numerous incidents of massive bee attacks in Mexico between 1987 and 1992. Fatalities have been mentioned, but whether they resulted from multiple stings or anaphylaxis is not clear. Since Mexico and the southern United States have many feral and domestic honey bee populations, the aggressiveness of the African bees was thought to be possibly dampened by hybridization. However, recent studies[69,70,174] indicate that European bee populations become rapidly Africanized with little reciprocal gene flow.

Other bees, such as the giant bee *(Apis dorsata)* of southeast Asia, may be important locally. This large feral species has a reputation for savagery, and deaths from multiple stings have occurred. Bumblebees (*Bombus* and related genera) are a largely holarctic group often found in quite cold environments. Small colonies usually nest just under the surface of the ground, often in mammal burrows. Some species are aggressive if disturbed, although most are quite mildly disposed.

Sweat bees (family Halictidae) are small bees of cosmopolitan distribution. They are attracted to sweaty skin and ingest perspiration. They nest in burrows, often in clay banks. Females sting if squeezed or trapped under clothing. The sting itself is not very painful, but anaphylactic reactions have been reported. The allergens are immunologically unrelated to those in other bee and wasp venoms.[134]

Wasps

Social wasps occur throughout most of the world but are recognized chiefly as a medical problem in the United States and Europe. They often establish colonies close to human dwellings. Paper wasps *(Polistes)* suspend their nests in shaded places, often in shrubbery near houses or below eaves, gutters, or window frames. Old World hornets (*Vespa* spp.) and white-faced hornets *(Dolchiovespula maculata)* create large paper nests that may be plastered to buildings but more typically are hung from tree branches (Fig. 31-2). Yellowjackets (*Vespula* spp.) make underground nests in rotted-out tree stumps, mammal burrows, and cavities under stones.

Solitary wasps are predators, feeding largely on other insects and spiders. However, adults often do not eat the prey but carry it alive and paralyzed to the nest, where it serves as food for the larvae. Some wasps excavate burrows, while others make mud nests that may be plastered on shaded walls of buildings or under bridges. Although many nests may be grouped together, they have no social organization, and adults make little effort to defend them. The cicada-killers *(Specius speciosus)* and tarantula hawks (*Pepsis* species) are among the largest North American wasps. Velvet ants (family Mutillidae) are actually wingless wasp females that are nest parasites of other Hymenoptera. They prefer dry and open habitat, such as deserts, and can inflict a painful sting.

Ants

Ants are social insects, worldwide in distribution over a wide range of habitats. Many ants sting, while others have repugnant secretions. The ant species of greatest importance in the United States is the imported fire ant, *Solenopsis invicta* (Fig. 31-1, *E*). It apparently was introduced from South America into Mobile, Alabama, about 1930 and has subsequently spread throughout the southern states from eastern North Carolina to central Texas, largely eliminating another introduced fire ant *(S. richteri)* and two native species. Mound nests are usually found in open grass settings, often in urban areas (Fig. 31-3). Worker colonies reach maximum size in 2 years and rapidly give rise to satellite colonies. *S. invicta* is an extremely irritable insect.

Harvester ants *(Pogonomyrmex)* of the southwestern United States and Mexico are of some medical importance. Entrances to the underground nests are usually surrounded by clear zones and sometimes by rings of soil. Some species re-

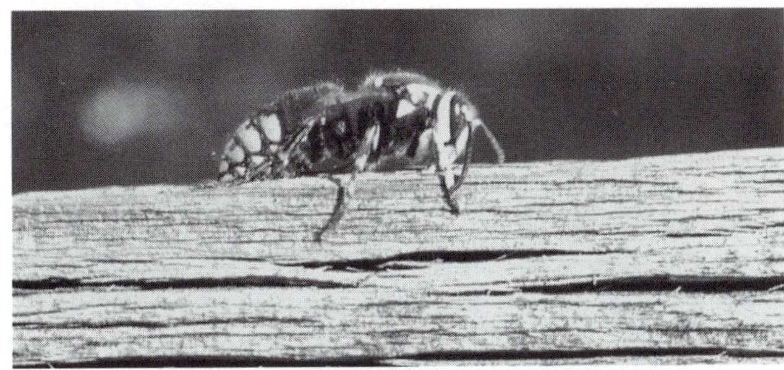

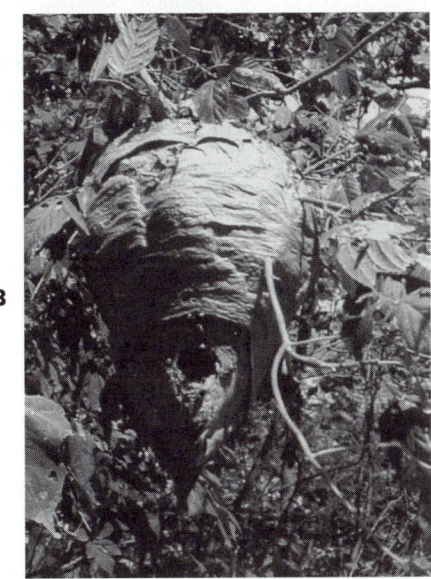

Fig. 31-2 **A,** White-faced hornet, *Dolchiovespula maculata,* largest of the common social wasps in the United States. **B,** Typical nest of the white-faced hornet.

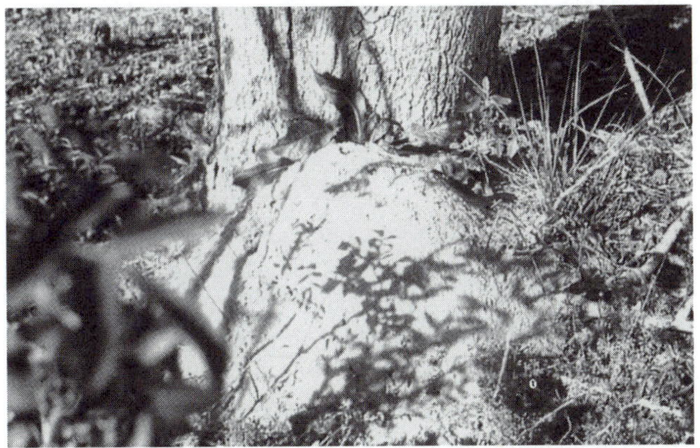

Fig. 31-3 Typical fire ant mound nest photographed near Valdosta, Georgia.

act aggressively to disturbance of the nest. The stings are painful and may be accompanied by systemic symptoms; anaphylaxis has been reported.[138] Australian bull ants *(Myrmecia)* are large insects with prominent jaws. They are common in suburban localities of southeastern Australia, and reports of allergic reactions to their stings are increasing (Fig. 31-4). Tropical American ants of the genus *Paraponera* are large and aggressive. Stings are reported to be painful and often are accompanied by systemic symptoms.

Stinging Patterns

Multiple stings often result from disturbance of a nest, as the first insects encountered release alarm pheromones that incite aggressive behavior in other members of the colony. With large species such as the white-faced hornet, 40 to 50 stings may create a life-threatening injury. Fatalities have resulted from 300 to 500 honey bee stings. In the United States and other Western nations the incidence of serious insect stings is higher in adults than in children and higher in males than in females. Most persons are stung while engaged in outdoor work or recreation. Beekeeping is a high-risk occupation; however, many beekeepers develop considerable immunity as a result of frequent stings. Other relatively high-risk occupations, as regards bee stings, are farmer, house painter, carpenter, and bulldozer operator. Fire ants may invade houses during periods of heavy rain. Wasps and bees sometimes are swept into the interior of a moving automobile, exposing the occupants to risk of both a sting and a highway accident. Many foods, particularly meats, ripe fruit, or fruit syrups, attract yellowjackets; syrups, flowers, and some perfumes attract bees. In temperate zones, incidence of hymenopteran stings is highest in late summer and early fall, when insect populations are highest.

Venom and Venom Apparatus

Venom is present in many hymenopteran species and is used for both defense and subjugation of prey. The venom apparatus is located at the posterior end of the abdomen and consists of venom glands, a reservoir, and structures for piercing the integument and injecting venom. Venoms of most medically important Hymenoptera are mixtures of protein or polypeptide toxins, enzymes, and pharmacologically active low–molecular weight compounds such as histamine,

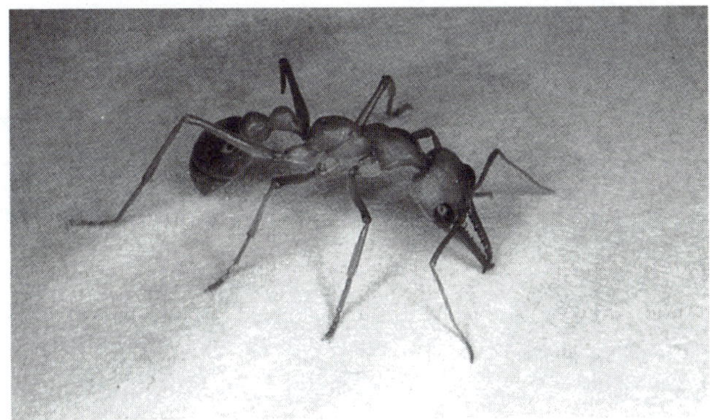

Fig. 31-4 Red bull ant or bulldog ant, *Myrmecia* species. These large ants are common in suburban areas of eastern Australia.

serotonin, acetylcholine, and dopamine. Melittin, a strongly basic peptide, is the principal component of honey bee venom. It damages cell membranes through detergent-like action, with liberation of potassium and biogenic amines. Peptides with similar activity occur in bumblebee venom.[8] Histamine release by bee venom appears to be largely mediated by mast cell degranulating (MCD) peptide. A third peptide, apamin, is a neurotoxin that acts principally on the spinal cord. Adolapin, a recently described bee venom peptide, has antiinflammatory activity[173] that may explain the effectiveness of bee venom in treating some forms of arthritis. The chief enzymes of bee venom are phospholipase A and hyaluronidase. The former is believed to be one of the major venom allergens.[79,172,175] Histamine makes up about 3% of the dry weight of bee venom. The LD_{50} of honey bee venom for mice (IV) is 6 mg/kg. An average sting injects about 50 μl of venom containing approximately 0.05 mg solids.

Intense pain following stings by hornets and other social wasps is largely caused by serotonin and acetylcholine, which comprise 1% to 5% dry venom weight. Wasp kinins (peptides) contribute to pain production and have strong, brief hypotensive effects. Mastoparans are similar in action to MCD peptide but are weaker.[8] Phospholipase A, phospholipase B, and hyaluronidase are present in relatively large amounts. Unidentified proteins, some of which appear to be major allergens, are also present. A lethal protein in *Vespa basalis* venom releases serotonin from tissue cells and has hemolytic and phospholipase A activity.[78] The LD_{50}s of hornet venoms for mice (IV) range from 1.6 to 4.1 mg/kg.[160]

Less is known of venoms of solitary wasps. The venom of *Sceliphoron caementarium,* a mud dauber, is comparatively low in protein and contains no acetylcholine, histamine, serotonin, or kinins, but contains several unidentified low–molecular weight compounds. Its proteins are immunologically different from those of honey bee, yellowjacket, and paper wasp venoms.[154] Philanthotoxin (molecular weight 435) from venom of the beewolf *(Philanthus triangulum)* acts at the insect's myoneural junction and has potential value as an insecticide.[8]

Ant venoms show great variation. Those of more primitive ants (subfamilies Ponerinae, Myrmicinae, and Dorylinae) resemble venoms of social wasps, containing kininlike peptides, enzymes, and unidentified proteins. In more highly evolved ants (subfamilies Dolichoderinae, Formicinae) a variety of low–molecular weight compounds (terpenes, ketones, and organic acids) make up the bulk of the secretion, which may be sprayed rather than injected. Venoms of fire ants (*Solenopsis* spp.) are composed largely of piperidine alkaloids, which cause histamine release and necrosis in human skin.[143] Proteins make up only 0.1% of dry weight of fire ant venoms; however, these proteins are highly allergenic.[7,133,148] Hyaluronidase and phospholipase activities have been demonstrated.

Clinical Aspects

Hymenoptera stings are most commonly inflicted on the head and neck, followed by the foot, leg, hand, and arms. Stings in the mouth, pharynx, and esophagus may occur when bees or yellowjackets in soft drink or beer containers are accidentally ingested. A single wasp, bee, or ant sting in an unsensitized individual usually causes instant pain, followed by a wheal and flare reaction, with variable edema. Fire ants typically grasp the skin with their mouthparts and inflict multiple stings. These produce vesicles that subsequently become sterile pustules (Color Plate 39). Multiple Hymenoptera stings may cause vomiting, diarrhea, generalized edema, dyspnea, hypotension, collapse, and oliguria. Widespread necrosis of skeletal muscle with hyperkalemia and acute tubular necrosis with renal failure, as well as hepatorenal syndrome with hemolysis, have been reported following multiple hornet stings.[13,171,192] Myocardial and cerebral infarction in previously healthy individuals may follow multiple hymenopteran stings.[35,94,95]

Large local reactions spreading more than 15 cm beyond the sting site and persisting more than 24 hours are relatively common.[194] They represent a cell-mediated (type IV) immunologic reaction, although more than half these patients also have IgE antibody against venom or show a positive skin test. Later stings in these individuals usually result in another large local reaction; systemic reactions are rare.[28,65,109]

Allergy is the most serious aspect of hymenopteran stings. Anaphylaxis and related syndromes from this source are relatively common outdoor emergencies. It is estimated that between 0.4% and 4% of the U.S. population shows some clinical degree of allergy to insect venoms, and 40 to 50 deaths are reported annually.[189] Asymptomatic sensitization, as shown by positive venom skin test, was observed in 15% of 269 randomly selected subjects with no history of allergic sting reaction.[60] Sudden death from insect sting may not always be recognized. Of 142 sera obtained post mortem in cases of sudden, unexpected death, 23% contained elevated levels of IgE to at least one insect venom. In contrast, 6% of sera from 92 blood donors contained comparable IgE levels.[167] In eight fatal cases of Hymenoptera sting anaphylaxis, IgE to the putative venom source was elevated in all, although levels were not higher than those of some healthy individuals in the same population.[80]

Wasp and bee venoms contain 9 to 13 antigens, some of which are potent allergens. Available evidence indicates little cross-sensitization between honeybee and wasp venoms. About 50% cross-sensitization occurs between *Polistes* and other social wasp venoms, and nearly 100% between yellowjacket and hornet venoms.[64] Positive radioallergosorbent test (RAST) reactions to imported fire ant venom were seen in 51% of patients allergic to bee and wasp venoms but without exposure to fire ants. A 37,000 dalton molecular weight allergen was identified as the cross-reactive antigen.[81]

Examination of sera of hypersensitive individuals for IgE and IgG antibodies against purified venom proteins indicates that phospholipase A, melittin, and acid phosphatase are important in honeybee venom, while phospholipase A, antigen 5 (a protein of unknown activity), and hyaluronidase are important in yellowjacket venom.[87,90] Antigen 5 from hornet venom is reported to have sequence similarity to certain plant leaf proteins and may explain anaphylactic reactions to first insect stings.[191] Despite the small amount of protein in fire ant venoms, about 12% of persons treated for fire ant stings show systemic allergic reactions, and 32 anaphylactic deaths have been confirmed.[85,149,177] Four antigens in *Solenopsis invicta* venom have been reported to be allergenic.[27]

Allergic sting reactions occur remote from the sting site and typically include pruritus, hives, difficulty in breathing, and nausea. In life-threatening reactions, marked respiratory distress, hypotension, loss of consciousness, and cardiac arrhythmias may be seen. At least half the severe reactions occur within 10 minutes after a sting, and virtually all occur within 5 hours. Most fatalities occur within 1 hour. The interval between the first known sting and the reaction-producing sting is usually less than 3 years but may be as long as 48 years. In a group of 3236 Hymenoptera-allergic individuals, 61.5% were males and 32.3% had a history of atopy. The mean age was 30.5 years. No correlation existed between systemic reactions and number of stings in the past or number of stings per incident and severity of a systemic reaction.[98] In sensitive adults, later stings tend to be increasingly severe. In children 10 years and younger, life-threatening reactions are less frequent than in adults, and repeated sting episodes do not tend to be increasingly severe.[163] Fatalities that occur within the first hour after a sting result from airway obstruction or hypotension or both. In 69% of fatal cases, obstruction of the respiratory tree by edema or secretions was the principal finding at autopsy; in 12%, vascular pathology was the principal finding; and 7% of the victims had primary central nervous system involvement such as petechial hemorrhages, infarction, and cerebral edema.[11] Hemostatic defects, including reduction of all clotting factors and release of a thrombin inhibitor, may be seen with insect sting anaphylaxis.[142] Severe fetal brain damage, presumably associated with hypoxia, has been reported.[47] A wide variety of delayed (3 to 14 days) atypical reactions have been reported following hymenopteran stings. These include serum sickness (Color Plate 40) and Arthus reaction, which are caused by systemic and local effects of antigen-antibody complexes[95]; nephrotic syndrome[10,126]; thrombocytopenic purpura[10,180]; grand mal and focal motor seizures[57]; transient cerebral ischemic attacks[114]; Guillain-Barré syndrome[6]; and progressive demyelinating neurologic disease.[112] Most appear to be immunologically mediated. In one series, elevated IgE to bee or yellowjacket venom was observed in 6 of 13 such patients.[95]

Identification of the individual with potentially dangerous allergy to hymenopteran sting is not always possible. Skin testing with hymenopteran venoms is the most sensitive method; RAST for IgE antibody to venoms is less sensitive.[97] A small but significant number of individuals with no history of sting reactions have IgE antibody specific for hymenopteran venoms; prevalence of this antibody is higher in summer.[199] These methods do not identify all at risk, and antibody levels do not correlate with severity of sting reactions.[61] In a significant number of individuals, particularly children, clinical sensitivity disappears and IgE levels fall virtually to zero 3 to 18 months after a reaction-producing sting. In perhaps 40% of cases, sensitivity may disappear within 3 years.[93,125] Venom antibody (both IgE and IgG) may be found in healthy individuals (40% of beekeepers, 12% of blood donors) with no history of systemic reaction to insect stings.[117] One study suggests that hyperreactivity is related to spontaneous kinin system hyperactivity and complement system defects.[124]

Therapy

Treatment of anaphylaxis is conventional. Aqueous epinephrine 1:1000 should be administered subcutaneously at the first indication of serious hypersensitivity. The dose for adults is 0.3 to 0.5 ml and for children under age 12, 0.01 ml/kg, not to exceed 0.3 ml. When symptoms are predominantly respiratory, epinephrine by inhalation (10 to 20 puffs for an adult; 2 to 4 puffs per 10 kg body weight for a child) may provide more rapid relief.[119] In the presence of profound hypotension, 2 to 5 ml of 1:10,000 epinephrine solution may be given by slow intravenous push, or an infusion may be initiated by mixing 1 mg in 250 ml and infusing at a rate of 0.25 to 1 ml/min. In infants and children the infusion should start at 0.025 ml/kg/min, not to exceed 0.375 ml/kg/min.[9] Aminophylline 5 mg/kg as a loading dose, followed by 0.9 mg/kg/hr as an infusion, may relieve bronchospasm not relieved by epinephrine, although its use has largely been replaced by β_2-selective inhaled agents, such as albuterol.

In the presence of hypotension, intravenous crystalloid solutions should be infused; pressor agents such as dopamine may be required. The military antishock trousers (MAST) garment may be helpful if rapid correction of decreased lower extremity peripheral resistance makes therapeutic sense. Oxygen, intubation, and mechanical ventilation may be needed to correct airway obstruction. Antihistamines and corticosteroids are of little value in acute, severe reactions. Propranolol is contraindicated. Patients under therapy with β-adrenergic blockers may respond poorly to epinephrine. Intravenous glucagon (1 mg) or isoproterenol in carefully titrated doses may be effective in counteracting shock. Atropine (1 mg IV) may be used for heart block and refractory bronchospasm.[4,84,187] Patients with insect sting anaphylaxis require close observation, preferably in the hospital, for about 24 hours.

For mild hymenopteran stings, application of ice packs often gives relief. Honeybees frequently and yellowjackets occasionally leave their stinger in the wound. Stingers should be scraped or brushed off with a sharp edge, not removed with forceps, because the latter may squeeze the attached venom sac and worsen the injury. Home remedies, such as baking soda paste or meat tenderizer applied locally to stings, are of dubious value although the latter is often thought to be effective. Topical anesthetics in commercial "sting sticks" are also of little value. Local application of antihistamine lotions or creams such as tripelennamine may be helpful. An oral antihistamine such as diphenhydramine 25 to 50 mg every 6 hours, pediatric dose 1 mg/kg, is often effective. No therapy is very effective against local effects of fire ant stings. However, oral antihistamines and corticosteroids may give some relief in severe cases. Since infection is common, topical use of antimicrobials such as mupirocin is advisable and prophylactic use of oral antibiotics has been recommended.[32,131] Breaking fire ant blisters should be avoided.

Corticosteroids, such as methylprednisolone 24 mg/day initially then tapered off over 4 to 5 days, often hasten resolution of large local reactions to bee and wasp stings. This may be combined with cold packs.

Envenomation from multiple hymenopteran stings may require more aggressive therapy. Intravenous calcium gluconate (5 to 10 ml of 10% solution) in conjunction with a parenteral antihistamine and corticosteroid may be helpful in relieving pain, swelling, nausea, and vomiting. Hypovolemic shock is managed conventionally. Patients should be observed for 12 to 24 hours for coagulopathy and evidence of renal and neurologic damage. Urinary output is monitored and urine tested for hemoglobin and myoglobin. Serum potassium levels should be monitored. Oliguria with myoglobinuria, azotemia, and hyperkalemia are indications for initiating hemodialysis.

Immunotherapy

Desensitization with purified venoms produces an excellent blocking antibody response and prevents anaphylaxis in more than 95% of patients. A protective antiidiotypic antibody to honey bee venom has been identified.[88] Venoms for desensitization generally available in the United States are honey bee, yellowjacket, wasp *(Polistes)*, and mixed vespid. A whole body extract of fire ant containing at least three venom antigens is also available. No firm guidelines are available for selecting patients to receive immunotherapy. Skin test results and IgE levels in RAST tests are not highly reliable. Adults with a history of systemic allergic reactions should be considered for immunotherapy. Those receiving β-blockers should be shifted to other appropriate medications if possible. Children under 16 who have suffered only cutaneous or mild systemic allergic reactions do not need immunotherapy, nor do patients with a history of only large local reactions.

The numerous regimens for desensitization aim to achieve tolerance to venom doses of about 100 μg. About 95 days is required to achieve a maintenance level of immunity. Rapid programs requiring 3 to 7 days for initial immunization have been described and appear to be effective.[17,122] Some programs make use of both active and passive immunotherapy.[118] Systemic reactions during treatment were experienced by 12% of a series of 1410 patients; no fatalities were reported.[97] Experience of 26 women with 43 pregnancies does not suggest significant increased risk from venom immunotherapy during pregnancy.[166] Maintenance doses are required at intervals after basic immunization. Neither skin test nor determination of IgG and IgE antibody levels against venom will reliably indicate success of immunization, although the majority of patients will be protected by a specific IgG antibody level of 400 RAST units/ml of serum.[188] Actual sting challenge is the most reliable test of desensitization, but it is not widely used.[130] If the skin test is negative after 3 years of immunotherapy, patients may be put on immunologic surveillance. Few patients require more than 5 years of immunotherapy.[146] For unknown reasons, desensitization to wasp venoms is achieved more quickly than to honey bee venom.[19]

Prevention and Preparedness

Patients with a history of allergic reactions to insect stings (including large local reactions) should carry an emergency kit containing epinephrine and should wear medical identification tags. Kits should be available in work or recreation areas where the risk of insect sting is high. Two kits widely available in the United States are EpiPen (Center Laboratories) (Fig. 31-5) and Ana-Kit (Miles Pharmaceutical). EpiPen and EpiPen Jr. are autoinjectors that deliver a 0.3 mg or 0.15 mg dose of epinephrine, respectively. They are quick and easy to use; however, patients should be cautioned against injecting the material into fingers or buttocks or directly over veins. Ana-Kit contains two doses of 0.3 mg of epinephrine in a conventional syringe, plus chewable an-

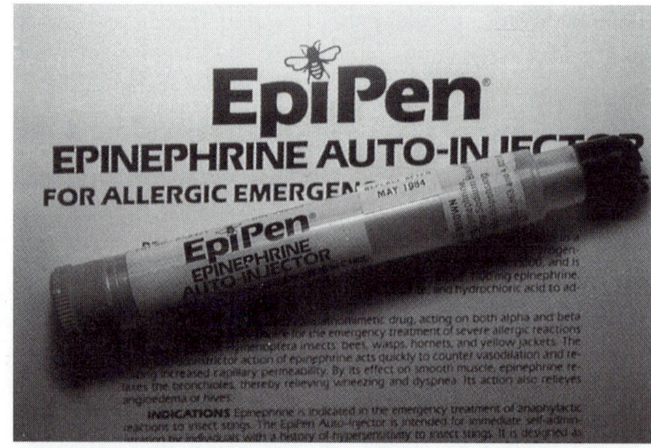

Fig. 31-5 EpiPen (Center Laboratories) preloaded delivery system for injection of aqueous epinephrine.

tihistamine tablets and a tourniquet. It is more versatile but requires more instruction for the user.

Frequent cleaning of garbage cans and disposal of decaying fruit will make premises less attractive to bees and wasps. The Hymenoptera are highly susceptible to many insecticides, and their control around dwellings and other inhabited buildings is rarely difficult. Spraying the nests after dark is safer. Many Hymenoptera are economically valuable as pollinators of plants or predators on other insects, so their control on a wide scale is rarely desirable. The fire ant in the southern United States has been the target of massive but marginally effective control campaigns that have had undesirable effects on local ecosystems. A new approach makes use of grain baits containing synthetic insect growth hormones. They are carried into the nests where they disrupt ant caste differentiation and inhibit egg production.[37] However, arrays of thousands of hormone-baited traps placed in selected areas of Mexico failed to stop the northward spread of Africanized bees.

LEPIDOPTERA

Venomous Species and Venoms

Insects of the order Lepidoptera commonly cause human envenomation, although generally less seriously than do hymenopteran species. Injury usually follows contact with caterpillars, less frequently with the cocoon or adult stage. The larval lepidopteran (caterpillar) is usually free living, is moderately active, and feeds on plants, although a few are parasites of insect nests or eat food of animal origin. The pupal stage may be free or encased in a silk cocoon. Wintering over in cold climates is usually in the pupal stage. Adults (butterflies and moths) are nearly always winged, with wings completely or partly covered with microscopic chitinous scales. They feed largely on nectar and other plant juices, but some feed on semiliquid mammalian feces and urine, and one genus of tropical moths feeds on ocular secretions of domestic mammals. Tropical moths of the family Pyralidae feed on ocular secretions of mammals including humans, and moths of the genus *Calyptera* feed on mammalian blood.[137] The adult provides no care or protection of immature stages, nor does a true social organization exist, although larvae and adults of some species assemble in large aggregations.

Venomous species occur in at least 10 families of Lepidoptera, without general rules for recognition. Many venomous caterpillars are broad, flat, and sluggish. Some have the dorsal surface densely covered with long hairs. Others are markedly spiny and may have bright, conspicuous colors and markings. Still others are highly cryptic.

Venoms in Lepidoptera are purely defensive. The venom apparatus consists of spines that may be simple or branched and are frequently barbed. They may be scattered widely over the surface of the insect or arranged in clumps, and often are intermixed with nonveniferous hairs or spines. In the most venomous caterpillars the spines are hollow and brittle with venom glands at the bases. No muscles or other structures for expelling venom have been described. In some other Lepidoptera the spines are solid and function primarily as mechanical irritants or contain surface toxicants. Little is known of the chemistry of caterpillar venoms. Some are heat labile and known or suspected to contain proteins. Venom of South American *Lonomia* species activates prothrombin, producing coagulopathy.[66] Histamine and serotonin have been found in a few caterpillar venoms but are not of general occurrence.

Venomous Lepidoptera occur on all continents, but the greatest concentration of species causing clinical envenomation occurs in the American tropics. The most dangerous are caterpillars of the genus *Lonomia*. They are large with tufts of stout spines. *Dirphia* and *Automeris* are similar and often brightly colored, but with less toxic venom. *Megalopyge* caterpillars are large, stout, and often densely covered with hair that accounts for such local names as *perrito* (little dog). Moths of the genus *Hylesia* have a tuft of venomous spines at the posterior end of the abdomen and occur through much of tropical South America.

Probably the most important venomous caterpillar in the United States is the puss caterpillar or woolly slug (*Megalopyge opercularis*), which occurs in the southern states west through most of Texas and north to Maryland and Missouri. This hairy, flat, and ovoid caterpillar reaches a length of 30 to 35 mm and feeds on a wide variety of shade trees, including elm, oak, and sycamore. Some years it may be plentiful enough to be a nuisance. In southeast Texas in 1958, 2130 persons were treated for stings and eight were hospitalized.[110] A related species, the flannel moth caterpillar (*M. crispata*), occurs in the eastern states north to New England. Its sting is less severe than that of *M. opercularis*. The large, spiny caterpillar of the io moth (*Automeris io*) is pale green with red and white lateral stripes (Fig. 31-6). It is widely distributed in the eastern United States, but rarely plentiful. The saddleback caterpillar (*Sibine stimula*) and oak slug (*Euclea delphinii*) are flat and almost rectangular.

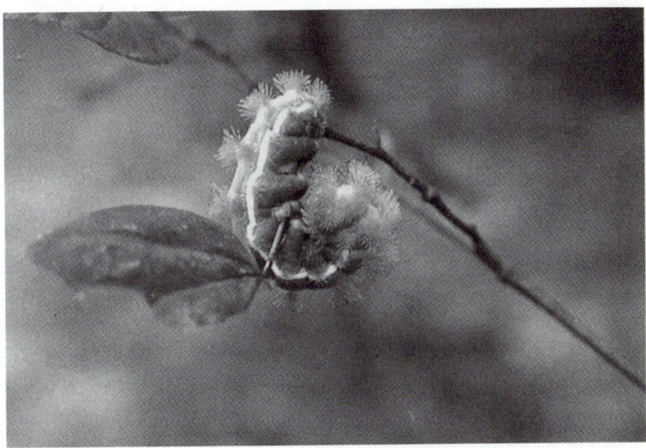

Fig. 31-6 Caterpillar of the io moth, *Automeris io*. A widespread species in the eastern United States, it can inflict a very painful sting.

Each species can deliver a painful injury. The gypsy moth *(Lymantria dispar)* feeds on a wide variety of plants and has caused thousands of cases of dermatitis in the northeastern United States.[15,168] Other common nettling caterpillars are the browntail moth *(Euproctis chrysorrhea)*, which also occurs in Europe, and the tussock or tooth-brush caterpillar *(Hemerocampa leucostigma)*, with its conspicuous red head and four tufts of bristles. Another tussock caterpillar, *Oryia pseudotsuga*, causes numerous cases of dermatitis and conjunctivitis among lumbermen and foresters in the northwestern states.[135]

Caterpillars of the genus *Euproctis* have been involved in large outbreaks of dermatitis in China and Japan. An outbreak at Shanghai in the late summer of 1972 affected about 500,000 individuals.[36] A moth of this genus *(E. flava)* caused hundreds of cases of dermatitis among the military in Korea.[16] Cases have also been reported in Australia.[176] Processionary caterpillars (*Thaumetopoea* spp.) and their cocoons frequently cause dermatitis and conjunctivitis in the Mediterranean region and Near East. Envenomations from about 20 species of caterpillars and four species of moths have been reported from the Nansei Islands of Japan.[86]

Stinging Patterns

Caterpillar envenomation usually occurs when living insects are touched as they cling to vegetation. Persons cutting branches, picking fruit, or climbing trees are likely to be stung. However, the largest outbreaks have been associated with spines detached from live or dead caterpillars and cocoons. These may be airborne or deposited on bedding or laundry hung outdoors. Moths are attracted in large numbers to lights. Outbreaks of *Hylesia* dermatitis sometimes occur among crews of ships loading cargo at South American ports.[41,77] In temperate regions, caterpillar stings are most frequent from August to early November. In the American tropics, envenomation is most prevalent during the rainy season. Heavy caterpillar infestations seem to occur during favorable weather, and decreases in populations of parasites serve as natural controls.

Clinical Aspects

Two general syndromes are associated with lepidopteran envenomations. In the case of caterpillars with hollow spines and basal venom glands (such as *Automeris, Megalopyge,* and *Dirphia*), direct contact with the live insect causes instant nettling pain, followed by redness and swelling. In ordinary cases, no systemic manifestations occur and symptoms usually subside within 24 hours. However, pain may be intense with central radiation, accompanied by nausea, headache, fever, vomiting, and lymphadenopathy.[34,82] Hypotension, shock, and convulsions have been reported.[110] A hemorrhagic syndrome with generalized ecchymosis, bleeding from mucous membranes, melena, and hematuria has been reported following stings by *Lonomia obliqua* and *L. achelous*. Coagulopathy may last 2 to 5 weeks. Acute renal failure, pulmonary hemorrhage, and cerebral hemorrhage may occur. In a series of 33 cases, 4 were fatal. Treatment with prednisone, plasma, and whole blood is ineffective.[3,44]

The second syndrome is associated with caterpillars with a less highly developed venom apparatus (for example, *Lymantria, Euproctis,* and *Thaumetopoea*) or moths such as *Hylesia*. Contact with the living insect is not necessary; detached spines are often involved. Little or no immediate discomfort is experienced. An itching, erythematous, papular, or urticarial rash develops within a few hours to 2 days and persists for up to a week. Rarely, the lesions may be bullous. Conjunctivitis, upper respiratory tract irritation, and rare asthmalike symptoms may be seen with or without dermatitis.[73,106,195] Ophthalmia serious enough to require enucleation may be caused by detached spines lodged in the eye.

Acute anaphylactic reactions have not been reported to follow lepidopteran stings. Both immediate and delayed hypersensitivity has been demonstrated by patch testing.[135] Some residents of the Peruvian jungle appear to develop immunity to caterpillar stings with regular and repeated exposure.[136] A chronic granuloma of the hands of Brazilian rubber workers, known as *pararama,* follows repeated contact with caterpillars and cocoons.[39]

Therapy

Treatment of lepidopteran envenomations is symptomatic. Prompt application and stripping of adhesive tape or a commercial facial peel at the site of the sting may remove many spines and serve as a diagnostic procedure, since the spines can be identified by microscopy. Patients with local symptoms usually get relief from group I corticosteroid creams and ointments. Over-the-counter preparations containing corticosteroids and antihistamines are not significantly better than simpler preparations such as calamine lotion with phenol. Oral antihistamines such as terfenadine (60 mg three times a day) or antiinflammatory drugs such as tolmetin sodium (400 mg three times a day) are often effective in more severe cases. Occasionally codeine (30 to 50 mg), meperidine (50 mg), or oxymorphone (1.5 mg) in combination with an antiemetic may be needed to control pain and vomiting.

Trees on which caterpillars feed may be sprayed with appropriate insecticides to control species such as the puss caterpillar. Near Shanghai, where chemical insecticides would have been harmful to silkworm culture, *Euproctis* caterpillars were controlled by spraying with an insect virus. Screens on windows and doors protect against moths with toxic spines.

HEMIPTERA (SUCKING BUGS)

The Hemiptera are a large order of insects characterized by sucking mouthparts, generally in the form of a beak, and a life cycle in which there are no well-demarcated larval and pupal stages, but a gradual transition from the hatchling nymph to adult. Most hemiptera are winged as adults, with the anterior wings generally divided into a chitinized and membranous section. Most feed on plant juices, but several families are predators, and two feed on the blood of humans and other vertebrates.

The assassin-bugs (family Reduviidae) are generally recognizable by the long and narrow head, a stout and three-jointed beak, long antennae, and typical hemipteran wings (Fig. 31-7). Most are of a dark color; a few are brightly marked or have a checkerboard pattern along the posterior edge of the abdomen. Some species attach fragments of their prey, sand grains, or other debris to their backs. Reduviidae occur on all continents. They frequent a variety of habitats and are often nocturnal.

The triatomids (kissing bugs, flying bedbugs, Mexican bedbugs, *barberos*) are a subfamily of the Reduviidae adapted for feeding on blood. They feed on a wide range of mammals and often live in the nests or burrows of their hosts. Armadilloes, opossums, and pack rats are common hosts in the southern United States and Mexico. Some triatomids adapt readily to life in human dwellings, particularly those of adobe construction. Triatomids are primarily a neotropical group with species ranging northward in the United States to Utah and southern Indiana. *Triatoma protracta* and *T. sanguisuga* are among the better known species. The family Cimicidae, or bedbugs, are flat, ovoid, reddish brown insects whose wings are reduced to a pair of functionless pads. Lack of large terminal claws distinguishes them from lice. Bedbugs are cosmopolitan in distribution. Two species, *Cimex lectularius* and *C. hemipterus,* feed primarily on humans and live in dwellings where they hide in bedding, under wallpaper, behind baseboards, and in window frames. Homes of the economically and socially disadvantaged are more likely to be heavily infested, but the insects may be carried into well-appointed residences, hospitals, and hotels. Other species of *Cimex,* normally parasitic on bats and swallows, occasionally attack humans.

Venomous aquatic Hemiptera include the giant waterbugs (family Belostomatidae) (Fig. 31-8), back-swimmers (family Notonectidae), and water scorpions (family Nepidae). The first are distinguished from aquatic beetles by their beak and hemipteran wings, the back-swimmers have a greatly elongated hind pair of legs, and the water scorpions have a slender body with long terminal breathing tubes. These insects are widely distributed in freshwater habitats.

The hemipteran venom apparatus consists of two or three pairs of glands in the thorax whose secretions are ejected through half of a double tube formed by the interlocking of the very elongate maxillae and mandibles, whose distal tips are modified for piercing. Few hemipteran venoms have been studied. Those of two reduviids, *Platymeris rhadamanthus* of Africa and *Holotrichus innesi* of the Middle East, contain several enzymes as well as some nonenzymatic proteins.[45,197] Venom serves primarily for subjugation and probably digestion of prey, but the insects may defend themselves by biting. Salivary secretions of blood-sucking hemipterans presumably have anticoagulant and vasodilating activity; they are also potent allergens.

Clinical Aspects

Triatomids usually bite at night on exposed parts of the body. Feeding may last from 3 to 30 minutes. Bites are painless. On initial exposure there is usually no reaction. Repeated bites are followed by reddish, itching papules that may persist for up to a week. Bites are often grouped in a cluster or line (Color Plate 41) and may be accompanied by giant urticarial wheals, lymphadenopathy, hemorrhagic bullae, fever, and lymphocytosis.[83,104,170] Systemic anaphylactoid reactions with respiratory or gastrointestinal manifestations are not rare.[176] Entomologists and small children are the groups most frequently bitten by assassin-bugs, for it takes rather rough handling of the insect to induce it to bite. Bites of several U.S. species, such as the wheel-bug *(Arilus cristatus),* black corsair *(Melanolestes picipes),* and masked

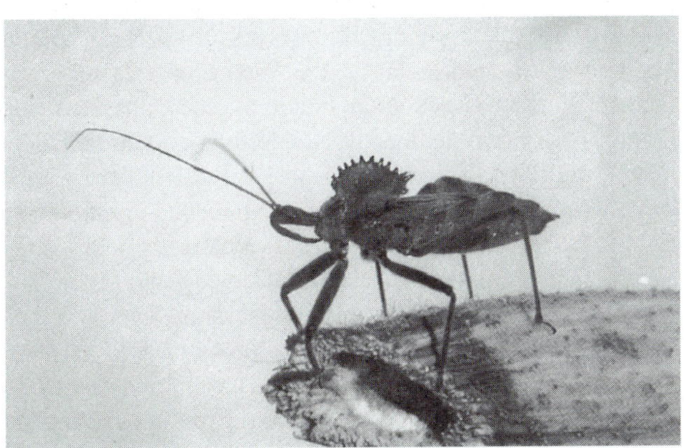

Fig. 31-7 Wheel-bug, *Arilus cristatus,* a large assassin-bug common in the eastern United States.

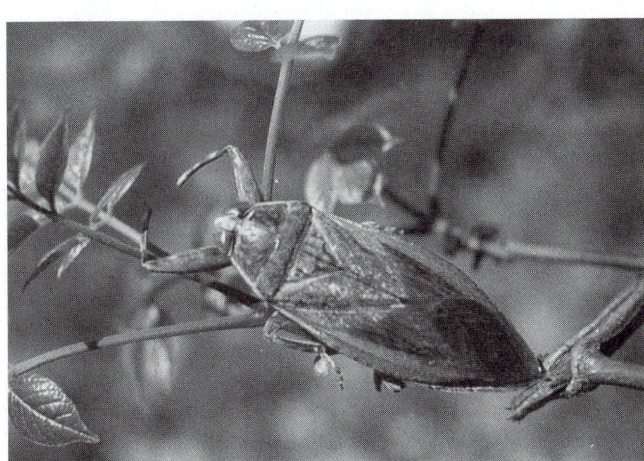

Fig. 31-8 Giant waterbug, *Benacus griseus,* a large insect common in aquatic habitats in the eastern United States.

bedbug hunter *(Reduvius personatus),* have been described as painful as the sting of a hornet and accompanied by local swelling lasting several hours. Bedbug bites usually raise a pruritic wheal with central hemorrhagic punctum, followed by a reddish papule that persists for several days. Bullae, generalized urticaria, arthralgia, asthma, and anaphylactic shock are rare sequelae of bedbug bites.[25,132] Bites of the African reduviid *Platymeris* may be followed by local necrosis; moreover, this species can eject its venom as a spray, causing irritation to eyes and mucous membranes. Bites by aquatic Hemiptera apparently are much like those of assassin-bugs; however, few cases have been described in detail.

Treatment and Prevention

Treatment is symptomatic and not particularly effective. Various antipruritic preparations are helpful in mild cases. Topical or intralesional steroids have generally been disappointing. Immobilization, elevation, and local heat are helpful in severe limb bites. Desensitization with triatomid salivary gland extract has been effective in a small series of patients with history of life-threatening anaphylactic reactions.[153]

Triatomids and bedbugs are more difficult to eradicate by insecticides than are many household insects. Benzene hexachloride has been effective against triatomids in Latin America.

BEETLES AND OTHER INSECTS

Beetles (order Coleoptera) are the largest group of insects, with at least 250,000 species. The prothorax of beetles is generally very distinct, while the two posterior thoracic segments are more or less fused to the abdomen. In most beetles the anterior wings are heavily chitinized, acting as covers for the posterior membranous wings used in flight. Mouthparts are of the chewing type. The life cycle involves larval and pupal stages before emergence of the adult. Many beetles feed on plants throughout their life cycle, many are predators or scavengers, and a few are parasitic. No beetles have a bite or sting venomous to humans. However, bites producing papules with small necrotic centers have been inflicted by a species of ladybug found in Australia and New Zealand.[139] Several families have toxic secretions that may be deposited on the skin. The blister beetles (family Meloidae) are a cosmopolitan group with numerous representatives in deserts and semiarid regions. A species may suddenly appear by the thousands, especially after rains, persist for a few days, and be replaced by another. The majority are of medium size (about 15 mm) and have soft, leathery forewings (elytra). Some are brilliantly colored. They are plentiful on vegetation, and some species are attracted to lights. A low–molecular weight toxin, cantharidin, is present in the hemolymph and most of the insect's tissues. It is exuded from multiple sites if the beetle is gently pressed or otherwise disturbed.

In the eastern United States, blister beetle dermatitis is usually caused by *Epicauta* species, which occur on many garden plants. Contact with the beetle is painless and seldom remembered by the patient. Blisters appear 2 to 5 hours after contact and may be single or multiple, ordinarily 5 to 50 mm in diameter and thin walled. Unless broken and rubbed, they are not painful. Cantharidin nephritis has been reported following unusually heavy vesication[21] but more frequently is the result of using a cantharidin preparation as an aphrodisiac.

Another type of beetle vesication is caused by small rove beetles. These are slender insects with elongate abdomens and very short, rectangular elytra. Most of the vesicating species belong to the genus *Paederus,* found in many tropical and warm temperate regions, but not in the United States. They usually fly during the evening in hot and humid weather. The vesicant substance is not cantharidin; it is reported to be an alkaloid. It is present in greatest concentration in hemolymph, but is not exuded spontaneously. If the beetles are crushed or rubbed on the skin, erythema appears after a period of several hours, followed by a crop of small blisters that persist for 2 to 3 days. Conjunctivitis occurs if the secretion is rubbed into the eyes.[50] A small fungus beetle *Orthoperus* is reported as the cause of "Christmas eye" conjunctivitis in parts of Australia.[176]

Darkling ground beetles are moderately large, dark, heavily chitinized insects that assume a characteristic posture with head down and tail up when disturbed. They are found worldwide in arid regions, where they live under stones and other cover and crawl about at night. Most species can spray irritant secretions, mostly benzoquinones, from the tip of the abdomen to a distance of 30 to 40 cm. These secretions are generally harmless to humans, but blistering of the skin has been reported and eye injury is possible.

No special treatment for beetle vesication is available. The injuries are best treated as superficial chemical burns. Local preparations containing corticosteroids or antihistamines are not particularly effective.

Other types of insect envenomation are sporadic. Many insects that normally feed on plant juices occasionally inflict annoying bites. This behavior may be initiated by dehydration of the insect or by unknown factors. In Kuwait about a hundred cases of dermatitis ranging from itching macules to lesions resembling erythema multiforme and granuloma annulare were attributed to the small hemipteran *Leptodemus minutus.*[158] Similar skin lesions have been ascribed to thrips.[120] Small predatory insects such as lacewing larvae, anthocorids, and *Sclerodermus* species occasionally attack humans instead of their normal arthropod prey. The stick insect, *Anisomorpha buprestoides,* a common species in Florida and adjacent states, ejects a noxious fluid from its thoracic region that deters birds and other predators. According to regional folklore, this fluid can be directed toward human eyes with painful consequences.

DIPTERA (TWO-WINGED FLIES)

Insects of the order Diptera are characterized by one pair of wings. The second pair is usually modified to form a pair of drumsticklike structures known as halteres. A typical life cycle consists of eggs, limbless larvae, pupae, and winged adults, but numerous variations exist. Mouthparts are of the sucking type. Females of many species, while free living, take blood or other tissue fluids from vertebrates. In doing so, they inject salivary secretions that do not seem to be intrinsically toxic but are potent sensitizing agents for most human beings. Larvae of some Diptera are human parasites. Other adult Diptera feed indiscriminately on feces and human foodstuffs. These habits make them by far the most important arthropod vectors of human disease. A list of the major groups of biting dipterans, their principal features, and the habitat of larval and pupal stages is given in Table 31-1.

Most of these insects are cosmopolitan in distribution, the exceptions being tsetse flies, which are restricted to Africa, and tropical and subtropical sand flies. Some species of mosquitoes and blackflies are adapted to cold temperate, sub-Arctic, and alpine environments, where they may occur in such numbers as to make areas virtually uninhabitable during the peak of their activity. Other mosquitoes and biting midges are equally abundant and annoying in some coastal areas and on islands.

Carbon dioxide and human sweat are attractants for at least some mosquitoes; certain skin lipids are repellent. It has been shown that children under 1 year of age rarely show a skin reaction to mosquito bites, but by age 5 nearly all are reactors. Both immediate and delayed types of hypersensitivity are induced. Typically, immediate pruritic wheals are followed after 12 to 24 hours by red, swollen, and pruritic lesions. The early lesions are associated with antibodies and are believed to be histamine induced.[147]

All the classic types of immunologic injury have been reported following mosquito bites, including injury from circulating immune complexes,[176] asthma,[59] and Arthus reaction.[76] Seasonal bullous eruptions in a coastal area of Britain were ascribed to *Aedes detritus*. Most of those affected were women with varicose veins or deep venous thromboses.[190] Intense skin reactions accompanied by fever, lymphadenopathy, and hepatosplenomegaly have been described and are associated with infiltration of skin lesions with natural killer lymphocytes.[186] Nodular skin lesions lasting up to a month have been reported following mosquito bites in AIDS patients receiving zidovudine.[42] Among 21 Japanese patients with severe local and constitutional reactions to mosquito bites, seven died of malignant histiocytosis before age 28. Nine others retained hypersensitivity; three lost it.[76]

Treatment of mosquito bites consists of local application of antipruritic lotions or creams. Antihistamines relieve the itching of early lesions but have no effect on later ones. Group I corticosteroid creams and ointments may be helpful. Desensitization with insect whole body extract is difficult but occasionally successful. Prolonged heavy exposure to mos-

Table 31-1 Major Groups of Biting Dipterans

Insect	Recognition Features of Adult	Larval and Pupal Stages
Mosquitoes (Culicidae, subfamily Culicinae)	Prominent proboscis; wings with scales; palps of female much shorter than proboscis; usually rests with body parallel to substrate	Aquatic in great variety of habitats; both larval and pupal stages motile
Mosquitoes (subfamily Anophelinae)	Prominent proboscis; wings with scales and often with dark mottling; palps of female about as long as proboscis; usually rests with head down and body held at angle to substrate	Same as above
Blackflies, buffalo gnats (family Simuliidae)	Stout; hump-backed; short antennae; wings broad with most of veins faint; body length >2.5 mm	Sessile in flowing water; usually attached to rocks and logs, sometimes to crustaceans
Sand flies (family Psychodidae)	Small (usually >2 mm body length); hairy; wings with straight, prominent veins	In damp crevices, animal burrows, leaf litter
Biting midges, sand flies, no-see-ums (family Ceratopogonidae)	Small (>2 mm body length); wings often mottled; most of wing veins faint	In mud, wet sand, rotting vegetation; larvae very motile
Horseflies, deerflies (family Tabanidae)	Large (5-25 mm body length) with large eyes; usually brilliantly colored; body stout; wings with prominent veins	In mud or shallow water
Stable flies (family Muscidae)	Similar to housefly in size and general appearance; sharp-pointed proboscis projects downward and backward	In decaying vegetable matter or urine-soaked straw
Tsetse flies (family Glossinidae)	Large (6-14 mm); proboscis projects forward; wings fold scissorlike over back	Larvae complete most of development in female; pupate in soil a few hours after birth
Snipe flies (family Rhagionidae)	Long legs; relatively slender body; large eyes; wings with prominent veins	Aquatic, in moist soil or rotten wood

quito bites causes some individuals to lose both immediate and delayed sensitivity, occasionally in less than 1 year.[89]

Refer to Chapter 34 for detailed information on protection from blood-feeding arthropods.

Biting Midges (Culicoides)

Biting midges are very small flies that have a bite out of proportion to their size. Only females feed on blood. The wormlike aquatic larvae develop in water-saturated soil rather than in open water. Mangrove swamps are a favorite habitat. The genus is cosmopolitan but presents the greatest problem in subtropical and tropical coastal regions. Activity is often seasonal. The flies bite most intensely in still air and reduced light.

Bites are immediately painful and result in raised, red, and pruritic lesions that persist from a few hours to a week or more. Some individuals develop vesicles, pustules, and superficial ulcers, particularly if bitten by the genus *Leptoconops*. Hypersensitivity is involved, although some persons seem to develop intense reactions on first exposure to the insects.

Treatment of bites is symptomatic and similar to that for mosquito bites. Artificial hyposensitization has not been successful; however, spontaneous decrease in skin reactivity may occur in some individuals.

See Chapter 34 for information on protection.

Sand Flies (Phlebotomus and Related Genera)

These are very small biting flies quite distinct from *Culicoides* and its relatives (see Table 31-1). They live in damp shaded places such as rock crevices, cracks in walls of houses and other structures, and mammal burrows. Favorite habitats in Central America are *gambas,* deep clefts between the buttresses of large forest trees. Larval and pupal stages are found in moist detritus in holes and crevices. The adults usually emerge at night during periods of still air and temperature of less than 13° C (56° F). They are poor fliers and are mostly confined to the tropics and subtropics.

Blackflies (Simuliidae)

Blackflies are small stocky flies that have a characteristic hump-back appearance. Adults prefer open and sunny situations and are good fliers. Not all species are anthropophilic. The sessile larvae and pupae are found in flowing water, from large rivers to small brooks. Blackflies are cosmopolitan, but their abundance and medical significance vary widely. They range well into the Arctic and constitute a major problem for both humans and domestic animals in parts of Europe, Canada, and the northern United States. In the tropics they tend to be more localized, often remaining close to streams.

Blackfly bites are more common on the upper half of the body. They snip the skin and suck the pooled blood, leaving relatively large punctures that may bleed, a symptom rarely seen with bites of other small flies. The local pain, swelling, and redness that follow blackfly bites are unusually intense and persistent. Vesicles and weeping, crusted lesions may last for weeks. Systemic symptoms such as malaise, fever, and leukocytosis are not uncommon. Enlarged indurated lymphatics, particularly in the posterior cervical region, are common in Canadian children living where blackflies are abundant.[111] Hemorrhagic symptoms have been reported in Brazil.[91] Generalized urticaria, bleeding, angioneurotic edema, cough, wheezing, toxemia, and even death may occur.[193]

No specific treatment for blackfly bites is available. Hyposensitization has been attempted with little success. Neither repellents nor ordinary clothing provides satisfactory protection against blackflies when they are present in large numbers. Avoidance of heavily infested areas during fly season is often the most practical solution. Control measures have not proved highly effective.

See Chapter 34 for further information on protection.

Horseflies and Deerflies (Tabanidae)

Horseflies and deerflies are medium to large (10 to 25 mm body length) stocky flies whose large eyes often are brightly colored. They are strong fliers and prefer open and sunny habitats. They attack a variety of large mammals, including humans. The predacious maggotlike larvae live in water-soaked soil or shallow water.

Bites from these large flies, predominantly the deerfly (*Chrysops* spp.), are painful and may cause both external and subcutaneous bleeding. An itching wheal up to 1 inch in diameter develops but usually does not last long. In some individuals, severe and prolonged swelling of an extremity develops. Systemic anaphylactoid reactions have been reported.[58,107]

As with other fly bites, treatment is symptomatic. Hyposensitization has been attempted in a few cases, apparently with some success.[58]

See Chapter 34 for information on protection.

Other Biting Diptera

Tsetse flies (*Glossina* spp.) are of great importance as vectors of human and domestic animal trypanosomiasis in sub-Saharan Africa. Although not closely related, they are similar to tabanid flies in appearance and habits. Their life history is peculiar in that a single large larva develops in the uterus of the female and is expelled shortly before pupation, which takes place in the soil. Tsetse bites are said to produce comparatively little local reaction, other than brief pain and itching.

Snipe flies are for the most part predators on insects. A few, such as *Symphoromyia,* feed on the blood of mammals. Their habits and life history are similar to those of tabanids. Reactions to snipe fly bites are varied, ranging from pain to anaphylaxis. A person who reacts severely may be bedridden for days.

The stable fly *(Stomoxys calcitrans)* is related to the housefly, which it closely resembles. It is plentiful throughout most of the United States, particularly in agricultural districts. Eggs are deposited in piles of decaying vegetation, where the larvae develop. Thunderstorms seem to stimulate fly activity, which accounts for the widespread belief that houseflies bite just before a storm. Bites cause a sharp stinging sensation, but dermal lesions are uncommon. Itching is brief.

Louse flies (Hippoboscidae) are peculiar Diptera that may lack wings entirely or have them for only part of their adult life. The wingless forms are flat leathery insects that resemble lice or ticks. They are ectoparasites of birds and mammals. Larvae are carried in the uterus until development is almost complete; the pupal stage may be spent in the soil or on the host. The sheep ked *(Melophagus ovinus)* is a common species in the United States and sometimes bites sheep shearers and handlers. The related deer ked *(Lipoptena cervi)* is a seasonal pest in wooded sections of northern Europe, causing hundreds of cases of dermatitis annually.[141] The pigeon fly *(Pseudolynchia canariensis)* is an avian parasite that sometimes infests buildings and bites the occupants.[159]

Lesions from hippoboscid bites appear 1 to 24 hours after the bites as reddish itching papules that may persist for up to 3 months. Topical corticosteroids may afford symptomatic relief and hasten resolution of the lesions. Repellents are reported to be ineffective against these insects. See Chapter 34 for information on protection.

Cutaneous Myiasis

The term "myiasis" for parasitism by fly larvae was introduced into the medical literature in 1840, although the condition has been observed since antiquity. More than a hundred species of Diptera have been reported to cause human myiasis. Some are obligate parasites for which humans are one of several hosts; some are opportunistic invaders that find parasitism an alternative to feeding on decaying tissue or its products. Nevertheless, humans are not a particularly good host for most species of fly larvae, and many infections terminate prematurely. Sensitization of host tissues to fly larvae does not occur as readily as with many other arthropod and helminth parasites.

Myiasis may be classified by clinical manifestations or etiologic agents; neither method is wholly satisfactory. In this chapter we consider only dermal and wound myiasis. Myiasis primarily involving the gastrointestinal tract, urinary tract, eye, and nasopharynx is not covered.

Furuncular Myiasis. The classic agent of furuncular myiasis is the so-called human botfly, *Dermatobia hominis*. Actually, humans are but one of a large number of mammals that serve as suitable hosts for the obligately parasitic larval stage of this fly. It is widely distributed in the American tropics and is an important parasite of domestic cattle in many places. Human infections appear to be most prevalent in Central America and northern South America. Adult flies resemble a bumblebee (body length about 15 mm). They do not feed and are infrequently seen. The life cycle of this fly is unique and remarkable in that the female attaches her eggs to the body of another arthopod for transport to the host. Large mosquitoes of the genus *Psorphora* are often used (8% were found bearing *Dermatobia* eggs in one study), but some 40 species of insects and ticks have been reported to be egg carriers.[14] When the carrier alights on a mammal, the eggs hatch immediately and the larva enters the skin through the bite of the carrier or some other small trauma. Very small larvae are fusiform and later become pyriform to ovoid as they reach full development at lengths of 15 to 20 mm (Fig. 31-9). They are encircled by several rings of spines. The larval stage lasts 6 to 7 weeks, after which the larva emerges from the skin and drops to the ground where pupation occurs.

Infection is fairly common among rural people in Central America. Cases in returned tourists and visitors from Latin America have been diagnosed in many parts of the United States.[51,53,128] Six cases occurred in one group of tourists visiting archeologic sites in Guatemala.[43] Lesions may be on any part of the body exposed to insect bites and may be single or multiple. An initial pruritic papule becomes a furuncle with a characteristic central opening from which serosanguineous fluid exudes. Pain often accompanies movements of the older larvae, but the lesion is not particularly tender to palpation. Lymphadenopathy, fever, and secondary infection are rare.

This form of myiasis should be suspected in patients with furuncular lesions and history of residence or travel in endemic areas (Color Plate 42). It must be differentiated from leishmaniasis and onchocerciasis, which have quite different prognoses and treatments. The sensation of movement within the lesion accompanied by pain but little tenderness or inflammation suggests myiasis. The tip of the larva may protrude from the central opening or bubbles produced by its respiration may be seen. Sometimes simple pressure will extrude the organism, particularly if it is small. Occlusion of the breathing hole with heavy oil or nail polish may cause the

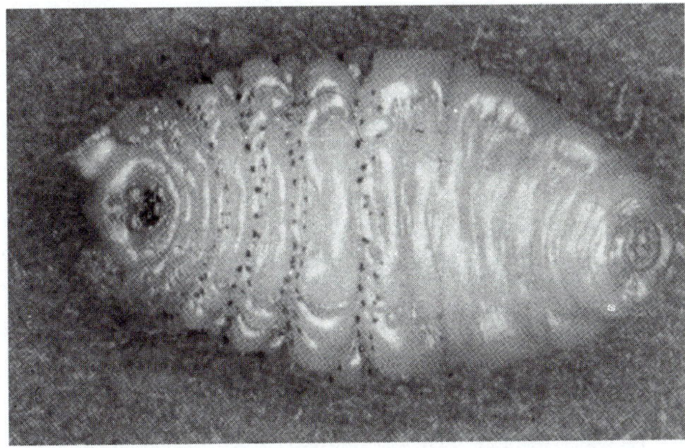

Fig. 31-9 Mature larva of the botfly *Dermatobia hominis* recovered from a lesion on the ankle of a U.S. engineer working in Venezuela. (Photo by Illustration Department, Indiana University Medical Center.)

larva to emerge sufficiently for it to be grasped and withdrawn. An effective folk remedy is binding a piece of pork fat over the opening. This often causes the larva to leave its burrow (Color Plates 43 and 44). Another technique is injection of about 2 ml of a local anesthetic into the base of the lesion, thus extruding the larva by fluid pressure.[51] If these methods are unsuccessful, surgical excision under local anesthesia is indicated. Whatever method is used, care should be taken not to break or rupture the larva. This may result in a strong inflammatory reaction, often followed by secondary infection. Repeated infections tend to confer some degree of immunity that may abort larval development. Screening, clothing, and use of insect repellents are helpful in preventing infection.

Furuncular myiasis in tropical Africa is usually caused by the tumbu fly, *Cordylobia anthropophaga.* The larval stage of this fly is an obligate parasite, parasitizing many mammals; rats and dogs are most important epidemiologically. The adult is about the size of a housefly but stockier. It prefers shade and is most active in early morning and afternoon. Females lay eggs on dry, sandy soil or on clothing. They are attracted by the odor of urine. The eggs hatch in 1 to 3 days, and hatchling larvae can survive up to 2 weeks waiting for contact with skin of a suitable host. They can penetrate unbroken skin. They become fusiform to ovoid and reach a length of 13 to 15 mm. The larval stage is completed in 9 to 14 days.

Human infections are known from most nations of sub-Saharan Africa and are reported to have increased with displacement of populations by war and famine.[68] Transmission increases during the rainy season. Among indigenous peoples, infection is most frequent in children; adults evidently acquire some immunity. Infections among Americans and Europeans visiting Africa are reported regularly.[67,106,161] Lesions may be on any part of the body but more frequently on the legs and buttocks. The furuncles are discrete, elevated, and nontender and have a central opening. The number of lesions, up to about 50, is greater than with *Dermatobia* infections. The course of the infection is much shorter. An exceptionally heavy infection (about 150 larvae) was caused by *C. rodhaini,* normally a parasite of forest mammals. It was accompanied by lymphadenopathy, leukocytosis, and elevated IgA. Clothing left to dry on the ground was the presumed source of the parasites.[129]

Principles of diagnosis and treatment are much the same as for *Dermatobia.* Avoidance of skin contact with potentially contaminated soil, ironing of clothing and bedding after open-air drying, and rodent control are preventive measures that are often difficult to achieve.

Autochthonous furuncular myiasis may be seen in the United States, particularly in children. Some cases are caused by larvae of botflies of the genus *Cuterebra* whose normal hosts are chipmunks and rabbits. Infection seems to be acquired from fly eggs attached to low vegetation that hatch on contact with skin of the host. Larvae penetrate directly, but human skin normally seems to be impermeable to them. Lesions resemble those produced by *Dermatobia.*[156] The same syndrome may be caused by larvae of *Wohlfahrtia vigil,* a large fly native to Canada and the northern United States. Its normal hosts are newborn mammals, particularly the mink, dog, and fox. The female fly deposits larvae on the skin; these penetrate within an hour or so. Human infections are almost always in infants under 9 months, and the furuncular lesions are usually on the face. Fever, irritability, and loss of appetite are common. Larvae can usually be expressed from the lesion; surgery rarely is necessary. Netting over the crib or pram when outdoors usually affords protection.

Migratory Myiasis. One type of migratory myiasis is caused by flies of the genus *Hypoderma.* Adult flies are large and hairy, somewhat resembling bumblebees. Normal hosts for the parasitic larvae are cattle, deer, and horses. The flies attach their eggs to hairs. Hatchling larvae penetrate the skin and wander extensively through the subcutaneous tissues, eventually locating under the skin of the back, where they produce furuncular lesions. The condition is one of considerable veterinary importance. Humans are abnormal hosts in which the parasite is unable to complete its development. Human infections usually occur in rural areas where cattle and horses are raised and are more common in winter. Larvae migrate rapidly (as much as 1 cm/hr) and erratically through subcutaneous tissues, producing intermittent painful swellings over a period of months. The sensation of larval movement is often noticed by the patient. Larvae respond negatively to gravity, so the last lesions are usually on the head or shoulders. Eosinophilia (35% eosinophils) and angioneurotic edema may be seen.[116] Larvae may emerge spontaneously from furuncles or may die in the tissues. Rare cases of invasion of the pharyngeal region, orbit, and spinal canal are on record.

Another form of migratory myiasis is caused by larvae of *Gastrophilus,* which normally are gastrointestinal or nasal parasites of horses (Fig. 31-10). In human infections, which are reported more frequently from Europe than from

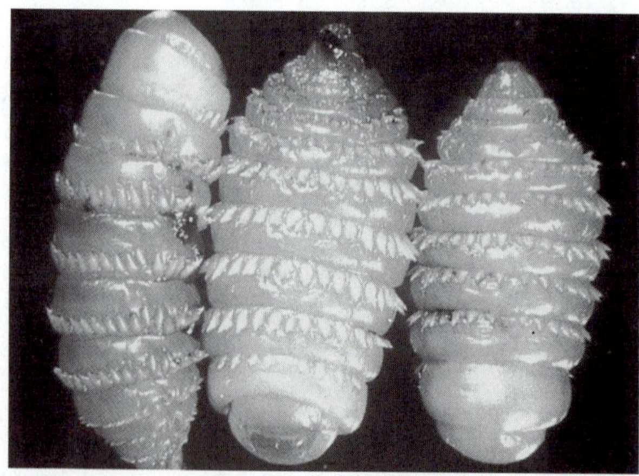

Fig. 31-10 Larvae of the botfly *Gastrophilus haemorrhoidalis* from a horse's stomach.

the United States, the young larvae burrow in the skin producing narrow, tortuous, reddish linear lesions with intense itching. Lesions usually advance 1.5 cm/day, but more rapid progress has been reported. Death of the larvae terminates the infection in a week or two without sequelae. This infection is clinically similar to creeping eruption, an invasion of the skin by larvae of the hookworms *Ancylostoma braziliense* and *A. caninum.* The helminthic parasitosis is more frequent in warm, moist regions, including the southern United States, and is associated with dogs and cats. The myiasis is more frequent in cooler regions and is associated with horses. Definitive diagnosis can be made only by removal of the parasite from its burrow and microscopic examination.

Removal of the larvae by surgery or expression is the only effective treatment for migratory myiasis, although local freezing of cutaneous burrows is sometimes successful. The most effective prevention is control of the infections in domestic animals.

Hematophagous Myiasis. The sole cause of this condition is the Congo floor maggot, *Auchmeromyia luteola.* It is dark, distinctly segmented, ovoid, 15 to 18 mm long, and the larval stage of a moderate-size yellowish fly. It is widely distributed in sub-Saharan Africa and is essentially a human parasite. It is unique among parasitic fly larvae in living apart from its host in the earthen floor of native dwellings. It seeks persons lying or sitting on the floor or on mats and feeds intermittently on blood, usually at night. The bites are trivial but may interfere with sleep. Sensitization appears to be uncommon.

Wound Myiasis. About 85% to 90% of cases are caused by larvae of flies of the family Calliphoridae, which includes both obligate parasites and opportunists. Probably the most dangerous type of myiasis is that caused by larvae of the screw-worm flies, *Callitroga americana* in the Americas and *Chrysomya bessiana* in Asia and Africa. The adults are rather stocky flies 8 to 12 mm in body length and metallic blue-green to purplish-black. The parasitic larvae are pinkish, fusiform, and strongly segmented, hence the common name. Length at maturity is 12 to 15 mm. They are obligate parasites whose chief hosts are cattle, sheep, and goats. They are a major cause of economic loss among livestock. Enzootic areas are mostly in the tropics and subtropics, but summer infections occur as far north as Colorado and Nebraska. Female flies deposit eggs near any break in the skin or around the nose, mouth, or ears if a discharge is present. Larvae invade healthy tissue, often causing considerable damage. The larval stage lasts 4 to 8 days, and the entire cycle 15 to 20 days in enzootic areas.

Human cases are nearly always associated with outbreaks of the disease in livestock. Cases in a Texas outbreak were north and northwest of a stockyard, indicating dispersal of flies by prevailing winds.[106] Infection is often acquired while sleeping or resting outdoors during the day. Lesions may appear on any exposed part of the body. Those on the scalp may be associated with pediculosis capitis. Typical dermal lesions are ulcers or sinuses that may contain up to 200 larvae. These are surrounded by a zone of induration. Pain is variable. Secondary bacterial infection is common. There may be extensive tissue destruction, and appreciable mortality is associated with nasopharyngeal invasion.[162]

Topical application of 5% chloroform in olive oil followed by irrigation and manual removal of larvae is often sufficient in dermal infections. Deeper nasopharyngeal and orbital infections require surgery. Antimicrobial therapy as dictated by culture and sensitivity tests is often necessary. The most effective prevention is elimination of the disease in domestic animals. Screw-worm has been virtually eradicated in the southern United States and some other regions largely by release of large numbers of laboratory-reared male flies sterilized by gamma irradiation. Females mate only once, so mating with a sterile male nullifies the female's reproductive effort. The result is a drastic reduction in population.

Opportunistic invasion of wounds by fly larvae is commonly seen during war and natural disasters, when injured persons are exposed to flies and medical facilities are inadequate to cope with the emergency. It may also be seen sporadically in nursing homes and hospitals and often is not reported for cultural and medicolegal reasons.[24] Six of 14 cases in one series were acquired in the hospital. Eleven of the 14 patients were over 63 years of age, and nearly all had underlying problems such as diabetes or peripheral vascular disease. Most of the infested lesions were on the feet or ankles.[101]

Numerous fly species may be involved. Most common are *Phaenicia* species (green-bottle flies), *Calliphora* species (blue-bottle flies), *Phorima regina* (black blowfly), *Sarcophaga haemorrhoidalis* (flesh fly), and *Musca domestica* (housefly). The flies, whose larvae normally feed on decaying animal tissues, often deposit eggs in wounds or around body orifices if a malodorous discharge is present. The larvae feed on necrotic tissue, and damage to healthy tissues and secondary infection are uncommon. They actually may debride wounds, and "maggot therapy" using aseptically reared larvae had a brief period of popularity in the 1930s. Laboratory-reared *Calliphora* larvae were used in two patients to debride massive superficial necrotic areas where antibiotic therapy and surgical debridement had been unsuccessful.[184] In two other reports, maggots serendipitously present were used to debride lesions.[23,144] Diagnosis is usually obvious on inspection of the wound. Species identification may require rearing the larvae to maturity. If this is not feasible, examination of the spiracular plates on the last segment of the larva and the chitinized oral structures usually permits adequate identification. Irrigation of the wound and mechanical removal of larvae are all that are generally required for treatment.

LICE (ORDER ANOPLURA)

Species, Life Cycle, and Distribution

Lice are small wingless insects that are ectoparasites of mammals. They are mostly host specific, and two species are human parasites: *Pthirus pubis* (the pubic louse) and *Pediculus humanus,* with two varieties, *Pediculus h. capitis* (the head louse) and *Pediculus h. corporis* (the body louse). They are obligatory parasites, subsisting on blood from the host, and have mouthparts modified for piercing and sucking. The mouthparts are drawn into the head of the louse when not in use.

The adult head louse is about 2 to 4 mm long with body elongated and flattened dorsoventrally (Fig. 31-11). The head is only slightly narrower than the thorax. The three pairs of legs are all of about equal length and possess delicate hooks at the distal extremities. The entire life is spent on the host's body. The eggs (nits) are deposited on hair shafts, generally one nit to a shaft. The nits hatch in about 1 week, and the freshly hatched larvae, which must feed within 24 hours of hatching or die, mature in about 15 to 16 days. The adult female lives for approximately 1 month and may deposit well over 100 eggs during her reproductive life. Body lice are slightly larger than head lice, but similar in appearance and with a similar life cycle, although the nits are deposited on fibers of clothing. Head lice and body lice interbreed.

Adult pubic lice are about 1 to 2 mm long, the head is much smaller than the thorax, and the broadly oval body is flattened dorsoventrally (Fig. 31-12). The anterior legs are much shorter than the second and third pairs, and the insect has a distinctive appearance suggestive of a miniature crab. Nits are deposited on hair shafts, often several per shaft, and the life cycle egg-to-egg is approximately 1 month.

Lice are found wherever people are found. Unable to exist for more than a brief time away from the human body, lice are spread by close personal contact and by sharing of clothing and bedding. The various species not only have a particular host, but often prefer a particular part of the host's body, so that generalizing about transmission of the three varieties that parasitize humans is impossible. During biting and feeding, secretions from the louse cause a small red macule. Severe pruritus and marked inflammatory responses to bites are caused by sensitization that occurs after repeated exposure to bites. Thus a victim may be lousy for weeks before pruritus becomes marked. Not all people are equally attractive to lice, possibly because of differences in odor and chemical composition of sweat.

Lice are medically important as vectors of systemic illnesses, as well as for dermatitis and discomfort.

Clinical Aspects

The head louse localizes on the scalp and rarely on other hairy areas of the body. Children are most frequently affected, but adults, particularly women, may also be affected. Lice are particularly common in young girls, possibly because of their long hair. Infestation is uncommon in blacks, at least in the United States, probably because the shaft of African hair has an oval cross section that makes it difficult for the louse to grip while depositing eggs. However, pediculosis capitis is found in Africa, where the indigenous head louse is adapted to grip the oval hair shafts. Since nits initially attach to the hair shaft close to the skin and are carried higher as the hair grows, the presence of nits near the tips indicates a long-standing infestation.

Itching is the principal symptom, and physical findings vary with such factors as duration and extent of the infestation, cleanliness, excoriations, and degree of secondary infection. Diagnosis is established by identifying nits and lice. It is not always simple to find lice, especially in early and mild cases where they may be few in number. Lice are very active, but nits are always present and easy to identify. Nits are whitish ovals, about 0.5 mm long, and attached firmly to

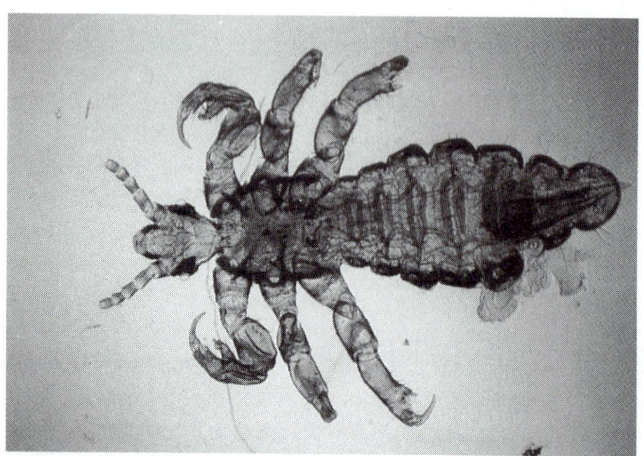

Fig. 31-11 Male of the human head louse, *Pediculus humanus capitis.*

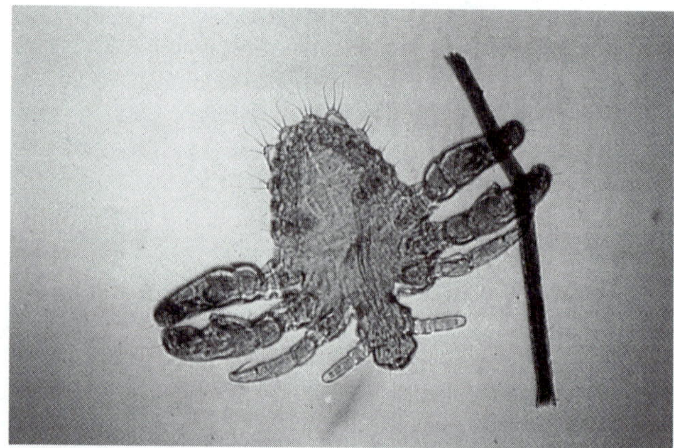

Fig. 31-12 The pubic or crab louse, *Phthirus pubis,* grasping a hair.

one side of the hair. Flakes of dandruff, which resemble nits superficially, are not attached to the hair shafts. Occipital and posterior cervical adenopathy is common and may be present even in less severe cases. A pruritic scalp accompanied by adenopathy should prompt a thorough search for lice and nits. In severe cases oozing and crusting may be present, sometimes with matting of the hair, and lice may be numerous.

The body louse lives chiefly in the seams of clothing and is rarely seen on the skin. These lice leave clothing to feed on the skin, or remain attached to the clothing while feeding, and thus are most abundant where clothing abuts the skin, as at the beltline. The bite results in a small red macule with characteristic central hemorrhagic punctum. Excoriations, crusts, eczematization, and other secondary lesions generally obscure the primary lesions by the time the victim is seen for medical attention. Shoulders, trunk, and buttocks are favorite sites for bites, and parallel scratch marks on the shoulders are a common finding. The diagnosis is confirmed by identifying parasites or nits from the clothing. Bands of trousers, side seams, and underarm seams are sites of preference. Untreated cases may persist indefinitely, and massive infestations are sometimes seen in vagabonds who have no ready access to frequent laundering or change of clothing, or who cannot bathe regularly.

Pediculosis pubis is ordinarily acquired during sexual activity, although it may be acquired from unchanged bedding or nonsexual activity, either from lice that live briefly away from the human body or from egg-infested pubic hairs that are shed. The lice localize principally in the pubic hair, but they are found occasionally in eyebrows, eyelashes, and axillary hairs. Adult pubic lice are not active and hug the skin at the base of the hair shafts, with their heads buried in the follicular orifice. They are not easy to find, but one or more can usually be found if suspicion of the diagnosis is strong enough to prompt a thorough search. A loupe is helpful. Nits are more easily found. Primary bite lesions are almost never seen, but the intense pruritus and pubic scratching are pathognomonic. Secondary infection, crusting, oozing, excoriations, and eczematization that often accompany head and body lice are rarely seen with pubic lice. Peculiar steel gray macules (maculae caeruleae) may appear in association with some cases of pubic lice. These lesions do not appear until the infestation has been present for several weeks and are most common on the trunk and thighs.

Treatment and Prevention

Treatment of all types of lice is aimed at eradication of lice and nits and at prevention of reinfestation.

Head lice may be treated with gamma benzene hexachloride shampoo. This is applied to the wet hair, lathered, and left in place 4 minutes before being rinsed out. A fine-toothed comb may be used to remove nits following rinsing. The treatment may be repeated 7 to 10 days later as a precaution in case some nits are not killed by the first shampoo. Other pediculicides are available if gamma benzene hexachloride is contraindicated or if the lice are resistant. Several alternative treatments contain pyrethrums and piperonyl butoxide as active ingredients. Family members and contacts should be treated simultaneously.

Body lice may be treated with the same medications, but parasites and nits are not generally found on the skin. Eradication of these from the clothing is the primary objective. Treatment includes a good bath, laundering of all clothing, and a change to fresh clothing that is free of lice and nits. Dry cleaning eradicates lice and nits, as does ordinary laundering with settings at hot for washing and drying. Malathion preparations and gamma benzene hexachloride formulations may be used for mass delousing.

Pubic lice may be treated with 1% gamma benzene hexachloride lotion or shampoo used as for head lice, or with other preparations used for head lice. Crotamiton lotion rubbed into the affected area daily for several weeks to destroy hatching ova may be used also. Eyelash infestations may be managed by careful application of physostigmine ophthalmic ointment, using a cotton-tipped applicator. Machine washing of sheets and clothing at the hot setting for washing and drying will kill lice and nits.

FLEAS (ORDER SIPHONAPTERA)

Species, Life Cycle, and Distribution

Fleas are small ectoparasites of mammals and birds. The wingless body, which is covered by a hard shiny integument, is compressed laterally, enabling the fleas to scurry easily among the hairs and feathers of the hosts. They are active insects with legs adapted for jumping, capable of prodigious leaps. Adult fleas subsist on blood. Some species must obtain blood from one particular host, others are less host specific, and all have mouthparts adapted for piercing and sucking. The eggs are laid on or near the host and drop to the ground as the host moves about or shakes itself, where they hatch into small wormlike larvae that feed on droppings from adult fleas and on other organic matter. The life cycle varies among species and may vary considerably within the same species, as each developmental stage is influenced by prevailing temperature and humidity. The customary larval stage of 9 to 15 days may be prolonged for months by adverse conditions, and the pupal stage varies from a week to nearly a year. Individual adult fleas may live for years when circumstances are favorable and can live for months without feeding.

Fleas exist universally, although the distribution of various species is restricted by climate and host. They are of medical importance because of the discomfort resulting from their bites, as a cause of papular urticaria, and as vectors of disease. They are more active in warm weather and more of a problem in warmer climates, such as the southwestern United States with its longer breeding season. They are a particular nuisance in California.[102] High standards of sanitation and personal hygiene in developed countries have discouraged the human flea, *Pulex irritans,* while the same popularity of household pets has been conducive to the proliferation of dog and cat fleas, *Ctenocephalides canis* and *Ctenocephalides felis.* The incidence of other species in mammals and birds remains high. Since dog, cat, and many other fleas are only partially host specific, the fleas associated with many mammals and birds cause disease in humans. In fact, most of the present-day flea bite problems are caused by animal fleas. Hungry fleas are more often attracted to people from an area frequented by an animal than from the animal itself. If the family dog is absent, hordes of hungry fleas may persist for months.[40] Consequently, anyone with pet cats or dogs, or near domesticated animals, is more likely to be bitten, but outbreaks in the absence of pets are common. One epidemic of flea bites among children in a day nursery was traced to dog fleas in a deserted fox nesting area beneath the building.[155] Another outbreak among poultry workers was caused by an infestation of hen fleas, *Ceratophyllus gallinae.*[185] Fleas from flying squirrels also have been documented as the source of bites.[73]

Clinical Aspects

The appearance of flea bites is not diagnostic, and the clinical features depend on degree of sensitivity. A bite produces a small central hemorrhagic punctum surrounded by erythema and urticaria. A small wheal at the bite site may be nonallergic because of primary urticogenic substances in the flea saliva, but increasingly severe reactions are caused by sensitization to substances in the saliva. Bullae or even ulceration may result from flea bites in highly sensitive individuals. Flea bites are intensely pruritic, and scratching often results in crusting and impetiginization. Fleas have a habit of sampling several adjacent areas while feeding, and bites characteristically appear in irregular groups. Feet, ankles, and legs are favorite targets, as well as the hips and shoulder areas, where clothing fits snugly. While an individual lesion produced by a flea bite is not diagnostic, the typical clinical picture of grouped multiple bites is generally sufficient to establish a diagnosis, which is usually confirmed by locating and identifying fleas.

Papular urticaria is a dermatologic manifestation of sensitivity to insect bites, most frequently fleas, although bedbugs, *Cimex lectularius,* and possibly other repeated insect bites may result in the same hypersensitive state. The condition is most prevalent in children 2 to 7 years and almost never occurs in infants, who have not yet been sensitized by repeated bites. The characteristic lesions are pruritic wheals and papules that often are scratched and excoriated, with resulting secondary infection and lichenification. Lesions tend to occur on the arms and legs, especially the extensor surfaces. Papular urticaria is almost always seen during the summer and fall months when insect activity is greatest. Victims generally become desensitized spontaneously after several summers.

One flea, *Tunga penetrans,* is responsible for a distinctive infestation known as tungiasis. The flea has a number of common names: burrowing flea, chigo, sand flea, and jigger. Infestation is common in Central and South America and in Africa, where the burrowing flea is widely distributed, but more cases are seen in the United States as increasing numbers of tourists visit exotic places. One woman resident of New York City developed lesions of tungiasis on her toes after visiting several countries in East Africa, where she frequently wore sandals in rural areas.[196] The primary lesions of tungiasis are produced by the female flea. As soon as it is impregnated, it burrows into the skin until only the posterior end protrudes. Sucking blood, the insect becomes as large as a small pea and deposits eggs that fall to the ground. Lodged in the skin, the gestating female produces a firm itchy nodule, with the posterior end of the flea visible as a dark plug or spot in the center of each nodule. Lesions occur most often on the feet, buttocks, or perineum of persons who wear no shoes or frequently squat, since the burrowing flea is not a good jumper and abounds in the dusty soil surrounding human habitations. If the infestation is extensive, numerous papules may aggregate into plaques with a honeycomb appearance. Secondary infection around each flea is inevitable, resulting in suppuration, ulceration, and rarely gangrene. The lesions become painful or even crippling, and severe infections may lead to death. If the burrowing flea is not removed, the pustule ruptures, leaving an ulcer.

Treatment and Prevention

Ordinary flea bites require syptomatic treatment directed at relief of pruritus and prevention of secondary infection. Corticosteroid creams or calamine lotion with phenol, systemic antihistamines, and antibiotics are helpful when indicated, but the management of flea bites consists largely of prevention. Not only must the animals that host the fleas be treated, but also such places as chicken coops, rat nests, sleeping sites for dogs and cats, and often the entire inside of dwellings where pets live. Many effective insecticides are available. Typically, *N,N*-diethyl-meta-toluamide (DEET), pyrethrins, piperonyl butoxide, and *d*-trans allethrin are ingredients in sprays and foggers. A recently introduced insect spray containing permethrin (a new synthetic pyrethroid) is said to be effective. Spraying or dusting must eradicate not only adult fleas, but also the many larvae and pupae in grass, carpet, spaces between floor boards, crevices in furniture, and beds. Lindane, carbaryl, and malathion are the active ingredients in many sprays and dusts, and the services of professional exterminators may be necessary.

Wearing shoes will prevent most cases of tungiasis. Cases should be treated promptly. One method is curettage of each nodule under local anesthesia, with concomitant use of systemic antibiotics to prevent secondary infection. Ether pledgets applied to the skin will kill the fleas before curettage is begun. Where burrowing fleas are endemic, eradication is important. Floors must be swept free of dust, and insecticides may be sprayed or dusted.

MITES (CLASS ARACHNIDA, ORDER ACARINA)

Species, Life Cycle, and Distribution

Mites make up the largest group in the class. Most are small arthropods, many barely visible to the naked eye. Mites have two body regions, a small cephalothorax and a larger, unsegmented abdomen. The cephalothorax and abdomen are broadly joined, giving most mites an oblong to globular appearance. Newly hatched larvae have three pairs of legs, and larvae acquire a fourth pair after the first molt. Mites are highly diverse. Some are parasitic, with both vertebrates and invertebrates serving as hosts; some are scavengers, some feed on plants, and many are free living and predaceous. While most species are oviparous, some are ovoviviparous, and a few are viviparous. They occur worldwide and frequently in great numbers. Mites have been associated with disease transmission, allergies, and dermatologic manifestations. Of the approximately 35,000 species, about 50 are known to cause human skin lesions, and most of the cutaneous lesions are caused by mites feeding or burrowing in the skin.[78] Since children and adults of all races are susceptible to these ubiquitous arthropods, they are responsible for considerable morbidity. The mites of medical importance are some of the sarcoptic mites, some of the trombiculid mites, a number of other acariform mites that infest organic substances such as grains and produce, and the gamasid mites that are vectors of several rickettsial and viral diseases. Dermatologic manifestations of mite bites may be seasonal, as in the case of the trombiculids; individual cases or outbreaks of varying magnitude may be related to contact with mites that infest animals or various foods. Epidemics may occur, as is currently the case with scabies.

Scabies

Life Cycle. The human scabies mite is *Sarcoptes scabiei* var. *hominis,* an obligate human parasite that completes its entire life cycle in and on the epidermis of humans. Unless treated, scabies can persist indefinitely. The adult female is responsible for the symptoms accompanying the infestation. Following impregnation, she burrows into the epidermis and remains in the burrow for a life span of about 1 month. She slowly extends the burrow, feeding during travel, during which time several eggs are deposited daily. The ovoid female mite is approximately 0.3 to 0.4 mm long. Numerous transverse corrugations and a large number of dorsal spinous processes are adaptations to prevent backward movement in the burrow. The males are much smaller than females, spend more time on the surface, and are short lived, dying shortly following copulation. The mite is passed in the vast majority of cases by intimate contact, but adult human scabies mites can survive off the host for 24 to 36 hours at room conditions and still remain infestive.[2] Consequently, it is possible to acquire scabies from infested bedding, furniture, and clothing. In fact, outbreaks not related to sexual activity occur frequently among nursing home patients and personnel; epidemics in schools for small children are also common. Scabies became uncommon following World War II (during the war it was a common problem), but the disease has increased in frequency since 1964 to epidemic proportions worldwide.[127,169]

Clinical Aspects. Severe nocturnal pruritus is the hallmark of scabies. Itching also may be provoked by any sudden warming of the body and generally does not involve the face. A warm bath or radiant heat from a fire may cause a paroxysm of itching. Since the pruritus is caused by sensitization, 4 to 6 weeks may elapse between infestation and the onset of severe pruritus. Reinfestation is common, since eradicating the disease from all contacts simultaneously is often difficult and reinfestation following cure results in prompt recurrence of symptoms. Cutaneous manifestations are varied. The primary lesion is the epidermal burrow, a tiny linear or serpentine track, rarely longer than 5 to 10 mm. While the female mite may burrow anywhere on the body, sites of predilection include the interdigital spaces, palms, flexor surfaces of the wrists, elbows, feet and ankles, beltline, anterior axillary folds, lower buttocks, and penis and scrotum. The distribution of burrows in infants may be atypical, with burrows frequently found in the scalp and on the soles. In the present epidemic, involving many people with excellent hygiene, cutaneous changes may be almost absent and burrows difficult to find. On the other hand, after the disease has been present for some time, eczematization, lichenification, impetiginization, myriad nonspecific papules and excoriations, and even urticaria may be present. The burrows are often the least conspicuous of various skin changes. The clinical picture varies with differences in personal hygiene, topical treatments used before diagnosis, and individual scratch threshold.

Diagnosis is based on the combination of nocturnal pruritus and cutaneous findings, and is confirmed by microscopic examination of burrow contents. The burrow and contents may be collected for examination by scraping with a scalpel blade or by pinching the skin to elevate it and shaving off a superficial layer. Burrows are often inflamed and no longer typical after the disease has been present for some time. The most productive sites to find burrows for examination are finger webs, sides of fingers, wrists, and elbows. Ectoparasites, ova, egg castings, feces, or pieces of mites are diagnostic.

Norwegian scabies is a term describing a particularly severe form of scabies occasionally seen in senile and mentally retarded patients, patients with debilitating illnesses, and immunosuppressed patients. Extensive crusting, particularly of the hands and feet, occurs. There may be erythema and scaling on the body, and patients are literally "crawling with mites." This form of scabies is highly contagious.[92,157]

Nodular scabies is another troublesome clinical variation. Persistent pruritic nodules develop, particularly on the male genitalia or in the groin, but usually on some covered part. Nodules may be the only finding and may persist for months after adequate antiscabetic therapy.

Treatment and Prevention. A number of topical treatments are available. In most cases a single overnight application of 1% gamma benzene hexachloride cream or lotion is curative, although symptoms may persist for over a month until the mite and mite products are shed with the epidermis. The chemical must be applied even beneath the fingernails, since ova and live mites are frequently lodged there as a result of frenzied scratching. If the itching has not abated in several weeks, the patient should be reexamined for treatment failure or reinfestation. Gamma benzene hexachloride has a potential for central nervous system toxicity, and percutaneous absorption does occur.[52] Alternative scabicides may be desired for use in infants and pregnant women or in patients known to be allergic to gamma benzene hexachloride. Permethrin cream (5%) has recently been approved for antiscabetic therapy. It has very low mammalian toxicity in studies to date, is reported to have a 91% cure rate,[181] and is approved for use in infants 2 months old. It is used in the same regimen as gamma benzene hexachloride cream. Infants should be treated on scalp, temple, and forehead. Sulfur in petrolatum (5% to 10%) or another suitable vehicle applied for three consecutive nights is a suitable alternative. Ten percent crotamiton cream or lotion applied for two consecutive nights is also used. In the treatment of Norwegian scabies, salicylic acid ointment may be needed to soften scales and permit penetration of the scabicide. Nodular scabies can be a perplexing therapeutic problem and may necessitate intralesional injections of corticosteroids, or occlusive corticosteroid creams or ointments, in addition to adequate antiscabetic therapy. Application of crude coal tar to the nodules may be effective.

Contacts must be treated simultaneously. Clothing and linens should be laundered the morning following treatment, to kill mites that may have strayed from the skin. When many members of a household are infested, live mites may be on the furniture. Gamma benzene hexachloride sprays are available.

Zoonotic Scabies. Other burrowing mites similar to the human scabies mite infest animals such as swine, cattle, horses, mules, sheep, dogs, and wild animals. They are relatively host specific but under conditions of close contact may cause self-limited dermatitis in humans. Because of humans' close association with dogs, the most common animal scabies is canine, caused by *Sarcoptes scabiei* var. *canis*. Studies indicate that the dog scabies mites are able to survive for at least 96 hours on human skin, even burrowing and laying eggs, but whether a perpetual life cycle can be established is not yet determined.[48] Infested dogs have reddish papules, scaling, crusting, and evidence of scratching. Humans develop itchy papules, often with some urtication, and scratching may give rise to varying degrees of secondary infection. The initial lesions are most commonly on areas of skin that come in contact with dogs: forearms, chest, anterior abdomen, and anterior thighs. Outbreaks are frequently traced to a kennel or litter of puppies. In one case, 15 patients developed an itchy dermatitis from five puppies in a single litter.[31] Human infestation with dog scabies mites subsides spontaneously when contact with dogs is discontinued or when the dogs are cured. The dogs must be treated with scabicides, and the human victims with symptomatic therapy for pruritus.

Cats, also closely associated with humans, have been known to harbor mites that can infest humans. *Notoedres cati* infestation is seen more commonly in Czechoslovakia and Japan than the dog sarcoptic scabies.[29]

Trombiculid Mites

Mites of the family Trombiculidae are distributed worldwide. In the United States the most important species is *Eutrombicula alfreddugesi* (red bug, chigger, harvest mite). Adults are free living and predaceous on small arthropods and their eggs, but the larvae are ectoparasites of vertebrates. Wild and domestic mammals, as well as reptiles, serve as hosts. The larval bite causes human dermatitis. Adult mites lay their eggs among vegetation, and newly hatched larvae crawl up on the vegetation, waiting to attach themselves to a passing host. They attach themselves to the skin with hooked mouthparts and feed on blood, falling off when full. However, humans are not good hosts, and larvae usually do not stay long. The typical bite is a maddeningly pruritic hemorrhagic punctum that usually becomes surrounded by intense erythema within 24 hours. Bites may number in the hundreds and can be associated with an allergic reaction. Hypersensitivity causes blisters and clear fluid weeping with crusting. The surrounding area may be purplish in color, with severe swelling, particularly of the feet and ankles (Fig. 31-13). The lesions regress in 1 to 2 weeks, but pruritus is persistent and often paroxysmal during this time, with secondary infection in excoriated skin.

Treatment is symptomatic. Superpotent topical corticosteroid creams and ointments (group I) alleviate pruritus when massaged sparingly into the individual lesions, and 1% phenol in calamine is sometimes effective. Systemic antihistamines may be prescribed, and severe infestations may require pulse therapy with systemic corticosteroids. As is the case in all self-limited conditions for which there is no satisfactory cure, home remedies abound, such as meat tenderizer rubbed into the moistened skin. Application of clear nail polish to the individual lesions is a favorite home remedy even though no evidence suggests that this is effective.

Preventive measures consist of avoidance and insect repellents used on skin and clothing. Clothing pretreated with permethrin has resulted in 74.2% increase in protection compared with unprotected controls.[20] Other repellents sug-

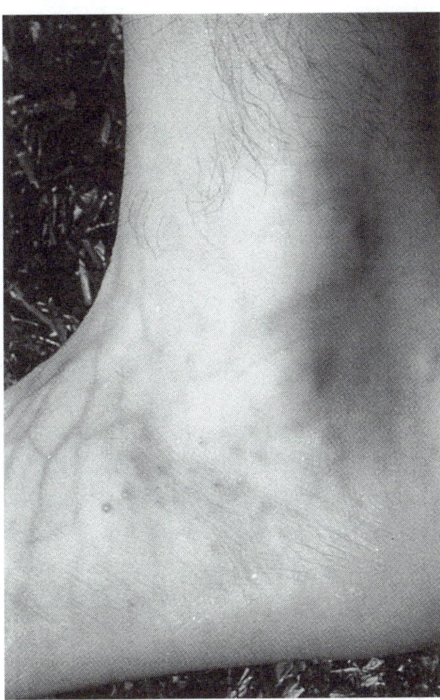

Fig. 31-13 Chigger bites on the ankle.

gested for treating clothing are ethyl hexandiol, DEET, and flowers of sulfur. Sulfur–cream of tartar, one tablet daily, is also used. The symptoms are allergic, and permanent residents in infested areas may develop tolerance to repeated bites.

Miscellaneous Mites

Parasitiformes. This group contains gamasid mites that are parasites of birds, mammals, snakes, insects, and rarely humans. In addition to being vectors of disease, gamasid mites are responsible for some cases of dermatitis.

The chicken mite, *Dermanyssus gallinae,* is responsible for most of the dermatitis caused by this group. This pest of poultry is widespread and is associated with both domestic and wild birds. While poultry workers are common targets, others may be infested from insidious sources, such as a pet canary or bird nest near an intake for ventilation or air conditioning. The clinical picture is nonspecific, but the diagnosis may be made by identifying the mite. Treatment consists of symptomatic therapy and eradication of the mite source.

The tropical rat mite, *Ornithonyssus bacoti,* has also been reported to cause dermatitis, from such diverse sources as a rat nest in the attic or a colony of laboratory mice.[31,55] Snake mites have been implicated as a cause of dermatitis. Four members of one family developed a vesicobullous eruption from *Ophionyssys natricis* harbored by a pet python.[164]

Acariniformes. This huge group includes mites that infest foods, feathers, and furs. Individual infestations and larger outbreaks are frequent, with increased exposure by occupation, resulting in such terms as grocer's itch, miller's itch, and copra itch.

Dogs, cats, and rabbits are primary hosts for mites of the genus *Cheyletiella,* and domestic pets are increasingly the source of mite dermatitis. Pet house cats are often involved.[33,56,152]

Dermatophagoides scheremetewskyi is an unusual mite that has been found in kapok and feather pillows, in a sparrow's nest, in monkey food, and on rats and other animals. This mite has been reported as the cause of feather pillow dermatitis.[5] Mites of this genus are said to be the principal inhaled allergen in house dust.

The most common cause of dermatitis in this group is *Pyemotes ventricosus.* This tiny mite parasitizes various insects often found in and around grain and straw. It attacks humans when a large mite population has no ready access to normal hosts, causing grain itch. Grain itch implies an occupational bias, but outbreaks not involving farmers or rural workers have been described. During a widespread epidemic of *Pyemotes* infestation of farm workers in the midwestern United States in 1950 to 1951, straw used at the Indiana State Fair was infested. During a 2-year period, 642 visitors were treated for grain itch at a dispensary maintained on the fairgrounds, and about 1100 animal attendants and fair workers were treated over the same period at a separate facility.[18] The reservoir of infestation by *Pyemotes* may be quite obscure. Several cases have been reported associated with the common furniture beetle, *Anobium punctatum,* in the floor joists of a house.[54] Therapy is symptomatic. Large-scale eradication measures may require services of professional exterminators.

Delusions of Parasitosis

Patients with delusions of parasitosis are convinced, against all evidence to the contrary, that parasites infest their skin, and often their homes and clothing as well. No single cause is known for this condition, although some cases may be associated with proven parasitic infestation. The idea may also be suggested by infestations of relatives or acquaintances. Patients over 50 years are most often female; patients under 50 are equally male and female.

Most cases of delusions of parasitosis commence with pruritus, which may be accompanied by crawling, creeping, stinging, and burning sensations. The initial reaction is to scratch, replaced soon by digging to remove the "parasites." Self-mutilation and suicidal behavior may develop. Generally, the first contact with a physician is to bring in evidence of the "infestation." Evidence consists typically of scales, lint, crusts, hairs, dust, and small pieces of skin, carefully collected and stored in a small box or folded in facial tissue. Medical attention is often sought not so much to relieve the symptoms as to get rid of the parasites. The sufferer may take the evidence to a professional entomologist for identification, and patients may employ professional exterminators for repeated fumigation. Patients may be so convincing that household members or acquaintances come to share the delusion.[38,49]

Many patients with parasitophobia know that their fear is groundless but are nevertheless unable to overcome it. On the other hand, patients with delusions of parasitosis are convinced that they have an infestation and regard as incompetent the physician who makes the correct diagnosis of no infestation. A complete examination of the patient and the evidence is essential, and investigation of the home or workplace may be indicated. Other medical conditions that may produce cutaneous sensations include liver and renal disease, alcoholism and toxic states, diabetes mellitus, cardiovascular disease, lymphoma, anemia, sideropenia, vitamin B_{12} deficiency, pellagra, peripheral neuritis, dermatitis herpetiformis drug reactions, and environmental irritants (including arthropods and fiberglass).[103,195]

Psychiatric intervention is often unsatisfactory to both patient and physician. Convinced that the physician is wrong, patients often seek repeated opinions and finally become despondent. Pimozide, a neuroleptic medication used to treat other monosymptomatic hypochondriacal psychoses, has been found useful in treating this condition.[121,145,151] In one group of 14 patients treated with pimozide and followed for an average of 34 months, seven had complete remissions at the end of the follow-up time, three had relapses that responded to repeat treatment with pimozide, and four were treatment failures.[96]

Centipedes and Millipedes

Centipedes are elongate, flattened arthropods with one pair of legs for each of the typical body segments, which may number from 15 to more than 100. The first segment bears a pair of curved hollow fangs with venom glands at the bases. The last segment bears a pair of filamentous to forcepslike caudal appendages not associated with venom apparatus. The largest species reach lengths of about 25 to 35 cm. Most centipedes live in crevices or beneath objects on the ground. Some are burrowers, while others are able to climb quite well. Many are nocturnal. *Scutigera coleoptrata,* with body length of 25 mm and long thin legs, is a common house arthropod in much of the United States. Centipedes are predators chiefly on invertebrates, but larger species occasionally eat small vertebrates. Female centipedes of some species curl around their egg clusters and newly hatched young and may actively defend them.

Centipedes use venom primarily to kill prey and only secondarily for defense. Venom may also have a digestive function. Enzymes including acid and alkaline phosphatase and amino acid naphthylamidase, lipoproteins, histamine, and serotonin are variably present.[115] Venom of *Scolopendra subspinipes* produces hypotension followed by hypertension. The major lethal toxin is an acidic protein with molecular weight of 60,000 daltons. It produces vasoconstriction, increased capillary permeability, and cardiac arrest.[62,63]

As with spiders, any centipede whose fangs can penetrate human skin can cause local envenomation. Contrary to popular folklore, centipedes do not inject venom with their feet or caudal appendages. Centipede bites have been reported from numerous tropical and subtropical regions, but never as a serious medical problem. Most have been ascribed to species of *Scolopendra,* which has a wide distribution with several species in the southern United States (Fig. 31-14).

Burning pain, local swelling, erythema, lymphangitis, and lymphadenopathy are common manifestations of a centipede bite. Swelling and tenderness may persist for as long as 3 weeks or may disappear and recur.[71] Superficial necrosis may occur at the site of fang punctures. Few bites with serious systemic reactions have been reported in detail. In one case ascribed to *Scolopendra heros* of the southwestern United States, a woman suffered massive edema of the leg, necrosis of the peroneal muscles, loss of motor function in the foot, myoglobinuria, and azotemia.[100] Other cases have been characterized by rapid onset of dizziness, nausea, collapse, and pyrexia.[26] An infant that ingested a centipede identified as *Scutigera morpha* developed hypotonia, vomiting, and lethargy presumably from being bitten in the mouth or pharynx. The child recovered spontaneously after about 48 hours.[12]

Treatment of centipede envenomation is symptomatic. Infiltration of the bitten area with lidocaine or another anesthetic promptly relieves pain. Antihistamines and steroids have been suggested for more severe reactions.[1,71] Tetanus prophylaxis is routine.

Millipedes differ from centipedes in having two pairs of legs per body segment and in lacking apparatus for injecting venom (Fig. 31-15). Some species are broad and short and roll into a ball when disturbed. Millipedes are generally ground dwelling and secretive. Occasionally they aggregate in enormous numbers. They generally feed on decaying vegetation.

Millipedes are exceptionally well endowed with defensive chemical secretions that include hydrogen cyanide, organic acids, phenol, cresols, benzoquinones, and hydroquinones.[46] These effectively deter most predators. Some large species can eject secretions for distances up to 80 cm.

Human injury from millipede secretions has been reported from a number of tropical regions. The most common injury is dermatitis that begins with a brown-stained area, which burns and may blister and exfoliate. Millipede secretion in the eye causes immediate pain, lacrimation, and blepharospasm. This may be followed by chemosis, periorbital edema, and corneal ulceration. Blindness has been reported.[72,140] Individuals exposed to large millipede aggregations may complain of nausea and irritation of the nose and eyes. No specific treatment is available. Prompt irrigation with water or saline should be followed by analgesics,

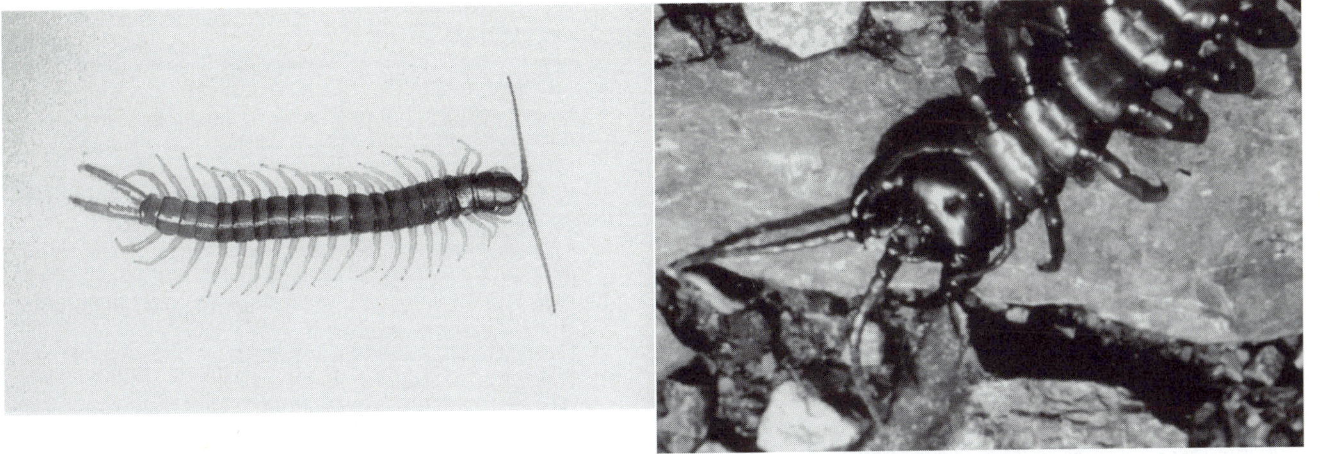

Fig. 31-14 **A,** *Scolopendra* species, a typical large centipede (body length about 150 mm) collected near Armidale in eastern Australia. **B,** Anterior end of large *Scolopendra* showing fangs.

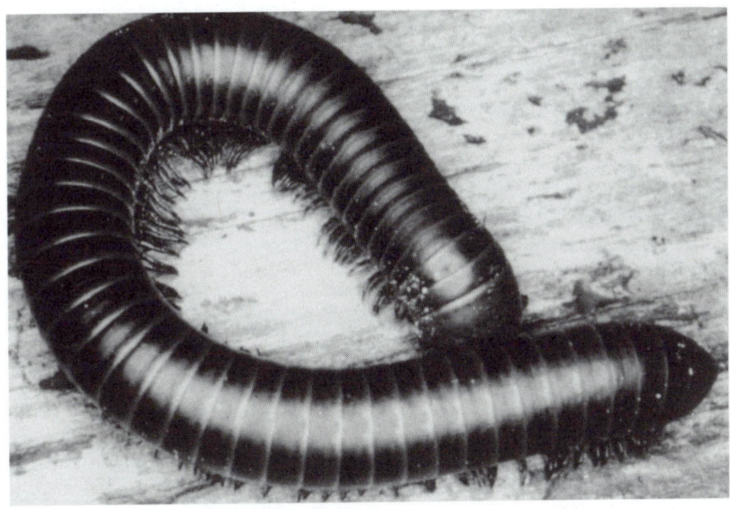

Fig. 31-15 Large millipede (*Spirobolus* species) photographed in central Arkansas.

antimicrobials, and other measures appropriate for superficial chemical burns. Ophthalmologic evaluation is mandatory for eye injuries.

REFERENCES

1. Ariff AW: Cortisone for centipede bites, *Br Med J* 1:986, 1956.
2. Arlian LG et al: Survival and infestivity of *Sarcoptes scabei* var. *canis* and var. *hominis, J Am Acad Dermatol* 11:210, 1984.
3. Arocha-Pinango CL, Layrisse M: Fibrinolysis produced by contact with a caterpillar, *Lancet* 2:810, 1969.
4. Awai LE, Mekori YA: Insect sting anaphylaxis and beta-adrenergic blockade: a relative contraindication, *Ann Allergy* 53:48, 1984.
5. Aylesworth R, Baldridge D: Feather pillow dermatitis caused by an unusual mite *Dermatophagoides scheremetewskyi, J Am Acad Dermatol* 13:680, 1985.
6. Bachman DS, Paulson GW, Mendell JR: Acute inflammatory polyradiculoneuropathy following Hymenoptera sting, *JAMA* 247:1443, 1982.
7. Baer H et al: Protein components of fire ant venom, *Toxicon* 17:397, 1979.
8. Banks BEC: The composition of Hymenoptera venoms with particular reference to venom of the honey bee. In Kornalik F, Mebs D, editors: Proceedings of the 7th European Symposium on Animal Plant & Microbial Toxins 1986, Prague, p 41.
9. Barach EM et al: Epinephrine for treatment of anaphylactic shock, *JAMA* 251:2118, 1984.
10. Barnard JH: Severe hidden delayed reactions from insect stings, *NY State Med J* 66:1206, 1966.
11. Barnard JH: Studies of 400 Hymenoptera sting deaths in the United States, *J Allergy Clin Immunol* 52:259, 1973.
12. Barnett PL: Centipede ingestion by a six-month-old infant: toxic side effects, *Pediatr Emerg Care* 7:229, 1991.
13. Barss P: Renal failure and death after multiple stings in Papua New Guinea, *Med J Aust* 151:659, 1989.

14. Bates M: Mosquitoes as vectors of *Dermatobia* in eastern Colombia, *Ann Entomol Soc Amer* 36:21, 1943.
15. Beaucher WN, Farnham JE: Gypsy-moth-caterpillar dermatitis, *N Engl J Med* 306:1301, 1982.
16. Berger TG: Korean yellow moth dermatitis: report of an epidemic, *J Assoc Mil Dermatol* 12:31, 1986.
17. Bernstein DI et al: Clinical and immunologic studies of rapid venom immunotherapy in Hymenoptera-sensitive patients, *J Allergy Clin Immunol* 84:951, 1989.
18. Booth BH, Jones RW: Epidemiological and clinical study of grain itch, *JAMA* 150:1575, 1952.
19. Bousquet J et al: Evolution of sensitivity to Hymenoptera venom in 200 allergic patients followed for up to 3 years, *J Allergy Clin Immunol* 84:944, 1989.
20. Breeden GC, Schreck CE, Sorensen AL: Permethrin as a clothing treatment for personal protection against chigger bites, *Am J Trop Med Hyg* 31:589, 1982.
21. Browne SG: Cantharidin poisoning due to a "blister beetle," *Br Med J* 2:1290, 1960.
22. Brummer-Korvenkontio H et al: Immunization of rabbits with mosquito bites: immunoblot analysis of IgG antimosquito antibodies in rabbit and man, *Int Arch Allergy Appl Immunol* 93:14, 1990.
23. Bunkis J, Gherini S, Walton RL: Maggot therapy revisited, *West Med J* 142:554.
24. Burgess I, Davies EA: Cutaneous myiasis caused by the housefly *Musca domestica, Br J Dermatol* 125:377, 1991.
25. Burnett JW, Calton GJ, Morgan RJ: Bedbugs, *Cutis* 38:20, 1986.
26. Burnett JW, Calton GJ, Morgan RJ: Centipedes, *Cutis* 37:241, 1986.
27. Butcher BT, Reed MA: Crossed immunoelectrophoretic studies of whole body extracts and venom from the imported fire ant *Solenopsis invicta, J Allergy Clin Immunol* 81:33, 1988.
28. Case RL, Altman LC, VanArsdel PP: Role of cell-mediated immunity in Hymenoptera allergy, *J Allerg Clin Immunol* 68:399, 1981.
29. Chakrabarti A: Human notoderic scabies from contact with cats infested with *Notoedres cati, Int J Dermatol* 25:646, 1986.
30. Charlesworth EN, Clegern RW: Tropical rat mite dermatitis, *Arch Dermatol* 113:937, 1977.
31. Charlesworth EN, Johnson JL: An epidemic of canine scabies in man, *Arch Dermatol* 110:572, 1974.
32. Cohen PR: Imported fire ant stings: clinical manifestations and treatment, *Pediatr Dermatol* 9:44, 1992.
33. Cohen SR: *Cheyletiella* dermatitis, *Arch Dermatol* 116:435, 1980.
34. Daly JJ, Derrick BL: Puss caterpillar sting in Arkansas, *South Med J* 68:893, 1975.
35. Day JM: Death due to cerebral infarction after wasp stings, *Arch Neurol* 7:184, 1962.
36. Delong S: Mulberry tussock moth dermatitis: a study of an epidemic of unknown origin, *J Epidemiol Community Health* 35:1, 1981.
37. De Shazo RD, Butcher BT, Banks WA: Reactions to stings of the imported fire ant, *N Engl J Med* 323:462, 1990.
38. Dewhurst K, Todd J: The psychosis of association—folie a deux, *J Nerv Mental Dis* 124:451, 1956.
39. Dias LB, Azevedo MC: Pararama doenca causada por larvas de Leipdoptera, *Bol Ofic Sanit Panam* 75:3, 1973.
40. Dickey RF: Papular urticaria—hordes of fleas in the living room, *Cutis* 3:345, 1967.
41. Dinehart SM et al: Caripito itch: dermatitis from contact with *Hylesia* moths, *J Am Acad Dermatol* 13:743, 1985.
42. Diven DG, Newton RC, Ramsey KM: Heightened cutaneous reaction to mosquito bites in patients with acquired immune deficiency syndrome receiving zidovudine, *Arch Intern Med* 148:2296, 1988.
43. Dondero TJ et al: Cutaneous myiasis in visitors to Central America, *South Med J* 72:1508, 1979.
44. Duarle A, Duarle G, Barros E: Acute renal failure in accidents caused by caterpillars, *Toxicon* 31:124, 1993.
45. Edwards JS: The action and composition of the saliva of the assassin bug *Platymeris rhadamanthus* Gaerst (Hemiptera Reduviidae), *J Exp Biol* 38:61, 1961.
46. Eisner T et al: Defensive secretions of millipedes, *Handbook Exp Pharmacol* 48:41, 1978.
47. Erasmus C, Blackwood W, Wilson J: Infantile multicystic encephalomalacia after maternal bee sting anaphylaxis during pregnancy, *Arch Dis Child* 57:785, 1982.
48. Estes SA, Kummel B, Arlain L: Experimental canine scabies in humans, *J Am Acad Dermatol* 9:397, 1983.
49. Evans P, Merskey H: Shared beliefs of dermal parasitosis: folie partagee, *Br J Med Psychol* 45:19, 1972.
50. Fain A: Toxic action of rove beetles (Coleoptera, Staphylinidae), *Mem Inst Butantan Simp Internac* 33:835, 1966.
51. Farrell LD et al: Cutaneous myiasis, *Am Fam Physician* 35:127, 1987.
52. Feldman FJ, Maibach HI: Percutaneous penetration of some pesticides and herbicides in man, *Toxicol Appl Pharmacol* 28:126, 1974.
53. File TM et al: *Dermatobia hominis* dermal myiasis, a furuncular lesion in a world traveler, *Arch Dermatol* 121:1195, 1985.
54. Fine R, Scott HG: Straw itch mite dermatitis caused by *Pyemotes ventricosus, J Med Assoc Ga* 52:162, 1963.
55. Fox JG: Outbreak of tropical rat mite dermatitis in laboratory personnel, *Arch Dermatol* 118:676, 1982.
56. Fox JG, Reed C: *Cheyletiella* infestation in cats and their owners, *Arch Dermatol* 114:1233, 1978.
57. Fox RW, Lockey RF, Bukantz SC: Neurologic sequelae following imported fire ant sting, *J Allergy Clin Immunol* 70:120, 1982.
58. Frazier CA: Biting insects, *Arch Dermatol* 107:400, 1973.
59. Gluck JC, Pacin MP: Asthma from mosquito bite; a case report, *Ann Allergy* 56:492, 1986.
60. Golden DBK et al: Epidemiology of insect venom sensitivity, *JAMA* 262:240, 1989.
61. Golub JR, Kaplan SR, Mascia AV: Stinging insect hypersensitivity: safety and efficacy of venom immunotherapy, *NY State J Med* 84:66, 1984.
62. Gomes A et al: Pharmacodynamics of venom of the centipede *Scolopendra subspinipes dehaani, Ind J Exp Biol* 20:615, 1982.
63. Gomes A et al: Isolation, purification and pharmacodynamics of a toxin from the venom of the centipede *Scolopendra subspinipes dehaani, Ind J Exp Biol* 21:203, 1983.
64. Grant JA et al: Diagnosis of *Polistes* wasp hypersensitivity, *J Allergy Clin Immunol* 72:399, 1983.
65. Green AW, Reisman RE, Arbesman CE: Clinical and immunological studies of patients with large local reactions following insect stings, *J Allergy Clin Immunol* 66:186, 1980.
66. Guerro B, Arocha-Pinango CL: Activation of human prothrombin by the venom of *Lonomia achelous* caterpillars, *Thrombin Res* 66:169, 1992.
67. Guillozet N: Diagnosing myiasis, *JAMA* 244:698, 1980.
68. Gunther S: Clinical and epidemiological aspects of the dermal tumbufly myiasis in equatorial Africa, *Br J Dermatol* 85:226, 1971.
69. Hall HG: Parental analysis of introgressive hybridization between African and European honeybees using nuclear DNA, *Genetics* 125:611, 1990.
70. Hall HG, Smith DR: Distinguishing African and European honeybee matrilines using amplified mitochondrial DNA, *Proc Natl Acad Sci USA* 88:4548, 1991.
71. Haneveld GT: Beten door reuzenduizendpoten van Niew-Guinea *(Scolopendra morsitans* en *Sc. subspinipes), Ned Tijdschr Geneesk* 100:2906, 1956.
72. Haneveld GT: Eye lesions caused by the exudate of tropical millipedes: report of a case, *Trop Geogr Med* 10:165, 1958.
73. Headlee WH: Some unusual cases of arthropod infestation, *Proc Ind Acad Sci* 62:298, 1953.
74. Heilsen B: Studies on mosquito bites, *Acta Allergol* 2:245, 1949.
75. Hellier FF, Warin RP: Caterpillar dermatitis, *Br Med J* 2:346, 1967.

76. Hidano KA, Kawakami M, Yago A: Hypersensitivity to mosquito bite and malignant histiocytosis, *Jpn J Exp Med* 52:303, 1982.
77. Hill WR, Rubenstein AD, Kovacs J: Dermatitis resulting from contact with moths (genus *Hylesia*), *JAMA* 138:737, 1948.
78. Ho CL, Hwang LL: Local edema induced by the black-bellied hornet *(Vespa basalis)* venom and its components, *Toxicon* 29:1033, 1991.
79. Hoffman DR, Shipman WH: Allergens in bee venom. I. Separation and identification of major allergens, *J Allergy Clin Immunol* 58:551, 1976.
80. Hoffman DR, Wood CL, Hudson PD: Demonstration of IgE and IgG antibodies against venoms in the blood of fatal sting anaphylaxis, *J Allergy Clin Immunol* 71:193, 1983.
81. Hoffman DR et al: Allergens in Hymenoptera venom XXI: cross-reactivity and multiple reactivity between fire ant and bee and wasp venoms, *J Allergy Clin Immunol* 82:828, 1988.
82. Hughes G, Rosen T: *Automeris io* caterpillar dermatitis, *Cutis* 26:711, 1980.
83. Hunt GR: Uncommon insect bites: the reduviid bite, *Tex Med* 73:45, 1977.
84. Ingall M, Goldman G, Page LB: β-Blockade in stinging insect anaphylaxis, *JAMA* 251:1432, 1984.
85. James FK et al: Imported fire ant sensitivity, *J Allergy Clin Immunol* 58:110, 1976.
86. Kano R: Lepidoptera. In Sasa M et al, editors: *Animals of medical importance in the Nansei Islands of Japan,* Tokyo, 1977, Shinjuku Shobo.
87. Kemeny DM et al: Antibodies to bee venom proteins and peptides, *J Allergy Clin Immunol* 72:376, 1983.
88. Khan RH, Szewcauk MR, Day JH: Bee venom anti-idiotypic antibody is associated with protection in beekeepers and bee-sting-sensitive patients receiving immunotherapy against allergic reactions, *J Allergy Clin Immunol* 88:199, 1991.
89. Kilby VA, Silverman PH: Hypersensitive reactions in man to specific mosquito bites, *Am J Trop Med Hyg* 16:374, 1967.
90. King TP et al: Immunochemical studies of yellowjacket venom proteins, *Mol Immunol* 20:297, 1983.
91. Lacey LA: Anthropophilic blackflies (Diptera:Simuliidae) in Amazon National Park and their effects on man, *Bull Pan Am Health Organ* 15:26, 1981.
92. Lang E, Humphries DW, Jaqua-Stewart MJ: Crusted scabies: a case report and review of the literature, *SD J Med* 42:15, 1989.
93. Lantner R, Reisman RE: Clinical and immunologic features and subsequent course of patients with severe insect-sting anaphylaxis, *J Allergy Clin Immunol* 84:900, 1989.
94. Levine HD: Acute myocardial infarction following wasp sting, *Am Heart J* 91:365, 1976.
95. Light WC et al: Unusual reactions following insect stings, *J Allergy Clin Immunol* 59:391, 1977.
96. Lindskov R, Baadsgard O: Delusions of infestation treated with pimozide: a follow-up study, *Acta Dermatol Venereol* 65:267, 1985.
97. Lockey RF: Immunotherapy for allergy to insect stings, *N Engl J Med* 323:1627, 1990.
98. Lockey RF et al: The Hymenoptera venom study I, 1979-1982: demographics and history-sting data, *J Allergy Clin Immunol* 82:370, 1988.
99. Lockey RF et al: The Hymenoptera venom study III: safety of venom immunotherapy, *J Allergy Clin Immunol* 86:775, 1990.
100. Logan DL, Ogden DA: Rhabdomyolysis and acute renal failure following the bite of the giant desert centipede *Scolopendra heros, West J Med* 142:549, 1985.
101. Lukin LG: Human cutaneous myiasis in Brisbane: a prospective study, *Med J Aust* 150:237, 1989.
102. Lunsford CJ: Flea problem in California, *Arch Dermatol Syph* 60:1184, 1949.
103. Lyell A: Delusions of parasitosis, *J Am Acad Dermatol* 8:895, 1983.
104. Lynch PJ, Pinnas JL: Kissing bug bites, *Cutis* 22:585, 1978.
105. Macias EG et al: Cutaneous myiasis in south Texas, *N Engl J Med* 289:1239, 1973.
106. March DH: A case of "ver du cayor" in Manhattan, *Arch Dermatol* 90:32, 1964.
107. Maretic Z, Zekic R, Bujan M: Bites of gad flies (Tabanidae) in humans, *Medicina* 10:43, 1973.
108. Maretic Z, Ladavac J: The *Thaumetopoa pityocampa* caterpillar—a contribution to the study of venom apparatus, pathology, epidemiology, and clinical effects of its sting, *Period Biol* 80:145, 1978.
109. Mauriello PM et al: Natural history of large local reactions from stinging insects, *J Allergy Clin Immunol* 74:494, 1984.
110. McGovern JP et al: *Megalopyge opercularis,* observations on its life history, natural history of its sting in man, and report of an epidemic, *JAMA* 175:737, 1961.
111. McKiel JA, West AS: Nature and causation of insect bite reactions, *Pediatr Clin North Am* 8:795, 1961.
112. Means ED, Barron KD, Van Dyne BJ: Nervous system lesions after sting by yellowjacket, *Neurology* 12:881, 1973.
113. Mejia G et al: Acute renal failure due to stings by Africanized bees, *Ann Intern Med* 104:210, 1986.
114. Meszaros I: Transient cerebral ischemia attack caused by Hymenoptera stings, *Eur Neurol* 25:248, 1986.
115. Mohamed AH et al: Proteins, lipids, lipoproteins and some enzyme characterizations of the venom extract from the centipede *Scolopendra morsitans, Toxicon* 21:371, 1983.
116. Morgan RJ, Moss HB, Honske WL: Hypoderma myiasis occurrence in Oklahoma, *Arch Dermatol* 90:180, 1964.
117. Mosbech H: Insect allergy, *Allergy* 39:543, 1984.
118. Muller UR et al: Combined active and passive immunotherapy in honeybee sting allergy, *J Allergy Clin Immunol* 78:115, 1986.
119. Muller UR et al: Emergency treatment of allergic reactions to Hymenoptera stings, *Clin Exp Allergy* 21:281, 1991.
120. Mumcouglu KY, Volman Y: Thrips stings in Israel, a case report, *Isr J Med Sci* 24:715, 1988.
121. Munro A: Monosymptomatic hypochondriacal psychosis manifesting as delusions of parasitosis, *Arch Dermatol* 114:940, 1978.
122. Nataf P, Guinnepain MT, Herman D: Rush venom immunotherapy: a 3-day program for Hymenoptera sting allergy, *Clin Allergy* 14:269, 1984.
123. Nelson DR et al: Biochemical and immunochemical comparison of Africanized and European honeybee venoms, *J Allergy Clin Immunol* 85:80, 1990.
124. Neuman I, Ishay JS, Creter D: Hyperreactivity to bee stings: reevaluation, *Ann Allergy* 50:410, 1983.
125. Nusslein HG, Baenkler HW: Spontaneous loss of hypersensitivity in patients allergic to bee or wasp stings; detection by venom-induced histamine release, *Ann Allergy* 54:516, 1985.
126. Olivero JJ, Ayus JC, Eknoyan G: Nephrotic syndrome developing after bee stings, *South Med J* 74:82, 1981.
127. Orkin M, Maibach HI: Current concepts in parasitology: this scabies pandemic, *N Engl J Med* 298:496, 1978.
128. Pallai L et al: Case report: myiasis—the botfly boil, *Am J Med Sci* 303:245, 1992.
129. Pampiglione S, Schiavon S, Fioravanti ML: Extensive furuncular myiasis due to *Cordylobia roshaini* larvae, *Br J Dermatol* 126:418, 1992.
130. Parker JL et al: Evaluation of Hymenoptera-sting sensitivity with deliberate sting challenges: inadequacy of present diagnostic procedures, *J Allergy Clin Immunol* 69:200, 1982.
131. Parrino J, Kandawalla NM, Lockey R: Treatment of local skin response to imported fire ant sting, *South Med J* 74:1361, 1981.
132. Parsons DJ: Bedbug bite anaphylaxis misinterpreted as coronary occlusion, *Ohio Med J* 51:669, 1955.
133. Paull BR: Imported fire ant allergy, *Postgrad Med J* 16:76, 1984.
134. Pence RL et al: Evaluation of severe reactions to sweat bee stings, *Ann Allergy* 66:399, 1991.
135. Perlman F et al: Tussockosis: reactions to Douglas fir tussock moth, *Ann Allergy* 36:302, 1976.
136. Pesce H, Delgado A: Lepidopterismo y erucismo, *Mem Inst Butantan Simp Internac* 33:829, 1966.

137. Peters W: *A colour atlas of arthropods in clinical medicine,* London, 1992, Wolfe Publishing, p 269.
138. Pinnas JL et al: Harvester ant sensitivity: in vitro and in vivo studies using whole body extracts and venom, *J Allergy Clin Immunol* 59:10, 1977.
139. Poskitt L, Duffill MB: Sleeping with a ladybird: suspected bites from *Diomus notescens, NZ Med J* 105:132, 1992.
140. Radford AJ: Millipede burns in man, *Trop Geogr Med* 27:279, 1975.
141. Rantanen T et al: Persistent pruritic papules from deer ked bites, *Acta Derm Venerol* 62:307, 1982.
142. Ratnoff OD, Nossei HL: Wasp sting anaphylaxis, *Blood* 61:132, 1983.
143. Read GW, Lind NK, Oda CS: Histamine release by fire ant *(Solenopsis)* venom, *Toxicon* 16:361, 1978.
144. Reames MK, Christensen C, Luce EA: The use of maggots in wound debridement, *Ann Plast Surg* 21:388, 1988.
145. Reilly TM: Pimozide in monosymptomatic psychosis, *Lancet* 1:1385, 1975.
146. Reisman RE, Lantner R: Further observations of stopping venom immunotherapy, *J Allergy Clin Immunol* 83:1049, 1989.
147. Reunala T et al: Cutaneous reactivity to mosquito bites: effect of cetirizine and development of anti-mosquito antibodies, *Clin Exp Allergy* 2:617, 1991.
148. Rhodes RB et al: Hypersensitivity to the imported fire ant, *J Allergy Clin Immunol* 56:84, 1975.
149. Rhodes RB, Stafford CT, James PK: Survey of fatal reactions to imported fire ant stings, *J Allergy Clin Immunol* 84:159, 1989.
150. Ribeiro JM, Rossignol PA, Spielman A: Role of mosquito saliva in blood vessel location, *J Exp Biol* 108:1, 1984.
151. Riding J, Munro A: Pimozide in the treatment of monosymptomatic hypochondrical psychosis, *Acta Psychiatr Scand* 52:23, 1975.
152. Rivers JK, Martin J, Pukay B: Walking dandruff and *Cheyletiella* dermatitis, *J Am Acad Dermatol* 15:1130, 1986.
153. Rohr AS, Marshall NA, Saxon A: Successful immunotherapy for *Triatoma protracta* induced anaphylaxis, *J Allergy Clin Immunol* 73:369, 1984.
154. Rosenbrook W, O'Conner R: The venom of the mud-dauber wasp *Sceliphron caementarium.* II. Protein content, *Can J Biochem* 42:1005, 1964.
155. Rothenborg HW: Of fleas and foxes, *Arch Dermatol* 111:1215, 1975.
156. Ryan ME: Cutaneous myiasis in Pennsylvania, *Pediatr Infect Dis J* 3:135, 1984.
157. Sadick N et al: Unusual features of scabies complicating human T-lymphotropic virus type III infection, *J Am Acad Dermatol* 15:482, 1986.
158. Salim MM et al: Insect bite lesions in Kuwait possibly due to *Leptodemus minutus, Int J Dermatol* 29:507, 1990.
159. Sanders DP, Peterson JL: The occurrence of the pigeon fly *Pseudolynchia canariensis* in Indiana, *Proc Ind Acad Sci* 84:287, 1975.
160. Schmidt JO, Blum MS, Overal WL: Comparative lethality of venoms from stinging Hymenoptera, *Toxicon* 18:469, 1980.
161. Schorr WF: Tumbu-fly myiasis in Marshfield, Wisconsin, *Arch Dermatol* 95:61, 1967.
162. Schreiber MM, Schuckmell N, Sampsel J: Human myiasis, *JAMA* 188:828, 1964.
163. Schuberth KC et al: An epidemiologic study of insect allergy in children. I. Characteristics of the disease, *J Pediatr* 100:546, 1982.
164. Schultz H: Human infestation by *Ophionyssus natricis* snake mite, *Br J Dermatol* 93:695, 1975.
165. Schumacher MJ et al: Quantity, analysis and lethality of European and Africanized honey bee venoms, *Am J Trop Med Hyg* 43:79, 1990.
166. Schwartz HJ, Golden DB, Lockey RF: Venom immunotherapy in the Hymenoptera-allergic pregnant patient, *J Allergy Clin Immunol* 85:709, 1990.
167. Schwartz HJ et al: Hymenoptera venom-specific IgE in post-mortem sera from victims of sudden and unexpected death, *Clin Allergy* 18:461, 1988.
168. Shama SK et al: Gypsy-moth-caterpillar dermatitis, *N Engl J Med* 306:1300, 1982.
169. Shaw PK, Juranek DD: Recent trends in scabies in the United States, *J Infect Dis* 134:414, 1976.
170. Shields TL, Walsh EN: Kissing bug bite, *Arch Dermatol* 74:14, 1956.
171. Shilkin KB, Chen BTM, Khoo OT: Rhabdomyolysis caused by hornet venom, *Br Med J* 1:156, 1972.
172. Shkenderov S: Anaphylactogenic properties of bee venom and its fractions, *Toxicon* 12:529, 1974.
173. Shkenderov S, Koburova A: Adolapin—a newly isolated analgetic and anti-inflammatory polypeptide from bee venom, *Toxicon* 20:317, 1982.
174. Smith DR, Taylor OR, Brown WM: Neotropical Africanized honey bees have African mitochondrial DNA, *Nature* 339:213, 1989.
175. Sobotka AK et al: Allergy to insect stings. II. Phospholipase A: the major allergen in honeybee venom, *J Allergy Clin Immunol* 57:29, 1976.
176. Southcott RV: Some harmful Australian insects, *Med J Aust* 149:656, 1988.
177. Stafford CT et al: Imported fire ant as a health hazard, *South Med J* 82:1515, 1989.
178. Suzuki S et al: A case of mosquito allergy, *Acta Allergol* 2:245, 1976.
179. Swezey RL: Kissing bug bite in Los Angeles, *Arch Intern Med* 112:977, 1963.
180. Tanphaichitr VS, Tuchinda M: Severe thrombocytopenic purpura following a bee sting, *Ann Allergy* 49:229, 1982.
181. Taplin D et al: Permethrin 5% dermal cream: a new treatment for scabies, *J Am Acad Dermatol* 15:995, 1986.
182. Taylor OR: African bees: potential impact in the United States, *Bull Entomol Soc Am* 39:15, 1985.
183. Taylor OR: Health problems associated with African bees, *Ann Intern Med* 104:267, 1986.
184. Tiech S, Myers RAM: Maggot therapy for severe skin infections, *South Med J* 79:1153.
185. Titchener RW: Infestation of broiler breeder houses with hen fleas, *Parasitology* 79:xiii, 1979.
186. Tokura Y et al: Severe hypersensitivity to mosquito bites associated with natural killer cell lymphocytosis, *Arch Dermatol* 126:362, 1990.
187. Toogood JH: The risk of anaphylaxis in patients receiving beta-blocker drugs, *J Allergy Clin Immunol* 81:1, 1988.
188. Urbanek R et al: Venom-specific IgE and IgG antibodies as a measure of the degree of protection in insect-sting-sensitive patients, *Clin Allergy* 13:229, 1983.
189. Valentine MD: Insect venom allergy: diagnosis and treatment, *J Allergy Clin Immunol* 73:299, 1984.
190. Walker GB, Harrison PV: Seasonal bullous eruption due to mosquitoes, *Clin Exp Dermatol* 10:127, 1985.
191. Warpinski JR, Bush RK: Stinging insect allergy, *J Wilderness Med* 1:249, 1990.
192. Weizman Z et al: Multiple hornet stings with features of Reye's syndrome, *Gastroenterology* 89:1407, 1985.
193. Wirtz RA: Allergic and toxic reactions to non-stinging arthropods, *Annu Rev Entomol* 29:47, 1984.
194. Wright DN, Lockey RF: Local reactions to stinging insects (Hymenoptera), *Allergy Proc* 11:23, 1990.
195. Wykoff RF: Delusions of parasitosis: a review, *Rev Infect Dis* 9:433, 1987.
196. Zalar GL, Walther RR: Infestation by *Tunga penetrans, Arch Dermatol* 116:80, 1980.
197. Zerachia T, Bergmann F, Shulov A: Pharmacological activities of the predacious bug *Holotrichus innesi, Toxicon* 10:537, 1972.
198. Ziprkowski L, Hofshi E, Tahari AS: Caterpillar dermatitis, *Isr Med J* 18:26, 1959.
199. Zora JA, Swanson MC, Yunginger JW: A study of the prevalence and clinical significance of venom-specific IgE, *J Allergy Clin Immunol* 81:77, 1988.

32 SPIDER BITES

Leslie V. Boyer Hassen
Jude T. McNally

Brown spiders
Widow spiders
Funnel-web spiders
Banana spiders (armed spiders)
Wolf spiders
Tarantulas
Hobo spiders
Running spiders and sac spiders
Other spiders

Of approximately 60,000 species in phylum Arthropoda, class Arachnida, 30,000 are spiders.[133] Most species have venom glands, whose ducts open through piercing fangs for injection into prey or predator. However, only a few dozen are considered harmful to people, because in most either the quantity of venom is insufficient or the fangs cannot penetrate human skin.

Like ticks, mites, scorpions, and other arachnids, spiders have a body consisting of an abdomen and an unsegmented cephalothorax with chelicerate jaws, pedipalps, and four pairs of legs (Fig. 32-1). Spider fangs are located on the chelicerae, which open sideways in the "true spiders" of suborder Labidognatha *(Latrodectus, Loxosceles, Phoneutria, Chiracanthium)* and move diagonally in the "mygales" of suborder Orthognatha *(Atrax, Aphonopelma, Trechona)*, requiring them to rear back for a downward, snakelike strike. On the abdomen, spiders have a silk-producing organ and a set of spinnerets.

Spider venom has a variety of purposes. Spiders that hunt, such as *Loxosceles* and *Phoneutria* species, rely on a variety of neurotoxic and proteolytic venom components to incapacitate insects and other prey. Most web-spinners, which incapacitate their prey by envelopment in silk, do not require strongly neurotoxic venom and are relatively harmless to man; an exception is the *Latrodectus* genus, which can produce a painful neurologic syndrome.[133] Digestive juices from most species' venom liquefy food so that it can be sucked out of an immobilized victim; in a few cases, this is of sufficient quantity and potency to cause cell necrosis and systemic toxicity in humans.

Spiders such as tarantulas produce urticating hairs, which irritate skin or mucous membranes of animals or humans. Exposure may result from direct contact with the spider or its web or from proximity to airborne hairs launched by an aggravated arachnid.

Although many spider species have a relatively well-defined geographic distribution (*Atrax robustus* in Australia, *Phoneutria nigriventer* in Brazil), others, such as the black widow *(Latrodectus mactans)*, are cosmopolitan (Table 32-1). The sections that follow consider the most common spiders of medical importance.

Brown Spiders

LOXOSCELES SPECIES AND NECROTIC ARACHNIDISM

Necrotic arachnidism, or "loxoscelism" in the case of bite by spiders of the genus *Loxosceles*, is a term applied to the clinical syndrome that follows envenomation by a variety of spiders for which *Loxosceles reclusa*, the brown recluse spider, is the prototype. The bites of these spiders often result in serious cutaneous injuries, with subsequent necrosis and tissue loss. Less often, there may be severe systemic reactions with hemolysis, coagulopathy, renal failure, and even death.[118,191]

Reports of severe reaction to spider bites possibly or probably attributable to brown spiders date to as early as 1872, in a report of a 45-year-old Texas woman who suffered a febrile illness accompanying a large necrotic lesion of her thigh.[34] In 1896 a death was reported with a case of renal failure accompanying another bite in Texas.[134] Spider bite was reported as a cause of blackwater fever (massive hemoglobinuria) in Tennessee in 1940.[70] The first documented case of loxoscelism (from *L. refuscens*) was reported by Schmaus in Kansas in 1929.[158] *Loxosceles laeta* was identified as the cause of similar lesions in South America in 1937, and *L. reclusa* was demonstrated to be the cause of necrotic arachnidism in the midwestern United States by 1958.[6,7] Since that time, numerous cases of cutaneous and more severe "viscerocutaneous" reactions have been reported and attributed to spiders of the genus *Loxosceles*.

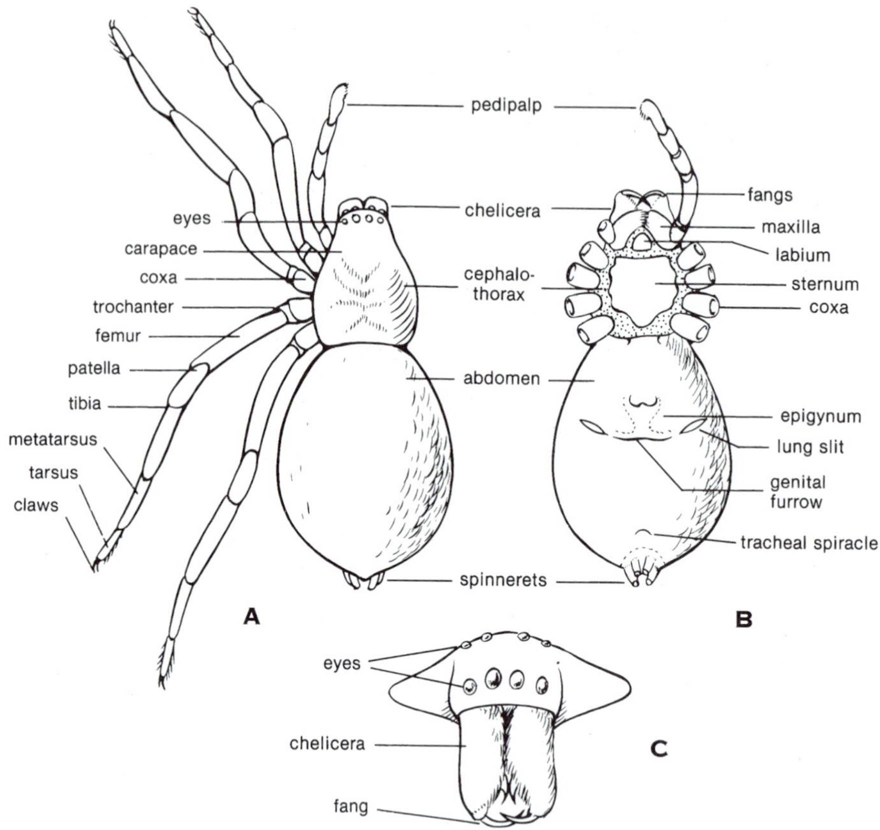

Fig. 32-1 External anatomy of a spider. **A,** Dorsal. **B,** Ventral, legs omitted. **C,** Frontal view of face and chelicerae, to note relationship of eyes.

Loxosceles Spiders

Spiders of genus *Loxosceles,* commonly known as brown or fiddle spiders, are found worldwide.[12,46,107,150,157] From the South American *L. laeta* to the South African *L. spinulosa,* these small arachnids have been associated with human pathologic conditions. At least five species in the genus have been associated with necrotic arachnidism in the United States, including *L. reclusa* (the true "brown recluse" spider), *L. refuscens, L. arizonica, L. unicolor,* and *L. laeta.* These spiders are native to all of the southernmost states of the United States. In the Mississippi River valley, their territory extends as far north as southern Wisconsin. Species native to one region or habitat may adapt successfully to new locations after transport by humans.[125,192]

The brown spiders are 8 to 15 mm in body length, 2 to 3 cm in leg length, and fawn to dark brown in color. Characteristically, they are marked with a dark, violin-shaped spot centered anterodorsally, such that the neck of the fiddle extends backward across the cephalothorax (Color Plate 45).[27,86,157] Magnified, the anterior margin of the fiddle mark is composed of three pairs of eyes, a distinguishing characteristic of the genus. Paired, segmented chelicerae inject venom from endocephalic venom sacs, which are modified salivary glands. Males have more slender abdomens and more prominent pedipalps than do females.

Brown spiders are most active at night from spring through fall, emerging from woodpiles and rats' nests to hunt insects and other spiders. South African savanna species have been observed under stones and logs and in the tunnels of old termite nests; spelean species are found naturally in caves but have also appeared in homes and export warehouses.[122,126,127] In endemic areas, brown spiders may infest homes, generally preferring warm, undisturbed environments such as vacant buildings and storage sheds. In Chile the tendency to inhabit human dwellings has earned *L. laeta* the names *araña de los rincones* (corner spider) and *araña de detrás de los cuadros* (spider behind the pictures).[155] "Molts" or shed exoskeletons may mark infested areas; the web, when present, may be limited to a small, flocculent structure alongside the egg sac. Females may live 1 to 3 years, longer in captivity.[65,87] Naturally unaggressive toward humans, brown spiders are not prone to bite unless threatened or trapped against the skin. Bites commonly follow the retrieval of old bedsheets or jackets from storage.

Table 32-1 Some Spiders (Order Araneae) of Clinical Importance

Suborder/Family	Genus and Species	Where Found	Clinical Pattern
ORTHOGNATHA (MYGALES)			
Dipluridae (funnel spiders)	*Atrax robustus* (Sydney funnel-web)	Australia	Presynaptic neurotoxin
	Hadronyche formidabilis (northern funnel-web)	Australia	Presynaptic neurotoxin
	Trechona venosa	South America	Neurotoxin
Grammostolinae	*Aphonopelma, Dugesiella henzi*	New World	Urticating hairs, local cytotoxin
LABIDOGNATHA (TRUE SPIDERS)			
Scytodidae (fiddle spiders)	*Loxosceles laeta*	South America	Local necrosis, edema, hematotoxicity, fever
	L. reclusa (brown recluse)	North America	Hematotoxicity, fever
	L. spinulosa	South Africa (savanna)	Hematotoxicity, fever
	L. parrami	South Africa (caves)	Hematotoxicity, fever
	L. refuscens	Israel and Middle East	Hematotoxicity, fever
Therididae (widow spiders)	*Latrodectus* spp.		
	L. mactans mactans (black widow)	Cosmopolitan	Presynaptic neurotoxin
	L. m. tridecimguttatus	Europe, South America	Presynaptic neurotoxin
	L. m. hasselti (redback spider)	Australia	Presynaptic neurotoxin
	L. pallidus	Middle East, Asia	Presynaptic neurotoxin
	L. indistinctus (black button spider)	South Africa	Presynaptic neurotoxin
	L. geometricus (brown button spider)	Cosmopolitan	Presynaptic neurotoxin
Lycosidae (wolf spiders)	*Lycosa tarentula*	Europe	Local cytotoxin
	L. raptoria	South America	Local cytotoxin
Clubionidae (sac spiders, running spiders)	*Chiracanthium* spp.	Europe, Africa, North America, Australia	Local necrosis, occasional systemic
Ctenidae	*Phoneutria nigriventer* (banana spider)	South America	Sodium channel toxin

Venom

Loxosceles venom normally serves as digestive juice, which digests prey tissues enzymatically in situ in preparation for sucking by the spider. Some vertebrate species, such as rats and fish, are essentially unaffected by the venom; others, such as rabbits, mice, and dogs, are highly susceptible to its effects.[156] Injected into humans, the venom is a hemolysin and cytotoxin, with a variety of enzymatic activities whose combined effect may bring about dermonecrosis and hemolysis. Pathogenesis of the human lesion is not well understood but is known to depend in part on the functions of complement and polymorphonuclear leukocytes.[11,157]

Fractionated venom contains at least eight or nine major protein bands and three or four minor bands identifiable by gel electrophoresis.[141] Hyaluronidase was first identified as a component by Wright and associates.[205] Hyaluronidase probably plays a facilitating role in lesion development, encouraging the gravitational spread of other venom components; however, it is not itself a cytotoxin. Hydrolytic enzyme activities include esterase,[205] alkaline phosphatase,[82] lipase,[92] and 5′-ribonucleotide phosphorylase,[64] but none of these appears by itself to explain cytotoxicity. Sphingomyelinase D, a protein fraction of molecular weight 32,000, appears to be the most important dermonecrotic factor in *L. reclusa* venom. Injection of the purified fraction produces characteristic lesions in rabbits.[98,185] A protein of similar molecular weight to sphingomyelinase D has been shown to have dermonecrotic activity in the venom of *L. gaucho* of Brazil.[13] Sphingomyelinase D is postulated to operate by a variety of mechanisms, among them cell membrane binding and polymorphonuclear leukocyte chemotaxis.[62,140,163] Lesions are inhibited in rabbits by pretreatment with nitrogen mustard to deplete polymorphonuclear neutrophils. Histologic studies suggest similarities between venom-induced lesions and those seen with the Arthus and Shwartzmann phenomena.[163]

Venom from *L. reclusa* has been shown to have a direct hemolytic effect on human erythrocytes; this process depends on the presence of serum components that include C-reactive protein and calcium.[88,185] Platelet aggregation, also calcium dependent, can also be induced in vitro with sphingomyelinase D; this process may activate the prostaglandin cascade. Platelet aggregation appears to depend on serum amyloid protein, a serum glycoprotein of previously unknown significance.[61,143,185]

Presentation

The clinical spectrum of loxoscelism runs from mild and transient skin irritation to severe local necrosis accompanied by dramatic hematologic and renal injury. Isolated cutaneous lesions are the most common presentation, and it has been suggested that most bites resolve spontaneously without the need for medical intervention.[18,19] Many authors distinguish between simple local presentation and more severe systemic, or "viscerocutaneous," loxoscelism.

Local symptoms usually begin at the moment of the bite, with a sharp stinging sensation, although it is not uncommon for a patient to report no awareness of having been bitten. Frequently the bite site corresponds to a portal of entry or a region of constriction of clothing, such as cuff, collar, waistband, or groin. The stinging usually subsides over 6 to 8 hours and is replaced by aching and pruritus as the lesion becomes ischemic from local vasospasm. The site then becomes edematous, with an erythematous halo surrounding an irregular violaceous center of "incipient necrosis" (actually hemorrhage and thrombosis[28,185]; a white ring of vasospasm and ischemia may be discernible between these two). Often the erythematous margin spreads irregularly, in a gravitationally influenced pattern that leaves the original center eccentrically placed near the top of the lesion (Color Plates 46 to 48). In more severe cases, serous or hemorrhagic bullae may arise at the center within 24 to 72 hours and an eschar forms beneath (Fig. 32-2). After 2 to 5 weeks this eschar sloughs, leaving an ulcer of variable size and depth through skin and adipose tissue, but sparing muscle.[84] Lesions involving adipose tissue may be extensive, perhaps as a result of lipolytic action of the venom.[92] The ulcer may persist for many months, leaving a deep scar.[1,148,194] Local sequelae in part depend on the anatomic location. Persistent segmental cutaneous anesthesia has been attributed to nerve injury after a recluse bite on the side of the neck.[77] Epiglottic and periepiglottic swelling severe enough to require endotracheal intubation has been reported in a recluse bite involving a child's ear.[83]

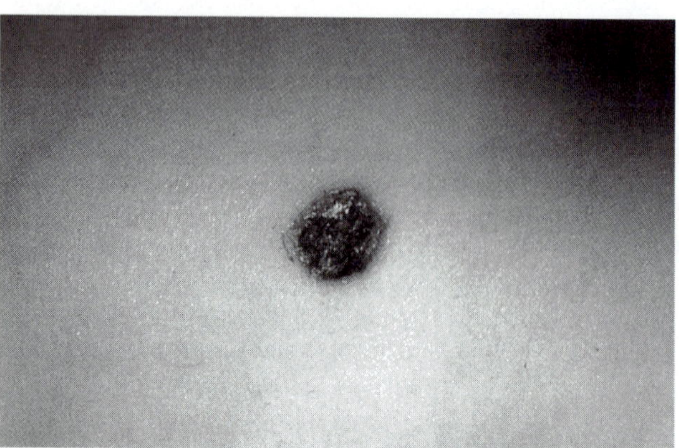

Fig. 32-2 Brown recluse spider bite at 48 hours, demonstrating central necrotic ulcer.

The bite of the somewhat larger South American spider *Loxosceles laeta* is reported to cause intense pain and extensive edema, with proportionately less necrosis than that caused by *L. reclusa*. The edema is notoriously prominent with facial bites and resolves over 2 to 4 weeks.[157]

Systemic involvement is less common but may occur in combination with cutaneous injury from any *Loxosceles* species; it occurs more frequently in children, but may be seen in adults.[135,183] Systemic reaction may develop in cases with minor-appearing local findings, making diagnosis difficult.[185] When there is systemic involvement, hemolytic anemia with hemoglobinuria is commonly the prominent feature, usually beginning within 24 hours of envenomation and resolving within 1 week. During this time, measured hemoglobin may drop markedly. The anemia is usually Coombs' negative, but two cases of Coombs'-positive anemia have been reported.[191] Fever, chills, maculopapular rash, weakness, leukocytosis, arthralgias, nausea, and vomiting may all occur, also usually within a day or two of the bite. Thrombocytopenia and disseminated intravascular coagulation have been reported.[191] In severe cases, hemoglobinuria and proteinuria have led to renal failure and even death.[43,67,121]

A series of five proved or suspected *L. reclusa* bites to women in the second and third trimesters of pregnancy has been reported. Despite significant local injuries, rash, and microhematuria, no fetal injury was noted.[2]

The diagnosis of loxoscelism is based on spider observation and identification, typical history, and local and systemic signs. The differential diagnosis of the local injury includes bacterial and mycobacterial infection,[177] herpes simplex, decubitus ulcer, third-degree burn, and pyoderma gangrenosum.[94,136,137] Systemic involvement may manifest as hemolytic anemia,[48] declining hemoglobin level and hematocrit value, thrombocytopenia, jaundice, and hemoglobinuria.

Loxosceles venom is known to provoke an immune response in experimental animals, so efforts have been made to develop diagnostic tests based on antigen or antibody detection in human blood. In 1973, Berger reported an in vitro lymphocyte transformation assay for *L. reclusa* venom, which turned positive in the lymphocytes of exposed individuals within 4 to 6 weeks of initial exposure. This test may help to document prior exposure, but not to diagnose envenomation at the time of the initial bite.[19] Barrett and coworkers[14] reported a passive hemagglutination inhibition test using rabbit antibody and human erythrocytes incubated in vitro with venom from *L. reclusa*. Cardoso and associates, observing that efforts to detect antigen in human serum may fail because of insufficient antigenemia, have demonstrated the presence of *L. gaucho* venom in biopsy homogenate using enzyme-linked immunosorbent assay. More recently, Barbaro and colleagues[13] have demonstrated circulating IgG against *L. gaucho* venom in 4 out of 20 patients, detectable between 9 and 120 days after the bite.

Treatment

Treatment of loxoscelism depends on its severity. Cutaneous loxoscelism can usually be managed on an outpatient basis. Most mild cutaneous envenomations respond to application of local cold compresses,[95] elevation of the affected extremity, and loose immobilization of the part. Tetanus prophylaxis should be provided where indicated. Necrotic lesions may need debridement after erythema has subsided to define the margins of the central eschar. This commonly involves significant debridement 1 or 2 weeks after the bite, with close follow-up for several weeks thereafter. In severe cases this can be followed with skin grafting or plastic surgery when the wound is stable. Severe necrotic or infected lesions may lead to hospitalization.

Recently the use of dapsone has gained popularity for the prevention of lesion progression in potentially necrotic wounds seen within 48 to 72 hours of a bite.[57,63] Dapsone is a leukocyte inhibitor that in theory can minimize the local inflammatory component of cutaneous loxoscelism, thereby preventing or lessening subsequent skin necrosis. In 1983, King and Rees[96] reported the use of dapsone for envenomation in a human bitten by *L. reclusa,* based on a successful trial of dapsone pretreatment in guinea pigs injected with recluse venom. Since that time, no prospective, controlled human trial has proved dapsone efficacy, but a variety of case reports and series have been put forward in support of its use in the treatment of potentially necrotic wounds treated in the first days after envenomation.[1,16,83,104,200] Typical dosage recommendations are for 50 to 100 mg orally, twice daily. Risks of dapsone therapy include hypersensitivity,[202] methemoglobinemia, and hemolysis in the presence of glucose-6-phosphate dehydrogenase (G-6-PD) deficiency.

Patients with systemic symptoms should be considered for admission when there is evidence of coagulopathy, hemolysis and hemoglobinuria, or rapid progression of other systemic signs. Care is mainly supportive, commonly involving wound care, fluid management, presumptive treatment for bacterial superinfection, and occasionally blood transfusion. Rarely, hemodialysis has been required for oliguric renal failure.[68] Discharge is appropriate when renal and hematologic statuses are stable.

For patients with significant local or systemic signs or symptoms, laboratory evaluation should include peripheral blood cell count, basic coagulation screening, and urinalysis. Liver and renal function tests are indicated in severe poisonings. When use of dapsone is considered, a screening test for G-6-PD deficiency may be indicated. The frequency of follow-up testing depends on the course and severity of envenomation. Hospitalized patients may need close follow-up of anemia and renal function over the course of several days.

In the past, several authors have reported the use of corticosteroids injected either at the wound site or systemically* but this remains of questionable benefit.[17,139] Antihistamines may help control itching but do not change the lesion.[101] Early surgical excision of the wound site has been advocated by some,[5,10,50,85] but others have demonstrated that outcomes are better with early medical management in human patients,[42,141] as well as in experimental animals.[139] Hyperbaric oxygen (HBO) treatment has been tried empirically in uncontrolled human trials with reports of good outcome.[182] Comparison of HBO with no treatment in rabbits showed enhanced recovery at 24 days at the histologic level, but there was no apparent clinical difference between the two groups.[166]

Loxosceles-specific antivenom has been tried both in the United States and in South America. In the early 1980s Rees and colleagues reported a protective effect of treatment with antivenom in rabbits before or up to 12 hours after envenomation. Small vessel occlusion, leukocyte infiltration, and necrosis all occurred but were diminished in antivenom recipients.[139] Pretreatment in a separate study abolished symptoms of systemic loxoscelism.[138] In 1987 these authors reported experience with 17 patients separated randomly into dapsone, antivenom, and combination therapy groups; all patients received erythromycin. Individual results suggested that the antivenom was efficacious when given early, but the overall trial was inconclusive, indicating the need for further study.[142]

In South America an antivenom to *L. laeta* was developed in 1954 by Vellard using immune serum of the donkey. Furlanetto developed *L. laeta* antivenom using immune serum of horses. Reports of the efficacy of systemically administered *L. laeta* antivenom are mixed.[157]

Widow Spiders

LATRODECTUS SPECIES

Spiders of genus *Latrodectus* are common worldwide. Latrodectism, the syndrome commonly resulting from *Latrodectus* envenomation, does not resemble the cytotoxic and hematotoxic consequences of brown spider bite. Victims of black widow bite suffer instead from the painful consequences of a neurotoxic venom best known for the induction of sustained muscle spasm. Although long-term outcomes are usually excellent, patients may in the short term have significant hypertension, autonomic and central nervous dysfunction, and abdominal pain severe enough to be mistaken for acute abdomen.

Latrodectus Spiders

Latrodectus (Latin for "robber-biter") spiders are worldwide in distribution, most plentiful in temperate and subtropical regions, and most abundant during summer.[20]

*References 18, 44, 45, 89, 91, 108, 134.

Latrodectus mactans mactans, the black widow, is cosmopolitan and occurs in every state of the United States except Alaska. In North America, species include *L. geometricus* (the brown widow), *L. bishopi* (the red-legged widow), *L. variolus,* and *L. hesperus*. Subspecies of *L. mactans* known to envenom humans are endemic to Australia *(L. m. hasselti)* and to Europe and South America *(L. m. tridecimguttatus)*. Related species are found in Asia and the Middle East *(L. pallidus)* and in Africa *(L. indistinctus)*.

The male black widow, half the size of the female, is nondescript brown and does not envenom humans. The female, at 2 to 2.5 cm, is shiny black with a characteristic red "hourglass" marking on the ventral abdomen (Color Plate 49). This feature becomes more prominent with maturity. She spins an irregular web in sheltered corners of fields, gardens, and vineyards and under stones, logs, and vegetation. Uncommon in occupied dwellings, the spiders may be plentiful in barns, garages, trash heaps, and outbuildings. A few *Latrodectus* species (such as *L. variolus*) are arboreal. The web's tattered "cobweb" appearance may belie an ongoing state of occupation, particularly during the daytime when the spider is out of sight. The female seldom ventures far from the web, in which she suspends an ovoid or tear-shaped whitish egg case.

The variation of *L. mactans* known as *tridecimguttatus* is most important in the Mediterranean region, the Middle East, and parts of the former Soviet Union. It may have red or orange spots or be pure black and is known as *kara kurt,* or "black wolf" in Russian. *L. indistinctus,* the black button spider of South Africa, has a narrow or broken red dorsal band or may be entirely black. The red-backed spider *(L. hasselti)* is medically important in Australia, New Zealand, and southern Asia (Color Plate 50). It has a dorsal red band similar to that of *L. indistinctus,* and the female has in addition a ventral red hourglass reminiscent of *L. m. mactans. L. geometricus* is brown with black, red, and yellow markings and is common in southern Africa and warmer parts of the Americas.

Widow spiders tend to bite defensively when a web is disturbed. In the Mediterranean basin, southern Russia, and South Africa, bites are associated with grain harvesting and threshing and with grape picking. In the United States, most bites occur in rural and suburban areas of southern and western states, with no special age, sex, or occupational predilection. In regions where outdoor privies are in common use, human envenomations are likely to involve the buttocks or genital area.[23,67,112,203] Outbreaks of latrodectism may occur locally in epidemic fashion, lasting several years, and depend on changes in spider predator and parasite balance and on occupational variations in human-spider contact.[20] Apparent outbreaks may also result from sudden increases in publicity and reporting.[20,93]

Venom

Unlike many other arthropod venoms, that of the widow spiders appears to lack locally active toxins capable of provoking inflammation. It contains several toxic components, including a potent mammalian neurotoxin, α-latrotoxin, which induces neurotransmitter release from nerve terminals.

In 1964, Frontali and Grasso[55] demonstrated three electrophoretically and toxicologically distinct fractions of *Latrodectus* venom. In 1976 Frontali and associates[56] further purified and defined these fractions, encountering one major constituent (the B5 fraction, later renamed α-latrotoxin) with significant toxicity in mice and frogs (other fractions have effects more specific to insect physiology). α-Latrotoxin, a protein mix with an average molecular weight of 130,000, caused profound depletion of presynaptic vesicles with swelling of the presynaptic terminal at frog neuromuscular junctions; complete blockade of neuromuscular transmission followed within 1 hour. The toxin binds irreversibly with the lipid bilayer of the cell membrane, producing cation-selective channels and interfering with the endocytosis of vesicle membranes.[35,51] The mechanism of action is not fully understood, but multivalent cations, including calcium, may enter the presynaptic nerve terminal by way of these channels, interfering with calcium-dependent intracellular processes.[72,116] These effects appear to be specific to presynaptic nerves but independent of the transmitter involved. Acetylcholine, noradrenaline, dopamine, glutamate, and enkephalin systems are all susceptible to the toxin.[145]

Presentation

The initial bite may be sharply painful, but many bites are not recognized initially, so diagnosis is often presumptive and based on local and systemic signs. Local reaction is commonly trivial, with only a tiny papule or punctum visible on examination. The surrounding skin may be slightly erythematous and slightly indurated. In many cases symptoms do not progress beyond this point.

In some cases, however, neuromuscular symptoms can become dramatic within 30 to 60 minutes as involuntary spasm and rigidity affect the large muscle groups of the abdomen, limbs, and lower back. Rhabdomyolysis has rarely been reported.[59] A predominantly abdominal presentation may closely mimic acute abdomen. Associated signs include fasciculations, weakness, ptosis, priapism, thready pulse, fever, salivation, diaphoresis, vomiting, and bronchorrhea. Pulmonary edema has been described in Europe[115] and in South Africa.[99,190] Respiratory muscle weakness combined with pain may lead to respiratory arrest. Hypertension with or without seizures may complicate management in elderly or previously hypertensive individuals. Isolated (normotensive) seizures do not appear to be a feature of latrodectism. Intractable crying may be the predominant feature in neonates.[29] Pregnancy may or may not be complicated by uterine contractions and, potentially, premature delivery.[12,86,114,148,149] A characteristic pattern of facial swelling, known as *Latrodectus* facies, may occur hours after the bite and is sometimes mistaken for an allergy to drugs used in treatment. The natural course of an envenomation is to achieve complete recovery after a few days, although pain may last a week or more.

The clinical picture of *Latrodectus* poisoning is similar around the world. In California the most common site of envenomation referred to a toxicology service in the 1980s was the lower extremity (48%), followed by upper extremities (28%), trunk (18%), and head or neck (5%). The most common systemic symptom was abdominal or back pain (58%), followed by extremity pain (38%), hypertension (29%), and diaphoresis (22%).[37] In Australia, a 1961 survey showed 37% of victims were bitten on the upper extremities, 27% on the lower extremities, 22% on the buttock or penis, 17% on the trunk, and 4% on the head or neck.[197] A report in 1978 showed a decline in incidence of genital and buttock involvement (9.7%), perhaps related to a decrease in the use of outdoor lavatories.[181] Australian envenomations showed a similar pattern of pain and diaphoresis, with more prominent local inflammation and lymphadenopathy and less hypertension than reported in the United States.[181] In South Africa, envenomation by *L. geometricus* results mainly in local pain, whereas *L. indistinctus* provokes a syndrome of generalized pain, diaphoresis, and muscle rigidity similar to that seen in the United States.[119] Victims bitten by *L. tridecimguttatus* show more spasm of facial muscles, swollen eyelids, lacrimation, and photophobia, more commonly resulting in recognized *Latrodectus* facies. A rash may appear 2 to 11 days after envenomation.

Treatment

Care of the local site commonly includes routine cleansing, intermittent application of ice, and tetanus prophylaxis. Severe pain and muscle spasm usually respond to intravenous narcotics or benzodiazepines. Careful observation of respiratory status is vital when either or both of these are used. Calcium gluconate infusion, advocated in the past, has proved only minimally useful and is no longer recommended. Hypertension may be treated with an infusion of sodium nitroprusside or nifedipine if it does not respond to pain control with narcotics or antivenom.

Laboratory evaluation may include complete blood cell count, electrolytes, blood glucose, and urinalysis. Common findings include leukocytosis and albuminuria. In the presence of severe muscle spasm, creatine phosphokinase levels may be elevated. Abdominal films and stool examination for occult blood, both of which should be normal after widow spider envenomation, may help with the differential diagnosis of abdominal pain. A pregnancy test should be done where clinically indicated. No specific antigen or antibody detection technique is currently available for clinical diagnosis.

Antivenom active against *Latrodectus* venom is available in the United States from Merck, Sharp, and Dohme, in Australia from Commonwealth Serum Laboratories, and in South Africa from the South African Institute of Medical Research. Standards for *Latrodectus* antivenom use vary around the world, as do guidelines for its administration.[37,119,178] In general, antivenom should be used in cases involving respiratory arrest, seizures, uncontrolled hypertension, or pregnancy.[149] In less severe settings its value must be weighed against the risks of acute hypersensitivity and of delayed serum sickness. In Australia 0.5% of cases result in anaphylaxis and an unknown number develop serum sickness[181]; death from anaphylaxis has been reported in the United States.[37] The usual therapeutic antivenom dose is one to three vials or ampules.

Although the worst pain usually occurs during the first 8 to 12 hours after a bite, symptoms may remain severe for several days. All symptomatic children, pregnant women, and patients with a history of hypertension should be admitted to the hospital. Discharge is usually possible within 1 to 3 days, when hypertension and muscle spasm have subsided. A patient with a satisfactory response to antivenom may be sent home after several hours' observation.

Funnel-Web Spiders

ATRAX SPECIES AND OTHERS

Funnel-web spiders are large, aggressive spiders belonging to a variety of genera within the family Dipluridae. Although many species have venom with significant in vitro toxicity, few have been implicated in human illness. The best described of these is *Atrax robustus* of Australia, the Sydney funnel-web spider. *Atrax* venom is a neurotoxin that causes release of various neurotransmitters, with painful, and potentially rapidly fatal, consequences in the human victim. Because symptoms may occur in rapid sequence, first aid recommendations have included limb immobilization and pressure wrapping, to minimize lymphatic return before emergency medical treatment (see Fig. 29-2). Antivenom specific to *Atrax* envenomation has been developed and successfully used in Australia.

Funnel-Web Spiders

The family Dipluridae, unlike *Loxosceles* and *Latrodectus* genera, is in the suborder Mygalomorphae. Mygales are sometimes referred to collectively as tarantulas or mygalomorph spiders. In mygales, fang position is vertical relative to the body, requiring them to rear back and lift the body to attack, inflicting a snakelike bite.

Funnel-web spiders have a glossy ebony cephalothorax and velvety black abdomen. The abdominal undersurface may have brushes of red hair. The fangs reach 4 to 5 mm in length and are capable of penetrating a fingernail or a chicken's skull, sometimes making removal of the spider difficult (Fig. 32-3).[154] Females are somewhat larger than males, with a body length of 4 cm. Mature males are more delicate with a tibial spur on the second pair of legs and pointed pedipalps. Like all mygales, they have two pairs of book lungs and long spinnerets.[90,154]

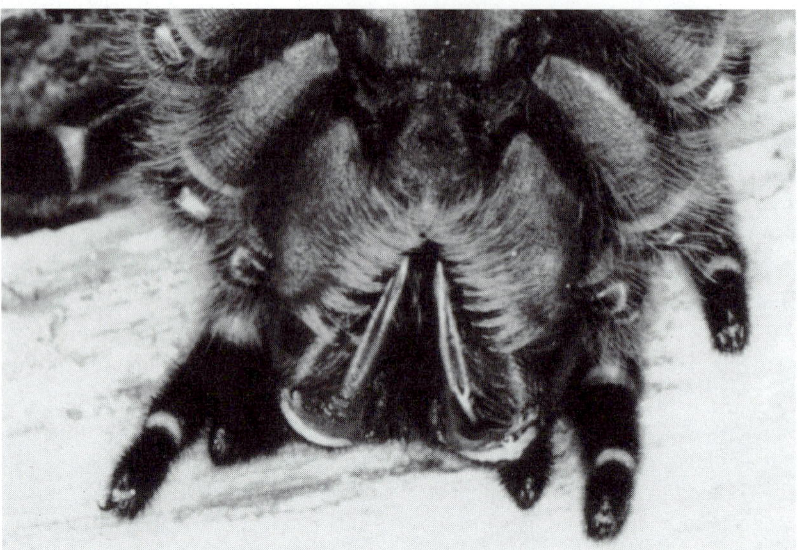

Fig. 32-3 Head of a mygalomorph spider (*Atrax* species) showing obliquely oriented fangs.

Within the Dipluridae are the *Atrax, Hadronyche,* and *Trechona* genera.[154] Among these, the species *Atrax robustus* is best known and most carefully studied. *Atrax* and *Hadronyche* species, all of which are believed to be dangerous, have been described in southern and southeastern Australia, Tasmania, Papua New Guinea, and the Solomon Islands. As a group they prefer cool, moist coastal and mountain regions.[74,75,159]

Atrax robustus, the Sydney funnel-web spider, is limited to a 160 km range around the center of Sydney, Australia (Color Plate 51). The spider creates a tubular or funnel-shaped, silk-lined shallow burrow under rocks, logs, fences, stumps, thick vegetation, or around foundations of houses.[38,60,74] Colonies of up to 150 spiders have been found. Females rarely roam far from their webs; males live a vagrant life after reaching maturity. Wandering males may enter houses or other areas of human habitation, especially during the summer months after a heavy rain. Its aggressive behavior and potent venom make the male Sydney funnel-web one of the most dangerous spiders in the world. It is responsible for all known fatal *Atrax* envenomations.*

Hadronyche formidabilis (formerly *Atrax formidabilis*), the northern funnel-web spider, is found in the central coastal region of New South Wales and the adjacent Blue Mountains. Its tree-dwelling habit was once thought to be unique, but it is now known that other species also live in trees. The webs may be camouflaged in rough-barked trees such as melaleuca (paper bark), banksia, and eucalyptus. No fatalities caused by this spider have been recorded. However, several severe envenomations have occurred.[74]

Trechona venosa is a large South American funnel-web tarantula with neurotoxic venom potentially dangerous to humans.[26,65,78] Like all *Trechona,* it is sedentary, living in holes or on plants in tropical forests along the Atlantic coast. The spider may be black or gray-brown with yellow stripes on the abdomen. Mature body length may be 3 to 4.5 cm, with 6 to 7 cm legs and 3 to 4 mm fangs. The venom is extremely toxic to rats. No cases of human envenomation have been reported.

Atrax Venom

Atrax venom is a neurotoxin believed to cause widespread release of neurotransmitters.[47,74,80,164,170]

Between 1956 and 1963, Wiener[195-197,199] demonstrated significant differences in the venom of male and female *Atrax* spiders. Males had an average venom yield of 1.01 mg, less than the 1.84 average from females. On the other hand, guinea pig lethality was much greater after a bite by a male (75% to 90%) than by a female spider (20%). He concluded that there was a significant qualitative difference between the venoms of males and females.

Animal species vary in susceptibility to *Atrax* venom. Rabbits given 15 mg of crude venom intravenously and cane toads given 12 mg of female venom show no effects after envenomation. Primates, including humans, are among the most susceptible species. Newborn mice, also highly susceptible, have been used as an in vivo biologic assay for venom toxicity.[74,171] Sutherland[174] found that a lethal dose of venom from a male *A. robustus* could be neutralized in

*References 38, 60, 74, 154, 181, 195.

newborn mice by nonimmune sera from rabbits and other nonprimate vertebrates. Scheumack and co-workers[161] later demonstrated that the active fraction of nonimmune rabbit sera contained IgG and IgM immunoglobulins.

Early efforts to purify the active component of *Atrax* venom resulted in reports of neurotoxins of various molecular weights purified from venom preparations in separate experiments. These were termed "atraxotoxin" (molecular weight 10,000 to 25,000, from "milked" venom),[74] "robustoxin" (molecular weight 4887, also from "milked" venom),[160] and "atraxin" (molecular weight 9800, from ground venom glands).[76] The relationships among these toxins are not entirely clear. It is possible, for instance, that atraxotoxin or atraxin may be a precursor of robustoxin.

The best characterized of these toxins is robustoxin, whose 42–amino acid sequence was determined in 1985.[160] It is the sole lethal toxin that can be isolated by cation-exchange chromatography, and its effects in monkeys duplicate the effects of crude venom preparations. A 5 μg/kg intravenous dose of robustoxin causes dyspnea, blood pressure fluctuations culminating in severe hypotension, lacrimation, salivation, skeletal muscle fasciculation, and death within 3 to 4 hours of administration to monkeys.[120]

A purified IgG antivenom protective against *Atrax* envenomation was developed in rabbits by Sutherland[172] at the Commonwealth Serum Laboratories in 1980. To date, it has been used with good effect in over 40 humans bitten by *Atrax* species.[178] More recently, Sheumack and colleagues[162] developed a toxoid from robustoxin by polymerization with glutaraldehyde. Immunization with the toxoid conferred protection against the lethal effects of 50 μg/kg *Atrax* venom in monkeys for at least 26 weeks after toxoid injection.

Atrax venom is believed to cause widespread release of neurotransmitters.[47,74,80,164,170] This may occur by a direct action of the venom on nerve membranes, producing spontaneous action potentials[164] and consequently provoking a global outpouring of transmitters that may account for the neuromotor and autonomic stimulation seen clinically.

Hypertension in *Atrax* toxicity may have several causes. Morgans and Carroll[117,118] demonstrated direct α-adrenergic stimulation with vasoconstriction of isolated arterial preparations exposed to *A. robustus* venom. An initial decrease, followed by an increase, in cardiac inotropy and chronotropy, observed in rabbit atria, may be explained by vagal acetylcholine and myocardial norepinephrine releases, respectively.[33] The combination of myocardial responses and peripheral vasoconstriction may explain the hypertensive response.

Isolated human intercostal muscles were studied to determine the etiology of muscle fasciculations in humans and monkeys. Intercostal muscles treated with *A. robustus* venom developed marked contractions, which were abolished by *d*-tubocurarine.[32] Muscles treated with venom for more than an hour stopped contracting and could be stimulated only by increasing the stimulus duration. These results suggested that after initially causing the release of acetylcholine, the venom blocked release.[32] *A. robustus* venom has already been shown to lack anticholinesterase activity,[167] and contractions are not a direct venom action on the muscle fiber, so acetylcholine appears to have been released from the presynaptic terminals.[58] Muscle fasciculations were apparently caused by abnormal repetitive firing of motor neurons. It was hypothesized that the venom changes the membrane's electrical field, activating sodium channels without altering the transmembrane potential or damaging the neuronal membrane ultrastructurally.[47,74,164]

Presentation

Humans bitten by the Sydney funnel-web spider complain of intense pain at the bite site. This is probably from direct trauma and low venom pH (4.5). *Atrax* venom does not provoke cutaneous necrosis. Wiener studied the cutaneous effects of the venom on himself by injecting 0.5 mg intradermally. Local pain and a wheal surrounded by erythema lasted for 30 minutes, followed by localized sweating and piloerection. No systemic effects occurred.

Systemic envenomation by male *Atrax* spiders causes a severe, rapidly progressive neuromotor syndrome that, untreated, may lead to death within 2 hours of the bite. Monkeys, which have a pattern of envenomation similar to that of humans, provide a model in which Sutherland has described a biphasic clinical syndrome.[171,178]

Phase I begins minutes after venom injection, with local piloerection and muscle fasciculation. This extends proximally, becoming generalized over the next 10 to 20 minutes. After another 5 minutes, severe hypertension, tachycardia, hyperthermia, and coma with increased intracranial pressure may occur. These are followed by diaphoresis, salivation, lacrimation, diarrhea, sporadic apnea, borborygmi, and grotesque muscle writhing. Death may occur at this point from asphyxia resulting from laryngeal spasm combined with copious respiratory secretions, apnea, or pulmonary edema. Laboratory evaluation reveals metabolic acidosis and elevated plasma creatine phosphokinase.

Phase II begins 1 to 2 hours after envenomation, as the phase I symptoms subside. There may be return of consciousness and appearance of recovery. In severe cases, hypotension gradually worsens over 1 to 2 hours, with periods of apnea. Pulmonary edema and death may occur despite ventilatory support.

Thirteen fatalities from *A. robustus* envenomation have been recorded since 1927. Children are particularly susceptible; those under 12 years may die within 4 hours of the bite.[54,81,175] Before the development of specific antivenom in 1980, severe envenomations resulted in a minimum 8-

hour critical period, followed by a 9- to 21-day hospital course.[53,175,178]

Treatment

A number of pharmacologic interventions have been attempted to reverse the clinical syndrome of envenomation. Survival was not improved in mice treated with antihistamines, adrenocorticotropic hormone, atropine, or mephenesin. Gallamine blocked hyperthermia and fasciculations in monkeys but did not alter the cardiovascular response. Diazepam, atropine, and furosemide were found to increase survival in monkeys, but this may not be the case in humans.[52,74,184] Other than antivenom, no consistently effective agent has been found to enhance survival.

Prehospital first aid has been modeled in *Macaca fascicularis* monkeys. Noting that a significant amount of venom moves centrally by the lymphatics, studies were conducted to evaluate methods to retard the movement of venom. In conscious monkeys, application of a crepe bandage and immobilization of the bitten extremity (termed the pressure immobilization technique) delayed the movement of subcutaneously injected radioactive iodine.[180] An occlusion cuff proximal to the bite inflated to 35 mm Hg delayed venom flow in anesthetized monkeys.[171] A monkey had crepe bandages and a splint applied to the envenomed limb 5 minutes after injection with a lethal dose (2 mg) of venom. It remained free of any systemic signs or symptoms until the bandage was removed 90 minutes later, at which time it developed the full syndrome of envenomation.[180] These data led to the first aid recommendations described below, which should reduce both superficial capillary and lymphatic flow, postponing most systemic manifestations during transport.

Immediate treatment after a bite consists of four steps: wrap the length of the bitten extremity with an elastic bandage, splint to immobilize the extremity, immobilize the victim, and transport to the nearest hospital with the bandage in place.[129,176,180] A human case report has illustrated the utility of this method, with occurrence, disappearance, recurrence, and reresolution of symptoms coinciding with compression wrap removal and replacement in a man bitten by a male *A. robustus*.[71]

Specific antivenom is the mainstay of treatment for *Atrax* envenomation. The antivenom is a purified IgG product produced by immunizing rabbits with a combination of male *Atrax* venom and Freund's adjuvant. The antivenom was demonstrated to neutralize *Atrax* venom in vitro and to reverse symptoms in monkeys before its introduction for human use in 1981.

If a tourniquet or bandage is in place when the patient presents, it should be removed in an intensive care setting, with careful observation for development or progression of symptoms. If systemic signs or symptoms occur, patients are commonly pretreated with antihistamine. Two ampules of antivenom (100 mg of purified IgG per ampule) are then administered intravenously every 15 minutes until symptoms improve. During a 10-year period the antivenom was given to at least 40 patients, with no reported adverse effects of the antivenom and no deaths reported.[178]

General management in addition to antivenom administration is symptomatic and supportive. Oxygen, mechanical ventilation if indicated, and intravenous fluid support may be needed in severe cases. Atropine 0.6 mg may be used to lessen salivation and bronchorrhea. β-Blockers may be indicated for severe hypertension and tachycardia.

Banana Spiders (Armed Spiders)

PHONEUTRIA SPECIES OF SOUTH AMERICA

The *Phoneutria* spiders of South America are large nocturnal creatures notorious for their aggressive behavior and painful bite. Humans bitten by *Phoneutria* species may experience pain, profound systemic symptoms, and occasionally death from respiratory paralysis within 2 to 6 hours. A polyvalent antivenom effective against *Phoneutria* and *Loxosceles* venoms is available from the Instituto Butantan in São Paulo, Brazil.

The best known representative of this genus is *P. nigriventer*. It is known in Brazil as *aranha armadeira,* meaning "spider that assumes an armed display," because of its characteristic defensive-aggressive display. Other names include wandering spider and banana spider.[154]

Banana Spiders

P. nigriventer is the largest, most aggressive true spider found in South America, with an average body length of 35 mm, leg length of 45 to 60 mm, and fangs 4 to 5 mm in length for females. Males are slightly smaller.[153] The body is gray to brown-gray with white marks forming a longitudinal band on the dorsal abdomen. The eyes are in three rows of two, four, and two, the last two being the largest. A distinguishing characteristic is the red-brown brush of hairs around the chelicerae. *P. nigriventer* is mainly found in southern Brazil, Argentina, and Uruguay. Other species have been found in Bolivia and Colombia. The spiders do not construct a web, since they are nocturnal hunters, often traveling several hundred meters in search of prey. They may enter houses during this time, hiding in clothes in the light of day. According to Bucherl,[25] 600 to 800 spider bites occur each year around the city of São Paulo alone.

Phoneutria Venom

Phoneutria venom is a complex mixture of histamine, serotonin, glutamic acid, aspartic asid, lysine, hyaluronidase, and other polypeptides. Histamine, serotonin, and incompletely characterized kallikrein-kinin activating fractions contribute to local tissue swelling from the increased vascular permeability that may occur with envenomation.[3] In addition, the venom contains at least six neurotoxic polypeptides, with molecular weights between 3500 and 8500.[41]

The neurotoxic components are sodium channel poisons that appear to potentiate action potentials along axons, provoking erratic or rapid uncontrolled muscle twitches in invertebrates[49] as well as vertebrates.[4,102] Microscopically, it causes acute transient swelling of axons, particularly at the nodes of Ranvier, in a pattern similar to that caused by the venoms of scorpions *Centruroides exilicauda* and *Leiurus quinquestriatus.* The axons recover within a few hours of exposure, but return of nodal width to normal takes several days.[102]

The effects of the venom have been studied in mice, rats, guinea pigs, rabbits, pigeons, and dogs. The venom has little or no effect on frogs and snakes, and it has four times greater toxicity in dogs than in mice. Rats and rabbits are very resistant to the venom's effects. Dogs developed intense pain, manifested by yelping, followed by sneezing, lacrimation, mydriasis, hypersalivation, erection, ejaculation, and death after 200 μg/kg of venom was injected subcutaneously.[154] This is well within the dose that a single spider may inject. Electrical stimulation yields an average of 1.6 to 3.2 mg venom per spider.[25]

Presentation

Phoneutria nigriventer venom acts on both the peripheral and central nervous systems.[78] Humans bitten by *P. nigriventer* immediately develop severe local pain that radiates up the extremity into the trunk, followed within 10 to 20 minutes by tachycardia, hypertension, hypothermia, profuse diaphoresis, salivation, vertigo, visual disturbances, nausea and vomiting, priapism, and occasionally death in 2 to 6 hours. Respiratory paralysis is generally the cause of death. Priapism is predominantly observed in boys less than 10 years old with severe envenomation. Fatalities may occur in the debilitated or the young, but most people recover in 24 to 48 hours. Workers who handle bananas are frequently bitten because the spider hides in bunches of bananas. Bites have been reported in Switzerland and Argentina in produce workers inadvertently encountering these traveling spiders.[78,153,154]

Treatment

A polyvalent antivenom (Sero Antiaracidico Polivalente, Instituto Butantan) active against *Phoneutria* and *Loxosceles* species is available in Brazil. Skin testing and antihistamine prophylaxis are recommended before its use. One to five ampules of antivenom are injected intramuscularly and intravenously, and clinical response is judged by the relief of pain or resolution of priapism. Milder envenomations are treated symptomatically by infiltrating the bite site with local anesthesia or by achieving peripheral vasodilation with warm water. Opiates may potentiate the venom's effects on respiration and should generally not be used.[78,153,154]

Wolf Spiders

LYCOSA SPECIES

The family Lycosidae includes hunting spiders, many of which are wandering predators. They are found from beaches to grassy fields and pastures. At one time it was believed that they hunted in packs, hence the Greek name *lycosa* (wolf).[39,204]

The family includes various middle-sized to large spiders with mildly cytotoxic venom capable of provoking transient inflammation in humans. The most famous wolf spider species is *Lycosa tarentula,* to which the term "tarantula" was first applied. Its bite was once believed to cause tarantism, a syndrome of stupor, the desire to dance, and sometimes death, but this historical syndrome is now attributed to *Latrodectus tridecimguttatus,* and the wolf spider bite is now known to cause little more than stinging pain. The South American *Lycosa raptoria* has been reputed to be more dangerous than other wolf spiders, provoking necrosis at the site of envenomation. It now appears likely that this, too, was based on a misunderstanding. Necrotic arachnidism in South America is now attributed mainly to *Loxosceles* species. Treatment is symptomatic.

Wolf Spiders

Wolf spiders are diurnal predators with strong front legs and stout chelicerae used to hold and crush prey. They may be moderately large, with body length 3 to 35 mm. Eight eyes are distinctively arranged in three rows of four, two, and two. Four small eyes are located on the lower part of the cephalothorax, looking forward and to the sides. Two very large eyes sit above these, pointing forward, followed by two large ones that look upward. The spiders can see for several feet in four directions simultaneously. Color is usually a mottled dark gray or brown. In general, the spiders do not spin webs.

Lycoside Venom

Lycoside venom is thought to be primarily cytotoxic, without hemolytic or anticoagulant activity.[204] Although there have been few, if any, scientific reports of necrosis after envenomation by the Australian wolf spider *L. godeffroyi,* occasional reports in the popular press have suggested that bites may lead to necrosis. Atkinson and Wright have demonstrated that the raw venom of *L. godeffroyi* causes a strong inflammatory response and cutaneous necrosis when injected into mice.[8] They further hypothesize that this action may be the result of contamination of the venom with digestive juices, since electrically collected raw venom caused necrosis, whereas venom gland extract did not.[9]

Presentation

A series of 515 cases of confirmed *Lycosa* bites in Brazil showed that most bites occur between the hours of 6 AM and 6 PM, at a fairly consistent rate year round. The most common bite sites were feet (40%) and hands (39%). The most common signs and symptoms were all local, with pain in 83%, swelling in 19%, and erythema in 14%. No local necrosis was described.[144]

In the United States five cases of Lycosidae bites have been documented, with one resulting in skin necrosis at the bite site.[31] This was probably from the combined results of envenomation and infection.

Treatment

Although South American antivenom active against *Lycosa* venom was available in the past, it was only rarely used (1 case out of 515 reviewed by Ribeiro[144]). Since 1985 the polyvalent Butantan Institute spider antivenom has not included the anti-lycosid fraction.[103] Most *Lycosa* cases can be managed with tetanus immunization and ice or oral analgesics; occasionally, local anesthetic block has been used for pain management.[144]

Tarantulas

APHONOPELMA AND OTHERS

The term "tarantula" was first applied to *Lycosa tarentula,* a species of European spider actually belonging to the wolf spider family. There are more than 1500 tarantula species, with approximately 40 species in the United States. In the United States, the term "tarantula" usually refers to the large spiders of the Orthognatha (Mygalomorphae) suborder, which does not include the wolf spiders.

Tarantulas tend to be large, slow, long-lived spiders capable of inflicting a painful bite when threatened. Although most genera inflict a bite no more dramatic than most Hymenoptera stings, a few can cause more severe pain and swelling, numbness, or lymphangitis. Several Latin American varieties possess urticating hairs, which they may flick by the thousands through the air into an attacker's skin and eyes; these cause intense inflammation, which may remain pruritic for weeks.

Tarantulas

Bird spiders, funnel-web spiders, and trapdoor spiders all belong to the Orthognatha suborder and are often called tarantulas. Their average body length is around 2 to 3 cm. *Grammostola mollicoma* is the largest tarantula known, with a body length of 7 to 10 cm and leg spread of 21 to 27 cm.[26,65] Tarantulas may live for 1 to 25 years. As a group, they are found mainly in tropical and subtropical areas. They are distinguished by two pairs of book lungs and a vertical alignment of the chelicerae with the body.

Tarantula Venom

Except for funnel-web spider venom, which has been detailed separately, few tarantula venoms have been studied systematically. In the United States, *Dugesiella henzi* and members of the genus *Aphonopelma* have venom containing hyaluronidase, nucleotides (adenosine triphosphate [ATP]), and polyamines (principally spermine).[30,36,100,151,152] The role for the polyamines is unclear, hyaluronidase is postulated to be a spreading factor, and ATP potentiates the major effects of the venom on mice. Both venoms cause rapid, irreversible necrosis of skeletal muscle when injected intraperitoneally into mice.[131] *Dugesiella* venom was found to have a necrotoxin with several similarities to sea snake venoms.[100] *Aphonopelma* venom resembles scorpion *(Centruroides exilicauda)* venom in composition and biologic effect.[100]

Presentation

Several species of tarantula have been implicated as causes of human illness, including the previously detailed funnel-web spiders of genera *Atrax, Hadronyche,* and *Trechona,* as well as genera *Sericopelma* of Panama, *Pterinochilus* of Africa, *Bothriocyrtum* of the southwestern United States, *Ummidia* of the eastern United States, *Aphonopelma* of Mexico and the United States, *Pamphobeteus* of South America, and *Avicularia* of the southwest United States. With the exception of the first three, however, envenomation usually resembles a bee or wasp sting, occasionally followed by some redness and swelling and usually without necrosis or serious sequelae.*

Four genera of tarantulas *(Lasiodora, Grammastola, Acanthoscurria,* and *Brachypelma)* possess urticating hairs irritative to skin and mucous membranes. These genera are located throughout the Western Hemisphere, with many species indigenous to the United States. When one of these spiders is threatened, it rubs its hind legs across the dorsal surface of its abdomen and flicks thousands of hairs toward the aggressor. In humans, these barbed hairs can penetrate the skin, causing edematous, pruritic papules. The itching may persist for weeks. There are four morphologic types of urticating hairs. Tarantulas within the United States possess only type I hairs, which do not penetrate the skin as deeply as type III hairs. Type III hairs can penetrate up to 2 mm into human skin; this is the type of hair most likely to cause inflammation. They are commonly found on Mexican, Caribbean, and Central and South American species. Type II hairs are incorporated into the silk web retreat but are not thrown off by the spider. Type IV hairs, which belong to the South American spider *Grammastola,* are able to cause inflammation of the respiratory tract in small mammals. Rats and mice have been reported to die of asphyxia within 2 hours after exposure to the hairs.[20,40,204]

Treatment

Except for funnel-web envenomations, described earlier, tarantula bite management is purely symptomatic. Elevation and immobilization of the extremity and oral analgesics may help reduce pain. Topical or systemic corticosteroids and oral antihistamines can be used for urticating hair exposure. All bites should receive local

*References 26, 30, 36, 65, 97, 151.

wound care; the victims require appropriate prophylaxis against tetanus.

Hobo Spiders

TEGENARIA AGRESTIS

The hobo spider, also called the Northwestern brown spider *(Tegenaria agrestis),* has recently been implicated in several cases of necrotic arachnidism similar to that seen in *Loxosceles* envenomation. Systemic effects reported include headache, visual disturbances, hallucinations, weakness, and lethargy. Hemorrhagic complications have been reported in experimental animals. Since relatively little experience with this bite has been documented, treatment is uncertain. It has been suggested that these be treated in a similar fashion to *Loxosceles* envenomations.

Hobo Spiders

The hobo spider is a 10 to 15 mm, nondescript brown spider originally from Europe and first noted in the northwestern United States in 1936. By the mid-1960s it had become established in Washington, Oregon, and Idaho.[189]

Tegenaria Agrestis Venom

Experimental envenomation of rabbits by live male spiders resulted in extensive cutaneous injury and clear evidence of systemic poisoning. Local erythema appeared and faded within the first day; discolored patches were visible by day 4 and sloughed by day 6. Autopsy revealed petechial hemorrhages on the surfaces of the lungs, liver, and kidneys.[188]

Presentation

According to Vest, who studied 22 cases of "highly probable" *T. agrestis* envenomation, the local lesion follows a pattern reminiscent of that with loxoscelism. The initial lesion appeared as a small reddened induration, often with a large zone of erythema around it. Vesicles occurred within 36 hours, then burst; marked necrosis developed in 50% of cases. The most common symptoms included headache, weakness, and lethargy.

Treatment

No studies of treatment have been published for envenomation by *Tegenaria* species. As with mild cases of loxoscelism, these patients should be treated supportively, with tetanus prophylaxis, careful wound debridement as needed, and observation.

Running Spiders and Sac Spiders

CHIRACANTHIUM SPECIES

Spiders belonging to the genus *Chiracanthium* have had a documented history of human envenomation since the eighteenth century. *Chiracanthium* species are found worldwide and known for their tenacious, painful bite. A pruritic, erythematous wheal appears within 30 minutes. Nausea, abdominal cramps, headache, and local necrosis have been reported.

Chiracanthium Spiders

The genus *Chiracanthium* as a whole has no distinctive marks or patterns.[69,204] Members may be pale yellow, brown, green, or olive (Color Plate 52). The dorsal abdomen may have a median longitudinal stripe. Body size ranges from 7 to 15 mm, with a total diameter of 3 cm, including long, slender legs.

In the United States, *C. inclusum* is the only indigenous species. *C. diversum* is widely found in the Pacific islands. It was transported into Hawaii from Australia approximately 45 years ago. *C. mildei* was introduced from Europe and is now found from New England to Alabama and Utah. It is a common biting spider in Boston; it is most abundant in autumn, when most bites occur.[165]

The South African sac spider *C. lawrencei* is a common nocturnal house spider that forages at night and may become trapped in bedding.[126] During the day these spiders hide in the concavities of leaves, curtains, or windowsills, encased in a silk sac. They are fast-moving and aggressive when threatened.[124]

Chiracanthium Venom

Limited research has been carried out on *Chiracanthium* venom. Seventy-five percent of guinea pigs bitten by *C. mildei* for the first time developed a wheal within 5 minutes, with 60% developing an eschar within 1 day.[165] Fractionation of dissected venom gland extracts from *C. japonicum* resulted in five fractions with lethal activity in mice. These were considered neurotoxic based on symptoms of dyspnea, flaccid paralysis, and death after intraperitoneal injection.[130]

Presentation

In 1901, Kobert described local swelling, erythema, pain, and fever after the author's third *C. punctorium* envenomation.[21] Maretic[112,113] has seen local redness, pain, and edema, but never necrosis after *C. punctorium* envenomation. *C. inclusum* caused local pain that radiated from the forearm bite site up the arm, associated with nausea. No other signs developed.[21]

The Australian species *C. mordax* and *C. longimanus* caused local swelling, erythema, and pain associated with malaise, headache, dizziness, and nausea. Symptoms receded within 36 hours after treatment with antihistamines and local anesthetics.[21] Ori[130] found similar signs and symptoms after envenomation by *C. japonicum.*

In South Africa, most *C. lawrencei* bites occur at night during sleep.[126] Paired bite marks 6 mm apart are evident within the first few hours. Local edema and erythema may be slight. By the third day the marks may become necrotic, with more edema, erythema, and pain; headache and fever may accompany this stage. Seven to 10 days after the bite the small ulcer begins to heal.[125]

Treatment

The lesion usually heals without problems provided secondary infections are avoided. Treatment consists of cool compresses, elevation, immobilization, analgesics, and tetanus prophylaxis.

Other Spiders

A number of other spiders have been implicated in medically notable bites (Color Plate 53). A short description of each is presented in the following paragraphs. Treatment, unless otherwise noted, is symptomatic and may include elevation and immobilization, cool compresses, analgesics, antihistamines, tetanus prophylaxis, and antibiotics as needed for signs of infection.

Argiope aurantia, known as the golden orb weaver or black and yellow garden spider, is common in California, Oregon, and the eastern United States. Other species in this genus are found throughout the United States, the Orient, and Australia.[65] It is a large, brightly colored spider with a large, symmetric orb web and a leg spread of up to 7.5 cm. Bites may cause local pain and erythema.[69] Bites by a related species, *A. argentata,* cause local pain, erythema, and vesicle formation, which resolve within 24 hours except for the bite marks.[69,204] Although the venom appears to be cytotoxic in vivo, research indicates the venom has neurotoxic effects in vitro. Venom gland extracts from *A. trifasicata* are postsynaptic blockers of neuromuscular transmission at locust glutamate receptors.[187]

Badumna insignis (Ixeuticus robustus), a common window spider in Australia, caused local pain, itching, and swelling followed by regional lymph node tenderness and discoloration of the area around the bite. Over the following 2 weeks, the lesion resolved with some tissue necrosis and sloughing centrally.[105]

Harpactirella lightfooti, the baboon spider or bobbejaan-spinnekop, is a megalomorph spider found in South Africa. Body length is 3 cm; the cephalothorax is brown with a yellowish border. Although no fatalities have been reported, localized pain followed by several bouts of emesis, weakness, and collapse has been noted after envenomation.[26,78,123]

Herpyllus ecclesiasticus, the parson spider, lives widely throughout the United States under rocks and rubbish and in houses. One case report described pruritus, arthralgia, malaise, and nausea beginning 1 hour after the bite. There was no necrosis.[106,204]

Lampona cylindrata, the white-tailed spider, was identified as the spider involved in eight cases in Australia. Symptoms included a mild stinging sensation followed by 1 to 10 days of itching, redness, and swelling. In one case a small blister was present for a few hours, and in no case was there necrosis. The authors suspected that most *L. cylindrata* bites may be benign, despite earlier reports of ulceration after suspected *L. cylindrata* envenomations.[201] Gray[73] reported a case of more significant illness, with nausea, lethargy, and a small zone of necrosis after a known white-tailed spider bite.

Palystes natalius, the lizard-eating spider, is one of the largest true spiders in South Africa. It has a brownish-gray body with bright yellow and black striped legs. The female is larger than the male, with body length up to 4 cm. Only localized burning accompanied by slight swelling was noted after a female spider bite to the left wrist.[123,128]

Peucetia viridans, the green lynx spider of the United States and Mexico, is a diurnal hunting spider whose bite results in a burning sensation, pruritus, erythema, and induration. *P. viridans* is translucent green, with red eyes and joints.[79]

Phidippus spiders, such as the jumping spider of the United States, can cause pain, erythema, pruritus, and sometimes minor ulceration. The swelling usually subsides within 2 days.[147]

Sicarius species, or six-eyed crab spiders, are occasionally implicated in human bites in South Africa. They tend to bite only when provoked and are rarely implicated in human poisonings despite fairly high toxicity of the venom in laboratory animals. Envenomation reportedly can cause edema, erythema, and necrosis, occasionally associated with disseminated intravascular coagulation. Care is supportive.[124-126]

Steatoda paykulliana of Europe and *S. grossa,* the false black widow of the United States, bear an external resemblance to the black widow. In humans, *S. nobilis* of southern England has caused brief local pain and slight swelling, followed by local sweating and piloerection, facial flushing, and feverishness.[193]

Supunna picta, a common leaf litter–dwelling spider of Australia, caused a transient erythematous rash and slight itch in a woman bitten at home. The lesion resolved uneventfully.[24]

Trachelas volutus and several other species of the *Trachelas* genus have been reported to cause mild local reactions without necrosis. These spiders are commonly encountered in houses in late summer and fall. Bites are painful initially and may swell. No systemic effects have been reported.[132,186]

REFERENCES

1. Alario A et al: Cutaneous necrosis following a spider bite: a case report and review, *Pediatrics* 79:618, 1987.
2. Anderson PC: Loxoscelism threatening pregnancy: five cases, *Am J Obstet Gynecol* 165:1454, 1991.
3. Antunes E et al: *Phoneutria nigriventer* (armed spider) venom induces increased vascular permeability in rat and rabbit skin in vivo, *Toxicon* 30:1011, 1992.

4. Araújo DAM et al: Effects of a toxic fraction, $PhTx_2$, from the spider *Phoneutria nigriventer* on the sodium current, *Arch Pharmacol* 347:205, 1993.
5. Arnold RE: Brown recluse spider bites: five cases with a review of the literature, *JACEP* 5:262, 1976.
6. Atkins JA et al: Necrotic arachnidism, *Am J Trop Med Hyg* 7:165, 1958.
7. Atkins JA, Wingo CW, Sodeman WA: Probable cause of necrotic spider bite in the Midwest, *Science* 126:73, 1957.
8. Atkinson RK, Wright LG: A study of the necrotic actions of the venom of the wolf spider, *Lycosa godeffroyi,* on mouse skin, *Comp Biochem Physiol* 95C:319, 1990.
9. Atkinson RK, Wright LG: Studies of the necrotic actions of the venoms of several Australian spiders, *Comp Biochem Physiol* 98C:441, 1991.
10. Auer AI, Hershey FB: Surgery for necrotic bites of the brown spider, *Arch Surg* 108:612, 1974.
11. Babcock JL et al: Systemic effect in mice of venom apparatus extract and toxin from the brown recluse spider *(Loxosceles reclusa), Toxicon* 19:463, 1981.
12. Banner W: Bites and stings in the pediatric patient, *Curr Probl Pediatr* 8:69, 1988.
13. Barbaro KC et al: Dermonecrotic and lethal components of *Loxosceles gaucho* spider venom, *Toxicon* 30:331, 1992.
14. Barrett SM et al: Passive hemagglutination inhibition test for diagnosis of brown recluse spider bite envenomation, poster presentation at the Society for Academic Emergency Medicine, San Diego, Calif, May 23, 1989.
15. Barron WE: Spider bites, *J Med Assoc Ga* 49:511, 1980.
16. Benavides MI, Moncada X: Tratamiento de loxocelismo cutaneo con dapsona, *Rev Med Chile* 118:1247, 1990.
17. Berger RS: A critical look at therapy for the brown recluse spider bite, *Arch Dermatol* 107:298, 1973.
18. Berger RS: The unremarkable brown recluse spider bite, *JAMA* 225:109, 1973.
19. Berger RS, Millikan LE, Conway F: An in vitro test for *Loxosceles reclusa* spider bite, *Toxicon* 11:465, 1973.
20. Bettini S: Epidemiology of latrodectism, *Toxicon* 2:93, 1964.
21. Bettini S, Brignoli PM: Review of the spider families, with notes on the lesser known poisonous forms. In Bettini S, editor: *Arthropod venoms, handbook of experimental pharmacology,* vol 48, Berlin, 1978, Springer-Verlag.
22. Bettini S, Maroli M: Venoms of Theridiidae, genus *Latrodectus.* In Bettini S, editor: *Arthropod venoms, handbook of experimental pharmacology,* vol 48, Berlin, 1978, Springer-Verlag.
23. Binder LS: Acute arthropod envenomation: incidence, clinical features and management, *Med Toxicol Adverse Drug Exp* 4:163, 1989.
24. Boyle CF: Spider bite by a female *Supunna picta, Med J Aust* 153:239, 1990.
25. Bucherl W: Biology and venoms of the most important South American spiders of the genera *Phoneutria, Loxosceles, Lycosa,* and *Latrodectus, Am Zool* 9:157, 1969.
26. Bucherl W: Spiders. In Bucherl W, Buckley EE, editors: *Venomous animals and their venoms,* New York, 1971, Academic Press.
27. Butz WC: Envenomation by the brown recluse spider (Aranae, Scytodidae) and related species: a public health problem in the United States, *Clin Toxicol* 4:515, 1971.
28. Butz WC, Stacy LD, Heryford NN: Arachnidism in rabbits: necrotic lesions due to the brown recluse spider, *Arch Pathol* 91:97, 1971.
29. Byrne GC, Pemberton PJ: Red-back spider *(Latrodectus mactans hasselti)* envenomation in a neonate, *Med J Aust* 2:665, 1983.
30. Cabbiness SG et al: Polyamines in some tarantula venoms, *Toxicon* 18:681, 1980.
31. Campbell DS, Rees RS, King LE: Wolf spider bites, *Cutis* 39:113, 1987.
32. Carroll PR, Morgans D: The effect of the venom of the Sydney funnel web spider *(Atrax robustus)* on isolated human intercostal muscles, *Toxicon* 14:487, 1976.
33. Carroll PR, Morgans D: Responses of the rabbit atria to the venom of the Sydney funnel-web spider *(Atrax robustus), Toxicon* 16:489, 1978.
34. Caveness WA: Insect bite, complicated with fever, *Nash J Med Surg* 10:333, 1872.
35. Ceccarelli B, et al: Freeze-fracture studies of frog neuromuscular junctions during intense release of neurotransmitter. I. Effects of black widow spider venom and Ca^{2+}-free solutions on the structure of the active zone, *J Cell Biol* 81:163, 1979.
36. Chan TK et al: Adenosine triphosphate in tarantula spider venoms and its synergistic effect with the venom toxin, *Toxicon* 13:61, 1975.
37. Clark RF et al: Clinical presentation and treatment of black widow spider envenomation: a review of 163 cases, *Ann Emerg Med* 21(7):782, 1992.
38. Clyne D: *A guide to Australian spiders,* Australia, 1969, Thomas Nelson.
39. Comstock JH: *The spider book,* New York, 1912, Doubleday, Page.
40. Cooke JAL, Miller FJ, Grover RW: Urticaria caused by tarantula hairs, *Am J Trop Med Hyg* 22:130, 1973.
41. Cordeiro MdoN et al: Purification and amino acid sequences of six TX3 type neurotoxins from the venom of the Brazilian "armed" spider *Phoneutria nigriventer* (Keys), *Toxicon* 31:35, 1993.
42. DeLozier JB et al: Brown recluse spider bites of the upper extremity, *South Med J* 81(2):181, 1988.
43. Denny WF, Dillaha CJ, Morgan PN: Hemotoxic effect of *Loxosceles reclusa* venom: in vivo and in vitro studies, *J Lab Clin Med* 64:291, 1964.
44. Dillaha CJ et al: The gangrenous bite of the brown spider in Arkansas, *J Arkansas Med Soc* 60:91, 1963.
45. Dillaha CJ et al: North American loxoscelism—necrotic bite of the brown recluse spider, *JAMA* 188:153, 1964.
46. Duffey PH, Limbacher HP: Brown spider bites in Arizona, *Ariz Med* 28:89, 1971.
47. Duncan AW, Tibballs J, Sutherland SK: Effects of Sydney funnel-web spider envenomation in monkeys, and their clinical implications, *Med J Aust* 2:429, 1980.
48. Eichner ER: Spider bite hemolytic anemia: positive Coombs' test, erythrophagocytosis, and leukoerythroblastic smear, *Am J Clin Pathol* 81(5):683, 1984.
49. Entwistle ID et al: Isolation of a pure toxic polypeptide from the venom of the spider *Phoneutria nigriventer* and its neurophysiological activity on an insect femur preparation, *Toxicon* 20:1059, 1982.
50. Fardon DW et al: The treatment of brown spider bite, *Plast Reconst Surg* 40(5):482, 1967.
51. Finkelstein A, Rubin LL, Tzeng MC: Black widow spider venom: effect of purified toxin on lipid bilayer membranes, *Science* 193:1009, 1976.
52. Fisher M, Carr GA: *Atrax robustus* envenomation, *Med J Aust* 2:643, 1972.
53. Fisher M et al: *Atrax robustus* envenomation, *Anaesth Intens Care* 8:410, 1980.
54. Fisher M et al: Funnel-web spider *(Atrax robustus)* antivenom, *Med J Aust* 2:525, 1981.
55. Frontali N, Grasso A: Separation of three toxicologically different protein components from venom of the spider *Latrodectus tredecimguttatus, Arch Biochem Biophys* 106:213, 1964.
56. Frontali N et al: Purification from black widow spider venom of a protein factor causing the depletion of synaptic vesicles at neuromuscular junctions, *J Cell Biol* 68:462, 1976.
57. Futrell JM: Loxoscelism, *Am J Med Sci* 304:261, 1992.
58. Gage PW, Spence I: The origin of the muscle fasciculation caused by funnel-web spider venom, *AJEBAK* 55:453, 1977.

59. Gala S, Katelaris CH: Rhabdomyolysis due to redback spider envenomation, *Med J Aust* 157:66, 1992.
60. Garnet JR, editor: *Venomous Australian animals dangerous to man,* Melbourne, 1968, Commonwealth Serum Laboratory.
61. Gates CA, Rees RS: Serum amyloid P component: its role in platelet activation stimulated by sphingomyelinase D purified from venom of the brown recluse spider *(Loxosceles reclusa), Toxicon* 28:1303, 1990.
62. Gebel HM, Campbell BJ, Barrett JT: Chemotactic activity of venom from the brown recluse spider *(Loxosceles reclusa), Toxicon* 17:55, 1979.
63. Gendron BP: *Loxosceles reclusa* envenomation, *Am J Emerg Med* 8:51, 1990.
64. Geren CR et al: Isolation and characterization of toxins from brown recluse spider venom *(Loxosceles reclusa), Arch Biochem Biophys* 174:90, 1976.
65. Gertsch WJ: *American spiders,* ed 2, New York, 1979, Van Nostrand Reinhold.
66. Ginsburg CM, Weinberg AG: Hemolytic anemia and multiorgan failure associated with localized cutaneous lesion, *J Pediatr* 112:496, 1988.
67. Ginsburg HM: Black widow spider bite, *Calif West Med* 46(6):381, 1937.
68. Gonzalez C et al: Insuficiencia renal aguda en loxocelismo cutaneovisceral: 11 casos, *Rev Med Chile* 114:1155, 1986.
69. Gorham JR, Rheney TB: Envenomation by the spiders *Chiracanthium inclusum* and *Argiope aurantia:* observations on arachnidism in the United States, *JAMA* 296:158, 1968.
70. Gotten HB, MacGowan JJ: Blackwater fever (hemoglobinuria) caused by spider bite, *JAMA* 114:1547, 1940.
71. Grant SJB, Loxton EH: Effectiveness of a compression bandage and antivenene for Sydney funnel-web spider envenomation, *Med J Aust* 156:510, 1992.
72. Grasso A, Mastrogiacomo A: Alpha-latrotoxin: preparation and effects on calcium fluxes, *FEMS Microbiol Immunol* 105:131, 1992.
73. Gray M: A significant illness that was produced by the white-tailed spider, *Lampona cylindrata, Med J Aust* 151:114, 1989.
74. Gray MR, Sutherland SK: Venoms of the Dipluridae. In Bettini S, editor: *Arthropod venoms, handbook of experimental pharmacology,* vol 48, Berlin, 1978, Springer-Verlag.
75. Gray RR: Getting to know funnel-webs, *Aust Nat Hist* 20:256, 1981.
76. Gregson RP, Spence I: Isolation and characterization of a protein neurotoxin from the venom glands of the funnel-web spider *(Atrax robustus), Comp Biochem Physiol* 74:125, 1983.
77. Gross AS et al: Persistent segmental cutaneous anesthesia after a brown recluse bite, *South Med J* 83(11):1321, 1990.
78. Habermehl GG: *Venomous animals and their toxins,* Berlin, 1981, Springer-Verlag.
79. Hall RE, Madon MB: Envenomation by the green lynx spider, *Peucetia viridans* (Hentz, 1932), in Orange County, California, *Toxicon* 11:197, 1973.
80. Harriss JB: Toxic constituents of animal venoms and poisons. 2. Spiders, scorpions, marine animals, nonvenomous animals, reactions to antivenoms, *Adverse Drug React Acute Poisoning Rev* 1:143, 1982.
81. Hartman LJ, Sutherland SK: Funnel-web spider *(Atrax robustus)* antivenom in the treatment of human envenomation, *Med J Aust* 141:796, 1984.
82. Heitz JR, Norment BR: Characteristics of an alkaline phosphatase activity in brown recluse venom, *Toxicon* 12:181, 1974.
83. Herman TE, McAlister WH: Epiglottic enlargement: two unusual causes, *Pediatr Radiol* 21:139, 1991.
84. Hershey FB, Aulenbacher CE: Surgical treatment of brown spider bites, *Ann Surg* 170:300, 1969.
85. Hollabaugh RS, Fernandes ET: Management of the brown recluse spider bite, *J Pediatr Surg* 24(1):126, 1989.
86. Horen WP: Arachnidism in the United States, *JAMA* 185:839, 1963.
87. Horner NV, Steward KW: Life history of the brown spider, *Loxosceles reclusa, Tex J Sci* 19:333, 1967.
88. Hufford DC, Morgan PH: C-reactive protein as a mediator in the lysis of human erythrocytes sensitized by brown recluse spider venom, *Proc Soc Exp Biol Med* 167:493, 1981.
89. Ingber A et al: Morbidity of brown recluse spider bites: clinical picture, treatment and prognosis, *Acta Derm Venereol (Stockh)* 71:337, 1991.
90. Ingram WW, Musgrave A: Spider bite (arachnidism): a survey of its occurrence in Australia with case histories, *Med J Aust* 2:10, 1933.
91. Jansen GT et al: The brown recluse spider bite: controlled evaluation of treatment using the white rabbit as an animal model, *South Med J* 64(10):1194, 1971.
92. Jong Y-S, Norment BR, Heitz JR: Separation and characterization of venom components in *Loxosceles reclusa.* III. Hydrolytic enzyme activity, *Toxicon* 17:539, 1979.
93. Kaston BJ: Is the black widow spider invading New England? *Science* 119, 1954.
94. Kemp DR: Inappropriate diagnosis of necrotizing arachnidism: watch out Miss Muffet but don't get paranoid, *Med J Aust* 152:669, 1990.
95. King LE, Rees RS: Brown recluse spider bites: stay cool, *JAMA* 254:2895, 1986.
96. King LE, Rees RS: Dapsone treatment of a brown recluse bite, *JAMA* 250:648, 1983.
97. Kunkel DB: Arthropod envenomations, *Emerg Med Clin North Am* 2:579, 1984.
98. Kurpiewski G et al: Platelet aggregation and sphingomyelinase D activity of purified toxin from the venom of *Loxosceles reclusa, Biochem Biophys Acta* 678:467, 1981.
99. LaGrange MAC: Pulmonary oedema from a widow spider bite (letter), *South Afr Med J* 77:110, 1990.
100. Lee CK et al: The purification and characterization of a necrotoxin from tarantula, *Arch Biochem Biophys* 164:341, 1974.
101. Lessenden CM Jr, Zimmer LK: Brown spider bites: a survey of the current problem, *J Kans Med Soc* 61:379, 1960.
102. Love S, Cruz-Hölfling MA: Acute swelling of nodes of Ranvier caused by venoms which slow inactivation of sodium channels, *Neuropathol (Berl)* 70:1, 1986.
103. Lucas S: Spiders in Brazil, *Toxicon* 26:759, 1988.
104. Mack RB: The bite of the spider woman, *NC Med J* 53(5):200, 1992.
105. Macmillan DL: Envenomation by a widow spider, *Med J Aust* 150:163, 1989.
106. Majeski JA, Durst GG: Bite by the spider *Herpyllus ecclesiasticus* in South Carolina, *Toxicon* 13:377, 1975.
107. Majeski JA, Durst GG: Necrotic arachnidism, *South Med J* 69:887, 1976.
108. Mara JE, Myers BS: Brown spider bites: treatment with hydrocortisone, *Rocky Mt Med J* 74:257, 1977.
109. Maragoni RA et al: Activation by *Phoneutria nigriventer* (armed spider) venom of tissue kallikrein-kininogen-kinin system in rabbit skin in vivo, *Br J Pharmacol* 109:539, 1993.
110. Maragoni S et al: Biochemical characterization of a vascular smooth muscle contracting polypeptide purified from *Phoneutria nigriventer* (armed spider) venom, *Toxicon* 31:377, 1993.
111. Maran B: Pathologic reactions associated with bite of *Latrodectus tredecimguttatus, Arch Pathol (Chicago)* 59:727, 1955.
112. Maretic Z: Epidemiology of envenomation, symptomatology, pathology and treatment. In Bettini S: *Arthropod venoms,* New York, 1978, Springer-Verlag.
113. Maretic Z: Some clinical and epidemiological problems of venom poisoning today, *Toxicon* 20:345, 1982.
114. Maretic Z: Latrodectism: variations in clinical manifestations provoked by *Latrodectus* species of spiders, *Toxicon* 21(4):457, 1983.
115. Maretic Z, Lebez D: *Araneism with special reference to Europe,* Belgrade, 1979, Nolit.

116. Misler S, Falke L: Dependence on multivalent cations of quantal release of transmitter induced by black widow spider venom, *Am J Physiol* 253:C469, 1987.
117. Morgans D, Carroll PR: A direct acting adrenergic component of the venom of the Sydney funnel-web spider, *Atrax robustus, Toxicon* 14:185, 1976.
118. Morgans D, Carroll PR: The responses of the isolated human temporal artery to the venom of the Sydney funnel-web spider *(Atrax robustus), Toxicon* 15:277, 1977.
119. Müller GJ: Black and brown spider bites in South Africa, *South Afr Med J* 83:399, 1993.
120. Mylecharane EJ et al: Actions of robustoxin, a neurotoxic polypeptide from the venom of the male funnel-web spider *(Atrax robustus),* in anaesthetized monkeys, *Toxicon* 27:481, 1989.
121. Nance WE: Hemolytic anemia of necrotic arachnidism, *Am J Med* 31:801, 1961.
122. Newlands G: A revision of the spider genus *Loxosceles* Heinecken & Lowe, 1835 (Araneae: Scytodidae) in southern Africa with notes on the natural history and morphology, *J Ent Soc S Afr* 38(2):141, 1975.
123. Newlands G: Review of the medically important spiders in southern Africa, *S Afr Med J* 49:823, 1975.
124. Newlands G, Atkinson P: Review of southern African spiders of medical importance, with notes on the signs and symptoms of envenomation, *SAMT* 73:235, 1988.
125. Newlands G, Atkinson P: A key for the clinical diagnosis of araneism in Africa south of the equator, *S Afr Med J* 77:96, 1990.
126. Newlands G, Atkinson P: Behavioural and epidemiological considerations pertaining to necrotic araneism in southern Africa, *S Afr Med J* 77:92, 1990.
127. Newlands G, Isaacson C, Martindale C: Loxoscelism in the Transvaal, South Africa, *Trans R Soc Trop Med Hyg* 76(5), 1982.
128. Newlands G, Martindale CB: Wandering spider bite—much ado about nothing, *S Afr Med J* 60:142, 1981.
129. Noel V: Funnel-web antivenom, *Med J Aust* 142:328, 1985.
130. Ori M: Envenomation of *Chiracanthium japonicum* and the properties of the spider venom (proceedings), *Jpn J Med Sci Biol* 31:200, 1978.
131. Ownby CL, Odell GV: Pathogenesis of skeletal muscle necrosis induced by tarantula venom, *Exp Mol Pathol* 38:283, 1983.
132. Pase HA, Jennings DT: Bite by the spider *Trachelas volutus* Gertsch (Araneae, Clubionidae), *Toxicon* 16:96, 1978.
133. Peters W: *Zoology of the arthropods: a colour atlas of arthropods in clinical medicine,* London, 1992, Wolfe.
134. Presley TE: A case of spider bite, *Memphis Med Monthly* 16:520, 1896.
135. Prince GE: Arachnidism in children, *J Pediatr* 49:101, 1956.
136. Rand RP et al: Pyoderma gangrenosum and progressive cutaneous ulceration, *Ann Plastic Surg* 20:280, 1988.
137. Rees RS, Fields JP, King LE Jr: Do brown recluse spider bites induce pyoderma gangrenosum? *South Med J* 78(3):283, 1985.
138. Rees RS, O'Leary JP, King LE: The pathogenesis of systemic loxoscelism following brown recluse spider bites, *J Surg Res* 35:1, 1983.
139. Rees R et al: Management of the brown recluse spider bite, *Plast Reconstr Surg* 68(5):768, 1981.
140. Rees RS et al: Interaction of brown recluse spider venom on cell membranes: the inciting mechanism? *J Investig Derm* 83:270, 1984.
141. Rees RS et al: Brown recluse spider bites: a comparison of early surgical excision versus dapsone and delayed surgical excision, *Ann Surg* 202(5):659, 1985.
142. Rees R et al: The diagnosis and treatment of brown recluse spider bites, *Ann Emerg Med* 16:9, 1987.
143. Rees RS et al: Plasma components are required for platelet activation by the toxin of *Loxosceles reclusa, Toxicon* 26:1035, 1988.
144. Ribeiro LA et al: Wolf spider bites in São Paulo, Brazil: a clinical and epidemiological study of 515 cases, *Toxicon* 28:715, 1990.
145. Rosenthal L, Meldolesi: Alpha-latrotoxin and related toxins, *Pharmacol Ther* 42:114, 1989.
146. Russell FE: Muscle relaxants in black widow spider *(Lactrodectus mactans)* poisoning, *Am J Med Sci* 243:81, 1962.
147. Russell FE: Bite of the spider *Phidippus formossus:* case history, *Toxicon* 8:193, 1970.
148. Russell FE: Venomous arthropods. In Schachner LA, Hansen R, editors: *Pediatric dermatology,* New York, 1988, Churchill Livingstone.
149. Russell FE, Marcus P, Streng JA: Black widow spider envenomation during pregnancy: report of a case, *Toxicon* 7:188, 1979.
150. Russell FE, Waldron WG, Madon MB: Bites by the brown spiders *Loxosceles unicolor* and *Loxosceles arizonica* in California and Arizona, *Toxicon* 7:109, 1969.
151. Schanbacher FL et al: Composition and properties of tarantula, *Dugesiella hentzi* (Girard) venom, *Toxicon* 11:21, 1973.
152. Schanbacher FL et al: Purification and characterization of tarantula, *Dugesiella hentzi* (Girard) venom hyaluronidase, *Comp Biochem Physiol* 44:389, 1973.
153. Schenberg S, Lima FA: *Phoneutria nigriventer* venom—pharmacology and biochemistry of its components. In Bucherl W, Buckley EE, editors: *Venomous animals and their venoms,* vol 3, New York, 1971, Academic Press.
154. Schenberg S, Pereira Lima FA: Venoms of Ctendiae. In Bettini S, editor: *Arthropod venoms, handbook of experimental pharmacology,* vol 48, Berlin, 1978, Springer-Verlag.
155. Schenone H, et al: Prevalence of *Loxosceles laeta* in houses in central Chile, *Am J Trop Med Hyg* 19(3):564, 1970.
156. Schenone H, Letonja T, Knierim F: Algunos datos sobre el aparato venenoso de Loxosceles laeta y toxicidad de su veneno sobre diversas especies animales, *Bol Chile Parasit* 30:37, 1975.
157. Schenone H, Suarez G: Venoms of scytodidae: genus *Loxosceles.* In Bettini S: *Arthropod venoms, handbook of experimental pharmacology,* ed 48, Berlin, 1978, Springer-Verlag.
158. Schmaus LF: Case of arachnidism (spider bite), *JAMA* 92:1265, 1929.
159. Sheumack DD et al: A comparative study of properties and toxic constituents of funnel-web spider *(Atrax)* venoms, *Comp Biochem Physiol* 78:55, 1984.
160. Sheumack DD, et al: Complete amino acid sequence of a new type of lethal neurotoxin from the venom of the funnel-web spider, *Atrax robustus, FEBS Lett* 181:154, 1985.
161. Sheumack DD et al: An endogenous antitoxin to the lethal venom of the funnel web spider *Atrax robustus* in rabbit sera, *Comp Biochem Physiol* 99C:157, 1991.
162. Sheumack DD et al: Protection of monkeys against the lethal effects of male funnel-web spider *(Atrax robustus)* venom by immunization with a toxoid, *Toxicon* 29:603, 1991.
163. Smith CW, Micks DW: The role of polymorphonuclear leukocytes in the lesion caused by the venom of the brown spider, *Loxosceles reclusa, Lab Invest* 22:90, 1976.
164. Spence I, Adams DJ, Gage PW: Funnel web spider venom produces spontaneous action potentials in nerve, *Life Sci* 20:243, 1977.
165. Spielman A, Levi HW: Probable envenomation by *Chiracanthium mildei:* a spider found in houses, *Am J Trop Med Hyg* 19:729, 1970.
166. Strain GM et al: Hyperbaric oxygen effects on brown recluse spider *(Loxosceles reclusa)* envenomation in rabbits, *Toxicon* 29(8):989, 1991.
167. Sutherland SK: The Sydney funnel-web spider *(Atrax robustus).* 1. A review of published studies on the crude venom, *Med J Aust* 2:528, 1972.
168. Sutherland SK: The Sydney funnel-web spider *(Atrax robustus).* 2. Fractionation of the female venom into five distinct components, *Med J Aust* 2:643, 1972.
169. Sutherland SK: The Sydney funnel-web spider *(Atrax robustus).* 3. A review of some clinical records of human envenomation, *Med J Aust* 2:643, 1972.
170. Sutherland SK: Venomous Australian creatures: the action of their toxins and the care of the envenomated patient, *Anaesth Intensive Care* 2:316, 1974.

171. Sutherland SK: Primum non nocere and the Sydney funnel-web spider, *Med J Aust* 2:105, 1978.
172. Sutherland SK: Antivenom to the venom of the male Sydney funnel-web spider *Atrax robustus:* preliminary report, *Med J Aust* 2:437, 1980.
173. Sutherland SK: The management of bites by the Sydney funnel-web spider, *Atrax robustus, Med J Aust* 1:148, 1978.
174. Sutherland SK: *Australian animal toxins,* Melbourne, 1980, Oxford University Press.
175. Sutherland SK: *Venomous creatures of Australia: a field guide with notes on first aid,* London, 1981, Oxford University Press.
176. Sutherland SK: Sydney funnel web spider bite, *Aust Fam Physician* 14:316, 1985.
177. Sutherland SK: Inappropriate diagnosis of necrotising arachnidism (letter), *Med J Aust* 153:499, 1990.
178. Sutherland SK: Treatment of arachnid poisoning in Australia, *Aust Fam Phys* 19:47, 1990.
179. Sutherland SK, Duncan AW, Tibballs J: Local inactivation of funnel-web spider *(Atrax robustus)* venom by first-aid measures: potentially lifesaving part of treatment, *Med J Aust* 2:435, 1980.
180. Sutherland SK, Tibballs J, Duncan AW: Funnel-web spider spider *(Atrax robustus)* antivenom. 1. Preparation and laboratory testing, *Med J Aust* 2:522, 1981.
181. Sutherland SK, Trinca JC: Survey of 2144 cases of red-back spider bites, *Med J Aust* 2:620, 1978.
182. Svendsen FJ: Treatment of clinically diagnosed brown recluse spider bites with hyperbaric oxygen: a clinical observation, *J Ark Med Soc* 83:199, 1986.
183. Taylor EH, Denny WF: Hemolysis, renal failure and death, presumed secondary to the bite of brown recluse spider, *South Med J* 59:1209, 1966.
184. Torda TA, Loong E, Greaves T: Severe lung oedema and fatal consumptive coagulopathy after funnel-web bite, *Med J Aust* 2:147, 1980.
185. Truett AP III, King LE: Sphingomyelinase D: a pathogenic agent produced by bacteria and arthropods, *Adv Lipid Res* 26:275, 1993.
186. Uetz GW: Envenomation by the spider *Trachelas tranquillas* (Hentz), *J Med Entomol* 10:227, 1973.
187. Usherwood PNR, Duce IR, Boden P: Slowly reversible block of glutamate receptor channels by venoms of the spider, *Argiope trifasciata* and *Araneus gemma, J Physiol (Paris)* 79:241, 1984.
188. Vest DK: Envenomation by *Tegenaria agrestis* (Walckenaer) spiders in rabbits, *Toxicon* 25:221, 1987.
189. Vest DK: Necrotic arachnidism in the northwest United States and its probable relationship to *Tegenaria agrestis* (Walckenaer) spiders, *Toxicon* 25:175, 1987.
190. Visser LH, Khusi SN: Pulmonary oedema from a widow spider bite, *S Afr Med J* 75:338, 1989.
191. Vorse H et al: Disseminated intravascular coagulopathy following fatal brown spider bite (necrotic arachnidism), *J Pediatr* 80:1035, 1972.
192. Waldron WG, Madon MB, Suddarth T: Observations on the occurrence and ecology of *Loxosceles laeta* (Araneae: Scytodidae) in Los Angeles County, California, *California Vector Views* 22(4):29, 1975.
193. Warrell DA et al: Neurotoxic envenoming by an immigrant spider *(Steatoda nobilis)* in southern England, *Toxicon* 29:1263, 1991.
194. Wasserman GS, Anderson PC: Loxoscelism and necrotic arachnidism, *J Toxicol Clin Toxicol* 21:451, 1983.
195. Wiener S: The Sydney funnel-web spider *(Atrax robustus).* I. Collection of venom and its toxicity in animals, *Med J Aust* 2:377, 1957.
196. Wiener S: The Sydney funnel-web spider *(Atrax robustus).* II. Venom yield and other characteristics of spider in captivity, *Med J Aust* 2:269, 1959.
197. Wiener S: Observations on the venom of the Sydney funnel-web spider *(Atrax robustus), Med J Aust* 2:293, 1961.
198. Wiener S: Red back spider bite in Australia: an analysis of 167 cases, *Med J Aust* 6:44, 1961.
199. Wiener S: Primum non nocere and the Sydney funnel-web spider, *Med J Aust* 2:104, 1978.
200. Wesley RE et al: Dapsone in the treatment of presumed brown recluse spider bite of the eyelid, *Ophthalmic Surg* 16(2):116, 1985.
201. White J, Hirst D, Hender E: 36 cases of bites by spiders, including the white-tailed spider, *Lampona cylindrata, Med J Aust* 150:401, 1989.
202. Wille RC, Morrow JD: Case report: dapsone hypersensitivity syndrome associated with treatment of the bite of a brown recluse spider, *Am J Med Sci* 296(4):270, 1988.
203. Wilson H: Acute abdominal symptoms in arachnidism, *Surgery* 13:924, 1943.
204. Wong RC, Hughes SE, Voorhees JJ: Spider bites, *Arch Dermatol* 123:98, 1987.
205. Wright RP et al: Hyaluronidase and esterase activities of the venom of the poisonous brown recluse spider, *Arch Biochem Biophys* 149:415, 1973.

33 TICK-BORNE DISEASES

Douglas A. Gentile

- Tick envenomation
- Tick paralysis
- Ticks as vectors
  - *Borrelia* infections
  - Tick-borne rickettsial diseases
  - Tick-borne viral diseases
  - Babesiosis
- Prevention and prophylaxis

Ticks are familiar pests to those who frequent wilderness or rural areas. They inhabit forests, marshes, deserts, steppes, mountains, and high meadows and have few natural enemies. Most feed on an extremely wide range of hosts, including humans. Ticks are most noted for their high nuisance potential, but they are also efficient vectors for a large number of zoonoses. In fact, ticks transmit a greater variety of infectious agents than any other group of arthropods and run a close second to mosquitoes as vectors of human disease worldwide.[86] In the United States, ticks outrank even mosquitoes as vectors, and tick-borne illnesses constitute an important infectious disease problem, particularly in wilderness and other outdoor recreational areas.

Ticks belong to the class Arachnida, which also includes spiders and scorpions, and they are closely related to mites. Taxonomists divide ticks into two major families: Ixodidae (hard ticks) and Argasidae (soft ticks). Argasid ticks are covered with a leathery integument, and the capitulum (head) is subterminal and not visible from above. Ixodid ticks possess a hard, shieldlike scutum, which covers the entire dorsal surface in males but only the anteromedial portion in females (Fig. 33-1). The head of ixodid ticks is anterior and visible from above.

Hard ticks have three feeding stages: larva, nymph, and adult. If molting through all stages occurs on the same host, the tick is referred to as a one-host tick. Most Ixodidae are three-host ticks, with each stage feeding on a different host. Hard ticks feed on mammals, reptiles, and birds, and virtually all feed slowly over the course of days. Most take a single adult blood meal, and engorgement with blood is a prerequisite to egg laying. Females may ingest over 50 times their body weight in blood and other fluids.

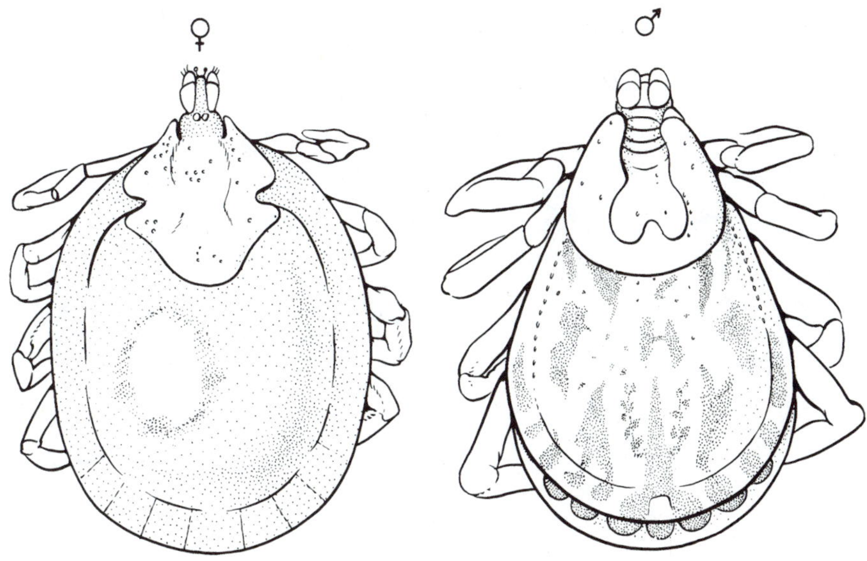

Fig. 33-1 *Dermacentor andersoni,* the tick that causes Rocky Mountain spotted fever, demonstrating the difference in appearance between males and females.

All the major tick-borne diseases in North America are transmitted by ixodid ticks, with the exception of relapsing fever.

A typical ixodid life cycle is illustrated by *Dermacentor andersoni,* a major vector for Rocky Mountain spotted fever. The tick hatches as a six-legged larva and actively attaches to a small mammal, often a rodent. After feeding for 3 to 5 days, it drops off and molts to the eight-legged nymph. The nymph hibernates in soil, becoming active again in the spring. After feeding for 4 to 9 days on a larger animal, it again drops off and undergoes a second molt to the adult stage. The mature tick attaches to a third host on which mating may occur. *D. andersoni,* like many ticks, is capable of surviving for extended periods (over a year in adults) without a blood meal.

While ixodid ticks are wide ranging, most argasids are nidicolous, or nest loving. Nymph and adult Argasidae generally inhabit the host lair, hiding in cracks and crevices when not feeding. They usually have several nymphal stages (instars), with each stage taking a blood meal. Adults may take several blood meals, feeding rapidly over the course of hours when the host returns.

While some ticks are host specific, most are opportunists feeding on a variety of hosts. Appendages on the capitulum, the chelicerae (Fig. 33-2), function as piercing and tearing structures, enabling the entire capitulum to be inserted into the host's integument. Retrose teeth on the chelicerae help anchor the tick to the host; many ixodid species also secrete a cementlike substance that seals the wound and further secures the attached tick. Salivary glands secrete an anticoagulant, allowing the host's blood to be easily ingested.

Tick Envenomation

Ticks cause human disease either by transmitting microorganisms or by secreting toxins or venoms. The nature of most tick toxins is poorly understood. Many appear to be secreted by the tick salivary glands. Some stimulate potent host immune responses; others appear to have direct tissue toxicity. Clinical effects range from localized reactions to anaphylaxis, paralysis, and death.[11]

Local reactions vary from formation of a small pruritic nodule to development of extensive areas of ulceration, erythema, and induration. Lesions may be accompanied by

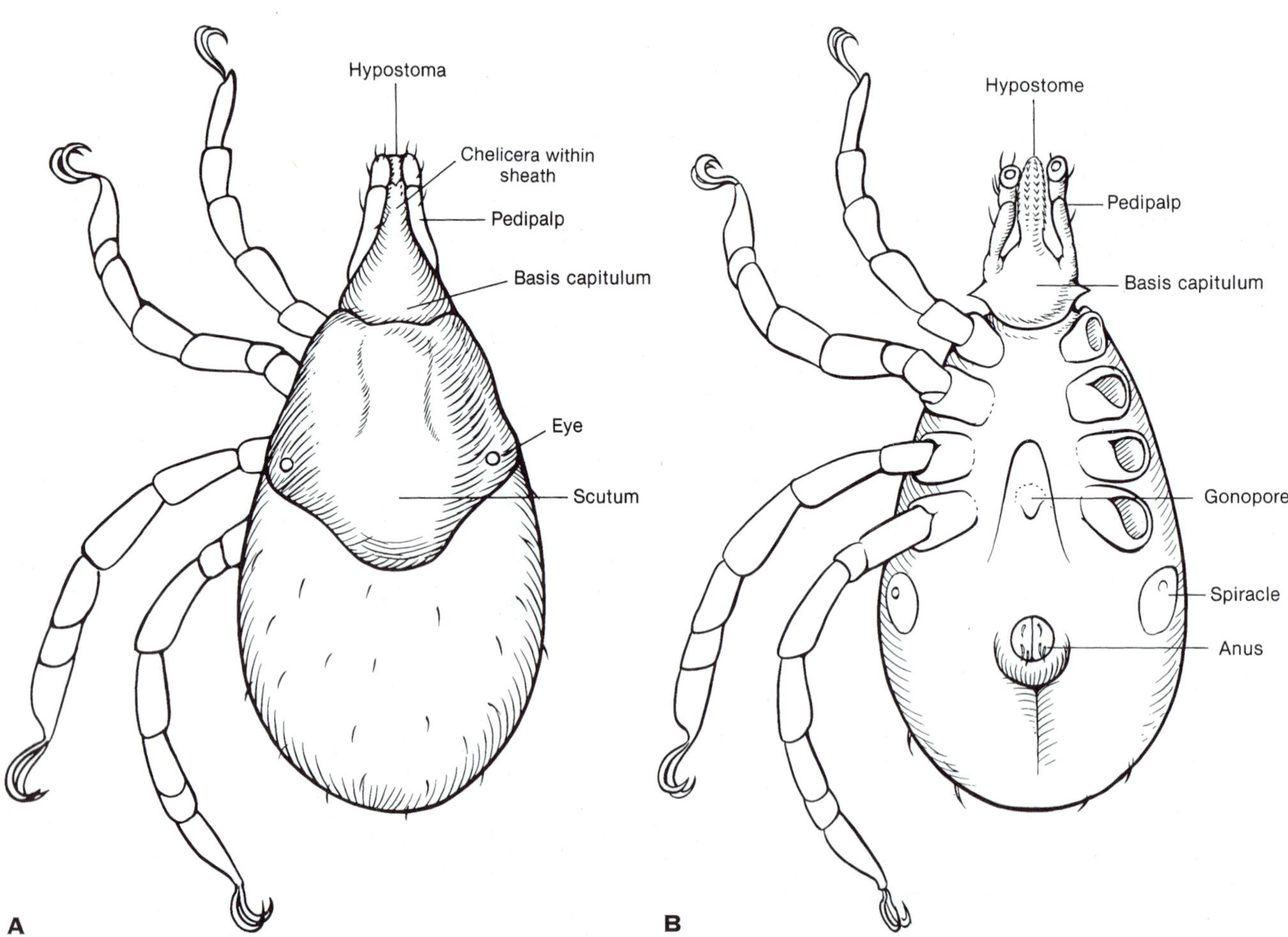

Fig. 33-2 **A,** Dorsal aspect of tick, to show anatomic features. **B,** Ventral surface of tick, to show anatomic features.

fever, chills, and malaise unrelated to infection. The severity of the reaction varies with both host susceptibility and tick species. A granuloma histologically resembling a lymphoma may develop at the site of a tick bite as long as 6 weeks after the tick is removed.[73] The lesion is believed to be caused by a salivary toxin. Treatment is surgical excision.

Pajaroello Tick Bites

According to local folklore of southern California and Mexico, the bite of the pajaroello tick *Ornithodoros coriaceus* is more feared than the bite of a rattlesnake. In fact, pajaroello bites usually result in a 10 to 30 mm erythematous papule with minimal associated pain and itching. The papule gradually resolves over the subsequent 3 to 4 weeks. Severe local and systemic reactions have been reported but are rare and probably occur in persons sensitized by previous bites. Local erythema, pain, and edema develop rapidly, followed by tissue necrosis and ulceration. Fever, chills, rigors, and hypotension occur rarely. Severe reactions are probably caused by sensitization to a salivary toxin.[54,67]

Treatment of pajaroello bites includes wound disinfection and administration of tetanus toxoid. The rare severe allergic reaction may require epinephrine, antihistamines, and corticosteroids. When tissue necrosis occurs, consideration should be given to excision and primary closure.

Tick Paralysis

As early as 1912, Todd[215] recognized that paralysis occurred in humans and animals following the bite of certain species of ticks. Tick paralysis has been observed only sporadically in humans since that time but has on occasion constituted a serious veterinary problem.[139] Although uncommon, familiarity with the clinical features of the disease is important, since prompt diagnosis and removal of the tick are curative.

Tick paralysis has been reported worldwide, but most human cases occur in North America and Australia.[182,230] Forty-three species of ticks, both Ixodidae and Argasidae, have been reported to cause tick paralysis.[34] Human cases in North America are usually caused by *Dermacentor andersoni* or less commonly *D. variabilis,* although *Amblyomma americanum* (Color Plate 54), *A. maculatum,* and *Ixodes scapularis* have also been incriminated.[79] The Pacific Northwest and Rocky Mountain areas account for most of the cases. In Australia, *Ixodes holocyclus* is primarily associated with the disease, although *I. cornuatus* has been implicated.[214]

Tick paralysis occurs during the spring and summer months when ticks are feeding. Children are affected more commonly than adults, and girls twice as often as boys, probably because ticks on the female scalp are hidden in longer hair.[1] Men account for most of the adult cases, presumably because of increased occupational and recreational exposure to tick habitats.

Tick paralysis in humans develops 5 to 6 days after an adult female tick attaches (male ticks do not cause paralysis). Initially, the patient may be restless, irritable, and complain of paresthesias in the hands and feet. Over the ensuing 24 to 48 hours, an ascending, symmetric, and flaccid paralysis develops with loss of deep tendon reflexes. Weakness usually is initially greater in the lower extremities; within 1 to 2 days, severe generalized weakness may develop, accompanied by bulbar and respiratory paralysis. Some patients develop cerebellar dysfunction with incoordination and ataxia.[1,79] Facial paralysis as an isolated finding has occurred in patients with ticks embedded behind the ear.[1,138] In uncomplicated cases, fever and chills are absent and the white blood cell count and cerebrospinal fluid (CSF) analyses remain normal.

Resolution of paralysis when the tick is removed establishes the diagnosis. Laboratory aids to diagnosis are not available. In North America, recovery after removal of the tick is quite rapid, with most patients showing improvement within hours and complete resolution within several days. Undiagnosed, however, tick paralysis may be fatal; mortality in children was 12% in a large Canadian series.[169]

Australian tick paralysis differs from North American in several aspects. Patients often appear more acutely ill, and paralysis may continue to progress for 48 hours after tick removal.[11,138] Recovery may be prolonged.

A venom secreted from the tick salivary glands during a blood meal causes the paralysis. The mechanism of action of the venom is not completely understood, but it appears to produce a conduction block in the peripheral branches of motor fibers resulting in failure of acetylcholine release at the neuromuscular junction.[79,132] Electrophysiologic measurements in humans consistently demonstrate motor conduction slowing and reduction in muscle action potential amplitude.[47,129,210] A central effect of the toxin has been postulated to explain the cerebellar dysfunction observed in some patients.

Aside from removal of the tick, treatment is supportive. Tick antivenom from hyperimmunized dogs has been developed for Australian tick paralysis and may be beneficial in patients with severe disease.[138] The most important aspect of treatment is to consider tick paralysis in any patient with ascending paralysis. Once considered, it is a simple matter to search for and remove the concealed tick.

Ticks as Vectors

Ticks transmit a wide variety of infectious agents, all of which cause zoonoses. Ticks may act either as amplifiers or as reservoirs for a given agent.[87] In the agent-tick *amplifier* system, the reservoir for the agent is a vertebrate. An immature tick ingests the microorganism while feeding on an infected vertebrate or while feeding concurrently on a vertebrate host with an infected tick. The pathogen replicates in the tick and is passed transstadially, from larval to nymphal to adult stage. The maturing tick transmits the agent to other vertebrate hosts when it feeds. A key epidemiologic feature of this system, transstadial survival of microorganisms, is common in argasid and ixodid ticks but rare in hematophagous insects. This important difference is primarily due to the relatively insignificant anatomic changes that occur in the tick during molting.[87]

In the agent-tick *reservoir* system, the microorganism is passed transovarially from one generation of ticks to the next. The agent replicates within the tick and depends solely on the tick population for survival. The agent may also replicate within the vertebrate host of the tick, allowing amplification of the cycle, thereby increasing the density and prevalence of the microorganism.

The major tick-borne diseases occurring in the United States are listed in Table 33-1. Lyme disease, babesiosis, and ehrlichiosis have only recently been recognized in this country. Lyme disease and babesiosis constitute important infectious disease problems in endemic areas, and Lyme disease is now the most common tick-borne illness in the United States and throughout the world. Tularemia and Rocky Mountain spotted fever are observed throughout the United States and continue to produce significant morbidity and mortality. Tick-borne relapsing fever and Colorado tick fever occur in the western states and are particularly likely to affect campers, hikers, hunters, and others who frequent wilderness areas.

BORRELIA INFECTIONS

Borreliae are bacteria belonging to the order Spirochaetales, which also includes the treponemes and leptospires. *Borrelia* species can be stained with aniline dyes, including routine blood stains (such as Wright and Giemsa); this feature allows easy differentiation from the other two genera.[178] They are helical, actively motile spirochetes, usually 10 to 20 μm long, with 3 to 10 spirals.[59] Strains cannot be differentiated on the basis of morphology but are classified according to specificity of the tick-spirochete relationship, the range of animals susceptible to infection, and cross-immunity.[14]

Table 33-1 Major Tick-Borne Diseases in the United States

Disease	Organism	Major Vectors
Lyme disease	*Borrelia burgdorferi*	*Ixodes scapularis, I. pacificus*
Rocky Mountain spotted fever	*Rickettsia rickettsii*	*Dermacentor andersoni, D. variabilis*
Relapsing fever	*Borrelia hermsii, B. turicatae, B. parkeri*	*Ornithodoros hermsi, O. turicata, O. parkeri*
Colorado tick fever	Orbivirus	*Dermacentor andersoni*
Ehrlichiosis	*Ehrlichia chaffeensis*	*Ixodes scapularis? Amblyomma americanum?*
Babesiosis	*Babesia microti*	*Ixodes scapularis*
Tularemia	*Francisella tularensis*	*Amblyomma americanum*

Human *Borrelia* infections occur worldwide, with the possible exception of parts of the southwestern Pacific.[59] All are transmitted by hematophagous arthropods. *Borrelia recurrentis* causes an epidemic form of relapsing fever that is transmitted by the human body louse *Pediculus humanus*. A group of closely related *Borrelia* species causes tick-borne or endemic relapsing fever. A third borrelial disease was recognized in 1982 with the identification of *B. burgdorferi* as the etiologic agent of Lyme disease.

Lyme Disease

An epidemic form of oligoarticular arthritis, originally diagnosed as juvenile rheumatoid arthritis, was recognized in 1975 in the area around Lyme, Connecticut.[198] However, subsequent clinical observations revealed a complex, multisystem disorder with dermatologic, cardiac, and neurologic complications. The disorder was termed Lyme disease.

The rural setting in which most cases occurred, the close geographic and temporal clustering of cases, and the clinical response to penicillin suggested an arthropod-borne infection. The presence of a distinctive erythematous skin lesion, erythema migrans, preceding the arthritis pointed to a tick vector.[190] Erythema migrans had been observed in Europe since 1910, where it was associated with the bite of the sheep tick *Ixodes ricinus*.[4]

Epidemiologic evidence implicated the deer tick *Ixodes scapularis (dammini)* as the likely vector of Lyme disease. In 1982 the spirochete *Borrelia burgdorferi* was isolated from the midgut of *I. scapularis* ticks collected from a known endemic focus of Lyme disease,[28] and patients with Lyme disease were soon shown to have antibodies to *B. burgdorferi*. Isolation of *B. burgdorferi* from the blood, cerebrospinal fluid, and skin lesions of affected patients subsequently confirmed the spirochetal etiology of Lyme disease.[18,194]

Epidemiology. The overall frequency of Lyme disease is unknown. In 1992, 45 states reported a provisional total of 9677 cases, accounting for more than 90% of all reported vector-borne illnesses in the United States. Over 90% of cases were acquired in the 19 states in which established enzootic cycles of *B. burgdorferi* exist (Box 33-1).[37] The ages of patients range from 1 to 81 years (median 34 years), and the male/female ratio is nearly 1:10. Eighty percent of cases occur during the period from May to August, with peak incidence in July.

The principal vectors of Lyme disease are several closely related ticks of the genus *Ixodes*. The deer tick *I. scapularis (dammini)* is the best documented vector; its geo-

BOX 33-1

REPORTED CASES OF LYME DISEASE IN STATES WITH ESTABLISHED ENZOOTIC FOCI, 1992

New York	3370
Connecticut	1760
Pennsylvania	1119
New Jersey	681
Wisconsin	525
Rhode Island	274
California	231
Delaware	218
Massachusetts	212
Minnesota	201
Maryland	183
Virginia	123
North Carolina	65
Illinois	41
Michigan	35
Florida	24
Georgia	23
Oregon	13
Maine	1

graphic distribution correlates with endemic foci of Lyme disease in the northeastern and midwestern United States.[170,195,223] The range of *I. scapularis* extends from the northeastern United States to the southeastern states. The northern form of *I. scapularis* was originally thought to be a separate species and was named *Ixodes dammini*. However, recent studies have demonstrated mating compatibility and genetic similarity, and the two forms are now considered to be the same species.[14] The southern form of *I. scapularis* appears to be responsible for Lyme disease cases in the southeast United States.[27,142]

Northern *I. scapularis* larvae, abundant in late summer and fall, and nymphs, numerous in spring and summer, are aggressive and parasitize a number of vertebrate species.[27] The preferred host is the deer mouse *Peromyscus leucopus,* which serves as an important reservoir for *B. burgdorferi.*[21,180,185] Transovarial transmission in ticks occurs but appears to be unusual.[24] Adult *I. scapularis* ticks, abundant in spring and fall, have a narrow host range, feeding primarily on deer, which are key hosts in the life cycle of the tick. The high incidence of Lyme disease in the northeastern United States has been linked to increases in the deer population.[202,232] In some focal endemic areas, up to 60% of *I. scapularis* ticks are infected with *B. burgdorferi,* and tick populations may be high even on well-kept lawns.[55]

Spirochetal development in most ticks is limited to the midgut, but the organisms disseminate during feeding and appear in saliva, providing the likely mechanism for disease transmission.[21,153] This phenomenon also explains the relationship between duration of tick feeding and *B. burgdorferi* transmission. In one study, nymphal *Ixodes scapularis* transmitted *Borrelia burgdorferi* to 1 of 14 rodents exposed for 24 hours, 5 of 14 rodents exposed for 48 hours, and 13 of 14 rodents exposed for 72 hours.[141] While all three stages of the tick may bite humans, the nymph is primarily responsible for transmission of Lyme disease.[195] The small size of nymphs accounts for the fact that only about 30% of patients with Lyme disease recall a tick bite.

A third endemic focus in the United States has been identified on the West Coast (California and Oregon), where the vector is the western black-legged tick *Ixodes pacificus,* another member of the *I. ricinus* complex. The zoonotic transmission cycle for *I. pacificus* differs from *I. scapularis,* as evidenced by the fact that only 1.5% of *I. pacificus* surveyed in northern California and southwestern Oregon are infected with *B. burgdorferi,*[29] a fraction too small to maintain an animal reservoir. In addition, the major hosts for immature *I. pacificus* are species of lizards, which are not competent hosts for *B. burgdorferi.*[100] Instead, the enzootic cycle is maintained by a second tick, *Ixodes neotomae*, which does not bite humans.[13] Up to 15% of *I. neotomae* ticks are infected with *B. burgdorferi,* which is enough to maintain endemic disease. The primary host for *I. neotomae* is *Neotoma fuscipes,* the dusky-footed woodrat, which is a competent reservoir for *B. burgdorferi.*[23] Larval *I. pacificus* ticks will feed on a variety of vertebrates, and become infected when they feed on *N. fuscipes*. Transmission to humans may then occur from an infected nymph or adult.

Cases of Lyme disease in states outside the range of *I. scapularis* and *I. pacificus* suggest that additional vectors are involved. Ticks from five genera *(Amblyomma, Dermacentor, Haemaphysalis, Ixodes, Rhipicephalus)* and other arthropods, such as mosquitoes, horseflies, and deerflies, have been found naturally infected with *B. burgdorferi,* but only members of the *I. ricinus* complex appear to be competent vectors for the disease.[97,109,131,142]

Lyme disease or similar syndromes also occur in Europe, Asia, and Australia. Garin and Bajadoux[68] in France recognized as early as 1922 that neurologic abnormalities occasionally followed erythema migrans. This symptom complex has been described variously as Bannwarth's syndrome, tick-borne meningopolyneuritis, and meningopolyneuritis.[68] The neurologic features of the syndrome include intense radicular pains, chronic lymphocytic meningitis, and involvement of the peripheral nervous system, particularly facial palsies. The full description of Lyme disease in the United States has led to the recognition of other erythema migrans–associated manifestations (arthritis and cardiac symptoms) in Europe,[70,161,225] and patients with European erythema migrans–associated diseases (arthritis, carditis, and meningoradiculitis) demonstrate raised antibody titers against *B. burgdorferi.*[92,161,167,206]

The established vector for European erythema migrans, *I. ricinus,* is closely related to the common vectors for Lyme disease in the United States, *I. scapularis* and *I. pacificus,* and the major reservoirs in Europe are species of rodents.[117] *B. burgdorferi* isolated from *I. ricinus* shows minor differences from United States strains in morphology, outer surface proteins, plasmids, and DNA homology.[2,160,187]

Lyme disease cases have also been reported from China, Japan, and Russia, where the principal vector is *Ixodes persulcatus,* and from Australia in the Hunter Valley[205] and along the New South Wales coast.[118] No ticks of the *I. ricinus* complex have been found in Australia, suggesting that other vectors are likely to be identified.

Clinical Manifestations. Lyme disease is multisystemic and multiphasic. It can be divided into three stages, each with different clinical manifestations. The disorder usually begins as a localized infection with erythema migrans and associated symptoms (stage I). Within days to weeks, spirochetes may disseminate via blood or lymph, and neurologic, cardiac, or joint abnormalities may develop (stage II). Finally, chronic, persistent infection (stage III) of the joints, nervous system, skin, or eyes may occur months to years after the onset of Lyme disease. However, marked variation in clinical expression is possible. Incomplete disease presentations occur, and virtually any clinical feature may be present in isolation or recur at intervals, complicating clinical diagnosis.

Although the exact roles of the infecting spirochete, spirochetal antigens, and host immune responses are unclear, many later manifestations of Lyme disease are probably caused by tissue invasion and persistence of the organism. This concept is supported by the isolation of *B. burgdorferi* from blood, skin lesions (erythema migrans), and cerebrospinal fluid.[20,194] The organism has also been visualized in the eye,[191] myocardium,[110] and synovium.[177] In addition, all stages of disease respond to antimicrobial therapy.

Stage I. Erythema migrans is the most characteristic clinical manifestation of Lyme disease, but it develops in only 60% to 80% of patients (Color Plate 55). An average of 7 days (range 3 to 32 days) after inoculation from a tick bite, *B. burgdorferi* spreads locally in the skin, producing an expanding, annular, and erythematous lesion. Initially a central red macule or papule may be present. As the lesion expands, partial central clearing usually is seen, while the outer borders remain bright red. The borders are usually flat but may be raised. The center of some early lesions becomes intensely red and indurated or may even become vesicular or necrotic. In some instances multiple red rings form within the outside margin, or the central area turns blue before clearing. The lesion often reaches a diameter of 15 cm (range 3 to 68 cm) and may appear anywhere on the body, although the thigh, groin, and axilla are the most common sites. The lesion is warm to the touch and usually described by the patient as burning, but occasionally as itching or painful. Biopsy of erythema migrans shows dermal and epidermal involvement at the center, but only dermal changes in the periphery, which are findings suggestive of an arthropod bite.[188] Constitutional symptoms may accompany erythema migrans, but are usually mild and consist of regional lymphadenopathy, fever, and malaise. Annular erythematous lesions occurring hours after a tick bite represent hypersensitivity reactions and should not be confused with erythema migrans.

Erythema migrans fades after an average of 28 days (range 1 to 14 weeks) without treatment; with antibiotics the lesion resolves after several days. Recurrent lesions may develop from 1 to 14 months after the initial lesion in patients who do not receive antibiotic therapy. These take the form of erythema migrans, secondary lesions, or both. Rarely, evanescent small red circles and blotches may develop. Patients treated with appropriate antibiotics rarely have recurrent skin lesions.[188]

Stage II. Within days or weeks after infection, the *B. burgdorferi* may spread from the skin to other organs via the blood or lymph. During this stage, spirochetes can be recovered from patients' blood. *B. burgdorferi* probably spreads initially to all organs, but like its spirochetal cousin *Treponema pallidum* (syphilis), it appears to sequester in certain niches.[187]

During hematogenous spread, multiple, annular secondary skin lesions develop in 20% to 50% of patients in the United States. The secondary lesions are generally smaller, migrate less, and lack indurated centers. They may be located anywhere except the palms and soles. Ten to fifteen percent of patients have more than 20 such lesions; rarely, the lesions exceed 100 in number. Blistering and mucosal involvement do not occur; this is an important feature in differentiating the lesions from erythema multiforme. Other skin manifestations include a malar rash (10% to 15%) and, rarely, urticaria.[188]

Constitutional symptoms commonly accompany stage II Lyme disease. Malaise and fatigue are most common, may be severe, and are usually constant throughout the duration of the illness. Fever, typically low grade and intermittent, is common. In children, temperature elevations may be constant and reach 40° C. Tender regional lymphadenopathy in the distribution of erythema migrans or the posterior cervical chains is frequent, and generalized lymphadenopathy and splenomegaly may occur.[188]

Symptoms of meningeal irritation predominate in some patients. Severe headaches are typically intermittent and localized. Stiff neck with extreme forward flexion occurs, but Kernig's and Brudzinski's signs are negative, with no associated cerebrospinal fluid pleocytosis. Some patients have evidence of mild encephalopathy with somnolence, insomnia, memory disturbances, emotional lability, dizziness, poor balance, or clumsiness. Dysesthesias, most commonly of the scalp, may be particularly bothersome.[188]

Musculoskeletal complaints are common. Arthralgias, myalgias, and pain in tendons, bursae, or bones are typically migratory, sometimes lasting only hours in one location. Patients may complain of generalized stiffness or severe cramping pain, particularly in the calves, thighs, and back. Frank arthritis is uncommon in the first several weeks of illness.[188]

Symptoms of hepatitis (such as anorexia, nausea, vomiting, right upper quadrant pain, and weight loss), hepatomegaly, and generalized abdominal pain may occur. Respiratory symptoms are generally minor. Conjunctivitis occurs in 10% to 15% of patients.[188]

During this phase of the illness, Lyme disease might easily be confused with a viral or collagen-vascular disease, especially if there was no preceding skin rash. A distinguishing feature of Lyme disease is that early signs and symptoms are intermittent and rapidly changing. Such a pattern in a patient from an endemic area should suggest Lyme disease.

After dissemination, *B. burgdorferi* typically produces sequestered infection, most commonly of the nervous system, heart, and joints. Neurologic manifestations develop in 10% to 15% of patients with erythema migrans who are not treated with appropriate antibiotics.[137] Symptoms begin an average of 4 weeks (range 0 to 10 weeks) after the onset of erythema migrans, usually after a latent period. However, neurologic signs and symptoms may be the presenting manifestations of Lyme disease. In untreated persons, symptoms usually resolve after several months (median duration 30 weeks).[137]

Meningoencephalitis is the most common neurologic presentation. Headache, typically fluctuating in intensity, is the predominant symptom. Subtle symptoms of encephalitis, including sleep disturbances, poor concentration, memory loss, irritability, and emotional lability, may develop. Unlike stage I disease, cerebrospinal fluid examination in stage II often shows a pleocytosis with an average of 100 cells/mm^3, predominantly lymphocytic, usually with elevated protein level but with normal glucose level and opening pressure.[137]

Facial nerve palsy develops in 50% of patients with Lyme disease meningitis and may occur as an isolated finding. This is similar to Bell's palsy, except that it is frequently bilateral. Duration is from weeks to months, and return of function is almost always complete.[38] Involvement of other cranial nerves occurs but is unusual.

The third common neurologic manifestation of Lyme disease is radiculoneuritis, including thoracic sensory radiculitis, motor radiculoneuritis in extremities, brachial plexitis, mononeuritis, and mononeuritis multiplex. Outcome is generally favorable with complete recovery, although a few patients have had residual weakness.[137]

The triad of meningitis, cranial neuritis, and radiculoneuritis presents a unique clinical picture. However, any neurologic manifestation of Lyme disease may occur alone and may be the presenting manifestation. Other neurologic abnormalities described in association with Lyme disease include chorea,[152] cerebellar ataxia,[152] myelitis,[151,152] dementia,[151] and optic atrophy.[165]

Cardiac abnormalities develop in 4% to 10% of patients with untreated Lyme disease.[156,189] The most common abnormality is fluctuating atrioventricular block, including first-degree, Wenckebach, or complete heart block.

Progression to symptomatic complete heart block is common and frequently requires treatment with a temporary transvenous pacemaker. Electrophysiologic studies suggest the block is at the level of the atrioventricular node. The block does not respond to atropine, suggesting a direct effect on the atrioventricular node.[156] Evidence for more diffuse cardiac involvement, most commonly electrocardiographic changes compatible with myopericarditis, is found in about one half of patients with carditis. Left ventricular dysfunction can be shown by radionuclide angiography in some patients, but is rarely clinically significant. Cardiomegaly rarely develops, and valvular involvement is not a feature. At least one death has been linked to cardiac involvement,[110] but abnormalities usually resolve completely, often within 1 to 2 weeks.[189]

In approximately 60% of untreated persons with erythema migrans, arthritis develops a few weeks to 2 years (median 4 weeks) after the onset of illness. The typical pattern is brief, recurrent episodes of asymmetric, oligoarticular swelling and pain in large joints, separated by longer periods of complete remission. Arthritis may be monarticular or migratory, usually one joint at a time, in as many as 10 different joints. Arthritis in a single joint is usually of short duration (median 8 days) but may persist for months. The knee is most commonly affected, followed by the shoulder, elbow, temporomandibular joint, ankle, wrist, hip, and small joints of the hands and feet.[231] Frank arthritis with joint swelling usually does not begin until months after the onset of illness, and it is unusual for any joint other than the knee to swell. Affected knees are commonly much more swollen than painful. Baker's cysts may develop and rupture, simulating thrombophlebitis. Most patients have recurrent attacks of arthritis, with a tendency over time toward less frequent and less severe episodes.[196]

Synovial fluid in Lyme disease is inflammatory, with a median white blood cell count of 25,000, predominantly polymorphonuclear leukocytes. Higher white blood cell counts may simulate septic arthritis.[89] Complement level is generally greater than one-third that of serum, and protein level ranges from 3 to 8 g/dl. Synovial biopsy reveals hypertrophy, vascular proliferation, and a mononuclear cell infiltrate.[193]

A number of other manifestations of stage II Lyme disease have been reported, but they occur much less frequently. A solitary lymphocytoma, borrelial lymphocytoma, may develop in patients with Lyme disease from Europe; it occurs rarely in patients in the United States. The lesion is characterized histologically by a dense polycolonal lymphocytic infiltrate in the dermis or cutis. Clinically, it presents as a red to dark bluish red nodule a few centimeters in diameter, most commonly on the earlobe in children and the nipple in adults. Untreated, borrelial lymphocytoma may persist for many months.[208] Other findings associated with *B. burgdorferi* infection include adult respiratory distress syndrome (ARDS),[96] hepatitis,[71] myositis,[10] osteomyelitis,[89] and iritis.[191]

Stage III. Late or persistent infection usually begins a year or more after the onset of erythema migrans, although patients may present with stage III disease as the initial manifestation of Lyme disease. In about 10% of patients with arthritis, involvement of the knees or other large joints becomes chronic. Radiographically, juxtaarticular osteoporosis, cartilage loss, cortical or marginal bone erosions, and joint effusions may be seen. Features of degenerative arthritis, cartilage loss, subarticular sclerosis, and osteophytosis are less commonly found.[100] Patients do not usually have continual joint inflammation for more than several years.[200] Rheumatoid and antinuclear antibodies are generally absent,[193] although there appears to be an increased incidence of B cell alloantigens DR2 and DR4 in patients with chronic Lyme arthritis.[192]

Patients with Lyme disease may develop chronic persistent nervous system involvement months to years after becoming infected. Several distinct, but often overlapping, syndromes have been described. The best established syndrome is a severe, progressive encephalomyelitis characterized clinically by spastic paraparesis, ataxia, cognitive impairment, bladder dysfunction, and cranial neuropathy, particularly of the seventh and eighth cranial nerves.[2a] Cerebrospinal fluid examination typically shows a lymphocytic pleocytosis and intrathecal production of anti–*B. burgdorferi* antibody. Magnetic resonance imaging of the brain may show abnormalities of the white matter.

Chronic involvement of the peripheral nervous system also occurs in Lyme disease. Patients may have painless distal paresthesias or painful radiculopathy. The distal paresthesias are generally intermittent, are often symmetric, and involve the legs more frequently than the upper extremities. Radicular pain is more frequently asymmetric and may involve the cervical, thoracic, or lumbosacral segments, often in combination. The pain is typically spinal with radiation into the affected limbs or trunk.[104] Nerve conduction and electromyographic studies suggest a mild axonal polyneuropathy with reductions in motor or sensory nerve conduction velocities and denervation of spinal and limb muscles.[105] The underlying pathophysiologic mechanism appears to be mononeuritis multiplex.[62]

Several syndromes have also been described in which the association with infection by *B. burgdorferi* is less certain. Some patients with serologic evidence of *B. burgdorferi* infection develop a mild encephalopathy with memory difficulties, depression, mood swings, language disturbance, and fatigue. Most of these patients do not have increased intrathecal production of antibodies to *B. burgdorferi*, although some of them do show improvement with antibiotic treatment.[104] More problematic is the group of syndromes that have been termed postborreliosis disorders. Following treatment for Lyme disease many patients note persistent fatigue, sleep disorder, depression, or cognitive difficulties. The cause of this disorder is unknown, and it does not appear to respond to antibiotics.[62]

Acrodermatitis chronica atrophicans is the best example of prolonged latency followed by persistent infection in Lyme disease. Observed primarily in Europe, it may begin years after the onset of illness. It begins with an inflammatory phase with bluish red discoloration, often at the same site as a previous erythema migrans lesion, preferentially involving the extensor surfaces of the extremities. The inflammatory phase may persist for years or decades, with gradual conversion to atrophy of the skin.[9] Several patients with a history of Lyme disease have also been described with keratitis similar to syphilitic keratitis beginning years after their initial infection.[187]

Lyme Disease During Pregnancy. The risk of adverse outcome for pregnancies complicated by Lyme disease is not currently known. However, other spirochetes cause congenital infections, and cases of human transplacental transmission of *B. burgdorferi* have been documented.[107,114,166,224] In each case the infant was either stillborn or died shortly after birth; in one case the mother had been treated with an orally administered penicillin for Lyme disease early in pregnancy.[224] In another report of 19 pregnancies complicated by Lyme disease, five had an adverse outcome, although several were minor with no permanent sequelae, no two outcomes were the same, and none were documented to be caused by *B. burgdorferi*.[114] Although data are limited, women who acquire Lyme disease during pregnancy should be treated promptly with penicillin. For patients with localized disease, treatment with oral amoxicillin appears adequate. For patients with disseminated disease, the authors who reported the failure of an orally administered penicillin to prevent transplacental infection now recommend intravenous penicillin (20 million units/day in divided doses for 10 to 14 days).[224] In patients allergic to penicillin, erythromycin (500 mg four times daily) might be an alternative, although clinicians have had little experience with this regimen.

Diagnosis. The diagnosis of early Lyme disease requires careful consideration of clinical and epidemiologic data. Erythema migrans or typical organ involvement that develops after exposure in an endemic area strongly suggests Lyme disease. However, incomplete cases without erythema migrans may prove difficult to diagnose, presenting as a viral-like illness.[57] Arthritis or neurologic involvement may develop months after the cutaneous eruption, which the patient may not remember. Most patients do not recall a tick bite.

Routine laboratory studies add little to the early diagnosis of Lyme disease. Most patients have a mildly elevated erythrocyte sedimentation rate and decreased absolute lymphocyte count, and some are mildly anemic.

Culture for *B. burgdorferi* is difficult, and direct visualization techniques have yields too low to be clinically useful.[174] This leaves detecting indirect evidence of infection—antibodies to *B. burgdorferi*—as the only practical laboratory aid to diagnosis.

Unfortunately, antibody response to *B. burgdorferi* develops slowly. Serologic studies are usually negative in the first few weeks of illness, particularly in patients with limited manifestations. However, patients with complicated Lyme disease (neurologic, cardiac, or joint involvement) or patients in remission nearly always have elevated specific antibody titers.[124,174] IgM antibody titers generally peak between the third and sixth weeks after the onset of illness; IgG antibody titers rise slowly and are highest months later when arthritis is present. Early treatment with antibiotics may blunt or completely suppress antibody formation. Both IgM and IgG antibodies may persist for months or years following clinical resolution, even after treatment with appropriate antibiotics.[56]

Current methods for detecting antibodies to *B. burgdorferi* include indirect immunofluorescent assay (IFA), enzyme-linked immunosorbent assay (ELISA), and Western blot or immunoblot. In most laboratories, ELISA appears to be the test of choice for evaluation of suspected Lyme disease, although IFA can be comparable when performed by experienced technicians.[74] Western blot can be used to increase the specificity of serologic testing when results are equivocal by demonstrating the presence of antibodies to epitopes that are unique to *B. burgdorferi*.[50] False-positive results are common in patients with other treponemal diseases, including syphilis, yaws, and pinta, and have been reported in patients with leptospirosis and relapsing fever.[124] Patients with Lyme disease, however, do not have positive Venereal Disease Research Laboratories (VDRL) tests.

Considerable caution must be exercised in interpreting the results of serologic testing in Lyme disease. In a recent study only 23% of patients referred to the Lyme Disease Clinic at New England Medical Center had active Lyme disease, and a majority of those without Lyme disease had been treated inappropriately with antibiotics.[201] In this study, by far the most common reason for lack of response to antibiotics was misdiagnosis. The limitations of laboratory testing in Lyme disease include lack of sensitivity and specificity of serologic tests and considerable interlaboratory and intralaboratory variability in test results.[171] An additional problem stems from the persistence of antibodies in patients with past or asymptomatic infection with *B. burgdorferi*. If another illness develops, which was the case in 20% of patients referred to the New England Medical Center clinic, it may be incorrectly attributed to Lyme disease. This is particularly problematic in patients with nonspecific symptoms of chronic fatigue or fibromyalgia.

Diagnosis of Lyme disease requires careful consideration of epidemiologic and clinical information, supplemented by serologic testing when appropriate. For patients in nonendemic areas the pretest probability of Lyme disease is low. Serologic testing will be useful only in patients with symptoms specific for Lyme disease; in patients with nonspecific symptoms a positive test is more likely to represent a false positive than a true positive. The tests should be done in a reference laboratory and confirmed with a Western blot.

In patients from endemic areas who have erythema migrans, serologic tests are not indicated. The patient should be assumed to have Lyme disease whether or not serologic tests are positive. Many patients with localized Lyme disease will not have developed antibodies at the time of testing. Convalescent titers are not helpful, since early antibiotic treatment may prevent seroconversion. If doubt exists about whether a lesion is erythema migrans, careful observation is indicated. A lesion that resolves in 1 to 2 days, that does not expand centrifugally, or that is less than 5 cm in diameter is unlikely to be erythema migrans.[69]

Most patients with symptoms of early disseminated Lyme disease have positive serologic tests. However, if clinical and epidemiologic data strongly support the diagnosis of Lyme disease, antibiotic treatment is appropriate even with negative findings, since some patients will not have seroconverted. Patients with possible central nervous system involvement should have a lumbar puncture performed, and the cerebrospinal fluid tested for *B. burgdorferi* antibodies.[69] In patients with established cardiac, neurologic, or joint manifestations of Lyme disease, serologic tests are almost always positive. A negative serologic test makes Lyme disease extremely unlikely. As previously noted, however, a positive test does not establish the diagnosis of Lyme disease, but merely indicates that infection has occurred at some time in the past.

In patients with isolated nonspecific symptoms such as chronic fatigue, transient musculoskeletal pain, or difficulty concentrating, Lyme serologic tests should not be performed. These symptoms are rarely if ever the sole manifestation of Lyme disease. The pretest probability of Lyme disease in this situation is so low that a positive test is likely to be a false positive.

Treatment. Treatment of the early manifestations of Lyme disease with antibiotics will significantly shorten the duration of erythema migrans and its associated symptoms and largely prevent major complications.[164,195] However, the optimal drug, dose, and treatment duration are still unknown. One recent treatment regimen for stage I disease is amoxicillin 1 g orally three times a day for 4 weeks. An alternative is doxycycline 200 mg orally twice a day for 3 days, then 100 mg orally twice a day to a total of 4 weeks. Amoxicillin and doxycycline have well-established efficacy in early Lyme disease, and several other oral agents (cefuroxime axetil, cefixime, azithromycin) have high in vitro activity against *B. burgdorferi*.[5,186] Small controlled trials suggest that cefuroxime and azithromycin (200 mg orally twice a day for 2 weeks; not yet approved by the Food and Drug Administration for this indication) are also effective in vivo.[133,186] Erythromycin also has good in vitro activity, but is not as effective as amoxicillin or doxycycline in vivo. The recommended duration of therapy is at least 10 days and up to 4 weeks if symptoms persist or recur. Because *B. burgdorferi* is very slow growing, prolonged antibiotic exposure may be necessary to kill the organism.[5] This, combined with some treatment failures with shorter course therapy, has led many clinicians to recommend a minimum of 21 days of therapy. Another important consideration in choosing an antimicrobial agent for early Lyme disease is attainable cerebrospinal fluid levels, since *B. burgdorferi* can invade the central nervous system early in the course of infection, even in the absence of symptoms of its involvement.[106] Patients may develop a Jarisch-Herxheimer reaction (higher fever, redder rash, or greater pain) in the first 24 hours of therapy.[133,195]

Intravenous penicillin (in meningeal dose), ceftriaxone (1 g every 12 to 24 hours for 2 to 4 weeks), and cefotaxime have been shown to be effective in treating central nervous system involvement (meningitis, cranial neuritis, or radiculoneuritis) in Lyme disease.[139] Ceftriaxone has been found in some studies to be more effective than penicillin,[42,43] and the once daily dose schedule makes outpatient treatment feasible. Meningitic symptoms usually resolve with therapy in 1 week, although complete recovery of motor deficits may require 7 to 8 weeks.[199] In chronic, persistent infection (stage III), the outcome after antibiotic treatment is usually favorable, but incomplete resolution is common.[104] In isolated facial nerve palsy, treatment with an oral regimen may be adequate.[145]

Although cardiac manifestations of Lyme disease usually resolve within 1 to 2 weeks, even without antibiotic treatment, *B. burgdorferi* can directly invade the myocardium and produce a cardiomyopathy.[183] In addition, other manifestations of disseminated infection commonly occur in patients with cardiac involvement.[145] For these reasons patients with Lyme carditis should be treated with intravenous antibiotics.

Optimal therapy for Lyme arthritis has not been established. Several oral and parenteral regimens have been used successfully, but failures occur with any of them. A reasonable approach for patients without evidence of neurologic involvement is to use an oral regimen initially.[198] If an adequate clinical response is not obtained, a parenteral regimen can be tried. However, clinicians should keep in mind that the response to antibiotics may not occur for 3 months or longer after completion of therapy.[145]

Antibiotic prophylaxis for tick bites does not appear to be warranted, even in endemic areas. The risk of serious late sequelae in untreated patients bitten by a tick is extremely low.[6,173] This is probably because of two factors. First, most patients who find an attached tick remove it before transmission of *B. burgdorferi* occurs; this accounts for the low incidence of infection in controlled trials of antibiotic prophylaxis. Second, most patients who become infected develop erythema migrans and can be treated effectively. The major area of concern is that patients who become infected and do not develop erythema migrans may develop the late and more difficult to treat manifestations of Lyme disease. However, in the more than 400 patients given placebo after a deer tick bite, none have developed late Lyme disease.[173]

Relapsing Fever

Relapsing fever is an acute borrelial disease characterized by recurrent paroxysms of fever separated by afebrile periods. It occurs in both endemic and epidemic forms (Table 33-2). The endemic or sporadic form occurs worldwide and is caused by a group of closely related *Borrelia* species. Argasid ticks belonging to the genus *Ornithodoros* are the vectors. The epidemic form of relapsing fever is transmitted by the human body louse; it has not been reported in the United States in recent years.

The *Ornithodoros* ticks that transmit relapsing fever act as both vectors and reservoirs for *Borrelia* organisms. Transovarial transmission allows all developmental stages to be potentially infective. The ticks generally feed at night and attach themselves to the host for a short time, usually for less than 1 hour. The bite is seldom painful and frequently goes unrecognized. The ticks are extremely resilient and may survive for years between feedings.

Ticks ingest *Borrelia* organisms while feeding on an infected vertebrate, most commonly a rodent. Borreliae enter the tick hemocele and then spread to other tick tissues, including the salivary glands, coxal organs, and reproductive

Table 33-2 Tick-Borne Relapsing Fever Borreliae

Arthropod Vector	*Borrelia* Species	Geographic Distribution
Ornithodoros hermsi	*B. hermsii*	Western United States and Canada
O. turicata	*B. turicatae*	Southwestern United States and Mexico
O. parkeri	*B. parkeri*	Western United States and Mexico
O. moubata	*B. duttoni*	Tropical Africa
O. tholozani	*B. persica*	Central Asia, Middle East, Greece
O. tartakovskyi	*B. latyschevi*	Iran, Central Asia
O. erraticus	*B. crocidurae*	Russia, Middle East, East Africa, Turkey
O. graingeri	*B. graingeri*	Kenya
O. talaje	*B. mozzottii*	Mexico, Central America
O. rudis	*B. venezuelensis*	Central and South America
O. asperus	*B. caucasica*	Iraq and Russia
O. marocianus	*B. hispanica*	Northern Africa, Southern Europe

organs. The coxal organs in argasid ticks are specialized tissues for excretion of excess fluids and solutes accumulated during feeding. In some *Ornithodoros* species, the coxal fluid is released near the mouthparts during feeding, allowing transmission of spirochetes to vertebrate hosts. Transmission may also occur via saliva or regurgitated gut contents.[14] *Borreliae* remain infective within ticks for many months.[178]

A high degree of specificity exists between the major strains of relapsing fever *Borrelia* and associated tick vectors. For instance, the three *Borrelia* species found in the United States—*B. hermsii, B. turicatae,* and *B. parkeri*—show complete specificity for their respective vectors, which are *O. hermsi, O. turicata,* and *O. parkeri. B. hermsii* can be transmitted only by *O. hermsi,* and not by *O. turicata* or *O. parkeri.* This specificity is used extensively in classification of *Borrelia* species.[44]

Epidemiology. *Ornithodoros* ticks generally inhabit rodent burrows and nests, cracks and crevices in human and animal habitats, caves, and similar locations. Habits and patterns of infection vary between tick species. In parts of Africa, ticks live in the dust and cracks of earthen floored huts, and sporadic cases are seen throughout the year. In the Middle East, Mexico, and southwestern United States, ticks live in the guano of cave floors, and human infection is often associated with visiting or camping in caves.

The majority of cases of relapsing fever in the United States are attributed to *B. hermsii.* Its vector, *O. hermsi,* inhabits the coniferous forest biome of the western United States and Canada, where it lives in remains of dead trees and burrows inhabited by mice, rats, and chipmunks. Ticks are carried by rodents into poorly maintained cabins and huts; lodging in such shelters by hikers and hunters is a major factor in acquiring relapsing fever.[61,88] Occasional cases are also caused by *O. turicata* in Texas and adjacent areas of the Southwest; *O. parkeri* rarely bites humans.[87]

Relapsing fever in the United States has been reported from Colorado,[51,88] California,[51] the Pacific Northwest,[61] and several other western states. In California, where reporting of relapsing fever is encouraged, 2 to 12 cases are reported per year.[51] Large outbreaks have been reported from Spokane County, Washington,[213] and the north rim area of the Grand Canyon.[33] The disease is more common in men, presumably because of increased exposure to tick vectors, and occurs primarily during summer months. Tick-borne relapsing fever is rarely fatal in adults, but in infants less than 1 year of age, case fatality rates may be 20% or higher.[101,178]

Clinical Features. The characteristic clinical feature of relapsing fever is the abrupt onset of fever lasting about 3 days, an afebrile period of variable duration, and then relapse with return of fever and other clinical manifestations. A pruritic eschar may appear at the site of the tick bite but is usually absent by the onset of clinical symptoms. After an incubation period of approximately 7 days, patients develop fever, frequently accompanied by shaking chills, severe headache, myalgias, arthralgias, upper abdominal pain, nausea, and vomiting. The temperature is usually high (over 39° C), and patients may manifest extreme muscular weakness and lethargy. Splenomegaly develops in approximately 40% of cases of tick-borne relapsing fever, and hepatomegaly in 17% to 18%. Neurologic involvement occurs in less than 10% of cases. Abnormalities include altered sensorium, peripheral neuropathy, pupillary abnormalities, and pathologic reflexes. A rash, ranging from a macular eruption to petechiae and erythema multiforme, develops in 25% to 30% of patients.[178]

The initial febrile period averages 3 days but may last from 1 to 17 days. It terminates with rapid defervescence or a "crisis," accompanied by drenching sweats and intense thirst. The subsequent afebrile period is of variable duration but averages 6 to 7 days. An average of three relapses is observed in tick-borne disease, and as a rule, each succeeding relapse is less severe.[178]

Mortality rates have been as high as 40% in some epidemics of louse-borne relapsing fever,[178] but tick-borne disease is generally self-limited, although clinical features may be severe and prolonged. Iritis or iridocyclitis occurs in up to 15% of untreated cases, and formation of adhesions between the iris and anterior lens capsule frequently leads to visual defects.[178] Neurologic complications generally resolve spontaneously, but severe depression may persist for months. Hemorrhagic complications, pneumonia, adult respiratory distress syndrome, or myocarditis may develop rarely.[45,61,228]

Relapsing fever in pregnancy results in a high incidence of spontaneous abortion.[178] Fetal death is probably caused by direct placental invasion by spirochetes.[184] Infection in the neonatal period usually occurs by placental transmission and presents as overwhelming sepsis with very high mortality.[237]

Antigenic Variation. The phenomenon of relapse in relapsing fever is caused by the ability of borreliae to undergo antigenic variation in an infected host. The organisms are capable of spontaneous conversion to a large number of serotypes. Clinically, defervescence occurs when the dominant serotype is eradicated by interaction with host antibody. Spirochetemia probably persists at undetectable levels during the afebrile period and consists of mixed serotypes. Relapse occurs when a variant population reaches detectable levels. Antigenic variation is under complex genetic control and does not appear to require contact of the organism with host antibody.[12,207]

Diagnosis. The clinical diagnosis of tick-borne relapsing fever requires thorough knowledge of the epidemiology of the disease and a high index of suspicion. Routine laboratory tests are of little utility. The leukocyte count is usually normal but may be increased or decreased. Thrombocytopenia is common but nonspecific. A false-positive serologic test for syphilis (Wassermann) occurs in about 5% of cases.[178]

The diagnosis of relapsing fever is confirmed by demonstrating spirochetes on peripheral blood smears. A routine peripheral blood smear (Wright-Giemsa stain) from a febrile patient is initially positive in 70% of cases.[178] The diagnostic yield can be increased by examining thick smears and by staining with acridine orange.[172] Inoculating laboratory animals (rats, mice) with blood and examining blood smears from the animals will also increase the diagnostic yield. Serologic tests are difficult to perform and are not yet of practical utility.

Treatment. Tetracycline and erythromycin are both effective in treating relapsing fever. A single oral dose of 500 mg of either drug is effective in louse-borne relapsing fever.[31] However, a 5- to 10-day course (500 mg orally four times a day) is generally recommended in tick-borne disease.[87,178] The borreliae are also sensitive to penicillin and chloramphenicol, but treatment failures have been reported with penicillin.[31]

A Jarisch-Herxheimer reaction is common following the first dose of antibiotics. It is often severe and may be fatal. The reaction begins with a rise in body temperature and exacerbation of existing signs and symptoms; vasodilation and a fall in blood pressure follow. This complex reaction is mediated, in part, by products of mononuclear leukocytes. The leukocytes are stimulated by increased contact with antibiotic-altered spirochetes. Neither endotoxin nor complement appears to be necessary in the pathogenesis of the reaction.[30]

Waiting to begin treatment until the patient is afebrile does not prevent a Jarisch-Herxheimer reaction,[88] and pretreatment with acetaminophen and hydrocortisone results in only a mild reduction of hypotension and does not prevent rigors.[31] Patients who are receiving the initial dose of antibiotics for relapsing fever should receive an intravenous infusion of isotonic saline in anticipation of a possible Jarisch-Herxheimer reaction. This is generally sufficient to counteract the hypotension. Lower initial doses of tetracycline or erythromycin may reduce the frequency of this reaction.[88]

TICK-BORNE RICKETTSIAL DISEASES

Bacteria of the family Rickettsiaceae are small, fastidious intracellular parasites with gram-negative bacterium-like cell walls, typical prokaryotic DNA arrangement, and considerable independent metabolic activity. There are six major antigenic groups, which cause a variety of human diseases worldwide (Table 33-3). Three are potentially transmissible to humans by ticks: spotted fever group diseases, Q fever, and *Ehrlichia* infections. Organisms from the genus *Rickettsia* cause the various spotted fevers. *Coxiella burnetii* is the etiologic agent of Q fever. *Ehrlichia* are intraleukocytic Rickettsiaceae that infect humans and a variety of wild and domestic animals.

Spotted Fever Group Diseases

Rickettsia of the spotted fever group (SFG) share intracellular growth characteristics and a group-specific antigen. They are distributed worldwide and with the exception of *Rickettsia akari* (rickettsial pox) are transmitted by the bite of ixodid ticks (Table 33-4). Ticks serve as the natural hosts, reservoirs, and vectors for the rickettsiae.[120] The organisms replicate freely within the tick host and are passed transovarially and transstadially. Amplification of the cycle occurs when uninfected ticks feed on an infected vertebrate host or concurrently with an infected tick.

In most natural vertebrate hosts, the SFG rickettsiae induce an inapparent infection with transient rickettsemia. Human infection occurs through accidental intrusion into the natural cycle of infection, or when ticks are transferred into human environments. Humans are incidental and

Table 33-3 Human Rickettsial Diseases

Disease	Organism	Arthropod Vector	Geographic Distribution
TYPHUS GROUP			
Murine typhus	*Rickettsia mooseri*	Flea	Worldwide
Epidemic typhus	*R. prowazekii*	Body louse	Worldwide
Scrub typhus	*R. tsutsugamushi*	Chigger	Asia, Australia, Southeast Asia
SPOTTED FEVER GROUP			
Rocky Mountain spotted fever	*R. rickettsii*	Ticks	Western Hemisphere
Eastern spotted fevers	*R. conorii*	Ticks	Eastern Hemisphere
	R. sibirica		
	R. australis		
Rickettsial pox	*R. akari*	Mites	United States, Russia
Q fever	*Coxiella burnetii*	Ticks	Worldwide
Trench fever	*Rochalimaea quintana*	Body louse	Africa, Mexico
Ehrlichia	*E. sennetsu*	Ticks	Japan
	E. canis		Worldwide

Table 33-4 Spotted Fever Group Diseases

Disease	Etiologic Agent	Major Vector	Geographic Distribution	Primary Lesion	Usual Severity
Rocky Mountain spotted fever	*Rickettsia rickettsii*	*Dermacentor andersoni, D. variabilis*	Western Hemisphere	None	Moderate-severe
North Asian tick typhus	*R. sibirica*	*Dermacentor, Haemaphysalis*	Europe to Russian Far East	Often present	Mild
Mediterranean spotted fever	*R. conorii*	*Rhipicephalus sanguineus, Haemaphysalis*	Mediterranean littoral, South Africa, Kenya, India	Often present	Moderate
Queensland tick typhus	*R. australis*	*Ixodes holocyclus*	Australia	Often present	Mild

"dead-end" hosts not involved in sustaining the life cycle of the organism.

Pathogenesis. The tick-borne SFG diseases share a similar pathogenesis. The usual route of infection is by direct inoculation through the skin via the bite of a tick vector. However, infection may also develop after contamination of broken skin with infected tick parts or feces, after blood transfusion from an infected donor,[227] or through aerosol transmission among laboratory personnel working with pathogenic rickettsiae.[136]

Local proliferation of rickettsiae probably occurs at the site of the tick bite, and a primary lesion or eschar (absent in Rocky Mountain spotted fever) frequently develops. Regional lymphadenitis may develop in the distribution of the eschar, suggesting early lymphatic spread. Rickettsemia is typically present at the onset of clinical illness and persists throughout the febrile period.[233]

The SFG diseases are characterized by disseminated vasculitic lesions.[221] The rickettsiae invade, proliferate within, and ultimately destroy capillary and precapillary endothelial cells. In Rocky Mountain spotted fever (RMSF), the organisms spread into larger arterioles and arteries and invade medial smooth muscle cells. Medial necrosis and destruction of the vascular wall may follow. At sites of endothelial cell damage, a perivascular inflammatory response ensues, and platelet and fibrin thrombi tend to form and occlude the vessel lumen. In severe cases, vascular thrombi lead to necrosis of peripheral parts, including fingers, toes, the external ear, and scrotum. Antibodies develop 5 to 7 days after the onset of illness, but do not appear to play a significant role in the pathogenesis of the vasculitis.[235] Immunity develops with clinical recovery, tends to be long-lasting, and appears to involve both antibody- and cell-mediated mechanisms.

Clinical Manifestations and Diagnosis. The SFG diseases display similar clinical manifestations, including fever, chills, headache, and myalgias. Three to 5 days after the onset of illness a characteristic maculopapular rash develops on the ankles, feet, wrists, and hands, then spreads centripetally to involve the entire body, including the palms and soles. With the exception of RMSF, the SFG diseases are generally mild, self-limited illnesses, with deaths seen primarily in elderly or debilitated patients. Untreated RMSF, however, may be severe, with a case-mortality rate approaching 30%.[24]

Early diagnosis and treatment virtually eliminate mortality and reduce morbidity in SFG diseases. However, at the onset of illness, signs and symptoms are frequently nonspecific, leading to diagnostic confusion with viral or other infectious diseases.[94] Rash, the most characteristic feature of the illness, may develop late or rarely not at all. Identification of the eschar is helpful, but its presence is variable and it is absent altogether in RMSF. Only 60% to 70% of patients recall a tick bite. Laboratory data may provide clues to the diagnosis (hyponatremia, thrombocytopenia) but are nonspecific. Serologic evidence of infection develops late in the illness. Early diagnosis therefore is based primarily on clinical evidence and relies on the ability of physicians to correlate clinical signs and symptoms with epidemiologic features.

Rickettsial infection is confirmed by identification of rickettsiae in tissues (not widely available), by isolation of rickettsiae from infected blood or tissues (difficult and hazardous to laboratory personnel), or by demonstrating antibody rise in paired sera. The widely used Weil-Felix test is based on the unique sharing of polysaccharide antigens between certain *Proteus* strains (OX-19, OX-2) and the SFG rickettsiae. However, this agglutination test lacks both sensitivity and specificity and should be abandoned where other serologic methods are available. Newer and more sensitive serologic methods include complement fixation, microimmunofluorescence, IFA tests, microagglutination, indirect hemagglutination, and ELISA.[39,93,140]

Treatment. Early treatment of the spotted fevers is the most important factor in speeding convalescence and reducing mortality. Antibiotic therapy begun early in the course results in rapid resolution of clinical abnormalities. Tetracycline and chloramphenicol are both very effective, although neither drug is rickettsicidal. The antibiotics inhibit the rickettsiae until an adequate immune response by the patient eradicates the infection. Tetracycline is given orally at a dosage of 25 to 50 mg/kg/day in four divided doses (2 g/day in adults); the dose of chloramphenicol is 50 and 75 mg/kg/day for adults and children, respectively. Appropriate intravenous doses of both drugs may be substituted. Penicillins, streptomycin, and sulfonamides are ineffective. Treatment should be continued until the patient is afebrile for 48 hours, or for a minimum of 5 to 7 days. Relapses are uncommon but may be treated with the same drug when they occur.[235]

Rocky Mountain Spotted Fever

Epidemiology. RMSF was first recognized in the northwestern United States in the latter part of the eighteenth century, and may have been prevalent even earlier in native Americans of that region. It has since been identified throughout the Western Hemisphere. Human infections have been reported in all 48 contiguous states except Maine. The disease is also seen in Canada, Mexico, and parts of Central and South America.

A major shift in the demographics of RMSF has occurred during this century. Before 1930, most cases were reported from the mountainous areas of the western United States; in recent years more than 90% of cases have been reported from southern and eastern states. Reported cases in the mountain states have actually decreased more than tenfold.[119] "Rocky Mountain" spotted fever has thus become somewhat of a misnomer.

In the early 1970s a marked increase in the reported cases of RMSF was seen in this country, reaching a peak in 1981 of 1192 cases, for an incidence rate of 0.51 cases/100,000 population. Reported cases have gradually declined since that time, with a provisional total of 628 cases reported in 1991 (0.25 cases/100,000 population).[36] Most of this decline has occurred in the South Atlantic states, although they still account for a majority of the cases reported each year. States with the most cases in 1991 were North Carolina (159 cases), Oklahoma (71 cases), Tennessee (58 cases), and Georgia (41 cases).[36]

The changes in the incidence and endemicity of RMSF have been attributed to cyclical changes in tick populations, changes in the virulence of infecting rickettsiae, and the process of suburbanization.[19,82,119] A convincing explanation, however, is still lacking.

RMSF is caused by *Rickettsia rickettsii*. Many species of ixodid ticks have been implicated as vectors of the disease,[24,98,119] but by far the most important in the United States are *Dermacentor andersoni*, the wood tick, and *Dermacentor variabilis*, the American dog tick. *D. andersoni* is the principal acarine host of *R. rickettsii* in the western United States and Canada; it feeds on virtually any available warm-blooded animal. *D. variabilis* is the primary host in the eastern United States and Canada. The domestic dog is the major host of adult *D. variabilis*, but the tick will feed on a variety of large and medium-sized animals. Nymphal and larval *D. variabilis* feed on various mice, voles, and rabbits. Serosurveys have indicated that a broad range of vertebrate hosts are infected with *R. rickettsii*, although not all sustain rickettsemia of sufficient magnitude to transmit the infection to feeding ticks. *R. rickettsii* occurrence in the United States does not depend on the presence of any given order of mammal.[119]

Domestic dogs become infected with *R. rickettsii* and may become acutely ill with fever and rash. Dogs probably do not play an important role in the amplification cycle of RMSF, but may be important in transporting infected ticks into proximity to humans.[24] Several studies have shown an association between domestic dogs and RMSF.[24,77,116] An infected tick may detach from a dog and complete its engorgement on a human, thereby transmitting *R. rickettsii*. Alternatively, infection through abraded skin or conjunctivae may occur during manual deticking of dogs.

Transmission by a tick vector delimits the clinical epidemiology of RMSF. It is a seasonal disease occurring when ticks are active—95% of the cases in the United States occur between April 1 and September 30, and the majority occur in May, June, and July. RMSF also tends to be focally endemic with a high proportion of cases occurring in small, circumscribed areas. This may be the clinical expression of "islands" of infected ticks.[116] It is more common in males (60%) and young people (50% less than 20 years of age), who are more likely to be exposed to tick habitats.[212]

Clinical manifestations. RMSF ranges from mild, even subclinical, illness[115] to fulminant disease with vascular collapse and death occurring within 3 to 6 days of onset. The incubation period ranges from 2 to 14 days, with severe disease associated with a shorter incubation period. Typically there is a sudden onset of fever, chills, headache, and myalgias. The fever is usually high (greater than 39° C), and myalgias and headache may be severe. The most characteristic feature, the rash, usually develops 2 to 5 days after the onset of illness. Other signs and symptoms, including abdominal pain, vomiting, diarrhea, confusion, conjunctivitis, and peripheral edema, are common (Table 33-5).

The rash in RMSF results from injury to dermal capillaries and small blood vessels. It typically develops first on the wrists, hands, ankles, and feet, spreading rapidly in centripetal fashion to cover most of the body, including the palms, soles, and face. Initially the lesions are pink macules, 2 to 5 mm in diameter, which readily blanch with pressure. After 2 to 3 days the lesions become fixed, darker red, papular, and finally petechial. The hemorrhagic lesions may coalesce to form large areas of ecchymoses. In its classic form, the rash occurring during the summer months in an endemic area is almost pathognomonic for RMSF. Unfortunately, it is often absent on initial patient presentation, making diagnosis more difficult. The rash usually develops within 2 to 5 days of the onset of illness, but its onset is delayed in approximately 10% of patients.[83] In an additional 10% to 15% of laboratory-confirmed cases of RMSF, no rash is noted

Table 33-5 Clinical Findings in Rocky Mountain Spotted Fever

Clinical Finding	Percent of Cases
Fever	99
Headache	80-90
Any rash	85-90
Myalgias	70-85
Petechial rash	45-60
Nausea and vomiting	56-60
Abdominal pain	34-50
Conjunctivitis	30
Stupor	21-37
Diarrhea	19-20
Edema	18
Meningismus	17-18
Splenomegaly	14-29
Hepatomegaly	12-15
Pneumonitis	13-17
Coma	10
Jaundice	8-9
Seizures	8

("spotless" fever).[64,82,84] In other patients it is evanescent, occurring only with fever spikes.

Neurologic involvement in RMSF ranges from mild headache to serious focal or generalized disorders of cerebral function. Headache is very common. Meningismus occasionally develops but does not correlate well with cerebrospinal fluid findings, which may be normal or show modest protein elevation and pleocytosis of both lymphocytes and polymorphonuclear cells (usually 8 to 35 cells/cm³).[125] Cerebral vasculitis may manifest with focal neurologic deficits, which are quite variable but usually transient.[16,125] Seizures may develop during the acute phase of the illness but rarely persist.[78,125] Lethargy and confusion are common and may progress to stupor or profound coma. Generalized cerebral dysfunction may be secondary to vasculitic lesions, especially in the reticular network of the brainstem, or to toxicity from severe rickettsial infection (fever, hypotension, hyponatremia, and thrombocytopenia with intracranial hemorrhage).[16,125] Children with RMSF who develop coma have an increased risk of subsequent behavioral disturbances and learning disabilities.[78]

Myocarditis is frequently found at necropsy in fatal RMSF; however, the clinical significance of the cardiac involvement is unclear. Pathologic study shows a patchy, interstitial, mononuclear infiltrate that appears to coincide with the distribution of rickettsiae in myocardial capillaries, venules, and arterioles.[222] Abnormal left ventricular function can frequently be demonstrated echocardiographically in hospitalized patients,[60,112] but overt clinical manifestations of left ventricular dysfunction are uncommon and hypotension and pulmonary edema are generally attributable to noncardiogenic causes. Cardiac enlargement rarely may be seen on chest radiographs.[102,113] Electrocardiographic abnormalities include nonspecific ST-T changes, conduction abnormalities (primarily first-degree atrioventricular block), and arrhythmias (paroxysmal atrial tachycardia, nodal tachycardia, and atrial fibrillation).[113] Most patients have complete resolution of cardiac abnormalities with clinical improvement, but persistent echocardiographic abnormalities have been noted.[112]

Infection of the pulmonary microcirculation by *R. rickettsii* results in interstitial pneumonitis and increased pulmonary vascular permeability. Although pulmonary involvement is not usually a prominent aspect of RMSF, a significant number of patients complain of cough, chest pain, dyspnea, or coryza.[48] Patchy infiltrates may occasionally be seen on chest radiographs, and in severe cases noncardiogenic pulmonary edema may develop with potential progression to ARDS.[48,102,162]

Gastrointestinal symptoms are common in RMSF and are prominent complaints in some patients. At autopsy, rickettsial vascular lesions are found throughout the gastrointestinal tract and pancreas, although actual necrosis appears to be a rare event.[146] Occasionally RMSF presents as an acute abdomen, suggesting appendicitis or cholecystitis.[220]

In the kidneys a focal perivascular interstitial nephritis is concentrated near the corticomedullary junction. Clinically, however, significant renal involvement is usually caused by prerenal azotemia or acute tubular necrosis following a hypotensive episode.[221]

In late stages of the disease, diffuse vasculitic lesions cause increased systemic capillary permeability leading to hypovolemia and vascular collapse. Disseminated intravascular coagulation (DIC), metabolic acidosis, and cardiorespiratory dysfunction may ensue and often presage death.

Diagnosis and treatment. In the prechemotherapy era, RMSF was frequently a fatal disease. Even with effective antibiotic agents the mortality rate remains approximately 5%.[63,83] Patients older than 30 years, males, and nonwhites are at higher risk.[63,82,83] Elderly patients appear more likely to have a severe course of illness and to have atypical features, including delayed or absent rash.[130] In susceptible individuals, such as those with glucose-6-phosphate dehydrogenase (G-6-PD) deficiency, RMSF may be fulminant and rapidly fatal.[219]

The most significant factor in deaths from RMSF is delay in diagnosis and initiation of appropriate antibiotic therapy. Unfortunately, early diagnosis in RMSF is often difficult. The classic triad of rash, fever, and tick bite is actually rare during the first 3 days of illness,[84] and confirmatory laboratory evidence is usually lacking early in the disease. Factors commonly leading to delay in diagnosis include absence or late appearance of the rash, lack of a history of tick bite or tick exposure, and nonspecific or unexpected initial symptoms leading to an incorrect initial diagnosis.

The diagnosis of RMSF must generally be made on clinical grounds, which requires careful consideration of epidemiologic data and both typical and atypical clinical findings. RMSF should be suspected and antibiotic treatment strongly considered in any patient who resides in or has recently visited an endemic area during the summer months and who has fever, headache, and myalgias even in the absence of a rash. Symptoms referable to the pulmonary, gastrointestinal, and central nervous systems commonly occur in RMSF and should not delay diagnosis.

The differential diagnosis of RMSF is extensive and includes meningococcemia, measles, enteroviral infections, leptospirosis, and murine typhus. Meningococcemia may be impossible to differentiate initially, but chloramphenicol is effective therapy for both diseases. The rash of atypical measles may mimic that of RMSF.[135]

Routine laboratory values are nonspecific but may provide some clues to diagnosis. Thrombocytopenia has been reported in over 50% of patients in some series,[219] although the actual incidence may be closer to 35%.[82,84] Hyponatremia is also common and is probably a result of antidiuretic hormone (ADH) secretion in response to intravascular volume depletion.[95] Other laboratory abnormalities include azotemia, hypoalbuminemia, and elevated bilirubin level and liver function tests.

Laboratory confirmation of RMSF has generally relied on serologic techniques detecting antibody increases in paired sera. Even with the most sensitive tests, antibody rises are not seen until 5 to 6 days after the onset of symptoms; early antibiotic therapy may delay titers even longer.[140] The widely used Weil-Felix test is neither sensitive nor specific for RMSF and should not be relied on where other tests are available. The complement fixation test is widely available but also lacks sensitivity.[140] False-positive results can occur during pregnancy with latex agglutination assays.[226] The most sensitive and specific serologic tests currently in use appear to be the IFA and indirect hemagglutination tests.[93]

The most promising method for early laboratory diagnosis of RMSF is immunofluorescent identification of *R. rickettsii* in biopsy specimens of the skin rash. Rickettsiae have been identified as early as the fourth day of illness with this method.[236]

Mortality is largely eliminated in RMSF by early treatment with tetracycline or chloramphenicol. In severe cases supportive therapy is also essential to a favorable outcome. Fluid replacement is critical in the hypotensive patient but must be monitored closely because of the risk of fluid extravasation through damaged vessels. Measurement of pulmonary capillary wedge pressures with a Swan-Ganz catheter may be necessary, especially if pulmonary edema develops. Use of corticosteroids has not been adequately evaluated, but may be beneficial in patients with widespread vasculitis or encephalitis.[121,235]

Prophylactic use of antibiotics after a tick bite is not recommended because of the low incidence of infection and risk of adverse reactions. Routinely testing ticks for rickettsial antigen has been evaluated but found to be of no benefit.[163]

Eastern Spotted Fever. Three other diseases in the spotted fever group are transmitted to humans by tick bite: Mediterranean spotted fever (MSF), North Asian tick typhus, and Queensland tick typhus. The three diseases closely resemble one another and have many similarities to RMSF. Generally, the course of illness in all three is milder than in RMSF, although complications and death may occur in susceptible patients. They are characterized by the abrupt onset of fever, headache, and malaise following a short (5 to 7 days) incubation period. Unlike in RMSF, a primary lesion (eschar, tache noire) is often present at the site of the tick bite and may be associated with regional lymphadenitis. The lesion is classically a small ulcer, 2 to 5 mm in diameter, with a black center and red areola. A rash that varies from maculopapular to petechial usually develops 3 to 5 days after the onset of illness. Untreated, the fever and other symptoms resolve after several days to 2 weeks. Treatment with tetracycline or chloramphenicol significantly shortens the course of illness and, if instituted early, prevents complications.

MSF is caused by *Rickettsii conorii* and has been described under various names, often reflecting its geographic occurrence: Marseille fever, South African tick bite fever, Kenya tick bite fever, India tick typhus, and Boutonneuse fever. As the names indicate, it is endemic in areas bordering the Mediterranean Sea, as well as parts of Africa and India. The major vector of MSF in the Mediterranean countries is the dog tick *Rhipicephalus sanguineus.* Several tick species have been implicated as vectors in other areas: *Haemaphysalis leachi* (Kenya, South Africa), *Rhipicephalus simus, Dermacentor reticulatus,* and *Ixodes hexagonos.*[58] All stages of *R. sanguineus* occasionally attach to humans, and dogs may be important in transporting the ticks into the vicinity of humans.[216]

Like other SFG diseases, MSF occurs during the warm weather months. Seasonal occurrence, geographic location, and the presence of a tache noire (noted in 50% to 75% of cases)[128,148] are the most helpful criteria for early diagnosis. Although the disease is usually mild in children and young adults, a malignant form resembling severe RMSF has been described.[149,218]

The elderly, alcoholics, and patients with G-6-PD deficiency appear particularly at risk.[143,149] The diagnosis can be confirmed by specific serologic testing or by immunofluorescent demonstration of *R. conorii* in cutaneous lesions.[147]

North Asian tick typhus or Siberian tick typhus is endemic throughout Siberia, from European Russia to the Soviet Far East. It is seen primarily in agricultural areas and is closely associated with steppe landscapes.[25] The causative organism, *Rickettsia siberica,* is transmitted to humans by several species of *Dermacentor* and *Haemaphysalis* ticks. In the natural cycle, adult ticks feed on large wild and domestic animals, especially cattle and dogs. As for other SFG rickettsiae, humans are accidental and dead-end hosts.

Queensland tick typhus is caused by *Rickettsia australis.* It is endemic to southern and northern Queensland, and the major vector is the scrub tick, *Ixodes holocyclus.*[25] Both Queensland tick typhus and North Asian tick typhus are benign illnesses of mild-to-moderate severity with typical rickettsial manifestations: fever, headache, variable appearance of an eschar at the site of the tick bite, and a rash.

Spotted fever group rickettsiosis also occurs in Japan, where the causative agent appears to be a distinct serotype of spotted fever group rickettsiae.[211]

Q Fever. Q fever is a worldwide zoonosis affecting both wild and domestic animals. It was first described in 1937 as an occupational disease of abattoir workers and dairy farmers in Australia.[46] Aerosol spread of *Coxiella burnetii,* the causative organism, is the usual mode of transmission to humans. Although ticks may become infected with *C. burnetii* after feeding on an infected vertebrate, tick-borne transmission to humans appears to be very rare.

The most common clinical presentation of Q fever is an influenza-like illness with fever, headache, myalgias, and pneumonitis. Abnormal liver function tests, jaundice, and hepatomegaly may develop. In most patients the illness resolves spontaneously within 2 to 4 weeks of onset; tetracycline (500 mg orally four times a day) hastens the resolution.

Q fever may also be a chronic infection, with or without a history of an acute episode. Granulomatous hepatitis and culture-negative endocarditis are the chronic forms of the disease. Endocarditis most commonly involves the aortic valve, but others, including prosthetic valves, may be affected.[72]

Diagnosis of Q fever depends primarily on serologic testing. Two specific complement-fixing antibodies, phase 1 and phase 2, develop after infection with *C. burnetii.* In patients with acute Q fever, phase 2 antibody is usually detectable by the second week of illness; phase 1 is not detectable. The finding of phase 1 antibody indicates chronic infection.

Treatment of chronic Q fever is not always successful. Patients probably need to be treated with tetracycline for at least 12 months.[52] Some authors recommend adding another drug, such as lincomycin or cotrimazole, but their efficacy is unproven.[66,217]

Ehrlichia Infections. Ehrlichiae are tick-borne rickettsial organisms that cause disease in humans and animals throughout the world. *Ehrlichia sennetsu* was isolated in Japan in 1954 and causes an infectious mononucleosis–like syndrome.[126] *Ehrlichia canis,* which causes an illness in dogs, was associated with human illness in the United States by Maeda and colleagues in 1987.[64,108] However, subsequent investigations have concluded that ehrlichiosis in the United States is caused by *Ehrlichia chaffeensis,* a closely related species.[7]

Ehrlichiosis has been reported in over 20 states, but most cases occur in the south central and southern Atlantic states (Oklahoma, Missouri, Virginia, Georgia).[119] Both *Dermacentor variabilis* and *Amblyomma americanum* have been implicated as vectors for the disease, but further work is needed to fully characterize the host-vector relationships for *E. chaffeensis.*[8] Patients with ehrlichiosis tend to be older than patients with RMSF, and males contract the disease more commonly than females. Over 70% of cases occur between May and July.

Human ehrlichiosis has a broad clinical spectrum ranging from a subclinical infection to a mild viral-like illness to a life-threatening disease. Most patients report a tick bite or tick exposure before the onset of illness. After an average incubation period of 7 days (range 1 to 21 days), a high fever, headache, chills or rigors, malaise, myalgia, and anorexia typically develop. A rash, which may be maculopapular or petechial, develops in 20% to 40% of patients, a median of 8 days after the onset of illness.[120] The rash appears to be more common in children than adults.[15]

Severe and even fatal complications develop in some patients and are more likely in older persons. Respiratory complications may be relatively common; cough, pulmonary infiltrates, dypsnea, and respiratory failure have all been reported. Other serious complications include encephalopathy and renal failure.

Leukopenia and thrombocytopenia are common during the first week of illness, as are elevated alanine and aspartate aminotransferase values. These abnormalities are usually mild and of short duration.[53a] A lymphocytic cerebrospinal fluid pleocytosis is often present in patients with encephalopathy.

As with RMSF, the diagnosis of ehrlichiosis depends on clinical findings. Serologic tests can be used to confirm the diagnosis. Indirect immunofluorescent antibody testing against *E. chaffeensis* is now available from the Centers for Disease Control and Prevention. Antibody levels rise rapidly during the first 3 weeks and peak after approximately 6 weeks.

Controlled trials of antibiotic therapy have not been conducted for ehrlichiosis. However, tetracycline (or doxycycline) appears to be effective. Chloramphenicol has been used to treat ehrlichiosis, but treatment failures have been reported, and *E. chaffeensis* is resistant to chloramphenicol in vitro.[22] Rifampin is bactericidal against *E. chaffeensis* in vitro, but no published experience with its use in treating human ehrlichiosis is available. Currently tetracycline (doxycycline) should be considered the drug of choice for ehrlichiosis. The optimal dosage and duration of treatment have not been established, but 5 to 10 days of therapy is usually sufficient.

TICK-BORNE VIRAL DISEASES

Ticks transmit a wide variety of viruses to humans. Like other tick-borne diseases, the viral illnesses are zoonotic. Ticks ingest the organisms while feeding on a viremic host; the virus replicates within the tick and is passed transstadially. Transovarial transmission has been documented for tick-borne encephalitis virus and Crimean-Congo hemorrhagic fever virus; the role of transovarial passage in maintaining these viruses in nature is unknown.[87] Amplification occurs when the infected tick feeds on an uninfected vertebrate. Humans usually are accidentally infected after intrusion into the natural tick-vertebrate cycle.

Tick-borne viruses cause clinical syndromes in humans that can be classified into four broad groups: influenza-like febrile illness with malaise, headache, myalgias, and arthralgias; febrile illness with hemorrhagic complications; febrile illness associated with meningoencephalitis; and subclinical or very mild illness. A specific virus may produce any or all of these syndromes depending on the virulence of the organism, host susceptibility, and the stage of the illness.

For example, Colorado tick fever (CTF) virus usually causes an influenza-like febrile illness, but in susceptible hosts it may produce meningoencephalitis or, rarely, a hemorrhagic diathesis.

Diagnosis of tick-borne viral diseases relies on the clinical acumen of the physician and requires interpretation of epidemiologic and clinical information. Isolation of the virus, usually by intracerebral inoculation in suckling mice, or demonstration of a rise in antibody titers, confirms the diagnosis. As with most viral diseases, treatment is primarily supportive.

Only CTF occurs with any frequency in the United States. Other tick-borne viruses are listed in Table 33-6.

Colorado Tick Fever

A small RNA virus of the genus *Orbivirus,* family Reoviridae, causes CTF. Endemic to mountain or highland regions of the western United States and Canada, its distribution largely corresponds to that of the major vector *Dermacentor andersoni.* However, CTF virus has been found in small mammals in California outside the known range of *D. andersoni,* suggesting that other tick species are capable of transmitting the virus.[99]

CTF virus is maintained in its natural cycle by transmission between ticks and rodents.[122] Larval stages of *D. andersoni* ingest the virus while feeding on a viremic rodent host and pass it transstadially. Hibernating nymphs and adults carry the virus through the winter. Infected ticks emerge in the spring and feed on susceptible animals, renewing the cycle. Nymphal and adult ticks may also acquire the virus by feeding on viremic hosts. The virus does not appear to cause disease in its natural hosts[122]; humans are incidental and "dead-end" hosts.

CTF is usually a benign, self-limited febrile illness. Over 200 cases of CTF are reported annually in the United States, but the actual incidence is probably much higher; many cases are not brought to medical attention or are diagnosed simply as a viral illness. It is a seasonal disease occurring from late March to early October, with a peak incidence in May and June. All age groups are susceptible to CTF, but it occurs most commonly in young men, reflecting their greater recreational and occupational activities in outdoor mountain areas. A history of tick exposure can be obtained in approximately 90% of patients with CTF; the usual time between the tick bite and the onset of symptoms is 3 to 6 days (range 0 to 14 days).[76,181]

CTF usually begins with the abrupt onset of fever. Most patients experience severe headaches, myalgias, and lethargy; complaints of photophobia, ocular pain, anorexia, nausea and vomiting, and abdominal pain are common.[76] A macular or maculopapular rash is reported in 5% to 12% of patients but is not a prominent feature.[76,181] The most characteristic feature of the illness is a biphasic or "saddle-backed" temperature pattern. Patients initially experience 2 to 3 days of fever, followed by a 1- to 2-day remission, and then an additional 2 to 3 days of fever. This pattern is helpful when present but cannot be relied on for diagnosis, since it is observed in only about 50% of patients.[76,181]

CTF is usually mild, but severe complications do occur, particularly in children under the age of 10. Meningoencephalitis has been described in several children,[33,49,175,181] and at least two cases have been reported in which a child developed a hemorrhagic diathesis leading to death.[76] Other unusual complications associated with CTF include pericarditis,[85] myocarditis,[53] hepatitis,[103] epididymoorchitis,[76] and pneumonitis.[76] Information on CTF contracted during pregnancy is inconclusive, but of five cases reported, one terminated in a spontaneous abortion and in another a liveborn infant had multiple congenital anomalies.[127] CTF virus is teratogenic in mice.[81]

Nearly half the patients with CTF require 3 weeks or longer to recover fully from the illness. The most common persistent symptoms are malaise and weakness. Prolonged symptoms occur most frequently in patients over age 30.[76] Treatment of CTF is supportive; infection generally confers lifelong immunity.

CTF virus circulates free in the plasma and bone marrow of infected patients until the end of the first week of illness, when it is neutralized by antibodies. In the bone marrow the virus infects erythrocyte precursors and persists within mature erythrocytes, where it is protected from antibodies. This allows viremia to persist for a prolonged period, even when clinical recovery is complete. Infective virus can be recovered from the blood for a month or longer in nearly 50% of patients.[76] Persistent viremia in blood donors poses a risk to recipients of blood transfusions; transfusion-acquired infection has been reported.[36]

Other hemopoietic cells may also be affected in CTF. Leukopenia involving both granulocytes and lymphocytes is

Table 33-6 Tick-Borne Viral Diseases

Virus	Taxonomic Group	Major Vector	Animal Hosts	Geographic Distribution	Human Illness	Frequency of Recognized Disease	Risk Factors
Colorado tick fever	Reoviridae, genus *Orbivirus*	*Dermacentor andersoni*	Rodents, other small mammals	Mountain highland areas of western United States and Canada	Biphasic FI, ME especially in children, prolonged viremia	Sporadic, common in endemic areas	Occupational and recreational pursuits in mountain areas
Kemerovo	Reoviridae, genus *Orbivirus*	*Ixodes ricinus, I. persulcatus*	Domestic and wild mammals, birds	Siberia, Czechoslovakia	Mild FI, occasional ME, not fatal	Sporadic, rare	Occupational and recreational pursuits in forested areas
TICK-BORNE ENCEPHALITIS COMPLEX							
Powassan encephalitis	Togaviridae, genus *Flavivirus* ↓ (Powassan through Omsk hemorrhagic fever)	*I. marxi, I. cookei*	Small mammals	Northern United States, Canada	FI, ME—sequelae and death may occur, especially in young children	Sporadic, rare	Rural areas, pets?
Louping-ill		*I. ricinus*	Sheep, cattle, grouse	Great Britain	Biphasic ME, sequelae uncommon	Rare in humans	Shepherds, laboratory workers
Tick-borne encephalitis		*I. ricinus*	Goats, sheep, cattle, small mammals	Central and eastern Europe	Biphasic ME	Sporadic, common in endemic areas	Agricultural and forestry workers, drinking goats' milk
Russian spring-summer encephalitis		*I. ricinus, I. persulcatus*	Goats, sheep, cattle, small mammals	Siberia	Biphasic ME, may be severe, with 20% case fatality	Sporadic, common in endemic areas	Agricultural and forestry workers
Kyasanur Forest disease		*Haemaphysalis spinigera*	Monkeys, small mammals	Southern India	FI, ME, hemorrhagic complications may develop	Sporadic, epidemics occur	Residence in or travel to endemic areas
Omsk hemorrhagic fever		*? Dermacentor pictus*	Muskrats	Western Siberia	FI, hemorrhagic complications	Rare	Direct contact with muskrats
Crimean-Congo hemorrhagic fever	Bunyaviridae, genus *Nairovirus*	*Hyalomma marginatum, H. anatolicum,* others	Domestic and wild mammals	Southern USSR, Middle East, India, Pakistan, Central Africa	FI, petechial-ecchymotic rash, hemorrhage, case fatality 3%-30%	Sporadic, epidemics occur	Agricultural workers
Dugbe	Bunyaviridae, genus *Nairovirus*	Ixodid species	Cattle	Nigeria, Central African Republic	Acute FI	Rare, primarily children	Herding or caring for livestock
Bhanja	Probably Bunyaviridae	Ixodid species	Domestic and mammals	Yugoslavia, Italy, Kenya, Nigeria, India	FI, ME	Rare	Agricultural workers
Thogoto	Possibly Orthomyxoviridae	Ixodid species	Ruminants	Egypt, Kenya, Nigeria	FI, ME, optic neuritis	Rare	Herding or caring for livestock
Quaranfil	Unclassified	*Argas arboreus*	Pigeons, wild birds	Africa, Iran, Afghanistan	FI	Rare	Residence in endemic areas

FI, Febrile illness; *ME*, meningoencephalitis.

common and may be helpful diagnostically, although one third of patients have normal leukocyte counts.[79] Thrombocytopenia may also develop; anemia associated with the virus is rare.

Isolation of CTF virus from blood or cerebrospinal fluid by inoculating suckling mice or cell cultures confirms the diagnosis. A fluorescent conjugate prepared against CTF viral antigen can be used to stain erythrocyte smears, but the test lacks sensitivity.[76] Serologic tests are available (neutralizing antibody, complement fixation, IFA), but titers rise slowly and are not generally diagnostic during the clinical illness.

BABESIOSIS

Babesia, like malarial organisms, are intraerythrocytic protozoan parasites. Over 70 distinct species have been described from various vertebrate hosts.[154] Some of the most important species include *B. bigemina, B. bovis,* and *B. divergens* (all in cattle); *B. caballi* and *B. equi* (horses); *B. canis* (dogs); and *B. microti* (rodents). *Babesia* are transmitted to vertebrates primarily via the bite of ixodid ticks.

Epidemiology

Babesiosis has been recognized as an important veterinary disease for many years, but human disease was originally limited to rare reports of infection in splenectomized individuals. Five cases of human infection with bovine *Babesia (B. bovis, B. divergens)* were reported from Europe between 1957 and 1976; two cases of babesiosis of unknown species were reported from California in 1968 and 1981; a human case of *B. gibsoni* infection was reported in California in 1993; and a single *B. caucasia* infection was reported from the USSR in 1978.[91,154,155] These cases were widely separated geographically, and all occurred in splenectomized individuals.

Since 1970 the incidence of human babesiosis has accelerated, primarily because of an outbreak of *B. microti* infections in the northeast United States; since 1968 over 450 confirmed cases have occurred in the United States.[40,123] *B. microti* is endemic to the coastal regions of southern New England, where the principal vector is the northern deer tick *Ixodes scapularis.* Most cases are contracted on Cape Cod and the offshore islands of Massachusetts (Nantucket, Martha's Vineyard), New York (Shelter Island, Long Island), and Rhode Island (Block Island).[40] Cases have also been reported from Wisconsin, a known focus of *I. scapularis.*[204] The high incidence of *B. microti* infection is caused by its ability to produce disease in individuals with intact spleens. Recently a distinct but as yet unidentified species of *Babesia* was isolated from an immunocompetent patient with an intact spleen in Washington State.[144]

The ecology of *B. microti* parallels that of *Borrelia burgdorferi,* the agent of Lyme disease. The major vector in both diseases is *Ixodes scapularis.* White-footed mice *(Peromyscus leucopus)* constitute the major reservoir for *B. microti.* Larval or nymphal ticks ingest the parasite during a blood meal from an infected rodent. *Babesia* replicate within the tick and are passed transstadially; unlike *Borrelia burgdorferi,* no evidence for transovarial passage is available. Amplification of the cycle occurs when the infected tick transmits the organism to a vertebrate host during the next blood meal. White-tailed deer *(Odocoileus virginianus)* are the principal hosts for adult ticks; larvae and nymphs feed on deer, mice, and other small mammals.[179]

Human babesiosis occurs when humans accidentally intrude on the natural cycle and are bitten by an infected tick. Like other tick-borne diseases, the peak incidence is during the warm weather months from May to September, when ticks are actively feeding.

Pathogenesis

Ticks inoculate *Babesia* into vertebrate hosts when taking a blood meal. The organisms rapidly invade erythrocytes and multiply asexually by asynchronous budding. The predominant forms are ring-shaped and ameboid trophozoites, but great pleomorphism is displayed.[209] After the parasite multiplies, the infected erythrocyte ruptures, freeing the organisms to invade other red blood cells; a severe hemolytic anemia may ensue. Despite extensive study the mechanism of hemolysis in babesiosis remains unknown.

Prolonged parasitemia is common in babesiosis.[157] Persistence of *B. microti* for as long as 4 months in an otherwise healthy patient has been demonstrated.[229] Parasitemia may persist after clinical recovery or may develop in asymptomatic individuals. Prolonged, subclinical infection creates the potential for transmission of *B. microti* through blood donation; several cases of transfusion-acquired babesiosis have been reported.[98,111,176,234]

The presence of an intact spleen appears to play an important role in resistance to *Babesia* organisms. Although the presence of a spleen is not protective against *B. microti,* the disease is often more severe or fatal in splenectomized patients. Age also appears to be an important factor in susceptibility to babesiosis. Children and young adults usually have subclinical or mild, self-limited infections, whereas older adults are more likely to have severe, clinically apparent disease.[17,159] Chronic medical disorders may be an additional risk factor for severe babesiosis.[18]

Clinical Manifestations

Acute *B. microti* infection is characterized by the gradual onset of malaise, anorexia, and fatigue followed within several days to a week by fever, sweats, and myalgias. Other, less common symptoms include headache, nausea and vomiting, depression, and shaking chills. Most patients do not recall a tick bite, and rash is not a feature of the illness. Physical examination is usually normal except for fever and mild splenomegaly in some patients. Laboratory evaluation reveals a mild-to-moderate hemolytic anemia; normal to slightly reduced leukocyte counts; and, in some patients mild-to-moderate thrombocytopenia. Serum LDH and bilirubin levels are mildly elevated in most patients, reflecting the hemolytic anemia.[75,157]

Although most patients with spleens recover without specific therapy, prolonged fatigue and malaise are common.[157] Splenectomized patients generally have more severe clinical disease with higher levels of parasitemia and more severe hemolytic anemia.[159] Recovery, however, is the rule.

Clinical infection with *B. divergens* or *B. bovis* has been reported only in splenectomized patients. The illness is characterized by high fever, chills, headache, and severe hemolytic anemia, often resulting in hemoglobinuria, jaundice, and renal insufficiency. Major findings on physical examination include fever, hepatomegaly, jaundice, and hypotension. Most human infections with bovine *Babesia* have been fatal.[154]

Only one case of human babesiosis during pregnancy has been reported to date.[150] The patient recovered without specific therapy, and the infant did not develop babesiosis. Cases of intrauterine infection in animals, however, have been reported.

Diagnosis

The diagnosis of babesiosis can be confirmed by identifying the intraerythrocytic parasites on thick or thin Giemsa-stained blood smears. Patients with intact spleens usually have low levels of parasitemia (less than 5% parasites), so that examination of repeated smears may be necessary.[75,157] The predominant forms of *B. microti* closely resemble the small rings of *Plasmodium* species. A later tetrad form may be seen and is positive morphologic evidence of babesiosis. Differentiating *Babesia* from *Plasmodium* may be difficult but should be possible by noting the absence of pigment deposits in erythrocytes parasitized with the older stages of *Plasmodium* species.

In cases in which organisms cannot be detected on blood smears, the diagnosis can made by intraperitoneal inoculation of the patient's blood into splenectomized hamsters. Serologic studies may also be helpful in confirming the diagnosis[158] but are performed in only a few laboratories. No test for circulating *Babesia* antigen is available.

Treatment and Prevention

Treatment of babesiosis with antimalarial agents such as chloroquine and quinacrine has shown limited or no efficacy. Clinical improvement occurred in patients treated with the antitrypanosomal drug pentamidine, but it did not eradicate the parasitemia, and side effects were significant.[65] The combination of quinine (650 mg) and clindamycin (600 mg), both given every 6 hours, has been shown to be effective in patients with severe disease.[41] Parasites appear to be eradicated from the blood with this therapy, although a treatment failure has been reported.[176] In seriously ill patients with high levels of parasitemia, exchange transfusion may also produce rapid clinical improvement.[90,209] Many patients with babesiosis, however, have a mild clinical illness and recover without specific anti-*Babesia* chemotherapy. Currently, treatment is recommended only for seriously ill patients.[41]

Avoidance of ticks is the only currently effective method of preventing babesiosis. Splenectomized patients should probably be advised to avoid visiting areas endemic for babesiosis.

Prevention and Prophylaxis

Prevention of tick-borne diseases is directed toward preventing tick bites. Protective clothing (long pants cinched at the ankles or tucked into boots or socks) should be worn when in tick-infested areas. Spraying clothes with an insect repellent may provide an additional barrier against ticks. Most repellents contain *N,N*-diethyl-meta-toluamide (DEET), which repels ticks but does not kill them. A new tick repellent, Permanone, is an aerosol spray for use on clothing. Its active ingredient, permethrin, kills ticks on contact. Field tests have shown Permanone to be 90% to 100% effective in preventing tick bites. Permethrins as a class have very low toxicity in mammals.

Close and regular (at least twice daily) inspection of all parts of the body should be performed when traveling in tick-infested areas. Adult ixodid ticks are generally on the body for an hour or two before attaching. Even after a tick attaches, disease transmission may be prevented by prompt removal. Proper removal of the tick is important, since infection may be acquired by careless handling of infected ticks, even without a bite. The tick should be grasped as close to the skin surface as possible with blunt curved forceps, tweezers, or fingers protected with tissue. The tick should be pulled out with steady pressure, taking care not to crush or squeeze the body, since expressed fluid may contain infective agents. After the tick is removed, the bite site should be disinfected. Traditional methods of tick removal, such as applying fingernail polish, isopropyl alcohol, or a hot match head, do not effect tick detachment and may induce the tick to salivate or regurgitate into the wound.[134]

In general, prophylactic antibiotics are not recommended for tick bites. Clinical trials of antibiotic prophylaxis for RMSF or Lyme disease demonstrate that the risk of infection in a patient who seeks medical treatment for a tick bite is very low. In most areas of the country the chances are small that a tick harbors an infectious agent. Even if the tick is infected, the agent probably will not be transmitted if the tick is found and removed promptly. Added together, these facts suggest that the risk/benefit ratio of an adverse reaction to the antibiotic versus disease prevention will be high.

REFERENCES

1. Abbott KH: Tick paralysis: a review, *Proc Mayo Clin* 18:39, 1943.
2. Ackermann R et al: *Ixodes ricinus* spirochete and European erythema chronicum migrans disease, *Yale J Biol Med* 57:573, 1984.

2a. Ackermann R et al: Chronic neurologic manifestations of erythema migrans borreliosis, *Ann NY Acad Sci* 539:16, 1988.

3. Ackley A, Lupovici M: Lyme-disease meningitis treated with tetracycline, *Ann Intern Med* 105:630, 1986.
4. Afzelius A: Erythema chronicum migrans, *Acta Derm Venereol* 2:120, 1921.
5. Agger WA, Callister SM, Jobe DA: In vitro susceptibilities of *Borrelia burgdorferi* to five oral cephalosporins and ceftriaxone, *Antimicrob Agents Chemother* 36:1788, 1992.
6. Agre F, Schwartz R: The value of early treatment of deer tick bites for the prevention of Lyme disease, *Am J Dis Child* 147:945, 1993.
7. Anderson BE et al: *Ehrlichia chaffeensis,* a new species associated with human ehrlichiosis, *J Clin Microbiol* 29:2838, 1991.
8. Anderson BE et al: Detection of the etiologic agent of human ehrlichiosis by polymerase chain reaction, *J Clin Microbiol* 30:775, 1992.
9. Asbrink E, Hovmark A: Lyme borreliosis: aspects of tick-borne *Borrelia burgdorferi* infection from a dermatologic viewpoint, *Semin Dermatol* 9:277, 1990.
10. Atlas E et al: Lyme myositis: muscle invasion by *Borrelia burgdorferi, Ann Intern Med* 108:245, 1988.
11. Banfield JF: Tick bites in man, *Med J Aust* 2:600, 1966.
12. Barbour AG: Molecular biology of antigenic variation in Lyme borreliosis and relapsing fever: a comparative analysis, *Scand J Infect Dis (Suppl)* 77:88, 1991.
13. Barbour AG, Fish D: The biological and social phenomenon of Lyme disease, *Science* 260:1610, 1993.
14. Barbour AG, Hayes SF: Biology of *Borrelia* species, *Microbiol Rev* 50:381, 1986.
15. Barton LL, Rathore MH, Dawson JE: Infection with *Ehrlichia* in childhood, *J Pediatr* 120:998, 1992.
16. Bell WE, Lascare AD: Rocky Mountain spotted fever, *Neurology* 20:841, 1970.
17. Benach JL, Habicht GS: Clinical characteristics of human babesiosis, *J Infect Dis* 144:481, 1981.
18. Benach JL, Habicht GS, Hamburger MI: Immunoresponsiveness in acute babesiosis in humans, *J Infect Dis* 146:369, 1982.
19. Benach JL et al: Changing patterns in the incidence of Rocky Mountain spotted fever on Long Island (1971-1976), *Am J Epidemiol* 106:380, 1977.
20. Benach JL et al: Spirochetes isolated from the blood of two patients with Lyme disease, *N Engl J Med* 308:740, 1983.
21. Bosler EM et al: Natural distribution of the *Ixodes dammini* spirochete, *Science* 220:321, 1983.
22. Brouqui P, Raoult D: In vitro antibiotic susceptibility of the newly recognized agent of ehrlichiosis in humans, *Ehrlichia chaffeensis, Antimicrob Agents Chemother* 36:2799, 1992.
23. Brown RN, Lane RS: Lyme disease in California: a novel enzootic transmission cycle of *Borrelia burgdorferi, Science* 256:1439, 1992.
24. Burgdorfer W: A review of Rocky Mountain spotted fever (tick-borne typhus), its agent, and its tick vectors in the United States, *J Med Entomol* 12:269, 1975.
25. Burgdorfer W: The spotted fever group diseases. In Steele JH, editor: *CRC handbook series in zoonoses, section A: bacterial, rickettsial, and mycotic diseases,* vol II, Boca Raton, Fla, 1980, CRC Press, pp 279-300.
26. Burgdorfer W: Discovery of the Lyme disease spirochete and its relation to tick vectors, *Yale J Biol Med* 57:515, 1984.
27. Burgdorfer W, Gage K: Susceptibility of the black-legged tick, *Ixodes scapularis,* to the Lyme disease spirochete, *Borrelia burgdorferi, Zbl Bakt Hyg* 263:15, 1986.
28. Burgdorfer W et al: Lyme disease—a tick-borne spirochetosis? *Science* 216:1317, 1982.
29. Burgdorfer W et al: The western black-legged tick, *Ixodes pacificus:* a vector of *Borrelia burgdorferi, Am J Trop Med Hyg* 34:925, 1985.
30. Butler T: Relapsing fever: new lessons about antibiotic action, *Ann Intern Med* 102:397, 1985.
31. Butler T, Jones PK, Wallace CK: *Borrelia recurrentis* infection: single-dose regimens and management of the Jarisch-Herxheimer reaction, *J Infect Dis* 137:573, 1978.
32. Centers for Disease Control: Relapsing fever, *MMWR* 22:242, 1973.
33. Centers for Disease Control: Transmission of Colorado tick fever virus by blood transfusion, *MMWR* 24:422, 1975.
34. Centers for Disease Control: Tick paralysis—Wisconsin, *MMWR* 30:217, 1981.
35. Centers for Disease Control: Update: Lyme disease and cases occurring during pregnancy—United States, *MMWR* 34:376, 1985.

35a. Centers for Disease Control: Rocky Mountain spotted fever—United States, 1985, *MMWR* 35:247, 1986.

36. Centers for Disease Control: Summaries of notifiable diseases in the United States, *MMWR* 40:1, 1991.
37. Centers for Disease Control: Lyme disease, 1991-1992, *MMWR* 42:345, 1993.
38. Clark JR et al: Facial paralysis in Lyme disease, *Laryngoscope* 95:1341, 1985.
39. Clements ML et al: Serodiagnosis of Rocky Mountain spotted fever: comparison of IgM and IgG enzyme-linked immunosorbent assays and indirect fluorescent antibody test, *J Infect Dis* 148:876, 1983.
40. Dammin GJ et al: The rising incidence of clinical *Babesia microti* infection, *Hum Pathol* 12:398, 1981.
41. Dammin GJ et al: Clindamycin and quinine treatment for *Babesia microti* infections, *MMWR* 32:65, 1983.
42. Dattwyler RJ et al: Ceftriaxone as effective therapy in refractory Lyme disease, *J Infect Dis* 155:1322, 1987.
43. Dattwyler RJ et al: Treatment of late Lyme borreliosis—randomized comparison of ceftriaxone and penicillin, *Lancet* 1:1191, 1988.
44. Davis GE: The relapsing fevers: tick-spirochete specificity studies, *Exp Parasitol* 1:406, 1952.
45. Davis RD, Burke JP, Wright LJ: Relapsing fever associated with ARDS in a parturient woman, *Chest* 102:630, 1992.
46. Derrick EH: Q fever, a new fever entity: clinical features, diagnosis and laboratory investigation, *Med J Aust* 2:281, 1937.
47. Donat JR, Donat JF: Tick paralysis with persistent weakness and electromyographic abnormalities, *Arch Neurol* 38:59, 1981.
48. Donohue JF: Lower respiratory tract involvement in Rocky Mountain spotted fever, *Arch Intern Med* 140:223, 1980.
49. Draughn DE, Sieber OF, Umlauf HJ: Colorado tick fever encephalitis, *Clin Pediatr* 4:626, 1965.
50. Dressler F et al: Western blotting in the serodiagnosis of Lyme disease, *J Infect Dis* 167:392, 1993.
51. Edell TA et al: Tick-borne relapsing fever in Colorado—historical review and report of cases, *JAMA* 241:2279, 1979.
52. Editorial: Chronic Q fever, *J Infect* 8:1, 1984.
53. Emmons RW, Schade HI: Colorado tick fever simulating acute myocardial infarction, *JAMA* 222:87, 1972.

53a. Eng TR et al: Epidemiologic, clinical, and laboratory findings of human ehrlichioses in the United States, 1988, *JAMA* 264:2251, 1990.

54. Failing RM, Lyon CB, McKittrick JE: The pajaroello tick bite—the frightening folklore and the mild disease, *Calif Med* 116:16, 1972.
55. Falco RC, Fish D: Prevalence of *Ixodes dammini* near the home of Lyme disease patients in Westchester county, New York, *Am J Epidemiol* 127:826-830, 1988.
56. Feder HM et al: Persistence of serum antibodies to *Borrelia burgdorferi* in patients treated for Lyme disease, *Clin Infect Dis* 15:788, 1992.
57. Feder HM et al: Early Lyme disease: a flu-like illness without erythema migrans, *Pediatrics* 91:456, 1993.

58. Feldman-Muhsam B: Ixodid tick attacks on man in Israel: medical implications, *Isr J Med Sci* 22:19, 1986.
59. Felsenfeld O: Borreliae, human relapsing fever, and parasite-vector-host relationships, *Bacteriol Rev* 29:46, 1965.
60. Feltes TF et al: M-mode echocardiographic abnormalities in Rocky Mountain spotted fever, *South Med J* 77:1130, 1984.
61. Fihn S, Larson EB: Tick-borne relapsing fever in the Pacific Northwest: an under-diagnosed illness? *West J Med* 133:203, 1980.
62. Finkel MJ, Halperin JJ: Nervous system Lyme borreliosis—revisited, *Arch Neurol* 49:102, 1992.
63. Fishbein DB et al: Surveillance of Rocky Mountain spotted fever in the United States, 1981-1983, *J Infect Dis* 150:609, 1984.
64. Fishbein DB et al: Unexplained febrile illnesses after exposure to ticks: infection with an *Ehrlichia? JAMA* 257:3100, 1987.
65. Francioli PB et al: Response of babesiosis to pentamidine therapy, *Ann Intern Med* 94:326, 1981.
66. Freeman R, Hodson ME: Q fever endocarditis treated with trimethoprim and sulphamethoxazole, *Br Med J* 1:419, 1972.
67. Furman DP, Loomis EC: The ticks of California, *Bull Calif Insect Survey* 25:13, 1984.
68. Garin C, Bujadoux: Paralysie par les tiques, *J Med Lyon* 3:765, 1922.
69. Gerber MA, Shapiro ED: Diagnosis of Lyme disease in children, *J Pediatr* 121:157, 1992.
70. Gerster JC et al: Lyme arthritis appearing outside the United States: a case report from Switzerland, *Br Med J* 283:951, 1981.
71. Goellner MH et al: Hepatitis due to recurrent Lyme disease, *Ann Intern Med* 108:707, 1988.
72. Goffin Y et al: Chronic Q fever, *Lancet* 1:1421, 1981.
73. Goldman L, Johnson P, Ramsey J: The insect bite reaction, *J Invest Dermatol* 18:403, 1984.
74. Golightly MG: Laboratory considerations in the diagnosis and management of Lyme borreliosis, *Clin Pathol* 99:168, 1992.
75. Gombert ME et al: Human babesiosis—clinical and therapeutic considerations, *JAMA* 248:3005, 1982.
76. Goodpasture HC et al: Colorado tick fever: clinical, epidemiologic, and laboratory aspects of 228 cases in Colorado in 1973-1974, *Ann Intern Med* 88:303, 1978.
77. Gordon JC et al: Epidemiology of Rocky Mountain spotted fever in Ohio, 1981: serologic evaluation of canines and rickettsial isolation from ticks associated with human case exposure sites, *Am J Trop Med Hyg* 33:1026, 1984.
78. Gorman RJ, Saxon S, Snead OC: Neurologic sequelae of Rocky Mountain spotted fever, *Pediatrics* 67:354, 1981.
79. Gorman RJ, Snead C: Tick paralysis in three children—the diversity of neurologic presentations, *Clin Pediatr* 17:249, 1978.
80. Gresikova M, Beran GW: Tick-borne encephalitis. In Steele JH, editor: *CRC handbook series of zoonoses, section B: viral zoonoses,* vol I, Boca Raton, Fla, 1981, CRC Press, p 201.
81. Harris RE, Morahan P, Coleman P: Teratogenic effects of Colorado tick fever virus in mice, *J Infect Dis* 131:397, 1975.
82. Hattwick MAW, O'Brien RJ, Hanson BF: Rocky Mountain spotted fever: epidemiology of an increasing problem, *Ann Intern Med* 84:732, 1976.
83. Hattwick MAW et al: Fatal Rocky Mountain spotted fever, *JAMA* 240:1499, 1978.
84. Helmick CG, Bernard KW, D'Angelo LJ: Rocky Mountain spotted fever: clinical, laboratory, and epidemiological features of 262 cases, *J Infect Dis* 150:480, 1984.
85. Hierholzer WJ, Barry DW: Colorado tick fever pericarditis (letter), *JAMA* 217:825, 1971.
86. Hoogstaal H: Tick-borne Crimean-Congo hemorrhagic fever. In Steele JH, editor: *CRC handbook series in zoonoses, section B: viral zoonoses,* vol I, Boca Raton, Fla, 1981, CRC Press, p 267.
87. Hoogstaal H: Argasid and nuttalliellid ticks as parasites and vectors, *Adv Parasitol* 24:135, 1985.
88. Horton JM, Blaser MJ: The spectrum of relapsing fever in the Rocky Mountains, *Arch Intern Med* 145:871, 1985.
89. Jacobs JC, Stevens M, Duray PH: Lyme disease simulating septic arthritis, *JAMA* 256:1138, 1986.
90. Jacoby GA et al: Treatment of transfusion-transmitted babesiosis by exchange transfusion, *N Engl J Med* 303:1098, 1980.
91. Jerant AF, Arline AD: Babesiosis in California, *West J Med* 158:622, 1993.
92. Kahan A et al: Meningoradiculitis associated with infections by *Borrelia burgdorferi, Lancet* 1:148, 1985.
93. Kaplan JE, Schonberger LB: The sensitivity of various serologic tests in the diagnosis of Rocky Mountain spotted fever, *Am J Trop Med Hyg* 35:840, 1986.
94. Kaplowitz LG, Fischer JJ, Sparling PF: Rocky Mountain spotted fever: A clinical dilemma. In Remington JS, Swartz MN, editors: *Current clinical topics in infectious diseases,* vol 2, New York, 1981, McGraw-Hill, p 89.
95. Kaplowitz LG, Robertson GL: Hyponatremia in Rocky Mountain spotted fever: role of antidiuretic hormone, *Ann Intern Med* 98:334, 1983.
96. Kirsch M et al: Fatal adult respiratory distress syndrome in a patient with Lyme disease, *JAMA* 259:2737, 1988.
97. Lane RS, Peisman J, Burgdorfer W: Lyme Borreliosis: relation of its causative agent to its vectors and hosts in North America and Europe, *Annu Rev Entomol* 36:587, 1991.
98. Lane RS et al: Ecology of tick-borne agents in California—I. Spotted fever group rickettsiae, *Am J Trop Med Hyg* 30:239, 1981.
99. Lane RS et al: Survey for evidence of Colorado tick fever virus outside of the known endemic area in California, *Am J Trop Med Hyg* 31:837, 1982.
100. Lawson JP, Steere AC: Lyme arthritis: radiologic findings, *Radiology* 154:37, 1985.
101. Le CT: Tick-borne relapsing fever in children, *Pediatrics* 66:963, 1980.
102. Lees RF et al: Radiographic findings in Rocky Mountain spotted fever, *Radiology* 129:17, 1978.
103. Loge RV: Acute hepatitis associated with Colorado tick fever, *West J Med* 142:91, 1985.
104. Logigian EL, Kaplan RF, Steere AC: Chronic neurologic manifestations of Lyme disease, *N Engl J Med* 323:1438, 1990.
105. Logigian EL, Steere AC: Clinical and electrophysiologic findings in chronic neuropathy of Lyme disease, *Neurology* 42:303, 1992.
106. Luft BJ et al: Invasion of the central nervous system by *Borrelia burgdorferi* in acute disseminated infection, *JAMA* 267:1364, 1992.
107. MacDonald AB, Benach JL, Burgdorfer W: Stillbirth following maternal Lyme disease, *NY J Med* 615, 1987.
108. Maeda K et al: Human infection with *Ehrlichia canis,* a leukocytic rickettsia, *N Engl J Med* 316:853, 1987.
109. Magnarelli L, Anderson JF: Ticks and biting insects infected with the etiologic agent of Lyme disease, *Borrelia burgdorferi, J Clin Microbiol* 26:1482, 1988.
110. Marcus LC et al: Fatal pancarditis in a patient with coexistent Lyme disease and babesiosis: demonstration of spirochetes in the myocardium, *Ann Intern Med* 103:374, 1985.
111. Marcus LC et al: A case report of transfusion-induced babesiosis, *JAMA* 248:465, 1982.
112. Marin-Garcia J, Barrett FF: Myocardial function in Rocky Mountain spotted fever: echocardiographic assessment, *Am J Cardiol* 51:341, 1983.
113. Marin-Garcia J, Gooch WM, Coury DL: Cardiac manifestations of Rocky Mountain spotted fever, *Pediatrics* 67:358, 1981.
114. Markowitz LE et al: Lyme disease during pregnancy, *JAMA* 255:3394, 1986.
115. Marx RS et al: Rocky Mountain spotted fever—serological evidence of previous subclinical infection in children, *Am J Dis Child* 136:16, 1982.

116. Massachusetts Department of Public Health: On the alert for Rocky Mountain spotted fever, *N Engl J Med* 292:1127, 1975.
117. Matuschka F et al: Capacity of European animals as reservoir hosts for the Lyme disease spirochete, *J Infect Dis* 165:479, 1992.
118. McCrossin I: Lyme disease on the NSW south coast, *Med J Aust* 144:139, 1986.
119. McDade JE: Ehrlichiosis—a disease of animals and humans, *J Infect Dis* 161:609, 1990.
120. McDade JE, Newhouse VF: Natural history of *Rickettsia rickettsii, Annu Rev Microbiol* 40:287, 1986.
121. McHugh TP, Ruderman AE, Gibbons TE: Rocky Mountain spotted fever, *Ann Emerg Med* 13:1132, 1984.
122. McLean RG et al: The ecology of Colorado tick fever in Rocky Mountain National Park in 1974, *Am J Trop Med Hyg* 30:483, 1980.
123. Meldrum SC et al: Human babesiosis in New York State: an epidemiological description of 136 cases, *Clin Infect Dis* 15:1019, 1992.
124. Mertz LE et al: Ticks, spirochetes, and new diagnostic tests for Lyme disease, *Mayo Clin Proc* 60:402, 1985.
125. Miller JQ, Price TR: The nervous system in Rocky Mountain spotted fever, *Neurology* 22:561, 1972.
126. Misao T, Kobayashi Y: Studies on infectious mononucleosis (glandular fever). I. Isolation of etiologic agent from blood, bone marrow, and lymph node of a patient with infectious mononucleosis by using mice, *Kyushu J Med Sci* 6:145, 1955.
127. Monath TP: Orbivirus (Colorado tick fever). In Mandell GL, Douglas RG, Bennett JE, editors: *Principles and practice of infectious diseases*, New York, 1985, Wiley, p 931.
128. Moraga FA et al: Boutonneuse fever, *Arch Dis Child* 57:149, 1982.
129. Morris HH: Tick paralysis: electrophysiologic measurements, *South Med J* 70:121, 1977.
130. Morrison RE et al: Rocky Mountain spotted fever in the elderly, *J Am Geriatr Soc* 39:205, 1991.
131. Mukolwe SW et al: Attempted transmission of *Borrelia burgdorferi* (Spirochaetales: Spirochaetaceae) (JDI strain) by *Ixodes scapularis* (Acari: Ixodidae), *Dermacentor variabilis*, and *Amblyomma americanum*, *J Med Entomol* 29:673, 1992.
132. Murnaghan MF: Site and mechanism of tick paralysis, *Science* 131:418, 1960.
133. Nadelman RB et al: Comparison of cerfuroxime axetil and doxycycline in the treatment of early Lyme disease, *Ann Intern Med* 117:273, 1992.
134. Needham GR: Evaluation of five popular methods for tick removal, *Pediatrics* 75:997, 1985.
135. Nieburg PI, D'Angelo LJ, Herrmann KL: Measles in patients suspected of having Rocky Mountain spotted fever, *JAMA* 244:808, 1980.
136. Oster CN et al: Laboratory-acquired Rocky Mountain spotted fever—the hazard of aerosol transmission, *N Engl J Med* 297:859, 1977.
137. Pachner AR, Steere AC: The triad of neurologic manifestations of Lyme disease: meningitis, cranial neuritis, and radiculoneuritis, *Neurology* 35:57, 1985.
138. Pearn J: Neuromuscular paralysis caused by tick envenomation, *J Neurol Sci* 34:37, 1977.
139. Pfister HW et al: Randomized comparison of ceftriaxone and cefotaxime in Lyme neuroborreliosis, *J Infect Dis* 163:311, 1991.
140. Philip RN et al: A comparison of serologic methods for diagnosis of Rocky Mountain spotted fever, *Am J Epidemiol* 105:56, 1977.
141. Piesman J et al: Duration of tick attachment and *Borrelia burgdorferi* transmission, *J Clin Microbiol* 25:557, 1987.
142. Piesman J, Sinsky RJ: Ability of *Ixodes scapularis, Dermacentor variabilis*, and *Amblyomma americanum* to acquire, maintain, and transmit Lyme disease spirochetes, *J Med Entomol* 25:336, 1988.
143. Piras MA et al: Glucose-6-phosphate dehydrogenase deficiency in male patients with Mediterranean spotted fever in Sardinia, *J Infect Dis* 148:607, 1983.
144. Quick RE et al: Babesiosis in Washington State: a new species of *Babesia? Ann Intern Med* 119:284, 1993.
145. Rahn DW, Malawista SE: Lyme disease: recommendations for diagnosis and treatment, *Ann Intern Med* 114:472, 1991.
146. Randall MB, Walker DH: Rocky Mountain spotted fever gastrointestinal and pancreatic lesions and rickettsial infection, *Arch Pathol Lab Med* 108:963, 1984.
147. Raoult D et al: Laboratory diagnosis of Mediterranean spotted fever by immunofluorescent demonstration of *Rickettsia conorii* in cutaneous lesions, *J Infect Dis* 150:145, 1984.
148. Raoult D et al: Mediterranean spotted fever: clinical, laboratory and epidemiological features of 199 cases, *Am J Trop Med Hyg* 35:845, 1986.
149. Raoult D et al: Incidence, clinical observations and risk factors in the severe form of Mediterranean spotted fever among patients admitted to hospital in Marseilles, 1983-1984, *J Infect* 12:111, 1986.
150. Raucher HS, Jaffin H, Glass JL: Babesiosis in pregnancy, *Obstet Gynecol* 63:7S, 1984.
151. Reik L, Burgdorfer W, Donaldson JO: Neurologic abnormalities in Lyme disease without erythema chronicum migrans, *Am J Med* 81:73, 1986.
152. Reik L et al: Neurologic abnormalities of Lyme disease, *Medicine* 58:281, 1979.
153. Ribeiro JMC et al: Dissemination and salivary delivery of Lyme disease spirochetes in vector ticks, *J Med Entomol* 24:201, 1987.
154. Ristic M, Healy GR: Babesiosis. In Steele JH, editor: *CRC handbook series in zoonoses, section C: parasitic zoonoses,* vol I, Boca Raton, Fla, 1981, CRC Press, p 151.
155. Rosner F et al: Babesiosis in splenectomized adults—review of 22 reported cases, *Am J Med* 76:696, 1984.
156. Rubin DA et al: Prospective evaluation of heart block complicating early Lyme disease, *Pace* 15:252, 1992.
157. Ruebush TK et al: Human babesiosis on Nantucket Island—clinical features, *Ann Intern Med* 86:6, 1977.
158. Ruebush TK et al: Development and persistence of antibody in persons infected with *Babesia microti, Am J Trop Med Hyg* 30:291, 1981.
159. Ruebush TK et al: Human babesiosis on Nantucket Island—evidence for self-limited and subclinical infections, *N Engl J Med* 297:825, 1977.
160. Ryberg B: Bannwarth's syndrome (lymphocytic meningoradiculitis) in Sweden, *Yale J Biol Med* 57:499, 1984.
161. Ryberg B et al: Antibodies to Lyme-disease spirochaete in European lymphocytic meningoradiculitis (Bannwarth's syndrome), *Lancet* 2:519, 1983.
162. Sacks HS, Lyons RW, Lahiri B: Adult respiratory distress syndrome in Rocky Mountain spotted fever, *Ann Rev Respir Dis* 123:547, 1981.
163. Sacks JJ, Pinner TAF, Parker RL: Tick testing as a method of controlling Rocky Mountain spotted fever, *Am J Public Health* 73:903, 1983.
164. Salazar JC, Gerber MA, Goff CW: Long-term outcome of Lyme disease in children given early treatment, *J Pediatr* 122:591, 1993.
165. Schechter SL: Lyme disease associated with optic neuropathy, *Am J Med* 81:143, 1986.
166. Schlesinger PA et al: Maternal-fetal transmission of the Lyme disease spirochete, *Borrelia burgdorferi, Ann Intern Med* 103:67, 1985.
167. Schmedding E et al: Lymphocytic meningoradiculitis (Garin-Bujadoux Bannwarth): from syndrome to disease? *Eur J Pediatr* 144:497, 1986.
168. Schmid GP et al: Surveillance of Lyme disease in the United States, 1982, *J Infect Dis* 151:1144, 1985.
169. Schmitt N, Bowmer EJ, Gregson JD: Tick paralysis in British Columbia, *Can Med Assoc J* 100:417, 1969.
170. Schrock CG: Lyme disease: additional evidence of wide spread distribution, *Am J Med* 72:700, 1982.

171. Schwartz BS et al: Antibody testing in Lyme disease—a comparison of results in four laboratories, *JAMA* 262:3431, 1989.
172. Sciotto CG et al: Rapid identification of *Borrelia* in blood and tissue with acridine orange, *Lab Invest* 46:74, 1982.
173. Shapiro ED et al: A controlled trial of antimicrobial prophylaxis for Lyme disease after deer-tick bites, *N Engl J Med* 327:1769, 1992.
174. Shrestha M, Grodzicki RL, Steere AC: Diagnosing early Lyme disease, *Am J Med* 78:235, 1985.
175. Silver HK, Meiklehogn G, Kempe CH: Colorado tick fever, *Am J Dis Child* 101:56, 1961.
176. Smith RP et al: Transfusion-acquired babesiosis and failure of antibiotic treatment, *JAMA* 256:2726, 1986.
177. Snydman DR et al: *Borrelia burgdorferi* in joint fluid in chronic Lyme arthritis, *Ann Intern Med* 104:798, 1986.
178. Southern PA, Sanford JP: Relapsing fever—a clinical and microbiological review, *Medicine* 48:129, 1969.
179. Spielman A et al: Human babesiosis on Nantucket Island, USA: description of the vector, *Ixodes (Ixodes) dammini*, n. sp. (Acarina: Ixodidae), *J Med Entomol* 15:218, 1979.
180. Spielman A, Levine JF, Wilson MI: Vectorial capacity of North American *Ixodes* ticks, *Yale J Biol Med* 57:507, 1984.
181. Spruance SL, Bailey A: Colorado tick fever—a review of 115 laboratory confirmed cases, *Arch Intern Med* 131:288, 1973.
182. Stanbury JB, Huyck JH: Tick paralysis: a critical review, *Medicine* 24:219, 1945.
183. Stanek G et al: Isolation of *Borrelia burgdorferi* from the myocardium of a patient with long-standing cardiomyopathy, *N Engl J Med* 322:249, 1990.
184. Steenbarger JR: Congenital tick-borne relapsing fever: report of a case with first documentation of transplacental transmission, *Birth Defects* 18:39, 1982.
185. Steere AC: Conference summary, *Yale J Biol Med* 57:711, 1984.
186. Steere AC: Effectiveness of early Lyme disease treatment (letter), *Am J Med* 94:553, 1993.
187. Steere AC: Lyme disease, *N Engl J Med* 321:586, 1989.
188. Steere AC et al: The early clinical manifestations of Lyme disease, *Ann Intern Med* 99:76, 1983.
189. Steere AC et al: Lyme carditis: cardiac abnormalities of Lyme disease, *Ann Intern Med* 93:8, 1980.
190. Steere AC, Broderick TF, Malawista SE: Erythema chronicum migrans and Lyme arthritis: epidemiologic evidence for a tick vector, *Am J Epidemiol* 108:312, 1978.
191. Steere AC et al: Unilateral blindness caused by infection with the Lyme disease spirochete, *Borrelia burgdorferi, Ann Intern Med* 103:382, 1985.
192. Steere AC, Dwyer E, Winchester R: Association of chronic Lyme arthritis with the HLA-DR4 and HLA-DR2 alleles, *N Engl J Med* 323:219, 1990.
193. Steere AC et al: Chronic Lyme arthritis—clinical and immunogenetic differentiation from rheumatoid arthritis, *Ann Intern Med* 90:896, 1979.
194. Steere AC et al: The spirochetal etiology of Lyme disease, *N Engl J Med* 308:733, 1983.
195. Steere AC et al: Treatment of the early manifestations of Lyme disease, *Ann Intern Med* 99:22, 1983.
196. Steere AC, Malawista SE: Cases of Lyme disease in the United States: locations correlated with distribution of *Ixodes dammini, Ann Intern Med* 91:730, 1979.
197. Steere AC et al: Erythema chronicum migrans and Lyme arthritis—the enlarging clinical spectrum, *Ann Intern Med* 86:685, 1977.
198. Steere AC et al: Antibiotic therapy in Lyme disease, *Ann Intern Med* 93:1, 1980.
199. Steere AC et al: Lyme arthritis—an epidemic of oligoarticular arthritis in children and adults in three Connecticut communities, *Arthritis Rheum* 20:7, 1977.
200. Steere AC, Pachner AR, Malawista SE: Neurologic abnormalities of Lyme disease: successful treatment with high-dose intravenous penicillin, *Ann Intern Med* 99:767, 1983.
201. Steere AC, Schoen RT, Taylor E: The clinical evolution of Lyme arthritis, *Ann Intern Med* 107:725, 1987.
202. Steere AC et al: The overdiagnosis of Lyme disease, *JAMA* 269:1812, 1993.
203. Steere AC et al: Longitudinal assessment of the clinical and epidemiological features of Lyme disease in a defined population, *J Infect Dis* 154:295, 1986.
204. Steketee RW et al: Babesiosis in Wisconsin—a new focus of disease transmission, *JAMA* 253:2675, 1985.
205. Stewart A et al: Lyme arthritis in the Hunter Valley, *Med J Aust* 1:139, 1982.
206. Stiernstedt GT et al: Chronic meningitis and Lyme disease in Sweden, *Yale J Biol Med* 57:491, 1984.
207. Stoenner HG, Dodd Y, Larsen C: Antigenic variation of *Borrelia hermsii, J Exp Med* 156:1297, 1982.
208. Strle F et al: Solitary borrelial lymphocytoma: report of 36 cases, *Infection* 20:201, 1992.
209. Sun T et al: Morphologic and clinical observations in human infection with *Babesia microti, J Infect Dis* 148:239, 1983.
210. Swift TR, Ignacio OJ: Tick paralysis: electrophysiologic studies. *Neurology* 25:1130, 1975.
211. Takanori O, Tange Y, Kobayashi Y: Causative agent of spotted fever group rickettsiosis in Japan, *Infect Immun* 58:887, 1990.
212. Tanaka R: Rocky Mountain spotted fever—United States, 1986, *JAMA* 258:25, 1987.
213. Thompson RS et al: Outbreak of tick-borne relapsing fever in Spokane County, Washington, *JAMA* 210:1045, 1969.
214. Tibballs J, Cooper SJ: Paralysis with *Ixodes cornuatus* envenomation, *Med J Aust* 145:37, 1986.
215. Todd JL: Tick bite in British Columbia, *Can Med Assoc J* 2:1118, 1912.
216. Tringali G et al: Epidemiology of boutonneuse fever in western Sicily—distribution and prevalence of spotted fever group rickettsial infection in dog ticks *(Rhipicephalus sanguineus), Am J Epidemiol* 123:721, 1986.
217. Turck WPG et al: Chronic Q fever, *Q J Med* 45:193, 1976.
218. Walker DH, Gear JHS: Correlation of the distribution of *Rickettsia conorii,* microscopic lesions, and clinical features in South African tick bite fever, *Am J Trop Med Hyg* 34:361, 1985.
219. Walker DH, Hawkins HK, Hudson P: Fulminant Rocky Mountain spotted fever—its pathologic characteristics associated with glucose-6-phosphate dehydrogenase deficiency, *Arch Pathol Lab Med* 107:121, 1983.
220. Walker DH et al: Rocky Mountain spotted fever mimicking acute cholecystitis, *Arch Intern Med* 145:2194, 1985.
221. Walker DH, Mattern WD: Rickettsial vasculitis, *Am Heart J* 100:896, 1980.
222. Walker DH, Paletta CE, Cain BG: Pathogenesis of myocarditis in Rocky Mountain spotted fever, *Arch Pathol Lab Med* 104:171, 1980.
223. Wallis RC et al: Erythema chronicum migrans and Lyme arthritis: field study of ticks, *Am J Epidemiol* 108:322, 1978.
224. Weber K et al: *Borrelia burgdorferi* in a newborn despite oral penicillin for Lyme borreliosis during pregnancy, *Pediatr Infect Dis* 7:286, 1988.
225. Weber K, Puzik A, Becker T: Erythema-migrans krankheit: Beitrag zur klinik und besiehung zur Lyme-krankheit, *Dtsch Med Wochenschr* 108:1182, 1983.
226. Welch KJ, Rumley RL, Levine JA: False-positive results in serologic tests for Rocky Mountain spotted fever during pregnancy, *South J Med* 84:307, 1991.
227. Wells GM et al: Rocky Mountain spotted fever caused by blood transfusion, *JAMA* 239:2763, 1978.

228. Wengrower D et al: Myocarditis in tick-borne relapsing fever, *J Infect Dis* 149:1033, 1982.
229. Western KA et al: Babesiosis in a Massachusetts resident, *N Engl J Med* 282:854, 1970.
230. Wilkinson PR: Tick paralysis. In Steele JH, editor: *CRC handbook series in zoonoses, section C: parasitic zoonoses,* vol III, Boca Raton, Fla, 1981, CRC Press, p 275.
231. Williamson PK, Calabro JJ: Lyme disease—a review of the literature, *Semin Arthritis Rheum* 13:229, 1984.
232. Wilson ML, Adler GH, Spielman A: Correlation between abundance of deer and that of the deer tick *Ixodes dammini, Ann Entomol Soc Am* 78:172, 1985.
233. Wisseman CL: Rickettsial diseases. In Wyngaarden JB, Smith LH, editors: *Cecil textbook of medicine,* Philadelphia, 1985, WB Saunders, p 1672.
234. Wittner M et al: Successful chemotherapy of transfusion babesiosis, *Ann Intern Med* 96:601, 1982.
235. Woodward TE: Rocky Mountain spotted fever: epidemiological and early clinical signs are keys to treatment and reduced mortality, *J Infect Dis* 150:465, 1984.
236. Woodward TE et al: Prompt confirmation of Rocky Mountain spotted fever: identification of rickettsiae in skin tissues, *J Infect Dis* 134:297, 1976.
237. Yagupsky P, Moses S: Neonatal *Borrelia* species infection (relapsing fever), *Am J Dis Child* 139:74, 1985.

34 PROTECTION FROM BLOOD-FEEDING ARTHROPODS

Carl E. Schreck

Blood-Feeding Arthropods

On a preference scale of 1 to 10, with 10 the most attractive, people probably rank second or third as the preferred hosts of blood-feeding arthropods (insects, mites, and ticks). Nevertheless, these creatures have had a tremendous impact on the health and welfare of humankind. As a result, people through the ages have attempted to shield themselves from the pain and itch of bites. In modern entomologic terms this is called personal protection. It is accomplished by using clothing, screens, nets, enclosures, and chemicals or by avoiding or leaving infested areas. Often, coexistence with blood feeders can be accomplished without undue hardship. This chapter is written for the benefit of those with a stalwart spirit who are willing to risk exposure to blood-feeding arthropods and for those who have suffered the consequences of ill preparation. Further clinical information concerning arthropods is found in reference 50 and in Chapters 31 to 33, 35, and 41.

Of all insects, mosquitoes are the foremost disease vectors and pests affecting people. They belong to the order Diptera, or two-winged flies. Other two-winged flies that bite humans are blackflies, biting midges, deerflies, horseflies, green heads, tsetse, stable flies, sand flies, snipe flies, and a few others of lesser numerical importance, although they may bite fiercely. The remaining taxonomic groups of importance include lice, fleas, chigger mites, ticks, kissing bugs, and bedbugs. Lice and bedbugs are discussed in Chapter 31.

MOSQUITOES (FAMILY CULICIDAE)

More people are bitten by mosquitoes (Fig. 34-1, *D*) than by any other blood sucker. Mosquitoes usually can be separated into daytime or nighttime biters. Most bite at twilight, which is a good time to be indoors or provided with some form of personal protection. Vertebrate hosts include mammals, birds, reptiles, and amphibians. One species, *Uranotaenia lateralis,* feeds on a fish, the mud skipper. Blood feeding takes only a few minutes for most species. Mosquito saliva is released into the wound, which causes the victim's capillaries to dilate; blood pools, and the mosquito rapidly pumps its stomach full. Anticoagulant is not always present in the saliva and is not vital to the feeding process.[32]

Only female mosquitoes bite. They feed every 3 or 4 days, but someone is unlikely to be bitten twice by the same female because after feeding, mosquitoes tend to disperse, sometimes great distances, depending on proximity of oviposition sites, prevailing winds, population density, longevity, and presence of suitable hosts. Male mosquitoes are distinguished by their bushy antennae and feed solely on plant juices and nectars. Anopheline, or malaria, mosquitoes have long thin legs. They rest with the head positioned close to the skin surface and with the posterior portion of the body raised above the skin surface, almost standing on their heads. Most other species rest with the body parallel to the skin surface, with their hind legs raised as if they were testing the air. Nonbiting midges, sometimes called blind mosquitoes, are similar, but they rest with their front legs raised and do not have mouthparts for blood sucking.

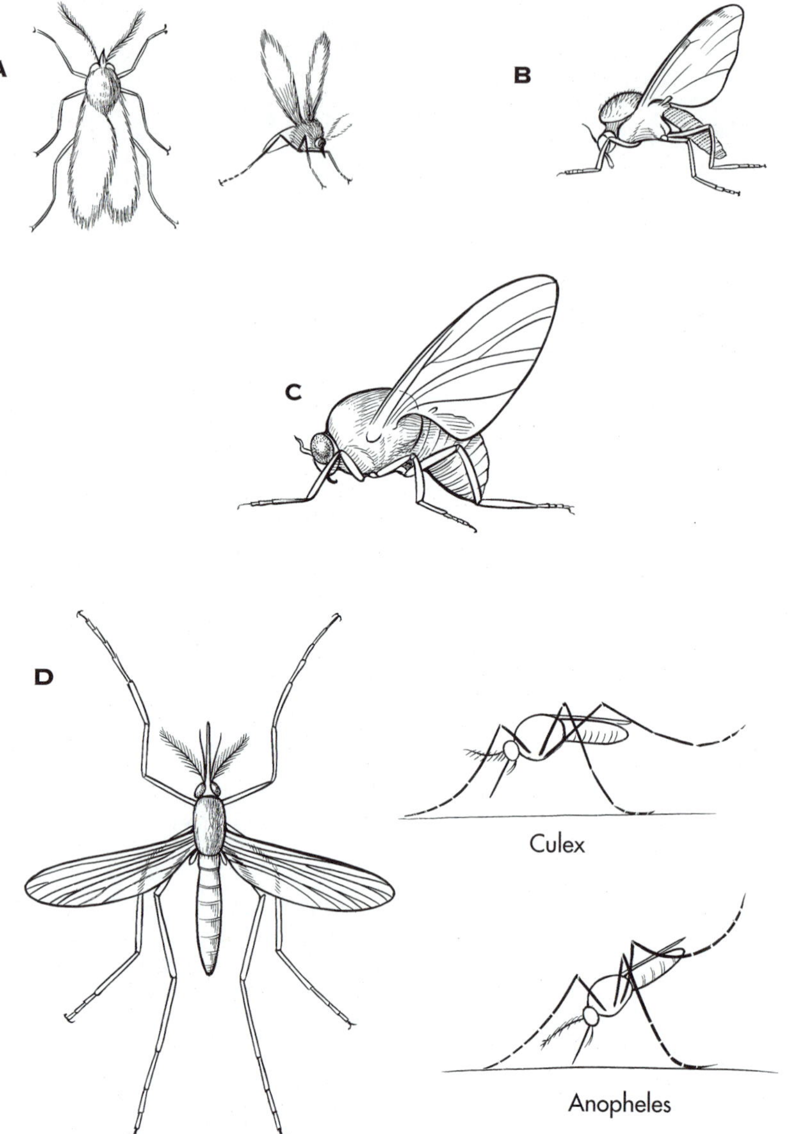

Fig. 34-1 Blood-feeding biting flies (not drawn to scale). **A,** Sand fly. **B,** Biting midge. **C,** Blackfly. **D,** Mosquito.

Daytime resting sites for mosquitoes are cool, dark places, including caves, animal burrows, hollow logs or trees, and the shade of lush bushes and tall grasses. Campsites should be as far from these resting places as practical to minimize exposure to bites.

Mosquitoes rely primarily on their olfactory senses rather than sight to find a blood meal. They can detect the presence of a large animal such as a calf in darkness at a distance of up to 40 yards.[20] Metabolic carbon dioxide exhaled from the lungs and secreted from the skin is thought to be a primary chemical signal by which a host is sensed, but as the insect approaches, other chemical cues emanating from the host probably provide information about whether it is a favored food source. One chemical cue is lactic acid.[1] At very close range, heat induces probing by some species. Attractiveness of individual persons to mosquitoes varies.[74]

The intensity of an attack may depend on the physical state of the mosquito. Researchers have suggested that reduced carbohydrate reserves can limit frequency of attempts to feed on a host[78]; thus a mosquito repeatedly thwarted in attempts to feed may yield to fatigue. Unfortunately, rested mosquitoes are usually nearby to act as stand-ins.

Periodic occurrences of dense mosquito populations (Fig. 34-2) result from several natural or human-induced conditions. Natural population fluctuations are directly related to the interaction of a complex of environmental and biologic factors. These include time of year, weather, habitat type and availability, predators, insect pathogens, and breeding potential. Seasonally, tremendous numbers of

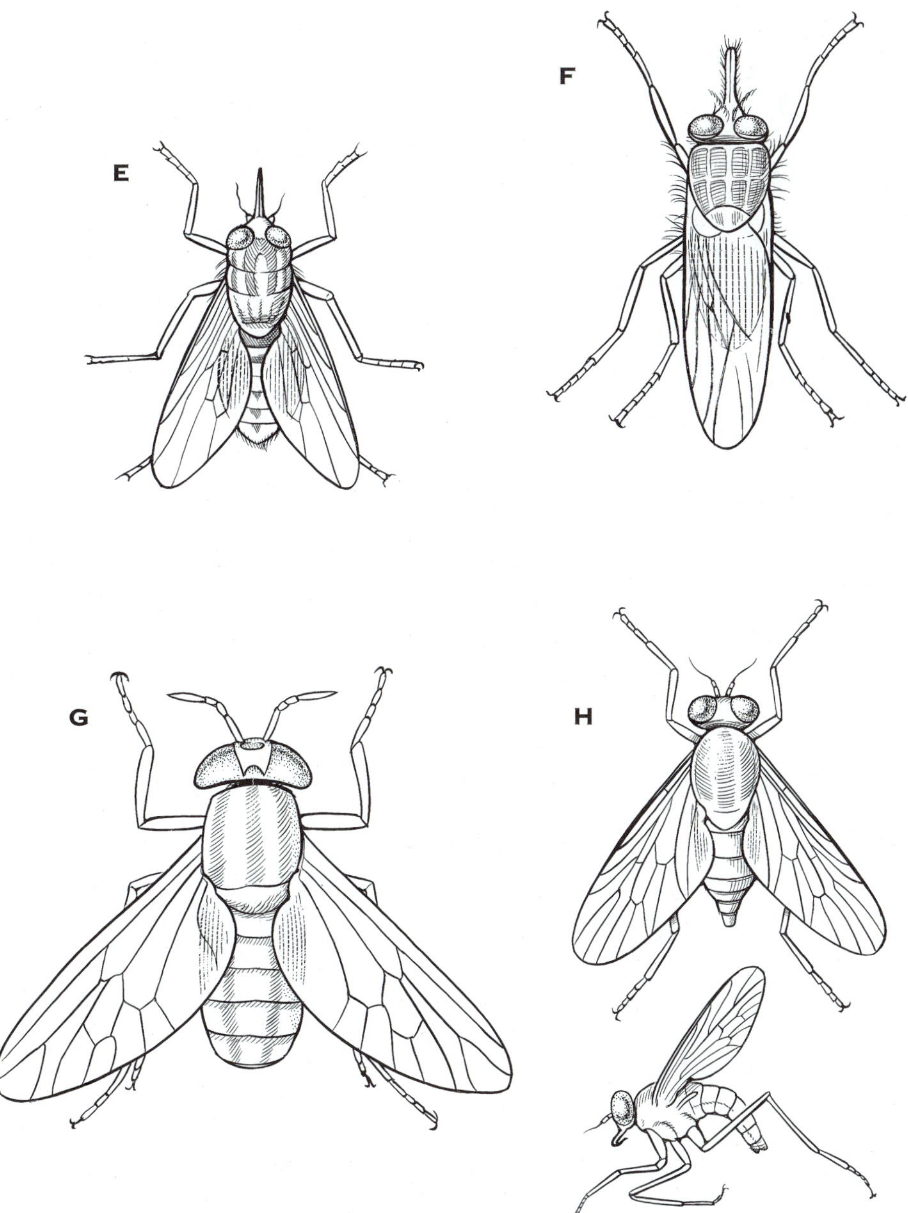

Fig. 34-1, cont'd. E, Stable fly. **F,** Tsetse fly. **G,** Tabanid fly. **H,** Snipe fly.

mosquitoes are found in tidal marshes, the sub-Arctic north, and flooded lowlands bordering lakes and rivers.

Humans can alter densities of mosquitoes by manipulation of environmental conditions. Agricultural operations can be responsible for spectacular population increases. Irrigation practices in western U.S. semidesert areas produce large numbers of mosquitoes that formerly were rare or not found in these habitats. Artificially raising and lowering water levels over vast areas during rice production augments species that breed in flood water and permanent water in the lower Mississippi valley and delta regions.

A worrisome new pest and potential disease vector recently introduced into the Western Hemisphere is the Asian tiger mosquito *Aedes albopictus*.[25] Experts believe that this mosquito will become established in both North and South America. It is especially annoying because it is small, feeds readily on humans, and bites in daylight. While feeding, it is easily disturbed. Hence a person may receive multiple bites from a single persistent mosquito and be convinced that swarms are present.

BLACKFLIES (FAMILY SIMULIIDAE)

Blackflies (Fig. 34-1, *C*) are small (2 to 4 mm), thick bodied, hump backed, and mostly black. Unlike most mosquitoes, they are largely daytime biters and rely primarily on

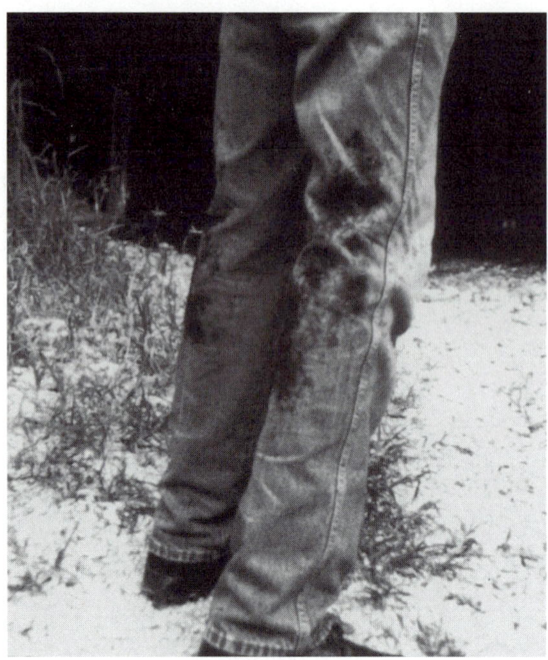

Fig. 34-2 Clusters of salt marsh mosquitoes attacking the lower legs.

vision to locate a potential host, although they are also attracted to carbon dioxide and warm objects. They are widely distributed on every continent and usually breed in fast-flowing waters. Only the female bites, taking 4 to 5 minutes to feed roughly every 5 days.[32] Many species prefer to feed on birds rather than mammals, and some are particularly annoying because they are attracted to the eyes, nostrils, and ears. Blackflies often crawl under clothing to feed. Although the bite is relatively painless, it is regarded as among the worst inflicted by blood-sucking arthropods[80]; it can cause intense itching, raw lesions that are slow to heal, scarring, fevers, anaphylaxis, and in rare cases death.

Blackflies tend to be attracted to dark, moving objects. Although they are more apt to hover over and crawl on a person wearing dark- rather than light-colored clothing, they avoid dark places such as the insides of buildings or cars. If trapped, they fly and crawl upward on windows ceaselessly, trying to escape.

BITING MIDGES (FAMILY CERATOPOGONIDAE)

The town name of Punxsutawney, Pennsylvania (pronounced Punks-a-tawny and famous for Groundhog Day), reportedly was originated by the Delaware Indians and means "Land of Biting Midges." Biting midges (the name may be misleading, for only the female [Fig. 34-1, *B*] bites) are less than 2 mm long. Although they are barely visible, their bite is not quickly forgotten. With worldwide distribution, they have been bestowed with more local names than any other hematophagous (blood-feeding) arthropod. Examples include "punkies" (United States and Canada), "no-see-ums" (United States and Canada), "moose flies" (Alaska), "sand flies," "sand gnats," "sand fleas" (United States Atlantic and Gulf Coasts, Australia, and Caribbean Islands), "flying teeth" (U.S. Marines, Guantanamo Bay), "majes" (Puerto Rico), "mimes" (Spanish origin), "punchins" (Holland), "maruins" (Brazil), "biting midges" (Scotland), "jejenes" (West Indies), "no-nos" (Polynesia), and "valley black gnats" or "Bodega black gnats" (Arizona, New Mexico, and California). Members of the genus *Culicoides* are distributed from tropics to tundra and from sea level to over 13,000 feet on Mt. Everest.[32] The genus *Leptoconops* is found largely in the warmer regions of the world. Biting midges breed in salt marshes, freshwater wetlands, and plant debris. Adults may be active day or night, depending on the species. Activity is governed by wind speed, temperature, and time of day, but midges may be induced to bite at an unusual time for them if a host disturbs them at rest. They are troublesome mainly in calm weather and decline in number as wind speed increases. In winds over 5 m/sec (11 mph),[32] nearly all biting ceases.

Usually attacking in swarms, midges inflict large numbers of bites within a few minutes (Fig. 34-3). Several species may feed on a host simultaneously. Some prefer arms to legs and light areas to dark, or vice versa. They often crawl into the hair and bite.

Some evidence suggests that an individual's attractiveness to midges is changeable,[32] but when midge densities are high, this phenomenon may be of little consequence. "One midge is an entomological curiosity, a thousand can be hell. . . ."[31]

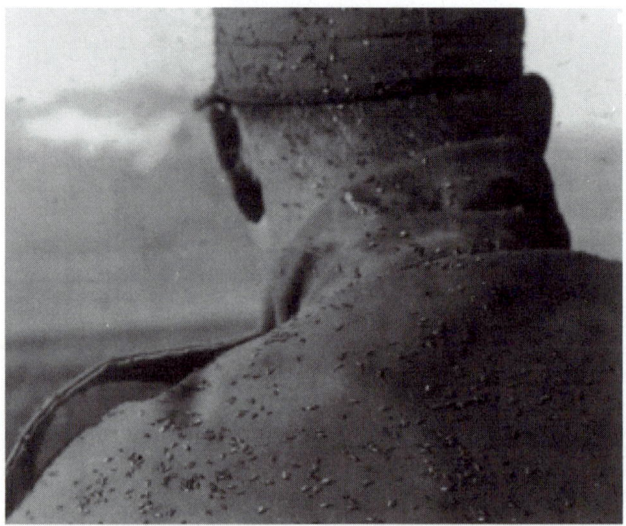

Fig. 34-3 Alaskan biting midges *(Culicoides tristriatulus)* attacking a man's back.

TABANIDS (FAMILY TABANIDAE)

Tabanids (Fig. 34-1, *G*) are insects of worldwide distribution. Relatively large (10 to 15 mm), stoutly built, and strong fliers, they include the horseflies, deerflies, greenheads, and yellow flies. In Europe the group is sometimes called gadflies.[7] Most species breed in aquatic or semiaquatic habitats. Emerging adults usually occur for a limited period in late spring or early summer. Most are active in daylight. Only females bite, feeding mainly on mammals. Despite their size they attack silently. The bite is vicious; the slashing action of the mouthparts causes a large bleeding puncture that may ooze blood for some time. Their host-seeking activity is temperature dependent. Tabanids are especially active on bright, warm, overcast days. Their very large eyes orient them to visual stimuli such as movement of people, cattle, and cars. Odor and carbon dioxide also are used in host finding, but to a lesser degree. The human upper body is attacked when the host is moving; when the host is still, the lower body may be preferred. Tabanids have been known to fly 30 miles and have been found at altitudes up to 9000 feet. Fortunately, their adult lives last only 3 to 4 weeks and usually only one generation emerges each year; thus, although densities may be high and at times intolerable, the duration of exposure to bites is limited.

OTHER BITING FLIES

The stable fly (family Muscidae) (Fig. 34-1, *E*), dog fly, or "biting" housefly, as it is sometimes called for its resemblance to the common housefly, is most familiar as a pest found at beaches. It is easily distinguished from the housefly because it rests with its head held high while the rear of the body is low; the housefly rests with the body parallel to the surface. Close examination reveals a stiletto-like piercing organ at the front of the head. Preferred hosts are horses and cattle, but humans, dogs, and other animals are readily attacked. Stable flies breed in decaying vegetation and in the dung of herbivores. They congregate in sunny places on walls and fences and may live 3 to 4 weeks in summer and longer during cooler weather. Both sexes take blood and are vicious biters, perhaps because they must feed every 48 hours to survive. Feeding is accomplished by rasping a puncture wound with the mouthparts and then pumping up the blood. Stable flies are active in the daytime and may feed more than once, preferring to attack ankles and legs. They are persistent, often engaging in successive feeding attempts because of the host's response to the painful bite (a sharp pricking sensation). They are particularly apt to bite before and during storms, a phenomenon caused perhaps by changes in atmospheric pressure together with darkened skies. From breeding sources, stable flies can travel many miles on prevailing winds to aggregation areas, sometimes coastal, where their numbers may have a substantial economic impact by reducing tourist trade. Interestingly, while near horses or cattle people are rarely bitten because they are not preferred hosts. As a result they may be unaware of the flies' presence.

Tsetse, African flies of the family Glossinidae (Fig. 34-1, *F*), are not found in the Western Hemisphere, but fossil evidence shows they were once residents of North America. They are now confined to tropical Africa. Both sexes of this brownish fly take blood, and the female may live for several months. Like the tabanids, they feed mostly in daylight. Large eyes are used to detect hosts, particularly those in motion. When hungry, tsetse will attack large mammals and passengers in vehicles with equal ferocity. Tsetse have a 2- to 3-day feeding cycle, are particularly vicious when blood starved, and can bite through heavy clothing.

Phlebotomine sand flies (family Psychodidae), not to be confused with biting midges, breed in forest litter of mostly subtropical and tropical areas of the world (Fig. 34-1, *A*). Dinosaurs were their contemporaries and are suspected to have been among their earlier hosts.[32] Sand flies are important vectors of severe cuticular and systemic disease in both the Eastern and Western Hemispheres. At least three species occur in the southern United States, and one, found as far north as Delaware, feeds on human blood.[24] Reported encounters are rare, and bites are likely to be blamed on other pests such as mosquitoes. Sand flies are tiny (2 mm), hairy, delicate mothlike insects with long legs. Only females suck blood, feeding mostly during calm nights. Very sensitive to wind speed, they fly low and hop from place to place. Resting sites are in crevices at the base of large trees and in rodent burrows and caves.[18,32] Bites from phlebotomine sand flies, although rare in North America, are painful. They usually occur on the face, ears, and neck of a person sleeping on or near the ground.

Snipe flies (family Rhagionidae) are little known except in mountain and coastal areas of western North America (Fig. 34-1, *H*). Although some biting species occur in the east, they are seldom a problem except in isolated areas. Somewhat smaller than houseflies, snipe flies are black with color markings that vary with species. Only the females feed on blood. Somewhat like deerflies, they alight quietly and inflict sudden painful bites, even through clothing.[49] Allergic reactions to the bite occur, although rarely. Breeding in moist soil, they are active from late spring through August, but little else is known of their habits and host preferences.

KISSING BUGS (FAMILY REDUVIIDAE)

Kissing bugs (Fig. 34-4, *B*), sometimes called Texas bedbugs, are night feeders like bedbugs. These insects received their name because of the frequency of attack in the mouth area. Adults of both sexes are poor fliers and are about 1 inch (25 cm) long, achieving this size through five intermediate (nymphal) growth stages, during all of which they feed on blood. Both nymphs and adults hide during the

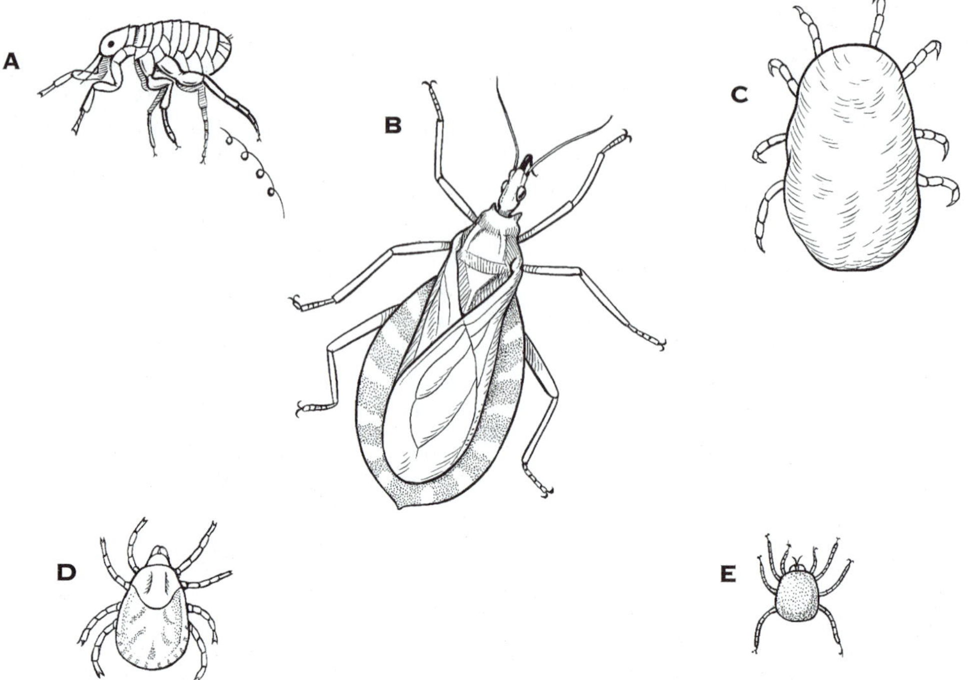

Fig. 34-4 Various blood-feeding arthropods (not drawn to scale). **A,** Flea. **B,** Kissing bug. **C,** Soft tick. **D,** Hard tick. **E,** Chigger mite.

day and emerge at night. They can survive without blood for 4 to 6 months. Kissing bugs are attracted to warmth, carbon dioxide, host odor, and light.[42] Favorite resting sites are palm trees, hollow trees, under tree bark, in walls and roofs, and underneath built-up houses. Kissing bugs are a problem mostly in the western states. It is estimated that if bitten, as many as 30,000 people living in California would be subject to a serious or life-threatening hypersensitivity reaction.[43]

FLEAS (FAMILY PULICIDAE)

Fleas (Fig. 34-4, *A*) are capable of transmitting sylvatic plague, a disease now established on all continents except Australia. Sylvatic plague is of limited sporadic occurrence in forests and open country of the western one third of the United States. Fleas attack rodents, particularly ground squirrels, and are often found in close association with people at campgrounds and recreational areas. Hungry fleas (both sexes) feed on the nearest warm-blooded animal whether or not it is a preferred host, hence the risk of plague transmission to humans. A flea does not normally feed in one place until satiated, but moves about, biting and feeding several times.

MITES AND TICKS (ORDER ACARINA)

Trombiculid mites (Fig. 34-4, *E*) are widely distributed around the world and are found at altitudes up to 16,000 feet in warmer climates. The larvae are barely visible animals commonly referred to as chiggers. They are called redbugs in the southern states and harvest mites in Europe. Their presence can be detected by placing a black flat surface, such as a piece of floor tile, in the leaf litter. If present, they will be seen as tiny, rapidly moving reddish specks against the black background. Localized mite infestations may contain many thousands; however, just one bite can cause considerable discomfort. Only the larvae are parasitic, feeding on a variety of amphibians, reptiles, birds, and mammals. Chigger mites do not suck blood, but rather secrete salivary fluid that contains a proteolytic enzyme into the host's skin to digest tissue. Chiggers may feed on a single host for several days.

Chigger mites usually infest people by crawling onto the shoes, then up the legs (they move rapidly for their size). They attach in a skin fold, in a hair follicle, or at the juncture of clothing and skin, such as the top of stockings, the waistline, or the elastic edge of undergarments. Chiggers are most active in summer and early fall. They are encountered in diverse places, especially within or along the margins of forests, at edges of wetlands, and in blackberry patches. It is unclear why some people become heavily infested while others are virtually immune to attack. A person who cannot recognize a chigger habitat and take precautions is likely to become a victim. Unfortunately, the unprotected usually are not aware of acquired bites until hours after exposure, when it is too late.

TICKS

Ticks (Fig. 34-4, *C* and *D*) lead the list of least-tolerated blood suckers because of their crablike appearance, persistent attachment, and predilection for the perineum.

Ticks are classified as hard ticks (family Ixodidae) and soft ticks (family Argasidae). Both have worldwide distribution, but North Americans are more familiar with hard ticks because of their wide distribution and the common occurrence of these pests on domestic animals. Soft ticks are found mainly in western states, where they have less economic importance than hard ticks.

Few creatures are more successfully adapted to their environment than ticks. They attack all vertebrates except fish and are particularly troublesome to mammals. A leathery exterior renders them resistant to environmental stresses; they are relatively free from natural enemies, can regenerate lost parts, and have been known to survive without feeding for over 4 years.[32]

Both sexes, and in most species the larval and nymphal life stages, are blood feeders. Soft ticks feed mainly at night, with meals lasting only minutes. Hard ticks most actively seek hosts during the day and may feed for several days. "Questing" describes activity in which a tick climbs to the end of a blade of grass or other upright object and rests with forelegs extended in an open, searching posture. Vibrations set up by a potential host moving into range reinforce the questing habit. When fur or cloth touches the upraised forelegs, the tick readily secures a ride. It then crawls about on a host until it locates a suitable feeding site. Bites are nearly painless, so the tick attachment is not noticed until later.

Difficulty in removing a well-attached tick can be attributed to the hypostome, a barbed feeding device that is thrust into a wound made by tiny teeth on other mouthparts. The hypostome anchors the tick tightly into the flesh. Ticks with short mouthparts secrete a cement that anchors them to the host. When the tick is fully fed, a process that may take several hours to days, the mouthparts are slowly relaxed and the tick drops to the ground. Inflammation, itching, swelling, and ulcerations may be part of a sensitive person's reaction. Early removal of a tick can help to minimize these symptoms. Improper or partial removal of tick mouthparts may cause lesions that become infected or are slow to heal and can lead to a granuloma of many months' duration.[18] Localized larval and nymphal tick infestations may be enormous. Thus an intruder into this habitat can quickly become heavily infested. The larvae are tiny, and nymphs are not easily seen except by close inspection of the environment.

Common suggestions for removing attached ticks rival hiccup cures. The following removal procedures have proved successful. Forceps, if available, or tissue-protected fingers are applied to the tick as close to the skin and mouthparts as possible. An evaluation of adult tick removal devices showed that medium-tipped angled forceps gave the best overall results.[6] Sharp forceps can puncture engorged ticks, and straight ones make the angle of approach to grasp the tick more difficult. The technique is to pull straight back, gently but firmly, counter to the direction that the mouthparts are entered into the skin. If the tick is not embedded tightly, it should come out with little resistance. If it is well embedded, the force should be gradually increased. If the pulling force is too great or applied too rapidly, the tick may be decapitated and the mouthparts left buried in the skin. If this happens, they should be removed as a splinter would be to prevent infection. During the procedure the tick should not be squeezed or crushed because the gut contents may contain pathogens that can be released into the wound. After the tick has been removed, an antiseptic should be applied to the attachment site. The tick should be saved for species identification in case a disease has been transmitted.

Reaction to Arthropod Bites

Aside from pain, reactions to bites vary widely, depending on the number of previous bites, the species, and a person's sensitivities. Sensitivity may develop on initial exposure, but for most people, symptoms are less after subsequent encounters with an offending arthropod.

Feingold, Benjamini, and Michaeli[15] suggest that reactions to bites are caused by antigenic and nonantigenic irritating substances contained in the oral secretions. Repeated bites over time may produce a sequential effect on skin that can be characterized in consecutive stages of reactivity: (1) no observable skin reactions (initial bites), (2) delayed skin reactions, (3) immediate skin reactions followed by delayed reactions, (4) immediate reactions only, and (5) no reactions. Stage 5 supports subjective observations of persons who have long-term exposure to bites and who appear to have been desensitized. For further information on arthropod bite reactions see reference 50 and the discussions in Chapters 31 and 32.

Disease

For the most part, commercial advertising of insect repellents in North America highlights protection against discomfort, rather than against disease. Nevertheless, vector-borne diseases are endemic in North America and persons should be aware that they are at risk when they fail to protect themselves in areas indigenous to infective arthropod populations. A wise traveler is familiar with these diseases and their vectors. Early diagnosis and swift treatment could mean the difference between a brief illness and one with serious long-term complications.

Table 34-1 provides a general introduction to some important diseases, their associated parasites, the kinds of arthropod vectors, and the regions of the United States where they are likely to be encountered.

Visitors to other countries, particularly in subtropical and tropical regions, should also become familiar with the diseases listed in Table 34-2. For further reading on the diseases given in both tables and the associated vector species, see references 4, 27, 32, 50, and 55 and Chapters 33, 41, 44, and 45.

Table 34-1 Arthropod-Borne Diseases and Their Encounter Sites

Disease	Causal Agent	Vector	Distribution (States)
Encephalitis	Virus	Mosquito	All
Lyme disease	Spirochete	Tick	All*
Rocky Mountain spotted fever	*Rickettsia*	Tick	South Atlantic, West South Central
LaCrosse virus	Virus	Mosquito	East North Central
Colorado tick fever	Virus	Tick	Mountain
Sylvatic plague	Bacteria	Flea	Mountain, Pacific
Relapsing fever	Spirochete	Tick	Mountain
Tularemia	Bacteria	Deerfly	Mountain
Leishmaniasis	Protozoa	Sand fly	West South Central
Babesiosis	Protozoa	Tick	New England

*Lyme disease has been reported in all states except Montana.[9]

Table 34-2 Subtropical and Tropical Diseases

Disease	Causal Agent	Vector	Distribution
Malaria	Protozoa	Mosquito	Tropical, subtropical, temperate
Dengue	Virus	Mosquito	Tropical, subtropical
Filariasis	Microfilariae	Mosquito	Tropical, subtropical
Yellow fever	Virus	Mosquito	Tropical, subtropical
Leishmaniasis	Protozoa	Sand fly	Tropical, subtropical
Onchocerciasis	Microfilariae	Blackfly	Tropical
Chagas' disease	Trypanosome	Kissing bug	Tropical America
Plague	Bacteria	Flea	Tropical, subtropical
Trypanosomiasis	Trypanosome	Tsetse	Tropical Africa
Scrub typhus	*Rickettsia*	Chigger mite	Tropical, subtropical

Personal Protection

Personal protection is achieved in three ways: by avoiding infested areas, by use of physical barriers, and by use of chemicals. This discussion stresses physical and chemical methods of personal protection.

PHYSICAL PROTECTION

For outdoor protection against biting arthropods, a proper wardrobe can provide an excellent physical barrier. The objective is to prevent access of the pest to the skin. Ankle-high footwear, pant cuffs tucked into socks, pants with zipper fly, and a long-sleeved shirt tucked into pants will keep most ticks and chigger mites outside the clothing. Light-colored clothing makes it easier to spot ticks and is less attractive to biting flies.[2] Loose-fitting clothing made with tightly woven fabric coupled with a T-shirt undergarment reduces the likelihood of bites on the upper body, particularly the shoulder area. A light-colored, full-brimmed hat provides protection for the head and neck. Deerflies land on the hat instead of the head and neck, and blackflies and biting midges are less likely to crawl into hair and bite because the shaded area under the hat brim is less attractive. The outfit just described provides complete skin coverage except for the hands, face, and neck. Further protection is attained by wearing a head net, which is especially important with high densities of flying pests.

Garments designed for protection against insects are available. One hooded jacket and pants outfit (Bug Out Outdoor Wear, Wauwatosa, Wisc.; 414-258-1654), is made of polyester netting fine enough to exclude tiny biting midges and ticks; it is said to be a "protective billowy screen around the body" (Fig. 34-5).

With any clothing, crouching or bending may draw the fabric tight to parts of the body where mosquitoes might bite through. Another manufacturer (Shannon Outdoors, Winnsboro, S.C.; 800-852-8058) approaches this problem with clothing constructed of double-layered mesh that is supposed to be amply spaced to prevent mosquito penetration (Fig. 34-6).

Although all of these suggestions are effective, the garments may be uncomfortable to wear in hot weather or during vigorous activity.

Persons in suspected tick habitats should check their clothing often. At the end of the day, companions should inspect the head, back, and body carefully. Ticks, like lint on clothing, are easily trapped on a ring of cellophane tape over the fingers with the sticky side out. Sticky tape is particularly useful for rapid removal if a person is heavily infested; hundreds can be picked up quickly (Fig. 34-7). A variation of this idea is to use a lint roller with layers of removable sticky tape. When this device is rolled on infested clothing, ticks become stuck fast. A fresh sticky surface is exposed when the old layer with ticks is peeled off.

Mosquitoes and other nocturnal blood suckers are active at dusk, when it is wise for people to be indoors. Screens over windows, screened enclosures, or bed nets can provide protection. People on the move are best protected both indoors and outside with lightweight self-supported portable insect nets, in sizes that sleep one or two adults (Fig. 34-8).

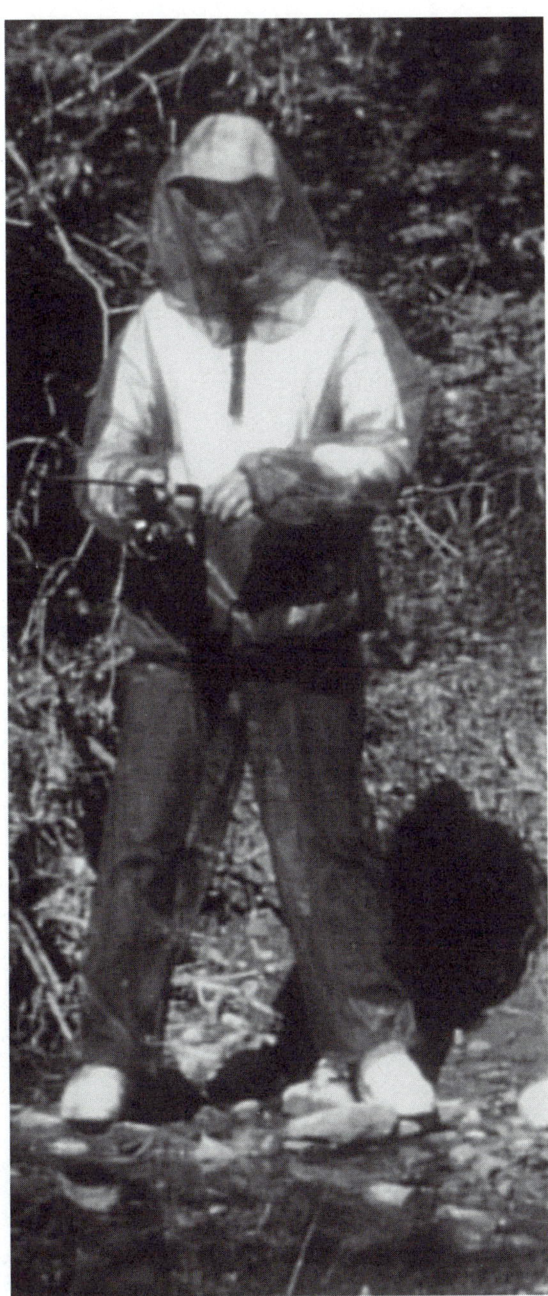

Fig. 34-5 Bug Out protective clothing of polyester mesh fine enough to prevent tiny biting midges from passing through. (Courtesy Bug Out Outdoor Wear, Wauwatosa, Wisc.)

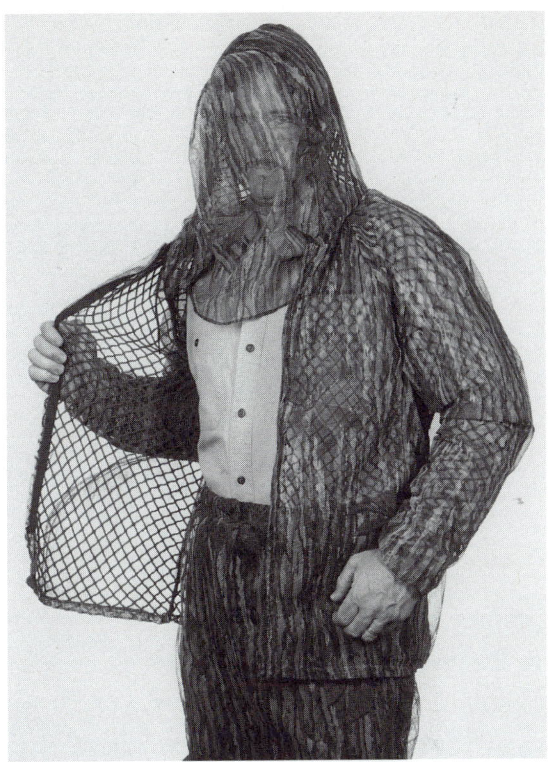

Fig. 34-6 Bug Tamer double-mesh clothing, which prevents mosquitoes from reaching the skin. (Courtesy Shannon Outdoors, Winnsboro, S.C.)

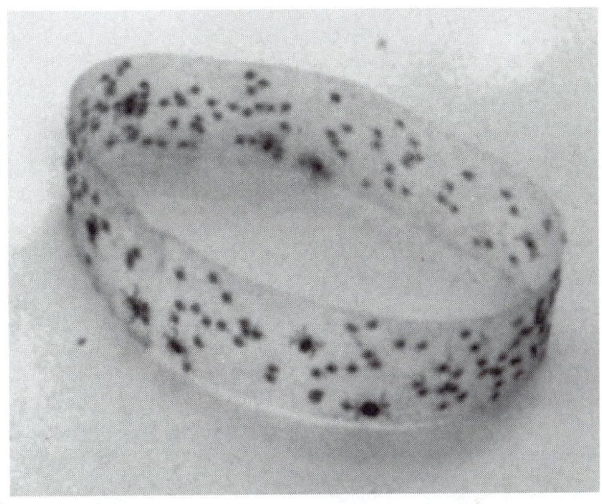

Fig. 34-7 Adult and juvenile ticks taken from clothing with cellophane tape, sticky side out.

These nets are lightweight (10 to 45 ounces) and compact for travel. A variety of designs and features are available at outdoor recreation stores in the United States and Canada. Further information can be obtained from Long Road Travel Supplies, Berkeley, Calif. 800-359-6040 (Fig. 34-8, *A* to *C*) and EPCO Design, 119 Seward St., Juneau, Alaska, 907-586-1622 (Fig. 34-8, *D* to *F*).

Avoid unnecessary use of lights. Along with myriad other insects, lights attract biting midges small enough to pass through standard mosquito screen. Campers should look for a site that is high, dry, open, and uncluttered. It makes little sense to camp in places where biting arthropods rest during the daytime.

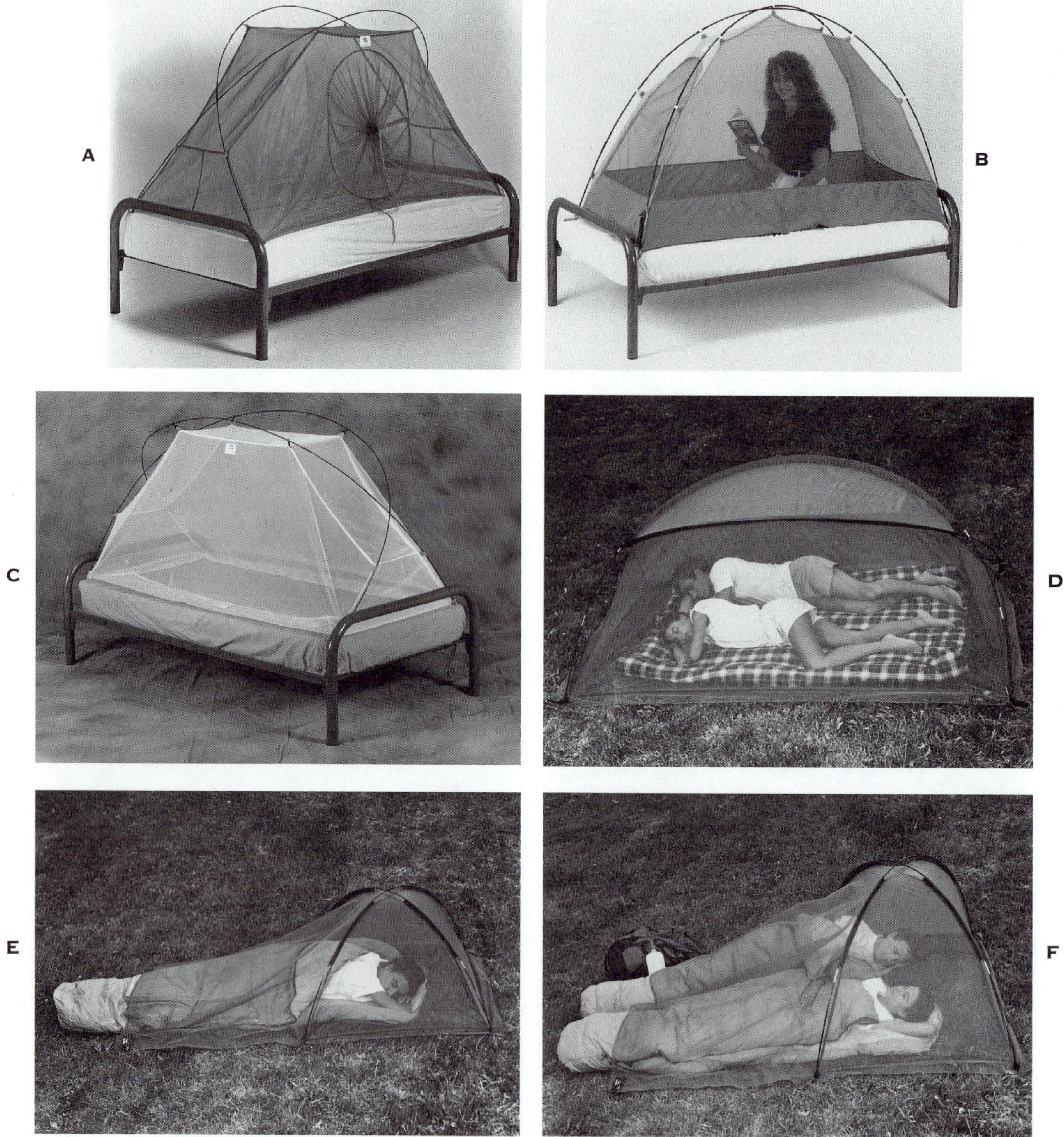

Fig. 34-8 Types of portable insect nets that can be used on a bed or on the ground. (**A** to **C** courtesy Long Road Travel Supplies, Berkeley, Calif.; **D** to **F** courtesy EPCO Design, Juneau, Alaska.)

CHEMICAL PROTECTION

Repellents

Three essential requisites for a good repellent are the number of different pests it repels, the duration of protection from bites, and acceptance by the user.

A January 1993 list of 27 active ingredients found in 212 products registered by the Environmental Protection Agency (EPA) for human use as arthropod repellents or feeding depressants included octyl bicycloheptene dicarboximide, dimethyl phthalate, oil of citronella, dipropyl isocinchomeronate, cedarwood oil, pyrethrins, and pine tar oil. None of these or the remaining 20 active ingredients totally fulfills the three requirements for a good repellent. One, however, clearly outperforms the rest as an all-purpose repellent: *N,N*-diethyl-meta-toluamide, recently renamed *N,N*-diethyl-3-methylbenzamide, but more commonly called DEET.[8,46,77] DEET is the major active ingredient in 90% of commercial repellent formulations marketed worldwide and is in 192 of the 212 products mentioned previously. It is effective against mosquitoes (including the Asian tiger mosquito), blackflies, biting midges, various biting flies, fleas, mites, and ticks. In more than 40 years since the discovery of DEET, no superior replacement has been developed, and no significant breakthrough is expected in the immediate future. This is in part because of the enormous cost of developing and registering a new repellent, currently estimated at $25 million.

DEET is a clear yellowish liquid, soluble in ethanol but not in water. Its chemical structure is:

O
N C_2H_5
C_2H_5
CH_3

DEET is a mixture of ortho, para, and meta isomers, of which the meta form is most active. Standard technical DEET is composed of 95% meta isomer. For example, if the label on a repellent product reads DEET and other isomers 50%, it means that 47.5% is meta and 2.5% is collectively ortho and para isomers. DEET can be applied directly to skin, clothing, screens, tents, and bedrolls. However, since DEET can soften or dissolve some materials, the label of the product should be consulted before it is applied to surfaces.

The length of time a repellent gives full protection from bites depends on several factors, the most important of which are the application rate, uniformity of coverage, pest species and population density, rate of absorption into the skin, user's attractiveness as a host, user's activity level, rate of evaporation, and weather. A truly effective repellent can be applied in relatively small amounts, provided it is spread evenly and completely over all exposed skin. DEET and other available repellents lack strong spatial activity; consequently, untreated skin proximate to treated skin is vulnerable to attack (Fig. 34-9).

Arthropod sensitivity to repellents varies. For example, DEET poorly repels some anopheline mosquitoes[65] but is very effective against the coastal salt marsh and woodland mosquitoes of North America. Repellents are used extensively for protection from a species before the effectiveness against that species has been evaluated scientifically. For example, the efficacy of commercial repellents is known for only a fraction of approximately 170 mosquito species believed to live in North America.[77]

After application the period of protection a repellent provides is often related to pest population density. The greater the density, the shorter the duration of repellency. This does not mean that the repellent suddenly and completely fails to protect. Instead, some bites might be experienced sooner than would normally occur with a smaller pest population. Reapplication usually will solve this problem.

Early attempts at controlling the absorption rate of repellents into skin by use of polymers, encapsulation, and various additives were unsuccessful. However, new formulation technology allows a smaller amount of the active ingredient to provide protection for the same duration of time. An example is the DEET-based repellent recently developed for the U.S. Armed Services.[64] This formulation uses less than half as much DEET (35%) as was in the original, with better results.

Individual attractiveness, activities that cause abrasion and sweating, and meteorologic conditions also influence the effectiveness of a repellent. Chemicals emanating from the body may determine attractiveness to the pest. The more attractive the host, the more likely that duration of repellency is reduced. Any excessive sweating and wiping or other abrasive action that depletes the supply of available repellent on skin reduces its effectiveness.[75] Rain will easily wash DEET-based repellents off skin and clothing. These conditions may justify more frequent reapplication.

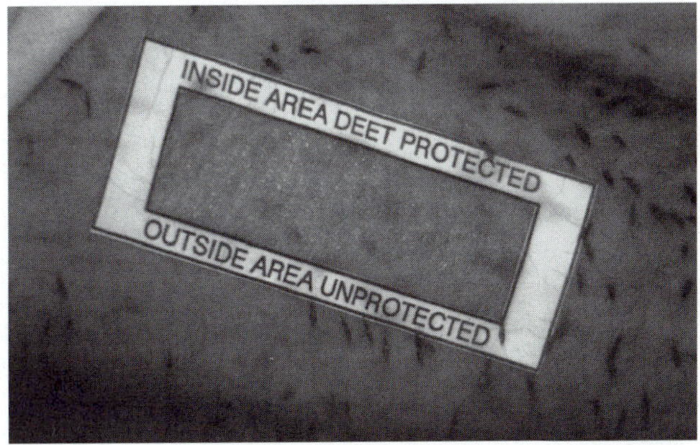

Fig. 34-9 Mosquito response to untreated skin of the arm when the indicated area has been treated with the repellent DEET. The close proximity of treated skin does not protect untreated skin.

Consumer acceptance of DEET varies because of its odor, oiliness, and solvent effect (it softens and damages some plastics, paints, vinyl, and waxed surfaces). These objectionable characteristics are minimized by controlling the amount of DEET and by adding perfumes or other materials to mask its presence. Formulations containing up to 35% DEET appear to be acceptable to most people. Higher concentrations are generally less well tolerated[28] but normally do not require reapplication as often.

Choosing a suitable repellent from the large number of products available can be bewildering to the consumer. For example, at this writing 35 repellents are registered by the EPA that are simply technical DEET with different trade names. Others contain the same active ingredients in proportions so nearly identical that only the packaging and added fragrances are different. Moreover, various products can have from 2% to 100% DEET in the formulation. A compendium of some currently available over-the-counter insect repellent formulations was tabulated to familiarize the reader with the variety of choices (Table 34-3). They all contain DEET, whether in spray, lotion, gel, cream, towelette, or stick form. As a rule, the higher the concentration,

Table 34-3 DEET Content of Some Over-the-Counter Insect Repellents

Manufacturer	Product Name	Formulation	Percent
Miles Inc., Chicago, Illinois	Cutter Evergreen Scent	Cream	35
	Cutter Insect Repellent	Stick	33
	Cutter Insect Repellent	Spray	18
	Cutter Maximum Strength Formula 100	Lotion	100
	Cutter for Kids	Spray	8
Wisconsin Pharmacal Co., Jackson, Wisconsin	Repel Insect Repellent Towelette	Wipe	55
	Repel 100	Lotion	100
	Repel Scented Family Formula	Spray	35
	Repel Insect Aerosol	Spray	55
Hysan Corp., Chicago, Illinois	Adios Insect Repellent	Spray	7
Reckitt & Coleman Household Products, Wayne, New Jersey	Insect Repellent Spray For Personal Use	Spray	7
Whitmire Research Laboratories, Inc., St. Louis, Missouri	P/P Outdoor Lotion	Lotion	19.4
	Whitmire Insect Repellent Stick No. 1	Stick	14
Fuller Brush Co., Great Bend, Kansas	Insect Repellent	Gel	7
	Ful-Scat Insect Repellent	Spray	8
D-Con Co. Inc., Montvale, New Jersey	6-12 Super Strength Premium	Spray	26.3
	6-12 Plus Brand	Spray	5
	Sportsmate II Premium	Cream	45
Pete Rickard Inc., Cobleskill, New York	Ole Time Woodsman Kampers	Lotion	50
	Ole Time Woodsman Jungle Formula	Spray	60
S.C. Johnson & Son Inc., Racine, Wisconsin	Off Insect Repellent	Spray	15
	Maximum Strength Deep Woods Off 100	Lotion	100
	Off Towelette	Wipe	25
	Off Skintastic II	Lotion	7.5
	Unscented Off	Spray	15
Schering-Plough Health Care Products Inc., Liberty Corners, New Jersey	Muskol Insect Repellent	Lotion	100
	Muskol Insect Repellent	Spray	25
ARI, Inc., Griffin, Georgia	Bug Barrier 100%	Lotion	100
	Bug Barrier	Spray	7
	Bug Barrier II	Spray	25
AMREP, Inc., Marietta, Georgia	Misty Insect Repellent	Spray	7
	Misty Extra-Strength	Spray	25
Woodlands Products, Ormond Beach, Florida	Woodlands Insect Repellent	Lotion	10
CCL Custom C.C.L. Manufacturing Inc., Danville, Illinois	Personal Insect Repellent I	Spray	10.5
	CCL Quick Breaking Insect Repellent	Foam	8.9
Winsol Labs, Seattle, Washington	Eddie Bauer Insect Formula	Lotion	100
3M Co., St. Paul, Minnesota	3M Ultrathon	Lotion	33.3
	3M Ultrathon	Spray	9.6
Olson Outdoor Laboratory, Freehold, New Jersey	One + One	Lotion	11.2
Littlepoint Corp., Cambridge, Massachusetts	Littlepoint Insect Repellent	Lotion	10

the longer the duration of activity. For normal use, however, choosing the lower concentrations is preferable. Where arthropod pest attacks may be more severe or disease is a concern, products with a higher percentage of DEET are favored. Nonetheless, full-strength DEET should not be needed, even under extreme conditions.

To some consumers odor is important; to others the application method, such as spray, is important; and to still others it is how the repellent feels on the skin that matters most. *Read the label and use only as directed.*

The newest products contain considerably less DEET. Because of certain objectionable characteristics of DEET and the possible adverse reactions from overexposure to DEET, consumers prefer these newer products. The repellents provide an alternative for children and for adults with sensitive skin. They also offer a choice of more pleasant products that protect for a few hours over less pleasant products that may last all day. The user benefits by having a wider selection of repellents.

Hazard Assessment of DEET

An estimated 50 to 100 million people use DEET each year. Although serious adverse reactions are thought to be rare, occasional toxic and allergic reactions to DEET have been reported.[77] Studies have been conducted to determine how rapidly DEET is absorbed and metabolized and whether adverse effects may result from chronic use. The data suggest that dermal absorption is rapid but that excretion rates vary.

DEET is not usually a dermal irritant or a sensitizer, but in selected cases and under some circumstances it can cause skin reactions. For example, red, raised lesions developed in a 35-year-old woman who had applied an unspecific amount of DEET. Tests revealed hypersensitivity to DEET, indicating that the response was immunologic.[41] Also, in soldiers using a high concentration of DEET (50% to 75%), burning, erythema, and blisters of the antecubital fossa developed.[38]

In a health hazard evaluation report on use of repellents by Park Service employees at Everglades National Park, the National Institute for Occupational Safety and Health recommended limiting the amount of DEET used to that absolutely necessary for repellency.[45] An EPA study of DEET[77] reported that its general toxicity is low and that local skin reactions are infrequent. However, individual responses can be severe, depending on the area of application. Slight temporary eye irritation occurs frequently. The report added that inadequate information exists to judge potential effects in persons with preexisting allergic conditions or to determine if specific groups (such as children or pregnant women) are at risk.

Since 1961, six children, all girls from 1 to 8 years of age, have been reported to have toxic encephalopathy associated with use of products containing DEET.[23,26,53,54,81] Exposure to the repellent ranged from a few days to 3 months. In one case, exposure was by ingestion. Three deaths occurred,[53] but the causes of death were not resolved because of varying circumstances and case histories. One physician reported that an enzyme deficiency may have precipitated the attack[26]; in the other two cases, fatalities were suspected to be caused by hypersensitivity to DEET.[51,81] These observations emphasize the need for extreme care in the use of repellents around young children. Prolonged and excessive use of high concentrations of DEET by adults should also be avoided.

Clothing composed of wide-mesh polyester-cotton netting treated with DEET was developed by the Department of Defense and the U.S. Department of Agriculture for use as a lightweight overgarment for protection mainly against flying insects (Fig. 34-10).[22] The cotton fibers act as a wick that, unless washed, will continue to release the protective vapors of DEET for many weeks. Cole Outdoor Products of America (Lincoln, Nebraska) offers protective pants and jackets of this mesh fabric that may be worn over short-sleeved shirts and shorts during the warm summer months. This DEET-treated apparel is effective against some biting pests without the need for application of repellents directly to exposed skin.

Repellents clearly provide only temporary protection. Following the guidelines in Box 34-1 will improve efficacy and help prevent undesirable effects.

Insecticides

Chemical repellents applied to skin and clothing provide effective and reliable short-term protection but are quickly lost from the skin and easily washed from clothing. Another approach is the use of clothing treated with a contact insecticide, or one that kills insects that alight upon it. One such compound, permethrin, is (3-phenoxyphenyl) methyl (±) *cis*/*trans* 3-(2,2-dichloroethenyl) 2,2-dimethylcyclopro-

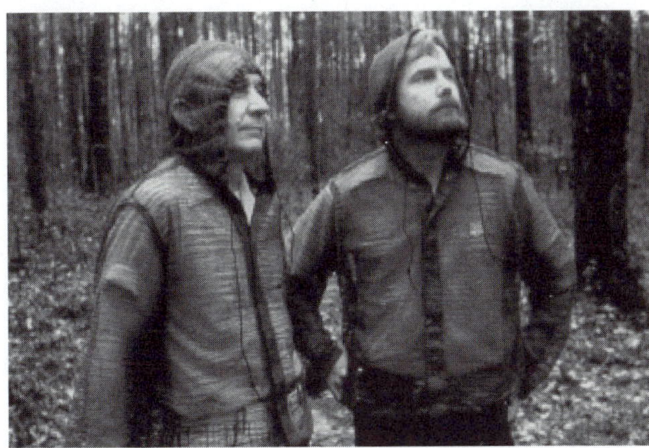

Fig. 34-10 A DEET-treated lightweight polyester-cotton hooded overjacket, developed by the Agricultural Research Service of the U.S. Department of Agriculture and military scientists, provides long-term protection against a variety of flying insects, including mosquitoes, biting midges, and blackflies.

BOX 34-1

GUIDELINES FOR USE OF INSECT REPELLENTS

DO:

Read the entire label carefully.
Choose a product that contains DEET and is easy to apply.
Look for an EPA registration label.
Follow use directions carefully.
Apply to *all* exposed skin.
Spray repellent on clothing where it fits tightly and insects can bite through.
Apply to lower pant legs and socks.

DON'T:

Apply unless needed.
Apply close to eyes, lips, cuts, sunburn, or rashes.
Apply excessive amounts, particularly on children.
Apply to children's hands.
Spray directly on the face (instead, spray onto hands and apply sparingly to face).
Spray near vinyl, plastics, paints, or waxed surfaces.

panecarboxylate. Its use has many advantages over conventional repellents. As a clothing impregnant, it is safe and long lasting; it persists after extensive wear and washing and is stable in light.[67] Even after 20 washings, permethrin-impregnated fabric worn on the skin prevents mosquitoes from biting. Also, permethrin is not greasy, is not a plasticizer, and is nearly odorless. Because permethrin protects by insecticidal action rather than by repellency, its use can noticeably reduce the density of the biting population in the immediate area.[62]

Permethrin has been tested worldwide as a U.S. military clothing impregnant to help guard troops against arthropod-borne diseases. It is recognized by the World Health Organization (WHO) as a highly effective chemical for treatment of bed nets to protect against malaria mosquitoes.[56,68] A pressurized spray formulation for ticks and mosquitoes of 0.5% permethrin in a water base was more effective than DEET-based repellents against tick species known to transmit Rocky Mountain spotted fever and Lyme disease.[14,69] The same spray is now EPA registered, available in the military supply system, and sold commercially under such trade names as Duranon Tick Repellent, Permanone Tick Repellent, and Coulston's Permethrin Arthropod Repellent. The term "repellent" appears to be a misnomer when used regarding this insecticide. Nevertheless, like repellents, its function is to prevent bites. After contact, pests drop or fly from treated clothing but are not necessarily killed.

Further evidence of the effectiveness of permethrin is its persistence in preventing mosquito bites over a 9-month period in a tent exposed to year-long weathering.[60] Permethrin is also registered by the EPA under the trade name Expel for use against ticks, mosquitoes, and other flying and crawling insects and in coatings applied to fabrics for tents, shelters, truck covers, awnings, hunting blinds, and netting.

ELECTRONIC, SYSTEMIC, BOTANICAL, AND OTHER PRODUCTS AS REPELLENTS

For over a decade, various electronic devices have been sold with assurances that they protect against mosquitoes and other insects. Of the four or five different original types, essentially three continue to be marketed: light traps with electrocution grids, ultrasound devices, and audible sound devices. Light traps use household current and contain black, fluorescent, or incandescent lights. Consumers seem to prefer electrocution traps because they see piles of dead insects under the trap. What they do not realize is that few of these dead insects are mosquitoes or other blood suckers. Hungry mosquitoes are not preferentially attracted to lights; they are attracted to carbon dioxide and the odors of a host. In studies to determine if mosquito biting could be reduced by use of these traps, it was found that humans near the electrocuting devices were consistently more attractive than the device. Even after 11 days of continuous operation, the electrocuting devices failed to reduce the mosquito biting rate.[47] Most of the dead mosquito-like insects found beneath these traps are harmless midges and crane flies. Actually, light traps attract *more* insects into the area; this is especially true of traps baited with black light because the vision of many insects is better in the ultraviolet spectrum. An estimated 95% of the insect population is either beneficial or innocuous to people, so the traps may actually have a negative effect by eliminating large numbers of helpful predators and parasites.

Ultrasound devices using household current are said to repel a variety of pests, including mosquitoes and fleas. Investigations with seven different devices reveal they had little or no effect on mosquitoes seeking a blood meal.[17,70] The devices were also ineffective in repelling or removing flea infestations from indoors.[36] Scientific data fail to show that the devices repel fleas and ticks from an animal's body. The Federal Trade Commission has charged one ultrasonic manufacturer with making false and unsubstantiated claims, maintaining that "the devices do not eliminate rodent and flea infestation in the home."[30]

It is claimed that hand-carried battery-powered devices producing audible sound repel female mosquitoes from large areas and prevent bites. They are said to simulate the male mosquito sound (with no supporting scientific evidence, the claim is that mated females are repelled by male wingbeat sound) and the sound of bats. These devices vary in size from that of a lipstick to a pack of cigarettes and range in price from $4 to $30. Investigations of a large variety of these devices against many different mosquito species have been conducted in Alaska,[21] California,[19] Canada,[39] Delaware,[37] Denmark,[3] England,[10,12] Florida,[71] Gambia,[12] Russia,[52] and Zaire.[12] The results consistently confirmed that the devices neither repel mosquitoes nor prevent them from biting.

Although such scientific evidence should be sufficiently persuasive, the following quotation from *National Geographic Magazine*[59] probably paints a more vivid picture:

> During all my years in the far north I have never encountered such a plague of mosquitoes as we suffered on Knud Peninsula. Most of us resorted to nets and repellent, but Tore put his trust in the electronic age. As we unpacked our gear at the base camp, he produced a device about the size of a pack of cigarettes, equipped with a cord to be worn around the neck. "It's a battery-powered sonic mosquito guard," he announced. "It gives off a signal so high you can barely hear it, and mosquitoes hate it." Poor Tore. Whoever designed the device must have chosen the wrong frequency. The mosquitoes loved it, and they flocked to Tore in such droves it almost seemed that the best spot to be was roughly 10 feet away from him so that he acted as a lure. Within a week the sonic guard quietly disappeared, and Ellesmere Island's brief electronic age came to an end.

Sales promotions of both ultrasound and audible sound devices appear to fluctuate. After sales drop following initial performance failure and the advertising ceases, the shape, color, or size of the product is altered, and new promotional strategies are contrived. With the emergence of a fresh crop of unwary consumers, the marketing cycle begins anew.

It is always wise to request scientific evidence of efficacy and consult a county cooperative extension service agent or a representative of another consumer-oriented organization before purchasing any new-theory pest control merchandise.

The concept of ingesting a pill to protect against biting arthropods has great appeal. It would eliminate the need to apply chemicals to the skin and clothing, wear extra garments during warm weather, and be subjected to other inconveniences. Unfortunately, no such medication yet exists. In 1943, oral thiamine chloride was reported to reduce the itch, welts, and biting of mosquitoes.[73] Additional studies in 1945[13] and 1972[57] seemed to substantiate these findings, but when subjective observations were challenged with objective data in 1944,[79] 1952,[35] 1969,[33] and 1973,[40] researchers unanimously found no repellent effect on mosquitoes. Still, at least two products containing thiamine chloride appeared on the market. They were widely advertised as being the most effective and least expensive of all mosquito repellents, with claims for repelling mosquitoes for up to 24 hours. In part because of misleading advertising, the products were investigated by the Food and Drug Administration. On June 10, 1983, the following statement appeared in the Federal Register, Part III, p. 26987[16]:

> There is a lack of adequate data to establish the effectiveness of this or any other ingredient for OTC (over the counter) internal use as an insect repellent. Labeling claims for OTC orally administered insect repellent drug products is either false, misleading, or unsupported by scientific data.

In earlier times, somewhat protective plant-derived repellents were available. Later, these were replaced by more effective synthetic chemicals. More recently, however, people have been searching for natural product supplements or so-called substitutes for chemical repellents. Also, natural products are of interest in developing countries where industrial resources are limited and botanical repellents may be developed inexpensively and made readily available. For example, Quwenling, an insect repellent product of China derived from extracts of the lemon eucalyptus plant *(Eucalyptus maculata citriodon),* has largely replaced dimethyl phthalate as the repellent of choice in that country.[11]

Unfortunately, no repellents of plant origin, including Quwenling,[65] have been found that provide the duration of protection and spectrum of effectiveness that are available with DEET. A publication listing 677 plant species reported to have been used in different parts of the world for pest control identifies nearly 200 plants said to protect against mosquitoes, mites, ticks, fleas, and biting flies. However, actual efficacy data are not given.[72] Two technical publications from the U.S. Department of Agriculture[34,44] report results of laboratory tests against mosquitoes with over 600 botanical samples, of which only about 4% were found to have some repellent effect. The common names of the plants reported to have repellent properties are allspice, bay, camphor, cedar, cinnamon, citronella, geranium, lavender, nutmeg, pennyroyal, peppermint, pine, thyme, and verbena (for technical names see reference 29). The data suggest that the plants may provide some protection from mosquitoes for up to 2 hours, depending on mosquito species.

Oil of garlic applied to the skin in tests against blackflies in India[5] was reported to be very effective, but its obnoxious odor doomed its common use. Laboratory and field tests in India[48] indicated up to 4 hours of protection when a cream containing 19% citronella oil was used, but it caused slight facial irritation.

The effects of two EPA-registered U.S. products and one Australian unregistered product containing botanicals were compared with 15% DEET in ethanol in repelling two mosquito species (Table 34-4). Based on these data, a person using the natural product would have to reapply the repellent up to 28 times to equal one application of a relatively low concentration of DEET formulation. Furthermore, little is known about the potential health risk of frequent use of these natural products.

Consumers should beware of marketing ploys used to promote some of these products. One children's lotion is claimed to be chemical and DEET free. It is the blend of at least 17 chemicals, but nowhere on the label does it claim to

Table 34-4 Comparison of Chemical and Botanical Repellents

	Minutes of Complete Protection from Bites			
Mosquito Species	**Product A***	**Product B†**	**Product C‡**	**15% DEET**
Aedes aegypti (yellow fever mosquito)	10	13	9	260
Aedes taeniorhynchus (salt marsh mosquito)	19	16	20	335

*Contains undisclosed amounts of citronella, pennyroyal, sassafras, cajuput, lavender, bergamot, calendula, and soy and tea tree oils.
†Citronella 10% plus inert ingredients 90%.
‡Oil of citronella 19%, oil of cedar 19%, oil of lavender 4.8%, oil of geranium 1.2%, plus inert ingredients 56%.

repel insects. The DEET-free message implies that it has repellency and probably sells the product.

Another lotion is advertised to "not attract mosquitoes" but does not claim to repel them either. Neither product has an EPA registration number confirming that it is a repellent. The EPA cautions *not* to use unregistered pesticides.

The available evidence suggests that an all-purpose naturally occurring repellent may not exist. On the other hand, the isolation and identification of promising materials of plant origin may reveal superior repellents that can be chemically synthesized. For example, oxazolidine derivatives of citronellal, a commercially available chemical derived from citronella oil, have been reported to be significantly more effective as fabric treatments than either DEET or dimethyl phthalate.[76]

The concentrated bath oil Skin-So-Soft (marketed by Avon Products, Inc.) is being widely used at full strength as a skin application to protect against biting midges and mosquitoes. Tests with biting midges demonstrated that much of its effectiveness was the result of a mechanical factor—the midges became trapped on the skin surface because it was so oily.[63] However, some fractions of the product have been reported to have repellent properties.[34,58] In tests against mosquitoes in the laboratory[66] and field (unpublished data), duration of protection for Skin-So-Soft at full strength ranged from 0.6 to 1.3 hours, whereas DEET at 25% ranged from 6 to 8 hours; the bath oil would have to be reapplied up to 11 times to achieve the protection provided by DEET. These tests were against high densities of insect population. At low densities, a longer duration of protection would be expected. Skin-So-Soft might provide several hours of protection when only a small number of mosquitoes are present.

In spite of the endorsements of repellency given to Skin-So-Soft, it is not EPA registered for this use.

INTEGRATED APPROACH TO PERSONAL PROTECTION

An integrated approach is rewarded by excellent protection nearly anywhere against a broad spectrum of blood-feeding arthropods. Field clothing that is carefully chosen, properly worn, and pretreated with permethrin, plus an effective all-purpose DEET-based repellent on exposed skin, is environmentally safe and not only protects the individual, but also kills or disables only attacking pests. The repellent applied on skin drives pests to the treated clothing that is toxic to them; thus the wearer becomes a walking insect trap.

Each personal protection strategy has a limited protective value. Combined they become a potent defense. For example, proper application of repellent to only exposed skin may protect against blackflies and biting midges but not mosquitoes, because mosquitoes repelled from treated skin will bite through untreated clothing. Treating exposed skin and wearing treated clothing can protect against all three insects, but often not against ticks and chigger mites. Thus, to ensure protection against all of the above pests, a person must use repellent on exposed skin, wear treated clothing, and tuck pant cuffs into stockings. One further suggestion is to wear a treated hat. Deerflies, biting midges, and some blackflies seem to favor the head and will readily crawl into the hair and bite where there is no protection.

Being prepared is important. Before a wilderness trek, other outdoor activity, or trip to unfamiliar territory, the traveler should learn what arthropod pests and diseases may be encountered. The essentials for protection should be packed, since they may not otherwise be available in the area traveled. These include a repellent, a bed net or tent treated with permethrin, proper clothing, clothing treatment, and, where mosquito-borne diseases occur, the currently recommended immunizations (such as for yellow fever) and drug prophylaxis (such as for malaria).

A PERSPECTIVE ON PERSONAL PROTECTION

After nearly a century of enormous advances in the study and treatment of arthropod-borne diseases, personal protection endures as an indispensable means of preventing host-vector contact. However, the essentials of this discipline have remained largely unchanged, probably because in the past a disproportionate amount of support for scientific research has been devoted to medical cures for diseases rather than preventive approaches to managing arthropods that transmit disease agents.

Personal protection techniques have been improved mostly by the borrowing of materials and knowledge from unrelated fields. For example, dimethyl phthalate was used as a plasticizer in the chemical industry before it was discovered to have repellent properties. Advances in cosmetics formulation technology helped to extend the persistence of

DEET on skin.[64] Agricultural chemicals (permethrin and other pyrethroids) were adopted for impregnating clothing and netting, and textile industry methods and materials have been applied to the treatment and design of protective clothing and netting.

Although the repellency of DEET and other chemicals has been known for 40 years or more, the biologic basis for repellent activity has never been determined. Also not yet determined is why people differ in attractiveness to biting arthropods, or how mosquitoes distinguish a preferred animal host from other animals. Admittedly these are complex questions, but within the answers lie exciting new areas of study.

One area being explored is the identification of chemicals emanating from human skin that attract mosquitoes. These investigations might reveal if preferred and fortuitous hosts differ chemically, if diet is a factor in host attractiveness, if systemic repellents are a realistic goal, and if natural repellents occur on human skin.

Success would mean that powerful new strategies against mosquito-borne diseases could be developed before the end of this century. Meanwhile, protection from blood-feeding arthropods must continue to rely on the knowledge and materials at hand.

REFERENCES

1. Acree F Jr et al: L-Lactic acid: a mosquito attractant isolated from humans, *Science* 161:1346, 1968.
2. Anderson JF: The control of horse flies and deer flies (Diptera: Tabanidae), *Myia* 3:547, 1985.
3. Arevad K: Evaluation of an electronic mosquito-repelling device. In *Danish Pest Infestation Laboratory annual report,* Lyngby, Denmark, 1981, Statens Skadedyrlaboratorium Arsberentning.
4. Benenson AS, editor: *Control of communicable diseases in man,* ed 15, Washington, DC, 1990, American Public Health Assoc.
5. Bhuyan M, Saxena BN, Rao KM: Repellent property of oil of garlic, *Allium sativum* Liun, *Ind J Exp Biol* 12:575, 1974.
6. Bowles DE, McHugh CP, Spradling SL: Evaluation of devices for removing attached *Rhipicephalus sanguineus* (Acari: Ixodidae), *J Med Entomol* 29:901, 1992.
7. Burgess NRH, editor: *John Hull Grundy's arthropods of medical importance,* Watch Cottage, Chilbolton, Eng, 1981, Noble Books.
8. Carlson DA: Repellents. In Eckroth D, editor: *Kirk-Othmer encyclopedia of chemical technology,* ed 3, New York, 1984, John Wiley.
9. Craven R, Dennis D, editors: *Lyme disease surveillance summary,* March 1992, 3:1, Fort Collins, Colo, Centers for Disease Control Division of Vector-Borne Infectious Diseases.
10. Curtis CF: Fact and fiction in mosquito attraction and repulsion, *Parasitol Today* 2:316, 1986.
11. Curtis CF, editor: *Appropriate technology in vector control,* Boca Raton, Fla, 1990, CRC Press.
12. Curtis C, White G: Once bitten, twice shy, *New Sci,* Feb 4, 1982, p 328.
13. Eder HL: Flea bites, prevention and treatment with thiamine chloride, *Arch Pediatr* 62:300, 1945.
14. Evans SR, Korch GW Jr, Lawson MA: Comparative field evaluation of permethrin and DEET-treated military uniforms for personal protection against ticks (Acari), *J Med Entomol* 27:829, 1990.
15. Feingold BF, Benjamini E, Michaeli D: The allergic responses to insect bites, *Annu Rev Entomol* 13:137, 1968.
16. Food and Drug Administration: Drug products containing active ingredients offered over-the-counter (OTC) for oral use as insect repellents, *Fed Reg* 48:26987, 1983.
17. Foster WA, Lutes KR: Tests of ultrasonic emissions on mosquito attraction to hosts in a flight chamber, *J Am Mosq Control Assoc* 1:199, 1985.
18. Frazier CA: *Insect allergy: allergic and toxic reactions to insects and other arthropods,* St Louis, 1969, Warren H Green.
19. Garcia R, Rochers BD, Voigt WG: Evaluation of electronic mosquito repellers under laboratory and field conditions, *Calif Vector Views* 23:21, 1976.
20. Gillies MT, Wilkes TJ: A comparison of the range of attraction of animal baits and of carbon dioxide for some West African mosquitoes, *Bull Entomol Res* 59:441, 1969.
21. Gorham JR: Tests of mosquito repellents in Alaska, *Mosq News* 34:409, 1974.
22. Grothaus RH et al: Insect repellent jacket: status, value and potential, *Mosq News* 36:11, 1976.
23. Gryboski J, Weinstein D, Ordway NK: Toxic encephalopathy apparently related to the use of an insect repellent, *N Engl J Med* 264:289, 1961.
24. Gustafson HE et al: Human cutaneous leishmaniasis acquired in Texas, *Am J Trop Med Hyg* 34:58, 1985.
25. Hawley WA: The biology of *Aedes albopictus, J Am Mosq Control Assoc* 1(suppl):1, 1988.
26. Heick HMC et al: Reye-like syndrome associated with use of insect repellent in a presumed heterozygote for ornithine carbamoyl transferase deficiency, *J Pediatr* 97:471, 1980.
27. Hoogstraal H: Tickborne diseases of humans—a history of environmental and epidemiological changes. In *Proceedings of the Medical Entomology Centenary Symposium,* London, 1978, Royal Society of Tropical Medicine and Hygiene.
28. Hooper RL, Wirtz RA: Insect repellent used by troops in the field: results of a questionaire, *Milit Med* 148:34, 1983.
29. Jacobson M: *Glossary of plant-derived insect deterrents,* Boca Raton, Fla, 1990, CRC Press.
30. *Kansas Pesticide News Letter,* April 14, 1992, 15:24.
31. Kettle DS: The bionomics and control of *Culicoides* and *Leptoconops* (Diptera, Ceratopogonidae = Heleidae), *Annu Rev Entomol* 7:401, 1962.
32. Kettle DS: *Medical and veterinary entomology,* New York, 1985, John Wiley.
33. Khan AA et al: Vitamin B1 is not a systemic mosquito repellent in man, *Trans St John's Hosp Dermatol Soc* 55:99, 1969.
34. King WV: Chemicals evaluated as insecticides and repellents at Orlando, Fla, In: *USDA Handbook, 69,* Washington, DC, 1954,
35. Kingscote AA: Orally administered insect repellents: approaches and problems related to the search, *Proc 10th Int Congr Entomol,* 3:799, 1958.
36. Koehler PG, Patterson RS, Webb JC: Efficacy of ultrasound for German cockroaches and oriental rat flea control, *J Econ Entomol* 79:1027, 1986.
37. Kutz FW: Evaluations of an electronic mosquito repelling device, *Mosq News* 34:369, 1974.
38. Lamberg SI, Mulrennan JA Jr: Bullous reaction to diethyltoluamide (DEET): resembling a blistering insect eruption, *Arch Dermatol* 100:582, 1969.
39. Lewis DJ, Fairchild WL, Leprince DJ: Evaluation of an electronic mosquito repeller, *Can Entomol* 114:699, 1982.
40. Maasch HJ: Investigations on the repellent effect of vitamin B1, *Z Tropen Med Parasit* 4:119, 1973.
41. Maibach HI, Johnson HL: Contact urticaria syndrome: contact urticaria to diethyltoluamide—immediate-type hypersensitivity, *Arch Dermatol* 111:726, 1975.
42. Marshall NA, Street DH: Allergy to *Triatoma protracta* (Heteroptera: Reduviidae) I. Etiology, antigen preparation, diagnosis and immunotherapy, *J Med Entomol* 19:248, 1982.

43. Marshall NA et al: The prevalence of allergic sensitization to *Triatoma protracta* (Heteroptera: Reduviidae) in a southern California, USA, community, *J Med Entomol* 23:117, 1986.
44. Materials evaluated as insecticides, repellents, and chemosterilants at Orlando and Gainesville, Florida, 1952-1964. In *USDA-ARS Agriculture Handbook 340,* Washington, DC, 1967, Superintendent of Documents.
45. McConnell R, Fidler AT, Chrislip D: *Health hazard evaluation report,* US Dept of Health and Human Services, CDC, HETA 83-085-1757, Cincinnati, 1986, National Institute for Occupational Safety and Health.
46. Metcalf RL: Repellents to bloodsucking insects. In *Encyclopedia of chemical technology,* vol 13, New York, 1977, John Wiley, p 475.
47. Nasci RS, Harris CW, Porter CK: Failure of an insect electrocutor device to reduce mosquito biting, *Mosq News* 43:180, 1983.
48. Osmani Z, Anees I, Naidu MB: Insect repellent creams from essential oils, *Pesticides* 6:19, 1972.
49. Pechuman LL: *Symphoromyia* biting in New York State (Diptera, Rhagionidae), *Mosq News* 27:183, 1967.
50. Peters W: *Color atlas of arthropods in clinical medicine,* ed 3, London, 1992, Wolfe.
51. Pronczuk de Garbino J, Laborde A, Fogel de Korc E: Toxicity of an insect repellent: *N,N*-diethyltoluamide, *Vet Hum Toxicol* 25:422, 1983.
52. Rasnitsyn SP et al: Negative results of a test of examples of sound generators intended to repel mosquitoes, *Meditsinskaya Parazitologiya i Parazitarnye Bolezni* 43:706, 1974.
53. Robbins PJ, Cherniack MG: Review of the biodistribution and toxicity of the insect repellent *N,N*-diethyl-*m*-toluamide (DEET), *J Toxicol Environ Health* 18:503, 1986.
54. Roland EH, Jan JE, Rigg JM: Toxic encephalopathy in a child after brief exposure to insect repellent, *Can Med Assoc J* 132:155, 1985.
55. Rose SR: *International travel health guide,* ed 4, Northampton, Mass, 1992, Travel Medicine.
56. Rozendaal JA: Impregnated mosquito nets and curtains for self-protection and vector control, *Trop Dis Bull* 86:1, 1989.
57. Ruiz-Maldonado R, Tamayo L: Treatment of 100 children with papular urticaria with thiamine chloride, *Int J Dermatol* 12:258, 1973.
58. Rutledge LC, Wirtz RA, Buescher MD: Repellent activity of a proprietary bath oil (Skin-So-Soft), *Mosq News* 42:557, 1982.
59. Schledermann P: Eskimo and Viking finds in the Arctic, *National Geographic* 159:585, 1981.
60. Schreck CE: Permethrin and dimethyl phthalate as tent fabric treatments against *Aedes aegypti, J Am Mosq Control Assoc* 7:533, 1991.
61. Schreck CE: The status of DEET *N,-N*-diethyl-*m*-toluamide as a repellent for *Anopheles albimanus, J Am Mosq Control Assoc* 1:98, 1985.
62. Schreck CE, Haile DG, Kline DL: The effectiveness of permethrin and DEET, alone or in combination, for protection against *Aedes taeniorhynchus, Am J Trop Med Hyg* 33:724, 1984.
63. Schreck CE, Kline DL: Repellency determinations of four commercial products against six species of ceratopogonid biting midges, *Mosq News* 41:7, 1981.
64. Schreck CE, Kline DL: Personal protection afforded by controlled-release topical repellents and permethrin-treated clothing against natural populations of *Aedes taeniorhynchus, J Am Mosq Control Assoc* 5:77, 1989.
65. Schreck CE, Leonhardt BA: Efficacy assessment of Quwenling, a mosquito repellent from China, *J Am Mosq Control Assoc* 7:433, 1991.
66. Schreck CE, Mc Govern TP: Repellents and other personal protection strategies against *Aedes albopictus, J Am Mosq Control Assoc* 5:247, 1989.
67. Schreck CE, Mount GA, Carlson DA: Wear and wash persistence of permethrin used as a clothing treatment for personal protection against the lone star tick, *J Med Entomol* 19:143, 1982.
68. Schreck CE, Self LS: Bed nets that kill mosquitoes, *World Health Forum* 6:342, 1985.
69. Schreck CE, Snoddy EL, Spielman A: Pressurized sprays of permethrin or DEET on military clothing for personal protection against *Ixodes dammini* (Acari: Ixodidae), *J Med Entomol* 23:396, 1986.
70. Schreck CE, Webb JC, Burden GS: Ultrasonic devices: evaluation of repellency to cockroaches and mosquitoes and measure of sound output, *J Environ Sci Health [A]* 19:521, 1984.
71. Schreck CE, Weidhaas DE, Smith N: Evaluation of electronic sound-producing devices against *Aedes taeniorhynchus* and *Ae. sollicitans, Mosq News* 37:529, 1977.
72. Secoy DM, Smith AE: Use of plants in control of agricultural and domestic pests, *Econ Bot* 37:28, 1983.
73. Shannon WR: Thiamine chloride—an aid in the solution of the mosquito problem, *Minn Med* 26:799, 1943.
74. Skinner WA et al: Human sweat components attractancy and repellency to mosquitoes, *Experientia* 24:679, 1968.
75. Smith CN: Factors affecting the protection obtained with insect repellents, *Trans Int Congr Entomol* 2:482, 1962.
76. Taylor WG, Schreck CE: Chiro-phase capillary gas chromatography and mosquito repellent activity of some oxazolidine derivatives of (+) and (−)-citronellal, *J Pharm Sci* 74:534, 1985.
77. US Environmental Protection Agency: *N,N diethyl-m-toluamide (DEET),* Pesticide Registration Standard, Washington, DC, 1980, US Environmental Protection Agency, Office of Pesticide and Toxic Substances.
78. Walker ED, Edman JD: The influence of host defensive behavior on mosquito (Diptera: Culicidae) biting persistence, *J Med Entomol* 22:370, 1985.
79. Wilson CS, Mathieson DR, Jachowski LA: Ingested thiamine chloride as a mosquito repellent, *Science* 100:147, 1944.
80. Wirtz RA: Allergic and toxic reactions to non-stinging arthropods, *Annu Rev Entomol* 29:47, 1984.
81. Zadjkoff CM: Toxic encephalopathy associated with use of insect repellent, *J Pediatr* 95:140, 1979.

35 SCORPION ENVENOMATION

David A. Connor
Brad S. Seldon

Scorpions were one of the first land animals. These arthropods have a fossil record that dates back 430 million years to the Silurian period. There are approximately 650 known living species, with almost all the lethal species in the Buthidae family.[62] These lethal scorpions are distributed worldwide in desert or semiarid regions.

The genera of the family Buthidae include *Centruroides* and *Tityus* in the Western Hemisphere and *Leuirus, Androctonus, Buthus,* and *Parabuthus* in the Eastern Hemisphere. These age-old arthropods have been documented to have envenomed humans since biblical times: "My father hath chastised you with whips, but I will chastise you with scorpions" (I Kings 12:11). King Mithirates of Pontus in Asia Minor (132-63 BC) is reported to have developed an antidote for the venom of the Middle Eastern scorpion. Fortunately, morbidity and mortality from scorpion stings today can be reduced with good supportive care and antivenin.

Epidemiology of Human Envenomation

Scorpion envenomations are a public health concern worldwide. In the Western Hemisphere, severe envenomations with significant morbidity and mortality have occurred in Arizona, Mexico, Brazil and other parts of South America, and Trinidad in the West Indies.[7,22,59,89] In the Eastern Hemisphere, scorpion envenomations have caused deaths in the deserts of northern Africa and in the Middle East, Iran, South Africa, and India.[5,14,43,66,71]

Scorpion envenomation, primarily from the *Androctonus* genus, is a significant health problem in Tunisia in northern Africa. Scorpion stings between the years 1967 and 1977 in the Sanitary District of Sfax, Tunisia, were reported at between 1930 and 3467 stings a year with a mortality rate of 0.3% to 0.9%.[43] In the Middle East, mortality rates have decreased with improved care. *Leiurus quinquestriatus* is the predominant offending scorpion in the area. In Jordan, a series of hospitalized children under 10 years old in 1965 had a mortality rate of 18%, while in 1984 a review of 51 scorpion stings in Israel reported a mortality rate of 3.9%.[5,91] A study in India of 121 hospital admissions between 1986 and 1989 for scorpion stings revealed a mortality rate of 8.5%.[14] In Spain 100 envenomations from the *Buthus* scorpion between 1974 and 1978 yielded no deaths.

In Brazil in 1980 Campos and associates reported only 3 deaths out of 1173 cases of *Tityus* scorpion stings (mortality rate 0.26%) after aggressive treatment, including intensive care unit support and administration of antivenin.[22,34] In Trinidad envenomations reported in 1970 from the *Tityus* scorpion caused 24 cases of acute pancreatitis with no deaths.[7] Mexico is home to several dangerous species of *Centruroides.* The morbidity and mortality from *Centruroides* envenomation are on the decline. However, a total of 20,352 deaths during the years between 1940 to 1949 and 1957 to 1958 were reported in Mexico.[59]

The American Association of Poison Control Centers reported 6765 scorpion stings from 75 poison centers throughout the United States in 1991, 2968 within Arizona alone.[55] *Centruroides* stings caused 75 deaths in Arizona between 1929 to 1965. This was twice as many deaths as from all other venomous animals combined, including the rattlesnake. Most of the victims were under 16 years of age. Much of the mortality has been caused by a lack of availability of modern intensive care support or antivenin and by iatrogenic causes such as oversedation.[87] The last verified death from a scorpion sting in Arizona was that of a 5-month-old child in 1968.[54]

Classification

Scorpions are grouped in the phylum Arthropoda (Fig. 35-1).[6] The arthropods, which are joint-legged animals with an external skeleton, are further subdivided on the basis of the morphology of their feeding apparatus: arthropods with a mandible (Mandibulata) and those with the first set of appendages (or chelicerae) forming the mouth (Chelicerata). The subphylum Chelicerata is further divided into three classes, including the Arachnida class, of which the order Scorpionida is a member. In addition to scorpions, this class includes spiders, mites, and ticks. The Scorpionida order contains six families, including Buthidae (Fig. 35-2). This family is associated with the most significant morbidity and mortality in humans and is characterized by a triangular sternum. Members of the other five families (Scorpionidae, Diplocentridae, Chactidae, Vejovidae, and Bothruridae) have a pentagonal sternum (Fig. 35-3).[6,50]

Anatomy

Scorpions of the southwestern United States are crablike in body shape with a segmented abdomen (opisthosoma) and a cephalothorax (prosoma). The body has four pairs of attached legs, two pincerlike pedipalps, and small chelicerae (Fig. 35-4), which are located between the bases of the pedipalps and are used to tear apart food. The tail has five segments and terminates in a bulbous structure (telson), which contains the stinger at its end. The body size of a mature scorpion varies from 2 to 20 cm, depending on the species.[50]

Centruroides, the bark scorpion of Arizona, is usually less than 5 cm in length (Fig. 35-5, *A;* Color Plate 56). *Centruroides* is yellow to brown, may be striped, and has the identifying subaculear tooth (Fig. 35-5, *B*) beneath its stinger. The presence and size of the subaculear tooth may vary within the species and in both the adult and immature stages. Scorpion sensory organs include up to six

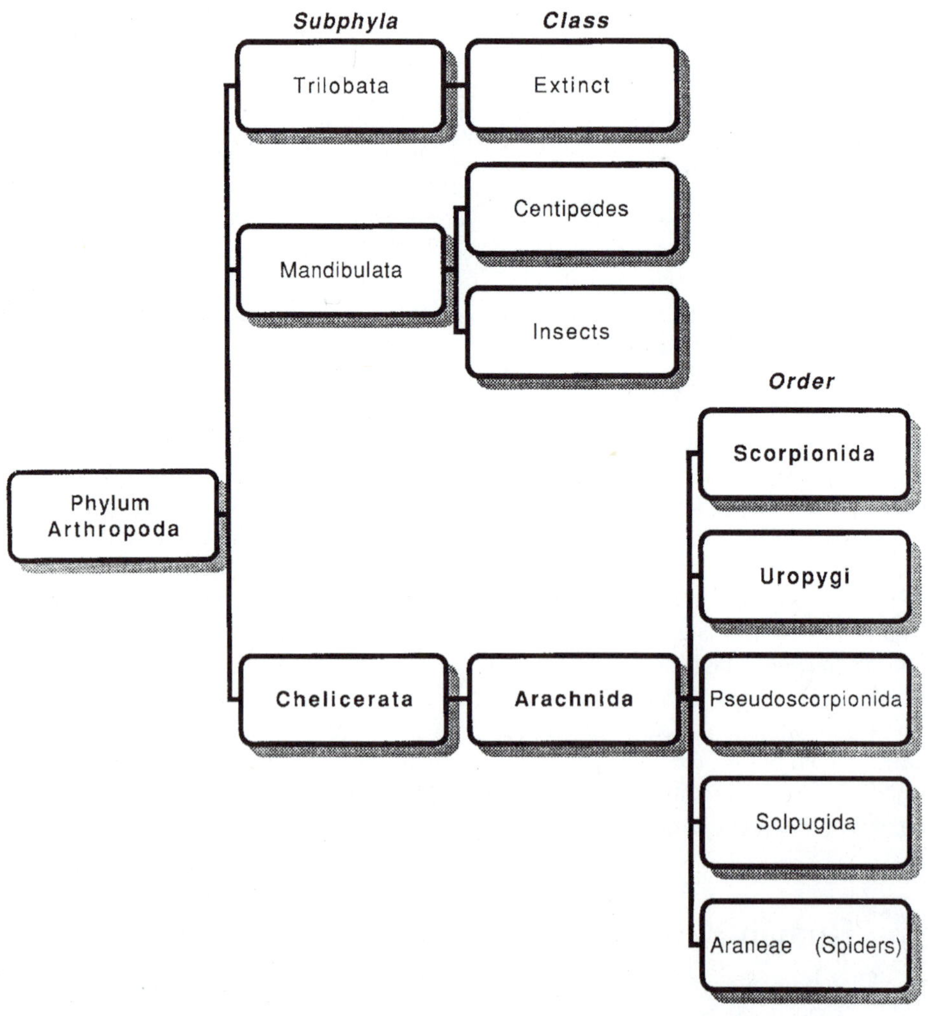

Fig. 35-1 The organization of the phylum Arthropoda, showing the relationship of scorpions to spiders and more distantly related insects.

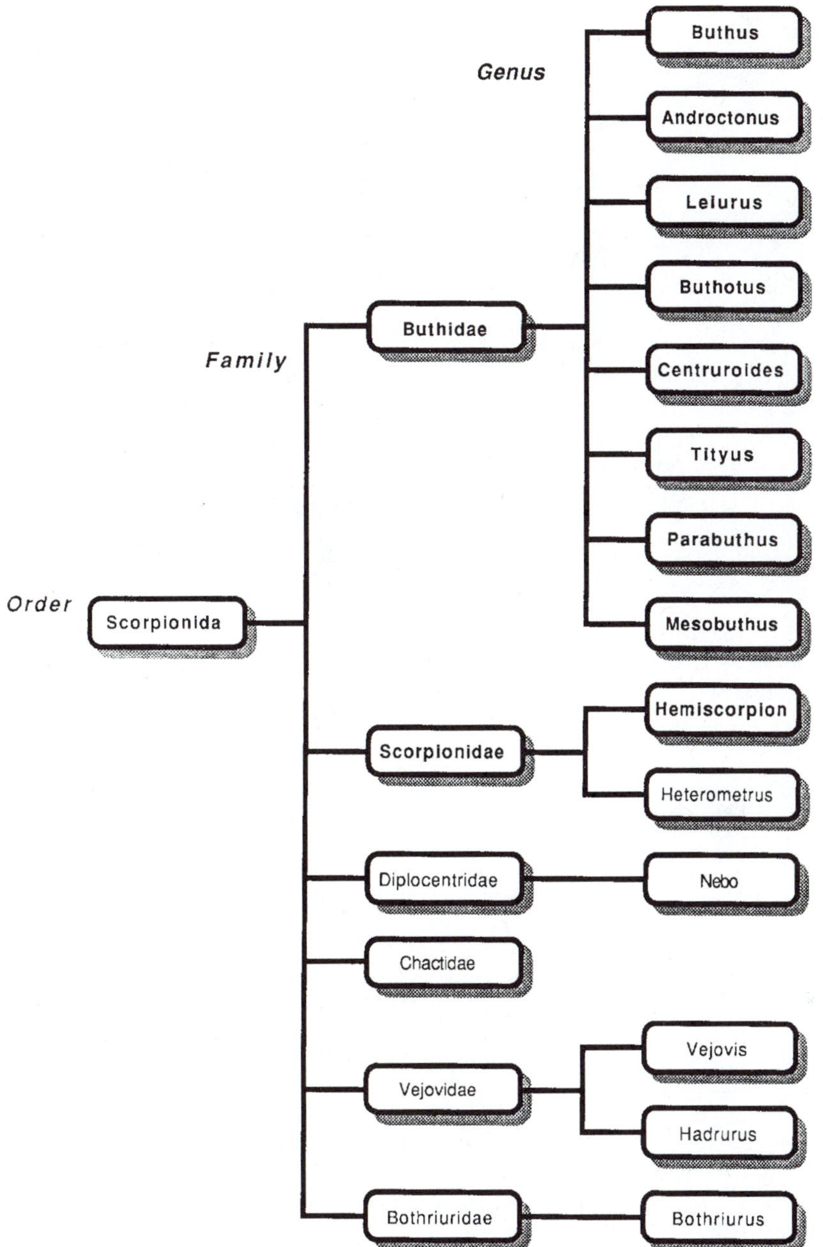

Fig. 35-2 The order Scorpionida has six principal families; however, the Buthidae family contributes the largest number of genera significant in human envenomations, as indicated by the bold type.

pairs of eyes, which are thought to play only a minor role in prey location. *Centruroides* appears to use a pair of comblike structures called pectines as chemoreceptors to locate its prey. Bristles (trichobothria) on the body and pedipalps are also thought to serve the function of detecting prey. Venom is located within two glands of the ampulla of the telson. The venom is injected into the scorpion's prey through duct openings lateral to the stinger tip. The scorpion delivers its venom by stinging, not biting, its victim.[50]

Habits

Scorpion young climb onto their mother's back after a period as embryoes within brood chambers in the mother's body (Fig. 35-6). The young may stay on the mother's back for weeks until their first molt. They take approximately six molts to reach adulthood. Scorpions are nocturnal feeders and have a negative response to high-intensity light. Some burrow, but most live above ground, including *Centruroides,* which hides under wood (old stumps, lumber piles, firewood, loose bark on fallen trees), in ground debris, or in

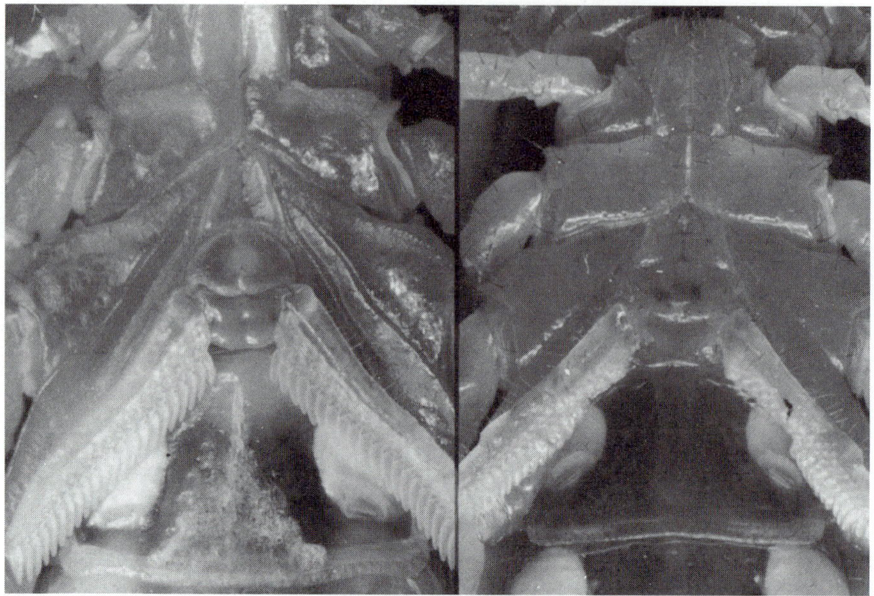

Fig. 35-3 The central sternal plate of the genus *Centruroides (left)* is more triangular in appearance than that of other common southwestern U.S. scorpions such as *Vejovis spingeris (right),* which is more truly pentagonal. Note the sensory hairs, especially on the winglike pecten.

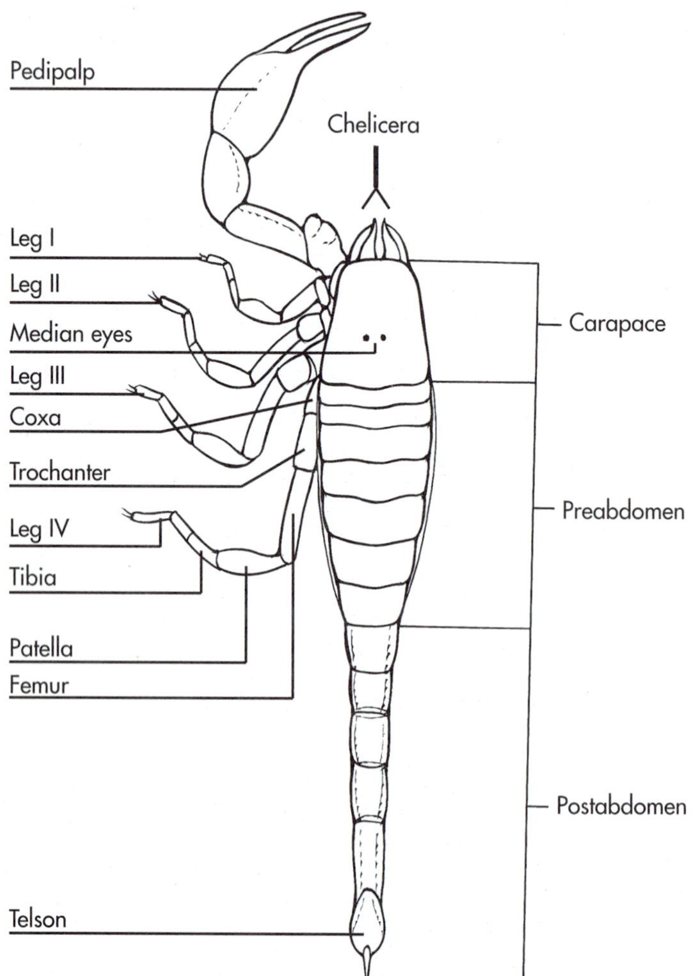

Fig. 35-4 Anatomy of a scorpion. (Redrawn from Keegan HL: *Scorpions of medical importance,* Oxford, 1980, University Press of Mississippi.)

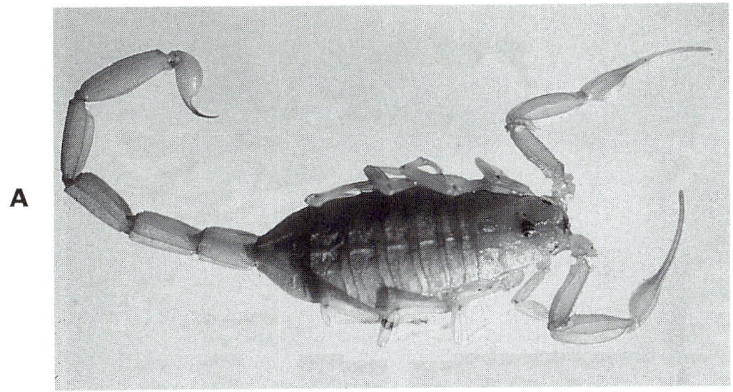

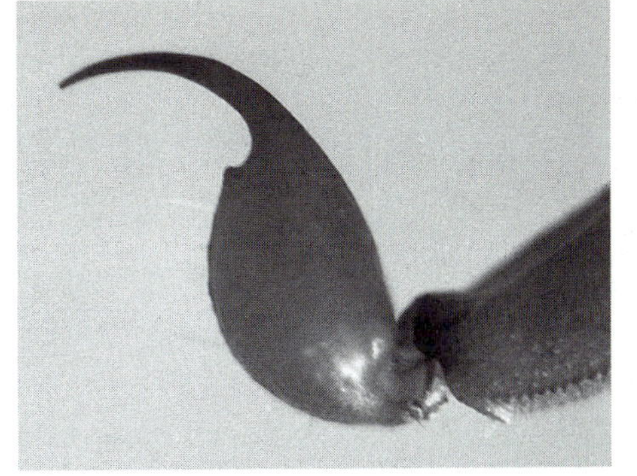

Fig. 35-5 **A,** *Centruroides,* the bark scorpion of Arizona. **B,** Subaculear tooth beneath stinger of *Centruroides.*

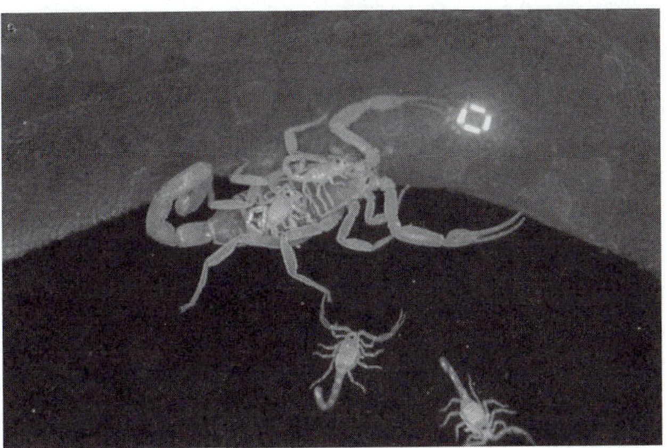

Fig. 35-6 Newborn members of the species *Centruroides exilicauda* cling to the back of the mother until after their first molt.

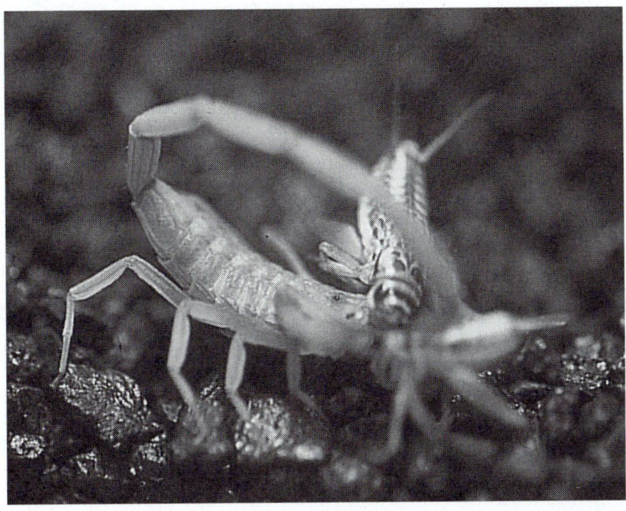

Fig. 35-7 Prey grasped and stung by scorpion.

crevices during the daytime.[90] This is troublesome to humans, since the scorpions may hide in shoes, blankets, or clothing left on the floor during daylight hours, as well as under common ground cover (tents).[77]

Scorpions feed primarily on ground-inhabiting arthropods (crickets, roaches) and small lizards. The scorpion first grasps its prey with the pedipalps and then stings by rapidly bringing the tail forward directly over the body (Fig. 35-7). The scorpion consumes only the juices and liquefied tissues of its prey. Solid material is discarded as pellets.[50]

Geographic Distribution, Clinical Effects, and Treatment

SCORPIONS OF THE UNITED STATES

Scorpions of the United States can be divided into two groups based on the clinical severity of human envenomation: scorpions whose venom can be lethal and scorpions whose venom is not. The potentially lethal scorpion found in the United States is *Centruroides sculpturatus ewing,* also known as *Centruroides exilicauda* (see Box 35-1).[77,88]

C. exilicauda resides in the southwestern United States and northern Mexico. The venom contains neurotoxins that produce systemic effects as well as local paresthesias and pain, which can be accentuated by tapping over the envenomed area (tap test). All other scorpions within the United States produce a local reaction that consists only of painful swelling and burning with ecchymosis (Color Plate 57). Tissue does not slough. The venom of *C. exilicauda* acts by stabilizing the Na^+ channel in an open position, resulting in repetitive firing of the neuronal axon. Symptoms begin immediately after envenomation and progress to maximum severity in approximately 5 hours. Death has been commonly attributed to exhaustion, but the cause probably has been respiratory arrest.

Lethal scorpions are found in the desert areas of the southwestern United States (Arizona, New Mexico,

BOX 35-1

NORTH AMERICAN SCORPIONS DANGEROUS TO HUMANS (GENUS CENTRUROIDES)

C. elegans
C. infamatus infamatus
C. infamatus ornatus
C. limpidus limpidus
C. limpidus tecomanus
C. suffusus suffusus
C. exilicauda
C. noxius

BOX 35-2

GRADES OF ENVENOMATION

I Local pain and/or paresthesias at site of envenomation

II Pain and/or paresthesias remote from the site of the sting in addition to local findings

III *Either* cranial nerve or somatic skeletal neuromuscular dysfunction:
1. *Cranial nerve dysfunction:* blurred vision, wandering eye movements, hypersalivation, trouble swallowing, tongue fasciculation, problems with upper airway, slurred speech
2. *Somatic skeletal neuromuscular dysfunction:* jerking of extremity(ies), restlessness, severe involuntary shaking and jerking that may be mistaken for a seizure

IV *Both* cranial nerve and somatic skeletal neuromuscular dysfunction

Modified from Curry S et al: *J Toxicol Clin Toxicol* 21(4&5):417, 1983-1984.

California, Texas, along the northern shore of Lake Mead in Nevada, and northern Mexico).[29,77] *Centruroides* does not display strutting behavior before delivering its sting, and after stinging in defense it beats a hasty retreat. The number of reported *Centruroides* stings increases in the summer months.[54]

The clinical findings after an acute envenomation have been reviewed by Curry and associates.[29] A scale was developed reflecting four grades of envenomation and recommended treatment for each grade (Box 35-2).[29] Grade I envenomation is characterized by local pain and paresthesias at the sting site, with the "tap test" nearly always eliciting severe pain. Grade II envenomations have local findings plus pain and paresthesias remote from the sting site. Cranial nerve or somatic skeletal neuromuscular dysfunction occurs in grade III. Cranial nerve dysfunction can be demonstrated as blurred vision, abnormal eye movements, slurred speech, and hypersalivation with difficulty maintaining an adequate airway. Abnormal eye movements most often are involuntary, conjugate, slow, and roving. Opsoclonus (chaotic multidirectional conjugate saccades) and unsustained primary position nystagmus can also be seen.[26] Somatic skeletal neuromuscular dysfunction can cause restlessness, fasciculations, arching of the back (opisthotonos), and jerking and shaking of extremities that at times can be so severe as to be mistaken for a seizure. Grade IV envenomation is characterized by *both* cranial nerve *and* somatic skeletal neuromuscular dysfunction.

True seizures can be caused by other scorpion species, such as from the genera *Leiurus* (Color Plate 58), *Androctonus,* and *Mesobuthus*.* There are several reasons that seizures are seen with these three species but not with *Centruroides*. It is possible that *Centruroides* venom does not cross the blood-brain barrier as well as the venom of these other scorpions. It is also possible that the true seizures are secondary to hypoxic brain injury, hypertensive encephalopathy, ischemia from cardiac arrhythmias or cerebral thrombosis, or shock. Perhaps somatic neuromuscular dysfunction is mistaken for seizures in victims of a *Centruroides* sting.

Other complications seen with *Centruroides* envenomation include nausea, vomiting, rhabdomyolysis, metabolic acidosis, hyperthermia, tachycardia, hypertension, and respiratory distress and arrest.[17,54,75]

The respiratory arrest is thought to be secondary to loss of the airway from hypersalivation and the inability to clear secretions caused by cranial nerve dysfunction and fatigue. Although death from scorpion envenomation in Arizona has not occurred in years, prior fatalities in infants and children were probably from respiratory arrest.

Today, death from the sting of the *Centruroides* scorpion is preventable with good supportive care. Symptoms in grades III and IV can be rapidly reversed with administration of scorpion antivenin. After envenomation by *C. exilicauda,* symptoms may begin immediately and progress to maximum severity in approximately 5 hours. Infants can reach grade IV in 15 to 30 minutes. The symptoms abate at a rate dependent on the age of the victim and grade of envenomation. However, most persons improve without antivenin within 9 to 30 hours.[19,29,69,75] Paresthesias and pain are the exception and have been known to persist for days to 2 weeks.

Treatment for grade I and II envenomations is supportive. Local pain can be controlled with ice, which may be applied for 30 minutes each hour with a cloth between the ice and the skin. Oral analgesics are also useful. Patients whose symptoms are within grades I and II are not referred to the emergency department by our poison center (Good

*References 2, 5, 31, 46, 58, 70, 74.

Samaritan Regional Poison Center, Phoenix). These patients should see a physician for tetanus immunization if needed. The major caveat regarding triage is that a rare patient with grade I or II envenomation can rapidly progress through grades III and IV, which may require aggressive airway management. Therefore all patients should be instructed to watch for symptoms of grade III and IV envenomation and go to the emergency department if symptoms worsen.

Narcotics, barbituates, benzodiazepines, or other potent analgesics to control symptoms of agitation or motor hyperactivity should be avoided. Increasingly large amounts of these medications are generally ineffective in controlling motor activity and can lead to apnea, loss of protective airway reflexes, leading to respiratory arrest and an otherwise unnecessary endotracheal intubation.[75]

Hyperthermia from uncontrolled muscular activity should be treated with cooling as needed to keep the patient normothermic.

Antivenin administration is controversial. Our center recommends it for reversal of grade III envenomations with respiratory distress or grade IV envenomation. An alternative to antivenin administration is intensive care unit observation and support, which might require pharmacoparalysis, endotracheal intubation, and ventilation. If antivenin will not be given and the patient is to be hospitalized in the intensive care unit, benzodiazepines may be given to make the patient amnestic.

Antivenin is effective in reversing cranial nerve dysfunction and somatoskeletal symptoms. However, it is not effective in reversing pain and paresthesias after a scorpion sting. Antivenin administration carries with it the risk of anaphylaxis, a type I hypersensitivity reaction, although this is an extremely rare occurrence. Serum sickness, a type III hypersensitivity reaction, is a more common side effect of antivenin administration.[19,78,89] Since the antivenin is derived from goat serum, a contraindication to antivenin use is an allergy to goat serum. As with many other animal proteins and drugs, patients with a history of asthma or atopy have a higher incidence of allergic reactions. The antivenin has been prepared since 1965 at the Antivenin Production Laboratory at Arizona State University. It has special dispensation by the Arizona Board of Pharmacy for use in Arizona, but has not been approved by the Food and Drug Administration. Administration of *Centruroides* antivenin requires that the clinician anticipate anaphylaxis. The patient should be monitored in a critical care area, and the clinician should be prepared to perform endotracheal intubation. Two intravenous lines should be in place, with extra intravenous fluids at the bedside. Additional necessary materials in preparation for treatment of anaphylaxis include an epinephrine infusion, steroids, and histamine-1 and -2 blockers.

Before administration of a therapeutic dose, a small test dose of the antivenin is prepared by taking 0.1 ml of a mixed vial of antivenin and diluting this 1:10 in saline solution. No more than 0.02 ml of this test solution is used to raise a small intradermal wheal. A positive reaction is an urticarial wheal with a zone of surrounding erythema. If no reaction to the test dose is seen within 10 minutes, the antivenin can be given, although a patient with a negative skin test for goat serum may still have an anaphylactic reaction. We have found that a more reliable risk indicator for anaphylaxis to goat serum scorpion antivenin is a history of ingestion of goat milk or goat products or being raised near goats, such as on a farm or ranch. The test dose should not be applied to the conjunctivae.

Centruroides antivenin for therapeutic infusion is prepared by mixing one vial of antivenin in 50 ml of normal saline. The volume is given intravenously over 20 to 30 minutes. It should never be given intramuscularly. The clinician should start the infusion slowly, watching for signs or symptoms of an allergic reaction. If the patient tolerates the antivenin, the infusion rate can be increased. Severe symptoms from the sting should begin to abate almost immediately; however, it usually takes a little more than 1 hour for complete resolution of the most severe symptoms. At times a second vial may be needed, but this depends on the effectiveness of the particular batch of antivenin. At least 1 hour should pass after the completion of the antivenin infusion before the decision is made to administer a second vial for persistent disabling grade III and IV symptoms. The patient may be discharged home after the administration of antivenin once symptoms have resolved and tetanus immunization is updated.

The patient should be instructed to watch for signs of serum sickness and to return if they develop. Serum sickness from scorpion antivenin was rare at one time. Today, it occurs with some consistency.[19,29] This may be a result of the antigenic differences within each batch of goat antivenin.

At the University of Arizona, Fab antibody fragments specific for *Centruroides* venom are being developed. It is hoped that the use of a Fab fragment–based antivenin will lead to fewer type III allergic reactions. In addition, purification of the antivenin and removal of goat serum proteins will decrease the number of type I allergic reactions.

SCORPIONS OF MEXICO

Centruroides scorpions are the lethal scorpions of Mexico. The clinical presentation and treatment of envenomations are similar to those for the *Centruroides* of the southwestern United States. Antivenin is available for *Centruroides* envenomation in Mexico.

SCORPIONS OF THE MIDDLE EAST AND NORTH AFRICA

The Middle East and northern Africa are home to several species of potentially lethal scorpions. The lethality of these scorpions is attributed to massive release of endogenous catecholamines into the victim, which affect target organs such as the heart. *Leiurus quinquestriatus* (yellow scorpion) is a significant medical hazard throughout the area. The effects of its venom are more severe depending on the age and size of the victim. Smaller victims and those at the extremes of age are the most susceptible, with a higher incidence of death in children.

The venom of *Leiurus quinquestriatus* is rapidly distributed, with the highest concentration in the liver, lungs, and heart. The overall clinical presentation after a sting reflects an acute massive release of catecholamines from the sympathetic nervous system and the adrenal glands, and catecholamine effects on target organs.[38-41,63,64] Elevated renin activity has also been observed.[44] In addition, the parasympathetic branch of the autonomic nervous system can be activated, releasing acetylcholine at postganglionic nerve endings.[45]

Initially the sting produces intense local pain, erythema, and edema. This can be followed by an outpouring of catecholamines and acetylcholine from nerve endings. Clinical signs of sympathetic overload predominate, with severe hypertension, tachyarrhythmias including ventricular tachycardia and fibrillation, and pulmonary edema.[1,9,72] Parasympathomimetic action of the venom also may cause bradyarrhythmia or atrioventricular block, which usually precedes the sympathetic overload.[23,72] Cardiomyopathy and myocardial damage with electrocardiographic changes have been reported.[5,21,38,52,94]

Severe hypertension may lead to acute hypertensive encephalopathy with agitation, convulsions, and decreased level of consciousness. Cerebral infarctions with focal neurologic findings have also occurred in victims of *Leiurus quinquestriatus*. The mechanism, although not definitively known, could be cerebral thrombosis, cerebral hemorrhage secondary to hypertension, hypoxia, or ischemia from cardiac arrhythmias.[1,32] Hypersalivation, diaphoresis, priapism, and gastrointestinal symptoms including acute pancreatitis also occur.[84]

Treatment for minor envenomations is supportive care. Local pain can be treated with ice for 30 minutes per hour with cloth between the ice and skin, as well as with oral analgesics.

Treatment of severe hypertension may require vasodilators. Sofer and Gueron[85] reviewed 23 pediatric cases of scorpion envenomation associated with severe hypertension between 1987 and 1988. They found that hypertension was controlled in 65% of the patients with analgesics and sedation (meperidine and diazepam). The remaining patients required vasodilator therapy. Hypertension and pulmonary edema respond to afterload reduction with vasodilators such as nifedipine, nitroprusside, hydralazine, or prazosin. Diuretics may be of some use in the absence of hypovolemia. Angiotensin converting enzyme (ACE) inhibitors were shown to improve the clinical condition of 5 patients with pulmonary edema.[49] Severe bradyarrhythmias with atrioventricular block from the parasympathomimetic action of venom have been effectively treated with atropine. Caution is recommended here because the vagolytic effect of atropine may exacerbate the sympathetic effects of the venom.[23] In general, the use of vasodilators has decreased morbidity and mortality from the sting of *Leiurus quinquestriatus*. An excellent review of the effects of scorpion venom on the cardiovascular system has been written by Gueron, Reuben, and Sofer.[36]

The use of antivenin for *Leiurus quinquestriatus* stings is controversial because it is less efficacious than antivenin therapy for *Centruroides* stings.[34,36] The immunoglobulins within the antivenin take 40 times longer to reach peak tissue concentration than does the venom. Therefore, at the time of peak tissue venom concentration, antivenin is only minimally distributed and the cardiac protection afforded by neutralization of the venom is small. This has focused clinicians on preventing the end organ effects of catecholamines released by the venom, rather than on neutralizing the venom itself.[37,47,48] However, when Dudin and associates[31] reviewed 54 cases of scorpion stings in Jordan, they found that intravenous antivenin quickly reversed central nervous system and cardiovascular symptoms of scorpion envenomations.

Symptoms caused by *Androctonus crassicauda* envenomation are similar clinically to those of *Leiurus quinquestriatus* envenomation and have also been reported to be reversed by *Leiurus quinquestriatus* antivenin.[1,43,68] Other dangerous scorpions in the Middle East include *Buthus occitanus* and *Buthus judaicus* (black scorpion). *Buthus judaicus* has been reported to cause not only local symptoms, but also cardiotoxicity and convulsions.[4,18]

SCORPIONS OF INDIA

The only lethal scorpion found in India is *Mesobuthus tamulus* (red scorpion, *Buthus tamulus,* or *Buthotus tamulus*). *Palamneus gravimanus* (black scorpion) also is an inhabitant of India, but its envenomation does not result in systemic effects.[14] Envenomation by *Mesobuthus tamulus* produces a clinical picture similar to that induced by scorpions of the Middle East and northern Africa. Release of catecholamines is the primary effect, with major morbidity and mortality resulting from cardiopulmonary toxicity.*

Treatment is similar to that for envenomations by scorpions of the Middle East and northern Africa. Atropine use for bradyarrhythmias and other transient cholinergic effects produced by *Mesobuthus tamulus* envenomations has been shown to increase morbidity by exacerbating the sympathetic effects of the venom through the drug's vagolytic effect.[16] The development of pulmonary edema in five of seven male patients stung by *Buthus tamulus* was preceded by priapism, which may be a clinical sign of autonomic dysfunction that predicts severe toxicity.[11]

---

*References 2, 3, 10, 12-15, 51, 74, 80, 81.

Autopsy examination in humans and experimental evidence in animals has shown that the venom of *Buthus tamulus* can cause a defibrination syndrome with disseminated intravascular coagulopathy, independent of hyperthermia and shock. In animals pretreated with heparin before venom administration, the coagulation dysfunction was prevented and outcome improved.[31,57] This coagulopathy, although rare, is thought to be responsible for a reported case of cerebral infarction after a scorpion sting. However, intracerebral hemorrhage has also occurred secondary to severe hypertension.[73] Hemiplegia has also been reported from a scorpion sting in India.[2,53,86] The hemiplegia was thought to be caused by venom-induced cerebral thrombosis, although cerebral ischemia secondary to cardiac dysfunction and arrhythmias is also possible.[86] Antivenin is not available for Indian scorpion envenomation.[14]

SCORPIONS OF IRAN

Androctonus and *Mesobuthus* of the Buthidae family account for most of the scorpion stings during the summer months and cause severe morbidity.[70,71] *Hemiscorpion lepturus* (family Scorpionidae) is reported to be the most dangerous scorpion in Khuzestan in southwestern Iran. This species accounts for 10% to 15% of the total scorpion stings during the warmest part of the year and nearly all cases during the winter in southwestern Iran. Envenomation by *Hemiscorpion lepturus* has been reported to cause central nervous system toxicity (confusion, delirium, restlessness, and seizures), cardiovascular symptoms (hypotension, myocarditis, and cardiopulmonary arrest), gastrointestinal symptoms, fatal hemolysis with secondary renal failure, necrotic ulcers, and ankylosis of the joints.[71] The development of severe skin lesions at the sting site is an indication of a severe envenomation and a predictor of systemic derangements.

Treatment includes dexamethasone to prevent local tissue destruction, diazepam and phenobarbital for seizures, blood transfusions for hemolysis, hydration and urine alkalinization to prevent kidney damage from hemolysis and hemoglobin deposition within the renal tubules, and intensive supportive care. No antivenin is available for *Hemiscorpion lepturus* at this time.[71]

Iran is also home to the scorpion *Buthus sauloci,* whose venom is thought to have caused hemolysis with resulting renal failure in a 28-year-old female victim.[25]

SCORPIONS OF SOUTH AFRICA

The *Parabuthus* and *Buthotus* scorpions of South Africa deliver toxins that produce primarily central nervous system toxicity. Cranial nerve dysfunction, convulsions, muscular rigidity, paralysis, and death from asphyxiation thought to be secondary to muscular paralysis have been described. However, the majority of the stings result in minor discomfort only. Some species of *Parabuthus* can squirt their venom up to 1 m from an apparatus within the distal tail segment. If the venom reaches the eyes, it can cause severe conjunctivitis. However, most envenomations occur from the species that sting their victims.[65] The venom has been seen to produce delayed effects, so observation of envenomed victims for 24 hours is recommended. Antivenin for South African scorpion envenomation is recommended only for patients with systemic symptoms. The antivenin is prepared by the South African Institute for Medical Research in Johannesburg.[62,82]

SCORPIONS OF SOUTH AMERICA AND THE CARIBBEAN

Lethal scorpions of the genus *Tityus* can be found throughout South America. Brazil is inhabited by several species of these dangerous scorpions. The size, habits, and general appearance of *Tityus* are similar to those of *Centruroides. T. serrulatus* can produce sympathetic and parasympathetic symptoms as well as intense local pain and erythema. *T. serrulatus* venom given intravenously to rats produced an increase in serum catecholamines and sustained hypertension.[64] It has also been demonstrated to exert a sympathetic effect in isolated guinea pig heart.[27] Thus the venom of *T. serrulatus* exerts an effect similar to that of the scorpions of the Middle East, North Africa, and India, with release of catecholamines affecting target organs. *T. trinitatis* has been reported to cause acute pancreatitis in 24 of 30 patients admitted to the hospital over a 2-month period in Trinidad. All patients made an uneventful recovery.[7] In animal studies, *Tityus* toxin induced pancreatic exocrine secretion and increased the volume, pepsin, and acid output of gastric juice, causing a significant decrease in gastric pH.[8,28] The treatment recommended by Campos and co-workers,[22] who have treated over 1000 *Tityus* envenomations, includes aggressive intensive supportive care and, in cases of severe envenomation, antivenin.

Venom

Scorpion venom is characteristically a neurotoxin that contains low–molecular weight proteins of approximately 7000 to 8000 daltons. *Centruroides* venom has been well described and can serve as a prototype. This venom has been purified by McIntosh and Watt.[60] They have characterized four toxins (I to IV), although at least eight different polypeptide toxins have been isolated.[93] A three-dimensional model of scorpion toxin has been developed.[33]

Most scorpion venom does not contain enzymes, so no extensive tissue inflammation and destruction are seen at the sting site. Serotonin is found in scorpion venom and may contribute to the pain of the sting. *Centruroides sculpturatus* and *Leiurus quinquestriatus* venoms elevate plasma renin activity, which is thought to contribute to the hypertensive response produced by the venom along with elevation in circulating catecholamines.[35] *Centruroides* venom at high concentrations also has been shown to inhibit ACE.[56]

The scorpion toxins are composed of a single chain of basic proteins with approximately 60 to 70 amino acids that are cross-linked with four disulfide bridges. Reduction of the disulfide bonds in vitro destroys the lethality of the venom.[60]

Multiple studies have demonstrated that the major neurotoxic effects of scorpion venom are caused by slowed and incomplete Na^+ channel inactivation.[61,67,76] Wang and Strichartz[92] isolated neurotoxins from the venom of both *Leiurus quinquestriatus* and *Centruroides sculpturatus*. The neurotoxins isolated from *Leiurus* slowed the rate of inactivation of Na^+ channels. Such slowing resulted in a prolonged action potential. Five neurotoxins were isolated from the venom of *Centruroides*. One of these neurotoxins produced similar slowing of the inactivation of the Na^+ channels, with a prolonged action potential. These toxins are called "stabilizers" because of their ability to maintain the Na^+ channel in an ion conduction state and thus a steady state of Na^+ current. Four toxins act primarily on the activation process of the Na^+ channels, producing increased Na^+ permeability on repolarization of the membrane following a depolarizing pulse. This results in a greater Na^+ channel activation at a given negative membrane potential than would be present without the toxin. This is further accompanied by attenuation of the height of the action potential, but the impulse can still propagate down the axon. The "inducers," which can modify Na^+ channel activation, also cause and enhance repetitive firing of axons. Scorpion toxins that inactivate and prolong the closing of Na^+ channels bind in a voltage-dependent manner. Scorpion toxins that activate Na^+ channels bind in voltage-independent manner and at a different site than the toxins that inactivate the closing of the Na^+ channels.[29,60,92] Scorpion toxin also contains a minor toxin, charybdotoxin, which blocks K^+ channels.[20,24,69,79,83]

Antivenin

The use of antivenin for several of the world's most toxic species of scorpion has been noted. Table 35-1 contains a partial listing of commercially prepared antivenins.[6] Some may be effective in neutralizing venom from other scorpion species. Mexican *Centruroides* antivenin neutralizes North African *Buthus occitanus* and South American *Tityus* venoms effectively, but does not neutralize *Androctonus crassicauda* venom. The clinical effects of *A. crassicauda* venom have been reported to be reversed with *Leiurus quinquestriatus* antivenin.[62] Antivenin administration for a particular scorpion species should be undertaken with direction from local medical experts skilled in its use.

Prevention

Prevention is of extreme importance in reducing morbidity and mortality from scorpion envenomation. Organophosphates, pyrethrins, and chlorinated hydrocarbons (DDT, chlordane, lindane, dieldrin) kill scorpions. Home spraying is ineffective because of the lack of contact between the body of the scorpion and the insecticide. However, spraying insectides decreases the number of other insects in the area and removes the scorpion's food supply. The natural enemies of scorpions include cats, solfugids, and certain lizards.[49]

Prevention should include removal of dead wood, firewood, and leaves that provide an excellent habitat for scorpions. In scorpion-infested areas, clothing, shoes, and camping gear left outside should be shaken and checked for scorpions before being used. Footwear is recommended in scorpion-prone areas. *Centruroides exilicauda* is fluorescent under an ultraviolet light and can be more easily located at night with a Wood's lamp.

Table 35-1 Commercially Prepared Antivenins

Organization	Species Used	Host	Also Useful in Treating
Iatric Laboratories, Phoenix, Arizona	*Centruroides exilicauda*	Goat	
Laboratories Myn, Avenida Coyoacan #1707, Mexico 12 DF	*Centruroides*	Horse	*C. exilicauda*
Institut Pasteur of Tunis	*Androctonus australis, Buthus occitanus*	Horse	
Hebrew University, Jerusalem	*Leiurus quinquestriatus*	Donkey	*A. crassicauda*
Institut Pasteur d' Algerie, Algiers, Algeria	*A. australis, B. occitanus*		
State Serum and Vaccine Institute, Agouza, Cairo, Egypt	*L. quinquestriatus*		
Central Institute of Hygiene, Ankara, Turkey	*A. crassicauda*		*A. australis, B. occitanus, T. serrulatus, T. bahiensis*
South African Institute for Medical Research (SAIMR), Johannesburg, South Africa	*Parabuthus*		
Instituto Butantan, São Paulo, Brazil	*Tityus serrulatus, T. bahiensis*	Horse	

REFERENCES

1. Abroug F et al: Cardiac dysfunction and pulmonary edema following scorpion envenomation, *Chest* 100(4):1057, 1991.
2. Ahmed B: Studies on scorpion stings, *East Afr Med J* 60(6):402, 1983.
3. Alagesan R et al: Transient complete right bundle branch block following scorpion sting, *J Ind Med Assoc* 69(5):113, 1977.
4. Amitai Y et al: Convulsions following a black scorpion *(Buthus Judaicus)* sting, *Isr J Med Sci* 17:1083, 1981.
5. Amitai Y et al: Scorpion sting in children: a review of 51 cases, *Clin Pediatr* 24(3):136, 1985.
6. Banner W: Scorpion envenomation. In Auerbach P, Geehr E, editors: *Management of wilderness and environmental emergencies,* ed 2, St Louis, 1989, Mosby, p 603.
7. Bartholomew C: Acute scorpion pancreatitis in Trinidad, *Br Med J* 1:666, 1970.
8. Bartholomew C et al: Experimental studies on the aetiology of acute scorpion pancreatitis, *Br J Surg* 63:807, 1976.
9. Barzilay Z: Myocardial damage with life-threatening arrhythmia due to a scorpion sting, *Eur Heart J* 3:191, 1982.
10. Basu P: Observations on scorpion-sting and snake-bite, *Am J Trop Med* 19:385, 1939.
11. Bawaskar H: Diagnostic cardiac premonitory signs and symptoms of red scorpion sting, *Lancet* 1:552, 1982.
12. Bawaskar H, Bawaskar P: Prazosin in management of cardiovascular manifestations of scorpion sting, *Lancet* 1:510, 1986.
13. Bawaskar H, Bawaskar P: Stings by red scorpions *(Buthotus tamulus)* in Maharashtra State, India: a clinical study, *Trans R Soc Trop Med Hyg* 83:858, 1989.
14. Bawaskar H, Bawaskar P: Scorpion sting: a review of 121 cases, *J Wilderness Med* 2:164, 1991.
15. Bawaskar H, Bawaskar P: Consecutive stings by red scorpions evoke severe cardiovascular manifestations in the first, but not in the second, victim: a clinical observation, *J Trop Med Hyg* 94:231, 1991.
16. Bawaskar H, Bawaskar P: Role of atropine in management of cardiovascular manifestations of scorpion envenoming in humans, *J Trop Med Hyg* 95:30, 1992.
17. Berg R, Tarantino M: Envenomation by the scorpion *Centruroides exilicauda (C sculpturatus):* severe and unusual manifestations, *Pediatrics* 87(6):930, 1991.
18. Blum A, Lubezki A, Sclarovsky S: Black scorpion envenomation: two cases and review of the literature, *Clin Cardiol* 15:377, 1992.
19. Bond R: Antivenin administration for *Centruroides* scorpion sting: risks and benefits, *Ann Emerg Med* 21(7):788, 1992.
20. Bontems F et al: Refined structure of charybdotoxin: common motifs in scorpion toxins and insect defensins, *Science* 254:1521, 1991.
21. Brand A et al: Myocardial damage after a scorpion sting: long-term echocardiographic follow-up, *Pediatr Cardiol* 9:59, 1988.
22. Campos J et al: Signs, symptoms and treatment of severe scorpion poisoning in children. In Eaker D, Wadstrom T, editors: *Natural toxins,* Oxford, Eng, 1980, Pergamon Press, p 61.
23. Cantor A et al: Parasympathomimetic action of scorpion venom on the cardiovascular system, *Isr J Med Sci* 13(9):908, 1977.
24. Castle N, Strong P: Identification of two toxins from scorpion *(Leiurus quinquestriatus)* venom which block distinct classes of calcium-activated potassium channel, *FEBS Lett* 209(1):117, 1986.
25. Chadha J, Leviav A: Hemolysis, renal failure, and local necrosis following scorpion sting, *JAMA* 241(10):1038, 1979.
26. Clark R et al: Abnormal eye movements encountered following severe envenomations by *Centruroides sculpturatus* (letter), *Neurology* 41:604, 1991.
27. Corrado A, Antonio A, Diniz C: Brazilian scorpion venom *(Tityus serrulatus),* an unusual sympathetic postganglionic stimulant, *J Pharmacol Exp Ther* 164(2):253, 1968.
28. Cunha-Melo et al: Effects of purified scorpion toxin (tityustoxin) on gastric secretion in the rat, *Toxicon* 21(6):843, 1983.
29. Curry S et al: Envenomation by the scorpion *Centruroides sculpturatus, J Toxicol Clin Toxicol* 21(4&5):417, 1983-1984.
30. Devi C et al: Defribrination syndrome due to scorpion venom poisoning, *Br Med J* 1:345, 1970.
31. Dudin A et al: Scorpion sting in children in the Jerusalem area: a review of 54 cases, *Ann Trop Paediatr* 11:217, 1991.
32. Elitsur et al: Localized cerebral involvement caused by a yellow scorpion sting on the face: two case reports, *Isr J Med Sci* 20:160, 1984.
33. Fontecilla-Camps: Three-dimensional model of the insect-directed scorpion toxin from *Androctonus australis hector* and its implication for the evolution of scorpion toxins in general, *J Mol Evol* 29:63, 1986.
34. Freire-Maia L, Campos J: On the treatment of the cardiovascular manifestations of scorpion envenomation (Response to the letter to the editor, by Gueron and Ovsyshcher), *Toxicon* 25(2):125, 1987.
35. Gueron M, Ovsyshcher: What is the treatment for the cardiovascular manifestations of scorpion envenomation? (letter to the editor), *Toxicon* 25(2):121, 1987.
36. Geuron M, Reuben I, Sofer S: The cardiovascular system after scorpion envenomation: a review, *Clin Toxicol* 30(2):245, 1992.
37. Geuron M, Sofer S: Scorpion envenomation and the heart, *J Wilderness Med* 2:175, 1991.
38. Geuron M, Stern J, Cohen W: Severe myocardial damage and heart failure in scorpion sting (report of five cases), *Am J Cardiol* 19:719, 1967.
39. Gueron M, Weizmann S: Catecholamine excretion in scorpion sting, *Isr J Med Sci* 5(4):855, 1969.
40. Geuron M, Yarom R: Cardiovascular manifestations of severe scorpion sting, *Chest* 57:156, 1970.
41. Geuron M et al: Hemodynamic and myocardial consequences of scorpion venom, *Am J Cardiol* 45:979, 1980.
42. Gonzalez D: Epidemiological and clinical aspects of certain venomous animals of Spain, *Toxicon* 20(5):925, 1982.
43. Goyffon M, Vachon M, Broglio N: Epidemiologic and clinical characteristics of scorpion envenomation in Tunisia, *Toxicon* 20:337, 1982.
44. Grange R: Elevation of blood pressure and plasma renin levels by venom from scorpions, *Centruroides sculpturatus* and *Leiurus quinquestriatus, Toxicon* 15:429, 1977.
45. Grupp I et al: Effects of the venom of the yellow scorpion *(Leiurus quinquestriatus)* on the isolated work-performing guinea pig heart, *Toxicon* 18:261, 1980.
46. Hershkovich Y et al: Criteria map audit of scorpion envenomation in the Negev, Israel, *Toxicon* 23(5):845, 1985.
47. Ismail M, Abd-Elasalam M: Are the toxicological effects of scorpion envenomation related to tissue venom concentration? *Toxicon* 26(3):233, 1988.
48. Ismail M et al: Pharmacokinetics of 125I-labelled antivenin to the venom from the scorpion *Androctonus amoreuxi, Toxicon* 21(1):47, 1983.
49. Karnad D et al: Captopril for correcting diuretic-induced hypotension in pulmonary edema after scorpion sting, *Br Med J* 289:1430, 1989.
50. Keegan H: *Scorpions of medical importance,* Jackson, 1980, University Press of Mississippi.
51. Kothari U et al: Myocarditis from scorpion sting, a clinical and electrocardiographic study of 50 cases, *Ind Heart J* 28(2):88, 1976.
52. Kumar E et al: Scorpion venom cardiomyopathy, *Am Heart J* 123:725, 1992.
53. Lath G, Bhattacherjee A: Hemiplegia following scorpion sting, *J Ind Med Assoc* 53(3):148, 1969.
54. Likes K, Banner W, Chavez M: *Centruroides exilicauda* envenomation in Arizona, *West J Med* 141(5):634, 1984.
55. Litovitz T et al: 1991 annual report of the American Association of Poison Control Centers National Data Collection System, *Am J Emerg Med,* vol 10, no 5, 1992.

56. Longenecker G, Longenecker J: *Centruroides sculpturatus* venom and platelet reactivity: possible role in scorpion venom-induced defibrination syndrome, *Toxicon* 19:153, 1980.
57. Longenecker G et al: Inhibition of the angiotensin converting enzyme by venom of the scorpion *Centruroides sculpturatus, Toxicon* 18:667, 1980.
58. Mahadevan S et al: Scorpion envenomation and the role of lytic cocktail in its management, *Ind J Pediatr* 48:757, 1981.
59. Mazzotti L, Bravo-Becherelle: Scorpionism in the Mexican Republic. In Keegan H, Macfarlane W, editors: *Venomous and poisonous animals and noxious plants of the Pacific region.* A collection of papers based on a symposium in the public health and medical science division at the Tenth Pacific Science Congress, New York, 1963, Pergamon Press, p 119.
60. McIntosh M, Watt D: Purification of toxins from the North American scorpion *Centruroides sculpturatus.* In DeVries A, Kochva E, editors: *Toxins of animal and plant origin 2,* New York, 1972, Gordon & Breach, p 529.
61. Meves H, Rubly N, Watt D: Effect of toxins isolated from the venom of the scorpion *Centruroides sculpturatus* on the Na currents of the node of Ranvier, *Pflugers Arch* 393:56, 1982.
62. Milton S: *Venom diseases,* Springfield, Ill, 1974, Charles C Thomas.
63. Moss J, Colburn R, Kiopin: Scorpion toxin-induced catecholamine release from synaptosomes, *J Neurochem* 22:217, 1974.
64. Moss J, Thoa N, Kopin I: On the mechanism of scorpion toxin-induced release of norepinephrine from peripheral adrenergic neurons, *J Pharmacol Exp Ther* 190:39, 1974.
65. Newlands G: The venom-squirting ability of *Parabuthus* scorpions (Arachnida: Buthidae), *S Afr J Med Sci* 39(4):175, 1974.
66. Newlands G: Review of southern African scorpions and scorpionism, *S Afr Med J* 154:613, 1978.
67. Okamoto H, Takahashi K: One to one binding of a purified scorpion toxin to Na^+ channels, *Nature* 266:456, 1977.
68. Pomeranz A: Scorpion sting: successful treatment with nonhomologous antivenin (short communication), *Isr J Med Sci* 20(5):451, 1984.
69. Rachesky I et al: Treatments for *Centruroides elixicauda* envenomation, *Am J Dis Child* 138:1136, 1984.
70. Radmanesh M: *Androctonus crassicauda* sting and its clinical study in Iran, *J Trop Med Hyg* 93:323, 1990.
71. Radmanesh M: Clinical study of *Hemiscorpion lepturus* in Iran, *J Trop Med Hyg* 93:327, 1990.
72. Rahav G, Weiss A: Scorpion sting–induced pulmonary edema, *Chest* 97:1478, 1990.
73. Rai M et al: Intracerebral hemorrhage following scorpion bite, *Neurology* 40:1801, 1990.
74. Rajarajeswari G, Sivaprakasam S, Viswanathan J.: Morbidity and mortality pattern in scorpion stings, *J Ind Med Assoc* 73(7 & 8):123, 1979.
75. Rimsza M, Zimmerman D, Bergeson P: Scorpion envenomation, *Pediatrics* 66(2):298, 1980.
76. Romey G, Chicheportiche R, Lazdunske M: Scorpion neurotoxin-A presynaptic toxin which affects both Na^+ and K^+ channels in axons, *Biochem Biophys Res Commun* 64(1):115, 1975.
77. Russell F, Madon M: The introduction of the scorpion *Centruroides exilicauda* into California and its public health importance, *Toxicon* 22:658, 1984.
78. Schnur L, Schnur P: A case of allergy to scorpion antivenin, *Ariz Med* 413, 1968.
79. Schweitz H et al: Charybdotoxin is a new member of the K^+ channel toxin family that includes dendrotoxin I and mast cell degranulating peptide, *Biochemistry* 28, 9708, 1989.
80. Singh D, Bisht D, Muralidhar K: Scorpion stings in adult south Indians at Pondicherry, *J Ind Med Assoc* 72(10):234, 1979.
81. Sinha A: Cardiovascular manifestations of scorpion sting in a case of congenital complete atrioventricular block, *J Ind Med Assoc* 87(10):237, 1989.
82. Smith L, Potgieter P, Chappell W: Scorpion sting producing severe muscular paralysis, *S Afr Med J* 64(2):69, 1983.
83. Smythies J et al: A molecular mechanism of action of scorpion neurotoxins, *Ala J Med Sci* 14(1):68, 1977.
84. Sofer S: Acute pancreatitis in children following envenomation by the yellow scorpion *Leiurus quinquestriatus, Toxicon* 29(1):125, 1991.
85. Sofer S, Gueron M: Vasodilators and hypertensive encephalopathy following scorpion envenomation in children, *Chest* 97:118, 1990.
86. Solanki S, Kothari U, Dave D: Hemiplegia following scorpion sting, *J Ind Med Assoc* 77(9&10):155, 1981.
87. Stahnke H: *The treatment of venomous bites and stings,* Phoenix, 1966, Arizona State University Bureau of Publications.
88. Stahnke H: Arizona's lethal scorpion, *Ariz Med* 29:490, 1972.
89. Stahnke H, Stahnke J: The treatment of scorpion sting, *Ariz Med* 14(10):577, 1957.
90. Torres F, Heatwole H: Orientation of some scorpions and tailless whipscorpions, *Eingegangen* 12(11):546, 1966.
91. Wahbeh Y: A study of Jordanian scorpion, *Jordan Med J* 2:85, 1976.
92. Wang G, Strichartz G: Purification and physiological characterization of neurotoxins from venoms of the scorpion *Centruroides sculpturatus* and *Leiurus quinquestriatus, Mol Pharmacol* 23:519, 1982.
93. Watt D, Babin D, Mlejnek R: The protein neurotoxins in scorpion and elapid snake venoms, *J Agr Food Chem* 22(1):43, 1974.
94. Yarom R, Braun K: Cardiovascular effects of scorpion venom, morphological changes in the myocardium, *Toxicon* 3:41, 1970.

36 PLANT-INDUCED DERMATITIS

William L. Epstein
John H. Epstein

- Irritation
- Allergy
- Phytophotodermatitis
- Granulomas

Advertent or inadvertent exposure to plants is one of the common causes of skin eruptions. Because the reactions are often acute, the victims frequently seek emergency care. This subject has been reviewed in detail.[9,39] This chapter considers plant dermatitis from the emergency perspective. Although most acute, itchy eruptions share clinical features, not every rash is poison ivy dermatitis. Plant dermatitis is discussed under four major headings: irritation, allergy, phytophotodermatitis, and granulomas. Similarities, distinctions, and different plans for management are emphasized. Proper recognition and adequate early treatment often lead to a cure with no further recurrence, whereas failure to diagnose and less optimal management can result in chronic, disabling dermatosis.

Irritation

Primary irritation is the most frequent cutaneous response to vegetation. The majority of these injuries are sufficiently mild to be ignored or self-treated. Many wild plants, such as brambles and berries, have sharp thorns that can inflict significant skin trauma. The typical appearance is of linear scratches or excoriations. The area can be swollen and red with a weeping or bloody crust. Fever and adenopathy are uncommon. Pruritus, when present, is mild.

Treatment consists mostly of cool soaks, or compresses with soft gauze or soft linen with aluminum acetate solution diluted 1:20 for use. The lesions usually heal in a few days. Secondary infection relates to the environment and personal hygiene. Uncommonly, these wounds allow entry of microorganisms that cause systemic diseases such as sporotrichosis. In addition to inflicting gross mechanical damage, many plants, weeds, and fruits have fine hairs (trichomes) and barbed hairs (glochids), which cause more subtle and annoying forms of irritation. The trichome-glochid response is acute development of wheals with itching and occasionally intense pain. Large blisters may form. While this irritation appears to have a mechanical origin, the reaction is produced by natural substances in the trichomes or glochids. Low–molecular weight acids, glycosides, proteolytic enzymes, and crystals are among the major plant chemicals that cause primary skin irritation. These lesions can occur on skin or mucous membranes and are classified as nonimmunogenic urticaria. An example is itch powder, from dried cowhage *(Mucuna pruriens),* which contains a proteolytic enzyme and causes intense pruritus.[133,134] Other irritant enzymes include bromelin from pineapples, papain from papaya, and ficin from figs.

Many species of flowering plants, shrubs, and trees induce primary skin irritation, but most of the irritant species belong to the spurge family (Euphorbiaceae). Spurge is a huge and diverse family of over 7000 species, for practical purposes classified into five subfamilies and about 50 tribes,[148] only three of which (Acalyphoteae, Crotonoideae, and Euphorbioideae) produce significant irritation in humans (Color Plates 59 to 61). Euphorbiaceae flourish primarily in tropical and subtropical climates. In rainforests they may grow as tall trees, but usually they are found in arid areas, as small trees and shrubs.[150] In North America the varieties are limited and populate mainly southern Florida and the southwestern United States; varieties grow in Europe, where they are commonly called wolfsmilk. Honey made from these plants causes burning mouth irritation accentuated by drinking water. Table 36-1 lists the more commonly recognized irritant plants of the spurge family. One of the most poisonous is the manchineel tree *(Hippomane mancinella)* or beach apple, which inhabits the Caribbean and at one time was the scourge of south Florida.[94] Every part of the plant, including the fruit, contains a milky latex that is extremely irritating and causes burning, swelling, blisters, and even blindness when rubbed into the eyes. The most irritating ingredients are diterpene esters similar to phorbol esters.[1]

Other well-known members of the spurge family are of the genus *Croton,* which contains up to 750 species distributed throughout the tropics. Croton oil is an extract of the seed of the croton plant *(Croton tiglium).* Croton oil was

Table 36-1 Some Common Irritant Plants in the Spurge Family (Euphorbiaceae)

Subfamily	Tribe/Genus	Common Names	Mechanisms or Irritant Chemical
Crotonoideae	*Croton*	Croton bush	Phorbol esters (croton oil)
	Jatropha	Coral plant	Thioglycoside (mustard oil)
	Cnidoscolus	Spurge nettle, tread softly	Stinging hairs
Euphorbioidae	*Hippomane*	Manchineel, beach apple	Diterpenes and alkaloid
	Sapium	Aurou-wood	Terpenes
	Hura	Sandbox tree	Ricinlike toxalbumin and triterpenes
	Euphorbia	Beach spurge, red spurge, milkweed, wolfsmilk, asthma plant, candelabra cactus, caper spurge, snow-on-the-mountain, crown-of-thorns	Diterpenes and triterpenes; terpenoids
	Poinsettia	Poinsettia	Phorbol esters
	Pedilanthus	Slipper bush	Terpenes?
Acalyphoideae	*Tragia*	Nose-burn	Stinging hairs

exported from the Caribbean and South America to the United States in the last century in large quantities to be used as a purgative and to treat warts, skin growths, and superficial fungal infections. When croton oil was purified, it was found to be a mixture of diterpenes called phorbol esters, which are well known cocarcinogens[17] and have been used extensively in recent years in cell biology and cell differentiation experiments. Phorbol esters appear to be the irritant chemicals in most members of the genus *Croton.* The majority of irritating euphorbs secrete a white, milky, or viscous latex composed of a mixture of polycyclic diterpenes or triterpenes and terpenoids, which can polymerize into rubber. These complex irritant terpenes may be cocarcinogens.[72] Many are related to the phorbol esters. Poinsettia, a member of the genus *Euphorbia,* is considered by some to have relatively low irritant potential, while others have reported up to 10% irritant responses.[127,148]

Stinging hairs are found in many species of plants and produce injury by different mechanisms. The clinical presentation is usually an explosive onset of painful urticaria, limited or extensive, that in some geographic regions can result in tissue necrosis. In the United States the genus *Tragia* of the spurge family is a prominent offender; more than 100 species are found, mainly in southern states. The stinging mechanism is complex and involves insertion into the skin of a long crystal that releases caustic chemicals. The exact nature of the injected material remains unclear,[144] but it is considered to be a mixture of amines, possibly including histamine. Other plants with stinging hairs in the spurge family are found throughout the tropics in the genera *Cnidoscolus* and *Jatropha*. Their mechanism of stinging is similar to that of the stinging nettles, which are seen commonly in Europe and throughout North America. Plants of the genus *Urtica* produce injury when the tip of the nettle breaks off in the skin and syringelike action forces chemicals into the dermis. There is evidence that histamine and similar amines are responsible for this contact urticaria.[103,143]

Another family of irritant plants, Brassicaceae, contains the mustard seed plant and radishes (Color Plate 62). Contact with these odoriferous plants tends to cause blisters rather than hives. A third family of irritant plants is the buttercups (Ranunculaceae) (Color Plates 63 and 64). Table 36-2 lists common plants in this family. The irritant chemical appears to be a glycoside, ranunculin, protoanemonin, or a dimer, anemonin.[9] Many other families contain a few species of irritant plants (such as cereal grasses and dogwood leaves), which produce mechanical irritation.

The pathogenesis of primary irritation from plants has not been fully elucidated. In the case of nonimmunologic urticaria, release of histamine from mast cells with vasodilation and leakage of fluid appears to be an early direct chemical change leading to hives.[30,131] The molecular events in mast cell degranulation are thought to be similar to those described for immunogenic urticaria, with certain discrete differences. Thus there is no evidence for a selective membrane receptor, such as the high-affinity IgE receptor that is

Table 36-2 Some Irritant Plants in the Family Ranunculaceae (1900 Species)

Botanical Name	Common Name
Aconitum napellus	Wolfsbane
Anemone nemorosa	Windflower
Clementis vitalba	Traveler's joy
Delphinium (250 species)	Staves-acre
Helleborus niger	Christmas rose
Pulsatilla vulgaris	Pasque flower
Ranunculus (400 species)	Buttercup
Thalictrum foliosum	Meadow rue

now well characterized and required for immunologic degranulation of mast cells.[131,138] Instead, current information suggests that a receptor-independent mode of action occurs for all nonimmunologic histamine liberators, acting directly on a pertussis toxin–sensitive G protein to initiate a signal through phospholipase C activation, which degranulates mast cells of their histamine content.[95] Furthermore, there does not seem to be a requirement for methylation of the membrane phospholipids. Rather, a high intracellular calcium accumulation must occur, and the reaction is rapidly terminated without delayed mediator release.[123] Furthermore, arachidonic acid metabolites are not formed in any amount.[10] The role of other mediators, such as biologically active cytokines, has not been fully investigated. Evidence suggests that primary irritation alters the function of other cells, particularly epidermal cells. This may well constitute the initial event that then nonspecifically amplifies vascular alterations by release of vasoactive cytokines.

TREATMENT

Treatment of primary irritant dermatoses is often unsatisfactory. The patient must be removed from exposure to irritant chemicals and treated conservatively with rest, medicated soaks, and compresses, such as aluminum acetate solution (1:20), dilute potassium permanganate solution (1:16,000 in water), acetic acid solution (1:100), or Dalibour solution (copper and zinc sulfate and camphor, supplied commercially as Dalidane). Antihistamines usually have minimal effect. The dermatitis heals in less than 5 days if no complications develop and if tissue damage is minimal. Corticosteroids are of no use in controlling primary irritation.

Allergy

As with conventional contact dermatitis, irritant reactions far outnumber allergic responses elicited by vegetation. Although irritation can be severe, it is often so trivial that no medical help is sought. However, distinguishing irritation from allergy is important clinically because treatment varies considerably according to diagnosis. Allergic responses are more likely to evoke a reaction severe enough that the patient seeks help. Plants cause all varieties of allergic reactions. Immediate hypersensitivity reactions with angioedema, urticaria, and anaphylaxis from ingestion of foods, especially nuts, are well recognized.[14,90,125] (See Chapter 31 for management of anaphylaxis.)

Contact urticaria, or hives from exposure to plants, is fairly common and increasingly recognized as a major cause of immunogenic contact urticaria.[78] The patient observes redness, itching, and swelling, which can develop as discrete wheals or widespread edema 1 to 2 hours after exposure. Usually the eruption is linear or grouped at sites of contact, but extreme swelling and edema of an extremity can develop, depending on level of antigen exposure and the patient's degree of sensitivity, not unlike the range of responses in bee venom hypersensitivity. Thus an oral reaction may be minimal with simple burning and tingling, especially in the mouth, or massive, with edema of the lips, oral mucous membranes, and pharynx noted after eating fruit and vegetables. With chronic low-grade exposure, the eruption is a prominent occupational problem of field workers, packers, grocery workers, cooks, and bakers who handle raw fruits and vegetables.[64] Long lists of offending agents have been published.[54,78] Box 36-1 is a partial list of plants and plant products that cause immunogenic contact dermatitis.

The pathogenesis of immunogenic contact urticaria is a variation of immediate type I hypersensitivity. The central cytologic reactor in skin is the mast cell, which has high-affinity IgE receptors in its membrane. An IgE molecule binds to the receptor by its Fc portion, exposing the Fab segments as recognition sites. When a divalent protein antigen appropriately bridges two IgE molecules, a series of biochemical events transpires that leads to mast cell degranulation. The plasma membrane is perturbed. Several lipids are phosphorylated and G proteins are activated, which in turn activate phospholipase C to hydrolyze phosphatidylinositol-4,5-bisphosphate (PIP_2) and yield two messengers: diacylglycerol (DG) and inositol triphosphate ($InsP_3$).[12] $InsP_3$ binds to its receptor on the endoplasmic reticulum, forming a calcium channel to release free calcium ions (Ca^{++}) into the cytosol.[7,12,66,102] Simultaneously, DG activates protein kinase C in the plasma membrane, opening calcium channels and allowing entrance of extracellular Ca^{++}, which further loads the cytosol with free Ca^{++}, an important "messenger" in the stimulus secretion process.[82] G proteins interact with and

BOX 36-1

SOME PLANTS AND PLANT PRODUCTS CAUSING IMMUNOGENIC URTICARIA

FRUITS
Apple
Carrot
Celery
Parsley
Parsnip
Potato
Tomato

VEGETABLES
Chives
Grains
Lettuce
Onion

SPICES
Cinnamon
Garlic
Mustard
Rapeseed

PLANTS
Tulips

TREES
Birch pollen
Teak
Western red cedar
Various nuts

release the nucleotide complexed to protein α-chains,[140] some of which probably inhibit or stimulate cyclic adenosine phosphate and its actions as a second messenger.[16]

The result of the extensive alteration in intracellular milieu is activation of a serine proteinase and exocytosis of mast cell granule contents.[30,131] These come in three forms: preformed and rapidly released; preformed, bound to the granule matrix of heparin, and slowly released; and newly formed mediators. In addition, mast cells produce a variety of cytokines, including interleukins (ILs) 1, 3, 4, 5, and 6, granulocyte-macrophage colony-forming units, and tumor necrosis factor-alpha (TNFα),[139] and these cytokines interact with cells and structures such as endothelium in the skin to amplify the various inflammatory responses.[30,131,139] In acute urticaria the rapidly released preformed mediators account for most of the signs and symptoms. These mediators include histamine, some chemotactic factors, and arylsulfatase. If the lesions persist or extend, other mediators, such as newly formed leukotrienes, heparin (or heparin fragments), cytokines, and a number of proteases, may be involved in the continuing tissue damage.

The sequence of inflammatory events leading to acute urticaria is most likely to occur in patients with an atopic background, especially those with pollen allergies.[78] This is the same group of people, mainly women and especially health care workers, who have been found in recent years to be exquisitely sensitive to latex rubber gloves[18,80,135,145] and sensitive to proteins in the natural latex from rubber trees in Asia.[96] In addition to fruit and nuts, mustard in pizza has been implicated in anaphylaxis.[107] In less severe cases, vesicular, eczematous rashes have been noted within hours of eating mustard or rapeseed, which is used widely in production of vegetable oils and margarine.[88] Erythema multiforme–like eruptions are well recognized after contact with bracelets and ornamental necklaces made of exotic woods, such as *Dalbergia nigra*.[48] Erythema multiforme has also been seen after exposure to more common plants, such as poison ivy, primula, and mugwort.[48] It is theorized that multiforme lesions result from vasculitis caused by deposition of immune complexes in or around the vessels, but no formal proof has been published.

Diagnosis of immunogenic contact urticaria can be confirmed by simple tests. As a use test, application of the suspected plant product to the antecubital fossa twice a day for several days may reproduce the wheal response. Open and closed patch tests, with examination of test sites in 2 to 6 hours, can be useful, as can more conventional prick, scratch, or scratch-chamber tests, in which the results are read in 15 to 20 minutes.[78] It is most important to determine whether urtication is immunologic or nonimmunologic in nature.[54,78] For complete evaluation an allergist obtains radioallergosorbent tests to quantify specific IgE in the patient's serum. More refined serologic tests include crossed radioimmunoelectrophoresis (CRIE) and CRIE inhibition.[19]

Patients with contact urticaria visit the emergency department when an eruption is extensive or extreme, or if it is associated with stridor, wheezing, and collapse. Since mast cell degranulation is the central problem, and because epinephrine stimulates cyclic adenosine monophosphate formation that opposes degranulation, it is logical to use this drug. Other supportive treatment for anaphylactic shock may be required, such as albuterol, aminophylline, oxygen, or intravenous hydrocortisone. In less severe cases, antihistamines are valuable. Intramuscular or intravenous diphenhydramine (Benadryl) in adult doses of 50 to 100 mg usually stops progression of wheal formation and can be followed by oral hydroxyzine (25 to 50 mg three times a day) or cyproheptadine (4 to 8 mg four times a day) for 2 to 5 days. Pure H_1 blockers such as terfenadine (60 mg two or three times a day) are also effective and do not depress the central nervous system, although the prescriber has to be aware of their unusual adverse reactions, such as inducing cardiac arrhythmias and drug interactions. It is important to make certain the patient has not inadvertently hidden parts of the plant on the body, in clothing, or in a towel, blanket, or knapsack. Recrudescence of the urticarial response usually can be traced to continuing unknown contact with the offending agent.

Delayed hypersensitivity or type IV allergy of the contact hypersensitivity variety occurs more frequently as a result of contact with plants than does type I contact urticaria. Sensitivity to poison ivy or poison oak is undoubtedly the single most common cause of allergic skin reactions in the United States and, along with contact allergy to sesquiterpene lactones ("compositae"), probably worldwide (Color Plate 65). When a distraught young person arrives in the emergency department with a rip-roaring, acute, edematous, erythematous skin eruption and a history of consorting with nature in outdoor activity, it is correct to conclude that this is probably a serious bout of poison ivy or poison oak dermatitis. Approximately 50% of the U.S. adult population is clinically sensitive to poison ivy, poison oak, and poison sumac. If a sensitive individual brushes against the plant or comes in contact with the heavy, nonvolatile oil in the resin canals, he or she will acquire poison ivy or poison oak dermatitis. In the natural state the oil is colorless or slightly yellow. On exposure to air, however, it oxidizes, polymerizes, and turns black. This is a way to recognize the weeds, especially in the autumn when the leaves fall off.

Contrary to popular belief, urushiol is present in poison ivy and poison oak in roughly equal amount year round, even when they are only sticks without leaves in the winter. It appears that as the leaves turn red and start to dry up in the fall, important nutrients, including urushiol, return to the stem and roots through the subepidermal resin canals.[53] Thus, when the dead leaves fall to the ground, they are virtually devoid of urushiol. The amount of purified urushiol (the active allergenic principle) required to elicit a reaction is 2 to 2.5 μg.[45] Another group of people (about 35%) are considered subclinically sensitive because they have negative skin test reactions to 2.5 μg urushiol but are reactive to higher concentrations such as 5, 10, and 50 μg.[34,45] Clinically this group is very interesting. They invariably did not have poison ivy dermatitis as teenagers and often plucked the weeds with apparent impunity. However, usually in midlife after a bout of weed pulling, a rash spreads explosively. For unknown reasons the victims have crossed the line into clinical sensitivity. If patch tested with dilutions of urushiol, they are often exquisitely sensitive and do not appear to lose their reactivity. The flare-up may last for several weeks, probably because of prior contamination of the home and workplace with urushiol oil. Treatment must be aggressive and more prolonged than usual.

A smaller group (10% to 15%) does not react to the higher concentrations and cannot be sensitized by 1000 μg. This group was first detected and studied in passive transfer experiments in the 1950s.[43] These individuals are considered to be naturally tolerant, but it remains unclear whether they achieved that state by early antigenic exposure or by genetic luck of the draw. They do not have an inherent resistance to contact sensitization with other chemicals[44] and otherwise appear healthy. Perhaps they hold a clue to the molecular basis for immunologic tolerance.

The weeds are surprisingly fastidious. They do not grow in Alaska and Hawaii, nor do they survive well above 4000 feet, in deserts, or in rainforests. They grow best along cool streams and lakes and luxuriate if it is also sunny and hot. In the California hills they grow like a forest, but in cooler, dry climates they remain isolated in small patches. Nevertheless, they are found in every state of the continental United States. The plants have different configurations in different regions, but generally speaking, poison ivy grows east of the Rockies, poison oak grows west, and poison sumac grows best in the southeastern United States. Since avoidance is the best prevention, it is important to learn what the plant looks like in a given area (Fig. 36-1). No universal picture or

A

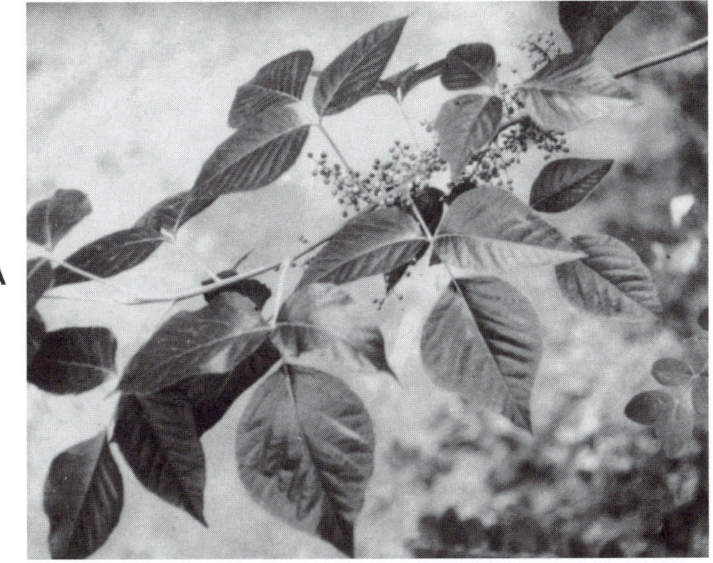

C

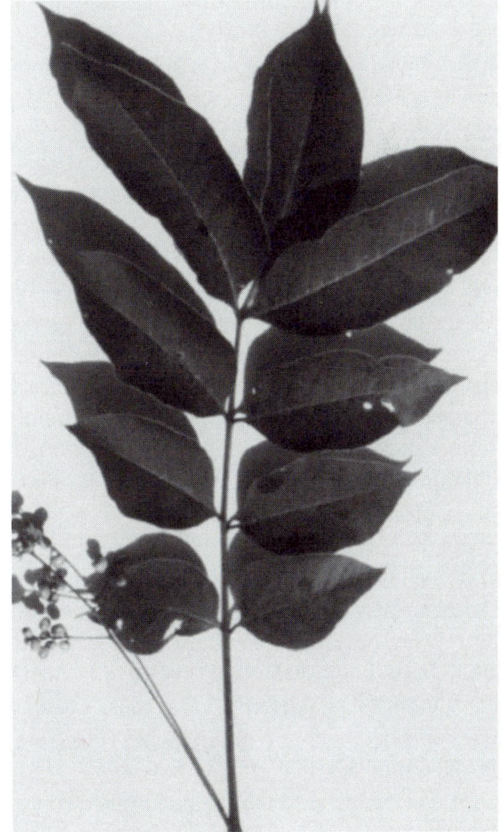

B

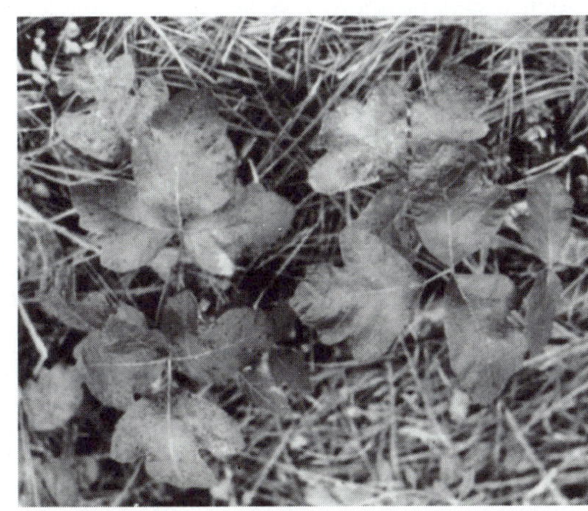

Fig. 36-1 **A,** Poison ivy *(Toxicodendron radicans).* **B,** Poison oak *(Toxicodendron diversiloba).* **C,** Poison sumac *(Toxicodendron vernix).* (From Ellis MD: *Dangerous plants, snakes, arthropods and marine life—toxicity and treatment,* Hamilton, Ill, 1964, Drug Intelligence Publications.)

description is adequate. Once contaminated with the oil, an average person has 1 to 4 hours to wash it off if the dermatitis is to be prevented. Very sensitive individuals are probably doomed to a reaction within minutes of contact.

From a practical standpoint, only 10% to 15% of Americans (up to 40 million persons) can be categorized as exquisitely sensitive, and generally these are the patients who seek and need emergency medical care. They typically have had prior unpleasant experiences. Within 2 to 6 hours after exposure, swelling is accompanied by an erythematous, intensely pruritic, edematous, vesicular, and ultimately bullous eruption that can be associated with fever, malaise, and prostration. This true dermatologic emergency should be treated immediately and vigorously.

The genetics of extreme susceptibility are incompletely understood. Such sensitivity tends to be familial; if one parent is supersensitive, children are likely to be as well. If both parents are sensitive, the chance of sensitive offspring is about 80%.[147] The level of individual sensitivity is not determined by the severity of the initial bout of dermatitis. Although almost half of patients admit to a memorable bout of dermatitis as a teenager, no more than 25% to 35% of victims at age 30 to 40 were stricken within the previous year.[34] There are many reasons for this, not the least being avoidance. If these subjects are patch tested with weak dilutions of urushiol, less than half react as might be expected from their histories. An individual's level of reactivity does not change appreciably if he or she is tested monthly over a year[45]; testing at less frequent intervals in very sensitive subjects over 3 to 4 years has shown little or no change in the level of reactivity. The complete biologic factors that modify a person's level of sensitivity over a lifetime remain obscure. Repeated mild to moderate bouts of dermatitis maintain the sensitive state, while a single severe bout may produce a prolonged period of anergy or refractoriness,[33,34] not unlike the clinical condition of "hardening" or unresponsiveness, well described in the industrial setting.[130]

The chemistry of urushiols, the allergenic principle in poison ivy and poison oak dermatitis, has been studied extensively. Early in this century the study of lacquer in Japan led to isolation and characterization of these catechols with a long carbon side chain at ring position 3 (Fig. 36-2). In the 1950s, Dawson and his group[23] investigated poison ivy urushiols and synthesized the saturated side chain molecule, 3-*N*-pentadecylcatechol (PDC). Ready availability of this chemical allowed the first thorough and systematic review of poison ivy reactivity.[75] In the past quarter century much has been learned of the molecular structure and immunologic binding properties of urushiol.[2,37] The urushiols in poison ivy, poison oak, and poison sumac differ only slightly in structure and biologically cross-react, so that a person sensitive to poison ivy also reacts to poison oak and poison sumac. Poison ivy urushiol generally has a C-15 carbon side chain that can be completely saturated or has one, two, or three double bonds. Poison oak mainly has a C-17 side chain, which is seldom fully saturated (Fig. 36-2). Poison sumac seems to have a C-13 side chain. Of these molecules, saturated PDC is the least reactive on skin and the diene yields the most severe responses on a molar basis. This suggests that earlier investigations with PDC probably underestimated the level of skin reactivity in individual subjects. Furthermore, it has been amply confirmed that the side chain determines specificity of sensitivity to poison ivy and poison oak. For instance, shortened side chains below 10 carbon atoms or altered configurations do not show cross-reactivity.[3,4] Urushiol by itself is not very reactive chemically. In tissue in the presence of oxygen, the hydroxyl groups at ring sites 1 and 2 convert spontaneously or by enzyme action to a quinone, which is a highly reactive molecular species. This change allows nucleophilic attack by proteins at ring positions 4, 5, and 6. An amino attack preferentially occurs at site 5 and a sulfhydryl attack at site 6 (Fig. 36-3), and the differences determine whether animals can be sensitized or made tolerant.[27,28] Plants, shrubs, and trees with cross-reacting catechols are found throughout the world, arising either indigenously or by transplantation.[37,118] The most common cross-reacting plants are mango, cashew nut shell, India marking nut, and Japanese lacquer. Increasing numbers of cross-reacting plants are reported from South America.[68] A chemical curiosity is the cross-reaction with resorcinols from cashew nut shell oil.[71] Similar cross-reacting resorcinol-containing plants have been observed in Australia[89] and more recently in Hawaii.[76]

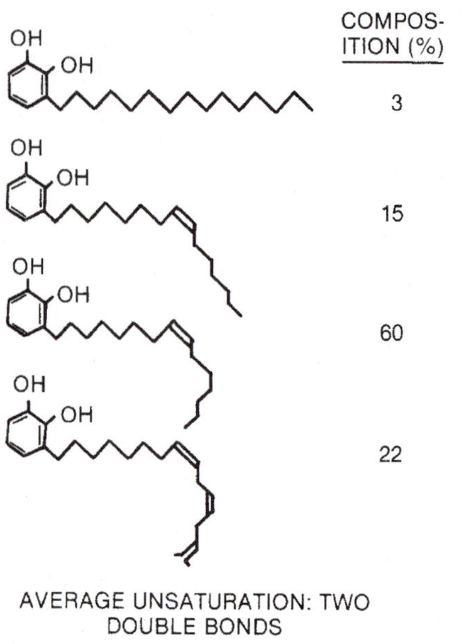

Fig. 36-2 General structure and composition of poison ivy urushiol.

The immunologic mechanism for allergic contact dermatitis is generally conceded to be type IV cell-mediated delayed hypersensitivity.[38] However, in skin it is now clear that the keratinocytes also are part of the immune surveillance

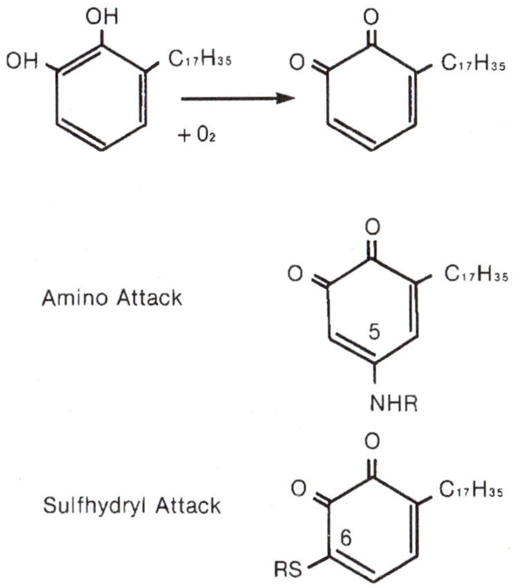

Fig. 36-3 Chemical reactivity of urushiol in skin. In the presence of oxygen the hydroxyl groups open up to become quinones, which allows a preferential amino attack at ring position 5 or a sulfhydryl attack at position 6.

system. They respond quickly to every chemical insult, either irritant or allergenic, in an antigen-independent fashion to produce a variety of cytokines. These function mainly to amplify future inflammatory responses.[6,101] Early on, they secrete TNFα and intercellular adhesion molecule 1. Somewhat later, they release IL-1, 6, 8, and 10, and still later a macrophage chemotactic factor and other cytokines.[5,56,57,101,115] These may in turn release acute-phase reactants from mast cells and endothelial cells, as seen in irritant responses.[6,101] Current research is attempting to identify which keratinocyte cytokines specify the allergic reaction, as distinct from simple injury. Nevertheless, it is known that the catechol molecules of poison oak and poison ivy enter the skin and bind through nucleophilic attack at benzene ring positions 4, 5, or 6 to surface proteins on antigen-presenting cells (APCs), which are primarily Langerhans' cells in the epidermis. The molecules are then internalized and processed in the APCs, which leave the epidermis and travel to regional lymph nodes, where they present their processed antigen on the cell surface in context with a major histocompatibility complex class II molecule to the T cell receptor complex on a CD4 T-helper cell. To complete the sensitization signal, another surface protein (the B7 antigen) forms a costimulatory signal by binding to the CD28 ligand on the T cell. This then activates the T cell, which divides repeatedly to form a clone of urushiol-specific CD4 cells. These subsequently expand into clones of circulating activated T-effector and T-memory lymphocytes.

Upon a new challenge by urushiol, the lymphocytes elicit a cell-mediated cytotoxic immune response characterized by erythema, edema, and vesiculation resulting from destruction of epidermal cells and activation of the dermal vasculature. Simultaneously, urushiol molecules bind to other carrier proteins and stimulate T8 suppressor cells, so that in effect the clinical reaction seen is a balance between T4 and T8 responses. In an individual patient this determines the severity of the dermatitis after exposure to the poisonous weeds. This logical formulation, however, does not completely explain acute poison oak or poison ivy dermatitis. An acute eruption tends to begin within hours of exposure and is primarily edematous. Some workers have emphasized the presence of basophils in acute poison oak and poison ivy lesions and have proposed a role for basophil mediators in the pathogenesis of an early-onset acute reaction.[31] Certainly the clinical presentation in these cases favors a late-phase reaction[80] and a mechanism possibly involving mast cell degranulation, as mentioned previously,[73] as well as other cytokine mediators.

The mast cell is probably responsible for this late-phase type of inflammation. Almost certainly the same initial cell membrane and cytosol perturbations occur as in type I urticaria. However, the final effect is a more delayed (late-phase) degranulation with release of preformed mediators (bound firmly to the granule matrix) and newly formed mediators, including leukotrienes, other eicosanoids, proteases, platelet activating factor, and lipid chemotactic factors.

Late-phase inflammation also involves T lymphocytes and mononuclear macrophages. While the membrane signals are similar to those for mast cells,[47] there are some differences. Inositol triphosphate directly activates calcium ion channels in the plasma membrane of T lymphocytes[77]; the generation and release of cytokines and mediators are considerably slower. In this system in monocytes, phospholipase A_2 hydrolyzes phospholipids in the plasma membrane to yield free arachidonic acid, which is further metabolized to yield prostaglandins, leukotrienes, and other metabolites that contribute to the delayed inflammatory response.

Some believe that this process is down-regulated by a family of intracellular proteins, lipocortins/annexins, one of which, lipocortin/annexin 1, appears to be secreted. There are putative lipocortin receptors on select cells such as the epidermis and monocytes that would facilitate a buildup of these molecules in the cells of inflammation to down-regulate proinflammatory lipid synthesis.[55] Initially it was believed that lipocortin 1 directly inhibited phospholipase A_2, but that does not seem to be the case,[5,55] and its effects, if any, are far more complex.[5] Nevertheless, it is possible to envision a tight regulatory cycle in or near the plasma membrane, where a specific signal transduces a receptor-effector message through calcium, nucleotide, protein, and lipid interactions that results in selective exocytosis of a variety of mediators of inflammation. An important concept is that corticosteroids readily induce gene transcription of the lipocortin/annexin family of proteins, albeit by indirect induction of synthesis of transcriptional factors.[5] This mechanism partially explains the dramatic effect of corticosteroids in treating acute poison ivy dermatitis. The bottom line in understanding the antiinflammatory effect of glucocorticoids appears to be an absolute block in translation of the mRNA of prostaglandin synthase, which appears to be the rate-limiting enzyme step in the synthesis of these biologically active proinflammatory lipid molecules. However, the complexity of the glucocorticoid effect is indicated by the fact that these hormones also block nitric oxide synthase in monocytes,[22] another proinflammatory pathway in cells.

TREATMENT

Systemic corticosteroids are widely accepted as the first line of treatment, especially when given early and in large, therapeutic doses. If the reaction is of less than 2 hours' duration, intravenous hydrocortisone or methylprednisolone can be curative. After a patient has suffered 4 to 6 hours with massive edema, erythema, and pruritus, intravenous therapy is highly effective, but it must be followed by more prolonged oral or intramuscular administration of corticosteroids (Fig. 36-4). Most patients in this category seek help after 8 to 16 hours of discomfort, at which point intravenous therapy is less effective. Intramuscular methylprednisolone sodium succinate (Solu-Medrol), 40 mg, combined with betamethasone sodium phosphate (Celestone), 4 to 8 mg, should give relief for 7 to 14 days. Adrenocorticotropic hormone (ACTH) gel, 80 units intramuscularly with a repeat in 8 to 12 hours, often is curative. Prednisone, 100 to 120 mg divided in four equal doses daily for 2 days, may achieve the same salubrious effect. At the same time, patients are instructed to rest at home for 3 or 4 days. If a flare-up starts, another dose of ACTH gel or a repeat regimen of prednisone is prescribed. Subsequent exacerbations are usually caused by reexposure to urushiol that has contaminated the patient's local environment, so that the patient must be warned to thoroughly wash all clothing and other articles that might have been exposed during the initial contact.

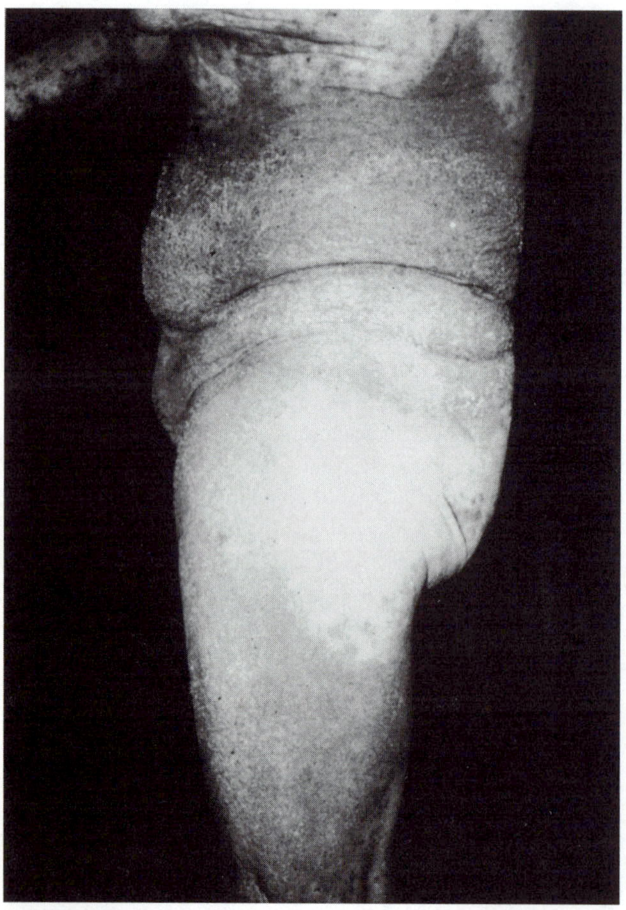

Fig. 36-4 Generalized poison ivy dermatitis.

If the dermatitis has been present for more than 24 hours, the aggressive regimen just detailed is less successful (Fig. 36-5). Under these circumstances many physicians prefer a more conservative approach. Oral prednisone, 80 to 100 mg/day for 3 to 4 days with a 10- to 14-day every-other-day taper, helps many patients, but the danger lies in a sudden flare-up at the end of therapy, which becomes poorly responsive to steroids. Whenever considering systemic corticosteroids for acute allergic contact dermatitis, the physician must be certain that the patient is otherwise healthy, without active infections, vascular accidents, endocrinopathies, or a familial history of glaucoma.

When the onset of dermatitis is delayed for several days and the eruption is mild or moderate, systemic therapy offers little benefit. Antihistamines, aspirin, or nonsteroidal antiinflammatory drugs are without effect. Results of systemic corticosteroids, even in large doses, are disappointing. Topical application of soothing aluminum acetate (1:20) soaks, calamine lotion, or tepid baths, with one cup Aveeno oatmeal or two cups linnet starch per tub, relieves pruritus and allows healing to occur uneventfully. Although field workers have mentioned that aloe vera latex empirically improves wound healing, a prospective trial has not been conducted. Topical lotions with anesthetics or antihistamines offer no additional benefit and may induce contact sensitization to the chemical additives. Allergic contact dermatitis is a self-healing disease that resolves over 10 to 14 days if iatrogenic influences are avoided. Secondary superficial infections may occur in children or during hospitalization. Cleanliness usually prevents this complication.

Topical corticosteroids are highly touted for treatment of allergic contact dermatitis and are sold for this purpose over the counter. However, they are expensive and do not work well. In only two situations do these preparations justify the expense. In the mild to moderately sensitive person when the eruption is beginning (red and itchy, but not yet blistered), potent, fluorinated steroids in a gel or optimized vehicle can prevent spread of the rash and speed healing. Many such preparations are available; an example is fluocinonide 0.05% gel (Lidex). Since topical steroids are readily absorbed and can cause adrenal suppression, they should be

A

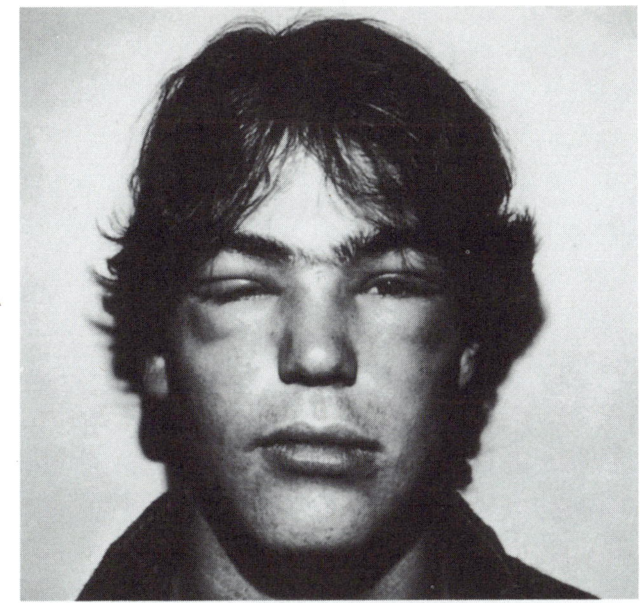

B

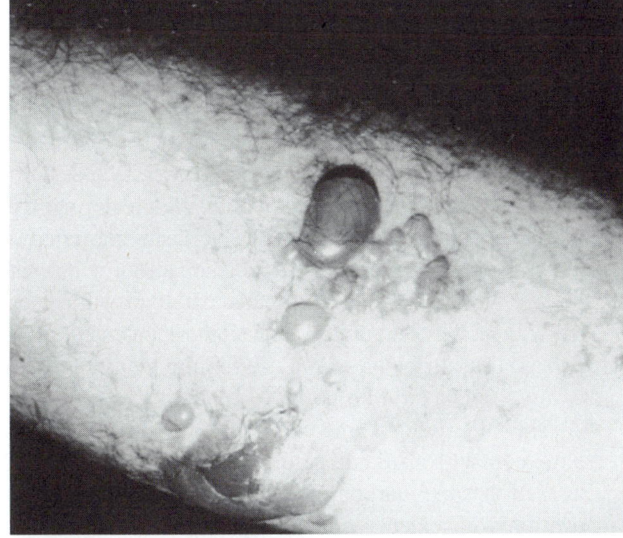

C

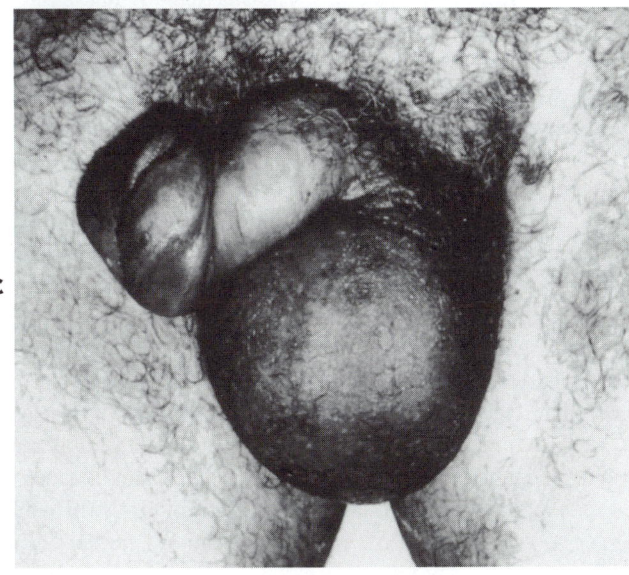

Fig. 36-5 Acute poison oak dermatitis. **A,** Facial edema. **B,** Blisters. **C,** Penile edema. (Courtesy Dr. Axel Hoke.)

restricted to limited amounts (less than 15 g) for a brief period (2 to 3 days). Generally the opportunity to use this approach does not occur in an emergency department, but it can be very effective in helping persons repeatedly exposed to poison ivy or poison oak in the course of their work.

The other circumstance amenable to topical steroids occurs more commonly. As the dermatitis heals and scales after 10 to 14 days, the patient may note a resurgence of pruritus, which untreated can lead to a patch of subchronic lichenoid neurodermatitis (Fig. 36-6). Judicious use of almost any steroid cream or ointment alleviates the symptoms. Examples include triamcinolone acetonide 0.025%, desonide 0.025%, and hydrocortisone 1%.

The best approaches to prophylaxis come from an intimate understanding of the chemistry of urushiol and the biology of the weeds[37] and reside mainly in recognition and avoidance. Where this is not possible, protective clothing that is either disposable or washable should be worn. Water rapidly inactivates urushiol, and organic solvents such as alcohol, gasoline, and acetone can extract it from contaminated surfaces. The idea of using barrier preparations has become popular again, even though in the past such creams and ointments proved disappointing.[105] One effective barrier preparation that is currently on the market[106] is a linoleic acid dime ester (Stokogard Outdoor Cream). It can be ordered through a pharmacy or obtained from industrial medical suppliers. Experimental barrier preparations that are effective include chitosan and organoclay.[37] Hyposensitization by oral ingestion of gradually increasing amounts of the active urushiol allergen in olive oil can be considered,[36] but should be done under the direction of a dermatologist or allergist skilled in the procedure.

COMPOSITAE DERMATITIS

Although poison oak and poison ivy are the most common causes of allergic contact dermatitis in the United States, supremacy for this distinction worldwide is challenged by the enormous plant family Compositae. This family contains more than 20,000 species in 1000 genera and consists of many commonly recognized plants, vegetables, wildflowers, weeds, and commercially useful plants (Color Plates 66 to 68).[129] Listed in Box 36-2 are a number of these plants and species. Fortunately, casual exposure is usually insufficient to induce contact sensitization, or the quality of outdoor life would be greatly compromised. Most Compositae dermatitis is reported as an occupational hazard by florists, horticulturists, forestry workers, food handlers, and similar workers. However, it occasionally affects home gardeners and recreational nature enthusiasts. In India the weed

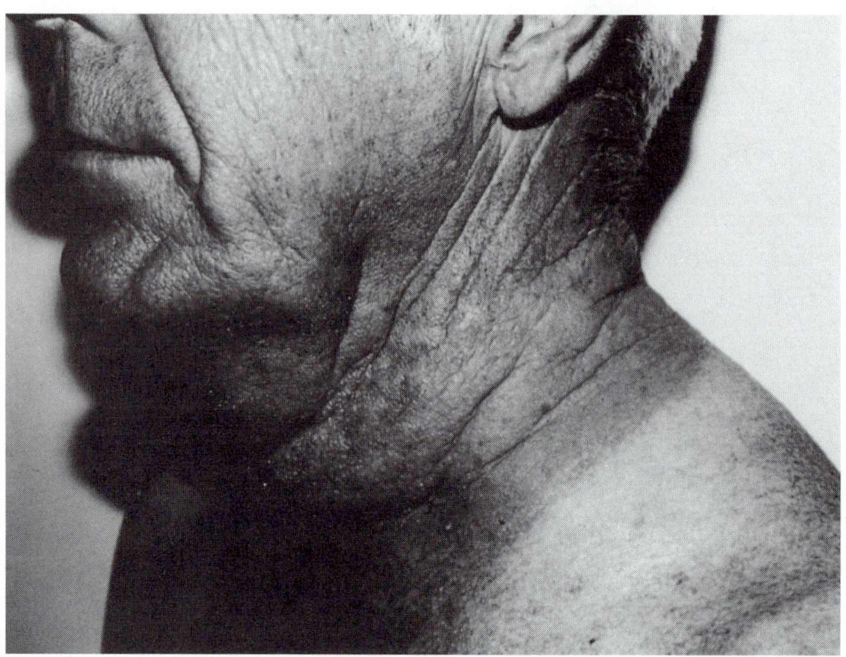

Fig. 36-6 Airborne poison oak dermatitis from a brush fire. (Courtesy Dr. Axel Hoke.)

BOX 36-2

SOME COMPOSITAE THAT CAUSE ALLERGIC CONTACT DERMATITIS

VEGETABLES

Artichoke
Chicory
Endive
Lettuce
Yarrow

WEEDS

Burweed
Cocklebur
Dog fennel
Goldenrod
Mugwort
Sneezeweed
Stinking mayweed

PERFUMERY

Costus

FLOWERS

Black-eyed Susan
Cardoon
Chamomile
Chrysanthemum
Dahlia
Daisy
Dandelion
Elecampane
Gaillardia
Mountain tobacco
Sunflower
Tansy

Parthenium hysterophorus (Congress grass, feverfew), which was incidentally imported from the United States with loads of grain, subsequently created an epidemic of Compositae dermatitis.[84]

The eruption generally spares children and affects predominantly young and middle-aged men. The dermatitis involves the face, neck, arms, and exposed areas in airborne or photocontactant patterns, so that both allergic dermatitis and photoallergic contact dermatitis have been suggested.[65,114] When the eruption presents as an acute airborne dermatitis, the patient is often severely affected and likely to seek emergency help. The dermatitis can become subacute or chronic, as has been attributed to ragweed in the Midwest and to a variety of plants in Europe.[25]

The underlying theme that links the Compositae species is the contact-sensitizing sesquiterpene lactones. More than 3000 of these 15-carbon ringed structures of complex organization with extensive ligand substitutions have been extracted from plant products. They have many important biologic properties, such as their use in antitumor, cytotoxic, antiinflammatory, antimicrobial, and antiparasitic drugs. Only some of the structures are contact sensitizers. One problem with use of the term "Compositae dermatitis" is that cross-reacting allergens are found in plants and weeds of other plant families. Species of the Magnoliaceae, Lauraceae, and Liliaceae families have been implicated. Liliaceae is a very large family containing such diverse, useful, and ornamental plants as aloe, asparagus, colchicum, hyacinth, and tulip. Certain species can be both irritating and sensitizing. "Hyacinth itch" is a primary irritant dermatitis probably caused by calcium oxalate crystals in the bulb scales, which may also contain an unknown sensitizer. "Tulip fingers" can be caused by irritation but usually results from contact sensitization to the sesquiterpene lactones tulipan A or tulipan B. In addition, at least three families of liverworts contain cross-reacting sesquiterpene lactones.[129]

Forestry workers sensitized to frullanolide in the liverwort genus *Frullania* show cross-contact reactivity to sesquiterpene lactones in plants of the families Compositae and Asteraceae.[91]

The chemical structure in sesquiterpene lactones responsible for contact sensitization appears to be an α-methylene–γ-butyrolactone arrangement, which is available for nucleophilic attack by amino groups in proteins.[29] Experimental contact sensitization has been accomplished in guinea pigs with four sesquiterpene lactones devoid of the exocyclic α-methylene grouping on the lactone ring.[62] This does not invalidate the pattern observed in the natural state; it simply means that many chemicals can be sensitizers. At one time it was proposed that alantolactone be used to detect sesquiterpene lactone hypersensitivity because of its propensity for cross-reactivity with other related compounds. However, it has become clear that patterns of cross-reactivity vary extremely, so a simplistic approach is not acceptable[122] and a sesquiterpene lactone mix has proved useful in diagnosing apparent airborne or generalized eczema.[26] In a molecular analysis of the pattern of cross-reactivity in *Costus*-sensitized patients, we reported that sesquiterpene lactones with the lesser degree of oxygenated substituents close to the α-methylene–γ-butyrolactone ring gave the highest frequency of cross-reactivity.[8] Furthermore, we observed that sesquiterpene lactones belonging to any one of the six skeletal classes (Fig. 36-7) contain sensitizers that would not be expected to cross-react with those from a different class, and this might explain some of the discrepancies in cross-reactivity patterns described in the literature.[8] The emergency physician who is familiar with the Compositae family and sesquiterpene lactones may help sort out the correct offending agent in the unusual case of "poison ivy" dermatitis when that diagnosis does not clearly fit. This knowledge is critical in distinguishing between airborne and phototoxic allergic contact dermatitis.[65,114]

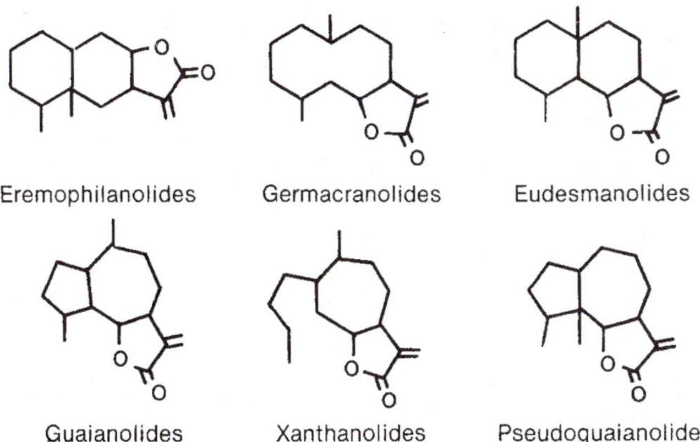

Fig. 36-7 The six skeletal backbones of sesquiterpene lactones. Note the methylene configuration on the lactone ring, which is responsible for contact sensitization and contributes to other biologic activities.

TOXIC WOODS

Toxic woods also contain plant chemicals that produce allergic contact dermatitis (Fig. 36-8). Most of these are exotic tropical woods with great commercial value.[61] They are crafted into a wide variety of common objects such as furniture, musical instruments, boats, cabinets, walking sticks, jewelry, and art forms.

Table 36-3 lists some common sensitizing trees. The main problem with wood dermatitis occurs in an occupational setting with forestry workers, lumber workers, carpenters, and craftspeople, but it can affect the souvenir hunter or art aficionado. Chemical sensitizers in woods have been studied in detail[60] and are numerous and diverse. Many are quinones and can cause cross-sensitivity with primin found in some species of *Primula* (such as *P. obconica*).[9] One of the best known is Brazilian rosewood *(Dalbergia nigra),* which has been nearly depleted by its wide decorative use. The sensitizing chemical is R-4-methoxydalbergione, a complex quinone. Because of the scarcity of rosewood in recent years, it has been replaced by pao ferro wood from South America. Unfortunately, pao ferro contains an even more potent sensitizer and may be the most hazardous tim-

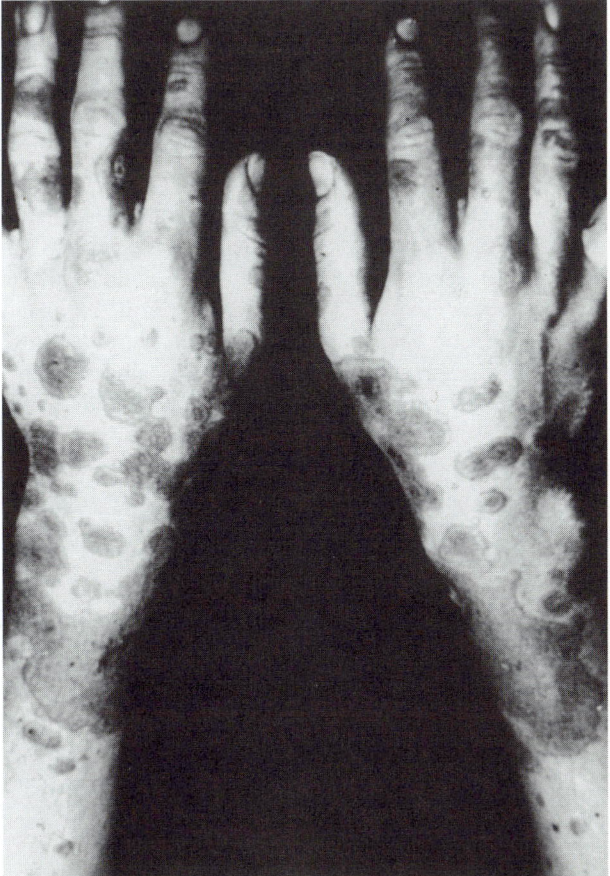

Fig. 36-8 Contact erythema multiforme, usually caused by contact with exotic woods.

Table 36-3 Some Trees That Cause Allergic Contact Dermatitis

Common Name	Botanical Name
African blackwood	*Dalbergia latifolia*
Australian blackwood	*Acacia melanoxylon*
California redwood	*Sequoia sempervirens*
Cocobolo	*Dalbergia retusa*
Mansonia	*Mansonia altissima*
Pao ferro	*Machaerium scleroxylum*
Pine	*Pinus* (about 80 species in North America)
Rosewoods	*Dalbergia* species
Silky oak	*Grevillea robusta*
Spruce	*Picea* species
Teak	*Tectona grandis*
Western red cedar	*Thuja plica*

ber in commercial use.[61] Australian silky oak *(Grevillea robusta)* is grown as a shade tree but is also used for plywood and furniture. Grevillol (5-*N*-tridecylresorcinol) is the sensitizer and may cross-react with urushiol.[89] Pines contain several terpenes that are used commercially as crude balsams or purified colophony (rosin) and turpentine. All can cause allergic contact dermatitis. California redwood *(Sequoia sempervirens)* can induce allergic alveolitis and contact dermatitis.[87] Along the Pacific coast, western red cedar *(Thuja plicata)* is a well-known cause of "cedar poisoning." It can elicit immediate hypersensitivity with allergic rhinitis, allergic alveolitis,[137] and allergic contact dermatitis.[61] The tree contains at least two quinones that act as contact sensitizers. One of these, β-thujaplicin, is reputed to be responsible for the trees' natural resistance to decay and is used in Japan to manufacture cosmetics.[51] There are many sensitizing plants whose allergenic chemicals have not yet been identified. Reynolds, Epstein, and Rodriguez[120] have identified prenyl chain–substituted hydroquinones called phacelioids in the family Hydrophyllaceae, a woody shrub that grows wild in the Southwest. These plants produce allergic dermatitis in botanists and field workers. The phacelioids structurally resemble urushiol but do not show cross-reactivity. In humans the most potent sensitizer of the phacelioid group is geranyl hydroquinone.[120] The creosote bush, *Larrea,* is responsible for an airborne weed dermatitis rash pattern, but whether the bush is a contact sensitizer or photosensitizer is uncertain.[81] Although more than 100 chemicals have been isolated, the actual sensitizer remains unknown.[81] English ivy, a common ground cover over much of the United States, can induce allergic contact dermatitis, usually in epidemics. Recently the principal contact-sensitizing chemical has been detected and identified as falcarinol.[52,63]

Treatment for plant-induced allergic contact dermatitis is the same as described for poison ivy or poison oak dermatitis. The majority of eruptions from other plant sources would be considered mild to moderate and deserve conservative, not aggressive, therapy.

Phytophotodermatitis

Phytodermatitis is the term used for adverse photoreactions to plants. Phytophotodermatitis denotes adverse reactions to nonionizing rays from the sun induced by plants.[74]

In general, two types of phytophotodermatitis occur. The reaction may be phototoxic or photoallergic in nature.[32] Phototoxic reactions are much more common than photoallergic responses. They occur in anyone if sufficient amounts of offending wavelengths arrive at the skin in the presence of enough of the photosensitizing molecules. The reaction is characterized by erythema with or without edema, followed by hyperpigmentation and desquamation.

Photoallergic reactions are generally uncommon. Like all allergies, they represent an acquired altered reactivity that depends on an antigen-antibody relationship or a cell-mediated delayed hypersensitivity response. Morphologically, they are characterized by an immediate wheal and flare or a delayed papular to eczematous eruption. In general, it requires less energy to induce a photoallergic reaction than to induce a phototoxic response.

Sun-induced plant dermatitis reactions are not rare. They may be induced by internal ingestion or topical applications of plants or plant products. The former is quite rare because of the large amount of plant material that must be eaten to sensitize an individual. However, such events have been reported with the ingestion of relatively large amounts of psoralen contained in vegetables and prolonged exposure to intense UVA radiation (long-wave ultraviolet rays between 320 and 400 nm) as would occur in a suntan salon.[83] Photoreactions to topical applications are not uncommon.

The major photoactive chemicals in plants are furocoumarins (psoralens), which are found in plant families such as Umbelliferae (for example, celery, giant ragweed, parsnip, fennel, dill, wild carrot); Rutaceae (for example, lime, citron, lemon, bergamot, gas plant, and Persian lime); and Leguminosae (for example, scurf-pea and bavchi) (Table 36-4) (Color Plates 69 and 70). Contact with the plant followed by exposure to UVA often leads to a phototoxic response.

The reaction is characterized by erythema with or without edema, followed by dense hyperpigmentation with unusual patterns and distribution. The lesions may be linear, irregular blotches, or confluent. All are confined to areas contacted by the plant and exposed to the sun or artificial irradiators such as those used in UVA suntan salons (Fig. 36-9).

Bullae may occur if the reaction is severe. A linear bullous eruption apparently induced by photosensitizers in "meadow grass" was described six decades ago as "dermatitis bullosa striata pratensis."[104]

Plant-induced photosensitization has caused industrial problems. For example, severe vesiculobullous eruptions in-

Table 36-4 Common Plants Implicated in Causing Phytophotodermatitis

Family	Botanical Name	Common Name
Umbelliferae	*Anthriscus sylvestris*	Cow parsley, wild chervil
	Apium graveolens	Celery
	Heracleum mantegazzianum	
	Heracleum maximum (H. dulce)	Giant hogweed
	Pastinaca sativa (P. urens)	Parsnip (garden variety)
	Heracleum laciniatum	Tromsopalm
	Angelica sylvestris	
	Heracleum spondylium	Cow parsley
	Heracleum giganteum	Parsnip (wild parsnip)
	Foeniculum vulgare	Fennel
	Anethum graveolens	Dill
	Peucedanum oreoselium	
	Daucus carota	Wild carrot, garden carrot
	Peucedanum ostruthium	Masterwort
	Ammi majus	
	Angelica archangelica	Angelica
Rutaceae	*Citrus aurantifolia*	Lime
	Citrus medica (C. acida)	Citron
	Citrus sinensis	
	Citrus aurantium	Bitter orange
	Citrus limon	Lemon
	Citrus bergamia	Bergamot
	Dictamnus albus (D. fraxinella)	Gas plant, burning bush
	Ruta graveolens	Common rue
	Phebalium argenteum	Persian lime (Tahitian)
Moraceae	*Ficus carica*	Fig
Compositae	*Achillea millefolium*	Milfoil, yarrow
	Anthemis cotula	Stinking mayweed
Ranunculaceae	*Ranunculus* spp.	Buttercup
Cruciferae	*Brassica* spp.	Mustard
Convolulaceae	*Convolvulus arvensis*	Rindweed
Rosaceae	*Argrimonia eupatoria*	Agrimony
Chenopodiaceae	*Chenopodium* spp.	Goosefoot
Leguminosae	*Psoralea corylifolia*	Scurf-pea, bavchi
Hypericaceae	*Hypericum perforatum*	St. John's wort
Anacardiaceae	*Hypericum crispum*	Red quebracho
	Schinopsis quebracho-colorado (S. lorentzii)	

From Pathak MS, Worden LR, Kaufman KD: *J Invest Dermatol* 48:103, 1967.

volving sun-exposed areas were reported in a large number of field workers harvesting celery in Michigan in 1961.[13] The cause of this response was contact with a psoralen compound elaborated by celery infected by pink rot *(Sclerotinia sclerotinorum)* and exposure to sunlight. Normally, noninfected celery contains some 5-methoxypsoralen (5-MOP). When it is infected with the fungus, the combination produces 8-methoxypsoralen (8-MOP) and trimethylpsoralen.[116,117,121,128] The infected celery also contains higher than normal concentrations of 5-MOP.

More recently, phytophotodermatitis developed in several grocery workers handling produce in a chain of supermarkets in 13 different states.[11] This reaction apparently was induced by contact with a newly developed disease-resistant brand of celery. In at least one location the eruption was related to handling the produce and subsequent tanning in a UVA suntan salon.[21]

Another example of industrially induced phytophotodermatitis, noted in Florida, resulted from bartenders' squeezing Persian limes *(Citrus aurantifolia)* into cocktails.[126] The rind contains a photosensitizing psoralen compound released by the squeezing.

Other persons at occupational risk are dairy workers (from plants eaten by cows), farmers, gardeners, and can-

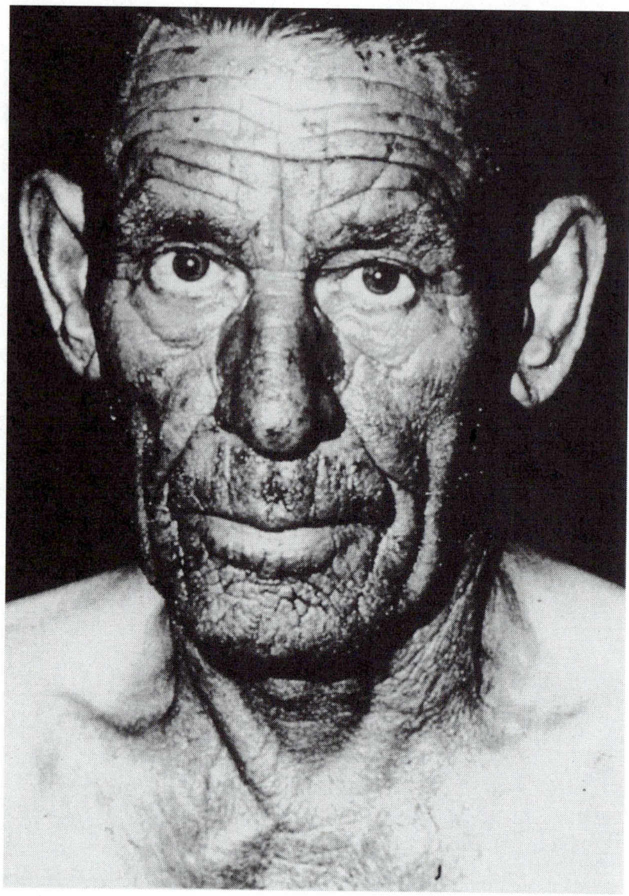

Fig. 36-9 Phototoxic eczematous dermatitis caused by furocoumarins.

nery workers who pack carrots, parsnips, figs, celery, or limes. Recently a rare industrially related photoeruption caused by topical contact with celery was reported in a chef.[86] It should be noted that recreational exposures to limes and other plants can also induce phytophotodermatitis.[58,149]

Perfume-induced berloque dermatitis is a special form of phytophotodermatitis. It is characterized most notably by bizarre pigmentation with or without preceding erythema involving areas contacted by the perfume and exposed to the sun.[50] The name "berloque" derives from the frequent pendant configuration of the hyperpigmentation.[124]

Oil of bergamot extracted from the rind of fresh bergamot oranges *(Citrus bergamia)* is a common ingredient in several commercial perfumes and colognes. This oil contains a number of furocoumarins.[85] The most potent photosensitizer appears to be bergapten, which is 5-MOP.[99,110,112] Phytophotodermatitis follows contact with offending plants and subsequent exposure to UVA (320 to 400 nm). Oral plant intake rarely induces photosensitization because a very large amount of plant must be ingested to attain high blood and skin levels of the photosensitizing furocoumarins, which are also readily metabolized to nonphotosensitizing molecules.

When photosensitizing furocoumarins are raised to an excited state (usually a triplet state) by exposure to UVA, they form photoaddition products with pyrimidine bases in the cellular DNA.[99,100,110-112] The first reaction appears to be monoadduct formation to one strand of the DNA material, with some conversion to DNA interstrand cross-links by a second photon reaction. This is a type I reaction that does not require oxygen.

There is evidence that a type II reaction also occurs.[108] This is a so-called photodynamic reaction, which depends on the presence of oxygen. After UVA irradiation the psoralen compound in the triplet state induces singlet oxygen, superoxide anions, and hydroxy radicals, which are responsible for cell membrane damage, erythema, and edema. The type I reaction results in nuclear and RNA damage. Keratinocytes, Langerhans' cells, melanocytes, mononuclear cells, fibrocytes, and endothelial cells can be involved in these phototoxic events.

Photoallergic reactions are rarely induced by psoralen compounds.[70] Plant-induced photoallergic responses appear to relate to chemicals other than psoralens.[70,92]

Dense hyperpigmentation is characteristic of the psoralen-induced photoreaction. This appears to be related to increased numbers of melanocytes, melanocytic hypertrophy, increased arborization of melanocytic dendrites, increased number of melanosomes, changed pattern of melanosomes, hyperplasia of the keratinocytes, and resultant increased transfer of melanosomes into keratinocytes.[108]

A distressing eruption occurs in patients who present a clinical picture of airborne contact sensitivity, but who actually have a phototoxic or even photoallergic component to the response.[49,109] These patients demonstrate a mixture of acute and subacute dermatitis with pruritic, erythematous, edematous, scaly, and lichenified eruptions distributed over the face, back of the neck, and exposed regions of the extremities. Areas shielded by glasses, the nose, and the chin often are spared, so the dermatitis in its initial presentation is fairly distinctive. However, with severe reactions the lesions often become disseminated to the trunk and elsewhere. Thus it is important to obtain a history of the original pattern of distribution. The dermatitis can be explosive and incapacitating. The key to good care is rapid recognition and prompt institution of therapy. Unfortunately, the correct diagnosis is often not made early and the skin disease progresses to a chronic, more slowly evolving generalized dermatitis with limited remissions and frequent exacerbations.

While furocoumarins may cause the preceding type of reaction, they more often are responsible for acute reactions. More likely culprits include aromatic lichen compounds such as usnic acid[142] and atranorin,[141] the Compositae oleoresins, and other sesquiterpene lactones such as parthenin and ambrosin.[49] Parthenin has been demonstrated during an epidemic of airborne contact, and presumably photocontact dermatitis, after inadvertent importation of feverfew *(Parthenium hysterophorus)* into India.[84] These cases unfortunately can eventuate as persistent light reactors,[20,49,67,141,142] and can even develop with granulomatous skin inflammation.[140]

The pathophysiologic mechanisms behind some phytophotodermatitis remain unresolved. The phototoxic mechanisms of furocuomarin effects have been delineated,[109] but how the aromatic lichen compounds and Compositae oleoresins effect these changes is unclear. Towers and associates[146] reported phototoxic effects of polyacetylenes and thiophene, which are present in Compositae plants. α-Terthienyl from marigold *(Tagetes erecta,* a member of the Compositae family) has been shown to act as a nonphotodynamic photosensitizer in vitro and in vivo.[69]

Rarely, cases are considered to be caused by photoallergy (Fig. 36-10). It has been proposed that plant chemical adducts on body proteins are altered further by UV exposure to become foreign haptens that initiate a cell-mediated immune response through conventional type IV delayed hypersensitivity mechanisms.[38,48] Uncertainty exists as to what role prior contact sensitization to ubiquitous sesquiterpene lactones might play in perpetuating the phototoxic photoallergic responses to Compositae.[109] It has been argued that because a relatively large number of photosensitive patients are also contact sensitive to sesquiterpene lactones, repeated exposure to these common allergens might predispose persons to become perennial and persistent light reactors.[49] This state of perennial or persistent light reactivity has become well recognized and is called chronic actinic dermatitis.[22] It is characterized by a severe eczematous eruption involving primarily sun-exposed areas but spreading to covered sites at times. This eruption predominantly affects older men, a significant number of whom are contact allergic to Compositae oleoresins.[49] A relationship between the contact allergy and the development of chronic actinic dermatitis has not been definitively demonstrated. However, Murphy and her coworkers recently reported a gardener who progressed from a state of proven contact allergy to Compositae resins to a state of proven photosensitivity.[97] The patient had a chronic eczematous eruption of his hands and face for 12 months with positive patch tests to sesquiterpene lactone mix and negative phototests. Six months after the initial phototesting, he was retested and found to have a significant eczematous reaction to UVA radiation as well as being contact sensitive to Compositae resins. The authors suggest that the initial contact allergy could enable the formation of an endogenous photoallergen that would be responsible for a chronic photo-induced delayed-type hypersensitivity reaction.

The management of phytophotodermatitis depends on a number of factors, including the extent and severity of the process; the identity, amount, and potency of the photosensitizer; and the nature of the photosensitive eruption.

The initial approach is to discontinue contact with the photosensitizing plant, avoid sun exposure, or both. The vast majority of these reactions are phototoxic. Thus the offend-

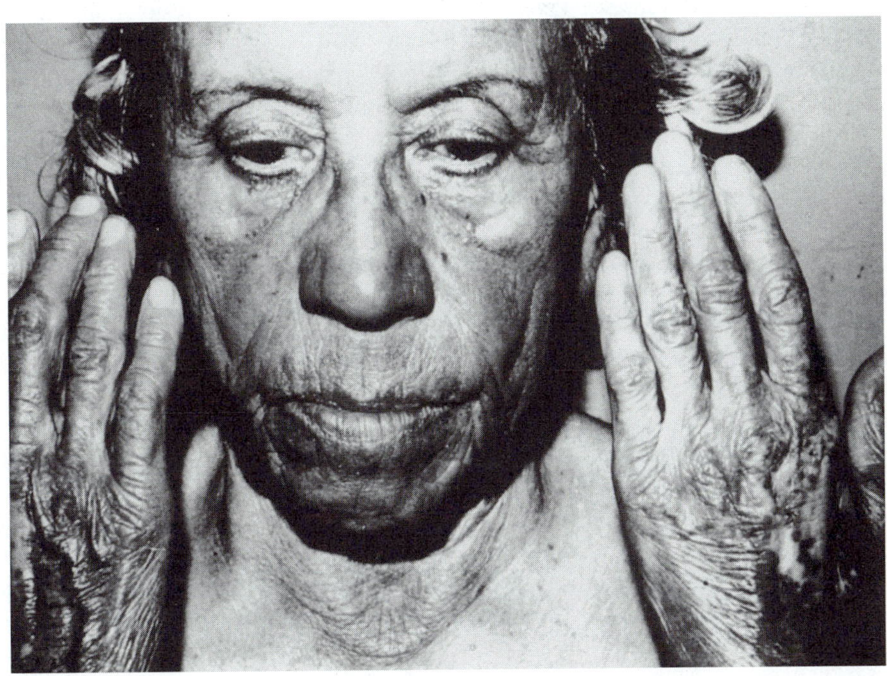

Fig. 36-10 Persistent light eruptions that can eventuate from acute photoallergic contact dermatitis.

ing plant is usually identified from the history of contact with a known photosensitizing plant and the distribution and character of the eruption. If the contactants are not known photosensitizers, epidemiologic and photopatch testing procedures are needed to identify the offending plant. If the problem is photoallergic in nature, photopatch testing may also be needed.

The acute inflammatory aspects of the responses are treated with appropriate dermatologic measures. The intensity of treatment depends on the severity and extent of the dermatitis. Cool tap water wet dressings applied every 2 hours when awake for 2 to 3 days reduce inflammation and discomfort. Ice and ice water should be avoided. Topical fluorinated corticosteroids such as fluocinonide 0.05% cream, ointment, or gel may be useful. If the process is severe or extensive, systemic corticosteroids may be needed. Thus betamethasone suspension, 6 mg; methylprednisolone, 40 to 80 mg; or triamcinolone acetonide, 40 mg intramuscularly, is equally effective.

In general, a phototoxic event is self-limited and subsides within a week if further insult does not occur. Hyperpigmentation may persist for several months and frequently is unsightly. Topical application of 5% hydroquinone cream once or twice a day for several weeks may lighten the hyperpigmentation. Treatment of the chronic actinic dermatitis state has been most difficult. Complete elimination of light exposure temporarily ameliorates the photodermatosis. However, exacerbations generally occur with return to even minimal exposures. Photochemotherapy with 8-methoxypsoralen and UVA radiation has been helpful in a few cases.[93] However, recent studies indicate that azathioprine, generally in daily doses of 100 mg for several months, is quite effective in inducing remissions.[98] The appropriate laboratory evaluation must be performed periodically to detect azathioprine toxicity.

Granulomas

Penetration and breakage of thorns, spines, and spicules in the skin can lead to a subacute or foreign body granuloma. When a young person has an infiltrated and erythematous plaque or patch on the buttocks or an exposed part of the body and gives a history of having fallen in the desert from a horse, motorcycle, or all-terrain vehicle 7 to 10 days previously, the clinical diagnosis of cactus granuloma is not difficult. However, when an urban inhabitant arrives in the emergency department during or after recovery from a prolonged domestic bout of substance abuse with grouped erythematous papulopustules on the same exposed areas, the diagnosis may not be so apparent. Cacti abound throughout urbia and conurbia.

Cactus lesions generally evolve over a matter of days to weeks but can take years to appear.[59] All lesions seem to be roughly the same age at the time of presentation. They do not develop explosively. Nevertheless, various infections must be considered, so a Gram-stained smear and culture are often indicated, although most lesions are aseptic. Plant-associated pathogens, such as *Mycobacterium* spp., should be considered. If the lesions are fairly firm and more papular than pustular, a biopsy should be performed. Sometimes a member of the party can provide the necessary botanical clue, but it is the essential observation that lesions are in groups or patches on extremities that leads to the suspicion that a victim might have fallen or been thrust inadvertently into a cactus. In Israel and other parts of the world, where edible cacti (prickly pears of the *Opuntia* spp.) are cultivated, a somewhat more acute papulopustular eruption is seen (Color Plate 71).[132,151] So-called sabra dermatitis is caused by implantation of detachable glochids of the cactus,[143] which can be blown by wind onto the skin or into the eyes to cause an annoying keratoconjunctivitis.[150]

Although the basic histologic features are those of a foreign body granuloma, with periodic acid–Schiff–positive spicules detected in giant cells,[35] lesions are clearly more inflammatory than simple foreign body reactions. The predominant cells are type 1 epithelioid cells with both secretory rough endoplasmic reticulum and dense lysosomal bodies in the cytoplasm.[41,42] This implies that an element of hypersensitivity also exists. Although T lymphocytes and dendritic mononuclear cells are present in the area of chemically induced hypersensitivity granulomas,[40] it is not yet clear whether this type of granuloma requires an intact cell-mediated immune system to initiate granuloma formation.[40,46] However, it is generally agreed that granulomas are fully formed in the presence of a cell-mediated immune response.[15,35,40,42,151] Emergency department treatment of cactus-induced skin lesions must remain conservative because final diagnosis cannot be achieved without histologic interpretation. Systemic corticosteroids are effective in reducing inflammation and relieving discomfort. However, failure to recognize an active infection or an infectious granuloma could lead to aggravation by overzealous corticosteroid treatment. Topical corticosteroids offer little help. The patient should be treated with cool compresses of aluminum acetate and systemic medication for pain or discomfort until a diagnosis can be made and definitive treatment (surgical, supportive, or specific) is initiated. Surgical removal of solitary or small grouped granulomas is recommended where feasible. Incision and drainage may help expose the inciting agent. If the glochids are visible in the skin, removal with sterile splinter forceps in the reverse direction of penetration usually leads to rapid healing, but this procedure can be difficult and tedious. Removal of large spines may require localization using soft tissue radiographic techniques. Small spines in groups within the skin may be peeled off using water-soluble facial gel or rubber cement, taking care to avoid contact with sensitive mucous membranes. These procedures are gratifying when they work, but they often fail. The primary reason for failure is that the tiny barbs on the glochids point backward like barbed fishhooks and hold the dart into the skin.[136] At times, watchful waiting and supportive care are all that work.[136]

REFERENCES

1. Adolf W, Hecker E: On the active principles of the spurge family. X. Skin irritants, cocarcinogens and cryptic cocarcinogens from the latex of the manchineel tree, *J Nat Prod* 47:482, 1984.
2. Baer H: Chemistry and immunochemistry of poisonous Anacardiacae, *Clin Dermatol* 4:152, 1986.
3. Baer H, Dawson CR, Kurtz AP: Delayed contact sensitivity to catechols IV, *J Immunol* 101:1243, 1968.
4. Baer H et al: Delayed contact sensitivity to catechols, *J Immunol* 99:370, 1967.
5. Bailey JM: New mechanisms for effects of anti-inflammatory glucocorticoids, *Bio Factors* 3:97, 1991.
6. Barker JW et al: Keratinocytes as initiators of inflammation, *Lancet* 337:211, 1989.
7. Bell RM: Protein kinase C activation by diacylglycerol second messengers, *Cell* 45:631, 1986.
8. Benezra C, Epstein WL: Molecular recognition patterns of sesquiterpene lactones in *Costus*-sensitive patients, *Contact Dermatitis* 15:223, 1986.
9. Benezra C et al: *Plant contact dermatitis,* Toronto, 1985, BC Decker.
10. Benyon RC, Robinson C, Church MK: Differential release of histamine and eicosanoids from human skin mast cells activated by IgE dependent and nonimmunological stimuli, *Br J Pharmacol* 97:898, 1989.
11. Berkley SF et al: Dermatitis in grocery workers associated with high natural concentrations of furocoumarins in celery, *Ann Intern Med* 105:351, 1986.
12. Berridge MJ: Inositol triphosphate and calcium signalling, *Nature* 361:315, 1993.
13. Birmingham DJ et al: Phototoxic bullae among celery harvesters, *Arch Dermatol* 83:73, 1961.
14. Bock SA, May CD: Adverse reactions to food caused by sensitivity. In Middleton E Jr et al, editors: *Allergy: principles and practice,* ed 2, St Louis, 1993, Mosby.
15. Boros DL: Immunopathology of *Schistosoma mansoni* infection, *Clin Microbiol Rev* 2:250, 1989.
16. Bourne HR, Masters SB, Sullivan KA: Mammalian G proteins: structure and function, *Biochem Soc Trans* 15:35, 1987.
17. Boutwell RK: The function and mechanisms of promotors in carcinogenesis, *CRC Crit Rev Toxicol* 2:419, 1974.
18. Bubak ME et al: Allergic reactions to latex among health care workers, *Mayo Clinic Proc* 47:1075, 1992.
19. Carrillo T, Cuenoas M, Munoz T: Contact urticaria and rhinitis from latex surgical gloves, *Contact Dermatitis* 15:69, 1986.
20. Castro JLC et al: Musk ambrette and chronic actinic dermatitis, *Contact Dermatitis* 13:302, 1985.
21. Centers for Disease Control: Phototoxic dermatitis in grocery workers, *MMWR* 34:11, 1984.
22. Cutaneous photosensitivity, *Lancet* 1:1317, 1988.
23. Dawson C: The chemistry of poison ivy, *Trans NY Acad Sci* 18:427, 1956.
24. DiRosa M, et al: Glucocorticoids inhibit induction of nitric oxide synthase in macrophages, *Biochem Biophys Res Commun* 172:1246, 1990.
25. Dooms-Goosens A, Deleu H: Airborne contact dermatitis: an update, *Contact Dermatitis* 25:211, 1991.
26. Ducombs G et al: Patch testing with the "sesquiterpene lactone mix": a marker for contact allergy to Compositae and other sesquiterpene-lactone-containing plants; a multicentre study of the EECDRG, *Contact Dermatitis* 22:249, 1990.
27. Dunn IS et al: Contact sensitivity to urushiol: role of covalent bond formation, *Cell Immunol* 74:220, 1982.
28. Dunn IS et al: Influence of chemical reactivity of urushiol-type haptens on sensitization and induction of tolerance, *Cell Immunol* 97:189, 1986.
29. Dupuis G, Mitchell JC, Towers GHN: Reaction of alantolactone, and allergenic sesquiterpene lactone with some amino acids, *Can J Biochem* 52:575, 1974.
30. Dvorak AM: Human mast cells, *Adv Anat Embryol Cell Biol* 114:1, 1989.
31. Dvorak HF, Mihm MC: Basophilic leukocytes in allergic contact dermatitis, *J Exp Med* 135:235, 1972.
32. Epstein JH: Photoallergy and photoimmunology. In Stone J, editor: *Dermatologic immunology and allergy,* St Louis, 1985, Mosby.
33. Epstein WL: Rhus dermatitis, *Pediatr Clin North Am* 6:843, 1959.
34. Epstein WL: Poison oak and poison ivy dermatitis as an occupational problem, *Cutis* 13:544, 1974.
35. Epstein WL: Granulomatous inflammation in skin. In Ioachim HL, editor: *Pathology of granulomas,* New York, 1983, Raven Press.
36. Epstein WL: Allergic contact dermatitis to poison oak and ivy: feasibility of hyposensitization, *Dermatol Clin* 2:613, 1984.
37. Epstein WL: The poison ivy picker of Pennypack Park, *J Invest Dermatol* 88:7s, 1987.
38. Epstein WL: Allergic contact dermatitis. In Fitzpatrick TB et al, editors: *Dermatology in general medicine,* ed 3, New York, 1987, McGraw-Hill.
39. Epstein WL: Plant-induced dermatitis, *Ann Emerg Med* 16:950, 1987.
40. Epstein WL: Mechanisms of granuloma formation. In Norris DA, editor: *Mechanisms in cutaneous disease,* New York, 1989, Marcel Dekker.
41. Epstein WL: Ultrastructural heterogeneity of epithelioid cells in cutaneous organized granulomas of diverse etiology, *Arch Dermatol* 127:821, 1991.
42. Epstein WL: *Pathogenesis of granulomatous inflammation in skin.* In Moschella SL, Hurley HJ, editors: *Dermatology,* ed 3, Philadelphia, 1993, WB Saunders.
43. Epstein WL, Kligman AM: Transfer of allergic contact-type delayed hypersensitivity in man, *J Invest Dermatol* 28:291, 1957.
44. Epstein WL, Kligman AM: The interference phenomenon in allergic contact dermatitis, *J Invest Dermatol* 31:103, 1958.
45. Epstein WL et al: Poison oak hyposensitization, *Arch Dermatol* 109:356, 1974.
46. Epstein WL et al: T-cell independent transfer of organized granuloma formation, *Immunol Lett* 14:59, 1986.
47. Evans SW, Farrar WL: Identity of common phospho-protein substrates stimulated by interleukin-2 and diacylglycerol suggests a role of protein kinase C for IL-2 signal transduction, *J Cell Biochem* 34:47, 1987.
48. Fisher AA: Erythema multiforme–like eruptions due to exotic woods and ordinary plants, *Cutis* 37:101, 1986.
49. Frain-Bell W: Photosensitivity and Compositae dermatitis, *Clin Dermatol* 4:122, 1986.
50. Freund E: Uber bisher noch nicht beschribene Kunstliche Hautverfarbungen, *Dermatol Wochenschr* 63:931, 1916.
51. Fujita M, Auki T: Allergic contact dermatitis to pyridoxine ester and hinokitiol, *Contact Dermatitis* 9:61, 1983.
52. Gafner F et al: Human maximization test of falcarinol, the principal contact allergen of English ivy and Algerian ivy, *Contact Dermatitis* 19:125, 1988.
53. Gartner BL et al: Seasonal variation of urushiol content in poison oak leaves, *Am J Contact Dermatitis* 4:33, 1993.
54. Gollhausen R, Kligman AM: Human assay for identifying substances which induce non-allergic contact urticaria, *Contact Dermatitis* 13:98, 1985.

55. Goulding JJ, Guyre PM: Regulation of inflammation by lipocortin-1, *Immunol Today* 13:295, 1992.
56. Griffiths CEM, Nickoloff BJ: Keratinocyte intercellular adhesion molecule-1 expression precedes dermal T lymphocytic infiltration in allergic contact dermatitis (rhus dermatitis), *Am J Pathol* 135:1045, 1989.
57. Griffiths CEM et al: Modulation of leukocyte adhesion molecules, a T-cell chemotaxin and a regulatory cytokine in allergic contact dermatitis (*Rhus* dermatitis), *Br J Dermatol* 124:519, 1991.
58. Gross TP et al: An outbreak of phototoxic dermatitis due to limes, *Am J Epidemiol* 125:509, 1987.
59. Gutierrez-Ortega MC et al: Facial granuloma caused by cactus bristles, *Med Cutan Ibero—Latin Am* 18:197, 1990.
60. Hausen BM: Woods injurious to human health, New York, 1981, deGruyter.
61. Hausen BM: Contact allergy to woods, *Clin Dermatol* 4:65, 1986.
62. Hausen BM, Schmalle HW: Structure-activity aspects of 4 allergenic sesquiterpene lactones lacking the exocyclic α-methylene at the lactone ring, *Contact Dermatitis* 13:329, 1985.
63. Hausen BM et al: Allergic and irritant dermatitis from falcarinol and didehydrofalcarinol in common ivy, *Contact Dermatitis* 17:1, 1987.
64. Hjorth N, Roed-Petersen J: Occupational protein contact dermatitis in food handlers, *Contact Dermatitis* 2:28, 1976.
65. Hjorth N, Roed-Peterson J, Thomsen K: Airborne contact dermatitis from Compositae oleoresins simulating photo-dermatitis, *Br J Dermatol* 95:613, 1976.
66. Holub BJ: The cellular forms and functions of the inositol phospholipids and their metabolic derivatives, *Nutr Rev* 45:65, 1987.
67. Horio T: Actinic reticuloid via persistent light reaction from photoallergic contact dermatitis, *Arch Dermatol* 118:339, 1982.
68. Hurtado I: Poisonous Anacardiaceae of South America, *Clin Dermatol* 4:183, 1986.
69. Kagan J, Gabriel R, Reed SA: Alpha-terthienyl, a nonphotodynamic phototoxic compound, *Photochem Photobiol* 31:465, 1980.
70. Kavli G et al: In vivo and in vitro phototoxicity of different parts of *Heracleum laciniatum, Contact Dermatitis* 9:269, 1983.
71. Keil H, Wasserman D, Dawson CR: Relationship of hypersensitiviness to poison ivy and to the pure ingredients in cashew nut shell liquid and related substances, *Indust Med* 14:825, 1945.
72. Kinghorn AD: Cocarcinogenic irritant Euphorbiaceae. In Kinghorn AD, editor: *Toxic plants,* New York, 1979, Columbia University Press.
73. Kishimoto T et al: The role of basophils and mast cells in cutaneous basophil hypersensitivity reaction, *Clin Exp Immunol* 67:611, 1986.
74. Klaber R: Phyto-photo-dermatitis, *Br J Dermatol* 54:193, 1942.
75. Kligman AM: Poison ivy dermatitis, *Arch Dermatol* 77:149, 1958.
76. Knight TE: Philodendron-induced dermatitis, *Cutis* 48:375, 1991.
77. Kuno M, Gardner P: Ion channels activated by inositol 1,4,5-triphosphate in plasma membrane of human T-lymphocytes, *Nature* 326:301, 1987.
78. Lahti A: Contact urticaria to plants, *Clin Dermatol* 4:127, 1986.
79. Larsen GL: Late-phase reactions: observations on pathogenesis and prevention, *J Allergy Clin Immunol* 76:665, 1985.
80. Layier F, et al: Prevalence of latex allergy in operating room nurses, *J Allergy Clin Immun* 90:316, 1992.
81. Leonforte JF: Contact dermatitis from *Larrea* (creosote bush), *J Am Acad Dermatol* 14:202, 1986.
82. Linau M, Fernandex JM: IgE-mediated degranulation of mast cells does not require opening of ion channels, *Nature* 319:150, 1986.
83. Ljunggren B: Severe phototoxic burn following celery ingestion, *Arch Dermatol* 126:1334, 1990.
84. Lonker A, Mitchell JC, Calnan CD: Contact dermatitis from *Parthenium hysterophorus, Trans St Johns Hosp Dermatol Soc* 60:43, 1974.
85. Marzulli FN, Maibach HI: Perfume phototoxicity, *J Soc Cosmet Chem* 21:685, 1970.
86. Maso MJ et al: Celery phytophotodermatitis in a chef, *Arch Dermatol* 127:912, 1991.
87. McCord CP: The toxic properties of some timber woods, *Indust Med Surg* 27:202, 1958.
88. Meding B: Immediate hypersensitivity to mustard and rape, *Contact Dermatitis* 13:121, 1985.
89. Menz J et al: Contact dermatitis from Grevillea "Robyn Gordon," *Contact Dermatitis* 15:126, 1986.
90. Metcalfe DD: Food hypersensitivity, *J Allergy Clin Immunol* 73:749, 1984.
91. Mitchell JC et al: Allergic contact dermatitis from Frullania and Compositae: the role of sesquiterpene lactones, *J Invest Dermatol* 54:233, 1970.
92. Möller H: Contact and photocontact allergy to psoralens, *Photoderm Photoimmunol Photomed* 7:43, 1990.
93. Morrison WL et al: Oral methosalen photochemotherapy of uncommon photodermatoses, *Acta Derm Venerol (Stockh)* 59:366, 1979.
94. Morton JF: *Plants poisonous to people in Florida and other warm areas,* ed 2, Miami, 1982, JF Morton.
95. Mousli M et al: G-proteins as targets for non-immunological histamine releasers, *Agents Actions* 33:81, 1991.
96. Mukinen-Kiljunen S et al: Characterization of latex antigens and allergies in surgical gloves and natural rubber by immunoelectrophoretic methods, *J Allergy Clin Immunol* 90:230, 1992.
97. Murphy GM, White IR, Hawk JLM: Allergic airborne contact dermatitis to Compositae with photosensitivity—chronic actinic dermatitis in evolution, *Photodermatol Photoimmunol Photomed* 7:38, 1990.
98. Murphy GM et al: Azathioprine treatment in chronic actinic dermatitis: a double-blind controlled trial with monitoring of exposure to ultraviolet radiation, *Br J Dermatol* 121:639, 1989.
99. Musajo L, Rodighiero G, Caporale G: Relation between constitution and photodynamic properties of furocoumarins (Italian), *Farmaco (Ed Sci)* 13:355, 1958.
100. Musajo L et al: Photoreactions between skin photosensitizing furocoumarins and nuclei acid. In Pathak MA et al, editors: *Sunlight and man,* Tokyo, 1974, University of Tokyo Press.
101. Nickoloff BJ: Role of epidermal keratinocytes as key initiators of contact dermatitis due to allergic sensitization and irritation, *Contact Dermatitis* 3:65, 1992.
102. Nishizuka Y: Studies and perspectives of protein kinase C, *Science* 233:305, 1986.
103. Oliver F et al: Contact urticaria due to the common stinging nettle *(Urtica dioica)*—histological, ultrastructural, and pharmacological studies, *Clin Exp Dermatol* 16:1, 1991.
104. Oppenheim M: Dermatite bulleuse striee consecutive aux bains de soleil dans les pres (dermatitis bullosa striata pratensis), *Ann Dermatol Syphiligr* 3(series)7:1, 1932.
105. Orchard S: Barrier creams, *Dermatol Clin* 2:619, 1984.
106. Orchard SM, Fellman JH, Storrs FJ: Poison ivy/oak dermatitis use of polyamine salts of linoleic acid dimer for prophylaxis, *Arch Dermatol* 122:783, 1986.
107. Panconesi E et al: Anaphylactic shock from mustard after ingestion of pizza, *Contact Dermatitis* 6:294, 1980.
108. Pathak MA: *Photobiologic toxicology and pharmacologic aspects of psoralens,* Monograph 66, Washington, DC, 1984, US Dept of Health and Human Services, National Institutes of Health.
109. Pathak MA: Phytophotodermatitis, *Clin Dermatol* 4:102, 1986.
110. Pathak MA, Fellman JH, Kaufman KD: The effect of structural alterations on the erythemal activity of furocoumarins, *J Invest Dermatol* 35:165, 1960.
111. Pathak MA, Kramer DM: Photosensitization of the skin in vivo by furocoumarins (psoralens), *Biochim Biophys Acta* 195:197, 1969.
112. Pathak MS, Worden LR, Kaufman KD: Effect of structural alterations on the photosensitizing potency of furocoumarins (psoralens) and related compounds, *J Invest Dermatol* 48:103, 1967.

113. Paulson E: Compositae dermatitis: a survey, *Contact Dermatitis* 26:76, 1992.
114. Pecequeiro M, Menezes-Brandae F: Airborne contact dermatitis to plants, *Contact Dermatitis* 13:277, 1985.
115. Pequet et al: Tumor necrosis factor is a critical mediator in hapten-induced irritant and contact hypersensitivity reactions, *J Exp Med* 173:673, 1991.
116. Persone VB: The natural occurrence and uses of the toxic coumarins. In Kadis S et al, editors: *Microbial toxins,* vol 8, New York, 1972, Academic Press.
117. Persone VB, Scheel LD, Meitus RJ: A bioassay for the quantitation of cutaneous reaction associated with pink-rot celery, *J Invest Dermatol*, 42:267, 1964.
118. Powell SM, Barrett DK: An outbreak of contact dermatitis from *Rhus verniciflua, Contact Dermatitis* 14:288, 1986.
119. Rasmussen H: The calcium messenger system, *N Engl J Med* 314:1094, 1986.
120. Reynolds GW, Epstein WL, Rodriguez E: Unusual contact allergens from plants in the family Hydrophyllaceae, *Contact Dermatitis* 14:39, 1986.
121. Richards DE: The isolation and identification of the toxic coumarins. In Kadis S et al, editors: *Microbial toxins,* vol 8, New York, 1972, Academic Press.
122. Roed-Peterson J, Hjorth N: Compositae sensitivity among patients with contact dermatitis, *Contact Dermatitis* 2:171, 1976.
123. Rosengard BR, Mahalik C, Cochrane DE: Mast cell secretion: differences between immunologic and non-immunologic stimulation, *Agents Actions* 19:133, 1986.
124. Rosenthal O: Berloque dermatitis: Berliner Dermatologische Gesellschaft, *Dermatol Z* 42:295, 1925.
125. Sach MI, Gleich GJ, Yunginger JW: Adverse reactions to food. In Franklin EG, editor: *Clinical immunology update,* New York, 1983, Elsevier.
126. Sams WM: Photodynamic action of lime oil *(Citrus aurantifolia), Arch Dermatol Syphilol* 44:571, 1941.
127. Santacci B, Picardo M, Cristaudo A: Contact dermatitis from *Euphorbia pulcherrima, Contact Dermatitis* 12:285, 1985.
128. Scheel LD et al: The isolation and characterization of two phototoxic furocoumarins (psoralens) from diseased celery, *Biochemistry* 2:1127, 1963.
129. Schmidt RJ: Compositae, *Clin Dermatol* 4:46, 1986.
130. Schwartz L: Allergic occupational dermatitis in our war industries, *Ann Allergy* 2:387, 1944.
131. Schwartz LB: Mast cells and their role in urticaria, *J Am Acad Dermatol* 25(suppl):190, 1991.
132. Shanon J, Sagher F: Sabra dermatitis, *Arch Dermatol* 74:269, 1956.
133. Shelley WB, Arthur RP: Mucunain, the active pruritogenic proteinase in cowhage, *Science* 122:469, 1955.
134. Shelley WB, Arthur RP: Studies on cowhage and its pruritogenic proteinase, mucunain, *Arch Dermatol* 72:399, 1955.
135. Smart ER, Macleod RI, Lawrence CM: Allergic reactions to rubber gloves in dental patients, *Br Dental J* 172:445, 1992.
136. Snyder RA, Schwartz RA: Cactus bristle implantation, *Arch Dermatol* 119:152, 1983.
137. Sosman AJ et al: Hypersensitivity to wood dust, *N Engl J Med* 281:977, 1969.
138. Spoerke DG, Spoerke SE: Granuloma formation induced by spines of the cactus, *Opuntia acanthocarpa, Vet Hum Toxicol* 33:342, 1991.
139. Stevens RL, Austen KF: Recent advances in the cellular and molecular biology of mast cells, *Immunol Today* 10:381, 1989.
140. Sullivan KA et al: Identification of receptor contact site involved in receptor-G protein coupling, *Nature* 330:758, 1987.
141. Thune P, Eeg-Larsen T: Contact and photocontact allergy in persistent light reactivity, *Contact Dermatitis* 11:98, 1984.
142. Thune PO, Solberg YJ: Photosensitivity and allergy to aromatic lichen acids, Compositae oleoresins and other plant substances, *Contact Dermatitis* 6:81, 1980.
143. Thurston EL: Morphology, fine structure and ontogeny of the stinging emergency of *Urtica dioica, Am J Bot* 61:809, 1974.
144. Thurston EL, Lersten NR: The morphology and toxicology of plant stinging hairs, *Bot Rev* 35:393, 1969.
145. Tomazic VJ et al: Latex-associated allergies and anaphylactic reactions, *Clin Immunol Immunopathol* 64:89, 1992.
146. Towers GNH et al: Phototoxic polyacetylenes and their thiophene derivatives (effects on human skin), *Contact Dermatitis* 5:140, 1979.
147. Walker FB, Smith PD, Maibach HI: Genetic factors in human allergic contact dermatitis, *Int Arch Allergy* 32:453, 1967.
148. Webster GL: Irritant plants in the spurge family, *Clin Dermatol* 4:36, 1986.
149. White W: Club Med dermatitis, *N Engl J Med* 314:319, 1986.
150. Whiting DA, Bristow JH: Dermatitis and keratoconjuctivitis caused by prickly pear, *South Afr Med J* 49:1445, 1975.
151. Williams GT, Jones Williams W: Granulomatous inflammation, *J Clin Pathol* 36:723, 1983.

37 TOXIC PLANT INGESTIONS

George Braitberg
Donald B. Kunkel
Michele Adler
Edward C. Geehr

As both poisons and medicines, plants figure prominently in the history of religious ritual, political intrigue, and the healing arts. For centuries, South and Central American Indians invoked mystical visions through the use of mushrooms. North American Indians still employ peyote buttons as part of their magico-religious rites. Socrates succumbed to a fatal draught of hemlock, and Alexander died from the treacherous use of plant poisons. In the eighteenth century, William Withering keenly recognized both the toxic effects of foxglove and its efficacy as a cure for dropsy[79]:

> I found him incessantly vomiting, his vision indistinct, his pulse 40 in a minute. Upon inquiry it came out that his wife had stewed a large pail full of foxglove leaves in half a pint of water, and given him the liquor, which he drank at one draught. This good woman knew the medicine of her country, but not the dose of it, for her husband narrowly escaped with his life.

Thus, Withering astutely observed that plants bring us the mixed blessing of important therapeutic agents and some of our most dangerous toxins.

Today, toxic plants are ingested mostly by curious children attracted to bright berries or houseplants, by hikers and foragers mistaking poisonous roots and berries for edible fare, by self-taught herbalists looking for natural remedies, and by pleasure seekers attempting to discover natural highs.

Phytotoxicology, the study of plant poisoning, is a field founded in botany, chemistry, and physiology that has not yet achieved true clinical sophistication. This has much to do with the disparity among botanists, pharmacologists, and physicians; few scholars have interdisciplinary training in all of these fields. Thus there is generally poor recording and follow-up of plant poisoning, often a result of improper identification of plants, use of common names, and mixing of scientific facts with myth.

The 1992 *Annual Report* of the American Association of Poison Control Centers (AAPCC) noted that over 106,000 plant ingestions or exposures were reported to 68 poison control centers serving 196.7 million people.[45] Plant exposures represented 5.7% of total exposures reported in 1992. This is the fifth most frequently reported category after cleaning substances, analgesics, cosmetics, and cough and cold preparations. Eight percent of ingestions resulted in treatment at a health care facility. No deaths were reported. However, one must be cautious when interpreting these data because deaths have been reported in previous years and AAPCC data may not necessarily reflect the true incidence of morbidity or mortality. Over 81% of all plant ingestions were reported in children under 6 years of age. Unfortunately, data regarding specific plant ingestions are unavailable.

This chapter focuses on recognition and treatment of plant poisoning, with emphasis on known chemistry and physiology. Plants used as herbal remedies or recreational drugs are only briefly mentioned (but their importance is recognized with the growing number of imported and indigenous plants now used for self-medication[43]), while those encountered and ingested in their natural form are stressed. With few exceptions,[2,16,18] North American species are considered. It is not the intent of this chapter to provide details of botanical description, since amateur attempts to distinguish poisonous species may lead to disaster. Definitive identification should always be left to a trained botanist. Guidelines are provided, however, to help classify certain categories of ingestions, stressing unique features of treatment. This will facilitate the institution of appropriate care before absolute identification can be obtained. The two hallmarks of management are that few specific antidotes are available and that one must treat the patients and their symptoms, not necessarily the historical ingestion. Aggressive supportive care, precise fluid and electrolyte management, and careful monitoring should prevent most fatalities.

The chapter is divided into three major sections: "General Considerations," a discussion of principles of history taking, physical examination, and management; "Plants: The Toxic Principles," a discussion of the major plant toxins by chemical grouping, which details physiologic effects and specific treatments; and "Organ System Effects."

General Considerations

PATIENT HISTORY

An accurate history gives the clinician significant clues about the nature of the plant ingested. The time of the ingestion, amount and number of plants consumed, initial symptoms, and time between ingestion and onset of symptoms are fundamental toxicologic questions. Inquiry should include the method of preparation of the plant, such as drying, cooking, or boiling as a stew or tea, and the number of people who ate the same plant and their symptoms.

Every effort should be made to obtain as much of the original plant or plants as possible. The clinician should not rely on common names as a guide to treatment, but rather should determine the scientific name by taxonomic identification. Past medical history and current medications are helpful guides to therapy in any symptomatic patient.

PHYSICAL EXAMINATION

The physician should be attuned to certain syndromes that may develop after plant ingestion. An anticholinergic crisis induced by certain alkaloid components is easily distinguished by the combination of tachycardia, mydriasis, hot dry skin, decreased bowel sounds, altered vision, and abnormal mental status. Nicotinic alkaloids may act as stimulants at first, soon followed by depression and weakness. In many cases a mixture of syndromes may occur with no definite pattern. Thus a rush to therapy using an "antidote" based on inadequate assessment and physical examination may exacerbate a major and unanticipated aspect of the intoxication.

Changes in behavior should not automatically be attributed to plant toxins. Alterations in mental status mandate a thorough neurologic examination. Focal signs may point to an intracranial lesion, the result of a fall or other injury. Table 37-1 provides a symptoms and signs–oriented guide to the diagnosis of toxic plant ingestions.

MANAGEMENT

After the basic ABCs of airway, breathing, and circulation are ensured, removal of the toxin is the highest priority. In patients with depressed gag reflex, unresponsiveness, or seizures, an endotracheal airway is inserted before a large-bore Ewald tube is inserted to perform gastric lavage. Gastric lavage, even using a wide-bore tube, may fail to remove significant amounts of toxin because of the size and nature of plant material.[37] After lavage, activated charcoal (0.5 to 1 g/kg in 8 ounces of water) should be given in a slurry to absorb any toxin left in the upper gastrointestinal tract. Most alkaloids are bound by activated charcoal.[37] Dialysis has not yet been shown to be effective in removing any plant toxin. Meticulous attention should be paid to urinary output and specific gravity as measures of the adequacy of hydration and volume replacement.

Baseline laboratory evaluation in symptomatic patients should include urinalysis, complete blood count, electrolytes, blood urea nitrogen (BUN), and glucose. If hepatotoxins or other specific organ toxins are suspected, appropriate laboratory data should be obtained, as suggested in later sections on management.

Mixed ingestions require greater vigilance because confusing physical signs may evolve or earlier mild signs may give way to serious illness. As previously mentioned, it is prudent to treat the patient, not the suspected ingestion. Specific antidotes are few and may be deleterious as the clinical pattern changes.

Plants: The Toxic Principles

The toxic principles underlying all major poisonous plant ingestions are organized by chemical and physical properties. Although the human physiologic response tends to be fairly consistent within each group of toxic principles, disparities exist, as we discuss. Toxic principles and therapeutics are presented in Appendix A at the end of this chapter. A list of nontoxic plants is provided in Appendix B.

In a consideration of plant toxicity, the toxic principles involved may be viewed as one or a combination of the groups listed: the alkaloid group, the glycoside group, the resin group, the oxalate group, and the phytotoxin (also known as toxalbumin) group.[16,17]

ALKALOIDS

Alkaloids are found in 10% of plant species; about 5000 types are known to exist. Alkaloids are principally distributed in the families Apocynaceae (dogbane), Berberidaceae (mayapple), Fabaceae (pea), Papaveraceae (poppy), Ranunculaceae (buttercup), and Solanaceae (potato).

Chemical similarities exist among all alkaloids. They are nitrogen-containing organic compounds that act as bases and form salts with acids. In plants, alkaloids are present as soluble organic acid-alkaloid salts.[33] These complex structures all contain nitrogen in a ring structure that is heterocyclic or aromatic or both. Alkaloids are generally distributed throughout the plant, rendering all ingested parts toxic.

The major types can be divided into chemical groups, with physiologic activity based on ring structure.[16]

Table 37-1 Signs and Symptoms of Common and/or Serious Plant Intoxications

		Dieffenbachia, Philodendron	*Colchicum, Gloriosa*	*Euphorbia, Hippomane*	*Actaea, Anemone, Ranunculus*	*Convallaria, Digitalis, Nerium*	*Aconitum*	*Solanum*	*Pieris, Rhododendron, Veratrum*	*Conium, Laburnum, Nicotiana, Sophora*	*Cicuta*	*Taxus*	*Gelsemium*	*Brugmansia, Datura*	*Amaryllis, Narcissus, Wisteria*	*Ilex*	*Abrus, Ricinus*	*Prunus*	*Phytolacca*	*Podophyllum*	*Karwinskia*
Mouth & Throat	Burning, irritation	++	++	D	++	+	+	D	+	+											
	Increased salivation	+		D	++		+		D	+	+	D									
	Dry mouth											+	+	++							
	Dysphonia, dysphagia	+		D			±						+	+							
Gastroenteric Tract	Nausea		+			+	±		D	+	+				+	+	DD				
	Vomiting		+	+	+	+	±		D	+	±	D			++	++	DD	D	++	+	
	Diarrhea		++	+	+	+		D	D	+					±	DD		D	+		
	Abdominal pain		++	++	+	+		D	D			D			+			D	+		
	Decreased bowel sounds													++						±	
Cardiovascular	Tachycardia									+				+							
	Bradycardia					+			+			D									
	Arrhythmias					±	++					D									
	Conduction defects					++															
	Hypertension													+							
	Hypotension								++			D									
Nervous & Neuromuscular	Dizziness				±		+		+	+		+	+								
	Weakness, lethargy						+			+		D						D			
	Syncope				±																
	Delirium, psychosis				±										+						
	Tremors, convulsions				±				D±				±					D±			
	Depression, coma								D	+		D						D±		±	
	Headache								+	±			+								
	Paresthesias						++		D												
	Muscle weakness, paralysis		±						D	+			+					D±		±	DD
Visual	Mydriasis						+			±		+		+							
	Visual disturbances						+		D				+	+							
Cutaneous	Increased sweating								+	+								D	++		
	Dry skin													++							
	Flushing, rash											D		+							
	Cyanosis											D						D±			
Misc.	Hyperthermia							+						+							
	Painful, bloody micturition		+		+																

From Lampe KF, McCann MA: *AMA handbook of poisonous and injurious plants,* Chicago, 1985, American Medical Association, pp 6-7.
+, Commonly occurs; + +, pronounced or persistent; ± occasionally reported; *D,* delayed onset; *DD,* occurrence significantly delayed.

GLYCOSIDES

Glycosides are substances in which an alcohol or hydroxyl group is replaced by a glycosyl group. The glycoside-producing plants constitute a second major group of poisonous principles consisting of cardioactive, cyanogenic, saponin, anthraquinone, and coumarin glycosides. On hydrolysis the glycosides yield sugars (glycones) and aglycone compounds. The aglycone moiety accounts for the major toxic effects of the group.[16]

RESINS

Resins are a group of highly toxic compounds of diverse chemical and plant origin. They are united by the physical characteristics of insolubility in water, absence of nitrogen, and solid or semisolid state on extraction at room temperature. Resins are usually found in mixtures with other compounds, such as volatile (essential) oils (oleoresins), gum (gum resins), and sugars (glycoresins). Common examples of plants that elaborate their toxic properties through resin are the water hemlock *(Cicuta maculata)* and chinaberry *(Melia azedarach)*. These are considered later.

The term "latex" refers to the chemicals located in the emulsion present in the plant ducts that cause toxicity only after plant tissue has been damaged. An example of this group is the *Rhus* species plants of the Anacardiaceae family.

OXALATES

Oxalates occur naturally in plants in the form of soluble (sodium and potassium) (see p. 879) or insoluble calcium oxalates or acid oxalates.[16] Their toxicity is related to corrosive effects and ability to bind serum calcium, with resultant hypocalcemia. Insoluble calcium oxalate crystals (raphides) are abundant in leaves of common houseplants of *Dieffenbachia* and *Caladium* species. Biting into the leaves induces mechanical and chemical injuries, with severe burning of the mouth and throat and occasional marked swelling of the lips, mouth, and tongue.[18] Airway obstruction may result.

PHYTOTOXINS

Phytotoxins are among the most toxic substances of plant origin. Composed of large protein molecules, phytotoxins resemble bacterial toxins in structure and in their ability to act as antigens, eliciting an antibody response. An example to be considered later is ricin, the phytotoxin of the castor bean *(Ricinus communis)*.[11]

Organ System Effects

Like a grouping of plant toxicity according to the active principle involved, a classification of clinical syndromes may be useful to the physician when dealing with a known or suspected plant exposure. In this manner, toxic effects of certain plants can be grouped in categories designated by the major effect on organ systems. Once the toxicity of the active compounds is appreciated, management can be more specifically directed.

This section considers effects on the following organ systems: central nervous system, gastrointestinal system, cardiovascular system, and renal-metabolic system. It also considers local and miscellaneous effects.

CENTRAL NERVOUS SYSTEM

Many plants exhibit toxic effects on the central nervous system. The plants to be considered here are alkaloids in the tropane alkaloid group, pyridine-piperidine alkaloid group, quinolizidine alkaloid group, and indole-derivative alkaloid group. Also considered is a resin, water hemlock–cicutoxin.

Alkaloids

Tropane Alkaloids. The tropane alkaloids are found in many plants (25 genera, 2000 species), but only plants commonly encountered in human toxicity are singled out here. All the plants mentioned previously are members of the Solanaceae family. In addition to these poisonous or medicinal plants, a number of food staples such as potato, tomato, eggplant, and chili pepper are family members. Although atropine can be isolated from the green, unripened skins of these plants, toxicity is seldom a problem.

Anticholinergic syndrome. Anticholinergic plant poisoning can occur commonly with *Datura stramonium* (known as jimsonweed, Color Plate 72), *Mandragora officinarum* (known more commonly as mandrake), and *Hyoscyamus niger* (henbane). Less common toxicity occurs with exposure to *Atropa belladonna* (deadly nightshade).[18]

The plants contain tropane alkaloids, often called belladonna alkaloids. These alkaloids include atropine (hyoscyamine), scopolamine (hyoscine), and ecgonine (cocaine) compounds. Ecgonine is mentioned here only because of its structural similarity to atropine. It has little antimuscarinic effect, while atropine causes few of the anesthetic effects of cocaine. *Datura* species typically contain 0.25% to 0.7% alkaloids by weight.[35,62]

The structures of the tropane alkaloids follow:

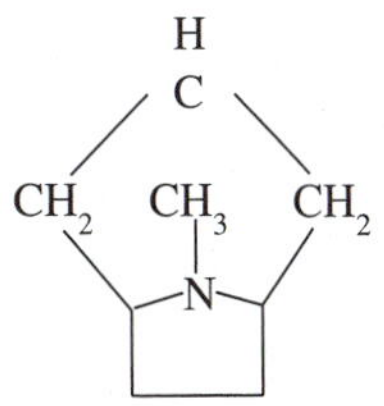

Tropane

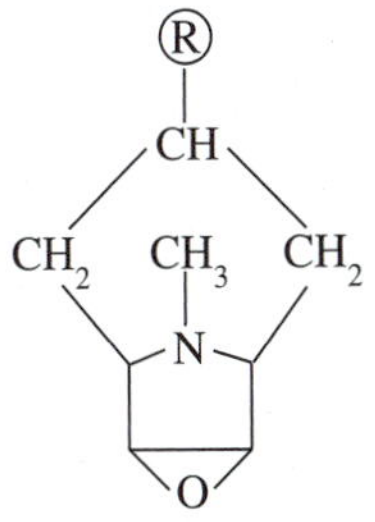

Scopolamine

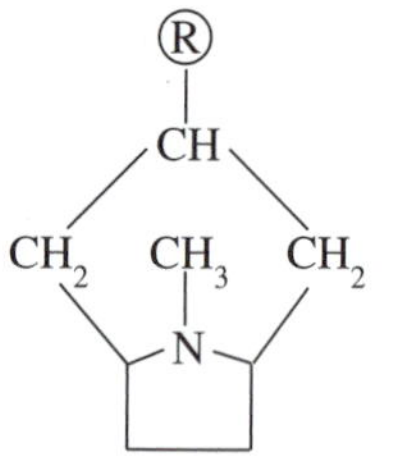

Atropine 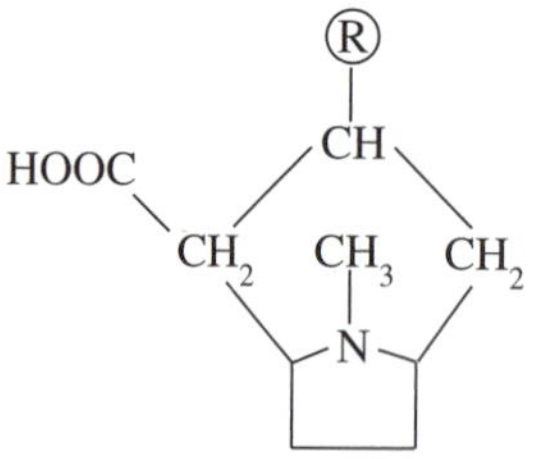 **Cocaine**

BOX 37-1

CHARACTERISTICS OF CENTRAL ANTICHOLINERGIC SYNDROME

Biphasic effect of central nervous system (CNS) excitation followed by depression leading to sedation and coma.

Distinctive mumbling or fragmentary speech pattern. Patients may begin to answer questions clearly at first but trail away to incomprehensible words by the end of a sentence.

Atypical behavior. For example, undressing is common in children and less commonly occurs in adults.

Repetitive "picking" movements are common. The patient is constantly picking at the bed sheets, smoothing out items of clothing, or even picking repetitively at the air.

Hallucinations may occur. These are typically visual but may be auditory.

Movement disorders are of an ataxic or clonic nature.

Hyperthermia, caused by a combination of decreased ability to sweat and increased motor activity, is commonly seen and is a potential problem that can lead to worsening of CNS toxicity.

BOX 37-2

CHARACTERISTICS OF PERIPHERAL ANTICHOLINERGIC SYNDROME

In order of effect, ability to salivate, to sweat, and to lacrimate is decreased initially.

Then, with increasing toxicity, ocular effects are noticed, manifesting as blurred vision with decreasing ability to accommodate and associated with pupillary mydriasis.

After this, an increase in heart rate occurs, which is then followed by decrease in bladder and intestinal motility at high toxic exposure.

Plants with anticholinergic (atropine-like) properties give characteristic central and peripheral anticholinergic syndromes (Boxes 37-1 and 37-2).[48] These syndromes result from the competitive inhibition of acetylcholine at the autonomic muscarinic receptor leading to receptor blockade.

One of the clinical signs most useful for detecting peripheral anticholinergic toxicity is discovered through examination of the patient's axillae. A dry axilla in the presence of the signs and symptoms outlined in Box 37-2 is almost pathognomonic for anticholinergic toxicity.[66]

The symptoms of anticholinergic poisoning are often remembered using the following mnemonic:

Hot as a hare,
Blind as a bat,
Dry as a bone,
Red as a beet,
Mad as a hatter.

In a series of 27 cases of jimsonweed poisoning, all the victims had mental status changes and mydriasis.[41] There may be electroencephalogram abnormalities, which resolve rapidly with recovery. Abnormal liver function tests may occur transiently.[50] Death occurs rarely; when it does, it is usually secondary to misjudgment while under the influence of the alkaloid.[24] In a case report of datura poisoning, a 20-year-old man drowned after ingesting a brew derived from the flowers of *Datura arborea*. The deceased had been in a party of seven who became intoxicated on 50 flowers gathered from a datura shrub. The author describes in some detail the observed behavior of the surviving members of the party.[25] According to the police report, one young man was "disoriented, with dilated pupils and obviously terrified." On recovery he described how he imagined he had been chased by trees and people, armed with guns and spears. He had imagined that these "people" had shot his brother, who in fact had drowned in shallow water in a nearby creek bed while under the influence of the datura brew. These hallucinations continued for a further 48 hours after exposure to a diminishing degree.

Children seem to be more sensitive to atropine poisoning and more commonly eat the seeds and the flowers.[53] Adult poisonings are usually the result of ingesting tea made from the flowers or leaves of the jimsonweed or henbane plant, as described in the case documented previously. It is noteworthy that pupillary dilation, or atropine mydriasis, is not reversed by application of 1% pilocarpine.[73]

Jimsonweed has been used historically to treat asthma, heralding the current use of ipratroprium bromide. The seeds are the most highly concentrated part, and only 4 or 5 g (2 teaspoons) of the leaf may be fatal to a child.

Treatment. The treatment of belladonna alkaloid intoxication requires the removal of toxin from the gastrointestinal tract via gastric lavage, followed by instillation of activated charcoal as described previously. Removal of seeds from the stomach may not preclude serious toxicity, since alkaloids are rapidly leached into the gastric contents.[41]

Many authorities recommend treatment of the "full-blown" central anticholinergic syndrome with carefully titrated physostigmine.[41,49,50,75] The pharmacology is appealing. By using an anticholinesterase to block acetylcholine degradation, the physician can override competitive inhibition of atropinic agents and rapidly reverse peripheral and central nervous system effects. However, reports of asystole, ventricular arrhythmia, hypotension, bronchospasm, difficulty in clearing secretions, and seizures after rapid intravenous administration of physostigmine to treat anticholinergic syndromes mandate caution in the use of this drug compared with supportive treatment.[42,60,74] Thus we recommend consultation with a toxicologist before the use of physostigmine in this setting. The most useful application of physostigmine is in the evaluation of a comatose patient when central anticholinergic poisoning is suspected and the use of physostigmine is limited to a diagnostic role in a crisis situation.

Isotonic fluid volume replacement is the first-line treatment for hypotension. Vasopressors such as dopamine may be used if volume challenge does not reverse hypotension. Phenothiazines should not be used because their antimuscarinic properties may enhance toxicity.

Chronic exposure. The similarity of symptoms chronically induced by anticholinergics and those of schizophrenia, including one of Kraepelin's diagnostic criteria for dementia praecox, *gedankenlautwerden* (audible thoughts), was noted previously.[21] Unlike acute intoxication, chronic exposure may not resolve by abstinence alone and may require the use of psychotropics to reestablish baseline functioning.

Pyridine-Piperidine and Quinolizidine Alkaloid Groups. The pyridine-piperidine group contains the major alkaloids nicotine, coniine (found in the poison hemlock plant, Color Plate 73), lobeline, aercoline, piperine, and isopelletierine.

Nicotine alkaloids are found mainly in the Solanaceae family of plants. Other families containing nicotine alkaloids include the horse chestnut (a member of the Hippocastanaceae) and the milkweed (a member of the Asclepiadaceae), among many diverse groups.

The classic source of nicotine has been the Solanaceae, in particular the tobacco plant. Tobacco contains not only nicotine, but also other related alkaloids with similar pharmacologic properties such as anabasine, which is found in the wild tree tobacco, *Nicotiana glauca* (Color Plate 74). The other tobacco family members include *N. rustica, N. tabacum, N. trigonophylla,* commonly known as desert tobacco, and *N. attenuata,* known as coyote tobacco. *N. tabacum* is the major source of commercial tobacco and contains between 0.5% and 9% nicotine.

Lobeline, derived from the Indian tobacco plant, *Lobelia inflata,* is thought to be less toxic than nicotine and is sometimes used as a nicotine substitute in such products as Bantron Smoking Deterrent Tablets, Lobidram Computabs, and Nikoban lozenges and gum.[36] Concentrations range from 0.5 to 2 mg/dose. Lobelia herbal teas are reported to produce euphoria.

The pyridine/piperidine alkaloids are shown below:

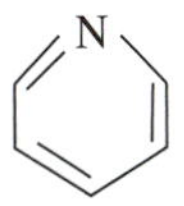

N

Pyridine

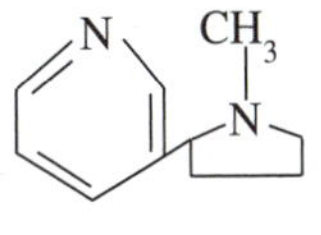

N CH$_3$ N

Nicotine

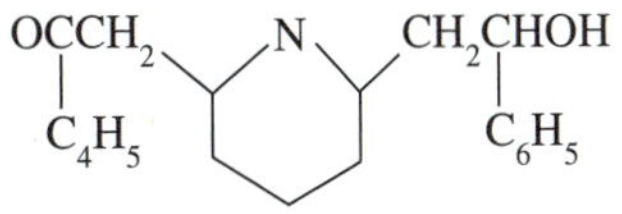

OCCH$_2$ N CH$_2$CHOH
C$_4$H$_5$ C$_6$H$_5$

Lobeline

N CH$_2$-CH$_2$-CH$_3$

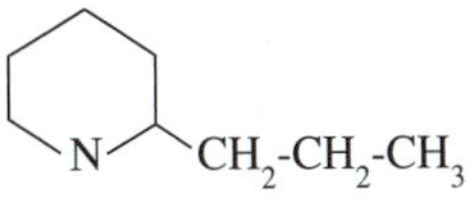

Coniine

The quinolizidine alkaloids, cytisine and lupinine, act much like nicotinic ganglionic stimulating agents. Common toxic plants in this group include golden chain tree *(Laburnum anagyroides),* Kentucky coffee tree *(Gymnocladus dioica),* and lupine (*Lupinus* species), the necklace pod sophora *(Sorphora tomentosa),* and the mescal bean bush *(Sophora secundiflora)* (Color Plate 75) (this last plant is considered in more detail in the section on psychoactive plants).[14,36]

Because toxicity from these plants resembles nicotine toxicity, they are considered together. Special mention is made of poison hemlock at the end of this section.

Structures of the quinolizidine alkaloids follow:

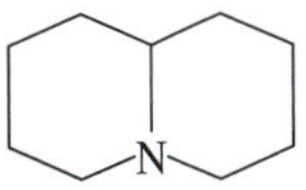

N

Quinolizidine

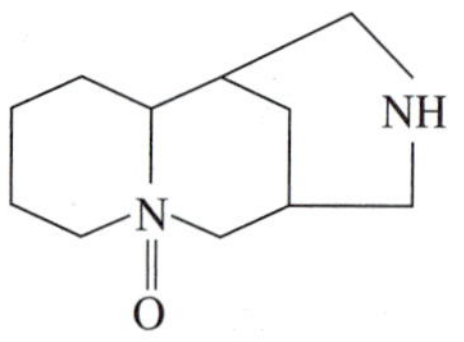

Cytisine

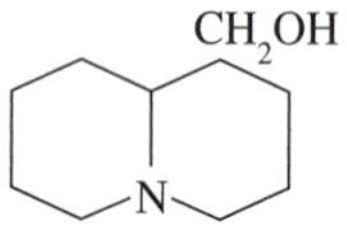

Lupinine

Nicotinic syndrome. In the previous section the anticholinergic syndrome was described in terms of stimulation of the muscarinic receptors of the parasympathetic nervous system. Nicotinic receptors exist within the brain as central nicotinic receptors and peripherally in both the autonomic nervous system (Nn type) and the somatic nervous system (Nm type).[23]

Nicotine markedly stimulates the CNS. Tremor and convulsions can be produced. Increased respiration by direct stimulation of the medulla oblongata occurs, as can vomiting by stimulation of the chemoreceptor trigger zone directly or via activation of vagal afferent pathways.

In the sympathetic nervous system the Nn receptor resides in the paravertebral ganglion and modulates the conduction of electrical impulses of the sympathetic outflow to effector organs through the release of biogenic amines and catecholamines (such as norepinephrine, epinephrine, dopamine, serotonin).[28,39] In the parasympathetic chain the nicotinic Nn receptors are also located in ganglia (although not within anatomic chains). In response to a craniosacral outflow from the CNS, nicotine receptors, once stimulated, modulate electrical activity down the nerve to cause an increase in acetylcholine release to act on postganglionic muscarinic receptors.[29,40]

In addition, Nn receptors are located within the adrenal glands and when stimulated cause release of catecholamines.

In the somatic nervous system the nicotinic Nm receptors are postganglionic and respond to the acetylcholine released at the motor end plate.[29,40] Hence an increase in nicotinic receptor stimulation may cause a combination of the following:

In the autonomic nervous system:

- Increased release of catecholamines and acetylcholine with stimulation of their respective postganglionic receptors
- Increased release of catecholamines from the adrenal medulla[29]

In the somatic system:

- Increased stimulation of postganglionic receptors at the motor end plate

Thus nicotine poisoning may present a combined picture of autonomic and motor dysfunction mediated by central or peripheral effects or both. The autonomic receptor sites are shown in Fig 37-1.

TOXICOLOGIC EFFECTS. The action of nicotine on a variety of neuroeffector junctions is rapid and variable because of the biphasic effect of the alkaloid and the dose to which

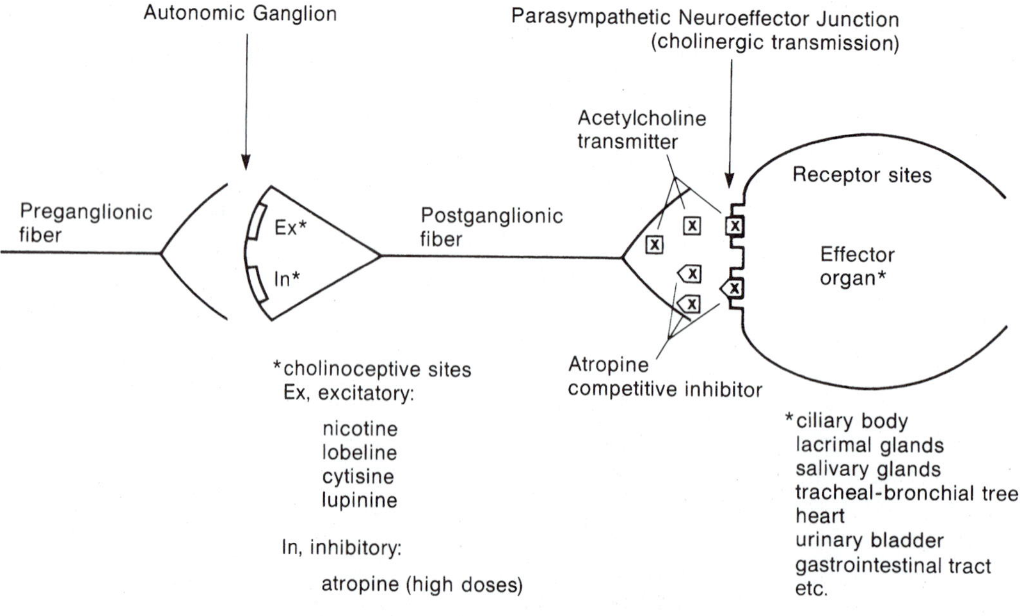

Fig. 37-1 Autonomic receptor sites.

the patient is exposed. In general, the larger the dose, the more rapidly the patient progresses to neuromuscular blockade.[23,40] The clinical syndromes produced by pyridine-piperidines are mixed.

Poisoning is heralded by abdominal pain, nausea, and vomiting. There is initial stimulation of most autonomic ganglia, both central and peripheral, followed by depression of transmission. Nicotine similarly affects the neuromuscular junction, with a stimulant phase followed rapidly by paralysis (Fig. 37-2).[22,39,46]

Peripheral nervous system. In the excitatory phase, augmented acetylcholine effect on postganglionic muscarinic receptors produces hypersalivation, increased bronchial secretions, diaphoresis, bradycardia, bowel hyperactivity, diarrhea, and pupillary constriction. Tachycardia and hypertension may be seen during this phase because of sympathetic nervous stimulation or increased adrenal medulla output. After initial stimulation, prolonged ganglionic blockade and adrenal medulla inhibition ensue. At this time, bradycardia and hypotension predominate. Thus tachycardia, bradycardia, hypertension, and hypotension may all be seen in a progressive pattern of toxicity, or because of the brief nature of the stimulatory phase, the patient may have only the signs and symptoms of neurologic depression.[23,36,40,47]

Central effect. Initial stimulation leads to tremor and convulsion with particular stimulation of the chemoreceptor trigger zone leading to vomiting. Confusion, agitation, restlessness, and incoordination may then be seen. This is followed by central nervous system depression with onset of decreased mental state and coma.[23,33,36,40,47]

Although small doses may augment respiration in the manner described previously, respiratory blockade follows higher doses, secondary to central nervous system depression and peripheral neuromuscular junction paralysis of the muscles of respiration.[23,33,36,40,47]

Neuromuscular symptoms. Hypotonia, decreased deep tendon reflexes, fasciculation, and motor paralysis sequentially occur.[36,40,47]

Toxicity. Nicotine is water soluble and can accumulate in water droplets and dew on tobacco leaves. Contact with the wet plants can transfer nicotine percutaneously to humans, causing a mild form of toxicity known as "green tobacco illness."[35] Nicotine is also readily absorbed through the oral mucosa and respiratory tract. Gastrointestinal absorption may be somewhat delayed by the "ion trapping" effect in the acid gastric juice, given the high pKa of nicotine.[36]

Nicotine is excreted fairly rapidly by the kidneys after biotransformation in the liver and lungs. The half-life is ½ to 2 hours. Conitine, the major urinary metabolite, can be measured in the urine if quantification of excretion is needed.[23,40,47]

The lethal dose of ingested nicotine has not been well determined. It is estimated in humans that 2 to 5 mg may cause nausea, while 40 to 60 mg may be lethal. One to two cigarettes if ingested and absorbed could be lethal to a child.[23,36,40]

TREATMENT. Therapy consists of supportive care with particular attention to protecting the airway, removing the toxin from the stomach with gastric lavage, and instilling activated charcoal. Syrup of ipecac is contraindicated because of the anticipation of protracted vomiting and depressed conscious state with a significant ingestion.[47]

Treating initial excessive adrenergic stimulation with phentolamine is ill advised because this compounds the effect of nicotinic blockade that is expected to follow a significant exposure. Symptomatic bradycardia should be treated

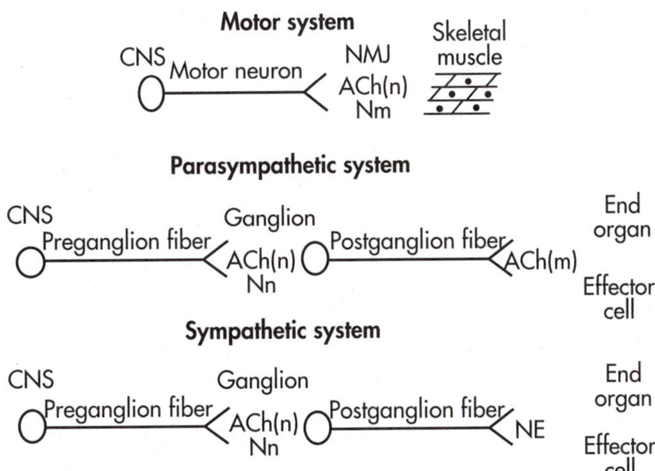

Fig. 37-2 Locations of nicotinic receptors. *CNS*, Central nervous system; *NMJ*, neuromuscular junction; *ACh*, acetylcholine; *n*, nicotine subset; *m*, muscarinic subset; *NE*, norepinephrine. (Modified from Lavoie FW, Thomas TM: *J Emerg Med* 9:133, 1991.)

with atropine. Hypotension should be treated with intravenous fluids and inotropic agents such as dopamine.[40]

In the presence of liver or renal failure, supportive treatment may be required for days. There is no evidence that dialysis is effective in removing the toxins. Airway control with endotracheal intubation and mechanically assisted ventilation is the mainstay of therapy, and properly managed patients should survive.

Poison hemlock. Coniine, the principal alkaloid in *Conium maculatum* (poison hemlock), is a pyridine derivative similar to nicotine. It also works as a ganglionic stimulating agent, producing transitory parasympathetic and central nervous system stimulation, followed by mental status depression and respiratory paralysis. The alkaloid is volatile and lost by drying or heating. As in nicotine poisoning, biphasic central nervous system effects may be observed, but death ultimately results from central nervous system depression and respiratory failure. Seizures may also occur as a terminal event.[33,36]

Poison hemlock has been romanticized through the ages. It is thought to be the means by which Socrates met his fate. John Keats referred to the neurologic manifestations of hemlock in his "Ode to a Nightingale"[31]:

> My heart aches and a drowsy numbness pains
> My sense as though of hemlock I have drunk.

Psychoactive Plants. Hallucinogens occur throughout the plant kingdom. Approximately 90 of the 800,000 plant species are hallucinogenic. Human history is replete with rituals and religious ceremonies using these plants, which have been practiced on every continent.[67,68]

Many psychoactive plants are indole derivatives (see below), which are among the most potent psychoactive compounds in nature:

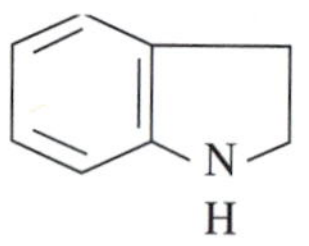

Indole nucleus

The active component of the naturally occurring hallucinogen found in the seeds of the morning glory *(Ipomoea violacea)* (Color Plate 76) is ergin, or *d*-lysergic acid diethylamide an indole derivative.[19] About 300 seeds, or enough to fill a cupped hand, is the equivalent of 200 to 300 μg of *d*-LSD, with similar systemic and hallucinatory effects.

Striking structural similarities exist between the most potent psychoactive plant compounds and biochemically important neurotransmitters. Chemical relationships exist among serotonin, psilocybin (*Psilocybe* spp.), and *d*-LSD (see below).[69] LSD is synthesized from ergometrine, one of the ergot alkaloids derived from *Claviceps purpurea*. Chemical similarities between hallucinogens and neurotransmitters are illustrated above right:

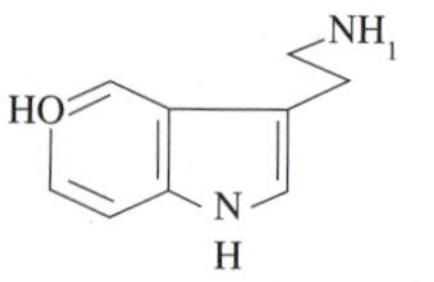

Serotonin 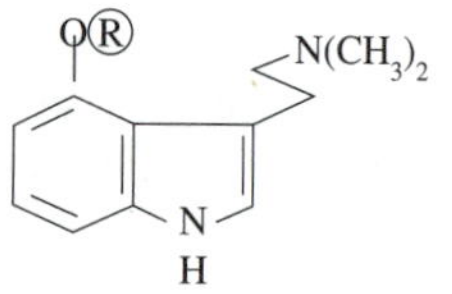 **Psilocybin**

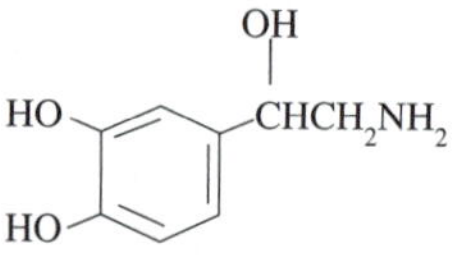

Norepinephrine 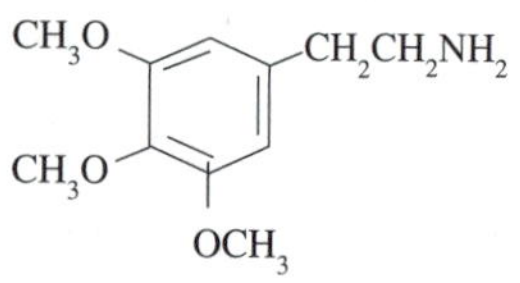 **Mescaline**

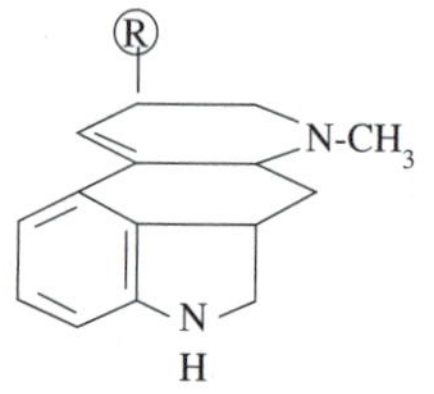

Lysergic acid diethylamide 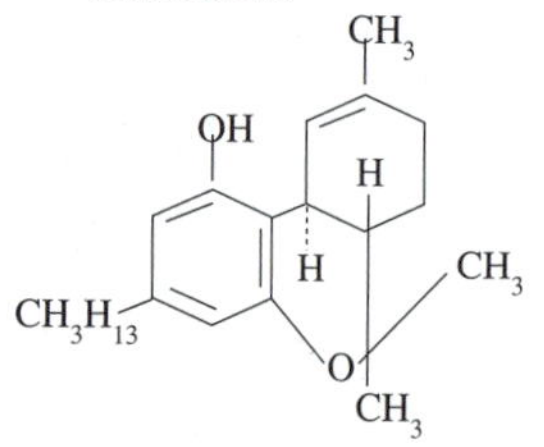 **Tetrahydrocannabinol**

The most characteristic effects of these alkaloids, natural or derived, are visual deceptions and feelings of depersonalization. Acute psychosis has been described.[69]

Scopolamine-rich plants of the tropane alkaloid group, including henbane *(Hyosyamus niger)*, jimsonweed *(Datura stramonium)*, trumpet lily *(Datura arborea)*, and mandrake *(Mandragora officinatum)*, have depressant or euphoric effects or both. A tea may be made from leaves, flowers, or roots. Eating the flowers and seeds directly may induce similar effects, occasionally resulting in anticholinergic crisis (see the section on tropane alkaloids).

Ingestion of large amounts of the common household spice nutmeg *(Myristica fragrans)* may mimic the anticholinergic crisis seen with tropane alkaloids. Dry mouth, thirst, tachycardia, and hot, dry skin are typical clinical signs. Ten grams or more produces a brief euphoria followed by a floating, dreamlike sensation, hallucinations, and drowsiness. The psychoactive component is thought to be the aromatic fraction containing myristicin, elemicin, and safrole.[44]

Marijuana *(Cannabis sativa)* is one of few psychoactive plants that possess nitrogen-free compounds. The active ingredients are derivatives of tetrahydrocannabinol (THC). THC is believed to be the most psychoactive isomer (see above). Much is known about the behavioral, systemic, and neurophysiologic effects of THC. The drug is found in abundance in the flowering tops, or "buds," of the plant.

The THC concentration may range from less than 1% in home-grown varieties, with mild mood-altering qualities, to 10% in Hawaiian, South American, and Southeast Asian varieties, with powerful psychoactive and hallucinatory effects. Potency depends on the growing season, climate, soil, cultivation, and other agricultural factors.

THC is easily volatilized and may be inhaled with prompt effect. The drug may also be ingested, with a delay in effect of 30 to 40 minutes. The effective dose on smoking is 200 to 250 μg/kg and on ingestion is 300 to 480 μg/kg.[44] THC is known to alter brain levels of 5-hydroxytryptamine (serotonin) and norepinephrine, although the true mechanism of toxicity is unknown.

Observed effects are mood alteration with either euphoria or depression, a sense of dissociation from surroundings, and altered perceptions of time and distance, combined with atropine-like effects of dry mouth, thirst, and tachycardia. Toxic psychosis and panic reactions are occasionally seen and probably represent the major known risks. Clinical cases of pulmonary aspergillosis have been ascribed to smoking contaminated marijuana.[27]

Another striking chemical similarity exists between the phenylethylamine derivative mescaline (from peyote, *Lophophora williamsii*) (Color Plate 77) and the neurotransmitter norepinephrine (see p. 870). At a dose of about 5 mg/kg, mescaline induces sympathomimetic effects, followed by marked visual hallucinations.[3] Thus compounds that cause marked perceptual alterations tend to resemble structurally important neurohumoral substances, while non-nitrogen-containing derivatives, such as the tropane alkaloids and THC (see p. 870), have less specific depressant or euphoric effects.[69]

The Texas mountain laurel, *Sophora secundiflora,* contains dark red beans, known as mescal beans, that are hallucinogenic. The "red bean dance" of Mexico and Texas was based on this hallucinogenic bean. Necklaces made from the bean were thought to ward off evil. The psychoactive nature is attributed to a toxic pyridine, cytisine. It is estimated that one seed thoroughly chewed is enough to kill a child.[14,69]

The evergreen tree khat *(Catha edulis)* contains a potent amphetamine-like constituent, cathinone. In addition to cathinone, the khat leaf contains two further alkaloids of the phenylpropylamine group, cathine and norephedrine.[28]

A recent analysis of 22 khat samples of different origin showed that, on average, 100 g of fresh khat contains 36 mg cathinone, 120 mg cathine, and 8 mg norephedrine. However, cathinone is the major psychoactive constituent. As the leaf wilts, cathinone is metabolized to cathine, explaining why only fresh leaves are chewed to achieve the desired stimulating effect. Methcathinone is a synthetic derivative of cathinone. Currently there is an increase in the use of this stimulant in the Midwest of the United States, but most experience with the synthetic "street drug" derivative comes from Russia, where it first surfaced in 1982.[15]

The structures of methcathinone and related drugs follow:

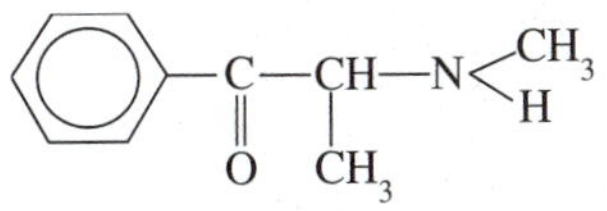

C_6H_5—C(=O)—CH(CH_3)—N<CH_3, H

Methcathinone

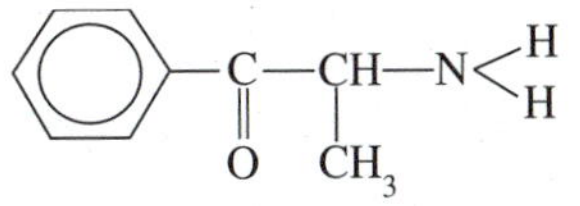

C_6H_5—C(=O)—CH(CH_3)—N<H, H

Cathinone

C_6H_5—CH(OH)—CH(CH_3)—N<CH_3, H

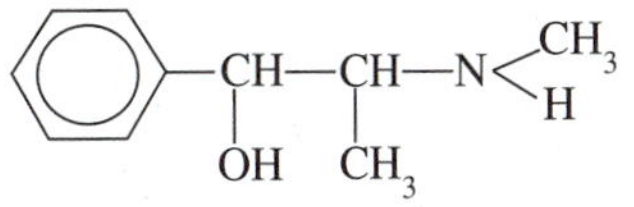

Ephedrine

Treatment of psychoactive plant intoxication. Treatment is supportive. Unless there is a firm clinical suspicion that the patient has a central anticholinergic syndrome, physostigmine should be withheld. First-line treatment for agitation is benzodiazepines, but haloperidol may be used for refractory agitation.

Extensive discussions of psychoactive plants may be found in the work of Schultes and Hofmann.[69]

Other Central Nervous System Toxins. The remaining indole derivatives include gelsemine and sempervine, found in *Gelsemium sempervirens* (Carolina or yellow jessamine). These act as neuromuscular blocking agents and can cause death by respiratory paralysis.[26]

The ergot alkaloids, ergonovine and ergotamine, are indole derivatives but have little relevance to modern poisons. Historically, the fungus *Claviceps purpurea* (the source of ergonovine and ergotamine) infected rye and other grains, which, when consumed, caused a burning sensation and necrosis in the extremities known as St. Anthony's fire and produced a convulsive disorder.[69]

Commercial grains are now inspected for the presence of ergot, and inadvertent poisoning is rare. Ergot derivatives, which are potent vasoconstrictors and oxytocic agents, are used in therapy for vascular headaches and obstetric and gynecologic disorders.

Strychnine, found in seeds of the tree *Strychnos nux-vomica,* is a powerful central nervous system stimulant and convulsant. This indole derivative may be ingested accidentally by children who mistakenly consume rat poison. We have treated several persons who attempted suicides by taking strychnine-impregnated grain baits.

Treatment consists of supportive measures. Endotracheal intubation and mechanically assisted ventilation may be required, but recovery is expected and mortality is low.[26]

Resin

Water Hemlock. Unlike the other plants mentioned in this section, water hemlock *(Cicuta maculata)* (Color Plate 78) exerts toxicity through elaboration of a resin and not through alkaloids. It is considered here because of the parasympathomimetic nature of its resin, an unsaturated aliphatic alcohol, cicutoxin. It has a characteristic and dramatic physiologic action, starting 15 to 60 minutes after ingestion with initial muscarinic effects of salivation, abdominal pain, vomiting, and diarrhea, followed by central nervous system depression and respiratory distress. Seizures may be a prominent feature of water hemlock poisoning.[52] Death is usually secondary to respiratory arrest.[39,55]

Treatment is symptomatic and supportive with particular attention to the airway. Benzodiazepines are recommended for control of seizures. It has been hypothesized that seizures may be caused by overstimulation of central cholinergic pathways. Animal experiments do not demonstrate any benefit from treatment with anticholinergics.[57] Gastrointestinal fluid losses from cicutoxin may require vigorous fluid replacement to maintain adequate blood pressure.

The structure of cicutoxin is shown below.

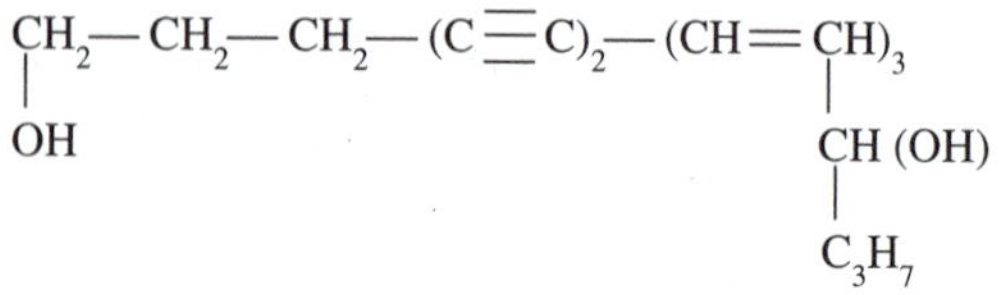

$$\underset{\displaystyle \text{OH}}{\text{CH}_2}\text{—CH}_2\text{—CH}_2\text{—(C}\equiv\text{C)}_2\text{—(CH=}\underset{\displaystyle \underset{\displaystyle \text{C}_3\text{H}_7}{\text{CH (OH)}}}{\text{CH}}\text{)}_3$$

Cicutoxin

GASTROINTESTINAL SYSTEM (BOX 37-3)
Alkaloids

Isoquinoline and Quinoline Group. These contain such divergent species as *Papaver somniferum* (opium poppy), *Cephaelis ipecacuanha* (ipecac), and *Cinchona* spp. (quinine). The major toxicity is gastrointestinal and mucous membrane irritation, with few reported poisonings from plant ingestions in this group. Cardiac toxicity at higher doses has been reported.

The isoquinoline and quinoline nucleus is shown below.

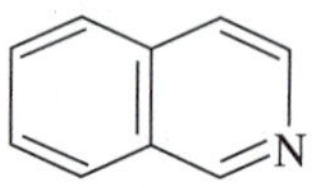

N

BOX 37-3

PLANTS PRODUCING GASTROINTESTINAL SYSTEM TOXICITY

ALKALOIDS

Isoquinoline and quinoline group
Pyrrolizidine group
Amine alkaloid group

GLYCOSIDES

Saponin glycosides
Anthraquinone glycosides
Coumarin glycosides

RESIN

Cicutoxin

PHYTOTOXIN

Ricin
Abrin
Curcin

The most commonly ingested isoquinoline derivative is emetine in the form of syrup of ipecac.[19] It is mentioned here to highlight the gastrointestinal manifestations of this group of compounds.

Pyrrolizidine Alkaloids. Ingestion of pyrrolizidine alkaloids usually involves consumption of mislabeled herbal medicines or teas. For example, gordolobo yerba, which contains the harmless herb, *Gnaphalium,* closely resembles groundsel *(Senecio longilobus)* and toxicity may occur with teas made from the substituted brew.[17] Other natural sources are *Amsinckia* spp. (fiddle neck or tar weed) and *Crotalaria* spp. (rattlebox).

The principal alkaloids are heliotrine, lasiocarpine, and retronecine, which may be hepatotoxic and carcinogenic. The structure of retronecine is shown below.[9]

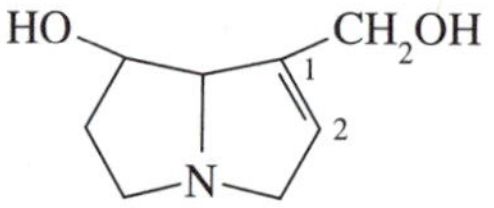

HO CH_2OH 1 2 N

Retronecine

These alkaloids are capable of causing both acute hepatitis and chronic venoocclusive liver disease resembling Budd-Chiari syndrome or cardiac cirrhosis. Venoocclusive disease is endemic in Jamaica and is thought to be secondary to the consumption of "home brew" containing these alkaloids.[7]

Case reports note deaths from hepatic failure in a person who consumed large amounts of matte tea[1] and acutely in a child who drank groundsel tea.[17] The herbal tea Russian comfrey contains at least eight known pyrrolizidine alkaloids. Hepatomas and pancreatic tumors have been produced in rats fed retronecine. The mechanisms of carcinogenesis and hepatotoxicity are unknown, but it is thought that the alkaloids are activated in the liver by the P_{450} and mixed-function oxidase systems to reactive pyrrolic metabolites that alkylate proteins and DNA.[51] Young victims seem to be more susceptible than adults to the effects of acute ingestions.

Toxicity may be delayed by weeks or months.[17] An exact toxic dose has not been established, although case reports indicate that toxicity can occur with 10 to 30 mg/kg.

Treatment is supportive.

Amine Alkaloids. The amine alkaloids are important for the medicinal derivatives ephedrine and colchicine. Plant ingestions occur from intentional use of peyote *(Lophophora williamsii),* discussed under "Psychoactive Plants," and accidental ingestion of the garden ornamental autumn crocus *(Colchicum autumnale),* which contains colchicine. Although accidental plant poisoning is rare, a brief discussion of colchicine and its toxicity illustrates its unique biochemical effect.

Colchicine directly affects cell mitosis by arresting cell division in metaphase and dissolving the microtubular system necessary for cell division and polymorphonuclear mobility.[26] Acute poisoning may occur after a latent period of several hours. Initial effects are gastrointestinal, with severe abdominal pain, nausea, vomiting, and diarrhea. The diarrhea may induce volume depletion and shock. Muscular weakness and ascending paralysis culminate in respiratory arrest, which may occur in the presence of a clear sensorium.[18]

Treatment is symptomatic and supportive. Parenteral analgesics may be given to relieve severe abdominal pain, keeping in mind that the patient is sensitized to central nervous system depressants by colchicine. Early and vigorous fluid replacement with monitoring of central venous pressure and urine output is essential. Pulmonary function tests should be used to monitor respiratory function, particularly fatigue and ascending paralysis. Assisted ventilation should be employed as long as necessary, since spontaneous resolution may occur.

Glycosides

Saponin Glycosides. Saponin glycosides are found throughout the plant kingdom, contained within English ivy *(Hedera helix),* pokeweed *(Phytolacca americana),* tung tree (*Aleurites* spp.), ginseng *(Panax ginseng* or *quinquefolium),* and licorice *(Glycyrrhiza glabra).* After hydrolysis, saponin glycosides yield an aglycone (sapogenin), which is responsible for the toxicity, and a sugar, usually glucose, galactose, rhamnose, or arabinose, which may enhance solubility and absorption of the aglycone.[34]

Saponins may induce lysis of erythrocytes, causing hemolytic anemia. In addition, there are gastrointestinal irritants that appear to facilitate their own intestinal absorption. Most saponins are found in combination with other toxins, including gastrointestinal irritants and phytotoxins, which contribute to a widely varying clinical picture.

Pokeweed may be mistaken for horseradish, parsnips, or Jerusalem artichoke. Pokeberries typically leave a purple stain. The root is the most toxic part of the plant, and parboiling does not necessarily offer protection. A fulminant gastroenteritis with vomiting and diarrhea is described and may be delayed for 2 to 4 hours.[22] The diarrhea may appear foamy from the sudsing effect of the saponin glycosides on the bowel contents. Severe ingestions may result in respiratory depression, weakness, or seizures. A nonspecific pokeweed mitogen may induce morphologic changes in lymphocytes and plasma cells and can induce lymphocytosis that may last for weeks.[64]

Treatment should be supportive to prevent dehydration from gastrointestinal fluid loss. Respiratory depression and seizures should be treated in standard fashion, with recovery expected. Hematologic changes are thought to be transient.[64]

Anthraquinone Glycosides. The aglycone moiety of this group is anthraquinone, known to have cathartic activity. Buckthorn *(Rhamnus frangula)* is the only significant toxin in natural form, although herbal teas that contain senna leaves, flowers, and bark *(Cassia senna),* aloe leaves *(Aloe barbadensis),* and buckthorn bark have caused severe diarrhea.[1]

Treatment is supportive, emphasizing adequate volume and electrolyte replacement.

Coumarin Glycosides. Coumarin glycosides act much the same as irritant glycoalkaloids of the steroid-alkaloid group. The only plant of significance is daphne *(Daphne mezereum),* with its fragrant succulent berries. The fruits contain a coumarin glycoside and a diterpene that cause irritation of mucous membranes, with swelling of the tongue and lips. Severe gastroenteritis with gastrointestinal bleeding may occur.[16] In addition, progressive weakness, paralysis, seizures, and coma may develop. Blisters will form if berries are rubbed on the skin.

The widely cultivated daphne represents a significant risk to curious children, in whom only a few ingested berries may be lethal.[44]

No antidote is known; treatment is supportive.

Resins

Water Hemlock and Chinaberry. Water hemlock *(Cicuta maculata)* and chinaberry *(Melia azedarach)* (Color Plate 79) are two of the most toxic resin-containing plants. Water hemlock is discussed earlier. Chinaberry tree (also known as China tree or Texas umbrella tree) also contains an unknown alkaloid that contributes to its toxicity.[16] Gastroenteritis can occur after ingestion of any part of the plant, but typically it is the berries that are ingested by children.

The berries are green but turn yellow and wrinkle with age. After ingestion of as little as one berry a severe gastroenteritis and often bloody diarrhea may ensue. Symptoms may be rapid or delayed for several hours after ingestion. Central nervous system depression or excitation, dyspnea, and diaphoresis are less commonly observed.[14]

Phytotoxins

Ricin and Abrin. Ricin, the phytotoxin of the castor bean, is a glycoprotein composed of two peptide chains. The larger chain binds to cell surfaces. The chains uncouple and the smaller chain is taken up by the cell, where it interferes with protein synthesis, leading to cell death.[11] The oral lethal dose is estimated to be 1 mg/kg or as little as one bean in a child and eight to ten in an adult.[77]

Phytotoxins are grouped exclusively in the families Fabaceae, including jequirity bean *(Abrus precatorius),* containing the phytotoxin abrin, and Euphorbiaceae, including the castor bean *(Ricinus communis)* (Color Plate 80), containing the phytotoxin ricin, and purging nut *(Jatropha curcas)* containing the phytotoxin curcin. Poisoning results from eating or chewing on the nut or seed. Castor oil, made from pressing castor beans at temperatures less than 50° F, is a nontoxic cathartic.[72]

Local effects are prompt and include burning of the mouth and throat, accompanied by abdominal pain. Headache, nausea, vomiting, diarrhea, and hemorrhagic gastritis occur hours later.[6] The seeds are highly allergenic and may cause urticaria, dermatitis, or anaphylaxis secondary to contact alone.[46]

Systemic effects may be delayed as much as a day or more as inhibition of protein synthesis occurs. Target organs are principally the heart and central nervous system. Tachyarrhythmias and hypotension may be features of the clinical course. Alterations in mental status are characterized by stupor and coma. Seizures may occur. Terminally, liver enzyme abnormalities may arise, indicating hepatic necrosis and liver failure.[57] Although the mechanism is unknown, renal failure may be present and has been characterized as a transient elevation of serum creatinine.[5,11,44,76]

Treatment is supportive. Dehydration is common and may be the only significant effect. Fluid losses must be closely followed and aggressively replaced. Challoner and McCarron[11] reviewed the literature on *Ricinus communis* poisoning. They reported a mortality of between 2% and 4% and noted that before the introduction of intravenous fluid resuscitation in World War II the mortality was as high as 8%. If swallowed intact, mature seeds are often harmless because of their thick coat, which allows them to pass undigested. Efforts should be made to remove chewed or immature (soft) seeds from the stomach. It has been suggested that alkalinization of the urine may help promote excretion of the toxin, although this is anecdotal advice.[5]

CARDIOVASCULAR SYSTEM (BOX 37-4)

Alkaloids

Purine Alkaloids. The purine alkaloids caffeine and theobromine are found in a variety of plants. The derivative beverages and stimulants, not the plants themselves, represent a toxic risk.

Steroid Alkaloids. Veratrum alkaloids as found in *Veratrum viride* (American hellebore) are extremely toxic substances that act by increasing the permeability of cell membranes to sodium ions, causing initial depolarization and subsequent loss of membrane potential.[10] The net result is depression of impulses from central and peripheral vasomotor centers, leading to a decrease in heart rate and blood pressure.[26] Although intoxication is rare, these alkaloids are of interest because of their once widespread medicinal use as antihypertensives.

Previously restricted to use in preeclampsia, veratrum alkaloids have a narrow therapeutic margin, and severe gastrointestinal side effects preclude continued use.

In a published review of intoxication from *Veratrum album,* Quatrehomme and co-workers[61] reviewed the caseload at the Lyon (France) Poison Control Center over a 10-year period and noted that *Veratrum album* represented 0.06% of all intoxications registered.

In a review of the world literature of 30 published cases of toxicity,[61] the features of note are as follows:

1. Poisoning is often inadvertent, as a result of confusion in identification of the plant with *Gentiana lutea,* which is used in herb tea or homemade liquor.
2. After a short time (30 minutes to 3 hours) the onset of symptoms occurs in the following order: nausea, vomiting and abdominal pain, and a fall in blood pressure and pulse.
3. In more serious intoxications, electrocardiographic abnormalities, including QT prolongation, are characteristically seen.
4. Neurologic signs are more rarely seen.

Glycosides

Digitalis, a pharmaceutical of extraordinary medical significance, is the most famous member of the cardiac glycoside group. Its parent plant, *Digitalis purpurea* (foxglove) (Color Plate 81), grows wild in parts of the United States and is cultivated as a garden ornamental. Digitalis plant ingestion is rarely a problem, although children have been poisoned by sucking the leaves or seeds. Highly toxic common oleander *(Nerium oleander)* (Color Plate 82), which grows in abundance along highways and in gardens; yellow oleander *(Thevetia peruviana)* (Color Plate 83), the principal cause of plant poisoning in India; and lily of the valley *(Convallaria majalis)* (Color Plate 84), an attractive garden plant, are more commonly implicated in poisons and death in the United States than is foxglove. *N. oleander* is believed to contain at least five potent glycosides, including oleandrin, digitoxin, and nerium.

The aglycones are released by acid and enzymatic hydrolysis. The attached sugar moiety has no inherent cardiac action but may enhance solubility, absorption, and toxicity of the aglycone moiety.[16]

The mechanism of toxicity of cardiac glycosides is incompletely understood. It is believed to be associated with inhibition of a sodium- and potassium-stimulated, magnesium- and adenosine triphosphate (ATP)–dependent,

BOX 37-4
PLANTS EXHIBITING CARDIOVASCULAR TOXICITY

ALKALOIDS

Purine alkaloid group
Steroid alkaloids

GLYCOSIDES

Cardiac glycosides

RESIN

Grayanotoxin

Table 37-2 Antibodies Used for Cardiac Glycoside Assay

Antibody	Hapten	Source	Cross-Reactivity (%)	
			Digoxin	Digitoxin
A	12-Acetyl-3-succinyl digoxigenin	Goat	100	350
B	3,12-Disuccinyl digoxigenin	Goat	100	100
C	Digoxin	Cow	100	23
D	Unknown (commercial laboratory)	Rabbit	100	1.6

From Radford DJ et al: *Med J Aust* 144:540, 1986.

Table 37-3 Cardiac Glycoside Level in Oleander Measured by Radioimmunoassay as Apparent Digoxin Level

Source	Apparent Digoxin (μg/g)			
	A*	B*	C*	D*
Thevetia peruviana (yellow oleander)				
Leaves		52	36	7.6
Fruit		24		
Nerium oleander (oleander)				
Stem	430	620	33	17.0
Leaves			22	5.0

From Radford DJ et al: *Med J Aust* 144:540, 1986.
*Antibody used; see Table 37-2.

sodium-potassium transport enzyme complex.[26] As a result of inhibition of this transport mechanism, the extracellular potassium and intracellular sodium concentrations rise. The enzyme complex appears to be protected by high concentrations of potassium and transiently by magnesium. High concentrations of calcium and low serum potassium levels enhance toxicity of the cardiac glycosides.

Clinical signs of acute digitalis ingestion, first described by Withering in 1785,[79] consist of gastrointestinal disturbance with nausea and vomiting, alteration of vision, changes in mental status, and symptomatic bradycardia. The onset of action is well known for certain glycoside preparations, such as digoxin, digitoxin, and ouabain, but may be highly variable after plant ingestions, depending on the species. The clinical signs and symptoms are similar for all cardiac glycosides ingested in their natural form.

Effects on cardiac rate and rhythm are potentially the most dangerous sequelae and tend to fall into one or a combination of extrasystoles, tachyarrhythmias, bradyarrhythmias, and varying degrees of atrioventricular block. Central nervous system effects tend to be minimal until late in the course, when dizziness, disorientation, and stupor may occur.

Factors that may enhance systemic and cardiac toxicity include hypoxia, hypercalcemia, renal insufficiency, hypothyroidism, recent myocardial infarction, and old age. Most cardiac glycosides are excreted in the urine. A notable exception is digitoxin, largely metabolized by the liver.

Therapy is directed at removing the toxin and controlling cardiac arrhythmias. Although gastrointestinal absorption is usually completed in 2 hours, every effort should be made to recover the toxin by the use of gastric lavage and activated charcoal. Cholestyramine may help block enterohepatic recirculation but is unproven in this regard. Dialysis is probably ineffective in removing the highly protein-bound aglycone moiety.

Careful potassium administration is warranted if hypokalemia is accompanied by tachyarrhythmias or extrasystoles. Potassium should not be given with existing atrioventricular block or hyperkalemia. Magnesium infusion has also been advocated because of its transient protection of the sodium-potassium transport enzyme complex.

Recent reports of successful treatment with digoxin antibodies (Digibind)[78] have been published. One such case is a report of a patient with third-degree heart block from oleander ingestion, suggesting that digoxin-specific antibody fragments are useful for oleander poisoning.

Digoxin assays may help confirm the diagnosis of oleander ingestion in persons not taking digitalis preparations. The amount of cross-reactivity is unknown; thus the digoxin immunoassay predicts only the presence of the glycoside, not the degree of toxicity.[59]

Radford and associates[63] reviewed the toxicity of the naturally occurring glycosides using radioimmunoassay technique and established a table of relative potency and cross-reactivity to digoxin (Table 37-2). They found that the yellow oleander contained the equivalent of 36 μg of digoxin per gram of plant (Table 37-3).

Resin

Although they do not contain steroid alkaloids, rhododendrons, mountain laurel, and azaleas may contain grayanotoxins that exhibit similar toxicity.[10] Poisoning may result from the ingestion of leaves, flowers, or nectar but most commonly is caused by the ingestion of grayanotoxin-contaminated honey.[38,80] This substance is a resinoid, andromedotoxin. Symptoms include salivation, emesis, and circumoral and extremity paresthesias. Marked hypotension, bradycardia, incoordination, muscular weakness, and arrhythmias may result. Intoxication is rarely fatal and usually resolves within 24 hours with supportive treatment as described for steroid alkaloids.[18]

DERMATOTOXICITY AND LOCAL EFFECTS

Resin and Latex

The irritant constituents of the *Rhus* plants are the highly allergenic substances urushiols, which are catechol derivatives. These compounds are constituents of the latexlike emulsion present in the leaf ducts and therefore cause toxicity if the plant tissue has been damaged. It has been estimated that up to 70% of the population in the United States is sensitized to the skin irritant constituents of the *Rhus toxicodendron* species.

Insoluble Oxalates

Ingestions involving the *Philodendron* and *Dieffenbachia* members of the arum family group accounted for 188 exposures in a 2-year period reported to the Pittsburgh Poison Center.[54] These plants contain complex oxalate crystals arranged in linear spicules (see p. 879 for structure of simple oxalates) that are well documented as causing local mucous membrane irritation. In fact, the common name for the dieffenbachia is dumbcane. This name originated from the practice of Jamaican slave traders of torturing their slaves by rubbing *Dieffenbachia* onto their mouths as a punishment.[18]

Topical measures may be helpful in managing severe burning associated with oropharyngeal contact.

MISCELLANEOUS EFFECTS

Many plants exhibit syndromes that cannot be predominantly confined to one organ system or another.

Alkaloids

Steroid Alkaloids. Steroid alkaloids form the principal toxic components of several common plant poisons: American hellebore *(Veratrum viride)*, discussed previously, death camas (*Zigadenus* spp.), monkshood (*Aconitum* spp.) (Color Plate 85), and *Solanum* spp., including black nightshade *(S. americum*, not to be confused with deadly nightshade, *Atropa belladonna)*, horse nettle *(S. carolinense)*, and Jerusalem cherry *(S. pseudocapsicum)*.[33]

The plant-derived toxic steroid alkaloids are composed of several distinct glycoalkaloids. On hydrolysis the glycoalkaloids yield a sugar and an alkamine. The intact glycoalkaloid is a severe irritant to the mucous membranes and gastrointestinal tract, while the alkamine accounts for the effects on multiple organ systems, principally the cardiovascular and central nervous systems.

The glycoalkaloids cause burning of the mouth and throat, nausea, vomiting, abdominal pain, and diarrhea.

The alkamines' cardiovascular effects include hypotension and bradycardia, probably mediated through stimulation of afferent nerve fibers (the Bezold-Jarisch reflex).[23] Bradycardia can be reversed by atropine, but hypotension is refractory to vagal blockade, probably because of direct effects on the carotid sinus.

Digitalized patients may be at increased risk for cardiac arrhythmias.[23] Chest pain, paresthesias, muscle cramps, sweating, salivation, headache, hallucination, and altered mental status have been observed. Pupils may or may not be dilated.[33,44] Death camas and monkshood are especially toxic; the latter, often found as a garden ornamental, may cause death from arrhythmias in a few hours. A fairly constant pattern of mucous membrane and gastrointestinal irritation, followed by progressive systemic symptoms of chest pain, paresthesias, muscle cramps, headache, and altered mental status, is observed.[33]

The *Solanum* spp. are the largest group of steroid alkaloid–containing plants. Symptoms depend on the balance between the glycoalkaloid irritant effects and the alkamine systemic effects.

Treatment is supportive. Hypotension usually responds to fluid administration. Atropine may be helpful for bradycardia. Spontaneous recovery usually occurs in 1 to 3 days.

Glycosides

Cyanogenic Glycosides. Glycosides that yield hydrocyanic acid on hydrolysis are known as cyanogenic glycosides. The only toxicologically important glycoside in this group is amygdalin, which is abundant in the Rosaceae family.

The seeds of apples, *Malus* spp., and the pits of *Prunus* spp., including cherries, peaches, plums, and apricots (the commercial source of laetrile), are rich in amygdalin. The black or wild cherry *(P. serotina)* is considered the most dangerous of the group. Deaths have been reported from the ingestion of apricot, apple, cherry, and other fruit seeds.[44,65]

Poisonings have resulted from milkshakes that include apricot kernels.[1] Chronic cyanide toxicity causing goiter, ataxia, and amblyopia has been reported from ingestion of cassava *(Manihot esculenta)*.[1]

After ingestion, hydrocyanic acid is liberated from amygdalin by enzymatic action (β-glucosidase) or mild acid hydrolysis in a two-step process (p. 877). Cyanide readily combines with the trivalent ion of cytochrome oxidase in mitochondria, blocking the supply of oxygen for

(1) $Cyt\text{-}Fe^{3+}$ + HCN $\rightleftharpoons$ Cyt-FeCN
(cytochrome oxidase) + (hydrocyanic acid) (cytochrome oxidase-cyanide complex)

(2) $Hb\text{-}Fe^{2+}$ + $NaNO_2$ $\rightleftharpoons$ $Hb\text{-}Fe^{3+}$
(hemoglobin) + (nitrites) (methemoglobin)

(3) $Hb\text{-}Fe^{3+}$ + Cyt-FeCN $\rightleftharpoons$ Hb-FeCN + $Cyt\text{-}Fe^{3+}$
(methemoglobin) + (cytochrome oxidase-cyanide complex) (cyanomethemoglobin) + (cytochrome oxidase)

(4) $Na_2S_2O_3$ + CN $\underset{SCN^- \text{ - oxidase}}{\overset{\text{rhodanese}}{\rightleftharpoons}}$ SCN^- + Na_2SO_3
(sodium thiosulfate) + (cyanide) (thiocyanate) + (sodium sulfate)

Fig. 37-3 Principal steps in hydrocyanic acid poisoning and detoxification. *1,* Breakdown of cellular respiration resulting from the binding of cyanide to cytochrome oxidase. *2,* Conversion of the ferrous (Fe^{2+}) form of hemoglobin to the ferric (Fe^{3+}) form (methemoglobin) by the use of nitrites. *3,* Preferential binding of cyanide with methemoglobin, liberating cytochrome oxidase and restoring cellular respiration. *4,* Providing exogenous thiosulfate to aid in the formation of nontoxic thiocyanate via the enzyme rhodanese. Thiocyanate is then excreted from the body. The reaction is slowly reversible via the enzyme SCN-oxidase, so rebound may occur if a person is inadequately treated.

metabolic respiration and causing cytotoxic hypoxia (Fig. 37-3).

The body is normally capable of liberating cytochrome oxidase from the cyanide-cytochrome oxidase complex through action of the mitochondrial enzyme rhodanese.

Rhodanese provides sulfur from endogenous thiosulfate to cyanide, releasing cytochrome oxidase. The resulting thiocyanate ion is relatively nontoxic and readily excreted in urine.

Hydrolysis of amygdalin, leading to hydrocyanic acid production, is illustrated below.

Some doubt has been cast on the role of rhodanese, since thiosulfate is thought to be unable to penetrate the inner mitochondrial membrane where rhodanese is located.[12]

At present, although the exact mechanism of provision of a sulfane sulfur (such as thiosulfate) is unclear, all agree that thiosulfate is necessary to detoxify cyanide, in the method described previously. The body's ability to handle cyanide is limited, however, by the rate of cleavage of the sulfur-sulfur bond in thiosulfate and the available supply of the thiosulfate, a system that may be rapidly overwhelmed.

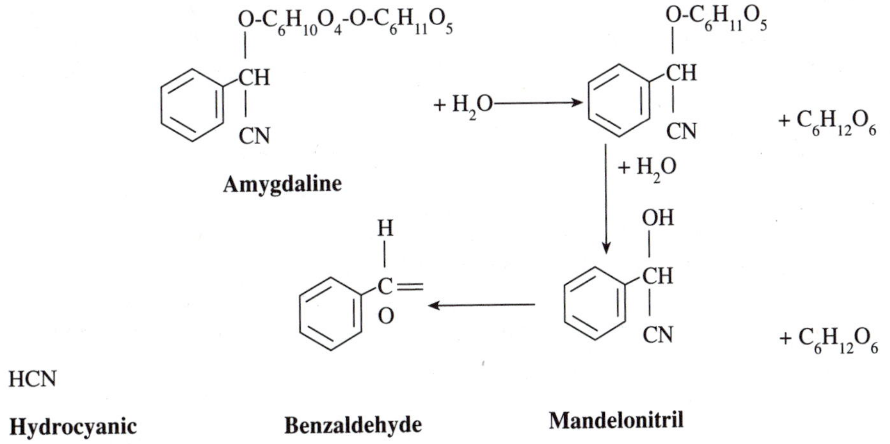

$O\text{-}C_6H_{10}O_4\text{-}O\text{-}C_6H_{11}O_5$ — CH — CN (phenyl)
Amygdaline

$+ H_2O \longrightarrow$ $O\text{-}C_6H_{11}O_5$ — CH — CN (phenyl) $+ C_6H_{12}O_6$

$+ H_2O$

OH — CH — CN (phenyl) $+ C_6H_{12}O_6$
Mandelonitril

$\longleftarrow$ H — C=O (phenyl)
Benzaldehyde

HCN
Hydrocyanic

The clinical signs of cyanide poisoning include agitation, excitement, gasping, hyperpnea, dyspnea with cyanosis, rapid decline in mental status, and death. There may be a characteristic breath odor of bitter almonds. However, wide individual variations in odor threshold and rapid olfactory fatigue make it very possible for individuals to be exposed to toxic concentrations of hydrogen cyanide without noticing any abnormal odor. Metabolic acidosis is the most common laboratory finding.[12]

Treatment must be prompt. It is based on the principle that cyanide preferentially combines with methemoglobin, breaking up the dissociable cyanide-cytochrome oxidase complex and liberating the respiratory enzyme (Fig. 37-3). Methemoglobin is rapidly formed on administration of sodium nitrite and, after combining with cyanide, forms cyanomethemoglobin. Exogenous thiosulfate is then administered to complete the detoxification.[12]

The oxygen-carrying capacity of blood is not affected by cyanide, and Po_2 may remain normal in the face of marked cyanosis. Oxygen should be administered, however, because cellular hypoxia and induced methemoglobinemia shift the oxygen-dissociation curve to the left, further impairing cellular oxygen delivery.[12]

The cyanide treatment kit by Eli Lilly and Company should be readily available. Treatment begins with inhalation of vials of amyl nitrite while an intravenous line is placed. Sodium nitrite in a 3% solution is given intravenously based on hemoglobin and weight. Methemoglobin levels and clinical response should be monitored to prevent treatment excess.

Others

Irritant and Essential Oils. Irritant oils are a problem only to livestock and to persons who overindulge at the delicatessen. Various mustards (*Brassica* spp.), horseradish *(Amoracia lapathifolia),* and protoanemonin from the buttercup family (Ranunculaceae) induce gastroenteritis.

Essential oils, often found in combination with resins (oleoresins), are extracted commercially for use as rubifacients, salves, and liniments. Essential oils are mentioned here to warn of their extreme toxicity and to condemn their use as folk medicines.

Methyl salicylate, or wintergreen, is the methyl ester of salicylic acid, derived from *Gaultheria procumbens.* It was widely used as an antirheumatic agent in the nineteenth century but fell into disfavor because of its extreme side effects and the availability of more effective acetylsalicylic acid.[13]

Poisoning now occurs most often in children who are attracted to the color, smell, and flavor of wintergreen oil, resulting in the usual features of salicylism, including central nervous system excitation, hyperventilation, hyperthermia, and metabolic acidosis.

The structures of salicylic acid and methyl salicylate follow:

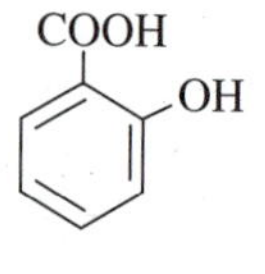

COOH, OH — **Salicylic acid**

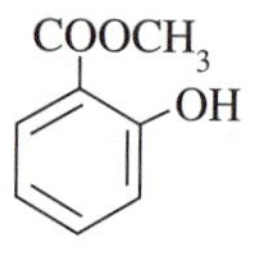

$COOCH_3$, OH — **Methyl salicylate**

Pulegone, an essential oil, is the primary component in pennyroyal oil derived from *Hedeoma pulegioides* or *Mentha pulegium.* As an herbal medicine, it has been used as an over-the-counter abortifacient.[13] One of us (E.G.) observed a patient in the emergency department who had ingested 1 ounce of pennyroyal oil. Initial signs of urticaria, bronchospasm, and delirium progressed to disseminated intravascular coagulation, hepatic necrosis, and death within 4 days.[71]

Hypoglycemic Agents. Eating unripe Caribbean akee fruit *(Blighia sapida)* produces a unique metabolic effect. Hypoglycin A, the toxic component, blocks hepatic gluconeogenesis, resulting in hypoglycemia. It also interferes with long-chain fatty acid oxidation.[32] The latter is mediated by the metabolite methylenecyclopropylacetyl-coenzyme A and results in the accumulation of short-chain fatty acids, which is thought to contribute to observed central nervous system depression.[8]

Vomiting and mental status depression are the principal clinical features, accounting for the early designation "Jamaican vomiting sickness."[8] Onset begins promptly after ingestion, and deaths are frequent without adequate supportive care. Mortality ranges from 40% to 80%.

Treatment consists of activated charcoal to absorb the toxin, intravenous fluid replacement, frequent blood glucose determinations, and serum electrolyte measurements. Two 50 ml boluses of 50% dextrose are given, followed by a 10% dextrose infusion until repeated blood glucose estimations show normalization. Glycine has been advocated as an effective treatment in akee poisoning. The mechanism of action is thought to be inhibition of long-chain fatty acid oxidation blockade. Glycine therapy must be considered experimental at this stage.[70]

Licorice. A unique feature of licorice is that chronic excessive ingestion of the natural candy can cause a type of pseudoaldosteronism, with hypertension and hypokalemic alkalosis. Glycyrrhizin may mimic the action of aldosterone, leading to retention of sodium and free water and excretion of potassium. Heart failure and cardiac arrest have been attributed to licorice root ingestion.[1] Myopathy with reversible myoglobinuria and muscular weakness has been reported.[13,56]

Treatment consists of removing the offending agent from the diet. Commonly available "licorice" candies manufactured in the United States usually do not contain true licorice, *Glycyrrhiza glabra.*

Element and Nitrate Absorption. Many plants absorb or accumulate metallic compounds (selenium, molybdenum, arsenic, lead, cadmium), nitrites, and nitrates. They are generally of little importance in humans and constitute a danger only to grazing livestock. However, there are numerous case reports of methemoglobinemia in infants caused by the ingestion of vegetables high in nitrate content. Vegetables cited include spinach, beets, cabbage, and carrots grown in high-nitrate soils. Nitrates are converted to nitrites in the infant gastrointestinal system.[30]

Soluble Oxalates. Soluble oxalates found in the leaves of the common garden plant rhubarb *(Rheum rhaponticum)* are rapidly absorbed through the gastrointestinal tract and cause a prompt drop in serum-ionized calcium level. There appears to be a generalized disturbance of monovalent and divalent cation metabolism. Weakness, tetany, hypotension, and seizures may develop.

Acute renal failure may occur if calcium oxalate precipitates in urine and obstructs the renal tubules. Adjacent epithelial cells become necrotic on contact with the precipitate. Ureteral calculi may be formed.[33,34]

Treatment consists of removal of stomach contents and gastric lavage with 0.15% calcium hydroxide solution to precipitate the soluble oxalates. Sodium bicarbonate should not be used in the lavage fluid because of the formation of sodium oxalate, a toxic compound that may be rapidly absorbed. Intravenous calcium gluconate is indicated in the face of tetany, a prolonged QT interval on electrocardiogram, or depressed serum ionized calcium levels. From 10 to 20 ml of 10% calcium gluconate should be given intravenously over 10 to 15 minutes, followed by additional doses titrated to blood levels and symptoms.[26] Every effort should be made to maintain a brisk diuresis in order to prevent deposition of calcium oxalate crystals in the renal tubules.

The structure of oxalates is shown below:

COOH
|
COOH

Oxalic acid

COOK
|
COOH

Potassium oxalate

COONa
|
COONa

Sodium oxalate

APPENDIX A

Plants: Toxic Principles and Therapeutics

Common Name	Genus	Species	Poisonous Principle	Toxic Parts	Distribution*	Section† Therapeutic Reference
Akee	*Blighia*	*sapida*	Hypoglycin	Fruit wall, seeds, white aril	II, S. Fla., Carib.	Hypoglycemic agents
Anemone	*Anemone*	spp.	Protoanemonin	All parts	II	Irritant and essential oils
Angel's trumpet	*Datura*	*sauveolens*	Atropine, hyoscyamine, hyoscine	Leaves, flowers	II, VI, S.E. U.S., Hi.	Tropane alkaloids
Apple of Peru	*Nicandra*	*physalodes*	Unknown	Leaves, berries	I	General considerations
Apple seeds	*Malus*	spp.	Cyanogenic glycosides	Seeds	III	Cyanogenic glycosides
Apricot pits	*Prunus*	spp.	Cyanogenic glycosides	Pits	II	Cyanogenic glycosides
Arnica	*Arnica*	*montana fulgens*	Unknown	Flowers, roots	II, N. U.S., Can.	General considerations
Autumn crocus	*Colchicum*	*autumnale*	Colchicine	Seeds, corms	II	Amine alkaloids
Azalea	(See *Rhododendron*)					
Balsam pear	*Mamordica*	*balsimia*	Saponic glycoside	Seeds, wall of fruit	I, coastal Fla. to Tex.	Saponin glycosides
Baneberry	*Actaea*	spp.	Protoanemonin, unknown glycosides	Berries, rootstock	I, widely except S.W.	Irritant and essential oils
Beech	*Fagus*	spp.	Saponic glycoside	Nuts	III	Saponin glycoside
Belladonna	(See deadly nightshade)					
Bellyache bush	*Jatropha*	*gossypiifolia*	Curcin	Fruit, seeds, sap	I, V	Phytotoxins
Betel nut	*Areca*	*catechu*	Arecoline, arecaine	Seeds	II, Fla., Hi.	Pyridine-piperidine group
Bird of paradise	*Poinciana*	*gillesii*	Unknown	Green seed pods	II	General considerations
Black cherry	*Prunus*	*serotina*	Cyanogenic glycoside	Bark, leaves, seeds, "tea" of leaves	I, E. N.A.	Cyanogenic glycosides
Black locust	*Robinia*	*pseudoacacia*	Robin, robitin (glycoside)	Inner bark, young leaves, seeds	I, S. Can., E. N.A., Mid. W., roadsides	Phytotoxins
Black nightshade	*Solanum*	*nigrum*	Solanine	Unripened fruit	I, widely, roadsides	Steroid alkaloids
Black snake root	(See death camas)					
Bleeding heart	(See dicentra)					
Bloodroot	*Sanguinaria*	*canadensis*	Sanguinarine	All parts	I	Isoquinoline and quinoline group
Blister bush	*Phebolium*	*anceps*	Unknown	Leaves, fruit	I	General considerations
Blue cohosh	*Caulophyllum*	*thalactroides*	Unknown	Seeds, rootstock	I	General considerations
Boxwood	*Buxus*	*sempervirens*	Buxine, volatile oil	Leaves, twigs	II, V	Alkaloids, irritant and essential oils
Brazilian pepper, also: pink or red peppercorn, Florida holly	*Schinus*	*terebinthifolius*	Unknown	Berries, leaves, flowers	I, Fla.	General considerations
Broom, also: Scotch broom	*Cytisus*	*scoparius*	Cytisine	Branches	VI	Quinolizidine alkaloids

Buckeye	*Aesculus*	spp.	Aesculin	Leaves, flowers, young sprouts, seeds	III, widely	Coumarin glycosides
Buckthorn	*Rhamnus*	*cathartica, frangula*	Anthraquinones	Berries, leaves, bark	I, VI	Anthraquinone glycosides
Burning bush	*Euonymus*	spp.	Unknown	Leaves, bark, seeds	III	General considerations
Bushman's poison	*Acokanthera*	spp.	Ouabain, G-strophanthin, acokantherin	All	I	Cardiac glycosides
Buttercup	*Ranunculus*	spp.	Protoanemonin	All parts	III	Irritant and essential oils
Caladium	*Caladium*	spp.	Oxalates	Leaves	II, IV	Oxalates
Candle nut	(See lumbang nut)					
Caper spurge	*Euphorbia*	*lathyris*	Unknown alkaloid	Milky sap throughout plant	II	General considerations
Carolina jessamine, also: yellow jessamine	*Gelsemium*	*sempervirens*	Gelsemine, sempervirine	All parts	II	Psychoactive plants
Cassava, also: manioc, tapioca	*Manihot*	*esculenta*	Cyanogenic glycoside	Raw root	II, VI	Cyanogenic glycosides
Castor bean	*Ricinis*	*communis*	Ricin	Seeds	III	Phytotoxins
Catnip	*Nepeta*	*cataria*	Acetic, butyric and valeric acids, nepetalic acid, limonene	Leaves	VI	Psychoactive plants
Chalice vine	*Solandra*	*nitida*	(See trumpet flower)		II	
Cherry	*Prunus*	spp.	Cyanogenic glycoside	Pits	II	Cyanogenic glycosides
Chinaberry tree	*Melia*	*azederach*	Unknown resin	Fruit, tea from leaves	III	Resins
Christmas rose	*Helleborus*	*niger*	Hellebrin, helleborin, helleborein	Rootstocks and leaves	II	Cardiac glycosides
Clematis	*Clematis*	spp.	Steroid alkaloids	Seeds, young plants	II, widely	Steroid alkaloids
Coca	*Erythoxylon*	*coca*	Ecogonine	Extract of leaves	VI	Psychoactive plants
Coontie	*Zamia*	*floridana*	Unknown alkaloid	Fleshy seeds	II, S. U.S., Hi.	General considerations
Coral plant	*Jatropha*	*multifida*	Curcin	Fruit, seeds, sap of all parts	III, S. Fla. to Tex., Hi.	Phytotoxins
Corn cockle	*Agrostemma*	*githago*	Githagenin, sapogenin	All parts, especially seeds	I	Saponin glycosides
Cotoneaster	*Cotoneaster*	spp.	Unknown	Berries	II	General considerations
Coyotillo	*Karwinskia*	*humboldtiana*	Unknown	Fruit, seeds	I, S.W. U.S.	General considerations
Crepe jasmine	*Ervatamia*	*coronaria*	Unknown	Leaves, flowers	II	General considerations
Crownflower	*Calotropis*	*gigantea*	Unknown	All parts	II, V	General considerations
Crown of thorns	*Euphorbia*	spp.	Unknown alkaloid	Milky sap throughout plant	II, widely	General considerations

Continued.

Plants: Toxic Principles and Therapeutics—cont'd

Common Name	Genus	Species	Poisonous Principle	Toxic Parts	Distribution*	Section† Therapeutic Reference
Cup of gold	*Solandra*	*cuttata*	Solanine-like alkaloids	Leaves, flowers	II	Steroid alkaloids
Cycads	(See coontie)					
Cypress spurge	*Euphorbia*	*cyparissias*	Unknown alkaloids	Milky sap throughout plant	II	General considerations
Daffodils	*Narcissus*	spp.	Lycorine	Bulb	II	General considerations
Daphne	*Daphne*	*mezereum*	Dihydroxycoumarin, diterpene mezerein	Bark, leaves, fruit	II	Coumarin glycosides
Day jessamine	*Cestrum*	*diurnum*	Tropane alkaloids	All parts	III, Fla., Hi.	Tropane alkaloids
Deadly nightshade	*Atropa*	*belladonna*	Atropine	All parts, black berries	I	Tropane alkaloids
Death camas, also: black snakeroot	*Zigadenus*	spp.	Zygacine, zygadenine	Bulb	I, widely	Steroid alkaloids
Delphiniums	*Delphinium*	spp.	Delphinine, ajacine	Seeds, young plants	III	Steroid alkaloids
Desert potato	*Jatropha*	macrorhiza	Phytotoxin	Plant root	I	Phytotoxins
Devil's trumpet, also: hairy thorn apple	*Datura*	*metel*	Atropine, hyoscyamine, hyoscine	Leaves, flowers	II, VI, Coastal Fla. to Tex.	Tropane alkaloids hyoscine
Dicentra, also: bleeding heart, Dutchman's breeches	*Dicentra*	spp.	Protopine, apomorphine, protoberberine	All parts	I, widely	Isoquinoline and quinoline group
Dieffenbachia, also: dumbcane	*Dieffenbachia*	spp.	Oxalate, asparagine	Leaves	II, IV	Oxalates
Dogbane, also: Indian hemp	*Apocynum*	*cannabium*	Cymarin	Flowers, seeds, leaves	I, widely, roadsides	Cardiac glycosides
Duranta	(See sky flowers)					
Elderberry	*Sambucus*	spp.	Unknown alkaloids	Unripe berries, leaves, wood	III, all N.A. except Pac. Coast	General considerations
Elephant ear	*Colocasia*	*antiquorum*	Oxalates	Leaves	IV	Oxalates
English bean	(See fava bean)					
English ivy	*Hedera*	*helix*	Hederogenin	Berries and leaves	II, IV, V	Saponin glycosides
False hellebore, also: Indian poke	*Veratrum*	spp.	Veratrin	Leaves	I, E. N.A., Minn.	Steroid alkaloids
False sago palm	*Cycas*	*circinalis*	Alkaloids	Seeds	II, V, S. U.S., Hi.	General considerations
Fava bean	*Vicia*	*faba*	Hemolytic anemia in glucose-6-phosphate deficiency	Bean	II	General considerations
Finger cherry	*Rhodomyrtus*	*macrocarpa*	Saponin	Fruit	S. Pacific	Saponin glycosides
Fool's parsley	*Aethusa*	*cynapium*	Unknown	Leaves	I	General considerations
Four o'clock	*Mirabilis*	*jalapa*	Unknown	Roots or seeds	II	General considerations
Foxglove	*Digitalis*	*purpurea*	Digitoxin, gitaloxin, gitoxin	Leaves	III, W. U.S.	Cardiac glycosides

Ginseng	*Panax*	*quinque-folium*	Saponin glycosides	Root	VI	Saponin glycosides
	Panax	*ginseng*				
Glory lily	*Gloriosa*	*superba*	Colchicine-like alkaloids, superbine	Rhizomes	II	Amine alkaloids
Golden chain, also: golden rain	*Laburnum*	*anagyroides*	Cytisine	Flowers, seeds	II, N. U.S., S. Can.	Quinolizidine alkaloids
Golden seal	*Hydrastis*	*canadensis*	Steroid alkaloids	Seeds, young plants	I, N.E. U.S., VI	Steroid alkaloids
Ground cherry	*Physalis*	spp.	Unknown	Leaves, unripe fruit	I, widely	General considerations
Hill gooseberry	*Rhodomyrtus*	*tomentosa*	None—N. A. nontoxic (*Rhodomyrtus* spp.)		II, N. Am.	—
Holly	*Ilex*	spp.	Ilicin	Berries	III, V	General considerations
Horse chestnut	*Aesculus*	spp.	Aesculin	Sprouts, mature nuts	II	Coumarin glycosides
Horseradish	*Amoracia*	*rusticana*	Mustard oil	Roots	II	Irritant and essential oils
Horse bean	(See fava bean)					
Horse nettle, also: wild tomato	*Solanum*	*carolinense*	Solanine	Fruit	I, widely	Steroid alkaloids
Hyacinth	*Hyacinthus*	*orientalis*	Narcissine-like alkaloids	Bulb	II, IV	General considerations
Hyacinth bean	*Dolichos*	*lablab*	Cyanogenic glycosides	Pods, seeds	II	Cyanogenic glycosides
Hydrangea	*Hydrangea*	spp.	Cyanogenic glycosides	Leaves, buds	III	Cyanogenic glycosides
Inkberry	(See pokeweed)					
Iris (blue flag)	*Iris*	*versicolor*	Irisin, irigenin, iridin	Flowers, leaves	III	Resins
Jack-in-the-pulpit	*Arisaema*	spp.	Oxalate	Rhizome	I, N.E. U.S.	Oxalates
Jequirty pea, also: rosary pea, precatory bean	*Abrus*	*precatorius*	Abrin	Beans	I, V	Phytotoxins
Jerusalem cherry	*Solanum*	*pseudocapsicum*	Solanine	Fruit	II, V, widely	Steroid alkaloids
Jessamine	(See Carolina jessamine)					
Jessamines	*Cestrum*	spp.	Tropane alkaloids	All parts	III	Tropane alkaloids
Jetbead	*Rhodotypus*	*tetrapetala*	Cyanogenic glycosides	Berries	II, N. U.S.	Cyanogenic glycosides
Jimson weed	*Datura*	*stramonium*	Atropine, hyoscyamine, hyoscine	Leaves, flowers	I, VI	Tropane alkaloids
Jonquil	(See daffodil)					
Kentucky coffee tree	*Gymnocladus*	*dioica*	Cytisine	Seeds, pulp	III, E. N.A., Okla.	Quinolizidine alkaloids
Lantana	*Lantana*	*camara*	Lantanin, lantadene A	Unripe fruit	II, N. U.S., S.E. U.S.	General considerations
Larkspur	(See delphinium)					
Laurel	(See mountain laurel)					
Lignum vitae	*Guaiacum*	*officinale*	Unknown	Resin in wood and fruit	II, S. Fla., S. Cal., Hi.	General considerations

Continued.

Plants: Toxic Principles and Therapeutics—cont'd

Common Name	Genus	Species	Poisonous Principle	Toxic Parts	Distribution*	Section† Therapeutic Reference
Lily of the valley	*Convallaria*	*majalis*	Convallotoxin, convallarin, convallamarin	Rhizome, leaves, flowers	II, widely	Cardiac glycosides
Lobelia also: Indian tobacco	*Lobelia*	spp.	Lobelamine, lobeline	All parts	III, IV, VI	Pyridine-piperidine group
Lumbang nut	*Aleurites*	*trisperma*	(See tung oil tree)			
Manchineel tree	*Hippomane*	*mancinella*	Unknown	Milky sap	I	General considerations
Mandrake, also: Satan's apple	*Mandragora*	*officinarum*	Hyoscyamine, Scopolamine	Rhizome	VI	Tropane alkaloids
Marijuana, also: grass, dope, pot, ganja, pokololo	*Cannabis*	*sativa*	Tetrahydrocannabinol	Leaves	III, VI	Psychoactive plants
Mayapple	*Podophyllum*	*peltatum*	Podophyllotoxin	All parts except ripe fruit	I, widely	General considerations
Mescal bean	*Sophora*	*secundiflora*	Unknown alkaloids	Seeds	III, VI	General considerations
Mexican prickly poppy	(See prickly poppy)					
Milk bush, also: pencil tree	*Euphorbia*	*tirucallii*	Unknown alkaloids	Milky sap throughout plant	I	General considerations
Mistletoe (American)	*Phoradendron*	*serotinum*	Toxalbumin	Berries	I, V	General considerations
Mistletoe (European)	*Viscum*	*album*	Viscumin	Berries	I, V	General considerations
Monkshood, also: aconite, wolfsbane	*Aconitum*	spp.	Aconitine	All parts, especially roots	III	Steroid alkaloids
Moonseed	*Menispermum*	*canadense*	Dauricine	Berries	I	Isoquinoline and quinoline group
Morning glory	*Ipomoea*	*violacea*	*d*-Lysergic acid amide	Seeds	II, VI	Psychoactive plants
Mountain ash	*Sorbus*	spp.	Unknown	Berries	I	General considerations
Mountain laurel	*Kalmia*	*latifolia*	Andromedotoxin, arbutin, grayanotoxins	All parts	III	Steroid alkaloids
Narcissus	(See jonquil)					
Night-blooming jasmine	*Cestrum*	spp.	Tropane alkaloids	All parts	I, S. U.S.	Tropane alkaloids
Nightshade, also: woody nightshade, climbing nightshade, bittersweet	*Solanum*	*dulcamara*	Solanine	Fruit	I, V, widely	Steroid alkaloids
Nutmeg	*Myristica*	*fragrans*	Myristicine	Nut	VI	Psychoactive plants
Oak	*Quercus*	spp.	Tannin, unknown	Acorns	III, S.W.	General considerations
Ochrosia plum	*Ochrosia*	*elliptica*	Unknown	Fruit	II, Fla., Hi.	General considerations
Oleander	*Nerium*	*oleander*	Oleandrin oleandroside, nevioside	All parts	II, S. U.S., Cal., Hi., roadsides	Cardiac glycosides
Peach pits	*Prunus*	spp.	Cyanogenic glycosides	Pits	II, widely	Cyanogenic glycosides

Peyote	*Lophophora*	*williamsii*	Mescaline, lophophorine	Seeds, buttons	I, S. Tex.	General considerations, psychoactive plants
Philodendron	*Philodendron*	spp.	Oxalate	Leaves	IV	Oxalates
Physic nut also: purge nut	*Jatropha*	*curcas*	Curcin	Fruit, seeds	II	Phytotoxins
Pigeonberry	(See pokeweed)					
Plum pit	*Prunus*	spp.	Cyanogenic glycosides	Pit	II, widely	Cyanogenic glycosides
Poinsettia	*Euphorbia*	*pulcherrima*	Unknown alkaloid	Milky sap throughout plant	II, V	General considerations
Poison hemlock	*Conium*	*maculatum*	Coniine	Seeds, roots, young leaves	I	Pyridine-piperidine group
Pokeweed also: pokeberry, Virginia poke, scoke, garget, inkberry, caokum, American cancer, cancer jalap	*Phytolacca*	*americana*	Triterpene saponins	All parts	I	Saponin glycosides
Pongam	*Pongammia*	*pinnata*	Unknown	Seeds, roots	II, S. Fla., S. Cal., Hi.	General considerations
Potato	*Solanum*	*tuberosum*	Solanine	Unripe tubers	II, widely	Steroid alkaloids
Prickly poppy	*Argemone*	spp.	Sanguinarine, berberine, protopine	All parts, especially seeds	III, VI	Isoquinoline and quinoline group
Privet	*Ligustrum*	*vulgare, japonicum*	Unknown glycoside	Berries, leaves	II, widely	General considerations
Purge nut	(See physic nut)					
Rattlebox, also: coffee bean, sesbane, coffeeweed, rattlebrush	*Sesbania*	spp.	Saponins	Seeds, flowers	III, V, S.E. coastal	Saponin glycosides
Rayless goldenrod	*Haplopappus*	*heterophyllus*	Tremetol	The milk of cows grazing on this plant	I	Irritant and essential oils
Rhododendron, also: laurel, azalea	*Rhododendron*	spp.	Grayanotoxins	All parts	III, E. N.A., Pac. Coast	Steroid alkaloids
Rhubarb	*Rheum*	*rhabarbarum*	Oxalates	Leaves	II	Oxalates
Rock poppy	*Chelidonium*	*majus*	Sanguinarine, berberine, protopine	Leaves, seeds	I, E. N.A.	Isoquinoline and quinoline group
Rubber vine	*Cryptostegia*	*grandiflora*	Unknown	All parts	II, V, S. U.S., Hi.	General considerations
Sandbox tree	*Hura*	*crepitans*	Unknown	Milky sap	II, S. U.S.	General considerations
Senecio, also: threadleaf, groundsel	*Senecio*	*longilobus*	Pyrrolizidine alkaloids	Entire plant	I, VI	Pyrrolizidine alkaloids
Sky flower	*Duranta*	*repens*	Saponin	Berries	I	Saponin glycosides

Continued.

Plants: Toxic Principles and Therapeutics—cont'd

Common Name	Genus	Species	Poisonous Principle	Toxic Parts	Distribution*	Section† Therapeutic Reference
Snow-on-the-mountain	*Euphorbia*	spp.	Unknown alkaloids	Milky sap throughout plant	II	General considerations
Spring adonis	*Adonis*	*vernalis*	Steroid alkaloids	Seeds, young plants	II	Steroid alkaloids
Spurge	*Euphorbia*	spp.	Unknown alkaloids	Milky sap	III	General considerations
Squill	*Drimia*	*maritima*	Cardiac glycosides	Bulbs	II, S. Cal., S.W.	Cardiac glycosides
Star of Bethlehem	*Ornithogalum*	*umbellatum*	Cardiac glycosides, amine alkaloids	All parts	III, V, E. N.A., Mid. W., Hi.	Cardiac glycosides, amine alkaloids
Strawberry bush	(See burning bush)					
Sweet pea	*Lathyrus*	spp.	β(λ-L-glutamyl)-aminopropionitrile, L considerations α, λ-diaminobutyric acid	Peas	III	General considerations
Tobacco	*Nicotiana*	*tabacum*	Nicotine	Leaves	II, VI	Pyridine-piperidine group
Tomato	*Lycopersicon*	*esculenta*	Solanine	Leaves	II	Steroid alkaloids
Tree tobacco	*Nicotiana*	*glauca*	Anabasine	All parts	I, S.W., Hi., Carib.	Pyridine-piperidine group
Trumpet flower	*Solandra*	spp.	Solanine-like	Leaves, flowers	II	Steroid alkaloids
Trumpet lily	*Datura*	*arborea*	Atropine, hyoscyamine, hyoscine	Flowers, leaves	II, VI	Tropane alkaloids
Tulip bulb	*Tulipa*	*gesnariana*	Unknown	Bulb	II	General considerations
Tung oil tree	*Aleurites*	*fordii*	Saponins	Seed	II	Saponin glycosides
Virginia creeper, also: woodbine, American ivy	*Parthenocissus*	*quinquefolia*	Unknown	Berries	I, E. N.A., S.W.	General considerations
Water hemlock	*Cicuta*	*maculata*	Cicutoxin	Roots	I, widely in swamps	Resins
White snakeroot	*Eupatorium*	*rugosum*	Tremetol	The milk of cows grazing on this plant	I, N. Car., Ill., Ind., Oh.	Irritant and essential oils
Wild balsam apple	*Mamordia*	*charantia*	Saponin glycoside	Seeds and wall of fruit	I	Saponin glycosides
Wild cherry	(See black cherry)					
Wisteria	*Wisteria*	spp.	Resin	Seeds	II	Resin, general considerations
Woody nightshade	(See nightshade)					
Yellow allamanda	*Allamanda*	*cathartica*	Unknown	Fruit	II, S. U.S., Hi.	General considerations
Yellow jessamine	(See Carolina jessamine)					
Yellow nightshade, also: Wild allamanda	*Urechite*	spp.	Unknown	Seed pods	I, S. Fla.	General considerations

Yellow oleander also: Lucky nut	*Thevetia*	*peruviana*	Thevetin, thevetoxin	Flowers, seeds, leaves	II, Hi.	Cardiac glycosides
Yew	*Taxus*	spp.	Taxine	Berries	III, V., E. N.A., Pac. Coast	Steroid alkaloids

*Distribution key:

I Native or naturalized; found in fields, woods, and roadsides.
II Cultivated; found in gardens and yards.
III Found in both I and II.
IV Common houseplants.
V Found in decorations or as seasonal ornamentals.
VI Found in herbal or folk remedies or used for mood alteration.

Can.	Canada
Carib.	Caribbean
Coastal Fla. to Tex.	Coastal Florida to Texas
E. N.A.	Eastern North America
Fla.	Florida
Hi.	Hawaii
Ill.	Illinois
Ind.	Indiana
Mid. W.	Midwestern United States
Minn.	Minnesota
N.A.	North America
N. Car.	North Carolina
N.E. U.S.	Northeastern United States
N. U.S.	Northern United States
Oh.	Ohio
Pac. Coast	Pacific Coast States
Roadsides	Roadsides, waste areas, and swamps
S. Cal.	Southern California
S. Can.	Southern Canada
S.E. Coastal	Southeastern Coastal Plain
S.E. U.S.	Southeastern United States
S. Fla.	Southern Florida
S. Tex.	Southern Texas
S.W.	Southwestern United States
Widely	Distributed throughout the United States

†See appropriate section in text.

APPENDIX B

Nontoxic Plants*

African violet *(Saint pauliaionantha)*
Air plant *(Kalanchoe pinnata)*
Aluminum plant *(Pilea cadierei)*
Aralia, false *(Dizygotheca elegantissima)*
Aralia, Japanese *(Fatsia japonica)*
Asparagus fern *(Asparagus plumosus),* berry
Baby's breath *(Gypsophilia paniculata)*
Baby's tears *(Helxine* or *Soleirolia soleirolii)*
Begonia *(Begonia rex)*
Bird of paradise* *(Strelitzia reginae)*
Birdsnest fern *(Asplenium nidus)*
Boston fern *(Nephrolepsis exaltata bostoniensis)*
Bromeliad family
California poppy *(Eschscholzia californica)*
Camelia *(Camellia japonica)*
Chinese evergreen *(Aglaonema modestrum)*
Christmas cactus *(Schlumbergera bridgesii)*
Coffee tree *(Coffee arabica)*
Coleus
Cornstalk plant *(Dracaena fragrans)*
Coral berry* *(Aechamea fulgens, Ardisia crispa)*
Crape myrtle *(Lagerstromea indica)*
Creeping Charlie* *(Pilea nummularifolia)*
Crocus*—spring-blooming only
Croton* *(Codiaeum variegatum)*
Dahlia
Dandelion *(Taraxacum officinale)*
Dogwood *(Cornus)*
Donkey's tail *(Sedum morganianum)*
Dragon tree *(Dracaena draco, marginata)*
Easter cactus *(Schlumbergera bridgesii)*
Easter lily *(Lilium longiflorum)*
Echeveria: Mexican snowball, painted lady, plush plant
Emerald ripple *(Peperomia caperata)*
Fiddleleaf fig *(Ficus lyrata)*
Weeping fig tree *(Ficus benjamina)*
Forget-me-not *(Myosotis alpestris, sylvatica)*
Forsythia
Fuchsia
Gardenia
Geranium* *(Pelargonium)*
Gloxinia *(Sinningia speciosa)*
Grape ivy *(Cissus rhombifolia)*
Hawaiian ti plant *(Cordyline terminalis)*
Hawthorne *(Crataegus),* berry
Heavenly bamboo *(Nandina domestica),* berry
Hibiscus
Honeysuckle berry *(Lonicera)*
Ice plant
Impatiens walleriana
Jade plant *(Crassula argentea)*
Jasmine *(Jasminum rex),* Madagascar jasmine
Kalanchoe: maternity plant, monkey plant, panda bear plant
Lace plant, Madagascar *(Aponogeton senetralis)*
Lady, Lady's Slipper *(Cypripedium, Paphiopedilum)*
Lily-of-the-nile *(Agapanthus)*
Lipstick plant *(Aeschynanthus radicans)*
Maidenhair fern *(Adiantum)*
Marigold, African/American/tall *(Tagetes)*
Moon cactus *(Gymnocalycium)*
Mother-in-law's tongue or snake plant *(Sansevieria trifasciata)*
Mother of pearls *(Grapetopetalum paraguayense)*
Nandina berry
Natal plum *(Carissa grandiflora)*
Norfolk Island pine *(Araucaria heterophylla)*
Old man cactus *(Cephalocereus senilis)*
Olive tree *(Olea europaea)*
Orchid *(Cattleya, Cymbidium, Oncidium)*
Oregon grape *(Mahonia aquifolium)*
Palm: Bamboo *(Chamaedorea erumpeus),*
Paradise *(Howea* or *Kentia forsterana),*
Parlor *(Chamaedorea elegans* or *Kentia),*
Sentry *(Howea belmoreana)*
Pansy flower *(Viola)*
Passion vine *(Passiflora)*
Peanut cactus *(Chamaecereus sylvestri)*
Pellionia
Peony flower *(Paeonia)*
Peperomia
Petunia
Phlox
Piggy-back plant *(Tolmiea menziesii)*
Pigmy date palm *(Phoenix roebelenii)*
Pocketbook *(Calceolaria herbeohybrida)*
Polka dot or freckle face plant *(Hypoestes sanguinolenta)*
Prayer plant *(Maranta leuconeura)*
Pussy willow *(Salix discolor)*
Pyracantha berry
Queen's tears *(Billbergia nutans)*
Rabbit's foot fern *(Davallia fejeensis)*
Raphiolepsis
Rainbow plant *(Billbergia saundersii)*
Rattlesnake plant *(Calathea insignis)*
Ribbon plant *(Dracaena sandriana)*
Rock rose *(Cistus)*
Rosary pearls *(Senecio rowleyanus)*
Rosary vine *(Ceropegia woodii)*
Roses *(Rosa)*
Rubber plant *(Ficus elastica)*
Schefflera plant *(Brassaia* or *Schefflera actinophylia)*
Sedum
Sensitive plant *(Mimosa pudica)*
Silver heart *(Peperomia marmorata)*
Snake plant or mother-in-law's tongue *(Sansevieria trifasciata)*

Snapdragon *(Antirrhinum majus)*
Spider plant *(Anthericum, Chlorophytum comosum)*
Staghorn fern *(Platycerium bifurcatum)*
Starfish flower *(Stapelia)*
String of beads* *(Senecio rowleyanus* and *herreianus)*
String of hearts *(Ceropegia woodii)*
Swedish ivy *(Plectranthus australis)*
Sword fern *(Nephrolepsis cordifolia, exaltata)*
Tahitian bridal veil *(Gibasis geniculata, Tripogandra multiflora)*
Umbrella tree *(Schefflera actinophylla)*
Vagabond plant *(Vriesea)*
Velvet plant, purple *(Gynura aurantiaca)*
Venus fly trap *(Dionaea muscipula)*
Violet *(Viola)*
Wandering Jew *(Tradescantia albiflora)*
Wandering Jew—Red and White *(Zebrina pendulla)*
Wax plant *(Hoya exotica)*
Yucca
Zebra plant *(Aphelandre squarrosa)*
Zinnia

From *Your guide to plant safety,* courtesy San Francisco Bay Area Regional Poison Center.
*Have not been reported to cause illness. An asterisk (*) indicates that other species may be toxic.

REFERENCES

1. Abramowicz M, editor: Toxic reactions to plant products sold in health food stores, *Med Lett* 21(7):29, 1979.
2. Alpin TEH: *Poisonous garden plants and other plants harmful to man in Australia,* Perth, Australia, 1976, Western Australia Department of Agriculture.
3. Anderson EF: *Peyote, the divine cactus,* Tucson, 1980, University of Arizona Press.
4. Applefeld JJ: A case of water hemlock poisoning, *JACEP* 8(10):401, 1979.
5. Arena JM, Hardin JW: *Human poisoning from native and cultivated plants,* ed 2, Durham, NC, 1974, Duke University Press.
6. Balint GA: Ricin: the toxic protein of castor oil seeds, *Toxicology* 2:77, 1974.
7. Bras G, Jelliffe DB, Stuart KL: Veno-occlusive disease of liver with non portal type of cirrhosis, occurring in Jamaica, *Arch Pathol* 57:285, 1954.
8. Bressler R: The unripe akee—forbidden fruit, *N Engl J Med* 295:500, 1976.
9. Buel LB, Culvenor CI, Dick AT: *The pyrrolizidine alkaloids—their chemistry, pathogenicity and other biologic properties,* Amsterdam, 1968, North Holland Publishing Co.
10. Catterall W: Neurotoxins that act on voltage sensitive sodium channels in excitable membranes, *N Rev Pharmacol Toxicol* 20:15, 1980.
11. Challoner KR, McCarron MM: Castor bean intoxication, *Ann Emerg Med* 19(10):1177, 1990.
12. Curry SC: Hydrogen cyanide and inorganic cyanide salts. In Sullivan JB, Kreiger JR, editors: *Hazardous materials toxicology,* Baltimore, 1992, Williams & Wilkins.
13. Duke JA: *CRC handbook of medicinal herbs,* Boca Raton, Fla, 1987, CRC Press.
14. Ellis MD, editor: *Dangerous plants, snakes, arthropods and marine life: toxicity and treatment,* Hamilton, Ill, 1975, Drug Intelligence Publications.
15. Emerson TS, Cisek JE: Methcathinone: a Russian designer amphetamine infiltrates the rural Midwest, *Ann Emerg Med* 22:1897, 1993.
16. Everist SL: *Poisonous plants of Australia,* Sydney, Australia, 1981, Angus & Robertson.
17. Fox DW et al: Pyrrolizidine (senecio) intoxication mimicking Reye syndrome, *J Pediatr* 93:980, 1978.
18. Frohne D, Pfander HJ: *A colour atlas of poisonous plants,* London, 1984, Wolfe.
19. Fuller TC, McClintock E: *Poisonous plants of California,* Berkeley, 1986, University of California Press.
20. Geehr EC: Management of hydrocarbon ingestions, *Topics Emergency Med* 1(3):97, 1979.
21. Goates MG, Escobar JI: "Gedankenlautwerden" and datura intoxication, *J Clin Psychiatry* 53:4, 1992.
22. Goldfrank L et al: The pernicious panacea: herbal medicine, *Hosp Physician* 64:64, 1982.
23. Goodman LS, Gilman A: *The pharmacological basis of therapeutics,* ed 8, New York, 1990, Pergamon Press.
24. Gowdy JM: Stramonium intoxication—review of symptomatology in 212 cases, *JAMA* 221:585, 1972.
25. Haymon J: Datura poisoning—the angel's trumpet, *J Pathol* 17:465, 1985.
26. Hoelzer M: Mushroom and plant ingestion. In Reisdorff ES, Roberts MR, Weigenstin JG, editors: *Pediatric emergency medicine,* Philadelphia, 1993, WB Saunders.
27. Kagen SL: *Aspergillus:* an inhalable contaminant of marijuana (letter), *N Engl J Med* 304:483, 1981.
28. Kalix P: Cathinone, a natural amphetamine, *Pharmacol Toxicol* 70:77, 1992.
29. Katzung BG: Introduction to autonomic pharmacology. In Katzung BG, editor: *Basic clinical pharmacology,* ed 5, Norwalk, Conn, 1992, Appleton & Lange.
30. Keating JP et al: Infantile methemoglobinemia caused by carrot juice, *N Engl J Med* 288:824, 1973.
31. Keats J: Ode to a nightingale. In Harmon W, editor: *The top five hundred poems,* New York, 1992, Columbia University Press.
32. Keeler RF: Toxins and teratogens of higher plants, *Lloydia* 38(1):56, 1975.
33. Kingsbury JM: *Poisonous plants of the United States and Canada,* Englewood Cliffs, NJ, 1964, Prentice-Hall.
34. Kingsbury JM: Phytotoxicology. I. Major problems associated with poisonous plants, *Clin Pharmacol Ther* 10(2):163, 1969.
35. Klein-Schwartz W, Oderda GM: Jimsonweed intoxication in adolescents and young adults, *Am J Dis Child* 138:737, 1984.
36. Kunkel DB: The toxic emergency: tobacco and friends, *Emerg Med* 17(19):142, 1985.
37. Kunkel DB: Poisonous plants. In Haddad LM, Winchester JF, editors: *Clinical management of poisoning and drug overdose,* ed 2, Philadelphia, 1990, WB Saunders.
38. Lampe KF: Rhododendrons, mountain laurel, and madhoney, *JAMA* 259:2009, 1988.
39. Landers D, Seppi K, Blaner W: Seizures and death on a white river float trip—report of water hemlock poisoning, *West J Med* 142:637, 1985.
40. Lavoie FW, Harris TM: Fatal nicotine ingestion, *J Emerg Med* 9:133, 1991.
41. Levy R: Jimson seed poisoning—a new hallucinogen on the horizon, *JACEP* 6:58, 1977.
42. Levy R: Arrhythmias following physostigmine administration in jimsonweed poisoning, *JACEP* 6:107, 1977.
43. Lewis WH: Reporting adverse reactions to herbal ingestants (letter), *JAMA* 240:109, 1978.
44. Lewis W, Elvin-Lewis MPF: *Medical botany: plants affecting man's health,* New York, 1977, John Wiley.
45. Litovitz T et al: 1992 annual report of the American Association of Poison Control Centers' toxic exposure surveillance system, *Am J Emerg Med* 11:494, 1993.

46. Lockey SD: Anaphylaxis from an Indian necklace (letter), *JAMA* 206:2900, 1968.
47. McGuigan MA: Nicotine, *Clin Toxicol Rev* 4:6, 1982.
48. Mendelson G: Datura intoxication (letter), *Med J Aust* 3:163, 1976.
49. Mendelson G: Treatment of hallucinogenic plant toxicity (letter), *Ann Intern Med* 85:126, 1976.
50. Mikolich JR, Paulson GW, Cross CJ: Acute anticholinergic syndrome due to jimson seed ingestion, *Ann Intern Med* 83:321, 1975.
51. Miranda CL et al: The microsomal function of a pyrrolic alcohol glutathione conjugate of the pyrollizidine alkaloid senecionine, *Xenobiotica* 22(11):1321, 1992.
52. Mitchell MI, Routledge PA: Poisoning by hemlock water dropwort (letter), *Lancet* 1:423, 1977.
53. Morton JF: *Plants poisonous to people in Florida and other warm areas,* Miami, 1971, Hurricane House.
54. Mrvos R et al: Philodendron/dieffenbachia ingestions: are they a problem? *Clin Toxicol* 29(4):485, 1991.
55. Mutter L: Poisoning by western water hemlock, *Can J Public Health* 67(5):386, 1976.
56. Nielsen I, Pedersen RS: Life-threatening hypokalemia caused by liquorice ingestion, *Lancet* 1(8389):1305, 1984.
57. Niyogi S: Elevation of enzyme levels in serum due to *Abrus precatorius* (jequirity bean) poisoning, *Toxicon* 15:577, 1977.
58. North DS, Nelson RB: Anticholinergic agents in cicutoxin poisoning (letter), *West J Med* 143:250, 1985.
59. Osterloh J, Herold S, Pond S: Oleander interference in the digoxin radioimmunoassay in a fatal ingestion, *JAMA* 247:1596, 1982.
60. Pentel P, Peterson C: Asystole complicating physostigmine treatment of tricyclic antidepressant overdose, *Ann Emerg Med* 9:588, 1980.
61. Quatrehomme G et al: Intoxication from *Veratrum album, Hum Exp Toxicol* 12:111, 1993.
62. Quek KC, Cheah JS: Poisoning due to ingestion of *Datura fastuosa, J Trop Med Hyg* 77:111, 1974.
63. Radford DJ et al: Naturally occurring glycosides, *Med J Aust* 144:540, 1986.
64. Roberge R et al: The root of evil—pokeweed intoxication, *Ann Emerg Med* 15:470, 1986.
65. Sayre JW, Kaymakcalan S: Cyanide poisoning from apricot seeds among children in central Turkey, *N Engl J Med* 270:1113, 1964.
66. Seldon BS, Curry SC: Anticholinergics. In Reisdorff EJ, Roberts MR, Wiegenstein JG, editors: *Pediatric emergency medicine,* Philadelphia, 1993, WB Saunders.
67. Shepard SM, Jagoda AS: Phenylcyclidine and the hallucinogens. In Haddad LM, Winchester JF, editors: *Clinical management of poisoning and drug overdose,* ed 2, Philadelphia, 1990, WB Saunders.
68. Shultes RE, Hoffman A: *The botany and chemistry of hallucinogens,* Springfield, 1973, Charles C Thomas.
69. Schultes RE, Hofmann A: *Plants of the gods,* Rochester, Vt, 1992, Healing Arts Press.
70. Sherratt HS, Al-Bassam SS: Glycine in akee poisoning (letter), *Lancet* 2:1243, 1976.
71. Sullivan JB et al: Pennyroyal oil poisoning and hepatotoxicity, *JAMA* 242:2873, 1979.
72. Taylor N: *Plant drugs that changed the world,* New York, 1965, Dodd, Mead.
73. Thompson HS: Cornpicker's pupil: jimson weed mydriasis, *J Iowa Med Soc* 61:475, 1971.
74. Tong TG, Benowitz NC, Becker C: Tricyclic antidepressant overdose, *Drug Int Clin Pharmacol* 10:711, 1976.
75. Vanderhoff BT, Mosser MD: Jimsonweed toxicity: management of anticholinergic plant ingestion, *Am Fam Physician* 46(2):526, 1992.
76. Wedin GP: Castor bean poisoning, *EMS,* September 1987, p 30-A-C.
77. Wedin GP et al: Castor bean poisoning, *Am J Emerg Med* 4:259, 1986.
78. Wenger T: The data on Digibind, *Emerg Med* 19(11):109, 1987.
79. Withering W: *An account of the foxglove and some of its medical uses,* London, 1785, Robinson.
80. Yavuz H et al: Honey poisoning in Turkey (letter), *Lancet* 337:789, 1991.

ADDITIONAL RECOMMENDED READINGS

Angier B: *Field guide to edible wild plants,* Harrisburg, Pa, 1974, Stackpole Books.

Frohne D, Pfander HJ: *A colour atlas of poisonous plants,* London, 1983, Wolfe.

Fuller TC, McClintock E: *Poisonous plants of California,* Berkeley, 1986, University of California Press.

Kingsbury JM: *Poisonous plants of the United States and Canada,* Englewood Cliffs, NJ, 1964, Prentice-Hall.

Lampe KF, McCann MA: *AMA handbook of poisonous and injurous plants,* Chicago, Ill, 1985, American Medical Association.

Lewis W, Elvin-Lewis MPF: *Medical botany: plants affecting man's health,* New York, 1977, John Wiley.

Morton J: *Plants poisonous to people in Florida and other warm areas,* Miami, 1971, Hurricane House.

Shultes RE, Hofmann A: *Plants of the gods: their sacred healing and hallucinogenic powers,* Rochester, Vt, 1992, Healing Arts Press.

38 MUSHROOM TOXICITY

Sandra M. Schneider

Had nature any outcast face?
Could she a son condemn?
Had nature an Iscariot
That mushroom—it is him.

Emily Dickinson

Mushrooms are often considered the vermin of the vegetable world, likened to snakes, slugs, worms, and spiders. Other times they are viewed as mystical or as delicacies. The locations of tasty morels are passed from generation to generation, closely guarded from strangers. Each autumn and spring, foragers scour the woods for delicacies known and others untried. Some persons search for "little brown mushrooms" for the hallucinations they induce.

There is real danger in eating unidentified or misidentified mushroom species. Each year, there are 10,000 to 15,000 cases of human mushroom toxicity in the United States.[52] In the vast majority of these cases (perhaps up to 95%), the mushroom was misidentified by the picker.[86] Over 40,000 species of fungi are currently described, and a few thousand new ones are added each year. Of these, only a relatively small number are toxic.

Fungi are simple plants without chlorophyll or green color. The fungus family contains molds, smuts, rusts, mildews, yeast, toadstools, and mushrooms. The term "mushroom" is generally reserved for nontoxic fungi; "toadstool" is used to describe toxic mushrooms. The body of a fungus is a dense network of branching filaments or hyphae. The mushroom we see is the fruiting body of the fungus, containing the spores. The hyphae and mycelia generally occur in an underground network supporting the visible mushroom. This network of mycelia is in part responsible for the pattern of the growing mushroom. Mushrooms (the fruits) emerge in large rings radiating from a central network of mycelia. In some cultures these were called fairy rings and believed to possess mystical powers. Fungi are largely saprophytic, living on decaying organic material and accelerating the decomposition of trees. A host tree derives nitrogen, phosphorus, and other nutrients from the fungus; the fungus receives moisture and protection from the tree.

As a mushroom emerges from the ground, it generally looks like a small button covered with a membrane or veil (Fig. 38-1). As the mushroom grows, the membrane breaks and leaves residual marks (warts) on the cap of the mushroom. The warts may be firmly attached to the mushroom or there may be only a hint of residual spots, depending on the species of mushroom and on environmental conditions. The emerging cap takes on a shape consistent with the specific species, ranging from cylindrical to convex to funnel shaped.

Gills, located under the caps, contain the spore-producing bodies. Some gills are covered with a second membrane or partial veil that protects the cap, later pulling away to form an annulus or ring midway down the mushroom stalk. Gills may be attached firmly to the stalk, run down the stalk, or be attached only to the cap itself (free gills) (Fig. 38-2). Gill attachment is an important aid to identification of some poisonous mushrooms, such as *Amanita phalloides*.

The stalk (stipe) begins at the cap and ends either underground or in a cup (volva). A cup or volva at ground level is often seen in poisonous species. The stalk is generally centrally located and enters the middle of the cap, although occasionally it is off center. It may or may not be tapered. The stalk of many poisonous species enlarges below the cap, ending in a bulb. The stalk may have a ringed membrane as evidence of the partial veil once protecting the gills. Spores are produced by spore-forming bodies on the gills and are expelled into the air after they mature.

Spores vary in size, color, and shape but are usually unicellular. They average 5 to 10 μm in diameter. Spores are useful in identifying mushroom species. They can be obtained by cutting the stalk of a fresh specimen close to the gills and laying the cap gill-side down on white paper for a few hours at room temperature. The initial color seen after removal of the gills is used for identification. With drying, the color may fade or change. Additional information about spores can be acquired by staining with Melzer's reagent (a

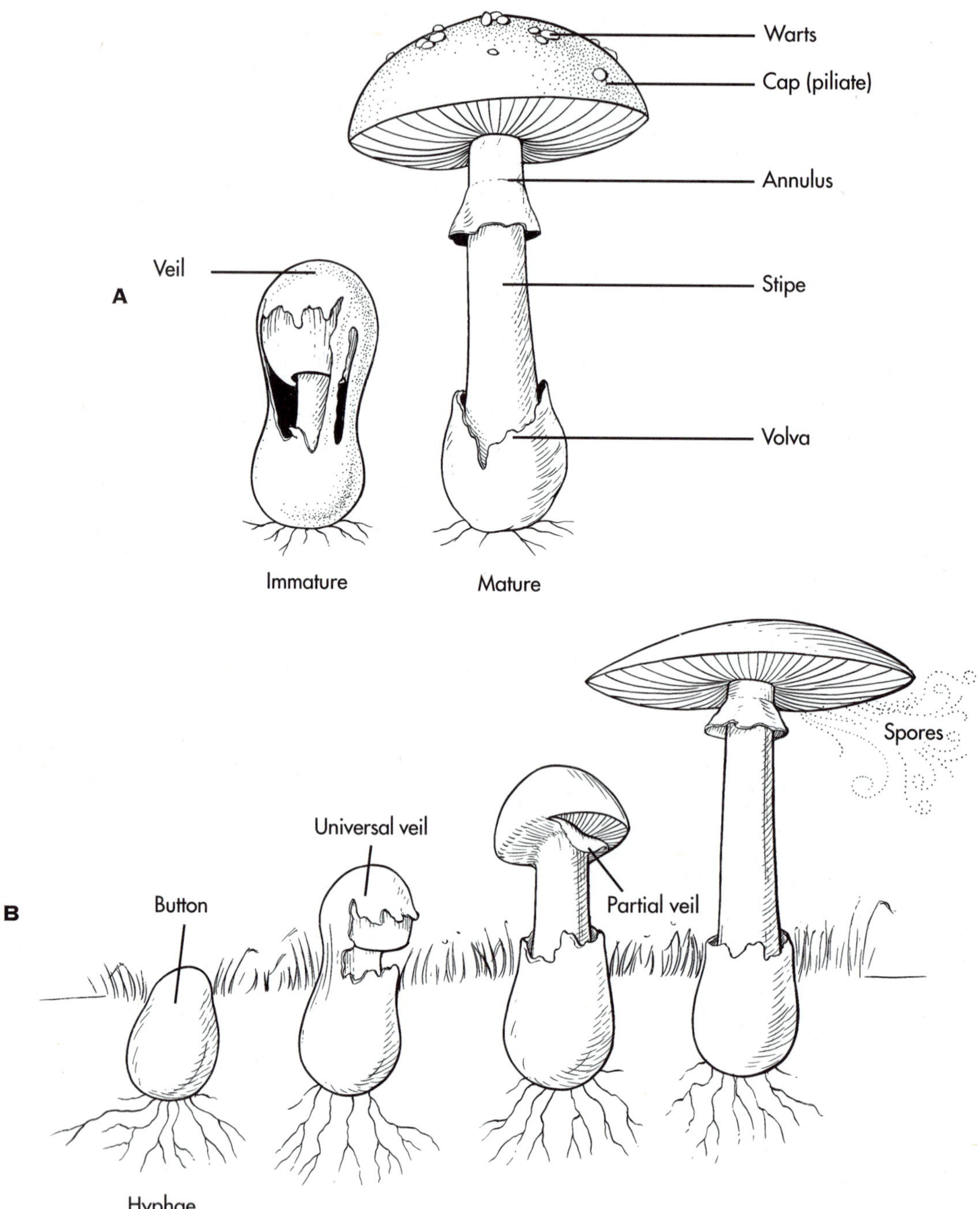

Fig. 38-1 **A,** Structural characteristics and, **B,** life cycle of mushrooms.

solution of iodine and chloral hydrate). Spores staining blue are called amyloid, indicating the presence of starch. This technique may be particularly useful in spore identification from gastric aspirates. The spores of *Amanita* species are amyloid. Thin-layer chromatography of spores is a more recent and more accurate aid to identification.

Mushrooms contain approximately 90% water and 3% proteins and other nitrogen-containing compounds. The remainder is largely carbohydrate, fat, and a few vitamins. Nutritionally unimpressive, mushrooms are consumed in great quantities, primarily for their taste and texture. Wild mushrooms have the additional allure of being free. Of the many varieties of wild mushrooms, few are deadly or cause serious pathophysiologic derangements.

Many immigrants to the United States fail to realize that the nontoxic mushrooms from their native lands have toxic look-alikes in the United States. This has been particularly true of Southeast Asian immigrants who are attracted to the

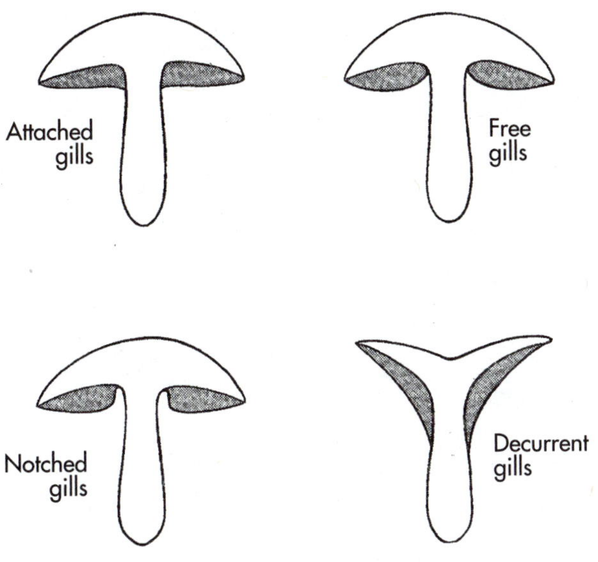

Fig. 38-2 Mushroom gill types.

large white *Amanita* species found on the West Coast. Entire families have been poisoned, with many fatalities. The Russian roulette played by mushroom foragers is statistically safe. Some self-proclaimed experts are simply lucky; occasionally they are not.

Nontoxic Mushrooms

The most common commercially available mushroom in the United States is *Agaricus bisporus*. It is cultivated in abandoned mine shafts and caves. This small white mushroom with dark gills is often picked before the gills are fully exposed. Although the mushroom is considered nontoxic, hypersensitivity reactions and gastrointestinal symptoms have been reported. Researchers have tried to link carcinogenesis to *A. bisporus*.[84] While tumors of the bone (osteomas, osteosarcomas) and stomach (papillomas and carcinomas) develop in mice fed large amounts of uncooked mushrooms, there is no direct link between human ingestion and cancer.[84]

A. bisporus can also be found in the wild. *Agaricus* species may be confused with the deadly *Amanita* species, as well as with some *Agaricus* species that cause gastrointestinal irritation. Nontoxic mushrooms may carry environmental toxins such as heavy metals and pesticides. Mushrooms with high lead concentrations have been gathered near highways.[49] High mercury concentrations are found in mushrooms from industrial sites.[49] Human toxicity has not been reported.

Mushrooms may cause allergic reactions. Acute anaphylaxis from mushroom ingestion is rare despite the presence of haptens capable of inciting an allergic response.[46] More often, symptoms develop from inhalation of spores.[62] Patients may present with anaphylaxis or, more commonly, with chronic hypersensitivity pneumonitis. Hypersensitivity reactions are described in workers exposed to cultivation of *A. bisporus* (the most popular commercially grown mushroom in the United States)[53] and shiitake *(Lentinus edodes)*, the popular Japanese mushroom.[73] Asthma symptoms developed in nearly 10% of shiitake-exposed workers.[79] In one study all workers had positive skin and inhalation-challenge tests.[79] Spore counts correlate with asthma symptoms.

Gastrointestinal symptoms after ingestion of mushrooms may not be due to toxins. Bacterial food poisoning may occur in foods that coincidentally contain mushrooms. Small bowel obstruction occurred in a patient who consumed 500 g of the edible mushroom *Cantharellus cibarius* (chanterelle).[31] This was largely a result of poor mastication, since entire mushrooms were recovered from his intestines.

Most wild mushrooms are nontoxic and many are delicious. Morels *(Morchella esculenta* or *deliciosa)* are highly prized delicacies. Chanterelles *(Cantharellus cibarius)* and several species of *Boletus* are particularly tasty. The chicken mushroom *(Laetiporus sulphures)* is often used in place of chicken in Chinese dishes.

Toxic Mushrooms

There are four major types of mushroom toxins: gastrointestinal toxins, disulfiram-like toxins, neurotoxins, and protoplasmic toxins.

GASTROINTESTINAL TOXINS

Most toxic mushrooms fall into the group of gastrointestinal irritants. This large, heterogeneous group of mushrooms causes gastrointestinal distress—nausea, vomiting, and diarrhea—beginning 1 to 2 hours after ingestion and resolving in 6 to 12 hours. Even *A. bisporus*, the common cultivated mushroom, may cause a brief gastroenteritis in some individuals.[80]

Causative Mushrooms

A large number of unrelated mushrooms (see Box 38-1) cause gastrointestinal symptoms with varying host response. *Chlorophyllum molybdites (Lepiota morganii)* (Color Plate 86) is the most frequently reported toxic mushroom ingested in the United States.[11,86] Most patients ingesting *C. molybdites* confuse it with *A. bisporus*, which it closely resembles. The common name for this species, green-spored parasol, describes the characteristics of this distinctive summer mushroom. The whitish cap is large (often 10 to 40 cm), initially smooth and round and becoming convex with maturity. Tan or brown warts may be present. The gills are free from the stalk, initially white to yellow and becoming green with maturity. The stalk is 5 to 25 cm long, smooth, and white. The ring is generally brown on the underside. Spores are green. The mushroom is common in most of eastern and southern North America and in

BOX 38-1
MUSHROOMS REPORTED TO CAUSE GASTROINTESTINAL IRRITATION

Agaricus albolutescens
Agaricus hondensis
Agaricus placomyces
Agaricus silvicola
Agaricus xanthodermus
Amanita brunnescens
Amanita chlorinosma
Amanita flavoconia
Amanita flavorubescens
Amanita frostiana
Amanita parcivolvata
Amanita spissa
Amanita spreta
Amanita volvata
Boletus luridus
Boletus pulcherrimus
Boletus satanus
Boletus sensibilis
Cantharellus bonari
Cantharellus floccosus
Cantharellus kauffmanii
Chlorophyllum molybdites (Lepiota morganii)
Entoloma (Rhodophyllus) lividum
Entoloma (Rhodophyllus) nidorosum
Entoloma (Rhodophyllus) rhodopolium
Entoloma (Rhodophyllus) salmoneum
Entoloma (Rhodophyllus) strictius
Entoloma (Rhodophyllus) vernum
Hebeloma crustuliniforme
Hebeloma fastibile
Hebeloma mesophaeum
Hebeloma sinapizans
Lactarius chysorheus
Lactarius glaucescens
Lactarius helvus
Lactarius representaneus
Lactarius rufus
Lactarius scrobiculatus
Lactarius torminosus
Lactarius uvidus
Lepiota clypeolaria
Lepiota cristata
Lepiota lutea
Lepiota morganii
Lepiota naucina
Lycoperdon marginatum
Lycoperdon subincarnatum
Morchella angusticeps
Morchella crassipes
Morchella deliciosa
Morchella esculenta
Morchella semilibera
Naematoloma (Hypholoma) fasciculare
Omphalotus illudens
Omphalotus olearius
Omphalotus olivascens
Paxillus involutus
Ramaria (Clavaria) formosa
Ramaria (Clavaria) gelatinosa
Russula emetica
Scleroderma aurantium
Scleroderma cepa
Tricholoma album
Tricholoma muscarium
Tricholoma pardinum
Tricholoma pessundatum
Tricholoma saponaceum
Tricholoma sejunctum
Tricholoma sulphureum
Tricholoma venenata
Verpa bohemica

California. In southern California it is one of the most common lawn mushrooms.

Another common mushroom causing gastrointestinal symptoms is the jack-o'-lantern (Color Plate 87). Its botanical classification is not completely settled. Most commonly it is referred to as *Omphalotus illudens, O. olearius,* or *O. olivascens.* The jack-o'-lantern mushroom is a bright orange-yellow mushroom with sharp-edged gills; it often grows in clusters at the base of stumps or on buried roots of deciduous trees. The cap is 4 to 16 cm in diameter on a stalk that is 4 to 20 cm long. Gills are olive to orange, with spores white to yellow. The mushroom has a characteristic luminescence that lasts 40 to 50 hours after collection. Members of this family are found in both eastern and western North America, generally in the autumn and early spring. It may be mistaken for the edible species *Cantharellus cibarius.* Some European reports have documented hepatic impairment and muscarinic effect following ingestion.[55,56] It is not clear whether the mushroom and its toxins are the same on both sides of the Atlantic.[3]

Although the genus *Amanita* is most famous for its deadly member *Amanita phalloides,* the genus also contains tasty nontoxic mushrooms *(A. caesarea* and *A. rubescens).* Several *Amanita* species cause gastrointestinal symptoms indistinguishable from those caused by jack-o'-lantern mushrooms or *Chlorophyllum molybdites. A. brunnescens* and *A. flavorubescens* are frequently listed as containing gastrointestinal toxins, although some list them as edible. These mushrooms resemble the edible *A. rubescens* ("the blusher"). Both have broad caps (3 to 15 cm) with loosely attached warts. The caps are yellowish to brown. The stalks are 3 to 18 cm long, enlarging toward the base with a superior ring. *A. brunnescens* stains reddish brown when bruised. Like their edible cousins, they are found in summer or fall associated with hardwoods or conifers.

Several members of the genus *Agaricus*—particularly *A. albolutescens, A. silvaticus,* and *A. xanthodermus*—cause gastrointestinal symptoms in some patients. They resemble the cultivated mushrooms in grocery stores. They are found in meadows and lawns in the summer or fall. Table 38-1 lists the look-alike toxic and nontoxic mushrooms in this group.

Toxins

A variety of toxins have been extracted from these mushrooms, although their structures are generally poorly described. Most are protein based and heat labile, although toxicity may not be completely eliminated with cooking. In some cases the toxin may be destroyed by heating, parboiling, or even preserving in salt. There is considerable variation in host response to the toxin; some patients can eat such mushrooms without harm, while others become quite ill. Some mushrooms also contain hemolysins and toxins that cause hemorrhage and hepatitis in animals.[47,83] Human hemolysis has not been reported.[47]

Clinical Presentation

Within 1 to 2 hours of ingestion of gastrointestinal irritant mushrooms, nausea, vomiting, intestinal cramping, and diarrhea develop. Stools are usually watery and occasionally bloody with fecal leukocytes. Chills, headaches, and myalgias may occur. Symptoms remit spontaneously in 6 to 12 hours. Most patients require only electrolytes and fluid replacement. The few serious cases reported in the literature have been associated with severe dehydration. In a review of 106 cases, all patients responded well to electrolyte replacement and occasional antiemetic or antidiarrheal medications.[15] Admitted patients were discharged in an average of 2 days.

Patients whose symptoms are delayed (beginning 4 hours or more after ingestion) probably have ingested a more toxic mushroom—either an *Amanita* or a *Gyromitra*. Such patients have severe gastrointestinal distress and may develop hepatic failure. Most mushroom fatalities occur from ingestion of these mushrooms.

Recent reports of ingestion of jack-o'-lantern mushrooms describe mildly elevated liver transaminases.[88] Cases of metabolic acidosis and dehydration, and even death, are attributed to *Chlorophyllum molybdites*.[11,82]

Table 38-1 Gastrointestinal Irritant Mushrooms Mistaken for Edible Species

Gastrointestinal Irritant	Edible Species
Amanita brunnescens	*Amanita rubescens, Amanita inaurata*
Chlorophyllum molybdites	*Lepiota* spp., *Agaricus bisporus*
Entoloma spp.	*Pluteus cervinus, Entoloma abortivum*
Hebeloma crustuliniforme	*Rozites caperata*
Naematoloma fasciculare	*Armillariella mellea, Naematoloma sublateritium, Naematoloma capnoides*
Omphalotus olearius	*Cantharellus cibarius, Laetiporus sulphureus, Armillaria mellea*
Paxillus involutus	*Lactarius* spp.
Ramaria formosa, Ramaria gelatinosa	*Ramaria* spp.
Scleroderma aurantium	*Lycoperdon perlatum*
Tricholoma pessundatum	*Tricholoma pessundatum*

Treatment

Treatment is largely supportive and not dependent on the type of mushroom ingested. Intravenous fluid and electrolyte replacement is frequently required. In severe cases antiemetics, such as prochlorperazine, 5 mg intravenously or 10 mg intramuscularly, prevent further emesis. Antidiarrheals are generally withheld unless diarrhea is prolonged or severe. Activated charcoal can be given, although there is no proof that it decreases toxicity.

Care should be taken not to dismiss early gastrointestinal symptoms when a mixed ingestion of unknown mushrooms has occurred. Individuals may ingest both gastrointestinal-irritant mushrooms *and* mushrooms containing amatoxins. Patients with prolonged gastroenteritis from unidentified mushrooms should be observed for later hepatic damage. In these patients a special effort should be made to identify the ingested mushrooms.

DISULFIRAM-LIKE TOXINS

A fascinating toxicity is caused by the *Coprinus* family—known as "inky caps" or "shaggy manes." Individuals who ingest these mushrooms and subsequently ingest alcohol have symptoms similar to those of an alcohol-disulfiram (Antabuse) reaction.

Causative Mushrooms

Several members of the *Coprinus* family may contain disulfiram-like toxins (see Box 38-2), but symptoms are most common with *C. atramentarius* ("inky cap") (Color Plate 88). The mushroom has a 2 to 8 cm cylindrical cap on a 4 to 5 cm thin stalk. The cap is white, occasionally orange or yellow at the top, with a surface that is characteristically shaggy. The mature cap often develops cracks at its margins,

BOX 38-2

MUSHROOMS SUSPECTED OR REPORTED TO CAUSE AN ALCOHOL-DISULFIRAM-LIKE REACTION

Clitocybe clavipes
Coprinus atramentarius
Coprinus comatus
Coprinus insignis
Coprinus micaceus

which turn up. The cap blackens as it matures and then liquefies, therefore the name "inky cap." A ring may be present low on the stalk. Spores are black. The mushroom grows throughout North America in clusters of three or more in grass or wood debris. It often appears overnight after a rain. Some members of the *Coprinus* family are edible, including *C. nivenus* and *C. disseminatus*. All members of this family are edible if no alcohol is ingested for the next 72 hours.

Toxin

Mushrooms causing disulfiram-like reactions contain the toxin coprine, isolated from the mushroom *Coprinus atramentarius* in 1975.[37] Coprine is distinct from disulfiram and is most likely a derivative of glutamine. It is probably not present in the raw mushroom, but rather a hydrolate created during cooking.[49]

Coprine (or its derivative L-aminocyclopropanol) inhibits acetaldehyde dehydrogenase, similar to the action of disulfiram. Acetaldehyde accumulates, leading to β-adrenergic stimulation and the typical vasomotor response of flushing, diaphoresis, headache, tachycardia, nausea, and vomiting. Some authors believe that coprine is a relatively poor inhibitor of acetaldehyde dehydrogenase and suggest that symptoms result from altered neurotransmitter levels.[14]

Clinical Presentation

Ingestion of the mushroom imparts sensitivity to alcohol, which begins 2 to 6 hours after ingestion and may last for up to 72 hours. Within 15 to 30 minutes of subsequent alcohol ingestion, the patient experiences severe headaches, flushing, and tachycardia. Hyperventilation, shortness of breath, and palpitations may be seen. In more severe cases, chest pain and orthostatic hypotension occur. Symptoms can be confused with an allergic reaction or acute myocardial infarction. Symptoms resolve spontaneously within 3 to 6 hours. A history of wild mushroom ingestion 3 days before symptoms is rarely offered.

Treatment

Supportive and symptomatic treatments are suggested. Baseline laboratory tests (blood urea nitrogen [BUN], creatinine, electrolytes, glucose) should be drawn. Urine output should be monitored. Activated charcoal is not beneficial. Charcoal does not adsorb alcohol; the coprine has already been absorbed by the time the reaction occurs. Hypotension generally responds to intravenous fluid administration. Severe hypotension refractory to fluid replacement should be treated with norepinephrine rather than an indirect vasopressor, since norepinephrine stores are depleted in a true disulfiram reaction. Propranolol has been suggested for the treatment of supraventricular tachycardia.[49]

NEUROLOGIC TOXINS

Muscarine

Muscarine was first isolated from the mushroom *Amanita muscaria* over 150 years ago. Classic muscarinic reaction includes salivation, lacrimation, urination, diaphoresis, gastrointestinal upset, and emesis (SLUDGE syndrome).

Causative Mushrooms. *Amanita muscaria* (Color Plate 89) has a cap 5 to 30 cm in diameter, which is scarlet red with white warts. The stalk is white, often hollow, and grows 15 to 20 cm long, tapering upward. It has a prominent cup and volva and numerous rings. Gills are free and white. Spores are white. The mushrooms grow in eastern North America and occasionally in California, often near *Boletus edulis*. They grow under hardwoods and conifers from spring to fall.

Potentially toxic amounts of muscarine are found in some members of the *Inocybe* and *Clitocybe* families (Table 38-2, Box 38-3). The *Inocybe* family (Color Plate 90) contains small brown mushrooms with conical caps up to 6 cm in diameter. Stalks are 2 to 10 cm long, covered with fine brown to white hairs. Gills are brown and notched; spores are brown. They are found typically under hardwoods and conifers in the summer and fall. All members of this family are considered poisonous.

In contrast, many members of the *Clitocybe* family are edible. *Clitocybe* mushrooms are whitish tan to gray mushrooms with 15 to 33 mm caps on hairless stalks 1 to 5 cm long. Gills are decurrent (run down the stalk); spores are white. They are usually single specimens (not clustered) found on lawns in summer and fall.

Many *Inocybe* and *Clitocybe* mushrooms contain larger concentrations of muscarine than does *A. muscaria*.[10] Several other toxins (such as ibotenic acid) are present in *A. muscaria* that contribute to toxicity.

Table 38-2 Look-Alikes with Mushrooms Causing Muscarine Poisoning

Toxic Species	Edible Species
Clitocybe dealbata	*Marasmius oreades*
Inocybe spp.	*Marasmius oreades*

BOX 38-3

MUSHROOMS REPORTED OR SUSPECTED TO CONTAIN MUSCARINE

Amanita gemmata
Amanita muscaria
Amanita pantherina
Amanita parcivolvata
Boletus calopus
Boletus luridus
Boletus pulcherrimus
Boletus satanus
Clitocybe aurantiaca
Clitocybe dealbata
Clitocybe nebularis
Hebeloma crustuliniforme
Inocybe fastigiata
Inocybe geophylla
Inocybe napipes
Inocybe patouillardii
Inocybe pudica
Mycena pura

Toxin. Muscarine is a quaternary trimethyl ammonium salt of 2-methyl-3-oxy-5-(amino)-tetrahydrofuram. Muscarine stimulates postganglionic cholinergic receptors (muscarinic receptors), mimicking the action of acetylcholine. Muscarinic stimulation of the gastrointestinal tract leads to increased secretory activity, contraction amplitude, and peristalsis. Stimulation of the urinary tract leads to bladder contraction and increased peristalsis of the ureters. Stimulation of the secretory tissue leads to salivation and lacrimation. Bronchoconstriction, flushing, and diaphoresis result from additional stimulation of the bronchial and vascular tissues. Cardiac effects include reflex tachycardia, or more commonly bradycardia, and decreased atrioventricular conduction. Central nervous system (CNS) effects include headache, ataxia, and visual disturbances. The sensorium is generally not affected (except in ingestion of *A. muscaria,* which contains other CNS toxins).

Clinical Presentation. After ingestion of muscarine-containing mushrooms, symptoms develop within 15 to 30 minutes. Typical symptoms include salivation, urination, lacrimation, diarrhea, diaphoresis, abdominal pain, gastrointestinal upset, and emesis. Bradycardia and bronchospasm are present and pupils are constricted. Copious bronchial secretions may cause respiratory failure requiring mechanical ventilation.

Symptoms remit spontaneously in 6 to 24 hours. In Europe, deaths have been reported from *Inocybe patouillardii.*[49] Although this mushroom is rarely eaten, ingestion carries a mortality rate of 6% to 12%, particularly among persons with preexisting pulmonary or cardiac disease. Most deaths occur within the first 12 hours as a result of respiratory failure or cardiovascular collapse.

Treatment. Most patients require supportive care with oxygen, suctioning, and intravenous fluid replacement. Activated charcoal and cathartics are rarely given because of the prominent emesis and diarrhea. Atropine antagonizes muscarine and should be used only to control secretions or profound bradycardia. It should not be given prophylactically because it may worsen the CNS effects associated with *A. muscaria.* Atropine doses of 0.01 mg/kg for children and 1 mg for adults can be repeated as needed until secretions are manageable. Symptoms resolve spontaneously within 24 hours.

Isoxazole Reactions

The isoxazole derivatives, ibotenic acid and muscimol, produce CNS symptoms, including excitement and alteration in visual perception.

Causative Mushrooms. Several mushrooms contain ibotenic acid (Table 38-3 and Box 38-4). *Amanita muscaria* (Color Plate 89) is described previously. *Amanita pantherina* (Color Plate 91) is 5 to 15 cm long with a cap 5 to 15 cm in diameter. The cap is generally white to pink in the young specimen but becomes reddish brown or brown with maturity, often darker at the rim. Fragments of the universal veil form warts on the cap but may be washed off by rain. The stalk has a distinct ring, with a volva or cup at the bottom. When the flesh is cut or injured (such as by insect larvae), it develops a pinkish tinge. Gills are free and produce

Table 38-3 Look-Alikes of Mushrooms Containing Isoxazole Toxins

Toxic Species	Edible Species
Amanita muscaria	*Amanita caesarea, Amanita rubescens, Armillariella mellea*
Amanita pantherina	*Amanita rubescens*
Amanita gemmata	*Russula* spp.

BOX 38-4

MUSHROOMS REPORTED OR SUSPECTED TO CONTAIN IBOTENIC ACID, MUSCIMOL, AND RELATED COMPOUNDS

Amanita cokeri
Amanita gemmata
Amanita muscaria
Amanita pantherina
Panaeolus campanulatus
Tricholoma muscarium

white spores. The raw mushroom itself has little smell, tasting much like a raw potato. It grows from June to November in woodlands throughout North America.

Toxin. Ibotenic acid is found in the bright red cap of *Amanita muscaria* and undergoes decarboxylation during drying to form muscimol, the more toxic of the compounds. The potency of the cap remains high despite drying for up to 7 years.[49] *A. muscaria* contains 0.17% to 1% isoxazole derivatives, while *Amanita pantherina* contains only 0.02% to 0.53%[36] and tends to lose potency with storage. Muscimol acts on γ-aminobutyric acid (GABA) receptors, possibly as a weak noncompetitive inhibitor of GABA uptake. Muscimol increases CNS serotonin levels and decreases catecholamine levels.

Clinical Presentation. Ingestion of 10 mg of *A. muscaria* produces mild intoxication, dizziness, and ataxia. Ingestion of 15 mg leads to pronounced ataxia and visual disturbances.[36,59] Delirium or manic behavior may develop after large ingestions. There is accelerated physical activity and inability to judge size. Visual hallucinations, seizures, and muscle twitching are common.[7] Some patients complain of residual headache.

Symptoms begin within 30 minutes of ingestion and generally last 2 hours. Fatalities have been reported but are rare. Some patients have been reported to have ataxia and paralysis of ocular convergence.[32] In rare cases symptoms last as long as 48 hours, depending on the dosage and individual host effect. Short-acting hypnotics are potentiated by muscimol in animals.[36] Phenobarbital or diazepam may lead to unexpected apnea, flaccid paralysis, or both.

Treatment. Treatment consists of supportive care. Emesis caused by the toxin is unusual. Gastric emptying and charcoal administration are difficult because of the CNS disturbances and have not been proven to be effective. Appropriate sedation with intravenous phenobarbital (30 mg intravenously hourly) or diazepam (5 mg repeated every 10 to 15 minutes in adults as needed or 0.1 to 0.3 mg/kg in children) is often necessary but should be used with caution. Airway support and ventilatory assistance should be readily available. Atropine may cause worsening of the CNS symptoms associated with isoxazole derivatives and should therefore be withheld unless the muscarinic effects are serious.

Hallucinogenic Mushrooms

Perhaps the most sought-after mushrooms are "magic mushrooms," which are available in the wild and as spores available through mail-order catalogs to grow at home. These mushrooms have been used for centuries because of their hallucinogenic effects. Small stone mushroom icons were found in Meso-American ruins believed to be 3500 years old.[49]

Causative Mushrooms. The most common hallucinogenic mushrooms are members of the *Psilocybe* family (Table 38-4 and Box 38-5). This family includes over 100 species (Color Plate 92), not all of which cause hallucinations. These are little brown mushrooms (referred to in the vernacular as LBMs). The cap is 0.5 to 4 cm broad (depending on the species), is usually smooth, and becomes sticky or slippery when wet. The stalks are slender and 4 to 15 cm long. Gills are gray to purple gray; spores are dark, nearly

Table 38-4 Look-Alikes of Mushrooms Containing Psilocybin-Psilocin

Toxic Species	Edible Species
Panaeolus foenisecii	*Psathyrella candolleana, Agrocybe pediades, Marasmius oreades*
Panaeolus spp.	*Coprinus* spp.

BOX 38-5

MUSHROOMS REPORTED OR SUSPECTED TO CONTAIN PSILOCYBIN, PSILOCIN, OR BOTH

Amanita citrina
Amanita porphyria
Conocybe cyanopus
Conocybe siligineoides
Conocybe smithii
Gymnopilus aeruginosus
Gymnopilus purpuratus
Gymnopilus spectabilis
Gymnopilus validipes
Naematoloma popperianum
Panaeolus campanulatus
Panaeolus castaneifolius
Panaeolus cyanescens
Panaeolus fimicola
Panaeolus foenisecii
Panaeolus phalaenarum
Panaeolus semiovatus
Panaeolus sphinctrinus
Panaeolus subbalteatus
Psathyrella sepulchralis
Psilocybe baeocystis
Psilocybe caerulescens
Psilocybe caerulipes
Psilocybe cubensis
Psilocybe cyanaescens
Psilocybe pelliculosa
Psilocybe semilanceata
Psilocybe strictipes
Psilocybe stuntzii
Stropharia aeruginosa
Stropharia coronilla
Stropharia hornemannii
Stropharia squamosa

black. The flesh of these mushrooms turns blue or greenish when bruised or cut. They are often mistaken for more poisonous species (such as *Galerina* or *Inocybe*). These mushrooms also resemble *Agaricus bisporus.* Regular grocery store mushrooms laced with lysergic acid diethylamide (LSD) or other hallucinogens are sold on the street as *Psilocybe.* Hallucinogenic mushrooms ("shrooms") grow primarily on dung and are found in warmer climates of North America.

Other mushrooms, including members of the *Panaeolus* and *Gymnopilus* families, may contain psilocybin. *Panaeolus* mushrooms are also little brown mushrooms about the same size as *Psilocybe.* Gills are dark gray or black with black spores. They also grow on dung throughout the tropics and subtropics of North America. Unlike *Psilocybe,* their caps are not sticky or slippery when wet. The hallucinogenic effect and quantity of toxin vary among the species.

Some *Gymnopilus* (such as *G. aeruginosus*) contain hallucinogens. These are medium-size mushrooms (cap 5 to 15 cm, stalk 5 to 12 cm) and variable in color (green, yellow, salmon, red) with yellowish gills and rusty spores. They grow on stumps or sawdust in the Pacific Northwest.

Visual hallucinations and ataxia were recently reported in a patient ingesting *Laetiporus sulphureus,* previously thought to be a safe and harmless mushroom.[4] It is not clear whether this mushroom contained hallucinogenic material or the individual ingested an additional mushroom as well.

Toxin. Psilocybin and its somewhat unstable metabolite psilocin are indole compounds derived from tryptamine. These two toxins were first isolated by Albert Hofmann,[38] known as the father of LSD. Chemically, the toxins resemble 5-hydroxytryptamine and LSD and have similar effects. They maintain their potency in dried specimens.

Psilocybin, as well as LSD, inhibits the firing rate of serotonin-dependent neurons, particularly at the presynaptic receptors. It induces a strange euphoria, hallucinations, and a loss of time sensation. Many of these symptoms are similar to those seen with LSD.

Clinical Presentation. Ingestion of 5 mg psilocybin (10 mg fresh *P. cubensis*) causes moderate euphoria. Ingestion of 10 mg leads to hallucinations and a loss of time sensation.

A heightened imagination develops within 15 to 30 minutes of ingestion. Hallucinations may last for 4 to 6 hours. Serious side effects are rarely seen, but fever and seizures have been reported in children.[58] Up to 50% of patients have tachycardia and hypertension.[66] Flashbacks have been reported to occur in some patients for up to 4 months after ingestion.[6]

Treatment. Initially the patient should be placed in a quiet supportive environment. Gastric emptying and activated charcoal administration are often impossible and may only enhance the hallucinations. They should be considered in patients with very large ingestions who are brought for treatment early. Sedation can be accomplished when necessary with benzodiazepines (diazepam, 0.1 mg/kg in children, or in adults 5 mg intravenously, repeated every 5 minutes as needed), phenobarbital (0.5 mg/kg in children, 30 to 60 mg in adults intravenously repeated every 10 minutes as needed), chlorpromazine (50 to 100 intramuscularly), or haloperidol (5 mg intramuscularly). Seizures can be controlled with diazepam in the doses above. Hyperpyrexia, seen primarily in children, is best treated with external cooling, avoiding antipyretics.

PROTOPLASMIC POISONS

Gyromitra Toxin

False morels *(Gyromitra esculenta)* were once thought to be edible. Even today they are collected, sold fresh or canned ("morschels"), and exported throughout eastern and central Europe.[61] Since 1793 they have been suspected of causing toxicity, and since World War II they have been known to cause hepatic failure, neurologic symptoms, and death.[35] Symptoms appear 4 to 50 hours (usually 5 to 12 hours) after ingestion, timing similar to that of *A. phalloides* poisoning. Since *Gyromitra* grow primarily in the spring and *A. phalloides* grows in the fall, there is rarely confusion of the two mushrooms.

Causative Mushrooms. *Gyromitra esculenta* (Color Plate 93) is approximately 5 to 16 cm in height with a reddish brown to dark brown, irregularly shaped cap. The cap's surface is curved and folded, resembling a human brain. The stalk is often as thick as the cap. The inside of the cap and stalk are hollow. This mushroom grows in the spring near pines and in sandy soil throughout North America. It is particularly common in Germany, Poland, and other Eastern European areas. Mature species, particularly those with cap decay, may have increased toxicity. These mushrooms may be mistaken for morels, which are considered among the most delicious wild mushrooms (Table 38-5).

Other members of the *Gyromitra* family contain gyromitrins. None of these mushrooms have been reported to cause toxicity in humans.

Toxin. Gyromitrin (*N*-methyl-*N*-formylhydrazone) was first isolated in 1967.[51] This substance is moderately volatile and heat sensitive. Cooking thoroughly and discarding the cooking liquid decrease or eliminate the toxin. Symptoms have occurred despite proper cooking.[33]

Once gyromitrin enters the stomach, hydrolysis yields *N*-methyl-*N*-formylhydrazine (MFH) and then *N*-methylhydrazine or monomethylhydrazine (MH).[61] MH is a compo-

Table 38-5 Look-Alikes of Mushrooms Containing Gyromitrin

Toxic Species	Edible Species
Gyromitra esculenta	*Morchella esculenta*

nent of rocket fuel. Workers in rocket fuel plants exposed to the very volatile MH develop central nervous system toxicity and nephrotoxicity.[44,81] MH is a competitive inhibitor of pyridoxal phosphate, which interferes with enzyme systems requiring pyridoxine as a cofactor, including decarboxylases, deaminases, and transaminases.[5] As a result, levels of GABA fall, interfering with neurotransmission.[45] This may lead to altered mental status, seizures, or both. Recent questions have been raised about this widely accepted theory, since MH may cause seizures without a change in brain GABA levels.[57]

MFH and MH undergo oxidation in the liver to two highly reactive intermediates—a free methyl radical and an unstable diazonium compound.[61] These substances appear to produce local hepatic necrosis by blocking the activity of cytochrome P_{450} systems, glutathione, and other hepatic biomolecules.

Gyromitrin causes tumors in a variety of animals.[85] There are significant concerns about long-term toxicity associated with repeated consumption of this mushroom. It has been included in the list of naturally occurring carcinogens.[41]

Each kilogram of fresh *Gyromitra esculenta* contains 3 to 100 mg gyromitrin. Fresh mushroom contains 50 to 300 mg of MH per kilogram and dried mushroom up to 400 mg.[61] The human LD_{50} of gyromitrin is suspected to be 20 to 50 mg/kg for adults and 10 to 30 mg/kg for children, or 0.4 to 1 kg of fresh mushrooms for adults (average 30 mushrooms) and 0.2 to 0.6 kg for a child.[61]

Clinical Presentation. Symptoms are generally delayed for 4 to 50 (average 5 to 12) hours after ingestion. Initial symptoms include nausea, vomiting, and severe diarrhea. Some patients have dizziness, weakness, muscle cramps, and loss of coordination. In severe ingestions, delirium, seizures, and coma develop. Hepatic failure develops over several days after ingestion, although hepatic damage is generally mild. Hypoglycemia, hypovolemia, severe hepatic failure, and death may occur.

Symptoms from gyromitrin toxin are highly variable. As with other mushroom toxins, variability depends on amount consumed, toxin concentration, nature of the mushrooms, and other factors. The variability of symptoms after ingestion of gyromitrin mushrooms is much greater than that seen with other mushroom species. Some individuals can consume large quantities of *Gyromitra* with few or no symptoms. A second meal by the same person may lead to severe toxicity. Some believe repeated consumption increases the risk of a severe reaction.[12]

Several drugs, including isoniazid, hydralazine, and probably MH,[13] are metabolized through acetylation of a hydrazine or amino group by the liver. Individuals vary markedly in the rapidity of acetylation. Two major human groups are termed "fast" and "slow" acetylators, with slow acetylation being an autosomal recessive trait. Slow acetylators in general have greater and more prolonged toxicity after ingestion of these drugs. Similar variation in fast and slow acetylators is seen when *Gyromitra* mushrooms are ingested.

Treatment. Symptoms develop several hours after ingestion of *Gyromitra.* Activated charcoal is generally given but is of little proven value. Gastric emptying is of little value. Pyridoxine has been useful in patients suffering neurologic disorders from MH toxicity and is of theoretical benefit in victims of gyromitrin toxicity. High-dose pyridoxine therapy may cause peripheral neuropathies.[1] Patients who ingest gyromitrin mushrooms and develop significant neurologic symptoms should receive pyridoxine (25 mg/kg up to 25 kg/day orally).[44,93] There is no evidence that pyridoxine alters the course of hepatic disease.

Baseline measurements of liver transaminases, prothrombin time, partial thromboplastin time, BUN, creatinine, complete blood cell count, platelet count, glucose, and electrolytes should be performed. Liver transaminases, prothrombin time, partial thromboplastin time, BUN, and creatinine should be monitored at least daily for 3 to 4 days. Patients with significant hepatic failure may require monitoring of blood glucose every 2 to 4 hours and supplemental glucose administration for symptomatic hypoglycemia.

No specific antidote or treatment is available for the fulminant hepatic failure. Patients with severe hepatic failure should be transferred to facilities capable of performing liver transplantation. No good studies have been performed to determine the appropriate timing or necessity of liver transplantation. In patients with fulminant hepatic failure from infectious causes, the presence of prolonged prothrombin time (unresponsive to fresh-frozen plasma) and the development of hepatorenal syndrome, grade II hepatic encephalopathy, hypoglycemia, and uncorrectable metabolic acidosis are used as signs that transplantation is needed on an emergency basis. In patients with fulminant hepatic failure from toxic ingestion, elevated bilirubin level and young age are important indicators of a poor prognosis.[28,64] Mortality from gyromitrin poisoning is reported to be 15% to 35%.[29,65]

Orellanine Poisoning

Although originally thought to be an edible mushroom, *Cortinarius orellanus* was associated with 81 cases of late renal toxicity in the 1950s.[34] This led to the isolation of the toxin orellanine, which is found in the mushrooms *C. orellanus, C. speciosissimus,* and *C. gentilis.* Most cases occur in Europe and Japan.

Causative Mushroom. The mushroom *C. orellanus* has a brownish to brownish red smooth cap 30 to 80 cm in diameter. The stalk is somewhat yellow, often darker toward the soil. Gills are orange to rust with rust-colored spores. It grows in deciduous woods, most commonly in sandy soil underneath oaks and birches. It is ubiquitous throughout Europe. Some other species of *Cortinarius* are found in the United States and may be toxic (see Box 38-6).

Toxin. The two toxins isolated from *C. orellanus,* orellanine and orelline, are structurally related to paraquat and diquat. Their mechanism of action remains a mystery. They are heat-stable compounds, unaffected by cooking. Considerable host variability is noted. The toxin appears to cause an intense interstitial nephritis with early fibrosis.[39]

Clinical Presentation. Patients who ingest the mushroom are generally asymptomatic for 2 to 20 days. After this latent period, acute renal failure develops. Some patients have neurologic changes, including paresthesias, taste impairment, and cognitive disorders.

The occurrence of symptoms is highly variable. One case report described 26 soldiers who ate soup made of *C. orellanus* in nearly identical quantities.[8] In 12 of these individuals acute renal failure developed on or around day 11. Eight later recovered normal renal function; 4 required long-term dialysis or kidney transplantation. The other 14 soldiers showed no rise in BUN or creatinine levels but developed leukocyturia and hematuria that persisted for more than 1 month. Renal failure reportedly occurs in 30% to 46% of patients. Renal function returns in 46% to 66% of affected patients.[8]

Renal biopsy in patients with orellanine-induced renal failure shows tubule lesions with epithelial necrosis and disruption of the tubular basement membrane. These biopsy changes may persist for up to 3 months.[8]

Treatment. In most persons who ingest orellanine, unexplained acute renal failure develops many days later. If a person sought treatment early after eating orellanine-containing mushrooms, gastric emptying and activated charcoal administration might prevent some absorption, decreasing the resultant toxicity. Early presentation is rare, however.

Once acute renal failure develops, baseline and repeated monitoring of BUN, creatinine, electrolytes, CBC, differential, and urinalysis should be performed. Urinary output should be monitored, and if it decreases, a fluid bolus should be tried. Serum potassium, calcium, and magnesium should be monitored closely. If renal failure progresses, the patient should be transferred to a facility for hemodialysis and possible renal transplantation. Renal function may return to normal after months of dialysis dependency. Steroids seem to have no effect on the course of the disease—but they may have been given too late.

Amatoxin

The mushrooms that contain amatoxins are responsible for 90% to 95% of fatalities caused by mushrooms (Table 38-6 and Box 38-7). *A. phalloides* is most common in central and eastern Europe. It is thought that the mushroom *A. phalloides* may have originated in Europe and been carried with immigrants to the United States. One theory suggests that the mushroom spores were carried in wood products during the emigration from eastern Europe. *Amanita verna* and *Amanita virosa* are more common in the United States.

Causative Mushrooms. The common names of *A. phalloides* and its relatives *A. verna* and *A. virosa* are death cap, death angel, and destroying angel, which reflects their association with fatal outcome. *A. phalloides* (Color Plate 94) has a white to greenish cap 4 to 16 cm in diameter, often with remnants of the veil (warts). The stalk is generally thick, 5 to 18 cm long, with a large bulb at the base, often with a volva or cup. A thin ring is usually present on the stalk. Gills are generally free and white to green in color; spores are white. The mushrooms grow under deciduous trees in the fall.

A. virosa (Color Plate 95) is more common in the United States. It has a similar appearance, but the cap is more yel-

Table 38-6 Look-Alikes of Mushrooms Containing Amatoxin

Toxic Species	Edible Species
Amanita phalloides	*Amanita fulva*
Amanita virosa	*Agaricus bisporus*
Amanita verna	*Lepiota flavovirens*

BOX 38-6

MUSHROOMS REPORTED OR SUSPECTED TO CONTAIN ORELLINE OR ORELLANINE

Cortinarius gentilis
Cortinarius orellanus
Cortinarius speciosissimus
Cortinarius splendena
Cortinarius venenosus

BOX 38-7

MUSHROOMS REPORTED OR SUSPECTED TO CONTAIN AMATOXINS

Amanita phalloides
Amanita verna
Amanita virosa
Galerina autumnalis
Galerina marginata
Galerina venenata

lowish or white. *A. verna* is characteristically white. Both grow in deciduous woods. Even self-proclaimed knowledgeable mushroom pickers have been known to be tempted by the large white mushroom, which is said to be tasty. However, the fatality rate of 35% for adults and 50% for children demonstrates that eating these mushrooms is highly dangerous.

Mushrooms that contain amatoxin may have a positive Meixner test. This test was first described by Wieland in 1949[92] and popularized by Meixner.[60] A drop of liquid is expressed from a fresh mushroom onto print-free (ligand-free) newspaper and allowed to dry. A drop of concentrated (10 to 12 N) hydrochloric acid is added. A blue color develops within 1 to 2 minutes in the presence of amatoxins. A control test of newspaper without mushroom juice and a piece of paper containing ligand should be conducted. False-positive results are common and can be elicited from excessive drying temperatures (greater than 63° C) or exposure to sunlight. False-positive tests also occur from mushrooms containing psilocybin, terpenes, and bufotenin. Nearly 20% of gilled mushrooms that did not contain amatoxins tested positive in one study.[78] The usefulness of this technique is therefore in doubt. Thin-layer chromatography more accurately identifies the presence of amatoxin and can be done on mushroom liquid, patient serum, or urine.[69] Radioimmunoassay of serum or urine can detect amatoxins in the body.

Toxin. The mushroom *A. phalloides* contains two groups of toxins: amatoxins and phallotoxins. Each group contains several toxins. There are now eight amatoxins identified—α-amanitin, β-amanitin, γ-amanitin, ε-amanitin, amanin, amaninamide, amanullinic acid, and amanullin.[90] Of these, α-amanitin is thought to be primarily responsible for human disease. α-Amanitin injected into animals produces hepatic toxicity characteristic of human ingestion of *A. phalloides*. Phallotoxins include phalloidin, phalloin, phallisin, phallacidin, phallacin, phallisacin, and prophalloin.[90] Phalloidin is the primary phallotoxin. Phallotoxins bind to F-actin, disrupting plasma membranes and causing massive efflux of calcium and potassium. Phallotoxins cause death in animals within 2 hours and are not believed to play a role in human toxicity.[30] It is possible that humans do not even absorb these toxins or that they may be responsible for local gastric irritation. *A. virosa* contains amatoxins and virotoxins—the latter resembling phallotoxin biochemically. Like phallotoxins, virotoxins bind F-actin and cause death within hours. Six different virotoxins have been isolated, but none are thought to play a role in human *Amanita* hepatotoxicity.[90]

After ingestion, amatoxins are absorbed from the gut and actively transported into the liver through transport systems shared by bile acids and xenobiotics.[91] There they bind to RNA polymerase II and inhibit the formation of messenger RNA.[50] This in turn inhibits transcription as the reservoir of messenger RNA is depleted.[21] Amatoxin is excreted into the bile where it is reabsorbed and once again transported into the liver.[9] Interruption of this enterohepatic circulation may be an important therapeutic tool.

Within the liver, α-amanitin most likely undergoes some metabolism through the cytochrome P_{450} system. Animal studies suggest that a more toxic metabolite is produced through this metabolism.[75,77] Nuclear fragmentation and condensation of chromosomal material have been observed within 15 hours of injection.[20] Glycogen is rapidly depleted, and fatty degeneration occurs within the liver parenchymal cells.[16] Mitochondria become swollen, and microvesicules appear throughout the cytoplasm.[75] Direct renal toxicity may occur, but renal failure is more likely to be caused by hepatorenal syndrome (10% of cases).

Clinical Presentation. Persons who ingest the mushroom *Amanita phalloides* feel well for 4 to 16 hours. This characteristic latent period is followed by severe nausea, vomiting, abdominal cramps, and diarrhea. Early complications include fluid and electrolyte imbalance (hypernatremia, hypokalemia, elevated BUN level) and hypoglycemia. Patients in whom symptoms develop earlier (between 4 and 10 hours) are more likely to experience severe hepatotoxicity. Over the next 12 to 24 hours the patient's gastrointestinal symptoms abate. The second latent period is followed by hepatic failure, which develops between 48 and 72 hours after ingestion in most patients. Hypoglycemia can be severe. Hepatic failure may be of varying severity; it is frequently worse in children and only mildly dependent on the amount of mushroom ingested.

It is unclear why children have greater toxicity and higher mortality. In part, it may be a result of the relative quantity of mushrooms ingested or of the varying metabolism in young children (differing levels of P_{450}-metabolizing enzymes). Previous experiments showed that ethanol ingestion concurrent with *A. phalloides* (whole mushroom lyophilized) decreased hepatotoxicity.[26] It was therefore theorized that one reason for decreased toxicity in adults could be ingestion of ethanol with an *Amanita* mushroom dinner. More recently, however, ethanol failed to alter the hepatotoxicity in an animal model poisoned with α-amanitin, which raises doubts about this explanation for increased toxicity in children.[74]

In addition to hepatic failure, endocrinopathies can develop, reflected by hypocalcemia, decreased thyroid function, and elevated insulin level in the presence of hypoglycemia.[43] The reason for these laboratory abnormalities is not clear. Hypocalcemia may be caused in part by loss of calcium through diarrhea or a direct effect on osteoclasts. Renal failure may contribute to the hypocalcemia. The thyroid abnormalities are probably decreased hormone synthesis caused by overwhelming illness and blocked peripheral conversion of T_4 to T_3. Thyroid stimulating hormone depression may result from decreased synthesis caused by the inhibition of RNA polymerase II by amatoxin. The hypothyroidism has not been clinically significant. The hypoglycemia is probably the result of several processes including impaired hepatic gluconeogenesis, increased insulin release from the initial hyperglycemia, or tissue destruction of the pancreas.[43] Bone marrow toxicity with decreased neutrophils, lymphocytes, and platelets has been noted.[72] Disseminated intravascular coagulation and coagulopathies secondary to hepatic dysfunction are common.[72] Pancreatitis occurs in up to 50% of patients.[24] Hypophosphatemia is particularly common in children, for unknown reasons.

Hepatic biopsy shows diffuse and severe steatosis with periportal inflammation and necrosis. Extremely high levels of hepatic transaminases are seen. The level of liver transaminase is not helpful in predicting the patient's prognosis. A precipitous drop in levels may occur just before death.

Treatment. Attempts to treat *A. phalloides* poisoning have ranged from scientific to purely empirical. Noting that rabbits were able to eat the *A. phalloides* mushroom with impunity, clinicians fed ground raw rabbit to victims of *Amanita* poisoning, without success.[87] Hemodialysis was long recommended but now has been shown to be ineffective, since the toxin is rapidly cleared. Amatoxin is taken up in liver cells within 5 hours after intravenous administration.[18] In a retrospective study of 205 cases of amatoxin ingestion,[28] hemodialysis worsened the prognosis and charcoal hemoperfusion did not provide any improvement in outcome. Plasmapheresis has been used, but this appears to be ineffective for similar reasons.[68]

Amatoxins are enterohepatically circulated. Attempts have been made to divert the enterohepatic circulation using a fistula. Although animal studies showed some benefit with this treatment,[19] it is not recommended. Multidose activated charcoal (every 4 hours) should be used, since the charcoal may adsorb the amatoxins and interrupt the enterohepatically circulated drug.

Fab monoclonal antibodies against amatoxin were developed by immunizing rats and fusing their spleen cells to mouse myeloma cells. The amatoxin-specific clones were selected and their immunoglobulin separated into Fab fragments. When this Fab antibody was used in α-amanitin-poisoned mice, renal toxicity was 50 times greater and all animals died of renal failure.[17] Interestingly, these animals had no hepatic damage. It is thought that the Fab-amatoxin compound may have disassociated in the kidney, leading to severe local damage.

Thioctic acid is used throughout Europe as a treatment for *A. phalloides* poisoning. Although its exact mechanism is unknown, it may act as a free radical scavenger or interfere with the hepatic transport of toxin. In animal studies, thioctic acid has been ineffective against α-amanitin or extracts of the mushroom.[2] In the large retrospective study it was more frequently associated with a fatal outcome in humans.[28] Its use is not recommended.

Silymarin is the active component of the milk thistle *Silybum marianum*. A water-soluble preparation (silibinin) has been developed that has been shown to be effective against amatoxin in both animals and humans. Silibinin is thought to interrupt the enterohepatic circulation, or it may act as a free radical scavenger. Patients treated with silibinin were more likely to survive in one study.[40] In a retrospective study its use was associated with increased survival.[28] Silibinin is not available in the United States but can be obtained from European sources.

High-dose penicillin was noted in an animal study to decrease toxicity.[27] This finding came during an experiment to look at the utility of hemodialysis, with penicillin used prophylactically. The control group (penicillin alone) showed a decrease in toxicity. Other animal studies have indicated its effectiveness in reducing hepatotoxicity.[23,76] In humans it has been very effective.[28] Other antibiotics, including rifampin and cephalosporins, have been shown to protect against amatoxin poisoning.[22,63] The exact mechanism by which penicillin acts is unclear. There may be sterilization of the intestines leading to decreased GABA production, which may diminish ensuing cerebral encephalopathy. Another hypothesis is that penicillin may share a common transport system with amatoxin and that this interferes with uptake.[25] Regardless of the mechanism, large doses of benzylpenicillin (300,000 to 1 million units per kg per day) are recommended. This dose may be associated with seizures.

The French have used hyperbaric oxygen as a treatment for *Amanita* toxicity.[48] Hyperbaric oxygen may assist in hepatic regeneration, as well as lessen toxicity. It is most commonly used with high-dose penicillin.

Other therapies have been suggested by animal data. High-dose cimetidine (4 to 10 g/day in adults) appears to inhibit formation of more toxic metabolites by blocking the cytochrome P_{450} system.[75] Other drugs under investigation in animals include vitamin C,[89] zinc, and thiol compounds.[25]

Gastric aspirate or emesis can be sent for spore analysis if mushroom specimens are not available for identification. Patients with documented or suspected amatoxin ingestion should receive activated charcoal repeated every 4 to 6 hours, if necessary by duodenal tube. Repeated administration should bind drug that is enterohepatically circulated. Cathartics are generally not necessary, since diarrhea is prominent. Intravenous normal saline or Ringer's lactate is needed to replace gastrointestinal losses. Electrolyte losses (particularly potassium) may be great. BUN, creatinine, CBC, differential, platelet count, electrolytes, glucose, calcium, phosphorus, magnesium, urinalysis, prothrombin time, partial thromboplastin time, fibrinogen, amylase, protein, and albumin should be initially measured and repeated at least daily. Hyperglycemia is common on the first day, but insulin is generally not required. Hypoglycemia occurs after 24 hours and may be significant, requiring concentrated intravenous glucose. Bedside determinations of glucose should be performed at least every 6 hours. Tests of liver function, including serum glutamic oxaloacetic transaminase (SGOT), serum glutamic pyruvate transaminase, alkaline phosphatase, prothrombin time, and partial thromboplastin time, should be repeated at least daily and with increased frequency if findings become abnormal.

To confirm the diagnosis of amatoxin ingestion, a red-top glass tube blood sample drawn on admission can be sent for serum radioimmunoassay for amatoxins. Urine can also be studied. The nearest laboratory performing this assay is usually known to the regional poison information center.

Specific treatment should begin as soon as diagnosis is suspected (either by symptoms or confirmed by the fresh specimen or spores). Benzylpenicillin (penicillin G), 300,000 to 1 million U/kg/day, should be given intravenously in divided doses. Silibinin, if available, can be given intravenously, 20 to 40 mg/kg/day in divided doses. Hyperbaric oxygen treatments (dives to 2 atm for 30 minutes once or twice a day) can be tried. Consideration should be given to using intravenous cimetidine (4 to 10 g intravenously for adults for 3 days).

Once liver failure begins, hypoglycemia becomes more likely. Supplemental glucose should be readily available. Dietary protein should be limited and thiamine and multivitamin supplementation given. Oral lactulose, 30 to 45 ml every 6 to 8 hours, may reduce hepatic encephalopathy. Clotting studies should be performed several times a day and vitamin K or fresh-frozen plasma (or both) used to correct abnormalities.

Once acute hepatic failure has progressed, patients may require liver transplantation. The timing of transplantation is highly debated, and appropriate criteria have not been established. Criteria for transplant in other forms of fulminant hepatic failure are often applied to this setting. Factors associated with poor prognosis in acetaminophen-induced hepatic damage include metabolic acidosis, elevated prothrombin time, and elevated serum creatinine level.[64] However, in viral hepatitis and other drug reactions, factors such as bilirubin, patient age, and the duration of jaundice before encephalopathy appears are important.[64] In the few studies of *A. phalloides* ingestions that are pertinent, poor outcome is related to age less than 10 years old, a short latent period, and the severity of the coagulopathy.[28] The best study suggests that patients with SGOT levels greater than 2000 IU, grade II hepatic encephalopathy, or prothrombin time greater than 50 seconds are at serious risk for death and should be considered for emergency liver transplantation.[15] Patients who met these criteria and survived have been described.[54,71] Because hepatic failure develops rapidly, it is imperative that patients with significant hepatic dysfunction be transferred early to sites where transplantation can be performed. Patients undergoing liver transplantation for fulminant hepatic failure (not caused by *A. phalloides*) have a 62% survival rate.

Patients who survive the acute hepatic failure without needing transplantation may have persistent elevation in liver transaminases. In one study of 14 patients with severe hepatotoxicity, 8 showed persisted elevation in transaminases with no normalization over a 1-year follow-up period.[15] These patients all had biopsy evidence of chronic active hepatitis with positive anti–smooth muscle antibody and positive cryoglobulins. It is not known whether these patients will have an increased risk of hepatoma or develop more serious complications of chronic active hepatitis.[67]

Approach to the Patient

Four types of individuals develop mushroom toxicity: foragers, children, those seeking hallucinogenic "highs," and, in rare instances, victims of attempted homicide. Most patients seek medical care only after symptoms develop. Caretakers of small children observed chewing on lawn mushrooms should be advised to call the nearest regional poison information center. Children who have ingested an entire lawn mushroom or more should receive ipecac and be observed for symptoms at home. Follow-up calls should be made to ensure that emesis has occurred and at 1, 4, and 24 hours to assess symptoms.

Patients with agitation, altered perceptions, or frank hallucinations temporally related to mushroom ingestion are probably intoxicated with isoxazole or hallucinogenic mushrooms. The former are usually picked accidentally, the latter either intentionally or grown at home from mail order spores. Regardless of the source, the treatment and clinical course are identical.

Patients who develop muscarinic symptoms (salivation, urination, diaphoresis, gastrointestinal upset, and emesis) present such a classic picture that it is rarely confused with other syndromes. Some drugs (such as bethanechol) may give similar symptoms when taken in overdose. Patients generally remain mentally clear and should be able to relate the appropriate history.

Patients who with gastrointestinal symptoms can be divided into early and delayed presentations. Those with gastrointestinal symptoms early (within 2 hours) generally have a benign course, *except* for persons with mixed ingestions. Most guidebooks for mushroom hunters suggest eating only one variety of mushrooms at a time, but more daring or foolish individuals mix multiple mushrooms and eat them frequently over a day. This makes diagnosis based on time of onset of symptoms difficult. Early onset of gastrointestinal symptoms may mask more significant delayed symptoms. In these cases, identification of ingested mushrooms becomes essential to planning therapy.

Accurate botanical identification of the mushroom can be difficult. Only 800 of the 3000 species found in Europe can be identified without a microscope.[87] When multiple mushrooms are eaten together, the residual specimens brought from home may not be those causing toxicity. Cooking and refrigeration alter identifying features. Fresh mushroom specimens should be transported in a paper bag rather than in a plastic container to limit the effects of humidity. Finally, precise identification of even a good specimen can be difficult and time consuming and is best left to a expert. Mycologists can be contacted through a regional poison information center, university, museum, or commercial mushroom grower.

In difficult cases, spores can be obtained from emesis or gastric emptying procedures. Specimens should be refrigerated while awaiting analysis. More specific diagnosis can be made through thin-layer chromatography or radioimmunoassay techniques. Botanical identification and the patient's symptoms may not agree. The patient should be treated according to time of onset and symptoms when examined.

Patients with early-onset gastrointestinal symptoms require supportive care with fluid and electrolyte replacement. For those with delayed gastrointestinal symptoms or mixed ingestions containing amatoxin or gyromitrin mushrooms, treatment should begin as soon as possible. It is generally possible to differentiate amatoxin- and gyromitrin-containing mushrooms by description of the mushroom or by the season (spring—*Gyromitra,* fall—*Amanita*).

Patients who have disulfiram-like reactions to alcohol but who are not taking disulfiram should be questioned about prior mushroom ingestion. In such patients the condition is rarely correctly diagnosed; their symptoms are thought to result from panic attacks, alcohol intoxication, or even allergic reactions. Patients seldom relate these symptoms to the dinner of mushrooms eaten days before.

All patients with unexplained acute renal failure should be questioned about prior wild mushroom ingestion. Although *Cortinarius orellanus* is more common in Europe and Japan, it has been found with increasing frequency in the United States. Because of the long delay before the onset of renal failure (1 to 2 weeks), the history of mushroom ingestion may be missed.

The incidence of mushroom toxicity is increasing. Mushroom foraging is becoming more popular in the United States. The incidence of children poisoned by mushrooms is also increasing. While the United States has only a few fatal cases of mushroom poisoning each year, the incidence in Europe is higher. Mushroom poisoning is also a problem in countries in the Far East, including Japan (average 70 cases per year with three or four deaths)[42] and China (where deaths are reported from *A. phalloides*),[94] and in South Africa.[70] The clinician should be aware of the variety of toxicities associated with mushrooms, particularly those with delayed symptoms that may not be temporally related to the ingestion (disulfiram-like reactions and acute renal failure).

REFERENCES

1. Albin RL, et al: Acute sensory neuropathy-neuronopathy from pyridoxine overdose, *Neurology* 37:1729, 1987.
2. Alleva FR et al: *Failure of thioctic acid to cure mushroom-poisoned mice and dogs,* 14th Annual Meeting of the Society of Toxicology, vol 33, Williamsburg, Va, 1975, p 184.
3. Ammirati JF, Traquair JA, Horgen PA: *Poisonous mushrooms of Northern United States and Canada,* Minneapolis, 1985, University of Minnesota Press, p 290.
4. Appleton RE, Jan JE, Kroeger PD: *Laetiporus sulfureus* causing visual hallucinations and ataxia in a child, *Can Med Assoc J* 139:48, 1988.
5. Azar A et al: Pyridoxine and phenobarbital as treatment of aerozine-50 toxicity, *Aerospace Med* 4:1, 1970.
6. Benjamin C: Persistent psychiatric symptoms after eating psilocybin mushrooms, *Br Med J* 1:1319, 1979.
7. Benjamin DR: Mushroom poisoning in infants and children: the *Amanita pantherina/muscaria* group, *J Toxicol Clin Toxicol* 30:13, 1992.
8. Bouget J et al: Acute renal failure following collective intoxication by *Cortinarius orellanus, Intensive Care Med* 16:506, 1990.
9. Busi C et al: *Amanita* toxins in gastroduodenal fluid of patients poisoned by the mushroom *Amanita phalloides* (letter), *N Engl J Med* 300:800, 1979.
10. Catalfomo P, Eugster C: Muscarine and muscarine isomers in selected *Inocybe* species, *Helv Chim Acta* 53:848, 1970.
11. Chestnut VK: Poisonous properties of the green spored *Lepiota, ASA Gray Bull* 8:87, 1900.
12. Coulet M, Guillot J: Poisoning by *Gyromitra:* a possible mechanism, *Med Hypoth* 8:325, 1982.
13. Coulet M et al: A propos des intoxications par *Gyromitra esculenta* Pers ex Fr, *Acta Mycol* 4:379, 1968.
14. Ellenhorn MJ, Barceloux DG: *Medical toxicology: diagnosis and treatment of human poisoning,* New York, 1988, Elsevier.
15. Fantozzi R et al: Clinical findings and follow-up evaluation of an outbreak of mushroom poisoning—survey of *Amanita phalloides* poisoning, *Klin Wochenschr* 64:38, 1986.
16. Faulstich H: New aspects of *Amanita* poisoning, *Klin Wochenschr* 57:1143, 1979.
17. Faulstich H, Kirchner K, Derenzini M: Strongly enhanced toxicity of the mushroom toxin α-amanitin by an amatoxin-specific FAB or monoclonal antibody, *Toxicon* 26:491, 1988.
18. Faulstich H, Talas A, Wellhoner HH: Toxicokinetics of labeled amatoxins in the dog, *Arch Toxicol* 56:190, 1985.
19. Fauser U, Faulstich H: Beobachtungen zur therapie der Knollenblattenpilzvergiftung, *Dtsch Med Wochenschr* 98:2259, 1973.
20. Fiume L, Lachi R: Lesioni ultrastrutturali prodotte nelle cellule parenchimal epa tiche dalle phalloidina e dalla α-amanitin a, *Sperimentale* 115:288, 1965.
21. Fiume L, Stripe F: Decreased RNA content in mouse liver nuclei after intoxication with α-amanitin, *Biochim Biophys Acta* 123:643, 1966.
22. Floersheim GL: Antagonistic effects against single lethal doses of *Amanita phalloides, Naumyn-Schmiedeberg Arch Pharmacol* 273:171, 1976.
23. Floersheim GL: Experimentille Grundlagen zur Therapie von Vergiftungen durch den grunen Knollenblatterpilz *(Amanita phalloides), Schweiz Med Wochenschr* 108:185, 1978.
24. Floersheim GL: Treatment of mushroom poisoning, *JAMA* 253:3252, 1985.
25. Floersheim G: Treatment of human amatoxin mushroom poisoning: myths and advances in therapy, *Med Toxicol* 2:1, 1987.
26. Floersheim G, Bianchi L: Ethanol diminishes the toxicity of the mushroom *Amanita phalloides, Experimenta* 40:1268, 1984.
27. Floersheim GL, Schneiberger J, Bucher K: Curative potencies of penicillin in experimental *Amanita phalloides* poisoning, *Agents Actions* 213:138, 1971.
28. Floersheim GL et al: Die Klinische Knollenblatterpilzvertigiftung *(Amanita phalloides):* Prognostiche faktoren und Therapeutische massahmen, *Schweiz Med Wochenschr* 112:1164, 1982.
29. Franke S et al: Uber die Giftigkeit der Fruhjahrslorchel *Gyromitra esculenta* Fr, *Arch Toxicol* 22:293, 1967.
30. Frimmer M: What we have learned from phalloidin, *Toxicol Lett* 35:169, 1987.

31. Gerber P: Pilzileus ohne vorbestehendes Passagehindernis, *Schweiz Med Wochenschr* 119:1479, 1989.
32. Gilad E, Biger Y: Paralysis of convergence caused by mushroom poisoning, *Am J Ophthalmol* 102:124, 1986.
33. Giosti GV, Carnevale A: A case of fatal poisoning by *Gyromitra esculenta, Arch Toxicol* 33:49, 1974.
34. Grzymala S: Erfahrung en mit Dermacybe orellana (Fr.) in Polen. B. Massenvergiftung durch den orange fuchsigen. Hautkopf, *Z Pilzk* 23:137, 1957.
35. Grzymala S: Les recherches sur la frequence des intoxications par les champignons, *Bull Med Leg Toxicol Med* 2:200, 1965.
36. Hatfield GM: Toxins of higher fungi, *Lloydia* 38:36, 1975.
37. Hatfield GM, Schaumberg JP: Isolation and structural studies of coprine, the disulfiram-like constituent of *Coprinus atramentarius, Lloydia* 38:489, 1975.
38. Hofmann A et al: Psilocybin ein psychotropen Winkstoff aus dem Mexikanischen Rauschpitz *Psilocybe mexicana* Heim, *Experientia* 14:107, 1958.
39. Holmdahl J et al: Isolation and nephrotoxic studies of orellanine from the mushroom *Cortinarius speciosissimus, Toxicon* 25:195, 1987.
40. Hruby K et al: Chemotherapy of *Amanita phalloides* poisoning with intravenous silibinin, *Hum Toxicol* 2:183, 1983.
41. International Agency for Research on Cancer: Gyromitrin (acetaldehyde formylmethylhydrazone)—on the evaluation of carcinogenic risk of chemicals to man, *IARC Monogr* 31:163, 1983.
42. Ishihara Y, Yamaura Y: Descriptive epidemiology of mushroom poisoning in Japan, *Nippon Eiseigaku Zasshi* 46:1071, 1992.
43. Kelner MJ, Alexander NM: Endocrine hormone abnormalities in *Amanita* poisoning, *Clin Toxicol* 25:21, 1987.
44. Kirklin JK et al: Treatment of hydrazine induced coma with pyridoxine, *N Engl J Med* 294:938, 1976.
45. Klosterman HJ: Vitamin B_6 antagonists of natural origin, *J Agric Food Chem* 22:13, 1974.
46. Koivikko A, Savolainen J: Mushroom allergy, *Allergy* 43:1, 1988.
47. Kretz O, Creppy EE, Dirheimer G: Characterization of bolesatine, a toxic protein from the mushroom *Boletus satanas* Lenz and its effects on kidney cells, *Toxicology* 66:213, 1991.
48. Larcan A et al: Les indications de l'oxygenotherapie hyperbare en reanimation medico-chirurgicale, *Ann Med Nancy* 13:476, 1981.
49. Lincoff G, Mitchel DH: *Toxic and hallucinogenic mushroom poisoning,* New York, 1977, Van Nostrand Reinhold.
50. Lindell TJ et al: Specific inhibition of nuclear RNA polymerase II by α-amanitin, *Science* 170:447, 1970.
51. List PH, Luft P: Gyromitrin, das Gift der Fruhjahrslorchel *Gyromitra (Helvella) esculenta* Fr, *Tetrahedron Lett* 20:1893, 1967.
52. Litovitz TL et al: 1991 annual report of the American Association of Poison Control Centers National Data Collection System, *Am J Emerg Med* 10:452, 1992.
53. Lockey R: Mushroom workers' pneumonitis, *Ann Allergy* 34:282, 1974.
54. Lopez A et al: Fulminant hepatitis and liver transplantation, *Ann Intern Med* 108:769, 1988.
55. Maretic Z: Poisoning by the mushroom *Clitocybe olearia* Maire, *Toxicon* 4:263, 1967.
56. Maretic Z, Russell FE, Golobie V: Twenty-five cases of poisoning by the mushroom *Pleurotus olearius, Toxicon* 13:379, 1975.
57. Maynert EJ, Kaji K: On the relationship of brain gamma-aminobutyric acid to convulsions, *J Pharmacol Exp Ther* 137:114, 1963.
58. McCawley EL, Brummett RE, Dana GW: Convulsions from*Psilocybe* mushroom poisoning, *Proc West Pharmacol Soc* 5:27, 1962.
59. Mendelson G: Treatment of hallucinogenic plant toxicity, *Ann Intern Med* 85:126, 1976.
60. Meixner A: Amatoxin nochwers, *Pilzen Z Mykol* 45:137, 1979.
61. Michelot D, Toth B: Poisoning by *Gyromitra* esculenta—a review, *J Appl Toxicol* 11:235, 1991.
62. Nakazawa T, Tochigi T: Hypersensitivity pneumonitis due to mushroom *(Pholiota nameko)* spores, *Chest* 95:1149, 1989.
63. Neftel K et al: Sind Cephalosporine bei der Intoxikation mit Knollenblatterpilz besser wirksam als Penicillin-G? *Schweiz Med Wochenschr* 118:49, 1988.
64. O'Grady JG et al: Early indications of prognosis in fulminant hepatic failure, *Gastroenterology* 97:439, 1989.
65. Orlav NI: *Sjedobuye i jadovitye griby gribenye ostravlenjia i ich profilaktica,* Moscow, 1953, Megdiz, p 44.
66. Peden NR, Pringle SD, Crooks J: The problem of psilocybin mushroom abuse, *Hum Toxicol* 1:417, 1982.
67. Pinson CW et al: Liver transplantation for severe *Amanita phalloides* mushroom poisoning, *Am J Surg* 159:493, 1990.
68. Piqueras J et al: Mushroom poisoning: therapeutic apheresis or forced diuresis (letter), *Transfusion* 27:116, 1987.
69. Reick W, Platt D: High-performance liquid chromatographic method for the determination of α-amanitin and phalloidin in human plasma using the column-switching technique and its application in suspected cases of poisoning by the green species of *Amanita* mushroom *(Amanita phalloides), J Chromatogr* 425:121, 1988.
70. Rivett MJ, Boon GPG: Mushroom *(Amanita phalloides)* poisoning in Ciskei (letter), *S Afr Med J* 73:317, 1988.
71. Ronzoni G et al: Recovery after serious mushroom poisoning (grade IV encephalopathy) with intensive care support without liver transplantation, *Minerva Anestesiol* 57:383, 1991.
72. Sanz P et al: Disseminated intravascular coagulation and mesenteric venous thrombosis in fatal *Amanita* poisoning, *Hum Toxicol* 7:199, 1988.
73. Sastie J et al: Respiratory and immunological reactions among shiitake *(Lentinus edodes)* mushroom workers, *Clin Exp Allergy* 20:13, 1990.
74. Schneider SM: The effect of ethanol on alpha amanitin hepatotoxicity (abstract), *Vet Hum Toxicol* 34:352, 1992.
75. Schneider SM, Borochovitz D, Krenzelok EP: Cimetidine protection against alpha-amanitin hepatotoxicity in mice: a potential model for the treatment of *Amanita phalloides* poisoning, *Ann Emerg Med* 16:1136, 1987.
76. Schneider SM, Vanscoy GJ, Michelson EA: Penicillin and cimetidine in *Amanita* toxicity in mice (abstract), *Vet Hum Toxicol* 30:364, 1988.
77. Schneider SM et al: P_{450} inducer increases toxicity of alpha-amanitin (abstract), *Vet Hum Toxicol* 32:369, 1990.
78. Seeger R: Zweitungspapiertest for Amanitin-falsch-positive Erge bnisse, *Z Mykol* 50:353, 1984.
79. Shichijo K et al: A case of bronchial asthma caused by spores of *Lentinus edodes* (Berk) Sing, *Jpn J Allergy* 18:35, 1969.
80. Simons DM: The mushrooms toxins, *Del Med J* 43:177, 1971.
81. Sotaniemi E et al: Hydrazine toxicity in the human: report of a fatal case, *Ann Clin Res* 3:30, 1971.
82. Stenklyft PH, Augenstein WL: *Chlorophyllum molybdites*—severe mushroom poisoning in a child, *J Toxicol Clin Toxicol* 28:159, 1990.
83. Suzuki K et al: Purification and some properties of a hemolysin from the poisonous mushroom *Rhodophyllus rhodopolius, Toxicon* 9:1019, 1990.
84. Toth B, Erikson J: Cancer induction in mice by feeding of the uncooked cultivated mushroom of commerce *Agaricus bisporus, Cancer Res* 46:4007, 1986.
85. Toth B, Patel K: The tumorigenic effect of low dose levels of *N*-methyl-*N*-formyl hydrazine in mice, *Neoplasma* 27:25, 1980.
86. Trestrail JH: Mushroom poisoning in the United States—an analysis of 1989 United States Poison Center Data, *Clin Toxicol* 29:459, 1991.
87. Tyler VE: Poisonous mushrooms, *Prog Chem Toxicol* 6:339, 1963.
88. Vanden Hoek TL et al: Jack o'lantern mushroom poisoning, *Ann Emerg Med* 20:559, 1991.
89. Vanscoy GJ, Schneider SM: Cimetidine and ascorbic acid in the treatment of alpha-amanitin toxicity in mice (abstract), *Vet Hum Toxicol* 30:368, 1988.

90. Wieland T: The toxic peptides from *Amanita* mushrooms, *Int J Peptide Protein Res* 22:257, 1983.
91. Wieland T, Faulstich H: Fifty years of amanitin, *Experientia* 47:1186, 1991.
92. Wieland TH: Uber die Gifstoffe des Knollenblatterpilzes VII. β-Amanitin, eine dritte Komponente des Knollenblatterpilz giftes, *Justus Liebigs Ann Chem* 564:152, 1949.
93. Wright AV et al: Amelioration of toxic effects of ethylidene gyromitrin (false morel poison) with pyridoxine chloride, *J Food Safety* 3:199, 1981.
94. Yi-gu Z, Guang-zhao H: Poisoning by toxic plants in China: report of 19 autopsy cases, *Am J Forensic Med Pathol* 9:313, 1988.

39 PLANT MEDICINE

Kevin Jon Davison

Historical Aspects

The history of herbally based medicines begins before the advent of written records. In all ancient civilizations plants served as important elements of food, shelter, dyes, ornamentation, religious rituals, and medicines. The term "herb" is broadly defined as a nonwoody plant that dies down to the ground after flowering. However, the most commonly used interpretation is any plant used for medicinal therapy, nutritional value, food seasoning, or dyeing another substance.

Humans' precise medicinal discovery of the uses of plants remains conjectural. Many scenarios probably occurred. Perhaps, in a prehistoric jungle of South America, a pool of water containing fallen plant material leached out some of the precious medicinal constituents of leaves, flowers, stems, and bark. Tannins, glycosides, sugars, and alkaloids from the bark were infused into the waters. We can envision an extremely ill native passing that way; because of his burning fever and severe dehydration, he drank from the pool and his fever miraculously disappeared. The pond became known for its magical healing powers. If the water held bark from the cinchona tree, the native may have serendipitously discovered quinine.

Archeologic evidence shows that prehistoric humans used plants extensively to treat physical ailments. Instinct and trial and error led to the realization that, for example, cinchona bark controlled intermittent fevers, animals fed on ergotized grain aborted their fetuses, and latex from the opium poppy could be eaten to alleviate pain. Innumerable medicinal plant traditions that remain intact to the present originated as far back as 2700 BC. Ethnobotanically, it is evident that the use of plant-based medicines represented far more than individual efforts to survive. Analyzing the methods and degrees of use of indigenous medicines reveals much about cultural philosophy, ingenuity, and sophistication. The Chinese developed an extensive and elaborate system for prescribing, classifying, and processing of herbs, which dates back to the third millennium BC. The formulas used carefully identified the specific effect of each herb, as well as interactions with other herbs. Less tolerable herbs were blended with those that would counteract undesirable effects. Formulas were custom blended, taking into account a patient's constitution and the stage of the disease. Some of the ancient knowledge from these writings is being used in many contemporary herbal preparations commercially sold as "patent" (readily available in pill form) medicines.

Many native tribes of New Guinea, Indonesia, and the Amazon use single-herb formulations as they did thousands of years ago to treat nearly all of their medical conditions. In the West, written records dating to the Sumerians accurately describe the medicinal uses of specific plants.[99] In the same period of about 3000 years ago, the first Asian written record, the *Ben Tsao Gan Mu,* was compiled by the Chinese. It listed more than 360 medicinal plants and their classification, uses, contraindications, and methods of action as perceived at that time. Roman and Greek herbal remedies were described in the writings of Hippocrates and later in those of Galen, providing a pattern for the development of the Western medical tradition. Hippocrates was an advocate of using a few simple plant preparations along with fresh air, rest, and proper diet to help the body's own "life force" eliminate problems. Conversely, Galen promoted the use of direct intervention, employing large doses of complicated "drug" mixtures that included animal, plant, and mineral ingredients to correct the imbalances that cause disease.[112]

The earliest European compendium that listed the uses and properties of medicinal plants, *De Materia Medica,* was written by the Greek physician Dioscorides in the first century AD. He described about 600 plants, and his work remained the authoritive herbal medicinal resource into the seventeenth century.

Herbalism was practiced in many different ways during and after the Middle Ages. There were learned traditional herbalists and lay practitioners, as well as wandering herbalists who professed pagan animism or Christian superstitions that often were more influential in healing than the herbs' actual properties. Little was added to the knowledge of herbalism during this period. After the Middle Ages and the invention of the printing press in the 1400s, hundreds of herbal publications were compiled. Most early works were available only in Latin or Greek; it was not until the fifteenth, sixteenth, and seventeenth centuries that the great age of herbalism was appreciated in English.[99]

Tides changed in European herbalism when a Swiss pharmacist-physician named Theophrastus Bombastis von Hohenheim, better known as Paracelsus (1490-1541), introduced a new dimension. He advocated chemistry and chemical processing and used mineral salts, acids, and other preparations in medicinal therapies. This was a departure from the plant-based medicinal methods of the past. During the latter seventeenth century the predominance of plant medicines slowly eroded. In 1806, Freidrich Serturner, a small town German pharmacist, became known for his efforts to isolate organic acids from plants in an attempt to find the active ingredient in opium. He discovered organic alkaloids, which became known as the first set of active plant constituents.[147] Because of their physiologic activity, the search for plant alkaloids continued into the twentieth century.

Discoveries quickly followed. The bronchodilator and antitussive ephedrine, which comes from the herb *Ephedra sinica,* became commonly used in Chinese medicinal formulas for bronchial asthma. The discovery of morphine led to creation of all the narcotic analgesics. The bark of cinchona was found to contain quinine in 1819, which led to development of antimalarial drugs.

The traditional herbal extract from rhubarb (*Rheum* spp.) has several active compounds. These compounds mediate many of the pharmacologic effects, such as its purgative action (from sennosides); antibacterial, antifungal, and antitumor activities (from anthroquinones); antiinflammatory and analgesic activities; and improvements of lipid metabolism (from stilbenes). Treatment of leukemias from an extract of Madagascar periwinkle *(Catharanthus roseus),* known as vincristine, has been highly effective.[42]

Discoveries in the mid to late nineteenth century included atropine (from belladona leaves, *Atropa belladona*) in 1831, cocaine (from coca leaves, *Erythoxylum coca*) in 1860, ergotamine (from *Claviceps purpurea*) in 1918, and tubocurarine in 1935.[112]

As settlers from Europe came to the Americas, they brought herbal knowledge and many of their medicinal methods. Because of the abundance and wide use of plants on the new continents, they also learned much from the indigenous peoples. The colonists found that conditions afflicting them, such as malaria and scurvy, were treated effectively with herbs by the Native Americans.[112]

In the 1700s, herbal medicine continued to have popular applications in lay circles, but it also began to be investigated by the medical establishment that was beginning to form. Although the creation of a small elite group of learned professionals was thought to violate the political and constitutional concepts being developed by the early American democratic movement, the practice of medicine was carried over from England and Scotland during prerevolutionary days. Before a professional medical class was established, most illness in America was treated within the family or extended family network.

Many concepts were modified in the colonies between 1765, when the first medical school opened, and 1850, when over 42 schools of medicine were recognized. The inquiry into *Digitalis purpurea* (foxglove) by William Withering exemplified the change in perspective from anecdotal folk medicine to a critical examination for specific uses of botanicals from a biochemical point of view. During the early 1800s the trend was to look at the efficacy of botanicals and their intrinsic value from a more scientific perspective.

Several developments delayed the appreciation of herbalism by physicians in the colonies. For instance, Samuel Thomson promoted a system of herbal medicine by proselytizing about his patented method of herbal prescribing, which used many native American herbs. A central theme in his approach was the advocacy of self-prescribing based on the philosophies and herbal prescriptions found in his book, *New Guide to Health.* The right to sell "family franchises" for use of the Thomsonian method of healing was the basis of a widespread lay movement between 1822 and Thomson's death in 1843. Thomson adamantly believed that no professional medical class should exist and that democratic medicine was best practiced by lay persons within a Thomsonian "family unit."[38] Although his methods were considered crude and unscientific, he had over 3 million faithful followers in 1839. Founded on ignorance, prejudice, and dogma, the Thomsonian school did little to lead the professional physician to accept many of the herbal medicines being used in Europe and America. Some of the professionally trained European physicians who had become part of the Thomsonian movement wished to separate themselves from the lay practitioners by creating requirements and standards for the practice of Thomsonian medicine. Thomson was adamantly against this, so it was not until a decade after his death that the Thomsonian doctors helped to form what became known as the Eclectic School of Medicine. The Eclectic School of Medicine attempted to bridge the gap between "professional physicians," Thomsonianism, and traditional herbal medicine. The establishment of several Eclectic medical schools was a step toward validating herbal medicine, but it failed to bring herbalism into the mainstream medical establishment. The founding of the American Medical Association and the Flexner Report on medical education in 1910 thoroughly established the modern pharmaceutical industry in the medical education system.[38]

Because of the availability of pure, active constituents from plant drugs and the synthetic drugs that began to appear on the market toward the end of the nineteenth century, the prescribing habits of physicians began to change. The sensibility and predictability of administering exact doses were appealing. It was possible, for example, to prescribe the pure alkaloid of quinine for malaria rather than a foul-tasting extract of cinchona bark containing variable percentages of quinine and other alkaloids with different physiologic properties.

Many "crude drugs" were standardized for therapeutic activity. Digitalis, which still retains its status in the United States Pharmacopeia (USP), is one example. It is interesting to note that of the 200 plant drugs officially listed in the USP in 1936, about 19% are still official today.[147] It has been estimated that 25% of all prescriptions dispensed in community pharmacies between 1959 and 1980 contained ingredients extracted from higher plants. For a significant number of synthetic drugs, natural drug products continue to serve as either models or starting points for synthesis.

Evolution of Phytopharmaceuticals

The drive toward patenting and ownership in the pharmaceutical industry has been a strong incentive to research and develop plant-based products. However, because a plant per se cannot be patented, comparatively little U.S. effort has gone into developing herbal medicines during the last century. What occurs is investigation of active principles of botanicals for their biological activity, although in many cases, the active constituent is less effective than the whole crude extract of a herb.[112]

One problem in the development of the botanical pharmaceutical industry in the United States has been quality control. In addition, lack of standardization plagues plant-based products. Quality control and standardization of crude plant extracts for herbal medicines were virtually nonexistent until recently.[112] Were this not the case, we might be using more botanical medicines for common ailments. In Europe and Asia, where pharmaceutical firms have been producing standardized phytopharmaceuticals (plant-based standardized extracts) for decades, research and development have demonstrated economic and medical sense. Europeans use phytopharmaceuticals as part of their "mainstream" medical practice. In hospitals, they are used primarily as adjuvant therapies. More that 70% of general practitioners in Germany prescribe phytopharmaceuticals, and most of these prescriptions are paid for by the public health insurance system.[128] The total annual market for phytopharmaceuticals in Germany alone is $1.7 billion.[128] Beginning in 1993 the licensing procedure for German physicians required a knowledge of phytotherapy.[128]

Improvement in production and evaluation of botanical medicines has been significant in the past six decades. In crude plant evaluation, modern laboratory analysis can determine the percentage of active principles, as well as solubility, specific gravity, melting point, optical rotation, and water content. Scientists detect resins, alkaloids, flavonoids, enzymes, essential oils, fats, carbohydrates, and protein content.

Through the use of liquid, high-pressure liquid, paper, and thin-layer chromatographies, spectrophotometry, atomic absorption, and nuclear magnetic resonance imaging, quality, purity, potency, and uniformity can be precisely assayed. These methods improve the predictability and therapeutic effectiveness of standardized crude botanical medicines, which are then evaluated for their efficacy in animal studies to determine pharmacologic potency, activity, and toxicity. In the areas of quality control and cultivation techniques, companies in the United States and Europe have set strict guidelines to ensure optimum yields of pharmacoactive principles and sanitation. This includes guidelines for acceptable levels of impurities, bacterial counts, pesticides, residual solvents, and heavy metals.

Specific cultivation and harvesting techniques affect the therapeutic value of a given herb, which is related to the amount of active constituents in a specific medicinal plant. Methods of packaging, storage, and transport can dramatically affect the stability of active compounds.

Major innovations have been made in extraction and concentration processes in the past few decades. Both extracts and concentrates are obtained by adding appropriate solvents to raw herbs, which removes the active constituents. The most commonly practiced and familiar method is infusion. As a tea bag is steeped in hot water to make a cup of tea, the water acts as a solvent. If the water were slowly evaporated, the concentrate would contain the active constituents.

Pure ethanol is an effective solvent commonly used to concentrate active herbal constituents. Immersing a high-quality bulk or raw herb in pure ethanol for hours or days, depending on the herb and the part used, then pressing it out, yields an herbal tincture. The alcoholic tincture is remixed with water to yield a 20% alcohol tincture. In another method, a 20% alcohol mixture is the solvent. Fluid extracts are made by distilling off some of the alcohol with vacuum distillation to avoid elevating the temperature, which may affect some of the active constituents. Another concentration process, solid extraction, yields a solid or semisolid product that can then be powdered or granulated for administration.

Once an extract is produced, qualitative and quantitative analyses can be performed to assist in standardization. The percentage of known active constituents is assayed, so that predictable clinical results can be obtained.

An herbal infusion is generally a better source of active compounds than is an air- or sun-dried powdered herb (Color Plate 96), but it may not be as strong in action as concentrates such as tinctures, solid extracts, and fluid extracts. Generally the potency of an extract can be defined in two ways. One is by the percentage of active constituents; another is by concentration. Herbalists express concentration as an equivalency. For instance, a four-to-one extract is equivalent to or derived from four parts of the crude herb to yield one part extract. This is usually written as "4:1 solid extract." Longer shelf life, greater effectiveness, and higher concentration of active constituents make a more standardized (better) product than does the raw powdered herb; however, efficacy is difficult to compare.

An example of a product that is standardized to the percentage concentration of pharmacoactive glycosides is the extract of *Ginko biloba,* marketed in Europe under the trade names Tanakan, Rokan, and Tebonin. It is typically standardized as 24% flavonoid glycoside. *G. biloba* extract has been shown to prevent metabolic and neuronal disturbances of cerebral ischemia and hypoxia in experimental models.[85,95]

The issue of quality control has been addressed for many herbal products when the known clinical effectiveness can be attributed to a specific active constituent. With improved analytic methods and the use of high-quality herbs (high in active principles), the standardization problem can be addressed. In Europe the dosage is expressed in milligrams of active constituents, which favors consistency. The main difference of this method of administration from the process of chemical isolation or synthesis is that the extracts still contain all the synergistic cofactors that enhance the function of the active ingredient. This is believed to be an important aspect of herbal medicine, which is lost once the active constituent is removed from the whole plant.

Herbal Preparation for Modern Clinical Use and in the Wilderness Setting

Botanical preparations are readily applicable in acute prescribing for travelers and wilderness enthusiasts. Throughout the ages, botanicals have been useful adjunctive therapeutic agents. Knowing how and what preparations from the natural pharmacopeia can be used can give us a sense of integration with our natural environment. The indigenous peoples of the world who have depended on the botanical world throughout their existence hold a vast amount of untapped knowledge. It should be a goal for wilderness enthusiasts to help engender and preserve this understanding of our natural world and help save natural habitats. Further investigation into the plant kingdom for useful medicinal agents will aid in these efforts.

Herbal medicines can be prepared by decoction or infusion of bulk or raw herbs, or by the use of extracts, concentrates, and tinctures.

Infusions are prepared like a standard tea. The soft parts of plants—flowers, stems, and leaves—are placed in a warmed pot. Boiling water is poured over the herb, and the pot is covered to prevent beneficial essential oils from evaporating. The mixture infuses for about 10 minutes, then is strained. The supernatant can be used immediately or be refrigerated in an airtight container for as long as 2 days. A standard adult dose of an herbal preparation would be 1 ounce (28 g) of dried herb to 1 pint (or 500 ml) of water, or a teaspoon per cup. The amount is doubled if the herb is fresh.

Generally, it is best to take infusions hot by the cupful three times daily for a chronic problem and up to every hour or two during an acute illness. To make infusions palatable, many herbalists have added licorice, aniseed, or honey. The hard or woody parts of plants, such as bark, seeds, roots, rhizomes, and nuts, have tough cell walls that must be broken down by great heat before they can impart their constituents to water. The herbs can be broken into small pieces by chopping, crushing, or hammering.

Traditionally, a decoction was prepared in an earthen crock reserved especially for making herbal preparations. In the past, herbalists believed that some of the quality of the medicine was affected by the type of vessel or container in which the brew was prepared. Contemporary practitioners generally recommend the use of stainless steel, ceramic, or enamel, and specifically discourage the use of aluminum or other alloyed metal pots. The herb is placed in an appropriate container and covered with cold water. The mixture is brought to a boil, covered, and simmered for 10 to 45 minutes, depending on the type and part of the herb being used. A decoction can be strained, flavored, or sweetened like an infusion, and it is consumed while hot.

Modern practitioners use the most efficient and predictable forms of specific herbal medicines. Many producers have found that concentrates in capsule form are most effective and easiest to administer. The standard herbal concentrate found in the marketplace is in the ratio of 4:1. Ease of administration and dosage and the predictable clinical effects have made this the industry standard. Herbal tinctures are extracted into a specific percentage of alcohol and can be mixed easily by practitioners to make formulas tailored to personal conditions. A combination may be many times more effective than a single herb. Formula prescribing is an art. Classic formulas for common ailments have been cataloged since the first herbal compendiums were recorded centuries ago. However, for the purposes of this chapter, single herbs and their specific uses, identifications, and preparation are detailed.

Homeopathic Use of Botanicals

Samuel Hanhaman, a medical pioneer, developed a radically different system of medicine nearly 200 years ago. Homeopathy is derived from the Greek words *homoios,* which means "similar," and *pathos,* which means "disease" or "suffering." The "Law of Similars" states that a substance that causes a set of symptoms in large doses can create a cure for similar symptoms (even if the etiologic agent is different) if that substance is given in a homeopathic dilution.

Most homeopathic remedies are prepared from plant, mineral, and animal products. In homeopathic medicine the medicine is a perfectly matched similimum (the most effective medicine) if the predominant symptoms of a disease or illness match the symptoms produced when the substance is taken in large doses in a healthy individual. For example, the herb *Atropa belladona,* which contains atropine, is poisonous. In excessive doses the herb causes death, in moderate doses it creates hot, feverish states, and in tiny (homeopathic) doses it can effectively treat certain types of fevers, viral syndromes, and inflammatory states.

A homeopathic dilution is created by taking a prepared tincture of a botanical or an extract from nonplant sources and diluting it in a sequential method. The dilution can range from a 1× potency, which is a decimal dilution of a given ingredient (one part per nine parts solute) to an extremely dilute 200 c (one part per 99 solute, serially diluted 200 times). A high-potency dilution (serially diluted more than 30 times) would be taken much less frequently than a low-potency (serially diluted less than 30 times). This is contrary to our pharmacologic understanding of drug dynamics.

The actual mechanisms by which homeopathy works have yet to be elucidated, even though it has been practiced effectively for several hundred years. At the turn of this century, it was estimated that 15% of the practicing physicians in the United States were prescribing homeopathic remedies.[103] Recent studies have shown effective results in clinical trials using homeopathic medicines.[28,80,91] Although a complete explanation of the effects of homeopathic techniques has not been given, mechanisms of action for many commonly prescribed traditional pharmaceuticals also remain unknown. Indeed, many theories in medicine are still based largely on empirical observations rather than theoretical understanding.

One herbal folk remedy for bruises, sprains, strains, and rheumatism in European and native American medicine was topical application of the plant *Arnica montana* (leopard's bane). Consistent with the homeopathic principle, the toxic effects of the whole-plant extract of *Arnica* produce the same set of symptoms it is intended to cure when administered internally in a homeopathic dosage or if the tincture or oil is applied topically to the affected area.

In *Homeopathic Materia Medica,* William Boericke described the systemic toxic affects produced by *Arnica* tincture: it "produces conditions upon the system quite similar to those resulting from injuries, falls, blows, contusions . . . Limbs and body ache as if beaten; joints as if sprained . . . Affects the venous system as inducing stasis, ecchymosis and hemorrhages."

Generally, the most commonly prescribed homeopathic remedy after any trauma is *Arnica.* It is contained in herbal and homeopathic dosages in numerous ointments, salves, and poultices from European and American phytopharmaceutical companies for the treatment of trauma resulting from localized sprains, strains, or contusions. Controlled studies in Germany have shown that effective products for sprains from athletic activity use an ointment that contains homeopathic *Arnica.*[156]

Topical Application

In the earliest times the method of plant administration used most often was topical application. Although many plants contain generalized moisture-enhancing properties, some were found to be particularly effective in ameliorating specific acute conditions when applied topically. There are two general methods of applying remedies to the skin. The endermatic method applies medicine on the skin without friction, as when applying a compress to the dermis and epidermis after an abrasion or laceration. The epidermatic method uses application with friction and is most effective when using botanical oils, liniments, ointments, and medicated warm and cold friction rubs. These are mostly applied for subdermal contusions and trauma, when circulatory changes are desired.[51]

Topical application of medicinal plants can be useful for a multitude of conditions, including abrasions, lacerations, burns, insect bites, infections, rashes, and varied dermatoses. Other applications include contusions, varicosities, joint pain, inflammation, musculotendinous aches, strains, and sprains.

Topical herbal remedies are applied with a poultice, compress, fomentation, or ointment. Probably the most common is the poultice. This is used to apply a remedy to a skin area with moist heat. A poultice is prepared by bruising or crushing the medicinal parts of the plant to a pulpy mass, then applying this to the affected area and covering it all with a moist heat source. If dried plants are used (or if necessary with fresh plants), the materials are moistened by mixing with a hot, soft, adhesive substance such as moist flour or corn meal. A good way to apply a poultice is to spread the paste or pulp on a wet and hot cloth, which is wrapped around the affected area to help retain moisture and heat. The cloth is moistened with hot water as necessary. Where irritant plants are involved (as in a mustard "plaster"), the paste is kept between two pieces of cloth to prevent direct contact with the skin. After the poultice is removed, the area is washed well with water to remove any residue. A poultice can be used to soothe, to irritate, or to draw impurities from the affected area, depending on which plant or plants are applied.

A fomentation is a hot cloth soaked with an herbal infusion or decoction. Fomentations are generally less active than poultices. A cold compress is used for conditions that require an antiinflammatory cure. A cold infusion- or decoction-soaked cloth is applied to an area and then removed when the body's circulation has warmed the cloth to body temperature. The botanicals' active principles determine what actions the external applications will impart. For example, a poultice with an astringent herb such as *Hammamelis* (witch hazel) has an entirely different effect than one made with a strong vasodilator and rubefacient, such as *Capsicum* (cayenne pepper).

Ointments are another method of topical administration. Most ointments are made in a base of petroleum jelly, stable vegetable oils, bees' wax, or a combination of these. The extract from the desired botanical is suspended within the base to create a stable solid product. Topical botanical products have the same function as topical pharmaceutical ointments and are used to treat lacerations, abrasions, infections, and insect bites. Other uses for botanical topicals include hemostatic, antiinflammatory, antihistamine, rubefacient, analgesic, emollient, and circulatory stimulant actions. Like pharmaceutical topical agents, herbal poultices, compresses, and ointments deliver their active compounds transdermally.

Some ethnobotanists think that the first uses of most medicinal plants were probably topical. In contemporary herbology, many of these plants are also used internally. Whole plants containing more than one ingredient with biologic activity generally invoke synergistic action of several components to produce the therapeutic action. Thus most botanicals have multiple applications for therapeutic purposes.

The major precaution needed in the field of medical botany is to identify toxicity. Some of the most effective topical agents can be toxic if ingested. Most of these plants found in the wild could not be taken in large enough doses to be fatal before causing gastrointestinal upset. However, a tincture, herbal concentrate, or powdered version of the plant could have deadly potential.

A method of treatment used by herbalists and homeopaths alike to treat trauma of the skin, muscles, tendons, ligaments, and joint tissue is to administer a topical agent in ointment or poultice form and give the same medicine internally in minute (homeopathic) doses to enhance the activity, as is done with concurrent use of *Arnica* ointment and homeopathic *Arnica*.

Considerations and Rationale for the Use of Herbal Medicine in the Wilderness

Travelers in the wilderness must choose either a preprocessed herbal preparation or what is naturally available in the immediate vicinity.

A surprisingly large number of minor medical conditions encountered in an outdoor setting can be treated by the use of plants found in that location. North American recreational areas are home to medicinal plants that have been used by Native Americans for centuries. Recreationists in desert, alpine, and river environments can find medicinal plants in abundance. Nearly all of the vegetation encountered during an alpine trek in North America has some medicinal property. In the tropical and subtropical regions are a plethora of plants with medicinal properties.

Some considerations for using herbal products in the wilderness are availability, ease of application, incidence of side effects, toxicity, spectrum of applicability, affordability, and effectiveness.

AVAILABILITY AND EASE OF APPLICATION

If a condition can be improved by application of a local botanical and it happens to be growing in the immediate vicinity, the pharmacy is immediately available. If plants are in season, plentiful, and easily harvested, all the better. Finding the appropriate plants can be challenging, depending on the location, season, the traveler's familiarity with botanicals, and the type of medical condition. During the popular mild seasons and at elevations conducive to plant growth in the continental United States, the chances of finding some of the common plants mentioned in this chapter are quite good. If not, standardized commercial preparations of these herbs can be carried. These are packaged for long storage life, sanitary and convenient application, and standardization of active ingredients. Some of the standardized preparations are mentioned in the following sections.

Hundreds of plants can be applied topically for a variety of conditions. Most of the readily available plants, even if properly identified, require some form of processing for the active constituents to be used fully. Furthermore, expertise in the field requires years of training by a knowledgeable botanist and herbalist. It also requires knowledge of plant seasonal variation, ecologic niches, and precise plant identification. However, it is not beyond the scope of a non-botanist-herbalist to gain a basic understanding of a few plant medicines that have a wide spectrum of applicability and a broad range of geographic distribution.

INCIDENCE OF SIDE EFFECTS AND TOXICITY

The American Association of Poison Control Centers annually reports plant ingestion as a significant category of accidental poisoning. In 1985 and 1986, 9.1% of U.S. poisonings came from plants and mushrooms. Only 7% of the victims were taken to a health care facility. There were six deaths, four from mushroom ingestion. Of the poisonings reported, nearly 90% were in children under the age of 6 years.[15]

Side effects or toxic reactions from botanicals are rarely experienced. In those covered in this chapter, toxicity is not a major consideration. It must be remembered that anything can be toxic when used excessively or indiscriminantly. Many toxic plants produce gastrointestinal distress, vomiting, or diarrhea before any severe neurologic or cardiorespiratory derangement. Quite often, toxic side effects are caused by one substance in a plant. When isolated, minute amounts of an alkaloid may be potentially dangerous, but when ingested in a form modified by other constituents present, a significant alteration of the drug effect occurs so that larger amounts of the toxic substance or substances may be tolerated.

Like any medication, medicinal plants should be applied with a degree of awareness, and dosages for internal use should not exceed recommendations. Pregnancy and nursing may pose contraindications. Dosages for almost any herb can be found in numerous references.[112] H.W. Felter stated, "As a rule, doses usually administered are far in excess of necessity and it is better to err on the side of insufficient dosage and trust to nature, than to overdose to the present or future harm or danger of the patient." In general, for the herbs presented in this chapter, it is safe to state that for those that are self-harvested, the dry crushed herbal adult dosage should be 1 teaspoon per pint of water; when the fresh herb is used, the amount should be twice that. While no absolute law can be laid down in administering medicines to children, Cowling's Rule takes the child's age at the next birthday and divides by 24, to determine what fraction of the adult dose should be given.[51]

SPECTRUM OF APPLICATION

Most herbal medicines that have been cataloged and used historically are specifically indicated for one condition, although additional therapeutic effects have been noted over time. All of the botanicals covered here have multiple uses. Comfrey *(Symphytum officinale)* may be used as a topical antiinflammatory agent; it also has principles that when taken internally are effective for certain gastrointestinal conditions.[99] *Aloe vera* gel is an excellent topical agent for abrasions and burns; when the latex portion is taken internally, it serves as an effective laxative.[99] *Calendula officianalis* has antimicrobial properties that make it an effective topical dressing for mild infectious conditions, while internally it has antipyretic effects.[99]

AFFORDABILITY

If the herbalist collects plants and processes them personally, the cost is minimal. The purchase price of botanicals depends on the rarity and origin. Some exotic and rare botanicals from Asia and the Amazon rainforest demand a high price on the world market. *Panax ginseng* has long been regarded by Asian peoples as a prized herbal tonic and can cost hundreds of dollars per root, depending on the size, origin, and age. *Panax quinquefolius* or American ginseng can cost as much as $52 per pound, and as a cash crop in 1992 was valued at $62 million.[15] Many exotic herbal and animal-derived medicines from China have prices as high as those of precious metals.

Most of the herbs used for common ailments produced in the continental United States average 20 to 30 cents per dose (equivalent to 1 teaspoon of herbal tincture). As yet there is little standardization of prices. Quality control for production and supply and demand seem to dictate the cost of the mass-marketed herbal products. The best way to get a standardized product that reflects a relationship between quality and price is to acquire the product from a botanical company that has been in business for at least 10 years and sells only to licensed health care practitioners.

Commonly Used Plant Medicines Found in North America

EPHEDRA (EPHEDRA SINICA)

Description and Habitat

Common names for *Ephedra* include Brigham Young weed, desert herb, Mormon tea, squaw tea, and teamsters' tea.

Ephedra species are shrubs with erect strawlike branches found in desert or arid regions throughout the world and in the southwestern deserts of the United States (Color Plate 97). The Chinese *Ephedra* called Ma Huang, *Ephedra sinica,* is found throughout Asia; *E. distacha* is found throughout Europe; *E. trifurca* or *E. viridis* (desert tea), *E. nevadensis* (Mormon tea), and *E. americana* (American *Ephedra*) are found in North America; and *E. gerardiana* (Pakistani *Ephedra*) is found in Pakistan and India. The 2- to 7-foot shrubs grow on dry, rocky, or sandy soils. The broomlike shrub has many jointed green stems with two or three small scalelike leaves that grow at the joint of stems and branches.

Pharmacology

Ephedra is generally utilized for its alkaloid content, which tends to be ephedrine, pseudoephedrine, and norpseudoephedrine. The various species vary significantly in both alkaloid type and content. In *E. sinica* the total alkaloid content can be from 3.3% to 20%, with 40% to 90% being ephedrine and the remainder pseudoephedrine.[46] The North American varieties, such as Mormon tea *(E. nevadensis),* are reported to contain no ephedrine.

Ephedra's pharmacology centers on the actions of ephedrine. Ephedrine and pseudoephedrine are used widely in prescription and over-the-counter drugs to treat asthma, hay fever, and rhinitis.[58]

The central nervous system effects of ephedrine are similar to those of epinephrine but are much milder and longer in duration of action. The cardiovascular effects are increased blood pressure, cardiac output, and heart rate. In addition, ephedrine increases brain, heart, and muscle blood flow while decreasing renal and intestinal circulation.[58] There is also relaxation of bronchial, airway, and uterine smooth muscles.[58]

Pseudoephedrine has weaker central nervous and cardiovascular system actions but has bronchial smooth muscle relaxation effects. Because of fewer side effects, it is used more often than ephedrine for asthma.[58] Pseudoephedrine also demonstrates significant antiinflammatory activity.[69,86] Per 100 g the dry leaf *Ephedra* is reported to contain 5 g protein, 5810 mg calcium, and 500 mg potassium.[46]

Native and European Medicinal Use

Ephedra has been used extensively both in the West and in Asia for conditions of the upper respiratory tract such as asthma, bronchitis, and hay fever. It has also been used to treat edema, arthritis, fever, hypotension, and urticaria.[33] It is said to be valuable as a diuretic, febrifuge, and tonic.[99]

The Navajo Indians used the dried, crushed long leaf *Ephedra* to apply to syphilitic sores, and the Hopi Indians drank a tea from the branches and twigs of a related species for the same condition.[150] Other tribes used the ground and roasted root for making bread.[46]

Mormon tea is a folk remedy for colds, gonorrhea, headache, nephritis, and syphilis.[46] Mexicans mix the leaves with tobacco and smoke them for headaches.[46]

Modern Clinical and Wilderness Applications

Ephedra has proved to be an effective bronchodilator for treating mild to moderate asthma and hay fever. The common preparations include other herbs that have antitussive and expectorant effects, such as licorice *(Glycyrrhiza glabra)* and grindelia *(Grindelia camporium).*

Studies in animals and humans have shown that ephedrine promotes weight loss.[112] Appetite suppression may be one mechanism, but an increase in metabolic rate of adipose tissue is the main mechanism.[7]

Other studies have shown that the weight reduction effects can be enhanced by up to 60% with the addition of methylxanthine.[47]

Clinically, standardized preparations are used because of the predictable alkaloid content. *E. sinica* extracts are available with a standardized 10% ephedrine alkaloid content. The dosage of a 10% alkaloid content extract would be 125 to 250 mg three times a day.

In the wilderness, specifically the desert, the raw herb Mormon tea from *E. nevadensis* or *E. viridis* can be quite useful for hay fever, mild asthma, bronchitis, or an upper respiratory tract infection (URI). These species contain minimal amounts of ephedrine and are principally pseudoephedrine containing; hence they can be used without some of the unpleasant side effects of the Asian species. They can also be used for mild fevers associated with influenza or URI.

The shrubs are typically found growing on dry, rocky, or sandy slopes. The leaves can be picked fresh or sun-dried for 6 to 8 hours and can be prepared as a steeped tea or an infusion. Generally, the dose should be the equivalent volume of 1 tablespoon of dried, crushed stems per 4 ounces of water, steeped for 10 minutes. The patient should not exceed a dosage given six times per day. Once harvested, the leaves can be kept for an indefinite period for later use if stored in an airtight container.

Toxicity

According to Duke, an infusion of *Ephedra* produced a "prompt and extensive contraction of uterine muscle when applied to smooth muscle strips of virgin guinea pig uteri." It may also elevate blood pressure. Frequent use may result in nervousness and restlessness. It should be used with caution if the patient has hypertension, heart disease, thyrotoxism, diabetes, or benign prostatic hypertrophy. Ephedrine should not be used while antihypertensive or antidepressant medications are being given.

GOLDENSEAL (HYDRASTIS CANADENSIS)

Description and Habitat

Hydrastis has a perennial root or rhizome, which is tortuous, knotty, and creeping in appearance. The internal color is bright yellow, with numerous long fibers. The stem is erect, simple, herbaceous, and rounded, from 6 to 12 inches in height, becoming purplish and bearing two unequal terminal leaves. The leaves are alternately palmate with three to five lobes, hairy, dark green, and cordate at the base. The flowers, which are evident in early spring, are solitary, terminal, small, and white or rose colored.

The plant is a native of eastern North America and cultivated in Oregon and Washington. The parts used are the dried rhizome and roots.

Pharmacology

The alkaloids derived from *Hydrastis* are hydrastine (1.5% to 4%), berberine (0.5% to 6%), berberastine (2% to 3%), canadine, hydrastinine, and other related compounds. Other constituents include meconin, chlorogenic acid, phytosterins, and resins.[112]

Native and European Medicinal Use and Folklore

Native Americans used *Hydrastis* extensively as an herbal medicine and clothing dye. The plant was used by a number of eastern North American Indian groups. The Cherokee Indians used the roots as a wash for local inflammations and as a decoction for general debility, for dyspepsia, and to improve appetite. The Iroquis Indians used a decoction of the root for whooping cough, diarrhea, liver trouble, fever, sour stomach, flatulence, pneumonia, and heart trouble.[106]

Early European uses date back to 1793, when it was noted in the *Collections for an Essay Towards a Materia Medica of the United States* by Benjamin Smith Barton to be useful as an eyewash for conjunctival inflammation and as a bitter tonic. In the pharmacy of the nineteenth century (1830), goldenseal was listed among the official remedies in the first revision of the New York edition of the United States Pharmacopeia. It was listed in the USP until 1926 and recognized in the National Formulary until 1955.[70]

Modern Clinical and Wilderness Application

Goldenseal is among the top sellers in the American herbal medicine market. It is used as an antiseptic, hemostatic, diuretic, laxative, tonic, and antiinflammatory for inflammation of the mucous membranes. It has also been recommended for hemorrhoids, nasal congestion, sore mouth and gums, conjunctivitis, external wounds, sores, acne, and ringworm.[97]

Modern research into the active ingredients berberine and hydrastine has yielded some interesting scientific evidence as to why some of the folk applications are effective. The most widely studied component is berberine. This isoquinoline alkaloid has demonstrated antibiotic, immunostimulatory, anticonvulsant, sedative, febrifugal, hypotensive, uterotonic, choleretic, and carminative (promoting the elimination of intestinal gas) activities.[112]

Berberine has been shown to have broad-spectrum antibiotic activity. The antimicrobial activity has been demonstrated on protozoa, fungi, and bacteria, both in vitro and in vivo. Antimicrobial action on the following organisms has been noted: *Staphylococcus, Streptococcus, Chlamydia, Corynebacterium diphtheriae, Escherichia coli, Salmonella typhi, Vibrio cholerae, Pseudomonas, Shigella dysenteriae, Entamoeba histolytica, Trichomonas vaginalis, Neisseria gonorrhoeae* and *N. meningitidis, Treponema pallidum, Giardia lamblia, Leishmania donovani,* and *Candida albicans.*[112] One mechanism of action of berberine antimicrobial activity involves its ability to inhibit the adherence of bacteria to host cells.[138]

Several capabilities of the active ingredients in the crude botanical may be responsible for the wide-spectrum effectiveness of *Hydrastis.* The antifungal properties, for example, prevent overgrowth of *Candida* that frequently occurs with the use of other antibiotic therapies.

Other studies have shown the immunostimulatory activity of berberine-containing plants. Berberine increases blood flow through the spleen,[123] and improved circulation may augment the immune function of this lymphoid organ. Berberine has also been shown to activate macrophages.[90] Historically, berberine-containing plants have been used as febrifuges, and in rat studies they have been shown to have an antipyretic effect three times as potent as aspirin.[112]

Plants such as goldenseal are very effective in treating acute gastrointestinal infections. In several clinical studies, berberine has shown significant success in treating acute diarrhea. It has been found effective against diarrheas caused by *E. coli, Shigella dysenteriae, Salmonella, Klebsiella, Giardia,* and *Vibrio cholerae.** The berberine-containing plants, in addition to their antimicrobial properties, influence the enterotoxins produced by the offending pathogens.[24,139,140]

Gastrointestinal illness is generally one of the major concerns of the traveler who ventures to areas where sanitation is questionable. Both water-borne and food-borne bacterial and protozoal infections are genuine concerns for persons in wilderness and Third World environments.

Some experts recommend that a berberine-containing botanical source be used as a prophylactic measure at least 1 week before a visit to questionable areas, extending the use to 1 week after return.[112]

Various eye complaints involving the conjunctivae and surrounding mucous membranes have been effectively treated with forms of berberine extract. Recent studies point to the effectiveness of berberine in treating the infection caused by *Chlamydia trachomatis.* Clinical trials found that a 2% berberine solution compared favorably to sulfacetamide. Although the symptoms resolved more slowly with the berberine extract, the rate of relapse was much lower in the berberine-treated group.[9,107]

For the traveler and wilderness enthusiast a berberine-containing botanical preparation would be a good provision. A standardized form of *Hydrastis canadensis* is beneficial for generalized digestive disorders (acute dysentery, gastritis) and infective, congestive, and inflammatory states of the mucous membranes (sinusitis, pharyngitis, stomatitis).

A typical dose for administration depends on the source and method of the extract. For the above-mentioned conditions the following three times a day dosage is recommended: dried root or as infusion, 2 to 4 g; tincture (1:5) 6 to 12 ml (1.5 to 3 teaspoons); or solid extract (4:1 or 10% alkaloid content) 250 to 500 mg.

In addition to being ingested, *Hydrastis* can be used as a wash or rinse for conjunctivitis, sinusitis, and pharyngitis. Eye drops, nasal lavage, and a gargle are applied in a 5% preparation of a 1:5 tincture, or ½ teaspoon powdered herb to 8 ounces water for the infusion for the inflamed mucous membranes. This can be repeated three times a day.

Toxicity

Berberine and berberine-containing plants are generally nontoxic. In recommended doses, berberine-containing plants have not been shown to be toxic in clinical trials. The LD_{50} of berberine sulfate in mice is approximately 25 mg/kg, while in dogs, intravenous doses of up to 45 mg/kg do not produce lethal or gross toxic effects.[123] It has been suggested that *Hydrastis* should not be used during pregnancy and that long-term ingestion may interfere with the metabolism of B vitamins.

ARNICA (ARNICA MONTANA)

Description and Habitat

Arnica is a perennial plant generally found in mountainous areas of Canada, the northern United States, and Europe. The plant reaches a height of 1 to 2 feet and generally contains from one to nine large daisylike flowerheads, which bloom in the summer months (Color Plate 98).

*References 11, 36, 45, 66, 84, 129.

Pharmacology

The flower is used both internally and externally for medicinal effects. The rootstock is used to make commercial preparations for tinctures and oils that are applied topically.

The active principles of the plant drug are flavonoids, volatile oils, and plant pigments (carotinoids).[151] Specific constituents include arnicine, formic acid, thymohydroquinone, lobelamine, and lobeline (piperidine alkaloid).[27]

Native and European Medicinal Use and Folklore

The Catawa Indians administered the tea of *Arnica* roots to treat back pain. In Europe the flowerheads have been used since the sixteenth century as an application for bruises and strains.[149] European *Arnica* was included in the U.S. Pharmacopeia from the early 1800s until 1960 and was recognized for its effects on the healing of bruises and sprains.

Specific instructions given in the *American Dispensory* in 1922 listed *Arnica* as effective for "muscular soreness and pain from strain or overexertion; advanced stage of disease, with marked enfeeblement, weak circulation, and impaired spinal innervation; . . . tensive backache, as if bruised or strained; [and] . . . headache with tensive, bruised feeling and pain on movement."[51] *Arnica* in tincture (concentrated) form has long been a popular, but not necessarily safe, medicine to treat inflammatory swellings and to relieve the soreness of myalgia and the effects of bruises and contusions. Doses above the therapeutic range cause vagal inhibition when ingested and may cause toxicity if the concentrated tincture is applied topically. Therefore the most common use has been fomentation of the flowers for topical applications in treatment of strains and sprains.

Modern Clinical and Wilderness Applications

Contemporary use of *Arnica montana* is generally limited to topical commercially prepared ointments and salves, in conjunction with internal homeopathic (low-dose) use for the same indications. Although its alkaloid (arnicine) and volatile oil (thymohydroquinone) are both relatively toxic, the actions of these constituents are extremely useful in resolving contusions and soft tissue injury. Most ointments are found to contain a 1× homeopathic dilution of *Arnica* tincture, which is about 4% by volume. Oral dosage is given in homeopathic potencies of 30× to 200 c depending on the severity of the condition.

For application in the wilderness, most naturopathic first aid kits include both the ointment and oral homeopathic forms of *Arnica*. For direct use of the plant in treating minor sprains and strains, 2 teaspoons of the dried flower tops can be steeped in 1 cup of water for 10 minutes, and the infusion in a compress can be applied cold to the affected area. This should be repeated each 2 hours in addition to standard first aid procedures. The infusion lasts a day if refrigerated and a few hours if not; therefore it is best to use a fresh infusion whenever possible. In addition, if available, the oral homeopathic (30× to 200 c) should be taken three times daily until the swelling is reduced significantly. A topical ointment can be applied each 2 to 3 hours for this condition in place of the compress.

According to Weiss, *Arnica* is safe and effective for topical contusions and for stimulating granulation and epithelialization. "Arnica is still the leader in the field . . . a truly excellent vulnerary, particularly for indolent wounds with a sticky deposit on the base and poor granulation."[150] A tablespoon of tincture is added to 500 ml of water, and the gauze compress is then placed on the wound. This stimulates local circulation and acts on the peripheral vasculature. After granulation has occurred, ointments may be applied.

Toxicity

The tincture or infusion can be toxic if taken in too high a concentration. Undiluted tincture should not be used internally or in compress form over an open wound. Vagus nerve inhibition is the primary toxic effect; gastrointestinal irritation is also noted. Toxic reactions include gastric burning; nausea; vomiting; headache; decreased temperature; dyspnea; cardiovascular collapse; convulsions; motor, sensory, and vagal paralysis; and death.[27]

GARLIC (ALLIUM SATIVUM)

Description and Habitat

Garlic is a member of the lily family. It is a perennial plant cultivated worldwide (Color Plate 99). The garlic bulb is composed of individual cloves enclosed in a white skin. The medicinal herb is found in the bulb and is used either fresh or dehydrated. Garlic oil, which also has medicinal value, is obtained by steamed distillation of the crushed fresh bulbs.[97]

Pharmacology

The medicinal compounds in garlic are generally those that contain sulfur, and these have been the subject of most research on garlic. Two primary compounds contained within garlic are an odorless chemical called alliin and the enzyme allinase, which begins a cascade of chemical reactions when the garlic clove is cut, crushed, or bruised. Alliin is converted to allicin, which is responsible for the characteristic odor of garlic. Allicin is strongly antibacterial and considered to be the major source of the antimicrobial effects of garlic. Diallyl sulfide, disulfide, and trisulfide are yielded from the breakdown of allicin. Heat speeds up the reaction, so cooked garlic and steamed distilled garlic oil contain little or no allicin. Within garlic, about 0.1% to 0.36% of the volatile oil is composed of sulfur-containing compounds (allicin, diallyl sulfide, diallyl trisulfide, and others). These volatile oils are considered to be responsible for most of the pharmacologic properties of garlic. Other constituents of garlic include s-methyl-L-cysteine sulfoxide, protein (16.8% dry weight basis), a high concentration of trace minerals (particularly selenium and germanium), vitamins, glucosinolates, and enzymes, which are composed of allinase, peroxidase, and myrosinase.[112,120]

Native and European Medicinal Use and Folklore

Throughout history, garlic has played an important part in medicinal herbology. Clay garlic bulbs dating back to 3750 BC were found in Egypt. Preserved garlic bulbs were discovered in the tomb of Tutankhamen. An entire basket of these bulbs from the tomb of Kha at Thebes is in the Turin Museum. The Greek historian Herodotus recorded that an enormous amount of money was spent on garlic for the builders of the great pyramids. One of the earliest Sanskrit manuscripts, *The Bower Manuscript,* devotes its entire first section to garlic. It describes the legendary origins of garlic, how "Vishnu cut off the head of Rahu, king of the demons, who had just stolen and drunk the elixir of mortality. Where drops of his blood mixed with the elixir fell, garlic first grew." That garlic is both demonic and beneficial is repeated in many cultures. In *The Bower Manuscript,* a fascinating account of the annual Indian Winter Garlic Festival is given. It says that garlic keeps in order the three fluids and can cure thinness, weakness of digestion, lassitude, coughs, inflammation of the skin, piles, glandular swellings in the abdomen and enlargement of the spleen, indigestion, constipation, excessive urination, worms, wind in the body (rheumatism), leprosy, epilepsy, and paralysis.

Within the traditional medical circles of Greece and Rome, medieval Europe, and the Far East, similar claims may be found. The great doctors Galen, Dioscorides, and Aristotle extolled garlic as an excellent medicine. Hippocrates recommended garlic as a diuretic; to regulate digestion; for bowel pains, inflammations, and infections of all kinds; and to regulate menstruation. Early Chinese and European herbalists found garlic to be useful for heating and drying. Therefore it was used to prevent and cure diseases arising from cold, poisons, excesses of diet and drink, and sluggish metabolism.

The folklore of garlic includes its alleged ability to ward off vampires. Sir John Herrington wrote in 1609 of garlic's virtues and faults: "Garlic then have power to save from death, bear with it though it may give unsavory breath, and scorn not garlic like some that think it only maketh men wink and drink and stink." Antibiotic properties were noted by Pasteur in 1858. Garlic was used by Albert Schweitzer in Africa to treat amebic dysentery. It was also used as an antiseptic to prevent gangrene during both world wars.

Modern Clinical and Wilderness Applications

The pharmacologic effects of garlic are based on its activity as a hypoglycemic and hypolipemic regulating agent,* anticoagulant,† antihypertensive,[101,122] antimicrobial,‡ detoxifier of heavy metals,[2] and immune system modulator.[81]

*References 6, 8, 12, 17, 18, 20, 21, 26, 34, 35, 65, 73, 74, 77-79, 82, 83, 87, 88, 114.

†References 5, 16, 19, 24, 25, 57, 76, 100, 117, 125, 135.

‡References 3, 4, 31, 53, 92, 100, 113, 142, 144.

Animal and human studies have substantiated that garlic lowers serum cholesterol and triglyceride levels and increases the amount of high-density lipoproteins. Dietary atherosclerosis was significantly reduced in rabbits when fed garlic consistently for a few weeks; also, extract of garlic and onions was more effective against hyperlipidemia and subsequent lipid deposition within the aorta than was clofibrate.[23] This study showed that after 4 months of feeding the rabbits a high-cholesterol diet, the average lipid content in the aorta of the control animals rose from 5.95 to 13.75 mg/100 g dry weight. Animals taking clofibrate after 4 months showed 7.95 mg/100 g dry weight, while for the same time period the garlic-fed animals showed 6.23 mg/100 g dry weight of lipid content in the aorta.[23] Other studies by investigators of experimental atherosclerosis in rabbits support these findings.[75,87] Decreased atheromatous lesions seem to be a consistent finding in rabbits fed high-cholesterol diets supplemented with garlic.

Of various sulfur-containing amino acids isolated from garlic, s-methylcysteine and s-allylcysteine have been shown to exert the greatest antilipidemic effects.[73] Components of garlic have been ascribed the properties of combining with the sulfhydryl group, the functional part of coenzyme A that is necessary for the biosynthesis of fatty acids, cholesterol, triglycerides, and phospholipids. The lipid-lowering effect may best be attributed to inactivation of the sulfhydryl group.[8] In both in vitro and in vivo tests, reduced conversion of acetate into cholesterol by liver tissues has been reported.[34] Since the sulfhydryl groups are involved at all levels of metabolic activity, the impact of garlic could be more extensive. Studies suggest that garlic may exert its ability to lower blood pressure by acting like prostaglandin E_1, which decreases peripheral vascular resistance.[116]

As a nutritional supplement, garlic is composed of magnesium, iron, copper, zinc, selenium, calcium, potassium chloride, germanium, sulfur compounds, amino acids, and vitamins A, B_1, and C. Garlic increases the body's capacity to assimilate thiamine by enhancing its absorption. Thiamine is a key part of the cocarboxylase enzyme system that acts beneficially on liver cells, which may help to explain claims that garlic is prophylaxis against liver and gallbladder damage. In one study, garlic was shown to protect hepatocytes in tissue culture from the damage of carbon tetrachloride.[116]

Antioxidant activity has also been attributed to garlic and garlic derivatives. The free radical scavenger action of garlic can be probably explained by its germanium, glutathione, selenium, and zinc content. The last three are key components of the antioxidant enzyme superoxide dismutase and glutathione peroxidase. Animal studies show that feeding garlic oil enhanced physical endurance in normal rats and also reduced the decrease in physical endurance induced by isoproterenol, a synthetic catecholamine that induces necrosis of the myocardium.[127]

Garlic inhibits platelet aggregation in animals; similar effects can be demonstrated in vitro and in vivo in humans.[43,135] An antiplatelet extract of garlic, ajoene, was found to potentiate the antithrombotic effect of antiinflammatory drugs. A number of investigators have observed that, under fasting conditions, the inhibition of platelet aggregation by garlic or its extracts is dose related.[136] The garlic effect may be linked to inhibition of thromboxane synthesis or to altered properties of the plasma membrane. Methyl (2-propenyl) trisulfide, another component of garlic, is 10 times more potent relative to platelet aggregation inhibition than is diallyl disulfide or trisulfide.[5] Thrombocyte aggregation inhibition is enhanced by two other compounds, 2-vinyl-1,3-dithiene and allyl-1,5-hexidienyl-trisulfide.[14]

Enhancement of fibrinolytic activity has also been studied in relation to garlic ingestion. Garlic and its juice or oil enhance fibrinolysis.[22] Cycloalliin, the component of garlic given in a double-blind placebo-controlled trial to volunteers and patients following myocardial infarction, induced a significant increase in fibrinolysis 1½ hours after medication.[49] Chutani and Bordia observed that the increase took place 6½ to 12 hours after garlic intake. Daily garlic ingestion for 1 month generated a 72% to 85% increase in fibrinolysis in patients with ischemic heart disease.[37]

The pharmacologic versatility of garlic is best reflected by its antiviral, antifungal, antiprotozoan, antiparasitic, and antibacterial activities.* Laymen is credited with being the first to describe the scientific basis for the medicinal use of garlic extract.[153] Huddleson and Cavallito demonstrated in 1944 that garlic juice and allicin inhibited the growth of *Staphylococcus, Streptococcus, Bacillus, Brucella,* and *Vibrio* species at low concentrations.[32,71] Recent studies using serial dilutions and filter paper disk techniques have shown that fresh garlic, powdered garlic, and vacuum-dried preparations were effective antibiotic agents against many bacteria, including *Staphyloccus aureus,* α- and β-hemolytic *Streptococcus, Escherichia coli, Proteus vulgaris, Salmonella enteritidis, Citrobacter,* and *Klebsiella pneumoniae.*[112] In these studies, antibiotics including penicillin, streptomycin, chloramphenicol, erythromycin, and tetracycline were compared in antimicrobial effects with garlic. Besides confirming garlic's well-known antibacterial effects, studies demonstrated the effectiveness in inhibiting the growth of some bacteria that had become resistant to many commonly used antibiotics.[1,48,130] Garlic has also demonstrated significant antifungal activity against a wide range of fungi.†

From a wilderness perspective, inhibition of fungi that can affect the skin *(Microsporum, Trichophyton, Epidermophyton,* and *Candida albicans)* can be significant. Garlic juice applied topically is an effective alternative in treating a wide variety of fungal skin diseases.[3] It was found that garlic compares well with nystatin, gentian violet, and six other reputed antifungal agents to treat *Candida albicans.*[1,108,119,126]

Garlic has long been associated with prophylaxis against the influenza virus. In vivo studies with mice revealed that garlic administration protected mice against intranasal inoculation with influenza viruses and enhanced the reproduction of neutralizing antibodies after vaccine administration.[113] In vitro studies have shown that garlic has antiviral activity against influenza B virus and herpes hominis virus type I.[143] Preliminary studies have revealed significant enhancement of natural killer (NK) cell activity in humans administered raw or cold aged whole clove garlic preparations daily for 3 weeks.[81] It has been hypothesized that the antiviral activity of garlic in humans may be secondary to the direct toxic effect on viruses and enhanced NK cell activity that destroys virus-infected cells.

Wilderness Medical Applications

The use of garlic in the outdoor setting can be extensive. Its use as a food should be encouraged despite its odor, particularly in people with elevated cholesterol levels, heart disease, hypertension, diabetes, asthma, fungal infections, respiratory tract infections, and gastrointestinal disorders (intestinal parasites and dysentery). A macerated garlic poultice and garlic slices serve as readily applied topical agents in the cases of fungal infections, ulcerated wounds, pyoderma, and other skin infections. The poultice can be used directly on the dermatologic problem, and as a suppository can be used to treat vaginitis, particularly infections caused by *C. albicans.* For this application, one to two fresh chopped cloves can be made into a poultice. This should be kept on the affected site for several hours and changed at least once each 6 hours with a fresh preparation. If the garlic causes epidermal irritation, its use is discontinued.

Prophylactic use during the flu season can reduce the incidence of infection. Within the first 48 hours of onset of a flu or URI, one or two cloves can be consumed with a carbohydrate source to prevent stomach irritation. Alternatively, two or three oil of garlic capsules can be taken with the same frequency. For persons concerned about the social segregating aspect, extracts that preserve the allicin content but remain odorless can be used.

Toxicity

For the vast majority of individuals, garlic is nontoxic at dosages commonly used. However, some people develop allergic contact dermatitis or irritation of the digestive tract. Apparently, they are unable to effectively detoxify allicin and other sulfur-containing components. Prolonged consumption of large amounts of raw garlic by rats results in anemia, weight loss, and failure to grow.[115]

*References 3, 4, 31, 53, 113, 141, 155.

†References 1, 3, 55, 72, 108, 119, 126.

GINGER (ZINGIBER OFFICINALE)

Description and Habitat

Ginger is an upright perennial herb with tuberous rhizomes (underground roots or stems), from which grows an aerial stem to 1.5 m in height. It is native to southern Asia, although it is cultivated in the tropics. Extracts and dried ginger are produced from dried unpeeled ginger; peeled ginger loses much of its essential oil content.[145]

Pharmacology

Ginger is composed of a rich variety of nutrients and enzymes. The general composition is starch (50%); protein (9%); lipid (6% to 8%) composed of phosphatidic acid; lecithin; free fatty acids; triglycerides; protease (up to 2.26%); volatile oils (1% to 4%), the principal components of which are three sesquiterpenes (bisabolene, zingiberene, zingiberol); vitamins, especially niacin and vitamin A; and resins.[145]

Native and European Medicinal Use

Z. officinale is native to southern Asia and tropical Africa. Therefore it did not have a role in the early herbal preparations of European and native American herbal medicine.

Modern Clinical and Wilderness Applications

Clinical use of ginger for antiinflammatory action, liver and serum cholesterol lowering effects, and its ability to relieve dizziness and motion sickness is most noted in herbal texts.* A choleretic effect (the promotion of bile flow to the gallbladder and small intestine) and the conversion of cholesterol into bile acids are enhanced by ginger ingestion and may be responsible for its overall cholesterol-lowering effect.

In an early eclectic medical text, ginger was noted as an admirable local stimulant, sialogogue, diaphoretic, and carminative.[51] Powdered ginger in a large quantity of cold water taken before sleep frequently "breaks up" a severe cold, and a hot infusion of ginger tea is a popular remedy for similar use to mitigate the pains of dysmenorrhea.[51] It was noted in the same text that ginger remedies painful spasmodic contractions of the stomach and intestine. The antiinflammatory action of ginger is thought to be caused by potent inhibition of inflammatory compounds such as prostaglandins and thromboxanes.[89] Ginger is also known to contain strong plant proteases such as bromelain, ficaine, and papain, which may explain some of its antiinflammatory action.[145]

Ginger has been used historically for major complaints concerning the gastrointestinal system. It is generally regarded as an excellent carminative (promotes the elimination of intestinal gas) and intestinal spasmolytic.[112]

*References 51, 52, 62-64, 89, 111, 132, 136, 137, 145.

One of the most noted uses of ginger in contemporary herbal medicine that applies to wilderness medicine is its action on the symptoms of motion sickness and seasickness.[62,63,111] Ginger is also a significant antiemetic. It has long been used in the treatment of nausea and vomiting associated with pregnancy. In a recent study the efficacy of ginger was confirmed in hyperemesis gravidarum, a severe form of nausea and vomiting during pregnancy. Ginger root powder at a dose of 250 mg four times a day brought a significant reduction in both the severity of nausea and the number of attacks of vomiting during pregnancy.[52]

The general dose applied to the treatment of motion sickness, vertigo, and nausea is two 500 mg capsules of powdered ginger root eaten 20 to 30 minutes before the event that would cause motion sickness, or the same dose for the nausea of pregnancy during the acute attack. The raw ginger root can be grated using 1 teaspoon in 4 ounces of water, steeped for 10 minutes, and taken every 30 minutes until the symptoms of motion sickness abate.

Toxicity

There appears to be no toxicity associated with ginger root ingestion.

COMFREY (SYMPHYTUM OFFICINALE)

Description and Habitat

Comfrey is a perennial herb with a stout spreading root that is essentially divisible for propagation. Comfrey grows approximately 3 feet high and has coarse, bristly, oblong, lanceolate leaves. The tubular flower can be purplish, blue, white, red, or yellow (Color Plate 100). About 25 *Symphytum* species are described in the literature; they are indigenous to countries around the Mediterranean Sea and in northern Asia. Comfrey is commonly found in moist meadows and other wet places in the United States and Europe.

Pharmacology

The chemical constituents of *Z. officinale* roots can be summarized: the carbohydrate is predominantly sucrose; the amino acids are serine and asparagine; the phenolic acids are chlorogenic acid, caffeic acid, and *p*-coumaric acid; the alkaloids are choline, allantoin, and the pyrrolizidine alkaloids viridiflorine, echinatine, heliosupine, symphytine, echimidine, and lasiocarpine.[148] The most concentrated alkaloid, allantoin (0.88% to 1.71%), is generally credited with the beneficial effects of comfrey's application.

Native and European Medicinal Use

In Europe, comfrey is a common perennial grown in the garden for animal fodder. Russian comfrey is often promoted as a medicinal herb for use as a tonic. Comfrey is also cultivated in Japan as a green vegetable and tonic and has been used in American herbal medicine for hundreds of years.[94]

Comfrey has long been known as an external agent for the rehabilitation of musculoskeletal and orthopedic injuries. Its old name, bone knit, derives from the external use of poultices of leaves and roots, which were believed to help heal burns, sprains, swellings, and bruises. Comfrey has been claimed to heal gastric ulcers and hemorrhoids, suppress bleeding, and relieve bronchial congestion and inflammation.[13] The healing action of a poultice derived from the roots and leaves is probably related to the presence of allantoin, an agent that promotes cell proliferation. The underground parts contain 0.6% to 1.3% allantoin and 4% to 6.5% tannin.[29,104] Comfrey extracts applied topically have been reported to heal wounds and bones in about half of the normal time. In herbology there is a general rule that if anything is broken, use comfrey.[154] Herbalists have also found that the allantoin concentration from a fluid extract of comfrey can increase the rate of wound healing of lacerations sufficiently to avoid the use of sutures.[152]

In European folklore, comfrey was regarded as an herb having unsurpassed ability to heal any tissue that was either injured or broken. The mucilage (gelatinous mucopolysaccharide) of the comfrey root has been named "the great cell proliferator," helping new flesh and bones to grow.

In old folklore and European herbal medicine, comfrey was one of the main herbs found in any poultice or fomentation. European herbalists considered comfrey exceptional for coughs and for soothing inflamed tissues in a remarkable way. Comfrey is effective for treating upper respiratory inflammation and has been used successfully to treat hemorrhagic conditions of the lungs.

Modern Clinical and Wilderness Applications

Comfrey lotions and salves containing 0.5% to 2.5% allantoin have been used for sprains, strains, and contusions. In the 1980s, comfrey became controversial because of potential hepatotoxicity. Members of the family Boraginaceae *(Heliotropium* and *Symphytum)* contain a variety of related pyrrolizidine alkaloids that have been reported to cause hepatotoxicity in animals. Although no hepatotoxic episodes from the ingestion of comfrey have been reported in humans, the potential exists, so caution is advised when using comfrey for internal consumption.[94] The topical use of comfrey products as yet poses no concern for toxicity.

There are many wilderness medical applications for comfrey. As a topical agent after acute trauma for musculoskeletal injuries, strains and sprains, or contusions, comfrey is an exceptional medicine. A prepared gel of comfrey with a standardized allantoin concentration should be carried during travel or camping expeditions in the wilderness.

The raw herb can be used if one is in the plant's environment. The herb is readily identifiable, although it should not be confused with foxglove *(Digitalis purpurea)* and should be used with caution when taken internally in its raw state. For use in a poultice or compress, the leaves may be picked damp, macerated, and applied topically for up to 24 hours.

Toxicity

Comfrey is not recommended for internal ingestion on a routine basis; animal studies indicate that hepatic damage is an eventual outcome if the herb is consumed over a long period.

ALOE (ALOE VERA)

Description and Habitat

The aloe is a perennial plant native to South and East Africa and is also cultivated in the West Indies and other tropical and temperate areas. The leaves, which emerge from a central rosette produced by a central fibrous root, are 1 to 2 feet long, narrow, fleshy, and light green with spiny teeth on the margins (Color Plate 101). Aloe is easily cultivated as a houseplant and can be grown in a sunny warm spot with good drainage.

The genus *Aloe* comprises more than 300 species, which are members of the Liliaceae (lily) family. *Aloe* species are perennial succulents native to Africa. They are not cacti and should not be confused with American aloe, the century plant.

Pharmacology

Two important products are derived from aloe. One is aloe gel, a clear gelatinous material extracted from the mucilagenous cells found in the inner tissue of the leaf. The gel is obtained by crushing the leaves and repeated straining to remove cellular debris. The result is a clear gel, which is the product most frequently used in the health food and cosmetic industries. It is generally devoid of anthroquinone glycosides. A variety of compounds have been identified in the aloe species, including polysaccharides, tannins, organic acids, enzymes, vitamins, minerals, saponins, and steroids.[94]

The other product is a bitter yellow latex that contains cathartic anthroquinone glycosides, mostly barbaloin, as the active principles. The concentrations of the glycosides vary with the type of aloe, ranging from 4% to 25% of aloe in concentration. The water-soluble fraction of aloe is called aloin and is a mixture of active glycosides. Cathartics have been derived from extracts of the latex and can create strong purgative effects by stimulating the large intestine.

Native and European Medicinal Use and Folklore

Fresh *Aloe vera* gel is well known for its domestic medicinal values.[59,96,109,118] Aloe has been dubbed the burn plant, first aid plant, and medicine plant. When fresh, the gel relieves thermal burns and sunburns and promotes wound healing. It also has moisturizing and emollient properties. Because of these effects, aloe is widely used as a home remedy.

Aloin and other anthroquinone derivatives of aloe are extensively used as active ingredients in laxative preparations. Aloin is also used as an antiobesity preparation.[97]

Aloe or aloin extracts are also used in sunscreens and other cosmetic preparations and in drugs for moisturizing, emollient, or wound-healing purposes.

In folk medicine, aloe is used for a number of conditions, such as condylomas, warts, abnormal skin growths, and cancers of the lip, anus, breast, larynx, liver, nose, stomach, and uterus.[46] Other folklore suggests that parts of the plants be chewed to purify the blood. The pulp is said to possess wound-healing hormonal activities and "biogenic stimulators" and is used for intestinal ailments, sore throat, and ulcers. In India it is used to treat piles and rectal fissures. Slukari hunters in Africa's Congo rubbed their bodies with the gel to eliminate the human scent, making them less likely to disturb prey. During epidemics of influenza, Lesotho natives take a public bath in an infusion of *Aloe latifolia*.[46]

Modern Clinical and Wilderness Application

Although numerous claims have been made for aloe gel, its most common lay use is in the treatment of minor burns and skin irritations. In 1935 a report described the use of aloe in the treatment of radiation-induced dermatitis.[39] This study followed a 5-week course of topical applications of either the whole leaf or leaf macerated into gel, resulting in complete wound healing after 4 months. In 1937, studies using a calamine- and lanolin-based aloe preparation treated skin irritations resulting from burns, pruritus vulvae, and poison ivy. The results suggested that aloe stimulated tissue granulation and accelerated wound healing.[94]

Barnes evaluated the effect of 5% aloe ointment on sandpaper-abraded human fingertips and found that the wound-healing rate was two to three times that of control subjects as measured by decrease in electrical potential of the wound.[10] Other studies measured tensile strength of the healed surgical wounds of mice. Healing occurred within 9 days, an improvement over the control mice.[60]

Studies of antibacterial activity of aloe extracts have been attempted several times, yielding mixed results. In 1963, studies of the antibacterial effect of macerated *Aloe vera* gel found no activity against *S. aureus* and *E. coli*.[54] Other studies have determined that *Aloe chinensis* is effective against *S. aureus, E. coli,* and *Mycobacterium tuberculosis,* although *Aloe vera* showed no inhibitory effect.[61] On the other hand, the latex possesses in vitro activity against several pathogenic strains of bacteria, although the whole leaf minus the latex from the leaf epidermis and mesophyll of aloe showed no activity.[98] Two commercial preparations of aloe gel were found to exert antimicrobial activity against gram-negative and gram-positive bacteria and *C. albicans* when used in concentrations greater than 90%.[67]

It has been hypothesized that the moisturizing effect could be beneficial in the treatment of burns. It has been thought that the healing process is related to mucopolysaccharides in combination with sulfur derivatives and nitrogen compounds contained within the gel, but this has not been well substantiated in documented studies.[93] There have been attempts to document the antiinflammatory effects of aloe. In 1976 a study found that *Aloe vera* had bradykinase activity in vitro, but this was not confirmed in vivo.[56]

Evidence for the internal use of aloe has been limited to studies involving mucous membrane tissue repair. Corneal ulcers treated with aloe extracts had more healing, less cellular reaction, and fewer signs of irritation than in control groups.[94] Topical application of *Aloe vera* gel after periodontal flap surgery reduced postoperative pain more than the saline control, and swelling of the treated tissue was less marked than with the control.[68]

Because of easy recognition and administration, use of the aloe plant in the wilderness environment is practical. The wild plant can yield an excellent preparation for dermal abrasions, cuts, and superficial wounds. A leaf cut from the base of a healthy plant can be conveniently carried. This allows the gel to remain intact, protected by the outer skin of the leaf. It can be squeezed from the inside through the cut portion directly onto superficial wounds with or without a gauze dressing. A standardized preparation of *Aloe vera* may be used as an antibacterial agent and an emollient for superficial wounds or dermatitis.

In the event of constipation the mixture of aloe gel and latex can be scraped or squeezed from the leaf cortex and ingested at 1 tablespoon three times per day or until a mild laxative effect is noted. This allows the collection of a gel and latex mixture that produces less of a cathartic effect than the straight latex. Because of the bitterness of the gel and the latex, it should be taken with food or a flavored beverage.

Toxicity

Because of its cathartic effects, aloe is not advised if gripping pain is associated with constipation and is contraindicated in pregnancy. Otherwise it has no reported toxicity.

PLANTAIN MAJOR (PLANTAGO MAJOR)

Description and Habitat

The common broadleaf plantain is a familiar perennial "weed" that may be found along roadsides and in meadowlands. Plantain belongs to the order Plantaginaceae, which contains more than 200 species, 25 or 30 of which have a domestic use. The plant is a small weed with a rosette of ribbed leaves and small projecting seed stalks. Its seeds, known as psyllium seeds, resemble those of another species, *Plantago psyllium.* The leaves contain 84% water, 2.5% protein, 0.2% fat, and 14% carbohydrate, trace amounts of calcium, phosphorus, iron, sodium, and potassium, as well as β-carotene, riboflavin, niacin, and ascorbic acid. The following compounds have been biochemically identified: allantoin, adenine, baicalein, baicalin, benzoic acid, chlorogenic acid, choline, cinnamic acid, ferulic acid, L-fructose, fumaric acid, gentisic acid, D-glucose, *p*-hydroxy-benzoic acid, indicain, lignoceric acid, neochlorogenic acid, oleanolic acid, plantagonine, planteose, saccharose, salicylic acid, scutellarein, sitosterol, sorbitol, stachyose, syringic acid, tyrosol, ursolic acid, vanillic acid, and D-xylose.[46]

Native and European Medicinal Use and Folklore

Historically the plant has been used for stings, bites, and irritations from venomous insects or reptiles. The folk medicine of the eastern United States suggests using crushed plantain leaves to stop the itching of poison ivy. It has also been reported to help relieve toothache. Ancient herbalists maintained that plantain had refrigerant (an agent that imparts a cooling sensation to the mucosa and allays thirst), diuretic, and astringent properties. When the leaves are applied to a bleeding surface wound, there is some diminution of hemorrhage. In the highlands of Scotland, it is still called *slan-lus,* or plant of healing.

In the United States plantain has been known as snake weed, from the belief that it is effective for bites from venomous creatures. Felter[51] noted that "the crushed leaves were very effective for the distressing symptoms caused by puncture by the horny appendages of larvae of Lepidoptera and the irritation produced by certain caterpillars as well as the stings of insects and bites of spiders." In native American folklore the plant was known as white man's foot, in reference to its trait of growing in the settlements of white men. It was used by the Shoshoni Indians, who heated the leaves and applied them in a wet dressing for wounds.[151]

Modern Clinical and Wilderness Application

Plantain is readily available in the recreational areas of North America. This plant is extremely useful for various superficial wounds, abrasions, stings, and bites of mildly venomous insects. It appears that the constituents in the crushed leaves have an antihistamine effect, as well as an anesthetic-like quality. In the event of a tooth fracture, a compress or poultice of ½ teaspoon of fresh leaves may be used on the exposed nerve root of a tooth. The seeds of the plantago plant are quite useful for spastic colon, an effect that appears to be related to their mucilagenous properties. The seeds, known on the Asian continent as flea seed husk and in North America as psyllium seed, are used commonly as a bulk laxative. The seeds can be collected from the stalk and 1 teaspoon fresh seeds mixed into 4 ounces water taken twice a day for mild constipation. It is advised that water be taken throughout the day to alleviate the condition and assist the laxative effect.

Because of its astringent effects, an infusion of the leaves is recommended to treat diarrhea and may be prepared in the following manner: pour 1 pint of boiling water on 1 ounce of the herb and let it stand in a warm place for 20 minutes. Afterward, strain and leave to cool, then take ½ cup three or four times a day.

Toxicity

No known toxicities are attributed to *Plantago.*

CHAMOMILE (MATRICARIA CHAMOMILLA)

Description and Habitat

Chamomile is a low-growing perennial with a hairy prostrate branching stem. It blooms late in July through September and is found growing throughout North America and Europe. The word "chamomile" is derived from the Greek *chamos* (ground) and *melos* (apple), which refer to the plant's low growing habit and the fact that the scent of fresh blooms is somewhat reminiscent of apples.[133] The flower head is about 1 inch in diameter, has a conical receptacle, and is covered by yellow disk flowers surrounded by 10 or 20 white down-curving ray flowers.

Pharmacology

The most important chemicals associated with chamomile are the volatile oils containing tiglic acid esters, chamazulene, farnesene, and α-bisabolol oxide. These volatile oils are destroyed if the herb is boiled.[134]

Native and European Medicinal Uses and Folklore

A distinction should be made between German and Roman chamomile, which have been used interchangeably for centuries. The German is preferred on the European continent, while the Roman chamomile has been used widely in Great Britain. In the United States, German chamomile is by far the more widely consumed of the two species.[102]

German chamomile has a long tradition as a folk or domestic remedy. It has been used for a wide variety of purposes, including external compresses or fomentations for gout, sciatica, inflammations, lumbago, rheumatism, and skin ailments. Infusions, decoctions, and tinctures have long been used internally to treat colic, convulsions, croup, diarrhea, fever, indigestion, insomnia, teething, toothaches, bleeding or swollen gums, and as folk cancer remedy. Historically, Roman chamomile was used in a similar fashion.[46,97]

Modern Clinical and Wilderness Applications

The biochemical constituent of chamomile is chamazulene. It is found in both species of chamomile and is reported to have antihistamine properties.[50] Both histamine release and inhibition of histamine discharge have been considered mechanisms for the potential antiallergic action of chamazulene.

In Germany, chamomile products include tinctures, extracts, teas, and salves. These are widely used as antiinflammatory, antibacterial, antispasmodic, and sedative agents.[102] Studies have shown that both chamazulene and α-bisabolol have antiinflammatory activities. Chamazulene may comprise as much as 5% of the essential oil. Other studies have shown that α-bisabolol has a protective effect against peptic ulcer, as well as antibacterial and antifungal activities. α-Bisabolol has also been shown to reduce fever and to shorten the healing time of skin burns in laboratory animals.[44] Most commercial European chamomile preparations have been standardized with regard to the chamazulene and α-bisabolol content.[147]

According to Rudolph Weiss, one action of chamomile is to reduce gastric motility and secretions, which would alleviate colic and painful spasm. Some 20 flavones and flavonols, such as apingenin, are found in the aqueous portion of the distillation process. Investigations have shown these to be three times as effective at spasmolytic activity as the opium alkaloid papaverine.[150] Chamomile has also been shown to have a significant calming affect on the nerves and has been traditionally applied as a mild sedative.

Chamomile is a good botanical to have on hand when traveling or camping. For infants experiencing restlessness and discomfort from teething, one third of the adult dosage may provide relief. For the treatment of conditions that may arise from excessive nervous tension (intestinal gas, colic, and peptic ulcers), 2 teaspoons (or one standard teabag) of the flower tops can be added to a cup of boiling water and infused for 5 to 10 minutes; 2 to 3 cups may be taken in 30 minutes for acute intestinal colic.

REFERENCES

1. Adetumbi MA, Lau BH: *Allium sativum*—a natural antibiotic, *Med Hypotheses* 12(3):227, 1983.
2. Airolo P: *The miracle of garlic,* Phoenix, 1983, Health Plus Publisher.
3. Amer M, Taha M, Tosson Z: The effect of aqueous garlic extract on the growth of dermatophytes, *Int J Dermatol* 19:285, 1980.
4. Appleton JA, Tansey MR: Inhibition of growth of zoopathogentic fungi by garlic extract, *Mycopathologia* 67:882, 1975.
5. Ariga T, Oshiba S, Tamada T: Platelet aggregation inhibitor in garlic, *Lancet* 1:150, 1981.
6. Arora RC, Arora S: Comparative effect of clofibrate, garlic and onion on alimentary hyperlipemia, *Atherosclerosis* 39(4):447, 1981.
7. Astrup A et al: The effect of chronic ephedrine treatment on substrate utilization, the sympathoadrenal activity and expenditure during glucose-induced thermogenesis in man, *Metabolism* 35:260, 1986.
8. Augusti KT, Matthew PT: Lipid-lowering effect of allicin (diallyl disulphide-oxide) on long-term feeding to normal rats, *Experientia* 30:468, 1974.
9. Babbar OP et al: Effect of berberine chloride eye drops on clinically positive trachoma patients, *Ind J Med Res* 70:233, 1979.
10. Barnes: *Am J Bot* 34, 1937.
11. Bhakat MP et al: Therapeutic trial of berberine sulphate in non-specific gastroenteritis, *Ind Med J* 68:19, 1974.
12. Bhushan S et al: Effect of garlic on normal blood cholesterol level, *Indian J Physiol Pharmacol* 23(3):211, 1979.
13. Bianchini F, Corbetta R: *Health plants of the world,* New York, 1975, Newsweek Books.
14. Block E et al: Ajoene: a potent antithrombotic agent from garlic, *J Am Chem Soc* 106:8295, 1984.
15. Blumenthal M: Ginseng takes root in *Wall Street Journal, J Am Botan Council* 28:10, 1993.
16. Bordia A: Effect of garlic on human platelet aggregation in vitro, *Atherosclerosis* 30:355, 1978.
17. Bordia A: Effect of garlic on blood lipids in patients with coronary heart disease, *Am J Clin Nutr* 34:2100, 1981.
18. Bordia A, Bansal HC: Essential oil of garlic in prevention of atherosclerosis, *Lancet* 2:1491, 1973.
19. Bordia A, Joshi JK: Garlic on fibrinolytic activity in cases of acute myocardial infarction, Part II, *J Assoc Physicians India* 26(5):323, 1978.
20. Bordia AK, Verma SK: Garlic on the reversibility of experimental atherosclerosis, *Ind Heart J* 30:47, 1978.
21. Bordia A, Verma SK: Effect of garlic feeding on regression of experimental atherosclerosis in rabbits, *Artery* 7:428, 1980.
22. Bordia A et al: Effect of the essential oils of garlic and onion on alimentary hyperlipemia, *Atherosclerosis* 21:15, 1975.
23. Bordia A et al: The protective action of essential oils of onion and garlic in cholesterol-fed rabbits, *Atherosclerosis* 22:103, 1975.
24. Bordia AK et al: Effect of essential oil of garlic on serum fibrinolytic activity in patients with coronary artery disease, *Atherosclerosis* 28:155, 1977.
25. Bordia AK et al: The effectiveness and active principle of garlic and onion on blood lipids and experimental atherosclerosis in rabbits and their comparison with clofibrate, *J Assoc Physicians India* 25:509, 1977.
26. Bordia A et al: Protective effect of garlic oil on the changes produced by 3 weeks of fatty diet on serum cholesterol serum triglycerides, fibrinolytic activity, and platelet adhesiveness in man, *Ind Heart J* 34(2):86, 1982.
27. Brinker F: *An introduction to the toxicology of common medicinal substances,* National College of Naturopathic Medicine course in postgraduate program in botanical medicine, 1983, National College of Naturopathic Medicine.
28. *Br J Clin Pharmacol* 9:453, 1980.
29. *British Pharmaceutical Codex,* London, 1934, The Pharmaceutical Press.
30. Britz JJ et al: *J Am Osteopath Assoc* 62:731, 1963.
31. Caporaso N, Smith SM, Eng RH: Antifungal activity in human urine and serum after ingestion of garlic, *Antimicrob Agents Chemother* 23(5):700, 1983.
32. Cavallito CJ, Bailey JH: Allicin, the antibacterial principle of *Allium sativum.* I. Isolation, physical properties and antibacterial action, *J Am Chem Soc* 66:1950, 1944.
33. Chang HM, But PP: *Pharmacology and applications of Chinese materia medica,* vol 2, Teaneck, NJ, 1987, World Scientific.
34. Chang MLW, Johnson MA: Effect of garlic on carbohydrate metabolism and lipid synthesis in rats, *J Nutr* 110:931, 1980.
35. Chaudhuri BN et al: Hypolipidemic effect of garlic and thyroid function, *Biomed Biochim Acta* 43(7):1045, 1984.
36. Choudry VP, Sabir M, Bhide BN: Berberine in giardiasis, *Ind Pediatr* 9:143, 1972.
37. Chutani SK, Bordia A: The effect of fried vs. raw garlic on fibrinolytic activity in man, *Atherosclerosis* 38:417, 1981.
38. Cody G: *History of natural medicine, a textbook of natural medicine,* Seattle, 1985, John Bastyr College Publications.
39. Collins CE, Collins C: *Am J Roentgenol Rad Ther* 33:396, 1935.
40. Crellin JK, Philpott J: *Herbal medicine: past and present,* vol 2, London, Duke University Press.
41. Reference deleted in proofs.
42. Cunnick J, Takamoto D: Research review of bitter melon *(Momordica charantia), J Naturopath Med* (4)1:16, 1993.
43. Deboer LWV, Folts JD: Garlic extract limits acute platelet thrombus formation in canine coronary arteries, *Clin Res* 34:292A, 1986.
44. Der Marderosian AD, Liberti LE: *Natural product medicine: a scientific guide to foods, drugs, cosmetics,* Philadelphia, 1988, George F Stickley.
45. Desai AB, Shah KM, Shah DM: Berberine in the treatment of diarrhea, *Ind Pediatr* 8:462, 1971.
46. Duke J: *CRC handbook of medicinal herbs,* Boca Raton, Fla, 1985, CRC Press.
47. Dulloo AG, Miller DS: The thermogenic properties of ephedrine/methylxanthine mixtures: animal studies, *Am J Clin Nutr* 43:388, 1986.
48. Elnima EL et al: The antimicrobial activity of garlic and onion extracts, *Pharmazie* 38(11):747, 1983.

49. Ernst E: Cardiovascular effects of garlic: a review, *Pharmatherapeutica* 5(2):83, 1987.
50. Farnsworth NR, Morgan BM: Herb drinks: chamomile tea, *JAMA* 221:410, 1972.
51. Felter HK: The eclectic materia medica pharmacology and therapeutics, 1983, *Eclectic Medical Publications.*
52. Fischer-Tasmu S et al: Ginger treatment of hyperemesis gravidarum, *Eur J Obstet Gynecol Reprod Biol* 38:19, 1990.
53. Fliermans C: Inhibition of *Histoplasma capsulatum* by garlic, *Mycopathol Mycol Appl* 50:227, 1973.
54. Fly, Kiem: *Econ Bot* 14:46, 1963.
55. Fromtling R, Bulmer GS: In vitro effect of aqueous extract of garlic *(Allium sativum)* on the growth and viability of *Cryptococcus neoformans, Mycolagia* 70:397, 1978.
56. Fugita et al: *Biochem Pharmacol* 25:205, 1976.
57. Gaffen JD, Tavares IA, Bennett A: The effect of garlic extracts on contractions of rat gastric fundus and human platelet aggregation, *J Pharm Pharmacol* 36(4):273, 1984.
58. Gilman AG, Goodman AS, Gilman A: *The pharmacologic basis of therapeutics,* New York, 1980, Macmillan.
59. Gjerstad, Riner TD: *Am J Pharm* 140:58, 1968.
60. Goff S, Levenstein I: *J Soc Cosm Chem* 15:509, 1964.
61. Gottshall et al: *J Clin Invest* 28:920, 1949.
62. Grontved A et al: Ginger root against seasickness: a controlled trial on the open sea, *Acta Otolaryngol* 105:45, 1988.
63. Grontved A, Hentzer E: Vertigo reducing effect of ginger root, *ORL* 48:282, 1986.
64. Gujaral S, Bhurmara H, Swaroop M: Effects of ginger oleoresin on serum and hepatic cholesterol levels in cholesterol-fed rats, *Nutr Rep Intl* 17:183, 1978.
65. Gupta NN, Mehrota RML, Sircar AR: Effect of onion on serum cholesterol blood coagulation factors and fibrinolytic activity in alimentary lipemia, *Ind J Med Res* 54:48, 1966.
66. Gupta S: Use of berberine in the treatment of giardiasis, *Am J Dis Child* 129:866, 1975.
67. Haggers JP et al: *J Am Med Technol* 41:293, 1979.
68. Henry R: *Cosmetics Toiletries* 94:42, 1979.
69. Hikino H et al: Anti-inflammatory effects of ephedra herbs, *Chem Pharm Bull* 28:2900, 1980.
70. Hobbs C: Goldenseal in early American medical botany, *Pharmacy History* 32(2):79, 1990.
71. Huddleson IF et al: Antibacterial substances in plants, *J Am Vet Med Assoc* 105:394, 1944.
72. Hunan Medical College, China: Garlic in cryptococcal meningitis: a preliminary report of 21 cases, *Chinese Med J* 93:123, 1980.
73. Itokawa Y et al: Effect of S-methylcysteine sulfoxide, S-allylcysteine sulfoxide and related sulfur-containing amino acids on lipid metabolism of experimental hypercholesterolemic rats, *J Nutr* 103:88, 1973.
74. Jain RC: Onion and garlic in experimental cholesterol atherosclerosis in rabbits. I. Effect of serum lipids and development of atherosclerosis, *Artery* 1:115, 1975.
75. Jain RC: Onion and garlic in experimental cholesterol induced atherosclerosis, *Ind J Med Res* 64:1509, 1976.
76. Jain RC: Effect of garlic on serum lipids, coagulability and fibrinolytic activity, *Am J Clin Nutr* 30:1380, 1977.
77. Jain RC: Effect of alcoholic extraction on garlic in atherosclerosis, *Am J Clin Nutr* 31:1982, 1978.
78. Jain RC, Konar DB: Effect of garlic oil in experimental cholesterol atherosclerosis, *Atherosclerosis* 29:125, 1978.
79. Jain RC, Vyas CR: Garlic in alloxan-induced diabetic rabbits, *Am J Clin Nutr* 28:684, 1975.
80. *J Am Inst Homeopathy* 62: 1969.
81. Kadil O, Abdullah TH, Elkadi A: Garlic and the immune system in humans: its effect on natural killer cells, *Fed Proc* 46(4):1222, 1987.
82. Kamanna VS, Chandrasekhara N: Effect of garlic on serum lipoproteins and lipoprotein cholesterol levels in albino rats rendered hypercholesteremic by feeding cholesterol, *Lipids* 17:483, 1982.
83. Kamanna VS, Chandrasekhara N: Hypocholesteremic activity of different fractions of garlic, *Ind J Med Res* 79:580, 1984.
84. Kamat SA: Clinical trial with berberine hydrochloride for the control of diarrhoea in acute gastroenteritis, *J Assoc Physicians India* 15:525, 1967.
85. Karcher L, Zagerman P, Krieglstein K: Effect of an extract of *Ginkgo biloba* on rat brain energy metabolism in hypoxia, *Naunyn-Schmiedeberg's Arch Pharmacol* 327:31, 1984.
86. Kasahara Y et al: Anti-inflammatory action of ephedrines in acute inflammations, *Planta Medica* 54:325, 1985.
87. Kritchevsky D: Effect of garlic oil on experimental atherosclerosis, *Artery* 1:319, 1975.
88. Kritchevsky D et al: Influence of garlic oil on cholesterol metabolism in rats, *Nutr Rep Int* 22:641, 1980.
89. Kuichi F, Shibuyu M, Sankawa U: Inhibitors of prostaglandin biosynthesis from ginger, *Chem Pharm Bull* 30:754, 1982.
90. Kumazawa Y et al: Activation of peritoneal macrophages by berberine alkaloids in terms of induction of cytostatic activity, *Int J Immunopharmacology* 6:587, 1984.
91. *Lancet* Oct 18:885, 1986.
92. Lau BHS, Keeler WH, Adetumbi MA: Antifungal effect of garlic, *Ann Am Soc Microbiol* 387, 1983.
93. *Lawrence review of natural products,* vol 3, no 21, Collegeville, Penn, 1982, Pharmaceutical Information Associates.
94. *Lawrence review of natural products,* vol 3, nos 23/24, Collegeville, Penn, 1982, Pharmaceutical Information Associates.
95. Le Poncin, Lafitte M, Rapin JR: Effect of *Ginko biloba* on changes induced by quantitative cerebral microembolization in rats, *Arch Int Pharmacodyn Ther* 243:236, 1980.
96. Leung AY: *Drug Cosm Ind* 120(6):34, 1977.
97. Leung AY: *Encyclopedia of common natural ingredients used in foods, drugs, and cosmetics,* New York, 1980, Wiley.
98. Lorenset LJ et al: *J Pharm Sci* 53:1287, 1964.
99. Lust J: *The herb book,* New York, 1980, Bantam Books.
100. Makheja AN, Vanderhoek JY, Bailey JM: Inhibition of platelet aggregation and thromboxane synthesis by onion and garlic, *Lancet* 1:781, 1979.
101. Malik SA, Siddiqui S: Hypotensive effect of freeze-dried garlic sap in dogs, *J Pakistan Med Assoc* 31:12, 1981.
102. Mann C, Staba E: The chemistry, pharmacology, and commercial formulations of chamomile. In Cracker LE, Simon JE, editors: *Herbs, spices, and medicinal plants,* vol 1, 1986, Ory Press.
103. Manning C: *Bioenergetic medicines east and west,* Berkeley, Calif, 1988, North Atlantic Books.
104. *Merck Index,* ed 5, 1940, Merck.
105. Mishra SB, Dixit SN: Fungicidal spectrum of the leaf extract of *Allium sativum, Ind Phytopathol* 29:448, 1976.
106. Moerman DE: *Medicinal plants of native America,* Technical report No 19, Research Reports in Ethobotany, Contribution 2, Ann Arbor, 1986, University of Michigan, Museum of Anthropology.
107. Mohan M et al: Berberine in trachoma, *Ind J Ophthalmol* 30:69, 1982.
108. Moore GS, Atkins RD: The fungicidal and fungistatic effects of an aqueous garlic extract on medically important yeast-like fungi, *Mycopathologia* 69:341, 1977.
109. Morton JF: *Econ Bot* 15:311, 1961.
110. Reference deleted in proofs.
111. Mowrey D, Clayson D: Motion sickness, ginger, and psychophysics, *Lancet* i:655, 1982.
112. Murray M: *The healing power of herbs,* Rocklin, Calif, 1992, Prima Publishing.
113. Nagai K: Experimental studies on the preventive effect of garlic extract against infection with influenza virus, *Jpn J Infect Dis* 47:321, 1973.
114. Nagai K, Osawa S: Cholesterol-lowering effect of aged garlic extract in rats, *Basic Pharmacol Ther* 2:41, 1974.
115. Nakagawa S et al: Effect of raw and extracted-aged garlic juice on growth of young rats and their organs after peroral administration, *J Toxicol Sci* 5:9, 1980.

116. Nakayama S et al: Cytoprotective activity of components of garlic, ginseng, and ciuwjia on hepatocyte injury induced by carbon tetrachloride in vitro, *Hiroshima J Med Sci* 8:803, 1985.
117. Nasada KK et al: Effect of onion and garlic on blood coagulation and fibrinolysis in vitro, *Ind J Physiol Pharmacol* 27:141, 1983.
118. Nieberding JF: *Am Bee J* 114:15, 1974.
119. Prasad G, Sharma VD: Efficacy of garlic *(Allium sativum)* treatment against experimental candidiasis in chicks, *Br Vet J* 136:448, 1980.
120. Raj KP, Parmer RM: Garlic—condiment and medicine, *Ind Drugs* 15:205, 1977.
121. Rashid A, Khan HH: The mechanism of hypotensive effect of garlic extract, *JPMA* 35:357, 1985.
122. Ruffin J, Hunter S: An evaluation of the side effects of garlic as an antihypertensive agent, *Cytobios* 37:85, 1983.
123. Sabir M, Bhide N: Study of some pharmacologic actions of berberine, *Ind J Physiol Pharm* 15:111, 1971.
124. Sack RB, Froehlich JL: Berberine inhibits intestinal secretory response of *Vibrio cholera* toxins and *Escherichia coli* enterotoxins, *Infect Immun* 35:471, 1982.
125. Sainani GS et al: Effect of garlic and onion on important lipid and coagulation parameters in alimentary hyperlipemia, *J Assoc Physicians India* 27(1):57, 1979.
126. Sandrhu DK, Warraich MK, Singh S: Sensitivity of yeasts isolated from cases of vaginitis to aqueous extracts of garlic, *Kykosen* 23(12):691, 1980.
127. Saxena KK et al: Effect of garlic pretreatment on isoprenaline-induced myocardial necrosis in albino rats, *Ind J Physiol Pharmacol* 24:223, 1980.
128. Schilcher H: The significance of phytotherapy in Europe, an interdisciplinary and comparative study, *Z Phytother* 14:132, 1993.
129. Sharma R, Joshi CK, Gjoyal RK: Berberine tannate in acute diarrhea, *Ind Pediatr* 7:496, 1970.
130. Sharma VC et al: Antibacterial property of *Allium sativum:* in vivo and in vitro studies, *Indian J Exp Biol* 15:446, 1977.
131. Ship, *JAMA* 238:1770, 1970.
132. Shoji N et al: Cardiotonic principles of ginger *(Zingiber officinale), J Pharm Sci* 10:1174, 1982.
133. Smith AW: *A gardener's book of plant names,* New York, 1963, Harper & Row.
134. Spoerke DG: *Herbal medications,* Santa Barbara, Calif, 1980, Woodbridge Press.
135. Srivastava KC: Aqueous extracts on onion, garlic and ginger inhibit platelet aggregation and alter arachidonic acid metabolism, *Biomed Biochem Acta* 43:s335, 1984.
136. Srivastava KC: Effects of aqueous extracts of onion, garlic, and ginger on platelet aggregation and metabolism of arachidonic acid in the blood vascular system: in vitro study, *Prostaglandins Leukotrienes Med* 13:227, 1984.
137. Srivastava KC, Mu S, Tafa T: Ginger and rheumatic disorders, *Med Hypothesis* 29:25, 1989.
138. Sun D, Courtney HS, Beachey EH: Berberine sulfate blocks adherence of *Streptococcus pyogenes* to epithelial cells, fibronectin, and hexadecane, *Antimicrob Agents Chemother* 32:1370, 1988.
139. Swabb EA, Tai YH, Jordan L: Reversal of cholera toxin-induced secretion in rat ileum by luminal berberine, *Am J Physiol* 248, 1981.
140. Tai YH et al: Antisecretory effects of berberine in rat ileum, *Am J Physiol* 241:253, 1981.
141. Tansye MR, Appleton JA: Inhibition of fungal growth by garlic extract, *Mycopathologia* 67:409, 1975.
142. Tariq H et al: *J Nat Med Assoc* 80(4):441, 1988.
143. Tsai Y et al: Antiviral properties of garlic: in vitro effects on influenza B, herpes simplex I, and Coxsackie viruses, *Planta Med* 5:460, 1985.
144. Tutakne MA et al: Sporotrichosis treated with garlic juice: a case report, *Indian J Dermatol* 28(1):41, 1983.
145. Tyler V, Brady L, Roberts J: *Pharmacology,* ed 8, Philadelphia, 1981, Lea & Febiger.
146. Tyler V: An overview: natural products and medicine, *Herbal Gram* 28:40, 1993.
147. Tyler VE: *The new honest herbal,* Philadelphia, 1987, George F Stickley.
148. University of Illinois at the Medical Center, Dept. of Pharmacognosy and Pharmacology, abstract prepared for the Herb Trade Association.
149. Weiner M: *Earth medicine, earth food,* New York, 1980, Ballantine Books.
150. Weiss R: *Herbal medicine,* 1991, Beaconsfield Publisher.
151. Weiss S, Weiss G: *Growing and using the healing herbs,* Emmays, Pa, 1985, Rodale Press.
152. Willard T: *The Wild Rose scientific herbal,* Calgary, Alberta, Canada, 1991, Wild Rose College of Natural Healing.
153. Willis ED: Enzyme inhibition by allicin, the active principle of garlic, *Biochem J* 63:514, 1956.
154. Wren RC: *Potter's new encyclopaedia of botanical drugs and preparations,* Rustington, Sussex, UK, 1975, Health Science Press.
155. Yamada Y, Azuma K: Evaluation of the in vitro antifungal activity of allicin, *Antimicrob Agents Chemother* 11:713, 1977.
156. Zell J et al: Treatment of acute sprain of the ankle: a controlled double blind trial to test the effectiveness of homeopathic ointment, *Biol Ther* v VII, (1):1, 1989.

40 BITES AND INJURIES INFLICTED BY MAMMALS

Michael L. Callaham
Section on bear attacks contributed by Steven P. French

Mammalian bites possess some unique characteristics that distinguish them from the other assorted injuries suffered by human beings. Tearing, cutting, and crushing injuries are combined in animal bites. While it is true that animal bites* may develop local infection, this complication is hardly unique; many of the offending bacteria are present in numerous environmental sources. However, few traumatic lacerations are as regularly contaminated with as broad a variety of pathogens as animal bites.

Animal bites have special features that warrant attention. First, many victims are understandably terrorized by an attacking animal. Second, animals are capable of transmitting a wide variety of systemic diseases, many of which induce substantial morbidity and mortality. Finally, and perhaps most important, in contrast to the large and detailed scientific literature on nonbite traumatic injuries, the literature on animal bites is largely unscientific and often simply anecdotal. As a result, rational treatment decisions must often be made without a completely satisfactory scientific basis. This chapter interprets the present state of knowledge to make logical specific recommendations.

Incidence of Bites

The true incidence of animal bites will always be unknown. Neither the annual number of bites nor the base population at risk can be reliably estimated. The world supports approximately 4400 species of mammals, 8600 species of birds, 6000 species of reptiles, and 35 to 40 species of domestic animals.[137] None of these species is subject to census. The actual number of wild animals in the world is estimated to be in the billions, including 3 billion domestic animals in 1968.[367] In 1991, 57 million cats and 53 million dogs were estimated to be in the United States.[211,440] Even dog and cat population figures are unreliable, since no method of enumeration is available in the United States other than county pet license statistics, which are known to be incomplete. Even pets such as purebred dogs are poorly counted; the only available figures come from the registry of

*Throughout this chapter, animal bites will be used to refer specifically to mammalian bites, although most of the statements are applicable to bites inflicted by birds and reptiles as well.

the American Kennel Club (AKC), which in 1976 totaled only 386,000 dogs. This is obviously a small proportion of the total canine population.

Accurate figures for the total number of bites inflicted in any given year are also unavailable. Many people who suffer relatively minor injuries from pets, laboratory animals, or farm animals do not seek medical attention unless infection or some other complication occurs. Since reporting the bites of pets can have negative consequences for both owners (financial responsibility, violation of local ordinances) and victims (angry owners), these factors probably also contribute to underreporting.

Few studies have examined the incidence of animal bites. In Sweden 3 of 1000 inhabitants were injured in some way by animals each year.[29] Dogs accounted for 42% of the total, cats 9%, horses 31%, cattle 8%, moose 6% (almost all involved in auto accidents), and all other animals 4%. However, bites were not separately examined in this study; many of the injuries occurred in accidents caused by animals.

Some cities, such as New York, Los Angeles, and Baltimore, mandate reporting of animal bites (Table 40-1). In these locations the incidence of dog bites has tended to run between 300 and 700 per 100,000 population.[23,187,401] In rural Ohio the rate was 271 per 100,000 in 1966, as compared with 2059 per 100,000 in West Texas in 1977.[228,367] In Sweden the incidence of dog bite was 0.7 per 1000 inhabitants in 1985.[29] The 1970s witnessed an increase of up to 186% in the reported incidence of urban dog bite in the United States, although this seems to have leveled off recently. Extrapolating these data to the entire United States yields an annual incidence of at least 1.5 million dog bites. Estimates from the Humane Society of the United States are 1 to 3 million dog bites a year.[368] About 1.2% of postal letter carriers in the United States are bitten by dogs every year.[368] In a survey of schoolchildren, 45% had been bitten by a dog and 30% of these were bitten by their own dog.[441]

Persons in certain occupations in developed countries, such as postal workers, veterinary and animal control workers, and laboratory workers, are at greatest risk of animal bite. Nonetheless, these individuals—at least partly because of professional experience, training, and prevention—do not incur the greatest absolute number of bites.[49] Instead, the greatest number of victims are children, often in poorly supervised situations. In undeveloped countries this is not the case; many persons are exposed on an everyday basis to bites from species considered "exotic" in the developed world or to rabid dogs.

Special risk groups, such as veterinarians, may have a high exposure. Sixty-four percent of veterinarians have sustained a major animal-related injury at some time in their careers, and 17% have been hospitalized. Thirty-five percent have suffered lacerations, 10% have had fracture-dislocations, and a few have incurred major head and abdominal trauma.[238] Incidence of biting species varies with exposure; among veterinarians the greatest number of injuries are inflicted by cattle, followed by dogs and then horses. Twelve percent have been bitten by pigs. The average veterinarian loses 1.3 days from work in 1 year because of animal injury. Interestingly, 4% of veterinarians reduced their own fractures and dislocations, and 20% sutured their own lacerations.

Table 40-1 Incidence (Percent) of Bites by Species in the United States

	Reference					
Species	**267**	**367**	**108**		**410**	**228**
Dog	89	91.6	63	50	83	
Cat	4.6	4.5	15	14	1	
Human	3.6	0.03	15	23	0	
Rodent	2.2	3	0.6	12	3.4	65
Monkey	0.1*	0.2	2.4		2.2	15
Skunk		0.02			2.2	
Lagomorph	0.2	0.5	0.6			
Horse	0.1	0.06				6
Large mammal	0.03†	0.01‡		1.2		3§
Reptile	0.1				8	
Bat		0.004	0.6			6
Raccoon		0.08	0.7			3‖

*Includes 21 monkeys, 4 raccoons, 3 ferrets, 1 weasel, 1 coatimundi, 1 skunk, and 1 goat.
†Includes 3 lions, 1 ocelot, 1 leopard, 1 polar bear, and 1 anteater.
‡Includes 1 goat, 1 ocelot, 1 jaguar, and 1 groundhog, which inflicted a bite on Groundhog Day.
§One coyote.
‖One kinkajou.

Extensive information is available regarding the incidence of animal bites by species in the United States (Table 40-1). In New York City, dogs accounted for 89% of all animal bites, cats 4.6%, humans 3.6%, rodents 2.2%, and other species for very small percentages.[267] Since the United States has more cats than dogs, the low percentage of the total number of bite wounds attributed to cats is surprising. Also surprising is that rodents, which are ubiquitous in city, country, pet, and laboratory environments, produce few treatable bites. By contrast, mandatory reporting in a largely rural area of Ohio demonstrated that dogs accounted for 91.6% of all bites, cats 4.5%, rodents 3%, and skunks, rabbits, horses, bats, and raccoons less than 1% each; humans accounted for only 0.03%.[367] Presumably, the figure for human bites represents either different methods of handling aggression in a rural population or a greater reluctance to report such incidents.

In every statistical series of bites, small numbers of exotic animals such as ocelots, jaguars, lions, leopards, polar bears, wolves, anteaters, ferrets, and weasels are represented. These occur from exposure to wild and zoo animals, and from the increasing popularity of wild animals as pets, usually kept illegally and without adequate understanding and training regarding animal care and behavior. All too often this results in harsh or even fatal attacks for the owners and in misfortune for the animal.[66] In a series reported from 1971 to 1981—before exotic pets became popular—73 such bites were reported in the United States, which clearly represents only a fraction of the real total.[342] Five timber wolves were involved, as were seven lions, four tigers, two leopards, and one Malayan sun bear.

All the preceding figures represent only reported bites. Doubtless, many bites in homes, barns, zoos, and laboratories are not reported and therefore are never reflected in the data. The data cited on veterinarians suggest that this is the case.[238] Therefore the incidence of infection and other complications from animal bite wounds suggested by the reported data is probably significantly greater than the true incidence, since logically many of the unreported bites remain so because of lack of complications.

The cost of bites in time, money, and disability is great. Modern laboratory, zoo, and farm workers are injured fairly frequently in their work, while in many underdeveloped countries, animals remain the daily threat to health and existence that they were in prehistoric times. In Britain 21% of those injured had to take sick leave, averaging 45 days per person, and the costs averaged 450 British pounds per person in 1985.[29] Dog bites account for 1% of all emergency department visits made in the United States.[108] Of these patients, 10% require suturing and 1% require hospitalization.[23] In 1974 the average outpatient charge for a dog bite wound was $38; medical costs have inflated drastically since then, but no more recent study figures are available.[23] These figures do not include time lost from work and other pursuits. On a rubber plantation in Sumatra, animal-inflicted injuries (including nonmammalian) regularly accounted for 1% to 2% of hospital admissions annually.[378]

Several thousand people a year are killed by mammalian bites, with most of the wounds inflicted by man-eating lions and tigers in Africa and Asia (Table 40-2). However, these figures must be kept in perspective. The World Health Organization estimates that roughly 60,000 people a year are killed by snakes and that additional millions are killed by insect-borne diseases.[69]

One must wonder, however, at the rationality of worrying (as people often do) about being bitten or killed by animals (wild or domestic), when statistics clearly identify that humans are by far the most dangerous animal (Table 40-2). It would be unfair to the other animals not to point out that in World War II, humans killed 22 million of their own kind, including 6 million in programs of genocide. Individual acts of murder currently account for more than 200,000 annual worldwide deaths, and suicide accounts for more than 400,000. In the United States alone, currently 49,000 people a year are killed in traffic accidents, and 38,000 a year by firearms.[244] Another 235,000 a year are injured by gunshot in the United States, and homicide has become the eleventh most common cause of death, killing 21,000 in 1985.[244] Each year 500,000 Americans go to an emergency department for treatment of injuries inflicted by other humans.

By comparison, an estimated 200 Americans are killed by animals each year; 131 of these die in traffic accidents involving deer.[191] Bees killed 43 persons, dogs 14, and rattlesnakes 10, and wild animals such as bears and cougars killed fewer people than did goats, rats, jellyfish, and a captive elephant. One can only conclude from these figures that although death from animal attack has at times been a major problem, we are in much greater danger at the hands of our own aggressive species.

Circumstances and Prevention of Animal Bites

ANIMAL BEHAVIOR

Prevention of animal bites requires a thorough knowledge of the behavior, personalities, and patterns of various species of animals. This information is available more in the form of folk wisdom and personal experience than as published text. A person wishing to avoid the bite of a particular species will often be able to gain expertise about that species' behavior only from those who work with it regularly. For example, the behavior of domestic farm animals is best learned from farm workers and veterinarians. Such information can be critical. For example, horses bite frequently, cattle almost never. Horses tend to kick backward with both rear feet; cows tend to kick forward with only one foot. Some small species of deer have large canines and bite; most do not. The various attack and defense pat-

Table 40-2 Human Deaths from Animal Attacks

Species	Annual Estimated Deaths	Annual Estimated Attacks	Predominant Area	Comments
Humans	200,000		Worldwide	Individual murders only; excludes 1 million/year by war in recent decades
Humans	21,000	500,000	United States only	Homicides and deliberate assaults only; most murders by firearms; firearm injuries alone estimated to cost $429 million a year[20]
Snake	50,000		Worldwide	
Crocodile	1000		Africa	Man-eating predominantly
Domestic horse, cow, pig	800	39,549	Europe alone	Mostly accidental; goring injuries cause evisceration
Tiger	600-800		India	Frequently man eaters
Lion	300-500		Africa	Frequently man eaters
Leopard	400		Africa, India	Frequently man eaters
Elephant	200-500		Central Africa, India	Occasionally rogue man killers; incidence increasing because of environmental pressures
Hippopotamus	200-300		Africa	Unpredictable; bites and tramplings common
Buffalo	20-100		Africa	Only if cornered or wounded
Hyena	10-50	Hundreds	Africa	Frequently bites off face of sleeper
Wolf	20-50	200-500	Eurasia (none in North America)	Hundreds per year in previous centuries
Domestic dog	10	1,500,000	United States only	Most dangerous to infants, disabled; pit bulls most common breed
Indian sloth bear	5-10	50?	India, Ceylon	Severe facial injuries common
Gorilla	0	2-3	Africa	Only if cornered; injuries usually not severe
Baboon	0	1-2	South Africa	Usually pets
Ostrich	1-2		South Africa	Disembowelment, kick to head
Grizzly bear	Rare	<1	North America	Occasional attacks on campers; most attacks provoked or avoidable
Black rhinocerus	<1		Africa	Easily provoked

terns of animals are well described by Fowler.[138] Detailed information on behavior and attack patterns of animals in the wild (particularly African and Asian animals) is available from Clarke.[69]

BASIC PRINCIPLES FOR AVOIDING ANIMAL BITES

Recognition of a few simple principles may help a person avoid animal bites. Animals rarely attack people without provocation. Exceptions are large carnivores, which may be relatively unafraid of humans, and creatures clinically infected with rabies. However, carnivores do not commonly hunt humans as preferred prey. In the vast majority of cases involving domestic and wild animals, bite injury is provoked, although the animal's perception of provocation may differ from that of the human. Patterns of behavior and attack differ, and details are discussed in the sections on the relevant species (especially the sections on dogs, big cats, and bears).

People often capture or restrain animals, wild or domestic. In this stressful situation, even the most benign of animals may turn on its owner. Wild animals that are allegedly tame are very likely to struggle. Even a shy animal, such as an antelope, being captured for a benign purpose such as treatment of an injury, may attempt to defend itself and can inflict a life-threatening injury such as goring. Therefore all situations of animal restraint and capture should be considered high risk, and careful study of the behavior of the species, the individual animal, and the physical environment and resources should precede actual attempts at restraint.

Important distinctions exist between domestic and wild animals, but this is increasingly forgotten by people in modern developed countries, who seem unable to differentiate between theme parks and wilderness. Also an increasingly popular and unfortunate trend is the raising of wild animals as pets.[256] A large and lucrative market exists for these animal victims of urban fantasies, particularly in the United States. No matter how raised, the animals remain wild and will never be as predictable, trustworthy, and nonaggressive as animals that have been domesticated for centuries. Most "domesticated" wild creatures cause problems as they grow older, often injuring their owners, who then lose enthusiasm and want to be rid of their pet instantly.[356] In many cases owners demonstrate a remarkable lack of common sense, as in the case of a pet wolf that was allowed access to a 10-week-old infant, with fatal results.[66] Similarly, the owner of a pet buffalo was not persuaded to get rid of his pet until it gored him, a year after it had gored his son.[330] Many of these mistakes probably stem from the fact that, unlike their rural and Third World counterparts, most modern urban dwellers have an almost total lack of firsthand experience with wild animals or even domestic ones other than dogs and cats.

Most wild species have a strong sense of territoriality.[2,212] Individuals, pairs, or larger groups stake off territory that ranges in size from square feet to square miles and aggressively prevent any intrusion into that territory, particularly by members of their own species. During the mating season this drive may stimulate even small animals to threaten or attack humans, particularly in protection of the nest and young. Some species, such as dogs, are selected by humans for their particularly strong territorial instincts. Depending on the size and type of dog and whether the terrain is rural or urban, the dog's territory may vary from a small yard to several city blocks. Intrusion into this territory may trigger an attack.

A major principle of animal behavior is that physical attack is often the animal's last resort. This may not be obvious when observing some of the spectacular contests that occur in the wild. However, these confrontations are governed by elaborate rituals and rules that encourage a nonviolent solution, so that the victor may successfully defend his territory and himself with little or no injury. When humans encounter animals, they can often avoid attack and injury by successful interpretation of visual, auditory, and olfactory warning signs.

Animals generally give ample warning of their intentions, which are to repel the intruder or to permit its escape, rather than to inflict damage. If a human slowly and carefully backs off without making sudden or threatening gestures, usually no harm will be done. The ideal reaction may depend on the species. For example, man-eating lions and tigers have been turned from a full charge by an angry human being who attacked or advanced rather than fled.[69] Given a choice of victims, such a predator prefers the fleeing, panicky victim who demonstrates expected flight rather than unexpected behavior. Nonpredator species such as cattle and deer are extremely susceptible to human intimidation, while dogs can be provoked to attack by a direct stare, which is regarded as a challenge.

Humans may provoke attack by attempting to capture or corner an animal. Even the most timid creature will kick, bite, or scratch if cornered in a small space or if physically restrained. This desperate behavior should be expected when an animal is inadvertently trapped. If the creature is allowed to escape without threat, the human will usually not be attacked. If capture of an animal is essential, detailed preparation should be undertaken. For small animals, using nets or heavy cloth and wearing extremely heavy gloves with other protective clothing are advisable. Desperate animals can bite with tremendous force; large carnivores can easily amputate a gloved digit. A wolf can tear apart a stainless steel bowl with its teeth, while a hyena can bite through a 2-inch plank.[69] Four men are needed to subdue an adult chimpanzee; an orangutan can maintain a one-fingered grip that an adult human cannot break.[138] A camel can break a 4 × 4 inch wooden beam with one kick.[138] Larger animals will generally require a team approach, nets, barriers, cages, and immobilizing drugs. Ideal immobilization techniques for various species have been detailed in several veterinary texts.[138,139] Behavioral modification to prevent dog attacks is discussed in the section on that species.

An increasing number of animal-induced injuries can only be classified as bizarre. The reason for these probably is that the average human is considerably less familiar with animal behavior than was true even 50 years ago and therefore is more likely to do careless things. Examples are given in the discussions of the various species. One such foolish victim was a man who was illegally hunting turkey. He shot a large bird and put it in the trunk of his automobile next to his loaded shotgun. When later he tried to take it out to show it off, the bird (wounded, not dead) struggled and its claw fired the gun, wounding the hunter in the leg.[260]

Prehospital Considerations

Domestic and farm attacks are fairly predictable and preventable. Unfortunately, wilderness attacks are not always avoidable, as shown by grizzly bears' behavior in Glacier and Yellowstone National Parks. In other countries, life-threatening attacks by large animals such as water buffalo, lions, tigers, and elephants are common. Attacks by larger animals should be considered as major blunt or penetrating trauma, with possible major arterial blood loss, airway damage, broken ribs, pneumothoraces, and intraperitoneal bleeding.[378] Victims of such attacks should be managed in the same way as victims of nonanimal major trauma. The victim's condition and the availability of rapid evacuation determine the extent of treatment in the field. In many situations in which wild animals are encountered, medical personnel or supplies are not on the scene. Thus the patient should be moved to a hospital or clinic as soon as possible.

Local wound treatment should be initiated at the scene of the bite (Box 40-1). This is often more important in determining the course of healing than any later therapy. Medical and lay personnel should be aware of the usefulness of simple first aid measures, which must be initiated immediately unless definitive or better treatment is available within a short time. Pressure on the wound or pressure points controls most bleeding; tourniquets should be avoided unless blood loss cannot be otherwise controlled. If the victim is more than an hour from treatment, the wounds should be cleansed at the scene as soon as the ABCs of resuscitation

BOX 40-1

SUMMARY OF ANIMAL BITE WOUND TREATMENT

MANDATORY (ALL WOUNDS)

1. Evaluate for potential blunt trauma and injury to deeper and vital structures by penetrating canine teeth.
2. Ensure appropriate tetanus immunization.
3. Irrigate wound with several hundred milliliters of normal saline or 5% povidone-iodine solution using a 12 ml syringe and 19-gauge needle or similar irrigation device.
4. Debride obviously crushed and devitalized tissue where possible.
5. If the animal is suspected to be rabid (atypical behavior, high-risk species):
   a. Infiltrate wound edges with 1% procaine hydrochloride.
   b. Swab wound surface vigorously with cotton swabs and 1% benzalkonium chloride (Zephiran) solution.
   c. Rinse out wound with normal saline.
   d. Assess need for rabies immune globulin and vaccine.
6. Assess risk factors to decide on further (selective) treatment (see Box 40-3).
7. Do not culture fresh wounds.
8. Do not give prophylactic antibiotics for routine low-risk bite wounds.

SELECTIVE TREATMENT (WOUNDS SELECTED BY RISK FACTORS)

1. Suture or staple all skin wounds in the usual fashion unless high risk (hand wounds, high-risk species, immunosuppressed patient).
2. Culture infected wounds only if they fail to respond to initial antibiotic therapy, they are very high risk (see Box 40-3), or there is evidence of systemic sepsis.
3. Consider: delayed primary closure of high-risk wounds, prophylactic antibiotics in high-risk wounds.

are completed. Early cleansing reduces the chance of bacterial infection and is extremely effective in killing rabies and other viruses. Using potable water, preferably boiled or treated with germicidal agents, is adequate. Ordinary hand soap adds some bactericidal, virucidal, and cleansing properties. If a 1% povidone-iodine (Betadine) solution is available, it should be used as an irrigant. However, alcohol, hydrogen peroxide, and other disinfectants, which in their commonly available concentration are harmful to normal tissue, should be avoided. The wound should be thoroughly irrigated with at least a pint of soap and water and then gently debrided of dirt and foreign objects by swabbing with a soft, clean cloth or sterile gauze. Simple irrigation without actual swabbing of the wound edges will not remove rabies virus.[222] (Irrigation with a syringe is much better, but syringes are seldom available.) If available, topical external antibiotic ointments such as gramicidin-neomycin-bacitracin (Neosporin) may be helpful for abrasions but should not be used in open wounds.[364]

After the wound has been cleansed thoroughly, it should be covered with sterile dressings or a clean, dry cloth. Wounds of the hands or feet require immobilization of the wound after cleansing. If the wounds are substantial, treatment is hours away, and antibiotics such as penicillin, a cephalosporin, or erythromycin are available, it is reasonable to start immediate treatment with a large oral dose (0.5 to 1 g). To be most effective in preventing subsequent wound infection, this should be done within an hour of wounding. However, with severe wounds it is worthwhile even many hours later. In circumstances in which antibiotics are not available, the wound is infection prone, and medical care is hours or days away, simple remedies such as filling the wound with honey may be effective antibacterial strategies.[315]

When definitive medical care cannot be obtained for a day or more, cleansing and irrigating the wound thoroughly and in some wounds attempting closure are reasonable. In general, since suturing requires suture equipment, a trained person, and local anesthesia and has an increased risk of infection, it should be avoided in this setting. However, good closure can often be obtained with the use of tape, Steri-Strips, or a tape-suture device (Ready-Stitch, Med United Ltd., London, U.K.).[424] This provides reasonably good cosmetic results, protection of deep tissues such as cartilage or bone, and minimal risk of infection.

Many if not most of the complications and serious infections from animal bites are caused by inadequate first aid and significant delays (which in developing countries can be days or weeks) in receiving medical care. Unscientific local folk remedies, such as soaking bitten extremities in extremely hot water, also worsen the prognosis.

In addition to treating the bite victim, rescuers should try to capture the offending animal for examination, if this can be done without risk of further injury. Unusual behavior, such as unprovoked attack by a wild animal in broad daylight or a complete absence of fear of humans, should raise the suspicion of rabies. Live capture is optimal, but freshly killed animals are usually satisfactory for examination for fluorescent rabies antibody (FRA). Damage to the animal's head and brain should be avoided because brain tissue is needed for analysis. The availability of the animal can eliminate the need for costly and uncomfortable rabies prophylaxis. If more than an hour will elapse before the animal can be transported to a hospital or public health department, the body should be refrigerated. Use of preservatives should be avoided; this is discussed in Chapter 41.

Examination of the animal is not useful for most other diseases and will not help predict local wound infections. Therefore good judgment must be used in deciding how much time and energy to expend on capture.

Evaluation of Injuries

All victims of animal bites should be evaluated for blunt trauma and internal injuries that may be less obvious than the bite wound itself (see Box 40-1). Many animals are large, strong, and heavy, and patients should be treated like any other victim of blunt or penetrating trauma. Details of injuries are given in the sections on particular species, but internal organ damage, deep arterial and nerve damage, and penetration of joints are all possible. Particularly in children, animal bites can penetrate vital structures such as joints or the cranium[426]; radiographs should be taken whenever these injuries are suspected. In an infant the attacking animal need not even be particularly large. Roosters have caused skull fractures with their beaks in this age group.[328] Therefore a complete head-to-toe evaluation for trauma is advised in all but the most trivial and isolated bite injuries.

The principles of wound care for injuries caused by inanimate objects apply to bite wounds as well. Many bite injuries are simple contusions that do not break the skin. The infection potential of these injuries is low; superficial wound cleansing and symptomatic treatment of pain and swelling suffice. In the case of large herbivores, most of the injury may consist of severe contusion and the skin is usually not broken (Fig. 40-1).[268] Treatment should include prompt and liberal application of ice or other cold packs during the first 24 hours. However, this is not beneficial in snakebite and is obviously impractical in many undeveloped locations. (Snakebite is discussed in detail in Chapters 28 and 29.)

When skin is broken, the risks of local wound infection or the transmission of systemic disease are incurred. Infection can be caused by organisms carried in the animal's saliva or nasal secretions, by skin microbial flora that are carried into the wound, or by environmental organisms that enter the wound during or after the attack. Virtually any bacterium, virus, or fungus can become a contaminant in bite wounds, and despite such folklore as the belief that tetanus is likely only after puncture with a rusty nail, virtually any type of infection can occur after even minor skin trauma.

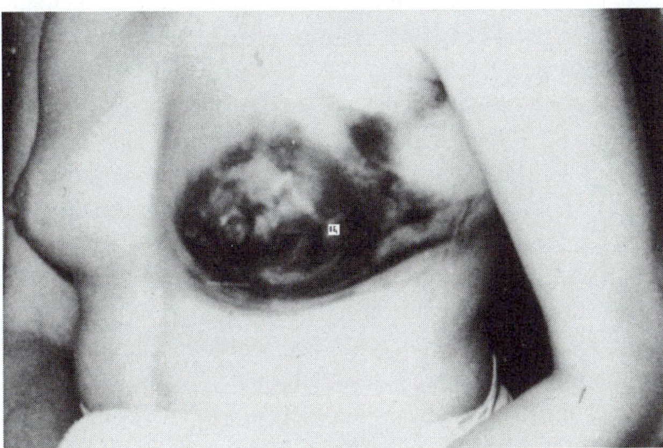

Fig. 40-1 Soft tissue injury after horse bite. (Photograph by Murray Fowler, D.V.M., University of California, Davis.)

Fortunately, most wounds do not become infected, and observance of a few general principles of wound care can significantly reduce infection rates (see Box 40-1). Unfortunately, the topic is so undramatic that it is frequently ignored.

Very few laboratory tests are of use in the evaluation of animal bite injuries (see Box 40-2). X-ray examinations should be performed as needed. Unless hematocrit is being assessed for evidence of blood loss from occult trauma, the CBC is not useful because it is a nonspecific and unreliable gauge of infection. Cultures are discussed later in the chapter.

Mandatory Basic Wound Care

SOAKING THE WOUND

Normal skin contains both resident and transient bacterial flora. The transient flora reflect continuous exposure to various environmental microorganisms. Healthy skin is quite efficient at microbe control, and bacteria planted on normal skin rapidly disappear. The resident bacteria consist of very few species, chiefly aerobic *Staphylococcus epidermis* and *Micrococcus* species, as well as anaerobic *Propionibacterium acnes,* which may outnumber aerobic bacteria by 10 to 1 on most surfaces.[18] These resident bacteria, which inhabit the sweat and sebaceous glands, persist even when the surface of the skin is sterile. Pathogenic *Staphylococcus aureus* and occasionally *Streptococcus pyogenes* can be

BOX 40-2

INDICATIONS FOR LABORATORY TESTS IN BITE WOUNDS

X-RAY EXAMINATION

Deep bite wounds of the hand (fractures, osteomyelitis, air in joint)
Cranial and facial bites in infants (bony penetration)
Any suspected fight-bite (clenched fist) injury

WOUND CULTURES

Never indicated in fresh uninfected wounds
Infected wounds: only if resistant to initial antibiotic treatment or multiple risk factors

BLOOD CULTURES

Only in patients with sepsis after bite wounds

WHITE BLOOD CELL COUNT OR SEDIMENTATION RATE

Not indicated: management should be based on clinical factors recovered from normal skin at the site of fresh wounds and are often the offending organisms in local wound infection. Other species, including gram-negative bacteria and *Pseudomonas,* can be found on the skin of up to 11% of healthy individuals.[333]

Elimination of these pathogens is desirable.[213] However, removing resident skin flora is no simple matter. An isolated traditional 2-minute surgical scrub of the hands does not reduce the number of bacteria significantly,[254] and nearly all of the benefit occurs in the first 30 seconds. Repeated scrubs performed several times a day over a period of days can markedly reduce but not eliminate the resident flora, but this is obviously not relevant to acute wound care. Twenty percent of the flora can never be eliminated because of its residence in sebaceous glands.[375] Thus a single superficial wound scrub is probably not helpful, and simple rinsing with antiseptic preparations has no effect.[254]

For disinfecting intact skin, chlorhexidine is superior to hexachlorophene (pHisoHex) and povidone-iodine but can damage tissue if it enters the wound itself.[375] Alcohol is one of the more effective agents—even in the form of convenient alcohol wipes.[47] When wipes are used, however, povidone-iodine commercial wipes are much more effective than alcohol wipes.[63] However, fluid from the wipes cannot be allowed to enter the wound because of its potential for tissue damage. Even the most effective agents, such as chlorhexidine, vary in their effectiveness against different species of bacteria.[297]

Soaking fresh traumatic wounds in fluid (usually containing povidone-iodine solution) to cleanse and disinfect the wound itself (separate from the surrounding skin) is common practice. The effectiveness of this practice has been little tested. Some surgeons believe that it is harmful, claiming that it breaks down the skin's protective mantle.[113] Wound soaking possibly washes large numbers of transient microflora off the skin, suspends them in solution, and redistributes them throughout the wound. In one study of 80 nonbite wounds, although 57% had a decrease in bacteria after being prepared with povidone-iodine, hexachlorophene, or green soap solution, 25% showed no change and 18% had an increase in the number of bacteria per gram of wound tissue.[112] This last parameter is the only accurate predictor of wound infection.[233] In this study, however, the method of wound preparation was not specified. The most thorough study demonstrated that a povidone-iodine soak (compared with no soaking at all) had no effect on quantitative bacterial wound counts, whereas a saline soak increased them significantly.[237] Thus there seems to be no experimental basis for this common practice.

Soaking and scrubbing the skin around the wound have only a moderate effect on the bacterial population.[91] Furthermore, they occasionally increase wound contamination. An acceptable procedure for removing excess dirt is to scrub the surrounding skin gently with a surgical sponge and normal saline or a 1% povidone-iodine solution for 5 minutes (see the section on irrigation).[375] *The wound itself should not be scrubbed with a common surgical sponge,* and contamination of the wound with scrub solution should be avoided. Preliminary irrigation and scrubbing in the wilderness are described in the previous section and are recommended whenever definitive medical care will not be provided within 2 hours.

IRRIGATION

Irrigation of nonbite traumatic wounds has been studied extensively and has consistently been shown to substantially decrease infection. Other techniques, such as scrubbing wound surfaces, are damaging to tissues and actually increase infection.[89,350,351,386] However, prophylactic antibiotics become ineffective within a few hours of wounding because the bacteria are encased in and protected by a coagulum of blood and fibrin.[119] If this coagulum is removed by scrubbing, antibiotics are once again effective in killing bacteria in the wound. Thus the question of exactly when and how to scrub has not really been resolved.

Irrigation removes bacteria, debris, and soil that have been introduced into the wound. The last two are deleterious to tissue healing even when they are sterile.[351] Irrigation cannot remove devitalized tissue; this must be carried out by debridement. In dog bites an infection rate of 12% in irrigated wounds was noted compared with 69% in those not irrigated.[53] Irrigation is clearly a useful technique.

The ideal irrigation method should produce enough pressure to dislodge the bacteria and debris without inducing tissue damage. At any given pressure, pulsatile jet irrigation has no advantage over steady-stream application.[351] At 90 pounds per square inch (PSI), irrigation fluid applied to a skin wound on the back of an animal disseminates into the pleural and peritoneal cavities.[99] At 70 PSI, irrigating fluid spreads into surrounding soft tissue for distances of up to 14 mm from the wound edge, but bacteria in the wound are not disseminated into the tissues along with the fluid.[428] High-pressure irrigation used experimentally on clean wounds may greatly increase the incidence of infection, so it should be used only in heavily contaminated wounds where its benefit outweighs this risk.[428]

At the low end of the pressure spectrum, irrigation at less than 5 PSI provides little or no benefit. This includes gravity and bulb syringe techniques, which generate about 0.05 PSI.[351] A pressure of 10 PSI removes approximately 80% of the soil in a wound and lowers the infection rate from 100% at 1 PSI to 21% at 10 PSI (and 7% at 15 PSI).

A 19-gauge needle on a 12 ml syringe will deliver a pressure of approximately 20 PSI when the plunger is depressed with moderate force.[396] Using a smaller syringe increases the pressure but is impractical for delivering irrigating quantities of 100 ml or more. A 19-gauge needle or plastic intravenous catheter on a 35 ml syringe delivers approximately 7 to 8 PSI and decreases the infection rate of lacerations fivefold.[396] The 35 ml syringe requires less frequent filling and is more practical. The pressure it generates should suffice unless a wound is heavily contaminated, in which case a 12 ml syringe should be used to generate higher pressures. This technique does not damage tissues or increase the likelihood of infection in relatively clean wounds. In addition, it has the advantage of using equipment that is extremely inexpensive, disposable, and readily available. Greater convenience at low cost is offered by 12 ml ring-handle syringes with built-in one-way valves, intravenous tubing, and blunt irrigating tips (Travenol Pressure Irrigation Set, Code No. 2D2113). These irrigate with fluid from standard intravenous bags. The least labor-intensive method uses commercial saline canisters pressurized to 8 PSI, which are faster than all other methods and achieve similar results.[61]

The optimal quantity of irrigation fluid appears to be between 100 and 200 ml for wounds a few inches long. Greater quantities provide no further benefit.[117,351] When saline is used, the time necessary to irrigate the wound is not important, but when antibacterial agents are added, a minimum duration of irrigation may be crucial. A 1% povidone-iodine (Betadine) solution requires 5 minutes to kill all bacteria, although most are killed within 30 seconds.[201] Weaker solutions are not advised, since they require contact times in excess of 10 minutes.

The irrigating fluid must not be toxic to the tissues. Because normal saline possesses no bactericidal or surfactant cleansing properties, it functions only as a mechanical dislodger of particles. Normal saline irrigation effectively reduces infection, and it does not injure tissues or increase inflammation.[35,117,128,396] However, *scrubbing* a contaminated wound with a surgical sponge and irrigating with normal saline may result in more infection than irrigation alone.[350] Fresh saline should always be used, since bacteria can grow in previously opened containers.[219]

An irrigating fluid possessing antibacterial and detergent properties would be ideal. Pluronic F-68 (ShurClens) is a nonirritating surfactant that is effective in removing debris from wounds and decreasing infection, although it completely lacks intrinsic antibacterial activity.[350] When a scrubbing technique is used experimentally, it is more effective than normal saline. It appears to be completely nontoxic to tissue, leukocytes, and red blood cells, and this is a particularly attractive quality when used for irrigation of wounds about the eye, since it causes no damage or irritation to the cornea.[41] However, this new agent has had only a few clinical trials and is very expensive. In a large recent trial it was no more efficacious than saline or 1% povidone-iodine, and it cost 22 times more than either of these alternatives.[104]

Many other potential irrigants possess antibacterial activity in commonly available concentrations. These include tincture of iodine, povidone-iodine, hexachlorophene, benzalkonium chloride solution, Dial soap, green soap, 70% ethyl alcohol, quaternary ammonium compounds, chlorhexidine, hydrogen peroxide, and hand soap.[117,180,386] Unfortunately, most of these are toxic to tissue at all concentrations.[35] Treatment of wounds with any of these agents causes almost immediate abnormality of vascular flow on the edge of the wound and a complete standstill of blood in the microvascular bed to a depth of 300 to 400 μm, as well as extensive local hemolysis and intravascular disruption of granulocytes. This is followed by endothelial leakage with edema, hemorrhage, and deposition of fibrin microthrombi. Eventually, because of the disruption of nutrition, cells in the immediate region exhibit different stages of cellular damage. In most cases the tissue does not regain normal function within the first 6 hours. Hydrogen peroxide in any concentration is particularly destructive to tissues, does not penetrate well, and is a weak germicide.[188] Silver nitrate is also extremely damaging to tissues; it almost universally causes infection in treated wounds.[117] Agents that contain detergents, such as povidone-iodine *scrub* solution or 3% hexachlorophene solution, cause significant damage when injected into joint spaces.[128] A 1% chlorhexidine-gluconate (Hibiclens) solution also may have significant harmful tissue effects.[350] Thus many agents that are clearly bactericidal are so damaging to open tissue and wound healing that their routine use is contraindicated.

The one agent that has proved both bactericidal and nondamaging to tissues is povidone-iodine *solution* (*not* the frequently used surgical scrub), which is supplied in a stock concentration of 10%. This is an excellent bactericidal, fungicidal, and virucidal agent to which few bacteria develop resistance.[201] However, a contact time of at least 2 minutes is needed for full efficacy because release of free iodine is needed to actually kill organisms.[239] Some controversy exists over which concentration is ideal. The 1% solution (dilution of the stock solution in a ratio of 1:10 with normal saline) has been proven to have no ill effects on wound healing and to reduce wound infection.[421] Another study of 500 patients with traumatic nonbite lacerations found a significantly lower infection rate in wounds treated with a 60-second scrub with 1% povidone-iodine.[177] Five and ten percent solutions of povidone-iodine (Betadine) have been better studied than the 1% solution. The consensus of several major studies is that these higher concentrations also have no deleterious effect on tissue, wound healing, or wound strength and decrease wound infection.[117,128,290,346,385] One study, however, found the higher concentration to be harmful to wound healing.[421] Therefore the traditional teaching has been that 1% solution was safe and effective, while 10% might be harmful to wound tissue.

Two new studies have suggested that this teaching may be wrong and that 1% povidone-iodine may not be effective in the traumatic lacerations typically seen in the emergency department. In a large recent study of nonbite lacerations, both 1% povidone-iodine and ShurClens were no more efficacious than saline.[104] One percent povidone-iodine combined with scrubbing was effective in reducing infection in contaminated experimental wounds that were not treated until 12 hours after injury, but showed no benefit when scrubbing was omitted.[205] These new studies lead to the conclusion that in most clean wounds (in which the likelihood of infection is low) and in those in which cosmetic considerations are extremely important (such as on the face), a 1% solution should be used to be completely certain of causing no tissue injury. In wounds thought to be heavily contaminated with soil or bacteria, effective killing of bacteria probably takes precedence over issues of tentative wound injury, and a 5% or 10% solution may be used.

Povidone-iodine solution must not be confused with surgical scrub solution, which contains a detergent and doubles the infection rate.[89] A further caution is that 1% povidone-iodine solution has not been specifically proven effective against rabies virus, although it is virucidal. Therefore benzalkonium chloride should be used to cleanse wounds inflicted by animals suspected of being rabid, since this agent has been proven effective. Finally, prolonged application of high concentrations of povidone-iodine to wounds results in systemic absorption of iodine. This has been a problem only with repeated applications over a period of days in burns and in peritonitis involving a large percentage of the external body or peritoneal surfaces.[188,318,422] Systemic effects of one-time use in lacerations are unknown and unlikely to be significant because of the brevity of application and the relatively small surface area.

Wound irrigation with topical antibiotics is a well-studied and much used technique in major surgery and orthopedics, so considering wound irrigation with these agents in cutaneous trauma is logical.[105] Antibiotics possess the attractive qualities of killing bacteria without harming tissues. Topical antibiotics are as effective against infection in experimental wounds as systemic antibiotics, and the two methods combined are synergistic in heavily contaminated experimental wounds.[369] This is explained by the fact that antibiotics in the wound not only produce very high wound tissue concentrations (greatly exceeding those achieved by intravenous antibiotics), but also within an hour match the serum levels produced by intravenous administration.[271,402] Systemic toxicity from the use of large amounts of aminoglycoside antibiotics in the operating room has been reported.[188,318,422]

Irrigation of experimental cutaneous wounds with antibiotic solutions such as kanamycin, neomycin, vancomycin, ampicillin, tetracycline, cefamandole, cefazolin, and streptomycin has generally been more effective than irrigation with saline.* Flooding of nonbite lacerations with 5% penicillin solution reduced purulent wound infection to 1%, compared with 9% with saline.[249] Topical penicillin applied within 1 hour of contamination prevented infection experimentally and was superior to parenteral penicillin.[249] In an experimental model of irrigation 12 hours after contamination of a wound, cefazolin irrigation alone was ineffective, when combined with wound scrubbing was only slightly more effective than the control, and was less effective than povidone-iodine irrigation and scrubbing.[205] Topical cefamandole applied to experimental wounds in animals was more effective than intravenous antibiotics.[271] However, use of modern antibiotics for cutaneous wounds has not been extensively studied. Much variation is seen in techniques of irrigation, concentration of antibiotics, and type of wounds in these studies.

Although the use of agents such as penicillin, ampicillin, or a cephalosporin in low concentrations seems rational, normal saline or povidone-iodine has been proven effective and safe. Thus recommendations for antibiotic irrigation of cutaneous wounds await further study.

DEBRIDEMENT

Dog and other animal bites are not clean lacerations, but crush injuries that usually contain devitalized tissue. Adult dog teeth can exert a great deal of pressure, enough to perforate sheet metal.[309] Debridement is a well-proven means of reducing infection in all types of wounds.[99,190,206,386] It has been proven particularly effective in dog bites, in which it decreases infection 30 fold.[51] No other technique removes the crushed, torn, or devitalized tissue present in animal bites, which so greatly increases the propensity for infection. Debridement removes bacteria, clots, and soil far more effectively than irrigation. Although irrigation can remove surface bacteria, it cannot remove organisms embedded in dead tissue. In addition, debridement creates new, cleaner surgical wound edges that are easier to repair, heal faster, and produce a smaller scar. Once the physician becomes adept at using a scalpel to debride several millimeters of tissue from wound edges, debridement becomes a time-saving procedure. The only limitations of this technique are those imposed by anatomy, where skin tautness (such as on fingers or the pretibial region) or the presence of vital structures (such as tendons, nerves, and vessels) precludes debridement. In such cases the wound should be unusually well irrigated and debrided to whatever degree anatomy permits.

A number of the advantages of debridement derive from other conservative therapy that usually accompanies such wounds. In a controlled trial in promptly treated low-velocity gunshot wounds, patients were assigned randomly to either a debridement or a no debridement group.[40] In all cases, wounds were thoroughly irrigated, were packed open with sterile gauze to heal, did not receive antibiotics, and were not sutured. Both groups did equally well and had very low infection rates. Therefore the key ingredient may not be debridement so much as secondary or delayed primary closure. The physician should use this technique liberally in wounds thought to be at high risk for infection or in those where

*References 39, 90, 205, 206, 271, 386, 402.

traditional debridement is difficult or contraindicated. However, this issue has not yet been studied in bite wounds.

SCRUBBING THE WOUND

Scrubbing of the actual wound surface is a different matter than that of scrubbing the skin around the wound. Vigorous scrubbing of wounded surfaces with coarse materials does not decrease wound infection and may in fact increase it.[89,350,386] However, use of a fine-pore sponge to scrub the wound has been beneficial in other studies.[118,352] In the most recent large study of the topic, scrubbing grossly contaminated wounds with a finely porous sponge (Optipore, Calgon Vestal Laboratories, St. Louis, Mo.) with irrigating solution, 2.7% of scrubbed wounds became infected versus 6.1% of those not scrubbed, but this difference was not significant.[104] In an animal model, 1% povidone-iodine was effective in reducing infection in contaminated experimental wounds that were not treated until 12 hours after injury, but only when the wounds were scrubbed as well; irrigation alone provided no benefit.[205]

The actual wound surface should be scrubbed, but only with the proper fine-mesh sponge. Commercial surgical brushes should not be used because they are much too coarse (and traumatic), and many of them are already contaminated with bacteria.[300] Scrubbing is of maximal benefit in wounds that are very contaminated, or when initial treatment has been delayed.

SHAVING SKIN AROUND THE WOUND

Shaving the skin around the wound has been shown to increase wound infection because it inflicts microscopic nicks in the skin.[280] It is not recommended under any circumstances. If long hairs close to the wound are thought to interfere with visualization or pose a risk of creating a foreign body in the wound, they should be carefully clipped short with scissors.

TETANUS PROPHYLAXIS

In recent years in the United States, approximately twice as many cases of human tetanus from animal bites have been seen each year as cases of human rabies.[81,401] The spores of *Clostridium tetani* are ubiquitous in the soil, on the teeth, and in the saliva of animals. Therefore the risk of tetanus may be present from any animal injury that penetrates the skin. However, bites may not be particularly tetanus-prone wounds; they account for about 4% of human cases of tetanus, far less than causes such as abscesses or skin ulcers.[81] Seventy-eight percent of tetanus cases occur after an acute injury.[332] Failure to provide proper tetanus immunization after acute injury was present in 42% of those who contracted tetanus in the United States.[332] Since tetanus is a preventable disease, and many patients still do not receive tetanus immunoprophylaxis according to guidelines of the Centers for Disease Control and Prevention (CDC), proper emergency prophylaxis against tetanus remains an important, but often underappreciated, intervention.

Tetanus prophylaxis is administered in standard fashion (Table 40-3). In the case of a clean wound that contains little devitalized tissue and that can be easily irrigated and debrided, a previous full course of immunization plus a booster within the last 10 years is sufficient. In deep punctures or wounds with much devitalized tissue that are difficult to irrigate and debride (predisposing to anaerobic growth), a full series of previous immunizations plus a booster within the last 5 years is sufficient. Regardless of the patient's prior immunization status, those with high-risk wounds should receive an intramuscular injection of 250 to 500 units of tetanus human immune globulin, as well as 0.5 ml of diphtheria tetanus (dT) toxoid booster vaccine. The

Table 40-3 Tetanus Prophylaxis

	Clean Minor Wounds		Major Dirty Wounds	
History of Immunization (Doses)	**Toxoid***	**TIG†**	**Toxoid**	**TIG**
Unknown	Yes	No	Yes	Yes
None to one	Yes	No	Yes	Yes
Two	Yes	No	Yes	No (unless wound older than 24 hr)
Three or more				
Last booster within 5 years	No	No	No	No
Last booster within 10 years	No	No	Yes	Yes
Last booster more than 10 years ago	Yes	No	Yes	Yes

*Toxoid: Adult: 0.5 ml dT intramuscularly (IM).
Child less than 5 years old: 0.5 ml DPT IM.
Child older than 5 years: 0.5 ml DT IM.

†Tetanus immune globulin (TIG): 250 to 500 units IM in limb contralateral to toxoid.

latter contains one-twentieth the amount of diphtheria toxoid contained in the pediatric (DT) version (to diminish the increased reactions to diphtheria toxoid seen in adults) and elicits a good booster response with few local reactions. Diphtheria immunization is recommended every 10 years throughout life, so the dT combination should be used after the age of 7 years.

Because many patients do not have full prior immunization against tetanus, questioning the patient thoroughly on this point is critically important. The risk of inadequate prior immunization is particularly high for the elderly and those reared in underdeveloped countries. With the increasing levels of immigration into the United States, many patients in this country now fall into the latter category, and either they do not know if they have been immunized or they have been incompletely immunized. Unfortunately, many inner city children in the United States also no longer receive routine immunization, although by school age this has been remedied in nearly all, at least as far as tetanus is concerned. More than half of persons over 60 years of age lack protective levels of circulating tetanus antibody (in marked contrast to younger age groups), and 60% of human tetanus cases occur in those over the age of 50.[20,81,332]

If the patient has not been immunized in the previous 10 years, tetanus immune globulin (TIG) is recommended because most such patients have no significant antibody response to a booster dose for at least 4 days.[323] If a definite history of prior immunization cannot be elicited, the patient must be treated with 250 to 500 units of human TIG intramuscularly in one arm and 0.5 ml of the adult DT toxoid in the other. Booster doses of tetanus toxoid are administered at 30 and 60 days after the initial injection to complete the course of immunization. Tetanus antibody titers are not a guarantee of immunity against tetanus.[86]

The only contraindication to tetanus toxoid is a history of severe hypersensitivity reaction or neurologic reaction to previous injections; these reactions are extraordinarily rare. A history of local swelling, redness, tenderness, fever, malaise, and nonspecific rash is not a contraindication. If the patient is thought to have true severe hypersensitivity, an allergist or infectious disease specialist should be consulted, but the patient should receive TIG regardless.

TOPICAL ANTISEPTICS

Topical antiseptic ointments, such as neomycin-bacitracin-polymyxin, have been demonstrated to be highly effective in promoting healing in minor skin wounds.[151,247] This action may be related more to the stimulation of reepithelialization than to antibacterial activity.[341] In addition, a regimen of topical Neosporin cream plus parenteral prophylactic antibiotics has been proven more effective at reducing infection in experimental heavily contaminated wounds than either treatment alone.[21] Povidone-iodine ointment has no effect, and nitrofurazone ointment slows healing.[151] Despite the widespread belief, based on early reports, that neomycin is highly sensitizing, at least one recent evaluation recorded sensitivity to this agent in only 2 of 2175 subjects.[247] Five percent povidone-iodine cream is even more effective than Neosporin cream, killing most organisms in 1 minute versus 15 minutes and speeding wound healing.[391] However, topical ointments are appropriate only in abrasions produced by animal bites; punctures and sutured lacerations would not be expected to benefit.

DRESSINGS

In most cases a simple sterile dry dressing is sufficient to protect the wound. In the case of sutured wounds, even this is not needed, unless to protect the wound from the rubbing of clothing or other minor trauma. Delayed primary closure requires that the wound be kept moist; this is usually done with a wet saline dressing. Using even dilute povidone-iodine solution for wet dressings in delayed primary closure is not recommended because of the likelihood of systemic absorption of significant amounts of the antiseptic.

Occlusive dressings have improved greatly in the last decade, and now a number of semipermeable ones are available, (such as Tegaderm, Op-Site, Biobrane, and Duoderm).[224,341] Although these dressings speed reepithelialization and exclude bacteria from the wound, they tend to accumulate fluid under the dressing that must be aspirated to prevent infection. Since most animal bites do not cause large epithelial losses, simple application of a topical antiseptic and a dry sterile dressing is sufficient.

Further Wound Treatment

WOUND CLOSURE AND INFECTION RISK FACTORS

Three major considerations govern the decision of whether to suture a wound: cosmetics, function, and risk factors. Cosmetic appearance virtually mandates suturing all facial wounds, which are low risk anyway. Similar reasons may dictate closure of wounds elsewhere on visible portions of the body. Function is of critical importance in wounds of the hand and foot, which are high-risk areas where infection has disastrous consequences. Thus wounds of the hand should in general be left open.

Risk factors are many and complex and provide a useful logical framework in making the decision whether to suture, start antibiotics, or undertake other treatments (see Box 40-3).[53] The risk factors for dog bites were first described by Callaham and have been further elaborated recently by Dire.[53,101] In Dire's study of 802 dog bite wounds, risk factors for infection included advancing age, delays to initial treatment, deeper wounds, and wounds requiring debridement (5 times higher) or suturing (2.5 times higher). The best predictors were full-thickness wound (odds ratio [OR] .09), male sex (OR 2.7), and use of antibiotics (OR 2.6).

BOX 40-3
ANIMAL BITE RISK FACTORS

HIGH RISK

Location
- Hand, wrist, or foot
- Scalp or face in infants (high risk of cranial perforation; skull x-ray examination mandatory)
- Over a major joint (possibility of perforation)
- Through-and-through bite of cheek

Type of wound
- Punctures (impossible to irrigate)
- Tissue crushing that cannot be debrided (typical of herbivores such as cows and horses)
- Carnivore bite over vital structure (artery, nerve, joint)

Patient
- Older than 50 years
- Asplenic
- Chronic alcoholic
- Altered immune status (chemotherapy, AIDS, immune defect)
- Diabetic
- Peripheral vascular insufficiency
- Chronic corticosteroid therapy
- Prosthetic or diseased cardiac valve (consider systemic prophylaxis)
- Prosthetic or seriously diseased joint (consider systemic prophylaxis)

Species
- Domestic cat
- Large cat (canine teeth produce deep punctures that can penetrate joints, cranium)
- Human (hand wounds only, particularly with delayed medical care)
- Primates (anecdotal evidence only)
- Pigs (anecdotal evidence only)

LOW RISK

Location
- Face, scalp, ears, and mouth (all facial wounds should be sutured)
- Self-bite of buccal mucosa that does not go through to skin

Type of wound
- Large clean lacerations than can be thoroughly cleansed (the larger the laceration, the lower the infection rate)
- Partial-thickness lacerations and abrasions

Species
- Rodents

However, most of these factors are almost circular in their relationship to causation.

Time since wounding is a crucial risk factor; the longer the interval, the more likely an infection. After the first few hours, adequate wound toilet is unlikely to be carried out. In developed countries, many patients are seen within hours of wounding, and the results are usually very good. In remote and undeveloped areas and countries, wounds commonly do not receive medical attention for half a day or more. This alone puts them into a high-risk category that may eliminate the possibility of suturing.

Certain species, including humans and other primates, domestic and wild cats, pigs, and large wild carnivores, seem to have a propensity for inflicting infection-prone wounds, although the evidence is incomplete. Cases must be assessed individually; the presence of one or more risk factors may preclude suturing or may suggest the use of delayed primary closure (discussed below). However, the vast majority of fresh bites of most species, including dogs, can be safely sutured after proper wound preparation.

In recent years the consensus has changed from that of never suturing animal bite wounds to that of closing most of them with good surgical technique, if optimal conditions are present and risk factors are absent. Optimal conditions include prompt medical treatment, which is seldom available in remote and undeveloped areas. In those locations, leaving bite wounds open (or with a drain, although this is also controversial) is the more prudent course. The discussion below pertains only to situations allowing prompt medical care. Adequate data exist only for dog bite wounds, and the following comments are based on that species.

Opponents of suturing have only one small study to cite, consisting exclusively of wounds selected for study because they were thought to be heavily contaminated.[243] In this 27-year-old study, wound irrigation was not routinely carried out. Two large studies of typical emergency department dog bite wounds have shown a lower infection rate in wounds sutured than in those left open, even though all wounds were irrigated with saline and all puncture wounds were excluded.[51,53] As in other studies reporting less infection in larger dog bite wounds, these results were attributed to better surgical wound toilet received by larger (and sutured) wounds.[410] Dog bites of the face and neck, all sutured and none treated with antibiotics, had an infection rate of only 1.4%.[184]

Alternative methods of wound closure have not been studied specifically for bites. In all likelihood the following findings would apply to bite wounds. In nonbite wounds, cutaneous staples are much faster to apply than sutures and produce a superior result in most areas.[345] Wound infection rates are slightly lower than with sutures, and because the staple touches the skin only at two entry points, it does not produce the transverse cross-hatch scar frequently seen if sutures are not removed within a few days.[120] Staples also produce less discomfort on removal, although unlike sutures their removal requires a special tool that a typical patient does not own. Since most caregivers prefer to see a patient during his or her return visit, this is not a significant drawback. Probably the greatest single advantage of using staples is that the stapling device applies the staple in a uniform and accurate manner, producing optimal closure results. The technique is thus not operator dependent. Suturing, by contrast, is highly operator dependent, and minor variations such as in suture placement and tightness of sutures can significantly increase infection rates.

Tape closure is another simple and effective method, requiring no foreign body placement in the wound edges and thus having a much lower infection rate than suturing or stapling. The lower infection rate is particularly noteworthy in experimental models using contaminated wounds, and the protection occurs whether the contamination originates in the wound or later on the surface of the wound. Tape occlusion also increases the rate of closure of superficial skin wounds.[120] Tape is best suited to linear lacerations on the relatively lax skin of the face and abdomen. The extremities, with their taut skin and frequent movement, and the axillae, palms, and soles with their skin secretions, are more difficult areas for adhesion. Since tape cannot close deep layers, deep lacerations require suturing. Areas of significant skin tension may require supplementation with cutaneous sutures, but use of tape allows a smaller number of sutures and their earlier removal.

The basics of proper suturing are well reviewed elsewhere.[288] When sutures are used, they should be removed as soon as possible, preferably within 3 days. This greatly increases the subsequent tensile strength of the wound, as compared with leaving them in place for 7 to 10 days or more.[120] Of course, the problem here is that the wound's tensile strength at this point is weak, provided almost exclusively by fibrin clot (fibroblasts have not yet begun to migrate into the wound itself). Thus this approach requires that tape or other closures be applied to provide reinforcement of the closure. Because of this, leaving sutures in place longer in parts of the anatomy that see a great deal of movement or skin stress is often more convenient. This allows more rapid and complete return to normal use of the injured area, although it does increase the likelihood of cutaneous scarring from the sutures themselves.

Bites of the Hand

Bites of the hand are common, and infection can be disastrous. As a result, this location is considered a risk factor for complications (see Box 40-3). The hand contains many poorly vascularized structures and tendon sheaths that poorly resist infection. The fascial spaces and tendon sheaths of the hand communicate with each other. Movement seals off the wound from external drainage and spreads bacteria and soil internally. About 10% of serious hand infections result in tenosynovitis; the remainder are fascial space infections or felons.[273] Because of the unique anatomy of the hand, irrigating hand wounds adequately is often impossible. The laceration may be irrigated or debrided to the subcutaneous level, but deeper layers are already sealed and cannot be entered. However, irrigation of nonbite lacerations of the hand with povidone-iodine solution has been shown to reduce infection, so this is worth attempting.[346]

In nonbite lacerations of the hand, infection rates vary from 1.1% to 8.5%—not significantly different from those of other areas of the body. Sutured nonbite lacerations of the feet and legs are more likely than hand and arm wounds to become infected.[209,359] The response of hand wounds to suturing is variable; this suggests an increase in infectious complications.[181,189,363] However, a study of 108 hand wounds, most sutured after careful wound toilet, showed an infection rate of only 6% in tidy wounds, compared with 32% in unsutured untidy wounds.[299]

For animal bites, data on wound infection have been collected only for dog bites. Although dog bites have an infection rate of 6% to 13%, dog bite wounds of the hand have an infection rate of 30% to 36%, even when promptly treated.[51,53,350] Human bites of the hand present other unique problems and are discussed in a separate section.

Because of the high morbidity and permanent residual impairment of hand infections, treating them aggressively is best (see Box 40-1). Hand bite wounds should be irrigated, debrided if possible, and initially left open. The hand should be immobilized with a bulky mitten dressing in an elevated position, and the patient usually should be started promptly on antibiotics, as discussed in the sections on prophylactic antibiotics and human bites. Patients with an established infection should be admitted to the hospital and started on intravenous antibiotics.[273,313] X-ray examination should be performed on all injured extremities. Signs of localized pus, devitalized tissue, joint or bone penetration, gas in the soft tissue, or foreign body on the radiographs necessitate admission to the hospital and surgical drainage. Repeat incision and drainage with irrigating catheters are needed in about 10% of established infections.[273] Patients not hospitalized should be rechecked daily until signs of infection clear. In the patient without initial evidence of infection, 5 to 7 days of splinting and oral antibiotics should suffice if no complications develop.

Punctures

Up to half of dog bite wounds are punctures, which have an infection rate of about 20% to 25%.[51,53] The infection rate is related to the difficulty of irrigating them properly.[51,53,410] Usually, attempts to irrigate simply result in rapid development of tissue edema from infused saline, which does not achieve the goal of wound cleansing. However, if the wound is large or can be held open wide enough to permit fluid to escape, irrigation is worth the effort. Although total excision of puncture wounds has been attempted, it is time consuming, expensive to the patient in physician time, often prohibited by anatomy, and of no proven benefit. Suturing of puncture wounds is often proscribed, although the only study that specifically addressed this issue did not support such a ban.[51]

Puncture wounds should be irrigated or debrided as well as possible, sutured only if cosmetic or functional considerations require it, and treated as at high risk for infection. The technique of delayed primary closure should be used liberally.

Facial and Scalp Wounds

Facial and scalp wounds are most common in small children[58] and tend to heal rapidly with little risk of infection.[184] They are generally sutured primarily and do not require prophylactic antibiotics; good wound toilet is easy to achieve, since debridement is usually feasible. Typical dog bites of the face and neck (including punctures) have an infection rate of only 1.4%, even when sutured.[184] They can be closed up to 12 or 18 hours after the injury, although the risk of infection is somewhat higher.[308,444] Very severe wounds may warrant hospital admission and operative repair; their infection rate is about 12%.[308]

If necessary, delayed primary closure can be used for full-thickness facial wounds, but choosing healing by secondary intention in this category of wound is unacceptable. This approach not only takes much longer, but also produces a disfiguring scar. The wound should be closed primarily, usually in the most simple fashion possible, which produces satisfactory results the majority of the time. In the few cases where it does not, the wound can be revised by a plastic surgeon a few months later under optimal and sterile circumstances.

Intraoral wounds of the lips and buccal mucosa self-inflicted by teeth during seizures or trauma are discussed in the section on human bites.

A major risk associated with facial and scalp wounds in children, particularly infants, is that the large teeth of animals such as dogs can easily perforate the cranium, producing depressed skull fractures, brain laceration, intracranial abscess, or meningitis.[227,319,393,426,429] In young children with such wounds, skull films should be routine, looking for evidence of perforation that would mandate immediate neurosurgical consultation and admission to the hospital (see Box 40-2). Other bony injuries, such as mandible fracture, have been also reported in young children bitten by dogs[336] and can occur in adults bitten by large and powerful animals.

INDICATION FOR CULTURES

Cultures of fresh wound surfaces have been shown to be useless as predictors of infection whether judged quantitatively or qualitatively,[117,258,271,301,322] because pathogens are present in all lacerations even when fresh and "clean."[112] Some of the pathogens of greatest concern (such as *Eikenella*) can take 10 days to grow out in culture, by which time most therapeutic decisions are long ago made. Other organisms (such as *Pasteurella*) are fastidious, hard to identify, and frequently missed by the laboratory technician, who rarely sees them. Gram stains are similarly useless.[129] Only quantitative cultures of homogenized tissue samples are useful predictors of infection, but this is an unwieldy and expensive procedure, done in few institutions.[112] The specific bacteriology of bites has been well studied only in dog bites and is discussed in that section and the one on antibiotics.

Once infection is established, cultures are indicated only with failure of initial antibiotic therapy or in very high-risk wounds or patients (see Box 40-2). Only about 5% of infecting organisms in dog and cat bites fail to respond to initial treatment with a penicillinase-resistant penicillin, cephalexin, cephradine, or erythromycin; thus about 95% of cultures taken at the time of initiating antibiotic therapy contribute nothing to patient care.[53,301] Gram stains of pus (or, better yet, aspirated fluid) from an established infection are useful only if one predominant bacterial type is seen. Therefore most therapeutic decisions about treatment of infection are made before any culture results could be obtained or used. On the other hand, if the patient or wound is very high risk, or if animal bite sepsis is suspected (see section on sepsis), obtaining cultures would be prudent to guide subsequent antibiotic therapy.

If cultures are indicated, both aerobic and anaerobic cultures should be obtained (see Boxes 40-4 and 40-5). Many of

BOX 40-4

TYPICAL AEROBIC BACTERIA FOUND IN ANIMALS' MOUTHS AND AS PATHOGENS IN INFECTED BITE WOUNDS

Actinobacillus lignieresii	*Actinobacillus suis*
Micrococcus spp.	*Moraxella* spp.
Staphylococcus intermedius	*Staphylococcus epidermidis*
Staphylococcus aureus	*Acinetobacter calcoaceticus*
Streptococcus	*Enterobacter* spp.
Bacillus subtilis	*Serratia marcescens*
Corynebacterium spp.	*Proteus mirabilis*
Eubacterium	*Aeromonas hydrophila*
Pasteurella aerogenes	*Pasteurella dagmatis, canis*
Pseudomonas	*Pasteurella multocida*
Eikenella corrodens	*Haemophilus aprophilus*
Peptostreptococcus	*Klebsiella*
Clostridium perfringens	CDC alphanumerics:
Brucella canis	II-J
Bordetella spp.	EF-4
Haemophilus haemolyticus	NO-1 (nonoxidizer 1)*
Neisseria spp.	DF-2 *(Capnocytophaga canimorsus)*

*Newly described, clinical significance unknown.

BOX 40-5

TYPICAL ORGANISMS (ANAEROBIC OR RARE) FOUND IN ANIMALS' MOUTHS AND AS PATHOGENS IN INFECTED BITE WOUNDS

ANAEROBIC BACTERIA

Bacteroides spp.
Fusobacterium spp.
Leptotrichia
Peptococcus
Peptostreptococcus anaerobius
Propionibacterium acnes
Veillonella parvula

OTHER PATHOGENS (RARE)

Actinobacillus lignieresii or *suis*
Aeromonas spp.
Afipia felis
Blastomyces dermatitidis
Cat-scratch disease organism
Citrobacter freundii
Clostridium tetani
Cowpox and catpox virus
Erysipelothrix spp.
Eubacterium plautii
Hepatitis virus
Herpesvirus
Leptospira interrogans
Mycobacterium bovis
Mycobacterium marinum
Nocardia brasiliensis
Rabies virus
Rio Bravo virus
Rochalimaea henseleae
Seal finger agent
Simian herpes B virus
Spirillum minus
Sporothrix schenckii
Streptobacillus moniliformis

the bacterial species in animal mouths are anaerobic, and some of these (such as *Bacteroides*) have caused fatal sepsis.[131] In adults, locally infected wounds produce no purely anaerobic cultures, but 75% of wounds contain anaerobes in combination with aerobes.[162,166] In children, 8% of infected wounds yielded only anaerobes; 74% grew aerobes and anaerobes.[38] If unusual or fastidious species (such as *Pasteurella* or *Capnocytophaga canimorsus,* formerly CDC alphanumeric strain DF-2) are suspected, the laboratory should be advised in advance. Many of these pathogens require special media, tests, or vigilance for successful detection. In certain cases, cultures should be sent to reference laboratories such as those in state health departments or at the CDC in Atlanta.

PROPHYLACTIC ANTIBIOTICS

In bite wounds, treatment can begin only *after* wounding and bacterial inoculation; thus antibiotics are never truly prophylactic. Prophylactic antibiotics are a much overused form of therapy. In theory, they should be useful in virtually all wounds. However, in major surgery, they are of proven value only in carefully selected high-risk procedures and only if begun *before* surgery.[258,423] In nonbite outpatient lacerations, prophylactic antibiotics either demonstrate no benefit or actually increase the infection rate, even in wounds of the hand.*

*References 12, 95, 181, 189, 209, 285, 438.

In animal bite wounds, only dog bites have been studied prospectively in blinded clinical trials. Thus all conclusions are based on dog bite studies, and we can only assume that the same results would pertain to other species.

In dog bites, prophylactic antibiotics were of no benefit in many double-blind studies, including one with 280 patients.* In one controlled study of outpatient dog bite wounds, all irrigated by syringe-and-needle technique, prophylactic penicillin V-K lowered the infection rate in trunk, limb, and particularly hand wounds, but not at a statistically significant level.[51] Penicillin provided no benefit in low-risk facial and scalp wounds.[51] A similar study using oxacillin (predicted to eliminate more organisms) found no benefit.[122] A well-controlled study using currently recommended antibiotics (dicloxacillin and cephalexin) also found no significant benefit.[103] In three of these studies a trend toward benefit from prophylactic antibiotics in hand wounds only was seen, although the groups were too small for the studies to be of statistical significance.[51,214,354]

Why do prophylactic antibiotics seem not to work? After all, therapeutic antibiotics for established infection are certainly effective. Several explanations are possible. For one thing, all studies to date have been limited in their statistical power and could well have missed a small but significant subgroup of patients who benefitted from treatment. Some of these studies have shown a trend for lower infection rates with prophylactic antibiotics, but it was never

*References 31, 51, 103, 122, 214, 217, 354, 387.

statistically significant.[103] Thus prophylactic antibiotics might work for a carefully selected group of patients.

Another explanation is that patient compliance may be poor. Typical practice is that patients are perhaps given a few pills in the emergency department and then a prescription to fill. In the only study to examine compliance, even when all patients were given a free supply of pills in the emergency department, about half of them took only half or less of the prescribed tablets.[392] Although prophylactic antibiotics were not effective in this overall population, they were effective when the subpopulation of compliant patients was examined separately.

A third factor is that prophylactic antibiotics are typically administered orally, usually many hours after wounding. Research shows a latency period before active microbial multiplication occurs in the wound.[445] At least for staphylococci, if antibiotics are not given within 6 hours of original wound contamination, they have no effect on subsequent multiplication. This may be because bacteria in wounds become encapsulated within a few hours in a coagulum of blood and fibrin that protects them from antibiotics.[119] If that coagulum is physically scrubbed and removed, antibiotics are effective many hours after wounding. However, physical scrubbing of the wound is not common clinical practice. More recent studies show that most bacteria also bind to host proteins, and that this binding is rapid and irreversible.[423] Once bound, antibiotics have no effect. In most of the studies in the literature, patients were given oral antibiotics, which even if taken promptly might not produce effective tissue levels soon enough, or at all.

Prophylactic antibiotics must be given early to be effective. The offending bacteria are already present in the wound when the patient is first seen. Three hours is generally considered the maximum acceptable delay, although treatment should not be withheld if more time has elapsed.[3] Oral administration is markedly less efficacious than parenteral, taking several hours to demonstrate a useful serum level. Intravenous administration is 4 to 12 times faster than intramuscular administration in developing a useful wound fluid antibiotic concentration, although intramuscular doses are effective in maintaining a sustained level.[4] Antibiotics differ in the speed with which they enter the wound; ampicillin is one of the fastest, exceeding the serum concentration within 1 hour.[4] Oxacillin, penicillin, and the cephalosporins are also rapid. Erythromycin and gentamicin take 2 to 4 hours for wound concentration to match serum concentrations, while tetracycline and clindamycin never reach serum levels. Even different drugs within the same family (for example, quinolones) may have very different half-lives, which are different in serum than in wound tissue fluid. These half-lives can make the difference between success and failure of prophylactic antibiotics.[423]

The bite victim needing prophylactic antibiotic treatment should be identified early, preferably during triage on entry to the emergency department. The patient should receive immediate antibiotics by protocol; the intravenous or intramuscular route is by far the quickest. The common practice of giving the patient a written prescription to fill hours or days after the injury is useless. Although previous practice has led to prescription of prophylactic antibiotics for 7 to 10 days, current knowledge in the surgical literature is that prophylaxis is needed only for a few days after surgery. In animal bites, oral antibiotics are not expensive to continue for a few extra days; thus a maximal period of 5 days of prophylaxis should be more than sufficient with uninfected bites.

Surgical wound toilet, not antibiotic treatment, remains the most important factor in decreasing infection. In addition to the usual irrigation and debridement, physicians concerned about high-risk wounds may wish to add the procedure of scrubbing the wound margins themselves with a finely porous sponge, since this will break up coagulum and reduce bacterial numbers. The weight of the evidence at this time does not support the use of prophylactic antibiotics in other than high-risk wounds. The use of antibiotics is most advisable in wounds of the hand; the speed of development, frequency, severity, and complications of hand wound infections can be impressive.[273,313] Patients with other risk factors, particularly asplenia, diabetes mellitus, or immune deficiency, may benefit from prophylactic antibiotics (see Box 40-3).

The cost and side effects of such focused use of antibiotics are relatively small, and the potential benefits great. Such focused use will ensure that only a relative small percentage of bite victims are treated with prophylactic antibiotics. No indication exists for their use in ordinary animal bites in normal patients.

One final remark is needed concerning studies of prophylactic antibiotics in dog bites. Although the studies cited previously all failed to show any statistically significant trend in favor of patients given prophylaxis, the trend in a number of these studies favored prophylaxis. Recently a metaanalysis was performed of the eight randomized clinical trials of prophylactic antibiotics, which reported all the necessary information and controls.[87] The relative risk for infection in patients given antibiotics compared to control subjects was 0.56 (95% CI 0.38 to 0.82). This means that about 14 patients must be treated to prevent one infection. This metaanalysis does not radically change recommendations because treating 14 patients with antibiotics to avoid one infection may not be a cost-effective strategy, especially in low-risk wounds where the consequences of wound infection are not severe.[52] In addition, this metaanalysis included treatment with a variety of antibiotics, and one of the weaknesses of metaanalysis is that negative clinical trials are less likely to be published and thus are not included.

General Principles for Choosing an Antibiotic

Whether an antibiotic is given prophylactically or in response to established infection, choosing the medication presents a major problem. No single antibiotic is effective against all possible pathogens (see Table 40-4 and Boxes 40-4 and 40-5).

Most authors recommend antibiotics based on their in vitro effectiveness against a particular organism, because no studies compare the effectiveness of different antibiotics in a true clinical setting. This approach has many failings, and in vitro sensitivities correlate poorly with in vivo effectiveness. This is particularly true for local superficial cutaneous infection. In vitro sensitivities were developed as a useful simple model of antibiotic effectiveness against single organisms in human serum in systemic infection. They were not developed as models of complex wound component interactions. In vitro sensitivities are not determined in the complex real-life wound environment of tissue fluids, fibrin coagulum, contaminated skin, interacting bacterial species, neutrophils, local tissue factors, and complex immune response, but in the sterility of a glass container containing only nutrient media.

The in vitro environment is artificial and simple compared with the real world. Bacteria exhibit different sensitivities to antibiotics when isolated, as compared with the bacteria-laden skin squames, detached bacterial clumps, and isolated bacteria floating in skin fluids that cause infection in real life.[15,423] In fact, bacteria grown in vitro may not even be exactly the same as the "wild" bacteria in vivo; certainly the antigenic properties vary depending on the environment.[73] The activities of many antibiotics are significantly affected by pH, which varies widely in tissues but is not examined in the in vitro method.

The discussion in the previous section on prophylactic antibiotics and their timing also hints at another contributory factor: the different behavior of antibiotics in living systems versus a nutrient broth. In vitro sensitivities are based entirely on concentrations in serum, but animal bite wound infections do not take place in serum, but in tissue. The concentration of drug in in vitro models is uniform and determined by nothing but passive diffusion through a homogeneous medium. In tissue, however, drug distribution varies widely according to factors including type of tissue, local pH, and presence of infection. In vivo and in vitro environments resemble each other less than a living animal and a hamburger in the refrigerator.

Drugs behave very differently in vivo. For example, for the new macrolide azithromycin, the ratio of tissue fluid concentration to serum concentration after oral administration is 35 to 1 in skin.[316] Even different drugs within the same family (such as quinolones) may have different rates of absorption and very different half-lives, which are different in serum versus wound tissue fluid; these different half-lives can make the difference between success and failure of prophylactic antibiotics.[185,423] Drug concentrations in tissue are quite different than they are in serum, and they are achieved at different times. Low concentrations of antibiotics may not kill organisms, but they can profoundly affect cell wall characteristics, with a resultant impact on adherence and virulence.[241] Drugs in vivo also exert synergism; two drugs, neither effective alone, can be quite effective when combined.[44] Drug combinations are not tested in the usual laboratory methods.

Although these differences have been well demonstrated in experimental models, they are never even mentioned in most discussions of antibiotic efficacy in cutaneous wounds, and there has been almost no examination of these principles in realistic clinical situations. Most clinicians, however, are quite familiar with the manifestations of this problem in actual patients.[347] The available literature, although not extensive, documents the discrepancy between in vivo and in vitro results. Some studies have reported in vitro insensitivity of an organism but nonetheless also reported that patients treated with the "wrong" antibiotic recovered without other treatment.[427] The only study of prophylactic antibiotics in cat bite that found them effective used oxacillin, a drug considered only marginally effective against *Pasteurella* (a common pathogen in cat bite, and one for which oxacillin is not a recommended treatment).[121] In a study of hand infections after human bite, 95% of organisms were sensitive to cefamandole in vitro and only 67% to nafcillin.[394] Despite this, the complication rate in wounds was 3.2 times higher in the cefamandole group than in the nafcillin group. In another large series of infections of the hand (many from human bites), many resistant organisms were present in infected wounds but responded well to intravenous antibiotics that theoretically should not have been effective.[98] Twenty-five percent of isolates in one group of patients were resistant to administered methicillin, but the incidence of failure or success did not relate to the incidence of resistance. Thirty-two percent of patients receiving methicillin had resistant organisms present on culture, but only 13% had an unsatisfactory response to antibiotics. Only 7% of patients had organisms resistant to cefamandole, but 14% had an unsatisfactory response to the antibiotic. Overall, the difference in outcome was not statistically significant when resistant bacteria were isolated versus when they were not.[98]

Further limiting the usefulness of in vitro sensitivities is the fact that different institutions and regions report different sensitivities for the same organism, and these sensitivities change from year to year, leaving the clinician to guess as to which one is correct at that time for the particular patient he or she is treating. Individual authors reporting in vitro sensitivities give differing results for the same species and strains on different occasions.[164,165] Part of the reason for this is that many of these pathogens come from animals that are exposed routinely to "prophylactic" antibiotics in feed, and therefore resistance may be widespread but varies according to the brand of feed being used and the antibiotic it contains.

In vitro results are often difficult to translate into clinical terms; a 98% kill rate of one species of bacteria at 2 hours of exposure to 2 μg/ml might be considered resistance, whereas a 99% kill rate at 4 μg/ml is considered sensitivity. Although having a drug and a concentration that promptly kills all bacteria is certainly optimal, recent studies show that bacteria grown in subeffective minimum inhibitory concentrations of antibiotics are still profoundly affected. "Nontherapeutic" concentrations have profound effects on cell surface characteristics (such as surface antigens), with concomitant effects on adherence and other characteristics determining virulence.[241]

Even if in vivo results did correlate with in vitro results, another problem exists. The potential range of bacteria in any bite wound is vast, and no one antibiotic is fully effective against all of them. The best antibiotic for a particular pathogen is seldom the best antibiotic for the greatest variety of possible pathogens. The clinician virtually never knows the offending organism when initiating treatment of infection in an individual patient. Therefore even the most "scientific" choice can be completely wrong in an individual case.

Therapy should be tailored to the largest variety of most likely pathogens for a particular type of bite. No drug has been proven superior in the actual clinical conditions in which physicians practice. Clinicians should be wary of a recommendation for the latest high-price antibiotic based on in vitro analysis. The reality is that many tried and true, less expensive antibiotics are effective in the great majority of cases. This is particularly true when the indication is "prophylaxis," because in most situations bite victims will not become infected whether treated or not.

Follow-up and Indications for Hospital Admission

Assuming the possibility of major or occult trauma has been ruled out, follow-up of animal bites depends on the risk factors present (see Box 40-3) and the patient's response to treatment. With only a superficial abrasion, infection is unlikely, and in most cases no return visit is needed. In the case of an ordinary low-risk bite wound, one follow-up visit (in 2 days, to assess any infection) is all that is needed. If the patient is very reliable and no sutures have been placed, even one visit is not necessary.

Infected wounds dictate much closer follow-up, the frequency of which depends on the wound's response to treatment and the patient's risk factors. In a high-risk patient the initial follow-up should be on the next day. Again, this must be tailored to the reliability of the patient and social circumstances (distance, transportation, availability of telephone). If an infected wound fails to respond to 5 days of initial antibiotic treatment, it may be time to culture the wound. However, simply switching to another, broader spectrum antibiotic is reasonable (see Tables 40-4 and 40-8). In most cases cultures are not cost effective and do not aid in patient management.

In a few cases the patient will need hospitalization, as summarized in Box 40-6. Along with the obvious indications, failure of a wound to respond to appropriate initial or secondary antibiotic treatment (particularly in a high-risk patient) should be a possible indication for admission. Again, patient characteristics are crucial. An elderly chronic alcoholic living alone may need hospitalization for a cellulitis that could easily be treated on an outpatient basis in a 30-year-old healthy person.

BOX 40-6

INDICATIONS FOR HOSPITAL ADMISSION

Hand bite
- Involvement of bone, joint, tendon
- Deep space infection or tenosynovitis

Sepsis from animal bite
Severe wound infection causing systemic toxicity in immunocompetent patient
Cellulitis or local infection in severely immunocompromised patient (diabetes, AIDS, chronic alcoholism, asplenia)*
Cranial injuries in an infant
Major trauma inflicted by large animal

*Possible indication, depending on patient circumstances.

Complications of Bite Wounds

WOUND INFECTION

Immense numbers of bacteria inhabit animals' mouths and can be inoculated into a bite wound. The exact pathogens vary depending on what is doing the biting and are discussed in the sections on the offending species. The major aerobic and anaerobic species are listed in Boxes 40-4 and 40-5. If inoculated in sufficiently large numbers, these bacteria can cause localized cellulitis and abscess formation, the most common forms of infection. Wound infection is generally diagnosed on the basis of increasing redness, swelling, and tenderness of the wound margins, eventually progressing to production of pus, spreading cellulitis, lymphangitis, and local lymphadenopathy. Lymphadenitis and lymphangitis are much less common but can occur as local defenses are overwhelmed. Systemic symptoms of infection are rare and suggest bacteremia or sepsis.

The treatment of wound infection from animal bites is the same as that for other traumatic wounds—elevation of the wound, immobilization of the affected part, removal of sutures or staples if present, and antibiotic therapy (see Box 40-1). The diversity of pathogens in animals' mouths is incredibly large and is discussed in more detail under antibiotic choices. However, most infection is caused by common gram-positive organisms such as *Streptococcus* or *Staphylococcus*. Even less common pathogens, such as *Pasteurella* or *Eikenella,* are within the normal experience of most clinicians and are effectively treated by common antibiotics (Table 40-4).

However, the clinician should not forget that extremely rare and unusual pathogens can cause infection (see Box 40-

Table 40-4 Relative Merits of Various Oral Antibiotics for Bite Wounds

Antibiotic	Advantages	Disadvantages	Daily Cost* ($)	Strepto-coccus	Staphy-lococcus	Gram Negative	Pasteu-rella	Eike-nella	Anaer-obes	DF-2 (Capno-cytophaga)
Ampicillin-amoxicillin			0.13	S	R	V-R	S	S	S	S
Amoxillin-clavulanate		High incidence of GI side effects	2.39	S	S	S	S	S	S	S
Azithromycin	Once a day dose		7.80	S	S	V	S†		V	
Cefixime	Once a day dose	High incidence of GI side effects	5.60	S	S	S	S	S	V	S
Cefuroxime	Twice a day doses	No oral suspension available‡	2.75	S	S	S	S	S	S	S
Cephalexin			2.41	S	S	V	V-R	R	V-R	S
Cephalosporins—third generation (all parenteral)	Eliminate compliance problems	Requires injection and office visit; expensive	8.77 (cefotaxime)	S	S	S	S	S	S	S
Ciprofloxacin	Twice a day doses	Contraindicated in children, pregnant women	2.15	V	S	S	S	S	V	
Clarithromycin	Twice a day doses		2.67	S	S	M	S	S†	S	
Dicloxacillin			1.76	S	S	R	V-R	R	V	S
Erythromycin		GI complications, poor effectiveness	0.43	S	V	R	V	V	V-R	S
Penicillin V			0.07	S	R	R	S	V†,§	R‖	S
Tetracycline		Contraindicated in children, pregnant women	0.03	V	V	S	V	S	R	S
Trimethoprim-sulfamethoxazole	Twice a day doses	Contraindicated in term pregnancy, nursing, <2 mo old (kernicterus)	0.08	S	S	S	S	V	R	R

R, Resistant; *V,* variable (80% or less sensitivity); *M,* most species sensitive; *S,* sensitive (90% or better) *GI,* gastrointestinal.

Few antibiotics are effective against all organisms, and therapy should not be aimed at this goal; for example, DF-2 infection is very rare, and anaerobes are of unknown clinical significance in local infection. See cautionary note regarding costs below. All sensitivities are derived from in vitro data, whose relevance to actual clinical infection is unknown.

*Cost based on lowest daily cost to pharmacist, generic rather than brand name drug if available, and highest recommended dose.[183] Actual costs to patient are greatly higher than these costs and vary dramatically even within one locality. Clinicians must check local pharmacy charges on a regular basis to determine cost effectiveness of local practice.

†In all likelihood; not actually tested yet.

‡If a child cannot swallow pills, pills must be crushed and have very bitter taste.

§Previously *Eikenella* was believed to always be sensitive to penicillin, but new studies indicate 18% of strains are resistant.

‖Pen V not effective; Pen G is very effective for anaerobes.

5). Cutaneous blastomycosis has been reported after dog bite, demonstrating that virtually any organism can be present.[154] Unusual species, such as *Capnocytophaga canimorsus,* cause sepsis. Some animal species (especially marine ones) harbor unusual mycobacteria, which are also ubiquitous in the environment.[92,134,321] These bacteria should be suspected when indolent ulcers are present that do not respond to the usual measures. The ulcers usually have nongranulating bases and rolled margins with violaceous coloration and satellite lesions. Subcutaneous infection and necrosis are extensive, but revealed only by debridement. Culture of debrided tissue is the only reliable identification technique, and sensitivity testing may take weeks. Surgical debridement of all infected tissue is crucial. The organisms are usually sensitive to ciprofloxacin, cefoxitin, and perhaps rifampin.[321]

SEPTIC COMPLICATIONS

Bacteremia and sepsis, although theoretical risks with any animal bite pathogen, have so far been reported with only a limited number of species (see Box 40-7). Shock, disseminated intravascular coagulation, symmetric peripheral gangrene, and adult respiratory distress syndrome have been attributed to gram-negative bacillemia from *C. canimorsus* (formerly CDC alphanumeric strain DF-2) in an asplenic woman following a dog bite.[132] More than 60 similar cases have been identified so far,[60,235,314] 38% of them in patients who were not known to have any immune suppression. Even nonbite exposure to a dog seems to be a source of transmission.[372] However, transmission has occurred from cats in a few cases, including one case of cat scratch.[57,257] A number of cases have been unrelated to any animal exposure.[211]

Clinical manifestations include cellulitis, endocarditis, meningitis, pneumonitis, Waterhouse-Friderichsen syndrome, renal failure, shock, and death. Purpuric lesions are seen in one third of cases and may progress to symmetric peripheral gangrene and amputation. In some cases cutaneous gangrene develops at the site of the bite, a finding unique to this species of bacteria.

C. canimorsus is a fastidious, gram-negative, nonmotile, filamentous facultative aerobe that grows poorly in most standard media, making identification difficult. Growth of *C. canimorsus* from blood often takes a week, making Gram stain of the blood buffy coat a useful diagnostic test.[235] The organism is found in the peripheral blood smears of 17% of patients. It is susceptible to penicillin, ampicillin, cefuroxime, erythromycin, vancomycin, and cephalosporins but is resistant to aminoglycosides. In one case, plasmapheresis and leukopheresis were carried out in an attempt to remove toxins, cytokines, and activated granulocytes and monocytes.[235] If this infection is suspected, the laboratory should be alerted to look for unusual species in cultures, and additional cultures should be sent to reference laboratories (for example, the CDC in Atlanta).

A case of fatal *Bacteroides* sepsis accompanied by coagulopathy and renal thrombotic microangiopathy after a dog bite occurred in an alcoholic patient.[131] A generalized Shwartzman reaction secondary to dog bite and sepsis has been reported.[276] Sepsis with secretory bacteria from unknown organisms has been reported as well.[311]

Pasteurella multocida can also produce bacteremia.[287] Usually the source is a cat bite, but dog bites also contribute. Most patients who develop bacteremia, like those dying of *Capnocytophaga* infection, have cirrhosis, HIV infection, or malignancy or are otherwise immunosuppressed. The mortality rate can be as high as 36%. Treatment is usually with penicillin, but resistant strains have been described.

When sepsis or shock is potentially related to an animal bite, the wound discharge and blood should be cultured for aerobes and anaerobes. The laboratory should be notified of the source of infection so they can seek out uncommon pathogens. Tender, inflamed lymph nodes should be aspirated and cultured. If there is no obvious source of culture material, normal saline can be injected into areas of cellulitis and then aspirated for culture, although getting fluid back is usually difficult.[415] The same material should be examined by Gram stain in an effort to identify the offending organism (Box 40-7). If one predominant type of organism is identified, the indicated antibiotics for that specific organism should be initiated. However, in most cases organisms will not be found, will be mixed, or will be difficult to identify. In such cases the optimal adult antibiotic therapy is intravenous broad-spectrum coverage, such as a third-generation cephalosporin,[383] penicillinase-resistant synthetic penicillins, ticarcillin-clavulanate, or aztreonam.[365] Antipseudomonal penicillins should be added intravenously if needed. Another new broad-spectrum antibiotic for sepsis of unknown etiology is imipenem–cilastatin sodium, which is effective against gram-positive bacteria, *Staphylococcus,* coliform bacteria and gram-negative rods, *Pseudomonas, Bacteroides,* clostridia, and many others.[182,234,298] Although no clinical experience has been published so far with imipenem–cilastatin sodium in animal bite sepsis, it covers all possible pathogens. Within 24 hours, preliminary identification by culture should be possible and the patient can be switched to optimal antibiotic therapy based on the specific organism and its sensitivity.

In the last few years the introduction of many new broad-spectrum antibiotics has greatly increased the choices available to clinicians. Because of the rarity of some organisms, occasional discovery of new organisms, complexity of antibiotic coverage, and rapid evolution of new antibiotics, immediate consultation (within hours) with an infectious disease specialist is strongly recommended in all cases of sepsis suspected to be related to animal bite.

BOX 40-7

POTENTIAL BACTERIAL PATHOGENS IN SEPSIS FROM DOG BITES

Aeromonas hydrophila
*Bacteroides**
CDC alphanumeric species: II-J*
DF-2* *(Capnocytophaga canimorsus)*
EF-4*
Eikenella corrodens
Enterobacter spp.*
Eubacterium plautii
Hemophilus aprophilus
Klebsiella spp.
*Pasteurella multocida**
Proteus mirabilis
*Staphylococcus aureus**
*Streptococcus pyogenes**

*Proven cases of sepsis reported in literature.

ALLERGIC REACTIONS

Allergic reactions to animal bites are virtually unheard of. However, up to 11% of laboratory workers have allergic reactions to laboratory animal dander, hair, and urine.[434] One case of proven hypersensitivity to rat saliva after a bite has been reported.[434] The patient was subsequently proven allergic to the saliva (presumably because of saliva proteins) and not to other portions of the rat. The bite produced lymphangitic swelling and itching that subsided within 24 hours.

A letter that alleged an allergic reaction and mild anaphylaxis after a gerbil bite was followed by an unreferenced editorial comment that "allergic reactions to the bites of nonvenomous animals are very common."[84] However, the case reported was anecdotal and the allergic etiology unproven.

TRANSMISSION OF SYSTEMIC INFECTION

Approximately 150 systemic diseases of mammals can be transmitted in some fashion to humans. However, relatively few of these have been documented to occur through a bite or scratch (Table 40-5). The list includes pasteurellosis, leptospirosis, rat-bite fever, cat-scratch fever, tularemia, fish handler's disease, hepatitis B, bubonic plague, tetanus, gas gangrene, rabies, and sporotrichosis.[228,370] Pathogens may be secreted in saliva, nasal secretions, or tears or reach the animal's mouth through cleaning activities. In parts of the world many exotic diseases are endemic in domestic and wild animal populations. However, no proof supports the belief that they are transmitted by bite and they occur rarely in humans.

Table 40-5 lists most of the diseases theoretically transmitted by lick, bite, or scratch. For example, tularemia is almost invariably contracted by the skinning of infected rabbits, not by bites. Leptospirosis is usually transmitted through the urine of infected animals. Some of the really rare diseases, such as simian herpes, simian AIDS, foot-and-mouth disease, lymphocytic choriomeningitis, simian hepatitis, and Rio Bravo infection, are limited to occupational exposures of laboratory workers handling animals, to pet owners, and to veterinarians. Excluding *Clostridium, Staphylococcus, Streptococcus,* and *Bacteroides* infections, cat-scratch fever is by far the most frequent disease, yet only a few hundred cases have been reported. Thus, although systemic disease is a valid consideration, 99% of mortality and morbidity arises from local wound infection, including rabies and tetanus.

With the exception of unusual entities such as rat-bite fever and cat-scratch fever, most systemic infections caused by animal bites do not come to medical attention with the bite as the chief complaint. Generally the bite is completely forgotten by the patient or overlooked by the physician in the history and examination. Workups proceed in standard fashion for fevers, rashes, and other systemic complaints. If animal disease transmission is suspected, the differential diagnosis must be extensive.

NEUROTROPIC DISEASE

Rabies

Rabies is discussed in detail in Chapter 41. Coverage in this chapter is limited to brief remarks about assessment of risk in the bite victim, and local wound treatment at the scene.

Rabies is a rhabdovirus of the genus *Lyssavirus,* which also includes two other viruses (Mokola and Duvenhage) that infect humans.[270] Rabies occurs in wild and domestic animals; migrating epidemics alternate with periods of endemicity. Differing antigenic strains of the virus exist and can be identified by monoclonal antibody typing, which is of increasing importance in understanding the epidemiology of the disease.[79,133] It is generally believed that no true reservoir host exists for rabies; that is, no species harbors a latent and nonfatal infection. However, rabies can be latent and nonfatal in individuals of a species.

Epidemiology of Rabies. The epidemiology of rabies varies widely in different parts of the world. In the United States, western Europe, and Canada, wild animals are by far the main vectors of rabies; in 1988 they accounted for 88% of all rabid animals,[124] and skunks, raccoons, and bats accounted for 96% of wild animals rabies in the United States.[305] Foxes are the primary offenders in Europe, although some countries have succeeded in eliminating rabies in wild populations using innovative vaccination programs.[62] The focus of rabies investigation has increasingly been directed to animal epidemics, such as the growing spread of rabies in raccoons in the Central Atlantic United States after the introduction of infected animals from Florida by hunters.[14,62,126,435] A similar epidemic is growing among coyotes in Texas. Such epidemics change the distribution and likelihood of rabies exposure from year to year. Fortunately, in the United States (and most other countries), cases of rabies in various species are tabulated annually by the CDC and published in *Morbidity and Mortality Weekly Report.* Such geographic incidence figures are a crucial resource for the physician assessing the risk of a particular exposure.

People do not usually associate cats with rabies, but this will probably change. Because the population of domestic cats now exceeds 90 million in the United States and because 15 to 35 million of these are strays, some people are proposing licensing and leashing of cats.[397] The very large proportion of the cat population (over 25%) that consist of strays is of great concern in rabies prophylaxis. Most cats are not vaccinated, and strays frequently come into contact with wild animal vectors of rabies; feral cats have even been known to nest with skunks.[397] As a result, the chance of a cat being rabid in the United States now exceeds the likelihood of that of a rabid dog. Rabid cats outnumber rabid dogs, of which only 155 were reported in 1991. Nonetheless, most localities require that dogs, not cats, be vaccinated.[72]

Simultaneous with the increase of rabies in wild animals, the number of cases in dogs and domestic animals in the United States has steadily declined. Surprisingly, cattle are the most common domestic animals to have rabies in the United States.[72] Many counties in the United States have not seen canine rabies in decades. This compares with an annual figure of almost 5000 dogs proven rabid in the United States in 1950.[335] Thus, while vaccination of domestic animals continues, prevention now focuses on educating the public to avoid wild animals, which are illegal as pets in many states because of their ability to harbor rabies virus while remaining asymptomatic for periods averaging a month.[435] Exposures to a single wild animal can be expensive, necessitating rabies prophylaxis for up to 174 people and costing up to $64,000.[435]

Rabies in humans has become an extremely rare disease in the United States in recent years. Cases now number less than one a year, most of them originating outside of the United States, often from dogs.[305] Only 3 cases occurred in the 1980s that originated in the United States, compared with 55 a year in the early part of the century.[133] No human has been infected by a dog in the United States since 1979.[208] The other 9 cases in the United States during the 1980s were acquired abroad; in 3 cases genetic analysis of the virus strains demonstrated that the disease had been acquired in the patients' native countries with minimum incubation periods of 1, 5, and 7 years.[388] Although the number of human cases has declined, about 18,000 people a year receive postexposure prophylaxis in the United States.[133]

In the rest of the world, virtually all rabies occurs in dogs. Worldwide, dogs account for 91% of all human rabies cases, cats 2%, other domestic animals 3%, bats 2%, foxes 1%, and all other wild animals only 1%.[62,420] Each year, 35,000 humans die from rabies and 30 million doses of rabies vaccine are administered to 5.4 million people.[62] In Africa, Latin America, and most of Asia, dogs are the principal vector, although jackals are also a factor. In South America and Mexico, rabid vampire bats cause occasional infection of humans. In recent years, disruption of the natural ecology by introduction of humans and domestic animals in the rainforest has produced epidemics of rabies caused by vampire bats. In these settings, up to 22% of inhabitants are routinely bitten by vampire bits and overall mortality from rabies is 5% (as high as 17% in adolescents).[351] In India and Israel, wolves and jackals are the chief vectors, and the mongoose prevails in Puerto Rico. In Eastern and central Europe, the raccoon dog *(Nyctereutes procynoides)* is an increasingly common vector.[62]

Transmission of Rabies. Rabies virus is excreted in the saliva of infected animals. Direct bite wounds account for the vast majority of human and animal cases. Infections can also occur when saliva or infected tissues make contact with fresh, open wounds or mucosal membranes, although this risk is estimated at only 0.1%.[7] Rabies can be transmitted by aerosol, which was the case in persons who contracted the disease after visiting a cave full of infected bats, and by transplantation of tissues from infected persons.[381]

Not every animal that has rabies can transmit it. From 50% to 90% of animals dying of rabies excrete virus in the saliva.[381] The titer of virus in the saliva also varies greatly and determines infectivity. Bites by a proven rabid animal carry a risk of transmission that ranges from 5% to 80%.[7] Skunks tend to secrete more virus than other species for a longer time, and they also bite readily.[138] Although rodents (most frequently woodchucks) are susceptible to rabies infection, they account for only 16 rabid animals a year and are thought virtually never to excrete the virus in their saliva.[305] Therefore the CDC rates a rodent bite as carrying extremely low risk and not warranting treatment with vaccine or immune globulin. However, a recent rash of bites by rabid woodchucks in the eastern United States has prompted more frequent rabies prophylaxis.

Although the amount of virus present in the saliva is the chief concern, the virus replicates in kidneys, mammary glands, nasal mucosa, and muscle and has been shown to be present occasionally in maternal milk.

An extremely important factor in the transmission and severity of disease is the location of the wound. Rabies virus ascends to its target organ, the central nervous system, by traveling up peripheral nerves. The farther the bite is from the brain, the more time the victim has to develop antibodies in response to a course of vaccination. Wounds of the face have a 20-day incubation period with an ultimate mortality of 1 in 160, whereas wounds to the leg have a 60-day incubation period with an ultimate mortality of 1 in 6670.[381] Thus a facial wound carries the highest risk and should receive much more aggressive treatment.

Risk Factors for Rabies. The judgment of risk rests on several factors. The incidence of rabies in local species is important; in the United States, urban dogs and cats, domestic ferrets, rodents, and lagomorphs (rabbits and hares) are at low risk. However, domestic ferrets that escape can easily contract rabies in the wild and are thus a risk if recaptured. The behavior of the animal is a sometimes helpful sign. This is easily evaluated in wild animals, since most tend to shun humans. The urban appearance of a skunk, fox, or bat in broad daylight, showing no fear of human beings, is abnormal and should raise the index of suspicion.

Assessing provocation and unusual behavior in domestic species, such as dogs under crowded urban conditions, is often impossible. Classic rabies with unprovoked attack, foaming at the mouth, and laryngospasm is seldom seen in developed countries. Recent cases of human rabies caused by dogs were often transmitted by pets with normal behavior.[305] Species not previously thought to carry rabies are occasionally found to do so after unusual attacks, so the index of suspicion should be high and laboratory examination should be carried out early whenever rabies is a possibility.[79]

Knowing if a pet animal has been fully and recently vaccinated is helpful; unfortunately, most dogs and cats are not. For some animals, such as ferrets, no effective vaccine exists, so their safety is impossible to ensure. Vaccination does

Table 40-5 Summary of Diseases Transmitted from Mammals to Humans by Bite, Scratch, or Lick

Disease	Organism	Proven Transmission	Possible Transmission	Dog	Cat	Rodents	Lagomorphs
GRAM-NEGATIVE BACTERIA							
Bacteroides infection (B)	*Bacteroides* spp.	X					
Brucellosis (C)	*Brucella* spp.	X		X	X	X	X
Melioidosis (C)	*Pseudomonas pseudomallei*		X	X			
Glanders (C)	*Pseudomonas mallei*		X			X	
Pasteurellosis (B, C)	*Pasteurella multocida*	X		X	X		
	Pasteurella hemolytica		X				
	Pasteurella pneumotropica	X		X	X	X	
Plague (C)	*Yersinia pestis*		X		X	X	X
Yersiniosis (B)	*Yersinia enterocolitica*						
	Yersinia pseudotuberculosis	X		X			
Rat-bite fever (B)	*Spirillum minus*	X			Very rare	X	
	Streptobacillus moniliformis	X				X	
Tularemia (C)	*Francisella tularensis*	X		X	X	X	X
GRAM-POSITIVE BACTERIA							
Tetanus (B, C)	*Clostridium tetani*	X		X	X	X	X
Corynebacterium infections (C)	*Corynebacterium* spp.	X					
Erysipeloid (B, C)	*Erysipelothrix rhusiopathiae*	X		X	X		
Staphylococcus infections (B)	*Staphylococcus aureus*	X					
Streptococcus infections (B)	*Streptococcus* spp.	X					
Tuberculosis (C)	*Mycobacterium* spp.		X				
RICKETTSIA							
Q fever (C, A)	*Coxiella burnetii*		X				
Murine typhus (A, C)	*Rickettsia typhi*		X			X	
SPIROCHETES							
Leptospirosis (B, C)	*Leptospira interrogans*	X		X		X	
VIRUSES							
Simian herpes (B)	Herpesviruses B and T	X					
Foot-and-mouth disease (C)	Virus		X				
Rabies (B)	Virus	X		X	X	X	X
Cat-scratch disease (B)	Unknown bacterium	X		X	X		
Lymphocytic choriomeningitis (C)	Arenavirus		X	X		X	X
Simian hepatitis (C)	Virus		X				
Rio Bravo infection (B)	Arbovirus B	X					
FUNGI							
Sporotrichosis (B)	*Sporothrix schenckii*	X				X	
Blastomycosis	*Blastomyces dermatitidis*	X		X			

A, Normally transmitted from animal to human by arthropod vector; *B,* normally transmitted from animal to human by bite, scratch, or abrasion with saliva contact; *C,* normally transmitted from animal to human by nontraumatic contact with excretions, or direct contact with skin, fur, feathers, or secretions.

Horse	Cow	Goat, Sheep	Fox, Coyote	Pig	Raccoon	Bat	Monkey	Other
								All species—normal oral flora
X	X	X	X	X	X	X		Proven only in dog bite
	X							Virtually all species
X								Virtually all species except cows and pigs
								Virtually all species
								Virtually all species
								Skinning infected rabbits
								All mammals; rare
								Also carnivores
								Rats only
	X	X						
X	X	X	X		X			All species and soil contaminants
X	X	X						Bites rare
				X				Especially pigs
								All species; normal human skin flora
								All species
X	X	X						Dogs and cats resistant; monkeys have highest rate
	X	X						All species; rarely, through abrasion
	X							Rare
								Monkey bites; usually fatal
X	X	X		X				Low infectivity
X	X	X	X	X		X		Excreted in saliva 50%-90%
								Low infectivity; monkey also
								Low infectivity
								Monkey only; unproven
						X		Rare; laboratory acquired
								All species; common in nature

not guarantee immunity; about 5% of reported cases were in vaccinated animals.[223] The vaccination status of the victim is also important; many persons whose profession involves animal handling receive preexposure immunization with human diploid cell vaccine (HDCV). This is very effective but requires a booster dose at the time of being bitten. Omitting the booster can have fatal consequences.[305]

Future control of rabies will almost certainly involve large-scale vaccination of wild animal populations by oral baits, which has been quite successful.[37,353]

Local Wound Treatment for Rabies. Local wound treatment is extremely important in rabies prophylaxis. Rabies virus is easily killed by sunlight, ultraviolet radiation, air, drying, heat, formalin, and strong acids and bases. It has a half-life in vitro of 24 hours at 4° C, 4 hours at 40° C, 30 minutes at 54° C, and 35 seconds at 60° C.[437] Wound swabbing with 20% soap solution or 2% benzalkonium chloride reduces ultimate mortality by about 50%.[222] However, simple flushing is not in itself protective, regardless of the solution used. For unknown reasons, protection is provided experimentally only by physical swabbing of the wound, a practice not otherwise recommended in wound care. The effectiveness of syringe-needle irrigation remains untested. Antirabies immune globulin is also useful as a swabbing solution but is more effective when infiltrated locally around the wound.[222] The best location for infiltration is proximal to the wound, which presumably blocks migration of virus to the central nervous system. Other agents that are effective when used with the scrubbing technique include warm tap water, 20% soap solution, 1% aqueous benzalkonium chloride, and Ivory soap. Benzalkonium chloride 1% to 2% equals or outperforms the rabies antiserum[222] but may produce severe local tissue reactions, so it should be flushed from the wound with saline solution after use. Substances that have not been found useful in killing rabies virus are 5% Lugol's aqueous iodine solution, 7% tincture of iodine, and 1:1000 tincture of thimerosal. Unfortunately, no one has studied the effectiveness of iodine or povidone-iodine as swabbing solutions or for syringe irrigation; both have excellent virucidal qualities, and the latter is nonirritating to tissues.[188,201] However, since they have not been studied, they should not be relied on, particularly since other iodine solutions were ineffective.[222]

Almost complete protection is seen experimentally when effective agents are applied with scrubbing within 1 to 3 hours after inoculation. Experimental mortality increases markedly when treatment is delayed, going from 10% at 3 hours to 60% at 6 hours and 100% at 24 hours.[96] Equine rabies immune globulin is most effective when administered within the first 6 hours of inoculation.

One percent procaine hydrochloride infiltration of the wound edge (especially proximally) also provides some protective effect against the rabies virus.[222] Lidocaine and bupivicaine are more commonly used local anesthetics that would be predicted to have the same effect, but they have not been studied for antirabies activity.

Thorough and rapid early treatment of wounds from animals suspected of being rabid is mandatory. Within the first 3 hours the wound should be irrigated and scrubbed gently with a gauze sponge or cotton swabs using whatever solution is at hand. Plain tap water or handsoap and water are effective, readily available, and not damaging to tissue. In the hospital the wound edges should be anesthetized with 1% procaine hydrochloride, which exerts a protective effect. A benzalkonium chloride (Zephiran) solution should be applied with a gauze sponge scrub and then rinsed from the wound with saline. Scrubbing to the depths of puncture wounds by rotating cotton swabs against the wound surfaces is extremely important. This is not the preferred treatment for optimal wound healing, since it is irritating and mildly damaging to tissues. However, since high-pressure irrigation or povidone-iodine has not been proved to be effective against rabies virus, high-risk wounds should continue to be treated in this fashion. If rabies immune globulin is immediately available and can be used to irrigate and swab the wound, this is even better because it is as effective as benzalkonium chloride but not irritating to tissues.

All patients exposed to a possibly rabid animal need evaluation for rabies immunoprophylaxis, which is discussed in Chapter 41.

Other Neurotropic Infections

A single case of progressive motor neuron disease similar to amyotrophic lateral sclerosis has been reported to follow a cat bite and was thought to be caused by an unidentified virus.[207] Although not caused by bites or wounds, oral transmission of Creutzfeldt-Jakob disease has been reported from the regionally common practice of eating the brains of wild goats, pigs, or squirrels, even when cooked.[220] Creutzfeldt-Jakob disease is characterized by progressive dementia, ataxia, and myoclonus and is untreatable. It is caused by a virus that has also been identified in the brains of sheep and mule deer.[220]

Bacterial Systemic Infection. Animal bites can penetrate vital structures or seed infection to distant parts of the body such as distant arthritic and prosthetic joints, or even cause mycotic thoracic aortic aneurysm.[171] *Pasteurella multocida* was cultured from a brain abscess in a 19-month-old girl bitten 3 weeks earlier by a dog, with perforation of the skull not observed at the initial presentation.[230] Meningitis caused by CDC alphanumeric group II-J occurred in a 5-year-old girl after she was bitten on the head and neck by a dog.[34] *Pasteurella* and *Haemophilus canis* have also been responsible for inoculation osteomyelitis, which is not always associated with the typical fever and toxicity of gram-positive hematogenous osteomyelitis of childhood.[240,405] *Haemophilus aprophilus* has caused vertebral osteomyelitis after a self-inflicted accidental lip bite.[195] These various infections are discussed at greater length under the sections on the offending species.

Infection with *Sporothrix schenckii,* a ubiquitous saprophytic fungus found on vegetation, soil, and timber in warmer climates, has been reported after contact with an infected cat.[55] Similar infection has been reported after injuries inflicted by dogs, horses, and rats.

Mention should be made of other infections transmitted by cats in special circumstances, particularly to the immunosuppressed. In the era of AIDS, this has included *Pasteurella* peritonitis[123] and pneumonia.[109] However, these infections are transmitted by other animals as well, and exposure is most often nontraumatic. Cat-scratch disease in AIDS patients is discussed below.

Cat-Scratch Disease. Cat-scratch disease is uncommon but after rabies accounts for more wound infections than most of the other diseases listed in Table 40-5. It is probably the most common cause of unilateral lymphadenopathy in children.[390] Research in the early 1980s tentatively suggested that it was caused by a pleomorphic gram-negative bacillus[158,265] initially identified as *Rothia dentocariosa* (a common resident of the human mouth, previously known as *Leptotrichia*).[149] In 1988 the organism was positively identified and named *Afipia felis.*[125] Nonetheless, some uncertainty remains as to its role relative to other organisms.

A. felis can be visualized frequently in lesions of cat-scratch disease but is extraordinarily difficult to culture.[27] Many believe it to be the causative agent of cat-scratch disease, but the picture is not entirely clear. Eighty-eight percent of patients with cat-scratch disease have high antibody titers to *Rochalimaea henselae* (see later section on bacillary angiomatosis), but their sera do not react with *A. felis* antigen or vice versa.[373] The absence of antibody to *Afipia* in some persons with cat-scratch disease casts the causative relationship into doubt. In addition, *Rochalimaea* has been cultured from the lymph nodes of immunocompetent patients with cat-scratch disease and from the blood of cats.[106]

Ninety percent of cases are caused by scratches from cats, but dog and monkey bites, as well as thorns and splinters, have also been implicated.[82] Most cases occur in children. The average incubation period is 3 to 10 days. The characteristic feature is regional lymphadenitis, usually involving lymph nodes of the arm or leg. In a recent series, 54% of lymphadenopathy occurred in the axilla, and the remainder in the neck.[390] Often only one node is involved. The nodes are often painful and tender, and about 25% of them suppurate.[425] Adenopathy may spread proximally; occasionally, cervical adenopathy is mistaken for Hodgkin's disease. In most cases a characteristic raised, erythematous, slightly tender, and nonpruritic papule with a small central vesicle or eschar that resembles an insect bite is seen at the site of primary inoculation. Constitutional symptoms are mild, with approximately two thirds of patients manifesting fever, which is rarely greater than 102° F. Chills, malaise, anorexia, and nausea are common. Infrequent evanescent morbilliform and pleomorphic skin rashes lasting for 48 hours or less have been reported. Eighty-eight percent of patients have this typical clinical course; the remainder seek medical treatment for complications such as encephalopathy, atypical pneumonia, and severe systemic disease.[264] Parinaud's oculoglandular syndrome of granulomatous conjunctivitis and an ipsilateral, enlarged, tender preauricular lymph node occurs in about 6% of cases.[264]

Serious complications are rare and include encephalitis, seizures, transverse myelitis, osteolytic bone lesions, arthritis, splenic abscess, mediastinal adenopathy, optic neuritis, and thrombocytopenic purpura.[36,264,292,317] Although encephalopathy is rare, cat-scratch disease is becoming a more common cause of encephalopathy as other viral infectious diseases disappear; its incidence of neurologic complications now ranks with varicella and herpes simplex infections, Lyme disease, Rocky Mountain spotted fever, and Kawasaki disease.[56] Cat-scratch disease encephalopathy should enter the differential diagnosis of patients (especially young ones) with unexplained coma or seizures (half of whom were afebrile in one series). The prognosis of encephalopathy seems to be generally good.

Results of routine laboratory studies, including urinalysis and complete blood cell count, are normal, although mild leukocytosis may be seen. An indirect fluorescence antibody test to *Rochalimaea henselae* is now commercially available (EIA for *Rochalimaea henselae,* test code 8851, Specialty Laboratories, 2211 Michigan Ave., Santa Monica, CA 90404-3900, telephone 800-421-7110).

Immunity is thought to be largely cell mediated.[150] An intradermal skin test of 0.1 ml of cat-scratch disease antigen is positive in approximately 95% of victims, although 10% of the population reacts in a false-positive fashion. In confusing cases, biopsy of lymph nodes can yield characteristic findings of areas of granulomatous change and necrosis with central neutrophilic infiltration, a peripheral zone of histiocytic cells, and an outermost zone infiltrated by small lymphocytes and plasma cells.[262] However, this picture is not diagnostic; it is also seen in lymphogranuloma venereum, histoplasmosis, tularemia, brucellosis, sarcoidosis, and tuberculosis. Thus lymph node biopsy is most useful to rule out malignancy. Warthin-Starry or Brown-Hopps staining of the nodes or the primary skin lesion usually demonstrates the small, pleomorphic bacilli.[264]

In most cases clinical diagnosis is based on finding three of the following four criteria: (1) single or regional lymphadenopathy without obvious signs of cutaneous or throat infection, (2) contact with a cat (usually an immature one), (3) detection of an inoculation site, and (4) a positive skin test for cat-scratch disease.[56]

Cat-scratch disease usually resolves spontaneously in weeks to months, although in 2% of persons (usually adults) the course is prolonged and with systemic complications.[264] Systemic cat-scratch disease in an adult has been successfully treated with gentamicin[246] and, in a child, with cefuroxime.[144] Trimethoprim-sulfamethoxazole was used in a retrospective series of 71 patients with good results; this was not the case with other antibiotics.[71] The best study, of 202 patients, is also retrospective but found a response rate of 87% with rifampin, 84% with ciprofloxacin, 73% with intramuscular gentamicin, and 58% with trimethoprim-sulfamethoxazole.[263] Antibiotics that were of no benefit included amoxicillin-clavulanate, erythromycin, dicloxacillin, cephalexin, tetracycline, cefaclor, ceftriaxone, and cefotaxime.

Antibiotics should be reserved for persons with severe or very prolonged disease.[263] Symptomatic treatment and reassurance that the prognosis is excellent are the best therapies. No sequelae of cat-scratch disease other than the rare complications mentioned are known.

The workup should exclude other causes of regional lymphadenopathy, such as tuberculosis, tularemia, lymphogranuloma venereum, lymphoma, brucellosis, and sporotrichosis.[370] In general, only sporotrichosis and lymphogranuloma venereum demonstrate localized unilateral lymphadenopathy; lymphogranuloma venereum usually occurs in the groin. Cat scratches are normally found on the upper extremities. Skin tests, cultures, serologic tests, and biopsies are available for the differentiation of these other diseases.

Rochalimaea Infection (Bacillary Angiomatosis). In recent years the widespread HIV epidemic has introduced bacillary angiomatosis, which consists of vascular proliferative lesions of skin, bone, lymph node, brain, liver, and spleen.[408] Because of initial similarities and the fact that bacteria are observed in the lesions, the disorder was initially attributed to *A. felis*. However, the bacteria are now known to be *Rochalimaea henselae* and *Rochalimaea quintana* (the agent of trench fever). All three of these closely related organisms belong to the tribe Rickettsieae. Despite the different organism, bacillary angiomatosis is also closely associated with exposure to cats; recent cat scratch or cat bite was associated with an odds ratio of about 4:1.[408] The vast majority of patients are HIV positive, but a few are not and appear otherwise well. In 34% of cases this infection was the first one to establish the diagnosis of AIDS in a given patient. AIDS patients with bacillary angiomatosis can die if untreated, but the organism almost always responds favorably to erythromycin.[22]

R. henselae is a small, curved, and fastidious gram-negative rod that is extremely difficult to culture or isolate. It may take 6 weeks to grow; in fact, it was identified by polymerase chain reaction of its genetic material.[373] The most common skin lesions of bacillary angiomatosis are elevated, friable, red granulation tissue papules resembling pyogenic granulomas, numbering from a few to thousands. The second most common lesions are deeper nodules, seen in about half of the patients. Similar lesions can occur in tissues virtually anywhere in the body.[22] Visceral lesions may be the first sign of infection.[97] Patients often have fever, weight loss, and malaise. Hepatic involvement can lead to hepatic failure or even rupture. The organism can also cause bacteremia, even in immunocompetent patients. Treatment is with erythromycin. If patients cannot tolerate this therapy, rifampin and doxycycline or trimethoprim-sulfamethoxazole should be given. Norfloxacin, gentamicin, and ciprofloxacin are also clinically effective.[373] Penicillin and first-generation cephalosporins are not beneficial. Therapy is for a minimum of 6 weeks and may have to continue indefinitely in an immunosuppressed patient.

Cowpox and Catpox Infection. Poxvirus infection in the domestic cat has only been recently discovered, but the incidence has increased steadily and cats are now the most commonly reported hosts of poxvirus in Britain.[419] The infection occurs mostly among hunting cats in the late summer and early autumn; infection in humans has also been reported, usually after close contact or scratch from a sick cat.[419] The infection is manifested as an inflamed vesicular nodule with lymphadenitis, systemic symptoms including fever, and a rapid but self-limited course, similar to the orf poxvirus carried by sheep, cattle, and goats. The catpox virus is immunologically related to vaccinia, raising the question of whether more human cases will be seen now that smallpox vaccination has been abandoned.[419] This disease has not yet been reported in immunosuppressed patients. No effective treatment is available, but normally the disease is self-limited.

Rat-Bite Fever. Rat-bite fever is an acute illness caused by *Streptobacillus moniliformis* or *Spirillum minus,* which are part of the normal oral flora of rodents, including squirrels. It may also result from bites by wild and domestic carnivores such as weasels, dogs, cats, and pigs, which may have been infected when hunting rats and mice.[377] Carrier rates among wild rats vary from none to 50%.[25,404] Fewer than 70 cases have been reported in the North American literature.[159] Victims are chiefly children of lower socioeconomic groups with poor sanitation and heavy rodent populations.[274] The streptobacillary form is an occupational hazard of laboratory workers[80]; at least 10% and perhaps up to 100% of rats are nasopharyngeal carriers of the *Streptobacillus* variety.[6] Although relatively rare, cases can occur in any setting and can easily be fatal, particularly when the proper diagnosis is not suspected.[274]

Streptobacillary rat-bite fever. Streptobacillary rat-bite fever (Haverhill fever) is caused by *S. moniliformis,* an aerobic, nonmotile, gram-negative bacillus. The onset usually occurs within a week of the bite, but the incubation period may extend to several weeks, during which time the original wound usually heals completely. A bite need not be present, since the disease can also be transmitted by contaminated food, milk, or water.[136] It has also been transmitted by simply playing with pet rats, with no history of bite or injury.[360] Initial symptoms include fever, chills, cough, malaise, headache, and, less frequently, local lymphadenitis. These are followed by a nonpruritic morbilliform or petechial rash, which frequently involves the palms and soles. Migratory polyarthritis develops in approximately 50% of patients. Generalized lymphadenitis may be present; splenomegaly and hepatomegaly are rare.[404] Twenty-five percent of patients have a false-positive Venereal Disease Research Laboratories (VDRL) test. Leukocytosis with left shift is common, and agglutinating antibodies for the bacillus appear during the course of the disease. On autopsy, interstitial pneumonia, fibrinous endocarditis, mononuclear meningitis, hepatosplenomegaly, and mononuclear cell infiltrates in regional lymph nodes have been found.[376]

When a history of animal bite is lacking, the differential diagnosis must include rickettsial and viral infections. The fever and rash may suggest meningococcemia, but meningeal signs are lacking in rat-bite fever. Definitive diagnosis requires demonstration of rising antibody titers or culture of the bacillus from the blood, joint fluid, pustules, or original bite location. This can present a difficult differential diagnosis, as suggested by a pig farmer hospitalized for fever, malaise, and arthritis, whose cultures were identified only after 12 days of hospitalization and without any history of rat bite.[136] Typically, identification by culture is difficult and requires experienced laboratory workers who are seeking the organism.

Untreated, the disease runs a course of several weeks; prolongation of symptoms should raise the suspicion of endocarditis. The mortality in untreated persons is 10%, with most deaths caused by endocarditis and pneumonia. Although mortality is low, the disease can be fulminant; an infant bitten by a wild rat died 4 days after the bite and 2 days after the onset of symptoms.[376] The drug of choice is procaine penicillin in a dose of 600,000 units intramuscularly twice a day for 7 to 10 days.[404] Effective alternatives for penicillin-allergic patients are tetracycline, 30 mg/kg/day orally in four divided doses, or streptomycin, 15 mg/kg/day intramuscularly in two divided doses. Erythromycin is not effective. Complications such as endocarditis should be treated with high-dose intravenous potassium penicillin G (10 to 20 million units a day). The organism has both a bacillary and a cell wall–deficient L phase, which is thought to account for some of the antibiotic failures. The bacterial phase responds to penicillin, streptomycin, and tetracycline, whereas the L phase is resistant to penicillin.[376]

Spirillar rat-bite fever. Spirillar rat-bite fever is caused by *Spirillum minus,* a gram-negative, tightly coiled, spirillar microorganism. It is usually transmitted by infected wild rats, although cats have also been implicated. The general setting of socioeconomic deprivation in which this disease occurs is the same as in the streptobacillary form; cases in laboratory animals are unusual. Reported cases are rare. The incubation period is between 7 and 21 days, during which the bite lesion heals. The onset of illness is heralded by chills, fever, lymphadenitis, and a dark red macular rash. Myalgias are common, but arthritis is absent, which helps in the differentiation from streptobacillary fever. Leukocytosis and a false-positive VDRL test are often present. The disease is episodic and relapsing, with a 24- to 72-hour cycle. The differential diagnosis includes rickettsial and viral diseases when the history of animal bite is not present. In addition to the absence of arthritis, the manifestations at the bite site are more pronounced than in the streptobacillary variety (usually involving lymphadenitis, and still present when systemic illness occurs), and the fever and illness are relapsing in nature.[404] Definitive diagnosis rests on demonstrating the presence of *S. minus* in a dark-field preparation of exudate from an infected site. The patient's blood can be inoculated into mice, which may be tested for subsequent infection. The mortality of untreated disease is considerably lower than for streptobacillary fever. The untreated course spans several months; antibiotic therapy is the same as for streptobacillary fever.[159]

Tularemia. Tularemia represents a variety of syndromes caused by *Francisella tularensis,* a small, gram-negative coccobacillus. This bacterium normally parasitizes about 100 different mammals and arthropods, most commonly cottontail rabbits, rodents, hares, moles, beavers, muskrats, squirrels, rats, and mice. The primary mode of transmission to humans is via a bloodsucking arthropod, such as a tick, or by skin or eye inoculation resulting from skinning, dressing, or handling diseased animals. Other routes of infection include ingestion of water contaminated by urine or feces and inhalation of dust. Infection following bites or scratches from dogs, cats, skunks, coyotes, foxes, and hogs has been reported, although it is rare.[334] The disease is an occupational hazard of hunters, butchers, cooks, campers, and laboratory technicians. Humans are quite susceptible, and several hundred cases a year are reported in the United States.[200]

Tularemia is manifested by an abrupt onset of fever, often with chills and temperatures of up to 106° F. Headache is common and may mimic meningitis in severity. Hepatomegaly and splenomegaly are present in most patients. The exact symptom pattern depends on whether the disease is transmitted cutaneously (ulceroglandular form), by inhalation (pulmonary form), or by ingestion (enteric form). Of all cases, 80% take the ulceroglandular form, in which the skin is ulcerated at the point of entry and regional lymph nodes are enlarged. Bacteremia, pneumonitis, and, more rarely, meningitis, osteomyelitis, and endocarditis may occur. The oculoglandular form occurs in 1% of cases and is marked by extreme ocular pain, photophobia, itching, lacrimation, and mucopurulent discharge. Ulceration and corneal perforation may take place. When pneumonia occurs, mortality increases from 5% to 30%.

Diagnosis depends on a thorough history that elicits admission of contact with an infected animal, since patients usually seek treatment for a fever of unknown origin. The differential diagnosis of regional lymphadenopathy must entertain plague, cat-scratch disease, sporotrichosis, mononucleosis, and ecthyma. The accurate diagnosis of tularemia depends on a positive Foshay skin test (usually not commercially available) and rising agglutination titers, which appear by the second week. The organism can also be isolated by blood culture and animal inoculation, but both of these techniques pose a risk of infection to laboratory personnel.

The treatment of choice is streptomycin 30 to 40 mg/kg/day, given intramuscularly in two divided doses. Kanamycin or gentamicin should be equally effective, although they have not been used extensively.[404] Chloramphenicol and tetracycline are clinically useful but are not as effective in eradicating the organism.

Leptospirosis. Leptospirosis is caused by *Leptospira interrogans,* an organism of many serotypes that infects virtually every wild and domestic species at some time and is shed in large quantities in the urine. Among pets, the disease is common in dogs but rare in cats. The vast majority of cases are transmitted by contact or ingestion of material contaminated by urine, where the organisms can survive for weeks.[404] Transmission by bite has occurred in dogs, mice, and rats but is extremely rare, since leptospires are not secreted in the saliva; therefore the mouth would have to be contaminated with urine.[100] Farm workers and slaughterhouse workers have traditionally been at high risk of occupational exposure, but the disease now occurs more commonly in children, students, and housewives and is most commonly contracted during swimming, hunting, and fishing. Dogs are the most common vector. About 100 cases a year are reported in the United States.

The disease occurs in both an anicteric form and the more severe icteric form (Weil's disease). It carries a mortality of 3% to 6% overall and 15% to 40% in patients who have severe renal and hepatic involvement.[100,404] The illness is characterized by an initial phase of abrupt high fever, headache, prostration, myalgia, and prominent conjunctival injection; 25% have cough and chest pain. Relative bradycardia, calf, thigh, and lumbar muscle tenderness, and neck stiffness are prominent. A maculopapular, petechial, or purpuric rash may be present. Apparent recovery is seen for a few days, followed by the return of fever associated with meningitis and the appearance of IgM antibodies. In Weil's disease, jaundice, petechial hemorrhages, and renal insufficiency caused by interstitial nephritis are noted; the serum glutamic oxaloacetic transaminase (SGOT) level is only mildly elevated, even when bilirubin is very high.[404] Most cases are initially interpreted as septic meningitis, infectious hepatitis, or fever of unknown origin.[100] Elevated blood urea nitrogen (BUN) levels, hematuria, and proteinuria occur in about 20% to 25% of patients, 28% have elevated cerebrospinal fluid protein concentrations, and 44% have increased white cells in the cerebrospinal fluid. The glucose level in cerebrospinal fluid is usually normal. Congestive heart failure and arrhythmias may appear. Clinically different forms of the disease were formerly attributed to different varieties of *Leptospira* (recently renamed), but this is no longer believed to be true.[404]

In the early stages of leptospirosis, other infectious causes of fever, such as malaria, typhoid, typhus, and brucellosis, are included in the differential diagnosis. The correct diagnosis is usually not entertained at first, and aseptic meningitis, encephalitis, hepatitis, viral syndrome, or fever of unknown origin may be diagnosed. Definitive diagnosis rests on the demonstration of a fourfold rise in antibody titers by the microscopic slide agglutination test, which is rapid and simple but not of high specificity. If positive results are obtained, further experimental tests such as fluorescent antibody staining should be conducted at the CDC. Rising agglutination titers are seen after the first week. The organism requires special care and many weeks to culture,[404] and infectious disease consultation is recommended.

The efficacy of specific antibiotic treatment has not been proved, although treatment within the first few days seems to reduce the severity of the disease. Procaine penicillin G, 50,000 units/kg/day in four divided doses intramuscularly, is the preferred treatment and is continued for 7 to 10 days. Intravenous penicillin has not been studied. Tetracycline, 20 mg/kg/day in four divided oral doses, is used as an alternative. A Jarisch-Herxheimer-type reaction may be seen within a few hours of treatment.

Brucellosis. Brucellosis is caused by a number of species of *Brucella,* a small, gram-negative bacterium. The disease usually results from the ingestion of contaminated milk or milk products or by direct skin contact. *Brucella* organisms are carried chiefly by swine, cattle, goats, and sheep and may be recovered from almost all tissues. Most animals used as livestock are susceptible to brucellosis, while the occurrence in wild animals is rather small. Infection may occur accidentally in the laboratory or occupationally; today most cases occur in those who work in meat packing.[404] A proven case of transmission by dog bite has been reported,[348] and dogs carry their own species that is pathogenic.[140]

The incubation period in humans is 1 to 15 weeks. The disease ranges from mild to severe; it is frequently recurrent and can persist for years. No specific symptoms or signs are seen; hence the illness has been nicknamed mimic disease.[192] The most characteristic clinical manifestation is undulating fever.[192] Others include fever, chills, weakness, malaise, headache, muscle and joint pains, backache, and loss of weight. Bacteremia in the early stages almost always induces lesions of the viscera, bones, and joints; osteomyelitis, particularly spondylitis, is a common complication. Because of the nonspecific clinical syndrome, diagnosis rests on demonstrating rising agglutination titers.

The treatment is oral tetracycline, 50 mg/kg/day in four divided doses for 21 days. In very severe cases, streptomycin,

20 to 40 mg/kg intramuscularly once a day for 1 week, is added to this regimen. The next week, streptomycin is continued at a level of 15 mg/kg. Trimethoprim-sulfamethoxazole has been used, but its effectiveness is not certain. The prognosis is generally excellent, with only two deaths reported in several thousand cases.[140]

Plague. Plague is caused by the bacterium *Yersinia pestis*. It once had a dread reputation, but in recent centuries it has had much less deadly results. Wild plague is endemic in many parts of the world, chiefly among rats, mice, moles, marmots, squirrels, hares, cats, and mongooses. Dogs, cats, bobcats, and coyotes can also be affected.[404] More than 200 species of rodents and lagomorphs are naturally infected. Major plague areas include parts of China, Afghanistan, and South Africa. Recent cases in India highlight the risk. One of the larger areas of endemic plague is the western United States, where voles, field mice, ground squirrels, prairie dogs, and pack rats carry the infection. The infection is usually transmitted to humans by the bite of arthropods from infected animals. Handling infected animals allows *Yersinia pestis* to enter cuts and abrasions; this has been reported in veterinarians and in hunters who skin and clean infected rabbits.[94] Transmission by bite or scratch has never been reported. The disease is mentioned here because of its historical significance and the frequency of occurrence in wild animals. Further details can be found in Chapter 41.

Dog Bites

Dogs are the only species whose bites have been well studied in large numbers. They account for about 90% of all reported bites (Table 40-1). At the turn of the century, stray dogs were greatly feared because of their high incidence of rabies, and bounties were offered for their slaughter.[187] Such procedures are not warranted today because stray dogs account for only 15% to 20% of bites and are virtually never rabid.

Since dogs are territorial, are bred to protect territory, and remain the most common animals inflicting bites on humans, their behavior deserves special comment. Invasion of their territory may trigger attack. Dogs are hunting carnivores and pack animals, characteristics that are frequently inconsistent with peaceful human cohabitation. They are prone to attack and bite, which they do liberally to friend and foe alike. Indeed, the majority of cases occur when a dog bites someone it knows or lives with (Table 40-6). Eye contact with dogs should be avoided, since it will be interpreted as a threat or challenge.[368] Running away is a bad idea because it often provokes a chase and a human cannot outrun a dog (or almost any other animal, for that matter; the speed of human runners is considered an achievement only by other, slower humans). Particularly for dogs of herding or working breeds such as collies or sheepdogs, movement is a real trigger. Such dogs almost invariably want to chase (and "herd") running humans. If a dog does start to attack, the best reaction is to freeze. Some experts believe the next step is to face the dog frontally, look it in the eye, and issue a command (such as "No" or "Go home"). Others believe this is a mistake, and that a submissive posture should be adopted; in dog body language, this means making no noise, not looking at the dog directly, turning sideways, and leaning away from the dog.[368] All these activities signal to the dog that the person has given up, and usually the dog will simply growl or sniff, then leave. At that point the person should move away to the side, slowly and cautiously. A person should not turn his or her back on the dog.

If a dog launches a full attack or knocks someone to the ground, the person should curl up in a ball with fists covering the ears (to protect these vulnerable parts). If possible, the dog should be given something (like a piece of clothing) instead of flesh to bite. When the attack is over, the dog should be reported to local authorities; many areas have leash laws and ordinances to curb vicious dogs, and reporting a problem dog may prevent another (and worse) attack. As discussed in the section on fatal dog attacks, most dogs who seriously wound or kill humans have a long history of aggressive behavior. Prevention is the best course, and advance training in avoidance is a good idea, especially for children. Such courses are offered by animal control associations, veterinary societies, and the Humane Society.[441]

A dog's tendency to bite is based on the interaction of five factors: heredity, early experience, later socialization and training, health, and victim behavior.[441] Obviously a combination of approaches is needed to minimize biting. Early identification of problem dogs needs to be combined with better education of children and parents. More stringent

Table 40-6 Relationship of Biting Animal to Victim (Percent) in Various Studies

Relationship	Dog[187]	Dog[23]	Dog[228]	Cat[228]	Cat[440]	Miscellaneous[228]
Victim's or family pet	16	18	30	60	21	38
Friend's pet	0	42	55	20	21	40
Stranger's pet	62	22	0	0		0
Stray	22	17	15	20	57	22
Wild			15	20		22
Total number of cases	186	214	189	34	623	32

animal control legislation is probably needed. Courses on canine behavior should be offered to those at risk, such as children, animal control officers, and postal workers.

Young dogs (under 1 year of age) seem to produce the highest incidence of bites; this is an age when they are developing dominance aggression, that is, biting directed primarily at family (pack) members in situations where they are protecting resources or resisting dominant gestures by a family member.[441] Large dogs (weighing more than 50 pounds) account for about 43% of all bites, medium-sized dogs (15 to 20 pounds) for about 26%, and small dogs (less than 15 pounds) for only about 5%.[187] The incidence of biting increases substantially during the warm summer months. Most bites occur between 1 and 9 PM, which is probably related to the number of people on the street at those hours.[187] Most bites are inflicted on children coming home from school or playing outdoors. An estimated 1% of all children are injured by dog bites each year; animal bites are the fourth leading cause of accidents in this age group.[228] The increased susceptibility of children is caused by their smaller size, relative inability to defend themselves, interest in animals, and frequent abuse of animals because of inexperience. Hand and arm bites are the most common in all groups, although facial wounds are frequent in smaller children.[23,76,200] Virtually all severe facial injuries (estimated at 16,000 a year) occur in children under the age of 10 years; the highest incidence of facial wounds is 152 per 100,000 for children under age 4.[58]

Drawing confident conclusions regarding the likelihood of biting by breed is difficult (Table 40-7). Only 4% of the total dog population, all purebred, are registered; thus the sample population is very small and probably not representative. In almost all series, German shepherds were responsible for the largest proportion of bite wounds, both fatal and nonfatal. In a study that controlled for population by breed, only German shepherds bit at a disproportionately high rate.[178] Contrary to their reputation for viciousness, Dobermans contributed only a very small number of nonfatal attacks and 2.4% of fatal attacks. This may reflect precautions taken on the basis of their reputed behavior. The category of sporting dogs, which includes the golden and Labrador retrievers, known for their unaggressive nature, represents 17% of total American Kennel Club (AKC) registration but contributed only 0.4% of nonfatal bites and 5% of fatal bites. In contrast, the St. Bernard and Great Dane represent only 4.4% and 5% of AKC registration, respectively, but contribute 10% and 7.4% of fatal attacks, respectively. Although none of these data are comprehensive, they do suggest that some breeds of purebred are more prone to attack behavior.

None of the earlier studies reported on pit bulls, a loosely defined type of dog (not an official breed) that has become popular in the last decade and is bred for aggressive behavior. Episodic attacks, particularly on infants and children, are reported in the news; in one county in California, pit bulls contributed 9.5% of all attacks in 1984-1985.[64] Of 14 fatal dog attacks in the United States in 1986, 9 were attributed to pit bulls, and another 5 had occurred by June 1987.[226] In recent years, fatal attacks from pit bulls have increased from 20% of the total to 62%, and attacks by pit bulls were twice as likely to be caused by strays as other species.[362] This reflects not only a dramatic rise in the proportion of attacks by pit bulls, but a dramatic increase in fatal attacks. Many towns and counties are passing legislation limiting or outlawing ownership of pit bulls, and owners have even been formally charged with murder after fatalities.[225] However, the pro-

Table 40-7 Incidence of Dog Bites by Breed

Breed	Percent of Total AKC Registrations, 1976	Bites	Percent of All Licensed Dogs*	Reference 228	Reference 320†
Mixed	0.0	37.0	28.0	31.0	12.3
German shepherd	19.0	44.0	44.0	28.0	20.0
Terrier	5.4			5.0	8.6
Cocker spaniel				4.0	
Doberman	19.0	1	1.7	4.0	2.4
St. Bernard	4.4			4.0	10.0
Great Dane	5.0			4.0	7.4
Poodle				4.0	
Collie	6.0	2.6			2.4
Sporting dogs‡	17.0	0.4			5.0
Other		13.6	18.6	16.0	
Total number of cases	386,000	2921		135	81

*Percent of total Baltimore dog license registrations, by breed, 1976.
†All fatal attacks.
‡Golden and Labrador retrievers.

portion of pit bulls in the dog population is also unknown, and no doubt some of these dismal statistics reflect the popularity of the breed among owners who train them exclusively for viciousness and attack purposes.

FATAL ATTACKS BY DOGS

Like all other larger animals, large dogs can easily inflict severe injury. For example, right cerebral infarction from carotid artery injury in a patient bitten by a rottweiler (but whose wounds were initially thought to not even have penetrated the platysma muscles) has been reported.[278] With such potential, the fact that deaths occur is not surprising. Of course, more bizarre episodes are possible; people have died from a dog preventing efforts at cardiopulmonary resuscitation or from being pushed into a mound of fire ants by a dog and developing anaphylaxis.[362]

Fatal attacks by dogs in the United States cause many more deaths than rabies. At least 51 such cases occurred in the years 1975 to 1980 (Table 40-2).[320,432] During this same period, only one person acquired rabies from a dog bite in the United States. The incidence is estimated at 1 fatal attack per 5 million dogs per year, or 2 fatalities per 1000 bites.[320,439] However, 14 fatal attacks occurred in 1986 alone, suggesting that the rate may be increasing (owing primarily to the contributions of pit bulls).[226] A more recent review identified 157 fatalities between 1979 and 1988, for a rate of 6.7 deaths per 100 million population per year.[362] However, for infants less than 1 year, the death rate was 68 per 100 million population per year.

Only about one fourth of these fatal attacks were caused by stray dogs; most dogs were owned either by the victim's family or by an immediate neighbor or friend, and many attacks occurred in the victim's home or yard. Many of the dogs had previously been friendly and without a history of attacks. Ten of the cases involved attacks by three or more dogs, including one attack by 20 to 40 dogs. In several cases of pack attacks the dogs were small and knew the victim well.[32] The victims ranged in age from infancy to old age, and most died at the scene of the attack. However, infants and small children, particularly those left unattended for even short periods, are frequent victims, accounting for 70% of victims in the largest series.[68,362]

Injuries were markedly concentrated about the head and neck, as opposed to the extremity distribution usually seen in nonfatal dog bites. This suggests that the triggering and intent of these attacks differ in some critical fashion from the usual nonfatal biting episode. Similar characteristics occur in nonfatal severe attacks in which the head and neck are attacked in a virtual frenzy.[439] The beginning of the attack was unwitnessed in most fatal cases, but in nonfatal cases there was seldom much warning and little if any provocation.[439]

Attacks on infants were the most frequent. All involved pet dogs (not strays), and all but one occurred in the home and involved only one dog. Half occurred while the infant was sleeping in a crib.[362] In children over the age of 1 year, 36% of deaths occurred when a child gained unauthorized access to a fenced yard, and 28% resulted from a child wandering too close to a chained dog.

Fatal attacks and vicious attacks cannot be predicted from a dog's prior behavior, and most offending dogs revert to normal, friendly behavior after the episode. In recent years, fatal attacks from pit bulls have increased from 20% to 62% of the total.[362] German shepherds, huskies, malamutes, and wolf-hybrids are the next most common.[362] Packs of aggressive dogs should be avoided carefully, and aggressive and pack behavior toward humans punished by the owner.[32]

Dogs represent a significant potential cause of death for infants and small children. Children and the disabled should *never* be left alone with a dog regardless of the dog's reputation and prior behavior. Certain breeds such as pit bulls seem to contribute far more than their share of cases and should be considered for more effective supervision and controls.

OTHER COMPLICATIONS

Certain situations produce greater injuries. Police dogs, for example, are not only large, but also trained to bite and hold on to the victim until commanded to release. This is not the normal pattern for an attacking dog. In a 3-year period, of 486 patients evaluated on a jail ward for police dog bites, 7.2% required angiography to rule out arterial injury to an extremity, and 21% of these were found to have arterial injury.[389] This incidence is roughly similar to that found in nonbite trauma patients evaluated by angiography. All the patients who had angiograms had multiple puncture wounds, but only half of those with arterial injury were lacking a distal pulse. These results suggest that patients bitten by a large dog and with proximity of injury to a major vessel, absent or decreased pulse, sensory or motor deficit, large or expanding hematoma, and active bleeding should receive this evaluation.[389] Similar conclusions could be made for bites from any large carnivore, although the "bite and hold" training of police dogs may increase the incidence of injury. However, a similar injury to an artery has been reported with a delayed presentation after a trivial dog bite injury in a child.[355]

WOUND INFECTION IN DOG BITES

Overall, wound infection rates for dog bites vary in the literature from 0.5% to 29%.* The latter rate was reported only in a small study of atypical, heavily contaminated wounds,[243] although a rate of 25% was reported in a very

*References 51, 53, 108, 174, 243, 400, 411, 446.

large series from France.[400] However, this report spanned the last 30 years and was probably atypical in many regards, particularly its definition of wound infection and its very high usage of prophylactic antibiotics (52%).

Nonbite lacerations treated in the emergency department have had a 5% infection rate in two studies.[104,145] Another recent study of nonbite lacerations reported 9% of routinely treated wounds to have nonpurulent infection and 6% to have purulent infection, for a total of 15%.[177] In a pediatric population, however, the infection rate of nonbite lacerations was only 1.2%.[12] No doubt, much of the variation depends on treatment technique, but typical nonbite lacerations in the emergency department seem to have an infection rate of about 5% to 10%.

In typical outpatient-treated dog bite wounds, which are managed properly with irrigation and debridement, a wound infection rate of 5% to 10% is usual. This compares favorably with the nonbite infection rates cited previously. Dog bites of the head and neck, all sutured and none treated with antibiotics, have an infection rate of only 1.4%.[184] Bites of the face and ears, although often requiring extensive plastic surgery, also heal well when treated aggressively and with antibiotics.[403] Those around the eyes almost always involve children and are usually punctures, but do well with aggressive treatment.[172] Dog bites of the genitalia, although sometimes requiring surgery, are reported to heal well with antibiotic coverage.[107,433] Therefore dog bite wounds in general are probably no more infection prone than nonbite accidental cutaneous lacerations.

The bacteriology of dog bite wound infections is complex. More than 64 species of bacteria are part of the normal flora of a dog's mouth (see Boxes 40-4 and 40-5).[11] Most wound infections are caused by organisms (see Boxes 40-5 and 40-7) that originate in the dog's mouth, not on the patient's skin.[166] Cultures of fresh wounds have no predictive value; all wounds contain bacteria, the bacteria cultured are not predictive of subsequent infection, and 28% of infected wounds grow no bacteria.[11,301] In 25% to 36% of wound infections, cultures grow more than one species; no single organism accounts for more than 15% of infections.[51,301]

Although *Pasteurella multocida* is commonly mentioned in the literature, only 22% or less of dogs carry this organism.[366] A larger recent series found that *P. multocida* was present in the mouths of 13% of dogs versus 77% of cats.[146] Although some particular *Pasteurella* species were found in 66% of dogs and 87% of cats, most of the species in dogs were less virulent (or even nonpathogenic) varieties, such as *P. stomatis, canis,* and *dagmatis.*[146] These differences probably account for the fact that *Pasteurella* is not often found in wound infections from dog bites. In recent studies of dog bite wounds, *Pasteurella* was not cultured at all.[50,141,301] (In the largest of these series, this absence may well have been caused by poor laboratory techniques.) The vast majority of *Pasteurella* infections follow cat bites.[198] Thus this is an unlikely pathogen in the dog bite victim, which makes therapy simpler, since neither erythromycin nor oral first-generation cephalosporins are highly effective against it. *P. multocida* and antibiotic therapy against it are discussed in detail in the section on cat bites.

Pseudomonas and *S. aureus* are each seen in 10% to 15% of infections. *S. epidermidis* has been reported in 11.5% of infected dog bites; whether it is a pathogen or contaminant in this role is not known.[301] *S. intermedius* has recently been reported; up to 20% of staphyloccocal infections may actually be caused by this organism, which is usually susceptible to a wide variety of antibiotics, often including penicillin G.[406] *S. intermedius* can be cultured from 39% of dogs, whereas only 10% carry *S. aureus;* this may help explain why most wound infections respond even to drugs not effective against penicillinase-resistant drugs.[407] Many anaerobic species are commonly present (Table 40-8) but are almost invariably mixed with aerobic species.[38,166] Anaerobes seldom cause infection alone, so both aerobic and anaerobic species should be cultured and covered with antibiotics when infection is severe. This is particularly important with sepsis.

Other pathogens are possible; one case of human blastomycosis following a dog bite has been reported.[154] *Blastomyces dermatitidis* was demonstrated in the poorly healing wound, and therapy was successfully undertaken with ketoconazole. Infection (usually systemic) with *Capnocytophaga canimorsus* (formerly DF-2) occurs rarely; sepsis caused by dog bite pathogens is discussed in the section on systemic infections (see Box 40-7). The CDC has recently isolated a new fastidious, nonoxidative, gram-negative rod (thought to be related to the *Acinetobacter* species) from infected human bite wounds. It has been named NO-1 (nonoxidizer 1).[196] Its clinical significance is unknown; 50% of isolates were resistant to trimethoprim but sensitive to ciprofloxacin, amoxicillin-clavulanate, cefuroxime, cephalothin, and the tetracyclines. *Veillonella parvula* is moderately commonly found and is sensitive to penicillin.[340]

ANTIBIOTIC RECOMMENDATIONS FOR DOG BITES

The recommendations given here apply to dog bites (the most common type) and most other animal bites. Special considerations are necessary for cat bites and human bites; these are discussed in detail in the sections on those topics. Prophylactic antibiotics of any kind are not indicated in ordinary low-risk dog bites.

Penicillin, although used in a number of the studies cited, is not adequate initial coverage because organisms in 46% of infected wounds in one series had β-lactamase activity.[38] Cloxacillin, dicloxacillin, and an oral cephalosporin are all reasonable choices, although none is optimal against *Pasteurella* (seen most commonly in cat bites) or against anaerobes that may be particularly found in hand infections (Table 40-4, Box 40-5). When one of these is used, dicloxacillin is preferred because it produces the highest serum concentrations. The higher dose (500 mg in adults) is recommended because serum levels may be too low with lower doses.

Of the oral first-generation cephalosporins available, cephalexin and cephradine are most commonly used and require doses four times a day; cefadroxil is given every 12 to 24 hours (Table 40-4).[365,383] Cefadroxil is much more expensive than cephalexin and costs the same as oral second-generation cephalosporins such as cefuroxime, which offer superior coverage and twice a day doses.

In most cases, oral cephalexin or dicloxacillin is inexpensive and effective. An alternative that is also inexpensive and effective is trimethoprim-sulfamethoxazole, which is seldom discussed but is a good choice if the patient is penicillin allergic. Erythromycin is also inexpensive but is somewhat less effective against *Staphylococcus* than trimethroprim-sulfamethoxazole.

Special comment must be made about amoxicillin–clavulanic acid, since it has been heavily promoted for animal bites. This antibiotic possesses attractive efficacy against a broad spectrum of pathogens, such as *Eikenella corrodens* and *Staphylococcus,* but is less effective against other common bite pathogens. It has been studied only once in an unblinded and uncontrolled protocol funded by the manufacturer; the study was too small to accurately detect statistical differences between treatments.[168,170] Patients included those with human and animal bites and those with fresh and infected wounds; results were not reported separately for these very different clinical groups. The authors found the "cure rate" of amoxicillin–clavulanic acid to be the same as that for penicillin or dicloxacillin, although since most of the wounds were uninfected, how they measured "cure" is unknown. The authors strongly advocated use of amoxicillin–clavulanic acid even though this treatment was no more effective than penicillin or dicloxacillin and produced adverse reactions in 46% and diarrhea in 30% of the patients who received it. In addition, vaginitis developed in one patient and bacterial colitis in another which could be life threatening in an immunocompromised patient. Virtually none of these complications occurred in the other treatment groups.

Amoxicillin–clavulanic acid was no more effective than the other regimens in the study, but at the time of the study it was less expensive than dicloxacillin or cephalosporins. The design and size of this study make drawing any conclusions impossible. Nonetheless, aggressive marketing has led some clinicians to consider amoxicillin–clavulanic acid an acceptable alternative treatment.[38] Currently it costs the same as cefuroxime, which only has to be given twice a day, has the same spectrum, and has far fewer side effects. Cefuroxime seems to be the better drug.

Other bacteria are not optimally covered by the preceding regimen. *Pasteurella* is optimally treated with penicillin, but the incidence of *Pasteurella* is so low in dog bites that it should not be a major consideration in initial treatment.[130] It is much more likely in cat bites, and antibiotic selection is discussed in that section. Most cases of *Pasteurella* infection reported are in cat bites. *Pseudomonas* is a possibility that is not covered by most oral antibiotics. The new oral quinolone antibiotic ciprofloxacin is effective against *Pseudomonas.*[365] *Pseudomonas* infection is very rare in animal bites and need be addressed only when its presence is proven (or in cases of sepsis; Box 40-7).

Although many theoretical problems exist in using cloxacillin or a cephalosporin, in clinical practice the drugs are highly effective against the vast majority of bite wound infections. The risk status of the wound should be decided by the factors listed in Box 40-3, and prophylactic antibiotics given to the small subset of patients in whom the possible benefit of antibiotics outweighs the risk of side effects. Antibiotic choices are listed in Table 40-4, and recommended antibiotics are listed in Table 40-8.

Western medicine has become increasingly conscious of the costs of health care, and therefore concern about the cost of antibiotics is appropriate. Costs are often cited as a reason not to use one of the newer antibiotics (which generally have a broader spectrum). However, costs fluctuate constantly. After a few years, costs of newer drugs often approximate those of old ones. Large institutions often get competitive bids that make the cost of new drugs reasonable. In addition, the figures quoted for costs (even in Table 40-4) are wholesale costs to the hospital or pharmacy; the additional markup and fees added to these by the dispenser may completely change the cost equation. Therefore the clinician should not rely on published (and already out of date) recommendations based on cost, but must investigate the local cost of the drug as delivered to patients.

The least expensive drug is not necessarily the most cost effective. The cost of even expensive antibiotics, at least in Western society, is usually much less than the cost of the physician visit, x-ray studies, or hospitalization. The least expensive antibiotic (such as penicillin) may cost only $10 for the actual prescription, which is no contest against an antibiotic costing $45. However, if a more expensive and better antibiotic prevents infection and precludes a follow-up physician visit costing $75 or more, it is clearly the more cost effective of the two. Therefore, in particularly high-risk situations, prescribing the best—not the least expensive—antibiotic is usually cost effective. This should be the case particularly when several risk factors are present, for example, a bite of the hand in an elderly diabetic.

Asplenic or severely immunosuppressed patients who are bitten by dogs are at increased risk of life-threatening infection by *C. canimorsus.* They should be treated with penicillin or cephalosporin antibiotics parenterally. Some authors have recommended a short hospitalization for all such patients (even without any clinical signs of infection), but this seems unnecessary in reliable, well patients with good follow-up.[203]

Table 40-8 Recommended Initial Oral Antibiotics for Bite Wounds

Drug	Child	Adult
ORGANISMS KNOWN		
Treat according to specific antibiotic sensitivities of cultured organism		
ORGANISMS UNKNOWN*,†		
Dog and most other bites		
Dicloxacillin (least expensive) or cephalexin	500-100 mg/kg/day in 4 divided doses	500 mg po qid
Cefuroxime (best coverage, not needed in most cases)	250 mg po bid	500 mg po bid
If penicillin allergic:		
Erythromycin	30-50 mg/kg/day in 4 divided doses	500 mg po qid
or		
Trimethoprim/sulfamethoxazole	40 mg/200 mg per 10 kg bid (5 m/suspension/10 kg bid)	160 mg/800 mg (DS) bid
Cat bites (high likelihood of *Pasteurella multocida*‡)		
Penicillin plus dicloxacillin (least expensive)	50-100 mg/kg/day in 4 divided doses	500 mg po qid
Cefuroxime (best coverage)	250 mg po bid	500 mg po bid
If penicillin allergic:		
Trimethoprim/sulfamethoxazole	40 mg/200 mg per 10 kg bid (5 suspension/10 kg bid)	160 mg/800 mg (DS) bid
or		
Ciprofloxacin (nonpregnant adults only)	Contraindicated	500 mg bid
Human bites of hand (organisms of concern include *Streptococcus, Staphylococcus,* and *Eikenella corrodens*)		
Dicloxacillin plus ampicillin (least expensive)	50-100 mg/kg/day in 4 divided doses	500 mg po qid
or		
Cefuroxime (best coverage)	250 mg po bid	500 mg po bid
If penicillin allergic:		
Ciprofloxacin plus erythromycin	Contraindicated	500 mg bid

Listed are antibiotics chosen for efficacy against most likely organisms at lowest cost. See Table 40-4 for details of possibly resistant organisms and special clinical situations.

Which antibiotic is the cheapest varies greatly over time and by locality; these choices are based on average U.S. wholesale prices in 1993. The difference between lowest and moderately priced antibiotics typically averages $25 to $35 cost to the patient, which is not warranted in low-risk cases but in high-risk cases may be cost-effective if the antibiotic prevents infection and additional physician visits.

*This regimen is effective for most potential pathogens. No one antibiotic covers all.

†Most patients can take an oral cephalosporin such as cephalexin without adverse effect. Erythromycin is not effective against *Staphylococcus.*

‡Penicillin is excellent for *Pasteurella* but is not optimal for many other significant pathogens; dicloxacillin has a much broader spectrum but slightly less efficacy against *Pasteurella.*

Bites of the Cat Family

DOMESTIC CATS

Domestic cats are becoming an increasingly significant problem in the United States. The population has exploded and is now estimated to total over 90 million; of these, 15 to 35 million are strays.[397] (This may be of particular significance because of the opportunity for these strays to be exposed to wild vectors of rabies; see section on rabies.) In the past, cats caused few complaints, but they now account for 50% of animal control calls, which is leading to proposals for leash and licensing laws for cats (Table 40-1). The increase in population has not only increased complaints, but also greatly increased the population of stray and feral cats.

Cat bites vary in many important variables from those of dogs. Domestic cat bites tend to be wounds of the hand. Although few cats attack passers-by on the legs, some go much further than that, chasing children on bicycles and actually crashing through a skylight to attack a family in their home.[397] Sixty-three percent of bites are on a hand or finger, usually the right (dominant) hand.[440] Seventy-six percent of those receiving bites on these two locations either treated the wound themselves at home or obtained no treatment. Fifty-seven percent of bites were inflicted by stray cats, perhaps because only one third of cats stay with the same owner for more than 3 years. Seventy percent of wounds are scratches, and 27% are punctures of the skin.[440]

Cat bites are notorious in the literature for their high infection rate. However, as in human bites, selection bias may be at work. The United States has more cats than dogs, yet dogs account for 80% to 90% of bites seen by physicians, while cats account for 5% to 15%. Surveys of reported bites also suggest that the biting rate of dogs is up to five times higher than that of cats, regardless of subsequent treatment.[306] Either cats inflict fewer bites and scratches on their owners, or the vast majority of these wounds are relatively minor and cause no sequelae. In the only survey of cat bites, 57% of victims treated the bites at home, and only 15% went to an emergency department.[440]

Because cats have small, sharp fangs and do not slash, their bite is much more likely than that of a dog to produce a small, deep puncture wound, often involving joint spaces and tendons. Thus cat bites frequently possess two risk factors for infection: location on the hand and depth of puncture. As a result, the reported infection rate ranges from 29% to 50%, although these figures are from older studies skewed toward infected patients.[108,228] This rate is comparable to that of dog bite puncture wounds, but much higher than the rate for dog bites in general. In a more recent study of 180 emergency department patients with cat bites, the infection rate was 16%, and most of these infections were present when the patient sought medical care.[102]

Other risk factors associated with wound infections in cat bite include older age, longer time intervals until emergency department treatment, wounds inflicted by "pet" cats rather than strays, attempting wound care at home, having a more severe wound, and having a deeper wound. Wound infections are more likely to develop in uninfected patients with lower extremity wounds who did not receive prophylactic oral antibiotics and in those with puncture wounds who did not receive prophylactic oral antibiotics. Scratches very seldom become infected.[102]

Cat bite puncture wounds of the hand are high risk (Table 40-6) and should receive prophylactic antibiotics, which have been proven effective with oxacillin (a drug not very effective against *Pasteurella*).[122] Cat bites and scratches elsewhere on the body have not been proven to carry a high risk and should receive standard wound care. In addition, cat bites and scratches have been known to seed distant arthritic and prosthetic joints and cause *Pasteurella* septic arthritis and even mycotic thoracic aortic aneurysm.[167] Patients with such predisposing conditions (or prosthetic heart valves) deserve antibiotic prophylaxis.[303,430] Two cases of DF-2 bacteremia (usually seen after dog bite) have been reported after cat bites.[57]

The bacteriology of a cat bite is somewhat different from that of other species. Samples from the gingival margins of normal healthy cats produced a mean number of bacterial species per sample of 11 with a range of 7 to 16 isolates. Seventy-three percent of isolates were obligate anaerobes. Of the facultatively anaerobic species, *Actinomyces* (including *A. viscosus, A. hordeovulneris,* and *A. denticolens*) comprised 12% of isolates, *Pasteurella multocida* 9%, and *Propionibacterium* species 6%. Gram-negative bacilli belonging to the genera *Bacteroides* and *Fusobacterium* comprised 77% of the obligate anaerobes isolated. *Clostridium villosum* comprised 10% of obligately anaerobic isolates, *Wolinella* species 6%, and *Peptostreptococcus anaerobius* 5%. The most commonly isolated obligate anaerobic species was *Clostridium villosum,* and the most commonly isolated facultative anaerobic species was *Pasteurella multocida.* This bacterial flora is very similar to that of cat bite abscesses and is somewhat different (particularly in the incidence of *Pasteurella*) from that of dogs.[253]

The choice of antibiotic in cat bite infections poses real problems when, as is usual, the specific pathogen is unknown, because of the potential presence of *P. multocida* (Tables 40-4 and 40-8). A large study found that *P. multocida* was present in the mouths of 13% of dogs versus 77% of cats.[146] Most of the species in dogs were less virulent (or even nonpathogenic) varieties such as *P. stomatis, canis,* and *dagmatis.*[146] *Pasteurella* is not often found in wound infections from dog bite but is a frequent pathogen in infected cat bites.[304] In fact, the vast majority of all reported *Pasteurella* infections in the literature are secondary to bites of the cat family.[198,436] *Pasteurella* must be considered in virtually any animal bite; it has even been reported after a bite by a Tasmanian devil.[148] Nonetheless, even in cat bites, other pathogens such as *Staphylococcus aureus* may be present and must be covered by any proposed antibiotic treatment.[418]

Pasteurella is such a significant pathogen because of the rapidity with which it causes cellulitis (and worse complications) in infections of the hand, its potential for infectious complications elsewhere in the body, and the complexity it introduces into antibiotic choices. Septic complications from this organism include septic arthritis after cat scratch in a patient with rheumatoid arthritis[202] and meningitis after cat bite.[236] As mentioned previously, cat bites and scratches may seed distant prosthetic joints and even cause *Pasteurella* mycotic thoracic aortic aneurysm.[167] Endocarditis has been reported.[199]

Pasteurella introduces complexity into antibiotic decisions because it is variably sensitive to the normal antibiotic choices for the wide variety of organisms that may be present (Table 40-9). Penicillin is very effective against *Pasteurella* but of course does not provide anti-*Staphylococcus* coverage. The usual drug of choice when the pathogen is unknown—dicloxacillin—has not been tested clinically.[165] However, oxacillin has been proven effective in cat bite prophylaxis.[122] Oral cephalosporins have been reported to be ineffective against *Pasteurella* because of low serum levels.[427] Cefuroxime is moderately active against *Pasteurella,* and cephalexin is the least active cephalosporin in human isolates.[197] In human bite isolates, cefuroxime was generally more than four times more active than cephalexin and cefadroxil against all aerobic isolates, including *P. multocida.*[169,197] In veterinary isolates, in more than 90% of cases a kill of more than 99% was achieved within 4 hours of antibiotic treatment at concentrations of 2 or 4 μg/ml with either cefuroxime or cephalexin. Although cefuroxime was effective at lower concentrations than cephalexin, the rates of kill of the two antibiotics were comparable.[382] (These are the types of levels typically achieved by oral first-generation cephalosporins). Amoxicillin-clavulanate is effective (as is amoxicillin alone) but is expensive and has a high incidence of side effects. Also, it is inferior to second-generation cephalosporins. Cefuroxime, a second-generation oral cephalosporin, is the same price as amoxicillin-clavulanate but very effective, has few side effects, and is taken only twice a day (Table 40-4). Cefixime is a new oral third-generation cephalosporin that should be very effective; it is about twice as expensive as cefuroxime but is given only once a day.

The literature on this topic is obviously complex and contradictory but suggests that an inexpensive first-generation cephalosporin such as cephalexin will be effective (particularly in larger doses) against many *Pasteurella* isolates, while still effective against *Staphylococcus*. Cefuroxime, an oral second-generation cephalosporin, is much more effective but also more expensive (Table 40-4). Cefuroxime is the best compromise, but if cost is a primary consideration, a combination of penicillin and dicloxacillin is inexpensive and effective against both *Staphylococcus* and *Pasteurella*.

If the patient is allergic to penicillin, the choices get harder. Erythromycin would be logical, but a variety of reports suggest that sensitivity of *Pasteurella* to this drug is poor. *P. multocida* meningitis developed in a 73-year-old woman compliant with oral erythromycin; her organism showed intermediate sensitivity to erythromycin.[245] The results of in vitro sensitivity testing is mixed. Shikuma tested 15 isolates and found a wide variation in sensitivity. Weber studied 19 clinical isolates and found only 32% of isolates susceptible to erythromycin. Goldstein found 14% of 22 clinical isolates resistant to erythromycin.[164,165] Another study found 22 animal bite isolates of *Pasteurella* very sensitive to both erythromycin and cephalexin.[165]

An older review has stated that for patients who are penicillin allergic and are suspected or known to have infection with *Pasteurella*, erythromycin should not be used because it is ineffective against this species; tetracycline should be used instead.[427] Using tetracycline in the cat bite victim allergic to penicillin is wrong for several reasons. First, in vitro results have notoriously poor correlation with in vivo results, and in this paper, of the seven patients with bites infected with *Pasteurella* "improperly" treated with erythromycin, all responded to therapy. More important, the mean inhibitory concentrations commonly achieved with oral antibiotics still exceed by fivefold the level for inhibition with erythromycin.[165] In addition, research shows that although low levels of antibiotic may not kill *Pasteurella*, they have a very significant effect on its adherence and virulence.[241] Tetracycline is a poor antibiotic for cellulitis, achieves low tissue levels at a very slow rate,[4] and has very low effectiveness against many common pathogens, especially *Streptococcus*, *Staphylococcus*, diphtheroids, *Bacteroides*, and anaerobic gram-positive cocci.[164] In many animal populations *P. multocida* is resistant to tetracycline (no doubt because of its common use in animal feeds).[324] In addition, tetracycline cannot be used safely in children or pregnant women.[383] However, tetracycline has been found to have a synergistic treatment effect against *Pasteurella* when combined with erythromycin (other combinations are not synergistic).[44]

One reason that *Pasteurella* is so variably resistant to so many older antibiotics is its natural history as a common pathogen among farm animals, including swine, cattle, sheep, and poultry. As a result, this is one of the best studied bacterial pathogens known to science. Since so many commercial animals are prey to *Pasteurella* infections, and since these infections have dire financial implications for farmers, treating animals with prophylactic antibiotics through their feed or otherwise is commonplace. As a result, many isolates of *Pasteurella* have acquired resistance through antibiotic exposure.[26] The resistance of *Pasteurella* natural populations to antibiotics fluctuates constantly according to the antibiotics of choice.[431] This means that the antibiotic resistance of the pathogens in a particular animal's mouth is variable and hard to predict, although knowing the species and local farming practice provides cues. For example, in wild animals *Pasteurella* has not been exposed to antibiotics and thus is susceptible to most, including cephalexin at low levels. In pet cats, antibiotic resistance is higher, but is by far the highest in farm animals.

Fortunately, the difficulty of choosing an antibiotic has decreased with the introduction of new drugs (Tables 40-4 and 40-8). *Pasteurella* is quite susceptible to ciprofloxacin, a good choice for those allergic to penicillin, but contraindicated in children and pregnant women.[327] Ciprofloxacin is generally more active than either enoxacin or ofloxacin[161] and effective against *Pasteurella* and *Staphylococcus*, which make up the majority of pathogens in infected cat bites, but it is not very reliable for *Streptococcus*. The new macrolide antibiotics also offer some good choices. Azithromycin inhibits *Pasteurella* and need be taken only once a day, but its effectiveness has not been well studied, and it costs twice as much as clarithromycin.[296] Clarithromycin is taken only twice a day and is effective against *Pasteurella* (as well as a number of other gram-negative bacteria) and all gram-positive bacteria such as *Streptococcus* and *Staphylococcus*.[295] Trimethoprim-sulfamethoxazole is also a good choice.[186]

In short, the new drugs have made the treatment of the penicillin-allergic victim of cat bites easy, because any one of these drugs is a superior replacement for erythromycin. They are a bit more expensive, but the cost difference is about $3 per day of treatment, which is trivial compared with the cost of physician visits (and complications) in developed countries. In settings where the cost of medication is crucial, trimethoprim-sulfamethoxazole is an inexpensive and effective alternative; in its absence, reliance on high doses of cephalexin is reasonable.

Infection with *Sporothrix schenckii,* a ubiquitous saprophytic fungus found on vegetation, soil, and timber in warmer climates, has been reported after contact with an infected cat.[55] Similar infection has been reported after injuries inflicted by dogs, horses, and rats. Lymphocutaneous *Nocardia brasiliensis* has been reported after a cat scratch; this ubiquitous aerobic filamentous gram-positive bacterium is also common in soil.[361] Sulfonamides and trimethoprim-sulfamethoxazole remain the drugs of choice, although amoxicillin–clavulanic acid is effective; penicillin is usually not. Both of these organisms infect humans more commonly after puncture wounds than after animal injury.

Special mention should be made of other infections transmitted by cats in special circumstances, particularly to the immunosuppressed. In the era of AIDS, these have become commonplace, including *Pasteurella* peritonitis[123] and pneumonia.[109] However, these infections are transmitted by other animals as well, and exposure is most often nontraumatic. The possibility of transmission of cat-scratch disease should be remembered, although antibiotic prophylaxis is not recommended for this (see section on cat-scratch disease).

WILD (BIG) CATS

Adult cats have 30 permanent teeth, arranged in rows of 16 upper and 14 lower. The upper teeth overlap the lower, resulting in an overbite.[68] This helps the animal lock its teeth into the prey and exert severe twisting and tearing forces. The feline bite is much shorter and more rounded than that of a dog.

Big cats typically attack from behind, biting the neck and occiput of their prey and attempting to maneuver their canine teeth between the victim's cervical vertebrae and into the spinal cord.[70] Proprioceptors in the cat's tooth allow it to detect when it has encountered bone. The goal of rapidly paralyzing the prey is also accomplished by a violent shake of the cat's head, which fractures the cervical spine. In a study of jaguar fatalities, 77% of victims were bitten on the nape of the neck and half of the bites were made to the base of the skull.[70] In 20% of cases the killing bite was to the head, with at least one canine piercing the skull or ear canal. Cheetahs prefer to attack the throat of their prey, a method occasionally used by jaguars and leopards. Big cats also claw their prey, producing deep parallel incised wounds.

Wound care is the same as for other species, with special attention paid to the occurrence of major internal injury. In particular, penetration of deep structures of the cranium and neck should be sought, and injuries of the cervical spine and deep cervical vessels ruled out (Box 40-1).[70] Typical is a patient with an apparently trivial puncture wound after a bite to the neck from a pet cougar; she was discharged from the emergency department.[229] Within hours her voice was hoarse; on return she recalled that the cougar had shaken her in its jaws when it bit her, and air was found in the prevertebral and retropharyngeal spaces on x-ray examination.

Like domestic cats, big cats usually carry *Pasteurella* as normal flora, and because of the deep penetration of their large teeth, *Pasteurella* septic arthritis, meningitis, and other serious deep infections can occur.[43,232,436] Most information about bites from large feline carnivores is anecdotal. Tiger bites, for example, seem commonly to become infected with *Pseudomonas* (E. Fowler, personal communication, 1980).

Thanks to the growing propensity for people of developed countries to keep exotic animals as pets (or raise them for profit for hunting purposes), injuries by big cats can occur anywhere. In a series reported from 1971 to 1981, before this practice became popular, seven lion bites were posted in the United States, four bites by tigers, and two by leopards.[342] Since no systematic method of collecting these data is available, this probably represents significant underreporting, since in recent years the raising of big cats has exploded in popularity.

Tigers

Adult tigers are so powerful that the victim is often killed instantly. It is not unusual for a limb to be severed with a single bite. A swiping blow to the human head can cause a skull fracture.[326] Like many of the big cats, tigers typically strike without warning from behind, biting the head and neck and often shaking their head violently to sever the victim's spinal cord.[232]

The big cats are a major threat to the lives of humans in the cats' native regions.[69] Although the number of tigers in the world is dwindling rapidly, they still remain the number one animal killer of humans (Table 40-2). Nonetheless, man-killing is almost invariably the result of stress, such as wounds or old age, that forces the animal to adopt this alien diet. A tiger subsisting solely on human meat would have to kill approximately 60 adults a year, and documented cases in selected regions have approached this rate over periods of up to 8 years. Man-eaters in India between 1906 and 1941 ate an estimated average of 125 persons each, and one had killed 436 persons. However, unlike lions, tigers are not thought to become exclusive man-eaters.

Over the last five centuries an estimated 1 million people have been eaten by tigers. Entire districts have been depopulated and villages abandoned. In the nineteenth century the tigers' toll in India averaged 2000 victims a year. From 1930 to 1940 the annual number never dropped below 1300. In the late 1940s this rate dropped to about 800 a year, where it remains. At the same time, approximately 17,000 people per year are killed in India by other wild beasts, which include nonmammalian species.

Lions

Despite their appearance and reputation, lions are not as greatly feared or respected by experienced hunters as tigers. Recent studies in Zimbabwe have shown that lions are primarily scavengers, making fewer original kills than hyenas.

A threatening gesture or shout may repel a lion, although a lioness guarding her cubs is more likely to attack. Experienced hunters find that when a charging lion is faced head on and confronted, it will often turn tail and run.[69] An intended victim who flees is most likely to be attacked. Walking unarmed in lion country is usually safe; the majority of hunters who succumb to lions are killed by wounded or sorely provoked animals, usually in dense brush. Many who survive the initial mauling die later of infection. Details of their treatment are not available. Persons who have survived attacks state that it is unwise to struggle and that the cat should be allowed to chew on an arm or other extremity. With luck, it will lose interest and leave.

Occasionally, man-eating lions appear, particularly in central Africa. Lions are estimated to eat 300 to 500 Africans a year. This cat is ranked second to tigers among man-eaters. Conversion to man-eating has been blamed on drought, famine, and human epidemics in which large numbers of corpses are abandoned in the bush. Lions that become man-eaters and subsist exclusively on human flesh need approximately 40 victims a year to stay alive. They usually kill instantly with one bite in the head or neck or with a swipe of the paw, which can break an ox's neck. Lions have tremendous strength and can easily carry victims for a mile without rest.

Although most lions in captivity become passive and dull, circus and zoo lions periodically kill attendants. Many such deaths have occurred when keepers accidentally have backed into or trod on an animal.

Leopards

Most leopard attacks are provoked by wounds or by a dog attack. When wounded, trapped, or cornered, a leopard is unpredictable and ruthless, attacking the first person to come within striking distance. Unmolested and in normal health, it is a shy and nervous animal with a marked fear of humans. Unlike a lion or tiger, which often kills by cuffing a victim with a tremendous blow, the leopard relies on fast clawwork and biting. Like the jaguar, the leopard may go for the neck (in an effort to sever the spinal cord) or attempt disemboweling by raking at the victim's abdomen with the claws. The leopard seems inclined to retreat when much resistance is offered, even in encounters with baboons. There are some well-documented instances of an unarmed man fighting and killing an attacking leopard. Before the era of antibiotics, three fourths of people mauled by leopards died from wound infection, but today morbidity is estimated to be less than 10%.[69]

Mauling is much more common than killing; estimated casualties are 400 a year, mostly in Africa. The leopard does not often turn man-eater; when it does, it attacks mainly children or sick adults. In the state of Bihar in India, leopards ate 300 people in 1959 and 1960.[69] The man-eating leopard of Rudraprayag in India killed 150 people between 1918 and 1926. Becoming increasingly bold, it eventually took its prey by banging down doors, leaping through windows, or clawing its way through the walls of mud huts. Like man-eating lions, man-eating leopards completely change their normal hunting pattern when their prey becomes exclusively human.

Cougars and Other Big Cats

The North American cougar (mountain lion or puma) is a clever and basically shy cat. It is the most widely distributed large animal on the American continent. However, in recent years cougars are encroaching with increasing frequency into populated areas of the western United States, probably because of both human expansion into the wilderness and the increased population of protected cougars.[231] The cougar population in California alone is now estimated at 5000, and humans with increasing frequency live, exercise, or picnic in cougar country. The result is that modern suburban dwellers (who typically are ignorant of wild animal behavior) are now in regular close contact with cougars in their homes and parks—whether they know it or not.

Only 66 cougar attacks on humans were documented between 1750 and 1985; a third were fatal.[229] Most of these attacks occurred in the western United States and Canada. Throughout the United States, cougars took sixteenth place as causes of death in recent years, just behind jellyfish or goats.[337] In California, no attacks occurred from 1925 to 1986, when two children were attacked in a regional park in southern California.[229] In 1989 a 5-year-old in Montana was killed by a 60-pound "kitten." Young animals that are forced out by adults and must find their own turf are the most frequent offenders in attacks on humans.[231] Hunters or joggers have been attacked by cougars who probably mistook them for nonhuman prey. Children are the preferred victims, and frequently the offending animal is a pet cougar.[175,229] This emphasizes again the risk of wild animals as pets, and perhaps the cougar in particular. There has been only one alleged report of a cougar as a primary man-eater, but cougars have sometimes partially eaten victims of their attacks.

Despite the rarity of attacks, cougars receive a great deal of attention in the popular press, which has led to demands for their elimination. A 5-year-old in California who wandered off in a park and was mauled by a cougar was the focus of a lawsuit in which the court found that visitors had not been adequately warned of the dangers and awarded the victim \$2 million.[337] The result has been that the park must now post signs advising visitors that actual wild animals live there, and children are banned from the park.

Like other big cats, the cougar hunts like a domestic cat: crouching, slinking, sprinting, pouncing, and then breaking the prey's neck. The types of injuries to the neck are similar to those described for lions and tigers. Like many potentially dangerous wild animals, the cougar can often be scared off by the victim's aggressive behavior, even after the attack has begun.[191]

As is the case with all cats, big and small, *Pasteurella* is a frequent pathogen in cougar bite.[229]

The jaguar is a shy animal that usually avoids humans, although it has killed humans.[70] The cheetah is the most amiable of all the large cats and has reportedly never killed a human. A few attacks have been reported, but none with severe effects.

Human Bites

Although humans would not be considered to fall into the category of domestic feral animals, human bite injury certainly can occur in any environment in which this aggressive species is endemic. Human bites account for 3.6% to 23% of all bites seen by urban physicians (Table 40-1). By contrast, in a rural population only 0.03% of bites are human. Human bites differ from others in that they may be more contaminated, and their circumstances lead to bites in high-risk areas of the body and to delayed treatment.

At least 42 different species of bacteria have been reported in human saliva[261]; total anaerobes measure 1×10^8/ml of saliva, while streptococci measure 2×10^7, and *Staphylococcus* and *Bacteroides* measure 5×10^3. Coliform bacteria measure 2×10^2, and *Actinomyces* and *Proteus* number fewer than 100.[255] One hundred ninety species have been found when gingivitis or periodontitis is present.[282,283] *Eikenella corrodens,* a fastidious, slow-growing, gram-negative anaerobic rod, is found in 59% of plaque samples in humans, but only 0.3% of saliva samples.[169] Plaque is found deep in the gingiva and probably is seldom transmitted via a bite, so tooth scrapings (8.2% *Eikenella*) and saliva (0.6%) are much more representative of the typical human population.[339] *Veillonella parvula* is a common isolate.[340]

Virtually all bacteriologic studies of actual infection caused by human bites are of the hand, which follow a different clinical course than human bites elsewhere on the body. These studies suggest that hand infections from human bites usually involve a wider spectrum of pathogens than other animal bites. Thirty-one percent of human bite wounds of the hand are infected with gram-negative organisms, and 43% are infected with mixed gram-positive and gram-negative organisms. In some series up to 89% of infections have been with multiple organisms.[98] In a recent large series human bite infections were polymicrobial in 92% of cases, with an average of five isolates per wound.[98] Although *Staphylococcus* or β-hemolytic *Streptococcus* were found in 72% of bite infections (no different from nonbite hand infections), the incidence of aerobic and facultative gram-negative rods (25%) and anaerobic bacteria (43%) was much higher in the former.[98] Gram-negative bacilli are found in 30% to 60% of wounds in diabetics with hand infection.[153,261]

The single most frequent aerobic organism is *Streptococcus,* and the next most frequent is *S. aureus,* which has been most strongly associated with the major infectious complications in older case series.[153,259] However, one bacteriologic study found streptococci in 50%, *S. aureus* in 38%, and *E. corrodens* in 29% of human bite wounds of the hand.[160] Another study found that *S. aureus* and *Peptostreptococcus anaerobius* accounted for 42% of infections.[349] A variety of other organisms have been seen in smaller numbers, including *E. corrodens, Bacteroides,* anaerobic cocci, *Fusobacterium* species, and *Peptostreptococcus.*[38,166] *Pasteurella, Bacteroides,* and *Pseudomonas* are uncommon.[38]

A number of studies suggest that human bite wounds in the hand are more likely to involve anaerobic pathogens than other causes of hand infection. Eighty-three percent of infections yielded both aerobic and anaerobic bacteria in one study,[38] but a larger series found such combinations in only 26%.[394] Infection is thought to be more virulent when anaerobes are present[163]; 26% of wounds with mixed aerobes and anaerobes developed complications in one large series, but only 10% of those with aerobes alone.[394] Another series found a worsened outcome when either anaerobes or *Eikenella* was present.[98] The clinical significance of this is uncertain, however, because none of these studies compared this bacteriologic spectrum to that in hand infections from nonbite injuries. In the only large study that did, the incidence of pure anaerobic infection was higher in traumatic, drug injection, and animal bite hand wounds than in human bite wounds; the incidence of mixed aerobic and anaerobic infection was only slightly higher in human bite wounds, and the incidence of gram-negative and gram-positive organisms did not differ significantly.[394] The relationship of anaerobes in these wounds may be opportunistic because it is commonly observed that antibiotics do not need to cover every single pathogen present to be clinically effective in resolving infection (Table 40-4).

Human bites can transmit systemic diseases. Transmission of actinomycosis, syphilis, tuberculosis, herpes, hepatitis C, and hepatitis B has been documented by the human bite route.[284,344,399] Herpetic whitlow (infection of the distal phalanx) from herpes simplex virus is a well-known occupational hazard of nurses, physicians, dentists, and oral hygienists.[215] Although herpetic whitlow can be acquired by fingernail biting and from salivary excretions of others, bites by infected children (in particular) are a common source of infection. Health care workers are at high risk for this infection because of their exposure and the fact that they are less likely to have antibodies to herpes virus than the general population. Toxic shock has also been reported after a clenched fist injury.[250]

Although human immunodeficiency virus (HIV, HLTV-III) is secreted at some time in the saliva of up to 44% of patients infected with this organism, human bites are not considered by the CDC to carry a risk of transmission.[179,242] Chiefly, this is because HIV is not usually present in the saliva of infected patients, and when it is, the titer of virus is very low.[344] A factor that reduces the risk of transmission is that most persons with AIDS secrete antibody to the virus in their saliva.[8,9] So far no cases of transmission by bite wound have been reported. Small numbers of patients have been bitten by HIV-positive individuals, none of whom have become infected.[344] Probably the most reassuring fact is that even after parenteral exposure to blood via needlestick wounds (which contains up to 20 HIV-infected lymphocytes, far more than any saliva sample ever could), the HIV infection rate is extremely low—less than 1%.[344]

Unfortunately, in the past authorities have had the same view of several other potential exposures that eventually turned out to be documented routes of transmission, and transmission of simian AIDS by saliva from infected animals has been proved.[176] Recent studies have shown that cell-free HIV exists in the plasma of infected persons. Furthermore, particularly in a fight or with physical contact, saliva can easily be contaminated with blood, which clearly is infectious. Toothbrushing or kissing can cause blood to appear in saliva, but the amount of blood is small and theoretically could expose the victim to only one HIV-infected lymphocyte.[344] HIV transmission through skin contact with blood during fights or soccer matches has been reported.

The prudent conclusion seems to be that bites from infected or high-risk persons (homosexual men, intravenous drug users, hemophiliacs, recipients of multiple transfusions before 1985, and possibly prostitutes) should be considered a low but real risk for HIV and AIDS transmission. Victims of such bites should receive unusually vigorous and thorough wound irrigation with virucidal agents such as 1% povidone-iodine, and it may be worth considering a baseline HIV blood test and a follow-up test in 6 months for medicolegal purposes and for reassurance. Human bites inflicted by the low-risk population do not warrant such testing. Also worth repeating is that the physician working on any bite victim should be fully gloved, wear protective eyewear, and avoid unprotected contact with body fluids, since virtually any patient may be seropositive for HIV.

As with other types of bites, recommending that all human bite wounds be treated in one particular fashion is simplistic. Human bite wounds have long had a bad reputation for infection.[183,261] However, this reputation is not fully deserved, since it is largely dependent on selection bias in the reported studies. In most of the cases reported over the years, human bites involved predominantly the hand, their treatment was markedly delayed (24 hours to 6 days), and they were already infected when treatment was sought.[261] All these factors dramatically increase the risk of infection in any wound and have not been characteristic of reported series of animal bites; thus these results may not be related directly to the human mouth and teeth.

Children are frequently both the inflicters and the recipients of bite wounds; in a study of day care centers, 46% of children were bitten in a year's time.[147] The vast majority of these bites occur on an upper extremity, and 75% are superficial abrasions, none of which become infected.[13] In this series of 322 bites, punctures and lacerations both had an infection rate of 37%, but almost all the infections were already present when the patient first sought care. Eighty percent of these children were seen within 12 hours of injury, and in this group of patients the infection rate was only 1.6%.[13] Human bites in children in another study had an infection rate of only 3.4%, probably also because most of the bites are superficial and most are seen by physicians in less than 12 hours.[374]

However, human bites in adults seem to have a much higher incidence of mixed aerobic and anaerobic infections (83% compared to 66% in animal bites[38]), which may contribute to more virulent infection. Nonetheless, a recent and definitive study of 434 human bites found an infection rate of 17.7% compared with 13.4% in 803 lacerations in the same patient group—a higher rate of infection, but not dramatically so.[248] The infection rate was slightly higher in sutured wounds in both groups, but the authors concluded that it was still reasonable to suture human bite wounds. Like other experienced clinicians, they also concluded that there are really two groups of human bite wounds: simple bites, which are no more malignant than any other bite or laceration, and the closed fist injury, or "fight bite." The latter has a high infection rate and morbidity, but because of the anatomy of the wounded area as much as the bacteriology of the wound. Human bites in locations other than the hand do not have an unusually high infection rate,[248,259,374] This is true even in complex human bite wounds of the face and ears, when they are treated aggressively with surgery and antibiotics.[403]

To the categories of fight-bite clenched fist injuries and uncomplicated bites elsewhere on the body (especially in children) should be added the category of bites in Third World countries, particularly Africa. Several unique characteristics apply to these. For one, as with many injuries in underdeveloped countries, the time before medical treatment is long, with delay of 1 to 3 weeks in published series.[93,252,275,289] As a result, patients have established and well-advanced infections and other complications when brought to medical attention. (This is reminiscent of the situation with fight-bite injuries, also largely a phenomenon of lower socioeconomic groups.) Second, many of these bites are inflicted by and on women, and many are disfiguring (sometimes amputating) bites of the lip, nose, ears, and face. The reason for this is that most are inflicted in quarrels between lovers or husbands and wives, or between rivals for another's love, and are often intended to be disfiguring. The injuries carry significant social stigma, further delaying treatment. The third important factor is that immediate first aid in many developing countries is not in accordance with First World medical principles and may worsen the situation. For example, in Africa it is customary to treat fresh bites with very hot water; patients have the finger covered with husks soaked with boiling water.[252] All of these factors produce complicated, infected wounds that require aggressive antibiotic and surgical treatment.

Traumatic love bites occur in First World countries as well, but as might be expected they come under medical care early and thus have better results. As in Africa, they tend to involve potentially disfiguring bites of face, breasts, or genitalia.

HUMAN BITES OF THE HAND (FIGHT-BITE INJURIES)

The fight-bite injury is the most common and the most high risk of human bites. From 60% to 80% of closed fist injuries are seen in males, and most occur in the dominant fist as a result of the fist's striking an opponent's tooth. In this position the extensor tendon and its underlying bursa are pulled distally over the metacarpophalangeal joint. The result is a deep laceration that can disrupt superficial and deep fasciae, the extensor tendon and its bursa, and the joint capsule. When the fingers are extended, the skin and tendon retract proximally, sealing off the contaminated wound. These anatomic relationships set the stage for the characteristic spread of infection. The sites of infection in order of frequency are the subcutaneous space of the dorsum of the hand, the fascial space of the dorsum of the proximal phalanx, the metacarpophalangeal joint, the palmar fascial spaces, and the flexor tendon sheaths.

Any penetrating injury in the vicinity of the metacarpophalangeal joint should be considered a human bite closed fist injury wound until proven otherwise. Radiographs should be obtained to look for foreign bodies, fractures, and air in joints. Up to 70% of patients undergoing x-ray examination may have positive findings.[110] Films should be obtained in a lateral or steep oblique attitude, since this is the best view for initial soft tissue swelling.[343] The ideal view is the skyline view of the metacarpal head, taken with the x-ray beam in the same plane as the proximal phalanx with the metacarpophalangeal joint fully flexed. This fully exposes the articular surface of the metacarpal head itself. In one series, half of standard finger films showed no joint involvement, but vertical articular fractures of the metacarpal head were seen in all with the skyline view.[127] Small defects in the subchondral bone plate of the metacarpal head are important early clues to penetration of bone by a tooth, and may require magnified views to be seen well. Common x-ray findings, especially with late presentation, include soft tissue swelling, periarticular osteoporosis, narrowing of the joint space, bony erosions, periostitis, air, and bone fragments in the joint. Fourth and fifth metacarpal fractures may point to punching activity and be a further clue to the origin of wounds.

Morbidity seems to be most clearly related to the delay until medical care. Treatment should optimally be initiated as soon as possible and no later than 12 hours after injury.[412] Of all human bite wounds of the hand, 60% are uninfected when originally seen; 21% are superficially infected with local tenderness or inflammation; 15% are moderately infected with a stiff, swollen, tender finger or hand, cellulitis, lymphangitis and purulent drainage; and only 1% are severely infected, with inability to move a hand or fingers and involvement of deep hand structures.[259] Tenosynovitis and septic arthritis are serious complications.

Treatment of clenched fist injuries should be aggressive. Although debriding them significantly is generally not possible, they should be thoroughly irrigated with 5% povidone-iodine solution and should not be sutured. Although it is reasonable to suture human bites elsewhere on the body for cosmetic reasons,[248,374] tradition has dictated avoidance of suturing on the hand. However, in a study of infected human bites of the hand, sutured wounds had no difference in complications or eventual outcome from those not sutured, putting this practice in some question.[28] Since few cosmetic indications for primary repair of hand bites exist, suturing should probably be avoided until a definitive study is reported in the literature. Soaks and compresses of 1% povidone-iodine solution three to four times a day are useful adjuncts for particularly large, open wounds. (Continued exposure to povidone-iodine carries little risk of significant systemic absorption in this case because of the small surface area of the wounds.) The affected extremity should be elevated with a sling and immobilized by packing the palm of the hand with bulky gauze and wrapping the hand in a mitten-type dressing.

Subsequent treatment depends largely on the time since wounding and the likelihood of compliance by the patient. Wounds seen less than 24 hours after injury and with no overt signs of infection can be treated on an outpatient basis.[409] Oral antibiotic therapy has been shown to be just as effective as parenteral therapy in this clinical situation and should result in a very low infection rate.[447] Patients with any degree of infection beyond very limited local wound cellulitis should be hospitalized with the same treatment plus intravenous antibiotics. In the majority of patients with established infection, surgical procedures are needed as well.[98] In particular, redness, swelling, and tenderness of large areas of the hand, as well as pain on passive range of motion, indicate the need for admission. (However, one experienced physician hospitalized only 6% of patients despite infection in more than 50%, and reported good results.[110])

Patient compliance is an important factor; many of the classic studies have been done in inner city hospitals on patients with poor compliance and low educational status. Such patients may warrant admission for social rather than medical reasons. However, in several large studies, up to half of the patients were treated within 12 hours of injury as outpatients and no complications developed.[67,259] By contrast, wounds treated late usually have complications at the first visit and have an average morbidity of 87 days.[110] Even established hand infections can be treated on an outpatient basis if patients are reliable in following the treatment regimen. In a series of 160 cases, a third of which were caused by bites and half of which needed outpatient surgery such as incision and drainage, all persons were treated as outpatients with oral antibiotics and did well.[395] None had to be admitted for treatment of further complications, and no osteitis, septic arthritis, or tendon sheath infection developed.

Controlled studies of prophylactic antibiotics in nonbite wounds of the hand show no benefit.[181,189,285,438] However, no controlled studies have been done in human bites of the hand, and most authors are emphatic in recommending prophylactic antibiotics. Nonetheless, large series in the literature report good results with no antibiotics.[110] Since *Staphylococcus* and *Streptococcus* account for most of the infections, cephalosporins appear to be a rational initial antibiotic choice for outpatients; they cover many gram-negative bacteria as well.[28]

A cephalosporin regimen would not be effective against *Eikenella corrodens,* an unusual fastidious anaerobe seen in 7% to 29% of human bite hand infections (Tables 40-4 and 40-8).[98,160] (In a much larger series of infections from a variety of trauma including bites, *Eikenella* was found in less than 1% of wounds.[395]) *Eikenella* produced serious complications in 80% of patients with significant infection; 10% required amputation.[371] Conventional wisdom has stated, based on older studies, that penicillin should be added to the antibiotic regimen because *Eikenella* is resistant to dicloxacillin, clindamycin, aminoglycosides, clindamycin, and many first-generation cephalosporins and is always sensitive to penicillin or a second-generation cephalosporin (Tables 40-4 and 40-8). It is also sensitive to tetracycline, ampicillin, and carbenicillin.[160] However, recent studies call this into question, because up to 18% of *Eikenella* is now penicillin resistant.[340] These studies also found that 82% of *Eikenella* was susceptible to cephalothin (the same as penicillin), and 100% to second- and third-generation cephalosporins (including cefuroxime, cefoxitin, ceftazidime, and ceftriaxone). Sensitivity was also 100% to ampicillin and ciprofloxacin and 91% to erythromycin.

Thus, when antibiotics are used in human hand bite wounds, dicloxacillin plus penicillin is no longer the best choice for full coverage of both aerobic and anaerobic pathogens. Instead, a second- or third-generation cephalosporin should be used alone (Table 40-8). Cefuroxime can be given orally and is taken only twice a day; cefixime is more expensive and has a high incidence of gastrointestinal side effects, but is taken only once a day.

Antibiotic regimens in underdeveloped countries differ; cost and availability of drugs are crucial. A common and successful regimen in Africa is the use of penicillin and metronidazole,[93] sometimes with the addition of gentamicin or intravenous cloxacillin.[275] The recommended low-cost regimen in the United States would be dicloxacillin plus ampicillin.

If a patient is allergic to penicillin, the best combination in adults would be ciprofloxacin (effective against all relevant pathogens except *Streptococcus*) plus erythromycin or trimethoprim-sulfamethoxazole (Table 40-4). Another possibility is clarithromycin alone.

Culturing all infected human bite injuries of the hand is a wise practice, particularly in hospitalized or immunocompromised patients such as diabetics. When infection is already established, getting a specimen from deep within the wound, lymph nodes, or cellulitis, is important since contamination with many other organisms occurs in more superficial specimens. The commonly obtained cultures of pus from the wound are pointless because multiple contaminants that have no clinical significance are obtained. Cultures of human hand bite wounds must always include anaerobic cultures, and the laboratory should be informed of the suspected organism. *Eikenella,* for example, is very slow growing and requires special media.[160]

HUMAN BITES IN OTHER LOCATIONS

Human bite injuries in locations on the body other than the hand appear no more likely to become infected than animal bite injuries. A large series of sutured facial human bites treated in a plastic surgery clinic had an infection rate of only 2.5%,[115] compared with 14.7% in a large series of facial dog bites.[308] Even when the ear was involved, virtually no infection was present, an experience cited by other authors.[16]

Treatment includes aggressive debridement, irrigation, and suturing if anatomy permits and cosmetic considerations are important, as they invariably are on the face. Antibiotics are indicated for the same risk factors as in animal bites. Although no prospective study has been done, a retrospective study of low-risk human bite wounds in children found no benefit with prophylactic antibiotics.[374]

Facial wounds are generally of low risk. However, intraoral self-inflicted bite wounds constitute another special situation that is not well studied. Self-inflicted accidental bites of the mouth and lips may have low infection rates, possibly because of protective effects from saliva and resistance of mucosal tissues to the patient's own flora. However, a case of *Haemophilus aphrophilus* vertebral osteomyelitis has been reported in a healthy 36-year-old secondary to an accidental lip laceration of just this sort, despite his having received prophylactic antibiotics.[195] Shallow avulsion injuries with up to 40% partial-thickness loss of the lip vermilion can be treated conservatively with healing by secondary intention with good results.[444]

In one small series of patients with bites of the oral or buccal mucosa, 22% of wounds became infected.[248] In older studies, completely intraoral wounds had an infection rate of 12%, which was not affected by prophylactic antibiotics, but oral-cutaneous (through-and-through) wounds had an infection rate of 33%, which was reduced by half with antibiotics.[157] Another study from this era found no benefit to antibiotics but found a similar high infection rate in through-and-through wounds.[310] A more recent uncontrolled randomized trial of mostly minor intraoral lacerations in children found an infection rate of only 6% but noted that infection was more likely in wounds needing suturing.[5] In this study the infection rate in patients receiving prophylactic penicillin was 4%, only half that of children not receiving antibiotics, but the difference was not statistically significant.

Only one double-blinded prospective randomized trial of prophylactic antibiotics in intraoral wounds has been done, using oral penicillin given just before suturing in adults with wounds up to 24 hours old.[392] Nineteen percent of patients treated with placebo versus 7% treated with penicillin became infected, but this difference is not statistically significant. Interestingly, however, when patients with poor compliance are eliminated, the results were 18% versus none, respectively, which is statistically significant. As in previous studies, the infection rate in untreated through-and-through wounds is 20%, twice as high as in mucosa-only wounds. Among the small number of infected wounds, *Streptococcus* was present in 63%, *Staphylococcus aureus* in 38%, *S. epidermidis* in 38%, *Bacteroides* in 38%, *Corynebacterium* in 25%, *Neisseria* species in 13%, and *Haemophilus haemolyticus* in 13%.[392]

The literature therefore suggests that oral-cutaneous wounds are high risk and may benefit from penicillin prophylaxis. Lacerations that involve only the buccal mucosa, particularly those that do not need suturing, do not require prophylaxis. Larger randomized trials are needed to resolve the uncertainty still present. Penicillin is the recommended antibiotic because it is the only one studied, and most of the organisms are sensitive. However, *Staphylococcus* is the second most common pathogen in through-and-through lacerations and would not be treated effectively by penicillin.[392] A second-generation cephalosporin or one of the new macrolide antibiotics (such as clarithromycin) would be effective against both *Staphylococcus* and anaerobes.

FORENSIC CONSIDERATIONS OF HUMAN BITES

Human bite marks are relatively distinctive, although particularly after a delay they can mimic certain dermatologic conditions such as drug eruptions, pityriasis rosea, tinea corporis, and granuloma annulare.[156] Acute bites are distinctive and have considerable forensic significance, since in many cases assault or abuse of children, a spouse, or the elderly may be at issue. The examining physician should document the appearance of the bite carefully, including its shape, color, and size. Determining the age of the bite can be difficult and is often a critical legal issue; accurate description is better than unsupported speculation. The physician must determine at this point if he or she thinks a criminal act may have occurred; if so, evidence should be collected in the form of photographs of the wound area, salivary swabbings from the wound, tissue samples, and dental impressions from the bite surface if necessary.[155] Since most physicians are not familiar with these procedures, consultation with a forensic pathologist or dentist is recommended and may be arranged through the local police department.

Rodent Bites

Rodents do not tend to bite unless severely provoked; their bites are usually small and do not cause much disability. The exact number of rodents in the world is unknown, but they probably number in the hundreds of millions, with 1500 species of laboratory and pet rodents. Despite these numbers they account for only 1.7% to 10% of animal bites brought to medical attention.[302] The reasons for poor reporting may be that such bites are infrequent in occurrence, seldom cause any problems for the victim, or often occur among lower socioeconomic groups that do not have good access to medical attention. The other human populations at risk are owners of pet rodents and laboratory workers who handle rodents used in research. Insufficient data exist to determine any difference in outcome between wild and domestic rat bites.

Rat bites show an infection rate of 2% to 10%, even without treatment, and the rate is usually on the low end of this spectrum.[143,228,302] Other than bites inflicted by laboratory animals, the vast majority occur in poverty areas while the victim is sleeping and involve the face and neck, usually in infants.[302] Sometimes these can be severe; a week-old infant was bitten around the eyes by a rat, resulting in perforations of the globe, an estimated vascular loss of 55% of red blood cell mass (with an initial hematocrit value of 20%), and eventual blindness.[293] Despite the rat's reputation for spreading disease, however, infection did not occur. Similar bites in infants have resulted in loss of more than three fourths of the eyelids.[443]

The bacteriology is the same as for other animal species, and the various systemic diseases transmitted by rats are summarized in Table 40-5. Rat-bite fever was discussed earlier. Sporotrichosis has been reported; this widely distributed saprophyte is found on a variety of plants, in the soil, and on many animals.[142,357]

Although rodents can occasionally become infected with rabies, they seldom secrete this virus in saliva; therefore they inflict extremely low-risk bites for transmission of the disease. However, local epidemics do occur, as is currently taking place among rodents and lagomorphs on the east coast of the United States.[286] In that epidemic, woodchucks constituted 80% of all rabid animals; the remainder were squirrels, beavers, rabbits (lagomorphs, not rodents), and one rat. Some of these rabid animals were very aggressive; a woodchuck attacked and knocked down an elderly woman in her garden, biting her repeatedly. Rabies was isolated from the buccal cavity. A reasonable current recommendation is that a biting wild rat in the United States should be caught and examined for rabies and rabies immunoprophylaxis initiated only if the rabies test is positive; rabies immunoprophylaxis is probably appropriate for bites of uncaptured rodents inflicted outside of the United States and Canada.[302]

A case has been reported of a cowpox virus–like infection transmitted by a probable rat bite.[325] Rodents are believed to be the natural reservoir for cowpox virus.

Ferret Bites

European ferrets *(Mustela putorius)* are descended from the polecat, a member of the weasel, mink, and wolverine family with a reputation for being extremely bloodthirsty.[74] (The European ferret should not be confused with the black-footed ferret, an endangered species indigenous to the United States.) Ferrets were bred to hunt and kill rats and rabbits in their holes, so the ferocity of the polecat was a desirable feature that in fact is regularly cross-bred back into ferrets. In addition to being bred for hunting ability and bloodthirstiness, ferrets were bred to return to their owners and thus to have no fear of humans. They therefore must be actively trained not to bite their owners or keepers, a characteristic they share with other wild species with similar upbringing, such as wolves, coyotes, raccoons, and ocelots. All of these have a very high incidence of biting relative to dogs and have killed humans.

Ferrets pose a particular problem because they have been bred not only to be unafraid of humans, but also to be extremely ferocious and tenacious with prey.[74] This means that when intent on attacking prey or when cornered, members of this family show no fear and aggressively approach even an armed human, an experience unnerving even when it involves only a 6-pound animal. Because of its speed, an attacking ferret can easily run over the shoulders and head of an adult human and inflict 20 to 40 bites without stopping.[74]

Until recently, ferrets were kept largely by hunters who appreciated their killer instincts and who had no illusions about their trustworthiness. Recently, however, ferrets have joined the list of wild animals being kept as fashionable pets by city dwellers in developed countries with little or no understanding of the spectrum of animal behavior. Ferrets are an increasingly popular urban pet, with about 50,000 to 75,000 being bred annually in the United States for that purpose.[416] An estimated 100,000 or more pet ferrets live in California alone,[74] and an estimated 1 million are kept in the entire United States as pets.[306] Unfortunately, like many other largely wild animals, they have far less predictable behavior than those that have been domesticated for tens of thousands of years, and they have a number of characteristics that make them remarkably unsuitable for pets.

The rate of ferret bites in California (where they are illegal) is about 27 per year; it is about 25 times higher in states where they are legal. The ferret lobby (consisting of loyal owners and breeders who profit from their sales) is constantly lobbying to make them legal everywhere. Whether their incidence of biting is greater than housecats is not known, but one survey suggests that it is the same (0.3% of the ferret population inflicting bites during approximately 1 year).[306]

However, it is the characteristics of ferret bites that raise concern. Ferrets seem to have a particular propensity for unprovoked attacks on the faces of unattended infants.[416] In a comprehensive review of 452 ferret attacks over 10 years, virtually all the unprovoked attacks fell into this category.[74] Most victims were less than 3 years of age, and 91% of the victims were attacked while sleeping or lying down, one with fatal consequences and several nearly fatal. Forty-eight percent were bitten on the head only, and 71% on the head or neck and limbs. The face was the most frequent location for bites of the head. Only 5% of victims were bitten only once; many victims had dozens of bites, and several had 80 to 200 bites. In several cases this number of bites occurred despite the efforts of a witnessing adult to prevent them.[306] People lost entire noses, ears, lips, or eyelids. Tissue is frequently eaten. In at least three cases the ferret's jaws had to be pried open to release the victim; in other cases the ferret had to be killed to remove it.[306] Twenty-eight percent of the victims required major plastic and reconstructive surgery. Thirty-three percent of the biting ferrets were pets in the victim's own household, and the vast majority of the remainder were also pets (not strays).[74]

Why ferrets have such a propensity for attacking infants is unknown, but this resembles their completely instinctive killing of infant animals, which is unaffected by previous training. Sucking or squeaking sounds that resemble those of rabbits in pain stimulate attacks by many kinds of predators, including ferrets. Suckling rabbits are a favorite prey of ferrets in the wild. Similarly, ferrets instinctively go for the neck of prey, often tenaciously holding on while drinking blood, regardless of previous training. Ferrets and polecats sometimes display frenzy behavior in nature, slaughtering animals regardless of number, hunger, or ability to eat.

Provoked attacks generally occur in awake older humans and frequently involve feral or stray animals, consisting of just a single bite to an extremity.

Ferrets are unusually adept at escaping from cages and enclosures, guaranteeing that they will occasionally be loose unsupervised in the house and also that they can escape to the wild, where they will be exposed to endemic rabies. On recapture or return they often bite, necessitating rabies prophylaxis in 22%. Four percent of biting ferrets were positive for rabies virus.[74] Not only can ferrets transmit rabies, but as yet no effective and approved rabies vaccine exists for them. Therefore they cannot be prevented from becoming infected. Live rabies vaccines cannot be used, since they produce rabies in some wild carnivores. The incubation period of rabies in ferrets is unknown (as are the clinical signs), so any biting animal should be destroyed and examined immediately. This is particularly true because facial bites are more likely to induce rabies than are bites at other locations, and the incubation period is dramatically shortened.

Unfortunately, as is the case with other exotic wild animal pets, owners of ferrets (whose ownership is illegal in California and many other states) have agitated aggressively in the press for the legal right to raise these animals. Human loyalty to pets sometimes seems to overcome common sense; a mother whose ferret had attacked both her newborn infant and the face of a neighbor's infant succeeded in preventing the destruction of the animal by state authorities, reportedly declaring that she would rather destroy the child because she had possessed the ferret longer.[74]

In addition to the fact that they are bloodthirsty and essentially untamed, ferrets pose serious threats to native wildlife and small livestock when they escape, which they do frequently. They also pose a risk as a significant rabies vector. Therefore their use as pets is strongly discouraged by a wide variety of wildlife, veterinary, and humane organizations.

Nothing is specifically known of infection rates or bacteriology in ferret-inflicted wounds, despite the extensive data on bites. Presumably, treatment would be the same as for dog bites. Unusual species such as *Mycobacterium bovis*, seldom anticipated by physicians, may be pathogens.[216] Owners of ferrets should be advised to get rid of them (humanely, not by releasing them), and this should be mandatory and immediate with small children in the home.

Opossum Bites

The American opossum *(Didelphis virginiana)* inflicts bite injuries both when hunted for food and when accidentally provoked while handled in captivity. Aerobically cultured organisms from the mouths of seven wild opossums included streptococci, coagulase-positive and coagulase-negative staphylococci, *Aeromonas* species, *Citrobacter freundii*, *E. corrodens*, and *Escherichia coli*.[204] No literature is available on the bites themselves.

Monkey and Ape Bites

Monkeys and other primates have an informal reputation for inflicting vicious bites, which virtually always become infected (M.E. Fowler, University of California–Davis, personal communication, 1981). Although in developed countries this is largely an issue for laboratory workers, in tropical undeveloped countries, large apes (such as baboons) are not only common, but often aggressive. Weighing up to 90 pounds, a large baboon can be dangerous and lethal. These animals have frequent contact with humans and lose most fear of them. A similar situation occurs in parks and memorials where monkeys or apes are tolerated and large numbers of tourists come to visit. Here a situation of exposure (and ignorance on the part of tourists) arises that is reminiscent of the bear and buffalo problem in North America. In Malaysia a band of 60 monkeys at the botanical gardens attacked joggers and visitors who were wearing yellow clothing, because the previous day youths wearing yellow shirts had stoned a baby monkey to death.[281]

Monkeys often bite the hands and have been known to amputate parts of fingers. Unfortunately, the credible published reports cover only 13 patients, 15% of whom became infected.[108,228] Like much of the literature on uncommon animal bites, many of the studies suffer from poor scientific quality and follow-up rates as low as 3%.[54] Infecting organisms have not been reported.[378] The sole exception was a laboratory worker with a rapidly progressing cellulitis after a finger bite, from whom *E. corrodens* was cultured.[210] At the present time these bites should be considered relatively high risk and treated in the same fashion as human bites.

Old World macaque monkeys (rhesus macaques, cynomolgus, and other Asiatic macaque monkeys) are often infected with simian herpes virus (B virus); the classic symptoms are the same as human herpes virus type I, but infection and carrier state can be undetectable clinically.[307] Transmission to humans is rare and only 24 cases are reported, but most of them developed encephalitis, and 18 have died.[77,307] One case of person-to-person transmission has been reported.[77] Only a few human victims have had a total recovery from the illness, and the impression is that infection is nearly always fatal.[307] However, as with rabies, local wound treatment may be important; in a series of 61 persons bitten by probably infectious monkeys and receiving wound cleansing with cetrimide and iodine solution, none became infected.[413]

Exposed humans treated with acyclovir have had a mild course with full recovery, and as a result, the CDC recommends that humans with bite exposure to monkeys with this virus or with clinical syndromes suggestive of herpes virus be treated prophylactically with acyclovir 400 mg, five times a day[33] (unpublished guidelines, Jonathan Kaplan, M.D., CDC). They also recommend that even if the monkey appears asymptomatic, a victim with a deep penetrating wound that cannot be cleansed thoroughly should receive prophylactic acyclovir, 800 mg orally five times a day, unless the entire monkey colony is known and certified to have been tested for herpes B and to be virus free. Immune globulin has not been shown to be effective. The biting monkey should be quarantined, examined, and tested for active infection; if none, the acyclovir can be stopped. If the animal is positive, continuing the acyclovir indefinitely may be necessary to continue suppression of the virus. However, this is a controversial area, and infectious disease consultation should be obtained. Physicians should contact the Viral Exanthem and Herpesvirus Branch of the CDC, 404-639-3532, for further details. Testing of human or monkey mucosa and secretions for the virus can be arranged through the Southwest Foundation for Biomedical Research, San Antonio, Texas, 512-674-1410.

Since few physicians are familar with simian herpes B virus, and the treatment decisions are complex and immediate, any institution handling Old World macaque monkeys should have a full protocol developed describing screening and treatment in the case of human exposure, based on CDC recommendations.[78] Most animal laboratories and the veterinarians in charge of them are familiar with this problem and have such protocols; they are an excellent source of information for the treating physician. The local medical treatment facility should participate in developing this protocol, which should be available at nights and on weekends when consultants are not.

The wild gorilla, despite its reputation and appearance, is shy and takes any opportunity to avoid humans. Although it may charge in defense, it seldom attacks and can be easily confronted and forced to retreat. When a gorilla attacks, it takes one bite and runs. In Africa, gorillas are responsible for two to three attacks per year, none of which are fatal and few of which are severe. Chimpanzees occasionally attack humans, usually only if provoked or cornered. Rare instances of chimpanzees eating children and women have been reported. The baboon is responsible for one to two attacks per year, almost all in South Africa; these are usually by pets. Occasionally, man-eating has been reported. The incidence of hunting and meat eating by these animals has increased over the last century, perhaps paralleling the evolution of humans into hunters and meat eaters.[69]

Attacks by Coyotes, Wolves, and Hyenas

The coyote has not only survived the onslaught of civilization in the United States, but has thrived and multiplied. Perhaps as a result, more and more coyote attacks on people have been reported, even in urban areas such as Los Angeles.[65] Occasionally these animals are rabid, but most are not, and some attacks (especially on small children) are fatal.[414]

As a predator of humans, the wolf has a contradictory history. No significant problems or killings have been reported in North America, where wolves are traditionally timid. However, throughout Europe and Asia the wolf has a well-documented history of cunning behavior, pack attacks, and human-killing. European wolves tend to hunt in packs and attack women and children. In 1712, 100 persons in France were killed by wolves, a typical toll for the time. In December 1927 the Siberian village of Pilovo was besieged by hundreds of starving wolves that not only attacked and ate all the human beings and animals found outdoors but actually broke down doors of homes to attack and kill humans in their cottages. Only the arrival of the army prevented total extermination of the inhabitants. In a single year in the 1960s, wolves killed 10,000 horses, 35,000 head of livestock, and 26,000 poultry in Russia. That same year, 168 people were attacked, 112 of whom were killed.[69] In 1968, in one winter week in Iran, 18 people were eaten by hungry wolves. Rabid wolves are still seen; a substantial number of attacks by rabid wolves in Iran in the last 10 years provided the clinical population on which the human diploid cell vaccine for rabies was tested.[10]

Two other canines that traditionally hunt in packs are the cape hunting dog of Africa and the Indian "devil dog." Although both are feared in their respective environments, they are not deliberate attackers of humans.

Hyenas have tremendously strong jaws and can leave teeth marks in forged steel. In a circus act a hyena was able to chew up and eat a 2-inch wooden plank covered with horse fat.[69] The hyena frequently attacks humans in Africa. In certain areas Africans leave the dead or dying in the bush for predators (hyenas) to eat, which accustoms the animals to the taste of human meat. Hyenas forage around campsites and villages and are wary of awake people. During the summer months when Africans sleep outside their huts, many of them are assaulted with one clean, massive bite that removes the face or the entire head. Campers too are frequently bitten on the face or limbs while they sleep at night, particularly if they have left food around. They usually survive but are massively disfigured. As with other species, an occasional hyena becomes a man-eater. In some parts of Africa the hyena is a more consistent man-eater than the leopard or lion.

Bear Attacks

The public's image of bears is complex, in part because of the varied behavior of bears. They can be delightful, entertaining, playful, caring, doleful, intelligent, powerful, and vicious.[379] The latter characteristics are both fascinating and terrifying, for the image of the bear as a "man-eater" ignites our most primitive and visceral emotion toward the feared bear.

Although bear-inflicted injuries are rare, the psychologic impact of widespread media that sensationalize the horror and gore appears to inflate their frequency and significance.[85,221] Every attack, regardless of the extent of injuries, is traditionally referred to as a "mauling," and this term itself supports the "bearanoia" that many people have, particularly when they visit bear country.

Being injured and sometimes killed by a wild animal is not considered an acceptable form of injury by most members of modern American society. This attitude and the fear of bears may affect how people use wilderness areas where bears typically live, or their attitudes toward the conservation of bears and their habitat. Having a better understanding of bear attacks not only helps reduce these incidences, but also assists in managing bears and their habitat and assists physicians in treating bear attack victims.

Bears are one of the most widely distributed animals in the world. As a result of its evolutionary adaptation to a variety of habitats, at least one of the eight bear species can be found on every continent, with the exception of Australia. (The koala bear is actually a marsupial, not a true bear.) The current North American bear taxa are limited to the subfamily Ursinae and include the black *(Ursus americanus),* brown *(Ursus arctos),* and polar bears *(Ursus maritimus).* The brown bear is found in two subspecies: the grizzly bear *(U. a. horribilis)* and the Kodiak bear *(U. middendorfi)* of the Alaskan islands of Kodiak, Shuyak, and Afognak.[338]

NORTH AMERICAN BEARS

Grizzly bears are larger and more heavily built than most other ursids, with adults weighing 147 to 386 kg.[45] Polar bears are similar in size and weight but are more elongated in shape. Black bears have the same general shape of grizzly bears but are generally smaller than both polar and grizzly bears. Average weights range from 60 to 140 kg for adult females and 250 to 300 kg for adult males.

Dentition in these three species is bunodont and reflects their omnivorous diet, although polar bears are the most carnivorous of the three. Their canine teeth are sturdy and can reach a length of 7 cm. Their legs are of approximately equal length and taper to large plantigrade feet. The foreclaws of a grizzly bear are heavier, longer, and straighter than those of a black bear and can reach a length of 83 mm measured along the external curvature.[398] A large muscular hump overlies the scapulae of grizzly bears, giving additional strength to the forelimbs for digging.

The physical strength of bears is well known, and they can run up to 40 mph over irregular terrain. They have a keen sense of hearing and an even keener sense of smell, but their eyesight has been described as poor.[193] However, many field researchers believe that bears can actually see quite well, perhaps as well as humans, and are especially adept at detecting movement. Some evidence suggests that grizzly bears have good night vision.[143]

Grizzly and black bears hibernate about 5 months during the winter, an evolutionary adaptation to reduced food availability. The hibernation of polar bears is slightly different, since their primary food (seals) is available during the winter.[294] Adult male polar bears tend to hibernate for short periods each winter in response to severe storms, whereas pregnant females have a more extended period of hibernation. During the active (nondenning) season, all bear species wander throughout a general home range in search of seasonal foods.

Grizzly Bears. The grizzly bear symbolizes wilderness in North America. It ranges from Alaska down through western Canada and into the lower 48 states in remnant populations located in relatively undeveloped federal lands, primarily in the northern Rocky Mountains.

Attacks by grizzly bears are relatively rare and sporadic. A total of 162 bear-inflicted injuries were reported from 1900 through 1985 in Canadian and North American national parks.[193,194] In Alaska, an increase in the number of people injured by grizzly bears has been seen in recent times.[277] This increase may be a result of an increase in recreational use of grizzly habitat; this trend will probably continue as more people invade grizzly habitat throughout North America.

Calculation of an accurate injury rate remains elusive. Not only were earlier records incomplete, but also defining and quantifying those at risk have always been difficult. Nonetheless, injury rates are reported based on total visitation days to the national parks in Canada and North America.[194] The average number of grizzly bear–inflicted injuries is 1 in 2,260,276 visitors to these parks combined, with a high of 1 in 317,700 visitors in Kluane National Park and a low of 1 per 6,693,859 visitors in Banff.[194] During this same time period the grizzly bear–inflicted injury rate for Yellowstone National Park was 1 in 1,543,287 visitors and for Glacier National Park was 1 in 848,180 visitors.

Obviously, not every visitor to a national park is exposed to the same risk of being attacked by a grizzly bear. To more accurately calculate an injury rate for visitors with a higher and more uniform exposure, similar rates are reported based on registered backcountry users. However, they are no more reliable for an injury index because some parks do not register backcountry use, and when they do, generally underestimate it. More important, a significant amount and perhaps majority of backcountry use (and therefore exposure) occurs from day hikers who are unregistered.

There is a seasonal variation in bear attacks (both black and grizzly) that correlates with human use of bear habitat during the active (nondenning) period for bears. The greater the number of people seeking recreation in bear country, generally from midsummer to early fall, the greater the opportunity for human-bear encounters.

Native peoples and grizzly bears occupied the same land for thousands of years in North America in what was probably a neutral coexistence, since neither side had a profound influence on the lives of the other. However, the European expansion into the west following Lewis and Clark's expedition in the early 1800s tipped the scales heavily in favor of humans, both in sheer numbers and technology, such as guns, traps, and poisons. Bears were killed in large numbers, out of fear and hatred and for protection of life and property. Most of their original habitat was occupied by either people or livestock or was dramatically altered by ranching and agricultural development.

Selection pressures that began with European expansion into the grizzly bears' habitat has probably been altering their behavior. Since that early period and even today in protected areas such as national parks, aggressive bears have been removed at a higher rate than nonaggressive bears. Bears curious about humans and human developments and those that do not readily flee the presence of humans have also been removed at a higher rate. Therefore bears that avoid humans have survived at a higher rate than these other bears and probably pass this trait on to their offspring, through either genetics or learning.

Bears' avoidance behavior is a built-in safety factor for people entering grizzly country because the vast majority of bears avoid a confrontation if given the opportunity. This fact probably explains why grizzly bear attacks on humans are so rare. Nonetheless, they occasionally occur and sometimes produce serious and even fatal injuries. Unfortunately the available data on grizzly attacks do not give an accurate description. The specific sequence of events is not always known and is subjectively reconstructed. Nonetheless, a systematic review of case histories reveals certain patterns that give insight into the nature of these incidences.

A sudden and close encounter between a grizzly bear and a person is the primary event leading to human injury. These attacks are often brief, and the bear generally leaves after it responds to a perceived threat. Although injuries are typically described as a mauling, they are generally far less severe than the bear has the potential to inflict, and victims are rarely killed after a close encounter incident. This is further evidence that the behavior of the bear in response to a close encounter is to remove a perceived threat.

A close encounter with a female with cubs is considered more dangerous, since she is more aggressive in defense of her young and is more likely to attack and cause injury. Evidence to support this hypothesis is strong. Females with young represent about 20% of a bear population but account for more than 80% of the bears that injure humans. However, another explanation to account for this disproportion is that females with young are more likely to be active during daylight hours, when humans are active; males are active primarily in the predawn hours and after dusk (S.P. French and M.G. French, Yellowstone Grizzly Foundation, unpublished data).

Grizzly bear attacks sometimes occur near a carcass on which the bear has been feeding. Grizzly bears may be more aggressive under these circumstances in defense of the carcass. However, grizzly bears of all age and sex classes have been observed to be readily displaced when they sense people approaching (S.P. French and M.G. French, Yellowstone Grizzly Foundation, unpublished data). Some bears aggressively defend a prime food source such as a carcass, but in many of these incidences the carcass simply creates an opportunity for a close encounter by keeping the bear anchored to a fixed location for prolonged periods and by keeping it preoccupied.

Another class of grizzly bear–inflicted injuries is that resulting from provoked attack. This most commonly occurs when a grizzly is injured by a hunter. Once the bear is injured, its behavioral response is no longer one of removing a threat but perhaps fighting for its life. These attacks tend to be more prolonged and aggressive, resulting in more severe injuries and deaths than close encounter attacks. Provoked attacks can also result from the direct harassment of bears by aggressive photographers trying to get too close or trying to follow a bear. Although such incidences are rare and therefore the data are too scant to draw firm conclusions, these attacks tend to resemble the response of an injured bear rather than one responding to a close encounter. The injuries photographers receive tend to be more severe, and a disproportionate number of them are killed. Up to 1985 at least ten photographers were injured, one fatally,[193] and from 1986 to 1992 at least four were injured, two fatally.

Most people attacked by grizzly bears are injured but not killed. This is important to understand because the intent of the bear is simply to remove a perceived threat, *not* to prey on the individual. From 1900 to 1979, 19 human deaths resulted from grizzly attacks documented in the national parks in North America and an additional 22 deaths occurred in Alaska outside the parks.[193,221] Some were victims of defensive attacks and probably would have survived if current medical management techniques had been available. However, some of these deaths occurred as a result of predatory attacks. The most puzzling point is not that grizzlies (or other large predators) occasionally prey on humans, but why they do not do it more often. As a potential prey species, humans are predictable and abundant, are easy to catch and kill, and are easy for a grizzly to consume. So why do bears not prey on us as part of their routine feeding behavior?

Little historical evidence suggests that grizzly bears preyed on humans except in unusual circumstances. In 1860 a smallpox epidemic struck a small band of Stonie Indians (Assiniboin Tribe) who were camped in the Yarrow Creek drainage in Alberta, Canada.[358] Grizzlies began scavenging on the dead who were left on the ground as the tribe moved to the next drainage. Grizzlies followed them to their next encampment and began preying on those who had survived. For several years thereafter the Indians avoided this area for fear of being eaten by grizzlies who had learned to prey on humans.

A major circumstance associated with grizzly bear–inflicted injuries is a history of the bear being conditioned to human foods (regularly seeking out and receiving human foods) or habituated to human presence (not readily fleeing the presence of humans). Incidences involving bears with these behavioral traits appear to have developed only in recent times, when bears have been protected from hunting in national parks and human garbage was readily available. Between 1967 and 1986, 12 deaths were inflicted by grizzly bears in Banff, Glacier, and Yellowstone National Parks. In all cases the bear was considered to be either conditioned or habituated.[193] Nine of the victims were partially consumed, and eight deaths were classified as predatory events.

The relationship between conditioning and habituation appears strong but is not conclusive. The exact bear involved in each instance was not always known, and the terms "conditioned" and "habituation" are borrowed from learning theory and have never been precisely defined by wildlife biologists. Much remains to be learned about this relationship in regard to bears that feed on human foods and do not readily flee the presence of humans. The worst-case scenario is that these bears appear to place humans within their image of prey under certain but still unknown circumstances. This potential relationship has had a significant influence on how grizzly bears are managed.

Since the time reasonably accurate records were first kept (roughly 1900), predatory attacks on humans by grizzly bears have been generally rare, sporadic, and isolated events.* However, a disturbing trend appears to have begun in recent times. Since 1967 there have been eight cases of predation on humans in or adjacent to Glacier and Yellowstone National Parks in the United States and Banff National Park in Canada.[194] In all cases the grizzly involved was judged to be either habituated to the presence of humans or conditioned to human foods. During this same time period, however, perhaps thousands of bears with these same behavioral traits did not prey on humans. Nonetheless, conditioned or habituated behavior possibly predisposes some grizzlies to prey on humans under certain circumstances.

Another interesting but much less common circumstance associated with grizzly bear–inflicted injuries is when bears mistakenly perceive a person as one of their normal prey species and attack. Five incidences have been documented in which people were seriously injured (two were killed) after they made prey calls (such as the call of a wounded rabbit or a deer), as they were bent over field-dressing a game animal, or when they were carrying the hide of a game animal through the woods. Clearly, looking, sounding, or smelling like a prey species is risky for a human.

Black Bears. Black bears are the most numerous and widely distributed of all North American bears. They occur in more than 30 of the lower 48 states, from Maine to Florida and from California to Washington. They occur throughout Canada and Alaska, extending up to treeline below the Arctic Circle.

Between 1960 and 1980 more than 500 people were injured by black bears,[193] but at least 90% of these episodes resulted in minor scratches or bites inflicted by bears that were either conditioned to human foods or habituated to human presence. Injuries as a result of close encounters are extremely rare, and in contrast to female grizzly (brown) bears, female black bears display little aggression in defense of their young and rarely cause injury.

Whereas grizzly (brown) bears prey on humans as a nighttime event, black bears occasionally prey or attempt to prey on humans during the daytime. From 1900 through 1980, 20 people were killed by black bears, and in 18 cases predation was considered to be the bears' motivation.[193] All but one case occurred in remote areas outside park boundaries, indicating that neither conditioning nor habituation was a major factor.

Since 1985 black bears attempted to prey or preyed on humans in 15 episodes (J.C. Pederson, Utah Division of Wildlife Reserves, personal communication), with 2 fatalities and 7 major injuries.[193] Reported details of these events are scant, but at least 4 occurred at night while the victims were asleep. In one case the bear broke into a camper and pulled the victim out, and in another case the bear entered a wooden wickiup and dragged the victim out by her foot.

In the majority of cases of black bear aggression, the bears were frightened away relatively easily by aggressive actions by the victim and his or her companions.

Polar Bears. Polar bear–inflicted injuries are much less frequent than those by grizzly (brown) or black bears primarily because of their remote and harsh environment with relatively little human intrusion. From 1973 through 1987 three people were injured (one fatally) in Norway,[152] and from 1965 through 1985 20 people were injured (six fatally) by polar bears in Canada.[194] The number of injuries would probably be much higher except that most people who are in polar bear habitat are armed, and in the majority of aggressive encounters the bear is killed before causing human injury.

Polar bear–inflicted injuries have been classified into two general categories. The larger is predation, primarily by subadult and adult males. In these instances five of the six victims who died were probably killed instantly. The other category is by adult females thought to be defending their young.[194] These episodes are typically brief and nonfatal, which supports the theory that the bear is only trying to remove a perceived threat. In more than 90% of the incidences of aggressive encounters with polar bears, an attractant, such as food, garbage, or carcasses, was considered contributory.

BEAR ATTACKS ON OTHER CONTINENTS

The available data on attacks by bears on other continents are much less complete than those on North American bear attacks. In Europe the brown bear has coexisted with humans much longer than its American counterpart. As a result, its behavior is less aggressive and more like that of black bears. Numbers of bears are extremely low, and the

*References 173, 277, 279, 358, 398, 442.

animals are highly cryptic and nocturnal and thus are rarely seen or encountered. Human injury by black and brown bears in Europe is almost nonexistent.

The brown bears in the former Soviet Union live in vast, relatively undeveloped wild areas and appear to have aggressive responses against humans similar to those of North American brown bears. Several instances of human injuries from brown bear attacks, including deaths, have been reported, but many of these may be related to bears injured by hunters (I. Chestin, University of St. Petersburg, Russia, personal communication, 1992).

The spectacled bear *(Tremarctos ornatus)* of South America is rarely seen and appears nonaggressive. It lives in dense forest and is primarily cryptic, so that encounters are rare events, even for researchers trying to study them.

The panda bear *(Ailuropoda melanoleuca)* of China is perhaps the most docile of bear species. This, combined with their low numbers, makes human injury in the wild improbable.

The Asiatic black bear *(Ursus thibetanus)* is distributed throughout most of southern Asia but is concentrated in low numbers in isolated regions. These bears are hunted extensively for illegal trade of bear parts and represent almost no threat to human safety.

The sun bear *(Helarctos malayanus)* is distributed in Southeast Asia and the Malay archipelago. It is perhaps the least known bear species, but because of its low numbers, illegal harvest, and forested habitat, it represents little or no significant threat to human safety.

The sloth bear *(Melursus ursinus)* is found in Sri Lanka, India, Nepal, Bhutan, and Bangladesh. Although the data are limited primarily to anecdotal reports, the sloth bear appears to be the most dangerous bear species in Europe or Asia next to the Russian brown bears. Approximately one native is seriously injured or killed by a sloth bear in Chitwan National Park in Nepal each year (D.L. Garshelis, Minnesota Department of Natural Resources, personal communication). In the remote regions of western Nepal, at least one villager is seriously injured by a sloth bear every other year. Most of these injuries are the result of close encounter, and the victims receive wounds to the head and neck. No predatory behavior has been reported.

The aggression of the sloth bear has been estimated to be somewhere between that of the American black bear and grizzly bear. In fact, sloth bear researchers in Nepal do their work exclusively while riding elephants because of their concern of attacks from rhinos, sloth bears, and tigers, in that order.[218]

AVOIDING BEAR ATTACKS

A significant amount of literature concerning safety in bear country is written about attack victims.[85,193,194,221,277] But what can be learned from others' mistakes? Realizing that such information is gathered from victims who generally are inexperienced with respect to bear behavior and whose interpretations of the events reflect their cultural biases is important. Also, victims often become instant media celebrities. Several cases have occurred in which the circumstances surrounding the attack changed significantly with each telling, usually with the effect of reducing the victim's own culpability. Because of potential litigation, some victims have told their stories only through an attorney.

Our notions of how best to avoid bear attacks have been drawn primarily from what attack victims did "wrong." But because most people who live, work, and vacation in bear country for a significant part of their lives are never injured, it is equally important to understand what they have done "right." Unlike bear attack victims, these people have successfully navigated grizzly country without being injured. How have they done it? Unfortunately, this information is not as readily available as attack records, but it nonetheless remains critical to our knowledge of grizzly-human interactions.

From 1900 to 1985, 115 human injuries were reported from black, polar, and grizzly bear attacks combined in Alaska, but only two victims were natives.[277] This strongly suggests that the behavior of people is important in determining how they coexist with bears safely.

Concerning safety in bear country, four levels of interaction warrant special attention[45]: avoiding an encounter,[48] reducing the chances of being attacked after an encounter, reducing the severity of injuries received if attacked, and reducing the chances of becoming prey to a bear.

Avoiding an Encounter

The chances of having a close encounter with a bear can be significantly reduced by doing three simple things:

1. Make noise so that the bear knows a person is present. This requires no more than conversation along the trail, but voices may have to be amplified somewhat while traveling along a noisy stream or a windy ridge.
2. Remain alert in bear country. Be aware that the terrain and environment may hamper a bear's ability to detect a human by sight, smell, or sound.
3. Use good judgment to avoid a potentially dangerous situation. If fresh bear signs are seen, such as tracks, droppings, or a carcass (or even scavenger activity indicating a carcass nearby), consider that a bear is somewhere nearby and take an alternate route. If the bear is seen first, slowly and quietly retreat to safety and either abort the trip or take an alternate route.

Not Provoking an Attack

Even in a close encounter, several things should be considered that may reduce the chance of being attacked. However, these considerations vary depending on the species of bear.

Persons should identify themselves to the bear to let it know they are human and not a prey species. They should step away from any visual obstructions to let the bear clearly see them and should talk to allow the bear to hear the human voice. Any attempt to hide once the bear is aware of a human's presence will only confuse it, and it may approach closer to identify the disturbance, resulting in an even closer encounter.

Although remaining calm is difficult, a person should not make sudden movements or yell out, particularly with a grizzly bear. The bear may view this as an aggressive action and deal with it by an aggressive response. The person should also not stare directly at the bear but should look to the side or look at the bear sideways for the same reason.

Once the close encounter is under way, it is too late to consider climbing a tree or running away. Not only is outrunning a bear impossible, but also it may prevent the bear from identifying a human and initiate a charge. Attempting to climb a tree may also prevent the bear from correctly identifying a human. If the bear charges at that point, climbing a tree to a safe height is difficult, given the bear's ability to accelerate quickly. Therefore the best defense is to stand quietly and nonaggressively and allow the bear to identify the presence of a human. Once the bear departs, the person should quickly leave the area.

If the bear charges, chances are great that it is either bluffing or trying to get closer to see who the human is. In either event the best defense is still to stand still. However, what to do if the bear continues to charge depends on the species of the bear. This is where the data from attack victims are most beneficial.

Damage Control when Attacked

If attacked a person can take several important steps to minimize injury. If an attack is imminent, important actions must be considered. What a person does immediately before, during, and after an attack will influence the type and severity of the injuries.

Humans are rarely killed during an attack precipitated by a surprise close encounter even though bears are physically capable of easily and quickly doing so. During these types of attacks, grizzlies are only trying to remove a perceived threat, and their intent is to use only as much force as necessary. When interacting with others of their species, grizzly bears are head oriented, and they commonly direct their aggression toward humans in the same manner—toward the head. Therefore the general rules to follow during an attack are to "help" the bear remove the perceived threat and to protect vital body parts:

1. Do not run, try to climb a tree, fight, or scream.
2. Protect the head and neck by interlocking the hands behind the head (ear level) and flexing the head forward, either in the fetal position or flat on the ground face down. Use elbows to cover the face if the bear turns you over.
3. Do not hold out a forearm or hand to ward off the attack. Bears can readily cause significant neurovascular injuries to these structures.
4. *Never* look at the bear during an attack.
5. After the attack, stay down until sure the bear has completely left the area. *This is an extremely important point.* Persons who have gotten up before the bear has left generally received more severe injuries during the second attack.
6. When you believe the bear has left the area, peek around while moving as little as possible, try to determine which way the bear went, evaluate your options, and then leave the area.

Victims who, when attacked from a close encounter situation, immediately protect themselves and do not try to resist typically receive injuries that can be treated on an outpatient basis. However, those who try to get up and leave after the initial attack but before the bear leaves the area typically receive much more severe injuries during a second attack, requiring multiple surgical procedures that result in permanent cosmetic or functional disabilities.

If the attack is by a black bear, a different set of considerations apply. Black bear aggression should be countered with aggression such as shouting, yelling, throwing rocks or sticks, or whatever means are available. The victim should never lie down in a protective, submissive position because black bears are more likely to prey on humans during daytime than are grizzly bears.

The data on polar bears are less complete but suggest that attacks by females with offspring are behavioral responses similar to those of grizzly females with offspring. That is, the attacks are defensive in nature, are brief, and result in nonlethal injuries; the bear typically leaves shortly after the incident. However, if the polar bear is alone it should be assumed to be a male whose behavioral response is predation, so any and all aggressive responses available at the time should be employed.

Avoiding Predation by Bears. The most important means of reducing the chance of being preyed on by a bear is to avoid anything that may attract a bear to the campsite while the occupants are sleeping:

1. Avoid camping along bear travel corridors or at seasonal feeding sites.
2. Avoid campsites littered with human refuse.
3. Use proper food storage to render human food unavailable to bears.
4. Reduce food odors by cooking and eating at a site different from the sleeping area. Also sleep in different clothes from those worn when cooking and eating.
5. Do not leave garbage or food buried or poured into the ground at the campsite. This can cause problems for future campers at this site.

Even though the chances of a bear entering the campsite in an attempt to prey on humans is small, a contingency plan should always be kept in mind when camping in bear country:

1. Become familiar with the area because it will probably be dark when a bear enters the campsite with the intent to prey on one of the campers. Be familiar with escape options such as trees or rocky ledges.

2. Sleep in a tent. The tent appears to offer some boundary of protection and may deter an inquisitive bear from walking directly to the campers. In several instances a victim trapped inside a sleeping bag has been dragged away from a campsite by a bear. Keeping the bag at least partially unzipped increases the chance of a quick exit.
3. Always keep a flashlight readily available. This is a situation in which bear spray or a gun may be beneficial. Remember that a bear that enters a tent or picks up a sleeping camper is trying to prey on that person. Therefore any available defense should be applied.

The actions of companions can make an important difference if a bear pulls one of the campers away from the camp. The data about such incidences are gruesome but significant. Predatory grizzly and black bears rarely kill their victims before consuming them. After dragging their victims away from camp, usually less than a few hundred feet, they concentrate their efforts toward soft tissue or visceral consumption and the victims frequently remain alive for an hour or more. Therefore a quick, aggressive, unified response by companions may save the victim's life. Approaching a predatory bear in the dark while it is trying to feed on a human victim is not without risk but is probably the victim's only chance for survival. This action has been successful on several occasions.

In contrast, the victim of a predatory attack by a polar bear is typically killed instantaneously, so prevention of such attacks is the best and only chance for survival. In all predatory attacks, any and all defensive measures must be considered, including guns where they are permitted.

Protective Devices

Bear spray. A commercially available aerosol bear spray containing capsaicin, a red pepper derivative, is marketed as a "grizzly-proven self-defense" and "the best life insurance you can carry" into bear country. Unfortunately, nothing offers complete protection against bears (or anything else, for that matter).

Bear spray was developed by testing on captive, caged grizzly bears. Under these conditions, bears that charged the cage were repelled when they were sprayed in the face at close range with a capsaicin aerosol. Unfortunately, such a test fails to duplicate real-life conditions, so such marketing claims are hard to justify. Conducting adequate scientific studies testing the real-life effectiveness of bear spray is impossible. However, many persons who enter bear country are so afraid of the prospect of being mauled by a bear they are desperate to try anything, especially a product billed as having such all-encompassing potential. If bear spray is carried into bear country for protection, several key points about its use should be considered.

Bear encounters are usually sudden and unexpected, and even persons who have had bear spray with them note that they could not get to it in time to use it. Therefore the spray is not likely to be available when really needed. Although the manufacturers of bear spray point out that it has a range of up to 30 feet, this is rarely the effective range under the field conditions of a close encounter. If a person is traveling with the wind, the bear can readily detect his or her presence well in advance, and this precludes a sudden, unexpected close encounter situation. The chances of having a close encounter are much greater when the person travels into the wind. Under such circumstances the effective range of bear spray is significantly diminished.

Two more points about bear spray should be considered. When holding a can of bear spray out in front of the body to spray a charging bear, a person leaves himself or herself in a vulnerable position for injury if the charge is not halted, such as misfiring the spray, having a defective can, or missing the bear entirely. And if bear is hit with the spray, instead of deterring a charge, the irritating reaction may convert the bear's defensive attack to a more offensive attack, resulting in more significant injury.

Bear spray is not a substitute for the good judgment needed to avoid the close encounter to begin with and should not be considered an option for tough situations.

Guns. Many people consider carrying guns for protection when they enter bear country. Guns certainly are useful in some situations. However, many concerns about the use of guns for protective purposes are similar to those regarding the use of bear spray. Two additional points should be considered. First, the kill target for a grizzly is small. The brain is narrow and long, and the bear is a quickly accelerating moving target. Second, an enraged wounded bear is likely to deliver a more severe, if not fatal, injury. Most attacks are so sudden that people relying on guns do not have a chance to fire them. Persons who decide to use a gun must make sure the bear is killed before it gets to them. This is a huge gamble, and a person's life is at stake.

Menstruation. In August 1967, two women were killed in separate events on the same night by different grizzly bears in Glacier National Park. The postmortem examination showed that one had been menstruating. That menstruation may be a precipitating factor in attacks or predation has unfortunately become solidly ingrained into popular opinion. Hysterical coverage by the mass media has enhanced the role of this factor, and the scientific question has been left unanswered by both scientists and bureaucrats.[48]

A study of polar bear response to menstrual odors was published in 1985,[88] and although it was not designed to adequately test the hypothesis that menstruating women were more likely to be either attacked or preyed on by bears, the press came to this conclusion. The Interagency Grizzly Bear Committee then gave an ambivalent caution in the government's official grizzly bear pamphlet *Bear Us In Mind* that said, "Women may choose to stay out of bear country during their menstrual period." Fortunately, this has recently been removed from the pamphlet because *no* scientific evidence even suggests that menstrual odors precipitate grizzly bear attacks. The attack mentioned previously is the only serious attack on a known menstruating woman that has been documented in North America, and even the official investigating team concluded that menstruation did not appear to have played a major role.[193]

BEAR-INDUCED INJURIES

Injuries inflicted by bears range from superficial and trivial, typically treated on an outpatient basis, to severe, requiring hospitalization and surgery and resulting in significant cosmetic and functional disability. In this regard, bear attacks are similar to most other animal attacks, particularly those inflicted by large animals.

The character of such injuries is determined in part by the three main sources: teeth, claws, and paws. The teeth of bears, especially the canines, are large and sturdy. Although the teeth are not particularly sharp, the power of the jaw muscles allows the teeth to penetrate deep into soft tissues and to fracture facial bones and bones of the hand and forearm with ease. The resulting trauma is characteristically a result of punctures with shearing, tearing, and crushing forces.

The claws are another important source of trauma. Although the claws on the front pads can be as long as human fingers, they are not particularly sharp on grizzly and polar bears. Nonetheless, the power of the bear's shoulders produces the force and speed that allow claws to cause significant soft tissue damage in a scraping maneuver that results in deep, parallel gashes.

The bear paw is capable of delivering powerful force, resulting in significant blunt trauma, particularly to the head and neck, ribcage, and abdominal viscera. Therefore, as with all large animals, the patient needs a complete evaluation for occult blunt trauma.

Another set of injuries associated with bear attacks has to do with ballistics and gravity. Several victims have been inadvertently shot by a companion who was trying to shoot the attacking bear. Several cases are known of people suffering long bone fractures when they fell out of trees they were climbing to avoid a bear attack. At least two people in North America were killed by such falls, and in both incidents the attacking bear did not additionally injure the victim.

WOUND MANAGEMENT

The specifics of initial wound treatment are determined in part by the available medical equipment and location in which the victim is first received. Stabilization of the patient remains the primary objective. All cases of bear attack should be considered major trauma, and the patient should be transported to the most appropriate facility.

Bear-inflicted injuries are often occult, producing greater tissue necrosis than initially expected. Deep structure involvement is typically more prevalent than is apparent initially. Internal injuries from either direct penetration (claws, teeth) or blunt trauma are common. Neurovascular injuries must be considered with trauma to the extremities, and neurosensory and cosmetic injuries are common with trauma to the face. When brought to medical attention, wounds are usually "old" and contaminated.

ANTIBIOTICS

Little information is available about the organisms likely to be encountered in bear-inflicted wounds, but anecdotal evidence suggests that bear attack victims do not develop unusual or rare septic complications from unknown pathogens. In one study, culture of the mouths of black bears revealed a bacterial spectrum similar to that in dogs, with the majority of species being *Micrococcus* and *Streptococcus*.[135] *S. aureus* was found in only 8%, and *Pasteurella* and *Eikenella* were not found.

The use of antibiotics shortly after the injury but before clinical evidence of infection remains controversial. The usual risk factors should be assessed (see Box 40-3). However, the blunt trauma, deep punctures, and shearing-tearing forces that are typical of bear attacks create significant tissue ischemia and necrosis that are not apparent on the initial examination. Therefore antimicrobial prophylaxis should be considered for all bear-inflicted wounds pending culture results and before clinical evidence of infection.

Before culture results are available, penicillin is suggested for relatively clean superficial injuries. A third-generation cephalosporin should be added to cover gram-negative organisms for deeper and more contaminated wounds.[135] However, adequate wound debridement and cleansing are the primary means of reducing the infection rate among these victims.

No cases of rabies have been documented in any bear species, wild or captive. However, the CDC recommends rabies immunization for victims attacked by wild carnivores. Therefore all victims should have the standard informed consent discussion of the risks and benefits of rabies immunization.

Injury from Skunks

Skunks bite readily when captured and are frequent carriers of rabies.[138] No data exist concerning the likelihood of other wound infections after skunk bite; in one series only 21 bites were reported for the entire United States for a 10-year period.[342] Skunks' most frequent means of defense is spraying the secretions of anal sacs.

A skunk ready to spray directs its hindquarters to the enemy, feet firmly planted and tail straight in the air, often stamping the front feet in warning. The spray is accurate to 13 feet, and contrary to popular belief, can be discharged when the animal is lifted by the tail.

Skunk musk causes skin irritation, keratoconjunctivitis, temporary blindness, nausea, and occasional convulsions and loss of consciousness.[138] The chief component of the musk is butyl mercaptan. This can be neutralized by strong oxidizing agents, such as sodium hypochlorite in a 5.25% solution (household bleach), further diluted 1:5 or 1:10 in water. The chlorine forms odorless sulfate or sulfone compounds by oxidizing the mercaptan and breaking the sulfur free from the carbon chain. This solution can be cleansed with a tincture of green soap, followed by a dilute bleach rinse. Tomato juice shampoo has been advocated for deodorizing hair, which can be washed and mildly bleached or cropped short.

Injury from Porcupines

Porcupines (a species of rodent) are virtually never reported to bite, but their quills frequently are embedded in the skin of humans. Because of the structure of quills, they not only embed themselves and are extremely difficult to extract, but also can migrate—as much as 10 inches under the skin in some cases. The average porcupine has 30,000 quills, which range from less than an inch to 4 inches in length. The quills are barbed and their cores are spongy, so if they are not removed immediately, they absorb body fluid and expand, which causes the barbs to flare even further outward. Thus each movement of the victim's body or muscles helps a quill work its way in deeper. Allegedly, in rare cases such migration has led to injury to internal organs and death in humans. Infection seldom results because the quills have mild antiseptic properties, presumably to protect the porcupines themselves, which sometimes fall on them.

No medical reports are available of appropriate treatment or complications of porcupine quill injuries.

Injury from Swine

Although domestic pigs are common, pig bites are as rare in developed countries as lion and monkey bites, probably because the total number of farmers in those countries is small.[17] Domestic swine can be aggressive and inflict deep goring or bite injuries, often on the posterior thigh.[17] The location is because of their practice of approaching from behind. Wounds tend to be deep (particularly when the boar, with deep penetrating tusks, is involved), although sometimes deceptively small on the surface.[417] Treatment is at least as much surgical as antibiotic; wounds must be carefully and thoroughly explored and debrided.

Twelve percent of veterinarians have been bitten by a pig, placing it fourth behind dogs (63%), cats (81%), and horses (87%).[238] The usual wide range of bacterial pathogens is reported, including *Pasteurella aerogenes, Bacteroides, Proteus,* and α- and β-hemolytic streptococci.[416] Like many domestic animals, pigs often carry *Pasteurella multocida,* but pigs accounted for only 5 of 3700 cases of *Pasteurella* infection from animals in one series.[17] Unusual gram-negative bacteria have been isolated, and probably many other poorly understood species are present.[171] Among veterinarians, pigs have a reputation of inflicting bites of high-infection risk (M.E. Fowler, personal communication, 1980). Wound infection is common despite debridement and antibiotics.

Wild pigs are even more likely to inflict injury. In Melanesia, typical wounds in 20 victims included abdominal injuries with prolapse and strangulation of the intestine; "sucking" chest wounds; bilateral pneumothoraces; two infected open fractures of the radius and ulna; perforating injury of the knee with septic arthritis; hand injury with laceration of multiple tendons; arterial injury of the wrist; injury of a tibial nerve with footdrop; and severe scrotal injury with exposure of the testicles.[19] Swine wounds should be treated as high risk, warranting broad-spectrum prophylactic antibiotics (perhaps parenterally) and close follow-up if the victim is not admitted to hospital.

Vampire Bat Bites

Vampire bats are a vector of rabies in Central and South America, inducing one to two deaths per year in those regions. Sometimes small epidemics occur in isolated villages in the jungle; these can infect (and kill) up to 5% of the population, up to 17% of children, and 22% of all families.[272,351] Sometimes such epidemics are triggered by destruction of wild or domestic hosts (such as pigs) of the bats.[272] Vampire bats feed at night on animal blood, including humans, by making an incision in the skin to lap up the blood on the lips, earlobes, forehead, or fingers or between the toes. One bat can eat a maximum of 1 ounce of blood per night, which is clearly not enough to cause death. However, a cave of 1000 bats needs 15 gallons each night, which amounts to more than 5750 gallons per year.[69,83] Protection against vampire bats is effectively provided by mosquito nets.

Other species of bats are noteworthy chiefly for the high risk of rabies transmission. All bats should be considered high risk, and exposure—even to sick or "pet" bats that have been in captivity—should be avoided. Some of the situations mandating rabies prophylaxis are bizarre and reveal more about human nature than about either rabies or bats. For example, rabies prophylaxis has been initiated after a patient dunked a dead bat in his beer, chewed on the bat's ear, and then drank the beer.[111] In a similar case, prophylaxis was needed when a miner swallowed a live bat on a bet.[24]

Most bats have small teeth that often cannot penetrate human skin, so risks of bacterial wound infection are low.

Bites of Venomous Mammals

Only two types of venomous mammals are known. The short-tailed shrew *(Blarina brevicauda)* of the northeastern United States secretes a protein venom from its maxillary gland and injects it with the lower incisors. The venom may cause edema, a few days of burning sensation, and pain lasting up to 2 weeks.[59] No specific antivenin is available and treatment is symptomatic. No bites have been reported since the 1930s. A similar venom is possessed by the European water shrew *(Neomys fidiens)* and the primitive Cuban insectivore *(Solenodon paradoxus)*.[42] Documented bites are exceedingly rare.

A second type of venomous mammal is the male platypus *(Ornithorhynchus anatinus)*, which injects venom from a hollow spur in its hind leg. This appears to resemble viperine snake venom and causes local pain, edema, and lymphangitis.[42] The pain can be excruciating and completely unresponsive to intravenous narcotics. Regional nerve block has been reported to be effective.[130] Localized edema also occurs; no specific treatment is available, and the exact pathophysiology is unknown. Reports of such injuries are exceedingly rare. The echidna, or spiny anteater, possesses a similar spur and venom, but envenomation has not been reported.[138]

Injury from Large Wild and Domestic Herbivores

Cattle are usually docile but are capable of inflicting a variety of injuries. Cows typically weigh 1400 pounds, and bulls can exceed 3000 pounds. Accidental treading on the human victim or butting can cause major crush injuries and fractures.[378] Deer, gazelle, and antelope are also capable of delivering damaging kicks. Domestic animals, such as cows, bulls, and horses, are estimated to kill 800 people a year in Europe alone.[69,75] About 120 persons a year were gored in Great Britain in the early 1960s, 5 fatally.[380] About six people a year are killed by farm animals in Wisconsin.[46] In one hospital in rural Wisconsin an average 22 patients a year were treated for horse and cattle injuries, most of them inflicted by kick or other assault.[46] Domestic cattle and horses are fairly frequently infected with rabies, but because of immunization of veterinary workers seldom account for human infection.

Cattle horn injuries (or gorings) present a typical and unique damage pattern. The horns are used in an inward hooking motion to butt and fling the victim, or the horn tip can be used for goring. Goring injuries seen in bullfighting typically involve the perineum and thigh; they tend to be deep and sometimes fatal. Scrotal skin avulsion is common in bullfight gorings.[380] By contrast, bull horn injuries from domestic cattle involve a sweeping arc at the level of the bull's head, which is at the level of the human abdomen. The semicircular motion of the horn often produces a relatively superficial laceration, leaving deeper structures of the abdomen intact. In one series of 29 cases in which the peritoneum was breached, usually producing prolapse of bowel or omentum, 27 laparotomies demonstrated no additional injuries. In only a few cases was the bowel itself damaged.[380] The wound infection rate in this series was high (54%), probably because of the 9-hour delay to treatment (typical of underdeveloped countries).

The horse is inclined both to bite and to kick, whereas cattle, lacking upper incisors, virtually never bite. The soft tissue contusions inflicted by a horse can be severe (Fig. 40-1). However, in a series of 24 horse bites, 21 healed uneventfully.[116] A death has been reported from fat embolism caused by fractures after a donkey bite.[30] Rams have killed farmers by repeated blunt trauma.[291]

Horse injuries are common, especially in farm and stable employees and patrons. At one hospital serving a racehorse training area, many of these injuries involved falls from the horse, injury against the neck of the horse when rearing, crush injuries when the horse rolled over on its rider, and kick injuries from horses' hooves.[116] Many of these injuries were severe and resulted in fractures and internal injuries. Particular note should be made of the fact that a half-ton horse falling onto the rider frequently results in pelvic ring injuries and knee ligament injuries.[116]

Since such injuries are relatively frequent, prevention is essential. Horseback riders, especially novices, should wear protective helmets (many injuries occur when teen-age girls fall from horses).[29] Farmers or veterinarians examining a sick animal should always have a second person present to assist and warn them. Bulls should be approached only with a protective device (such as a heavy stick) and a preplanned exit. A ring in the bull's nose gives a victim something to hang onto besides the horns and a way to yank the bull's nose up, which may stop the attack. Dehorning the bull eliminates goring injury but not the potential for crushing. If struck by a bull or cow, the victim should not attempt to stand (since this will provoke being thrown to the ground again) but should try to crawl to safety. Children (and naive city dwellers and suburbanites) must be educated about the risks of large animals and kept away from them whenever possible.

Little about wound infection from herbivore-inflicted injuries is known or reported. Species of *Actinobacillus lignieresii* and *A. suis*, as well as *Pasteurella multocida*, have been isolated from infected horse and sheep bites.[312] All are common organisms in the mouths of herbivores. *Actinobacillus* and *Pasteurella* are closely related genera, distinguished chiefly by biochemical tests. Thus inexperienced laboratories may confuse them. Not only do most domestic herbivores carry *Pasteurella*, but most are given frequent and regular doses of various antibiotics (especially in their feed), leading to antibiotic resistance among the bacteria.[324] Resistance to ampicillin, penicillin, tetracycline, and sulfadimethoxine is common in isolates from such sources.

The African buffalo is a threat chiefly when provoked, but it accounts for many deaths and maimings. Left alone, it does not attack, but when shot or cornered, it charges, is difficult to avoid or stop, and can hook the victim 10 feet into the air with its horns. Buffalo charging humans are usually old single bulls that have left the safety of the large herds, most often because of wounds from poachers' snares, spears, or lion attacks. They are thus not in a good frame of mind when encountered in the bush. The buffalo is also wily and intelligent; wounded buffalo may lay in wait for trackers or may double around and come up behind them on the trail, often with fatal consequences for the humans. Buffaloes' hatred of hunters is legendary in Africa; one hunter was treed but could not get his feet high enough to keep them clear of the animal. The buffalo repeatedly hooked the man's feet with his horns, eventually cutting them to ribbons so that the hunter bled to death, still hanging in the tree.

Once the victim is prostrate, the buffalo gores into the ground with its horns and the heavy horny boss across its forehead and then whips its head from side to side, disemboweling the victim with the sharp horn tips. Such injuries are estimated to be responsible for 20 to 100 deaths per year, mostly in Africa. The horns are always covered with mud, so goring wounds must be laid open and cleansed. However, patients who do not have major traumatic injuries generally do well.[378]

The North American bison and the musk ox have been responsible for occasional accidental deaths.

Camels have a bad reputation as foul-tempered animals that work up a deep hatred for persons who overload them; they have bitten handlers to death.[69] Unlike most other herbivores, the camel has canine teeth and its bite can sever a person's limb.[75] The camel can also use a biting technique in which it lifts its head up and back, whipping the victim about strongly enough to break his or her neck (M.E. Fowler, personal communication, 1980).

Other wild species, such as the giraffe, may turn rogue, but this is exceedingly rare. The black wildebeest has killed one or two zookeepers, as have the spiral-horned kudo and the bushbuck. Other antelopes have killed or wounded hunters or zookeepers with their sharp horns.

The elephant can be one of the most dangerous of wild animals and was until recently probably the greatest killer of hunters. Statistics are hard to come by, but the annual death toll in Central Africa was probably between 200 and 500.[69] In defense of the elephant, the majority of injuries occur when humans accidentally approach elephants too closely, which the animals interpret as a threat. However, elephants turn rogue from time to time, deliberately attacking and killing humans. The incidence of such deaths might be expected to decrease as the world becomes progressively less wild, but the unfortunate human population explosion is making such encounters increasingly frequent as humans and elephants compete for the same space and humans despoil and devastate the forest. In Sri Lanka, for example, such encounters force some families to sleep in trees, and at least four people a year are killed by elephants in one area with a population of only 25,000.[331]

Elephants kill by trampling, goring with the tusks, or striking or throwing with the trunk. Once the victim has been run over or skewered with the tusks, the elephant kneels on them and crushes them. Elephants have been known to use weapons in their attacks; a villager who retreated safely up a baobab tree was hit by a tree branch the bull elephant picked up in its trunk and used as a club. The villager's back was broken, and he was paralyzed. Elephants frequently rip the victim's body apart and scatter the pieces, later covering them with grass and branches. Another elephant tactic is to toss the victim into the trees or straight over the pachyderm's back; a number of victims have survived this experience. Some hunters pursued by elephants have diverted them by throwing off items of clothing. Elephants were used extensively as war machines in the past; this period reached its golden age under the Romans, who, after consolidating their victories, insisted on international elephant disarmament. Having made sure that all war elephants in neighboring countries were eliminated, they then retired their own. As history shows, this rational gesture did not deter their ultimate downfall at the hands of barbarians unequipped with elephants.

Many rogue elephants seem to be injured; others have become intoxicated by eating fermenting marula berries. Persistent hunting has made the elephant more wary and irritable than it was 100 years ago. Its traditional feeding and migration ground is increasingly invaded by farmers, leading inevitably to negative interactions. The elephant is under ever-increasing pressure from humans. The elephant is incredibly destructive of plants and trees, and its future in this escalating conflict is in grave doubt.

A few rare stories suggest that an elephant may actually be a man-eater; one of these occurred in 1944 at the Zurich zoo. A person who had a particularly close relationship with an elephant, and actually slept in a room next to its stall, disappeared; all that was found was a human hand and toe. Similarly, authorities in India's state of Meghalaya reported an elephant that killed and ate five people.[329]

Elephants captive in zoos and circuses may cause deaths while temporarily deranged. Man-killing in trained work elephants in India is frequently tolerated, since the country has only approximately 7000 trained elephants, while elephant handlers are plentiful.[69] Indian elephants tend to be more docile than African ones, but they too occasionally turn rogue. An estimated 50 people annually in India are killed in elephant attacks.

The black rhinoceros has been represented as one of the meanest animals in Africa because it charges any moving object, including trains. The click of a camera, a gentle movement, or a scent is enough to induce a charge. Because the rhinoceros has poor eyesight but excellent hearing, it may well be running toward sounds to investigate them. Contrary to the popular belief that, owing to its nearsightedness, it can be easily sidestepped, it can turn on a dime.[69] At the end of its charge it usually hooks right and left with its horns and is generally satisfied with tossing the victim high (12 feet) in the air. However, like so many large wild animals, it probably does not have a malicious intent in many cases. Rhinoceroses often flee once they have identified a sound as originating from something dangerous (such as,

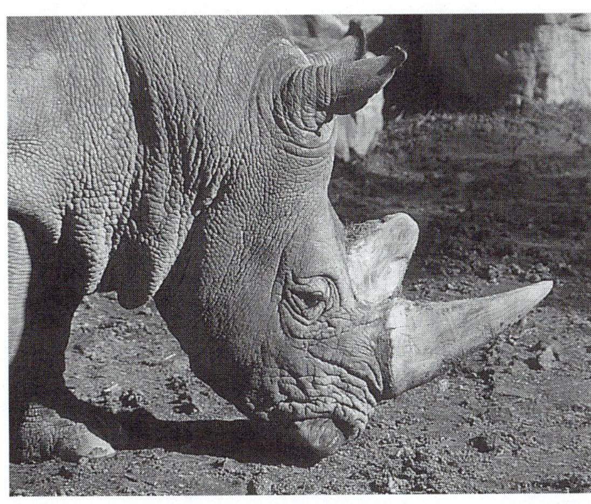

Fig. 40-2 The rhinoceros is a formidable foe when it tramples and gores. (Photo by Paul Auerbach, M.D.)

humans), and persons who have fallen while running from a charge have been investigated with a few typical snorts and then ignored. However, severe injuries can result if the human fails to get out of the way of the rhino; as with the hippopotamus, injuries and death may have more to do with being in the path of a very large fast-moving object than with malicious intent (Fig. 40-2). The white rhinoceros is docile and has killed few, if any, people.

The hippopotamus is a frequent killer in Africa. Its placid and indolent appearance in zoos completely belies its activity and personality in the wild. A hippo can travel at up to 45 mph on land. It is relatively unpredictable and made irritable by people, and it will attack boats and people in the water if it feels that it is trapped (between a boat and deep water, for example) or if its calf is threatened. With its large canine teeth, it is capable of chopping canoes (and the people in them) in half, and it does so several times a year on the Zambezi River in Zimbabwe. However, these attacks are usually in self-defense, and hippos will get out of the way if they can; they certainly do not seek out and attack canoes or people who do not intrude upon them. Hippopotamuses graze on land and habitually run along established narrow tracks back to the river, mostly at night but also in the day. They will not change course for anything, and humans who make the mistake of staying in the tracks may be trampled. Since their browsing often takes place in dense stands of reeds, and their paths are the only practical means of getting through such vegetation, humans not surprisingly frequently use these paths and occasionally get run down.

Injury from Birds

Birds are of course not mammals, but they do inflict injuries. The ostrich is responsible for one to two deaths a year, mostly in Africa, where it is raised commercially.[69] Most of the fatal attacks are kicks to the head and abdomen. The ostrich can kick only forward, but when it does, a sharp toenail flicks out like a switchblade and can penetrate the abdomen. Since the ostrich can easily outrun a human being, the only protection is to lie prone to protect against disembowelment and to cover the neck to protect against pecks. Eventually the ostrich loses interest and allows the victim to escape. The cassowary (common in New Guinea) can easily disembowel a hunter with a single kick from its long sharp toe claws. Birds of paradise have been found to secrete a venom on their feathers, although cases of human toxicity from this have not been reported and the phenomenon is little studied.

Injury from Other Nonmammalian Species

The Nile crocodile accounts for 1000 human deaths a year in Africa.[69] Individual crocodiles have been responsible for up to 400 deaths. Most attacks take place in the water where crocodiles are accustomed to scavenging for the dead, sick, and deformed human babies who are tossed into the water to be disposed of by these reptiles. The crocodile has tremendous grip strength and locks this grip by slotting two lower teeth into holes in the upper jaw. When unable to drag the victim completely underwater, it may grip a limb and then spin over until the limb is detached.

Happily, the American crocodile has not yet been documented to be responsible for any cases of man-eating, and the American alligator has also caused few problems. However, the American alligator is thriving in the southern United States, and its habitat is so greatly threatened that incidents of alligators appearing in suburban backyards and swimming pools are now common. Attacks on children and pets are not unknown, and sooner or later this will probably end in a human fatality (it has already ended in many alligator fatalities).

Medicolegal Implications

Unlike many other traumatic injuries, bites have a host of medicolegal implications. In some cities and regions, animal bites must be reported to public health authorities. Reporting of suspected exposure to rabies is mandatory in most regions, and failure to report could become the basis for legal action. Reporting often leads to examination of the offending animal by public health authorities and sometimes to quarantining or even killing the animal. The owner's failure to meet local regulations regarding licensure and vaccination can lead to legal consequences. In addition, the victim may seek compensation from the owner of the animal, with the result that the health care provider and possibly the medical record will be summoned to court. The injury may be related to the victim's employment, generating worker's compensation or other insurance claims. Therefore injuries and their circumstances should be documented as fully as possible, with line drawings or photographs added to the medical record whenever possible. Certain types of animal bites, particularly those of the hand, are prone to infection and can lead to permanent, litigation-associated complications. A complete medical record is the best protection against such issues, as well as the more ordinary matter of malpractice claims made against the health care provider.

Human bites add another layer of legal ramifications because they are commonly inflicted in assaults or fights or may be a marker for child, spousal, or elder abuse. All these conditions must be reported to police in most jurisdictions. Subsequent criminal investigations may depend heavily on the initial medical record. Again, line drawings and photographs are helpful. Precise molds of bite marks can be taken by forensic pathologists and may help in subsequent identification of assailants. In addition, human bites of the hand have a propensity for infection and complications, so a malpractice suit is possible if a bad result is obtained. In addition to providing and documenting thorough and appropriate care of the wounds, the physician should warn the patient of the possibility of complications despite the best treatment available.

Acknowledgments

I would like to thank Peter Tetlow and Dr. Philip H. Rees for their review of the text on exotic animals.

REFERENCES

1. Aghababian R, Conte J: Mammalian bite wounds, *Ann Emerg Med* 9:79, 1980.
2. Alcock J: *Animal behavior: an evolutionary approach,* ed 2, Sunderland, Mass, 1979, Sinauer Association.
3. Alexander J, Alexander N: Influence of route of administration on wound fluid concentration of prophylactic antibiotics, *J Trauma* 16:488, 1976.
4. Alexander J, Sykes N, Mitchell M: Concentration of selected intravenously administered antibiotics in experimental surgical wounds, *J Trauma* 13:423, 1973.
5. Altieri M, Brasch L: Antibiotic prophylaxis in intraoral wounds, *Am J Emerg Med* 4:507, 1986.
6. Anderson L, Leart S, Manning P: Rat-bite fever in animal research laboratory personnel, *Lab Anim Sci* 33:292, 1983.
7. Anderson J, Winkler W, Hafkin B: Clinical experience with a human diploid cell rabies vaccine, *JAMA* 244:781, 1980.
8. Archibald D, Zon L, Groopman J: Antibodies to human T-lymphotropic virus type III (HTLV-III) in saliva of AIDS patients and in persons at risk for AIDS, *Blood* 67:831, 1986.
9. Archibald D, Zon L, Groopman J: Salivary antibodies as a means of detecting HLTV-III/lymphadenopathy associated virus infection, *J Clin Microbiol* 24:873, 1986.
10. Bahmanyar M, Fayaz A, Nour-Salehi S: Successful protection of humans exposed to rabies infection, *JAMA* 236:2751, 1976.
11. Bailey W, Stowe E, Schmit A: Aerobic bacterial flora of oral and nasal fluids of canines with reference to bacteria associated with bites, *J Clin Microbiol* 7:223, 1978.
12. Baker MD, Lanuti M: The management and outcome of lacerations in urban children, *Ann Emerg Med* 19(9):1001, 1990.
13. Baker MD, Moore SE: Human bites in children: a six-year experience, *Am J Dis Child* 141(12):1285, 1987.
14. Ban BD: Rabies epizootic continues to grow (news), *J Am Vet Med Assoc* 202(2):203, 1993.
15. Baquero F et al: Laboratory and in-vitro testing of skin antiseptics: a prediction for in-vivo activity? *J Hosp Infect* 18:5, 1991.
16. Bardsley A, Mercer D: The injured ear: a review of 50 cases, *Br J Plast Surg* 36:466, 1983.
17. Barnham M: Pig bite injuries and infection: report of seven human cases, *Epidemiol Infect* 101(3):641, 1988.
18. Barry A: Clinical specimens for microbiologic exams. In Hubbert W, McCulloch W, Schnurrenberger P, editors: *Diseases transmitted from animals to man,* ed 6, Springfield, Ill, 1975, Charles C Thomas.
19. Barss P, Ennis S: Injuries caused by pigs in Papua New Guinea, *Med J Aust* 149(11-12):649, 1988.
20. Bentley DW: Vaccinations, *Clin Geriatr Med* 8(4):745, 1992.
21. Bergamini T et al: Combined topical and systemic antibiotic prophylaxis in experimental wound infection, *Am J Surg* 147:753, 1984.
22. Berger TG, Perkocha LA: Bacillary angiomatosis, *AIDS Clin Rev* (81):81, 1991.
23. Berzon D, DeHoff J: Medical costs and other aspects of dog bites in Baltimore, *Public Health Rep* 89:377, 1974.
24. Bettor eats a live bat, *San Francisco Chronicle* Aug 31, 1989, p A13.
25. Biberstein E: Rat bite fever. In Hubbert W, McCulloch W, Schnurrenberger P, editors: *Diseases transmitted from animals to man,* ed 6, Springfield, Ill, 1975, Charles C Thomas.
26. Biberstein EL: Our understanding of the Pasteurellaceae, *Can J Vet Res* 54(suppl):S87,1990.
27. Birkness K et al: Intracellular growth of *Afipia felis,* a putative etiologic agent of cat scratch disease, *Infect Immun* 60(6):2281, 1992.
28. Bite U: Human bite injuries of the hand, *Can J Surg* 27:616, 1984.
29. Bjornstig U, Eriksson A, Ornehult L: Injuries caused by animals, *Injury* 22(4):295, 1991.
30. Bloch B: Fatal fat embolism following severe donkey bites, *J Forensic Sci* 16:231, 1977.
31. Boenning D, Fleisher G, Campos J: Dog bites in children: epidemiology, microbiology, and penicillin prophylactic therapy, *Am J Emerg Med* 1(1):17, 1983.
32. Borchelt P, Lockwood R, Beck A: Attacks by packs of dogs involving predation on human beings, *Public Health Rep* 98:57, 1983.
33. Boulter E et al: Successful treatment of experimental B virus infection with acyclovir, *Br Med J* 280:681, 1980.
34. Bracis R, Seibers K, Julien R: Meningitis caused by group II-J following a dog bite, *West J Med* 131:438, 1979.
35. Branemark P, Ekholm R: Tissue injury caused by wound disinfectants, *J Bone Joint Surg* 49A:48, 1967.
36. Brazis P, Stokes H, Ervin F: Optic neuritis in cat scratch disease, *J Clin Neuroophthalmol* 6:172, 1986.
37. Brochier B et al: Large-scale eradication of rabies using recombinant vaccinia-rabies vaccine (comments), *Nature* 354(6354):520, 1991.
38. Brook I: Microbiology of human and animal bite wounds in children, *Pediatr Infect Dis J* 6:29, 1987.
39. Brote L, Elfstrom J, Hojer H: Treatment of *Pasteurella multocida* infection after dog bite by ampicillin wound irrigation, *Acta Chir Scand* 143:485, 1977.
40. Brunner RG, Fallon W Jr: A prospective, randomized clinical trial of wound debridement versus conservative wound care in soft-tissue injury from civilian gunshot wounds, *Am Surg* 56(2):104, 1990.
41. Bryant C, Rodeheaver G, Reem E: Search for a nontoxic surgical scrub solution for periorbital lacerations, *Ann Emerg Med* 13:317, 1984.
42. Bucherl W, Buckley E, Deulofeu V: *Venomous animals and their venoms,* New York, 1968, Academic Press.
43. Burdge D, Scheifele D, Speert D: Serious *Pasteurella multocida* infections from lion and tiger bites, *JAMA* 253:3296, 1985.
44. Burrows GE, Ewing P: *In vitro* assessment of the efficacy of erythromycin in combination with oxytetracycline or spectinomycin

against *Pasteurella haemolytica, J Vet Diagn Invest* 1(4):299, 1989.

45. Burt W, Grossenheider R: *A field guide to the mammals,* ed 2, Boston, Mass, 1964, Houghton-Mifflin, p 284.
46. Busch H et al: Blunt bovine and equine trauma, *J Trauma* 26(6):559, 1986.
47. Butz AM et al: Alcohol-impregnated wipes as an alternative in hand hygiene, *Am J Infect Control* 18(2):70, 1990.
48. Byrd CP: *Of bears and women: investigating the hypothesis menstruation attracts bears,* M.S. thesis, University of Montana, 1988.
49. California, State of: *Guidelines for the treatment, investigation, and control of animal bites,* 1992, Department of Health Services, Veterinary Public Health Section.
50. Callaham M: Emergency medical management: dog bite wounds, *JAMA* 244:2327, 1980.
51. Callaham M: Prophylactic antibiotics in common dog bite wounds: a controlled study, *Ann Emerg Med* 9:410, 1980.
52. Callaham M: Prophylactic antibiotics in dog bite wounds: nipping at the heels of progress, *Ann Emerg Med* 23(3):577, 1994.
53. Callaham M: Treatment of common dog bites: infection risk factors, *JACEP* 7:83, 1978.
54. Campbell AC: Primate bites in Gibraltar—minor casualty quirk? *Scott Med J* 34(5):519, 1989.
55. Caravalho J et al: Feline-transmitted sporotrichosis in the Southwestern United States, *West J Med* 154:462, 1991.
56. Carithers HA, Margileth AM: Cat-scratch disease: acute encephalopathy and other neurologic manifestations, *Am J Dis Child* 145(1):98, 1991.
57. Carpenter P, Heppner B, Gnann J: DF-2 bacteremia following cat bites, *Am J Med* 82:621, 1987.
58. Center for Health Systems Research and Analysis, University of Wisconsin: The incidence of facial injuries from dog bites, *JAMA* 251:3265, 1984.
59. Chadwick J: New England's venomous mammals, *N Engl J Med* 281:274, 1969.
60. Check W: An odd link between dog bites, splenectomy, *JAMA* 241:225, 1979.
61. Chisholm CD et al: Comparison of a new pressurized saline canister versus syringe irrigation for laceration cleansing in the emergency department, *Ann Emerg Med* 21(11):1364, 1992.
62. Chomel BB: The modern epidemiological aspects of rabies in the world, *Comp Immunol Microbiol Infect Dis* 16(1):11, 1993.
63. Choudhuri M et al: Efficiency of skin sterilization for a venipuncture with the use of commercially available alcohol or iodine pads, *Am J Infect Control* 18(2):82, 1990.
64. Chronicle: Beware of dog, *San Francisco Chronicle,* May 27, 1987.
65. Chronicle: L.A. County's war against killer coyotes, *San Francisco Chronicle,* Oct 8, 1981.
66. Chronicle: Pet wolf kills little girl at grandma's, *San Francisco Chronicle,* May 29, 1982.
67. Chuinard R, Ambrosia R: Human bite infections of the hand, *J Bone Joint Surg* 59A:416, 1977.
68. Clark MA et al: Fatal and near-fatal animal bite injuries, *J Forensic Sci* 36(4):1256, 1991.
69. Clarke J: *Man is the prey,* London, 1969, Andre Deutsch.
70. Cohle SD, Harlan CW, Harlan G: Fatal big cat attacks, *Am J Forensic Med Pathol* 11(3):208, 1990.
71. Collipp P: Cat-scratch disease: therapy with trimethoprim-sulfamethoxazole, *Am J Dis Child* 146:397, 1992.
72. Compendium of animal rabies control, 1993, National Association of State Public Health Veterinarians, Inc (news), *J Am Vet Med Assoc* 202(2):199, 1993.
73. Confer AW, Durham JA, Clarke CR: Comparison of antigens of *Pasteurella haemolytica* serotype 1 grown *in vitro* and *in vivo, Am J Vet Res* 53(4):472, 1992.
74. Constantine D, Kizer K: *Pet European ferrets: a hazard to public health, small livestock, and wildlife,* Sacramento, 1988, California Department of Health Services.
75. Consul B: Orbital fracture due to camel bite, *J All India Ophthalm Soc* 16:245, 1968.
76. Control CfD: Annual summary, 1979, *MMWR* 28:47, 1980.
77. Control CfD: B-virus infection in humans—Pensacola, Florida, *MMWR* 36:289, 1987.
78. Control CfD: Guidelines for prevention of herpesvirus simiae (B virus) infection in monkey handlers, *MMWR* 36:680, 1987.
79. Control CfD: Rabies in a javelina—Arizona, *MMWR* 35:555, 1986.
80. Control CfD: Rat-bite fever in a college student—California, *MMWR* 33:318, 1984.
81. Control CfD: Tetanus in the U.S., 1982-84, *MMWR* 34:606, 1985.
82. Corey L: Cat-scratch disease. In Isselbacker K, Adams R, Brauwald E, editors: *Harrison's textbook of medicine,* ed 11, New York, 1986, McGraw-Hill, p 1176.
83. Corey L, Hatwick M, Baer G: Serum neutralizing antibody after rabies postexposure prophylaxis, *Ann Intern Med* 85:170, 1976.
84. Corkum D: Mild anaphylactic reaction from a gerbil bite, *Ann Emerg Med* 13:210, 1984.
85. Crammond M: *Killer bears,* New York, 1981, Scribner's.
86. Crone NE, Reder AT: Severe tetanus in immunized patients with high anti-tetanus titers, *Neurology* 42(4):761, 1992.
87. Cummings P: Antibiotics to prevent infections in patients with dog bite wounds: a meta-analysis of randomized trials, *Ann Emerg Med* 23(3):535, 1994.
88. Cushing BS: Responses of polar bears to human menstrual odors. In *Proceedings of International Conference on Bear Research and Management,* vol 5, p 270, 1983.
89. Custer J, Edlich R, Prusak M: Studies in the management of the contaminated wound, *Am J Surg* 121:572, 1971.
90. Cutwright D, Bhaskar S, Gross A: Effect of vancomycin, streptomycin, and tetracycline pulsating jet lavage on contaminated wounds, *Milit Med* 20:810, 1971.
91. Dagher F: Cutaneous wounds, *Contemp Surg* 17:73, 1980.
92. Dalovisio JR, Stetter M, Mikota-Wells S: Rhinoceros' rhinorrhea: cause of an outbreak of infection due to airborne *Mycobacterium bovis* in zookeepers, *Clin Infect Dis* 15(4):598, 1992.
93. Datubo BD: Human bites of the face with tissue losses, *Ann Plast Surg* 21(4):322, 1988.
94. Davis D et al: In Hubbert W, McCulloch W, Schnurrenberger P, editors: *Diseases transmitted from animals to man,* ed 6, Springfield, Ill, 1975, Charles C Thomas.
95. Day T: Controlled trial of prophylactic antibiotics in minor wounds requiring suture, *Lancet* 4(7946):1174, 1975.
96. Dean D, Baer G, Thowpson W: Studies on the local treatment of rabies-infected wounds, *Bull WHO* 28:477, 1963.
97. Delahoussaye PM, Osborne BMS: Cat-scratch disease presenting as abdominal visceral granulomas, *J Infect Dis* 161(1):71, 1990.
98. Dellinger EP et al: Hand infections: bacteriology and treatment; a prospective study, *Arch Surg* 123(6):745, 1988.
99. Dhingra J, Schauerhamer R, Wangenstein O: Peripheral dissemination of bacteria in contaminated wounds: role of devitalized tissue, *Surgery* 80:535, 1976.
100. Diesch S, Ellinghaufen H: Leptospirosis. In Hubbert W, McCulloch W, Schnurrenberger P, editors: *Diseases transmitted from animals to man,* ed 6, Springfield, Ill, 1975, Charles C Thomas.
101. Dire D, Hogan D, Riggs M: A prospective evaluation of risk factors for dog bite wound infections (abstract), *Ann Emerg Med* 19(9):961, 1990.
102. Dire DJ: Cat bite wounds: risk factors for infection, *Ann Emerg Med* 20(9):973, 1991.
103. Dire DJ, Hogan DE, Walker JS: Prophylactic oral antibiotics for low-risk dog bite wounds, *Pediatr Emerg Care* 8(4):194, 1992.
104. Dire DJ, Welsh AP: A comparison of wound irrigation solutions used in the emergency department, *Ann Emerg Med* 19(6):704, 1990.

105. Dirschl DR, Wilson FC: Topical antibiotic irrigation in the prophylaxis of operative wound infections in orthopedic surgery, *Orthop Clin North Am* 22(3):419, 1991.
106. Dolan M et al: Syndrome of *Rochalimaea henselae* adenitis suggesting cat scratch disease, *Ann Intern Med* 118:331, 1993.
107. Donovan JF, Kaplan WE: The therapy of genital trauma by dog bite, *J Urol* 141(5):1163, 1989.
108. Douglas L: Bite wounds, *Am Fam Physician* 11:93, 1975.
109. Drabick J et al: *Pasteurella multocida* pneumonia in a man with AIDS and nontraumatic feline exposure, *Chest* 103:7, 1993.
110. Dreyfuss U, Singer M: Human bites of the hand: a study of one hundred six patients, *J Hand Surg* 10:884, 1985.
111. Drinking man nibbles bat ear, *San Francisco Chronicle,* Sept 30, 1988.
112. Duke W, Robson M, Krizek T: Civilian wounds, their bacterial flora and rate of infection, *Surg Forum* 23:518, 1972.
113. Dushoff I: Handling the hand, *Emerg Med* 8:26, 1976.
114. Eadie PA et al: Seal finger in a wildlife ranger, *Ir Med J* 83(3):117, 1990.
115. Earley M, Bardsley A: Human bites: a review, *Br J Plast Surg* 37:458, 1984.
116. Edixhoven P, Sinha S, Dandny D: Horse injuries, *Injury* 12:279, 1981.
117. Edlich R, Custer J, Madden J: Studies in management of the contaminated wound. III. Assessment of irrigation with antiseptic agents, *Am J Surg* 118:21, 1969.
118. Edlich R, Madden J, Prusak M: The therapeutic value of gently scrubbing in prolonging the limited period of effectiveness of antibiotics in contaminated wounds, *Am J Surg* 121:668, 1971.
119. Edlich R, Smith Q, Edgerton M: Resistance of the surgical wound to antimicrobial prophylaxis and its mechanisms of development, *Am J Surg* 126:583, 1973.
120. Edlich RF et al: Scientific basis for selecting staple and tape skin closures, *Clin Plast Surg* 17(3):571, 1990.
121. Elenbaas R, McNabney W, Robinson W: Prophylactic oxacillin for cat bite wounds (letter), *Ann Emerg Med* 13:1083, 1984.
122. Elenbaas R, McNabney W, Robinson W: Prophylactic oxacillin in dog bite wounds, *Ann Emerg Med* 11:248, 1982.
123. Elsey RM, Carson RW, DuBose TJ: *Pasteurella multocida* peritonitis in an HIV-positive patient on continuous cycling peritoneal dialysis, *Am J Nephrol* 11(1):61, 1991.
124. Eng TR et al: Rabies surveillance, United States, 1988, *MMWR CDC Surveill Summ* 38(1):1, 1989.
125. English CK et al: Cat-scratch disease: Isolation and culture of the bacterial agent, *JAMA* 259(9):1347, 1988.
126. Extension of the raccoon rabies epizootic—United States, 1992, *MMWR* 41(36):661, 1992.
127. Eyres KS, Allen TR: Skyline view of the metacarpal head in the assessment of human fight-bite injuries, *J Hand Surg* 18(1):43, 1993.
128. Faddis D, Daniel D, Boyer J: Tissue toxicity of antiseptic solutions, *J Trauma* 17:895, 1977.
129. Feder H, Shanley J, Baerbera J: Review of 59 patients hospitalized with animal bites, *Pediatr Infect Dis J* 6:24, 1987.
130. Fenner PJ, Williamson JA, Myers D: Platypus envenomation—a painful learning experience, *Med J Aust* 157(11-12):829, 1992.
131. Fiala M, Bauer H, Khaleel M: Dog bite, *Bacteroides* infections, coagulopathy, renal microangiopathy, *Ann Intern Med* 87:248, 1977.
132. Findling J, Pohlmann G, Rose H: Fulminant gram-negative bacillemia (DF-2) following a dog bite in an asplenic woman, *Am J Med* 60:154, 1980.
133. Fishbein D: Rabies, *Infect Dis Clin North Am* 5(1):53, 1991.
134. Flowers D: Human infection due to *Mycobacterium marinum* after a dolphin bite, *J Clin Pathol* 23:475, 1970.
135. Floyd T, Manville AM, French SP: Normal oral flora in black bears: guidelines for antimicrobial prophylaxis following bear attacks, *J Wilderness Med* 1:47, 1990.
136. Fordham JN et al: Rat bite fever without the bite, *Ann Rheum Dis* 51(3):411, 1992.
137. Fowler M: Diseases of children acquired from nondomestic animals, *Curr Probl Pediatr* 4:1, 1975.
138. Fowler M: *Restraint and handling of wild and domestic animals,* Ames, 1978, Iowa State University Press.
139. Fowler M: *Zoo and wild animal medicine,* Philadelphia, 1978, WB Saunders.
140. Fox M, Kaufmann A: Brucellosis in the United States, 1965-1974, *J Infect Dis* 136:312, 1977.
141. Francis D, Holmes M, Brandon G: *Pasteurella multocida* infections after domestic animal bites and scratches, *JAMA* 233:42, 1975.
142. Frean JA et al: Sporotrichosis following a rodent bite: a case report, *Mycopathologia* 116(1):5, 1991.
143. French S, French M: Predatory behavior of grizzly bears feeding on elk calves in Yellowstone National Park, 1986-88. In *Proceedings of International Conference on Bear Research and Management,* vol 9, p 335, 1990.
144. Fretzayas A et al: Multiorgan involvement in systemic cat-scratch disease, *Scand J Infect Dis* 25(1):145, 1993.
145. Galvin R, Desimon D: Infection rate in simple suturing, *JACEP* 5:332, 1976.
146. Ganiere JP et al: Characterization of *Pasteurella* from gingival scrapings of dogs and cats, *Comp Immunol Microbiol Infect Dis* 16(1):77, 1993.
147. Garrard J, Leland N, Smith DK: Epidemiology of human bites to children in a day-care center, *Am J Dis Child* 142(6):643, 1988.
148. Georghiou PR, Mollee TF, Tilse KW: *Pasteurella multocida* infection after a Tasmanian devil bite (letter; comment), *Clin Infect Dis* 14(6):1266, 1992.
149. Gerber M, Sedgwick A, MacAlister T: The aetiological agent of cat scratch disease, *Lancet* 1(8440):1236, 1985.
150. Gerber M et al: Cell-mediated immunity in cat-scratch disease, *J Allergy Clin Immunol* 78:887, 1986.
151. Geronemus R, Mertz P, Eaglstein W: Wound healing: the effects of topical antimicrobial agents, *Arch Dermatol* 115:1311, 1979.
152. Gjertz I, Persen E: Confrontations between humans and bears in Svalbard, *Polar Res* 5:253, 1987.
153. Glass K: Factors related to the resolution of treated hand infections, *J Hand Surg* 7:388, 1982.
154. Gnann J, Bressler G, Bodet C: Human blastomycosis after a dog bite, *Ann Intern Med* 98:48, 1983.
155. Gold KW et al: Evaluation and treatment of patients with human bite marks, *Am J Forensic Med Pathol* 10(2):140, 1989.
156. Gold KW et al: Human bite marks: differential diagnosis, *Clin Pediatr* 28(7):329, 1989.
157. Goldberg M: Antibiotics and oral and oral-cutaneous lacerations, *J Oral Surg* 23:117, 1965.
158. Goldsmith M: Has AFIP debugged the cat scratch mystery? *JAMA* 250:2745, 1983.
159. Goldstein E: Rat-bite fever. In Hoeprich P, editor: *Infectious disease: a modern treatise of infectious processes,* Hagerstown, Md, 1977, Harper & Row.
160. Goldstein E, Barones M, Miller T: *Eikenella corrodens* in hand infections, *J Hand Surg* 8:563, 1983.
161. Goldstein EJ, Citron DM: Comparative activities of cefuroxime, amoxicillin–clavulanic acid, ciprofloxacin, enoxacin, and ofloxacin against aerobic and anaerobic bacteria isolated from bite wounds, *Antimicrob Agents Chemother* 32(8):1143, 1988.
162. Goldstein E, Citron D, Finegold S: Dog bite wounds and infection: a prospective clinical study, *Ann Emerg Med* 9:508, 1980.
163. Goldstein E, Citron D, Finegold S: Role of anerobic bacteria in bite-wound infections, *Rev Infect Dis* 6(suppl 1):S177, 1984.
164. Goldstein E, Citron D, Richwald G: Lack of in vitro efficacy of oral forms of certain cephalosporins, erythromycin, and oxacillin against *Pasteurella multocida, Antimicrob Agents Chemother* 32:213, 1988.

165. Goldstein E, Citron D, Vagvolgyi A: Susceptibility of bite wound bacteria to seven oral antimicrobial agents, including RU-985, a new erythromycin: considerations in choosing empiric therapy, *Antimicrob Agents Chemother* 29:556, 1986.
166. Goldstein E, Citron D, Wield B: Bacteriology of human and animal bite wounds, *J Clin Microbiol* 8:667, 1978.
167. Goldstein R, Goodhart G, Moore J: *Pasteurella multocida* infection after animal bites (letter), *N Engl J Med* 315(7):460, 1986.
168. Goldstein E, Reinhardt J, Murray P: Animal and human bite wounds: a comparative study, Augmentin vs. penicillin +/– dicloxacillin: a special report, *Postgrad Med* 56(suppl):105, 1984.
169. Goldstein E et al: Prevalence of *Eikenella corrodens* in dental plaque, *J Clin Microbiol* 17:636, 1983.
170. Goldstein E et al: Outpatient therapy of bite wounds: demographic data, bacteriology, and a prospective randomized trial of amoxicillin/clavulanic acid versus penicillin +/– dicloxacillin, *Int J Dermatol* 26:123, 1987.
171. Goldstein EJ et al: Recovery of an unusual *Flavobacterium* group IIb-like isolate from a hand infection following pig bite, *J Clin Microbiol* 28(5):1079, 1990.
172. Gonnering R: Ocular adnexal injury and complications in orbital dog bites, *Ophthalm Plast Reconstr Surg* 3(4):231, 1987.
173. Gowans F: *Mountain man and grizzly,* Orem, Utah, 1986, Mountain Grizzly Publications.
174. Graham W, Calabretta A, Miller S: Dog bites, *Am Fam Physician* 15:132, 1977.
175. Grant D: Massive trauma to the head and face, attack by a cougar: report of a case, *ASDC J Dent Child* 46:226, 1979.
176. Gravell M, London W, Lecatsas G: Transmission of simian acquired immunodeficiency syndrome with type D retrovirus isolated from saliva or urine, *Proc Soc Exp Biol Med* 177:491, 1985.
177. Gravett A, Sterner S, Clinton J: A trial of povidone-iodine in the prevention of infection in sutured lacerations, *Ann Emerg Med* 16:167, 1987.
178. Greenhalgh C, Cockington RA, Raftos J: An epidemiological survey of dog bites presenting to the emergency department of a children's hospital, *J Paediatr Child Health* 27(3):171, 1991.
179. Groopman J, Salahuddin S, Sarngadharan M: HTLV-III in saliva of people with AIDS-related complex and healthy homosexual men at risk for AIDS, *Science* 226:447, 1984.
180. Gross A, Cutwright E, Larson W: Effect of antiseptic agents and pulsating jet lavage on contaminated wounds, *Milit Med* 21:145, 1972.
181. Grossmann J, Adams J, Kurec J: Prophylactic antibiotics in simple hand lacerations, *JAMA* 245:1055, 1981.
182. Group SS: Imipenem/cilastatin vs. gentamycin/clindamycin for treatment of serious bacterial infections: report from a Scandinavian study group, *Lancet* 1(8382):868, 1984.
183. Guba A, Mulliken J, Hooper J: Selection of antibiotics for human bites of the hand, *Plast Reconstr Surg* 56:538, 1975.
184. Guy R, Zook E: Successful treatment of acute head and neck dog bite wounds without antibiotics, *Ann Plast Surg* 17:45, 1987.
185. Halstead SL et al: Pharmacokinetic evaluation of ceftiofur in serum, tissue chamber fluid and bronchial secretions from healthy beef-bred calves, *Can J Vet Res* 56(4):269, 1992.
186. Harari J et al: Bacterial isolates from blood cultures of dogs undergoing dentistry, *Vet Surg* 22(1):27, 1993.
187. Harris D, Imperato P, Oken B: Dog bites: an unrecognized epidemic, *Bull NY Acad Med* 50:981, 1974.
188. Harvey S: Antiseptics and disinfectants, fungicides, ectoparasticides. In Gilman A, Goodman L, Rall T, Murad F, editors: *Goodman and Gilman's the pharmacological basis of therapeutics,* ed 7, New York, 1980, Macmillan.
189. Haughey R, Lammers R, Wagner D: Use of antibiotics in initial management of soft tissue hand wounds, *Ann Emerg Med* 10:187, 1981.
190. Haury B, Rodeheaver G, Vensko J: Debridement: an essential component of traumatic wound care, *Am J Surg* 135:238, 1978.
191. Haynes J: Wildlife encounters seldom fatal, *San Francisco Examiner,* May 24, 1992.
192. Hendricks S, Meyer M: Brucellosis. In Hubbert W, McCulloch W, Schnurrenberger P, editors: *Diseases transmitted from animals to man,* ed 6, Springfield, Ill, 1975, Charles C Thomas.
193. Herrero S: *Bear attacks—their causes and avoidance,* 1985, Winchester Press.
194. Herrero S, Fleck S: Injury to people inflicted by black, grizzly, and polar bears: recent trends and new insights. In *Proceedings of International Conference on Bear Research and Management,* vol 8, p 25, 1990.
195. Ho J et al: *Hemophilus aphrophilus* osteomyelitis, *Am J Med* 76:159, 1984.
196. Hollis DG et al: Characterization of Centers for Disease Control group NO-1, a fastidious, nonoxidative, gram-negative organism associated with dog and cat bites, *J Clin Microbiol* 31(3):746, 1993.
197. Holst E, Rollof J, Miorner H: In vitro activities of cefcanel and some other cephalosporins against *Pasteurella multocida, Antimicrob Agents Chemother* 33(12):2142, 1989.
198. Holst E et al: Characterization and distribution of *Pasteurella* species recovered from infected humans, *J Clin Microbiol* 30(11):2984, 1992.
199. Hombal SM, Dincsoy HP: *Pasteurella multocida* endocarditis, *Am J Clin Pathol* 98(6):565, 1992.
200. Hornick R: Tularemia. In Hoeprich P, editor: *Infectious diseases: a modern treatise of infectious processes,* ed 2, Hagerstown, Md, 1977, Harper & Row.
201. Houang E, Gilmore O, Reid C: Absence of bacterial resistance to povidone-iodine, *J Clin Pathol* 29:752, 1976.
202. Houtman PM: Septic monarthritis due to *Pasteurella multocida* after a cat scratch in a patient with rheumatoid arthritis, *Netherlands J Med* 36(3-4):207, 1990.
203. Howell J, Woodward G: Precipitous hypotension in the emergency department caused by *Capnocytophaga canimorsus, J Emerg Med* 8:312, 1990.
204. Howell JM, Dalsey WC: Aerobic bacteria cultured from the mouth of the American opossum *(Didelphis virginiana)* with reference to bacteria associated with bite infections, *J Clin Microbiol* 28(10):2360, 1990.
205. Howell JM et al: The effect of scrubbing and irrigation with normal saline, povidone iodine, and cefazolin on wound bacterial counts in a guinea pig model, *Am J Emerg Med* 11(2):134, 1993.
206. Howes E: Topical use of streptomycin in wounds, *Am J Med* 3:449, 1947.
207. Hudson A, Vinters H, Povey R: An unusual form of motor neuron disease following a cat bite, *Can J Neurol Sci* 13:111, 1986.
208. Human rabies—Texas, Arkansas, and Georgia, 1991, *MMWR* 40(44):765, 1991.
209. Hutton P, Jones B, Law D: Depot penicillin as prophylaxis in accidental wounds, *Br J Surg* 65:549, 1978.
210. Janda DH et al: Nonhuman primate bites, *J Orthop Res* 8(1):146, 1990.
211. Job L et al: Dysgonic fermenter-2: a clinico-epidemiologic review, *J Emerg Med* 7:185, 1989.
212. Johnsgard P: *Animal behavior,* ed 2, DuBuque, Ia, 1972, William C Brown.
213. Johnson J: Wound infections, *Postgrad Med* 50:126, 1971.
214. Jones D, Stanbridge T: A clinical trial using co-trimoxazole in an attempt to reduce wound infection rates in dog bite wounds, *Postgrad Med J* 61:593, 1985.
215. Jones J: Herpetic whitlow: an infectious occupational hazard, *J Occup Med* 27(10):725, 1985.
216. Jones JW et al: Recurrent *Mycobacterium bovis* infection following a ferret bite (letter), *J Infect* 26(2):225, 1993.
217. Jorden R, Walls R, Vellman P: Antibiotic prophylaxis for dog bites: a prospective controlled study, 1987.
218. Joshi AR, Garshelis DL, Smith JLD: Seasonal movements and variation in habitat use of sloth bears in the lowlands of Nepal: implica-

tions for conservation. In *Proceedings of International Conference on Bear Research and Management,* in press.

219. Kaczmarek E, Sula J, Hutchinson R: Sterility of partially used irrigating solutions, *Am J Hosp Pharm* 39:1534, 1982.
220. Kamin M, Patten B: Creutzfeldt-Jakob disease: possible transmission to humans by consumption of wild animal brains, *Am J Med* 76:142, 1984.
221. Kaniut L: *Alaska bear tales,* Anchorage, 1989, Alaska Northwest Publishing.
222. Kaplan M, Cohen D, Koprowski H: Studies on local treatment of wounds for the prevention of rabies, *Bull WHO* 26:765, 1962.
223. Kappus K: Canine rabies in the U.S. 1971-73: a study of reported cases with reference to vaccination history, *Am J Epidemiol* 103:242, 1976.
224. Katz S, McGinley K, Leyden J: Semipermeable occlusive dressings: effects on growth of pathogenic bacteria and reepithelialization of superficial wounds, *Arch Dermatol* 140:58, 1986.
225. Keane T: Killer pit bull's owner blames parents of dead 2-year-old, *San Francisco Chronicle,* June 16, 1987.
226. Keane T: Pit bulls, stars of a bloody sport, fight and die in secret, *San Francisco Chronicle,* June 18, 1987.
227. Kenevan R, Gottleib V, Rich J: A dog bite injury with involvement of cranial content: case report, *Milit Med* 150:502, 1985.
228. Kizer K: Epidemiologic and clinical aspects of animal bite injuries, *JACEP* 8:134, 1979.
229. Kizer KW: *Pasteurella multocida* infection from a cougar bite: a review of cougar attacks, *West J Med* 150(1):87, 1989.
230. Klein D, Cohen M: *Pasteurella multocida* brain abscess following perforating cranial dog bite, *J Pediatr* 49:588, 1970.
231. Knox ML: Close encounters of the feline kind: big cats on the prowl. *San Francisco Examiner,* Jan 6, 1991.
232. Kohout MP et al: Tiger mauling: fatal spinal injury, *Aust NZ J Surg* 59(6):505, 1989.
233. Krizek T, Robson M: Evolution of quantitative bacteriology in wound management, *Am J Surg* 130:579, 1975.
234. Kropp H: Antibacterial activity of imipenem: the first thienamycin antibiotic, *Rev Infect Dis* 7(suppl):S389, 1985.
235. Kullberg BJ et al: Purpura fulminans and symmetrical peripheral gangrene caused by *Capnocytophaga canimorsus* (formerly DF-2) septicemia—a complication of dog bite, *Medicine* 70(5):287, 1991.
236. Kumar A, Devlin HR, Vellend H: *Pasteurella multocida* meningitis in an adult: case report and review, *Rev Infect Dis* 12(3):440, 1990.
237. Lammers RL et al: Effect of povidone-iodine and saline soaking on bacterial counts in acute, traumatic, contaminated wounds, *Ann Emerg Med* 19(6):709, 1990.
238. Landercasper J et al: Trauma and the veterinarian, *J Trauma* 28(8):1255, 1988.
239. Laufman H: Current use of skin and wound cleansers and antiseptics, *Am J Surg* 157:359, 1989.
240. Lavine L, Isenberg H, Rubins W: Unusual osteomyelitis following superficial dog bite, *Clin Orthop Rel Res* 98:251, 1974.
241. Lebrun A, Caya M, Jacques M: Effects of sub-MICs of antibiotics on cell surface characteristics and virulence of *Pasteurella multocida, Antimicrob Agents Chemother* 36(10):2093, 1992.
242. Lecatsas G, Houff S, Macher A: Retrovirus-like particles in salivary glands, prostate and testes of AIDS patients, *Proc Soc Exp Biol Med* 178:653, 1985.
243. Lee J, Buhr A: Dog bites and local infection with *Pasteurella* species, *Br Med J* 248(1):169, 1960.
244. Leighty J: Doctors declare war on violence, *San Francisco Chronicle,* Sept 26, 1993.
245. Levin JM, Talan DA: Erythromycin failure with subsequent *Pasteurella multocida* meningitis and septic arthritis in a cat-bite victim, *Ann Emerg Med* 19(12):1458, 1990.
246. Lewis DE, Wallace MR: Treatment of adult systemic cat scratch disease with gentamicin sulfate, *West J Med* 154(3):330, 1991.
247. Leyden J, Sulzberger M: Topical antibiotics and minor skin trauma, *Am Fam Pract* 23:121, 1981.
248. Lindsey D, Chrisopher M, Hollenbach J: Natural course of the human bite wound: incidence of infection and complications in 434 bites and 803 lacerations in the same group of patients, *J Trauma* 27:45, 1987.
249. Lindsey D, Nava C, Marti M: Effectiveness of penicillin irrigation in control of infection in sutured lacerations, *J Trauma* 22:186, 1982.
250. Long WT et al: Toxic shock syndrome after a human bite to the hand, *J Hand Surg* 13(6):957, 1988.
251. Lopez A et al: Outbreak of human rabies in the Peruvian jungle, *Lancet* 339(8790):408, 1992.
252. Loro A, Franceschi F: Human bites and finger infections: a survey at Dodoma Regional Hospital, Tanzania, *Trop Doct* 22(1):24, 1992.
253. Love DN, Vekselstein R, Collings S: The obligate and facultatively anaerobic bacterial flora of the normal feline gingival margin, *Vet Microbiol* 22(2-3):267, 1990.
254. Lowbury E, Lilly H, Bull J: Methods for disinfection of hands and operation sites, *Br Med J* 257(3):531, 1964.
255. Lynch M: Laboratory procedures. In *Burket's oral medicine,* Philadelphia, 1977, JB Lippincott.
256. Lyons R: 90's pets, the more exotic the better, *New York Times* 140:34(L) col 1, 22 col in, June 23, 1991.
257. Mahrer S, Raik E: *Capnocytophaga canimorsus* septicemia associated with cat scratch, *Pathology* 24(3):194, 1992.
258. Maki D: Lister revisited: surgical antisepsis and asepsis, *N Engl J Med* 294:1286, 1976.
259. Malinowski R, Strate R, Perry J: Management of human bite injuries of the hand, *J Trauma* 19:655, 1979.
260. Man hunting out of season shot by turkey, *San Francisco Chronicle,* Apr 25, 1992.
261. Mann R, Hoffeld T, Farmer C: Human bites of the hand: twenty years of experience, *J Hand Surg* 2:97, 1977.
262. Margileth A: Cat scratch disease in 65 patients, *Clin Proc Child Hosp DC* 27:213, 1971.
263. Margileth AM: Antibiotic therapy for cat-scratch disease: clinical study of therapeutic outcome in 268 patients and a review of the literature, *Pediatr Infect Dis J* 11(6):474, 1992.
264. Margileth A, Wear D, English C: Systemic cat scratch disease: report of 23 patients with prolonged or recurrent severe bacterial infection, *J Infect Dis* 155:390, 1987.
265. Margileth A, Wear D, Hadfield T: Cat-scratch disease: bacteria in skin at the primary inoculation site, *JAMA* 252:928, 1984.
266. Markham R, Polk B: Seal finger, *Rev Infect Dis* 1(3):567, 1979.
267. Marr J, Beck A, Lugo J: An epidemiologic study of the human bite, *Public Health Rep* 94:514, 1979.
268. Marrie T, Bent J, West A: Extensive gas in tissues of the forearm after horsebite, *South Med J* 72:1473, 1979.
269. Mass D, Newmeyer W, Kilgore E: Seal finger, *J Hand Surg* 6(6):610, 1981.
270. Matthews R: Classification and nomenclature of viruses, *Intervirology* 17:109, 1982.
271. Matushek KJ, Rosin E: Pharmacokinetics of cefazolin applied topically to the surgical wound, *Arch Surg* 126(7):890, 1991.
272. McCarthy TJ: Human depredation by vampire bats *(Desmodus rotundus)* following a hog cholera campaign, *Am J Trop Med Hyg* 40(3):320, 1989.
273. McConnell C, Neale H: Two-year review of hand infections in a municipal hospital, *Am Surg* 45:643, 1979.
274. McHugh T, Bartlett R, Raymond J: Rat bite fever: report of a fatal case, *Ann Emerg Med* 14:1116, 1985.
275. Mennen U, Howells CJ: Human fight-bite injuries of the hand: a study of 100 cases within 18 months, *J Hand Surg* 16(4):431, 1991.
276. Meyers B, Hirschmann S, Sloan W: Generalized Shwartzmann reaction in man after a dog bite, *Ann Intern Med* 73:33, 1970.

277. Middaugh J: Human injury from bear attacks in Alaska, 1900-1985, *Alaska Med* 29(4):121, 1987.
278. Miller SJ et al: Stroke following rottweiler attack, *Ann Emerg Med* 22(2):262, 1993.
279. Mills E: *The grizzly,* 1919, Comstock.
280. Mishriki SF, Law DJ, Jeffery PJ: Factors affecting the incidence of postoperative wound infection, *J Hosp Infect* 16(3):223, 1990.
281. Monkeys out for revenge in Malaysia, *San Francisco Chronicle,* May 13, 1988.
282. Moore W, Holdeman L, Smibert R: Bacteriology of experimental gingivitis in young adult humans, *Infect Immun* 38:651, 1982.
283. Moore W, Holdeman L, Smibert R: Bacteriology of severe periodontitis in young adult humans, *Infect Immun* 38:1137, 1982.
284. Morgan MG, Mardel SN: Clenched fist actinomycosis in a penicillin-allergic female (letter), *J Infect* 26(2):222, 1993.
285. Morgan W, Hutchison D, Johnson H: Delayed treatment of wounds of the hand and forearm under antibiotic cover, *Br J Surg* 67:140, 1980.
286. Moro KW et al: The epidemiology of rodent and lagomorph rabies in Maryland, 1981 to 1986, *J Wildlife Dis* 27(3):452, 1991.
287. Morris JT, McAllister CK: Bacteremia due to *Pasteurella multocida, South Med J* 85(4):442, 1992.
288. Moy RL, Lee A, Zalka A: Commonly used suturing techniques in skin surgery, *Am Fam Physician* 44(5):1625, 1991.
289. Muguti GI, Zvomuya NM, Bvuma ET: Experience with human bites in Zimbabwe, *Cent Afr J Med* 37(9):294, 1991.
290. Mulliken J, Healey N, Glowacki J: Povidone-iodine and tensile strength of wounds in rats, *J Trauma* 20:323, 1980.
291. Murray L, Sivaloganathan S: Rambutt—the killer sheep, *Med Sci Law* 27:95, 1987.
292. Muszynski M, Eppes S, Riley H: Granulomatous osteolytic lesion of the skull associated with cat scratch disease, *Pediatr Infect Dis J* 6:199, 1987.
293. Myers CB, Christmann LM: Rat bite—an unusual cause of direct trauma to the globe, *J Pediatr Ophthalmol Strabismus* 28(6):356, 1991.
294. Nelson R et al: Behavior, biochemistry, and hibernation in black, grizzly, and polar bears In *Proceedings of International Conference on Bear Research and Management,* vol 5, p 284, 1983.
295. Neu HC: The development of macrolides: clarithromycin in perspective, *J Antimicrob Chemother* 27(suppl A):1, 1991.
296. Neu HC et al: Comparative in vitro activity of the new oral macrolide azithromycin, *Eur J Clin Microbiol Infect Dis* 7(4):541, 1988.
297. Nicoletti G, Boghossian V, Borland R: Hygienic hand disinfection: a comparative study with chlorhexidine detergents and soap, *J Hosp Infect* 15(4):323, 1990.
298. Norrby S, Eriksson M, Ottosson E: Imipenem/cilastatin versus gentamycin/clindamycin: a cost effectiveness study, *Scand J Infect Dis* 18:371, 1986.
299. Nylen S, Carlsson B: Time factor, infection frequency and quantitative microbiology in hand injuries, *Scand J Plast Reconstr Surg* 14:185, 1980.
300. Oie S, Kamiya A: Microbial contamination of brushes used for preoperative shaving, *J Hosp Infect* 21(2):103, 1992.
301. Ordog G: The bacteriology of dog bite wounds, *Ann Emerg Med* 15:1324, 1986.
302. Ordog G, Balasubramanium S, Wasserberger J: Rat Bites: fifty cases, *Ann Emerg Med* 14:126, 1985.
303. Orton D, Fulcher W: *Pasteurella multocida:* bilateral septic knee joint prostheses from a distant cat bite, *Ann Emerg Med* 13:1065, 1984.
304. Owen C, Buker E, Bell J: *Pasteurella multocida* in animals' mouths, *Rocky Mt Med J* 65:45, 1968.
305. Pacer R, Fishbein D, Baer G: Rabies in the U.S. and Canada, 1983, *MMWR* 34:1SS, 1985.
306. Paisley J, Lauer B: Severe facial injuries to infants due to unprovoked attacks by pet ferrets, *JAMA* 259(13):2005, 1988.
307. Palmer A: B virus, herpesvirus simiae: historical perspective, *J Med Primatol* 16:99, 1987.
308. Palmer J, Rees M: Dog bites of the face: a 15 year review, *J Plast Surg* 36:315, 1983.
309. Parks B, Hawkins L, Horner P: Bites of the hand, *Rocky Mt Med J* 71:85, 1974.
310. Paterson J, Cardo V, Stratigos G: An examination of antibiotic prophylaxis in oral and maxillofacial surgery, *J Oral Surg* 28:753, 1970.
311. Peek RJ, Truss C: Secretory diarrhea following a dog bite, *Dig Dis Sci* 36(8):1151, 1991.
312. Peel MM et al: *Actinobacillus* spp. and related bacteria in infected wounds of humans bitten by horses and sheep, *J Clin Microbiol* 29(11):2535, 1991.
313. Peeples E, Bowick J, Scott F: Wounds of the hand contaminated by human or animal saliva, *J Trauma* 20:383, 1980.
314. Pers C, Kristiansen J, Scheibel J: Fatal septicemia caused by DF-2 in a previously healthy man, *Scand J Infect Dis* 18:265, 1986.
315. Phuapradit W, Saropala N: Topical application of honey in treatment of abdominal wound disruption, *Aust NZ J Obstet Gynecol* 32(4):381, 1992.
316. *Physicians' Desk Reference,* ed 47, Montvale, NJ, 1993, Medical Economics Data.
317. Picker R, Milder J: Transverse myelitis associated with cat-scratch disease in an adult, *JAMA* 246:2840, 1981.
318. Pietsch J, Meakins J: Complications of povidone-iodine absorption in topically treated burn patients, *Lancet* 1(7954):280, 1976.
319. Pinckney L, Kennedy L: Fractures of the infant skull caused by animal bites, *Am J Radiol* 135:179, 1980.
320. Pinckney L, Kennedy L: Traumatic deaths from dog attacks in the United States, *Pediatrics* 69:193, 1982.
321. Plaus W, Hermann G: The surgical management of superficial infections caused by atypical mycobacteria, *Surgery* 110:99, 1991.
322. Pollack A, Kroome K, Evans M: Bacteriology of primary wound sepsis in potentially contaminated abdominal operations, *Br J Surg* 65:76, 1970.
323. Porter JD et al: Lack of early antitoxin response to tetanus booster, *Vaccine* 10(5):334, 1992.
324. Post KW, Cole NA, Raleigh RH: In vitro antimicrobial susceptibility of *Pasteurella haemolytica* and *Pasteurella multocida* recovered from cattle with bovine respiratory disease complex, *J Vet Diagn Invest* 3(2):124, 1991.
325. Postma BH et al: Cowpox-virus-like infection associated with rat bite (letter), *Lancet* 337(8743):733, 1991.
326. Prasad A, Madan VS, Buxi TB: Tiger assault: an unusual mode of head injury (letter), *Clin Neurol Neurosurg* 93(2):171, 1991.
327. Prescott JF, Yielding KM: In vitro susceptibility of selected veterinary bacterial pathogens to ciprofloxacin, enrofloxacin and norfloxacin, *Can J Vet Res* 54(1):195, 1990.
328. Presier G, Lavell T: Rooster attacks on children, *Pediatrics* 79(3):426, 1987.
329. Press A: Big hunt for elephant that ate five Indians, *San Francisco Chronicle,* 1986.
330. Press A: Pet buffalo must die, *San Francisco Chronicle,* Dec 24, 1988.
331. Press A: Humans and elephants battle for survival: 8 people, 10 animals dead in Sri Lanka, *San Francisco Chronicle,* Sept 27, 1993.
332. Prevots R et al: Tetanus surveillance—United States, 1989-1990, *MMWR CDC Surveill Summ* 41(8):1, 1992.
333. Puckett A, et al: Post transfusion septicemia 1980-1989: importance of donor arm cleansing, *J Clin Pathol* 45(2):155, 1992.
334. Quenzer R, Mostow S, Emerson J: Cat-bite tularemia, *JAMA* 238:1845, 1977.
335. Rabies prevention—United States, 1991. Recommendations of the Immunization Practices Advisory Committee (ACIP), *MMWR* 3:1, 1991.
336. Rapuano R, Stratigos G: Mandibular fracture resulting from a dog bite, *J Oral Surg* 34:359, 1976.

337. Rauber P: When nature turns nasty, *Sierra,* Nov/Dec 1993, p 46.
338. Rausch R: Geographic variation in size in North American brown bears, *Ursus arctos* L., as indicated by condylobasal length, 41:33, 1963.
339. Rayan GM et al: *Eikenella corrodens* in human mouth flora, *J Hand Surg* 13(6):953, 1988.
340. Rayan G et al: A comparison of human and animal mouth flora, *J Okla State Med Assoc* 84:510, 1991.
341. Reed B, Clark R: Cutaneous tissue repair: practical implications of current knowledge, *J Am Acad Dermatol* 13:919, 1985.
342. Reported human injuries or health threats attributed to wild or exotic animals kept as pets (1971-1981), *J Am Vet Med Assoc* 180(4):382, 1982.
343. Resnick D et al: Osteomyelitis and septic arthritis of the hand following human bites, *Skel Radiol* 14:263, 1985.
344. Richman KM, Rickman LS: The potential for transmission of human immunodeficiency virus through human bites, *J AIDS* 6(4):402, 1993.
345. Ritchie AJ, Rocke LG: Staples versus sutures in the closure of scalp wounds: a prospective, double-blind, randomized trial, *Injury* 20(4):217, 1989.
346. Roberts A, Roberts F, Hall R: A prospective trial of prophylactic povidone-iodine in lacerations of the hand, *J Hand Surg* 10:370, 1985.
347. Roberts J: Cat bites, *Emerg Med Amb Care News* 10-11, Dec 1988.
348. Robertson M: *Brucella* infection transmitted by dog bite, *JAMA* 225:750, 1973.
349. Robson M, Heggers J: Cefamandole therapy in hand infections, *J Hand Surg* 8:560, 1983.
350. Rodeheaver G, Kurtz L, Kircher B: Pluronic F-68: a promising new skin wound cleanser, *Ann Emerg Med* 9:572, 1980.
351. Rodeheaver G, Pettry D, Thacker J: Wound cleansing by high pressure irrigation, *Surg Gynecol Obstet* 141:357, 1975.
352. Rodeheaver G, Smith S, Thacker J: Mechanical cleansing of contaminated wounds with a surfactant, *Am J Surg* 129:241, 1975.
353. Rosatte RC et al: Trap-vaccinate-release and oral vaccination for rabies control in urban skunks, raccoons and foxes, *J Wildlife Dis* 28(4):562, 1992.
354. Rosen R: The use of antibiotics in the initial management of recent dogbite wounds, *Am J Emerg Med* 3:19, 1985.
355. Rothrock SG, Howard RM: Delayed brachial artery occlusion owing to a dog bite of the upper extremity, *Pediatr Emerg Care* 6(4):293, 1990.
356. Rowley B: Born cages (wild animal pets), *Sierra* 77:14, 1992.
357. Rugiero J, Gozalez C, Yerga M: Sporotrichosis transmitted by rat bite, *Rev Asoc Med Argent Microbiol* 75:491, 1961.
358. Russel A: *Grizzly country,* New York, 1985, Alfred A Knopf.
359. Rutherford W, Spence R: Infection in wounds sutured in the accident and emergency department, *Ann Emerg Med* 9:350, 1980.
360. Rygg M, Bruun CF: Rat bite fever *(Streptobacillus moniliformis)* with septicemia in a child, *Scand J Infect Dis* 24(4):535, 1992.
361. Sachs MK: Lymphocutaneous *Nocardia brasiliensis* infection acquired from a cat scratch: case report and review, *Clin Infect Dis* 15(4):710, 1992.
362. Sacks JJ, Sattin RW, Bonzo SE: Dog bite–related fatalities from 1979 through 1988, *JAMA* 262(11):1489, 1989.
363. Samson R, Altman S: Antibiotic prophylaxis for minor lacerations, *NY State J Med* 77:1728, 1977.
364. Sande M, Mandell G: Antimicrobial agents: the aminoglycosides. In Gilman A et al, editors: *Goodman and Gilman's the pharmacological basis of therapeutics,* ed 7, New York, 1980, Macmillan.
365. Sanford J: *Guide to antimicrobial therapy 1993,* Dallas, 1993, Antimicrobial Therapy.
366. Saphir D, Carter G: Gingival flora of the dog with special reference to bacteria associated with bites, *J Clin Microbiol* 3:344, 1976.
367. Scarcella J: Management of bites, *Ohio State Med J* 65:25, 1969.
368. Schelkun P: Fearsome Fido: how to handle canine aggression while exercising, *Physician Sportsmed* 21(4):142, 1993.
369. Scher KS, Peoples JB: Combined use of topical and systemic antibiotics, *Am J Surg* 161(4):422, 1991.
370. Schiappacasse R, Colville J, Wong P: Sporotrichosis associated with an infected cat, *Cutis* 268, 1985.
371. Schmidt D, Heckman J: *Eikenella corrodens* in human bite infections of the hand, *J Trauma* 23:478, 1983.
372. Schoen R, Wohlgelernter D, Barden G: Infection with CDC Group DF-2 gram-negative rod, *Arch Intern Med* 140:657, 1980.
373. Schwartzman W: Infections due to *Rochalimaea:* the expanding clinical spectrum, *Clin Infect Dis* 15:893, 1992.
374. Schweich P, Fleisher G: Human bites in children, *Pediatr Emerg Care* 1:51, 1985.
375. Sebben J: Surgical antiseptics, *J Am Acad Dermatol* 9:759, 1983.
376. Sens MA et al: Fatal *Streptobacillus moniliformis* infection in a two-month-old infant, *Am J Clin Pathol* 91(5):612, 1989.
377. Shackelford P: Rat bite fever. In Feigin RD, editor: *Pediatric infectious disease,* Philadelphia, 1981, WB Saunders.
378. Shattock F: Injuries caused by wild animals, *Lancet* 1(539):412, 1968.
379. Shepard P, Sanders B: *The sacred paw,* New York, 1985, Viking Penguin.
380. Shukla H, Mittal D, Naithani Y: Bull horn injury: a clinical study, *Injury* 9:164, 1978.
381. Sikes R: Rabies. In Hubbert W, McCulloch W, Schnurrenberger P, editors: *Diseases transmitted from animals to man,* ed 6, Springfield, Ill, 1975, Charles C Thomas.
382. Silley P, Brewster G: Kill kinetics of the cephalosporin antibiotics cephalexin and cefuroxime against bacteria of veterinary importance, *Vet Rec* 123(13):343, 1988.
383. Simon H, Swartz M: Chemotherapy for microbial diseases. In Rubenstein E, Federman D, editors: *Scientific American medicine,* New York, 1993, Scientific American.
384. Sims J et al: Marine bacteria complicating seawater near-drowning and marine wounds: a hypothesis, *Ann Emerg Med* 12:212, 1983.
385. Sindelar W, Mason R: Irrigation of subcutaneous tissue with povidone-iodine solution for prevention of surgical wound infection, *Surg Gynecol Obstet* 148:227, 1979.
386. Singleton A, Julian J: An experimental evaluation of methods used to prevent infection in wounds contaminated with feces, *Ann Surg* 151:912, 1960.
387. Skurka J, Willert C, Yogev R: Wound infection following dog bite despite prophylactic penicillin, *Infection* 14:134, 1986.
388. Smith JS et al: Unexplained rabies in three immigrants in the United States: a virologic investigation, *N Engl J Med* 324(4):205, 1991.
389. Snyder KB, Pentecost MJ: Clinical and angiographic findings in extremity arterial injuries secondary to dog bites, *Ann Emerg Med* 19(9):983, 1990.
390. Spires J, Smith R: Cat-scratch disease, *Otolaryngol Head Neck Surg* 94:622, 1986.
391. Stahl-Bayliss CM et al: The comparative efficacy and safety of 5% povidone-iodine cream for topical antisepsis, *Ostomy Wound Manage* 31:40, 1990.
392. Steele M et al: Prophylactic penicillin for intraoral wounds, *Ann Emerg Med* 18:847, 1989.
393. Steinbrook P, Flodmark O, Scheifele D: Animal bites causing central nervous system injury to children, *Pediatr Neurosci* 12:96, 1986.
394. Stern P et al: Established hand infections: a controlled prospective study, *J Hand Surg* 8:553, 1983.
395. Stevenson J, Anderson I: Hand infections: an audit of 160 infections treated in an accident and emergency department, *J Hand Surg* 18B:115, 1993.
396. Stevenson J, Thatcher J, Rodeheaver G: Cleansing the traumatic wound by high pressure irrigation, *JACEP* 5:17, 1976.

397. Stipp D: Tabbies terrorize our towns, landing cats in the doghouse. Garfield, from Massachusetts, crashes through skylights and stalks his neighbors, *Wall Street Journal,* Aug 18, 1993.
398. Storer T, Trevis L: *California grizzly,* Berkeley, 1955, University of California Press.
399. Stornello C: Transmission of hepatitis B via human bite (letter), *Lancet* 338(8773):1024, 1991.
400. Strady A et al: Morsures d'animaux (animal bites), *Presse Med* 17(42):2229, 1988.
401. Strassburg M et al: Animal bites: patterns of treatment, *Ann Emerg Med* 10:193, 1981.
402. Stringel G et al: Topical and systemic antibiotics in the prevention of wound infection, *J Pediatr Surg* 24(10):1003, 1989.
403. Stucker FJ et al: Management of animal and human bites in the head and neck, *Arch Otolaryngol Head Neck Surg* 116(7):789, 1990.
404. Swartz M, Calin A: Leptospirosis, relapsing fever, rat-bite fever, and Lyme disease. In Rubenstein E, Federman D, editors: *Scientific American medicine,* New York, 1993, Scientific American.
405. Szalay G, Sommerstein A: Inoculation osteomyelitis secondary to animal bites, *Clin Pediatr* 11:687, 1972.
406. Talan DA et al: *Staphylococcus intermedius:* clinical presentation of a new human dog bite pathogen, *Ann Emerg Med* 18(4):410, 1989.
407. Talan DA et al: *Staphylococcus intermedius* in canine gingiva and canine-inflicted human wound infections: laboratory characterization of a newly recognized zoonotic pathogen, *J Clin Microbiol* 27(1):78, 1989.
408. Tappero J et al: The epidemiology of bacillary angiomatosis and bacillary peliosis, *JAMA* 269:770, 1993.
409. Taylor G: Management of human bite injuries of the hand, *Can Med Assoc J* 133:191, 1985.
410. Thomson H, Svitek V: Small animal bites: the role of primary closure, *J Trauma* 13:20, 1973.
411. Tindall J, Harrison C: *Pasteurella multocida* infections following animal injuries, especially cat bites, *Arch Dermatol* 105:412, 1972.
412. Tomasetti B, Walker L, Gormley M: Human bites of the face, *J Oral Surg* 37:565, 1979.
413. Tribe G, Noren E: Incidence of bites from cynomolgus monkeys in attending animal staff 1975-80, *Lab Animals* 17:110, 1983.
414. Tribune: Man bitten by coyote gets rabies shot, *Oakland Tribune,* Sept 12, 1982.
415. Uman S, Kunin C: Needle aspiration in the diagnosis of soft tissue infections, *Arch Intern Med* 135:423, 1973.
416. Van J: Ferret fad dangerous, vets warn. *Chicago Tribune,* Sept 6, 1986.
417. Van Demark RES, Van Demark REJ: Swine bites of the hand, *J Hand Surg* 16(1):136, 1991.
418. Veitch J, Omer G: Case report: treatment of catbite injuries of the hand, *J Trauma* 19(3):201, 1979.
419. Vestey JP, Yirrell DL, Aldridge RD: Cowpox/catpox infection, *Br J Dermatol* 124(1):74, 1991.
420. Veterinary Public Health Unit: World Survey of Rabies XXII (years 1984/85) (WHO RABILES 87.189), Geneva, 1987, World Health Organization.
421. Vijanto J: Disinfection of surgical wounds without inhibition of normal wound healing, *Arch Surg* 115:253, 1980.
422. Vorherr H, Vorherr U, Mehta P: Vaginal absorption of povidone-iodine, *JAMA* 244:2628, 1980.
423. Waldvogel F et al: Perioperative antibiotic prophylaxis of wound and foreign body infections: microbial factors affecting efficacy, *Rev Infect Dis* 13(suppl):S782, 1991.
424. Warren RA, Roomi R: Ready-Stitch: a new device for the closure of skin wounds, *Ann Plast Surg* 25(3):230, 1990.
425. Warwick W: Cat scratch disease. In Hubbert W, McCulloch W, Schnurrenberger P, editors: *Diseases transmitted from animals to man,* ed 6, Springfield, Ill, 1975, Charles C Thomas.
426. Watson D: Severe head injury from dog bites, *Ann Emerg Med* 9:28, 1980.
427. Weber D, Wolfson J, Swartz M: *Pasteurella multocida* infections: report of 34 cases and review of the literature, *Medicine* 63:133, 1984.
428. Wheeler C, Rodeheaver G, Thacker J: Side effects of high pressure irrigation, *Surg Gynecol Obstetr* 143:775, 1976.
429. Wilberger J, Pang D: Craniocerebral injuries from dog bite in an infant, *Neurosurgery* 9:426, 1981.
430. Williams R, Fincham W: Septic arthritis due to *Pasteurella multocida* complicating rheumatoid arthritis, *Ann Rheum Dis* 38:394, 1979.
431. Willson PJ: *Haemophilus, Actinobacillus, Pasteurella:* mechanisms of resistance and antibiotic therapy, *Can J Vet Res* S73, 1990.
432. Winkler W: Human deaths induced by dog bites, United States, 1974-75, *Public Health Rep* 92:425, 1977.
433. Wolf J Jr et al: Dog bites to the male genitalia: characteristics, management and comparison with human bites, *J Urol* 149(2):286, 1993.
434. Wong A: Hypersensitivity to rat saliva, *J Am Acad Dermatol* 4:606, 1984.
435. Woodruff R, Jones J, Eng T: Human exposure to rabies from pet wild raccoons in South Carolina and West Virginia, 1987 through 1988, *Am J Public Health* 81(10):1328, 1991.
436. Woolfrey B, Quall C, Lally R: *Pasteurella multocida* in an infected tiger bite, *Arch Pathol Lab Med* 109:744, 1985.
437. World Health Organization expert committee on rabies. Sixth report. Geneva: World Health Organization Technical Report series 1973; 523 12.
438. Worlock P, Boland P, Darrell J: The role of prophylactic antibiotics following hand injuries, *Br J Clin Pract* 34:290, 1980.
439. Wright J: Severe attacks by dogs: characteristics of the dogs, the victims, and the attack settings, *Public Health Rep* 100:55, 1985.
440. Wright JC: Reported cat bites in Dallas: characteristics of the cats, the victims, and the attack events, *Public Health Rep* 105(4):420, 1990.
441. Wright JC: Canine aggression toward people: bite scenarios and prevention, *Vet Clin North Am Small Anim Pract* 21(2):299, 1991.
442. Wright W: *The grizzly bear,* Lincoln, 1977, University of Nebraska Press.
443. Wykes WN: Rat bite injury to the eyelids in a 3-month-old child, *Br J Ophthalmol* 73(3):202, 1989.
444. Zackowski D, Lehman J, Tantri M: Management of dog bite avulsions of the lip vermilion, *Pediatr Emerg Care* 2:85, 1986.
445. Zimmerli W et al: Pathogenesis of foreign body infection: description and characteristics of an animal model, *J Infect Dis* 146:487, 1982.
446. Zook E, Miller M, Van Beek A: Successful treatment protocol for canine fang injuries, *J Trauma* 20:243, 1980.
447. Zubowicz VN, Gravier M: Management of early human bites of the hand: a prospective randomized study, *Plast Reconstr Surg* 88(1):111, 1991.

41 WILDERNESS-ACQUIRED ZOONOSES

Leonard C. Marcus

Zoonoses with a minor wildlife reservoir for human infection
Rabies
Leptospirosis
Hantavirus pulmonary syndrome
Tularemia
Plague
Glanders
Melioidosis
Trichinosis

This chapter reviews selected infectious diseases likely to be acquired by contact with wild animals in a wilderness setting. The risk of acquiring such zoonoses increases proportionately with the frequency and intensity of contact. For example, hunters and trappers who handle and are exposed to the blood, viscera, secretions, and excretions of wild animals are at much greater risk than recreational campers.

In this chapter we emphasize diseases in which wildlife plays a significant role in transmission to humans. Although glanders and melioidosis do not fit this pattern, they are also discussed. Zoonoses acquired primarily from domestic animals that also have a minor reservoir in wildlife are mentioned briefly, but for full discussion, standard texts of veterinary public health[96,166,174] or infectious disease[83,118] should be consulted.

Zoonoses with a Minor Wildlife Reservoir for Human Infection

Brucella abortus occurs in bison in the American West, and *Brucella suis* can be found in wild swine. However, in most of the world, brucellosis is acquired primarily from domestic livestock.

Rat-bite fever (see Chapter 40) is a theoretical risk from the bite of any wild rodent and some carnivores, but most cases are associated with the bite of laboratory rats or peridomestic rodents such as the black rat *(Rattus rattus)* and the sewer rat *(Rattus norvegicus)*. Cat-scratch disease can be acquired from the scratch or bite of various animals but is most commonly associated with injuries inflicted by the domestic cat. Psittacosis or ornithosis can be carried and transmitted by hundreds of different species of birds, but people usually acquire the infection from pet parrots, other caged birds, pigeons, or poultry.

Toxoplasmosis can be acquired by ingestion of oocysts passed in the stool of felids. Usually, domestic cats are involved in this form of transmission to humans, but wild felids can also harbor the intestinal stages of this parasite. An outbreak of toxoplasmosis in American soldiers in Panama may have been caused by drinking water from a stream contaminated by the feces of a jungle cat.[17] People can also acquire toxoplasmosis by ingesting raw or undercooked meat and organs from various wild birds and mammals, but many more cases are acquired by ingestion of food products from domestic animals than from game.

Rabies

HISTORICAL ASPECTS[172]

Rabies is one of the most ancient and feared diseases. The first apparent reference to rabies is found in the Eshnunna Code of Mesopotamia, circa 2000 BC, which provides for fining the owner of a dog that kills a person through its bite. Aristotle (322 BC) recognized that dogs transmitted the infection to other dogs through bites. Galen (200 AD) recommended surgical excision of bite wounds to prevent rabies. Celsus (100 AD) recommended that wounds be cauterized to prevent the infection; this remained the prophylactic treatment of choice until 1885, when rabies immunization was introduced by Louis Pasteur.

Transmission of rabies by inoculation of saliva from a rabid dog into a normal dog was demonstrated by Zinke in 1804. Control of stray dogs and quarantine of suspected rabid animals resulted in elimination of canine rabies in Denmark, Norway, and Sweden by 1826.

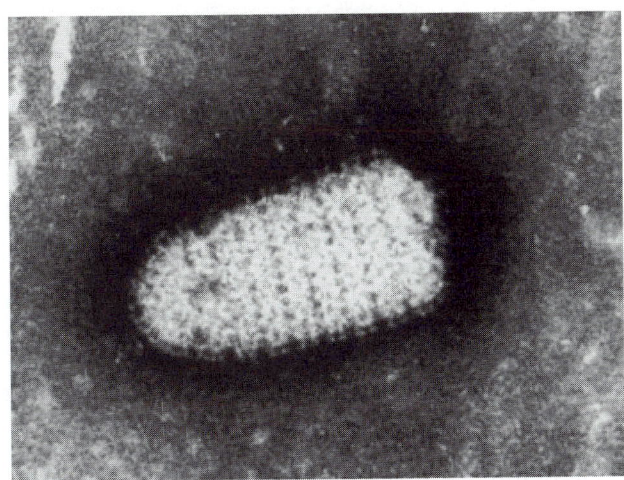

Fig. 41-1 Electron micrograph of rabies virus, demonstrating the bullet shape and capsular spikes. (Courtesy Merieux Institute.)

Several excellent reviews of rabies have been published.*

VIROLOGY

Rabies is caused by an RNA virus in the family Rhabdoviridae. Rhabdoviruses are bullet shaped, with RNA coiled inside an outer envelope covered with surface spikes (Fig. 41-1).[127] The rabies virus contains five proteins, including a glycoprotein and a nucleocapsid protein[164]; each of the latter two has a molecular weight of 60,000. The glycoprotein constitutes the major part of the capsular spikes. This protein induces neutralizing antibody, which can confer immunity and protection against the disease. The nucleocapsid protein induces antibodies that do not appear to be protective but are useful diagnostically. The fluorescent antibody technique, widely used to demonstrate rabies antigen in tissues, is directed largely against the nucleocapsid protein.

TRANSMISSION

Rabies is usually transmitted by the bite of an infected animal. There have been a few cases of rabies transmission to humans by corneal transplantation from donors who died of rabies, which was unknown at the time of surgery.[35,39,94] Rabies has been transmitted by accidental aerosol in a laboratory[200] and by inhalation in a bat-infested cave.[58] In this cave, aerosols of rabies virus are created from the saliva, secretions, and excretions of large numbers of infected bats concentrated in a dark, humid environment that favors survival of the virus outside the host. Transmission occurs via the nasal neuroepithelium. The virus is destroyed in the presence of fresh air and sunshine.

*References 8, 19, 77-79, 147, 198.

Carnivorous animals can acquire rabies by eating infected prey.[18,59] Skunks can transmit rabies to their young transplacentally,[95] and one probable case of congenital rabies has been reported in a calf.[121] A congenital human case has also been reported, with mother and child dying of rabies within 48 hours of delivery.[169] The mother had been bitten by a dog 33 days before she became ill. The diagnoses were made by finding Negri bodies in the brain of mother and child and by unspecified animal studies.

EPIDEMIOLOGY

Although all mammals are experimentally susceptible to rabies, the major reservoir and vectors of transmission are wild and domestic carnivores, particularly the dog (Canidae), cat (Felidae), weasel (Mustelidae), mongoose (Viveridae), raccoon (Procyonidae), and bat (Chiroptera) families. In the United States, Canada, and most of Europe, the principal reservoir is wildlife (Figs. 41-2 and 41-3). Between 1980 and 1991, approximately 90% of rabies cases reported in the United States and Puerto Rico occurred in wild animals. In 1985, 44.8% of these cases occurred in skunks and 26.5% in raccoons.[48] A rabies epizootic in the Northeast caused reversal of these statistics 6 years later. Of the 6354 cases reported to the Centers for Disease Control and Prevention (CDC) in 1991, 44.1% occurred in raccoons, 29.7% in skunks, 4.9% in bats, and 4.6% in foxes. In Canada, foxes account for more than 40% and skunks for approximately 20% of rabies cases.[110]

Vaccination and leash law enforcement have greatly reduced the incidence of rabies in dogs in the United States and Canada. Cattle are now more frequently reported rabid than are dogs in these countries. From 1981 through 1991, rabid cats outnumbered rabid dogs in the United States (Fig. 41-4).[110] In many developing countries, dogs remain the principal reservoir of rabies. In 1991, 81.6% of 8528 reported rabies cases in Mexico occurred in dogs.[110]

The significant wildlife reservoirs of rabies vary geographically. The mongoose is important in Puerto Rico, the jackal in much of Africa, the red fox in Europe, the wolf in Iran and neighboring countries, the raccoon dog in Eastern and Central Europe, and the vampire bat in certain Latin American countries. More than 50 countries reportedly have no rabies cases, including most islands in Pacific Oceania, most Caribbean islands, the United Kingdom, Cyprus, Finland, Iceland, Norway, Portugal, Spain, Sweden, Japan, Korea, Malaysia, Singapore, New Zealand, and Taiwan. The largest land mass reported free of rabies is Australia.[53]

Because human contact with dogs is much more intimate than with wildlife, dogs offer a greater threat of rabies transmission. Countries with significant domestic canine rabies also have the highest incidence of human rabies. Thus there have been no more than five reported cases of human rabies in any year since 1960 in the United States. Twenty (36%) of the 55 human cases of rabies reported in the United

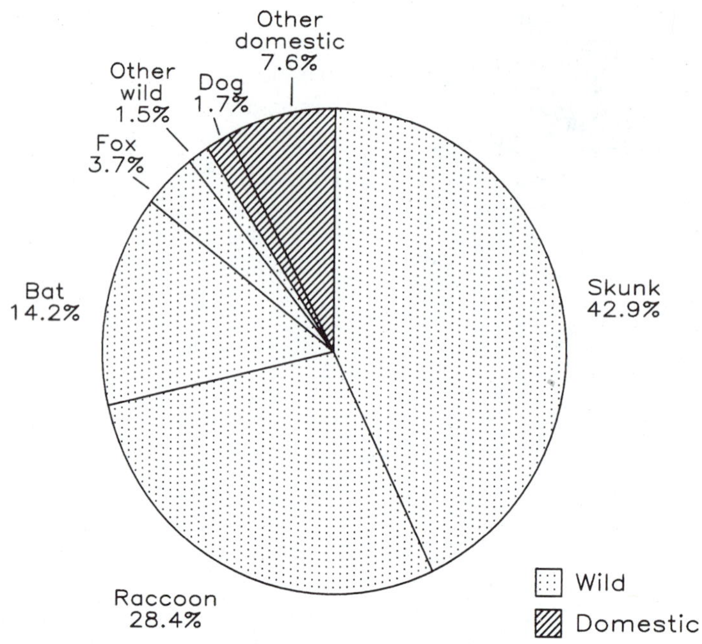

Fig. 41-2 Animal rabies, United States including Puerto Rico, 1986. Five thousand five hundred fifty-one cases were reported. (From Centers for Disease Control: *MMWR* 36, No. 3S, 1987.)

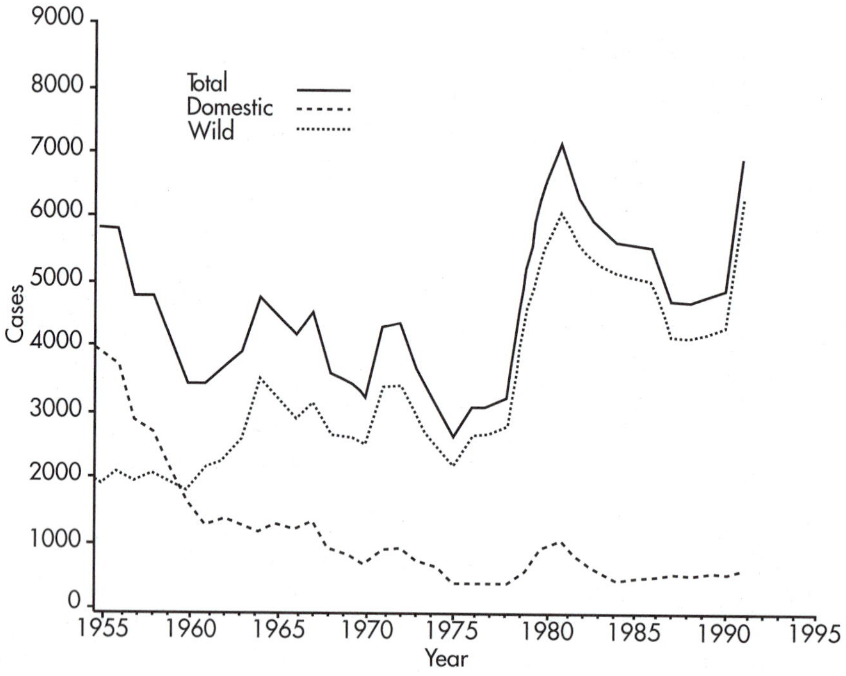

Fig. 41-3 Cases of rabies in the United States by year, 1955 to 1991. (From Krebs JW et al: *J Am Vet Med Assoc* 201:1836, 1992.)

States (including two Americans who acquired and died of rabies abroad) from 1960 to 1991 were acquired in foreign countries, most resulting from dog bites (Fig. 41-5).[77] Forty-eight human cases were reported in Mexico in 1991.[110] In India, another country where canine rabies is endemic, estimates of annual human rabies cases range from 15,000 to more than 25,000.[198] Defining the local reservoir of infection helps define the manner in which the disease is maintained in a given country or region and the people at high risk. A significant risk of being exposed to rabies in the United States occurs in wildlife handlers such as trappers, hunters, and wildlife biologists. People in many developing

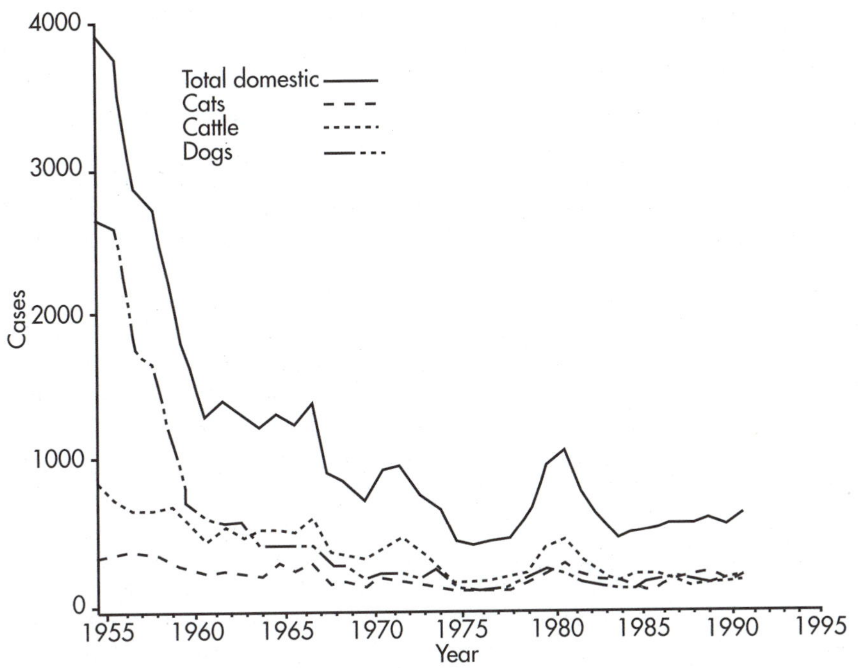

Fig. 41-4 Cases of rabies in domestic animals in the United States, by year, 1955 to 1991. (From Krebs JW et al: *J Am Vet Med Assoc* 201:1836, 1992.)

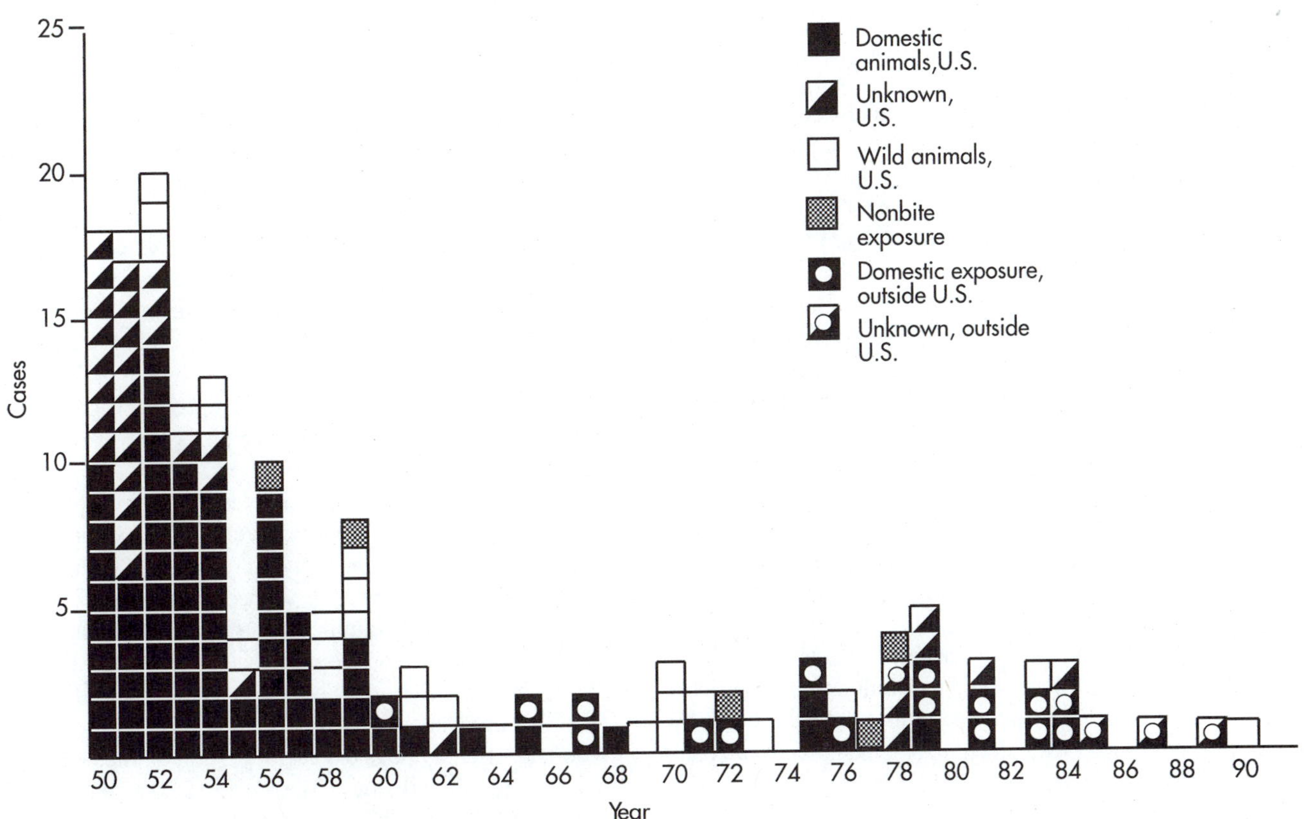

Fig. 41-5 Human rabies in the United States from 1950 to 1989. Figure includes two Americans who contracted and died of rabies outside the United States (1981 and 1983). (From Fishbein DB: *Infect Dis Clin North Am* 5:53, 1991.)

countries, including foreign tourists, are more at risk from local dogs than from wildlife.

Mammalian species vary in their susceptibility to rabies.[18] In general, the animals most susceptible also have the shortest course of infection. Wolves, foxes, and jackals, which are highly susceptible, generally suffer acute disease. Skunks and raccoons are somewhat less susceptible, and the duration of illness tends to be more prolonged. Opossums are very resistant to infection, and the only consistent way to induce rabies in them is by intracerebral inoculation.

Although rabies is considered an almost uniformly fatal infection once symptoms have developed, some cases of spontaneous recovery or of chronic, asymptomatic infection have been recorded in various wildlife species and dogs.[6,15,18,64,74] Bats that harbor and shed the virus may not be overtly ill, especially to the casual observer.

The pattern of human rabies reflects the epidemiology of animal bites.[14] As is true for animal bites in general, a disproportionately large number of rabies occurs in males less than 18 years of age. All cases of animal bites and of rabies in people or animals should be reported to local public health authorities.

PATHOGENESIS[10,128]

After the rabies virus is inoculated by a bite, it is first sequestered in skeletal muscle. The virus travels via neuromuscular spindles and motor end plates to the peripheral nervous system, then travels in the axons of peripheral nerves at an estimated rate of 3 mm/hr to the central nervous system. Thus rabies resulting from a bite on the foot has an average incubation period of 60 days, but 30 days after an infective bite to the face. With superficial bites, movement of the virus to the central nervous system may be via sensory nerves.

The virus moves across synapses and multiplies within neurons. The brain may be diffusely involved or there may be relative concentration in different parts of the brain, depending on species. For example, the hippocampus is frequently involved in carnivores and humans; Purkinje cells of the cerebellum are commonly involved in herbivores, such as cattle. After multiplication within the central nervous system, there is centrifugal spread along cranial and peripheral nerves out to the skin, cornea, salivary glands, and other tissues. Terminally, rabies virus can be found in many organs of the body, including the nervous system, skin, eyes, salivary glands, pancreas, kidney, and myocardium. Saliva can contain up to 1 million virus particles per milliliter. Rabies is not disseminated in the body by viremia, and contact with blood of a rabid animal is not considered an exposure risk.

Clinical rabies develops in approximately 15% of untreated persons bitten by rabid dogs. The probability of the disease developing varies with the size and depth of the inoculum, from 0.1% with salivary contamination (such as licking) of a minor wound, to 80% after a severe rabid wolf bite.

SYMPTOMS[18,19]

The incubation period of rabies varies from as little as 9 days to more than 1 year. For the great majority of human cases the incubation period is between 2 and 16 weeks. Claims of incubation periods as long as 19 years are difficult to substantiate. Proof of long incubation periods is provided by identifying the strain of virus as coming from an area where the patient last visited or resided a long time ago. For example, in three immigrants to the United States who died of rabies, the viral nucleic acid pattern matched strains from their native countries, the Philippines, Laos, and Mexico, which they had left 6 years, 4 years, and 11 months before, respectively.[171]

The initial symptoms of rabies are usually nonspecific and include malaise, fatigue, anxiety, agitation, irritability, insomnia, depression, fever, headache, nausea, vomiting, sore throat, abdominal pain, and anorexia. Pain or paresthesias at the site of the bite occur early in approximately half the patients.

After the prodromal period, which lasts approximately 2 to 10 days, more specific neurologic symptoms develop related to localization of the infection to the limbic system, with relative sparing of the neocortex. In lower animals and in people this can take one of two forms, either furious or paralytic (dumb) rabies. Furious rabies is characterized by increasing agitation, hyperactivity, seizures, and episodes in which the animal or person may thrash about, bite, and become aggressive, alternating with periods of relative calm. Rabid human patients may hallucinate. Severe pharyngeal spasm or spasms of respiratory muscles may occur when the individual attempts to drink. Later in the disease this reaction may be excited merely by the sight of water, giving rise to the synonym "hydrophobia." A truly rabid patient often attempts to drink because of thirst. A hysterical patient mimicking rabies does not make the attempt. Pharyngeal spasm and choking may also occur when air is blown on the patient's face (aerophobia).

In the initial phases of furious rabies, animals may appear unusually alert and responsive. Later they show some discomfort and restlessness and may vocalize with unusual frequency. Animals become hypersensitive and hyperresponsive to external stimuli, such as sound or touch. Certain behavioral changes develop, so that wild animals that normally shun association with humans may appear unusually friendly and approach people without apparent fear. Normally friendly dogs or cats may begin to bite. They may appear and act ferocious. They may salivate excessively, "foaming at the mouth" (Fig. 41-6). The key to maintenance of this infection in nature is the behavioral change in animals that causes them to bite. Skunks are particularly dangerous because they tend to bite and hold on viciously.

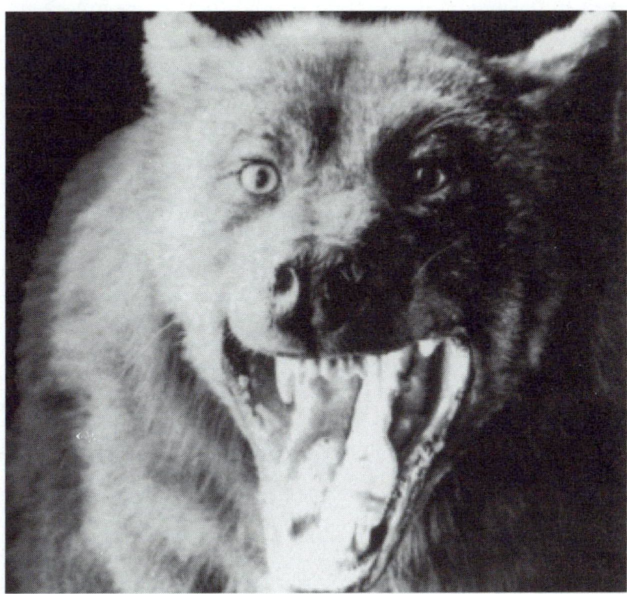

Fig. 41-6 A dog-wolf cross from Canada with furious rabies. It has a ferocious appearance, excess salivation, and anisocoria. (Courtesy Merieux Institute.)

Eventually, animals and people die, for example, with a convulsive or paralytic disorder, in coma, of cardiac arrhythmias, or of secondary complications such as aspiration pneumonia.

In dumb rabies there is progressive lethargy, incoordination, and ascending paralysis, starting as posterior paraplegia. In animals, cranial nerve palsies can result in protrusion of the tongue and nictitating membrane and abnormal vocalization. The tone and pitch of the animal's voice may change, probably because of involvement of laryngeal muscle innervation. Dumb or paralytic rabies in animals and humans follows a progressive course, with eventual coma and death.

Because of progressive paralysis without biting behavior, dumb rabies is usually not transmitted further in nature. However, people may be exposed while taking care of such patients, whether animal or human, through exposure to saliva, for example, in clearing oral secretions.

PREVENTION AND CONTROL OF RABIES IN ANIMALS

Close to 90% of reported animal bites in the United States are caused by dogs. Therefore it is important to maintain an immune canine population to act as a barrier against rabies, even in the United States, where most rabies occurs in wildlife. Without canine herd immunity, it is likely that rabies would spill over from the wildlife population to dogs. Because there are now more reported cases of rabies in cats than in dogs in the United States, it is also important to maintain immunization in the feline population.

There are 23 commercially available rabies vaccines available in the United States for dogs and cats.[130] They all contain inactivated virus. They provide immunity for either 1 or 3 years. Local ordinance may dictate which type of vaccine is to be used, or it may be left to the veterinarian's discretion.

In addition to immunization, control of rabies in cats and dogs depends on enforcement of leash laws, quarantine of imported animals, and other animal control programs. Stray animals should be picked up and removed from the community as efficiently as possible. It is especially important to keep dogs used for hunting currently immunized and to give them booster doses of rabies vaccine as needed after possible or proven exposure. People who camp or hike with their dogs should keep them immunized and appropriately restrained. Current certificates of vaccination should accompany dogs or cats that are transported across state or international boundaries.

Immunization of farm livestock (such as horses, cattle, sheep, and goats) is not routine but may be advisable when outbreaks of rabies occur in pastoral areas. Immunization of cattle is advisable in parts of South and Central America, where there are vampire bats.

At the present time there is no commercially approved vaccine for rabies in wildlife in the United States.[62] A modified live rabies vaccine, distributed in baits, was used with considerable success in controlling an epizootic in foxes in Europe.[187] It is not universally applicable to the control of wildlife rabies, however, because it is pathogenic for striped skunks[153] and some rodents, and it is not very immunogenic in some other species, such as raccoons.

A live vaccine that incorporates the rabies glycoprotein into the vaccinia virus (VRG) provides protective immunity in raccoons[152,196] and is nonpathogenic for a variety of wild, laboratory, and domestic animals.[24] Initial field trials indicate that VRG is ecologically safe.[54] Additional field trials are currently being conducted to determine its efficacy in controlling the epizootic of raccoon rabies now occurring in the northeastern United States.

Rabies viruses occur in different strains, which tend to be host specific. There are five strains in terrestrial animals in the United States (Fig. 41-7) and eight strains in American bats.[78] Although all strains of rabies are considered pathogenic for all mammals, the tendency is for the disease to be maintained within one kind of animal in a given area. Some scientists have advocated population control of a given carrier species within a geographic area to control the spread of rabies. Probably widespread immunization of wildlife would be more effective than population control, because as animals are killed in a given area, others enter from surrounding areas to fill the ecologic void.[129]

One situation in which controlled killing of wildlife may be useful in reducing human exposure and in limiting epizootic spread is in parks or campgrounds where wild animals have become used to the presence of people. If a host-specific outbreak of rabies has occurred in such an area, exercising population control within the park boundary may be useful.

In parts of Central and South America, vampire bats are a significant reservoir of rabies and frequently transmit the disease to cattle. A unique mechanism for controlling this problem has been developed. A jelly containing anticoagulant is smeared on captured bats[115] or on the backs of cattle.[81] In the latter situation, bats get this jelly on their bodies when they feed. They lick the anticoagulant off in grooming and subsequently bleed to death. This technique has been effective in reducing vampire bat populations because the bats nest in colonies and contaminate one another with the compound. It is also possible to give anticoagulants orally or parenterally to cattle, so their blood has enough anticoagulant activity to be lethal to feeding vampire bats but tolerable for cattle.[181]

If it becomes necessary to eliminate a colony of insectivorous bats that has a high prevalence of rabies, DDT is the pesticide of choice.[190] Because of adverse ecologic effects on birds and other creatures, DDT is strictly regulated in the United States. A special permit is required to use it for bat control. Extermination of bats should be discouraged because they fill a valuable ecologic niche, destroying mosquitoes and other harmful insects. Killing wildlife should be allowed only when they threaten human or domestic animals and cannot otherwise be controlled or avoided.

Wild animals should not be kept as pets. Many instances of human exposure to rabies have resulted from keeping raccoons, skunks, ferrets, and other wild animals, including animals purchased from commercial sources.[25,33,36]

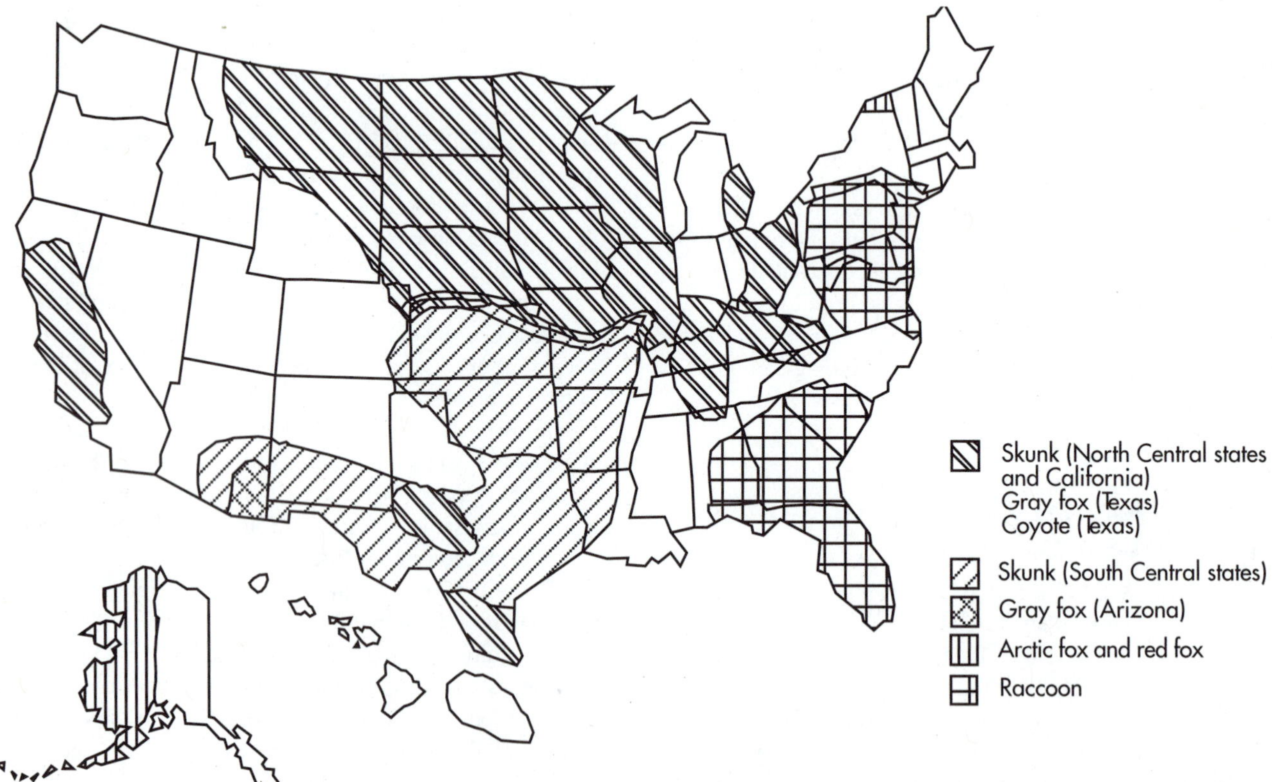

Fig. 41-7 Distribution of five antigenically distinct rabies virus strains and the predominant wildlife species affected in the United States during 1991. (From Krebs JW et al: *J Am Vet Med Assoc* 201:1836, 1992.)

PREEXPOSURE IMMUNIZATION OF HUMANS

People at high risk for rabies, such as veterinarians, wildlife biologists, trappers, taxidermists, and laboratory personnel working with the virus, should be immunized before exposure. Other possible candidates for preexposure immunization include spelunkers, avocational hunters, and long-term travelers (especially hikers and bikers) to intensely enzootic areas. The CDC recommends preexposure rabies immunization "for persons living in or visiting (for more than 30 days) areas of the world where rabies is a constant threat."[53] This recommendation should be followed more aggressively if the individuals' activities are likely to put them at significant risk of exposure, or if they are likely to have difficulty getting appropriate medical care, including safe, effective vaccines administered with a sterile needle and syringe, within a few days of exposure. If appropriate care is available, it may be more cost effective to forgo preexposure immunization and to just administer postexposure treatment to persons who need it.[163]

A theoretical advantage of preexposure immunization is that it could protect against inapparent or unknown exposure. This is more likely to occur in occupational settings, such as among veterinarians, biologists, taxidermists, or butchers who work on an animal with undiagnosed rabies than in a travel setting, where possible exposure, usually a bite, is more likely to be noticed and brought to medical attention.

The two vaccines approved for human use in the United States are human diploid cell vaccine (HDCV) (Imovax), produced by Pasteur Merieux Serum et Vaccins and distributed by Connaught Laboratories, and rabies vaccine adsorbed (RVA), made by the Michigan Department of Public Health and distributed by SmithKline Beecham. Both contain virus inactivated with β-propiolactone.[52] Preexposure immunization consists of three injections given on days 0, 7, and 21 or 28. HDCV and RVA can be given intramuscularly, 1 ml in the deltoid muscle (or anterior thigh muscle in children). An alternative route for preexposure HDCV (only) is intradermal, 0.1 ml in the lateral aspect of the upper arm.[21,26,47,65] The intradermal dosage for HDCV is significantly less expensive than the intramuscular. Unfortunately, the intradermal commercial product is poorly packaged and difficult to dissolve and administer.

The frequency of booster doses for preexposure immunization depends on the antirabies titer of the individual and the likelihood of exposure to infection.[52,76] For individuals whose activity puts them at continuous risk (such as workers in rabies biologics production and research laboratories), the titer should be checked every 6 months and a booster dose given if the titer drops below 0.5 IU per milliliter (1:5 dilution) by the rapid fluorescent focus inhibition test (RFFIT). For those who have frequent exposure risk, such as veterinarians and wildlife workers in enzootic areas, RFFIT titers should be checked and boosters given as needed every 2 years. Two percent to 7% of individuals receiving the three-dose preexposure HDCV series intramuscularly and 5% to 17% receiving it intradermally have a titer of less than 1:5 after 2 years.[80] Three percent of individuals given the three-dose RVA preexposure series did not have an adequate titer after 9 to 12 months. Routine testing and booster administration are not recommended for individuals who are at low risk of infection, such as veterinarians in a nonenzootic area.

Pain, erythema, or pruritus occurs at the injection site in a majority of those receiving primary immunization with HDCV or RVA.[21,52] Malaise, headache, dizziness, fever, and nausea occur in 5% to 40% of vaccinees. Vomiting occurs in approximately 0.5% of patients receiving primary preexposure vaccination with RVA (author's observation). Marked local induration and regional lymphadenopathy are occasionally seen. Booster doses with HDCV at 1 year can cause malaise, headache, fever, myalgia, and arthralgias in 26% of recipients.[21] Boosters with HDCV can also cause an immune complex–like disease characterized by urticaria, macular rash, angioedema, or arthralgia in 10% of patients.[66] Similar delayed hypersensitivity reactions are seen in 1% of patients receiving a booster dose of RVA. I observed generalized urticaria in a 26-year-old man with Hashimoto's thyroiditis given the primary intradermal immunization series with HDCV. Three cases of Guillain-Barré paralytic syndrome with complete recovery within 3 months have been reported associated with HDCV.[20,22,52] Immediate hypersensitivity reactions with bronchospasm, laryngeal edema, and rashes have followed primary immunization with HDCV but are rare.

Concurrent use of immunosuppressive drugs, such as corticosteroids, interferes with immunization. If possible, such drugs should not be given at the time of immunization. Chloroquine has an immunosuppressive effect and can interfere with immunization. Peace Corps workers who were treated with chloroquine malarial prophylaxis failed to respond adequately to preexposure immunization with rabies vaccine.[47] One such person died of rabies after a dog bite, even though she had been given preexposure rabies prophylaxis.[42] Phenytoin can also be immunosuppressive and theoretically could interfere with rabies immunization.[43] If preexposure immunization must be given to someone while that person is taking an immunosuppressive drug, the vaccine should be given by the intramuscular rather than the intradermal route, and titers checked to determine if immunization is effective (see p. 1003).

POSTEXPOSURE PROCEDURES

Because no specific or effective antirabies treatment is available for symptomatic disease, all effort should be directed at prevention, which consists of adequate wound cleansing and prompt immunization. Sometimes, evaluating exposure and the need for prophylactic immunization is difficult, which results in considerable overtreatment.[92]

However, considering the grim prognosis of the disease and the relative safety of prophylaxis, overtreatment is understandable and inevitable.

Significant exposure risk is associated with bites that penetrate the epidermis or contact of saliva, other secretions, cerebrospinal fluid, or animal tissue with open wounds or mucous membranes. In general, the deeper the inoculation (for example, by bite or scratch) and the bigger the inoculum, the greater the risk of contracting rabies.

If a dog or cat bites an individual, the animal should be quarantined for a 10-day period.[130] Rabies prophylaxis can be started and discontinued if the animal remains well for 10 days. If the animal dies or neurologic symptoms develop within that time, the brain should be examined. The brain should be double bagged in plastic and sent refrigerated (for example, on ice, not chemically fixed, frozen, or on dry ice) in a leakproof container to an appropriate diagnostic laboratory, such as that maintained by the state department of health. If quarantine is not possible or practical, the dog or cat can be killed immediately and the brain sent for examination. Any wild animal that bites a person should be killed immediately and the brain sent for diagnostic laboratory studies.[130] Wild animals are not kept under observation because their period of infectivity is usually unknown, and some species, such as skunks and bats, may shed virus in saliva for 2 weeks or more before they appear ill. If the biting animal is proven rabid, postexposure prophylaxis should be continued or instituted immediately.

If the biting animal is not available for examination, the physician should act on the statistical probability that it was or was not rabid. If rabies is known to occur locally in that species, the person should be treated. If rabies has not occurred in the region for many years and there is no likelihood that the animal was exposed to rabies, rabies treatment should be withheld. There are parts of the United States where rabies has not infected dogs or cats for decades and where their exposure to infected wildlife is highly unlikely. Although this line of reasoning is usually correct, its fallibility is demonstrated by a rabid cat found in Boston in 1980. No rabies in a terrestrial animal had been recorded in Boston for more than 40 years. Monoclonal antibody testing of the rabies virus from this cat revealed that it was probably of bat origin. Bat rabies is fairly common in New England but is rarely transmitted to a terrestrial animal. Fortunately, no human case of rabies resulted from exposure to the cat. If someone had been bitten by that cat and it had escaped, public health officials might not have advised postexposure prophylaxis because of the extreme unlikelihood that a cat in Boston at that time would have been rabid. (In 1992 the rabies epizootic in raccoons reached the Boston area and it would no longer be surprising to find a rabid cat there.)

Unvaccinated dogs and cats bitten by a rabid animal should be destroyed immediately. If the owner is not willing to have this done, the unvaccinated animal should be kept in strict isolation for 6 months and vaccinated 1 month before being released.[130] Dogs and cats that were currently and appropriately vaccinated before exposure should be given a booster dose immediately and kept in confinement for 45 days.[56a] Local authorities will define the exact conditions of quarantine.

Domestic livestock such as sheep, cattle, and goats exposed to rabid animals should be slaughtered immediately. If they are slaughtered within 7 days of being bitten, their tissues can be eaten without risk of infection, providing that the area around the bite is discarded. Animals that were exposed to rabies more than 7 days and less than 8 months previously should not be used for food. Meat, milk, or any other organ product of a clinically rabid animal should not be consumed; however, pasteurization or adequate cooking kills the virus, and inadvertent consumption of properly heated food should not be considered a rabies exposure.[130]

Although rodents are experimentally susceptible to infection, naturally acquired rabies is extremely rare in small rodents such as mice, rats, gerbils, hamsters, guinea pigs, and squirrels, and in lagomorphs such as rabbits and hares. Exceptional cases in rabbits and a squirrel have been reported.[25] With rare exceptions a bite from a lagomorph or a small rodent should not be considered a rabies exposure, and postexposure prophylaxis should usually be withheld. Local public health officials or infectious disease specialists should be consulted about individual problem cases.

Some cases of rabies in woodchucks and beavers, which are large rodents, have been reported recently in the United States.[44,48] Most of these cases have occurred in the Middle Atlantic states, probably from exposure to raccoons. Bites from bats and wild carnivores, such as skunks, foxes, and raccoons in the United States, and jackals, wolves, and mongooses in other enzootic countries, should be considered possible exposures. Prophylaxis should be given if the biting animal escapes.

It is helpful to acquire as much information as possible about the biting animal and incident to determine the likelihood of rabies exposure. The risk is greater if the biting incident was unprovoked. The question of provocation should be asked from the perspective of the animal rather than of the victim. For example, feeding a wild animal or attempting to separate fighting animals is likely to result in a bite. An unprovoked attack is one in which the person did not intrude on the animal's territory or behave in a manner that a normal animal might find hostile or aggressive and would probably respond to with an attack. The question of provocation indicates relative risk because a rabid animal can bite when provoked; a normal animal is not likely to bite unless provoked.

A description of the animal's behavior and appearance should be obtained. Most rabid animals have obvious behavioral and neurologic abnormalities, such as staggering gait, excess salivation, uncontrolled rage, abnormal eye movements or pupillary reflexes (Fig. 41-6), altered vocalization, bizarre behavior (for example, wild animals approaching humans), convulsions, or paralysis.

The physician should inquire about the animal's vaccination history. No vaccine is perfect, but the likelihood of rabies is reduced if the animal was given an appropriate vaccine within the proper time frame. Rabies has occurred in immunized dogs[49] and in two people bitten by dogs that supposedly had been immunized in Nigeria[44] and Mexico.[114]

A history taken on the animal should include whether it has been bitten recently or been involved in a fight with another animal, and whether it has traveled out of the region within the past year. For example, the likelihood of a dog that stays in a nonenzootic area being rabid is small, but the risk increases considerably if it is taken periodically to enzootic areas to hunt.

Postexposure prophylaxis consists of three steps. The first is adequate wound washing with soap and water.[61] This should be done as soon as possible, preferably within minutes after the bite or scratch, and before seeking medical attention. Immunization can be delayed for hours or 1 or 2 days; washing a wound cannot.

The second component of postexposure prophylaxis is administration of rabies antiserum. In some parts of the world, this product may be of equine origin. Modern purified equine antirabies serum (SCLAVO, Italy; Pasteur Merieux Institute, France; Swiss Serum and Vaccine Institute, Switzerland) is much safer than the earlier products, which carried a high risk of serum sickness.[197] Equine antirabies serum currently available in various countries could be of either the newer, nonreactive type or the older, more dangerous variety. Review of the package insert is recommended. It may also be advisable to test for hypersensitivity by intradermally injecting 0.1 ml of the product diluted 1:10 with saline before giving the full dose. The principal advantage of equine antirabies serum over human rabies immune globulin is cost, a major factor in the Third World countries, where rabies is most common.

In many Western countries, including the United States, rabies antiserum is made from the blood of immunized human donors. Human rabies immune globulin (HRIG) is commercially available as Imogam from the Pasteur Merieux Institute (distributed by Connaught Laboratories) and as Hyperab (Miles, Inc.). HRIG contains 150 IU of neutralizing antibody per milliliter. It is given as a single dose of 20 IU/kg body weight. Approximately half the dose should be infiltrated around the bite wound. If the wound is in a small site, such as the finger, as much as feasible should be injected in that area. The remainder is given intramuscularly, in the upper outer quadrant of the buttocks in adults or the anterolateral aspect of the thigh in small children. HRIG is a safe product, not associated with anaphylaxis, serum sickness, or transmission of hepatitis or human immunodeficiency virus.

Theoretically, antiserum may be effective at any time before development of symptoms and should be given no matter how much time has expired since the biting incident. The antiserum is given at the same time that active immunization is started, as described below. With recommended doses, no interference between passive and active immunization should take place. If HRIG was not given when active immunization was started, it can be given up to 7 days after the first vaccine dose.[52]

The third component of postexposure prophylaxis is active immunization with rabies vaccine. The only vaccines currently available for humans in the United States are HDCV (Imovax, Pasteur Merieux Institute, distributed by Connaught Laboratories) and RVA made by the Michigan Department of Public Health and distributed by SmithKline Beecham. HDCV contains rabies virus grown on MRC-5 human diploid cells. RVA is grown on fetal rhesus monkey lung cells. HDCV and RVA are inactivated by β-propiolactone. Although intradermal vaccination with HDCV is acceptable for preexposure prophylaxis, this vaccine should be administered in the deltoid muscle for postexposure prophylaxis. RVA should always be given in the deltoid muscle, whether used before or after exposure. HDCV or RVA can be given in the midanterior thigh muscles of infants and small children. Either vaccine is given on days 0, 3, 7, 14, and 28 as a 1 ml dose, regardless of the age or size of the patient. The vaccines should not be given with the same syringe or in the same site as HRIG. They should *not* be given in the gluteal region, since the vaccine might be deposited in fat and be poorly immunogenic. Rabies has occurred in a person given postexposure prophylaxis using gluteal injections.[168]

After exposure, individuals previously immunized should receive booster doses of HDCV or RVA on days 0 and 3. Such individuals should not receive antiserum. An effective booster response has been documented in people given primary immunization many years earlier,[72] including those given duck embryo vaccine, providing they had an appropriate immune response after the primary series.

After vaccination, antirabies titers need to be checked only on individuals who may be immunosuppressed. A person who does not show a satisfactory antibody response (a titer of at least 1:25 or 0.5 IU by RFFIT 2 to 4 weeks after the immunization series is completed) should receive additional booster doses of rabies vaccine at weekly intervals until a satisfactory antibody response is obtained. Obviously, this is more important for postexposure than for preexposure immunization. Nursing and pregnancy do not contraindicate postexposure rabies prophylaxis.

Adverse reactions to HDCV and RVA are described on p. 1001.

In developing countries, HDCV and RVA as used in the United States may be prohibitively expensive for general use, and modified protocols for these products or other vaccines may be used. None of these other methods are approved for use in the United States. In one protocol, 0.1 ml intradermal doses of HDCV are given at multiple sites during four visits over a 3-month period.[52,77,198] Another protocol decreases the number of 1 ml intramuscular doses of HDCV to four, given in three visits over a 21-day course.[52,77,198]

A purified Vero cell rabies vaccine has been used with success in Thailand.[52,77,198] Purified duck embryo cell rabies vaccine is more immunogenic and safer than the duck embryo vaccine widely used in the United States in the 1960s.[198] A purified chick embryo fibroblast rabies vaccine is made in Japan, and a hamster kidney cell vaccine is made in China.[198]

Inactivated rabies vaccines prepared in animal brains, collectively known as Semple vaccines, are used for 93% of all postexposure rabies treatment worldwide because they are relatively cheap. They have relatively low immunogenicity and a high incidence of significant side effects, the most serious being neuroparalytic reactions because they induce antineural antibody and cellular response.[198]

The treatment of people who have clinical rabies is directed toward the symptoms and consists of intensive care support of vital functions. α-Interferon, vidarabine, ribavirin, corticosteroids, inosine pranobex, multiple doses of vaccine, antithymocyte globulin, and large doses of rabies immune globulin have been used unsuccessfully in treating rabid persons.[198] Three persons (two with major neurologic sequelae) known to have survived clinically evident rabies had received at least partial preexposure or postexposure immunization before they became symptomatic.[89,140,200]

DIAGNOSIS

The differential diagnosis of rabies is extensive. In a review of diagnoses considered for patients with rabies in the United States and territories for the years 1960 to 1979, the following were recorded: rabies, viral encephalitis, poliomyelitis, postinfectious encephalitis, vaccine reaction, Guillain-Barré syndrome, brain abscess, cerebrovascular accident, brain tumor, tetanus, phenothiazine toxicity, psychosis, rabies phobia, respiratory tract infection, pneumonia, sinusitis, otitis media, viral infection, gastroenteritis, myocardial infarction, hypertension, dissecting aortic aneurysm, arteritis, dehydration, lumbago, and headache.[4]

Presumptive diagnosis of rabies depends on getting an exposure history and observing compatible neurologic signs. The source of infection was not identified in 6 of 38 (16%) U.S. human rabies cases reported from 1960 to 1979[4] and in 6 out of 10 (60%) cases from 1980 to 1989.[51]

Definitive diagnosis is made by demonstrations of the virus before or after death from saliva, neurologic tissue, cerebrospinal fluid, urine sediment, or other body tissues. One of the most reliable means of demonstrating the infection before death in the symptomatic individual is by direct immunofluorescent staining of skin biopsy specimens from the back of the neck.[75] The biopsy sample should contain as many hair follicles as possible because the virus reaches the site by peripheral nerves to these follicles. Direct immunofluorescent staining of corneal impression smears may also be positive.[75] Rabies viruses can be isolated from saliva or cerebrospinal fluid by culture on murine neuroblastoma cells or inoculation of mice.[198] These tests have great specificity but limited sensitivity. They become positive a week or more after the onset of illness.

Rabies can be indirectly diagnosed by antibody studies on serum or cerebrospinal fluid.[75] The RFFIT, an in vitro neutralization procedure, is the standard diagnostic test used in the United States. Approximately half of persons with untreated rabies show antibody by day 8 and close to 100% do by day 15. Titers resulting from actual rabies infection are generally much higher than those attained after immunization. No currently available diagnostic technique used before death can be absolutely relied on to rule out rabies.

Definitive diagnosis of rabies is usually made by a direct immunofluorescent antibody test on brain tissue. This test demonstrates fluorescent viral antigen particles within neurons (Color Plate 102). Confirmatory testing can be done by intracerebral inoculation of mice with saliva, brain, or other tissue from suspect human or animal patients.[75] Infected mice die in approximately 2 to 3 weeks. The diagnosis is confirmed by using the direct immunofluorescent test on the brains of any mice that die or show neurologic signs. Although mouse inoculation is very reliable, one obvious disadvantage is the time required for results. Virus isolation on murine neuroblastoma cells takes only 24 hours but is not widely available.

Rabies can be diagnosed by immunofluorescence and by peroxidase-antiperoxidase techniques on formalin-fixed brain tissue.[133] These methods should be used when only formalin-fixed tissues are available and should not be considered substitutes for the immunofluorescence technique and mouse inoculation with fresh brain tissue.

PATHOLOGY OF RABIES

On gross examination the brain may appear normal or slightly swollen and hyperemic. Histologic features include multifocal polioencephalomyelitis. Perivascular cuffing by lymphocytes is common, and there may be diffuse glial proliferation. Neurons may appear swollen, and some may be undergoing neuronophagia. Glial cells may accumulate in clusters called Babe's nodules.

Negri bodies are intracytoplasmic inclusion bodies, 0.25 to 27 μm in diameter, containing nucleocapsid material. They are diagnostic of rabies when correctly identified (Color Plate 103). They are absent in approximately 20% of cases, and some animals, such as cats, have neuronal changes associated with aging that can be mistaken for Negri bodies. Seller's stain is used to demonstrate Negri bodies in impression smears of brain.[75] Several special stains have been used for tissue sections, but the inclusion bodies are usually demonstrable with standard hematoxylin and eosin staining.

Pathologic changes are best seen in the brainstem, including the substantia nigra, periaqueductal gray matter, and hypothalamus. The hippocampus (Ammon's horn) is commonly affected in humans and carnivores. Purkinje cells of the cerebellum are commonly affected in ruminants.

Pathologic changes are also commonly found in the gasserian ganglion. This may be a useful site for examination if the rest of an animal's brain has been destroyed.

INFECTION CONTROL

Human-to-human transmission of rabies by bite, scratch, or aerosol has not been documented. Nevertheless, medical personnel should avoid contact with secretions from patients suspected of being rabid. Gloves, masks, and eye protection should be worn for such procedures as tracheal intubation. Rabid patients may have to be sedated and restrained if they attempt to engage in dangerous behavior, such as biting. Postexposure prophylaxis should be given only to personnel who are involved in the care of a rabies patient and had percutaneous or mucous membrane contact with saliva, respiratory secretions, tears, cerebrospinal fluid, or tissue.[146]

There must be some reasonable index of clinical suspicion to avoid transmission by organ donation, as has happened with corneal transplants.[35,39,94] The CDC has published safety procedures to reduce exposure in the laboratory.[28]

Leptospirosis

Leptospirosis is an infectious disease caused by *Leptospira interrogans.* More than 170 serotypes are known. Formerly these serotypes were given separate species status, and for the sake of simplicity and brevity they are so designated here. *Leptospira* organisms are spirochetes with hooked or curved ends, 6 to 20 μm long by 0.1 μm wide. They can grow on artificial media containing rabbit serum, such as Fletcher's semisolid and Stuart's liquid media, or containing albumin and fatty acids, such as Ellinghausen, McCullough, Johnson, Harris (EMJH) medium.[176]

In describing outbreaks with shared epidemiologic or clinical features, several syndromes were ascribed to different serotypes, such as Fort Bragg fever caused by *L. autumnalis,* swine herd disease caused by *L. pomona,* and Weil's disease caused by *L. icterohaemorrhagiae.* Such terms are no longer commonly used because there is considerable overlap in the symptoms and epidemiology associated with various *Leptospira* serotypes.

HISTORY[61]

Adolf Weil first described the clinical picture of human leptospirosis in 1886. The term "Weil's disease" was coined by F. Goldschmidt in 1887. A.M. Stimson described the organism for the first time in a human kidney in a person suspected of dying of yellow fever in 1907. The carrier status was described in asymptomatic field mice by Ido and coworkers in 1915. These early references were cited by Diesch and Ellinghausen.[63] Since 1915 the infection has been recognized both as a disease and as an asymptomatic carrier state in hundreds of animal species. The history of leptospirosis in the United States was reviewed by C.W. Heath and associates.[90]

EPIDEMIOLOGY

Leptospirosis is found throughout tropical and temperate areas of the world. It is particularly common in Southeast Asia and parts of Latin America, including some Caribbean islands.[70] Approximately 40 to 100 cases are reported annually in the United States (Fig. 41-8). Undoubtedly, many cases are unreported. Active surveillance on Kauai and the east coast of the big island of Hawaii revealed a high incidence, accounting for a large proportion of flulike illness.[156]

Leptospirosis is a zoonosis, with a tendency for certain serotypes to have host specificity. The serotypes often responsible for human infection in the United States, and their usual animal sources, are listed in Table 41-1. Dogs are usually associated with *L. icterohaemorrhagiae* and *L. canicola;* swine and cattle are more frequently involved with *L. pomona* and *L. grippotyphosa,* although all four of these serovars or serotypes have been isolated from each host species. The major reservoir for *Leptospira* infections for humans and domestic animals is wildlife.

While wild and domestic mammals are commonly recognized sources of leptospirosis, the organism has also been isolated from frogs and snakes; serologically positive fish and turtles have been found.[119] The role of these poikilotherms in transmission or maintenance of the infection is unknown. Public health and certain veterinary aspects of leptospirosis were reviewed by Hanson.[87]

Animals contaminate the environment by shedding organisms in urine. Many human cases are environmentally acquired by contact with contaminated water or soil. In such cases it is often difficult or impossible to discover the original animal source. Infection is also acquired by contact with infected animal blood and tissues. Factors strongly associated with acquiring leptospirosis in Hawaii include household use of rainwater catchment systems and the presence of skin cuts at the presumed time of exposure.[156]

Leptospirosis is an occupational problem for veterinary, agricultural, sewer, slaughterhouse, laboratory, and military personnel.[71,90,156] Dairy farmers are at risk in milking parlors, probably through exposure to cows' urine.[5,100] Leptospirosis poses an avocational risk for hunters, trappers, hikers, and persons who swim in nonchlorinated fresh water such as ponds and streams. It is acquired by ingestion or by entry through abraded skin or through the mucous membranes of the eye and mouth.

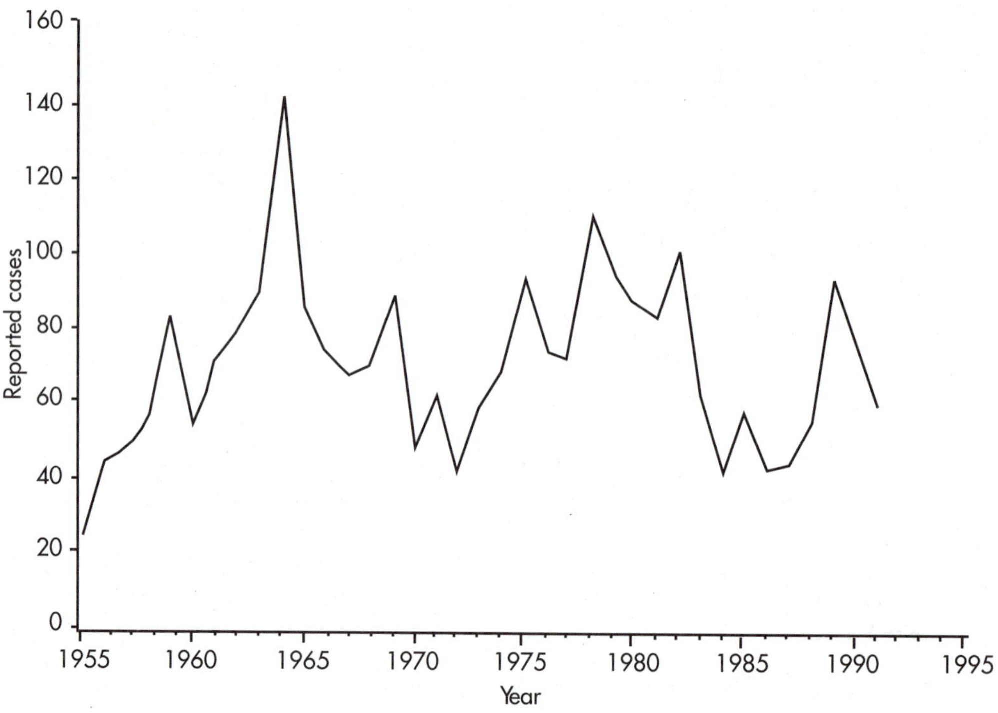

Fig. 41-8 Reported annual cases of leptospirosis in the United States, 1955 through 1991. (From *MMWR* 40, No 53, 1991.)

Table 41-1 Leptospires Isolated from Humans in the United States, and Their Animal Reservoirs

Serogroup	Serovar	Domestic Animals	Wildlife
Icterohaemorrhagiae	*Icterohaemorrhagiae*	Dogs, cattle, swine	Brown rat, house rat, cotton rat, Pacific rat, house mouse, muskrat, gray fox, red fox, opossum, striped skunk, woodchuck, nutria
Canicola	*Canicola*	Dogs, cattle, swine	Striped skunk, raccoon, armadillo, mongoose
Pomona	*Pomona*	Dogs, cattle, swine, goats, sheep, horses	Striped skunk, raccoon, wildcat, opossum, woodchuck, red fox, deer, armadillo
Grippotyphosa	*Grippotyphosa*	Dogs, cattle, swine	Muskrat, fox squirrel, gray squirrel, bobcat, cottontail rabbit, swamp rabbit, raccoon, striped skunk, red fox, gray fox, vole, opossum
Hebdomidis	*Hardjo*	Cattle	None

Modified from Hanson LE: *J Am Vet Med Assoc* 181:1505, 1982.

SYMPTOMS[90]

The incubation period is usually 7 to 12 days (range 1 to 26 days).[155] The disease characteristically is biphasic.[101,148] The primary stage lasts 4 to 7 days and is characterized by the presence of organisms in blood, cerebrospinal fluid, and various body tissues. During the initial phase more than half of patients show fever, chills, severe malaise, myalgias, headache, lymph node enlargement, and conjunctival suffusion, usually without exudate. There may be nausea, vomiting, and abdominal pain. A nonproductive cough is common.

After the primary stage there is usually an afebrile period of 1 to 2 days. The onset of the second stage coincides with development of IgM antibodies. The organisms usually cannot be cultured from blood or spinal fluid during this phase, but can be isolated from urine for weeks or months. During the second stage there may be fever, but it is lower than in the primary stage. Headache is persistent, severe, and unresponsive to analgesics. It often heralds the onset of meningitis, one of the common complications of the secondary stage.

Myalgias, abdominal pain, nausea, and vomiting can occur in the second as well as in the primary stage. In addition to conjunctival suffusion seen in the the primary stage, uveitis (iridocyclitis) can be seen in the secondary stage. This can leave persistent ocular damage.[165] Occasionally, pharyngitis and a macular, purpuric, or ecchymotic rash occur (Fig. 41-9). Rarely, endocarditis or myocarditis occurs. In a clinical study of leptospirosis on Barbados, cardiac arrhythmias and myocarditis occurred in 18% and pericarditis in 6% of patients.[67]

Splenic enlargement develops in approximately 20% of patients in the second stage. Hepatomegaly is sometimes found, especially if the patient is icteric.

Jaundice is a serious prognostic sign. Mortality in cases with jaundice exceeds 15%, but is rare in anicteric cases. The overall case-fatality rate is approximately 5%. Mortality depends, in part, on the prior condition of the patient. It is higher in aged individuals than in young adults. Death can occur from hemorrhagic manifestations as a result of vasculitis, renal or hepatic failure, cardiogenic shock, or myocarditis.

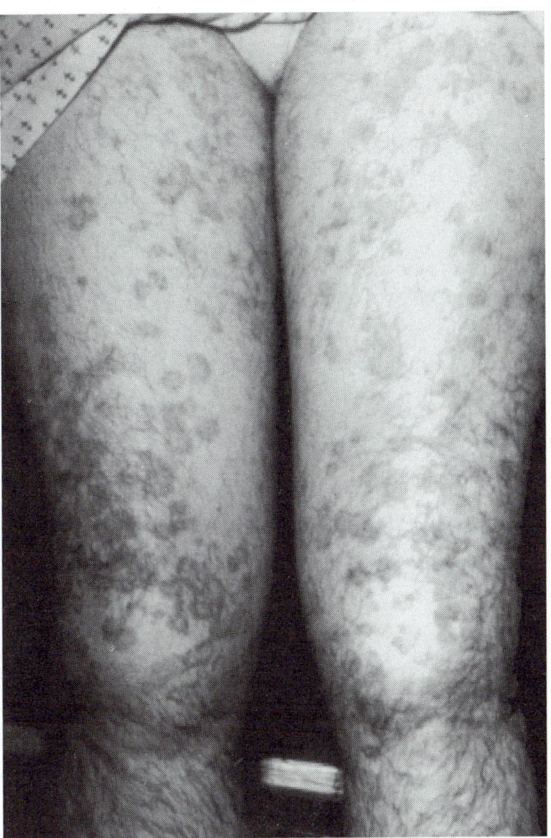

Fig. 41-9 Hemorrhagic macular rash in a case of leptospirosis. (Courtesy University of Massachusetts Medical School.)

LABORATORY STUDIES

Laboratory findings in leptospirosis include moderate leukocytosis, usually caused by an increase in neutrophils, elevated erythrocyte sedimentation rate, and thrombocytopenia. The presence of an elevated bilirubin level (up to 65 mg/dl, mainly direct bilirubin), greatly increased serum creatine phosphokinase level (often five times normal), and a less than fivefold increase in aspartate aminotransferase is suggestive of the diagnosis. Elevated blood urea nitrogen level is a common finding. The serum amylase concentration may also be elevated.

Definitive diagnosis of leptospirosis can be made by culture of the organism on Fletcher's, Stuart's, EMJH,[176] or Tween 80-albumin medium. Blood and cerebrospinal fluid should be cultured during the first week of illness; urine should be cultured thereafter. The likelihood of obtaining a positive culture is greatly diminished once antibiotics have been given. Oxalated blood samples can be sent to the laboratory for culture because the organisms can remain viable in oxalated blood for up to 11 days.

Some physicians have relied on dark-field examination for identification of the organisms, but this method is not considered reliable. Artifacts such as fibrin are readily mistaken for leptospires. The spirochetes can be demonstrated in tissue sections with silver stains (Color Plate 104).

Leptospirosis can be diagnosed serologically.[186] The macroscopic slide agglutination test, using killed organisms, or the complement fixation test is useful for screening purposes. The macroscopic agglutination test may become positive within the first week of illness and can persist for several months. Complement-fixing antibodies are detectable between days 10 and 21. Acute and convalescent sera should be tested 2 weeks apart because false-positive reactions can occur in single samples. A fourfold or greater rise in titer suggests active leptospirosis.

Serologic diagnosis of serogroup or serotype of infection can be made with the microscopic agglutination (MA) test, which uses live organisms but is available in relatively few reference laboratories. A genus-specific microscopic agglutination test employs a single broadly reactive antigen.[188] An IgM-specific dot-enzyme-linked immunosorbent assay is comparable to the MA test in its ability to detect recent exposure to leptospires and is rapid and simpler.[134] Latex agglutination and indirect hemagglutination have high specificity and sensitivity and are especially useful early in the infection.[138]

TREATMENT

Treatment of leptospirosis with antibiotics is most effective when begun during the first week of illness. Although most older articles state that antibiotics have little value after this time, recent studies indicate that they may still have some usefulness.[189] The treatment of choice is doxycycline, 100 mg orally twice a day for 7 days.[125] Alternative antibiotics include tetracycline, 2 g/day orally in three or four divided doses, or penicillin G, 3 million units/day parenterally.

Amoxicillin, ampicillin, a cephalosporin, or erythromycin could also be used. Doxycycline and tetracycline should not be given to pregnant women or to children less than 8 years old.

A Jarisch-Herxheimer reaction may occur after treatment. This is a response to release of endotoxins, usually occurring within 2 to 6 hours after initiating therapy, with sudden onset of fever, chills, malaise, headache, and tachycardia. The reaction typically resolves spontaneously within 24 hours.

Other than antibiotic treatment, therapy for leptospirosis is supportive, including fluid therapy, dialysis for renal failure,[103] and transfusion for hemorrhagic complications.

PREVENTION

Prevention of human leptospirosis depends on avoiding infected animal tissues and areas contaminated by animal urine, blood, or tissue. Individuals who are at particularly high risk should be educated about prevention and encouraged to wear protective clothing, such as rubber gloves, when handling infective material. Swimming in freshwater ponds and streams likely to be heavily contaminated by urine from livestock or wildlife should be discouraged.

Doxycycline, 200 mg once a week, was found effective in preventing infection in U.S. soldiers training in Panama.[179] Such prophylactic treatment could be given to individuals at unusually high risk.

Although *Leptospira* vaccines have been experimentally produced for human use, no product is approved and commercially available in the United States. Vaccines are available for animals. Immunization of domestic animals primarily has a veterinary benefit, in that the animals are protected from clinical disease. Immunity lasts about 6 months, but immunization does not guarantee that the animal cannot become infected. Several human cases have been traced to immunized dogs that apparently were still able to shed organisms.[73] Since then, some veterinary vaccines have been shown experimentally to reduce the renal carrier state.[104]

VETERINARY SYMPTOMS

Leptospirosis may be asymptomatic in animals. This is usually the situation in wild animals, including rodents. Animals that acquire clinical disease have fever, appear depressed, lose appetite, may become jaundiced, develop hemorrhages on mucous membranes, and in late stages of the disease may suffer renal failure.[87]

In cattle, leptospirosis can cause stillbirths, hemoglobinuria, and thickened yellowish or blood-tinged milk. Leptospires have been isolated from the milk of cattle and goats. A theoretical risk exists that leptospirosis could be transmitted by consuming such milk. Pasteurization should destroy organisms. Stillbirths or delivery of weak piglets is a common sign of leptospirosis in swine.

Cats are rarely affected by leptospirosis. They must be resistant to the disease because presumably they are frequently exposed to infection through catching mice and other rodents.

Leptospirosis has been suspected as a cause of recurrent uveitis in horses. This is more of interest in comparative pathology than in public health, since horses infrequently transmit the infection to humans.

PROGNOSIS

Recovery from leptospirosis apparently leaves serotype-specific immunity. Individuals can become infected with other serotypes. Assuming that the infection and hemorrhagic complications can be controlled, the long-term prognosis after successful treatment is good. There is usually complete return of renal and hepatic function, but headache and ocular damage may persist.[165]

Hantavirus Pulmonary Syndrome

Hantavirus pulmonary syndrome (HPS) is a severe respiratory illness caused by a hantavirus most closely related to the Prospect Hill strain. The causative agent has been identified by serologic tests, polymerase chain reaction (PCR) to ribonucleic acid, and immunohistochemistry.[56,113]

Hantaviruses of the Bunyaviridae family have been known to cause the hemorrhagic fever with renal disease syndrome. This is predominantly a disease of East Asia, where it has been called Korean hemorrhagic fever or epidemic hemorrhagic fever.[111] Wild rodents are the vectors of Hantaan, Puumala, Prospect Hill, and Seoul viruses. Hantaviruses have been isolated from the lung tissues of bats.[106]

Although most cases of HPS have been clustered in the western United States, particularly the Four Corners area (Arizona, New Mexico, Colorado, and Utah), reports of the disease indicate that the virus may be present across the entire country.[131,141] The sin nombre (formerly Muerto Canyon) virus variant has been the most virulent. Rodents are the major reservoir hosts for the recognized hantaviruses.[55] The major vector for the virus that causes HPS is the deer mouse *Peromyscus maniculatus,* which inhabits all areas of the United States except the southeastern and the Atlantic Coast states. However, at least one case has been investigated in Florida. Other small mammals may be infected, such as piñon mice, brush mice, and western chipmunks.

The hantaviruses do not cause apparent illnesses in the reservoir hosts, but the animals shed virus in saliva, urine, and feces for weeks. Human infection probably occurs when infective saliva or excreta are inhaled as aerosols, or when excreta are directly inoculated through the skin or perhaps ingested. Persons have been infected with hantavirus via rodent bite. There is no known transmission from arthropods or human to human.

The clinical syndrome is typified by a prodrome of fever, myalgia, and variable respiratory symptoms, which may include cough and shortness of breath with minimal bronchospasm. Acute respiratory distress rapidly follows. Other symptoms reported in the early phase of illness include headache, chills, abdominal pain, nausea, and vomiting. Patients have often shown hemoconcentration and thrombocytopenia, leukocytosis, hypoalbuminemia, and lactic acidosis.

Rapid deterioration occurs, coincident with marked bilateral pulmonary infiltrates identified on chest x-ray examination. Fever, hypoxia, and hypotension may culminate in death; survivors have few or no sequelae. Autopsies have demonstrated intense pulmonary infiltration, with marked accumulations of hantavirus antigens in the endothelial cells.

Treatment is supportive. Previously isolated hantaviruses have demonstrated in vitro sensitivity to ribavirin. The CDC has made the drug available as an investigational agent through an open-label protocol for treatment of patients with HPS. The protocol calls for administration of a 2 g loading dose of intravenous ribavirin, followed by 15 mg/kg body weight every 6 hours for 4 days and then 7.5 mg/kg every 8 hours for another 4 days. There has been at least one reported case of administration that may have contributed to survival of a patient.[143]

Laboratory evidence of acute hantavirus infection can be obtained by any of the following tests: IgM antibodies to hantavirus antigens, fourfold or greater increase in antibody titers to hantavirus antigens in paired serum specimens, positive immunohistochemical stain for hantavirus antigen in formalin-fixed tissues, or positive PCR from frozen tissue specimens (usually lungs).

Any person with a severe and sudden respiratory illness should be suspected to have been infected with hantavirus. The CDC has published screening criteria for hantavirus pulmonary syndrome in persons with unexplained respiratory illness, which state that there must be a febrile illness in a previously healthy person characterized by unexplained adult respiratory distress syndrome *or* bilateral interstitial pulmonary infiltrates developing within 1 week of hospitalization with respiratory compromise requiring supplemental oxygen.

According to the CDC, hantavirus transmission to humans may be epidemiologically associated with planting or harvesting field crops, occupying previously vacant dwellings, disturbing rodent-infested areas while hiking or camping, inhabiting dwellings with indoor rodent populations, or residing in an area with an increasing rodent density.

The hantaviruses are susceptible to most disinfectants. Since a wide-scale rodent roundup is not feasible, the following suggestions[55] may prove useful to modify habitat:

1. Eliminate rodents and reduce the availability of food sources and nesting sites used by rodents inside the home.
2. Keep food and water covered and stored in rodent-proof metal or thick plastic containers.
3. Dispose of clutter.
4. Remove food sources that might attract rodents.
5. Spray dead rodents, nests, and droppings with a general-purpose disinfectant before handling. Always wear rubber or plastic gloves.
6. Avoid coming into contact with rodents and rodent burrows or disturbing dens (such as pack rat nests).
7. Do not use cabins or other enclosed shelters that are rodent infested until they have been appropriately cleaned and disinfected.
8. Do not pitch tents or place sleeping bags in areas close to rodent feces or burrows or near possible rodent shelters (garbage dumps or wood piles).
9. If possible, do not sleep on the bare ground. Use a cot with the sleeping surface at least 12 inches above the ground. Use tents with floors.
10. Burn or bury all garbage promptly.
11. Use only bottled water or water that has been disinfected by filtration, boiling, chlorination, or iodination for drinking, cooking, washing dishes, and brushing teeth.

Tularemia

HISTORICAL ASPECTS[16,69]

Tularemia was first described in 1837 by Homma Soken, a Japanese physician who wrote of a febrile illness with generalized lymphadenopathy in persons who had eaten infected rabbit meat. In 1911, McCoy described a disease resembling plague in California ground squirrels. In the following year, McCoy and Chapin isolated the organism from rodents in Tulare County, California; this geographic site gave rise to the name of the disease. Edward Francis did much of the landmark bacteriologic and clinical investigation, and the genus of the causative organism, *Francisella*, is named after him. The role of ticks as vectors of the disease was discovered by Parker and Spencer in 1924. In 1929, they described transovarial transmission of the bacterium in ticks.

MICROBIOLOGY

Francisella tularensis is a nonmotile, gram-negative coccobacillus measuring 0.2 by 0.3 to 0.7 μm. It must be grown aerobically on media containing cysteine or other sulfhydryl compounds. The organism is best grown on glucose cysteine agar with thiamine or on cysteine glucose blood agar. The organism has also been isolated in thioglycollate broth, charcoal yeast extract, and Thayer-Martin agar.

Two varieties of the organism are recognized in North America. Type A can ferment glycerol and has citrulline ureidase activity. It generally causes more severe disease than does type B, which is found in Europe and Asia as well as North America. Type B does not ferment glycerol and does not have citrulline ureidase activity. Type A is more commonly recovered from rabbits and various blood-sucking arthropods. Type B is often recovered from water, voles, muskrats, and beavers. However, the two varieties sometimes share an ecologic niche.[120]

TRANSMISSION

Before 1950, most reported cases of tularemia were associated with contacting rabbits. Tularemia is now most commonly transmitted by ticks.[23] Many different species of ticks are potential or proven vectors. A common vector in the United States is the dog tick, *Dermacentor variabilis*. The lone star tick, *Amblyoma americanum,* is the main vector in the southern United States. Because the infection can be transmitted transovarially, ticks are an important natural reservoir. It is thought that ticks transmit the bacteria through their feces because the organism has not been isolated from their salivary glands. Deerflies and other biting flies may also be suitable vectors.[108] In the United States, the second most common source for human infection is rabbits. The infection can be acquired by skinning, eviscerating, or handling the tissues of infected rabbits or by eating improperly cooked infected meat.

Transmission can also occur by direct contact with or ingestion of infected soil, water, or fomites. Infection can occur by inhalation of dust or water aerosol,[60] or in the laboratory. Organisms remain viable in mud samples stored as long as 14 weeks, in tap water for 3 months, in dry straw for 6 months, and in salted meat for 31 days.[16]

Occasional cases of tularemia have been transmitted by cat bite[41,144] or by handling infected tissue from animals other than rabbits, such as bear,[37] deer,[32] beaver, and muskrat.[201] Person-to-person transmission is rare.

EPIDEMIOLOGY

Transmission by ticks and other arthropods usually occurs in the spring and summer. Transmission from rabbits most commonly occurs during the fall and winter hunting seasons.

The reported incidence of tularemia has been steadily decreasing in the United States. It peaked at 2291 cases in 1939. A steady decline in the incidence of this disease has occurred since 1950, with fewer than 200 cases reported annually since 1967 (Fig. 41-10). This decline is not easy to explain because tularemia is so widespread in nature. Other tick-borne infections, such as Rocky Mountain spotted fever and Lyme disease, have increased. Perhaps the empirical use of antibiotics has aborted undiagnosed cases.

Most cases in the United States have been reported from the South and Midwest, particularly Arkansas, Illinois, Missouri, Oklahoma, Texas, and Tennessee. The disease is also widespread in Europe, Canada, the Middle East, Russia, and Japan.

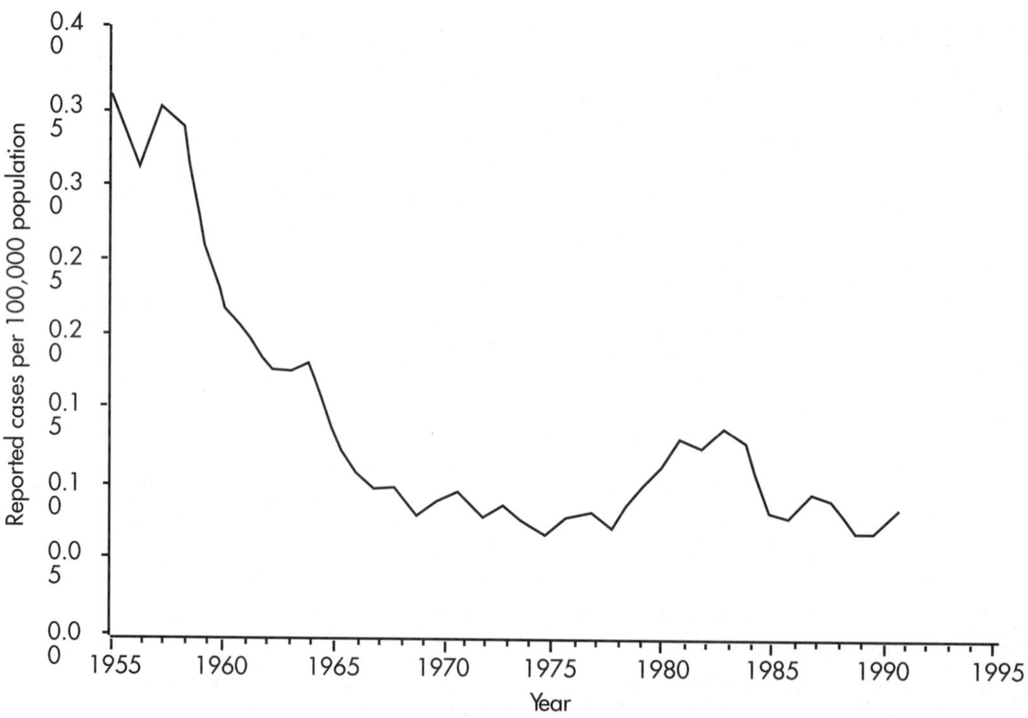

Fig. 41-10 Reported cases of tularemia in the United States, 1955 through 1991. (From *MMWR* 40, No 53, 1991.)

SYMPTOMS

Classically, tularemia occurs in one of six clinical presentations: glandular, ulceroglandular, oculoglandular, oropharyngeal, pneumonic, or typhoidal.[16,120] Evans and associates[69] simplified this classification into two major categories: ulceroglandular and typhoidal. Patients are considered to have ulceroglandular disease if they have lesions of the skin or mucous membranes, with or without associated lymphadenopathy, with affected lymph nodes at least 1 cm in diameter. Patients without lesions of the skin or mucous membranes and with lesser enlargement of lymph nodes are considered to have typhoidal tularemia. In this classification, pharyngitis or pneumonia can occur in either the ulceroglandular or the typhoidal form of the disease.

The ulceroglandular form accounts for approximately 80% of tularemia cases. The typical skin lesion begins as an erythematous papule or nodule that indurates and ulcerates. It is frequently painful and tender. Ulcers associated with handling infected animals are usually located on the hand, with associated lymphadenopathy found in the epitrochlear or axillary regions. Infections transmitted by tick bites are usually located on the lower extremities, associated with inguinal or femoral lymphadenopathy.

So-called glandular tularemia is characterized by the presence of enlarged, tender lymph nodes without an associated skin lesion. However, the skin lesion may have healed or gone unnoticed before the development of lymphadenopathy.

In the oculoglandular form of the disease, unilateral conjunctivitis occurs with concentration of inflammatory response in and around a nodular lesion on the conjunctiva and with enlargement of the ipsilateral preauricular lymph node.[86] The oculoglandular form constitutes 1% to 2% of tularemia cases.

The typhoidal form of the disease occurs in approximately 10% of tularemia cases. It is characterized by fever, chills, and debility. As the disease progresses, there may be significant weight loss. Hepatosplenomegaly can occur, especially in children.[99] Pericarditis occurs rarely.[69]

Exudative pharyngitis can occur with either the typhoidal or the ulceroglandular form of the disease. There is usually associated cervical lymphadenitis.

Pneumonia is a fairly common complication of tularemia. The pulmonary infection can be acquired by inhalation of aerosol or from bacteremia. Symptoms include cough, chest pain, shortness of breath, production of sputum, and hemoptysis. Radiographic abnormalities of the chest may be found in patients without pulmonary symptoms. Chest films may reveal infiltrates, most commonly of the lower lobe, hilar lymphadenopathy, and pleural effusion. Tularemia patients with pneumonia are more likely to be older, less likely to have a known source of infection, and more likely to die than those without pulmonary infection.[167]

Severe complications of tularemia, such as bacteremia, pneumonia, and rhabdomyolysis, are most likely to be seen in patients with significant underlying disease, such as lymphoma, other forms of cancer, or diabetes.[137] From 1981 through 1987 the case-fatality rate of tularemia in the Southwest-Central United States was 2%.[180]

Chronic illness, characterized by lassitude, weakness, and weight loss, has been described. Cough and pleural pain can persist for months, even after treatment. Relapsing episodes of fever, diaphoresis, malaise, weakness, and lymph node enlargement are also known.[69]

DIFFERENTIAL DIAGNOSIS

Ulceroglandular tularemia can be confused with cat-scratch disease, streptococcal and staphylococcal skin diseases, sporotrichosis, and plague. Typhoidal tularemia can mimic septicemic plague, brucellosis, salmonellosis, typhoid fever, other forms of gram-negative sepsis, and leptospirosis. Tularemic pneumonia can appear similar to other forms of bacterial and nonbacterial pneumonias, including Q fever, psittacosis, and Legionnaires' disease.[150,167]

Oculoglandular tularemia resembles Parinaud's syndrome (granulomatous conjunctivitis with preauricular lymphadenitis) caused by other bacteria, such as *Leptothrix* species, *Mycobacterium tuberculosis,* syphilis, and cat-scratch disease.[86]

The differential diagnosis of oropharyngeal tularemia includes infectious mononucleosis, streptococcal pharyngitis, and plague pharyngitis. The disease most likely to be confused with tularemia is plague, because both diseases occur under similar epidemiologic circumstances and are characterized by certain similar clinical syndromes.[30,170] The bacteria causing plague and tularemia share common morphologic and cultural features. However, they can be differentiated serologically and with appropriate microbiologic techniques.

Infectious mononucleosis can be differentiated by hematologic findings (atypical lymphocytosis) and serologic studies. The other bacterial infections that can be mistaken for tularemia are differentiated on the basis of appropriate cultures and immunologic studies.

Definitive diagnosis of tularemia is usually based on antibody studies.[109,178] The method most commonly used is agglutination, which can be run as a tube agglutination or microagglutination test.[161] Enzyme-linked immunosorbent assay (ELISA) is also used for diagnosis. An advantage of ELISA is that it can be used to identify IgM, IgA, and IgG antibodies.

Diagnosis is established serologically by demonstrating a fourfold or greater rise in titer between acute and convalescent sera taken 1 or more weeks apart. Titers of 80 or greater are generally considered significant in the agglutination test. Values rarely reach that level during the first week of infection, but usually reach or exceed that by the sixteenth day of infection. Agglutinating antibodies remain detectable for 10 to 30 years after infection. IgM, IgA, and IgG antibodies also remain detectable by the ELISA technique for at least 11 years after infection. Because of this long persistence of antibody, single titers cannot be relied on for definitive diagnosis.

Tularemia can also be definitively diagnosed by isolation and identification of the organism from blood or lesions. Samples for culture, however, are not routinely taken in suspect cases and indeed are not encouraged because of the high frequency of contamination and infection of workers in the laboratory when working with this organism in vitro.

TREATMENT[69,137]

Streptomycin, the drug of choice, should be given in a dose of 30 to 40 mg/kg/day, in two divided portions intramuscularly every 12 hours for 3 days, followed by half that dose for another 4 to 7 days. The smaller dosage may be adequate for the entire course of therapy in mild cases. Kanamycin and gentamicin are alternative drugs, but there is less experience with their use.

A recommended dose for gentamicin is 1 to 1.5 mg/kg/day, in three divided doses intravenously, adjusted for serum creatinine concentration. If the use of aminoglycosides is contraindicated because of problems with toxicity or hypersensitivity, tetracycline or chloramphenicol can be used at a dosage of 50 to 60 mg/kg/day in four divided doses orally every 6 hours for 14 days. Relapses frequently occur with this alternative therapy, but if the same regimen is repeated, cure can usually be achieved. Relapses are particularly likely when chloramphenicol or tetracycline is used early in the course of the disease. Success with these agents is more likely if they are instituted during the second or third week of illness. A favorable clinical response should occur within 48 hours of starting an appropriate antibiotic.

F. tularensis is sensitive in vitro to fluoroquinolone antibiotics. A small number of patients with tularemia have been treated successfully with ciprofloxacin or norfloxacin.[177]

PREVENTION

Prevention of tularemia includes avoidance of ectoparasites and appropriate hygiene in the handling of infected animal tissues. Insect repellents should be applied when going into areas where ticks, deerflies, and other possible vectors are found (see Chapter 34). Persons walking in tick-infested brush should wear long pants, with the bottoms of trouser legs tucked into socks or boot tops. Individuals should check frequently for the presence of ticks while in the field, and any ticks that have become attached should be removed as quickly as possible, preferably with pointed forceps grasping the mouthparts, taking care not to break them or to squeeze the body of the tick in the removal process (see Chapter 33).

Persons handling suspect animals should wear rubber or plastic gloves. Reservoir animals such as rabbits or muskrats that appear ill should not be handled. When handling sick animals is necessary, infection control procedures should include the use of gloves, face masks, and disposable gowns.

Attempts at culturing the organism should be done only in laboratories that have appropriate containment facilities for handling such dangerous organisms. Laboratory work with *F. tularensis* should always be conducted under an appropriate microbiologic hood. Standard halogen-containing phenol or alcohol-based antiseptics can be used for disinfecting surfaces.

Although person-to-person transmission is rare, reasonable infection control measures should be taken to reduce exposure to aerosols from patients with oropharyngeal or pneumonic tularemia, and exposure to exudates should be avoided.

A live attenuated vaccine is available as an investigational new drug from the U.S. Army Medical Research Institute for Infectious Diseases at Fort Detrick, Maryland. Physicians using this vaccine must register as collaborative investigators and follow a prescribed protocol in advising the patient, administering the vaccine, and reporting on its use. The vaccine is made available only for those who are at high risk, such as laboratory personnel who frequently work with the organism. The vaccine is effective in preventing the typhoidal form of tularemia,[157-160] but will not prevent cutaneous lesions forming at the site of an inoculation. The vaccine, when administered by scarification, induces humoral and cell-mediated immune responses.[185]

Plague

HISTORICAL ASPECTS

Plague, a bacterial disease caused by *Yersinia pestis,* has occurred in explosive epidemics, leaving great misery, death, and destruction in its wake. Probable epidemics of plague occurred during the Peloponnesian War as described by Thucydides, approximately 400 BC. It ravaged the Roman Empire and western Europe during the age of Justinian and continued through the seventh century. The best-known and most devastating epidemic started in 1348. Known as the Black Death, the infection spread from Asia throughout western Europe, killing one third of the population.[82] Plague is carried by various rodent reservoir hosts and transmitted by rodent fleas. Most of the outbreaks in Europe have been ascribed to importation of plague from enzootic foci in Asia, by ships bringing infected rats and people to port cities. A matter of considerable historical and epidemiologic interest is how and why the various epidemics eventually subsided. Theories include development of mutant bacteria; changes in patterns of shipping, building, and hygiene; replacement of *Rattus rattus* by *R. norvegicus;* and development of immunity in animals and humans. A review of some of these concepts has been published by Ell.[68] This article contains a useful bibliography for persons interested in historical aspects of plague.

BACTERIOLOGY

Y. pestis is a gram-negative, nonmotile, nonsporulating rod with a bipolar, or safety-pin, appearance in smears stained with Giemsa's or Wayson's stain.[27] The appearance is somewhat variable by Gram's technique.

Most standard bacteriologic media support the growth of the organism aerobically or under facultative anaerobic conditions. Optimal in vitro growth occurs at 28° C, at which temperature colonies become visible on plain agar in approximately 48 hours.

Virulence factors encoded by the bacterial chromosome include surface capsular material that is antiphagocytic, ability to synthesize purines even if phagocytosed, and a surface component needed for iron uptake. Virulence factors mediated by a plasmid include dependence on environmental calcium for growth at 37° C and production of V and W antigens. The relationship between calcium dependence and virulence is under investigation.[82]

EPIDEMIOLOGY

The epidemiology of plague is complex. Various fleas can transmit the infection between reservoir rodent hosts and humans. In some of the major epidemics that have swept through the civilized world, the prominent actors were the tropical rat flea *(Xenopsylla cheopis)* and the black rat *(R. rattus)*.

The bacteria multiply so extensively in *X. cheopis* that they block its proventriculus or foregut. The flea cannot feed effectively, becomes ravenously hungry, and regurgitates large numbers of bacilli when it bites.

The black rat is highly susceptible to plague and dies with severe septicemia. The concentration of organisms in the rat's blood ensures infection of the biting flea. When the rat dies, the flea leaves to seek other hosts. This cycle is unusual in that the infection kills the reservoir host and vector, but the nature of the infection in the flea and rat guarantees further transmission and survival of the microorganism.

Smoldering foci of infection are maintained in nature in wild rodents and their fleas. In the United States, enzootic (maintenance) hosts include deer mice *(Peromyscus maniculatus)* and various voles (*Microtus* species). Epizootic (amplifying) hosts include the prairie dog (*Cynomys* species) (Fig. 41-11) and ground squirrel (*Spermophilus* species). Other rodents and lagomorphs that maintain infection include chipmunks (*Eutamias* species), marmots (*Marmota* species), wood rats (*Neotoma* species), rabbits (*Sylvilagus* species), and hares (*Lepus* species).[139]

Enzootic foci of plague remain in parts of Asia, Africa, and South America[27,139] as well as the western United States. The major enzootic states in the United States are New Mexico, Arizona, California, Colorado, Oregon, Nevada, and Utah. In many foreign areas the exact species of rodents and fleas involved in transmission and maintenance are not known. Vietnam is the only country considered a threat for the international introduction of plague. Trong, Nhu, and Marshall[182] reviewed plague outbreaks in Vietnam from 1898 to 1965. Recent cases in India are of great concern.

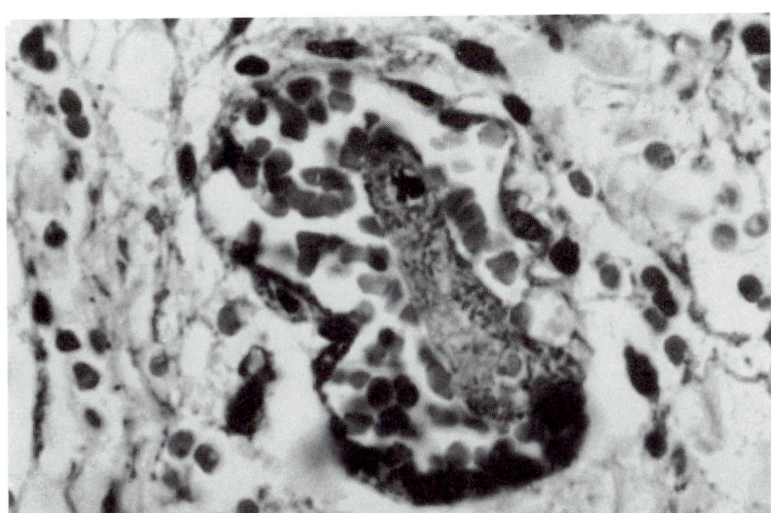

Fig. 41-11 A thrombus in a vein in the subcutis of a prairie dog naturally infected with plague. Many organisms *(fine stippling)* are present in the thrombus. (Hematoxylin and eosin, original magnification 1000×.)

Carnivorous mammals can acquire plague by ingesting infected rodents or by being bitten by their fleas. Dogs usually do not become very ill with plague, but cats can acquire severe, often fatal, forms of infection, resembling syndromes seen in humans.[102,149] Bubonic plague in cats is usually manifested as severe submandibular lymphadenopathy. Cats can also acquire pneumonic plague, characterized by a subacute febrile course with cough and respiratory distress. Cats can transmit plague to humans by bite, respiratory droplets, or carrying fleas to people. Plague is an occupational risk for veterinarians who handle sick cats or their tissues.[102,149]

Although dogs are usually not as severely affected as cats, at least one human case was associated with a dog that apparently died of plague.[154] Dogs may be significantly involved in the epidemiology of plague in Tanzania, as reservoirs of vector fleas or bacterial infection.[105] In the United States, one person acquired plague while skinning an infected coyote[31] and two from skinning bobcats.[38] Other carnivores, such as skunks, badgers, and raccoons, have been found with antibody to the plague bacillus and presumably were exposed while hunting infected rodents. Exposure to infected rabbits, their fleas, or both has been associated with human plague.[29]

Ancient literature describing medieval outbreaks of plague described widespread morbidity and mortality among farm animals. Plague is not generally recognized as a disease of such animals in modern times, but a recent report ascribed one outbreak of plague in a Libyan village to contact with a sick camel, and another to contact with two goats.[57]

In the United States the major epidemiologic factor associated with acquiring plague is living in a rural or suburban area where the enzootic disease occurs. People who hike, camp, or perform field studies in such areas are subject to this disease. Its diagnosis should be considered in anyone with a compatible history who has recently been in an enzootic area. The incidence in the United States is shown in Fig. 41-12.

SYMPTOMS[97,98,139,191,192]

The three most common forms of plague are bubonic, pneumonic, and septicemic. Less common forms are meningeal, pharyngeal, and ophthalmic.

The most common form is bubonic. Buboes are greatly enlarged and very tender lymph nodes proximal to the point of percutaneous entry, such as a flea bite or a cut infected by handling infected tissues. Inguinal nodes are the most commonly involved because fleas most commonly bite on the legs. Skinning an infected animal or handling its tissues often results in axillary buboes. Less commonly the cervical, hilar, or mesenteric lymph nodes are enlarged.

The incubation period for bubonic plague is usually 2 to 6 days. In mild or early stages of infection, seeding of the blood occurs intermittently. Later, if disease becomes severe, all blood cultures are positive. Patients usually have high fever, chills, severe malaise, headache, and myalgias.

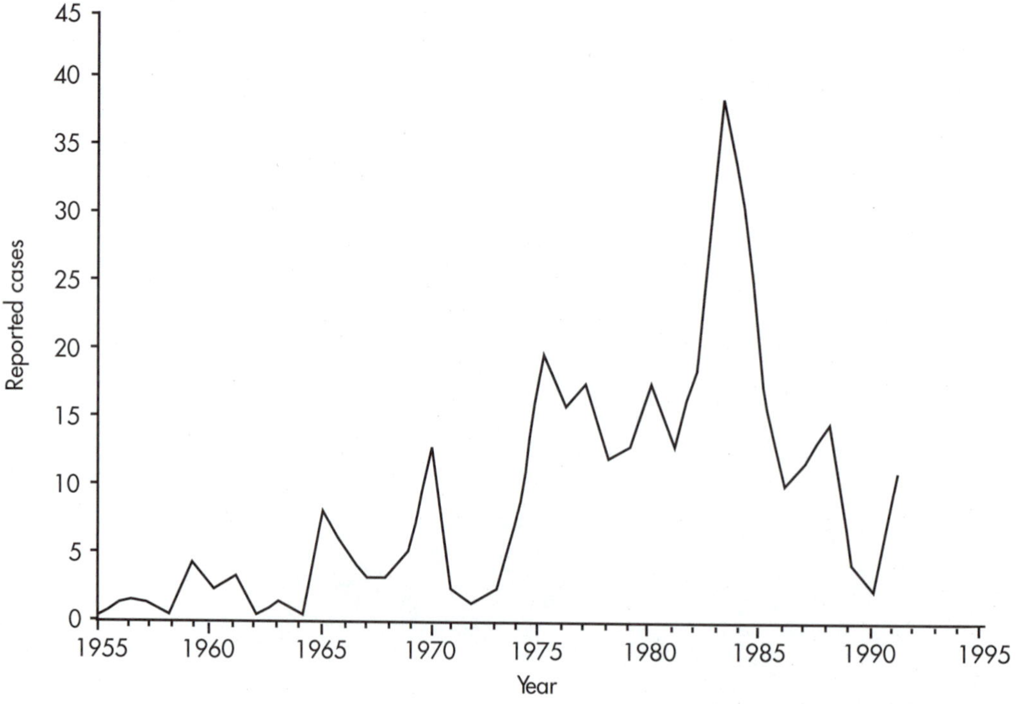

Fig. 41-12 Reported cases of plague in humans in the United States, 1955 to 1986. (From *MMWR* 40, No 53, 1991.)

Toxicity, cardiovascular collapse with shock, and hemorrhagic phenomena may occur. Blackened hemorrhagic skin lesions gave rise to the name "Black Death" during the pandemic of the fourteenth century.

Victims may have a septicemic form of disease without bubo formation. Such cases may be difficult to diagnose unless the physician suspects plague based on epidemiology. As with other forms of gram-negative sepsis, patients have fever, chills, malaise, headache, and gastrointestinal symptoms such as nausea, vomiting, and diarrhea, and the disease can result in cardiovascular collapse. Thrombosis (Fig. 41-11) and disseminated intravascular coagulopathy may be present.

The pneumonic form can result from inhalation of droplets from another pneumonic patient or by pulmonary seeding from the blood. Pneumonic plague runs an acute and fulminant course and is almost uniformly fatal if not treated. Coughing often produces bloody sputum. Radiographs reveal progressive consolidation of pneumonic patches in the lung, often with pleural effusion.

Of 71 cases of plague reported in New Mexico between 1980 and 1984, 18 were septicemic.[98] The victims were significantly older and more likely to die than those with bubonic plague. The white blood cell counts in the New Mexican septicemic cases were low, normal, or elevated (range 3000 to 68,700/mm^3), but all patients had relative or absolute neutrophilia with a left shift. Bacteria were demonstrable on direct blood smears in 3 of 17 septicemic patients.

Statistics gathered in New Mexico indicate that while plague is most common in persons less than 40 years old, perhaps because of their greater outdoor activity, the risk of the septicemic form increases in individuals over 40 years of age. However, among patients with septicemic plague, mortality was greater in younger patients, perhaps because of greater delay in diagnosis and decreased likelihood that they would receive antibiotic therapy on an empirical basis.[98]

Abdominal pain was present in almost 40% of the patients in New Mexico. Hepatosplenomegaly has been reported to occur in plague and could be a possible source of abdominal pain, but it was not found in the patients reported in this series. The presence of abdominal symptoms in plague should be emphasized because the disease could be mistaken for other forms of gastrointestinal illness. A review of the 71 plague cases in New Mexico from 1980 to 1984 revealed that gastrointestinal symptoms occurred in 57% of patients, with vomiting (39%) the most frequent symptom. Nausea (34%), diarrhea (28%), and abdominal pain (17%) were also observed.[97]

Plague should be suspected in patients who have various combinations of lymphadenopathy, high fever, malaise, tachycardia, tachypnea, hypotension, and abdominal symptoms and who have come from an endemic area. If the suspicion is reasonable, antibiotic therapy should be instituted immediately. Treatment should not be delayed to await laboratory confirmation of the diagnosis.

Rare forms of plague include pharyngeal, meningeal, and ophthalmic. Pharyngeal and ophthalmic plague can be acquired by exposure to droplets expelled by a pneumonic patient. Endophthalmitis can also be secondary to septicemia. Meningitis is acquired hematogenously.

Definitive diagnosis is based on culture of the organism from sputum, transtracheal aspirate, blood, or aspirates of buboes. The best staining technique to demonstrate bipolar morphology of the organism is Giemsa's or Wayson's.

Direct fluorescent antibody (FA) stain of aspirates and smears provides a reasonably rapid diagnostic technique. Although cross-reactions with *Yersinia pseudotuberculosis* have been recorded, and occasional strains of the plague bacillus do not stain well with FA, a positive FA test in a patient with a compatible epidemiologic and clinical picture is a reasonable basis for making a diagnosis of plague and instituting therapy.

Material from buboes should be obtained by fine-needle aspiration rather than excision or incision and drainage. This reduces risks of transmission to medical personnel and of iatrogenic septicemia.

TREATMENT[139,191]

Patients with suspected plague should be treated immediately without awaiting definitive laboratory studies. The best available drug is streptomycin. However, if this drug is given too rapidly, it can cause a severe reaction as a result of rapid killing of organisms and release of endotoxin. The recommended dosage is 30 mg/kg/day intramuscularly in four divided doses every 6 hours for 5 days. A less preferred alternative to streptomycin is gentamicin, 5 mg/kg/day intravenously in four divided doses every 6 hours, reduced to 3 mg/kg/day after clinical improvement. Patients with impaired renal function should have their dosage of streptomycin or gentamicin modified appropriately.

Tetracycline is often used concurrently with streptomycin. The recommended loading dose is 15 mg/kg up to 1 g total dose given orally. This is followed by 40 to 50 mg/kg in six divided doses every 4 hours on the first day. Thereafter, 30 mg/kg is administered orally in four divided doses every 6 hours for 10 to 14 days. If the patient cannot tolerate treatment by mouth, tetracycline can be given intravenously, using one third of the calculated oral dose until oral therapy is tolerated.

An alternative to tetracycline is chloramphenicol, administered in a loading dose of 25 mg/kg (up to 3 g total) orally, followed by 50 to 75 mg/kg orally in four divided doses for 10 to 14 days. If the patient does not tolerate oral therapy, chloramphenicol can be given intravenously, 50 mg/kg in four divided doses every 6 hours until oral therapy is tolerated. It is preferable to use chloramphenicol in the event of meningitis or endophthalmitis because of good penetration into affected tissues. Whichever drug combination is selected, antibiotic therapy should be given for at least 10 days, or for 3 or 4 days after clinical recovery.

Sulfadiazine is a less satisfactory alternative. A loading dose of 25 mg/kg is given orally followed by 75 mg/kg orally in four divided doses every 6 hours for 10 to 14 days. Cotrimoxazole (320 mg of trimethoprim and 1600 mg of sulfamethoxazole) twice or three times a day for 10 to 17 days was found effective in treating plague,[2] but much less experience has been accumulated with this medication than with other antibiotics.

Infants born to plague-infected mothers may have congenital infection. They should be treated with kanamycin, 15 mg/kg/day intravenously or intramuscularly in four divided doses every 6 hours, or streptomycin, 10 to 20 mg/kg/day in four divided doses every 6 hours.

QUARANTINE AND INFECTION CONTROL[193]

The greatest risk of contagion is by aerosol transmission from patients with the pneumonic form of plague. All persons with suspected plague should be placed in strict quarantine and isolation for a minimum of 48 hours of specific antibiotic treatment. If no respiratory signs develop within 48 hours, wound and skin precautions will suffice for the rest of his or her hospitalization. Patients with plague pneumonia or pharyngitis should be kept under strict respiratory quarantine for at least 4 days of antibiotic treatment, until the pharyngeal culture is negative for the organism or respiratory signs abate. Contact personnel should wear gloves, gowns, masks, and eye protection. Dramatic illustrations of effective protective clothing are shown in the report by Strong on his work during a pneumonic plague epidemic in Manchuria in 1911.[175]

The greatest risk of acquiring plague from a patient with the septicemic or bubonic form is by inoculation of blood or exudate; therefore strict needle precautions should be taken. Buboes should not be incised and drained. In theory, fleas harbored by a septicemic patient should be capable of transmitting the disease, but official recommendations from the CDC for the control of plague do not cover eradication of fleas from human patients. No pesticides have been specifically approved for this use by the U.S. Food and Drug Administration. Products that are effective against lice could be used, but they may have limited effectiveness because most fleas do not remain long on a human host.

Individuals exposed face to face to patients with plague pneumonia should be prophylactically treated with antibiotics. Tetracycline, 500 mg orally every 6 hours for 6 days, can be given to adults. Trimethoprim-sulfamethoxazole can be given to children under 8 years of age and to pregnant women. Streptomycin, chloramphenicol, and sulfadiazine are alternative prophylactic medications, given in doses indicated for therapy for 1 week to 10 days.

Household contacts of individuals with bubonic plague do not have to be treated prophylactically. They should have their temperature recorded twice daily, and if it exceeds 37.7° C (100° F) orally, they should report immediately to a physician for evaluation.

Careful surveillance is indicated for persons who have had face-to-face contact with patients with pneumonic plague. Their well-being should be confirmed daily, for example, by telephone contact.

The incubation period for primary pneumonic plague is 1 to 3 days, and for pharyngeal plague, 3 to 6 days. Precautionary follow-up observation of contacts should be maintained throughout this time. All cases of suspected or confirmed plague should be reported to the state health department.

PREVENTION

Residents and visitors to plague endemic areas should be advised of the risks of infection. They should avoid contact with rodents and other possible animal reservoirs of infection that are found sick or dead in the wild. Disposable plastic or rubber gloves should be worn when skinning or dressing a possibly infected animal. Cats and dogs should be kept indoors, leashed, or otherwise restrained. Owners of pets that have access to wild rodent populations must maintain flea control. Veterinary personnel working on animals that could have plague should follow strict infection control procedures.

Health departments in enzootic areas should maintain surveillance for plague in local reservoir species. At times of increased plague activity, insecticide sprays and powders can be applied to rodent burrows. It is important that ectoparasite control be exercised before any attempt to kill the rodents, because killing the rodents without control of their ectoparasites causes fleas to seek other hosts, including dogs, cats, and people.

IMMUNIZATION[40]

A killed bacterial vaccine (Plague vaccine, USP, Miles Biological) is available in the United States but is rarely used. Its application is limited to persons who have intensive, usually occupational exposure to the infection. Many of these persons prefer to rely on sanitation, protective clothing, and prophylactic or therapeutic treatment rather than use the vaccine, since it has short-term (6- to 12-month) efficacy and has a significant incidence of side effects such as fever, malaise, and pain at the site of injection.

Clinical and epidemiologic assistance for problems relating to plague can be obtained from the Plague Branch, Centers for Disease Control and Prevention, P.O. Box 2087, Fort Collins, CO 80522, phone 303-221-6400. After-hours consultation can be obtained from the CDC in Atlanta, phone 404-639-8107.

Glanders

Glanders is a zoonotic disease, primarily involving equine animals, caused by *Pseudomonas mallei*.

HISTORY[199]

Glanders, although little known in the Western world today, is one of the classic infectious diseases. Its greatest historical impact has been through its effect on cavalry horses during military campaigns, influencing battles from before the time of Christ through the Crusades and World War I.

One of the earliest descriptions of the disease is attributed to Aristotle. Apsyrtus in the third century and Vegetius in the fifth century recognized the contagious nature of glanders and recommended that affected animals be isolated to prevent spread of the infection.

Theories and disputes about the origin, nature, transmission, and treatment of glanders figured prominently in the development of veterinary science in Europe in the latter half of the eighteenth century. In 1795, Erik Viborg published an account that is remarkably close to our understanding of the disease today. He demonstrated that equine farcy, characterized by cutaneous lymphangitis, and the respiratory form of the disease in horses, classically referred to as glanders, were different manifestations of the same infection. He demonstrated that the disease was transmissible from one horse to the next by infectious exudates, and that the causative organism could be carried by fomites and killed by heat.

Transmission of glanders from horses to humans was documented in France and Germany during the first three decades of the nineteenth century. The causative organism was isolated by Loeffler and Schütz, and also by Bouchard, Capiton, and Charrin in 1882, the same year that Robert Koch isolated *Mycobacterium tuberculosis*. In 1891, a year after Koch discovered tuberculin, Kalning and Helmann independently discovered an analogous substance, mallein, derived from the glanders bacillus. Like tuberculin, mallein was thought to have therapeutic or prophylactic value. This turned out to be erroneous, but both substances have proved to be of great diagnostic value. Mallein provided a means of diagnosing the infection in clinically ill and carrier animals and provided a basis for test and slaughter techniques, which have largely eliminated glanders from most of Europe, North America, and most other parts of the world where it occurred in the past. Kalning, Helmann, and five other European scientists working on glanders died of the disease, acquired during their investigations.

BACTERIOLOGY[145,173]

The causative organism is *Pseudomonas mallei,* a member of the Pseudomallei group of *Pseudomonas,* which includes *P. pseudomallei,* the cause of melioidosis, and *P. cepacia*. It is a gram-negative, nonsporulating, obligate aerobic, and nonmotile bacillus. It requires glycerol for optimum growth in vitro.

EPIDEMIOLOGY[145,173]

Glanders occurs in a few Asian and African countries, such as India, China, Mongolia, Egypt, and Mauritania. It is primarily a disease of equids and is spread most rapidly when large numbers of horses, mules, or donkeys are kept in close proximity. Many carnivorous mammals are also susceptible to infection, and outbreaks have occurred when infected horse meat was fed to lions, tigers, and other wild animals in zoos. Occasionally, infections occur in dogs, cats, sheep, and goats.

Humans are usually infected by exposure to sick horses. Infection can occur by inhalation of respiratory droplets or by contact with infected discharges. Human infections have also occurred by the respiratory route, from direct contact in the laboratory, and in dealing with human patients.

SYMPTOMS IN EQUIDS[145,173]

Horses may suffer unilateral or bilateral mucopurulent nasal discharge (Fig. 41-13). There may be enlargement and

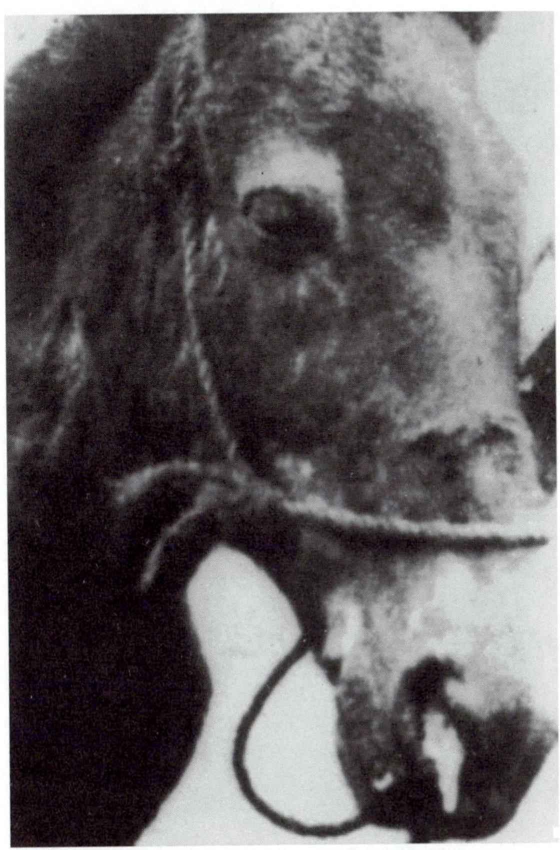

Fig. 41-13 Mucopurulent nasal discharge from a horse with glanders. (Courtesy Armed Forces Institute of Pathology.)

induration of lymphatics, with ulceration and discharge, especially involving the legs. Nodules, pustules, and ulcers may be seen on the horse's skin (Fig. 41-14). The cutaneous form of the disease is often referred to as farcy, the thickened, inflamed lymphatics as farcy pipes, and the enlarged lymph nodes as farcy buds. Horses also suffer pneumonia, with mild respiratory embarrassment in early stages of the disease, and more severe respiratory difficulties and cachexia in later stages. Septicemia with lesions in multiple internal organs can occur.

Glanders can run an acute and fulminant course in equids, most commonly seen in donkeys and mules, or a more chronic course, more often seen in horses. The case-fatality rate is high, especially with more virulent strains of the organism.

SYMPTOMS IN HUMANS[145,173]

The incubation period of glanders in humans can be as short as 1 to 5 days. Cases with apparent incubation periods of several months may have represented instances of smoldering, unrecognized infection. The severity of disease can vary from mild to fatal, and the course can be acute and fulminant or chronic. Relapses can occur after quiescent periods of up to 10 years. As in horses, manifestations in humans usually involve the skin and respiratory tract. There may be pustular cutaneous eruptions, thick, indurated lymphatics that may ulcerate, mucopurulent discharge from the eyes or nose, pneumonia, and metastatic abscesses in internal organs. Depending on the severity of disease, the patient may have anorexia, fever, weight loss, headache, nausea, diarrhea, or septicemic shock. Lobar pneumonia, bronchopneumonia, or nodular densities may be seen on chest radiographs. Cases recently reported from Southeast Asia have been relatively mild, indicating that the local strain of the organism appears to have moderate pathogenicity for people.

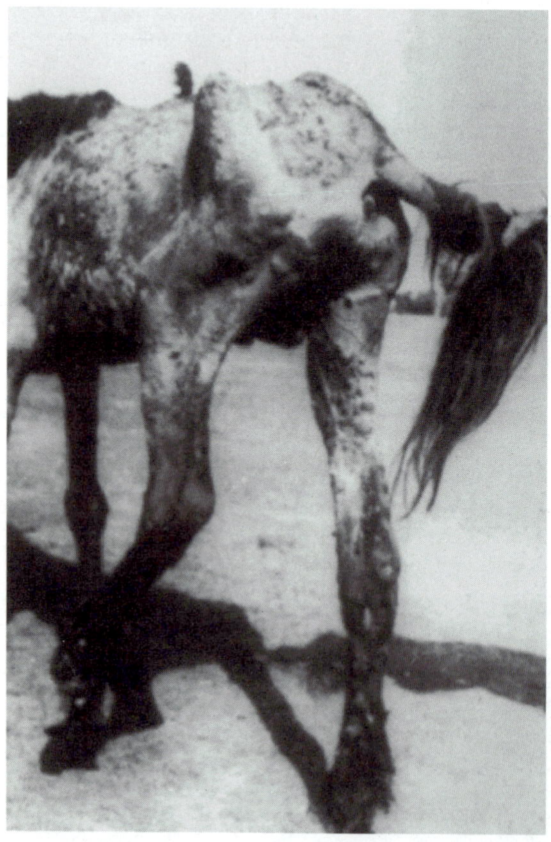

Fig. 41-14 Marked cachexia and cutaneous nodules in a horse with glanders. The cutaneous form of this disease in horses is often called farcy. (Courtesy Armed Forces Institute of Pathology.)

DIAGNOSIS[145,173]

Clinical diagnosis in horses based on symptoms can be confirmed by reaction to mallein with a cutaneous hypersensitivity test. Mallein, a filtrate derived from culture of the organism, is injected into the eyelid of a horse. A positive reaction, read 48 hours later, consists of marked local swelling and purulent conjunctivitis. Several serologic tests are also available. Complement fixation is commonly used. A dot-enzyme-linked immunosorbent assay is a more sensitive test.[184]

Clinical diagnosis in humans is based on compatible symptoms in an individual exposed to horses in an endemic area. The diagnosis can be confirmed by culture of the organism from lesions or by serologic testing, using complement fixation (CF) or agglutination tests. Agglutination titers are often detectable by the second week of infection. The CF test is less sensitive but more specific than agglutination. CF tests become positive during the third week of infection.[145]

Laboratory diagnosis can be made by injection of infected material intraperitoneally into male guinea pigs or hamsters. The animals develop peritonitis that extends into the scrotal sac with severe inflammation, the Strauss reaction.

PATHOLOGY

In acute phases of the disease, abscessation occurs. Later, the inflammatory focus is surrounded by a granulomatous reaction, but central karyorrhexis remains a prominent feature of the lesion. The lungs are the internal organs most typically involved (Figs. 41-15 and 41-16), but septicemic glanders can involve liver, spleen, bone, or brain. With chronic infection, multiple subcutaneous and intramuscular abscesses may develop.

TREATMENT

Early studies indicated that sulfadiazine, 100 mg/kg/day in three divided doses given for 3 weeks, is effective.

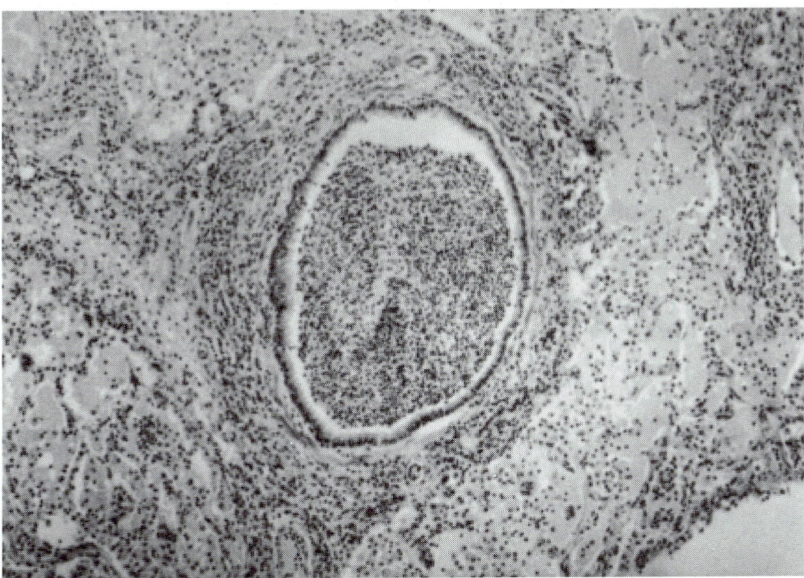

Fig. 41-15 A bronchus filled and surrounded by pus in the lung of a horse with glanders. (Hematoxylin and eosin, original magnification 100×.)

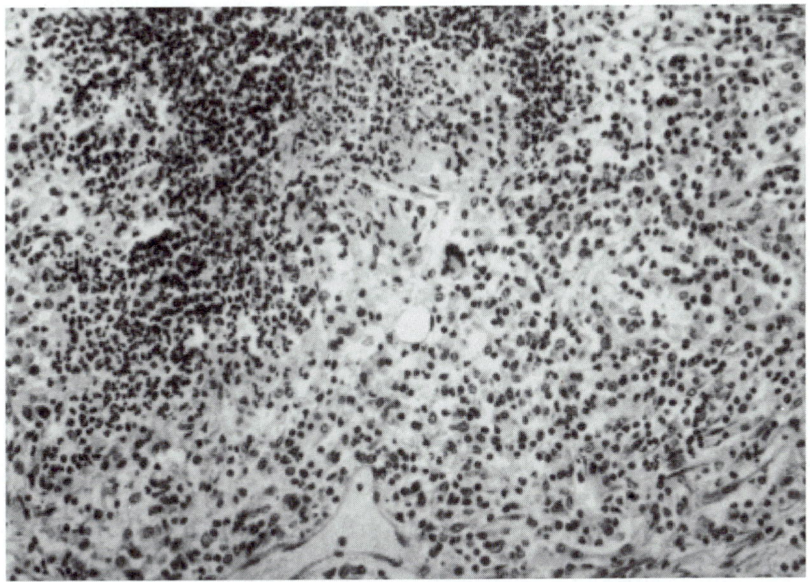

Fig. 41-16 Gangrenous pneumonia with characteristic karyorrhexis in the lung of a horse with glanders. A multinucleated giant cell is in the center of the figure. (Hematoxylin and eosin, original magnification 250×.)

Treatment with tetracyclines and streptomycin is also recommended.[145] The organism is sensitive in vitro to sulfamethizole, sulfathiazole, trimethoprim-sulfamethoxazole, gentamicin, kanamycin, streptomycin, and tetracycline.[3] Ciprofloxacin and ofloxacin, but not norfloxacin, were found to be effective in treating experimentally infected guinea pigs and hamsters.[13] Therapy should be based on culture and sensitivity testing of isolates and on clinical response to treatment.

PROGNOSIS

Acute septicemic cases are almost uniformly fatal within 7 to 10 days.[145] The prognosis is better in chronic forms of the disease, which can last for years, but deaths are still likely to occur without adequate treatment.

PREVENTION AND CONTROL[145,173]

The only significant reservoir of infection in nature is equids. If the disease were eradicated in them, it would disappear. National programs should be instituted in enzootic countries to eradicate the infection, by mallein or serologic tests of all horses, donkeys, and mules and slaughter of reactive animals. Persons who handle horses in enzootic countries, including trekkers who pack gear into the wilderness on these animals, should be advised of the signs of glanders in equids and warned to avoid contact with sick animals.

Glanders can be transmitted from one person to another, so strict infection control should be exercised with suspect infected patients. Personnel should avoid contact with all secretions and respiratory droplets. There is also risk of transmission in the laboratory, so if this organism is being cultured, all laboratory work should be done under appropriate microbiologic hoods.

Melioidosis

Melioidosis is an infection caused by the bacterium *Pseudomonas pseudomallei.* The causative agent and disease process in humans were first described by Whitmore and Krishnaswami[195] in Rangoon, Burma, in 1912. Leelarasame and Bovornkitt[112] have written a useful review of the disease.

BACTERIOLOGY

P. pseudomallei is a bipolar, gram-negative, aerobic rod approximately 0.5 to 1 µm in width and 3 to 5 µm in length. It is readily grown on standard laboratory media at 37° C. After 48 to 72 hours of growth, distinctive wrinkled colonies with a "daisy head" appearance are formed. They give off a pungent, putrefactive odor.[112] The organism is oxidase positive and nonpyocyanogenic. It is resistant to colistin and gentamicin in vitro.[85]

TRANSMISSION AND EPIDEMIOLOGY

Melioidosis is a saprozoonosis transmitted to animals and humans from the environment; transmission does not generally occur between living organisms. There is a singular case of presumed transmission by the venereal route.[126] Disease is much more commonly reported in adults than in children.

Most cases of melioidosis have been reported in areas between 20° north and 20° south of the equator.[84] A majority of cases have been reported from Southeast Asia and tropical Australia. The most heavily endemic areas include Myanmar (Burma), Malaya, Vietnam, Singapore, Cambodia, Thailand, Java, Borneo, New Guinea, and northern Australia. Occasional human and animal cases have been reported from Central India, Sri Lanka, Niger, Madagascar, Ecuador, Panama, Aruba, and Mexico. Cases reported from the Western Hemisphere were recently reviewed.[12] *P. pseudomallei* is a free-living inhabitant of soil and water. It survives in the dry season in Australia in the clay layer of the soil, 25 to 30 cm below the surface, and can be brought to the surface and distributed by water seeping through this layer during the wet season.[85]

Clinical and subclinical infections occur in a variety of animals, most commonly sheep, goats, and swine. Infections in animals offer no direct threat to human health but are epidemiologic indicators that the organism is in a given geographic area.[84]

Transmission is thought to occur by direct percutaneous inoculation through wounds contaminated with soil or water, by ingestion, or by inhalation of infective droplets. A high incidence of pulmonary melioidosis in helicopter crew members in Vietnam was ascribed to inhalation of dust and aerosols raised by the helicopters operating in highly endemic areas.[84]

SYMPTOMS

The majority of human infections are asymptomatic, as indicated by the high prevalence of seropositivity in the absence of clinical disease within endemic areas. Active disease is most likely to be seen in individuals with predisposing conditions, particularly diabetes mellitus, alcoholism, neoplasms, malnutrition, and various forms of immunodeficiency.

Clinical disease can occur in acute, subacute, or chronic forms. The lungs are the organs most frequently involved. Pulmonary melioidosis can mimic tuberculosis in that the upper lobes are most frequently involved, there is a productive cough, sputum often contains blood, and patients complain of chest pain and fever. However, calcifications in the lung and hilar lymph nodes commonly seen in tuberculosis are rarely seen with melioidosis. An entire lobe or major segment of a lobe may be consolidated, and multiple pulmonary abscesses may be scattered in the lung parenchyma.

Septicemia can develop in the acute form of the disease and may mimic other forms of gram-negative sepsis in its manifestations. Multiple abscesses can form in skin, lungs, liver, spleen, kidney, and bone, but the central nervous system is rarely involved. Without treatment the case-fatality rate exceeds 90%.

In the subacute and chronic forms of disease, abscesses can form in internal organs and may drain through sinus tracts.

Melioidosis has been referred to as a medical time bomb because infection can lie dormant for months or years, only to become manifest when resistance is lowered. An incubation period as long as 26 years has been reported.[122] The infection should be suspected in anyone with a compatible clinical picture, including fever of unknown origin, who ever resided in an endemic area.

DIAGNOSIS

The only definitive diagnostic procedure is culture of the organism from blood, bone marrow, sputum, pus, or infected tissue. Several serologic tests are available but are not reliable because many individuals from endemic areas have antibodies to the organism without any evidence of clinical disease. An indirect hemagglutination antibody titer of 1:40 or greater is considered compatible with infection, as is a complement fixation titer of 1:10 or greater. Rising titers by IgM-indirect fluorescent antibody are probably the best immunologic indication of infection.

No pathognomonic lesions are seen histologically. The abscesses consist of central areas of necrosis without unique or distinctive features permitting definitive histopathologic diagnosis.

TREATMENT

Combinations of antibiotics have been used to treat melioidosis. Combination therapy almost always includes chloramphenicol, 40 mg/kg/day in adults and 50 to 75 mg/kg/day in children.[135] Tetracycline is also commonly used in adults and in children over 7 years of age, 50 mg/kg/day in four divided doses six times a day orally. Kanamycin, 15 to 20 mg/kg/day in two divided doses intramuscularly, and amikacin, 15 to 20 mg/kg/day in two divided doses every 12 hours intramuscularly, have also been recommended for treatment. Cotrimoxazole may prove useful, but experience is too limited to define its appropriate dosage and role in treatment. The antibiotic treatment should be given for several weeks in acute cases and for approximately 6 months in chronic cases. Dosage of kanamycin and amikacin should be modified appropriately if there is renal impairment. These drugs may have to be discontinued if eighth cranial nerve damage is present.

Ceftazidine has largely replaced combination antibiotic therapy and is now generally recognized as the drug of choice.[194]

In vitro sensitivity tests do not always correlate with clinical response to antibiotics. Therapy must be given at a high enough dosage and for a sufficiently prolonged time to avoid recurrence of infection and emergence of resistant organisms.

PREVENTION AND CONTROL

In the field, prevention consists of avoiding ingestion or inhalation of potentially infective soil or water. Wounds, burns, and other injuries should be thoroughly cleaned to avoid infection through contamination. No evidence exists that transmission is likely to occur from person to person, so isolation of hospitalized patients is not necessary. Reasonable care and precautions should be taken in handling purulent drainage of blood, sputum, and other materials from patients with melioidosis.

Trichinosis

Trichinosis is an infection caused by nematodes in the genus *Trichinella.* In the past, only one species, *T. spiralis,* was recognized. Isoenzyme and DNA analysis indicate that the genus is polyspecific.[142] Eight gene pools, T_1 through T_8, have been identified. T_1 is classic *T. spiralis;* the principal reservoir is in domestic swine, but some wild animals can also be infected. T_2, *T. nativa,* is found primarily in terrestrial mammals, rarely in sea mammals, in Arctic and sub-Arctic regions. Most human infections are caused by T_1, fewer by T_2. Relatively few data are available on how frequently the other species infect people. T_3 occurs in bears (Ursidae), T_7 and T_8 in African Hyenidae and Felidae. Only T_4, *T. pseudospiralis,* can infect mammals and birds.

Unless stated otherwise, the rest of this discussion relates to trichinosis generically or to *T. spiralis* specifically.

LIFE CYCLE

The life cycle is unusual in that every host is necessarily both a definitive host, harboring the adult stage of the parasite, and an intermediate host, harboring the larval stage.

The infection is acquired by ingestion of larvae encysted in skeletal muscle. The worms mature within a few days in the small intestine. The female burrows into the mucosa and deposits larvae in the tissue, starting around the fifth day after infection. Most larvae are deposited within 4 weeks, but they can be produced for as long as 4 months. The larvae enter the circulation and invade skeletal muscle within 7 to 14 days (Fig. 41-17). They become encapsulated around day 21 after infection and are then infective for the next host that ingests them.

EPIDEMIOLOGY

All carnivorous and omnivorous mammals are susceptible to trichinosis, but the majority of human infections are acquired by eating raw or undercooked pork. Game animals can harbor the parasite. Trichinosis was found in 1.3% of black bears in New England.[88] It can infect other species of bears, raccoons, opossums, seals, walruses, peccaries, and wild swine.

Rodents such as mice and rats are commonly infected in nature. Except in certain cultures, these small rodents are rarely eaten by people, but their larger cousins, squirrels, woodchucks, muskrats, agoutis, and capybaras, find themselves on dinner plates with some regularity. These larger

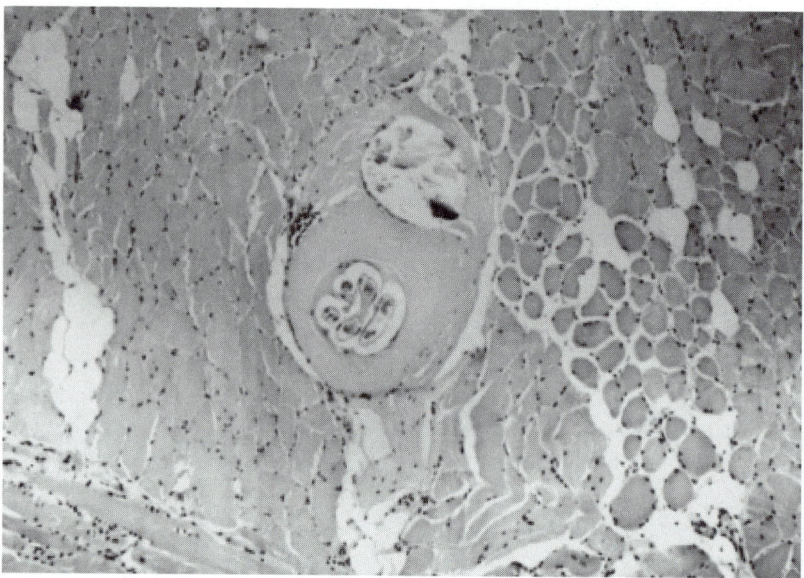

Fig. 41-17 Trichinosis in a polar bear. A larva is seen within a muscle fiber in the center of the picture. The parasite found in Arctic mammals is highly resistant to freezing and has been given a separate species status, *Trichinella nativa*. (Hematoxylin and eosin, original magnification 100×.)

rodents are mostly, but not exclusively, herbivorous, and they could be an occasional source of human infection.

Although experimentally susceptible to trichinosis, herbivores, such as members of the deer and antelope families, are almost never infected naturally, and consumption of their flesh is not associated with this infection. Interestingly, some outbreaks of trichinosis have occurred in people who consumed horseflesh.[46] It is theorized that the horses could have become infected by consuming mice, dead or alive, in their feed. Alternatively, larvae passed in the stool of infected rodents could have been ingested in the horses' grain or hay.

Passing laws that forbid the feeding of raw garbage to swine, developing techniques for detecting infection in swine carcasses in slaughterhouses, freezing pork, and educating the public to cook pork products have greatly reduced the incidence of trichinosis in humans in most Western countries. The declining incidence in the United States is shown in Fig. 41-18. Swine that are privately raised and slaughtered are a continuing source of human infections in many areas, including the northeastern United States.[11] Bears, walruses, and feral swine are the principal nondomestic sources of trichinosis in the United States.[123] Wild boars are a source of infections in Germany.[93]

Twenty-six cases of trichinosis reported in the United States from 1975 to 1989 were acquired during foreign travel. Seventeen of these persons had traveled to Mexico or Asia.[124]

SYMPTOMS

The signs and symptoms of trichinosis are closely related to the activities of the parasite in its life cycle. The severity of disease is proportional to the number of adult and larval worms present. Gastrointestinal symptoms predominate during the first week after ingestion of infective meat. The worms mate and invade the intestinal mucosa during the first 48 hours. Larvae are deposited starting on approximately the fifth day after ingestion. This activity results in irritation of the bowel, with nausea, vomiting, variable diarrhea, and abdominal pain. Fever may occur. These symptoms are often mistaken for various forms of food poisoning. Gastrointestinal symptoms may continue until the females are cleared from the intestinal tract at approximately 4 to 6 weeks after infection.

Larval production reaches a peak during the second week after infection. The larvae start to invade skeletal muscle as early as the seventh day. During the time of larval migration, capillary damage occurs, resulting in facial edema, especially involving the periorbital area, which may be accompanied by photophobia, blurred vision, diplopia, and complaints of pain on moving the eyes. Splinter hemorrhages may appear in the nailbeds, and there may be cutaneous petechiae. Hemorrhagic lesions can also occur in the conjunctivae and retinae. The temperature may reach 105° F.

Eosinophils start to increase in peripheral blood during the second week, often exceeding 20% of the total white blood cell count after the third week of infection. The

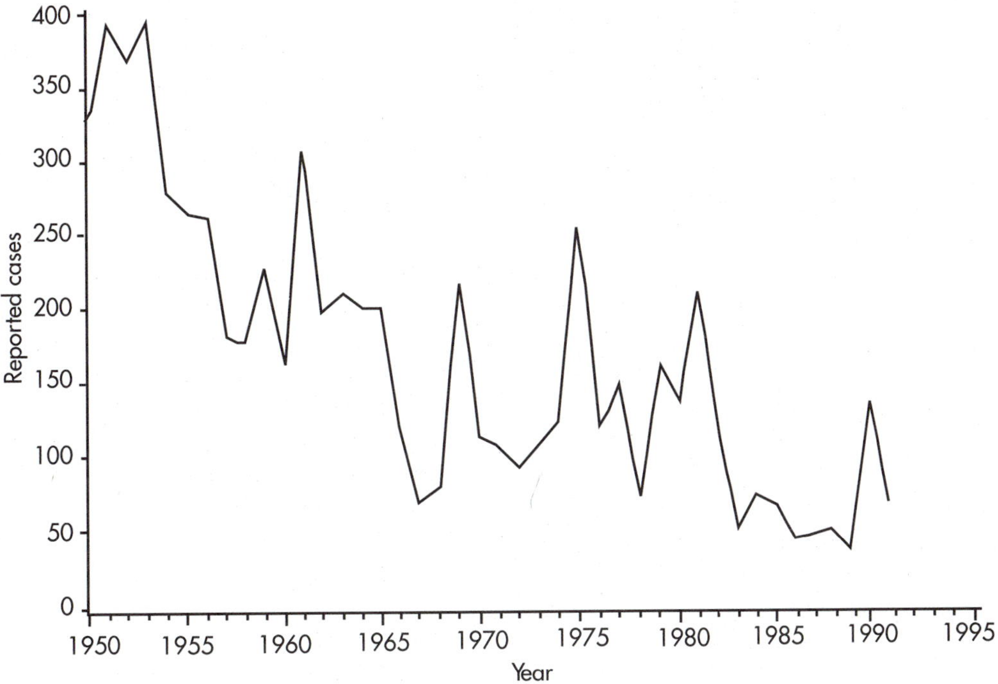

Fig. 41-18 Reported cases of trichinosis in the United States, 1950 to 1991. (From *MMWR* 40, No 53, 1991.)

eosinophil count returns to normal from 6 to 12 months after infection. Gastrointestinal symptoms may continue during this period, until the females are cleared from the intestinal tract approximately 4 to 6 weeks after infection.

During the second phase of infection, migrating larvae can cause pulmonary damage, resulting in cough, dyspnea, and pleuritic pain. There may be hemoptysis. Myocarditis can occur and may be life threatening. Damage to the brain or meninges by migrating larvae can cause encephalitic or meningitic symptoms. A spinal tap may reveal eosinophils in cerebrospinal fluid.

The third phase of infection is encystment of the larvae within skeletal muscle, starting around the second or third week after infection. This can cause significant myalgias and stiffness in affected muscle groups.

The final phase of infection occurs as the larvae die and become calcified. This is a period of convalescence, which is usually asymptomatic, and typically occurs between 6 and 18 months after infection.

Trichinosis in the Inuit population of northeastern Canada, associated with eating raw walrus, is characterized by prolonged diarrhea and brief muscle symptoms. A high peripheral eosinophilia and high *Trichinella* antibody titers occur. The disease is probably caused by *T. nativa,* and at least some cases may be associated with reinfection.[116]

DIAGNOSIS

Larvae are sometimes passed in the stool in the early stages of infection, but this occurs infrequently and inconsistently and cannot be relied on for diagnosis.

Trichinosis is definitively diagnosed by biopsy of the gastrocnemius muscle or of clinically affected (painful, tender) muscles. The larvae are demonstrable in muscle beginning about the seventh day after infection. Diagnosis can also be made serologically, using bentonite flocculation, latex particle agglutination, or countercurrent immunoelectrophoresis. These tests usually do not become positive until 3 to 4 weeks after infection. ELISA tests are available that measure reaction by different immunoglobulin classes. Most ELISA tests offer greater specificity and sensitivity and become positive earlier than many of the other tests.[7,162,183] An ELISA IgG test had a specificity and sensitivity of 100% at days 57 and 120 after infection but was negative at day 23[117] using the excretory-secretory antigen of *T. spiralis* larvae.

PREVENTION

Trichinosis is prevented by cooking meat to an internal temperature of 150° F (65.6° C). Most *Trichinella* larvae are killed by freezing. The time required depends on the thickness of the meat, but holding meat at 20° F for 6 to 12 days,

10° F for 10 to 20 days, or 0° to 5° F for 20 to 30 days is recommended. *T. nativa* found in Arctic mammals (Fig. 41-12), however, is resistant to freezing.[34]

TREATMENT

No satisfactory, safe, and effective drug is available for elimination of larvae, which are responsible for most of the pathologic changes and symptoms of trichinosis. Thiabendazole (25 mg/kg twice a day for 5 days, maximum 3 g/day) is effective against adult worms in the intestine, but its efficacy against larvae is questionable, and it can cause allergic reactions, such as fever, increased edema, and myocarditis.[107] Mebendazole (200 to 400 mg three times a day for 3 days, then 400 to 500 mg three times a day for 10 days) has been recommended,[132] but is considered an investigational drug for this purpose by the FDA. Albendazole or flubendazole may be effective, but these are not commercially available in the United States.

Steroids, for example, prednisone 30 to 60 mg/day orally for 10 to 30 days, can be given for relief of severe illness, such as myocarditis caused by migrating larvae.[107] The dose and duration of treatment are individually determined by clinical response. Steroids reduce the inflammatory response to larvae but can also interfere with rejection of adult females in the intestine, thus prolonging the period of larva deposition.

REFERENCES

1. Ahuja S et al: Epidemiology of rabies in India. In Kuwert E et al, editors: *Rabies in the tropics,* Berlin, 1985, Springer-Verlag.
2. Ai NV et al: Co-trimoxazole in bubonic plague, *Br Med J* 4:108, 1973.
3. Al-Izz SA, Al Bassam LS: In vitro susceptibility of *Pseudomonas mallei* to antimicrobial agents, *Compar Immunol Microbiol Infect Dis* 12:5, 1989.
4. Anderson LJ et al: Human rabies in the United States, 1960 to 1979: epidemiology, diagnosis and prevention, *Ann Intern Med* 100:728, 1984.
5. Andrew ED, Marrocco GR: Leptospirosis in New England, *JAMA* 238:2027, 1977.
6. Arko RJ, Schneider LG, Baer GM: Non-fatal canine rabies, *Am J Vet Res* 34:937, 1973.
7. Au ACS et al: Study of acute trichinosis in Ghurkas: specificity and sensitivity of enzyme-linked immunosorbent assays for IgM and IgE antibodies to *Trichinella* larval antigens in diagnosis, *Trans R Soc Trop Med Hyg* 77:412, 1983.
8. Baer GM, editor: *The natural history of rabies,* ed 2, Boca Raton, Fla, 1991, CRC Press.
9. Baer GM, Fishbein DB: Rabies post-exposure prophylaxis, *N Engl J Med* 316:1270, 1987.
10. Baer GM, Lentz TL: Rabies pathogenesis to the central nervous system. In Baer GM, editor: *The natural history of rabies,* ed 2, Boca Raton, Fla, 1991, CRC Press.
11. Bailey TM, Schantz PM: Trends in the incidence and transmission patterns of trichinosis in humans in the United States: comparisons of the periods 1975-1981 and 1982-1986, *Rev Infect Dis* 12:5, 1990.
12. Barnes PF, Appleman MD, Cosgrove MM: A case of melioidosis originating in North America, *Am Rev Respir Dis* 134:170, 1986.
13. Batmanov VP: Sensitivity of *Pseudomonas mallei* to fluoroquinolones and their efficacy in experimental glanders (Russian), *Antibiot Khimioter* 36:31, 1991.
14. Beck AM: The epidemiology of animal bite: compendium on continuing education, *Practic Vet* 3:254, 1981.
15. Bell JF et al: Non-fatal rabies in an enzootic area: results of a survey and evaluation of techniques, *Am J Epidemiol* 95:190, 1972.
16. Bell JF: Tularemia. In Steele JH, editor: *Handbook series in zoonoses, section A: bacterial, rickettsial and mycotic diseases,* vol 2, Boca Raton, Fla, 1980, CRC Press.
17. Benenson MW et al: Oocyst-transmitted toxoplasmosis associated with ingestion of contaminated water, *N Engl J Med* 307:666, 1982.
18. Beran GW: Rabies and infections by rabies-related viruses. In Steele JH, editor: *CRC handbook series in zoonoses, section B: viral zoonoses,* vol 2, Boca Raton, Fla, 1981, CRC Press.

18a. Berlin BS et al: Rhesus diploid rabies vaccine (adsorbed), a new rabies vaccine: results of initial clinical studies of preexposure vaccination, *JAMA* 247:1726, 1982.

19. Bernard KW, Fishbein DB: Rabies virus. In Mandell GL, Douglas RG, Bennett JE, editors: *Principles and practice of infectious diseases,* ed 3, New York, 1990, Churchill Livingstone.
20. Bernard KW et al: Neuroparalytic illness and human diploid cell rabies vaccine, *JAMA* 248:3136, 1982.
21. Bernard KW et al: Pre-exposure immunization with intradermal human diploid cell rabies vaccine: risks and benefits of primary and booster vaccination, *JAMA* 257:1059, 1987.
22. Boe E, Nyland H: Guillain-Barré syndrome after vaccination with human diploid cell rabies vaccine, *Scand J Infect Dis* 12:231, 1980.
23. Boyce JM: Recent trends in the epidemiology of tularemia in the United States, *J Infect Dis* 131:197, 1975.
24. Brochier B et al: Use of recombinant vaccinia rabies glycoprotein virus for oral vaccination of wildlife against rabies: innocuity to several nontarget bait consuming species, *J Wild Dis* 25:540, 1989.
25. Burridge MJ: Wildlife rabies in the United States, *Avian/Exotic Pract* 1:17, 1984.
26. Burridge MJ et al: Intradermal immunization with human diploid cell rabies vaccine: serological and clinical responses of persons with and without prior vaccination with duck embryo vaccine, *JAMA* 248:1611, 1982.
27. Butler T, Mahmoud AAF, Warren KS: Algorithms in the diagnosis and management of exotic diseases. XXV. Plague, *J Infect Dis* 136:317, 1977.
28. Centers for Disease Control: Rabies exposure in laboratories—a statement of safety, *MMWR* 21:179, 1972.
29. Centers for Disease Control: Human plague—New Mexico, *MMWR* 23:425, 1974.
30. Centers for Disease Control: Tularemia mimicking plague—New Mexico, *MMWR* 23:299, 1974.
31. Centers for Disease Control: Human plague case—Bernalillo County, New Mexico, *MMWR* 24:90, 1975.
32. Centers for Disease Control: Tularemia—California, *MMWR* 24:126, 1975.
33. Centers for Disease Control: Oklahoma reports third case of rabies in pet skunk, *Vet Pub Health Notes,* Aug 1977, p 3.
34. Centers for Disease Control: Trichinosis—United States, 1978, *MMWR* 28:541, 1979.
35. Centers for Disease Control: Human to human transmission of rabies via a corneal transplant—France, *MMWR* 29:25, 1980.
36. Centers for Disease Control: Rabies in pet raccoons, *MMWR* 29:177, 1980.
37. Centers for Disease Control: Tularemia acquired from a bear—Washington, *MMWR* 29:57, 1980.
38. Centers for Disease Control: Human plague—Texas, New Mexico, *MMWR* 30:137, 1981.
39. Centers for Disease Control: Human to human transmission of rabies via corneal transplant—Thailand, *MMWR* 30:473, 1981.

40. Centers for Disease Control: Plague vaccine, *MMWR* 31:301, 1982.
41. Centers for Disease Control: Tularemia associated with domestic cats—Georgia, New Mexico, *MMWR* 31:39, 1982.
42. Centers for Disease Control: Human rabies—Kenya, *MMWR* 32:494, 1983.
43. Centers for Disease Control: Rabies post-exposure prophylaxis with human diploid cell rabies vaccine: lower neutralizing antibody titers with Wyeth vaccine, *MMWR* 34:90, 1985.
44. Centers for Disease Control: *Rabies surveillance summary, 1983,* issued Nov 1985, p 3.
45. Centers for Disease Control: *Rabies surveillance summary, 1983,* issued Nov 1985, p 6.
46. Centers for Disease Control: Horsemeat associated trichinosis—France, *MMWR* 35:291, 1986.
47. Centers for Disease Control: Rabies prevention: supplementary statement on the pre-exposure use of human diploid cell rabies vaccine by the intradermal route, *MMWR* 35:767, 1986.
48. Centers for Disease Control: *Rabies surveillance, annual summary, 1985,* issued Dec 1986.
49. Centers for Disease Control: An imported case of rabies in an immunized dog, *MMWR* 36:94, 1987.
50. Centers for Disease Control: Imported dog and cat rabies—New Hampshire, California, *MMWR* 37:559, 1988.
51. Centers for Disease Control: Human rabies—Oregon, 1989, *MMWR* 38:335, 1989.
52. Centers for Disease Control: Rabies prevention—United States, 1991, Recommendations of the Immunization Practices Advisory Committee (ACIP), *MMWR* 40/No RR-3:1.
53. Centers for Disease Control: Health information for international travel 1992.
54. Centers for Disease Control: Extension of the raccoon rabies epizootic—United States, 1992, *MMWR* 41:661, 1992.
55. Centers for Disease Control: Hantavirus infection—southwestern United States: interim recommendations for risk reduction, *MMWR* 42/No RR-11:1, 1993.
56. Centers for Disease Control: Hantavirus pulmonary syndrome—United States, *MMWR* 43(3):45, 1994.
56a. Centers for Disease Control: Compendium of animal rabies control, *MMWR* 43/No RR-10:8, 1994.
57. Christie AB, Chen TH, Elberg SS: Plague in camels and goats: their role in human epidemics, *J Infect Dis* 141:724, 1980.
58. Constantine DG: Rabies transmitted by the non-bite route, *Public Health Rep* 77:287, 1962.
59. Correa-Giron EP, Allen R, Sulkin SE: The infectivity and pathogenesis of rabies administered orally, *Am J Epidemiol* 91:203, 1970.
60. Dahlstrand S, Ringertz O, Zetterberg B: Airborne tularemia in Sweden, *Scand J Infect Dis* 3:7, 1971.
61. Dean DJ, Baer GM, Thompson WR: Studies on the local treatment of rabies infected wounds, *Bull WHO* 28:477, 1963.
62. Debbie JG: *Rabies control in wildlife, report on rabies,* Princeton Junction, NJ, 1983, Veterinary Learning Systems.
63. Diesch SL, Ellinghausen HC: Leptospirosis. In Hubbert WT, McCulloch WF, Schnurrenberger PR, editors: *Diseases transmitted from animals to man,* Springfield, Ill, 1975, Charles C Thomas.
64. Doege TC, Northrop RL: Evidence for inapparent rabies infection, *Lancet* 2:826, 1974.
65. Dreesen DW et al: Intradermal use of human diploid cell vaccine for pre-exposure rabies immunizations, *J Am Vet Med Assoc* 181:1519, 1982.
66. Dreesen DW et al: Immune complex–like disease in two groups of persons following a booster dose of rabies human diploid cell vaccine In *Proceedings of the 89th Annual Meeting, US Animal Health Association,* 1985.
67. Edwards CN et al: Leptospirosis in Barbados: a clinical study, *W Ind Med J* 39:27, 1990.
68. Ell SR: Immunity as a factor in the epidemiology of medieval plague, *Rev Infect Dis* 6:866, 1984.
69. Evans ME et al: Tularemia: a 30-year experience with 88 cases, *Medicine* 64:251, 1985.
70. Everard CO, Maude GH, Hayes RJ: Leptospiral infection: a household serosurvey in urban and rural communities in Barbados and Trinidad, *Ann Trop Med Parasitol* 84:255, 1990.
71. Everard CO et al: An investigation of some risk factors for severe leptospirosis on Barbados, *J Trop Med Hyg* 95:13, 1992.
72. Fayaz A et al: Booster effect of human diploid cell antirabies vaccine in previously treated persons, *JAMA* 246:2334, 1981.
73. Feigin RD et al: Human leptospirosis from immunized dogs, *Ann Intern Med* 79:777, 1973.
74. Fekadu M, Baer GM: Recovery from clinical rabies of two dogs inoculated with a rabies virus strain from Ethiopia, *Am J Vet Res* 41:1632, 1980.
75. Fekadu M, Smith JS: Laboratory diagnosis of rabies. In Fishbein DB, Sawyer LA, Winkler WB, editors: *Rabies concepts for medical professionals,* ed 2, Miami, 1986, Merieux Institute.
76. Fishbein DB: Pre-exposure and post exposure immunization against rabies. In Fishbein DB, Sawyer LA, Winkler WG, editors: *Rabies concepts for medical professionals,* ed 2, Miami, Fla, 1986, Merieux Institute.
77. Fishbein DB: Rabies, *Infect Dis Clin North Am* 5:53, 1991.
78. Fishbein DB, Robinson LE: Rabies, *N Engl J Med* 329:1632, 1993.
79. Fishbein DB, Sawyer LA, Winkler WG, editors: *Rabies concepts for medical professionals,* ed 2, Miami, Fla, 1986, Merieux Institute.
80. Fishbein DB et al: Human diploid cell rabies vaccine purified by zonal centrifugation: a controlled study of antibody response and side effects following primary and booster pre-exposure immunization, *Vaccine* 7:437, 1990.
81. Flores-Crespo R et al: Vampirinip II: un producto utilizable en tres metodos para el combate del murcielago hematofago, *Tecnica Pecuaria Mexico* 30:67, 1976.
82. Ganem DE: Plasmids and pestilence—biological and clinical aspects of bubonic plague—Medical Staff Conference, University of California, San Francisco, *West J Med* 144:447, 1986.
83. Gorbach SL, Bartlett JG, Blacklow NR: *Infectious diseases,* Philadelphia, 1992, WB Saunders.
84. Groves MG: Melioidosis. In Steele JH, editor: *Handbook series in zoonoses, section A: bacterial, rickettsial and mycotic diseases,* vol 1, Boca Raton, Fla, 1979, CRC Press.
85. Guard RW et al: Melioidosis in far north Queensland, a clinical and epidemiological review of twenty cases, *Am J Trop Med Hyg* 33:467, 1984.
86. Halperin SA, Gast T, Ferrieri P: Oculoglandular syndrome caused by *Francisella tularensis, Clin Pediatr* 24:520, 1985.
87. Hanson LE: Leptospirosis in domestic animals: the public health perspective, *J Am Vet Med Assoc* 181:1505, 1982.
88. Harbottle JE, English DK, Schultz MG: Trichinosis in bears in northeastern United States, *HSMHA Health Rep* 86:473, 1971.
89. Hattwick MAW et al: Recovery from rabies: a case report, *Ann Intern Med* 76:931, 1972.
90. Heath CW, Alexander AD, Galton MM: Leptospirosis in the United States: analysis of 483 cases in man, 1949-1961, *N Engl J Med* 273:857, 1965.
91. Heath CW, Alexander AD, Galton MM: Leptospirosis in the United States (concluded): analysis of 483 cases in man, 1949-1961, *N Engl J Med* 273:915, 1965.
92. Helmick CG: The epidemiology of human rabies post-exposure prophylaxis, 1980-1981, *JAMA* 250:1990, 1983.
93. Hinz E: Trichinellosis and trichinellosis control in Germany, *Southeast Asian J Trop Med Pub Health* 22(suppl):329, 1991.
94. Houff SA et al: Human to human transmission of rabies virus by corneal transplant, *N Engl J Med* 300:603, 1979.

95. Howard DR: Transplacental transmission of rabies virus from a naturally infected skunk, *Am J Vet Res* 42:691, 1981.
96. Hubbert WT, McCulloch WF, Schnurrenberger PR: *Diseases transmitted from animals to man,* ed 6, Springfield, Ill, 1975, Charles C Thomas.
97. Hull HF, Montes JM, Mann JM: Plague masquerading as gastrointestinal illness, *West J Med* 145:485, 1986.
98. Hull HF, Montes JM, Mann JM: Septicemic plague in New Mexico, *J Infect Dis* 155:113, 1987.
99. Jacobs RF, Condrey YM, Yamauchi T: Tularemia in adults and children: a changing presentation, *Pediatrics* 76:818, 1985.
100. Jamieson S et al: Leptospirosis du New Zealand, *Bull Off Int Epizoot* 73:81, 1970.
101. Jevon TR et al: A point source epidemic of leptospirosis: description of cases, cause, and prevention, *Postgrad Med* 80:121, 1986.
102. Kaufmann AF et al: Public health implications of plague in domestic cats, *J Am Vet Med Assoc* 179:875, 1981.
103. Kennedy ND et al: Leptospirosis and acute renal failure—clinical experience and a review of the literature, *Postgrad Med J* 55:176, 1979.
104. Kerr DD, Marshall V: Protection against the renal carrier state by a canine leptospirosis vaccine, *Vet Med/Small Anim Clin* 69:1157, 1974.
105. Kilonzo BS, Makundi RH, Mbise TJ: A decade of plague epidemiology and control in the western Usambara mountains, north-east Tanzania, *Acta Trop* 50:323, 1992.
106. Kim GR, Lee YT, Park CH: A new natural reservoir of hantavirus: isolation of hantaviruses from lung tissues of bats, *Arch Virol* 134:85, 1994.
107. Klein JS: Treatment of severe trichinellosis. In Kim CW, Pawlowski ZS, editors: *Trichinellosis,* 1978, University Press of New England.
108. Klock LE, Olsen PF, Fukishima T: Tularemia epidemic associated with the deerfly, *JAMA* 226:149, 1973.
109. Koskela P, Salminen A: Humoral immunity against *Francisella tularensis* after natural infection, *J Clin Microbiol* 22:973, 1985.
110. Krebs JW et al: Rabies surveillance in the United States during 1991, *J Am Vet Med Assoc* 201:1836, 1992.
111. LeDuc JW, Childs JE, Glass GE: The hantaviruses, etiologic agents of hemorrhagic fever with renal syndrome: a possible cause of hypertension and chronic renal disease in the United States, *Annu Rev Pub Health* 13:79, 1992.
112. Leelarasame A, Bovornkitt S: Melioidosis: review and update, *Rev Infect Dis* 11:413, 1989.
113. Le Guenno B: Identifying a hantavirus associated with acute respiratory illness: a PCR victory? (letter), *Lancet* 342:1438, 1993.
114. Libby J, Meislin HW: Human rabies, *Ann Emerg Med* 12:217, 1983.
115. Linhart SB et al: Control of vampire bats by topical application of an anticoagulant, chlorophacinone, *Bull Pan Am Health Organ* 6:31, 1972.
116. MacLean JD et al: Trichinosis in the Canadian Arctic: report of five outbreaks and a new clinical syndrome, *J Infect Dis* 160:513, 1989.
117. Mahannop P et al: Immunodiagnosis of human trichinellosis using excretory-secretory (ES) antigen, *J Helminth* 66:297, 1992.
118. Mandell GL, Douglas RG, Bennett JE: *Principles and practice of infectious diseases,* ed 4, New York, 1995, Churchill Livingstone.
119. Marcus LC: *The veterinary biology and medicine of captive amphibians and reptiles,* Philadelphia, 1981, Lea & Febiger.
120. Markowitz LE et al: Tick-borne tularemia: an outbreak of lymphadenopathy in children, *JAMA* 254:2922, 1985.
121. Martell MA, Montes FC, Alcocer R: Transplacental transmission of bovine rabies after natural infection, *J Infect Dis* 127:291, 1973.
122. Mays EE, Ricketts EA: Melioidosis: recrudescence associated with bronchogenic carcinoma 26 years following initial geographic exposure, *Chest* 68:261, 1975.
123. McAuley JB, Michelson MK, Schantz PM: Trichinosis surveillance, United States, 1987-1990, *MMWR* 40:ss-3, 35, 1991.
124. McAuley JB, Michelson MK, Schantz PM: Trichinella infection in travelers, *J Infect Dis* 164:1013, 1991.
125. McClain JBL et al: Doxycycline therapy for leptospirosis, *Ann Intern Med* 100:696, 1984.
126. McCormick JB et al: Human to human transmission of *Pseudomonas pseudomallei, Ann Intern Med* 83:512, 1975.
127. Murphy FA: Rabies virus morphology and morphogenesis. In Baer GM, editor: *The natural history of rabies,* vol 1, New York, 1975, Academic Press.
128. Murphy FA: The rabies virus and pathogenesis of the disease. In Fishbein DB, Sawyer LA, Winkler WG, editors: *Rabies concepts for medical professionals,* ed 2, Miami, Fla, 1986, Merieux Institute.
129. Murray JD: Modeling the spread of rabies, *Am Sci* 75:280, 1987.
130. National Association of State Public Veterinarians, Inc: Compendium of animal rabies control, 1993, *MMWR* 42, RR3.
131. Nerurkar VR et al: Genetically distinct hantavirus in deer mice (letter), *Lancet* 342:1058, 1993.
132. Ozeretskovskaya NN et al: Benzimidazoles in the treatment and prophylaxis of synanthropic and sylvatic trichinellosis. In Kim CW, Pawlowski ZS, editors: *Trichinellosis,* 1978, University Press of New England.
133. Palmer DG et al: Demonstration of rabies viral antigen in paraffin tissue sections: comparison of the immunofluorescence technique with the unlabeled antibody enzyme method, *Am J Vet Res* 46:283, 1985.
134. Pappas MG et al: Rapid serodiagnosis of leptospirosis using the IgM-specific dot-ELISA: comparison with the microscopic agglutination test, *Am J Trop Med Hyg* 34:346, 1985.
135. Patamasucon P, Urs BS, Nelson JD: Melioidosis, *J Pediatr* 100:175, 1982.
136. Peck FB, Powell HM, Culbertson CG: Duck embryo rabies vaccine: study of fixed virus vaccine grown in embryonated duck eggs and killed with beta-propiolactone, *JAMA* 162:1373, 1956.
137. Penn RL, Kinasewitz GT: Factors associated with a poor outcome in tularemia, *Arch Intern Med* 147:265, 1987.
138. Petchclai B et al: Evaluation of two screening tests for human leptospirosis, *J Med Assoc Thailand* 73:64, 1990.
139. Poland J, Barnes AL: Plague. In Steele JH, editor: *CRC handbook series in zoonoses,* Boca Raton, Fla, 1979, CRC Press.
140. Porras C et al: Recovery from rabies in man, *Ann Intern Med* 85:44, 1976.
141. Posson SC, Told TN, Hollar GF: Recognition of hantavirus infection in the rural setting: report of first Colorado resident to survive, *J Am Osteopath Assoc* 93(10):1061, 1993.
142. Pozio E, La Rosa G: General introduction and epidemiology of trichinellosis, *Southeast Asian J Trop Med Public Health* 22(suppl):291, 1991.
143. Prochoda K, Mostow SR, Greenberg K: Hantavirus-associated acute respiratory failure (letter), *N Engl J Med* 329(23):1744, 1993.
144. Quenzer RW, Mostow SR, Emerson JK: Cat bite tularemia, *JAMA* 238:1845, 1977.
145. Redfearn MS, Palleroni NJ: Glanders and melioidosis. In Hubbert WT, McCulloch WF, Schnurrenberger PR, editors: *Diseases transmitted from animals to man,* Springfield, Ill, 1975, Charles C Thomas.
146. Remington PL, Shope T, Andrews J: A recommended approach to the evaluation of human rabies exposure in an acute-care hospital, *JAMA* 254:67, 1985.
147. *Report on rabies,* Princeton Junction, NJ, 1983, Veterinary Learning Systems.
148. Robertson MH: Leptospirosis, *Practitioner* 226:1552, 1982.
149. Rollag OJ et al: Feline plague in New Mexico: report of five cases, *J Am Vet Med Assoc* 179:1381, 1981.
150. Roy TM, Fleming D, Anderson WH: Tularemic pneumonia mimicking Legionnaire's disease with false positive direct fluorescent antibody stains for *Legionella, South Med J* 82:1429, 1989.

151. Rubin RH et al: Adverse reactions to duck embryo vaccine: range and incidence, *Ann Intern Med* 78:643, 1973.
152. Rupprecht CE et al: Efficacy of a vaccinia-rabies glycoprotein recombinant virus vaccine in raccoons *(Procyon lotor), Rev Infect Dis* 10(suppl 4):S803, 1988.
153. Rupprecht CE et al: Ineffectiveness and comparative pathogenecity of attenuated rabies virus vaccines for the striped skunks *(Mephitis mephitis), J Wildl Dis* 26:99, 1990.
154. Ryan CP: Selected arthropod-borne diseases: plague, Lyme disease, and babesiosis. In The veterinary clinics of North America, Small animal practice, vol 17, *Zoonotic diseases,* Philadelphia, 1987, WB Saunders.
155. Sanford JP: Leptospirosis—time for a booster, *N Engl J Med* 310:524, 1984.
156. Sasaki DM et al: Active surveillance and risk factors for leptospirosis in Hawaii, *Am J Trop Med Hyg* 48:35, 1993.
157. Saslaw S, Carhart S: Studies with tularemia vaccines in volunteers. III. Serological aspects following intracutaneous or respiratory challenge in both vaccinated and nonvaccinated volunteers, *Am J Med Sci* 241:689, 1961.
158. Saslaw S, Carlisle HN: Studies with tularemia vaccines in volunteers challenged with *Pasteurella tularensis, Am J Med Sci* 242:166, 1961.
159. Saslaw S et al: Tularemia vaccine study. I. Intracutaneous challenge, *Arch Intern Med* 107:121, 1961.
160. Saslaw S et al: Tularemia vaccine study. II. Respiratory challenge, *Arch Intern Med* 107:134, 1961.
161. Sato T et al: Microagglutination test for early specific serodiagnosis of tularemia, *J Clin Microbiol* 28:2372, 1990.
162. Schantz PM: Improvements in the diagnosis of helminthic zoonoses, *Vet Parasitol* 25:95, 1987.
163. Schlim DR, Schwartz E, Houston R: Rabies immunoprophylaxis strategy in travelers, *J Wilderness Med* 2:15, 1991.
164. Schneider LG, Diringer H: Structure and molecular biology of rabies virus, *Curr Top Microbiol Immunol* 75:153, 1976.
165. Shpilberg O et al: Long term follow-up after leptospirosis, *South Med J* 83:405, 1990.
166. Schwabe CW: *Veterinary medicine and human health,* ed 3, Baltimore, 1984, Williams & Wilkins.
167. Scofield RH, Lopez EJ, McNabb SJ: Tularemia pneumonia in Oklahoma, 1982-1987, *J Okla State Med Assoc* 85:165, 1992.
168. Shill M, Baynes RD, Miller SD: Fatal rabies encephalitis despite appropriate post-exposure prophylaxis: a case report, *N Engl J Med* 316:1257, 1987.
169. Sipahioghi U, Alpaut S: Insanda transplacental kuduz (transplacental rabies in human), *Mikrbiyol Bult* 19:95, 1985 (Turkish, English abstract).
170. Sites VR, Poland JD, Hudson BW: Bubonic plague misdiagnosed as tularemia: retrospective serologic diagnosis, *JAMA* 222:1642, 1972.
171. Smith JS et al: Unexplained rabies in three immigrants in the United States: a virological investigation, *N Engl J Med* 324:205, 1991.
172. Steele JH: History of rabies. In Baer G, editor: *The natural history of rabies,* vol 1, New York, 1975.
173. Steele JH: Glanders. In Steele JH, editor: *CRC handbook series in zoonoses, section A: bacterial, rickettsial and mycotic diseases,* vol 1, Boca Raton, Fla, 1979, CRC Press.
174. Steele JH: *CRC handbook series in zoonoses,* Boca Raton, Fla, 1979, 1980, 1981, 1982, CRC Press.
175. Strong RP: Studies on pneumonic plague and plague immunization. I. Introduction: the expedition to Manchuria and the conditions under which the work was performed there, *Philippine J Sci* 7B:131, 1912.
176. Sulzer CR, Jones WL: Leptospirosis: methods in laboratory diagnosis (rev ed), Publication No (CDC) 74-8275, Washington, DC.
177. Syrjala H, Schildt R, Raisainen S: In vitro susceptibility of *Francisella tularensis* to fluoroquinolones and treatment of tularemia with norfloxacin and ciprofloxacin, *Eur J Clin Microb Infect Dis* 10:68, 1991.
178. Syrjala H et al: Agglutination and ELISA methods in the diagnosis of tularemia in different clinical forms and severities of the disease, *J Infect Dis* 153:142, 1986.
179. Takafuji ET et al: An efficacy trial of doxycycline chemoprophylaxis against leptospirosis, *N Engl J Med* 310:497, 1984.
180. Taylor JP et al: Epidemiologic characteristics of human tularemia in the southwest-central states, 1981-1987, *Am J Epidemiol* 133:1032, 1991.
181. Thompson RD, Mitchell GC, Burns RJ: Vampire bat control by systemic treatment of livestock with an anticoagulant, *Science* 177:806, 1972.
182. Trong P, Nhu TQ, Marshall JD: A mixed pneumonic bubonic plague outbreak in Vietnam, *Milit Med* 132:93, 1967.
183. Van Knapen F et al: Detection of specific immunoglobulins (IgG, IgM, IgA, IgE) and total IgE levels in human trichinosis by means of the enzyme-linked immunosorbent assay (ELISA), *Am J Trop Med Hyg* 31:973, 1982.
184. Verma RD et al: Development of an avidin-biotin dot enzyme-linked immunosorbent assay and its comparison with other serological tests for diagnosis of glanders in equines, *Vet Microbiol* 25:77, 1990.
185. Waag DM et al: Vaccination of human volunteers with a new lot of the live vaccine strain of *Francisella tularensis, J Clin Microbiol* 30:2256, 1992.
186. Waitkins S: Laboratory diagnosis of leptospirosis, *Lab Technol* 17:178, 1983.
187. Wandeler AI: Oral immunization of wildlife. In Baer GM, editor: *The natural history of rabies,* ed 2, Boca Raton, Fla, 1991, CRC Press.
188. Watt G et al: The rapid diagnosis of leptospirosis: a prospective comparison of the dot-ELISA and genus-specific microscopic agglutination test at different stages of illness, *J Infect Dis* 157:840, 1988.
189. Watt G et al: Placebo-controlled trial of intravenous penicillin for severe and late leptospirosis: demonstration of efficacy by a double-blind, placebo-controlled study, *Lancet* 1:433, 1988.
190. Wells LF, Girard KF: Bats, rabies, and DDT, *N Engl J Med* 297:390, 1977.
191. Welty TK: Plague, *Am Family Physician* 33:159, 1986.
192. Welty TK, Grabman J, Kompare E: Nineteen cases of plague in Arizona: a spectrum including ecthyma gangrenosum due to plague and plague in pregnancy, *West J Med* 142:641, 1985.
193. White ME et al: Recommendations for the control of *Yersinia pestis* infections, recommendations from the CDC, *Infect Control* 1:324, 1980.
194. White NJ et al: Halving of mortality of severe melioidosis by ceftazidime, *Lancet* 2:697, 1989.
195. Whitmore A, Krishnaswami CS: An account of the discovery of a hitherto undescribed infective disease occurring among the population of Rangoon, *Ind Med Gaz* 47:262, 1912.
196. Wiktor TJ et al: Protection from rabies by a vaccinia virus recombinant containing the rabies virus glycoprotein gene, *Proc Natl Acad Sci* 81:7194, 1984.
197. Wilde H, Chutivongse S: Equine rabies immune globulin: a product with an undeserved poor reputation, *Am J Trop Med Hyg* 42:175, 1990.
198. Wilkerson JA: Rabies: epidemiology, diagnosis, prevention and prospects for worldwide control, *J Wilderness Med,* in press.
199. Wilkinson L: Glanders: medicine and veterinary medicine in common pursuit of a contagious disease, *Med History* 25:363, 1981.
200. Winkler WG et al: Airborne rabies transmission in a laboratory worker, *JAMA* 226:1219, 1973.
201. Young LS et al: Tularemia epidemic: Vermont, 1968; Forty-seven cases linked to contact with muskrats, *N Engl J Med* 280:1253, 1969.

42 INFECTIOUS DIARRHEA FROM WILDERNESS AND FOREIGN TRAVEL

Herbert L. DuPont
Howard D. Backer

Acute diarrhea is one of the two most common medical complaints in all populations. In many regions of the developing world it is the most important cause of hospitalization and mortality among children. More than 1 billion episodes of acute diarrhea occur annually in the developing world, which result in death in over 5 million.[192] The rates of illness among children in these areas range from 5 to 15 bouts per child per year. Now that oral rehydration solutions are available to prevent dehydration-associated deaths, invasive bacterial enterocolitis, caused by *Shigella* species and *Campylobacter jejuni,* and persistent diarrhea (defined as illness lasting 14 days or longer) are the major enteric problems.[32]

A number of U.S. populations have diarrhea rates not unlike those seen in the developing tropical world. They include travelers, gay males, non-toilet-trained toddlers in day care centers, and residents of custodial institutions for the mentally retarded.

This discussion is oriented primarily to infectious diarrhea likely to result from wilderness or foreign travel and methods of evaluation in a remote setting. In formulating an approach, the goals are to provide information that would decrease exposure to enteropathogens or reduce the chance of acquiring illness and to furnish a clinical approach to self-therapy that is likely to minimize the complications and suffering caused by illness that does occur. Acute diarrheal illnesses often do not allow strict categorization by clinical features. Fortunately, the vast majority of these infections do not require etiology-specific treatment. In the following discussion the term "traveler" indicates business or pleasure travelers as well as wilderness venturers.

General Principles of Enteric Infections

EPIDEMIOLOGY

Transmission

Enteric pathogens for the most part are spread by fecal-oral contamination; water and food are the most common vehicles. The relative importance of food and water may be difficult to determine for traveler's diarrhea, depending mainly on location and precautions taken (see section on prophylaxis). Water-borne pathogens account for most infectious diarrhea acquired in the U.S. wilderness.[42] Inadvertent ingestion during water recreational activity has resulted in enteric infections. Diseases spread by fecal contamination of drinking water include typhoid, cholera, *Campylobacter* enteritis, giardiasis, and hepatitis A infection. Water-borne diseases are usually preventable by proper sanitation and water disinfection. Person-to-person transmission is seen in select populations whose habits expose them to high levels of pathogens (such as infants in day care centers, homosexuals, and those with minimal access to water). Prevention of these illnesses includes adequate hand washing and personal hygiene.

Reservoirs of Infection

Organisms are shed in the stools during asymptomatic and symptomatic infection and for a period after illness. Long-term or chronic carrier states are seen only with typhoid fever, amebiasis, and giardiasis. In areas where direct fecal contamination of drinking water is unlikely, these cases may act as a reservoir for spreading infection. Animals are the reservoir for some enteric pathogens (collectively called zoonoses). Animals have been implicated as reservoirs for *Salmonella, Yersinia, Campylobacter, Giardia, Balantidium coli, Entamoeba,* and *Cryptosporidium.*

Etiology

Most diarrhea cases are caused by enteric pathogens, including bacteria, viruses, and protozoa. Table 42-1 lists the etiologic agents often associated with travel to developing tropical areas or wilderness travel in an industrialized region. Enteric bacteria, such as enterotoxigenic *Escherichia coli,* invasive *E. coli, Aeromonas* species, *Plesiomonas shigelloides, Shigella, Vibrio cholerae, Campylobacter jejuni,* and *Yersinia enterocolitica,* can be food borne as well as water borne. Food-borne illness may consist of food "poisoning" or food "infection." In food poisoning an intoxication results when toxins produced by bacteria are found in food in sufficient concentrations to produce symptoms. The major forms of intoxication or poisoning result from *Staphylococcus aureus* or *Bacillus cereus.* A rare cause of food poisoning is botulism, caused when the neurotoxin of *Clostridium botulinum* is ingested. Other causes of diarrhea include the viruses, including rotavirus and small round viruses (Norwalk virus, astrovirus), and the intestinal protozoal agents, including *G. lamblia, E. histolytica,* and *Cryptosporidium.*

MORBIDITY, MORTALITY, AND IMMUNITY

Although travelers rarely die of diarrhea,[198] this is not the case among infants in the developing world. Worldwide, diarrhea remains an important cause of morbidity, while in Africa, Asia, and Latin America, where sanitation is lacking, diarrhea is the leading cause of infant morbidity and mortality.[212] Malnutrition and diarrhea form a vicious cycle in underdeveloped areas, greatly increasing the morbidity and mortality of diarrheal illness. Countries with good sanitation, such as the United States and those in northern and western Europe, have a markedly lower incidence of infectious diarrhea.

New research techniques are beginning to identify the range of immune responses to these infections, but the mechanisms remain to be completely elucidated. Significant advances may result from understanding intestinal immunity, which appears to be more important than humoral immunity in enteric diseases.[104] Complete immunity is unusual for most infections; strain-specific immunity often results from enteric infection or from repeated exposure to the agent. Certain infections, such as rotavirus and giardiasis, are more commonly found in children. Acquired resistance may be related to the development of immunity or to loss of intestinal receptors to the pathogen.

Vaccines are available for typhoid, hepatitis A and B, and cholera. Vaccines for other enteric bacterial infections, such as rotavirus and enterotoxigenic *E. coli* (ETEC), are not yet available. Because of the economic incentive, and in the cases of rotavirus and ETEC disease, the impact on children's health in the developing world, vaccine development is being pursued actively.[104,219]

Table 42-1 Enteric Pathogens Found in Tropical and Wilderness Travel

Agent	Travel to Developing Tropical Regions	Wilderness Travel in Industrialized Regions
BACTERIA		
Enterotoxigenic *Escherichia coli*	Yes	Rarely
Shigella spp.	Yes	Yes
Salmonella spp.	Yes	Yes
Campylobacter spp.	Yes	Yes
Vibrio cholerae	Limited	Not currently
Aeromonas spp.	Yes	Yes
Plesiomonas shigelloides	Yes	Occasionally
Yersinia enterocolitica	Rare	In Scandinavia, Canada
VIRUSES		
Norwalk and other small round viruses	Yes	Yes
Rotavirus	Yes	Rarely
Hepatitis A	Yes	Yes
PROTOZOA		
Giardia lamblia	Yes	Yes
Entamoeba histolytica	Yes	Rarely
Cryptosporidium	Yes	Yes
Isospora belli	Limited	Rarely
Blastocystis hominis	Limited	Rarely
Balantidium coli	Limited	Rarely
Dientamoeba fragilis	Limited	Rarely
Entamoeba polecki	Rarely	Probably not
Cyclospora	Limited	Rarely

Traveler's Diarrhea

Approximately 50% of short-term (less than 3 weeks) travelers from low-risk countries (industrialized countries such as the United States and Canada, countries in northwestern Europe, South Africa, Australia, New Zealand, and Japan) to high-risk countries (developing tropical regions of Latin America, southern Asia, or Africa) experience at least one diarrheal illness during their trip. Persons who drink domestic surface water in recreational and wilderness areas are also at increased risk for infectious diarrhea. Travelers to foreign countries and the wilderness often leave behind sanitation associated with flush toilets and safe tap water, as well as proximity to advanced medical care. Diarrhea is virtually always a nuisance and in as many as one third of cases can be debilitating for a period of time. Prevention of these illnesses in remote areas depends on a combination of dietary precautions and disinfection of drinking water. Water disinfection is discussed in Chapter 43.

Traveler's diarrhea (TD) is a syndrome, not a specific disease.[117] Although a large percentage of cases are caused by strains of *E. coli,* TD may be caused by any of the water-borne or food-borne enteric pathogens. The bacterial flora of the bowel changes rapidly after arrival in a country with high rates of TD. At least 15% of travelers remain asymptomatic despite the presence of pathogenic organisms, including ETEC and *Shigella.*[63,179,205] However, most become ill.

DEFINITION

TD refers to an illness contracted while traveling, although in 15% of patients symptoms begin after the return home.[117] Point of origin, destination, and host factors are the main risk determinants.[57,118] International travel is more commonly associated with enteric infection and diarrhea, particularly when the destination is a developing tropical region, although the same infections can be contracted domestically. Different studies variously define TD as one to three unformed stools in one day, or a doubling or tripling of "normal" stool frequency, associated with one or more enteric symptoms, such as abdominal cramps, fever, nausea, and vomiting.[127] Typically, diarrheal stools are watery; however, dysentery may occur in 10% to 15% of cases, particularly when certain etiologic agents, such as *Shigella, C. jejuni,* or *Salmonella,* are the causes of the illness.

RISK

The number of persons at risk for TD is enormous. Of 300 million international travelers in 1986, 16 million traveled to developing countries; half of these visitors originated in the United States.[117] Attack rates of illness are highest (average 40%) among people from the industrialized or "developed" countries in North America and northern Europe who travel to developing tropical regions of Africa, southern Asia, and Latin America.* Intermediate risk occurs for short-term travelers to resorts in the Caribbean, the northern Mediterranean countries, the Middle East, China, and Russia.[196,199] For the traveler to an intermediate area, the risk of acquiring diarrhea is about 10%. Travelers between two high-risk areas or between two low-risk areas have attack rates of about 2% to 4%. These low rates may be caused by consuming food from a variety of sources, altered levels of alcohol consumption, or stress. Multiple episodes of diarrhea may occur on the same trip.[62] Attack rates remain high for up to 1 year, then decrease, but not to the levels of local inhabitants.[60,62,127] Immunity to ETEC infection, either asymptomatic[163] or symptomatic,[67] occurs after repeated or chronic exposure, which supports the development of a vaccine.

*References 18, 73, 116, 127, 138, 189, 199, 204.

ETIOLOGY

Since the incidence of TD reflects in part the extent of environmental contamination with feces, the etiologic agents are pathogens found as causative agents of illness in local children. The list of etiologic agents changes as laboratory techniques identify new enteric pathogens (Table 42-2). Twenty years ago, specific pathogens were found in only 20% of cases.[116,117] Since that time ETEC has proved to be the most common cause of TD worldwide.[93,138,189] Approximately one third to one half of cases appear to be caused by this agent. The organism shows a seasonal variation. ETEC is more common during rainy summer seasons and may be reduced in dryer winters, at least in semitropical countries such as Mexico and Morocco.[134] Currently, etiologic agents can be identified in up to 80% of TD episodes.[205] However, in most studies, causative pathogens are not identified in 20% to 40% of cases.[18,138] Overall, the major etiologic agents and their frequency of isolation are remarkably similar when one world region is compared with another. Given the favorable effect of antibacterial agents in the therapy of

Table 42-2 Important Pathogens in Traveler's Diarrhea (Travel in Developing Tropical Regions)

Etiologic Agent	Approximate Frequency (%)
Enterotoxigenic *Escherichia coli*	5-40*
Shigella	10
Salmonella	7
Clostridium jejuni	3-15†
Aeromonas	1-8
Plesiomonas	1-4
Enteropathogenic *E. coli* (classic serotypes)	<1
Rotavirus	<10
Giardia lamblia	<2
Unknown	20

*Lower frequency in rainy summer, higher in dryer winter.
†Lower frequency in winter, higher in summer.

illness,[65,70,78] it appears that a majority of the undiagnosed disease is caused by bacterial agents. Regardless of the similarities of enteropathogens causing traveler's diarrhea, certain differences exist in the occurrence of agents.

The traveler's risk of significant illness from cholera is estimated to be only 1:500,000 for a journey to an endemic area.[140,191,198] The risk of typhoid fever is 1:25,000 for a visit to most developing countries, but higher in India.[196]

CLINICAL SYNDROMES

Table 42-3 outlines the major syndromes in patients with enteric infection. The typical clinical syndrome experienced by travelers with ETEC (and diarrhea of many other causes) begins abruptly with watery diarrhea and abdominal cramping. Most cases are mild, consisting of two to four unformed stools per day with cramping but few other symptoms.[117,127,196,199] Another 30% of victims experience moderate illness with malaise, nausea, and vomiting accompanying the diarrhea. Only 10% to 20% experience severe illness with more than five unformed stools passed per day, malaise, myalgias, nausea, vomiting, chills, and fever. While the average duration is 3 days, half of cases resolve within 48 hours, 10% last longer than 1 week, and 1% to 2% last 1 month or longer.[146] An extensive study among Swiss travelers serves as the basis of much of the clinical information available on the disease.[196] Ten percent to 15% of affected persons experience dysenteric symptoms of fever and passage of bloody stools. Less than 1% were admitted to a local hospital while traveling, and only 4% consulted a local physician. No deaths were reported. Approximately one third of travelers are confined to bed or need to alter their travel plans when a diarrheal illness develops.[116,127,138]

DIETARY PRECAUTIONS

Food and water transmit the pathogens causing TD.[11,49,76,208,221] Dietary habits cannot always be rigidly controlled, and when diarrhea occurs, it is not possible to determine the source. Food in developing countries can be shown to be contaminated with fecal coliforms and enteric pathogens.[208] *Vibrio cholerae* remains viable on food for 1 to 3 weeks.[82] *Salmonella* can survive 2 to 14 days in water or in the environment in a desiccated state.[126]

Risk of illness appears to be lowest when the majority of meals are self-prepared and eaten in a private home, highest when obtained from street vendors, and intermediate when food is consumed at public restaurants.[21,76,208] Guests staying at four-star hotels have only slightly reduced risk.[199] Except in one instance,[120] most studies evaluating risk have found little correlation between routine precautions and illness.[22,127] Thus the following standard dietary recommendations for prevention are based more on known potential vehicles for transmission of illness than on strong evidence[22,127,146]:

1. Avoidance of tap water and ice made from untreated water and suspect bottled water is advised. Bottled and carbonated drinks, beer, and wine are probably safe. Boiled or otherwise disinfected water is safe. Water-borne epidemics of almost all of the enteric pathogens have been demonstrated.[42] Tap water in high-risk countries is difficult to implicate in traveler's diarrhea but has been shown to contain enteric bacteria[149] and pathogenic viruses[49] and to be responsible for giardiasis and cryptosporidiosis in travelers to St. Petersburg (former Leningrad).[113] Tap water and occasionally even bottled water may be unsafe. Noncarbonated bottled spring water has been associated with cholera in Portugal and typhoid in Mexico City[22,118] and found to contain protozoa in Mexico.[173] Bottled carbonated beverages are considered safe because of the antibacterial effects of the low acidity.[22] Alcohol in mixed drinks does not disinfect, so these may not be safe, but bottled beer and wine have not been found to be contaminated.[22] Home-made beverages cannot be guaranteed. Most enteric organisms can survive freezing and melting in common drinks,[51] so ice is not considered safe unless made from treated or previously boiled water. Ice in block form is often handled with unsanitary methods.[208]

2. Avoidance of unpasteurized dairy products is suggested. These may be the source of infection with *Salmonella, Campylobacter, Brucella, Listeria monocytogenes, Mycobacterium tuberculosis,* and others.[167]

Table 42-3 Pathophysiologic Syndromes in Diarrheal Disease

Syndrome	Agent
Acute watery diarrhea	Any agent, especially the toxin-mediated diseases (e.g., enterotoxogenic *Escherichia coli*)
Febrile dysentery	*Shigella, Clostridium jejuni, Salmonella;* less commonly, invasive *E. coli, Aeromonas* spp., *Vibrio* spp., *Yersinia enterocolitica, Entamoeba histolytica,* inflammatory bowel disease
Vomiting (as predominant symptom)	Viral agents, preformed toxins of *Staphylococcus* or *Bacillus cereus*
Persistent diarrhea (>14 days' duration)	Protozoa, especially *Giardia lamblia;* small bowel bacterial overgrowth; invasive enteropathogens; when longer than 30 days: small bowel injury, inflammatory bowel disease, irritable bowel syndrome, Brainerd diarrhea

Pasteurization renders dairy products safe if properly refrigerated.

3. Avoidance of raw vegetables, salads, meats, and uncooked seafood is advisable. Eating peeled fruits and properly washed vegetables is important, as is eating food served steaming hot. Raw vegetables in salads may be contaminated by fertilization with human waste or by washing in contaminated water.[22,127,138] Anything that can be peeled or have the surface removed is safe. Fruits and leafy vegetables can also be disinfected by immersion and washing in iodinated water or by washing thoroughly with dilute soap and previously boiled water, or by exposure to boiling water for 30 seconds.[82] Raw seafood has been associated with increased risk of diarrheal illness in travelers[22] and is suspected to be the cause of *Vibrio parahaemolyticus* infection in Asiatic travelers.[195,204] Shellfish concentrate enteric organisms from contaminated water and can carry hepatitis A, Norwalk virus, *Aeromonas hydrophila, Yersinia enterocolitica, Vibrio cholerae,* and *Vibrio parahaemolyticus.* Raw fish can carry parasites such as *Anisakis simplex, Clonorchis sinensis,* and *Metagonimus yokogawai.*[31] Raw crustaceans are the source of *Paragonimus westermani.* Raw meat is a source of *Salmonella* and *Campylobacter* and the vehicle for *Trichinella, Taenia saginata* and *T. solium* (beef or pork tapeworm), and *Sarcocystis.* Adequate cooking kills all microorganisms and parasites. However, if food is left at room temperature and recontaminated before serving, it can incubate *Salmonella, E. coli,* or *Shigella.* Travelers leaving a country should remember that the food served on an airplane, train, boat, or bus probably has been catered in the country of origin. The problems of food hygiene pertain to these forms of public transportation, even if the employees handling the food are from the United States.

The safe foods are those served steaming hot, items that are dry (such as bread), foods that have high sugar content (such as syrups and jellies), and fruits that have been peeled. Foods such as hamburgers that have been cooked once but may have remained stored at room temperature for a prolonged period may have been recontaminated and be dangerous. Cooked items require terminal heating (just before consumption).[11]

PROPHYLACTIC MEDICATION FOR PREVENTION OF TRAVELER'S DIARRHEA

Ten percent to 25% of European travelers[198] to high-risk areas and one third of U.S. travelers to Mexico[116] take prophylactic medication to prevent TD. In one survey, 42% took prophylactic or therapeutic intestinal drugs and 22% took more than one agent.[199] Lactobacilli have been tested on the assumption that they favorably modify intestinal flora, but they did not reduce the incidence of TD.[198] Antimotility drugs such as loperamide may be beneficial in treatment of symptoms but have adverse effects when used for prophylaxis.[197] Hydroxyquinolones, mainly iodochlorhydroxyquin or clioquinol (available commercially as Entero-vioform) are widely available in some parts of the world. While primarily used as amebicides, they have been used to prevent and treat TD. Available studies have shown mixed results; the best designed showed no significant protective effect.[116,198] This medication is not recommended because of its association with subacute myelooptic neuropathy leading to blindness.

Bismuth Subsalicylate Prophylaxis of Traveler's Diarrhea

Of the nonantibiotic drugs, only bismuth subsalicylate (BSS) has been shown by controlled studies to offer reasonable protection and safety. The first study for prevention used liquid BSS, 4.2 g/day in four divided doses (60 ml/dose) for 3 weeks in Mexico.[63] Those taking BSS experienced lower rates of diarrhea (23% versus 61%) for a protection rate of 62%, as well as fewer abdominal symptoms and soft stools not meeting the criteria for TD. Since the volume required is quite large with the liquid preparation, BSS in tablet form was evaluated in volunteers challenged with ETEC; this resulted in a protection rate of 77% with fewer symptoms when diarrhea did develop in subjects taking BSS.[96] Two studies attempting to find the minimal effective dosage regimen and the optimal administration schedule evaluated efficacy using 1.05 or 2.1 g/day of BSS tablets in divided doses twice or four times a day.[68,200] Diarrhea incidence was reduced at both dosages, but the higher dose when given four times a day was most effective (65% protection versus 40% protection). The currently recommended dose of BSS is 2 tablets four times a day (2.1 g/day).[68] Mild side effects include constipation, nausea, and blackened tongue or stools. BSS concurrent with doxycycline should be avoided, since BSS may bind to the antimicrobial and prevent absorption.[77] The potential toxicity of both active ingredients (bismuth and salicylate) in BSS has been questioned.[121,176] Ninety percent of salicylate from liquid BSS is absorbed and excreted in the urine of children.[164] Using 4.2 g/day of liquid BSS is the equivalent of 8.3 325 mg aspirin tablets, which is consistent with adult therapeutic doses. Although whether this salicylate cross-reacts with aspirin is unknown, BSS should not be used by someone with a history of aspirin allergy. Caution is recommended in small children, patients with gout or renal insufficiency, and those taking anticoagulants, probenecid, methotrexate, or other aspirin-containing products. Although bismuth was not detected in the urine or serum of children given multiple doses of BSS,[164] levels averaging 10 parts per billion (ppb) were detected in travelers using BSS tablets for 2 to 3 weeks.[200] This is well below the average level of 100 ppb found in cases of bismuth toxicity. The precise mechanism by which BSS prevents diarrhea is unknown. There is also bactericidal activity; patients taking BSS have decreased recovery of enteric pathogens from the stool,[63,68] and BSS inhibits growth of bacterial enteropathogens in vitro.[96] In addition, salicylate exhibits antisecretory activity after exposure to bacterial enterotoxins.[75] Adherence of bacteria to intestinal mucosa may be affected.

Antimicrobial Prophylaxis of Traveler's Diarrhea

Several antimicrobial agents have been shown to be highly effective in preventing traveler's diarrhea when given over short periods at risk. The most experience has been obtained with doxycycline, trimethoprim-sulfamethoxazole (TMP-SMX), and the fluoroquinolones. Other antimicrobials have shown significant protection but have not been well studied.[182] These include streptotriad (streptomycin and sulfonamides), erythromycin, and mecillinam. Doxycycline (200 mg on the day before first exposure, then 100 mg/day) resulted in 81% to 86% protection in areas where antibiotic resistance was low.[86,179,180] In areas with antibiotic-resistant ETEC, protection was considerably less.[183] Studies of U.S. students in Mexico taking trimethoprim 160 mg and sulfamethoxazole 800 mg twice daily for 3 weeks[64] or once daily for 2 weeks[66] demonstrated 71% and 95% protection, respectively. Trimethoprim 200 mg/day was less effective.[66] Ciprofloxacin[168] and norfloxacin[109] have been shown to be highly protective when employed as prophylactic agents. With the antibiotics evaluated, the effect lasted only as long as the drug was continued. Subjects who remained in a high-risk area experienced an increased incidence of diarrhea during the week after cessation of prophylaxis.[63,64,180] Because of the emergence of resistance among enteropathogens to tetracyclines, doxycycline can no longer be recommended for prophylaxis unless the susceptibility of prevalent organisms is known. Similarly, TMP-SMX resistance has been reported in many regions of the developing world. At present, TMP-SMX is recommended for use in prophylaxis only in the interior of Mexico during summer rainy months, when ETEC is the major cause of illness.[12] In all other regions and seasons a fluoroquinolone is suggested. The fluoroquinolones (such as norfloxacin, ciprofloxacin, ofloxacin, pefloxacin, and fleroxacin) all seem to have equal effectiveness.

Despite dramatic protection against diarrhea, investigators do not recommend widespread use of these medications by travelers.[55,146] Several reasons are cited:

1. Side effects. These include gastrointestinal symptoms, photosensitivity, and other cutaneous eruptions and reactions. Pregnant women and children cannot use fluoroquinolones and doxycycline. With larger numbers of people using these drugs, more serious side effects (such as Stevens-Johnson syndrome and hemolytic or aplastic anemia, antibiotic-associated colitis, and anaphylaxis) will undoubtedly result.
2. Alteration of normal bacterial flora. Alteration of bacterial flora with broad-spectrum antimicrobials may increase risk of infection with other antibiotic-resistant bacteria.[143] Severe pseudomembranous colitis caused by colonic overgrowth with *Clostridium difficile* has occurred after therapy with most antibiotics. Vaginal candidiasis and gastrointestinal side effects, including diarrhea, are common with antibiotic therapy. Changes in anaerobic flora can cause long-term alterations in the metabolism of bile acids and pancreatic enzymes, although clinical effects are unknown. A 2-week trial of norfloxacin for TD prophylaxis demonstrated complete eradication of gram-negative bacteria from the stool, but no evidence of complications.[109]
3. Tendency to lower one's guard. Travelers taking antibiotics may relax their vigilance of dietary precautions and increase their risk of acquiring other infections.

Recommendations for Prophylaxis

Although the consensus is that not all travelers should use antibiotic prophylaxis, the approach may be appropriate for some.[54] Potential candidates would be residents of a low-risk country going to a high-risk area for less than 3 weeks who have one or more of the following conditions or requirements:

1. An important underlying illness, such as gastric achlorhydria (from surgery or taking omeprazole); AIDS; inflammatory bowel disease; or a cardiac, renal, or central nervous system disorder.
2. An itinerary that is so rigid and critical to the overall mission that they would not tolerate even the minor changes caused by illness rendered short-term by effective therapy.
3. Those who prefer prophylaxis after hearing the pros and cons of the approach. No studies have evaluated prophylaxis of TD in young children, although they may be at higher risk for infectious diarrhea. Because of the potential side effects, prophylaxis with BSS or antibiotics cannot be recommended in children under 5 years of age.

CLINICAL ASSESSMENT OF DIARRHEAL ILLNESS

History

A patient's history of foreign or wilderness travel helps to determine potential etiologic agents. Association with eating a specific food, such as raw seafood, especially with a cluster of cases, suggests the etiologic agents of food poisoning. Aside from prior medical problems, other significant history includes recent antibiotic use (antibiotic-associated colitis) and homosexuality (high incidence of many enteric pathogens).

Pathophysiologic Syndromes

Enteric pathogens can be divided into noninvasive and invasive groups according to their pathophysiologic mechanisms. Table 42-3 gives the general syndromes produced by the etiologic agents that cause diarrhea. Noninvasive organisms primarily colonize the proximal small bowel and cause symptoms by altering water and electrolyte transport in epithelial cells (secretory diarrhea) without disruption of the mucosal surface. The soft to watery stools that result are often voluminous and rarely bloody. Upper abdominal and midabdominal cramping, nausea, and vomiting are common, but high fever is not. The bacterial pathogens in this group include *Vibrio cholerae* and enterotoxigenic *E. coli,* which exert their effects via enterotoxin; *Vibrio parahaemolyticus;* preformed food toxins; Norwalk virus; rotavirus; *Giardia lamblia;* and *Cryptosporidium.* Dehydration is the major complication of illness; potassium depletion and renal failure can follow. Although cholera may cause the highest fluid losses, significant dehydration is most often associated with ETEC diarrhea and rotavirus gastroenteritis, especially in infants.[20]

Invasive organisms chiefly involve the distal ileum and colon, damaging cell membranes and eliciting an inflammatory response, including ulceration, gross inflammation, and microabscesses. Stools are typically liquid and of small volume, containing gross blood and leukocytes. Fever, lower abdominal cramps, and tenesmus are common. Illness with this combination of signs and symptoms, when combined with the passage of bloody stools, is called dysentery.

Enteric bacteria that cause this syndrome include *Shigella, Salmonella,* invasive *E. coli, Yersinia enterocolitica, Campylobacter jejuni, Aeromonas* species, *Vibrio parahaemolyticus, Entamoeba histolytica,* and, rarely, *Balantidium coli.* Enterotoxins and cytotoxins may play a major role in the pathophysiology of the invasive organisms.[141] In addition to dehydration, the major complications from invasive infection, occurring characteristically in children with malnutrition, are septicemia, disseminated intravascular coagulation, pneumonia, hemolytic-uremic syndrome, and metastatic abscesses. In some infections, such as typhoid fever, septicemia may result with more systemic than enteric symptoms. Poorly understood reactions, probably immune mediated, can result in reactive arthritis (Reiter's syndrome), and when caused by a Shiga toxin or Shiga-like toxin producing bacteria such as *S. dysenteriae* 1 or *E. coli* 0157:H7, the hemolytic-uremic syndrome.

Clinical differentiation of illnesses within either group is not reliable. Although noninvasive organisms rarely cause dysentery, invasive organisms commonly cause watery diarrhea without dysentery, or a sequential illness beginning with watery diarrhea and progressing to bloody dysentery. If multiple people acquire the illness at the same time, food poisoning caused by ingestion of preformed toxins in food can usually be distinguished by a short incubation period (4 hours or less), the predominance of vomiting, and resolution within 24 hours.

Clinical Examination

Most important is assessment of level of hydration: vital signs with orthostatic pulse and blood pressure, mental status, skin turgor, hydration of mucous membranes, and urine output. The abdominal examination often shows mild tenderness but should not demonstrate signs of peritoneal irritation. A rectal examination may reveal tenderness in enterocolitis. The patient may have painful external hemorrhoids, a result of the excess stooling.

Diagnosis by Clinical Means

Studies have attempted to determine the reliability of clinical factors to predict which patients will have a positive stool culture.[50,148] Bacterial pathogens are suspected when the patient has a large number of stools per day (more than six),[50] has a fever,[148] and has had the ailment more than 24 hours but less than 1 week. Better correlation has been found with stool examination. Grossly bloody stools correlated with bacterial pathogens (mostly *Shigella* or *Campylobacter*) in several studies,[148,202] but the majority of stools with blood were not found to contain invasive pathogens.[202] The presence of fecal leukocytes is a reliable indicator of invasive and inflammatory distal gastrointestinal infection.

LABORATORY FINDINGS

In Table 42-4 the various laboratory tests or procedures useful in evaluating patients with diarrheal disease are listed along with their indication for performance. The laboratory tests available include procedures for fecal leukocytes, bacteriologic culture, parasite identification, and special tests. For most traveler's diarrhea, use of the laboratory is reserved for continuing illness after the patient returns home. For all moderate to severe illness the fecal leukocyte test is the ideal screening procedure. The test should be performed on a fresh sample. A mucus strand, if available, or liquid stool is mixed on a slide with a drop of dilute methylene blue and observed under a microscope. The stool can be heat fixed and examined under oil immersion, or a wet mount can be prepared with observation over a coverslip by use of the "high dry" objective of the microscope. Leukocytes are easily seen, although they can be confused with protozoal cysts. A large number of polymorphonuclear leukocytes (PMNLs) per high-power field (hpf) correlates most significantly with invasive bacterial infection caused by *Shigella, Salmonella,* or *Campylobacter.*[50,98,162,202] A count of more than 50 PMNLs/hpf helps distinguish bacterial from amebic dysentery (Color Plate 105).[202] Fecal leukocytes are less likely to be seen in noninvasive infections, such as diarrhea caused by ETEC, *G. lamblia,* and viral pathogens,[98] yet they are often observed in culture-negative stools.[202]

Bacterial infection is specifically diagnosed by stool culture. However, relatively few pathogens are identified by routine stool testing. In the United States, only about 10% of stool cultures are positive. The percentage is higher (12% for adults and about 50% for children or travelers) among patients in developing countries when research laboratories are looking for all of the important agents including ETEC.[202] The major indications for stool culture in a patient

Table 42-4 Diagnosis Using the Laboratory

Laboratory Test or Procedure	Indication	Etiologic Agents Identified
Fecal leukocytes	All moderate to severe diarrhea	Invasive agents and others that produce diffuse colonic inflammation
Stool culture	High fever, severe or persistent diarrhea, presence of fecal leukocytes	*Shigella, Clostridium jejuni, Salmonella, Aeromonas, Yersinia, Plesiomonas,* invasive *Escherichia coli*
Parasite examination	Persistent diarrhea, diarrhea in gay male, association with a day care center, travel to mountainous areas or to St. Petersburg	Protozoa (see text)
SPECIAL TESTS		
Rotavirus antigen	Infants <2 yr old, persistent diarrhea, gay male	Rotavirus, *Giardia,* colitis versus proctitis versus enteritis
String test		
Sigmoidoscopy		
Amebic serology	Liver abscess, persistent diarrhea	*Entamoeba histolytica*

with diarrhea are diarrhea lasting 1 week or longer, high fever or intense diarrhea, or presence of fecal leukocytes in fecal smears.

When microscopy is used for parasites, multiple samples may have to be examined to identify the causative agent. Parasitic examination is indicated when patients have diarrhea lasting more than 1 week, when diarrhea occurs during or shortly after travel to the mountainous areas of the United States or to St. Petersburg, Russia, when diarrhea occurs in someone who works in or attends an infant day care center, or when diarrhea occurs in a gay male.

Special diagnostic procedures include the Enterotest for small bowel protozoa, including *Giardia.* A gelatin capsule affixed to a nylon string is swallowed after the end of the string is taped to the cheek. After the patient consumes a meal, or after the string has been attached to the cheek overnight, it is carefully and slowly removed so that the mucus and secretions can be scraped off and studied for enteropathogens. The pH of the string confirms that it had reached the alkaline small bowel. Rotavirus antigen testing of stool can be done in hospitalized infants less than 2 years of age to help guide therapy (fluids without antimicrobials when positive). In a patient with a typhoidlike systemic illness who has taken one or more doses of an antimicrobial, a bone marrow aspiration and blood sample should both be obtained for culture. In selected cases, sigmoidoscopy or colonoscopy are employed to study colonic lesions and collect samples for culture and microscopy. Antibody-specific serologic tests are now widely used for invasive amebiasis and will become available for other infections in the future.

DIAGNOSTIC AND TREATMENT CONSIDERATIONS

Even among potentially severe infections, almost all are self-limited, requiring nonspecific treatment to prevent dehydration. Only 4% of travelers consult a local doctor for diarrheal illness,[196] and most of those seeking treatment wait until after a self-administered therapeutic trial of symptomatic or antimicrobial therapy.[199] Culture results are not conclusive for at least 24 to 48 hours. By this time, most patients have begun treatment or spontaneously improved, so therapy is frequently not changed by culture results. The illness, not the infection, should be treated, so most can be managed on the basis of symptoms, and in the case of dysentery, on the basis of stool appearance. In certain situations, empirical therapy may be given without establishing an etiologic agent; in other cases, specific therapy follows laboratory confirmation of an etiologic agent (see Tables 42-5 to 42-7).

Acute Diarrhea

Where routine laboratory evaluation is available, logical approaches to patients with acute diarrhea vary with the situation. When the symptoms include watery diarrhea, no fever, and duration of less than 1 week, laboratory testing is not done and treatment is symptomatic. When a patient has bloody diarrhea or fever and fecal leukocytes, a stool culture is taken and antibacterial drugs are begun pending culture results. When the patient has a high fever and toxic

Table 42-5 Antimicrobial Therapy for Diarrheal Disease

Therapy	Disease
Empirical antimicrobial therapy	Traveler's diarrhea (see text), febrile dysenteric syndromes, suspected bacteremia or sepsis, persistent diarrhea
Specific therapy	Giardiasis, shigellosis, bacteremic salmonellosis, amebiasis, cholera, campylobacteriosis

Table 42-6 Empirical Therapy for Traveler's Diarrhea

Clinical Syndrome	Pharmacologic Agent	Dose and Duration
Mild diarrhea without fever or dysentery	Symptomatic treatment	Loperamide 4 mg initially, then 2 mg after each unformed stool not to exceed 16 mg/d (prescription dose) or 8 mg/d (over-the-counter dose); or bismuth subsalicylate 30 ml (or 2 tabs) each 30 minutes for eight doses; both can be given for 2 days
Moderate to severe diarrhea*	Antimicrobial therapy	Trimethoprim-sulfamethoxazole (160 mg/800 mg) bid for 3 days for travel to interior of Mexico in summer; for other areas and times, use one of the following: norfloxacin 400 mg, ciprofloxacin 500 mg, ofloxacin 300 mg bid, or fleroxacin 400 mg qd for 3 days
Vomiting as predominant symptom	Bismuth subsalicylate	Dose given above

*If the patient has a fever, the antimicrobial treatment is given alone. If there is no fever and stools do not contain blood or mucus, loperamide may be combined with the antimicrobial for faster relief. Antimicrobials are advised with the passage of the third unformed stool in 24 hours.

Table 42-7 Therapy for Established Bacterial Diarrhea

Etiologic Agent	Antimicrobial Agent	Duration of Therapy (Days)
Shigella spp.	TMP-SMX	3-5
Bacteremic salmonellosis	Fluoroquinolone*	10
Campylobacter jejuni	Erythromycin	5
Aeromonas spp.	TMP-SMX	5
Plesiomonas shigelloides	TMP-SMX	5
Vibrio cholerae	Tetracycline	2
Noncholera vibrios	None or tetracycline or furazolidone	5
Yersinia enterocolitica	Tetracycline or fluoroquinolone	5

TMP-SMX, Trimethoprim-sulfamethoxazole.
*Daily dose given in Table 42-6.

appearance, stool and blood cultures are taken and antibacterial drugs are begun (Table 42-6) pending culture results.

Persistent and Chronic Diarrhea

Diarrhea may persist after the traveler returns home. Persistent diarrhea is defined as illness lasting 14 days or longer. Diarrhea is considered chronic when the illness has lasted 30 days or longer. The etiology of persistent or chronic diarrhea often differs from that seen in the patient with acute diarrhea. Important causes of persistent diarrhea include bacterial infection *(Salmonella, Shigella, Campylobacter, Yersinia enterocolitica),* a parasitic agent *(G. lamblia, Cryptosporidium, Cyclospora,* and *E. histolytica),* lactase deficiency induced by a small bowel pathogen (*G. lamblia* or a viral enteropathogen such as rotavirus or Norwalk virus), or a small bowel bacterial overgrowth syndrome secondary to small bowel motility inhibition (as a result of enteric infection). Occasionally, other parasitic enteric infections can cause more persistent illness, including *Strongyloides stercoralis, Trichuris trichiuria,* and severe *Necator americanus* or *Ancylostoma duodenale.* In rare cases, more protracted diarrhea may be a prominent symptom in patients with schistosomiasis, *P. falciparum* malaria, leishmaniasis, or African trypanosomiasis.

After eradication of microbial pathogens, bowel habits may not return to normal for several weeks. Postdysenteric colitis resembling ulcerative colitis occasionally follows infection with invasive pathogens, especially infection caused by *E. histolytica.* This could represent slow repair of damage to the intestinal mucosa.

When chronic diarrhea occurs, additional possibilities should also be considered. Postinfective malabsorption can persist for weeks to months after acute diarrhea; it is especially common after giardiasis. Giardiasis itself can last for a number of months.

A poorly defined condition, tropical jejunitis, also known as tropical sprue, may explain prolonged diarrhea in a traveler. Onset usually follows an episode of acute enteritis. It is associated with substandard hygiene and longer stay, thus is not common in short-term travelers. The cause is thought to involve small bowel bacterial overgrowth, since small bowel intubation may yield a heavy growth of bacteria and patients often respond to antimicrobial agents, including tetracycline or metronidazole.

An underlying condition such as inflammatory bowel disease, irritable bowel syndrome, or celiac sprue may worsen after an episode of acute enteritis. Finally, Brainerd diarrhea may be the explanation for chronic diarrhea. This condition, named after a community outbreak in Brainerd, Minnesota, follows the consumption of raw (unpasteurized) milk[152] or untreated water.[154] It may last months and even years.[152] There is no diagnostic test and no therapy. The diagnosis is suspected based on the epidemiologic history (exposure to unpasteurized milk or untreated water just before onset of illness).

The approach to persistent or chronic diarrhea in travelers should begin with stool culture for all of the organisms listed previously, as well as for *Clostridium difficile* (culture and toxin assay), since many patients will have taken antibiotics. If any cultures are positive, the patient should be treated with the appropriate antibiotic. Optimally, three stools should be examined for ova and parasites. If all tests to this point are negative and stools contain leukocytes, sigmoidoscopy or colonoscopy should be performed, along with empirical treatment for *Shigella* or *Campylobacter* infection. If there are no leukocytes, duodenal mucus is examined for *G. lamblia,* followed by empirical treatment for *Giardia*. Dietary modification in all cases should include avoidance of lactose. The next step is to perform tests for malabsorption and biopsy of the small bowel mucosa. Most of these chronic forms of diarrhea are self-limiting. It is unwise to keep treating these patients with multiple antibiotics such as metronidazole, which only alters the gut ecology and encourages diarrhea.

INFECTIOUS DIARRHEA

Outpatient treatment with instructions for oral rehydration can be used in the vast majority of adults and children. Significant dehydration from diarrhea in travelers is unusual. Inpatient treatment with intravenous fluids is indicated for the very rare patient with hypotension, inability to retain oral fluids, septicemia (high fever and toxicity), or moderate toxicity or dehydration in patients with severe underlying disease or for patients at extremes of age.

Fluid and Dietary Treatment

The major cause of morbidity and mortality from acute diarrheal disease is depletion of body water and electrolytes. The most significant advance in the field of diarrhea in the past 25 years has been the development of the concept of oral rehydration. Oral rehydration solution (ORS) was first developed for treatment of cholera. This simple form of treatment has saved countless lives, mostly of children. ORS obviates extensive use of scarce and expensive intravenous fluids in developing countries. Oral rehydration is the cornerstone of the World Health Organization (WHO) program to combat diarrheal diseases worldwide.

Two discoveries led to the development of ORS. The first was that glucose enhanced absorption of sodium through the intestinal mucosa. The second was the finding that this absorption remained intact despite the presence of enterotoxin and concurrent secretory losses of water and electrolytes.[160] Other electrolytes are also absorbed nonselectively when ORS is administered.

Watery diarrhea, often caused by production of an enterotoxin, has an electrolyte composition similar to plasma, varying somewhat with the type of infection and the age of the patient. The formula packaged and promoted by the WHO and UNICEF contains powder to be mixed with 1 L of disinfected water: sodium 90 mEq, potassium 20 mEq, chloride 80 mEq, bicarbonate 30 mEq, and glucose 111 mmol. Although this concentration of electrolytes is ideal for treating purging diarrhea associated with cholera and other dehydrating forms of diarrhea, most traveler's diarrhea can be adequately managed with readily available flavored mineral water taken with saltine crackers. In addition to flavored soft drinks, fruit juice, coconut milk, simple sugar and salt solutions,[44] or diluted cola drinks[101] are adequate for mild dehydration, partial maintenance, or supplementation or for use if nothing else is available.

Supplemental nutrition is beneficial and can be given as soon as fluid deficit losses are replaced, usually after the first 4 hours. Breast feeding of infants should be resumed as soon as possible. Except for an occasional patient with carbohydrate intolerance, staple foods such as cereals, bananas, lentils, potatoes, and other cooked vegetables are well tolerated and can be continued during diarrhea. Foods high in starch may even decrease diarrhea.[13] Only foods and drinks that prolong diarrhea or increase intestinal motility should be avoided. These are foods that contain lactose, caffeine, alcohol, high fiber, and fats.

Nonspecific Therapy

Nonantibiotic therapies that may be used in addition to fluids are best considered by their effects on pathophysiologic mechanisms.

Alteration of Intestinal Flora. Lactobacillus preparations and yogurt are safe, but there is little evidence that they have any important effect on acute diarrhea.[146]

Adsorbents. Adsorbent agents bind nonspecifically to water and other intraluminal material, including bacteria and toxins, and potentially to other medications such as antibiotics. The most common medication in this group is attapulgite. Other examples are kaolin and pectin and activated charcoal. By adsorbing water, these agents give stools more form or consistency, but do not decrease stool frequency, cramps, or duration of illness. However, they are completely safe.[54,146]

Antimotility Drugs. Narcotic analogs related to opiates are the major drugs in this group. In addition to inhibiting intestinal motility, these drugs alter water and electrolyte transport, probably having effects on both secretion and absorption.[52] They are the most widely prescribed drugs for diarrhea. The most commonly used product is loperamide (Imodium) taken in a dose of 2 capsules or caplets (both 2 mg each), followed by 1 capsule or caplet after each unformed stool, not to exceed 4 caplets (8 mg) per day (over-the-counter dose) or 8 capsules (16 mg) per day (prescription dose). Diphenoxylate with atropine (Lomotil) is less expensive but has greater central opiate effects in case of accidental overdose by a child and more side effects without antidiarrheal benefits because of the atropine (which is added only to prevent overdoses). Diphenoxylate is given in a dose of 2 tablets (2 mg each) four times a day (maximum daily dose 16 mg). Tincture of opium or paregoric opium preparations are rapidly and equally effective. This class of drugs decreases the number of stools passed and offers a modest reduction in associated symptoms. The drugs should never be used in patients who have fever or are passing bloody stools, since inhibition of gut motility may facilitate intestinal infection by invasive bacterial enteropathogens.[56] They should not be given to children under the age of 3 years because of the danger of central nervous system depression.[175] The antimotility drugs should not be administered for more than 48 hours. Compared with a placebo, these drugs reduce the number of stools passed by about 80% during their administration.

Anticholinergics and Antispasmodics. Although occasionally used, anticholinergic and antispasmodic drugs have not been shown to be effective in treating diarrhea.[171]

Antisecretory Drugs. Since increased secretion of water and electrolytes is the major physiologic derangement in acute watery diarrhea, therapy aimed at this effect is appealing. Although aspirin and other nonsteroidal antiinflammatory agents have been found to inhibit secretion, their usefulness is still limited, primarily because of mucosal toxicity.[52] BSS is the best studied antisecretory drug.[61,108] BSS reduces the number of stools passed and duration of diarrhea by about 50%. The drug is not as effective as the motility-inhibiting agents in relieving diarrhea.[108] Novel compounds are being developed that have antisecretory properties without motility effects.[71] These compounds should become important forms of therapy for acute diarrhea.

To treat milder forms of traveler's diarrhea (one or two unformed stools per 24 hours), symptomatic treatment (bismuth subsalicylate or loperamide) alone is recommended (Table 42-6).

Antimicrobial Treatment. Most enteric infections do not require antibiotics, and antibiotics are not useful in a majority of diarrhea cases in view of the low frequency of bacterial agents in naturally occurring diarrhea (Tables 42-5 and 42-6). However, considerably better results are achieved in acute traveler's diarrhea because bacterial agents cause most cases. Therapy for specific infections is discussed in the corresponding sections.[54] At times, treatment is indicated regardless of symptoms, to prevent person-to-person spread (for example, for food handlers, day care center workers) or to eradicate pathogenic strains when infection can be converted from asymptomatic to symptomatic illness (for example, *E. histolytica*).

In TD the diagnosis is rarely established. This, plus the fact that most cases are caused by bacterial agents, supports the use of antibacterial drugs on an empirical basis. Trimethoprim-sulfamethoxazole (TMP-SMX) 160/800 mg and trimethoprim 200 mg twice a day for 5 days were equally effective in reducing the number of unformed stools, duration of illness, and abdominal symptoms compared with placebo in a study carried out in Mexico.[65] In infections caused by ETEC, illness was reduced from an average of 93 hours in the placebo group to 30 hours in the treated group. For shigellosis, illness was reduced from a mean of 110 hours to 16 hours. Reduction was also seen in the group without identifiable stool pathogens, which suggested a probable bacterial origin even in culture-negative cases. Fluoroquinolones, including those that have been evaluated in TD (norfloxacin, ciprofloxacin, ofloxacin, and fleroxacin), represent the treatments of choice for TD when individuals are traveling to areas where TMP resistance among bacterial enteropathogens is common or has not been determined. Potential advantages of the quinolones include a high degree of in vitro activity against virtually all bacterial etiologic agents (including *Campylobacter*) and the potential for less bacterial resistance.[61,161] Ciprofloxacin 500 mg twice a day was equally effective in treating TD compared with TMP-SMX in an area where TMP resistance was unusual.[78] In a separate study it appeared to decrease the duration of fever and diarrhea in patients with campylobacteriosis, salmonellosis, and shigellosis.[161] The duration of antimicrobials needed in TD appears to be short. No person needs more than 3 days, and many respond to single-dose treatment.[79] It is probably advisable to give patients with milder disease single-dose treatment and more severely ill persons 3 days of the antimicrobial.

We believe that the optimal approach for travelers to high-risk regions is to carry an antibacterial drug and a symptomatic drug such as loperamide (Table 42-6). Persons should be instructed to take their temperature with the passage of the third unformed stool and to take the antimicrobial[55] in all cases (fever or no fever); they should take the loperamide also if there is no fever.[79,206] In such patients who pass a third stool in less than 24 hours, illness is likely to progress without therapy. Loperamide induces more rapid relief of symptoms, while the antimicrobial exerts curative effects. The added benefit of combining the drugs may depend on the severity of the diarrhea and the antimicrobial agent employed.[79,206]

The antibiotic regimens would not be effective against diarrhea caused by viruses, *Campylobacter* (in the case of TMP-SMX or TMP therapy), *Salmonella, G. lamblia, E. histolytica,* or other protozoa or noninfectious causes. Therefore antibiotics should not be continued in the face of persistent or worsening diarrhea.

Specific Enteric Pathogens

ESCHERICHIA COLI

The diarrheagenic *E. coli* is a heterogeneous group of organisms that differ in their virulence properties, disease epidemiology, and clinical features. At least four groups have been characterized, at least partially. The first is enteropathogenic *E. coli* (EPEC), which is an important cause of hospital nursery outbreaks. While the organisms are usually detected by their characteristic serotypes, the major virulence property of these organisms is enterocyte attachment[74,131,132] and selective damage at the site of attachment. Screening for this property of adherence can be performed by looking for attachment to HEp-2 cells, a continuous cell line that is used in respiratory virology culture.[131] HEp-2 cell–adherent *E. coli,* called enteroadherent *E. coli* (EAEC), has been shown to be an important cause of TD and is considered separately from EPEC.

Strains of Escherichia Coli

Enterotoxigenic Escherichia Coli. ETEC produces one, or in many cases, two enterotoxins, which both act on the small intestine to produce diarrhea with the same electrolyte concentration, but by different physiologic mechanisms and with different time responses.[58,181] One of these enterotoxins is a high–molecular weight protein, immunologically similar to and with the same mode of action as cholera toxin, and identifiable via the same assay techniques. It is referred to as heat-labile toxin (LT). Another important virulence property in human ETEC strains is a low–molecular weight, poorly antigenic toxin that is heat stable (ST). The net result of both enterotoxins is inhibition of sodium reabsorption and increased secretion of anions and fluid into the intestinal lumen, resulting in diarrhea without inflammatory exudate. Because genes encoding for enterotoxin production have been found to reside on plasmids, they can be transferred to other strains.[181] ETEC has been identified as the major cause of traveler's diarrhea, accounting for 20% to 50% of cases in series from all parts of the world.[93,189] It also accounts for a large percentage (frequently the majority) of enteritis in local pediatric populations of developing countries, where contaminated food and water are the primary sources of infection. Most outbreaks of ETEC in the United States have been water borne.[42] The first well-documented event occurred in 1975 within Crater Lake National Park and affected more than 2000 individuals. It was attributed to sewage contamination of the water supply with inadequate disinfection.[174] Person-to-person spread is infrequent because of the large infectious dose (10^6 to 10^{10} organisms).[58] Attack rates and clinical illness increase with increasing dose.[124]

Enteroadherent Escherichia Coli. EAEC shows a characteristic adherence to the villi of the small intestine with localized damage to the enterocyte. The pathophysiology of these strains as it relates to diarrhea production is unknown, but mucosal invasion and focal injury may be sufficient to produce diarrhea. Infectious dose and clinical illness in adult subjects resemble those of ETEC.[132] Prolonged illness lasting weeks and dysenteric disease may occur.[177]

Enteroinvasive Escherichia Coli. EIEC has been associated with food-borne outbreaks, which may be extensive. The organism has been implicated as a moderately important cause of traveler's diarrhea.[216] The bacteria invade bowel mucosa, resulting in microabscesses and ulcer formation resembling *Shigella* infection.[58] Invasive strains of *E. coli* are more likely to cause fever, tenesmus, and mucopurulent bloody stools. Other invasive organisms that should be considered in the differential diagnosis include *Shigella, Salmonella, E. histolytica,* and *Vibrio parahaemolyticus.*

Enterohemorrhagic Escherichia Coli. EHEC produces copious bloody diarrhea with mucus, but unlike *Shigella* and EIEC infection, the stool does not contain numerous fecal leukocytes and fever is either low grade or absent. The major source is beef, often obtained at a "fast food" hamburger chain. Because of the production of Shiga or a similar toxin, a complication of the illness is the hemolytic-uremic syndrome.

Diagnosis

Laboratory culture cannot differentiate the various diarrheagenic strains of *E. coli* from normal bowel flora or from one another. For research purposes, specialized assays are used for this purpose. In the future, it is hoped that serologic techniques will become available for the practitioner. The presence of antibody to enterotoxin is not a sensitive indicator of infection.

Treatment

Treatment of *E. coli* diarrhea, other than that produced by invasive strains, is primarily supportive with oral fluid replacement and maintenance. Since most cases are brief and self-limited, routine treatment is not needed. Moreover, since the diagnosis of *E. coli* diarrhea cannot be confirmed by most laboratories, therapy is based on the setting and clinical syndrome. In developing tropical countries, traveler's diarrhea with watery stools and associated symptoms is most often caused by ETEC; antibiotics shorten the duration of illness, especially when started within 48 to 72 hours of symptom onset.[65,70,78] Dysenteric illness should be treated with antibacterial drugs in all settings (whether a developing country or industrialized region). Susceptibility of ETEC to TMP-SMX depends on the region. In many areas, such as the interior of Mexico, this is the drug of choice; in many others the fluoroquinolones are required for therapy of adult cases. EPEC strains are invariably resistant to a broad range of drugs. With geography and time, resistance patterns vary, necessitating ongoing surveillance of susceptibility.

Immunology

There is great interest in a vaccine against ETEC. Differences in frequency and duration of illness in adults from industrialized and underdeveloped countries indicate that repeated infections offer protection.[20,60,174,223] Immunity from enteropathogenic *E. coli* infections has been demonstrated for homologous strains but may not cross over for heterologous strains. Because of the similarity of ETEC LT and cholera toxin, there is great interest in developing vaccines that might prevent both after oral administration. The most promising vaccine so far developed is a whole-cell *V. cholerae* purified binding subunit of LT given in two or three oral doses. It appears that preventing both cholera and ETEC infection[158] might be possible with such a preparation.

SALMONELLA (NONTYPHOIDAL)

Definition

Salmonella infections may result in four different clinical syndromes: gastroenterocolitis, enteric (typhoid) fever, septicemia and focal extraintestinal infection, and asymptomatic carriage.[185] The type of infection depends on organism and host characteristics. Gastroenterocolitis is usually a mild to moderately severe, self-limited illness; it is more correctly termed enterocolitis than gastroenteritis because of the preferential involvement of the lower intestine. Enteric fever is characterized by septicemia with a prolonged toxic course if not treated. In patients infected with *S. choleraesuis* strains, in those with sickle cell disease or previous splenectomy, in newborns or the elderly, or in persons with malignancies, nontyphoid salmonellae may disseminate and produce localized infection including osteomyelitis, meningitis, or an infected aortic aneurysm. In as many as 1% to 3% of persons who have experienced typhoid fever, the organism may continue to be shed in the intestinal tract for 1 year or longer. These persons are chronic carriers. Characteristically, the chronic typhoid carrier is a woman with cholelithiasis.

Microbiology

Salmonellae are nonsporulating, facultatively anaerobic, gram-negative rods. The genus *Salmonella* is composed of more than 2000 serotypes, which are further broken down into phages or serotypes. *S. typhi,* the cause of typhoid fever, is the most virulent. Paratyphoid fever is a similar but generally milder illness caused by *S. paratyphi* A, B, and C. These enteric fever organisms are further distinguished by their adaptation to humans as the primary host. Although numerous other serotypes are capable of causing enteric fever, illness is usually limited to gastroenteritis.[37,185] New serotypes occasionally become prominent, but the majority of human infections are caused by only 10 serotypes; the most common is *S. typhimurium.*[185]

Distribution and Incidence

Nontyphoid salmonellal organisms infect nearly all animal species, including wild, farm, and household animals. Thus a zoonosis of immense proportions exists. Although salmonellae do not form spores, they may remain dormant in a desiccated state.[126] In fresh water they behave like other enteric bacteria, persisting 2 to 14 days.[40] Human infection from *Salmonella* is a global problem. In the United States the reported incidence of *S. typhi* infection has decreased to about 500 cases per year; most are imported by travelers to endemic areas, and only one fourth are domestically acquired from common source outbreaks.[42] This species remains endemic in large areas of the developing world, where it is passed primarily through contaminated water. Nontyphoidal *Salmonella* enteritis continues to be a major problem worldwide, but particularly so in industrialized countries. The Centers for Disease Control and Prevention (CDC) estimates that the 25,000 human cases of nontyphoid salmonellosis reported annually in the United States represent less than 1% of the actual number of clinical cases.[39] Water-borne outbreaks generally account for 1% of these infections, underscoring the point that food is the major source of infection.

Transmission and Epidemiology

Salmonella is the most common identifiable cause of food-borne illness. Contamination may occur from the animal feed, at slaughter, or most commonly, during food preparation. Because the infectious dose is relatively high, averaging 10^3 to 10^6 organisms (much lower in water),[23] the bacteria must multiply on or in food. This accounts for the high summer case incidence, when refrigeration may not be adequate.[39] The foods most commonly implicated are meat, dairy products (especially unpasteurized), poultry, and eggs. Person-to-person spread accounts for 10% of cases, but 20% to 35% of household contacts may become infected.[42,126] *Salmonella* is an occasional cause of traveler's diarrhea; its incidence ranges from zero to 15%.[18,204]

Salmonellosis primarily affects children and the elderly. Of reported isolates in the United States, 55% are from persons under 5 years of age. The organism has an unexplained propensity to infect infants under 1 year of age, and these infants may experience a serious systemic infection including sepsis and meningitis. Greater susceptibility has also been observed in patients with gastrectomy, hemolytic disorders (sickle cell anemia), parasitic infections (such as malaria and schistosomiasis), and chronic illness (such as malignancies and liver disease).[39,126] Normal gastric acid, gut motility, bacterial flora, and poorly understood immune factors are elements in host resistance. Bacterial virulence factors, the vehicle of transmission, and infectious dose are the major determinants of infection. Higher doses result in higher attack rates, lower rates of asymptomatic infection, and shorter incubation periods.[23]

Pathogenesis and Pathophysiology

Salmonella infections involve mucosal invasion and possibly enterotoxin production.[141] After surviving the gastric acid barrier, the organisms reproduce in the gut, where they attach to the wall of the ileum and colon, inducing local degeneration of the microvilli. Invasion occurs via vacuolization, which transports the organism through the mucosal cell, discharging it into the lamina propria. Presumably, entry into the bloodstream occurs here. At this point, *Salmonella* organisms that cause enteric fever (but not those causing enterocolitis) enter and multiply within lymphatic tissue and phagocytic cells.[39] The mechanism of diarrhea in enterocolitis is not clear. A heat-stable enterotoxin has been identified that acts in a different fashion from that of *E. coli* or *V. cholerae*. In most cases, local inflammation of the bowel wall is not severe enough to cause mucosal sloughing and dysentery.

Clinical Syndromes

The incubation for typhoid fever is 1 to 2 weeks; for intestinal infections it is only 8 to 48 hours.[39,185] In cases of food-borne infection by nontyphoid *Salmonella*, the patient often is awakened with symptoms from food eaten the day before or the symptoms begin on rising in the morning. Nausea, vomiting, malaise, headache, and low-grade fever may precede abdominal cramps and diarrhea. Stools are usually foul, green-brown to watery, with variable amounts of mucus, blood, and leukocytes. Cholera-like fluid loss occurs rarely, as does dysentery with grossly bloody and mucoid stools. The acute phase lasts only a few days. Asymptomatic excretion of organisms in the stool continues for 4 to 8 weeks, but chronic carriers are extremely rare. Children and infants routinely experience longer illnesses (average 8 days) with more complications. Among all ages, transient bacteremia is common, accounting for a significant isolation of *Salmonella* types from blood.[39,185] Fever and malaise occurring more than 1 week after resolution of enterocolitis symptoms suggest a suppurative complication or another diagnosis.[126,185] *Salmonella* bacteremia occurs in 5% to 10% of infections and is not distinguishable from other causes of sepsis. Focal infections may be seen in any organ.[39,185] Sites adjacent to bowel are most common; meningitis, pneumonia, osteomyelitis, pyelonephritis, and endocarditis are rare.[185] Mortality is highest at the extremes of age, but deaths occur in all age groups, even in the United States.

Diagnosis

Diagnosis of enterocolitis can be made by clinical presentation and isolation of *Salmonella* organisms from stool or rectal swabs cultured onto selective media (MacConkey or *Salmonella-Shigella* agar). Blood cultures (or bone marrow aspirates) for *S. typhi* are used to diagnose enteric or typhoid fever. Stool cultures are often negative early in the disease. The Widal serologic test is useful to diagnose typhoid fever in endemic countries. In industrialized areas it is not useful because of the more frequent occurrence of antibody development to cross-reacting nontyphoid gram-negative antigens.

Treatment

Supportive treatment with fluids is sufficient therapy for most cases of *Salmonella* enterocolitis. In uncomplicated infections, antibiotics are not indicated. They do not shorten the illness but prolong the carrier state, with excretion of organisms in the stool, and encourage development of resistant strains.[7] Patients with underlying debility that may dispose to septicemia or localized infection (immunocompromised persons or very young infants) are generally treated with antibiotics, as in enteric fever. The new fluoroquinolones probably shorten the duration of fever and diarrhea in salmonellosis[67,161] and should be used in patients with severe or toxic illness. All patients with enteric (typhoid) fever or septicemic salmonellosis and those in whom local tissue suppuration is diagnosed are treated with antibiotics. As for typhoid fever, the drug of choice is chloramphenicol 25 to 50 mg/kg/day in divided doses every 6 hours. Alternative therapy is ampicillin (100 mg/kg/day in three or four divided doses) or trimethoprim (160 mg) with sulfamethoxazole (800 mg) twice daily for 2 weeks. In our opinion the drugs of choice for enteric fever in the United States are the fluoroquinolones. These drugs can be given for a shorter duration (10 versus 14 days), resistance to them is essentially nil, and posttreatment carriage of *S. typhi* is probably reduced.[80] Local suppuration may require 2 to 6 weeks of antibiotics, depending on the adequacy of surgical drainage.[126]

Immunology

Immunity to *Salmonella* is serotype specific. Vaccines have not been successful for nontyphoid *Salmonella* because of the number of serotypes. For typhoid fever, immunoprophylaxis is possible. Currently there are two commercially available and protective vaccines. The first is a live attenuated strain Ty21a that is given as one oral dose every other day for four doses.[91] The second is a Vi polysaccharide preparation given as a single parenteral immunization.[1] Both preparations are of approximately equal cost and effectiveness.

SHIGELLA

Microbiology

Dysentery has been described since biblical times. At the end of the nineteenth century, Shiga first identified *Shigella dysenteriae* as the cause of epidemic disease in Japan. Shigellosis has since become synonymous with bacterial dysentery, although other bacteria and protozoa are capable of causing the bloody and mucoid stools that define the dysentery syndrome.

Shigellae are thin, nonmotile, nonsporulating, and gram-negative rods in the Enterobacteriaceae family. There are four species or groups: A *(S. dysenteriae)*, B *(S. flexneri)*, C *(S. boydii)*, and D *(S. sonnei)*; the first three contain numerous serotypes.

Distribution

Shigellosis occurs worldwide. *S. dysenteriae* 1 (the Shiga bacillus), which produces an especially severe disease, is most common in developing countries. An unusually severe epidemic affected large parts of Central America and Asia in the late 1960s and early 1970s. In the United States, *Shigella* remains endemic, with *S. sonnei* the most common etiologic agent. *S. sonnei* is replacing *S. flexneri* as the most common isolate in the United States and in many other areas of the world, particularly in more industrialized regions.

Transmission and Epidemiology

Humans and certain primates are the only hosts for *Shigella*. Fecal-oral contamination is the mode of spread. Common source infections occur via fecally polluted water or food prepared by contaminated hands. Shigellae can survive freezing and thawing in ice cubes. With an infectious dose as low as 10 to 200 organisms,[69] person-to-person spread is common. This accounts for persistent endemic foci (even in countries with good sanitation) and high rates of transmission among groups in close physical contact (such as homosexuals and children), groups with poor hygiene (such as mentally retarded patients and children), and those who lack sanitary facilities and wash water (such as populations in developing countries and Native Americans on reservations). Long-term carriage of *Shigella* is unusual. *Shigella* is a potential pathogen in the American wilderness. Environmental persistence averages 3 to 4 weeks, with best survival in cool fresh water. Two documented outbreaks of dysenteric illness caused by *S. sonnei* occurred among Grand Canyon river rafting crews and passengers in 1972 and 1979.[38,137] A common source was never found, but the epidemics were halted by improved sanitary practices (hand washing) among guides and passengers and careful attention to water disinfection.

Pathogenesis and Pathophysiology

The essential virulence factor of *Shigella* is invasiveness associated with a large (120 to 140 megadaltons) plasmid. *Shigella* organisms invade and proliferate within the epithelium of the large bowel, producing well-demarcated ulcers with cellular infiltrates (chiefly polymorphonuclear) and an overlying suppurative exudate. Organisms have also been demonstrated in the small bowel, but these have reduced potential for invasion or marked changes in the mucosa. Here they cause profuse watery fluid loss, possibly mediated by an enterotoxin.

Clinical Syndromes

Attack rates in nonimmune volunteers are dose dependent. As with most enteric pathogens, infection with *Shigella* may be asymptomatic, mild, or severe, depending on a combination of host and organism factors. Two distinct diarrheal syndromes may occur separately or sequentially in shigellosis. After an incubation period, which averages 1 to 3 days, illness begins with malaise, headache, nausea, fever, abdominal cramps, and watery diarrhea. This illness represents small bowel infection, so clinically it resembles other forms of acute watery diarrhea. In certain children with this form of the disease, the presentation is fever with or without a febrile seizure; diarrhea occurs only later. In the second and classic form of shigellosis, usually following the first small bowel phase of the disease, colonic involvement causes progression to clinical dysentery after 1 to 3 days' illness.[57] In the dysenteric form of the illness, stools decrease in volume and increase in frequency, with passage of up to 20 to 30 movements a day; gross blood is found in stool. These patients complain of fecal urgency and often tenesmus. Fever is seen in most of the dysenteric cases and between one third and one half of cases of shigellosis overall. Vomiting is seen in about half. Mild abdominal tenderness is common, but peritoneal signs are not. The natural course of shigellosis is as varied as the illness. Most cases resolve spontaneously within 7 days, but others may persist for weeks.[57] *S. dysenteriae* occurring in developing tropical countries may result in a mortality rate as high as 25% when untreated.[130] With treatment, mortality is less than 1%.

Complications

Several potential complications may occur. Febrile convulsions are seen in young children with shigellosis.[97] Pneumonitis may complicate *Shigella* infection. A severe leukemoid reaction with white cell count up to 50,000 may occur after apparent clinical improvement in patients who have manifested high fever and severe colitis. In some patients hemolytic-uremic syndrome associated with disseminated intravascular coagulation develops, probably induced by immune complexes. This complication is characteristic of infection caused by strains that produce Shiga *(S. dysenteriae* 1*)* toxin. Manifestations of Reiter's syndrome are occasionally seen. Septicemia follows in less than 5% of *Shigella* infections; metastatic abscesses occur but are rare. Severe anemia and hypoalbuminemia may result from bowel blood and protein losses.

Laboratory

Laboratory tests often show a mild leukocytosis with a shift to the left (increase in number of immature granulocytes). If dysentery is present, microscopic examination of the stool shows countless white (polymorphonuclear) and red blood cells, but this is not specific to shigellosis. Diagnosis is made by stool culture on selective media (MacConkey or *Salmonella-Shigella* agar), which is positive in most symptomatic patients.[57] Fresh stools or sigmoidoscopic scrapings are the best source of culture material; saturated cotton swabs from the rectum, although not as reliable, can be used if plated rapidly or placed in a holding media. In patients with toxic conditions and where hospitalization is planned, blood cultures should be obtained.

Treatment

Therapy is first oriented toward fluid replacement. Although large-volume diarrhea is unusual, significant dehydration may occur, especially in children. Antimotility drugs should be avoided in patients with signs of toxicity; however, these medications are unlikely to be detrimental in mild to moderate cases without fever and dysentery. Normal motility is believed to be protective to the bowel.[56] Patients with fever and dysentery should be treated with antimicrobial agents, since these drugs decrease the duration of fever, diarrhea, and excretion of *Shigella* in stool. Conventional therapy is with TMP-SMX, although in some parts of the world TMP resistance is occurring with important frequency. Known community patterns and in vitro susceptibilities should guide antibiotic use. The dose of trimethoprim-sulfamethoxazole for adults is 160 mg/800 mg (one double-strength tablet) twice a day for 3 to 5 days, and for children, 10 mg/kg/day of trimethoprim and 50 mg/kg/day of sulfamethoxazole in two divided doses per day for 3 to 5 days. Recommended therapy for adult patients infected with TMP-resistant strains or when illness occurs in areas where susceptibility to TMP is unknown is with the fluoroquinolones: norfloxacin 400 mg, ciprofloxacin 500 mg, or ofloxacin 300 mg twice a day or fleroxacin 400 mg/day for 3 to 5 days. Single-dose therapy is probably effective in milder forms of illness. The newer quinolones cannot be used in children because of possible damage to articular cartilage. For children in areas where TMP resistance occurs, nalidixic acid, furazolidone (not effective in severe illness), or TMP-SMX plus erythromycin may be used.

Immunology

Immunity to homologous strains follows natural infection.[59] Attempts to develop an effective anti-*Shigella* vaccine are under way, aided by the limited number of serotypes involved in cases of illness.

CAMPYLOBACTER

Microbiology

The organism is a small, curved, gram-negative rod, formerly classified as *Vibrio. Campylobacter jejuni* strains are widespread in the environment. The major reservoir is animals, including dogs, cattle, birds, horses, goats, pigs, cats, and sheep. The most important source for human illness is poultry. Epidemics have been associated with ingestion of raw milk.[25] *C. jejuni* has been isolated from surface water and can survive up to 5 weeks in cold water, ensuring its potential for wilderness water-borne spread.

Transmission and Epidemiology

Most epidemics of gastroenteritis have been through food or, less commonly, water. Person-to-person spread occurs but is uncommon. During the summers of 1980 and 1981, *C. jejuni* was isolated from 23% of persons with diarrheal disease acquired in the area of Grand Teton National Park, associated with ingestion of untreated surface water. This was the leading identifiable cause of diarrhea, followed by *G. lamblia,* which was identified in 8% of diarrhea cases. The organism has been cultured from populations worldwide.[22,33] Traveler's diarrhea is caused by *C. jejuni* in about 3% of cases in rainy summertime and in 15% of cases during dryer wintertime.[134] In the largest American water-borne epidemic the attack rate was 20%. Studies in the United States and abroad have demonstrated that *C. jejuni* can explain up to 25% of patients with gastroenteritis, which is nearly always more frequent than *Salmonella* (except during the time of extensive food-borne outbreaks) and often more common in occurrence than *Shigella* species.[26,27,83] The organism has emerged as the leading identifiable cause of bacterial enteritis in the United States. Rates are highest among children and young adults.[27,83]

Pathogenicity

The pathogenic mechanism is unclear. All segments of the small and large intestine may be affected, accounting for the variety of diarrheal symptoms. There is evidence of tissue invasion, since the organism may be cultured from blood. Colitis with cellular infiltration is characteristically noted on biopsy. A heat-labile enterotoxin produced by *C. jejuni* strains may play a role in disease pathogenesis.

Clinical Syndromes

The incubation period of *C. jejuni* enteritis is 2 to 7 days, averaging 4 days. The clinical symptoms are extremely variable and nonspecific. There is often a 1-day prodrome of general malaise and fever before diarrhea begins. Abdominal cramps and pain herald the onset of diarrhea, with up to eight bowel movements a day, which are initially watery and frequently turn bile stained or bloody. The frequencies of reported symptoms are diarrhea (75% to 95%), cramps and abdominal pain (80% to 90%), nausea (20% to 50%), headache (50%), fever (50% to 80%), vomiting (20%), and bloody diarrhea (10% to 50%).[24-27,150] Tenesmus is unusual. Examination is nonspecific, with variable degrees of fever (averaging 40° C), abdominal tenderness, and dehydration. Microscopic evaluation of stool shows blood and polymorphonuclear cells in 60% to 75% of samples.[26,33] The enteric symptoms subside in 2 to 4 days, and the entire illness resolves spontaneously within 1 week. Organisms are shed in the stool for 3 to 5 weeks after resolution of symptoms, but chronic carrier states have not been described. Twenty percent of patients suffer relapse, usually less severe than the original symptoms.[26] Chronic diarrhea caused by *C. jejuni* has been reported in children and adults but is usually associated with important underlying disease. *C. jejuni* infection has been associated with Guillain-Barré syndrome.

Diagnosis

Diagnosis is made by culturing stool on a selective medium (such as Skirrow, Butzler, or Campy-BAP). Severe cases with fever and bloody diarrhea are more likely to be positive by culture. Extraintestinal sources account for 0.4% of positive *Campylobacter* cultures in the United States. Blood is the most common site, followed by the gallbladder and cerebrospinal fluid (in children). Most cases of septicemia are preceded by gastroenteritis, but since blood cultures are rarely drawn in the evaluation of gastroenteritis, the frequency of bacteremia is unknown. Predisposing factors are usually present in septicemic patients.

Treatment

Treatment is primarily supportive with oral fluids; dehydration is usually mild. Most patients have improved by the time the culture results return and do well without antibiotics. Antibiotic treatment has not been proven conclusively to be effective in improving *C. jejuni* gastroenteritis. One study demonstrated no significant effect when antibiotics were started 4 days after the onset of symptoms,[5] but earlier therapy appears to be effective.[161] Antibiotic therapy eradicates the organism from the stool within 48 hours. The antibiotic of choice is probably erythromycin: for adults, 250 to 500 mg every 6 hours for 5 days, and for children, 20 to 50 mg/kg every 6 hours. Alternative therapy for adults is the fluoroquinolones (norfloxacin, ciprofloxacin, ofloxacin, or fleroxacin) given in the same doses as outlined in the section on therapy for shigellosis (above). A major advantage of quinolones for therapy is that they can be given to patients with febrile dysentery in view of the drugs' activity against the major causes: *C. jejuni, Shigella,* and less commonly, *Salmonella.*

VIBRIOS

Microbiology

Vibrio cholerae 0 group 1 (01) is responsible for cholera. The organism is a motile, curved, gram-negative rod. Pathogenic strains have two major biotypes, classic and El Tor, which produce similar clinical illness; each contains two main serotypes, Ogawa and Inaba. Non-01 *V. cholerae* strains also produce diarrheal illness, but they show less potential for epidemic disease. Nine species of *Vibrio* other than *V. cholerae* have been associated with human disease. Most are associated with gastroenteritis: *V. parahaemolyticus, V. fluvialis, V. mimicus, V. hollisae,* and *V. furnissii.* Others, mainly *V. vulnificus,* are associated with wound infections and septicemia (see Chapter 53). All are halophilic, gram-negative rods that reside in seawater and on marine organisms. Infection is acquired by ingesting infected and undercooked seafood or by contamination of a wound with infected water. The most significant gastrointestinal pathogen in this group is *V. parahaemolyticus.*[28,195] For a full discussion of *Vibrio* species, see Chapter 53.

Epidemiology

V. cholerae has accounted for seven deadly worldwide pandemics since the early 1800s. The last began in 1961 in Indonesia and spread throughout Southeast Asia, the Middle East, Africa, parts of the Pacific and Europe, and then to South America. In 1973, cholera resurfaced in the United States after an absence since 1911. Since the early 1970s, small numbers of cases have occurred along the Gulf Coast of Louisiana and Texas. New domestic cases continue to be reported.[35] It is of interest that between 1961 and 1981, only 10 cases of cholera were reported in travelers returning from endemic areas. In January 1991, cholera was reported in the coastal regions of Peru and in Lima. Over the next 2 years it progressed to many regions of Latin America, moving as close to the United States as northern Mexico. The infection has been associated with the consumption of uncooked or poorly handled seafood. Cholera continues to be a disease of the poor and lower socioeconomic groups; provided some care is exerted in the foods consumed, it should be a minimal risk to travelers. The risk to travelers has been estimated to be approximately 1:500,000 during a journey to an endemic area.[140,191,199]

V. parahaemolyticus causes 70% of food-borne gastroenteritis in Japan, where large amounts of raw seafood are eaten, and sporadic outbreaks in the United States.[28] It has been found to be a common cause of traveler's diarrhea in Thailand. Transmission has been associated with a variety of seafood, but drinking water and person-to-person spread have not been implicated.

Distribution and Transmission

Humans are not the sole reservoir for *V. cholerae* 01; environmental habitation exists, especially in marine or brackish waters.[135] As with related vibrios (*Vibrio parahaemolyticus* and non-01 *V. cholerae* strains), shellfish ingest and carry these organisms (see Chapter 53). Fecal-oral spread is the major mechanism of transmission, and water is the most common vehicle, followed by food.[42] The organism remains viable for days to weeks in various foods. The infective dose is large, requiring between 10^6 to 10^{10} organisms,[40,105] so person-to-person spread is uncommon. Gastric acid acts as a barrier; ingestion of bacteria with food, milk, or bicarbonate lowers the infectious dose.[40,105]

Most cases of gastroenteritis caused by noncholera vibrios have been associated with ingestion of raw oysters and other seafoods. Cases have been reported from travelers, particularly after visits to coastal areas of Southeast Asia and Latin America. Like other vibrios, the bacteria are commonly found in bays, estuaries, and brackish inland lakes. Some strains produce an enterotoxin, but generally it is not cholera-like toxin. Intestinal illness is associated with diarrhea, abdominal cramps, and fever. Nausea and vomiting occur in about 20% of cases. Diarrhea may be severe, with up to 20 to 30 watery stools per day. In 25% of cases, diarrhea is bloody. Duration of illness averages less than 48 hours in some outbreaks, and up to 6 days (range 2 to 12) in others. Treatment considerations are the same as for cholera.

Pathophysiology

After passing through the stomach, the organism multiplies and colonizes the small bowel. In cholera, no pathologic changes are noted in the bowel wall. The local effects of enterotoxin account for the pathophysiology of cholera. Cholera enterotoxin has been studied extensively.[141]

Binding subunits attach the toxin to the cell membrane of the mucosa, after which the cyclase-activating unit enters the cell. The enzyme acts inside the serosal cell, enhancing production of cyclic adenosine monophosphate. This produces a 70% reduction in influx of water, saline, and a wide range of other molecules into the gut mucosal cells, resulting in watery diarrhea. Glucose, potassium, bicarbonate, and most significantly, glucose-linked enhancement of sodium and water absorption remain intact. Thus, while plain water worsens cholera diarrhea, the addition of glucose renders the water and essential electrolytes absorbable, forming the basis for oral rehydration therapy.[44,160]

Details of the pathogenesis of infection by the noncholera vibrios are unclear. In the case of *V. parahaemolyticus,* a hemolytic toxin was thought to explain its effects, but dysenteric illness implies invasion and another enterotoxin has been found in some strains.[28] As yet, there is no reliable test to separate enteropathogenic from harmless marine strains.

Clinical Syndromes

Some cholera infections are asymptomatic, and 60% to 80% of clinical cases are mild diarrheal illnesses that never raise suspicion for cholera.[105,110] After an incubation period of 2 days (range 1 to 5 days), fluid accumulates in the gut, causing intestinal distention and diarrhea. Diarrhea may begin as brown colored but soon assumes the translucent gray appearance known as rice-water stools. In serious cases, stool volume may reach 1 L/hr, leading to severe dehydration, acidosis, shock, and death. Vomiting may occur as a result of gut distention or acidosis.

The clinical syndrome caused by noncholera vibrios is not highly characteristic. In outbreaks of *V. parahaemolyticus* infection, explosive diarrhea associated with abdominal cramps and nausea is often described. Vomiting occurs in about 50% and fever in about 30% of cases. In Asia a dysentery-like syndrome with mucoid bloody diarrhea is commonly seen, but this presentation has been infrequent in infections acquired in the United States.[15,28] Infections are usually brief, lasting an average of 3 days, with spontaneous resolution.

Diagnosis

Infection by a vibrio can be diagnosed in several ways. In the case of *V. cholerae,* darkfield microscopic examination of fresh stools may reveal the characteristic helical vibrio motion. More commonly, diagnosis for any of the vibrios is made by stool culture on suitable media (such as TCBS). Vibrios survive for 1 week on a stool-saturated piece of filter paper sealed in a plastic bag.

Treatment

Severe untreated cholera has a 50% mortality, which may be reduced to 1% with appropriate treatment. Children are at higher risk for complications and death. Fluid and electrolyte replacement must be aggressive. With fluid replacement, most cases of cholera last 3 to 5 days, with the peak fluid losses 24 hours after the onset of illness. When hypotension or persistent vomiting is present, intravenous fluids are necessary. As soon as initial rehydration is complete, oral rehydration solutions are used for maintenance. Less than 5% of patients require intravenous maintenance after initial rehydration. Oral rehydration alone is successful in 90% of cholera cases without shock. With voluminous losses, rehydration fluid can be given by nasogastric tube to continue fluids during the night. A normal or light diet should be resumed early in the course of treatment, after initial rehydration. Antibiotics shorten the duration of diarrhea and excretion of organisms in severe cholera and reduce fluid losses but are not as important as fluid therapy.[142] Oral antibiotics can be started within a few hours of initial rehydration. The drug of choice is tetracycline, 500 mg every 6 hours for 2 days for adults, and 50 mg/kg/day in four divided doses for children. This is perhaps the only indication for the use of tetracycline in children; a short course (2 to 4 days) is unlikely to stain teeth. Furazolidone (100 mg every 6 hours for adults and 5 mg/kg/day in four divided doses for children) for 2 days may be used. *V. cholerae* strains are also susceptible to the new fluoroquinolones.

Treatment of patients infected with noncholera vibrios should also focus on fluid replacement. Little information exists on the benefit of antibiotic therapy for gastrointestinal disease, but it is reasonable in dysentery-like cases or prolonged illness. Tetracycline, furazolidone, or a quinolone is the drug of choice.

Immunology

Immunity exists to homologous but not to heterologous strains of cholera.[104] The current parenteral vaccine is only about 50% effective in reducing attack rates over a 3- to 6-month period for those living in endemic areas; it has no antitoxin activity. It is recommended for persons who live and work under poor sanitary conditions in highly endemic areas and for those with compromised gastric defenses. Vaccination of residents is not practical in endemic areas, and the current vaccine is not recommended for travelers to endemic areas.

YERSINIA ENTEROCOLITICA

Microbiology and Epidemiology

Y. enterocolitica is a facultative, anaerobic, gram-negative rod in the Enterobacteriaceae family. The major natural reservoir of the organism is animals. Human disease strains have been isolated from wild, farm, and domestic animals; rodents and rat fleas can also harbor the organism. The organism resides in United States and European surface and unchlorinated well waters. In a California wilderness area, 10 strains were recovered from 34 high-elevation lakes and streams. The source was likely to be animals, since some of the lakes were infrequently visited by humans. The evidence, which is scant, indicates that persistence in warm water is fairly brief, ranging from days to weeks, with longer survival at colder temperatures. Human isolates of *Y. enterocolitica* are found worldwide but have been most frequently reported from Canada and northern European countries, with an incidence equal to or greater than those of *Salmonella* and *Shigella*.[129] Transmission occurs from fecal-oral contamination, via food and water, and probably via person-to-person or animal-to-person contact.[40,42,129] Transmission of *Y. enterocolitica* from surface water was suspected in an outbreak of gastrointestinal illness at a Montana ski resort and in a case of septicemia from an Adirondack hunting camp. Untreated spring water used to package tofu accounted for 87 cases of illness in Washington State. Raw milk and oysters have also been implicated as vehicles for transmission. The infectious dose and attack rate are not well studied. Patterns of common source transmission suggest a large infectious dose. The incubation period averages 3 to 7 days.

Clinical Syndromes

Illness caused by *Y. enterocolitica* may involve three mechanisms: bowel mucosa invasion, a heat-stable enterotoxin similar to that produced by ETEC, and a cytotoxin.[210] The organism multiplies in the small bowel and invades the mucosa at the terminal ileum and colon. The mucosa may be diffusely inflamed with small and shallow ulcerations. Some bacteria migrate through lymphatics to mesenteric lymph nodes, producing adenitis with focal areas of necrosis. The most common clinical presentation is gastroenteritis, characterized by diarrhea, fever, and abdominal pain. Nausea and vomiting occur in 20% to 40% of patients. About 10% to 25% of affected persons report bloody stools.[35,129,209] Fever or abdominal pain without much diarrhea may be the most prominent sign. In 20% of patients with positive stool cultures, the symptoms and signs mimic appendicitis, more commonly in adolescents.[209,210] Although acute appendicitis has been associated with serologic evidence of *Y. enterocolitica* infection, the usual operative findings are mesenteric adenitis or terminal ileitis. In some adults prominent symptoms of colitis develop, with blood and pus in the stools. Severe colitis rarely results in extensive necrosis, perforation, and septicemia. Numerous extraintestinal manifestations of *Y. enterocolitica* infection include skin rash (erythema nodosum or maculopapular) and arthritis, probably related to an immune reaction. Extraintestinal infection involving lung, joints, lymph nodes, wounds, or septicemia may occur with or without enteritis. In one outbreak of 56 culture-positive patients, 38 had enteritis, 6 had only extraintestinal infection, and 4 had both enteritis and extraintestinal infection. In the majority of infections, illness is mild and self-limited, with duration averaging 1 week, but some patients experience prolonged symptoms.[34,129,209,210] Excretion of the organism in stool continues for a few weeks to months. Complications may be related to particularly severe disease or misdiagnosis of Crohn's disease or appendicitis.

Diagnosis

The diagnosis of yersiniosis is usually made by stool culture. The organism grows better at lower (22° to 25° C) temperatures, which inhibit most other enteric bacteria. Abnormalities related to ileitis or colitis seen on contrast radiography and endoscopy may be mistaken for other causes of colitis.[209,210] Occasionally, blood or surgical specimen cultures identify the organism. Serologic tests by agglutination titer or the enzyme-linked immunosorbent assay (ELISA) are also diagnostic and especially helpful to diagnose *Yersinia* arthritis.

Treatment

Tetracycline has been suggested as the drug of first choice for chronic or fulminant infections.[8] Most isolates are sensitive in vitro to streptomycin, chloramphenicol, aminoglycosides, tetracyclines, the fluoroquinolones, and TMP-SMX. Most are resistant to penicillins and cephalosporins and variably resistant to erythromycin and sulfonamides.[209]

AEROMONAS SPECIES AND PLESIOMONAS SHIGELLOIDES

Aeromonas and *Plesiomonas shigelloides* are gram-negative, facultatively anaerobic, nonsporulating rods that are members of the Vibrionaceae family (commonly misidentified as Enterobacteriaceae). They have recently been placed into separate genuses. Like the noncholera vibrios, their normal habitats are water and soil. They have been implicated in a variety of human illnesses, most commonly gastroenteritis.[48,211] *Aeromonas* contains three species, two of which are associated with human disease. *A. hydrophila* is most commonly isolated. It has been found in 3% of asymptomatic patients' stools in the United States and in 30% in Thailand. It has been associated with diarrheal illness in the United States, Australia, travelers from Asia, and Peace Corps members in Thailand.[89,102] Association of illness with drinking untreated spring or well water was demonstrated in the United States. Pathogenicity has been shown in the laboratory to result from an enterotoxin with cytotoxic and hemolytic effects.[36,43,125,166] *A. sobria* has been isolated in cases of human diarrheal illness and found to have pathogenic properties similar to those of *A. hydrophila*. Infections of soft tissue and septicemia have yielded *Aeromonas,* usually associated with submersion incidents or exposure of wounds to water.[42,211] Clinical illness associated with enteric infection by *A. hydrophila* varies from acute to chronic, and from watery stools to dysentery with colitis.[48,89,102,148,166] Median duration of diarrhea is 2 weeks with occasional cases that persist a month or longer.[89,94,102] Treatment trials in enteritis have not been conclusive[48]; good response to TMP-SMX (160/800 mg twice daily for 5 days) has been noted.[89,95,102] Isolates are usually susceptible to chloramphenicol, tetracycline, TMP-SMX, fluoroquinolones, and aminoglycosides. They are resistant to penicillin and ampicillin and variably sensitive to erythromycin and cephalothin.

P. shigelloides has been isolated from patients with gastroenteritis[103,159] and is associated with foreign travel and ingestion of raw shellfish. It may cause a self-limited dysenteric illness suggestive of an invasive organism. However, laboratory studies have failed to demonstrate pathogenic mechanisms and adult volunteer studies have not established organism pathogenicity.[166]

VIRAL GASTROENTERITIS

Recent advances in detection have identified viruses as major causes of diarrheal disease (acute nonbacterial gastrointestinal infections) that had formerly been classified as of unknown etiology.[10,21] The most important defined agents are Norwalk virus and rotavirus. They cause watery diarrhea, frequently associated with vomiting. Transmission occurs via fecal-oral contamination. Although airborne spread has been suspected, it has not been proven. Respiratory symptoms are common in patients with viral gastroenteritis. Many viruses have been suspected or implicated in diarrheal disease, but their incidence is low or proof is lacking. Diagnosis of viral gastroenteritis is made by detecting antigens in stool (in the case of rotavirus infection) or immune electron microscopy of feces, radioimmunoassay or ELISA of stool and blood, and paired serologic titers for Norwalk virus and the other small round viral particles. Rotavirus testing reagents are commercially available, while for the small round particles, the diagnostic reagents are limited to research laboratories. Norwalk virus testing reagents may be available soon for routine use.

Norwalk and the Norwalk-Like Viruses

Norwalk agents and related viruses are 27 nm particles related to caliciviruses. They cause epidemic outbreaks of gastrointestinal illness previously called "winter vomiting disease" because of the seasonal incidence and prominence of vomiting. The CDC found that 40% of nonbacterial gastroenteritis outbreaks investigated between 1976 to 1980 were caused by Norwalk virus. Infection is spread by common-source vehicles with secondary person-to-person spread.[42,115,207] So far, humans are the only known carriers of these viruses. An outbreak of diarrheal illness, presumed to be of viral etiology, was linked to water consumption from a spring in Yellowstone National Park. Norwalk gastroenteritis has been implicated as a cause of traveler's diarrhea,[107] as well as diarrhea from recreational area water ingestion and contact. Electron microscopy demonstrates changes in the mucosal surface of the proximal small intestine, concurrent with diarrhea, which return to normal within 1 to 2 weeks. Malabsorption of fat, lactose, and xylose occurs in conjunction with these histologic changes. The mechanism of diarrheal production in viral gastroenteritis is unknown. Small numbers of viral particles are shed in the stool during the acute illness, but prolonged carrier states are not seen. Attack rates of 50% to 75% are commonly seen during outbreaks.[21,42,207] After an incubation period of 24 to 48 hours, illness begins abruptly with vomiting, abdominal cramps, and diarrhea.[21] Among children, vomiting occurs in the majority of cases more frequently than does diarrhea. Stools do not contain blood or leukocytes. Other common symptoms include low-grade fever, malaise, myalgias, respiratory symptoms, and headache. Illness is almost always mild, lasting 1 to 2 days, and recovery is without sequelae.

Supportive treatment with oral fluids is sufficient in the vast majority of cases. Some malabsorption of fats and disaccharides persists after the acute illness. Deaths involve elderly and debilitated patients. In the United States, antibodies commonly appear during late adolescence, but in tropical, developing countries, children experience infection and acquire antibodies at a young age. Although antibodies persist in most people, they do not provide protection from clinical illness. Reinfection and illness occur in persons with demonstrable serum antibodies, while those without the antibodies may not become infected. This has suggested that certain persons are resistant to Norwalk infection, based on the lack or absence of intestinal receptors for the virus. Vaccine development is not currently feasible because of difficulties culturing the virus, lack of animal models, and the low level of excretion in stool.

Rotavirus

Rotaviruses are 70 nm RNA viruses. Infection tends to be endemic, with peak incidence during the winter months in temperate climates. Transmission is by person-to-person contact. Common-source outbreaks are uncommon, but a water-borne outbreak was reported in a Colorado ski resort in 1981. Rotavirus has been found in almost every animal species, and transmission of illness from human to animal has also been shown. Rotavirus is the most frequently isolated pathogen in infantile diarrhea[19,20,90,223] and is responsible for a disproportionate amount of hospitalization for dehydration.[20,190] The majority of symptomatic infections occur in children under 5 years old with peak incidence in children 6 months to 2 years of age. Rotavirus can also cause illness in adults, usually associated with secondary spread within a family. It has been implicated in traveler's diarrhea occurring in Mexico.[29,178] Nonspecific pathologic changes are seen in small bowel epithelial cells with particles identified intracellularly. The exact mechanism of diarrhea is unknown, but a net secretion of water, sodium, and chloride occurs during the illness. Diarrheal losses contain 30 to 40 mEq/L each of sodium and potassium. Lactose malabsorption may persist for 1 to 2 weeks, associated with continued viral excretion in stool. Large numbers of virus particles are shed in the stool of ill patients, but prolonged excretion is unusual. After an incubation period of 24 to 72 hours, illness begins with vomiting, followed by diarrhea associated with abdominal cramps, low-grade fever, and malaise. Vomiting usually resolves within 2 days (range 1 to 5), but the diarrhea lasts 3 to 8 days and occasionally longer. Severity of illness usually decreases with age. Adults are more likely to have asymptomatic or mild illness with less vomiting; however, one study in Thailand showed that adult patients with rotavirus diarrhea were second only to cholera patients in numbers of watery stools and degree of dehydration. In children, dehydration frequently occurs, accounting for appreciable mortality in developing countries. Fortunately, oral electrolyte solutions can be successfully used in the majority of cases.

Serum antibody levels are demonstrated within the first few years of life and in almost all adults but do not appear to be protective. Reinfection occurs at all ages, in some cases caused by different serotypes, yet resistance to infection does occur beyond age 2 or 3 years. Because of the high incidence and morbidity associated with this virus, a vaccine would be beneficial.[219]

INTESTINAL PROTOZOA

Protozoal infections are always beneficial to the protozoa, but may be pathogenic or commensal (little or no effect) to the human host. Pathogenicity has been difficult to prove for some of these protozoa (such as *Giardia*) and is still actively debated in others (such as *Blastocystis hominis*) because even those known to be pathogenic result in commensal infections most of the time. Most protozoal infections are suspected on the basis of subacute or chronic gastrointestinal symptoms, which may fluctuate over time.

Although acute self-limited diarrheal illness may occur, the symptoms are nonspecific and diagnosis is often made fortuitously by stool examination. As with enteric bacteria, symptoms depend on the level of bowel colonized. Those colonizing the small intestine, such as *Giardia* and coccidia, cause a wide spectrum of gastrointestinal complaints, including symptoms of malabsorption (foul stools and flatulence). Weight loss is frequently seen in persistent infections. Although many protozoa are capable of superficial mucosal invasion, only *Entamoeba histolytica* and *Balantidium coli,* which colonize the colon, can ulcerate the bowel wall, cause dysentery, and metastasize to other tissues.

All intestinal protozoa are transmitted by fecal-oral contamination, so infection rates are highest in areas and groups with poor sanitation, close contact, or particular customs favoring transmission. In addition to food, water, and person-to-person contact, mechanical vectors such as flies may spread these organisms. Transmission of intestinal protozoa is favored by a hardy cyst, which is passed in the feces of an infected host. In addition to an infective cyst, the life cycle for most intestinal protozoa includes a trophozoite, which is responsible for reproduction and pathogenicity. Only a single host is required, except for *Sarcocystis,* which requires ingestion of raw meat from an intermediate host. However, zoonoses exist for *Giardia, Cryptosporidium, Entamoeba polecki,* and *B. coli,* with cross-infectivity between humans and animals.

Treatment of intestinal protozoan infections is summarized in Table 42-8.

Giardia Lamblia

G. lamblia is a flagellate protozoan that was observed in 1681 by Leeuwenhoeck. In the last 20 to 30 years it has gained recognition as an important human pathogen.[30,119,153] Agreement of species designation will be decided by application of new biochemical and genetic techniques. The life cycle of *Giardia* involves two forms. Trophozoites are responsible for symptomatic illness. The organisms grow in the duodenum and proximal jejunum, where they attach to the mucosa with an adhesive disk and multiply rapidly via binary fission. Trophozoites are rarely infective because they rapidly die outside the body. Responding to unknown stimuli, some trophozoites encyst and are passed in the stools of infected hosts. Cysts are infectious as passed in the host stool; no period of maturation or intermediate development stage is required. Furthermore, they are very hardy in the external environment. When ingested by a potential host, excystation is stimulated by passage through the stomach, and the motile trophozoite migrates to the small bowel to complete the cycle. All age groups are affected; children have a higher incidence of infection because of lack of hygiene or immunity.[119] Examination of wild and domestic animal feces in Colorado wilderness areas found *Giardia* cysts morphologically similar to *G. lamblia* in beavers, cattle, dogs, and cats. Human-passed cysts have infected beavers, dogs, rodents, and bighorn sheep, while cysts from beavers, dogs, and mule deer have infected humans. Beavers have been blamed for multiple water-borne human epidemics of giardiasis based on finding cyst-passing beavers in the watershed.[16,72] Cross-species transmission experiments can be criticized for lack of controls, failure to ensure absence of natural *Giardia* infection, inability to differentiate brief cyst passage from true infection, and inability to morphologically distinguish various *Giardia* strains.[16,220] Still, giardiasis probably represents a zoonosis with cross-infectivity from animals to humans.

The infective dose of *Giardia* for humans is low[169]; 10 to 25 cysts caused infection in 8 of 25 subjects; more than 25 cysts caused infection in 100%. Person-to-person may be the most common means of transmission. Areas and populations with poor hygiene and close physical contact have higher rates of infection. Venereal transmission occurs among homosexuals through direct fecal-oral contamination.[139] Twenty-five percent of family members with infected children become infected.[30,163] Epidemics and carrier rates of 30% to 60% have been found among children in day care centers, institutions, and Native American reservations. Water is a major vehicle of infection.[41,42] Cysts retain viability in cold water for as long as 2 to 3 months. In the United States from 1964 to 1984, 90 outbreaks (24,000

Table 42-8 Therapy for Parasitic Infections

Etiologic Agent	Indication	Drug and Duration
Giardia lamblia	Proven disease	Quinacrine* 100 mg tid for 7 days for adults, 7 mg/kg/day in three divided doses for for 7 days for children
	Infants	Furazolidone 1.5 mg/kg qid for 7 days
	Empirical (unproven)	Metronidazole 250 mg tid for 7 days for adults, 15 mg/kg/day in three divided doses for 7 days for children
Entamoeba histolytica	Carrier/no symptoms	Diiodohydroxyquin 650 mg tid for 10 days for adults and 40 mg/kg/day in three divided doses for 7 days for children or diloxanide furoate (unlicensed)
	Intestinal disease	Metronidazole 750 mg tid for 5-10 days plus diiodohydroxyquin 650 mg tid for 21 days for adults or metronidazole 50 mg/kg/day in three divided doses for 10 days plus diiodohydroxyquin 40 mg/kg/day in three divided doses for 21 days
Dientamoeba fragilis or *Balantidium coli*	Intestinal disease	Tetracycline 250-500 mg qid for 7 to 10 days or diiodohydroxyquin 650 mg tid for 20 days for adults
Entamoeba polecki	Intestinal disease	Metronidazole 750 mg tid for 10 days followed by diloxanide furoate 500 mg tid for 10 days for adults
Blastocystis hominis	Intestinal disease	Diiodohydroxyquin 650 mg tid for 20 days or metronidazole 750 mg tid for 10 days for adults
Cryptosporidium parvum	Intestinal disease	Paromomycin 500 mg tid for 5 to 7 days for adults
Isospora belli	Intestinal disease	TMP/SMX 160 mg/800 mg bid for 3 to 4 weeks
Cyclospora or *Sarcocystis*	Intestinal disease	Uncertain

*If available; otherwise use tinidazole or metronidazole.

cases) of giardiasis were linked epidemiologically to water, making it the most frequently identified cause of water-borne diarrhea outbreaks. Most of these occurred in small water systems that used untreated or inadequately treated surface water.[41,42] Clear and cool mountain water has been so often associated with giardiasis that the illness has been called "backpacker's diarrhea" or "beaver fever." An outbreak in Aspen, Colorado, in 1964 was the first well-documented water-borne outbreak in the United States. More recent outbreaks in Aspen, Vail, and Estes Park, Colorado, indicate that this area remains endemically infected with *Giardia*.[106] In Camas, Washington, infected beavers were first implicated as a reservoir of infection. In the northeastern states, large outbreaks have occurred in the mountain communities of Rome, New York, and Berlin, New Hampshire.[42] Every region of the United States has experienced water-borne outbreaks, but the western mountain regions (Rocky Mountains, Cascades, and Sierra Nevada) have reported the majority, and giardiasis must be considered endemic.[30,40,42] *Giardia* accounts for a small percentage of traveler's diarrhea.[18,204] In certain locations it has occurred more commonly. It has been identified in a large percentage of cases among travelers to St. Petersburg, Russia, where tap water is the usual source. Because of the relatively long incubation period and persistent symptoms, *Giardia* is more likely to be found as the cause of diarrhea that occurs or persists after returning home from travels to any developing region.[111,139]

The pathophysiology of giardiasis remains an enigma.[30,139] Reversible malabsorption of fats, vitamins B and A, folate, and disaccharides has been demonstrated in some, but not all, patients with diarrhea. Several explanations of malabsorption have been proposed: physical blockade by large numbers of trophozoites blanketing the intestinal mucosa; deconjugation of bile acids; bacterial or fungal overgrowth in the small intestine; increased turnover of cells on the mucosa of the villi, which do not absorb normally; and epithelial damage. Histologic changes of villous atrophy and inflammatory infiltrates with epithelial cell destruction have been observed. In some series these changes correlated with degree of malabsorption and reverted to normal after treatment. However, most small bowel biopsies in human patients demonstrate minimal or no changes.[30,139] Mucosal invasion has been shown, with trophozoites found intracellularly and extracellularly, but this is not a consistent feature and does not elicit a local inflammatory response.[30,139] Enterotoxins have not been found, although cytotoxic changes have been observed in cell culture.[139] Altered gut motility and hypersecretion of fluids, perhaps via increased adenylate cyclase activity, may play a role.[30] Most likely more than one mechanism is involved. Infectivity depends on host and, presumably, parasite factors. Most infections are asymptomatic. In endemic areas the role of *Giardia* in diarrhea can be confusing; in rural Egypt *Giardia* was found in 45% of patients with diarrhea but in 65% of controls.[223] In some human transmission studies a few persons experienced mild and transient changes in stool consistency but none felt ill.[169] The attack rate for symptomatic infection in the natural setting varies widely, from 5% to 70%.[14,30,40,105,213] Asymptomatic carrier states with high numbers of cysts excreted in stools are common.[111,119] Correlation between inoculum size and infection rates has been noted, but these do not correlate with numbers of cysts passed or severity of symptoms.[106,139,169] Hypochlorhydria, certain immunodeficiencies, blood group A, and malnutrition dispose to symptomatic infection.[119,139] Pathogenicity is also strain specific.

The incubation period averages 1 to 3 weeks with a mean of 9 days.[30,111,214] A wide array of clinical syndromes may occur.[14,30,214] A small number of people experience abrupt onset of explosive watery diarrhea accompanied by abdominal cramps, foul flatus, vomiting, fever, and malaise. This commonly lasts 3 to 4 days before transition into the more common subacute syndrome. In most patients the onset is more insidious and symptoms are persistent or recurrent. Stools become mushy, greasy, and malodorous. Watery diarrhea may alternate with soft stools and even constipation. Upper gastrointestinal symptoms, typically exacerbated postprandially, accompany stool changes but may be present in the absence of soft stool. These include mid and upper abdominal cramping, substernal burning, acid indigestion, sulfurous belching, nausea, distention, early satiety, and foul flatus.

Dysenteric symptoms are not a feature of giardiasis. Constitutional symptoms of anorexia, fatigue, and weight loss are common, but fever and vomiting are infrequent except during acute onset of illness. Unusual presentations include allergic manifestations such as urticaria, erythema multiforme, and bronchospasm. Some *Giardia* infections are associated with a chronic illness. Adults may have a long-standing malabsorption syndrome and marked weight loss.[30,139] Children may have a failure-to-thrive syndrome.

The differential diagnosis includes the entire spectrum of gastrointestinal illnesses. The acute phase may be similar to amebiasis, bacterial enterocolitis, food poisoning, and viral gastroenteritis. The absence of blood and pus in the stool helps separate giardiasis from the dysenteric conditions.

Laboratory confirmation of giardiasis can be difficult.[139] Stool examination remains the primary means of diagnosis (Color Plate 106). Trophozoites may be found in fresh, watery stools but disintegrate rapidly. Cysts are passed in soft and formed stools. Although they remain in fresh stools for at least 24 hours, stools should be preserved in a fixative such as polyvinyl alcohol or a formalin preparation if not immediately examined. Cyst passage is extremely variable and not related to clinical symptoms.[45,145] Mean prepatency period is 2 weeks, meaning that appearance of cysts in stool may lag behind clinical symptoms by 1 week or more.[111,145] Irregular and cyclical shedding have been demonstrated.[45,111] In the office, fresh stool can be mixed with an iodine solution (such as Gram's iodine) or methylene blue and examined for cysts on a wet mount. Many antibiotics, enemas, laxatives, and barium studies mask or cause disappearance of parasites from the stools, so examinations should be delayed for 5 to 10 days after these interventions. The yield on stool examination depends not only on excretion patterns but also on the ability and perseverance of the technologist. Trichrome stain is better than the formalin-ether concentration technique for identification of protozoal cysts and trophozoites.[87] The current recommendation is to examine three samples taken at intervals of 2 days. Another noninvasive office test is duodenal mucus sampling.[139] Tube aspiration has been replaced by the string test (Enterotest). A weighted gelatin capsule containing a string is swallowed with one end taped to the cheek. After 4 to 6 hours, the other end of the string is retrieved from the duodenum and the bile-stained mucus is scraped onto a slide and immediately examined for trophozoites. Positive yields of 80% have been reported, but one well-conducted study found positive results in only 1 of 10 infected patients. Mixed results have been found in the patients with negative stools.[114] Duodenal biopsy should rarely be necessary but may be the most sensitive test.[114] Other laboratory aids are not diagnostic. Hematologic tests usually result in normal findings. Eosinophilia is not present normally in giardiasis, and when present it should be attributable to other conditions. Radiologic findings with barium studies may show spasm and irregular thickening of mucosal folds in the duodenum and proximal jejunum.[30] Serologic tests using three methods (ELISA, immunodiffusion test, and indirect immunofluorescent antibody test) have been applied to investigation of immunologic responses and diagnosis of *Giardia* infections. Counterimmunoelectrophoresis and immunofluorescence techniques have been applied to detect cysts in stools, which could increase the yield of these examinations.[172]

Immunologic responses to *Giardia* infection appear complex.[92,139,145] Acquired resistance has been demonstrated by epidemiologic studies showing lower rates of infection and illness among residents of endemically infected areas compared with visitors[106] and among adults compared with children. However, reinfection certainly occurs. Levels of IgG antitrophozoite antibodies rise with both symptomatic and asymptomatic infections. While these may help clear infection, they do not offer lasting protection. On the other hand, hypogammaglobulinemic patients have a higher incidence of symptomatic giardiasis, implying an important protective function of immune globulins.[139,217] Levels of IgM antibodies also rise with infection, but the elevations are short lived, suggesting that they may be useful for diagnosing acute infections. Effects of mucosal secretory antibodies in humans have not been clearly demonstrated, although mouse studies show a protective effect of IgA secretory antibodies. Both cellular and humoral responses to *Giardia* have been demonstrated. T cell–deficient mice do not clear *Giardia* infections as well as do normal mice. Mononuclear leukocytes and granulocytic cells infiltrate the intestinal mucosa during *Giardia* infection and can pass to and from the gut lumen. Macrophages phagocytose *Giardia* on contact, probably representing an early line of defense, while granulocytes kill only in the presence of antibody.

Whatever the mechanism, immunologic responses are effective in the majority of infections because spontaneous clinical recovery with or without the disappearance of organisms is common. In the classic volunteer studies of Rendtorff,[169] experimentally infected adults cleared the organisms from the stools within 40 days, except for two men who continued to shed for at least 4 months. Infected children have been observed to excrete cysts for months or years, but like adults, most clear organisms within 6 weeks. Average duration of symptoms in all ages ranges from 3 to 10 weeks.[139,213] In one study of travelers with giardiasis, however, the average length of symptoms before treatment was 12 weeks, and the majority of patients in an Indian study were symptomatic for more than 6 months. New immunologic tests are being developed and will probably replace stool examination in the future. Techniques to culture trophozoites and in vitro hatching of cysts cannot yet replace stool examinations but may become useful adjuncts, in addition to helping provide a source of antigen for immunologic tests.[139]

Given the difficulty and expense of confirming the diagnosis in some patients, a therapeutic trial of drugs may be attempted when suspicion is high. Symptomatic improvement concurrent with a course of quinacrine suggests the diagnosis of giardiasis. Imidazole derivatives, like metronidazole, affect bacterial flora as well, so they are less specific but better for empirical (unproven diagnosis) therapy because of their wide activity.

Cure can be achieved with one of several drugs. Symptomatic patients should be treated for comfort and to prevent the development of chronic illness. Asymptomatic carriers in nonendemic areas should be treated when identified because they may transmit the infection or develop symptomatic illness.[136] No drug is effective in all cases. In resistant cases, longer courses of two drugs taken concurrently have been suggested. Relapses occur up to several weeks after treatment, necessitating a second course of the same medication or an alternative drug. Malabsorption usually resolves with treatment; persistent diarrhea may result from lactose intolerance or a syndrome resembling celiac disease rather than treatment failure.[139] Stool samples taken 1 to 2 weeks after treatment help distinguish persistent infections. Three groups of drugs are currently being used: nitroimidazoles (metronidazole, tinidazole, ornidazole, and nimorazole), nitrofuran derivatives (furazolidone), and acridine compounds (mepacrine and quinacrine). Quinacrine (Atabrine, 100 mg three times a day for 7 days for adults and 7 mg/kg/day in three divided doses for children for 7 days), with cure rates around 95%, has been considered the drug of first choice in adults, although it produces more frequent side effects, especially in children.[53] It is not always available. Also, a pediatric liquid form does not exist to help with the treatment of young children. The most serious side effect is toxic psychosis, which occurs in 1 to 4:1000 patients. Symptoms may appear after the last dose has been taken and persist for 8 to 85 days (average 23 days). Metronidazole (Flagyl) is commonly used in the United States, although not formally approved for this use. Cure rates of 85% to 90% are comparable to those with quinacrine, but in the recommended dosage (250 mg three times a day for 7 to 10 days for adults), tolerance is better.[47] Perhaps the best cure rates would be achieved with two complete courses separated by 1 week. Single- and double-dose therapy of 2 to 2.5 g has not been as effective and produces more side effects. Newer derivatives (tinidazole, ornidazole, and nimorazole) are currently being tested around the world and show promise.[9] Considerable experience has been obtained with tinidazole (Fasgyn, Tiniba). Reported success rates are 90% to 95% when a single oral dose of 50 mg/kg in children and 2 g in adults is used.[6,9,136] Side effects with single-dose tinidazole are comparable to those with other common regimens. Although not released in the United States, this is the drug of choice for giardiasis in other parts of the world. Furazolidine (Furoxone 6 mg/kg/day in four divided doses for 7 days), available in suspension, is convenient for small children. Reports of cure rates average 80% to 85%, and side effects, although common, are mild.[47] Serious infection during pregnancy presents a special problem, since the issue of mutagenicity of imidazoles is not yet resolved. When possible, treatment should be withheld until after delivery. In severely symptomatic individuals, paromomycin (Humatin 25 to 30 mg/kg in three divided doses for 5 to 10 days), a poorly absorbed broad-spectrum antibiotic related to aminoglycosides, has been successful.

Entamoeba Histolytica

As with *Giardia,* the life cycle of *E. histolytica* involves two forms and one host. The reproductive form is the trophozoite, which resides in the host and can cause illness. Being delicate, the trophozoite cannot long survive the external environment or gastric acid and therefore is unlikely to transmit infection. Encystment occurs in the gut, and cysts pass in the stool. The early cyst matures within the host or externally by undergoing two nuclear divisions. Usually the cysts are infectious when passed. Although sensitive to boiling, adequate chlorination, and complete desiccation, cysts may survive drying or freezing and persist for months in a moist environment.[40] When a cyst is ingested through fecal contamination of food, water, or person-to-person contact, it undergoes nuclear division in the small intestine, resulting in eight trophozoites. Humans are the primary reservoir of *E. histolytica.* Infected individuals may pass up to 45 million cysts per day. Other species of amebae infect animals, but cross-transmission has not been found. Insects such as flies and cockroaches can spread infection by contact with feces.

E. histolytica is found worldwide. Approximately 10% of the world's population carry the parasite. The higher prevalence in tropical countries (30% to 50%) is related to increased risk of fecal-oral contamination, which depends on sanitation, cultural habits, crowding, and socioeconomic status.[212] Similar conditions create pockets of endemic infection in the United States among institutional inmates, Native Americans on reservations, and homosexuals. Surveys have found that 20% to 30% of homosexuals are infected with amebae. Importation of infections by travelers and immigrants accounts for most cases in the United States and other temperate countries.[122,123,157] Amebiasis accounts for less than 1% of traveler's diarrhea.[85,133] Earlier in this century, 10% to 15% of the U.S. population was infected with *E. histolytica,* but that has decreased to 1% to 5% overall,[123] primarily because of adequate water and sewage treatment. The last reported water-borne outbreak, in 1953, affected only 31 people. The largest, in Chicago in 1933, caused by sewage contamination of hotel water, resulted in 1409 cases of amebiasis and 98 deaths.

Attempts have been made to subdivide *E. histolytica* into different groups corresponding to pathogenicity. This may explain geographic differences in rates of invasive disease. Recently, isoenzyme analysis has recognized 22 different zymodemes of *E. histolytica,* which appear to correspond to pathogenic and commensal strains of the organism.[3,186] This distinction would be significant in determining the need for treatment of asymptomatic carriers. Arguments for no treatment of carriers with nonpathogenic zymodemes may be premature, since it is unclear whether this is a phenotypic or genotypic trait.

Infectivity and infectious dose are not well understood. Attack rate and prevalence are difficult to determine because the majority of infections are asymptomatic and screening with single stool samples is likely to identify only 20% to 50%.[3,100,156] Pathogenicity is not well understood.[156,187] Invasion may be a function of motility or lytic enzymes. The mechanism of diarrhea in noninvasive cases is still a mystery. Pathologic lesions in the bowel are well described. The cecum and ascending colon are most frequently involved, followed by the rectum and sigmoid colon. Five lesions of increasing severity can be distinguished in the colon. There may be diffuse inflammation with cellular infiltrate and an intact epithelium; superficial erosions; early invasion followed by shallow ulceration; late invasive lesions forming the classic flask ulcers with skip lesions; and loss of mucosa and muscularis resulting in exposure of underlying granulation tissue. Extraintestinal spread is hematogenous. Abscesses containing acellular debris develop primarily in the liver but may involve the brain and lung.

Although 80% to 99% of infections result in asymptomatic carriers, a spectrum of gastrointestinal diseases may result, corresponding to the pathologic lesions. Most commonly, colonic inflammation without dysentery causes lower abdominal cramping and altered stools, sometimes containing mucus and blood.[157,212] Weight loss, anorexia, and nausea may be present. Symptoms commonly fluctuate and continue for months. The subacute infection may evolve into a chronic, nondysenteric bowel syndrome with symptoms consisting of intermittent diarrhea, abdominal pain, weight loss, and flatulence.

Dysentery may develop suddenly after an incubation period of 8 to 10 days or after a period of mild symptoms. Affected persons may appear quite ill with frequent bloody stools, tenesmus, moderate to severe abdominal pain and tenderness, and fever. There is considerable variation in severity.

Humoral antibodies rise with invasive disease and persist for long periods. Although they do not protect against reinfection or bowel invasion, they show antiamebic action in vitro and may prevent recurrent liver infection, which is uncommon.[155,187] Asymptomatic cyst shedding and active gastrointestinal illness may persist for years, indicating lack of consistent immune response in the intestinal lumen.[119,155] Prevalence rates show a steady level in adults, but severity of infection increases with age. Groups without prior infection also have a higher rate of symptomatic illness.

The fatality rate for amebic dysentery and its complications is about 2%. Complications of intestinal involvement develop in 1% to 4% of cases and include perforation, toxic megacolon, and development of strictures or an ameboma. An ameboma is an annular inflammatory lesion containing live trophozoites that develops on the ascending colon. It may be manifested as a pyogenic abscess or resemble a carcinoma. A postdysenteric syndrome has been described after acute amebic dysentery that can be confused with ulcerative colitis.

Amebiasis accounts for 40,000 to 75,000 deaths annually, making it the third leading parasitic cause of death in the world. Deaths still occur in the United States because of complications or failure to consider the diagnosis. The diagnosis of intestinal amebiasis is made by identification of cysts or trophozoites in stool. Mucus from fresh stools or sigmoidoscopic scrapings and aspirates mixed with a drop of saline may show trophozoites if examined within an hour.[122] For delayed examination, stool must be preserved in polyvinyl alcohol or other fixative and may later be examined by formalin-ether suspension or trichrome stain; the latter has the best yield.[87] The same limitations and problems discussed with *Giardia* apply to *E. histolytica.* Fecal shedding of cysts is irregular. Three stools on alternate days identify most, but not all, infections.[4,123,157] Overdiagnosis may result from misidentification of leukocytes. Sigmoidoscopy or colonoscopy is useful for viewing the pathologic lesions and obtaining selective samples of mucus and biopsies of mucosal ulcers that commonly contain organisms.[157,212] Unlike the situation in giardiasis, cathartic purging may improve the yield of parasites in the stool. Barium enema is rarely helpful and obscures parasites in the stool for at least a week. Culture techniques have been developed that identify infection in some cases when small numbers of cysts are missed in stool examinations.[3] This is expensive and time consuming, so it is not widely used. Serologic tests are not useful for identifying asymptomatic carriers but are positive in 85% to 95% of patients with dysentery and 90% to 100% of patients with liver abscess.[100,123,155] They help to distinguish amebic dysentery from ulcerative colitis, diagnose extraintestinal amebiasis, and they assist epidemiologically. The hemagglutination inhibition assay is most commonly used, but other diagnostic tests (indirect immunofluorescence, ELISA, latex agglutination, immunodiffusion, and immunoelectrophoresis) have been developed.[155,156]

Treatment of amebiasis is based on the location of infection and degree of symptoms (Table 42-8).[53] Medications are divided into tissue amebicides (well-absorbed drugs that combat invasive amebiasis in the bowel and liver) and poorly absorbed drugs for luminal infections. Metronidazole, tinidazole, emetine, dehydroemetine, and chloroquine are tissue amebicides; iodoquinol, paromomycin, and diloxanide furoate are luminal agents. In general, treatment is effective for invasive infections but disappointing for luminal infections; no regimen is completely effective in eradicating intestinal infection. Asymptomatic carriers should be treated in the United States. The rationale is that a cyst passer represents a potential health hazard to others and, except in certain groups, reinfection is not likely. In addition, unless nonpathogenic strains are reliably differentiated, long-term carriage can result in active intestinal disease or hepatic abscess.[122,156] Some argue that asymptomatic carriers do not become ill, their infections clearing in less than 1 year. Routine screening of asymptomatic members of high-risk groups is not cost effective, except for food handlers.

The current drug of choice for asymptomatic carriers is iodoquinol (650 mg three times a day for 10 days for adults and 40 mg/kg/day in three divided doses for children).[53] Although related to iodochlorhydroxyquin, it does not cause optic atrophy in doses recommended for intestinal amebae. Side effects are mild and consist of abdominal pain, diarrhea, and rash. Diloxanide furoate (Furamide) is an alternative, considered the drug of choice by some (500 mg three times a day for 10 days for adults and 20 mg/kg/day in three divided doses for children). In the United States, it is classified as investigational, available through the CDC. Side effects are limited to flatulence and other mild gastrointestinal symptoms. Paromomycin is also effective (500 mg three times a day for 7 to 10 days for adults and 30 mg/kg/day in three divided doses for children). Although metronidazole has been used in asymptomatic carriers with 90% success, most reserve this drug for invasive and symptomatic infections because of the risk of side effects. Mildly symptomatic patients without dysentery may also respond to a luminal-acting drug such as diloxanide furoate or paromomycin. The latter was recently shown to be quite effective and well tolerated in a study among homosexual men with mild to moderate intestinal amebiasis. Invasive disease is treated with a tissue-active drug, followed by a luminal agent (in the same doses as above for 21 days). For oral therapy, metronidazole is the drug of choice (750 mg three times a day for 10 days for adults and 50 mg/kg/day in three divided doses for children), followed by iodoquinol.[53] Side effects are listed under treatment of giardiasis. Tinidazole, not yet available in the United States, appears to be quite successful and is well tolerated for intestinal and hepatic amebiasis. Regimens include 600 mg twice a day for 5 days and 2 g in a single dose once daily for 3 days. Emetine and dehydroemetine (1 mg/kg/day, maximum 90 mg/day) are used parenterally in severe cases of amebiasis, primarily extraintestinal, followed by iodoquinol for 20 days. They have frequent systemic side effects, including cardiac arrhythmias requiring hospital treatment and cardiac monitoring. Since they are related to ipecac, they also cause vomiting. Tetracycline has indirect amebicidal action in the bowel and is sometimes used in conjunction with iodoquinol for nondysenteric intestinal amebiasis.[2]

Cryptosporidium Parvum and Isospora Belli

The intestinal pathogens *Cryptosporidium* and *Isospora* are important human pathogens. These intestinal coccidia have attracted renewed interest recently because of an increase in the number of reported cases, especially in AIDS patients. While these represent opportunistic infections among immunosuppressed patients, increased surveillance and new identification techniques are discovering other reservoirs of infection. Treatment recommendations are summarized in Table 42-8.

Cryptosporidium

Cryptosporidium is a common enteric pathogen in humans. The infection has been described as important in certain patient groups: those with contact with animals such as veterinarians, infants in day care centers, travelers to St. Petersburg, Russia, patients with AIDS, and large numbers of individuals in community-wide water-borne outbreaks.[46,113,193] *Cryptosporidium* infects a wide variety of animals, including domestic calves, horses, pigs, kittens, puppies, and wild mammals such as raccoons, beavers, squirrels, and coyotes.[147] An outbreak of illness among animal handlers demonstrated transmission between calves and humans. Subsequently, experimental transmission was accomplished between multiple animal strains. Clearly, a zoonosis exists as a reservoir for human infections, and there may be only a single species. The brush border of the jejunum is the usual site of infection. The trophozoite attaches to epithelial cells, possibly invading the cell membrane but definitely remaining extracytoplasmic.[17,147] Successful development of *Cryptosporidium* in cell culture assists further study. Sporulated oocysts are infective as passed in the stool, so fecal-oral contamination is the mode of transmission.[147] The thick-walled and hardy oocyst is capable of persisting in the environment. Ingestion of untreated surface water, well water, and raw milk has been implicated as a vehicle of transmission; food-borne transmission is suspected.

The frequency of occurrence of cryptosporidiosis in patients with diarrhea varies by geography. The organism was found in 4% of patients with diarrhea seen in Australia, 3% in Finland, and 1% to 2% in England. Serologic evidence suggests that between one third and two thirds of people have been exposed to the organism based on baseline serum antibody levels. The attack rate of illness in several outbreaks among immunocompetent persons was high: 9 of 12 infected animal handlers developed symptoms; all Finnish travelers with cryptosporidia in their stools were symptomatic; 37% of residents infected from a water-borne epidemic were symptomatic. However, it is likely that many infections will prove to be asymptomatic like those from other intestinal protozoa. The incubation period is 1 to 2 weeks.[112]

The pathophysiologic mechanisms of diarrhea and malabsorption are unknown. The clinical illness depends on immune status.[147] In immunocompetent persons, symptoms consist of watery diarrhea (without blood or leukocytes) associated with cramps, nausea, flatulence, and sometimes vomiting and low-grade fever.[147] The syndrome is generally mild and self-limited. Diarrhea averaged 5 to 6 days in some groups, but 12 days (range 2 to 26) in others.[112,193] Children more often become significantly dehydrated. Since the symptoms are nonspecific and flulike, a specific diagnosis is not likely to be made. In contrast, immunocompromised hosts experience profuse watery diarrhea with malabsorption and weight loss lasting months to years.[147,218] Fluid losses can be overwhelming. Most patients die before clearing their infections. While cryptosporidiosis has not been associated directly with this mortality, dehydration and malnutrition were thought to be contributory. Cyst passage in stool usually ends within 1 week of symptom resolution but has persisted for up to 2 months after recovery.[46,112,201] The vastly different response to infection between immunocompetent and compromised hosts suggests that functional cellular and humoral immunities are necessary to clear an infection. However, reinfection of an immunocompetent person has been documented.

Diagnosis in initial case descriptions was made by small bowel biopsy, but oocysts can be found in the stools routinely in intestinal infections, even though shedding may be intermittent. Concentration techniques, such as formalin-ether or sugar flotation, and subsequent staining with acid-fast, Giemsa, or Ziehl-Neelsen techniques facilitate identification of *Cryptosporidium* oocysts.[112,147,218] The organism has also been found in duodenal mucus using the string test (Enterotest). Serologic techniques have been developed, but their specificity and temporal relation to infection are not yet known.

While no clearly effective treatment has been found,[53,147,192] paromomycin may be effective in eradicating the infection and improving symptoms in immunocompetent persons and in decreasing the intensity of intestinal infection in immunocompromised persons. Spiramycin has been used with mixed success in the therapy of cryptosporidiosis.[53,218]

Isospora Belli

I. belli is an uncommon cause of diarrhea in humans, but like *Cryptosporidium,* it has been appearing in immunocompromised patients with diarrhea. Humans are the only host, and infections are transmitted by fecal-oral contamination through direct contact or food and water. The organism invades mucosal cells of the small intestine, causing an inflammatory response in the submucosa and variable destruction of the brush border.[218] Infection rates are usually low. Most cases have been identified in tropical regions among natives, travelers, and the military.[81] In immunocompetent persons the infection may be asymptomatic or the cause of mild transient diarrhea and abdominal cramps. Others symptoms include significant watery diarrhea, flatulence, anorexia, weight loss, low-grade fever, and signs of malabsorption.[218] While the illness is generally self-limited, ending in 2 to 3 weeks, some affected patients have symptoms lasting months to years, clinically similar to giardiasis. Infections in immunocompromised patients tend to be severe and follow a more protracted course.[84,218]

Diagnosis can be made by identification of immature oocysts in the stool. However, excretion may occur sporadically and in small numbers, so concentration techniques are usually required. When stools are negative, the organism can be recovered from the jejunum via biopsy, aspiration, or string test.[218] Unlike the other intestinal protozoa, *I. belli* may cause eosinophilia.[84,218] Successful treatment has recently been reported with TMP-SMX (160/800 mg four times a day for 10 days, then two times a day for 3 to 4 weeks).[84,53,218]

Miscellaneous Parasitic Agents

Cyclospora species, previously described as blue-green algae or cyanobacteria-like organisms, have been shown to cause protracted diarrhea in immunocompetent travelers to developing countries including Nepal, Mexico, and Haiti and in patients with AIDS.[151] The illness in healthy travelers averaged 43 days.[188] The importance of the organism in patients with AIDS is less clear.[99] The small spherical organisms resemble *Cryptosporidium,* yet in contrast to *C. parvum,* they show variable staining when examined by light microscopy after acid-fast staining.[151]

Although few human infections with *Sarcocystis* have been reported, infection rates in pigs and cattle reach 100% in some areas. Earlier studies combined *Sarcocystis* with *I. belli,* confusing the epidemiology.[81] Stool surveys and volunteer studies indicate asymptomatic infections in some. In others, symptoms appeared within 8 hours of ingesting cysts in raw meat and included diarrhea, abdominal pain, nausea, and bloating. Symptoms improve within 48 hours. Peak shedding of sporocysts in the stool occurs 14 to 18 days after ingestion of cysts and is associated with diarrhea and abdominal pain. Reports from Thailand found *Sarcocystis* parasites in segments of resected bowel in six cases of intestinal obstruction. Diagnosis is based on identification of cysts in feces. Concentration techniques are necessary because the number of cysts shed is small. No specific treatment has been determined, but TMP-SMX and furazolidone have been suggested. Human intestinal infection with *Sarcocystis* is probably self-limited.

Balantidium coli is pathogenic in humans, but infection is rare.[88,203,215] Although many aspects of the epidemiology are unclear, pigs appear to be the primary reservoir and source of human infection. The overall prevalence of infection is low except in areas where humans and pigs live together and hygiene is poor; in Papua New Guinea an incidence of 20% to 30% has been reported. Cysts can be transmitted by direct contact or through ingestion of water or food. The largest reported epidemic (110 cases) occurred on the Pacific island of Truk.[215] In the United States 16 cases were reported in 1950 from New Orleans. Most were rural residents, and at least half were farmers. *B. coli* inhabits the colon and can invade the bowel wall, causing ulcerations that remain superficial or extend into the submucosa and muscularis. Clinical features also resemble amebiasis with a spectrum including asymptomatic infection, chronic intermittent diarrhea of variable intensity, acute dysentery with mucosal invasion, and rarely, metastatic abscesses. In the Truk outbreak, symptoms among the infected did not differ significantly from those in controls, but poor records were kept and most patients harbored multiple pathogens. Patients in the New Orleans series experienced diarrhea with abdominal pain, occasional fever, and other constitutional symptoms; half had dysentery and colonic lesions. Duration of symptoms in this group before treatment ranged from 1 week to 2 years, with most exceeding 1 month. Diagnosis is made by observing the organism in stool. Trophozoites are seen much more often than cysts. A saline wet preparation of fresh stool observed under low power should suffice for visualization of the large, motile organisms. Recommended treatment is tetracycline (500 mg four times a day for 7 days) or iodoquinol (650 mg three times a day for 20 days).[53] Metronidazole (750 mg three times a day for 10 days) is an alternative.[88,53] Paromomycin (500 mg three times a day for 7 days) may also be effective.

Blastocystis hominis still creates debate concerning both classification and pathogenicity. Formerly classified as a nonpathogenic yeast, it has characteristics of protozoa (Sporozoa group). *B. hominis* is commonly identified in stool samples in Nepal and California.[128] A direct correlation with symptoms has not been possible, and it may be argued that symptoms were caused by other undetected pathogens. When found in large numbers, *B. hominis* is suspected of causing diarrheal illness.[224] Little is known about the pathogenic mechanisms. Optimal treatment has not been determined, but antiprotozoal drugs may prove effective.

Dientamoeba fragilis is most commonly observed in asymptomatic persons or in conjunction with other pathogenic parasites, but it is capable of causing illness.[194,222] It inhabits the crypts of the colon but is not invasive. Symptoms include mild intermittent diarrhea, abdominal pain, anorexia, flatulence, fatigue, and weight loss. Cyst forms have not been observed, so the mode of transmission is unknown. Because only the fragile trophozoites are passed in stool, organisms are most frequently identified from immediately preserved specimens viewed on fixed stained smears.[222] Symptomatic infections usually respond to treatment with iodoquinol or tetracycline, alone or in combination (the same doses as for amebiasis and balantidiasis).[53,194] Paromomycin is an alternative.

Entamoeba polecki, usually nonpathogenic, has been suspected of causing lower intestinal symptoms in sporadic cases involving heavy infection.[184] *E. polecki* is commonly found in pigs, which probably act as a reservoir for human infections, accounting for the high incidence of infection in Papua New Guinea, where people and pigs live in close contact. Cysts are passed in stool and may be confused with *E. histolytica,* which they closely resemble.[184] Successful resolution of symptoms has been reported with metronidazole followed by diloxanide furoate in the same doses as for amebiasis and balantidiasis.

REFERENCES

1. Acharya IL et al: Prevention of typhoid fever in Nepal with the Vi capsular polysaccharide of *Salmonella typhi, N Engl J Med* 317:1101, 1987.
2. Adams EB, MacLeod IN: Invasive amebiasis. I. Amebic dysentery and its complications, *Medicine* 56:315, 1977.
3. Allason-Jones E et al: *Entamoeba histolytica* as a commensal intestinal parasite in homosexual men, *N Engl J Med* 315:353, 1986.
4. American Society of Parasitologists: Procedures suggested for use in examination of clinical specimens for parasitic infection, *J Parasitol* 63:959, 1977.
5. Anders BJ et al: Double-blind placebo controlled trial of erythromycin for treatment of *Campylobacter* enteritis, *Lancet* 1:131, 1982.
6. Apte VV, Packard RS: Tinidazole in the treatment of trichomoniasis, giardiasis, and amoebiasis: report of a multicenter study, *Drugs* 15(suppl 1):43, 1978.
7. Aserkoff B, Bennett JV: Effect of antibiotic therapy in acute salmonellosis on the fecal excretion of salmonellae, *N Engl J Med* 281:636, 1969.
8. Attwood SEA et al: *Yersinia* infection and acute abdominal pain, *Lancet* 1:529, 1987.
9. Bakshi JS, Ghiara JM, Nanivadekar AS: How does tinidazole compare with metronidazole? A summary report of Indian trials in amoebiasis and giardiasis, *Drugs* 15(suppl 1):33, 1978.
10. Banatvala JE: The role of viruses in acute diarrhoeal disease, *Clin Gastroenterol* 8:569, 1979.
11. Bandres JC, Mathewson JJ, DuPont HL: Heat susceptibility of bacterial enteropathogens: implications for the prevention of travelers' diarrhea, *Arch Intern Med* 148:2261, 1988.
12. Bandres JC et al: Trimethoprim/sulfamethoxazole remains active against enterotoxigenic *Escherichia coli* and *Shigella* species in Guadalajara, Mexico, *Am J Med Sci* 303:289, 1992.

13. Banwell JG: Treatment of travelers' diarrhea: fluid and dietary management, *Rev Infect Dis* 8(suppl 2):182, 1986.
14. Barbour AG, Nickols CR, Fukushima T: An outbreak of giardiasis in a group of campers, *Am J Trop Med Hyg* 25:348, 1976.
15. Barker WH, Gangarosa EJ: Food poisoning due to *Vibrio parahaemolyticus, Annu Rev Med* 25:75, 1974.
16. Bemrick WJ: Some perspectives on the transmission of giardiasis. In Erlandsen SL, Meyer EA, editors: *Giardia and giardiasis: biology, pathogenesis and epidemiology,* New York, 1984, Plenum Press.
17. Bird RG, Smith MD: Cryptosporidiosis in man: parasite life cycle and fine structural pathology, *Pathology* 132:217, 1980.
18. Black RE: Pathogens that cause travelers' diarrhea in Latin America and Africa, *Rev Infect Dis* 8(suppl 2):131, 1986.
19. Black RE et al: A two-year study of bacterial, viral, and parasitic agents associated with diarrhea in rural Bangladesh, *J Infect Dis* 142:660, 1980.
20. Black RE et al: Incidence and severity of rotavirus and *Escherichia coli* diarrhoea in rural Bangladesh, *Lancet* 1:141, 1981.
21. Blacklow NR, Greenberg HB: Viral gastroenteritis, *N Engl J Med* 325:252, 1991.
22. Blaser MJ: Environmental interventions for the prevention of travelers' diarrhea, *Rev Infect Dis* 8(suppl 2):1142, 1986.
23. Blaser MJ, Newman LS: A review of salmonellosis. I. Infective dose, *Rev Infect Dis* 4:1096, 1982.
24. Blaser MJ, Reller LB: *Campylobacter* enteritis, *N Engl J Med* 305:1444, 1981.
25. Blaser MJ, Sazie E, Williams P: The influence of immunity on raw milk–associated *Campylobacter* infection, *JAMA* 257:43, 1987.
26. Blaser MJ et al: *Campylobacter* enteritis: clinical and epidemiological features, *Ann Intern Med* 91:179, 1979.
27. Blaser MJ et al: *Campylobacter* enteritis in the United States: a multicenter trial, *Ann Intern Med* 98:360, 1983.
28. Bolen JL, Zamiska SA, Greenough WB: Clinical features in enteritis due to *Vibrio parahaemolyticus, Am J Med* 57:638, 1974.
29. Bolivar R et al: Rotavirus in travelers' diarrhea: study of an adult student population in Mexico, *J Infect Dis* 137:324, 1978.
30. Brandborg LL, moderator: Giardiasis and travelers' diarrhea, *Gastroenterology* 78:1602, 1980.
31. Brown HW: *Basic clinical parasitology,* ed 5, Norwalk, Conn, 1983, Appleton & Lange.
32. Butler T et al: Causes of death in diarrhoeal diseases after rehydration therapy: an autopsy study of 140 patients in Bangladesh, *Bull WHO* 65:317, 1987.
33. Butzler JP, Skirrow MB: *Campylobacter* enteritis, *Clin Gastroenterol* 8:737, 1979.
34. Centers for Disease Control: Outbreak of *Yersinia enterocolitica*—Washington State, *MMWR* 31:562, 1982.
35. Centers for Disease Control: Toxigenic *Vibrio cholerae* 01 infections—Louisiana and Florida, *MMWR* 35:606, 1986.
36. Champsaur H et al: Cholera-like illness due to *Aeromonas sobria, J Infect Dis* 145:248, 1982.
37. Cherubin CD et al: Septicemia with non-typhoid *Salmonella, Medicine* 53:365, 1974.
38. Cococino Country (Arizona) Dept Public Health reports: *Outbreak of S. sonnei gastroenteritis on Colorado River raft trips, 1979.*
39. Cohen ML, Gangarosa EJ: Nontyphoidal salmonellosis, *South Med J* 71:1540, 1978.
40. Cooper RC et al: *Infectious agent risk assessment water quality project,* UCB/SEEHRL Reps No 84-4 and 84-5, Berkeley, 1984, University of California.
41. Craun GF: Waterborne giardiasis in the United States 1965-84 (letter), *Lancet* 2:513, 1986.
42. Craun GF: *Waterborne disease in the United States,* Boca Raton, Fla, 1986, CRC Press.
43. Cumberbatch N et al: Cytotoxic enterotoxin produced by *Aeromonas hydrophila:* relationship of toxigenic isolates to diarrheal disease, *Infect Immun* 23:829, 1979.
44. Cutting WAM: Oral rehydration in diarrhoea: applied pathophysiology, *Trans R Soc Trop Med Hyg* 74:30, 1980.
45. Dancinger M, Lopez M: Numbers of *Giardia* in the feces of infected children, *Am J Trop Med Hyg* 24:237, 1975.
46. D'Antonio RG et al: A waterborne outbreak of cryptosporidiosis in normal hosts, *Ann Intern Med* 103:886, 1985.
47. Davidson RA: Issues in clinical parasitology: the treatment of giardiasis, *Am J Gastroenterol* 79:256, 1984.
48. Davis WA, Kane JG, Garagusi VF: Human *Aeromonas* infections: a review of the literature and case report of endocarditis, *Medicine* 57:267, 1978.
49. Deetz TR et al: Occurrence of rota- and enteroviruses in drinking and environmental water in a developing nation, *Water Res* 18: 567, 1984.
50. DeWitt TG, Humphry KM, McCarthy P: Clinical predictors of acute bacterial diarrhea in young children, *Pediatrics* 76:551, 1985.
51. Dickens DL, DuPont HL, Johnson PC: Survival of bacterial enteropathogens in the ice of popular drinks, *JAMA* 253: 3141, 1985.
52. Donowitz M, Wicks J, Sharp GW: Drug therapy for diarrheal diseases: a look ahead, *Rev Infect Dis* 8(suppl 2):188, 1986.
53. Drugs for parasitic infections, *Med Lett* 28:9, 1986.
54. DuPont HL: Nonfluid therapy and selected chemoprophylaxis of acute diarrhea, *Am J Med* 78:81, 1985.
55. DuPont HL, Ericsson CD: Prevention and treatment of traveler's diarrhea, *N Engl J Med* 328:1821, 1993.
56. DuPont HL, Hornick RB: Adverse effect of Lomotil therapy in shigellosis, *JAMA* 226:1525, 1973.
57. DuPont HL et al: The response of man to virulent *Shigella flexneri* 2a, *J Infect Dis* 119:296, 1969.
58. DuPont HL et al: Pathogenesis of *Escherichia coli* diarrhea, *N Engl J Med* 285:1, 1971.
59. DuPont HL et al: Immunity in shigellosis. II. Protection induced by oral live vaccine or primary infection, *J Infect Dis* 125:12, 1972.
60. DuPont HL et al: Comparative susceptibility of Latin American and United States students to enteric pathogens, *N Engl J Med* 295:1520, 1976.
61. DuPont HL et al: Symptomatic treatment of diarrhea with bismuth subsalicylate among students attending a Mexican university, *Gastroenterology* 73:715, 1977.
62. DuPont HL et al: Diarrhea of travelers to Mexico: relative susceptibility of United States and Latin American students attending a Mexican university, *Am J Epidemiol* 105:37, 1977.
63. DuPont HL et al: Prevention of travelers' diarrhea (emporiatic enteritis): prophylactic administration of subsalicylate bismuth, *JAMA* 243:237, 1980.
64. DuPont HL et al: Prevention of travelers' diarrhea with trimethoprim-sulfamethoxazole, *Rev Infect Dis* 4:533, 1982.
65. DuPont HL et al: Treatment of travelers' diarrhea with trimethoprim/sulfamethoxazole and with trimethoprim alone, *N Engl J Med* 307:841, 1982.
66. DuPont HL et al: Prevention of travelers' diarrhea with trimethoprim-sulfamethoxazole and trimethoprim alone, *Gastroenterology* 84:75, 1983.
67. DuPont HL et al: Current problems in antimicrobial therapy for bacterial enteric infection, *Am J Med* 82(suppl 4A):324, 1987.
68. DuPont HL et al: Prevention of travelers' diarrhea by the tablet formulation of bismuth subsalicylate, *JAMA* 257:1347, 1987.
69. DuPont HL et al: Inoculum size in shigellosis and implications for expected mode of transmission, *J Infect Dis* 159:1126, 1989.
70. DuPont HL et al: Five versus three days of ofloxacin therapy for traveler's diarrhea: a placebo-controlled study, *Antimicrob Agents Chemother* 36:87, 1992.

71. DuPont HL et al: Zaldaride maleate (Zm), an intestinal calmodulin inhibitor, in the therapy of travelers' diarrhea, *Gastroenterology* 104:709, 1993.
72. Dykes AC et al: Municipal waterborne giardiasis: an epidemiologic investigation, *Ann Intern Med* 92:165, 1980.
73. Echeverria P et al: Travelers' diarrhea among American Peace Corps volunteers in rural Thailand, *J Infect Dis* 143:767, 1981.
74. Edelman R, Levine MM: Summary of a workshop on enteropathogenic *Escherichia coli* (from the National Institute of Allergy and Infectious Diseases), *J Infect Dis* 147:1108, 1983.
75. Ericsson CD et al: Bismuth subsalicylate inhibits activity of crude toxins of *Escherichia coli* and *Vibrio cholerae, J Infect Dis* 136:693, 1977.
76. Ericsson CD et al: The role of location of food consumption in the prevention of travelers' diarrhea in Mexico, *Gastroenterology* 79:812, 1980.
77. Ericsson CD et al: Influence of subsalicylate bismuth on absorption of doxycycline, *JAMA* 247:2266, 1982.
78. Ericsson CD et al: Ciprofloxacin or trimethoprim-sulfamethoxazole as initial therapy for travelers' diarrhea, *Ann Intern Med* 106:216, 1987.
79. Ericsson CD et al: Treatment of traveler's diarrhea with sulfamethoxazole and trimethoprim and loperamide, *JAMA* 263:257, 1990.
80. Eykyn SJ, Williams H: Treatment of multiresistant *Salmonella typhi* with oral ciprofloxacin, *Lancet* 2:1407, 1987.
81. Faust EC et al: Human isosporosis in the Western Hemisphere, *Am J Trop Med Hyg* 10:343, 1961.
82. Felsenfeld O: Notes on food, beverages and fomites contaminated with *Vibrio cholerae, Bull WHO* 33:725, 1965.
83. Finch MJ, Riley LW: *Campylobacter* infections in the United States: results of an 11 state surveillance, *Arch Intern Med* 144:1610, 1984.
84. Forthal DN, Guest S: *Isospora belli* enteritis in three homosexual men, *Am J Trop Med Hyg* 33:1060, 1984.
85. Frachtman RL et al: Seroconversion to *Entamoeba histolytica* among short-term travelers to Mexico, *Arch Intern Med* 142:1299, 1982.
86. Freeman LD et al: Brief prophylaxis with doxycycline for the prevention of travelers' diarrhea, *Gastroenterology* 84:276, 1983.
87. Garcia LS, Brewer TC, Bruckner DA: A comparison of the formalin-ether concentration and trichrome-stained smear methods for the recovery and identification of intestinal protozoa, *Am J Med Technol* 45:932, 1979.
88. Garcia-Laverde A, De Bonilla L: Clinical trials with metronidazole in human balantidiasis, *Am J Trop Med Hyg* 24:781, 1975.
89. George WL et al: *Aeromonas*-related diarrhea in adults, *Arch Intern Med* 145:2207, 1985.
90. Georges MC et al: Parasitic, bacterial, and viral enteric pathogens associated with diarrhea in the Central African Republic, *J Clin Microbiol* 19:571, 1984.
91. Germanier R, E Fürer: Isolation and characterization of *galE* mutant Ty21a of *Salmonella typhi:* a candidate strain for a live oral typhoid vaccine, *J Infect Dis* 131:553, 1975.
92. Gillon J: Giardiasis: review of epidemiology, pathogenic mechanisms and host responses, *Q J Med* 209:29, 1984.
93. Gorbach SL et al: Travelers' diarrhea and toxigenic *Escherichia coli, N Engl J Med* 292:933, 1975.
94. Gracey M, Burke V, Robinson J: *Aeromonas*-associated gastroenteritis, *Lancet* 2:1304, 1982.
95. Gracey M et al: *Aeromonas* spp in travellers' diarrhoea, *Br Med J* 289:658, 1984.
96. Graham DY et al: Double-blind comparison of bismuth subsalicylate and placebo in the prevention and treatment of enterotoxigenic *Escherichia coli*–induced diarrhea in volunteers, *Gastroenterology* 85:1017, 1983.
97. Haltalin KC et al: Treatment of acute diarrhea in outpatients: double-blind study comparing ampicillin and placebo, *Am J Dis Child* 124:554, 1972.
98. Harris JC, DuPont HL, Hornick RB: Fecal leukocytes in diarrheal illness, *Ann Intern Med* 76:697, 1972.
99. Hart AS et al: Novel organisms associated with chronic diarrhoea in AIDS, *Lancet* 335:169, 1990.
100. Healy GR: Immunologic tools in the diagnosis of amebiasis: epidemiology in the United States, *Rev Infect Dis* 8:239, 1986.
101. Hefelfinger DC: More on cola drinks and rehydration in acute diarrhea (letter), *N Engl J Med* 316:280, 1987.
102. Holmberg SD et al: *Aeromonas* infections in the United States, *Ann Intern Med* 105:683, 1986.
103. Holmberg SD et al: *Plesiomonas* infections in the United States, *Ann Intern Med* 105:690, 1986.
104. Holmgren J, Svennerholm AM: Vaccine development for the control of cholera and related toxin-induced diarrheal diseases. In Evered D, Whelan J, editors: *Microbial toxins and diarrheal disease,* Ciba Symposium 112, London, 1985, Pitman.
105. Hornick RB et al: The Broad Street pump revisited: response of volunteers to ingested cholera vibrios, *Bull NY Acad Med* 47: 1181, 1971.
106. Istre GR et al: Waterborne giardiasis at a mountain resort: evidence for acquired immunity, *Am J Public Health* 74:602, 1984.
107. Johnson PC et al: Occurrence of Norwalk virus infections among adults in Mexico, *J Infect Dis* 162:389, 1990.
108. Johnson PC et al: Comparison of loperamide with bismuth subsalicylate for the treatment of acute travelers' diarrhea, *JAMA* 255:757, 1986.
109. Johnson PC et al: Lack of emergence of resistant fecal flora during successful prophylaxis of traveler's diarrhea with norfloxacin, *Antimicrob Agents Chemother* 30:671, 1986.
110. Johnston JM et al: Cholera on a Gulf Coast oil rig, *N Engl J Med* 309:523, 1983.
111. Jokipii AMM, Jokipii L: Prepatency of giardiasis, *Lancet* 1:1095, 1977.
112. Jokipii L, Jokipii MM: Timing of symptoms and oocyst excretion in human cryptosporidiosis, *N Engl J Med* 315:1643, 1986.
113. Jokipii L, Pohjola S, Jokipii AMM: Cryptosporidiosis associated with traveling and giardiasis, *Gastroenterology* 89:838, 1985.
114. Kamath KR, Murugasu R: A comparative study of four methods for detecting *Giardia lamblia* in children with diarrheal disease and malabsorption, *Gastroenterology* 66:16, 1974.
115. Kaplan JE et al: Epidemiology of Norwalk gastroenteritis and the role of Norwalk virus in outbreaks of acute nonbacterial gastroenteritis, *Ann Intern Med* 96:756, 1982.
116. Kean BH: The diarrhea of travelers to Mexico, *Ann Intern Med* 59:605, 1963.
117. Kean BH: Travelers' diarrhea: an overview, *Rev Infect Dis* 8(suppl 2):111, 1986.
118. Kean BH, Gorbach SL, editors: International conference on the diarrhea of travelers—new directions in research: a summary, *J Infect Dis* 137:355, 1978.
119. Knight B: Epidemiology and transmission of giardiasis, *Trans R Soc Trop Med Hyg* 74:433, 1980.
120. Kozicki M, Steffen R, Shär M: "Boil it, cook it, peel it, or forget it": does this rule prevent travellers' diarrhoea? *Int J Epidemiol* 14:169, 1985.
121. Kreuse M: Bismuth preparations for diarrhea (letter), *JAMA* 244:1435, 1980.
122. Krogstad DJ, Spencer HC, Healy GR: Current concepts in parasitology: amebiasis, *N Engl J Med* 298:262, 1978.
123. Krogstad DJ et al: Amebiasis: epidemiologic studies in the United States, 1971–1974, *Ann Intern Med* 88:89, 1978.
124. Levine MM et al: Immunity to enterotoxigenic *Escherichia coli, Infect Immun* 23:729, 1979.
125. Ljungh A, Popoff M, Wadstrom T: *Aeromonas hydrophila* in acute diarrheal disease: detection of enterotoxin and biotyping of strains, *J Clin Microbiol* 6:96, 1977.

126. Longfield R: Nontyphoidal *Salmonella* infections. In Strickland GT, editor: *Hunter's tropical medicine,* ed 6, Philadelphia, 1984, WB Saunders.
127. MacDonald KL, Cohen ML: Epidemiology of travelers' diarrhea: current perspectives, *Rev Infect Dis* 8(suppl 2):117, 1986.
128. Markell EK, Udkow MP: *Blastocystis hominis:* pathogen or fellow traveler? *Am J Trop Med Hyg* 35:1023, 1986.
129. Marks MI et al: *Yersinia enterocolitica* gastroenteritis: a prospective study of clinical, bacteriologic and epidemiologic features, *Pediatrics* 96:26, 1980.
130. Mata LJ et al: Epidemic Shiga bacillus dysentery in Central America. I. Etiologic investigations in Guatemala, 1969, *J Infect Dis* 122:170, 1970.
131. Mathewson JJ et al: A newly recognized cause of travelers' diarrhea: enteroadherent *Escherichia coli, J Infect Dis* 151:471, 1985.
132. Mathewson JJ et al: Pathogenicity of enteroadherent *Escherichia coli* in adult volunteers, *J Infect Dis* 154:524, 1986.
133. Mathewson JJ et al: Risk of acquisition of *Entamoeba histolytica* infection during long-term travel to Mexico, *Travel Med Internat* 8(2):65, 1990.
134. Mattila L et al: Seasonal variation in etiology of travelers' diarrhea, *J Infect Dis* 165:385, 1992.
135. McIntyre RC: Modes of transmission of cholera in a newly infected population on an atoll: implications for control measures, *Lancet* 1:311, 1979.
136. Mendelson RM: The treatment of giardiasis, *Trans R Soc Trop Med Hyg* 74:488, 1980.
137. Merson MH et al: An outbreak of *Shigella sonnei* gastroenteritis on Colorado river raft trips, *Am J Epidemiol* 100:186, 1974.
138. Merson MH et al: Travelers' diarrhea in Mexico, *N Engl J Med* 294:1299, 1976.
139. Meyer EA, Radulescu S: *Giardia* and giardiasis, *Adv Parasitol* 17:1, 1979.
140. Morger H, Steffen R, Schär M: Epidemiology of cholera in travellers, and conclusions for vaccination recommendations, *Br Med J* 286:184, 1983.
141. Moriarty KJ, Turnberg LA: Bacterial toxins and diarrhoea, *Clin Gastroenterol* 15:529, 1986.
142. Morris JG, Black RE: Cholera and other vibrioses in the United States, *N Engl J Med* 312:343, 1985.
143. Murray BE, Rensimer ER, DuPont HL: Emergence of high-level trimethoprim resistance in fecal *Escherichia coli* during oral administration of trimethoprim or trimethoprim-sulfamethoxazole, *N Engl J Med* 306:130, 1982.
144. Nanda R, Baveja U, Anand BS: *Entamoeba histolytica* cyst passers: clinical features and outcome in untreated subjects, *Lancet* 2:301, 1984.
145. Nash TE et al: Experimental human infections with *Giardia lamblia, J Infect Dis* 156:974, 1987.
146. National Institutes of Health (Gorbach SL, Edelman R, editors): Travelers' diarrhea: consensus development conference, *Rev Infect Dis* 8(suppl 2): 1986.
147. Navin TR, Juranek DD: Cryptosporidiosis: clinical, epidemiologic, and parasitologic review, *Rev Infect Dis* 6:313, 1984.
148. Nelson JD, Haltalin KC: Accuracy of diagnosis of bacterial diarrheal disease by clinical features, *J Pediatr* 78:519, 1971.
149. Neumann HH: Bacteriological safety of hot tapwater in developing countries, *Public Health Rep* 84:812, 1969.
150. Nolan CM et al: *Campylobacter jejuni* enteritis: efficacy of antimicrobial and antimotility drugs, *Am J Gastroenterol* 78:621, 1983.
151. Ortega YR et al: *Cyclospora* species—a new protozoan pathogen of humans, *N Engl J Med* 328:1308, 1993.
152. Osterholm MT et al: An outbreak of a newly recognized chronic diarrhea syndrome associated with raw milk consumption, *JAMA* 256:484, 1986.
153. Owen RL: Direct fecal-oral transmission of giardiasis. In Erlandsen SL, Meyer EA, editors: *Giardia and giardiasis: biology, pathogenesis and epidemiology,* New York, 1984, Plenum Press.
154. Parsonnet J et al: Chronic diarrhea associated with drinking untreated water, *Ann Intern Med* 110:985, 1989.
155. Patterson M, Healy GR, Shabot JM: Serologic testing for amoebiasis, *Gastroenterology* 78:136, 1980.
156. Patterson M, Schoppe LE: The presentation of amoebiasis, *Med Clin North Am* 66:689, 1982.
157. Pehrson PO: Amoebiasis in a non-endemic country, *Scand J Infect Dis* 15:207, 1983.
158. Peltola H et al: Prevention of travellers' diarrhoea by oral B-subunit/whole-cell cholera vaccine, *Lancet* 338:1285, 1991.
159. Penn RG et al: *Plesiomonas shigelloides* overgrowth in the small intestine, *J Clin Microbiol* 15:869, 1982.
160. Phillips RA: Water and electrolyte losses in cholera, *Fed Proc* 23:705, 1964.
161. Pichler HET et al: Clinical efficacy of ciprofloxacin compared with placebo in bacterial diarrhea, *Am J Med* 82(suppl 4A):329, 1987.
162. Pickering LK et al: Fecal leukocytes in enteric infections, *Am J Clin Pathol* 68:562, 1977.
163. Pickering LK et al: Isolation of enteric pathogens from asymptomatic students from the United States and Latin America, *J Infect Dis* 135:1003, 1977.
164. Pickering LK et al: Absorption of salicylate and bismuth from a bismuth subsalicylate–containing compound (Pepto-Bismol), *J Pediatr* 99:654, 1981.
165. Pickering LK et al: Diarrhea caused by *Shigella,* rotavirus and *Giardia* in day care centers: prospective study, *J Pediatr* 99:51, 1981.
166. Pitarangsi C et al: Enteropathogenicity of *Aeromonas hydrophila* and *Plesiomonas shigelloides:* prevalence among individuals with and without diarrhea in Thailand, *Infect Immun* 35:666, 1982.
167. Potter ME et al: Unpasteurized milk; the hazards of a health fetish, *JAMA* 252:2050, 1984.
168. Rademacher CM et al: Results of a double-blind placebo-controlled study using ciprofloxacin for prevention of travelers' diarrhea, *Eur J Clin Microbiol Infect Dis* 8:690, 1989.
169. Rendtorff RC: The experimental transmission of human intestinal protozoan parasites. II. *Giardia lamblia* cysts given in capsules, *Am J Hyg* 59:209, 1954.
170. Rendtorff RC: The experimental transmission of human intestinal protozoan parasites. IV. Attempts to transmit *Entamoeba coli* and *Giardia lamblia* cysts by water, *Am J Hyg* 60:327, 1954.
171. Reves R et al: Failure to demonstrate effectiveness of an anticholinergic drug in the symptomatic treatment of acute travelers' diarrhea, *J Clin Gastroenterol* 5:223, 1983.
172. Riggs JL et al: Detection of *Giardia lamblia* by immunofluorescence, *Appl Environ Microbiol* 45:698, 1983.
173. Rivera F et al: Bottled mineral waters polluted by protozoa in Mexico, *J Protozool* 28:54, 1981.
174. Rosenberg ML et al: Epidemic diarrhea at Crater Lake from enterotoxigenic *Escherichia coli, Ann Intern Med* 86:714, 1977.
175. Rosenstein G et al: Warning: the use of Lomotil in children, *Pediatrics* 51:132, 1973.
176. Rossi JG, Mangione RA: Travelers' diarrhea (letter), *N Engl J Med* 3018:464, 1983.
177. Rothbaum R et al: A clinicopathologic study of enterocyte-adherent *Escherichia coli:* a cause of protracted diarrhea in infants, *Gastroenterology* 83:441, 1982.
178. Ryder RW et al: Travelers' diarrhea in Panamanian tourists in Mexico, *J Infect Dis* 144:442, 1981.
179. Sack DA et al: Prophylactic doxycycline for travelers' diarrhea: results of a prospective double-blind study of Peace Corps volunteers in Kenya, *N Engl J Med* 298:758, 1978.

180. Sack DA et al: Prophylactic doxycycline for travelers' diarrhea: results of a prospective double blind study of Peace Corps volunteers in Morocco, *Gastroenterology* 76:1368, 1979.
181. Sack RB: Human diarrheal disease caused by enterotoxigenic *Escherichia coli, Annu Rev Microbiol* 29:333, 1975.
182. Sack RB: Antimicrobial prophylaxis of travelers' diarrhea: a selected summary, *Rev Infect Dis* 8(suppl 2):160, 1986.
183. Sack RB et al: Doxycycline prophylaxis of travelers' diarrhea in Honduras, an area where resistance to doxycycline is common among enteropathogenic *Escherichia coli, Am J Trop Med Hyg* 33:460, 1984.
184. Salaki JS, Shirey JL, Strickland GT: Successful treatment of symptomatic *Entamoeba polecki* infection, *Am J Trop Med Hyg* 28:190, 1979.
185. Saphra I, Winter JW: Clinical manifestation of salmonellosis in man, *N Engl J Med* 256:1128, 1957.
186. Sargeaunt PG, Jackson TFHG, Simjee A: Biochemical homogeneity of *Entamoeba histolytica* isolates, especially those from liver abscess, *Lancet* 1:1386, 1982.
187. Sepulveda B: Amebiasis: host-pathogen biology, *Rev Infect Dis* 6:1247, 1982.
188. Shlim DR et al: An algae-like organism associated with an outbreak of prolonged diarrhea among foreigners in Nepal, *Am J Trop Med Hyg* 45:383, 1991.
189. Shore EG et al: Enterotoxin-producing *Escherichia coli* and diarrheal disease in adult travelers: a prospective study, *J Infect Dis* 129:577, 1974.
190. Shukry S et al: Detection of enteropathogens in fatal and potentially fatal diarrhea in Cairo, Egypt, *J Clin Microbiol* 24:959, 1986.
191. Snyder JD, Blake PA: Is cholera a problem for US travelers? *JAMA* 247:1168, 1982.
192. Snyder JD, Merson MH: The magnitude of the global problem of acute diarrhoeal disease: a review of active surveillance data, *Bull WHO* 60:605, 1982.
193. Soave R, Ma P: Cryptosporidiosis: travelers' diarrhea in two families, *Arch Intern Med* 145:70, 1985.
194. Spencer MJ, Garcia LS, Chapin MR: *Dientamoeba fragilis:* an intestinal pathogen in children? *Am J Dis Child* 133:390, 1979.
195. Sriratanaban A, Reiprayoon S: *Vibrio parahaemolyticus:* a major cause of travelers' diarrhea in Bangkok, *Am J Trop Med Hyg* 31:128, 1982.
196. Steffen R: Epidemiologic studies of travelers' diarrhea, severe gastrointestinal infections, and cholera, *Rev Infect Dis* 8(suppl 2):122, 1986.
197. Steffen R, Gsell O: Prophylaxis of travellers' diarrhea, *J Trop Med Hyg* 84:239, 1981.
198. Steffen R, Heusser R, DuPont HL: Prevention of travelers' diarrhea by nonantibiotic drugs, *Rev Infect Dis* 8(suppl 2):151, 1986.
199. Steffen R et al: Epidemiology of diarrhea in travelers, *JAMA* 249:1176, 1983.
200. Steffen R et al: Prevention of travelers' diarrhea by the tablet form of bismuth subsalicylate, *Antimicrob Agents Chemother* 29:625, 1986.
201. Stehr-Green JK et al: Shedding of oocysts in immunocompetent individuals infected with *Cryptosporidium, Am J Trop Med Hyg* 36:338, 1987.
202. Stoll BJ et al: Value of stool examination in patients with diarrhea, *Br Med J* 286:2037, 1983.
203. Swartzwelder JC: Balantidiasis, *Am J Dig Dis* 17:173, 1950.
204. Taylor DN, Echeverria P: Etiology and epidemiology of travelers' diarrhea in Asia, *Rev Infect Dis* 8(suppl 2):136, 1986.
205. Taylor DN et al: Polymicrobial aetiology of travellers' diarrhoea, *Lancet* 1:381, 1985.
206. Taylor DN et al: Treatment of travelers' diarrhea: ciprofloxacin plus loperamide compared with ciprofloxacin alone: a placebo-controlled, randomized trial, *Ann Intern Med* 114:731, 1991.
207. Taylor JW, Gray GW, Greenberg HB: Norwalk-related viral gastroenteritis due to contaminated drinking water, *Am J Epidemiol* 114:584, 1981.
208. Tjoa WS et al: Location of food consumption and travelers' diarrhea, *Am J Epidemiol* 106:61, 1977.
209. Vantrappen G et al: *Yersinia* enteritis and enterocolitis: gastroenterological aspects, *Gastroenterology* 72:220, 1977.
210. Vantrappen G et al: *Yersinia* enteritis, *Med Clin North Am* 66:639, 1982.
211. von Graevenitz A, Mensch AH: The genus *Aeromonas* in human bacteriology, *N Engl J Med* 278:245, 1968.
212. Walsh JA: Problems in recognition and diagnosis of amebiasis: estimation of the global morbidity and mortality, *Rev Infect Dis* 8:228, 1986.
213. Walsh JA, Warren KS: Selective primary health care: an interim strategy, for disease control in developing countries, *N Engl J Med* 301:967, 1979.
214. Walzer PD (Center for Disease Control): Giardiasis in travelers, *J Infect Dis* 124:235, 1971.
215. Walzer PD et al: Balantidiasis outbreak in Truk, *Am J Trop Med Hyg* 22:33, 1973.
216. Wanger AR et al: Enteroinvasive *Escherichia coli* in travelers' diarrhea, *J Infect Dis* 158:640, 1988.
217. Webster ADB: Giardiasis and immunodeficiency disease, *R Soc Trop Med Hyg* 74:440, 1980.
218. Whiteside ME et al: Enteric coccidiosis among patients with the acquired immunodeficiency syndrome, *Am J Trop Med Hyg* 33:1065, 1984.
219. WHO Working Group: Intestinal immunity and vaccine development, *Bull WHO* 57:719, 1979.
220. Woo PK: Evidence for animal reservoirs and transmission of *Giardia* infection between animal species. In Erlandsen SL, Meyer EA, editors: *Giardia and giardiasis: biology, pathogenesis and epidemiology,* New York, 1984, Plenum Press.
221. Wood LV et al: Incidence of bacterial enteropathogens in foods from Mexico, *Appl Environ Microbiol* 46:328, 1983.
222. Yang J, Scholten TH: *Dientamoeba fragilis:* a review with notes on its epidemiology, pathogenicity, mode of transmission, and diagnosis, *Am J Trop Med Hyg* 26:16, 1977.
223. Zaki AM et al: The detection of enteropathogens in acute diarrhea in a family cohort population in rural Egypt, *Am J Trop Med Hyg* 35:1013, 1986.

43 FIELD WATER DISINFECTION

Howard D. Backer

Water-borne disease is a risk for international travelers who visit undeveloped countries that have poor hygiene and inadequate sanitation, and for wilderness users in developed countries, including the United States. Natural water may be contaminated with organic or inorganic material from land erosion, dissolution of minerals, decay of organic vegetation, biologic organisms that reside in soil and water, industrial chemical pollutants, and microorganisms from animal or human biologic wastes.[37,66] Fecal pollution with enteric pathogens is the primary reason for disinfecting drinking water. However, chemical contamination of groundwater is increasing at an alarming rate in the United States and around the world from industrial, agricultural, and individual sources. Natural organic and inorganic material may not cause illness but can impart unpleasant turbidity, color, and taste to the water. Water safety cannot be estimated by look, smell, or taste. Of the 1700 million square miles of water on earth, less than 0.5% is potable.[220]

Etiology and Risk in Underdeveloped Countries

In tropical areas and developing countries, water has a complex relationship with spread of disease. A useful classification from Bradley[20] is summarized in Table 43-1. Worldwide, 1.5 billion rural people and 200 million urban people in the world suffer from the lack of safe drinking water and adequate sanitation. Some estimates suggest that 80% of the world's diseases are linked to inadequate water supply and sanitation. Between 10 and 25 million people die each year (28,000 to 68,000 persons each day) from diseases caused by contaminated water and unsanitary conditions. In undeveloped countries these illnesses account for 1 billion cases of diarrhea every year and 95% of the deaths in children under 5 years of age.[212,215]

The sanitary situation in many undeveloped countries is illustrated by current statistics from Peru evaluated during a recent cholera epidemic. Only 73% of the urban population have access to a water distribution system and only 50% have access to sanitation services. In rural areas only 23% have access to a water supply and 6% have access to a sanitation system. In urban areas over the past 5 years the quality of water has deteriorated because of the lack of water treatment chemicals, laboratories for monitoring, and operators to control the processes. Institutional barriers impede improvements for adequate water and sanitation systems.[43]

Infectious agents found in contaminated drinking water worldwide with the potential for water-borne transmission include bacteria, viruses, protozoa, and parasites (Box 43-1). This list is similar to that of potential etiologic agents of traveler's diarrhea. Separating the contribution of water-borne transmission of these pathogens from food-borne and person-to-person transmission is impossible. The latter two are probably more common. The source of fecal contamination may be either human or animal. Some bacterial pathogens occur exclusively in human feces *(Shigella, Salmonella typhosa),* while others may be present in wild or domestic animals *(Yersinia, Campylobacter).* The enteric viruses occur exclusively in human feces, as far as is known.[86] No viruses excreted by animals have been shown to be pathogenic to humans.[153] In any case the major source of these enteric pathogens is fecal contamination from infected residents.

No evidence exists of human immunodeficiency virus (HIV) transmitted via a water-borne route, and no epidemiologic evidence exists of casual transmission by fomites or by any environmentally mediated mode.[161] *Legionella* can be isolated from a variety of aquatic sources and is a common inhabitant of natural surface waters, but the mode of transmission appears to be inhalation of aerosolized water.[189] One report found *Legionella* pneumonia from aspiration during near drowning.[42]

Table 43-1 Water and Spread of Disease

Type	Mechanism	Examples	Prevention
Water borne	Fecal contamination of drinking water by infectious organisms	Typhoid fever, cholera, campylobacteriosis, giardiasis, hepatitis A	Sanitation and disinfection of water
Water washed	Person-to-person fecal-oral spread via direct contact, food, water (all these are also water borne)	Shigellosis, amebiasis, ascariasis, eye and skin infections	Hand washing and personal hygiene
Water based	Organism or agent that lives in water	Schistosomiasis, dracunculosis, parasitic worms	Prevention of exposure from bathing or collecting water
Water related	Spread by insects that breed in water	Malaria, sleep sickness, yellow fever, dengue	Insect protection and piped water

BOX 43-1

WATER-BORNE ENTERIC PATHOGENS

BACTERIAL

Escherichia coli
Shigella
Campylobacter
Vibrio cholerae
Salmonella
Yersinia enterocolitica
Aeromonas

VIRAL

Hepatitis A
Hepatitis E
Norwalk virus
Poliovirus
Miscellaneous enterics (more than 100 types: adenovirus, enterovirus, calcivirus, ECHO, astrovirus, coronavirus, etc.)

PROTOZOAL

Giardia lamblia
Entamoeba histolytica
Cryptosporidium
Blastocystis hominis
Isospora belli
Balantidium coli
Acanthamoeba
Cyclospora coccidian-like body

PARASITIC

Ascaris lumbricoides
Ancylostoma duodenale (hookworm)
Taenia spp. (tapeworm)
Fasciola hepatica (sheep liver fluke)
Dracunculus medinensis
Strongyloides stercoralis
Trichuris trichiura (whipworm)
Clonorchis sinensis (Oriental liver fluke)
Paragonimus westermani (lung fluke)
Diphyllobothrium latum (fish tapeworm)
Echinococcus granulosus (hydatid disease)

Data from Drinking Water Health Effects Task Force, U.S. Environmental Protection Agency: *Health effects of drinking water treatment technologies,* Chelsea, Mich, 1989, Lewis Publishers (Originally published Washington DC, USEPA, 1988); and Gelreich EE: Microbiological quality of source waters for water supply. In McFeters GA, editor: *Drinking water microbiology,* New York, 1990, Springer-Verlag.

In certain tropical countries the influence of high-density population, rampant pollution, and absence of sanitation systems means that available raw water is virtually wastewater.[35] Contamination of tap water must be assumed because of antiquated and inadequately monitored disposal, disinfection, and distribution systems.

Water-Borne Risk in the United States

Water-borne pathogens account for most infectious diarrhea acquired in U.S. wilderness and recreation areas. From 1920 to 1980, 178 water-borne outbreaks were reported in systems serving parks, campgrounds, and recreation areas.[42] Most of these were caused by use of contaminated, untreated surface water or groundwater. Between 1970 and 1980, gastroenteritis of undefined etiology accounted for the largest number of cases, but *Giardia* caused the most cases of defined etiology.[42] During the 2-year period from 1989 to 1990, *Giardia* continued to be the most commonly identified cause of all water-borne disease outbreaks in the United States.[81] A distinct seasonal variation is seen, with the majority of cases from recreational areas occurring during the summer months.[42] This is probably a result of both increased contamination and number of persons at risk.

Since the source of *G. lamblia* in surface water is fecal contamination of water, other enteric organisms are to be expected. The other most commonly identified causes of water-borne outbreaks of illness in the United States between 1976 and 1980 were chemical poisoning (3081 cases), *Shigella* (2392 cases), viral gastroenteritis (3147 cases), *Salmonella* (1113 cases), *Campylobacter* (3821 cases), and hepatitis A virus (HAV) (95 cases).[42] Several other enteric organisms have been implicated in illness from ingestion of wilderness or recreational water (Box 43-2). *Campylobacter* enteritis was found to be more prevalent than giardiasis among campers in Grand Teton National Park during one summer and was ascribed to untreated surface water.[195] Water-borne *Cryptosporidium* epidemics are being identified with increasing frequency, and the organism appears to be ubiquitous (see later discussion).[79,166] Hepatitis E has occurred in travelers, mainly from Asia, and water-borne transmission is suspected.[29,99] Some common, well-known enteric pathogens, such as *Vibrio cholerae, Entamoeba histolytica,* and *Shigella dysenteriae,* and some lesser known, such as *Aeromonas hydrophila,* have been implicated in past water-borne epidemics and clearly have the potential for wilderness outbreaks.[41-43,87] Two new organisms have been implicated recently in U.S. water-borne outbreaks of disease: enteropathogenic *Escherichia coli* (which caused four deaths in 1989 and 1990) and a cyanobacterium (blue-green, algalike), whose role in causing diarrheal illness is being studied.[81]

BOX 43-2

ENTERIC PATHOGENS IN U.S. WILDERNESS OR RECREATIONAL WATER

COMMONLY REPORTED

Giardia
- Numerous outbreaks in recreational areas and mountain resort communities[41,42,90]
- Campers in Utah[6]

Campylobacter
- Grand Teton National Park campers[195]

OCCASIONALLY REPORTED WITH FIRM EVIDENCE FOR WATER BORNE

Hepatitis A
- Various water-borne outbreaks[41,42,129]
- Recreational water[70]

Hepatitis E
- Kathmandu, contaminated surface waters[99]

E. coli
- Crater Lake National Park[171]

Shigella
- Colorado River rafters[121]
- Recreational water[81,170,187]

Enteric viruses
- Yellowstone National Park[25]
- Recreational water[7,81]
- Campground well, stream[27]
- Lake, pool, recreation area, well[70]

Cryptosporidium
- Untreated surface water[26]
- Public water supply[48,79]

SUSPECTED

Yersinia enterocolitica[177]
- Montana ski resort[54]
- Hunting camp[78]

RECREATIONAL CONTACT

Inadvertent drinking during recreational water contact is a risk for swimmers and white-water boaters. Recreational water activities have resulted in typhoid fever, salmonellosis, shigellosis, viral gastroenteritis, and hepatitis A, as well as in wound infections, septicemia, and aspiration pneumonia.[42,168,226] From 1989 to 1990, 17 outbreaks of infectious diseases caused by the use of recreational water (excluding hot tub dermatitis) were reported in the United States, including 13 of swimming-associated gastroenteritis, 5 outbreaks of shigellosis (3 in lakes, 1 in a pond), a hepatitis A outbreak from a swimming pool, and 3 cases of primary amebic meningoencephalitis caused by *Naegleria* from a lake or pond.[81] *Giardia* has also been acquired while swimming.[145]

EVALUATING RISK

Water-borne outbreaks do not give a complete picture of the potential for water-borne illness. Most outbreaks of water-borne disease are not identified unless at least 1% of the population becomes ill within a few months, providing an insensitive mechanism for detecting water contamination. Risk of water-borne illness depends on the number of organisms consumed, which depends on the volume of water, concentration of organisms, and treatment system efficiency.[41] Infectious dose data (Table 43-2) and several statistical techniques have been used to devise models for determining risk. These cannot be applied unless the microbial

Table 43-2 Estimated Infectious Levels of Enteric Organisms

Organism	Infectious Dose
Coliform bacteria	10^5
Enteric viruses	1-10
Giardia	10-100
Cryptosporidium	(?)10-100

content of water is known. Pathogenic microorganisms clearly exist in most raw source waters, especially in surface waters.[51] One investigator found significant numbers of pathogenic *Salmonella* bacteria in high-quality surface water in the Colorado mountains, presumably from animal contamination.[58]

Levels of coliform bacteria have historically been used as an indicator of microbiologic contamination, and they remain the worldwide standard indicator organism for determining potable water. *Escherichia coli* inhabits predominantly the intestines of warm-blooded animals, so its presence is assumed to indicate recent fecal contamination.[80] While compelling reasons exist for testing for other organisms before determining the safety of drinking water, cost and relative difficulty in testing for viruses and protozoa are major obstacles to expanding routine water testing.

Most microbiologic testing is done on community water intake sources and sewage treatment effluent. Sewage discharges contain a variety of pathogens related to the size of population, seasonal patterns of disease, and the extent of community infection.[66] The concentration of coliform bacteria in raw sewage is 10^9/100 ml, and the concentration of enteroviruses is estimated at 10^3/L to 10^4/L. In polluted stream water, coliform bacteria have been found to exceed 10^5/100 ml and viruses may be found in concentrations of 10 to 100/L.[207] Water plant intakes from U.S. midwestern rivers commonly contain up to 2000 fecal coliform bacteria/100 ml.[67] Overall, surface waters for U.S. public water intakes were found to contain the following coliform bacteria counts: 14% contained 200 to 2000/L, 23% contained 21 to 200/L, 30% contained 1 to 20/L, and 44% contained less than 1/L.[66] Less information is available for more remote water sources.[41]

BACTERIAL SPORES

Bacterial spores can cause serious wound and gut infections but are not likely water-borne enteric pathogens. *Clostridium* is ubiquitous in soil, lake sediment, tropical water sources, and the stool of animals and humans.[80,175] *C. perfringens* type C causes enteritis necroticans, probably through in vivo production of an enterotoxin, and thus has the potential for water-borne transmission in the tropics. However, the epidemiology of these infections is related to food-borne sources; infections occur in small children and malnourished adults. *C. botulinum* and *C. perfringens* type A food poisoning requires germination of spores in food by inadequate cooking, then production of an enterotoxin, which is ingested.

VIRUSES

The most frequent water-borne illness (acute infectious nonbacterial gastroenteritis of unknown etiology) in the United States may be caused by undetected viruses.[42,119,183,219] Hepatitis A virus, Norwalk virus, and rotavirus are the main concerns for potable water supplies; the last two are responsible for about 77% of acute water-borne gastroenteritis.[220] Many others are capable and suspected of water-borne transmission, and more than 100 different virus types are known to be excreted in human feces.[76,226] Furthermore, the infectious dose of enteric viruses is thought to be only a few infectious units in the most susceptible people.[119,213,226] Testing in the United States, Europe, and developing countries shows consistent, sometimes astounding, degrees of viral contamination of drinking and surface water.* Even remote surface lakes and streams tested in California showed disturbing levels of viral contamination.[69] Widespread enteric viral contamination was found at multiple sites in a popular recreation canyon in Arizona. Viruses included polio, ECHO, Coxsackie, rotavirus, and other unidentifiable viruses, exceeding the recommended state level for recreational water use in several areas. Virus levels correlated with human activity but did not correlate well with excess levels of standard coliform indicators.[168] A consensus of virologists is that all surface water supplies in the United States and Canada contain naturally occurring human enteroviruses.[220]

GIARDIA

New methods to detect *Giardia* cysts in surface water have found widespread contamination.[91,162,186] Recent surveys have found 0.6 to 5 cysts/100 L (average) in pristine surface waters and 0.33 to 104 cysts/100 L in unprotected watersheds.[167] Surface water samples for 301 municipalities in the United States had *Giardia* cysts present in 798 of 4423 samples. Repeated sampling of "negative" sources invariably produced positive results. Hibler and Hancock[82] have also found cysts as frequently in pristine water and protected sources as in unprotected waters. Samples from Rocky Mountain National Park[109,123] and the California Sierra Nevada[186,192] show a direct correlation between numbers of cysts and levels of human use or beaver habitation. In high-use areas, 44% of samples were positive. An average of 3 to 10 cysts/1000 L water was detected, but in some instances 100 to 600 cysts/1000 L were found. (The laboratory recovery rate for the technique used is 10% to 30%.) One high-use stream drainage in the California Sierra Nevada found mean cyst concentration of 2.0 to 4.5/100 gallons of water filtrate, with a range of 0 to 25/100 gallons.[189,227]

Ongerth[137] tested three pristine rivers and 12 tributaries in the Pacific Northwest, examining 222 samples over 9 months. *Giardia* cysts were found in 94 (43%) samples at a concentration of 0.1 to 5.2 cysts/L, adjusted for a 22% recovery rate by the immunofluorescence procedure. No sig-

*References 40, 66, 69, 84, 119, 147, 183, 205, 226.

nificant variability between sites and no seasonal variation were seen. Ongerth[136] also tested water draining from three surface creeks in California and Washington (considered relatively remote high-quality sources) that provided community water sources, and found 1.3 to 6 cysts/gallon. The source was presumed to be animal, since human access is restricted in these watersheds.

Water testing in Yukon, Canada, yielded *Giardia* cysts in 7 of 22 samples from pristine areas. Of 61 scat samples from various wild animals, 13 yielded *Giardia* cysts.[163]

A zoonosis with *Giardia* is known, but at least three different species of *Giardia* exist and the extent of cross-species infection is not clear.[11,223] Many of the species apparently capable of passing *Giardia* cysts to humans, including dogs, cattle, ungulates (deer), and beaver, are present in wilderness areas. Forty percent of beaver in Colorado were found to be infected and shedding 1×10^8 cysts per animal per day. All of 386 muskrats were found to be infected. Up to 20% of cattle examined were infected.[82] Beaver have been implicated in multiple municipal outbreaks of giardiasis.

Ten *G. lamblia* cysts may result in infection, although the infections in this widely quoted study were asymptomatic.[157] Even with a low infectious dose, the cyst recovery data indicate that the risk of ingesting an infectious dose of *Giardia* cysts is small.[230,231] However, the likely model that poses a risk to campers is pulse contamination—a brief period of high cyst concentration from fecal contamination. Beaver stool and human stool may contain 1×10^6 cysts/g. Stream contamination from a beaver has been calculated to reach 245 cysts/gallon.[91] In this instance, small amounts of water may cause infection, similar to an outbreak among lap swimmers from inadvertent water ingestion in a fecally contaminated pool.[145]

CRYPTOSPORIDIUM[165,166]

Cryptosporidium is a newly recognized enteric pathogen. Many aspects of the epidemiology and transmission appear similar to *Giardia*. Large water-borne outbreaks of *Cryptosporidium* have been documented.[26,48,79] The largest took place in Milwaukee in 1993. The oocysts are found widespread in surface water, and the cyst is durable in the environment. A large zoonosis is evident, and the infectious dose is also unknown. Thus the protective nature of antibodies is uncertain.

Environmental occurrence appears ubiquitous, with an average of 5180 oocysts/L in raw sewage with agricultural runoff, an average of 1063 oocysts/L in treated sewage, and up to 40 oocysts/L in effluents. In the western United States, oocysts were found in 77% of rivers, 75% of lakes, and 28% of treated drinking water samples. The average level in surface waters ranged from 0.02 to 1.3 oocysts/L, in pristine areas from 0.02 to 0.08/L, in reservoirs and lakes from 0.58 to 0.91/L, and in streams and rivers from 0.94 to 1.2/L. These data probably underestimate the levels because of insensitivity of sampling techniques.[138,166] Oocysts were found in Yukon water that received sewage effluent, but not in remote pristine water.[163]

Although the evidence is mounting for a significant role in water-borne gastroenteritis, the overall significance of water-borne cryptosporidiosis is unknown.

PARASITES

Parasitic organisms other than *Giardia* and *Entamoeba histolytica* are seldom considered in discussions of disinfection. Infectious eggs or larvae of many helminths are found in sewage, even in the United States.[156,180] The frequency of infection by water-borne transmission is unknown, since food and environmental contamination or skin penetration is more prevalent.[22,227]

The most obvious risk is from nematodes with no intermediate host that are infectious immediately or soon after eggs are passed in stool with no intermediate host. *Ascaris lumbricoides* (roundworm) is transmitted by ingestion of the eggs in contaminated food or drink. In endemic areas 85% of the population is infected; this leads to daily global environmental contamination by 9×10^{14} eggs.[227] *Ancylostoma duodenale* (hookworm) usually infects as larvae penetrate the skin of the foot, but it also may be acquired by mouth. Oral entry of the larvae causes pulmonary (Wakana) disease.[227] *Necator americanus* does not appear to be infectious via the oral route.

Taenia solium (pork tapeworm) is infectious to humans in cyst or egg form. Eggs passed in stool are ingested in food or water and develop into tissue cysts, often in the brain, resulting in cysticercosis.

Echinococcus granulosus (dog tapeworm) can use humans as an intermediate host. Eggs from the feces of an infected dog or other carnivore are ingested in food and water. Hydatid disease generates cysts in the liver, peritoneum, and other sites.

Isle Royale National Park in Lake Superior has issued a warning to disinfect water to remove or destroy echinococcal parasites because of infection in the local population of wolves. However, no human cases have been reported.

Fasciola hepatica (liver fluke of herbivores and humans) is normally acquired by ingestion of encysted metacercariae on water plants or free organisms in water.

Cercariae of schistosomiasis, which live in fresh water and normally enter through skin, can enter through the oral mucosa. Normally, the cercariae are killed by stomach acid.

Dracunculus medinensis (Guinea tapeworm) is a tissue nematode of humans and is the only such disease transmitted exclusively through drinking water.[215] *Dracunculus* larvae are released in water from subcutaneous worms on the legs of infected bathers or water-gatherers. Larvae are ingested by a tiny crustacean (*Cyclops* species), which acts as the intermediate host and releases infectious larvae when ingested by humans.

Persistence of Enteric Pathogens in the Environment

Once environmental contamination has occurred, enteric pathogens can retain viability for long periods (Table 43-3).[51] Factors promoting survival of microorganisms are pH near neutral (between 6 and 8) and cold temperatures, which explains the risk of transmission in mountain regions. In temperate and warm water, survival is measured in days, with densities of infectious agents decreasing by 90% every 60 minutes. However, tropical water differs from temperate in nutrients and microbiologically rich environment. Coliform bacteria can survive several months in natural tropical river water and may even proliferate. Survival of other bacteria is also much longer (about 200 hours in tropical compared with 30 hours in temperate water). *E. coli* and *Vibrio cholerae* may occur naturally in tropical waters and be capable of surviving indefinitely.[43,80,141]

Most enteric organisms, including *Shigella,* resist freezing.[50,52] *S. typhosa* can survive for up to 5 months in frozen debris and ice.[220] Hepatitis A virus survives 6 months at below freezing temperatures.[199] Potentially water-borne parasitic eggs and larvae are also long lived in the environment; *Ascaris* eggs remain viable for 6 to 9 years and are resistent to desiccation,[227] hookworm larvae retain infectivity for 122 days during the rainy season, and *Echinococcus* eggs remain viable for 5 to 12 months.[22]

Standards

Water standards in the United States still require microbiologic testing only for enteric bacteria; the Public Health Service recommendations for potable water specify a mean of 1 coliform organism/100 ml water or 10 organisms/L. Absolute limits are 3 coliform bacteria/50 ml, 4/100 ml, and 13/500 ml.[209] These standards acknowledge the impracticality of trying to eliminate all microorganisms from drinking water; they allow a small risk of enteric infection.[183] In 1989 the standards for detection of fecal coliform bacteria in drinking water were relaxed slightly in recognition that coliform bacteria occur in large numbers in many water distribution systems that have no problem with water-borne disease.[207] Generally the goal is to achieve a 3 to 5 log reduction in the level of microorganisms. In 1986 an amendment to the Safe Drinking Water Act required the Environmental Protection Agency (EPA) to establish drinking water regulations for treatment of surface waters that include *Giardia* and enteric viruses. Treatment must reduce *Giardia* by 99.9% (3 log) and enteric viruses by at least 99.99% (4 log).[153] Risk models can be used to predict levels of illness and desired levels of reduction. For example, EPA guidelines suggest *Giardia* cyst removal with the goal of ensuring high probability that consumer risk is no more than 1 infection per 10,000 people per year.[154] *Cryptosporidium* was added to the Drinking Water Priority List in 1988, meaning that the EPA must provide regulations for its control.

Table 43-3 Viability of Enteric Pathogens in Water

Organism	Conditions	Survival	Reference
Giardia	Cold	2-3 months	14, 49
Giardia	15° C lake, river	10-28 days	49
Entamoeba histolytica	Cold	3 months	33
Vibrio cholerae	Cold	4-5 weeks	59
V. cholerae	Tropical	>1 year	141
Campylobacter	Cold	3-5 weeks	17
Campylobacter	Temperate stream	3-10 days	181
Escherichia coli	Temperate stream	13 hours	181
E. coli	Tropical	>1 year	141
Salmonella	Temperate stream	Half-life 16 hours	141
Yersinia	Temperate stream	540 days	181
Shigella	Temperate stream	Half-life 22 hours	181
Shigella	Freeze/thaw	Yes	52
Enteric pathogens	Freeze/thaw	Yes	50
Salmonella typhosa	Ice/frozen debris	5 months	220
Viruses	Cold	17-130 days	173,226
Hepatitis A virus	Cold	1 year	15, 199
Hepatitis A	Fresh, sea, wastewater	12 weeks	15
Hepatitis A	<0° C	6 months	199
Cryptosporidium	Cold	12 months	47
Ascaris eggs	Wet or dry	6-9 years	227
Hookworm larvae	Wet sand	122 days	22

Benefits of Treatment

Virtually all enteric pathogenic microorganisms are killed or inactivated by chlorine and other disinfection processes. Disinfection alters the incidence of certain enteric diseases but does not eliminate diseases. In general, commonly used drinking water treatment processes provide enormous benefits with minimal risk. Without disinfection and filtration, water-borne disease would spread rapidly in most public water systems served by surface water.[51]

In an attempt to see whether treatment standards are generally adequate for preventing disease, Payment and associates[140] studied two large population bases (N = 1026 in each group), one supplied with under-sink reverse osmosis filters capable of removing all microorganisms and the other supplied with a dummy filter yielding regular tap water. A higher incidence of mild gastrointestinal illness was found in the tap water group. However, no organisms were detected at the municipal treatment plant output, so there was no speculation as to the cause.[140]

In remote settings in developing countries, potable water alone does not necessarily make a substantial difference in the incidence of many gastrointestinal diseases. A study in a Brazilian village showed no reduction in incidence of diarrhea with use of disinfected water. This emphasizes the importance of general hygiene, which requires education and sanitation, plus many other variables that have an impact on health and nutrition, all of which influence susceptibility to diarrhea.[35]

Poor local hygiene has a direct effect on wilderness travelers. A *Shigella* outbreak among river rafters on the Colorado river was investigated and assumed to be water borne from adjacent Native American communities, but no source was found in the tributaries. Finally it was traced to infected guides who were shedding organisms in the stool and contaminating clients' food through poor hygienic practices.[121]

Natural Purification Mechanisms of Surface Water

A widespread belief is that streams purify themselves and that certain places are safe for drinking. While these concepts have some truth, they do not preclude the need for further disinfection to ensure water quality.

Surface water is subject to frequent, dramatic changes in microbial quality as a result of activities on a watershed. Stormwater causes deterioration of source water quality by increasing suspended solids, organic materials, and microorganisms. Some of these contaminants are carried by rain from the atmosphere, but most come from ground runoff. In water sources downstream from towns or villages, storms may overload sewage facilities and cause them to discharge directly into the receiving water. However, rainwater can also flush steams clean by dilution and by washing microbe-laden bottom sediments downstream.[66,80]

Every stream, lake, or groundwater aquifer has limited capacity to assimilate waste effluents and stormwater runoff entering the drainage basin. Self-purification is a complex process that involves settling of microorganisms after clumping or adherence to particles, sunlight providing ultraviolet destruction, higher temperatures causing increased metabolic rates and die-off, predators eating bacteria, and dilution. Environmental factors include water volume and temperature, hydrologic effects, acid soil contact, and solar radiation. The process is time dependent and less active during wet periods and winter conditions. Hours needed in flow time downstream to achieve a 90% bacterial kill by natural self-purification vary with pollution inflow and rate of water flow. They have been measured at approximately 50 hours in the Tennessee River in summer, 47 hours in the Ohio River in summer, and 32 hours in the Sacramento River.[66]

Storage in reservoirs or lakes also improves microbiologic quality, with sedimentation as the primary process. A 100- to 1000-fold increase in fecal coliform bacteria can be found in bottom sediments compared with overlying water. This removal must be considered temporary, influenced by recirculation of organisms trapped in bottom sediments.[51,66] In optimal conditions, 10 days of reservoir storage can result in 75% to 99% removal of coliform bacteria and 30 days can produce safe drinking water. Generally, 80% to 90% of bacteria and viruses are removed by storage, depending on inflow and outflow, temperature, and no further contamination. Cysts, with a larger size and greater weight, should settle even faster than bacteria and viruses.[3]

Groundwater is generally cleaner than surface water because of the filtration action of overlying sediments, but wells and aquifers can be polluted from surface runoff. Spring water is generally of higher quality than surface water, provided that the true source is not surface water channeling underground from a short distance above the spring.

Given the preceding factors, drawing conclusions is difficult. The major factor governing the amount of microbe pollution in surface water is human and animal activity in the watershed. The settling effect of lakes may make them safer than streams, but care should be taken not to disturb bottom sediments when obtaining water.

Chemical Hazards

Chemical hazards are also becoming an alarming source of pollution in surface water. Industrialization proceeds worldwide without adequate environmental protection. A vast array of toxins are sold with little concept of safe use and no means of safe disposal. Inorganic chemicals in drinking water include common salts, heavy metals, asbestos, fluorides, nitrates, radionuclides, and some heavy metals (arsenic, copper, iron, lead, selenium). Natural organic chemicals predominate from soil runoff, forest canopy aquatic biota, and human and animal wastes. Synthetic organic matter includes pesticides, herbicides, and chemicals from industrial or human activities.[51] Major underground aquifers are becoming contaminated. Streams and rivers in rural areas are contaminated by individual carelessness, leaching landfills, and agricultural runoff. Atmospheric spread has resulted in pesticides being found in remote wilderness lakes and in the well-publicized acid rain. From 1981 to 1983, chemical-induced gastroenteritis was the third leading cause of water-borne illness outbreaks in the United States.[89] Numerous pesticides have been found in runoff and rivers in agricultural areas of the Midwest.[122] Wilderness users may soon need to ensure removal of chemical, as well as microbiologic, contaminants.

Definitions

Disinfection removes or destroys harmful microorganisms. Technically, the term refers only to chemical means such as halogens, but it can be applied appropriately to heat and filtration. It should not be confused with *sterilization,* which is defined as the destruction or removal of all lifeforms.[111] Water sterilization is not necessary, since not all organisms are enteric human pathogens.[84] *Purification* (a term frequently used interchangeably with "disinfection") is the removal of organic or inorganic chemicals and particulate matter, including radioactive particles. While purification can eliminate offensive color, taste, and odor, it may not remove or kill microorganisms. *Potable* indicates only that a water source, on average over a period of time, contains a "minimal microbial hazard," so the statistical likelihood of illness is acceptable.[215]

Field Water Treatment Methods

HEAT

Heat is the oldest means of water disinfection. The old recommendation for treating water is to boil for 10 minutes and add 1 minute for every 1000 feet in elevation. However, available data indicate this is not necessary for disinfection. The boiling time required is important when fuel is limited. One kilogram of wood is required to boil 1 L of water.[35]

Heat inactivation of microorganisms is exponential and follows first-order kinetics. Time plotted against temperature yields a straight line when plotted on a logarithmic scale.[74,96] Thus the thermal death point is reached in shorter time at higher temperatures, while lower temperatures are effective with a longer contact time. Pasteurization uses this principle to kill enteric food pathogens and spoiling organisms at temperatures between 60° and 70° C, well below boiling.[63] Therefore the minimum critical temperature is well below the boiling point at any terrestrial elevation.

Heat resistance varies with different microorganisms.[2] Common enteric pathogens are readily inactivated by heat. Bacterial spores (such as *Clostridium* species) are the most resistant; some can survive 100° C for long periods[64] but, as previously discussed, are not likely to be water-borne enteric pathogens.

Protozoa and Parasites

Protozoal cysts, including *Giardia* and *E. histolytica,* are the most susceptible to heat. Jarroll, Hoff, and Meyer[95] showed that *Giardia* cysts are inactivated after 5 minutes in 55° C (131° F) water or immediately in boiling water.[14] Ongerth and associates[139] achieved similar results: heating to 50° C for 10 minutes produced 95% inactivation of *Giardia* cysts, 60° C produced 98% inactivation, and 70° C produced 100% inactivation. In a biologic model, Aukerman and Monzingo[5] demonstrated cyst inactivation by heating water to 55° C, then cooling, but 40° and 50° C were not effective. *E. histolytica* and parasitic nematode cysts are also killed at these temperatures.[32,130,180] *Cryptosporidium* is also inactivated at pasteurization levels: 45° C for 5 to 20 minutes, or by warming to 55° C gradually over 20 minutes.[4]

Parasitic eggs, larvae, and cercariae are all susceptible to heat. For most helminth eggs and larvae (which are more resistant than cercariae and *Cyclops*), the critical lethal temperature is 50° to 55° C.[180]

Bacteria

Common bacterial enteric pathogens *(E. coli, Salmonella, Shigella)* are killed by standard pasteurization temperatures of 55° C (131° F) for 30 minutes or 65° C (149° F) for less than 1 minute.[63,130] Recent studies confirmed safety of water contaminated with *V. cholerae* and *E. coli* after 10 minutes at 60° to 62° C or after boiling water for 30 seconds.[160]

Viruses

Viruses are more closely related to vegetative bacteria than to spore-bearing organisms[96] and are generally inactivated at 56° to 60° C in less than 20 to 40 minutes.[2,142,194] Inactivation at higher temperatures is similar to that of vegetative bacteria. Death occurs in less than 1 minute above 70° C (158° F).[97] This has been confirmed in milk products, despite some degree of thermal protection from particles.[193] Lymphadenopathy-associated virus (LAV), an experimental model for HIV virus, is inactivated at 56° C after 30 minutes.[188]

Hepatitis A Virus. Given its environmental stability and clinical virulence, hepatitis A virus causes special concern. It should respond to heat like other enteric viruses,[72] but data indicate that it has greater thermal resistance than some other enteric viruses. Widely varying data are probably the result of variation in models for infectivity and destruction and in testing media. Hepatitis A virus maintained infectivity after exposure to 56° C for 30 minutes but was uninfective and nonimmunogenic after exposure to 98° C for 1 minute.[108] Heat treatment of infected shellfish at 60° C (140° F) for 19 minutes decreased infectivity and immunogenicity in monkeys.[143] Fifty percent of hepatitis A virus particles disintegrated after 10 minutes at 61° C, compared with 43° C for similar destruction of poliovirus.[199] Using new cell culture and radioimmunoassay, researchers found that hepatitis A virus completely lost infectivity after heating to 85° C for 1 minute.[176,199] Hepatitis B virus, which has greater thermal resistance than hepatitis A, can be inactivated in vaccine preparation at 98° C for 1 minute or 101° C for 90 seconds.[149] Hepatitis E virus, which can be water borne, is inactivated at 60° C for 30 minutes.[199]

Recommendation

In summary, enteric pathogens are killed within seconds by boiling water and rapidly at temperatures above 60° C. In the wilderness the time required to heat water from 55° C to boiling temperature works toward disinfection. Therefore any water brought to a boil should be adequately disinfected. An extra margin of safety can be added by boiling for 1 minute or by keeping the water covered and allowing it to cool slowly after boiling. Although the boiling point decreases with increasing altitude, this is not significant compared with the time required for thermal death at these temperatures (Table 43-4). In recognition of the difference between pasteurizing water for drinking purposes and sterilizing for surgical purposes, many other sources now agree with this recommendation to bring water to a boil or to boil it for 1 minute. However, to give a wide margin of safety, many still suggest 3 minutes' boiling time at high altitude.[28,65,88,160]

When no other means are available, the use of hot tap water has been suggested to prevent traveler's diarrhea in developing countries.[130,131] Ciochetti and Metcalf[36] experimented with a solar cooker constructed from a foil-lined cardboard box with a glass window in the lid for disinfecting large amounts of water by pasteurization. They were able to obtain bottom temperatures of 65° C for at least 1 hour in up to three 3.7 L jugs; the temperature was much higher if only one jug was used or if the box was rotated to follow the sun.[37]

PHYSICAL REMOVAL

Filtration

The size of a microorganism determines its susceptibility to filtration (Table 43-5). Filters may be rated by absolute retention; by the maximum size of any particle that can pass through; or by industrial or "nominal" standards, which represent a reduction level somewhere above 90% and which allow a small number of larger particles in the effluent. Ratings are determined with hard particles (beads of known diameter), while microorganisms are soft and compressible under pressure.

Table 43-4 Boiling Temperatures at Various Altitudes

Altitude (ft)	Boiling Point (°C)
5,000	95
10,000	90
14,000	86
19,000	81

Table 43-5 Average Size of Water-Borne Pathogens

Organism	Size (μm)
Giardia cyst	6-10 × 8-15
Entamoeba histolytica cyst	5-30 (average 10)
Cryptosporidium oocyst	2-6
Escherichia coli	0.5 × 3-8
Campylobacter	0.2-0.4 × 1.5-3.5
Viruses	0.03
Nematode eggs	30-40 × 50-80
Schistosome cercariae	50 × 100
Dracunculus larvae	20 × 500
Fasciola hepatica metacercariae	200
Hookworm larvae	16 × 275-500

Filters can be constructed with various architecture and materials, and many filters are available for field use. Surface, membrane, or mesh filters are very thin with a single layer of fairly precise pores, whose size should be equal to or less than the smallest dimension of the organism. These filters provide little volume for holding contaminants, so they will clog rapidly but can be cleaned easily by washing and brushing without destroying the filter. Maze or depth filters depend on a long, irregular labyrinth to trap the organism, so they may have a larger pore or passage size. Contaminants adhere to the walls of the passageway or are trapped in the numerous dead-end tunnels. Granular media, such as sand or charcoal, diatomaceous earth, or ceramic filters function as maze filters. Depth filters are commonly used in municipal plants to remove particles, the majority of cysts, and a large number of bacteria.[46,116] A depth filter has a large holding capacity for particles, so it lasts longer before clogging. However, they are hard to clean effectively, since many particles are trapped deep in the filter. Surface cleaning is partially effective but tends to destroy some of the filter medium. As the filter clogs, it requires increasing pressure to drive the water through, which can force microorganisms throught the filter. Bacteria may grow within a depth filter.

Filters have the advantage of being simple, not requiring a holding time, and not being dependent on water quality. They do not add any unpleasant taste, and if the filter contains charcoal, the taste may be improved. But several potential problems exist with filters. A crack or eroded channel allows passage of unfiltered water. Effective filters need a pump or substantial standing pressure; even laboratory filter paper with pores small enough to exclude bacteria is impermeable to water without back pressure. All filters eventually clog from suspended particulate matter (present even in clear streams), requiring cleaning or replacement of the filter.

A membrane with pore size of 0.2 μm is required for removal of enteric bacteria. *Giardia* and *E. histolytica* cysts are easily filtered, requiring a maximum filter size of 5 μm. *Cryptosporidium* cysts are somewhat smaller than *Giardia* and more flexible; 57% are able to pass through a 3 μm membrane filter, so a filter with 1 to 2 μm pore size is recommended.[166] Helminth eggs and larvae, which are much larger, can be removed by a 20 μm filter. *Cyclops* carrying dracunculosis can be removed by passage through a fine cloth.

While most filters sold for field disinfection meet these requirements, they are not small enough to reliably remove viruses, which are another order of magnitude smaller than bacteria. The back pressure required to pump water through such small pores limits field filter design; only the semipermeable membranes in reverse osmosis filters are inherently capable of removing viruses. However, reduction of viruses by mechanical filters is accomplished by adsorption and aggregation. Virus particles may adhere to the walls of diatomite (ceramic) or charcoal filters by electrostatic chemical attraction.[57,148,155] Viruses in heavily polluted water often aggregate in large clumps and become adsorbed to particulates or enmeshed in colloidal materials, making them amenable to filtration.[51,150] Thus turbidity (cloudiness from contaminants) may help remove pathogens with filtration, while it inhibits halogens. However, in one study, only 10% of total virus particles detected were recovered on 3 to 5 μm pore prefilters, suggesting that most were not associated with the suspended sediment.[133] Furthermore, adsorbed viral particles can be subsequently dislodged and eluted from a filter.[148,202] Therefore filters should not be considered adequate for complete removal of viruses, except with special equipment.[216] Additional treatment with heat or halogens before or after filtration is essential for effective virus removal.[153]

For domestic use and in pristine protected watersheds where pollution and viral contamination are minimal and the main concerns are bacteria and cysts, filtration is feasible as the only means of disinfection. However, for foreign travel and for surface water with heavy levels of fecal or sewage contamination, filters should not be used as the sole means of disinfection.[57] One rational use of filtration is to clear the water of sediment and organic debris, allowing more accurate, lower doses of halogens.[127] Filters are also useful as a first step to remove parasitic and *Cryptosporidium* organisms that have high resistance to halogens.

Filtration using simple, available products is of interest for use in developing countries and in emergency situations. Sand filtration is still used widely in municipal plants. A column of fine sand 60 to 75 cm deep that permits no more than 200 L/m^2/hr is capable of removing turbidity and greater than 99% of organisms.[153] Rice hull ash filters are moderately effective. The United Nations International Children's Emergency Fund has devised a filter containing crushed charcoal sandwiched between two layers of fine sand that can filter 40 L/day and requires cleaning only once a year, but it has not been well tested.[35]

Reverse Osmosis. A reverse osmosis filter uses high pressure (100 to 800 PSI) to force water through a semipermeable membrane that filters out dissolved ions, molecules, and solids.[51] Thus it can desalinate water, as well as remove microbiologic contamination. If pressure or degradation causes breakdown of the membrane, treatment effectiveness is lost.[67] Even *Giardia* cyst passage has been shown to occur in a reverse osmosis unit.[43]

Small hand pump units have been developed. Their high price currently prohibits large-scale use by wilderness travelers, but they are important survival items for ocean travelers. Battery-operated units are commonly used on boats.

The U.S. Department of Defense is converting their large-scale mobile units from mechanical filtration to reverse osmosis water purification units because these are the only units capable of producing potable water from fresh, brackish, or salt water, as well as from water contaminated by nuclear, biologic, or chemical agents. Moreover, these are considered the most fuel-efficient mobile units, producing the highest quality water from the greatest variety of raw water qualities. The units use pretreatment, filtration and desalination, and then disinfection for storage.[216]

Granular Activated Carbon. Granular charcoal has been used as an adsorbent for water purification since biblical times and was used medicinally by ancient Egyptians as early as 1550 BC.[113] It is still in use for water treatment and for medical detoxification. When activated, charcoal's regular array of carbon bonds are disrupted, yielding free valences that are highly reactive and adsorb dissolved chemicals.[66,169] Granular activated carbon (GAC) is the best means to remove organic and inorganic chemicals from water.[51,127,226] Thus it is widely used in municipal disinfection plants and in home undersink devices to remove chemical contaminants and disinfection by-products, improving odor and taste. It is also a common component of field units as a filter and water purifier. Many, but not all, viral particles and bacteria adhere to GAC,[127] and some cysts are trapped in the matrix.[116] However, using a bed of GAC to filter particles and microorganisms results in more rapid saturation of binding sites and clogs the bed. GAC also removes radioactive contamination.

An alternative means of disinfection should always be used. GAC does not kill microorganisms, so it does not disinfect. In fact, bacteria colonize beds of GAC and slough off into the effluent water. Bacteria attached to charcoal are resistant to chlorination because the chlorine is adsorbed by the GAC.[51,113,127] This bacterial contamination has not been found to be harmful because the usual heterophilic bacteria are not enteric pathogens. Enteric pathogens have been shown to survive on GAC, but if an active biofilm exists, the pathogens are rapidly displaced by heterophilic bacteria and fail to become established. Therefore nonpathogenic bacterial colonization is encouraged in municipal plants.[117,155]

GAC can be used rationally before or after disinfection. Used before disinfection, it will remove many organic impurities that result in bad odor and taste and that are precursors to trihalomethane formation. GAC is best used after chemical disinfection to make water more palatable by completely removing the halogen[127,220] and other chemical impurities. With increasing industrial and agricultural contamination of distant groundwater, final treatment of drinking water with GAC may become a necessity. Although GAC is most often used as a pour-through filter unit, adsorption (but not filtration) also occurs if granular or powdered charcoal is stirred in the water.[127]

Eventually the binding sites on the carbon particles become saturated and do not adsorb any more; competitive binding occurs with some molecules released as others preferentially bind.[127] Unfortunately, no reliable means are available to determine precisely when saturation is reached. Filters using charcoal in compressed block form as the filter element may clog before the charcoal is fully adsorbed. Presence of unpleasant taste or color in the water can be the first sign that the charcoal is spent. To test the charcoal, filter iodinated water or water tinted with food coloring to ensure that all color is removed. With regular use the lifetime of GAC is probably measured in months; it is substantially longer with infrequent use. GAC can be "recharged," but this is not practical for small-quantity use. Ingested particles of charcoal are harmless.

Silver Impregnation. Silver impregnation of filters neither prevents microbial contamination of the filter nor sustains its action as a bactericide in the effluent water.[10,38] While silver has slow antibacterial effect on coliform organisms, filter cartridges impregnated with silver typically become contaminated with heterotrophic bacteria, which increase the total bacterial count in the effluent water but have not been linked to increased illness.[10,57,67,155] In GAC filters designed to operate in line with chlorinated tap water, silver merely exerts selective pressure on the kinds of bacteria that will colonize the filter.[117] Silver is known to be effective against *E. coli* and may be effective within filters to prevent colonization or survival of enteric pathogens. While colonization of filters with pathogenic coliforms has not been demonstrated, a protective effect cannot be attributed to silver impregnation.[57,155]

Commercial Devices Using Mechanical Filtration or Charcoal. Many filters are available for field use during camping or travel. Some are designed as purely mechanical filters, while others combine filtration with GAC. Filters that contain iodine resins are considered in the discussion on halogens. Appendix A at the end of the chapter enumerates details on filter design and function and provides photographs for identification of products. Of course, products constantly change; some are discontinued, and new ones evolve.

Environmental Protection Agency Registration. Until recently, no testing criteria were mandated for EPA registration. As of this writing, the EPA still does not endorse, test, or approve mechanical filters; it merely assigns registration numbers.[39] However, registration requirements distinguish between two types of filters: those that use mechanical means only and those that use a chemical(s), which is designated as a pesticide. Units containing halogens ("pesticides") must demonstrate compliance with proposed standards that were developed to act as a framework for testing and evaluation of water purifiers for EPA registration, as a testing guide to manufacturers, to assist in research and development of new units, and as a guide to consumers.[207] Under the standards, to be called a microbiologic water purifier the unit must remove, kill, or inactivate all types of disease-causing microorganisms from the water, including bacteria, viruses, and protozoan cysts, so as to render the processed water safe for drinking. An exception for limited claims may be allowed for units removing specific organisms to serve a definable environmental need, such as to remove *Giardia.* The standards include microbiologic reduction requirements, chemical health limits, and stability of the chemical(s). The unit should signal the end of effective lifetime by terminating discharge of treated water or other recognizable sign, or give simple instructions for servicing or replacing within measurable volume throughput or time frame. Testing with bacteria, viruses, and *Giardia* is required; *Cryptosporidium* is not currently included as a challenge organism but will be in the future. Testing is done at 20° and 5° C with worst-case scenarios of high levels of pollution and turbidity. A 3 log reduction is required for viruses and cysts, and 5 to 6 log reduction for bacteria. Testing is done or contracted by the manufacturer; the EPA neither tests nor specifies laboratories.

The standards were also intended to be applied to mechanical filters for those microorganisms against which claims are made (such as *Giardia* and bacteria, excluding viruses). However, current registration of mechanical filters requires only that the product make reasonable claims and that the location of the manufacturer be listed; no disinfection studies are required.[24] Many companies are beginning to use the standards as their testing guidelines. Data provided by the companies may be derived in good laboratories and be valid, or they may not be reproducible, poorly reflect true operating conditions, and avoid worst-case scenarios.

Filter Testing. Consideration of examples of filter testing shows the difficulty in attempting to draw comparisons based on data. The Environmental Health Department (EHD) of Canada rigorously tested a silver-impregnated ceramic candle filter with enteric bacteria in high concentrations and under various conditions of prolonged use.[57] Only one colony was recovered during all tests. Silver content was below 50 ppb except when stagnant for a time. Ninety percent of flow was reestablished after cleaning with a brush. However, when a portable hand pump version was tested, removal was complete until days 19 to 22, then both units being tested failed to maintain water quality. The problem was thought to be caused by improper sealing by the washer, which might have allowed some water to bypass the filter.

The EHD also tested a carbon depth-filter that makes bacterial claims. These filters failed continuous flow tests, passing large numbers of bacteria, and clogged well before their claimed capacity of 100 L. The EHD concluded that "while the filter may remove most bacteria when 1 L of sample is poured in and the effluent is collected, it cannot support a continuous challenge for any extended length of time."

Ongerth[135] tested four filters for *Giardia* removal: First Need and Katadyn removed 100% from 1 L volumes with 30,000 cysts. Both performed as efficiently for cyst removal after use approximating several months of weekend use (88 L for First Need, more for Katadyn).[139]

A Katadyn ceramic filter was tested by Schmidt with *Giardia* cysts at a concentration of 10^5/L. None passed through. Tobin found ceramic candle filters very effective at removing bacteria and cysts, but not viruses.[202] Ceramic candle filters tested in India with artificially contaminated well water markedly lowered bacteriologic content but never reduced the coliform count to zero.[35] The bacterial count in the effluent was not dependent on input.

Kerasote[103] reported that independent testing demonstrated the effectiveness of the Katadyn filter in removing all bacteria and cysts. One independent test of the First Need filter demonstrated breakthrough of 1% of fecal coliform bacteria after 10 L.

Strum[191] tested the Katadyn and First Need filters with challenges of *Giardia* cysts, bacteria, and poliovirus. Both filters removed 100% of cysts. The First Need filter allowed a few colonies of bacteria to pass, but no poliovirus. The Katadyn filter removed all bacteria and allowed a few of the viruses to pass.

A drink-through straw containing a 10 μm filter, iodine, resin, and charcoal (Pocket Purifier) has not performed well on testing. Ongerth[139] found only 50% cyst removal. Extensive testing sponsored by the company indicated excellent disinfection capabilities, but small amounts of breakthrough of cysts and bacteria after 10 to 30 L. However, two other independent tests showed passage of *Giardia* cysts and bacteria through the straw.[38,103] These tests are not completely valid, since cyst viability testing is necessary to determine whether the iodine resin was able to inactivate the microorganisms.

Until standard test protocols are uniformly used, varying test results will be difficult to interpret. Companies market affirmatively and stand proudly behind their products, but this, unfortunately, does not always ensure efficacy.

Turbidity and Clarification

River, lake, or pond water is often quite cloudy and unappealing. Turbidity (cloudiness) is an optical measurement of light scattering as it passes through water. Turbidity is caused by the presence of suspended organic and inorganic matter such as clay, silt, plankton, and other microscopic organisms. High turbidity is often associated with unpleasant odors and tastes, most often caused by organic compounds and metallic hydroxides with a much smaller particle size.[37,112] Clay-organic complexes may also carry pesticides or heavy metals. Bacteria, as well as viruses, may be adsorbed to particulate matter or be embedded in it, and in highly contaminated water, microorganisms tend to aggregate and clump. In one study 17% of turbidity particles contained attached microbes, averaging 10 to 100 bacteria per particle.[112] Organisms in the center of these conglomerates are afforded some protection from disinfectants. Thus removing particulate matter also decreases the number of microorganisms and decreases halogen demand.[127]

Removal of turbidity and particulates may be important in preventing chemical or infectious illness. Even if the turbidity is caused by benign inorganic particles, such as clay, removal is desirable for improving the esthetic quality of the water. Filtration can remove larger particles, but cloudy water can rapidly clog a filter. Sedimentation and coagulation-flocculation are other clarification techniques routinely used in municipal disinfection plants that can be easily applied in the wilderness for pretreatment of cloudy water, which is then disinfected by filtration or halogenation. Coagulation-flocculation and filtration are also used to remove *Giardia* and especially *Cryptosporidium* cysts that are more resistant to chlorine. Early experiments with water heavily contaminated with feces containing hepatitis A virus demonstrated that filtration and sedimentation alone did not prevent infection, but reduced the severity of the illness. However, water pretreated with coagulation, settling, and filtration was subsequently disinfected with 0.4 ppm residual chlorine, whereas water chlorinated to 1 mg/L without pretreatment remained infectious.[128,129]

Sedimentation. Sedimentation is the separation of suspended particles large enough to settle rapidly by gravity—for instance, sand and silt. The time required depends on the size of the particle. Generally, 1 hour is adequate if the water is allowed to sit without agitation. After sediment has formed on the bottom of the container, the clear water is decanted or filtered from the top. Microorganisms, especially protozoal cysts, eventually settle, but this takes longer and the organisms are easily disturbed during pouring or filtering. In one test in Tanzania, 4 days was required for sedimentation to improve microbiologic quality of the water.[35] Sedimentation should not be considered a means of disinfection.

Coagulation-Flocculation. Smaller suspended particles and chemical complexes too small to settle by gravity are called colloids. Most of these can be removed by coagulation-flocculation. It has been used to remove unpleasant color, smell, and taste in water since 2000 BC.

Coagulation is achieved with addition of an appropriate chemical that alters the physical state of dissolved and suspended solids, causing particles to stick together on contact because of electrostatic and ionic forces.[37,51] Lime (alkaline chemicals principally containing calcium or magnesium and oxygen) and alum (an aluminum salt) are commonly used, readily available coagulants. Rapid mixing is important to obtain dispersion of the coagulant. The second stage, flocculation, is a purely physical process obtained by prolonged gentle mixing to increase interparticle collisions and promote formation of larger particles. The flocculate particles can be removed by sedimentation and filtration. Coagulation-flocculation removes most coliform bacteria (60% to 98%), viruses (65% to 99%),[46,150,183] *Giardia* (60% to 99%), helminth ova (95%),[180] heavy metals, dissolved phosphates, and minerals.[37,51,115,226,228] However, a subsequent disinfection step is advised. Organic and inorganic compounds may be removed by forming a precipitate or by adsorbing onto aluminum hydroxide or ferric hydroxide floccular particles.[51] Coagulation-flocculation also works in cold water.

To clarify water by this means in the field, a person adds 10 to 30 mg of alum per liter of water.[228] The exact amount is not important, so it can be done with a pinch of alum, lime, or both for each gallon of water—more if the water is very cloudy. The person stirs or shakes briskly for 1 minute to mix the coagulant, then agitates gently and frequently for at least 5 minutes to assist flocculation. Settling requires at least 30 minutes, after which the water is carefully decanted or poured through a cloth or paper filter. Finally, disinfection can be ensured by filtration or halogenation.

Toxicity of coagulation-flocculation. Most of the aluminum in alum is removed with the floc. Questions have been raised concerning the association of aluminum with central nervous system toxicity in mammals, but these effects have been observed only following exposures other than ingestion. A report from the National Academy of Sciences concluded that aluminum in drinking water does not present a significant risk.[51] Alum is a common chemical used by the food industry in baking powder and for pickling. It can be found in some food stores or at chemical supply stores.

Alternative agents for coagulation-flocculation. Many substances can be used as a coagulant (for example, lime or potash); baking powder or even the fine white ash from a campfire can be used in an emergency.[204] Other coagulation-flocculation agents used traditionally by native peoples include seeds from the nirmali plant in southern India and rauwaq (a form of bentonite clay) and seeds from moringa plants in Sudan.[35]

HALOGENS

Aside from heat, chemical disinfection is the primary method for improving microbiologic quality of drinking water. Halogens, chiefly chlorine and iodine, are the most effective chemical disinfectants. Germicidal activity results from oxidation of essential cellular structures and enzymes.[32,111,127,132,220] Some evidence shows that halogenated amines may be synthesized by white blood cells as part of the body's natural defenses to destroy microorganisms.[218] The disinfection process is determined by characteristics of the disinfectant, the microorganism, and environmental factors.[34,54,87,110,126] Dilute solutions do not sterilize water.

Environmental Protection Agency Registration of Halogen Techniques

Registration by the EPA Pesticide Branch required for all disinfectants, including chlorine, signifies the following:

1. Its composition is such as to warrant the proposed claims for it.
2. Its labeling and other material required to be submitted comply with the requirements of the act.
3. It will perform its intended function without unreasonable adverse effects on the environment.
4. When used in accordance with widespread and commonly recognized practice, it will not generally cause unreasonable adverse effects on the environment.

Thus the only thing implied by EPA registration is that the bacteriostatic agent is not released into the water at unsafe levels.[24,39] This is less stringent than for filters that contain halogens.

Variables with Halogenation

Concentration and Contact Time. The major variables in the disinfection reaction with chlorine or iodine are the amount of halogen (concentration) and the exposure time of the microorganism to the halogen disinfectant (contact time). Concentration of halogen in water is measured in parts per million (ppm) or milligrams per liter (mg/L), which are equivalent. Contact time is usually measured in minutes but ranges from seconds to hours. In field disinfection, concentrations of 1 to 10 mg/L for 10 to 60 minutes are generally effective (Tables 43-6 and 43-7).

Ct Constant. Theoretically the disinfection reaction follows first-order kinetics. The rate of the reaction is determined by the initial concentration of reactants, and a given proportion of the reaction occurs in any specified time interval.[8,32,86,220] Mathematically, this means a reaction constant should result in a specified percentage reduction of viable microorganisms for each disinfectant and organism under given conditions of water temperature and pH: concentration × time = constant (Ct = K) (Fig. 43-1).[8,12,33,220] When concentration and contact time are graphed on logarithmic coordinates, a straight line results. Practically, this means that concentration and time can be varied to achieve the same results.[8,219] In field disinfection this can be used to minimize halogen dose and improve taste.

In reality, the disinfection reaction deviates from first-order kinetics, and Ct values do not follow the exponential rates described by the empirical equation because microor-

Table 43-6 Disinfection Data for Chlorine

Halogen*	Organism	Concentration (mg/L)	Time (min)	pH	Temp. (°C)	Disinfection Constant (Ct)	Reference
HOCl	*Escherichia coli*	0.1	0.16	6.0	5	.016	174
FAC	*Campylobacter*	0.3	0.5	6.0-8.0	25	.15	18
Free Cl	Bacteria	0.2	10	7.0	25	2	111
FRC	20 enteric virus	0.5	60	7.8	2	30	21
Free Cl	Enteric viruses	0.3	30	7.0	25	9	101
Free Cl	Enteric viruses	0.5	20	7.8	2	10	127
Free Cl	6 enteric viruses	0.5	4.5	6.0-8.0	5	2.5	55
FRC	Hepatitis A virus	0.5	1	6.0	25	0.5	76
Free Cl	Hepatitis A virus	0.5	5	6.0	5	2.5†	184
HOCl	Amebic cysts	3.5	10		25	35	32
FRC	Amebic cysts	3.0	10	7.0	30	30	190
Free Cl	*Giardia* cysts	1.5	10	6.0-8.0	25	15	94
Free Cl	*Giardia* cysts	2.0	60	6.0-8.0	5	120	94
Free Cl	*Giardia* cysts	2.5	60	6.0-8.0	5	150	159
Free Cl	*Giardia* cysts	0.5	180	6.5	3	90	135
Free Cl	*G. lamblia* cysts	0.85	90	8.0	2-3	77	211
Free Cl	*G. muris* cysts	3.05	50	7.0	5	153	172
		5.87	25	7.0	5	139	172
Free Cl	*Giardia*			6.0	0.5	170	83
				6.0	5	120	83
FRC	Schistosome cercariae	1.0	30	7.0	28	30	222
Free Cl	Nematodes	2-3	120	(not lethal)			127
Free Cl	Nematodes	95-100	30	(95% lethal)			127
FRC	*Ascaris* eggs	200	20	5.0	37	2000	107
Free Cl	*Cryptosporidium*	80	90			7200	220

HOCl, Hypochlorous acid; *FAC,* free active chlorine; *Free Cl,* free chlorine; *FRC,* free residual chlorine.
*These represent nearly equivalent measurements of the residual concentration of active chlorine disinfectant compounds.
†Four log reduction. Most experiments use 2 to 3 log (99% to 99.9%) reduction as endpoint.

Table 43-7 Disinfection Data for Iodine

Halogen*	Organism	Concentration (mg/L)	Time (min)	pH	Temperature (°C)	Disinfection Constant (Ct)	Reference
FRI	All bacteria	1.0	5	7.0	?	5	46
FRI	*Escherichia coli*	1.3	1	6.0-7.0	2-5	1.3	127
I_2	Amebic cysts	3.5	10		25	35	32
I_2	Amebic cysts	6.0	5		25	30	31
I_2	Amebic cysts	12.5	2		25	25	31
I_2	Viruses	6.3	10		25	63	31
FRI	Poliovirus 1	1.25	39	6.0	25	49	12
FRI	Poliovirus 1	12.7	5	6.0	25	63	12
I_2	Poliovirus 1	1	6	7.0	18	6	12
I_2	Coxsackie virus	0.5	30	7.0	5	15	12
Added I_2	Amebic cysts	8	10	4.0-8.0	23	80	31
	Bacteria, viruses	8	20		0-5	160	34
FRI	*Giardia* cysts	4	15	5.0	30	60†	62
FRI	*Giardia* cysts	4	45	5.0	15	170†	62
FRI	*Giardia* cysts	4	120	5.0	5	480†	62

*FRI (free residual iodine) and I_2 (elemental iodine) are nearly equivalent measurements of the residual concentration of active iodine disinfectant compounds. Added I (added iodine) indicates initial dose.
†100% kill; viability tested only at 15, 30, 45, 60, and 120 minutes.

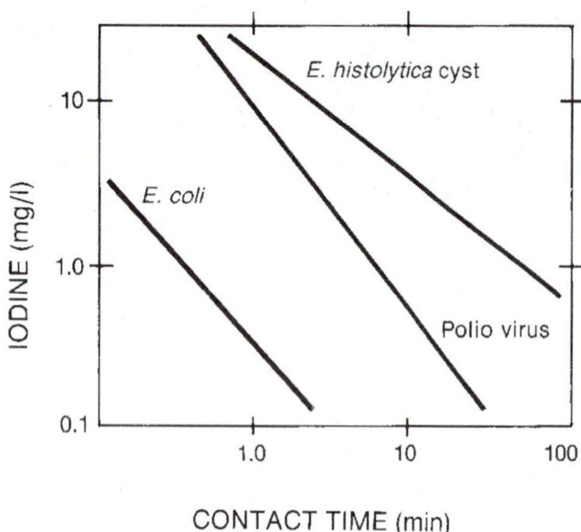

Fig. 43-1 Relationship of halogen concentration and contact time for a given temperature and pH. The first-order chemical reaction results in a straight line over most values for each microorganism and halogen compound. (Data from Chang SL: *J Am Pharm Assoc* 47:417, 1958; and Water and Sanitation for Health [WASH] Project: *Report on mobile emergency water treatment and disinfection units,* WASH Field Report No 217, Arlington, Va, 1980.)

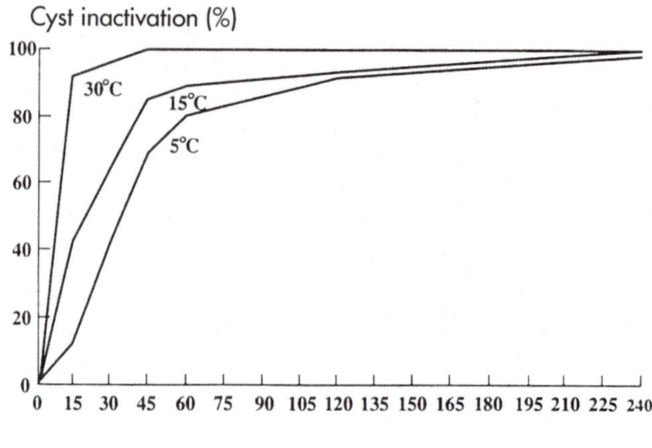

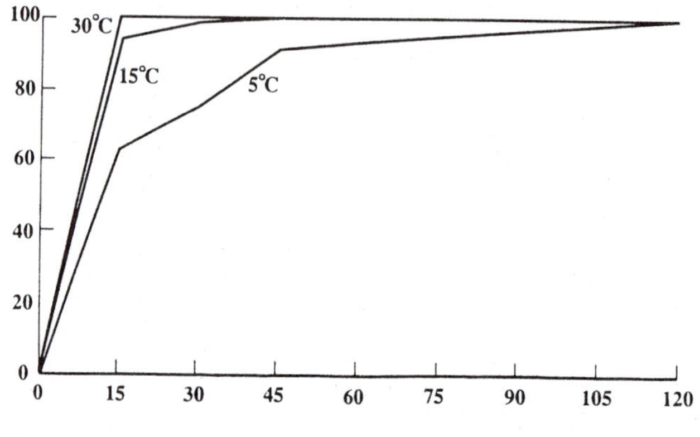

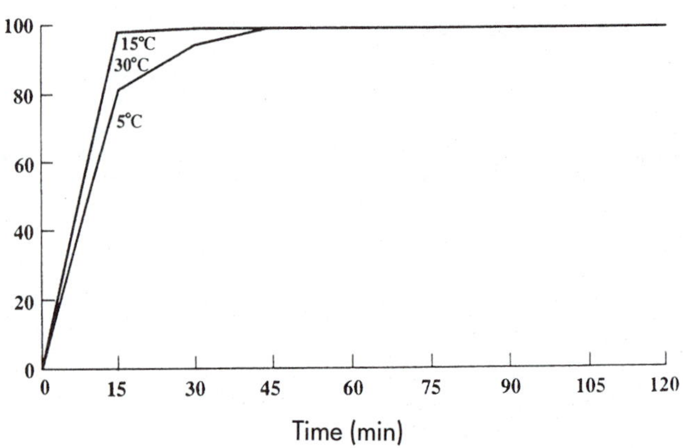

Fig. 43-2 Effect of concentration and temperature on *Giardia* cyst inactivation by iodine. Low concentrations are effective at cold temperatures with prolonged contact time. (From Fraker LD et al: *J Wilderness Med* 3:351, 1992.)

ganisms do not act like chemical reagents ($C^n t = K$). An initial lag period may be seen before inactivation begins (for example, because of penetration of the cyst wall), as well as a tailing off of inactivation for those organisms that are more resistant or protected by aggregation of association with other particulate matter (Fig. 43-2).[77,82,86,178]

Halogen Demand. Several other variables complicate disinfection with halogens and must be considered in field water treatment. The most important is the presence of nitrogen compounds: organic (amino acids, proteins [fecal matter, urea]) and inorganic (ammonia, nitrites and nitrates [decomposition of organisms and their wastes]). Vegetable matter, ferrous ions, nitrites, sulfides, and humic substances also exert demand for oxidizing disinfectants.[53,127,220] These contaminants react with halogens (especially chlorine) to form compounds with little or no disinfecting ability, effectively decreasing the concentration of available halogen.

Halogen demand is the amount of halogen reacting with impurities. Residual halogen concentration is the amount of active halogen remaining after halogen demand of the water is met. To achieve microbial inactivation in aqueous solution with a chemical agent, a residual concentration must be present for a specified contact time. Failure of chlorination in municipal systems to kill cysts or other microorganisms is usually caused by difficulty maintaining adequate residual halogen concentration and contact times, rather than by extreme resistance of the organism.[190]

Halogen demand and residual concentration of surface water are the greatest uncertainties in field disinfection. Nitrogen appears in most natural waters in varying amounts, which relate directly to the sanitary quality of water. Cysticidal dose of halogens is strongly affected by the level of contamination (cyst or viral density) in otherwise clean water.[33,76,190] Scant data are available on halogen demand for surface water (Table 43-8). Clear water is assumed to have minimal demand, while cloudy water is assumed to have high halogen demand. Surface water that is used in the wilderness contains 10 times the organic carbon content of aquifer groundwater. The green or brown color in stagnant ponds or lakes or in tropical and lowland rivers is usually

Table 43-8 Halogen Demand of Surface Water

Source	Halogen Demand (mg/L)	Reference
Cloudy river water, Portland, Oregon	3-4	92
Cloudy water from clay particles	none	34
Clear water with 10% sewage added	2	34
Lily pond and turbid river water	5-6	34
Colorado River; cloudy from inorganic sand, clay	0.3	203
Unspecified surface waters	2-3	45
Municipal wastewater	20-30	45
High-elevation spring	0.3	137
Western river	0.7	137
Six watersheds in western Oregon	0.4-1.6	112

caused by organic matter with considerable halogen demand. In some cases, such as runoff after storms and snowmelt, cloudy water may be caused by inorganic sand and clay that exerts little halogen demand. Chlorine demand has been shown to rise with increased turbidity.[112] In addition, particulate turbidity can shield microorganisms and interfere with disinfection.[45,46,112,113]

The initial dose of halogen must take halogen demand into consideration. For clear alpine waters, 1 mg/L demand can be assumed; for cloudy waters the assumption is 3 to 5 mg/L. If a method is used that adds 4 mg/L to clear water, extra time can compensate for the lower expected residual concentration. However, in cloudy water, where the demand may be nearly 4 mg/L, an increased dose of halogen, rather than prolonging the contact time, is needed to ensure free residual. The usual field recommendation to compensate for the unknown demand of cloudy water is a double dose of halogen (to achieve 8 to 16 mg/L). This crude means of compensation often results in a strong halogen taste on top of the taste of the contaminants. If the cause of turbidity is uncertain, the water should be allowed to sit; inorganic clay and sand will sediment, clarifying the water considerably. Other means of clarification, such as coagulation-flocculation or filtration, significantly reduce halogen demand.

Several simple color tests measure the amount of free (residual) halogen in water, using the oxidation-reduction potential of halogens.[53,75,106,111,220] These are most commonly used to test swimming pools and spas but can be applied to field water disinfection.[164] Testing in the wilderness for halogen residual may be reasonable for large groups but is not practical for most. Smell of chlorine usually indicates some free residual, although it may be combined with amines. Color and taste of iodine can be used as indicators. Above 0.6 ppm, a yellow to brown tint is noted.[220]

pH. Two other variables in the disinfection reaction are pH and temperature.[53,74,111,127,219] Halogen oxidizes water to form several compounds, each with different disinfection capabilities. The percentage of each halogen compound is determined by pH. The optimal pH for halogen disinfection is 6.5 to 7.5.[34,125] As water becomes more alkaline, approaching pH 8.0, much higher doses of halogens are required.[8,111]

The pH could be measured in the field, but the relationship is too complex to allow meaningful use of the information. Most surface water pH is neutral to mildly acidic, which is within the effective range of the halogens used. Granite keeps many alpine waters mildly acidic. Unfortunately, acid rain is affecting some high mountain lakes.[120] The EPA found the average pH in western alpine lakes to be no less than 5.5; lakes in other parts of the country are beginning to show lower pH levels. Some surface water with pH 7.0 to 8.0 begins to affect the chemical species of chlorine, favoring less active forms.[86] Certain desert water is so alkaline that halogens would have little activity; however, these waters are usually not palatable. At this time, compensating for pH is not necessary. Tablet formulations of halogen have the advantage of some buffering capacity.

Temperature. Temperature influences the rate of the disinfection reaction. Cold water affects germicidal power and must be compensated by longer contact time or higher concentration to achieve comparable disinfection (Fig. 43-2, Table 43-9).[75] In general, the common rule of a twofold to threefold increase in inactivation rates per 10° C increase in temperature seems fairly well substantiated. Unusual retardation of rates as temperatures approach 0° C has not been seen.[86]

Temperature can be estimated with reasonable accuracy in the field. Some treatment protocols recommend doubling the dose of halogen in cold water, but if time allows, time can be increased, instead of dose. New data for killing *Giardia* in very cold water (5° C) with both chlorine and iodine indicate that contact time must be prolonged three to four times, not merely doubled, to achieve high levels of inactivation.[62,83] Raising the temperature by 10° to 20° C allows a lower dose of halogen and more reliable disinfection at a given dose.

Susceptibility of Microorganisms. The final variable is the target microorganism. Sensitivity to halogen is determined by the diffusion barrier of the cell wall or capsule and the relative susceptibility of proteins and cellular respiration to denaturation and oxidation.[32,127] Organisms, in order of increasing resistance to halogen disinfection, are enteric (vegetative) bacteria, viruses, protozoan cysts, bacterial spores, and parasitic ova and larvae (Tables 43-6 and 43-7); for example, *E. histolytica* cysts are 160 times as resistant as *E. coli* and 9 times as resistant as hardier enteroviruses to chlorine (HOCl). Virucidal residuals of I_2 and HOCl are 5 to 70 times higher than bactericidal residuals.[32,127] Relative resistance between organisms is similar for iodine and chlorine.

Table 43-9 Temperature Effects on Disinfection

Halogen	Organism	Temperature Change (°C)	Effect	Reference
Chlorine		+10 (20-50)	Decrease in contact time 60%-65%	53
		−10	2.2 times increase in contact time	53
Chlorine	Coxsackievirus	+25	1/10 chlorine residual	8
Chlorine	Virus	+10	2-3 times increase in inactivation rate	127
Iodine	Bacteria	+10	2-3 times increase in inactivation rate	31
Chlorine	Cysts	+20	½ concentration needed	33
Chlorine	Virus	+10 (5-25)	75% less contact time	12
		−10	4-5 times increase in contact time	12
Chlorine	*Giardia*	+10	Ct decrease twofold	83

Bacteria. All vegetative bacteria are extremely sensitive to halogens. Inactivation involves oxidation of enzymes on the cell membrane and does not require penetration.[220] Little modern work has focused on bacterial agents because they are more sensitive than viruses and cysts, and little difference is evident between the bacterial pathogens.[86] Although halogens were first used to disinfect water during cholera epidemics in 1850, recent cholera epidemics prompted review of data to ensure the susceptibility of *V. cholerae* to low levels of chlorine and iodine.[43] *Campylobacter* and *Legionella* have susceptibility similar to that of other enteric pathogens.[18,220]

Viruses. Enteroviruses are more resistant than enteric bacteria,[127] but they constitute such a large and diverse group of organisms that generalization is especially difficult.[32,51,111] Most studies have used polio, a phage virus, or Coxsackievirus.[127,220] The mechanism of action for halogen inactivation of viruses has not been resolved. It is not clear whether the oxidant injures protein on the shell, a process similar to bacterial inactivation,[23] or penetrates the protein capsid by chemical transformation and then attacks the nucleic acid core, as in cyst inactivation.[220]

Most viruses tested against chlorine have shown resistance 10 times greater than that of enteric bacteria, but inactivation is still achieved rapidly (0.3 to 4.5 minutes) with low levels (0.5 mg/L) of chlorine.[55,205] Current data suggest that hepatitis A virus is not significantly more resistant than other enteric viruses.[76,144,185,199] Norwalk virus may be more resistant to chlorine than several other viruses, which may account for its importance in water-borne outbreaks.[104] Clumping and association of viruses with cells and particulates are thought to be significant factors affecting viral disinfection, causing departure from first-order kinetics.[55,184,205] Cell-associated hepatitis A virus was 10 times more resistant than dispersed hepatitis A virus. But these differences are minor compared with that inherent in protozoal cysts; if disinfection is aimed at the more resistant cysts, 99.99% viral inactivation will be achieved when only 68% of cysts have been killed.[153]

Cysts and parasites. Protozoal cysts are considerably more resistant than enteric bacteria and significantly more resistant than enteric viruses. This is probably due to the physiologically inactive outer shell, which the disinfectant must penetrate to be effective.[32,220] Early data exist for *E. histolytica,* but recent work on *G. lamblia* indicates similar sensitivity to both iodine and chlorine.[95] Higher pH and lower temperature decrease the effectiveness of halogens on *Giardia*.[25,59,82,91,184] Review literature frequently attributes exaggerated resistance of *Giardia* to halogens; Hoff[85] traced this to misquoted data. Jarrol, Bingham, and Meyer[92,93] tested two chlorine methods and four iodine methods for effectiveness against *Giardia* cysts. They found all methods effective in warm water, but only two methods destroyed all cysts in cold water. They concluded that recommended doses for certain techniques in cold water were inadequate. Either higher doses or longer contact times would have made all of these methods effective. Other excellent data show that halogens can be used in the field to inactivate *Giardia* cysts (Fig. 43-2).[62,83,86,91,172]

Acanthamoeba and *Naegleria* cysts are more sensitive than *Giardia* to chlorine.[220]

Limited data on parasitic helminth larvae and ova indicate such high levels of resistance that chemical disinfection is not useful.[107,111,127,180] Likewise, the disinfection constant values for chlorine disinfection of *Cryptosporidium* oocysts are too high for this technique to be used in the field.[47,166,220] Bacterial spores, such as those of *Bacillus anthracis,* are relatively resistant to halogens, but in the case of chlorine, not much more than *Giardia* cysts.[8,220] Quantitative data are not available for iodine solutions, but iodine does kill spores. Fortunately, sporulating bacteria do not normally cause water-borne enteric disease.[84] Schistosome cercariae are susceptible to low concentrations of chlorine.[222]

The best comparison of disinfection power is the disinfection constant (Ct). Tables 43-6 and 43-7 give representative data, and Fig. 43-1 shows this graphically. However, meaningful comparison is limited by disparate results. This may be caused by lack of standardized experimental conditions of pH, temperature, chemical species of halogen, and species of microorganism, or by different techniques for concentrating, counting, and determining viability of organisms.[86,127,172] The latter is especially a problem for cysts and viruses, which cannot easily be cultured. The usual endpoint for disinfectant effectiveness is 99.9% of organisms killed, but some experiments use 99% or 99.99%. Standardization is important, since the infectious dose for *G. lamblia* and viruses is as low as 1 to 10 organisms. Despite variation, Ct remains a useful and widely used concept; values provide a basis for comparing the effectiveness of different disinfectants for inactivation of specific microorganisms and for comparing the relative resistance of different microorganisms to specific disinfectants.[86,153] To use halogens for disinfection, a "consensus organism" (the most resistant target) determines the Ct.[31,86,111,220] For wilderness water this is protozoan cysts. Differences between laboratory and field conditions also make extrapolation from data to practice inaccurate. This indicates the need for safety factors when establishing Ct disinfection criteria for use in the field.

Chlorine

Chlorine has been used as a disinfectant for 200 years. Hypochlorite was first used for water disinfection in 1854 during cholera epidemics in London and was first used continuously for water treatment in Belgium in 1902. It is currently the preferred means of municipal water disinfection worldwide, so extensive data support its use.[220]

Chemistry. Chlorine reacts in water to form the following compounds[53,111,182,220]:

$$Cl_2 + H_2O \leftrightarrow HOCl + H^+ + Cl^-$$

$$HOCl \leftrightarrow OCl^- + H^+$$

At neutral pH, negligible amounts of diatomic chlorine are present. The major disinfectant is hypochlorous acid (HOCl), which penetrates cell and cyst walls easily. Dissociation of HOCl to the much weaker disinfectant hypochlorite (OCl^-) depends on temperature and pH. In pure water at pH 6.0, 97% of chlorine is HOCl; at pH 7.5, the ratio of $HOCl/OCl^-$ is 1:1; and above pH 7.5, OCl^- predominates.[220] The combination of these two compounds is defined as free available chlorine. Both calcium hypochlorite ($Ca[OCl]_2$) and sodium hypochlorite (NaOCl) readily dissociate in water, allowing the same equilibrium to form as when elemental chlorine is used.[111,220] Chloride ion (Cl^-, NaCl, or $CaCl_2$) is germicidally inactive. In addition, chlorine readily reacts with ammonia to form monochloramines (NH_2Cl), dichloramines, or trichloramines, referred to as combined chlorine. In field disinfection, these compounds are not considered and only free residual chlorine should be measured. However, chloramines have weak disinfecting power and are calculated as a disinfectant in municipal sewage plants.[86,125,127,220]

The disinfection constants for various organisms with chlorine at specific pH and temperatures have been compiled.[86,127,220] Selected experimental results for pH near 7.0 and representative organisms are shown in Table 43-6.

Toxicity. Acute toxicity to chlorine is limited; the main danger is irritation and corrosion of mucous membranes if concentrated solutions (for example, household bleach) are ingested. Numerous cases have been reported of short-term ingestion of very high residuals (50 to 90 ppm) in drinking water; one military study used 32 ppm for several months without adverse effects.[220] Animal studies using long-term chlorination of drinking water at 100 to 200 ppm have not shown toxic effects.[127]

Sodium hypochlorite is not carcinogenic; however, reactions of chlorine with certain organic contaminants yields chlorinated hydrocarbons, chloroform, and other trihalomethanes, which are considered carcinogenic.[51,127] The public health department limits residual chlorine in public systems to decrease ingestion of trihalomethane. The concern is now fueled more by public fears than by scientific conclusion.[220] The risk of death from infectious diseases if disinfection is not used is far greater than any risk from chlorine disinfection by-products.[51] These compounds are not likely to form in clean wilderness surface water, since the organic precursors would not be present.

Formulations. Chlorine is available in liquid and tablet forms for field use (Tables 43-10 and 43-11 and Appendix B at end of chapter).

Bleach. Liquid household bleach is a hypochlorite solution that comes in various concentrations, usually 5.25%. This has the convenience of easy availability, low cost, high stability, and administration with a dropper. If bleach containers break or leak in a pack, the liquid is corrosive and stains clothing.

Table 43-10 Water Disinfection Techniques

Technique	Amount Added to 1 L of Water*
IODINATION	
Iodine tabs	½ tab†
Tetraglycine hydroperiodide	
EDWGT (emergency drinking water germicidal tablet)	
Potable Aqua	
Globaline	
2% iodine solution (tincture)	0.25 ml 5 gtts
5%-7% iodine solution	0.1 ml 2-3 gtts
10% povidone-iodine solution	0.35 ml 8 gtts
Saturated iodine crystals in water	13 ml
Saturated iodine crystals in alcohol	0.1 ml
CHLORINATION	
Halazone tabs	2 tabs
Mono- or dichloraminobenzoic acid	
Household bleach 5%	0.1 ml
Sodium hypochlorite	2 gtts

*Amount added equals 4 ppm with iodination technique, 5 ppm with chlorination technique.

†Tablets cannot be divided; example is for equipotent dose.

Table 43-11 Field Halogenation

Concentration of Halogen (ppm)	Contact Time in Minutes at Various Water Temperatures		
	5° C	15° C	30° C
2	240	180	60
4	180	60	45
8	60	30	15

Sodium hypochlorite solutions are vulnerable to significant loss of available chlorine over time. Stability is greatly affected by heat and light. Lower concentrations (less than 10%) are more stable. Five percent solution loses about 10% available chlorine over 6 months at 70° F. Five percent solution freezes at 24° F.

Tablets. Halazone tablets contain a mixture of monochloraminobenzoic and dichloraminobenzoic acids.[53] Each tablet releases 2.3 to 2.5 ppm of titratable chlorine.[134] These tablets have been criticized because the alkaline buffer necessary to improve halazone dissolution decreases disinfectant efficiency, requiring unacceptably high concentrations and contact times (6 tablets = 15 mg/L for 60 minutes) for reliable disinfection under all conditions.[164] Tablets have the advantage of easy administration and can be salvaged if the container breaks. However, they lose effectiveness with exposure to heat, air, or moisture. Although no significant loss of potency results from opening a glass, wax-dipped bottle intermittently over weeks,[188] 75% of activity is lost after 2 days of continuous exposure to air with high heat and humidity. The shelf life is 6 months; potency decreases 50% when stored at 40° to 50° C (104° to 122° F). A new bottle should be taken on each major trip or changed every 3 to 6 months.

Superchlorination-dechlorination. The Sanitizer (Appendix B) is a method of field chlorination that uses first superchlorination and then dechlorination. High doses of chlorine are added to the water in the form of calcium hypochlorite crystals. Concentrations of 30 to 200 ppm of free chlorine are reached at the recommended doses. These extremely high levels are above the margin of safety for field conditions and rapidly kill all bacteria, viruses, and protozoa. After at least 10 to 15 minutes, several drops of 30% hydrogen peroxide solution are added. Hypochlorite is reduced to chloride and forms calcium chloride (a common food additive), which remains in solution.

$$Ca(OCl)_2 + 2\,H_2O \rightarrow 2\,HOCl + Ca^{++}\,(OH^-)_2$$
$$Ca(OCl)_2 + 2\,H_2O_2 \leftrightarrow CaCl_2 + 2\,H_2O + 2\,O_2$$

Excess hydrogen peroxide reacts with water to form oxygen and water. Chloride has no taste or smell. Hydrogen peroxide is also a weak disinfectant,[229] although not in common use.

The minor disadvantage of a two-step process is compensated by excellent taste, often improved by the superchlorination and oxygenation. Measurements to titrate peroxide to the estimated amount of chlorine do not need to be exact, but some experience is needed to balance the two and achieve optimal results. This is a good technique for highly polluted or cloudy waters and for disinfecting large quantities. It is by far the best technique for storing water on boats: a high level of chlorine prevents growth of algae or bacteria during storage; water is then dechlorinated in needed quantities when ready to use.

Both calcium hypochlorite and hydrogen peroxide lose potency over time, although if they are kept sealed in original containers, the shelf life of each should be years. Calcium hypochlorite loses 3% to 5% of available chlorine per year. The two reagents must be kept tightly sealed; calcium hypochlorite can ignite spontaneously if in contact with an oxidizing substance. Thirty percent peroxide is extremely corrosive and burns skin, so it should be used cautiously.

The process of superchlorination-dechlorination with different reagents is used in some large-scale disinfection plants to avoid long contact times and to remove tastes and smells. High doses of chlorine remove or oxidize hydrogen sulfide and some other chemical contaminants that contribute to poor taste and odor. Chlorine bleaches organic matter, giving a sparkling blue look to water, as in swimming pools.[220]

Chlorination-flocculation. AquaCure tablets (see Appendix B) were devised for the military in South Africa and are now becoming widely available in the United States. They contain alum and 1.4% available chlorine in the form of sodium dichloro-s-triazinetrione. Bicarbonate in the tablets promotes rapid dissolution. When used in cloudy water, the tablets release alum to coagulate-flocculate and yield 8 mg/L free chlorine. In clear water without enough impurities to flocculate, the alum causes some cloudiness and leaves a strong chlorine residual. However, this is an excellent one-step technique for cloudy and highly polluted water.

Iodine

Iodine has been used as a topical and water disinfectant since the beginning of the century.[71,111] During World War II its efficacy was demonstrated on a wide range of organisms at concentrations of a few parts per million.[33] Iodine has been used successfully in low concentrations for continuous water disinfection of small communities.[106] Despite several advantages over chlorine disinfection, it has not gained general acceptance, probably because of concern for its physiologic activity.

Chemistry. Iodine is the only halogen that is a solid at room temperature. Of the halogens, it has the highest atomic weight, lowest oxidation potential, and lowest water solubility. Its disinfectant activity in water is quite complex because of formation of various chemical intermediates with variable germicidal efficiencies. Seven different ions or molecules are present in pure aqueous iodine solutions, but only elemental (diatomic) iodine (I_2) and hypoiodous acid (HOI) play major roles as germicides. Diatomic iodine reacts in water to form the following compounds[34,75]:

$$I_2 + H_2O \leftrightarrow HOI + I^- + H^+$$

I_2 is two to three times as cysticidal and six times as sporocidal as HOI, because it more easily diffuses through the cyst wall. Conversely, HOI is 40 times as virucidal and three to four times as bactericidal as I_2, since inactivation of organisms depends directly on oxidation potential, without involving cell wall diffusion.[32] Their relative concentrations are determined by pH and concentration of iodine in solution.[34] At pH 7.0 and 0.5 ppm of iodine, the concentrations of I_2 and HOI are approximately equal, resulting in a broad spectrum of germicidal action. At pH 5.0 to 6.0, most of the iodine is present as I_2, whereas at pH 8.0, 12% is present as I_2 and 88% as HOI. At higher concentrations of iodine, more HOI is present. Under field conditions, I_2 is the major disinfectant for which doses are calculated.[34]

Triiodide (I_3^-), which has mild cysticidal but no virucidal or bactericidal efficacy, may be present in significant quantities in solutions containing iodide, such as tincture of iodine or Lugol's solution.[34] At pH 6.5 to 8.0 and I_2 levels of 1 to 2 ppm, the formation of triiodide can be ignored.[220] Above pH 8.5, hypoiodous acid decomposes to form a nongermicidal iodate (HIO_3) and iodide (I^-).[34,46] Iodide ion is without any effect for water disinfection. Iodine is effective in low concentrations for killing bacteria, viruses, and cysts, and in higher concentration against fungi and even bacterial spores, but it is a poor algicide.[34,73,75,127] Selected experimental results are shown in Table 43-7 and Fig. 43-2.

Toxicity. The main issue with iodine is its physiologic activity, potential toxicity, and allergenicity. Iodine is required in the human body in doses of 100 to 300 µg/day; the recommended dietary allowance of iodine is 400 µg/day. Toxicity of large doses is caused mainly by corrosive effects in the gastrointestinal tract, leading to hemorrhagic gastritis and gastrointestinal fluid losses. Poisonings are not uncommon; fatalities are rare but have occurred from ingestion of 30 to 250 ml of tincture of iodine.[73] Mean lethal dose is probably about 2 to 4 g of free iodine or 1 to 2 ounces of strong tincture.[61,74] Toxicity is limited by rapid conversion of iodine to iodide by food (especially starch) in the stomach and early reflex vomiting. Little iodine reaches the bloodstream. Iodide is absorbed into the bloodstream but has minimal toxicity. Acute toxicity to iodide is rare and manifests as individual hypersensitivity, such as angioneurotic and laryngeal edema.[73] Iodide compounds are widely used intravenously for radiographic imaging, but they have no other therapeutic benefit. Previously they were widely used as expectorants because of their stimulatory effects on bronchial secretion.

Chronic iodide poisoning, or iodism, occurs in anyone after prolonged ingestion of sufficiently high doses, but marked individual variation is seen. Symptoms simulate an upper respiratory illness, with irritation of mucous membranes, mucus production, and cough. Skin lesions are common and variable, and gastrointestinal symptoms may occur.[73,74]

In water disinfection the concern is long-term use of iodine for pregnant women and those with thyroid disease. Iodine given during pregnancy is taken up by the fetal thyroid after about the twelth week of gestation. Chronic ingestion of large amounts of iodine can result in neonatal goiter, which can lead to asphyxia during birth, or hypothyroidism with mental retardation. Daily intakes as small as 12 mg have been reported to produce congenital iodide goiters, but generally much higher doses are required.[214,223] The military performed several studies on long-term toxic effects of iodine used in concentrations similar to field disinfection.[124,134] In the most comprehensive study, sodium iodide was added to drinking water at a naval base for a 6-month period. The estimated daily dose of iodine per person was 12 mg for the first 16 weeks and 19.2 mg for the next 10 weeks. No evidence of functional changes or damage in the thyroid gland, cardiovascular system, bone marrow, eye, or kidneys was noted. Neither an increase in skin diseases or sensitization to iodine nor any indication of impaired wound healing or resolution of infections was evident.[123]

Three prisons in Florida with about 750 persons had continuous water disinfection with iodine beginning in 1963, with 15-year surveillance of health effects.[16,198] During the first 6 years, 1 ppm of elemental iodine was added to the water, with the exception of one 3-month period during which 5 ppm was added. Subsequently the dose was decreased to 0.5 ppm. No toxic effect, evidence of hypersensitivity to iodine, or thyroid gland enlargement was noted. Thyroid function tests revealed a decrease in radioactive iodine uptake from 17% to 7% and a slight increase in protein-bound iodine, but no appreciable change in serum thyroxine concentration.[64,197,198] Patients with prior thyroid disease had no recurrence with iodinated water; four patients with active hyperthyroidism were treated in standard fashion, and their condition remained well controlled despite the extra iodine intake. One hundred seventy-seven inmates gave birth to 181 full-term infants. No neonatal goiters were detected.[197]

In Tasmania, where goiter is endemic, the incidence of thyrotoxicosis doubled after the iodization of bread, with an average daily intake of only 0.08 to 0.27 mg. This increase was predominant in the older age groups among persons with toxic nodular goiter.[214]

These studies have not been sufficient to alleviate professional concerns about possible toxicity with medium- to long-term use of iodine, and the question of iodide toxicity remains controversial. Insufficient data are available to state that long-term consumption will definitely produce problems. However, few authorities will make categorical statements, and responsible agencies are sufficiently concerned to discourage its use as anything but a short-term emergency measure. Opinions as to the length of time that iodine can be safely used vary from 3 weeks to 2 months or longer.[214]

A technical paper from the World Health Organization[233] has stated,

> It is clear that a prolonged administration of several milligrams of iodine per day can have adverse effects to individuals with a history of thyroid disease. The health hazards for healthy individuals seem to be low, although no data are available on the physiological effect of prolonged use over many years, especially in children.

EPA officials who registered triiodide resin believed that normal individuals could not tolerate the residual for 2 years, but they could not offer an opinion about 2 months. The EPA stated that emergency use and use for up to 3 weeks should not present a problem, but that iodine disinfection of public water supplies with a largely permanent population is not recommended because of risk to individuals with impaired thyroid function or to the unborn child.[51,214]

Continuous use for years appears unwise in the face of existing evidence and uncertainty. Where to draw the line depends on local conditions and the feasibility of alternative means of disinfection.[214] Use for intermediate periods of 3 to 6 months has been demonstrated safe in the studies discussed previously and is commonly adopted by travelers. It would be prudent for the following persons to avoid the use of iodine: pregnant women, people with known or stated allergy to iodine, and those with unstable thyroid disease.

Formulations. Several forms of iodine are available for field use (Table 43-10 and Appendix B).

Iodine solutions. Iodine solutions commercially sold as topical disinfectants have the advantage of being inexpensive, available, and measured accurately with a dropper,[28] but are staining and corrosive if spilled. These contain iodine and potassium or sodium iodide in water, ethyl alcohol, or glycerol (Table 43-12). Iodide improves stability and solubility but has no germicidal activity and adds to the total amount of ingested iodine.

Iodophors are solutions in which diatomic iodine is bound to a neutral polymer of high molecular weight, giving the iodine greater solubility and stability with less toxicity and corrosive effect.[34,75] Povidone-iodine is a 1-vinyl-2-pyrrolidinone polymer with 9% to 12% available iodine.

Table 43-12 Iodine Solutions

Preparation	Iodine (%)	Iodide (%)	Type of Solution
Iodine topical solution	2.0	2.4 (sodium)	Aqueous
Lugol's solution	5.0	10.0 (potassium)	Aqueous
Iodine tincture	2.0	2.4 (sodium)	Aqueous-ethanol
Strong iodine solution	7.0	9.0 (potassium)	Ethanol (85%)

The iodophors are routinely used for topical disinfection, since they have less tissue toxicity than iodine solutions. Although they are not approved for water disinfection in the United States, they are used in other countries for this purpose.[9] A representative from Purdue-Frederick (the manufacturer of Betadine) explained that approval for this use in the United States was not pursued because the anticipated use did not justify the expense. Povidone is nontoxic and was used as a blood extender during World War II.[110]

In aqueous solution, povidone-iodine provides a sustained-release reservoir of halogen; free iodine is released in water solution depending on the concentration (normally, 2 to 10 ppm is present in solution). In dilutions below 0.01%, povidone-iodine solution can be regarded as a simple aqueous solution of iodine.[75] One report found these compounds similar in germicidal efficiency to other iodine-iodide solutions.[34] Data indicate persistence of about 2 ppm of free iodine at a 1:10,000 dilution,[75] which corresponds to a 0.001% solution made by adding 0.1 ml (2 drops) to 1 L of water. However, another study found conflicting values for available iodine and free iodine (measured by different techniques). Bactericidal effect on *Pseudomonas* and *Staphylococcus* bacteria increased at dilutions of 1:100, compared with 10% stock solutions, but dilutions of 1:10,000 were not bactericidal.[13] The complex chemistry of povidone-iodine solutions accounts for these conflicting data. Since free residual iodine can be measured at the concentration used for water disinfection, it should be effective. My experience and that of others attest to its effectiveness in field use.[9]

Tablets. Iodine tablets used by the military and sold in the United States for water disinfection contain tetraglycine hydroperiodide, which is 40% I_2 and 20% iodide (Appendix B).[34,126] They are sold as Globaline, Potable Aqua, and EDWGT (emergency drinking water germicidal tablet). Each tablet releases 8 mg/L of elemental iodine into water. An acidic buffer provides a pH of 6.5, which supports better cysticidal than virucidal capacity but should be adequate for both.[32,134,164] Tablets have the advantages of easy handling and no danger of staining or corroding if spilled. They are stable for 4 to 5 years under sealed storage conditions and for 2 weeks with frequent opening under field conditions, but lose 30% of the active iodine if bottles are left open for 4 days in high heat or humidity.[34,126,134,164]

Tetraglycine hydroperiodide was originally developed and chosen as a preferred technique by the military for individual field use because of its broad-spectrum disinfection effect, ease of handling, rapid dissolution, stability, and acceptable taste.[34,100,126,134,164] The military requirements dictated a short contact time (10 minutes in clear, warm water)—thus the relatively high concentration of iodine (8 ppm) compared with other iodination techniques. One tablet can be added to 2 quarts of water to yield 4 ppm of free iodine, with extension of the contact time.

Crystals (saturated solution). Because of limited solubility in water, iodine crystals may be used for disinfection.

One technique for field use is to put 4 to 8 g of crystalline iodine in a 1 to 2 ounce bottle, which is then filled with water.[98] A small amount of elemental iodine goes into solution (no iodide is present); the solution is used to disinfect drinking water. Water can be added to the crystals hundreds of times before they are completely dissolved.

Since the amount of iodine dissolved depends on the temperature of the solution (200 ppm at 10° C, 300 ppm at 20° C, 400 ppm at 30° C),[34,75,220] the bottle should be kept warm or the amount added to drinking water adjusted for temperature of the iodine crystal solution. In the field it may be easier to warm the bottle in an inner pocket than to estimate temperature and adjust the dose. The supernatant should be carefully decanted or filtered to avoid ingestion of the crystals[232]; this is aided by the weight of the crystals, which causes them to sink. Many people prefer crystalline iodine because of its large disinfectant capacity, small size, and light weight. A commercial product (Polar Pure) has made iodine crystals readily available in camping supply stores (Appendix B).

An alternative technique is to add 8 gm of iodine crystals to 100 ml of 95% ethanol.[221] Increased solubility of iodine in alcohol makes the solution less temperature dependent, and allows much smaller doses to be used (8 mg/0.1 ml), which can be measured with a 1 ml syringe or dropper (2 drops).

The stability and simplicity of iodine crystals have led to their testing for in-line systems that provide continuous water disinfection for remote households and small communities. In these designs, residual iodine is removed with GAC.[56,200]

Resins. Iodine resins containing complexed molecules of iodine, triiodine and pentaiodine are a fascinating new technique for water disinfection. They are one form of solid-phase disinfectant with which a solution containing the pathogenic microorganism contacts a biocidal surface. Some are strictly contact disinfectants with no measurable release of chemical. Others are specifically fabricated to release traditional disinfecting agents slowly to the aqueous environment (constant release). Others, including the iodine resins being used for field water disinfection, release disinfectant to microorganisms or organic molecules in solution with very little residual in the water, known as demand release.[117] This is the profile of the ideal chemical water disinfectant.

Although the exact mechanism of action has yet to be determined, apparently when a microorganism comes into contact with the resin, iodine binds to the wall or capsule, penetrating and killing the organism.[60,118,196] Transfer of iodine to the microorganism probably depends on electrical charge and the reducing properties of iodine. Contact is necessary; microorganisms in a dialysis bag were not killed when placed in aqueous solution with triiodide resin beads, and disinfectant activity of I_3 and I_5 is out of proportion to the concentration of I_2 in solution. Significant measurable iodine is attached to the organism after treatment. The percent kill is proportional to the number of iodine atoms bound per cyst.[117] Full resin effect requires close contact between the beads and organisms. Calculations from dropping beads through a bacterial suspension suggest[33] that collisions are necessary to kill. Collisions are encouraged by electrostatic factors. I_5 resin is slightly more reactive than I_3, releasing more iodine. I_5 can kill 10^9 organisms per milliliter compared with 10^7 for I_3, but this is not likely to be significant for water disinfection with a resin device.

The amount of dissolved iodine can be controlled by properties of the resin and varies between 0.02 and 5.0 ppm, increasing slightly as temperature increases. Bactericidal activity of resins is not influenced by pH, suggesting that I_2 is the disinfecting species and transferred directly to microorganisms.

Resins are chemically and physically stable during conditions of dry storage at room temperature. Aqueous suspensions or resins retain biocidal potential for 15 years. No alteration in activity was observed after dry storage for 1 month at 50° C.[117]

Iodine resin filters. Iodine resins have been incorporated into a broad line of filters for field use (Appendix A). Some incorporate filters to remove cysts and eggs, such as *Cryptosporidium,* that are more resistant to iodine. Many incorporate charcoal filters to remove the small residual concentration of iodine. Not all iodine is removed; some is converted to iodide, which remains in the water. While a residual may be desirable, theoretically this should not decrease effectiveness if disinfection does not rely on the dissolved iodine, but rather on iodine bound to the microorganisms. However, the resins have not been tested with charcoal. Iodine appears to be covalently associated with cellular molecules and resists removal by repeated washing, so the iodine bound to microorganisms is not likely to be removed by charcoal. The removal of residual iodine also makes those filters safe for long-term use.

Resins have proved effective against bacteria, viruses, and cysts, but not against *Cryptosporidium parvum* oocysts.[117] When *Cryptosporidium* oocysts were passed through a triiodide resin column, most were retained in the resin column, probably by electrostatic attraction to the resin. Of those that passed through, only a small percentage were inactivated within 30 minutes by the iodine.[210] The EPA conducted tests of triiodide resin against *E. coli,* but not against other organisms, for which it relied on independent testing. It concluded that the product depends on a 0.2 ppm residual and that additional testing would be necessary below this level. The resins are used in the space shuttle and have been used in large-scale units for international disasters.

Iodine resins and contact time. The necessary contact time with iodine resins is not clearly elucidated but is less than that required with dilute iodine solutions.[60,117,196] *Giar-*

dia was killed within 3 minutes at room temperature.[118] Consistent with other methods of halogen disinfection, *Giardia* cysts in cold water require longer contact time. Viable cysts could be recovered in 4° C water 40 minutes after passage through an iodine resin.[118]

PUR (Recovery Engineering) Traveler cup filters (I_2 and I_3 resin) were tested according to EPA guidelines against *Klebsiella,* poliovirus, and *G. lamblia* cysts up to the filter's 100-gallon lifetime. At 0% and 50% lifetime, greater than 99.9999% of bacteria, 99.9% of *Giardia,* and 99.99% of viruses were removed. At 75% and 100% lifetime, worst-case water required two passages. Holding water for 5 to 10 minutes after it passed through the units resulted in a further reduction of the test bacteria and viruses. This filter had a residual of about 0.6 to 0.7 ppm of iodine.[69]

An in-line resin triiodide unit with a 10 μm prefilter was tested by the Canadian Health Department with "worst-case scenario" conditions (sewage diluted to give 1000 to 5000 coliform bacteria per 100 ml at 17.8 L/min for 455,000 L over 28 days with water temperature of 5° to 8° C). Without contact time, essentially no reduction of coliform bacteria was seen after passing through the resin (residual concentration of 0.35 mg/L). The conclusion was that a holding, contact time was necessary and possibly that an adequate residual was needed. In warm water 0.5 to 1.0 mg/L for 15 minutes should be sufficient, but for cold water (below 7° C), 30-minute contact was optimal.[56] Neutralization of disinfection effect is not considered likely with ingestion before this time, since iodine apparently penetrates the organisms within minutes.[117] However, since the effect of iodine on microorganisms can be neutralized after passage through the resin, a 15- to 30-minute contact time is recommended before drinking, unless cysts are filtered out during passage through the unit. This raises questions about the efficiency of drink-through straws.

In conclusion, iodine resins are effective disinfectants that can be engineered into attractive field products. This type of disinfectant may be useful for small communities in undeveloped and rural areas where chlorine disinfection is technically and economically unfeasible. However, more testing is needed on specific products to ensure adequate resin contact, to define the need for contact time, and to confirm whether a residual iodine concentration is needed.

Solid-phase disinfectants are attractive for remote, small communities because of their simplicity of use and minimal monitoring required. Activated rice husk adsorbed with chlorine or iodine was tested in India. Chlorine did not de-adsorb and was not effective, but iodine was released.[35] Silver can also be used as a constant release disinfectant (see later discussion).

Chlorine Versus Iodine. A few investigators have reported data suggesting ineffectiveness of common halogen preparations. Jarroll, Bingham, and Meyer[92,93] tested six methods of field disinfection and found that none achieved high levels of *Giardia* inactivation at the recommended dose and times. However, this failure simply reflected the need for longer contact times in cold water.[114] Ongerth[139] tested seven chemical treatments for *Giardia* inactivation in clear and turbid water at 10° C. None achieved 99.9% reduction in 30 minutes. All iodine-based chemical methods were effective at 8 hours, but none of the chlorine preparations were effective, even after this extended time. While these results after 30 minutes in cold water are to be expected, the 8-hour results do not conform with other experimental data on chlorine. Unfortunately, the authors did not test for residual halogen, although initial levels achieved should have been effective, and they did not test at time intervals to determine when iodine methods were effective.

A large body of data proves that both iodine and chlorine are effective disinfectants with adequate concentrations and contact times (cold temperatures equate with slow disinfection time for both). Comparing effectiveness between chlorine and iodine is difficult because of the different ionic species and compounds that may exist under varying conditions.[84] Amounts of halogen and recommended contact times for various preparations are listed in Table 43-10. These contact times are extended from the previous recommendations for treatment in cold water to provide a margin of safety and to ensure high levels of cyst destruction.

Iodine has several advantages over chlorine. Of the halogens, iodine has the lowest oxidation potential, reacts least readily with organic compounds, is least soluble, and is least hydrolyzed by water, all of which indicate that low iodine residuals should be more stable and persistent than corresponding concentrations of chlorine.* Although iodine is pH dependent, it is less sensitive than chlorine, so a constant disinfecting efficiency of iodine in aqueous solutions over a broad range of pH can be expected (from a combination of I_2 and HOI).[75,106]

Taste tolerance or preference for iodine over chlorine is individual. At levels commonly used in the field, most persons prefer the taste of iodine. In cysticidal doses the taste of iodine was more acceptable than that of chlorine.[132] Since organic compounds with halogens produce highly objectionable taste and smell, and since iodine reacts less readily than chlorine with these chemicals, iodine solutions are more acceptable under similar conditions.

Taste of Halogens and Halogen Administration. Objectionable taste and smell are the major problems with acceptance of halogens. These depend on specific chemical compounds. Most people are familiar with the taste of chlorine (hypochlorite); tap water usually contains 0.2 to 0.5 ppm of chlorine, swimming pools 1.5 to 3.0 ppm, and hot tubs 3.0 to 5.0 ppm. Most persons note a distinct taste at 5 ppm and a strong, unpleasant taste at 10.0 to 15.0 ppm.[164] Hypochlorous acid and chloride have no taste or odor.[220] Most objectionable tastes in treated water are derived from

*References 31, 46, 60, 75, 106, 127, 146.

dissolved minerals, such as sulfur, and from chlorine compounds, chloramines, and organic nitrogen compounds, even at extremely low levels.

Elemental iodine at 1 mg/L is undetectable. Most persons can detect iodine solutions at 1.5 to 2 mg/L but do not find it objectionable.[16,46,65] Eight ppm of iodine produces a distinct taste and odor; however, tablets yielding these concentrations were preferred by military personnel over tincture of iodine in equivalent doses.[34,126] Iodide ion has no color or taste.

Minimal dosage. Taste can be improved by several means (Box 43-3). One method is to use the relationship between halogen concentration and time and to give the minimum necessary dose, allowing a longer contact time (Table 43-11). Wilderness travelers usually can allow a longer contact time for water disinfection.

Giardia cysts and viruses can be killed with doses of chlorine or iodine of 2 ppm or less (Fig. 43-2).[62,83,111,135] Concentrations of chlorine as low as 0.2 mg/L have been shown effective for *Giardia* cyst destruction if the contact time is at least 12 to 18 hours.[135] In 1965 the National Research Council investigated minimum chlorine residuals for military water supplies from existing experimental data, using a 30-minute contact time in 20° to 25° C water. The recommendations were bactericidal—0.2 mg/L residual free chlorine, and cysticidal—1.5 to 2 residual free chlorine (pH 7.0).[111]

Theoretically, doubling the contact time allows a 50% reduction of halogen dose at any level. While this relationship holds true at the higher field doses of halogens, as the levels drop, the reaction departs from mathematical models, and the straight line graph illustrated in Fig. 43-1 has a "tail." For amebic cysts in fairly heavily polluted water, Chang and Fair[33] found that whenever the contact time was doubled, the cysticidal dose of chlorine decreased by 25%. This departure from strict first-order kinetics and the uncertainty of halogen demand in field disinfection mean that a margin of safety must be incorporated into contact times at lower doses.

BOX 43-3

IMPROVING THE TASTE OF HALOGENS

- Use the Ct constant: decrease dose and increase contact time.
- Clarify cloudy water before adding halogen.
- Use iodine resin.
- Use dehalogenation:
  - Granular-activated charcoal
  - Chemical techniques
  - Zinc brush
  - Chlorination-dechlorination (Sanitizer)
  - Ascorbic acid
  - Sodium thiosulfate
- Use alternative techniques:
  - Heat
  - Filtration

Of all standard iodine doses, iodine tablets yield the highest dose (8 mg/L with an intended contact time of 10 minutes in warm water). While the tablets cannot be broken in half, they can be added to 2 quarts instead of 1 to yield concentrations consistent with the other preparations. Chang, who developed the iodine tablets, noted that 2 to 3 ppm should be effective for cysts and viruses after 30 minutes in warm, relatively clean water (rather than 8 ppm for 10 minutes).[31] The liquid preparations of iodine add 4 mg/L. Since even clear surface water has some halogen demand, this dose of 4 mg/L should generally not be reduced when treating surface water. The exception would be high-quality, but very cold, water with an extended contact time (4 to 6 hours or overnight). For backing up tap water in developing countries, the dose may routinely be cut in half for an added dose of 2 ppm with a few hours of contact time. For chlorination methods that add 5 mg/L, adding half the amount to clean surface water should be adequate if the contact time is tripled. Even less could be used for tap water.

Effective disinfection with low iodine residual can also be achieved by use of iodine resins.

Temperature and organic matter in the water may be manipulated. Increasing the temperature of the water, especially when near 5° C, allows for shorter contact times for a given halogen concentration (Table 43-11 and Fig. 43-2). Filtering water before adding halogen improves the reliability of a given halogen dose by decreasing halogen demand, allowing a lower dose of halogen.[127] Sedimentation or coagulation-flocculation cleans cloudy water and lowers the required halogen dosage considerably, in addition to removing many of the contaminants that contribute to objectionable taste.

Dehalogenation. Halogen can be removed from water after the required contact time. Activated charcoal removes iodine or chlorine, allowing standard or even high doses to be used without residual taste.[220]

The relative instability of chlorine in dilute solutions can be used to decrease taste over time. Chlorine residual in an open container decreases 1 mg/L in the first hour, then 0.2 mg/L in the next 5 to 8 hours, for a total of 2.0 to 2.5 mg/L in 24 hours. Ultraviolet light also depletes free chlorine.[220]

Several chemical means are available to reduce free iodine or chlorine to iodide or chloride products that have no color, smell, or taste. These forms also have no disinfection action, so the techniques should be used only after the required contact time. The Sanitizer, discussed previously, uses hydrogen peroxide to "dechlorinate" the water by forming calcium chloride. This reaction with hydrogen peroxide works best if calcium hypochlorite is used as a disinfectant. If bleach (sodium hypochlorite) is used, hydrogen peroxide reacts with chlorine in water to form hydrochloric acid in harmless amounts:

$$Cl_2 + H_2O_2 \rightarrow 2HCl + O_2$$

Two other chemicals that may be safely used with any form of chlorine or iodine are ascorbic acid (vitamin C) and sodium thiosulfate. Ascorbic acid is widely available. Using the crystalline or powder form is preferable to grinding up tablets, which have binders that may cloud the water. A potential disadvantage of ascorbic acid is that it has a tart taste. It is a common ingredient of flavored drink mixes, which accounts for their usefulness to cover up the taste of halogens.[134,164]

Sodium thiosulfate neutralizes iodine and chlorine and is used routinely for this purpose in disinfection experiments. A few granules in 1 quart of iodinated water decolorizes and removes the taste of iodine by converting it to iodide. In reaction with chlorine, it forms hydrochloric acid, which is not harmful or detectable in such dilute concentration:

$$Na_2S_2O_3 + Cl_2 + H_2O \rightarrow 2\,NaHSO_4 + 8\,HCl$$

Sodium thiosulfate is available at chemical supply stores. Thiosulfate salts are inert in vivo and poorly absorbed from the gastrointestinal tract. They can be injected intravenously, as for cyanide poisoning, without ill effect, and are recommended for iodine poisoning because they combine with iodine to form relatively harmless sodium iodide.[105]

Zinc acts as a catalyst to reduce free iodine and chlorine through an electrochemical reaction. It also removes or reduces dissolved metals such as copper and heavy metals such as lead, selenium, and mercury. Some products have incorporated zinc into the bristles of a small brush to be stirred in the water after halogen disinfection. It is effective, but slow, which limits its use to small volumes of water. It removes 10 mg/L chlorine in 250 ml after 1 minute of stirring.

Finally, alternative techniques such as filtration or heat can be used in many situations without imparting any taste to the water.

MISCELLANEOUS DISINFECTANTS

Silver

Silver ion has bactericidal effects in low doses. The literature concerning antimicrobial effects of silver is voluminous, but confusing and contradictory.[25,89,127,220,225] Concentrations in water below 100 ppb are effective against enteric bacteria. The reaction follows first-order kinetics and is temperature dependent. Calcium, phosphates, and sulfides interfere significantly with silver disinfection. Organic chemicals, amines, and particulate or colloidal matter may also interfere, but no more than with chlorine.

Silver is physiologically active. Acute toxicity does not occur from small doses used in disinfection, but argyria, which is permanent discoloration of the skin and mucous membranes, may result from prolonged use. For this reason, a maximum limit of 50 ppb of silver ion in potable water is recommended. At this concentration, disinfection requires several hours.

Experimental results indicate 18% survival of *E. coli* at 3 hours at 40 µg/L. *Salmonella typhi* was reduced more than 5 log at 50 µg/L with a 1-hour exposure; poliovirus was not reduced at 50 µg/L with a 1-hour exposure.[10]

Water disinfection systems using silver have been devised for spacecraft, swimming pools, and other settings.[220] The advantage is absence of taste, odor, and color; persistence of residual concentrations allows reliable storage of disinfected water. Silver can be supplied through a silver nitrate solution, desorption from silver-coated materials, or electrolysis. When coated on surfaces, silver acts as a constant-release disinfectant that produces aqueous silver ion concentrations of 0.006 to 0.5 ppm, which are sufficient to disinfect drinking water.[117] Because of this attractive feature, silver-based devices are being designed and tested in developing countries. In Pakistan a nylon bag with silver-coated sand was designed to be placed in earthenware pitchers that store water. Silver incorporated into alum is also being tested in India.[35]

Filters and granular charcoal media are sometimes coated with silver to prevent bacterial growth on the surface, but this does not maintain sterility. A slow, selective action against total coliform count is noted, but none against total bacterial count. Long use might overcome any bacteriostatic action initially shown.[67] In an EPA study, effluent populations from the silver-containing units were about as large as those from the nonsilver units.[10] Bacteria can develop resistance to silver ions through generation of silver reductase.

Large-scale use of silver for water disinfection has been limited by cost, difficulty controlling and measuring silver content, and physiologic effects. Short-term field use is limited by silver's marked tendency to adsorb onto the surface of any container (resulting in unreliable concentrations) and interference by several common substances. Furthermore, the scant data on silver for disinfection of viruses and cysts indicate limited effect, even at high doses.[32,127]

The use of silver as a drinking water disinfectant has been much more popular in Europe than in the United States. Silver tablets for field water disinfection (MicroPur) are sold widely. They have not been approved by the EPA for sale in the United States (Appendix B).

Potassium Permanganate

Potassium permanganate is a strong oxidizing agent with some disinfectant properties. It was used extensively before hypochlorites as a drinking water disinfectant.[126,150] It is still used for this purpose and also for washing fruits and vegetables in parts of the world. It is used in municipal disinfection to control taste and odor and is usually employed in a 1% to 5% solution for disinfection. Bacterial inactivation can be achieved with moderate concentrations and contact times (45 minutes at 2 mg/L, 15 minutes at 8 mg/L). A 1:5000 (0.5%) solution controlled *V. cholerae* and *Salmonella typhosa* contamination of fruits and vegetables. The virucidal action has been tested, but without titrations of virus that remained after various periods of contact time, so the rate of action is not known. However, in most instances, a 1:10,000 solution destroyed the infectivity of virus suspensions in ½ hour at room temperature; 30 mg/L was effective in inactivating hepatitis A virus within 15 minutes.[199] Although potassium permanganate clearly has disinfectant action, it cannot be recommended for field use, since quantitative data are not available for viruses and no data are available for protozoan cysts. More data would be welcome, given the chemical's frequent use in some parts of the world. Packets of 1 g to be added to 1 L of water are sold in some countries.

The solutions are deep pink to purple and stain surfaces. The chemical leaves a pink to brown color in water at concentrations above 0.05 mg/L.

Hydrogen Peroxide

Hydrogen peroxide is a strong oxidizing agent but a weak disinfectant.[19,127,229] Small doses (1 ml of 3% H_2O_2 in 1 L water) are effective for inactivating bacteria within minutes to hours, depending on the level of contamination. One million colony-forming units/ml of seven bacterial strains were killed overnight, with 80% kill in 1 hour. Viruses require extremely high doses and longer contact times. Although information is lacking on the effect of hydrogen peroxide on protozoa, it is a promising sporicidal agent in high (10% to 25%) concentrations.

Hydrogen peroxide was popular as an antiseptic and disinfectant in the late nineteenth century and remains popular today as a wound cleanser; for odor control in sewage, sludges, and landfill leachates; and for many other applications. It is considered safe enough for use in foods. In fact, it is naturally present in milk and honey, helping to prevent spoilage. It yields the innocuous end products oxygen and water. However, direct ingestion of solutions can be fatal.[61] Solutions lose potency in time, but stabilizers can be added to prevent decomposition.[19]

Although hydrogen peroxide can sterilize water, lack of data for protozoal cysts and quantitative data for dilute solutions prevents it from being useful as a field water disinfectant. Its application for superchlorination-dechlorination is an excellent one.

Ultraviolet Light

The germicidal effect of ultraviolet (UV) light is the result of action on the nucleic acids of bacteria and depends on light intensity and exposure time. It is well established that UV light can inactivate bacteria, viruses, and protozoans when administered in sufficient dose. However, cysts should probably be removed by filtration. UV treatment does not require chemicals and does not affect the taste of the water. It works rapidly, and an overdose to the water presents no danger; in fact, it is a safety factor. UV light has no residual disinfection power, so water may become recontaminated or regrowth of bacteria may occur.[56] Particulate matter can shield microorganisms from UV rays.

UV disinfection units are cumbersome and require power, so they are not well adapted to use by small groups in the wilderness. However, an intriguing question is whether direct sunlight can disinfect small quantities of water. One investigation tested the ability of sunlight to disinfect oral rehydration salt solution in clear polyethylene bags or plastic containers contaminated by sewage.[1] After 1 hour in sun the coliform bacteria count was zero. Certainly, this could be helpful for reducing contamination of water in an emergency situation, but insufficient data are available to quantitate the results.

Other Disinfectant Products

A few other products being marketed for water disinfection for travelers cannot be recommended until more data become available. These were initially introduced into the health food market but are now being offered to the general travel market.

Aerobic Oxygen is advertised not only as a water disinfectant, but also as a cure for headaches and tropical fish diseases. The company claims that the active disinfectant is a trade secret and will say only that it is a molecular form of oxygen. It could be chlorine dioxide, a known and tested disinfectant, but this has not been confirmed. Company-sponsored testing demonstrates activity against bacteria and viruses, but not against cysts. No dose/time response has been developed to compare the product against other disinfectants.

Traveler's Friend contains citrus extract, which is known to have some antimicrobial activity. A concentrated form is being used as a topical disinfectant. Company-sponsored data are convincing for antibacterial and antiviral activity. However, the product was not tested against *Giardia* cysts. The active chemical disinfectant has not been identified, and a time/dose response has not been generated.

Preferred Technique

The optimal technique for an individual or group depends on the number of persons to be served, space and weight available, quality of source water, personal taste preferences, and availability of fuel. For alpine camping with high-quality source water, mechanical or iodine resin filtration or halogens in low doses can be used. Heat is limited by fuel supplies. Filtration has the advantage of imparting no taste and requiring no contact time. Halogens can be applied with equal ease to large quantities of water. For small groups, collapsible plastic containers can be used to disinfect water with low doses of iodine during the day or overnight, or higher doses can be used, followed by chemical reduction to improve taste. The only limitation for halogens are *Cryptosporidium* cysts, but in high-quality, pristine surface water they have not been found to be present in high enough numbers to cause a problem.

Water from cloudy, low-elevation rivers, ponds, and lakes in developed or undeveloped countries should be pretreated with coagulation-flocculation, then disinfected with heat or halogens. Iodine resin filters with microfiltration and activated charcoal are a simple alternative but become clogged much more rapidly with this kind of water.

Water in undeveloped countries should be treated with halogens or heat, not just filtration, to ensure viral destruction. The iodine resin filters are well designed for this. Those with microfilters in addition to the resin give added protection against halogen-resistant cysts and eggs.

Halogens have a distinct advantage in systems where the water will be stored for a period of time, such as on a boat or in a large camp. When only heat or filtration is used before storage, the water can become recontaminated or bacterial regrowth can occur. Superchlorination-dechlorination is especially useful in this situation because high levels of chlorination can be maintained for long periods, and when ready for use, the water can be poured into a smaller container and dechlorinated. If another means of chlorination is used, a minimum residual of 3 to 5 mg/L should be maintained in the water. Iodine works for short-term but not prolonged storage, since it is a poor algicide. Iodine resins leave a small amount of residual iodine unless they are combined with activated charcoal to remove all residual.

On long-distance, ocean-going boats where water must be desalinated during the voyage, only reverse osmosis membrane filters are adequate. Halogens should then be added to the water in the storage tanks.

Prevention and Sanitation

Water disinfection plays an indispensable role in preventing spread of enteric disease.[42] However, other measures are also important. Personal hygiene—mainly hand washing—prevents spread of infection from food contamination during preparation of meals.[121] No one with a diarrheal illness should prepare food. Dishes and utensils should be disinfected by rinsing in chlorinated water prepared by adding enough household bleach to achieve a marked chlorine odor.

The ultimate responsibility is proper sanitation to prevent contamination of water supplies from human waste. Ubiquitous toilet paper litter is proof that Westerners in the wilderness take as little responsibility for their waste as inhabitants of "undeveloped" countries. Jonathon Waterman writes in *Surviving Denali* that at the higher elevations where gale-force winds regularly scour all fresh snow from the slopes soon after it falls, climbers must "select cooking snow very carefully from among the wasteland of brown turds . . . Fortunately, sometimes below 15,000 feet, snowfall will cover the excrement. . . ."[217]

Ultraviolet rays in sunlight eventually inactivate most microorganisms, but rain may first wash pathogens into a water source. In the soil, microorganisms can survive for months.[206] A study sponsored by the Sierra Club found more prolonged survival in alpine environments.[152] The investigator marked group latrines in alpine terrain and returned 1 to 2 years later to dig test trenches. He found a thin crust of decomposition covering unaltered raw waste with high coliform bacteria counts. Microorganisms may percolate through the soil. Most bacteria are retained within 50 cm of the surface, but in sandy soil this increases to 75 to 100 feet[206]; viruses can move laterally 75 to 302 feet.[173] When organisms reach groundwater, their survival is prolonged, and they often appear in surface water or wells.[206]

It has been suggested that campers smear feces on rocks to aid in desiccation and UV disinfection. This is a reasonable suggestion if it is done in arid areas away from camping sites and trails, but it will be repulsive to most campers. In the Sierra, feces left on the ground generally disappeared within 1 month, but it was not known whether disinfection occurred before decomposition or whether the feces washed away, dried, or were blown in the wind.[152] Despite more rapid decomposition in sunlight rather than underground, burying feces is still preferable in areas that receive regular use. The U.S. Forest Service recommends burial of human waste 8 to 12 inches deep and a minimum of 100 feet from any water.[204,208] Judgment should be used to determine a location that is not likely to allow water runoff to wash organisms into nearby water sources. Groups larger than three persons should dig a common latrine to avoid numerous individual potholes and inadequate disposal. To minimize latrine odor and improve its function, it should not be used for disposal of wastewater.

In some areas the number of individual and group latrines is so great that the entire area becomes contaminated. Therefore sanitary facilities (outhouses) are becoming common in high-use wilderness areas. Popular river canyons require camp toilets, and all waste must be carried out in sealed containers.

REFERENCES

1. Acra A et al: Disinfection of oral rehydration solutions by sunlight (letter), *Lancet* 2:1257, 1980.
2. Alder VG, Simpson RA: Sterilization and disinfection by heat methods. In Russel AD, Hugo WB, Ayliffe GAJ, editors: *Principles and practice of disinfection, preservation, and sterilization,* Oxford, Eng, 1982, Blackwell, p 433.
3. Amirtharajah: Variance analyses and criteria for treatment regulations, *J Am Water Works Assoc* 78:34, 1986.
4. Anderson BC: Moist heat inactivation of *Cryptosporidium* sp., *Am J Public Health* 75:1433, 1985.
5. Aukerman R, Monzingo DL Jr: Water treatment to inactivate *Giardia, J Forestry,*1989, p 18.
6. Barbour AG, Nichols CR, Fukushima T: An outbreak of giardiasis in a group of campers, *Am J Trop Med Hyg* 25:348, 1976.
7. Baron RC et al: Norwalk gastroenteritis illness: an outbreak in a recreational lake and secondary person-to-person spread, *Am J Epidemiol* 115:163, 1982.
8. Baumann ER, Ludwig DD: Free available chlorine residuals for small nonpublic water supplies, *J Am Water Work Assoc* 54:1379, 1964.
9. Beal CB: Another method of water purification for travelers (letter), *West J Med* 135:341, 1981.
10. Bell FA: Review of effects of silver-impregnated carbon filters on microbial water quality, *J Am Water Works Assoc* 83:74, 1991.
11. Bemrick WJ: Some perspectives on the transmission of giardiasis. In Erlandsen SL, Meyer EA, editors: *Giardia* and giardiasis: biology, pathogenesis and epidemiology, New York, 1984, Plenum Press.
12. Berg G, Chang SL, Harris EK: Devitalization of microorganisms by iodine, *Virology* 22:469, 1964.
13. Berkelman RL, Holland BW, Anderson RL: Increased bactericidal activity of dilute preparations of povodone-iodine solutions, *J Clin Microbiol* 15:635, 1982.
14. Bingham AK, Jarroll EL, Meyer EA: *Giardia* sp.: physical factors of excystation in vitro and excystation vs. eosin exclusion as determinants of viability, *Exp Parasitol* 47:284, 1979.
15. Biziagos E et al: Long-term survival of hepatitis A virus and poliovirus type 1 in mineral water, *Appl Environ Microbiol* 54:2705, 1988.
16. Black AP et al: Use of iodine for disinfection, *J Am Water Works Assoc* 1401, 1965.
17. Blaser MJ et al: Survival of *Campylobacter fetus* subsp. *jejuni* in biological milieus, *J Clin Microbiol* 11:309, 1980.
18. Blaser MJ et al: Inactivation of *Campylobacter jejuni* by chlorine and monochlorine, *Appl Environ Microbiol* 51:307, 1986.
19. Block SS: Peroxygen compounds. In Block SS, editor: *Disinfection, sterilization, and preservation,* ed 4, Philadelphia, 1991, Lea & Febiger, p 182.
20. Bradley DJ: Health aspects of water supplies in tropical countries. In Feachem R et al, editors: *Water, wastes and health in hot climates,* New York, 1977, Wiley, p 3.
21. Briton G: *Introduction to environmental virology,* New York, 1980, Wiley.
22. Brown HW, Neva FA: *Basic clinical parasitology,* ed 5, New York, 1983, Appleton & Lange.
23. Butler M: Virus removal by disinfection of effluents. In Goddard M, Butler M, editors: *Proceedings of international symposium on viruses and wastewater treatment,* Oxford, Eng, 1980, Permagon Press, p 145.
24. Castillo AE: Federal regulation of antimicrobial pesticides in the United States. In Block SS, editor: *Disinfection, sterilization, and preservation,* ed 4, Philadelphia, 1991, Lea & Febiger, p 977.
25. Centers for Disease Control: Epidemiologic notes and reports: gastroenteritis—Yellowstone National Park, *MMWR* 26:283, 1977.
26. Centers for Disease Control: Cryptosporidiosis—New Mexico, 1986, *MMWR* 36:561, 1987.
27. Centers for Disease Control: Viral gastroenteritis—S. Dakota and New Mexico, *MMWR* 37:69, 1988.
28. Centers for Disease Control: *Health information for international travel,* HHS Pub No (CDC) 94-8280, Washington, DC, 1994, US Department of Health and Human Services.
29. Centers for Disease Control: Hepatitis E among US travelers, 1989-1992, *MMWR* 42:1, 1993.
30. Chambers CW, Proctor CM, Kabler PW: Bactericidal effect of low concentrations of silver, *J Am Water Works Assoc* 54:208, 1962.
31. Chang SL: The use of active iodine as a water disinfectant, *J Am Pharm Assoc* 47:417, 1958.
32. Chang SL: Modern concepts of disinfection: water treatment in the seventies. In *Proceedings of National Specialty Conference on Disinfection,* 1970, Am Soc Civ Engineers, p 635.
33. Chang SL, Fair GM: Viability and destruction of the cysts of *Entamoeba histolytica, J Am Water Works Assoc* 33:1705, 1941.
34. Chang SL, Morris JC: Elemental iodine as a disinfectant for drinking water, *Ind Engineer Chem* 45:1009, 1953.
35. Chaudhuri M, Sattar SA: Domestic water treatment for developing countries. In McFeters GA, editor: *Drinking water microbiology,* New York, 1990, Springer-Verlag, p 168.
36. Ciochetti DA, Metcalf RH: Pasteurization of naturally contaminated water with solar energy, *Appl Environ Microbiol* 47:223, 1984.
37. Cohen JM, Hannah SA: Coagulation and flocculation. In *American Water Works Association: Water quality and treatment: a handbook of public water supplies,* New York, 1971, McGraw-Hill, p 66.
38. *Consumer Reports,* Water filters, Feb 1983, p 68.
39. *Consumer Reports,* Jan 1990, p 28.
40. Cookson JT: Virus and water supply, *J Am Water Works Assoc* 66:707, 1974.
41. Cooper RC et al: *Infectious agent risk assessment water quality project.* UCB/SEEHRL Report No. 84-4 and 84-5, Berkeley, 1984, University of California.
42. Craun GF: *Waterborne disease in the United States,* Boca Raton, Fla, 1986, CRC Press.
43. Craun G et al: Prevention of waterborne cholera in the United States, *J Am Water Works Assoc* 83:40, 1991.
44. Cullimore DR, Jacobsen H: The efficiency of point of use devices for the exclusion of *Giardia muris* cysts from a model water supply system. In Wallis PM, Hammond BR, editors: *Advances in Giardia research,* Calgary, 1988, University of Calgary Press, p 107.
45. Culp RL: Breakpoint chlorination for virus inactivation, *J Am Water Works Assoc* 66:699, 1974.
46. Culp RL, Wesner GC, Culp GL: *Handbook of advanced wastewater treatment,* New York, 1978, Van Nostrand Reinhold.
47. Current WL: *Cryptosporidium:* its biology and potential for environmental transmission, *Crit Rev Environ Cont* 17:21, 1985.
48. D'Antonio RG et al: A waterborne outbreak of cryptosporidiosis in normal hosts, *Ann Intern Med* 103:886, 1985.
49. DeRegnier DP et al: Viability of *Giardia* cysts suspended in lake, river, and tap water, *Appl Environ Microbiol* 55:1223, 1989.
50. Dickens DL, DuPont HL, Johnson PC: Survival of bacterial enteropathogens in the ice of popular drinks, *JAMA* 253:3141, 1985.
51. Drinking Water Health Effects Task Force, US Environmental Protection Agency: *Health effects of drinking water treatment technologies,* Chelsea, Mich, 1989, Lewis Publishers (originally published Washington, DC, USEPA, 1988).
52. DuPont HL et al: The response of man to virulent *Shigella flexneri* 2a, *J Infect Dis* 119:296, 1969.
53. Dychdala GR: Chlorine and chlorine compounds. In Block SS, editor: *Disinfection, sterilization, and preservation,* Philadelphia, 1983, Lea & Febiger.
54. Eden KV et al: Waterborne gastrointestinal illness at a ski resort: isolation of *Yersinia enterocolitica* from drinking water, *J Public Health Rep* 92:245, 1977.
55. Engelbrecht RS et al: Comparative inactivation of viruses by chlorine, *Appl Environ Microbiol* 40:249, 1980.

56. Environmental Health Directorate Health Protection Branch: *Laboratory testing and evaluation of iodine-releasing point-of-use water treatment devices,* Ottawa, 1979, Department of National Health and Welfare.
57. Environmental Health Directorate Health Protection Branch: *Assessing the effectiveness of small filtration systems for point-of-use disinfection of drinking water supplies (80-EHD-54),* Ottawa, 1980, Department of National Health and Welfare.
58. Fair JF, Morrison SM: Recovery of bacterial pathogens from high quality surface water, *Water Res* 3:799, 1967.
59. Felsenfeld O: Notes on food, beverages and fomites contaminated with *Vibrio* cholera, *Bull WHO* 33:725, 1965.
60. Fina LR et al: Virucidal capability of resin I_3 disinfectant, *Appl Environ Microbiol* 44:1370, 1982.
61. Finkelstein R, Jacobi M: Fatal iodine poisoning: clinicopathologic and experimental study, *Ann Intern Med* 10:1283, 1937.
62. Fraker LD et al: *Giardia* cyst inactivation by iodine, *J Wilderness Med* 3:351, 1992.
63. Frazier WC, Westhoff DC: Preservation by use of high temperatures. In *Food microbiology,* New York, 1978, McGraw-Hill.
64. Freund G: Effect of iodinated water supplies on thyroid function, *J Clin Endocrinol Metab* 26:619, 1966.
65. Geldreich EE: Drinking water microbiology—new directions toward water quality enhancement, *Int J Food Microbiol* 9:295, 1989.
66. Geldreich EE: Microbiological quality of source waters for water supply. In McFeters GA, editor: *Drinking water microbiology,* New York, 1990, Springer-Verlag, p 3.
67. Geldreich EE, Reasoner DJ: Home treatment devices and water quality. In McFeters GA, editor: *Drinking water microbiology,* New York, 1990, Springer-Verlag, p 147.
68. Gerba CP, Nakhforoosh M: *Evaluation of iodine (I_2) as tri-iodine (I_3) resin for inactivation of enteric bacteria and viruses, and of microfiltration for removal of Giardia cysts as incorporated in the Recovery Engineering antimicrobial water purifier for world travelers: efficacy of antimicrobial agents,* Tucson, 1990, University of Arizona.
69. Gerba CP, Rose JB: Viruses in source and drinking water. In McFeters GA, editor: *Drinking water microbiology,* New York, 1990, Springer-Verlag, p 380.
70. Gerba CP, Rose JB, Singh SN: Waterborne gastroenteritis and viral hepatitis. In Straub CP, editor: *Crit Rev Environ Cont* 15:213, 1985.
71. Gershenfeld L, Witlin B: Iodine as an antiseptic, *Ann NY Acad Sci* 53:172, 1950.
72. Ginoza W et al: Mechanisms of inactivation of single stranded virus nucleic acids by heat, *Nature* 203:606, 1964.
73. Goodman LS, Gilman A: *The pharmacological basis of therapeutics,* ed 7, New York, 1985, Macmillan.
74. Gosselin RE, Smith RP, Hodge HC: *Clinical toxicology of commercial products,* ed 5, Baltimore, 1984, Williams & Wilkins.
75. Gottardi W: Iodine and iodine compounds. In Block SS, editor: *Disinfection, sterilization, and preservation,* ed 4, Philadelphia, 1991, Lea & Febiger, p 152.
76. Grabow WOK et al: Inactivation of hepatitis A virus and indicator organisms in water by free chlorine residuals, *Appl Environ Microbiol* 46:619, 1983.
77. Haas CN, Heller B: Kinetics of inactivation of *Giardia lamblia* by free chlorine, *Water Res* 24:233, 1990.
78. Harvey S et al: Recovery of *Yersinia enterocolitica* from streams and lakes of California, *Appl Environ Microbiol* 32:352, 1976.
79. Hayes EB et al: Large community outbreak of cryptosporidiosis due to contamination of a filtered public water supply, *N Engl J Med* 320:1372, 1989.
80. Hazen TC, Toranzos GA: Tropical source water. In McFeters GA, editor: *Drinking water microbiology,* New York, 1990, Springer-Verlag, p 32.
81. Herwaldt BL et al: Waterborne disease outbreaks 1989-1990, *MMWR* 40(SS-3):1, 1991.
82. Hibler CP, Hancock CM: Waterborne giardiasis. In McFeters GA, editor: *Drinking water microbiology,* New York, 1990, Springer-Verlag, p 380.
83. Hibler CP et al: *Inactivation of Giardia cysts with chlorine at 0.5° C to 5.0° C,* AWWA Research Report, Denver, 1987, AWWA Research Foundation.
84. Hoehn RC: Comparative disinfection methods, *J Am Water Works Assoc* 68:302, 1976.
85. Hoff JC: Disinfection resistance of *Giardia* cysts: origins of current concepts and research in progress. In Jakubowski W, Hoff JC, editors: *Waterborne transmission of giardiasis. Proceedings of a symposium (EPA-600/9-79-001),* Cincinnati, 1979, US Environmental Protection Agency.
86. Hoff JC: *Inactivation of microbial agents by chemical disinfectants (EPA/600/2-86/067),* Cincinnati, 1986, US Environmental Protection Agency.
87. Holmberg SD et al: *Aeromonas* infections in the United States, *Ann Intern Med* 105:683, 1986.
88. How long to boil water, *Foreign Service Med Bull,* 23, Oct-Dec 1992.
89. Hurst CJ: Disinfection of drinking water, swimming pool water and treated sewage effluents. In Block SS, editor: *Disinfection, sterilization, and preservation,* ed 4, Philadelphia, 1991, Lea & Febiger, p 713.
90. Istre GR et al: Waterborne giardiasis at a mountain resort: evidence for acquired immunity, *Am J Public Health* 74:602, 1984.
91. Jakubowski W: Detection of *Giardia* cysts in drinking water. In Erlandsen SL, Meyer EA, editors: *Giardia and Giardiasis: biology, pathogenesis and epidemiology,* New York, 1984, Plenum Press, p 263.
92. Jarroll EL, Bingham AK, Meyer EA: *Giardia* cyst destruction: effectiveness of six small water disinfection methods, *Am J Trop Med Hyg* 29:8, 1980.
93. Jarroll EL, Bingham MS, Meyer EA: Inability of an iodination method to destroy completely *Giardia* cysts in cold water, *West J Med* 132:567, 1980.
94. Jarroll EL, Bingham MS, Meyer EA: Effect of chlorine on *Giardia lamblia* cyst viability, *Appl Environ Microbiol* 41:483, 1981.
95. Jarroll EL, Hoff JC, Meyer EA: Resistance of cysts to disinfection agents. In Erlandsen SL, Meyer EA, editors: *Giardia and giardiasis: biology, pathogenesis and epidemiology,* New York, 1984, Plenum Press, p 311.
96. Joslyn L: Sterilization by heat. In Block SS, editor: *Disinfection, sterilization, and preservation,* Philadelphia, 1983, Lea & Febiger.
97. Joslyn L: Personal communication, 1986.
98. Kahn FH, Visscher BR: Water disinfection in the wilderness—a simple, effective method of iodination, *West J Med* 122:450, 1975.
99. Kane MA et al: Epidemic non-A, non-B hepatitis in Nepal, *JAMA* 252:3140, 1984.
100. Kapoor SK, O'Connor JT: Emergency disinfection. In *Water treatment in the seventies. Proceedings of National Specialty Conference on Disinfection,* 1970, Am Soc Civ Engineers, p 179.
101. Kelly S, Sanderson WW: The effect of chlorine in water on enteric viruses, *Am J Public Health* 48:1323, 1958.
102. Kelly S, Sanderson WW: The effect of combined chlorine on poliomyelitis and coxsackie virus, *Am J Public Health* 50:14, 1960.
103. Kerasote T: Drops to drink, *Audobon* 88:28, 1986. (Research by Standridge JH, Wisconsin State Laboratory of Hygiene, University of Wisconsin, Madison.)
104. Keswick BH et al: Inactivation of Norwalk virus in drinking water by chlorine, *Appl Environ Microbiol* 50:261, 1985.
105. Kim S: Sodium thiosulfate. In Olson SR, editor: *Poisoning & drug overdose,* San Mateo, Calif, 1990, Appleton & Lange.
106. Kinman RN, Black AP, Thomas WC: Disinfection with iodine. In *Water treatment in the seventies. Proceedings of National Specialty Conference on Disinfection,* 1970, Am Soc Civ Engineers, p 11.

107. Krishnaswami SK: Effect of chlorine on *Ascaris* eggs, *Health Lab Sci* 5:225, 1968.
108. Krugman S, Giles JP, Hammond J: Hepatitis virus: effect of heat on the infectivity and antigenicity of the MS-1 and MS-2 strains, *J Infect Dis* 122:432, 1970.
109. Kunkle S et al: *Field survey of Giardia in streams and wildlife of the Glacier Gorge and Loch Vale basins, Rocky Mountain National Park,* Natural Resources Report Series 85-3, Fort Collins, Colo, 1985, National Park Service.
110. Lange WE: Personal communication, 1987.
111. Laubusch EI: Chlorination and other disinfection processes. In American Water Works Association: *Water quality and treatment: a handbook of public water supplies,* New York, 1971, McGraw-Hill, p 160.
112. LeChevallier MW, Evans TM, Seidler RJ: Effect of turbidity on chlorination efficiency and bacterial persistence in drinking water, *Appl Environ Microbiol* 42:159, 1981.
113. LeChevallier MW, McFeters GA: Microbiology of activated carbon. In McFeters GA, editor: *Drinking water microbiology,* New York, 1990, Springer-Verlag, p 104.
114. Lin SD: *Giardia lamblia* and water supply, *J Am Water Works Assoc* 77:40, 1985.
115. Logsdon GS: Microbiology and drinking water filtration. In McFeters GA, editor: *Drinking water microbiology,* New York, 1990, Springer-Verlag, p 120.
116. Logsdon GS et al: Alternative filtration methods for removal of *Giardia* cysts and cyst models, *J Am Water Works Assoc* 73:111, 1981.
117. Marchin GL, Fina LR: Contact and demand-release disinfectants, *Crit Rev Environ Control* 19:227, 1989.
118. Marchin GL et al: Effect of resin disinfectants I_3 and I_5 on *Giardia muris* and *Giardia lamblia, Appl Environ Microbiol* 46:965, 1983.
119. McDermott JH: Virus problems and their relation to water supplies, *J Am Water Works Assoc* 66:693, 1974.
120. Melack JM, Stoddard JL, Dawson DR: *Acid precipitation and buffer capacity of lakes in the Sierra Nevada, California.* Presented at International Symposium on Hydrometeorology, 1982, American Water Resources Association.
121. Merson MH et al: An outbreak of *Shigella sonnei* gastroenteritis on Colorado river raft trips, *Am J Epidemiol* 100:186, 1974.
122. Miltner RJ et al: Treatment of seasonal pesticides in surface waters, *J Am Water Works Assoc* 83:43, 1989.
123. Monzingo DL, Stevens DR: *Giardia contamination of surface waters: a survey of three selected backcountry streams in Rocky Mountain National Park,* Water Resources Report No. 86-2, Fort Collins, Colo, 1986, National Park Service.
124. Morgan DP, Karpen RJ: Test of chronic toxicity of iodine as related to the purification of water, *US Armed Forces Med J* 4:725, 1953.
125. Morris JC: Chlorination and disinfection—state of the art, *J Am Water Works Assoc* 63:769, 1971.
126. Morris JC et al: Disinfection of drinking water under field conditions, *Ind Engineer Chem* 45:1013, 1953.
127. National Academy of Sciences, Safe Drinking Water Committee: The disinfection of drinking water. In *Drinking water and health,* vol 2, Washington, DC, 1980, National Academy Press.
128. Neefe JR et al: Disinfection of water containing causative agent of infectious hepatitis, *JAMA* 128:1076, 1945.
129. Neefe JR et al: Inactivation of the virus of infectious hepatitis in drinking water, *Am J Public Health* 37:365, 1947.
130. Neumann HH: Bacteriological safety of hot tapwater in developing countries, *Public Health Rep* 84:812, 1969.
131. Neumann HH: Alternatives to water chlorination (correspondence) *Rev Infect Dis* 3:1255, 1981.
132. Neuwirth M et al: Effects of chlorine on the ultrastructure of *Giardia* cysts. In Wallis PM, Hammond BR, editors: *Advances in Giardia research,* Calgary, 1988, University of Calgary Press, p 133.
133. O'Connor JT, Hemphill L, Reach CD: *Removal of virus from public water supplies,* EPA-600/2-77-087, Cincinnati, 1982, US Environmental Protection Agency.
134. O'Connor JT, Kapoor SK: Small quantity field disinfection, *J Am Water Works Assoc* 62:80, 1970.
135. Olsen KE: *An evaluation of low chlorine concentrations on Giardia cyst viability,* ED&T Project 1150A, January 1982, USDA Forest Service.
136. Ongerth J: *A study of water treatment practices for the removal of Giardia lamblia cysts.* In Proceedings of Conference on Current Research in Drinking Water Treatment, EPA/600/9-88/004, Cincinnati, 1987, Cincinnati, 1988, US Environmental Protection Agency.
137. Ongerth JE: *Giardia* cyst concentrations in river water, *J Am Water Works Assoc* 83:81, 1989.
138. Ongerth JE, Stibbs HH: Identification of *Cryptosporidium* oocysts in river water, *Appl Environ Microbiol* 53:672, 1987.
139. Ongerth JE et al: Backcountry water treatment to prevent giardiasis, *Am J Public Health* 79:1633, 1989.
140. Payment P et al: A randomized trial to evaluate the risk of gastrointestinal disease due to consumption of drinking water meeting current microbiological standards, *Am J Pub Health* 81:703, 1991.
141. Perez-Rosas N, Hazen TC: In situ survival of *Vibrio cholerae* and *Escherichia coli* in a tropical rain forest watershed, *Appl Environ Microbiol* 55:495, 1989.
142. Perkins JJ: Thermal destruction of microorganisms: heat inactivation of viruses. In *Principles and methods of sterilization in health sciences,* Springfield, Ill, 1969, Charles C Thomas, p 63.
143. Peterson DA et al: Thermal treatment and infectivity of hepatitis A virus in human feces, *J Med Virol* 2:201, 1978.
144. Peterson DA et al: Effect of chlorine treatment on infectivity of hepatitis A virus, *Appl Environ Microbiol* 45:223, 1983.
145. Porter JD et al: *Giardia* transmission in a swimming pool, *Am J Public Health* 78:659, 1988.
146. Poynter SFB, Slade JS, Jones HH: The disinfection of water with special reference to viruses, *Water Treatment Exam* 22:194, 1973.
147. Poyry T, Stenvik M, Hovi T: Viruses in sewage waters during and after a poliomyelitis outbreak in Finland, *Appl Environ Microbiol* 54:371, 1988.
148. Preston DR et al: Novel approach for modifying microporous filters for virus concentration from water, *Appl Environ Microbiol* 54:1325, 1988.
149. Purcell RH, Gerin JL: Hepatitis B vaccines: a status report. In Vyas GN, Cohen SN, Schmidt R, editors: *Viral hepatitis,* Philadelphia, 1978, Franklin Institute Press, p 492.
150. Rao VC et al: Removal of hepatitis A virus and rotavirus by drinking water treatment, *J Am Water Works Assoc* 82:59, 1988.
151. Reddish GF, editor: *Antiseptics, disinfectants, fungicides and chemical and physical sterilization,* Philadelphia, 1954, Lea & Febiger.
152. Reeves H: Human waste disposal in the Sierran wilderness. In Stanley JT, Harvey HT, Hartesveldt RJ, editors: *A report on the wilderness impact study: the effects of human recreational activities on wilderness ecosystems with special emphasis on Sierra Club wilderness outings in the Sierra Nevada,* San Francisco, 1979, Sierra Club, p 129.
153. Regli S: *Regulations on filtration and disinfection.* In Proceedings of a Conference on Current Research in Drinking Water Treatment, Cincinnati, 1987, EPA/600/9-88/004. Cincinnati, 1988, US Environmental Protection Agency, p 151.
154. Regli S et al: Modeling the risk from *Giardia* and viruses in drinking water, *J Am Water Works Assoc* 83:76, 1991.
155. Regunathan P, Beauman WH: Microbiological characteristics of point-of-use precoat carbon filters, *J Am Water Works Assoc* 79:67, 1987.
156. Reimers RS et al: *Investigation of parasites in sludges and disinfection techniques,* USEPA Project Summary EPA/600/s1-85/022, Cincinnati, 1986, US Environmental Protection Agency.

157. Rendtorff RC: The experimental transmission of human intestinal protozoan parasites. II. *Giardia lamblia* cysts given in capsules, *Am J Hyg* 59:209, 1954.
158. Rendtorff RC: The experimental transmission of human protozoan parasites. IV. Attempts to transmit *Entamoeba coli* and *Giardia lamblia* cysts by water, *Am J Hyg* 60:327, 1954.
159. Rice EW, Hoff JC, Schaefer FW: Inactivation of *Giardia* cysts by chlorine, *Appl Environ Microbiol* 43:250, 1982.
160. Rice EW, Johnson CH: Cholera in Peru (letter), *Lancet* 338:455, 1991.
161. Riggs JL: AIDS transmission in drinking water: no threat, *J Am Water Works Assoc* 81:69, 1989.
162. Riggs JL et al: Detection of *Giardia lamblia* by immunofluorescence, *Appl Environ Microbiol* 45:698, 1983.
163. Roach PD et al: Waterborne *Giardia* cysts and *Cryptosporidium* oocysts in the Yukon, Canada, *Appl Environ Microbiol* 59:67, 1993.
164. Rogers MR, Vitaliano JJ: Military and small group water disinfecting systems: an assessment, *Milit Med* 7:267, 1979.
165. Rose JB: Occurrence and significance of *Cryptosporidium* in water, *J Am Water Works Assoc* 82:53, 1988.
166. Rose JB: Occurrence and control of *Cryptosporidium* in drinking water. In McFeters GA, editor: *Drinking water microbiology,* New York, 1990, Springer-Verlag, p 294.
167. Rose JB, Haas CN, Regli S: Risk assessment and control of waterborne giardiasis, *Am J Public Health* 81:709, 1991.
168. Rose JB et al: Occurrence of rotaviruses and enteroviruses in recreational waters of Oak Creek, Arizona, *Water Res* 21:1375, 1987.
169. Rosen AA, Booth RL: Taste and odor control. In American Water Works Association: *Water quality and treatment: a handbook of public water supplies,* New York, 1971, McGraw-Hill.
170. Rosenberg ML et al: Shigellosis from swimming, *JAMA* 236:1849, 1976.
171. Rosenberg ML et al: Epidemic diarrhea at crater lake from enterotoxigenic *Escherichia coli, Ann Intern Med* 86:714, 1977.
172. Rubin AJ et al: Inactivation of gerbil-cultured *Giardia lamblia* cysts by free chlorine, *Appl Environ Microbiol* 55:2592, 1989.
173. Sattar SA: *Viruses, water and health,* Ottawa, Canada, 1978, University of Ottawa Press.
174. Scarpino PV et al: A comparative study of the inactivation of viruses in water by chlorine, *Water Res* 6:959, 1972.
175. Schaffner W: Gas gangrene (other *Clostridium*-associated diseases). In Mandell GL, Douglas RG, Bennett JE, editors: *Principles and practice of infectious disease,* New York, 1990, Churchill Livingstone, p 1850.
176. Scheid R et al: Inactivation of hepatitis A and B viruses and risk of iatrogenic transmission, *Int Symp Viral Hepatitis* 23:627, 1981.
177. Scheimann DA: *Yersinia enterocolitica* in drinking water. In McFeters GA, editor: *Drinking water microbiology,* New York, 1990, Springer-Verlag, p 322.
178. Schmidt SD, Meier PG: Evaluation of *Giardia* cyst removal via portable water filtration devices, *J Freshwater Ecol* 2:435, 1984.
179. Reference deleted in proofs.
180. Shephart M: Helminthological aspects of sewage treatment. In Feachem R, McGarry M, Mara D, editors: *Water, wastes and health in hot climates,* New York, 1977, Wiley, p 299.
181. Singh A, McFeters GA: Injury of enteropathogenic bacteria in drinking water. In McFeters GA, editor: *Drinking water microbiology,* New York, 1990, Springer-Verlag, p 368.
182. Sletten O: Halogens and their role in disinfection, *J Am Water Works Assoc* 66:690, 1974.
183. Sobsey MD: Enteric viruses and drinking water supplies, *J Am Water Works Assoc* 67:414, 1975.
184. Sobsey MD, Fuji T, Hall RM: Inactivation of cell-associated and dispersed hepatitis A virus in water, *J Am Water Works Assoc* 83:64, 1991.
185. Sobsey MD, Fuji T, Shields P: *Inactivation of hepatitis A virus and model viruses in water by free chlorine.* In Proceedings of Conference on Current Research in Drinking Water Treatment, Cincinnati, 1987, EPA/600/9-88/004, Cincinnati, 1988, US Environmental Protection Agency, p 230.
186. Sorenson SK et al: Isolation and detection of *Giardia* cysts from water using direct immunofluorescence, *Water Resources Bull* 22:843, 1986.
187. Sorvillo FJ et al: Shigellosis associated with recreational water contact in Los Angeles County, *Am J Trop Med Hyg* 38:613, 1988.
188. Spire B et al: Inactivation of lymphadenopathy-associated virus by heat, gamma rays, and ultraviolet light, *Lancet* 1:188, 1985.
189. States SJ et al: *Legionella* in drinking water. In McFeters GA, editor: *Drinking water microbiology,* New York, 1990, Springer-Verlag, p 340.
190. Stringer R, Kruse CW: Amoebic cysticidal properties of halogens in water. In *Water treatment in the seventies.* Proceedings of National Specialty Conference on Disinfection, New York, 1970, American Society of Civil Engineers, p 319.
191. Strum WH: *Techniques of water disinfection,* LaJolla, Calif, 1991 (unpublished data).
192. Suk TJ, Sorenson SK, Dileanis PD: The relation between human presence and occurrence of *Giardia* cysts in streams in the Sierra Nevada, California, *J Freshwater Ecol* 4:71, 1988.
193. Sullivan R et al: Thermal resistance of certain oncogenic viruses in milk, *Appl Microbiol* 22:315, 1971.
194. Sykes G: *Disinfection and sterilization,* London, 1965, JB Lippincott.
195. Taylor DN et al: *Campylobacter* enteritis from untreated water in the Rocky Mountains, *Ann Intern Med* 99:38, 1983.
196. Taylor SL, Fina LR, Lambert JL: New water disinfectant: an insoluble quaternary ammonium resin-triiodide combination that releases bactericide on demand, *Appl Microbiol* 20:720, 1970.
197. Thomas WC et al: Iodine disinfection of water, *Arch Environ Health* 19:124, 1969.
198. Thomas WC et al: Effects of an iodinated water supply, *Trans Am Clim Assoc* 90:153, 1978.
199. Thraenhart O: Measures for disinfection and control of viral hepatitis. In Block SS, editor: *Disinfection, sterilization, and preservation,* ed 4, Philadelphia, 1991, Lea & Febiger, p 445.
200. Tobin RS: *Performance of point-of-use water treatment devices.* In Proceedings of the First Conference on Cold Regions Environmental Engineering, Fairbanks, Alaska, 1983, p 312.
201. Tobin RS: Water treatment for the home or cottage, *Can J Public Health* 75:79, 1984.
202. Tobin RS: Testing and evaluating point-of-use treatment devices in Canada, *J Am Water Works Assoc* 79:42, 1987.
203. Tunnicliff B et al: *Drinking water treatment and procedures for Colorado River corridor raft trips,* Grand Canyon National Park, 1984, (unpublished manuscript).
204. US Army: *Sanitary control and surveillance of field water supplies,* Department of Army Technical Bulletin (TB Med 577), 1986, Department of Army.
205. US Environmental Protection Agency: *Human viruses in the aquatic environment,* EPA-570/9-78-006, Cincinnati, 1978.
206. US Environmental Protection Agency: *Health effects of land treatment: microbiological,* USEPA-600/1-82-007, Cincinnati, 1982.
207. US Environmental Protection Agency: *Guide standard and protocol for testing microbiological water purifiers: report to task force,* Cincinnati, revision 1987.
208. US Forest Service: *Back country safety tips,* United States Department of Agriculture, Forest Service (public information pamphlet).
209. US Public Health Service: *Drinking water standards,* 1962. USPHS Pub No 956.
210. Upton SJ et al: Efficacy of a pentaiodide resin disinfectant on *Cryptosporidium parvum* oocysts *in vitro, J Parasitol* 74:719, 1988.

211. Wallis PM et al: Removal and inactivation of *Giardia* cysts in a mobile water treatment plant under field conditions: preliminary results. In Wallis PM, Hammond BR, editors: *Advances in Giardia research,* Calgary, 1988, University of Calgary Press, p 137.
212. Walsh JA, Warren KS: Selective primary health care: an interim strategy for disease control in developing countries, *N Engl J Med* 301:967, 1979.
213. Ward RL, Akin EW: Minimum infective dose of animal viruses, *Crit Rev Environ Control* 14:297, 1984.
214. Water and Sanitation for Health (WASH) Project: *Triocide questions and answers,* Arlington, Va, 1980, WASH.
215. Water and Sanitation for Health Project: *Water supply and sanitation in rural development: proceedings of a conference for private and voluntary organizations,* WASH Technical Report No 14, Washington, DC, 1981, WASH.
216. Water and Sanitation for Health Project: *Report on mobile emergency water treatment and disinfection units,* WASH Field report no 271, Arlington, Va, 1989, WASH.
217. Waterman J: *Surviving Denali,* New York, 1983, American Alpine Club.
218. Weiss SJ, Lampert MB, Test ST: Long-lived oxidants generated by human neutrophils: characterization and bioactivity, *Science* 222:625, 1983.
219. White GC: Disinfection: the last line of defense for potable water, *J Am Water Works Assoc* 67:410, 1975.
220. White GC: *Handbook of chlorination,* ed 3, New York, 1992, Van Nostrand Reinhold.
221. Wilkerson JA: *Medicine for mountaineering,* ed 3, Seattle, 1985, The Mountaineers.
222. Witenberg G, Yofe J: Investigation on purification of water with respect to *Schistomoma cercariae, Trans R Soc Trop Med Hyg* 31:549, 1938.
223. Wolff J: Iodide goiter and the pharmacologic effects of excess iodide, *Am J Med* 47:101, 1969.
224. Woo PK: Evidence for animal reservoirs and transmission of *Giardia* infection between animal species. In Erlandsen SL, Meyer EA, editors: *Giardia and giardiasis: biology, pathogenesis and epidemiology,* New York, 1984, Plenum Press, p 341.
225. Woodward RL: Review of the bactericidal effectiveness of silver, *J Am Water Works Assoc* 55:881, 1963.
226. World Health Organization Technical Report Series: *Human viruses in water, wastewater, and soil,* Series 639, Geneva, 1979, World Health Organization.
227. World Health Organization Technical Report Series: *Intestinal protozoan and helminthic Infections,* Geneva, 1981, World Health Organization.
228. York DW, Drewry WA: Virus removal by chemical coagulation, *J Am Water Works Assoc* 66:711, 1974.
229. Yoshpe-Purer Y, Eylan E: Disinfection of water by hydrogen peroxide, *Health Lab Sci* 5:233, 1968.
230. Zell S: Epidemiology of wilderness-acquired diarrhea: implications for prevention and treatment, *J Wilderness Med* 3:241, 1992.
231. Zell SC, Sorenson MS: Cyst acquisition rate for *Giardia lamblia* in backcountry travelers to Desolation Wilderness, Lake Tahoe, *J Wilderness Med* 4:147, 1993.
232. Zemlyn S et al: A caution on iodine water purification, *West J Med* 135:166, 1981.
233. Zoeteman BCJ: *The suitability of iodine and iodine compounds as disinfectants for small water supplies,* Technical Paper No 2, *WHO International Reference Centre for Community Water Supplies,* The Hague, 1972, World Health Organization, p 17.

APPENDIX A

Water Disinfection Products

Product/Manufacturer	Price	Structure/Function
KATADYN FILTERS		
Katadyn U.S.A., Inc. 3020 N. Scottsdale Rd. Scottsdale, AZ 85251 602-990-3131		All filters contain 0.2 μm ceramic candle filter, silver impregnated to decrease bacterial growth; large units also contain silver quartz in center of filter
Katadyn pocket filter (Fig. 43-3)	$225	Hand pump; 40-inch intake hose and strainer, zipper case; size: 10 × 2 inches; weight: 1 lb 9 oz; flow: ¾ qt/min
Replacement filter element	$120	
Minifilter (Fig. 43-4)	$140	Smaller, lighter hand pump; 31-inch intake hose and strainer, hard plastic enclosure and pump; size: 7 × 3.5 × 1.75 inches; weight: 9 oz; flow: 0.5 L/min; capacity: approx 7000 L
Hand pump filter KFT (Fig. 43-5)	$725	Large hand pump with steel stand; size (packed in case): 23 × 6 × 8 inches; weight: 10 lb, 13 oz; flow: 1.5-3 qt/min
Replacement filter element	$40	
Drip filter TRK (Fig. 43-6)	$395	Gravity drip from one plastic bucket to another with three ceramic candle filter elements (same filter element as hand pump); size: 18 × 11 inch diameter (26 inches high when assembled); weight: 9 lb 4 oz; flow: 1 pt/hr

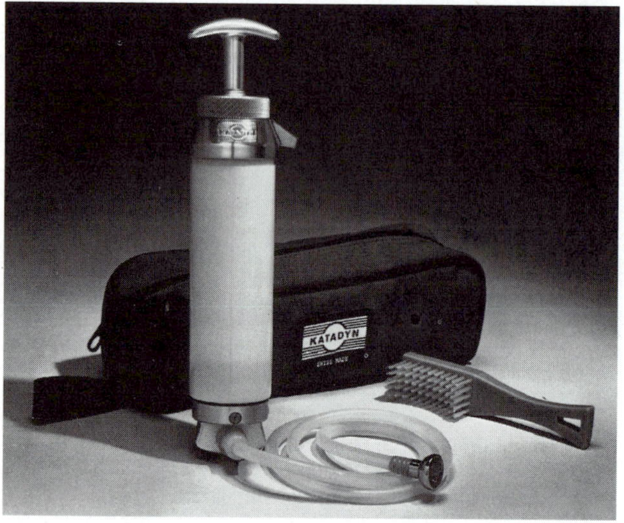

Fig. 43-3 Katadyn pocket filter.

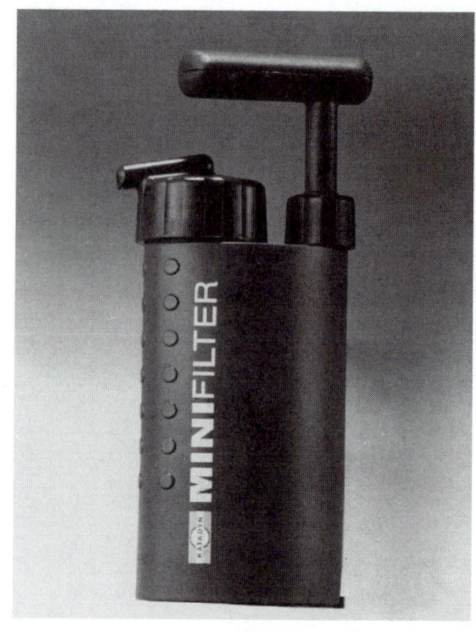

Fig. 43-4 Katadyn minifilter.

Claims	Comments
Removes bacterial pathogens, protozoan cysts, parasites, nuclear debris. Clarifies cloudy water. If filter clogs, flow can be restored by brushing filter element. This can be done hundreds of times before needing to replace filter element. Claims for removal of viruses not made in United States, although testimonials imply effectiveness in all polluted waters.	Well-designed, durable products. Effective for claims. Pocket filter is the original, individual, or small group filter. Minifilter was designed to be lighter and more cost competitive. Hand pump filter is popular for larger groups, especially river trips where weight is not a factor. Complete virus removal cannot be expected, although viruses usually clump to larger particles that can be filtered. Silver impregnation does not prevent bacterial growth in filters. With any filter, dilute bleach solution should be pumped through the unit after each trip, before storage.

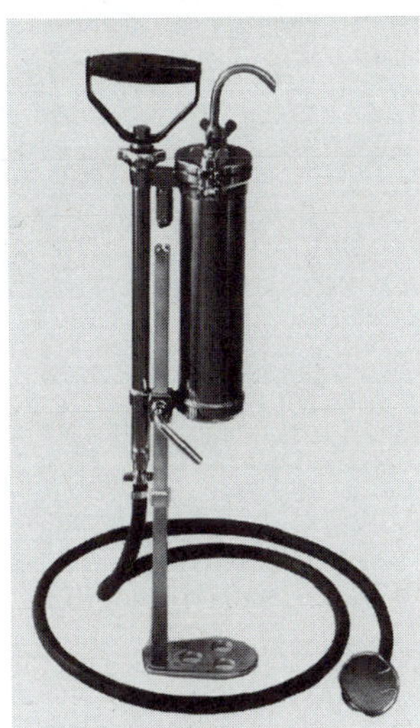

Fig. 43-5 Katadyn hand pump filter KFT.

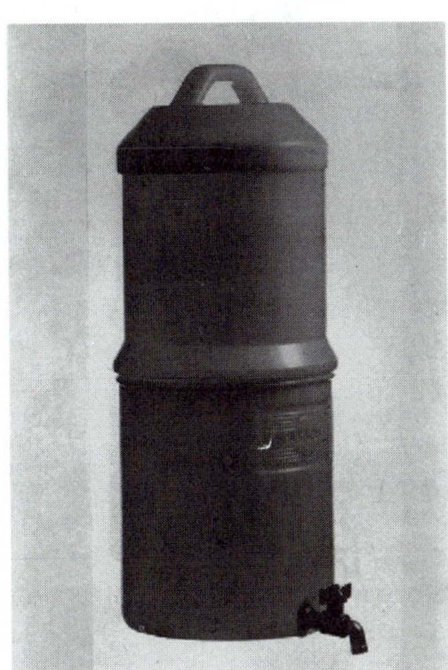

Fig. 43-6 Katadyn drip filter TRK.

Continued.

Water Disinfection Products—cont'd

Product/Manufacturer	Price	Structure/Function
TIMBERLINE FILTERS		
Timberline Filter 211 Pawnee Dr. Boulder, CO 80303 800-777-5996		
Timberline filter (Fig. 43-7) Replacement element	$24 $12	2 μm fiberglass and polyethylene matrix; hand pump; size: 9 × 1-3 inches; weight: 6 oz; flow: 1 qt in 1.5 min
Base Camp (Fig. 43-8) Replacement filter	$50 $25	Gravity-drip unit with filter in-line between input and reservoir bag; size: 5 × 10 inches empty and folded; weight: 12 oz; flow: 0.8 L/min; capacity: approx 50 gal
Quick-Sip (manufactured by Kenyon)	$20	Drink-through, filter unit in water bottle

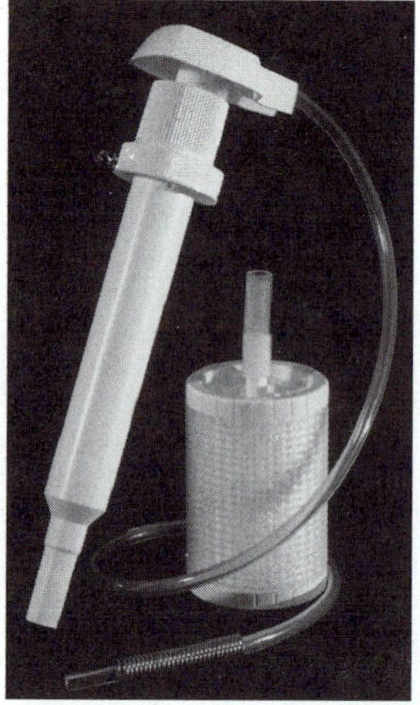

Fig. 43-7 Timberline filter.

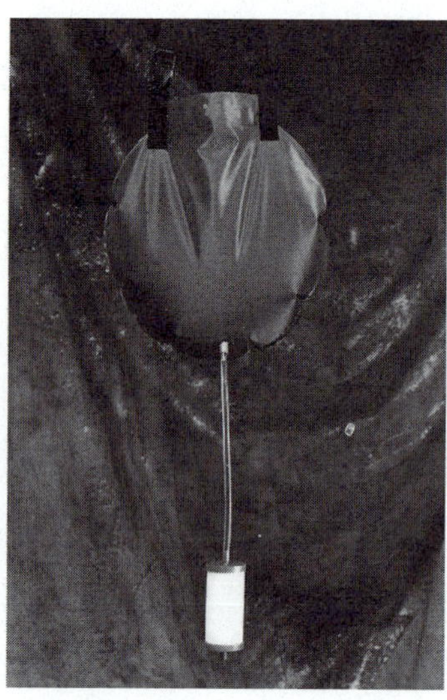

Fig. 43-8 Timberline Base Camp.

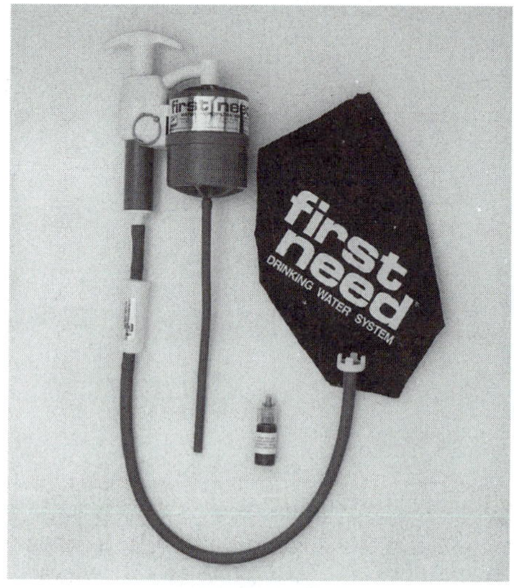

Fig. 43-9 General Ecology First Need deluxe unit.

Product/Manufacturer	Price	Structure/Function
GENERAL ECOLOGY FILTERS		
General Ecology, Inc. 151 Sheree Blvd. Lionville, PA 19353 215-363-0412		All filters (except Microlite) contain 0.1 μm (0.4 μm absolute) carbon matrix filter in removable canister
First Need purifier deluxe unit (Fig. 43-9)	$49 $60	Hand pump with intake strainer; size: 6 × 6 inches; weight: 12 oz; flow: 1 pint/min; capacity: 100-400 L individual replacement parts available
Matrix pumping system	$9	2 L carry bag, polyethylene liners, 18-inch hose and hose adapter for creating gravity filter unit from one of filter elements above
Trav-L-Pure (carrying case included) (Fig. 43-10) Replacement canister	$120 $30	Filter and hand pump in rectangular housing (1.5-pint capacity); pour water into housing, then pump through prefilter and microfilter; size: 4.5 × 3.5 × 6.75 inches; weight: 22 oz; flow: 1-2 pint/min; capacity: 100-400 L
Base Camp (carrying case included) (Fig. 43-11) Replacement cartridge	$500 $60	Stainless steel casing and hand pump connected with tubing; capacity 1000 gal; canister size 4.8 × 5.4 in; pump 1.5 × 10.5 inches; weight: 3 lb; flow: 1.5 L/min
Microlite Replacement cartridges (set of two)	$30 $10	Structured matrix filter 0.5 μm (nominal) with activated carbon; hand pump, 24-inch intake hose and strainer; attaches directly to wide-mouth or bike bottle or use outlet spout; size: 5.5 inches high × 2.5 inches diameter; weight: 8oz; flow: 0.5 L/min; capacity: 50 L/cartridge

Claims	Comments
Removes *Giardia* cysts. No claims for bacteria or viruses.	Effective for claims; intended only for North American backcountry use where *Giardia* is the primary contaminant, but should also remove *Cryptosporidium*. Lightest pump filter available.

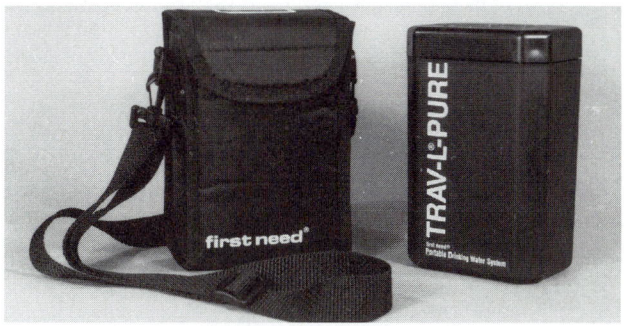

Fig. 43-10 General Ecology Trav-L-Pure with carrying case.

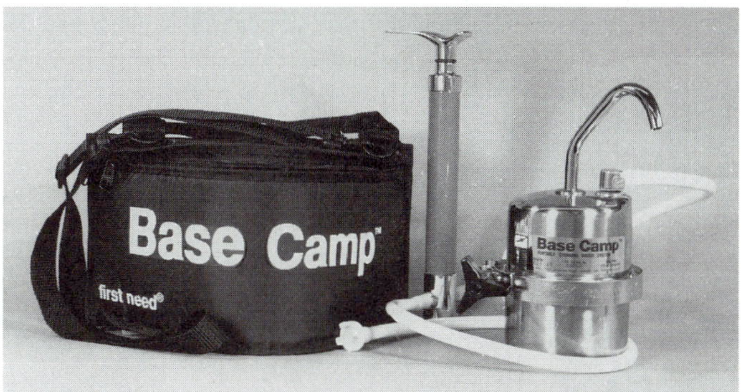

Fig. 43-11 General Ecology Base Camp with carrying case.

Claims	Comments
"Microfiltration" with 0.1 μm retention (0.4 absolute) "removes bacteria and larger pathogens" (cysts, parasites). No claims for viruses: Trav-L-Pure comes with iodine tablets for pretreatment if viral contamination suspected. "Adsorption and molecular seiving": carbon adsorbers remove chemicals and organic pollutants that cause color and taste. Does not remove all dissolved minerals or desalinate. "Ionic charges remove colloids and ultra-small particles." Microlite removes sediment, protozoal cysts, algae, and chemicals (including iodine) and improves color and taste of water. Iodine tablets are included for bacterial and viral elimination.	Reasonable design, cost, and effectiveness. Most testing of First Need with *E. coli* and *Giardia* cysts shows complete removal. Charcoal matrix removes chemical pollutants. Clarifies cloudy water. Despite testimonials for effectiveness in underdeveloped countries, recommend caution where viruses may be a problem; prior disinfection with halogen would guarantee disinfection, and carbon would remove hallogen. "Ionic surface charges" are not likely to play significant role. Microlite is designed primarily for day use or light backpacking. Halogen pretreatment would be used for all water except pristine alpine water in North America. This filter is compact, lightweight, and well designed for low-volume use. Filter cartridges are inexpensive and easily changed.

Continued.

Water Disinfection Products—cont'd

Product/Manufacturer	Price	Structure/Function
WATER ONE FILTER		
Calco Ltd. 7011 Barry Ave. Rosemont, IL 60018 708-296-6615		
Water One Filter	$50	Cartridge containing charcoal block, 0.4 μm filter; prefilter sponge 30-50 μm; bulb hand or foot pump generates 3-5 lb pressure; can back-wash to unclog; size: 3 × 6 in cartridge with about 7 ft of tubing and bulb pump; weight: 1 lb; capacity 400 gal or 3 yr
BASIC DESIGNS FILTERS		
Basic Designs Santa Rosa, CA 95404 707-575-1220		
Basic Designs ceramic water filter (Fig. 43-12)	$69	Ceramic candle filter with 0.9 μm absolute retention size and carbon center; filter is at bottom of heavy plastic reservoir bag with outflow tube connected to collection bag; gravity drip, or squeeze bag to increase flow rate; packing size: 4 × 4 × 8 inches; weight: 13 oz; flow (if bag is squeezed): 1 L/4 min; capacity: up to 1000 L
High flow ceramic water filter (Fig. 43-13)	$89	Gravity filter with larger capacity bag (7.5 L) and 6-ft tubing providing 2-3 lb hydrostatic pressure through in-line ceramic and carbon filter; flow rate: 10 L/hr
Ceramic filter pump (Fig. 43-14)	$29	Hand pump with ceramic cartridge at end of intake tubing and polyurethane prefilter; size: pump 8 × 1 inches; filter 4 × 3 in, 18 in tubing; weight: 7 oz; flow: 1 oz per stroke; capacity: 500 gal

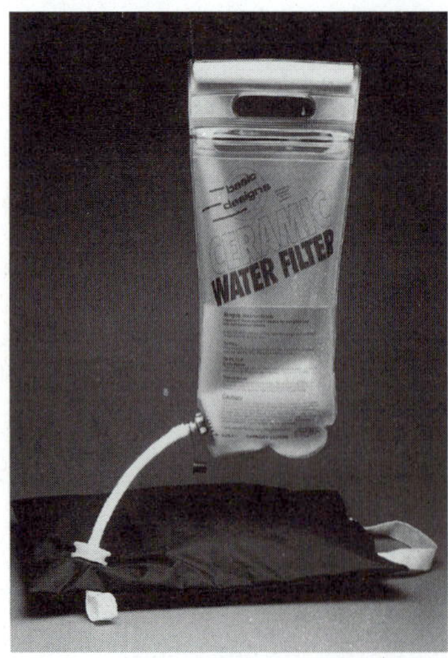

Fig. 43-12 Basic Designs ceramic water filter.

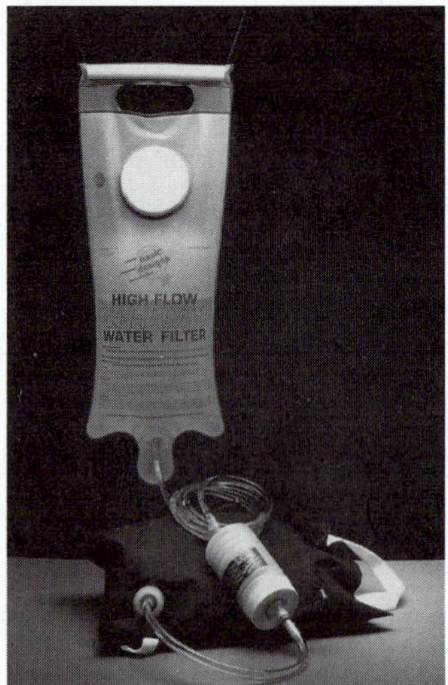

Fig. 43-13 Basic Designs high flow ceramic water filter.

Claims	Comments
Removes *Giardia;* no claims for bacteria or viruses. Unbreakable, 2-year guarantee. Comes with dye to test filter integrity.	Should be effective for claims made. Charcoal will remove most chemical pollutants and halogens, so filter could be used as second stage after halogen disinfection of water that may contain bacteria and viruses. Bulb pump is too stiff for hand pumping and is actually intended for foot use. Filter plus tubing is heavy and bulky compared with other filters with similar capacity.
Ceramic filter removes *Giardia,* bacteria, *Cryptosporidium,* cysts, tapeworm, flukes, other harmful pathogens larger than 1 μm, and bad taste. Carbon removes color, tastes, and odors. Filter can be cleaned with abrasive pad. Pump is easily serviced in the field; ceramic cartridge is replaceable.	Ceramic candle filters are effective filtering elements, and charcoal is an effective adsorbent. No claims for virus removal. 0.9 μm is large for bacterial removal, although a low-pressure depth filter this size could trap most of them. The simple gravity design decreases cost and moving parts. Filtration rate is slow, and filter could clog rapidly, since there is no prefilter for larger particulates. Basic filter is too slow, and squeezing bag is poor solution. High flow filter is more practical than basic filter because of faster filtration rate and larger reservoir capacity. Filter pump is the most practical and is reasonably priced.

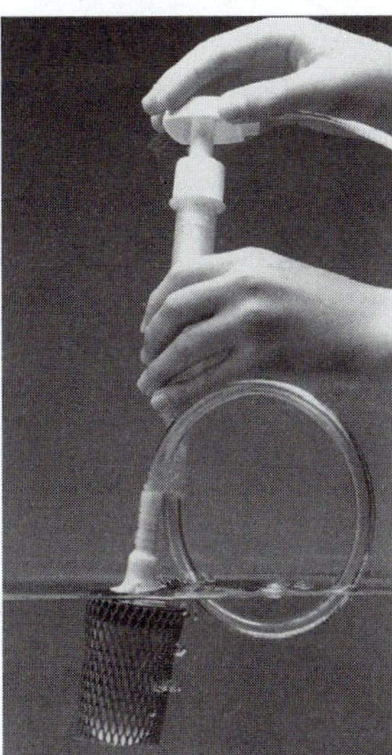

Fig. 43-14 Basic Designs ceramic filter pump.

Continued.

Water Disinfection Products—cont'd

Product/Manufacturer	Price	Structure/Function
MOUNTAIN SAFETY RESEARCH FILTERS		
Mountain Safety Research Box 3978 Terminal Station Seattle, WA 98124 206-624-7948		
MSR waterworks total filtration system (Fig. 43-15) (all filter elements and parts replaceable.)	$140	Four filter elements of decreasing pore size: porous foam, 10 µm stainless steel wire mesh screen, activated carbon filter (ceramic/carbon filter optional, may soon be standard), then 0.1 µm absolute membrane filter; hand pump with intake tubing; storage bag (2 or 4 L) attaches directly to outlet of pump; size: 9 × 4 × 3 inches; weight: 18.4 oz; flow rate: 1 L/90 sec
Dromedary beverage bag	$13-20	

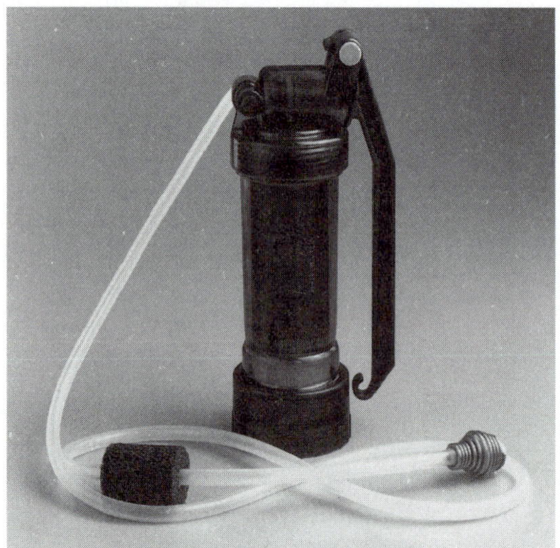

Fig. 43-15 Mountain Safety Research (MSR) waterworks filtration system.

Claims	Comments
Removes protozoa (including *Giardia* and *Cryptosporidium*), bacteria, pesticides, herbicides, chlorine, discoloration. Design and ease of use are distinct advantages. Filter can be easily maintained in the field; maintenance kit and all replacement parts available.	Excellent filter design and function. Prefilters protect more expensive inner, fine-pore filters. Should be effective for claims made. No claims made for viruses. Many would be removed by clumping and adherence to larger particles, but this should not be considered reliable for highly polluted waters in developing countries. Attaching reservoir bag is a nice addition.

Continued.

Water Disinfection Products—cont'd

Product/Manufacturer	Price	Structure/Function
WATER TECHNOLOGIES IODINE RESIN FILTERS		
Water Technologies Corp. 14405 21st Ave. N., Suite 120 Plymouth, MN 55447 800-627-0044		All products use Pentacide iodine resin under trade name of PentaPure
Travel Cup (Fig. 43-16)	$30	Gravity pour-through; size: 3 × 4 inches; weight: 3.5 oz; flow: 6 oz in 45 sec; capacity 100 gal
PentaPure water jug (Fig. 43-17)	$22	Collapsible 2-gal container with iodine resin cartridge at outpour spout; size: collapses to 8.5 × 8.5 × 7 inches; weight: 13 oz; flow: 20-30 oz/min; capacity: 20 gal
Replacement cartridge	$17	
The straw (Fig. 43-18)		Drink-through straw; cartridge with prefilter, granular activated carbon filter sandwiched between two stages of PentaPure resin; size: 5.5 inches long; weight: 1 oz; capacity: 25 gal

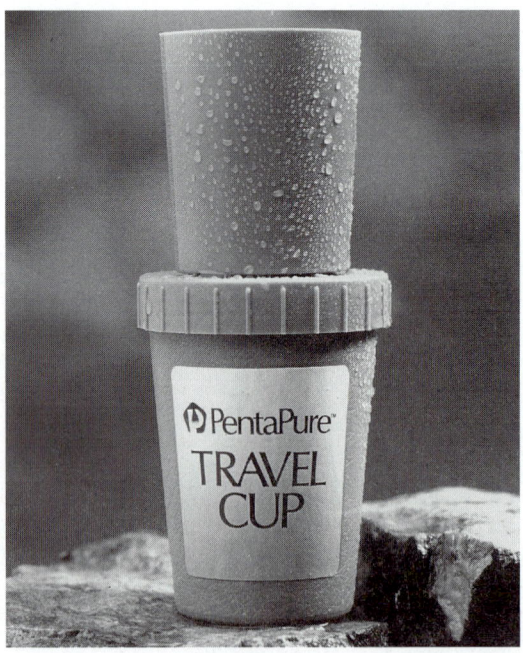

Fig. 43-16 Water Technologies Corporation PentaPure travel cup.

Claims	Comments
Resin releases iodine "on demand," on contact with microorganisms; minimal iodine dissolves in water: effluent 1-2 ppm iodine. Charcoal removes any residual dissolved iodine. Tested effective for bacteria, *Giardia,* schistosomiasis, and viruses, including hepatitis.	(See text for discussion of iodine resins.) The company has developed a large number of new products applicable to different size groups and various settings. The effectiveness of individual products depends on effectiveness of filter matrix assuring contact of every microorganism with iodine resin (no channeling of water). Carbon to remove residual dissolved iodine is an excellent addition that apparently does not decrease the effectiveness of the resin, but original resin testing was not done with residual iodine removed by charcoal. The removal of residual iodine makes the water unsuitable for storage, since microorganisms could subsequently contaminate the stored water. While all these products are already produced and sold in Europe, many are not yet available in the United States. Most are available through the company; contact the sales department. The most rational products are the hand pump models, the water jug and bucket, and the faucet filter. In general, these products tend to be heavy and bulky and are not as well engineered as others using iodine resin technology. The travel cup is much too slow and gives only small quantities. The straw has limited applications. The bulb (hand pump) is quite stiff and not as easy as a pump handle, and its cartridge and tubing are fairly bulky. The collapsible water jug is an excellent design, except for the valve, which seems fragile and does not work smoothly. The faucet filter is also an excellent design, but a little heavy for hotel travelers or short-term foreign residents. The bucket would work well for longer residence.

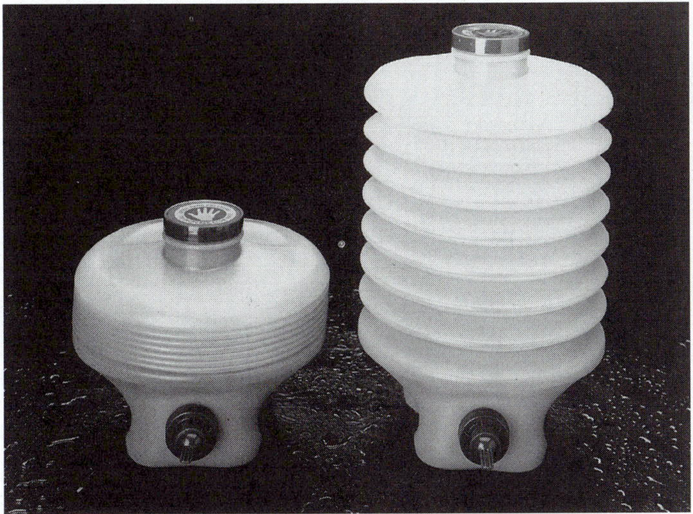

Fig. 43-17 Water Technologies Corporation PentaPure water jug.

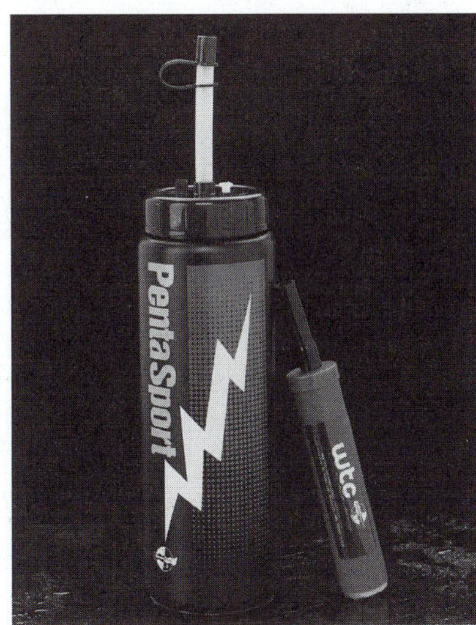

Fig. 43-18 Water Technologies Corporation Penta Sport and straw.

Continued.

Water Disinfection Products—cont'd

Product/Manufacturer	Price	Structure/Function
WATER TECHNOLOGIES IODINE RESIN FILTERS—cont'd		
(EPA registration submitted but not obtained for products below, so currently sold only outside United States. Contact company for these products.)		
MicroPure hand pump (Fig. 43-19)	$130	Hand- or foot-operated bulb pump; sediment filter, PentaPure and carbon cartridge; size: 7 × 2 inches cartridge, 50-inch tubing; weight: 1 lb 12 oz; flow: 1.5 qt/min; capacity: 500 gal
Replacement cartridge	$90	
Penta-Pour bucket (Fig. 43-20)	$200	Gravity drip bucket with 3-gal holding capacity; sediment filter, pentacide, and carbon cartridge; size: 12 × 30 inches; weight: 2.5 kg; flow: 10 gal/hr; capacity: 2000 gal
Replacement cartridge	$100	
Travel Tap Faucet Filter (Fig. 43-21)	$80	Sediment filter, Pentacide, and carbon cartridge; attaches to any faucet without tools; length: 6 inches; flow: 0.5 gal/min; capacity: 200 gal or 12 mo

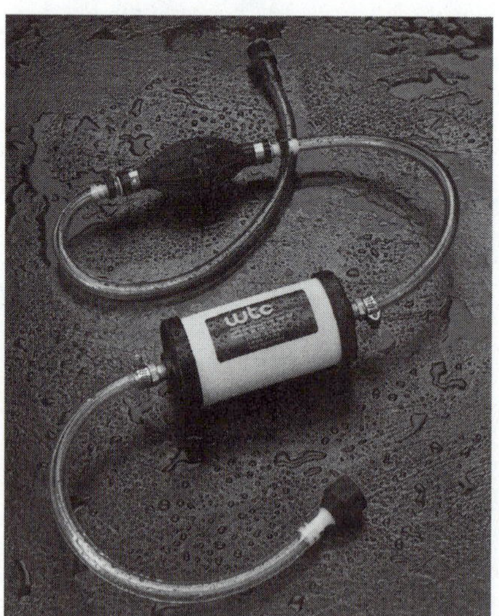

Fig. 43-19 Water Technologies Corporation MicroPure hand pump.

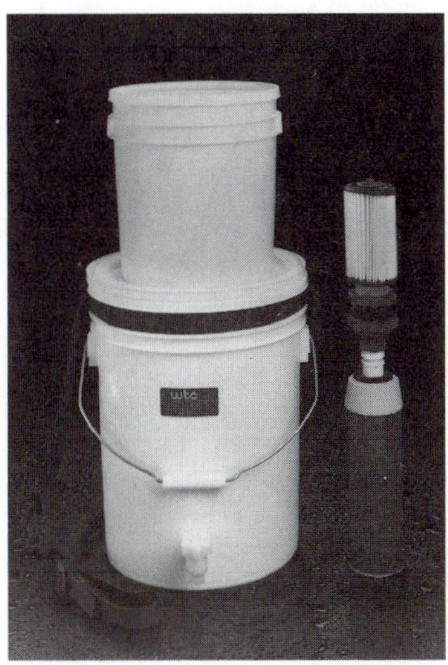

Fig. 43-20 Water Technologies Corporation Penta-Pour bucket.

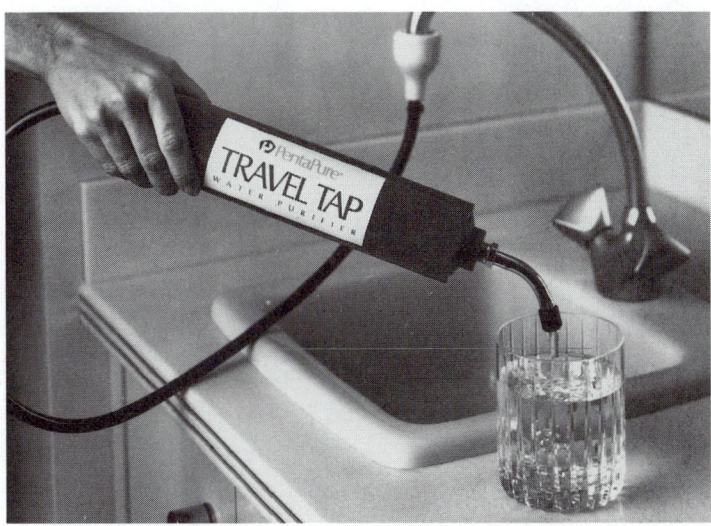

Fig. 43-21 Water Technologies Corporation PentaPure travel tap.

Water Disinfection Products—cont'd

Product/Manufacturer	Price	Structure/Function
RECOVERY ENGINEERING FILTERS		
Recovery Engineering, Inc. 2229 Edgewood Ave. South Minneapolis, MN 55426 800-845-7873		
PUR water filters		
PUR Explorer (Fig. 43-22)	$140	Hand pump with 130 μm prefilter, and replaceable cartridge with 1 μm pore size fiber/membrane filter and triiodine resin matrix; self-contained brushes clean filter with twist of handle; optional carbon cartridge attaches to effluent end to remove residual dissolved iodine and other chemicals; size: 10.75 × 2.25 inches; intake and output hoses: 3 ft; weight: 21 oz; flow 1 L/min; capacity: 500 gal/cartridge
Replacement parts		
Tritek cartridge	$45	
pump	$45	
intake filter/hose	$16	
PUR Scout (Fig. 43-23)	$64	Hand pump with 150 μm intake filter, 1 μm membrane filter and triiodine resin; optional carbon cartridge; size: 9 × 2.25 inches; weight: 12 oz; flow: 0.5 L/min; capacity: 200 gal
Replacement cartridge	$35	
Carbon cartridge	$20	
PUR Traveler (Fig. 43-24)	$70	Small filter/purifier designed for travelers to disinfect one glass of tap or well water at a time; no prefilter; pour water into 135 ml chamber, then press hand piston to pump into cup provided: 1 μm fiber/membrane filter and triiodine resin matrix; compact and lightweight; capacity: 100 gal/cartridge
Replacement cartridge	$30	
PUR Hiker	$45	Hand pump with 0.5 μm pleated glass fiber microfilter and activated carbon core (no iodine resin); intake filter for particulates; 7.5 × 2.5 × 3.5 inches; tubing 3 feet long; flow 1 L/min; capacity: 200 gal

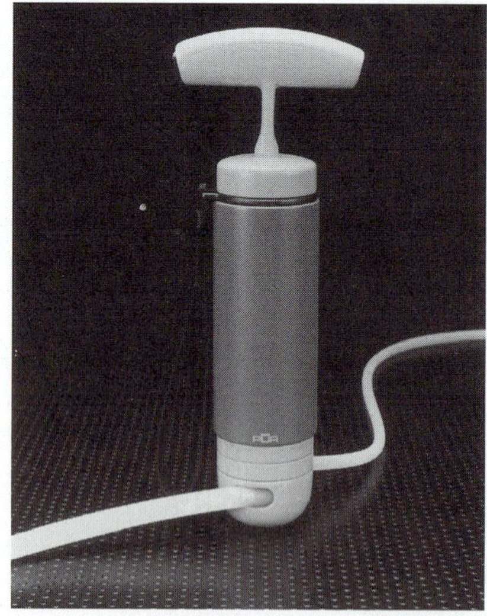

Fig. 43-22 Recovery Engineering, Inc., PUR Explorer.

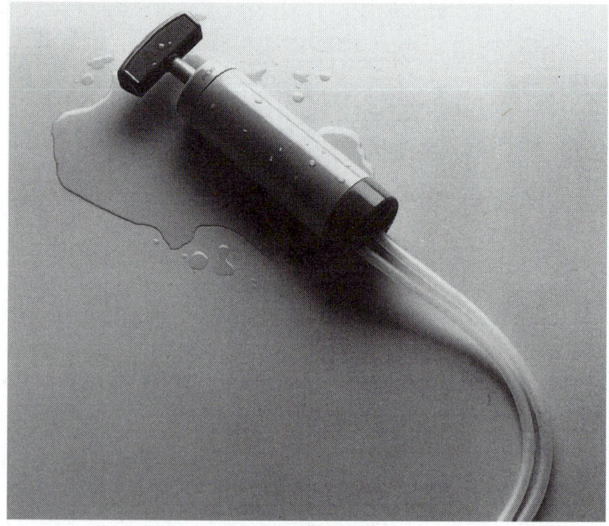

Fig. 43-23 Recovery Engineering, Inc., PUR Scout.

Claims	Comments
Microfilter removes cysts, and iodine resin kills bacteria and viruses on contact. Explorer has unique self-contained brush to clean filter without disassembling. Leaves no iodine taste. Two passages through the filter are recommended for "worst-case" water (below 5° C and highly polluted). Filter will clog before resin is exhausted. The Hiker is designed for higher quality surface water, not international travel. It will "eliminate *Giardia* and most bacteria"; activated carbon core "reduces chemicals and pesticides, plus improves taste of water." Filter surface area of 126 square inches is "quaranteed not to clog for 1 year."	(See text.) Iodine resins have been shown to be effective disinfectants leaving minimal residual iodine in the water. Although the resins are effective for *Giardia* cysts, the microfilter should effectively remove them, as well as *Cryptosporidium* and any other parasitic eggs or larva. Since bacteria and viruses are killed rapidly by iodine resins, no significant contact time is required. The Explorer is a well-designed, lightweight unit for individual or small group use in any wilderness environment. The pumping action is easy, and the internal brush is a great idea that seems to effectively clean the membrane and restores flow. The Scout is less expensive and slightly smaller without the internal brush. The antimicrobial water purifier has narrow applications. Instructions advise passing cold highly polluted water through filter twice, but an alternative would be to allow 30 to 40 minutes of contact time. This limitation indicates the need for further testing of these products. The Hiker was designed for the domestic backpacking market.

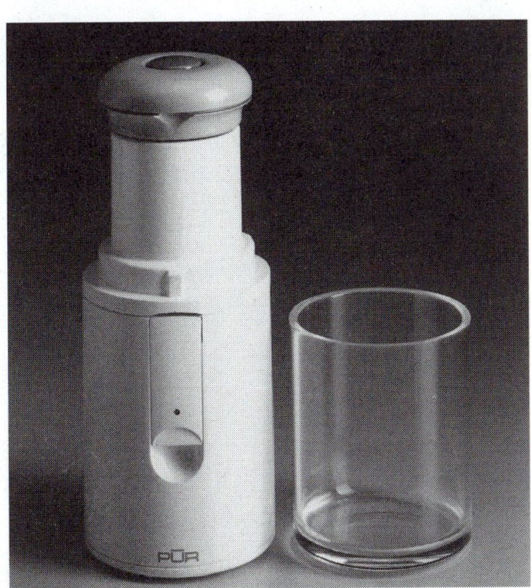

Fig. 43-24 Recovery Engineering, Inc., PUR Traveler.

Continued.

Water Disinfection Products—cont'd

Product/Manufacturer	Price	Structure/Function
Reverse osmosis filters		
PUR Survivor-06 (Fig. 43-25)	$550	Hand-operated pump, reverse osmosis membrane filter with prefilter on intake line; size: 2.5 × 5 × 8 inches; weight: 2.5 lb; flow: 1 L/hr
PUR Survivor-35 (Fig. 43-25)	$1425	Hand-operated pump, reverse osmosis membrane filter with prefilter on intake line; size: 3.5 × 5.5 × 22 inches; weight: 7 lb; flow: 1.2 gal/hr

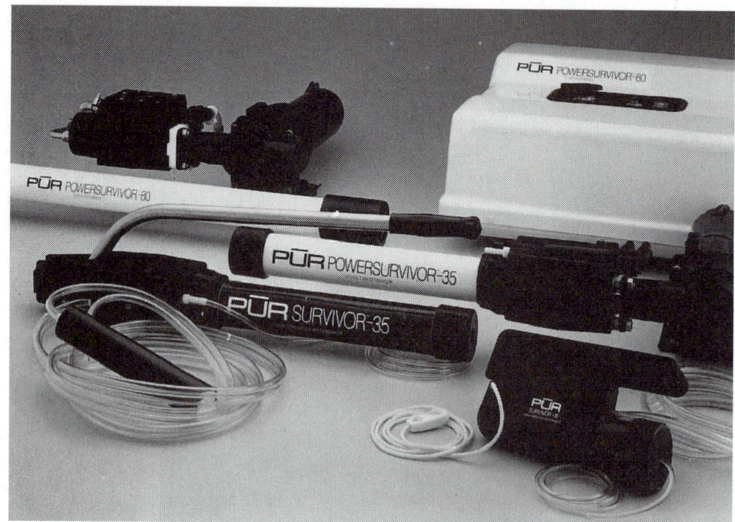

Fig. 43-25 Recovery Engineering, Inc., PUR Survivor-06 (manual), PUR Survivor-35 (manual), PUR Powersurvivor-35, and PUR Powersurvivor-80.

SWEET WATER FILTERS

SweetWater Filter
2525 Arapahoe, Suite E4-404
Boulder, CO 80302
303-444-5865

The Guardian microfiltration system (Fig. 43-26)	$50	Lexan body and pump handle; 100 μm metal prefilter; in-line 4 μm secondary filter; 0.5 μm labyrinth filter cylinder of borosilicate fibers; granular-activated carbon; safety pressure relief valve; outflow tubing has universal adaptor that fits all water bottles; optional biocide cartridge containing iodinated resin attaches to filter. Water passes through resin first, then filter cartridge, then GAC; optional input adaptor that attaches to sink faucet while traveling; size: 7.75 × 3.5 inches; weight: 8 oz; flow: 1 L/min; capacity: 200 gal
Replacement filter	$20	
Biocide cartridge	$15	
Tap-Adapt	$10	

Claims	Comments
Reverse osmosis units desalinate, removing 98% salt from seawater by forcing water through a semipermeable membrane at 800 PSI. In the process, bacteria are filtered out. The manual operation of these units makes them unique and useful for survival at sea or for use in small craft without power source. Larger, power-operated units also available. (Note that flow rates are per hour, not per minute.)	Reverse osmosis units are included here because sea kayaking and small boat journeys in open water are becoming more popular. These units can obviate the need for large water storage containers or add a margin of safety. I do not have good test data for these products, but desalinators should remove microorganisms, including viruses. The company does not make claims for viral removal because they assume that the membrane is imperfect and some pores will be imprecise, perhaps allowing viral passage. Reverse osmosis filters could be used for land-based travel, but are very expensive with low flow.
Eliminates *Giardia, Cryptosporidium,* and other critical pathogens, pollutants, heavy metals, pesticides, and flavors. Kills viruses when used with the Biocide cartridge accessory. Lighter, more compact and durable than comparable models, and easiest to clean or replace. Filter cartridges will be recycled by the company.	Well-designed filter at reasonable price. The three major water treatment components—filtration, GAC, and iodine resin — offer broad protection and maximum flexibility. Some unique design features, such as universal bottle adaptor. Filter component tested, but needs further bacterial challenges. I have not seen testing of the Biocide cartridge; however, iodine resins have been well tested. If filter lives up to its performance specifications, it will be an excellent product.

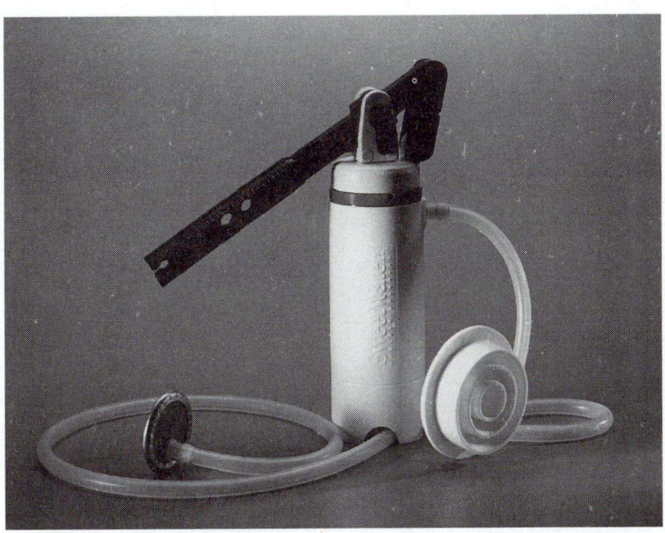

Fig. 43-26 SweetWater Filter, The Guardian microfiltration system.

Continued.

Water Disinfection Products—cont'd

Product/Manufacturer	Price	Structure/Function
ACCUVENTURE FILTERS		
Accuventure, Inc. 9915 S.W. Arctic Dr. Beaverton, OR 97005 800-422-1820		Drink-through products in three forms: straw, military canteen, and sport bottle insert; three-stage products use mechanical filtration through coconut shell, carbon matrix, and membrane filter with final pore size of 4 μm; five-stage product line contains three filtration stages with iodine resin and activated charcoal; the Fountain connects to a water faucet, producing a stream of water. Straw: size: 8.5 × 75 inches; weight: 0.5 oz; capacity: 40 gal. Bottle: size: 10 × 2.75 inches; weight: (filter only) 2 oz; capacity 80 gal. Canteen: US military specifications; capacity 20 gal.
AccuFilter straw		
AccuFilter mini straw	$10	
AccuFilter 5 straw	$20	
AccuFilter canteen insert	$8	
AccuFilter sport bottle (Fig. 43-27)	$18	
The Fountain 3-stage	$30	
5-stage	$50	

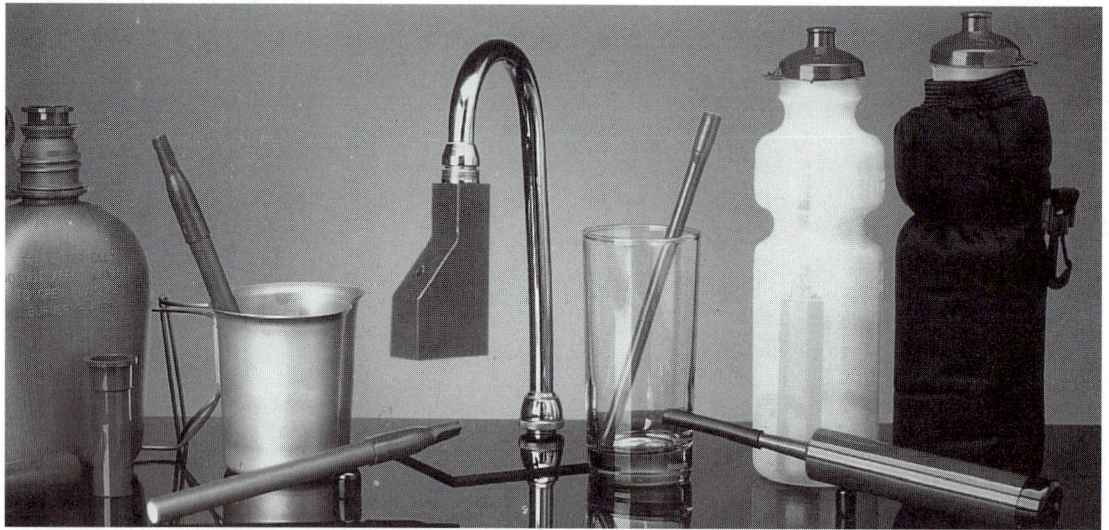

Fig. 43-27 Accuventure, Inc., AccuFilter canteen and insert, AccuFilter sport bottle, AccuFilter straw, and AccuFilter fountain.

Claims	Comments
Three-stage filters remove particulate matter, and activated carbon "removes the taste of chlorine, heavy metals, herbicides, pesticides, organic poisons, and other particulate matter causing bad taste, odor, and color." For use in domestic wilderness or hotel travel. Five-stage filters include PentaPure iodine resin that "kills bacteria viruses and parasites by contact." Three-stage products are designed for use with water having little or no bacterial, viral, or parasitic contamination, whereas the five-stage products are designed for use with water having suspected or known bacterial, viral, or parasitic contamination. Drink-through products require suction pressure of 1.5 inches of mercury. They are designed so that water circulates internally and contacts resin for 3 minutes during use to ensure disinfection when water is ingested.	Rational combination of treatment steps in interesting designs. The convenience of drink-through products is theoretically an advantage but could become a liability if easy flow is not maintained, requiring high oral suction pressures. None of these products (except the Fountain) allows disinfection for a group unless the bottle is shared. Straws have even more limited applications. A filter pore of 4 μm removes *Giardia* but is borderline for *Cryptosporidium*. The removal of protozoal cysts obviates the need for contact time, since bacteria and viruses can be killed quickly after contact with iodine resin. The 3-minute circulation claim is interesting but difficult to imagine. The three-stage filters could be used for North American alpine water where *Giardia* is the main concern or to improve taste of some municipal waters. These products also could be very useful for day hikers and bikers who carry only one bottle or canteen and can refill with surface water.

APPENDIX B

Halogen Products

(See text for discussion of these products.)

Polar Equipment
12881 Foothill Lane
Saratoga, CA 95070

Polar Pure ($9) (Fig. 43-28):
Iodine crystals, 8 g in 3-oz bottle; 30-50 µm fabric prefilter provided; "trap" in bottle to catch crystals when pouring off water; bottle cap used to measure; directions and color dot thermometer on bottle (temperature affects iodine concentration in bottle); capacity: 2000 qt; weight: 5 oz; yields 4 ppm iodine when appropriate dose is added to 1 qt clean water

Polar Pure Plus (new product in development):
2-oz plastic dropper bottle of concentrated iodine-alcohol solution; thermometer and graph for determining dosage and contact time

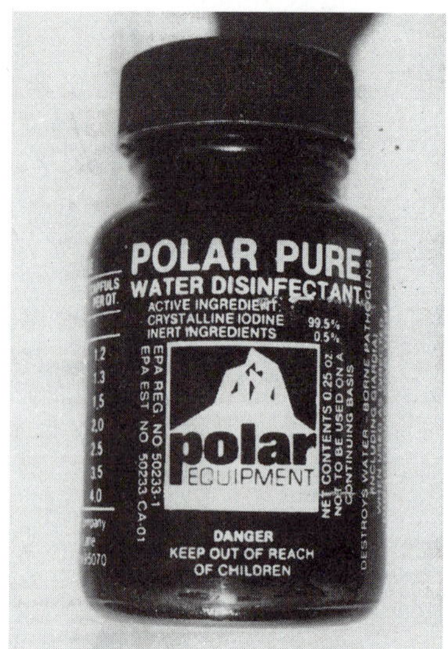

Fig. 43-28 Polar Equipment Polar Pure water disinfectant.

Emergency germicidal drinking water tablets (50 tablets, $5):
Sold widely with camping supplies under several different brand names (e.g., Potable Aqua)

Micropur tablets (not licensed or sold in United States; marketed by Katadyn in Europe, England, Australia):
Silver tablets in individual bubble packing; add 1 tablet to 1 quart of water; mix thoroughly and allow 2 hr contact time; product claims: "For the disinfection and storage of clear water. Reliably kill bacterial agents of enteric diseases but *not* worm eggs, ameba, viruses. Neutral to taste, simple to use and innocuous. Treatment of water will ensure protection against reinfection for 1-6 months"; package insert does not state residual concentration

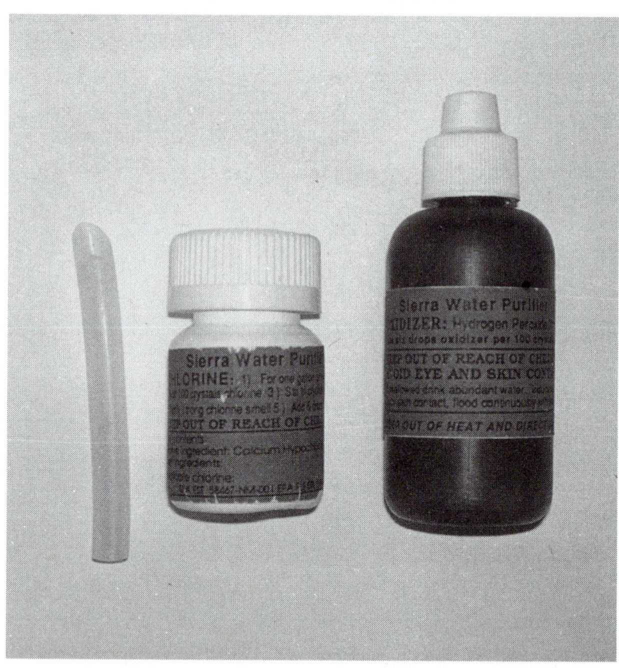

Fig. 43-29 The Sanitizer (formerly Sierra Water Purifier)—calcium chloride crystals with scoop and hydrogen peroxide squeeze bottle.

The Sanitizer
(formerly Sierra Water Purifier)
1430 Willamette, Suite 237
Eugene, OR 97401

Mail order from:
Wilderness Exchange
513 West Cordova Rd.
Santa Fe, NM 87502
Attn: Randy

Sanitizer (Fig. 43-29):

Starter kit (hikers)	$13 (treats 160 gal)
Marine and RV kit	$15 (treats 720 gal)

Refills available at reduced price
Unrestrained chlorination and dechlorination; chlorine crystals (calcium hypochlorite) and 30% hydrogen peroxide in separate small plastic bottles with dropper and scoop; total weight: 5 oz.

Safesport Manufacturing Co.
Box 11811
Denver, CO 80211
800-433-6506

AquaCure ($7.95):
Tablets contain alum as flocculating agent and 1.4% available chlorine in form of sodium dichloro-s-triazinetrione; cloth provided for simple straining of flocculation sediment; 30 tablets individually sealed in foil packets; wgt 1.6 oz; capacity: 30 L (8 gal)

44 TRAVEL MEDICINE

Elaine C. Jong

When individuals and groups travel to foreign destinations to participate in wilderness and outdoors activities, exposure to unfamiliar people, food, sanitation, and environments may have a deleterious effect on health and interfere with the purpose and enjoyment of the trip. Travel medicine is a multidisciplinary specialty that encompasses subjects from the fields of public health, infectious diseases, tropical medicine, and environmental and wilderness medicine. From this broad body of knowledge, prevention and treatment recommendations have been developed to address the unique health needs of international travelers. This chapter serves as a basic introduction to travel medicine, focusing on public health and communicable diseases. Closely related topics are covered extensively in other chapters in this book.

Sources of Information

A publication of the Centers for Disease Control and Prevention (CDC), *Health Information for International Travel* (the "yellow book"), is an authoritative source of information on travel medicine and is updated annually. Two other periodicals published by the CDC, *Morbidity and Mortality Weekly Report* and *Summary of Health Information for International Travel* (the "blue sheet," published biweekly), provide current information on the status of worldwide disease outbreaks and changes in health conditions. Subscribers to the *Summary* also receive copies of the *CDC Advisory Memorandum* (the "tan sheet"), issued on an as-needed basis, which inform about specific outbreaks of disease that relate to CDC policies.

Travel health information, including vaccine requirements, malaria chemoprophylaxis, and disease outbreaks for various regions of the world, can be obtained by telephone through the CDC audiolibrary and facsimile transmission services. Professional societies, foundations, and private publishers are additional sources of telephone advice and printed materials, including current lists of travel medicine clinics in the United States and abroad, English-speaking physicians worldwide, and newsletters with updated information on travel medicine topics and lists of relevant meetings and continuing education courses. A list of resources for travel medicine information is given in Appendix A at the end of the chapter.

Standard textbooks on infectious diseases and tropical medicine, as well as a number of monographs on travel medicine, provide in-depth information on travel medicine–related subjects; these are given in the suggested readings at the end of the chapter. A number of computer data bases and interactive programs for travel medicine are commercially available. They are not listed here because the software and vendors are rapidly changing; the best sources of current information on travel medicine software are reviews published in some of the newsletters listed in Appendix A and "hands-on" demonstrations at medical and scientific meetings.

Travelers abroad who experience an emergency of any sort should contact the nearest U.S. consulate or embassy or call the U.S. Department of State Citizen's Emergency Center (see Appendix A). If an extended stay in a given country is planned, the Citizen's Emergency Center suggests that the traveler register with the consulate or embassy shortly after arrival in the country.

Travelers should ascertain several months in advance of departure whether their regular health insurance policy covers the costs of treatment and hospitalization for illness or injuries occurring abroad, and the costs of emergency medical evacuation back to the United States, if necessary. Medicare usually covers only health care expenses arising in the United States and its territories. Some credit card services provide worldwide medical referrals and arrangements for emergency transportation for their cardholders but do not actually cover the costs incurred. What the traveler needs is a short-term health insurance policy that specifically covers medical expenses and medical evacuation during foreign travel. Depending on the insurer, chronic medical conditions may be excluded or covered only if they are certified to be under control for 60 to 90 days before departure. Travelers older than 70 years of age may find it more difficult to get medical insurance of this kind. Some companies offering short-term health insurance for travelers are listed in Appendix A.

Travel Health Risk Assessment

Pretravel medical preparation appropriate for a given traveler and trip is determined by a review of the geographic destinations, the duration of the trip, the style of travel, the purpose of the trip, the underlying health of the traveler, and access to medical care during the trip (Box 44-1). In this context, immunizations, malaria chemoprophylaxis, traveler's diarrhea, and parasitic infections must be addressed. Prevention and treatment of common ailments such as jet lag, motion sickness, sun exposure, altitude illness, insect bites, and animal bites should be reviewed. Some attention should be given to personal safety, sexually transmitted diseases, prevention of motor vehicle injury, and emergency medical evacuation. Information about the level of sanitation and environmental hazards at the destinations can be used to identify special health concerns in tropical climates and areas of extreme weather conditions, high altitude, or aquatic activities.[38,39]

An itinerary with multiple destinations in several countries and travel lasting more than 3 weeks both tend to increase the complexity of the medical preparation with regard to vaccination and malaria recommendations. In addition, the content of the travel medical kit becomes more inclusive as a greater number of health needs over time are anticipated.

BOX 44-1

APPROACH TO MEDICAL PREPARATION FOR TRAVEL

TRAVEL INFORMATION

Geographic itinerary (countries in order of travel)
Month(s) and duration of travel in each country
Urban versus rural travel
Style of travel (hotel or resort versus hut or camping)
Purpose of travel
Access to medical care during travel

PERSONAL HEALTH

General health status
Allergies to drugs and vaccines
Age and weight
Pregnant or lactating
Impaired immune response resulting from disease, medications, or treatment
Medications taken on a regular basis
History of previous immunizations
Medical or physical conditions requiring special care

Modified from Jong EC: *Med Clin North Am* 76:1277, 1992.

The style of travel is an important factor in travel risk assessments. Travelers staying in urban air-conditioned hotels or well-developed resorts have less exposure to mosquitoes carrying malaria and other diseases than those living among residents in small villages or camping. If accommodations in malarious areas are likely to be in unscreened rooms, travelers should plan to take with them portable mosquito bed nets and insect repellents.

The purpose of the trip is another factor that influences exposure of the traveler to potential health hazards. Teachers, students, missionaries, relief workers, agricultural consultants, field biologists, and adventure travelers are more likely than sight-seeing tourists and business travelers to be exposed to endemic infectious diseases transmitted by the local residents (such as hepatitis B, tuberculosis, and meningitis), insects (such as malaria, yellow fever, leishmaniasis, and filariasis), and animals (such as rabies and plague).

All travelers, however, should be cautioned about the infectious hazards of sexual activity with strangers, especially prostitutes. Gonorrhea and chlamydia are common in the industrialized world and also have a worldwide distribution. Other sexually transmitted diseases, such as human immunodeficiency virus (HIV) infection, syphilis, chancroid, and lymphogranuloma venereum, are more prevalent in the developing world.[36,45]

Although surveys and case reports of returned travelers confirm that attention to vaccine-preventable diseases (for example, diphtheria, measles, polio, hepatitis, typhoid fever, and cholera) and exotic infectious diseases (such as malaria, schistosomiasis, leishmaniasis, and trichinosis) is appropriate, the importance of the traveler's underlying health and accidental injuries must also be emphasized.* Cardiovascular diseases, motor vehicle accidents, and injuries accounted for more morbidity and mortality among American travelers and expatriates than did infectious diseases.[28,29]

Most international travelers should begin pretravel medical preparation 4 to 6 weeks before the date of departure, so that immunization schedules can be adequately spaced and appropriate medications and special supplies obtained (Table 44-1). While the medical preparation for an international trip may be straightforward for people in good health, advance planning and consultation with a travel medicine expert are recommended for people with allergies, special health needs (pregnancy, infancy, handicaps), or underlying health conditions (such as cardiovascular disease, respiratory conditions, immunocompromising conditions, diabetes, renal failure, organ transplants, and seizure disorders).

Immunizations for Travel

Immunizations may be divided into three categories: routine, required, and recommended.[38] Primary vaccine schedules and booster intervals are given in Tables 44-2 and 44-3.

*References 4, 7, 8, 12, 13, 25, 31, 33, 48, 58, 63, 71.

Table 44-1 Vaccine Interactions

Vaccine	Interaction	Precaution
Immune globulin	Measles/mumps/rubella (MMR) vaccine	Give these vaccines at least 2 wk before immune globulin (IG) or 3-5 mo after IG, depending on dose received
Oral typhoid vaccine	Antibiotic therapy	Administer oral typhoid vaccine (OTV) at least 1 wk after antibiotic therapy is completed; do not take antibiotics for at least 3 wk after OTV is completed
Oral typhoid vaccine	Mefloquine malaria chemoprophylaxis	Schedule an interval of at least 8 hr between oral typhoid dose and mefloquine dose
Oral typhoid vaccine	Oral polio vaccine	Oral polio vaccine (OPV) should not be taken at same time as OTV; OPV can be given 7-10 days before or 10-14 days after OTV
Rabies vaccine (HDCV) intradermal series	Chloroquine malaria chemoprophylaxis	Complete rabies vaccine (intradermal series) at least 3 wk before starting chloroquine; use rabies vaccine intramuscular series if 3-wk interval is not possible
Virus vaccines, live (MMR, OPV, yellow fever vaccine)	Other live virus vaccines	Give live virus vaccines on same day, or separate doses by at least 1 mo
Virus vaccines, live (MMR, OPV, yellow fever vaccine)	Tuberculin skin test (PPD)	Do skin test on same day as receipt of a live virus vaccine, or 4-6 wk after, because virus vaccines can impair the response to PPD skin test
Yellow fever	Cholera vaccine	Give the two vaccines on same day or at least 3 wk apart

From Jong EC: Immunizations for international travelers. In *The Travel Medicine Advisor,* Atlanta, 1993, American Health Consultants.

The international traveler should have all current immunizations recorded in *The International Certificates of Vaccination* as approved by the World Health Organization (WHO), a document in booklet form printed on yellow paper.[37] The booklet has a special page for official validation of the yellow fever vaccine. Recent copies of the document (after 1988) do not contain a separate page for cholera vaccine validation because the WHO officially removed cholera vaccination from the International Health Regulations in 1973. If given, the cholera vaccination can be recorded in the space provided for "Other Vaccinations" in the newer booklets.

In general, live virus vaccines and attenuated bacterial vaccines are contraindicated during pregnancy and in persons with altered immunocompetence.[15]

REQUIRED TRAVEL IMMUNIZATIONS

The required immunizations refer to those regulated by the WHO. Yellow fever vaccine may be required for entry into member countries according to current WHO regulations. Smallpox vaccine and cholera vaccine are no longer required for international travel according to WHO regulations.

Yellow Fever Vaccine

Yellow fever is a viral infection transmitted by *Aedes aegypti* mosquitoes in equatorial South America and Africa. The endemic zones are shown in Fig. 44-1.

The yellow fever (YF) vaccine is a live attenuated viral vaccine that is highly immunoprotective. The YF vaccine is given as a single dose for primary immunization; the booster interval is 10 years. The vaccine is contraindicated in infants less than 4 months of age because of the age-related risk of encephalitis after immunization. If possible, YF immunization should be delayed until the infant is 9 months of age or older. The vaccine is generally not recommended during pregnancy except when travel to a highly endemic area cannot be avoided or postponed by the pregnant traveler, and the risk of the actual disease is thought to be greater than the theoretical risk of adverse effects from the vaccine.

Additional contraindications to receiving the vaccine include immunosuppression caused by underlying disease (for example, malignancy, HIV infection, congenital immune deficiency) or by medical therapy (for example, corticosteroids, cancer chemotherapy, radiation therapy, organ transplant therapy). The vaccine virus is cultured in eggs and is not recommended for persons with a history of severe allergy to eggs. The package insert contains instructions for skin-testing persons with an uncertain history of allergy to eggs.

If a person for whom the vaccine is contraindicated must travel to a country where yellow fever vaccine is required for entry, a signed statement on letterhead stationery that the yellow fever vaccine could not be given to the traveler because of medical contraindications will be accepted in lieu of the vaccination statement, according to WHO regulations.

Cholera Vaccine

The injectable cholera vaccine in current use is not highly efficacious, even when the primary series of two

Table 44-2 Dosage Schedules for Routine Immunizations (1993)

Vaccine	Primary Series	Booster Interval
Diphtheria and tetanus toxoids and pertussis vaccine adsorbed (DTP) (use in children <7 yr old)	4 doses* IM of vaccine: first 3 doses given 4-8 wk apart; dose 4 given 6-12 mo after dose 3	Booster at 4-6 yr of age
Haemophilus B conjugate		
(Hib conjugate vaccines are not considered interchangeable for the primary immunization series)		
PRP-HbOC	3 doses* IM or SC at 2, 4, 6 mo	Booster at 15 mo
PRP-OMP	2 doses* IM or SC at 2, 4 mo	Booster at 15 mo
PRP-D, PRP-HbOC, or PRP-OMP	1 dose* IM or SC at ≥15 mo up to 5th birthday	None
Hepatitis B (Engerix B) (accelerated schedule)	3 doses at 0, 30, and 60 days (1 ml IM in deltoid area)	4th dose is recommended at 12 mo if still at risk for hepatitis B exposure
Hepatitis B (Engerix B) (standard schedule)	3 doses at 0, 1, and 6 mo (1 ml IM in deltoid area)	Need for booster not determined
Hepatitis B (Recombivax) (standard schedule)	3 doses at 0, 1, and 6 mo (1 ml IM in deltoid area)	Need for booster not determined
Influenza virus	1 dose* IM or SC annually	
Measles/mumps/rubella (MMR)†	1 dose* SC at 15 mo of age or older	Boost measles vaccine at 12 yr old; boost measles vaccine *once* in adult life before international travel for people born after 1957 and before 1980
Pneumococcus (23-valent)	1 dose* SC	None (see text)
Poliomyelitis, enhanced inactivated (E-IPV) (killed vaccine, safe for all ages)	Give doses* 1 and 2 SC or IM 4-8 wk apart; give dose 3 6-12 mo after dose 2; give dose 4 to children 4-6 yr of age	Give dose *once* to people before travel in areas at risk
Poliomyelitis, oral (OPV) (attenuated live virus)†	Give doses* 1 and 2 po 6-8 wk apart; give dose 3 at 6 wk after dose 2 (customarily at 8-12 mo after dose 2); give dose 4 to children 4-6 yr of age	Give dose *once* to people less than 18 yr before travel in areas of risk
Tetanus and diphtheria toxoids adsorbed (Td) (for children >7 yr of age and for adults)	3 doses (0.5 ml SC or IM), doses 1 and 2 given 4-8 wk apart, dose 3 6-12 mo later	Routine booster dose every 10 yr

From Jong EC: Immunizations for international travelers. In *The Travel Medicine Advisor,* Atlanta, 1993, American Health Consultants.
*See manufacturer's package insert for recommendations on dosage.
†May be contraindicated in patients with any of the following conditions: pregnancy, leukemia, lymphoma, generalized malignancy, immunosuppression from HIV infection or treatment with corticosteroids, alkylating drugs, antimetabolites, or radiation therapy.

doses given a week or more apart is received. The WHO no longer endorses a requirement for this vaccine for entry into any country. Nonetheless, some countries still require a cholera vaccine for travelers arriving from cholera-endemic areas.[26] If this situation is anticipated, a single cholera dose should meet this requirement and should be recorded in the traveler's *International Certificates of Vaccination* (see earlier discussion).

Travelers going to cholera-endemic or cholera-epidemic areas are encouraged to follow food and water precautions as recommended to prevent all forms of travel-associated diarrhea. Some practitioners recommend that people with underlying gastric conditions, such as achlorhydria or partial gastric resection, which may increase susceptibility to cholera infection, be immunized with the full two-dose series of cholera vaccine.

Smallpox Vaccine

Although the last case of smallpox acquired through natural transmission was reported in 1977 and the requirement for smallpox vaccine for international travel was removed from the WHO regulations in 1982, health care providers still receive sporadic inquiries about smallpox vaccine. The vaccine is no longer available commercially. Limited supplies are released on a case-by-case basis from the CDC based on individual review. Research scientists and health care workers who work with the smallpox (vaccinia) and closely related viruses are candidates for immunization.[14]

RECOMMENDED TRAVEL VACCINES

The recommended vaccines are those given to travelers depending on the travel risk assessment. Vaccines in this

Table 44-3 Dosage Schedules for Travel Immunizations (1993)

Vaccine	Primary Series	Booster Interval
Cholera	2 doses 1 wk or more apart (0.5 ml SC or IM); pediatric dose 0.3 ml for 5-10 yr of age, 0.2 ml for 6 mo-4 yr of age	6 mo
Immune globulin (hepatitis A protection)	1 dose IM in gluteus muscle (2 ml dose for 3 mo protection; 5 ml divided dose for 5 mo); pediatric dose 0.02 ml/kg for 3-mo trip, 0.06 ml/kg for 5-mo trip	Boost at 3- to 5-mo intervals depending on initial dose received
Japanese encephalitis	3 doses given on days 0, 7, and 30 (1 ml SC ≥3 yr old; 0.5 ml SC <3 yr old)	Booster dose may be given after 2 yr
Meningococcus (A/C/Y/W-135)	1 dose* SC	None (variable immunogenic response in children <4 yr of age: revaccination for this group recommended after 2-3 yr for those who continue to be at high risk)
Plague	1st dose (1 ml IM); 2nd dose (0.2 ml IM) 4 wk later; dose 3 (0.2 ml IM) 3-6 mo after dose 2	Boost if risk of exposure persists: give first 2 booster doses (0.1-0.2 ml) 6 mo apart, then give 1 booster dose at 1- to 2-yr intervals as needed
Rabies, human diploid cell vaccine (HDCV)	3 doses (0.1 ml ID) on days 0, 7, and 21 or 28	Boost after 2 yr or test serum for antibody level (must not use chloroquine prophylaxis until 3 wk after completion of ID vaccine series)
Rabies (HDCV) or rabies vaccine absorbed (RVA)	3 doses (1 ml IM in the deltoid area) on days 0, 7, and 28	Boost after 2 yrs or test serum for antibody level
Tick-borne encephalitis	3 doses given SC on days 0, 30, and 180 days	Boost at 3- to 5-year intervals
Tuberculosis (BCG vaccine)†	1 dose percutaneously with multiple-puncture disk; ½ strength for infants <1 mo old	Revaccination after 2-3 mo in those who remain tuberculin neg to 5 TU skin test
Typhoid, injectable	2 doses (0.5 ml SC or IC) 4 or more wk apart; pediatric dose (<10 yr old) 0.25 ml	Boost after 3 yr for continued risk of exposure
Typhoid, injectable (not acetone-killed and dried vaccine)		Boost with 0.1 ml ID every 3 yr
Typhoid, oral	1 capsule po every 2 days for 4 doses (>6 yr old)	5 yr
Yellow fever†	1 dose (0.5 ml SC); pediatric dose 0.5 ml SC for >6 mo old	10 yr

From Jong EC: Immunizations for international travelers. In *The Travel Medicine Advisor,* Atlanta, 1993, American Health Consultants.
*See manufacturer's package insert for recommendations on dosage.
†Caution, may be contraindicated in patients with any of the following conditions: pregnancy, leukemia, lymphoma, generalized malignancy, immunosuppression from HIV infection or treatment with corticosteroids, alkylating drugs, antimetabolites, or radiation therapy.

category include typhoid fever, immune globulin (for hepatitis A), meningococcal meningitis, Japanese encephalitis B virus, rabies, plague, and tick-borne encephalitis. Immunization against hepatitis B and tuberculosis (bacillus Calmette-Guerin [BCG] vaccine) or a tuberculosis skin test (purified protein derivative [PPD]) may also be recommended for some travelers.

Typhoid Fever Vaccine

The incidence of typhoid fever among American travelers is relatively low (58 to 174 cases per 1 million travelers), but among reported cases in the United States, 62% were acquired during international travel.[58] Mexico, Peru, India, Pakistan, and Chile are countries where the risk of transmission appears particularly high. Sub-Saharan Africa and Southeast Asia are also regarded as areas of increased risk for typhoid fever.

Avoidance of potentially contaminated food and drink during travel is important, even if the typhoid vaccine is received. The protection against typhoid fever afforded by immunization with the currently available parenteral vaccine ranges from 51% to 76%. Although protection rates of 43% to 96% were reported in field trials with the oral live-attenuated typhoid vaccine among residents of endemic areas, limited data are available for protection rates in people from nonendemic areas who travel to endemic areas.[8]

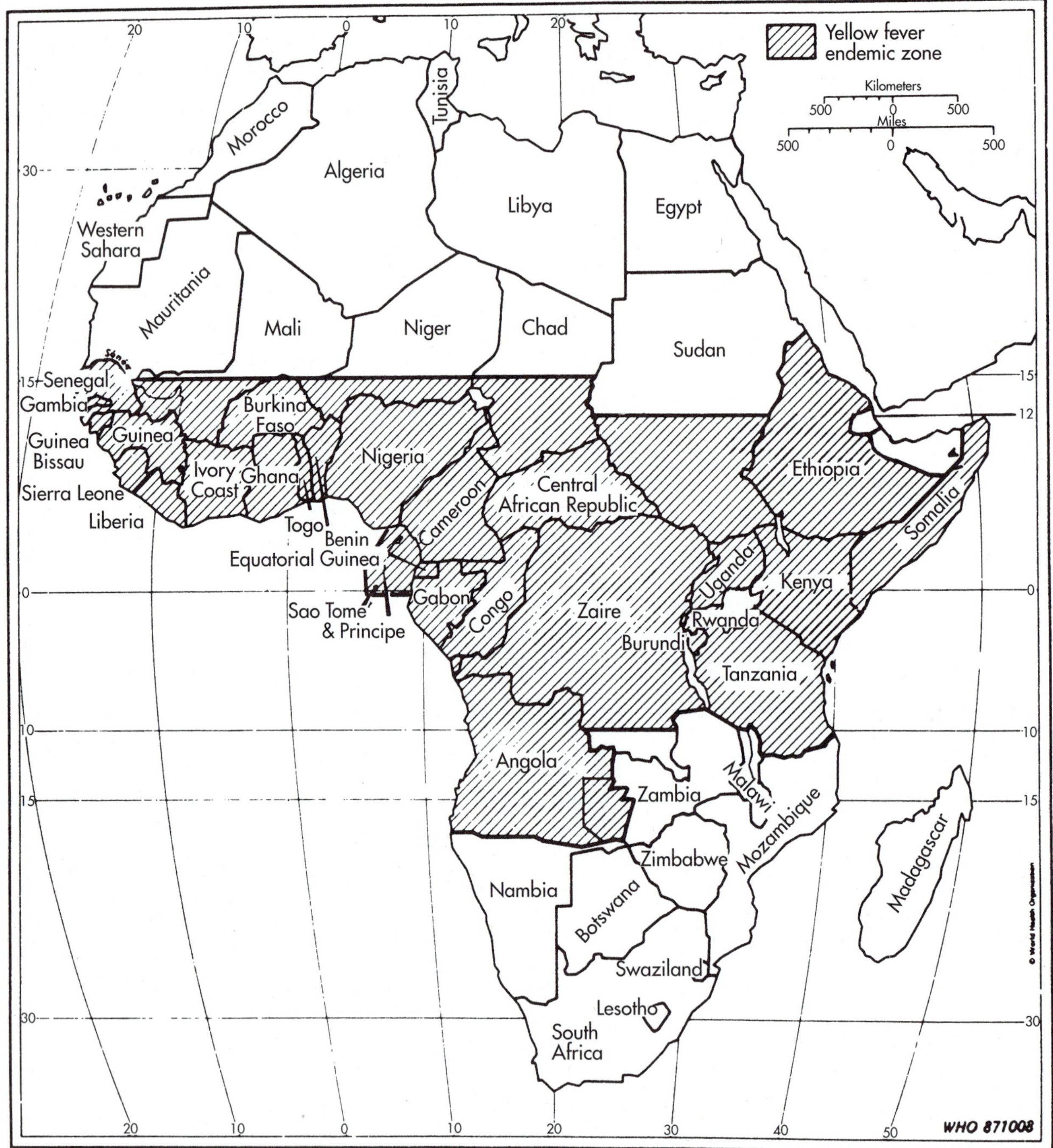

Fig. 44-1 Yellow fever endemic zones. (From Centers for Disease Control: *Health information for international travel, 1992*, Washington, DC, 1992, US Government Printing Office.)

The injectable heat-phenol-inactivated whole-cell typhoid vaccine requires two doses given 4 weeks apart for primary immunization, and a booster dose after 3 or more years. The injectable vaccine has been associated with troublesome side effects; most recipients complain of soreness at the injection site, headache, low-grade fever, and general malaise for 1 or 2 days after immunization.

The oral typhoid vaccine contains a live attenuated strain of *Salmonella typhi* bacteria (Ty21A). The vaccine is in capsule form and is recommended for people 6 years of age and older. A primary (or booster) series consists of four capsules, one taken every other day over the course of a week. The booster interval is 5 years. A liquid suspension form of this vaccine is expected in the near future;

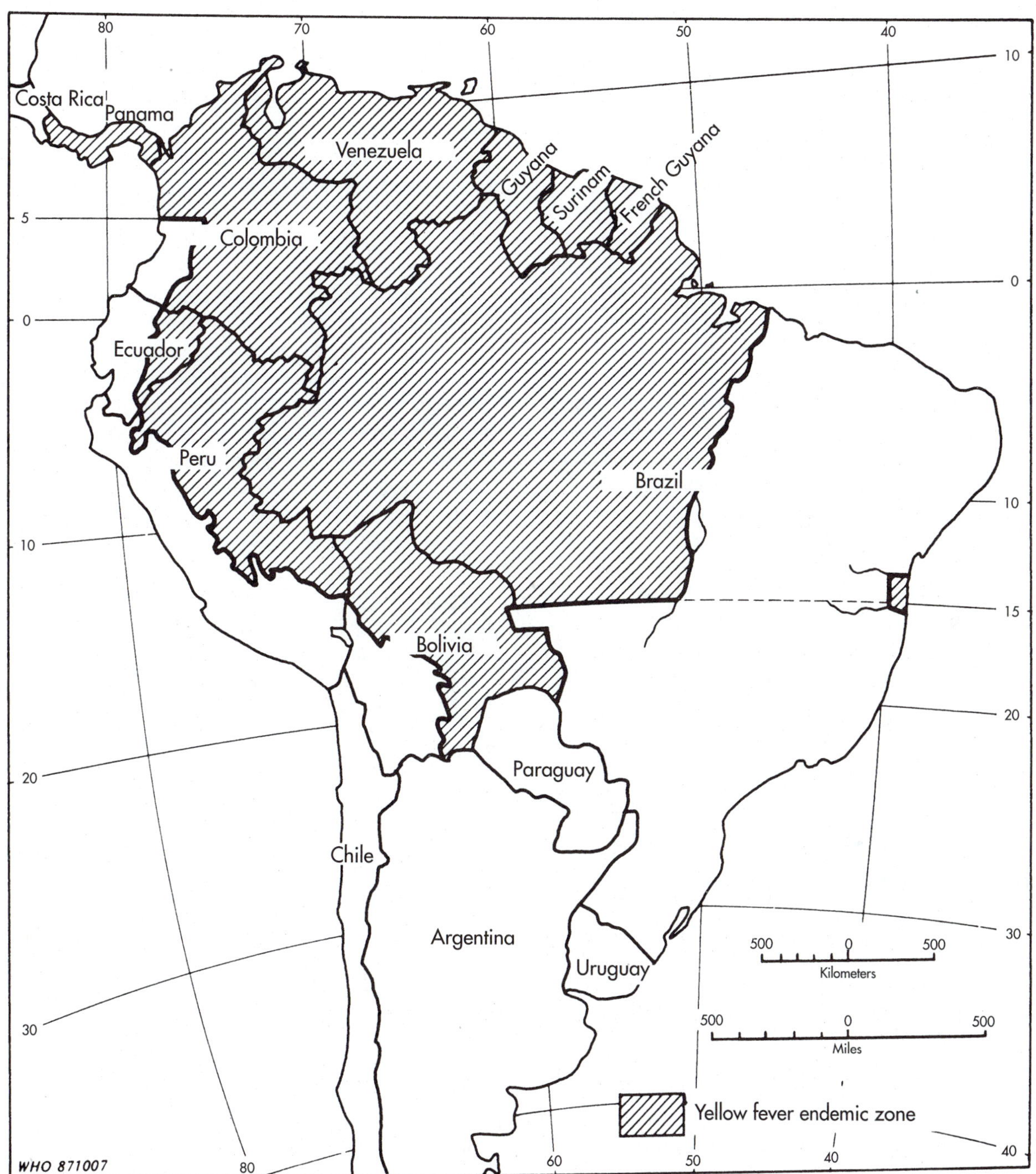

Fig. 44-1, cont'd. For legend see opposite page.

this will facilitate administration of the vaccine to young children and to others who have difficulty swallowing capsules.

Persons who have previously received the injectable typhoid vaccine series and who now desire immunization with the oral vaccine should receive the full four-capsule series because limited data on alternative regimens are available.

Hepatitis A Vaccine

Hepatitis A is a serious viral infection with a transmission similar to polio, cholera, typhoid, and traveler's diarrhea: that is, fecal contamination of food and water. Although up to 60% of adults over 40 years of age from industrialized countries may have immunity to hepatitis A through clinical or subclinical infection, most travelers less than 40 years old are susceptible.[49] Protection against hepatitis A can be obtained from an intramuscular dose of immune globulin (gamma globulin). If time allows, a serum test for hepatitis A antibody should be performed in people who travel frequently, who are of foreign birth, or who are over age 40; unnecessary immunization may be avoided if a person has protective antibodies from an inapparent hepatitis A infection in the past.

At least two new hepatitis A inactivated viral vaccines are awaiting licensure and release in the United States at the time of this writing. The new vaccines are most likely to benefit people who are susceptible to hepatitis A and travel frequently or are going abroad for longer than 5 months.

Meningococcal Vaccine

Vaccine protection against meningococcal meningitis is recommended for people going trekking in Nepal or traveling to Tanzania or Burundi, where outbreaks have been reported. The meningococcal vaccine is required for travel to Saudi Arabia during the time of the annual religious pilgrimage (the Hadj) to Mecca in late spring. The vaccine is also recommended for people going to live and work in certain areas of Africa (sub-Saharan) and South America (Brazil) where outbreaks of the disease are frequent among the residents.

The meningococcal polysaccharide vaccine is a quadrivalent vaccine inducing immunity against serogroups A, C, Y, and W-135. A single dose appears to provide immunity for at least 3 years. Vaccine efficacy is variable in young children, and a second dose of vaccine after 2 or 3 years is recommended for children living in high-risk areas who received the first vaccine dose at less than 4 years of age.

Japanese Encephalitis Virus Vaccine

Japanese encephalitis (JE) is a viral infection transmitted by *Culex* mosquitoes in Asia and Southeast Asia. Transmission is year round in the tropical and subtropical areas and during the late spring, summer, and early fall in temperate climates. Pigs and some species of birds are natural reservoirs of the virus, while the mosquito vectors breed extensively in flooded rice fields and irrigation projects.

JE virus is not considered a risk for short-term travelers visiting the usual tourist destinations in urban areas and developed resort areas. For visitors to rural areas during the transmission season, the estimated risk for JE during a 1-month period is 1:5000 or 1:20,000 per week.[16]

The risk of infection can be greatly decreased by personal measures that prevent mosquito bites: wearing protective clothing, using insect repellents, and sleeping under bed nets. Nonetheless, since JE has been acquired by short-term travelers to endemic rural areas, and since agricultural projects bordering on urban areas can bring infected mosquitoes into the proximity of susceptible urban dwellers, the vaccine should be offered to travelers going on trips of any length to rural areas (especially areas of pig farming), and to expatriate workers, missionaries, and students who plan to live in endemic areas.[68]

An inactivated viral vaccine (JEV) consisting of three doses given by injection over the course of a month is available for administration to travelers determined to be at significant risk. A schedule consisting of doses at 0, 7, and 30 days appears to result in a higher seroconversion rate and geometric mean titer of antibody among recipients than does a 2-week accelerated schedule consisting of doses at 0, 7, and 14 days.[3,16,56,68] A booster dose of vaccine may be given 2 to 3 years after the primary immunization for continued risk of exposure.

Adverse reactions to JEV include local pain and swelling at the site of injection in about 20% of recipients, systemic symptoms (fever, headache, malaise, rash) in about 10% of recipients, and hypersensitivity reactions (mainly urticaria, angioedema, or both) in 15 to 62 per 10,000 American vaccinees. The hypersensitivity reactions reported occurred after the first, second, or third dose of vaccine, either almost immediately afterward or with delays of up to 2 weeks after receipt of the vaccine dose. Limited data suggest that persons who have had urticarial reactions to Hymenoptera envenomation and to other stimuli might be at greater risk of JEV-induced hypersensitivity reactions. The CDC recommends that vaccinees be directly observed for 30 minutes after receipt of JEV and that they not depart on their travel until 10 days after the last JEV dose, so that delayed adverse reactions can be detected and treated.[16]

Rabies Vaccine

Animal bites, especially dog bites, present a potential rabies hazard to international travelers who travel to rural areas in Central and South America, the Middle East, Africa, and Asia.[11,70] Preexposure rabies immunization is recommended for rural travelers, especially adventure travelers who go to remote areas, and for expatriate workers, missionaries, and their families living in countries where rabies is a recognized risk.

The rabies vaccine is an inactivated virus vaccine used for preexposure and postexposure immunization. Preexposure rabies immunization consists of three doses of human diploid cell vaccine (HDCV) over the course of 1 month, given by intramuscular (1 ml dose) or intradermal (0.1 ml dose) injection. The smaller dose used for the intradermal series is less expensive but requires advance planning; vaccine efficacy is compromised if chloroquine prophylaxis against malaria is started within 3 weeks after the third dose of intradermal vaccine.[55] If there is not sufficient time before departure, the intramuscular series should be given. The usual booster interval for rabies vaccine is 2 years; however, if time permits, serologic testing may show persistence of protective levels of antibody and so the booster dose may be delayed to 3 or even 4 years after the last dose on the basis of annual testing. This sparing of vaccine doses received could be beneficial to recipients who have a long-term need for protection (veterinarians, field biologists, laboratory workers, and expatriates living in high-risk areas).

Mild local reactions to rabies vaccine are common and consist of erythema, pain, and swelling at the injection site. Mild systemic symptoms—headache, dizziness, nausea, abdominal pain, and myalgia—may develop in some recipients. In approximately 5% of people receiving booster doses of HDCV for preexposure prophylaxis and in a few receiving postexposure immunization, a serum sickness–like illness characterized by urticaria, fever, malaise, arthralgias, arthritis, nausea, and vomiting may develop 2 to 21 days after a vaccine dose is received.

Rabies vaccine adsorbed (RVA) is a newer rabies vaccine produced by the Michigan Department of Public Health. This inactivated virus vaccine is derived from virus grown in tissue culture cells in medium free of human albumin. The RVA vaccine may be used for intramuscular administration only. Data are accumulating on the incidence of reactions after immunization with this preparation.

Receipt of preexposure rabies immunization simplifies the care of a person if a high-risk bite is sustained; in addition to immediate wound care (vigorous cleansing, debridement, loose approximation of skin edges, and antibiotics to prevent wound infection), two additional 1 ml intramuscular doses of rabies vaccine on days 0 and 3 are recommended for optimal protection.

If a person who has not received preexposure rabies vaccine is bitten while in a rabies-endemic area, postexposure care for the bite includes a dose (20 IU/kg) of rabies immune globulin (RIG), with one-half the dose infiltrated at the wound site if possible and the remainder given by intramuscular injection. In addition, five doses (1 ml) of rabies vaccine should be given by intramuscular injection on days 0, 3, 7, 14, and 28.

Safe supplies of rabies immune globulin and rabies vaccine (HDCV) are difficult to obtain in many rabies-endemic areas. The supply of RIG in developing countries is likely to be derived from horse serum (in contrast to the human-derived RIG product available in industrialized countries). Administration of horse-derived RIG is accompanied by a significant risk of serum sickness. The rabies vaccines available in developing countries are often Semple-type vaccines, derived from infected brain tissue of laboratory animals. Such preparations have a potential for adverse side effects and decreased protective efficacy compared with the modern tissue culture–derived rabies vaccines.

Hepatitis B Vaccine

Hepatitis B vaccine has been added recently to the list of vaccines recommended for routine immunization of children in the United States.[10,17] However, immunization of American adults continues to target persons at risk because of occupation, personal activities (travel, close contact with infected people, institutionalization), or medical treatment with blood or tissue products.

In many parts of Asia and Africa, up to 15% of the general population may be asymptomatic carriers of hepatitis B virus. Travelers to countries in Asia and Africa who will live and work among the residents, such as missionaries, volunteer relief workers, teachers, students, adventure travelers, and other travelers who might have intimate or sexual contact with the residents, should consider immunization against hepatitis B.

Two recombinant vaccines are available, Recombivax and Engerix B. The standard dosage schedule for both vaccines consists of injectable doses at 0, 1, and 6 months. Engerix B vaccine has an approved accelerated dosage schedule of 0, 1, and 2 months. This may allow full immunization of a traveler with limited time before departure; however, a booster dose at 12 months is recommended if risk of infection continues.[10,13]

Plague Vaccine

Plague, a bacterial disease caused by *Yersinia pestis,* is enzootic among wild rodents in countries of Africa, Asia, and the Americas. Plague is transmitted to humans by fleas or direct contact with infected animals. Person-to-person spread is common through respiratory secretions. International travelers going on standard tourist itineraries to countries where plague is reported are unlikely to be at risk. Persons who are at high risk of exposure include field biologists and those who will reside or work in rural mountainous or upland areas, where avoidance of rodents and fleas is difficult.

Plague vaccine is a killed bacterial vaccine with poorly documented protective efficacy. Primary immunization consists of 3 doses of vaccine given by intramuscular injection over 10 months. Side effects include pain, redness, and induration at the site of injection. Systemic symptoms consisting of fever, headache, and malaise may occur after repeated doses. An alternative to plague vaccination is the use of prophylactic tetracycline (500 mg by mouth four times a day) during periods of active exposure to plague-infected animals or humans. The efficacy of using tetracycline prophylaxis is unproven by controlled clinical trial, but inferred from use of the drug in the treatment of plague.

Tick-Borne Encephalitis Vaccine

Tick-borne encephalitis (TBE) is a viral disease spread by ticks in Europe (Austria, Czechoslovakia, Germany, Hungary, Poland, Switzerland, northern Yugoslavia) and the Commonwealth of Independent States (the former Soviet Union) during the months of April through August. TBE is transmitted to humans by bites from infected *Ixodes ricinus* ticks usually found in forested areas of endemic regions. However, systemic infection after ingestion of unpasteurized dairy products from infected cows, goats, or sheep can also occur.[50]

Vaccination against TBE is not available in the United States. A vaccine manufactured by Immuno (Vienna, Austria) is available in Europe. The vaccine is produced in chick embryo cell cultures; primary immunization consists of three doses given by subcutaneous injection over 6 months. The limited availability of the vaccine and the relatively long immunization schedule mean that most travelers from North America who anticipate a need for protection against TBE will not be able to obtain the vaccine.[3,50]

Travelers planning outdoor activities (hiking, biking, camping) in areas where TBE is endemic need to rely on personal measures to prevent tick bites. They should wear protective clothing when outdoors, use insect repellents containing *N,N*-diethyl-meta-toluamide (DEET) on exposed areas of skin, and treat their outer clothing with a permethrin-containing insecticide. All travelers to such areas should be advised to avoid ingestion of unpasteurized dairy products.

Tuberculosis (BCG Vaccine)

People going on short trips for tourism or business to countries where tuberculosis is much more common among the general population than in the United States are not considered to be at great risk of contracting this infection, which is commonly spread from person to person by inhalation of infected respiratory droplets in closed environments.

However, travelers who will live among foreign residents or who will work in foreign orphanages, schools, hospitals, or other facilities may be at significant risk of exposure to infection with tuberculosis. Such travelers should be skin tested with tuberculin (PPD) and control antigens (such as *Candida* and *Trichophyton*) before the trip, and afterward if the original test was negative. People who convert to skin test positivity can be treated with isoniazid or other drugs to prevent tuberculosis.[6]

The BCG vaccines around the world were originally derived from in vitro attenuation of a bovine tubercle bacillus *(Mycobacterium bovis)* strain in the early 1900s in France. Subsequently, the organisms have been maintained by several laboratories under varying conditions, so currently available vaccines are not considered microbiologically identical.

The BCG vaccines are used widely all over the world for childhood immunization against tuberculosis, although this has never been a public health policy in the United States. There is no consensus on the protective efficacy of BCG vaccines, and estimates of protection have varied from study to study. BCG strain differences, regional differences in mycobacterial ecology, and differences in trial methods have all contributed to the observed variation in studies of vaccine efficacy.[6,24]

Epidemiologic data suggest that the vaccine may be more useful in protecting children from disseminated extrapulmonary complications of tuberculosis than in protecting adults from primary pulmonary infection. Persons immunized with BCG vaccine become PPD skin test positive for many years afterward, regardless of the degree of protection conferred by the vaccine. As a result, the PPD skin test cannot be used as a reliable indicator of infection in recipients, and this situation can contribute to a delay in diagnosis in people who have contracted tuberculosis infection despite BCG vaccination.

Occasionally, children in families going abroad for extended residence are requested by the receiving country to provide proof of BCG vaccination to qualify for a visa. A BCG vaccine is commercially available in the United States and is approved by the American Academy of Pediatrics Committee on the Control of Infectious Diseases for use in children going to live in areas where tuberculosis is prevalent or where there is a likelihood of exposure to adults with active or recently arrested tuberculosis. The vaccine is also recommended for children of tuberculous mothers. The vaccine might be considered appropriate in the case of uninfected (PPD skin test–negative) health care workers who are going to work in areas where there is a high endemic prevalence of tuberculosis in the population and who will have limited access to medical diagnosis and treatment.[6]

Like other live attenuated vaccines, BCG vaccine is contraindicated in people with immunosuppression caused by congenital conditions, chemotherapy, radiation therapy, HIV infection, or another condition resulting in impaired immune responses. Pregnancy is considered a relative contraindication.[15]

ROUTINE IMMUNIZATIONS

The routine immunizations are those customarily given in childhood and updated in adult life, usually regardless of travel.[13,17] The assessment of immunization needs for international travel provides an opportunity for individuals to receive "missed" booster doses of the routine immunizations. This is a special concern among middle-aged and older people.[34,40]

The routine vaccines currently recommended in childhood include those against tetanus, diphtheria, pertussis, measles, mumps, rubella, poliovirus, *Haemophilus influenzae* type b (Hib), and hepatitis B.[13,17] After 7 years of age, booster doses for tetanus, diphtheria, measles, and poliovirus are given as indicated below.

The recommendation for universal pediatric immunization against hepatitis B is relatively recent (see previous section on hepatitis B vaccine).[10] Recommendations for immunization against viral infuenza and pneumococcal pneumonia are based on underlying health and age.

Tetanus and Diphtheria Vaccine

The tetanus/diphtheria vaccine (Td) is used for primary immunization and booster doses in older children and adults. Booster doses of Td vaccine given at 10-year intervals throughout life are recommended to maintain immunity. The diphtheria-pertussis-tetanus vaccine is used for immunization of children less than 7 years of age and contains different proportions of the tetanus and diphtheria vaccine antigens than those present in the Td.[9,13]

Poliomyelitis Vaccine

Poliomyelitis vaccine is usually not boosted after childhood in the United States, except for anticipated high-risk exposure through work or travel to areas where polio is endemic or epidemic. Although the risk of polio transmission is greatest in the developing countries, sporadic outbreaks have occurred in industrialized countries among unvaccinated subpopulations, usually religious groups.

The attenuated live-virus oral polio vaccine (OPV) is recommended for a primary immunization series given before 18 years of age. The enhanced inactivated (killed) virus polio vaccine (e-IPV) is recommended for primary immunization and for booster doses in people 18 years of age and older, because of a higher risk of complications associated with OPV in older patients.[13]

Measles, Mumps, and Rubella Vaccine

A single dose of measles, mumps, rubella (MMR) vaccine is recommended for all infants at 15 months of age. The Immunization Practices Advisory Committee recommends a second dose of measles vaccine in childhood on entry into grade school, middle school, or high school; this is required by law in many states. Also, persons born after 1957 but before 1980 should receive a second dose of measles vaccine. The second dose of measles vaccine may be given either as the monovalent vaccine or as the MMR vaccine; there is no contraindication to reimmunization with the MMR vaccine.[13,17]

Haemophilus Influenzae B Vaccine

The risk for invasive *H. influenzae* disease, including meningitis, is greatest in children less than 7 years old, and the infection is common among children in the developing world. Primary immunization is recommended at 2 months of age or as soon as possible thereafter.

Three different conjugate vaccines are commercially available against *H. influenzae* type b (Hib). The vaccines contain the antigenic polyribosyl-ribitol (PRP) moiety conjugated to a carrier protein. Two doses of PRP-OMP vaccine or three doses of HbOC vaccine given 2 months apart are recommended for all children less than 12 months of age. After 12 months of age, a single dose of either vaccine is sufficient for immunization. The third Hib conjugate vaccine, PRP-D, is approved for use only in children 15 months or older and is given as a single dose.

Influenza Vaccine, Pneumococcal Vaccine

Annual immunization against viral influenza is recommended for all people over 65 years of age. Influenza vaccine is also recommended for special groups of patients at increased risk from complications of viral influenza. These patients include those with chronic respiratory disease (emphysema, asthma), ischemic heart disease, transplanted organs, renal failure, and impaired immune response from congenital conditions, acquired illness, or immunosuppressive therapy. The 23-valent polysaccharide vaccine against pneumoccal pneumonia is a one-time-only injection and is recommended for the same groups mentioned.[13]

In addition to the elderly and the ill, "flu" vaccine is also recommended for all health care workers and for international travelers because prolonged air travel and exposure to crowded or extreme environments predispose them to respiratory infections.

Malaria

Malaria is a mosquito-transmitted blood-borne parasitic infection present throughout tropical and developing areas of the world, including Mexico, Haiti, Central and South America, Africa, the Middle East, the Indian subcontinent, Asia, Southeast Asia, and Oceania (Fig. 44-2). The estimated worldwide incidence is 280 million cases a year. Approximately 1000 cases a year are reported in the United States to the CDC. Although the risk to travelers is relatively low compared with other medical problems (diarrhea, respiratory problems) in travelers, malaria infection causes a severe febrile illness that is potentially fatal.

Four species of malaria commonly cause disease in humans: *Plasmodium vivax* (worldwide distribution), *P. falciparum* (worldwide distribution), *P. ovale* (western Africa), and *P. malariae* (worldwide distribution). The protozoan malaria parasites are transmitted by female *Anopheles* mosquito vectors, which tend to bite between dusk and dawn.

The incubation period for malaria is usually 1 or more weeks after the mosquito injects malaria sporozoites into the human host during a blood meal. The malaria parasites incubate, then multiply in hepatocytes. The infected hepatocytes rupture, releasing thousands of malaria merozoites into the bloodstream. The merozoites invade circulating red blood cells (RBCs) and develop into the next developmental stage, trophozoites. Ring-shaped trophozoites within RBCs can be seen on peripheral blood smears, as can later parasite stages: schizonts (asexual reproduction) or male and female gametocytes (sexual reproduction). Diagnosis of malaria is based on recognition of characteristic trophozoites, schizonts, and gametocytes on peripheral blood smears. Schizonts rupture, releasing new crops of merozoites that can infect other RBCs. Male and female gametocytes are taken up by the female mosquito during a blood meal and propagate infection in the mosquito.[35,73]

MALARIA CHEMOPROPHYLAXIS

Travelers to malarious areas are usually prescribed one of several drug regimens to prevent malaria (chemoprophylaxis). However, in *P. falciparum* strains development of drug resistance to chloroquine and other drugs has made the selection of appropriate chemoprophylaxis for some travel-

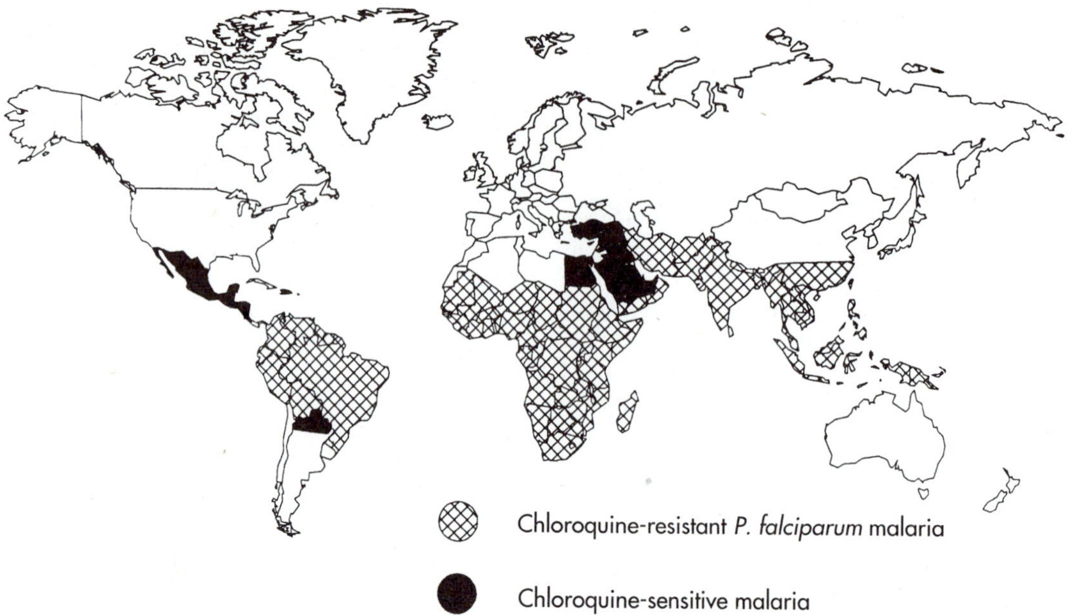

Fig. 44-2 Map of worldwide malaria transmission. (From Centers for Disease Control: *Health information for international travel, 1992,* Washington, DC, 1992, US Government Printing Office.)

ers a difficult process.* Drug allergies, contraindications, drug toxicity, drug interactions, underlying medical conditions, access to recommended drugs, and compliance with recommended regimens all contribute to the problem.[2,47,54,69]

Rapidly developing drug resistance among malarial parasites worldwide means that no current antimalarial drug regimen can be considered to provide complete protection. Use of personal insect precautions (repellents, protective clothing, and bed nets) and behavioral modification (limiting time outdoors) are two important adjuncts to malaria chemoprophylaxis.

Selection of malaria chemoprophylaxis is determined by the geographic destination (Table 44-4). The drug regimen is based on the risk of chloroquine-resistant falciparum malaria (CRPF). Chloroquine is efficacious and relatively nontoxic in the few areas where malaria is still sensitive to the drug. Mefloquine is generally the drug of choice for malaria chemoprophylaxis in CRPF areas; however, in some places, such as certain border areas in Thailand where CRPF strains have developed resistance to mefloquine, or in some patients who cannot take mefloquine, doxycycline is recommended for prophylaxis against CRPF. Doses and schedules for malaria chemoprophylaxis are given in Table 44-5.

Chloroquine-resistant *Plasmodium vivax* has been reported in Irian Jaya and Sumatra, Indonesia, and Papua New Guinea.[2,59,60] Mefloquine chemoprophylaxis recommended for the CRPF present in these areas is also adequate for resistant *P. vivax.*

*References 35, 41, 43, 44, 64, 72.

Travelers should be aware that some regimens against CRPF recommended by experts are not licensed or available in the United States; even if these are not standard recommendations, the alternative regimens may be considered in special cases. For instance, standard regimens of mefloquine or doxycycline are not recommended for use in pregnant women. Mefloquine is not recommended for children weighing less than 15 kg, and doxycycline is not recommended for children less than 8 years of age. In travelers unable to take either drug, a combination of chloroquine plus proguanil may give some protection against CRPF in east Africa, and this alternative regimen is considered safe in pregnant women and young children. Proguanil is not licensed or marketed in the United States and must be purchased abroad.

Travelers who are going to other CRPF areas (where chloroquine plus proguanil is not effective) and are unable to take mefloquine or doxycycline may be advised to take weekly pyrimethamine plus dapsone. This drug combination is marketed under the brand name Maloprim in many malaria-endemic areas outside the United States. Travelers electing to take this alternative regimen should be warned about dose-related bone marrow suppression and the possibility of idiosyncratic hypersensitivity reactions. This regimen cannot be used by pregnant women because of the risk of fetal toxicity from pyrimethamine. Travelers taking Maloprim chemoprophylaxis for more than a month should have periodic peripheral blood counts to monitor for potential toxicity. Although Maloprim is not licensed or marketed in the United States, both pyrimethamine and dapsone are available and may be prescribed separately at the appropriate doses.

Table 44-4 Malaria Chemoprophylaxis Based on Geographic Risk

Geographic Area	Drug of Choice	Alternative
CHLOROQUINE-SENSITIVE AREAS LOCATED WITHIN:		
Mexico	Chloroquine	Standby*
Caribbean	Chloroquine	Standby*
Central America (west of Panama Canal)	Chloroquine	Standby*
Middle East (Egypt, Turkey, Iraq, Syria, United Arab Emirates)	Chloroquine	Standby*
CHLOROQUINE-RESISTANT AREAS LOCATED WITHIN:		
Central America (east of Panama Canal)	Mefloquine	Chloroquine + standby*
South America	Mefloquine	Chloroquine + standby*
South America (Amazon Basin)	Mefloquine	Doxycycline
Middle East	Mefloquine	Chloroquine + standby*
Africa (sub-Saharan)	Mefloquine	Doxycycline (or C+P+SB)†
Southeast Asia	Mefloquine	Doxycycline
Thailand (border areas along Cambodia and Burma)	Doxycycline	(Proguanil + sulfa or dapsone)‡
Oceania	Mefloquine	Doxycycline

From Jong EC, White NJ: *The travel and tropical medicine manual,* ed 2, Philadelphia, WB Saunders.
*Standby malaria treatment: take a treatment dose of the antimalarial when experiencing signs and symptoms of malaria, and prompt medical attention is not available:

1. Pyrimethamine plus sulfadoxine (Fansidar), or
2. Halofantrine (Halfan)

†*C+P+SB,* Chloroquine plus proguanil (Paludrine) plus carry standby malaria treatment.
‡See text.

Another approach for travelers to CRPF areas who are unable to take the optimal chemoprophylactic drugs would be to take weekly chloroquine prophylaxis, use good personal insect precautions, and carry standby drug treatment for CRPF malaria (see later discussion). Chemoprophylactic regimens using proguanil plus sulfonamide, proguanil plus dapsone, and mefloquine plus sulfadoxine-pyrimethamine have been studied in areas where there is intense transmission of multidrug-resistant falciparum malaria, but there are limited data about the efficacy and tolerance of these regimens in civilian travelers.[42,53,64]

Travelers should start taking any antimalarial drug selected for prophylaxis at least 1 or 2 weeks before departure. This allows time for familiarity with the side effects of the drug while the drug builds up to steady-state levels in the body, enables the traveler to habituate to the timing of doses, and gives the traveler time to contact his or her health care provider and switch to an alternative drug if necessary while still at home.

Travelers should be warned not to switch antimalarial regimens during the trip without the specific advice of a knowledgeable health care provider. Casual advice given by travelers from other countries or recommendations by personnel in drugstores where many antimalarials are available over the counter should not be the basis for medication changes.

Antimalarial chemoprophylaxis should be continued for 4 weeks after the person leaves the malarious area to prevent attacks of malaria in the immediate posttravel period. The usual incubation periods for malaria are 8 to 11 days for *P. falciparum,* 10 to 17 days for *P. vivax* and *P. ovale,* and 18 to 40 days for *P. malariae.* Prolonged latent incubation times of up to 3 years or more have been reported rarely, especially with the *P. malariae* species. Among cases reported in Americans, over 90% of *P. falciparum* infections and 50% of *P. vivax* infections cause clinical attacks during the first 4 to 8 weeks after return from a malarious area.

STANDBY DRUG TREATMENT FOR MALARIA

In some cases a prescription for standby drug treatment for CRPF malaria in addition to chemoprophylaxis should be given to travelers, especially adventure and outdoor travelers going to remote areas known to have highly resistant strains of malaria. Standby drug treatment should also be given to other travelers who for any reason must take a regimen of malaria chemoprophylaxis that is suboptimal for the geographic region. Drugs and doses used for standby treatment of malaria are given in Table 44-6.

Travelers need to familiarize themselves with the signs and symptoms of the clinical illness, so they can recognize a possible attack of malaria and treat themselves if necessary (Table 44-7). In case of an illness accompanied by high fever similar to a bad case of viral influenza, the traveler

Table 44-5 Malaria Chemoprophylaxis*

Drug	Dose
ADULTS	
Chloroquine phosphate (Aralen)	250 mg, 2 tab/wk 500 mg, 1 tab/wk
Mefloquine (Lariam)	250 mg, 1 tab/wk
Doxycycline (Vibramycin)	100 mg, 1 tab/day
Proguanil (Paludrine) (in addition to weekly chloroquine)	100 mg, 2 tab/day
Pyrimethamine-dapsone (Maloprim)	12.5 mg pyrimethamine, 100 mg dapsone, 1 tab/wk
CHILDREN	
Chloroquine phosphate	8.3 mg/kg/wk po
Hydroxychloroquine sulfate	6.5 mg/kg/wk po
Proguanil	<2 yr: 50 mg/day po 2-6 yr: 100 mg/day po 7-10 yr: 150 mg/day po >10 yr: 200 mg/day po
Pyrimethamine-dapsone	<2 yr: ¼ tab/wk po 3-10 yr: ½ tab/wk po >10 yr: 1 tab/wk po
Mefloquine (not FDA approved)	15-19 kg: ¼ tab/wk po 20-30 kg: ½ tab/wk po 31-40 kg: ¾ tab/wk po

From Jong EC, White NJ: *The travel and tropical medicine manual,* ed 2, Philadelphia, WB Saunders.
*See general remarks and precautions in the text.

should seek immediate medical care. A traveler who becomes ill while remote from health care should be instructed to use standby malaria treatment as prescribed. Because of drug resistance among *P. falciparum* parasites from most malarious areas of the world, the standby treatment (regardless of which drug regimen is selected) may result only in temporary or partial improvement from a malaria attack, thus allowing evacuation from a distant area. However, further definitive treatment of malaria as soon as possible may be necessary to eradicate the infection.

Pyrimethamine plus sulfadoxine (Fansidar) is currently recommended by the CDC as a standby treatment for a malaria attack and can be used if the person is not allergic to sulfa drugs. Although serious and potentially fatal hypersensitivity reactions were reported in travelers taking this drug combination for CRPF prophylaxis on a weekly basis (1 case per 5000 to 8000 users), the remote risk of a significant adverse effect after taking a single treatment dose would be outweighed by the seriousness of an untreated CRPF attack. Thailand is reported to have a high prevalence of *P. falciparum* infections resistant to Fansidar, so other drugs should be considered for standby treatment of malaria acquired there.

Mefloquine may be used in treatment doses as a standby regimen if the traveler is not already taking mefloquine for malaria chemoprophylaxis. Serious adverse side effects, including seizures and cardiac arrest, have been reported rarely for mefloquine given at treatment doses, but again, the remote risk of a significant adverse effect after taking the drug in treatment doses would be outweighed by the seriousness of an untreated CRPF attack.[69] Mefloquine-resistant *P. falciparum* infections are being reported sporadically from countries in Southeast Asia and Africa but appear to be of most concern along the Thai-Burma (Myanmar) border.

Halofantrine, which is pending release in the United States, is already available in some countries of Western Europe, Africa, and Asia. Halofantrine is an effective oral drug for treatment of CRPF and Fansidar-resistant CRPF and may be prescribed as a standby treatment. The incidence of side effects is low but includes abdominal pain, pruritus, vomiting, diarrhea, headache, and rash. The drug is contraindicated in pregnant women because animal data show embryotoxic effects.

Higher-than-conventional doses of halofantrine appear to be required for successful treatment of mefloquine-resistant *P. falciparum* strains being reported along the Thailand-Cambodia (Democratic Kampuchea) and the Thailand-Burma (Myanmar) borders. However, recent reports of cardiac conduction disturbances with prolongation of the PR and QT intervals on electrocardiograms of malaria patients treated with halofantrine, especially after mefloquine treatment failure, have raised concerns about the drug's safety.[54] Some experts recommend that physicians obtain a pretravel electrocardiogram from travelers who will be prescribed halofantrine standby treatment to document that there is no underlying conduction defect that might be exacerbated by the drug.

The regimen of oral quinine sulfate plus a second drug (tetracycline, doxycycline, clindamycin, or Fansidar) remains one of the most effective treatments for CRPF. However, this regimen should not be recommended to travelers as a standby treatment if other options are available. The development of cinchonism (ringing in the ears, headache, nausea, visual disturbance) from quinine is almost predictable during the first 3 days of treatment, and many travelers would be unable to complete the 7-day therapeutic quinine course (recommended for malaria acquired in South east Asia) in the field without medical assistance and support.

Qinghaosu (artemisinin) and its derivatives artemether, artesunate, and arteether are a group of antimalarial drugs derived from a Chinese medicinal herb, *qing hao*. The compounds have shown remarkable efficacy during clinical trials in the treatment of severe chloroquine-resistant falciparum malaria and can rapidly clear parasites without apparent significant toxicity. Artemisinin compounds are available for clinical use in China, Vietnam, and other malarious areas of Southeast Asia.[32]

Table 44-6 Malaria Drugs for Standby Treatment*

Drug	Adult Dose	Pediatric Dose
Pyrimethamine 25 mg/sulfadoxine 500 mg (Fansidar)	3 tab po as single dose	2-11 mo: ¼ tab 1-3 yr: ½ tab 4-8 yr: 1 tab 9-14 yr: 2 tab >14 yr: 3 tab po as single dose
Mefloquine, 250 mg tab (Lariam)	2 tab as single dose, followed by 2 tab after 8-12 hr: reduce 2nd dose to 1 tab for adults <60 kg	15 mg/kg po as single dose (do not use in infants <15 kg)
Halofantrine, 250 mg tab (Halfan)	2 tab in one dose + 2 tab after 6 hr + 2 tab after 6 more hr (total dose of 6 tab in 12 hr); *repeat therapy in 7 days in nonimmune patients*	
Halofantrine, 2% suspension (Halfan)		8 mg/kg po × 3 doses, each dose 6 hr apart; *repeat therapy in 7 days in non-immune patients*
Quinine sulfate tab	650 mg 3 times a day for 3 days (continue for 7 days in Southeast Asia)	10 mg/kg 3 times a day for 3 days (continue for 7 days in Southeast Asia)
Plus tetracycline	250 mg 4 times a day for 7 days	>8 yr of age: 5 mg/kg of body weight po 4 times a day for 7 days
Or plus doxycycline	100 mg twice a day po for 7 days	>8 yr of age: 2 mg/kg of body weight po twice a day for 7 days
Or plus clindamycin	10 mg/kg 3 times a day for 5 days	10 mg/kg 3 times a day for 5 days
Or plus Fansidar	Fansidar dose above	Fansidar dose above

From Jong EC, White NJ: *The travel and tropical medicine manual,* ed 2, Philadelphia, WB Saunders.
*See general remarks and precautions in the text.

Table 44-7 Clinical Illness in Malaria and Dengue Fever

Signs and Symptoms	Malaria	Dengue Fever
Fever	+++	+++
Chills	+++	++
Headache	+++	+++
Malaise		++
Anorexia		++
Nausea, vomiting	++	++
Abdominal pain	++	
Myalgia	++	++
Arthralgia		++
Backache	+	
Dark urine	+	

+++, >90% of patients; ++, >50% of patients; +, <10% of patients.

Artesunate may be given by intravenous or intramuscular injection, artemether can be given by intramuscular injection only, and various artemisinin compounds are available for administration by mouth or by suppository. At the time of writing, dosage and toxicity parameters for the oral compounds are still under investigation, so the artemisinin compounds cannot be considered in the category of standby treatment for malaria. Travelers developing severe febrile illness in multidrug-resistant malarious areas of Asia who reach medical assistance might be treated effectively with artemisinin compounds, however.[32,35]

PERSONAL INSECT PRECAUTIONS

Personal insect precautions are just as important as drugs for preventing malaria, especially if the traveler must take one of the suboptimal antimalarial drug regimens. Prevention of itching skin lesions caused by insect bites (and the possibility of secondary skin infections) and prevention of other insect-borne infections for which there are no prophylactic drugs or vaccines are other considerations.

In regard to malaria prevention, exposure to mosquito vectors of malaria can be decreased by limiting time outdoors between dusk and dawn, by wearing protective clothing while outdoors, and by applying insect repellents to exposed areas of skin while outdoors.

The most effective insect repellents for skin application contain *N,N*-diethyl-meta-toluamide (DEET). Older formulations of repellents containing DEET depended on high concentrations and frequent applications to the skin for effectiveness. Concerns about DEET toxicity and the inconvenience of frequent applications led to development of repellent formulations that rely on new technology to keep repellent chemicals on the surface of the skin for longer periods. Newer insect repellents have lower concentrations of DEET and a longer duration of skin adherence and are claimed to have decreased absorption through the skin (Box 44-2).

Mosquito bed nets should be used when sleeping in unscreened rooms. The protection afforded by bed nets can be increased by application of a pyrethrum-based insecticide. Pyrethrums are insecticides related to naturally occurring alkaloids in the chrysanthemum plant family. Permethrin is a chemical derivative and is relatively nontoxic. Permethrin insecticides are suitable for treatment of external clothing and mosquito nets but are not recommended for direct skin application because they may induce skin hypersensitivity reactions.

Bed nets and external clothing can be treated by spraying or soaking with a permethrin solution and letting it air dry before use (Fig. 44-3; Box 44-2). Treated bed nets and clothing retain residual insecticide activity for weeks (sprayed) to months (soaked).[61] In addition to repelling mosquitoes, permethrin insecticides are effective against gnats, ticks, chiggers, bedbugs, scorpions, centipedes, beetles, and flies (see Chapter 34). Permethrin insecticide coils and electric vaporizers can augment the use of bed nets indoors.

BOX 44-2

INSECT REPELLENTS AND INSECTICIDES*

INSECT REPELLENTS CONTAINING DEET

Ultrathon Insect Repellent: 35% DEET in polymer formulation, up to 12-hr protection against mosquitoes, also effective against ticks, biting flies, chiggers, fleas, gnats (3M, Minneapolis, MN)

DEET Plus Insect Repellent: 17.5% DEET with 2.5% R 326, apply every 4 hr for mosquitoes, every 8 hr for biting flies (Sawyer Products, Safety Harbor, FL 34695)

Skedaddle Insect Protection for Children: 10% DEET using molecular entrapment technology (Little Point Corp., Cambridge, MA)

PERMETHRIN-CONTAINING INSECTICIDES

Permanone Tick Repellent: Contains permethrin in a pressurized spray can, repels ticks, chiggers, mosquitoes, and other bugs (Coulston International Corp., Easton, PA 18044)

Duranon Tick Repellent: Contains permethrin in a formula lasting up to 2 wk, supplied in a pressurized spray can (Coulston International Corp., Easton, PA 18044)

PermaKill 4 Week Tick Killer: 13.3% permethrin liquid concentrate supplied in 8-oz bottle, can be diluted (⅓ oz permethrin concentrate in 16 oz water) to be used with a pump spray bottle, or be diluted 2 oz in 1½ cups of water to be used to impregnate outer clothing, bed nets, and curtains (see Fig. 44-3) (Coulston International Corp., Easton, PA 18044)

From Jong EC, McMullen R: *The travel and tropical medicine manual,* ed 2, Philadelphia, WB Saunders.

*Brand names are given for identification purposes only and do not constitute an endorsement.

DENGUE FEVER

Dengue fever is a mosquito-transmitted viral infection that occurs worldwide in tropical and subtropical zones. The areas of dengue virus transmission overlap malaria endemic areas in many parts of the world, although the vector mosquitoes are different: *Aedes aegypti* and *Aedes albopictus.*

An attack of dengue fever may be clinically indistinguishable from a malaria attack, especially as assessed by travelers in the field. Acute dengue fever is characterized by high fever, headache, and severe myalgias and arthralgias, similar to malaria (Box 44-2). Thus, if a traveler is stricken while in a malarious area with an illness accompanied by a high fever, he or she should be instructed to seek medical care for diagnosis and treatment of possible malaria, or to take standby drug treatment for malaria if remote from medical care. No specific treatment is recommended for dengue fever, but if the cause of the febrile illness is malaria, early medication with antimalarial drugs may be lifesaving.

The incidences of dengue fever and other arboviral infections acquired by travelers abroad are not known because they may not come to medical attention or be diagnosed. Many arboviral illnesses are mild and self-limited. However, diagnosis and treatment in returned travelers with a febrile illness who do seek medical attention can be hampered by limited diagnostic tools (serologic tests, cultures) and a lack of specific therapeutic agents.[3,5,46,68]

Of the more than 530 arboviruses registered in the International Catalogue of Arboviruses, more than 150 are known to infect humans. Effective vaccines are available for yellow fever, Japanese encephalitis, and tick-borne encephalitis. Vaccines for other arboviral infections have been produced but are limited to investigational use. Personal behavior and practices that limit exposure to arthropod vectors (see earlier discussion of insect precautions) are an important health measure for all travelers.

Traveler's Diarrhea

The term "traveler's diarrhea" usually refers to an acute syndrome of watery diarrhea, which may be accompanied by nausea, loss of appetite, abdominal cramps, low-grade fever, and malaise (see Chapter 42). The risk of traveler's diarrhea is high (20% to 50%) among short-term travelers going from industrialized areas and northern temperate zones to tropical and developing areas. The risk of traveler's diarrhea is high wherever food storage, fuel for cooking, and sanitation are inadequate. Latin America, the Caribbean island of the Dominican Republic and Haiti, north, east, and west Africa, India, and south Asia are recognized high-risk areas for acquisition of traveler's diarrhea. Seasonal or climatic factors may also contribute to the risk of traveler's diarrhea.

Diarrhea associated with travel can result from any of multiple causes, including a change in the normal diet, food poisoning (toxins), and infection with viruses (rotavirus and Norwalk virus), bacteria (enterotoxigenic *E. coli, Shigella, Campylobacter, Aeromonas, Salmonella,* and *Vibrio,* among others), and parasites (including *Giardia lamblia, Entamoeba histolytica,* and *Cryptosporidium*). The worldwide prevalence of *Cyclospora,* the recently described cyanobacterium-like microorganism, as a causative agent of traveler's diarrhea is unknown.[18,20,27]

Traveler's diarrhea usually runs a self-limited course lasting less than a week. In one study only 8% to 15% of persons had an episode of illness lasting longer than 1 week.[20] Recovery without antimicrobial treatment is usual in healthy adults; however, most travelers want to avoid the inconvenience and discomfort of diarrhea and ask for medications to terminate an attack as soon as possible. Dehydration from loss of fluids and decreased oral intake is the biggest risk to health, and young children and debilitated or older people are most susceptible to this complication.[20,23,30,65]

Food and water precautions recommended against traveler's diarrhea aim to decrease the risk of diarrhea from all possible causes. Antimicrobial therapy is directed against the bacterial pathogens implicated most often in cases of traveler's diarrhea. Presumably such antimicrobial therapy will not alter the course of illness if the cause is toxin, virus, or parasite. If the antimicrobial used for empirical treatment of traveler's diarrhea is active against the bacteria involved, a rapid recovery may be obtained.

PREVENTION OF TRAVELER'S DIARRHEA

Prevention of traveler's diarrhea can be divided into three categories: food and water precautions, bismuth subsalicylate prophylaxis, and antimicrobial prophylaxis (Table 44-8).

Food and water precautions include drinking only disinfected water or bottled carbonated or canned beverages; eating well-cooked foods served piping hot, baked goods, or fruits with thick skins that can be peeled by the traveler; avoiding ice cubes in beverages; and not eating salads, raw or undercooked fish and shellfish, or cheese and dairy products made from unpasteurized milk. Despite good intentions, most travelers eventually face situations in which they have no choice but to eat and drink whatever is available.

Bismuth subsalicylate (BSS) can be used to prevent

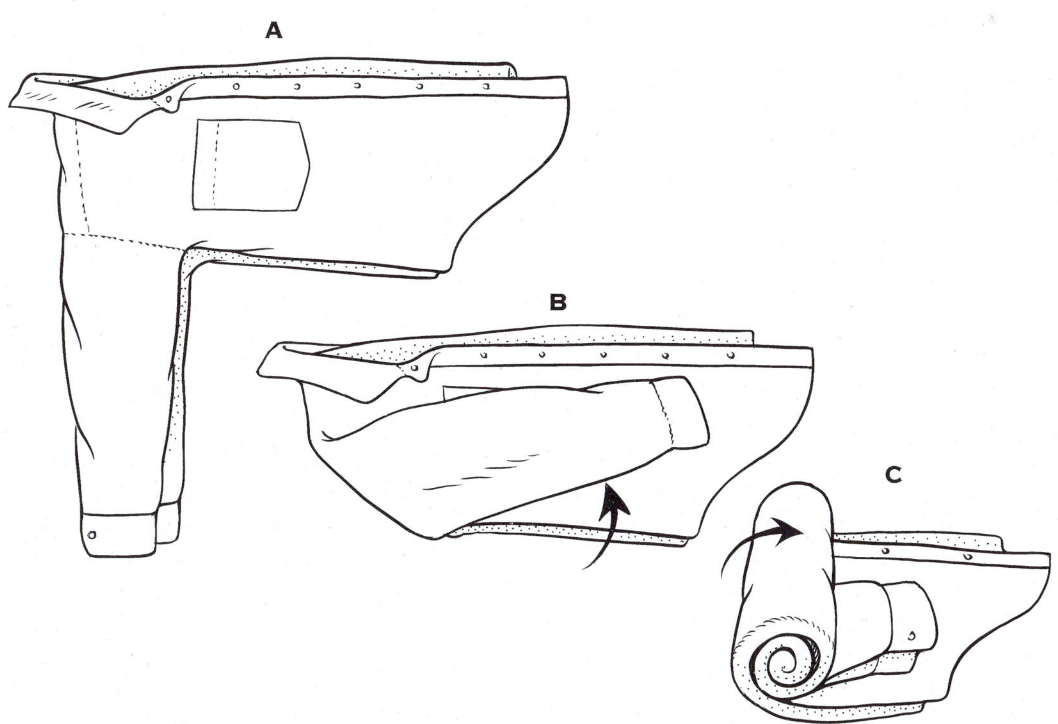

Fig. 44-3 Technique for impregnating clothing or mosquito netting with permethrin solution. **A** to **C,** Lay jacket flat and fold it shoulder to shoulder. Fold sleeves to inside, roll tightly, and tie middle with string. For mosquito net, roll tightly and tie. *Continued.*

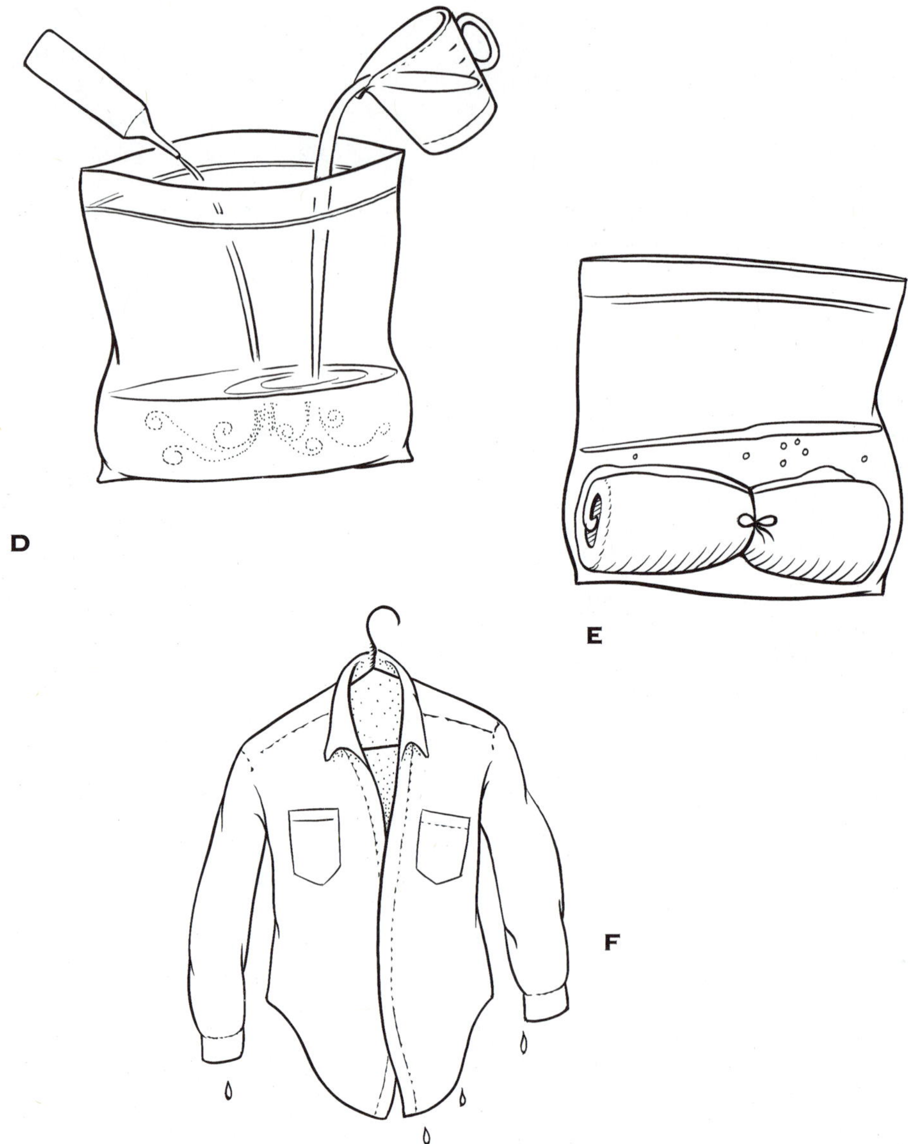

Fig. 44-3, cont'd. D, Pour 2 ounces of permethrin into plastic bag. Add 1 quart water. Mix. Solution will turn milky white. **E,** Place garment or mosquito netting in bag. Shut or tie tightly. Let rest 10 minutes. **F,** Hang garment or netting for 2 to 3 hours to dry. Fabric can also be laid on clean surface to dry. (Redrawn from Rose S: *International travel health guide,* Northampton, Mass, 1993, Travel Medicine.)

traveler's diarrhea by persons going on trips of 3 weeks or less. A regimen of two tablets of BSS four times a day appears to significantly reduce the incidence of diarrhea among travelers to Mexico. Disadvantages to this regimen include cost, the bulk of the BSS in luggage, the risk of salicylism, development of a black tongue, and possible constipation.[18,20]

Some experts concede that taking a broad-spectrum antibiotic during travel can be an effective way to avoid becoming ill; this might be a reasonable strategy for a traveler who is taking a brief trip (1 week or less) to a high-risk area and cannot afford to be ill for even a single day. Travelers falling into this category might include competitive athletes, politicians, sales representatives, and people going to special events.[18,20,52] However, prophylaxis with antimicrobials may be unnecessary now that recent studies have shown that relief of diarrhea within a few hours can be obtained after a high dose of an oral antibiotic taken immediately after the onset of symptoms.[19,22,67]

The antibiotics trimethoprim-sulfamethoxazole (Bactrim, Septra), norfloxacin (Noroxin), ciprofloxacin (Cipro), and ofloxacin (Floxin) have been studied as prophylactic agents. Table 44-9 summarizes antibiotic doses. The quino-

Table 44-8 Prevention of Traveler's Diarrhea: Drug Regimens for Adults

Drug	Dosage	Comments
Bismuth subsalicylate (Pepto-Bismol)	2 tab qid	Less effective than antibiotic prophylaxis; contraindicated in people allergic to aspirin, in people on other salicylate-containing drugs, and during pregnancy; not recommended for children
Trimethoprim 160 mg and sulfamethoxazole 800 mg (Bactrim, Septra)	1 tab/day	Contraindicated in people allergic to sulfa; may not be as effective as the quinolones in some parts of the world
Doxycycline 100 mg (Vibramycin, Doryx, etc.)	1 tab/day	Contraindicated in pregnancy, age <8 yr; efficacy shown in Africa only
Norfloxacin 400 mg (Noroxin)	1 tab/day	Contraindicated in pregnancy, age <18 yr, and in people allergic to quinolones; drug interaction with theophylline and caffeine
Ciprofloxacin 500 mg (Cipro)	1 tab/day	Contraindicated in pregnancy, age <18 yr, and in people allergic to quinolones; drug interaction with theophylline and caffeine
Ofloxacin 200 mg (Floxin)	1 tab/day	Contraindicated in pregnancy, age <18 yr, and in people allergic to quinolones; no significant drug interaction with theophylline and caffeine

From Jong EC, McMullen R: *The travel and tropical medicine manual,* ed 2, Philadelphia, WB Saunders.

lone antibiotics are contraindicated in pregnancy and in persons less than 18 years of age.

SYMPTOMATIC TREATMENT OF TRAVELER'S DIARRHEA

Fluid replacement is the cornerstone of therapy for traveler's diarrhea. Correcting dehydration significantly lessens the general malaise of the stricken person, whether or not antimicrobial therapy is used. Oral fluid intake should be pushed to approximate fluid losses in the stools. Maintenance of normal urine frequency, color, and volume can serve as a marker of adequate rehydration.

Generally, fruit juices or flavored mineral water can be used for oral rehydration during mild to moderate diarrhea. Packets of oral rehydration salts, which can be reconstituted to make oral rehydration solution according to WHO guidelines, are increasingly available in pharmacies throughout the world. Sports electrolyte solutions also provide adequate replacement if diluted to approximately one half to two thirds strength.

BSS in large doses (30 ml of BSS liquid or two BSS tablets by mouth every 30 minutes for eight doses) has been reported to relieve diarrhea and cramps.[18,20] A recent study suggests that in infants and young children with acute watery diarrhea, BSS at weight-adjusted doses (100 or 150 mg/kg body weight/day for up to 5 days) may be a useful adjunct to oral rehydration therapy.[23]

The over-the-counter antiperistaltic drugs loperamide (Imodium) and diphenoxylate plus atropine (Lomotil) may offer some relief to people with watery diarrhea and cramps but should be avoided in those with blood or mucus in the stool or with signs of serious illness (high fever, recurrent vomiting, and increasingly severe abdominal pain).

ANTIBIOTIC TREATMENT OF TRAVELER'S DIARRHEA

Traveler's diarrhea can be relieved within hours after empirical antibiotic therapy is instituted with or without the concurrent use of the antiperistaltic drug loperamide. The drug regimens studied included the antibiotics trimethoprim-sulfamethoxazole and ciprofloxacin. With reports of increasing resistance to trimethoprim-sulfamethoxazole among bacterial enteropathogens such as *Shigella* species and *Campylobacter jejuni,* many experts recommend ciprofloxacin or one of the other quinolones as the drug of choice for empirical diarrhea treatment. Recommended dosages are shown in Table 44-9.[18-22,65-67] If the traveler has started initial treatment of watery diarrhea with BSS therapy, at least 8 hours should elapse before antimicrobial therapy because BSS can impair absorption of the orally administered antimicrobial.[57]

If blood or mucus is present in the stool, travelers should be advised to take the antibiotic prescribed for diarrhea but to refrain from using an antiperistaltic medication. If the diarrhea is caused by a susceptible bacterial species, the patient may obtain relief within a few hours after empirical treatment but should continue to take the given antibiotic for a minimum of 3 days to prevent relapse.

If the patient is ill with a bacterial pathogen resistant to the antibiotic taken, with a viral or parasitic infection, or with toxin-induced gastroenteritis, the antibiotic therapy usually does not alter the outcome of the illness, although the possible risk of antibiotic-associated side effects must always be considered. Travelers who do not respond to empirical antibiotic treatment or who have persistent diarrhea of more than 1 week's duration should have a complete workup for bacterial and parasitic pathogens so that specific treatment may be instituted.

Table 44-9 Drugs for Adult Self-Treatment of Traveler's Diarrhea

Drug	Dosage*	Comments†
Bismuth subsalicylate (Pepto-Bismol)	30 ml (or 2 tabs) every 30 min for 8 doses	Maximum recommended dose is 240 ml (16 tablets) per day
Diphenoxylate plus atropine (Lomotil)	2 tab for first dose, then 1 after each loose bowel movement; do not exceed 8 tabs in 24 hr	Antiperistaltic drug; do not use in dysentery; available by prescription
Loperamide (Imodium)	2 caplets (2 mg each) for first dose then 1 after each loose bowel movement, do not exceed 8 caplets (16 mg) in 24 hr	Antiperistaltic drug; do not use in dysentery; sold over the counter; liquid form available for pediatric doses—use dose adjusted for weight as described on package insert
Tetracycline	2.5 g as a single oral dose	Antibiotic; do not use during pregnancy or for children <8 yr old
Doxycycline (Vibramycin, Doryx, etc.)	100 mg po every 12 hr for 6 doses	Antibiotic; do not use during pregnancy or for children <8 yr old
Trimethoprim/sulfamethoxazole (Bactrim, Septra)	160 mg/800 mg tab (one double-strength tab) every 12 hr for 6 doses	Antibiotic; do not use in sulfa-allergic patients
Norfloxacin‡ (Noroxin)	400 mg tab every 12 hr for 6 doses	Antibiotic; do not use during pregnancy or for teenagers <18 yr old.
Ciprofloxacin (Cipro)	500 mg tab every 12 hr for 6 doses	Antibiotic; do not use during pregnancy or for teenagers <18 yr old
Ciprofloxacin‡ (Cipro)	750 mg tab once at start of diarrhea symptoms	Antibiotic; do not use during pregnancy or for teenagers <18 yr old
Ofloxacin§ (Floxin)	200 mg or 300 mg tab every 12 hr for 6 doses§	Antibiotic; do not use during pregnancy or for teenagers <18 yr old
Furazolidone	100 mg qid for 7-10 days	Antibiotic; also has activity against *Giardia*

From Jong EC, McMullen R: *The travel and tropical medicine manual,* ed 2, Philadelphia, WB Saunders.
*Adult doses given.
†See comments in Table 44-8 also.
‡Unlabeled use.
§This drug has been studied for this use at both doses.

Table 44-10 Short-Acting Benzodiazepine Medications for Jet Lag

Drug	Adult Dose*	Elimination Half-Life
Triazolam (Halcion)	0.25 mg hs	1.5-5.5 hr
Temazepam (Restoril)	30 mg hs	8-12 hr
Estazolam (ProSom)	1-2 mg hs	10-24 hr

From Jong EC, McMullen R: *Infect Dis Clin North Am* 6:285, 1992.
*Use half the usual dose for elderly patients or first-time users.

Travel Medical Kit

Traveling patients are advised to prepare a travel medicine kit appropriate to their itinerary (see Chapter 17). Such a kit should contain adequate supplies of all prescription medications normally taken, the medications for malaria and diarrhea as discussed previously, and some remedies for common problems such as headache, musculoskeletal pain, allergies, nasal and sinus congestion, cough, jet lag, and constipation. Medications used to help travelers cope with jet lag are listed in Table 44-10. Persons prescribed one of these drugs should be warned not to ingest alcoholic beverages concomitantly.[51] Travelers should be instructed to carry their prescription medications in their hand-held luggage to avoid loss, and to carry copies of their prescriptions in case replacements are needed.[39]

Depending on the travel itinerary, insect repellent, sunscreen, topical antibiotic ointment, antifungal cream or powder, and medications for motion sickness, allergic reactions, and high-altitude illness might be included. Female travelers should be reminded to carry personal sanitary supplies; disposable tampons and pads may be difficult to obtain in developing countries. Sexually active travelers of both sexes should take along a supply of high-quality latex condoms; those available abroad may be of lesser quality and more susceptible to leaks and rupture.

Follow-up After Travel

Travelers should be reminded of the importance of continuing malaria chemoprophylaxis for 4 weeks after leaving a malarious area to decrease the possibility of a clinical attack. Travelers should be instructed to alert their health care providers about the possibility of malaria in case a severe illness accompanied by high fever develops weeks, months, or even years after travel in a malaria-endemic area. Many physicians in geographic areas where malaria is not endemic are unfamiliar with the clinical signs and symptoms of a primary malaria attack and may fail to include malaria in the differential diagnosis.[25,44,71] A person who has traveled in a malaria-endemic area and who has taken malaria chemoprophylaxis may not donate blood for 3 years, according to current blood-banking practice.

Diarrhea or any change in normal bowel habits that persists after empirical treatment for traveler's diarrhea should prompt a thorough diagnostic workup. Drug-resistant bacterial infections, intestinal parasites, dietary changes, or hepatitis may account for the prolonged symptoms after return home.[4,7,27,48] However, coincidental manifestations of biliary tract disease, inflammatory bowel disease, or intestinal malignancy must be considered in cases of gastrointestinal illness that elude diagnosis after the first round or two of diagnostic tests have been done.

Unusual skin lesions in returned travelers are often misdiagnosed in medical facilities that do not routinely see immigrants, refugees, and returned travelers. Common exotic infections in returned travelers seeking medical care include cutaneous myiasis (subcutaneous fly larvae), cutaneous larva migrans (migrating dog or cat hookworm larvae), and cutaneous and mucocutaneous leishmaniasis (protozoan parasitic infection).

Secondary bacterial infection is common with all these conditions, and the appearance of the skin lesion may initially seem to improve after institution of standard antibiotic therapy for bacterial skin infection. However, if the skin lesion fails to completely resolve, consultation with a tropical medicine specialist might be helpful. In a series of cases reported to the CDC of cutaneous leishmaniasis in American returned travelers, the average time between seeking initial medical care for a nonhealing skin lesion and the correct diagnosis was 5 months.[31]

Intestinal parasites, especially helminthic or worm infections, can manifest their presence by spontaneous passage of adult worms from the rectum after dwelling for months in an unsuspecting, asymptomatic host. However, a systemic parasitic infection may have signs and symptoms that are not referable to a particular organ system: fever, headache, myalgia, malaise, fatigue, and nausea. The initial differential diagnosis may be broad and includes viral, bacterial, and parasitic infections. The differential diagnosis can be narrowed after the clinician takes into account incubation time, geographic area, immunizations received, malaria chemoprophylaxis taken, dietary habits, insect and rodent exposure, animal bites, and intimate or sexual contact with foreign residents or fellow travelers.

SUMMARY

While the potential for travel-acquired illness during or after travel exists, it appears that pretravel medical preparation and behavior modification can promote travel in good health by reducing risk of many health hazards and enabling the traveler to cope with common travelers' ailments, thus increasing the overall enjoyment of the trip.

APPENDIX A

Resources for Travel Medicine Information

TELEPHONE INFORMATION, HOTLINES, AND AUDIO LIBRARIES

Centers for Disease Control and Prevention
Traveler's Health Hotline: 404-332-4559
Centers for Disease Control and Prevention
FAX Information Number: 404-332-4565
United States Department of State
Citizen's Emergency Center: 202-647-5225
University of Washington Medical Center
Travel Medicine Service Audio Library: 206-548-4888

OFFICIAL REFERENCES

Centers for Disease Control: *Health Information for International Travel,* Washington, DC, U.S. Government Printing Office (revised annually). 202-738-3238.

World Health Organization: *International Travel and Health, Vaccination Requirements and Health Advice,* World Health Organization Publications Center USA, 49 Sheridan Avenue, Albany, NY 12210 (revised annually).

BULLETINS, DIRECTORIES, AND NEWSLETTERS

Alert Diver, The Magazine of the Diver's Alert Network: Wachholz C, editor, D.A.N., Box 3823, Duke University Medical Center, Durham, NC 27710. Telephone 919-684-2948; FAX 919-490-6630.

American Committee on Clinical Tropical Medicine and Traveler's Health Directory of Travel Medicine Clinics: Marcus L, editor: American Society of Tropical Medicine and Hygiene, 148 Highland Avenue, Newton, MA 02165.

Commodores' Bulletin; Seven Seas Cruising Association, Inc., 500 SE 17th Street, Fort Lauderdale, FL 33316.

International Association for Medical Assistance to Travellers Directory of English-Speaking Physicians: IAMAT, 40 Regal Road, Guelph, Ontario, N1K 1B5 (revised periodically). Telephone 519-836-0102; FAX 519-836-3412.

International Association for Medical Assistance to Travellers World Malaria Risk Chart 1993: IAMAT, 40 Regal Road, Guelph, Ontario, N1K 1B5 (revised annually). Telephone 519-836-0102; FAX 519-836-3412.

International Association for Medical Assistance to Travellers World Status of Malaria Medication Availability: IAMAT, 40 Regal Road, Guelph, Ontario, N1K 1B5, July 1991.

International Society of Travel Medicine International Register of Travel Clinics and Advisors: ISTM, P.O. Box 15060, Atlanta, GA 30333-0060.

Morbidity and Mortality Weekly Report, Centers for Disease Control and Prevention, Atlanta, GA 30333. Subscriptions are available through the Massachusetts Medical Society, P.O. Box 9120, Waltham, MA 02254-9120.

The Travel Medicine Advisor Update: Bia F, editor, American Health Consultants, P.O. Box 740056, Atlanta, GA 30374. Telephone 404-262-7436; FAX 404-262-7837.

Travel Medicine News, official publication of the International Society of Travel Medicine: Kozarsky P, editor, P.O. Box 15060, Atlanta, GA 30333-0060.

Tropical Medicine and Hygiene News, official bulletin of the American Society of Tropical Medicine and Hygiene: Western KA, editor, 64343 First Street N.W., Washington, DC 20015. Telephone 202-364-5969; FAX 202-364-5969.

Wilderness Medicine Letter: Wilderness Medical Society, P.O. Box 2463, Indianapolis, IN 46206. Telephone 317-631-1745; FAX 317-634-7817.

TRAVEL HEALTH INSURANCE COMPANIES

Access America: 800-284-8300
Health Care Abroad, Wallach and Co.: 800-237-6615
Tele-Trip: 800-228-9792
Travel Assistance International: 800-821-2828
Travel Guard International: 800-782-5151

REFERENCES

1. Baird JK, Basri H, Purnomo: Resistance to chloroquine by *Plasmodium vivax* in Irian Jaya, Indonesia, *Am J Trop Med Hyg* 44:547, 1991.
2. Bern JL, Kerr L, Stuerchler D: Mefloquine prophylaxis: an overview of spontaneous reports of severe psychiatric reactions and convulsions, *J Trop Med Hyg* 95:167, 1992.
3. Brandt WE: From the World Health Organization: development of dengue and Japanese encephalitis vaccines, *J Infect Dis* 162:577, 1990.
4. Centers for Disease Control: Enterically transmitted non-A non-B hepatitis—Mexico, *MMWR* 36:597, 1987.
5. Centers for Disease Control: Management of patients with suspected viral hemorrhagic fever, *MMWR* 37(S-3):1, 1988.
6. Centers for Disease Control: Use of BCG vaccines in the control of tuberculosis: a joint statement by the ACIP and the Advisory Committee for Elimination of Tuberculosis, *MMWR* 37:663, 1988.
7. Centers for Disease Control: Acute schistosomiasis in U.S. travelers returning from Africa, *MMWR* 39:140, 1990.
8. Centers for Disease Control: Typhoid immunization: recommendations of the Immunization Practices Advisory Committee (ACIP), *MMWR* 39(RR-10):1, 1990.
9. Centers for Disease Control: Diphtheria, tetanus, and pertussis: recommendations for vaccine use and other preventive measures: recommendations of the Immunizations Practices Advisory Committee (ACIP), *MMWR* (RR-10):1, 1991.
10. Centers for Disease Control: Hepatitis B virus: a comprehensive strategy for eliminating transmission in the United States through universal childhood vaccination: recommendations of the Immunization Practices Advisory Committee (ACIP), *MMWR* 40:1, 1991.
11. Centers for Disease Control: Rabies prevention—United States, 1991: recommendations of the Immunization Practices Advisory Committee (ACIP), *MMWR* 40(RR-3):1, 1991.
12. Centers for Disease Control: Update: cholera—Western hemisphere, 1991, *MMWR* 40:860, 1991.
13. Centers for Disease Control: Update on adult immunization: recommendations of the Immunization Practices Advisory Committee (ACIP), *MMWR* 40(RR-12):1, 1991.
14. Centers for Disease Control: Vaccinia (smallpox) vaccine. Recommendations of the Immunization Practices Advisory Committee (ACIP), *MMWR* 40(RR-14):1, 1991.
15. Centers for Disease Control and Prevention: Committee on Immunization Practices (ACIP): use of vaccines and immune globulins in persons with altered immunocompetence, *MMWR* 42(RR-4): 1, 1993.
16. Centers for Disease Control and Prevention: Inactivated Japanese encephalitis virus vaccine: recommendations of the Advisory Committee on Immunization Practices (ACIP), *MMWR* 42(RR-1):1, 1993.
17. Centers for Disease Control and Prevention: Standards for pediatric immunization practices recommended by the National Vaccine Advisory Committee, approved by the U.S. Public Health Service, *MMWR* 42(RR-5):1, 1993.
18. DuPont HL, Ericsson CD: Prevention and treatment of traveler's diarrhea, *N Engl J Med* 328:1821, 1993.
19. DuPont HL et al: Five versus three days of ofloxacin therapy for traveler's diarrhea: a placebo-controlled study, *Antimicrob Agents Chemother* 36:87, 1992.
20. Ericsson CD, DuPont HL: Travelers' diarrhea: approaches to prevention and treatment, *Clin Infect Dis* 16:616, 1993.
21. Ericsson CD et al: Ciprofloxacin or trimethoprim-sulfamethoxazole as initial therapy for traveler's diarrhea, *Ann Intern Med* 106:216, 1987.
22. Ericsson CD et al: Treatment of traveler's diarrhea with sulfamethoxazole and trimethoprim and loperamide, *JAMA* 63:257, 1990.
23. Figueroa-Quintanilla D et al: A controlled trial of bismuth subsalicylate in infants with acute watery diarrheal disease, *N Engl J Med* 328:1653, 1993.
24. Fine PEM, Rodrigues LC: Modern vaccines: mycobacterial diseases, *Lancet* 335:1016, 1990.
25. Froud JRL et al: Imported malaria in the Bronx: review of 51 cases recorded from 1986-1991, *Clin Infect Dis* 15:774, 1992.
26. Gellert G, Wagner G, Ehling LR: Risks of cholera immunisation at port of entry, *Lancet* 337:552, 1991.
27. Guerrant RL, Bobak DA: Bacterial and protozoal gastroenteritis, *N Engl J Med* 325:327, 1991.
28. Hargarten SW, Baker SP: Fatalities in the Peace Corps: a retrospective study: 1962-1983, *JAMA* 254:1326, 1985.
29. Hargarten SW, Baker T, Guptill K: Overseas fatalities of United States citizen travelers: an analysis of deaths related to international travel, *Ann Emerg Med* 20:622, 1991.
30. Hayani KC, Ericsson CD, Pickering LK: Prevention and treatment of diarrhea in the traveling child, *Semin Pediatr Infect Dis* 3:22, 1992.

31. Herwaldt BL, Stokes SL, Juranek DD: American cutaneous leishmaniasis in U.S. travelers, *Ann Intern Med* 118:779, 1993.
32. Hien TT, White NJ: Qinghaosu, *Lancet* 341:603, 1993.
33. Hill D: Illness associated with travel to the developing world. In Lobel HO, Steffen R, Kozarsky P, editors: *Travel medicine 2,* Atlanta, 1992, International Society of Travel Medicine.
34. Hilton E et al: Status of immunity to tetanus, measles, mumps, rubella, and polio among U.S. travelers, *Ann Intern Med* 115:32, 1991.
35. Hoffman SL: Diagnosis, treatment, and prevention of malaria, *Med Clin North Am* 76:1327, 1993.
36. Holmes KK: The changing epidemiology of HIV transmission, *Hosp Pract*, Nov 1991, p 153.
37. *International certificates of vaccination,* Washington, DC, US Government Printing Office.
38. Jong EC: Immunizations for international travelers, *Med Clin North Am* 76:1277, 1992.
39. Jong EC, McMullen R: General advice for the international traveler, *Infect Dis Clin North Am* 6:275, 1992.
40. Jong EC, McMullen R: Immunization needs of Americans attending a university-based travel medicine clinic from July 1980 to June 1990. In Lobel HO, Steffen R, Kozarsky P, editors: *Travel medicine 2,* Atlanta, 1992, International Society of Travel Medicine.
41. Kamolratanakul P et al: The effectiveness of chemoprophylaxis against malaria for non-immune migrant workers in eastern Thailand, *Trans R Soc Trop Med Hyg* 83:313, 1989.
42. Karwacki JJ et al: Proguanil-sulphonamide for malaria chemoprophylaxis, *Trans R Soc Trop Med Hyg* 84:55, 1990.
43. Keystone JS: Prevention of malaria, *Drugs* 39:337, 1990.
44. Lackritz EM et al: Imported *Plasmodium falciparum* malaria in American travelers to Africa—implications for prevention strategies, *JAMA* 265:383, 1991.
45. Laga M: Risk of HIV infection and other STDs for travelers. In Lobel HO, Steffen R, Kozarsky P, editors: *Travel medicine 2,* Atlanta, 1992, International Society of Travel Medicine.
46. LeDuc JW: Epidemiology of hemorrhagic fever viruses, *Rev Infect Dis* 11(suppl 4):S730, 1989.
47. Lobel HO et al: Effectiveness and tolerance of long-term malaria prophylaxis with mefloquine—need for a better dosing regimen, *JAMA* 265:361, 1991.
48. McAuley JB, Michelson MK, Schantz PM: Trichinella infection in travelers, *J Infect Dis* 164:1013, 1991.
49. McMullen R, Jong EC: Incidence of antibody to hepatitis A among employees of a multinational corporation: implications for immunoglobulin prophylaxis. In Steffen R et al, editors: *Travel medicine,* Berlin, 1989, Springer-Verlag.
50. McNeil JG et al: Central European tick-borne encephalitis: assessment of risk for persons in the armed services and vacationers, *J Infect Dis* 152:650, 1985.
51. Morris HH, Estes ML: Traveler's amnesia: transient global amnesia secondary to triazolam, *JAMA* 258:945, 1987.
52. National Institutes of Health Consensus Development Conference: Travelers' diarrhea, *JAMA* 253:2700, 1985.
53. Navaratnam U et al: Chemosuppression of malaria by the triple combination mefloquine/sulfadoxine/pyrimethamine: a field trial in an endemic area in Malaysia, *Trans R Soc Trop Med Hyg* 83:755, 1989.
54. Nosten F et al: Prospective electrocardiogram study of Karen patients with falciparum malaria, *Lancet* 341:1054, 1993.
55. Pappaioanou M et al: Antibody response to pre-exposure human diploid cell rabies vaccine given concurrently with chloroquine, *N Engl J Med* 314:280, 1986.
56. Poland JD et al: Evaluation of the potency and safety of inactivated Japanese encephalitis vaccine in US inhabitants, *J Infect Dis* 161:878, 1990.
57. Radandt JM, Marchbanks CR, Dudley MN: Interactions of fluoroquinolones with other drugs: mechanisms, variability, clinical significance, and management, *Clin Infect Dis* 14:272, 1992.
58. Ryan CA, Hargrett-Brown NT, Blake PA: *Salmonella typhi* infections in the United States, 1975-1984: increasing role of foreign travel, *Rev Infect Dis* 11:1, 1989.
59. Schuurkamp GJ, Spicer PE, Kereu RK: Chloroquine-resistant *Plasmodium vivax* in Papua New Guinea, *Trans R Soc Trop Med Hyg* 86:121, 1992.
60. Schwartz IK, Lackritz EM, Patchen LC: Chloroquine-resistant *Plasmodium vivax* from Indonesia (letter), *N Engl J Med* 324:927, 1991.
61. Sexton JD et al: Permethrin-impregnated curtains and bed-nets prevent malaria in western Kenya, *Am J Trop Med Hyg* 43:11, 1990.
62. Shanks GD et al: Malaria chemoprophylaxis using proguanil/dapsone combination on the Thai-Cambodian border, *Am J Trop Med Hyg* 46:643, 1992.
63. Steffen R et al: Health problems after travel to developing countries, *J Infect Dis* 156:84, 1987.
64. Steffen R et al: Malaria chemoprophylaxis among European tourists to tropical Africa: use, adverse reactions and efficacy, *Bull WHO* 68:313, 1990.
65. Swerdlow DL, Ries AA: Cholera in the Americas: guidelines for the clinician, *JAMA* 267:1495, 1992.
66. Tauxe RV et al: Antimicrobial resistance of Shigella isolates in the USA: the importance of international travelers, *J Infect Dis* 162:1107, 1990.
67. Taylor DN et al: Treatment of travelers' diarrhea: ciprofloxacin plus loperamide compared with ciprofloxacin alone, *Ann Intern Med* 114:731, 1991.
68. Tsai TF: Arboviral infections: general considerations for prevention, diagnosis, and treatment in travelers, *Semin Pediatr Infect Dis* 3:62, 1992.
69. Weinke T et al: Neuropsychiatric side effects after the use of mefloquine, *Am J Trop Med Hyg* 45:86, 1991.
70. Wilde H et al: Rabies in Thailand: 1990, *Rev Infect Dis* 13:644, 1991.
71. Winters RA, Murray HW: Malaria—the mime revisited: fifteen more years of experience at a New York City teaching hospital, *Am J Med* 93:243, 1991.
72. Wyler D: Malaria chemoprohylaxis for the traveler, *N Engl J Med* 329:31, 1993.
73. Wyler D: Malaria: Overview and update, *Clin Infect Dis* 16:449, 1993.

ADDITIONAL RECOMMENDED READINGS

Centers for Disease Control: *Health Information for International Travel, 1992,* Washington, DC, 1992, US Government Printing Office.

Gardner P, editor: Infectious diseases in international travelers, *Infect Dis Clin North Am,* vol 6, June, 1992.

Goldsmith R, Heyneman D, editors: *Tropical medicine and parasitology,* San Mateo, Calif, 1989, Appleton & Lange.

Jong EC, editor: *The travel and tropical medicine manual,* Philadelphia, 1987, WB Saunders.

Jong E, Keystone J, McMullen R, editors: *The travel medicine advisor,* Atlanta, 1991, American Health Consultants.

Lobel HO, Steffen R, Kozarsky P, editors: *Travel medicine 2,* Atlanta, 1992, International Society of Travel Medicine.

Steffen R et al, editors: *Travel medicine,* Berlin, 1989, Springer-Verlag.

Strickland GT: *Hunter's tropical medicine,* Philadelphia, 1991, WB Saunders.

Wilson ME: *A world guide to infections,* New York, 1991, Oxford University Press.

Wolfe MS, editor: *Health hints for the tropics,* ed 11, 1993, American Society of Tropical Medicine and Hygiene.

Wolfe MS, editor: Travel medicine, *Med Clin North Am,* vol 76, November 1992.

45 FOREIGN TRAVEL AND EXOTIC DISEASES

Jay D. Wenger
James W. Kazura

Major viral infections
Major bacterial infections
Major protozoan infections
Major helminthic infections

Travel to many tropical or subtropical areas of the world and to those with poor hygienic conditions exposes the traveler to many infectious diseases that are uncommonly or never encountered in the United States, Canada, and most areas of Europe.[61,111] This chapter focuses on infections with the greatest clinical significance in terms of morbidity and mortality, such as falciparum malaria and Japanese B encephalitis. Other chapters discuss additional important infections (for example, amebiasis in water-borne diarrhea and trichinosis as a zoonosis) and specific sources of information for travelers.

Major Viral Infections

A vast number of viral agents cause disease. This section describes the serious viral infections still prevalent overseas for which appropriate preventive and therapeutic measures can be taken. These include the viral hemorrhagic fevers, viral hepatitis, and Japanese B encephalitis.

VIRAL HEMORRHAGIC FEVERS

A diverse group of RNA viruses can produce the hemorrhagic fever syndrome (see Box 45-1). Although clinical presentations vary with different etiologic agents, the syndrome is usually characterized by fever, headache, myalgias, and malaise, which develop over several hours to 3 to 4 days. In the full-blown hemorrhagic fever syndrome, these early disease manifestations are followed by hemorrhagic signs, including petechiae and bleeding from the gums and gastrointestinal tract.[50,71] Loss of plasma volume is usually manifested by an increased hematocrit value, although hypotension and shock may occur in some individuals. Elevated blood urea nitrogen and creatinine levels herald renal dysfunction. Death most often follows intractable hypotension, bleeding, electrolyte disturbances, and renal failure.

YELLOW FEVER

The clinical syndrome now known as yellow fever was not recognized by European physicians until the late 1490s. Initially described by Columbus in the West Indies, large-scale epidemics were later observed throughout the Americas and tropical Africa in the 1700s and 1800s.[86] After epidemic yellow fever in Texas, Louisiana, and Tennessee took 20,000 lives in the 1880s, the Yellow Fever Commission was organized to study the problem. Identification of the mosquito vector, *Aedes aegypti,* was followed by massive campaigns to eradicate breeding sites. This led to virtual elimination of urban yellow fever from the Americas. The last endemically acquired case of yellow fever in the continental United States was reported in 1911. However, the impossibility of eradicating jungle virus reservoirs has resulted in 50 to 300 and 100 to 200 cases reported annually from South America and tropical Africa, respectively.[32,88] Larger outbreaks secondary to resurgent vector populations have occurred in recent years in tropical West Africa.[81,123a]

Virology and Pathophysiology

Yellow fever is a single-stranded RNA flavivirus. Strain differences are of little clinical relevance, although they may be of use in epidemiologic studies. The pathophysiologic mechanisms operating in viral hemorrhagic fevers are not well defined. In general, viral replication occurs at the site of inoculation. After the virus spreads to lymph nodes and monocyte-rich organs, further reproduction results in massive viremia.

The liver is the principal target organ. Pathologic studies show coagulative necrosis of hepatocytes and the appearance of various markers of cell involvement (Councilman

BOX 45-1
MAJOR VIRAL HEMORRHAGIC FEVERS

Yellow fever
Dengue fever
Hemorrhagic fever and renal syndrome nephropathia epidemica
Lassa fever; Argentine and Bolivian hemorrhagic fevers
Ebola virus
Marburg virus
Crimean-Congo hemorrhagic fever

and Torres bodies). However, physiologic derangements are usually much more severe than expected for the extent of hepatic damage seen on pathologic examination. Perivascular edema and occasional focal bleeding occur in kidney, heart, and brain, but these changes are less severe than expected for the degree of clinical disease.

Ecology and Epidemiology

In the Americas, primates in the forest canopy serve as hosts of the yellow fever virus. Infection is transmitted by mosquitoes of the genus *Haemogogus*. Since this vector does not travel far from the forest, jungle yellow fever occurs when humans enter jungle areas or the forest border zones. Urban yellow fever involves a different vector, *A. aegypti*. This mosquito is highly anthropophilic, lives in and around human habitations, and prefers domestic water storage containers for breeding. The presence of a large population of *A. aegypti* places an urban area at significant risk for epidemic spread of yellow fever once the virus is introduced from a nearby forest area. In Africa the presence of larger numbers of mosquito species that can serve as vectors has hindered a complete understanding of the ecology of the disease.

At present, both the Americas and Africa have a constant low level of jungle yellow fever (5 to 500 cases per year) because of the inability to eradicate either the monkey reservoir or the mosquito vector. Some suggest that these rates are underestimated by at least tenfold.[32,71,81] Persons at risk include workers or travelers in or near the tropical rainforest canopy. Urban yellow fever has been eliminated in the Western Hemisphere through massive anti-*Aedes* campaigns. Less intense vector control measures and a more complex ecology make eradication of urban yellow fever in Africa less certain. Introduction of *Aedes albopictus,* an aggressive anthropophilic dengue vector from Southeast Asia, and reemergence of *A. aegypti* into the Americas[25a,80] raise the specter of increased yellow fever (and dengue fever) transmission in the Western Hemisphere.

Clinical Presentation

Although yellow fever may appear as an undifferentiated viral syndrome, classic disease is characterized by a triphasic pattern. The infection phase begins with sudden onset of headache, fever, and malaise, often accompanied by bradycardia and conjunctival suffusion. After approximately 3 to 4 days, patients often experience a brief remission. Within 24 hours, however, the intoxication phase develops, characterized by jaundice, recrudescent fever, prostration, and, in severe cases, hypotension, shock, oliguria, and obtundation. Hemorrhage is usually manifest as hematemesis; however, bleeding from multiple sites may occur. Signs of a poor prognosis include early onset of the intoxication phase, hypotension, severe hemorrhage with disseminated intravascular coagulation (DIC), renal failure, shock, and coma. Diagnosis in the infection phase is difficult. With development of the classic syndrome, the differential diagnosis narrows somewhat but still includes malaria, leptospirosis, typhoid fever, typhus, Q fever, viral hepatitis, and other viral hemorrhagic fevers. The standard means of diagnosis is evaluation for neutralizing antibodies in acute and convalescent sera (available through state health departments in the United States). Several new systems for early detection of IgM or viral antigen are now being evaluated for more rapid diagnosis.[82] A specimen of whole blood (at –70° C on dry ice) should be sent to the state health laboratory for isolation. Growth of the virus is possible in a number of systems, including Vero cells and infant mice. The virus is most easily isolated in the first 4 days of fever.

Management

Appropriate management of viral hemorrhagic fevers requires awareness of the geographic distribution of the disease and travel history of the patient. In the first several days of infection, differentiation of a viral hemorrhagic fever from other infectious diseases is nearly impossible. However, the occurrence of an undifferentiated febrile syndrome in a traveler from a yellow fever endemic area warrants a careful physical examination, thick and thin blood smears to rule out malaria, and blood cultures for bacterial pathogens *(Salmonella typhi)*. Progression to the intoxication phase or any sign of volume disturbance, renal failure, or hemorrhage mandates immediate admission to an intensive care unit.

There are no effective antiviral therapies for yellow fever. Supportive care should address several important problem areas. Fever should be controlled with acetaminophen, not with salicylates. Evaluation of volume status should include Swan-Ganz or central venous pressure monitoring to direct volume expansion and use of vasopressor agents. Calculation of fractional excretion of urinary sodium may help to differentiate prerenal azotemia (for which volume expansion is appropriate) from acute tubular necrosis (which may require temporary dialysis). Plasma volume loss may contribute to serious electrolyte disturbances, necessitating close observation of serum electrolytes and arterial blood gases. Rapid correction of these abnormalities, which commonly include hyperkalemia and acidosis, is essential. Hypoglycemia is presumably a result of impaired hepatic gluconeogenesis.

Serial coagulation studies (including platelet count, prothrombin time, partial thromboplastin time, fibrinogen, and fibrin degradation products) should be obtained.[5,24,30] Whole blood or fresh-frozen plasma is indicated to maintain the prothrombin time and hematocrit at reasonable levels. If DIC is documented, the use of heparin may be considered. No controlled trials have documented the effectiveness of heparin in yellow fever, but the benefit of heparin was suggested in a small number of patients with DIC.[5,104] This approach remains controversial. To reduce the risk of upper gastrointestinal hemorrhage, H_2 blockers have been suggested. Although the efficacy of intensive care treatment has not been studied in patients with yellow fever, clinical experience with dengue shock syndrome suggests that similar benefits might be obtained.

Prevention

Avoidance of this potentially fatal infection is possible through use of the yellow fever vaccine. The vaccine strain 17D is an attenuated live virus grown in chicken embryoes. Greater than 95% of vaccinees achieve significant antibody levels. Repeat vaccinations are recommended every 10 years, although persistent antibody titers have been detected as long as 30 to 40 years after vaccination.[22a] The vaccine is well tolerated, with headache or malaise occurring in less than 10% of vaccinees. Rare allergic side effects occur primarily in persons with hypersensitivity to eggs. The vaccine is not recommended in the first 6 months of life or in other situations where live virus vaccines are contraindicated. Although pregnant women have received the vaccine without adverse effect to themselves or their infants, it is not recommended for use in this group because of the theoretical risk of interference with embryogenesis. Other means of reducing the risk of yellow fever (and any mosquito-borne disease) include liberal use of mosquito repellent and netting in endemic areas.

Treatment of severe yellow fever is difficult and often unsuccessful. Avoidance through mosquito protection measures and administration of the highly effective vaccine before entry into endemic areas is of utmost importance.

DENGUE

Dengue fever has been reported since the late 1700s. Since World War II, increased attention has been focused on the dengue virus, largely as a result of recognition of dengue hemorrhagic fever (DHF) and dengue shock syndrome (DSS). First noted in Southeast Asia, DHF and DSS have attained worldwide distribution in the last 30 years.[18,25a,50]

Virology and Pathophysiology

The etiologic agent is a single-stranded RNA flavivirus, which may be one of four serotypes, denoted dengue 1 through 4. As with yellow fever, local viral replication is followed by dissemination to lymphocyte- and macrophage-rich areas, where most of the reproductive activity occurs. Infection with one virus serotype provides long-lasting protection against that type only. For the dengue 2 serotype, previous infection with a heterologous serotype may result in a more severe clinical course than noted in those experiencing dengue 2 infection without such a history. Nonneutralizing antibodies produced in response to infection with other dengue serotypes aid entrance of the virus into host macrophages.[33] Although much of DHF and DSS may result from "immune enhancement,"[49] it is clear that severe DHF and DSS occur with other serotypes and do not require previous infection with a heterologous dengue virus serotype.[83,102,103] Pathologic studies of DHF and DSS show hemorrhage, congestion, and perivascular edema of multiple organs. The liver may show areas of focal necrosis. As with yellow fever, the extent of pathologic findings does not correspond to severity of the clinical course.

Ecology and Epidemiology

A. aegypti is the principal vector for dengue viruses worldwide. In the Americas and Asia, viral transmission is maintained through a mosquito-human cycle without a major animal reservoir. Monkey carriers have been identified in Africa and Asia, but their importance in transmission is unclear. *A. albopictus,* an anthropophilic dengue vector from Southeast Asia, has also been recognized recently in the Western Hemisphere. Both of these mosquitoes are capable of large-scale transmission to humans in endemic areas. At present dengue is endemic in tropical and subtropical Asia, Africa, South America, and the Caribbean basin. In the early 1920s, large epidemics occurred in Texas, where dengue infections were reported in 500,000 inhabitants. In the last 30 years endemic transmission on the mainland United States has been documented only in Texas; however, between 1986 and 1992, 157 cases of dengue were confirmed in U.S. travelers by the Centers for Disease Control and Prevention (CDC).[25a]

Clinical Presentation

Most dengue infections appear either as an undifferentiated viral syndrome with fever and mild respiratory or gastrointestinal symptoms or as dengue ("break-bone") fever with fever, severe headache, and myalgias. After several days, dengue fever is often accompanied by a maculopapular or morbilliform rash spreading outward from the chest. Lymphadenopathy and leukopenia occur during this phase of the illness. More severe cases of dengue disease are referred to as either DHF or DSS. These syndromes are classified grades I to IV, according to World Health Organization (WHO) guidelines.[122] In cases of grade I DHF, the only hemorrhagic manifestation is a positive tourniquet test, in which inflation of a tourniquet to midway between systolic and diastolic pressure leads to development of petechiae distal to the tourniquet. A complete blood cell count shows a decreased platelet count and an increase in hematocrit value. Grade II DHF is defined as the above plus hemorrhage from any site. DSS (grade III) includes clammy skin, hypotension, or a narrow pulse pressure (less than 20 mm Hg) in a patient with DHF. An undetectable blood pressure defines grade IV DHF and DSS. Most studies have noted DHF and DSS primarily in infants and young children, usually with a history or serologic evidence of previous heterologous dengue infection.[50] Two cases of DSS in American travelers involved young children (ages 7 years and 16 months).[83,102,103] However, DHF and DSS may occur in adults. Of the 10 cases in the 1986 Puerto Rico outbreak, four were in adults, and of the two deaths, one was in an adult.[18]

Management

Awareness of the local epidemiology of DHF and DSS, especially the occurrence of other cases, is important in establishing the diagnosis. The diagnosis may be confirmed by a fourfold rise in antibodies detected in acute and convalescent sera or by measurement of antidengue IgM antibodies. In the United States, virus isolation from serum can be arranged through state health departments.[25a] Management is symptomatic. In the dengue fever syndrome, acetaminophen may be given for fever and myalgias. Salicylates should not be used. Hydration should be vigorously maintained.

Selected patients with grade I or II DHF may be managed as outpatients. However, outpatient care requires careful monitoring of hematocrit value, platelets, and electrolytes. If significant bleeding develops, hospitalization is appropriate for rapid and continuous assessment. Progression to DSS (grade III or IV) is a medical emergency and requires immediate hospitalization. There is no specific therapy, and supportive measures described in the section on treatment of severe yellow fever are appropriate.

LASSA FEVER

Lassa fever was first recognized in 1969, when several nurses caring for febrile patients at a mission hospital in Nigeria became ill.[37] Since that time, seroepidemiologic studies have established a large area of endemicity and a broad spectrum of clinical manifestations of infection.

Epidemiology

The principal animal host for this virus is a rat, *Mastomys natalensis,* which prefers living in and around human dwellings. The rodents become chronically infected, secreting viral particles for long periods. Natural infection in humans occurs after rodent contamination of food and drink, inhalation of aerosolized rodent secretions, or contact with rodent material through skin abrasions. Lassa fever has been reported in several areas of sub-Saharan West Africa, and large outbreaks have been noted in Nigeria, Sierra Leone, and Liberia.[71,74] Complete seroprevalence data are lacking, making definition of an endemic area impossible at this time. Secondary human infection has been reported and may occur after contact with infected secretions.

Virology and Pathophysiology

Lassa virus is a single-stranded RNA arenavirus. Proliferation and dissemination presumably occur after initial replication at the inoculation site. As with the flaviviral diseases, the extent of end organ involvement noted at autopsy does not account for the rapid death of infected patients. Recent work in an animal model provides evidence for platelet dysfunction and an endothelial cell defect in shock caused by Lassa fever virus.[34,35] DIC, believed to be a major cause of bleeding and death in patients with other viral hemorrhagic fevers, appears to play a relatively minor role in arenavirus infections.[5,29]

Clinical Presentation

A seroepidemiologic study indicates that most seroconversions to Lassa virus are not accompanied by any obvious symptoms.[74] Only 5% to 14% of seroconverters experienced a febrile illness, and the fatality/infection ratio was 1 to 2:100. Patients hospitalized with Lassa fever show a distinct clinical syndrome. After insidious onset of headache, fever, and malaise, purulent pharyngitis often develops. A complaint of retrosternal chest pain, possibly a result of pharyngitis and esophagitis, suggests the diagnosis. A recent case-control study found the combined presence of retrosternal chest pain, fever, pharyngitis, and proteinuria to be the best predictor of Lassa fever.[73] Hemorrhagic complications (hematemesis, vaginal bleeding, hematuria, lower gastrointestinal bleeding, and epistaxis) were seen in less than 25% of patients with Lassa fever. Nonfatal disease usually begins to resolve in 8 to 10 days. The combined presence of fever, sore throat, and vomiting was associated with a poor prognosis (relative risk of death equals 5.5). Terminal stages of fatal disease were accompanied by hypotension, encephalopathy, and often respiratory distress caused by stridor (presumably secondary to laryngeal edema). Laboratory indicators of poor prognosis include an admission serum aspartate aminotransferase (AST) of greater than 150 IU/L (55% death rate) and viremia greater than 10^4 $TCID_{50}$ ($TCID_{50}$ is the titer at which virus will infect 50% of tissue culture test plates).

Diagnosis

In the early stages of Lassa fever establishing an accurate diagnosis is extremely difficult. As the classic clinical syndrome develops, differentiation from other viral hemorrhagic fevers still depends on serologic confirmation. Serologic diagnosis is made by indirect fluorescent antibody analysis of acute and convalescent sera or detection of Lassa-specific IgM. Clotted whole blood may be sent to the

CDC for viral culture if handled appropriately. If the diagnosis is suspected, the CDC should be contacted immediately for assistance in diagnosis, isolation, and management.

Management

Four viral hemorrhagic fevers—Lassa, Marburg, Ebola, and Crimean-Congo—have been associated with outbreaks of fatal person-to-person spread.[21,39] Secondary infection occurs through direct contact with infected persons or their secretions. The role of aerosols in person-to-person spread is unclear. Blood and body fluids should be considered infectious. In light of the potentially fatal outcome of Lassa fever and the relative ease of transmission, the CDC has published specific recommendations for management of possible or confirmed cases.[21] If a person has (1) a compatible clinical syndrome (especially pharyngitis, vomiting, conjunctivitis, diarrhea, and hemorrhage or shock); (2) a relevant travel history, including time spent in an endemic area; and (3) prior contact within 3 weeks of presentation with a person or animal from an endemic area suspected of having a viral hemorrhagic fever, he or she should be isolated and local, state, and federal (CDC) health officials contacted. Ideally, an isolation unit with negative air pressure vented outside the hospital should be employed. However, lack of a negative-pressure room is not a reason for transfer to another medical care facility.

Transmission of Lassa fever virus to medical and nursing staff can be prevented by the use of routine blood and body fluid precautions (such as those employed in caring for patients infected with human immunodeficiency virus [HIV]) and strict barrier nursing.[52] Barrier nursing includes wearing gloves, gown, mask, shoe covers, and, if there is risk of splashing fluids, goggles whenever entering the patient's room. Decontamination of solid articles and rooms may be accomplished with 0.5% sodium hypochlorite solution. Full recommendations for the management of patients with viral hemorrhagic fever have been published by the CDC.[21]

Supportive care as described in the treatment section for severe yellow fever is indicated for patients with signs and symptoms suggestive of a poor prognosis, including manifestations of significant hemorrhage, volume disturbance, or hypotension. In addition to supportive measures, an effective antiviral compound, intravenous ribavirin, is now available.[72] This drug should be administered as soon as the diagnosis is suspected and is significantly more effective if given during the first 6 days of fever. Ribavirin should be administered as a 30 mg/kg intravenous loading dose, followed by 16 mg/kg intravenously every 6 hours for 4 days. Then 8 mg/kg is given intravenously every 8 hours for 6 days. Persons having significant contact with a patient with Lassa fever (mucous membrane contact or a penetrating wound contaminated with infected material) should receive prophylactic ribavirin, 250 mg by mouth three times a day for 10 days.[21]

Argentine and Bolivian hemorrhagic fevers are endemic to the Pampas of Argentina and the Bolivian plateau, respectively.[71,79] Both are arenaviruses causing infection of humans through contact with infected rodents. Disease occurs primarily in rural areas. The clinical symptoms are similar to those of other viral hemorrhagic fevers. Management guidelines given for yellow fever may be followed. Person-to-person spread has not been significant. Strict isolation (such as is suggested for Lassa, Ebola, Marburg, and Crimean-Congo hemorrhagic fevers) is not required, although instituting enteric precautions may be advisable.

EBOLA AND MARBURG VIRUSES

Ebola and Marburg viruses are closely related large RNA viruses. They cause severe viral hemorrhagic fever syndromes with high mortality rates. Both are endemic in areas of central and southern Africa, with Ebola virus seropositivity noted in Sudan, Zaire, the Central African Republic, and Kenya. Marburg disease is found in South Africa, Zimbabwe, and Kenya. Although Marburg disease was associated with contact with African green monkeys during the initial outbreak in 1967,[75] no clear animal reservoir has been defined for either virus. Person-to-person transmission, primarily through contaminated needles and contact with infected persons, has been well documented.[2,53,75]

Pathophysiology and Clinical Presentation

Marburg and Ebola viruses presumably act through pathophysiologic mechanisms similar to other viral hemorrhagic fevers. Work with a primate model of Ebola virus infection found no evidence for DIC and suggested the possibility of platelet dysfunction and endothelial cell defects as important in the creation of a capillary leak syndrome leading to multisystem failure.[35]

Patients have fever, headache, and myalgias. Diarrhea and abdominal pain occur commonly. In many patients, rash, conjunctivitis, sore throat, and chest pain appear early in the disease. As in other hemorrhagic fevers, fatal courses are marked by hemorrhage, hypotension, shock, and electrolyte abnormalities. The striking mortality noted in various outbreaks (25% for Marburg virus and 55% to 88% for Ebola virus) emphasize the need for intensive supportive care.

Diagnosis

If these diseases are suspected, strict isolation procedures should be instituted and the local health authorities and CDC notified immediately. Although anecdotal reports have suggested efficacy of administration of immune sera, this has not been consistently seen in experimental studies, and at present no specific antiviral therapy exists for Marburg or Ebola virus infection.[21] Care is supportive, and the therapeutic considerations given for treatment of severe yellow fever should be followed. Two patients with documented DIC and Marburg virus infection were given heparin and survived.[39]

CRIMEAN-CONGO HEMORRHAGIC FEVER

Virology and Epidemiology

The etiologic agent of Crimean-Congo hemorrhagic fever (CCHF) is a bunyavirus. Ixodid ticks serve as both reservoirs and vectors of the virus. Infection in humans results from tick bites or direct contact with infected secretions from crushed ticks, animals, or humans. Most naturally acquired cases occur in persons working with or spending time near domestic goats, sheep, or cattle, on which ticks usually feed.[26,44] Disease has been identified in southeastern Europe, south central Asia, the Middle East, and much of Africa.[1,44] Nosocomial transmission through contact with infected body fluids has been well documented.[1,115]

Pathophysiology and Clinical Presentation

Pathophysiologic mechanisms are presumably similar to those of other hemorrhagic fevers. One in five infections results in clinical disease.[44] Among those clinically ill, mortality ranges from 15% in sporadic cases to 70% in rare hospital outbreaks.[1,44]

Diagnosis

The diagnosis can be confirmed with acute and convalescent serologic evaluation for a fourfold rise in IgG antibody titers as measured by the CDC. The virus can be cultured from whole blood if it is drawn during the first week of symptoms and kept on dry ice (or at –70° C) during shipment.

Management

Initial management is similar to that for Lassa, Marburg, and Ebola viruses, with strict patient isolation and notification of health authorities. Supportive therapy should be instituted as discussed for yellow fever. Although not confirmed in clinical trials, ribavirin has good activity in vitro against CCHF virus. The CDC recommends that patients believed to have CCHF receive intravenous ribavirin in the doses suggested for the treatment of Lassa fever.[21] Persons in contact with CCHF patients should receive prophylactic ribavirin as suggested for Lassa fever contacts.

HEMORRHAGIC FEVER WITH RENAL SYNDROME

Hemorrhagic fever with renal syndrome (HFRS) first came to the attention of Western medical science during the Korean War, when febrile illness accompanied by bleeding and renal failure developed in 3000 United Nations troops.[123] Mortality ranged from 5% to 10%. A similar, although much less severe, syndrome ("nephropathia epidemica") had been recognized in Scandinavia since the 1930s.

Epidemiology

The agent of HFRS causes chronic nondebilitating infections of rodents, and human infection is initiated by contact with rodent secretions or inhalation of aerosolized rodent material. The disease occurs most commonly in rural areas, although occasional urban outbreaks, presumably with the common house rat as vector, have been described.[68,123] Cases have been described most frequently from the Far East, including China, Korea, Japan, and the Soviet Union, but the disease also occurs in eastern Europe. A recent epidemiologic study from China found the highest rates of infection in men who engaged in heavy farm work and slept on the ground (rather than on raised wooden beds).[125]

Virology and Pathophysiology

The etiologic agent of HFRS is the prototype hantavirus, Hantaan virus, a member of the bunyavirus family. A related hantavirus, the Puumala agent, is the apparent cause of the more benign nephropathia epidemica. Other closely related viruses can cause similar, although less frequently recognized syndromes. Seoul virus causes a milder form of HFRS in the Far East, and a recently described severe HFRS-like syndrome in eastern Europe has been attributed to a related virus.[75]

Clinical Presentation

As with most viral hemorrhagic fevers, infection may be asymptomatic or accompanied by a mild nonspecific illness. In the classic severe form the initial febrile phase is associated with petechiae, proteinuria, and abdominal pain. After 3 to 5 days a hypotensive phase occurs with decreased platelet counts and more significant hemorrhagic phenomena. An oliguric phase follows with concomitant electrolyte abnormalities. Subsequently a diuretic phase develops, which usually begins 10 days after the onset of illness. Death occurs with hemorrhage, hypotension, and pulmonary edema, presumably secondary to fluid overload and renal failure. With modern management the case-fatality rate of classic HFRS is about 5%.[123] The more benign nephropathia epidemica syndrome has a case-fatality rate of less than 1%. In this disease hypotension, shock, and hemorrhagic manifestations are rare.

Diagnosis

The diagnosis of HFRS or nephropathia epidemica is confirmed by indirect fluorescent or enzyme-linked immunosorbent assay (ELISA) serum antibody studies of acute and convalescent sera. Specific IgM antibody determination may also be useful. These studies are performed by the CDC. Virus isolation is difficult and not recommended.

Management

Care of patients with HFRS is supportive and should follow the guidelines given for yellow fever. With HFRS, renal dysfunction occurs early and may require institution of dialysis soon after diagnosis to prevent fluid overload and to correct electrolyte disturbances. Patients' secretions should be handled with care, and enteric precautions (but not strict isolation) are prudent. Controversy exists about the possibility of person-to-person transmission through direct inoculation. For the hantaviruses, viremia recedes as the clinical phase appears, as evidenced by rising antibody levels. As a result, nosocomial transmission or hematogenous transmission with hantavirus infections has not been documented.[125]

JAPANESE B ENCEPHALITIS

Japanese B encephalitis has been known in Japan since the 1920s. It is the only arboviral encephalitis for which an effective inactivated vaccine has been developed. The use of vaccine in Japan since the 1960s has resulted in a significant decrease in the disease rate.

Epidemiology

Rice field–breeding mosquitoes serve as the vectors for Japanese B encephalitis. In addition to humans, birds and pigs can be infected. Pigs play an important role as amplifying hosts, producing high-grade viremias from which mosquitoes are infected in large numbers, facilitating infection in humans. Most infections in endemic areas are in children, whereas infection may occur in all age groups of previously unexposed populations. At present, Japanese B encephalitis transmission may occur in India, Southeast Asia, China, Korea, Indonesia, the far western Pacific region, eastern Russia, and Japan.[114]

Virology and Pathophysiology

Japanese B encephalitis is caused by a neurotropic flavivirus. After initial replication near the mosquito bite, viremia occurs, which if prolonged may seed infection to the brain.[10] The cytopathologic effect of the flavivirus is believed to cause nerve cell destruction and necrosis.

Clinical Presentation

Most infections do not cause clinical illness, and it has been suggested that only 1 in 300 infections results in encephalitis. Many patients recall a mild undifferentiated febrile illness, which probably coincides with the viremic phase of infection. Patients experiencing encephalitis often report a similar prodrome. The encephalitis syndrome is not easily distinguishable from other arboviral encephalitides. The patient usually complains of headache, lethargy, fever, and confusion and may display tremors or seizures. Reported mortality of persons with clinical encephalitis ranges from 10% to 50%.[114] One clinical series suggested that the presence on admission of (1) unresponsiveness to pain; (2) low levels of anti–Japanese B encephalitis virus IgG or IgM antibodies (in serum or cerebrospinal fluid [CSF]); or (3) virus in CSF culture were associated with subsequent death.[10] Of the 16 patients with fatal disease in this series, all died within 7 days of hospitalization.

Diagnosis

Acute and convalescent serologic studies for antibody (virus neutralization or hemagglutination inhibition assays) provide the only reliable method of diagnosis. Paired sera should be sent for these assays through state health departments. Sensitive assays for determinations of IgG and IgM antibodies in serum and CSF have been developed[8,9] but are not yet widely available. Since most patients seek treatment long after the viremic phase, blood cultures are rarely positive for the virus and CSF cultures are often positive only in patients with a very poor prognosis.

Management

There is no specific therapy for this disease. Supportive care may require an intensive care unit. Since the virus is present in body fluids, especially CSF, blood and body fluid precautions should be considered. An effective inactivated vaccine, used successfully for 20 years in Japan, is recommended for travelers to endemic areas in the transmission season who will be staying for a month or longer. The vaccine must be given in three doses, at 0, 7, and 30 days.[25]

HEPATITIS

Although infectious hepatitis has been a well-known clinical entity for hundreds of years, only in the last few decades has identification of specific viral pathogens been possible. Since widespread use of the anti–hepatitis A antibody test for diagnosis of hepatitis A became a reality in the early 1980s, the spectrum of disease has been increasingly understood.

Epidemiology

Hepatitis A virus is transmitted primarily through the fecal-oral route, either by person-to-person contact or by ingestion of contaminated food or water. Popular food items associated with outbreaks are raw or undercooked clams and shellfish. Cohorts of homosexual males have higher rates of seropositivity for hepatitis A virus, which may represent another form of fecal-oral spread. Occasional cases are associated with exposure to nonhuman primates. Transmission by blood transfusion has been reported,[85] but this is an uncommon source of infection. Hepatitis A is endemic worldwide, but underdeveloped nations have a significantly higher prevalence. The majority of persons in these areas show serologic evidence of past infection with hepatitis A virus. Several recent studies suggest that hepatitis is the most common serious viral infection occurring in travelers and that hepatitis A virus is the most common clearly identified cause.[28,43,47]

Virology and Pathophysiology

Hepatitis A virus is a picornavirus with a single-stranded RNA genome. Although the complete pathophysiologic mechanism has not been delineated, most infections begin with introduction of viral particles into the proximal gastrointestinal tract. Brief viremia precedes seeding of hepatocytes, where viral replication has been documented.[43] With replication, hepatocellular necrosis is accompanied by lymphocytic infiltrates. In the vast majority of cases, hepatic regeneration occurs after acute disease and no significant sequelae are observed.

Clinical Manifestations

The incubation period ranges from 2 to 7 weeks. The infection may be asymptomatic or mild, primarily in children, but also in a minority of adults. The classic syndrome includes early onset of anorexia, followed by nausea, vomiting, fever, and abdominal pain. These symptoms may be accompanied by hepatosplenomegaly. AST and alanine aminotransferase (ALT) levels rise within a few days of the onset of symptoms. In children, AST and ALT return to normal levels in 2 to 3 weeks, whereas in adults, resolution of elevated serum aminotransferase levels may take several months. The bilirubin level rises shortly after AST and ALT elevations. As noted, jaundice usually follows gastrointestinal symptoms by several days to a few weeks. Resolution of jaundice may take another 3 to 4 weeks. The entire syndrome is occasionally preceded by arthralgias and rash, but these prodromal symptoms are uncommon.[60] In most instances resolution of acute disease is permanent, but rare cases of relapse have been noted.[92] It has become clear in recent years that death after acute hepatitis A is not as rare as initially believed.[43] The fatality rate in cases reported to the CDC is 0.6%.[22] After natural infection, anti–hepatitis A antibody (primarily IgG) is detectable in the blood for many years. The presence of the antibody confers immunity, and reinfection with hepatitis A virus is not believed to occur.

Diagnosis

Although the clinical presentation of hepatitis A is often milder than the other types of viral hepatitis, the symptoms are not distinctive enough to allow a firm diagnosis, which requires detection of hepatitis A antigen in the stool or serologic evaluation for hepatitis A–specific IgM or total anti–hepatitis A virus antibody. Stool antigen is maximal before the onset of symptoms but occasionally is detected as long as 2 weeks after the onset of disease. A more practical test is measurement of hepatitis A–specific IgM, which is usually present by the time symptoms are recognized and is generally absent 6 months later. Measurement of total anti–hepatitis A antibodies may be helpful in evaluating possible causes of past icteric episodes, or for seroepidemiologic studies, but their presence does not differentiate recent from past infection.

Management

No specific therapy exists for hepatitis A. Affected persons are usually managed as outpatients and should be instructed on enteric precautions to avoid transmission to others. Although infectivity drops sharply soon after the onset of jaundice, it is prudent to maintain enteric and blood-drawing precautions for about 2 weeks after jaundice appears. Nosocomial transmission has been documented, but most spread probably occurs before jaundice and diagnosis.[45]

Prevention

Although no effective therapy is available for hepatitis A, effective prophylactic measures may be taken.[22] Human immunoglobulin (IG) is effective for both preexposure and postexposure prophylaxis. IG is concentrated human immunoglobulin prepared by ethanol fractionation of pooled human sera. Although HIV contamination is a theoretical risk, epidemiologic studies show no increased risk of acquired immunodeficiency syndrome (AIDS) in recipients of IG, and laboratory evaluations confirmed that the IG manufacturing process inactivates HIV.[19] Thus IG is safe for use as prophylaxis.

Prophylaxis is recommended for persons traveling to developing countries if they anticipate eating in or visiting areas with poor sanitation. The recommended dose of IG is 0.02 ml/kg body weight by intramuscular injection if the length of stay is less than 3 months and 0.06 ml/kg body weight for longer periods. If the traveler will be overseas for 5 months or longer, repeat injections should be given every 5 months unless the traveler has adequate titers of anti–hepatitis A antibodies before initial immunization. Persons having intimate contact (household or sexual) with infected individuals or who have been exposed to a common source of hepatitis A virus should receive 0.02 ml/kg body weight of IG intramuscularly if it can be given within 2 weeks of exposure. IG is of unproven value if given more than 2 weeks after exposure. At the time of printing no hepatitis A vaccines had been licensed in the United States. However, the vaccines being developed are promising, and it is likely that licensure is imminent. Hepatitis A vaccine will probably be recommended for travelers to endemic areas.

HEPATITIS B

The spread of hepatitis by parenteral means was noted in 1885. Recognition in the 1960s of specific viral particles (the Australia antigen) in the serum of hepatitis patients led to identification of the responsible agent.

Epidemiology

With the widespread use of serologic markers for hepatitis B disease, it became apparent that spread occurs through exchange of blood, semen, or, rarely, saliva of infected people. Although spread is possible from persons with acute disease, the primary sources of viral particles are chronic carriers. Persons are defined as carriers if blood samples obtained 6 months apart contain hepatitis B surface antigen particles (HBsAg). The carrier state follows acute infection in up to 90% of infected infants and 10% of adults.[38] Risk factors for acquisition of hepatitis B infection in the United States include intravenous drug use, homosexual activity, and working in health care. In the United States, most patients are adults, and the carrier rate in the general population is less than 0.5%. In many areas of the developing world, most infections occur in infancy or childhood, and chronic carriers may comprise as much as 10% to 20% of the total population. Thus travelers are more likely to be exposed to carriers than is the nontraveling population. The risk is higher in persons regularly exposed to body fluids, including medical personnel and those with sexual contact abroad.

Virology and Pathophysiology

Hepatitis B virus is a DNA virus unrelated to the agent responsible for hepatitis A. Infection occurs naturally in humans and can be induced easily in some nonhuman primates. The virus cannot be grown in vitro. The majority of hepatitis B infections are subclinical. In those resulting in clinical disease, entry of the virus into the liver is followed by viral replication and hepatocyte necrosis. Viral particles, HBsAg, and hepatitis B core antigen (HBcAg) appear in the bloodstream within 3 months of infection. In most cases the first antibody to appear is to the core antigen, followed by anti-HBsAg antibody. Antibody to a third hepatitis antigen, the e antigen (HBeAg), is present for variable periods. The course of the disease varies widely, depending on a number of factors that are not well defined. In brief, most cases are self-limited and resolve in 4 to 6 months. In these patients, anti-HBsAg or anti-HBcAg antibody can be detected for years after the episode of hepatitis. Chronic carriers do not develop anti-HBsAg antibody, but rather maintain measurable levels of HBsAg. Similarly, carriers with persistent HBeAg detectable in blood samples appear to be more infectious than carriers without circulating HBeAg. The intricate network of antibody-antigen relationships in hepatitis B is believed to play a role not only in development of acute and chronic hepatitis, but also in the many extrahepatic syndromes associated with hepatitis B.[92] Immune complex formation has been suggested as etiologic in hepatitis B–associated arthritis, rash, arteritis, and renal disease.[42]

Clinical Presentation

The incubation period for hepatitis B ranges from 7 to 22 weeks, although the patient may be antigenemic for a large portion of that time. The manifestations of hepatitis B infection are similar to hepatitis A, with the presence of fever, anorexia, nausea, vomiting, and abdominal pain. However, a prodrome of rash, arthralgias or arthritis, and fever is seen in up to 20% of hepatitis B patients, compared to rare occurrence with hepatitis A. Glomerulonephritis is occasionally seen. Jaundice usually appears a short time after onset of gastrointestinal symptoms. In the self-limited disease, recovery is complete by 6 months. Some infections follow a fulminant course; case-fatality rates are 2% or less in most series. In addition to complete resolution or death, three other sequelae are possible with acute hepatitis B. A person may become an asymptomatic chronic carrier and remain HBsAg positive, but have no detectable ongoing hepatitis. Chronic persistent hepatitis is a term used to describe persistent, but not progressive, hepatic inflammation (usually monitored by serum transaminase levels), often with HBsAg in the serum. Persons with chronic active hepatitis may be HBsAg positive and have progressive hepatitis, which may result in cirrhosis and death directly related to liver disease. Any of these three conditions results in the presence of hepatitis B viral particles in the blood.

Diagnosis

A wide variety of antigen and antibody tests have been developed for the diagnosis and monitoring of hepatitis B disease. The most practical and widely available test for diagnosis of acute disease is the assay for HBsAg. Antigen will usually be present before the onset of symptoms and will persist during symptomatic disease. Occasionally, HBsAg may be undetectable in patients with clinical disease caused by hepatitis B. In these cases, antibody to HBcAg is often present. Later, antibody to HBsAg will appear, but this is often long after the episode of clinical hepatitis.

Management

Management is similar to that for hepatitis A. Prolonged and sometimes persistent viremia makes blood and body fluid precautions necessary until the absence of HBsAg antibodies and the presence of antibody to HBsAg are established.[22]

Prevention

Travelers to highly endemic areas who may stay for 6 or more months or who have close contact with inhabitants or travelers who may have contact with body fluids of inhabitants should be vaccinated. Two types of vaccine have been available for use. The first vaccine was prepared from pooled human plasma using several biochemical and physical procedures that result in a suspension of HBsAg particles. The processes used in manufacturing this vaccine inactivate blood-borne human viruses,[19,22] including HIV. This vaccine is no longer produced in the United States, and its use is generally restricted to persons with allergies to yeast and severely immunocompromised hosts. The newer hepatitis vaccines are produced using recombinant DNA technology by introduction of a plasmid containing the gene for HBsAg into baker's yeast. After the yeast has grown, the cells are lysed and HBsAg is separated from the lysate. The recombinant HBsAg is suspended to a concentration of 10 µg/ml. The recommended dose is 1 ml (10 μg) intramuscularly, with repeat doses at 1 and 6 months. Immunogenicity is similar for both vaccine preparations if used as directed.[22] Injections into subcutaneous fat are poorly immunogenic, so either vaccine should be given in the deltoid muscle.[119] Hepatitis B immune globulin (HBIG) is available for certain postexposure situations. HBIG is prepared from pooled sera by ethanol fractionation and contains high titers of antibody to HBsAg. Use of HBIG is not associated with risk of transmission of AIDS.[22] In brief, if an unvaccinated person is exposed to blood or has sexual contact with a person known to be HBsAg positive, he or she should receive HBIG (0.06 ml/kg body weight, intramuscularly) and the complete vaccine series (first shot in a different site from the HBIG). This should be done within 7 days of exposure. If only HBIG is available, then the initial HBIG dose should be followed in 1 month by another HBIG injection. This second dose of HBIG is not required if the patient is receiving the vaccine series.

The remaining recommendations assume availability of vaccine. If the exposed person has been vaccinated and serologic testing is available, nothing need be done if anti-HBsAg antibody is adequate. If levels of this antibody are inadequate, a routine dose of HBIG and a booster dose of vaccine (1 ml, intramuscularly) should be given. If there is uncertainty of the HBsAg status of the source, HBsAg testing should be done. In the unvaccinated person, the vaccine series should be given immediately, and if the source proves to be HBsAg positive, HBIG should be administered as previously described. In vaccinated persons with adequate vaccine response, no action should be taken. If the vaccine response was inadequate and the source was HBsAg positive, HBIG and a booster of vaccine should be given. If the source was unknown, the vaccine series should be given to the unvaccinated, and nothing need be done for the vaccinated person.[22]

DELTA HEPATITIS

Hepatitis with the delta agent was first suspected in 1977, when cases of severe hepatitis B disease and exacerbations of hepatitis were being evaluated.

Epidemiology

Delta virus infection is found only in patients concomitantly or previously infected with hepatitis B.[99] Transmission seems to follow similar patterns.[100] In the United States, affected populations are intravenous drug abusers and multiply transfused hemophiliacs.[101] Serologic evidence of delta virus disease has been documented in the Mediterranean basin, West Africa, and parts of South America.[99]

Virology and Pathophysiology

The delta agent has been termed a "defective" virus, since it requires hepatitis B virus activity for its own replication.[98,101] The agent itself is a single strand of RNA and a 68 kd protein enclosed in a protein coat of HBsAg. The agent may infect cells at approximately the same time as does hepatitis B virus (coinfection), or it may be introduced much later in the course of persistent hepatitis B infection (superinfection). In coinfected patients, the clinical picture may not differ from hepatitis B, but coinfection with both agents may lead to a higher percentage of patients with severe disease. Patients superinfected with delta agent develop flare-ups of hepatitis, which may become fulminant. After the acute infection, the delta agent can cause progressive disease in previously stable hepatitis B patients. In general, infection with the delta agent worsens the prognosis of hepatitis B disease. The diagnosis can be made by detection of antibody to the delta antigen in the serum[100] or less commonly by detection of free delta antigen in serum.[98]

Management and Prevention

Management consists of supportive care. Precautions against transmission are the same as for hepatitis B. There is no specific vaccine or IG for the delta agent. The best preventive measure is to be vaccinated for hepatitis B because delta agent infection cannot occur in the absence of hepatitis B. No preventive measures exist for chronic hepatitis B patients other than avoidance of exchange of body fluids with infected persons.

NON-A, NON-B HEPATITIS

With serologic methods available for the diagnosis of hepatitis A, B, and delta agent disease, it has become apparent that a fourth grouping of clinical hepatitis occurs for which no etiologic agent has been identified. This disease has been termed non-A, non-B (NANB) hepatitis.[107]

Epidemiology

Two distinct forms of NANB hepatitis have been characterized based on epidemiologic patterns: parenterally transmitted (PT) NANB disease and enterically transmitted (ET) NANB hepatitis. PT NANB hepatitis was studied extensively in the United States, and the genome of an RNA virus was cloned from infected chimpanzees and patients (hepatitis C).[27] Risk factors for hepatitis C include parenteral drug abuse, blood transfusion, and multiple sexual partners, all consistent with parenteral transmission.[63,64] Although it appears that most PT NANB hepatitis in the United States is caused by hepatitis C, additional studies suggest that other as yet unidentified agents may also cause PT NANB hepatitis. ET NANB hepatitis was originally recognized as hepatitis A antibody–negative ET (usually waterborne) outbreaks of hepatitis. A new virus was cloned from infected patients and is now referred to as hepatitis E.[98] As with PT NANB hepatitis, it is likely that other viral agents may also cause this syndrome.[112,126]

Virology and Pathophysiology

As noted previously, several agents may be responsible for PT NANB hepatitis and liver pathologic studies do not differentiate between infection caused by different viral agents. Much remains to be learned about the clinical spectrum of hepatitis C disease, but it is clear that, similar to hepatitis B disease, infection may range from asymptomatic disease to fulminant, fatal infections. In addition, a small proportion of cases progress to chronic hepatitis. Less is known about hepatitis E disease. However, studies of ET NANB outbreaks suggest that, compared to hepatitis A, infection may strike a somewhat older population and lead to substantial mortality in pregnant women.

Diagnosis

Patients with clinical and laboratory evidence of hepatitis who have had other infections or toxic causes ruled out may be considered to have NANB hepatitis. Sensitive and specific tests are available for measurement of anti–hepatitis C antibody, and a positive test in the setting of acute illness may be helpful; however, the serologic assay does not differentiate acute infection from chronic exposure. No test is currently available for hepatitis E virus. Further evidence of NANB hepatitis can be obtained by transmitting the disease to a subhuman primate, but this is available only in research laboratories.

Management and Prevention

Management of NANB hepatitis is the same as that for hepatitis A and B. No effective vaccine or prophylaxis preparations are currently available for these infections, and although one may wish to administer IG to persons with percutaneous exposure to blood from a person with PT NANB hepatitis, no data support the efficacy of this procedure. The best method of prevention is avoidance of infected body fluids and prudent selection of food and water when traveling.

Major Bacterial Infections

This section reviews several bacterial diseases of relevance to the overseas traveler and includes discussions of typhoid fever, meningococcal disease, pertussis, diphtheria, and tetanus. Other chapters in this text deal specifically with bacterial causes of gastroenteritis and diarrheal disease, tick-borne diseases, and zoonoses.

TYPHOID FEVER

Typhoid fever was recognized as a clinical entity in the 1800s and was first associated with transmission by the fecal-oral route in the 1870s. Although effective treatment with chloramphenicol became possible in 1948, the disease continues to be a major cause of morbidity and mortality in the developing world.[31]

Epidemiology

Typhoid fever occurs worldwide, but its prevalence and attack rates are much higher in underdeveloped countries. Humans are the only host for *Salmonella typhi,* the most common cause of the typhoid fever syndrome. Nearly all cases are contracted through ingestion of contaminated food or water. Transmission occurs through a variety of mechanisms, the most common of which include contact with a chronic carrier of the organism or ingestion of untreated waste material or sewage. One expert has estimated an incidence rate of 12.5 million cases a year in the developing world (excluding China).[31] Improved sewage systems and tracking of chronic carriers have markedly reduced the incidence in developed countries, although several hundred cases a year are reported to the CDC in the United States. Evaluation of cases reported between 1975 and 1984 revealed that 62% of typhoid fever cases in the United States were acquired during foreign travel. The highest attack rates occurred in persons traveling to India, Pakistan, Peru, and Chile (58 to 174 cases/1 million travelers).[113]

Bacteriology and Pathophysiology

Salmonella species are gram-negative enteric bacilli. *S. typhi* is the prime cause of typhoid fever, but other species, including many of the *S. enteritidis* serotypes and some non-*Salmonella* enteric organisms such as *Yersinia* or *Campylobacter,* may cause a typhoid fever–like syndrome. *Salmonella* species are easily grown on routine bacterial culture plates, but if multiple organisms are present, media with selective growth inhibitors may be needed for optimal sensitivity. After ingestion of food or water containing the pathogen, organisms are subjected to the acid stomach environment, which results in significant bacterial killing. If the organisms get through the small intestine, several processes may occur. The bacteria may simply pass through, causing few clinical symptoms. If the bacteria multiply and invade the mucosa, a gastroenteritis-like syndrome will result. Typhoid fever requires penetration of the intestinal mucosa and intestinal lymphatics, where replication of *S. typhi* occurs intracellularly. Soon thereafter, bacteria seed the bloodstream and are transported to reticuloendothelial cells throughout the body, where further intracellular replication can take place. After the acute episode of infection is over, *Salmonella* species may remain and asymptomatically reproduce in scarred or chronically inflamed tissues. Persons may persistently shed organisms from such foci for years and serve as a source of outbreaks while they themselves are asymptomatic. The most common site for such colonization is the chronically diseased gallbladder.

Clinical Presentation

After exposure to the pathogen, 10 to 14 days usually passes before the onset of clinical illness. Some patients may experience gastroenteritis early in the course of disease, and abdominal pain or diarrhea may be present at the time the classic typhoid fever picture develops. Fever is usually the first sign of disease. Fever increases slowly over several days[59] and may remain constant for 2 to 3 weeks, after which time defervescence begins. With antibiotic therapy, fever resolves more rapidly, often within 3 to 4 days.[59] Relative bradycardia may accompany fever. Most patients also report headache, malaise, and anorexia. Rose spots (2 to 4 mm maculopapular blanching lesions) are classically described on the trunk, although they are not seen in the majority of patients. Hepatomegaly and splenomegaly have been reported in a large number of patients.[58,96] Laboratory examination early in the course may show a high white blood cell count (WBC), anemia, and mild elevations of serum hepatic enzyme levels, including AST, lactate dehydrogenase, and alkaline phosphatase.[58] Later in the course of the disease, leukopenia (WBC <3500/mm^3) develops.

Uncomplicated and untreated typhoid fever resolves in 3 to 4 weeks. Several complications may herald or contribute to death. Intestinal perforation, presumably secondary to necrosis of lymphoid areas of the bowel wall, may lead to peritonitis and death. Significant gastrointestinal hemorrhage may occur, but rarely is fatal. Secondary pneumonia is common. A subgroup of patients have more severe disease, which may include myocardial involvement, mental status changes, hyperpyrexia, and multisystem failure. The overall case fatality rate has ranged from 12% to 32% in the developing world but is less than 2% in industrialized nations.[31]

Diagnosis

The diagnosis is made by culturing a bacterial species associated with the syndrome (most likely *S. typhi*) from a normally sterile fluid. Multiple studies have evaluated the usefulness of various diagnostic tests. In general, bone marrow culture is the most sensitive method, detecting up to 90% of cases, whereas blood cultures are somewhat less sensitive.[31] Both these methods are most useful in the first week of disease. Stool cultures (and string test cultures) may be positive later in the course of disease but provide only circumstantial evidence of the causative agent. Much work is currently being done on serodiagnostic methods, but no clear consensus has been reached on the relative usefulness of any test.[31]

Management

Chloramphenicol (50 mg/kg/day in four divided doses for 2 weeks) has been the mainstay of treatment for typhoid fever since the late 1940s. Although chloramphenicol resistance has been noted, it has remained at relatively low frequencies in most series. Ampicillin (100 mg/kg/day in four divided doses for at least 2 weeks) is an appropriate alternative. Trimethoprim-sulfamethoxazole (80 mg trimethoprim plus 400 mg sulfamethoxazole/day in two divided doses for at least 2 weeks) may also be used and is helpful for *S. typhi* resistant to both chloramphenicol and ampicillin. Relapse can occur after 2 weeks of therapy and necessitates retreatment.

Other treatment measures include fluid support and adequate nutrition. Corticosteroids have been used empirically for many years. A randomized, double-blind study showed that administration of high-dose dexamethasone (3 mg/kg for the first dose, followed by 1 mg/kg every 6 hours for eight more doses) with chloramphenicol resulted in significantly lower mortality in patients with severe typhoid fever than was noted in those treated with chloramphenicol alone.[57] Severe typhoid fever was defined as present if the patient was obtunded, delirious, stuporous, comatose, or in shock (systolic blood pressure less than 90 mm Hg for those 12 years or older and less than 80 mm Hg in children). High-dose steroids were not recommended for those with less severe disease.

Prevention

Vaccination with the heat-killed, acetone-precipitated vaccine is indicated for persons traveling to areas with increased risk of typhoid fever. Efficacy in Americans, however, is only about 50%, and significant incidences of local inflammatory reactions and febrile responses occur in persons receiving the vaccine. Two doses of 0.5 ml are given subcutaneously separated by a 4-week interval. An oral vaccine was licensed for use in the United States in 1989. The vaccine contains the Ty21a strain of *S. typhi* and is associated with minimal side effects. The Ty21a vaccine is licensed for use in persons under 6 years old and is given as a four-dose series, with 2 days between each dose.[121] Even when the vaccine is given before travel, it is important to observe routine precautions for ingestion of food and water.

MENINGOCOCCAL DISEASE

Meningococcal meningitis classically attacks children and young adults and is often seen in epidemic form. Although the advent of effective antibiotic therapy and a useful vaccine have greatly improved the ability to deal with this disease, it remains a major problem in many parts of the world.

Epidemiology

Cases of meningococcal disease occur sporadically worldwide, with epidemic disease generally limited to developing nations. Epidemic situations clearly pose the greater health problem to both travelers and resident populations. Since 1970, large outbreaks have occurred in Brazil; China; the Sahel region of sub-Saharan Africa (from Mali and Burkino Fasa to Ethiopia and northwestern Somalia); New Delhi, India; and Nepal.[29] Particularly in sub-Saharan Africa and China, the disease demonstrates yearly incidence peaks and periodic massive outbreaks, the exact determinants of which are unknown. Transmission of the organism occurs by exchange of respiratory secretions; thus close contact is believed to be important in the spread of the disease. Asymptomatic transient nasopharyngeal carriage of the meningococcus, occurring with a baseline prevalence of 5% to 10%,[6] may increase during epidemic periods and in close contacts of cases. The secondary attack rate among household contacts of patients with sporadic disease is 2 to 4:1000, whereas that in epidemics ranges from 11 to 45:1000 household contacts.[77]

Bacteriology and Pathogenesis

Neisseria meningitidis is a gram-negative diplococcus that grows easily on several common media, including chocolate and blood agar. The organism is characterized further on the basis of serologic analysis of capsular antigens. The most common serogroups are A, B, C, Y, and W135. Serogroups A and C are often associated with epidemic disease, whereas serogroup B is the major cause of sporadic disease in the United States.[22a] Asymptomatic persons may carry various serotypes of *N. meningitidis* in the nasopharynx for short periods of time. An antibody response is often generated to these strains during asymptomatic carriage. The conditions that cause one person to become clinically ill with invasive disease while another carrier remains well are not well understood. The route of entrance of the organism to the bloodstream and central nervous system (CNS) is presumably through the nasopharynx or respiratory tract.

Clinical Presentation

Meningococcal disease may appear in a variety of forms, including, but not limited to (1) bacteremia with septic shock; (2) meningitis, often accompanied by bacteremia; and (3) pneumonia. Sustained meningococcemia may lead to severe toxemia with hypotension, fever, and DIC. In the fulminant presentation, adrenal hemorrhage may lead to Waterhouse-Friderichsen syndrome and death may follow intractable shock. In the United States the case-fatality rate for sustained meningococcemia is generally higher than for meningococcal meningitis.[120]

Meningitis caused by *N. meningitidis* classically begins with fever, headache, and a stiff neck. It may also be accompanied by bacteremia and any of several skin manifestations, including petechiae, pustules, or maculopapular rash. In either meningitis or bacteremia, progression of petechiae to broad ecchymoses is a poor prognostic sign. As with septic meningococcemia, severe meningitis may progress with mental status deterioration, hypotension, congestive heart failure, DIC, and death. The case fatality rate of meningococcal meningitis with or without bacteremia is now estimated to be about 10%.[120] In classic cases of meningitis or bacteremia with sepsis, the peripheral WBC count is elevated, with a polymorphonuclear cell predominance. CSF typically is purulent, usually with more than 500 polymorphonuclear cells/mm^3. There may be a more heterogeneous cell population and fewer cells if CSF is obtained early in the course or if the patient has been treated with antibiotics. The CSF glucose level is usually low and protein high, as in other bacterial meningitides. Gram's stain of CSF may show the gram-negative diplococci. Meningococcal pneumonia is a well-known but less common clinical entity,[95] most recently described in military recruit populations involving serogroup Y organisms.[65]

Diagnosis

The presumptive diagnosis in an epidemic can be made on the basis of clinical presentation and purulent spinal fluid. The presence of characteristic bacterial forms on Gram's stain is also suggestive. A definitive diagnosis requires culture of the organism from CSF or a normally sterile fluid (usually peripheral blood). This may be impossible in the case of a patient who was previously treated. Several commercial kits for measuring meningococcal antigen are now available for use on CSF or blood samples.

Management

Treatment of meningococcal meningitis or sepsis is a medical emergency. Fortunately, the organism remains sensitive to a large number of antibiotics. The treatment of choice is penicillin G, 300,000 units/kg/day (up to 24 million units a day), given intravenously in divided doses every 2 hours. Seven to 10 days of therapy for serious disease is appropriate. Ceftriaxone is an alternative antimicrobial agent. If the patient is allergic to penicillin, chloramphenicol (100 mg/kg/day) may be given.

Supportive care should include close monitoring for hypotension and cardiac failure. Fluids and vasoactive and cardioselective agents may be important. This type of support necessitates invasive monitors and intensive care unit technology. Development of DIC is an ominous sign. The role of heparin in this disease is still debated. Although focal bleeding and adrenal necrosis may lead to acute adrenal insufficiency, the role of replacement steroids in the treatment of Waterhouse-Friderichsen syndrome is unclear.[3] Since the infectious agent has been found in household contacts and in those with exposure to oral secretions, contacts should receive prophylaxis to eradicate the organism. Rifampin, 600 mg by mouth every 12 hours for four doses, is standard adult prophylaxis. Children should receive 10 mg/kg of rifampin every 12 hours for four doses if they are older than 1 month and 5 mg/kg every 12 hours for four doses if they are less than 1 month of age.[15]

Prevention

An effective meningococcal vaccine has been available in the United States for several years. The vaccine contains purified polysaccharide from the bacterial capsule of *N. meningitidis* serogroups A, C, Y, and W135. The recommended dose is one injection of 0.5 ml subcutaneously.[15] Clinical efficacy of more than 65% is maintained for at least 3 years in persons immunized at 4 years of age or older, although protection wanes more rapidly in children vaccinated at less than 4 years of age.[97] Although the incidence of meningococcal disease in the United States is so low that mass administration of the vaccine is inappropriate, vaccination is recommended for persons without spleens, with specific complement deficiencies, or planning to travel to certain high-risk areas.[14,15] Epidemics have occurred since 1980 in sub-Saharan Africa, New Delhi, India, Nepal, and Saudi Arabia. From January 1984 to January 1985, six foreign hikers in Nepal developed meningococcal disease and two died.[15] A large number of pilgrims to the 1987 Hadj in Mecca, Saudi Arabia, developed meningococcal meningitis after arrival. Since the areas in which epidemic meningococcal disease occurs change, it is prudent to check with local and federal health officals to determine current recommendations for meningococcal vaccination (see Chapter 44).

PERTUSSIS

Pertussis, or whooping cough, was first recognized as a major threat in the 1500s. After the introduction of a vaccine in the 1940s, the incidence of pertussis dropped sharply among immunized populations. However, since recognition of rare side effects to the pertussis vaccine, immunization rates have fallen. The age-specific incidence of pertussis in all age groups increased between 1981 and 1985 in the United States, with rates in persons 20 years and older increasing by 13-fold during that period.[20]

Epidemiology

Pertussis is found throughout the world. At the present time the incidence is highest in undeveloped countries, where immunization rates are low and socioeconomic conditions predispose to many communicable diseases. Pertussis is highly infectious, with attack rates of greater than 90% in unvaccinated household contacts. In the United States, most infections and the most severe disease occur in children under 5 years old. Transmission is by airborne particles from respiratory secretions of infected persons.

Bacteriology and Pathophysiology

Bordetella pertussis is a gram-negative coccobacillus, isolation of which usually requires Bordet-Gengou medium supplemented with methicillin. The organism produces several toxins when present in the respiratory tract. Pertussigen stimulates lymphocytosis and hemagglutination. Dermonecrotic toxin and tracheal cytotoxins damage respiratory epithelium. In addition, endotoxin is produced. During the course of the somewhat protracted disease, complications can occur that may cause death. The most serious of these are secondary pneumonia or fulminant encephalopathy. In addition, fits of coughing often result in pneumothorax, hemorrhage (facial, conjunctival, and CNS), and aspiration.

Clinical Presentation

Classic pertussis develops after an incubation period of 7 to 10 days. The disease appears in three stages: catarrhal, paroxysmal, and convalescent. The catarrhal stage lasts 1 to 2 weeks and resembles an undifferentiated upper respiratory tract infection with cough and mild fever. Progression of the cough to yield the classic whoop (which results when the patient gasps for breath after a prolonged coughing episode) marks the paroxysmal stage, which again can last as long as 2 weeks. During this stage the peripheral white blood cell count may show marked lymphocytosis. Finally, the cough resolves during the convalescent stage. Death may occur from pertussis alone or from the complications. Recent case fatality rates for Americans were 0.4% for all persons and 1% for patients less than 1 year old.[20] The disease in adults is often milder, although it may show a severe classic pattern.[69] Some investigators believe mild or atypical disease in adults may serve as a reservoir for infection of susceptible children.[84]

Diagnosis

Culture of the organism from a nasopharyngeal swab is the most efficient way to diagnose pertussis; however, the culture is positive most frequently early in the illness, and late cultures (after the second week of illness) are rarely helpful. For optimal recovery, Bordet-Gengou media should be used with methicillin added to reduce overgrowth by other bacteria present in the nasopharyngeal flora. Direct fluorescent antibody techniques may also be used to evaluate nasopharyngeal swabs or sputum samples for the presence of organisms.

Management

Treatment with antibiotics, unless begun in the incubation or catarrhal period, has little effect on the course of the disease. Antibiotics can reduce subsequent transmission to contacts, however, and should be instituted as soon as the diagnosis is made. Erythromycin, the drug of choice, should be given for at least 2 weeks. Other useful agents include doxycycline, trimethoprim-sulfamethoxazole, and chloramphenicol. In patients with severe disease, corticosteroids may provide some improvement.[127] Perhaps more important than specific antibiotics is supportive care, including hydration, nutrition, care to maintain adequate ventilation, and supplemental oxygen. In addition, external stimuli, which seem to exacerbate symptoms, should be kept to a minimum.

Prevention

Immunization of children with diphtheria-pertussis-tetanus (DPT) vaccine is recommended by the CDC, since the benefits of immunization are greater than the risk of neurologic damage from the vaccine.[23,55,56] Introduction of new acellular pertussis vaccines may reduce this risk even further.[23a] Vaccination is not recommended for persons older than 7 unless there is specific risk. The goal of treatment is to reduce secondary transmission. Close contacts under 7 years old who are unimmunized should be immunized, and persons who have not had a dose of DPT in 3 years should receive one. Furthermore, all close contacts under 1 year old should receive a 14-day course of erythromycin or trimethoprim-sulfamethoxazole, as should unimmunized contacts under 7 years old.[23]

DIPHTHERIA

Diphtheria, once a highly feared cause of morbidity and mortality in young people, can be controlled with appropriate use of a vaccine. However, according to some surveys, waning immunity has left more than 40% of American adults (18 years or older) with inadequate circulating levels of antitoxin against diphtheria. Of 15 cases of respiratory diphtheria occurring in the United States between 1980 and 1983, 11 occurred in persons 20 years of age or older.[23] Endemic diphtheria is present in the developing world and a cause for concern among travelers. A recent outbreak in the Russian Federation primarily involving persons older than 14 highlights the need for up-to-date immunization in travelers.[24]

Epidemiology

Humans are the natural host for *Corynebacterium diphtheriae*. Person-to-person spread occurs through contact with respiratory secretions or diphtheritic skin lesions. A carrier state exists in which people who have either been immunized or previously infected harbor the organism and asymptomatically transmit it to others. Evidence suggests that diphtheria can be transmitted through food or water, but this is not a major route of transmission.

Bacteriology and Pathogenesis

C. diphtheriae is a gram-positive, club-shaped bacillus. On Gram's stain the clustered bacteria have the characteristic "Chinese letter" configuration. The organisms grow on standard media, but to avoid overgrowth of other oral flora, selective media (Loeffler's culture medium or cysteine-tellurite agar) are suggested. The presence of a lysogenic bacteriophage in some *C. diphtheriae* organisms induces production of diphtheria toxin. The toxin is produced as a single molecule with two sections, fragments A and B. Fragment B facilitates attachment to the cell membrane of host cells, and after attachment, fragment A enters the cell. Cell death results from large-scale disruption of protein synthetic capabilities.

Clinical Presentation

The most important manifestation of diphtheria is respiratory tract infection. Illness begins after an incubation period of about a week with nonspecific symptoms of malaise, fatigue, mild sore throat, and slight fever. The classic lesion is exudative pharyngitis progressing to a greenish gray membrane that is difficult to dislodge. This membrane may spread over the posterior pharynx, tonsils, and uvula and down the respiratory tree to involve the larynx and trachea. Any one of these areas may be involved selectively, and the severity of illness is to some extent related to the area grossly involved.

In severe disease, swollen tissues may result in a bull neck appearance. Major complications include obstruction of the respiratory tract, which may result from direct parapharyngeal swelling or laryngeal involvement in young children, and sloughing of the tracheobronchial membrane in older patients. In addition to respiratory tract damage, toxin directly injures myocardial and neural tissue. Endocarditis occurs in some patients. Early signs in the first week of disease include ST-T wave depression and atrioventricular conduction abnormalities on the electrocardiogram. Congestive heart failure and cardiac enlargement may develop. Neurologic deficits usually begin with pharyngeal and cranial nerve paralysis. Cranial nerve paralysis may progress to bilateral motor paralysis, which generally resolves over a period of 3 to 6 months.[48] In the tropics, cutaneous diphtheria is seen frequently. The skin lesions are not consistent in appearance and range from very superficial impetigo-like lesions to deep ulcers. In most cases of cutaneous disease, absorption of toxin is not great enough to cause the multisystem involvement seen in respiratory tract disease. The prevalence of skin lesions increases the overall likelihood of coming in contact with toxigenic *C. diphtheriae*.

Diagnosis

Reliable isolation of the organism requires a selective medium and several days of culture. Treatment should be started as soon as the patient is evaluated and should be guided by clinical manifestations.

Management

Since life-threatening clinical manifestations of diphtheria are mediated by the toxin and not the organism per se, neutralization of absorbed toxin is crucial.[48] A horse-derived antitoxin is available and should be administered as soon as the diagnosis is seriously considered. A test dose of intradermal 0.1 ml antitoxin diluted to a 1:1000 concentration (with a saline control) is observed for 20 minutes. If no reaction occurs, full doses can be given intravenously. Antitoxin should be diluted to 1:20 in saline and given no faster than 1 ml/min. For mild cases, 20,000 units may be adequate, 40,000 units for moderate cases, and as much as 80,000 to 120,000 units for severely ill patients. Erythromycin or penicillin may be given to eradicate the carrier state, although their use has no effect on the clinical course of disease. Close observation is crucial to evaluate the need for respiratory support, especially in young children. Serial electrocardiograms and neurologic evaluation establish the onset of complications. If significant conduction abnormalities are present, continuous heart monitoring should be undertaken. Strict bed rest is recommended for all patients for 2 to 3 weeks.

Prevention

Close contacts of patients with respiratory diphtheria should receive diphtheria vaccine if they have not received at least three doses previously or if 5 or more years have elapsed since the last dose.[23] In addition, unimmunized or partially immunized contacts should receive either intramuscular benzathine penicillin (600,000 units if less than 6 years old and 1.2 million units if more than 6 years old) or 7 to 10 days of erythromycin (40 mg/kg/day for children or 1 g/day for adults, in four divided doses). Antitoxin is not recommended for contacts. The most important way to prevent diphtheria in adults, however, is to ensure that all adults receive a booster dose of diphtheria-tetanus toxoid every 10 years.

TETANUS

Tetanus was recognized by the early Greeks and continues to be a feared cause of infant and adult mortality. Today the mortality approaches 90% and 40% for untreated infants and adults, respectively.[105] Tetanus toxoid immunization has drastically reduced the incidence of disease in populations with high coverage rates.

Epidemiology

The bacterium and its spores are ubiquitous. Approximately 10% of all people carry *Clostridium tetani* in fecal flora.[94] Person-to-person spread is not important in this disease. Disease occurs when the organism is introduced into an environment suitable for its growth, specifically, wound sites with an anaerobic environment. In the United States, most of the 75 to 90 cases each year occur in persons over 50 years old.[108] In the developing world, the vast majority of cases are in neonates.

Bacteriology and Pathophysiology

C. tetani is a gram-positive, anaerobic, spore-forming rod. The spores are hardy and can occasionally survive boiling for short periods. After proliferating in an appropriate anaerobic environment, *C. tetani* releases the toxin, tetanospasmin, which in generalized disease reaches the spinal column and CNS by hematogenous spread. The toxin is taken up by inhibitory neurons, where it interferes with release of inhibitory neurotransmitters, resulting in disinhibition of motor groups. Disinhibition of the sympathetic nervous system neurons occurs through a similar mechanism. The result is muscular spasm of varying severity and signs of sympathetic nervous system hyperactivity, including tachycardia, sweating, arrhythmias, and high blood pressure.

Clinical Presentation

Most adult disease is preceded by a tetanus-prone wound, which may not be evident at the time of presentation. Localized tetanus, with spasm of a focal set of muscle groups, may occur and remain localized for weeks, then slowly resolve. This form of tetanus is much less common than the generalized form, which often begins with trismus, or spasm of the masticator muscle group. Gradual onset of spasm of other muscle groups usually involves the trunk and extremities. Since the posterior muscles are stronger during spasms, the patient exhibits lumbar lordosis, with the neck and legs extended and arms flexed at the elbows (opisthotonos). Spasms seem to be exacerbated by external stimuli, such as sudden sound or light. The primary danger is loss of ability to breathe, especially during prolonged spasms. Respiratory failure is the main cause of death. The clinical picture in neonatal tetanus is similar but begins with restlessness and failure to nurse, with progression to tetany and sympathetic overactivity. The common source of infection is the umbilical stump. There is no laboratory test to confirm the diagnosis of tetanus, but the clinical picture is adequate in the majority of cases.

Management

Specific emergency medical treatment of tetanus patients should include (1) excision of the wound, (2) administration of human tetanus IG (at least 500 units,[4] but a range of 500 to 3000 has been frequently used), and (3) administration of an antibiotic effective against *C. tetani,* such as penicillin or metronidazole.[105] Depending on the severity of the case, different levels of supportive care and sedation may be appropriate. Diazepam may be given to mildly affected patients for sedation. Patients should be evaluated carefully for dysphagia by testing with a drink of water. If dysphagia is present or other respiratory difficulties arise, endotracheal intubation or a tracheostomy should be performed. With prolonged spasms, hypoxia and cyanosis may occur. At this point, mechanical ventilation with pharmacologic paralysis is appropriate. At the same time, attention must be given to fluid balance and nutrition. Enteral feeding by a nasogastric tube is the least invasive way to supply both. β-Blockers have been suggested to relieve symptoms of autonomic overactivity, such as tachycardia and hypertension. An effort should also be made to reduce sources of sensory stimulation when the spasms are uncontrolled.

Prevention

Although rare cases of tetanus have occurred in apparently immunized persons,[89] immunization is considered at least 99.9% effective.[23] Several vaccine formulations are now available in the United States. Children under 7 years old may receive either DTP or DT (diphtheria and tetanus toxoid only) vaccine. A third vaccine, Td, is manufactured for use in persons at least 7 years old and consists of tetanus toxoid and a smaller amount of diphtheria toxoid than is present in the pediatric vaccines. A reduced amount of diphtheria toxoid is used in the adult preparation, since both the amount of toxoid and increasing age were found to be associated with more severe reactions to vaccination. Adults who are unimmunized should be given a series of three doses (0.5 ml intramuscularly) of Td, with the second dose 4 to 8 weeks after the first and the third dose 6 to 12 months after the second. A booster should be given every 10 years thereafter. All travelers should be urged to be certain of their primary immunization and stay up to date with booster doses. From the standpoint of tetanus prevention, care of wounds is crucial. The tetanus-prone wound, contaminated with dirt or feces or caused by puncture, crush, avulsion, or frostbite, should be cleaned and debrided appropriately. Persons with tetanus-prone wounds should receive 250 to 500 units of human tetanus IG if their immunization history is unknown or their immunization series is incomplete. These persons should also receive a dose of Td and complete an immunization series. Persons fully immunized and given an appropriate booster before a tetanus-prone wound should not receive tetanus IG. If they have not received a booster within 5 years, however, they should get a dose of Td.[23]

Major Protozoan Infections

MALARIA

Malaria, or "ague" in previous centuries, is a major cause of childhood mortality in developing countries. Travelers who are not immune (that is, most North Americans and Europeans) are at great risk for the disease.

Epidemiology

The four major human malaria parasites, *Plasmodium falciparum, P. vivax, P. ovale,* and *P. malariae,* are found in most tropical developing countries where the appropriate anopheline vector exists. The degree of endemicity in a specific region may be judged by the proportion of residents who have enlarged spleens. The degree varies from a hypoendemic area, in which less than 10% of children have enlarged spleens, to hyperendemic, in which more than 50% of children have enlarged spleens.

Persons are inoculated by sporozoites when a mosquito releases the parasite during a blood meal. Sporozoites rapidly invade liver cells, where they proliferate into multiple merozoites. After 1 to 2 weeks, merozoites rupture from hepatocytes and invade red blood cells. A proportion of *P. vivax* and *P. ovale* organisms may enter a dormant phase in the liver and cause recrudescence of disease months to years later. *P. falciparum* does not enter this dormant phase. After merozoites enter a red blood cell, they may undergo asexual proliferation (schizogony) to eventually form more merozoites (which may invade other red blood cells) or sexual differentiation to form gametocytes. Merozoites cause red blood cell lysis, whereas gametocytes must be ingested by mosquitoes to continue the parasite life cycle. Development of fertilized eggs in the mosquito to form infective sporozoites takes 10 to 14 days. Travelers may be infected and develop disease from one sporozoite. Thus cases of malaria have been reported in individuals who presumably had contact only with mosquitoes that entered an aircraft in transit through endemic areas.

Pathogenesis and Clinical Manifestations

Rupture of erythrocytes by asexual schizonts containing merozoites is associated with fever, nausea, and severe myalgias.[110] Cerebral malaria and other evidence of organ dysfunction, such as renal failure in falciparum malaria, are presumably related to sludging in the microvasculature by poorly deformable red blood cells or erythrocytes with parasite-induced surface molecules that adhere to the endothelium. Anoxia of surrounding tissue results.[110] Anemia induced by all *Plasmodium* species is primarily secondary to hemolysis.

Clinical manifestations of malaria may first be evident within 1 to 2 weeks after the victim enters an endemic area, or sooner if infected blood obtained by transfusion or use of shared needles is the source. Although there are no pathognomic signs, many subjects report paroxysms of chills, followed by high fever and sweating. These may last several hours and recur every 2 to 3 days. It should be stressed that classic periodic attacks are often not observed in severe falciparum malaria and that fever may be constant. In addition, abdominal cramps and diarrhea may be presenting symptoms. Cerebral malaria, associated with high levels of parasitemia (usually more than 10% of red blood cells infected) is characterized by high fevers, confusion, and eventually coma and death.

Diagnosis

Malaria can be definitively diagnosed only by the presence of malaria parasite–containing red blood cells. Prophylactic medications do not exclude the possibility of being infected. Thick and thin blood smears should be made and stained with Giemsa stain for microscopic inspection. Thin films are prepared in a standard manner. Thick films are prepared by spreading a drop of blood in a 1 cm diameter circle. The blood is allowed to dry, red blood cells are lysed with water, and the slide is stained with Giemsa stain. Various intraerythrocytic forms (schizonts, trophozoites, merozoites) should be identified by an experienced person. Blood smears should be obtained on initial contact with the patient and every 12 hours until they show positive results. Speciation of malaria is important when falciparum infection is a possibility because this parasite may be resistant to chloroquine and cause lethal disease.

Management

Plasmodium Falciparum. A major issue involved in treating falciparum malaria is the sensitivity of the parasite to chloroquine.[92] Chloroquine-resistant strains of *P. falciparum* are found in all endemic areas of the world except Central America west of the Panama Canal, islands in the Caribbean Sea, and the Middle East, including Egypt. Since no laboratory tests can distinguish between sensitive and resistant strains, all persons diagnosed as having *P. falciparum* acquired outside these areas should be treated as having chloroquine-resistant malaria. There are multiple useful drug regimens. A commonly used regimen for adults is quinine sulfate, 600 mg orally three times per day for 7 days, plus tetracycline, 250 mg every 6 hours for 7 days. The dose of quinine salt for children is 10 mg/kg body weight. Pregnant women and children under 8 years should not be given tetracycline. In some parts of the world, mefloquine (Lariam) at a single dose of 1250 mg (the drug should not be administered if quinine has been given in the previous 12 hours) is used. In persons believed to have chloroquine-sensitive *P. falciparum* infection, chloroquine phosphate, 1000 mg initially, should be followed by 500 mg 6 hours later and 500 mg per day for an additional 2 days. In persons with severe and complicated *P. falciparum* infection, such as those with cerebral malaria, intravenous quinine should be used. For quinine, a loading dose of 16.7 mg base (suspended in isotonic saline) per kilogram of body weight is given intravenously over 4 hours. This is followed by an 8.3 mg base every 8 hours until oral medications can be taken and a full 3- or 7-day course (if infection was acquired in Southeast Asia) is completed. The loading dose is decreased to 8.3 mg/kg if mefloquine or quinine has been taken within the previous 12 hours. If intravenous quinine is unavailable, quinidine gluconate may be substituted. The loading dose is 10 mg/kg given in saline over 1 hour followed by continuous infusion of 0.02 mg/kg/min up to 3 days. The patient should be switched to oral quinine as soon as possible. These medications should be administered in an intensive care unit with continuous cardiac monitoring. Exchange transfusion to lower the level of parasitemia may also be useful in this setting. Corticosteroids are contraindicated, since controlled studies show that mortality is higher when they are given.[117]

Plasmodium Vivax, P. Ovale, and P. Malariae. These infections are treated as described for chloroquine-sensitive *P. falciparum*. Since *P. vivax* and *P. ovale* may have dormant hepatic forms, primaquine phosphate, 26.3 mg daily for 14 days, should follow administration of chloroquine to eliminate extraerythrocytic hypnozoites. Individuals given primaquine should first be screened for the presence of glucose-6-phosphate dehydrogenase (G-6-PD) deficiency, since this drug may cause oxidant-induced hemolysis. If G-6-PD deficiency is severe, primaquine should not be administered and the patient should be monitored periodically for symptoms of malaria. Individuals with mild G-6-PD deficiency may be given primaquine under close supervision because hemolysis is self-limited.

Proper precautions include avoidance of contact with mosquitoes through the use of nets, sprays, and long-sleeved clothing. Travelers to endemic areas should take prophylactic medications.[16] These are discussed in Chapter 44.

African Trypanosomiasis

Trypanosoma brucei rhodesiense and *T. brucei gambiense* have provided remarkable insights into the importance of antigenic variation as a strategy used by parasites to avoid the immune response.[116] *T. brucei gambiense* causes African sleeping sickness, and *T. brucei rhodesiense* causes an acute disease that may end in heart failure. The parasites are transmitted to humans by tsetse flies (*Glossina* species) in sub-Saharan Africa. Metacyclic promastigotes are injected into the bloodstream through the saliva of the biting tsetse and divide into long slender forms in the bloodstream. These eventually differentiate into short stumpy forms, which are taken up in the blood meal of the tsetse. Once in the fly, the parasite differentiates into procyclic forms. It takes approximately 3 weeks for the protozoa to develop into infective metacyclics within the tsetse.

Clinical Manifestations. In nonimmune individuals, the initial sign of infection is a nodule at the site of the tsetse bite. This lesion becomes erythematous and painful over a period of 1 week and recedes after several days. Dissemination of the trypanosome throughout the body occurs and causes clinical symptoms, notably fever, headache, and severe malaise. On physical examination, enlarged supraclavicular and posterior cervical lymph nodes are noted. This phase of illness lasts several days and is followed by an asymptomatic period of several weeks. The acute phase may then recur. In the case of *T. brucei gambiense* infection, symptoms are less severe and evolve into a syndrome characterized by behavioral changes and chronic somnolence. *T. brucei rhodesiense* infections cause severe anemia, frequent episodes of fever, and eventual heart failure and severe CNS involvement.

Diagnosis. The definitive diagnosis depends on identification of parasites in the blood, lymphatics, or CSF. Thick blood smears and buffy coat preparations should be stained with Giemsa and examined for the presence of trypanosomes. The CSF should be subjected to centrifugation and the sediment examined for parasites. Associated laboratory abnormalities include anemia, monocytosis, and elevated serum and CSF IgM levels.[36]

Management. Suramin* should be used for treatment of African trypanosomiasis, although the drug may cause proteinuria.[76] A test dose of 100 mg intravenously is first given to detect possible idiosyncratic reactions. If tolerated, 1 g should be given on the initial day of treatment and 3, 7, 14, and 21 days later. If CNS involvement is diagnosed or strongly suspected (CSF lymphocytosis and elevated IgM), melarsoprol (available from the CDC) should also be administered.[76] This drug is given at an initial dose of 1.5 mg/kg of body weight, with gradually increasing doses (e.g., increase every 48 hours to a dose of 3.6 mg/kg in 2 weeks). After a week with no drug given, additional injections of 3.6 mg/kg are given every other day three times. This arsenical compound is toxic, causing encephalopathy and exfoliative dermatitis, and should be used only in a controlled hospital setting.

*Available in the United States from the Parasitic Diseases Division of the CDC, 404-639-3670.

South American Trypanosomiasis (Chagas' Disease)

T. cruzi is transmitted to humans by triatomids that live in the cracks of mud-built homes in Central and Latin America. These insects are particularly common in areas of Brazil, Venezuela, and Argentina with poor socioeconomic development. The infection has been reported as far north as the southern United States. Affected individuals generally do not recall initial contact with the protozoan, during which time the organisms deposited on broken skin or mucous membranes in feces of the triatomid insect multiply within local macrophages. These macrophages rupture and elicit an inflammatory reaction characterized as a nodule with slightly painful satellite nodules or draining lymph nodes. A symptomatic phase characterized by fever and diffuse lymph node enlargement subsequently develops. Hepatosplenomegaly may also occur. In severe cases, acute myocarditis, pericarditis, or endocarditis is seen. After several months the acute phase resolves and chronic disease characterized by cardiomyopathy, megaesophagus, or megacolon appears.[66] It is rare for the traveler to develop these signs and symptoms. Diagnosis during the acute phase may be made by demonstration of the parasites in leukocytes in Giemsa-stained blood smears. Amastigotes of *T. cruzi* may also be present in biopsy specimens of lymph nodes or muscle. Elevated IgM antibody titers to *T. cruzi* (performed by the CDC) also support the diagnosis. In the chronic phases of Chagas' disease the clinical findings of cardiomyopathy, megaesophagus, or megacolon in concert with isolation of *T. cruzi* from blood support the diagnosis. To detect trypanosomes in blood, uninfected triatomids are permitted to feed on the patient's forearm for 30 minutes. The insects are then kept for 30 days and the intestinal contents of the insects examined for *T. cruzi*. If negative, the examination may be repeated after 60 days. This test is positive in about 50% of cases. Serologic tests, including complement fixation for anti–*T. cruzi* antibodies (done at the CDC), are also useful but may be positive in long-term residents of endemic areas. Acute Chagas' disease is treated with nifurtimox, 8 to 10 mg/kg orally in four divided doses per day for 120 days. The drug is available from the CDC.

Leishmaniasis

Humans may be infected by *Leishmania* species that cause skin, mucocutaneous, or visceral disease.[124] These intracellular parasites are transmitted by phlebotomine sandflies. Various forms of the infection occur throughout Latin and Central America, Africa, the Middle East, and Asia (Color Plate 107). Cutaneous lesions caused by *L. tropica* and *L. tropica major* are referred to as "Oriental sores" in Asia and the Middle East. In Central and South America, *L. mexicana* and *L. braziliensis* cause skin lesions characterized in the chronic phase as nonhealing ulcers that frequently become secondarily infected by bacteria. Espundia, or mucocutaneous leishmaniasis caused by *L. braziliensis*, begins as a single nodule and eventually involves the oropharyngeal or nasal mucosa, where it causes severe destruction. This disease occurs primarily in residents of the Amazon basin in Brazil. Kala azar, or visceral leishmaniasis, is caused by *L. donovani* in Africa and Asia. Affected individuals generally do not recall an initial skin lesion. Several months after inoculation, fever, abdominal discomfort, and weakness develop and become progressively more severe. Nausea and vomiting are protracted, the skin becomes dry and dark, and abdominal distention with hepatosplenomegaly eventually appears. This disease is rare in travelers and nonresidents of endemic areas.

Major Helminthic Infections

Worm infections are common among travelers to developing countries, especially among persons who spend time in rural areas. However, unlike many viral or protozoan infections, helminths rarely cause life-threatening disease and infested persons are often asymptomatic.

SCHISTOSOMIASIS

Three major species of schistosomes infect humans: *Schistosoma mansoni, S. haematobium,* and *S. japonicum*. *S. mansoni* infection occurs in South America and Africa. *S. haematobium* infection occurs primarily in Africa, especially Egypt and East Africa. *S. japonicum* infection is present exclusively in the Far East. Schistosomiasis is transmitted by freshwater snails. These snails release cercariae that penetrate the skin of humans. The cercariae rapidly transform into schistosomulae, which migrate to the lungs and eventually the portal (in the case of *S. mansoni* and *S. japonicum*) or vesical (in the case of *S. haematobium*) venous system to differentiate into adult worms. Fecund female worms release eggs, which may be passed in feces or urine. Miracidia released from this stage may then infect snails in water used for bathing, washing clothes, or other communal activities.

Signs and symptoms of infection vary among the three schistosome species. The initial presentation of *S. mansoni* infection in Puerto Rico has been reported to include fever, anorexia, weight loss, and abdominal pain.[54] Hepatomegaly and splenomegaly were observed in 33% and 20% of subjects, respectively. This unusual symptom complex, which occurs in individuals with heavy infection, has been referred to as Katayama fever and appears 18 to 60 days after exposure. Travelers with light or moderate exposure, however, usually have no specific signs or only mild local dermatitis associated with contact with cercariae, the infective stage of the parasite released by snails. In persons with established infections the prevalence of clinical manifestations is low. Most individuals have no signs specifically attributable to *S. mansoni* infection. Hepatomegaly or splenomegaly, attributable to portal hypertension following granulomatous reactions to eggs deposited in the liver, occurs in 15% of subjects.[109] Eggs may also embolize to the lungs and induce granulomatous lesions and cor pulmonale. Those at greatest risk are persons who have the heaviest intensity of infection as judged by fecal egg counts. These complications may ultimately result in esophageal and gastrointestinal varices, which cause acute blood loss. The manifestations of schistosomiasis japonicum are similar to schistosomiasis mansoni except that Katayama fever appears to be more frequent. In addition, there is a unique manifestation of *S. japonicum* infection attributable to embolization of eggs to the brain. Generalized or jacksonian seizures are the major signs of cerebral schistosomiasis. Since *S. haematobium* adult worms inhabit the venous system of the genitourinary tract, the signs and symptoms of this helminth infection are primarily secondary to granulomatous reactions to eggs present in the ureters and bladder wall. Dysuria and hematuria have been reported in many individuals who reside in endemic areas. The frequency and severity of hematuria and dysuria and associated complications (such as calcification of the bladder and lower ureters and hydronephrosis) correlate directly with the intensity of infection, as judged by urinary egg output. It should be stressed that these complications are unusual in the traveler who spends little time in fresh water in endemic areas.[118]

All three species of schistosome infections are diagnosed by identification of eggs in urine, feces, or tissue sections. In the cases of *S. mansoni* and *S. japonicum,* microscopic inspection of feces by the Kato or formol-ether methods is most widely available in hospital laboratories.[91] *S. haematobium* eggs may be seen in urinary sediment or by more sensitive filtration techniques.[91] The treatment of all three species of schistosome infections is with praziquantel (40 mg/kg body weight in two divided doses for *S. haematobium* and *S. mansoni,* 60 mg/kg for *S. japonicum*). To avoid infection, travelers should be advised against swimming in freshwater lakes and rivers in endemic areas.

FILARIASES

Three major types of human filariasis exist. Infections caused by *Onchocerca volvulus* are manifest primarily as skin and eye disease. *Brugia malayi* and *Wuchereria bancrofti* cause lymphatic filariasis. Loa loa infection may cause skin disease. Each of these is described separately, since their ecologies and manifestations are distinctive.

Onchocerciasis

O. volvulus is transmitted to humans by *Simulium* species of blackflies in Central America and West and Central Africa. Infective, or third-stage, larvae eventually develop into adult worms contained in deep subcutaneous nodules. These are asymptomatic and may be palpable. Microfilariae are released from adult female worms and cause dermatitis as they migrate through the skin. In Central and West Africa the organisms have a propensity to invade the eye (especially the anterior chamber and cornea), where they cause blindness. Diagnosis is based on prolonged residence in an endemic area (for example, Peace Corps volunteers) and parasitologic identification in skin snips or slit-lamp examination of the eye.[7]

Lymphatic Filariasis

B. malayi and *W. bancrofti* are transmitted by mosquitoes. Infective larvae eventually develop into lymphatic-dwelling adult worms, which release microfilariae into the bloodstream. Although chronic infection and recurrent exposure are associated with a wide variety of clinical manifestations, including tropical pulmonary eosinophilia, acute lymphangitis, and elephantiasis, these manifestations are rare in nonresidents of endemic areas.[87] The only definitive diagnostic test is identification of parasites in the bloodstream. Since nonresidents and many residents who are infected may not have detectable parasitemia, other laboratory studies (eosinophilia, elevated serum IgE level) must be used as aids in diagnosis. Diethylcarbamazine (cumulative dose of 72 mg/kg body weight given over 2 weeks) is the treatment.[51] Studies are under way to determine if single-dose diethylcarbamazine or ivermectin is efficacious.

Loiasis

Loa loa is transmitted to humans by the bites of tabanid flies that live along river edges in Central and West Africa. Microfilariae migrate in the bloodstream, whereas adult worms migrate in cutaneous tissues. The major disease manifestation is the Calabar swelling. These are characterized as egg-sized or smaller raised lesions, predominantly over the extremities, that are tender and surrounded by edematous skin. They may migrate and last several days. Their pathogenesis is unclear but may be related to migration of adult worms or release of antigens that elicit immunologic hypersensitivity reactions. Treatment is with diethylcarbamazine at a dose of 9 mg/kg body weight/day for 3 weeks.[51] Retreatment is required occasionally.

INTESTINAL HELMINTH INFECTIONS

Ascariasis

Approximately 25% of the world's population is infected with *Ascaris lumbricoides*.[67] Although this nematode contributes significantly to morbidity in children with poor nutrition, it generally does not cause significant health problems for the traveler. The helminth is transmitted by eggs contained in ingested pieces of soil, such as may be found on vegetables grown in many countries with poor hygienic conditions. It is not limited to tropical climates but occurs in North America and Europe. Ingested eggs enter the small intestine. Larvae leave the eggshell to penetrate the mucosa and eventually enter the bloodstream and lymphatics. One to 5 days after infection they enter the liver and, at about 14 days, the lungs. The larvae then rupture through the alveoli, ascend the trachea, and return to the intestine upon being swallowed. In the small intestine adult males and females develop into macroscopic worms (12 to 25 cm long). Eggs passed via feces continue the life cycle. Ascaris infection is often totally asymptomatic, but several syndromes are associated with tissue and intestinal phases of infection. Persons who are recurrently exposed may develop pulmonary ascariasis, characterized by cough, wheezing, eosinophilia, and fleeting pulmonary infiltrates on chest x-ray examination.[90] Children may suffer from intestinal or biliary tract obstruction if they repeatedly ingest eggs. Intestinal symptoms are seen mainly in persons with heavy infection, an uncommon situation in the traveler.

Diagnosis of ascariasis may be made by identification of one of several parasite stages. Adult ascarids occasionally migrate from the mouth or anus. *Ascaris* larvae may rarely be observed in sputum or gastric washings. The most common means of diagnosis is identification of eggs in feces. Eggs are ovoid, 35 to 70 mm in diameter, and consist of an outer white shell and brownish ovum internally. The eggs are not produced until approximately 9 weeks after infection. Intestinal ascariasis is treated with mebendazole, 100 mg twice daily for 3 days.

Hookworm

Ancylostoma duodenale and *Necator americanus* infections occur most commonly in the tropics but also exist in temperate climates where sanitation is poor.[78] Hookworm is second only to *Ascaris* in terms of the number of people infected. Humans are infected percutaneously by third-stage larvae in the soil. The larvae enter the bloodstream, pass to the lungs, and rupture the alveolar lining to eventually ascend the trachea and descend the esophagus to differentiate into adult worms. These stages contain cutting plates on the anterior end and feed on host blood obtained through their attachment sites in the upper small intestine. It has been estimated that each *N. americanus* causes 0.03 ml of blood loss per day,[62] whereas *A. duodenale* consumes 0.26 ml per day. Iron deficiency anemia, especially in persons with low iron intake, is the major clinical manifestation of hookworm infection.[40] The diagnosis may be made by identification of hookworm eggs in feces. The eggs are round, 40 to 60 mm in diameter, and have a "smoother" shell than do *Ascaris* eggs. Although multiple drugs are effective in treatment, mebendazole (300 mg for the first dose, followed by 100 mg twice daily for 2 days) is most readily available. Supplemental iron should be given to persons when necessary. Infection with hookworm is rare in the traveler from a developed country.

Strongyloidiasis

Strongyloides stercoralis infection occurs in tropical and temperate regions. The infection is initiated by contact with soil containing infective third-stage larvae. The helminth follows a route within the host similar to that described for hookworms. In addition, there is an autoinfection cycle in which larvae released in the intestine may penetrate the mucosa directly and then migrate through the liver and lungs. This occurs only in immunocompromised individuals.[106]

Many persons with *S. stercoralis* infection are asymptomatic. Some persons, however, have cutaneous or intestinal manifestations. The former are urticarial lesions around the buttocks and waist that last 1 to 2 days.[46] These are secondary to penetration of larvae present in the feces. Other symptoms include indigestion, abdominal cramps, and diarrhea. Diagnosis is made by identification of larvae in fresh stools or gastrointestinal washings. Rhabditiform larvae with a length of 250 mm and a width of 10 to 20 mm are most commonly observed, although filariform larvae (500 mm long) may also be present. Treatment is with thiabendazole at a dose of 25 mg/kg body weight twice daily for 2 days.

Enterobiasis

Enterobiasis, or pinworm infection, exists in all parts of the world. Eggs are passed from female worms in the colon. Infection is transmitted by ingestion of *Enterobius vermicularis* eggs, which develop into gravid adult female worms in the large bowel. The infection is especially common in crowded settings where sanitation is poor. The diagnosis may be made by identification of adult worms migrating along the perianal area or by eggs deposited in the same area. Eggs are detected by applying a piece of sticky cellophane tape to the area and inspecting it microscopically.[70] Treatment is with a single 100 mg dose of mebendazole.

REFERENCES

1. Al-Tikriti SK et al: Congo/Crimean haemorrhagic fever in Iraq, *Bull WHO* 59:85, 1981.
2. Baron RC, McCormick JB, Zubeir OA: Ebola virus disease in southern Sudan: hospital dissemination and intrafamilial spread, *Bull WHO* 61:997, 1983.
3. Belsey NA, Hoffpauir CW, Smith MHD: Dexamethasone in the treatment of acute bacterial meningitis: the effect of study design on the interpretation of results, *Pediatrics* 44:503, 1969.
4. Blake PA et al: Serological therapy of tetanus in the United States, 1965-1971, *JAMA* 235:42, 1976.
5. Borges APA et al: Estudo da coagulacao sanquinea na febre amarela, *Rev Patol Trop* 2:143, 1973.
6. Broome CV: The carrier state: *Neisseria meningitidis, J Antimicrob Chemother* 18(suppl A):25, 1986.
7. Buck AA et al: Onchocerciasis: some new epidemiologic and clinical findings, *Am J Trop Med Hyg* 18:217, 1969.
8. Burke DS, Nisalak A: Detection of Japanese encephalitis virus immunoglobulin M antibodies in serum by antibody capture radioimmunoassay, *J Clin Microbiol* 15:353, 1982.
9. Burke DS, Nisalak A, Ussery MA: Antibody capture immunoassay for detection of Japanese encephalitis virus immunoglobulin M and G antibodies in cerebrospinal fluid, *J Clin Microbiol* 16:1034, 1982.
10. Burke DS et al: Fatal outcome in Japanese encephalitis, *Am J Trop Med Hyg* 34:1203, 1985.
11. Cahill KM et al: Preparing patients for travel, *Patient Care,* p 217, June 15, 1987.
12. Centers for Disease Control: Bacterial meningitis and meningococcemia, United States, 1978, *MMWR* 28:277, 1979.
13. Centers for Disease Control: Dengue—Texas, *MMWR* 29:451, 1980.

14. Centers for Disease Control: Epidemic meningococcal disease: recommendations for travelers to Nepal, *MMWR* 34:119, 1985.
15. Centers for Disease Control: Meningococcal vaccines, *MMWR* 34:121, 1985.
16. Centers for Disease Control: Revised recommendations for preventing malaria in travelers to areas with chloroquine-resistant *Plasmodium falciparum, MMWR* 34:185, 1985.
17. Centers for Disease Control: Dengue in the Americas, *MMWR* 35:732, 1986.
18. Centers for Disease Control: Dengue hemorrhagic fever—Puerto Rico, *MMWR* 35:779, 1986.
19. Centers for Disease Control: Safety of therapeutic immune globulin preparations with respect to transmission of human T-lymphotropic virus type III/lymphadenopathy-associated virus infection, *MMWR* 35:231, 1986.
20. Centers for Disease Control: Pertussis surveillance, United States, 1984 and 1985, *MMWR* 36:168, 1987.
21. Centers for Disease Control: Management of patients with suspected viral hemorrhagic fever, *MMWR* 37:1, 1988.
22. Centers for Disease Control: Recommendations for protection against viral hepatitis, *MMWR* 39(RR-2):1, 1990.
22a. Centers for Disease Control: Yellow fever vaccine, *MMWR* 39(RR-2):1, 1990.
23. Centers for Disease Control: Diphtheria, tetanus and pertussis: guidelines for vaccine use and other preventive measures, *MMWR* 40(RR-10):1, 1991.
23a. Centers for Disease Control: Pertussis vaccination: acellular pertussis vaccine for reinforcing and booster use—supplementary ACIP statement, *MMWR* 41(RR-1):1, 1992.
24. Centers for Disease Control: Diphtheria outbreak—Russian Federation, 1990-1993, *MMWR* 42:840, 1993.
25. Centers for Disease Control: Inactivated Japanese encephalitis virus vaccine, *MMWR* 42(RR-1):1, 1993.
25a. Centers for Disease Control: Dengue surveillance—United States, 1986-1992, *MMWR* 43(SS-2):7, 1994.
26. Chapman LE et al: Risk factors for Crimean-Congo hemorrhagic fever in northern Senegal, *J Infect Dis* 164:686, 1991.
27. Choo Q-L et al: Isolation of a cDNA clone derived from a blood-borne non-A, non-B viral hepatitis genome, *Science* 244:359, 1989.
28. Christenson B: Epidemiological aspects of acute viral hepatitis A in Swedish travelers to endemic areas, *Scand J Infect Dis* 17:5, 1985.
29. Cochi SL et al: Control of epidemic group A meningococcal meningitis in Nepal, *Int J Epidemiol* 16:91, 1987.
30. Cosgriff TM et al: Studies of the coagulation system in arenaviral hemorrhagic fever—pichinde virus in guinea pigs, *Am J Trop Med Hyg* 36:416, 1987.
31. Edelman R, Levine MM: Summary of an international workshop on typhoid fever, *Rev Infect Dis* 8:329, 1986.
32. Editorial: Yellow fever in Africa, *Lancet* 2:1315, 1986.
33. Editorial: The known and the unknown about dengue fever, *Lancet* 1:488, 1987.
34. Fisher-Hoch SP et al: Pathophysiology of shock and hemorrhage in a fulminating viral infection (Ebola), *J Infect Dis* 152:887, 1985.
35. Fisher-Hoch SP et al: Physiological and immunologic disturbances associated with shock in a primate model of Lassa fever, *J Infect Dis* 155:465, 1987.
36. Foulkes JR: Human trypanosomiasis in Africa, *Br Med J* 283:1172, 1981.
37. Frame JD et al: Lassa fever, a new virus disease of man from West Africa. I. Clinical description and pathological findings, *Am J Trop Med Hyg* 19:670, 1970.
38. Francis DP et al: Occurrence of hepatitis A, B, and non-A/non-B in the United States, *Am J Med* 76:69, 1984.
39. Gear JSS et al: Outbreak of Marburg virus disease in Johannesburg, *Br Med J* 4:489, 1975.
40. Gilles HM, Watson-Williams EJ, Ball P: Hookworm infection and anemia, *Q J Med* 33:1, 1964.
41. Gimson AE et al: Clinical and prognostic differences in fulminant hepatitis type A, B, and non-A non-B, *Gut* 24:1194, 1983.
42. Gocke DJ: Immune complex phenomena associated with hepatitis. In Vyas GN, Cohen SN, Schmidt R, editors: *Viral hepatitis: a contemporary assessment,* Philadelphia, 1978, Franklin Institute Press.
43. Gocke DJ: Hepatitis A revisited, *Ann Intern Med* 105:960, 1986.
44. Goldfarb LG et al: An epidemiological model of Crimean hemorrhagic fever, *Am J Trop Med Hyg* 29:260, 1980.
45. Goodman RA et al: Nosocomial hepatitis A transmission by an adult patient with diarrhea, *Am J Med* 73:220, 1982.
46. Grove DI: Strongyloidiasis in Allied ex-prisoners of war in Southeast Asia, *Br Med J* 280:598, 1980.
47. Hall SM, Mortimer PP, Vanderveld EM: Hepatitis A in the traveler, *Lancet* 2:1198, 1983.
48. Halsey NA, Smith MHD: Diphtheria. In Warren KS, Mahmoud AAF, editors: *Tropical and geographical medicine,* New York, 1984, McGraw-Hill.
49. Halstead SB: The pathogenesis of dengue: molecular epidemiology in infectious disease, *Am J Epidemiol* 114:632, 1981.
50. Halstead SB: Selective primary health care: strategies for control of disease in the developing world. XI. Dengue, *Rev Infect Dis* 6:251, 1984.
51. Hawking F: Diethylcarbamazine and new compounds for the treatment of filariasis, *Adv Pharmacol Chemother* 16:129, 1979.
52. Helmick CG et al: No evidence for increased risk of Lassa fever infection in hospital staff, *Lancet* 2:1202, 1986.
53. Heymann NL et al: Ebola hemorrhagic fever: Tandala, Zaire, 1977-78, *J Infect Dis* 142:371, 1980.
54. Hiatt RA et al: Factors in the pathogenesis of acute schistosomiasis mansoni, *J Infect Dis* 139:659, 1979.
55. Hinman AR, Koplan JP: Pertussis and pertussis vaccine: reanalysis of benefits, risks and costs, *JAMA* 251:3109, 1984.
56. Hinman AR, Koplan JP: Pertussis and pertussis vaccine: further analysis of benefits, risks and costs, *Dev Biol Stand* 61:419, 1985.
57. Hoffman SC et al: Reduction of mortality in chloramphenicol-treated severe typhoid fever by high-dose dexamethasone, *N Engl J Med* 310:116, 1984.
58. Hoffman TA et al: Waterborne typhoid fever in Dade County, Florida: clinical and therapeutic evaluations of 105 bacteremic patients, *Am J Med* 59:481, 1975.
59. Hornick RB et al: Typhoid fever: pathogenesis and immunologic control, *N Engl J Med* 283:686, 1970.
60. Inman RD et al: Arthritis, vasculitis and cryoglobulinemia associated with relapsing hepatitis A infection, *Ann Intern Med* 105:700, 1986.
61. Jones TC: Health advice and immunizations for travelers. In Remington JS, Swartz MN, editors: *Current topics in infectious diseases,* New York, 1985, McGraw-Hill.
62. Kalkofen UP: Intestinal trauma resulting from feeding activities of *Ancylostoma caninum, Am J Trop Med Hyg* 23:1046, 1974.
63. Khuroo MS: Study of epidemic of non-A, non-B hepatitis: possibility of another human hepatitis virus distinct from post-transfusion non-A non-B type, *Am J Med* 68:818, 1980.
64. Khuroo MS et al: Failure to detect chronic liver disease after epidemic non-A, non-B hepatitis, *Lancet* 2:260, 1980.
65. Koppes GM, Lellenbogen C, Gephart RJ: Group Y meningococcal disease in United States Air Force Recruits, *Am J Med* 62:661, 1977.
66. Laranja FS et al: Chagas' disease: a clinical epidemiologic and pathologic study, *Circulation* 14:1015, 1956.
67. Lawlowski SW: Ascariasis: host pathogen biology, *Rev Infect Dis* 4:806, 1982.
68. Lee HW et al: Isolation of Hantaan virus, the etiologic agent of Korean hemorrhagic fever, from wild urban rats, *J Infect Dis* 146:638, 1982.
69. Linneman CC Jr, Nasenbeny J: Pertussis in the adult, *Annu Rev Med* 28:177, 1977.
70. Mayers CP, Pervis RJ: Manifestations of pinworms, *Can Med Assoc J* 103:489, 1970.

71. McCormick JB: Viral hemorrhagic fevers. In Warren KS, Mahmoud AAF, editors: *Tropical and geographical medicine,* New York, 1984, McGraw-Hill.
72. McCormick JB et al: Lassa fever: effective therapy with ribavirin, *N Engl J Med* 304:20, 1986.
73. McCormick JB et al: A case-control study of the clinical diagnosis and course of Lassa fever, *J Infect Dis* 155:445, 1987.
74. McCormick JB et al: A prospective study of the epidemiology and ecology of Lassa fever, *J Infect Dis* 155:437, 1987.
75. McKee KT, Le Duc JW, Peters CJ: Hantaviruses. In Belshe RB, editor: *Textbook of virology,* ed 2, St Louis, 1991, Mosby.
76. *The Medical Letter:* Drugs for parasitic infection, 24(601):5, 1982.
77. Meningococcal Disease Surveillance Group: Meningococcal disease secondary attack rate and chemoprophylaxis in the United States, 1974, *JAMA* 235:261, 1974.
78. Miller TA: Hookworm infection in man, *Adv Parasitol* 17:315, 1979.
79. Molinas FC, de Bracco MME, Maiztegui JI: Coagulation studies in Argentine hemorrhagic fever, *J Infect Dis* 143:1, 1981.
80. Monath TP: *Aedes albopictus,* an exotic mosquito vector in the United States, *Ann Intern Med* 105:449, 1986.
81. Monath TP: Yellow fever: a medically neglected disease, report on a seminar, *Rev Infect Dis* 9:165, 1987.
82. Monath TP et al: Indirect fluorescent antibody test for the diagnosis of yellow fever, *Trans R Soc Trop Med Hyg* 75:282, 1981.
83. Morens DM et al: Dengue shock syndrome in an American traveler with primary dengue 3 infection, *Am J Trop Med Hyg* 36:424, 1987.
84. Nelson JE: The changing epidemiology of pertussis in young infants, *Am J Dis Child* 132:371, 1978.
85. Noble RC et al: Post-transfusion hepatitis A in a neonatal intensive care unit, *JAMA* 253:2711, 1984.
86. Noguiera P: Early history of yellow fever. In *Yellow fever: a symposium in commemoration of Juan Carlos Finlay,* Philadelphia, 1955, Jefferson Medical College.
87. Ottesen EA: Immunopathology of lymphatic filariasis in man, *Semin Immunopathol* 2:373, 1980.
88. Pan American Health Organization: Present status of yellow fever: memorandum from a PAHO meeting, *Bull WHO* 64:511, 1986.
89. Passen EL, Anderson BR: Clinical tetanus despite a "protective" level of toxin-neutralizing antibody, *JAMA* 255:1171, 1986.
90. Pawlowski ZS: Ascariasis, *Clin Gastroenterol* 7:157, 1982.
91. Peters PA, Kazura JW: Update on diagnostic methods for schistosomiasis. In Mahmoud AAF, editor: *Balliere's clinical tropical medicine and communicable diseases,* London, 1988, WB Saunders.
92. Peters RL: Viral hepatitis: a pathologic spectrum, *Am J Med Sci* 270:17, 1975.
93. Phillips RE: Management of *Plasmodium falciparum* malaria, *Med J Aust* 141:511, 1984.
94. Press E: Desirability of routine use of tetanus toxoid, *N Engl J Med* 239:50, 1948.
95. Putsch RW, Hamilton JD, Wolinsky E: *Neisseria meningitidis,* a respiratory pathogen, *J Infect Dis* 121:48, 1970.
96. Ramachandran S, Godfrey JJ, Perera MVF: Typhoid hepatitis, *JAMA* 230:236, 1974.
97. Reingold AL et al: Age-specific differences in duration of clinical protection after vaccination with meningococcal polysaccharide A vaccine, *Lancet* 2:114, 1985.
98. Reyes GR et al: Isolation of a cDNA from the virus responsible for enterically transmitted non A, non B hepatitis, *Science* 247:1335, 1990.
99. Rizzetto M, Canese MG: Hepatitis delta virus disease, *Prog Liver Dis* 8:417, 1986.
100. Rizzetto M et al: Incidence and significance of antibodies to delta antigen in hepatitis B virus infection, *Lancet* 2:986, 1979.
101. Robinson WS: Delta agent hepatitis. In Remington JS, Schwartz R, editors: *Current clinical topics in infectious diseases,* vol 8, New York, 1987, McGraw-Hill.
102. Rosen L: The emperor's new clothes revisited, or reflections on the pathogenesis of dengue hemorrhagic fever, *Am J Trop Med Hyg* 26:337, 1977.
103. Rosen L: The pathogenesis of dengue hemorrhagic fever, *S Afr Med J* 70s:41, 1986.
104. Santos F et al: Intravascular disseminada aguda na febre amarela: dosagem dos factores da coagulacao, *Brasilia Med* 9:9, 1973.
105. Schofield F: Selective primary health care: strategies for control of disease in the developing world. XXII. Tetanus: a preventable problem, *Rev Infect Dis* 8:144, 1986.
106. Schumaker JD et al: Thiabendazole treatment of severe strongyloidiasis in a hemodialysed patient, *Ann Intern Med* 89:655, 1978.
107. Shih W-K, Estebon Mur JI, Alter HJ: Non-A non-B hepatitis: advances and unfulfilled expectations of the first decade, *Prog Liver Dis* 8:433, 1986.
108. Simonsen O et al: Immunity against tetanus and response to revaccination in surgical patients more than 50 years of age, *Surg Gynecol Obstet* 164:329, 1987.
109. Siongok TKA et al: Morbidity in schistosomiasis mansoni in relation to intensity of infection: study of a community in Machakos, Kenya, *Am J Trop Med Hyg* 35:273, 1976.
110. Spitz S: The pathology of acute falciparum malaria, *Milit Surg* 99:555, 1946.
111. Steffen R et al: Health problems after travel to developing countries, *J Infect Dis* 156:84, 1987.
112. Tabor L et al: Additional evidence for more than one agent of human non-A, non-B hepatitis: transmission and passage studies in chimpanzees, *Transfusion* 24:224, 1983.
113. Ryan CA, Hargrett-Bean NT, Blake PA: *Salmonella typhi* infections in the United States, 1975-1984, *Rev Infect Dis* 11:1, 1989.
114. Umenai T et al: Japanese encephalitis: current worldwide status, *Bull WHO* 63:625, 1985.
115. Van Eeden PJ et al: A nosocomial outbreak of Crimean-Congo haemorrhagic fever at Tygerberg Hospital. A. Clinical features, *S Afr Med J* 68:711, 1985.
116. Vickerman K: Antigenic variation in trypanosomes, *Nature* 273:613, 1978.
117. Warrel DA et al: Dexamethasone proves deleterious in cerebral malaria, *N Engl J Med* 306:313, 1982.
118. Warren KS: Regulation of the prevalence and intensity of schistosomiasis in man: immunology or ecology? *J Infect Dis* 127:595, 1973.
119. Weber DJ et al: Obesity as a prediction of poor antibody response to hepatitis B plasma vaccine, *JAMA* 254:3187, 1985.
120. Wenger JD et al: Bacterial meningitis in the United States, 1986: report of a multistate surveillance study, *J Infect Dis* 162:1316, 1990.
121. Woodruff BA, Pavia AT, Blake PA: A new look at typhoid vaccination: information for the practicing physician, *JAMA* 265:756, 1991.
122. World Health Organization: Hemorrhagic fever with renal syndrome: memorandum from a WHO meeting, *Bull WHO* 61:269, 1983.
123. World Health Organization: *Dengue hemorrhagic fever: diagnosis, treatment and control,* Geneva, 1986.

123a. World Health Organization: Yellow fever virus surveillance in western Africa, *Weekly Epi Rec* 69(13):93, 1994.

124. Wyler DJ, Marsden PA: Leishmaniasis. In Warren KS, Mahmoud AAF, editors: *Tropical and geographical medicine,* New York, 1984, McGraw-Hill.
125. Xu ZY et al: Epidemiological studies of hemorrhagic fever with renal syndrome: analysis of risk factors and mode of transmission, *J Infect Dis* 152:137, 1985.
126. Yoshizawa H et al: Demonstration of two different types of non-A, non-B hepatitis by reinjection and cross challenge studies in chimpanzees, *Gastroenterology* 81:107, 1981.
127. Zoombaulakis D et al: Steroids in the treatment of pertussis: a controlled clinical trial, *Arch Dis Child* 48:51, 1973.

46 EMERGENCY VETERINARY MEDICINE

Murray E. Fowler

The wilderness experience often involves animals other than humans. Such domestic animals as horses, llamas, elephants, camels, and yaks may be used for packing or pulling supplies, relieving hikers of this burden. Dogs may accompany owners into the wilderness as companions, as trackers of game, or in the Arctic and Antarctic as primary draft animals. Any of these animals may become injured or fatigued or fall ill with a variety of ailments that may require emergency treatment and management by trek personnel.

Observation of wild animals in their natural habitat enhances the wilderness experience, but encounters between wild animals and animals accompanying the trekkers may be less than pleasant. Healthy wild animals usually try to avoid humans, but this may not carry over to domestic animals.

The objectives of this chapter are to engender a greater appreciation for wild animals encountered in the wilderness; describe safety precautions and other methods to avoid conflict; describe medical problems that may affect support animals on the trail, with the goal of recognition of predisposing factors and ultimately prevention; and describe basic treatment procedures for dealing with emergencies.

Wild Animal Encounters

Medical and paramedical personnel who may be called to render emergency medical care or assist in the rescue of injured or diseased humans or support animals should recognize that wild animals may be involved. Experienced trekkers can usually recognize when they are intruding into an animal's domain. Unfortunately, some people lack a sense of courtesy for animals. When trekkers in the wilderness behave as if they are entering the home of a human friend, they show appreciation for the rights of wild animals and have less risk of injury or illness to themselves or their support animals. Understanding the biology and normal behavior of wild animals known to live in the wilderness areas to be visited enhances enjoyment and diminishes exposure to potentially dangerous situations.

Others who may be at risk are wildlife biologists, hunters, and people who choose to live in remote areas. Hunters come into intimate contact with wild animals as they pursue, dress, and eat game. Plant scientists, paleontologists, geologists, and other non–animal scientists may inadvertently encounter wild animals. Wild animal biologists conducting field investigations may capture or immobilize wild animals to collect data. Such individuals are at potential risk of injury or disease, not only as a result of wild animal contact, but also from drugs and firearms used to administer the drugs.

WHY AND WHEN WILD ANIMALS ARE DANGEROUS

See Chapter 40 for more details on this subject. Few wild animals deliberately stalk humans. This may not be true of support animals. Most wild animals fear humans and, given an opportunity, avoid human contact. Injuries to humans caused by wild animals are usually the result of judgment errors, such as approaching too closely, ill-advised handling of diseased wild animals, or unlucky exposure to highly aggressive or protective animals. Such animals may be natural predators seeking food, prey species fearful for their lives or the lives of their young, or diseased and irrational animals (such as those with rabies). Attacks on support animals usually occur at night or when humans are absent.

Animals are most likely to respond adversely if startled from sleep or if their flight distance is violated. Flight distance is that distance at which, if approached by an enemy, an animal will either fight (attack) or flee. The distance is species specific for a given region and may become greater if animals in the area have been recently hunted. Flight distance may be greater for a person walking or carrying a gun than for a person riding on horseback or in a vehicle. Animals that find themselves cornered occasionally attack or risk injury trying to escape. Any animal may attack if its offspring are in danger. With any large animal, accidental or intentional positioning between a mother and her infant invites attack.

Equal danger exists for a person who comes between a territorial male and one or more females. Many wild animals are territorial. Males and females may establish feeding, breeding, and home territories. An animal may share feeding territories with other members of the same species or different species, but home territories may be defended against any intruder, including humans.

Injuries have been inflicted on hunters who approached a recently shot animal, believing it to be dead, only to have the animal revive explosively in a final Herculean effort to fight or flee.

HOW WILD ANIMALS INFLICT INJURY

Offensive and defensive maneuvers evolved to enhance food gathering or to avoid being eaten. All wild animals have one or more anatomic or behavioral adaptations that allow them to cope with enemies. Humans are the most recently evolved enemy, and a wild animal may efficiently employ its entire repertoire against its most formidable enemy. See Chapter 40 for more details.

Most North American wild mammals have incisor teeth and bite if handled. Carnivores and wild pigs have large, dangerous canine teeth. Large hoofed animals (such as elk, moose, and deer) may strike with the forelimbs and either bruise or lacerate the victim. Carnivores, including raptors, have large claws or talons to adeptly grasp prey. Bears may scratch with claws and inflict severe injury with swipes from powerful paws. Even small rabbits and rodents can inflict serious scratches with their nails.

Horned or antlered hoofed animals use their cranial adornments to do battle. The bighorn sheep uses its massive horns as a battering ram. Females without horns or antlers may still butt with their heads.

INJURY PREVENTION

Humans should not fraternize with wild animals. Food scraps should not be left to tempt wild animals closer for photographs. Any wild animal that will allow touching is a spoiled park animal or is diseased. Neither type should be hand fed. Travelers in the wild should be observant for animal signs (such as feces, tracks, trails, and resting areas) and should respect the behavioral characteristics of animals. Knowledge of the biology and habits of local animals obviates most avoidable close encounters and dangerous situations.

Zoonoses are discussed in Chapters 40 and 41. Expedition leaders who will be in the field in unknown environments for a prolonged period should investigate the potential for zoonotic infectious and parasitic diseases, obtain appropriate immunizations, and carry proper medications. Two major concerns are tetanus and rabies. Protective immunization is available for both (see Chapters 40 and 41), and the expedition medical officer should require current vaccinations for all persons traveling to high-risk endemic regions.

DEALING WITH AN ATTACK

Bear attacks on hikers have generated a great deal of literature, and such attacks seem to be increasing in prevalence. There is little unanimity about recommendations for avoiding attack. Outrunning a bear is nearly impossible. A person who anticipates a charge should face the animal and back away slowly. Some individuals have saved themselves by playing dead. Adult black bears can climb trees, so a tree is not necessarily a suitable refuge. Adult grizzlies are not as likely to climb trees, but they have tremendous reach, so the escapee must climb above 15 feet.

A person charged by an elk or moose should hide behind a barrier (such as a tree or large rock) or wield a club or large stone. Attacks from most other animals result from having cornered the animal, in which case the best thing to do is to get out of the way quickly.

Wild animal attacks on support animals usually occur when the animal is tied on a picket line or staked out for grazing. The animal may injure itself trying to escape the attack or be bitten and mauled by its attacker. In one example, a frightened llama broke loose from a stake, but the lead rope suddenly caught between rocks and the animal's cervical spine was fractured by the abrupt stop.

TREATMENT OF ANIMAL-INFLICTED INJURIES

Wounds may be lacerations, contusions, punctures, or abrasions. Specific therapy is addressed in Chapter 40.

Support Animals

Expedition leaders and participants should consider the well-being of support animals and understand their physical capabilities. These include maximal load, speed, and endurance. Humans should also be able to recognize signs of exertional stress.

Exertional stress is more likely to occur in horses that are ridden than in packhorses that are led. A horse can generally match or exceed the physical endurance of a hiker. Adverse metabolic conditions may develop in horses pushed beyond their limits of endurance. The type of syndrome arising from excessive exercise depends on intensity and duration, degree of prior conditioning, and nutritional status. Mules, donkeys, and llamas are less prone than horses to develop problems, because they usually refuse to be pushed to extremes of exertion.

The animal best suited to the terrain, climate, and task to be performed should be selected. Horses, mules, and donkeys are traditional beasts of burden in North America, wherever sufficient forage and water are available. Each animal has both admirable and undesirable qualities. Horses are usually the largest and can carry the heaviest loads. Mules and burroes tend to be more difficult for novices to handle. No animal should be used on a trek unless at least one member of the party has considerable experience in handling and caring for the chosen animal.

In South America the llama is the beast of burden. Adventurers traveling into rugged and remote areas above 3000 m will probably use the llama for support. Llamas have also become popular support animals with backpackers in North America. The llama requires less feed, can subsist better on sparse native forages, and is less damaging to the environment than the horse.

Dogs are necessary support animals for winter travel in the Arctic. In other regions they function more as companions.

Many expeditions are mounted in countries unfamiliar to both leaders and participants. In various parts of Asia the horse is replaced by the elephant, water buffalo, Bactrian camel, or yak. In North Africa and the Middle East the dromedary camel carries the load. Each species has specialized requirements for handling, packing, and health care.

Expedition physicians may be asked to treat the ailments of support animals. Basic medical training provides the foundation necessary to diagnose and treat many conditions that may be encountered on the trail. This chapter provides an overview and specific anatomic and therapeutic information for some common problems. If in doubt, expedition members should handle an ailing support animal as if it were human. With support animals carrying all or part of the load, a more sophisticated emergency medical kit may be carried.

PRETRIP ANIMAL HEALTH CONSIDERATIONS

Health certificates are needed for travel and entry into the state or province of destination and possibly intervening states to be traveled through. Regulations are extremely variable, and inquiry about them should be made at least 4 weeks before departure. It is wise for each animal to receive a physical examination by a qualified veterinarian before an extended trip. Conditioning is as important for trek animals as for human participants. Training should be in terrain similar to that expected on the trek, with special attention given to toughening the footpads of llamas and dogs by appropriate exercise.

Immature animals should not be taken on expeditions. Dogs should be at least 1 year old. Llamas and equids should be 3 years old. Well-conditioned and trained horses, mules, donkeys, or dogs can carry approximately 30% of their body weight. Llamas usually carry only 25% of their body weight (Table 46-1).

Frequently arrangements are made to contract for sup-

Table 46-1 Vital Statistics of Trek Animals

Animal	Body Weight		Heart Rate/Min	Respiratory Rate/Min	Body Temperature		Weight Carried by Well-Conditioned Animals*	
	Pounds	Kg			°C	°F	Kg	Pounds
Horse	800-1200	360-540	28-40	10-14	37.2-38.0	99.0-100.5	110-136	240-300
Mule	600-1200	275-540	28-40	10-14	37.2-38.0	99.0-100.5	82-136	180-300
Donkey	300-600	136-275	28-40	10-14	37.2-38.0	99.0-100.5	40-82	90-180
Llama	300-450	136-200	60-90	10-30	37.2-38.7	99.0-101.8	34-50	75-110
Dog	20-100	9-45	65-90	15-30	37.5-38.6	99.5-101.5	3-14	6-30
Camel	880-1200	400-550	40-50	5-12	36.4-42.0	97.5-107.6	225	500
Elephant	5000-8000	2300-3700	25-35	4-6	36.0-37.0	97.5- 99.0	900	2000
Yak	2200	1000	55-80	10-30	37.8-39.2	100.0-102.5	235	550

*For sustained trekking: 15 to 25 miles per day on moderately difficult trails. This includes tack. Animals in training should be expected to carry only one half to two thirds of this weight.

port animal service from suppliers in the trek locale. Persons providing these services do not always understand the trek requirements and may supply animals that are poorly shod, unconditioned, poorly trained, or otherwise unsuitable for the needs of trek participants. Trek leaders must clearly describe specifications and be adamant about compliance, well in advance of the trek.

Horses, Mules, and Donkeys

A tetanus booster should have been given within the past year. Vaccination against rabies is appropriate if the trek itinerary includes traveling in an endemic area. Encephalomyelitis vaccines should be used in endemic areas, especially during the insect seasons of summer and fall. Internal parasite levels should be evaluated by fecal flotation and appropriate medication given to reduce the parasite burden.

The feet should be trimmed and shod properly at least 2 weeks and not more than 4 weeks before a trek begins. Extra shoes for fore and hind feet of different-sized horses should be carried, along with the appropriate nails and hammer to reattach a shoe, should one be cast.

Llamas

Llamas should have been given a tetanus toxoid booster within the past 6 months. Other basic immunizations should include *Clostridium perfringens* toxoid, type C and D, within the past 6 months, and vaccinations against leptospirosis and rabies if entering an endemic area.

Toenails should have been trimmed within the previous 2 months. Internal parasitism is debilitating in llamas. Ova levels should be checked, but usually treatment with an anthelminthic (ivermectin 0.2 mg/kg subcutaneously, or fenbendazole 5 mg/kg orally) is desirable within the previous 2 months.

Dogs

Dogs are routinely immunized against canine distemper, canine adenovirus, leptospirosis, and rabies. Vaccinations should be current. A check should be made for internal parasites and fleas and appropriate action taken. Although dog fleas do not permanently infest humans, they bite and may cause mild to severe local dermal reactions in sensitive individuals. Dogs should be bathed with a shampoo containing a pyrethrin insecticide before a trek. Any pyrethrin-containing dusting powder may be carried on an extended trek to relieve dogs of flea burdens. It is unlikely that the fleas involved in the sylvatic plague cycle will infest a dog, so the dog is not a source of plague infections for humans in a trek situation.

REST

Support animals require less sleep than human trekkers. Horses can sleep while standing because they have a special locking mechanism of the tendons and ligaments of the limbs. Horses may also lie in sternal or lateral recumbency. Llamas usually rest in a sternal position but may also assume lateral recumbency.

Llamas enjoy taking a "dust bath" by rolling in dirt soon after packs are removed. A few may try to roll with the pack still in place.

WATERING AND FEEDING

All animals require daily access to potable water. It is not possible to filter or disinfect water for large animals except in extremely filthy conditions. Dogs may be susceptible to giardiasis, and theoretically it is desirable to provide filtered water for them. However, preventing a free-running dog from drinking from a stream or lake is virtually impossible. Heavily mineralized or silted water may be as unpalatable for animals as for humans and may cause similar gastrointestinal upsets.

The basic fluid requirement for a horse or other large trek animal is approximately 40 ml/kg/day. This would amount to 18 L (5 gallons) for a 450 kg (1000-pound) horse. With work and heavy sweating the requirement may be tripled. Llamas and donkeys may require one third less water than a horse.

Llamas and donkeys tolerate dehydration better than other species, but they function better if well hydrated. The camel is noted for its ability to tolerate a number of days (2 to 7) without drinking water. Equids sweat profusely and should be given the opportunity to drink along the trail. Some llamas refuse to drink until evening.

Feeding Horses, Mules, and Donkeys

Equids consume approximately 2% to 2.5% of their body weight daily (for a 1000-pound horse, this amounts to 20 to 25 pounds of total feed). When the animals are working hard, half of this amount should be concentrates (grains such as rolled oats, barley, or cracked corn, or mixed grains and molasses in loose or pellet form). If forage is unavailable, alfalfa pellets should be carried. Animals should become accustomed to eating pellets before the journey begins. Concentrates should be reduced on days when the animals are not working.

Feeding Llamas

Llamas require only 1.5% to 2% of their body weight in food daily. Given the opportunity, llamas will graze and browse to satisfy their requirements. Many packers carry a supplement mixture consisting of half alfalfa pellets and half grain mix (same as for horses), used as required. Some llamas are reluctant and must be trained to eat pellets or grain. Training should take place at home, not during the trek.

Feeding Dogs

A dog should be accustomed to high-quality dry dog food. The quantity fed should increase by half when the dog is exercising.

EMERGENCY RESTRAINT

It is assumed that one or (preferably) more persons on the trek are acquainted with the general care and handling of any domestic species involved in the expedition. Methods of haltering and leading are specific for each animal. Securing animals at night may require hobbling or tethering. Skill and experience are necessary to accomplish this without risk of injury to the animal or handler. Animal handlers should be able to examine and clean the feet and hoofs of their charges. All people who deal with animals should know how to create a halter tie (Fig. 46-1) so that a safe and secure tie can be made at rest stops or whenever an animal is to be tethered. A knowledge of temporary rope halter construction is desirable in the event of loss or breakage of halters (Fig. 46-2).

Horses, Mules, and Donkeys

Large animals can inflict serious or lethal injuries on people. When in pain or panicked, they may not respond even to their accustomed handlers. If a horse is down and entangled in rope, wire, or bushes, it should be approached from its back and its head held down until it can be extricated. The handler should stay out of the reach of both fore and hind limbs.

A horse's defensive and offensive actions are to strike with the fore limbs, kick forward and backward with the rear limbs, and bite. The safest place to stand is close to the left shoulder. A person examining the feet and legs of a standing horse should keep his or her head above the lower body line to avoid having the horse reach forward with a rear limb and strike it.

Additional restraint for painful procedures may be accomplished by grasping one or both ears of the horse. The method of "earing" a horse is as follows: Stand at the left shoulder and grasp the halter or lead rope with the left hand. Place the right hand palm down with the fingers together and the thumb extended, on the top of the neck. Slide the hand up the neck until the thumb and fingers surround the base of the ear (Fig. 46-3). Squeeze tightly, but do not twist the ear. The horse usually tries to pull away as the ear is grasped. Be prepared to move with the horse while maintaining a firm grip.

Llamas

Pack llamas are usually docile. Although most allow the feet to be lifted for inspection or treatment, some try to lie down. One or two people should stand on the side opposite the limb being lifted, or the llama should be placed next to a tree or large rock to prevent the animal from moving away. The limb should be firmly grasped. It may be necessary to semisupport the body if the animal tries to lie down.

If a llama refuses to get up, the rear limbs should be pulled out behind it. If it still refuses to rise, an injury or illness that inhibits rising should be suspected.

Only rarely does a llama "spit" against an annoyance. The "spit" is actually stomach contents, the foul odor of

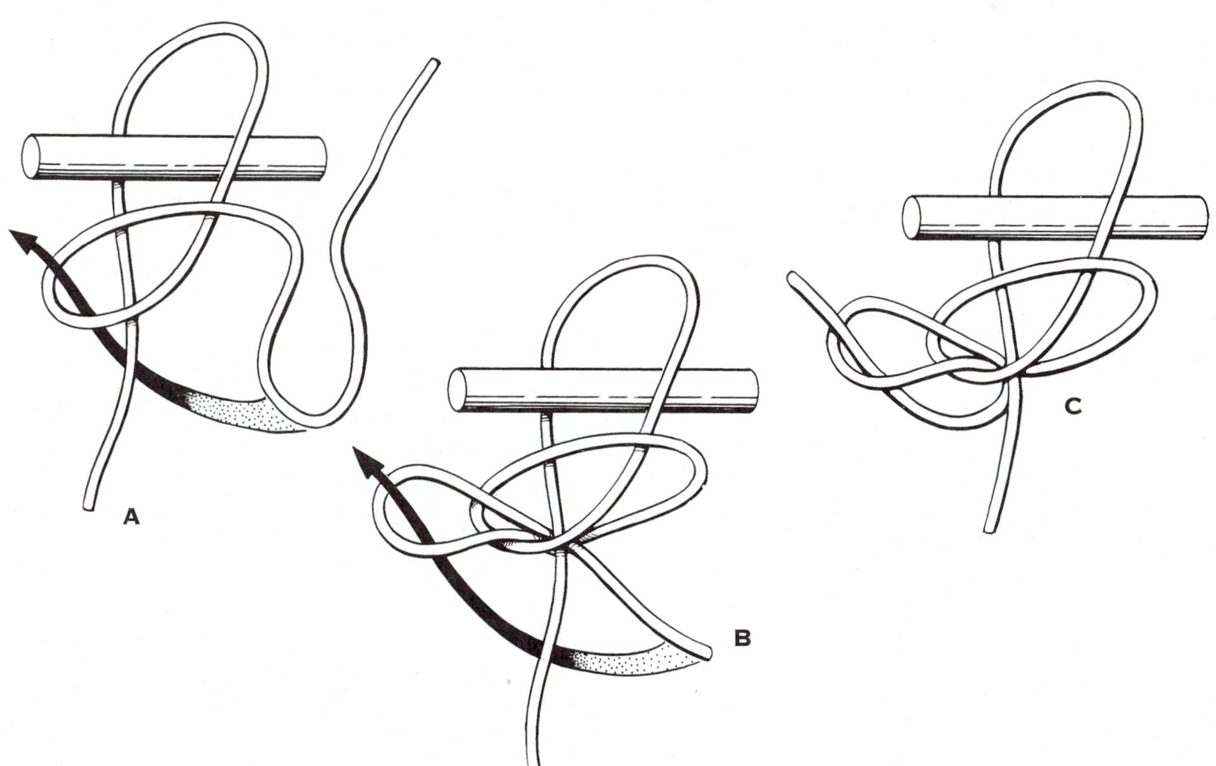

Fig. 46-1 Halter tie. **A, B, C,** Sequence.

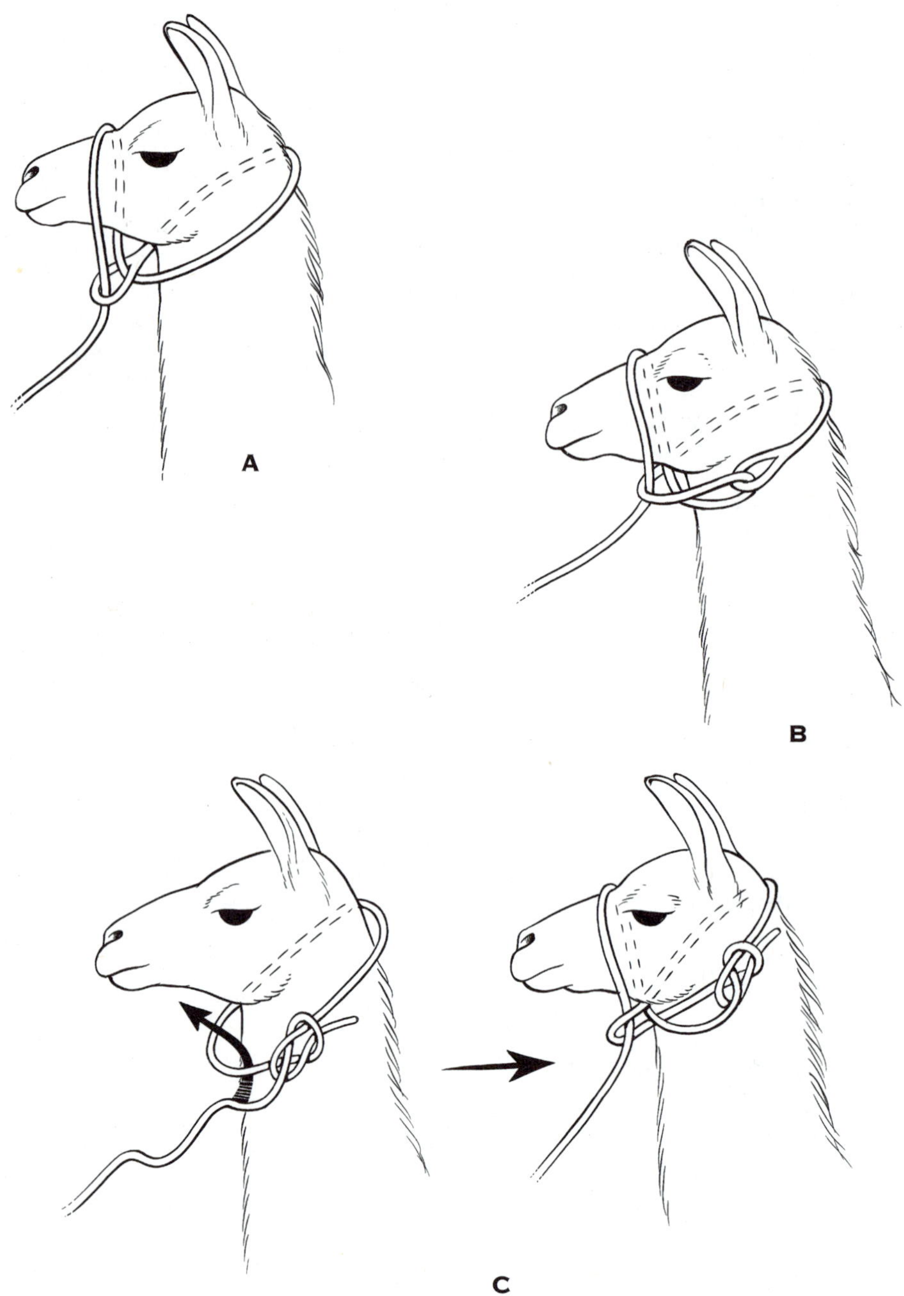

Fig. 46-2 Temporary rope halters.

which remains until thoroughly washed off. Spitting is usually directed toward other llamas to express displeasure, but handlers may be caught in the cross fire. If a llama becomes irritated during an examination or treatment procedure, spitting can be controlled by draping a cloth over the nose and tucking the top around the nose piece of the halter. Llamas also dislike the odor of stomach contents on their noses. Llamas can be "eared" in a manner similar to horses.

Dogs

Dogs usually accompany their owners, who are able to handle them under difficult circumstances. If mildly painful medical procedures must be performed, the head and mouth should be secured. The dog's body can be securely held against the handler's body by reaching across the back of the dog and grasping the base of the neck while pulling the opposite shoulder with the elbow toward the handler. The other hand should tuck the dog's head under the handler's arm.

Alternatively, a muzzle can be constructed from a nylon cord or even a shoelace. A loop should be formed with an overhand knot on one side. The loop is placed over the muzzle of the dog, with the knot on top, and tightened (Fig. 46-4). The ends of the loop should be wrapped around the muz-

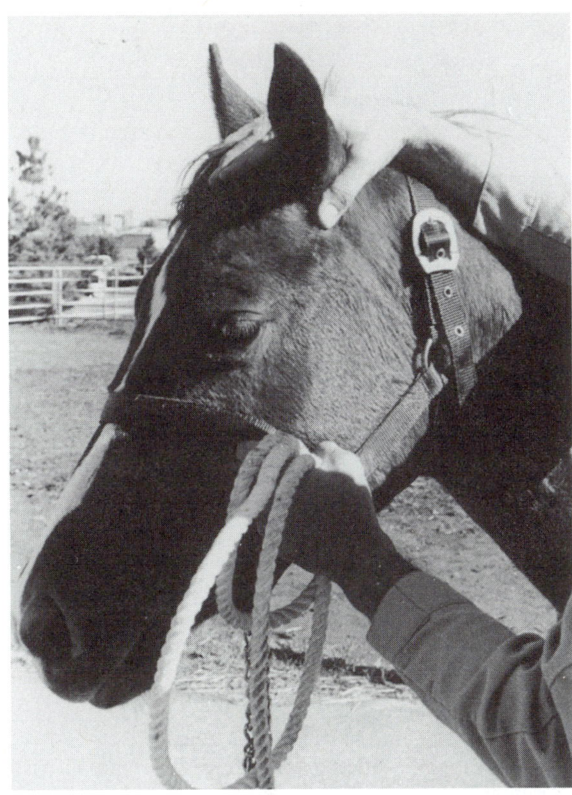

Fig. 46-3 Earing a horse.

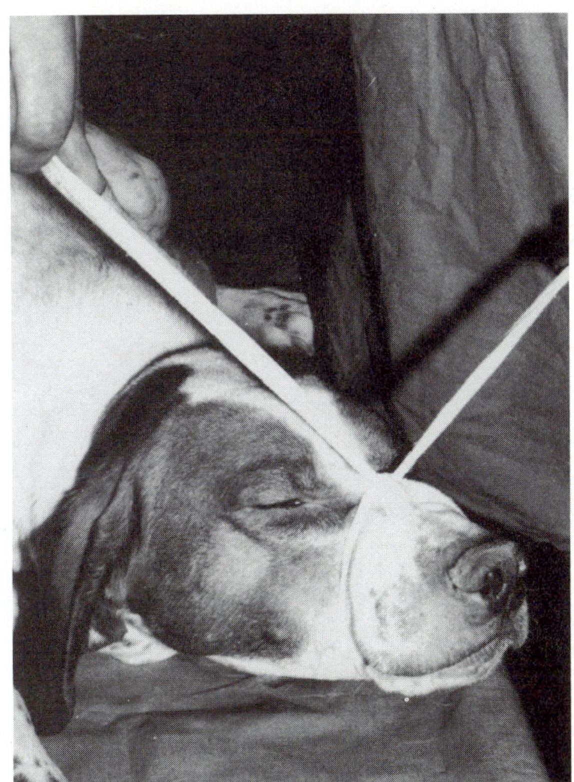

Fig. 46-4 Placing a muzzle on a dog.

zle, crossed beneath the jaw, and tied behind the ears (Fig. 46-5).

Conditions Common to All Species

Support animals may injure each other or their human handlers, or may spread disease (such as ringworm or lice). Human injuries are dealt with in other chapters.

TRAUMA

Contusions, abrasions, and lacerations are the most common ailments encountered in support animals. Falls, stumbling on sharp rocks, brushing against branches, and encounters with other animals are frequent causes of injury. Such wounds should be handled like similar human injuries. Hair or wool should be trimmed from the margins of wounds before treatment or suturing to prevent matting with exudate. The skin may be sutured with any suture material suitable for humans. Antibiotics are not necessary unless vital structures, such as synovial or serosal membranes, are exposed.

Rope burns may occur in all species but are more likely to occur in horses because they tend to struggle against entanglements and their skin is quickly burned by abrasive action. Therapy is similar to that for human burns. Thermal burns are unlikely unless animals are caught in brush or forest fires.

FOOT, HOOF, AND NAIL PROBLEMS[2]

Foot injuries may incapacitate an animal, and possibly the expedition. The hoof of the horse covers the distal extremity and third phalanx (P-3). The specialized horn of the hoof and nail is roughly analogous to the human nail. Horses are digitigrade, walking on the tip of P-3. In llamas, P-2 and P-3 lie in a horizontal plane within the foot, with only P-1 in the vertical position. The nails of the llama and dog are inconsequential in weight bearing, but if torn or contused are extremely painful.

The weight-bearing surface of the horse's hoof contains the firm sole and more flexible frog, overlying soft fibroelastic tissue called the digital cushion. Dogs have footpads similar to those of llamas.

The structures of the foot are subject to contusions, abrasions, lacerations, and penetration by foreign bodies (such as nails, stones, and sticks). Segments of the hoof wall and nail may be avulsed, exposing the sensitive laminae. Infection may invade the foot and undermine the outer layers, with abscess formation. Not all lesions are visible. Stone bruises of the sole or frog of a horse may be evident only when pressure is exerted on the site of the contusion.

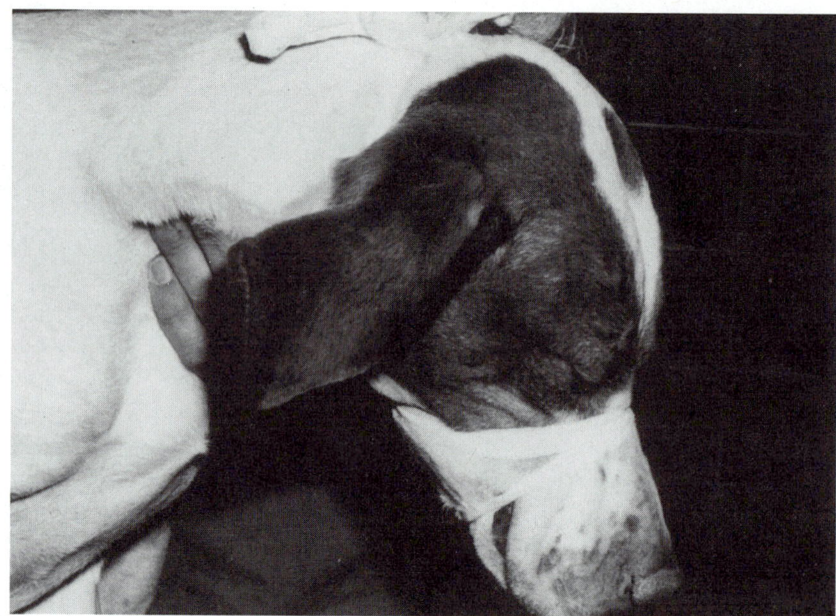

Fig. 46-5 Completed muzzle on a dog.

Foreign body penetrations and abscesses may cause reluctance to place any weight on the limb. The penetrating object may have been withdrawn or still be in place; in either case a discolored tract leads to the depth of the wound. Erosions and ulcerations of the footpads are common in unconditioned dogs and llamas. Dogs working in ice, snow, mud, and water may suffer from maceration, cracks, erosions, lacerations, and frostbite.

Foot and limb trauma is accompanied by varying degrees of lameness (limping). It may be difficult to establish which leg is painful, but the principles are similar to evaluation of such pain in humans, with the obvious differences of two extra limbs to evaluate and the animal's inability to communicate.

Cellulitis may develop on the limbs or body. The signs include heat, swelling, and redness and are the same in all species, as is therapy.

Therapy for foot injuries includes providing drainage of infected lesions, disinfection, and protection of exposed sensitive structures. Antibiotics are not indicated for most wounds unless a joint surface is exposed. It may be necessary to bandage the foot to provide protection while in camp, and to fashion special shoes or boots to keep an animal functioning on the trail. Special booties are available commercially for dogs, but a temporary moccasin may be constructed from soft leather (such as the leather used by crafts people to make moccasins).

HYPERTHERMIA (HEAT STRESS, HEAT EXHAUSTION)

Hyperthermia is elevation of the core body temperature above normal limits. Chapter 8 discusses hyperthermia in humans, but it is important to recognize that animals associated with a trek may become overextended as well.

Etiology

The primary cause of hyperthermia in pack animals on treks is excessive muscular exertion, especially during periods of high environmental temperatures and high humidity. Animals that struggle for prolonged periods in swampy terrain or in snow or mud may also produce excessive heat. Although high ambient temperature is a contributing factor, excessive muscle exertion in any climate may cause an elevation in body temperature. Pack animals may also develop fever as a result of infectious diseases. Dehydration from inadequate supplies of potable water exacerbates the problem.

Inadequate physical conditioning is a common problem and contributes to a cumulative heat load. Other contributing factors may include lack of salt in the diet, preexisting cardiovascular insufficiency, obesity, and trauma.

Clinical Signs

Signs may vary according to species and the stage of hyperthermia, but all affected animals have an increased heart and respiratory rate, usually accompanied by open-mouth breathing. Rectal temperatures may vary from 106° to 110° F (41.1° to 43.3° C). Horses, mules, donkeys, and llamas sweat in the early stages of hyperthermia, but sweating may cease if the animal becomes severely dehydrated. Sweating is evident in horses but imperceptible in llamas because most sweating occurs on the ventral abdomen in what is known as the thermal window, where the fibers are less dense and the staple is short.

Dogs cool themselves by evaporation of respiratory fluids while panting. The mouth is held open and the tongue lolls from the mouth. The respiratory rate increases from a normal of 30 breaths per minute up to 200 to 400. Moisture may be observed dripping from the tongue. As dehydration intensifies, salivation and dripping may slow or cease.

Hyperthermia causes a shift of blood volume from the viscera and muscles to the skin, resulting in hypovolemia and varying degrees of hypotension. Hypotension causes hypoxemia of the brain, resulting in dullness, restlessness, and incoordination. Hypoxemia may lead to convulsions and collapse. The shift of blood from the gastrointestinal tract may cause decreased motility and the potential for ileus and tympany. Colicky signs may be noted (kicking at the belly, looking back at the side, treading, attempting to lie down and roll).

A 1.8° F (1° C) rise in body temperature requires 10% more oxygen for proper function of the energy systems of the body. When body temperature reaches 105.8° F (41° F), the respiratory system is no longer able to supply sufficient oxygen by normal respiration. Respiratory acidosis and electrolyte imbalances associated with sweating may produce a syndrome similar to septicemia.

Hyperthermia may affect most of the organ systems of the body. The severity of the syndrome cannot be assessed in the field. It is important to recognize the conditions that lead to hyperthermia, watch for early signs of heat stress, and stop any activity that contributes to the problem. Mules and donkeys are not likely to become severely affected because they refuse to go on if stressed. Horses may be driven past their endurance and die of thermal stress.

Treatment

Cessation of excessive muscular activity may be all that is necessary if hyperthermia is mild. If streams or lakes are nearby, the animal can be walked into the water and water splashed on its underbelly. Contingencies for hyperthermia are part of all plans for capture operations for wildlife translocation and reintroduction projects. Water is carried for cooling and intravenous fluids to deal with heat stress. Cold water enemas are the most effective and rapid way to cool the body of a large animal.

PLANT POISONING[3-5,7]

It is unrealistic to expect to be able to identify all potentially harmful plants in every locale. However, certain highly toxic plants that grow in wilderness areas of the United States should be recognized (Table 46-2) (see Chapters 37 and 38). Cooperative extension offices at federal land grant institutions frequently publish booklets on local poisonous plants.

Horses may be less at risk than llamas because horses are primarily grazers and not likely to eat trees and shrubs. Llamas eat small quantities of almost anything within reach.

Animals are not affected by poison oak *(Rhus diversiloba)* or poison ivy *(Rhus toxicodendron)*. However, horses, dogs, and llamas may transmit the toxic oils of these shrubs to susceptible people via contact with contaminated hair.

Few specific antidotes are available for plant poisons. Symptomatic and supportive treatment includes removal of the poisonous material from the gastrointestinal tract by administration of a cathartic (Table 46-3) or adsorbing the toxin with a nonspecific substance such as activated charcoal.

EYE INJURIES

An abrasion, laceration, or penetrating wound of the cornea is serious, especially in a field situation. Dust and other foreign bodies within the conjunctival sac require prompt removal to avoid more serious injury to the cornea. The management of eye problems in animals is the same as for humans, with the added difficulty of restraint for examination and therapy.

Unique Disorders of Horses, Mules, and Donkeys

Common trail disorders encountered in horses may be classified as traumatic, metabolic, or digestive tract upsets.

LAMINITIS (FOUNDER)[6]

Etiology

Trauma is the most likely cause of inflammation of the foot in the trek horse. Horses should have been trained in a terrain similar to that to be found on the trek. However, even a trained horse occasionally encounters an excessively rocky path that traumatizes its feet, especially if the rider is unwise and fails to slow the pace when negotiating the trail. Leather or synthetic pads worn under the shoe may offer some protection, but new pads may be chewed off the foot by rocky trails after less than 50 miles.

Laminitis may be a sequel to severe digestive upset in a horse. Inflammation within the confines of an inflexible hoof causes malperfusion at the capillary level of the foot, which is accompanied by arteriovenous shunting.

Clinical Signs

Laminitis usually develops on both fore feet, but rear feet may also be affected in severe cases. The horse shifts its center of gravity to the hind limbs to minimize pressure on the fore feet, standing with the hind limbs forward under the body and the fore limbs extended in front of the body. The feet are hot to palpation, and there is a pounding digital artery pulse. The horse is reluctant to move.

Treatment

Therapy is directed at reestablishing circulation in the foot. Proper circulation of blood within the hoof depends partially on the pumping action of the foot while walking. It

Table 46-2 Poisonous Plants That May Affect Horses or Llamas on Trek

Plant Common Name	Plant Scientific Name	Poisonous Principle	Signs of Poisoning	Habitat	Species	Therapy
False hellebore, corn lily	*Veratrum californicum*	Alkaloids	Vomiting, salivation, convulsions, fast irregular pulse	High mountains, meadows	Llama	Symptomatic*
Death camas, sandcorn	*Zigadenus* spp.	Alkaloids	Foaming at mouth, convulsions, ataxia, vomiting, fast weak pulse	Hillsides, fields, meadows, in spring of year	Horse, llama	Symptomatic
Water hemlock	*Cicuta douglasii*	Resin	Frothing at mouth, muscle twitching, convulsions, death in 15-30 min	Standing or running water, obligate aquatic	Horse, llama	Symptomatic
Nightshade	*Solanum* spp.	Alkaloidal glycoside, solanine	Vomiting, weakness, groaning	Ubiquitous	Horse, llama	Symptomatic
Jimson weed	*Datura stramonium*	Alkaloid, atropine	Dry mucous membranes, dilated pupils, mania	Waste places	Horse, llama	Parasympathomimetics
Tobacco, tree tobacco	*Nicotiana* spp.	Alkaloid, nicotine	Stimulation of CNS, then depression; sweating, muscle twitching, convulsions	Waste places	Horse, llama	Symptomatic
Lupine, blue bonnet	*Lupinus* spp.	Alkaloid	CNS depression, dyspnea, muscle twitching, ataxia, frothing, convulsions	Ubiquitous	Horse, llama	Symptomatic
Dogbane, Indian hemp	*Apocynum cannabinum*	Cardioactive glycoside (digitoxin-like)	Dyspnea, cardiac arrhythmias, agonal convulsions, vomiting, diarrhea	Ubiquitous	Horse, llama	Symptomatic
Oleander	*Nerium oleander*	Same as dogbane	Same as dogbane	Ornamental	Horse, llama	Symptomatic and gastrotomy
Castor bean	*Ricinus communis*	Ricin, water soluble	Anaphylactic shock, diarrhea	Ornamental	Horse, llama	Treat for shock; fluids

CNS, Central nervous system.

*In most cases of poisoning from ingestion of poisonous plants, there is no specific antidote. It is necessary to treat symptomatically. The critical factor is to empty the digestive tract of the plant material with cathartics, parasympathomimetic stimulation, and enemas. Activated charcoal may be of value given orally.

is now thought that mild exercise is an important aid in preventing damage to the laminae. The horse should be exercised slowly on soft ground for 10 to 15 minutes every hour for 12 to 24 hours, then exercise should be stopped. Even slow walking may be quite painful, and an analgesic may be necessary (phenylbutazone, 2 to 4 g orally once daily). Corticosteroids are contraindicated.

Although soaking in cold water may give temporary relief to feet sore from laminitis, this practice is actually contraindicated in acute laminitis. Warm water soaks are appropriate, since they dilate the vascular tree and enhance circulation. A low volar block inhibits vascular constriction within the foot. This is accomplished by palpating the pulsating artery on the posterior lateral aspect of the fetlock (Fig. 46-6). The nerve lies posterior to the artery. With a 20- to 22-gauge needle 3 ml of 2% lidocaine is injected over each nerve. It may be necessary to repeat nerve blocks two or three times daily for several days.

Table 46-3 Medications for Trek Animals

Drug Generic Name	Trade Name and Company	Concentration in Vial	Route of Administration	Dosage and Interval: Horse	Dosage and Interval: Llama	Dosage and Interval: Dog	Indication for Use
Acepromazine maleate	Prom Ace (Fort Dodge)	10 mg/ml	IM or IV	0.04-0.1 ml/kg	Not indicated	5-10 mg/kg	Tranquilizer
Ampicillin sodium	Omnipen (Wyeth)		IM	10-100 mg/kg qid	10-25 mg/kg tid	25 mg/kg q 6 h	Infection
Atropine sulfate	Any pharmacy	2 mg/ml	IM, SC	0.04 mg/kg	0.04 mg/kg	0.04 mg/kg	Stinging nettle
Benzathine penicillin G	Benza Pen, (Beecham)	150,000 U/ml	IM	4000 U/kg q 2 days	5,000-15,000 U/kg q 2 days	40,000 U/kg q 5 days	Infection
Charcoal (activated)			po	60-250 g	100 g	3-5 g	Toxins
Dexamethasone	Azium (Schering)	2 mg/ml	IM	2-4 mg/kg	1-2 mg/kg	4 mg/kg q 8 hr	Shock
Diazepam	Valium (Roche)	5 mg/ml	IV, IM	0.2-4 mg/kg	0.2-4 mg/kg	0.25-1 mg/kg	Sedation
Epinephrine	Epinephrine (Haver-Lochart)	1:1000 1 mg/ml	IV, IM	0.1-0.4 mg/kg	0.1-0.5 mg/kg	0.1-0.5 ml	Anaphylaxis
Fenbendazole	Panacur (American Hoechst)		po		10-15 mg/kg single dose		Parasites
Flunixen meglumine	Banamine (Schering)		IM	1 mg/kg daily	1.0 mg/kg daily	0.3 mg/kg daily	Colic pain, inflammation
Ivermectin	Ivomec (MSD-Ag Vet)		po, SC	0.2 mg/kg single dose	0.2 mg/kg single dose	Not indicated	Parasites
Ketamine	Vetelar (Parke-Davis)	100 mg/ml	IV, IM	2.0 mg/kg	2-5 mg/kg	Not indicated	Anesthesia
Lidocaine	Xylocaine (Astra)	2%	SC	As needed	As needed	As needed	Local anesthesia
Magnesium oxide	Carmilax (Norden)	361 g/lb	po		10-20 g total dose		Cathartic
Magnesium sulfate	Any pharmacy		po	20-100 g animal	Not indicated	8-25 g per animal	Cathartic
Phenylbutazone	Butazolidin (Wellcome)	200 mg/ml 1 g tab	IV po	1-2 g/450 kg 2-4 g/450 kg daily	2-4 mg/kg daily	2.2 mg/kg q 8 hr	Pain, inflammation
Trimethoprim-sulfamethoxazole	Tribrissen (Wellcome)	24%	IV, SC	2 mg/kg bid	2 mg/kg bid	15 mg/kg q 12 hr	Infection
Xylazine	Rompun (Chemagro)	100 mg/ml	IV, IM	0.5-1.0 mg/kg	0.25-0.5 mg/kg	1.1 mg/kg	Sedation
	T-61 Euthanasia Solution (Taylor)		IV	40 ml total dose	25 ml total dose	0.3 ml/kg	Euthanasia

SADDLE, CINCH, AND RIGGING SORES[6]

Saddle sores are contusions, abrasions, or ulcerations of the skin and subcutis caused by friction or point pressure from the saddle, cinch, or rigging.

Etiology

Improperly fitted or maintained tack is the primary cause of saddle sores. A saddle tree may fit a horse properly at the beginning of a training period but become unsatisfactory after the horse has trimmed down.

Poorly distributed pressure is the primary cause of saddle sores. Spot pressure causes local ischemia. If pressure is prolonged, the capillary bed may be damaged. When the pressure is released rapidly, blood rushes into the blanched site, and extravasation may occur, causing swelling and pain.

If the lesion is rested and treated as inflamed tissue, complete healing may occur. However, if the saddle is reapplied, it overlies a lump that is subject to abrasion. The injury can extend through the dermis, resulting in severe ul-

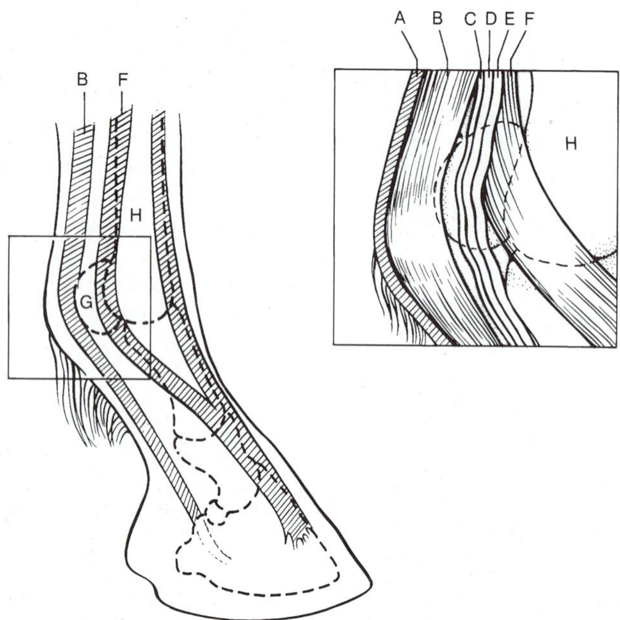

Fig. 46-6 Diagram of the anatomy of the equine fetlock. *A*, Skin. *B*, Flexor tendons. *C*, Volar nerve. *D*, Palmar digital artery. *E*, Digital vein. *F*, Suspensory ligament. *G*, Sesamoid bone. *H*, Metacarpal bone (cannon).

ceration. Cinch and rigging sores are usually caused by friction, leading to blister formation.

Clinical Signs

Hot and tender swellings are the primary signs of acute saddle sores. The hair or epidermis may be rubbed off. General sensitivity over the back is usually caused by muscle soreness.

Evidence of previous sores includes white hairs in spots over the withers or saddle bed, scars that may or may not be haired over, thickening of the dermis, and alopecia with or without swelling.

Treatment

Prevention is better than treatment. Toughening the backs of trail horses is a major job of the trainer. Proper pads or blankets must be selected for each horse.

Upon arrival at a rest area the girth should be slowly loosened at intervals of 10 to 15 minutes to prevent rapid flow of blood into ischemic areas.

Once a sore has developed, the horse must be rested or the tack changed to eliminate pressure or friction on the lesion. Holes are often cut in pads to accommodate a saddle sore, but spot pressure at the ring edge may be as detrimental as the original cause of the saddle sore. Obviously riders must keep tack cleaned and in good repair. When the saddle is removed, cold water poured over the back may minimize swelling.

MYOPATHY[1,6]

Exertional myopathies of horses vary from simple muscle soreness through the "tying up" syndrome to paralytic myoglobinuria (rhabdomyolysis, azoturia).

Etiology

Muscle integrity and function depend on proper mobilization and use of energy. Conditioned muscles may function vigorously for extended periods of time, but if either energy parameter is accelerated to the extreme, mild to severe muscle necrosis may occur.

Clinical Signs

Mild muscle soreness is characterized by alterations in gait that indicate muscle weakness. As severity increases, the gait becomes progressively altered until the horse is in obvious pain and is reluctant to move. The horse has an anxious expression and may sweat excessively. Affected muscles are painful to palpation and may be swollen. Skin temperature over the muscle may be elevated. Muscle spasms may occur, but not consistently. Myoglobinuria is observed grossly in moderate to severe cases and should be considered prima facie evidence for stopping and resting or treating the horse.

Treatment

Rest is paramount in all cases. A rider may have difficulty differentiating the pain associated with myopathy from that seen with colic. It is disastrous to force the severely myopathic horse to walk, as is done with a suspected case of colic. If there is doubt, the horse should not be exercised.

Horses in inaccessible locations should not be walked out until all possible recovery has taken place. Horses with mild muscle soreness may improve if walked slowly, but rest from ride exertion is the primary recommended therapy.

DEHYDRATION

Etiology

Fluid and electrolyte imbalances play a major role in all metabolic medical problems that develop in the horse as a result of exertional stress. The degree of dehydration is directly related to the amount of fluid loss through evaporative cooling (sweat), which in turn is related to the amount and rate of work performed and to ambient temperatures and humidity.

The horse must have an adequate amount (10 to 15 gallons) of water each day during a trek. The more strenuous the activity is, the more fluids the horse requires. Mules, and especially donkeys, are adapted to cope with mild dehydration.

Clinical Signs

Signs of mild dehydration (3% body weight loss) are low urine output, dry mouth, and mild loss of skin elasticity.

Moderate dehydration (5% body weight loss) is characterized by marked loss of skin elasticity. The eyes become sunken. Blood pressure may fall as a result of decreased plasma volume. Weakness, fever, and weak pulse may be observed. Sweating is not possible, even with elevated body temperature.

Marked dehydration (10% body weight loss) may involve circulatory failure from decreased plasma volume.

Treatment

During 3 hours of hard work, a 450 kg horse may lose as much as 45 L of fluid. If this degree of dehydration is not corrected quickly, death may result. The horse should be allowed to drink along the trail if water is available. Small amounts of cool, but not cold, water should be offered. If the horse refuses to drink, gastric intubation may be indicated. Fluid is also absorbed from the colon; thus enemas (200 to 500 ml water) are effective in rehydration.

Heat stress usually accompanies dehydration, so cooling (such as shade or a water bath) is important. Administration of intravenous fluids, if available, is routine therapy.

EXHAUSTED HORSE SYNDROME[1]

The term "exhausted horse syndrome" (EHS) was coined to describe a complex metabolic disease occurring when horses are pushed beyond endurance limits. The syndrome has no precise characterization because the initiating mechanism may vary with the prevailing conditions. The development of EHS depends on the condition and training of the horse, the pace set by the rider, the terrain traversed, and climatic factors such as temperature, wind, and humidity.

Clinical Signs

We present a composite picture, but the individual horse may show only a few signs. The severely affected horse is depressed and exhibits lethargic movements, holding its head low. The ears are expressionless. Facial grimacing gives an anxious expression that may progress to a painful expression if colic or muscle spasms accompany the syndrome. The horse takes no interest in its surroundings. Anorexia is typical, and frequently the horse has no inclination to drink, even though dehydrated. The corneas appear glazed.

Body temperature is usually elevated and may reach 41° C (106° F). The horse does not cool properly. Usually body temperature continues to rise. Temperature measured rectally may be inaccurate in the exhausted horse, since the anal sphincter loses tone and allows air to enter the rectum.

Cardiovascular and respiratory systems are markedly affected by endurance riding. Heart and respiratory rates are elevated. The degree depends on the prior condition of the horse, pace, length of action, and amount of work performed in climbing or walking on soft footing. Heart rates of 150 beats/min are not uncommon after a grueling climb. With 10 to 15 minutes of rest the heart rate of a conditioned horse should drop below 60 beats/min, whereas in the exhausted horse, tachycardia and tachypnea may persist. The exhausted horse may have a respiratory rate faster than the heart rate. Respiration under these circumstances is shallow and inefficient. Additional cardiopulmonary signs may include synchronous diaphragmatic flutter, arrhythmias, murmurs, and visible jugular pulses. Auscultation of the thorax may reveal moist rales and in extreme cases frank pulmonary edema.

Severe dehydration is the most consistent sign of EHS. Loss of skin elasticity, sunken eyeballs, and dry mouth and mucous membranes reflect a 7% to 10% loss of body weight, after loss of 30 to 40 L of fluid. Serious electrolyte and acid-base imbalances are associated with dehydration. Alkalosis is common.

Muscular manifestations of EHS include fatigue, trembling, spasm, stiffness, muscles painful to palpation, and, rarely, tying-up. Tying-up is usually a distinct entity.

Horses suffering from EHS are prone to colic, which also may occur independently. When colic accompanies EHS, it is of the spasmodic type, with diminished or absent borborygmus.

Treatment

Rest, rehydration, and electrolyte supplementation are the keys to recovery. If the horse is drinking and will take electrolytes in the water, the effect is nearly as beneficial as the administration of intravenous fluids. Packaged electrolyte powders can be carried.

If the horse is hyperthermic, shows evidence of shock, and refuses to drink, more drastic steps must be taken. The horse may require 40 to 50 L of fluid. Besides intravenous fluid administration, gastric intubation may be employed to give fluids orally. Enemas are also effective, since fluid is absorbed from the colon.

SYNCHRONOUS DIAPHRAGMATIC FLUTTER[1]

Synchronous diaphragmatic flutter (SDF) is a clinical sign observed in endurance horses while on long-distance rides and may be seen on an expedition. It is defined as a spasmodic contraction of the diaphragm synchronous with the heartbeat. It is not life threatening in itself, but it indicates mild to serious metabolic conditions that may be life threatening. Overexertion with excessive sweating produces metabolic alterations. The development of SDF at any point on a trek should be ample reason to prevent the horse from going further.

Contrary to what is seen in acute exertional stress characterized by acidemia, SDF is associated with alkalemia. Electrolyte imbalances may also be involved. Experimental work seems to indicate that hypocalcemia, hypokalemia, and alkalosis act in concert or, less likely, individually to cause equine SDF.

Clinical Signs

SDF may develop after 20 to 30 miles of riding. There is no sex, age, or breed predilection. The primary sign is spasmodic contraction in the flank area. The "thump" is easily felt by light palpation in the flank area. A person who auscultates the heart while holding a hand over the dorsocaudal rib area can tell that diaphragmatic contraction is synchronous with the heartbeat. SDF may be the only clinical sign noted, or it may be seen as part of EHS.

The degree of thumping may vary from a barely perceptible quiver to a contraction that seems to rock the horse's body and is observable from a distance. The flutter may be continuous or intermittent, especially in degree.

Treatment

Rest and rehydration are required.

COLIC

Colic is the clinical manifestation of abdominal pain, usually the result of a gastrointestinal disorder. It may also arise from the urinary system or peritoneum. Types of colic are numerous because of the unique and complex anatomy of the equine digestive system.

Etiology

Colic may be produced by gastric tympany, intestinal obstruction, or hyperspasticity. The most likely inciting causes on a trek are overeating of nonregular forages, ingestion of poisonous plants, or exhaustion. One illustrative tale is of a commercial packer who hobbled a pack string of horses to graze in a meadow for a noon rest stop. Two hours later, when it was time to begin the afternoon trek, two of the horses were colicky. In checking the meadow the packer saw many plants of death camas (*Zygadenus* species), some of which had been eaten. The colic was sufficiently severe to require a layover at the meadow for the rest of the day.

Clinical Signs

Horses express colic by looking back at one side, stamping the feet, getting up and down, rolling, and pressing the head against trees or rocks. The pulse rate may exceed 100 beats/min with severe pain. The conjunctival membranes are congested and cyanotic.

Treatment

Only superficial emergency measures are discussed. Treatment is variable, depending on the anatomic location of the obstruction or spasm. Mild obstructions may be relieved by hydration and administration of a cathartic. Cold water enemas may stimulate sluggish intestinal peristalsis and relieve impaction of the small (terminal) colon.

Pain and spasms may be relieved by administration of flunixen meglumine (Banamine), 1.1 mg/kg intramuscularly twice a day. Walking the horse may prevent it from lying down and injuring itself by rolling.

Unique Medical Problems of Pack Llamas

Most of the medical problems of llamas have been considered under headings of disorders common to all animals. Llamas are hardy animals and unlikely to allow themselves to be pushed to exhaustion. If fatigued, they simply lie down and refuse to rise. They will not tolerate excessive loads. One hundred pounds (45 kg) is an appropriate load for a well-trained and conditioned large llama.

Plant poisoning is more likely in llamas than in horses, but such incidents are rare. Rope burns from entanglement in tethers are less likely than in horses. The llama is less excitable, and if it becomes entangled, it usually lies quietly until help arrives.

North American venomous snakes pose minimal threat to large animals. However, llamas are curious and may be bitten on the nose while investigating the strange animal. Nose bites from rattlesnakes are especially hazardous to llamas, because local swelling may occlude the nostrils. Llamas are primarily obligate nasal breathers, so dyspnea and suffocation may ensue. Rattlesnake bites of the limbs cause edema and in severe cases local tissue necrosis and ulceration. Many cases are diagnosed as trauma unless the bite is observed. The signs of snakebite in llamas are essentially the same as for horses.

Therapy for a nose bite may require tracheostomy and insertion of an improvised tube to allow breathing. Edema may persist for 2 to 3 days. If the bite is observed and progressive swelling noted, a small tube (1 cm diameter) can be inserted 15 cm into the ventral meatus of the nasal passage and sutured to the nares. An alternative improvisation is to insert a woman's hollow plastic hair curler into the nostril. Swelling occurs around the tube or curler, but patency of the nasal passage is maintained.

Unique Problems of Dogs

EXERCISE STRESS

Dogs without adequate conditioning are frequently taken on a trek. Muscle soreness, fatigue, dehydration, and hyperthermia are common and are dealt with as for humans. Erosions of the footpads require special care. A sheet of soft leather out of which to fashion boots should be carried.

PORCUPINE QUILLS

When dogs are brought into porcupine country, the risk of an encounter is great. Some dogs fail to learn from experience and are repeatedly quilled. The dog must have physical contact with the porcupine for the tail to introduce the quills. The muzzle and face are the usual sites of penetration, and a dog can be blinded by perforation of the eyeball.

The quills must be removed physically. A pair of pliers should be included in supplies and equipment. The process is painful and sedation with diazepam is indicated. The quill should not be broken because the retrograde barbs on the quill foster migration and abscess formation.

GRASS AWNS

Numerous species of grass awns ("foxtails") may become attached to the dog's hair coat or lodged in the external ear canal, nasal passage, conjunctival sac, or interdigital space. Dogs that must travel at the time of year when plants are mature and awns are easily dislodged from the seed head should be inspected frequently for awns in these sites.

Signs depend on the location of the foreign body. When it is within the ear canal, the dog paws at its ear and shakes its head. The head may be held tilted. Exudate may flow from the ear. Awns in the nostril cause sneezing and nasal exudate. Awns in the conjunctival sac cause lacrimation, photophobia, and corneal edema and ulceration. The dog paws at the eye. Awn penetration between the digits and at other locations through the skin is more difficult to diagnose because the awn may be at some distance from the fistula.

Awns must be removed physically. Sedation, topical anesthesia, or both may be necessary. Although topical ophthalmic anesthetics are desirable in the eye, lidocaine may be used in an emergency. A pair of small alligator forceps is most suitable for reaching into otherwise inaccessible places. An otoscope may be necessary to visualize awns in the nostril or ear canal. Instillation of an antibiotic ointment is desirable after removal of the awn.

STINGING NETTLE POISONING

Stinging nettle (*Urtica* species) is common along streams and lakes in wilderness areas. Humans vary in sensitivity when the plants accidentally contact exposed skin. Leaves and stems are covered by harsh hairs, some of which have a tiny ball tip that breaks off just before penetration. The specialized hairs are hollow. A base gland produces histamines and acetylcholine, which are injected into the victim.

Short-haired dogs that move through patches of stinging nettle are at risk of poisoning from the cumulative effect of thousands of minute injections of acetylcholine. Weakness, dyspnea, and muscle tremors are characteristic of the action of acetylcholine on peripheral nerves. Parasympathomimetic effects include salivation, diarrhea, tachycardia, and pupillary dilation. Atropine sulfate (0.04 mg/kg) subcutaneously is a specific treatment.

SNAKEBITE

Dogs are at risk from venomous snakebite. The bite of the eastern diamondback rattlesnake *Crotalus adamanteus* is capable of killing a dog unless prompt therapy with antivenin and supportive treatment is carried out. Such therapy usually necessitates removal of the dog from the wilderness to a hospital environment. However, if the trek's medical supplies contain Wyeth's Antivenin (Crotalidae) in North America, this product may be administered to animals with minimal risk of anaphylaxis. A single vial administered intravenously is usually sufficient to counteract the venom from all but the largest rattlesnakes.

Bites from smaller snakes may also be life threatening. Tissue necrosis contiguous to the bite site may result in severe dermal ulceration and temporary or permanent nerve and tendon damage. The prompt administration of antivenin prevents development of the more severe responses.

HARNESS SORES

Improperly fitted harnesses of sled dogs may produce the same type of frictional lesions as occurs in horses or llamas.

Support Animal Escape

Support animals may escape from any type of restraint imposed and run away or simply wander off. More commonly, animals are tied with improper knots, or poor-quality snaps and halters are used that break when the slightest pressure is applied. A trekker may tie an animal to a shrub, bush, or branch that can be pulled up or broken off with a slight tug.

Animals that are frightened by predators or other wild animals wandering into an area where they are tied may bolt and exert tremendous pressure on tethers, picket lines, stakes, or branches.

Hobbling is a common technique used to allow horses and mules to graze. Trek leaders must know the habits of individual animals when hobbled. One horse may accept having the front feet hobbled together and graze peacefully, taking only the short steps possible. Another horse may learn how to gallop with the front feet hobbled. I once had to track a pair of packhorses for 5 miles to recapture them. They were heading home, and the only thing that stopped them was a stream they could not negotiate with the hobbles on. Some horses must be hobbled with three restrained legs.

Even experienced trekkers (such as commercial packers) may become overconfident and, placing misguided faith in an animal's willingness to stand quietly without wandering away, may leave just a lead rope dragging on the ground (ground tie). The animal may become frightened or bored and wander off. I am aware of a llama carrying a full pack that wandered off and was missing (pack and all) for a full month.

Contrary to popular belief, not all llamas are social, so they may not return to a herd that is securely tethered. Llamas, like horses and dogs, have homing instincts and may set off toward where they presume home to be.

STEPS TO TAKE IN THE EVENT OF AN ESCAPE

If a breakaway is observed, members of the party should not further frighten the animal by rushing at it. It should be given a chance to settle down and return to the group. The handlers can move around the animal to block obvious escape routes but should not try to chase it. All of these animals can run faster than a human. If the escapee has an animal buddy in the group or a favorite person, he or she can make an approach. A favorite treat in camp can be used to entice the animal back to the fold.

If an animal is discovered missing, an analysis of the situation to determine what caused the escape is needed. Was it frightened? Did it break tack? Is it dragging a log, branch, or rope? Is there evidence that other animals were nearby? Is blood or hair strewn about? In what direction did it probably go? Generally, animals return toward the direction from which they have come. Frightened animals or those escaping at night may not adhere to any rule. A search for tracks can be made, but llamas may not leave much of a track, particularly in rocky terrain.

Scanning the surroundings may result in a sighting of the animal. It may be in the vicinity of camp resting under a tree or in a clump of bushes. The search should be conducted in a planned fashion, using all persons possible. Unless tracks direct otherwise, the trail back toward a trailhead should be searched first. From firsthand experience, I can attest to the desirability of taking another animal, preferably a buddy of the escapee, along on the search. Even though the animal is sighted, it may not be caught unless a second animal is there to bait it in. Vantage points should be used, and searchers should consider where they might have gone under the circumstances. Lush meadows or other areas where there might be desirable feed should be checked.

Fellow hikers, and ultimately the Forest Service or other regulatory agencies, should be alerted about the missing animal.

Medication Procedures

A list of medications and indications for their use is provided in Table 46-3. In the horse, intramuscular injections are given in the neck or rump. Subcutaneous injections are given by lifting a fold of skin just cranial to the scapula. Intravenous injections are given in the jugular vein, which is easily distended along the jugular groove on the ventral aspect of the neck (Fig. 46-7).

In the llama, intramuscular injections are given in the relatively hairless area at the back of the upper rear leg, by standing against the body in front of the rear limb while facing the rear and reaching around the back of the animal to give the injection. Subcutaneous injections are given in the relatively hairless area of the caudal abdomen, just in front of the rear limb. It is difficult for an inexperienced individual to locate the jugular vein for intravenous administration in the llama. Intramuscular or subcutaneous routes are recommended.

In the dog, intramuscular injections may be administered in the triceps muscles caudal to the shoulder or in the muscle masses on the upper rear limb. Subcutaneous injections are made by lifting a fold of loose skin on the neck near the withers. Intravenous administration is via the jugular vein or the cephalic vein (Fig. 46-8). For the latter an assistant grasps the limb at the elbow to occlude the vein, which courses on the dorsal aspect of the forearm. The vein is more visible if the hair is wetted down with water.

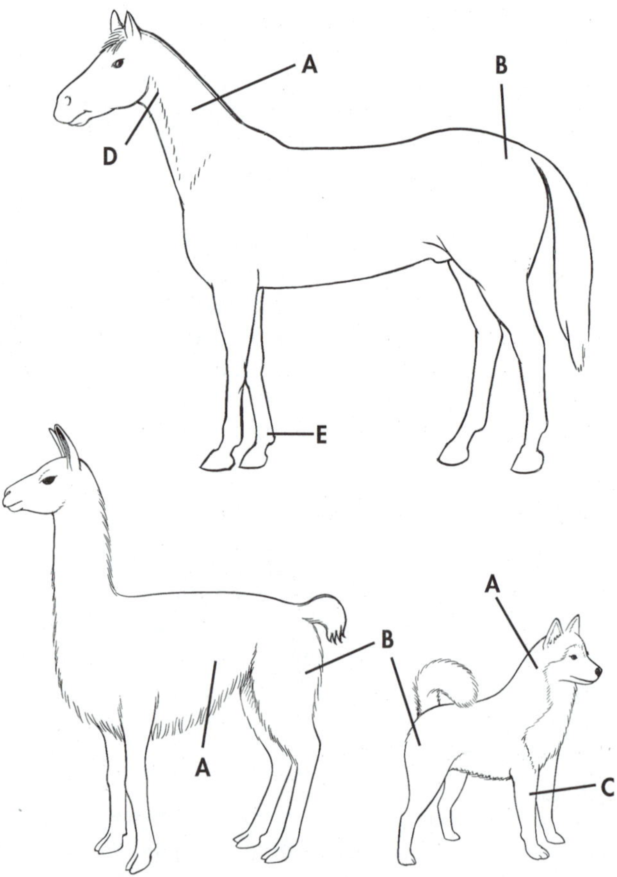

Fig. 46-7 Diagrams of medication sites in the horse, llama, and dog. *A*, Subcutaneous. *B*, Intramuscular. *C*, Cephalic vein for intravenous. *D*, Jugular vein. *E*, Site for low volar nerve block.

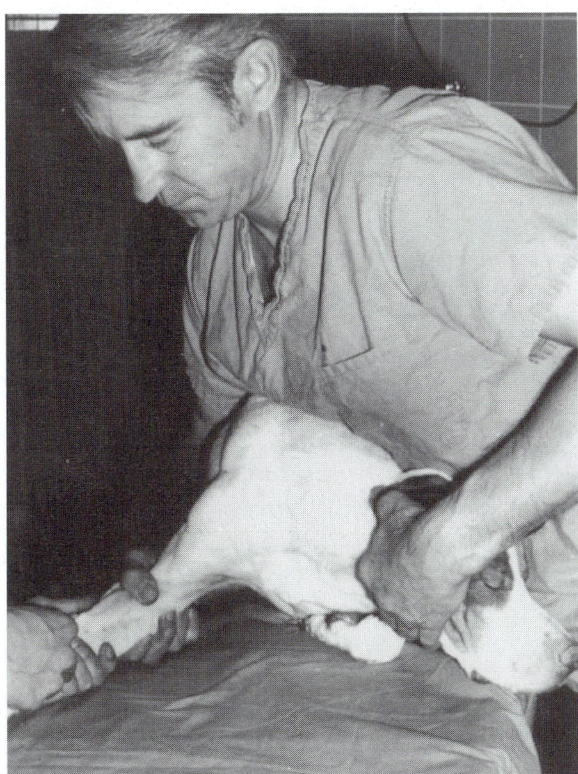

Fig. 46-8 Holding a dog for administration of intravenous medication.

EUTHANASIA

Euthanasia may become necessary in the event of injury or illness that cannot be corrected or when there is little likelihood of removing the animal to a location where remedial action can be taken. Horses, mules, donkeys, and llamas cannot be carried out of a wilderness area manually. Large animals can be airlifted out of the wilderness by helicopter, but obtaining such help may require great time and effort. All the while the animal is in pain, and it may have to be euthanized anyway. Dogs may be placed in an improvised stretcher and carried out.

Indications for euthanasia include compound and comminuted fractures of long bones, falling or sliding into inaccessible places from which the animal is unable to extricate itself or trek participants are unable to aid the animal, lacerations exposing abdominal or thoracic organs (such as wild animal attacks or ramming tree branches into the body), head injuries resulting in persistent convulsions or coma, and protracted colicky pain unrelieved by analgesics or mild catharsis, usually associated with a pulse rate greater than 100 beats/min, rolling, and congested conjunctival membranes.

The expedition may carry a bottle of euthanasia solution, which must be given intravenously or intraperitoneally (Table 46-3). If firearms are carried, a properly placed bullet to the head produces a fast and humane death. For placement, the shooter stands in front of the animal's head and draws an imaginary line from the medial canthus of each eye to the base of the opposite ear. The shot should be aimed where those lines cross and approximately perpendicular to the contour of the forehead (Fig. 46-9). The tip of the barrel should be no more than 6 inches from the head. A heavy blow to the head at the same location is equally effective. The blow may be administered with the blunt edge of a single-bladed ax or hatchet. A large rock held in the hand may also be used. A less desirable but sometimes expedient method is to sever the jugular vein to allow exsanguination. This would probably be used on an animal that is already unconscious.

Some vital statistics for support animals are provided in Table 46-1. Equipment for support animals and the sources are listed in Box 46-1, Table 46-4, and Appendix A.

The rectal body temperature of an animal is assessed by

BOX 46-1

EQUIPMENT AND SUPPLIES TO BE CARRIED FOR ANIMALS

1. Sterile pack
   Needle forceps
   Thumb forceps
   Scissors
   Scalpel handle and blades
   Hemostats (2)
2. Alligator forceps
3. Suture material (Vicryl), swedged—on needles, 4 packets, various sizes (0 to 4-0)
4. Gauze sponges, 4 × 4 (100)
5. Roll cotton, one pound
6. Vetrap bandages, 3 in, 6 rolls
7. Syringes, plastic, 12 ml (6)
8. Needles, 22-18 gauge (20)
9. Tubing:
   Silastic, 1 cm OD, 10 cm (4 in) long, for endotracheal tube
   Plastic flexible stomach tube, 1 cm ID, 100 cm (40 in) long
10. Funnel, plastic, to fit into stomach tube
11. Hose, garden, 20 cm (8 in), to serve as speculum for passage of stomach tube
12. Hoof knife
13. Hammer
14. Pliers
15. Horseshoes and nails
16. Pliable sheet of leather
17. Heavy needle and thread
18. Otoscope
19. Stomach pump

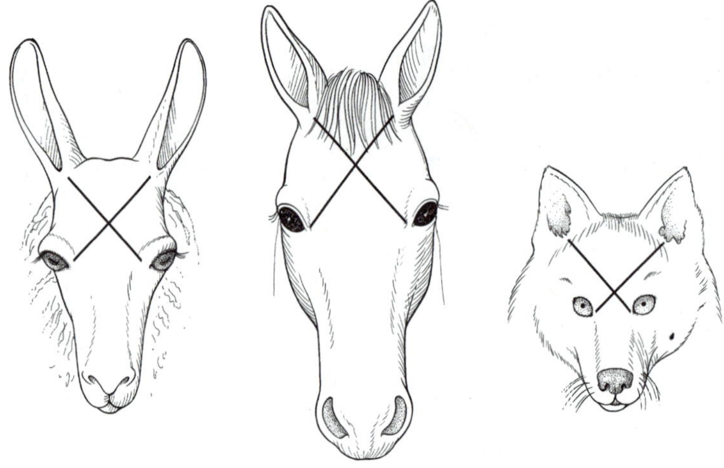

Fig. 46-9 Location for euthanasia blow or shot.

Table 46-4 Priority of Emergency Supplies (Listed in Box 46-1)

	Horse		Llama		Dog	
Priority	**1**	**2**	**1**	**2**	**1**	**2**
Drugs	1,2,4,7,9,10,12	5,11,14,15,16,17	2,4,7,8,9,10,11,12,17	6,13,15,16	3,4,7,8,9,12,16	11,15,17
Supplies	1,3,4,5,6,7,8,9,10,12,13,14,15	19	1,3,4,6,7,8,9,10,11,12,14	19	1,2,4,6,7,8,14,16,17	18

inserting a thermometer lubricated with water or spittle through the anus with a slight twisting motion. Heavy-duty glass veterinary clinical thermometers are available, but regular human clinical thermometers are equally useful. The use of the same thermometer for humans and animals is generally esthetically unacceptable, even though the thermometer can be cleansed and disinfected between uses. In hot climates, clinical thermometers must be kept in insulated containers; otherwise high temperatures render them useless.

APPENDIX A

Sources of Veterinary Drugs for Expeditions

American Hoechst
Somerville, NJ 08876

Astra Pharmaceuticals
7 Neponset Street
Worcester, MA 01606

Beecham Laboratories
501 Fifth Street
Bristol, TN 37620

Chemagro Agricultural Chem
Post Office Box 4913
Kansas City, MO 64120

Fort Dodge Laboratories
Post Office Box 518
Fort Dodge, IA 50501

Haver-Lochart
Box 390
Shawnee, KS 66201

MSD—Ag Vet
Post Office Box 2000
Rahway, NJ 07065

Norden Laboratories
Post Office Box 80809
Lincoln, NE 68501

Parke-Davis
201 Tabor Road
Morris Plains, NJ 07950

Roche Laboratories
Nutley, NJ 07110

Schering Corporation
Bloomfield, NJ 07003

Taylor Pharmaceutical Co.
Decatur, IL 62525

Wellcome Animal Health Division
520 West 21st Street
Kansas City, MO 61418

Wyeth Laboratories
Post Office Box 8299
Philadelphia, PA 19101

REFERENCES

1. Fowler ME: Veterinary problems during endurance trail rides, *S Afr Vet Assoc* 51:87, 1980.
2. Fowler ME: Hoof, claw and nail problems in nondomestic animals, *J Am Vet Med Assoc* 177:885, 1980.
3. Fowler ME: Plant poisoning in free-living wild animals: a review, *J Wildlife Dis* 19:34, 1983.
4. Fuller T, McClintock E: *Poisonous plants of California,* Berkeley, 1987, University of California Press.
5. James LF et al: *Plants poisonous to livestock in the western United States,* Agriculture Information Bull No 415, Washington, DC, 1980, US Department of Agriculture.
6. Mansman RA, McAllister ES, editors: *Equine medicine and surgery,* ed 3, Santa Barbara, Calif, 1982, American Veterinary Publications.
7. Schmutz EM, Freeman BN, Reed RE: *Livestock-poisoning plants of Arizona,* Tucson, 1968, University of Arizona Press.

47 SCUBA DIVING AND DYSBARISM

Kenneth W. Kizer

Approximately 70% of the earth's surface is covered by water, but relatively little is known about this underwater world. Only recently has this last frontier of the planet begun to be explored extensively. Much of this exploration has been made possible by the development of scuba diving.

Hazards include the problems found in other aquatic activities, such as near drowning, hypothermia, aquatic skin disorders, water-borne infectious diseases, and hazardous marine life, as well as some relatively unique problems related to the increased atmospheric pressure found under water.

Scuba diving is an exhilarating and generally safe activity for persons who are healthy, well trained, well conditioned, well equipped, and "water wise." It can, however, be a demanding and even dangerous sport because of the intrinsic hazards of the underwater environment.

Currently there are an estimated 4 million active recreational divers in the United States, and about 400,000 new divers are certified each year. In addition, tens of thousands of commercial and scientific divers are engaged in a wide array of underwater pursuits.

Despite the extent of diving activity, scuba diving fatalities and serious injuries are relatively infrequent. In recent years about 750 to 800 serious scuba diving accidents have occurred annually in North America.[36,79] Precise scuba diving risk calculations would require a denominator showing the number of actual dives each year by type of dive. The data are not available; however, existing data have shown an encouraging downward trend in fatalities despite steady growth in sport diving activities. Notwithstanding these encouraging data, concern about the safety of diving is increasing because of the changing character of the sport diving population.

In the past 40 years the nature of the scuba diving population has substantially changed. Scuba divers of the 1950s and early 1960s were generally "water people," well-trained athletes experienced in breath-hold diving and competitive swimming. To don a scuba tank, regulator, mask, fins, and snorkel was a natural extension of activity to persons already at home in the aquatic environment. These persons seldom encountered problems that required the attention of the general medical community. However, as more people became aware of scuba diving, and as scuba diving equipment became more readily available, adventure-minded people of all walks of life were attracted to the sport. The advent of underwater photography and cinema opened a new world of beauty and fascination to millions of people, attracting viewers to seek training in the sport, even though many had never been in the ocean.

The popularization of scuba diving in recent years has attracted participation by people who are often poorly conditioned, have little or no experience in aquatic sports, are of an advanced age, or have significant underlying medical conditions. Because of the often arduous nature of the environment in which scuba diving is done, such persons may be at increased risk for an accident. Many medical conditions are contraindications to diving.

Today almost every physician finds scuba divers among his or her patients and consequently should be prepared to answer questions about fitness for diving and to handle diving-related medical emergencies. Likewise, since scuba diving is conducted in lakes, rivers, quarries, and other aquatic settings, in addition to the ocean, each emergency medical facility must be prepared to assess and provide immediate care and transportation to a hyperbaric treatment facility (recompression chamber) for a victim of decompression sickness or arterial gas embolism. This chapter focuses primarily on the pressure-related diving syndromes collectively known as dysbarism.

Historical Perspective

While human beings did not evolve for an aquatic existence and are not well adapted to function in the aquatic environment, they have been breath-hold diving to gather food and other natural resources from the sea for thousands of years. There is archeologic evidence that Neanderthals breath-hold dived 40,000 years ago. The Ama of Japan and Hae-Nyu of Korea have been breath-hold diving to collect edible mollusks and seaweed for about 6000 years. The now extinct Alakaluf Indians of southern Patagonia engaged in similar diving practices. The fires along the shores of the Straits of Magellan built to warm these native American divers are believed to be the source of the name "Tierra del Fuego" (Land of Fire) given to the area by Ferdinand Magellan.

Written records of diving for salvage and military purposes date back to around 500 BC, when the Greek historian Herodotus recorded the feats of Scyllis as he dived in the Mediterranean Sea for the Persian king Xerxes during the 50-year war between Greece and Persia. Other colorful accounts of military and salvage divers dot the history of the Roman and other early cultures. However, humans' underwater exploits remained limited to breath-hold diving until about 300 years ago, when a series of technologic developments began to expand human underwater activity. These developments principally involved the use of different types of external air supply to prolong submergence.

In the seventeenth century, primitive bells containing air were carried from the surface, allowing Swedish divers to stay underwater longer than a single breath and to salvage cannons from Stockholm's harbor.[90] In 1690, Sir Edmund Halley (of astronomy and comet fame) devised a leather tube to carry surface air to barrels, which resupplied air to manned bells at a depth of 60 feet. These barrels were submerged, and the air they contained was compressed.[32]

The first practical diving suit was fabricated by Augustus Siebe in 1837.[1,32,90] Atmospheric air was supplied to the diver as compressed air from a manually powered pump on the surface. By 1841, French engineers had developed the technique of using compressed air to keep water and mud out of caissons sunk to the bottom of riverbeds for bridge footings and tunnels. Soon thereafter, it was noted that people working in a compressed air environment sometimes suffered joint pains, paralysis, and other medical problems after leaving the caisson. This poorly understood condition was called caisson disease and was the first recognition of what is now known as decompression sickness.

Underwater diving remained an esoteric activity having limited commercial and military utility until the 1930s. By this time, and increasingly during World War II, the military importance of an undersea capability became evident to navies throughout the world. With the development of submarine forces came the need to train men to escape from submarines that became disabled at depth. Given the shallow operational depths of these early boats, it was usually possible to escape by simply exiting the vessel and ascending to the surface. It was noted early that failure to exhale while ascending through the water led to pulmonary overpressurization accidents and a new and dramatic syndrome that we now know to be arterial gas embolism.

In 1865 the French engineers Rouquayrol and Denayrouse developed a device that could supply air on demand at ambient pressures different from the 1 atm of pressure found at sea level. These inventors were able to supply air on demand at appropriate breathing pressure to persons underwater with a "demand regulator," as it subsequently became known. This device originally required a surface air supply connection.[1] The demand valve regulator was later modified to supply auxiliary oxygen for pilots operating at high altitude. In 1943, as part of the French resistance activities against Nazi Germany, Jacques-Yves Cousteau and Emile Gagnon combined a demand valve regulator with a compressed air tank, giving rise to what they called self-contained underwater breathing apparatus, or "scuba."

The potential military usefulness of scuba was immediately recognized and led to a considerable amount of investigation during World War II. As initially configured, scuba was used in an open-circuit mode in which exhaled air was just vented into the water. This was wasteful of the compressed air supply and had other disadvantages for military uses. Further work led to the development of closed-circuit scuba devices, such as Lambertsen's amphibious respiratory unit, and a variety of semiclosed systems.[5] These types of breathing systems conserved the breathing gas by using a carbon dioxide scrubber and recirculating all or part of each exhalation. The specialized scuba systems were useful for military purposes because they allowed longer submergence times and could be used in clandestine operations. However, they had much greater risk of mishap and so were never popularized for general use.

After World War II the development and marketing of open-circuit scuba equipment to the general public made the underwater world accessible to growing numbers of people. In the last four decades, scuba diving has opened the underwater world to millions of divers and hundreds of millions of cinema observers. Scuba is now used as a basic tool with myriad commercial, military, scientific, and recreational applications (Box 47-1). The growth of sport diving has been especially noteworthy. For example, since scuba was first introduced into the United States in 1951, it is estimated that over 7 million Americans have been certified as recreational or sport divers.

Types of Diving and Diving Equipment

There are five general types of diving, each having increasingly sophisticated equipment requirements. From the least to the most sophisticated equipment used, the types of diving are breath-hold or free diving, scuba diving,

BOX 47-1

TYPES OF COMMERCIAL DIVING

- Harvest of natural resources
  - Oil and natural gas
  - Minerals
  - Fish and shellfish
  - Pearls, corals, and shells
  - Algae
  - Wood (logging)
  - Aquaculture
- Salvage and recovery operations
- Maintenance and construction
  - Ship hulls
  - Nuclear power plants
  - Bridges and tunnels
  - Piers and jetties
  - Aquariums
  - Water treatment plants
  - Dams
- Underwater photography and motion picture production
- Marine studies
  - Biology
  - Geology
  - Archeology
  - Other sciences
- Rescue operations
- Sport-diving instructors and tour guides

Modified from Kizer KW: Medical aspects of scuba diving. In Noble J, editor: *Textbook of general medicine and primary care,* Boston, 1987, Little, Brown.

surface-supplied or tethered diving, saturation diving, and one atmosphere diving.

BREATH-HOLD OR FREE DIVING

Breath-hold diving—also known as free diving, skin diving, or snorkeling—is the simplest and oldest form of underwater diving. It uses no external supply of air, so submergence time is limited to the length of time the diver can hold his or her breath. Generally, the breath-hold diver uses a face mask to allow underwater vision, fins for propulsion, a snorkel to breathe air while swimming face down on the water's surface, some sort of attire for thermal protection (for example, a neoprene wet suit), and sometimes lead weights to counterbalance the positive buoyancy of a wet suit.

SCUBA DIVING

Scuba is the acronym for self-contained underwater breathing apparatus. It uses a tank fitted with a pressure regulator that supplies compressed air to the diver at a pressure equal to ambient water pressure. In sport diving the diver's scuba tank is usually pressurized to between 2200 and 3000 PSIG with filtered, oil-free compressed air. The regulator employs two stages. The first stage is attached to the tank and makes an initial reduction in pressure to the lower pressure second stage, which is attached to the diver's mouthpiece and from which the diver actually breathes.

Like the snorkeler, the scuba diver wears a face mask covering the eyes and nose to allow underwater vision, fins for propulsion, a snorkel for surface swimming, a buoyancy-compensating vest and weight belt to adjust buoyancy under water and for flotation in case of an emergency, a watch and depth gauge to track time and depth (or a diving computer), and a tank pressure gauge to monitor air consumption. Because of the higher thermal conductivity of water, divers typically wear neoprene wet suits in all but warm tropical waters. These suits maintain a layer of water warmed by body heat between the skin and suit. A nonpermeable "dry suit" and warm undergarments are usually worn when diving in cold water.

In addition to the preceding, various equipment may be used for safety reasons, navigation, communication, or other special purposes. While recreational scuba diving is performed using compressed air in an open-circuit mode, special types of scuba gear may be worn for military, scientific, or commercial diving that use various helium-oxygen or nitrogen-oxygen mixtures in a semiclosed- or closed-circuit mode. In scientific and commercial work, diving is often done at depths deeper than would be safe in sport diving, and mixtures of helium and oxygen are used to avoid problems of nitrogen narcosis.

SURFACE-SUPPLIED OR TETHERED DIVING

Also known as hardhat diving, and sometimes called mud diving because it is done in harbors (which typically have muddy bottoms), surface-supplied diving is most often used for commercial or military purposes. It is frequently performed in arduous environments requiring special protective attire. In this form of diving the diver's breathing gases (such as compressed air or helium-oxygen mixtures) are supplied by hoses from the surface or from a diving bell at a pressure equal to water pressure. The techniques are quite different in scuba and surface-supplied diving, but the medical problems are similar.

SATURATION DIVING

Once under water, the diver begins to absorb increased amounts of nitrogen or another inert gas, depending on the breathing medium, until a new equilibrium is established according to the pressure of the depth attained. In certain deep-diving scenarios the time needed to off-gas, or "decompress," this inert gas on returning to normal atmospheric pressure may be much greater than the time spent at depth.

In the late 1950s, experiments by U.S. Navy diving medical officers George Bond and Robert Workman coincided with those of Jacques-Yves Cousteau and Edward Link, all of whom were working on ways to stay under water at great depths long enough to do useful work.[2] The need for prolonged decompression after deep diving led to the development of saturation diving. The basic concept of saturation diving is that after approximately 24 hours at any given depth, the diver's tissues have established equilibrium with the gases in the breathing mixture. From that point, the decompression obligation remains the same no matter how long the diver remains at that depth. If the diver can be kept "at pressure" for a prolonged period, the decompression is the same as if he or she were there for only a short time.

Modern saturation complexes allow divers to live for days in large chambers at the pressure of a given work site and to be transported to the underwater site by locking into a personal transfer capsule (PTC) or sealed diving bell. When depth is reached, the water pressure equals the gas pressure within the capsule and divers may exit the PTC into the water while breathing gas supplied by umbilical hoses. To maintain the diver's thermal balance in the very cold water found at great depths, heated water is circulated in special hot water suits.

Another application of saturation diving, used primarily for scientific purposes, is characterized by underwater habitats, steel chambers situated at a given depth of water and pressurized with a compressed gas atmosphere at the same pressure as the surrounding water. Divers may live for days or weeks in this environment, leaving the chamber with scuba equipment to perform studies or observe marine life in its natural state. In this specialized area of diving, special precautions are taken to avoid inadvertent surfacing, thermal stress, and skin and ear infections during prolonged stays in the saturation habitat. Prolonged saturation decompression schedules, often taking several days, are used to return divers safely to sea level pressure on completion of the mission.

ONE ATMOSPHERE DIVING

In recent years it has become clear that humans cannot reliably or safely function at the greatly elevated pressure of deep water, and this has become the limiting factor in human exploration of the ocean depths. This has led to numerous developments in one atmosphere diving systems. Leonardo da Vinci created schematic drawings that look similar to some of today's one atmosphere diving systems, but late twentieth century advances in metallurgy, engineering, and communications were required before these systems actually became a reality. In essence, 1 atmosphere absolute (ATA) diving systems are small submarines with various types of propulsion systems and manipulators that allow the operator to work at great depth. The interior of the unit is maintained with environmental control systems to retain safe physiologic parameters. These systems range from one-person 1 ATA suits (Fig. 47-1) to submersibles that accommodate two or more occupants.

Special Diving Situations

Diving in general, and scuba diving in particular, has become a tool that allows humans to engage in a wide array of underwater activities (Box 47-1). There are a number of special diving situations.

UNDER ICE AND POLAR DIVING

Diving under the ice in extremely cold environments is done for exploration, search and rescue, salvage, inspections, and other work. This takes place in lakes, rivers, and the polar regions. Besides meticulous preparation and provision of thermal protection for the diver under ice, the extremely low temperature, wind, and snow above water at the dive site necessitate careful planning for topside shelter. For diving in such cold water, dry suits or hot water suits are used. Dry suits are made of closed-cell foam neoprene, rubber, or rubberized canvas and fit loosely with seals at the wrists, ankles, and neck to keep the diver and insulating

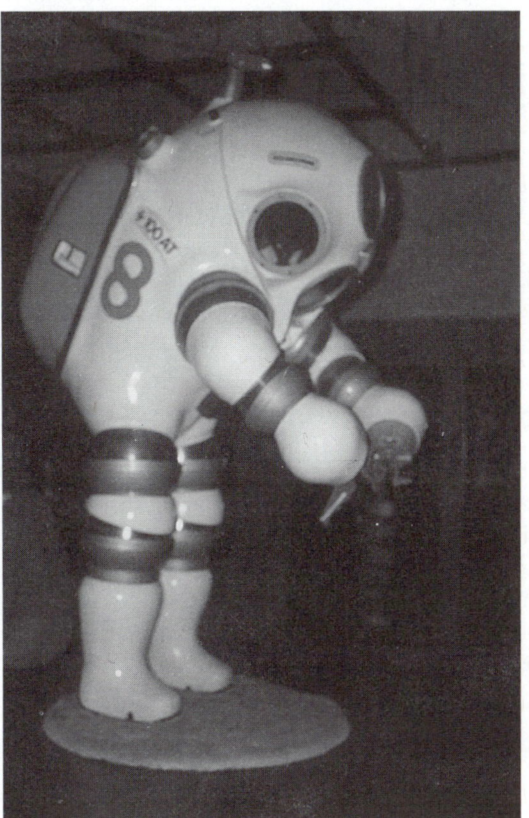

Fig. 47-1 JIM diving suit. The diver remains at 1 ATA inside the armor suit and can work while submerged in hundreds of feet of water.

underwear dry and to allow the admission of air to maintain equal suit volume during the dive. Free-flooding hot water suits are loosely fitted closed-cell foam neoprene suits with hoses inside to allow warm water to flow continuously over the diver's body and exit at the wrist and neck.[101] In this specialized type of diving, other considerations are provision of breathing regulators that are not likely to freeze, planning for immediate rescue and rapid rewarming of an individual who might fall into the frigid water without adequate protection, maintenance of adequate nutrition and hydration, and total prohibition of alcoholic beverages or mind-altering drugs at the dive operation, since these activities permit little margin for error.

CAVERN AND CAVE DIVING

The advent of scuba has allowed exploration of many underwater caverns and cave systems, leading to important archeologic and geologic discoveries. However, cave diving is the most dangerous form of diving.[52]

To trained, experienced, properly equipped cave divers, the number of cave diving fatalities (approximately 300 in Florida alone since 1960) is distressing, although generally explainable. Most fatalities have involved inexperienced open-water scuba divers who have never been trained in cave diving. Most often, the divers became lost and ran out of air while in a cave. The National Association of Cave Divers (NACD) and the National Speleological Society—Cave Diving Section (NSS-CDS) are the recognized training organizations for cave diving.

Because cave divers are separated from the outside world and cannot simply surface in case of an emergency, specific equipment and procedures are required. These include double tanks, meticulous planning of air consumption, backup lights, and guide cables to avoid becoming lost. No one should attempt cave diving without completing formal training approved by either the NACD or the NSS-CDS.

RIVER DIVING

Diving in rivers is often done by public safety personnel in search of evidence or to retrieve bodies (usually drowning victims). Because of the typically poor visibility, strong currents, and potential for entanglement in debris, this type of diving should be done only by persons who have been trained in the special techniques of river diving and who have proper surface support.

MISCELLANEOUS TYPES OF DIVING

Diving is undertaken for a variety of special purposes in settings that pose unique hazards. These settings include nuclear power plants, harbors with toxic chemical or infectious disease contamination, water treatment facilities, and dams generating electric power. Each of these settings requires special diving techniques, health monitoring, and safety precautions.

Dysbarism

Divers encounter many adverse environmental conditions underwater. These include cold, wetness, changes in light transmission and sound conduction, lack of air to breathe, increased density of the surrounding environment, and increased atmospheric pressure. Not surprisingly, diverse unique medical problems are related to diving (Box 47-2).

Of the various environmental factors affecting divers, pressure is by far the most important, since its effects directly or indirectly account for the majority of serious diving medical problems. Therefore understanding the basic

BOX 47-2

MEDICAL PROBLEMS OF SCUBA DIVERS

- Environmental exposure problems
  - Motion sickness
  - Near drowning
  - Hypothermia
  - Heat illness
  - Sunburn
  - Phototoxic and photoallergic reactions
  - Irritant and other dermatitides
  - Infectious diseases
  - Mechanical trauma
- Dysbarism
  - Barotrauma
  - Dysbaric air embolism
  - Decompression sickness
  - Dysbaric osteonecrosis
  - Dysbaric retinopathy
  - Hyperbaric cephalalgia
- Breathing gas–related problems
  - Inert gas narcosis
  - Hypoxia
  - Oxygen toxicity
  - Hypercapnia
  - Carbon monoxide poisoning
  - Lipoid pneumonitis
- Hazardous marine life
- Miscellaneous
  - Hyperventilation
  - Hearing loss
  - Carotid-related blackout
  - Panic and other psychologic problems

Modified from Kizer KW: *Emerg Med Clin North Am* 1:659, 1983.

physics and physiologic effects of pressure is essential to treating the pressure-related maladies that fall under the general term "dysbarism."

DEFINITIONS AND TERMINOLOGY

Dysbarism is a term that encompasses all pathologic changes caused by altered environmental pressure. It is primarily a disorder of divers and compressed air workers exposed to increased atmospheric pressure, but it may also occur in aviators, astronauts, and some industrial workers as a result of abrupt exposure to the reduced pressure found at actual or simulated high altitude.

Dysbarism most often develops acutely because of problems caused by the mechanical effects of pressure on closed air spaces (barotrauma) or problems caused by breathing gases at elevated partial pressure (such as nitrogen narcosis or decompression sickness). Less often the effects are delayed for months or years, as in the case of dysbaric osteonecrosis.

Pressure is defined as force per unit area. Atmospheric pressure is the pressure exerted by the air above the earth's surface. Atmospheric pressure varies with altitude. At sea level, atmospheric pressure is 760 millimeters of mercury (mm Hg) or 14.7 pounds per square inch (PSI). The barometric pressure at sea level is generally referred to as 1 atmosphere (atm).

Absolute pressure is the total barometric pressure at any point. With pressure gauges calibrated to read zero at sea level, gauge pressure is the amount of pressure greater than atmospheric pressure. In general, gauge pressure is 1 atm less than absolute atmospheric pressure. It is always important to specify whether pressure is expressed in terms of gauge or absolute pressure.

Except in situations requiring laboratory precision, the following units are commonly used to express water pressure:

1. Pounds per square inch gauge (PSIG)
2. Pounds per square inch absolute (PSIA)
3. Feet of seawater (FSW)
4. Feet of fresh water (FFW)
5. Atmospheres absolute (ATA)

As a diver descends under water, absolute pressure increases much faster than in air. Each foot of seawater exerts a force of 0.445 PSIG. Therefore, if the 14.7 PSI pressure of 1 atm is divided by 0.445 PSI per foot of seawater, at 33 FSW the absolute pressure will have doubled. In the ocean, each 33 feet of depth adds one additional atmosphere of pressure. The gauge pressure at 33 FSW is 14.7 PSIG (in excess of atmospheric pressure), and the absolute pressure is 29.4 PSIA.

Because of the weight of solutes in seawater, it is slightly heavier than fresh water. In fresh water, 34 feet equals one additional atmosphere of pressure.

Pressure change with increasing depth is linear, although the greatest relative change in pressure per unit of depth change occurs nearest the surface. Table 47-1 lists commonly used units of pressure measurement in seawater.

When a diver submerges, the force of the tremendous weight of the water above is exerted over the entire body. Except for air-containing spaces such as the lungs, paranasal sinuses, intestines, and middle ears, the body behaves as a liquid. The law that describes the behavior of pressure in liquids is named for the seventeenth century scientist Pascal. Pascal's Law states that a pressure applied to any part of a fluid is transmitted equally throughout the fluid. Thus, when a diver reaches 33 FSW, the pressure on the surface of the skin and throughout the body tissues is 29.4 PSIA or 1520 mm Hg (Fig. 47-2). The diver's body is generally unaware of this pressure, however, except in the air-containing spaces of the body. The gases in these spaces obey Boyle's Law (Fig. 47-3), which states that the pressure of a given quantity of gas whose temperature remains unchanged varies inversely with its volume. Hence, air in the middle ear, paranasal sinuses, lungs, and gastrointestinal tract is reduced in volume during compression or descent under water. Inability to maintain gas pressure in these body spaces equal to the surrounding water pressure leads to various untoward mechanical effects, which are discussed later.

Because of the weight of the water exerting pressure over the chest wall, humans can breathe surface air through a snorkel or tube connected to the surface for only a short distance underwater—typically only to a depth of 1 to 2 feet. Attempts to breathe at greater depths through the tube are not only impossible but dangerous, because the respiratory effort greatly augments the already physiologic negative-pressure breathing. In other words, when the respiratory muscles are relaxed at sea level, alveolar pressure equals surrounding air pressure. At a depth of 1 foot the total water pressure on the chest wall is nearly 200 pounds. Because of the loss of normal chest expansion and the pressurization of

Table 47-1 Commonly Used Units of Pressure in the Underwater Environment

Depth (FSW)	PSIG	PSIA	ATA	mm Hg (Absolute)
Sea level	0.0	14.7	1	760
33	14.7	29.4	2	1520
66	29.4	44.1	3	2280
99	44.1	58.8	4	3040
132	58.8	73.5	5	3800
165	73.5	88.2	6	4560
198	88.2	102.9	7	5320
231	102.9	117.6	8	6080
264	117.6	132.3	9	6840
297	132.3	147.0	10	7600

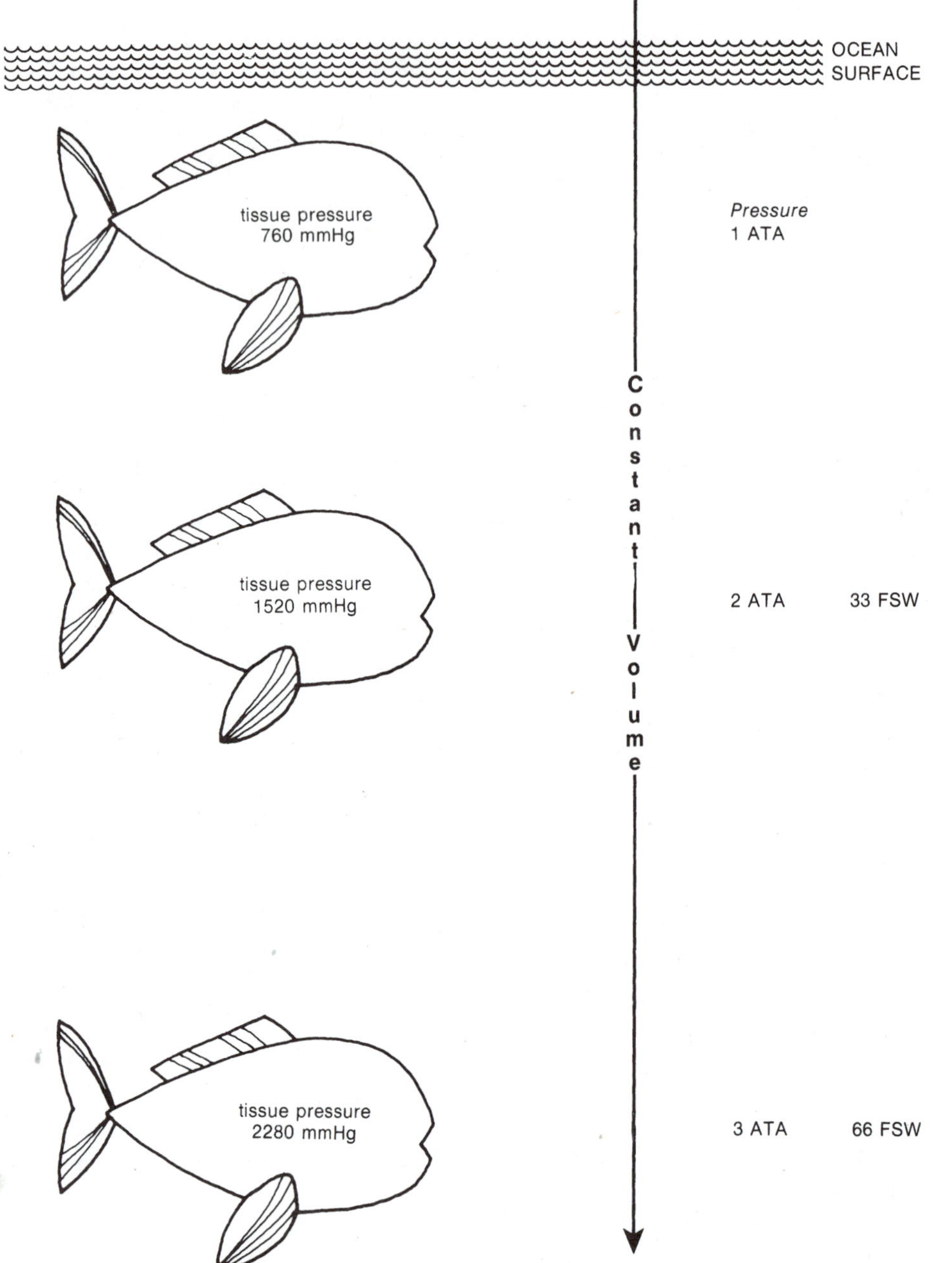

Fig. 47-2 Pascal's Law. Pressure applied to any part of a fluid is transmitted equally throughout.

intraalveolar air, the diver has to use forceful negative-pressure breathing to draw surface air into the lungs through the tube. Even at a depth of 1 foot the great respiratory effort required is rapidly fatiguing, and respiration becomes impossible at further depths of only a few inches. Forced negative-pressure breathing can ultimately result in pulmonary capillary damage, with intraalveolar edema or hemorrhage. Symptoms include dyspnea and hemoptysis. Should this occur, there is no specific treatment; therapy is purely supportive.

MECHANICAL EFFECTS OF PRESSURE (BAROTRAUMA)

Gas pressure in the various air-filled spaces of the body is normally in equilibrium with the environment. However, if anything obstructs the passageways of gas exchange for these spaces and a change in ambient pressure occurs, a pressure disequilibrium develops. The tissue damage resulting from such pressure imbalance is known as barotrauma. Overall, barotrauma is the most common medical problem in scuba diving, potentially involving any structure or com-

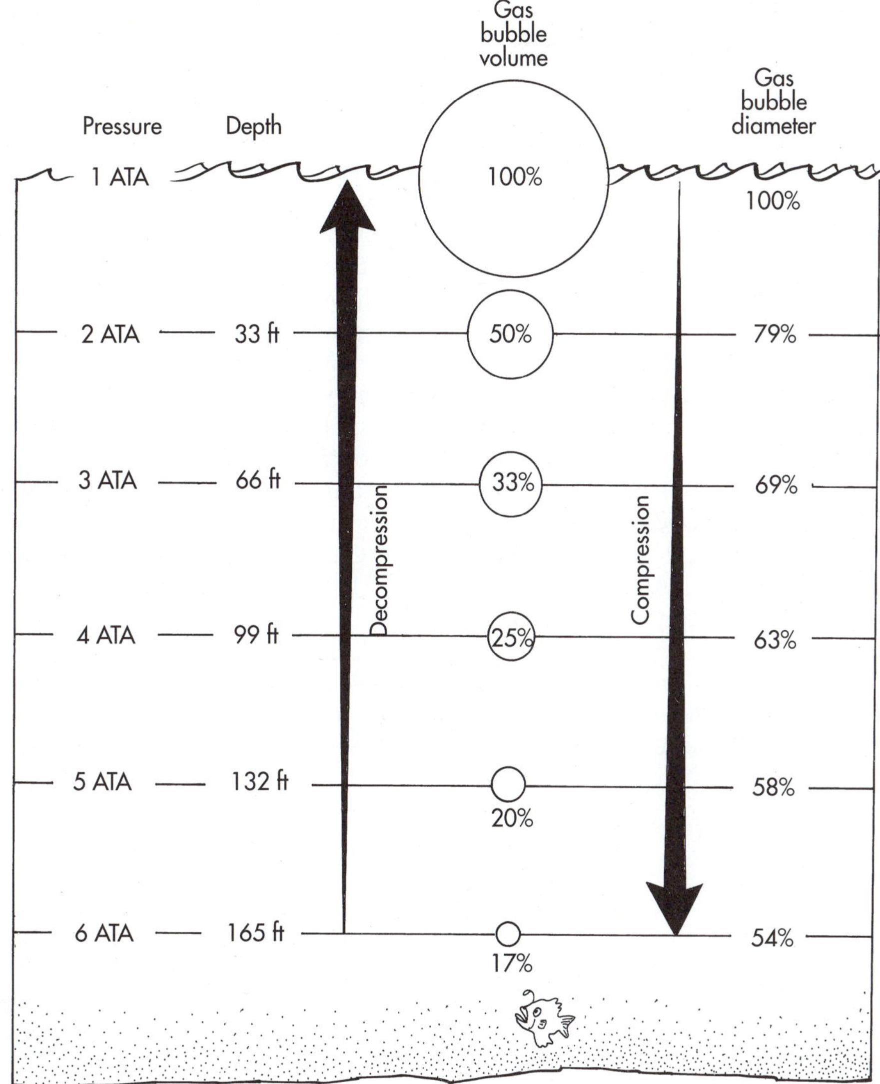

Fig. 47-3 Boyle's Law. The pressure of a given quantity of gas at constant temperature varies inversely as its volume: $P_1V_1 = P_2V_2$.

bination of structures that leads to entrapment of gas in a closed space. This may include skin trapped under a fold in a dry suit, the portion of the face under a face mask, or the ears, paranasal sinuses, lungs, and gastrointestinal tract.

Specific Types of Barotrauma

Mask Squeeze. For humans to see underwater, an airspace must be present between the eye and water. In scuba diving this is created by use of a face mask consisting of tempered safety glass in a soft malleable mask that seals across the forehead, on the sides of the face, and under the nose to allow nasal exhalations to maintain air pressure equal to water pressure during descent. If inexperience or inattention causes the diver to forget to maintain this balance, negative air pressure in the mask can cause capillary rupture, with skin ecchymoses and conjunctival hemorrhage (Color Plate 108). Such a pressure imbalance could be especially dangerous after keratotomy because of the slow healing rate of corneal incisions.[25]

Ear Canal Squeeze. A tight-fitting wet suit hood can trap air in the external auditory canal and potentially lead to a painful external ear squeeze during descent, as the volume of air is reduced according to Boyle's Law. This problem can be prevented by remembering to break the seal to allow water to fill the external ear canal before descent. An external ear squeeze also can occur if the canal is blocked by cerumen, exostoses, or ear plugs (which should never be used in diving).

Symptoms and signs of ear canal squeeze include pain, swelling, erythema, petechiae or hemorrhagic blebs of the ear canal wall, or actual hemorrhage. In very severe cases the tympanic membrane can rupture from the negative pressure in the ear canal. This is exceedingly rare, but if it occurs, further diving is contraindicated until the membrane has healed.

Barotitis Media or Middle Ear Squeeze. Referred to in diver parlance as "ear squeeze," barotitis media is the most common medical problem in scuba diving, probably affecting more than 40% of divers.[51] The physics and physiology of the problem are straightforward but are sometimes forgotten by the diver who eagerly jumps from a boat to explore the beauty beneath the surface. The problem is a direct application of Boyle's Law (Fig. 47-4), potentially compounded by the structure of the eustachian tube.

As previously noted, Boyle's Law describes the inverse relationship of pressure and volume in an enclosed airspace. It also explains why the greatest relative volume change for a given depth change occurs near the surface, which is why the greatest risk of middle ear squeeze occurs near the surface.

Since each foot of seawater exerts a pressure of about 23 mm Hg, a diver who descends 2.5 feet and does not equalize the pressure in his or her middle ear will develop a relative vacuum in the middle ear because of the contraction of air volume in the ear. Typically the diver notices slight pain at a 60 mm Hg pressure differential between air in the middle ear and ambient water pressure. This pressure differential causes the tympanic membrane to stretch and bulge inward, causing increasing discomfort and eventually severe pain. At a depth of 4 feet a 90 mm Hg pressure differential is generated, and the unsupported, flutter-valve medial third of the eustachian tube collapses and becomes obstructed. At this point, attempts to autoinflate the middle ear (as by Valsalva or Frenzel maneuvers) may be unsuccessful. The diver must ascend to equalize middle ear pressure with ambient environmental pressure.

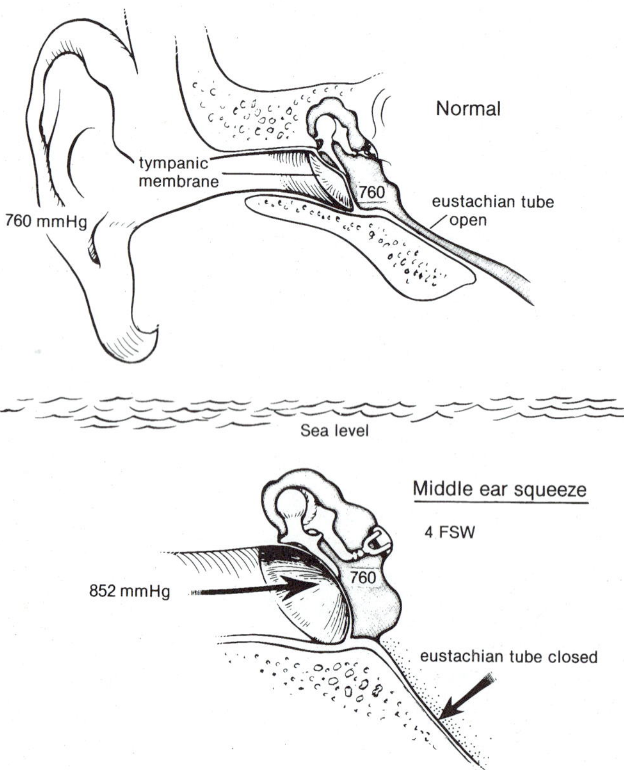

Fig. 47-4 Middle ear trauma. Symptoms include fullness and pain caused by stretching of the tympanic membrane.

The Valsalva maneuver involves blowing with an open glottis against closed lips and nostrils to increase pressure in the nasopharynx in order to inflate the middle ear through the eustachian tubes. This may force open a collapsed eustachian tube. The Frenzel maneuver is performed by swallowing with a closed glottis while the lips are closed and the nostrils are pinched.

If a diver does not heed the symptoms of barotitis media and allows the pressure differential to reach 100 to 400 mm Hg (that is, at depths of 4.3 to 17.4 feet), the pressure imbalance may be unsatisfactorily resolved by rupture of the tympanic membrane.[49] In such cases the problem for the diver may be compounded by entry of cold water into the middle ear, which will usually cause severe vertigo. Before this event, serum may have been drawn into the middle ear by the relative vacuum, with development of serous otitis media.

Prevention is the key element in dealing with barotitis media. Divers who understand the sequence just described generally take steps to inflate the middle ear immediately on submerging and thereby avoid the entire sequence as they descend in the water. If middle ear pressure is kept equal to or greater than water pressure, no problem should occur. However, if the diver forgets to inflate the middle ear or suffers from eustachian tube dysfunction (caused, for example, by mucosal congestion secondary to upper respiratory infection, allergies, or smoking; mucosal polyps; excessively vigorous autoinflation maneuvers; or previous maxillofacial trauma), middle ear barotrauma may occur. This most often happens just after the diver leaves the surface, with the diver complaining of ear fullness or pain. Generally the pain rapidly becomes severe enough that the diver either corrects the problem or aborts the dive.

The otoscopic appearance of the tympanic membrane in cases of barotitis media varies with the severity of the injury. A commonly used grading scheme is the Teed classification, which grades the severity according to the amount of hemorrhage in the tympanic membrane.[40] Grades are 0 for symptoms only; grade 1 for erythema over the malleus; grade 2 for erythema of the malleus plus mild hemorrhage of the tympanic membrane; grade 3 for gross hemorrhage throughout the tympanic membrane; grade 4 for free blood in the middle ear; and grade 5 for free blood in the middle ear plus perforation of the tympanic membrane. Use of this grading scheme facilitates communication when describing these injuries.

In addition to having an abnormal-appearing tympanic

membrane, persons with barotitis media occasionally have a small amount of blood around the nose or mouth, as well as a mild conductive hearing loss.

Middle ear squeeze should be treated with decongestants and analgesics. Antihistamines may be used if the eustachian tube dysfunction has an allergic component. Divers should abstain from diving until the condition has resolved. Combining an oral decongestant with a long-acting topical nasal spray (such as 0.5% oxymetazoline or phenylephrine) for the first few days is usually most effective. Repeated gentle autoinflation of the middle ear (as by use of the Frenzel maneuver) also can help to displace any collection of middle ear fluid through the eustachian tube. Antibiotics (such as amoxicillin–clavulanic acid) should be used when there is a tympanic membrane rupture or preexisting infection or if the dive was in "dirty" waters. If the tympanic membrane has ruptured, no diving should be done until it is fully healed or a surgical repair is successful, and until eustachian tube function allows easy autoinflation.

Most cases of barotitis media resolve without complication in 3 to 7 days, although occasionally it takes longer. The condition can be prevented if a diver refrains from diving when unable to easily equalize pressure in the ears and heeds the warning symptoms of ear pain.

Barosinusitis. Barosinusitis, or "sinus squeeze," results from essentially the same mechanism as barotitis media but is less common (Fig. 47-5). If there is inability to maintain the air pressure in any paranasal sinus during descent, a relative vacuum develops in the sinus cavity. This initially produces intense pain, then damage to the sinus wall mucosa, with bleeding into the sinus. Less commonly a "reverse sinus squeeze" can occur on decompression or ascent in the water. In this condition, pain is produced by relatively high air pressure in the sinus. This usually occurs in the setting of a diver who has an upper respiratory infection or allergies and who has taken a decongestant some time before diving but in whom the vasoconstricting effect wears off while at depth.

Prevention of barosinusitis requires avoidance of diving with an upper respiratory infection or while allergic rhinitis is causing edema of the mucosa about the sinus orifices, and when sinusitis, nasal polyps, or any other condition is present that impairs the free flow of air from sinus cavity to nose. Treatment involves the use of systemic (for example, pseudoephedrine) and topical (for example, phenylephrine or oxymetazoline) vasoconstrictors, analgesics, abstinence from diving until resolved, and antihistamines if needed. Antibiotics may be needed in the event of a severe squeeze with bleeding into the sinus cavity or in cases of frontal sinusitis.

Barodontalgia. One of the most infrequent types of barotrauma is barodontalgia or "tooth squeeze"; this is sometimes called aerodontalgia. This painful condition is caused by entrapped gas in the interior of a tooth or in the structures surrounding a tooth. The confined gas develops either positive or negative pressure relative to ambient pressure, which places force on the surrounding sensitive dental structures and causes pain.

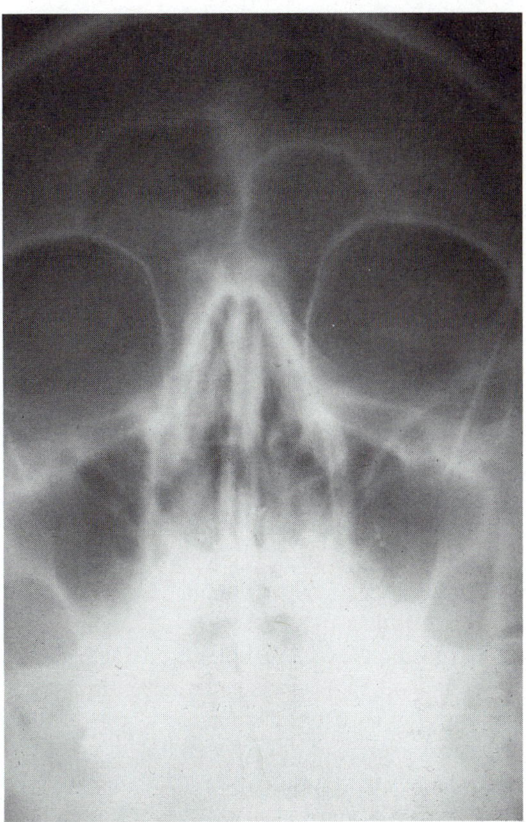

Fig. 47-5 Frontal sinus barotrauma. Note the air-fluid level. (Courtesy Kenneth W. Kizer, M.D.)

Barodontalgia may be caused by an array of dental conditions, including caries, defective restorations, oral tissue lacerations, recent extractions, periodontal abscesses, pulpal or apical lesions or cysts, and endodontal (root canal) therapy. If a pocket of trapped air remains at sea level pressure while ambient pressure increases during descent, the tooth can implode or the cavity can fill with blood. Conversely, air that is forced into a tooth during descent can expand during ascent, causing the tooth to explode. To prevent barodontalgia, a diver should wait at least 24 hours after dental treatment (including fillings) before diving.

Other causes of tooth pain associated with pressure changes are less well understood. Pulpitis or other dental infections can produce pain during a dive. Of course, upper tooth pain associated with pressure changes should raise a question about a pathologic condition in the maxillary sinus.

Labyrinthine Window Rupture. A serious form of aural barotrauma, although much less common than barotitis media, is inner ear barotrauma causing a labyrinthine window rupture. This is the most serious form of aural barotrauma because of possible injury to the cochleovestibular system that may lead to permanent deafness or vestibular dysfunction.[41,48]

Inner ear barotrauma results from rapid development of markedly different pressures between the middle and inner ear, such as may occur from an overly forceful Valsalva maneuver or an exceptionally rapid descent, during which the middle ear pressure is not adequately equalized. The pressure disequilibrium may cause several types of injury to the cochleovestibular apparatus, including hemorrhage within the inner ear; rupture of Reissner's membrane, leading to mixing of endolymph and perilymph; fistulation of the oval or round window, with development of a perilymph leak; or a mixed injury involving any or all of these things.[91]

The classic triad of symptoms indicating inner ear barotrauma is roaring tinnitus, vertigo, and hearing loss. In addition, a feeling of fullness or "blockage" of the affected ear, nausea, vomiting, nystagmus, pallor, diaphoresis, disorientation, or ataxia may be present in varying degree.

Symptoms of inner ear barotrauma may develop immediately after the injury or may be delayed for hours, depending on the specific damage and the diver's activities during and after the dive. Vigorous isometric exercise after a dive may complete an incipient membrane rupture. Findings on aural physical examination may be normal or may reveal signs of middle ear barotrauma or vestibular dysfunction. Audiometry may demonstrate a mild to severe sensorineural hearing loss.

Hemorrhage within the inner ear is usually associated with findings of middle ear barotrauma, absent or transient vestibular symptoms, and diffuse mild to severe sensorineural hearing loss. Patients should be treated with bed rest (with the head elevated to 30 degrees), avoidance of any strenuous activity, and symptomatic measures as needed. There is a good prognosis for full recovery of hearing in 3 to 12 weeks. Patients with a tear in Reissner's membrane have manifestations similar to those with inner-ear hemorrhage, although there is a persistent localized sensorineural hearing loss commensurate with the area of membrane tear. The management is unchanged.

A patient with a perilymph fistula usually has high-frequency sensorineural hearing loss or marked cochleovestibular dysfunction and little evidence of middle ear barotrauma. Initially he or she should be treated with bed rest, avoidance of strain, and symptomatic measures, although some authorities advocate immediate tympanotomy if severe symptoms are present. In all cases, however, deterioration of hearing, worsening of vestibular symptoms, or persistence of significant vestibular symptoms after a few days heralds the need for detailed otolaryngologic evaluation and probable surgical exploration and repair.

A diagnostic dilemma exists whenever a diver complains of vertigo, tinnitus, and hearing loss associated with a dive. These symptoms may indicate a diagnosis of inner ear decompression sickness, which requires expeditious treatment in a hyperbaric chamber. Conversely, symptoms may indicate labyrinthine rupture, in which case recompression is contraindicated because of potential further barotrauma. In such cases the most important differential feature for diagnostic use on a dive boat or other diving site is a careful history. If symptom onset was during descent and ear clearing was difficult or impossible, requiring forcible Valsalva maneuvers, perilymph fistula is more likely. If the onset was during or after a decompression dive, decompression sickness must be assumed and chamber treatment sought. In some cases, however, it simply is not possible to rule out decompression sickness or rarely, air embolism, and a "trial of pressure" in the recompression chamber may be necessary.

Alternobaric Vertigo. An unusual type of barotrauma is alternobaric vertigo (ABV). This usually occurs with ascent and is caused by sudden development of unequal middle ear pressure, which causes asymmetric vestibular stimulation and resultant pronounced vertigo.[77] Although usually only transient and requiring no treatment, ABV may precipitate a panic response leading to near drowning, pulmonary barotrauma and resultant air embolism, or other serious injury. Rarely, alternobaric vertigo lasts for several hours or days, in which case it should be treated symptomatically after excluding inner ear barotrauma.

Suit Squeeze. Should an area of diver's skin become trapped under a fold or wrinkle of a dry suit, causing a closed airspace, the pressure-induced contraction of air under the fold, and resulting partial vacuum, can cause transudation of blood through the skin. This is unusual and generally benign, although the resultant skin ecchymosis may make for a dramatic appearance. Generally, suit squeeze requires no treatment and resolves in a few days to a couple of weeks.

Lung Squeeze. Lung squeeze is an unusual form of barotrauma that has been observed with breath-hold diving. Persons having this syndrome typically complain of shortness of breath and dyspnea after surfacing from a deep (greater than 100 FSW) breath-hold dive. The diver may cough up frothy blood, and a chest radiograph may show pulmonary edema. The condition is treated with supplemental oxygen and respiratory support as needed, typically with complete resolution of symptoms within a few days.

The classic understanding of lung squeeze is that it occurs when a diver descends to a depth at which total lung volume (TLV) is reduced to less than residual volume (RV), at which point transpulmonic pressure exceeds intraalveolar pressure, causing transudation of fluid or frank blood (from rupture of pulmonary capillaries) and the overt manifestations of pulmonary edema and hypoxemia.

According to this scenario, a breath-hold diver with a TLV of 6000 ml and an RV of 1200 ml could dive to only 6000/1200 or 5 ATA (equal to 132 FSW) before lung squeeze would occur. However, breath-hold divers have dived much deeper without apparent problem.

In 1968, Schaefer and associates[4] reported that breath-hold divers pool their blood centrally, accumulating a central volume increase of as much as 1047 ml at 90 FSW. If it is assumed that this adjustment in pulmonary blood volume reduces the RV, then theoretically it should be possible for the diver with a TLV of 6000 ml to breath-hold to 6000/(1200 to 1047) or almost 40 ATA.[96] While Jacques Mayol's world record breath-hold dive to 316 FSW seems to support the beneficial effect of central pooling of blood, cases of lung squeeze continue to occur at much shallower depths. The exact pathophysiology of this condition remains unclear. Fortunately, it occurs infrequently.

Underwater Blast Injury. Barotrauma can be caused by underwater explosions. Shock waves from a blast are propagated farther in the dense medium of water than in air. Underwater explosions may result from ordnance or ignition of explosive gases during cutting or welding operations.

Underwater blasts can cause serious injuries to divers. Air-containing body cavities such as the lungs, intestines, ears, and sinuses are most vulnerable. Pneumothorax, pneumomediastinum, and air embolism may result from laceration of the lung and pleura.[59] There may be intestinal perforation, subserosal hemorrhage, and subsequent peritonitis. The occurrence of air embolism at depth, which worsens with decompression, requires treatment by recompression if possible. Otherwise, management of underwater blast injuries is no different than for terrestrial blast injury.

Gastrointestinal Barotrauma. Since the intestines are pliable, contraction of intraluminal bowel gas during descent does not cause barotrauma. In unusual situations, however, expanding gas can become trapped in the gastrointestinal tract during ascent and cause gastrointestinal barotrauma, which is also known as aerogastralgia or gas in the gut.[21,77] This infrequent condition has been noted most often in novice divers, who are more prone to aerophagia; in divers who repeatedly perform the Valsalva maneuver in the head-down position, which forces air into the stomach, or who chew gum while diving; and in divers who consume large quantities of carbonated beverages or legumes shortly before diving.

Divers with gastrointestinal barotrauma typically complain of abdominal fullness, colicky abdominal pain, belching, and flatulence. Rarely, syncope has been reported and is presumed to result from a combination of decreased venous return and vagal reflexes.

Most often the physical examination of divers having symptoms of gastrointestinal barotrauma is normal, since the condition typically resolves by the time medical care is obtained. However, abdominal distention, tympany, and abdominal tenderness may be seen. In extreme cases there may even be signs of cardiovascular compromise as a result of obstruction of venous return.

Gastrointestinal barotrauma is most often self-remedied by elimination of the excess gas. Recompression may be necessary in severe cases, but this is exceedingly rare.

Pulmonary Barotrauma of Ascent (the Pulmonary Overpressurization Syndrome). The most serious type of barotrauma is pulmonary barotrauma of ascent, which results from expansion of gas trapped in the lungs. If a diver does not allow the expanding gas to escape, it ruptures alveolae, producing a spectrum of injuries collectively referred to as the pulmonary overpressurization syndrome (POPS) or burst lung. Basically, the POPS is a dramatic clinical demonstration of Boyle's Law.

Divers suffering pulmonary overpressurization typically give a history of rapid and uncontrolled ascent to the surface before the onset of symptoms—for example, as a result of running out of air, panic, or sudden development of uncontrolled positive buoyancy (dropped weight belt or inadvertent inflation of the buoyancy compensator). However, localized overinflation of the lung from focally increased elastic recoil may also occur in divers who ascend at a proper rate.[20]

It is important to remember that the purpose of all diving regulators is to keep intrapulmonic pressure equal to surrounding water pressure, thus avoiding negative-pressure breathing. So long as these pressures are equal, the diver is relatively unaware of the surrounding crushing water pressure and no problems occur. In this regard, three additional factors have clinical importance:

1. There is significant change in barometric pressure in shallow water. Boyle's Law dictates greater volume changes for a given change in depth near the surface than at greater depths. Hence, shallow depths are the most dangerous for breath-holding ascents.
2. A pressure differential of only 80 mm Hg (alveolar air) above ambient water pressure on the chest wall, or about 3 to 4 feet of depth, is adequate to force air bubbles across the alveolar-capillary membrane.
3. Fatal pulmonary overpressure accidents have occurred from breath-holding during ascent from a depth as shallow as 6 feet of water.

If a given intrapulmonic gas volume is trapped by forcible breath-holding or a closed glottis, or even in a small portion of the lung by bronchospasm during ascent, intrapulmonic volume increases (according to Boyle's Law) until the elastic limit of the chest wall is reached. After that, intrapulmonic pressure rises until, at a positive differential pressure of about 80 mm Hg, air is forced across the pulmonary capillary membrane. This air usually enters either the pulmonary interstitial spaces or the pulmonary capillaries.

The diagnosis of the POPS is based on the development of characteristic symptoms after diving. The actual clinical manifestations may take several forms, including pneumomediastinum, subcutaneous emphysema, pneumopericardium, pneumothorax, pneumoperitoneum, and pulmonary interstitial emphysema. Recently, diffuse alveolar hemorrhage has been described as a manifestation of pulmonary barotrauma.[3] Systemic arterial gas embolism resulting from gas leaking into ruptured pulmonary veins is the most feared complication of the POPS.

The specific clinical manifestations of the POPS depend on the location and amount of air that escapes into an extraalveolar location.

Mediastinal emphysema. Mediastinal emphysema is the most common form of the POPS, resulting from pulmonary interstitial air dissecting along bronchi to the mediastinum. In these cases the diver usually has gradually increasing hoarseness, neck fullness, and substernal chest pain several hours after diving. Subcutaneous emphysema may be present. In severe cases the diver may complain of marked chest pain, dyspnea, and dysphagia. Syncope may occur. Radiographs may show extraalveolar air in the neck, mediastinum, or both, although radiographs are rarely necessary to make the diagnosis.

Treatment of mediastinal emphysema and most other forms of the POPS is conservative, consisting of rest, avoidance of further pressure exposure (including flying in commercial aircraft), and observation. Supplemental oxygen administration may be useful in severe cases. Recompression is indicated only in extraordinarily severe cases, since it carries a risk of causing further barotrauma and worsening the situation.

Pneumothorax. Pneumothorax is an infrequent manifestation of diving-related pulmonary overpressurization, since this requires that air be vented through the visceral pleura, a path generally having greater resistance than air tracking through the interstitium. Despite being infrequent, pneumothorax must be considered and excluded whenever the POPS is suspected.

In cases of diving-related pneumothorax the diver usually complains of pleuritic chest pain, breathlessness, and dyspnea, just as in cases of pneumothorax from another cause. Radiographs may confirm the diagnosis. It is treated in the standard fashion with tube thoracostomy in all but trivial cases.

A diver with an untreated pneumothorax should not be recompressed except in dire circumstances, and then only if tube thoracostomy will be completed before decompression begins. Since the intrapleural gas of a pneumothorax cannot be vented to the environment, it may convert to a lethal tension pneumothorax during depressurization from hyperbaric treatment.

ARTERIAL GAS EMBOLISM

Arterial gas embolism (AGE)—also known as dysbaric air embolism and cerebral air embolism—is the most feared complication of POPS. AGE is one of the most dramatic and serious injuries associated with compressed air diving and is a major cause of death and disability among sport divers.[69]

AGE results from air bubbles entering the pulmonary venous circulation from ruptured alveolae. When air is introduced into the pulmonary capillary blood, gas bubbles are showered into the left atrium, to the left ventricle, and subsequently into the aorta, where bubbles may enter the coronary arteries and produce myocardial infarction or cardiac arrest secondary to vessel occlusion.[16] Gas embolization to the coronary arteries also may induce arrhythmias, which may be exacerbated or independently generated by cerebral air embolism.[47,62]

Most of the bubbles entering the aorta pass into the systemic circulation, lodging in small arteries and occluding the more distal circulation. Bubbles most often pass up the carotid arteries to embolize the brain. They may also embolize the vertebral arteries, causing sudden cardiopulmonary arrest from brainstem ischemia.

Depending on the site or sites of circulatory occlusion, AGE produces myriad and often disastrous consequences. The neurologic pattern may be confusing, as showers of bubbles randomly embolize the brain's circulation, producing ischemia and infarction of diverse brain regions. Combined carotid and vertebral artery embolization may produce severe diffuse brain injury (Color Plate 109).[69]

Arterial gas embolism typically develops immediately after the diver surfaces, at which time the high intrapulmonic pressure resulting from lung overpressurization is relieved, allowing bubble-laden pulmonary venous blood to return to the heart and pass into the systemic circulation. *It is axiomatic that symptoms of AGE develop within 10 minutes of surfacing from a dive,* although most often they are clearly evident within the first 2 minutes. *Sudden loss of consciousness upon surfacing from a dive should be considered to represent air embolism until proven otherwise.*

In a pulmonary overpressure accident, as soon as normal breathing resumes at the surface of the water, the pressure differential that drives air bubbles into the pulmonary capillaries is equalized. From this point on, usually no further intraarterial air is introduced.

Clinical manifestations of cerebral air embolism are sudden, dramatic, and often life threatening. Probably many diver deaths officially listed as drownings are actually cases of cerebral air embolism in which the diver has been suddenly incapacitated (by a seizure or loss of consciousness) while in the water, leading to secondary drowning. Unfortunately, the accident investigation and postmortem evaluation of many diving accident victims are insufficient to establish the precise cause of death.

Neurologic manifestations of AGE are typical of an acute stroke, although hemiplegia and other purely unilateral brain syndromes are infrequent. Most often observed are loss of consciousness, monoplegia or asymmetric multiplegia, focal paralysis, paresthesias or other sensory disturbances, convulsions, aphasia, confusion, blindness or visual field defects, vertigo, dizziness, or headache (Table 47-2).[37,47,84]

The physical findings of AGE are extremely variable and depend on the specific site or sites of vascular occlusion. Neurologic findings generally dominate the clinical picture because of the frequency of cerebral involvement. All patients with suspected AGE should be carefully examined for neurologic deficits. Specific manifestations of POPS (such as subcutaneous or mediastinal emphysema) may or may not be present but should always be carefully sought.

Rarely it is possible to visualize air bubbles in the retinal arteries or see sharply circumscribed areas of glossal pallor

Table 47-2 Pulmonary Overpressure Accident: Typical Symptoms and Signs

Condition	Symptoms	Signs
Arterial gas embolism	Seizure (focal or general), unconsciousness, confusion, headache, visual disturbances, bloody sputum	Hemiplegia, monoplegia, altered level of consciousness, blindness, visual motor deficit, focal motor or sensory losses
Mediastinal-subcutaneous emphysema	Substernal pain, "brassy voice," neck swelling, dyspnea, bloody sputum	Subcutaneous crepitus, gas patterns on radiograph of mediastinum and neck
Pneumothorax	Chest pain, dyspnea, bloody sputum	Loss of breath sounds, hyperresonant chest percussion, tracheal shift

(Liebermeister's sign), but these findings cannot be relied on to make the diagnosis. The diagnosis is clinical and based on the diving history and symptoms.

Management of Arterial Gas Embolism

All cases of suspected arterial gas embolism must be referred for recompression treatment (hyperbaric oxygen therapy) as rapidly as possible. This is the primary and essential treatment for the condition.[39]

Before recompression, whether in the field, emergency department, or clinic or during transport to a recompression chamber, the affected diver should be given supplemental oxygen at a high flow rate, with other necessary supportive measures as indicated by the specific clinical condition.

Historically, much attention was directed toward keeping the AGE patient in the Trendelenburg position in the field. This was based on anecdotal reports and limited experimental data.[71] The rationale for keeping the patient with AGE head down was the belief that the weight of the column of blood would force bubbles through the cerebral capillary bed, that the buoyancy of the bubbles would keep them in the aorta or heart, and that the weight of the spinal fluid might compress bubbles in the cord. These benefits have never been well demonstrated. A recent study showed that the Trendelenburg position did not keep bubbles from being distributed to the systemic circulation.[13] Likewise, it is more difficult to oxygenate persons in a head-down position, and if one is maintained in this position for longer than 30 to 60 minutes, it may cause or worsen cerebral edema. Therefore, in contrast to prior recommendations, *it is now recommended that both in the field and during transport the patient with AGE be maintained in the supine position.*

Because the AGE event is so often acutely enacted in the water, the victim frequently suffers concomitant near drowning. Thus the rescuer must be prepared to provide cardiopulmonary resuscitation and to protect the airway from the aspiration of gastric contents secondary to vomiting.

While life support measures are being instituted, a member of the diving or rescue team should telephone the nearest civilian or military recompression chamber and contact an air ambulance if air evacuation is required. Aircraft selection is crucial because the stricken diver *should not be exposed to significant cabin altitude.* Ideally the diver should be transported by aircraft pressurized to sea level so that existing intraarterial bubbles do not expand further. In the case of helicopter evacuation or in the event that an unpressurized aircraft is required, the flight altitude must be maintained as low as possible, not to exceed 1000 feet above sea level.

An intravenous infusion of isotonic solution should be started and urine output maintained at 1 to 2 ml/kg/hr.[24] It is important to maintain adequate intravascular volume, since inert gas cannot be effectively eliminated from tissues or from intravascular bubbles at the arteriolar-capillary level unless adequate capillary perfusion is maintained.

The AGE-affected diver should be transported to the recompression chamber as quickly as possible. Delay prolongs cerebral ischemia and cellular hypoxia, resulting in significant cerebral edema, which typically leads to a more difficult course of therapy. Conversely, transport should still be undertaken even if delay is unavoidable. Remarkable improvement has been seen in cases in which treatment was delayed for more than 24 hours after the onset of neurologic manifestations.[66]

If the AGE-stricken diver is first seen at a hospital emergency department or clinic, and if transport to a hyperbaric treatment facility will not be delayed, baseline laboratory, radiographic, and other diagnostic tests (such as electrocardiography) should be obtained before the patient is sent to the chamber. Computed tomography or magnetic resonance imaging of the brain should be deferred until after initial hyperbaric treatment unless intracranial hemorrhage or other injury is thought more likely than AGE.

Hyperbaric treatment consists of rapidly increasing ambient pressure (recompression) to reduce intravascular bubble volume and to restore tissue perfusion, using oxygen-enriched breathing mixtures to enhance bubble resolution and to supply oxygen to ischemic and hypoxic nervous tissue, and providing slow decompression to avoid the reformation of bubbles.

Specific details about the hyperbaric regimens employed for treating AGE are beyond the scope of this discussion, especially with regard to whether these patients should be treated only in multiplace hyperbaric chambers (Fig. 47-6) capable of being pressurized to 6 ATA and in which both air and oxygen can be administered to the patient.* The minutiae of compression chamber treatment are well described in standard diving medicine references.†

Hyperbaric chamber treatment of air embolism should be performed only by specially trained diving medicine physicians or in their absence by trained divers skilled in hyperbaric chamber treatment and having physician consultation.

Although the majority of patients with AGE have neurologic deficits when examined, the initial manifestations may spontaneously resolve by the time the patient is seen. Occasionally a patient has symptoms but no reproducible neurologic deficits on physical examination.[69,72] Nonetheless, all patients must be referred for diving medicine consultation and hyperbaric treatment if the history is suggestive of AGE, since neurologic impairment is impossible to exclude in the acute care setting and waiting to complete definitive diagnostic studies may allow subtle neurologic injuries to become irreversible.[87]

*References 12, 55, 68, 72-74, 87.

†References 24-26, 28, 29, 42, 43.

Prevention of Pulmonary Overpressure Accidents

In view of the potentially catastrophic consequences of POPS, one of the key goals of scuba diving training is to prevent pulmonary overpressure accidents. Divers must be warned of the potentially great intrathoracic volume changes that can occur at shallow depths, as well as be trained to keep an open airway during ascent, particularly through the last 10 feet to the surface. If equipment malfunction or depletion of air supply at depth makes this impossible, the diver must make every attempt to exhale continuously during an "emergency swimming ascent." This is an attempt to vent the increasing volume of air in the lungs. With a satisfactory air supply the diver should simply breathe normally on ascent to the surface, taking care to ascend slowly near the surface.

INDIRECT EFFECTS OF PRESSURE

Several diving-related problems may develop as a result of breathing gases at higher than normal atmospheric pressure. Chief among these are nitrogen narcosis, oxygen toxicity, and decompression sickness.

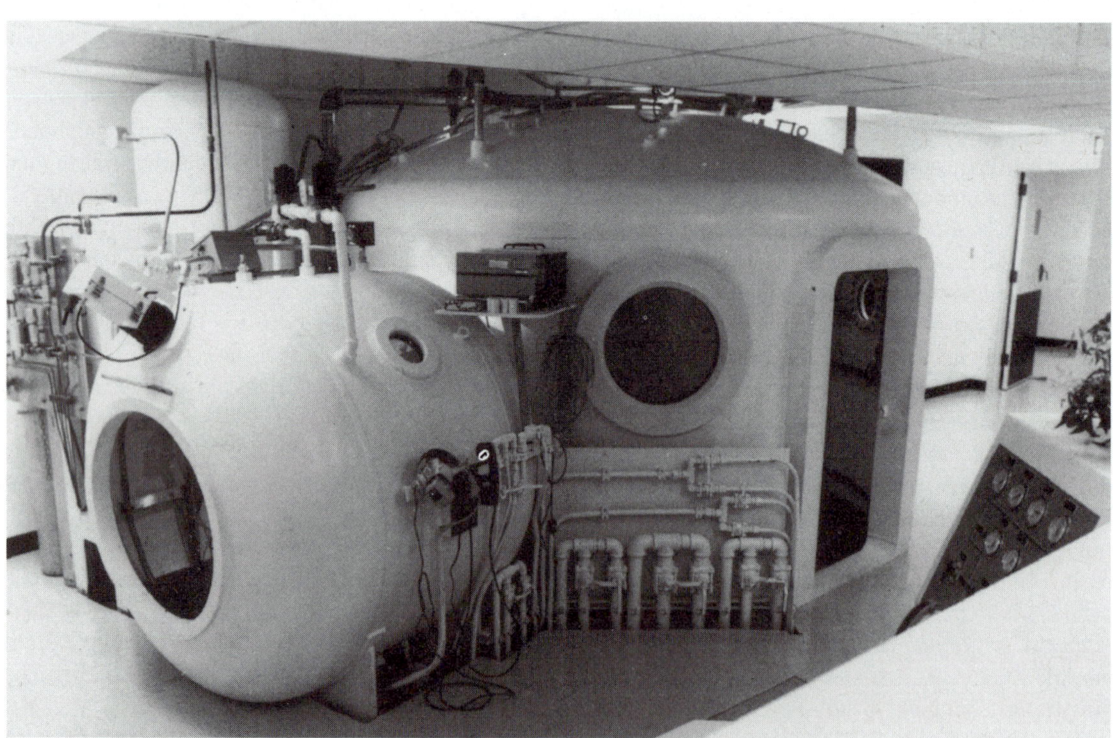

Fig. 47-6 Preferably, a hyperbaric chamber for treating decompression sickness or arterial gas embolism should have a pressure capability of at least 6 ATA (165 FSW). It should have space for an attendant to provide ongoing care and repeated neurologic examinations. It must have provisions for supplying 100% oxygen and other gases for treatment of the stricken diver.

Dalton's Law of Partial Pressures

Dalton's Law of Partial Pressures states that the total pressure exerted by a mixture of gases is the sum of the pressures that would be exerted by each of the gases if it alone occupied the total volume. The partial pressure of a gas in a mixture is the pressure exerted by that gas alone. The symbols for partial pressure of oxygen, nitrogen, carbon dioxide, and water vapor are PO_2, PN_2, PCO_2, and PH_2O, respectively. Dalton's Law states that in an air mixture the total pressure $(P_T) = PN_2 + PO_2 + PH_2O + P_{other}$. The partial pressure of each gas in the mixture is found by multiplying the percentage of that gas present by the total pressure. In Fig. 47-7, a mixture of air with nitrogen is assumed to be present in a proportion of 78%, oxygen 21%, carbon dioxide 0.03%, and the balance composed of water vapor and other trace gases.

The partial pressures of inspired gases in a gas mixture, not their percentages, are of prime importance in diving. For example, it has been shown that in hyperbaric chamber treatment of decompression sickness, 100% oxygen can be safely used at depth to 60 FSW (2.8 ATA) for 20-minute periods with the subject at rest in the dry chamber. On the other hand, even with 20% oxygen in a helium-oxygen mixture at 600 FSW (20 ATA), the diver would breathe 0.21 × 20 or 4.2 ATA of oxygen, which would rapidly produce central nervous system oxygen poisoning. This type of problem is avoided in deep diving by reducing the oxygen percentage in the gas mixture to maintain a PO_2 of 0.35 to 0.50 ATA of oxygen (266 to 380 mm Hg).

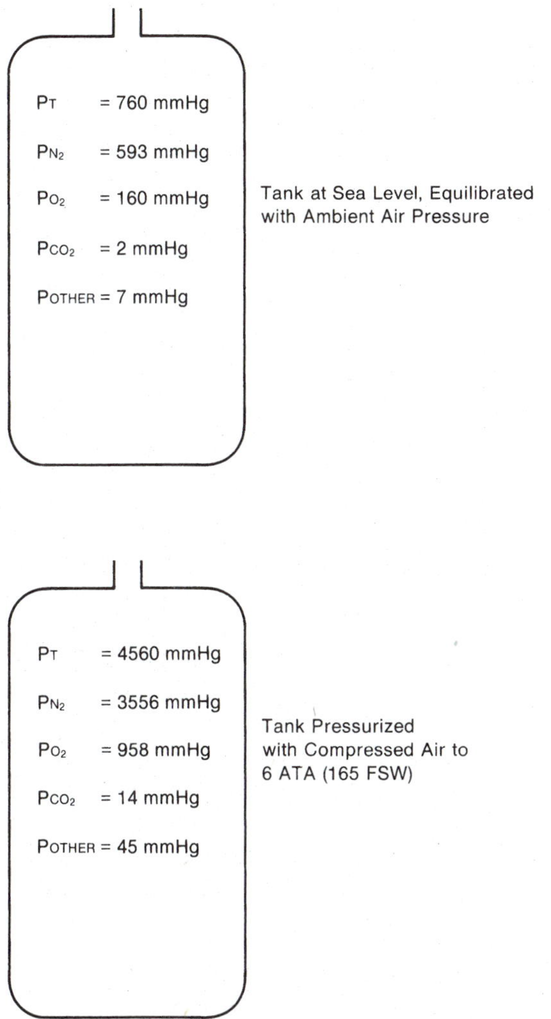

Fig. 47-7 Dalton's Law of Partial Pressures. The total pressure exerted by a mixture of gases is the sum of the pressures that would be expected by each of the gases if it alone were present and occupied the total volume.

The scuba diver who uses open-circuit compressed air is subject to the effects of the component gases in the air according to their partial pressures. Thus, even though the gas mixture is simply air with normal percentages of oxygen and nitrogen, the increases in partial pressures of these gases, along with multiplication of trace contaminants at sea level, create numerous potential problems. Most notable among these for scuba divers is the problem of nitrogen narcosis.

Nitrogen Narcosis

Nitrogen narcosis, also known as rapture of the deep, inert gas narcosis, or "the narcs," is the increasing development of anesthesia or intoxication as the partial pressure of nitrogen in inspired compressed air increases at depth. Nitrogen narcosis is important to divers because it causes anesthetic-like euphoria, overconfidence, and deterioration in judgment and cognition, all of which can lead to serious errors in diving techniques, accidents, and drowning. Many divers have died directly or indirectly as a result of nitrogen narcosis.

During the 1930s, Behnke and associates[5,6] first suggested that the mood changes described by divers breathing compressed air at 200 FSW were caused by high inspired PN_2. Much has been learned since that time, and a complete compilation of data on inert gas narcosis has been provided by Bennett.[8-10] The subject has been more recently reviewed by Hamilton and Kizer.[54]

Theories to explain the mechanism by which nitrogen causes its intoxicating effects center on the effects of gaseous anesthetics in general.[83,89] According to currently accepted theory, an alteration in electrical properties of cellular membranes is effected by absorption of gas molecules into their lipid component. Supporting this theory is the observation that the greater the lipid solubility of a given gas, the greater its narcotic potency. Thus higher partial pressures of pure nitrogen are required to produce an anesthetic effect than can be achieved by a much lower partial pressure of nitrous oxide, which is much more soluble in lipid than is nitrogen. Helium's lack of narcotic effect is in accord with its low lipid solubility. Indeed, substitution of helium for nitrogen as the inert gas in the diver's breathing gas prevents nitrogen narcosis and is the main reason helium-oxygen mixtures are used for deep diving.

Typically a scuba diver breathing compressed air develops symptoms of nitrogen narcosis at depths between 70 and 100 feet. These symptoms include lightheadedness, loss of fine sensory discrimination, giddiness, and euphoria. Symptoms progressively worsen at deeper depths. At depths over 150 FSW the diver becomes severely intoxicated, manifesting increasingly poor judgment and impaired reasoning, overconfidence, and slowed reflexes. At depths of 250 to 300 FSW, auditory and visual hallucinations may occur, along with feelings of impending blackout. Most divers lose consciousness by a depth of 400 FSW.

Of note, both individual and diurnal variability occurs in the depth of onset of symptoms, as well as in the severity of symptoms, in nitrogen narcosis. Also, some degree of acclimatization allows experienced divers to work more safely at greater depths than can inexperienced divers. Nonetheless, nitrogen narcosis is a major problem for all compressed air divers at depths greater than 100 FSW. This is one of the factors that has led to the recommendation that sport divers not dive deeper than 100 FSW.

Treatment of nitrogen narcosis requires ascent to a shallower depth (usually less than 70 to 100 FSW), where symptoms promptly clear. Of course, the condition can be prevented by avoiding deep dives. In commercial diving, where there may be reason to dive deeper than 100 FSW, the problem is prevented by substituting helium-oxygen for compressed air.

Oxygen Toxicity

While oxygen is essential for most life-forms on earth, it becomes a poison at elevated partial pressures, so oxygen toxicity is another indirect effect of pressure that divers need to understand. Oxygen toxicity in divers can affect either the central nervous or the pulmonary system.

High inspired Po_2 can occur in diving in two ways. Breathing 100% oxygen in underwater or hyperbaric chambers is one. The second results from Dalton's Law of Partial Pressures. If a normal 21% oxygen-gas mixture is breathed at 300 FSW (10 ATA), an inspired Po_2 of 2.1 ATA is generated, equivalent to breathing 100% oxygen at 36 FSW. Again, it is the partial pressure of a gas that determines its biologic effects.

Pulmonary Oxygen Toxicity. Retrolental fibroplasia in premature infants and pulmonary oxygen toxicity in adults are well-known problems associated with the use of therapeutic oxygen. Pulmonary oxygen toxicity is induced by breathing a relatively low Po_2 for prolonged periods. It is generally considered that the limit for indefinite exposure without demonstrable lung damage is a Po_2 of about 0.5 ATA, and that on a time-dose curve it is safe to breathe 100% oxygen at 1 ATA for up to about 20 hours or at 2 ATA for up to 6 hours. This time can be lengthened significantly by using intermittent exposures, such as interspersing a 5-minute air break between every 20 minutes of oxygen breathing.[56] At 2.8 to 3 ATA (60 to 66 FSW), where 100% oxygen is used to treat decompression sickness and gas gangrene, pulmonary oxygen toxicity is rarely a problem because central nervous system manifestations usually intervene before sufficient time elapses to induce pulmonary damage. A complete review of this subject has been provided by Clark and Lambertsen.[19] Use of hyperbaric oxygen according to U.S. Navy Treatment Table 6 (as is used in treating decompression sickness) does not produce clinical manifestations of pulmonary oxygen toxicity. However, animal studies with more extreme oxygen exposures have shown a pathologic sequence of alveolar capillary endothelial damage, with increased permeability leading to pulmonary edema and hemorrhage. While species variation in susceptibility occurs, interruption of exposure usually results in reversal of these pathologic changes.[19]

The most common clinical manifestation of pulmonary oxygen toxicity is substernal discomfort on inhalation. If exposure continues, this can progress to severe burning substernal pain and persistent coughing. Reduction of inspired oxygen partial pressure to 0.21 to 0.5 ATA usually results in prompt relief. Severe cases of pulmonary oxygen toxicity may require endotracheal intubation and positive end-expiratory pressure (PEEP) ventilation to achieve adequate arterial oxygenation at the required lower partial pressures of inspired oxygen.

Central Nervous System Oxygen Toxicity. During the 1880s the French physiologist Paul Bert described convulsions in animals breathing 100% oxygen at elevated chamber pressures. This work was confirmed by Behnke and others in human studies during the 1930s. The classic human observations on divers by Donald[37,38] in 1947 provided much of the current knowledge on predisposing factors and clinical manifestations of central nervous system oxygen toxicity. He found that, at a given duration and pressure of oxygen, a diver in the water was more susceptible than the same diver in a warm, dry hyperbaric chamber. This observation called for the limit of 25 FSW for special operations dives while breathing 100% oxygen from closed-circuit oxygen diving rigs. Most people can tolerate breathing 100% oxygen for 30 minutes at rest at 2.8 ATA in a dry chamber, although some manifest toxicity even at this exposure. Common symptoms and signs of central nervous system oxygen poisoning are shown in Box 47-3. Unfortunately, some persons may have no early warning symptoms, and the first manifestation of central nervous system oxygen toxicity may be a grand mal seizure.

Treatment for central nervous system oxygen toxicity in a hyperbaric chamber involves removal of the oxygen mask, maintenance of the airway, and keeping the patient from injuring himself or herself. Chamber pressure should be kept constant until the seizure activity ceases to avoid a pulmonary overpressure accident.

After a postictal period the patient recovers without sequelae. Recurrent seizures are rare. Although anticonvulsants used in seizure treatment theoretically should suppress oxygen-induced seizures, none has been tested to determine doses needed to produce this result. Anticonvulsant drug therapy is not usually necessary because termination of oxy-

BOX 47-3

TYPICAL MANIFESTATIONS OF CENTRAL NERVOUS SYSTEM OXYGEN POISONING

Apprehension
Feeling of air hunger
Sweating
Nausea
Focal muscle twitching
Isolated jerking of a limb
Auditory changes (such as "bells ringing")
Tunnel vision
Diaphragmatic flutter
Convulsion

gen breathing routinely stops the seizure activity. Removing oxygen at the first sign of central nervous system toxicity (for example, feelings of apprehension, sweating, nausea, twitching) has to date prevented any documented permanent central nervous system damage after an oxygen-induced seizure.

Contaminated Breathing Gas

As breathing gas cylinders are pressurized or filled, the sea level partial pressure of each gaseous component is multiplied. Thus any contaminant in the air source can become dangerous to the diver. Compressor motors must be free of oil that could be pumped into tanks; otherwise, the diver may suffer lipoid pneumonitis.[70]

The siting of compressed air inlets to avoid engine exhaust from the compressor, parking lots, or other sources of carbon monoxide is crucial. Engine exhaust contamination of the air supply can produce carbon monoxide poisoning. Since carbon monoxide is colorless, odorless, and tasteless, the diver cannot detect it unless it is accompanied by other contaminants.

The first warning of carbon monoxide poisoning may be headache, nausea, or dizziness during the dive. Examination at the surface may show lethargy, mental dullness, and nonspecific neurologic deficits, which may be confused with those accompanying decompression sickness or air embolism. The cherry-red skin color often mentioned in standard medical texts is actually rarely observed in carbon monoxide poisoning. Fortunately, the treatment of choice for serious carbon monoxide poisoning, decompression sickness, and air embolism is hyperbaric oxygen.

Carbon Dioxide

Another potential breathing gas problem involves carbon dioxide. Alveolar partial pressure of carbon dioxide (P_{ACO_2}) reflects arterial P_{CO_2}; hence even as ambient pressure increases at depth, P_{ACO_2} remains constant at about 40 mm Hg unless environmental or physiologic changes occur. Hypercapnia can occur because of increased P_{CO_2} in the breathing gas or decreased pulmonary ventilation. Unless there is regulator malfunction or contaminated breathing gas, hypercapnia is exceptionally rare in open-circuit scuba diving. Hypercapnia can occur in helmet or chamber diving if these closed spaces are inadequately ventilated or breathing gas becomes contaminated by carbon dioxide, and in close-circuit scuba diving if there is failure of the CO_2-absorbent (scrubbing) material.

At sea level, 5% to 6% inspired CO_2 leads to dyspnea, increased respiratory rate, and mental confusion. At 10% inspired CO_2, a drop in pulse rate and blood pressure with unconsciousness may occur. At 12% to 14% inspired CO_2, death by central respiratory and cardiac depression occurs with prolonged exposure, as P_{aCO_2} exceeds 150 mm Hg.[44] Again, in diving with compressed gas breathing, contaminants are magnified. For example, 3% CO_2 in breathing gas at sea level is equivalent to 12% CO_2 at 99 FSW or 4 ATA. It is also important to remember that elevation of P_{aCO_2} causes vasodilation with potentially increased susceptibility to nitrogen narcosis, oxygen toxicity, and possibly decompression sickness.

Hyperventilation. Hypocapnia can result from hyperventilation during diving. The well-known symptoms of hyperventilation—dizziness and paresthesias—have been postulated to cause unconsciousness among divers, but whether this actually occurs is unclear. In contrast, unconsciousness associated with hyperventilation before a breath-hold dive is caused by hypoxia, rather than hypocapnia.

In what is commonly described as shallow water blackout, a diver hyperventilates before a dive, driving alveolar P_{CO_2} down to 20 to 30 mm Hg. However, because hemoglobin is nearly saturated with oxygen during normal respiration, there is little gain in arterial P_{O_2}. In an underwater swim, even in a shallow swimming pool, exercise-induced hypoxia of a degree sufficient to cause unconsciousness may occur before arterial P_{CO_2} reaccumulates to provide a stimulus to breathe.

In a deep breath-hold dive the problem is compounded when hyperventilation precedes the dive. Besides the initial depression of arterial P_{CO_2} secondary to hyperventilation, elevations in alveolar and arterial P_{O_2} are noted. During the dive these serve to suppress the respiratory response to hypercarbia. During descent in the water, P_{aCO_2} increases from compression, but after oxygen consumption at depth, decompression on return to the surface causes a dramatic drop in alveolar and arterial P_{CO_2}. Even if P_{aCO_2} rises to the stimulatory breakpoint during ascent, hypoxemia may cause unconsciousness and near drowning. An expansion of Edmonds' "Commonest Causes of Unconsciousness in Divers" is presented in Box 47-4.[42]

DECOMPRESSION SICKNESS

In the mid-nineteenth century, tunnel and bridge workers who labored in caissons pressurized with compressed air

BOX 47-4

CAUSES OF UNCONSCIOUSNESS IN DIVERS

BREATH-HOLD DIVING

Underwater hypoxemia after hyperventilation before the dive ("shallow-water blackout")
Near drowning

COMPRESSED GAS EQUIPMENT

Hypoxic breathing gas
Contaminated breathing gas (such as carbon monoxide)
Equipment failure or exhaustion of breathing gas
Near drowning
Inert gas narcosis
Oxygen poisoning
Pulmonary overpressure accident with arterial gas embolism

REBREATHING EQUIPMENT

Carbon dioxide toxicity
Oxygen poisoning

were sometimes observed to suffer joint pains, paralysis, and various other medical problems after decompression. The condition was not understood and was dubbed caisson disease or compressed air illness. Of course, these early high-pressure workers were experiencing the same symptoms that were later observed in divers and aviators, and that we now know to be decompression sickness (DCS).

For many decades "caisson disease" remained a medical curiosity, but because of its occurrence in increasingly important areas of activity in the twentieth century, considerable research has been directed toward its causes and treatment.

Today, we know that DCS is caused by the formation of bubbles of inert gas (such as nitrogen) within the intravascular and extravascular spaces after a reduction in ambient pressure. This may occur during or after decompression after being underwater or in a caisson or hyperbaric chamber in which pressures are greater than at sea level, as well as in aviators, astronauts, or hypobaric (high-altitude) chamber workers who travel rapidly from sea level to pressures less than 0.5 ATA. While DCS is a major concern in commercial divers who breathe helium-oxygen mixtures for deep work, this discussion concentrates on compressed air diving situations likely to be encountered by sport divers.

Etiology

To understand the etiology of DCS, readers must understand the temporal uptake and elimination of inert gases supplied in the diver's breathing medium. Clearly, if it were possible for a diver to breathe 100% oxygen while underwater, there would be no problems with decompression, since oxygen is rapidly metabolized by the body and for practical purposes does not contribute to bubble formation on ascent from depth. Unfortunately, pure oxygen breathing at increased atmospheric pressure causes central nervous system toxicity and is thus never used in sport diving. The need for an inert gas diluent (nitrogen) in the diver's breathing medium is the crux of the problem in DCS.

As alveolar air pressure increases at depth, partial pressures of inspired gases increase. At 99 FSW (4 ATA), the absolute pressure is 3040 mm Hg (Table 47-1). Seventy-nine percent of this pressure is nitrogen (2400 mm Hg, as compared with 600 mm Hg P_{N_2} at sea level). Accounting for water vapor and carbon dioxide, this results in an alveolar partial pressure of nitrogen (P_{AN_2}) of about 2360 mm Hg. This P_{AN_2} is rapidly reflected across the alveolar-capillary membrane to the arterial blood, where according to Henry's Law nitrogen becomes physically dissolved in the blood. Henry's Law states that the amount of gas dissolved in a liquid at any given temperature is a function of the partial pressure of the gas in contact with the liquid and the solubility coefficient of the gas in that particular liquid. As this nitrogen-laden blood is presented to tissues at the capillary level, a complex set of variables dictated by perfusion, diffusion, and inert gas solubility results in a family of nitrogen uptake curves similar to the pharmacokinetic drug uptake curves commonly displayed for medications. Thus, tissue nitrogen saturations on any given dive are a function of depth (that is, pressure) and time.

Clinical Manifestations

DCS is a multisystem disorder caused by a rapid decrease in ambient atmospheric pressure such that inert gas comes out of solution, causing the formation of bubbles in tissue and venous blood. Conceptually, DCS is the same illness whether it occurs in high-altitude aviators or deep-sea divers, although there may be some differences in the specific clinical manifestations of the disease depending on whether it is caused by hyperbaric or hypobaric exposure.

The physiologic sequelae of bubble formation in tissue and venous blood are myriad. These effects include cellular distention and rupture; mechanical stretching of tendons or ligaments, producing pain; and intravascular or intralymphatic occlusion, resulting in congestive ischemia and infarction or lymphedema.

Intravascular bubbles also cause multiple biophysical effects at the blood-bubble surface interface. In brief, bubbles are viewed by the immune system as foreign matter and incite an inflammatory reaction. The key step in the process is activation of Hageman factor, which in turn activates the intrinsic clotting, kinin, and complement systems, producing platelet activation, cellular clumping, lipid embolization, increased vascular permeability, interstitial edema, and microvascular sludging. The overall effect is decreased tissue perfusion and ischemia.

As with arterial gas embolism, the diagnosis of DCS is a clinical diagnosis based on the history of diving with compressed air and subsequent development of characteristic symptoms and signs. The majority of patients with DCS become symptomatic in the first hour after surfacing from a dive, with most of the rest noticing symptoms within 6 hours after diving. One percent to 2% of patients with DCS may not note their symptoms until 24 to 48 hours after diving.

The clinical manifestations of DCS are protean (Table 47-3), with the neurologic and musculoskeletal systems most often affected. Symptoms of DCS are often categorized into types I and II, type I referring to the mild forms of DCS (cutaneous, lymphatic, and musculoskeletal) and type II including the neurologic and other serious forms. Although this categorization of DCS is firmly entrenched in the literature, its use is not advocated. It is clinically more meaningful to refer to the body systems affected when discussing patients with DCS, especially in light of the growing awareness that all DCS must be considered serious and treated vigorously.

Musculoskeletal Decompression Sickness or "Limb Bends." Periarticular joint pain is the most common symptom of DCS, occurring in about 70% of patients. This form of DCS is often referred to as limb bends, joint bends, or pain only bends.

The term "bends" originated at the turn of the century with caisson workers on the Brooklyn Bridge. Workers suffering from DCS of the hips were noted to walk stiffly, bending forward at the hips. Co-workers would describe the stricken men as walking as if they were trying to do the "Grecian bend," a forward bending, stiff-at-the-hips way that stylish women of the day would walk because of their tight corsets. Over time the term became shortened to just "bends."

The shoulders and elbows are the joints most often affected by DCS in scuba divers, but any joint may be involved. The pain may radiate to surrounding areas. It is usually described as a dull ache deep within the joint but may also be characterized as sharp or throbbing. It is sometimes described as feeling like tendinitis or bursitis. Movement of the joint worsens the pain. A vague area of numbness or dysesthesia may surround the affected joint, but this typically does not conform to any anatomic distribution and should not be confused with neurologic involvement. Palpable tenderness may be present.

Sometimes the differential diagnosis between limb bends and trauma may be assisted by inflation to 150 to 250 mm Hg of a sphygmomanometer cuff placed around the joint. By reducing the gas volume in tendons and ligaments, this may immediately relieve the pain directly under the cuff if it is caused by DCS. This relief suggests that the mechanism of pain is gas expansion (that is, bubbles) in tendons and ligaments that stretches nerve endings. The pain of limb bends recurs when the cuff is deflated. The test is helpful when it is positive. Failure to respond to the application of local pressure, however, should not be used to rule out the presence of DCS; this must be done with a "test of pressure" in a hyperbaric chamber.[95]

Limb bends pain itself is not threatening to life or function but indicates that bubbling may be occurring in venous blood. Often, patients who begin with musculoskeletal DCS and are left untreated progress to more serious forms of DCS.

Table 47-3 Common Signs and Symptoms of Decompression Sickness

Condition	Symptoms	Signs
Limb bends	Awareness of severe tendinitis-quality joint pain, single or multiple joints involved, paresthesias or dysesthesias about joint, lymphedema (uncommon), grating sensation on joint motion	Presence of tenderness, which may be temporarily relieved by local pressure with blood pressure cuff
Neurologic decompression sickness		
Spinal cord	Back pain, girdling abdominal pain, extremity heaviness or weakness, paresthesias of extremities, fecal incontinence, urine retention, paralysis	Hyperesthesia or hypoesthesia, paresis, anal sphincter weakness, loss of bulbocavernosus reflex, urinary bladder distention
Brain	Scotomata, headache, dysphasia, confusion	Visual field deficit, spotty motor or sensory deficits, disorientation or mental dullness
Fatigue	Profound generalized heaviness or fatigue	May precede signs of other forms
Cutaneous manifestations	Intense pruritus	No visible signs, mottling, local or generalized hyperemia or marbled skin
Chokes	Dyspnea, substernal pain that is worse on deep inhalation, nonproductive cough	Cyanosis, tachypnea, tachycardia
Vasomotor decompression sickness	Weakness, sweating, unconsciousness	Hypotension, tachycardia, pallor, mottling, hemoconcentration, decreased urine output

Fatigue. Profound fatigue that is out of proportion to the activity performed may be an early manifestation of decompression sickness. While its etiology is unknown, a feeling of severe fatigue after diving demands careful evaluation for other manifestations of DCS.

Skin Bends or Cutaneous Decompression Sickness. DCS may present a variety of cutaneous manifestations, including scarlatiniform, erysipeloid, or mottled rashes, pruritus, and formication. Localized swelling or peau d'orange may result from lymphatic obstruction.

Skin manifestations are relatively uncommon and in and of themselves are usually not serious. However, they are often a harbinger of more severe DCS. Mottling or marbling of the skin (cutis marmorata) is considered especially important, since it often heralds the delayed onset of neurologic problems. The exact physiologic basis of the mottled skin lesion is unknown.

Itches, "the creeps," or "skin bends," a pruritic skin reaction, is seen during decompression in hyperbaric chamber workers when the skin is exposed to the high partial pressure of nitrogen in compressed air. The concentrations of dissolved gases in ocean water are essentially constant at all depths, so that the skin is not exposed to elevated partial pressures of inert gases under water. In contrast, in chambers, inert gas from the external environment is absorbed directly into skin, and the itches represents bubble formation in the skin during decompression.

Chokes or Pulmonary Decompression Sickness. The "chokes" is a serious form of decompression sickness characterized by burning substernal pain, cyanosis, dyspnea, and nonproductive cough. Animal studies have demonstrated gas bubbles or foam in the pulmonary arteries, right atrium, and right ventricle after unsafe decompression. Chokes probably represents massive pulmonary gas embolism with mechanical obstruction of the pulmonary vascular bed by bubbles. Typically, symptoms of pulmonary venous air embolization begin when 10% or more of the pulmonary vascular bed is obstructed. Patients with chokes can progress rapidly to profound shock or neurologic decompression sickness. The specific clinical and radiologic manifestations of the chokes are similar to those seen with venous gas embolism (VGE) from other causes.[65]

Symptoms of VGE include air hunger, dyspnea, cough, and chest pain. Findings may include tachypnea, tachycardia, hypotension, cyanosis, expiratory wheezing, neurologic signs, and a "mill wheel" heart murmur. Victims may also exhibit increased central venous or pulmonary artery pressure, electrocardiographic changes of ischemia or cor pulmonale, decreased end-tidal carbon dioxide fraction, and precordial Doppler sounds of circulating gas bubbles. Visualization of air in the main pulmonary artery is pathognomonic of pulmonary air embolism.[59,65]

Neurologic Decompression Sickness. Neurologic impairment may occur as the sole manifestation of DCS or as part of a progressive dysbaric syndrome. Neurologic DCS is manifested by a myriad of symptoms and signs because of the random nature by which DCS affects the nervous system. While any level of the central nervous system may be affected, the most commonly involved site in divers is the spinal cord, specifically in the lower thoracic and lumbar regions.

Based on military experience, neurologic DCS was believed to occur in only 10% to 20% of DCS cases,[93] but neurologic manifestations of DCS have been found in 50% to 60% of scuba-diving casualties treated in Hawaii[46,61] and have been reported in alarmingly high frequencies in other populations of sport divers.[24,35]

Classically, dysbaric spinal cord injury occurs in the lower thoracic, lumbar, and sacral portions of the cord, producing low back pain, subjective "heaviness" in the legs, paraplegia or paraparesis, lower extremity paresthesias, and possible bladder or anal sphincter dysfunction. Absence of the bulbocavernosus reflex, elicited by gently squeezing and pulling the glans penis to seek reflex contraction of the anal sphincter, often foretells a poor prognosis, as does absence of the superficial anal reflex, which can be elicited in the male or female by stroking the perianal region. Involvement of the cervical and thoracic cord may cause chest or abdominal pain, as well as weakness or sensory disturbances in the upper extremities. The mechanism of spinal cord DCS is considered to be inert gas formation in the epivertebral venous system (Batson's plexus) with resulting congestive infarction of the spinal cord.[53]

DCS of the brain produces a variety of symptoms, most of which are indistinguishable from AGE. Involvement of the cerebellum or inner ear may produce a condition known as the staggers because of the resultant ataxia.

Vasomotor Decompression Sickness ("Decompression Shock"). This is an extremely rare, life-threatening form of DCS. The pathogenesis of this shock syndrome is not completely understood, but it is believed to be caused by a rapid shift of fluid from intravascular to extravascular spaces secondary to diffuse bubble embolization, ischemia, and hypoxia.[18] Hypotension may also result from massive venous air embolization of the lungs.

Despite adequate intravenous fluid replacement, the hypotension of decompression shock may not respond until recompression is undertaken. Unfortunately, the condition is highly lethal, and many patients do not survive to undergo recompression unless a hyperbaric chamber is immediately available.

Long-Term Sequelae of Decompression Sickness

Dysbaric Osteonecrosis. Dysbaric osteonecrosis (DON) is a form of avascular or aseptic necrosis of bone associated with pressure changes. The major joints are most often affected, but essentially any bone can be involved.

DON was first recognized in compressed air workers in

the early 1900s.[88] Since then, its incidence in professional divers has been found to range from less than 1% to over 80%, depending on the age of the divers and the type of diving done.* Its occurrence correlates well with deep diving, decompression diving, the occurrence of decompression sickness, and missed decompression. Most diving medicine experts consider DON a long-term sequela of inadequate decompression. Interestingly, fossil evidence of avascular necrosis has been found in some species of marine mosasaurs of the Cretaceous period, suggesting that at least some of these extinct giant marine lizards dived deeply.[94]

Dysbaric Retinopathy. Infrequently, DCS affects the eyes, producing a wide array of acute ophthalmic effects, including homonymous hemianopsia, cortical blindness, central retinal artery occlusion, retinal hemorrhage, nystagmus, convergence insufficiency, and optic neuropathy.[14,15] Recently, some long-term ophthalmic findings in divers have been observed.

A retinal fluorescein angiography survey of asymptomatic divers found a higher incidence of retinal pigment epithelium than in nondivers, as well as various capillary changes at the fovea.[92] The significance of these abnormalities is unclear, since none of the divers had visual loss. Similarly, the cause of such changes is unclear, although they are postulated to be the result of small bubble microembolization.

Diagnosis of Decompression Sickness

A variety of laboratory abnormalities may be demonstrated in DCS, but most have little or no usefulness in the immediate management of patients. Two tests that may be useful, however, are the urine specific gravity and the hematocrit, since intravascular volume depletion and hemoconcentration are common in serious DCS. These tests can help guide replacement fluid therapy. Hematocrit percentages are commonly in the high 50s or 60s in serious DCS.

As with laboratory tests, radiographic evaluation of patients with suspected DCS may yield various findings, but these are rarely useful in acute management of the patient. Bone radiographs of patients with acute joint bends do not show abnormalities. Months to years later, they may demonstrate findings of DON. Noncardiogenic pulmonary edema may be seen on chest radiographs of persons with pulmonary or vasomotor DCS.

Both computed tomography (CT) and magnetic resonance (MR) imaging have been used to evaluate neurologic DCS injury, although conventional CT suffers from poor sensitivity of early lesions and its inability to image spinal cord lesions.[57,64] Limited clinical data support the feasibility and efficacy of MR imaging of these conditions,[75,100] especially when intracranial injury is suspected, although the exigency of obtaining recompression treatment makes these modalities useful primarily in the postrecompression evaluation of residual deficits.

*References 17, 33, 45, 60, 82, 88, 99.

Treatment of Decompression Sickness

All patients with suspected DCS must be referred to a hyperbaric treatment facility as quickly as possible, since recompression is the primary and essential treatment for this condition. The physician must have a high index of suspicion for the often diverse and confusing clinical manifestations of DCS. The history of the dive profile is helpful if the diver knowingly violated decompression procedures, but as already discussed, DCS may occur on dives that should be safe according to current decompression schedules. Likewise, the reported depth and time of the dive may be erroneous for a number of reasons.

Management of DCS must be commenced as soon as the condition is suspected.[24] Sport divers are usually far from a recompression chamber when their symptoms develop, so treatment is often initiated in the field or at an outpatient acute care facility. One hundred percent oxygen should be administered by a tight oronasal mask to provide a favorable gradient for nitrogen washout. Of equal importance is maintenance of intravascular volume to ensure capillary perfusion for elimination of microvascular inert gas bubbles and for tissue oxygenation. An intravenous infusion of isotonic solution should be started and run at a flow rate sufficient to maintain urine output at 1 to 2 ml/kg/hr. With spinal cord involvement an indwelling urinary catheter may be needed because of sacral nerve root dysfunction. Intractable vomiting or vertigo should be treated with appropriate parenteral agents. Diazepam has been quite effective in providing relief from the vertigo associated with labyrinthine decompression sickness when other agents have failed. Oral aspirin (5 to 10 grains) also may be useful for its antiplatelet activity. Of course, advanced life support measures should be undertaken appropriate to the patient's clinical condition.

While these measures are undertaken, someone should arrange for emergency transportation to the nearest recompression chamber. Because of the large number and frequently changing status of recompression chambers, no list is provided here. Instead, the reader is referred to the national Divers Alert Network (DAN) at Duke University (Fig. 47-8). Help with the treatment of dive-related incidents may be obtained 24 hours a day by calling 919-684-8111 and requesting DAN. This telephone number should be readily available to all divers and medical facilities. DAN's diving medicine experts provide help with diagnosis and immediate care of the patient and provide information about the location of the nearest hyperbaric chamber.

Before a patient is transferred to the hyperbaric treatment facility, it is imperative to contact the chamber to determine its availability. The physician should never send a

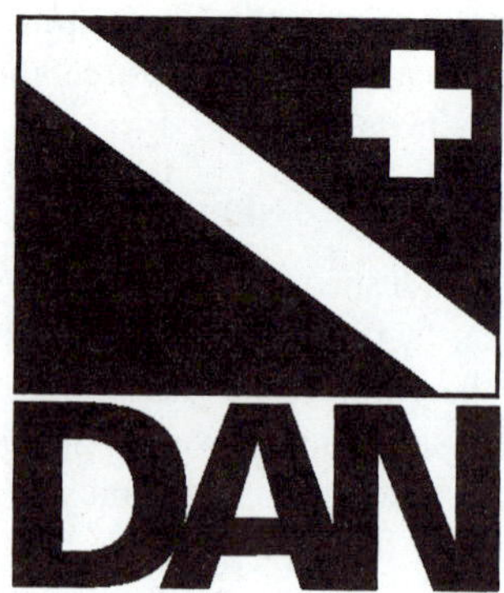

Fig. 47-8 Logo for Divers Alert Network. (Courtesy Divers Alert Network.)

patient without first discussing the transfer with the hyperbaric treatment personnel.

If airborne evacuation is required, it is critical to obtain an aircraft that can maintain sea level cabin pressurization during flight. Examples of such aircraft are the C-130 Hercules, Learjet, and Cessna Citation. If the patient is to be moved by helicopter, the crew must maintain the lowest possible flight altitude, but never greater than 1000 feet above the starting elevation. All resuscitative measures must be maintained in flight.

At the recompression chamber, one of several standard hyperbaric treatment protocols is followed. In a double-lock compressed air chamber, the patient and an attendant can be pressurized with compressed air and the patient given 100% oxygen by mask.

As with AGE, hyperbaric treatment of decompression sickness has undergone significant evolution during the past two decades and is not discussed in detail here. It is most often successful, but the likelihood of success is difficult to predict for any given diver. In one series of 92 sport scuba divers treated after a significant delay between the offending dive and the start of recompression treatment, 85% had good results when standard U.S. Navy treatment tables were followed.[24] Similar results were achieved in another series of 50 patients.[66] Such treatment is usually given according to U.S. Navy Tables 5 and 6 (Fig. 47-9). Any patient with neurologic or pulmonary DCS requires treatment with at least the protocol in Table 6 (Fig. 47-9, *B*), with extension of the hyperbaric oxygen periods depending on how the patient responds.

U.S. Navy Treatment Table 7 is an option for serious DCS cases; however, this treatment table should be reserved for patients with major deficits because of its length and commitment of resources. The diver and attendant are held at 2.8 ATA for at least 12 hours, and longer if needed, with the patient breathing oxygen in 30-minute periods as tolerated. A final slow 32-hour decompression follows, regardless of the time spent at 2.8 ATA. Details of Table 7 are found in the current edition of the *U.S. Navy Diving Manual*.[34]

Another potentially useful recommendation for dealing with the recurrence of neurologic symptoms and signs after apparently successful chamber treatment of neurologic DCS has been advanced by Edmonds.[43] Frequent postrecompression recurrence of neurologic manifestations led him to institute multiple 30-minute sea level oxygen breathing periods with 30-minute air breaks for 6 to 8 hours during posttreatment hospital observation, rechecking vital capacity frequently to prevent pulmonary oxygen toxicity.

While experimental proof of their efficacy is lacking, high-dose parenteral corticosteroids have been widely recommended and used in the past as an adjunct to recompression treatment of both neurologic DCS and arterial gas embolism. Rapid-acting hydrocortisone hemisuccinate (1000 mg) or methylprednisolone sodium succinate (125 mg) followed by dexamethasone 4 to 6 mg every 6 hours, with continuation of the dexamethasone for 72 hours, has been the standard regimen.

The use of steroids became prevalent based on the belief that they were beneficial in the treatment of cerebral edema, shock, and other conditions pertinent to DCS, although their benefit in many of these conditions is uncertain. Anecdotal data suggesting that steroids were beneficial, in combination with hyperbaric oxygen treatment, have been reported,[65,72] but there have been no published clinical series or controlled trials demonstrating their efficacy. In contrast, recent controlled studies of high-dose parenteral dexamethasone and methylprednisolone in DCS-affected dogs showed that the use of glucocorticoids as an adjunct to conventional hyperbaric oxygen therapy produced no benefit, and even suggested that the steroid-treated animals did less well.[50] Thus the benefit and role of steroids in the treatment of DCS are a matter of controversy at this time.

Because the outcome of recompression treatment is influenced by the time lapse from onset of symptoms to the start of treatment, every emergency department and every diver should know the location of the nearest recompression chamber. Spinal cord decompression sickness treated after a few hours of delay may result in residual deficits ranging from mild weakness or sensory changes to permanent paraplegia or worse. On the other hand, dramatic improvements have been witnessed even in persons arriving at a chamber many days after the insult.[66]

Prevention of Decompression Sickness

Decompression Tables. Navies and commercial diving companies around the world have developed various decompression schedules based on calculations and actual testing (animal and human) that allow divers to avoid exceeding safe rates of decompression after specified depth-time dive profiles. These listings of "safe" depth-time diving profiles are generally referred to as decompression tables. Many different sets of decompression tables exist, with the U.S. Navy Standard Air Decompression Tables being the most widely used.[34] Decompression tables continue to be

A 1. Treatment of type 1 decompression sickness when symptoms are relieved within 10 minutes at 60 feet and a complete neurologic exam is normal.

2. Descent rate — 25 ft/min.

3. Ascent rate — 1 ft/min. Do not compensate for slower ascent rates. Compensate for faster rates by halting the ascent.

4. Time at 60 feet begins on arrival at 60 feet.

5. If oxygen breathing must be interrupted, allow 15 minutes after the reaction has entirely subsided and resume schedule at point of interruption.

6. If oxygen breathing must be interrupted at 60 feet, switch to profile in part B of figure on arrival at the 30-foot stop.

7. Tender breathes air throughout unless he has had a hyperbaric exposure within the past 12 hours, in which case he breathes oxygen at 30 feet.

Depth (feet)	Time (min)	Breathing media	Total Elapsed Time (hr:min)
60	20	Oxygen	0:20
60	5	Air	0:25
60	20	Oxygen	0:45
60 to 30	30	Oxygen	1:15
30	5	Air	1:20
30	20	Oxygen	1:40
30	5	Air	1:45
30 to 0	30	Oxygen	2:15

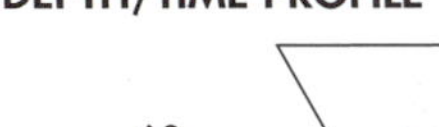

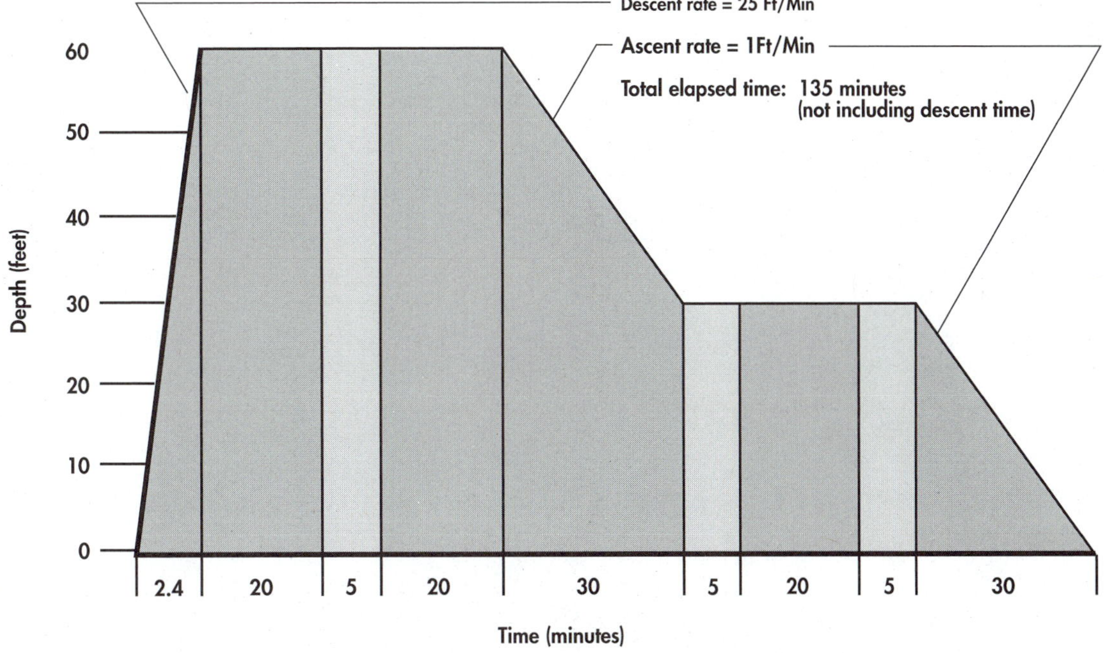

Fig. 47-9 U.S. Navy decompression tables. Dark shading represents air breathing; light shading represents oxygen breathing. **A,** Table 5. Oxygen treatment of type 1 decompression sickness.

the subject of considerable scientific controversy, however, resulting in periodic revision and continual search for improved safety.

Over the years the U.S. Navy decompression tables have been the ones most often used in recreational diving. Various rearrangements or modifications of these tables have been promulgated by sport diving groups in recent years in efforts to improve the safety of recreational diving, which is qualitatively different from military diving (for which the Navy decompression tables were developed). In general, these sport diving modifications have involved applying various safety factors to the standard Navy protocols.

Recent "multilevel" dive tables also have been developed to address the depth fluctuations that typically occur in

B 1. Treatment of type II or type I decompression sickness when symptoms are not relieved within 10 minutes at 60 feet.

2. Descent rate — 25 ft/min.

3. Ascent rate — 1 ft/min. Do not compensate for slower ascent rates. Compensate for faster rates by halting the ascent.

4. Time at 60 feet begins on arrival at 60 feet.

5. If oxygen breathing must be interrupted, allow 15 minutes after the reaction has entirely subsided and resume schedule at point of interruption.

6. Tender breathes air throughout unless the tender has had a hyperbaric exposure within the past 12 hours, in which case oxygen is breathed at 30 feet.

7. Profile can be lengthened up to two additional 25-minute periods at 60 feet (20 minutes on oxygen and 5 minutes on air), or up to two additional 75-minute periods at 30 feet (15 minutes on air and 60 minutes on oxygen), or both. If profile is extended only once at either 60 or 30 feet, the tender breathes oxygen during the ascent from 30 feet to the surface. If more than one extension is done, the tender begins oxygen breathing for the last hour at 30 feet during ascent to the surface.

Depth (feet)	Time (min)	Breathing media	Total Elapsed Time (hr:min)
60	20	Oxygen	0:20
60	5	Air	0:25
60	20	Oxygen	0:45
60	5	Air	0:50
60	20	Oxygen	1:10
60	5	Air	1:15
60 to 30	30	Oxygen	1:45
30	15	Air	2:00
30	60	Oxygen	3:00
30	15	Air	3:15
30	60	Oxygen	4:15
30 to 0	30	Oxygen	4:45

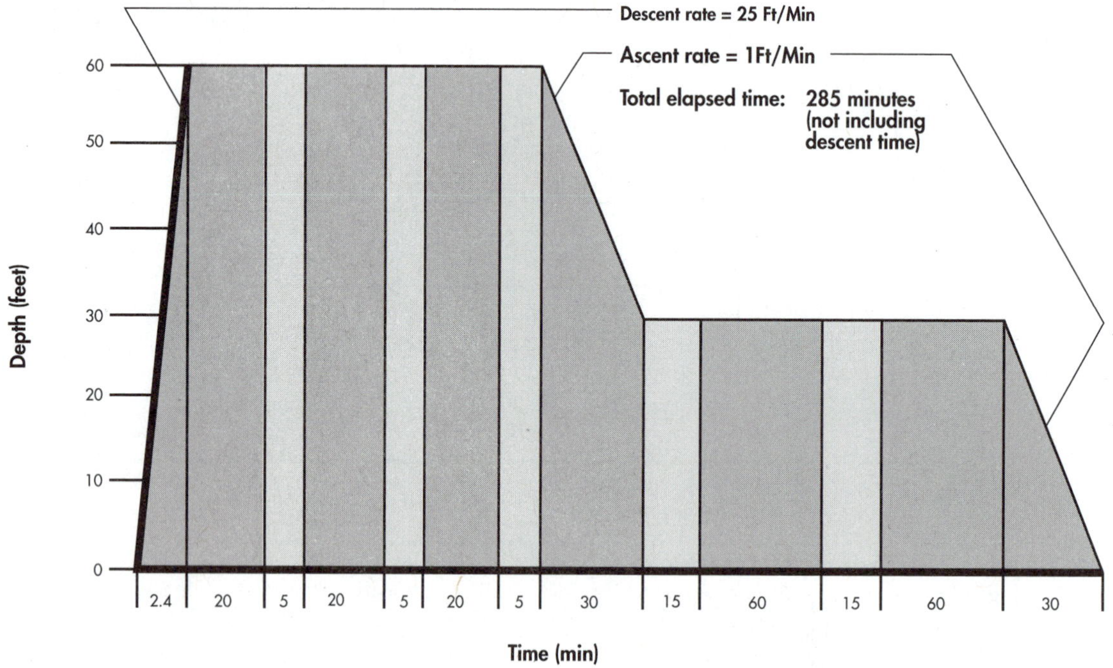

Fig. 47-9, cont'd B, Table 6. Oxygen treatment of type 2 decompression sickness. (Modified from Department of the Navy: *U.S. Navy diving manual,* vol 1, rev 2, Flagstaff, Ariz, 1988, Best Publishing Company.)

sport diving as the diver ranges from shallow to deep repetitively during the course of a dive. These multilevel tables give the diver decompression "credit" for the time spent at shallower depths, as opposed to the Standard U.S. Navy Tables, which require the diver to use the maximum depth of the dive to select no-decompression limits or decompression schedules and repetitive dive group designations. The reason for doing this has been the belief that the U.S. Navy tables are too restrictive and excessively limit the diver's time underwater. Multilevel tables allow a diver to spend more time underwater, although there continues to be concern that they provide less safety margin.

Dive Computers. Automatic decompression meters that measure and record time and pressure under water give the diver an indication of decompression status.[97] These "dive computers" track the exact dive profile and then calculate a decompression requirement according to the actual dive profile. The devices have used different physiologic and decompression models and technologies. Early automated decompression meters presented problems because their use was associated with an unacceptable rate of decompression sickness. Recent technologic innovations, however, have overcome many of the earlier difficulties.[58,76] The sport scuba diver now has access to a variety of devices that offer the convenience of automatic and accurate depth-time recording, together with accurately computed multilevel decompression schedules.

Modern dive computers typically use microprocessors with decompression tables stored in memory. The microprocessor in the dive computer quickly reads a pressure transducer (which converts pressure into electrical impulses) and applies nitrogen uptake and elimination algorithms to this information every few seconds. The computer tracks a diver's exact profile and calculates decompression requirements accordingly.

Use of dive computers has become common, although concerns about their safety remain. Clearly, these computers are accurate depth-time recorders and are convenient because they obviate the clerical aspect of diving (that is, the need to write down the depth and time of all dives, consult the decompression tables, calculate and record residual nitrogen time and surface intervals, and so on). Dive computers also offer advantages for some types of diving over use of the Standard U.S. Navy Decompression Tables. They are especially useful in multilevel diving because they give bottom time credit for time spent under water at depths shallower than the deepest depth attained. However, it must be remembered that dive computers calculate decompression status based on models designed to simulate nitrogen uptake and release in a diver's body. These models may or may not accurately predict gas flow into and out of a given diver's tissues. Human physiology is not always as predictable as the computer model, and many factors can influence the actual rate of inert gas uptake and elimination. Also, most computers have no built-in safety margin to compensate for the difference between predicted and actual gas uptake and elimination, in contrast to decompression tables, which usually contain an inherent safety margin and require "rounding up" intermediate depths and times, providing a further safety factor.

Because of the multiple-tissue compartment modeling that dive computers use, another concern with their use is that they integrate the entire depth-time profile, so that in cases of repetitive diving (multiple dives per day or multiple successive days of diving), dive computers would be more liberal than the Navy tables, allowing more time under water and potentially allowing a gradual unsafe accumulation of nitrogen in slow tissues. In such settings the risk of developing decompression sickness may be greater.

A number of other concerns are attendant to the use of dive computers, including their allowance of multiple "reverse profile" dives (shallow then deep dives—an inherently risky way to dive); the risk of equipment failure (such as battery failure or flooding of the battery compartment); loss of information by inadvertently turning off the computer; or failure to turn on the computer at the beginning of a dive. In the last three scenarios the safety of the dives done after the one in which the problem occurred would be jeopardized.

Despite the widespread use of dive computers in recent years, it is not possible at this time to say whether they are more or less safe than the U.S. Navy Standard Decompression Tables *when the tables are actually followed.* That substantial numbers of divers treated for decompression sickness in recent years (more than half of persons tested at some recompression chambers) were using dive computers underscores that they do not inherently protect a diver from getting the bends.[80,81,106] Based on experience, dive computers appear relatively safe *when used as directed.*

Safe Scuba Diving

Sport scuba divers are fortunate that the most colorful marine life and abundant natural light exist at shallow depths. This obviates the need to dive deep. Indeed, 100 FSW should be considered a deep dive for sport diving and, for all intents and purposes, the maximum depth for recreational diving.

Recreational diving is usually done hours to days away from the nearest recompression chamber, so the occurrence of decompression sickness or arterial gas embolism usually necessitates a major effort to evacuate an afflicted diver to the chamber. This often requires the use of special aircraft. Unfortunately, the delay between symptom onset and treatment may allow the damage to become fixed and poorly responsive to hyperbaric treatment. Therefore divers should do their best to avoid developing decompression sickness.

The need to take a conservative approach to depth and time is even clearer when one considers that individual variability in DCS susceptibility, workload during the dive, water temperature, and ill-advised postdive exercise or altitude exposure may confound any set of decompression tables or dive computers. Indeed, the potentially devastating consequences of DCS, even with the most vigorous hyperbaric treatment, mandate that divers always dive with the prevention of this disease foremost in their minds.

In this vein the following safe diving recommendations should be adhered to by recreational or sport divers:

1. Dive within the limits of "no-decompression" ("no-D") tables. When a decompression computer is used, do not approach the limits of no-decompression diving.

2. When using the decompression tables, always use the next greater depth to determine the "no-D" limits, then "jump" tables. For example, a dive with maximum depth of 68 feet is considered a 70-foot dive and the "no-decompression limit" should be determined for the next jump or, in this case, that of an 80-foot dive for 40 minutes. Ascent toward the surface at a rate no faster than 1 foot per second should begin at the end of the prescribed limit (40 minutes in this example) regardless of how much time was actually spent at shallower depths. This "penalty" for dive time spent at shallower depth is an important safety factor.
3. After any dive deeper than 60 FSW, and at the conclusion of all repetitive dives, make at least a 3- to 5-minute safety stop at 10 to 15 FSW.
4. When using the decompression tables, use the surface-to-surface time or "total time of dive" in selecting the repetitive group designation.
5. Carefully plan any repetitive dive so that it will be shallower than the previous dive and so that you stay well within "no-decompression" limits.
6. Remember that any device or table that allows prolonged time at shallow depths after a deeper excursion also allows continued uptake of inert gas.
7. Maintain hydration during diving days to ensure normal capillary perfusion for inert gas exchange. Remember that immersion diuresis and topside sweat loss in tropical regions can result in significant dehydration, which is often not overtly apparent. Keep the urine "clear and copious" on diving days.
8. Do not engage in heavy exercise, such as jogging or wind surfing, for at least 6 hours after a dive.
9. Do not fly, even in the pressurized cabin of commercial airlines, for at least 12 hours after "no-decompression" diving. If decompression stops were required, wait at least 24 hours before flying. If aircraft cabin altitude (for example, an unpressurized airplane) will exceed 8000 feet, wait 24 hours before flying after any compressed gas dive.
10. Diving in mountain lakes requires significant adjustments in decompression tables to account for the decreased atmospheric pressure at the surface of the lake. Dive computers must be calibrated for altitude. Boni and associates[11] pointed out that for the same depth and the same bottom time of a dive, surfacing at a lower ambient air pressure than sea level necessitates longer decompression times. Several decompression tables for altitude diving have been calculated and tested in the field.[7,22,86] The U.S. Navy Standard Decompression Tables can be used up to an altitude of 2300 feet.

Even when these safe diving practices are followed, unexplained DCS cases sometimes occur. Two mechanisms are postulated to account for these cases. After an otherwise safe dive, one well within the specified decompression procedure, elevated inert gas tensions exist in tissues and venous blood, which carry gas to the lungs for elimination. If all else is normal and conservative depths and times have been followed, the inert gas remains in solution or, at worst, "silent" or asymptomatic volumes of venous gas emboli are returned to the lungs. If a physiologically patent foramen ovale (PFO) allows intermittent retrograde flow from the right to the left atrium, bubbles can become arterial gas emboli. The potential for this type of paradoxical gas embolism to occur has been demonstrated in recent years for both PFO and other types of intracardiac shunts.[85,98,103-105] Whether the presence of a PFO should disqualify someone from diving is currently unclear, since conflicting data have been found as to the association of a PFO and the occurrence of neurologic DCS.[23,85,98]

Another plausible explanation for DCS occurring after safe diving postulates that focal pulmonary barotrauma, or inadvertent breath-holding during decompression, produces local air trapping during ascent and releases "microbubbles" into the systemic circulation. These microscopic "seed" bubbles in arterialized blood then pass through the capillary bed to become bubble nuclei in venous blood, precipitating overt bubble formation and the classic manifestations of DCS.

Dive Accident Investigation

When investigating a dive accident, whether for treatment purposes or as part of a forensic evaluation in the case of a fatal accident, the investigator begins by taking a detailed dive accident history. A number of specific details must be determined about the patient's diving activities, the time of symptom onset, and the nature and progression of the symptoms, in addition to past medical history and other information that should be obtained on any patient.[35] The diving-related history should specifically solicit information in the following areas[67]:

1. The type of dive engaged in and equipment used. Inquire specifically as to whether a decompression computer, a diving watch, and a depth gauge were used. Before referring a patient to a recompression chamber, always make sure the patient was diving with compressed air, and not just snorkeling or free diving.
2. The number, depth, bottom or total dive time, and surface interval or intervals between dives for all dives in the 72 hours preceding symptom onset. This information will be needed by the diving medicine consultant because it allows calculation of any omitted decompression and thus helps decide the likelihood of the patient having DCS or other problems. Unfortunately the diver's interpretation of whether required decompression was omitted cannot be the sole source of data; this is notoriously unreliable. If a decompression computer was used,

it should be checked for information about the need for recompression.

3. Whether in-water decompression was taken and if so how much. This is relevant to the likelihood of the diver having DCS. If a decompression computer was used, the diver should be asked whether the specified decompression profile was followed.
4. Whether in-water recompression with compressed air was attempted after the onset of symptoms. For all practical purposes this should never be done because it almost always leaves the diver in a worse condition than originally and is fraught with other hazards.
5. The site of diving (for example, ocean, lake, or quarry) and the environmental conditions (such as water temperature or presence of current or surge) associated with the dive. These factors enter into the differential diagnosis and may raise the possibility of the symptoms being caused by something other than a bubble-related problem. For example, DCS is more common after diving in cold water, other things being equal, or motion sickness may develop in a diver swimming back to shore on a choppy sea even if there was no problem with seasickness before or during the dive.
6. Primary diving activity (such as spearfishing, underwater photography, or shell collecting). Like knowledge of environmental conditions, this helps in the differential diagnosis. For example, DCS is more likely after an arduous dive.
7. Presence of predisposing factors for DCS. A number of factors have been associated with an increased risk of DCS, including dehydration, vigorous exercise under water, advanced age, obesity, poor physical conditioning, local physical injury, and multiple repetitive dives in unacclimatized individuals.
8. Whether the dive was complicated by running out of air, an untoward marine animal encounter, trauma, or another unexpected event. For example, low back pain suggestive of DCS may be caused by a muscle strain from lifting the scuba tank or climbing into the dive boat, and tingling or numbness in an extremity may be caused by jellyfish envenomation.
9. Whether the patient flew in an airplane, went jogging, or engaged in any other particular activity after diving but before the onset of symptoms. If so, the effect of the activity on the symptoms should be ascertained. Some activities (such as flying in an unpressurized aircraft or vigorously exercising immediately after diving) may precipitate DCS in someone who might otherwise not be affected, or trivial dysbaric symptoms may become severe after similar activities.
10. Time of symptom onset. Symptoms that began soon after getting in the water (for example, nausea from motion sickness), even if they worsen afterward, are not likely to be from DCS.

In fatal diving accidents, information gathered from the diving accident history should be supplemented with an appropriate diving accident autopsy, a thorough evaluation of the diving equipment used, and a detailed environmental history.[31]

Environmental factors, such as weather, currents, wave action, visibility, water temperature, potential for entanglement, and dangerous marine life, must be considered. The diving equipment should be carefully studied for proper function and amount of compressed air in the tanks, and the air should be analyzed for contaminants. The diver's medical and psychologic histories should be sought because they may contain clues to a coincidental medical event that led to the diver's death but was unrelated to the dive. Aside from the obvious psychosocial risk factors such as alcoholism, drug abuse, or propensity to panic, the use of a scuba dive for suicide or homicide must be considered.

Unique aspects of the diving victim autopsy should include a careful search for subcutaneous emphysema or other physical signs of the POPS and a search for signs of marine envenomation. For example, before the surface of the body is washed, it should be examined for evidence of nematocysts from coelenterate stings. In addition, in contrast to the thoracic incision being made first, the calvarium should be opened before other incisions to prevent accidental introduction of air into the intracranial circulation. A finding of gas bubbles in intracranial vessels may result from arterial gas embolism or decompression sickness. Postmortem introduction of gas into the cerebral veins can be avoided if the calvarium is opened under water.[29] Likewise, the initial thoracic incision must be made with care to determine whether pneumothorax is present. A careful search should be made for gas bubbles in the major blood vessels and the heart. The middle ear should be examined for presence of blood, and the tympanic membrane and paranasal sinuses should be examined for evidence of barotrauma.

Meticulous investigation of dive accidents is important to find equipment, procedural, or medical causes that could be useful in improving the safety of diving, as well as to gather information for legal procedures that often follow diving accidents.

Medical Fitness for Diving

Persons who want to take up scuba diving should first be cleared medically. The diving examination should focus on the pulmonary, otolaryngologic, cardiac, neurologic, and integumentary systems, as well as the person's psychologic stability.

Because of the changes in pressure that occur with excursions under water; the physical and sometimes psychologic stress of diving; the potential for nitrogen narcosis, altered sensory stimulation, and other factors to interact with pharmaceuticals; and the inherent nature of being underwater, many medical conditions are contraindications for diving. In general, these can be divided into five categories. People falling into any one of the following categories are at increased risk of a diving-related problem:

1. Persons who are unable to equalize pressure in one or more of the body's airspaces are at increased risk for barotrauma.
2. Persons who have a medical or psychiatric condition that may become manifest under water or at a remote diving site and endanger the diver's life because of the condition itself, because it occurs in the water, or because inadequate medical help is available.
3. Persons who have impaired tissue perfusion or diffusion of inert gases and thus have an increased risk of DCS.
4. Persons who are in poor physical condition and thus at increased risk of DCS or exertion-related medical problems. The factors compromising physical condition may be physiologic or pharmacologic.
5. Women who are pregnant, because the fetus may be at increased risk of dysbaric injury.

In accordance with the likelihood of causing a diving problem, as well as the potential seriousness of the problem, conditions falling into one of the preceding five categories may be absolutely, relatively, or temporarily disqualifying for scuba diving.

Based on the opinion of a multispecialty panel of diving medicine experts,[25] the following conditions are considered to be absolute disqualifications for diving:

1. History of epilepsy or other seizure disorder. Seizures occurring under water essentially always result in a catastrophic outcome. After head injury, diving should not be allowed during the time when the patient is at increased risk of seizures.
2. Insulin-dependent diabetes mellitus. The risk of a hypoglycemic reaction under water is increased by the possible need for sudden bursts of energy expenditure in emergencies. Underwater incapacitation not only endangers the life of the individual but may also cause the death of other persons during rescue attempts. Sport diving sometimes may be allowed for persons with adult-onset diabetes that can be controlled by diet and exercise programs.
3. Symptomatic coronary artery disease. In addition to the need for cardiac reserve in an in-water emergency, carrying tanks, donning equipment, and swimming against current entail significant physical stresses. A history of myocardial infarction is considered a disqualification for sport diving, except in the most unusual case of exceptional rehabilitation after revascularization procedures.
4. Sickle-cell disease or trait. The chances that a sport diver will breathe a hypoxic gas mixture are remote, but it is possible. Other concerns are heavy exertion in cold water or local compromise of microvascular blood flow by bubble evolution during decompression, which could lead to sickling and a vicious cycle of hypoxia with further sickling.
5. Unexplained syncope
6. Inability to equalize pressure in the middle ear by autoinflation. Of note, this may be caused by a correctable problem, such as polyps, allergic rhinitis, nasal septal deviation, or coryza, in which case the diver can be reevaluated after successful treatment.
7. Bullous lung disease. Air-containing pulmonary blebs or cysts can trap air and lead to local pulmonary overpressure accidents during decompression. If a ball-valve or flutter-valve effect allows such a bleb or cyst to equalize with the elevated breathing pressure during compression or descent but blocks the escape of air during decompression, rupture could cause POPS and air embolism.
8. Significant pulmonary obstructive disease
9. Substance abuse
10. Reactive airway disease (asthma). Because of the risk of local air trapping and pulmonary overpressure accidents, persons having asthma should not dive. Although scuba air is generally free of pollens, other stresses in diving (such as cold, heavy exertion, or psychic stress) could precipitate bronchospasm at depth, with resultant local air trapping during ascent. If there is any suggestion of bronchospastic tendencies, pulmonary function studies should be performed. Even minimal air trapping at sea level takes on great significance at depth.
11. Spontaneous pneumothorax. Even without the pressure variations of diving, a history of previous spontaneous pneumothorax carries a high incidence of recurrence, and the candidate must be advised against compressed gas diving. A pneumothorax that occurs while the diver is still at pressure underwater or in a recompression chamber can become a life-threatening tension pneumothorax as the pleural cavity air expands (Boyle's Law) during ascent. Persons who have had traumatic or surgical pneumothorax may be cleared for diving depending on the specific circumstances.
12. Perforation of the tympanic membrane. Until the eardrum is fully healed or successfully repaired and eustachian tube function is good, diving is contraindicated.

The following disorders require special consideration or represent subjects of controversy among diving physicians:

1. Migraine headaches. A migraine after diving could be misinterpreted, causing unnecessary recompression treatment. Scintillating scotomas and other neurologic symptoms associated with migraines may be confused with decompression sickness. Since commercial diving generally requires constant readiness to dive, migraine is often viewed as disqualifying for commercial diving.

2. Middle ear surgery with placement of a prosthesis in the conduction chain. The risk of displacement during pressure change and ear clearing is the determining factor in these cases.
3. History of overpressure accident in previous diving. The circumstances of the offending dive weigh heavily in these cases. For instance, if a diver suffers a "physiologically undeserved" or unexplained episode of POPS (that is, the diver breathes normally to the surface, yet suffers an air embolism), risk of recurrence would be a concern. On the other hand, a diver who suffers a pulmonary overpressure accident that is considered "physiologically deserved" (for example, rapid ascent after inadvertent inflation of a buoyancy compensator) could be considered for a return to diving after full neurologic recovery and with the determination of normal pulmonary function. However, some argue that even this diver is at greater risk because of potential pulmonary scarring and the inability to detect small airway air trapping.
4. Hypertension. The suitability of a hypertensive person for diving is based largely on the therapy required for blood pressure control. Diving has little effect on blood pressure, and when a regimen of weight control, diet, and mild diuretics is successful, diving usually can be allowed. If more potent antihypertensive agents are needed, diving may be contraindicated.
5. Decreased visual acuity. In sport diving, corrective lenses can be mounted in scuba face masks or contact lenses can be worn, so this is no longer as much a concern as in the early days of scuba diving. Soft contact lenses are preferable.

The following disorders are temporary disqualifications for diving:

1. Coryza or bronchitis. These conditions may cause inability to equalize pressure in the ears, sinuses, or lungs because of mucosal edema, mucus plugs, or bronchospasm.
2. Pregnancy. At present, there is near consensus that a woman who is or may be pregnant should suspend compressed air diving until after delivery. Animal studies have produced conflicting results in different species and laboratories, but the possibility of bubble formation in fetal or placental tissues is a concern, even on a dive that is safe for the mother.
3. Abdominal hernias. These present a potential risk of trapping expanding gas in a herniated loop of bowel during ascent. In general diving should be suspended until surgical repair is completed.
4. Physical fitness. Sport scuba diving is deceptively easy until an emergency occurs that requires swimming against a current, rescue of a buddy diver, or other vigorous activity. The diver should be capable of performing strenuous activity before entering the water. Regular swimming or other exercise programs to ensure cardiovascular fitness are encouraged.

Selection and Training of Disabled Divers

Interest is growing in the use of scuba diving in rehabilitation and recreation programs for disabled persons. When used in this context without expectation of unlimited diving certification, scuba diving can open exciting new vistas for some disabled persons. Williamson and co-workers[102] demonstrated significant improvement in self-concept and body image among a group of young people with disabilities ranging from post–head injury brain damage, congenital deafness, blindness, and spinal cord dysfunction to major limb amputations. They were examined according to standard diving medicine practice regarding pulmonary and ear, nose, and throat status and detailed psychologic testing. Motivation proved to be an important predictor of success. The subjects were given extensive scuba diving training with at least one-on-one instructor attention. A case of spinal cord DCS occurring in a person with postpoliomyelitis spinal cord syndrome evoked a strong recommendation for use of conservative no-decompression diving for such patients.

Flying After Diving

Since diving is often done at remote destinations, the question of when it is safe to fly after diving often comes up. Flying too soon after diving can seriously jeopardize decompression safety, leading to development of DCS during or after the flight. The normal commercial aircraft cabin pressure is equivalent to an altitude exposure of 5000 to 8000 feet, which is sufficient pressure reduction to cause dissolved nitrogen to come out of solution and form intravascular bubbles. The Divers Alert Network reports that about 5% to 7% of divers with DCS contacting them in recent years reported flying before the onset of their symptoms. (The actual significance of these statistics is uncertain, since the total number of divers who flew after diving is unknown, but it is estimated to be very large compared with the number who developed DCS.)

With the continued growth of the dive-travel vacation industry, the issue of when it is safe to fly after diving has become even more important. Unfortunately, not enough experimental or detailed experiential data on the subject are available to precisely quantitate the risks or to establish precise surface intervals for various types of diving profiles. However, this matter has been the subject of a number of workshops sponsored by the Undersea and Hyperbaric Medical Society and other concerned groups.

At present the generally accepted *guidelines* for flying after recreational diving are as follows:

1. The minimum surface interval should be 12 hours after the last dive before flying in a commercial jet.
2. Divers who make daily, multiple dives for several days or who make dives that require decompression stops should exercise special caution and wait for an extended surface interval *beyond 12 hours* before

flying in a commercial airliner. (Exactly what this extended surface interval should be is less well quantified, but many authorities suggest 24 hours.) The longer the interval between diving and flying, the less the likelihood of DCS.

Having noted the above, it is important to emphasize that no rule about flying after diving can be guaranteed to prevent DCS. These are guidelines that represent the best estimate of a safe surface interval for the majority of sport scuba divers.

REFERENCES

1. Bachrach AJ: A short history of man in the sea. In Bennett PB, Elliott DH, editors: *The physiology and medicine of diving and compressed air work,* ed 2, Baltimore, 1975, Williams & Wilkins.
2. Bachrach AJ: A short history of man in the sea. In Bennett PB, Elliott DH, editors: *The physiology and medicine of diving,* ed 3, London, 1982, Bailliere-Tindall.
3. Balk M, Goldman JM: Alveolar hemorrhage as a manifestation of pulmonary barotrauma after scuba diving, *Ann Emerg Med* 19:930, 1990.
4. Bayne CG: Breath-hold diving. In Davis JC, editor: *Hyperbaric and undersea medicine,* vol 1, San Antonio, 1981, Medical Seminars Publishing.
5. Behnke AR: The history of diving and work in compressed air. In Davis JC, editor: *Hyperbaric and undersea medicine,* vol 1, San Antonio, 1981, Medical Seminars Publishing.
6. Behnke AR, Thomson RMA, Motley EP: Psychological effects from breathing air at four atmospheres pressure, *Am J Physiol* 112:554, 1935.
7. Bell R, Borgwordt R: The theory of high-altitude corrections to the U.S. Navy Standard Decompression Tables: the cross corrections, *Undersea Biomed Res* 3:1, 1976.
8. Bennett PB: *Psychometric impairment in men breathing oxygen-helium at increased pressures,* Rep No 251, 1965, Medical Research Council, RN Personnel Research Committee, Underwater Physiology Subcommittee.
9. Bennett PB: Inert gas narcosis. In Bennett PB, Elliott DH, editors: *The physiology and medicine of diving,* ed 2, London, 1975, Bailliere-Tindall.
10. Bennett PB: The physiology of nitrogen narcosis and the high pressure nervous syndrome. In Strauss RH, editor: *Diving medicine,* New York, 1976, Grune & Stratton.
11. Boni M et al: Diving at diminished atmospheric pressure: air decompression tables for different altitudes, *Undersea Biomed Res* 3:189, 1976.
12. Bove AA et al: Successful therapy of cerebral air embolism with hyperbaric oxygen at 2.8 ATA, *Undersea Biomed Res* 9:75, 1982.
13. Butler BD et al: Effect of the Trendelenburg position on the distribution of arterial air emboli in dogs, *Ann Thorac Surg* 45:198, 1988.
14. Butler FK: Decompression sickness presenting as optic neuropathy, *Aviat Space Environ Med* 62:346, 1991.
15. Butler FK: Ocular manifestations of decompression sickness. In Gold D, Weinstein T, editors: *The eye in systemic disease,* Philadelphia, 1990, JB Lippincott.
16. Cales RH et al: Cardiac arrest from gas embolism in scuba diving, *Ann Emerg Med* 10:539, 1981.
17. Chryssanthou CP: Dysbaric osteonecrosis, *Clin Orthop* 130:94, 1978.
18. Chryssanthou CP et al: Studies on dysbarism. II. Influences of bradykinin and "bradykinin-antagonists" on decompression sickness in mice, *Aerospace Med* 35:741, 1964.
19. Clark JM, Lambertsen CJ: Pulmonary oxygen toxicity: a review, *Pharmacol Rev* 23:37, 1971.
20. Colebatch HJH, Smith MM, Ng CKY: Increased elastic recoil as a determinant of pulmonary barotrauma in divers, *Respir Physiol* 55:64, 1976.
21. Cramer FS, Heimback RD: Stomach rupture as a result of gastrointestinal barotrauma in a scuba diver, *J Trauma* 22:238, 1982.
22. Cross ER: Technifacts: high altitude decompression, *Skin Diver Magazine,* Nov 1970, p 17.
23. Cross SJ et al: Safety of subaqua diving with a patent foramen ovale, *Br Med J* 304:481, 1992.
24. Davis JC, editor: *Treatment of serious decompression sickness and arterial gas embolism,* Undersea Medical Society Pub No 34, WS (SDS), Bethesda, Md, 1979, The Society.
25. Davis JC: Hyperbaric medicine: critical care aspects. In Shoemaker WC, editor: *Critical care, state of the art,* 1984, Society of Critical Care Medicine.
26. Davis JC: Abnormal pressure. In Cralley LJ, Cralley LV, editors: *Industrial hygiene and toxicology,* ed 2, New York, 1985, Wiley.
27. Davis JC: *Medical examination of sport scuba divers,* San Antonio, 1986, Medical Seminars Publishing.
28. Davis JC, Elliott DH: Treatment of the decompression disorders. In Bennett PB, Elliott DH, editors: *The physiology and medicine of diving,* ed 3, London, 1982, Bailliere-Tindall.
29. Davis JC, Elliott DH: The causes of underwater accidents. In Bennett PB, Elliott DH, editors: *The physiology and medicine of diving,* ed 3, London, 1982, Bailliere-Tindall.
30. Davis JC, Youngblood DH: Definitive treatment of decompression sickness and arterial gas embolism. In Davis JC, editor: *Hyperbaric and undersea medicine,* vol 1, San Antonio, 1981, Medical Seminars Publishing.
31. Davis JH: The autopsy in diving fatalities. In Davis JC, editor: *Hyperbaric and undersea medicine,* vol 1, San Antonio, 1981, Medical Seminars Publishing.
32. Davis RH: *Deep diving and submarine operations,* ed 6, London, 1955, Siebe Gorman.
33. Decompression Sickness Central Registry and Radiological Panel: Aseptic bone necrosis in commercial divers, *Lancet* 2:384, 1969.
34. Department of the Navy: *U.S. Navy diving manual,* vol 1, rev 2, Flagstaff, Ariz, 1988, Best Publishing Company.
35. Dick APK, Massey EW: Neurological presentation of decompression sickness and air embolism in sport divers, *Neurology* 35:667, 1985.
36. Divers Alert Network: *1991 report on diving accidents and fatalities,* Durham, NC, 1993, Divers Alert Network.
37. Donald K: *Oxygen and the diver,* Worcester, UK, 1992, published by Kenneth Donald in conjunction with the Self Publishing Association, Ltd.
38. Donald KW: Oxygen poisoning in man, *Br Med J* 1:667, 1947.
39. Dutka AJ: A review of the pathophysiology and potential application of experimental therapies for cerebral ischemia to the treatment of cerebral gas embolism, *Undersea Biomed Res* 12:403, 1985.
40. Edmonds C et al: *Otological aspects of diving,* Glebe, New South Wales, Australia, 1973, Australasian Medical Publishing.
41. Edmonds C, Freeman P, Tonkin F: Fistula of the round window in diving, *Trans Am Acad Ophthalmol Otolaryngol* 78:444, 1974.
42. Edmonds C, Lowry C, Pennefather J: In *Diving and subaquatic medicine,* Mosman, New South Wales, Australia, 1976, Diving Medical Centre.
43. Edmonds C, Lowry C, Pennefather J: In *Diving and subaquatic medicine,* ed 2, Mosman, New South Wales, Australia, 1981, Diving Medical Centre.
44. Edmonds C, Lowry C, Pennefather J: In *Diving and subaquatic medicine,* ed 2, Mosman, New South Wales, Australia, 1981, Diving Medical Centre.
45. Elliott DH, Harrison JAB: Bone necrosis—an occupational hazard of diving, *J R Navy Med Serv* 56:140, 1970.
46. Erde A, Edmonds C: Decompression sickness: a clinical series, *J Occup Med* 17:324, 1975.

47. Evans DE et al: Cardiovascular effects of cerebral air embolism, *Stroke* 12:338, 1981.
48. Farmer JC: Diving injuries to the inner ear, *Ann Otol Rhinol Laryngol* 86(suppl 36, no 1, pt 3):1, 1977.
49. Farmer JC, Thomas WG: Ear and sinus problems in diving. In Strauss RH, editor: *Diving medicine,* New York, 1976, Grune & Stratton.
50. Francic TJR, Dutka AJ: Methyl prednisone in the treatment of acute spinal cord decompression sickness, *Undersea Biomed Res* 16:165, 1989.
51. Green SM et al: Incidence and severity of middle ear barotrauma in recreational scuba diving, *J Wilderness Med* 4:270, 1993.
52. Grey HV: Cave diving hazards and challenges, *Pressure* 16:5, 1987.
53. Hallenbeck JM: Cinephotomicrography of dog spinal vessels during cord-damaging decompression sickness, *Neurology* 26:190, 1976.
54. Hamilton RW, Kizer KW, editors: *Nitrogen narcosis,* Bethesda, Md, 1985, Undersea Medical Society.
55. Hart GB, Strauss MB, Lennon PA: The treatment of decompression sickness and air embolism in a monoplace chamber, *J Hyperbaric Med* 1:1, 1986.
56. Hendricks PL et al: Extension of pulmonary oxygen tolerance in man at 2 ATA by intermittent oxygen exposure, *J Appl Physiol* 42:593, 1977.
57. Hodgson M, Beran RG, Shirtley G: The role of computed tomography in the assessment of neurologic sequelae of decompression sickness, *Arch Neurol* 45:1033, 1988.
58. Huggins KE: Underwater decompression computers: actual vs. ideal. In Lang MA, editor: *Proceedings of the Eighth Annual Scientific Diving Symposium,* Costa Mesa, Calif, 1988, American Academy of Underwater Sciences.
59. Huller T, Buzini Y: Blast injuries of the chest and abdomen, *Arch Surg* 100:24, 1970.
60. Hunter WL et al: Aseptic bone necrosis among U.S. Navy divers: survey of 934 randomly selected personnel, *Undersea Biomed Res* 5:25, 1978.
61. Kizer KW: Dysbarism in paradise, *Hawaii Med J* 39:109, 1980.
62. Kizer KW: Ventricular dysrhythmia associated with serious decompression sickness, *Ann Emerg Med* 9:580, 1980.
63. Kizer KW: Corticosteroids in the treatment of serious decompression sickness, *Ann Emerg Med* 10:485, 1981.
64. Kizer KW: The role of computed tomography in the management of dysbaric diving accidents, *Radiology* 140:705, 1981.
65. Kizer KW, Goodman PG: Radiographic manifestations of venous air embolism, *Radiology* 144:35, 1982.
66. Kizer KW: Delayed treatment of dysbarism—a retrospective review of 50 cases, *JAMA* 247:2555, 1983.
67. Kizer KW: Management of dysbaric diving casualties, *Emerg Med Clin North Am* 1:659, 1983.
68. Kizer KW: Monoplace chamber treatment of dysbaric diving diseases, *J Hyperbaric Med* 1:137, 1986.
69. Kizer KW: Dysbaric cerebral air embolism in Hawaii, *Ann Emerg Med* 16:535, 1987.
70. Kizer KW, Golden JA: Lipoid pneumonitis in a commercial abalone diver, *Undersea Biomed Res* 14:545, 1987.
71. Kruse CA: Air embolism and other skin diving problems, *Northwest Med* 62:525, 1963.
72. Leitch DR, Green RD: Pulmonary barotrauma in divers and the treatment of cerebral arterial gas embolism, *Aviat Space Environ Med* 57:931, 1986.
73. Leitch DR, Greenbaum LJ Jr, Hallenbeck JV: Cerebral arterial air embolism. I. Is there benefit in beginning HBO treatment at 6 bar? *Undersea Biomed Res* 11(3):221, 1984.
74. Leitch DR, Greenbaum LJ, Hallenbeck JM: Cerebral arterial air embolism. III. Cerebral blood flow after decompression from various pressure treatments, *Undersea Biomed Res* 11:249, 1984.
75. Levin HS et al: Neurobehavioral and magnetic resonance imaging findings in two cases of decompression sickness, *Aviat Space Environ Med* 60:1204, 1989.
76. Lippmann J: Dive computers, *SPMMS J* 18:126, 1988.
77. Lundgren CEG, Ornhagen H: Nausea and abdominal discomfort—possible relation to aerophagia during diving: an epidemiologic study, *Undersea Biomed Res* 2:155, 1975.
78. Lundgren CEG, Tjernstrom O, Ornhagen H: Alternobaric vertigo and hearing disturbances in connection with diving: an epidemiologic study, *Undersea Biomed Res* 1:251, 1974.
79. McAniff JJ: *U.S. underwater diving fatality statistics, 1983-1984,* Washington, DC, 1986, US Dept of Commerce, NOAA Undersea Research Program.
80. McGough EK, De Santeles DA, Gallagher TJ: Dive computers and decompression sickness: a review of 83 cases, *J Hyperbaric Med* 5:159, 1990.
81. McGough EK, De Santeles DA, Gallagher TJ: Performance of dive computers during single and repetitive dives: a comparison to the U.S. Navy Diving Tables, *J Hyperbaric Med* 5:163, 1990.
82. Medical Research Council: Decompression sickness and aseptic necrosis of bone, *Br J Industr Med* 28:1, 1971.
83. Meyer HH: Theoris der alkoholnarkose, *Arch Exp Pathol Pharmacol* 42:109, 1899.
84. Miller J: Management of diving accident—author's reply, *Emerg Med* 13:23, 1981.
85. Moon RE, Camporesi EM, Kisslo JA: Patent foramen ovale and decompression sickness in divers, *Lancet* 1:513, 1989.
86. Morris B, McClellan M: *Practical altitude diving procedures,* Incline Village, Nev, 1986, Altitude Concepts.
87. Neuman TS, Hallenbeck JM: Barotraumatic cerebral air embolism and the mental status examination: a report of four cases, *Ann Emerg Med* 16:220, 1987.
88. Ohta Y, Matsunaga H: Bone lesions in divers, *J Bone Joint Surg* 56B:3, 1974.
89. Overton E: *Studien uber die narkose,* Jena, Germany, 1901, Fischer.
90. Paterson M: Underwater archeology. In Idyll CP, editor: *Exploring the ocean world,* New York, 1977, Thomas Y Crowell.
91. Parell GJ, Becker GD: Conservative management of inner ear barotrauma resulting from scuba diving, *Otolaryngol Head Neck Surg* 93:393, 1985.
92. Polkinghorne PJ et al: Ocular fundus lesions in divers, *Lancet* 2:1381, 1988.
93. Rivera JC: Decompression sickness among divers: an analysis of 935 cases, *Milit Med* 129:314, 1964.
94. Rothschild B, Martin LD: Avascular necrosis: occurrence in diving cretaceous mosasaurs, *Science* 236:75, 1991.
95. Rudge FW, Stone JA: The use of the pressure cuff test in the diagnosis of decompression sickness, *Aviat Space Environ Med* 62:266, 1991.
96. Schaefer KE et al: Pulmonary and circulatory adjustments determining the limits of depths in breath-hold diving, *Science* 162:1020, 1968.
97. Stubbs RA, Kidd DJ: Computer analogies for decompression. In Lambertsen CJ, editor: *Proceedings of the Third Underwater Physiology Symposium,* Baltimore, 1967, Williams & Wilkins.
98. Vik A, Jenssen BM, Brubakk AO: Arterial gas bubbles after compression in pigs with patent foramen ovale, *Undersea Hyperbaric Med* 20:121, 1993.
99. Wade CE et al: Incidence of dysbaric osteonecrosis in Hawaii's diving fishermen, *Undersea Biomed Res* 5:137, 1978.
100. Warren LP et al: Neuroimaging of scuba diving injuries to the CNS, *AJR* 142:1003, 1988.
101. Webb P: Thermal problems. In Bennett PB, Elliott DH, editors: *The physiology and medicine of diving,* ed 3, London, 1982, Bailliere-Tindall.

102. Williamson JA et al: Selection and training of disabled persons for scuba-diving, *Med J Aust* 141:414, 1984.
103. Wilmhurst PT, Byrne JC, Webb-Peploc MM: Neurological decompression sickness, *Lancet* 1:731, 1989.
104. Wilmhurst PT, Byrne JC, Webb-Peploc MM: Relation between interatrial shunts and decompression sickness in divers, *Lancet* 2:1302, 1989.
105. Wilmhurst PT, Ellis BG, Jenkins BS: Paradoxical gas embolism in a scuba diver with an atrial septal defect, *Br Med J* 293:1277, 1986.

48 SUBMERSION INCIDENTS

Andrew B. Newman
With Previous Contribution by Ronald D. Stewart, M.D.

A man who is not afraid of the sea will soon be drowned, he said, for he will be going out on a day he shouldn't. But we do be afraid of the sea, and we do only be drowned now and again.

John Millington Synge, *The Aran Islands*

Humans' ancestral home was the water, and we are often drawn back to the aquatic environment. Three fourths of our planet's surface is water, and the earliest records of human perception of life in and under the oceans indicate both fascination and fear. In eighteenth-century Europe, sudden death by drowning sparked the interest of humanitarians caught up by the idea that something could be done to restore life. The incidence of drowning on commercial waterways was probably high, since roads were nearly nonexistent and swimming as recreation was unknown among the general populace. Drowning became a significant public health issue.[8] In response to this fashionable humanitarian cause, the Society for the Recovery of Persons Apparently Drowned was formed in 1774. Their activities included research, public education, and treatment of victims. The organization survives today as the Royal Humane Society.[81] Techniques for resuscitating drowning victims developed after groups with a special interest in the problem of drowning were established. A particularly valuable summary of the approach to the victims of submersion was contained in a book published in 1796, *On the Treatment of Drowning*.[70] This remarkable work describes mouth-to-mouth ventilation and other techniques of resuscitation, among which is a detailed account of tactile endotracheal intubation.[70]

During the past decade, greater understanding of the pathophysiology and natural history of submersion incidents has allowed revised approaches to therapy, confirmed the importance of immediate care to eventual outcome, and permitted the adoption of more optimistic medical attitudes.[132]

Prevention

A study of drowning and near drowning shows that prevention is as important as anything that can be done after the fact. While survival may be serendipitous, premeditated attention to safety is not. No one who is going to be on or near the water should be without superb swimming, rescue, and lifesaving skills, including a working knowledge of cardiopulmonary resuscitation (CPR).

Swimming pools should be completely enclosed by a 5-foot-tall fence with self-closing and self-latching locks above the reach of small children. Lifesaving equipment should be close at hand—every pool should have a life preserver and a long pole for rescue attempts.

Parents should always be present to supervise children when they are in the water. After swimming, children should be dressed in clothing to discourage unsupervised returns to the swimming area. Children in families that have a pool or anticipate water-oriented vacations should have early swimming lessons. People prone to syncope or seizures should always be with someone when in the water. In addition, although alcohol and water mix well in cocktails, in the marine environment even a little alcohol may prove fatal.[65]

Everyone on a boat or raft should have a U.S. Coast Guard–approved life vest or life jacket that will support him or her with the head above water, even if the person becomes unconscious. Travelers on water should be aware of lifeboat and raft availability. Courses on safe boating, rescue, and navigation are offered by the local Coast Guard.

Emergency medical services systems in areas with lake, river, or ocean access should consider adopting a plan for a water rescue unit prepared to respond and deal immediately with accidents. These units include improved boat access and paramedics who are master divers.[186]

Terminology

Thirty years ago in a classic monograph on drowning, David Green succinctly summarized the problem: "Drowning is the process by which air-breathing animals succumb on submersion in a liquid. In the evolutionary process, water living species adapted to terrestrial life, lost their ability to breathe under water, and became susceptible to drowning."[59] Near drowning is a term introduced by Modell to indicate submersion with at least temporary survival.[115] Recent resistance to this terminology has developed because of growing knowledge of the pathophysiology of drowning and the success of many resuscitation efforts.[51,78,176] The terms "drowning" and "near drowning" depend on the ultimate outcome and therefore are of little immediate clinical value. It is often impossible to predict at the scene whether a patient will survive, particularly in light of advances in cerebral protection and resuscitation and the management of hypothermia. Use of these terms may create confusion both in the immediate-care period and ultimately in the medical record. According to a further modification of terms recently introduced,[73,168] a patient who dies within 24 hours is a victim of "drowning," while someone who dies after the first 24 hours is said to have died from "near drowning," although both patients are equally dead.

The whole matter of terminology is complicated further by use of the term "secondary drowning." This refers to the delayed death of a patient who dies of the complications of submersion, such as pulmonary failure.[34,48] This term is of little use and remains ill defined.[151]

A classification has been proposed in which a scoring system based on the organs adversely affected and the patient's physiologic problems more accurately define that patient's condition.[74] This system is cumbersome and has not gained wide acceptance. Most recently it has been proposed that the term "drowned" be used for patients who suffocate from submersion and that "near drowned" be reserved for those who survive, at least temporarily, the submersion episode. The use of a more neutral term without the implication of time, prognosis, or retrospective analysis is necessary to avoid confusion and to simplify classification. Indeed, a person who is adversely affected by being submersed in water has, simply put, suffered a "submersion incident." The term is descriptive, implies no particular prognosis, and can therefore be used in immediate care without the considerations of time or outcome.

Incidence

It is difficult to estimate accurately the total number of submersion incidents, since such accidents are not reportable. Two of the largest and most densely populated countries do not report statistics to the World Health Organization, and very little has been written about the morbidity of persons after submersion.[38] Retrospective studies are beginning to permit quantification of the problem and suggest directions for prevention and management. Drowning is now second only to motor vehicle accidents as the most common cause of accidental death. In states with seat belt laws, drowning has become the leading cause of accidental death in children.[21,20,111] It has been estimated that more than 140,000 deaths occur worldwide annually from drowning.[106,150] Nine thousand deaths occur each year in the United States, out of an estimated 80,000 submersion incidents.[7] These statistics probably underestimate the problem, since many incidents are unreported or classified in other categories, such as motor vehicle accidents, acute illnesses, and suicide.[12] Drowning kills mainly the young; 64% of all victims are less than 30 years of age, and 26% are under the age of 5.[50,135] The incidence of near drowning is thought to be 500 to 600 times the rate of drowning—a tremendous figure, especially given the expense of intensive care in attempting to save these victims.[85] The problem of submersion incidents is magnified in areas with abundant recreational waterways. However, it is in no way limited to these; the home swimming pool, or even the bathtub, can be the site of a lethal event.

Risk Factors

The problem of submersion incidents can often be related to risk factors (Box 48-1) or to certain behaviors or groups. This is particularly true of children.[143] An understanding of these factors can help in planning and instituting preventive measures and practices.

AGE

Age appears to be an indicator of risk. Drowning is a young person's accident. The most important age group is that of the toddler, with children under 1 year of age having the highest drowning rate, followed by that of teenage males.[80] In 1989, 1200 deaths occurred in the 10- to 19-year-old group.[162] In a survey of 9420 primary school children in South Carolina, it was estimated that up to 10% of children under the age of 5 had an experience judged as

BOX 48-1

FACTORS COMMON TO DROWNING INCIDENTS

Age—toddlers, teenage boys
Location—home swimming pools
Gender—males predominate in every age group
Race—black children most at risk
Drugs—particularly alcohol
Trauma—secondary to diving, falls, horseplay

constituting a "serious threat" of near drowning.[168] The highest risk of near drowning incidents is in the age group of 15 to 24 years, and the lowest in persons over the age of 65.[20,19,159]

Toddlers are at risk because of their inquisitive nature and the fact that they are often unsupervised, especially at home. Children frequently drown while bathing with a younger sibling without an adult at hand.[80] The high risk of a submersion incident among teenage boys reflects their mobility, their adventuresome nature, and the absence of adult supervision. The lowest risk of a serious submersion incident in the older age group reflects decreased exposure to water environments, increased experience, and mature judgment.

GENDER

Males predominate among the victims of drowning. In all age groups, males account for more than half the cases, with a male-to-female ratio of 12:1 for boat-related drownings and 5:1 for non-boat-related drownings.[7] For males the peak drowning incidence occurs at age 2 years, decreases until the age of 10, and then rises rapidly to a peak at age 18. The incidence in females peaks at age 1 year, then falls off and does not rise again.[7]

LOCATION

Drowning—that is, death by asphyxia resulting from submersion—is not necessarily a recreational accident. Incidents and deaths occur not only in the backyard swimming pool and in the ocean, but also in such unlikely places as the unsupervised bath and even the lowly cleaning bucket.[82,86,105,145,169] The location of the submersion incident is often determined by the geography and social aspects of the community. In water-oriented areas such as Florida, California, and Australia, submersion incidents are common year round and often occur in home swimming pools. It appears that the great majority of drowning deaths in children under the age of 4 take place at home.[159]

Domestic swimming pools are especially dangerous, particularly for young children. Approximately 300 children drowned in home swimming pools in the United States in 1981, and in 1983 about 2000 children were seen in emergency departments after submersion incidents.[181] Two of three victims of swimming pool drownings were under 3 years of age. While black children tend to drown in lakes, canals, and quarry sites, white children die more frequently in backyard swimming pools.[159] Public or motel pools are not frequently implicated. Despite ordinances defining safe operation of home swimming pools, records indicate that safety features were either faulty or ignored. Although all but 3% of home swimming pools in a Florida community were properly fenced and protected, 70% of the locks were found to be unfastened or nonfunctioning.[159] Worse yet, in a study of 700 pool owners in Florida, more than 40% did not know how to perform CPR.[98] In an Australian study of drowning incidents, only 1 of 66 swimming pool barriers was considered adequate, and in 76% of the incidents there was no fence.[150] The risk of drowning has been shown to be almost four times greater in unfenced pools.[148] The level of water in the pool may be important in the etiology of some deaths. The average distance from the water to the poolside lip is 12 to 14 inches (30 to 35 cm). This distance provides a significant barrier to young children who have fallen into a pool; they may reach the side but be unable to pull themselves out of the water. It has been recommended that the level of water in swimming pools be raised.[159]

While the incidence of drownings tends to be greater in coastal communities oriented to large bodies of water and the aquatic environment in general, most surveys indicate that drownings in salt water are relatively rare. Notable exceptions to this are in cold water fishing communities such as in Alaska, Nova Scotia, Maine, western New Zealand, and the North Sea, where the annual fatality rate may be as high as 415 drownings per 100,000 fisherman.[130,166] Submersion incidents that do not result in death or even in hospitalization may be quite common in these communities.[150] In my experience this is particularly true in Australia and California. This must be a result, at least in part, of effective surveillance and rescue efforts at public beaches by lifeguards and surf lifesaving societies.[106]

RACE

There is considerable evidence that race is a factor in the increased risk of exposure to submersion incidents, particularly in children. The incidence of both drowning and near drowning episodes appears to be greater in black children. The drowning rate of black male children has been estimated to be as much as three times that of white males.[167] In the United States, unsupervised swimming or accidental falls into unattended canals or quarries accounted for a large percentage of deaths in black males.[159] Such statistics probably reflect socioeconomic conditions in the affected communities.

ABILITY TO SWIM

The ability to swim does not appear to be consistently related to drowning rates unless gender differences are considered. White males have a higher incidence of drowning than do white females, yet reportedly have better swimming ability. On the other hand, black females are reported to have the lowest swimming ability but a very low rate of drowning.[167] In Florida, nonswimmers or beginners accounted for 73% of drownings in home swimming pools and 82% of incidents in canals, lakes, and ponds.[159]

Parental example is an important determinant of whether children can swim. Children whose parents can swim are most likely to be strong swimmers; those with parents who cannot swim are likely to be nonswimmers. Parents of white children are much more likely to be swimmers than are the parents of black children.[167]

DRUGS

Alcohol is the chief drug implicated in submersion incidents; the danger of its use in the aquatic environment cannot be overemphasized.[101] An Australian study reported that 64% of males who drowned had measurable levels of alcohol in blood samples taken after death, and 53% of those over the age of 26 years had blood alcohol levels greater than 100 mg/dl.[150] While it cannot be stated definitively that alcohol was the cause of these tragedies, the common association of intoxication with drowning argues strongly against the use of alcohol near the water.[37] Despite the sobering statistics a recent survey in Massachusetts revealed that 36% of men and 11% of women had consumed alcoholic beverages during their most recent aquatic activities.[1,76] Loss of judgment associated with the use of intoxicants is the most likely reason that they are so frequently associated with drowning incidents. In addition, alcohol increases heat loss, decreases laryngeal reflexes, and increases the incidence of vomiting—all factors that worsen the prognosis in submersion incidents.[38] Drugs such as phencyclidine (PCP), lysergic acid diethylamide (LSD), and marijuana alter the sensorium; their use undoubtedly increases the risk of accidents in the water. Up to 30% of adult drownings occur because of boating accidents in which occupants demonstrated poor judgment: overcrowding, speeding, use of boats for purposes not intended, failure to wear life jackets, and reckless handling of the craft. The incidence of drug use in these episodes is not known, but it can be assumed that intoxicants play a role in many such accidents.[37,150]

UNDERLYING DISEASE OR INJURY

Underlying injury or illness can account for loss of life in the water. Hypoglycemia, myocardial infarction, cardiac arrhythmias, depression and suicide, and syncope predispose to the drowning incident.[157] Persons with a history of seizures must be supervised at all times while on boats or while swimming and should be encouraged to shower (not take a bath) in a nonglass cubicle in an unlocked bathroom.[36,89,138] A search for an underlying cause of the tragedy should be made, particularly in those who are evaluated in the hospital after rescue.

Cervical spine injuries and head trauma should be suspected in all unwitnessed incidents, particularly in those involving surfers and in victims found near diving boards or rafts in shallow water. Possible damage to the cervical spine should be a consideration in both immediate on-scene and emergency department management.

CHILD ABUSE

Attention has been drawn to the problem of submersion incidents as a manifestation of child abuse. All suspicious incidents must have a thorough social service and legal investigation consistent with the obligations imposed by the laws of each community.[60,92,95] Frequently, however, this does not occur. In a study of 95 drownings and near drownings in Seattle, only 28% of the cases had a social service evaluation and only 8 drownings were reported to children's protective services.[42]

HYPOTHERMIA

Recent reports of children surviving after relatively long periods in very cold water have elicited medical and lay hypotheses regarding the possibility of survival, even after prolonged submersion.

Drowning may result directly from hypothermia.[26,73] Experiences with persons shipwrecked even in relatively warm water have shown that the body temperature of victims can be lowered to the point at which hypothermia threatens survival. Thermal conductivity of cold water is approximately 25 to 30 times that of air.[73,95,97] Thus, in very cold water, hypothermia may ensue rapidly and lead to drowning. This is particularly true in the case of children, who have less subcutaneous fat and a relatively greater body surface area than adults.[95] Survivors of a Canadian boating tragedy painted a vivid picture of the effects of hypothermia that resulted in the deaths of an instructor and 12 of his students.[180] "Gradually we could feel the sensation going out of our limbs, and we heard some of the boys starting to get paranoid about being in the water. . . . Some started to talk nonsense and then, one by one, their voices faded away as they lost consciousness."

Death in submersion-associated hypothermia can be attributed to three basic mechanisms.

Immersion Syndrome

Immersion syndrome is defined as cardiac arrest secondary to massive vagal stimulation.[53,87,95]

Excessive Fatigue and Confusion

The combination of hypothermia, exertion, panic, and confusion leads to poor judgment, which causes victims to endanger themselves further by swimming away from help, leaving an overturned canoe, or misjudging the distance to shore.

Direct Hypothermia

At or below a core temperature of 28° C (82° F), ventricular fibrillation is a real risk.[66,173] It has been estimated that at a water temperature of 0° C (32° F), the victim of submersion cannot survive for more than 1 hour; at a water temperature of 15° C (59° F), survival is not common after 6 hours.[25,52] However, several recent cases in Canada temper blind acceptance of any particular dogma. In one incident,[110] a pilot and passenger ditched their plane into a lake on final approach to an island airport. Air temperature was 2.2° C (36° F) and water temperature 4° C (39.2° F). Both men were similarly clothed and in the water for 60 minutes before being rescued. The passenger, a 48-year-old man, weighed 101 kg, was 190 cm in height, and had a core temperature of 32° C (89.6° F) on admission to the hospital. He was alert, complained only of being cold, was actively rewarmed, and left the hospital the next day. The pilot, a previously healthy 38-year-old man, was of medium body habitus and had little subcutaneous fat. He was admitted to the same regional trauma unit in ventricular fibrillation with a core temperature of 29.1° C (84.2° F). Despite core rewarming and vigorous resuscitative measures over 4 hours, he could not be revived. In view of the identical environmental conditions, clothing worn, and time in the water, the authors of this report concluded that skinfold thickness was the most important discriminating factor in the outcome of this tragedy.[110]

A second case illustrates the fact that preparation and protective clothing may lengthen survival time in cold water.[109] A married couple, both experienced sailors, began to take on water in their boat about 11 km from shore in a Canadian lake.[179] The boat sank after 40 minutes, during which time they were able to prepare for abandoning ship by lashing together life preservers and donning heavy parkas and special survival gear carried in the boat. The month was August, but a storm had developed with gale-force winds of 60 km/hr and high waves. Water temperature was estimated to be 18° C (64° F). Both persons spent over 18 hours in the water before rescue and helicopter transport to the regional trauma unit. Both were mildly hypothermic on admission; the husband's rectal temperature was 32° C (89.6° F), while his wife's was 36.4° C. Both were discharged the next day without complications, with survival attributed to survival preparedness and protective clothing.

In victims kept afloat by life preservers or other means, death may result directly from hypothermia. Although some people may appear to be dead after rescue, efforts to resuscitate and rewarm them may be rewarded with recovery. Still, the absolute effect of hypothermia on eventual survival after a submersion incident remains in doubt. In certain cases hypothermia appears to be protective, as in the case of the Norwegian child who survived neurologically intact after being rescued from an ice-laden stream in which he had been submerged for 40 minutes.[172] His temperature on admission to the hospital was 24° C (75° F), and after 1 hour of resuscitation, spontaneous circulation returned. He was discharged from the hospital 8 days later. Several similar cases were reported in the U.S. press in 1987; all involved submersion under ice with eventual survival.

Orlowski[135] reviewed the world literature on prolonged submersion with good outcomes. He reported 17 victims, most of whom were younger than 19 years of age, and almost all male. He concluded that no one factor correlated well with outcome. These factors included water temperature, core temperature, rewarming techniques, and duration of resuscitation. He further cautioned against assuming a good prognosis in the case of patients who suffer submersion in very cold water, citing several cases of children who, despite hypothermia and appropriate treatment, had poor outcomes.[191] One explanation for survival in some children after long periods of submersion in very cold water has focused on the possibility that the "diving reflex" present in lower mammals may be operative.[27,55,109] The mammalian diving reflex, especially impressive in seals, slows the heart rate, shunts blood to the brain, and closes the airway. However, recent evidence suggests that the diving reflex present in seals is active in only 15% to 30% of human subjects. This response, with its potential for improved brain circulation, may be a significant factor in why some persons survive and others drown.[54,64] After a study of breath-holding and bradycardia in children and adults, one group of investigators with significant expertise and interest in this question concluded that the diving reflex in children is weak and may not contribute significantly to survival after cold water submersion.[154]

Immersion in cold water may lead quickly to hypothermia because of surface heat loss and core cooling. In addition, swallowing or aspiration of cold water may contribute to rapid cooling.[64,135] Conn and Barker[28] recently reviewed the mechanism of cooling in submerged victims and reported that rapid onset of hypothermia during freshwater drowning resulted from core cooling from pulmonary aspiration and rapid absorption of cold water. Significant cerebral cooling was therefore likely before cessation of circulation.[28]

If the diving reflex is discounted, the most likely explanation for survival after prolonged submersion in cold water is that rapidly induced hypothermia reduces tissue oxygen demand and protects the brain. Perhaps catecholamine release is blunted in victims who quickly become hypothermic in very cold water, lessening the propensity to ventricular fibrillation that accompanies warm water submersion incidents.[135] Muscle movement is probably less in persons exposed suddenly to very cold water, further reducing oxygen demand.

In contradistinction to the possible protective effect of hypothermia in submerged victims, hypothermia can create grave problems for the victim struggling to survive in cold water. Specific patterns of heat loss can be demonstrated in subjects placed in water at temperatures as low as 4.5° C (40.1° F).[25] In these studies, thermograms have graphically recorded heat loss from various parts of the body, demonstrating preferential loss from the head and neck (up to 50%), thoracic cage, and inguinal area. Movement of any kind increases heat loss.

Collis[25] compared several options available to victims faced with the dilemma of cold water survival. He concluded that methods of survival that require much movement would be "suicidal" and, based on the observations of heat loss, devised preferred means of conserving body heat while immersed in cold water. These methods have been approved and adopted by the U.S. Coast Guard (Department of Transportation).

As summarized in Fig. 48-1, treading water, swimming, and drown-proofing all resulted in reduced survival time (less than 2 hours) at a water temperature of 10° C (50° F). Survival time was estimated to double if victims assumed a position designed to protect areas of body heat loss. In this position, dubbed the heat escape lessening posture (HELP), the arms are folded across the chest and pressed to the sides, the knees are drawn up to the chest, and the legs are crossed at the ankles. In this position, the victim attempts to keep still, maintaining the head out of water. To assume this position, the victim must be wearing a life jacket (Fig. 48-2). When this position was tested on members of the swim team at the University of Pittsburgh, they reported it as fatiguing at best.

Should there be more than one person in the water, the "huddle" position is recommended to lessen total body heat loss. Since children become hypothermic much more quickly than do adults, they should be placed in the middle of the huddle. In this position, it is necessary to tie life jackets behind the back to allow the groin and lower body regions to be pressed together (Fig. 48-3).[25]

Because hypothermia is not uncommon and alters the therapeutic approach to victims of submersion incidents, core temperatures should be determined in all potentially hypothermic patients brought to the emergency department. Resuscitation efforts must persist until normal core temperature is approached.[140,173] No decision on survival should be made until the patient is nearly euthermic. The management of hypothermia and immersion hypothermia is extensively discussed in Chapters 3 and 4.

TYPE OF WATER

Drowning may occur in almost any type of fluid, from the elegant swimming pool to the lowly puddle or gravel pit. Victims of submersion may aspirate salt or fresh water, sewage, wash water, or tap water.

Much discussion has been generated on the importance of the type of water in which the victim has been submersed.[123,124,178] Most victims of submersion injury aspirate impurities or foreign materials, including algae, bacteria, sewage, chemicals, and sand.[56] In animal experiments the osmolarity of water has been shown to cause biochemical changes in nonsurvivors.[123,124] While the difference between saltwater and freshwater submersion is not of immediate clinical importance, knowledge of the effect of aspiration of several kinds of fluids helps in the interpretation of laboratory and clinical findings seen in some patients.[161]

Theoretically, the changes that occur after aspiration of salt water and fresh water should be different, and the biochemical abnormalities secondary to such aspiration should play a role in management. This has not proved to be the case. Modell and associates[123,124,121] demonstrated convincingly that it is the amount of water aspirated, rather than the type, that is of prime importance.

Orlowski, Abulleil, and Phillips[137] studied pulmonary injury and the ability to resuscitate dogs after "drowning" produced by instilling fluids of varied tonicity into the lungs.

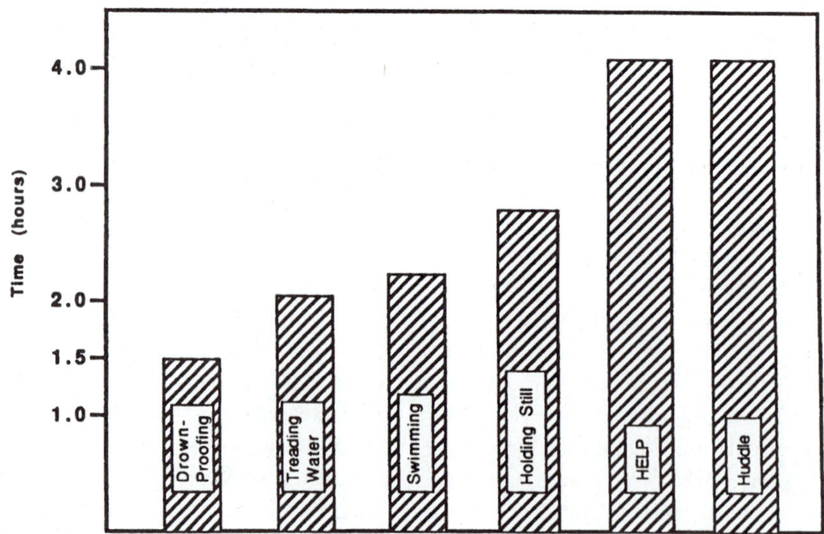

Fig. 48-1 Survival times in cool (50° F) water using various techniques in several situations. (Data from Collis ML: Survival behaviour in cold water immersion. In *Proceedings of the Cold Water Symposium*, Toronto, 1976, Royal Life-Saving Society of Canada.)

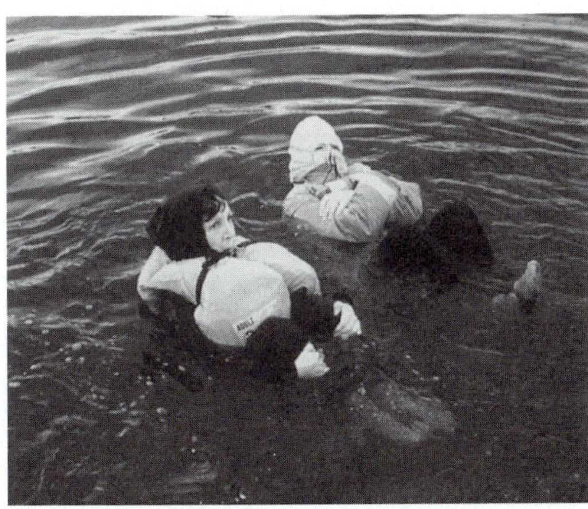

Fig. 48-2 The heat escape lessening posture (HELP). Heat loss is reduced by covering the head and neck, pressing the arms to the chest wall, and drawing the knees up to the chest. This requires a flotation device, despite which the position is still difficult to maintain. (Courtesy Alan Steinman, M.D.)

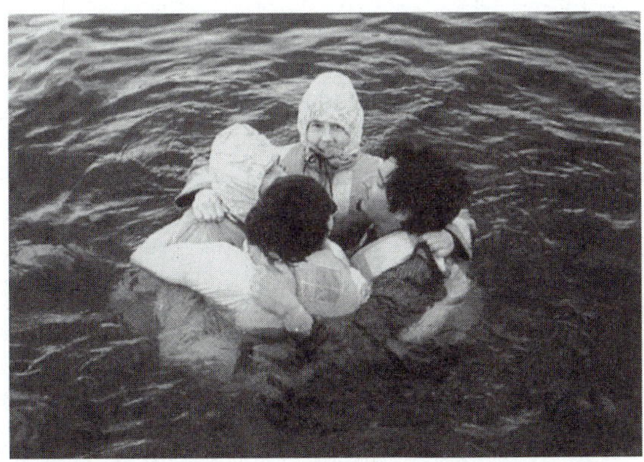

Fig. 48-3 The "huddle" technique. Three or more persons face one another with flotation devices tied on backward, pressing the chest, abdomen, and groin areas together. The victims hold one another around the neck. Children are placed in the middle. (Courtesy Alan Steinman, M.D.)

The six fluids used were sterile water and 0.225%, 0.45%, 0.9%, 2%, and 3% sodium chloride solutions. Each of these solutions was tested with and without additional chlorine. The dogs were anesthetized, intubated, and ventilated with room air; 20 ml/kg of each fluid was instilled into the endotracheal tube, which was then clamped for 5 minutes before resumption of ventilation with 100% oxygen and 10 cm of positive end-expiratory pressure (PEEP). Three control dogs were made anoxic for 5 minutes by occlusion of the endotracheal tubes, without fluid instillation.

When judged by the effect on pulmonary variables (A-a oxygen pressure difference, intrapulmonary shunt fraction, and Pa_{O_2}/Fi_{O_2} ratio), the 0.225% saline solution was less disruptive to lung function, particularly when compared with sterile water, with or without chlorine. Sterile water was found to be the most damaging to the lungs, whether chlorinated or not. No differences between solutions were seen in the ability to resuscitate dogs with cardiac arrest. The authors suggested that swimming pool water be salinated to 0.225% normal sodium chloride solution to reduce pulmonary injuries of persons who suffer submersion injuries. These studies clearly indicate that the cardiovascular changes that occur with drowning are really from anoxia and not dependent on the tonicity of the aspirated fluid.[139]

FRESHWATER ASPIRATION

Fresh water is hypotonic to plasma and passes readily out of the alveolus into the circulation. Theoretically at least, if a sufficient volume is aspirated (more than 22 mg/kg), blood volume can increase and hemolysis can result.[123] Hemolysis, along with hypoxia, can lead to hyperkalemia, high levels of circulating free hemoglobin, and lowered hematocrit value. Expansion of blood volume caused by fluid shifts from the alveoli to the intravascular compartment lowers the concentrations of serum sodium chloride, calcium, and magnesium.[123,124]

Hypokalemia has also been reported, but this may be caused by other factors such as administration of epinephrine, glucose, and bicarbonate during resuscitation.[24] Despite theoretical changes, few near drowning victims (survivors) have electrolyte abnormalities serious enough to warrant therapy. In survivors of a submersion injury, biochemical and blood volume changes are corrected quickly and should be considered transient.[121,119,161] Management efforts in both freshwater and saltwater submersion should be directed primarily toward the effects of aspiration on the lungs.

Aspiration of fresh water induces pulmonary changes, the most important of which is the "washout" of surfactant.[127] This leads to atelectasis, with consequent ventilation-perfusion imbalance and hypoxia.[114,125] In addition, direct destruction of alveolar cells may lead to accumulation of fluid within the lung and decreased compliance. Thus the overwhelming insult the clinician faces in the initial management of submersion injury is hypoxia.

SALTWATER ASPIRATION

Seawater has an osmolarity three to four times that of blood. The effect of aspiration of this hypertonic fluid is rapid shift of plasma fluid into the alveoli and interstitial spaces of the lung parenchyma, resulting in severe pulmonary edema.[22,95,114,124] Theoretically, loss of fluid from the circulation should produce a blood volume decrease and rise in serum electrolytes because of high concentrations of sodium, potassium, and magnesium in seawater. However, as with freshwater aspiration, electrolyte changes do not appear to be important in the early management of submersion casualties.[119,135]

Unusual exceptions to this rule occur. Near drowning episodes from bodies of water with high electrolyte content, such as the Dead Sea, are characterized by significant changes in concentrations of serum electrolytes, particularly calcium and magnesium. A recent report from Israel by Yagil and co-workers[188] confirms these findings, as well as a high mortality rate (50%) in eight treated patients. Experts still stress the importance of hypoxia and pulmonary injury caused by aspiration in the deaths of all victims of submersion.[117,142]

In a case of seawater aspiration, pulmonary edema results quickly, with outpouring of protein-rich fluid into the alveoli and interstitium, reduction of compliance, and direct parenchymal damage.[127] Hypoxia and metabolic acidosis remain the immediate concerns of the acute care physician.

CONTAMINANTS

Most water in which submersion incidents occur contains chemicals, contaminants, or particulates that may produce further pulmonary injury.[73,114] Calcium salts, frequently used near oil drilling equipment, may render near drowned divers hypercalcemic.[46] Although some maintain that pool water containing chlorine may be irritating to the tracheobronchial tree, recent animal studies indicate that it is the hypotonicity of the fluid, not the chlorine, that does the damage.[137] Water contaminated with chemical wastes, cleaning solvents, detergents, or disinfectants may induce further fluid accumulation in the already edematous lung.[123,169] Inhalation of mud, sand, and other particulates may require bronchoscopy to cleanse the airway. Although uncommon in survivors, "sand bronchograms" have been described on chest films of surfers and others who aspirated radiopaque calcium carbonate sand.[16]

The bacteriology of fresh water has been studied.[5,101,104,107] Persons suffering submersion in fresh water may be exposed to microbes, such as *Aeromonas hydrophila,* that are resistant to commonly employed antibiotics. In patients who develop lung infection, culture and sensitivity testing is essential to identify the causative agents and to choose the appropriate antibiotic.[156]

Classification and Types of Drowning

Death by submersion, or drowning, has historically been classified according to pathophysiology. Such classifications are usually made after the fact and are of little use in immediate management.

WET VERSUS DRY DROWNING

The term "wet drowning" refers to the great majority of patients who aspirate water; the lungs are wet, with pulmonary derangements resulting from the effect of the fluid. It is estimated that 85% to 90% of patients fall into this category.[73,114,142] The remaining 10% to 15% do not aspirate to a significant degree and have "dry" lungs. Such "dry drowning" cases may represent patients who develop laryngospasm in response to the cold water stimulus, mechanical irritation of swallowed water, or initial inhalation of fluid.[50,115] Although it might be reasonable to assume that patients who do not aspirate will respond better to resuscitation measures, there is no real evidence to support this notion. The response to resuscitation depends more on rapid reversal of hypoxia than on the type of submersion injury. Acute and chronic responses of the lungs to various amounts and types of fluids may range from mild to severe, as will be discussed. Patients with preexisting pulmonary disease are at greater risk for decompensation if they suffer submersion incidents.

SHALLOW WATER BLACKOUT

The phenomenon known as shallow water blackout predisposes to drowning in persons who hyperventilate before entering the water for an endurance underwater swim, a training method sometimes attempted by competitive swimmers. Hyperventilation substantially reduces arterial carbon dioxide pressure ($Paco_2$). Vigorous underwater muscular activity engenders hypoxia before enough CO_2 accumulates in the blood to provide a stimulus to return to the surface to breathe. Without sufficient hypercapnia to stimulate breathing, consciousness can be lost from hypoxia and the victim may drown. A case of apparent shallow water blackout is recorded in which the author of the report spent several days in his own intensive care unit.[188] His observations are well worth noting, as are those of a second clinician who warns against hyperventilation during training.[72]

IMMERSION SYNDROME AND THE DIVING REFLEX

Immersion syndrome is sudden death after contact with very cold water, presumably a result of vagal stimulation[53] and resultant cardiac arrest.[87] The exact mechanism of this phenomenon is not understood, but in the past it has been attributed to the mammalian diving reflex, also present in seals and lower mammals. Investigation into the nature of this reflex was reported in the early 1960s. Cold water stimulation of cutaneous receptors appears to trigger shunting of blood to the brain and heart from the skin, gastrointestinal tract, and extremities. Bradycardia results from the reflex vagal response to increased central volume. This allows increased cerebral circulation with longer breath-holding times because of lower peripheral oxygen use. The diving reflex does not occur to the same extent in all people. Work in humans suggests that the diving reflex is not a major mechanism of survival in cold water for all near drownings, but that it may be a significant factor for the 10% to 20% of victims who have a profound diving reflex response helping them to survive.*

POSTIMMERSION SYNDROME

"Postimmersion syndrome" is an unsatisfactory term referring to delayed development of the adult respiratory distress syndrome, which is preceded by a relatively asymptomatic interval of several hours to several days.[34,48] The term "secondary drowning" has been used to refer to delayed-onset pulmonary failure, but continued use of this term adds little to understanding of the problem of submersion injury and prolongs the chaos of varied terminologies.

Pathophysiology of Submersion

The effects of submersion on mammals were first reported in the scientific literature in the late 1800s. In his classic monograph, Greene noted that "inundation of the upper airway, the bronchial tree and segments of the alveolar spaces blocks gas exchange in the lung and produces asphyxia. Thus drowning involves the rapid development of hypoxia, hypercapnia and acidosis with the associated sequence of hypertension, bradycardia, arrhythmias, hypotension, hyperpnea, apnea, and terminal gasping." Findings in animals were consistent with drowning episodes later observed in humans.[73,102,129] The initial response in humans to submersion, particularly in cold water, includes a period of panic, accompanied by hyperventilation caused by stimulation of thermal receptors in the skin. Breath-holding may be attempted, but at some point in breath-holding the breaking point is reached. This is the point at which no voluntary efforts will prevent respiration and is determined by both the CO_2 and oxygen levels. Hyperventilation before diving or swimming may prolong this point, while it is also responsible for underwater blackout in swimmers attempting long underwater swims.[96] Hyperventilation is usually uncontrollable by the victim and can result in aspiration of significant quantities of water. If the water is very cold, it is likely that such aspiration hastens the onset of hypothermia and may explain the "protection" apparent in some cases of cold water immersion. Swallowing large amounts of water may lead to vomiting and subsequent aspiration of gastric contents.[95,109] It is this occurrence that may present difficulties to initial rescuers; gastric distention may make ventilation more difficult, and regurgitation is a constant danger.

In most victims of submersion, violent struggling occurs before loss of consciousness; exercise-induced acidosis leads to greater hyperventilation and risk of aspiration of water (Fig. 48-4).

*References 54, 64, 75, 114, 135, 153, 154, 175.

The common denominator of submersion is hypoxia, caused by either laryngospasm or water aspiration. Once the victim is unconscious, all airway reflexes are abolished and fluid is passively introduced into the airway. Cardiac arrest follows this sequence of events. Hypoxia and acidosis lead to derangements in many organ systems in those who have suffered serious incidents.[73]

PULMONARY SYSTEM

The target organ in submersion episodes is the lung (Fig. 48-5). Once aspirated, water evokes vagally mediated pulmonary vasoconstriction and pulmonary hypertension.[23,24] In cases of freshwater aspiration, fluid moves quickly across the alveolar-capillary membrane into the microcirculation, surfactant destruction or "washout" occurs, and high surface tensions in the lung lead to reduced compliance and atelectasis. Marked ventilation-perfusion mismatching occurs, with as much as 75% of blood flowing through hypoventilated lung tissue.[11,73,85,127] Seawater aspiration also leads to surfactant destruction and produces rapid exudation of protein-rich fluid into the alveoli and pulmonary interstitium, reduced compliance, and direct capillary damage.[77] These changes usually lead quickly to serious hypoxia. In some cases of near drowning, this may not occur until hours later, when alveolitis, atelectasis, and shunting show clinical effects.

Even in survivors of near drowning it may be days before normal ventilation-perfusion matching returns.[96] Nor-

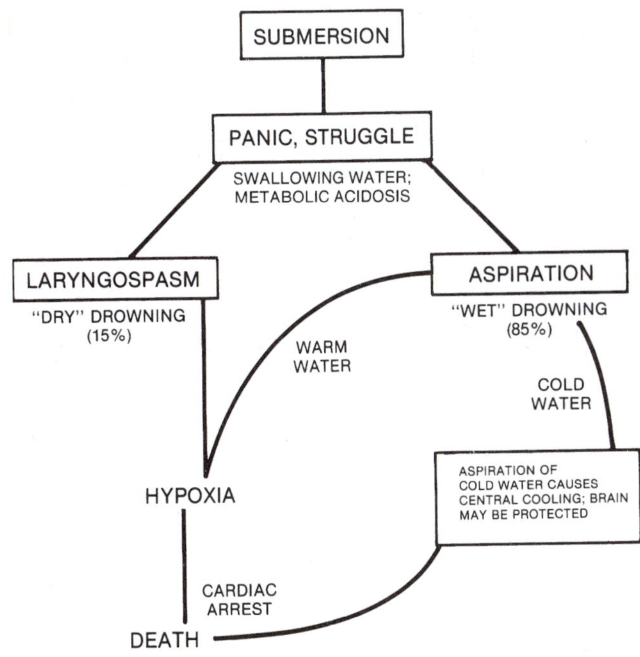

Fig. 48-4 Progression of the drowning incident.

mal lung function depends on alveoli that expand easily with inspiration (low surface tension) and recoil efficiently. These properties are facilitated by the presence of surfactant, a layer of fluid lining the alveolar walls. Fifty percent or more of this substance is dipalmitoyl phosphatidylcholine, a phospholipid; the rest is composed of other phospholipids and proteins. Surfactant is manufactured by alveolar epithelial type II cells, and its metabolism is under hormonal control as well as control through the interaction of β-adrenergic agonists, cyclic adenosine monophosphate, and prostaglandins.[90] Alveolar aspiration of water appears to destroy or "dilute" pulmonary surfactant.[49,50] When the substance is absent or does not function properly, atelectasis occurs and "stiff," noncompliant lungs result. The consequence in the nearly drowned patient is severe shunting and hypoxia.[73]

An important development in the treatment of premature infants who are surfactant deficient has been instillation of exogenous surfactant via an endotracheal tube.[47] The surfactant, which was first derived from bovine or human amniotic fluid, is now produced from artificial sources. Dramatic results have been reported in early studies with this replacement therapy, with improvement of pulmonary function and oxygenation evident within hours of treatment.[113] While no studies have yet been reported concerning the use of surfactant replacement in other than premature surfactant-deficient infants, this therapy in the injured lung of near drowning is a theoretical and logical extension of the experiences recently reported.[6]

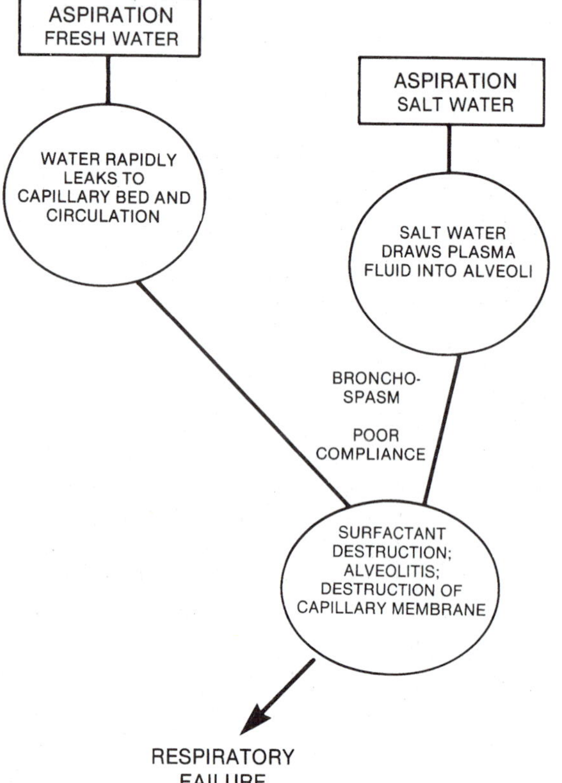

Fig. 48-5 Pulmonary effects of water aspiration.

Inhalation of particulate matter, contaminants, bacteria, or chemicals can produce irritation that results in more tracheobronchial fluid deposition or even alveolar destruction.[121,170] Despite the absence of direct evidence in humans, it is suspected that damage to the alveolar-capillary membrane may be produced by coagulation defects, platelet breakdown, microembolization, and other adverse effects initiated by fluid aspiration or hypoxia. While alveolar and surfactant destruction has been emphasized in most studies, recent animal research has suggested that the initial pulmonary insult may be damage to the vascular endothelium, rather than to the alveolar cells.[84]

Hypoxia in humans after submersion incidents is the result of fluid in the alveolar and interstitial spaces, loss of surfactant, proteinaceous material in the alveoli and tracheobronchial tree, damage to the alveolar-capillary membrane and vascular endothelium, and hypoxia-initiated central nervous system (CNS) reflex mechanisms.[73,95,115] Acute respiratory failure follows, with a reduction in compliance and an increase in ventilation-perfusion mismatching, resulting in an enhanced shunt.[38,73] The difference in oxygen tension between alveoli and arterial blood is increased with pulmonary failure after submersion. In normal subjects breathing 100% oxygen the difference is about 35 mm Hg; in human victims of submersion, differences as high as 600 mm Hg with 100% oxygen have been reported.[73]

In cases of prolonged submersion or significant aspiration, pulmonary derangements occur rapidly. In lesser insults the onset of symptoms may be delayed for as long as 24 hours. The phenomenon probably represents a delayed onset of the initial insult, rather than reflecting the severity of the injury or a different disease entity or syndrome.[116,151]

The type of water aspirated during a submersion incident may determine the extent of lung damage and degree of resultant hypoxia. In animal models, sterile water has produced the most profound changes in pulmonary function.[58,126] Isotonic sodium chloride solution (0.9%) has been shown to produce injury, but not as great as that produced by sterile water.[137] The presence of chlorine in 1 to 2 ppm apparently does not influence the degree of pulmonary injury or dysfunction.[137]

CARDIOVASCULAR SYSTEM

Cardiovascular derangements in cases of serious submersion injury are usually secondary to hypoxia, acidosis, or other indirect causes, rather than being caused by actual fluid aspiration. In the past, death was thought to be caused by induction of ventricular fibrillation by electrolyte changes, but this is now known not to be the case. Cardiac dysrhythmias and depression of myocardial function are caused by acidosis and hypoxia resulting from pulmonary injury.[62,73]

Supraventricular tachycardias are common.[38] Karch[83] reported that the myocardia of rabbits subjected to aspiration of fresh and salt water demonstrated focal areas of eosinophilia and disruption of some myocardial elements. The lesions resembled those produced in hearts exposed to very high levels of catecholamines. On the basis of this study and a review of other animal models, he suggested that cardiac derangements seen in near drowning may result from increased catecholamines secondary to the stress of the incident.[39,83]

Management requires close observation of the cardiovascular system. A delicate balance is often struck between pulmonary function and oxygenation versus cardiac output and right heart return. This has particular relevance to cases in which PEEP is used to improve oxygenation.

CENTRAL NERVOUS SYSTEM

The endpoint of successful resuscitation of victims of submersion incidents has heretofore been restoration of adequate perfusion and pulmonary function. With development of more sophisticated monitoring capabilities, attention is now directed toward preserving CNS function and preventing further damage once vascular perfusion has been restored. While much interest has been shown in the concepts of "cerebral resuscitation," most pharmacologic interventions are still experimental. The first and most important immediate steps toward cerebral preservation are rapid institution of rescue measures and basic life support, without which later measures may be futile.

Insults to the CNS include hypoxia and trauma to the spine and spinal cord. A search for other causes of CNS dysfunction is mandatory in persons who remain comatose after submersion incidents. All patients should be investigated for expanding intracranial lesions secondary to trauma or for damage to the spinal cord, which may occur in surfing mishaps, in platform diving accidents, or during horseplay.

The initial insult to brain tissue is hypoxia and ischemia, but evidence suggests that tissue damage can continue after restoration of cerebral blood flow.[30,164] Dysfunction of the CNS occurs rapidly after the onset of hypoxia; flattening of the electroencephalogram takes place within 20 seconds of total cerebral ischemia. Continued CNS injury after resuscitation results from edema, elevated intracranial pressure (ICP), and increased cerebral vascular resistance, which compromise oxygenation.[73,164] Hyperpyrexia that accompanies drowning increases cerebral oxygen consumption and tissue insult.[29,30]

Methods to monitor ICP are often promoted as essential guides to the success of measures directed toward cerebral resuscitation, but this has not been demonstrated definitively. Experimental and clinical evidence suggests that attempts to prevent postresuscitation cerebral injury will play a prominent role in management of patients who remain comatose after serious submersion accidents.[120,122,135]

RENAL SYSTEM

Acute renal failure is not common in victims of submersion incidents. When it occurs, the most frequent cause is destruction of tubules secondary to hypoxia. Reduced blood flow secondary to shock and acidosis increases the incidence of renal failure.[73,95]

METABOLIC CHANGES

Electrolyte changes in a survivor of a submersion incident do not appear to be either consistent or important in initial management. An unusual exception to this rule is near drowning in water with extremely high electrolyte concentrations such as are found in the Dead Sea.[189] Sodium concentrations are three times as high (1493 versus 531 mmol/L) in the Dead Sea as in the Mediterranean Sea; chloride 6092 versus 630 mmol/L; potassium 970 versus 11 mmol/L; calcium 1709 versus 48 mmol/L; and magnesium 6987 versus 273 mmol/L.[189]

Elevations of potassium levels in victims who have aspirated fresh water have been theoretically ascribed to hemolysis. Few patients who survive aspirate sufficient water to pose any problem; aspiration of quantities that would cause serious electrolyte imbalance usually results in death.[26,48] This applies equally to the aspiration of fresh and salt water. Postmortem measurements of electrolytes in experimental animals have uncovered increases in serum sodium, chloride, calcium, and potassium, presumably a result of the high concentrations in seawater. Again, these problems are not seen consistently in survivors of submersion incidents.

Respiratory acidosis is the main immediate problem in patients.[73,119,135,140] In most patients, severe metabolic acidosis develops, in part because of pulmonary failure with resultant cellular anaerobic metabolism. Persistent acidosis depresses myocardial function and leads to lethal arrhythmias.

HEMATOLOGIC CHANGES

Hemolysis has been described in both freshwater and saltwater aspiration, more commonly in the former, with levels of circulating free hemoglobin ranging from 8 to 500 mg/dl.[123] There is no consistent change in the level of hemoglobin or hematocrit after submersion in humans. Low values should initiate a search for underlying trauma with hemorrhage or a bleeding disorder. Disseminated intravascular coagulation has been described with submersion and aspiration.[32,73] Contributing to the genesis of this disorder are hypoxia, acidosis, sepsis, hemolysis, and low-perfusion states.

Predicting Outcome

It would be helpful to be able to predict the future course of patients, particularly those with severe injuries. Previous attempts to predict outcome were thwarted by lack of uniformity of terminology and of a standard classification of patients' conditions. Recent attempts have been more successful. The importance to eventual survival of rapid rescue and immediate CPR has been recognized by almost all authorities on the subject of near drowning.* The extent of cerebral recovery can be related to the factors (1) age and gender, (2) hypothermia, (3) submersion time, (4) initial resuscitation, and (5) critical care with special measures of cerebral salvage.[2,33,79,134] While some of these are more important than others, each should be considered an essential element in the overall evaluation of chances of recovery.

Predicting the outcome of patients is based largely on initial and serial examinations of cerebral function. Orlowski[134,135] has refined this principle and developed a "score" that, in conjunction with the Glasgow Coma Scale (GCS), permits a fairly accurate estimate of the likely outcome (Box 48-2). Unfavorable prognostic factors include young age, severe acidosis, submersion time longer than 5 minutes, coma on admission to the emergency department, and no attempt at CPR within 10 minutes of rescue. With one or two adverse factors present, a 90% change of recovery is indicated; three or more reduce the chances to less than 5%.

Biggart, Bahn, and Desmond[13] suggest that prolonged attempts to resuscitate victims who have not been hypothermic and who did not initially have vital signs will result in more deaths or more survivors with persistent vegetative states. The importance of initial assessment to predicting outcome cannot be overemphasized. Patients who are alert on admission, are in sinus rhythm, and have reactive pupils should do well, while those who are in coma with absent brainstem reflexes, unreactive pupils in the emergency department, or a GCS score of less than 5, or have been submerged more than 10 minutes and had resuscitation durations of more than 25 minutes, have a less than 5% chance of recovery.[44,54,88,94]

*References 41, 119, 135, 140, 143, 156.

Management

IMMEDIATE CARE

The scene of the submersion incident is often characterized by general chaos. Modell[114] notes that persons on the scene of the event rarely report seeing someone who was "flailing and screaming for help" while they "struggle to remain on the surface of the water." Instead, they found victims floating on the surface of the water, or saw swimmers suddenly become motionless or dive under water and never surface.[114] It is essential that attempts at rescue take into account the safety of rescuers, so that drownings of multiple persons do not occur. The Red Cross recommends that whenever possible, safety devices should be used to tow in the victim, or life preservers should be tossed to people in trouble before a lifesaver actually enters the water in a boat or on a board to attempt a rescue. Well-intentioned but ill-advised heroic efforts can create additional victims and compound the tragedy.

Recovery of victims still submerged should be the responsibility of professional or volunteer workers trained specifically in the art of water retrieval and rescue. Water rescue demands special equipment and expert personnel and may have to be carried out in extremely adverse circumstances, especially in winter weather (Fig. 48-6). An emergency medical services physician should be involved in consultation early during the incident, particularly in cases in which cold weather rescue and hypothermia are involved.

Until there is evidence that aggressive on-scene resuscitation does not help prevent loss of life, no effort should be withheld. Prehospital care workers should be given definitive guidelines that insist on prompt application of life support to all victims of submersion unless hypothermia is cer-

BOX 48-2

PROGNOSTIC SCORING SYSTEM FOR VICTIMS OF NEAR DROWNING

UNFAVORABLE PROGNOSTIC FACTORS

Age 3 years or less
Estimated submersion time longer than 5 minutes
No resuscitation attempts for at least 10 minutes after rescue
Patient in coma on admission to emergency department
Arterial blood gas pH 7.1 or less

Modified from Orlowski JP: *J Am Coll Emerg Phys* 8:176, 1979.

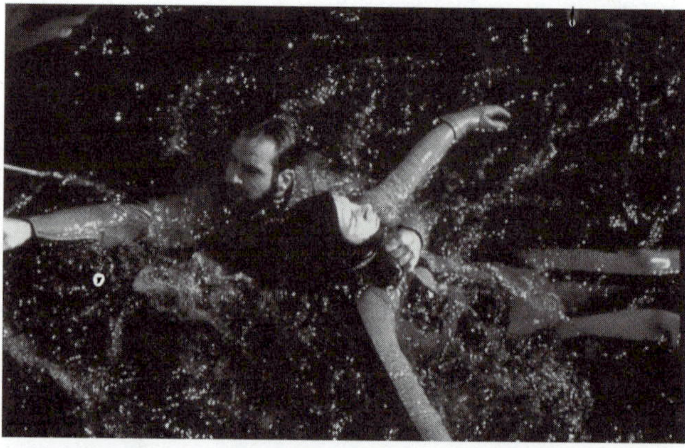

Fig. 48-6 Cold water rescue; both victim and rescuer are dressed in wet suits. (Courtesy Alan Steinman, M.D.)

tain not to be present and the duration of submersion is reliably known to be long. Thus rescuers must begin resuscitative measures and present the patient to the in-hospital team, who can decide on therapy. This is true especially in the case of winter or cold water conditions. The decision to withhold or cease resuscitation attempts is rarely made in the field, except in a remote wilderness area. Transport of the near-drowned victim from remote terrain has been made more expeditious with wider availability of helicopter evacuation.

Estimates of time under water are notoriously inaccurate when made by bystanders, parents, and even trained rescuers.[122] The history can be crucial in this regard. A publicized case occurred in which rescuers delayed instituting life support to a victim of submersion in a river with a water temperature of 11.7° C (53° F).[149] In a review of the problem it was found that the initial radio message relayed from the first unit receiving the call did not include information that the woman was struggling as she floated down the river. The rescuers removing her from the water assumed she had been submerged for some time and did not begin CPR until a rhythm was detected on the electrocardiographic monitor. As it happened, she was hypothermic, responded almost immediately to resuscitative measures, and survived to leave the hospital.

SPECIFIC THERAPY

Initial evaluation and resuscitation of any patient must include complete examination for obvious trauma, with appropriate stabilization and repeated examination. Thorough examination should minimize death from unrecognized trauma, such as ruptured spleen or fractured cervical spine. Appropriate intensive care monitoring should be part of the management routine.

The victims of submersion incidents may be classified into four groups: (1) the asymptomatic patient, (2) the symptomatic patient, (3) the patient in cardiopulmonary arrest, and (4) the obviously dead or still-submerged patient.

Asymptomatic Patients

The patient who has experienced a period of submersion or a near drowning episode and who remains asymptomatic presents a particular dilemma. The history is of prime importance. A description of the incident, an estimate of submersion time, and the past medical history of the patient should be obtained. All patients with any conceivable history of submersion who manifest shortness of breath (however slight) should be considered hypoxic; oxygen by simple face mask at 8 to 10 L/min should be given. It may be better to err on the safe side and administer oxygen to any patient seen in the field with a history of submersion, regardless of the time submerged or the absence of symptoms.

It has been frequently recommended that all patients with a history of submersion be treated as if a lung insult had occurred and that admission to a hospital for a period of observation be mandatory.[109,135,156] This recommendation is often made in the belief that in patients sustaining a near drowning episode with apparently successful resuscitation, an asymptomatic period sometimes precedes the onset of respiratory failure, a condition termed secondary drowning. Close examination of the patients on whom this belief is based indicates that patients who suffer significant pulmonary insults rarely fail to show signs or symptoms immediately after rescue and initial resuscitation.

In a survey of 52 swimmers who had suffered submersion incidents on California beaches, 31 of 52 persons declined medical attention and left the beach.[151] Telephone follow-up of 26 persons indicated that none had sought medical care subsequent to the incident and all returned to a normal state of health. Of 21 persons evaluated in a hospital, respiratory distress was manifested within 4 hours. Despite its obvious limitations and uncontrolled nature, this report suggests guidelines for the emergency management of the asymptomatic or minimally symptomatic patient with a history of near drowning (Table 48-1).

"Secondary drowning" probably represents evolution of preexisting lung injury, rather than sudden and unexpected occurrence in a patient exposed to near drowning. Most injured patients can be identified through careful evaluation and a 4- to 6-hour observation period in the emergency department combined with a plan for careful follow-up. No one recommends that asymptomatic survivors of a submersion incident be sent home from the site of the incident. All potential victims should be taken to a hospital for competent medical evaluation, or at least strongly encouraged to seek medical advice.[151]

Symptomatic Patients

Any patient who shows signs of distress (anxiety, tachypnea, dyspnea, syncope, persistent cough, or vital sign change) at the scene has suffered a significant submersion injury until serial observations in the hospital prove otherwise (Table 48-2). Two immediate problems will be hypoxia and acidosis. Correction involves respiratory manipulation. The airway must be kept patent, which can be a problem in patients who are vigorously vomiting. Emesis is frequent in submersion victims, especially in persons who have swallowed large amounts of seawater. If transport time is long, diarrhea caused by the laxative effect of swallowed seawater may add insult to injury.

Supplemental Oxygen. If the victim is breathing spontaneously, high flow rates should be provided by face mask (12 to 15 L/min via a nonrebreathing mask) or by demand valve, which gives 100% oxygen at the valve outlet. If available, pulse oximetry may be used to monitor oxygen saturation. Patients in respiratory distress who breathe spontaneously might benefit from continuous positive airway pressure using a tight-fitting mask. No prehospital experience has yet been reported with the use of this modality.

Any decrease in body temperature is unwelcome. All

Table 48-1 On-Scene Management of Asymptomatic Patients*

History	Baseline Examination	Intervention
Time submerged	Appearance	Oxygen by face mask, 8-10 L/min
Description of incident	Vital signs	Intravenous line at "keep-open" rate
Complaints	Chest examination	Reexamine patient as needed
Past health	Electrocardiographic monitor	Transport

*Patients refusing treatment should have telephone number and address taken and arrangement for follow-up made.

Table 48-2 Field Approach to the Symptomatic Patient*

History	Examination	Intervention
Description of incident	General appearance	Oxygen via mask (8-10 L/min) by demand valve
Time submerged, water temperature, water contamination, vomiting, type of rescue	Level of consciousness	Intravenous line at "keep-open" rate; consider intubation if patient is tachypneic or dyspneic with cyanosis or depressed mental status
Symptoms	Vital signs, electrocardiographic monitor	Transport patient

*Be prepared for vomiting. Take measures to prevent hypothermia and shivering. Treat cardiac arrhythmias as they arise, keeping in mind that hypoxia may be the underlying cause.

wet clothing must be removed and the patient wiped dry. If the patient continues to shiver, carefully wrapped hot packs may be placed in the axillae and inguinal areas and near the scalp and neck. A comprehensive discussion of hypothermia management is found in Chapters 3 and 4.

Attention to potential metabolic acidosis is given after establishment of a patent airway, oxygenation, and access to the intravascular space. Metabolic acidosis can exist even in relatively asymptomatic victims of submersion.[73,135] The first line of treatment is adequate ventilation and correction of hypoxia.[133] Administration of sodium bicarbonate has been advocated in patients with adequate circulation who are tachypneic or dyspneic with cyanosis.[112] Recent recommendations do not support this practice, particularly in the field environment.[119] Administration of bicarbonate should follow vigorous attention to ventilation and oxygenation and generally await arterial blood gas analysis.

For the most part, other drugs are administered in the hospital. Cardiac irritability usually responds to correction of hypoxia and acidosis. If significant ventricular irritability persists, judicious field use of lidocaine by multiple-bolus technique using an initial dose of 1 mg/kg over 2 minutes and 0.5 mg/kg every 5 to 10 minutes, not to exceed a total dose of 225 mg, is justified.

Patients in Cardiopulmonary Arrest (Box 48-3). Vigorous cardiopulmonary resuscitation can be initiated immediately, even with the victim in the water. This is the

BOX 48-3

FIELD INTERVENTION IN PATIENTS IN CARDIOPULMONARY ARREST*

BEGIN VENTILATION AND COMPRESSION

Use mouth-to-mouth, mouth-to-mask (preferably with oxygen supplementation), or bag-valve-mask (preferably with balloon mask or two-rescuer ventilation)
Use supplemental oxygen

ENDOTRACHEAL INTUBATION

Positive end-expiratory pressure at 5 to 10 cm may be useful
Intravenous line at "keep-open" rate

IF COPIOUS DRAINAGE FROM LUNGS OR STOMACH

Suction through endotracheal (ET) tube
Pass nasogastric tube
Apply abdominal thrusts between ventilations if ET tube in place and copious drainage persists

*Sodium bicarbonate ordered on advice of physician or according to protocol of the system. Treat dysrhythmias in standard fashion. If cervical injury is suspected, use collar and sandbags, etc.

most important survival factor in drownings.[111] Mouth-to-mouth ventilation should be attempted during extrication, but this may be difficult, depending on the strength of the rescuer and demands of the environment. As soon as shore, jetty, shallow water, surfboard, or a boat is reached, mouth-to-mouth ventilation should begin in earnest.

A suggestion has been made that closed-chest compressions be initiated in the water as soon as the victim is reached (Fig. 48-7).[108] Trials in which a recording manikin was ventilated and compressed, using a modified ventilator and posterior grasp position, demonstrated adequate chest compression and ventilation. However, these trials did not measure blood flow achieved when the patient was held in a nearly upright position. The likelihood of providing any circulation or even of keeping a victim afloat in the hypothetical circumstances described are at best remote. Other factors that argue against this technique include frigid water and rescuer fatigue; dangers from wave, surge, and current, wet suit and scuba apparatus obstruction; and the delay to definitive out-of-water cardiopulmonary resuscitation.[91,93] No reports have been published regarding the successful use of this technique in an actual submersion incident.

As soon as the patient is extracted from the water, he or she should be placed on a firm surface (float board, backboard, jetty, or boat deck) and appropriate resuscitation measures continued. Basic care given at the scene is thus far the most important treatment factor in determining survival.* A trial of cardiopulmonary resuscitation (CPR) with a pneumatic device appeared to produce better blood flow than did traditional CPR. Additional trials with this technique will suggest if it should become a new standard.[61] If rescue is performed on a sloping beach, the patient should be placed parallel to the water's edge (neither head up nor head down), theoretically to prevent a decrease in forward blood flow during chest compressions in the head-up position or an increase in intracranial pressure in the head-down position.

*References 43, 119, 135, 140, 143, 156.

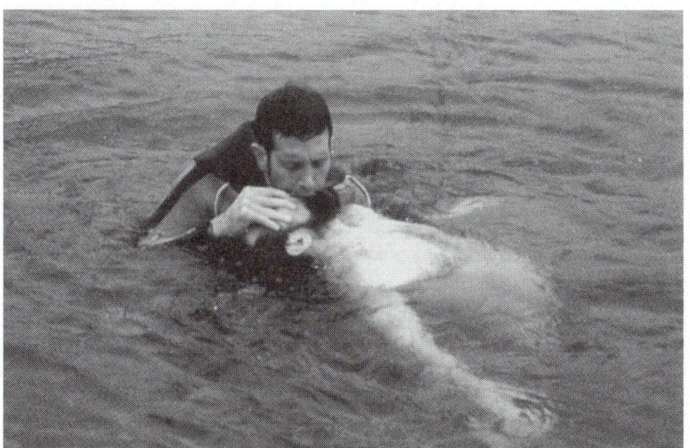

Fig. 48-7 Mouth-to-mouth ventilation in the water is difficult in the best of circumstances. (Courtesy Alan Steinman, M.D.)

An adequate airway provides access not only for positive-pressure ventilation, but also for clearing of copious secretions. This can be achieved only through the prompt insertion of an endotracheal tube, which should be placed after good initial ventilation. When only tank oxygen with a delivery hose, nasal cannula, or face mask is available, mouth-to-mouth or mouth-to-mask ventilation may be supplemented with oxygen by applying the nasal prongs to the rescuer (at 6 to 8 L/min). This increases the delivered oxygen concentration from 21% to 40%.[71] Proper mouth-to-mask rescue breathing is preferable to bag-mask ventilation in the hands of basic life support providers because it has been shown to deliver greater volumes with less mask leak.[40,63]

If a bag-valve-mask ventilator is used, it must have an oxygen reservoir to increase the percentage of oxygen delivered to the patient. This reservoir should be of the soft inflatable type with a capacity of at least 2.5 L.[3,18] It should be fitted with a newly designed balloon mask that provides a tight seal on the patient's face and reduces leak.[177] Without this mask, bag-valve-mask devices are not the preferred method of applying positive-pressure ventilation in a field setting because of the difficulty in achieving a mask seal and because of operator fatigue, both of which inevitably reduce delivered volumes.[3,40,63]

Lung Drainage. Frequent airway clearing is necessary with most victims of submersion. Vomiting and copious drainage from the lungs and stomach can occur. The issue of lung drainage is historically and currently controversial. Draining the lungs makes some sense, since submerged victims have been estimated to aspirate up to 2 L,[140] as well as to accumulate pulmonary edema fluid. The concept of draining water from the lungs dates back to the seventeenth and eighteenth centuries. The Dutch method consisted of rolling the victim over a barrel; another method advised flinging the victim over the back of a horse, which was then made to trot.[100] In 1975, Dr. Henry Heimlich introduced an abdominal compression maneuver (Heimlich maneuver), advocated for victims of food choking.[67] In the initial and subsequent reports, he suggested its use in the victims of drowning.[69,68]

Evidence for the effectiveness of the maneuver in drowning is anecdotal at best. It appears that the use of abdominal compression in victims of submersion may predispose to induced emesis of large amounts of swallowed water, thus exposing the patient to further aspiration, this time of gastric contents.[136]

Although one study demonstrated greater survival rates in animals subjected to drainage techniques,[127] the dogs used apparently did not require closed-chest cardiopulmonary resuscitation. It was concluded that drainage techniques were useful only in victims of seawater aspiration. Studies at the University of Pittsburgh demonstrated no difference in canine survival in groups treated without drainage, with the Heimlich maneuver, or with Trendelenburg positioning.[187] As far back as 1962, efforts to drain water from the lungs were condemned as "of no practical use" and "a waste of valuable time" in applying mouth-to-mouth ventilation.[160] The same investigators showed in cadavers that only small amounts of the 1 L of 1% saline solution instilled into the lungs could still be recovered by prone positioning, "jackknifing," or thoracic compression.[160] A delivered volume of up to 2 L of air could still be accomplished with higher ventilating pressures.[160]

No human studies of lung drainage in submersion have been reported, and descriptions of drainage procedures in recent works refer to *gastric* drainage.[164] The technique in these cases was to place the patient on the side and compress the abdomen, or to place the patient in a prone position, grasp him or her about the abdomen, and lift ("breaking" the victim, in older lay language). Whether these maneuvers led to drainage of water from the stomach or lungs is not clear.

Gastric drainage may be required in patients who have swallowed large amounts of water, since gastric distention may interfere with ventilation. If gastric distention is a problem, abdominal compression with adequate suction available (or gravity drainage) may suffice. Abdominal compression accomplishes drainage without the need to interrupt cardiac compressions or ventilation for as long a time as other methods. Whatever the method, it must be performed quickly so that basic life support can continue. A nasogastric tube is preferred to all other methods. Most clinicians and the official recommendations of the American Heart Association advise against the Heimlich maneuver except when the airway is obviously blocked with foreign material.[3,152] None of the methods suggested for gastric drainage should precede initial attempts at ventilation.

Endotracheal Intubation and Positive End-Expiratory Pressure. Endotracheal intubation controls the airway by reducing dead space, providing protection against aspiration, and facilitating pulmonary toilet. In apneic patients requiring positive-pressure ventilation, PEEP has been demonstrated to be of use in victims of submersion.[85,143,159,160] Although there is no decrease or is even an increase in total lung water, PEEP acts in several ways to improve ventilation patterns in the noncompliant lung: (1) by shifting interstitial pulmonary water into capillaries; (2) by increasing lung volume via prevention of expiratory airspace collapse; (3) by increasing the diameter of large and small airways to improve ventilation distribution; and (4) by decreasing alveolar capillary blood flow and providing better alveolar ventilation, and hence improved ventilation-perfusion ratio and Pa_{O_2}.

The use of PEEP in the field situation has been made possible with development of a small apparatus adaptable to manual self-inflating bag ventilation devices.[99] Experience with field PEEP is limited, and clinicians must be thoroughly familiar with its drawbacks. These include reduction of return to the right side of the heart, increase in fluid retention in an already stressed lung, increase in pulmonary artery pressure, decrease in cardiac output, and, at high levels, increased intracranial pressure.[4,35,171]

Drugs. In the past the standard drug therapy in cardiopulmonary resuscitation emphasized prompt attention to sodium bicarbonate administration. Severe metabolic acidosis may exist in a submersion victim because of circulatory arrest and the preceding muscular activity in the struggle for survival.[125] Administration of bicarbonate has potential disadvantages, which include increased sodium concentration with resultant fluid load that may not be beneficial to patients whose cardiovascular reserve is already limited.[174,185]

Other problems of bicarbonate use cited in the recent debate include impairment of oxygen delivery to the tissues, paradoxical increase in lactate production, and increase in CO_2 production that can worsen already profound metabolic and respiratory acidosis.[85,174,185] The possibility that bicarbonate administration in cardiac arrest may be inappropriate has led to reconsideration of this practice.[3,14] The decision to administer bicarbonate should be made by the in-hospital team after more data are available on which to base a decision. The most likely problems leading to acid-base imbalance are hypoxia and respiratory acidosis, which require effective ventilation before consideration of sodium bicarbonate.

Obviously Dead or Still-Submerged Patients. The term "obviously dead" refers to any patient who has a normal temperature and demonstrates asystole, absent respirations, postmortem lividity, or rigor mortis. In cases in which rescue operations have been in progress for more than 30 minutes, victims who are retrieved from warm water during summer months or in warm southern waters may be considered dead on the scene. Because cold water submersion for over 40 minutes has been associated with neurologic survival,[172] it is imperative that rescue crews institute life support measures in all patients who are not obviously dead, who may be hypothermic, and whose histories suggest recent signs of life.

In tragic cases in which the patients are obviously dead or are still submerged, the rescue team must comfort the family or friends and participate in recovery of the body. Once retrieved, the victim should be covered immediately and treated with proper dignity. Family members and friends should be escorted from the scene, if possible, before recovery. Most drownings are medical examiner cases, since the possibility of foul play must be investigated.

In-Hospital Management

Once the patient reaches the hospital, a brief but pertinent description of the event, an estimate of time submerged, and the extent of field intervention will provide team members with important information bearing on further treatment, as well as offer some basis for expectation of outcome.

Classification of Patients (Table 48-3). Patients may be classified on admission in a manner similar to that used in the field setting: asymptomatic, symptomatic, in cardiac arrest, or obviously dead. In 1980, Conn and Modell[120] suggested an ABC classification of patients based on presenting neurologic examination. This system has undergone revision, with the time of initial examination being changed to the emergency department after initial resuscitation, and usually within 1 hour of rescue. More aggressive resuscitation led to the introduction of a fourth subgroup under "C." Under this system, patients were "A"—alert, "B"—blunted in consciousness, or "C"—comatose. The comatose patients were further categorized according to their abnormal neurologic responses: C_1—flexor response; C_2—extensor response; or C_3—flaccid. A C_4 category was added to include patients in whom vigorous CPR was being applied that might result in a change in condition and therefore prognosis.[28]

In their series on children, Conn and his co-workers reported that all patients in category A survived and were normal and that all but one patient survived in category B. The patients in coma were most likely to benefit from therapy while being most at risk. The C group showed various responses, with increasingly bad outcomes. Similar studies in adults have not yet been reported.

Asymptomatic Patients (Box 48-4). Patients may arrive in the emergency department with little or no evidence of submersion injury. It is widely accepted that respiratory complications develop in some victims of submersion incidents 12 to 72 hours after the event.[34,140,141] This has led many to recommend that even asymptomatic patients be admitted for observation for this time period. A careful review of most of these cases indicates that almost all the patients had a history of severe insult (cardiopulmonary arrest requiring resuscitation) or had shown some abnormalities on arrival at the emergency department. Patients with minor symptoms who decline on-scene medical help probably do not deteriorate.[151] Most acute care clinicians, faced with a reliable history of submersion, elect to perform a physical examination, obtain arterial blood gas measurements, and acquire a chest x-ray study on even asymptomatic or minimally symptomatic victims of a near drowning.[93,119,135,143] Persons who show abnormalities or who deteriorate within 4 hours of admission to the emergency department should be admitted for observation and further management.

Table 48-3 Classification of Near Drowning Victims*

Category	Description
A	Awake—fully oriented
B	Blunted—arousable; purposeful response to pain
C	Comatose—not arousable; abnormal response to pain
C_1	Flexor response to pain
C_2	Extensor response to pain
C_3	Flaccid
C_4	Arrested

Modified from Conn AW, Barker GA: *Can Anaesth Soc J* 31:S38, 1984.
*Assessment is made in emergency department within 1 hour of rescue.

BOX 48-4

IN-HOSPITAL MANAGEMENT OF ASYMPTOMATIC PATIENTS

CHECK AIRWAY

Supplemental oxygen: nonrebreathing mask at 12 to 15 L/min or via demand valve pending oximetry or arterial blood gas determinations

Obtain history and estimate severity of incident, look for possible underlying causes, e.g., cerebrovascular accident, epilepsy, drugs, myocardial infarction, arrhythmia

TAKE VITAL SIGNS AND EXAMINE PATIENT

Draw and hold blood samples for complete blood count, electrolytes, blood urea nitrogen, platelets, prothrombin time, partial thromboplastin time; send if indicated

Arterial blood gases; consider pulse oximetry; consider blood alcohol level and toxicology screen

Urinalysis

Chest radiograph

DISPOSITION

Observe all patients for 4 to 6 hours; discharge home if completely asymptomatic and adequate telephone or medical follow-up can be guaranteed

Supportive therapy. The patient who remains asymptomatic may need attention because of the psychologic trauma of the near tragedy. This is frequently important when others have been involved in the incident, particularly when fatalities resulted.

Radiographic studies. Radiographic examination of the chest is performed on all patients with a history of submersion. The findings vary widely with the severity of the incident and other less well-identified factors. The usual pattern seen in patients suffering a significant insult is similar to that of noncardiogenic pulmonary edema. In mild cases fine alveolar infiltrates are found predominantly in the periphery. Patients who become symptomatic often demonstrate changes consistent with diffuse or localized intraalveolar or interstitial infiltrates, segmental atelectasis, or "shock lung." Air bronchograms are frequently seen in severely affected patients, and the lungs may appear opaque. An initial normal chest radiograph does not rule out a significant pulmonary insult. Depending on the duration of submersion, findings are usually seen within several hours of the incident, but changes have been delayed for as long as 24 hours after the patient became symptomatic.[77,158]

Spinal injury should be suspected in patients who have been platform diving or surfing or who may have fallen from a height into the water. A full radiographic series of all seven cervical vertebrae is standard before neck manipulation.

Symptomatic Patients (Box 48-5). Patients complain of combinations of coughing, sore throat, burning in the chest, and dyspnea. Patients who are dyspneic are almost always hypoxic and if severely affected (with cyanosis) are likely to be acidotic. Intervention must be aggressive and planned. Initial arterial blood gas and serum chemistry measurements should be performed. A chest radiograph may be taken by portable machine unless the patient receives priority in the main radiology department.

Blood gas determinations or pulse oximetry can be carried out rapidly in most modern emergency departments and in almost all cases should guide therapy. Oxygen is administered by demand valve (100%) or through a nonrebreathing mask at a rate of 12 to 15 L/min. This will suffice if the Pao_2 can be maintained at or above 90 mm Hg at an Fio_2 of 0.50 or less.[50] Maintaining positive pressure in the airway during expiration can be valuable. This is particularly indicated if the Pao_2/Fio_2 ratio is 300 or less.[135] In some patients who are able to hold a mask, continuous positive airway pressure (CPAP) can be provided via the tight-fitting mask, and intubation may be avoided.[57,171] Although experience with this method is growing, patients must be carefully chosen. In selected cases in the intensive care unit, use of mask CPAP has delayed or eliminated the need for intubation.[57] When provided by experienced personnel, it is an acceptable adjunct to emergency department therapy. Inability to maintain a Pao_2 of 55 mm Hg on an Fio_2 of 0.50 is one criterion for use of this method.[114] In addition, the patient must be able to respond to verbal commands, control his or her airway, and be nonhypercarbic ($Paco_2$ less than 45 mm Hg).[171] Pressures used within the system, as well as the Fio_2, vary according to the clinical and arterial blood gas response. Pressures may range from 0 to 4 cm H_2O on inspiration and 4 to 14 cm H_2O on expiration. Experience with this method is insufficient for it to be recommended definitively in the prehospital environment.

Irritation of the tracheobronchial tree by inhaled water and particles may evoke cough and bronchospasm. Bronchospasm may worsen hypoxia; aggressive management is essential in symptomatic patients. Aerosolized albuterol is the drug of choice for initial treatment of bronchospasm in the emergency department. It is a relatively selective β_2-adrenergic agonist, rapid acting, and with minimal side effects.[10,155] It is administered to spontaneously breathing patients via a nebulizer fitted with mouthpiece or face mask. The average dose for a single treatment is 1.25 to 2.5 mg (0.25 to 0.50 ml) diluted in 2 to 5 ml or more of sterile normal saline or sterile water. With severe bronchospasm the first dose may be increased to 5 mg, or the initial lower dose may be repeated if necessary. Albuterol may be administered to intubated patients using a nebulizer attached to a T-piece hooked to the endotracheal tube. Aminophylline, in an intravenous loading dose of 5.6 mg/kg over 20 to 30 minutes, may be added if bronchospasm is not relieved.[131,155] This is useful predominantly for persons who are already taking the medicine and in whom subtherapeutic blood levels are determined.

The decision to perform endotracheal intubation in patients is made on the basis of blood gas determinations and the following: (1) comatose patient unable to handle secre-

BOX 48-5

IN-HOSPITAL APPROACH TO THE SYMPTOMATIC PATIENT

CHECK AIRWAY

Supplemental oxygen: nonrebreathing mask at 12 to 15 L/min or via demand valve

CONSIDER ENDOTRACHEAL INTUBATION

For comatose patients
For patients unable to maintain a Pao_2 above 90 mm Hg on high-flow oxygen (nonrebreathing mask at 12 to 15 L/min), or unable to maintain a $Paco_2$ below 45 mm Hg

CHECK VITAL SIGNS

Start intravenous line: draw blood for complete blood count, electrolytes, blood urea nitrogen, platelets, prothrombin time, partial thromboplastin time
Arterial blood gas studies
Urinalysis
Administer bicarbonate according to blood gas results if acidosis is severe and cannot otherwise be corrected
Chest radiograph
Cervical spine radiograph if any doubt about circumstances of incident
Nasogastric tube
Indwelling urinary catheter if necessary

DISPOSITION

Admit all patients with abnormal vital signs, abnormal radiologic signs, or abnormal findings on blood gas measurements
Completely asymptomatic patients with no findings may be discharged after 4 to 6 hours' observation if adequate telephone or other medical follow-up can be guaranteed

tions; (2) comatose patient who requires a nasogastric tube; or (3) patient with a Pao_2 of 90 mm Hg or less on high-flow oxygen by nonrebreathing mask at 12 to 15 L/min or with a $Paco_2$ greater than 45 mm Hg.[69]

An intravenous line should be placed, as well as an external cardiac monitor, indwelling urinary catheter (as needed), and nasogastric tube.

Comatose Patients or Patients in Cardiac Arrest

Prognostic Signs. The guidelines discussed in the section "Predicting Outcomes" represent the experience of both Conn and Orlowski.[28,135] Such guidelines offer a uniform approach to management, allow for realistic expectations based on measurable data, and propose common terminology and nomenclature. Despite these advances, resuscitating patients who probably face serious central nervous system deficits often blunts the enthusiasm of the most ardent clinician. The traditional prognosis for persons resuscitated from serious accidents provides little comfort. In some pediatric studies, 21% of children who survived suffered severe encephalopathy.[146] Others report that the outlook, particularly in children, is good, with morbidity ranging from 3.5% to 5%.[29,122,144,184]

It seems clearer from recent data that in the absence of profound hypothermia, the neurologic status of a patient on admission to the emergency department is crucial in determining the patient's course. Patients who are alert when admitted should seldom die.[2,33,79,122,134] Prognostic indicators, particularly in pediatric patients, have included the Glasgow Coma Scale[33] and the presence of spontaneous respirations.[79] The duration of submersion, because of its unreliability, is not a helpful gauge of the outcome of resuscitation attempts. Full recovery of some patients with initial fixed and dilated pupils tempers the tacit acceptance of all factors historically outlined as prognostic signs. However, good and bad signs exist that bear significantly on the chances of recovery (Box 48-6).

BOX 48-6

PROGNOSTIC SIGNS IN SUBMERGED VICTIMS

GOOD

Alert on admission
Hypothermic
Older child or adult
Brief submersion time
On-scene basic or advanced life support (probably most important)
Good response to initial resuscitation measures

BAD

Age less than 3 years
Fixed, dilated pupils in emergency department
Submerged longer than 5 minutes
No resuscitation attempts for more than 10 minutes
Preexisting chronic disease
Arterial pH 7.10 or less
Coma on admission to emergency department

For emergency department personnel, initiation and continuation of resuscitation begun in the field should be automatic, except in the most unusual circumstances. Termination of efforts is entertained only after standard methods have been employed.

Hospital Management (Box 48-7). The airway is reevaluated. If the patient does not already have an endotracheal tube in place and is comatose without gag or cough reflexes, a nasotracheal or endotracheal tube should be inserted after initial hyperventilation with 100% oxygen via bag-valve device. Arterial blood gases should be measured immediately. Cervical spine precautions should be observed.

If the patient is not breathing spontaneously, 100% oxygen should be administered by volume ventilator. The object in these patients is to increase the functional residual capacity and to reduce ventilation-perfusion mismatching. PEEP may be necessary, beginning at 5 cm H_2O to increase the ratio of Pao_2/Fio_2 to 300 or greater.[135] Respiratory acidosis is managed with appropriate airway measures, including intubation, pulmonary toilet, and PEEP. Metabolic acidosis is often severe. Despite recent reluctance to administer bicarbonate during states of cardiac arrest,[3,174] most clinicians advise administration of sodium bicarbonate if the pH is less than 7.25 and not improving with vigorous respiratory management.[114] One formula for calculating the dose of bicarbonate is: sodium bicarbonate (mEq) = patient weight (kg) $\times$ base deficit $\times$ 0.2.[119] One-half the calculated dose is given initially and the effect on blood gases observed.

Hypoglycemia may be present as a result of marked fatigue and alcohol ingestion.[38] After initial resuscitation, treatment is directed toward correcting derangements in specific organ systems, including pulmonary, cardiovascular, and central nervous systems.

Pulmonary System. The major insult to the lung follows reduction of surfactant and accumulation of intrapulmonary and interstitial fluid.[49,50,73,95] The treatment of pulmonary failure caused either by salt or fresh water is mechanical ventilation with or without some form of continuous positive airway pressure (CPAP). The aim is to maintain a balance between adequate oxygenation, cardiac output, and reduction in intrapulmonary shunting. Continuous mechanical ventilation is appropriate for apneic patients or those who are spontaneously breathing but are unable to maintain a Pao_2 of at least 90 mm Hg while wearing a face mask delivering an Fio_2 of 0.50. Patients with a Pao_2/Fio_2 ratio less than 300 need positive airway pressure in addition to oxygen.[135] In comatose patients this requires intubation.

BOX 48-7

IN-HOSPITAL MANAGEMENT OF PATIENTS IN COMA OR CARDIAC ARREST*

AIRWAY CONTROL

Endotracheal tube; nasotracheal preferred
Supplemental oxygen or mechanical ventilation with intermittent mandatory ventilation (IMV), continuous positive airway pressure, or IMV with positive end-expiratory pressure
Bicarbonate therapy guided by arterial blood gas values
Treatment of cardiac arrhythmias according to protocol

DIAGNOSTIC

Arterial blood gases
Blood for complete blood count, electrolytes, coagulation baseline
Urinalysis
Chest x-ray examination
Cervical spine films (if indicated)
Electrocardiographic monitoring
Computed tomography or magnetic resonance imaging suggested in patients who remain comatose
No antibiotics
No steroids

FURTHER INTENSIVE CARE MEASURES

Arterial line
Swan-Ganz catheterization when fluid status in doubt
Diuretics
H_2 antagonists
Paralysis (pancuronium 0.1 mg/kg IV prn)
Maintain blood pressure: fluids if needed and vasopressors: dopamine, 1-20 μg/kg/min, dobutamine, 2-15 μg/kg/min

*Routine hypothermia is not recommended. Barbiturates after cardiac arrest are not proven effective. Intracranial pressure monitoring is suggested by some clinicians.

The most desirable form of ventilation in severely affected patients is intermittent mandatory ventilation, in which spontaneous breaths between mechanical inflations improve venous return and ensure adequate cardiac output. Most consultants recommend maintaining the $Paco_2$ at 40 mm Hg and the pH above 7.35[73] unless hyperventilation is undertaken for control of intracranial hypertension. The airway pressures required to provide a Pao_2 of at least 60 mm Hg with an Fio_2 of 0.45 vary according to the severity of the pulmonary insult and individual factors in different patients.[95]

In intubated patients whose ventilation is being controlled, PEEP may be used and should be maintained at a level that will ensure a balance between cardiac output and a reduction of shunt. After an adequate level of oxygenation is achieved, PEEP or CPAP should be maintained for at least 24 hours to foster the regeneration of surfactant.[95,140] Airway pressures with PEEP must be carefully monitored in postsubmersion patients, since increasing intrathoracic pressure leads to elevations in intracranial pressures.

Care must be exercised in removing patients from ventilatory support. Some respond dramatically to controlled ventilation, but 2 to 4 days may be required to replenish surfactant and resolve the problem of atelectasis. Premature removal from the ventilator may be followed by deterioration in pulmonary status, which could require reintubation and reintroduction of mechanical ventilation.[95] Generally, when a Pao_2 of 60 mm Hg or above can be supported with an Fio_2 of 0.40 or less in the absence of PEEP, the patient can be removed from the ventilator.

The use of steroids to prevent deterioration of lung function after submersion injury has few advocates.[73,119,135] No evidence shows a benefit in pulmonary failure, and good data suggest the progression of chemical aspiration to bacterial pneumonitis.[114,121]

Prophylactic antibiotics are not recommended. Daily Gram stains of sputum and frequent blood, urine, and sputum cultures may be required in the long-term management of these patients. Experimental studies are now looking into the use of butyl alcohol vapor or surfactant as an adjuvant to traditional respiratory support but are not yet far enough along to suggest routine use.[183]

Cardiovascular System. Cardiac dysrhythmias and arrest during the course of resuscitation often are corrected by improvements in oxygenation and acid-base status. Arterial pressure cannulas are helpful to monitor cardiovascular status and arterial blood gases.

The use of Swan-Ganz catheters is advisable in patients who develop hemodynamic instability or who require high levels of CPAP or PEEP to maintain oxygenation.[119] When shock is evident, pulmonary artery wedge pressures and cardiac output determinations allow a more rational approach to fluid administration. The Swan-Ganz catheter allows measurement of mixed venous oxygen saturation and can provide some information on oxygen transport and cardiac output. Pressor agents, such as dopamine and dobutamine, may be required if arterial hypotension and reduced cardiac output persist after adequate hydration is ensured. In most animal studies it is evident that cardiac output is best supported by fluids rather than inotropic agents.[38] The cause of most cases of postsubmersion pulmonary edema is altered permeability, rather than pump failure. However, dopamine in doses of 2 to 20 μg/kg/minute and dobutamine in doses of 2 to 15 μg/kg/minute have been reported effective in some patients.[71] Sepsis and shock are constant threats.

Renal and Metabolic Function. In patients who have suffered significantly from submersion, renal blood flow may decrease as a result of hypovolemia or hypotension. This can be detected by close attention to urine output. Renal failure is usually caused by hypoxia and acidosis with tubular damage.[56,83] Deposition of hemoglobin in the tubules from hemolysis of red blood cells is rarely a cause of renal failure. Maintenance of adequate circulating blood volume and restoration of renal perfusion are the best insurance against renal damage. An indwelling urinary catheter should be placed and urine production monitored and maintained at a minimum of 50 ml/hr. Mannitol in a dose of 0.25 g/kg intravenously has been used to maintain adequate urine flow and prevent obstruction of the tubules. This is given only after adequate intravascular volume is obtained.

Cerebral Resuscitation. Until recently, therapeutic measures were exclusively directed toward stabilizing the cardiovascular and pulmonary systems. Patients who were restored to adequate levels of cardiopulmonary function often died later from brain failure. Measures to protect the brain from postischemic insults have recently come into vogue, and many must be considered experimental. There is some evidence, however, that the outlook for patients with severe initial defects is improving.[28-30,120]

Measures directed toward cerebral salvage began with observations of the effect of hypothermia on brain metabolism. The initial enthusiasm and expectations for barbiturate "cerebral" resuscitation after cardiac arrest have not been justified, in light of the results of large international multicenter studies.[17,128,190]

It must be emphasized that the initial and most important approach to CNS "resuscitation" in postsubmersion patients is provision of an adequate airway and attention to ventilation and oxygenation. Patients who respond promptly to such measures are unlikely to require methods of cerebral preservation, probably because the cerebral insult has not been severe. Patients who remain comatose and who may have head trauma should be examined with computed tomography or magnetic resonance imaging as soon as practical. Scanning may reveal intracranial or intracerebral hemorrhage and provides an early picture of the extent of cerebral edema.

When the victim does not respond immediately to vigorous resuscitation measures, the practical approach suggested by Conn and co-workers[30] and recently revised[28,120] may be in order. The protocol for management requires the control of several elements, including ventilation, hydration, temperature, brain metabolism and edema, and muscular activity.

Ventilation. Hyperventilation is maintained to achieve a $Paco_2$ of about 30 mm Hg to balance cerebral vasoconstriction with cerebral blood flow. PEEP is used to maintain a high Pao_2 (150 mm Hg), since it is thought that this facilitates cerebral oxygen transport.

Hydration. Diuresis is promoted with a loop diuretic (furosemide 0.5 to 1 mg/kg). Fluid restriction is guided by laboratory and clinical measurements such as blood pressure, pulmonary wedge pressure, and occasionally blood volume measurements.

Temperature. Normothermia should be maintained and hyperpyrexia prevented with the use of cooling mattresses if necessary. The routine use of induced hypothermia is not recommended, particularly because hypothermia can induce neutropenia and lead to sepsis.[15,142,143] In the case of ICP uncontrolled by other measures, some clinicians advise reduction of core temperature to 30° C (86° F) while paralyzing the patient to combat shivering.[28] Recent revisions of this opinion urge caution, since the effect on outcome is uncertain.[118,119]

Cerebral Metabolism and Edema. Control of cerebral metabolism and reduction of edema are difficult and controversial areas of management. Patients who remain comatose and do not respond to adequate fluid balance and hyperventilation should have the management of presumed ICP elevation guided by clinical examination and direct monitoring using an epidural transducer, ventricular catheter, or subarachnoid bolt.

The use of barbiturates for cerebral protection after cardiac arrest has not been encouraging, but the ability of these drugs in certain circumstances to reduce ICP by cerebral vasoconstriction can be helpful to patients with an ICP above 20 cm H_2O.[119] A direct "protective" effect of barbiturates on nerve tissue has not been demonstrated. Difficulties with instituting barbiturate therapy and maintaining patients on the regimen include hypotension and inability to evaluate the patient clinically. Conn and his group used phenobarbital for a minimum of 4 days in children (50 mg/kg on day 1 in three divided doses, and half that dose subsequently). Daily determinations of barbiturate levels were required.[29,30] Recent reports of equivocal results in children treated with barbiturates and hypothermia indicate that these measures should not be employed routinely.[15,135]

If the decision to use barbiturates is made, the patient should be placed in an intensive care unit with staff fully skilled in the use of these agents. When pentobarbital is used, a constant infusion technique is guided by monitoring arterial pressure, ICP, and cardiac output. If blood pressure falls, the infusion rate should be decreased or an inotropic agent (dopamine, dobutamine) used to support myocardial function.[71,73] Whenever barbiturate therapy is considered, mass intracranial lesions should first be ruled out by computed tomography because of the possibility that any clinical signs caused by these lesions would be masked by the barbiturate. Sudden increases in ICP can be managed by hyperventilation and the use of mannitol (0.5 to 1 g/kg intravenous bolus). No comparative studies have demonstrated the success of therapy directed at reducing ICP and maintaining cerebral perfusion pressure.

The discovery that postischemic brain insult was associated with high intraneuronal calcium ion concentration led to the suggestion that calcium channel blocking agents be used to ameliorate the effects of ischemia on the central nervous system.[128] The use of these agents is under investigation, and they may prove useful in submersion victims who have suffered severe hypoxic insults.[128,165]

Corticosteroids found some proponents when steroid use was noted to improve the CNS function of patients with primary or secondary brain tumors.[9] The mechanism for this appeared to be reduction of cerebral reaction and consequent swelling around the mass lesions.[8] In an attempt to duplicate this beneficial effect in patients with acute intracranial hemorrhage, large doses of corticosteroids were administered to patients with head injury. No benefit was seen,[31] and corticosteroids for the reduction of ICP and for cerebral protection after ischemic brain insults are no longer recommended by most clinicians.[28,119] Steroids in high doses appear to be beneficial in selected cases of spinal cord injury.

Muscular Activity. Complete muscular paralysis is advocated by Conn and associates[28] to facilitate control of ventilation and to prevent ICP increase induced by muscle rigidity and restlessness. Muscle paralysis is achieved with pancuronium (0.1 mg/kg intravenously) hourly or as needed.

General Measures. Other measures for patient support during intensive postsubmersion therapy include placement of a nasogastric tube and selective administration of antacids or a histamine-2 antagonist, such as cimetidine, to prevent gastric hemorrhage.[135,147]

SUMMARY

While some progress has been made recently in management of the submerged patient, these improvements have resulted largely from better immediate rescue techniques and prehospital care. The key to reduction of tragic consequences of submersion incidents is prevention, and more vigorous programs in this regard are warranted. Combined with advances in emergency and critical care medicine, this approach may hold great hope for the future.

REFERENCES

1. Alcohol and aquatic activities—Massachusetts, 1988, *MMWR* 39(20): 1990.
2. Allman FD et al: Outcome following cardiopulmonary resuscitation in severe pediatric near-drowning, *Am J Dis Child* 140:571, 1986.
3. American Heart Association: Standards and guidelines for cardiopulmonary resuscitation and emergency cardiac care, *JAMA* 255:2841, 1986.
4. Ashbaugh DG, Petty TL: Positive end-expiratory pressure-physiology, indications and contraindications, *J Thorac Cardiovasc Surg* 65:165, 1973.
5. Auerbach PS et al: Bacteriology of the freshwater environment: implications for clinical therapy, *Ann Emerg Med* 16:1016, 1987.
6. Avery ME, Taeusch HW, Floros J: Surfactant replacement, *N Engl J Med* 315:825, 1986.
7. Baker SP, O'Neill B, Karpf RD: *The injury fact book,* Lexington, Mass, 1984, DC Heath.
8. Bartecchi CE: Cardiopulmonary resuscitation—an element of sophistication in the 18th century, *Am Heart J* 100:580, 1980.
9. Beks JWF, Doorenbos H, Walstra GJM: Clinical experiences with steroids in neurosurgical patients. In Reuben HJ, Schurmann K, editors: *Steroids and brain edema,* Berlin, 1972, Springer-Verlag.
10. Bennett P, Elliott D: *The physiology and medicine of diving,* ed 4, Philadelphia, 1993, WB Saunders.
11. Bergquist RE et al: Comparison of ventilatory patterns in the treatment of freshwater near-drowning in dogs, *Anesthesiology* 52:142, 1980.
12. Bierens JJLM et al: Submersion cases in the Netherlands, *Ann Emerg Med* 18:4, 1989.
13. Biggart MJ, Bahn DJ, Desmond J: Effect of hypothermia and cardiac arrest on outcome of near-drowning accidents in children, *J Pediatr* 117:179, 1990.
14. Bishop RL, Weisfeldt MZ: Sodium bicarbonate administration during cardiac arrest: effect on arterial pH, Pco_2 and osmolality, *JAMA* 235:506, 1976.
15. Bohn DJ et al: Influence of hypothermia, barbiturate therapy, and intracranial pressure monitoring on morbidity and mortality after near-drowning, *Crit Care Med* 14:529, 1986.
16. Bonilla-Santiago J, Fill WL: Sand aspiration in drowning and near-drowning, *Radiology* 128:301, 1978.
17. Brain Resuscitation Clinical Trial I Study Group: Randomized clinical study of thiopental loading in comatose survivors of cardiac arrest, *N Engl J Med* 314:440, 1986.
18. Campbell TP et al: Oxygen enrichment of bag-valve-mask units during positive pressure ventilation: a comparison of various techniques, *Ann Emerg Med,* in press.
19. Centers for Disease Control: Drowning—Georgia, 1981-1983, *MMWR* 34:281, 1985.
20. Centers for Disease Control: Drownings in a private lake—North Carolina, 1981-1990, *MMWR* 41(19):329, 1992.
21. Child drownings and near drownings associated with swimming pools, Maricopa County, Arizona, 1988 and 1989, *JAMA* 264(6): 1990.
22. Cohen DS et al: Pulmonary edema associated with salt water near-drowning: new insights, *Am Rev Respir Dis* 146(3):794, 1992.
23. Colebatch HJH, Halmagyi DFJ: Reflex pulmonary hypertension of fresh-water aspiration, *J Appl Physiol* 18:179, 1963.
24. Colebatch HJH, Halmagyi DJP: Effect of vagotomy and vagal stimulation on lung mechanics and circulation, *J Appl Physiol* 18:881, 1963.
25. Collis ML: Survival behaviour in cold water immersion. In *Proceedings of the Cold Water Symposium,* Toronto, 1976, Royal Life-Saving Society of Canada.
26. Conn AW: The role of hypothermia in near-drowning. In *Proceedings of the Cold Water Symposium,* Toronto, 1976, Royal Life-Saving Society of Canada.
27. Conn AW: Near-drowning and hypothermia (editorial), *Can Med Assoc J* 120:397, 1979.
28. Conn AW, Barker GA: Freshwater drowning and near-drowning—an update, *Can Anaesth Soc J* 31:S38, 1984.
29. Conn AW, Edmonds JF, Barker GA: Cerebral resuscitation in near-drowning, *Pediatr Clin North Am* 26:691, 1979.
30. Conn AW et al: Cerebral salvage in near-drowning following neurological classification by triage, *Can Anaesth Soc J* 27:201, 1980.
31. Cooper PR et al: Dexamethasone and severe head injury: a prospective double-blind study, *J Neurosurg* 51:307, 1979.
32. Culpepper RM: Bleeding diathesis in freshwater drowning (letter), *Ann Intern Med* 83:675, 1975.
33. Dean MJ, Kaufman ND: Prognostic indicators in pediatric near-drowning: the Glasgow Coma Scale, *Crit Care Med* 9:536, 1981.
34. Dick AE, Potgieter PD: Secondary drowning in the Cape Peninsula, *S Afr Med J* 62:803.
35. Dick W et al: The influence of different ventilatory patterns on oxygenation and gas exchange after near-drowning, *Resuscitation* 7:255, 1979.
36. Diekema DS, Quan L, Holt VL: Epilepsy as a risk factor for submersion injury in children, *Pediatrics* 91(3):612, 1993.
37. Drinking and drowning (editorial), *Br Med J* 2:1284, 1978.
38. Edmonds C, Lowry C, Pennefather J: Drowning. In *Diving and subaquatic medicine,* ed 3, Butterworth Heinemann.
39. Eliot RS, Todd GL, Pieper GM: Pathophysiology of catecholamine-mediated myocardial damage, *J SC Med Assoc* 75:513, 1979.
40. Elling R, Politis J: An evaluation of emergency medical technicians'

ability to use manual ventilation devices, *Ann Emerg Med* 12:765, 1983.
41. Emergency Cardiac Care Committee and Subcommittees, American Heart Association: Guidelines for cardiopulmonary resuscitation and emergency cardiac care. IV. Special resuscitation situations, *JAMA* 268(16):2242, 1992.
42. Feldman KW, Monastersky C, Feldman GK: When is childhood drowning neglect? *Child Abuse Negl* 17(3):329, 1993.
43. Fields AI: Near-drowning in the pediatric population, *Crit Care Clin* 8(1):113, 1992.
44. Fisher B, Peterson B, Hicks G: Use of brainstem auditory-evoked response testing to assess neurologic outcome following near drowning in children, *Crit Care Med* 20(5):578, 1992.
45. Frank BS: Hypokalemia following fresh-water submersion injuries, *Pediatr Emerg Care* 3(3):158, 1987.
46. Fromm RE: Hypercalcemia complicating an industrial near drowning, *Ann Emerg Med* 20:669, 1991.
47. Fujiwara T et al: Artificial therapy in hyaline membrane disease, *Lancet* 1:55, 1980.
48. Fuller RH: Drowning and the post-immersion syndrome: a clinicopathologic study, *Milit Med* 128:22, 1963.
49. Giammonna ST, Modell JH: Drowning by total immersion: effects on pulmonary surfactant of distilled water, isotonic saline, and seawater, *Am J Dis Child* 114:612, 1967.
50. Giammona ST: Drowning: pathophysiology and management, *Curr Probl Pediatrics* 3:3, 1971.
51. Golden FStC, Rivers JF: The immersion incident, *Anaesthesia* 30:364, 1975.
52. Golden FStC: Accident hypothermia, *R Naval Med Serv* 58:196, 1972.
53. Goode RC, Duffin J, Miller R: Sudden cold water immersion, *Respir Physiol* 23:301, 1975.
54. Gooden BA: Why some people do not drown: hypothermia versus the diving response, *Med J Aust* 157(9):629, 1992.
55. Gooden BA: Drowning and the diving reflex in man, *Med J Aust* 2:583, 1972.
56. Grausz H, Amend WJC Jr, Earley LE: Acute renal failure complicating submersion in seawater, *JAMA* 217:207, 1971.
57. Greenbaum DM et al: Continuous positive airway pressure without tracheal intubation in spontaneously-breathing patients, *Chest* 69:615, 1976.
58. Greenberg MI et al: Effects of endotracheally administered distilled water and normal saline on the arterial blood gases of dogs, *Ann Emerg Med* 11:600, 1982.
59. Greene DG: Drowning. In *Handbook of physiology, section 3: Respiration, vol II,* Washington, DC, 1965, American Physiological Society.
60. Griest KJ, Zumwalt RE: Child abuse by drowning, *Pediatrics* 83(1): 1989.
61. Halperin et al: A preliminary study of cardiopulmonary resuscitation by circumferential compression of the chest with use of a pneumatic vest, *N Engl J Med* 329:762, 1993.
62. Harries MG: Drowning in man, *Crit Care Med* 9:407, 1981.
63. Harrison RR, Maull KI, Keenan RL: Mouth-to-mouth ventilation: a superior method of rescue breathing, *Ann Emerg Med* 11:74, 1982.
64. Hayward JS et al: Temperature effect on the human dive response in relation to cold water near-drowning, *J Appl Physiol* 56:202, 1984.
65. Hazinski MF et al: Pediatric injury prevention, *Ann Emerg Med* 22(2, Pt 2):456, 1993.
66. Hegnauer HA, Angelakos ET: Excitable properties of the hypothermic heart, *Ann NY Acad Sci* 80:336, 1959.
67. Heimlich HJ: A life-saving maneuver to prevent food-choking, *JAMA* 234:398, 1975.
68. Heimlich HF: Subdiaphragmatic pressure to expel water from the lungs of drowning persons, *Ann Emerg Med* 10:476, 1981.
69. Heimlich JH, Hoffman KA, Canestri FR: Food-choking and drowning deaths prevented by external subdiaphragmatic compression, *Ann Thoracic Surg* 20:188, 1975.
70. Herholdt JD, Rafn CG: *Life-saving measures for drowning persons,* Copenhagen, 1796, H Tikiob.
71. Hess D, Kapp A, Kurtek W: The effect on delivered oxygen concentration of the rescuer's breathing supplemental oxygen during exhaled gas ventilation, *Respir Care* 30:691, 1985.
72. Higgins P, Siminski J, Pearson RD: "Hypoxic" lap swimming—a cause of near-drowning (letter), *N Engl J Med* 315:1552, 1986.
73. Hoff BH: Multisystem failure: a review with special reference to drowning, *Crit Care Med* 7:310, 1979.
74. Hoff BH: Drowning and near-drowning (letter), *Crit Care Med* 8:530, 1980.
75. Hong SK: Physical and physiologic adaptations to breath-hold diving in humans: a review, In *Proceedings of the 9th International Symposium on Underwater and Hyperbaric Physiology,* Bethesda, Md, 1987, Undersea and Hyperbaric Medical Society.
76. Howland J et al: A pilot survey of aquatic activities and related consumption of alcohol, with implications for drowning, *Pub Health Rep* 105(4):415, 1990.
77. Hunter TB, Whitehouse WM: Freshwater near-drowning: radiological aspects, *Radiology* 112:51, 1974.
78. Jacobsen JB et al: Drowning and near-drowning (letter), *Crit Care Med* 8:529, 1980.
79. Jacobsen WK et al: Correlation of spontaneous respiration and neurologic damage in near-drowning, *Crit Care Med* 11:487, 1983.
80. Jensen LR et al: Submersion injuries in children younger than 5 years in urban Utah, *West J Med* 157(6):641, 1992.
81. Julian DG: Cardiac resuscitation in the eighteenth century, *Heart Lung* 4:6, 1975.
82. Jumbelic MI, Chambliss, M: Accidental toddler drowning in 5 gallon buckets, *JAMA* 263(14): 1990.
83. Karch SB: Pathology of the heart in near-drowning, *Arch Pathol Lab Med* 109:176, 1985.
84. Karch SB: Pathology of the lung in near-drowning, *Am J Emerg Med* 4:4, 1986.
85. Karkal MB, Rasch DK, Gilbert J: Optimizing salvage in drowning and near drowning victims, *Emerg Med Rep* 10(16): 1989.
86. Kasian GF, O'Farrell NM, Linwood ME: Bathtub near-drowning of an infant in a flotation device, *CMAJ* 136: 1987.
87. Keatinge WR, Hayward MG: Sudden death in cold water and ventricular arrhythmia, *J Forensic Sci* 26:459, 1981.
88. Kemp AM, Sibert JR: Outcome in children who nearly drown: a British Isles study *Br Med J* 302(6782):931, 1991.
89. Kemp AM, Sibert JR: Epilepsy in children and the risk of drowning, *Arch Dis Child* 68(5):684, 1993.
90. King RJ: Pulmonary surfactant, *J Appl Physiol* 53:1, 1982.
91. Kizer KW: Resuscitation of submersion casualties, *Emerg Med Clin North Am* 1:643, 1983.
92. Knopp R: Near drowning, *J Am College Emerg Phys* 7:249, 1978.
93. Kram JA, Kizer KW: Submersion injury, *Emerg Med Clin North Am* 2:545, 1984.
94. Lavelle JM, Shaw KN: Near drowning: is emergency department cardiopulmonary resuscitation or intensive care unit cerebral resuscitation indicated? [see comments], *Crit Care Med* 21(3):368, 1993.
95. Levin DL: Near drowning, *Crit Care Med* 8:590, 1980.
96. Levin DL et al: Drowning and near-drowning, *Pediatr Clin North Am* 40(2):321, 1993.
97. Levinson R et al: Comparison of the effects of water immersion and saline infusion on central hemodynamics in man, *Clin Sci Mol Med* 52:343, 1977.
98. Liller KD et al: Risk factors for drowning and near-drowning among children in Hillsborough County, Florida, *Pub Health Rep* 108(3):346, 1993.
99. Lilly JK: An inexpensive portable positive end-expiratory pressure system, *Anesth Analg* 58:53, 1979.

100. Liss HP: A history of resuscitation, *Ann Emerg Med* 15:65, 1986.
101. Losonsky G: Infections associated with swimming and diving, *Undersea Biomed Res* 18:181, 1991.
102. Lougheed DW, James JM, Hall GE: Physiological studies in experimental asphyxia and drowning, *Can Med Assoc J* 40:423, 1939.
103. Mackie I: Alcohol and aquatic disasters, *Med J Aust* 1:652, 1978.
104. Mangge H et al: Late-onset miliary pneumonitis after near drowning, *Pediatr Pulmonol* 15(2):122, 1993.
105. Mann NC, Weller SC, Rauchschwalbe R: Bucket-related drownings in the United States, 1984 through 1990, *Pediatrics* 89(6, Pt 1):1068, 1992.
106. Manolios N, Mackie I: Drowning and near-drowning on Australian beaches patrolled by life-savers: a 10-year study, 1973-1983, *Med J Aust* 148:165, 1988.
107. Manser TJ, Warner JF: *Neisseria mucosus* septicemia after near drowning, *South Med J* 80(10):1323, 1987.
108. March NF, Matthews RC: New techniques in external cardiac compressions: aquatic cardiopulmonary resuscitation, *JAMA* 244:1229, 1984.
109. Martin TG: Near-drowning and cold water immersion, *Ann Emerg Med* 13:263, 1984.
110. McCallum AL et al: Two cases of accidental hypothermia with differing outcomes under identical conditions, *Aviation Space Environ Med,* 1988, in press.
111. Mebane GY: Drowning in a sea of tears, *Alert Diver* 4:8, 1993.
112. Medical news: *JAMA* 210:1683, 1969.
113. Merritt TA et al: Reduction of lung injury by human surfactant treatment in respiratory distress syndrome, *Chest* 83:27S, 1983.
114. Modell JH: Drowning, *N Engl J Med* 328(4):253.
115. Modell JH: *Pathophysiology and treatment of drowning and near-drowning,* Springfield, Ill, 1971, Charles C Thomas.
116. Modell JH: Drown versus near-drown: a discussion of definitions (editorial), *Crit Care Med* 9:351, 1981.
117. Modell JH: Serum electrolyte changes in near-drowning victims (editorial), *JAMA* 253:557, 1985.
118. Modell JH: Treatment of near-drowning: is there a role for H.Y.P.E.R. therapy? *Crit Care Med* 14:593, 1986.
119. Modell JH: Near-drowning. In Callaham ML, editor: *Current therapy in emergency medicine,* St Louis, 1986, Mosby.
120. Modell JH, Conn AW: Current neurological considerations in near-drowning (editorial), *Can Anaesth Soc J* 27:197, 1980.
121. Modell JH, Graves SA, Ketover A: Clinical course of 91 consecutive near-drowning victims, *Chest* 10:231, 1976.
122. Modell JH, Graves SA, Kuck EJ: Near-drowning: correlation of level of consciousness and survival, *Can Anaesth Soc J* 27:211, 1980.
123. Modell JH, Moya F: Effects of volume of aspirated fluid during chlorinated fresh-water drowning, *Anesthesiology* 27:663, 1966.
124. Modell JH et al: The effects of fluid volume in seawater drowning, *Ann Intern Med* 67:68, 1967.
125. Modell JH et al: Blood gas and electrolyte changes in human near-drowning victims, *JAMA* 203:99, 1968.
126. Modell JH et al: Changes in blood gases and A-aDO_2 during near-drowning, *Anesthesiology* 29:456, 1968.
127. Modell JH et al: Effects of ventilatory patterns on arterial oxygenation after near-drowning in seawater, *Anesthesiology* 40:376, 1974.
128. Newberg LA: Cerebral resuscitation: advances and controversies, *Ann Emerg Med* 13:853, 1984.
129. Noble CS, Sharp N: Drowning: its mechanism and treatment, *Can Med Assoc J* 89:402, 1963.
130. Norrish AE, Cryer PC: Work related injury in New Zealand commercial fishermen, *Br J Ind Med* 47(11):726, 1990.
131. Nowak RM: Acute adult asthma. In Rosen P et al, editors: *Emergency medicine: concepts and clinical practice,* St Louis, 1988, Mosby.
132. Oakes DD et al: Prognosis and management of victims of near-drowning, *J Trauma* 2:544, 1982.
133. Olshaker JS: Near drowning, *Emerg Med Clin North Am* 10(2):339, 1992.
134. Orlowski JP: Prognostic factors in drowning and near-drowning, *J Am Coll Emerg Phys* 8:176, 1979.
135. Orlowski JP: Drowning, near-drowning and ice-water submersions, *Pediatr Clin North Am* 34:75, 1987.
136. Orlowski JP: Vomiting as a complication of the Heimlich maneuver, *JAMA* 258:512, 1987.
137. Orlowski JP, Abulleil MM, Phillips JM: Effects of tonicities of saline solutions on pulmonary injury in drowning, *Crit Care Med* 15:126, 1987.
138. Orlowski JP, Rothner AD, Lueders H: Submersion accidents in children with epilepsy, *Am J Dis Child* 136:777, 1982.
139. Orlowski JP et al: The hemodynamic and cardiovascular effects of near drowning in hypotonic, isotonic, or hypertonic solutions, *Ann Emerg Med* 18:1044, 1989.
140. Ornato JP: The resuscitation of near-drowning victims, *JAMA* 256:75, 1986.
141. Pearn JH: Secondary drowning in children, *Br Med J* 281:1103, 1980.
142. Pearn J: The management of near-drowning, *Br Med J* 291:1447, 1985.
143. Pearn J: Why children drown, *Aust J Paediatr* 22:161, 1986.
144. Pearn JH, Bart RD, Yamaoka R: Neurologic sequelae after childhood near-drowning: a total population study from Hawaii, *Pediatrics* 65:187, 1979.
145. Pearn J, Nixon J: Bathtub immersion accidents involving children, *Med J Aust* 1:211, 1977.
146. Peterson B: Morbidity of childhood near-drowning, *Pediatrics* 59:364, 1977.
147. Peura DA, Johnson LF: Cimetidine for prevention and treatment of gastroduodenal mucosal lesions in patients in an intensive care unit, *Ann Intern Med* 103:173, 1985.
148. Pitt WR, Balanda KP: Childhood drowning and near-drowning in Brisbane: the contribution of domestic pools, *Med J Aust* 154(10):661, 1991.
149. *The Pittsburgh Press,* May 8, 1987, p 1.
150. Plueckhahn VD: Drowning: community aspects, *Med J Aust* 2:226, 1979.
151. Pratt FD, Haynes BE: Incidence of "secondary drowning" after saltwater submersion, *Ann Emerg Med* 15:1084, 1986.
152. Quan L: Drowning issues in resuscitation, *Ann Emerg Med* 22(2, Pt 2):366, 1993.
153. Quan L, Kinder D: Pediatric submersions: prehospital predictors of outcome, *Pediatrics* 90(6):909, 1992.
154. Ramey CA, Ramey DN, Hayward JS: The dive response of children in relation to cold water near-drowning, *J Appl Physiol* 63:665. 1987.
155. Robertson C, Levison H: Bronchodilators in asthma, *Chest* 87:64S, 1985.
156. Robinson MD, Seward PN: Submersion injury in children, *Pediatr Emerg Care* 3:44, 1987.
157. Rockett IR, Smith GS: Covert suicide among elderly Japanese females: questioning unintentional drownings, *Soc Sci Med* 36(11):1467, 1993.
158. Rosenbaum HT, Thompson WL, Ruller RH: Radiographic pulmonary changes in near-drowning, *Radiology* 83:306.
159. Rowe MI, Arango A, Allington G: Profile of pediatric drowning victims in a water-oriented society, *J Trauma* 17:587, 1977.
160. Ruben A, Ruben H: Artificial respiration: flow of water from lung and stomach, *Lancet* 1:780, 1962.
161. Rubenstein E: Water-related accidents, *Sci Am Med* 8(III):1, 1986.
162. Runyan CW, Gerken EA: Epidemiology and prevention of adolescent injury, *JAMA* 262(16): 1989.
163. Rutledge RR, Flor RJ: The use of mechanical ventilation with positive end-expiratory pressure in the treatment of near-drowning, *Anesthesiology* 38:194, 1973.

164. Safar P: *Cardiopulmonary cerebral resuscitation,* Stavanger, Norway, 1981, AS Laerdal.
165. Safar P: Recent advances in cardiopulmonary cerebral resuscitation: a review, *Ann Emerg Med* 13:856, 1984.
166. Schnitzer PG, Landen DD, Russell JC: Occupational injury deaths in Alaska's fishing industry, 1980 through 1988, *Am J Pub Health* 83(5):685, 1993.
167. Schuman SH et al: The iceberg phenomenon of near-drowning, *Crit Care Med* 4:127, 1976.
168. Schuman SH et al: Risk of drowning: an iceberg phenomenon, *J Am Coll Emerg Phys* 6:139, 1977.
169. Scott PH, Eigen H: Immersion accidents involving pails of water in the home, *J Pediatr* 92:282, 1980.
170. Segarra F, Redding RA: Modern concepts about drowning, *Can Med Assoc J* 110:1057, 1974.
171. Shelhamer JH, Nathanson C, Parilloje: Positive end-expiratory pressure in adults, *JAMA* 251:2692, 1984.
172. Siebke H et al: Survival after 40 minutes submersion without cerebral sequelae, *Lancet* 1:1275, 1975.
173. Southwick FS, Dalglish PH: Recovery after prolonged asystolic arrest in profound hypothermia, *JAMA* 243:1250, 1980.
174. Stacpoole PW: Lactic acidosis: the case against bicarbonate therapy (editorial), *Ann Intern Med* 105:276, 1986.
175. Sterba JA, Lundgren CEG: Breath-hold duration in man and the diving response induced by face immersion, *Undersea Biomed Res* 15(5):361, 1988.
176. Stewart RD: Drowning and near-drowning, *Top Emerg Med* 2:63, 1980.
177. Stewart RD et al: Influence of mask design on bag-mask ventilation, *Ann Emerg Med* 14:403, 1985.
178. Swann HG, Spafford NR: Body salt and water changes during fresh and seawater drowning, *Texas Rep Biol Med* 9:356, 1951.
179. *The Toronto Star,* August 10, 1987, p 1.
180. *The Toronto Sun,* June 16, 1978, p 2.
181. US Consumer Product Safety Commission and National Spa and Pool Institute: *National Pool and Spa Safety Conference: final report,* May 14, 1985.
182. Van Herringen JR et al: Treatment of the respiratory distress syndrome following nondirect pulmonary trauma with positive end-expiratory pressure, with special emphasis on near-drowning, *Chest* 66:305, 1974.
183. Waugh WH: Potential use of warm butyl alcohol vapor as adjunct agent in the emergency treatment of sea water wet near-drowning, *Am J Emerg Med* 11(1):20, 1993.
184. Wegener FH, Edwards RM: Cerebral support for near-drowned children in a temperate environment, *Med J Aust* 2:135, 1980.
185. Weil MH et al: Difference in acid-base state between venous and arterial blood during cardiopulmonary resuscitation, *N Engl J Med* 315:153, 1986.
186. Weiss LD et al: The development of a water rescue unit in an urban EMS system, *Ann Emerg Med* 18:884, 1989.
187. Werner JZ et al: No improvement in pulmonary status by gravity drainage or abdominal thrusts after sea water near-drowning in dogs, *Anesthesiology* 57:A81, 1982.
188. Westacott P: A most unlikely patient, *Med J Aust* 2:157, 1980.
189. Yagil Y et al: Near drowning in the Dead Sea: electrolyte imbalance and therapeutic implications, *Arch Intern Med* 145:50, 1985.
190. Yatsu F: Cardiopulmonary-cerebral resuscitation (editorial), *N Engl J Med* 314:440, 1986.
191. Young RSK, Zalneraitis EL, Dooling EC: Neurological outcome in cold water drowning, *JAMA* 244:1233, 1980.

49 WHITE-WATER MEDICINE AND RESCUE

Eric A. Weiss

Rivers have what man most respects and longs for in his own life and thought—a capacity for renewal and replenishment, continual energy, creativity, cleansing.

John M. Kauffman, *Flow East*

Rafting, canoeing, and kayaking have become the third largest outdoor recreation industry in the United States.[34] Over 19 million people go canoeing and kayaking each year, and more than 57 million enjoy rafting.[6] Combined participation in river sports is growing at a rate of 15% annually.[35,43] Kayaks and rafts are also being employed by law enforcement officers, park rangers, and game wardens to patrol and manage their territories.[29] New equipment designs, such as self-bailing inflatable rafts and polyethylene plastic kayaks, have opened up more difficult rivers for exploration and commercial recreation.

It is not surprising that the number of river-related accidents and deaths has also increased dramatically. The American Canoe Association reports that approximately 130 white-water fatalities occur each year.[43] This chapter examines the unique and dynamic hazards associated with rivers and white-water paddling. Safety equipment, accident prevention, common injuries, environmental hazards, medical management, and swift water rescue are also reviewed.

Historical Aspects

White-water boating as a recreational activity began in the United States in earnest during the late nineteenth century when adventurers attempted to emulate Major Wesley Powell's Colorado River expedition by rowing boats down many of the West's large rivers.[24] These heavy wooden boats were replaced by inflatable rafts after the Second World War, when surplus neoprene assault boats and life rafts became available for civilian use.[3] In 1966, fewer than 500 people boated the Colorado River through the Grand Canyon in an entire year. Recently, the figure exceeded 500 per day.[24]

Rafting did not become popular in the eastern United States until the early 1960s. In 1968, commercially guided raft trips were offered for the first time on the New River in West Virginia.[45] The Chattooga River in Georgia attracted many rafters after the movie *Deliverance* was filmed there in 1971. The Youghiogheny River in Pennsylvania and the South Fork of the American River in northern California have become the two most heavily rafted rivers in the country.

Technologic advances have revolutionized river running. Electronically welded plastic has largely replaced rubber as the primary material employed in raft construction, making the vessels lighter, stronger, and easier to repair. Self-bailing rafts, introduced in 1983, are now ubiquitous and provide greater maneuverability, allowing rafters to run rivers previously considered too difficult and dangerous. Unfortunately, greater mobility has been paralleled by an increase in the number of accidents occurring far from medical care.

A major innovation in kayaking was the development of the plastic kayak, first manufactured in 1972 by the Holloform Company.[45] (See Color Plate 110.) Kayaks had been previously constructed from resinous materials such as fiberglass and Kevlar, which were more fragile and less likely to "broach," or wrap around rocks. Paddlers were reluctant to run steep, rocky rivers for fear of breaking their boats. Most recreational white-water kayaks are now made of molded polyethylene plastic, which does not break apart and has the potential to fold when broached or pinned, trapping the paddler. Kayakers with "indestructible" boats are pushing the limits of navigable rivers. Even Niagara Falls has been successfully run by a kayaker!

The enormous popularity of rafting and kayaking has led to exponential growth of professional guide services. In 1990, 35 million people were taken down U.S. rivers by commercial companies.[43] Faced with increased competition, guide services have been leading inexperienced clients with little formal training and few practical skills into difficult and dangerous rivers (Fig. 49-1). In the summer of 1988, five U.S. executives died after their raft flipped on the Chilco River in British Columbia. One of the survivors was reported to have said, "We looked at white water as sort of a roller coaster ride."[41]

Equipment

The dynamic and unpredictable nature of rivers can turn any mishap into a tragedy. For this reason, the initial mission of white-water medicine is to emphasize safety and accident prevention.

According to the U.S. Coast Guard's boating accident statistics, the most common factor contributing to white-water-related deaths is failure to wear a personal flotation device (PFD, or life jacket).[43] Exposure to cold river water can stimulate respiratory and cardiovascular reflexes, making it difficult for a swimmer to keep his or her head above water (maintain freeboard) (see Chapter 4).[25] The Coast Guard is charged with regulating and testing life jackets and classifies PFDs into five types. Of these, only two types are commonly used in white-water sports.

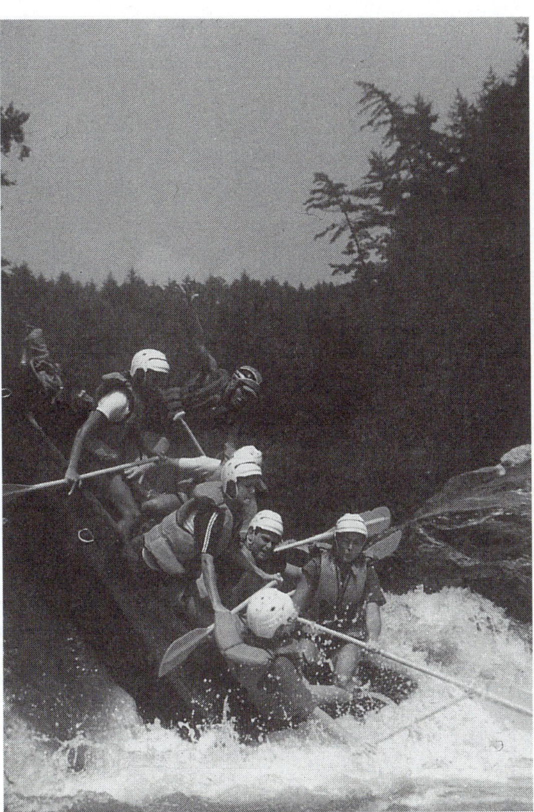

Fig. 49-1 Class V commercial rafting on the Chattooga River, Georgia. (Courtesy Robert Harrison, Whetstone Photography.)

The type III PFD, a vest-type jacket favored by most paddlers, permits greater mobility and comfort. The Coast Guard requires that type III PFDs have a minimum of 15½ pounds of flotation (lift). Because most adults effectively weigh between 10 and 12 pounds in the water, this allows at least 3½ pounds of effective required buoyancy.

Type V PFDs are used by commercial outfitters because they provide greater flotation and are constructed asymmetrically to turn an unconscious wearer face up.

A PFD should fit snugly and not ride up over the head when a person is in the water. Because even a well-fitting life jacket can be pulled off by turbulent water, some manufacturers now include crotch straps as an added safety feature. Testifying before a congressional subcommittee, the president of the National Transportation Safety Association cited the Chilco River accident to support his contention that crotch straps be made mandatory on all white water–use life jackets. Several survivors reported that their life jackets rode up over their heads and did not keep their faces above water.

Life jackets with built-in rescue harnesses, pioneered by the Europeans, are now widely available in the United States. A quick-release belt allows the wearer to attempt a strong swimmer rescue, but also to get free of the tethering line quickly in an emergency.

Beyond flotation, life jackets have other benefits that make them highly useful in wilderness settings. Their insulating properties help prevent hypothermia. The closed-cell foam flotation material acts as thoracic padding during falls on slippery rocks or when swimming rapids after exiting the craft. Life jackets also make excellent improvised splints; they can be fashioned into cervical collars, cylindrical knee braces, or padded ankle stirrups.

Helmets should be worn by all white-water boaters. Surveys have shown that head trauma after capsizing comprises 10% to 17% of all kayaking accidents.[29,44]

Another vital piece of safety equipment is a rope, which should be readily accessible and secured in a manner that facilitates rapid deployment and prevents entanglement. Throw ropes for river use should float, have a certain amount of dynamic stretch, and not absorb water. Self-contained throw bags have virtually replaced coiled ropes for river use and generally hold about 50 to 75 feet of ⅜-inch polypropylene rope inside a nylon stuff sack. Newer styles can be attached to life jackets for rapid access. They can also be thrown to rescuers by a paddler who is pinned or broached. Commercial outfitters and large groups of rafters should carry at least one 300-foot-long static rope to be used for Telfar lowers and Tyroleans and other rescue situations where mechanical advantages are employed.

Knives should be readily accessible. Fixed blades are preferable to folding ones unless the folded blade can be opened easily with one hand. Double-edged blades can cut in two directions and thus require minimal handling in precarious situations. Some modern knives designed for kayakers feature serrated edges that can cut through plastic boats during entrapment.

Whistles should be worn so paddlers can alert others that an accident has occurred. Paddlers are often spread out over the course of a rapid, and yelling over the roar of the water is usually a frustrating and fruitless endeavor.

Placing adequate barriers between the human body and the environment is of paramount importance in aquatic sports. Functional, insulated clothing should be considered a mandatory safety item to prevent hypothermia. Cotton is a poor choice for river wear; it loses all of its insulating properties when wet and dries slowly. Newer synthetics such as polypropylene and polyester pile absorb no more than 1% of their weight in water and maintain thermal insulating qualities when wet.[27] When combined with a nylon or Gore-Tex paddling jacket, a synthetic underlayer provides effective protection from cold and wind.

Wet suits, previously considered to be optimal garments for paddlers in extreme conditions, are stiff and somewhat constricting.[1] The dry suit, with tight-fitting latex seals at the wrist, ankle, and neck, is the new "gold standard" for cold water boating. By sealing water out and preventing evaporative heat loss, the dry suit can keep a paddler warm even during winter conditions.[17]

Overheating is occasionally a problem with dry suits. Recently a dry suit contributed to profound and unexpected hyperthermia in a kayaker who had suffered a submersion injury in cold water.[4]

River Hazards

The International Scale of River Difficulty grades rivers and rapids into classes I to VI. An American version of this rating has been adopted by the American Whitewater Affiliation (AWA) for most U.S. rivers (see Box 49-1).[42]

BOX 49-1
AMERICAN VERSION OF THE INTERNATIONAL SCALE OF RIVER DIFFICULTY*

CLASS I: EASY

Fast-moving water with riffles and small waves. Few obstructions, all obvious and easily avoided with little training. Risk to swimmers is slight; self-rescue is easy.

CLASS II: NOVICE

Straightforward rapids with wide, clear channels that are evident without scouting. Occasional maneuvering may be required, but rocks and medium-sized waves are easily avoided by trained paddlers. Swimmers are seldom injured, and group assistance, while helpful, is seldom needed.

CLASS III: INTERMEDIATE

Rapids with moderate, irregular waves that may be difficult to avoid and can swamp an open canoe. Complex maneuvers in fast current and good boat control in tight passages or around ledges are often required; large waves or strainers may be present but are easily avoided. Strong eddies and powerful current effects can be found, particularly on large-volume rivers. Scouting is advisable for inexperienced parties. Injuries while swimming are rare; self-rescue is usually easy, but group assistance may be required to avoid long swims.

CLASS IV: ADVANCED

Intense, powerful but predictable rapids requiring precise boat handling in turbulent water. The advanced river may feature large, unavoidable waves and holes or constricted passages that demand fast maneuvers under pressure. A fast, reliable eddy turn may be needed to initiate maneuvers, scout rapids, or rest. Rapids may require "must" moves above dangerous hazards. Scouting is necessary the first time down. Risk of injury to swimmers is moderate to high, and water conditions may make self-rescue difficult. Group assistance for rescue is often essential but requires practiced skills. A strong Eskimo roll is highly recommended.

CLASS V: EXPERT

Extremely long, obstructed, or violent rapids that expose a paddler to above-average danger. Drops may contain large, unavoidable waves and holes or steep, congested chutes with complex, demanding routes. Rapids may continue for long distances between pools, demanding a high level of fitness. Eddies may be small, turbulent, or difficult to reach. At the high end of the scale, several of these factors may be combined. Scouting is mandatory but often difficult. Swims are dangerous, and rescue is difficult even for experts. A very reliable Eskimo roll, proper equipment, extensive experience, and practiced rescue skills are essential for survival.

CLASS VI: EXTREME

Class VI runs exemplify the extremes of difficulty, unpredictability, and danger. The consequences of errors are very severe, and rescue may be impossible. For teams of experts only, at favorable water levels, after close inspection and taking all precautions. This class does not represent drops believed to be unrunnable, but may include rapids that are only occasionally run.

From *Safety code of the American Whitewater Affiliation,* Phoenicia, NY, 1989, American Whitewater Affiliation.

Some western rivers use the Grand Canyon System, which rates rapids on a scale from 1 to 10. Neither scale is a truly objective standard; individual and regional variations are common, and the margin of difficulty for a particular rapid may differ significantly for kayaks and rafts. Unfortunately, important safety parameters such as water temperature, remoteness, and evacuation potential are not taken into consideration.

The difficulty of a river generally increases with the volume of flow and the average gradient. As the water level rises, its speed and power increase exponentially, raising the difficulty of most rapids.[3] Occasionally, however, a rapid becomes easier as the added water submerges hazardous obstacles.

Hydraulics, also known as holes, reversals, rollers, suckholes, and pour-overs, are the most common hazards in rivers. A hydraulic is created when water flows over an obstacle, causing a depression that produces a relative vacuum within which the downstream water recirculates (Fig. 49-2). Rafts and kayaks can be turned upside down by the force of a hydraulic, and if the reversal currents are strong enough, crafts and people can become trapped in the recirculating flow. When proceeding into a rapid that contains a hazardous hydraulic, one of the group should preset a rope below the hole to facilitate rescue.

Hydraulics release water downstream from beneath the surface. This may be the only avenue of escape for a swimmer. Escape from a strong hydraulic may require a person to stay submerged and to resist the urge to return immediately to the surface. Surfacing too early can result in recirculation. Fortunately, most hydraulics eventually release people regardless of what action they take.

Novice paddlers often misjudge the force of hydraulics. It is not the height of the drop that generates the recirculating power, but rather the shape and angle of the obstruction, combined with water volume and adjacent eddy currents.

Low-head dams or weirs form massive hydraulics with enormous recirculating potential. In the Binghamton Dam disaster of 1975, a 13½-foot Boston whaler with a 20-horsepower engine was pulled into a hydraulic while attempting a rescue, resulting in the deaths of three firefighters.[39]

Undercut rocks are boulders or ledges that have been eroded just beneath the water surface. They can be difficult to recognize and pose significant risks for entrapment and drowning, even in class II rapids.

The potential for entrapment can also occur when swimmers attempt to stand up and walk in swift-moving currents. A foot can become wedged in an undercut rock or between rocks beneath the surface, causing the victim to lose his or her balance and fall face down into the river (Fig. 49-3, *A*). With the foot entrapped, the victim cannot regain an upright or even face-up position. This type of mishap has caused drownings in water less than 3 feet deep.

A swimmer in a rapid should assume a supine position, with feet at the surface and pointed downstream to serve as shock absorbers. This position minimizes the potential for both foot entrapment and head and neck trauma (Fig. 49-3, *B*).

Strainers are obstacles, such as fallen trees, bridge debris, or driftwood lodged between rocks or jutting out from the shore, that allow water to pass through (sieve effect) while trapping the swimmer or boater. Flooded rivers, a favorite of expert boaters, often develop many new strainers as riverbank debris is washed into the flow. In the summer of 1987, five paddlers drowned when their raft struck a large strainer on Canada's Ellaho River.[41]

Negotiating a strainer requires special tactics. The safest option for the swimmer is to swim aggressively into the strainer head first rather than feet first, and then attempt to climb over the debris (Fig. 49-4, *A*). Approaching a strainer feet first may lead to underwater entrapment (Fig. 49-4, *B*).

Human-made hazards can also pose a threat to river runners. Bridge pilings, submerged automobiles, dams, and low-hanging power lines can pin or injure boaters.

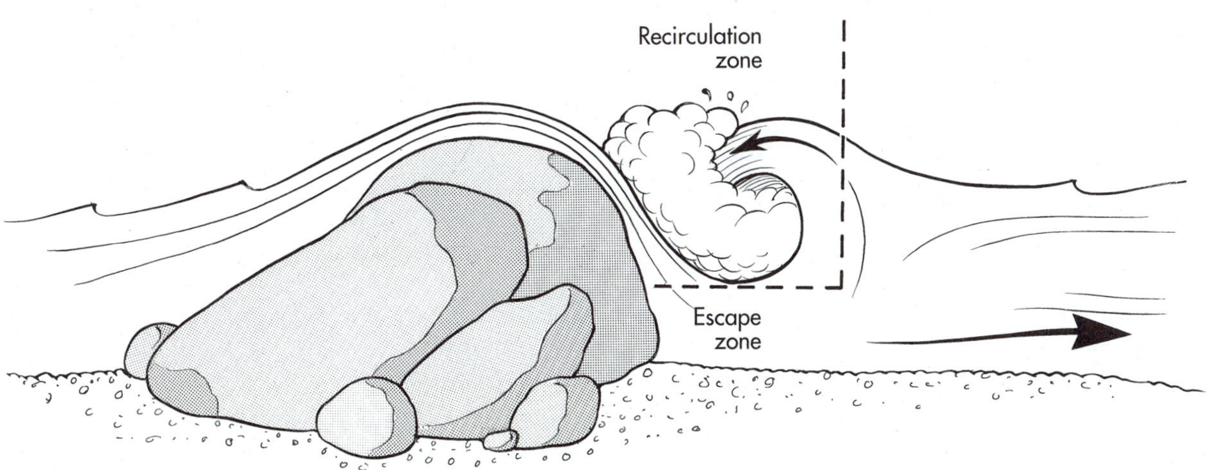

Fig. 49-2 Recirculating currents created by a hydraulic. Water and "swimmers" are released downstream beneath the surface.

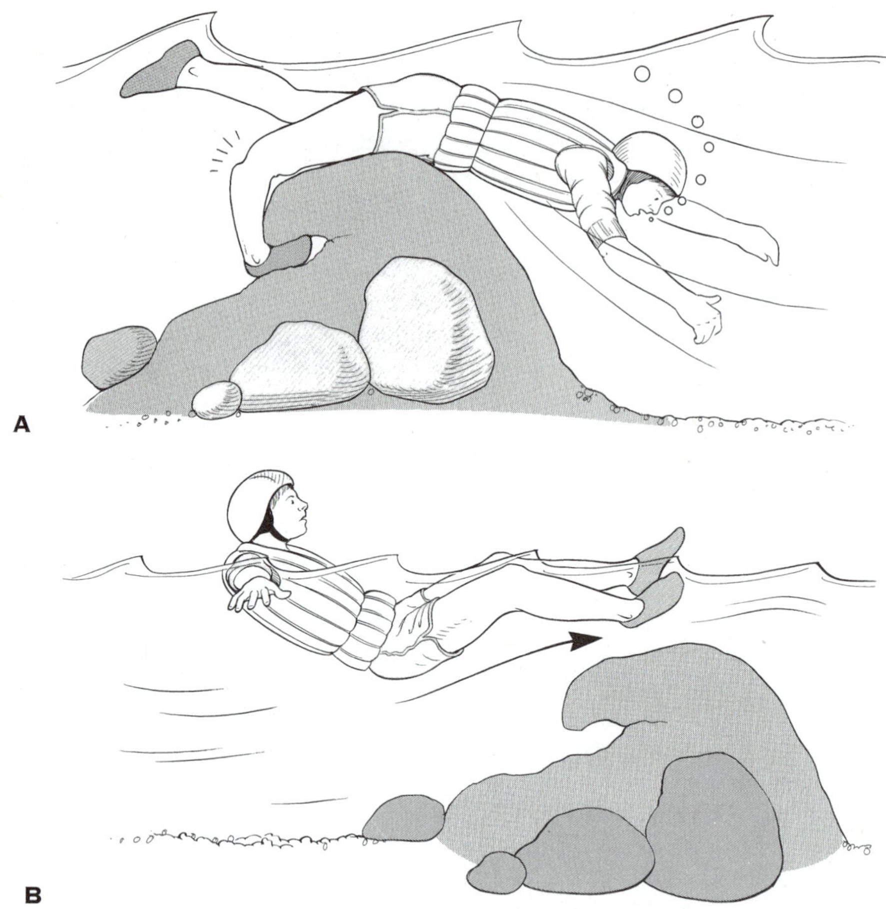

Fig. 49-3 **A,** Attempting to stand up in shallow water can produce foot entrapment in an undercut rock. **B,** Proper way to swim while in a rapid.

A broach occurs when a boat wraps sideways around an obstacle or when both bow and stern become stuck on separate obstacles simultaneously. Common obstacles include boulders, trees, bridge pilings, and ledges protruding from canyon walls. Drowning can occur if the paddler leans upstream away from the obstacle and flips upside down while still broached or if the boat collapses and entraps the victim (Fig. 49-5).

A vertical pin happens when a kayaker plunges over a drop and the end of the boat becomes trapped between rocks beneath the surface. The force of the water can fold a plastic kayak over on itself, trapping the occupant upside down beneath the surface (Fig. 49-6).

A survey of 365 members of the American Whitewater Affiliation revealed that 33% of serious kayaking incidents and 41% of open canoeing mishaps involved either pinning or broaching (Table 49-1).[44] In a separate survey of 500 paddlers between 1989 and 1993, 42% of kayaking fatalities resulted from vertical pins, broaches, or entrapments in strainers.

Kayak construction can have important safety implications in both broach and pin situations. The force of the current against the deck of the boat or back of the paddler can make it impossible for the victim to extract his or her legs and escape. European boat makers have developed kayaks with larger cockpits that make it easier to raise the knees out. Transverse bulkhead-type foot braces have replaced pedal-type braces to prevent the kayaker from being shoved forward in the boat. This feature ensures the escape potential offered by larger cockpits. One of the compromises of the larger cockpit, however, is that the sprayskirt is more likely to come off in turbulent water.

Another safety feature, the Safety Deck System (Outdoor Safety Systems, 140 Quaker Road, Princeton, NJ 08540), uses a manually releasable foredeck section that can be jettisoned by the paddler for emergency exit (Fig. 49-7). During normal use, this deckplate is securely fastened to the boat and does not alter its shape or performance. The Safety Deck System has been tested extensively with positive results, but unfortunately its cost has precluded commercial development.

Submersion Accidents

Almost all fatalities on rivers result from submersion. Each year the River Safety Task Force of the Ameri-

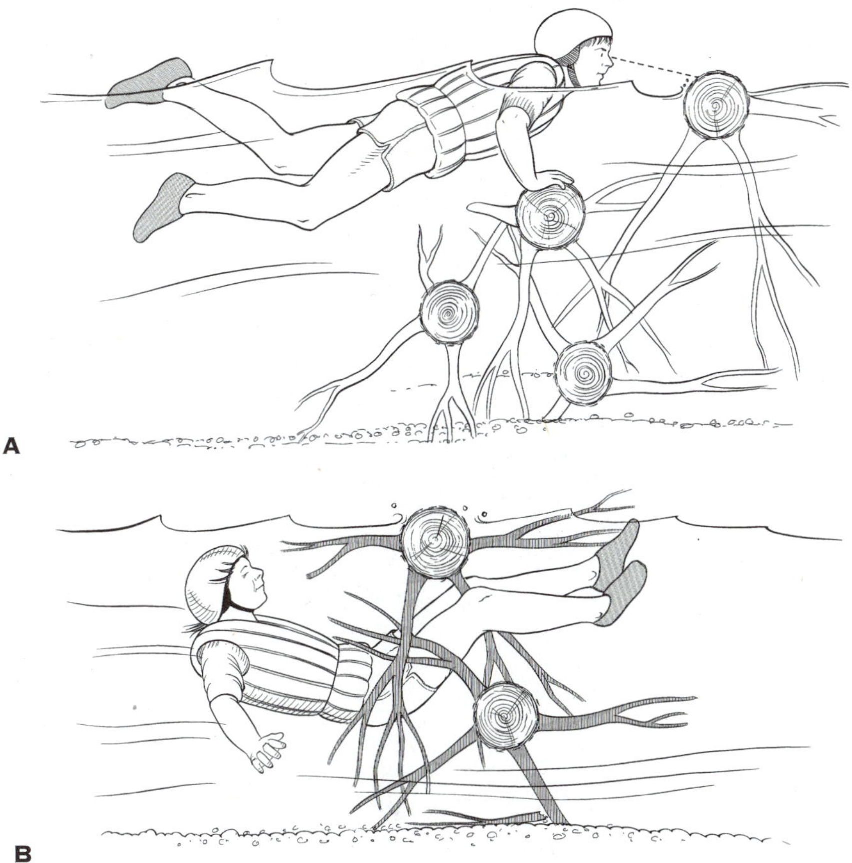

Fig. 49-4 **A,** Proper approach to a strainer. **B,** Incorrect approach to a strainer.

Table 49-1 Serious White-Water-Related Incidents

Incident	Number	Percentage of Accidents
Vertical pin entrapment	18	8
Broach entrapment	46	21
Rock sieve entrapment	16	7
Undercut rock entrapment	23	10
Recirculation in hydraulic	47	21
Long swim	42	19

From Wallace D: *AWA J* 3:27, 1991.

can Canoe Association compiles accounts of drownings and other accidents. Every 3 years it publishes the *River Safety Report,* which chronicles and analyzes these accidents.[39-41,43]

Most submersion fatalities occur after paddlers unexpectedly swim from their boats or become trapped in them underwater. The exact cause of drowning often remains unclear and is inexplicably blamed on immersion hypothermia. Although hypothermia induces impaired judgment and coordination and may be an important contributing factor, immersion hypothermia is probably never the sole cause of death.[46] Studies by Hayward and others have shown that seminude subjects are able to maintain normal core temperatures for 15 to 20 minutes in 10° C water.[19,20] Continuous immersion for up to 1 hour would be required to produce profound hypothermia.[20]

Cold water immersion precipitates drowning by three other mechanisms. Sudden cold water immersion produces profound cardiovascular and respiratory responses. Reflex sympathetic output can markedly increase blood pressure and heart rate, resulting in lethal arrhythmias.[16,25,26]

An immediate and involuntary gasp occurs after cold water immersion. This is followed by hyperventilation.[8] Pulmonary ventilation increases up to fivefold because of increased tidal volume and respiratory rate.[38] The initial gasp can result in aspiration of water and laryngospasm. Hyperventilation produces respiratory alkalosis with resultant muscle tetany and cerebral hypoperfusion.[8] This response can increase the risk of drowning in a person struggling to maintain an airway freeboard in rough water.

The respiratory stimulation produced by cold water immersion significantly decreases breath-holding duration.[21] This fact has enormous implications for kayakers who must hold their breath while attempting to roll up a boat after flip-

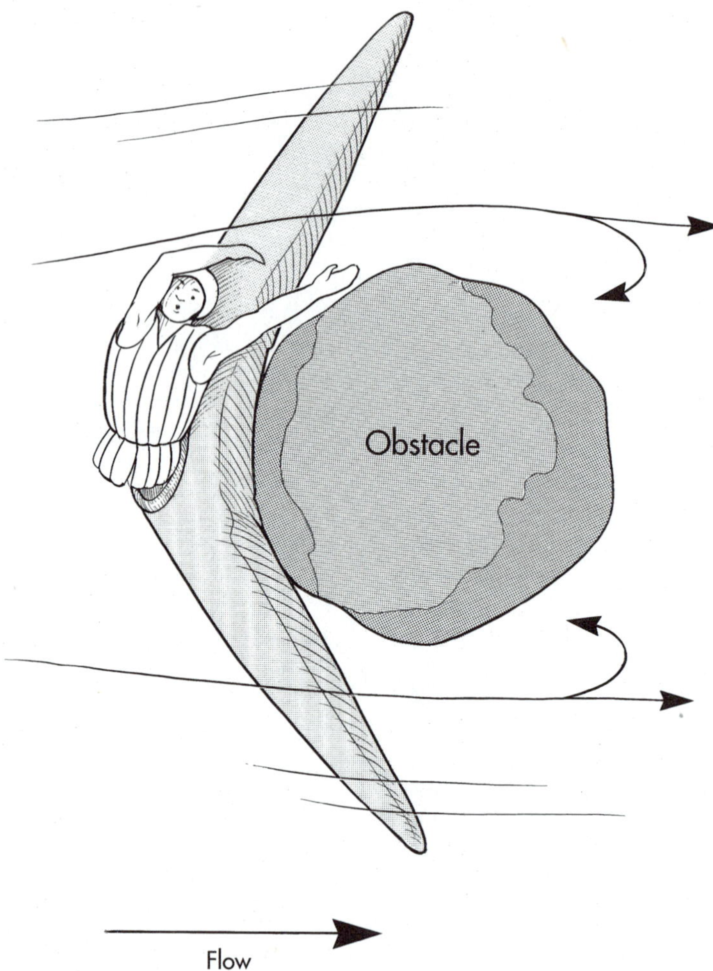

Fig. 49-5 Broach.

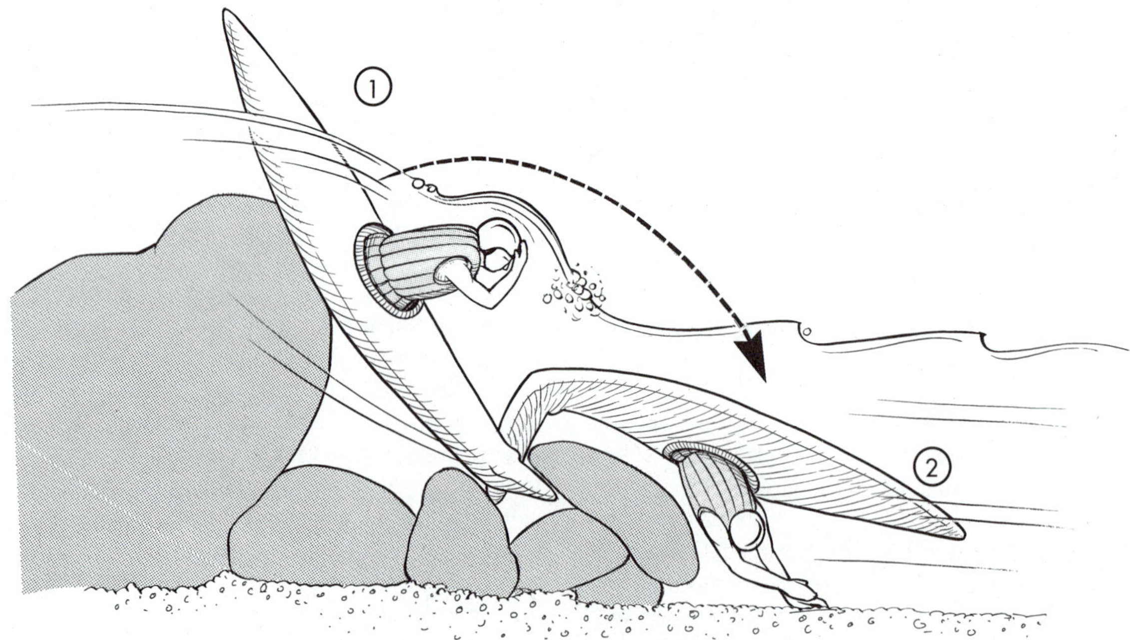

Fig. 49-6 *1*, Vertical pin. *2*, Pitchpole pin.

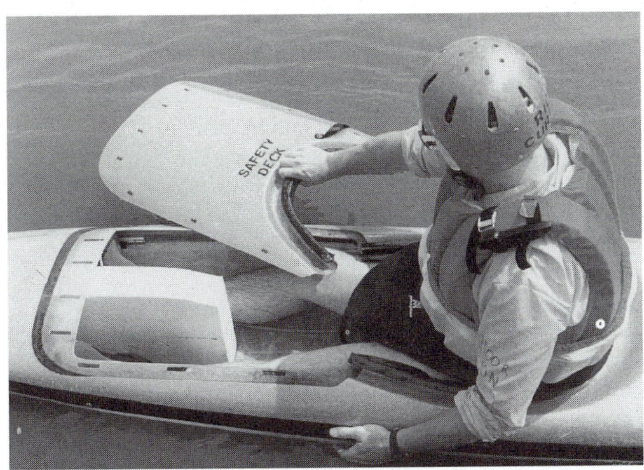

Fig. 49-7 Safety Deck system, which offers an emergency exit for a kayaker in distress.

ping upside down. This probably accounts for the unexplained swims by expert kayakers who sometimes fail to right themselves after flipping in cold water.

Peripheral cold water–induced vasoconstriction exacerbates rapid cooling of muscles and nerves in the extremities, resulting in loss of strength and coordination.[38] The ability to swim, maintain freeboard, avoid obstacles, and climb from the river may be greatly impaired.[28] Even when the air temperature is warm, paddlers running cold water rivers should wear sufficiently insulated clothing.

The combination of hyperventilation and muscle dysfunction can be lethal for a swimmer in rough water. A PFD helps but does not prevent even small waves from submerging a swimmer's head.[15] These dangers make imperative the need to preset safety systems in significant rapids and rescue swimmers first. Unfortunately, paddlers have drowned when their companions chased after equipment, assuming that the swimmer could climb out of the river without assistance.[40,42]

Safety kayaks with enhanced buoyancy are recommended on commercial raft trips, since they provide additional flotation for clients who fall overboard.

Although some maintain that the respiratory and cardiovascular reflexes can be abolished by repeated exposure of the face to cold water, there are currently no scientific data to support this theory of acclimatization.

Trauma

A survey of commercial raft clients revealed that the most common significant injury was a sprained or fractured ankle.[45] Ironically, these injuries usually occur out of the water when persons walk on loose, wet, and slippery rocks during scouting and portaging or when entering or leaving the river. Ankle and other lower extremity injuries also occur on the river when rafters are tossed onto each other in rapids.

Kayakers are prone to ankle injuries from forced dorsiflexion or inversion when the bow of the boat hits an obstruction. The feet are held against the narrow horizontal braces while the heels are pushed underneath, or the entire ankle is inverted. European- and some American-designed kayaks with bulkhead foot braces have reduced this problem.

Management of foot and ankle injuries should begin with ice, elevation, and compression to reduce swelling. Cold river water is usually substituted for ice. Compression wrapping is important after icing to prevent swelling from reflex vasodilation. Splinting is important to reduce pain and edema and to limit exacerbation of the injury during evacuation. Pneumatic splints, still carried by many raft companies, provide adequate support and compression but are prone to overinflation when heated by the sun. Zippers often malfunction when they rust or jam with sand. Neurovascular integrity must be checked frequently with an air splint. Ankle splints can be improvised from life jackets, kayak float bags, articles of clothing, or a SAM splint.

Strains are common in white-water sports. Researchers at Dalhousie University in Halifax, Nova Scotia, analyzed dynamic electromyographic potentials of the various muscle groups used in kayaking and then correlated them with videotaped sequences.[32] Muscles used most often in kayaking that are prone to strain injury are shoulder extensors (latissimus dorsi, teres major, pectoralis major). Medial scapula rotators (rhomboideus major and minor, pectoralis minor), lateral scapula rotators (pectoralis minor, serratus anterior), shoulder flexors and horizontal adductors (anterior deltoideus, pectoralis major, coracobrachialis), elbow extensors (triceps), and spine erector muscles. Any training program for kayakers needs to emphasize conditioning of these muscle groups.

Back strain afflicts rafters, kayakers, and canoers. Rafters are prone to back injuries while portaging, pushing stuck rafts off rocks, and carrying the crafts to and from the river. Raft guides are notorious for suffering back strain when pulling capsized customers, who often weigh more than they do, back into the rafts. Kayakers and canoers injure their backs lifting water-laden boats and loading their crafts onto automobile roofs. Sitting for prolonged periods with legs extended and minimal back support leads to muscle fatigue in kayakers, compounding the potential for injury.

Repetitive dorsiflexion of the wrist required to operate an offset (feathered) kayak paddle produces tendinitis and synovitis.[31] A paddle constructed with a 75- to 80-degree offset instead of the traditional 90 degrees can reduce wrist stress. Aspirin or nonsteroidal antiinflammatory agents ingested 30 minutes before paddling, combined with ice application afterward, may be beneficial. Wrist supports provide limited relief.

The injury most often associated with kayaking is anterior shoulder dislocation. Various surveys have placed its incidence in kayakers at 10% to 16%, making it the second most common white-water-related injury (Table

49-2).[5,30,44,45] The maneuver most notorious for precipitating this injury is the high brace. Often used while supporting the kayaker in a hydraulic, surfing on a wave, or rolling the kayak upright after a flip, the high brace entails abduction of the humerus, with external rotation of the glenohumeral joint (Fig. 49-8). If the arm becomes extended behind the midline plane of the body by the force of the current, the triad of abduction, external rotation, and extension of the shoulder can stretch or rupture the glenoid labrum and capsule, resulting in anterior subluxation or dislocation.[37] The paddle acts as a lever to increase the force on the glenohumeral joint.

To minimize the risk of shoulder dislocation, the preferred method of bracing is the "low brace," in which the arm is held in internal rotation and close to the body (adduction). While initially awkward for the novice paddler, this bracing maneuver is inherently stronger and more versatile because it allows backpaddling out of a hydraulic. Exercises that strengthen the rotator cuff and deltoideus, triceps, and pectoralis muscles reinforce the glenohumeral joint.

Table 49-2 Common White-Water-Related Injuries, 1980-1991 (N = 85)

Injury Type	Number	Percentage of Injuries
Shoulder dislocation	14	16.5
Near drowning	11	12.9
Fractures	15	17.6
Head and neck	6	7.0
Hypothermia	4	4.7
Leg injuries	11	12.9
Lacerations	9	10.5
Fatalities	7	8.2

From Wallace D: *AWA J* 3:27, 1991.

The paddler with a dislocation is usually aware that something has gone wrong and holds the extremity away from the body, unable to bring the arm across the chest.[37] The shoulder may appear square because of anterior, medial, and inferior displacement of the humeral head into a subcoracoid position.

Although on-scene reduction of shoulder dislocations is controversial, immediate relief of pain, curtailment of ongoing injury, and subsequent ability to function more actively in evacuation are strong reasons to do it. Several techniques have been advocated for reduction.[36] The key element is rapid initiation, since the longer a shoulder remains dislocated, the more difficult becomes the eventual reduction. Relocation is often delayed because river corridors rarely afford rapid access to a flat and comfortable area upon which to place a patient in the supine or prone position, a requirement for most techniques.

For river and other wilderness settings, I advocate reduction with the patient standing (Fig. 49-9). As soon as the diagnosis is made, the patient bends forward at the waist while the rescuer supports the chest with one hand. With the other hand, the rescuer grabs the patient's wrist and applies steady downward traction and external rotation. While maintaining traction, the rescuer can slowly flex the shoulder by moving it in a cephalad direction until reduction is obtained. If two rescuers are available, one should support the patient at the chest while the other pulls countertraction and flexion at the arm. Scapular manipulation by adducting the inferior tip using thumb pressure and stabilizing the superior aspect of the scapula with the cephalad hand may augment reduction (Fig. 49-10).[33,36] One should always monitor circulation and

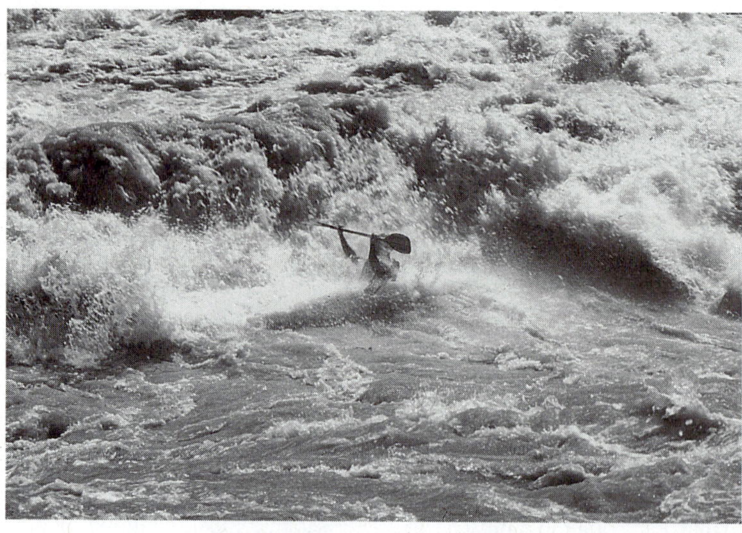

Fig. 49-8 High brace maneuver.

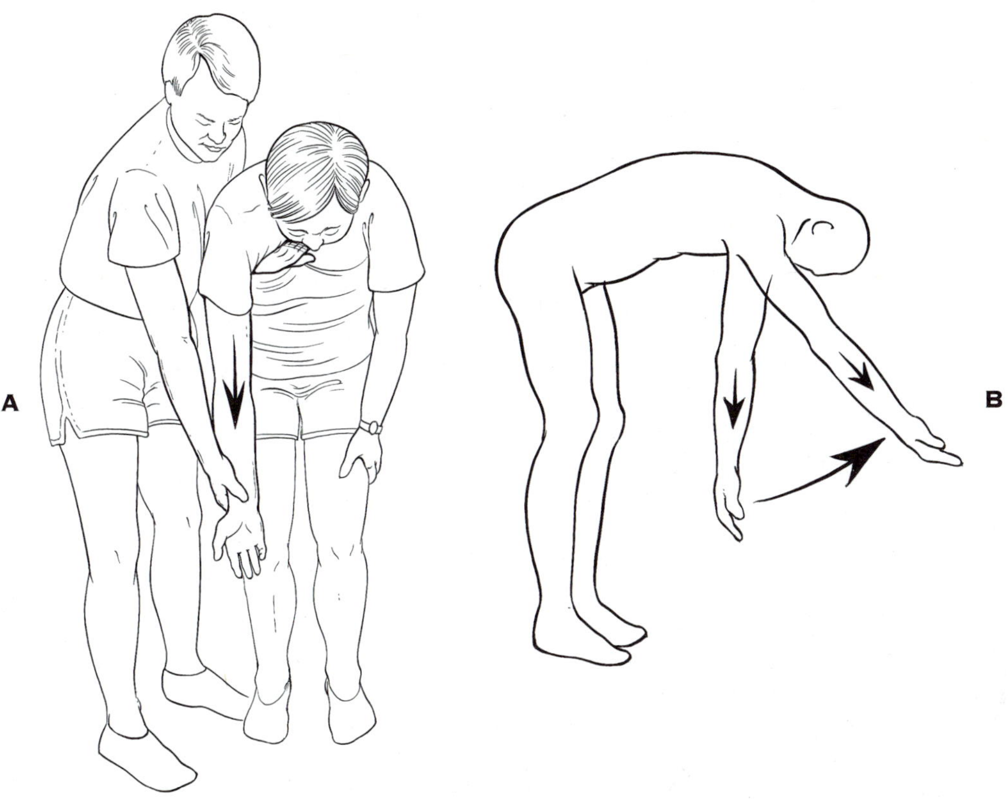
A
B

Fig. 49-9 Weiss technique for shoulder relocation with the victim standing. **A,** The rescuer supports the victim's chest with one hand and pulls down and forward (**B**) with the other hand.

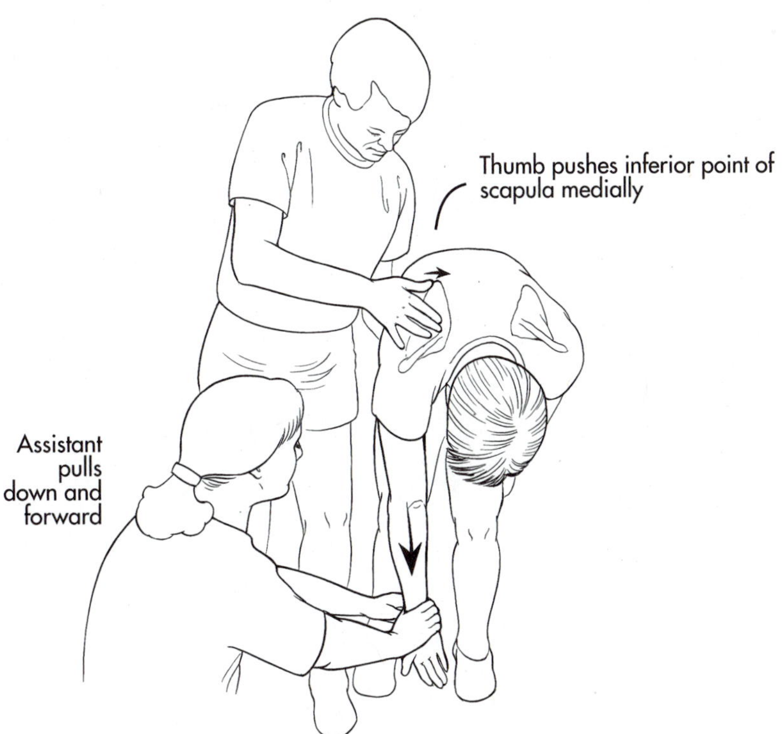
Thumb pushes inferior point of scapula medially
Assistant pulls down and forward

Fig. 49-10 If two rescuers are available, scapular rotation to assist shoulder relocation can be performed while the second rescuer pulls the arm down and forward. The inferior top of the scapula is pushed medially.

motor-sensory function to the wrist and hand before and after attempting a shoulder reduction.

To prevent a recurrent dislocation, the kayaker's arm should be splinted across the chest with a sling or swath or by safety pinning the sleeve of the arm across the chest. If circumstances preclude exiting the river without further kayaking, the shoulder can be partially stabilized by wrapping an elastic or neoprene wrap around the torso and involved arm to limit abduction and external rotation (Fig. 49-11).

Another relocation technique uses the victim's life jacket to allow one rescuer to apply both controlled traction and countertraction.[11] This technique requires that the patient be supine, with room for the rescuer to sit adjacent to the dislocated shoulder. The rescuer then slides his or her foot and leg through the life jacket's arm opening, under the neck, and out through the jacket's head opening. The rescuer's leg functions as a head rest, while the foot braced against the opposite shoulder strap of the life jacket provides countertraction. Holding the forearm of the affected side with the elbow bent at 90 degrees, the rescuer slowly leans back to apply traction while the leg exerts countertraction. The life jacket allows countertraction force to be distributed across the patient's chest. External and internal rotation can be applied to the humerus during traction to facilitate reduction (Fig. 49-12).

Head, facial, and dental trauma is more common in kayakers and decked canoeists than in rafters because of the potential for flipping upside down while still in the craft. Minor abrasions, lacerations, and contusions are common; serious head injury with loss of consciousness is rare. Head and facial trauma can be minimized by wearing a protective helmet and tucking forward, instead of leaning backward, while rolling.

Spine fractures have been reported in kayakers and canoers.[40-41,43] Cervical spine injuries have occurred in kayakers in conjunction with head trauma sustained after flipping upside down. Vertical compression fractures of the thoracolumbar spine have occurred from axial loading when a kayaker landed flat after paddling over a waterfall. One kayaker was rendered paraplegic after landing on his back on rocks while attempting to negotiate a waterfall.[43] Fortunately, his companions recognized the injury and kept him supported on minicell blocks from their kayaks until a backboard could be obtained.

Significant visceral and musculoskeletal injury can occur when a swimmer is sandwiched between a downstream boulder or obstruction and the upstream craft that has been exited. Swimmers should always stay upstream of their craft.

Many kayakers suffer abrasions and contusions to the fingers and knuckles while hanging upside down after flipping. Oar frames, oars, paddles, and the metal ammunition boxes used to keep supplies dry can all inflict injury when rafts are capsized or paddlers are tossed about in turbulent water.

Blisters on the hands are a frequently reported problem in paddling surveys.[45] Kayakers develop them at the metacarpophalangeal (MCP) joint of the thumb along the ulnar aspect. Common sites of blister formation in rafters and canoeists are the proximal palmar surfaces of the MCP joints. Taping and moleskin application reduce the incidence of this potentially incapacitating problem.

Infections

Blisters, abrasions, and lacerations are always at increased risk for infection in an aquatic environment. Maceration from prolonged immersion in water and exposure to atypical pathogens are contributing factors.

An outbreak of *Staphylococcus aureus* skin infections among raft guides in Georgia and South Carolina nearly led to the demise of two rafting companies.[10] Sharp grommets on the thwarts of the rafts had caused repeated lower ex-

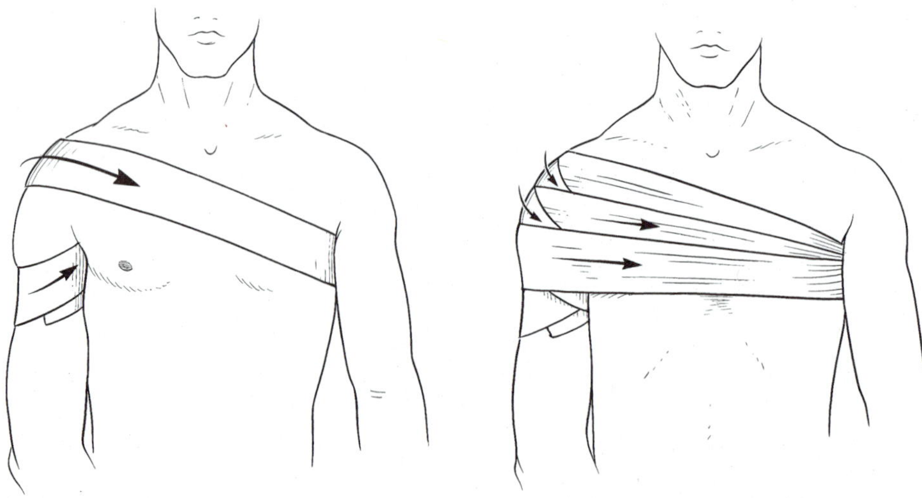

Fig. 49-11 Shoulder harness for support after shoulder dislocation.

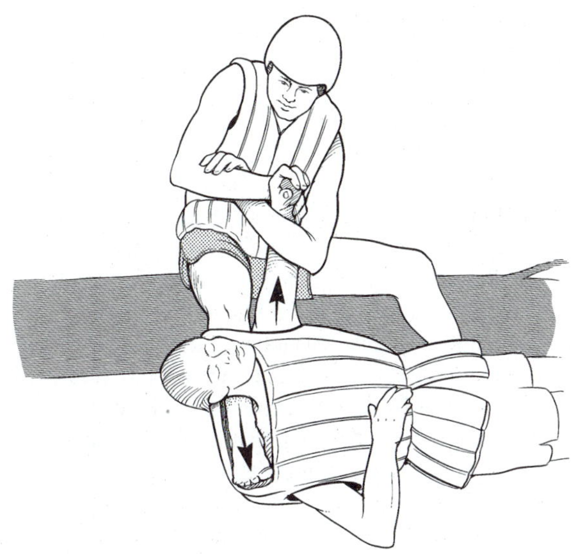

Fig. 49-12 Using a life jacket to assist in countertraction for shoulder relocation.

tremity abrasions. The causative organism was cultured from rafts up to 48 hours after use. Daily raft disinfection enabled the companies to remain in operation.

Otitis externa (swimmer's ear) is a common problem among paddlers. Water exposure to the ear canal macerates the epithelium and elevates the normally acidic pH of the canal, predisposing the ear to infection.[12] The bacteria most commonly cultured are *Pseudomonas aeruginosa, Proteus vulgaris,* and *Staphylococcus* species.[12,23] Antibiotic eardrops with or without hydrocortisone are widely available and very useful. Irrigation of the canal with commercially available solutions containing acetic acid and alcohol helps prevent infection by lowering the pH and drying the canal.[23] The drops should be applied after each outing (see Chapter 54).

Recent publicity given to water contamination by *Giardia lamblia* has been reinforced by statistics from the Centers for Disease Control, which report *Giardia* organisms to be the most common pathogenic intestinal parasite in the United States (see Chapters 42 and 43). *Giardia* cysts abound even in mountain streams and rivers once considered to be sources of pristine water (Color Plate 111). They persist in very cold water and have no detectable taste or smell. Rivers are contaminated by animals that defecate in or near the water. Studies by the Wild Animal Disease Center at Colorado State University, Ft. Collins, Colorado, have identified more than 30 species as *Giardia* carriers.

Paddlers who travel to foreign countries should seek information on local endemic diseases and relevant prophylactic measures. White-water rafting and kayaking in Third World countries subject paddlers to unusual aquatic-related infections. This is exemplified by a report of schistosomiasis in rafters returning from Ethiopia.[22] Schistosomiasis is endemic in large areas of Africa, South America, and the Caribbean and is transmitted to humans who swim or come into contact with fresh water containing the larval stage. Paddlers who return from endemic regions should be screened with serologic testing, since up to 50% of infections are asymptomatic.[31]

Malaria has been reported in rafters returning from New Guinea, and both leptospirosis and hepatitis have stricken kayakers venturing to Costa Rica.[2] In the United States, pulmonary blastomycosis was reported among canoeists in Wisconsin.[7]

Environmental Hazards

Although hypothermia is rarely the cause of death among white-water paddlers, hypothermia-induced impairment of judgment and coordination is a significant contributing factor in many fatalities and accidents.[18,28,39-41] The paddling season usually begins in early spring when air temperatures are cool and snow melt–swollen rivers run extremely cold. Paddlers with rusty skills are more prone to frequent swims and the effects of cold water immersion. Many rivers, especially in the western United States, are controlled by dams that release water from far beneath the surface and thus remain cold year round. Placing adequate barriers between the human body and the environment and carrying adequate food and waterproof matches are of paramount importance.

Another common environmental affliction suffered by paddlers is rhus dermatitis from poison oak or poison ivy. Most cases occur during spring paddling when the vines are potent but the characteristic leaves have not yet appeared. Barrier creams such as StokoGard Outdoor Cream and Tecnu Ivy Shield can be used by individuals highly sensitive to the plants. After plant contact occurs, the oil may be removed from the skin by washing within 30 minutes.[13] A commercial product, Tecnu Oak and Ivy Cleanser, can remove oil from the skin for up to 8 hours after exposure.

Treatment of rhus dermatitis consists of oral antihistamines and systemic corticosteroids. A 2-week course is needed to prevent recurrence of the rash (see Chapter 36).[13]

Sunburn and the effects of chronic exposure to solar radiation are compounded by water's ability to reflect up to 100% of ultraviolet radiation (UVR), depending on the time of day. Sand can reflect up to 17% of harmful UVR. Most rivers are situated in mountains, where UVR increases 4% to 5% with each additional 1000 feet of altitude.[9] Sunscreens must be applied frequently because they are prone to wash off in the water. Zinc oxide and other barrier creams are more resistant to water and are preferable on areas of intense exposure, such as the nose and lips. Paddlers with fair skin should consider using gloves to protect the hands from UVR exposure.

Eye protection from UVR is often overlooked or avoided by paddlers because sunglasses frequently fog while on the river. Application of Dawn dishwashing soap to the lenses prevents fogging for up to 30 minutes. Polarizing lenses reduce glare off the water but do not filter UVR and infrared radiation.

Venomous snakes, especially pit vipers, along with scorpions, spiders, and fire ants are frequently encountered by river enthusiasts and should be considered potential hazards. Paddlers should know appropriate first aid measures for envenomations.

Paddlers commonly consume wild foliage, which may produce severe illness. In one published report, six rafters were poisoned and one of them died after eating water hemlock, *Cicuta douglasili*.[31]

Swift Water Rescue

Time is the most important factor in river rescue and often precludes the use of technical rope-based systems. Basic equipment includes throw ropes, a rescue life jacket, and knife. Experience and an understanding of river dynamics are essential.

The most common rescue scenario involves a swimmer who has exited the craft. Swimmers can be pulled from the water by other rafts, safety kayaks, and canoes or with shore- or raft-based throw ropes.

Rescue from entrapment requires a higher level of skill and often presents greater potential risk to the rescuer. The method used depends on whether the victim can maintain adequate freeboard. If the entrapment site is accessible, direct contact with the victim is quickest and most effective. A rescuer may wade to the entrapment site or reach it by boat if there is a stable site to exit the craft. The river downstream should be scouted for hazards, and if possible a rope thrower should be stationed downstream in the event the rescuer loses footing.

A strong swimmer rescue is the next quickest method but entails significant risk to the rescuer (Fig. 49-13). The rescuer is tethered to a rope that provides added stability against the force of the current. If a quick-release harness is not available, a loose loop of rope can be passed under the rescuer's armpits.

A tag line rescue should be considered if the victim cannot be reached directly. A tag line is a rope stretched across the river downstream that is then brought upstream to the victim (Fig. 49-14). Getting the line across the river sometimes constitutes an insurmountable obstacle. If the river is narrow, it may be possible to throw the line across. Otherwise, it can be ferried across by a boat or team of swimmers. During a ferry, as much of the rope as possible should be kept out of the water to avoid drag.

There are two types of tag lines (Fig. 49-15). A floating tag line has a life jacket or some other flotation device attached to the middle to keep the rope on the surface, which helps support the victim. A snag tag is a weighted line submerged and walked upstream to snare a foot or other body part that has been trapped under the surface. A snag tag can be made by joining together two throw bags filled with rocks (Fig. 49-16).

The surge of interest in white-water sports and the regular occurrence of natural flooding have created the need for formal training of raft guides and emergency personnel in swift water rescue techniques. The Swift Water Rescue Technician course, designed and taught by Rescue 3 in Sonora, California, has become the industry standard. Guidelines have recently been established by the United States Life-Saving Association to certify basic and advanced swift water rescue technicians. Students learn techniques of shallow water crossings, tethered swimmer systems, vehicle rescue, and low-head dam survival.

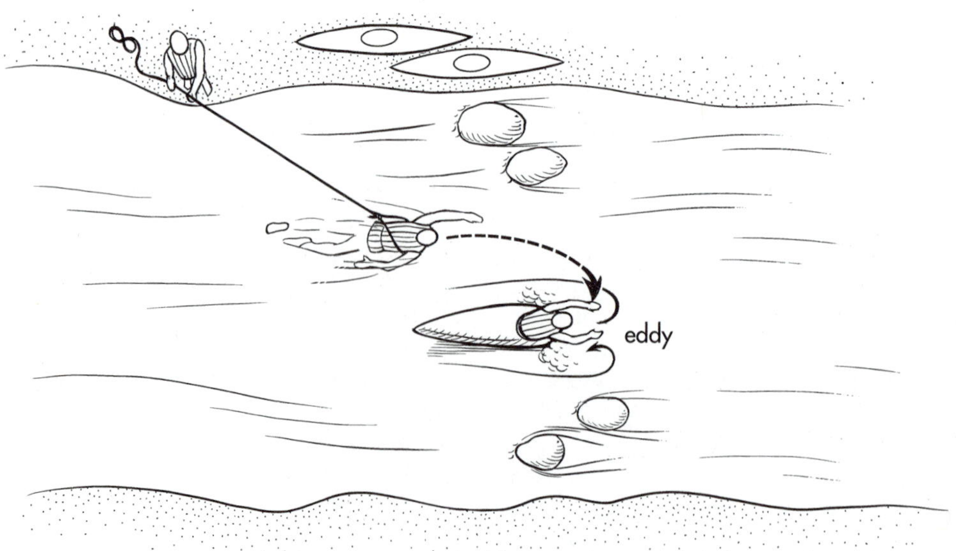

Fig. 49-13 Strong swimmer rescue.

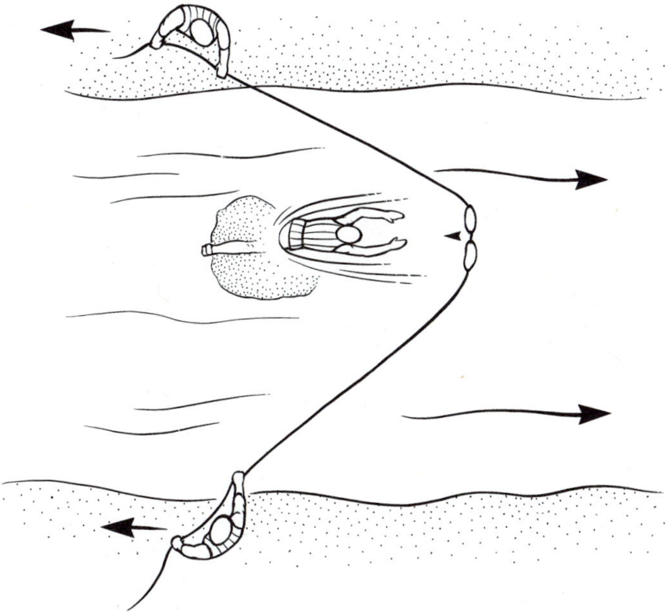

Fig. 49-14 Tag line.

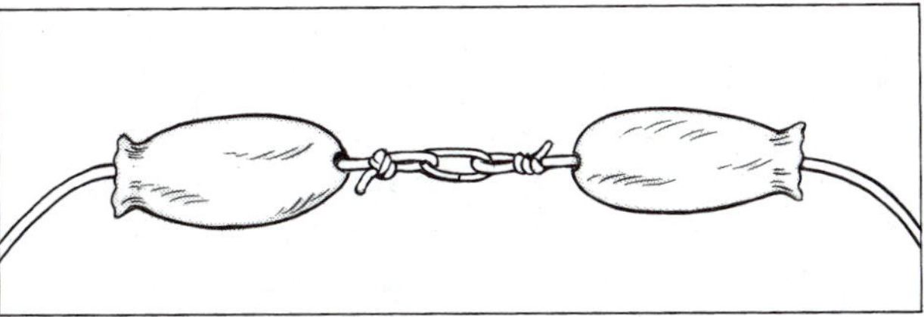

Fig. 49-15 Two throw bags connected with a carabiner to make a tag line.

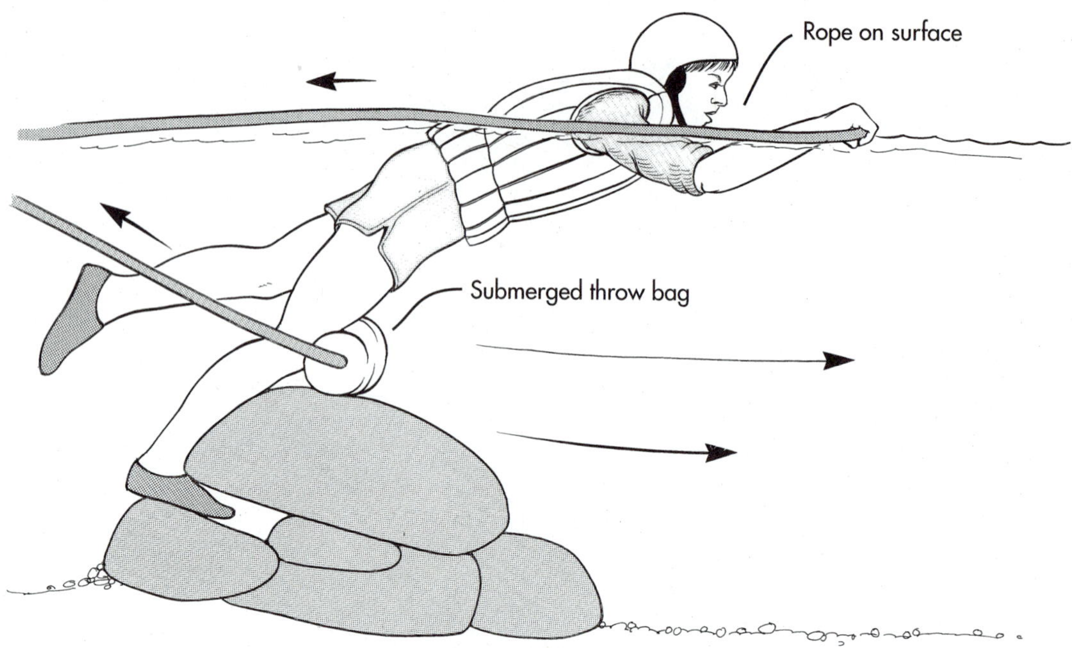

Fig. 49-16 Submerged snag tag.

SUMMARY

The beauty and adventure offered by rivers, combined with opportunities for athleticism and camaraderie, lure great numbers of people to white-water boating. The increased number of inexperienced river runners attempting more difficult rivers underscores the need for participants and their physicians to be aware of the inherent hazards and resultant medical problems. The remote and rugged environment in which white-water sports are undertaken compels responsible participants to acquire a foundation of wilderness medicine expertise and improvisational first aid skills.

APPENDIX A

White-Water First Aid Kits

The following variables should be considered when designing a white-water first aid kit: remoteness and accessibility of the river, Third World travel conditions, the number of people the kit will need to support, preexisting medical conditions; and space and weight restrictions. When assembling a kit, the following components are generally recommended for rafting and kayaking:

RAFTING KIT

Waterproof dry bag or Pelican box
Cardiopulmonary resuscitation mouth shield (CPR-Microshield
SAM Splint
Sawyer Extractor
Hypothermia/hyperthermia thermometer
Bandage scissors
Fine-point tweezers or forceps
Temporary dental filling (Cavit)
Glutose paste
Irrigation syringe with 18-gauge catheter
Povidone-iodine solution
3M surgical stapler (1 stapler holds 25 staples)
Cyanoacrylate glue (Crazy Glue)
Wound closure strips (Steri-Strips)
Tincture of benzoin
Polysporin ointment
Moleskin
Latex gloves
Antiseptic towelettes
Safety pins
Waterproof matches
Accident report form and pencil
Large garbage bag
4 × 4-inch sterile dressings
8 × 10-inch trauma pad or Bloodstopper dressing
Eye pads
Nonadherent dressing (Xeroform or Aquaphor)
Triangular bandage
3-inch conforming gauze bandage
3-inch elastic bandage with Velcro closure
1-inch × 10-yard surgical tape
Duct tape (can be wrapped around the paddle shaft)
Strip and knuckle bandages
Cotton-tipped applicators

Aloe vera gel
Diphenhydramine capsules
Cortisone cream
Acetaminophen tablets
Ibuprofen tablets
Eardrops
  Prophylactic eardrops (mixture of rubbing alcohol and white vinegar)
  Treatment eardrops (Cortisporin Otic Suspension)
Epinephrine injectable or Epi-Pen
Prochlorperazine suppository
Diazepam or midazolam
Oxycodone
Oxymetazoline nasal spray (Afrin)
Antibiotics (trimethoprim-sulfamethoxazole, ciprofloxacin, cephalexin)
Sunscreen (sun protection factor [SPF] of 15 or higher)
Insect repellent
Iodine tablets
Tampons
Tea bags

KAYAKING KIT

Waterproof dry bag or small Pelican box
Cardiopulmonary resuscitation mouth shield
Hypothermia/hyperthermia thermometer
Scissors
Fine-point tweezers or forceps
Small surgical stapler (3M)
Wound closure strips
Tincture of benzoin
Polysporin ointment
Latex gloves
Antiseptic towelettes
Safety pins
Waterproof matches
Accident report form and pencil
3 × 3-inch sterile dressings
Nonadherent dressings
2-inch conforming gauze bandage
Duct tape
Strip and knuckle bandages
Cotton-tipped applicators
Diphenhydramine
Acetaminophen
Ibuprofen
Prophylactic eardrops
Epinephrine
Prochlorperazine suppository
Diazepam or midazolam
Oxycodone
Sunscreen
Insect repellent
Iodine tablets

APPENDIX B
Organizations

American Canoe Association, Inc.
7432 Alban Station Boulevard
Suite B-226
Springfield, VA 22150-2311

American Whitewater Affiliation
P.O. Box 85
Phoenicia, NY 12464

Chinook Medical Gear
2805 Wilderness Place
Suite 700
Boulder, CO 80301

Rescue 3
P.O. Box 4686
Sonora, CA 95370

Safety Deck System
Outdoor Safety Systems
140 Quaker Road
Princeton, NJ 08540

REFERENCES

1. Allan JR, Elliot DH, Hayes PA: The thermal performance of partial coverage wet suits, *Aviat Space Environ Med* 57:1056, 1986.
2. Backer H: Malaria in returned travelers, *Wilderness Med* 4:11, 1987.
3. Bechdel L, Ray S: *River rescue,* Boston, 1989, Appalachian Mountain Club Books.
4. Brody AJ, Mitchell C, Springer M: Submersion injury complicated by hyperthermia in a kayaker wearing a dry suit, *J Wilderness Med* 4:198, 1993.
5. Burrell CL, Burrell R: Injuries in whitewater paddling, *Physician Sports Med* 10:119, 1982.
6. *Canoe Magazine,* Canoe America Associates, Kirkland, Wash, Dec 1993.
7. Centers for Disease Control: Blastomycosis in canoeists—Wisconsin, *MMWR* 29:450, 1979.
8. Cooper KE, Martins S, Riben P: Respiratory and other responses of subjects immersed in cold water, *J Appl Physiol* 40:903, 1976.
9. Daniels F: Physical factors in sun exposure, *Arch Dermatol* 85:98, 1962.
10. Decker MD et al: An outbreak of staphylococcal skin infections among river rafting guides, *Am J Epidemiol* 124:969, 1986.
11. Dutkly P: A simple method of treating shoulder dislocations for the whitewater enthusiast, *Wilderness Med* 5(3):9, 1988.
12. Ellison RT III, Zimner SH: Infectious disease emergencies. In Kravis TC et al, editors: *Emergency medicine: a comprehensive review,* ed 3, New York 1993, Raven Press.
13. Epstein WL: Plant-induced dermatitis, *Ann Emerg Med* 16:950, 1987.
14. Fraser RE: Paddling precautions advised, *Physician Sports Med* 10:16, 1982.
15. Girten TR, Wehr SE: An evaluation of the high-water performance characteristics of personal flotation devices, *USCG Report,* USCG-M-84-1 (167/4), Springfield, Va, 1984, National Technical Information Service.
16. Golden FS, Golden C: Problems of immersion, *Br J Hosp Med* 45:371, 1980.

17. Goldman RF et al: Wet versus dry suit approaches to water immersion protective clothing, *Aviat Space Environ Med* 37:485, 1966.
18. Harwett RM, Bijlani MG: The involvement of cold water in recreational boating fatalities. *I, Accid Anal Prevent* 14:147, 1982.
19. Hayward JS: The physiology of immersion hypothermia. In Pozos RS, Wittmers LE, editors: *The nature and treatment of hypothermia,* Minneapolis, 1983, University of Minnesota Press.
20. Hayward JS, Eckerson JD: Physiological responses and survival time prediction for humans in ice water, *Aviat Space Environ Med* 55(3):206, 1984.
21. Hayward JS et al: Temperature effect on the human dive response in relation to coldwater near drowning, *J Appl Physiol* 56:202, 1984.
22. Istre GR et al: Acute schistosomiasis among Americans rafting the Omo River, Ethiopia, *JAMA* 251:508, 1984.
23. Jenkins BH: Treatment of otitis externa and swimmer's ear, *JAMA* 175:402, 1961.
24. Jennings, AK: *Whitewater, wildwater,* Royal Oak Press, 1981, West Virginia.
25. Keatinge WR, Evans M: The respiratory and cardiovascular response to immersion in coldwater, *Q J Exp Physiol* 46:83, 1961.
26. Keatinge WR, Hayward MG: Sudden death in coldwater and ventricular arrhythmia, *J Forensic Sci* 16:459, 1981.
27. Keatinge WR et al: The effects of work and clothing on the maintenance of the body temperature in water, *Q J Exp Physiol* 46:69, 1961.
28. Keatinge WR et al: Sudden failure of swimming in coldwater, *Br Med J* 1:480, 1969.
29. Kizer KW: Medical aspects of whitewater kayaking, *Physician Sports Med* 15:128, 1987.
30. Kizer KW: Medical problems in whitewater sports, *Clin Sports Med* 6:663, 1987.
31. Kizer KW: Whitewater medicine, *Emerg Med Clin North Am* 29:91, 1987.
32. Mayer PJ: Helping your patients avert canoe and kayak injuries, *J Musculoskel Med* 4(8):31, 1987.
33. McNamara RM: Reduction of anterior shoulder dislocations by scapular manipulation, *Ann Emerg Med* 21:1140, 1993.
34. *National Sporting Goods Association survey,* Bellevue, Wash, 1989, GMA Research.
35. *Participation in sports activities by selected characteristics: 1990,* Mount Prospect, Ill, 1990, National Sporting Goods Association.
36. Reibel GD, McCabe J: Anterior shoulder dislocation: a review of reduction techniques, *Am J Emerg Med* 9:180, 1991.
37. Serra JB: Management of trauma in the wilderness environment, *Emerg Med Clin North Am* 2:3, 1984.
38. Steinman AM, Hayward JS: Coldwater immersion. In Auerbach PS, Geehr EC, editors: *Management of wilderness and environmental emergencies,* St Louis, 1989, Mosby.
39. Walbridge CW, editor: *Best of the river safety task force newsletter, 1976-1982,* Lorton, Va, 1983, American Canoe Association.
40. Walbridge CW, editor: *River safety report, 1982-1985,* Lorton, Va, 1986, American Canoe Association.
41. Walbridge CW, editor: *River safety report, 1986-1988,* Lorton, Va, 1989, American Canoe Association.
42. Walbridge CW, editor: *Safety code of the American Whitewater Affiliation,* Phoenicia, NY, 1989, American Whitewater Affiliation.
43. Walbridge CW, editor: *River safety report, 1989-1991,* Lorton, Va, 1992, American Canoe Association.
44. Wallace D: Scary numbers and statistics—results of AWA close calls and serious injuries survey, *AWA J* 3-4:27, 1991.
45. Weiss EA: Whitewater medicine, *J Wilderness Med* 2:245, 1991.
46. Wilkerson JA, Bangs CC, Haward JS: *Hypothermia, frostbite and other cold injuries,* Seattle, 1986, The Mountaineers.

50 SURVIVAL AT SEA

Scott A. Oslund
Christopher J. Brooks

- Mental preparation
- Physical preparation
- Preparation for emergencies
- Survival preparation
- Rescue preparation

He who commands the sea has command of everything.

Themistocles (c. 528-462 BC), quoted in Cicero, *Epistolae and Atticum, X.* 8[80]

The person preparing to go to sea must hope for the best but plan for the worst. This chapter describes the mental and physical preparations necessary before taking a sea voyage and the dynamics of rescuing a person overboard, saving a ship on fire or flooding, abandoning ship, launching a seaworthy life raft, desalinating water, procuring food, communicating in an emergency, signaling rescuers, navigating to safety, and conducting search and rescue operations. A glossary of terms and acronyms can be found in Appendix A at the end of the chapter.

Mental Preparation

PSYCHOLOGY OF SURVIVAL

Maritime literature is replete with stories of "superhuman" survivors. While physical stature and conditioning are important, most survival experts agree that a positive mental attitude and resolute will to survive are the keys to survival at sea. This thought was summed up by E.C.B. Lee and K. Lee[58]:

> No matter how much physical equipment the survivor has, his chances of survival are very much weakened if he does not have the right mental equipment with the power to adapt and the will to survive. Training in survival techniques, confidence in his equipment and in his own ability to survive are all essential. Men with a minimum of equipment, but with a strong will to live, have survived for long periods, whereas other men with ample equipment have succumbed in less.

Survival starts before going to sea. The motto of one sea survival training outfit is, "He failed to prepare, so he prepared to fail."[4] Unfortunately, some voyagers faced with a sea emergency have put themselves at a tactical disadvantage by not having acquired the necessary survival equipment before going to sea. One authority refers to this lack of physical preparedness as the "preimpact" phase of a sea emergency (personal communication, Professor John Leach, Lancaster University, United Kingdom). It is characterized by denial and disbelief. Common mental excuses for not being physically prepared include the following:

> My boat won't sink so I don't need any flares or a life raft. Besides, I'm only going a few miles offshore.
>
> I want to learn to swim, but my boat's so big I'll never fall overboard.
>
> I can't afford a good personal flotation device or life raft.

The "impact" stage occurs at the time of flooding, fire, or explosion. During this period 12% to 20% of victims remain calm and can assess the situation. From this group emerge spontaneous leaders with abilities not related to gender, profession, or training. Another 75% of people involved in a sea emergency are stunned and bewildered, demonstrating impaired reasoning and poor attention span. Some hyperventilate, tremble, or vomit. The final 10% to 20% of people weep, scream, and become confused and utterly paralyzed by anxiety and fear.

Specific training can help the born leaders to make informed decisions, but they will be leaders in a crisis regardless of the training received by the other two groups. The 75% of people who are neither leaders nor completely incapacitated can be trained to respond to simple survival commands. Ship abandonment drills are potentially lifesaving for this group of people. Unfortunately, some victims are virtually untrainable and will probably die regardless of "preimpact" interventions.

Following the impact stage of a sea emergency is a period of recoil during which a gradual realization occurs among the initial survivors of what has transpired. During this period, many maladaptive behaviors are seen.

Apathy, despair, and low morale are common. The Second Officer aboard the *MV Richmond Castle* endured a 7-day ordeal in a life raft after abandoning ship in the North Atlantic. In the beginning he was one of 23 castaways; at the end of 7 days only 14 survivors were left. He recorded the following observation[58]:

> The men who died all became apathetic and their morale became very low. I could not get them to move in an emergency or do anything to help themselves. They complained continually of thirst, but I could not spare them any more water.

Air Force Captain Paul Shook was forced to ditch his aircraft in the Gulf of Mexico. On the second day at sea, a search and rescue (SAR) aircraft flew within 500 feet of him. He later recorded these thoughts[58]:

> I moved, yelled, and kicked the water, but again he failed to see me. It was a terrible disappointment to see him fly away knowing that my chances of rescue were diminishing with each hour. Again I am at a loss for words to describe the feeling of despair I felt each time this happened during the second day. . . .

Depression is common at sea. Dr. David Lewis noted the following during a calm period while sailing his yacht in the North Atlantic[58]:

> Always in these calms a profound depression dominated me. Hour after hour the ship would wallow helplessly in the swell, rolling 20 degrees each way. There was a vicious brutality in the slap, slap, slap of the sails, something of the shock of a hand slapped to and fro across the face, and on it would go, on and on. . . . But until I started working, and this needed a great effort, it was impossible to overcome my depression.

Suicide is a distinct possibility. Lieutenant Ba Thaw penned these words while adrift in an inflatable raft in the Bay of Bengal[58]:

> On the seventh night, the First Lieutenant, Saw Oo, died. He had a gastric ulcer and had gradually been getting worse. He was in fearful pain. The skin was stretched tightly across his face and chest. He was retching nearly all the time. He had nothing to throw up. . . . He whispered to me, "Let me go. Let me go. It's better to go than suffer more." I nodded. He slipped over the side. . . . Two men died on the eighth day. One of them went mad. I think he had been drinking seawater. . . . The other man flopped over the side without making a sound. Before he went he just looked at me. I think he meant to say goodbye. . . . Another man died on the tenth day and another on the eleventh. They were both only skin and bone. Incredibly they did not die where they were. They found a sudden strength to go overboard. None of the others seemed to register any emotion. They were beyond that.

If a castaway survives beyond several weeks, the next common psychologic phase of survival is adaptation and consolidation. During this period a survivor's environment at sea is seen as the *real* and *correct* world. It is ultimately a period of survival by surrender and resignation. Maurice and Maralyn Bailey were at sea for 117 days and eventually referred to the turtles, fish, and sea as *their* world.[3]

E.C.B. Lee and K. Lee offer further insight into prolonged survival at sea[58]:

> As stress continues, his [the survivor's] powers of adaptation weaken, and he may unconsciously escape from harsh reality by day-dreaming, indulging in fantasies or lapsing into a stupor. He is then less able to exert self-control and he becomes irritable, selfish or aggressive.
>
> Complete mental exhaustion will eventually occur, accelerated by the physical effects of exposure, malnutrition, dehydration and loss of sleep. At this stage, he may be confused, delirious or hallucinate. True psychosis is unusual, but it may occur as a toxic effect, e.g., as a result of drinking seawater, severe wound infection . . . or any fever.
>
> Occasionally, in the extreme, the basic will for self-destruction or self-preservation may dominate his mental state, resulting in suicide or homicide, or rarely, cannibalism.

The authors quickly point out, however, that

> the survivor who adapts well to a change in his environment will set his mind to survival, work out the priorities of action, avoid panic, and make active and deliberate attempts to improve his morale by singing, conversation, prayer and preparations for his survival.

On the forty-eighth day adrift on a balsa raft in the South Pacific, William Willis stated[104]:

> There was a void, and then one day I started singing and realized that my soul had been hungering for this. What a joy to discover singing again. I knew that I had mastered the last big obstacle on my voyage.

Others have found solace in religious faith. While sailing single handed from Panama to Australia, John Caldwell, an atheist, ran intó serious trouble. Profaning God, out of food, and with his vessel, *Pagan,* dismasted, Mr. Caldwell humbly wrote on the one hundred and fifth day at sea[26]:

> And now, lost, foodless, without instruments, I humbly bent my knees to the deck and laid my folded hands upon the cabin. With eyes raised I read off a most heartfelt plea for forgiveness and piteous appeal to *Pagan's* real Captain.

At times a resolute will to survive can be enough to lift depressed spirits. Dougal Robertson and his family were at sea in a life raft and dinghy for 37 days. Their 43-foot schooner, *Lucette,* sank just west of the Galapagos Islands after being attacked by killer whales. The boat went down in less than 60 seconds, and they were left adrift in a 9-foot dinghy towing an inflatable raft. Without maps, compass, or navigational instruments, and having only enough emergency rations for 3 days, they set out for the Costa Rican coast, 1000 miles and an estimated 50 days away. After failing to attract the attention of a passing ship, Mr. Robertson had these thoughts[78]:

> I surveyed the empty flare cartons bitterly, and the one smoke flare which was damp and wouldn't work, and something happened to me in that instant, that for me changed the whole aspect of our predicament. If these poor bloody seamen couldn't rescue us,

then we would have to make it on our own and to hell with them. We would survive without them, yes, and that was the word from now on, "survival," not "rescue," or "help," or dependence of any kind, just survival. I felt the strength flooding through me, lifting me from the depression of disappointment to a state of almost cheerful abandon. I felt the bitter aggression of the predator fill my mind. . . . We would live for three months or six months from the sea if necessary. . . . From that instant on I became a savage.

Physical Preparation

PERSONAL FLOTATION DEVICES*[6,30,82,101,102]

On old-time sailors it was fashionable to tattoo a pig on one foot and a rooster on the other. An old-time bos'n claimed that anyone so marked could not drown, for these creatures despised the water.

Horace Beck, *Folklore and the Sea*[40]

Life jackets, life vests, life preservers, or Mae Wests are now referred to by the U.S. Coast Guard (USCG) as personal flotation devices (PFDs).[6] The ideal PFD is comfortable, well fitting, and highly visible, allows maximum freedom of movement with minimal bulk, provides substantial flotation, and, in the event of unconsciousness, turns the wearer face up.[52]

PFDs are constructed of several different materials. Kapok is organic fiber encased in vinyl. If the vinyl exterior is pierced, water-saturated kapok eventually rots, causing loss of buoyancy. Polyethylene foam is a commonly used material. When punctured or torn, it does not become waterlogged. It is lighter and less expensive than kapok, but because of its stiffness, it restricts movement. Aquafoam is closed-cell polyvinylchloride (PVC) that is soft and flexible. It preserves some body heat. If punctured or cut, it does not become waterlogged. PVC resists most chemicals, mildew, and ultraviolet radiation. Airex is also constructed of PVC. It is softer, more flexible, and therefore more comfortable than Aquafoam. Airex provides some thermal protection in cold water.

Five types of PFDs are approved by the USCG (Table 50-1). The type I PFD is designed for offshore use and survival when adrift in rough, open water. It is intended to be worn in the event of ship abandonment and, depending on the model, must provide a minimum of 22 pounds of buoyancy for an adult. Type I PFDs are designed to turn *most* unconscious wearers face up in the water. Some type I PFDs are reversible, which facilitates donning in an emergency.

*More information regarding PFDs and safe boating can be obtained by contacting the USCG toll-free Boating Safety Hotline: 800-368-5647. For information about free boating courses in specific areas, call 800-336-BOAT; in Virginia, call 800-245-BOAT.

Two types of USCG-approved type I PFDs are authorized for use aboard boats: the offshore jacket and the yoke or keyhole model. Both types consist of plastic foam buoyant material distributed to provide the flotation and buoyancy required to hold the wearer in an upright or slightly backward position with head and face clear of the water.[30] An offshore jacket PFD consists of several pieces of unicellular plastic foam (Fig. 50-1). A yoke or keyhole PFD consists of a large single piece of unicellular foam (Fig. 50-2).

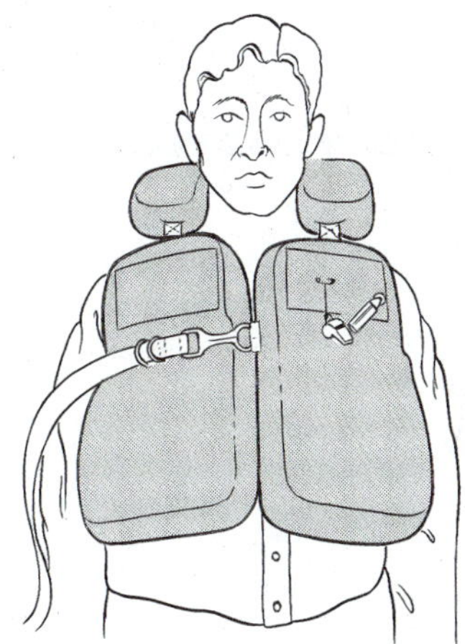

Fig. 50-1 Offshore jacket personal flotation device. (Courtesy U.S. Coast Guard.)

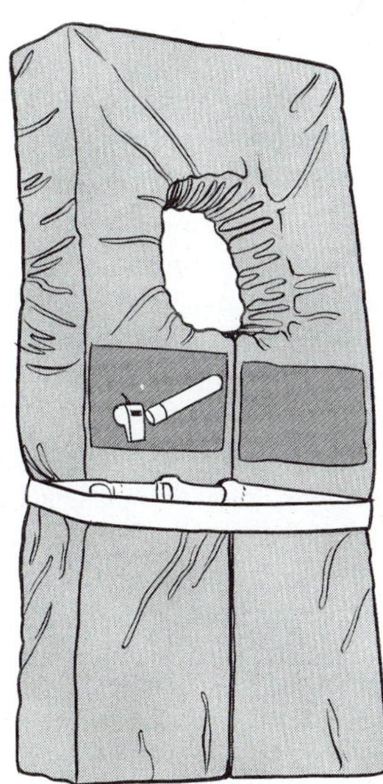

Fig. 50-2 "Keyhole" personal flotation device. (Courtesy U.S. Coast Guard.)

Table 50-1 Comparison of Personal Flotation Devices

Type/Characteristic	Wearability*	Buoyancy†	Freeboard‡	Righting Force§	Body Angle‖
Type I	Poor	Very good	Very good	Very good	Very good
Type II	Poor	Fair	Fair	Fair	Fair
Type III vest	Very good	Fair	Fair	Poor	Poor
Type III coat	Very good	Good	Fair	Poor	Fair
Type IV horseshoe	Horrible	Very good	Good	Poor	Poor
Type V hybrid	Excellent	Very good	Good	Fair	Fair
Inflatable vest	Very good	Excellent	Excellent	Excellent	Excellent

*Wearability: a qualitative term describing how much the personal flotation device (PFD) restricts activity.
†Buoyancy: the amount of force needed to submerge the PFD.
‡Freeboard: the distance from the water to the mouth.
§Righting force: the tendency of a PFD to right a man overboard from a face-down position.
‖Body angle: ideally, face plane measured at 30 to 80 degrees to the horizontal.

Most type I PFDs float an unconscious victim face up. The BOAT/U.S. Foundation for Boating Safety tested PFDs in an outdoor wave pool, attempting to simulate choppy waters found offshore. Investigators found that all volunteers preferred a type I PFD in the wave pool over all other USCG-approved models.[7] In particular, the offshore jacket was preferred over the yoke style. Wearers found that the yoke model was less comfortable and made swimming more difficult. In addition, it failed to right testers from the "deadman's float" to a face-up position in over half the trials. Because of its large bulky configuration, mobility is extremely limited and routinely wearing a type I PFD is difficult.

USCG approval means that the PFD has passed a series of tests conducted by Underwriters Laboratory. Many experts in the field of sea survival believe that USCG standards for PFD buoyancy are insufficient and recommend wearing PFDs that meet the more stringent criteria of Safety of Life at Sea (SOLAS). SOLAS is an international organization representing 137 maritime nations whose parent organization is the International Maritime Organization (IMO); it is under the auspices of the United Nations. SOLAS was established in 1914 after the sinking of the White Star liner *Titanic* in April 1912, in which all 1489 persons immersed in 32° F (0° C) water were found dead by rescuers who arrived 1 hour 50 minutes after the sinking; almost all of the people in lifeboats lived. SOLAS meets periodically to establish maritime regulations, including standards for ship construction, surveys, stability, machinery, fire protection, navigation, communication, cargo, dangerous goods, signaling, and lifesaving equipment.* A SOLAS-approved PFD must provide 35 pounds of buoyancy. PFDs with less than 35 pounds of buoyancy tend to float the wearer horizontally, as opposed to vertically, reducing freeboard (the distance between the mouth and level of the water).

The standard type II PFD (also called the near shore buoyancy aid) is shaped like a horseshoe collar (Fig. 50-3). A USCG-approved type II PFD must provide 15.5 pounds

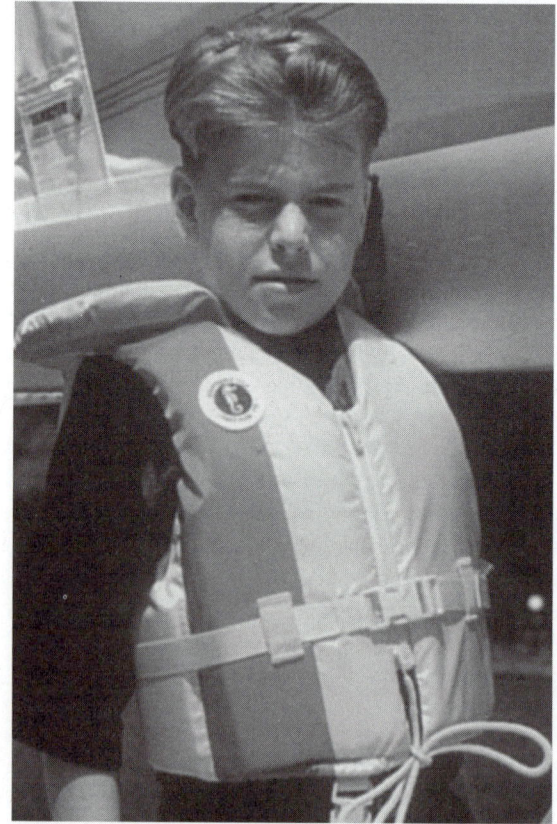

Fig. 50-3 Type II personal flotation device. (Courtesy U.S. Coast Guard.)

*For a complete listing of SOLAS and IMO publications, contact International Maritime Organization, 4 Albert Embankment, London, England, SE1 7SR; telephone 44-71-735-7611; FAX 44-71-587-3210. Chapter III of the publication *SOLAS*, which deals with lifesaving appliances, is being revised. The latest SOLAS standards for lifesaving appliances were established in 1983.

of buoyancy for an adult and is designed for use in calm, protected water with a good chance for rapid rescue. These devices are *not* designed for use in rough open water. A type II PFD may turn *some* unconscious wearers face up, but this is not assured. Type II PFDs are not reversible but are less bulky, allowing greater freedom of movement than type I PFDs. They are also less expensive than type I PFDs and for this reason are inappropriately purchased by some persons who sail in rough open water.

In the simulated rough conditions of the wave pool, a type II was found to be inadequate by investigators with the BOAT/U.S. Foundation for Boating Safety.[7] Volunteers found that significant treading of water was required to remain afloat and predicted that they would be unable to keep their heads above water for more than 30 minutes in such conditions. All the type II (and type III) PFDs tested floated volunteers vertically, causing them to bob up and down like corks in rough water. Volunteers discovered that downward inertia caused by each passing wave subjected them to significant dousing by the next wave, resulting in aspiration of water. The only PFD that prevented bobbing and dousing was a type I. Testers found that a type II PFD donned over a type III PFD increased buoyancy to at least 31 pounds, thereby reducing aspiration. Alternatively, two type II PFDs may be worn simultaneously. One expert believes that such combinations are dangerous and would not recommend them (personal communication, Kelsey Burr, Survival Technologies Group). Therefore mariners should don and test PFDs, ascertaining for themselves which flotation device maximizes freeboard (see later discussion). The key word in PFD is "personal."

A type III PFD is a flotation aid resembling a vest (Fig. 50-4). It is designed for use in calm water when the chance of being rescued quickly is good; it should never be relied on to provide prolonged flotation in rough water. Type III PFDs are usually quite comfortable, permitting continuous use by the wearer. In the water a type III PFD does not hold the head of an unconscious victim face up to ensure survival, hence the term "flotation aid." Like type II PFDs, a USCG-approved type III PFD must provide 15.5 pounds of buoyancy. It is designed to be worn when freedom of movement is needed and the risk of unconscious or extended immersion is minimal. This group includes flotation coats—a full-length jacket resembling an outerwear jacket. The coat has thin panels of closed-cell foam sewn into the lining for buoyancy. Type III PFDs come in a wide variety of colors and styles. A brightly colored PFD that enhances rescue in the event of falling overboard is recommended.

A type IV PFD is a throwable device such as a seat cushion, ring buoy, or horseshoe buoy. It is designed to be thrown to a victim who has fallen overboard but is able to assist with his or her own rescue. As such, it requires the cooperation of a person in the water and is not intended for use by nonswimmers, children, or exhausted or unconscious persons. A USCG-approved seat cushion must possess 18 pounds of buoyancy; ring and horseshoe buoys must possess 16.5 pounds of flotation. A ring or horseshoe buoy with attached marker light should be available topside at all times and attached to 100 feet of orange polypropylene line. The line should be sealed in an opaque plastic bag to prevent deterioration from ultraviolet light. As many seagoers can attest, type IV PFDs are difficult or impossible to throw a great distance because of their weight and bulk. This problem was addressed by one manufacturer that designed a throwable device called a Techfloat (Fig. 50-5). The Techfloat is a bag containing 75 feet of polypropylene line attached to a buoyancy aid that automatically inflates with carbon dioxide (CO_2) after contact with water. The inflatable

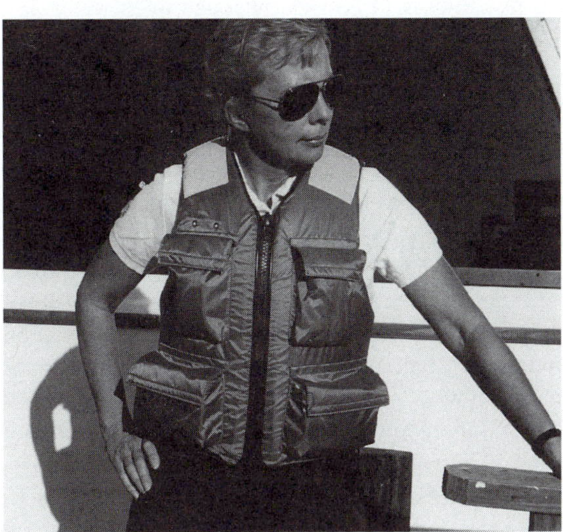

Fig. 50-4 Type III personal flotation device, vest model. (Courtesy Survival Technologies Group.)

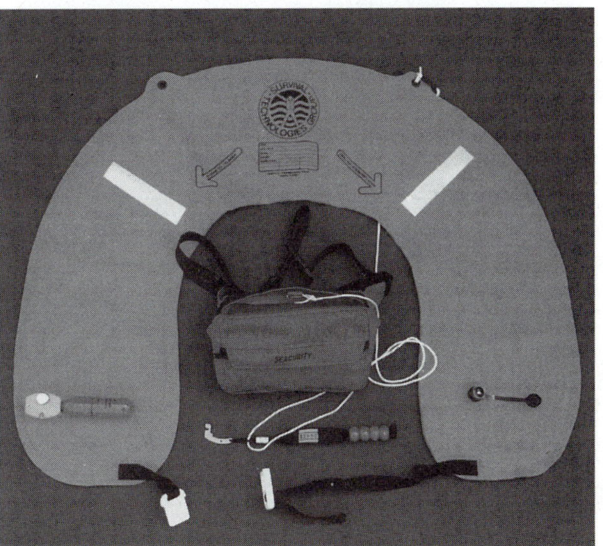

Fig. 50-5 Techfloat: inflatable type IV personal flotation device (not Coast Guard approved). (Courtesy Survival Technologies Group.)

horseshoe buoy provides 25 pounds of flotation. The entire bag is thrown underhand to maximize distance and accuracy.

Type V PFDs are special use items such as work vests with tether attachments, deck suits, and inflatable PFDs (see later discussion). All type V PFDs have some limitation on their approval and usage, but they contain features not available on other PFDs. PFDs are also made for pets, but these are not USCG approved.

The USCG rates and approves some inflatable PFDs. The only inflatable PFD approved by the USCG is a "hybrid." A hybrid is a type V PFD that must possess a minimum of 7.5 pounds of inherent buoyancy, which increases to a minimum of 22 pounds after CO_2 inflation. To satisfy USCG requirements, an inflatable PFD must be worn above deck when under way. The advantages of an inflatable over a noninflatable PFD are comfort, mobility, and in some cases buoyancy. Inflatable PFDs require more maintenance and are often more expensive than noninflatable PFDs. Increased maintenance and the possibility of CO_2 cartridge failure are the primary reasons given by the USCG for nonapproval. Some inflatable PFDs are automatically inflated after immersion in water for several seconds; others require that the wearer manually activate a CO_2 cartridge. Assured flotation in the event of unconsciousness is one advantage of an automatically inflated PFD. Each type can be orally inflated in the event of CO_2 cartridge failure.[103]

Many excellent inflatable PFDs are available that are not approved by the USCG (Fig. 50-6). They come in a variety of styles: pouch-belt, vest, and jacket types. In Europe inflatable PFDs have been used for years with good results. The Seavest and Crewsaver manufactured by Crewfit in England are not USCG approved but were noted by investigators in the United States to provide superior buoyancy, comfort, and fit.[8] In tests done by the BOAT/U.S. Foundation for Boating Safety, all volunteers wearing the Seavest or Crewsaver were immediately righted from the "deadman's float" position. The ultrabuoyant (35 to 40 pounds) devices enabled volunteers to float comfortably without treading water. Volunteers noted that they felt more confident in fully inflatable PFDs than in any other PFD tested. Modern inflatable PFDs are constructed of puncture-resistant, denier nylon that is often coated with urethane. A good discussion of required maintenance for inflatable PFDs is available.[92]

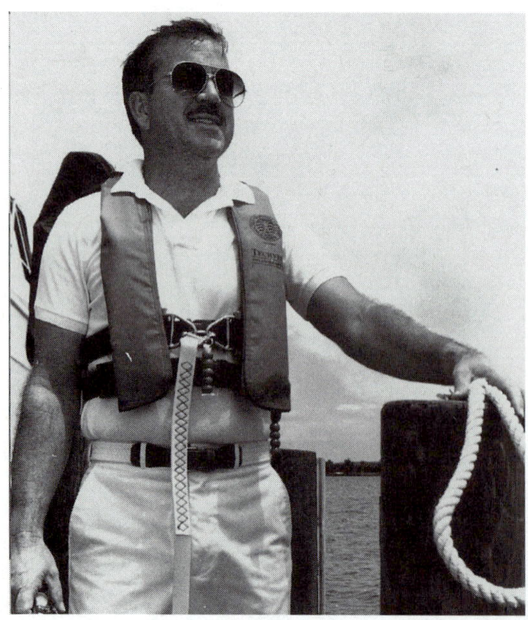

Fig. 50-6 Techvest: inflatable personal flotation vest with harness and lifeline (not Coast Guard approved). (Courtesy Survival Technologies Group.)

To meet current USCG regulations, all boats longer than 16 feet must come equipped with a type I, II, III, or V PFD for each person on board and have at least one type IV PFD available. Some type V PFDs must be worn when the boat is under way to meet minimum requirements. Boats under 16 feet must be supplied with one wearable or throwable PFD for each person on board. After May 1995, all boats (regardless of size) will be required to have a wearable PFD for each person on board. PFDs must be of the correct size, in good and serviceable condition, and readily accessible for each person aboard.[37,68,94] They should not be stowed in plastic bags or locked compartments or have other gear stowed on top of them. Type IV PFDs must be immediately available. A USCG-approved PFD must display a label documenting its authenticity.[95]

The fit and buoyancy of a PFD can be tested by wading slowly into the shallow end of a swimming pool. The PFD should fit comfortably and snugly. With the body relaxed and head tilted backward, the PFD should keep the chin well above water. If it fits well, the tester should jump off the edge of the pool. A PFD that fits properly will not ride up high on the trunk or make keeping the head above water difficult. If a PFD is to be used in rough open water, it must right the wearer from a "deadman's float" position.

Type I, II, III, and V PFDs are available for children.[9] A USCG-approved type I PFD must provide 11 pounds of buoyancy for a child. The USCG recommends that children always wear a PFD when aboard, even if not under way. In tests done by the BOAT/U.S. Foundation for Boating Safety, child-size type I PFDs were found to provide excellent flotation. They rolled all volunteer children tested face up and slightly backward from a "deadman's float" position. Each type I tested provided at least 5 inches of freeboard. Unfortunately, type I PFDs do not fit well on very small children and infants.

USCG-approved type II and III PFDs must provide 11 pounds of buoyancy for a medium-size child. Infant and small child sizes must provide at least 7 pounds of buoyancy. In tests done by the BOAT/U.S. Foundation for Boating Safety, type II PFDs with collars did not perform as well as expected. On average, they provided only 3½ inches of freeboard. When children leaned backward in the water to float more comfortably, most collars submerged, providing inadequate head support.

Infants are difficult to float in a stable position because of their body proportions. While testing type II PFDs for infants, investigators with the BOAT/U.S. Foundation for Boating Safety noted that most floating infants tended to arch backward when panicked. Arching backward forced the collars of type II PFDs downward, which in turn nearly forced the heads of such infants below water. In addition, type II PFDs did not prevent infants from rolling side to side. Despite these shortcomings, the USCG recommends that only type II PFDs be used on infants. One authority recommends that all children less than 2 years of age wear a PFD and be tethered to an adult fitted with an inflatable PFD (personal communication, Kelsey Burr, Survival Technologies Group). Finally, investigators note that a grab handle—a piece of reinforced fabric sewn onto the back of a child's PFD—is a useful feature that facilitates extraction of a child from the water.

Children's PFDs are sized according to weight: under 30 pounds (14 kg), under 50 pounds (23 kg), 30 to 50 pounds (14 to 23 kg), and 50 to 90 pounds (23 to 41 kg). Some manufacturers also specify chest size. For children, a PFD should be sized slightly smaller rather than bigger to ensure a tight fit. Several companies manufacture PFDs imprinted with popular cartoon and animation figures. Allowing a child to assist in the selection of the PFD may enhance compliance. To test the fit of a child's PFD, pick the child up by the PFD at the shoulders. The PFD should not come up over the child's chin or ears; if it does, the crotch strap should be adjusted or a smaller size selected. Most important, children should become accustomed to wearing a PFD in a swimming pool or by the shore. Familiarity with these devices provides a level of comfort and security in the event of a sea emergency.[71,96]

If a person falls overboard or abandons ship, the chances of being located in the water are improved through use of a plastic whistle, signaling mirror, waterproof light, orange smoke signal, or red flare attached to a PFD. When at sea, crew members should always wear PFDs unless authorized by the captain to remove them during nonhazardous operations associated with minimal chance of falling overboard. The USCG recommends that all PFDs be fitted with reflective material. A list of PFD manufacturers appears in Appendix B at the end of the chapter.

IMMERSION SUITS[30]

An immersion (survival or exposure) suit is not a PFD but is used when abandoning ship in cold water. It provides the greatest protection against hypothermia while in the water (Fig. 50-7). The term "immersion suit" is preferred over "survival" or "exposure suit." Survival suit fell out of favor because safety industry officials did not want to imply to the user that the suit would ensure survival. Immersion suits are designed to keep the wearer dry. By contrast, an exposure suit often refers to a work suit that gives some degree of thermal protection and buoyancy but does not keep the wearer dry.

Immersion suits are not designed to be worn routinely while working on deck. They are extremely bulky, brightly colored (international orange or yellow), and constructed of neoprene foam rubber. They provide approximately 35 pounds of buoyancy. The buoyancy of an immersion suit is distributed equally from head to toe, rather than being concentrated around the torso. Hence a wearer tends to float more horizontally than with a PFD of identical buoyancy.

An immersion suit is designed to keep the wearer entirely dry, reducing heat loss in cold water. To this end, the waterproof suit fabric is a highly efficient thermal insulator with sealed seams and a watertight front closure zipper. Neck, wrist, and ankle seals eliminate water influx. An immersion suit comes with hood, gloves, and boots. The hood and boots are usually permanently attached, but the gloves may be removable. Many hoods come equipped with a splash guard to prevent water spray from directly entering the nose and mouth. An immersion suit may have an auxiliary buoyancy device consisting of an orally inflated bladder or solid, foam-filled pillow located behind the head, designed to maximize freeboard and minimize exposure cooling. Ideally the wearer should float with a face plane angle

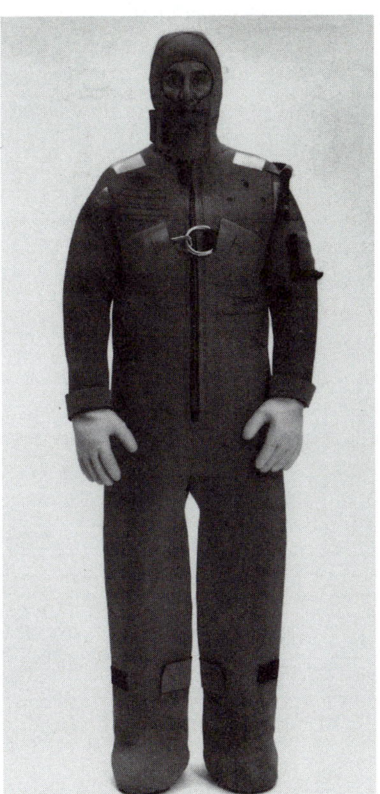

Fig. 50-7 Immersion suit. (Courtesy Stearns Manufacturing.)

between 30 and 80 degrees to the horizontal with the mouth located a minimum of 5 inches (13 cm) above the water.[4]

Immersion suits can be donned in less than 2 minutes by persons familiar with their use. They should be worn over warm clothing and, depending on the model, with socks or shoes. They are designed to provide flotation and thermal protection against hypothermia in extreme conditions. Tests done by the Hypothermia Water Safety Institute at the University of Minnesota demonstrated that a Stearns immersion suit could protect the wearer nearly indefinitely in 46° to 50° F (8° to 10° C) water.[93] Both USCG and IMO regulations specify that an immersion suit must prevent the wearer's core temperature from dropping more than 3.6° F (2° C) in 6 hours while he or she is immersed in calm 32° to 37° F (0° to 3° C) water at air temperature between 50° and 68° F (10° and 20° C). The USCG requires its cutters and inspected commercial vessels operating north or south of 32° latitude in the Atlantic Ocean or 35° latitude in the Pacific Ocean to carry immersion suits.

In an emergency an immersion suit should be donned only on an open deck. Because of its buoyancy an immersion suit donned below deck could prevent a person from diving or swimming out from beneath a capsizing vessel. Once it is donned, the wearer should never dive headfirst into water; doing so could cause the wearer to be suspended upside down in the water owing to redistribution of air within the suit. If "dry" boarding (see later discussion) a life raft is not possible, the wearer should jump feet first into the water with the legs twisted tightly together (Fig. 50-8). One hand should cover the face, and the other should hold the hood in place. The supplementary pillow should be inflated after the person gets clear of the ship. A list of immersion suit manufacturers appears in Appendix C at the end of the chapter.

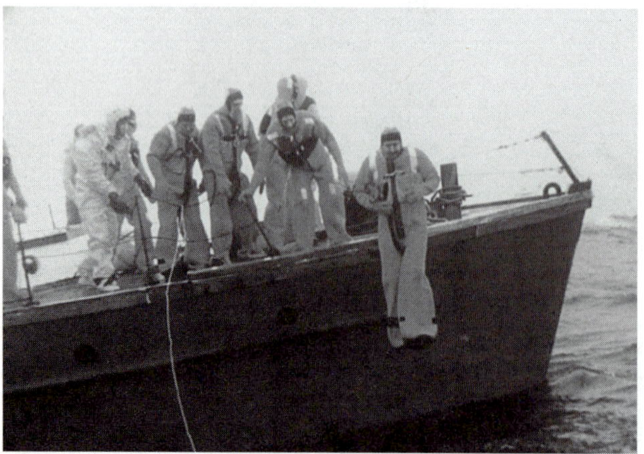

Fig. 50-8 Practice abandoning ship while wearing immersion suits; note the correct position of the legs. (Courtesy Survival Technologies Group.)

DRY SUITS[30]

Dry suits are constructed from vulcanized rubber, Gore-Tex, foam neoprene, crushed neoprene, urethane-coated fabrics, and trilaminates.[81] Currently a dry suit constructed of trilaminate or urethane-coated fabric (usually denier nylon) is the preferred thermal protection garment of the USCG when operating in cold water. The lightweight shell provides excellent mobility. The seams of a dry suit are sewn or glued and sealed with seam tape. The suit comes with attached boots and latex or neoprene neck and wrist seals. A front entry zipper is recommended to facilitate unassisted donning. For men an optional feature is a front relief zipper. Trilaminate and urethane-coated dry suits provide no inherent buoyancy or thermal protection and must be worn with thermal underwear (or warm clothing) and a PFD. All jewelry must be removed before donning the suit, which should be done with extreme care because a torn suit leaks, severely compromising its ability to protect the wearer from hypothermia. "Food-grade" silicon or unscented talcum powder applied to the neck and wrist seals facilitates donning and doffing. Paraffin or beeswax applied to the zippers retards corrosion, prolonging the life of the dry suit. A list of dry suit manufacturers appears in Appendix D at the end of the chapter.

WET SUITS[6,30]

A wet suit is effective, but not as good as a survival or dry suit, in prolonging survival and providing flotation for a person overboard. It is constructed of neoprene and should be at least 3⁄16 inch (7 to 8 mm) thick. A wet suit should be custom tailored for the wearer, since a loose fit increases cold water inflow, reducing the suit's effectiveness. It should fit snugly, but not be excessively tight. For added protection, a hood, gloves, and booties constructed of neoprene should be worn. Polypropylene underwear or a "diving skin" can be worn underneath for additional thermal protection. The USCG recommends that a rescue swimmer wear a wet suit (or dry suit) and rescue harness when assisting someone who has fallen overboard. All USCG boats operating in waters colder than 60° F (16° C) are required to carry wet suits, dry suits, or antiexposure coveralls for each crew member.

ANTIEXPOSURE SUITS

An antiexposure suit (coverall), also called a deck suit or work suit, is a type V PFD designed to be worn by boat crews exposed to intermittent cold spray and wind (Appendix E).[30] It provides significantly less thermal protection in the water than an immersion suit, dry suit, or wet suit. An antiexposure suit is brightly colored and constructed of nylon-covered, closed-cell foam. It provides about 17.5 pounds of buoyancy, slightly more than USCG-approved type II and III PFDs. A coverall allows full freedom of movement.

If an immersion suit, dry suit, wet suit, or antiexposure suit is unavailable, a PFD should be donned over heavy wool clothing. Swimming should not be attempted (unless back to a boat or raft), since it increases heat loss and reduces the boundary layers of warmer water around the body. Instead, the heat escape lessening position (HELP) should be assumed. If several people are in the water, they should huddle together for warmth, mutual support, and facilitation of rescue, since a larger group is more easily located (Fig. 50-9). To prevent hypothermia, every attempt should be made to get as much of the body out of the water as soon as possible (Fig. 50-10).

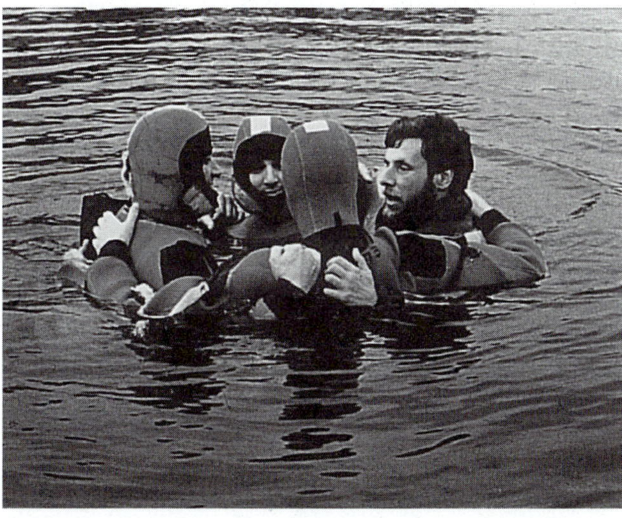

Fig. 50-9 Practicing the "huddle" while wearing immersion suits. (Courtesy Survival Technologies Group.)

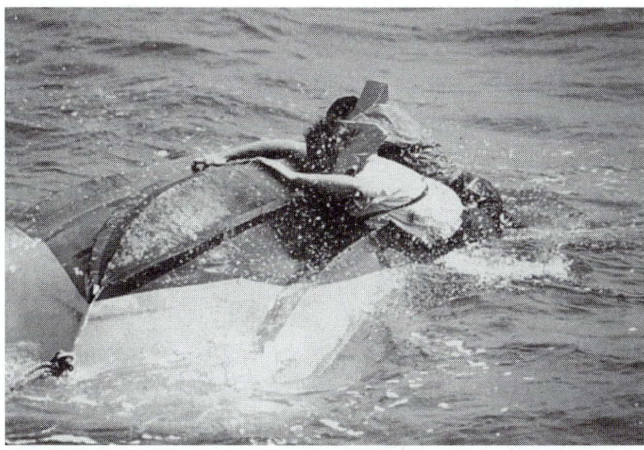

Fig. 50-10 Two survivors clinging to a capsized boat, attempting to get as much of the body out of the water as possible. (Courtesy U.S. Coast Guard.)

LIFE RAFTS*

Six types of life raft systems are available. Listed in descending order of sophistication and cost, they are the SOLAS approved, USCG approved, offshore, coastal, rescue platforms, and lifefloats (Appendix F). These definitions are not absolute and are used to facilitate discussion. Since noncommercial pleasure boats in the United States are not required by maritime law to carry a life raft, boat owners electing to carry a life raft may choose one not approved by the USCG. While USCG-approved rafts are designed to withstand harsh and prolonged survival conditions, many offshore and coastal rafts are sturdy and can adequately shelter survivors. SOLAS recommends that a life raft be able to remain afloat for a minimum of 30 days. Many stay afloat for much longer. With the advent of new SAR technology (such as 406.0 MHz EPIRB; see later discussion), some of the discussion of life raft longevity is artificial. If appropriately equipped with the proper electronic communication and signaling equipment, a survivor adrift at sea can usually expect to be rescued within days.

Some larger boats carry lifefloats (Fig. 50-11). These oval devices are constructed of rigid polyurethane or unicellular plastic foam coated with fiberglass or vinyl. They are designed to support 5 to 6 people. Strung from the perimeter of the lifefloat is a polyethylene mesh used to support the victims. The buoyancies of five-person and six-person lifefloats are 200 and 250 pounds, respectively.

A rescue platform resembles a child's play pool and does not have a canopy or ballast system. It is inflated with CO_2. On larger platforms the top and bottom are identical, ensuring that the platform always inflates with the appropriate side facing up. Rescue platforms come in a variety of sizes, the largest ones accommodating up to 50 persons. Many are equipped with a sea anchor, signal flares, flag, whistle, and repair kit. Use of a rescue platform is best confined to local waters where a higher density of boat traffic expedites rescue. Although rescue platforms are absolutely basic, they get victims out of the water, reducing the chances of drowning and hypothermia.

A coastal raft is the most basic type of life raft manufactured. A coastal raft should be used only when there is a high likelihood of being rescued rapidly. Coastal rafts have canopy and ballast systems but are not equipped with all the safety features routinely found on offshore, USCG- and SOLAS-approved rafts. In general, coastal rafts accommodate four to eight persons, but larger ones that hold up to 50 persons are available.

Offshore rafts are frequently carried by sailors traveling transcontinentally and are designed to shelter castaways awaiting rescue when adrift hundreds to thousands of miles offshore (Fig. 50-12). SOLAS- or USCG-approved rafts are required aboard commercial and large passenger ships in-

*References 4, 17, 29, 30, 43, 47, 48, 83.

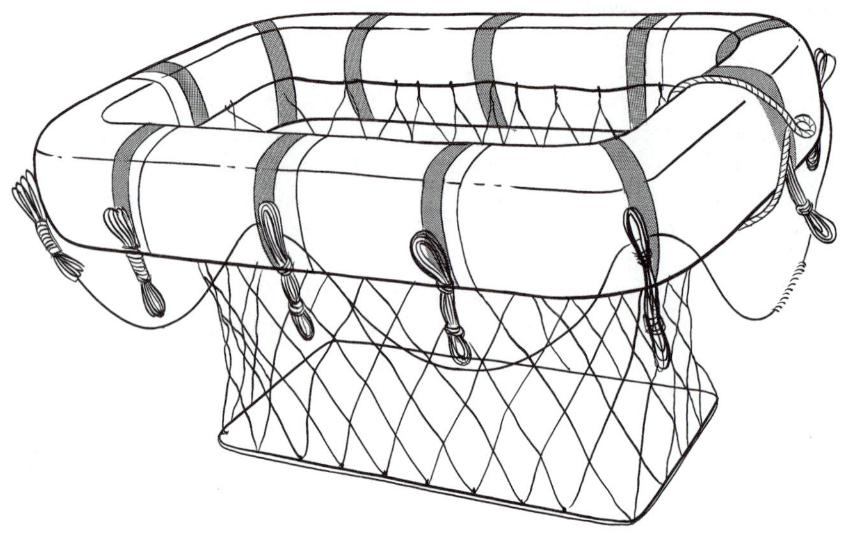

Fig. 50-11 Lifefloat. (Courtesy U.S. Coast Guard.)

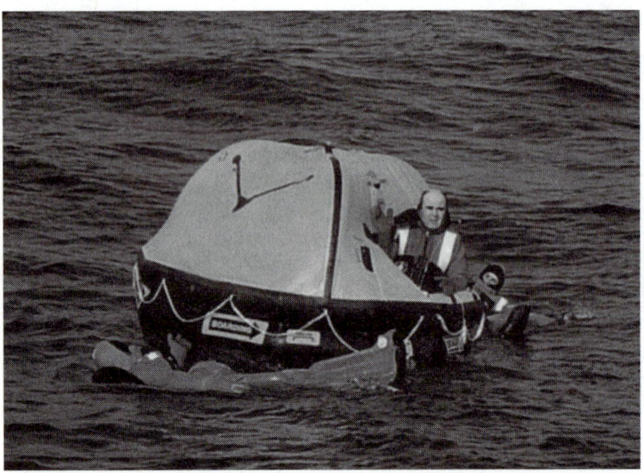

Fig. 50-12 Offshore life raft. (Courtesy Givens Life Raft.)

spected by the USCG. Given enough supplies, an offshore, USCG- or SOLAS-approved raft enables survivors to remain adrift at sea for weeks to months.

Life rafts are rectangular, circular, octagonal, dodecagonal, or oval in shape. Arguments favoring each type of design exist. Proponents of rectangular rafts argue that they provide more leg room, the lack of which is a frequent complaint by stranded castaways. A raft with corners may allow survivors to "wedge" or "lash" themselves into place, thereby increasing their stability within the raft. Those in favor of rafts without corners contend that they ride better in heavy seas.

Years ago, life rafts were constructed of rubber- or neoprene-coated cotton that quickly deteriorated. Modern life rafts are constructed of sturdy synthetic fabric (usually nylon), coated with urethane, neoprene, natural rubber, or polyvinylchloride. Most rafts are coated with neoprene, but those made by Viking are coated with natural rubber because of its ability to withstand colder temperatures. Seams are glued or heat sealed and reinforced with tape. The exterior of the raft is brightly colored to facilitate identification by SAR personnel. The interior surfaces of a raft should be darkly colored, which helps to prevent motion sickness and decreases glare associated with a bright canopy.

A well-designed raft has two or more nonconnected buoyancy chambers; this feature is important in the event that one chamber becomes punctured. With both buoyancy chambers 50% deflated or one chamber entirely deflated (simulating an irreparable leak or puncture), the raft should support a minimum of two thirds of its rated capacity.[17] On deployment, all life rafts inflate automatically with CO_2. Inflation canisters contain enough CO_2 to completely inflate the raft in Arctic conditions. In warmer climates, excess CO_2 is vented through high-pressure relief valves, thus preventing overinflation. When adrift at sea, castaways note that during the first few days following CO_2 inflation, the raft requires frequent air insufflations with a foot or hand pump to maintain inflation. Many consider hand pumps to be superior to foot pumps, which require a firm foundation to be used effectively. Gas leakage occurs because synthetic life raft materials are more permeable to CO_2 than air. Once air has largely replaced CO_2, the need for additional manual inflation decreases. Some seepage should still be expected on hot days.

A brightly colored canopy with affixed retroreflective material is an important part of a life raft system. Many manufacturers design canopies supported by arches automatically inflated coincident with raft inflation. When the raft and canopy arches are inflated, the canopy should be deployed in a furled position to facilitate boarding. When unfurled, the canopy covers the entire life raft to safeguard against falling overboard. In addition, the canopy protects survivors from the sun, wind, and rain. With the exception of coastal rafts, USCG- and SOLAS-approved rafts do not have furlable canopies. USCG- and SOLAS-approved rafts also have double canopies, designed to keep survivors warm in cold climates. Most coastal and offshore rafts have single-layer canopies. Although a canopy must be rugged enough to withstand heavy winds and high seas, it should ultimately be removable to facilitate watchkeeping, housekeeping, urination, defecation, and vomiting. A removable canopy or one containing viewing ports and furled panels reduces claustrophobia and motion sickness by providing a view of the horizon. Adequate ventilation also reduces feelings of nausea associated with the smell of synthetic raft and canopy materials. A rainwater collection apparatus attached to the canopy is useful in maintaining a supply of fresh water. The water collection device usually consists of a series of channels terminating in a water-collecting gusset fitted with a tube and plug protruding inside the raft. Many rafts have battery-operated, water-activated exterior and interior lights attached to the canopy. The water-activated cells are located just below the waterline.

To provide insulation from cold ocean temperatures capable of inducing hypothermia, a manually inflatable double floor should be strongly considered when purchasing a raft. A double floor that is permanently attached to the raft safeguards against flooding if the outer shell is punctured by flotsam (ocean debris) or marine animals. Less expensive rafts with removable outer floors are available. Most important, the floor should be designed in such a way as to shunt water away from raft occupants, thereby reducing the risk of hypothermia and decubitus ulcers. Raft floors fastened with buttons tend to accumulate small undesirable pools of water. In warmer climates the double floor can be deflated to facilitate cooling of the occupants. Most double floors are inflated manually after the raft is entered. If the cruising area is limited to warm water, a single floor is adequate.[21]

The bottom of a life raft has large, stabilizing ballast pockets that fill with water when the raft is deployed. Since water is weightless in water, the pockets do not function by "weighing" the raft down; instead, they act by resisting the lifting forces of wind and waves. At the time of this writing, three different ballast designs are in use: Icelandic, toroidal, and hemispheric. Icelandic ballast systems incorporate large, triangular, weighted pockets that are designed to fill rapidly with water. The Icelandic system also incorporates a special drogue, or sea anchor. The toroidal system is a patented design found on Switlik rafts. It consists of a deep, doughnutlike pocket that surrounds the rim of the raft and is divided into several chambers by internal baffles permeated by ports. The hemispherical bag patented by Givens holds the most water of any ballast system. It is a large, hemispheric dome that protrudes well below the surface of the raft. Water is admitted through small ports and a large opening in the bottom of the ballast system. The entire design is aptly referred to by the manufacturer as a hydrodynamic stabilizer. Although studies have shown that hemispheric and toroidal systems provided the most ballast, tests done by the British Board of Trade (equivalent to the USCG) and the Icelandic government found no difference in raft stabilization, as long as a proper drogue was deployed.[43,48]

For additional stabilization the raft should come equipped with several drogues that create drag, reducing the chance of capsizing (Fig. 50-13). In addition, a drogue deployed in front of the entrance will turn the raft door away from oncoming waves. If the sea anchor is lost or destroyed, one can be improvised from sail canvas (Fig. 50-14).

Grab handles and a grommeted (becketed) line attached to the outer and inner perimeters of the raft are features that facilitate "wet" boarding and righting. All modern rafts have a permanent righting strap attached to the bottom of the raft. A safety ladder and towing bridle enhance boarding and are standard equipment with most rafts. Plastic D rings and "patches" enable valuable anchors and lines to be attached to the raft. The raft should come with paddles and a bailer. Sponges should be included to assist bailing. Most life rafts come equipped with a floating safety knife stowed near the entrance of the raft. Some life rafts incorporate emesis receptacles within the raft so that castaways do not have to vomit over the side (inconvenient in cold, rough weather) or onto themselves and other castaways. If a raft is without this feature, plastic bags stowed in the abandon ship bag will suffice.

Most life rafts have basic survival equipment stowed inside, usually consisting of a small first aid kit, can opener, drinking cup, flashlight, pyrotechnics, signal mirror, and fishing kit. Most sea survival experts believe that additional survival equipment is necessary and recommend stowing an abandon ship bag (Fig. 50-15) containing other essential survival items (see later discussion).[21]

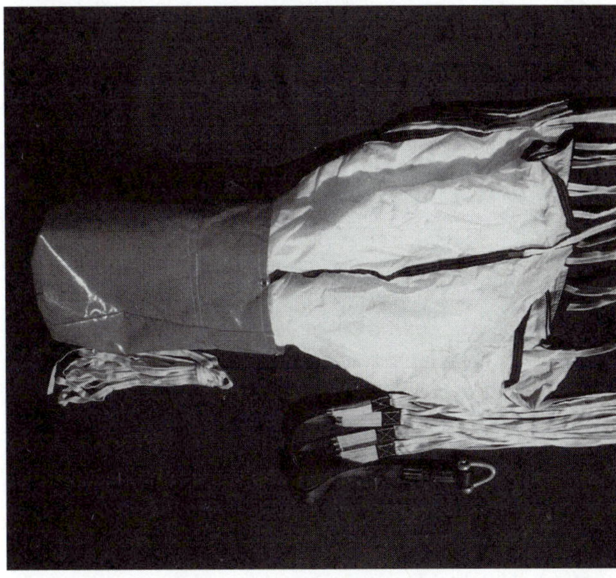

Fig. 50-13 Drogue. (Courtesy Survival Technologies Group.)

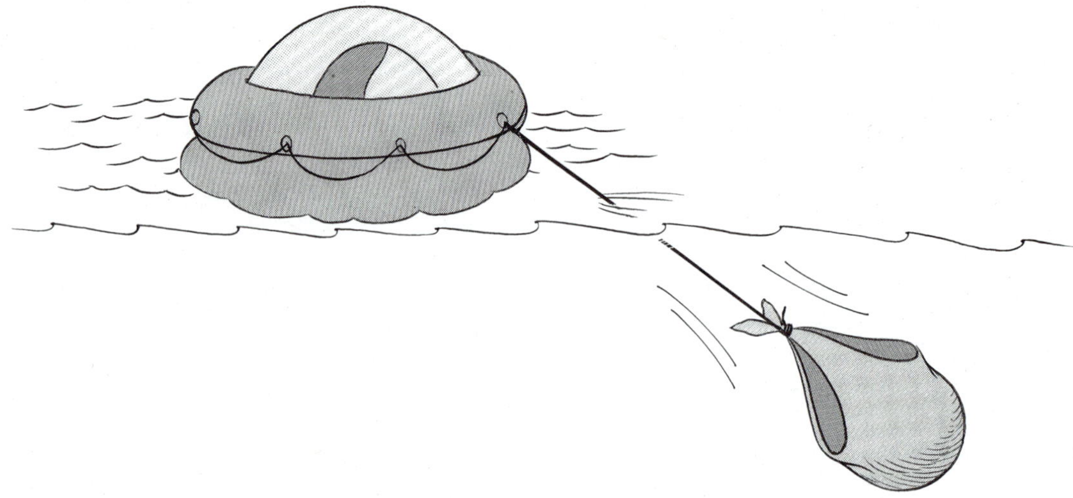

Fig. 50-14 Sea anchor (drogue) fashioned from sail canvas.

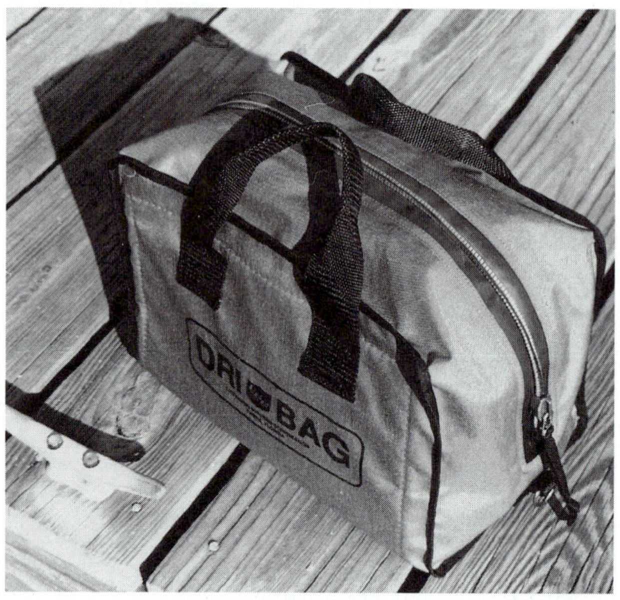

Fig. 50-15 Abandon ship bag. (Courtesy Survival Technologies Group.)

Since floor space within a raft is limited—less than 4 square feet per person—a raft should be selected that has a rated capacity of two more people than would actually be accommodated. Additional space is crucial if supplemental supplies and equipment are brought on board (such as an abandon ship bag; see later discussion) and water rations. Although a crowded raft facilitates ballasting, staying warm, and stabilizing passengers, these advantages can be obtained by other means. A sea anchor and ballast system amply stabilize the raft, and a thermal protection aid (see later discussion) helps to insulate cold castaways. In addition, the psychologic benefit of not sitting atop one's shipmates is invaluable.

Life rafts are stored in either a fiberglass canister or a fabric valise. The fiberglass canister is designed to be mounted on deck, allowing easy access to the raft in an emergency. However, the canister is vulnerable to theft in port and to being washed overboard in breaking seas. The canister's waterproof gasket must be routinely inspected to ensure a hermetic seal. A canister weighs approximately 10 to 20 pounds more than a comparably sized valise. A life raft must be easily deployed by even the weakest crew member under adverse conditions (for example, at night, in heavy seas, or while sinking or capsizing).

> I recall the life raft instructions: throw the [100 pound] life raft overboard before inflation. Who can maneuver such weight in the middle of a bucking circus ride? The first pull, then the second—nothing! This is it, the end of my life. The third pull comes up hard, and she blows with a bursting static shush![17]

A valise (soft, fabric container) and its raft are usually stowed below deck, protecting the raft from the elements. While less likely to be stolen in port, a raft stowed below deck can be rendered inaccessible by fire or serious flooding. Instead, a watertight topside compartment or locker, if available, should be used to stow the valise. Generally, a canister is preferable to a valise. If a valise is chosen, the crew *must* remember to tie the painter line (lanyard) to the ship before tossing the valise over the side. Valise-type life rafts have been found floating in the ocean undeployed, the unfortunate crew having forgotten to secure the lanyard to the boat.

Life rafts aboard noninspected vessels should be inflated, examined, and repackaged every 12 months by a USCG-authorized repacking station. Life rafts aboard inspected vessels must be serviced every 12 months. Failure to do so subjects the vessel to large fines and impoundment.[21] Owners should not conduct life raft tests by using CO_2 to inflate the raft. CO_2 canisters are expensive to refill, and raft fabric exposed to extremely cold CO_2 in dry air has a tendency to crack. Packing stations use compressed air to inflate rafts. Owners are encouraged to be present during raft inflation and inspection to gain additional familiarity with the raft. Additional survival gear can be added to the raft at this time.

If no life raft is available, improvisation may yield a suitable craft. While prawning off the coast of Australia, Jack Drinan's trawler sank early one morning. The following article appeared in *The Canberra Times,* May 13, 1963[58]:

> The prawning trawler . . . sank about 5 A.M. on April 24th. . . . As the trawler went down, the 7 foot × 8 foot icebox tore loose and bobbed up beside the swimming skipper . . . Jack Drinan. He broke a hole in one of the 3-foot deep compartments and stayed in it for the next twelve days. For water, he licked the moisture from the icebox lid, spending the days bailing salt water from the craft with a shirt. His only tools were a shovel and an eighteen-inch hammer. With these he cut the lid in half and made a flimsy raft measuring 6 feet 9 inches by 2 feet 4 inches. The first time he set out for the shore aboard the insulating foam-covered lid, he lost heart after one mile and returned to his icebox "mother ship." A day later he tried again and was on shore within twenty-four hours.

KNOTS

Survival at sea may be partly determined by one's skill in marlinspike seamanship (the art of handling and working line). In an emergency, "to be less than expert may be costly when the safety of life and property depends upon a few knots."[6] Line is used principally for four purposes: pulling, holding, lifting, and lowering. There are two types of line: natural fiber and synthetic.

Natural line is made from organic material. If not carefully stowed and protected, natural line deteriorates rapidly. Moisture causes mildew and rotting. Wearing of natural line is evidenced by a white powdery substance found between strands, representing small particles of line worn off by friction. Friction against the outer surface of the line causes chafing, evidenced by broken strands.

Synthetic line is constructed of inorganic materials. Nylon (double braided and three stranded), polypropylene, polyethylene, and Dacron polyester are common types of synthetic line. The USCG uses primarily double-braided nylon because of its high breaking strength. If polypropylene line is used, it should be stored in a black plastic bag to reduce damage by ultraviolet light. Synthetic line should be palpated; a line that feels hard has been overloaded. Chafing and fiber damage should be noted.

Line stretches when placed under tension. As line stretches and diameter decreases, breaking strength decreases. When line is stretched, it is said to elongate; its ability to recover from elongation is referred to as elasticity. Synthetic line has superior elongation and elastic properties and is better able to absorb the intermittent forces of sea motion (shockload). However, synthetic line is prone to slipping and does not hold knots as well as natural line. The best knot to use for securing or bending synthetic line is the bowline (see later discussion).

The breaking strength of a line is measured in pounds and is determined through stress tests conducted by the manufacturer. Shackles and hooks are also rated for load and should always be used with a line having a lower load rating. If given the choice between hardware breaking or line parting, the latter is preferable.[6]

The free or working end of a line is called the bitter end. The long or unused end is called the standing part. A loop formed by crossing the bitter end over the standing part is called an overhand loop; if the bitter end crosses under the standing part, it is called an underhand loop. A bight is a 180-degree half loop formed by turning the line back on itself. A loop or turn is a 360-degree turn. Two loops around an object is referred to as a round turn.

If a line is cut, it must be temporarily tied off with sail twine to prevent unraveling or fraying. This procedure is called whipping. Any time a line is cut, the new bitter end should be whipped. After whipping is completed, the excess ends should be trimmed (Fig. 50-16).

Knots are used to secure lines to one another or to other objects. When a knot is used to temporarily secure two lines together, it is referred to as a bend. A splice is used for permanent joining and is stronger than a bend. If a knot is used to secure a line to an object, the knot is called a hitch. Exceptions exist; a rolling hitch is commonly used to secure two lines together. If line becomes chafed, damaged, or distorted, it must be cut and spliced. All crew members should be adept at tying a few simple knots and have a knife in their possession when under way.[42]

A bowline is one of the most versatile knots (Fig. 50-17). It is used to quickly form a loop of almost any size and has a high breaking strength. A bowline will not slip or jam and is easy to untie. The most frequent use of a bowline is to create a large, permanent loop at the end of a docking line. If someone goes overboard, a bowline can be thrown into the bitter end of a heaving line and tossed to the victim. If tied properly, it will support the person being hauled aboard.

A hitch is used to secure line to objects. It is generally used to make a temporary fastening. If necessary, it can be untied quickly. The single half hitch is the smallest and simplest hitch but is prone to slipping (Fig. 50-18). Two half hitches may be used to reinforce a single half hitch (Fig. 50-19). This is a reliable knot and resists slipping. A round turn can be added for additional strength (Fig. 50-20).

An anchor bend or fisherman's bend is used to secure an anchor line to the anchor ring. It is similar to the round turn and two half hitches but is more secure; it is also slightly harder to tie and untie in an emergency.

A clove hitch is the best knot to use for securing a line to a ring or other round object. It is often used to secure a docking line (Fig. 50-21).

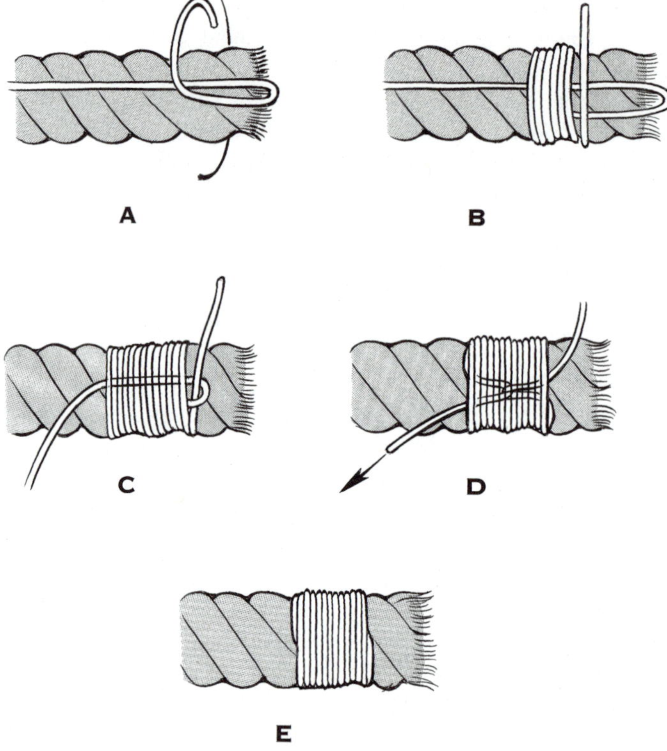

Fig. 50-16 Temporary whipping. (Courtesy U.S. Coast Guard.)

A single becket bend or sheet bend is used when two lines of the same diameter are temporarily joined together (Fig. 50-22). A double becket or double sheet bend is used to temporarily join together lines of unequal size (Fig. 50-23).

The double carrick bend is a traditional and effective means of tying together two lines of the same diameter. It is especially useful for heavy, stiff lines. It is slightly more difficult to tie than a single sheet bend but is more resistant to slipping. If a double carrick bend is subjected to strain and moisture, it can be difficult to untie (Fig. 50-24).

ABANDON SHIP BAG*

Every ship should have an abandon ship bag (bug-out or grab bag) containing a variety of items needed for survival at sea. Although most life rafts contain some survival supplies, they are usually insufficient for prolonged survival. The exact contents of an abandon ship bag vary depending on the size of the crew and characteristics of the sea voyage (length, location, and distance offshore). Once the ship is under way, all valuables and important survival gear should be stowed in the abandon ship bag. During a sea emergency it is impossible to gather such important items quickly.

All contents of the bag should be waterproof or placed in waterproof bags. Tupperware containers are rigid and take up valuable space within a raft; therefore they are not recommended. The bag itself should be inherently buoyant and constructed of brightly colored Cordura nylon with reinforced seams. Suitable bags may be purchased from marine supply retailers (Fig. 50-15).

In a sea emergency one of the crew members should be designated to locate the abandon ship bag and keep track of it at all times. It should be easily accessible and stowed in a convenient place. The list in Box 50-1 is meant to serve as a general guideline when selecting articles for an abandon ship bag.

*References 4, 22, 27, 43, 47, 48, 83, 84, 87, 88.

Preparation for Emergencies

MAN OVERBOARD*

Obscurest night involved the sky,
The Atlantic billows roared,
When such a destined wretch as I,
Washed headlong from onboard.
Of friends, of hope, of all bereft,
His floating home for ever left

William Cowper, *The Castaway*

Falling overboard is always unexpected. In rough cold water, shock, disorientation, and panic may quickly incapac-

*References 6, 18, 39, 40, 70, 75, 79, 97.

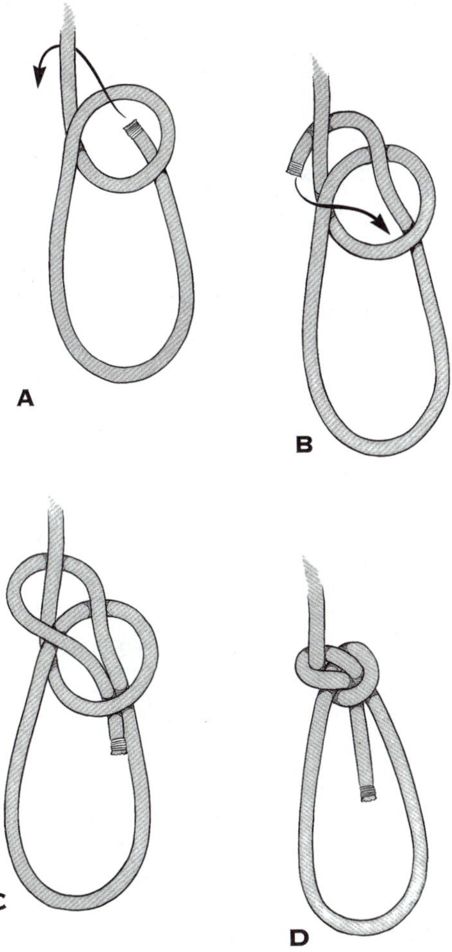

Fig. 50-17 Bowline. (Courtesy U.S. Coast Guard.)

itate the victim. Rescue efforts should be quick and decisive, since survival time may be measured in minutes. A boat moving at 6 knots travels 11 feet (3.4 m) per second. In just 1 minute the boat will be over 200 yards (183 m) away from a man overboard (MOB).

"The best protection against man overboard is anticipation and prevention by wearing a safety harness. Stay on the boat!" These words were spoken to the Wilderness Medical Society in Stratton, Vermont, on September 29, 1989, by Dr. Ray Brown, surgeon and veteran sailor from Annapolis, Maryland. On October 1, just 2 days later, Dr. Brown fell off his new boat and drowned. On this date, Dr. Brown had taken delivery of an Alden 50 in Portsmouth, Rhode Island, and was sailing home to Annapolis. During the midnight to 4 AM watch, Dr. Brown took off his harness and went below to consult his charts. Returning to the cockpit unharnessed, Dr. Brown went forward to inspect a fluttering jib. A large wave caused the boat to lurch suddenly and the main boom to jibe, knocking Dr. Brown over the side. Despite an exhaustive search by the crew and Coast Guard, his body was never recovered.[40]

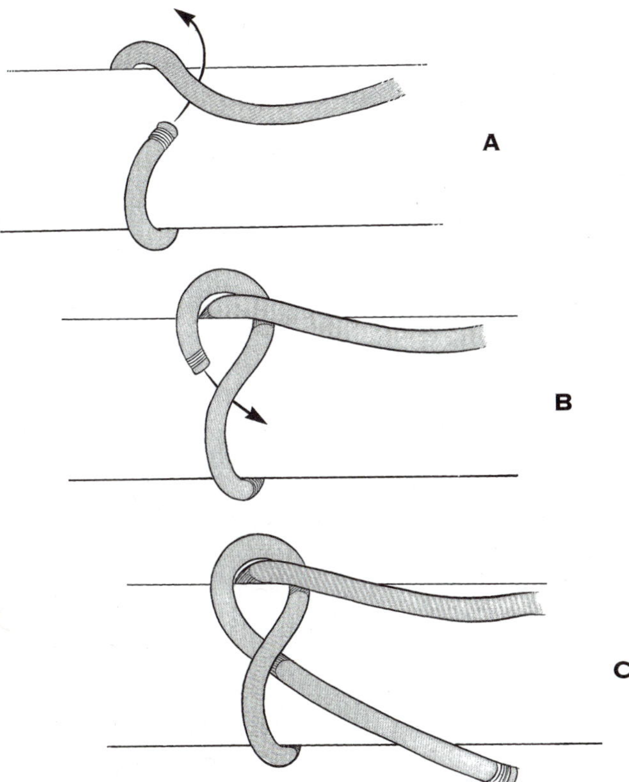

Fig. 50-18 Single half hitch. (Courtesy U.S. Coast Guard.)

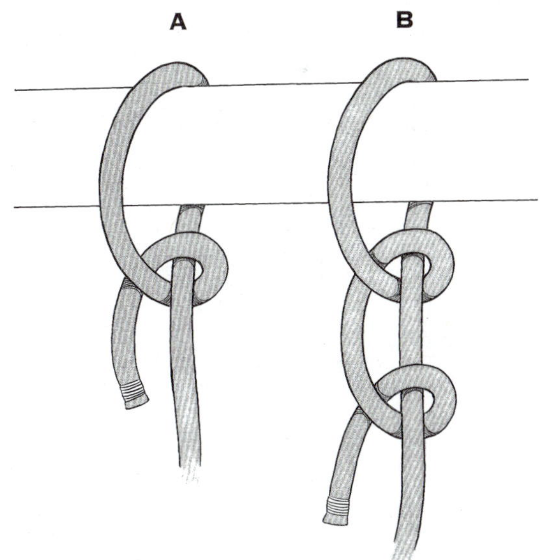

Fig. 50-19 Two half hitches. (Courtesy U.S. Coast Guard.)

Prevention against going overboard is vital. Several suggestions are offered: keep the deck and cockpit uncluttered, never urinate or vomit over the side at night or when a high sea is running, wear a PFD whenever on deck, wear good deck shoes with corrugated rubber soles, and use safety harnesses and jacklines. A harness is not foolproof. A sinking

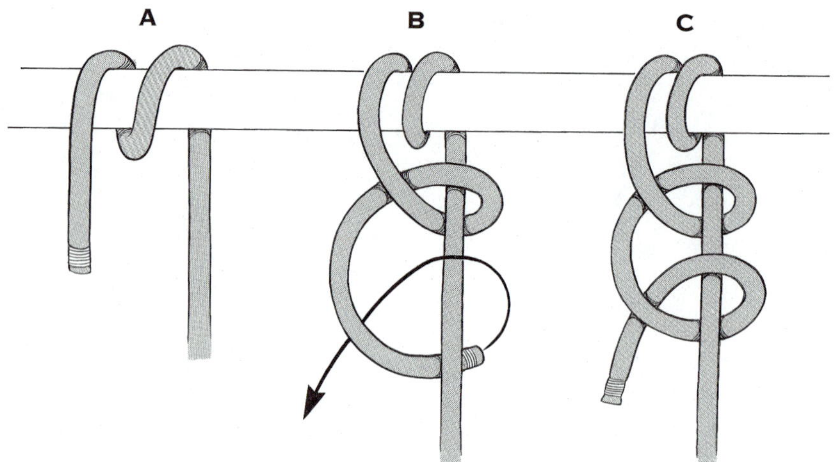

Fig. 50-20 Round turn with two half hitches.

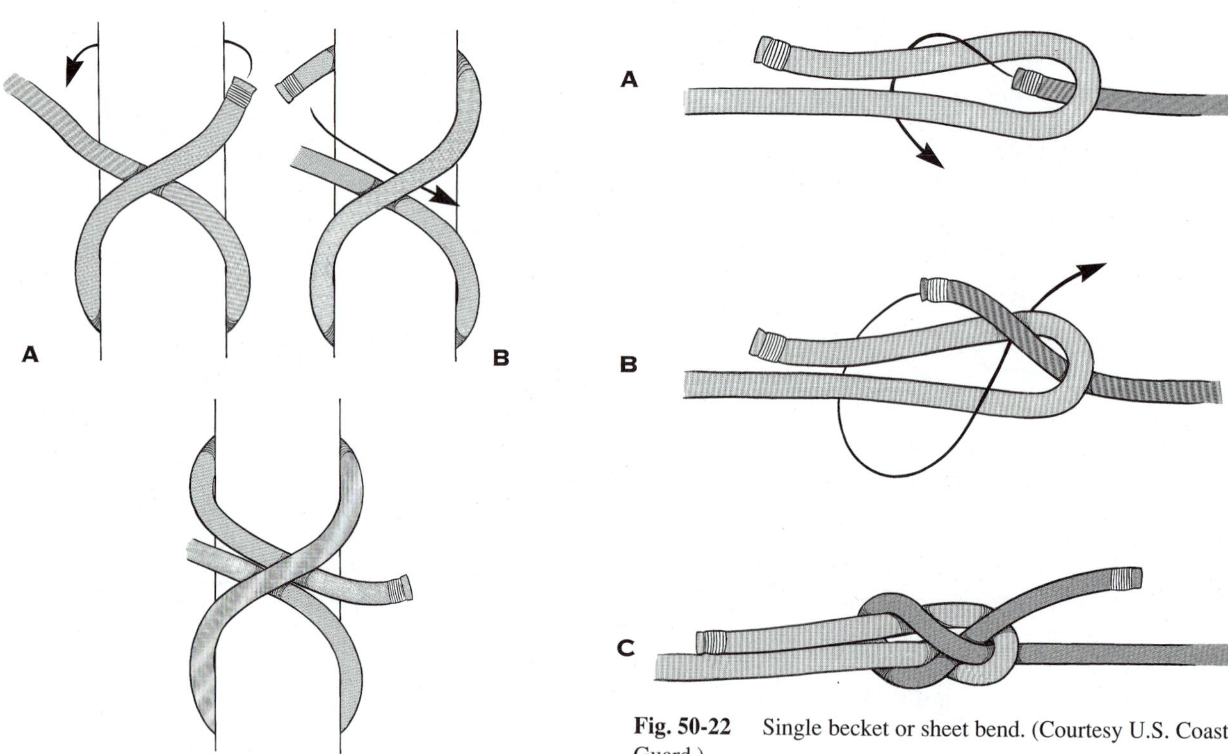

Fig. 50-21 Clove hitch. (Courtesy U.S. Coast Guard.)

Fig. 50-22 Single becket or sheet bend. (Courtesy U.S. Coast Guard.)

boat may pull a harnessed crew member underwater if the victim is unable to unclip from the lifeline. If the boat is moving, a harnessed MOB may be dragged underwater and drowned by its forward motion. Quick-release harnesses are available, but care should be exercised with their use to prevent accidental release.

No single best way exists to rescue a MOB. Methods vary depending on ocean and weather conditions, visibility, type of ship, and size of the crew. Each skipper should work out a plan and practice MOB drills. In general, three basic principles apply:

1. The victim must always be kept in sight and afloat.
2. A line, seat cushion, MOB pole, or anything that floats must be dispatched to the MOB as soon as possible.
3. The MOB must be hauled aboard.

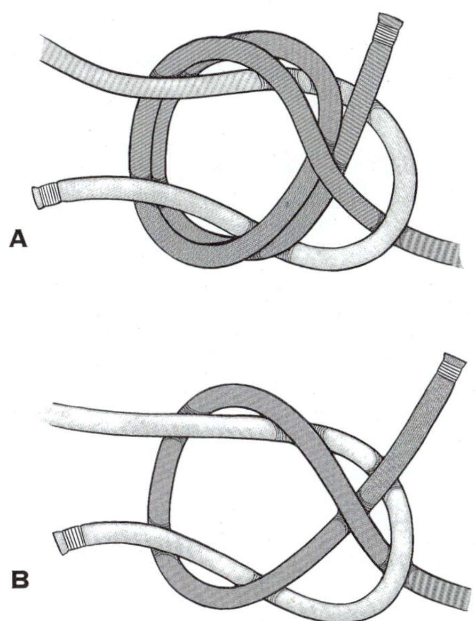

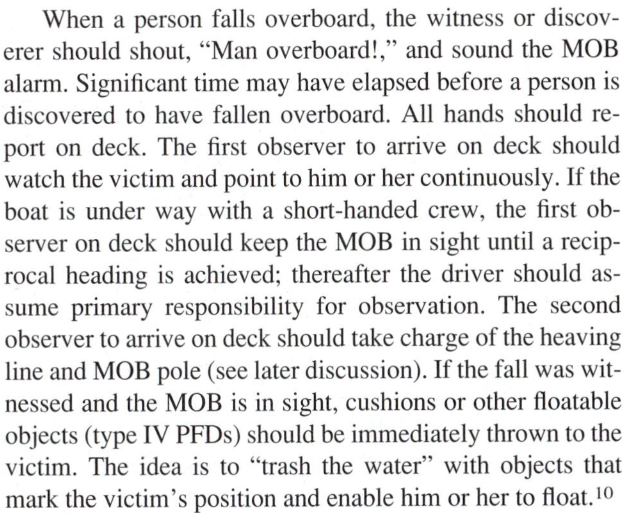

Fig. 50-23 Double becket or double sheet bend. (Courtesy U.S. Coast Guard.)

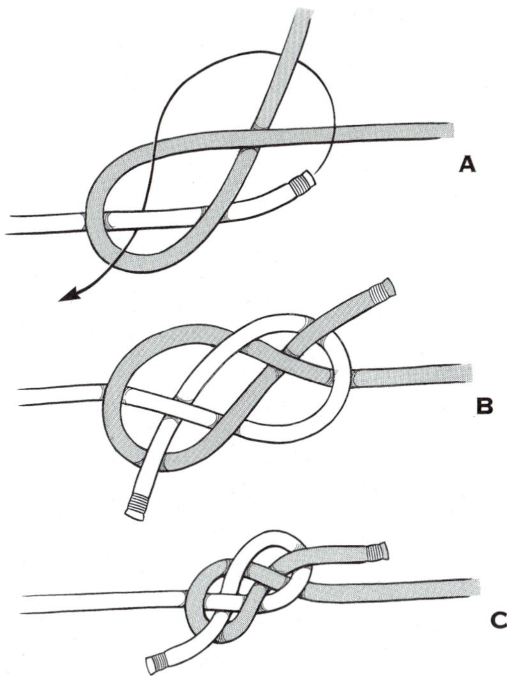

Fig. 50-24 Double carrick bend.

When a person falls overboard, the witness or discoverer should shout, "Man overboard!," and sound the MOB alarm. Significant time may have elapsed before a person is discovered to have fallen overboard. All hands should report on deck. The first observer to arrive on deck should watch the victim and point to him or her continuously. If the boat is under way with a short-handed crew, the first observer on deck should keep the MOB in sight until a reciprocal heading is achieved; thereafter the driver should assume primary responsibility for observation. The second observer to arrive on deck should take charge of the heaving line and MOB pole (see later discussion). If the fall was witnessed and the MOB is in sight, cushions or other floatable objects (type IV PFDs) should be immediately thrown to the victim. The idea is to "trash the water" with objects that mark the victim's position and enable him or her to float.[10]

An MOB pole is a 6-foot stiff or inflatable pole attached to a floating buoy (ring or horseshoe). It is used to provide emergency identification and flotation to a victim who has fallen overboard. Survival Technologies Group (STG) has developed a Man Overboard Module (MOM). The MOM is a canister containing a sea anchor, inflatable horseshoe buoy, and pole. The canister is usually attached to the stern rail. When a person falls overboard, the canister is quickly opened by removing a pin, allowing the MOM to fall into the water (Fig. 50-25). The horseshoe buoy and pole are fully inflated with CO_2 within 2 seconds after being released by gravity from the canister (Fig. 50-26). The purpose of the attached sea anchor is to allow the MOB module to drift at the same rate of speed as an MOB, maximizing the MOB's chances of reaching the module. In high seas a 6-foot pole is difficult for rescuers to see, and an MOB without a PFD stands a higher chance of drowning. Therefore STG recommends that an inflatable PFD, water-activated strobe light, hand smoke, whistle, and one red flare be attached to the MOM.

STG also manufactures an inflatable raft, pole, and vest packaged in a similar canister that can be attached to the stern rail. The raft and pole automatically inflate after being released from the canister. The advantage of a raft is that it gets the MOB out of the water (Fig. 50-27). In seas less than 6 feet the raft may be used as a reboarding platform.

At night a white parachute flare discharged by crew members searching for an MOB lights up 2 square miles for approximately 30 seconds. STG recommends that, when searching for an MOB at night, all shipboard lights be extinguished, including running lights, to optimize night vision. Extinguishing of lights should be undertaken carefully when traveling in busy shipping lanes. During extensive MOB testing at night, STG found it helpful if the victim splashed water when illuminated by a searchlight—the light reflected by the splashing water was notably bright.

Alternatively, a sling or inflatable horseshoe buoy can be attached to 100 to 150 feet of ½-inch polypropylene line and heaved to the MOB. Polypropylene is recommended because it floats. The heaving line is thrown underhanded to maximize accuracy and distance. Some experts believe that a "bagged" heaving line is more easily and accurately

BOX 50-1

ABANDON SHIP BAG

SIGNALING EQUIPMENT

1 406 or 121 EPIRB
1 SART
12 SOLAS red parachute flares
4 SOLAS white parachute flares
4 SOLAS red hand-held flares
2 SOLAS orange smoke canisters
2 colored dye markers
24 cyalume chemical light sticks
Waterproof halogen flashlight with extra flashlight batteries
Signaling mirror (heliograph)
Portable VHF radio in plastic bag with extra batteries
Cellular phone
Plastic whistle

FISHING EQUIPMENT

1 knife (dull tip, floatable) in scabbard
1 spool 80-pound test fishing line
20-foot wire leader
3 medium fishing spoons
75 fishing hooks
1 pair pliers
1 16-inch speargun
1 wire saw

MISCELLANEOUS EQUIPMENT

Log book with pen
Raft repair kit
Binoculars
Navigational equipment
50-foot polypropylene line stowed in a black plastic bag

PROVISIONS

Survivor-brand reverse-osmosis desalinator
Solar still
1-gallon plastic folding water jug
High-energy freeze-dried food

CLOTHING AND PERSONAL SUPPLIES

1 long-sleeved shirt and pants
1 pair shoes with wool socks
1 warm cap and hat
1 pair polypropylene underwear
1 pair sunglasses
1 thermal or Mylar-type blanket
2 rolls toilet paper in sealed plastic bag
Toothbrush
Passport
Money (American currency)
Credit cards
Ship's papers
Plastic emesis bags

MEDICAL SUPPLIES

First aid kit
Individual prescription medications
Prescription glasses
Sunglasses
Motion sickness medicine
Sunscreen
Petroleum jelly
Antiseptic ointment
Multivitamins
Nonsteroidal antiinflammatory medications
Narcotics
Antihistamine
Suture set with nylon suture, local anesthetic
Survival manual

thrown. These bags are often weighted to facilitate throwing. A strong swimmer on deck should be fitted with a type III PFD, dry suit or wet suit, diving fins, mask, and reverse harness attached to 100 feet of polypropylene line in case he or she is needed to assist the MOB. If the victim is helpless and unable to grab the line or buoy because of injury, confusion, weakness, or incoordination, the rescue swimmer may have to go over the side to assist. If the boat has a long range aid to navigation (LORAN) or global positioning system (GPS)—devices that continuously track a vessel's position—its memory should be activated to record the precise position where the MOB was last spotted. During the rescue the vessel's position should be updated continually.

An MOB is rarely able to swim back to the boat. Many maneuvers have been described to return a vessel quickly to a victim in the water. Whichever maneuver is chosen, it should be kept simple. With sailboats, a sailing text can be consulted for a detailed description of how to turn through the wind (spouse's maneuver), beat into the wind, run downwind (racetrack pattern), and "quick stop." For boats under power, four techniques are accepted for returning to an MOB: Williamson turn, racetrack turn, crash stop, and Anderson turn. These maneuvers are described in many books.

If the MOB has been thrown a line and is able to assist with the rescue, he or she should be maneuvered to a swimming platform or ladder using the heaving line. If a platform or ladder is not available, crew members must pull the victim on board. If the MOB cannot be fully pulled onto the

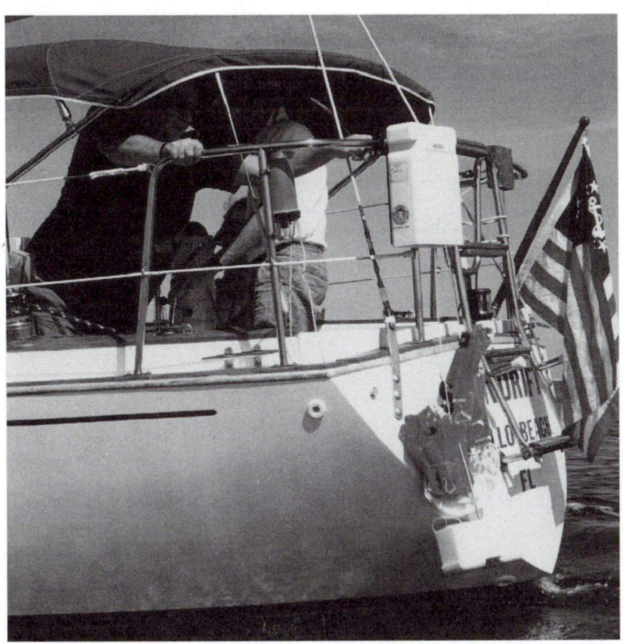

Fig. 50-25 Man Overboard Module (MOM) 8. Photo was taken 0.5 second after the MOM was released. (Courtesy Survival Technologies Group.)

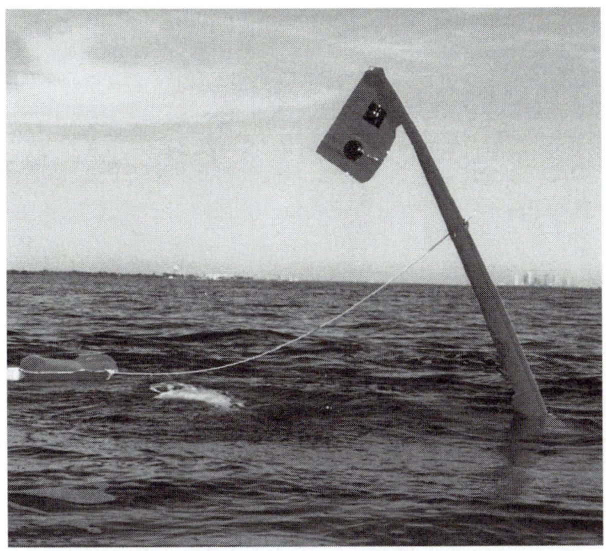

Fig. 50-26 Man Overboard Module (MOM) 8. Fully inflated; note the orange distress flag with black ball and square. (Courtesy Survival Technologies Group.)

ship, the victim should be hauled as high as possible out of the water and the heaving line tied to a cleat. A halyard winch or purchase can be used to complete hoisting of the MOB onto the ship. The reader should consult a boating guide for specific details on the application and rigging of this equipment.

If the MOB is lost at sea, the USCG and any nearby vessels should be notified immediately (see later discussion of

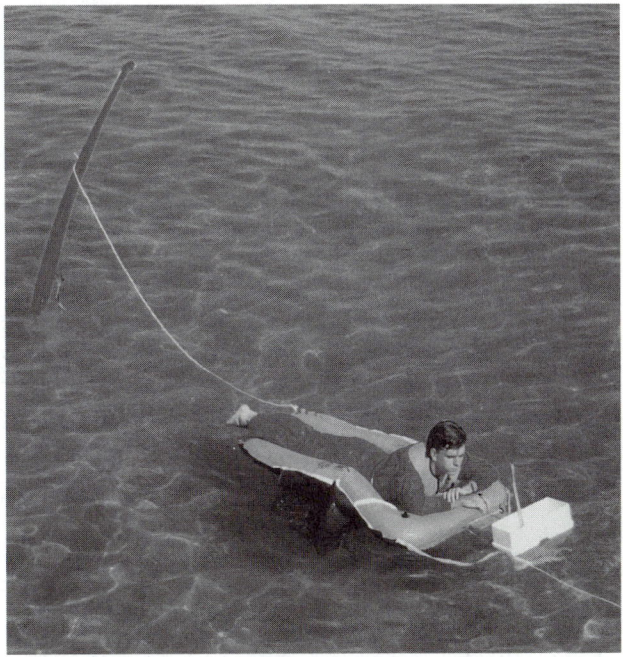

Fig. 50-27 Man Overboard Module (MOM) 9. Fully inflated; mechanism similar to MOM 8. (Courtesy Survival Technologies Group.)

Mayday procedures). In darkness the last known location of the MOB should be marked with a floating electrical marker light thrown into the water. These battery-powered lights are waterproof and emit a flashing light discharged from a xenon flashtube at approximately 60 flashes per minute. The battery should last 15 hours. The utility of marker lights is greatly reduced in high seas, but they should still be dispatched. A good navigational fix should be obtained using LORAN or GPS. VHF channel 16 should be monitored continuously. If the MOB's position is known within close limits, an expanding square search should be instituted (Fig. 50-28). A sector search is used when an MOB is difficult to detect (as in high seas) but his or her relative position is known (Fig. 50-29). If the MOB's location is known only to be somewhere along the boat's earlier course, a parallel trackline (Fig. 50-30) or creeping line search should be used (Fig. 50-31).[6,97]

The search for an MOB should "never" be stopped. Many victims have been rescued after hours or days at sea. In the mid-Atlantic, 1000 miles from the nearest land, Franz Strycharczyk, the third engineer on the German freighter *Freiberg,* fell overboard. Several hours passed before he was missed, at which time the *Freiberg* reversed course and began searching in the dark. Seventeen hours after falling overboard without any flotation, Strycharczyk was rescued by the Coast Guard cutter *Absecon,* which had responded to the report of an MOB. Under his own power, he was able to climb up a cargo net that had been lowered to him. The stocky, 185-pound German was returned to the *Freiberg,*

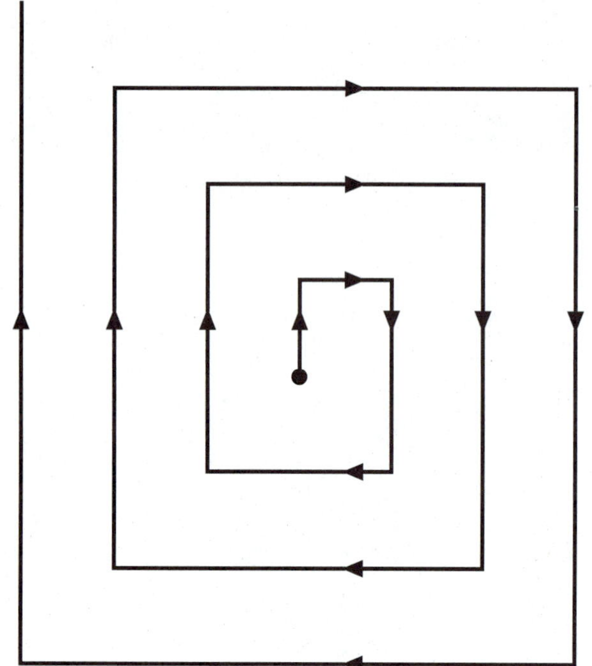

Fig. 50-28 Expanding square search. (Courtesy U.S. Coast Guard.)

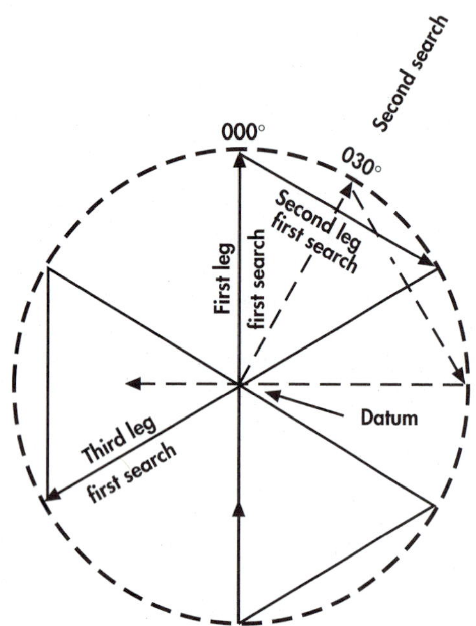

Fig. 50-29 Sector search. (Courtesy U.S. Coast Guard.)

which "paid" for his rescue with 185 pounds of German delicacies, including Lowenbraü beer![58]

FLOODING

In general, a ship should be abandoned only in the event of a consuming fire or imminent sinking. Some boats have

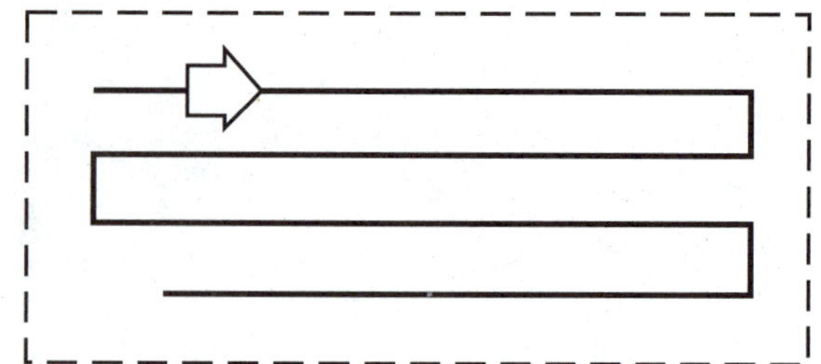

Fig. 50-30 Parallel track search. (Courtesy U.S. Coast Guard.)

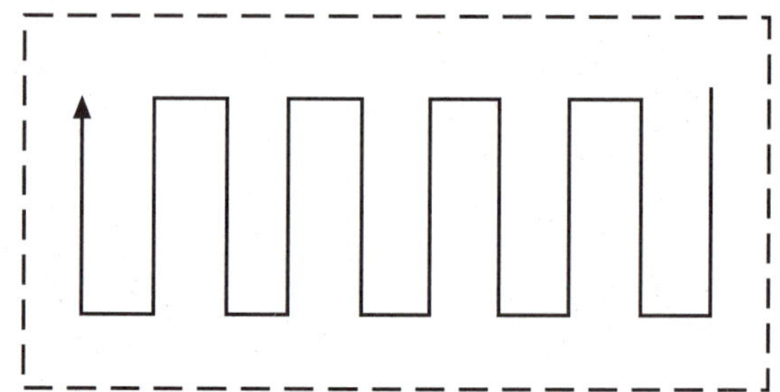

Fig. 50-31 Creeping line search. (Courtesy U.S. Coast Guard.)

been known to stay afloat for hours or days because of trapped air in the hull. The rate of flooding depends on the size and location of the hole. A 2-inch (5 cm) diameter hole located near waterline admits 7000 gallons (26,460 L) of water per hour. The same hole located 4 feet (122 cm) from the waterline admits 12,800 gallons (48,384 L) per hour. A 4-inch (10 cm) diameter hole located near waterline admits 9600 gallons (36,288 L) per hour. If the 4-inch hole is 4 feet below water, 18,900 gallons (71,442 L) per hour is admitted.[11] Since a 12-volt, battery-powered bilge pump on board a small boat pumps no more than approximately 1500 gallons of water per hour under ideal circumstances, sailors should make every attempt to slow flooding by plugging the hole. Bilge pumps are designed to control relatively minor accumulations of water, such as leaks around a shaft, hatch, or port. They are not designed to control flooding associated with hull damage. However, once the water level inside a damaged hull has risen above the level of the hole, the rate of water admission into the ship may slow by virtue of a reduced pressure head. With bilge pumps running, a point of zero net flooding may be reached. Failure to understand this principle has led to premature abandonments. Therefore the maxim "Never leave your ship until your ship leaves you" should be followed. Once a leak or flood is detected, all pumps must be started and the inflow of water reduced or stopped.[97] Discussion of a recent investigation of the top five bilge pumps is available.[12]

Since an electrical bilge pump is only as good as its battery supply and wire connections, which are frequently damaged by a large flood, a good manual pump should be on standby. Two basic types of manual pumps are available:

piston-cylinder and diaphragm. Although handy, the piston model is easily clogged by debris. The diaphragm pump is easier to operate for longer periods because of its shorter stroke. It also handles debris better and is capable of moving larger volumes of water.

A portable, gasoline-powered salvage pump kit is an invaluable resource in pumping out a boat in danger of sinking.[6] This is available to the public and used frequently by the USCG. A typical USCG pump contains a three-horsepower, four-cycle gasoline engine packaged inside a watertight, floatable aluminum container. This pump is capable of removing 7200 gallons (27,216 L) of water per hour at a 5- to 10-foot (1.5 to 3 m) suction lift—the distance from the base of the pump to the highest point in the discharge hose. Under a load the pump runs 4 to 5 hours on 1 gallon (3.8 L) of gasoline. In an emergency it can be airdropped to a flooding vessel by SAR helicopters or fixed-wing aircraft.[30]

A broken through-hull fitting or hose is a common cause of sinking in smaller boats. Corrosion, fire, vibration, and chafing can lead to failure of these materials. In many cases of hose failure, simply closing the seacock may stop the flooding. If this fails to counteract flooding, a soft, tapered, wooden expandable plug can be inserted into the fitting or hose. All through-hull fittings should have a wooden plug attached for easy access in case of a leak.

Underwater epoxy kits are available for repair of small holes in fiberglass boats. The epoxy is water activated and requires no mixing. Total setup time from application to hardening is less than 30 minutes.

A larger hole in the outer hull may be covered with a sail or collision mat (a prefabricated cover made of canvas or awning material) that is secured by lines to the boat; water pressure also helps keep it in place. Rigging it requires a couple of swimmers.[97]

An emergency flotation bag (EFB) is designed to provide emergency flotation to a small boat in danger of sinking. The EFB is a reusable, pillow-shaped bag that measures approximately 38 × 60 inches (97 × 152 cm). When inflated, it provides approximately 500 pounds of buoyancy. As a general rule, one EFB should support 1000 pounds of the boat's gross weight. Newer EFBs are constructed of urethane-coated fabric and inflated with compressed air or CO_2. For maximal performance the EFB should be positioned in the lowest part the boat.[97]

Many smaller vessels are now constructed with polyurethane foam incorporated into the boat. This adds approximately 4% to the purchase price of the boat and occupies roughly 6% of its interior space, but the result is a virtually unsinkable boat. Unfortunately, retrofitting a boat with this material is not cost effective.[97]

Finally, in the event of flooding, bailing should never be stopped; it may provide just enough time for deployment of a life raft or arrival of rescuers. A 3-gallon bucket of water emptied every 12 seconds equals the capacity of an average electric or manual diaphragm bilge pump. In October 1980 the 86-foot staysail schooner *Mariah* began taking on water in heavy weather. The electric bilge and gasoline-driven pumps failed. However, the crew bailed continuously for 30 hours, lending credence to the saying, "A frightened man with a bucket is a first-rate pump replacement." A Coast Guard helicopter and cutter finally rescued the weary crew.[97]

FIRE*

Few things are more terrifying than a fire at sea. Fires often force rapid abandonment and may cause injury or death before escape is possible. Fires at sea are often far more serious than fires ashore. Small boats are inherently flammable objects because of liquid fuel, wood, fiberglass, and paint. Smoke, intense fumes, and overwhelming heat often build up rapidly in the small confines of a boat, frequently forcing all aboard into an equally life-threatening abandonment predicament. In addition to the inherent dangers of a fire, flooding may occur because of burned hoses leading from through-hull fittings. Unless docked, boats have poor access to firefighting facilities. No outside help should be expected when fighting a boat fire. A crew must be prepared to battle a fire themselves.

A common cause of fire on board small boats is fuel leakage in the engine compartment or bilge. Ignition results from engine heat or fuel spillage onto hot engine parts. Faulty electrical wiring is a common source of fire aboard boats. Age, vibration, moisture, and heat cause cracking and chafing of wire, leading to short circuits and sparks. Electricity converted into heat can ignite wire insulation and circuit boards. Batteries under charge emit hydrogen gas, which is highly flammable and potentially explosive. Overcharging batteries leads to increased production of hydrogen gas. Accumulated hydrogen gas from a leaking battery in a nonventilated compartment can lead to an explosion if ignited by a spark. Lightning strikes, although uncommon, are a potential cause of fire on board any boat. Smoking is responsible for many fires aboard boats. It should be strictly forbidden below decks and allowed only on the lee side above deck. Smoking around batteries and fuel should be forbidden.

The galley stove is another source of many boat fires. Many different types of galley stoves are available. Electrical stoves are the safest but require an auxiliary generator for power. Liquid propane gas (LPG) is an excellent source of cooking fuel and is available in most ports. Its high molecular weight is the biggest drawback. If LPG leaks, it accumulates in engine compartments and bilges, making it susceptible to ignition. Compressed natural gas (CNG) is lighter than air, making it safer to use than LPG. Unfortunately, it is more expensive, is less readily available, and has

*References 4, 6, 13, 36, 38, 41, 51, 54, 64, 74, 94, 97, 100, 105.

only a fraction of the heat content of an equal volume of LPG. Alcohol is one of the most commonly used fuels in galley stoves. Cooking with alcohol is relatively safe, and an alcohol fire can be easily extinguished with water or a fireproof blanket. The disadvantages of cooking with alcohol are its cost (high-grade cooking alcohol is expensive) and the extensive maintenance required to prevent clogging of a highly pressurized alcohol stove.

A gasoline-fueled cabin heater should not be used, and portable kerosene or alcohol heaters should be used with extreme caution. All cabins should be well ventilated and, in general, any heater turned off before sleeping. A built-in electrical heater is the safest but requires an auxiliary generator when away from dock. All portable heaters should be well secured and have an automatic "tilt-switch" capable of turning off the heater in the event it is overturned.

For many years a "fire triangle" symbolized combustion. The three sides of the triangle were fuel, oxygen, and heat. Today a fourth element—the chain reaction—has been added, rendering combustion a tetrahedron. An extinguishing agent puts out a fire by eliminating one or more elements of the fire tetrahedron. Agents work specifically by cooling, smothering, and eliminating the chain reaction fueling combustion.

Four classes of fires are seen on board boats. Class A fires involve common combustible materials, such as wood, cloth, and paper. A class B fire is fueled by solvent, paint, fuel, and oil. Fuel should always be stored in plastic containers stowed on deck. Oily rags, paper towels, and similar highly flammable waste material should be disposed of immediately when on shore. While at sea, these should be kept in a closed metal container located on deck. Class C fires are caused by energized electrical equipment, conductors, and appliances. A class D fire involves combustible metals, such as sodium, potassium, magnesium, or titanium. The class of fire must be quickly ascertained to select the most appropriate means of extinguishing it.

Fire extinguishers are rated by a series of letters—A, B, and C—corresponding to the class or classes of fires for which they are approved. A series of numbers is added. A fire extinguisher bearing the letter "A" is approved for fighting a class A fire. The number preceding the "A" is the multiplier of the extinguishing power of 1.25 gallons of water. Thus 5-A equals 6.25 gallons of water. Every number preceding a "B" is equivalent to an ability to extinguish 1 square foot of flammable liquid from a class B fire. A fire extinguisher rated 10-B will effectively extinguish 10 square feet of flammable liquid. No number precedes the "C" designation. An extinguisher approved to combat class C fires means the agent is considered nonconductive and safe for extinguishing electrical fires. Class D fires are extinguished with sand.

All boats traveling in U.S. waters are required to carry USCG-approved fire extinguishers. These must be clearly marked. Boaters should consult the USCG regarding regulations for their particular boat. Boats should carry more than the minimum number of fire extinguishers required by law; no boat ever sank from having too many extinguishers. In tests of fire extinguishers the BOAT/U.S. Foundation for Boating Safety found that an experienced firefighter was barely able to extinguish a test fire using a 2.5-pound extinguisher. For an inexperienced person a 2.5-pound extinguisher was inadequate. Therefore a 6-pound extinguisher is recommended. Triclass (approved for class A, B, and C fires) extinguishers are highly recommended.

Fire extinguishers should be readily accessible and stored at temperatures below 130° F (54° C). At higher temperatures many pressurized extinguishers discharge their contents through a relief valve. All fire extinguishers bear a date of manufacture. Halon and CO_2 extinguishers are also imprinted with their weight. Fire extinguishers should be inspected at least once a year. A logbook should be kept for every extinguisher on board, noting its identification number and dates of purchase, inspection, maintenance, hydrostatic testing, and recharging. The extinguisher should be specifically checked for corrosion, with special attention paid to the hose and nozzle. If the extinguisher bears a gauge indicating its pressure, the gauge should be tapped lightly to be sure it is not stuck. If the extinguisher must be weighed, this should be done on an appropriate scale; bathroom scales are not sufficient. Fire departments and fire equipment dealers stock appropriate scales. If the weight of an extinguisher is less than 10% of its original weight, it must be recharged. Fire extinguishers must be hydrostatically (pressure) tested at an interval of time specified on the extinguisher. A cylinder under pressure should never be repaired without first discharging its contents. Some experts recommend discharging one of a ship's portable extinguishers each year. This ensures proper functioning of the extinguisher and allows for practicing of firefighting skills if a small fire is set ashore in a metal pan or tub.

Three chemical agents are commonly used to fight fires: CO_2, dry chemical, and Halon 1211/1301. CO_2 displaces oxygen and interrupts the chemical chain reaction of a fire. Once discharged, CO_2 leaves no messy residue. Because it is a gas, CO_2 can penetrate cracks and crevices, reaching fires behind obstructions. It does not damage sensitive electrical equipment or contaminate food. CO_2 is frequently used in "fixed," nonportable extinguishing systems commonly installed in engine compartments. The systems are activated manually or automatically in response to heat-sensitive detectors. After exposure to CO_2, an engine will stop. To be effective a portable CO_2 extinguisher must be discharged no more than 6 feet from the flames—a significant drawback when confronted with an intense fire. CO_2 extinguishers do not have pressure gauges to monitor fullness of their contents. Instead, the extinguisher must be weighed yearly to verify its contents.

The most common type of portable fire extinguisher found on boats is dry chemical. Standard dry chemical extinguishers are approved for combating class B and C fires. The chemical most often used is sodium bicarbonate (baking soda). The USCG frequently uses potassium bicarbonate. A multipurpose ("triclass") dry chemical extinguisher containing monoammonium phosphate is effective in combating class A, B, and C fires. When inspected, dry chemical extinguishers should be shaken to dislodge any clumps of material that may form if the extinguisher has been left undisturbed for several months. The dry chemical is dispensed from the extinguisher by means of a propellant gas under pressure. Portable dry extinguishers can be used effectively up to 15 feet from a fire. Once discharged, the dry chemical absorbs heat and interrupts the chemical reaction. Of note, dry chemicals damage equipment and contaminate food.

Halon 1211/1301 is composed of carbon, fluorine, chlorine, and bromine. The numeric designation on Halon extinguishers refers to the number of atoms of each element in a Halon molecule: 1211 contains one carbon, two fluorine, one chlorine, and one bromine atom. Halon 1211 is a liquid, and 1301 is a gas. Liquefied Halon 1211 is efficient at fighting fires 10 to 15 feet away. Halon 1301 is most often used in fixed, self-contained automatic extinguishing systems commonly found in engine rooms. Halon works by interrupting the reaction of fuel and oxygen. It is used primarily to combat class B and C fires, although it occasionally works on class A fires. Halon does not damage electronic equipment, but toxic and acidic products are formed that are noxious and dangerous if inhaled in sufficient quantities. In January 1994, worldwide production of Halon was halted because of environmental concerns about stratospheric ozone layer depletion. To date, no equivalent replacement has been found. Current investigators are considering using nitrogen, since it is nonpolluting, presents no health hazard, and would not impair the function of ship systems.

Aqueous film-forming foam (AFFF) is approved for combating class B fires and, as a last resort, against class C fires. It works by smothering the fire and depriving the chain reaction of oxygen. The foam consists of a blanket of bubbles and floats atop most flammable liquids, which facilitates smothering. The bubbles are formed by mixing water and a foam-making agent called foam concentrate. AFFF is most effective when the entire surface of a burning liquid is covered. It is used primarily by larger vessels and SAR craft when combating an oil fire.

Water efficiently extinguishes class A and class B fires caused by alcohol. Water works by cooling burning material below its ignition temperature. In addition, fires smothered by water are deprived of oxygen. Water should not be used on class B (except alcohol) or class C fires until after the power source has been disconnected.

Before sailing the crew should be briefed on their duties in an emergency and the location of fire extinguishing equipment. Smoke detectors and heat-activated extinguishing systems in closed compartments are useful. In the event of a fire the boat should be quickly maneuvered to minimize wind fanning. If the fire is in the bow, the stern should be turned into the wind, and vice versa. Afterward, the engines should be stopped and all fuel valves closed. Unessential electrical items should be turned off. All crew members should immediately don a PFD, and a Mayday call should be issued. If a life raft is available, it should be steadfastly protected from fire and launched if necessary.

A fire at sea is a dire emergency. Crew members should be prepared to crawl on their hands and feet to avoid inhalation of noxious fumes. Fires should be attacked at the source. When fighting a fire with a portable extinguisher, it is important to get as close as possible. The fire extinguisher propellant should be directed at the base of the fire and released in short blasts. Short blasts conserve the agent and allow better visualization of the fire. The extinguisher should always be held in an upright position but discharged into the fire from all sides and angles using a side-to-side motion. This ensures that hidden embers are extinguished. A fire should never be passed to get to an extinguisher; a dead-end passageway could lead to entrapment. Extreme caution should be used when opening a hatch. Fresh air admitted into a closed compartment containing a fire can initially accelerate the fire. Hatches are best opened while standing to the side and protecting the hands with gloves. If a compartment is entered, an escape route must be kept open; a fire should never be allowed to get between a firefighter and an escape. Alternatively, if all crew members are above deck and a compartment fire is under way, a compartment sealed with a hatch can be left sealed in the hope that oxygen deprivation will extinguish the flames. If a fire reaches the engine compartment and adjacent fuel tank, the likelihood of an explosion is high. All hands should be prepared to abandon ship.

FLOAT PLAN

Before a sea voyage, a float plan (Box 50-2) should be filed with a reliable onshore person giving a detailed description of the boat, voyage information, intended destination, crew list, instructions on when to alert authorities, and a list of survival equipment on board.[37,97] In the event of an emergency, such a list could prove invaluable.

Survival Preparation

ABANDONING SHIP

At the first hint of inclement weather, flooding, or fire, a PFD should be donned. All persons on board should remain fully clothed. If the situation becomes critical, a Mayday distress signal should be sent indicating the boat's position, nature of the emergency (such as fire, sinking, medical care needed), description of the vessel, and number of persons on board. Using the automated mutual-assistance vessel-rescue system (AMVER), the USCG tracks hundreds of ships at

BOX 50-2

FLOAT PLAN

BOAT DESCRIPTION: Type ________________________ Color ______________
Registration # ________________________ Length __________
Make __________________ Name __________________
Home port _______________ Radio type ______________
No. engines ______________ Engine type _____________

SURVIVAL EQUIPMENT: PFDs __________ Flares __________
Mirror __________ Smoke signals __________ EPIRB type __________
Flashlights __________ Life raft __________ Dinghy __________
Water __________ Food __________ SART __________

VOYAGE INFORMATION: Leave ____
(departure point)

at ______________ going to ____________________________ via ____________
(date/time) *(destination)*

____
(route)

Expect to arrive by ___________________
(date/time)

ALERTING INSTRUCTIONS: If not arrived by _________________________________
(date/time)

call Coast Guard at __________________________ or __________________________
(phone no.) *(local authority)*

at ___________________
(phone no.)

CREW LIST:

Name Phone number

____
____
____
____

CAR INFO: Where parked _______________ Color/Make/Model _______________
_________________ License _______________ Trailer license _______________

sea. AMVER consists of participating merchant vessels that report their identification, position, size, and onboard medical capabilities daily.[5] Typically the most suitable ship is notified and requested to assist with the rescue. In nearly all cases assistance is granted.

If ship abandonment occurs at night, a red parachute flare should be fired. In heavily traveled areas a pyrotechnic distress signal quite possibly will be recognized. Even if no other vessels are in sight, one could be just over the horizon or simply obscured by darkness and poor weather. If the first flare does not bring help, a second one should *not* be fired until rescuers are in sight.

Traditionally, life rafts have *always* been launched from the leeward side of a ship, regardless of sea conditions. However, recent research has shown that launching a raft from the leeward side during heavy sea and wind conditions can lead to raft destruction by the parent vessel, which often drifts at a greater rate of speed than a protected raft.[4] For this reason, whenever possible, life raft launching should be done from the windward side of a ship.

"Dry" boarding a life raft, that is, boarding without first jumping in the water, is always preferable. Although some authorities recommend jumping (even from significant heights) into a life raft to avoid wet boarding, this should be considered extremely dangerous and is not recommended. In addition to subjecting a life raft to damage from jumping survivors, the survivors already aboard the raft will probably be injured by jumping shipmates.[4]

Dry boarding a life raft during a heavy sea may be extremely difficult. In such conditions, strong consideration should be given to entering the water first. If wet boarding is done, the raft should be thrown over the windward side, but *not* inflated (see later discussion). After donning immersion suits and PFDs, crew members should jump into the water and grab hold of the painter line. Once clear of the ship, the raft is inflated and personnel are boarded. In this way any potential for life raft damage is reduced. Although this is a radical departure from conventional wisdom that states, "Never go into the water," this method of boarding has been well studied and proven to be effective in the cold, rough waters off Nova Scotia.[4] However, if the water is cold and immersion suits are not available, every effort should be made to dry board the raft. Under such circumstances survivors must judge for themselves which side of the parent vessel will facilitate dry boarding. For this reason, ship abandonment should be considered a series of choices based on existing conditions. Crew members must use good judgment and common sense when launching a raft, since each sea emergency is unique. If no survival craft is available, abandoning ship from the bow, stern, or windward amidships may be preferable to stay clear of the ship's drift.[69]

If water boarding of a raft is necessary, the strongest person should enter first to assist others into the raft. Jumping should be done from the lowest height possible. Before jumping feet first, the survivor must be certain that the water below is clear of survivors, debris, and survival craft.[4] Inherently buoyant PFDs should be securely fastened and held close to the body with one arm folded across the chest and the other used to hold the nose to prevent aspiration of water. Inflatable PFDs should *not* be inflated until the wearer is in the water. If the abandoned ship is entirely surrounded by burning oil, the USCG recommends donning an inflatable PFD, jumping feet first through the flames, and swimming windward underwater. When coming up to breathe, push flames away with a circular motion of the arms and hands, and take a deep breath with the back to the wind. Inherently buoyant PFDs do not permit swimming underwater and should not be worn when abandoning a ship surrounded by flames. If only noninflatable PFDs are available, a line should be attached to the PFD that is long enough to allow the swimmer to travel underwater beneath the flames while pulling the PFD along the surface. Although flames may damage the PFD, a damaged PFD is better than no PFD at all.

When launched, the entire canister or valise containing the raft should be thrown over the side. The inflation lanyard (painter line) of the CO_2 cartridge must be fully extended before it will inflate the raft. Crew members *must* be certain that the painter line is securely fastened to the parent vessel. Failure to do so results in an unattached life raft. Once inflation begins, the raft pops up out of its container. In less than 2 minutes the raft is completely inflated. At this time the abandon ship bag and additional survival equipment should be stowed in the raft and secured with retaining lines. Unsecured gear may be lost if the raft capsizes. To avoid damage to the raft from the parent vessel, enough slack in the heaving and painter lines should be left for the raft to drift several feet from the vessel's hull. However, because of the inherent difficulty in reeling in a deployed raft with full ballast bags, the raft should never be allowed to travel more than a few feet from the parent vessel unless such close proximity would pose a direct danger to the raft, as in a fire or explosion.[89] While waiting to board the raft, all hands should consume a large quantity of fresh water.

In heavy seas a boat may roll and capsize. If time permits, a Mayday signal should be dispatched and the engines secured or throttles left in neutral. A person trapped underneath the boat easily becomes disoriented because of minimal light and because the right side of the vessel is now on the left (and vice versa). Orientation is usually maintained through touch, rather than by sight. Most capsized boats will not right themselves, but they may float. Crew members trapped underneath the boat should seek out air pockets near the inverted bottom (now the top). Survival and signaling equipment should be gathered. Inherently buoyant PFDs may need to be doffed to egress from beneath a capsized boat. If a line is available, the best swimmer should exit first and attach the line to an outside fixture for the poorer swimmers to follow. If a line is unavailable, the poorest swimmer should go first, followed by the stronger swimmers. A poor swimmer left inside without a line may panic and fail to escape. The USCG recommends escaping from beneath a boat by using hand-over-hand motion. Both hands should never be released at the same time from a handhold or line. Survivors should make every effort to leave the capsized vessel. Staying inside a capsized vessel is a last resort. If egress from beneath a capsized boat is not possible, every attempt should be made to get as far above water as possible. Physical activity should be minimized to conserve heat and oxygen. The hull should be tapped on frequently to signal rescuers.

If egress is successful and no life raft is available, survivors should remain on the hull and stay out of the water if possible. A hull often remains afloat for a considerable time, providing a means of avoiding hypothermia and making a better target for rescuers. If available, a PFD should be donned.

Once all members of the parent vessel are aboard the life raft, the sea anchor (drogue) should be deployed and all castaways should spread their weight evenly to prevent the wind from lifting the raft in heavy seas.[4,50] These maneuvers help stabilize the raft and prevent capsizing. Some survivors have reported that a partially deflated raft rode better in higher seas. This may be true, but deflation will cause excessive wear on the raft and is not advised. The heaving and painter lines should remain attached to the parent vessel as long as possible. If the vessel is on fire or sinking rapidly, these lines should be cut immediately. However, if the vessel is only awash, remaining tied to it may permit retrieval of more supplies, and the combined larger surface area of the raft and sinking boat makes a better search and rescue target. If several rafts have been launched, they should remain tied to one another for the same reason. The emergency position indicating radio beacon (EPIRB; see below) should be activated and a Mayday signal broadcast every 30 minutes using a portable VHF radio. The physical and mental condition of each castaway should be assessed and appropriate first aid rendered.

Motion sickness is severely demoralizing and saps the will of the survivor. Unfortunately, life rafts are notorious for producing seasickness, even in seasoned sailors. In crowded conditions the initiation of vomiting by one castaway almost assuredly leads to vomiting by other castaways. Survivors with intractable vomiting are at increased risk for dehydration and hypothermia. In addition, prostrate survivors have great difficulty making and executing lifesaving decisions. Therefore all crew members *must* take antiemetics before or immediately after boarding the life raft.

To retard hypothermia, the floor of the raft should be inflated and the entrance and vents closed. Cold or hypothermic survivors can don a SOLAS-approved thermal protective aid (TPA). A TPA is a Mylar-type blanket or sleeping bag that reduces heat loss (Fig. 50-32). Folded, it is usually small enough to fit into a jacket pocket and should be part of any abandon ship bag.

In the event a life raft capsizes, the following maneuver helps right the raft. Attach a rope across the bottom of the raft (if one is not already present) to a D ring, loop patch, or grabline. While facing the wind, stand on the edge of the raft and lean back on the rope. The raft should right immediately (Fig. 50-33).

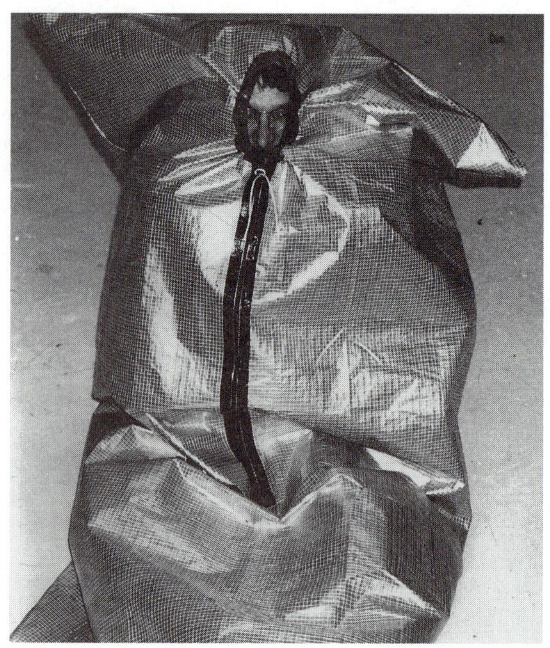

Fig. 50-32 Thermal protective aid (TPA). (Courtesy Survival Technologies Group.)

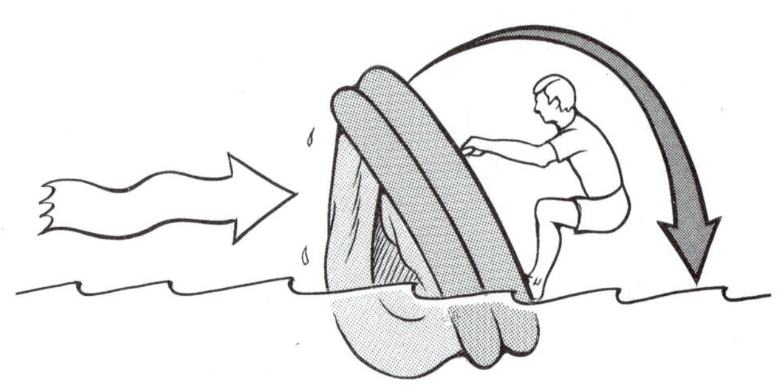

Fig. 50-33 Righting a capsized raft.

TRANSMITTING DISTRESS[4,6,33,89]

In radiotelephony, Mayday (French *M'aidez,* translated "help me") is the highest priority of urgency calls. It indicates that persons on board a vessel are threatened by grave or imminent danger and require immediate assistance. Since the International Radiotelegraphic Convention of 1912, the equivalent in radiotelegraphy is the SOS signal, represented by dot-dot-dot-dash-dash-dash-dot-dot-dot. SOS is a code signal only and not an abbreviation.[98] The urgency signal, Pan (pronounced Pahn), indicates that the transmitting station has an urgent message concerning the safety of a vessel, aircraft, or person. A Pan signal has priority over all other communications except Mayday. Securite (pronounced Say-Curitay) is the safety urgency signal. It indicates that the station is about to transmit a message concerning safety of navigation or important weather information. It has priority over all other types of routine communication.

A Mayday signal is composed of an alarm signal, distress call, and distress message (Box 50-3). It has priority over all other types of communications. During a Mayday signal, other boaters should listen only and not transmit. The alarm signal is used to indicate that an important Mayday signal is to follow and consists of two audio tones of different pitch lasting for 30 to 60 seconds (Box 50-4). A distress call confirms the Mayday alarm signal and identifies the craft in distress. A distress message confirms the ship's identity and conveys the position, nature of distress, type of assistance required, and physical description of the boat. For example:

> Mayday, Mayday, Mayday! This is the sailing yacht *Mr. Frisky,* WXG 5661 [repeat two more times]. Mayday, this is *Mr. Frisky,* WXG 5661. I am 1 mile southwest of Pinderski Point on a bearing of two-two-five degrees. I am holed, taking on water, and request immediate assistance. Three adult crew members and one child are on board, and we have put on PFDs. *Mr. Frisky* is a 32-foot sloop with a blue hull, white deck, sails furled. I will be standing by on 2182 kHz. Over.

BOX 50-3

MAYDAY/PAN DISTRESS CALL AND DISTRESS MESSAGE

DISTRESS CALL:

"Mayday, Mayday, Mayday! This is ____.
["Pan, Pan, Pan!] *boat name & call sign (say 3 times)*

DISTRESS MESSAGE:

Mayday, this is ________________________ . We are ________________________
[Pan] *boat name & call sign* *position in*

________________ , ________________ , requesting ________________________
latitude/longitude *nature of distress* *type of assistance requested*

________________ . Aboard are ________________ . ________________
 # adults/children *Boat name*

is ________________ with ________________ hull and ________________ trim.
length, type *color* *color*

I will listen on ________________ . Over."
specify channel

BOX 50-4

MAYDAY RADIO PROCEDURE

1. Press the alarm signal on the radio transmitter for 30 seconds at least 1 minute before transmitting the Mayday distress call.
2. If within 20 miles of shore, transmit first on VHF channel 16 (156.8 MHz). If no answer, proceed to step 3.
3. If offshore more than 20 miles, transmit first on SSB frequency 2182 kHz. If no answer, go to step 2.
4. If Mayday is not acknowledged within 30 seconds, reactivate the alarm signal of the radio transmitter and repeat steps 2 and 3.
5. If still no answer, transmit again (preceded by the radioalarm signal) on any channel or frequency used in the area.
6. If still no answer, try VHF channels 21 (157.05 MHz), 22A (157.1 MHz), or SSB 2670 kHz—primary Coast Guard working channels, or VHF channel 6 (156.3 MHz), SSB 2638 kHz, or SSB 2738 kHz, which at sea are used as international ship-to-ship channels.

The ship's call sign and any numerical information should be conveyed using the phonetic alphabet and numeral system (see later discussion).

A Pan signal is conveyed in a fashion similar to a Mayday call. For example:

> Pan, Pan, Pan! This is the sailing yacht *Mr. Frisky,* WXG 5661 [repeat two more times]. Pan, this is *Mr. Frisky,* WXG 5661 calling any vessel in the vicinity of Laura's Ledge. I am aground on a falling tide, but the boat is not holed. Aboard are three adult crew members and one child. *Mr. Frisky* is a 32-foot sloop with a blue hull, white deck, sails furled. I may need assistance and will be standing by on channel 16. Over.

A Securite safety call differs only slightly from a Mayday and Pan call. For example:

> Securite, Securite, Securite! This is the sailing yacht *Mr. Frisky,* WXG 5661 [repeat two more times]. Securite, this is *Mr. Frisky,* WXG 5661 calling any traffic in the Inland Passage. I am 1 mile north of Oso Tower and have sighted a half-submerged container. I am standing by on channel 16. Over.

As specified by international agreement, the first 3 minutes following each hour (00:00-00:03) and half hour (00:30-00:33) are designated as periods of radio silence in which distress signals issued on SSB 2182 kHz can be detected.

Using the International Code of Signs, distress can also be transmitted with a two-letter code (Table 50-2). Any ship hearing the distress signal can answer using a similar two-letter code (Table 50-3) This is particularly helpful in international waters where many languages are spoken.

Morse code (radiotelegraphy) is useful in maritime distress signaling. When a ship's batteries are low, a Morse code message may be transmitted farther and clearer than a voice signal. Morse code signals can be heard through heavy interference that might otherwise block a voice signal. International agreement specifies that the first 3 minutes beginning every fifteenth minute after each full and half hour (00:15-00:18 and 00:45-00:48) is a period of radio silence, designed to enhance detection of weak Morse code distress signals. Using an RDF, SAR craft can obtain a "fix" on a Morse code signal. Therefore any Morse code message should be followed by two very long dashes that allow a bearing to be taken, facilitating rescue.[4]

Table 50-2 Nature of Distress in Code from the International Code of Signs

Code Letters	Spoken Words	Text of Signal
AE	Alpha Echo	I must abandon my vessel.
CB	Charlie Bravo	I require immediate assistance.
CB6	Charlie Bravo Six	I require immediate assistance; I am on fire.
DX	Delta X-ray	I am sinking.
HW	Hotel Whiskey	I have collided with a surface craft.

Table 50-3 Answer to Ship in Distress Using the International Code of Signs

Code Letters	Spoken Words	Text of Signal
CP	Charlie Papa	I am proceeding to your assistance.
ED	Echo Delta	Your distress signals are understood.
EL	Echo Lima	Repeat the distress position.

The phonetic alphabet is used to spell words that are difficult to understand over the radio. The phonetic alphabet is composed of 26 words, each representing one of the 26 letters in the Roman alphabet. The concept behind the phonetic alphabet is that an agreed on spoken word is often easier to understand than a letter (Table 50-4). Difficult words within a message are spelled out using the phonetic alphabet preceded by the words, "I spell." For example, "I am afire off Point Cabrillo. I spell: CHARLIE, ALPHA, BRAVO, ROMEO, INDIA, LIMA, LIMA, OSCAR—Cabrillo."

To eliminate confusion, numbers are pronounced differently over the radio. The pronunciation for each number in the Arabic numbering system is listed below (Table 50-5). When a number consists of more than one digit, it is pronounced one numeral at a time with a short pause between digits. For example, the number "32" is spoken as THUH-REE TOO; do not say "thirty-two." Decimal points (for example, 156.8) are transmitted in the following manner: Wun Fi-Yiv Six Day-See-Mal Eight; do not say "one hundred fifty-six point eight."

When communicating by radio, certain words, called "prowords," have particular meaning and are important to learn. The most common prowords and their definitions are listed in Table 50-6.

When at sea, it is important that all radios are working properly. This is ensured by conducting a radio check. A radio check consists of a series of spoken numbers. For minor adjustments of the radio, a "short count" is used. It consists of the phonetic count from one to five and then from five back to one and should not exceed 10 seconds. Here is an example of a short count:

Wun, Too, Thuh-Ree, Fo-Wer, Fi-Yiv, Fi-Yiv, Fo-Wer, Thuh-Ree, Too, Wun

A "long count" is used for direction finding and making more technical adjustments of a radio. The long count uses the phonetic count from one to 10 and then from 10 back to

Table 50-4 Phonetic Alphabet

Roman Alphabet	Phonetic Alphabet
A	Alpha
B	Bravo
C	Charlie
D	Delta
E	Echo
F	Foxtrot
G	Golf
H	Hotel
I	India
J	Juliet
K	Kilo
L	Lima
M	Mike
N	November
O	Oscar
P	Papa
Q	Quebec
R	Romeo
S	Sierra
T	Tango
U	Uniform
V	Victor
W	Whiskey
X	X-ray
Y	Yankee
Z	Zulu

Table 50-5 Phonetic Numerals

Arabic Numeral	Radio Pronunciation
1	Wun
2	Too
3	Thuh-Ree
4	Fo-Wer
5	Fi-Yiv
6	Six
7	Seven
8	Eight
9	Niner
0	Zero
Decimal point (.)	Day-See-Mal

Table 50-6 Prowords

Proword	Meaning
Affirmative	Correct. What you have transmitted is correct.
Break	Term used to indicate the end of one message before commencing the transmission of a second
Correct	You are correct, or what you have transmitted is correct.
ETA	Estimated time of arrival
ETD	Estimated time of departure
I Spell	The preceding word will be spelled using the phonetic alphabet.
Negative	Incorrect. What you have transmitted is not correct.
Out	Used following the last line of a transmitted message
Roger	Indicates that a transmission has been received satisfactorily
Silence	Spoken three times, and pronounced See-Lons. Cease all transmissions immediately. Silence is maintained until instructed to resume.
Silence Fini	Pronounced See-Lons Fee-Nee. Silence is lifted. Indicates the end of an emergency and the resumption of normal traffic.
Wait	I must pause for a few seconds.
Wait Out	I must pause longer than a few seconds.

one. It is done in the same manner as the short count. After a radio check the receiving station should answer with signal strength (Table 50-7) and signal readability (Table 50-8) prowords.

In general, a radio check is necessary only once or twice a year.[33] It can be conducted on any locally available channel but should never be directed to the Coast Guard. It is done in the following manner:

Any vessel, any vessel, this is *Mr. Frisky,* WXG 5661, calling for a radio check, over.

The responding party should answer with signal strength and readability prowords. If it is necessary to contact the USCG, say:

Coast Guard radio, Coast Guard radio, this is *Mr. Frisky* WXG 5661, over.

While the USCG monitors channels 16 and 9, heavy traffic on these frequencies may necessitate calling on channel 22A, a USCG working channel.

ADRIFT

Once adrift, the castaway becomes occupied with four principal activities: avoiding hypothermia (or heat-related illnesses), collecting water, procuring food, and attracting the attention of rescuers. To these ends the captain should delegate responsibilities. If the captain of the ship is dead or incapacitated, a captain of the raft should be selected. His or her authority must be respected and supported. Daily duties, routines, and goals should be established and assigned for the purpose of ensuring that all necessary things are done and to provide a degree of orderliness to an otherwise chaotic situation. One of the essential duties is to inventory and dispense all rations and supplies. A daily log should be kept, noting wind and current direction, sunrise, sunset, and the last position and time of a Mayday transmission. Other duties include keeping lookout for rescue vessels or land, bailing out water, and ensuring that all aboard take antiemetics.

Table 50-7 Signal Strength Prowords

Proword	Meaning
Loud	Your signal is strong.
Good	Your signal is good.
Weak	Your signal can be heard with difficulty.
Very weak	Your signal can be heard with great difficulty.

Table 50-8 Signal Readability Prowords

Proword	Meaning
Clear	Excellent quality
Readable	Quality good, no difficulty in reading the transmission
Distorted	Quality poor, difficulty in reading the transmission

The raft should be inspected frequently. Chafing of the raft often occurs around flaps, handles, attachment points of towing, drogue, and grablines, and at the angle formed by the floor and walls of the raft. Lines causing chafing should be wrapped in soft cloth. All leaks must be taken seriously. Leaks are repaired by partially deflating the involved chamber and using a proper patching kit (standard equipment aboard all rafts and abandon ship bags). In the event that no effective patch is available, a beveled piece of soft wood or plastic wrapped in nonabrasive material can be inserted into the hole.

WATER PROCUREMENT

Water, water, everywhere,
And all the boards did shrink;
Water, water, everywhere,
Nor any drop to drink

Samuel Taylor Coleridge, *The Rime of the Ancient Mariner*

A person can survive for several weeks without food, but only 7 to 10 days without water. The average adult needs a minimum of 1 pint (472 ml) of water a day to survive. This is modified by air temperature, humidity, physical exertion, motion sickness, and hydration status at the time of ship abandonment. In warm climates castaways can minimize water loss by remaining beneath the raft's canopy during hot days, opening raft apertures at night, and wearing cooled, ocean-soaked clothing. During periods of severe thirst, castaways have reported an overwhelming desire to drink seawater. Since seawater contains 3.5% sodium chloride (versus 0.9% in the human body), drinking it accelerates death from hypernatremia. Under no circumstances should pure undesalinated seawater be consumed no matter how intense the desire. Drinking diluted seawater should also be forbidden, since the ultimate sodium content will be unknown. Although success with this method has been reported, it is still not recommended. Thor Heyerdahl on board the balsa raft *Kon-Tiki* noted[45]:

> Our water ration could be ladled into us till it squelched in our stomachs, but our throats malignantly demanded much more. On such days we added 20 to 40 per cent of . . . seawater to our fresh-water ration, and found to our surprise that this brackish water quenched our thirst. We had the taste of seawater in our mouths for a long time afterwards, but never felt unwell, and moreover, had our water considerably increased.

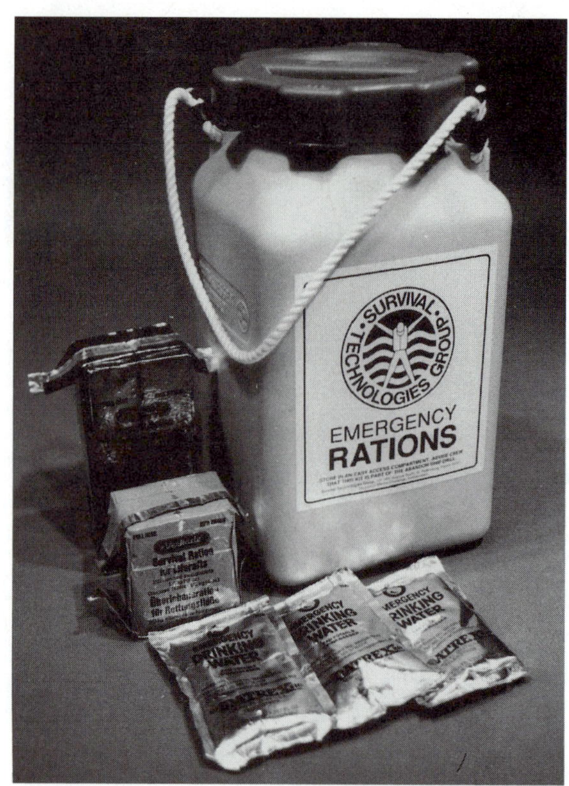

Fig. 50-34 Emergency water rations in individually sealed packets. (Courtesy Survival Technologies Group.)

One or two 5-gallon water containers per person should be on deck of the parent vessel at all times (space permitting), ready to be thrown into a life raft in an emergency. Filling them only three-quarters full will enable them to float. In the event of inadequate stowage space on board the raft for the water containers, they can be towed from the raft using polypropylene line. Some manufacturers make individually sealed water packets (Fig. 50-34). Each packet contains 4 fluid ounces (118 ml) and has a shelf life of 5 years. One advantage of individual water packets is prevention of contamination, which can ruin the entire contents of a 5-gallon water container. The trade-off is cost; a container of 64 4-ounce water packets costs approximately $75 at the time of this writing.

A portable desalinator is the most efficient and sophisticated means of obtaining fresh water when adrift. Three types are available: chemical, solar, and hand-powered reverse osmosis.

A chemical desalinator consists of a desalting briquet and filter. The chemical briquet binds and precipitates sodium chloride, which is then removed with a filter bag. The water produced is usually acrid and discolored, but safe to drink. It is estimated that each desalinating kit can produce seven times the amount of fresh water that could be stowed in the same space. Chemical desalinators can be used in overcast weather or at night when a solar still is impractical. Of the three types of desalinators, this is the least recommended.

A solar still requires sunlight. It is compact and reusable and requires no chemicals. It is capable of producing approximately 1 pint (472 ml) to 1 quart (944 ml) of water per day under ideal conditions in temperate climates. A variety of solar still designs exist, but the basic principle is as follows. Suspended inside a clear, plastic inflatable ball is a black cloth that is soaked with seawater admitted through an opening on top of the ball. When the moistened cloth is heated by sunlight, fresh water evaporates and the ensuing condensation is collected in a fresh water reservoir. Brand new and unused, a solar still has a virtually unlimited shelf life. After a short time (usually several days to 2 weeks), a still's efficiency is reduced because of excessive deposition of salt on the cloth. This type of desalinator is somewhat useful while adrift in warm, sunny conditions but is often inadequate if several survivors are present. Although its utility is limited, it should be included in an abandon ship bag, since it takes up little space.[47]

A manual reverse osmosis desalinator (MROD) is the most efficient means of obtaining fresh water while adrift. Reverse osmosis (RO) works by forcing water at high pressure through a series of filters that cull salts, bacteria, and viruses. Before the development of the Survivor series of MRODs, RO was not considered a viable alternative for manually converting seawater to fresh water. In RO, salt water is forced against a membrane at pressures approximating 800 PSI. About 10% of the seawater passes through the membrane as pure fresh water; the remaining 90% is expelled. Normally it would be difficult to manually generate pressures of this magnitude. Engineers at Recovery Engineering overcame this problem with a patented valve that uses stored energy in the waste brine. As a result, only several pounds of user force are needed to produce fresh water. The valve is incorporated into the Survivor-35, a 7-pound (3 kg), 22-inch (56 cm), portable MROD capable of producing 1.2 gallons (4.6 L) of fresh water per hour using 30 strokes per minute (Fig. 50-35). The Survivor-35 is recommended for large USCG- and SOLAS-approved life rafts. A smaller model, Survivor-06, is available that produces just over 1 pint of water in 30 minutes using 40 strokes per minute (Fig. 50-36). The Survivor-06 weighs only 2.5 pounds (1.1 kg) and is 8 inches (20 cm) long. It is recommended for 4- to 12-person life rafts. Both desalinators are USCG approved. The Survivor desalinators are the only MRODs available in the world.*

*References 1, 2, 20, 28, 60-62, 66, 72, 76, 86.

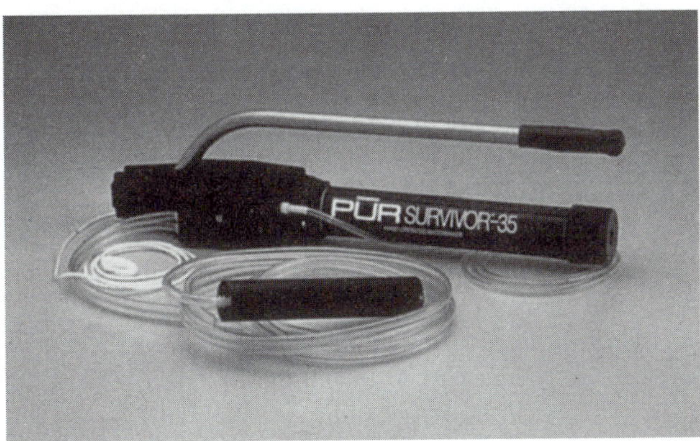

Fig. 50-35 Survivor-35 manual reverse osmosis desalinator. (Courtesy PUR, a division of Recovery Engineering.)

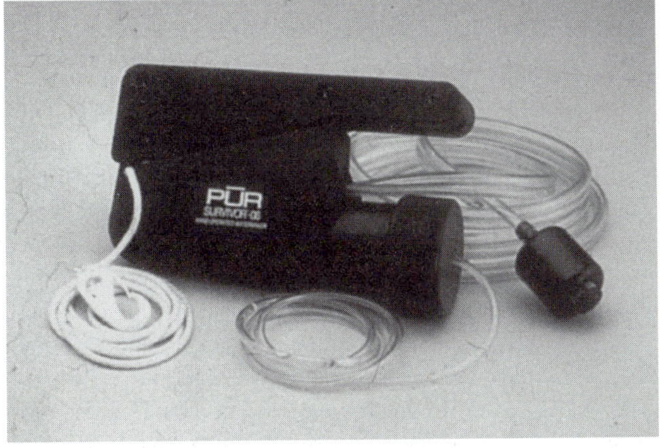

Fig. 50-36 Survivor-06 manual reverse osmosis desalinator. (Courtesy Recovery Engineering.)

Many castaways have greatly benefited from fresh water produced by storms. Rainwater should be collected in any potential container. Some life raft canopies employ a specially designed rainwater collection system.[67] If a warm, humid day is followed by a cool night, condensation forms on the raft canopy and can be collected in the morning using a designated fresh water sponge or rag.

If a castaway is shipwrecked in cold water, old sea ice collected from the sea can be melted and consumed. Old sea ice is ice from a glacier or iceberg that has lost its salt. It is blue, has round edges and a glossy surface, and breaks easily into flakes. Young sea ice has a milky appearance, angular corners and a rough texture, and is difficult to splinter; it cannot be used as a source of fresh water.

Dougal Robertson and his family survived for 38 days at sea without a desalinator. While adrift, they reported being able to obtain approximately 1¾ cups (400 ml) of water from 2 pounds of fish by sucking out the cerebrospinal fluid and aqueous and vitreous humors of the eyes. Others have reported success at squeezing juice out of fish. Thor Heyerdahl reported[45]:

> The old natives knew well the device which many shipwrecked men hit upon during the war—chewing thirst-quenching moisture out of raw fish. One can also press the juices out by twisting pieces of fish in a cloth, or, if the fish is large, it is a fairly simple matter to cut holes in its side, which soon become filled with ooze from the fish's lymphatic glands. It does not taste good if one has anything better to drink, but the percentage of salt is so low that one's thirst is quenched.

However, castaways should not depend on extracted fluid from fish as a primary source of hydration. In 1956 a subcommittee of the Royal Naval Personnel Research Committee on Survival at Sea reported that predicting how many fish might be caught by a survivor or how much juice might be obtained from them is impossible. Also, without mechanical aid, extracting juice from fish is very difficult. For centuries mariners have safely consumed turtle and bird blood.

Inability to replace free water ultimately leads to hypernatremia. The severity of consequences depends on the rate of development and degree of hypernatremia. If the serum sodium concentration rises gradually, individuals may remain conscious with serum sodium levels as high as 170 mEq/L. The primary insult of hypernatremia is on the central nervous system. Hyperactive deep tendon reflexes, muscular weakness, and seizures are common. Mental status changes range from lethargy and confusion to delirium and coma. After the *SS Empire Chaucer* went down in the South Atlantic and the crew abandoned ship into a lifeboat, the Third Officer noted[58]:

> Many of the crew drank salt water; although I threatened to stop their fresh water if they continued to do so, many of the men used to drink it at night. I could always tell when a man had been

drinking salt water because the guilty ones suffered from hallucinations. During the tenth day, the Second Cook became insane, probably through drinking seawater.

FOOD PROCUREMENT

For a month we'd neither wittles nor drink,
Till a-hungry we did feel,
So we drawed a lot, and accordin' shot
The captain for our meal.

Sir William S. Gilbert, *The Yarn of the Nancy Bell*

In preparation for a long stay at sea, food and water should be rationed. If the correct preparations have been made, the abandon ship bag should contain enough dehydrated food concentrates to last for a significant period. However, if a person is at sea for longer than anticipated, food may need to be harvested from the marine environment.

The most recent SOLAS recommendation for emergency life raft rations is 800 calories per day. Several companies make concentrated food bars.* These are generally composed of wheat flour, vegetable shortening, cane sugar, water, coconut, and salt. Ideally, food rations should be composed of complex carbohydrates and fats to avoid the nitrogenous wastes of protein and the associated higher urine volumes needed to excrete them.[32]

The fishing gear packed in the abandon ship bag is invaluable once prepackaged food rations are exhausted. If a fishing kit is unavailable, hooks can be fashioned from nails, safety pins, sharp pieces of wood, bone, or turtle shell. Lines can be made from any rope or cloth. Shiny lures can be improvised from buttons, bird feathers, turtle shell, or brightly colored cloth. Fishing is always easiest with bait. Suitable bait may come in the form of a captured flying fish or a small unsuspecting turtle that wanders close enough to the raft to be captured and killed. Since fish frequently feed at night and are attracted by light, fishing at night is frequently successful when aided by a signaling mirror used to reflect moonlight into the water.

When adrift, a castaway comes in contact with many marine animals and birds. Whales, sharks, turtles, and dolphins are drawn to the raft by curiosity. Schools of fish are attracted by the shadow of the raft. With time the raft becomes a floating marine ecosystem, its bottom covered with plants and barnacles.

Saltwater fish fillets can be eaten raw, but before any fish or marine creature is eaten, it should be tested for edibility by touching it to the tip of the tongue. If there is any stinging, burning, or bad taste, the food should be discarded and the hands thoroughly rinsed in seawater. If it tastes edible, a small piece may be left in the mouth for 5 minutes. If still no adverse reaction occurs, this piece can be swallowed and another small piece eaten. If one feels well after 1 hour, the specimen is probably edible.[47] Any fish that is not dried or eaten within 3 to 6 hours should be discarded or used for bait. The liver, head, intestines, genitals, or roe of any fish should not be eaten.

Sun-dried fish fillets may last for several days. Using whatever utensils are available, the fillets should be cut into slices no thicker than 1 inch and dried in the sun. They can be eaten at any point in the drying process, but since they are dehydrated, a small amount of water will be needed to aid in their consumption.

Some fish are inherently poisonous, while others become poisonous as a result of toxins ingested, most notably ciguatera (see Chapter 53). Since poisonous fish usually dwell in shallow waters, fish caught in the deep ocean are generally safe to eat. Inherently poisonous fish are pufferfish, porcupine fish, and sunfish (molas). Any fish with bristles or spines (instead of scales) should not be eaten.

Turtles are edible. They are frequently found sleeping on the surface of the ocean. Smaller turtles can be immediately brought aboard and killed, but larger ones need to be secured with a rope placed around the neck, weakened, and drowned. The claws and beak of a turtle are very sharp and can puncture a life raft. Once the turtle is on board, its neck should be severed and its blood collected. Turtle blood is an excellent source of hydration and nutrition. Turtle meat can be eaten raw or sun dried. In addition, the heart, bone marrow, and eggs can be eaten. The liver should not be eaten. The shell should be saved. Fat and oil from the turtle can be saved and used as a lubricant for chapped skin.

Marine birds are difficult to catch but, if caught, can all be eaten. A seabird can be caught by trolling a baited fishhook in the water. If a booby alights on the raft, passengers should grab it. If the bird is wary, a baited rope with a slip knot can be used. When the booby takes the bait, the bird is caught by pulling quickly on the knotted rope (hence the name "booby trap").

Castaways frequently report close encounters with sharks. Care should be taken when urinating, defecating, vomiting, or disposing of blood-soiled clothing over the side, since body fluids attract sharks. To reduce contact with these predators, erratic splashing should be avoided. Aggressive sharks may be deterred with bumps on the snout or gills with an oar. If one is fortunate enough to kill a small shark with a speargun, the meat can be eaten raw but spoils quickly. The flesh of the Greenland, hammerhead, white, six-gilled, seven-gilled, or black-tip sand shark should not be eaten.[47] Shark liver should never be eaten.

Seaweed is an excellent source of protein and carbohydrate. If water is not scarce, the seaweed should be washed in a small amount of fresh water before being eaten. Seaweed should be subjected to the same tasting techniques used for fish. It may be eaten raw or dried. High in cellulose,

*Datrex rations are available from STG. They have a 5-year shelf life.

seaweed should be ingested cautiously because of the laxative effect. Seaweed also attracts other edible creatures such as small crabs and fish.

After a few days adrift at sea, the life raft and drifting lines begin to attract barnacles. Barnacles are edible and contain fresh water. They may be eaten raw. Plankton may also be eaten but is usually reserved as a last alternative. Many species of plankton are poisonous (for instance, those that generate a red tide). Plankton are high in celluose and, like seaweed, should be eaten sparingly. They may be caught using a fine netting or cloth with care taken to discard jellyfish tentacles.

MEDICAL PROBLEMS

Medical illnesses suffered at sea are discussed in other chapters. Hypothermia, heat exhaustion, heatstroke, dehydration, frostbite, trench foot, ultraviolet exposure, motion sickness, orthopedic injuries suffered during ship abandonment, blisters, boils, and cramps are just a few of the possible ills befalling castaways adrift at sea. If survival at sea is prolonged, castaways note that urination and defecation become infrequent. Urine becomes concentrated, and bowel movements may occur only once every 10 days. Many good commercial medical first aid kits are available, or one can be assembled de novo.[40]

Rescue Preparation

EMERGENCY COMMUNICATION

An EPIRB is a small, portable, waterproof, floatable, and potentially lifesaving piece of survival equipment (Fig. 50-37). Depending on the model, an EPIRB will transmit on 121.5 MHz *and* 243.0 MHz (so-called 121 EPIRB), or on 406.0 *and* 121.5 MHz (so-called 406 EPIRB). The 121.5 MHz signal is the civilian VHF distress frequency; 243.0 MHz is the military distress frequency. The 406.0 MHz signal is for distress used in satellite communication (see later discussion). EPIRBs cannot receive. The effective range of an EPIRB depends on the model, transmission frequency, battery, and atmospheric conditions. Once activated, an EPIRB transmits continuously for the duration of its battery. It should never be turned off during an emergency. A fully charged battery must function for a minimum of 48 hours as specified by the Federal Communication Commission (FCC). Once an EPIRB battery has expired, the entire EPIRB must be returned to the factory for battery replacement. A 406 EPIRB signal allows SAR authorities to calculate a position within a radius of 2 to 3 miles of the survivor.

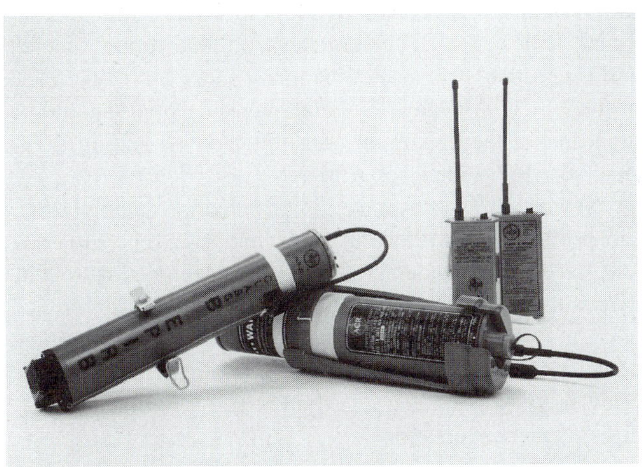

Fig. 50-37 Emergency position indicating radio beacons (EPIRBs). From left: RLB-20, RLB-14, RLB-21, and 21S. The two models on the far right are small enough to be attached to a PFD. (Courtesy ACR Electronics.)

All 406 EPIRBs transmit on 121.5 MHz. The 121.5 MHz signal of this EPIRB is not strong enough to reach a SARSAT/COSPAS satellite (see later discussion). In this regard the 121.5 MHz signal of a 406 EPIRB differs from a 121 EPIRB. The purpose of the 121.5 MHz signal on the newer 406 models is to facilitate rescue by SAR craft equipped with a radio direction finder (RDF). The 406.0 MHz signal provides an approximation of the survivor's location within a radius of 2 to 3 miles as calculated by a satellite. Using an RDF, mobilized SAR authorities can home in on the 121.5 MHz signal, providing an exact location of the survivor.

EPIRB signals can be detected by satellites, SAR ground stations, boats, and aircraft. Civilian and military aircraft are required by law to listen constantly for a 121.5 or 243.0 MHz distress signal. When a 121.5 or 243.0 MHz signal is detected, SAR personnel can home to the source using an RDF. The 406.0 MHz signal of a 406 EPIRB or the 121.5 MHz signal of a 121 EPIRB can be detected by SARSAT (Search and Rescue Satellite-Aided Tracking) or the Russian equivalent, COSPAS (Space System for Search of Vessels in Distress).[30] These satellites are capable of receiving EPIRB transmissions from virtually anywhere on earth, and calculate the position of the signal using the Doppler effect. When the distress signal of a 406 or 121 EPIRB is detected by satellite, the information is relayed to a ground station, called a local user terminal (LUT). After computer analysis the information is subsequently conveyed to a mission control center (MCC). Each participating country in the world has an MCC, which in turn alerts the nearest rescue coordination center (RCC). For a satellite to relay an EPIRB's signal, the satellite *must* be in the line-of-sight of an LUT. Unfortunately, not enough LUTs exist worldwide to ensure immediate broadcast of an EPIRB distress signal. If a satellite receives a distress signal from a *406* EPIRB and the satellite is not in immediate line-of-sight of a LUT, the message is "memorized" and broadcast later when line-of-sight is obtained. Therefore 406 EPIRBs provide *worldwide* coverage. Unfortunately, satellites are unable to memorize and rebroadcast a signal received from a 121 EPIRB. A SARSAT/COSPAS can, however, relay such a signal if an LUT is in line-of-sight at the exact moment the 121 EPIRB signal is received. This inability to receive, memorize, and rebroadcast the 121.5 MHz signal of a 121 EPIRB is a serious drawback to this type of EPIRB, which has contributed to delays in rescue.[5,19,31,55] Many survival experts, including the USCG, believe that the recent development of the 406 EPIRB represents one of the biggest and most important advances in SAR technology. If a survivor is in possession of a 406 EPIRB, his or her chances of being successfully rescued greatly increase.[23]

In addition to the advantages listed previously, a 406 EPIRB identifies the vessel as an aircraft, pleasure boat, commercial fishing boat, or other marine vessel. It also identifies the vessel's country of origin and registration number, allowing access to the U.S. National Oceanographic and Atmospheric Administration's (NOAA) data bank containing additional information on the vessel. The trade-off for the better performance of a 406 EPIRB is price, which is up to 10 times more than that of a 121 EPIRB. Once an EPIRB is purchased, the new owner must register it immediately with the NOAA. Failure to do so may have contributed to the death of an experienced transatlantic sailor.[49] EPIRBs can be purchased from a number of retailers and manufacturers (Appendix G).

Transponders are small electronic transmitters that broadcast on radar frequencies (Fig. 50-38). Their X-band signals are "captured" by searching radar and allow calculation of a position within several feet. When used in emergency situations, they are called search and rescue transponders (SARTs) (Appendix H). The range of a SART is 2 to 10 miles, depending on the height of the SART's signal above water. When activated, a SART remains in a "standby" mode. When a searching radar signal from rescuers is detected by the SART, it transmits an electronic response used by SAR authorities to pinpoint the exact source of transmission. Once activated, a SART operates for a minimum of 96 hours in a standby mode, and another 8 hours in a transmitting mode. It functions at temperatures as low as −4° F (−20° C) and floats in an upright position.[65]*

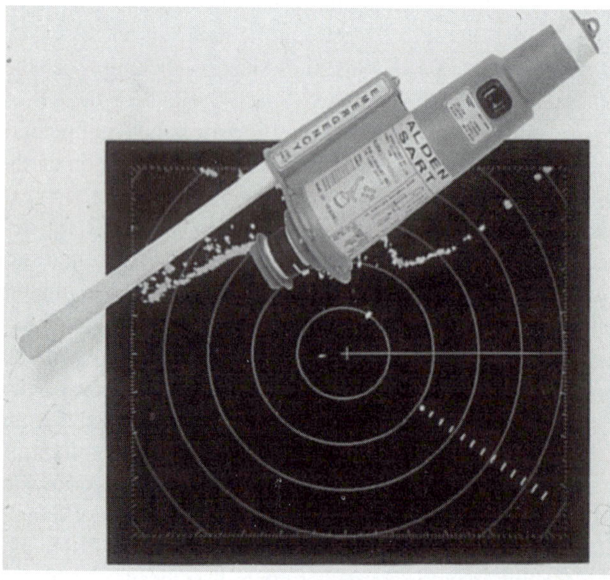

Fig. 50-38 Search and rescue transponder. (Courtesy Alden Electronics.)

A very high frequency/frequency modulation (VHF/FM) radio is an essential piece of equipment (Appendix I).† In highly traveled areas a VHF signal usually alerts authorities and other boats faster than using an EPIRB alone. Using an RDF, SAR authorities can pinpoint the source of its transmission. Hand-held, portable units are available that, when sealed in a waterproof plastic bag, make a great addition to an abandon ship bag (Fig. 50-39). A standard VHF radio has a maximal output of 25 watts. Hand-held VHF radios have outputs ranging from 1 to 7 watts. One expert recommends lower output (3- to 4-watt) models.[99] Extra watts do not significantly increase range of communication but do lead to rapid battery depletion. Extra battery packs should be purchased with hand-held VHFs. A telescopic antenna should be considered for additional range.

VHF radio uses line-of-sight principles. Practically speaking, this means that an antenna at sea level would have to be located within approximately 20 to 30 miles of a ship's transmitting radio. The range of a hand-held VHF is approximately 2 to 3 miles, but this range is extended significantly when communicating with an aircraft. Likewise, the range between a boat equipped with a 25-watt VHF radio and an aircraft can be extended up to 300 miles. This distance varies depending on the actual height of the radio antennas. All USCG cutters carry VHF, UHF, and single side band (SSB) radios. VHF channel 16 (156.8 MHz) is the international dedicated VHF emergency communication channel and is constantly monitored by many ships, including those of the USCG. Mayday, Pan, and Securite signals should be broadcast at the maximum transmitter power setting. VHF channels are listed in Table 50-9.

Newer VHF radios have digital selective calling (DSC) capability. DSC transceivers send bursts of numbers to other DSC receivers. In an emergency, VHFs equipped with DSC transmit the boat's identification, nature of the distress, and position using information from the LORAN or GPS. Three other useful features found on newer VHF radios are weather alert, automatic loud hailer, and scrambler permitting private conversations.

A citizens band (CB) radio is the least expensive option

---

*At present only one manufacturer is producing a SART. The SART is called ALDENSART and is available from Alden Electronics, 40 Washington St., Westborough, MA 01581; telephone 508-366-8851.

†References 6, 14, 33-35, 53, 56, 57, 59, 85, 91.

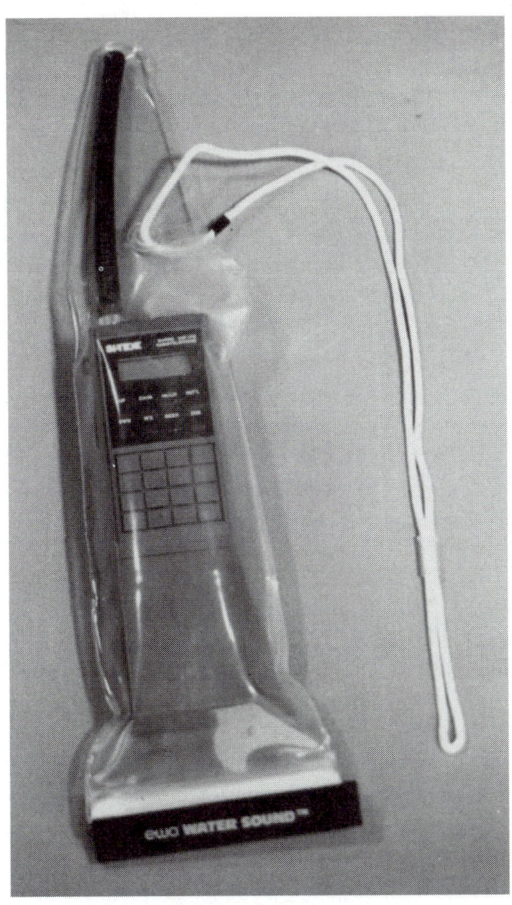

Fig. 50-39 Portable, hand-held VHF radio in waterproof bag. (Courtesy Survival Technologies Group.)

for short-range boat communications. It is easy to install and simple to operate. A CB operates at 5 watts, powered by a ship's batteries. In general, CBs transmit 5 to 15 miles. They are designed for personal and business communication and are frequently used for ship-to-shore conversation. Channel 9 is reserved for emergency communications, but USCG monitoring of this station is inconsistent.

An SSB radio is essential when a vessel is outside the effective range of VHF (Appendix J). SSBs transmit on frequencies of 2 to 23 MHz and are designed for long-range communication. If broadcasting on 2 MHz, coastal range is approximately 200 miles; at 4 MHz, range increases to 600 miles. During offshore communication at 22 MHz the effective range is from 10,000 miles to worldwide. SSB transmits great distances because the signal bounces off the ionosphere and ground. Accordingly, range does depend on atmospheric conditions. The distress calling frequency is 2182 kHz. Other important SSB frequencies are listed in Table 50-10. A facsimile (FAX) can be linked to an SSB, providing sailors with up-to-date weather printouts and charts. An SSB is not portable and requires a long antenna and use of ship batteries for operation.[6,73] Before an SSB radio can be installed, the vessel must have a VHF on board.

Ham or amateur radio is becoming increasingly popular with yacht owners, largely because it affords an informal link with the rest of the world. It is used primarily for socializing, since no business may be conducted on ham frequencies.[73] Many maritime ham "networks" (organizations of ham operators) now call for periods of radio silence, allowing detection of a faint Mayday signal from a distressed boat transmitting poorly because of low batteries or a damaged antenna. The Pacific Maritime Network keeps a daily log of each member boat checking in. Ham radios have three drawbacks. First, they have no designated emergency frequency.

Table 50-9 VHF Channels in the United States

Channel*	Use
6	Intership safety only, especially in search and rescue
9	Working channel and secondary calling channel, nationwide
13	Bridge-to-bridge navigation used in meeting and passing situations
16	Distress and safety
21	Intra–Coast Guard working frequency
22A	Coast Guard working channel
24, 25, 26, 27, 28, 84, 85, 86, 87	Public coast stations (telephones)
68, 69, 71, 78	Working channels for conversations
70	Digital selective calling
79, 80	Working channels for conversations in Great Lakes only
88	Public coast station, Puget Sound only
WX1, WX2, WX3	Marine weather broadcasts; receive only

Data from U.S. Coast Guard.
*Channel numbers followed by the letter "A" designate United States frequencies that differ from their international counterpart. Channels not listed are used in port and other commercial operations.

Table 50-10 Single Side Band Frequencies Used Worldwide

Frequency (kHz)	Use
2182	Medium-frequency band for calling and distress, monitored by all Coast Guard and commercial vessels while under way
2638, 2738	International ship-to-ship frequency
2670	Coast Guard working frequency available to public when Coast Guard requests shift to another frequency
3023.5	International search and rescue on-scene frequency
4125, 6215, 8291, 12290, 16420	High-seas frequencies for conducting distress and safety traffic; Coast Guard will be notified immediately if such traffic is received

Data from Dove T: *Sail,* May 1993; and Gooding B: *Cruising World,* Feb 1993.

Second, unlike VHF and SSB, they are not constantly monitored by the USCG. Third, a ham operator license is required. Additional information on amateur radio licensing is available.*

A cellular phone transmits up to 25 miles from offshore. In the near future, satellites will extend this range to several hundred miles. A cellular telephone should serve only as a backup to VHF, since it does not emit a directional signal useful in pinpointing its source. Cellular telephones are also extremely sensitive to moisture. However, they are still useful. In 1991 a fisherman's boat began sinking 17 miles off the coast of Maine. After grabbing his cellular phone, the man jumped into a life raft and dialed his wife at home. After looking up the phone number, she promptly contacted the USCG. Two aircraft and a boat were promptly dispatched, and the fisherman was subsequently rescued.[97]

In conclusion, for most boaters VHF is sufficient for safety and distress communications. A hand-held VHF stowed in a waterproof bag is probably adequate for a small boat with an open cockpit. A cellular phone is useful in areas where VHF traffic is heavy. For a larger boat, SSB offers hundreds more frequencies than VHF and allows sailors to take advantage of special features like weather FAX. Those who travel far out to sea and are communication hobbyists might consider using a ham radio. An EPIRB and SART should be carried by all offshore sailors who cruise out of sight of land. Additional information is available on maritime radio.†

VISUAL SIGNALING‡

Visual distress signals are an important part of a boat's safety equipment and are intended for emergency use only. USCG regulations state that "no person in a boat shall display a visual distress signal on water . . . under any circumstances except a situation where assistance is needed because of immediate or potential danger to the person aboard."[15] Since 1981 the USCG has required that boats over 16 feet in length used in U.S. coastal waters, the Great Lakes, territorial seas, and contiguous waters be equipped with day and night visual distress signals.* Recreational boats less than 16 feet in length; open sailboats less than 26 feet in length and not equipped with propulsion machinery; boats participating in organized events such as races, regattas, or marine parades; and manually propelled boats are not required to carry day signals but must carry night signals when operating from sunset to sunrise.[37]

Visual distress signals are divided into pyrotechnic and nonpyrotechnic devices. Pyrotechnic distress signals include flares and smoke. Nonpyrotechnic devices are flags, mirrors, flashlights, whistles, and hand-arm signals. In the United States, pyrotechnic devices must be USCG approved, in good condition (not moist or corroded), readily accessible, and not older than 42 months from the stamped date of the manufacturer. SOLAS-approved flares are valid for only 36 months from the date of manufacture. Expired flares do not count toward minimum requirements. Flare performance deteriorates with age, so expired flares should be kept on board as backups only. Flares should be stored in a waterproof container located in a cool, dry place shielded from direct sunlight. Expired flares may be disposed of by the fire department, police, or bomb squad. Under no circumstances should they be placed in the trash or thrown overboard. Expired, but unused, flares thrown into the sea may wash ashore and be found by children playing on the beach.

Boats are required to carry a minimum of three daylight and three nighttime signals. Some manufacturers make combined day and night distress signals; three of these satisfy

*For additional information on amateur radio licensing, contact the American Radio Relay League, Newington, CT 06111; 203-666-1541.

†For information on operating procedures, channels, FCC regulations, and so on, order the *Maritime Radio User's Handbook.* This can be obtained by calling BOAT/U.S. Foundation for Boating Safety at 703-823-9550.

‡References 4, 6, 15, 30, 44, 46, 47, 94.

*To receive a free brochure explaining the visual distress signal regulations, call the USCG Consumer Hotline at 800-368-5647.

USCG regulations. Distress signals approved for daylight use include floating or hand-held orange smoke and distress flags with a black square and ball on an orange background (3 square feet or larger). Electric distress lights that signal SOS are approved for night use only. Distress signals approved for day and night use are red hand-held flares, red meteor flares, and red parachute flares.*

Although federal regulations require vessels traveling in U.S. patrolled waters to carry USCG-approved flares, these devices often do not satisfy the more stringent SOLAS regulations. Signaling devices should meet SOLAS specifications. In 1983 SOLAS established the present criteria for flares and other signaling devices. Flares meeting these specifications are frequently designated "SOLAS 83." SOLAS standards exceed USCG standards for altitude; brightness (candela rating); and, except for red hand-held flares, burn time (Table 50-11). All SOLAS-approved flares are hand held and do not require pistol launchers. In 1989 the U.S. Foundation for Boating Safety conducted extensive day and night trials of 20 different models of visual distress signals. The tests evaluated altitude, burn time, brightness, reliability, and ease of deployment (Tables 50-12 and 50-13).†[46]

All flares will carry a candela rating (candle power, abbreviated cp). This is a measure of light given off by the flare. Before 1948, 1 candela was the light produced by a standard spermaceti (whale oil) candle burning at a specified rate. After 1948 this imprecise definition was replaced with a more precise one: 1 cm^2 of platinum heated to its melting point gives off 60 candela. One candela is easily visible at a distance of 1 mile on a clear, dark night.[24]

Survival Systems Limited has calculated air-to-surface sighting distance for visual signal aids.[4] Based on 30 miles (48 km) of visibility at 500 feet (152 m) altitude, the following observations were made for daytime (Table 50-14) and nighttime signaling (Table 50-15).[4] Of note, heliographs used in desert survival have been spotted by aircraft up to 100 miles away.

Many authorities believe that flare pistols are dangerous and do not recommend them. They are generally available in 12 gauge (Fig. 50-40) and 25 mm. Instead, SOLAS-approved, hand-held flares with self-contained ignition systems are preferred.[25]

Red parachute flares are designed to alert rescuers during the day or night, although they are significantly more effective at night (Fig. 50-41). Of all available emergency aerial flares, they burn the brightest and longest. At the apex of a parachute flare's ascent, a parachute opens, slowing the flare's descent and allowing more time for recognition. Both pistol-launched and hand-held rocket-propelled models are available. In gen-

*The USCG publishes a free brochure detailing visual distress signal regulations. They can be reached through the USCG Hotline at 800-368-5647.

†A full report of their findings can be obtained by writing or calling: BOAT/U.S. Foundation for Boating Safety, 880 South Pickett St., Alexandria, VA 22304; 703-823-9550. Request *Foundation Findings Report #6: Visual Distress Signals*. One way to observe signals in action is to attend a Safety at Sea seminar. For a schedule, contact *Cruising World,* 5 John Clarke Rd., Newport, RI 02840; 401-847-1588.

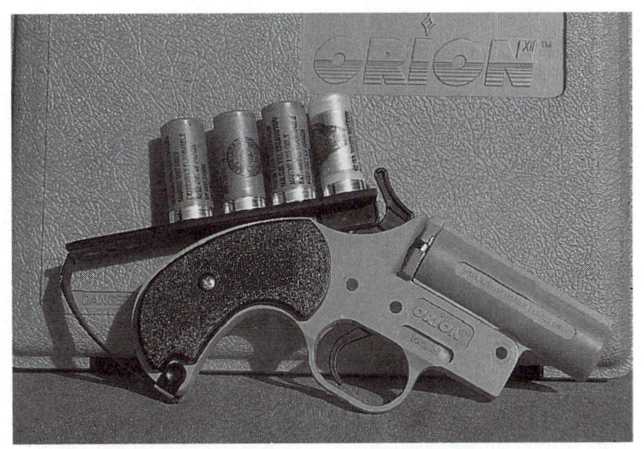

Fig. 50-40 Orion 12-gauge flare pistol.

Table 50-11 Comparison of USCG and SOLAS Specifications

	USCG Specifications			SOLAS Grade		
Pyrotechnic Device	**Altitude**	**Burn Time**	**Brightness**	**Altitude**	**Burn Time**	**Brightness**
Red hand-held flares	—	2 min	500 cp	—	1 min	15,000 cp
Orange smoke	—	50 sec	orange	—	3 min	Orange
Meteors (25 mm)	375 ft	5.5 sec	30,000 cp	*	*	*
Meteors (12 gauge)	250 ft	5.5 sec	10,000 cp	*	*	*
Red parachute flares	492 ft	30 sec	10,000 cp	984 ft	40 sec	30,000 cp

Data from *Boat crew seamanship manual,* COMDTINST M16114.5, Washington, DC, 1985, US Dept of Transportation.
*SOLAS grade does not include meteor flares because of their short burn time.

Table 50-12 Results of BOAT/U.S. Foundation for Boating Safety Pyrotechnic Trials

Device	Manufacturer's Brightness Rating in Candlepower (cp)	Burn Time (min:sec) (Manufacturer's Rating/Trial)	Maximum Height (ft) (Manufacturer's Rating/Trial)
Olin hand-held flare	500	2:00/3:16	—
Kilgore hand-held flare	500	2:00/2:11	—
SSI hand-held flare	500	2:00/3:00	—
Pains-Wessex hand-held flare (SOLAS)	15,000	1:00/1:27	—
Ikaros hand-held flare (SOLAS)	15,000	1:00/1:05	—
Olin orange smoke	—	0:50/0:45	—
Kilgore orange smoke	—	0:50/1:19	—
SSI orange smoke (not USCG-approved)	—	0:30/0:32	—
Pains-Wessex orange smoke (SOLAS)	—	3:00/3:32	—
Ikaros orange smoke (SOLAS)	—	4:00/3:25	—
Olin 12-gauge meteors	10,000	0:06/0:05	250/375
Kilgore 12-gauge meteors	10,000	0:05/0:06	325/425
SSI Skyblazer aerial flare	20,000	0:08/0:09	500/675
Kilgore six-shooter flare	10,000	0:05/0:07	250/350
Olin 25 mm meteor	30,000	0:08/0:06	375/550
Kilgore 25 mm meteor	30,000	0:05/0:06	325/450
Olin parachute flare	10,000	0:25/0:29	1000/1015
Kilgore parachute flare	20,000	0:25/0:19	200/775
Pains-Wessex parachute (SOLAS)	30,000	0:40/0:42	984/1175
Ikaros parachute flare (SOLAS)	40,000	0:40/0:45	984/1225

Data from Holman B: *Cruising World,* Dec 1989.

Table 50-13 Comments on Flares

Flare	Comments
Olin hand-held flare	Brightest of three USCG-approved types; dropped considerable ash and slag
Kilgore hand-held flare	Easy to ignite; considerable smoke
SSI hand-held flare	Least visible; dropped considerable ash and slag
Pains-Wessex hand-held flare (SOLAS)	(Firing mechanism redesigned since these tests); thick smoke
Ikaros hand-held flare (SOLAS)	Convenient pull-string ignition; thick smoke
Olin orange smoke	Hand-held strike ignition; did not meet USCG minimum burn time
Kilgore orange smoke	Hand-held; difficult to strike; more visible than Olin
SSI orange smoke (not USCG approved)	Floating canister; easy to strike; shortest burn time; least visible
Pains-Wessex orange smoke (SOLAS)	Floating canister; convenient pull-string ignition; longest burn time; most visible
Ikaros orange smoke (SOLAS)	Floating canister; convenient pull-string ignition; pinkish smoke less visible than bright orange smoke
Olin 12-gauge meteors	Pistol easy to fire; slight recoil
Kilgore 12-gauge meteors	Pistol launcher; not as bright as Olin 12-gauge
SSI Skyblazer aerial flare	Self-contained, compact, and easy to fire; strong recoil; bright; good value
Kilgore six-shooter flare	Easy to use, self-contained launcher
Olin 25 mm meteor	Good pistol launcher; strong recoil
Kilgore 25 mm meteor	Inadequate pistol launcher (being redesigned)
Olin parachute flare	Well-designed pistol launcher; strong recoil
Kilgore parachute flare	Pistol launched; did not meet USCG or manufacturer's specified minimum burn time
Pains-Wessex parachute (SOLAS)	Hand-held rocket launch; clear instructions; good launching mechanism
Ikaros parachute flare (SOLAS)	Hand-held rocket launch; difficult to fire; strong recoil; brightest of all parachute flares

Data from Holman B: *Cruising World,* Dec 1989.

Table 50-14 Daytime Signals

Signal Device	Distance (Miles)	Distance (km)
Orange smoke	12.0	19.3
Signal mirror	10.0	16.1
Water-soluble dye	8.0	12.9
Red life raft	3.5	5.6
Yellow life raft	2.0	3.0

Table 50-15 Nighttime Signals

Signal Device	Distance (Miles)	Distance (km)
Red flare (not otherwise specified)	22	36.4
Flashlight (not otherwise specified)	6	9.7

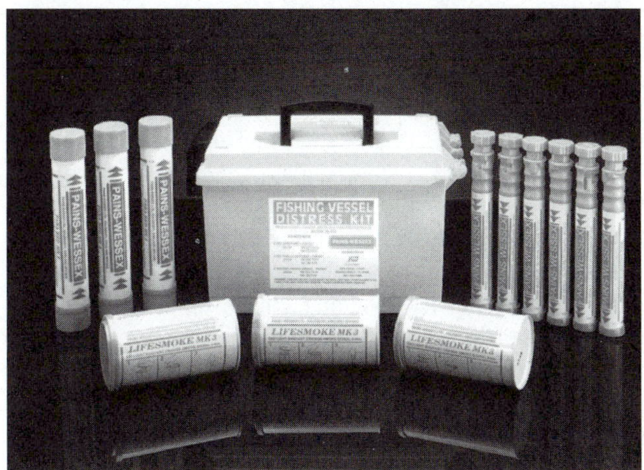

Fig. 50-41 Parachute flares *(far left),* hand-held flares *(far right),* and orange smoke generators *(center).* (Courtesy Simpson-Lawrence.)

eral, hand-held, rocket-powered flares achieve a significantly higher altitude than pistol-launched models. In calm winds the flares should be fired downwind with the arm held 60 degrees above horizontal. In stronger winds the arm angle should be increased to 80 to 85 degrees. Once launched, a parachute flare achieves an altitude of approximately 1000 feet (300 m) and burns for 20 to 40 seconds at 10,000 to 40,000 candela, depending on the model. SOLAS-approved parachute flares burn three to four times brighter and 30% to 50% longer than USCG-approved brands.

A white parachute flare is not a distress signal per se but is used primarily to illuminate dangerous shorelines and harbor entrances at night. It is also useful in locating an MOB at night. It attains an altitude of 1000 feet and a rated brightness of 80,000 candela. On a clear night it illuminates approximately 2 square miles of ocean for 30 seconds.

Meteor flares are short-lived red aerial devices designed for day and night use. They are fired by either pistol launchers or self-contained launching mechanisms. Depending on the model, a meteor flare achieves a maximal height of 250 to 500 feet and burns for 5 to 9 seconds.

One manufacturer produces a "six-shooter" distress signal that holds six preloaded cartridges. The self-contained launcher is easy to use. The six signals each burn for 6 to 7 seconds at 10,000 candela.[15]

Red hand-held flares are similar to automotive road flares (Fig. 50-42). However, they are safer, waterproof, and less messy to operate, with minimized dripping of heated material that could damage a raft or cause skin burning. Red hand-held flares are designed to assist SAR craft in pinpointing a final position. When ignited, they should be held over the side of the raft and pointed downwind to avoid damaging a boat or raft from dripping slag. Gloves should be worn whenever possible. Holding the flares at arm's length maximizes their visual range. Although most effective when used at night, they are approved for day use. A hand-held flare should burn for 1 minute at 15,000 candela.

Orange smoke is designed for daylight distress signaling and is the recommended choice for signaling on a clear day with low wind. In optimal conditions (clear day, minimal

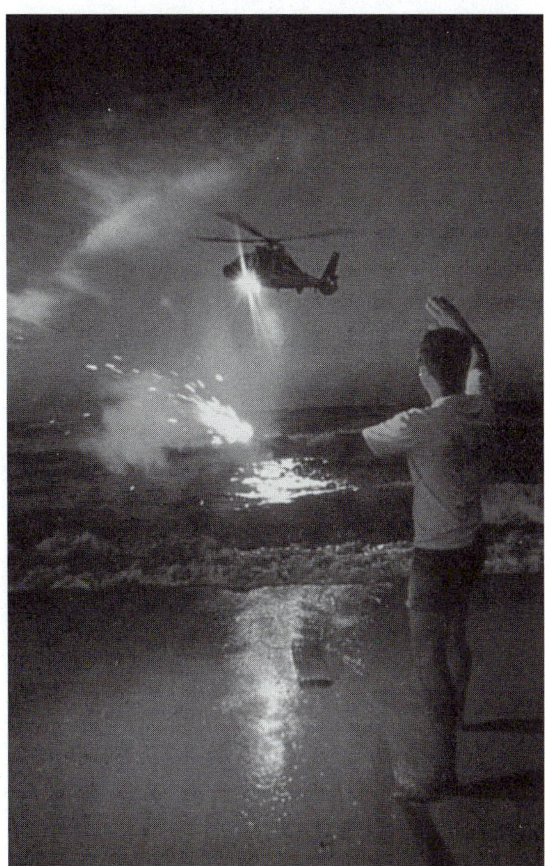

Fig. 50-42 Hand-held flare used to signal a Coast Guard helicopter. (Courtesy U.S. Coast Guard.)

wind), orange smoke can be identified by aircraft up to 12 miles (19 km) away. In high winds an alternative signaling device should be chosen, since smoke is kept close to the water and readily dispersed. Once ignited, a smoke canister should burn for a minimum of 50 seconds as specified by USCG regulations. Orange smoke is available in either hand-held or floating models. Hand-held smoke devices can burn the survivor, and for this reason some authorities recommend using a floating canister smoke system. The burn time of a floating canister is generally longer (about 3 minutes), but it costs approximately one and one half times as much as its hand-held counterpart. Most buoyant orange smoke signals are safe to operate on gasoline- or oil-covered water.

Combined day and night signals are available. They incorporate a red flare at one end for day or night signaling and an orange smoke explosive at the other end for daylight use. The end caps are coded for easy nighttime identification. Either end can be fired independently and the unused end stowed until required. The flare burns for approximately 20 seconds at 10,000 candela, and the orange smoke burns for approximately 18 seconds.[4]

Many different battery-operated, waterproof signaling lights are available (Fig. 50-43). They can be attached to a life raft, PFD, or MOB pole and generally operate on AA, C, or D batteries. Many signaling lights flash the SOS universal distress signal. The USCG rates these types of devices.

A personal marker light (PML) is a waterproof, windproof, nonflammable, disposable plastic tube designed to be worn on a PFD (Fig. 50-44). When the nontoxic chemical solutions are mixed and activated by depression of a lever, a yellow-green light is emitted. A PML emits light for over 8 hours that is visible up to 1 mile on a clear dark night. It is brighter, but only slightly more expensive, than a cyalume. Below 32° F (0° C) the light output of a PML or cyalume is diminished, so the USCG recommends that a battery-powered light be used under these conditions.

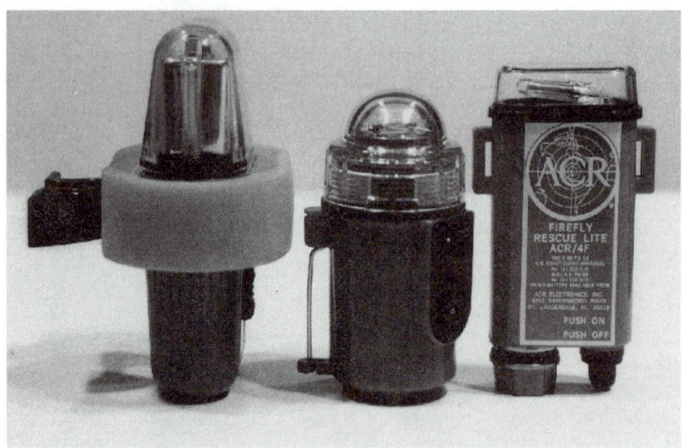

Fig. 50-43 Battery-operated distress signals. Mayday strobe *(far left),* ACR Firefly strobe *(far right),* and D-cell strobe *(center).* (Courtesy Survival Technologies Group.)

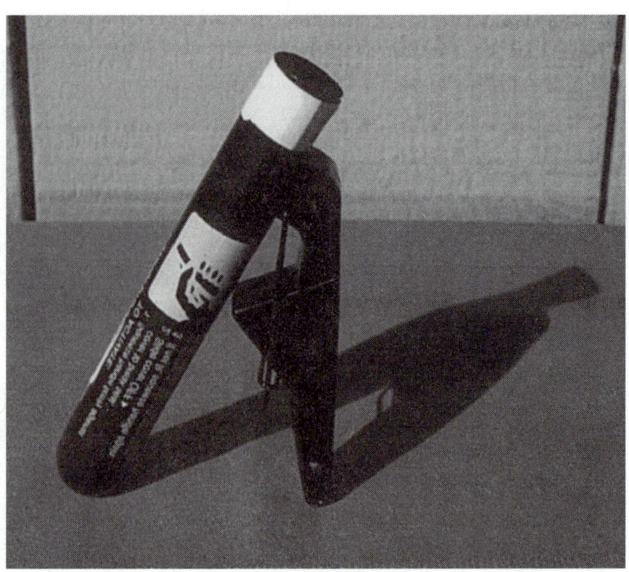

Fig. 50-44 Personal marker light. (Courtesy Survival Technologies Group.)

A chemical lightstick (cyalume) is a similar, portable, cost-efficient source of low-intensity luminescence. When the plastic lightstick is bent, a glass ampule containing one of the chemicals is broken and a chemical reaction occurs that converts energy to light without heat, flame, or sparks. Cyalume sticks come in a wide variety of colors and intensity. Once activated, they emit light for up to 12 hours and can be conveniently attached to a PFD.

Fluorescent green or orange water-soluble dye can be discharged into the sea during the daytime to signal aircraft. The dye comes in a waterproof, tear-open package (Fig. 50-45).

A signaling mirror (heliograph) is a simple and effective means of signaling distress (Fig. 50-46). It consists of a two-sided mirror with a hole in the middle. For it to work properly, a workable angle is needed between the sun, mirror, and rescue craft. Most heliographs have instructions printed on the back. Heliographs have been seen by SAR authorities up to 100 miles away in ideal conditions. When a heliograph is used, an SOS signal should be conveyed.

A whistle is inexpensive, small, and easily attached to a PFD. Plastic is preferred over metal to retard corrosion and prevent sticking to the lips under freezing conditions.

A variety of other means are available to signal distress: a gun fired at intervals of 1 minute, a continuously sounding fog horn, a hoisted flag with an attached round ball, a flag featuring a black ball and square against an orange background, and code flags "November" and "Charlie" (Fig. 50-47).

NAVIGATION[6,40,47]

Navigation in a raft is far from precise. Rafts are designed to float rather than sail. The effect of current and wind can be influenced, however, by using the drogue and

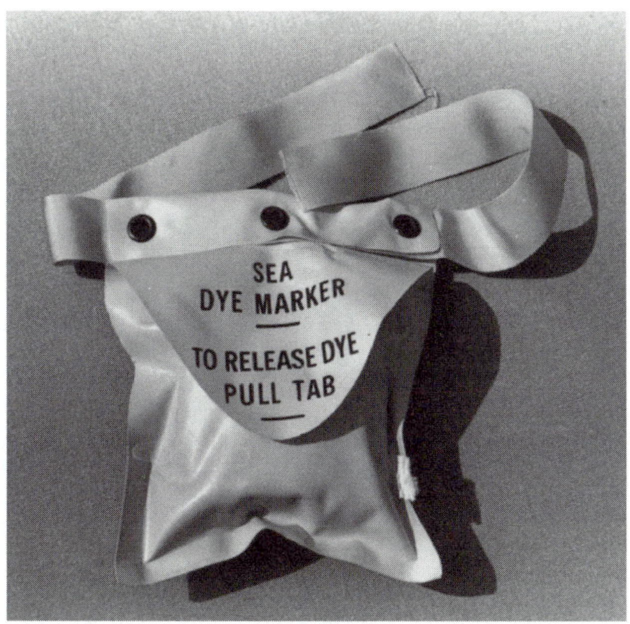

Fig. 50-45 Sea dye marker. (Courtesy Survival Technologies Group.)

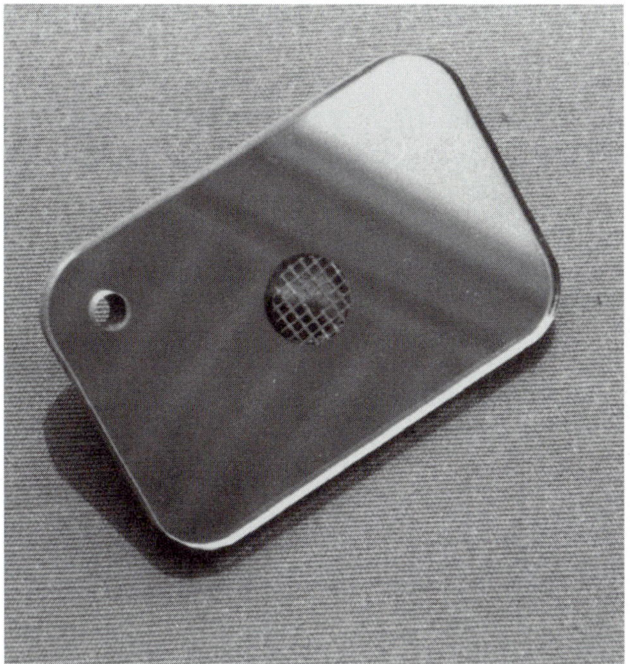

Fig. 50-46 Signaling mirror (heliograph). (Courtesy Survival Technologies Group.)

canopy. Ascertaining position at sea is important; it may influence decisions concerning whether to stay put or head for land, a shipping lane, or an area of greater rainfall. It may also influence decisions regarding rationing and gives the survivor something to do to improve his or her situation.

The following navigational gear stowed in the abandon ship bag enables determination of an approximate position: plastic sextant, nautical almanac, H0249 sight reduction tables, watch, world time zone chart, surface current chart of the world, universal plotting chart, navigational plotter, liquid compass, and charts providing an overview of the intended cruising areas.[47] Calculation of latitude and longitude is complex and beyond the scope of this chapter. The reader is encouraged to consult a text on navigation.

Sailors and castaways can now navigate electronically using hand-held global positioning system (GPS) units. GPS uses satellites and the principle of triangulation to calculate an accurate position at sea. Some GPS units calculate a position many times a minute, providing up-to-date information. With use of an adapter, hand-held units can be plugged into a ship's 12-volt power supply. A recent review rates the latest hand-held GPS units.[63]

Dead reckoning is the art and science of determining the direction of drift using a compass and speed through the water. If no compass is available, the prevailing wave pattern should be noted in its relationship to the sun, which is either due north or south at noon. At night the constellation Polaris bears roughly to the north and the Southern Cross to the south.

Following ship abandonment, castaways need to decide whether to stay put or travel. Several factors are important to consider. If a VHF or SSB distress signal was transmitted before the ship was abandoned, survivors should remain in the area where the vessel went down for at least 24 hours. If an EPIRB is activated, every effort should be made to remain in the area for *at least* 48 hours, which is the duration of an EPIRB battery. If help does not arrive within 72 hours after EPIRB activation, consideration should be given to striking out for a shipping lane or land. Factors important to consider are whether the craft can be sailed or rowed (less likely in a raft), amount of food and water, physical condition of the crew and craft, navigational skills of persons on board, availability of charts and instruments, and distance to land or shipping lanes.

If a raft is not well stocked with food, water, and equipment, or if no one on board has good navigational skills, the raft's drift should be slowed using the drogue until rescuers arrive. If the decision is made to travel, castaways should head for a busy shipping lane with a large land mass or island chain downwind and downcurrent in case the raft is not spotted by a ship.[40]

Old mariners claimed they could smell land before seeing it. While smelling, castaways should scan the horizon for stationary clouds that often indicate an underlying land mass. Sunlight reflected off a coral reef, shallow water, sandy beach, or snow-covered land may cause a bright aura on the horizon. Water color may lend a clue to the proximity of land; the deeper the water, the bluer the color. As water depth decreases, the color turns lighter shades of blue, green, brown, or black. Floating vegetation, driftwood, and

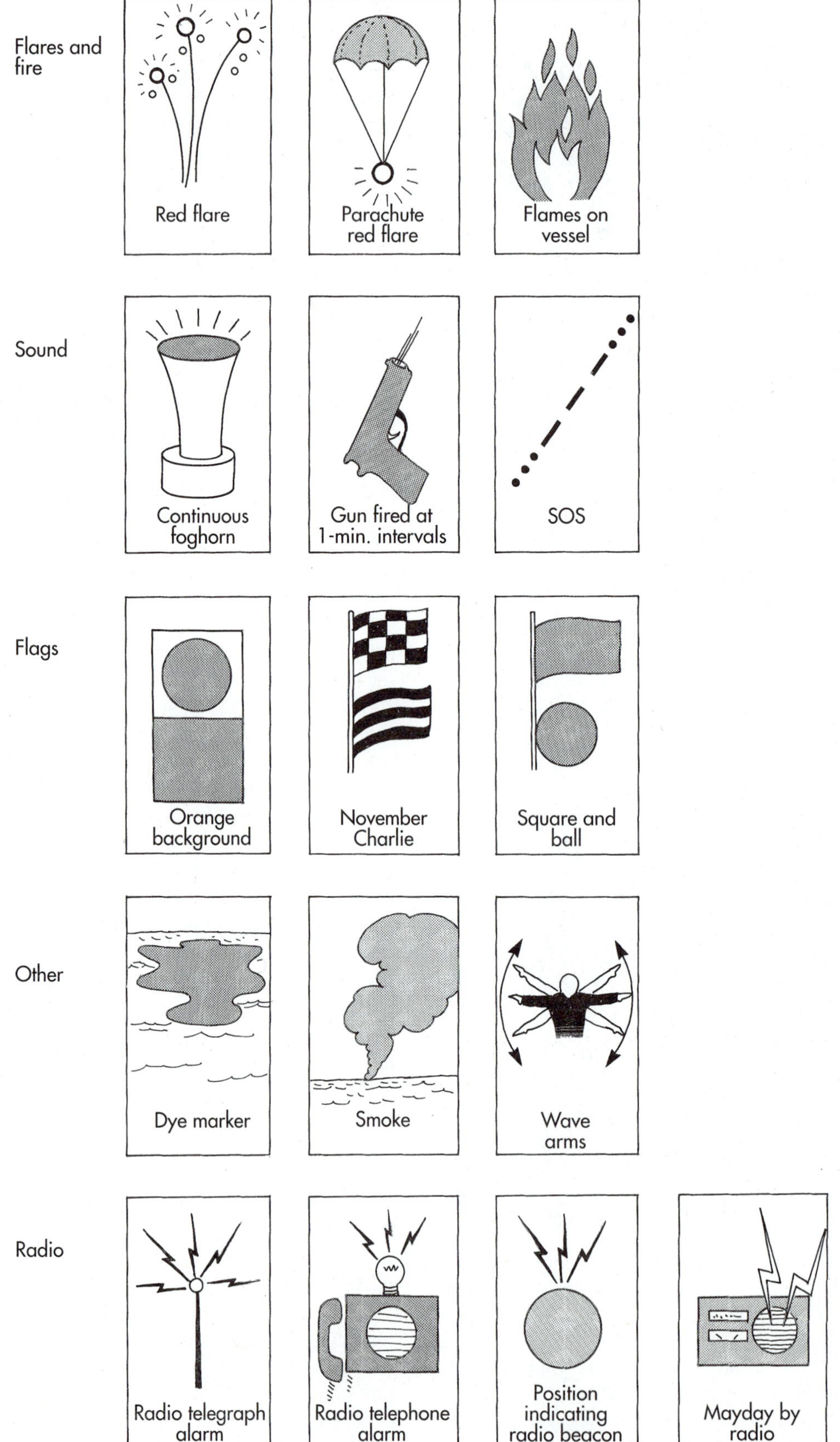

Fig. 50-47 Means to signal distress at sea. (Courtesy U.S. Coast Guard.)

human refuse are reliable signs of nearby land. While many believe that the presence of birds signifies nearby land, shore birds are often seen hundreds of miles from land and can be blown far out to sea by storms. However, the unidirectional sound of crying birds and crashing waves may indicate a nearby roost and, in foggy conditions, has guided many navigators to land.[40]

If possible, landings should not be attempted at night when surf condition and potential dangers are difficult to evaluate. Landing near the outlet of rivers often avoids the hazards of coral, which do not thrive in fresh water. Castaways should avoid landing where high spray and white water are produced by crashing waves; this usually indicates a shallow reef, rocky shore, or vertical cliff. The surf on the lee side of an island is often smaller than on the windward side. The physical condition of the crew should always be considered before attempting a landing. For an exhausted crew it might be better to travel by raft along the coast than to hike over rugged terrain and mountains.[47]

If a landing is attempted, all survivors should don PFDs. All clothing and shoes should be worn for protection against rocks and coral. The sea anchor should be deployed when surf is present to minimize the chance of capsizing. For additional stabilization the raft can be partially deflated and filled with water. The raft's center of gravity should be minimized by having all castaways seated low. If the raft is dangerously overcrowded, the stronger survivors can float outside the raft while holding onto the grommeted safety line and grab handles; this adds ballast to the raft as well. The canopy should be furled to facilitate escape in the event of capsizing.[47]

Waves should be studied before attempting a landing. Waves travel in groups called sets. A typical set is composed of five to nine waves. The ideal time to effect a landing is during the lull between sets. If the raft capsizes during landing, it is difficult to right in the surf. Castaways should, however, attempt to stay with the raft, since a capsized raft is nearly always carried toward shore. When close to shore, castaways should crawl out of the water, since crawling reduces the likelihood of being knocked over by a large wave. Castaways who have been adrift for a time may also find that leg strength is lacking.[47]

SEARCH AND RESCUE

In the United States the Coast Guard conducts most of the significant SAR operations at sea and on the navigable waters where the United States has jurisdiction. Their responsibilities include navigation, merchant marine inspection, small boat safety, maritime law enforcement, fishery and marine environmental protection, polar operations, and drug interdiction. In some distress situations the USCG calls on the U.S. Coast Guard Auxiliary. The Coast Guard Auxiliary is a voluntary civilian unit that, when under orders, has the same authority as the Coast Guard and often performs similar operations as the USCG. The Auxiliary is frequently dispatched to help mariners in nondistress situations. In addition to the USCG Auxiliary, marine towing companies may assist in rescues at sea. Licensed by the USCG, they are equipped to tow, dewater, fight fires, repair engines, and perform electrical work.[16]

A theoretical boating accident is presented to facilitate understanding of USCG SAR technique and equipment. A 30-foot sailboat located 100 miles offshore begins taking on water with bilge pumps unable to keep up with pumping demands. On board are five persons, including a child and a seriously injured person. They have no life raft on board. The crew on board render first aid to the injured victim, don PFDs, issue a Mayday distress signal, and activate a 406 EPIRB.

In all probability the first SAR craft seen will be a C-130 fixed-wing aircraft. If necessary, it may initially drop a gasoline-powered dewatering pump to help control flooding. Life rafts, survival gear, detection aids, portable radios, mechanical parts, and medications can also be dropped. Shortly afterward, a USCG helicopter may arrive. USCG helicopters can generally travel up to 250 miles offshore and are used when a victim is seriously injured and needs emergency medical attention. Depending on the situation the helicopter may be the first SAR craft sent. A surface vessel may also be sent to aid in rescue and possible towing of a disabled boat.[97]

The aircraft will attempt to contact the crew on VHF channel 16, so this channel should be constantly monitored. Using VHF the aircraft gets additional information about the nature of the emergency and uses the signal to pinpoint the location of the boat by means of a radio direction finder (RDF). In the meantime the crew must get the deck cleared and lashed in preparation for a helicopter, which is capable of generating rotor propwash winds over 100 mph. In anticipation of these high winds, crew members should be sufficiently dressed to combat the wind chill factor. Crew members on deck are advised to use a harness, tether, and jacklines, since propwash can blow a person overboard. All masts and booms should be lowered. After the deck is cleared, all unnecessary crew should get below deck. Approaching SAR craft should be signaled with orange smoke during the day and hand-held flares at night. Parachute and meteor flares should *never* be launched when survivors are approached by plane or helicopter. At night, the deck and any obstruction should be adequately lit by whatever means available, but no light should be shone upward into the eyes of rescue authorities.[89]

A helicopter usually approaches from aft and on the port side of the disabled boat, enabling maximal pilot view of the boat's forward superstructure and mast.[90] Hoisting is done on the starboard side of the airship. The injured person is the first crew member evacuated. Although a rescue basket is the preferred hoisting device, the transfer of an injured person is usually done with a Stokes litter. All persons evacuated by Stokes litter or rescue basket should wear a PFD. Once the litter or basket is lowered, the steadying line attached to the lowered device should be used to guide the litter to the boat. Because of potentially high-static electrical charges, the litter must first be allowed to touch (ground) either the water or the boat before being touched by a crew member. The steadying line attached to the litter does not develop a static electrical charge and is safe to handle immediately. At *no* time should a deployed line from a helicopter ever be attached to a boat. Lines should never be thrown from a boat toward a helicopter. The helicopter instructs the crew how to detach the Stokes litter and load the injured person. Uninjured and physically able crew members may be evacuated into the helicopter using a rescue basket. Horseshoe slings are used primarily when evacuating trained military personnel. A rescue basket is capable of lifting 600 pounds (273 kg) but can accommodate only one adult at a time. In this hypothetical situation the child should be placed in the rescue basket with one adult.

Acknowledgments

Special thanks to the following persons for their constructive criticism of this manuscript: Mark O. Hyde, Chief Warrant Officer and Rescue and Survival Systems Manager, Search and Rescue Division, United States Coast Guard Headquarters; Dave Comeau, Chief Instructor, Survival Systems Limited; and Kelsey Burr, Survival Technologies Group.

APPENDIX A

Glossary

Aft Near, toward, or in the stern (rear) of a vessel.

Amidships In or toward the middle of a ship between the bow and stern.

Ballast Any heavy substance (such as water) used in a vessel to improve its stability.

Bight A 180-degree half loop formed by turning a line back on itself.

Bilge The bottom of a hull; also short for bilge water, which is foul water that collects in the hull bottom.

Boom A long pole used to extend the bottom of a sail.

Bow The forward part of a vessel.

Bowsprit A large spar projecting forward from the bow of a vessel.

Compressed natural gas (CNG) A form of cooking fuel used on boats.

COSPAS A Russian satellite system, akin to SARSAT, translated Space System for Search of Vessels in Distress.

"Deadman's float" position The position commonly assumed by an unconscious victim floating in the water; typically, the victim is face down, with arms and legs abducted.

Doff To remove; used to describe the removal of a PFD or other survival attire.

Don To put on or dress; used to describe the application of a PFD or other survival attire.

Drogue A sea anchor; a miniparachute-like device deployed from a life raft, used in stabilization of the raft by resisting the lifting forces of wind and waves; also slows the drift of a raft.

Dry chemical A type of chemical used in fire extinguishers; the most common dry chemical is sodium bicarbonate (baking soda), but potassium bicarbonate and monoammonium phosphate are also used.

Emergency position indicating radio beacon (EPIRB) A small, electronic radio beacon used in an emergency to signal rescuers; its signal can be detected by satellites and SAR personnel.

Flotsam The wreckage of a ship or its cargo found floating on the sea.

Foremast The mast nearest the bow.

Freeboard The distance between the waterline and the deck; also used in reference to the distance between the waterline and a person's mouth when immersed in the ocean.

Furl To wrap or roll tightly; used in reference to the position of a canopy, an unfurled canopy is one in the open position.

Galley The kitchen and cooking apparatus of a vessel.

Halon Halogenated gas; a chemical used in fighting fires aboard boats.

Harness A device worn by a crew member while on board a vessel, designed to prevent falling overboard.

Heaving line Any line thrown from a boat or raft; commonly used in reference to a line dispatched to a person overboard.

Heliograph A two-sided signaling mirror.

Jackline A piece of reinforced line or wire, usually stretching from the cockpit to the bow; used by crew members wearing a harness and tether; allows for safer excursion atop the deck under rough conditions.

Jib A triangular sail extending from the head of the foremast to the bowsprit or jib boom.

Jibe To shift suddenly from one side to the other; said of a sail or its boom when the vessel is steered off the wind until the sail fills on the opposite side.

Lee The sheltered or protected side; the part of the ship that is farthest from the wind.

Leeward Opposite of windward; toward the lee side of the ship.

Liquid propane gas (LPG) A commonly used cooking fuel aboard ships.

Mae West A yellow inflatable PFD worn by pilots flying over bodies of water.

Man overboard (MOB) Any person who has fallen in the water.

Mayday The highest priority distress signal; indicates that a vessel or person is in grave danger and requires immediate assistance.

Painter line The line attached from the parent vessel to the life raft; when pulled taut, it activates the carbon dioxide inflation mechanism of the life raft.

Pan An urgency signal, pronounced "pahn," indicating that the transmitting station has an urgent message concerning the safety of a vessel, aircraft, or person.

Parachute flare A high-altitude pyrotechnic device, capable of reaching an altitude of 1000 feet.

Personal flotation device (PFD) Formerly called a life jacket, life vest, life preserver, or Mae West; now referred to collectively by the USCG as PFDs.

Port That side of a vessel on the left hand of a person who stands on board facing the bow; opposite of starboard.

Radio direction finder (RDF) A sophisticated electronic device used by SAR authorities to home in on a radio signal.

Retroreflective Special reflective tape used on survival gear to reflect light back to SAR authorities.

Safety of Life at Sea (SOLAS) An international organization consisting of 67 maritime nations whose parent organization is the International Maritime Organization; it is under the auspices of the United Nations. SOLAS meets periodically to establish maritime regulations, including standards for ship construction, surveys, stability, machinery, fire protection, navigation, communication, cargo, dangerous goods, signaling, and lifesaving equipment.

Sea anchor See Drogue.

Search and rescue (SAR) Those authorities, usually the USCG, designated to search for and rescue persons in need of immediate assistance at sea.

Search and rescue satellite (SARSAT) A low-altitude satellite system used to detect and relay the distress signal of an EPIRB.

Search and rescue transponder (SART) A small electronic device that emits a radar signal used by SAR personnel to pinpoint the exact location of a survivor at sea.

Securite Pronounced "say-curitay"; a safety urgency signal that indicates that the station is about to transmit a message concerning safety of navigation or important weather information.

Single side band (SSB) A radio used commonly at sea; can transmit thousands of miles; frequency 2182 kHz is monitored by the USCG and is used as a distress frequency.

SOS The universal distress signal composed of dot-dot-dot-dash-dash-dash-dot-dot-dot; is not an abbreviation, although mistakenly referred to as "Save Our Ship" or "Save Our Soul."

Spar A mast or boom.

Starboard That side of a vessel on the right hand of a person who stands on board facing the bow; opposite of port.

Stern The rear end of a vessel.

Stow To place or arrange in a compact mass; to pack; to hide.

Tether A piece of strong reinforced nylon attached from a harness to a jackline.

Thermal protective aid (TPA) A Mylar or aluminum covering designed to reflect the wearer's body heat; used in the prevention and treatment of hypothermia.

Under way Into motion from a standstill.

United States Coast Guard (USCG) That body of the United States military charged with conducting most of the significant SAR operations at sea and on the navigable waters where the United States has jurisdiction. Their responsibilities include navigation, merchant marine inspection, small boat safety, maritime law enforcement, fishery and marine environmental protection, polar operations, and drug interdiction.

Valise A soft fabric container that is used to protect a life raft and is usually stowed below deck.

Very high frequency (VHF) A commonly used form of radio when out at sea; channel 16 (156.8 MHz) is the distress frequency.

Windward The side from which the wind blows; toward the wind; opposite of leeward.

APPENDIX B

Personal Flotation Device Manufacturers and Distributors

Blue Water Marine Division
P.O. Box 1169
Pearland, TX 77588

Butler Parachute Systems Inc.
6399 Lindbergh Blvd.
California City, CA 93505

Cal-June
5328 Vineland Ave.
North Hollywood, CA 92601

Carlon Rubber Products
P.O. Box 377
Derby, CT 06418

Coleman Flotation
250 North Saint Francis St.
Wichita, KS 67202

Conax
2801 75th St. North
St. Petersburg, FL 33710

Ero Industries, Inc.
8130 North Lehigh Ave.
Morton Grove, IL 60053

Extrasport
5306 NW 35 Court
Miami, FL 33142

Giammanco
Route 6, P.O. Box 972
Palatka, FL 32177

Harishok Company Ltd.
RD w, P.O. Box 922
Canaan, NH 03741

Henri-Lloyd USA
P.O. Box 1039
Manhasset, NY 11030

Intamar Logistics Inc.
10-12 Union Hill Rd.
West Conshohocken, PA 19428

Landrigan Corp.
2-12 Jeffries St.
P.O. Box 444
East Boston, MA 02128

Mustang Technology Engineering Apparel Corp.
3810 Jacombs Rd.
Richmond, British Columbia V6V 1Y6
Canada

Noble Products
R.R. 6, County Rd. 13
Caldwell, OH 43724

Northwest River Supplies
P.O. Box 9186
Moscow, ID 83843-9186

Omega
130 Condor St.
East Boston, MA 02128

ParaGear International
3837 W. Oakton St.
Skokie, IL 60076

Rubber Crafters Inc.
P.O. Box 220
Grantsvill, WV 26147

Safegard Corporation
315 15th
Covington, KY 41011

Sea Safety International
10 Wood Ave.
Secaucus, NJ 07094

Seda Products
P.O. Box 997
Chula Vista, CA 92012

SoniForm Inc.
1908 Friendship Dr.
El Cajon, CA 92020

Stearns Manufacturing
P.O. Box 1498
St. Cloud, MN 56302

Survival Products
5614 SW 25th St.
Hollywood, FL 33023

Survival Technologies Group
6418 US Highway 41 North, Suite 266
Apollo Beach, FL 33572

Switlik Parachute Co., Inc.
P.O. Box 1328
East State St.
Trenton, NJ 08607

Taylortec Incorporated
2400 S. Range Rd.
Hammond, LA 70403

Wildwater Designs
230 Penllyn Pike
Penllyn, PA 19422

Wirt Inflatable
P.O. Box 520
Pike St.
Elizabeth, WV 26143

APPENDIX C

Immersion Suit Manufacturers and Distributors

Fitzwright Survival Systems, Inc.
Unit 150-5811 Cedarbridge Way
Richmond, British Columbia V6X 2A8
Canada

Harvey's Skin Diving Suits, Inc.
2505 South 252 St.
Kent, WA 98031

Lifesaving Systems Corp.
220 Elsberry Rd.
Apollo Beach, FL 33572-2289

Mustang Technical Engineering Apparel Corp.
3810 Jacombs Rd.
Richmond, British Columbia V6V 1Y6
Canada

Parkway/Imperial
241 Raritan St.
South Amboy, NJ 08879

Survival Technologies Group
6418 US Highway 41 North, Suite 266
Apollo Beach, FL 33572

APPENDIX D

Dry Suit Manufacturers and Distributors

Diving Unlimited International, Inc.
1148 Delevan Dr.
San Diego, CA 92102

Lifesaving Systems Corp.
220 Elsberry Rd.
Apollo Beach, FL 33572-2289

ML Lifeguard Equipment Ltd.
10627 Jones St.
Suite 101 B
Fairfax, VA 22030

O.S. Systems
P.O. Box 864
Scappoose, OR 97056

Typhoon Water Wares
1106 Market St.
Pocomoke City, MD 21851

Underwater Equipment Sales Corp.
3518 SE 21st Ave.
Portland, OR 97202-2909

APPENDIX E

Antiexposure Suit Manufacturers and Distributors

Lifesaving Systems Corporation
220 Elsberry Rd.
Apollo Beach, FL 33572-2289

Survival Technologies Group
6418 US Highway 41 North, Suite 266
Apollo Beach, FL 33572

APPENDIX F

Life Raft Manufacturers and Distributors

Air Cruisers Co.
P.O. Box 180
Belmar, NJ 07719

Aviation Marine Specialty Products
6626 Easton Rd., Route 611
Pipersville, PA 18947

Avon Seagull Marine
1851 McGaw Ave.
Irvine, CA 92714

Beaufort Air-Sea Equipment
12351 Bridgeport Rd.
Richmond, British Columbia
V6V 1J4, Canada

Blue Water Marine Division
P.O. Box 1169-T
Pearland, TX 77588

Butler Parachute Systems Inc.
6399-R Lindbergh Blvd.
California City, CA 93505

Datrex Inc.
P.O. Drawer 1150
Kinder, LA 70648-1150

Eastern Aero Marine Co.
3850-T NW 25th St.
Miami, FL 33142

Givens Ocean Survival Systems
1741 Main Rd.
Tiverton, RI 02878

Imtra Corp.
30 Barnet Blvd.
New Bedford, MA 02745

Intamar Logistics Inc.
10-12 Union Hill Rd.
West Conshohocken, PA 19428

Life Saving Equipment Repair Co.
P.O. Drawer 2725
Morgan City, LA 70381

Life Support International
200-T Rittenhouse Circle, Bldg. 4W
Bristol, PA 19007

Para-Gear International Sales Corp.
3837 W. Oakton St.
Skokie, IL 60076

Plastimo USA, Inc.
6605 Selnick Dr., Route 100
Business Park
Baltimore, MD 21227

Pugh, Billy, Co., Inc.
P.O. Box 802-T
Corpus Christi, TX 78403

RPR Industries, Inc.
Route 5, Old US Hwy. No. 1
Apex, NC 27502

Rubber Crafters Inc.
P.O. Box 220
Grantsvill, WV 26147

Samsel Supply Co.
1285-T Old River Rd.
Cleveland, OH 44113

Seaco-Elliot, Inc.
3874-T Fiscal Ct.
Route 200
Riviera Beach, FL 33404

Shoreline Aviation & Marine
8305-TR Monroe
Houston, TX 77061

SMR Technologies Inc.
Engineered Rubber Products Div.
P.O. Drawer 326-T
1420-T Wold Creek Trail
Sharon Center, OH 44274-0326

Survival Products Inc.
5614 SW 25th St., Dept. T
Hollywood, FL 33023

Survival Technologies Group
6418 US Highway 41 North, Suite 266
Apollo Beach, FL 33572

Switlik Parachute Co., Inc.
P.O. Box 1328
East State St.
Trenton, NJ 08607

USA Inflatable Inc.
2725 West 5th North St.
Summerville, SC 29483

Viking
1625 N. Miami Ave.
Miami, FL 33136

Winslow Marine Products Corp.
928 South Tamiami Trail
P.O. Box 888
Osprey, FL 34229

Wirt Inflatable Specialists
P.O. Box 520
Pike St.
Elizabeth, WV 26143

Zodiac of North America
1851 McGaw Ave.
Irvine, CA 92714

APPENDIX G

Emergency Position Indicating Radio Beacon Manufacturers and Distributors

ACR Electronics
5757 Ravenswood Rd.
Box 5247
Ft. Lauderdale, FL 33310-5247

Alden Electronics
40 Washington St.
Westborough, MA 01581

Clifford & Snell Ltd.
512 Purley Way
Croydon, Surrey CR0 4NZ
England

Electronics Safety Device Inc.
P.O. Box 1034
Manhasset, NY 11030

Jotron Electronics A.S.
P.O. Box 85
3280 Tjodalyng, Norway

Koden International
77 Accord Park Dr.
Norwell, MA 02061

Litton Special Devices
750 West Sproul Rd.
Springfield, PA 19064-4084

Lo-Kata N. America
950 Roosevelt Blvd.
Tarpon Springs, FL 34689

Modern Products Ltd.
Box 683
Victoria, British Columbia C Z8W 2P3
Canada

Radio-Holland USA
6033 S Loop E.,
Houston, TX 77033

Raytheon/Kannad
46 River Rd.
Hudson, NH 03051

Survival Technologies Group
6418 US Highway 41 North, Suite 266
Apollo Beach, FL 33572

World of Business
P.O. Box 17
Sequim, WA 98382-0017

APPENDIX H

Search and Rescue Transponder Manufacturers and Distributors

Alden Electronics
40 Washington St.
Westborough, MA 01581

Litton Special Devices
750 West Sproul Rd.
Springfield, PA 19064-4084

APPENDIX I

VHF Manufacturers and Distributors

Apelco Marine Electronics
1107 N. Ward St.
Tampa, FL 33607

Humminbird
c/o Techsonic Industries
#1 Humminbird Lane
Eufaula, AL 36027

Icom America Inc.
2380 116th Ave. N.E., P.O. Box C-9029
Bellevue, WA 98009-9029

IMI Kenyon Electronics
P.O. Box 308
New Whitfield St.
Guilford, CT 06437

Impulse
329 Railroad Ave.
Pittsburgh, CA 94565

Intech Inc.
Com/Nav Div.
282 Brokaw Rd, P.O. Box 58064
Santa Clara, CA 95052-8064

Kenwood
Communications & Test Equipment Group
2201 E. Dominguez St.
Long Beach, CA 90810

King Marine Electronics
5320 140th Ave. N
Clearwater, FL 33169

Lorad Corp.
14900 NW 159th St.
Miami, FL 33169

Marinetek
2239 Paragon Dr.
San Jose, CA 95131

Navico Inc.
7381 114th Ave. North, Suite 407
Largo, FL 34643

Panasonic
1 Panasonic Way
Secaucus, NJ 07094

Realistic
c/o Radio Shack
1800 One Tandy Center
Fort Worth, TX 76102

Raytheon Marine Co.
46 River Rd.
Hudson, NH 03051

Robertson-Shipmate Inc.
400 Oser Ave.
Hauppauge, NY 11788

Sailor
c/o RH Trading
19019 36 Ave., W., Bldg. A, Suite E
Lynwood, WA 98036

SMR Marine Electronics
1401 N.W. 89th CT
Miami, FL 33172

SEA Inc.
7030 220th S.W.
Mountlake Terrace, WA 98043

Sea Ranger Marine Inc.
201 Meadow Rd.
Edison, NJ 08818

Simrad, Inc.
620 N.W. Bright St.
Seattle, WA 98107

Si-Tex Marine Electronics
P.O. Box 6700
Clearwater, FL 33518

Uniden Corp. of America
2400 Amon Carter Blvd.
Fort Worth, TX 76155

West Marine Products
500 Westridge Dr.
Watsonville, CA 95076-4100

APPENDIX J

Single Side Band, Ham Radio Manufacturers and Distributors

Furuno
271 Harbor Way
South San Francisco, CA 94083

Glassmaster
P.O. Box 159
Newberry, SC 29108

Hull Electronics
1100-B.N. Magnolia Ave.
El Cajon, CA 92020-1953

ICOM
2380 116th Ave. NE
Bellevue, WA 98004

Kenwood USA
2201 E. Dominguez St.
Long Beach, CA 90810-5745

Morad Electronics
1125 NW 46th St.
Seattle, CA 98107

Panasonic Co.
1 Panasonic Way
Secaucus, NJ 07094

Raytheon Marine Co.
46 River Rd.
Hudson, NH 03062

Shakespeare Antennas
P.O. Box 733
Newberry, SC 29108

Yaesu
17210 Edwards Rd.
Cerritos, CA 90701

REFERENCES

1. A shipwrecked Miami couple owe their lives to a clever gadget that makes seawater drinkable, *People Weekly Magazine,* Oct 2, 1989.
2. Alper J: Survival at sea, *Chemmatters,* Oct 1992.
3. Bailey M, Bailey M: *Staying alive!* New York, 1974, McKay.
4. *Basic survival training,* Dartmouth, Nova Scotia, Canada, Survival Systems Limited.
5. Biewenga B, Pittman F: The offshore safety net, *Sail,* Sept 1991.
6. *Boat crew seamanship manual,* Washington, DC, 1985, US Department of Transportation.
7. BOAT/US Foundation for Boating Safety: *Foundation findings: life jackets,* Part II, Rep No 4, Alexandria, Va, The Foundation.
8. BOAT/US Foundation for Boating Safety: *Foundation findings: report on life jackets,* Rep No 3, Alexandria, Va, 1988, The Foundation.
9. BOAT/US Foundation for Boating Safety: *Foundation findings: children's life jackets,* Rep No 7, Alexandria, Va, 1990, The Foundation.
10. BOAT/US Foundation for Boating Safety: *Foundation findings: gearing up for man overboard,* Rep No 15, Alexandria, Va, The Foundation.
11. BOAT/US Foundation for Boating Safety: *Foundation findings: bilge pumps—on the level,* Rep No 13, Alexandria, Va, The Foundation.
12. BOAT/US Foundation for Boating Safety: *Foundation findings: bilge pump systems—it's all in your head,* Rep No 14, Alexandria, Va, The Foundation.
13. BOAT/US Foundation for Boating Safety: *Foundation findings: fire extinguishers,* Rep No 1, Alexandria, Va, The Foundation.
14. BOAT/US Foundation for Boating Safety: *Foundation findings: onboard communications,* Rep No 8, Alexandria, Va, The Foundation.
15. BOAT/US Foundation for Boating Safety: *Foundation findings: visual distress signals,* Rep No 6, Alexandria, Va, The Foundation.
16. BOAT/US Foundation for Boating Safety: *Foundation findings: help is on the way!* Rep No 11, Alexandria, Va, The Foundation.
17. BOAT/US Foundation for Boating Safety: *Foundation findings: survival rafts,* Rep No 12, Alexandria, Va, The Foundation.
18. Brennan B: A man overboard plan, *Cruising World,* Dec 1989.
19. Brennan B: New rules for faulty EPIRBs, *Cruising World,* Dec 1989.
20. Bright C: Water management, *Ocean Navigator,* Jan/Feb 1993.
21. Burr K: Life rafts: is there a right choice? *Newswave* 1(8), Winter 1988.
22. Burr K: Equipping your boat for safety, *Cruising World,* Dec 1989.
23. Burr K: The United States Coast Guard: they're always ready. We, usually, are not, *Newswave,* 1993.
24. Burr K: Candela, *Newswave,* 1993.
25. Burr K: Launching parachute flares, *Newswave,* 1993.
26. Caldwell J: *Desperate voyage,* Boston, 1949, Little, Brown.
27. Caprio D: Safety gear: the essentials, *Yachting,* July 1993.
28. Chesher R: Water, water, everywhere, *Cruising Helmsman,* June 1993.
29. *Coast Guard rescue and survival systems,* CIMDTINST M10470.10A, Washington, DC, 1982, US Department of Transportation.
30. *Coast Guard rescue and survival systems,* COMDTINST M10470.10C, Washington, DC, 1992, US Department of Transportation.
31. Day G: The new age of EPIRBs, *Cruising World,* Dec 1989.
32. Dhenin G, Sharp GR, Ernsting J: *Aviation medicine: physiology and human factors,* London, Tri-Med Books.
33. Dove T: Commonsense VHF, *Sail,* May 1993.
34. DSC: cutting through the clutter, *Sail,* March 1993.
35. Durkin JP: *Communication techniques,* presented at Marine Medicine Conference, July 12-16, 1993, San Diego, Calif.
36. Extinguished: a champion firefighter goes down for the count, *Scientific American,* June 1993.
37. *Federal requirements and safety tips for recreational boaters,* Washington, DC, 1992, USCG Boating Education Branch, US Dept of Transportation.
38. Fighting fire aboard, *Cruising World,* Dec 1992.
39. Fryer DM, Hayes FW: Swept away, *Yachting,* July 1991.
40. Gill PG Jr: *Waterlover's guide to marine medicine,* New York, 1993, Fireside.
41. Gladstone B: Preventing and fighting fires on board, *Motor Boating & Sailing,* July 1988.
42. Gladstone B: Boatkeeper's six essential knots, *Motor Boating & Sailing,* Nov 1990.
43. Gooding B: How safe are today's life rafts? *Cruising World,* Oct 1988.
44. Gooding B: Signaling distress, *Cruising World,* Feb 1992.
45. Heyerdahl T: *The "Kon-Tiki" expedition,* Chicago, 1950, Rand McNally.
46. Holman B: Visual distress signals, *Cruising World,* Dec 1989.
47. Huff R, Farley M: *Sea survival: the boatman's emergency manual,* Philadelphia, 1989, Tab Books.
48. Jacobs TR: The essential life raft, *Yachting,* July 1989.
49. Janssen PA: Lost at sea, *Motor Boating & Sailing,* Jan 1993.
50. Joughin RW: Survival techniques in lifeboats and liferafts, *Safety at Sea,* Dec 1987.
51. Kandebo SW: Navy to slash Halon 1211 use, *Aviation Week & Space Technology,* July 12, 1993.
52. Kimber R: Life jackets: choosing the proper one, *Country Journal,* May/June 1991.
53. Know the right signals, *Sail,* Feb 1993.
54. Knox S: Halon fire extinguishing system, *Sail,* May 1990.
55. Leaf JJ: EPIRBs: rescue by satellite, *Yachting,* April 1989.
56. Leaf JJ: The VHF handbook, *Yachting,* Jan 1991.
57. Leaf JJ: The communications handbook, *Yachting,* March 1991.
58. Lee ECB, Lee K: *Safety and survival at sea,* New York, 1971, WW Norton.
59. *Marine radiotelephone users handbook,* Washington, DC, Radio Technical Commission for Maritime Services.
60. Meluso D: Water-makers: get wet, *Boating,* Jan 1993.
61. Murray CJ: Manually powered system desalinates seawater, *Design News,* Apr 10, 1989.
62. Naranjo R: Water makers come of age, *Crusing World,* Nov 1993.
63. Naranjo R, Pittman F: GPS shoot-out, *Sail,* May 1993.
64. Navy seeks Halon replacement for firefighting, *Design News,* Apr 19, 1993.
65. Onboard electronics: so others can find us, *Motor Boating & Sailing,* Jan 1993.
66. OPTEVOR evaluation report: operational evaluation of the life raft reverse osmosis desalination unit, Rep No 3960, Norfolk, Va, Sept 1, 1989, US Dept of the Navy.
67. Pardey L, Pardey L: Sweet water from the skies, *Sail,* Nov 1991.
68. Personal Flotation Device Manufacturers Association: Choosing a PFD, *Trailer Boats,* April 1992.
69. *Personal survival at sea,* UK Dept of Transportation.
70. Pickthall B: Overboard, *Yachting,* July 1990.
71. Pint-size protection, *Trailer Boats,* Aug 1993.
72. Pizzino JF: *Technical evaluation test report of the pilot production of reverse osmosis desalinators for emergency application on Navy life boats,* Annapolis, Md, 1988, David Taylor Research Center.
73. Rains J, Miller P: Offshore communications connections, *Cruising World,* June 1993.
74. Rath D: Put out the fire, *Yachting,* July 1989.
75. Reekie S: Man overboard maneuvers, *Sail,* Dec 1989.
76. *Report of the evaluation of a water purifier from Recovery Engineering,* Baltimore, Md, 1991, Johns Hopkins University School of Hygiene and Public Health Division of Disease Control.

77. Reverse osmosis: slow, but effective, *Canadian Consumer,* Nos 7 & 8, 1990.
78. Robertson D: *Survive the savage sea,* New York, 1973, Praeger.
79. Rousmaniere J: Staying on board, *Cruising World,* Dec 1989.
80. Seldes G, editor: *The great thoughts,* New York, 1985, Ballantine Books.
81. Sleeper JB: Advanced diving. II. Drysuit diving materials and undergarments, *Skin Diver,* Dec 1992.
82. Smith M: Personal safety, *Yachting,* July 1989.
83. Smith M: Anatomy of a life raft, *Yachting,* 1992.
84. Stapleton S: Abandon ship, *Motor Boating & Sailing,* Dec 1988.
85. Stapleton S: Radio talk, *Motor Boating & Sailing,* May 1988.
86. Stapleton S: One couple survives 66 days on a raft, *Motor Boating & Sailing,* Nov 1989.
87. Stapleton S: What to grab when your boat sinks, *Motor Boating & Sailing,* Nov 1989.
88. Stapleton S: Abandon ship: suggested contents for an abandon ship bag, *Motor Boating & Sailing,* March 1990.
89. Stapleton S: Abandon ship: what to do when faced with the ultimate marine emergency, *Motor Boating & Sailing,* March 1990.
90. Stapleton S: How to be rescued by helicopter, *Motor Boating & Sailing,* March 1990.
91. *Stations and the maritime services,* Pub No 47, Code of Federal Regulations Part 80, Washington, DC, US Government Printing Office.
92. Sutphen H: Maintenance required: autoinflatable life vests provide plenty of buoyance, but need annual attention, *Ocean Voyager,* 1992.
93. Sutphen H: Immersion suits, *Ocean Voyager,* 1992.
94. *U.S. Coast Guard Auxiliary courtesy examiner manual,* COMDTINST M16796.2C, Washington, DC, 1985, US Dept of Transportation.
95. USCG Regulation, Title 33, Chapter 1, Part 175, Subpart B.
96. Vann J: Sailing with young children: boat proofing your toddler, *Sail,* Dec 1989.
97. Waters JM: *A guide to small boat emergencies,* Annapolis, Md, 1993, Naval Institute Press.
98. *Webster's new collegiate dictionary,* Springfield, Mass, 1959, G & C Merriam.
99. West G: Communication, *Motor Boating & Sailing,* Nov 1991.
100. Williams M: Fire prevention framework, *Cruising World,* Dec 1990.
101. Williams W: Safety equipment, *Cruising World,* Dec 1987.
102. Williams W: Fluid and flotation, *Cruising World,* Dec 1989.
103. Williams W: The life vests of the future, *Ocean Navigator,* March/April 1990.
104. Willis W: *The epic voyage of the "Seven Little Sisters,"* London, 1956, Hutchinson.
105. Woolridge J: Fire! *Motor Boating & Sailing,* April 1990.

51 INJURIES FROM NONVENOMOUS AQUATIC ANIMALS

Paul S. Auerbach
Bruce W. Halstead

The expanses of ocean and fresh water that cover the earth are the greatest wilderness. Seventy-one percent of the earth's surface is composed of ocean, the volume of which exceeds 325 million cubic miles. Within the undersea realm exists four fifths of all living organisms. Some aquatic microorganisms, plants, and animals can be hazardous to humans. This chapter and the next four classify and describe these unpleasant interactions between aquatic organisms and people.

The opportunity for direct encounters with aquatic organisms is also increasing with the number of recreational, industrial, scientific, and military oceanic and riverine activities. The underwater recovery of historical artifacts and treasures will accelerate in the 1990s. As fishermen harvest their catches, they handle animals that bite and sting in self-defense.

The year 2000 will see approximately 80% of the world's population living in coastal regions. It is estimated that 127 million U.S. citizens will live along the coasts by the year 2010. A significant proportion of this population will be directly involved as entrants into the aquatic world. Millions of sport scuba enthusiasts will venture into the undersea realm in the next decade. It is imperative that clinicians be familiar with hazards unique to the aquatic environment. Many diagnostic and therapeutic myths have been disproved through the development of the science of medicine since ancient mariners and shamanistic healers first proposed remedies for marine-acquired injuries, envenomation, and poisonings.

Although noxious marine organisms are concentrated predominantly in warm temperate and tropical seas, particularly in the Indo-Pacific region, hazardous animals may be found as far north as 50° latitude. The increasing number of saltwater aquaria in private homes and public settings, the intercontinental shipping of seafood, and the accessibility of air travel for the sport diver create additional risks. In pursuit of anatomic information that can elucidate the biology and ecology of fish, evolution, cellular physiology, and aquatic models of human disease, nuclear radiologists have performed in vivo nuclear magnetic resonance imaging and spectroscopy of anesthetized (tricaine methsulfonate [MS222]) aquatic organisms.[12]

As evidenced by increasing attendance at major urban aquaria and multimedia presentations, public fascination with marine fauna continues to increase.

Like the rainforest, the ocean depths have the potential to reveal virtually limitless active pharmaceutical agents. For example, genetically engineered reproduction of the adhesive protein of the marine mussel *Mytilus edulis* has created a tissue adhesive agent that may prove superior to a commonly used cyanoacrylic compound. Toxins isolated from ascidians (tunicates or sea squirts) include cyclic peptides, one of which (didemnin B) is undergoing clinical trials for cancer chemotherapy; it is also a potent immunosuppressive agent.[141]

For all the wonders of the deep, jeopardy still exists. The ubiquity of hazardous creatures and their propensity to appear at inopportune times make it imperative to be aware of them, to respect their territorial rights, and to avoid needless unpleasant contact with them.

Divisions and Definitions

Dangerous aquatic animals are divided into four groups: (1) those that bite, rip, puncture, or shock without envenomation; (2) those that sting (those that envenom); (3) those that are poisonous on ingestion; and (4) those that induce allergy. Aquatic plants and dermatology are discussed in Chapter 54. Freshwater hazards, which are in large measure parasitologic, are discussed in Chapters 43 and 49.

In Defense of the Fish

A word must be written in defense of the fish. As in all of nature (except for humans), indiscriminate aggression is rarely involved when injuries are inflicted by aquatic animals.[129] Most injuries result from gestures of warning or self-defense; with the exception of some sharks, few aquatic creatures attack humans without provocation.[119] Attacks are made in defense of young, in territorial disputes, or to procure food. It is hoped that better understanding will foster caution when dealing with potentially injurious aquatic creatures.

General Principles of First Aid

The physician must adhere to fundamental principles of medical rescue. While every injury or envenomation has a unique clinical presentation, the cornerstone of therapy is immediate attention to the airway, respiration, and circulation. Along with specific interventions directed against a particular venom or poison, the rescuer must simultaneously be certain that the victim maintains a patent airway, breathes spontaneously or with assistance, and is supported by an adequate blood pressure. Because marine attacks and envenomations may affect a scuba diver, the rescuer should anticipate near drowning (see Chapter 48), immersion hypothermia (see Chapter 4), and decompression sickness or arterial air embolism (see Chapter 47). Any victim rescued from the ocean should be thoroughly examined for external signs of a bite, puncture, or sting.

Wound Management

Whether the injury is a bite, abrasion, or puncture, meticulous attention to basic wound management is necessary to minimize posttraumatic infection.

WOUND IRRIGATION

All wounds acquired in the natural aquatic environment should be vigorously irrigated with sterile diluent, preferably a normal saline (0.9% sodium chloride) solution. Seawater is not a favorable irrigant because it carries a hypothetical infection risk. Sterile water or hypotonic saline is acceptable. Tap water appears to be a suitable irrigant and should be used when the alternative is delaying irrigation.[1] Irrigation should be performed before and after debridement to maximize the benefits. A 19-gauge needle or 18-gauge plastic intravenous catheter attached to a syringe that delivers a pressure of 10 to 20 PSI will dislodge most bacteria without forcing irrigation fluid into tissue along the wound edges or deeper along dissecting tissue planes.[36,128] Convenient ring-handle syringes with blunt irrigation tips and intravenous (IV) tubing that connects to standard IV bags are available. At least 100 to 250 ml of irrigant should be flushed through each wound. If a laceration is from a stingray, proteinaceous heat-labile venom may be present in the wound. In such a case the irrigant should be warmed to 113° F (45° C).

An antiseptic may be added to the irrigant if the wound appears to be highly contaminated. Povidone-iodine solution in a concentration of 1% to 5% may be used with a contact time of 1 to 5 minutes.[48,94,137] When antiseptic irrigation is completed, the wound should be thoroughly irrigated with normal saline to minimize tissue toxicity. Antiseptics that are particularly harmful to tissues include full-strength hydrogen peroxide, povidone-iodine scrub solution, hexachlorophene detergent, and silver nitrate.[18,38,98]

Scrubbing should be employed to remove debris that cannot be irrigated from the wound. Sharp surgical debridement is preferable to sponge scrubbing, which may increase infection rates, particularly when applied with harsh antiseptic solutions. Poloxamer 188 (Pluronic F-68) is a nontoxic nonionic surfactant skin wound cleanser that may be used to irrigate or scrub wounds. It does not have any significant advantage over traditional sterile saline irrigation.

WOUND DEBRIDEMENT

Debridement is more effective than irrigation at removing bacteria and debris. Crushed or devitalized tissue should be removed with sharp dissection to provide clean wound edges and encourage brisk healing with minimal infection risk. The limitations are those imposed by anatomy, specifically skin tautness or the presence of vital structures. Anesthesia of wound edges may be attained by regional nerve block or local infiltration with lidocaine, which do not damage local tissue defenses. A topical anesthetic mixture of tetracaine, epinephrine, and cocaine may be less desirable because of the vasoconstrictive effect of epinephrine and theoretical infection-potentiating effects.[37] Wound exploration, debridement, and repair should be undertaken in the appropriate sterile environment. It is inappropriate to explore complex wounds in the emergency department. Whenever necessary, operating loupes should be used to inspect the wound for residual foreign material, such as sand, seaweed, teeth, spine fragments, or integumentary sheath shards. Standard radiographs, static soft tissue techniques, or fluoroscopy may be used preoperatively or perioperatively to localize spines or teeth.

WOUND CLOSURE

The decision to close a wound weighs the cosmetic result against the risk of infection. The incidence of infection is high in wounds acquired in water because such wounds may be contaminated with venom, potentially virulent microorganisms, or both; because early adequate irrigation and debridement are often unavailable; and because definitive care is often delayed. Tight wound closure restricts drainage and promotes bacterial proliferation. Wounds at high risk in this regard include those on the hands, wrists, or feet; punctures and crush injuries; wounds into areas of fat with poor vascularity; and wounds to victims who are immunosuppressed. Whenever possible, the use of sutures to close dead space in contaminated wounds should be avoided because the absorbable sutures act as foreign bodies.

PROPHYLAXIS AGAINST TETANUS

Any wound that disrupts the skin can become contaminated with *Clostridium tetani*. Anaerobic bacteria, predominantly of the genus *Clostridium,* have been isolated in shark tissue and as part of the oral flora of alligators and crocodiles.[145] Proper immunization with tetanus toxoid virtually eliminates the risk of disease.[140] However, while it was previously accepted that the protective level of toxin-neutralizing antibody is 0.01 antitoxin unit/ml, it appears that clinical tetanus can develop despite an antibody level many times that amount.[97] Therefore it is imperative to provide an early and adequate booster injection. If the victim is over 50 years of age, is from an underdeveloped country, or cannot provide a definite history of tetanus immunization, prophylaxis should be provided according to the following scheme in Table 51-1.

Table 51-1 Prophylaxis Against Tetanus

History of Tetanus Immunization (Doses)	Clean Minor Wound		Other Wound	
	T/Td	**TIG**	**T/Td**	**TIG**
Uncertain	Yes	No	Yes	Yes
0-1	Yes	No	Yes	Yes
2	Yes	No	Yes	No*
3 or more	No†	No	No†	No

Modified from Immunization Practices Advisory Committee: *MMWR* 34:405, 1985.

T, Tetanus toxoid (0.5 ml); *Td,* tetanus/diphtheria toxoids (0.5 ml); *TIG,* tetanus immune globulin (250 to 500 units).

*Unless the wound is older than 24 hours.

†Unless it has been 10 or more years since the last dose.

Bacteriology of the Aquatic Environment

Wounds acquired in the aquatic environment are soaked in natural source water and sometimes contaminated with sediment. Penetration of the skin by the spines or teeth of animals, the razor-sharp edges of coral or shellfish, or the blades of a boat propeller may inoculate pathogenic organisms into a wound. Sports activities, such as surfing, snorkeling, and diving, lead to ubiquitous abrasions and minor lacerations that heal slowly and with marked soft tissue inflammation. Wounds acquired in the aquatic environment tend to become infected and may be refractory to standard antimicrobial therapy. Not infrequently, indolent or extensive soft tissue infections develop in the normal or immunocompromised host.[6,103] A clinician faced with a serious infection after an aquatic injury frequently needs to administer antibiotics to a patient before definitive laboratory identification of pathogenic organisms.

MARINE BACTERIOLOGY

Marine Environment

Ocean water provides a saline milieu for microbes. The salt dissolved in ocean water (3.2% to 3.5%) is 78% sodium chloride (sodium 10.752 g/kg; chlorine 19.345 g/kg). Other constituents include sulfate (2.791 g/kg), magnesium (1.295 g/kg), potassium (0.390 g/kg), bicarbonate (0.145 g/kg), bromine (0.066 g/kg), boric acid (0.027 g/kg), strontium (0.013 g/kg), and fluorine (0.0013 g/kg). The temperature of the surface waters varies with latitude, currents, and season. Tropical waters are warmer and maintain a more constant temperature than temperate and subtropical waters, which are subject to substantial meteorologic variation. Shallow and turbulent coastal waters are generally richer in nutrients than the open ocean, which is reflected in the diversity of life that can be identified in the intertidal zone. Although the greatest number and diversity of bacteria are found near the ocean surface, diverse bacteria and fungi are found in marine silts, sediments, and sand. In ocean waters having marked differences in density, the greatest concentration of bacteria is noted at the thermocline, where changes in both temperature and salinity are usually found.[107] This effect is lost in active coastal waters, where the constant admixture creates an even distribution of sediments, microbes, salinity, and temperature.[93] Microbes are most abundant in areas that have the greatest numbers of higher life-forms. Marine bacteria are generally halophilic, heterotrophic, motile, and gram-negative rod forms. Growth requirements vary from species to species with respect to use of organic carbon and nitrogen sources, requirements for various amino acids, vitamins and cofactors, sodium, potassium, magnesium, phosphate, sulphate, chloride, and calcium.[78] Most marine bacteria are facultative anaerobes, which can thrive in oxygen-rich environments. Few are obligatory aerobes or anaerobes. Some marine bacteria are highly proteolytic, and the proportion of proteolytic bacteria seems to be greater in the oceans than on land or in freshwater habitats.[107]

Diversity of Organisms

Although some scientists have questioned the existence of specific marine bacteria, it is now accepted that unique conditions of nutrient and inorganic mineral supply, temperature, and pressure have allowed the evolution of unique, highly adapted marine microbes.[78,146,147] In addition, numerous other bacteria, microalgae, protozoa, fungi, yeasts, and viruses have been identified in or cultured from seawater, marine sediments, marine life, and marine-acquired or marine-contaminated infected wounds or body fluids of septic victims.* In their natural environment the bacteria presumably serve to scavenge and transform organic matter in the intricate cycles of the food and growth chains. Some of these bacteria are listed in Box 51-1.

For practical purposes, most marine isolates are heterotrophic (require exogenous carbon and nitrogen-containing organic supplements) and motile gram-negative rods.[78] Previous opinions that enteric pathogens (associated with the intestines of warm-blooded animals) deposited into marine environments ultimately succumbed to sedimentation, predation, parasitism, sunlight, temperature, osmotic stress, toxic chemicals, or high salt concentration may be untrue.[46] Pathogens may accumulate in surface water in association with lipoidal particulates, from which they are rapidly dispersed toward shore by wave and wind activity. In addition, dredging, storms, upwellings, and other benthic disturbances may churn enteric organisms into the path of wastewater nutrients. Enteric pathogenic bacteria have been isolated from sharks.[47]

Growth in Culture

Although plating on standard clinical laboratory media may detect only 0.1% to 1% of the total number of microorganisms found in seawater or marine sediment, most marine bacteria that are pathogenic to humans can be readily recovered on standard media.[78] While pathogenic *Vibrio* species can grow on conventional blood agar media, other marine bacteria may require saline-supplemented media and incubation at 25° C instead of the standard 35° to 37° C. In culture, marine bacteria may grow at a slower rate than terrestrial bacteria, which delays identification. Pleomorphism in culture may be attributed to adaptation to small concentrations of nutrients in seawater. Most organisms require sodium, potassium, magnesium, phosphate, and sulfate for growth; a few require calcium or chloride.

Thiosulfate–citrate–bile salts–sucrose agar is selective and recommended for the detection of marine *Vibrio* organisms.[76] A useful identification scheme for pathogenic *Vibrio* species is found in the chapter on *Vibrio* in the most recent edition of the American Society for Microbiology's *Manual of Clinical Microbiology*. Mycobacteria must be cultured in media such as Middlebrook 7H10 or 7H11 agar or Lowenstein-Jensen medium; fungi require a medium such as Sabouraud dextrose or brain-heart infusion/Sabhi agar. Antibiotic susceptibility testing can be performed using established procedures, except for the addition of NaCl 2.3% to the Mueller-Hinton broth or agar used for disk diffusion.[4,9,11,64] Commercial test kits such as API-20E (Analytab Products) may not accurately identify marine organisms. In the setting of wound infection or sepsis, the clinician should alert the laboratory that a marine-acquired organism may be present.[74] If a laboratory does not have the time or resources to perform a complete identification, the bacteria may be sent to a reference laboratory.[2] Marine bacteria are kept in the American Type Culture Collection. Because of the diversity of species, complete agreement has not yet been reached on comprehensive taxonomic criteria for identification.[60,101]

Antibiotic Therapy

The objectives for the management of infections from marine microorganisms are to recognize the clinical condition, culture the organism, and provide antimicrobial therapy.[122] Management of marine-acquired infections should include therapy against *Vibrio* species. Third-generation cephalosporins (cefoperazone, cefotaxime, or ceftazidime) provide excellent coverage; first- and second-generation products (cefazolin, cephalothin, cephapirin, cefamandole, cefonicid, ceforanide, or cefoxitin) appear to be less effective in vitro. Oral cultures taken from two captive moray eels at the Chicago Shedd Aquarium demonstrated *V. fluvialis, V. damsela, V. vulnificus,* and *Pseudomonas putrefaciens* sensitive to cefuroxime, ciprofloxacin, tetracycline, and trimethoprim-sulfamethoxazole.[41] Imipenem-cilastatin is efficacious against gram-negative marine bacteria, as are trimethoprim-sulfamethoxazole, tetracycline, azlocillin, mezlocillin, and piperacillin. Gentamicin, tobramycin, and chloramphenicol have tested favorably against *P. putrefaciens* and *Vibrio* strains.[20] Nonfermentative bacteria (such as *Alteromonas, Pseudomonas,* and *Deleya* species) appear to be sensitive to most antibiotics.

Quantitative wound culture has no advantage before the appearance of a wound infection. Pending a prospective

*References 4, 6, 13, 14, 16, 17, 22, 29, 40, 43, 45, 52, 54, 60, 61, 63, 65-69, 75, 82, 92, 96, 99, 102, 103, 106, 112, 113, 115, 118, 120, 122, 125, 132, 133, 138, 144, 148.

BOX 51-1

BACTERIA AND FUNGUS ISOLATED FROM MARINE WATER, SEDIMENTS, MARINE ANIMALS, AND MARINE-ACQUIRED WOUNDS

Achromobacter
Acinetobacter lwoffi
Actinomyces
Aerobacter aerogenes
Aeromonas hydrophila
Aeromonas sobia
Alcaligenes faecalis
Alteromonas espejiana
Alteromonas haloplanktis
Alteromonas macleodii
Alteromonas undina
Bacillus cereus
Bacillus subtilis
Bacteroides fragilis
Branhamella catarrhalis
Chromobacterium violaceum
Citrobacter
Clostridium botulinum
Clostridium perfringens
Clostridium tetani
Corynebacterium
Deleya venustus
Edwardsiella tarda
Enterobacter aerogenes
Erysipelothrix rhusiopathiae
Escherichia coli
Flavobacterium
Fusarium solani
Klebsiella pneumoniae
Legionella pneumophila
Micrococcus sedentarius
Micrococcus tegragenus
Mycobacterium marinum
Neisseria catarrhalis
Pasteurella multocida
Propionibacterium acnes
Proteus mirabilis
Proteus vulgaris
Providencia stuartii
Pseudomonas aeruginosa
Pseudomonas beijerinckii
Pseudomonas cepacia
Pseudomonas iridescens
Pseudomonas maltophila
Pseudomonas marinoglutinosa
Pseudomonas marinum
Pseudomonas nigrifaciens
Pseudomonas putrefaciens
Pseudomonas stutzeri
Salmonella enteritidis
Serratia
Staphylococcus aureus
Staphylococcus citreus
Staphylococcus epidermidis
Streptococcus
Vibrio alginolyticus
Vibrio carchariae
Vibrio cholerae
Vibrio damsela
Vibrio fluvialis
Vibrio furnissii
Vibrio harveyi
Vibrio hollisae
Vibrio parahaemolyticus
Vibrio pelagius II
Vibrio mimicus
Vibrio splendidus I
Vibrio vulnificus

evaluation of prophylactic antibiotics in the management of marine wounds, the following recommendations are based on the indolent nature and malignant potential of soft tissue infections caused by *Vibrio* species:

1. Minor abrasions or lacerations (such as coral cuts or superficial sea urchin puncture wounds) do not require prophylactic antibiotics in the normal host. Persons who are chronically ill (as with diabetes, hemophilia, or thalassemia) or immunologically impaired (as with leukemia or AIDS, or undergoing chemotherapy or prolonged corticosteroid therapy), or who suffer from serious liver disease (such as hepatitis, cirrhosis, or hemochromatosis), particularly those with elevated serum iron levels, should be placed immediately after the injury on a regimen of oral ciprofloxacin, trimethoprim-sulfamethoxazole, or tetracycline because these persons appear to have an increased risk of serious wound infection and bacteremia.* Preliminary experience suggests that cefuroxime may be a useful alternative.[41] Penicillin, ampicillin, and erythromycin are not acceptable alternatives.[87,89] Norfloxacin may be less efficacious against certain vibrios.[88,104] Other quinolones (ofloxacin, enoxacin, pefloxacin, fleroxacin, lomefloxacin) have not been extensively tested against

*References 13, 17, 22, 42, 56, 62, 69, 70, 84, 86, 110, 124.

Vibrio; they may be useful alternatives, but this awaits definitive evaluation. The appearance of an infection indicates the need for prompt debridement and antibiotic therapy. If an infection develops, antibiotic coverage should be chosen that will also be efficacious against *Staphylococcus* and *Streptococcus* because these are still the most common perpetrators of infection. In general, the fluoroquinolones, which are particularly effective for treating gram-negative bacillary infections, may become less and less useful against resistant staphylococci.[136]

2. Serious injuries from an infection perspective include large lacerations, serious burns, deep puncture wounds, or a retained foreign body.[138] Examples are shark or barracuda bites, stingray spine wounds, deep sea urchin punctures, scorpaenid spine envenomations that enter a joint space, and full-thickness coral cuts. If the victim requires hospitalization and surgery for standard wound management, recommended antibiotics include imipenem-cilastatin, gentamicin, tobramycin, amikacin, trimethoprim-sulfamethoxazole, cefoperazone, cefotaxime, ceftazidime, and chloramphenicol. The clinician should note that patients who simultaneously receive imipenem or ciprofloxacin and theophylline may have an increased tendency to seizures.[116]

   If the victim is managed as an outpatient, the drugs of choice to cover *Vibrio* are ciprofloxacin, trimethoprim-sulfamethoxazole, or tetracycline. Cefuroxime is an alternative. It is a clinical decision whether oral therapy should be preceded by a single intravenous or intramuscular loading dose of a similar or different antibiotic, commonly an aminoglycoside.
3. Infected wounds should be cultured for aerobes and anaerobes. Pending culture and sensitivity results, the patient should be managed with antibiotics as described previously. In a person who has been wounded in a marine environment and has rapidly progressive cellulitis or myositis, *Vibrio parahaemolyticus* or *V. vulnificus* infection should be suspected, particularly in the presence of chronic liver disease.* (*Vibrio* infections are discussed in Chapter 53.) If a wound infection is minor and has the appearance of a classic erysipeloid reaction *(Erysipelothrix rhusiopathiae),* penicillin, cephalexin, or erythromycin should be administered.

FRESHWATER BACTERIOLOGY

Diversity of Organisms

Although it has not been as extensively studied as the marine environment, the natural freshwater environment of ponds, lakes, streams, rivers, lagoons, harbors, estuaries, and artificial bodies of water is probably as hazardous as the ocean from a microbiologic standpoint. Water-skiing accidents, propeller wounds, fishhook punctures, lacerations from broken glass and sharp rocks, fish fin or catfish stings, and crush injuries during white-water expeditions are increasingly commonplace. A large number of bacteria have been identified in water, sediments, animals, and wounds.[3] In fringe areas of the ocean that carry brackish water (NaCl content below 3%), marine bacteria, salt-tolerant freshwater bacteria, and brackish-specific bacteria such as *Agrobacterium sanguineum* are noted. The combined effects of human and animal traffic and waste disposal increase the risk for coliform contamination.[53] In Great Britain, antibiotic-resistant *Escherichia coli* have been documented in rivers and coastal waters.[125] Coxsackievirus A_{16} has been isolated from children stricken ill after bathing in contaminated lake water.[35] Of particular note is the presence of virulent species, such as *Chromobacterium violaceum, Vibrio parahaemolyticus,* and *Aeromonas hydrophila,* associated with serious and indolent wound infections.[83,139] The last can be cultured from natural bodies of water, as well as from the mouths of "domesticated" aquarium fish, such as the piranha.[108] Biologic control agents, such as guppy fish bred in wells to control mosquito proliferation, can carry bacterial pathogens such as *Pseudomonas.*[26]

One investigation sampled water, inanimate objects, and animals from freshwater environments in California, Tennessee, and Florida.[3] Bacteria isolated were predominantly gram negative and included *Aeromonas hydrophila, Flavobacterium breve, Pseudomonas* species, *Vibrio parahaemolyticus, Serratia* species, *Enterobacter* species, *Plesiomonas shigelloides, Bacillus* species, *Acinetobacter calcoaceticus,* and *Alcaligenes denitrificans.*

Antibiotic Therapy

Management of fresh water–acquired infections should include therapy against *Aeromonas* species. First-generation cephalosporins provide inadequate coverage against growth of freshwater bacteria. Third-generation cephalosporins provide excellent coverage, while second-generation products are less effective. Ciprofloxacin, imipenem, ceftazidime, gentamicin, and trimethoprim-sulfamethoxazole are superb antibiotics against gram-negative microorganisms.Trimethoprim alone may be inefficacious, as is ampicillin.

Whether to begin antimicrobial therapy before establishment of a wound infection is controversial. Pending a prospective evaluation of prophylactic antibiotics in fresh water–acquired wounds, the following recommendations are based on the potentially serious nature of soft tissue infections caused by *Aeromonas* species:

1. Minor abrasions or lacerations do not require the administration of prophylactic antibiotics in the normal host. Persons who have chronic illness, immunologic impairment, or serious liver disease, particularly those with elevated serum iron levels, should be

*References 29, 42, 69, 84, 109, 131.

placed immediately on a regimen of oral ciprofloxacin or trimethoprim-sulfamethoxazole (first choice) or tetracycline (second choice), because these persons appear to have an increased risk of serious wound infection and bacteremia. Doxycycline may be an acceptable alternative to tetracycline. Penicillin, ampicillin, erythromycin, and trimethoprim do not appear to be acceptable alternatives.[111] The appearance of an infection indicates the need for prompt debridement and antibiotic therapy. If an infection develops, antibiotic coverage that will be efficacious against *Staphylococcus* and *Streptococcus* should be chosen, since these are still the most common perpetrators of infection.

2. If the victim requires surgery and hospitalization for wound management, recommended antibiotics include ciprofloxacin, imipenem-cilastatin, ceftazidime, gentamicin, or trimethoprim-sulfamethoxazole. If the victim is to be managed as an outpatient, the oral drug of choice is trimethoprim-sulfamethoxazole or tetracycline. It is a clinical decision whether oral therapy should be preceded by a single intravenous or intramuscular loading dose of a similar or different antibiotic, commonly an aminoglycoside.
3. Infected wounds should be cultured. Pending culture and sensitivity results, the patient should be managed with antibiotics as outlined previously. If fever or rapidly progressive cellulitis characterized by bullae and large areas of necrosis develops, *Aeromonas hydrophila* infection should be suspected. Milder *Aeromonas* infections may have the appearance of streptococcal cellulitis.[67]

Sharks

Assume unidentified fish are sharks. Not all sharks look like sharks, and some fish which are not sharks sometimes act like sharks . . .
Do not bleed. Experience shows that bleeding prompts an even more aggressive attack. Admittedly, it is difficult not to bleed when injured. Indeed, at first this may seem impossible. Diligent practice, however, will permit the inexperienced swimmer to sustain a serious laceration without bleeding and without even exhibiting any loss of composure . . .
The control of bleeding has a positive protective element for the swimmer. This also has a profound effect on sharks. They begin questioning their own potency or, alternatively, believe the swimmer to have supernatural powers . . .
It is scarcely necessary to state that it is unethical for a swimmer under attack by a group of sharks to counter the attack by diverting them to another swimmer.

Voltaire Cousteau[32,58]

Your chances of being bitten are infinitesimally small. If you are worried about your life span, stop smoking, don't drive cars, never walk across a street, and do not fly in an aircraft.

G.D. Campbell and E.D. Smith[21]

Humor, myth, and folklore surround sharks, the most sinister of all sea creatures. These occasionally savage and highly feared animals are the subject of many behavioral investigations, but until more reproducible data are available, some degree of mystery will remain. Shark attacks on humans have always held enormous fascination for scientists, adventurers, and clinicians. The International Shark Attack File, initiated by Perry W. Gilbert and Leonard P. Schultz in 1958 for the American Institute of Biological Sciences and the Office of Naval Research and maintained at the Mote Marine Laboratory in Sarasota, Florida, remains the most authoritative collection of analyzed data available, containing a series of 1652 case histories. H. David Baldridge prepared a special technical report, *Shark Attack Against Man,* for the U.S. Navy Bureau of Medicine and Surgery in 1973.

Although dreaded, sharks are among the most graceful and magnificent denizens of the deep. Sharks may be found in oceans, tropical rivers, and lakes. The bull shark is a frequent river inhabitant.[31] Sharks range in size from 10 to 15 cm *(Squaliolus laticaudus)* to over 15 m and more than 18,144 kg (the whale shark *Rhiniodon typus,* fortunately a plankton feeder).

The world's shark population is in danger from overfishing (more than 100 million animals per year, or 10 million sharks for each human shark-related fatality), in large part for the heinous practice of "finning," in which a shark is captured, its fins are sliced off, and then it is returned to the water.[79] The fins are sold for the extraction of putative aphrodisiacs or to make shark-fin soup. Shark flesh is a major food source worldwide, particularly since, to date, sharks do not appear to carry ciguatera toxin except in the liver. Innumerable animals are ground into fertilizer. Although at least 7150 tons of sharks were harvested commercially in the United States in 1989, more than 90% of captured sharks are discarded. In Tahiti and other Polynesian locations, sharks are mercilessly slaughtered to acquire their teeth for jewelry manufacture. In 1991 the South African government declared the great white shark a protected species within 200 miles of its coast.

LIFE AND HABITS

Sharks have inhabited the oceans for at least 400 million years. They appeared on the planet during the Devonian period, approximately 200 million years before the dinosaurs. Ancestral sharks may have been enormous; *Carcharodon megalodon* ("Megalodon") probably grew to a length of more than 15 m, with teeth longer than 3.2 cm. This was a predator of astronomic proportions.

Approximately 32 of the at least 368 species of sharks have been implicated in the 50 to 100 shark attacks reported annually worldwide, and another 35 to 40 species are considered potentially dangerous. Six to 10 deaths from shark attacks are reported each year. The most frequently implicated offenders are the larger animals, such as the great white (Fig. 51-1), bull, tiger, and oceanic white tip sharks. Sporadic attackers include the gray reef, blue, mako, dusky, hammerhead, lemon, Ganges River, spinner, sand, nurse, blacktip, blue, bronze whaler, and ragged tooth sharks.[91] Tiger sharks were identified in a cluster of attacks around the Hawaiian Islands in the winter of 1993.

Sharks are carnivorous; many are apex predators. Their danger to humans results from the combination of size, aggression, and dentition. Some sharks, such as the giant whale shark (the largest fish at 50 feet in length and more than 40,000 pounds), eat plankton and use their teeth as filters. Even small sharks can be powerful and destructive. The white shark is responsible for more attacks than any other species, particularly in the waters of southern Australia, the east coast of South Africa, the middle Atlantic coast of North America, and the American Pacific coast north of Point Conception, California. In recent years an increase in attacks by the great white shark off the coast of northern California has led to the designation of a "red triangle" from Tomales Bay through the Farallon Islands down to Año Nuevo. This is a breeding area for elephant seals *(Mirounga angustirostris),* which yield 200-pound pups, perfect food for the immense predators.

The tiger *(Galeocerdo cuvieri)* (up to 18 feet and 2000 pounds) and bull *(Carcharinus leucas)* sharks are the next most dangerous with regard to attacks on humans. The great hammerhead *(Sphyrna mokarran)* has a reputation as a man-eater in equatorial waters. Scattered over its entire undersurface, the hammerhead has ampullae sensitive to electromagnetic fields, which in combination with its highly developed sense of smell may make it a superior predator (Fig. 51-2).

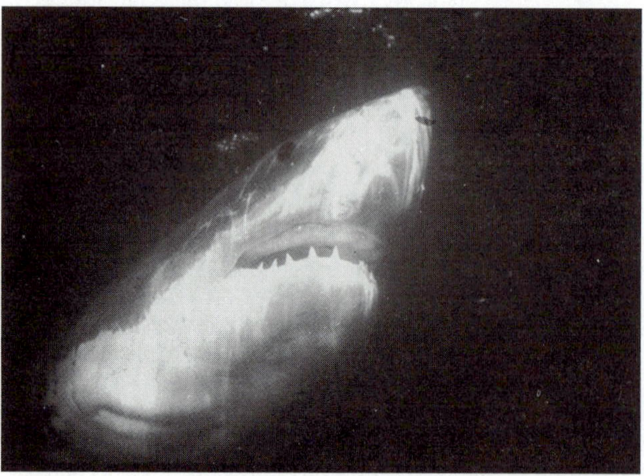

Fig. 51-1 Great white shark *(Carcharodon carcharias)*. This animal has been implicated in many attacks on humans. The most dangerous of sharks, it may attain a length of 25 feet and weigh 5500 pounds. (Photo by Carl Roessler.)

In an analysis of California attacks, Miller and Collier[85] attributed unprovoked attacks north of San Miguel Island to white sharks, while those south of this area involved members of the families Carcharhinidae (requiem sharks), Sphyrnidae (hammerheads), and possibly Squatinidae (angel sharks).

Sharks are members of the class Chondrichthyes, or cartilaginous fishes, which also includes rays and chimaeras, comprising approximately 780 species.[23] Unlike many bony fishes, sharks are not buoyant because they do not possess swim bladders for flotation. Thus sharks must stay in constant motion to keep from sinking and to drive water past the gills. Only a few bottom-dwelling species "rest." Although sharks are not highly intelligent, they are endowed with remarkable sensory systems. Their color vision is poor, but well compensated for by the acute perception of motion; the eye musculature is adapted for fixation with any body motion. The tapetum lucidum (responsible for the "eye shine" seen at night) is a series of reflecting plates containing silver guanine crystals in the choroidal layer behind the retina, which reflects light from a photoreceptor back along the same optical path to increase the sensitivity of the eye.[30] The eyes are protected by upper and lower eyelids and the nictitating membrane (except for the great white shark, which does not have the membrane; it rotates its eyes in the sockets to avoid injury). Keen olfactory and gustatory chemoreceptors permit taste and the recognition of blood, urine, or peritoneal fluid in the water (in some cases, 1 part blood in 100 million parts of water). Sharks are most sensitive to chemicals that are similar to those produced by normal prey, such as amino acids, amines, and small fatty acids.[91] Up to two thirds of the shark brain can be devoted to smell. The nostrils are the openings of the olfactory organs and do not take part in "breathing," which is accomplished by oxygen extraction from the water through a series of five to seven gill slits. Additionally, sharks possess skin chemoreceptors that detect chemical irritants. Perhaps the most important series of telereceptors is located about the head, within the ampullae of Lorenzini, which are extremely sensitive to electrical impulses. The lateral line system extending from the back along the side to the tail responds to sonic vibrations or pulsed low-frequency (20 to 60 cycles/sec) sound waves.[23] The lateral line organs are small holes along the sides of the shark's body that register motion in the water. These systems allow the shark to locate struggling fish, swimmers, or divers. Current research is directed at delineating the piscine ability to recognize electric fields.[114] For instance, the common smooth dogfish *(Mustelus canis)* can detect an electrical voltage gradient of 5/1000 of a microvolt. Sharks also have extremely sensitive hearing, which may detect prey under water from a distance of 3000 feet (914 m). Other research involves the isolation of antineoplastic agents from

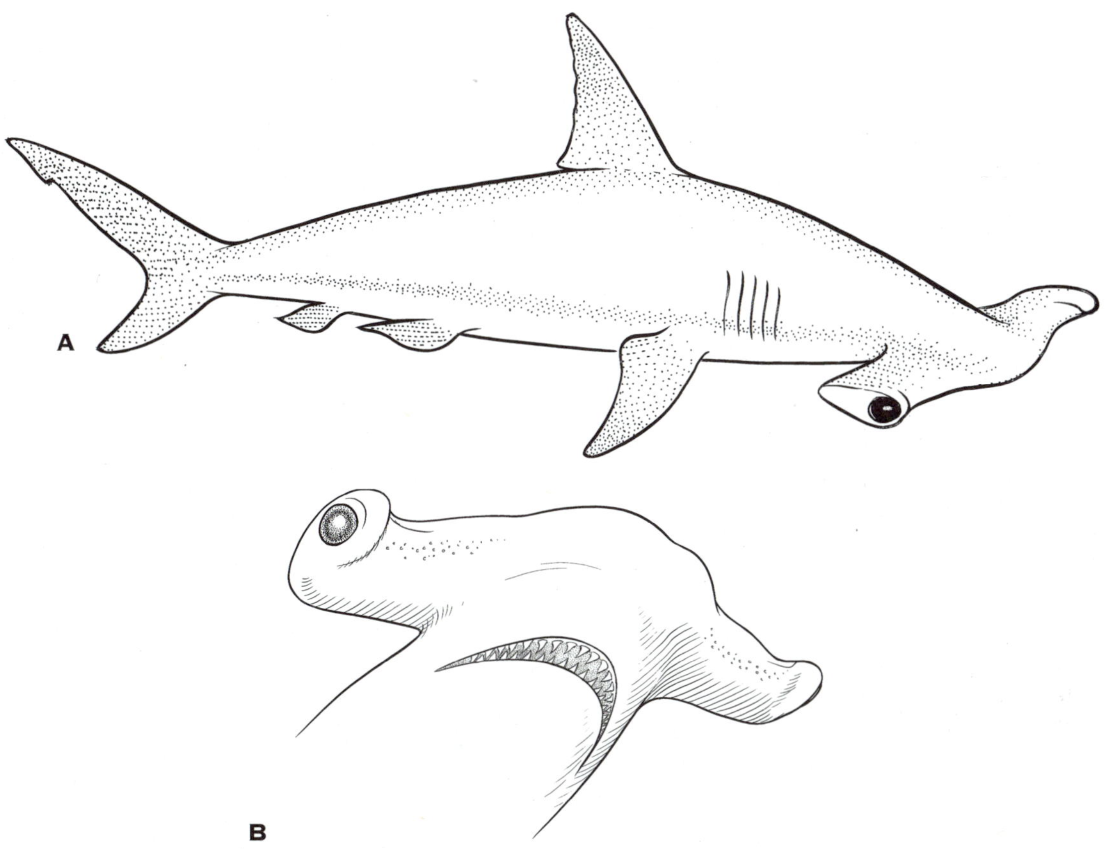

Fig. 51-2 Hammerhead shark. The positioning of the eyes is reputed to increase the peripheral vision of this apex predator.

shark cartilage, organs, and body fluids.[73,100] For instance, "sphyrnastatins" have been isolated from the hammerhead shark *Sphyrna lewini*.[100]

SHARK FEEDING AND ATTACK

As previously noted, sharks are well equipped in the sensory aspects of feeding.[90] They seem particularly able to avoid detection by potential prey, by virtue of coloration and a stealthy approach. Sharks feed in two basic patterns: (1) normal or subdued, with slow, purposeful group movements, and (2) frenzied or mob, as the result of an inciting event. The latter is precipitated by the sudden presentation of commotion or food/blood in the water. Frenzied behavior is enhanced by the proximity of other sharks in large numbers. In a frenzy, sharks become fearless and savage, snapping at anything and everything, including each other. After a shark decides to attack, it "postures," swimming erratically with elevated snout, arched back, pectoral fin depression, stiff lateral bending of the body, and rapid tail motion, in contrast to its normal sinuous and graceful swimming style.[59,90,95] In bursts of speed a shark can use its powerful caudal fin muscles and attain speeds in the water of 20 to 40 miles (32 to 64 km) per hour. As the Carchariniform shark prepares to strike, it rapidly opens and closes its jaws (up to three times each second), depresses the pectoral fins in a braking action, and elevates the head. During a bite the shark shakes its head and forebody in an effort to tear flesh from the victim. The shark may "bite and spit" to mortally wound the victim before eating it. Sharks swallow food whole without chewing it. It is difficult to postulate hunger as the sole attack motive, since more than 70% of victims are bitten only once or twice. "Hit and run" attacks are most common.[143] Usually the lower teeth are used first in feeding; solitary upper tooth slashes might indicate attacks unrelated to feeding. Up to 60% of wounds involve only the upper teeth.[91] At the moment of the strike the shark rolls its eyes back in the socket and uses the ampullae of Lorenzini to home in on the victim.

Sharks are selective feeders with clear dietary preferences. They commonly attack young, old, injured, or sick prey. Sea turtles, squid, penguins, seals, and stingrays are consumed in preference to humans. Sharks often eat other sharks.

It is difficult to generalize about shark attacks on humans. Current explanations suggest that frightened persons are more likely to be targets of aggression. This has been demonstrated in the case of the gray reef shark, *Carcharhinus amblyrhynchos*.[95] Aggression may be aggravated by purely anomalous behavior, the violation of courtship patterns, or territorial invasion.[8] More docile behavior tends to be the rule with other reef sharks, such as the silvertip *(Carcharinus albimarginatus),* blackfin *(C. melanopterus),* or whitetip *(Triaenodon obesus)* (Fig. 51-3).

The great white shark *(Carcharodon carcharias)* is a man-attacker but probably not a man-eater.[95] This statement reflects the observation that this highly feared animal (which has been captured at a length of 16 feet, 9 inches and a weight of 3450 pounds; it can probably attain a length of approximately 25 feet and a weight of 5500 pounds) usually releases its victim after a single bite, after it recognizes that a mouthful of neoprene, fiberglass, or lead weights is not normal dietary fare. This is small consolation to the unfortunate victim, who may have an entire hemithorax or limb removed (Fig. 51-4). The great white shark has not been closely observed and is thus the subject of much speculation about predation strategies.[81] Adults feed largely on pinnipeds; the bite-and-spit behavior is considered a means of avoiding injury from struggling prey. One theory is that a shark who largely consumes a human victim does so because the victim was solitary in the water.[39] Breath-hold diver behavior and the similarity of the silhouette of a contemporary surfboard to that of a surface seal may be responsible for attacks on humans. Most attacks on humans occur at the water's surface. One fatal attack in 1989 with two victims was on sea kayakers off the coast of southern California.

Shark attacks have occurred from the upper Adriatic Sea to southern New Zealand, with most between latitudes 46° N and 47° S (Fig. 51-5). The odds of being attacked by a shark along the North American coastline are approximately 1 in 5 million.[34] The danger is greater during the summer months (more persons in the water), in recreational areas, during late afternoon and nighttime feeding, and in murky warm (68° F or 20° C) water. White sharks frequently venture into colder water, and attacks have occurred in waters as cold as 50° F (10° C). The frequency of shark attacks off the northern California coastline appears to be increasing, particularly with respect to the great white shark. Contrary to the findings of worldwide shark attack analysis, attacks in northern California occur more frequently in clearer water at temperatures of less than 60° F (16° C).[85] Shark attacks in Hawaiian waters are relatively rare, with the exception of recent events.[142]

Although most attacks occur within 100 feet of shore, it is believed that the danger is greater further out, in deep channels or dropoffs. Because of their ability to detect contrasts, sharks have a predilection to attack bright, contrasting, or reflective objects. Movement is an added attraction to sharks, which have been known to bite surfboards, boats, and buoys. Recent shark attacks in northern California coastal waters involved swimmers on surfboards (black on white) who entered migratory elephant seal (shark food) habitats (Fig. 51-6).

Fig. 51-3 Adult whitetip shark. This species rarely if ever attacks humans unless cornered or otherwise provoked.

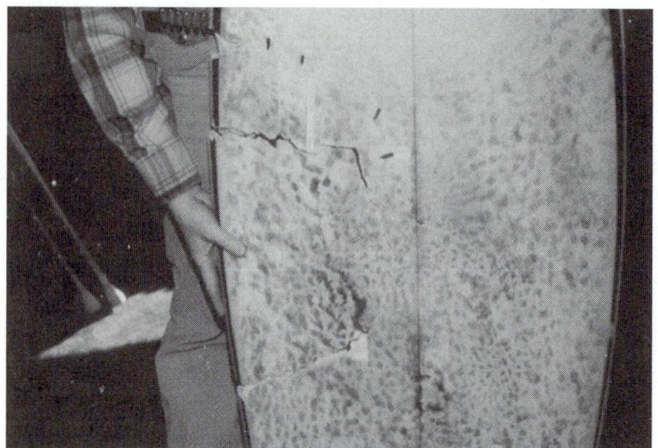

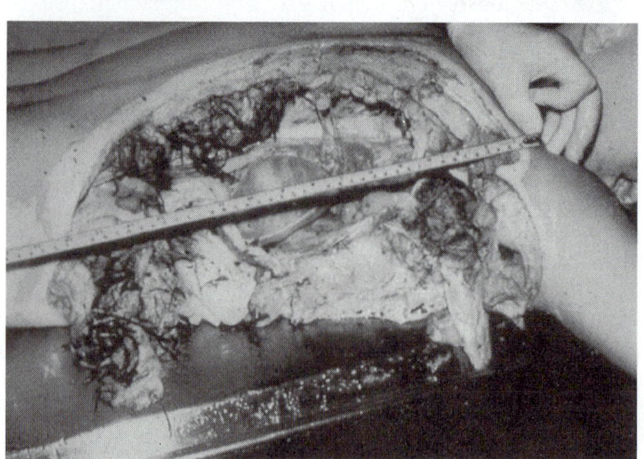

Fig. 51-4 Victim of great white shark attack. **A,** Damaged surfboard ridden by the victim. **B,** Massive thoracic injury after a single bite. It was estimated that the shark was 20 feet long. (Photos courtesy P. Crossman, Coroner's Division, Salinas, Calif.)

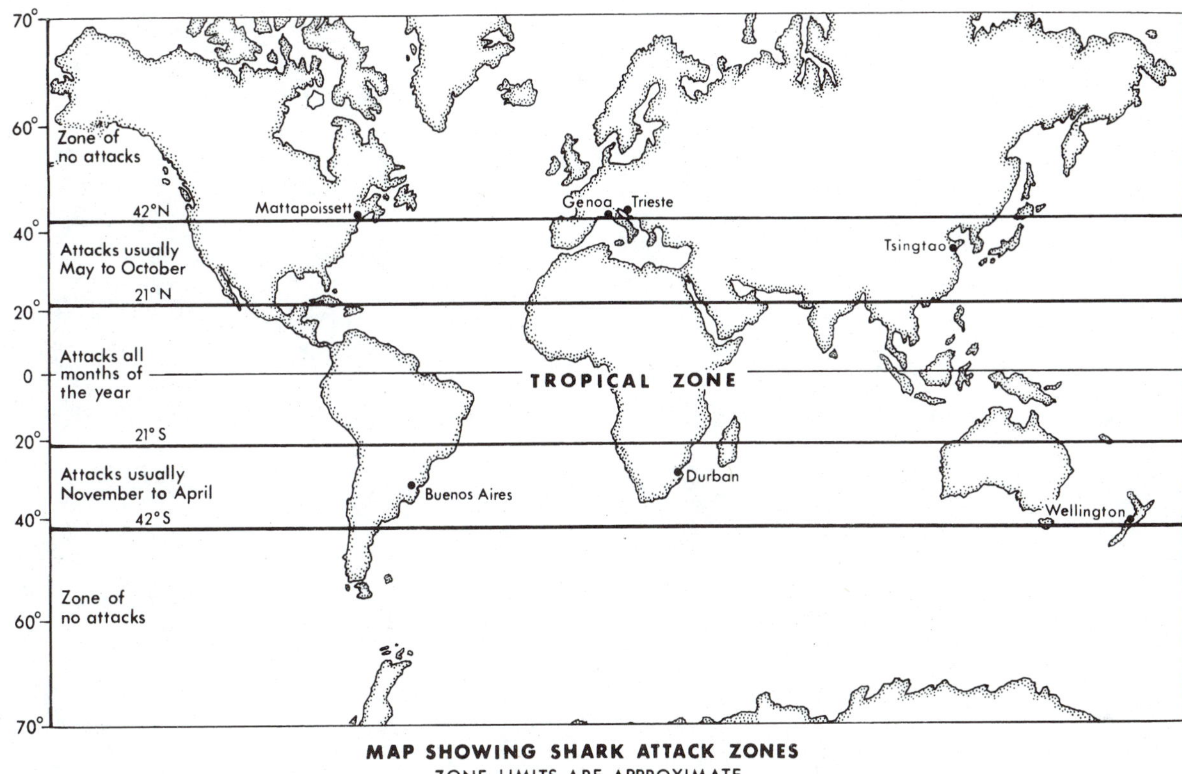

Fig. 51-5 Shark attack zones. (From Coppleson VM: *Med J Aust* 2:680, 1950.)

Most victims are attacked by single sharks, violently and without warning. In the majority of attacks the victim does not see the shark before the attack. The first contact may be a "bumping," or an attempt by the shark to wound the victim before the definitive strike. Severe skin abrasions from the shark skin (shagreen) placoid scales (denticles) are produced in this manner. These microscopic appendages have the same origin as teeth, with a pulp cavity, dentine, and vitreodentine ("enamel") covering.

CLINICAL ASPECTS

The jaws of the major carnivorous sharks are crescent shaped and contain up to five or six rows or series of razor-sharp ripsaw triangular teeth, which are replaced every few weeks by advancing inner rows. While normal tooth replacement takes 7 to 10 days, in some species a lost tooth can be replaced within 24 hours. The upper jaws generally have larger "cutting" teeth, while the sharp lower teeth are designed to fasten onto and hold prey during capture.[50] The teeth are cartilaginous, strengthened by the deposition of calcium phosphate crystals (apatite) in a protein matrix, all covered by an enameloid substance.[90] They are considered to be as hard as granite and as strong as steel. In a great white shark the largest serrated triangular teeth can grow to 2.5 inches. There are 26 upper and 24 lower teeth exposed in the front row. The height of the enamel of the largest tooth in the upper jaw is proportional to the animal's length, so a body length of up to 25 feet may be possible. The upper jaw is advanced forward and protruded to allow its participation in the biting action (Fig. 51-7). Incredibly, the biting force of some sharks is estimated at 18 tons per square inch.[19] Severe shark bites result acutely in massive tissue loss, hemorrhage, shock, and death. Even a smaller animal, such as a lemon shark, can bite with bone-crushing force.[51] The potential for destruction is unparalleled in the animal kingdom.

The human leg (or legs) is most frequently bitten, followed by the hands and arms, as the victim attempts to fend off the shark. Proximal femoral artery disruption carries a poor prognosis because of the torrential hemorrhage. Fractures are not uncommon, and broken ribs are often accompanied by intrathoracic, intraperitoneal, and retroperitoneal injuries. Because the victim is generally far from medical assistance, blood loss may be profound. The wounds have historically been fatal in 15% to 25% of attacks, with major causes of death listed as hemorrhage and drowning.[142] The advent of formal prehospital care and rapid response may diminish this somewhat.

TREATMENT

In most cases the immediate threat to life is hypovolemic shock. Thus it is occasionally necessary to compress wounds or manually to constrict arterial bleeding while the victim is

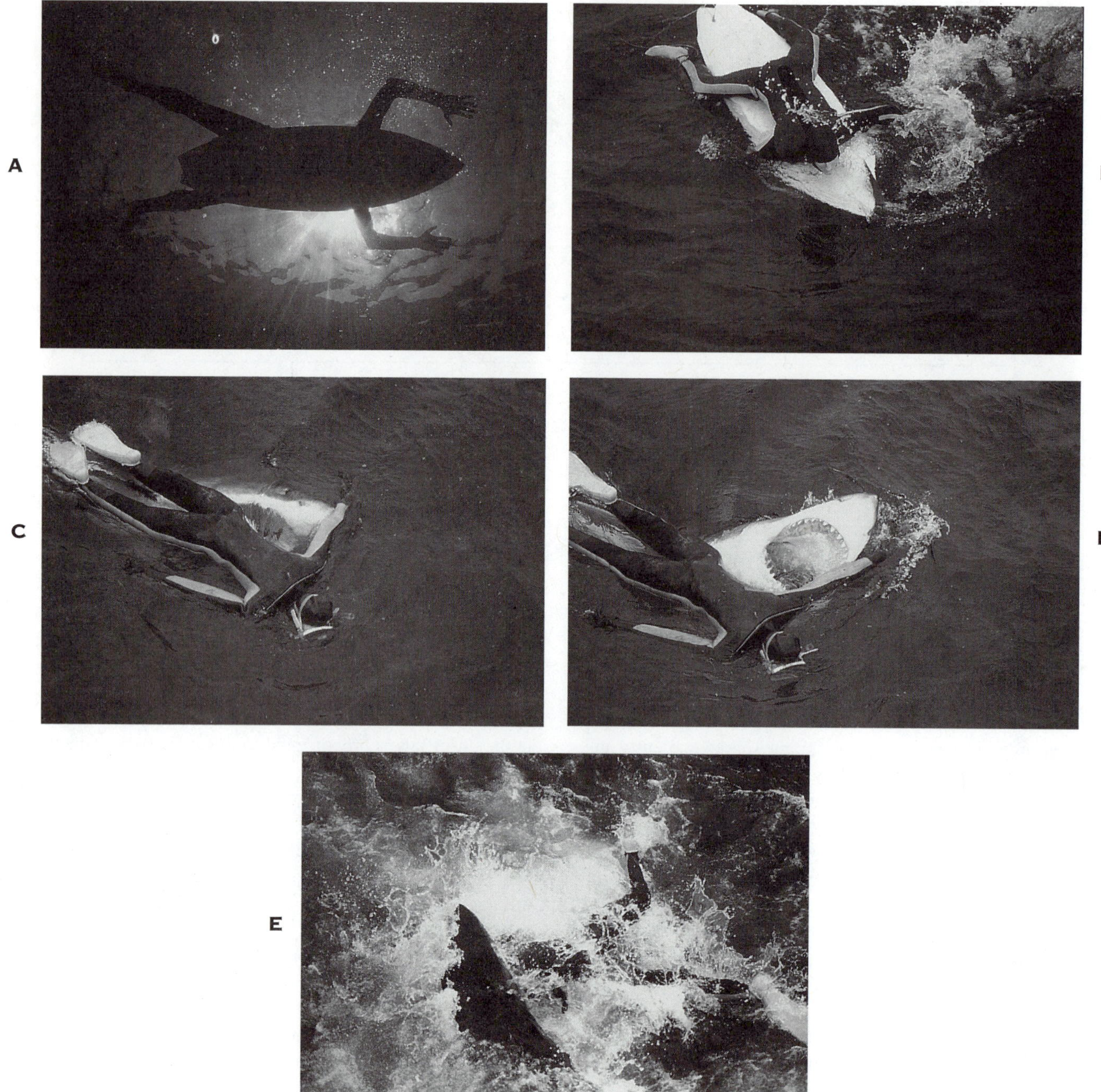

Fig. 51-6 **A,** Silhouette of diver on surfboard to demonstrate similarity in shadow and contour to a sea lion at the surface. **B,** A great white shark passes underneath a dummy on a surfboard before making an attack. **C,** The shark begins to elevate its head from the water. **D,** With jaws wide, the shark attacks the dummy. **E,** With great commotion the dummy and surfboard are dragged beneath the surface. (All photos from Images Unlimited, Inc. **A,** Al Giddings. **B,** Rosemary Chastney. **C** to **E,** Walt Clayton.)

in the water. As soon as the victim is out of the water, all means available must be used to ligate large, disrupted arteries or to apply compression dressings. If possible the injudicious use of pressure points or tourniquets should be avoided. If intravascular volume must be replaced in large quantities, at least two large-bore IV lines should be inserted into the uninvolved extremities to deliver crystalloid (lactated Ringer's solution, normal saline, or hypertonic saline), colloid, or blood products.[94,121,134] Central venous cannulation should be reserved for the emergency department.

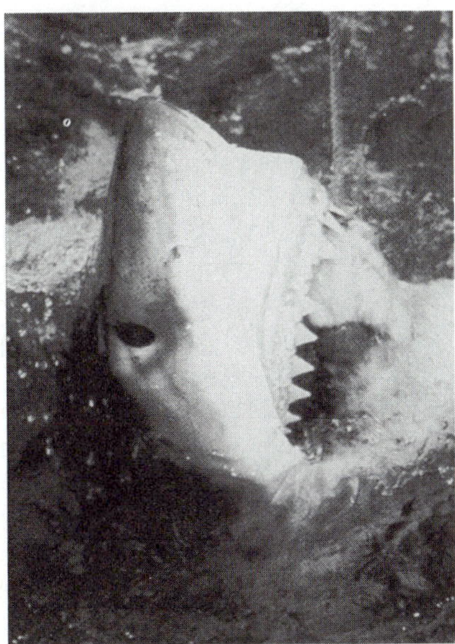

Fig. 51-7 Shark jaw advanced in biting. (Images Unlimited, Inc., Al Giddings.)

The patient should be kept well oxygenated and warm while being transported to a facility equipped to handle major trauma. Blood losses should be replaced with whole blood or packed red blood cells and fresh-frozen plasma.[135] The precise ratio of crystalloid to blood products and proper mean arterial blood pressure endpoint of primary resuscitation in the presence of a major vascular injury are the subjects of ongoing investigations.[127] The victim should be thoroughly examined for evidence of cervical, intrathoracic, and intraabdominal injuries. Because *Clostridium* can be cultured from ocean water, tetanus toxoid 0.5 ml intramuscularly (IM) and tetanus immune globulin (Hyper-Tet, Cutter) 250 to 500 units IM must be given. The administration of prophylactic antibiotics is more controversial. We recommend that the victim of a shark bite be treated with an IV third-generation cephalosporin, trimethoprim-sulfamethoxazole, chloramphenicol, an aminoglycoside, ciprofloxacin, or some reasonable combination of these agents. Imipenem-cilastatin should be reserved for established wound infections or early indications of septicemia, particularly in the setting of immunosuppression. The rationale for prophylactic antibiotics is that shark wounds are prone to heavy contamination with seawater, sand, plant debris, shark teeth, and shark mouth flora. After a clinical infection is recognized, wounds should be cultured for aerobes and anaerobes by insertion of sterile swabs deeply into available lesions.

Proper operative intervention is mandatory. It is inappropriate to attempt emergency department exploration of what often prove to be extensive and complicated wounds. In the operating room, devitalized tissue should be widely debrided and the wound irrigated copiously to remove all foreign material (Fig. 51-8). An x-ray may reveal one or

A

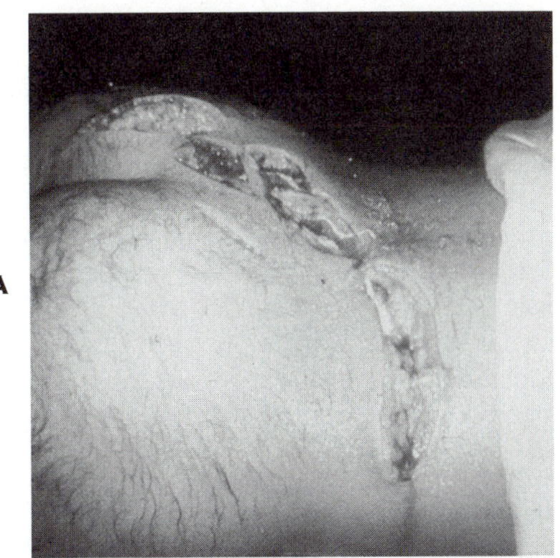

B

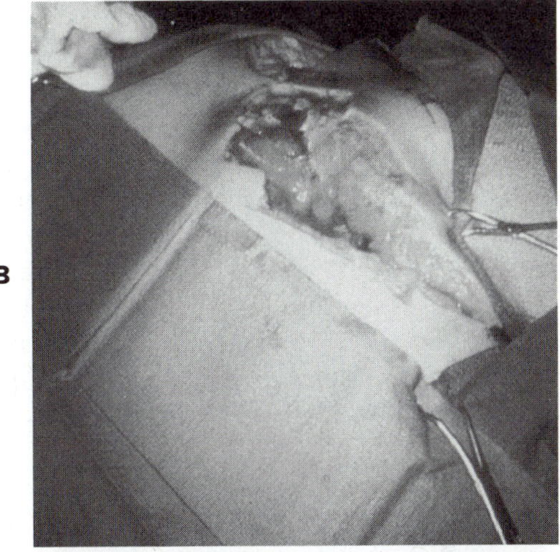

C

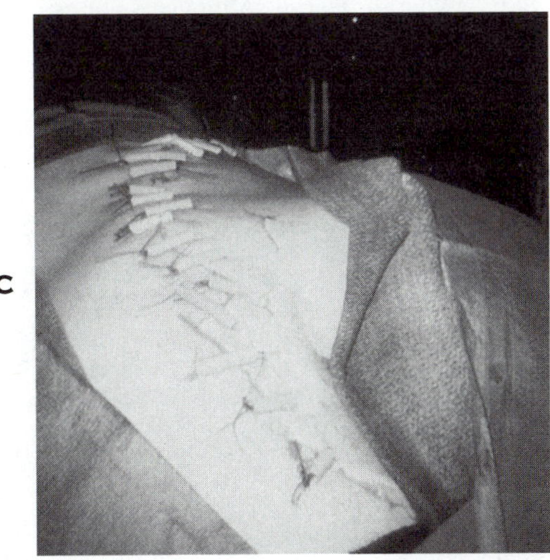

Fig. 51-8 Operative repair of shark bite wound. **A,** Multiple jagged crush lacerations from the bite of a large shark. **B,** Debridement and exploration of the wound in the operating room. **C,** Proper closure technique with tension-releasing sutures. (Photos courtesy T. Hattori, M.D.)

more shark teeth in the wound (Fig. 51-9). Unless it is absolutely necessary to achieve tight closure, the wound should be closed loosely around multiple drains (Jackson-Pratt closed systems or Penrose type) or packed open to await delayed primary closure. Although there is debate about whether to use internal or external fixation of grossly open and contaminated fractures, it seems logical to recommend surgical stabilization to facilitate vascular and soft tissue repair. In the pediatric population, damage to the physis and future limb length discrepancy should be anticipated.[51]

The abrasion associated with a shark "bumping" should be managed like a second-degree burn, with daily debridement and application of antiseptic ointment.

A reasonable "shark pack" should be available in emergency facilities and rescue vehicles near shark-infested waters. This must be portable and should include items necessary to control hemorrhage and initiate IV therapy.

PREVENTION

Every precaution should be taken to avoid shark attack, beginning with an intimate knowledge of the local waters. The following is precautionary advice and a list of alternatives for action in the event of a confrontation:

1. Avoid shark-infested water, particularly at dusk and at night. This fundamental rule is disregarded amazingly often. There is nothing heroic about losing life or limb to a shark. Do not enter posted waters. Surfers are generally at greater risk than divers. Do not disguise yourself as a pinniped (seal). Do not swim with animals (such as dogs or horses) in shark waters. Shark behavior can be unpredictable, so it is best not to remain in the water with sharks, particularly if you are fearful. Although some persons believe that sharks can be domesticated, there is no such thing as a "friendly" shark.

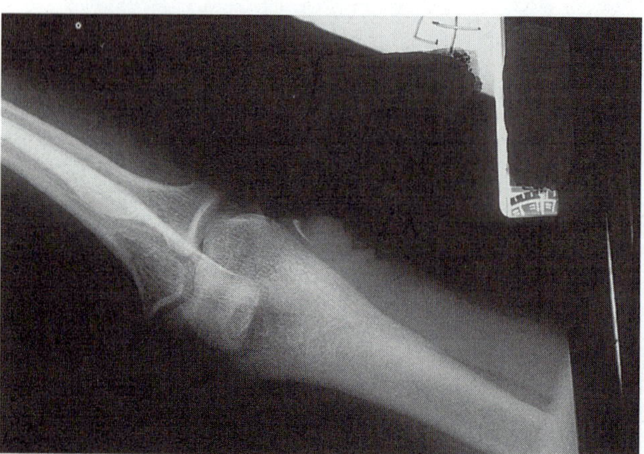

Fig. 51-9 The presence of a shark tooth in the arm is revealed by x-ray examination.

2. Swimmers should remain in groups. Isolation creates a primary target and eliminates companion surveillance. When diving, maintain constant vigilance.
3. Turbid water, dropoffs, deep channels, breeding inlets, and sanitation waste outlets are areas frequented by larger sharks and should be avoided. However, it appears that sharks attack at least half the time in clear water. Humans are most often attacked in shallow water or beyond the breakers.
4. Blood and other body fluids (including peritoneal fluid) attract sharks. No person should be in shark waters with an open wound. Women have historically been advised to avoid diving during menstruation, although there are no data to support attraction of sharks to the discharge of menstruation.
5. Brightly colored swimwear or diving equipment and shiny snorkeling gear attract certain sharks. Bright (international) orange appears to be particularly attractive to sharks. Flat black is probably the least attractive color. There is scant evidence that sharks are more attracted to light-skinned bathers.
6. Captured fish must be tethered at a distance from any divers. There is no greater chemical attractant for a shark than fish blood.
7. The presence of porpoises in the water does not preclude the presence of sharks. Be alert for the presence of a shark whenever schools of fish behave in an erratic manner.
8. Do not tease or corner a shark. This is particularly true with captive animals. If a shark begins to act in an erratic manner, do not photograph it at close range using a strobe flash apparatus.
7. If a shark appears in shallow water, swimmers should leave the water with slow, purposeful movements, facing the shark if possible and avoiding erratic behavior that could be interpreted as distress. If a shark approaches in deep water, the diver should remain submerged, rather than wildly surface to escape. The diver should move to defensive terrain with posterior protection to fend off, as best as possible, a frontal attack. It is inadvisable to trap a shark so that it must attack to obtain freedom. Fighting sharks is difficult; they are best repulsed with blunt blows to the snout, eyes, or gills. If possible the bare hand should not be used, to avoid severe abrasions or lacerations. A stream of air bubbles from a scuba regulator directed into the face of a shark may be sufficient deterrent. Although spears, knives, shotgun shell– or 30-.06-loaded powerheads, strychnine-filled spears, and carbon dioxide darts can kill small sharks, they can worsen the situation if they are misapplied or their application promotes frenzy in a school of sharks.[49]

Do not splash on the surface or create a commotion in a manner that might cause a shark to interpret your behavior as that of a struggling fish. Surface chop and perhaps the sounds created by helicopter rotor wash attract sharks.

8. Shark defense techniques and repellents are constantly evolving. In response to shark attacks on downed airmen and sailors during World War II, copper acetate blended with a water-soluble wax and nigrosine dye was packaged as a slowly dissolving waxy cake for deployment as "Shark Chaser" by the Office of Naval Research of the U.S. Navy.[7] It was theorized that the acetate resembled the decaying carcasses of sharks and sharks would thus be repelled. Unfortunately, while a morale booster, this was and is not a reliable deterrent. Its use was discontinued by the Navy in 1976. Limited progress has been made since that time. Recreational beaches in Australia and South Africa are protected with extensive gill net systems to trap overly curious animals. These work to a certain degree but are not foolproof. Electric shark barriers using 0.8 msec pulses 15 times per second to create a field of 4 volts per meter seem to generate a fright response in sharks longer than 1.2 m and are being investigated.[21,123] Their benefits include repulsion rather than shark capture or destruction. Abalone divers in South Australia work from one-person, self-propelled shark cages.

   Experimental devices for individuals include chain-mesh diving suits, inflatable dull-colored plastic protective bags (yellow is easy for aircraft to spot, but most attractive to sharks), acoustic and hand-held electrical field transmitters (thus far ineffective), surfactants and other chemical repellents (such as firefly and the Red Sea and western Indian Ocean Moses sole [flatfish; *Pardachirus marmoratus*] glandular extract [pardaxin]).[27] Pardaxin is a polypeptide neurotoxin that forms voltage-gated pores.[72] The ichthyotoxic secretion from the fish also contains shark repellent lipophilic constituents that appear to be steroid monoglycosides.[130] However, it has been estimated that about 24 kg of any effective drug would have to be contained in the volume of water through which a slowly approaching shark might swim as it attacked a human in the ocean.[7] For the exudate from the Moses sole, concentrations of 10 to 25 g/m^3 are needed to elicit an immediate indication of repellency. For more common synthetic detergents (sodium dodecylsulfate), the concentration needed is 800 g/m^3. These findings show that a chemical carried in a life jacket cannot be reliably useful against sharks, since it would have to be instantaneously effective at a concentration of no greater than 100 parts per billion. There is no question that shark avoidance is the most reliable maneuver.

Barracuda

To many divers the barracuda appears more sinister than the shark, and it is more highly feared. Barracuda are distributed from Brazil north to Florida, and in the Indo-Pacific from the Red Sea to the Hawaiian Islands. Of the 22 species of barracuda, only the great barracuda *(Sphyraena barracuda)* has been implicated in human attacks.

LIFE AND HABITS

The great barracuda is encountered in all tropical seas and can grow to 2.5 m and 50 kg, but is rarely sighted at a length greater than 1.5 m (Fig. 51-10). A solitary swimmer, the fish is extremely swift and swims in a disconcerting darting fashion. The barracuda possesses an elongated narrow

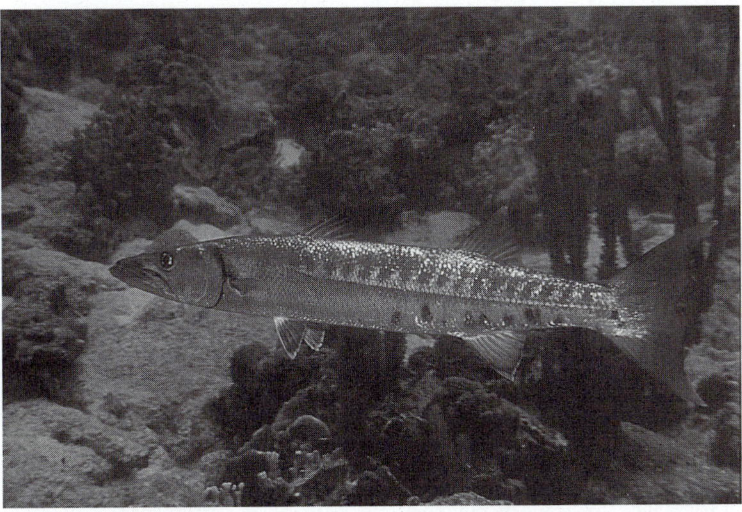

Fig. 51-10 Great barracuda *(Sphyraena barracuda).*

mouth filled with large knifelike teeth, similar in appearance to canines (Fig. 51-11). Smaller fish may be found in large schools.

Although great barracuda seldom attack divers, they do so rapidly and fiercely, often out of confusion in murky waters. More commonly the fish charges through or leaps from shallow water to bite the dangling legs of a boater, particularly if a shiny anklet (which resembles a fishing lure) is worn. Persons have been bitten on the face when trying to feed a barracuda by holding a dead fish bait in their mouths. Considering the frequency with which barracuda are encountered and the number of reported attacks, they do not pose nearly the hazard of sharks.

CLINICAL ASPECTS

Barracuda jaws contain two nearly parallel rows of teeth, which produce straight or V-shaped lacerations, in contradistinction to the crescent-shaped bite of the shark. Except for this difference and the magnitude of injury, the surgical problems generated by the barracuda do not differ from those of the shark. The clinician encounters tissue loss, moderate hemorrhage, and wound infections.

TREATMENT

Barracuda bites are treated identically to shark bites. If a barracuda is captured, it should not be eaten in ciguatera toxin–endemic regions.

PREVENTION

Barracuda are attracted to turbid waters, underwater commotion, irregular motion, surface splashing, shiny objects, and tethered fish. These should all be avoided. It is unwise to dangle a body part adorned with reflective jewelry before the jaws of a barracuda.

Moray Eels

LIFE AND HABITS

Moray eels are found in tropical, subtropical, and some temperate waters. In the family Muraenidae, some individuals of the larger species may attain lengths of 3.5 m and diameters of more than 35 cm. Morays are muscular, powerful, savage bottom dwellers, residing in holes or crevices or under rock and coral. The skin of the moray eel is leathery and mucus coated, not easily lacerated with a knife. Fortunately, the eel usually evades confrontation unless cornered or provoked. Bites occur when a diver intentionally probes into a coral bed or cave, or a fisherman reaches into a net and offers a hand to a feeding eel. Aquarium-housed morays may strike when handled improperly.[41] Most moray eels are easily intimidated and avoid confrontation unless cornered. An aggressive eel may strike out in competition for prey, particularly lobster. Elderly vision-impaired eels may attack without specific provocation, especially at night.

CLINICAL ASPECTS

Morays are forceful and vicious biters that can inflict severe puncture wounds with their narrow and viselike jaws, which are equipped with long, sharp, retrorse, fanglike teeth (Color Plate 112) (Fig. 51-12). A moray eel has the tenacity of a bulldog and will hold on to a victim, rather than strike and release. Multiple small puncture wounds are common after the bite of smaller eels, with the hand most commonly involved. If the eel is ripped forcefully from the victim, the resulting lacerations may be extensive.

TREATMENT

Moray bites are treated in a manner analogous to that of shark bites. If the eel remains attached to the victim, the jaws may need to be broken or the animal decapitated to ef-

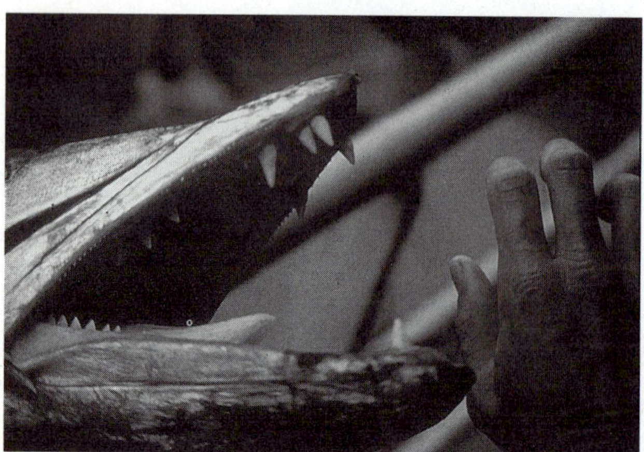

Fig. 51-11 Jaws of the great barracuda, with canine-configured teeth next to the senior author's hand.

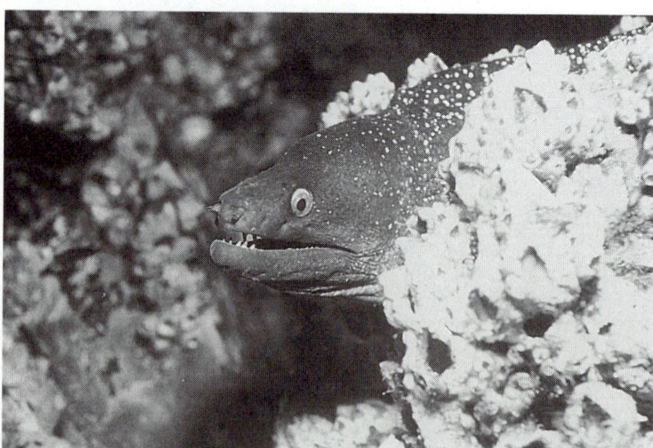

Fig. 51-12 Moray eel, demonstrating the sharp teeth and biting potential.

fect release. The primary wound should be irrigated copiously and explored to locate any retained teeth. The risk of infection is high, particularly in bites to the hand. The puncture wounds should be left unsutured to allow drainage and the victim given appropriate prophylactic antibiotics. If the wound is extensive and more linear in configuration (resembling a dog bite), the wound edges may be debrided and loosely approximated with nonabsorbable sutures or staples, and antibiotics may be administered. In all cases, it is prudent to inspect the wound at 24 and 48 hours to detect the onset of infection.

PREVENTION

It is unwise for a snorkeler or diver to place a hand underneath unexplored coral or rock unless it has been probed or otherwise disturbed specifically in search of an eel. All fishing nets should be handled carefully. A dive guide who feeds "friendly" moray eels by holding a loaf of bread or bait fish in his mouth is offering his nose and mouth as a meal for an unpredictable eel.

Giant Groupers

Some of the larger species of sea bass or grouper (family Serranidae) may grow to exceed 3.6 m and 227 kg (Fig. 51-13). Distributed in both tropical and temperate seas, they are curious, pugnacious, and voracious feeders. Although not aggressive like sharks, giant groupers should be respected for their fearlessness, bulk, and cavernous mouth. Groupers can be found frequenting shipwrecks; swimming in caves, caverns, and "holes"; and lurking behind large rocks and coral outcroppings. They are territorial and may become aggressive while protecting their domain. Bite wounds may be ragged with extensive maceration and are treated the same as shark bites. Large groupers should not be eaten in ciguatera toxin–endemic regions. It is always wise to visually survey an underwater cave before entering or exiting. The diver should not block the exit if a grouper is attempting to escape and should not carry speared fish. Most scare tactics used against sharks are of no avail with groupers.

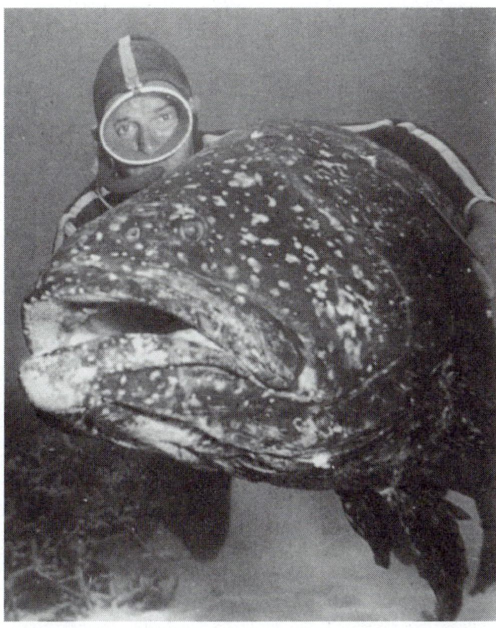

Fig. 51-13 Diver alongside a giant grouper.

Sea Lions

Sea lions (family Otaridae) and seals (family Phocidae) are mild-mannered mammals except during the mating season, when the males may become aggressive, and the breeding season, when both sexes attack in defense of their newborn pups. Divers have been seriously bitten and therefore should avoid ill-tempered and abnormally aggressive animals. There is nothing unique about the clinical aspects of these injuries, except for the posttraumatic infections. The bites are treated the same as shark bites.

Crocodiles and Alligators

Crocodiles (genus *Crocodylus*) and alligators (genus *Alligator*) are long-bodied loricates with reputations as ferocious aquatic reptiles. Considered to be less sluggish than alligators, crocodiles (*C. niloticus* in the Nile and the larger estuarine *C. porosus* of eastern Asia and the Pacific islands) may attack and severely injure a human. *C. porosus,* which ranges over an extensive geographic area including India, Sri Lanka, southern China, the Malay archipelago, Palau, the Solomon Islands, and northern Australia, has been claimed to be a prolific man-eater. Estimates of human fatalities may be exaggerated based on isolated reports of atrocities committed by this beast. An adult crocodile devours prey much larger in size than a human. According to one report the stomach of an Australian estuarine crocodile contained the remains of an aborigine and a 4-gallon drum containing two blankets. At a length greater than 20 feet and a weight exceeding 2500 pounds, the crocodile can travel in water at a speed of 20 mph and can charge a short distance over land at 15 to 30 mph. The enormous jaws and canine teeth can bite with sufficient force to sever an outboard boat propeller (Fig. 51-14). However, the teeth are not well suited for tearing apart or chewing, so most prey are allowed to rot, which makes them easier to swallow. Most crocodiles are content to eat fish, turtles, kangaroos, and wild pigs. However, excursions into freshwater rivers and onto land have introduced them to cows, horses, and humans. A crocodile attacks by grasping the victim in its powerful jaws and dragging it under water, where it drowns and dismembers the victim with a constant twirling motion ("death rolls"). In a series of 16 crocodile attacks reported from the Northern Territory of Australia, four fatalities involved transection of the torso or decapitation.[83] Most attacks (fatal and nonfatal) were on persons swimming or wading in shallow water.

Crocodile bites produce large crush injuries and lacerations. Surgical wound management is similar to that for dog bites. The bacteriologic considerations have not been extensively studied but should be assumed to be the same as for other animals that reside in the aquatic environment. Wound infections should be anticipated in the largely contaminated extensive crush injuries. Prophylactic antibiotics to cover *Aeromonas hydrophila, Pseudomonas,* and *Vibrio* should be administered. Coverage against anaerobes, such as *Bacteroides,* is prudent. Antitetanus primary or booster immunization is mandatory.

Needlefish

Marine needlefish (family Belonidae) are slender, tubular, silver, lightning-quick surface swimmers found in tropical seas. They resemble, but are not related to, the freshwater gar and may attain streamlined lengths of up to 2 m. Possessed of an elongated pointed snout, which comprises one quarter the length of the fish and contains small pointed teeth, the fish moves rapidly, often leaping out of the water in fear or when attracted to lights (Fig. 51-15). The needlefish, or garfish, is an occupational hazard for persons who fish from small canoes at night in tropical Indo-Pacific ocean waters.[10] On occasion they have flown into people, spearing them in the chest, abdomen, extremities, head, and neck. In one reported case a fish caused brain injury with an internal carotid-cavernous sinus fistula after orbitocranial perforation.[80] Exsanguination from a neck wound has been anecdotally reported from Papua New Guinea. A chest wound can be accompanied by a pneumothorax. Death may occur from chest or abdominal penetration. Treatment is according to the nature of the injury. All wounds should be debrided and irrigated, followed by a search for foreign material. A small superficial wound may cause the physician to underestimate an internal injury. The major risk is wound infection. Injury prevention is difficult, although it has been suggested that canoes be positioned in a circle to allow spearing of fish in a central pool of light.[10] Other species of flying fish pose less risk, since they have blunt heads.

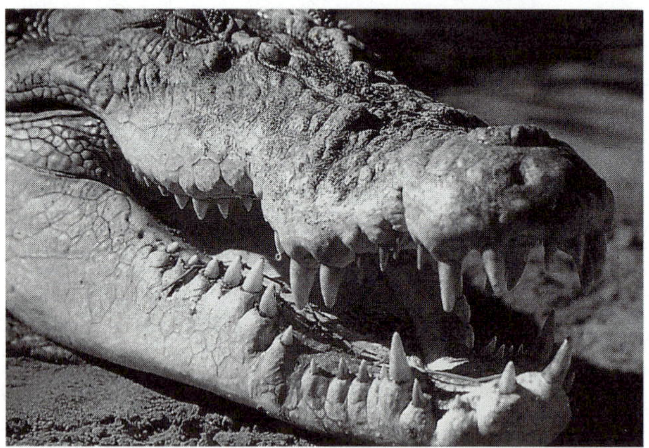

Fig. 51-14 The jaws of a saltwater crocodile. (Courtesy Allan P. Mekisic.)

Many other fishes leap from the water, but injuries are extremely uncommon. A single case of a wahoo (150 cm; 22.5 kg), family Scombridae, leaping from the water and biting a victim on the upper extremity has been reported.[55] The razor-sharp teeth generated extensor tendon lacerations on the dorsal hand and forearm that required surgical repair. As previously described, barracuda exit the water in pursuit of shiny metallic objects that resemble fishing lures. Bluefish *(Pomatomus saltatrix)* school and feed in a frenzy, but most bites occur as the fish are handled out of the water; in-water attacks on humans are theoretical.[71] The fish has sharp, conical canine teeth in both the upper and lower jaws and can grow to 1.2 m and over 12 kg.

Killer Whales

The killer whale, *Orcinus orca,* is probably not the ferocious killer it is reputed to be. The largest of the living mammalian dolphins, these magnificent animals grow to 33 feet and 10 tons and are found in all oceans. They usually travel in pods of up to 40 individuals. Swift and enormously powerful creatures, they feed on squid, fish, birds, seals, walruses, and other whales. Their powerful jaws are equipped with cone-shaped teeth directed back into the throat, designed to grasp and hold food. The killer whale can generate enough crushing power to bite a seal or porpoise in two with a single snap.

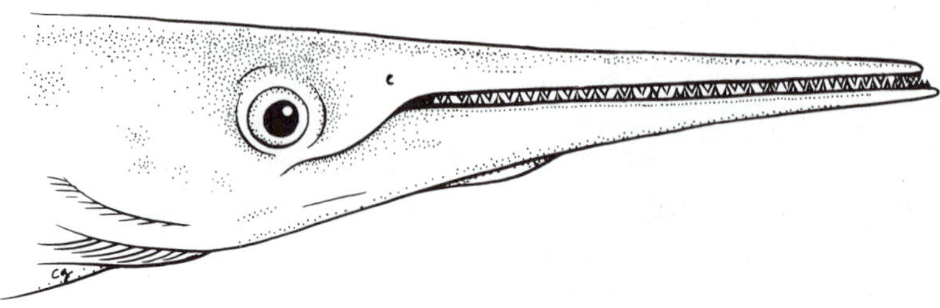

Fig. 51-15 Needlefish beak, capable of causing a penetrating injury.

In captivity, killer whales are playful creatures and seem intelligent, without the primal behavior of sharks. Nonetheless, although killer whales are believed not to prey on humans, they should be regarded with respect and at a distance in their natural habitat.[57] Mistaken for a sea lion, a human would be a nice snack for a killer whale.

Other whale species, such as the finback, have rammed boats, theoretically in defense of their young. Territorial behavior should be anticipated and respected.

Giant Clams

Although many adventure stories describe divers being caught in the clamp of a giant clam (family Tridacnidae), there are no verifiable reports of such a calamity resulting in a major injury.[126] *Tridacna gigas* can attain a length of 1 m and weigh as much as 300 kg.[33] The hazard to divers is hypothetical.

Giant Squid

The giant squid, possibly *Architeuthis,* grows to a length in excess of 20 m and weight of 38,000 kg, with long (10 m) menacing tentacles, eyes of nearly 35 cm, and a razor-sharp beak that it uses to eat prey.[28] The tentacles are armed with chitinous serrated rings equipped with teeth on each of the suckers. Sperm whales have been examined with sucker wounds of diameter 46 cm, which would extrapolate to a monstrous squid measuring at least 60 m in length. The battles between sperm whales and giant squid are legendary, but humans are unlikely to encounter this awesome animal, which is found at depths far beyond the range of a sport scuba diver. With increased deep sea exploration by small submersibles, we may learn more about this fascinating creature. It is likely that a hungry giant squid would not hesitate to ingest a human.

Giant Octopus

The Pacific giant octopus *Octopus dofleini* is a predator that has been captured at 272 kg with an arm span of over 30 feet. It ranges off the western North American coast from northern California to Alaska and off eastern Asia southward to Japan. The cephalopod is armed with suckers on eight arms and a parrotlike chitinous mouth located centrally underneath the head. Although it exhibits curiosity, it does not exhibit aggression directed against humans. However, it possesses the strength and agility to easily overwhelm a human. Anecdotes from the South Pacific tell of native breath-hold divers being subdued and drowned by angered captive octopuses.

Giant Manta Rays

The giant manta ray *Manta birostris* can have a "wing" span of more than 6 m and a weight of 1600 kg (Fig. 51-16).

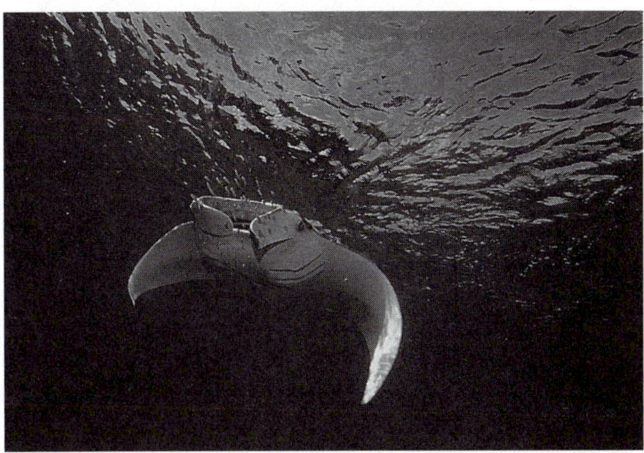

Fig. 51-16 Giant manta ray. The sting on the caudal appendage is vestigial, but the wings can "slap" and abrade the unwary individual.

The caudal appendage carries a vestigial stinger that poses no threat to humans. However, the coarse dermal denticles can create severe abrasions, which generally occur when divers attempt to ride the gentle and accommodating creatures.

Mantis Shrimp

The mantis shrimp *(Gonodactylus bredini)* resembles a miniature lobster (up to 18 cm) and is equipped with a pair of legs that serve as specialized jackknife claws.[77] The tail carries numerous sharp spines that may project beyond the edge of the sturdy tail fin. Lacerations may be induced by either the front claws or the tail, particularly when the shrimp attacks an unwary victim. It has been claimed that an attacking mantis shrimp struck with enough force to crack a diver's face mask.

Piranha

South American characins include the piranha *(Serrasalmus natterei)* equipped with a formidable set of razor-sharp teeth. These small fish attack in schools of several hundred and can theoretically reduce a human to a shiny skeleton in short order. They are attracted by blood or commotion.

Triggerfishes

The triggerfishes are usually shy and unimposing, but during mating season the females of at least two species *(Pseudobalistes fuscus* and *Balistoides viridescens)* can become extremely territorial in guarding a nest and thus aggressive, inflicting painful bites (Fig. 51-17, *A*). The former can grow to 55 cm and the latter to 75 cm. The strong jaws each carry eight long, protruding, chisel-like teeth in an outer row, backed by an inner row of six teeth.[105] Usually the fish "bites and runs," but the orange-striped triggerfish *(Balistoides undulatus)* has been reported to bite and not release (Fig. 51-17, *B*). It is common to have to strike the fish

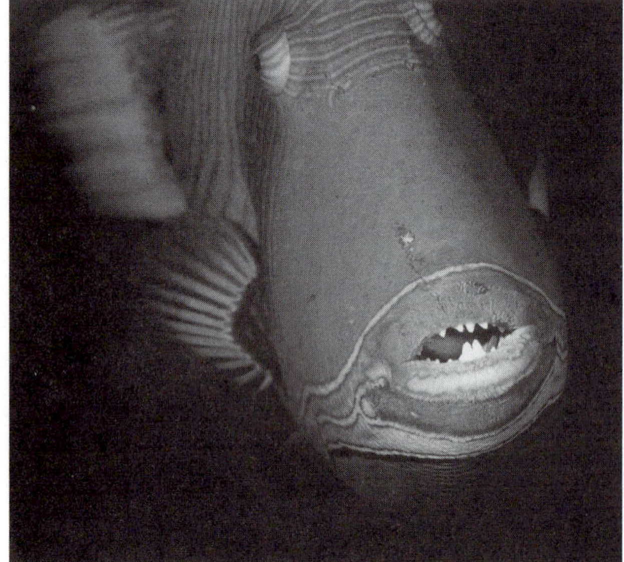

Fig. 51-17 **A,** Yellowspotted triggerfish *(Pseudobalistes fuscus),* Maldive Islands. **B,** Orange-striped triggerfish *(Balistoides undulatus),* Maldive Islands, demonstrating the chisel-like teeth. (Photos by J. Randall.)

in some manner to get it to release. In the Gilbert Islands a release technique is to bite the fish on the top of the head.

Stony Corals

LIFE AND HABITS

The anthozoan Madreporariae, or true (stony) corals, exist in colonies that possess calcareous outer skeletons with pointed horns, razor-sharp edges, or both (Fig. 51-18). They live in waters at temperatures of 20° C or higher, generally at depths of up to 20 fathoms. Rarer species have been noted at depths of more than 6000 fathoms. Certain coral species, such as *Plexaura hommomalla,* are under investigation as sources of prostaglandins and other pharmaceutical precursors.

CLINICAL ASPECTS

Snorkelers and divers, particularly photographers and spear fishermen, frequently handle or brush against these living reefs, resulting in superficial cuts and abrasions on the extremities (Fig. 51-19). Coral cuts are probably the most common injuries sustained underwater. The initial reaction to a coral cut is stinging pain, erythema, and pruritus, most commonly on the forearms, elbows, and knees. Divers without gloves frequently receive cuts to the hands. A break in the skin may be surrounded within minutes by an erythematous wheal, which fades over 1 to 2 hours. The red, raised welts and local pruritus are called coral poisoning. Low-grade fever may be present and does not necessarily indicate an infection. With or without prompt treatment, the wound may progress to cellulitis with ulceration and tissue sloughing. These wounds heal slowly (3 to 6 weeks) and result in prolonged morbidity. In an extreme case the victim develops cellulitis with lymphangitis, reactive bursitis, local ulceration, and wound necrosis.

TREATMENT

Coral cuts should be promptly and vigorously scrubbed with soap and water, then irrigated copiously with a forceful stream of fresh water or normal saline to remove all foreign particles. Using hydrogen peroxide to bubble out "coral dust" is occasionally helpful. Any fragments that remain can become embedded and increase the risk for an indolent infection or foreign body granuloma. If stinging is a major symptom, there may be an element of envenomation by nematocysts. A brief rinse with diluted acetic acid (vinegar) or isopropyl alcohol 20% may diminish the discomfort (after the initial pain from contact with the open wound). If a coral-induced laceration is severe, it should be closed with adhesive strips rather than sutures if possible; preferably it should be debrided for 3 or 4 days and closed in a delayed fashion.

A number of approaches can be taken with regard to wound care. The preferred method is to apply twice-daily sterile wet-to-dry dressings, using saline or dilute antiseptics (povidone-iodine solution, 1% to 5%). Alternatively, a nontoxic topical antibiotic ointment (bacitracin or polymyxin B–bacitracin–neomycin) may be used sparingly and covered with a nonadherent dressing (Metalline or Telfa). Secondary infections are dealt with as they arise. A final approach is to apply full-strength antiseptic solutions, followed by powdered topical antibiotics, such as tetracycline. No method has been supported by any prospective trial.

Despite the best efforts at primary irrigation and decontamination, the wound may heal slowly, with moderate to severe soft tissue inflammation and ulcer formation. All devitalized tissue should be debrided regularly using sharp dissection. This should be continued until a bed of healthy granulation tissue is formed. Wounds that appear infected should be cultured and treated with antibiotics as previously discussed.

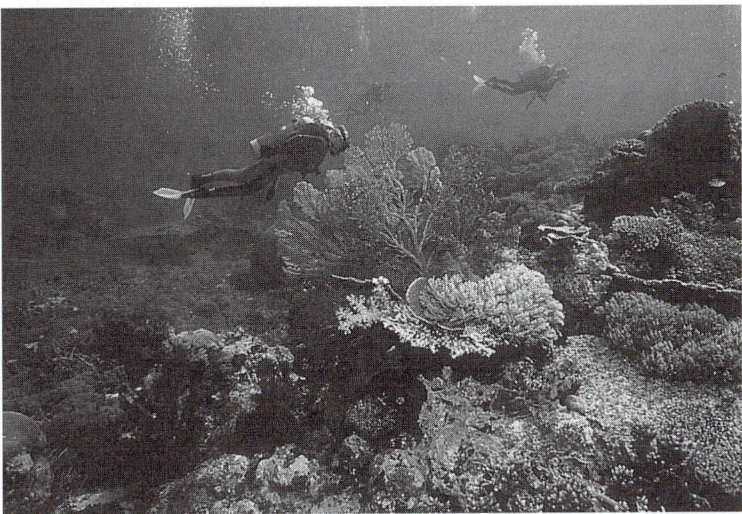

Fig. 51-18 Coral garden.

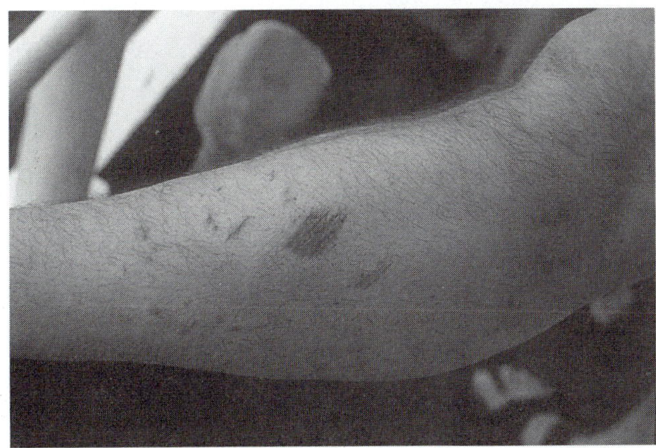

Fig. 51-19 Abrasions of the leg from bumping against sharp coral.

The patient who demonstrates malaise, nausea, and low-grade fever may have a systemic form of coral poisoning or be manifesting early signs of a wound infection. It is prudent at this point to search for a localized infection, procure wound cultures or biopsy specimens as indicated, and initiate antibiotics pending confirmation of organisms. If the patient is started on antibiotics and does not respond, a supplemental trial of systemic corticosteroids (prednisone 80 mg tapered over 2 weeks) is not unreasonable. In the absence of an overt infection, the natural course of the wound is to improve spontaneously over a 4- to 12-week period.

PREVENTION

Divers exploring near coral reefs must take every care to avoid coral cuts. Protective clothing and gloves should be impenetrable. Snorkelers and underwater photographers in shallow water should wear adequate hand, elbow, and knee protection.

Shocking Marine and Freshwater Animals

Only two groups of electric fish are marine; the remainder are freshwater animals. They rarely pose a health hazard but rather are curious creatures surrounded by superstition and folklore. The marine electric fish include the stargazers *(Astroscopus)* and the electric rays *(Torpedo)*. The electric eel is a freshwater Amazonian animal.

Electric rays are found in temperate and tropical oceans. Of the class Chondrichthyes, they are round bodied, with short tails and thick bodies (compared with stingrays). In California, *Torpedo californica* attains a length of 4 feet and weight of 80 to 90 pounds. They swim slowly and sluggishly and are usually found partially buried in bottom mud and sand. Well camouflaged, their dorsal surface is multicolored and their ventral surface creamy white. The externally visible electric organs are located on each side of the anterior part of the disk between the anterior extension of the pectoral fin and the head, extending from above the level of the eye backward past the gill region onto the ventral surface. They are composed of a honeycomb network of modified muscles organized into columnar prismlike structures and connective tissue, which generate an electrical charge by neuromuscular activity. The muscle cells ("electroplaques") are stacked 500 to 1000 deep, creating up to 500 cm^2 of surface area.[91] The electroplaques depolarize in series and in parallel simultaneously, producing amperage sufficient to stun prey.

Generally the ventral surface of the ray is negative and the dorsal side is positive. An electrical discharge is reflexively produced on contact, often in a series exhaustive for the fish. This necessitates a period of recharging. Electricity is delivered in doses of 8 to 220 volts.[44] The Atlantic *Torpedo nobiliana* produces 180 to 220 volts. Although the shock is of low amperage, it can stun a grown man and induce drowning. Recovery from the shock is usually uneventful. An electric ray should not be handled. The energy generated by skates is considerably less, measured in millivolts to 1 to 2 volts.

REFERENCES

1. Angerås MH et al: Comparison between sterile saline and tap water for the cleaning of acute traumatic soft tissue wounds, *Eur J Surg* 158:347, 1992.
2. Auerbach PS: Clinical therapy of marine envenomation and poisoning. In Tu AI, editor: *Handbook of natural toxins.* Vol 4. *Marine toxins and venoms,* New York, 1988, Marcel Dekker.
3. Auerbach PS et al: Bacteriology of the freshwater environment: implications for clinical therapy, *Ann Emerg Med* 16:1016, 1987.
4. Auerbach PS et al: Bacteriology of the marine environment: implications for clinical therapy, *Ann Emerg Med* 16:643, 1987.
5. Badhour LM: Extraintestinal *Aeromonas* infections—looking for Mr. Sandbar, *Mayo Clin Proc* 67:496, 1992.
6. Bailey JP et al: *Mycobacterium marinum* infection: a fishy story, *JAMA* 247:1314, 1982.
7. Baldridge HD: Shark repellent: not yet, maybe never, *Milit Med* 155(8):358, 1990.
8. Baldridge HD Jr, Williams J: Shark attack: feeding or fighting? *Milit Med* 134:130, 1969.
9. Barry AL, Thornberry C: Susceptibility tests: diffusion test procedures. In Lennette EH et al, editors: *Manual of clinical microbiology,* Washington, DC, 1985, American Society for Microbiology.
10. Barss PG: Injuries caused by garfish in Papua New Guinea, *Br Med J* 284:77, 1982.
11. Baumann H, Baumann L: The marine gram-negative eubacteria genera *Photobacterium, Benekea, Alteromonas, Pseudomonas,* and *Alcaligenes.* In Starr MP et al, editors: *The Prokaryotes: a handbook on habitats, isolation, and identification of bacteria,* New York, 1981, Springer-Verlag.
12. Blackband SJ, Stoskopf MK: In vivo nuclear magnetic resonance imaging and spectroscopy of aquatic organisms, *Magnet Reson Imag* 8(2):191, 1990.
13. Blake PA, Weaver RE, Hollis DG: Diseases of humans (other than cholera) caused by vibrios, *Annu Rev Microbiol* 34:341, 1980.
14. Blake PA et al: Disease caused by a marine vibrio: clinical characteristics and epidemiology, *N Engl J Med* 300:1, 1979.
15. Bloch S, Monteil H: Purification and characterization of *Aeromonas hydrophila* beta-hemolysin, *Toxicon* 27(12):1279, 1989.
16. Bonde GJ: The marine Bacillus. In Skinner FA Shewan JM, editors: *Aquatic microbiology,* New York, 1977, Academic Press.
17. Bonner JR et al: Spectrum of *Vibrio* infections in a Gulf Coast community, *Ann Intern Med* 99:464, 1983.
18. Branebark PI, Edholm R: Tissue injury caused by wound disinfectants, *J Bone Joint Surg* 49A:48, 1967.
19. Brown TW: *Sharks: the silent savages,* Boston, 1973, Little, Brown.
20. Buck JD, Spotte S, Gadbaw JJ: Bacteriology of the teeth from a great white shark: potential medical implications for shark bite victims, *J Clin Microbiol* 20:849, 1984.
21. Campbell GD, Smith ED: The "problem" of shark attack upon humans, *J Wilderness Med* 4(1):5, 1993.
22. Castillo LE, Winslow DL, Pankey GA: Wound infection and septic shock due to *Vibrio vulnificus, Am J Trop Med Hyg* 30:844, 1981.
23. Castro JI: *The sharks of North American waters,* College Station, 1983, Texas A & M University Press.
24. Centers for Disease Control: Aquarium-associated *Plesiomonas shigelloides* infection—Missouri, *MMWR* 38(36):617, 1989.
25. Centers for Disease Control: *Aeromonas* wound infections associated with outdoor activities—California, *MMWR* 39(20):324, 1990.
26. Chadee DD: Bacterial pathogens isolated from guppies *(Poecilia reticulata)* used to control *Aedes aegypti* in Trinidad, *Trans R Soc Trop Med Hyg* 86:693, 1992.
27. Clark E, Chao S: A toxic secretion from the Red Sea flatfish *Pardachirus marmoratus* (Lacepede), *Bull Sea Fish Res Sta (Haifa)* 60:53, 1973.
28. Clarke MR: A review of the systematics and ecology of oceanic squids, *Adv Marine Biol* 4:91, 1966.
29. Clarridge JE, Zighelboim-Daum S: Isolation and characterization of two hemolytic phenotypes of *Vibrio damsela* associated with a fatal wound infection, *J Clin Microbiol* 21:302, 1985.
30. Cohen JL: Vision in sharks, *Oceanus* 24:17, 1981-1982.
31. Compagno LJV: Legend versus reality: the Jaws image and shark diversity, *Oceanus* 24:5, 1981-1982.
32. Cousteau V: How to swim with sharks: a primer, *Perspect Biol Med* 16(4):525, 1973.
33. Crawford C, Nash W: Giant clams, *Oceanus* 29(2):60, 1986.
34. Davies DH, Campbell GD: The aetiology, clinical pathology and treatment of shark attack, *J R Naval Med Serv* 3:110, 1962.
35. Denis RA et al: Coxsackie A_{16} infection from lake water, *JAMA* 228:1370, 1974.
36. Dhingra J, Schauerhamer RR, Wangenstein OH: Peripheral dissemination of bacteria in contaminated wounds: role of devitalized tissue, *Surgery* 80:535, 1976.
37. Earampamoorthy S, Koff RS: Health hazards of bivalve-mollusk ingestion, *Ann Intern Med* 83:107, 1975.
38. Edlich RF: The biology of wound repair and infection: a personal odyssey, *Ann Emerg Med* 14:1018, 1985.
39. Engaña AC, McCosker JE: Attacks on divers by white sharks in Chile, *Calif Fish Game* 70(3):173, 1984.
40. English VL, Lindberg RB: Isolation of *Vibrio alginolyticus* from wounds and blood of a burn patient, *Am J Med Tech* 43:989, 1977.
41. Erickson T et al: The emergency management of moray eel bites, *Ann Emerg Med* 21(2):212, 1992.
42. Fernandez CR, Pankey GA: Tissue invasion by unnamed marine vibrios, *JAMA* 233:1173, 1975.
43. Fishbein M, Mehlman IJ, Pitcher J: Isolation of *Vibrio parahaemolyticus* from the processed meat of Chesapeake Bay blue crabs, *Appl Microbiol* 20:176, 1970.
44. Fisher AA: *Atlas of aquatic dermatology,* New York, 1978, Grune & Stratton.
45. Girard SM et al: *Clostridium perfringens* cultured from a Hawaiian sardine, *Sardinella marquesensis, Hawaii Med J* 38:327, 1979.
46. Grimes DJ et al: The fate of enteric pathogenic bacteria in estuarine and marine environments, *Microbiol Sci* 3:324, 1985.
47. Grimes DJ et al: *Vibrios* as autochthonous flora of neritic sharks, *Syst Appl Microbiol* 6:221, 1985.
48. Gruber RP, Vistnes L, Pardoe R: The effect of commonly used antiseptics on wound healing, *Plast Reconstr Surg* 55:472, 1975.
49. Gruber SH: Shark repellents: perspectives for the future, *Oceanus* 24:72, 1981-1982.
50. Gruber SH: Why do sharks attack humans? *Naval Res News* 90(1):2, 1988.
51. Guidera KJ et al: Shark attack: a case study of the injury and treatment, *J Orthop Trauma* 5(2):204, 1991.
52. Haghighi L, Waleh NS: Isolation of *Vibrio parahaemolyticus* from Persian Gulf, *J Trop Med Hyg* 81:255, 1978.
53. Hanson PG et al: Freshwater wound infection due to *Aeromonas hydrophila, JAMA* 238:1053, 1977.
54. Hiemenz JW, Kennedy B, Kwon-Chung KJ: Invasive fusariosis associated with an injury by a stingray barb, *J Med Vet Mycol* 28:209, 1990.

55. Hoffman J, Hack GR, Clark B: The man did fine, but what about the wahoo? (letter), *JAMA* 267(15):2039, 1992.
56. Howard RJ et al: Necrotizing soft-tissue infections caused by marine vibrios, *Surgery* 98:126, 1985.
57. Hoyt E: The whales called "killer," *National Geographic* 166:220, 1984.
58. Johns RJ: How to swim with sharks: the advanced course, *Trans Assoc Am Phys* 88:44, 1975.
59. Johnson RH, Nelson DR: Agonistic display in the gray reef shark, *Carcharhinus menisorrah,* and its relationship to attacks on man, *Copeia* 1:76, 1973.
60. Johnson RM, Katarski ME, Weisrock WP: Correlation of taxonomic criteria for a collection of marine bacteria, *Appl Microbiol* 16:708, 1968.
61. Johnston JM, Andes A, Glasser G: *Vibrio vulnificus:* a gastronomic hazard, *JAMA* 249:1756, 1983.
62. Johnston JM, Becher SF, McFarland LM: *Vibrio vulnificus:* man and the sea, *JAMA* 253:2850, 1985.
63. Johnston RG, Fung J: Bacterial flora of wild and captive porpoises, *J Occup Med* 11:276, 1969.
64. Jones RN et al: Susceptibility tests: microdilution and macrodilution broth procedures. In Lennette EH et al: editors: *Manual of clinical microbiology,* Washington, DC, 1985, American Society for Microbiology.
65. Joseph SW et al: *Aeromonas* primary wound infection of a diver in polluted waters, *J Clin Microbiol* 10:46, 1979.
66. Kaneko I, Colwell R: Distribution of *Vibrio parahaemolyticus* and related organisms in the Atlantic Ocean off South Carolina and Georgia, *Appl Microbiol* 28:1009, 1975.
67. Katz D, Smith H: *Aeromonas hydrophila* infection of a puncture wound, *Ann Emerg Med* 9:529, 1980.
68. Kelly MT, Avery DM: Lactose-positive *Vibrio* in seawater: a cause of pneumonia and septicemia in a drowning victim, *J Clin Microbiol* 11:278, 1980.
69. Kelly MT, McCormick WF: Acute bacterial myositis caused by *Vibrio vulnificus, JAMA* 246:72, 1981.
70. Kreger AS, Lockwood D: Detection of extracellular toxin(s) produced by *Vibrio vulnificus, Infect Immun* 33:583, 1981.
71. Lange WR: The perils of bluefish: handle with care! *Md Med J* 37(6):475, 1988.
72. Lazarovici P et al: Secondary structure, permeability and molecular modeling of pardaxin pores, *J Nat Toxins* 1(1):1, 1992.
73. Lee A, Langer R: Shark cartilage contains an inhibitor of tumor neovascularization. In Colwell RR, Sinskey AJ, Pariser ER, editors: *Biotechnology in the marine sciences,* Proceedings of the First Annual MIT Sea Grant Lecture and Seminar, New York, 1984, John Wiley & Sons.
74. Lennette EH et al, editors: *Manual of clinical microbiology,* Washington, DC, 1985, American Society for Microbiology.
75. Levin MA, Fisher JR, Cabielli VJ: Membrane filter technique for enumeration of enterococci in marine waters, *Appl Microbiol* 30:66, 1975.
76. Lotz MJ, Tamplin ML, Rodrick GE: Thiosulfate-citrate-bile salts-sucrose agar and its selectivity for clinical and marine vibrio organisms, *Ann Clin Lab Sci* 13:45, 1983.
77. Love HG Jr, Stephens LL: Dangerous marine life. In Ellis DM, editor: *Dangerous plants, snakes, arthropods and marine life,* Hamilton, Ill, 1978, Drug Intelligence Publications.
78. MacLeod RA: The question of the existence of specific marine bacteria, *Bacteriol Rev* 29:9, 1965.
79. Manire CA, Gruber SH: Anatomy of a shark attack, *J Wilderness Med* 3(1):4, 1992.
80. McCabe MJ et al: A fatal brain injury caused by a needlefish, *Neuroradiology* 15:137, 1978.
81. McCosker J: White shark attack behavior: observations of and speculations about predator and prey strategies, memoir No 9, *Calif Acad Sci* 9:123, 1985.
82. McSweeney RJ, Forgan-Smith WR: Wound infections in Australia from halophilic vibrios, *Med J Aust* 1:896, 1977.
83. Mekisic AP, Wardill JR: Crocodile attacks in the Northern Territory of Australia, *Med J Aust* 157:751, 1992.
84. Mertens A et al: Halophilic, lactose-positive *Vibrio* in a case of fatal septicemia, *J Clin Microbiol* 9:233, 1979.
85. Miller DJ, Collier RS: Shark attacks in California and Oregon, *Calif Fish Game* 67:76, 1980.
86. Morris JG, Black RE: Cholera and other vibrioses in the United States, *N Engl J Med* 310:343, 1985.
87. Morris JG, Tenney J: Antibiotic therapy for *Vibrio vulnificus* infection, *JAMA* 253:1121, 1985.
88. Morris JG, Tenney JH, Drusano GL: In vitro susceptibility of pathogenic *Vibrio* species to norfloxacin and six other antimicrobial agents, *Antimicrob Agents Chemother* 28:442, 1985.
89. Morse DL et al: Widespread outbreaks of clam- and oyster-associated gastroenteritis: association of Norwalk virus, *N Engl J Med* 314:678, 1986.
90. Moss SA: Shark feeding mechanisms, *Oceanus* 24:23, 1981-1982.
91. Moss SA: *Sharks: an introduction for the amateur naturalist,* Englewood Cliffs, NJ, 1984, Prentice-Hall.
92. Muic V et al: Infection and contamination of some edible animals in the polluted sea area of Pula, *Toxicon* 16:424, 1978.
93. Murakami-Walker A: High concentrations of marine bacteria pose health risk, *Makai* (U Hawaii Sea Grant College Program) 7(8):1, 1985.
94. Nakayama S et al: Small volume resuscitation with hypertonic saline (2400 mOsm/liter) during hemorrhagic shock, *Circ Shock* 13:149, 1984.
95. Nelson DR: Aggression in sharks: is the gray reef shark different? *Oceanus* 24(4):45, 1981-1982.
96. Ongibene AJ, Thomas E: Fatal infection due to *Chromobacterium violaceum* in Vietnam, *Am J Clin Pathol* 54:607, 1970.
97. Passen EL, Andersen BR: Clinical tetanus despite a protective level of toxin-neutralizing antibody, *JAMA* 255:1171, 1986.
98. Paunio KU, Knuttila M, Mielitynen H: The effect of chlorhexidine gluconate on the formation of experimental granulation tissue, *J Periodontol* 49:92, 1978.
99. Pavia AT et al: *Vibrio carchariae* infection after a shark bite, *Ann Intern Med* 111(1):85, 1989.
100. Pettit GR, Ode RH: Antineoplastic agents L: isolation and characterization of sphyrnastatins 1 and 2 from the hammerhead shark *Sphyrna lewini, J Pharm Sci* 66:757, 1977.
101. Pfister RM, Burkholder PR: Numerical taxonomy of some bacteria isolated from Antarctic and tropical seawaters, *J Bacteriol* 90:863, 1965.
102. Pien F, Lee K, Higa H: *Vibrio alginolyticus* infections in Hawaii, *J Clin Microbiol* 5:670, 1977.
103. Pien FD et al: Bacterial flora of marine penetrating injuries, *Diagn Microbiol Infect Dis* 1:229, 1983.
104. Qadri SM, Lee G, Brodie L: Antibacterial activity of norfloxacin against 1700 relatively resistant clinical isolates, *Drugs Under Exp Clin Res* 15:349, 1989.
105. Randall JE, Millington JT: Triggerfish bite—a little-known marine hazard, *J Wilderness Med* 1(2):79, 1990.
106. Reines HD, Cook F: Pneumonia and bacteremia due to *Aeromonas hydrophila, Chest* 30:264, 1981.
107. Rheinheimer G: *Aquatic microbiology,* New York, 1974, John Wiley & Sons.
108. Revord ME, Goldfarb J, Shurin SB: *Aeromonas hydrophila* wound infection in a patient with cyclic neutropenia following a piranha bite, *Pediatr Infect Dis J* 7(1):70, 1988.
109. Roland FP: Leg gangrene and endotoxin shock due to *Vibrio parahaemolyticus:* an infection acquired in New England coastal waters, *N Engl J Med* 282:1306, 1970.
110. Ronka EKF, Roe WF: Cardiac wound caused by the spine of the stingray (suborder-Masticura), *Milit Surg* 97:135, 1945.

111. Rosenthal SG, Bernhardt HE, Phillips AJ: *Aeromonas hydrophila* wound infection, *Plast Reconstr Surg* 53:77, 1974.
112. Rosenthal SI, Zuger JH, Apollo E: Respiratory colonization with *Pseudomonas putrefaciens* after near-drowning in salt water, *Am J Clin Pathol* 64:382, 1975.
113. Rubin SJ, Tilton RC: Isolation of *Vibrio alginolyticus* from wound infections, *J Clin Microbiol* 2:556, 1975.
114. Ryan PR: Electroreception in blue sharks, *Oceanus* 24:42, 1981-1982.
115. Schandevyl P, Van Dyk E, Piot P: Halophilic *Vibrio* species from seafish in Senegal, *Appl Environ Microbiol* 48:236, 1984.
116. Semel JD, Allen N: Seizures in patients simultaneously receiving theophylline and imipenem or ciprofloxacin or metronidazole, *South Med J* 84(4):465, 1991.
117. Semel JD, Trenholme G: *Aeromonas hydrophila* water-associated wound infections: a review, *J Trauma* 30(3):324, 1990.
118. Shandera WX et al: Disease from infection with *Vibrio mimicus,* a newly recognized *Vibrio* species, *Ann Intern Med* 99:169, 1983.
119. Shattock RM: Injuries caused by wild animals, *Lancet* 1:412, 1968.
120. Shewen JM: The strict anaerobes in the slime and intestines of the haddock *(Gadus aeglefinus), J Bacteriol* 35:397, 1938.
121. Shoemaker WC: Comparison of the relative effectiveness of whole blood transfusions and various types of fluid therapy in resuscitation, *Crit Care Med* 4:71, 1976.
122. Sims JK et al: Marine bacteria complicating seawater near-drowning and marine wounds: a hypothesis, *Ann Emerg Med* 12:212, 1983.
123. Smith ED: Electric shark barrier: initial trials and prospects, *Power Engineer J,* July 1991, p 167.
124. Smith GC, Merkel JR: Collagenolytic activity of *Vibrio vulnificus:* potential contribution to its invasiveness, *Infect Immun* 35:1155, 1982.
125. Smith HW: Incidence of R+ *Escherichia coli* in coastal bathing waters of Britain, *Nature* 234:155, 1971.
126. Southcott RV: Human injuries from invertebrate animals in the Australian seas, *Clin Toxicol* 3:617, 1970.
127. Stern SA et al: Effect of blood pressure on hemorrhage volume and survival in a near-fatal hemorrhage model incorporating a vascular injury, *Ann Emerg Med* 22:155, 1993.
128. Stevenson TR et al: Cleansing the traumatic wound by high pressure syringe irrigation, *JACEP* 5:17, 1976.
129. Strauss MB, Orris WL: Injuries to divers by marine animals: a simplified approach to recognition and management, *Milit Med* 139:129, 1974.
130. Tachibana K, Gruber SH: Shark repellent lipophilic constituents in the defense secretion of the Moses sole *(Pardachirus marmoratus), Toxicon* 26(9):839, 1988.
131. Tacket CO et al: Equine antitoxin use and other factors that predict outcome in type A foodborne botulism, *Am J Med* 76:794, 1984.
132. Taylor L: Tetanus from a marine sponge, *J Laryngol Otol* 72:762, 1958.
133. Thorsteinsson SB, Minuth JN, Musher DM: Clinical manifestations of halophilic non-cholera vibrio infections, *Lancet* 2:1283, 1974.
134. Traverso LW, Lee WP, Langford MJ: Fluid resuscitation after an otherwise fatal hemorrhage. I. Crystalloid solutions, *J Trauma* 26:168, 1986.
135. Traverso LW et al: Fluid resuscitation after an otherwise fatal hemorrhage. II. Colloid solutions, *J Trauma* 26:176, 1986.
136. Trucksis M, Hooper DC, Wolfson JS: Emerging resistance to fluoroquinolones in staphylococci: an alert (editorial), *Ann Intern Med* 144(5):424, 1991.
137. Viljanto J: Disinfection of surgical wounds without inhibition of normal wound healing, *Arch Surg* 155:253, 1980.
138. Von Graevenitz A, Carrington GO: Halophilic vibrios from extraintestinal lesions in man, *Infection* 1:54, 1973.
139. Voss LM, Rhodes KH, Johnson KA: Musculoskeletal and soft tissue *Aeromonas* infection: an environmental disease, *Mayo Clin Proc* 67:422, 1992.
140. Walton RL, Matory WE: Wound care. In Mills J et al, editors: *Current emergency diagnosis and treatment,* Los Altos, Calif, 1985, Lange Medical Publications.
141. Watters DJ, van den Brenk AL: Toxins from ascidians, *Toxicon* 31(11):1349, 1993.
142. Welch K, Martini FH: Non-fatal shark attack on Maui, *Hawaii Med J* 40:95, 1981.
143. White JAM: Shark attack in Natal: injury, *Br J Accident Surg* 6:187, 1974.
144. Wolff RL, Wiseman SL, Kitchens SC: *Aeromonas hydrophila* bacteremia in ambulatory immunocompromised hosts, *Am J Med* 68:238, 1980.
145. Youngren-Grimes BL, Gruber SH, Grimes DJ: *Anaerobic bacteria in shark tissue (abstract),* Victoria, BC.
146. ZoBell CE, Johnson FH: The influence of hydrostatic pressure on the growth and viability of terrestrial and marine bacteria, *J Bacteriol* 57:179, 1949.
147. ZoBell CE, Morita RY: Barophilic bacteria in some deep sea sediments, *J Bacteriol* 73:563, 1957.
148. ZoBell CE, Upham HC: A list of marine bacteria including descriptions of sixty new species, *Bull Scripps Inst Oceanogr Univ Calif* 5:239, 1944.

52 MARINE ENVENOMATION

Paul S. Auerbach

The science of poisons, biotoxicology, is divided into plant poisons, or phytotoxicology, and animal poisons, or zootoxicology. Naturally occurring aquatic zootoxins may be further designated as oral toxins (which are poisonous to eat and include bacterial poisons and products of decomposition), parenteral toxins (venom produced in specialized glands and injected mechanically (by spine, needle, fang, fin, or dart), and crinotoxins (venom produced in specialized glands and administered as slime, mucous, and gastric secretion). Within these three subdivisions, further classifications are by phylogeny, chemical structure, and clinical syndrome.

Although all venoms are poisons, not all poisons are venoms.[85] According to the theory that offensive venoms are generally oral (mouth and fang) and defensive venoms are aboral (tail and sting) or dermal (barb and secretion), the majority of marine venoms are defensive.[156] In the evolutionary scheme it appears that venomous fish seek specific self-defense, whereas poisonous fish are noxious in a nonspecific manner. A brief comparison of the features of venoms and poisons shows that poisons produced in skin, muscle, blood, or organs are generally heat stable (115° to 120° F), are gastric acid stable, and carry seasonal toxicity. They are not "released" and may lack a well-defined biologic function. Venoms are more commonly heat labile, gastric acid labile, and nonseasonal in toxicity. They can be released in varying amounts and have evolved for conquest and defense.

In snakes the latency, toxicity, and duration of a venom effect are related to the route of envenomation. Intravascular injection is significantly more lethal than intraperitoneal or transcutaneous injection, as determined by the measured lethal dose of 50% survival of the group (LD_{50}). This principle is not commonly applied to marine venoms because few encounters involve direct intravascular invasion.

Most venoms are high–molecular weight amalgams of vasoactive amines, proteolytic enzymes, and other biogenic compounds.[153] These substances denature membranes, catabolize cyclic 3′,5′-adenosine monophosphate, degranulate mast cells, provoke histamine release, initiate arachidonate metabolism, accelerate coagulopathy, interfere with cellular transport mechanisms, disrupt metabolic pathways, impede neuronal transmission, and evoke anaphylaxis and shock. Frustratingly, although many marine venoms are composed of protein and polypeptide subunits, they lack sufficient immunogenicity to allow development of antitoxins or antivenins.[121] Poisons represent metabolic by-products and are usually of smaller molecular weight.[68]

Anaphylaxis

An envenomation or administration of antivenin can elicit an allergic reaction. In the previously sensitized individual, the antigen (venom, aquatic protein, or animal serum) complexes with immunoglobulin E (IgE) and perhaps with IgG homocytotopic antibodies or activated complement cleavage products attached to the membranes of mast cells and basophils. This induces membrane permeability, which allows degranulation or membrane production of histamine, serotonin, kinins, prostaglandins, platelet-activating factor, eosinophil and neutrophil chemotactic factors, leukotrienes, and other bioactive chemical mediators.[6,9,18,46]

The signs and symptoms of anaphylaxis may occur within minutes of exposure and include hypotension, bronchospasm, tongue and lip swelling, laryngeal edema, pulmonary edema, seizures, cardiac arrhythmia, pruritus, urticaria, angioedema, rhinitis, conjunctivitis, nausea, vomiting, diarrhea, abdominal pain, gastrointestinal bleeding, and syncope. Most severe allergic reactions occur within 15 to 30 minutes of envenomation, and nearly all occur within 6 hours. Fatalities are related to airway obstruction or hypotension. Acute elevated pulmonary vascular resistance may contribute to hypotension that results from generalized arterial vasodilation.[11,14]

TREATMENT

Decisive treatment should be instituted at the first indication of hypersensitivity:

1. Maintain the airway and administer oxygen. If airway obstruction from laryngeal edema prevents visualization of the vocal cords, it may be necessary to perform a cricothyroidotomy. Percutaneous transtracheal jet ventilation may be used as a temporizing measure until a larger airway can be secured.

2. Obtain intravenous access and administer crystalloid to achieve a systolic blood pressure of 90 mm Hg in an adult. Blood pressure may be briefly augmented with application of the military anti-shock trousers (MAST), which increases systemic vascular resistance.[79] If the reaction is severe or the victim is older than 45 years, apply a cardiac monitor.

3. Administer epinephrine. Begin with administration of aqueous epinephrine 1:1000 subcutaneously in the deltoid region. The dose for adults is 0.3 to 0.5 ml and for children is 0.01 ml/kg. If the reaction is mild and the first injection provides partial relief, it may be repeated in 15 to 20 minutes. Aerosolized aqueous epinephrine is not adequate to abort systemic anaphylaxis.[94] If the reaction is limited to pruritus and urticaria, there is no wheezing or facial swelling, and the victim is older than 45 years, administer an antihistamine and reserve epinephrine for a worsened condition.

If the reaction is life threatening and there is no response to subcutaneous epinephrine, administer epinephrine intravenously. An adult should receive a 0.1 mg bolus of 1:1000 aqueous epinephrine (0.1 ml) diluted in 10 ml of normal saline (final dilution 1:100,000) infused over 10 minutes. A mixture for continuous infusion is prepared by adding 1 mg of 1:1000 aqueous epinephrine (1 ml) to 250 ml of normal saline, to create a concentration of 4 μg/ml. This infusion should be started at 1 μg/min (15 minidrops/min) and increased to 4 to 5 μg/min if the clinical response is inadequate. In children and infants, the starting dose is 0.1 μg/kg/min up to a maximum of 1.5 μg/kg/min, noting that infusion rates in excess of 0.5 μg/kg/min may be associated with cardiac ischemia and arrhythmias.[11]

4. Relieve bronchospasm. Inhaled nebulized bronchodilators may help to overcome reactive smooth muscle contraction. Widely employed agents are albuterol 0.5 ml or metaproterenol 0.3 ml in 2.5 ml normal saline administered by hand-held nebulizer. If a liquid β_2-sympathomimetic agent is not available, micronized versions may be administered by hand-held metered dose inhaler with spacer. Inhaled ipratropium may be added in refractory cases.

5. Administer antihistamines. A mild reaction may be managed with diphenhydramine 50 to 75 mg intravenously, intramuscularly, or orally. The dose for children is 1 mg/kg. Nonsedating antihistamines, such as terfenadine 60 mg orally or cimetidine 300 mg, are adjuncts.

6. Administer corticosteroids. If the reaction is severe or prolonged, or if the victim is regularly medicated with corticosteroids, administer hydrocortisone 200 to 300 mg, methylprednisolone 50 to 75 mg, or dexamethasone 10 to 25 mg intravenously with a 7- to 14-day oral taper to follow. The parenteral dose of hydrocortisone for children is 2.5 mg/kg. If therapy is initiated by mouth, administer prednisone 60 to 100 mg for adults and 1 mg/kg for children.

Antivenin Administration

A number of marine envenomations, such as those by the box-jellyfish and certain sea snakes, may require the administration of specific antivenin. Marine antivenins are raised in sheep and horses and therefore are antigenic in humans, inducing both immediate and delayed hypersensitivity. If the clinical situation permits after a sea snake envenomation, a skin test should be performed for sensitivity to horse serum. (There is rarely time with a *Chironex* envenomation, which requires immediate intervention.) This should be done only after deciding to administer antivenin and *not to determine whether antivenin is necessary*. The purpose of sensitivity testing is to allow adequate prophylaxis against anaphylaxis. The skin test is performed with an intradermal injection into the upper extremity of 0.02 ml of a 1:10 dilution of horse serum test material in saline, with 0.02 ml saline in the opposite extremity as a control. Erythema and pseudopodia are present in 15 to 30 minutes in a positive response. Because antivenin contains many times the protein content of horse serum used for skin testing, the use of antivenin for skin testing may increase the risk of anaphylactic reaction. If the skin test is positive, the antivenin should be diluted in sterile water to a 1:100 concentration for administration. Successive vials should be less dilute if the allergic reaction is minimal (controlled by antihistamines and epinephrine).

The rationale for administering antivenin is to provide early and adequate neutralization of the toxin at the tissue site of entry before it gains systemic dominance. It should be administered intravenously, taking care to provide adequate doses for children and the elderly, who have a decreased volume of distribution and increased sensitivity to venom effects. The antivenin should always be diluted with normal saline, Ringer's lactate, or dextrose 5% in water.[140]

Marine antivenins are currently produced and distributed in the Indo-Pacific regions.[199] They include the following:

1. *Chironex fleckeri* (box-jellyfish) antivenin, from Commonwealth Serum Laboratories (CSL), Melbourne, Australia. A hyperimmune sheep globulin preparation, this may be used to neutralize the stings of *Chironex fleckeri* and *Chiropsalmus quadrigatus*.
2. *Enhydrina schistosa* (beaked sea snake) and *Notechis scutatus* (terrestrial tiger snake) polyvalent sea snake antivenin, from CSL. A hyperimmune horse globulin preparation, this may be used to neutralize the bites of most sea snakes.
3. *Notechis scutatus* (tiger snake) antivenin, from CSL. This is the antivenin of second choice against the bites of most sea snakes.
4. *Enhydrina schistosa* (beaked sea snake) monovalent antivenin, from the Haffkine Institute in Bombay, India. This may be used to neutralize the bites of most sea snakes; it is most effective against the bite of *E. schistosa*.
5. *Synanceja trachynis* (stonefish) antivenin, from CSL. A hyperimmune horse globulin preparation, this may be used to neutralize the stings of stonefish and more virulent scorpionfish species.

A patient who is known to be sensitive to horse or sheep serum, has a positive skin test, or develops signs of an allergic reaction or anaphylaxis during antivenin therapy requires aggressive medical management.[141] A recipient of antivenin should be pretreated with 50 to 100 mg of intravenous diphenhydramine (1 mg/kg in children). After this the initial dose of antivenin is infused at a rate no faster than one vial each 5 minutes. If no allergic manifestations ensue, the antivenin can be administered at a more rapid rate. If signs of anaphylaxis develop, usually heralded by an urticarial eruption and pruritus, 0.1 to 0.2 ml aliquots of antivenin should be alternated with 3 to 10 ml (0.03 to 0.1 mg) intravenous doses of aqueous epinephrine 1:100,000 (infused over 5 to 10 minutes). Alternatively, an epinephrine drip may be prepared as previously described in the discussion on anaphylaxis. The patient should be managed in an intensive care unit, with electrocardiographic and blood pressure monitoring. The dose of epinephrine should not exceed that which elevates the pulse rate above 150 beats/min. The administration of intravenous epinephrine may cause transient hypokalemia as potassium is driven intracellularly; cessation of the epinephrine infusion may create a transient hyperkalemia as the potassium regains entry into the extracellular space. If a victim is highly allergic to antivenin, serious consideration should be given to supportive therapy (including hemodialysis) without antivenin administration.

SERUM SICKNESS

The formation of immunoglobulin G (IgG) antibodies in response to antigens present in antivenin (heterologous serum) results in the deposition of immune complexes in many tissue sites, notably in the walls of blood vessels. These complexes induce vascular permeability, activate the complement cascade and chemotactic factors, degranulate mast cells, and trigger the release of proteolytic enzymes. Decreased levels of C_3 and C_4 are accompanied by increased C_{3a}/C_{3a} des-arginine, a split product C_3.[73,111] Although immune complexes can be measured by various tests (Raji-cell IgG assay and C_{1q}-binding assay), levels of immune complexes may not correlate with the clinical presentation.[73,134] Dermal biopsy of lesional skin may reveal leukocytoclastic vasculitis.[21]

Symptoms are generally present within 8 to 24 days and include fever, arthralgias, malaise, urticaria, lymphadenopathy, urticarial and morbilliform skin rashes, peripheral neuritis, and swollen joints. It is not uncommon for the primary urticarial lesion to be noted at the injection site. Serum sickness is managed with the administration of corticosteroids. An initial loading dose of prednisone (40 to 60 mg for adults: 2 to 5 mg/kg, not to exceed 50 mg, for children) should be administered and maintained daily until symptoms markedly resolve. The corticosteroid should be tapered over a 2- to 3-week course to avoid induction of adrenal insufficiency. Aspirin or other nonsteroidal antiinflammatory agents are rarely helpful and may be contraindicated because of circulating immune complex–induced platelet dysfunction.[21]

Stinging Animals

The stinging animals constitute a large collection of marine organisms containing vertebrates and invertebrates, both primitive and extremely sophisticated organisms. These animals pose the most frequent hazards for swimmers and divers.

Invertebrates

SPONGES

Life and Habits

There are approximately 4000 species of sponges (phylum Porifera; predominately class Desmospongiae), which are composed of horny but elastic skeletons of "spongin," some forms of which we use as bath sponges.[83] Embedded in the connective tissue matrices are spicules of silicon dioxide (silica) or calcium carbonate, by which some sponges can be definitively identified.[19,50,51] In general, they are stationary animals that attach to the sea floor or coral beds and may be colonized by other sponges, hydrozoans, mollusks, coelenterates, annelids, crustaceans, echinoderms, fishes, and algae. These secondary coelenterate inhabitants are responsible for the dermatitis and local necrotic skin reaction termed sponge diver's disease.[121,171] In recognition of a medicinal property, the ancient Greeks burnt sea sponges and inhaled the vapors in prophylaxis against goiter.[53] Sponges harbor various biodynamic substances, with possible antineoplastic, antibacterial, growth-stimulating, antihypertensive, neuropharmacologic, psychopharmacologic, and antifungal properties.[85] A number of sponges produce crinotoxins that may be direct dermal irritants, such as subcritine, halitoxin (*Haliclonia* species), and okadaic acid.[161] Murine monoclonal antibodies against okadaic acid intended for use in an assay system for the detection of diarrhetic shellfish poisoning have been prepared from the sponge *Halichondria okadai.*[188]

Clinical Aspects

Two general syndromes, with minor variations, are induced by contact with sponges. The first is a pruritic dermatitis similar to plant-induced allergic dermatitis, although the dermatopathic agent has not been identified. Rarely, erythema multiforme or an anaphylactoid reaction may be present. A typical offender is the friable Hawaiian or West Indian fire sponge *(Tedania ignis),* a brilliant yellow-vermilion-orange organism with a "crumb-of-bread" appearance found off the Hawaiian Islands and the Florida Keys.[167] This sponge grows in branches extending from a larger base, which are easily broken off. Other culprits include *Fibula nolitangere,* the "poison bun sponge" (Fig. 52-1) and *Microciona prolifera,* the red moss sponge (found in the northeastern United States).[104] *F. nolitangere* is found in deeper water and grows in clusters, with holes (oscula) large enough to admit a diver's finger. It is brown and bready in texture, so it may crumble in the hands.

Within a few hours after skin contact the reactions are characterized by itching and burning, which may progress to local joint swelling, soft tissue edema, vesiculation, and stiffness, particularly if small pieces of broken sponge are retained in the skin near the interphalangeal or metacarpophalangeal joints. The skin may become mottled or purpuric.[167] Most victims of sponge-induced dermatitis have hand involvement, since they handle sponges without proper gloves. When the sponge is penetrated, torn, or crumbled, the skin is exposed to the toxic substances. Untreated, mild reactions subside within 3 to 7 days.[50] When large skin areas are involved the victim may complain of fever, chills, malaise, dizziness, nausea, muscle cramps, and formication. Bullae induced by contact with *Microciona prolifera* may become purulent. Systemic erythema multiforme or an anaphylactoid reaction may develop a week to 14 days after a severe exposure.[64,206]

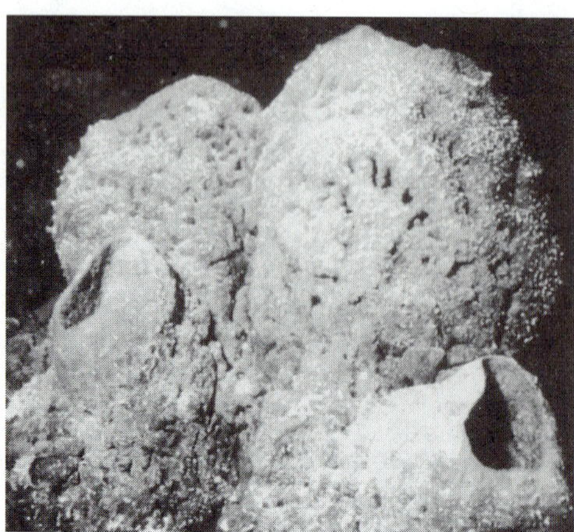

Fig. 52-1 The poison bun sponge *(Fibula nolitangere)* can produce sudden and intense skin inflammation.

The second syndrome is an irritant dermatitis and follows the penetration of small spicules of silica or calcium carbonate into the skin. Most sponges have spicules; "toxic" sponges may possess crinotoxins that enter microtraumatic lesions caused by the spicules.

In severe cases, surface desquamation of the skin may follow in 10 days to 2 months. No medical intervention can retard this process. Recurrent eczema and persistent arthralgias are rare complications.

Treatment

Because distinguishing clinically between the allergic and spicule-induced reactions is usually impossible, it is safest to treat for both. The skin should be gently dried. Spicules should be removed, if possible, using adhesive tape or a facial peel. As soon as possible, dilute (5%) acetic acid (vinegar) soaks for 10 to 30 minutes three or four times a day should be applied to all affected areas.[167,173,205] Isopropyl alcohol 40% to 70% is a reasonable second choice.[64] Although topical steroid lotions may help to relieve the secondary inflammation, they are of no value as an initial decontaminant. If they precede the vinegar soak, they appear to worsen the primary reaction. Delayed primary therapy or inadequate decontamination may result in the persistence of bullae, which may become purulent and require months to heal.

Erythema multiforme may require the administration of systemic corticosteroids, beginning with a moderately high dose (prednisone 60 to 100 mg) tapered over 2 to 3 weeks. Anecdotal remedies for the management of sponge envenomation that have been suggested without demonstration of efficacy include antiseptic dressings, broad-spectrum antibiotics, methdilazine, pyribenzamine, phenobarbital, diphenhydramine, promethazine, and topical carbolic oil or zinc oxide cream.[167]

After the initial decontamination a mild emollient cream or steroid preparation may be applied to the skin. If the allergic component is severe, particularly if there is weeping, crusting, and vesiculation, systemic corticosteroids (prednisone 60 to 100 mg, tapered over 2 weeks) may be beneficial. Severe itching may be controlled with an antihistamine.

Because *Clostridium tetani* has been cultured from sea sponges, they should not be used to pack wounds. Proper antitetanus immunization should be part of sponge dermatitis therapy. Frequent follow-up wound checks are important because significant infections sometimes develop.[105] Infected wounds should be cultured and managed with antibiotics (see Chapter 51). If sponge poisoning induces an anaphylactoid reaction, standard resuscitation using epinephrine, β-adrenergic bronchodilators, corticosteroids, and antihistamines should be undertaken.[206]

As mentioned previously, sponge diver's disease is not caused by any toxin produced by the sponge, but rather is a stinging syndrome related to contact with the tentacles of the small coelenterate anemone *Sagartia rosea* (family Sagartiidae) or anemones from the genus *Actinia* (family Actiniidae), which attach to the base of the sponge. Treatment should include that for coelenterate envenomation.

Prevention

All divers and net handlers should wear proper gloves. Sponges should not be broken, crumbled, or crushed with bare hands. If the victim brings a specimen, the physician should take care to document its appearance. Dried sponges may remain toxic.

COELENTERATES (CNIDARIA)

Coelenterates are an enormous group, comprising approximately 10,000 species, at least 100 of which are dangerous to humans. Coelenterates that possess the venom-charged stinging cells called nematocysts are known as cnidaria (nettle); those without nematocysts are acnidaria. For practical purposes the cnidaria can be divided into three main groups: (1) hydrozoans, such as the Portuguese man-of-war; (2) scyphozoans, such as true jellyfish; and (3) anthozoans, such as soft corals (alcyonarians), stony corals, and anemones. Gorgonians (order Gorgonacea, class Anthozoa, subclass Alcyonaria) secrete mucinous exudates having toxic effects in experimental animals that can be characterized as hemolytic, proteolytic, cholinergic, histaminergic, serotonergic, and adrenergic.[71]

Morphology, Venom, and Venom Apparatus

Coelenterates are predators that feed on other fish, crustaceans, and mollusks. They are radially symmetric animals of simple structure (95% water) and exist in two predominant life-forms, either as sedentary, asexual polyps (hydroids) or as free-swimming and sexual medusae. Generally the polyps are saclike creatures attached to the substrate at the caudal (aboral) end, with a single orifice or mouth at the upper end surrounded by stinging tentacles (dactylozooids). This form predominates in the hydrozoans and anthozoans. The medusa is a bell-shaped creature, with a floating gelatinous umbrella from which hang an elongated tubular mouth and marginal nematocyst-bearing tentacles. This form predominates in the scyphozoans and is also found in the hydrozoans.

The intracytoplasmic stinging organelles, or nematocysts (cnidocytes), are located on the outer epithelial surfaces of the tentacles or near the mouth and are triggered by contact with the victim's body surface. The nematocyst is contained within an outer capsule called the cnidoblast, to which is attached a single pointed "trigger" or cnidocil. The nematocyst is filled with fluid and contains a hollow, sharply pointed, coiled thread tube (nema) (Fig. 52-2). This tube may attain lengths of 200 to 400 μm and is sufficiently hardy to penetrate a surgical glove. The tube is lined with spines, which help it penetrate the victim. When the cnidocil is stimulated, either by physical contact or by a chemoreceptor mechanism, it causes the opening of a "trap door" (operculum) in the cnidoblast, and the venom-containing thread tube is everted (Fig. 52-3). This exocytosis has been hypothesized to occur because of osmotic swelling of the capsular matrix caused by influx of water, release of intrinsic tension forces, or defor-

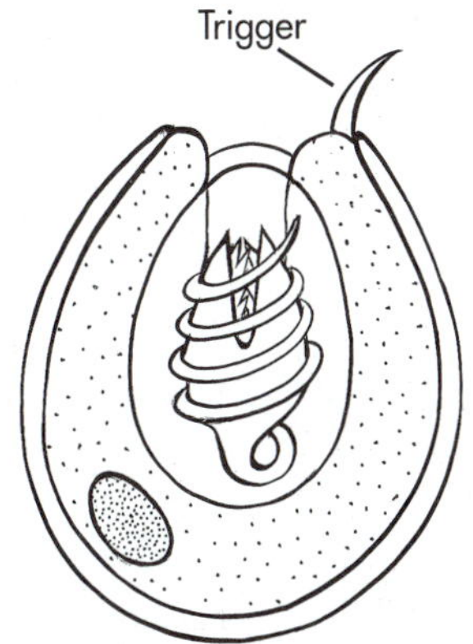

Fig. 52-2 Nematocyst before discharge.

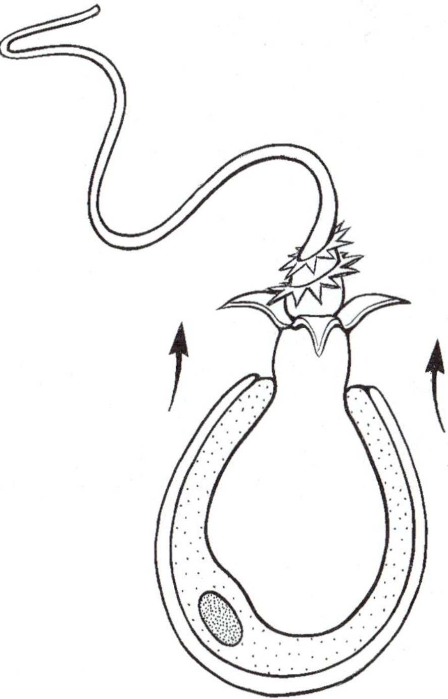

Fig. 52-3 Nematocyst after discharge.

mation of the wall-induced internal pressure. The sharp tip of the thread tube enters the victim's skin and envenomation occurs. It has been estimated that the velocity of ejection attains 2 m/sec, which corresponds to an acceleration of 40,000 g, with an estimated skin striking force of 2 to 5 PSI.[32,95] A human encounter with a large Portuguese man-of-war could conceivably trigger the release of several million stinging cells. The thread penetrates the epidermis and upper dermis, where the viscous venom diffuses into the general circulation. The agitated victim runs and assists the venom's distribution by the muscle-pump mechanism. Based on mouse studies, it appears that the rapid death of a victim is related to the discharge of venom directly into the capillaries, as opposed to that which must diffuse into the bloodstream from the dermis.[98]

In the case of the Indo-Pacific box-jellyfish *Chironex fleckeri,* it is the cigar-shaped microbasic p-mastigophores that are most important in human envenomation (Fig. 52-4). The capsule of the structure holds a hollow coiled tube and granular matrix. The thread tube has a thick butt end that is attached to the operculum. The tube contains three rows of helically arranged spines. When the nematocyst fires into the human victim, the tube everts through the opercular end of the nematocyst, with the butt anchoring first to keep the nematocyst adherent to the victim. The thread then everts through the hollow butt and uncoils, presenting the spines and accompanying toxins to the living tissue.

Coelenterate venoms are viscous mixtures of proteins, carbohydrates, and other nonproteinaceous components. To date, they have been difficult to fractionate. Although they are heat labile in vitro, this does not seem to apply in the clinical setting. The primary difficulties encountered in jellyfish venom purification are the lack of stability and the tendency of active toxins to adhere to each other and to support matrices.[139]

Clinical Aspects

For clinical purposes, a considerable phylogenetic relationship exists among all stinging species, so that the clinical features of the coelenterate syndrome are fairly constant,

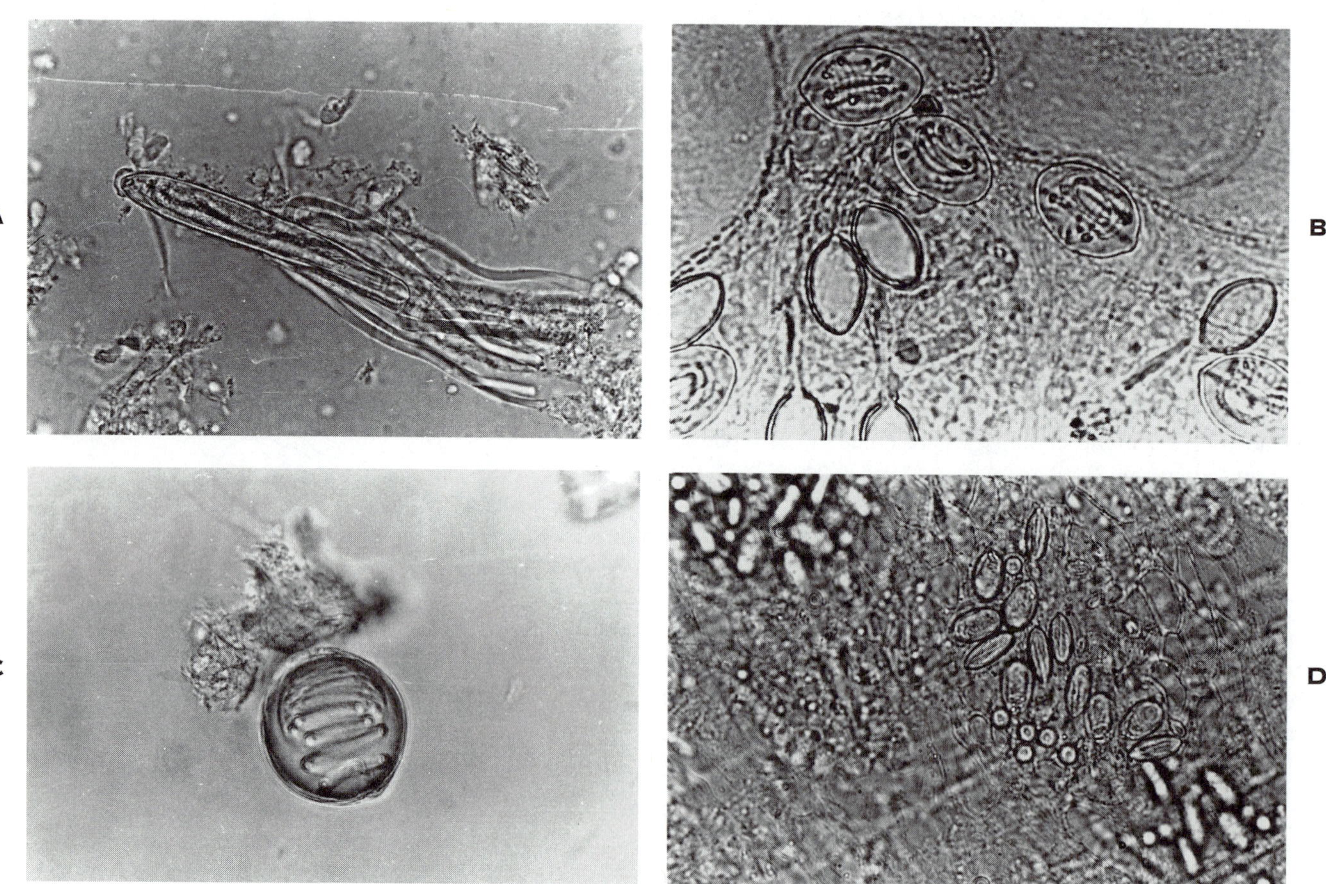

Fig. 52-4 Nematocyst identification guide **A,** Microbasic p-mastigophore (undischarged) of *Chironex fleckeri.* Capsule length 75 µm. **B,** Same (discharged and undischarged) of Irukandji. **C,** Isorhiza (undischarged) of "bluebottle"—*Physalia utriculus.* **D,** Clustered isorhizas and euryteles on tentacle of "hair jelly"—*Cyanea.* (All courtesy Bob Hartwick.)

with a spectrum of severity. This is related to the season and species (venom potency and configuration of the nematocyst), the number of nematocysts triggered and the size of the animal (venom inoculum), the size and age of the victim (the very young and old and the smaller person tend to be more severely affected), the location and surface area of the sting, and the health of the victim. The wise clinician suspects a coelenterate envenomation in all unexplained cases of collapse in the surf, diving accidents, and near drownings. Any victim in distress pulled from marine waters should be carefully examined for one or more cutaneous lesions that may provide the clue to a coelenterate envenomation. While the major toxic fractions appear to be present in the nematocysts, there appears to be toxic material present in tentacles denuded of such organelles.[26]

Mild envenomation may result only in an annoying dermatitis, whereas severe envenomation can progress rapidly to involve virtually every organ system, resulting in significant morbidity and mortality. Clinical envenomation is described here by severity, with the understanding that there is a fair amount of overlap.

Mild Envenomation

The stings caused by the hydroids and hydroid corals, along with lesser envenomations by *Physalia, Velella vellela,* scyphozoans, and anemones, result predominantly in skin irritation. There is usually an immediate pricking or stinging sensation, accompanied by pruritus, paresthesias, burning, throbbing, and radiation of the pain centrally from the extremities to the groin, abdomen, and axillae. The area involved by the nematocysts becomes red-brown-purple, often in a linear whiplike fashion, corresponding to "tentacle prints." Other features are blistering, local edema, and wheal formation, as well as violaceous petechial hemorrhages. The papular inflammatory skin rash is strictly confined to the areas of contact and may persist for up to 10 days. Areas of body hair appear to be somewhat more protected from contact than hairless areas. If the envenomation is slightly more severe, the aforementioned symptoms, which are evident in the first few hours, can progress over a course of days to local necrosis, skin ulceration, and secondary infection. This is particularly true of certain anemone *(Sagartia, Actinia, Anemonia, Actinodendron,* and *Triactis)* stings.

Untreated, the minor to moderate skin disorder resolves over 1 to 2 weeks, with occasional residual hyperpigmentation for 1 to 2 months. Rubbing can cause lichenification. Local hyperhidrosis, fat atrophy, and contracture may occur.[31] Permanent scarring may result. Persistent papules or plaques at the sites of contact may demonstrate a predominantly mononuclear cell inflammatory infiltrate, which may represent a delayed hypersensitivity response to an antigenic component of the coelenterate nematocyst or venom. This may be accompanied by localized arthritis and joint effusion. It has been suggested that sensitization may occur without a definite history of a previous sting, since coelenterates may release antigenic and allergenic venom components into the water. Granuloma annulare, which is usually both a sporadic and a familial inflammatory dermatosis, has been associated with a *Physalia utriculus* envenomation.[119]

Moderate and Severe Envenomation

The prime offenders in this group are the anemones, *Physalia* species, and scyphozoans. The skin manifestations are similar or intensified (as with *Chironex*) and are compounded by the onset of systemic symptoms, which may appear immediately or be delayed by several hours:

1. Neurologic—malaise, headache, aphonia, diminished touch and temperature sensation, vertigo, ataxia, spastic or flaccid paralysis, mononeuritis multiplex, parasympathetic dysautonomia, plexopathy, radial-ulnar-median nerve palsies, brainstem infarction (not a confirmed relationship), delirium, loss of consciousness, convulsions, coma, and death[40,63,128,144]
2. Cardiovascular—anaphylaxis, hemolysis, hypotension, small artery spasm, bradyarrhythmias (including electromechanical dissociation and asystole), tachyarrhythmias, congestive heart failure, and ventricular fibrillation[115,146,183]
3. Respiratory—rhinitis, bronchospasm, laryngeal edema, dyspnea, cyanosis, pulmonary edema, and respiratory failure
4. Musculoskeletal or rheumatologic—abdominal rigidity, diffuse myalgia and muscle cramps, muscle spasm, fat atrophy, arthralgias, reactive arthritis (seronegative symmetric synovitis with pitting edema),[191] and thoracolumbar pain
5. Gastrointestinal—nausea, vomiting, diarrhea, dysphagia, hypersalivation, and thirst
6. Ocular—conjunctivitis, chemosis, corneal ulcers, iridocyclitis, elevated intraocular pressure, synechiae, iris depigmentation, chronic unilateral glaucoma, and lacrimation[74,75]
7. Other—acute renal failure, chills, fever, and nightmares

The extreme example of envenomation occurs with *Chironex fleckeri,* the dreaded box-jellyfish. *Physalia* and anemone stings, although extremely painful, are rarely fatal. Death after *Physalia* stings has been attributed to primary respiratory failure or cardiac arrhythmia.[34,175]

Clinical reports and studies on the serologic response to jellyfish envenomation suggest that allergic reactions may play a significant pathophysiologic role in humans.[125] When crude or partially purified nematocyst venom and an antigen are used in an enzyme-linked immunosorbent assay (ELISA), both IgG and IgE can be detected.[72,158] Elevated specific antijellyfish IgG and IgE may persist for several years, recurrence of the clinical cutaneous reaction to jellyfish stings may occur within a few weeks without additional contact with the tentacles, and serologic cross-reactivity between the sea nettle *(Chrysaora quinquecirrha)* and *Physalia physalis* occurs.[36] In a case of significant envenomation by the moon jellyfish *Aurelia aurita,* the patient developed significant cross-reacting antibodies to *Chrysaora quinquecirrha* antigens.[33]

Persons with extracutaneous or anaphylactoid responses to a coelenterate sting have been noted to have higher specific IgG and IgE antibody levels.[158] However, elevated persistent specific antijellyfish serum IgG concentrations are not protective against the cutaneous pain resulting from a natural sting.[38] A false-positive ELISA serologic test to venom may occur, as demonstrated by negative skin testing.

A person recently stung by *Physalia physalis* may have recurrent cutaneous eruptions for 2 to 3 weeks after the initial episode, without repeated exposure to the animal. This may take the form of lichenification, hyperhidrosis, angioedema, vesicles, large bullae, nodules that resemble erythema nodosum, granuloma annulare, or a more classic linear urticarial eruption.[8,37,122] Recurrent eruptions have also followed a solitary envenomation by the cnidarian *Stomolophus meleagris.*[30] In a histologic study of delayed reaction to a Mediterranean Sea coelenterate, skin biopsy demonstrated grouping of human leukocyte antigen-DR-positive cells with Langerhans cells and helper/inducer T lymphocytes, which indicates the possibility of a type IV immunoreaction.[145]

Venom-specific IgG antibodies appear to persist for longer periods than IgM antibodies. The binding of brown recluse spider venom and purified cholera toxin to anti-*Chrysaora* and anti-*Physalia* monoclonal antibodies indicates that there may be a common or cross-reacting antigenic site or sites between these toxic substances and certain coelenterate venoms.[137]

Acute regional vascular insufficiency of the upper extremity has been reported after jellyfish envenomation. It can be manifested by acral ischemia, signs and symptoms of compartment syndrome, and massive edema.[202]

Treatment

Therapy is directed at stabilizing major systemic decompensation, opposing the venom's multiple effects, and alleviating pain.

Systemic Envenomation. Generally, only severe *Physalia* or Cubomedusae stings result in rapid decompensation. In both cases supportive care is based on the signs and symptoms. Hypotension should be managed with the prompt intravenous administration of crystalloid, such as lactated Ringer's solution.[186] This must be done in concert with detoxification of any nematocysts (particularly those of *Chironex* or *Chiropsalmus*) that are still attached to the victim, to limit the perpetuation of envenomation. Hypotension is usually limited to very young or elderly victims who suffer severe and multiple stings, the effects of which are worsened by fluid depletion that accompanies protracted vomiting. Hypertension is an occasional side effect of a cubomedusan envenomation, such as that of *Carukia barnesii.* Excessive catecholamine stimulation is one putative cause, which has prompted clinical intervention with phentolamine, an α-adrenergic blocking agent (5 mg intravenously as an initial dose). Bronchospasm may be managed as an allergic component. If the victim is in respiratory distress with wheezing, shortness of breath, or heart failure, arterial blood gas measurement may be used to guide supplemental oxygen administration by face mask.[107] Seizures are generally self-limited but should be treated with intravenous diazepam for 24 to 48 hours, after which time they rarely recur.

All victims with a systemic component should be observed for a period of at least 6 to 8 hours because rebound phenomena after successful treatment are not uncommon. All elderly victims should undergo electrocardiography and be observed on a cardiac monitor, with frequent checks for arrhythmias. Urinalysis demonstrates the presence or absence of hemoglobinuria, indicating hemolysis after the putative attachment of *Physalia* venom to red blood cell membrane glycoprotein sites.[81,115,174] If this is the case, the urine should be alkalinized with bicarbonate to prevent the precipitation of pigment in the renal tubules, while a moderate diuresis (30 to 50 ml/hr) is maintained with a loop diuretic (such as furosemide) or mannitol (0.25 g/kg intravenously every 8 to 12 hours). In rare instances of acute progressive renal failure, peritoneal dialysis or hemodialysis may be necessary.

If there are signs of distal ischemia or an impending compartment syndrome, standard diagnostic and therapeutic measures apply. These include Doppler ultrasound, angiography, or both for diagnosis, regional thrombolysis for acutely occluded blood vessels, measurement of intracompartmental tissue pressures to guide fasciotomy, and so forth. Reversible regional sympathetic blockade may be efficacious if vasospasm is a dominant clinical feature. However, the vasospasm associated with a jellyfish envenomation may be severe, prolonged, and refractory to regional sympathectomy and intraarterial reserpine or pentoxifylline.[2]

A small child may pick up tentacle fragments on the beach and place them into his or her mouth, resulting in rapid intraoral swelling and potential airway obstruction, particularly in the presence of exceptional hypersensitivity. In such cases an endotracheal tube should be placed before edema precludes visualization of the vocal cords. In no case should any liquid be placed in the mouth if the airway is not protected.

Chironex fleckeri, the box-jellyfish, produces the only coelenterate venom for which a specific antidote exists. To date, the venoms of *Physalia* and *Chrysaora* species have not been sufficiently purified as antigens to permit the production of an antitoxin. Antivenin administration may be lifesaving and should accompany the first aid protocol previously described.

Pain Control. Often the pain can be controlled by treating the dermatitis. However, if pain is excruciating and there is no contraindication (such as head injury, altered mental status, respiratory depression, allergy, profound hypotension), the administration of narcotics (morphine sulfate, 2 to 10 mg intravenously; nalbuphine, 2 to 10 mg intravenously or intramuscularly; meperidine, 50 to 100 mg, with hydroxyzine, 25 to 50 mg intramuscularly, or meperidine, 15 to 30 mg, with promethazine, 12.5 to 25 mg, or prochlorperazine, 2.5 mg intravenously) is often indicated. Severe muscle spasm may respond to 10% calcium gluconate (5 to 10 ml intravenous slow push), diazepam (5 to 10 mg intravenously), or methocarbamol (1 g, no faster than 100 mg/min through a widely patent intravenous line).

Treatment of Dermatitis. If a person is stung by a coelenterate, the following steps should be taken:

1. Immediately rinse the wound with seawater, *not with fresh water*. Do not rub the wound with a towel or clothing to remove adherent tentacles. Fresh water and abrasion will stimulate any nematocysts that have not already fired. Remove the gross tentacles with forceps or a well-gloved hand. The keratinized palm of the hand is relatively protected, but take care not to become envenomed.

Commercial (chemical) cold packs applied over a dry cloth have been shown to be effective when applied to mild or moderate *Physalia* stings.[58] Whether the direct application of ice to envenomed skin and the resulting freshwater melt stimulate the discharge of nematocysts has not been determined.

Application of hot packs or gentle rinses with hot water are not recommended because they may worsen the envenomation or in repeated applications lead to lymphangitis.[62] However, beach patrol members who have been stung by jellyfish (presumably, Portuguese man-of-war) report that an immediate hot shower with a forceful stream of water relieves the pain. This observation implies that a forceful jet of water that might dislodge tentacle fragments and nematocysts can supersede the deleterious effects of fresh (hypotonic) water that lead to nematocyst discharge.

2. Acetic acid 5% (vinegar) is the treatment of choice to inactivate the toxin. An alternative is isopropyl alcohol (40% to 70%). Perfume, aftershave lotion, and high-proof liquor are less efficacious and may be detrimental. The detoxicant should be applied continuously for at least 30 minutes or until the pain is relieved. Vinegar will not alleviate the pain from a *Chironex* sting but interrupts the envenomation. It may not be extremely effective against *Chrysaora* or *Cyanea*. Other substances reputed to be effective as alternatives are organic solvents such as formalin, ether, and gasoline (all to be condemned), dilute ammonium hydroxide, sodium bicarbonate (particularly for stings of the sea nettle, *Chrysaora quinquecirrha*), olive oil, sugar, urine, and papain (papaya latex [juice] or unseasoned meat tenderizer). The last is supposed to work by cleaving active polypeptides into nontoxic amino acids. There is recent evidence that alcohol may stimulate the discharge of nematocysts in vitro; the clinical significance is as yet undetermined. A commercial aqueous solution of aluminum sulfate 20% and 1.1% surfactant (Stingose) is an alternative. It has been proposed that the aluminum ion interacts with proteins and long-chain polysaccharide components to denature and inactivate the venom. Prior treatment with topical alcohol or methylated spirits reduces the effectiveness of the aluminum sulfate solution. This product seems to be falling out of favor with clinicians who are jellyfish experts in Australia. The pressure-immobilization technique for venom sequestration should not be used until after vinegar application; a venolymphatic occlusive "tourniquet" should be considered only if a topical detoxicant is unavailable, the victim suffers from a severe systemic reaction, and transport to definitive care is delayed.

3. No systemic drugs are of verifiable use. Ephedrine, atropine, calcium, methysergide, and hydrocortisone have all been touted at one time or another, but no proof exists that they help. Antihistamines may be useful if there is a significant allergic component. The administration of epinephrine is appropriate only in the setting of anaphylaxis.

4. Immersing the area in hot water is generally not recommended; the hypotonic solution causes nematocysts to fire.

5. Once the wound has been soaked with vinegar or alcohol, the remaining nematocysts must be removed. The easiest way to do this is to apply shaving cream or a paste of baking soda, flour, or talc and to shave the area with a razor or similar tool. If sophisticated facilities are not available, the nematocysts should be removed by making a sand or mud paste with seawater and using this to help scrape the victim's skin with a sharp-edged shell or piece of wood. The rescuer must take care not to become envenomed; bare hands must be rinsed frequently.

6. Local anesthetic ointments (lidocaine, 2.5%) or sprays (benzocaine, 14%), antihistaminic creams (diphenhydramine or tripelennamine), or mild steroid lotions (hydrocortisone, 1%) may be soothing. They are to be used after the toxin is inactivated. Paradoxical reactions to benzocaine are rarely noted.

7. Patients should receive standard antitetanus prophylaxis.

8. Prophylactic antibiotics are not needed. The wounds should be checked at 3 and 7 days after injury for infection. Any ulcerating lesions should be cleaned three times a day and covered with a thin layer of nonsensitizing antiseptic ointment. A jellyfish sting to the cornea may cause a foreign body sensation, photophobia, and decreased or hazy vision. Ophthalmologic examination reveals hyperemic sclera, chemosis, and irregularity of the corneal epithelium with stromal edema. Depending on the extent of the wound, the anterior chamber may demonstrate the inflammatory response of iridocyclitis ("flare" with or without cells).[204] The patient should be referred to an ophthalmologist, who may prescribe steroid-containing eye medications such as prednisolone acetate 1% with hyoscine 0.25%. Applying traditional skin detoxicants directly to the cornea is not recommended, since they are likely to worsen the tissue injury.

Delayed Reaction. A delayed reaction in areas of skin contact similar in appearance to erythema nodosum may be accompanied by fever, weakness, arthralgias, painful joint swelling, and effusions. This may recur multiple times over the course of 1 to 2 months. The treatment is a 10- to 14-day taper of prednisone, starting with 50 to 100 mg. This may need to be prolonged or repeated with each flare of the reaction.

Persistent Hyperpigmentation. Postinflammatory hyperpigmentation is common after the stings of many jellyfish and other lesser coelenterates. A solution of 1.8% hydroquinone in a glycol and alcohol base (70% ethyl alcohol and propylene glycol mixed at a 3:2 ratio) twice a day as a topical agent for 3 to 5 weeks has been used successfully to treat hyperpigmentation after a *Pelagia noctiluca* sting.

Prevention

Unfortunately, no agent that can be applied to the skin reliably protects the user from a sting. Failed topical barriers include petrolatum, mineral oil, silicone ointment, cocoa butter, and mechanic's grease. If jellyfish are sighted, they should be given a wide berth because the tentacles may trail great distances from the body. All swimmers and divers in hazardous areas should be on constant alert (Fig. 52-5). Persons should not dive head first into jellyfish-infested waters; it is far safer to walk in. Bathers should wear protective clothing in infested areas. This includes "stinger suits" or a double thickness of panty hose.[59] If "stinger enclosures" are present, bathers should stay within the netted barriers (Fig. 52-6). Divers should remain deeper than 20 feet to avoid surface concentrations of the animals and should always check snorkel and regulator mouthpieces for tentacle fragments in endemic areas. In areas inhabited by anemones and hydroid corals, protective gloves should be worn when handling specimens. Beached dead jellyfish or tentacle fragments washed up after a storm can still inflict serious stings. Any person stung by a jellyfish should leave or be assisted from the water because of the risk of drowning.

To gather prospective data, the International Consortium for Jellyfish Stings has been formed, with representatives largely from the United States and Australia (Fig. 52-7). At the time of this writing, a marine sting or bite report form can be obtained from Joseph W. Burnett, M.D., Department of Dermatology, 6th Floor, University of Maryland Hospital, 405 West Redwood Street, Baltimore, MD 21201-1703. The Australian contacts are John Williamson, M.D., Hyperbaric Medicine, Royal Adelaide Hospital, South Australia 5000, Australia, and Peter Fenner, M.D., P.O. Box 3034, North Mackay, Queensland 4740, Australia.

Hydrozoa

The hydrozoans range in configuration from the feather hydroids and sedentary *Millepora* hydroid coral to the free-floating siphonophore *Physalia* (Portuguese man-of-war). These are perfect examples of the class Hydrozoa.

Hydroids. Hydroids are the most numerous of the hydrozoans (Fig. 52-8). The feather hydroids of the order Leptomedusae, typified by *Lytocarpus philippinus* ("fire weed" or "fire fern"), are featherlike or plumelike animals that sting the victim who brushes against or handles them[150] (Color Plate 113). After a storm the branches may be fragmented and dispersed through the water, so that merely diving or swimming in the vicinity causes itching and burning and may induce a visible skin irritation.

Clinical aspects. Contact with the nematocysts of a feather hydroid induces a mild reaction, which consists of instantaneous burning, itching, and urticaria. If the exposure is brief, the skin rash may not be noticeable or it may consist of a faint erythematous miliary irritation (Fig. 52-9). A second variety of envenomation consists of a delayed papular, hemorrhagic, or zosteriform reaction with onset 4 to 12 hours after contact.[64] Rarely, erythema multiforme or a desquamative eruption may develop. In turbulent waters or in a strong current, fragments may be washed into a diver's mask or regulator mouthpiece; this will be evident as a burning sensation in the conjunctivae or oral mucous mem-

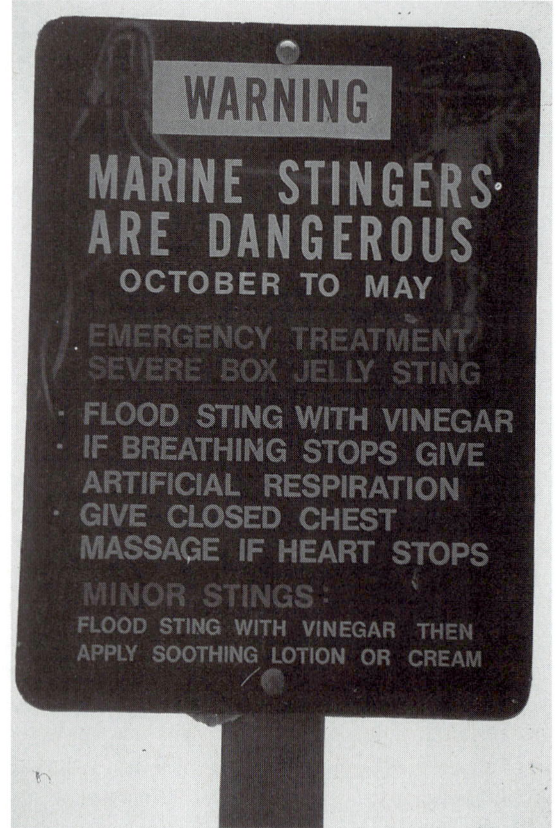

Fig. 52-5 Swimmers should obey posted warning signs developed for their protection.

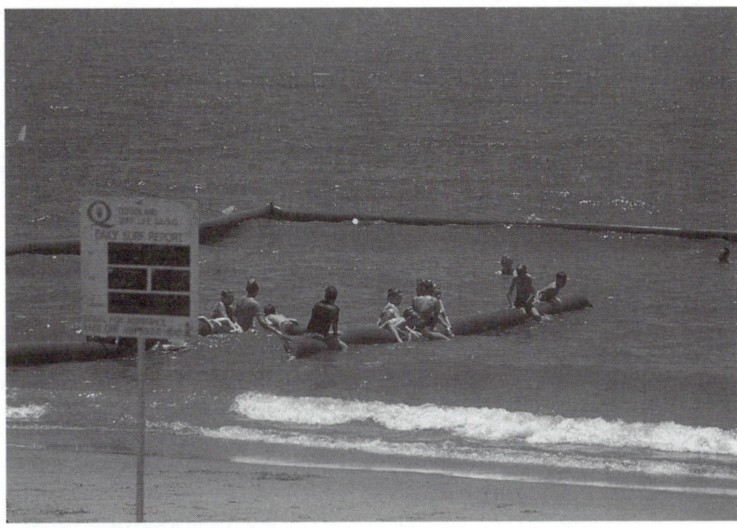

Fig. 52-6 Nets suspended from floating tubes provide some degree of protection in Cairns, Australia, for bathers during the box-jellyfish season.

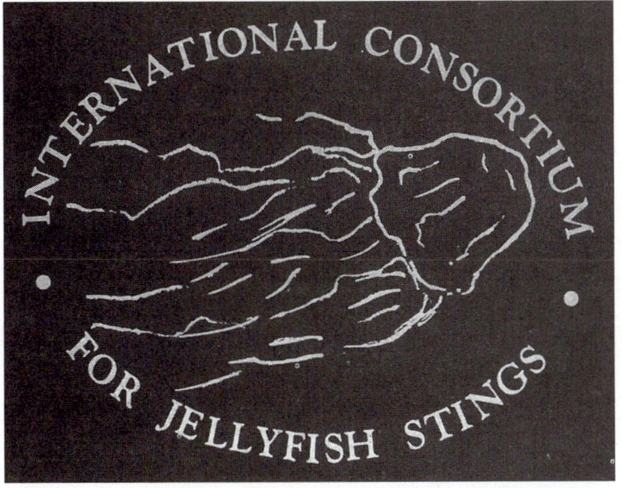

Fig. 52-7 Logo for the International Consortium for Jellyfish Stings.

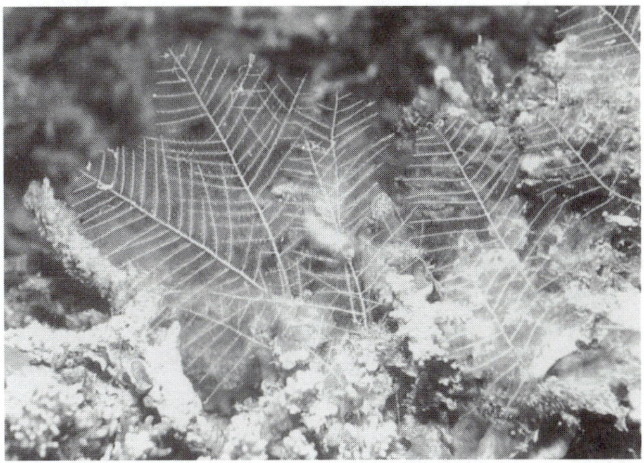

Fig. 52-8 Coelenterate hydroid.

branes. Systemic manifestations (such as abdominal pain, nausea, vomiting, diarrhea, muscle cramps, and fever) are rarely reported and are associated with large areas of surface involvement. Allergic sensitization and subsequent anaphylaxis have been proposed.

Treatment. The skin should be rinsed with seawater and gently dried without abrasive activity. Application of fresh water and brisk rubbing are strictly prohibited because they encourage any nematocysts remaining on the skin to discharge and thus worsen the envenomation. Acetic acid 5% (vinegar) or isopropyl alcohol 40% to 70% has been traditionally recommended for application to the skin for 15 to 30 minutes to relieve the cutaneous reaction. In an in vitro evaluation, vinegar and urine caused discharge of a few nematocysts in 10% to 15% of defensive tentacle polyps; methylated spirits were found to cause gross discharge of microbasic mastigophores in all defensive polyps.[150] Fresh water did not cause discharge. On the basis of this study the authors recommended that freshwater irrigation and the application of ice be used to treat acute stings. However, the clinical correlation remains to be described.

Alternative topical agents are discussed in the larger discussion on therapy for coelenterate stings. After pain relief is achieved, a mild steroid cream (hydrocortisone 1%) or moisturizing lotion may be applied.

Millepora (fire coral). The stony, hydroid, and coral-like *Millepora* species (for example, *M. alcicornis*), or fire corals, are not true corals. They are widely distributed in

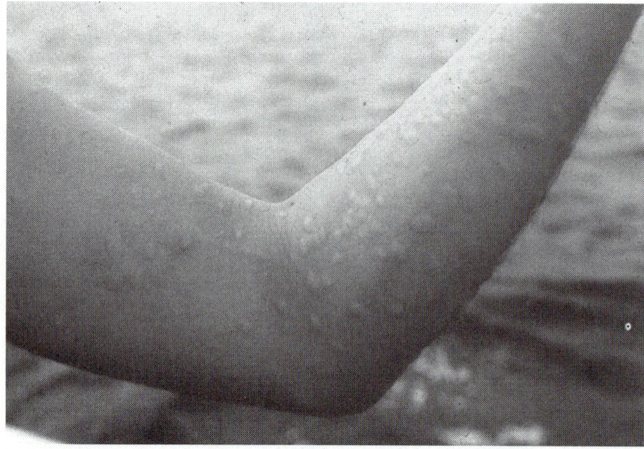

Fig. 52-9 Typical scattered miliary-urticarial rash from hydroids that have been fragmented in the water. (Courtesy John Williamson, M.D.)

shallow tropical waters. Sessile creatures, they are found attached to the bottom in depths of up to 1000 m. They are often mistaken for seaweed because they attach to pilings, rocks, shells, or coral. Although smaller segments resemble Christmas trees or bushes 3 to 4 inches in height, they may attain heights of 2 m (Fig. 52-10). The color ranges from white to yellow-green, with pale yellow most common. Fire coral is structured on a razor-sharp lime carbonate exoskeleton, which is an important component in the development of coral reefs. The outcroppings assume upright, clavate, bladelike, or branching calcareous growth structures that form encrustations over coral and objects such as sunken vessels. From numerous minute surface gastropores protrude tiny nematocyst-bearing tentacles, wherein lies the stinging apparatus. *M. alcicornis* probably accounts for more coelenterate envenomations than any other species. Unprotected and unwary recreational scuba enthusiasts handle, kneel, or lean on this marine stinger regularly.

CLINICAL ASPECTS. Immediately after contact with fire coral, the victim suffers burning or stinging pain, with, rarely, central radiation. Intense and painful pruritus follows within seconds, which frequently induces the victim to rub the affected area vigorously, worsening the envenomation. Over the course of 5 to 30 minutes, urticarial wheals develop, marked by redness, warmth, and pruritus (Fig. 52-11). The wheals become moderately edematous and reach a maximum size in 30 to 60 minutes. Untreated, they flatten over 14 to 24 hours and resolve entirely over 3 to 7 days, occasionally leaving an area of hyperpigmentation that may require 4 to 8 weeks to disappear. The pain generally resolves without treatment in 30 to 90 minutes. In the case of multiple stings, regional lymph nodes may become inflamed and painful. This does not necessarily indicate a secondary infection. Long thoracic mononeuritis with serratus anterior muscle paralysis has been described after *Millepora* sting confirmed by demonstrated presence of immune-specific IgG.[129]

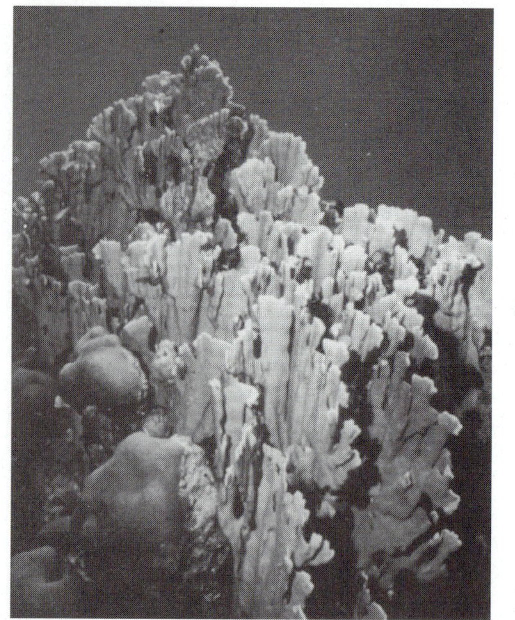

A

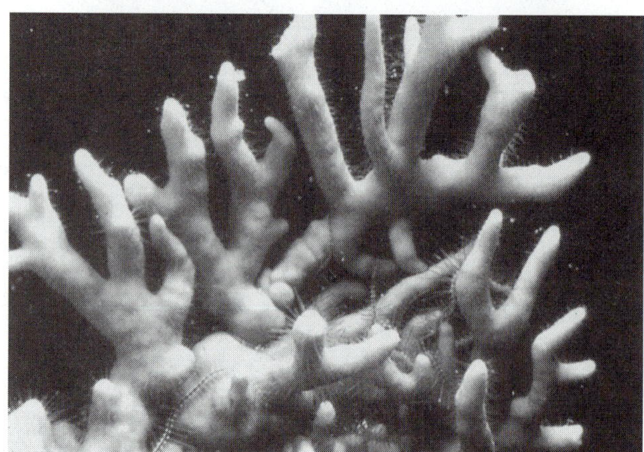

B

Fig. 52-10 Fire coral variations. **A,** Clavate blade form. **B,** Close view of branching form. (**A** Courtesy Dee Scarr.)

TREATMENT. The skin should be rinsed liberally with seawater and then immediately soaked with acetic acid 5% (vinegar) or isopropyl alcohol 40% to 70% until pain is relieved. Alternative topical agents are discussed in the larger coelenterate treatment section. Residual dermatitis is generally not very severe and can be managed in a fashion similar to that following a feather hydroid sting. If the rash becomes eczematous and indolent, it may respond to a course of systemic corticosteroids (prednisone 60 to 100 mg, tapered over 2 weeks).

Physalia (Man-of-War). The Atlantic Portuguese man-of-war *(Physalia physalis)* of the phylum Coelenterata, order Siphonophora, is a pelagic (open sea) polymorphic colonial siphonophore that inhabits the surface of the ocean. It is constructed of a blue or pink-violet and iridescent floating sail (pneumatophore), nitrogen and carbon monoxide

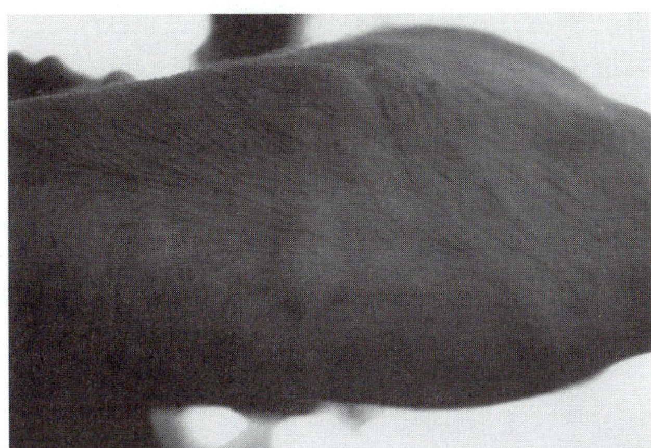

Fig. 52-11 Fire coral sting of the author. (Courtesy Kenneth Kizer, M.D.)

filled and up to 30 cm in length, from which are suspended multiple nematocyst-bearing tentacles, which may measure up to 30 m in length (Fig. 52-12). It has recently been reported that an Australian version of *Physalia physalis* is present in north Australian waters.[62] The smaller Pacific bluebottle *(Physalia utriculus)* usually has a single fishing tentacle, which attains lengths of up to 15 m (Fig. 52-13). In some species the sail can be deflated to allow the animal to submerge in rough weather.

The physaliae depend on the winds, currents, and tides for movement, traveling as individuals or in floating colonies that resemble flotillas. They are widely distributed but seem to abound in tropical waters and in the semitropical Atlantic Ocean, particularly off the coast of Florida and in the Gulf of Mexico. Their arrival at surf's edge can transform a halcyon vacation into a stinging nightmare. Unfortunately, peak appearance time for both the man-of-war and sea nettle is July through September, which is prime beach season.

As with icebergs, the scene above water conceals much of the story. Because the tentacles are nearly transparent, they pose a hazard to the unwary. As the animal moves in the ocean, the tentacles rhythmically contract, sampling the water for potential prey. If the tentacle strikes a foreign object, the nematocysts are stimulated and discharge their contents into the victim. Each tentacle in a larger specimen may carry more than 750,000 nematocysts. To increase the intensity of the "attack," the remainder of the tentacle shortens in such a way as to create loops and folds, presenting a greater surface area and number of nematocysts for offensive action in what are called "stinging batteries" (Fig. 52-14).

Detached moistened tentacles, often found by the thousands fragmented on the beach, carry live nematocysts capable of discharging for months. Air-dried nematocysts may retain considerable potency, even after weeks (Color Plate 114). The loggerhead turtle *(Caretta caretta)* feeds on *Physalia.* Like the clownfish with the sea anemone, the brightly colored fish *Nomeus gronovii* has a unique symbiotic relationship with the man-of-war, living freely among the tentacles. Two species of nudibranch (sea slug), *Glaucus atlanticus* and *G. glaucilla,* eat the tentacles and nematocysts of *P. physalis.* The nematocysts are not digested and ultimately reside in the dorsal papillae of the nudibranchs, where they may sting on contact.[64] Dermatitis can also result from contact with water containing venom that has already been released from stimulated nematocysts. The Mediterranean octopus *Tremoctopus violaceous* stores intact dactylozooid segments in its suckers for later use.[37]

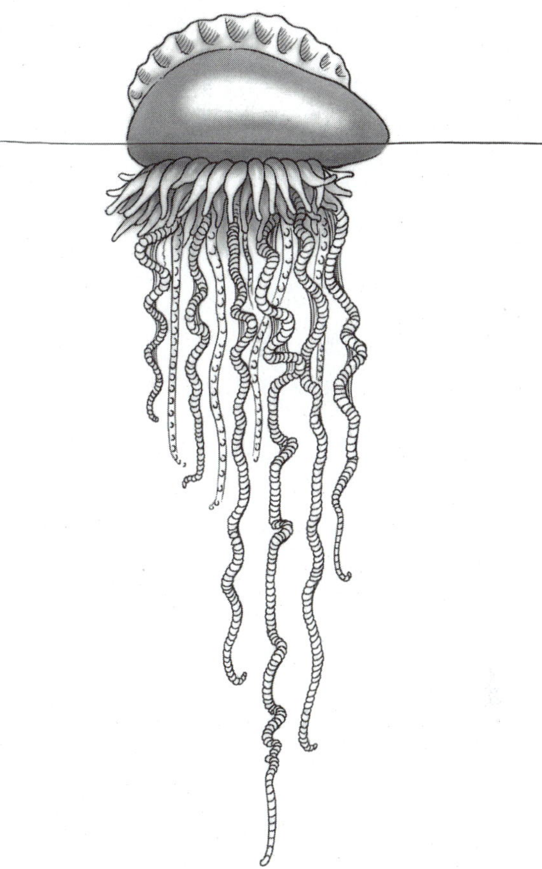

Fig. 52-12 Portuguese man-of-war, Atlantic Ocean version.

Sea Bather's Eruption

Sea bather's eruption, commonly termed "sea lice," refers to a dermatitis that results from contact with ocean water. In recent years it has become more of a problem afflicting ocean-goers in south Florida and across the Caribbean. It predominantly involves covered areas of the body and has been postulated, on the basis of epidemiologic analysis, to be caused by microscopic (0.5 mm) larvae of the thimble jellyfish *Linuche unguiculata* (Color Plate 115).[184] Another culprit off Long Island, New York, has been the planula larval form (visible at 2 to 3 mm) of the sea anemone *Edwardsiella lineata,* which carries hundreds of nematocysts.[66,67] Given the number of coelenterates that inhabit the oceans of the

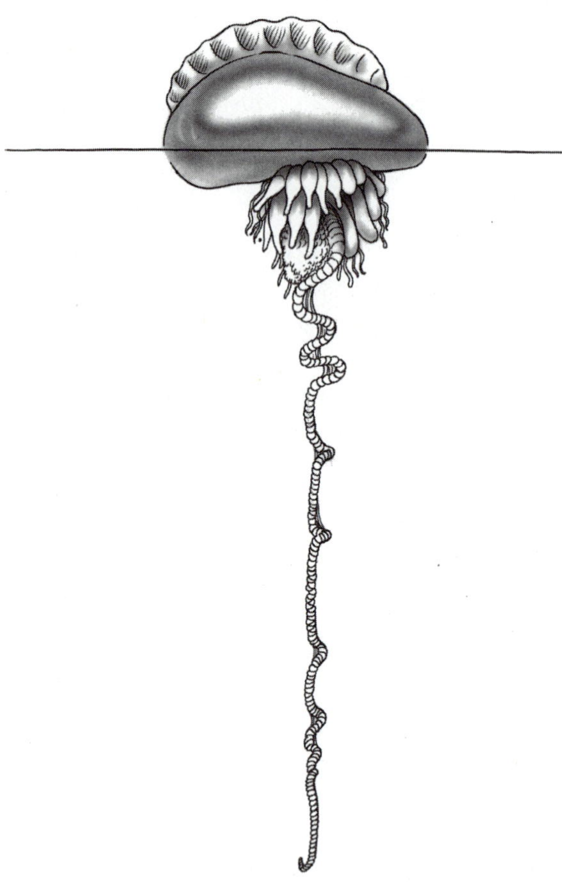

Fig. 52-13 Man-of-war, Pacific Ocean version.

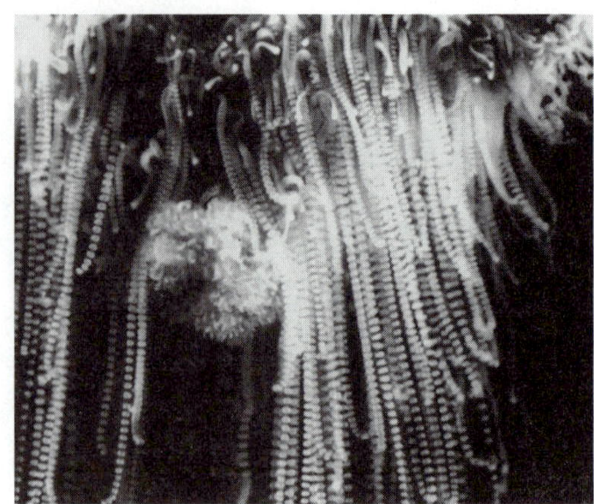

Fig. 52-14 Tentacles of the Atlantic Portuguese man-of-war. Nematocysts may number in the hundreds of thousands on tentacles coiled in "stinging batteries." (Courtesy Larry Madin, Woods Hole Oceanographic Institution.)

world and the cross-reactivity of antigens, it is likely that etiologic organisms are numerous.

A swimmer who encounters larvae usually complains of stinging soon after contact, often while in the water or soon after exiting. Application of fresh water may intensify the cutaneous reaction. The eruption occurs a few minutes to 12 hours after bathing and consists of pruritic, erythematous wheals, vesicles, or papules that persist for 2 to 14 days and then involute spontaneously. The areas involved include the buttocks, genital region, and breasts (women) (Color Plate 116). Coalescence indicates a large inoculum. Individual lesions resemble insect bites. Surfers develop lesions on areas that contact the surfboard (chest and anterior abdomen). The rash may also be seen under bathing caps and swim fins or along the edge of the cuffs of wet suits (Color Plate 117).[184] In children with extensive eruptions, fever is common. Other symptoms can include headache, chills, fatigue and malaise, vomiting, conjunctivitis, and urethritis. Itching is often pronounced at night and awakens the victim from sleep. Burnett and Burnett[25] reported blurred vision and left arm weakness in a teenager stung by "adult" *Linuche.* Persons who note a stinging sensation during the primary contact while still in the water may have a higher incidence of previous sensitization to the antigen or antigens. Persons who wear clothing that has been contaminated with the larvae may suffer recurrent reactions. Prior sensitization may precede prolonged (up to 6 weeks) reactions (rash and pruritus).

Elevated IgG levels specific for *Linuche unguiculata* can be measured by ELISA in the sera of patients who have suffered from sea bather's eruption.

The disorder is self-limited and rarely persists beyond 10 days. Treatment is palliative and consists of calamine lotion with 1% menthol. Because the lesions rarely extend into the dermis, topical corticosteroids may be helpful in mild cases. In more severe cases oral or parenteral antihistamines or systemic corticosteroids may be used. A thorough soap and water scrub (not a casual rinse) on leaving the water provides partial prophylaxis. Avoidance logically includes advice to ocean bathe in abbreviated swimwear, to maintain occlusive cuffs on dive skins and wet suits, to change swimwear as soon as possible after leaving the water, and to use caution during high season for *L. unguiculata* (April to July off south Florida) or *E. lineata* (August to November off Long Island) and when there are strong onshore winds. DermaShield (Benchmark Enterprises, Salt Lake City, Utah) is a barrier topical formulation that contains lanolin, aloe vera, and vitamin E. According to the manufacturer, this chemically inert (1-vinyl-2-pyrrolidione) protectant is hydrophobic (dimethicone and stearic acid) and does not wash off, but is shed as the epithelium sloughs naturally. It has been reported anecdotally by ocean bathers to protect against the agents of sea bather's eruption. At the time of this writing, no prospective evaluation of the use of DermaShield to protect against any coelenterate stings has been published.

True sea lice are parasites on marine creatures and do not cause this disorder (see Chapter 54).

Scyphozoa

This group of animals comprises the larger medusae or jellyfish, including the deadly box-jellyfish and sea wasps (for example, *Chironex, Cyanea,* and *Chiropsalmus*). These creatures are armed with some of the most potent venoms in existence. Jellyfish are mostly free-swimming pelagic creatures; however, some can be found at depths of more than 2000 fathoms. They may be transparent or multicolored and range in size from a few millimeters to more than 2 m in width across the bell, with tentacles up to 40 m in length. Like physaliae, the scyphozoans depend on the wind, currents, and tides for transport and are widely distributed. Some vertical motion may be produced by rhythmic contractions of the gelatinous bell, from which originate the feeding tentacles.

Some jellyfish contain less than 5% solid organic matter. Regardless, they can withstand remarkable temperature and salinity variations, although they do not fare well with violent activity and thus may descend to the depths during stormy surface weather. Some scyphozoans avoid sunlight; others follow an opposite pattern. Certain jellyfish have adapted to local nutrient (largely algal) supply and lost their ability to sting humans (Fig. 52-15).

In the eastern coastal waters of the North American continent, the creatures appear to grow larger as they progress north, so that true giant jellyfish, typified by *Cyanea capillata* (lion's mane), are found in arctic waters. Tentacles (which may number up to 1200) of larger specimens may exceed 100 feet in length (Fig. 52-16).[37] *Pelagia* species (purple-striped stingers) are commonly found in large numbers off the California coast. Australian jellyfish include the blubber jellyfish (*Catostylus* species), hair jellyfish (*Cyanea* species), little mauve stinger *(Pelagia noctiluca),* and the cuboid-shaped jellyfish *(Chironex fleckeri* and *Chiropsalmus quadrigatus).*[199] A number of cubomedusan ("box-shaped jellyfish") scyphozoans of highly toxic nature inhabit Indo-Pacific and, less frequently, Caribbean waters. These include *Carybdea rastoni* (jimble) and *C. marsupialis* (sea wasp), *Chiropsalmus quadrumanus* (box-jellyfish or sea wasp), *C. quadrigatus* (sea wasp), and *Chironex fleckeri* (box-jellyfish).[168]

Chironex (Box-Jellyfish). The dreaded box-jellyfish (*Chironex fleckeri* Southcott), often misnamed the "sea wasp," is the most venomous sea creature and can induce death in 30 seconds with its potent sting (Fig. 52-17). Like all other scyphozoans, it is a carnivore, adapted to deal rapidly with prey. It is a member of the group of Cubomedusae jellyfish and ranges in size from 2 to 10 cm across the bell (Color Plate 118). Although these creatures seem to prefer quiet, protected, and shallow areas, chiefly in the waters off northern Queensland, Australia, they can be found in the open ocean.[169] A seasonal alternation of polypoid and medusoid generations from winter to summer, respectively, appears to account for the shift in preferred habitat from tidal estuaries to the open eulittoral zone.[87] *Chironex* are fragile and photosensitive and thus are found submerged in bright sunlight, seeking the surface in the early morning, afternoon, and evening. They are swift and graceful travelers, capable of sailing along at a steady 2 knots.

An adult *Chironex* has enough venom (in excess of 10 ml) to kill three adults.[178] Two fractions have been isolated from the venom: a "lethal" fraction of molecular weight 150,000, and a lethal-hemolytic-dermatonecrotic fraction of molecular weight 79,000.[48,56,100,101] At least 72 fatalities have been verified in Australian and Southeast Asian waters, with greater numbers probably lacking official documentation.[195,199] Thus the box-jellyfish is a much greater true hazard than the more fearsome shark. Its lesser cohorts, such as *Carybdea rastoni* and *Pelagia noctiluca,* infrequently cause severe prolonged reactions and have rarely been reported to lead to death, but are capable of causing dramatic immediate reactions. Sudden death in a child has followed envenoma-

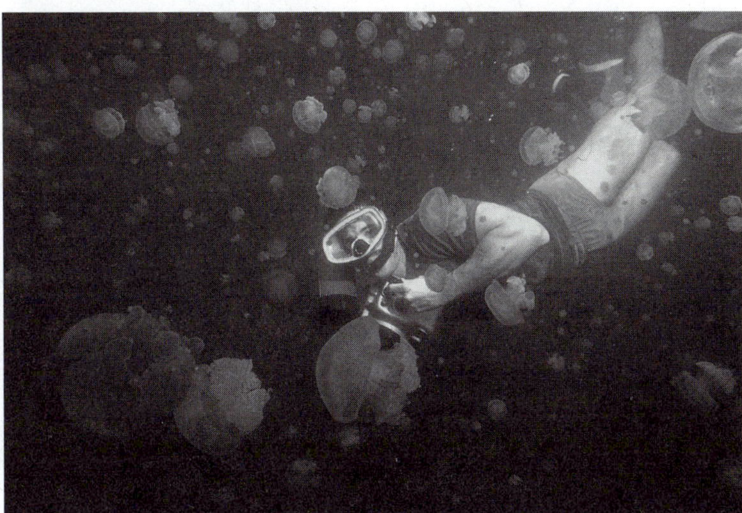

Fig. 52-15 The author snorkels in "Jellyfish Lake" in Palau. The jellyfish have evolved to subsist on algae and thus no longer pose a stinging hazard to humans. (Courtesy Avi Klapfer.)

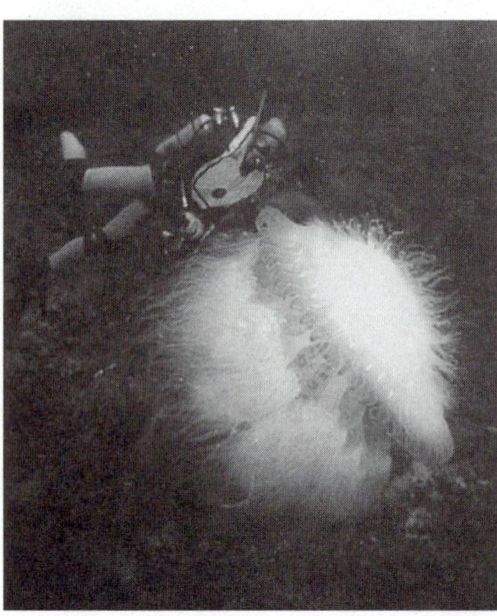

Fig. 52-16 Lion's mane jellyfish *(Cyanea capillata)*. (Courtesy Carl Roessler.)

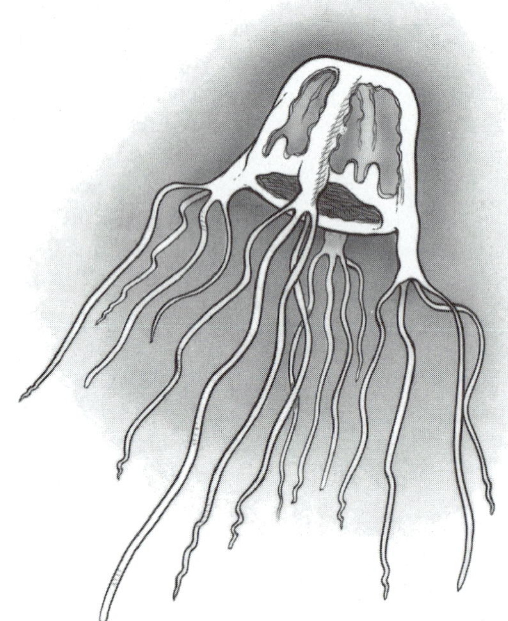

Fig. 52-17 The dreaded Indo-Pacific box-jellyfish *(Chironex fleckeri)*.

tion by *Chiropsalmus quadrumanus* in the Gulf of Mexico at Crystal Beach, Texas.[17] Death was attributed to acute arrhythmia after a catecholamine surge, followed by cardiogenic shock and pulmonary edema.

Clinical aspects. The extreme example of envenomation occurs with the chirodropid *Chironex fleckeri*. Death is attributed to hypotension, profound muscle spasm, muscular and respiratory paralysis, and subsequent cardiac arrest. The overall mortality after box-jellyfish stings may approach 15% to 20% in selected locales. Most commonly, bathers are stung, frequently aboriginal children in shallow and remote coastal waters who do not recognize the small, semitransparent, and submerged creature, which may approach as a member of a small armada. Most stings are minor; severe reactions or death follows skin contact with tentacles longer than 6 or 7 m.[179] The sting is immediately intensely painful, and the victim usually struggles purposefully for only a minute or two before collapse. The toxic skin reaction may be intense, with rapid formation of wheals, vesicles, and a darkened reddish brown or purple whiplike flare pattern with stripes 8 to 10 mm in width[101,103,207] (Fig. 52-18) (Color Plate 119). With major stings, skin blistering occurs within 6 hours, with superficial necrosis in 12 to 18 hours (Color Plate 120).[199] On occasion a pathognomonic "frosted" appearance with a transverse cross-hatched pattern may be present (Fig. 52-19) (Color Plate 121). More severe reactions and increased mortality in women and small children have been attributed to greater hairless body surface area and smaller body mass.[195]

Treatment. In the case of a known or suspected box-jellyfish envenomation, the victim must be assessed rapidly for adequacy of breathing and supported with an airway and artificial ventilation if necessary. The victim should be moved as little as possible. It is essential to immediately and liberally flood the skin surrounding any adherent tentacles

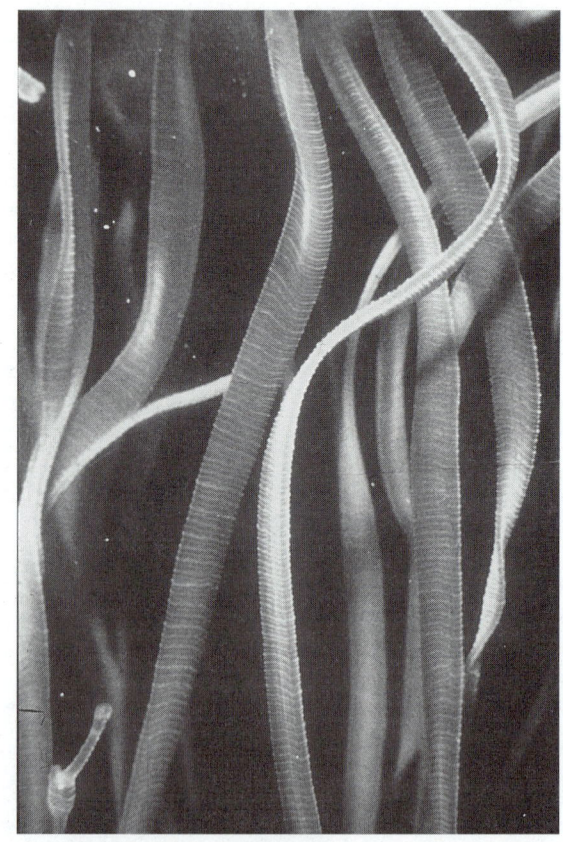

Fig. 52-18 Close-up view of the broad tentacles of *Chironex fleckeri*. (Courtesy John Williamson, M.D.)

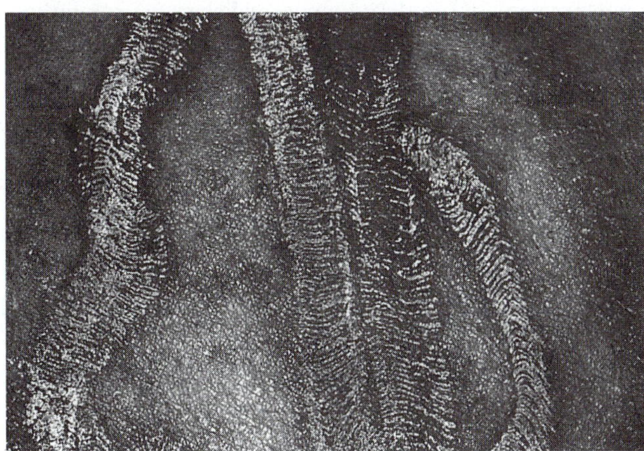

Fig. 52-19 Frosted cross-hatched skin pattern associated with box-jellyfish sting. (Courtesy John Williamson, M.D.)

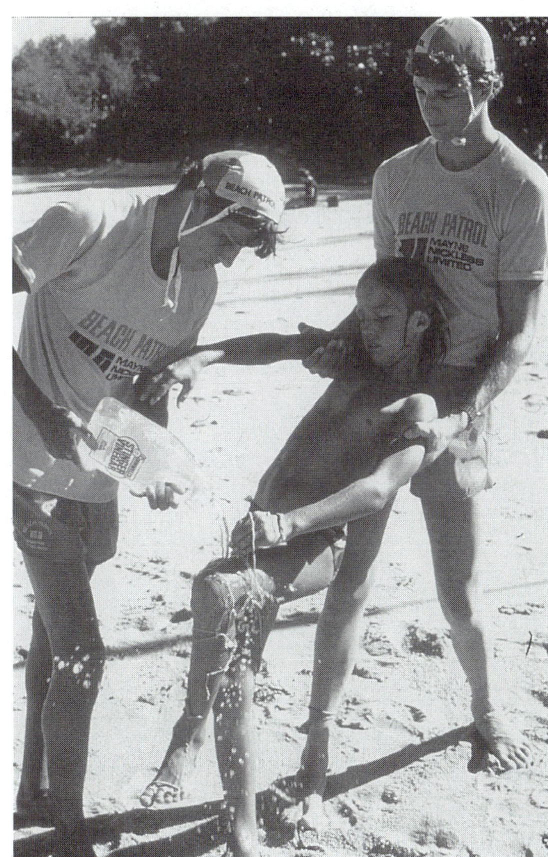

Fig. 52-20 Surf lifesavers pour vinegar on the leg of a child stung by a box-jellyfish. (Courtesy John Williamson, M.D.)

with acetic acid 5% (vinegar) before any attempt is made to remove them; this paralyzes the nematocysts and avoids worsening the envenomation (Fig. 52-20). Significant pain relief should not be expected from this maneuver. Although most nematocysts cannot penetrate the thickened skin of the human palm, the rescuer should pay particular attention to his or her own skin protection. If acetic acid is not available, aluminum sulfate surfactant (Stingose) may be used in substitution, although its efficacy has not been well demonstrated for a *Chironex* envenomation. Isopropyl alcohol 40% to 70% should be used as a last resort. A number of authors recommend that alcohol not be used, based on in vitro observations of inefficacy and nematocyst discharge after application of this detoxicant.[88,179]

Some authorities recommend immediate application of a constriction bandage proximal to the site of an extremity sting, to impede lymphatic and superficial venous return. The bandage should be loosened for 90 seconds every 10 minutes and should be completely removed after 1 hour. In no case should an arterial tourniquet be applied. The recently popularized pressure-immobilization bandaging technique could be used to prevent the absorption of *Chironex* venom, but it might also increase pain and skin damage by stimulating local nematocyst discharge.[178,200] If it is used, this should occur only after vinegar has been used to inactivate the nematocysts.

Chironex antivenin should be administered intravenously as soon as possible. The intramuscular route is less preferred. The antivenin is supplied in ampules of 20,000 units by Commonwealth Serum Laboratories, Melbourne, Australia (Fig. 52-21). The dose is one ampule (diluted 1:5 to 1:10 in isotonic crystalloid; dilution with water is not recommended) administered intravenously over 5 minutes, or three ampules intramuscularly. This has been administered successfully over the years by members of the Queensland Surf Life-Saving Association and the Queensland Ambulance Transport Brigade. Although the antivenin is prepared by hyperimmunizing sheep, the risk of anaphylaxis or serum sickness should be assumed to be the same as for equine hyperimmune globulin preparations. It cannot be overemphasized that the timely administration of antivenin can be lifesaving.[198] In addition to its lifesaving properties, the early administration of antivenin may markedly reduce pain and decrease subsequent skin scarring.[23,201] Antivenin administration may be repeated once or twice every 2 to 4 hours until there is no further worsening of the reaction (skin discoloration, pain, or systemic effects). A large sting in an adult may require the initial administration of two ampules. The antivenin may also used to neutralize the effects of a *Chiropsalmus* envenomation.[178] The antivenin should be stored in a refrigerator at 2° to 10° C and must not be frozen.[37] The concomitant administration of a corticosteroid (such as hydrocortisone 200 mg intravenously), is often recommended for its antiinflammatory activity but is no substitute for the administration of antivenin. Even with successful treatment, skin irritation may persist for months, marked by discolored striae, intermittent desquamation, and pruritus. Burnett and Calton[28] discovered that verapamil can prolong the life of mice challenged with box-jellyfish, sea nettle, or Portuguese man-of-war venom. Furthermore, it seems to enhance murine survival when administered antivenin after

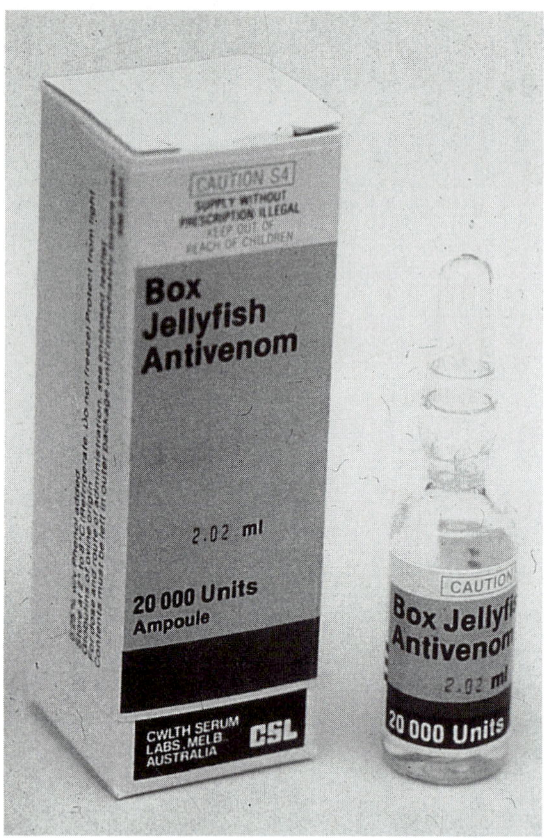

Fig. 52-21 Box-jellyfish antivenom. (Courtesy John Williamson, M.D.)

Chironex venom challenge.[39] The extrapolation of these data to the human condition is as yet untested. Sutherland[179] has noted that development of an immunizing vaccine against the sting of *Chironex fleckeri* has been abandoned because immunizing the right persons is not feasible. However, given the rapidity with which a victim can die after a box-jellyfish envenomation and the narrow temporal window of opportunity for administering antivenin, persons at high risk of being stung might receive better protection from an effective vaccine than by placing their reliance on swift rescue and the timely administration of antivenin.

Irukandji. *Carukia barnesii,* the jellyfish known as "Irukandji," is a small (1 to 2 cm across the bell) translucent jellyfish with four thin nematocyst-covered tentacles (2.5 to 4.5 cm in length at rest, and up to 65 cm extended) found off the coast of northern Australia in both inshore and open waters.[12,13,59,65,170] After causing a severe immediate skin reaction characterized by pain and erythema without wheal formation, the venom may induce muscle pain and spasm, back pain, abdominal pain, parasympathetic dysautonomia, respiratory difficulty, headache, nausea, and vomiting, which progress to profound weakness and collapse.[40] Localized piloerection and sweating have been reported.[59] Generally the discomfort remits in 6 to 24 hours; however, it occasionally recurs. The "Irukandji syndrome" presupposes massive catecholamine release, with abdominal and chest pain, vomiting, diaphoresis, hypertension (diastolic pressure to 140 mm Hg), tachycardia, severe pulmonary edema, and hypokinetic heart failure.[61,124] To date, death has not been reported.[196] It is interesting to note that many Irukandji-like stings occur inside "stinger enclosures" (bathing nets) designed to exclude *Chironex fleckeri.* Other carybdeid medusae that envenom with lesser severity include the jimble and fire jelly *(Tamoya haplonema).* The morbakka is a stinging creature that resembles the Irukandji but is larger. The bell, which measures up to 16 by 12 cm, is covered with clumps of nematocysts and may be as dangerous to handle as the meter-long tentacles. This animal may have been previously misidentified as *Tamoya.*[59]

Chrysaora (Sea Nettle). Sea nettles (such as *Chrysaora quinquecirrha* and *Cyanea capillata*) are considerably less lethal animals and can be found in both temperate and tropical waters, particularly in Chesapeake Bay. Not as dangerous as the Indo-Pacific box-jellyfish, they are still capable of inducing a moderately severe sting. *Chrysaora quinquecirrha* and similar species carry a proteinaceous venom that contains at least seven enzymes, with at least one antigenic and thermolabile component that is cardiotoxic, neurotoxic, and dermatonecrotic. The venom also contains histamine, histamine releasers, prostaglandins, serotonin, and kininlike factors; the last mentioned have also been found in venoms of *Chironex fleckeri* and *Physalia physalis.*[29,26] Large intradermal injections of crude sea nettle venom in normal saline produced immunosuppression (T cells) for several days, which was homologous against the same coelenterate antigen and heterologous against antigens contained within vaccinia and herpes simplex viruses and tetanus bacillus.[189]

Clinical aspects. The clinical presentation of a sea nettle envenomation is similar to that of *Physalia* species, with perhaps a greater incidence of systemic complications. Death is exceedingly rare. Elevated levels of serum anti–sea nettle venom IgM, IgG, and IgE may persist for years in patients who suffer exaggerated reactions to *Chrysaora quinquecirrha* stings. These antibodies cross-react with *Physalia* venom and have been postulated to be of value in identifying patients at risk for a severe reaction.[27] Currently this technique is not widely available or frequently employed, and its reliability and reproducibility require further verification.

The reaction after a sting by the blubber jellyfish (*Catostylus* species) is relatively mild, with the formation of wheals, erythema, and pruritus limited to the areas of contact.[203] Systemic effects are exceedingly rare. *Cyanea* species carry long thin tentacles that induce a similar effect, with occasional muscle aching, nausea, and drowsiness, particularly in small children. *Pelagia* species also induce wheals, which are more circinate or irregularly shaped and may not follow a linear pattern. The venom is sufficiently toxic to cause severe generalized allergy, with bronchospasm and pruritus.

Treatment. Treatment for a sea nettle envenomation is similar to that for the sting of *Physalia* species. Baking soda may be a more effective initial detoxicant than acetic acid or alcohol.[35] Monoclonal antibodies to jellyfish venoms have been developed that demonstrate cross-reactivity among venoms of a variety of coelenterates, which may allow the development of a single protective antivenin or vaccine.[29]

Anthozoa

The class Anthozoa includes the sea anemones, stony (true) corals (Zooantharia), and the soft corals (Alcyonaria). The anemones are considered here because they envenom.

Actinaria (Anemones). Actinarians (sea anemones) are abundant (1000 species) multicolored animals with sessile habits and a flowerlike appearance. They are composed of stalked, fingerlike projections capable of stinging and paralyzing passing fish (Fig. 52-22).[85,86,113] Their sizes range from a few millimeters to more than 0.5 m; they are found at depths of up to 2900 fathoms. The insides of some anemones can be eaten after they are dried.

Anemones are attractive creatures and are often found in tidal pools, where the unwary brush up against them or inquisitively touch them. Like other coelenterates, they possess tentacles loaded with one of two variations of the nematocyst, either the sporocyst or the basitrichous isorhiza (basitrich).[86] These wreak havoc once stimulated by an unfortunate victim. Some sporocysts are adhesive and act to hold as well as to envenom the prey. When an anemone wishes to present a greater number of nematocysts to the victim, it inflates the tentacles by filling them with water. While a number of sea animals, such as the clownfish, live in symbiosis with the anemone, humans are not so fortunate and are frequently stung when attempting to handle these not so delicate "flowers." The clownfish must acquire immunity to the anemone's sting by repeated contact and development of a mucous coat (Color Plate 122). Sea anemones contain biologically active substances, including neurotoxins (sodium channel interaction), cardiotoxins, hemolysins (for erythrocytes and platelets), and proteinase inhibitors.[127,164] A cytolytic toxin has been isolated from the Indo-Pacific sea anemone, *Stoichactis kenti*.[20] The anemone *Actinia equina* elaborates cytolytic polypeptide toxins known as equinatoxins, which may induce hemolysis as well as cardiorespiratory arrest in animals, attributed by some to coronary vasospasm.[118] Tenebrosin-C from the anemone *Actinia tenebrosa* is a positive inotrope that can be inhibited by the cyclooxygenase blockers indomethacin and aspirin, a lipooxygenase blocker and leukotriene antagonist, and mepacrine (a phospholipase A_2 inhibitor).[70] Potassium channel toxins have been isolated from the sea anemones *Bundosoma granulifera* and *Stichodactyla helianthus*.[89]

Clinical aspects. Most victims are stung when they handle or accidentally brush against the anemone in shallow water. Nudists may acquire genital injuries; small children may accidentally or intentionally ingest tentacles.[123] The dermatitis caused by contact with an anemone is similar in all regards to that from fire coral or a small man-of-war; it is often likened to a bee sting. The variation in skin reaction is related to the specific toxicity of the venom, so that while *Actinia* species produce painful urticarial lesions, *Anemonia* species induce paresthesias, edema, and erythema.[64] Most commonly the initial skin lesion is centrally pale with a halo of erythema and petechial hemorrhage. This is soon followed by edema and diffuse ecchymosis. If the envenomation is severe, intense local hemorrhage, vesiculation, necrosis, skin ulceration, and secondary infection may occur, par-

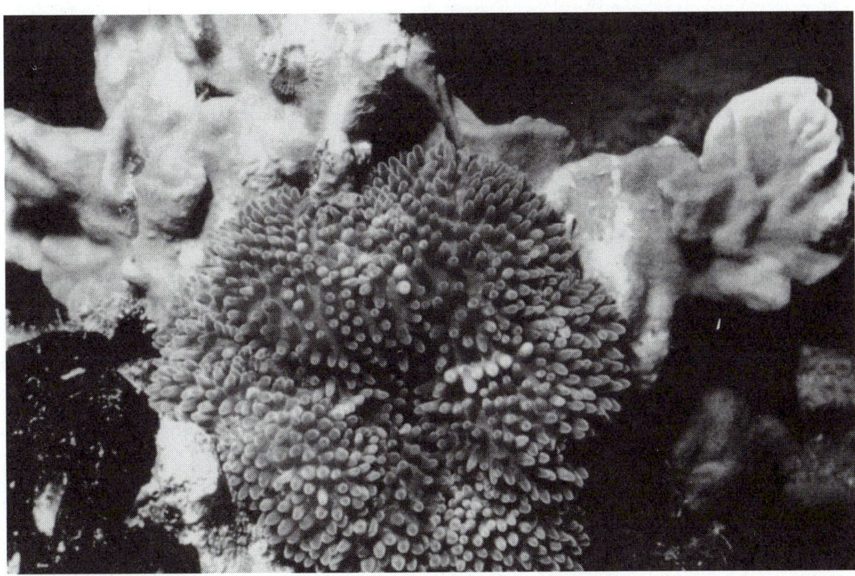

Fig. 52-22 Sea anemone *(Stoichactis helianthus)* coexisting with fire coral. (Courtesy Dee Scarr.)

ticularly after the stings of certain species *(Sagartia, Actinia, Anemonia, Actinodendron,* and *Triactis).*[86,113,123] The "Hell's fire sea anemone" *(Actinodendron plumosum)* is aptly named. Systemic reactions are less likely after the sting of an anemone than after that of a man-of-war; reactions include fever, chills, somnolence, malaise, weakness, nausea, vomiting, and syncope.

In most cases mild envenomations resolve within 48 hours. More severe reactions, characterized by discoloration and vesicle formation, may become indolent, with eschar leading to residual hyperpigmentation, hypopigmentation, or keloid formation.[123]

Sponge fisherman's (diver's) disease is caused by contact with an anemone *(Sagartia* or *Actinia)* that attaches itself symbiotically to the base of a sponge. A few minutes after contact with the sponge, the skin begins to itch and burn, with the development of erythema and small vesicles. As described previously, this transforms to a darkened purple appearance, with frequent systemic components (headache, nausea, vomiting, fever, chills, and muscle spasm).

Treatment. Treatment for an anemone envenomation is similar to that for the sting of *Physalia* species. The dermatitis is frequently more severe and may require prolonged wound care consisting of debridement and antibiotic therapy for secondary infection. The healing process is generally slower after an anemone sting than after a man-of-war envenomation.

ECHINODERMATA

The phylum Echinodermata has five classes: sea lilies, brittle stars, starfish, sea urchins, and sea cucumbers. Only the last three are of emergency medical interest.

Starfish

Life and Habits. Starfish are simple, free-living, stellate echinoderms covered with thorny spines of calcium carbonate crystals held erect by muscle tissue. The creatures move about over the ocean floor by means of tube feet located under the arms (rays). They eat other echinoderms, mollusks, coral, worms, and poisonous shellfish. Starfish proliferation and destruction of coral beds within the Great Barrier Reef off the coast of Australia is a conservation issue of international concern. The starfish everts its membranous stomach through its mouth and secretes digestive enzymes that destroy coral polyps. Only the stark white coral skeleton remains. The crown-of-thorns starfish *(Acanthaster planci)* is found in the coral reef communities of the Great Barrier Reef, throughout the Pacific and Indian Oceans, in the Red Sea, and in the Gulf of California.[117]

Venom and Venom Apparatus. Glandular tissue interspersed in or underneath the epidermis (integument) produces a slimy venomous substance. The carnivorous *Acanthaster planci* is a particularly venomous species normally 25 to 35 cm in diameter, which attains sizes of up to 70 cm in diameter, with 7 to 23 arms (Fig. 52-23).[130,131] The sharp, rigid, and venomous aboral spines of this animal may grow to 4 to 6 cm (Fig. 52-24). Potentially toxic saponins and histamine-like compounds have been isolated from the spine surfaces; crude venom extracts demonstrate hemolytic, capillary permeability–increasing, myotoxic (phospholipase A_2), myonecrotic, and anticoagulant effects.[57,90,131,135,181] *A. planci* lethal factor is a potent hepatotoxin in laboratory animals.[166]

The slime (cushion) star *Pteraster tessalatus* generates the unique defense of copious rubbery, poisonous mucus to repel natural enemies. No human injuries have been reported to date.

Clinical Aspects. The ice pick–like spine of *Acanthaster planci* can penetrate the hardiest of diving gloves (Color Plate 123). Most spines are composed of porous crystalline magnesium calcite, articulated at the base and extremely sharp, with three raised cutting edges at the tips. As the spine enters the skin, it carries venom into the wound, with immediate pain, copious bleeding, and mild edema. The pain is generally moderate and self-limited, with remission over a period of ½ to 3 hours. The wound may become dusky or discolored. Multiple puncture wounds may result in acute systemic reactions, including paresthesias, nausea, vomiting, lymphadenopathy, and muscular paralysis. If a spine fragment is retained, a granulomatous lesion may develop akin to that from a sea urchin puncture wound. If the victim has been previously sensitized, he or she may suffer a prolonged reaction lasting for weeks and consisting of local edema and pruritus. Contact with other less injurious starfish may induce a pruritic papulourticarial eruption (irritant contact dermatitis).

Treatment. Immersion therapy may provide some relief from the pain. The wound should immediately be immersed into nonscalding hot water to tolerance (113° F or 45° C) for 30 to 90 minutes or until there is significant pain relief. The pain is rarely severe enough to require local anesthetic infiltration. The puncture wound should be irrigated and explored to remove all foreign material. Because of the stoutness of the spines, it is rare to retain a fragment. However, if any question of a foreign body exists, a soft tissue radiograph often identifies the fractured spine. Not infrequently the victim suffers an indolent contact dermatitis from handling a starfish, such as *Solaster papposus,* the sun or rose star. The dermatitis may be managed in standard fashion with topical solutions, such as calamine with 0.5% menthol, or corticosteroid preparations. Systemic therapy is supportive. Granulomas from retained spine fragments may require excision. Starfish that have ingested poisonous shellfish are themselves toxic on ingestion.

Sea Urchins

Life and Habits. Sea urchins are free-living echinoderms that have an egg-shaped, globular, or flattened body. A hard shell (test) surrounds the viscera and is covered by regularly arranged spines and triple-jawed pedicellariae. Urchins are nocturnal and omnivorous eaters, yet are shy,

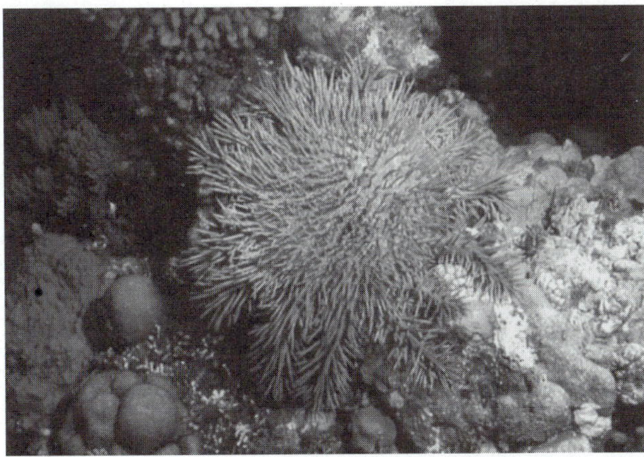

Fig. 52-23 Crown-of-thorns starfish *(Acanthaster planci).*

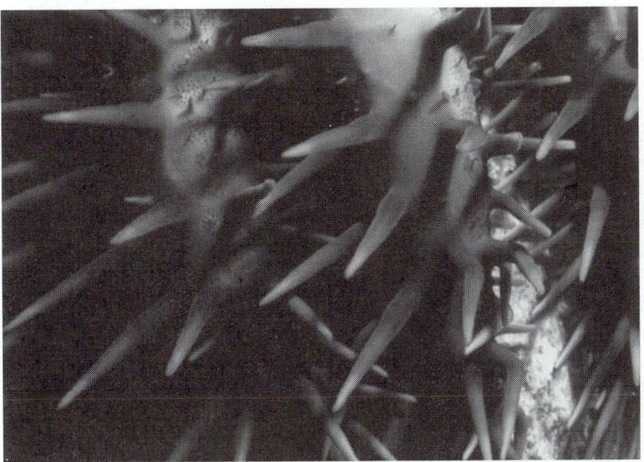

Fig. 52-24 Spines of the crown-of-thorns starfish may grow to 6 cm in length.

nonaggressive, slow-moving animals found on rocky bottoms or burrowed in sand and crevices (Color Plate 124). Their bathymetric range extends from the intertidal zone to great depths. The raw or cooked gonads of several species are eaten as great delicacies by humans.

Venom and Venom Apparatus. The venom apparatuses of sea urchins consist of the hollow, venom-filled spines and the triple-jawed globiferous pedicellariae. Generally only one or the other is present in a single animal.

The spines of sea urchins, formed by the calcification of a cylindrical projection of subepidermal connective tissue, may either be non-venom-bearing, with solid blunt and rounded tips (Fig. 52-25), or venom-bearing (such as families Echinothuridae and Diadematidae), with hollow, long, slender, sharp needles (Fig. 52-26). These are extremely dangerous to handle; the spines, which are attached to the shell with a modified ball-and-socket joint, are brittle and break off easily in the flesh, lodging deeply and making removal difficult. They are keen enough to penetrate rubber gloves and fins. *Diadema setosum* spines may exceed 1 foot in length. The genera *Asthenosoma* and *Aerosoma* have special venom organs (sacs) on the sharp tips of the aboral spines, which introduce the potent venom.

Pedicellariae are small, delicate seizing organs attached to the stalks scattered among the spines. One type are the globiferous pedicellariae, typified by those found in *Toxopneustes pileolus* and *Tripneustes* species, which have globe-shaped heads and serve as the venom organs (Fig. 52-27). The terminal head, with its calcareous pincer jaws, is attached by the stalk to the shell plates of the sea urchin. The outer surface of each jaw is covered by a large venom gland, which is triggered to contract with the jaw on contact. When the sea urchin is at rest in the water, the jaws are extended, slowly moving about. Anything that touches with them is seized. As long as the object is moving, the pedicellariae continue to bite and envenom. Once a pedicellaria attaches to a victim, it will be torn from the shell rather than let go. Detached pedicellariae may remain active for several hours.

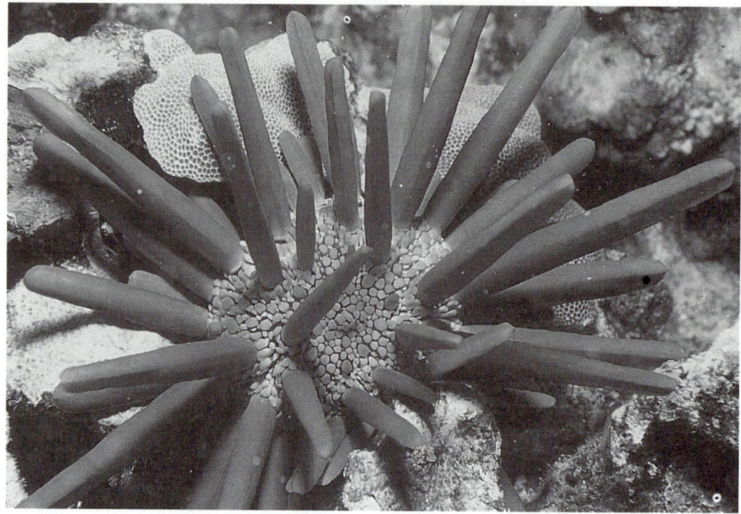

Fig. 52-25 Blunt spines of the "pencil urchin." These are not venom bearing and pose no hazard to humans.

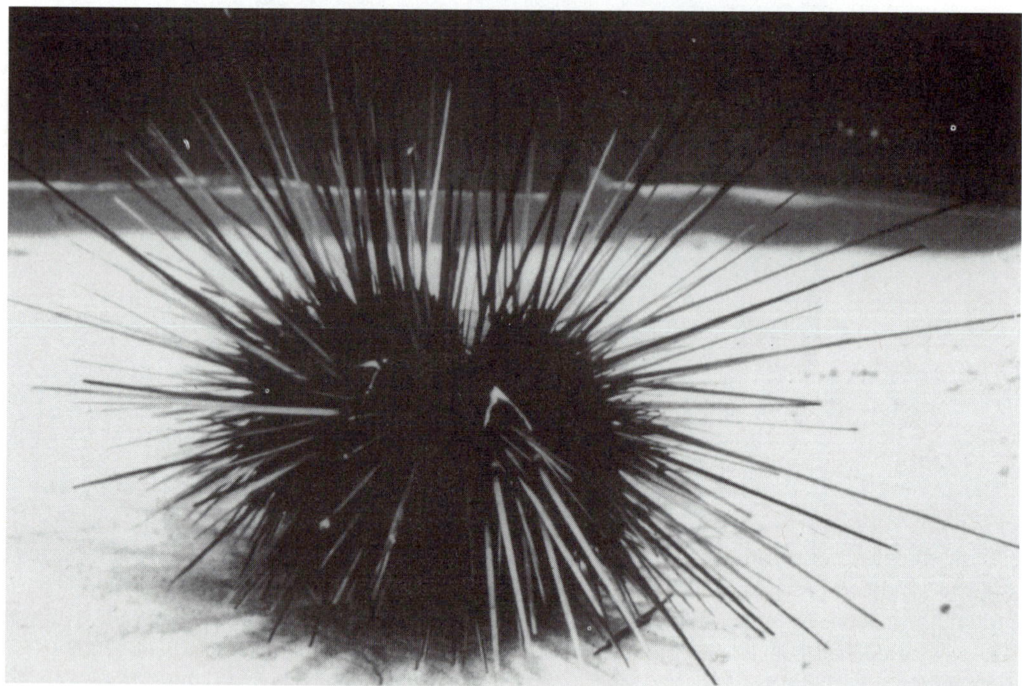

Fig. 52-26 Long, sharp spines of the black sea urchin, which bear venom and can easily penetrate human skin.

The venom of sea urchins contains various toxic fractions, including steroid glycosides, hemolysins, proteases, serotonin, and cholinergic substances. The Pacific *Tripneustes* urchin carries a neurotoxin with a predilection for facial and cranial nerves. A toxic substance from the sea urchin *Toxopneustes pileolus* induces histamine release from rat peritoneal mast cells.[182] Contractin A from the pedicellariae of the same species causes contraction of the isolated guinea pig tracheal smooth muscle.[133]

Two separate unusual cases were reported in 1993 to me by neurologists. In each case the victim sustained multiple punctures from one or several black sea urchins in Hawaiian waters. The immediate clinical reaction was typical, but it was followed in 6 to 10 days by severe bulbar polyneuritis with respiratory insufficiency. In one case the victim was hyporeflexic and appeared to suffer a Guillain-Barré variation with elevated protein levels in cerebrospinal fluid; in the other the victim manifested meningoencephalitis docu-

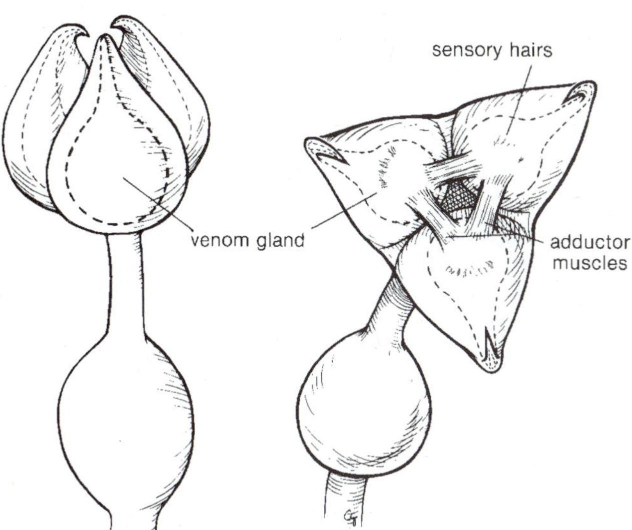

Fig. 52-27 Globiferous pedicellaria of a sea urchin, used to hold and envenom prey.

mented by magnetic resonance imaging. The relationship to the urchin stings suggests an autoimmune phenomenon, but this has not been proven.

Clinical Aspects. Most victims are envenomed when they step on, handle, or brush up against a sea urchin. Because the creatures tend to be nocturnal, divers are most commonly injured in dark waters during night diving activities, particularly in small caves or in shallow turbulent waters. Young inquisitive children who explore tidepools frequently handle urchins incorrectly and may be injured.

Venomous spines inflict immediate and intensely painful stings. The pain is initially characterized by burning, which rapidly evolves into severe local muscle aching with visible erythema and swelling of the skin surrounding the puncture site or sites. Frequently a spine breaks off and lodges in the victim. Some sea urchin spines (such as those of *Diadema setosum* or *Strongylocentrotus purpuratus*) contain purplish dye, which may give a false impression of spines left in the skin (Color Plate 125).[138] Soft tissue density x-ray techniques or magnetic resonance imaging may reveal a radiopaque foreign body. If a spine enters a joint, it may rapidly induce severe synovitis. If multiple spines have penetrated the skin, particularly if they are deeply embedded, systemic symptoms may rapidly develop, including nausea, vomiting, paresthesias, numbness and muscular paralysis, abdominal pain, syncope, hypotension, and respiratory distress.[116] The presence of a frank neuropathy may indicate that the spine has lodged in contact with a peripheral nerve. The pain from multiple stings may be sufficient to cause delirium. Secondary infections and indolent ulceration are common.

The stings of pedicellariae are often of greater magnitude, causing immediate intense radiating pain, local edema and hemorrhage, malaise, weakness, paresthesias, hypesthesia, arthralgias, aphonia, dizziness, syncope, generalized muscular paralysis, respiratory distress, hypotension, and rarely, death.[64,68,85] In some cases the pain may disappear within the first hour, while the localized muscular weakness or paralysis persists for up to 6 hours.

Treatment. The envenomed body part should immediately be immersed in nonscalding hot water (upper limit 113° F or 45° C) to tolerance for 30 to 90 minutes in an attempt to relieve pain. Any pedicellariae still attached to the skin must be removed or envenomation will continue. This may be accomplished by applying shaving foam and gently scraping with a razor. Embedded spines should be removed with care because they easily fracture. Black or purplish discoloration surrounding the wound after spine removal is often merely spine dye and of no consequence. Although some thin venomous spines may be absorbed within 24 hours to 3 weeks, it is best to remove those that are easily reached and leave the remainder for dissolution. All thick calcium carbonate spines should be removed because of the risk of infection, foreign body encaseation granuloma, or dermoid inclusion cyst. External percussion to achieve fragmentation may prove disastrous if a chronic inflammatory process is initiated in sensitive tissue of the hand or foot. If the spines have acutely entered joints or are closely aligned to neurovascular structures, the surgeon should take advantage of an operating microscope (in an appropriate setting) to remove all spine fragments. The extraction should be performed as soon as possible after the injury. If the spine has entered an interphalangeal joint, the finger should be splinted until the spine is removed to limit fragmentation and further penetration. This also may control the fusiform finger swelling commonly noted after a puncture in the vicinity of the middle or proximal interphalangeal joint.[138] It is inappropriate to rummage about in a hand wound in the emergency department, virtually looking for a needle in a haystack. If the presence of a spine is in question, soft tissue density radiographic techniques for a radiopaque foreign body may be diagnostic. Although the calcium carbonate is relatively inert, it is accompanied by slime, bacteria, and organic epidermal debris.[177] Therefore secondary infections are common and deep puncture wounds are an indication for prophylactic antibiotics.

Some sea urchin spines are phagocytosed in the soft tissues and ultimately dissolve. The granulomas caused by retained sea urchin spine fragments have sarcoidal histologic features and generally appear as flesh- or dye-colored surface or subcuticular nodules 2 to 12 months after the initial injury (Fig. 52-28).[103,151] In thin-skinned areas they are erythematous and rubbery, painless, and infrequently umbilicated. In thicker-skinned areas (palms, soles, knees) that are frequently abraded, they have a keratinized appearance. Although necrosis and microabscess formation may be evident microscopically, suppuration is unusual. Rarely, the destructive nature of the inflammatory process may be severe enough to necessitate amputation of a digit.[45] If a spine cannot be removed and becomes a nidus for cyst or granu-

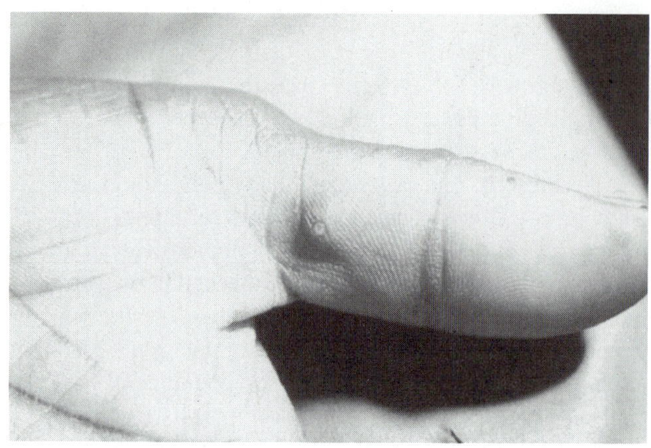

Fig. 52-28 Subcuticular nodule after a sea urchin puncture.

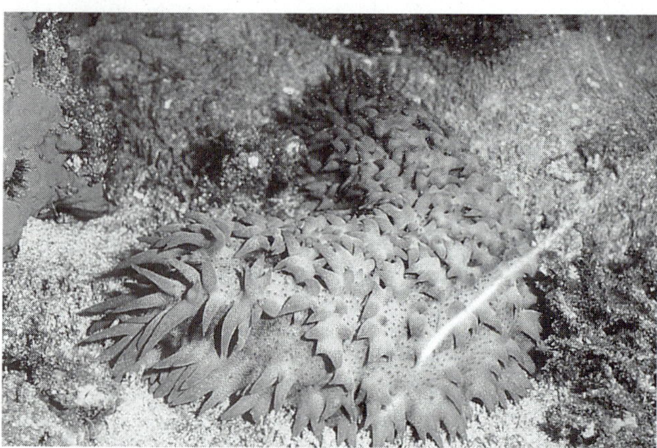

Fig. 52-29 Sea cucumber.

loma formation, the lesion may be removed surgically. Intralesional injection with a corticosteroid (triamcinolone hexacetonide 5 mg/ml) is less efficacious but may be successful. Systemic antiinflammatory drugs may be minimally helpful but are not substitutes for removal of the spine.[10,47] A diffuse delayed reaction, consisting of cyanotic induration, fusiform swelling in the digits, and focal phalangeal bony erosion, may be treated with systemic corticosteroids and antibiotics.

Sea Cucumbers

Life and Habits. Sea cucumbers are free-living worm- or sausage-shaped bottom feeders, of diverse external patterns and coloration, that are essentially scavengers. They are cosmopolitan in distribution, found in both shallow and deep waters.

Venom and Venom Apparatus. Cucumbers produce in their body walls a visceral cantharidin-like liquid toxin ("holothurin"). Holothurin is concentrated in the tentacular organs of Cuvier, which can be projected and extended anally when the animal mounts a defense (Figs. 52-29 and 52-30). Some cucumbers dine on nematocysts and thus can secrete coelenterate venom as well.

Clinical Aspects. Holothurin may induce contact dermatitis when the tentacular organs directly contact the skin. Generally the substance is diluted in the surrounding ocean water and the reaction is minimal. However, persons who dissect sea cucumbers topside in the preparation of food products may inadvertently handle the toxin and develop a papular skin irritation. The major risk under water is to the corneas and conjunctivae, which may become intensely inflamed if directly contacted by tentacular fragments or high concentrations of the toxin. This may occur if the mask is cleared in the immediate vicinity of recent sea cucumber manipulation. A severe reaction may lead to blindness.[64,68] Holothurin is a potent cardiac glycoside and may cause severe illness or death on ingestion.

Treatment. The management of holothurin-induced contact dermatitis is similar to that for starfish dermatitis. Topical or systemic corticosteroids may be necessary to manage a severe reaction. Because cucumbers that dine on nematocysts may secrete coelenterate venom, the initial skin detoxification should include topical application of 5% acetic acid (vinegar) or 40% to 70% isopropyl alcohol. If an eye is involved, it should be anesthetized with 1 or 2 drops of proparacaine 0.5% and then irrigated with 100 to 250 ml of normal saline to remove any residual foreign matter. The cornea should then be stained with fluorescein to identify corneal defects. A proper slit-lamp examination is optimal to determine whether inflammation extends into the anterior chamber or involves the iris. If there is no sign of infection, a moderate approach to the inflammatory keratitis includes regular instillation of cycloplegic, mydriatic, and corticosteroid ophthalmic solutions. Prompt referral to an ophthalmologist is essential.

Annelid Worms

Life and Habits. There are 6200 species of segmented marine worms (phylum Annelida, class Polychaeta), either free moving or sedentary. Some members of the former group are considered toxic and may attain 1 foot in length. The worms are predominantly carnivorous and exist in the tidal zone to depths of 5000 m, mostly as bottom feeders. Each segment of the worm possesses paddlelike appendages (parapodia) for locomotion. From these project numerous silky or bristlelike setae, which are capable of puncturing the victim (Fig. 52-31).

The chitinous bristles are arranged in soft rows about the body (Color Plate 126). When a worm is stimulated, its body contracts and the bristles are erected. Easily detached, the bristles penetrate skin like cactus spines and are difficult to remove. The ubiquitous bottom-dwelling bristleworm *Hermodice carunculata* is frequently handled in Floridian and Caribbean waters by snorkelers and divers. This worm

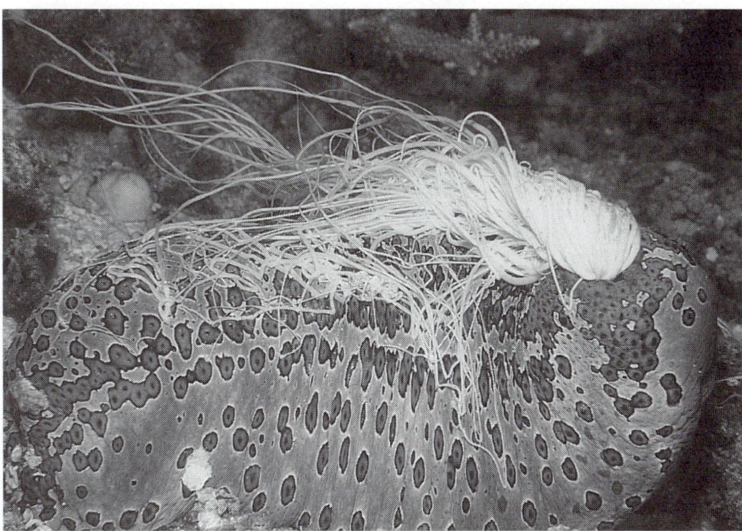

Fig. 52-30 Extruded tentacular organs of Cuvier from within a sea cucumber.

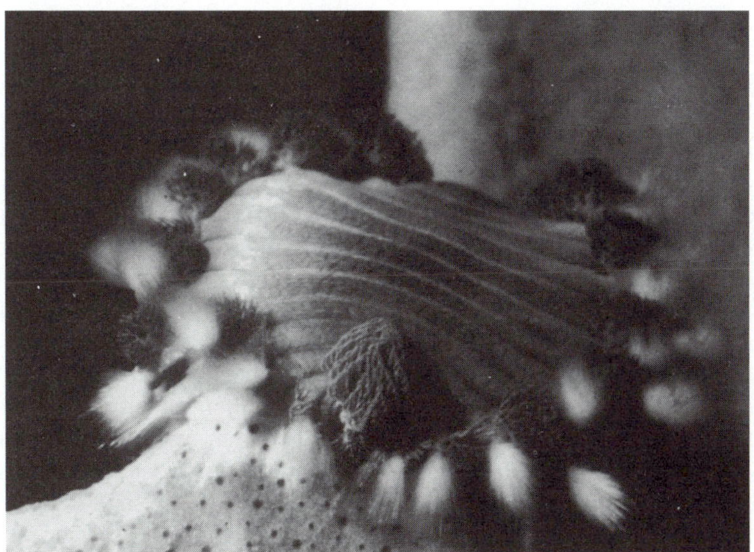

Fig. 52-31 Bristleworm eating fire coral. (Courtesy Dee Scarr.)

can attain a length of 1 foot and a width of 1 inch. It is found on coral, under rocks, and moving among sponges. The body is green or reddish with tufts of white bristles. *Chloeia flava* is found along the Malayan coast, *Chloeia viridus* in the West Indies, Gulf of California, and Gulf of Mexico south to Panama, and *Euythoe complanata* in Australia and other tropical seas. Other worms, such as *Chloeia euglochis ehlers,* are free swimming. Some marine worms possess strong chitinous jaws with pharyngeal teeth and can inflict painful bites.

Clinical Aspects. The bite or sting of an annelid worm may induce intense inflammation typified by a burning sensation with a raised, erythematous, urticarial rash, most frequently on the hands and fingers (Fig. 52-32). Edema and papules ensue, with rare necrosis. The setae are easily fractured into the skin and are generally not visible on external inspection, although the victim may report a sensation of pricking or abrasion. Untreated, the pain is generally self-limited over the course of a few hours, but the inflammatory component of erythema and urticaria may last for 2 to 3 days, with total resolution of the skin discoloration over 7 to 10 days. With multiple stings, marked local soft tissue edema and pruritus may develop. Secondary infections and cellulitis may occur if the eczematous component is severe.

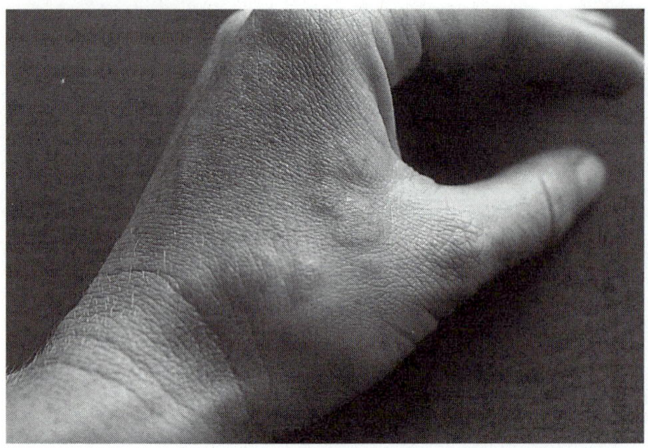

Fig. 52-32 Skin eruption caused by handling a bristleworm.

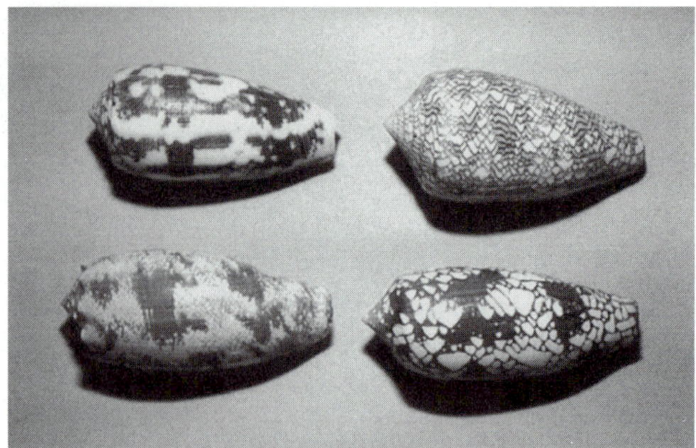

Fig. 52-33 Cone shells. The external appearance is deceiving, since these beautiful mollusks may envenom uncautious handlers.

Treatment. All large visible bristles should be removed with forceps. The skin should be dried (without scraping, to avoid breaking or embedding the spines further into the skin) so that a layer of adhesive tape may be applied to remove the remaining smaller spines, which are too tiny for individual extraction. Alternatively, a facial "peel" may be applied and removed. After this maneuver acetic acid 5% (vinegar), isopropyl alcohol 40% to 70%, dilute ammonia, or a paste of unseasoned meat tenderizer (papain) may provide some pain relief. If the inflammatory reaction becomes severe, the victim may benefit from the administration of topical or systemic corticosteroids.

MOLLUSKS

The phylum Mollusca (45,000 species) encompasses a group of unsegmented, soft-bodied invertebrates, many of which secrete calcareous shells. Generally a muscular foot is present with various modifications. There are five main classes, of which three predominate in their hazard to humans: the pelecypods (such as scallops, oysters, clams, and mussels), the gastropods (such as snails and slugs), and the cephalopods (such as squids, octopuses, and cuttlefish). Mollusks are often implicated as the transvectors in poisonous ingestions.

Cone Shells

Life and Habits. There are approximately 300 species of these circumtropical, beautiful, yet potentially lethal, univalve and cone-shaped shelled mollusks of the class Gastropoda, family Conidae, genus *Conus* (Fig. 52-33).[108] Most of these carnivores carry a highly developed venom apparatus, and at least 18 species have been implicated in human envenomations, with occasional fatalities (approximately 30 have been recorded).[80] These include *Conus aulicus* (court), *C. geographus* (geographer), *C. gloria-maris* (glory of the sea), *C. omaria* (marbled), *C. striatus* (striated), *C. textile* (textile), and *C. tulipa* (tulip).

Most harmful cone shells ("cones") are creatures of shallow Indo-Pacific waters; the variance in feeding habits and venom production accounts for the varying toxicity.[1] Apparently cones that feed on fish or mollusks are the most dangerous.[85] Less toxic stings are attributed to cones that feed on marine worms. Predominantly nocturnal creatures, cones burrow in the sand and coral during the daytime, emerging at night to feed.

Venom and Venom Apparatus. Cone shells are predators that feed by injecting rapid-acting venom by means of a detachable, dartlike radular tooth ("radula"). To do this, the head of the animal must extend out of the shell. The venom apparatus is composed of a set of minute, harpoonlike, chitinous radular teeth associated with a venom bulb, duct, and radular sheath (Fig. 52-34). The barbed teeth, which may attain a length of 1 cm, are housed within the radular sheath. The act of envenomation is performed by the release of a radular tooth from the sheath into the pharynx, where it is "charged" with venom from the venom duct and then transferred to the extensible proboscis. This appendage, which may extend in some species as far back as the spire of the shell, grasps the venom-impregnated and barbed tooth and thrusts it into the flesh of the victim. The venom is composed of biologically active peptides (to date, more than 100 "conotoxins" have been identified) of 13 to 35 amino acids in length.[136] The venom targets are neuromuscular transmission and ion channels.[80] At the same site as tetrodotoxin and saxitoxin, μ-conotoxins bind and modify muscle sodium channels.[82,133] Voltage-dependent calcium uptake at the presynaptic cleft and cholinergic transmission in avian and mammalian neuromuscular junctions are inhibited by ω-conotoxins like that from *Conus geographus*.[52] The α-conotoxins block the nicotinic acetylcholine receptor.[80,133] A "sleeper peptide" in *C. geographus* venom causes test animals to enter a deep sleeplike state.[80]

Clinical Aspects. Most stings occur on the fingers and hand, as the unknowledgeable fossicker incorrectly handles a hazardous specimen. Mild stings are puncture wounds that

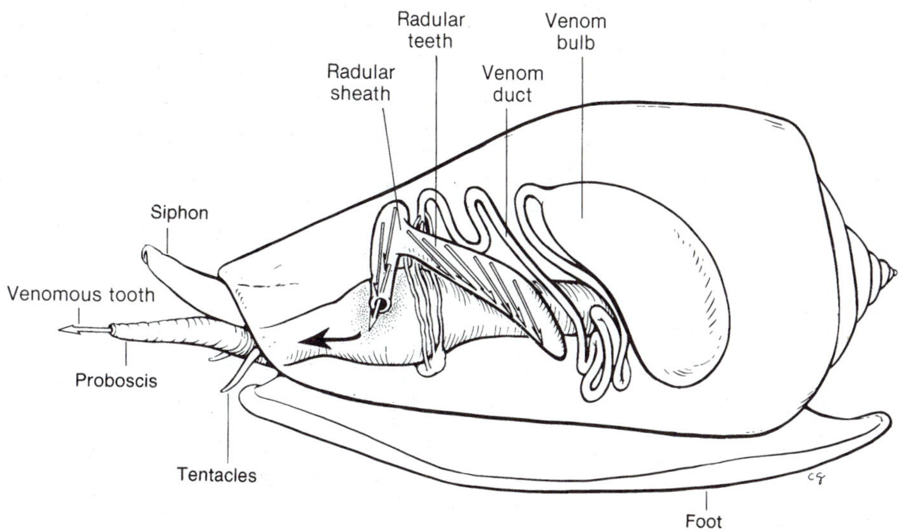

Fig. 52-34 Venom apparatus of the cone shell.

resemble bee or wasp stings. The initial symptoms may be localized ischemia, cyanosis, and numbness in the area about the wound but more commonly include a sharp burning or stinging sensation, much like a bee sting. More serious envenomations induce paresthesias at the wound site, which rapidly become perioral and then generalized. Generalized muscular paralysis may lead to respiratory failure; bronchospastic respiratory distress is not commonly seen. Coma has been observed, and death is attributed to cardiac failure.[149] Other symptoms include dysphagia, syncope, weakness, areflexia, aphonia, diplopia, blurred vision, and pruritus. The bite of *C. geographus* may be rapidly toxic, with progression to cerebral edema, coma, respiratory arrest, disseminated intravascular coagulopathy, and cardiac failure within a few hours. While mild stings may cause symptoms of nausea, blurred vision, malaise, and weakness for only a few hours, a severe envenomation may induce symptoms that require 2 to 3 weeks to achieve total resolution.

Treatment. No antivenin is available for a cone shell envenomation. Numerous therapies have been recommended, including application of a proximal lymphatic-venous occlusive bandage, incision and suction, soaking in nonscalding hot water to tolerance (upper limit 113° F or 45° C) until pain is relieved, injection of a local anesthetic (lidocaine 1% to 2% without epinephrine), and local excision. Although speculative, a reasonable theoretical approach appears to be the pressure-immobilization technique of venom containment. If practicable by virtue of location of the sting, a cloth or gauze pad of approximate dimensions 6 to 8 cm by 6 to 8 cm by 2 to 3 cm (thickness) should be placed directly over the sting and held firmly in place by a circumferential bandage 15 to 18 cm wide applied at lymphatic-venous occlusive pressure. The arterial circulation should not be occluded, as determined by the detection of arterial pulsations and proper capillary refill. The bandage should be released after the victim has been brought to proper medical attention and the rescuer is prepared to provide systemic support, or after 4 to 6 hours.

Cardiovascular and respiratory support are the usual priorities after a severe envenomation. In cases of severe persistent hypotension, naloxone 2 to 4 mg may be administered empirically to attempt to block the β-endorphin vasodepressor response. Edrophonium (10 mg intravenously in an adult) has been suggested as empirical therapy for paralysis. The cause of infrequently described coagulopathy after cone shell envenomation has not been well explained, and therapy varies with local custom. With regard to a general approach to marine toxin-induced coagulopathies, it is hoped that future investigations will estimate the extent of specific factor (II, V, VII, IX, X, XI) or antithrombin III deficiencies, autoimmune or functional disorders of platelets, or aberrations of hemostasis that allow the rational use of antivenin, heparin, single-donor plasma, fresh-frozen plasma, cryoprecipitate, arginine vasopressin, and fibrinolytic or antifibrinolytic agents.

Prevention. Cone shells should be handled only with the proper gloves; if the proboscis protrudes, the cone should be dropped. If the animal must be carried, it should always be lifted by the large posterior end of the shell, although this does not afford complete protection. A diver should never carry a live cone inside a wet suit or buoyancy compensator pocket.

Octopuses

Life and Habits. Octopuses and cuttlefish are cephalopods and are usually harmless and retiring. True octopuses are inhabitants of warmer waters and have little tolerance for extremes in salinity. They prefer rocky bottoms and rock pools in the intertidal zones. The entertainment media have created the image of a giant creature that envelops its victim in a maze of tentacles and suction cups. The truth is that most dangerous (envenoming) creatures are smaller than 10 to 20 cm and do not squeeze their victims at all. However, there are reports in the South Pacific of breath-hold spearfishermen drowned while hunting octopuses. The method used to kill the animals was to allow the octopus to cling to the diver, who would bite the animal between the eyes as they both surfaced. Apparently, the octopuses were large enough (4 m tentacle span) to resist the technique.

Octopus bites are rare but can result in severe envenomations. Fatalities have been reported from the bites of the Australian blue-ringed (or "spotted") octopuses, *Octopus (Hapalochlaena) maculosus* and *O. (H.) lunulata.* These small creatures, which rarely exceed 20 cm in length with tentacles extended, are found throughout the Indo-Pacific (Australia, New Zealand, New Guinea, Japan) in rock pools, under discarded objects and shells, and in shallow waters, posing a threat to curious children, tidepoolers, fossickers, and unwary divers.[54,180,193] Divers rarely spot them in water deeper than 3 m. In Australian waters, *Hapalochlaena maculosa,* the southern species, is smaller and yellow. *H. lunulata* is found in the north; larger, darker, and predominantly brownish, it favors the warmer tropical water.[199] When either animal is at rest, it is covered with dark brown to yellow-ochre bands over the body and arms, with superimposed blue patches or rings.[178] When the animal is excited or angered, the entire body darkens and the blue circles or stripes glow iridescent peacock blue (Fig. 52-35), a trait shared by other animals such as the peacock flounder *(Bothus lunatus)*. The colorful appearance is attractive to small children, who can easily handle the 25 to 90 g animal (Color Plate 127). *Octopus joubini* of the Caribbean is dangerous to a lesser degree. Many octopuses can release inky fluid into the water, which is used to confuse attackers; this mechanism is not present in the blue-ringed octopus. The chameleon-like changing of colors to match the surroundings is accomplished with pigment cells (chromatophores).

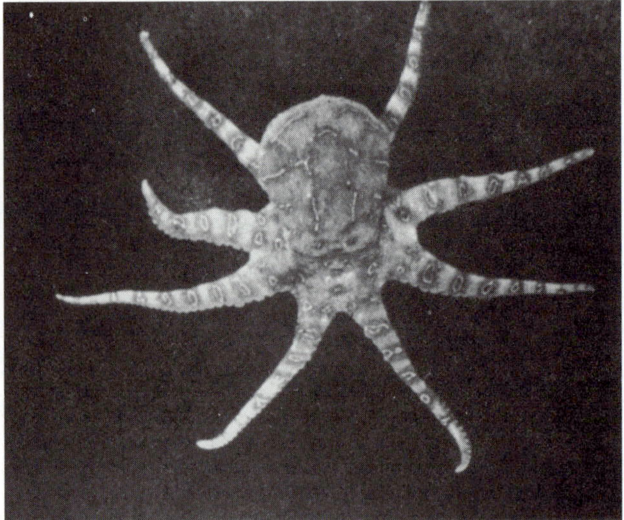

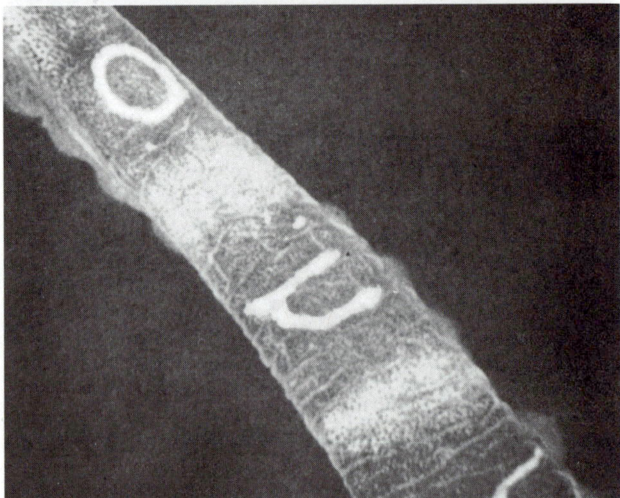

Fig. 52-35 Blue-ringed octopus. When the animal is excited, the markings glow iridescent peacock blue.

Venom and Venom Apparatus. The venom apparatus of the octopus consists of the anterior and posterior salivary glands, salivary ducts, buccal mass, and beak. The mouth is located ventrally and centrally at the base of the tentacles and is surrounded by a circular lip fringed with fingerlike papillae, leading into a muscular pharyngeal cavity. This complex (buccal mass), concealed by the tentacles, is fronted by two parrotlike, powerful, chitinous jaws (the beak), which bite and tear with great force at food held by the suckers. The salivary glands, particularly the posterior, secrete maculotoxin (or cephalotoxin) via the salivary ducts into the pharynx. This venom, normally released into the water to subdue crabs, may be injected into the victim with great force through the dermis down to the muscle fascia.[180] The toxin, maculotoxin (molecular weight less than 5000), contains at least one fraction identical to tetrodotoxin ($C_{11}H_{17}O_8N_3$) of molecular weight 319.3, which blocks peripheral nerve conduction by interfering with sodium conductance in excitable membranes.[85,163] This paralytic agent rapidly produces neuromuscular blockade, notably of the phrenic nerve supply to the diaphragm, without any apparent direct cardiotoxicity.[187] It has been estimated that enough venom (25 g) may be present in one adult octopus to paralyze 750 kg of rabbits or 10 adult victims.[178,180] An adult blue-ringed octopus can inject a second fatal dose of toxin after a 1-hour interval. The venom is active on ingestion or by parenteral administration, the latter being much more effective. Other components of the venom, which include hyaluronidase, histamine, tyramine, serotonin, and "hapalotoxin," are not thought to be major contributors to the clinical effects of an octopus bite.[159] Because most venoms and toxins with molecular weights less than 30,000 are poor antigens, octopus venom elicits no good antivenin.[68,180]

Clinical Aspects. Most victims are bitten on the hand or arm, as they handle the creature or "give it a ride." No blue-ringed octopus bites have yet been reported from an animal in the water.[197] An octopus bite usually consists of two small puncture wounds produced by the chitinous jaws. The bite goes unnoticed or causes only a small amount of discomfort, described as a minor ache, slight stinging, or a pulsating sensation.[64] Occasionally the site is initially numb, followed in 5 to 10 minutes by discomfort that may spread to involve the entire limb, persisting for up to 6 hours. Local urticarial reactions occur variably, and profuse bleeding at the site is attributed to a local anticoagulant effect or may rarely be a harbinger of coagulation abnormalities. Within 30 minutes, considerable erythema, swelling, tenderness, heat, and pruritus develop. By far the most common local tissue reaction is absence of symptoms, a small spot of blood, or a tiny blanched area.[194] More serious symptoms are related predominantly to the neurotoxic properties of the venom. Within 10 to 15 minutes of the bite, the patient notices oral and facial numbness, rapidly followed by systemic progression.[55,197] Voluntary and involuntary muscles are involved, and the illness may rapidly progress to total flaccid paralysis and respiratory failure. Other symptoms include perioral and intraoral anesthesia (classically, numbness of the lips and tongue), diplopia, blurred vision, aphonia, dysphagia, ataxia, myoclonus, weakness, a sense of detachment, nausea, vomiting, peripheral neuropathy, flaccid muscular paralysis, and respiratory failure, which may lead to death. Ataxia of cerebellar configuration may occur after an envenomation that does not progress to frank paralysis.[147] The victim may collapse from weakness and remain awake, so long as oxygenation can be maintained.[96,185] When breathing is disturbed, respiratory assistance may allow the victim to remain mentally alert, although paralyzed. Cardiac arrest is probably a complication of the anoxic episode.[190] Although tetrodotoxin is a potent vascular smooth muscle depressant, it does not appear to produce significant hypotension in humans.[99]

Treatment. First aid at the scene might include the pressure-immobilization technique described in the section on treatment of cone shell stings, although this is as yet unproven for management of octopus bites. If the location of the sting makes it practicable, a cloth or gauze pad of approximate dimensions 6 to 8 cm by 6 to 8 cm by 2 to 3 cm (thickness) should be placed directly over the bite and held firmly in place by a circumferential bandage 15 to 18 cm wide applied at lymphatic-venous occlusive pressure. The arterial circulation should not be occluded, as determined by the detection of arterial pulsations and proper capillary refill. One hypothesis holds that the pressure-immobilization technique devascularizes the area immediately below the pad and prevents the distribution of venom into the general circulation.[5] The bandage should be released after 4 to 6 hours or after the victim has been brought to proper medical attention and the rescuer is prepared to provide systemic support.

Treatment is based on the symptoms and is supportive. Prompt mechanical respiratory assistance has by far the greatest influence on the outcome. Respiratory demise should be anticipated early, and the rescuer should be prepared to provide artificial ventilation, including endotracheal intubation and the application of a mechanical ventilator. The duration of intense clinical venom effect is 4 to 10 hours, after which the victim who has not suffered an episode of significant hypoxia shows rapid signs of improvement. If no period of hypoxia occurs, mentation may remain normal. Complete recovery may require 2 to 4 days. Residua are uncommon and related to anoxia rather than venom effects.

Management of the bite wound is controversial. Some clinicians recommend wide circular excision of the bite wound down to the deep fascia, with primary closure or immediate full-thickness free skin grafts, while others advocate observation and a nonsurgical approach. Because the local tissue reaction is not a significant cause of morbidity, excision is putatively recommended to remove any sequestered venom. Kinetic studies of radiolabeled venom absorption are necessary to track the movement of octopus bite–introduced tetrodotoxin. As previously mentioned, there is no antivenin. Granuloma annulare of the hand developing over a 2-week period after an octopus (presumed to be *Octopus vulgaris* of the Florida Gulf Coast) bite of the hand has been reported.[69] On biopsy, histologic sections demonstrated superficial and deep dermal foci of altered dermis surrounded by histiocytes, lymphocytes, and fibroblasts. Intralesional triamcinolone acetonide injections were temporarily successful in treating the primary lesion.

Prevention. All octopuses, particularly those less than 20 cm in length (including *Octopus joubini* of the Caribbean), should be handled with gloves. Divers need to be familiar with the lethal creatures in their domain. Giving an octopus a ride on the back, shoulder, or arm is not recommended.

Vertebrates

STINGRAYS

The stingrays are the most commonly incriminated group of fishes involved in human envenomations. They have been recognized as venomous since ancient times, known as "demons of the deep" and "devil fishes."[64,154] Aristotle (384-322 BC) made reference to their stinging ability.[22]

Stingrays are members of the class Chondrichthyes (cartilaginous fish), subclass Elasmobranchii (plates and gills; with sharks and chimaeras), order Rajiformes (which contains stingrays [Dasyatidae], guitarfish [Rhinobatidae], skates [Rajidae], electric rays [Torpedinidae], eagle rays [Myliobatidae], mantas [Mobulidae], and freshwater rays [Potamotrygonidae]). There are 11 species of stingrays found in U.S. coastal waters, 7 in the Atlantic and 4 in the Pacific.[132] The family Dasyatidae includes most of the species that cause human envenomation. It is estimated that more than 1500 stingray injuries take place each year in the United States. On the west coast of the United States the round stingray *(Urolophus halleri)* is a frequent stinger; along the southeastern coast, it is the southern stingray *(Dasyatis amer-*

icana). Most attacks occur during the summer and autumn months, as vacationers venture into the surf.

Life and Habits

Stingrays are usually found in tropical, subtropical, and warm temperate oceans, generally in shallow (intertidal) water areas, such as sheltered bays, shoal lagoons, river mouths, and sandy areas between patch reefs.[121] Rays can enter brackish and fresh waters as well. Although rays are generally found above moderate depths, at least one deep-sea species has been discovered.

Rays are small (several inches) to large (up to 12 by 6 feet) creatures observed lying on top of the sand and mud or partially submerged, with only the eyes, spiracles, and part of the tail exposed (Fig. 52-36). Their flattened bodies are round or diamond or kite shaped, with wide pectoral fins that look like wings.[132] Rays are nonaggressive scavengers and bottom feeders that burrow into the sand or mud to feed on worms, mollusks, and crustaceans.[172] The mouth and gill plates are located on the ventral surface of the animal.

Venom and Venom Apparatus

The venom organ of stingrays consists of one to four venomous stings on the dorsum of an elongate, whiplike caudal appendage.[148] There are four different anatomic types of stingray venom organs, based on their adaptability as a defense organ (Fig. 52-37). Thus the stinging ability of rays may be divided into four categories: the gymnurid type (butterfly rays or Gymnuridae), with a poorly developed sting of up to 2.5 cm placed at the base of a short tail; the myliobatid type (eagle and bat rays or Myliobatidae), with a sting of up to 12 cm placed at the base of a cylindrical caudal appendage that terminates in a long whiplike tail; the dasyatid type (stingrays and whiprays or Dasyatidae), with a sting of up to 37 cm placed at the base or further out on the caudal appendage that terminates in a long whiplike tail; and the urolophid type (round stingrays or Urolophidae), with a sting of up to 4 cm located at the base of a short, muscular, well-developed caudal appendage.[84] The efficiency of the apparatus is related to the length and musculature of the tail and to the location and length of the sting. Eagle rays and some mantas (Atlantic *Mobular mobular* and Pacific *Mobula japanica*) have a stinging apparatus, but it is less of a threat because the spine is located at the base of the tail and is not well adapted as a striking organ. Although the manta may grow to a width of 20 feet and weight of 3000 pounds, it dines on small fish, crustaceans, and microorganisms (Fig. 52-38). Many divers have "hitched" a ride on the wings of a manta; there are no reports of envenomation. However, manta skin is rough and can abrade unprotected human skin.

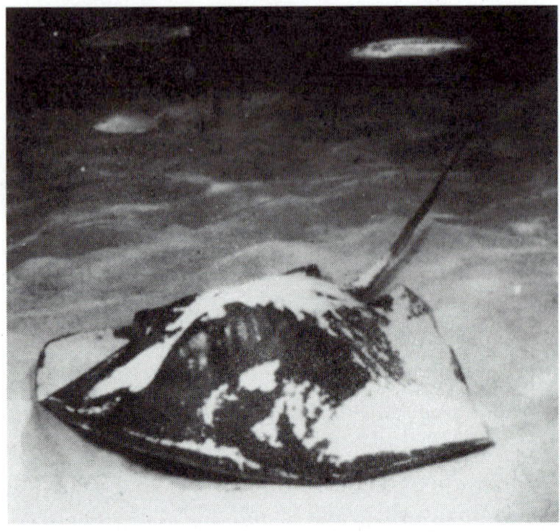

Fig. 52-36 Southern stingray nestles in the sand until disturbed. (Courtesy Dee Scarr.)

In all cases the venom apparatus of stingrays consists of a bilaterally retroserrate spine or spines and the enveloping integumentary sheath or sheaths.[22,85] The elongate and tapered vasodentine spine is firmly attached to the dorsum of the tail (whip) by dense collagenous tissue and is edged on either side by a series of sharp retrorse teeth. Along either edge on the underside of the spine are the two ventrolateral glandular grooves, which house the soft venom glands. The entire spine is encased by the integumentary sheath, which also contains some glandular cells. The sting is often covered with a film of venom and mucus. The spine is replaced if detached.

The venom contains various toxic fractions, including serotonin, 5′-nucleotidase, and phosphodiesterase.[85] Russell[155] investigated the pharmacologic properties of stingray venoms. In animal studies he demonstrated significant venom-induced peripheral vasoconstriction, bradycardia, atrioventricular block, ischemic ST-T wave abnormalities, asystole, central respiratory depression, seizure activity, ataxia, coma, and death. The venom did not appear to be a paralytic neuromuscular agent.

Clinical Aspects

Stingray "attacks" are purely defensive gestures that occur when an unwary human handles, corners, or steps on a camouflaged creature while wading in shallow waters. The tail of the ray reflexively whips upward and accurately thrusts the caudal spine or spines into the victim, producing a puncture wound or jagged laceration (Fig. 52-39). The integumentary sheath covering the spine is ruptured, and venom is released into the wound, along with mucus, pieces of the sheath, and fragments of the spine. On occasion the entire spine tip is broken off and remains in the wound.[157]

Thus a stingray wound is both a traumatic injury and an envenomation. The former involves the physical damage caused by the sting itself. Because of the retrorse serrated teeth and powerful strikes, significant lacerations can result. Secondary bacterial infection is common. Osteomyelitis may occur if the bone is penetrated. The lower extremities, particularly the ankle and foot, are involved most often, followed by the upper extremities, abdomen, and thorax. In rare cases

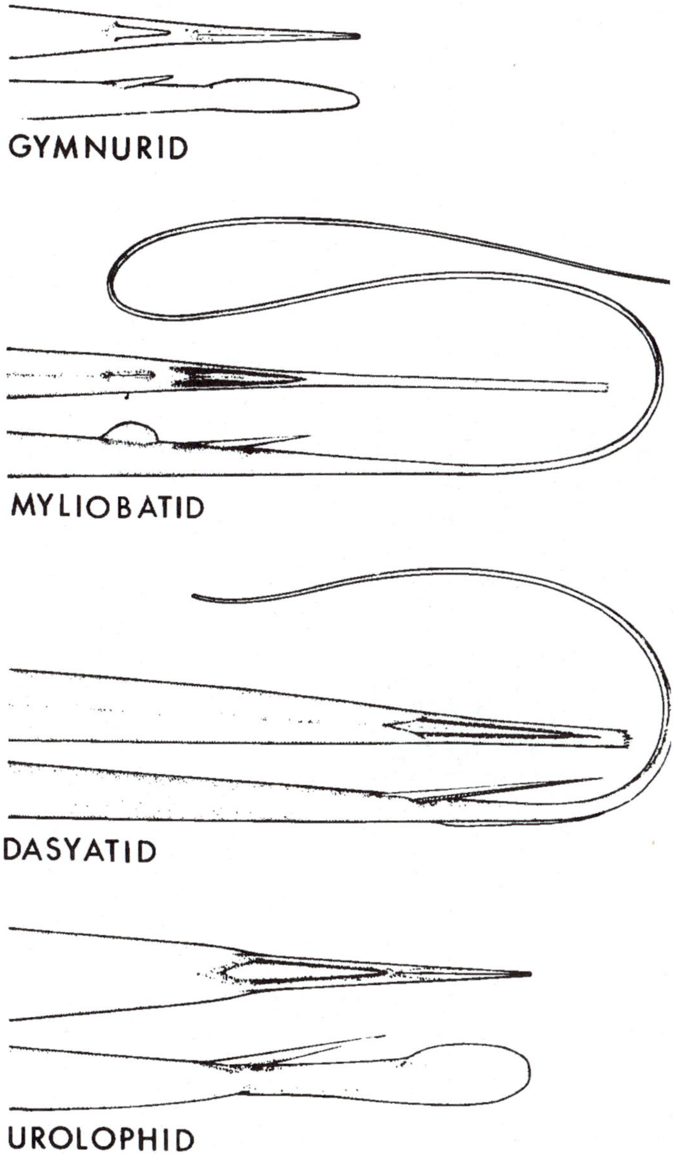

Fig. 52-37 Four anatomic types of stingray venom organs.

the heart may be directly injured.[152] Fatalities have been reported after abdominal or thoracic (cardiac) penetration, and from exsanguination from the femoral artery.*

The envenomation classically causes immediate local intense pain, edema, and variable bleeding. The pain may radiate centrally, peaks at 30 to 60 minutes, and may last for up to 48 hours. The wound is initially dusky or cyanotic and rapidly progresses to erythema and hemorrhagic discoloration, with rapid fat and muscle hemorrhage and necrosis.[15] If discoloration around the wound edge is not immediately apparent, within 2 hours it often extends several centimeters from the wound. Minor stings may simulate bacterial cellulitis. Systemic manifestations include weakness, nausea, vomiting, diarrhea, diaphoresis, vertigo, tachycardia, headache, syncope, seizures, inguinal or axillary pain, muscle cramps, fasciculations, generalized edema (with truncal wounds), paralysis, hypotension, arrhythmias, and death.[78,97] The paralysis may represent spastic muscle contractures induced by pain, which are a tremendous hazard for a diver or swimmer.

*References 44, 49, 60, 114, 121, 157.

Treatment

The success of therapy is largely related to the rapidity with which it is undertaken. Treatment is directed at combating the effects of the venom, alleviating pain, and preventing infection. The wound should be irrigated immediately with whatever cold diluent is at hand. If sterile saline or water is not available, tap or ocean water may be used. This removes some venom and mucus, provides mild anesthesia, and induces local vasoconstriction, possibly retarding the absorption of the toxin. In a rapid primary exploration of the wound, any visible pieces of the spine or integumentary sheath should be removed. Local suction, if applied in the first 15 to 30 minutes, may be of some value (this is controversial), as may a proximal constriction band (also controversial) that occludes only superficial venous and lymphatic return. This should be released for 90 seconds every 10 minutes to prevent ischemia.

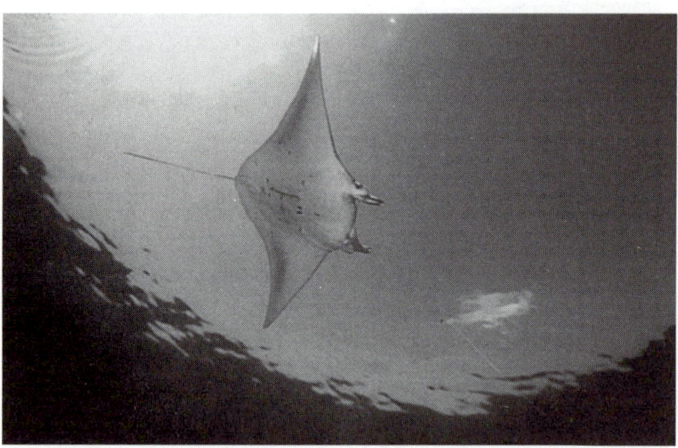

Fig. 52-38 Manta. This magnificent animal dines on small fish, crustaceans, and microorganisms. The stinging organ is vestigial. (Courtesy Carl Roessler.)

As soon as possible the wound should be soaked in nonscalding hot water to tolerance (upper limit 113° F or 45° C) for 30 to 90 minutes. This attenuates some of the thermolabile components of the protein venom and relieves pain. There is no indication for the addition of ammonia, magnesium sulfate, potassium permanganate, or formalin to the soaking solution. Under these circumstances they are toxic to tissue and may obscure visualization of the wound. During the hot water soak the wound should be explored and debrided of any readily visible pieces of the sting's integumentary sheath, which would continue to envenom the victim. Cryotherapy is disastrous, and no data support the use of antihistamines or steroids.

Pain control should be initiated during the first debridement or soaking period. Narcotics may be necessary. Local infiltration of the wound with 1% to 2% lidocaine (Xylocaine) without epinephrine may be useful.

After the soaking procedure the wound should be prepared in a sterile fashion, reexplored, and thoroughly debrided. Wounds should be packed open for delayed primary closure or sutured loosely around adequate drainage. Prophylactic antibiotics are recommended because of the high incidence of ulceration, necrosis, and secondary infection. If the abdominal cavity is penetrated, the victim should receive cefoxitin or clindamycin-gentamicin intravenously in addition to any antibiotics chosen to cover marine microbes.[92]

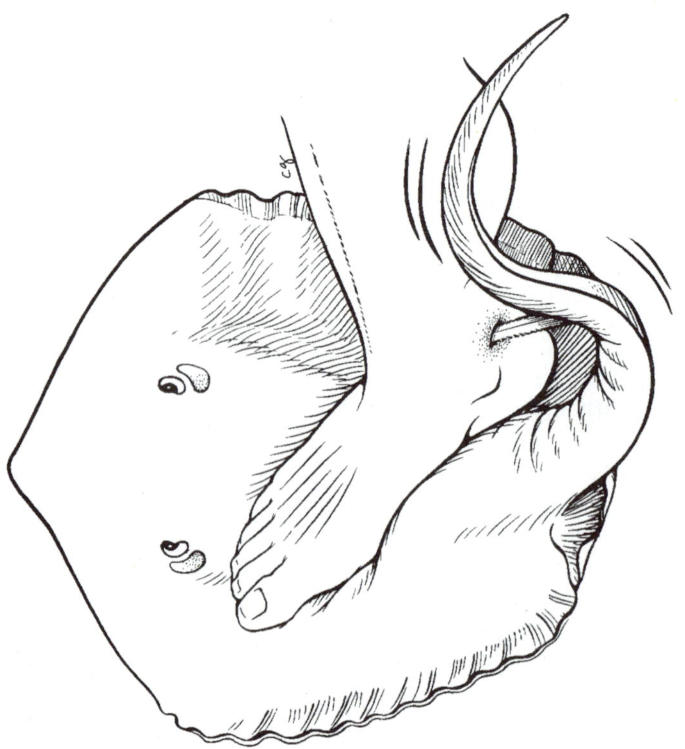

Fig. 52-39 The stingray lashes its tail upward into the leg and generates a deep puncture wound.

If a victim is to be treated and released, he or she should be observed for at least 3 to 4 hours for systemic side effects.

Wounds that are not properly debrided or explored and cleansed of foreign material may fester for weeks or months. Such wounds may appear infected, when what really exists is a chronic draining ulcer initiated by persistent retained organic matter. After a time, exploration may reveal erosion of adjacent soft tissue structures and the formation of an epidermal inclusion cyst or other related foreign body reaction.[16] As with other marine-acquired wounds, indolent infection should prompt a search for unusual microorganisms. A case of invasive fusariosis *(Fusarium solani)* after stingray envenomation responsive to sequential debridement and ketoconazole (the latter of indeterminant effect) has been reported.[93]

Prevention

The stingray spine can penetrate a wet suit, leather or rubber boot, and even the side of a wooden boat; therefore a wet suit or pair of sneakers is not adequate protection.[49,199] Persons walking through shallow waters known to be frequented by stingrays should shuffle along and create enough disturbance to frighten off any nearby animals.

SCORPIONFISH

Scorpionfish are members of the family Scorpaenidae and follow stingrays as perpetrators of piscine stings. Distributed in tropical and less commonly in temperate oceans, several hundred species are divided into three groups typified by different genera on the basis of venom organ structure: (1) *Pterois* (zebrafish, lionfish, and butterfly cod), (2) *Scorpaena* (scorpionfish, bullrout, and sculpin), and (3) *Synanceja* (stonefish). All have a bony plate (stay), which extends across the cheek from the eye to the gill cover. Each group contains a number of different genera and species; at least 80 species of the family Scorpaenidae have been implicated in human injuries or studied anatomically, biochemically, or physiopharmacologically.

Other venomous fish that sting in a manner similar to scorpionfish include the Atlantic toadfish (family Batrachoididae), with two venomous dorsal fin spines, and the Pacific ratfish *(Hydrolagus colliei)* and European ratfish *(Chimaera monstrosa),* both with a single dorsal venomous spine. Toadfishes hide in crevices and burrows, under rocks and debris, or in seaweed, sand, or mud. They may change coloration rapidly and remain superbly camouflaged. Rabbitfishes (family Siganidae), stargazers (family Uranoscopidae), and leatherbacks (family Carangidae) carry venomous spines and pose additional risks.

Life and Habits

The protective coloration and concealment in bottom structures make scorpionfish difficult to visualize. Some species bury themselves in the sand, and most dangerous types lie motionless on the bottom. In many regions scorpionfish are valuable as food fish. In the United States they are found in greatest concentration around the Florida Keys and in the Gulf of Mexico, off the coast of southern California, and in Hawaii.

Zebrafish (lionfish, firefish, or turkeyfish) are beautiful, graceful, ornate coral reef fish generally found as single or paired free swimmers or hovering in shallow water (Fig. 52-40) (Color Plate 128). They are increasingly popular as aquarium pets and are imported illegally as part of the "underground zoo."

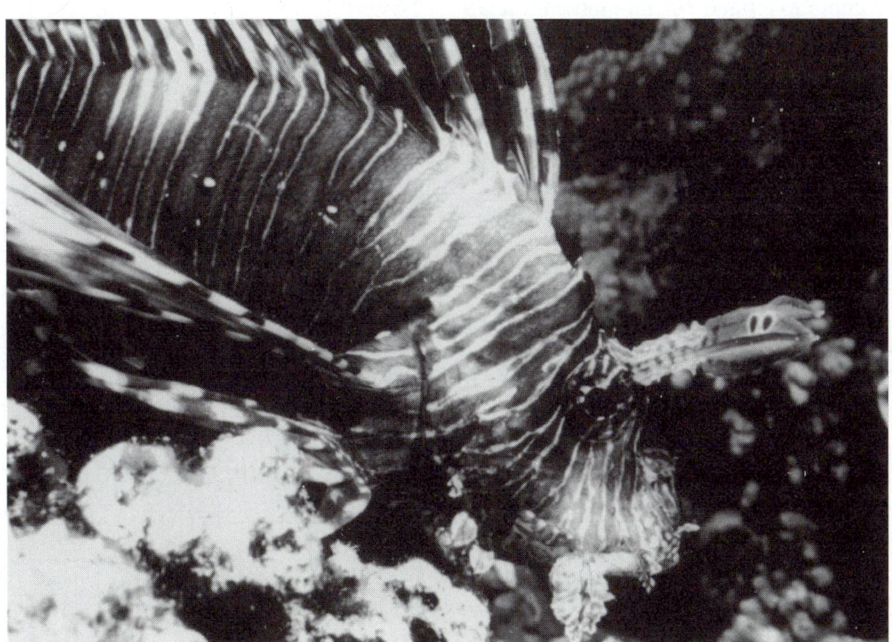

Fig. 52-40 Lionfish.

Scorpionfish proper *(Scorpaena)* dwell on the bottom in shallow water, bays, coral reefs, and along rocky coastlines, to a depth of 50 fathoms (Color Plate 129). Their shape and coloration provide excellent camouflage, allowing them to blend in with the ambient debris, rocks, and seaweed (Fig. 52-41). They can be captured by hook and line and serve as important food fish in many areas.

Stonefish live in shallow waters, often in tide pools and among reefs (Color Plate 130). They frequently pose motionless and absolutely fearless under rocks, in coral crevices or holes, or buried in the sand or mud (Fig. 52-42). They are so sedentary that algae frequently take root on their skin. They are usually 15 to 20 cm in length.

Venom and Venom Apparatus

The venom organs consist of 12 or 13 (of 18) dorsal, 2 pelvic, and 3 anal spines, with associated venom glands. Although they are frequently large, plumelike, and ornate, the pectoral spines are not associated with venom glands. Each spine is covered with an integumentary sheath, under which venom filters along grooves in the anterolateral region of the spine from the paired glands situated at the base or in the midportion of the spine. It is estimated that the two venom glands of a dorsal stonefish spine carry 5 to 10 mg of venom, closely associated with antigenic proteins of high molecular weight (between 50,000 and 800,000).[42,160,192] Scorpionfish venom contains multiple toxic fractions and, in the case of stonefish venom, has been likened in potency to cobra venom. The major toxic component of *Synanceja* venom (stonustoxin) is a protein of MW 150,000 that is both antigenic and heat labile.[199] The principal action of stonefish venom appears to be direct muscle toxicity, resulting in paralysis of cardiac, involuntary, and skeletal muscles.[76] In one analysis of biologic activity, stonefish *(Synanceja horrida)* venom exhibited edema-inducing, hemolytic, hyaluronidase, thrombinlike, alkaline phosphomonoesterase, 5′-nucleotidase, acetylcholinesterase, phosphodiesterase, arginine esterase, and arginine amidase activities.[102] Stonefish venom causes pulmonary edema in laboratory animals, which may reflect a general vascular permeability.[102,109] The neuromuscular toxicity appears to be a consequence of the venom's dose-dependent presynaptic and postsynaptic actions at the myoneural junction, which include release and depletion of neurotransmitter from the nerve terminal, followed by irreversible depolarization of muscle cells and microscopically observable muscle and nerve damage.[110] The nondialyzable opalescent venom retains full potency for at least 24 to 48 hours after death of a scorpionfish.[106,160] *Pterois* species carry long slender spines with small venom glands covered by a thin integumentary sheath. An extract of lionfish spine tissue contains acetylcholine and a toxin that affects neuromuscular transmission.[43] *Scorpaena* species carry longer heavy spines with moderate-sized venom glands covered by a thicker integumentary sheath. *Synanceja* species carry short, thick spines with large, well-developed venom glands covered by an extremely thick integumentary sheath (Fig. 52-43) (Color Plate 131). However, the skin over the venom gland is loosely attached, so when a human treads on the fish, the skin is pushed down the spine and the venom gland is compressed by the crumpled sheath. The pressure forces the venom gland to empty up the paired narrow ducts, so that venom and glandular tissue spurt into the wound.[77]

When any of these fish is removed from the water, handled, stepped on, or otherwise threatened, it reflexively erects the spinous dorsal fin and flares out the armed gill covers and pectoral and anal fins. If provoked while still in the water, it actually attacks. The venom is injected by a direct puncture wound through the skin, which tears the sheath and may fracture the spine, in a manner analogous to that of a stingray envenomation.

Clinical Aspects

Native residents of the Indo-Pacific islands have great fear of a sting from the dreaded venomous stonefish, such as the Tahitian "nohu" ("nofu" or "no'u") or the Australian

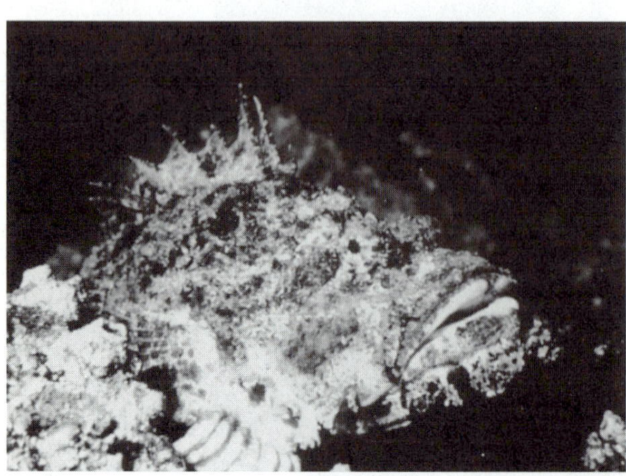

Fig. 52-41 Scorpionfish.

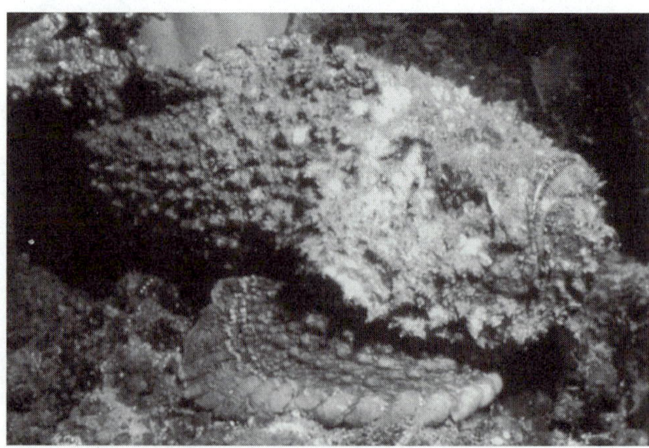

Fig. 52-42 Stonefish. (Courtesy Carl Roessler.)

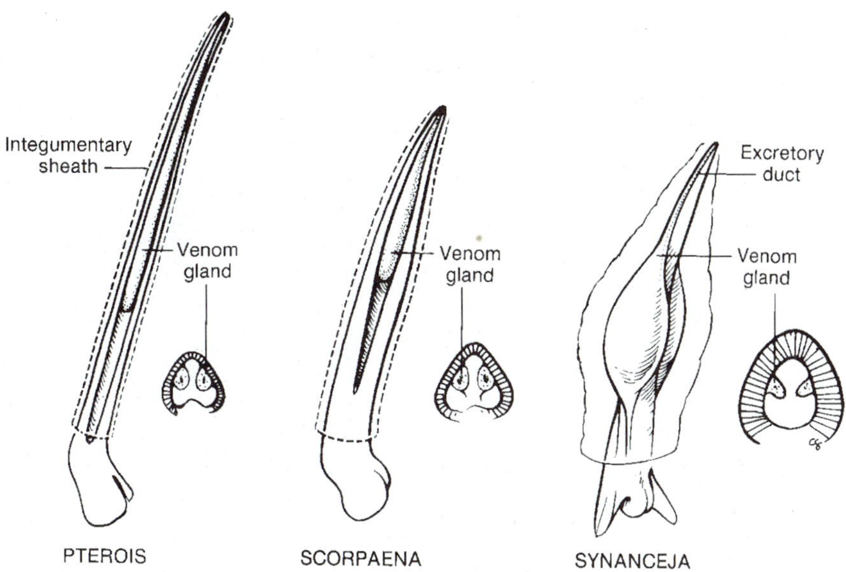

Fig. 52-43 Lionfish, scorpionfish, and stonefish spines with associated venom glands.

"warty ghoul." The presentation of the injury is similar to that of the stingray envenomation, in that the unwary diver or fisherman steps on or handles the fish. In the United States, marine aquarists and beneficiaries of illegal importation of tropical animals are increasingly envenomed as they unknowledgeably handle *Pterois volitans, P. radiata,* or *Scorpaena guttata.* In Indo-Pacific waters, envenomations of the foot and lower extremity are more commonly caused by the stonefish, such as *Synanceja horrida, S. trachynis,* or *S. verrucosa.* Scorpionfish stings vary according to the species, with a progression in severity from the lionfish (mild) through the scorpionfish (moderate to severe) to the stonefish (severe to life threatening).

The severity of the envenomation depends on the number and type of stings, species, amount of venom released, and age and underlying health of the victim. Pain is immediate and intense, with radiation centrally. Untreated, the pain peaks at 60 to 90 minutes and persists for 6 to 12 hours. In the case of the stonefish the pain may be severe enough to cause delirium and may persist at high levels for days. The wound and surrounding area are initially ischemic and then cyanotic, with more broadly surrounding areas of erythema, edema, and warmth. Vesicles may form (Color Plate 132). Human (hand) vesicle fluid after the sting of the lionfish *Pterois volitans* was analyzed for mediators of inflammation and demonstrated an appreciable quantity of prostaglandin $F_{2\alpha}$; thromboxane B_2, prostaglandin E_2, and 6-keto-prostaglandin $F_{1\alpha}$ were present in negligible quantities. Rapid tissue sloughing and close surrounding areas of cellulitis, with anesthesia adjacent to peripheral hypesthesia, may be present within 48 hours. Systemic effects include anxiety, headache, tremors, maculopapular skin rash, nausea, vomiting, diarrhea, abdominal pain, diaphoresis, pallor, restlessness, delirium, seizures, limb paralysis, peripheral neuritis or neuropathy, lymphangitis, arthritis, fever, hypertension, respiratory distress, bradycardia, tachycardia, atrioventricular block, ventricular fibrillation, congestive heart failure, pericarditis, hypotension, syncope, and death. Pulmonary edema is a bona fide sequel.[112] Death in humans, which is extremely rare, usually occurs within the first 6 to 8 hours. The wound is indolent and may require months to heal, only to leave a cutaneous granuloma or marked tissue defect, particularly after a secondary infection or deep abscess. Mild pain may persist for days to weeks. After successful therapy, paresthesias or numbness in the affected extremity may persist for a few weeks.

Treatment

As soon as possible, the wound or wounds should be immersed in nonscalding hot (upper limit 113° F or 45° C) water to tolerance to inactivate at least one of the thermolabile components of the protein venom that might otherwise induce a severe systemic reaction. Platelet aggregation in blister fluid is inhibited by heat treatment, which suggests that the venom or some other active component is neutralized. The soak should be maintained for a minimum of 30 minutes and may continue for up to 90 minutes. Recurrent pain that develops after an interval of 1 to 2 hours may respond to a repeat hot water treatment. During the soaking procedure, all obvious pieces of spine and sheath fragments should be gently removed from the wound. Vigorous irrigation should be performed with warmed sterile saline to remove any integument or slime. If pain is severe, local tissue infiltration with 1% to 2% lidocaine without epinephrine or regional nerve block may be necessary. Infiltration with emetine, hydrochloride, potassium permanganate, or Congo red has been largely abandoned, despite favorable experiences with acidic emetine. The biochemical bases for the success of folk remedies, such as the application of meat tenderizer, mangrove sap, or green papaya (papain), have yet to be confirmed. The effectiveness of alternative remedies may be related to the protein behavior of the venom, which is inactivated by heat, extremes of pH (it is partially inactivated at pH of greater than 8.6 and completely at a pH of less than 4), hydrogen peroxide, iodine, and potassium permanganate (which is, unfortunately, tissue toxic). Until further notice, no data are available to support the topical administration of empirical remedies, such as mineral spirits, organic dye, ground liver, or formalin. Cryotherapy is absolutely contraindicated.

Although the spine rarely breaks off into the skin, the wound should be explored to remove any spine fragments, which will otherwise continue to envenom and act as foreign bodies, perpetuating an infection risk and poorly healing wound. If the spine has penetrated deeply into the sole of the foot, surgical exploration should be performed in the operating room with magnification (Color Plate 133). Vigorous warmed saline irrigation should be performed. Wide excision and debridement are unnecessary. Because of the nature of the puncture wound, tight suture or surgical tape closure should not be undertaken; rather, the wound should be allowed to heal open with provision for adequate drainage. If the puncture wound is high risk (deep, into the hand or foot or both), prophylactic antibiotics should be administered.

A stonefish antivenin is manufactured by the Commonwealth Serum Laboratories, Melbourne, Australia (Fig. 52-44). In cases of severe systemic reactions from stings of *Synanceja* species, and rarely from other scorpionfish, it is administered intravenously. The antivenin is supplied in ampules containing 2 ml (2000 units) of hyperimmune Fab_2 horse serum, with 1 ml capable of neutralizing 10 mg of dried venom.[44] After skin testing to estimate the risk for an anaphylactic reaction to equine sera, the antivenin should be diluted in 50 to 100 ml of normal saline and administered slowly intravenously. Although the product may be given predilution intramuscularly, this route is not recommended in serious envenomations because absorption may be erratic. As a rough estimate, one vial should neutralize one or two significant stings (punctures). General guidelines for administration of antivenin have been previously discussed. When not in use, the antivenin should be protected from light and stored at 0° to 5° C, never frozen. Unused portions should be discarded. Physicians in the United States can obtain scorpionfish antivenin from the following sources: Health Services Department, Sea World, San Diego, California (619-222-6363, ext. 2201); Sea World, Aurora, Ohio (216-562-8101); and the Steinhart Aquarium, San Francisco, California (415-221-8014).

Prevention

The most effective way to prevent envenomation is to avoid handling a scorpionfish. A diver should make a careful inspection before setting down on the bottom. Amateur aquarists should be exceedingly cautious when handling exotic tropical fish. Seemingly dead fish may yield an unpleasant surprise for the unwary.

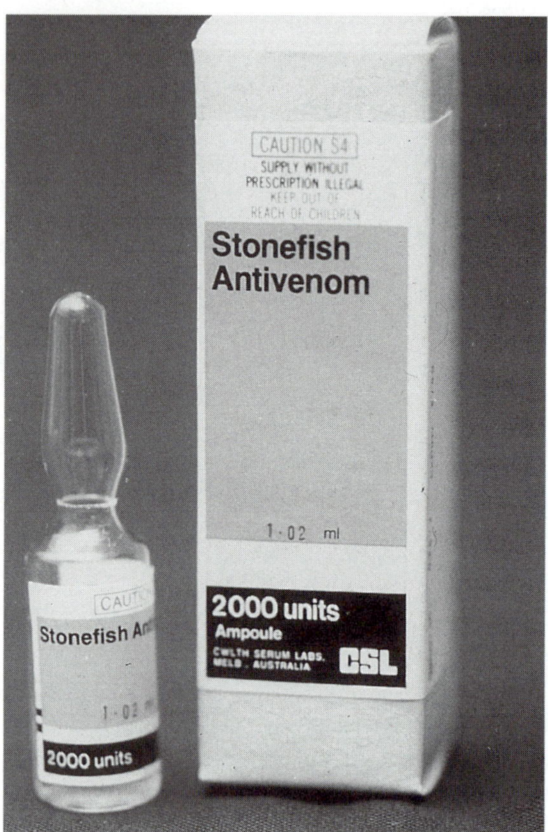

Fig. 52-44 Stonefish antivenom. (Courtesy John Williamson, M.D.)

CATFISH

Life and Habits

Approximately 1000 species of catfish inhabit both fresh and salt waters; many of these are capable of inflicting serious stings. Marine animals include *Plotosus lineatus* (oriental catfish), which lurks in tall seaweed and can inflict extremely painful stings, and the common sea catfish *(Galeichthys felis),* which hovers along the sandy bottom. The coral catfish *(Plotatus lineatus)* has also been reported to sting humans.[162] Freshwater catfishes of North America include the brown bullhead *(Noturus nebulosus),* Carolina madtom *(N. furiosus),* and channel *(N. punctatus),* blue *(N. furcatus),* and white *(N. catus)* catfish.

The catfish derives its name from the well-developed sensory barbels ("whiskers") surrounding the mouth. Catfish possess a slimy skin without any true scales. Marine catfish, unlike freshwater catfish, frequently travel in large schools. Most freshwater catfish are bottom feeders noted for their junkyard diet. They are poor swimmers and not very evasive.

The South American astroblepins have flattened suctorial lips that allow them to scale cliffs. Tiny South American (Amazonian) catfish of the genus *Vandellia* are known as "urethra fish" in English, "candirú" by Brazilians, and "canero" by Spanish speakers.[24] Approximately an inch long, they carry short spines on their gill covers (Fig. 52-45). The fish is putatively attracted to urine and can swim up the human urethra or other urogenital apertures, where it extends the gill covers and thus becomes embedded, preventing removal by pulling on the fish's tail. Since the animal normally seeks the outflow stream from a larger fish's gills, perhaps it is not urinophilic, but merely swimming upstream. Natives wear pudendal shields when urinating in natural bodies of water. A tight-fitting bathing suit is certainly prudent.

At best, extraction is painful. Amputation of the penis by natives has been described in the older literature. Ingestion of the green fruit of the jugua tree or buitach apple (*Genipa americana* L.) as a concoction (tea) apparently works to dispel the urethra-lodged candirú by the action of a large quantity of citric acid (mega-dose vitamin C), which softens calcium spines.[91]

Venom and Venom Apparatus

The venom apparatus of the catfish consists of the single dorsal and two pectoral fin spines ("stings") and the axillary venom glands. Both the dorsal and pectoral spines are exquisitely sharp and can be locked into an extended position by the fish when it is handled or becomes excited. The spines are enveloped by glandular tissue within an integumentary sheath; some spines have sharp retrorse teeth. Scattered reports note envenomation in persons who handled only the tail of the fish, such as the Arabian Gulf catfish *(Arius bilineatus),* which suggests the presence of a toxic skin secretion (crinotoxin). Oriental catfish toxin, which is poorly antigenic, contains vasoconstrictive, hemolytic, edema-forming, dermatonecrotic, and other biogenic fractions.[165] It behaves in vivo much like a milder version of stingray venom. In con-

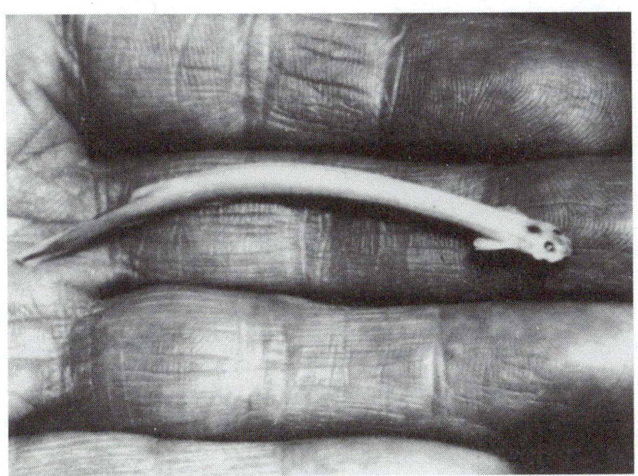

Fig. 52-45 Amazonian catfish (candirú), which can enter the human urethra.

crinotoxin of the Arabian Gulf catfish contracts smooth muscle and stimulates the release of prostaglandins; pretreatment with atropine and indomethacin attenuates the response.[3,162] Furthermore, wound healing responses are accelerated by repeated local application of preparations from the epidermal secretions of the Arabian gulf catfish (*Arius bilineatus,* Valenciennes).[4]

Clinical Aspects

Most stings are incurred when the fish are handled, which creates an injury out of proportion to the mechanical laceration. When the spine penetrates the skin, the integumentary sheath is damaged and the venom gland exposed. Catfish stings are described as instantaneously stinging, throbbing, or scalding, with central radiation up the affected limb. Normally the pain subsides within 30 to 60 minutes, but in severe cases it can last for up to 48 hours. The area around the wound quickly appears ischemic, with central pallor that gradually becomes cyanotic before the onset of erythema and edema. Swelling can be severe and secondary infections are frequent; gangrenous complications have been reported. Common side effects include local muscle spasm, diaphoresis, and fasciculations. Bleeding from the puncture wounds may be more severe than expected. Less common sequelae are peripheral neuropathy, lymphedema, adenopathy, lymphangitis, weakness, syncope, hypotension, and respiratory distress. Death is extremely rare. The sting of the marine catfish is usually more severe than that of its freshwater counterparts and may have a propensity to more local hemorrhage.[126]

Treatment

There are no specific antidotes. As with stingray and scorpionfish envenomations, the success of therapy is related to the rapidity with which it is undertaken. With catfish envenomations, in contrast to those of stingrays, constriction bandages have not been shown to be of value. The wound should be immediately immersed in nonscalding hot water to tolerance (upper limit 113° F or 45° C) for 30 to 90 minutes or until there is significant pain relief. This inactivates heat-labile components of the venom and perhaps helps to reverse local toxin-induced vasospasm. There is no evidence that adding mineral salts, solvents, antiseptics, or other chemicals to the water is of additional benefit. Cryotherapy is inefficacious. A popular and unstudied local (U.S. rural) remedy is to rub the sting with skin mucus (slime) from the catfish. If the hot water soak is not sufficient to control pain, local infiltration of the wound with buffered (alkalinized) bupivicaine or lidocaine without epinephrine or a regional nerve block may be necessary. It has been theorized that the pH alteration offered by the alkalinized local anesthetic may neutralize venom.[120] The wound should be explored surgically to remove all spine and sheath fragments. Standard radiographs or soft tissue exposures may locate a radiopaque foreign body. The wound should be left unsutured to heal, to allow adequate drainage and minimize the risk of infection. All wounds must be carefully observed for infection until healed. If the puncture wound is high risk (deep, into the hand or foot, or both), prophylactic antibiotics should be administered.

Prevention

Catfish should be handled without grabbing the dorsal or pectoral fins, preferably by using a mechanical instrument or gaff. If possible, *Plotosus lineatus* should not be handled at all.

WEEVERFISH

Life and Habits

The weeverfish (family Trachinidae) is the most venomous fish of the temperate zone. It is found in the Mediterranean Sea, eastern Atlantic Ocean, and European coastal areas. Common names for the weeverfish include the adderpike, sea dragon, sea cat, and stang. Weeverfish are small (10 to 53 cm) marine creatures that inhabit flat sandy or muddy bays, usually burying themselves in the soft bottom with only the head partially exposed (Fig. 52-46). They lead sedentary lives but when provoked can strike out with unerring accuracy. Weevers are terrors to fishermen working in shallow sandy areas.

Venom and Venom Apparatus

The venom apparatus consists of five to seven elongate and needle-sharp dorsal (up to 4.5 cm in length) and two opercular and daggerlike dentinal spines, associated holocrine glandular tissue, and the thin enveloping stratified squamous epithelium integumentary sheath. When excited, the fish extends the dorsal fin and expands the operculum, projecting the opercular spine out at a 35- to 40-degree angle from the longitudinal axis of the body. Weeverfish survive for hours out of the water, and the toxin remains potent for hours in dead animals, particularly when they are well refrigerated. Although incompletely characterized, the unstable (heat-labile) protein venom (ichthyoacanthotoxin) contains several peptides, at least one protein of high molecular weight (324,000), and possibly 5-hydroxytryptamine, epinephrine, norepinephrine, histamine, and mucopolysaccharide components. The greater weeverfish *(Trachinus draco)* releases a protein venom, dracotoxin, which has membrane depolarizing and hemolytic activities. It appears to be a single polypeptide of molecular weight 105,000.[41]

Clinical Aspects

Weeverfish stings usually afflict professional fishermen or vacationers who wade or swim along sandy coastal areas. The thrust of the spine is sufficient to penetrate a leather boot and creates a substantial puncture wound. The integumentary sheath is torn, and venom is injected into the wound. The onset of pain is instantaneous, described as intensely burning or crushing, spreading rapidly to involve the entire limb. The pain usually peaks at 30 minutes and subsides within 24 hours, but can last for days. Its intensity can induce irrational behavior and syncope; even narcotics are poorly effective. The puncture wound bleeds little and often appears pale and edematous initially. The sting of *Trachinus vipera* may bleed freely. Over the course of 6 to 12 hours the wound becomes erythematous, ecchymotic, and warm. The edema may increase for 7 to 10 days, causing the entire limb to become markedly swollen. Secondary bacterial infections are common, and gangrene has been reported. The indolent wound may require months to heal, depending on the nature of the sting and underlying health of the victim. Persistent edema has been noted to last for more than 1 year.

Systemic symptoms associated with weeverfish envenomations include headache, delirium, aphonia, fever, chills, dyspnea, diaphoresis, cyanosis, nausea, vomiting, seizures, syncope, hypotension, and cardiac arrhythmias. Death is rare.

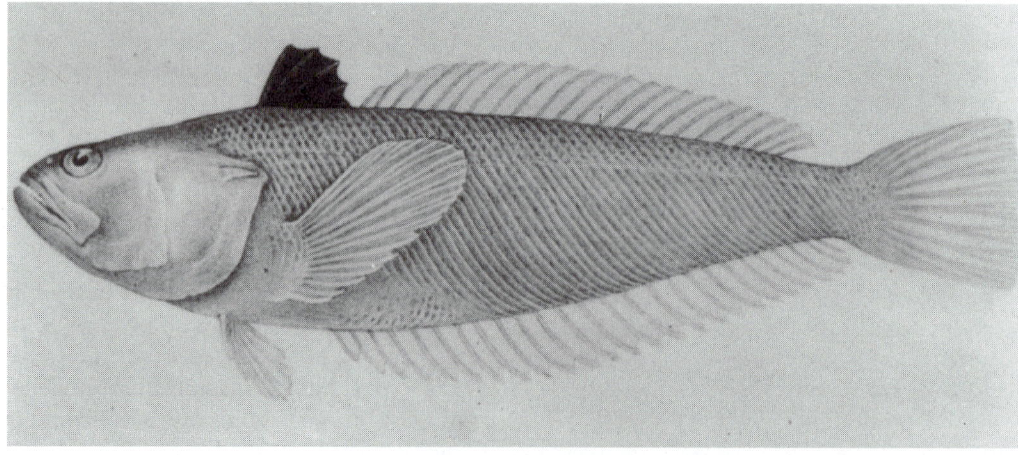

Fig. 52-46 Lesser weeverfish.

Treatment

The wound should immediately be immersed in nonscalding hot water to tolerance (upper limit 113° F or 45° C) for 30 to 90 minutes, or until there is significant pain relief. This inactivates heat-labile components of the venom and perhaps helps to reverse local vasospasm that might contribute to local sequestration of venom and the inhibition of free bleeding.[143] The addition of mineral salts, ammonia, vinegar, urine, or other substances to the water is of no proven value. Immersion in hot water is less often successful in therapy for a weeverfish sting than for that of a scorpionfish. When the heat inactivation method is inadequate to control pain, it is necessary to infiltrate the wound with a local anesthetic (1% to 2% lidocaine without epinephrine) or perform a regional nerve block. The liberal use of narcotics is often required. Cryotherapy is contraindicated.

Rarely, a spine breaks off into the skin. The wound should be gently explored, all fragments of sheath removed, and vigorous warmed saline irrigation performed. Wide excision and debridement are unnecessary. Because of the nature of the puncture wound, tight suture or surgical tape closure should not be undertaken; rather, the wound should be allowed to heal open with provision for adequate drainage. If the puncture wound is high risk (deep, into the hand or foot or both), prophylactic antibiotics should be administered. No commercial antivenin is currently available. An effective experimental *Trachinus* antivenin has been produced at the Institute of Immunology in Zagreb, Yugoslavia.

Prevention

Weeverfish hide in bottom sand and mud; thus persons must shuffle along with adequate footwear. These fish are easily provoked and should be avoided by scuba divers. They should *never* be handled alive and must be treated with extreme caution even when dead. Weeverfish survive for hours out of the water, and careless handling of a seemingly dead fish may result in an envenomation.

VENOMOUS (HORNED) SHARKS

Life and Habits

Horned sharks are species that possess dorsal fin spines. In the United States the group is essentially limited to the spiny dogfish *(Squalus acanthias)*. These and similar animals are distributed throughout sub-Arctic, temperate, tropical, and sub-Antarctic seas. The Port Jackson shark *Heterodontus portusjacksoni* is particularly dangerous.

The fish are sluggish and prefer cooler water and shallow protected bays. They are erratic in their migration and may be found singly or in schools. Voracious feeders, they eat other fishes, coelenterates, mollusks, crustaceans, worms, and fishing gear.

The venom apparatus consists of a spine anterior to each of two dorsal fins and the associated venom glands.

Clinical Aspects

As with other vertebrate stings, there is immediate intense stabbing pain that may last for hours and is accompanied by erythema and edema. Although systemic side effects are rare, fatalities are possible.

Treatment

Treatment is the same as for stingray envenomation.

SURGEONFISH

Life and Habits

The surgeonfish (doctorfish or "tang") is a tropical reef fish of the family Acanthuridae that carries one or more retractable jackknifelike spines on either side of the tail. When the fish is threatened, the spine may be extended out, where it serves as a blade (pointed in a forward direction) to inflict a laceration (Fig. 52-47). The spine may carry venom, which contributes to the pain.

Clinical Aspects

A victim cut by a surgeonfish notes a laceration or deep puncture wound that is immediately painful; it usually

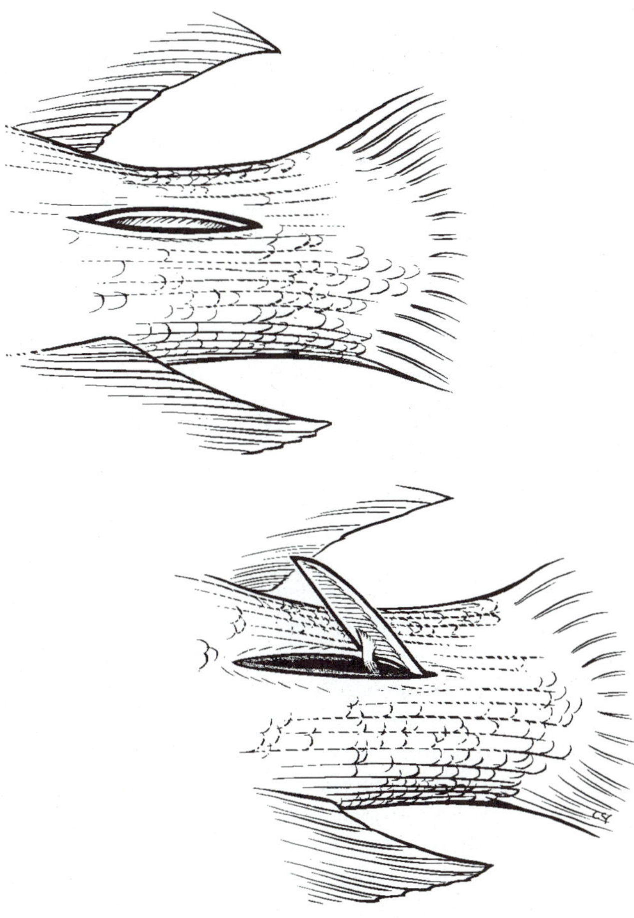

Fig. 52-47 "Blade" mechanism of the surgeonfish.

bleeds freely. The pain is moderate to severe and of a burning nature. Systemic reactions are infrequent and consist of nausea, local muscle aching, and apprehension.

Treatment

The wound should be irrigated and then soaked in nonscalding hot water to tolerance (upper limit 113° F or 45° C) for 30 to 90 minutes or until pain is relieved. It should be scrubbed vigorously to remove all foreign material and watched closely for the development of a secondary infection. Unless absolutely necessary for hemostasis, sutures should not be used to close the wound.

SEA SNAKES

Life and Habits

Sea snakes of the family Hydrophiidae (subfamilies Hydrophiinae [genera *Hydrelaps, Kerilia, Thalassophia, Enhydrina, Acalytophis, Thalassophis, Kolpophis, Lapemis, Astrotia, Pelamis, Microcephalophis*] and Laticaudinae [genera *Laticauda, Aipysurus, Emydocephalus*]) are probably the most abundant reptiles on earth. There are at least 52 species, all venomous. Species implicated in serious envenomations or human fatalities include *Astrotia stokesii, Enhydrina schistosa, Hydrophis ornatus, Hydrophis cyanocinctus, Lapemis hardwickii, Pelamis platurus,* and *Thalassophina viperina.*

The snakes are distributed in the tropical and warm temperate Pacific and Indian oceans, with the highest number of envenomations occurring along the coast of Southeast Asia, in the Persian Gulf, and in the Malay Archipelago. No sea snakes live in the Atlantic Ocean or in the Caribbean Sea. Hawaii is the only state that has sea snakes (predominantly *Pelamis platurus*). The Pacific snakes usually inhabit sheltered coastal waters and congregate about river mouths, but occasionally migrate far out to sea. *Pelamis platurus,* the most widely distributed sea snake, is pelagic and may be found in the Pacific coastal waters of Central and South America (Color Plate 134). It does not migrate to the Caribbean because of the freshwater barrier of Gatun Lake in the center of the Panama Canal.

Although sea snakes have the general appearance of land snakes, true sea snakes and sea kraits have valvelike nostril flaps and rudimentary ventral plates, without gills, limbs, ear openings, sternum, or urinary bladder. Most species of sea snakes are 3 to 4 feet long, but some attain lengths of up to 9 feet. They are sinuous scaled creatures whose bodies are compressed posteriorly into a flat, paddle-shaped tail designed for marine locomotion (Fig. 52-48). They swim in an undulating fashion and can move backward or forward in the water with equal speed. On land, however, they are awkward and do not survive readily. They may be brightly colored, as is the yellow-bellied sea snake, *Pelamis platurus.* With a single lung the sea snake is capable of diving to 100 m and remaining submerged for 2 hours. The sea snake can be distinguished from a sea eel by the presence of scales and the absence of gills and fins.

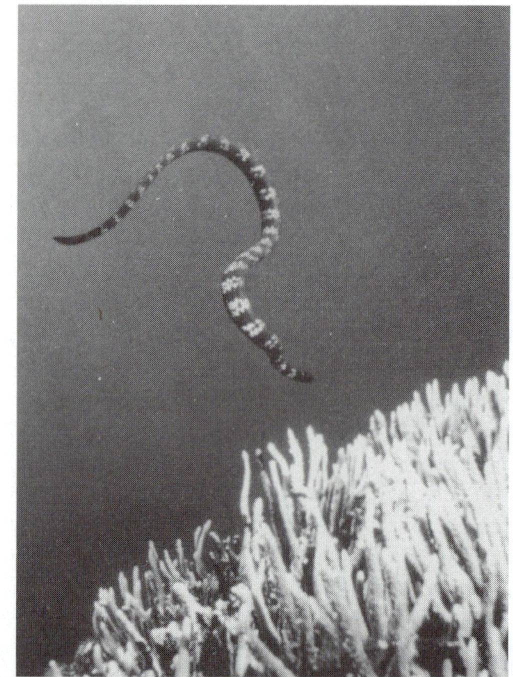

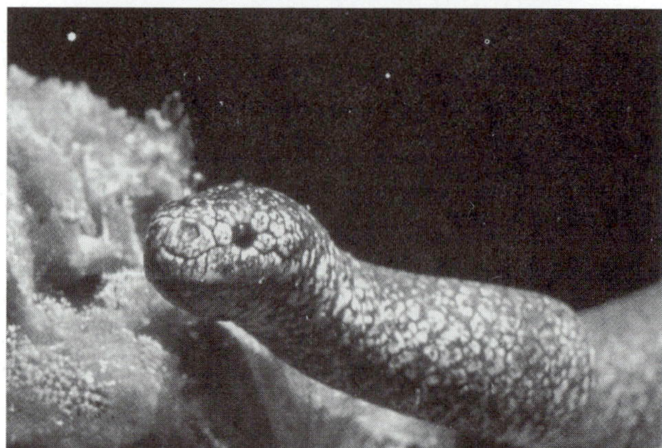

Fig. 52-48 Sea snakes in the Coral Sea. (Courtesy Carl Roessler.)

Sea snakes use an air retention mechanism in the lung to control buoyancy. Their food, small fish swallowed whole, is captured under water, usually around bottom rocks and coral. In general, sea snakes are docile creatures and flee when approached. However, when cornered or handled, they may become aggressive and strike out. During the reproductive season, some males adopt more irritable attitudes.

Venom and Venom Apparatus

The well-developed venom apparatus consists of two to four hollow maxillary fangs and a pair of associated venom glands. Fortunately, because the fangs are short and easily dislodged from their sockets, most bites (approximately 80%) do not result in significant systemic envenomation.

Most fangs, except for those of *Astrotia stokesii* and *Aipysurus laevii,* are not long enough to penetrate a wet suit. The venom yield of sea snakes varies with species and is largely related to the size of the venom glands.

The protein venom is highly toxic and includes stable peripheral neurotoxins more potent than those of terrestrial snakes. Neuromuscular transmission is blocked predominantly at the postsynaptic membrane and caused by attachment of toxin to the α subunit of the acetylcholine receptor. Presynaptic toxin in sea snake venom has been less well studied but appears to be related to inhibition of transmitter release by blocking resynthesis of acetylcholine from choline. It seems probable that the action of *Laticauda semifasciata* venom on excitable membranes is to alter ionic permeability, particularly that of sodium and chloride, without effect on Na^+,K^+ dependent adenosine triphosphatase activity. Calcium transport abnormalities are currently under investigation. Among other fractions of the venom are phospholipases, nerve growth factors, capillary permeability factor, anticomplement-active factor, enzymes (including acetylcholinesterase, hyaluronidase, leucine aminopeptidase, 5′-nucleotidase, phosphomonoesterase, phosphodiesterase), and hemolytic and myotoxic compounds, which result in skeletal muscle necrosis, intravascular hemolysis, and renal tubular damage. Myonecrosis is related to phospholipase A, which may inhibit calcium uptake into the sarcoplasmic reticulum. Neurotoxins are thought to exert their toxicity by binding in a nondepolarizing fashion to the nicotinic acetylcholine receptor and blocking neuromuscular transmission.[142]

The venoms of sea snakes are similar, as is reflected in positive reactions during immunodiffusion, immunoelectrophoresis, cross-neutralization by antivenin against heterologous venoms, and amino acid composition and sequences of neurotoxins. This is a reflection of phylogenetic relationships and is a logistic aid in the preparation of effective antivenin.

Although large venom yields have been obtained from *Astrotia stokesii, Enhydrina schistosa* is considered the most dangerous sea snake (Color Plate 135). *E. schistosa* is the most widely distributed sea snake in the Arabian sea. *Aipysurus duboisii* and *Acalyptophis peronii* from the Coral Sea have recently be shown to carry venoms of high human lethality potential.

Clinical Aspects

Bites are usually the result of accidental handling of snakes snared in the nets of fishermen, or of accidentally stepping on a snake while wading. Most sea snake poisonings occur in remote fishing villages and in boats at sea. Nearly all bites involve the extremities.

The diagnosis of sea snake bite is based on the following:

1. Location. A person must have been in the water or handling a fishing net containing a sea snake to have been bitten. Some snakes may foray briefly onto land, particularly in areas of heavy mangrove growth, but it is quite unusual for a bite to occur out of the water. Because snakes may inhabit sheltered coastal waters and frequently congregate near river mouths, a bite can occur in an estuarine setting.
2. Absence of pain. Initially, a sea snake bite does not cause great pain and may resemble no more than a pinprick.
3. Fang marks. These are multiple pinhead-sized hypodermic-like puncture wounds, usually one to four, but potentially up to twenty. If the skin is not broken, envenomation cannot occur. In some cases, particularly with a superficial injury through the arm or leg of a neoprene wet suit, the fang marks may be difficult to visualize because of the lack of a localized reaction.
4. Identification of the snake. Snakes should be captured or killed carefully with a nonmacerating blow behind the head and retained for identification by an expert.
5. Development of characteristic symptoms. These include painful muscle movement, lower extremity paralysis, arthralgias, trismus, blurred vision, dysphagia, drowsiness, vomiting, and ptosis. Neurotoxic symptoms are rapid in onset and usually appear within 2 to 3 hours. If symptoms do not develop within 6 to 8 hours, there has been no envenomation.

Envenomation by sea snakes characteristically shows an evolution of symptoms over a period of hours, with the latent period being a function of venom volume and patient sensitivity. The onset of symptoms can be as rapid as 5 minutes or as long as 8 hours. There is no appreciable local reaction to a sea snake bite other than the initial pricking sensation. The first complaint may be euphoria, malaise, or anxiety. Over 30 to 60 minutes, classic muscle aching and stiffness (particularly of the bitten extremity and neck muscles) develop, along with a "thick tongue" and sialorrhea, indicative of speech and swallowing dysfunction. Within 3 to 6 hours, moderate to severe pain is noted with passive movements of the neck, trunk, and limbs. Ascending flaccid or spastic paralysis follows shortly, beginning in the lower extremities, and deep tendon reflexes diminish and may disappear after an initial period of spastic hyperreactivity. Nausea, vomiting, myoclonus, muscle spasm, ophthalmoplegia, ptosis, dilated and poorly reactive pupils, facial paralysis, trismus, and pulmonary aspiration of gastric contents are frequent complications. Occasionally, bilateral painless swelling of the parotid glands develops.

Severe envenomations are marked by progressively intense symptoms within the first 2 hours of symptoms. Patients become cool and cyanotic, begin to lose vision, and may lapse into coma. Failing vision is reported to be a preterminal symptom. If peripheral paralysis predominates, the victim may remain conscious if hypoxia is avoided. Leukocytosis may exceed 20,000 white blood cells per milliliter; elevated plasma creatine kinase is variable. Elevated glutamic oxaloacetic transaminase reflects hepatic injury. Pathognomonic myoglobinuria becomes evident about 3 to 6 hours after the bite and may be accompanied by albuminuria and hemoglobinuria. Cerebrospinal fluid is normal. Respiratory distress and bulbar paralysis, pulmonary aspiration–related hypoxia, electrolyte disturbances (predominantly hyperkalemia), and acute renal failure (attributed in part to myonecrosis and pigment load) all contribute to the ultimate demise, which can occur hours to days after the untreated bite. Preterminal hypertension may occur. The mortality is 25% in patients who do not receive antivenin and 3% overall.

It is interesting to note the effects of sea snake *(Aipysurus laevis)* venom on prey fish.[208] The prey are subdued in six stages, which correlate roughly to certain aspects of a human envenomation: stage 1, increased ventilatory rate; stage 2, loss of mouth control, fin control, coordination, and buoyancy; stage 3, depressed ventilation, weakness, ineffective swimming; stage 4, apnea; stage 5, near paralysis, body color darkening; and stage 6, death.

Treatment

If possible, the offending snake should be captured for identification, taking care not to increase the number of victims. The therapy for bites by snakes of the family Hydrophiidae is similar to that for terrestrial snakes of the

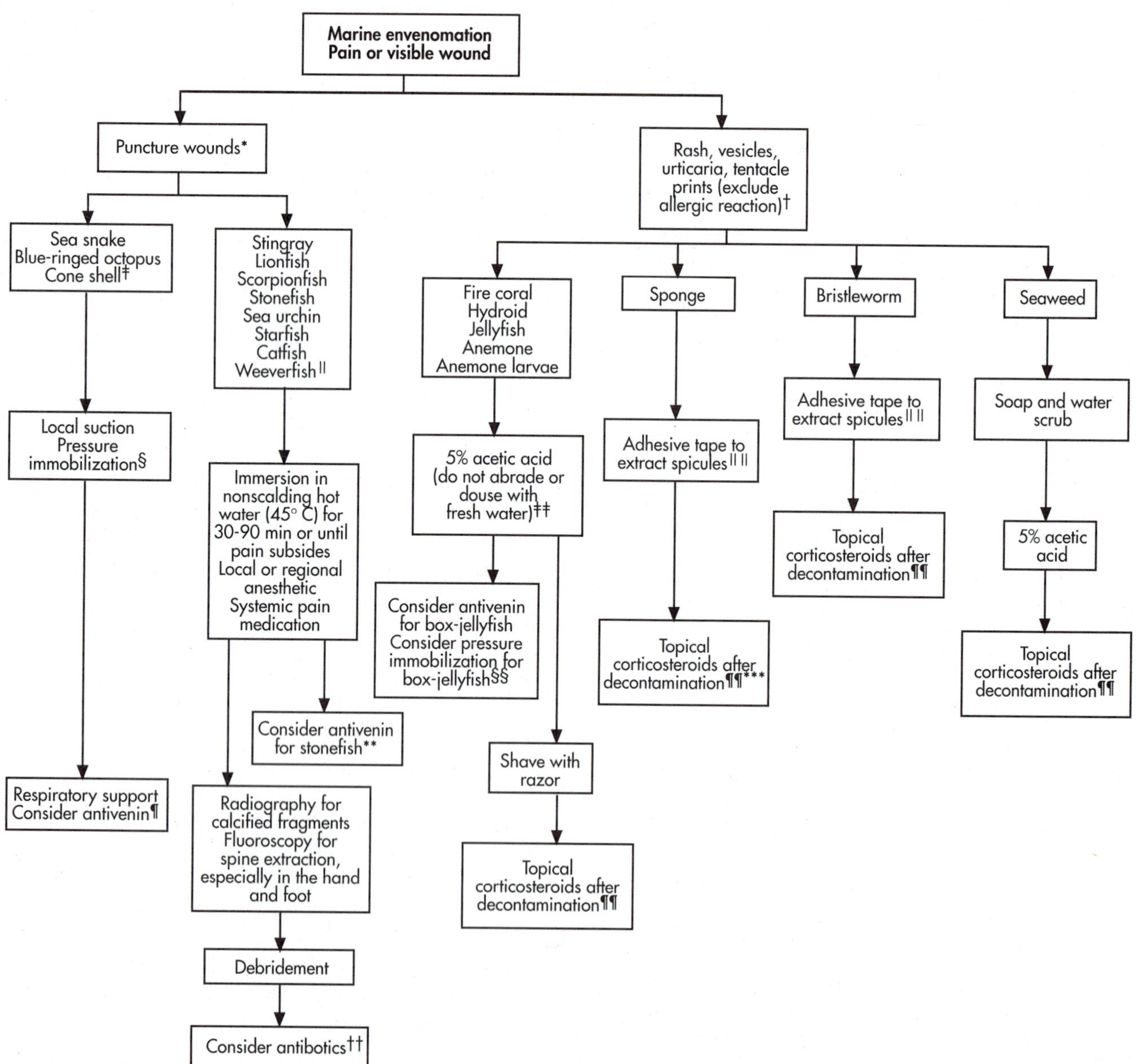

Fig. 52-49 For legend see opposite page.

family Elapidae. The affected limb should be immobilized and maintained in a dependent position while the victim is kept as quiet as possible. The pressure-immobilization technique for venom sequestration should be applied. If the location of the sting makes it practicable, a cloth or gauze pad of approximate dimensions 6 to 8 cm by 6 to 8 cm by 2 to 3 cm (thickness) should be placed directly over the fang marks and held firmly in place by a circumferential bandage 15 to 18 cm wide applied at lymphatic-venous occlusive pressure (70 mm Hg). The arterial circulation should not be occluded, as determined by the detection of arterial pulsations and proper capillary refill. The bandage should be released after 4 to 6 hours or after the victim has been brought to proper medical attention and the rescuer is prepared to provide systemic support. If the bite is on a digit where a compression bandage cannot be applied, a loose constriction bandage that constricts only the superficial venous and lymphatic flow may be applied proximal to the wound. This should be released for 90 seconds every 10 minutes and should be completely removed after 4 to 6 hours. If the bite is older than 30 minutes, neither technique may be very effective. Ice should not be directly applied to the wound.

Incision and suction therapy for snakebite is highly controversial. It should be employed only under the following

Fig. 52-49 Algorithmic approach to marine envenomation.
*A gaping laceration, particularly of the lower extremity, with cyanotic edges suggests a stingray wound. Multiple punctures in an erratic pattern with or without purple discoloration or retained fragments are typical of a sea urchin sting. One to eight (usually two) fang marks are usually present after a sea snake bite. A single ischemic puncture wound with an erythematous halo and rapid swelling suggests scorpionfish envenomation. Blisters often accompany a lionfish sting. Painless punctures with paralysis suggest the bite of a blue-ringed octopus; the site of a cone shell sting is punctate, painful, and ischemic in appearance.
†Wheal and flare reactions are nonspecific. Rapid (within 24 hours) onset of skin necrosis suggests an anemone sting. "Tentacle prints" with cross-hatching or a frosted appearance are pathognomonic for box-jellyfish *(Chironex fleckeri)* envenomation. Ocular or intraoral lesions may be caused by fragmented hydroids or coelenterate tentacles. An allergic reaction must be treated promptly.
‡Sea snake venom causes weakness, respiratory paralysis, myoglobinuria, myalgias, blurred vision, vomiting, and dysphagia. The blue-ringed octopus injects tetrodotoxin, which causes rapid neuromuscular paralysis.
§If *immediately* available (which is rarely the case), local suction can be applied without incision using a plunger device, such as The Extractor (Sawyer Products, Safety Harbor, Fla.). As soon as possible, venom should be sequestered locally with a proximal venous-lymphatic occlusive band of constriction or (preferably) the pressure immobilization technique, in which a cloth pad is compressed directly over the wound by an elastic wrap that should encompass the entire extremity at a pressure of 9.33 kPa (70 mm Hg) or less. Incision and suction are not recommended.
¶Early ventilatory support has the greatest influence on outcome. The mimimal initial dose of sea snake antivenin is one to three vials; up to ten vials may be required.
||The wounds range from large lacerations (stingrays) to minute punctures (stonefish). Persistent pain after immersion in hot water suggests a stonefish sting or a retained fragment of spine. The puncture site can be identified by forcefully injecting 1% to 2% lidocaine or another local anesthetic agent without epinephrine near the wound and observing the egress of fluid. Do not attempt to crush the spines of sea urchins if they are present in the wound. Spine dye from already-extracted sea urchin spines will disappear (be absorbed) in 24 to 36 hours.
**The initial dose of stonefish antivenin is one vial per two puncture wounds.
††The antibiotics chosen should cover *Staphylococcus, Streptococcus,* and microbes of marine origin, such as *Vibrio.*
‡‡Acetic acid 5% (vinegar) is a good all-purpose decontaminant and is mandated for the sting from a box-jellyfish. Alternatives, depending on the geographic region and indigenous jellyfish species, include isopropyl alcohol, bicarbonate (baking soda), ammonia, and preparations containing these agents.
§§The initial dose of box-jellyfish antivenin is one ampule intravenously or three ampules intramuscularly.
¶¶If inflammation is severe, steroids should be given systemically (beginning with at least 60 to 100 mg of prednisone or its equivalent) and the dose tapered over a period of 10 to 14 days.
***An alternative is to apply and remove commercial facial peel materials.
||||An alternative is to apply and remove commercial facial peel materials followed by topical soaks of 30 ml of 5% acetic acid (vinegar) diluted in 1 L of water for 15 to 30 minutes several times a day until the lesions begin to resolve. Anticipate surface desquamation in 3 to 6 weeks.

conditions: a mechanical suction extractor device is not available; the victim is seen within 5 minutes of the bite; the victim is elderly, chronically ill, or under 32 kg in body weight; the snake is positively identified as venomous; clear puncture marks are seen; the pressure-immobilization technique cannot be employed; and antivenin will be unavailable for 2 hours or longer. Two longitudinal parallel incisions should be made directly through the fang marks for a length of 5 mm to a depth of 5 to 10 mm. Cruciate incisions are improper. Suction is better applied with a rubber suction cup or commercial plunger-type venom extraction device; the mouth should be used only as a last resort because the introduction of mouth flora into the wound creates a contaminated human bite situation. Suction should be applied continuously for 30 to 60 minutes. A rescuer with denuded intraoral mucous membranes should take care to rapidly spit the mixture of blood and venom. There is little clinical enthusiasm for the perpetuation of incision and suction therapy, which may soon be relegated to therapeutic history.

The affected limb should be immobilized and maintained in a dependent position. The patient must be kept warm and as still as possible. As with terrestrial snakebite, cryotherapy is inefficacious and potentially harmful.

With any evidence of envenomation, polyvalent sea snake antivenin (an equine pepsin-digested immunoglobulin from Commonwealth Serum Laboratories, Melbourne, Australia) prepared against the venoms of *Enhydrina schistosa* and *Notechis scutatus* (terrestrial tiger snake) should be administered after appropriate skin testing for equine serum hypersensitivity. If this is not available, tiger snake *(Notechis scutatus)* antivenin should be used. Monovalent antivenin *(Enhydrina schistosa),* which is effective against the venoms of many species, is not yet widely available. Sea snake antivenin is specific and absolutely indicated in cases of envenomation. Supportive measures, while critical in management, are no substitute. The administration of antivenin should begin as soon as possible and is most effective if initiated within 8 hours of the bite. The minimum effective adult dosage is one ampule (1000 units), which neutralizes 10 mg of *E. schistosa* venom. The patient may require 3000 to 10,000 units (3 to 10 ampules), depending on the severity of the envenomation. The proper administration of antivenin is clearly described on the antivenin package insert.

Sea snake envenomation may induce severe physiologic derangements that require intensive medical management. Urine output and measured renal function should be closely monitored because hemolysis and rhabdomyolysis release hemoglobin and myoglobin pigments into the circulation, which precipitates acute renal failure. If hemoglobinuria or myoglobinuria is detected, the urine should be alkalinized with sodium bicarbonate and diuresis promoted with a loop diuretic (furosemide) or mannitol, as previously described for management of *Physalia* venom–induced nephropathy. Acute renal failure may necessitate a period of peritoneal dialysis or hemodialysis. Hemodialysis offers an alternative therapy that may be successful if antivenin is not available.

Respiratory failure should be anticipated as paralysis overwhelms the victim. Endotracheal intubation and mechanical ventilation may be required until antivenin adequately neutralizes the venom effects. Serum electrolytes should be measured regularly to guide the administration of fluids and electrolyte supplements. Hyperkalemia related to rhabdomyolysis and renal dysfunction must be promptly recognized and treated.

As previously mentioned, symptoms usually occur within 2 to 3 hours after envenomation. If there is no early evidence of envenomation, the victim should be observed for 8 hours before discharge from the hospital.

SUMMARY

A summary algorithmic approach to marine envenomation can be followed when the causative agent cannot be positively identified (Fig. 52-49).[7] Once the physician has made a commitment to a course of treatment based on a presumption of what creature has caused the injury, the subtleties of therapy can be employed.

REFERENCES

1. Abbott RT: Mollusks dangerous to scuba divers, *Del Med J* 45:161, 1973.
2. Abu-Nema T et al: Jellyfish sting resulting in severe hand ischaemia successfully treated with intra-arterial urokinase. Injury: *Br J Accident Surg* 19(4):294, 1988.
3. Al-Hassan JM et al: Vasoconstrictor components in the Arabian Gulf catfish *(Arius thalassinus)* proteinaceous skin secretion, *Toxicon* 24:1009, 1986.
4. Al-Hassan JM et al: Acceleration of wound healing responses induced by preparations from the epidermal secretions of the Arabian gulf catfish (*Arius bilineatus,* Valenciennes), *J Wilderness Med* 2:153, 1991.
5. Anker RL et al: Retarding the uptake of mock venom in humans: comparison of three first-aid treatments, *Med J Aust* 1:212, 1982.
6. Auerbach PS: Anaphylaxis. In Swartz MA, Moore ME, editors: *Emergency medical manual,* Baltimore, 1983, Williams & Wilkins.
7. Auerbach PS: Marine envenomations, *N Engl J Med* 325:486, 1991.
8. Auerbach PS, Hays T: Erythema nodosum following a jellyfish sting, *J Emerg Med* 5:487, 1987.
9. Bach MK: Mediators of anaphylaxis and inflammation, *Annu Rev Microbiol* 36:371, 1982.
10. Baden HP, Burnett JW: Injuries from sea urchins, *South Med J* 70:459, 1977.
11. Barach EM, et al: Epinephrine for treatment of anaphylactic shock, *JAMA* 251:2118, 1984.
12. Barnes JH: Observations on jellyfish stingings in North Queensland, *Med J Aust* 2:993, 1960.
13. Barnes JH: Cause and effect in Irukandji stingings, *Med J Aust* 1:897, 1964.
14. Barsan WG et al: A hemodynamic model for anaphylactic shock, *Ann Emerg Med* 14:834, 1985.
15. Barss P: Wound necrosis caused by the venom of stingrays, *Med J Aust* 141:854, 1984.
16. Bendt RR, Auerbach PS: Foreign body reaction following stingray envenomation, *J Wilderness Med* 2:298, 1991.

17. Bengston K et al: Sudden death in a child following jellyfish envenomation by *Chiropsalmus quadrumanus, JAMA* 266:1404, 1991.
18. Benoit E, Legrand AM, Dubois JM: Effects of ciguatoxin on current and voltage clamped frog myelinated nerve fibre, *Toxicon* 24:357, 1986.
19. Bergquist PR: Porifera. In Devaney DM, Eldredge LG, editors: *Reef and shore fauna in Hawaii. Section 1: protozoa through ctenophora,* Honolulu, 1977, Bishop Museum Press.
20. Bernheimer AW, Lai CY: Properties of a cytolytic toxin from the sea anemone, *Stoichactis kenti, Toxicon* 23:791, 1985.
21. Bielory L: A 17-year-old bitten by raccoon, *Consultant* 26(6):122, 1986.
22. Bitseff EL et al: The management of stingray injuries of the extremities, *South Med J* 63:417, 1970.
23. Boyd W: Sea-wasp antivenom in a toddler, *Med J Aust* 140:504, 1984.
24. Breault JL: Candirú: Amazonian parasitic catfish, *J Wilderness Med* 2:304, 1991.
25. Burnett HW, Burnett JW: Prolonged blurred vision following coelenterate envenomation, *Toxicon* 28:731, 1990.
26. Burnett JW, Calton GJ: The chemistry and toxicology of some venomous pelagic coelenterates, *Toxicon* 15:177, 1977.
27. Burnett JW, Calton GJ: Use of IgE antibody determinations in cutaneous coelenterate envenomations, *Cutis* 27:50, 1981.
28. Burnett JW, Calton GJ: Response of the box-jellyfish *(Chironex fleckeri)* cardiotoxin to intravenous administration of verapamil, *Med J Aust* 2:192, 1983.
29. Burnett JW, Calton GJ: Research in the Division of Dermatology of the University of Maryland, *Cutis* 33:387, 1984.
30. Burnett JW, Calton GJ: Recurrent eruption following a solitary envenomation by the cnidarian *Stomolophus meleagris, Toxicon* 23:1010, 1985.
31. Burnett JW, Calton GJ: Jellyfish envenomation syndromes updated, *Ann Emerg Med* 16:1000, 1987.
32. Burnett JW, Calton GJ, Burnett HW: Jellyfish envenomation syndromes, *J Am Acad Dermatol* 14:100, 1986.
33. Burnett JW, Calton GJ, Larsen JB: Significant envenomation by *Aurelia aurita,* the moon jellyfish, *Toxicon* 26(2):215, 1988.
34. Burnett JW, Gable WD: A fatal jellyfish envenomation by the Portuguese man-o'war, *Toxicon* 27:823, 1989.
35. Burnett JW, Rubinstein H, Calton GJ: First aid for jellyfish envenomation, *South Med J* 76:870, 1983.
36. Burnett JW et al: Studies on the serologic response to jellyfish envenomation, *J Am Acad Dermatol* 9:229, 1983.
37. Burnett JW et al: Local and systemic reactions from jellyfish stings, *Clin Dermatol* 5(3):14, 1987.
38. Burnett JW et al: Serological diagnosis of jellyfish envenomations, *Comp Biochem Physiol* 91C(1):79, 1988.
39. Burnett JW et al: Verapamil potentiation of *Chironex fleckeri* (box-jellyfish) antivenom, *Toxicon* 28(2):242, 1990.
40. Chand RP, Selliah K: Reversible parasympathetic dysautonomia following stinging attributed to the box-jellyfish *(Chironex fleckeri), Aust NZ J Med* 14:673, 1984.
41. Chhatwal I, Dreyer F: Isolation and characterization of dracotoxin from the venom of the greater weever fish *Trachinus draco. Toxicon* 30(1):87, 1992.
42. Choromanski JM, Murray TF, Weber LJ: Responses of the isolated buffalo sculpin heart to stabilized venom of the lionfish *(Pterois volitans), Proc West Pharmacol Soc* 27:229, 1984.
43. Cohen AS, Olek AJ: An extract of lionfish *(Pterois volitans)* spine tissue contains acetylcholine and a toxin that affects neuromuscular transmission, *Toxicon* 27(12):1367, 1989.
44. Cooper NK: Stone fish and stingrays—some notes on the injuries that they cause to man, *J R Army Med Corps* 137:136, 1991.
45. Cooper P, Wakefield MC: A sarcoid reaction to injury by sea urchin spines, *J Pathol* 112:33, 1974.
46. Corey EJ: Chemical studies on slow reacting substances/leukotrienes, *Experientia* 38:1259, 1982.
47. Cracchiolo A, Goldberg L: Local and systemic reactions to puncture injuries by the sea urchin spine and the date palm thorn, *Arthritis Rheum* 20:1206, 1977.
48. Crone HD, Keene TEB: Further studies on the biochemistry of the toxins from the sea wasp *Chironex fleckeri, Toxicon* 9:145, 1971.
49. Cross TB: An unusual stingray injury—the skindiver at risk, *Med J Aust* 2:947, 1976.
50. DeLaubenfels MW: The sponges of Kaneohe Bay, Oahu, *Pacific Sci* 4:3, 1950.
51. DeLaubenfels MW: The sponges of the Island of Hawaii, *Pacific Sci* 5:256, 1951.
52. DeLuca A et al: Differential sensitivities of avian and mammalian neuromuscular junctions to inhibition of cholinergic transmission by ω-conotoxin GVIA, *Toxicon* 29(3):311, 1991.
53. Dormandy TL: Trace element analysis of hair, *Br Med J* 293:975, 1986.
54. Edmonds C: A non-fatal case of blue-ringed octopus bite, *Med J Aust* 2:601, 1969.
55. Endean R: The venom of the blue-ringed octopus. In Pearn J, editor: *Animal toxins and man,* Brisbane, 1981, Division of Health, Education and Information, Queensland, Australia.
56. Endean R, Noble M: Toxic material from the tentacles of the cubomedusan *Chironex fleckeri, Toxicon* 9:255, 1971.
57. Everitt BJ, Jurevics HA: Some pharmacological properties of the crude toxin from the spines of the crown of thorns starfish *Acanthaster planci, Proc Aust Physiol Pharmacol Soc* 4:46, 1973.
58. Exton DR, Fenner PJ, Williamson JA: Cold packs: effective topical analgesia in the treatment of painful stings by *Physalia* and other jellyfish, *Med J Aust* 151:625, 1989.
59. Fenner P: The management of stings by jellyfish, other than *Chironex, J S Pacific Underwater Med Soc* 16(3):97, 1986.
60. Fenner PJ, Williamson JA, Skinner RA: Fatal and nonfatal stingray envenomation, *Med J Aust* 151:621, 1989.
61. Fenner PJ et al: The "Irukandji syndrome" and acute pulmonary edema, *Med J Aust* 149:150, 1988.
62. Fenner PJ et al: First aid treatment of jellyfish stings in Australia: response to a newly differentiated species, *Med J Aust* 158:498, 1993.
63. Filling-Katz MR: Mononeuritis multiplex following jellyfish stings, *Ann Neurol* 15:213, 1984.
64. Fisher AA: *Atlas of aquatic dermatology,* New York, 1978, Grune & Stratton.
65. Flecker H: Irukandji sting to North Queensland bathers without production of wheals but with severe general symptoms, *Med J Aust* 2:89, 1952.
66. Freudenthal AR: Seabather's eruption: range extended northward and a causative organism identified, *Rev Int Oceanographic Med* 137, 1991.
67. Freudenthal AR, Joseph PR: Seabather's eruption, *N Engl J Med* 329:542, 1993.
68. Freyvogel TA: Poisonous and venomous animals in East Africa, *Acta Trop (Basel)* 29:401, 1972.
69. Fulghum DD: Octopus bite resulting in granuloma annulare, *South Med J* 79:1434, 1986.
70. Galettis P, Norton RS: Biochemical and pharmacological studies of the mechanism of action of tenebrosin-C, a cardiac stimulatory and haemolytic protein from the sea anemone, *Actinia tenebrosa, Toxicon* 28(6):695, 1990.
71. Garcia-Alonso I et al: Biological activity of secretions and extracts of gorgonians from Cuban waters, *J Nat Toxins* 2(1):27, 1993.
72. Gaur PK, Calton GJ, Burnett JW: Enzyme-linked immunosorbent assay to detect anti–sea nettle venom antibodies, *Experientia* 37:1005, 1981.
73. Gilliland BC: Serum sickness and immune complexes, *N Engl J Med* 311:1435, 1984.

74. Glasser DV et al: Ocular jellyfish stings, *Ophthalmology* 92:1414, 1992.
75. Glasser DV et al: A guinea-pig model of corneal jellyfish envenomation, *Toxicon* 31(6):808, 1993.
76. Goetz CG: Pharmacology of animal neurotoxins, *Clin Neuropharm* 5:231, 1982.
77. Gopalakrishnakone P, Gwee MCE: The structure of the venom gland of stonefish *Synanceja horrida, Toxicon* 31(8):979, 1993.
78. Grainger CR: Occupational injuries due to sting rays, *Trans R Soc Trop Med Hyg* 74:408, 1980.
79. Granata AV, Halickman JF, Borak J: Utility of military anti-shock trousers (MAST) in anaphylactic shock—a case report, *J Emerg Med* 2:349, 1984.
80. Gray WR, Olivera BM, Cruz LJ: Peptide toxins from venomous *Conus* snails, *Annu Rev Biochem* 57:665, 1988.
81. Guess HA, Saviteer PL, Morris RC: Hemolysis and acute renal failure following a Portuguese man-of-war sting, *Pediatrics* 70:979, 1982.
82. Hahin R et al: Alterations in sodium channel gating produced by the venom of the marine mollusc *Conus striatus, Toxicon* 29(2):245, 1991.
83. Halstead BW: Marine pollution and the pharmaceutical scientist, *Am J Pharmacol Ed* 37:267, 1978.
84. Halstead BW: *Dangerous marine animals,* Centreville, Md, 1980, Cornell Maritime Press.
85. Halstead BW: *Current status of marine biotoxicology—an overview,* Colton, Calif, 1980, International Biotoxicological Center, World Life Research Institute.
86. Hansen PA, Halstead BW: The venomous sea anemone *Actinodendron plumosum* (Haddon) of South Vietnam, *Micronesia* 7:123, 1971.
87. Hartwick RF: Distributional ecology and behaviour of the early life stages of the box-jellyfish *Chironex fleckeri, Hydrobiologia* 216/217:181, 1991.
88. Hartwick R, Callahan V, Williamson J: Disarming the box-jellyfish, *Med J Aust* 1:15, 1980.
89. Harvey AL, Aneiros A, Casaneda O: Potassium channel toxins from marine animals (abstract), *Toxicon* 31(5):504, 1993.
90. Heiskanen LP, Jurevics HA, Everitt BJ: The inflammatory effects of the crude toxin of the crown of thorns starfish *Acanthaster planci, Proc Aust Physiol Pharmacol Soc* 4:47, 1973.
91. Herman JR: *Candirú:* urinophilic catfish: its gift to urology, *Urology* 1:265, 1973.
92. Heseltine PNR et al: The efficacy of cefoxitin vs. clindamycin/gentamicin in surgically treated stab wounds of the bowel, *J Trauma* 26:241, 1986.
93. Hiemenz JW, Kennedy B, Kwon-Chung KJ: Invasive fusariosis associated with an injury by a stingray barb, *J Med Vet Mycol* 28:209, 1990.
94. Hoehne JH, Lockey SD, Chosy JJ: Comparison of epinephrine excretion after aerosol and subcutaneous administration, *J Allergy* 46:336, 1970.
95. Holstein T, Tardent P: An ultrahigh-speed analysis of exocytosis: nematocyst discharge, *Science* 233:830, 1984.
96. Hopkins DG: Venomous effects and treatment of octopus bite, *Med J Aust* 1:81, 1964.
97. Ikeda T: Supraventricular bigeminy following a stingray envenomation: a case report, *Hawaii Med J* 48(5):162, 1989.
98. Ioannides G, Davis JH: Portuguese man-of-war stinging, *Arch Dermatol* 91:448, 1965.
99. Kao CY: Tetrodotoxin, saxitoxin, and their significance in the study of the excitation phenomena, *Pharmacol Rev* 18:997, 1966.
100. Keene TEB, Crone HD: The hemolytic properties of extracts of tentacles from the cnidarian *Chironex fleckeri, Toxicon* 7:55, 1969.
101. Keene TEB, Crone HD: Dermatonecrotic properties of extracts from the tentacles of the cnidarian *Chironex fleckeri, Toxicon* 7:173, 1969.
102. Khoo HE et al: Biological activities of *Synanceja horrida* (stonefish) venom, *Natural Toxins* 1:54, 1992.
103. Kingston CW, Southcott RV: Skin histopathology in fatal jellyfish stinging, *Trans R Soc Trop Med Hyg* 54:373, 1960.
104. Kizer KW: Marine envenomations, *J Toxicol Clin Toxicol* 21:527, 1984.
105. Kizer KW, Auerbach PS: Marine envenomations: not just a problem of the tropics, *Emerg Med Rep* 6:129, 1985.
106. Kizer KW, McKinney HE, Auerbach PS: Scorpaenidae envenomation: a five-year poison center experience, *JAMA* 253:807, 1985.
107. Kizer KW, Piel M: Arterial blood gas changes with bluebottle envenomation—a case report, *Hawaii Med J* 7:193, 1982.
108. Kohn AJ: Cone shell stings: recent cases of human injury due to venomous marine snails of the genus *Conus, Hawaii Med J* 17:528, 1958.
109. Kreger AS: Detection of a cytolytic toxin in the venom of the stonefish *(Synanceja trachynis), Toxicon* 29:733, 1991.
110. Kreger AS et al: Effects of stonefish *(Synanceia trachynis)* venom on murine and frog neuromuscular junctions, *Toxicon* 31(3):307, 1993.
111. Lawley TJ et al: A prospective clinical and immunologic analysis of patients with serum sickness, *N Engl J Med* 311:1407, 1984.
112. Lehmann DF, Hardy JC: Stonefish envenomation (letter), *N Engl J Med* 329(7):510, 1993.
113. Levy S, Masry D, Halstead BW: Report of stingings by the sea anemone *Triactis producta* Klunziger from Red Sea, *Clin Toxicol* 3:637, 1970.
114. Liggins JB: An unusual bathing fatality, *NZ Med J* 38:27, 1939.
115. Lin DC, Hessinger DA: Possible involvement of red cell membrane proteins in the hemolytic action of Portuguese man-of-war toxin, *Biochem Biophys Res Commun* 91:761, 1979.
116. Linaweaver PG: Toxic marine life, *Milit Med* 131:437, 1967.
117. Lucas J: The crown of thorns starfish, *Oceanus* 29(2):55, 1986.
118. Maček P, Lebez D: Isolation and characterization of three lethal and hemolytic toxins from the sea anemone *Actinia equina* L, *Toxicon* 26(5):441, 1988.
119. Mandojana RM: Granuloma annulare following bluebottle jellyfish *(Physalia utriculus)* sting, *J Wilderness Med* 1:220, 1990.
120. Mann JW, Werntz JR: Catfish stings to the hand, *J Hand Surg* 16A:318, 1991.
121. Manowitz NR, Rosenthal RR: Cutaneous-systemic reactions to toxins and venoms of common marine organisms, *Cutis* 23:450, 1979.
122. Mansson T et al: Recurrent cutaneous jellyfish eruptions without envenomation, *Acta Dermatol Veneriol (Stockh)* 65:72, 1985.
123. Maretic Z, Russell FE: Stings by the sea anemone *Anemonia sulcata* in the Adriatic Sea, *Am J Trop Med Hyg* 32:891, 1983.
124. Martin JC, Audley I: Cardiac failure following Irukandji envenomation, *Med J Aust* 153:164, 1990.
125. Matusow RJ: Oral inflammatory response to a sting from a Portuguese man-of-war, *J Am Dent Assoc* 100:73, 1980.
126. McKinistry DM: Catfish stings in the United States: case report and review, *J Wilderness Med* 4:293, 1993.
127. Mebs D et al: Hemolysins and proteinase inhibitors from sea anemones of the Gulf of Aqaba, *Toxicon* 21:257, 1983.
128. Meyer PK: Seastroke: a new entity? *South Med J* 86(7):777, 1993.
129. Moats WE: Fire coral envenomation, *J Wilderness Med* 3:284, 1992.
130. Moran PJ, Bradbury RH, Reichelt RE: Mesoscale studies of the crown of thorns/coral interaction: a case history from the Great Barrier Reef, *Proc Fifth Int Coral Reef Congr* 5:321, 1985.
131. Moran PJ, Williamson J: Toxic reactions to injuries caused by the spines of the crown of thorns starfish *(Acanthaster planci), J S Pacific Underwater Med Soc* 16(3):91, 1986.
132. Mullanney PJ: Treatment of sting ray wounds, *Clin Toxicol* 3:613, 1970.
133. Nakagawa H, Tu AT, Kimura A: Purification and characterization of contractin A from the pedicellarial venom of sea urchin, *Toxopneustes pileolus, Arch Biochem Biophys* 284(2):279, 1991.
134. Neale TJ, Theofilopoulos AN, Wilson CB: Methods for the detection of soluble circulating immune complexes and their application, *Pathobiol Annu* 9:113, 1979.

135. Odom CB, Fischelmann EA: Crown of thorns starfish wounds—some observations on injury sites, *Hawaii Med J* 31:99, 1972.
136. Olivera BM et al: Conotoxins and other biologically active peptides in *Conus* venoms (abstract), *Toxicon* 28:256, 1990.
137. Olson CE et al: Interrelationships between toxins: studies on the cross-reactivity between bacterial or animal toxins and monoclonal antibodies to two jellyfish venoms, *Toxicon* 23:307, 1985.
138. O'Neal RL, Halstead BW, Howard LD: Injury to human tissues from sea urchin spines, *Calif Med* 101:199, 1964.
139. Othman I, Burnett JW: Techniques applicable for purifying *Chironex fleckeri* (box-jellyfish) venom, *Toxicon* 28(7):821, 1990.
140. Otten EJ: Antivenin therapy in the emergency department, *Am J Emerg Med* 1:83, 1983.
141. Otten EJ, McKimm D: Venomous snakebite in a patient allergic to horse serum, *Ann Emerg Med* 12:624, 1983.
142. Pachner AR, Ricalton N: In vitro neutralization by monoclonal antibodies of α-bungarotoxin binding to acetylcholine receptor, *Toxicon* 27(12):1263, 1989.
143. Patkin M, Freeman D: Bullrout stings, *Med J Aust* 2:14, 1969.
144. Peel N, Kandler R: Localized neuropathy following jellyfish sting, *Postgrad Med* 66:953, 1990.
145. Piérard GE, Letot B, Piérard-Franchimont C: Histologic study of delayed reactions to coelenterates, *J Am Acad Dermatol* 22:599, 1990.
146. Portier H, Richet C: De l'action anaphylactique de certains venins, *Comp Rend Soc Biol (Paris)* 54:170, 1902.
147. Prescott BD: "Scombroid poisoning" and bluefish: the Connecticut connection, *Conn Med* 48:105, 1984.
148. Rathjen WF, Halstead BW: Report on two fatalities due to stingrays, *Toxicon* 6:301, 1969.
149. Rice RD, Halstead BW: Report of fatal cone shell sting by *Conus geographus* (Linnaeus), *Toxicon* 5:223, 1968.
150. Rifkin JF, Fenner PJ, Williamson JAH: First aid treatment of the sting from the hydroid *Lytocarpus philippinus:* the structure of, and in vitro discharge experiments with its nematocysts, *J Wilderness Med* 4:252, 1993.
151. Rocha G, Fraga S: Sea urchin granuloma of the skin, *Arch Dermatol* 85:406, 1962.
152. Ronka EKF, Roe WF: Cardiac wound caused by the spine of the stingray (suborder Masticura), *Milit Surg* 97:135, 1945.
153. Rosco MD: Cutaneous manifestations of marine animal injuries including diagnosis and treatment, *Cutis* 19:507, 1977.
154. Russell FE: Stingray injuries: a review and discussion of their treatment, *Am J Clin Pathol* 64:382, 1953.
155. Russell FE: Comparative pharmacology of some animal toxins, *Fed Proc* 26:1206, 1967.
156. Russell FE: *Snake venom poisoning,* Great Neck, NY, 1983, Scholium International.
157. Russell FE et al: Studies on the mechanism of death from stingray venom: a report of two fatal cases, *Am J Med Sci* 235:566, 1958.
158. Russo AJ, Calton GJ, Burnett JW: The relationship of the possible allergic response to jellyfish envenomation and serum antibody titers, *Toxicon* 21:475, 1983.
159. Savage IVE, Howden MEH: Hapalotoxin, a second lethal toxin from the octopus, *Hapalochlaena maculosa, Toxicon* 15:463, 1977.
160. Schaeffer RC Jr, Carlson RW, Russell FE: Some chemical properties of the venom of the scorpionfish *Scorpaena guttata, Toxicon* 9:69, 1971.
161. Schultz KE: Dangerous marine organisms. In Kravis TC, Warner CG, editors: *Emergency medicine. A comprehensive review,* 1983, Rockville, Md, Aspen Systems.
162. Shepherd S, Thomas SH, Stone CK: Catfish envenomation, *J Wilderness Med* 5(1):67, 1994.
163. Sheumack DD et al: Maculotoxin: a neurotoxin from the venom glands of the octopus *Hapalochlaena maculosa* identified as tetrodotoxin, *Science* 199:188, 1978.
164. Shiomi K et al: Isolation and characterization of a lethal hemolysin in the sea anemone *Parasicyonis actinostoloides, Toxicon* 23:865, 1985.
165. Shiomi K et al: Toxins in the skin secretion of the oriental catfish *(Plotosus lineatus):* immunological properties and immunocytochemical identification of producing cells, *Toxicon* 26:353, 1988.
166. Shiomi K et al: Liver damage by the crown-of-thorns starfish *(Acanthaster planci)* lethal factor, *Toxicon* 28(5):469, 1990.
167. Sims JK, Irei MY: Human Hawaiian marine sponge poisoning, *Hawaiian Med J* 9:263, 1979.
168. Southcott RV: Fatal stings to North Queensland bathers, *Med J Aust* 2:272, 1952.
169. Southcott RV: Studies on Australian Cubomedusae, including a new genus and species apparently harmful to man, *Aust J Mar Freshwater Res* 7:254, 1956.
170. Southcott RV: Revision of some Carybdeidae (Scyphozoa/ Cubomedusae), including a description of the jellyfish syndrome responsible for the "Irukandji syndrome," *Aust J Zool* 15:651, 1967.
171. Southcott RV: Human injuries from invertebrate animals in the Australian seas, *Clin Toxicol* 3:617, 1970.
172. Southcott RV: Australian venomous and poisonous fishes, *Clin Toxicol* 10:291, 1977.
173. Southcott RV, Coulter JR: The effects of the southern Australian marine stinging sponges, *Neofibularia mordens* and *Lissodendoryx* sp, *Med J Aust* 2:895, 1971.
174. Spielman FJ et al: Acute renal failure as a result of *Physalia physalis* sting, *South Med J* 75:1425, 1982.
175. Stein MR et al: Fatal Portuguese man-o'-war *(Physalia physalis)* envenomation, *Ann Emerg Med* 18:312, 1989.
176. Stiles BG, Sexton FW: Immunoreactivity, epitope mapping and protection studies with anti-conotoxin GI sera and various conotoxins, *Toxicon* 30(4):367, 1992.
177. Strauss BM, Macdonald RI: Hand injuries from sea urchin spines, *Clin Orthop Rel Res* 114:216, 1975.
178. Sutherland SK: *Venomous creatures of Australia,* Melbourne, Australia, 1981, Oxford University Press.
179. Sutherland SK: *Australian animal toxins,* Melbourne, Australia, 1983, Oxford University Press.
180. Sutherland SK, Lane WR: Toxins and mode of envenomation of the common ringed or blue-banded octopus, *Med J Aust* 1:893, 1969.
181. Taira E, Tananara N, Funatsu M: Studies on the toxin in the spines of the starfish *Acanthaster planci.* 1. Isolation and some properties of the toxin found in spines, *Sci Bull Coll Agr Univ Ryukus* 22:203, 1975.
182. Takei M et al: A toxic substance from the sea urchin *Toxopneustes pileolus* induces histamine release from rat peritoneal mast cells, *Agents Actions* 32(3/4):224, 1991.
183. Togias AG et al: Anaphylaxis after contact with a jellyfish, *J Allergy Clin Immunol* 75:672, 1985.
184. Tomchik RS et al: Clinical perspectives on seabather's eruption, also known as "sea lice," *JAMA* 269:1669, 1993.
185. Torda TA, Sinclair E, Ulyatt DB: Puffer fish (tetrodotoxin) poisoning: clinical record and suggested management, *Med J Aust* 1:599, 1973.
186. Traverso LW, Lee WP, Langford MJ: Fluid resuscitation after an otherwise fatal hemorrhage. I. Crystalloid solutions, *J Trauma* 26:168, 1986.
187. Trewethie ER: Tetrodotoxin in the blue-ringed octopus, *Med J Aust* 1:506, 1978.
188. Usagawa T et al: Preparation of monoclonal antibodies against okadaic acid prepared from the sponge *Halichondria okadai, Toxicon* 27(12):1323, 1989.
189. Wachsman M, Aurelian L, Burnett JW: Human immunosuppression induced by sea nettle *(Chrysaora quinquecirrha)* venom, *Toxicon* 29(3):386, 1991.
190. Walker DG: Survival after severe envenomation by the blue-ringed octopus *(Hapalochlaena maculosa), Med J Aust* 2:663, 1983.

191. Weinberg SR: Reactive arthritis following a sting by a Portuguese man-of-war (letter), *J Fla Med Assoc* 75(5):280, 1988.
192. Wiener S: Observations on the venom of the stone fish *(Synanceja trachynis), Med J Aust* 2:620, 1959.
193. Williamson JA: *Some Australian marine stings, envenomations and poisonings,* ed 2, Brisbane, 1981, Queensland State Centre, Inc. Surf Life Saving Association of Australia.
194. Williamson JA: The blue ringed octopus, *Med J Aust* 140:308, 1984.
195. Williamson JA: The box jelly fish sting, *S Pacific Underwater Med Soc J* 14:20, 1984.
196. Williamson JA: "Irukandji" syndrome, *S Pacific Underwater Med Soc J* 15:38, 1985.
197. Williamson JA: The blue-ringed octopus bite and envenomation syndrome, *Clin Dermatol* 5(3):127, 1987.
198. Williamson JA, Callahan VI, Hartwick RF: Serious envenomation by the northern Australian box-jellyfish *(Chironex fleckeri), Med J Aust* 1:13, 1980.
199. Williamson JA, Exton D: *The marine stinger book,* Queensland, 1985, The Surf Life Saving Association of Australia.
200. Williamson JA et al: Acute management of serious envenomation by box-jellyfish *(Chironex fleckeri), Med J Aust* 141:851, 1984.
201. Williamson JA et al: Box-jellyfish venom and humans, *Med J Aust* 140:444, 1984.
202. Williamson JA et al: Acute regional vascular insufficiency after jellyfish envenomation, *Med J Aust* 149:698, 1988.
203. Wolff RL, Wiseman SL, Kitchens SC: *Aeromonas hydrophila* bacteremia in ambulatory immunocompromised hosts, *Am J Med* 68:238, 1980.
204. Wong SK, Matoba A: Jellyfish sting of the cornea, *Am J Ophthalmol* 100:739, 1985.
205. Yaffee HS: Irritation from red sponge, *N Engl J Med* 282:51, 1970.
206. Yaffee HS, Stargardtner F: Erythema multiforme from *Tedania ignis, Arch Dermatol* 87:601, 1963.
207. Yasumoto T et al: Diarrhetic shellfish poisoning. In Ragelis EP, editor: *Seafood toxins,* Washington, DC, 1984, American Chemical Society.
208. Zimmerman KD, Gates GR, Heatwole H: Effects of venom of the olive sea snake, *Aipysurus laevis,* on the behaviour and ventilation of three species of prey fish, *Toxicon* 28(12):1469, 1990.

53 SEAFOOD TOXIDROMES

Paul S. Auerbach

- Monitoring programs for phycotoxin-producing marine algae, paralytic shellfish poisons, diarrheic shellfish poisons, and other phycotoxins
- Ichthyocrinotoxication
- Ichthyohemotoxication
- Ichthyohepatotoxication
- Ichthyootoxication
- Ichthyoallyeinotoxication
- Gempylotoxication
- Anemone poisoning
- Tridacna clam poisoning
- Cephalopod poisoning
- Whelk poisoning
- Ivory shell poisoning
- Abalone poisoning
- Grass carp gallbladder poisoning
- Sea cucumber poisoning
- Crab poisoning
- Ciguatera fish poisoning
- Clupeotoxin fish poisoning
- Scombroid poisoning
- Tetrodotoxin fish poisoning
- Paralytic and gastroenteric shellfish poisoning
- Other shellfish poisoning
- Seafood allergies*
- *Vibrio* fish poisoning, wound infections, and septicemia
- Fish tapeworm
- Trematodes
- Anisakiasis
- Eustronglylides
- Primary amebic meningoencephalitis
- Poisoning by environmental contamination
- Domoic acid intoxication
- Red seaweed *(Graciliaria tsudae)*
- Botulism
- Poisoning by sea hare ingestion
- Chelonintoxication
- Polar bear liver poisoning
- Blue-green algae

The world population is increasing, by some estimates, at a rate of 1 million persons a day, a rate that will overwhelm existing land-based food and energy resources. At present, 200 to 240 million tons of fish are harvested each year, with 50% of the total coming from coastal regions. Through the middle 1970s, at least 400,000 metric tons of sharks were harvested annually for food. Of the 25,000 classified species of fish, fewer than 15 species have heretofore provided the bulk of the world's catches, but this number is likely to increase dramatically. Americans consume on the order of 15 pounds of fish per person per year. It is becoming increasingly clear that the ocean is one of our last great food resources.

Marine creatures that are poisonous to eat include dinoflagellates, coelenterates, mollusks, echinoderms, crustaceans, fishes, turtles, and mammals. Because of increased use of marine nutrients, marine biotoxins are of increasing concern to the medical community. Geographic location, dietary and clinical histories, and appropriate index of suspicion figure prominently in the diagnosis and treatment.

Marine biotoxins most commonly are naturally occurring poisons derived directly from marine organisms.[33] These include phytotoxins (plant poisons) or zootoxins (animal poisons). Ingestible toxins may be classified by specific toxin or by the donor organ of origin ingested by the victim. "Ichthyosarcotoxin" is a general term for poison derived from the fresh flesh (that is, muscle, viscera, skin, or slime) of any fish. This is further defined by specific organ system.

Population growth has necessitated the development of marine fisheries for the production of harvestable protein, including fish, invertebrates, and plants. Epidemiologic data suggest that an inverse relationship exists between fish consumption and coronary heart disease; this is attributed to the protective effects of highly polyunsaturated omega-3 fatty acids (eicosapentaenoic and docosahexaenoic acids), which decrease levels of plasma cholesterol, triglycerides, and very-low-density lipoproteins.[31,154,244,445] In some analyses, dietary supplementation with fish oils decreases restenosis after percutaneous transluminal coronary angioplasty; in others the association is not demonstrated. Dietary enrichment may also favorably affect blood pressure, antiinflammatory mechanisms, and wound healing.[9,10,231,252]

*Text on seafood allergies contributed by Susan L. Hefle, Ph.D., and Robert K. Bush, M.D.

Monitoring Programs for Phycotoxin-Producing Marine Algae, Paralytic Shellfish Poisons, Diarrheic Shellfish Poisons, and Other Phycotoxins

It is a telling statistic that approximately 37% (up from 31% in 1985) of U.S. shellfish beds carry bans or limitations on harvesting because of high levels of fecal coliform bacteria.

Despite the increasing risk of human intoxication from contaminated seafood, standards and methods of screening and law enforcement vary. A survey of current worldwide regulations for marine phycotoxins portrayed the state of affairs in 47 countries.[433] Phycotoxin-producing marine algae yield *Alexandrium catanella, Dinophysis* species, *Protogonyaulax* species, and others to which the syndromes of paralytic or neurotoxic shellfish poisoning are attributed. The closure of fisheries (product harvest areas) depends on the density of algae, which may range from 200 to 10^6 per liter, depending on the species. In some cases the decision to close a fishery is based on the toxicity level in shellfish; in others, algae in the water and toxin in shellfish must both be found. In Florida, more than 5000 cells per liter of *Ptychodiscus breve* must be detected before fisheries are closed.

The threshold level of saxitoxin (or paralytic shellfish poisons) considered tolerable ranges across countries from 40 to 80 μg of toxin per 100 g seafood. The upper number, as determined by mouse bioassay, is used in the United States, as monitored by the Interstate Shellfish Sanitation Conference and the Food and Drug Administration.

Fewer countries monitor diarrheic shellfish poisonings. Those that do use 5 to 7 mouse units/100 g seafood as a threshold for toxicity. Countries (United States, Canada, Portugal) that monitor for domoic acid (cause of amnesic shellfish poisoning) use 2 mg/100 g seafood as the threshold. Ciguatoxins are monitored infrequently because of difficulties associated with the assay. In French Polynesia, 0.06 ng/g seafood as determined by mosquito bioassay is considered toxic; in the United States, detection of the toxin at any level by immunoassay (Florida, Hawaii) renders the fish unsaleable.

Two features render toxin surveillance difficult: the performance problems of the assays and the impracticality of surveying every fish. In French Polynesia the magnitude of the ciguatera problem is such that at least nine specific animals (including eels, jacks, barracuda, surgeonfish, and triggerfish) cannot be sold in the marketplace. Truly effective screening of seafood for toxicity will not be instituted until it is seen to be in the best interests of persons whose livelihood comes from the sale of seafood.

Ichthyocrinotoxication

Ichthyocrinotoxic fish poisoning is induced by the ingestion of glandular secretions not associated with a specific venom apparatus; this usually involves skin secretions, poisonous foams, or slimes. Examples of toxic fish are certain filefish, pufferfish, porcupine fish, trunkfish, boxfish, cowfish, lampreys, moray eels, and toadfish (see Box 53-1). Cyclostome poisoning (lampreys and hagfish) is of the ichthyocrinotoxic category. Pahutoxin and homopahutoxin found in the secretion of the Japanese boxfish *Ostracion immaculatus* contain hemolysins.[145]

A bitter taste may be associated with ichthyotoxic skin secretions, but this is not always present.[155] Gastrointestinal distress, which is evident within a few hours of ingestion, is characterized by nausea, vomiting, dysenteric diarrhea, tenesmus, abdominal pain, and weakness. Toxic slimes can also induce contact (irritant) dermatitis. While most victims recover within 24 hours, full reversal of the gastrointestinal syndrome requires 1 to 3 days. In addition, some slimes, such as "grammistin" from the soapfish (*Rypticus sapona-*

BOX 53-1

REPRESENTATIVE ICHTHYOCRINOTOXIC FISH HAZARDOUS TO HUMANS

Phylum Chordata
- Class Agnatha
  - Order Myxiniformes: hagfishes, lampreys
    - Family Myxinidae
      - *Myxine glutinosa:* Atlantic hagfish
      - *Petromyzon marinus:* sea lamprey, large nine-eyes
- Class Osteichthyes
  - Order Anguilliformes: eels
    - Family Muraenidae
      - *Muraena helena:* moray eel
  - Order Perciformes: perchlike fishes
    - Family Serranidae
      - *Grammistes sexlineatus:* golden striped bass
      - *Rypticus saponaceus:* soapfish
  - Order Tetrodontiformes: triggerfishes, puffers, trunkfishes
    - Family Canthigasteridae
      - *Canthigaster jactator:* sharp-nosed puffer
    - Family Diodontidae
      - *Diodon hystrix:* porcupinefish
    - Family Ostraciontidae
      - *Lactoria diaphana:* trunkfish
      - *Lactoria fornasini:* trunkfish, boxfish
    - Family Tetraodontidae
      - *Arothron hispidus:* puffer, toadfish, blowfish, rabbitfish
      - *Fugu xanthopterus:* puffer
  - Order Batrachoidiformes: toadfishes
    - Family Batrachoididae
      - *Opsanus tau:* oyster toadfish
      - *Thalassophyrne maculosa:* toadfish

ceous of the family Grammistidae), can cause a contact irritant dermatitis.[177]

Therapy is supportive and based on symptoms. The decision to replete fluids orally versus intravenously is based on the severity of symptoms, the degree of debilitation, and the victim's ability to ingest fluids without vomiting. The dermatitis is best managed with cool compresses of aluminum sulfate and calcium acetate (Domeboro).

All suspect fish should be washed carefully with water or brine solution and skinned before they are eaten. Puffer skin is extremely toxic. Care must be taken to avoid toxin contact with the eyes.

Ichthyohemotoxication

Ichthyohemotoxic fish are perfused with "poisonous blood," the toxicity of which is usually inactivated by heat and gastric juice. Examples are various eels, such as morays, anguilliformes, and congers. The syndrome is predominantly gastrointestinal and should be treated according to symptoms. Hematologic complications are rare. The risk of intoxication is increased by ingestion of undercooked fish.

Ichthyohepatotoxication

Ichthyohepatotoxic fish carry the toxin predominantly in the liver. The remainder of the fish may be nontoxic. Some observers believe that the toxicity may be partially caused by hypervitaminosis A, with seasonal variation. Fish that are always toxic fall into two basic groups: (1) Japanese perchlike fish (such as mackerel, sea bass, porgy, and sandfish), and (2) tropical sharks (such as requiem, sleeper, cow, great white, cat, hammerhead, angel, Greenland, and dogfish).[334] In addition, some skates and rays, which share a similar phylogeny with sharks, harbor ichthyohepatotoxins.

Ingestion of the Japanese perchlike fish group causes onset of symptoms within the first hour, with maximum intensity over the ensuing 6 hours.[389] These include nausea, vomiting, headache, flushing, rash, fever, and tachycardia. No fatalities have been reported. Delayed (24 to 48 hours) necrodermolysis is rare.

Ingestion of tropical shark liver, such as that of the Greenland shark *(Somniosus microcephalus),* and occasionally of the musculature results in "elasmobranch poisoning" (see Box 53-2).[33] Symptoms are noted within 30 minutes of ingestion and include nausea, vomiting, diarrhea, abdominal pain, malaise, diaphoresis, headache, stomatitis, esophagitis, muscular cramps, arthralgias, paresthesias, hiccoughs, trismus, hyporeflexia, ataxia, incontinence, blurred vision, blepharospasm, delirium, respiratory distress, coma, and death. Usually, if only the flesh is eaten, the symptoms are mild and gastroenteric, with spontaneous resolution. The intoxication induced by ingesting shark liver is probably not purely that of hypervitaminosis A. Recent information suggests that it may be caused by trimethylamine oxide, which is also found in the fish flesh (see later discussion).[18]

BOX 53-2

REPRESENTATIVE POISONOUS SHARKS (ELASMOBRANCHS) HAZARDOUS TO HUMANS

Phylum Chordata
- Class Chondrichthyes
  - Order Squaliformes: sharks
    - Family Carcharhinidae
      - *Carcharhinus melanopterus:* blacktip reef shark
      - *Carcharhinus menisorrah:* gray reef shark
      - *Galeocerdo cuvieri:* tiger shark
      - *Prionace glauca:* great blue shark
    - Family Dalatiidae
      - *Somniosus microcephalus:* Greenland shark, sleeper shark, nurse shark
    - Family Hexanchidae
      - *Hexanchus griseus:* cow shark, gray shark, mud shark
    - Family Isuridae
      - *Carcharodon carcharias:* white shark
    - Family Scyliorhinidae
      - *Scyliorhinus caniculus:* dogfish, lesser-spotted cat shark
    - Family Sphyrnidae
      - *Sphyrna diplana:* hammerhead
    - Family Squatinidae
      - *Squatina dumeril:* monkfish, angel shark
    - Family Triakidae
      - *Triaenodon obesus:* white-tip houndshark

Therapy is supportive and based on symptoms. If the victim is treated within 60 minutes of ingestion of shark liver or other viscera, gastric emptying or lavage followed by administration of activated charcoal (50 to 100 g) in 70% sorbitol may be of value. Fish liver should not be eaten; indeed, neither should any shark viscera. Drying the flesh properly may minimize the toxicity.

Ichthyootoxication

Ichthyootoxic fish possess toxic gonads, which may vary in toxicity with the reproductive cycle. The musculature is generally nontoxic. Examples are the sturgeon, alligator gar, salmon, pike, minnow, carp, catfish, killifish, perch, and sculpin. Sea urchins may be toxic during the reproductive period.[33] This toxicity is exemplified by *Paracentrotus lividus* (Europe), *Tripneustes ventricosus* (West Africa), and *Diadema antillarum* (West Indies).

Symptoms begin within an hour of ingestion and include nausea, vomiting, diarrhea, headache, dizziness, fever, thirst, xerostomia, bitter taste, tachycardia, seizures, migraine, paralysis, hypotension, and death. Treatment is supportive and based on symptoms. The roe of any fish should not be eaten during the reproductive season. Heat will not inactivate the toxin.

Ichthyoallyeinotoxication

Ichthyoallyeinotoxic fish induce hallucinatory fish poisoning. They are predominantly reef fish of the tropical Pacific and Indian reefs, which carry the heat-stable toxins mainly in the head parts, brain, and spinal cord, and in lesser amounts in the musculature. Typical species include surgeonfish, chub, mullet, unicornfish, goatfish, sergeant major, grouper, rabbitfish, rock cod, drumfish, rudderfish, and damselfish. Two representative species are the sea chup *(Kyphosus cinerascens)* and the goatfish *(Upenus arge)*.[171]

Hallucinatory mullet poisoning has been described as a seasonal condition that occurs only during the summer months in restricted areas on the Hawaiian islands of Kauai and Molokai.[179] Dangerous species include the mullet, surmullet or goatfish, rudderfish, and surgeonfish.

Symptoms can develop within 5 to 90 minutes of ingestion and include dizziness, circumoral paresthesias, diaphoresis, weakness, incoordination, auditory and visual hallucinations, nightmares, depression, dyspnea, bronchospasm, brief paralysis, and pharyngitis. [33,283,393] No fatalities have been reported.

Therapy is supportive and based on symptoms. If the victim is psychotic and violent, haloperidol may be used as an antipsychotic agent. Mild agitation may be eased with small graded doses of diazepam, particularly if the victim also suffers anticholinergic symptoms. The victim should be observed until a normal mental status is regained. The head, brain, or spinal cord of any tropical fish should not be eaten. Heat does not inactivate the toxin.

Gempylotoxication

Gempylotoxic fishes are the pelagic mackerels, which produce an oil with a pronounced purgative effect. The "toxin" is contained in both musculature and bones. No particular characteristic distinguishes a gempylotoxic fish from a nontoxic fish of the same species. The castor oil fish *(Ruvettus pretiosus)* is named for its purgative properties.

The victim suffers from abdominal cramping, bloating, mild nausea, and diarrhea, usually within 30 to 60 minutes of ingestion. The disorder is self-limited and resolves over 12 to 18 hours. The diarrhea often occurs without concomitant systemic effects. Fever, bloody or foul-smelling stools, or protracted vomiting suggests infectious gastroenteritis. No specific antidote is recommended. If diarrhea is profuse, the victim should maintain hydration by ingesting electrolyte-rich replacement fluids, such as commercial repletion formulas. If the victim cannot tolerate oral fluids because of nausea or severe abdominal cramping, intravenous supplementation may be initiated with lactated Ringer's solution. Antimotility agents, such as diphenoxylate with atropine, are not recommended unless the diarrhea is debilitating, because inhibition of peristalsis prolongs the transit time of the toxin through the gut and may increase the duration of the disorder.

Anemone Poisoning

In the South Pacific, ingestion of the green or brown anemones *Radianthus paumotensis* or *Rhodactis howesii (mata-malu samasama)* has been associated with severe illness and death. Accidental deaths generally involve small children, while adults may be the unfortunate recipients of improperly cooked anemone or even be intentionally stricken in acts of suicide. The toxic substances are found in the nematocysts and the tentacular tissues. Anemones have been used for criminal purposes in the South Pacific.[33] *Physiobranchia douglasi* is poisonous eaten raw but is reputedly safe if cooked.[173]

Ingestion of the raw anemone induces altered mental status within 30 minutes, often immediately after the ingestion. The victim becomes agitated or confused, delirious, and then comatose. Other symptoms reported include fever, seizures, myalgias, abdominal pain, respiratory failure, hypotension, and death. Contact with the skin, particularly mucous membranes, is extremely painful with rapid inflammation and vesiculation.

Treatment is symptomatic and supportive. Because of the rapid onset in symptoms the rescuer must be prepared to provide advanced life support within the first hour after ingestion. There is no known specific antidote, since the toxin or toxins are not well characterized.

Tridacna Clam Poisoning

Giant clams of the species *Tridacna maxima* are eaten in French Polynesia.[33] This causes a poisoning characterized by nausea, vomiting, diarrhea, paresthesias, tremor, and ataxia. Severe cases can be fatal. The toxin appears to be concentrated in the mantle and viscera of the clam. Therapy is supportive.

Cephalopod Poisoning

In certain areas of Japan, intoxications follow the ingestion of squid and octopus. Symptoms develop within 10 to 20 hours and consist of nausea, vomiting, diarrhea, abdominal pain, headache, weakness, paralysis, and seizures. Although most victims recover within 48 hours, deaths have occurred.[33] Therapy is supportive.

Whelk Poisoning

In Japan, poisoning has followed ingestion of mollusks of the genera *Neptunea, Buccinum,* and *Fusitriton* (whelks or ivory shells). The toxin is located in the salivary glands and has been characterized as tetramine. Symptoms include headache, dizziness, nausea, vomiting, blurred vision, and dry mouth. No fatalities have been reported. Therapy is supportive.

Ivory Shell Poisoning

Human intoxications have followed consumption of the ivory shell, *Babylonia japonica,* which is widely distributed along the coastline of Japan. The toxin, surugatoxin, located in the midgut of the animal, is reputed to be produced by a gram-negative bacterium on which the snail feeds. Surugatoxin and IS-toxin appear to have autonomic ganglionic blocking action. Symptoms include abdominal pain, diarrhea, nausea, vomiting, oral paresthesias, syncope, and seizures.[173] Tetrodotoxin has been identified in *B. japonica.*

Abalone Poisoning

Abalone poisoning follows ingestion of the viscera of certain Japanese abalone (tsunowata or tochiri), particularly from the Island of Hokkaido, where *Haliotis discus* and *Haliotis sieboldi* are found. Symptoms include severe urticaria, erythema, pruritus, edema, and skin ulceration. The reaction appears to be of a photosensitive nature, since the lesions are confined to areas of ultraviolet exposure. One theory holds that the toxin is derived from chlorophyll contained in the seaweeds on which the abalone feed.[31] A similar type of intoxication has been caused by ingestion of the Japanese turban shell, *Turbo cornutus.* Therapy is supportive.

Grass Carp Gallbladder Poisoning

Ingestion of the Asian freshwater grass carp *(Ctenopharyngodon idellus)* or other similar fishes *(Cyprinus carpio)* can lead to serious illness, attributed to the nephrotoxic and hepatotoxic properties of a toxin found in the bile.[83] The structure of the toxin in *C. carpio* has recently been characterized as 5∝-cholestane-3∝, 7∝, 12∝, 26,27-pentol 26-sulfate.[22]

People eat the raw gallbladder for its putative antirheumatologic properties. Several hours after ingestion, abdominal pain, nausea, vomiting, and watery diarrhea develop, which can be accompanied by marked elevations in concentrations of liver enzymes (aspartate and alanine aminotransferases). The hepatitis is transient and to date has not led to hepatic failure. Nephrotoxicity may be profound, leading to oliguric or nonoliguric renal failure within 48 to 72 hours after ingestion. Renal biopsy demonstrates acute tubular necrosis without evidence of rhabdomyolysis. Therapy is supportive and based on symptoms.

Sea Cucumber Poisoning

Sea cucumbers are eaten throughout Asia and in some Pacific islands, where they are known as trepang, sea slugs, cucumbers, erico, or hai shen. Gastroenteritis is induced by saponins of the triterpinoid variety, such as holothurin. The disorder consists chiefly of abdominal pain, nausea, and diarrhea and is self-limited.

Crab Poisoning

Human intoxications have followed ingestion of crabs in many Indo-Pacific islands. Most of the toxic crab species are members of the family Xanthidae and include the genera *Demania, Carpilius, Atergatis, Platypodia, Zosimus, Lophozozymus,* and *Eriphia.* Clinical symptoms develop 15 minutes to several hours after ingestion and include nausea, vomiting, diarrhea, perioral and extremity paresthesias, ataxia, aphasia, respiratory distress, altered mental status, coma, and rapid death. There is a marked similarity to the paralytic shellfish poisoning syndrome, which involves saxitoxin. Saxitoxin, neosaxitoxin, and gonyautoxins have been isolated from crab species in Okinawa and are attributed to a red algal food source. Similar toxins were extracted from *Eriphia sebana* and *Atergatis floridus* off Australian coral reefs.[268-271] Tetrodotoxin and palytoxin have also been characterized from poisonous crabs. The poisonous mosaic crab *Lophozozymus pictor* from the Indo-West Pacific region has caused several fatalities in the Philippines and Singapore. The toxicity (putatively palytoxin and paralytic shellfish toxins) has been found to be consistently high in the gut and hepatopancreas, while the muscle was less toxic. Captive crabs lose toxicity, such that it almost completely gone by 24 days.

Coconut crab *(Birgus latro)* poisoning is manifested as nausea, vomiting, headache, chills, myalgias, and exhaustion, with occasional deaths. Asiatic horseshoe crabs *(Carcinoscorpius rotundicauda)* are eaten in Thailand, where they cause mimi poisoning. Symptoms include nausea, vomiting, diarrhea, abdominal cramps, dizziness, palpitations, weakness, lower extremity paresthesias, aphonia, perioral burning, pharyngitis, sialorrhea, syncope, paralysis, and death. Again, the toxin appears highly similar to saxitoxin.[86]

Crab lung has followed the aspiration of tiny fragments of North American blue crab shells into the lung, necessitating removal with fiberoptic bronchoscopy.[110] The diagnosis of occult aspiration should be considered in anyone with an unexplained cough who has recently consumed cracked crab, particularly while intoxicated.

Ciguatera Fish Poisoning

Ciguatoxin derives its name from *cigua,* the word Spanish settlers used to describe poisoning from ingestion of the poisonous marine turban shell snail *(Turbo [Cittarium] pica)* found in the Caribbean Spanish Antilles.[283,420] Quite possibly it was ciguatera fish poisoning that was described by Captain James Cook, who sailed on the *Resolution* in the South Pacific in 1774.[331] In this episode, several of his officers were poisoned after eating fish from the island

Malicolo in the Pacific nation of Vanuatu. The poisoning involves almost exclusively tropical and semitropical marine coral reef fish and is a direct function of the food chain, initiated by the toxic dinoflagellate *Gambierdiscus toxicus*.[23,163,396] Ciguatoxic fish feed on certain plants or bottom fish, implicating specific species of algae.[336] No plankton feeders have been reported as ciguatoxic. The presence of *G. toxicus* in the gut content of fish relates in many cases to toxicity.[70] Undoubtedly other organisms, such as the cyanobacterium *Trichodesmium erythraeum,* can elaborate water- and lipid-soluble precursors to the toxins that generate the ciguatera syndrome.[125]

The food chain originates in sessile algae or microbial heterotrophs (such as *G. toxicus* Adachi and Fukuyo, which was identified from an investigation of coral reef biodetritus layers in the Gambier Islands and elaborates ciguatoxin and maitotoxin). These are consumed by herbivorous fishes, which in turn are ingested by carnivorous fishes.[34,348] As the fish within the food chain become larger, the toxin is accumulated, rendering larger (greater than 6 pounds) and elderly fish more toxic.[95,172,182,334] Experimental induction of ciguatera toxicity in surgeonfish *(Acanthurus xanthopterus)* has been achieved by a diet of ciguatoxic red snapper *(Lutjanus bohar)*.[180] Although the entire fish is toxic, the viscera (particularly the liver) and roe are considered to carry the highest concentrations of toxin.[33] In southwest Puerto Rico, ciguatoxicity in barracuda is seasonal; however, the most frequently toxic tissues are consistently the viscera and head.[428]

It has been suggested that the proliferation of toxic algae may be triggered by contamination of the water by industrial wastes, golf course runoff, metallic compounds, ship wreckage, or other pollutants.[170] These all contribute to the destruction of coral reefs, as do episodes of storms, earthquakes, tidal waves, and heavy rains.[356] In the Marshall Islands (Micronesia), consequent to nuclear testing, the incidence of toxin-producing plankton has tripled.[351] Similar observations have been made with respect to various military activities (dumping and explosives) in the Line and Gilbert Islands (Kiribati, Central Pacific), Hao Atoll (Tuamotu Archipelago, French Polynesia), Gambier Islands (thus *Gambierdiscus*—French Polynesia, 1968), and others.[356] Still another cause for toxic dinoflagellate proliferation is the transfer and dumping via ballast water in large oceangoing vessels.

Ciguatera poisoning is the most common nonbacterial food poisoning associated with fish in the United States.[311] In North America, cases have been reported in California, Florida, Louisiana, Texas, Hawaii, the Virgin Islands, Massachusetts, New York, Toronto, Vermont, and Washington, D.C.[148,184,437] Other dinoflagellates besides *Gambierdiscus toxicus* that may play a role in the production of the toxins associated with ciguatera poisoning include *Prorocentrum concavum, P. mexicanum, P. rhathymum, Gymnodinium sanguineum,* and *Gonyaulax polyedra*.[346,425] Ciguatera represents a class of diseases that appear to be growing in importance in most regions of the world, since the timing and occurrence of noxious phytoplankton are trending upward.[58] The ciguatera problem is an order of magnitude more pronounced in the South Pacific, with estimates of up to 70% of a local atoll human population being affected.

More than 400 species of benthic fish have been implicated, with the greatest concentration in the Caribbean Sea, in the Pacific Ocean around the Indo-Pacific islands, and along the continental tropical reefs. The most frequently implicated reef fishes include the families Muraenidae (moray eels), Mugilidae (mullets), Serranidae (groupers) (Fig. 53-1), Lutjanidae (snappers), Sparidae and Lethrinidae (porgies), Carangidae (jacks), Labridae (wrasses), Scaridae (parrotfishes), Acanthuridae (surgeonfishes), Balistidae (triggerfishes), and Sphyraenidae (barracuda).[30] Of reported cases, 75% (except in Hawaii) involve the barracuda, snapper, jack, or grouper. Hawaiian carriers include the parrot-beaked bottom feeders, particularly those that inhabit areas of high dinoflagellate population, such as disturbed coral reef waters, and surgeonfishes.[199] Ciguatoxic fish are rarely identified out of the zone defined by latitudes 35° north and south.[170] Other fishes that have been reported as ciguatoxic include Albulidae (ladyfishes), Chanidae (milkfishes), Clupeidae (herrings), Elopidae (tarpon), Engraulidae (anchovies), Synodontidae (lizardfishes), Congridae (true eels), Ophichthyidae (snake eels), Belonidae (needlefishes), Exocoetidae (flying fishes), Hemiramphidae (halfbeaks), Aulostomidae (trumpetfishes), Syngnathidae (seahorses), Holocentridae (squirrelfishes), Apogonidae (cardinalfishes), Arripidae (sea perches), Chaetodontidae (butterfly fishes), Cirrhitidae (hawkfishes), Coryphaenidae (dolphins), Gempylidae (oilfishes), Gerridae (silverfishes), Gobidae (gobies), Istiophoridae (sailfishes), Kuhliidae (bass), Kyphosidae (rudderfishes), Mullidae (goatfishes), Pempheridae (sweeperfishes), Pomacentridae (damselfishes), Pomadasyiidae

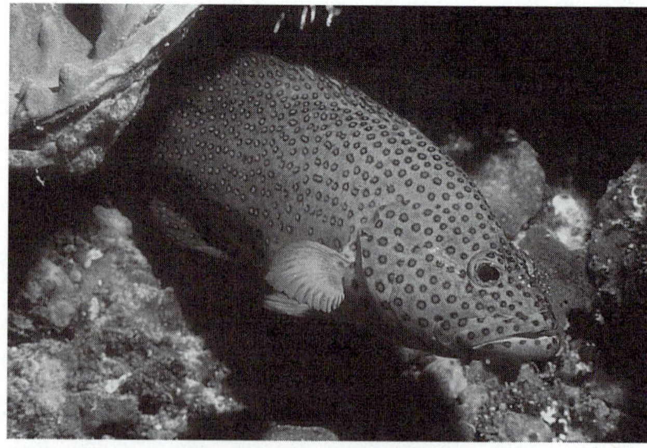

Fig. 53-1 Coral trout or grouper. This type of fish is often implicated in ciguatera fish poisoning. (Courtesy Carl Roessler.)

(grunts), Priacanthidae (snapper), Scatophagidae (spade fishes), Sciaenidae (croakers), Scombridae (tunas), Scorpaenidae (scorpionfish), Siganidae (rabbitfishes), Xiphiidae (swordfishes), Zanclidae (moorish idol), Bothidae (flounders), Aluteridae and Monacanthidae (filefishes), Ostraciontidae (trunkfishes), Batrachoididae (toadfishes), Antennariidae (sargassumfish), Lophiidae (goosefish), and Ogcocephalidae (longnose batfish).[376] Ciguatera toxin has recently been detected in the serum of a pediatric patient stricken ill after consuming an unknown jellyfish imported into the United States from Samoa.

Ciguatera fish poisoning is associated with more than five toxins, including fat-soluble quaternary ammonium compounds (ciguatoxins), a water-soluble component (maitotoxin, from the Tahitian vernacular name *maito* for the surgeonfish *Ctenochaetus striatus*), a maitotoxin-associated hemolysin (lysophosphatidylcholine or lysolecithin), and a ciguatoxin-associated adenine triphosphatase (ATPase) inhibitor.[174,301,350,371,455] Scaritoxin (isolated from *Scarus gibbus*) is similar to the fat-soluble component and is specific to parrotfishes.[89] Lipid-extracted toxins from *Gambierdiscus toxicus* have been designated GT-1, GT-2, and GT-3; a water-soluble toxin is designated GT-4.[107,298] Chemical analysis of ciguatoxins demonstrates that they closely resemble brevetoxin C (from *Ptychodiscus brevis*) and okadaic acid, isolated from marine sponges and the dinoflagellate *Prorocentrum lima*.[318,346] The identification of okadaic acid from the Caribbean dinoflagellate *Prorocentrum concavum* lends support to the notion that this toxin may be more significant in ciguatera poisoning than previously thought.[108]

Three major ciguatoxins are usually found in the flesh and viscera of ciguateric fishes. They are labeled CTX-1, 2, and 3. They are found in variable concentrations, which may account for the variability in the clinical syndrome.[264] Ciguatoxin-2 is a diastereomer of CTX-3.[267] The ciguatoxins may arise from the oxidation of gambiertoxins, possibly through the cytochrome system in the livers of fish.[266] The lipid components have been characterized as crystalline, colorless, heat-stable compounds of approximate molecular weight 1100 daltons, with functional hydroxyl and quaternary nitrogen groups. The water-soluble component (maitotoxin) has human erythrocyte and rabbit intestine anticholinesterase and neurotransmitter cholinomimetic activity.[272] However, there is some recent evidence that highly purified ciguatoxin preparations may not have anticholinesterase effects in vivo.[253,349] Respiratory failure cannot be attributed solely to the anticholinesterase action of ciguatoxin.

Ciguatoxins activate voltage-dependent Na^+ channels.[262] One mode of action of ciguatoxin may be the false occupation by the toxin of calcium receptor sites that modulate the sodium pore permeability in neural, muscle, and myocardial membranes.[41] This allows increased permeability to sodium and causes sustained depolarization.[349] Electrophysiologic studies of the sural and common peroneal nerves in humans with ciguatera poisoning who demonstrated reduced light touch, pain, and vibration appreciation in the extremities showed prolongation of the absolute refractory, relative refractory, and supernormal periods. These findings indirectly suggest that ciguatoxin causes an abnormally prolonged sodium channel opening in nerve membranes.[71]

Both ciguatoxin and brevetoxin compete for the same receptor site on the sodium channel, with the affinity being markedly greater for ciguatoxin. Maitotoxin may act by stimulating cellular uptake of calcium.

The clinical manifestations of hypertension and tachycardia, which can be suppressed in animal models by phentolamine, suggest α-adrenergic mimetic action. While purified ciguatoxin appears to have cardiac stimulatory effects (rate and inotropy), in vitro maitotoxin is a myocardial depressant, which may explain the variation in clinical presentation. Isolated human atrial trabeculae show concentration-dependent positive inotropy with ciguatoxin-1, which is not reversed with mannitol.[263] Calcium conductance is tentatively implicated in the activity of maitotoxin because its action is inhibited in the presence of verapamil, magnesium ions, or low-calcium solutions. In mice, injection of maitotoxin induced a marked increase in total calcium content of the adrenal glands as well as a rise in plasma cortisol concentration.[419] Ciguatoxin injected into mice targets the heart, adrenal glands, and autonomic nervous system.[420] Ciguatoxin and ciguatoxin-4c (a derivative) in repeated doses cause the mouse heart to suffer septal and ventricular interstitial fibrosis, accompanied by bilateral ventricular hypertrophy.[418]

Ciguatoxin is a potent substance, with an LD_{50} of 0.45 µg/kg (mouse intraperitoneal) in the purified form, which in a toxic fish would correlate with only 2 to 5 g of the original flesh. However, in most toxic fish flesh the concentration is 0.5 to 10 parts per billion. Maitotoxin is even more potent, with an LD_{50} of 0.13 g mouse intraperitoneal. It is interesting to note that ciguatoxins can be potent ichthyotoxins, which may impose an upper limit on the levels of ciguatoxin carried by fish.[261] However, the toxin or toxins may reside in the skeletal muscle or other fish tissues in association with proteins that protect the carrier from being affected.[167]

All toxins identified to date are unaffected by freeze-drying, heat, cold, and gastric acid and do not affect the odor, color, or taste of the fish.[13,95] Thus international trading patterns may go undetected unless a ciguatoxin assay is used routinely to reveal affected fish.[58] There is some evidence that cooking methods alter the relative concentrations of the various toxins; boiling the flesh removes water-soluble toxins, while frying or grilling may increase the toxicity attributable to lipid-soluble toxins as a result of conversion of water-soluble toxins or release of lipid-soluble toxins from cellular compounds that normally bind them.[124] The overall effect of cooking fish seems to be to lessen toxicity to a slight degree.

PALYTOXIN

Palytoxin has been isolated from various zoanthid "soft" corals of the genus *Palythoa,* but its true origin is unknown.[165] It is an extremely poisonous nonprotein agent of low molecular weight. In animal models it causes a fast potassium outflow from erythrocytes, increases the permeability of cell membranes to sodium and potassium but not calcium, and inhibits sodium-potassium ATPase.

Although palytoxin is presumed to originate with coelenterates or even bacteria, there has been some suggestion that it can be a causative agent for ciguatera poisoning.[234] Ingestion in humans reportedly causes abdominal cramps, nausea, diarrhea, paresthesias of the extremities, muscle spasm, and respiratory distress. Of these, the predominant physical findings among the cluster of others appeared to be respiratory distress and extreme tonic muscle contractions with massive accumulation of serum creatine kinase and myoglobinuria. Palytoxin has been found in mackerel *(Decapterus macrosoma),* triggerfish *(Melichtys vidua),* and crab *(Demania reynaudii).*[8,144,234] Since a rapid and sensitive hemolysis neutralization assay for palytoxin is now available, its presence in toxic seafood should become easier to determine.[45]

CLINICAL ASPECTS

The onset of symptoms may be within 15 to 30 minutes of ingestion, is generally within 1 to 3 hours of ingestion, and shows an increase in severity over the ensuing 4 to 6 hours. Most victims have symptom onset within 12 hours of ingestion, and virtually all are afflicted within 24 hours.[32] Symptoms, which have been reported to number over 150, include abdominal pain, nausea, vomiting, diarrhea, chills, paresthesias (particularly of the extremities and circumoral region), pruritus (particularly of the palms and soles after a delay of 2 to 5 days), tongue and throat numbness or burning, sensation of "carbonation" during swallowing, odontalgia or dental dysesthesias, dysphagia, dysuria, dyspnea, weakness, fatigue, tremor, fasciculations, athetosis, meningismus, aphonia, ataxia, vertigo, pain and weakness in the lower extremities, visual blurring, transient blindness, hyporeflexia, seizures, nasal congestion and dryness, conjunctivitis, maculopapular rash (erythematous, with occasional desquamation), skin vesiculations, dermatographia, sialorrhea, diaphoresis, headache, arthralgias, myalgias (particularly in the lower back and thighs), insomnia, bradycardia, hypotension, central respiratory failure, and coma, with an overall death rate of 0.1% to 12%.* The lower percentage seems more likely. Death is usually attributed to respiratory paralysis.[214] In a well-described clinical outbreak affecting a group of scuba divers who ate coral trout *(Cephalopholis miniatus),* the most common symptoms were weakness, cold sensitivity, paresthesias, a sensation of "carbonation," and myalgias.[6] Two men with ciguatera poisoning have been described who experienced painful ejaculation with urethritis, which in turn induced dyspareunia (pelvic and vaginal burning) in their female partners.[246] The variations in symptoms of ciguatera poisoning may result from different concentrations of specific toxins in different fishes.[232] Features associated with a severe attack include ingestion of a carnivorous fish and a history of previous ciguatoxism.[153] Possibly ciguatera poisoning can be transmitted by breast feeding an infant.[53,405]

Diarrhea, vomiting, and abdominal pain are usually seen approximately 3 to 6 hours after ingestion of a ciguatoxic fish and may persist for 48 hours. Using an extract from toxic *Ctenochaetus strigosus* applied to isolated rabbit ileal tissue, Fasano and associates[133] came to the conclusion that the toxins involved in ciguatera fish poisoning directly stimulate intestinal fluid secretion without accompanying tissue damage.

Tachycardia and hypertension have been described, in some cases after what can be severe transient bradycardia and hypotension.[84] Hallucinations, flushing, flaccid paralysis, and fever are uncommon. More severe reactions tend to occur in persons previously stricken with the disease. A pathognomonic symptom is the reversal of hot and cold tactile perception, which develops in some persons after 3 to 5 days and may last for months.[304] This peculiar symptom may have a delay in onset of from 2 to 5 days after ingestion and is only otherwise seen with neurotoxic shellfish poisoning (brevetoxins), caulerpicin (from the green alga *Caulerpa*) toxicity, or turban shell poisoning.[13,114,456] Pruritus may persist for weeks and be exacerbated by any activity that increases skin temperature (blood flow), such as exercise or alcohol consumption.[250] Severely affected persons may report intermittent myalgias, paresthesias, and pruritus for up to 6 months, with a gradual diminution in frequency and intensity. There may be some regional variability to the symptoms of presentation.[32,308] Persons who have ingested parrotfish (scaritoxin) may suffer from classic ciguatera poisoning as well as a "second phase" (5 to 10 days' delay) syndrome of disequilibrium with locomotor ataxia, dysmetria, and resting or kinetic tremor.[89] This affliction may persist for 2 to 6 weeks. It has been estimated that ciguatera poisoning may affect over 50,000 persons each year.

Maternal ciguatera toxin exposure during pregnancy may result in normal fetal outcome. Whether ciguatoxin crosses the placenta is not known.[376] However, the mother may note increased fetal movements immediately after the fish meal. Whether exposure to the toxins in the first trimester results in fetal demise is conjectural.

In small children the symptoms may be no more specific than irritability, sleep disturbance, nausea, and vomiting.[448] Other reported symptoms include carpopedal spasm, ptosis, and inconsolability.

Untreated, the gastroenteric syndrome of nausea and vomiting, which may be more common in victims of Asian descent, usually resolves within 24 to 48 hours. The differ-

---

*References 3, 6, 13, 30, 32, 36, 207, 353, 437.

ential diagnosis should include paralytic shellfish poisoning, eosinophilic meningitis, type E botulism, organophosphate insecticide poisoning, tetrodotoxin poisoning, and psychogenic hyperventilation.[32,207,237,354] It appears that the toxin can accumulate in humans as well as in fish, so that prior illness places a person at greater risk for a severe reaction on consumption of ciguatoxic fish. Coincidental ingestion of alcoholic beverages may also exacerbate the syndrome by an unknown mechanism. Recurrent symptoms may appear spontaneously during times of emotional or physical stress, malnutrition, or severe illness. Biopsy-proven polymyositis was demonstrated in two patients who were severely poisoned by ciguatera fish toxin.[398]

Because the severity of ciguatera fish poisoning is variable, two symptom checklist rating scales have been developed to quantify illness severity and to selectively monitor response to therapy in patients with chronic toxicity.[245] For recording *severity of poisoning at the time of peak symptoms,* the following symptoms are rated according to severity (none—0 points; minimal—1 point; mild—3 points; moderate—5 points; severe occasional—7 points; severe constant—9 points; and unbearable—10 points): diarrhea, abdominal pain, nausea, vomiting, tingling or numbness of legs, tingling or numbness of arms, tingling or numbness of mouth, hot and cold reversal, weakness of legs, weakness of arms, joint pain, muscle pain, headache, tooth pain, bad or metallic taste, chills, fever, sweating, itching, lightheadedness, vertigo, shakiness, incoordination, neck stiffness, watery eyes, skin rash, burning on urination, increased saliva, shortness of breath, and worsening of condition with alcohol. The disease severity is determined by totaling the points: mild less than 100 points; moderate 100 to 150 points; and severe more than 150 points. For recording *response to treatment in chronic cases,* the following symptoms are rated according to severity (none—0 points; minimal—1 point; mild—2 points; moderate—3 points; and severe—4 points): tingling or numbness of legs, tingling or numbness of arms, tingling or numbness of mouth, hot and cold reversal, weakness of legs, weakness of arms, joint pain, muscle pain, headache, tooth pain, sweating, itching, incoordination, burning on urination, and worsening of the condition with alcohol. The current status of the disease features is tracked numerically over time as a measure of progress.

DIAGNOSIS

Any person who arrives in the emergency department with acute gastroenteritis, particularly with an unusual constellation of neurologic symptoms, should provide a dietary history, which may yield the most important clue. Because freezing does not inactivate the toxin, any illness that originates after the ingestion of the appropriate (particularly imported) seafood is ciguatera poisoning until proven otherwise.

The diagnosis of ciguatera poisoning is clinical because currently no routinely used laboratory test identifies the presence of ciguatoxin in human blood. Hawaii Chemtect International (P.O. Box 92015, Pasadena, CA 91109), in cooperation with the University of Arizona, has developed an experimental method for testing human serum (Ciguatect-H) for the presence of ciguatoxins.[6]

The lipid-soluble component can be extracted from fish flesh with serial solvent (acetone, ether, methanol) elutions, to yield a transparent, light yellow, viscous oil.[371] A ciguatoxin enzyme immunoassay or radioimmunoassay may be used to test small portions of the suspected fish. In the enzyme immunoassay method, the sheep anticiguatoxin (antipolyether) IgG-horseradish peroxidase conjugate detects ciguatoxin and structurally related polyether toxins, such as okadaic acid and brevetoxin.[187] A stick enzyme immunoassay using monoclonal antibody to ciguatoxin is specific and sensitive.[188] However, it is not adaptable to field conditions where high temperatures and sunlight prevail.

In the radioimmunoassay, purified ciguatoxin is conjugated with human serum albumin. The ciguatoxin-albumin conjugate is mixed with Freund's adjuvant and administered subcutaneously to sheep to raise an antiserum, which is harvested from the animals. The sheep anticiguatoxin albumin is iodinated with ^{125}I to create ^{125}I sheep anticiguatoxin–human serum albumin, which is used to identify toxic fish.

In Hawaii a field bamboo "stick test" (coated with Liquid Paper) colorimetric immunoassay is available to detect ciguatoxin in fish, using the same substrates as the enzyme immunoassay.[186,317] Preliminary work indicates that the stick test may be oversensitive (10% to 15% false positives) because it detects polyethers related to ciguatoxin.[187] At the University of Arizona a commercial test kit for detecting ciguatoxins is under development, based on solid-phase immunobead technology.[6] This will be marketed by Hawaii Chemtect International (see above) for field (marketplace) detection of ciguatoxin-related compounds with a sensitivity of at least 1 ng/g fish. The test is performed by binding the toxins to a membrane attached to a plastic strip and exposing the toxin-laden membrane to a monoclonal antibody–colored latex bead complex that has a high specificity for the toxins (CTX and DSP). The intensity of the color indicates the presence of the toxins, which can then be quantified using specific extraction procedures. High-performance liquid chromatography (HPLC) is also available for ciguatoxins and okadaic acid. While such testing may be economically disadvantageous to local fishing industries, it may prove beneficial if other polyether toxins have adverse health effects.

The immunoassays have largely replaced determination of ciguatera toxicity by injection of fish tissue extracts into mice or by feeding fish to a mongoose or cat to observe for neurologic symptoms of drowsiness, weakness, limb flexion, hypersalivation, ataxia, coma, or death.[139,207] The traditional method of testing was to feed the liver or other portions of the viscera to a cat or mongoose in a dose of 10% of the test animal's weight, and then to watch for symptoms. Another bioassay uses mosquitoes; intrathoracic injection of serially diluted extracts from fish leads to a mosquito LD_{50}. Like the cat or mongoose tests, the assay is nonspecific and nonquantitative. Unreliable folklore includes the advice that a lone fish (separated from the school) should not be eaten; that ants and turtles refuse to eat ciguatoxic fish; that a thin slice of ciguatoxic fish does not show a rainbow effect when held up to the sun; and that a silver spoon tarnishes in a cooking pot with ciguatoxic fish.[95]

TREATMENT

If possible, a piece of the fish should be obtained for analysis. Therapy is supportive and based on symptoms. Gastric lavage or syrup of ipecac–induced emesis followed by the administration of a slurry of activated charcoal (100 g) in sorbitol may be of limited value if performed within 3 hours after ingestion. It has been suggested that the administration of magnesium-containing cathartics may augment a calcium channel blockade. Nausea and vomiting may be controlled with an antiemetic (prochlorperazine 2.5 mg intravenously or hydroxyzine 25 mg intramuscularly). The most worrisome systemic problem is hypotension, which may require the administration of intravenous crystalloid for volume replacement and, rarely, pressor drugs such as dopamine or dobutamine. Some investigators recommend the administration of calcium gluconate (1 to 3 g intravenously over 24 hours) to manage hypotension and myocardial failure, although clinical hypocalcemia is not a diagnostic standard. Bradyarrhythmias that lead to cardiac insufficiency and hypotension generally respond well to atropine (0.5 mg intravenously up to 2 mg). Cool showers or the administration of hydroxyzine (25 mg orally every 6 to 8 hours) has been recommended to relieve pruritus. Moderate headache may be extraordinarily responsive to acetaminophen. Other drugs that have been recommended at one time or another include edrophonium, neostigmine, corticosteroids, pralidoxime, ascorbic acid, pyridoxine (vitamin B_6), and salicylic acid–colchicine–vitamin B complex.[30,362] Although findings in some animal experiments support such therapies as pralidoxime, there is no current clinical support for these modalities.[308] Amitriptyline (25 mg orally twice a day) has been reported to be effective to ameliorate pruritus and dysesthesias, as has protamide. Depression caused by ciguatera poisoning has also been successfully treated with amitriptyline.[275] In three cases unresponsive to amitryptyline, tocainide appeared to be efficacious.[247] The authors postulated that the beneficial effect might result from the drug's ability to block axonal conduction by decreasing or preventing increased permeability of the nerve cell membrane to sodium. Nifedipine has been reported effective for ciguatera-associated headache.[69] No therapy has been shown incontrovertibly to have benefit.

Recent clinical evidence suggests that an intravenous infusion of mannitol may be beneficial in moderate or severe cases, particularly for distressing neurologic or cardiovascular symptoms.[259,329,397] The infusion is rendered initially as 1 g/kg over 45 to 60 minutes during the acute phase (days 1 to 5). Mannitol, the reduced form of mannose, exerts its effect by pulling intracellular water into the intravascular compartment. One theory is that the mechanism of the beneficial action in ciguatera intoxication is this hyperosmotic water-drawing action, which reverses ciguatoxin-induced Schwann cell edema.[332] Another is that mannitol acts in some poorly defined fashion as a "hydroxyl scavenger."[449] Neither theory has been confirmed. Curiously, mannitol therapy has no beneficial effect on mice administered a sublethal intraperitoneal dose of ciguatoxin (CTX-1).[265] In humans the empirical observation is that mannitol has greater benefit if administered early in the course.

Sims and Young[385] postulated that the syndrome of chronic ciguatera fish poisoning (symptoms with onset or persistence greater than 7 days after ingestion) may be related to the presence of prostaglandin precursors, such as arachidonic acid and the polycyclic ether thromboxane A_2, which may evoke an immune sensitization phenomenon. Although counterimmunoelectrophoresis of toxic (human reaction or in vivo mouse bioassay) fish extracts and human serum confirms toxic fish specimens, both immune and nonimmune human sera demonstrate precipitin reactions with toxic extracts. Therefore it is not yet possible to conclude that affected individuals possess ciguatera toxin–specific antibody.[123] It is unknown whether the observation that persons previously affected with ciguatera toxin tend to have more severe reactions on reexposure results from toxin accumulation or immune sensitization. In support of the hypothesis that prostaglandin formation may contribute to the clinical syndrome have been limited observations that victims appear extraordinarily responsive to the administration of acetaminophen (for headache) and indomethacin (for arthralgias, myalgias, pruritus, and temperature sensation reversal), and that cyproheptadine (antiserotonergic) ameliorates pruritus, while antihistamines and corticosteroids are relatively inefficacious.[385] During recovery from ciguatera poisoning the victim should exclude the following from the diet: fish (fresh or preserved), fish sauces, shellfish, shellfish sauces, alcoholic beverages, and nuts and nut oils, which may result in an exacerbation of the ciguatera syndrome.[383]

PREVENTION

Eating fish in ciguatera-endemic regions should be avoided. Because of the accumulation of toxin, all oversized fish of any predacious reef species (such as jack, snapper, barracuda, grouper, or parrot-beaked bottom feeder) should be suspected. The viscera of tropical marine fish should be discarded. Moray eels should never be eaten. If eating fish is necessary in a survival situation, a small portion of the fish in question may be fed to a sacrificial small animal, which is then observed for ill effects for 12 hours.

Clupeotoxin Fish Poisoning

Clupeotoxic fish poisoning involves plankton-feeding fish, which ingest planktonic blue-green algae and surface dinoflagellates. These fish of the order Clupeiformes are found in tropical Caribbean, Indo-Pacific, and African coastal waters. Examples include the families Clupeidae (herrings and sardines), Engraulidae (anchovies), Elopidae (tarpons), Albulidae (bonefishes), and Pterothrissidae (deep-sea slickheads).[33,295] Toxicity is reported to increase during the warm summer months. Viscera are considered to be highly toxic. The toxin is poorly characterized because of the infrequency of the syndrome and rare access to toxic animals.

CLINICAL ASPECTS

The onset of symptoms is rapid and characterized as "violent," often within 30 to 60 minutes of ingestion and rarely prolonged beyond 2 hours. Initial signs and symptoms include a marked metallic taste, xerostomia, nausea, vomiting, diarrhea, and abdominal pain. These are followed by chills, headache, diaphoresis, severe paresthesias, muscle cramps, vertigo, malaise, tachycardia, peripheral cyanosis, hypotension, and death, with a mortality of up to 45%. Severe debility leading to death may occur within 15 minutes of the onset of symptoms.[170] A postmortem examination in one case after ingestion of *Sardinella marquesensis* (Marquesan sardine) flesh and viscera demonstrated enterocolitis and the sequelae of hypotension and acute heart failure.[295] As with ciguatera toxin, the poison does not impart any unusual appearance, odor, or flavor to the fish.

TREATMENT

Therapy is supportive and based on symptoms. Because of the severe nature of the intoxication, early gastric emptying is desirable; however, the disease is so unusual and so rarely suspected (because of a lack of history) that gastric emptying is not often carried out. Aggressive management and early intensive care are essential.

PREVENTION

Clupeotoxic fish should be avoided, especially during summer months, in fish indigenous to the Caribbean, African coastal, or Indo-Pacific waters. The viscera of suspicious fish should be fed to experimental animals to see if an illness is generated.

Scombroid Poisoning

Fish of the families Scombridae and Scomberesocidae (suborder Scombroidei) include the albacore, bluefin and yellowfin tuna, mackerel, saury, needlefish, wahoo, skipjack, and bonito. Nonscombroid fish that produce scombroid (mackerel-like) poisoning include mahi-mahi (dolphin), kahawai, sardine, black marlin, pilchard, anchovy, herring, amberjack (yellowtail or kahala), and the Australian ocean salmon *Arripis truttaceus*.[138,378,387,414] In Hawaii, the most commonly implicated fish is the dolphin *Coryphaena hippurus*.[224] In the northeastern United States, bluefish *(Pomatomus saltratix)* has recently been linked to scombrotoxism.[342,344] Scombroid poisoning accounts for 5% of food-borne outbreaks reported to the Centers for Disease Control in Atlanta.[417] Because greater numbers of nonscombroid fish are now recognized as "scombrotoxic," Prescott[342] has suggested that the syndrome be more appropriately called pseudoallergic fish poisoning. On rare occasion, cheeses such as Swiss cheese (rarely, cheddar or gouda) can be implicated in histamine poisoning.[415]

During conditions of inadequate preservation or refrigeration (optimal temperatures for bacterial growth of 37 to 43° C), the musculature of these dark-fleshed or red-muscled fish undergoes bacterial decomposition.[4,21,40,296,334] The normal piscine surface bacteria *Proteus morganii, Klebsiella pneumoniae, Aerobacter aerogenes, Escherichia coli, Alcaligenes metalcaligenes,* and others have been implicated in the putrefactive process, which includes the decarboxylation of the amino acid L-histidine to histamine and saurine (histamine PO_4 and histamine HCl).[139,147,224,273,393] The term "saurine" originated because of the association of scombrotoxism with saury, a Japanese dried fish delicacy.[191] Evidence that histamine is the causative toxin of scombroid fish poisoning was provided in a landmark investigation of a small local outbreak.[312] The urinary excretion of histamine and its metabolite, *N*-methylhistamine, was measured in three persons who had scombrotoxism after ingestion of marlin. The marlin contained levels of histamine from 842 to 2503 μmol per 100 g of tissue. Urine samples collected 1 to 4 hours after fish ingestion demonstrated histamine and *N*-methylhistamine levels 9 to 20 times and 15 to 20 times the normal mean, respectively. The authors failed to measure any increase in 9α,1β-dihydroxy-15-oxo-2,3,18,19-tetranorprost-5-ene-1,20-dioc acid, which is the principal metabolite of prostaglandin D_2, a mast cell secretory product considered to indicate release of histamine from mast cells. This supports the notion that the excess histamine was from the fish rather than endogenously produced in the victims.

Histamine levels greater than 20 to 50 mg/100 g are noted in the toxic fish. It is not unusual to record levels in excess of 400 mg/100 g in scombrotoxic fish, while normal fresh fish contains less than 1 mg/100 g of histamine.[378] The toxin is heat stable and not destroyed by domestic or commercial cooking.[296]

Affected fish typically have a sharply metallic or peppery taste; however, they may be normal in appearance, color, and flavor. Not all persons who eat a contaminated fish become ill, possibly because of uneven distribution of decay within the fish.[259] It has been postulated that histamine alone is unlikely to be the sole causative agent of scombrotoxism because high doses of histamine can be administered orally without apparent effect as a result of poor absorption and conversion in the liver and bowel to *N*-acetyl histamine.[21,147,344] Potentiators of histamine toxicity in spoiled fish may include cadaverine or putrescine, which might inhibit intestinal histamine-metabolizing enzymes such as diamine oxidase or histamine-*N*-methyltransferase.[414]

CLINICAL ASPECTS

Symptoms occur within 15 to 90 (usually less than 60) minutes of ingestion and are mediated by histamine and its analogs. These include flushing (sharply demarcated, exacerbated by ultraviolet exposure, particularly of the face, neck, or upper trunk), a sensation of warmth without elevated core temperature, conjunctival hyperemia, pruritus, urticaria, angioneurotic edema, bronchospasm, nausea, vomiting, diarrhea, epigastric pain, abdominal cramps, dysphagia, headache, thirst, pharyngitis, burning of the gingiva, palpitations, tachycardia, dizziness, and hypotension.[110,170,222,224,296] This syndrome may mimic that of monosodium-L-glutamate sensitivity. Untreated, the symptoms generally resolve within 8 to 12 hours. The reaction may be markedly more severe in a person who is concurrently ingesting isoniazid (isonicotinic acid hydrazide [INH]) because of INH blockade of gastrointestinal tract histaminase.[431] Monoamine oxidase inhibitors pose a theoretical hazard. Death is unusual.

TREATMENT

Therapy is directed at reversing the histamine effect. Minor intoxications can be treated with the histamine-1 antagonist diphenhydramine (Benadryl) 25 to 50 mg orally or intravenously. Histamine-2 antagonists cimetidine (300 mg intravenously) or ranitidine (50 mg intravenously) are alternatives. Intravenous hydroxyzine (also an antiemetic) may be used if one of the previous drugs is not available, but it might be slightly less efficacious and is almost certainly more sedating. It has been suggested that a combination of H_1 and H_2 blockers is necessary to counteract the vascular effects of histamine and is more effective in situations of acute allergic urticaria.[312,358] However, unless scombrotoxism is refractory to unilateral therapy, there is no need to combine H_1 and H_2 blockers because, rarely, this causes hypotension. Although many newer H_2 blockers have not been specifically reported to be effective in the treatment of scombroid poisoning, cost might cause them to be considered for therapy. Nizatidine (Axid), 150 mg orally twice a day, is considerably less expensive than ranitidine, 150 mg orally twice a day, or famotidine, 20 mg orally twice a day. Terfenadine (60 mg twice a day) and astemizole (10 mg daily) are two newer ("second-generation") nonsedating H_1 antihistamines that have not yet been reported as therapies for scombroid poisoning. Antihistamine therapy may be supported as necessary with subcutaneous epinephrine, inhaled bronchodilators, and pressor agents. Corticosteroids are of no proven benefit. Anaphylaxis is uncommon and should be managed as outlined previously.

If large quantities of the tainted fish have been consumed within an hour before the patient's arrival at an emergency facility, emptying the stomach and administering activated charcoal with a cathartic (if the patient does not already have diarrhea) may have value. However, the disorder is virtually always self-limited and has never been reported as fatal. Nausea and vomiting are usually controlled by the antihistamine but occasionally require the addition of a specific antiemetic, such as prochlorperazine (2.5 mg intravenously). The persistent headache of scombroid poisoning may respond to cimetidine or a similar drug if standard analgesics are not effective.[24] If the allergic and gastroenteric components are severe, the cumulative effect may induce hypotension, which requires administration of intravenous crystalloid solutions and, rarely, pressor agents.

PREVENTION

Scombroid poisoning, ptomaine *(Staphylococcus, Streptococcus)* poisoning, enterotoxic poisoning, and botulism can all be avoided to a certain extent with proper refrigeration (below 15° C), preservation, and preparation of fish. All captured fish should be gutted, cooled, and placed on ice immediately. Recreational fishermen must pay particular attention to their coolers. No fish should be consumed if it has been handled improperly or has the smell of ammonia. Fresh fish generally has a sheen or oily rainbow appearance; "dull" packaged fish should be avoided.

Hawaii, California, and New York have the greatest number of outbreaks.[149] If an episode of scombroid poisoning is recognized, reporting it promptly to local public health authorities is important because it might prevent exposure of additional people, particularly if the food was served in a public eating establishment.[192]

Tetrodotoxin Fish Poisoning

Tetrodotoxin is one of the most potent nonprotein poisons found in nature and is characteristic of the order Tetraodontiformes.[403] The suborder Tetrodontoidei contains three families of fishes (Tetraodontidae, Diodontidae, and Canthigasteridae), including pufferfish (Fig. 53-2) (toadfish, blowfish, globefish, swellfish, balloonfish, toado) and porcupine fish. Sunfish (*Mola* species) are members of the suborder Moloidei.[393] Pufferfish are tropical and subtropical fish, some of which are prepared as delicacies (fugu) in Japan by specially trained and licensed chefs. Pufferfish can inflate their bodies to a nearly spherical shape using air or seawater. At least 50 of the more than 100 species of these fishes have been involved in poisonings of humans or may be intermittently toxic.[361]

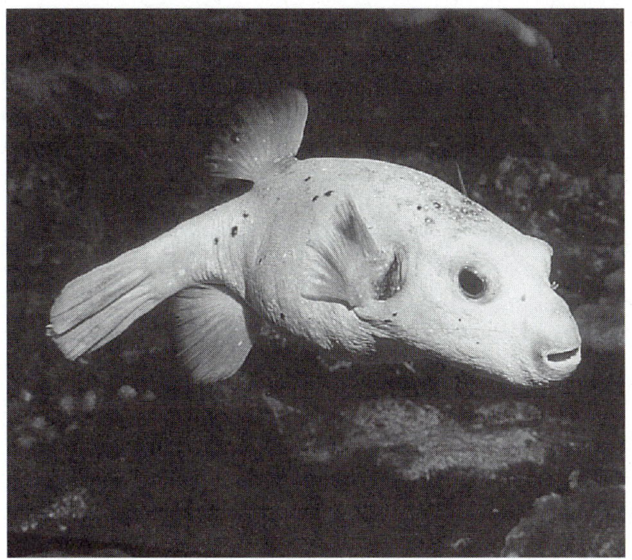

Fig. 53-2 Pufferfish (French Polynesia). (Courtesy Carl Roessler.)

The pufferfish has been recognized at least since Egyptian antiquity (2500 BC) as a toxic hazard and was almost certainly responsible for the nonfatal intoxication of Captain James Cook during his second voyage around the world in 1774.[299,436] Captain Cook's crew were also stricken with ciguatera poisoning. There has been some contention that the toxin ("puffer powder") was used as a component of Haitian voodoo potion in the zombie ritual.[428] This has been challenged on grounds, among others, that under the usual conditions of extreme alkaline storage, any tetrodotoxin in a "zombie potion" would be decomposed irreversibly into pharmacologically inactive products.[219,457]

Tetrodotoxin has been fully characterized and synthesized and is believed to be chemically identical to toxins (tarichatoxin) isolated from certain North American and Japanese newts (such as *Taricha granulosa, Notophthalmus viridescens,* and *Cynops ensicauda*); international salamanders of the family Salamandridae (such as *Triturus, Pleurodeles, Cynops, Paramesotriton,* and *Tylototriton*); the skin of central American frogs of the genus *Atelopus;* the goby *Gobius criniger;* shellfish (ivory shell, *Babylonia japonica;* lined moon shell, *Natica lineata;* calf moon shell, *Natica vitellus;* bladder moon shell, *Polinices didyma;* and trumpet shell, *Charonia sauliae*); the starfish *Astropecten polyacanthus;* the ribbon worm *Cephalothrix linearis;* the flatworm *Planocera multitentaculata;* the crab *Atergatus floridus;* the horseshoe crab *Carcinoscorpius rotundicanda;* and the Australian blue-ringed octopus *(Hapalochlaena maculosa).** Tetrodotoxin is also found in freshwater puffers and may be the cause of a number of tropical reef crab poisonings.[248] Structurally, it is amino-perhydroquinazolone ($C_{11}H_{17}N_3O_8$), a water-soluble and heat-stable compound of molecular weight 319 daltons.[427] The ichthyosarcotoxin is distributed throughout the entire fish, with the greatest concentrations in the liver, gonads (ovaries), intestine, and skin, and lesser amounts in the muscles and blood. There is some variability in toxicity among species and with reproductive and feeding cycles. Saxitoxin (the causal agent of paralytic shellfish poisoning) has been identified in pufferfish.[233]

The precise origin of the toxin may be production by *Pseudomonas* species that live on the skin of the pufferfish.[462] This would explain transmittal of toxicity between toxic and nontoxic fish through skin contact. Other investigators have found the production of tetrodotoxin by *Vibrio* and other species isolated from the intestines of pufferfish.[443] Radiolabeled tetrodotoxin injected into a puffer accumulated most in skin, liver, intestines, and muscle.

The poison interferes with central and peripheral neuromuscular transmission by altering sodium conductance. Although it is not a depolarizing agent, in animals it causes depression of the medullary respiratory mechanism, intracardiac conduction, and myocardial and skeletal muscle contractility. At the microcellular level the mechanism of action is linked to the axon, rather than to the nerve endplate. Tetrodotoxin blocks axonal transmission by interfering with sodium conductance within the depolarized regions of the cell membrane, perhaps by acting at a metal cation binding site in the sodium channel, without affecting the presynaptic release of acetylcholine or its effects on the neuromuscular junction.[7,181] Saxitoxin, implicated in paralytic shellfish poisoning, has essentially the same action as tetrodotoxin on the nerve membrane, although it is believed to have a discrete receptor.[220,326] There is no apparent effect on potassium permeability.[357] The LD_{50} for mice is 10 µg/kg when administration is intraperitoneal, intravenous, or subcutaneous.[325,427]

CLINICAL ASPECTS

The onset of symptoms can be as rapid as 10 minutes or can be delayed for up to 4 hours. Initially, oral paresthesias develop, with rapid progression to lightheadedness and generalized paresthesias. The following symptoms develop rapidly: hypersalivation, diaphoresis, lethargy, headache, nausea, vomiting, diarrhea, abdominal pain, weakness, ataxia, incoordination, tremor, paralysis, cyanosis, aphonia, dysphagia, seizures, dyspnea, bronchorrhea, bronchospasm, respiratory failure, coma, and hypotension. Nausea and vomiting are often marked.[384] Weakness and paralysis may appear in the upper extremities and descend to the lower extremities.[361] If mechanical ventilatory assistance is maintained and no anoxic brain injury is present, full mentation may be maintained in the face of total flaccid paralysis. Early miosis may progress to mydriasis with poor pupillary light reflex.[427] A disseminated intravascular coagulation–like syndrome is heralded by petechial skin hemorrhages, which may progress to bullous desquamation, along with

*References 12, 52, 59, 62-64, 195, 196, 225, 293, 315, 403, 440, 461, 463.

hematemesis and diffuse stigmata of prolonged coagulation. Sixty percent of victims die, most of these within the first 6 hours. Survival past 24 hours is a good prognostic sign.

In Japan, fugu is the ultimate gastronomic experience. Although fugu chefs are specially trained and licensed, occasional (currently up to 10 per year) fatal mishaps occur, particularly among epicures who insist on preparation of the highly toxic liver. Persons who ingest pufferfish intentionally as fugu seek a state of exhilaration characterized by the development of mild paresthesias, notably of the skin, tongue, and lips; flushing of the skin; generalized warmth; and mood elevation. Unfortunately, between 1955 and 1975 at least 3000 persons were poisoned in Japan by puffers, with an estimated mortality of 51%.[400]

TREATMENT

Early treatment is directed at eliminating the gastric acid–stable toxin, which is partially inactivated in alkaline solutions. Because the presence of tetrodotoxin may delay gastric emptying, if the patient arrives at an emergency facility within 3 hours of ingestion, gastric lavage with at least 2 L of 2% sodium bicarbonate solution in 200 ml aliquots should be performed, followed by intragastric placement of 50 to 100 g of activated charcoal in 70% sorbitol solution (or 30 g of "highly activated" charcoal in sorbitol). If the victim is obtunded or there is already evidence of dysphagia or respiratory insufficiency, this should be preceded by endotracheal intubation to protect the airway and prevent the pulmonary aspiration of gastric contents. Serial arterial blood gas measurements should be obtained to monitor base excess, carbon dioxide retention, and oxygenation. Supplemental oxygen therapy without mechanical ventilatory assistance is rarely adequate. Further therapy is supportive and usually involves advanced cardiac and ventilatory life support. The physician must remember that the paralyzed victim may be fully conscious and should take care to offer verbal explanations and reassurances.

Tetrodotoxin may induce hypotension, which is attributed to vasodilation and myocardial depression. This may require an infusion of crystalloid and, rarely, the addition of a pressor agent to achieve a systolic blood pressure of 100 mm Hg and a urine output of at least 40 ml/hr. Bradyarrhythmias are common and generally respond to atropine. Severe refractory heart block may necessitate temporary placement of a transvenous pacemaker. The use of cholinesterase inhibitors, such as edrophonium, is as yet empirical. Reports of improvement with anticholinesterase administration may be related to a phase during recovery when there is reduced quantal release of acetylcholine at the neuromuscular junction, so that cholinesterase inhibition would have clinical benefit.[427] The administration of veratrine-like agents, which prolong skeletal muscle contraction without dependence on intact neuromuscular transmission, provides prophylactic protection against the action of tetrodotoxin on sciatic nerve–anterior tibial muscle preparations from the rat.[357] Application to the human clinical situation is unclear.

A minor intoxication may be limited to paresthesias and mild dysphagia. In such a case the victim should be observed in the emergency department or intensive care unit for 8 hours to detect deterioration, particularly respiratory failure. Under no circumstances should anyone with dysphagia be given liquids by mouth. The victim should not be discharged from observation until the symptoms are clearly receding.

Unfortunately, no specific antidote has been identified. However, progress has been made. Tetrodotoxin was conjugated to keyhole limpet hemocyanin and the conjugate used as an immunogen in rabbits and mice. Mice immunized with the conjugate were protected from a lethal dose of toxin, and passive protection experiments using rabbit antiserum exhibited a dose-related therapeutic activity after toxin challenge.[143,404] The shore crab *Hemigrapsuss sanguineus* is highly resistant to tetrodotoxin by virtue of a toxin-binding substance.[380] Whether this natural phenomenon can be applied to the human situation remains to be seen.

PREVENTION

Although water soluble, the toxin is very difficult to remove from the fish, even by cooking. It is wisest to avoid all puffers, even when prepared by an expert.

Paralytic and Gastroenteric Shellfish Poisoning

Bivalve mollusks filter large quantities of water unselectively to gather plankton and extract oxygen, which allows concentration of bacteria, viruses, biologic toxins, pesticides, industrial chemicals, radioactive wastes, toxic metals, and hydrocarbon derivatives of oil spills in the viscera.[117] Standard depuration in purified (with ultraviolet light or ozone) water for 48 to 72 hours may not significantly reduce these contaminants, nor does it appear to remove viruses.[162]

TYPES OF SHELLFISH POISONING

Four types of illnesses can be related to the ingestion of shellfish: allergic or erythematous, bacterial choleratic or viral gastroenteric, diarrheic, and paralytic. Three types—gastroenteric, diarrheic, and paralytic—are discussed here. Allergic shellfish poisoning is discussed later in the chapter.

Gastroenteric Illness

Bacterial and viral enteric diseases may be caused by the consumption of contaminated shellfish, particularly raw clams and oysters, dried raw salt-fish, crabs, shrimp, or home-preserved fish products.[51,117,313,314] Illnesses from ingesting seafood, ocean water, or fresh water (by virtue of swimming or snorkeling) include typhoid fever, hepatitis A, and cholera; organisms include non-01 *Vibrio cholerae, Vibrio parahaemolyticus, Vibrio mimicus, E. coli, Salmonella, Shigella sonnei, Plesiomonas shigelloides,* Coxsackievirus B, Norwalk virus, calicivirus, other unidentified viruses, and *Campylobacter.* Steamed clams probably pose a significant risk because household cooking techniques are often insufficient to kill viruses. Although it takes 4 to 6 minutes of pressure-cooker steaming for the internal temperature of soft-shell clams ("steamers") to reach 100° to 106° C, it requires only 60 seconds for the shells to open, at which point they may appear cooked.[152,238,239] Poliovirus can survive (7% to 13%) in oysters that are steamed, fried, baked, or stewed.[112] Unfortunately, the relative absence of fecal coliform bacteria in areas of shellfish harvesting does not indicate freedom from viral contamination.[116,150,341] In addition, shellfish depuration processes that eliminate bacteria do not necessarily remove viral contaminants, particularly in the digestive glands.[72]

With regard to the 27 nm Norwalk virus (parvovirus), and probably to other viruses that express proliferation as a syndrome of gastroenteritis, the most common symptoms in descending order are generally diarrhea, abdominal cramps, nausea, vomiting, and fever.[313] The incubation period is usually 24 to 48 hours, with a similar duration of symptoms in a self-limited illness.[274] Seroconversion or elevated IgM antibody to the virus is diagnostic but not clinically useful except in epidemiologic investigations. A solid-phase microtiter radioimmunoassay can detect the Norwalk virus and its antibody.[46,157,164] This test is as sensitive and specific as immune electron microscopy.

Diarrheic Illness

Ingestion of shellfish contaminated with *Dinophysis fortii, D. acuminata,* or *Prorocentrum lima,* which generate dinophysistoxin-1 (a protein phosphatase inhibitor) and dinophysistoxin-3, the polyether okadaic acid and derivatives, and diarrheic toxins (which have many effects besides the induction of diarrhea), causes diarrheic shellfish poisoning (DSP).[276,283,458] The lipid-soluble toxins accumulate in shellfish in the fatty tissues. They exert their effects mainly on the small intestine, leading to diarrhea and degenerative changes of the absorptive epithelium.[434] Other DSP toxins exert various effects in experimental animals, including tumor promotion, liver necrosis (pectenotoxin-1), and cardiac necrosis (yessotoxin from the Japanese scallop *Patinopecten yessoensis*).[421] Symptoms include rapid onset (30 minutes to 2 hours) of diarrhea, nausea, vomiting, abdominal pain, and chills. Rarely, symptoms are delayed up to 12 hours. The syndrome is self-limited after 2 to 3 days. During the period 1976 to 1982, DSP was diagnosed in at least 1300 persons in Japan, particularly in the northeastern regions. The period of greatest toxicity appears to be May to August. In 1981, more than 5000 cases were reported in Spain.[458] Other outbreaks have occurred in the Netherlands and Chile.[173]

A radioimmunoassay has been developed to identify the presence of okadaic acid, using antibodies raised in rabbits.[260] A newer idiotypic-antiidiotypic competitive immunoassay may be useful in monitoring toxin levels.[379] A unified bioscreen for the detection of diarrheic shellfish toxins and microcystins (as from cyanobacteria *Microcystis aeruginosa* blooms) uses capillary electrophoresis coupled with a liquid chromatography–linked protein phosphatase bioassay.[56] The Japanese quarantine standard is 200 ng of okadaic acid per gram of shellfish tissue. Four times this amount of toxin has been identified recently in northeastern Pacific Ocean mussels. The presence of tumor promoters of the microcystin family in oceanic and coastal shellfish has been preliminarily termed hepatotoxic shellfish poisoning. This may be related to venerupin shellfish poisoning.[86]

Paralytic Illness

Paralytic shellfish poisoning (PSP) was first clearly described in 1793 in an attack on seamen who were exploring passages off the mainland coast of what is now British Columbia.[299] PSP is induced by ingesting any of a variety of filter-feeding organisms. These include familiar mollusks (such as clams, oysters, scallops, and mussels), chitons, limpets, murex, starfish, and sandcrabs. The affected seafoods may be feral or aquacultured as in the case of the purple clam of Taiwan.[197] In the Indo-Pacific, toxins have been isolated from tropical reef crabs and marine snails.[328] The origin of their toxicity is the biologic chemical toxin they accumulate and concentrate by feeding on various planktonic dinoflagellates and protozoan organisms, or in the case of toxic carnivorous mollusks, on contaminated bivalves. Outbreaks of shellfish poisoning have been reported in North America (the north Pacific coastline to Alaska and the northeast United States up into Canada), Europe, Africa, Asia, and the Pacific Islands. Five fatal cases of neurotoxic food poisoning have been reported after ingestion of *Oliva vidua fulminans* (or "olives," a marine mollusk) by natives in Sabah, Malaysia.[217]

The unicellular (*Protogonyaulax* is 0.03 mm in diameter) phytoplankton (phylum Protozoa, class Mastigophora, order Dinoflagellata) is the foundation of the food chain, and in warm summer months these organisms are noted to "bloom" rapidly in nutrient-rich coastal temperate and semitropical waters. They rank second in abundance to diatoms and are extremely important producers of marine carbohydrates, fats, and proteins. Typical species include *Alexandrium* species and *Gymnodinium catenatum.*

A number of dinoflagellates produce numerous toxins, of which saxitoxin is the most frequently identified. If a single organism predominates, it can discolor the water, creating a black, blue, pink, red, yellow, brown, or luminescent "tide."[90] Organisms can multiply rapidly from a concentration of 20,000 per liter to over 20,000,000 per liter. These plankton can release massive amounts of toxic metabolites into the water and with great rapidity cause enormous mortality in various bird and marine populations, including large mammals such as dolphins and even whales. Large numbers of dead animals on the beach suggest a colored tide. The trend to increased numbers and magnitude of blooms is attributed empirically to many factors, including coastal development, dumping of sewage, fertilizer runoff, and ocean warming. Kills by the dinoflagellate *Ptychodiscus* (formerly *Gymnodinium*) *breve* are estimated at 100 tons of fish per day. To date the magnitude of destruction has prompted multiple international congresses. The problem is increasing remarkably in Europe.[434] In California there is an annual 6-month quarantine (May through October) on mussels, clams, and oysters of local harvest. Paralytic shellfish poisoning has been a reportable condition in California since 1927, with more than 500 cases and 30 deaths reported since that time. The Alaska butter clam is virtually continually toxic.

A limited number out of approximately 1200 species of dinoflagellates have been implicated in toxic syndromes.[370] Paralytic shellfish poisoning can be can be linked to the dinoflagellate *Protogonyaulaux,* species *catanella* (U.S. Pacific coast) and species *tamarensis* var. *excavata* (U.S. Atlantic coast and Europe).[4,288,413] In northwestern Spain the organism that generates the toxins is *Gymnodinium catenatum.* These creatures are relatively fastidious and prefer warm, sunlit water of low salinity in which to bloom. The organisms release a number of toxic metabolites, including saxitoxin, into the water, where they are filtered through resident bivalves, which are subsequently ingested by humans.[392] Some of the algal organisms may release the toxin in the form of microscopic cysts, which can overwinter at the sediment-water interface. In mollusks the greatest concentration of toxin is found in the digestive organs (dark "hepatopancreas"), gills, and siphon.[370] Toxic benthic dinoflagellate cysts may be transported by dredging operations and potentially introduce a dinoflagellate population into a new region.[459]

Although the origin of PSP toxins is assumed to be dinoflagellates, the toxins have been isolated in both marine and freshwater bivalves that are not associated with dinoflagellates. It has not been determined how this has occurred.[327] The bacterium *Moraxella* isolated from *Protogonyaulax tamarensis* has been shown to produce PSP toxins in culture. Toxin production increased in nutritionally deficient environments.[235]

The paralytic shellfish toxins to date are 18 related tetrahydropurine compounds produced mainly by the dinoflagellates of the genus *Alexandrium.* The best characterized is saxitoxin.

Saxitoxin ($C_{10}H_{17}N_7O_4$), which takes its name from *Saxidomus giganteus,* the Alaskan butter clam, is also found in California sea mussels.[283,368] *Ptychodiscus* (formerly *Gymnodinium*) *breve* is a toxic dinoflagellate that produces a milder toxin. Other dinoflagellates considered poisonous to animals or humans include *Gonyaulax acatenella, Pyrodinium phoneus, Pyrodinium bahamense* var. *compressa, Gonyaulax monilata, Gonyaulax polyhedra, Gymnodinium veneficum,* and *Exuviaella mariaelebouriae.*[328,369] The taxonomic differentiation of *Protogonyaulax* from *Gonyaulax* species has only recently been appreciated, as has the relationship to the genus *Gessnerium.*[413] *S. giganteus* and the Washington clam *(S. nutalli)* may carry the toxin in their neck parts for up to 2 years; however, no physical characteristic distinguishes the carrier animal. A toxin concentration of greater than 75 to 80 μg/100 g foodstuff is considered hazardous to humans. In the 1972 New England red tide the concentration of saxitoxin in blue mussels exceeded 9000 μg/100 g foodstuff. More recently, after cases of paralytic shellfish poisoning in Massachusetts, saxitoxin concentrations of 24,400 μg/100 g were recorded in raw mussels. With oral ingestion the LD_{50} for mice is 263 μg/kg.

Unfortunately, a direct human serum assay is not as yet readily available to the clinician. Paralytic shellfish poison is assessed in foodstuff using the mouse bioassay, in which a 20 g mouse is injected with 1 ml of an acid extract of the shellfish and the time taken for the animal to die is recorded. One mouse unit (MU) or 0.18 μg is the amount of injected saxitoxin that kills a test mouse in 15 minutes.[434] In most countries the action level for closure of a fishery is 400 MU/100 g shellfish. Polyclonal enzyme-linked immunosorbent assays (ELISAs) that measure saxitoxin, neosaxitoxin, and gonyautoxins 1 and 3 may be refined soon to reasonable utility. Other testing methods under investigation include sodium channel–blocking assay, spectrometry, thin-layer chromatography, and high-performance liquid chromatography. The situation is analogous for DSP. An automated tissue culture (neuroblastoma cell) bioassay may become a valid alternative to live animal testing.[205]

The toxins are water-soluble heat- and acid-stable compounds. Twelve derivatives of saxitoxin (such as neosaxitoxin) that originate from dinoflagellates of the genus *Protogonyaulax* are formed by the addition to saxitoxin of *N*-1-hydroxyl, 11-hydroxysulfate, and 21-sulfo groups.[168] Like tetrodotoxin, they can be destroyed to a certain extent in an alkaline medium, but not by ordinary cooking. Saxitoxin appears to block sodium conductance, inhibiting neuromuscular transmission at the axonal and muscle membrane levels. Because of the similarity of the clinical syndrome to tetrodotoxication, it is inferred that the same receptors may be blocked. Saxitoxin suppresses atrioventricular nodal conduction, depresses the medullary respiratory center, and progressively reduces peripheral nerve excitability. The toxicity of saxitoxin is 5000 MU/mg (one MU will kill a 20 g mouse 15 minutes after intraperitoneal injection); in humans a lethal dose of purified saxitoxin is 0.1 mg. Although the illness-causing levels are not definitively known, it has been suggested that ingestion of 200 to 500 μg would cause at least mild symptoms, 500 to 2000 μg moderate illness, and more than 2000 μg serious or fatal illness. However, serious symptoms have followed ingestion of less than (reported) 100 μg in adults.

Within minutes to a few hours of ingestion of contaminated shellfish, there is the onset of intraoral and perioral paresthesias, notably of the lips, tongue, and gums. These progress rapidly to involve the neck and distal extremities. The tingling or burning sensation transforms to numbness. Other symptoms rapidly develop, including lightheadedness, "floating," disequilibrium, incoordination, weakness, hyperreflexia, incoherence, dysarthria, sialorrhea, dysphagia, thirst, diarrhea, abdominal pain, nausea, vomiting, nystagmus, dysmetria, headache, diaphoresis, loss of vision, a sensation of loose teeth, chest pain, and tachycardia. Flaccid paralysis and respiratory insufficiency may follow 2 to 12 hours after ingestion. Unless there is a period of anoxia, the victim often remains awake and alert, although paralyzed. Up to 25% of victims die of unsupported respiratory arrest within the first 12 hours. Children seem to be more sensitive to the saxitoxins than are adults, based on mortality figures from recent outbreaks.[434] Death has followed the ingestion of the viscera of a single purple-hinged rock scallop *(Hinnites multirugosa),* which probably contained saxitoxin at a level of approximately 600 μg/100 g in the adductor muscles and 26,000 μg/100 g in the viscera.[190] This is an unusual case, in that the adductor muscles of scallops are generally not involved. In milder cases, alcohol ingestion appears to increase toxicity.

Ingestion of the liver of the Japanese and Indo-Pacific parrotfish *Ypsiscarus ovifrons* causes a syndrome with symptoms of dyspnea, dysphonia, muscle rigidity, pain, paralysis, ataxia, paresthesias, tongue numbness, respiratory failure, and death. The toxin appears to be different from that of tetrodotoxin or saxitoxin and is concentrated in the viscera, with essentially the same distribution as tetrodotoxin. It is postulated that this represents a new marine toxin.

Neurotoxic Illness

As mentioned previously, *Ptychodiscus breve* is a toxic dinoflagellate that can "bloom" and create a colorful tide. Ingestion of shellfish contaminated with *P. breve* can induce a milder version of paralytic shellfish poisoning, known as "neurotoxic shellfish poisoning," with a delayed onset of up to 3 hours. The condition resembles ciguatera toxin poisoning in symptoms and does not have a major paralytic component.

A curious phenomenon occurs when large blooms of *P. breve* occur near the shoreline. If sea breezes blow the aerosolized toxin onshore, rapidly reversible rhinorrhea and bronchospasm with nonproductive cough can be expected to occur in sensitive individuals.[191] Severe respiratory distress is uncommon. The effects are similar to those of muscarinic stimulation.

P. breve produces at least 10 toxins, known as brevetoxins.[28,29] These polyethers are designated as PbTx-1, PbTx-2, and so on. In a canine model, Florida red tide brevetoxins produce depolarization of tracheal and bronchial smooth muscle.[352] The brevetoxins are potent ichthyotoxins. Signs and symptoms of intoxication in fish include violent twisting and corkscrew swimming, defecation and regurgitation, pectoral fin paralysis, caudal fin curvature, loss of equilibrium, quiescence, vasodilation, convulsions, and fatal respiratory failure.[28] An enzyme immunoassay has been developed to detect these brevetoxins, based on antibodies to PbTx-3.[429]

TREATMENT

Therapy is supportive and based on symptoms. If the victim of PSP comes to medical attention within the first few hours after ingestion, the stomach should be emptied with gastric lavage and then irrigated with 2 L in 200 ml aliquots of a solution of 2% sodium bicarbonate. The administration of activated charcoal (50 to 100 g) and a cathartic (sorbitol 30 to 50 g) makes empirical sense but is not documented as effective in the literature. Since the toxin is excreted in the urine, diuretics have been used, but as yet this has yielded no demonstrable benefit. Hemodialysis as a cure is unproven. Some authors advise against administration of magnesium-containing solutions, such as certain cathartics, with the explanation that hypermagnesemia can contribute to suppression of nerve conduction. The use of neostigmine to counteract the curare-like effects is empirical. Calcium supplementation is experimental. Antivenin raised in rabbits against a saxitoxin-bovine serum albumin conjugate is curative in mice, but the product has not yet been used in humans.

The greatest danger is respiratory paralysis. The victim should be closely observed in the hospital for at least 24 hours for respiratory distress. Supplemental oxygen should be administered and mechanical assistance applied if appropriate. With prompt recognition of respiratory failure, endotracheal intubation and mechanical ventilation prevent anoxic myocardial and brain injury.

Current research is directed at the development of polyclonal and monoclonal antibodies directed against saxitoxin and neosaxitoxin, for the purposes of diagnosis and therapy.

PREVENTION

With regard to PSP, although leeching of shellfish in fresh water for several weeks followed by vigorous cooking may remove up to 70% of the toxin, such procedures are recommended only for persons stranded on desert islands. To the old axiom "Don't eat shellfish in the Northern Hemisphere in months that contain the letter 'r'" should be added "It doesn't matter how you spell the month if the shellfish have been dining on *Gonyaulax*." Because fin fish do not accumulate the toxins in their muscle tissue, there is no risk of contracting PSP from eating them; a theoretical risk would involve consumption of an entire fish without processing.[447]

Shellfish gastroenteritis caused by viral agents has become a major health problem and may require the development of virologic water standards, increased health law enforcement, improved depuration procedures, regulations on harvesting and importing shellfish, and tagging requirements. Surveillance for fecal coliform bacteria in oyster-harvesting waters does not detect the presence of enteric viruses. The risks associated with the consumption of raw shellfish may soon become unacceptable.

Other Shellfish Poisoning

CALLISTIN SHELLFISH POISONING

The Japanese *Callista* clam *(C. brevisiphonata)* is toxic during the spawning months of May to September, at which time cholinergic compounds in the ovaries are increased. The intoxication resembles cholinergic crisis, with both muscarinic and nicotinic components. Within an hour of ingestion of the heat-stable toxin, generalized pruritus, urticaria, erythema, facial numbness and paralysis, hypersalivation, diaphoresis, fever, chills, nausea, vomiting, diarrhea, bronchorrhea, bronchospasm, and constrictive dyspnea develop. Therapy is supportive, and recovery is usually complete within 2 days. In severe cases of cholinergic crisis, particularly with marked bradycardia, atropine (0.5 mg intravenously every 5 minutes to a total dose of 2 mg) may be administered.

VENERUPIN SHELLFISH POISONING

The Japanese lake-harvested oyster *(Crassostrea gigas)* and clam *(Tapes semidecussata)* occasionally feed on toxic dinoflagellate species of the genus *Prorocentrum,* posing the greatest risk during the months of December through April.[33,172] The heat-stable toxin induces the rapid onset of gastrointestinal distress, headache, and nervousness, which are followed over 48 hours by hepatic dysfunction, manifested by elevation of liver enzymes, leukocytosis, jaundice, and profound coagulation defects. Delirium and coma may ensue, with death occurring in 33% of victims. Therapy is supportive and based on symptoms. Any victim who shows the early symptoms of gastroenteritis should be placed on a low-protein diet and observed for 48 to 72 hours for signs of liver failure. There is not yet clinical experience with exchange transfusion, chemotherapy, hemoperfusion, or liver transplantation in the management of profound liver failure associated with this disorder.

TETRAMINE AND TRIMETHYLAMINE POISONING

Tetramine (trimethylammonium) is a naturally occurring quaternary ammonium compound that has been identified in anemones, gorgonians, jellyfishes, and mollusks.[16] This includes the "edible" whelk *Neptunea antiqua.*[17] Although some variation exists depending on the species ingested, the victim of tetramine poisoning may suffer nausea, vomiting, headache, vertigo, transient blindness, photophobia, diplopia, ataxia, weakness, urticaria, and weakness. Symptoms occur within 30 minutes of ingestion and seem to disappear within a few hours.

The toxin is reputed to block the autonomic nervous system and is excreted predominantly by the kidneys. A lethal dose for humans is estimated at 250 to 1000 mg.[16]

Trimethylamine (TMA) poisoning may follow ingestion of the flesh of the Greenland shark *Somniosus microcephalus.*[18] The syndrome in sled dogs includes symptoms of nausea, vomiting, abnormal gait, hypersalivation, explosive diarrhea, muscular twitching, ophthalmoplegia, respiratory distress, and occasional seizures. Theoretically, trimethylamine oxide is metabolized to TMA, which exerts its effect by organ-selective muscarinic and nicotinic stimulation, followed by neuromuscular blockade.

In humans the only problems noted to date have been nausea and measurable TMA excretion in urine and sweat. However, as noted in the earlier section on ichthyohepatotoxication, human ingestion of Greenland shark liver can induce a syndrome similar to that seen in dogs that ingest large quantities of the same shark's flesh. The definitive link in humans or dog to TMA has not yet been made.

Seafood Allergies*

True seafood allergies are immunoglobulin E (IgE)-mediated reactions. Although allergic reactions can occur to all classes of seafoods, accurate epidemiologic data are difficult to obtain. Crustacean allergies are one of the most common types of food allergy in the U.S. adult population[257]; codfish allergy is probably the most common form of food allergy in Scandinavian countries.[1]

BIOLOGIC CLASSIFICATION

An understanding of the taxonomic relationships among different species of marine animals is important. While many seafood species may be allergenic, most allergic patients are not sensitive to all species. The degree of allergic cross-reactivity among the different fish species varies widely among patients. Thus selective avoidance diets are possible. The biologic classification of the edible species of fishes is given in Table 53-1. Most edible fishes belong to class Osteichthyes, although sharks are in a different class. The most commonly consumed fishes in the United States belong to only a few orders: Salmoniformes (salmons, trouts, whitefishes, smelts, and pikes), Perciformes (basses, perches, dolphins, snappers, groupers, redfishes, mackerels, and tunas), Gadiformes (codfishes, pollocks, haddocks, and hakes), Pleuronectiformes (flounders, halibuts, and soles), Clupeiformes (herrings, sar-

*Contributed by Susan L. Hefle, Ph.D., and Robert K. Bush, M.D.

Table 53-1 Taxonomic Relationships Among the Edible Fishes

Taxonomic Classification		
Class	**Subclass or Order**	**Common Name**
Chondrichthyes	Elasmobranchii	Sharks
Osteichthyes	Acipenseriformes	Sturgeons, paddlefishes
	Elopiformes	Tarpons, ten-pounders, bonefishes
	Anguilliformes	Common eels, morays
	Clupeiformes	Herrings, sardines, alewives, shad, menhaden, anchovies
	Salmoniformes	Trouts, salmons, whitefishes, graylings, discoes, pikes, lake herrings, pickerels, muskelunges, euchalons, capelins, smelts, saugers
	Gonorynchiformes	Milkfishes, awa
	Cypriniformes	Minnows, carps, suckers, catfishes
	Beloniformes	Sauries, needlefishes, flying fishes
	Mugiliformes	Mullets, barracudas, silversides, threadfishes
	Lambridiformes	Opah, mariposas
	Tetraodontiformes	Pufferfishes, boxfishes, trunkfishes
	Pleuronectiformes	Flounders, halibuts, soles, dabs, turbots
	Perciformes, suborder Percodei	Basses, crappies, bluegills, sea basses, sunfishes, perches, bluefishes, jacks, pompanos, dolphins, snappers, groupers, scups, grunts, porgies, pomfrets, sheepsheads, snooks, robalos, bigeyes, catalugas, croakers, spots, redfishes, tautogs, butterfly fishes, wrasses, spade fishes, goatfishes, mojarras, rudderfishes, surffishes, weakfishes, roaches, drums, cichlids
	Perciformes, suborder Scombroidei	Mackerels, tunas, cutlassfishes, albacores, bonitos, kingfishes
	Perciformes, suborder Xiphoidei	Swordfishes, marlins, sailfishes, spearfishes
	Perciformes, suborder Ammodytoidei	Sand lances
	Perciformes, suborder Stromateoidei	Butterfishes
	Scorpaeniformes	Rockfishes, scorpionfishes, greenlings
	Gadiformes	Codfishes, ling cods, pollocks, haddocks, tomcods, hakes, codlings
	Percopsoidei	Trout-perches, sand rollers

dines, anchovies, shad, menhadens, and alewives), Cypriniformes (carps and catfishes), and Scorpaeniformes (rockfishes). Since many of the edible fish species belong to the orders Salmoniformes, Perciformes, and Gadiformes, a more detailed breakdown of the relationships for those orders is provided in Tables 53-2 to 53-4.

The physician should be alert to the confusing common names of fishes. For instance, king mackerel may be sold as cero, silver cero, black salmon, cavalla, or kingfish. Kingfish can also mean king whiting, which itself is sold as ground mullet, whiting, gulf whiting, surf whiting, southern whiting, sand whiting, or silver whiting. Whiting may be a name used to describe hake. The identification of fish is often erroneous, particularly when performed by sport fishermen.

The biologic classification of the mollusks and crustacea is listed in Table 53-5. At least 30 edible species of crustacea are commonly consumed in the United States. More detailed lists of the edible species of mollusks and crustacea are given in Tables 53-6 and 53-7.

CLINICAL MANIFESTATIONS

Anaphylaxis is the life-threatening reaction that may follow the ingestion of allergens to which the patient has been previously sensitized. Food-dependent exercise-induced anaphylaxis is a condition wherein patients in the resting state can eat food without difficulty. However, if a patient eats a food to which he or she is allergic and exercises within 2 to 4 hours, the signs and symptoms of anaphylaxis develop. Shellfish are among the implicated foods.[286] Urticaria and angioedema are less severe manifestations of food allergy. Urticaria is epidermal, whereas angioedema is thought to arise from a similar pathologic process in the deeper dermis. Occupational asthma follows inhalation of airborne allergens in sensitive individuals. Seafood has often been implicated, including oysters,[215,323] shrimp,[146] fish,[115] snow crab,[76] lobster,[330] powdered marine sponges,[35] abalone,[91] and clam liver extract.[221] Immediate and late reactions may occur. Atopic dermatitis may be exacerbated by seafood allergies.[367]

DIAGNOSIS

Medical History

The diagnosis of food allergy may be simple or extremely complex. Guidelines are provided in Box 53-3. With seafoods it is particularly important to obtain correct identification of the offending food to determine if cross-

Table 53-2 Taxonomic Relationships Among Salmoniformes

Taxonomic Classification			
Suborder	**Family**	**Genus**	**Common Name**
Salmonoidei	Salmonidae	*Coregonus*	Whitefishes, ciscoes, bloaters, lake herrings
		Onchorhynchus	Pacific salmons
		Salmo	Trouts, Atlantic salmon
		Salvelinus	Chars, brook trout, Dolly Varden trout, lake trout
		Thymallus	Grayling
	Osmeridae	*Osmerus*	Smelts
		Mallotus	Capelins
		Thaleichthys	Euchalon
Esocoidei	Esocidae	*Esox*	Pikes, saugers, pickerels, muskelunges

Table 53-3 Taxonomic Relationships Among Perciformes

Taxonomic Classification		
Suborder	**Family**	**Common Name**
Percoidei	Centraranidae	Largemouth bass, black basses, breams, bluegill, sunfishes, crappie, Sacramento perch
	Percichthyidae	Striped bass, white bass, white perch, yellow bass
	Serranidae	Groupers, sea basses, jawfishes
	Percidae	Pikes, saugers, yellow perch, river perch
	Centropomidae	Snooks, robalos
	Priacanthidae	Cataluras, bigeyes
	Pomatomidae	Bluefish
	Coryphaenidae	Dolphin fish (mahi mahi)
	Carangidae	Jacks, pompanos, cavallas, moonfishes, scads, jack mackerel
	Bramidae	Pomfret
	Pomadasyidae	Grunts
	Lutjanidae	Snappers, mutton fish, rabirubias
	Chaetodontidae	Butterflyfishes
	Ephippidae	Spade fishes
	Labridae	Wrasses, tautog
	Cichlidae	Cichlids
	Sciaenidae	Drums, redfish, croakers, weakfishes, kingfishes
	Mullidae	Goatfishes
	Sparidae	Porgies, scups, spots, sheepsheads
	Gerridae	Mojarras
	Kyphosidae	Rudderfishes, sea chubs
	Embiotocidae	Surffishes
Scombroidei	Scombridae	Mackerels, tunas, bonitos, Spanish mackerels, sierra, kingfish, cero, cavalla, petos
	Trichiuridae	Cutlassfishes
Xiphioidei	Xiphiidae	Swordfishes
	Istiophoridae	Marlins, sailfishes, spearfishes
Ammodytoidei	Ammodytidae	Sand lances
Stromateoidei	Stromateidae	Butterfishes

reaction patterns can be established. An estimate of the quantity of the food needed to elicit the reaction may help to distinguish intolerance from allergy.

Skin Testing

If properly performed, skin testing with appropriate food allergens is useful in establishing an allergic etiology. There is some risk to patients who have experienced severe anaphylactic reactions. Food extracts for skin testing are obtained from commercial laboratories, usually in a 1:20 weight/volume concentration stabilized with 50% glycerine and 0.4% phenol. Control skin tests include a negative response to a solution of the diluent and a positive response to a solution of histamine (1 mg/ml). A positive response is the appearance

Table 53-4 Taxonomic Relationships Among Gadiformes

Taxonomic Classification			
Suborder	**Family**	**Genus**	**Common Name**
Gadoidei	Merlucciidae	*Merluccius*	Pacific hake
	Gadidae	*Pollachius*	Pollock
		Theragra	Walleye pollock
		Gadus	Codfishes
		Microgadus	Tomcods
		Lota	Turbot
		Melanogrammus	Haddock
		Urophycis	Atlantic hake, red hake, Gulf hake

Table 53-5 Taxonomic Relationships Among Edible Mollusks and Crustacea

Taxonomic Classification			
Phylum	**Class**	**Subclass**	**Common Name**
Mollusca	Gastropoda	Prosobranchi	Marine snails, abalone, periwinkles, whelks
		Pulmonata	Freshwater snails
	Bivalvia	Lamellibranchii	Mussels, cockles, oysters, scallops, clams
	Cephalopoda	Coleoidea	Squid, octopus
Arthropoda	Crustacea	Malacostraca	Shrimp, crabs, lobsters, crayfish

Table 53-6 Edible Bivalves and Cephalopods

Group	Common Name	Scientific Name
Clams	Surf or bar clam	*Mactra solidissima*
	Soft clam	*Mya arenaria*
	Hard clam or quahog	*Venus mercenaria*
	Atlantic razor clam	*Ensis directus*
	Pacific razor clam	*Siliqua patula*
	Stout razor clam	*Tagelus gibbus*
	Butter clam	*Saxidomus nuttali*
	Little neck clam	*Tapes staminea*
	Geoduck clam	*Panope generosa*
	Freshwater clam	*Corbicula leana*
	Pismo clam	*Tivela stultorum*
	Short-necked clam	*Venerupis japonica*
	Jackknife clam	*Tagelus californianus*
Mussels	European or Atlantic mussel	*Mytilus edulis*
	Pacific mussel	*Mytilus californianus*
	South Asian green mussel	*Mytilus smaragdinus*
Cockles	Common cockle	*Cardium corbis*
	Red cockle	*Cardium echinatum*
	Spiny cockle	*Cardium aculateum*
Scallops	Common scallop	*Pecten gibbus borealis*
	Deep water scallop	*Placopecten megallanicus*
	Japanese scallop	*Pecten yessoensis*
Oysters	Pacific oyster	*Ostrea gigas*
	Atlantic oyster	*Crassostrea virginica*
	Japanese oyster	*Crassostrea laperousei*
	Coon oyster	*Ostrea frons*
Squid	North American squid	*Loligo paeleii*
	North American squid	*Loligo opalescens*
	Japanese squid	*Ommastrephes sloani pacificus*
Octopus	Common octopus	*Octopus vulgaris*

of a wheal of 3 to 5 mm (minimum) at 15 minutes, which suggests an IgE-mediated reaction. Puncture tests should be used in preference to intradermal tests, since the latter create an excessive number of false-positive reaction.[54]

While the skin puncture test is extremely useful, commercial extracts are not available for all individual seafood species. Often, mixed extracts are used. Listed in Box 53-4 are the commonly available seafood extracts.

Radioallergosorbent Test

The radioallergosorbent test (RAST) is an in vitro test for detecting specific IgE antibodies in the serum.[365] Briefly, the test is conducted by incubating a patient's serum with a solid-phase support (paper disks, microcrystalline cellulose, sepharose) to which the allergen is covalently bound. If the patient's serum contains IgE antibody against the allergen, it attaches to the bound allergen. After several washes the solid-phase support is incubated with radioactively labeled anti-IgE. The number of counts of radioactivity bound to the solid-phase support provides a means of quantitating the amount of specific IgE in the serum. The RAST test is reserved for situations in which skin testing is inappropriate by virtue of previous severe reactions. For instance, it has been used successfully to demonstrate serum IgE binding in three individuals with hypersensitivity to bluegill *(Lepomis machrochirus)* skin mucin.[442] A list of commercially available RAST disks is provided in Box 53-4.

Double-Blind Food Challenges

The ultimate test to verify that a particular food causes a reaction is the double-blind food challenge.[44] This should not be performed in patients who have experienced life-threatening reactions and should be undertaken only under close physician supervision. Dried or freeze-dried foods are encapsulated in opaque, dye-free capsules. Appropriate identical placebo-control capsules are prepared. Although such testing is time consuming and expensive, it permits a precise diagnosis.

Table 53-7 Edible Crustacea

Group	Common Name	Scientific Name
Lobsters	Atlantic lobster	*Homarus vulgaris*
	European lobster	*Homarus gammarus*
	Northern lobster	*Homarus americanus*
	Spiny lobster	*Pancilirus argus*
Crabs	Blue crab	*Callinectis sapidus*
	Deep sea blue crab	*Portunus pelagicus*
	Dungeness crab	*Cancer magister*
	Jonah crab	*Cancer borealis*
	King crab	*Paralithodes camtschatica*
	Snow crab	*Chionoectes bairdi*
	Tanner crab	*Chionoectes tanneri*
	Spider crab	*Talvia maticum*
	Stone crab	*Menippe mercenaria*
Prawns and shrimp	Common prawn	*Palaemon serratus*
	Deep water prawn	*Pandalus bortalis*
	Pink Maine shrimp	*Pandalus borealis*
	Coon stripe shrimp	*Pandalus hypsinotus*
	Brown shrimp	*Panaeus aztecus*
	Pink shrimp	*Panaeus duorarum*
	White shrimp	*Panaeus indicus*
	Gamba shrimp	*Panaeus longirostris*
	Karuma prawn	*Panaeus japonicus*
	Giant tiger prawn	*Panaeus monodon*
	Common tiger prawn	*Panaeus esculentus*
	Indian prawn	*Panaeus indicus*
	Eastern king prawn	*Panaeus plebejus*
	Banana prawn	*Panaeus merguiensis*
	Brine shrimp	*Artemia salina*
	Rock shrimp	*Silyomia brevirostris*
	Sea bob shrimp	*Xiphophenaeus kroyeri*
	Royal red shrimp	*Hymenopenaeus robustus*
	Freshwater prawn	*Macrobrachium carcinus*

Elimination Diets

In situations where a seafood is suspected of producing symptoms, it may be eliminated from the diet. The patient then reintroduces the food after the initial complaints have resolved, to see if the reaction is reelicited.

Controversial Techniques

A number of clinical and laboratory tests are unreliable predictors of the presence of seafood allergy. These include pulse index, in vitro cytotoxic food tests, intracutaneous provocation, sublingual provocation, basophil degranulation, and sublingual neutralization.[14]

Diagnosis of Occupational Asthma

Although the measures described previously are useful in diagnosing cutaneous, gastrointestinal, or systemic manifestations of food allergy, the diagnosis of occupational asthma requires a different approach. If the patient notes the onset of asthma symptoms related to work exposure and improves on weekends or while on vacation, occupational asthma should be suspected. Asthma per se is verified by appropriate pulmonary function tests, such as spirometry with and without bronchodilators. If the history is suggestive but not corroborated by physical examination or simple spirometry, it may be necessary to perform provocation with inhaled methacholine or histamine to document airway hyper-

BOX 53-3

AN APPROACH TO THE DIAGNOSIS OF SEAFOOD ALLERGY

- Physical examination and clinical history with description of suspected food intolerance
- Time between food ingestion and onset of symptoms
- Description of the most recent reaction
- Estimate of the quantity of food necessary to cause a reaction
- Food and symptom diary to document food intake and frequency of symptoms
- Tests to rule out nonallergic food intolerance
- Elimination diet
- Strict avoidance diet
- When improvement seen, reintroduction of suspected foods under observation
- Double-blind allergen challenge under strict supervision
- Immunologic tests to determine if identified food intolerance is a food allergy

BOX 53-4

COMMERCIALLY AVAILABLE SEAFOOD EXTRACTS FOR SKIN TESTING AND RAST DISKS

SKIN TEST EXTRACTS

Fish: Bass, catfish, codfish, flounder, haddock, halibut, herring, mackerel, perch, pickerel, salmon, sardine, sole, trout, tuna, whitefish

Fish mixtures: 1. Codfish, flounder, mackerel, tuna
2. Codfish, halibut, mackerel, perch, salmon, trout, tuna

Crustacea: Crab, lobster, shrimp

Mollusks: Clam, oyster, scallop

Shellfish mixtures: 1. Clam, crab, oyster, scallop, shrimp
2. Clam, crab, lobster, oyster, shrimp, scallop

RAST DISKS

Crab, lobster, blue mussel, salmon, shrimp, tuna

reactivity. The diagnosis depends ultimately on the provocation of asthma by a bronchial inhalation challenge with the suspected allergen. Such evaluation should occur under close observation in a hospital setting.

Treatment and Prevention

The single best treatment for allergic reactions to seafood allergens is avoidance. To avoid unnecessary dietary restrictions, the proper diagnosis is extremely important. Occupational asthma may respond to cromolyn sodium prophylaxis. Atopic dermatitis requires diligent skin hydration with moisturizing lotions, control of the intense pruritus with antihistamines, and topical and systemic corticosteroids.

Identification and Characterization of Seafood Allergens

Fish. Allergists generally recommend removing all edible fish from a patient's diet, including both Osteichthyes (bony fish) and Chondrichthyes (shark), when the patient has a demonstrated history of allergic reaction to any fish or if there is a positive skin test or RAST to a fish extract. However, research using double-blind placebo-controlled fish challenges[42] and other tests[2,106] in fish-allergic children has shown that they are not uniformly sensitive to all species; hence hypersensitivity to one species does not automatically warrant dietary elimination of all fish. Fish challenges in children with negative skin tests were negative; therefore skin testing may be advisable first.[42]

Of the few seafood allergens that have been purified and characterized, the most notable is codfish allergen, *Gad c* I (allergen M), which belongs to a group of muscle tissue proteins known as parvalbumins.[121] The existence of structurally related parvalbumins in divergent fish species may offer an explanation of cross-reactivity to fish species in allergic individuals. *Gad c* I is an acidic protein of molecular weight 12,328 daltons, is composed of 113 amino acids and 1 glucose molecule, and has an isoelectric point of 4.75. It comprises three domains: AB, CD, and EF, consisting of three helices interspaced by one loop.[122] Each of the loops of the CD and EF domains coordinates one Ca^{+2}-binding site; these sites correspond to IgE-binding sites. It is stable to heat, extremes of pH, and mild proteolysis. Allergenicity of *Gad c* I is decreased by acetylation or polymerization of the tyr-30 residue,[19] modification of the arg-75 residue, or unchelating the two calcium ions,[120] but these methods cannot be used commercially. Lyophilization and canning seemed to decrease allergenicity of certain fish in a study of fish-sensitive subjects by Bernhisel-Broadbent, Straus, and Sampson.[43]

Protamine sulfate, a sperm protein of salmon, herring, and other species belonging to the families Salmonidae and Clupeidae, has been identified as an allergen in patients with sensitivities to salmon, herring, and related fish.[230] It is a low–molecular weight protein widely used as a heparin antagonist.

Crustacea. The crustacean family (order Decododa) includes shrimp, prawns, crabs, lobsters, and crayfish[464] and is a common reported cause of food hypersensitivity.[64] Research indicates that there are shared allergenic and antigenic determinants among the various members of the crustacea[169,256]; for example, individuals with shrimp sensitivity exhibit positive skin tests and RAST to other crustaceans.[102,441] In a study of crustacea-sensitive subjects, specific IgE binding was observed to six crayfish components and four spiny lobster components,[169] and other studies using RAST and additional immunochemical techniques indicate common antigenic or allergenic epitopes in shrimp and other crustacea.[254,256] However, some reactions are species specific.[254,302] Also, qualitative differences in the allergenic determinants of different shrimp extracts have been reported[302]; therefore use of extracts from more than one species in skin testing and RAST is recommended. Presence of IgE to either unique or shared allergens may explain an individual's clinical sensitivity to one or more members of this taxonomic class.

A study of the cross-reactivity of oyster (phylum Mollusca) and crustacea indicates some common antigenic or allergenic epitopes based on RAST inhibition studies.[253] Skin test and RAST reactivity to oysters did not appear to correlate with oyster sensitivity in this report, which should be a consideration when skin testing for shellfish sensitivity.

Shrimp is the most studied of the crustacea allergens. Hoffman, Day, and Miller[185] were the first to partially characterize allergens from shrimp; antigen I was isolated from raw shrimp and was found to be an acidic, heat-labile protein composed of two noncovalently bound polypeptide chains with a molecular weight of 21 kd. Antigen II, isolated from cooked shrimp, was found to be an acidic, heat-stable glycoprotein with a molecular weight of 38 kd and an isoelectric point of 4.5 composed of 341 amino acid residues and 4% carbohydrate. Antigen II appeared to be a major allergen for the subjects in this study.

An allergenic tRNA moiety from cooked prawns has been described[321]; however, the researchers were not able to isolate a preparation completely devoid of protein, so it is possible that the allergenicity was caused by RNA-associated proteins. Further work by this group[322] yielded the description of two allergenic polypeptides from cooked shrimp; SA-I had a molecular weight of 8.2 kd and was not analyzed further. The second allergen, SA-II, was composed of 301 amino acid residues, had a molecular weight of 34 kd, and appeared similar to antigen I isolated by Hoffman and colleagues.

Daul and co-workers[103] have described a major shrimp allergen of 36 kd that is readily isolated from the boiling water and meat of cooked shrimp. The protein was composed of 312 amino acid residues and 2.4% carbohydrate; protein sequencing indicated homology with the muscle protein tropomyosin. Monoclonal antibodies directed against the 36 kd shrimp allergen reacted to a 36 kd protein in crayfish, crab, and lobster extracts; this major shrimp allergen has been named *Pen a* I. Antigen I, SA-II, and *Pen a* I appear to be the same protein.

Shared antigenic and allergenic determinants between shrimp *Pen a* 1 and fruitfly extract have been found, with *Pen a* I sharing 87% homology with fruitfly tropomyosin.[101] This again illustrates the phylogenic conservation of certain allergenic epitopes.

Squid. IgE-mediated reactions have been documented in sensitive subjects after ingestion of squid or inhalation of vapors from cooking squid.[74] Almost all of these patients also experienced symptoms after ingesting shrimp and demonstrated strong positive skin test reactions to boiled squid extracts and various commercial crustacea extracts. RAST inhibition and other immunoassay studies showed cross-reactivity between shrimp and squid allergens, although cross-reactivity was not demonstrated between squid and octopus or squid and other mollusks.

Limpet and Abalone. Other mollusks causing reported moderate to severe anaphylactic reactions after ingestion are grand keyhole limpet and abalone.[73,281] Sensitive subjects had positive skin tests and RASTs to extracts of the offending shellfish. In one study the basophils of sensitive subjects released histamine in response to a cooked limpet extract.[73] By immunoblotting, the major allergens of grand keyhole limpet appear to have molecular weights of 38 and 80 kd.

Seafood-Insect Cross-Reactions. Patients allergic to chironomids (nonbiting midges) also often demonstrate positive skin tests to crustacea. Chironomid extracts have been found to inhibit RAST with shrimp and vice versa,[128] although other researchers report low cross-reactivity using this assay method.[454]

The invertebrate hemoglobin (erythrocruorin) molecule might be involved in the reported cross-reactivity of caddis fly and mollusk allergy. It is a potent allergen for chironomid, and serum from caddis-sensitive patients in one study reacted with a component of similar molecular weight in mollusk and bee venom extracts.[240] This raises the possibility that patients exposed to caddis fly antigens could develop allergic reactions during their first exposure to shellfish or their first bee sting.

Vibrio Fish Poisoning, Wound Infections, and Septicemia

Vibrio organisms can cause gastroenteric disease and soft tissue infections, particularly in immunocompromised hosts. Extraintestinal infections may be associated with bacteremia and death.[20] From April to December 1992, nine people in Florida died from *Vibrio vulnificus* infection after eating raw oysters; all but one had liver disease.[136] As discussed in the section concerning bacteriology of the aquatic environment (Chapter 51), the clinician must be alert to the possibility of infection with an aquatic organism to select appropriate antibiotics. *Vibrio* species are the most potentially virulent halophilic organisms that flourish in the marine environment. The teeth of a great white shark have been swabbed and yielded *V. alginolyticus, V. fluvialis,* and *V. parahaemolyticus.*[65] Mako shark tooth culture has yielded *V. damsela, V. furnisii,* and *V. splendidus I.*[25] *V. parahaemolyticus* has also been identified in freshwater habitats.[26,105,410] Water that is brackish (salinity of 15 to 25 parts per thousand) allows the growth of *Vibrio* species if appropriate nutrients are present; *V. vulnificus* infection has been documented after exposure to waters with salinities of 2 and 4 ppt.[55,410] The optimal season for disease appears to be summer, when water temperatures encourage bacterial proliferation. In most studies reported, infections seem to cluster during the summer months; this may be related to increased numbers of people at the seashore.[47,50,57,193] This has been corroborated to some degree by the observation that *V. parahaemolyticus* cultured from marine mammals was recovered only in the warmer months of the year in the Northeast or in animals from subtropical regions.[65] Sharks appear to develop some immunity to autochthonous *Vibrio* species, as suggested by the detection of a binding protein similar to the IgM subclass of immunoglobulin.[60,160] Allochthonous (for the shark) *Vibrio* species, such as *V. carchariae,* may be the agents of elasmobranch disease when the animal is under stress.[158,159]

Vibrio species are halophilic, gram-negative rods that are facultative anaerobes. They are part of the normal flora of coastal waters not only in the United States, but also in many exotic locations frequented by recreational and industrial divers and seafarers.[166,208,368] Vibrios are mesophilic organisms and grow best at temperatures of 24° to 40° C, with essentially no growth below 8° to 10° C.[57] Other marine bacteria are facultative psychrophiles, barophiles, or both.[280] *Vibrio* species seem to require less sodium for maximal growth than do other more fastidious marine organisms, a factor that allows explosive reproduction in the 0.9% saline environment of the human body. Gastrointestinal illness has been associated with *V. cholerae* 0 group 1, non-01, *V. parahaemolyticus, V. fluvialis, V. mimicus, V. hollisae, V. furnissii,* and *V. vulnificus.** Wound infections have been documented to yield *V. cholerae* 0 group 1 and non-01, *V. parahaemolyticus, V. vulnificus, V. alginolyticus,* and *V. damsela.*† Septicemia, with or without an obvious source, has been attributed to infections with *V. cholerae* non-01, *V. parahaemolyticus, V. alginolyticus, V. vulnificus,* and *V. metschnikoviii.*‡

Whenever a *Vibrio* species is suspected, the microbiology laboratory must be alerted to use an appropriate selective culture medium for stool cultures, such as thiosulfate–

*References 37, 135, 141, 210, 307, 309, 316, 377.

†References 92, 127, 134, 223, 291, 297, 307, 309, 337, 338, 353, 355, 364, 424, 438.

‡References 57, 127, 141, 204, 209, 223, 297, 307.

citrate–bile salts–sucrose (TCBS) agar or Monsur taurocholate-tellurite-gelatin agar.[276,303] A large clinical laboratory near the ocean might consider the use of TCBS agar routinely.[131] Pathogenic vibrios generally grow on MacConkey agar.

The stool specimen should be collected if possible within the first 24 hours of illness and before the administration of antibiotics; specimens should not be allowed to dry. The specimen may be transported in the semisolid transport medium of Cary and Blair; buffered glycerol-saline is not satisfactory because glycerol is toxic to vibrios. Tellurite-taurocholate-peptone broth is adequate. In a pinch, strips of blotting paper may be soaked in liquid stool and transported in airtight plastic bags.[131] All species except *V. cholerae* and *V. mimicus* require sodium chloride for growth.[48] Enrichment broth (alkaline peptone water with 1% NaCl) is recommended for isolation of vibrios from convalescent and treated patients.[200] All *Vibrio* species grow in routine blood culture mediums and on nonselective mediums such as blood agar.[307]

Key characteristics that aid in the separation of *Vibrio* species from other medically significant bacteria (Enterobacteriaceae, *Pseudomonas, Aeromonas, Plesiomonas*) are the production of oxidase, fermentative metabolism, requirement of sodium chloride for growth, and susceptibility to the 0/129 vibriostatic compound.[202] Species that cannot be identified in the hospital microbiology laboratory may be referred to a state laboratory or the Centers for Disease Control.

A superb review on the current epidemiology and pathogenesis of clinically significant *Vibrio* species is offered by Janda and associates.[202]

VIBRIO PARAHAEMOLYTICUS

Vibrio parahaemolyticus is a halophilic gram-negative rod to which is attributed a gastroenteric syndrome that has been reported in the United States, Japan, Great Britain, and Australia.[27,142,198,249] The organisms are found in waters along the entire coastline of the United States.[94,218,353] Generally the incidence of clinical disease is greatest in the warm summer months when the organism is commonly found in zooplankton. *V. parahaemolyticus* absorbs onto chitin and to minute crustacean copepods that feed on sediment.[47] It has been postulated that unusual warm coastal currents (such as *El Niño*) may contribute to increased proliferation of *Vibrio* species. The optimal growth temperature of *V. parahaemolyticus* is 35° to 37° C; under ideal conditions the generation time has been estimated at less than 10 minutes, with explosive population growth from 10 to 10^6 organisms in 3 to 4 hours.[37,218] Ingestion of raw or partially cooked contaminated shrimp, oysters, or fish is followed in 6 to 76 hours by explosive diarrhea, nausea, vomiting, headache, abdominal pain, fever, chills, and prostration. The stools may contain blood and classically demonstrate leukocytes on methylene blue staining. The syndrome generally resolves spontaneously in 24 to 72 hours but may be of a severity sufficient to cause significant fluid and electrolyte depletion. Stool cultures should be obtained before the initiation of antibiotic therapy. The laboratory should be alerted to the necessity for special culture media (TCBS with 0.5% NaCl). A course of oral trimethoprim-sulfamethoxazole or tetracycline may shorten the course of severe gastroenteritis.

Extraintestinal wound infections are most common in persons who suffer chronic liver disease or immunosuppression. Although over 95% of *V. parahaemolyticus* strains associated with human illness are positive, the relationship to pathogenicity of the Kanagawa reaction (production of a cell-free hemolysin on high salt–mannitol [Wagatsuma] agar), caused by a heat-stable direct hemolysin, is not yet clear.[47,202,307] Furthermore, most marine strains are not Kanagawa positive. Some primary soft tissue infections previously attributed to *V. parahaemolyticus* may theoretically be attributed to misidentified *V. vulnificus*.[134] Panophthalmitis requiring enucleation occurred in a man who suffered a corneal laceration.[406] The treatment of extragastroenteric syndromes should be the same as for *Vibrio vulnificus*.

In a review of seven fatal cases caused by *V. parahaemolyticus* or *V. cholerae* non-01 in Florida between 1981 and 1988, it was shown that although all patients died of sepsis, gastrointestinal signs and symptoms characterized the early illness in four patients and painful swelling and lesions of the lower extremities afflicted the others.[229] All patients had preexisting chronic diseases, and five had eaten seafood during the week before the onset of illness.

VIBRIO VULNIFICUS

Vibrio vulnificus (formerly known as a "lactose [fermenting]-positive" vibrio) is a halophilic gram-negative bacillus to which is attributed a syndrome of primary septicemia that occurs 12 hours to 7 days following the ingestion of raw oysters.* This is the presentation in approximately 60% of cases of illness associated with this organism.[229] It is not uncommon for oysters to undergo 5 to 10 days of transit after they have been harvested for consumption. The optimal temperature for growth (doubling time 15 minutes) for *V. vulnificus* is 35° C (95° F), but the organisms replicate nicely in the shell at 8° C (46.4° F). The peak incidence is in the summer months, which coincides with peak oyster-eating and ocean-bathing activities.[236] Summer crabs may also carry the organism. *V. vulnificus* is found in virtually all U.S. coastal waters and has been reported to cause infection worldwide.[78] Although it prefers a habitat of warm (at least 20° C or 68° F) seawater, it can be found in much

*References 50, 130, 189, 206, 307, 407.

colder water. It does not appear to be associated with fecal contamination of seawater.[411]

The organism may or may not have an acidic polysaccaride capsule (opaque colony), which confers protection against bactericidal activity of human serum and phagocytosis and thus renders the organism more virulent in animals. At extremely low frequency, some strains can shift between unencapsulated (avirulent; translucent colony) and capsulated (virulent) serotypes.[383,460] The encapsulated isolates show exquisite (positive) sensitivity to iron. Virulent isolates can use 100% but not 30% saturated (normal for humans) transferrin as an iron source, as well as iron in hemoglobin and hemoglobin-haptoglobin complexes.[310,453,465]

The classic syndrome evolves rapidly after the initiation of symptoms and has been noted most frequently in men over 40 years of age with preexisting hepatic dysfunction, leukopenia, or impaired immunity (malignancy, HIV infection, diabetes, long-term corticosteroids), although it has been reported in young, previously healthy individuals.[12,82,212] Persons with high serum iron levels (from chronic cirrhosis, hepatitis, thalassemia major, hemochromatosis) or achlorhydria (low gastric acid; may be iatrogenically induced with H_2 blockers) may be at greater risk for fulminant bacteremia.[340,453] This has been attributed in part to the protective effect of gastric acid, the iron requirement of the organism, and the effects of liver disease (decreased polymorphonuclear leukocyte and macrophage activity, flawed opsonization, shunting of portal blood around the liver).[82,306,347]

The syndrome consists of flulike malaise, fever, vomiting, diarrhea, chills, hypotension, and early skin vesiculation that evolves into necrotizing dermatitis, with vasculitis and myositis (Color Plates 136 and 137).[27,79] Hematogenous seeding of vibrios to secondary cutaneous lesions is probable. Primary wound infections (approximately 30% of cases) rapidly show marked edema, with erythema, vesicles, and hemorrhagic or contused-appearing bullae, progressing to necrosis.[49] This may require radical surgical debridement or amputation.[39,223] Up to 25% of these patients may have sepsis. Extracellular elastin-lysing proteases elaborated by the organism, as well as a potent collagenase, probably contribute to the rapid invasion of healthy tissue.[243,388] *V. vulnificus* also produces a cytotoxin-hemolysin and phospholipases.[78] The precise roles of these and other factors (pili, mucinase, chondroitinase, hyaluronidase) in the in vivo pathogenicity of the organism have yet to be determined.[203] Bleeding complications (which may include gastrointestinal hemorrhage and disseminated intravascular coagulation) are common and may be attributed in part to thrombocytopenia.[307] Gastroenteritis is more common (15% to 20%) with the septicemic presentation than with primary wound infection and may exist as an isolated entity (approximately 10% of cases), although it is debated that illness has been erroneously attributed to the asymptomatically carried organism.[203,210,229] *Vibrio vulnificus* endometritis has been reported after an episode of intercourse in the water of Galveston Bay, Texas.[426] Other presentations of *Vibrio vulnificus* infections have included meningitis, spontaneous bacterial peritonitis, corneal ulcers, epiglottitis, and infections of the testes, spleen, and heart valves.[111,236,294,430,452]

The explosive nature of the syndrome can lead to gram-negative sepsis and death, reportedly in up to 50% of cases.[126,306] The mortality rate may be as high as 90% in patients who become hypotensive within 12 hours of initial examination by a physician. Appropriate antibiotics should be administered as soon as the infection is suspected and include imipenem-cilastatin, trimethoprim-sulfamethoxazole, tetracycline, carbenicillin, chloramphenicol, tobramycin, gentamicin, and many third-generation cephalosporins. In an immunocompetent victim who acquired a *V. vulnificus* hand infection from peeling shrimps, treatment with oral ciprofloxacin was successful.[292]

The organisms can be cultured from the blood, wounds (bullae), and stool. The laboratory must be cautioned to use selective culture media with a high salt content (3% NaCl) for prompt identification. Suggestive features include positive fermentation of glucose, positive oxidase test, positive indole test, positive reaction for both lysine and ornithine decarboxylase, positive *o*-nitrophenyl-β-D-galactopyranoside, and inability to ferment sucrose.[223]

VIBRIO MIMICUS

Vibrio mimicus is a motile, nonhalophilic, gram-negative, oxidase-positive rod with a single flagellum. It can be distinguished from *V. cholerae* by its inability to ferment sucrose, inability to metabolize acetylmethyl carbonyl, sensitivity to polymyxin, and negative lipase test.[104] It has been identified as the causative agent in a syndrome of gastroenteritis (diarrhea, nausea, vomiting, abdominal cramps, fever, and headache) that follows the ingestion of raw oysters, crawfish, and perhaps crab or shrimp. The median incubation period is 24 hours, with delayed diarrhea noted up to 3 days after ingestion of contaminated seafood. In one series, heat-labile toxins were identified in 2 of 19 victims; heat-stabile toxin was absent.[377] An ear infection may follow exposure to ocean water.[377] Isolates are sensitive to tetracycline. Physicians who collect stool samples for culture to identify suspected *V. mimicus* must alert the laboratory to use appropriate culture media (TCBS agar).

VIBRIO ALGINOLYTICUS

Vibrio alginolyticus, found in seawater, has been implicated in soft tissue infections (such as those caused by coral cuts or surfing scrapes), sinusitis, and otitis, particularly after previous ear infections or a tympanic membrane perforation.[49,338,439] Although bacteremia has been reported in immunosuppressed patients and patients with burns, *V. alginolyticus* does not generally carry the virulent potential of *V. vulnificus*. Typical symptoms include cellulitis, with seropurulent exudate.

OTHER VIBRIOS

The dreaded diarrheal disease is cholera caused by infection with *Vibrio cholerae*. The recent scourge of South America, the disorder is commonly linked to ingestion of raw or inadequately cooked mollusks and crustaceans. The enteritis is secretory, with profound watery diarrhea, nausea, and vomiting. Since the stool is virtually isotonic, large amounts of fluid and electrolytes are lost at a rate that drives the victim into hypovolemic shock, acidosis, and renal failure. The treatment consists of aggressive fluid replacement, intravenous if available, combined with oral rehydration. Oral tetracycline may be beneficial if administered in the first 48 hours, but the key to survival is the administration of fluid. Recent preliminary studies suggest that normal saline is as effective as lactated Ringer's solution. Untreated, the disease remits in 3 to 8 days.

Non-01 *Vibrio cholerae* strains (biochemically identical to *V. cholerae*, but not agglutinating in vibrio 0 group 1 antiserum) cause gastroenteritis associated with the ingestion of mollusks (usually oysters and clams). Self-limited (24 to 48 hours) nausea, vomiting, abdominal cramping, and invasive diarrhea with blood and fecal leukocytes are typical.[49,193] The organisms have been isolated from the gastrointestinal tract in patients with ascending cholangitis, acute cholecystitis, acute appendicitis, cellulitis, otitis media, aspiration pneumonia, gram-negative sepsis, and meningitis.[193] Systemic infection appears to be associated with immunosuppression. *Vibrio metschnikovii* has caused bacteremia in a patient with cholecystitis; the authors postulated that it may have been associated with long-term carriage after seafood ingestion.[204] *Vibrio cincinnatiensis* has caused meningitis; a relationship to foreign travel, seawater exposure, or seafood ingestion has not been established.[55] *Vibrio fluvialis*, previously designated as enteric group EF-6 or group F, is common in the marine environment.[307,375] It causes diarrheal disease associated with vomiting, abdominal pain, dehydration, and fever.[194,408] It can be mistaken easily in the microbiology laboratory for *Aeromonas hydrophila*, from which it can be distinguished by growth in 6% to 7% sodium chloride.[251,307,375] *Vibrio hollisae* and *V. furnissii* have both been linked to gastroenteritis, putatively after seafood ingestion.[61,309] *V. hollisae* septicemia after consumption of catfish (captured in the Mississippi River) occurred in an elderly alcoholic man.[258] *Vibrio damsela*, formerly enteric group EF-5 and so named because it is pathogenic for the damselfish, causes wound infections similar to those attributed to other vibrios.[277] Rapidly progressive infection leading to muscle necrosis or to sepsis and death may transpire in an immunosuppressed victim.[92,93,242] This may be related to an extracellular cytolysin or other unidentified enzymes.[241] It has been proposed that *V. damsela* be placed into the new genus, *Listonella*.[279]

PREVENTION

Persons who are immunosuppressed or chronically ill, particularly with hepatic insufficiency, should not eat raw or partially cooked shellfish. All seafood should be cooked thoroughly, protected from cross-contamination after cooking, and eaten promptly or stored at temperatures above 60° C or below 4° C to prevent multiplication of *Vibrio* species.[48] Appropriate antibiotics for prophylaxis against wound infections are discussed in the previous section dealing with bacteriology.

The Food and Drug Administration (FDA) has prepared a series of four booklets for subpopulations of persons with altered immunity who may be susceptible to *Vibrio* infections. One set of booklets on seafood safety for high-risk individuals is available to health professionals free of charge from: FDA, Seafood Brochures, HFI-40, 5600 Fishers Lane, Rockville, MD 20857. They can be photocopied.[136]

Fish Tapeworm

In the United States the consumption of raw fish (sushi) is increasingly popular, which has led to more frequent recognition of infestation with the fish tapeworm, *Diphyllobothrium latum*. Salmon appears to be a popular culprit.[363] The fish tapeworm has a complex life cycle, in which a gravid egg released into fresh water releases a ciliated coracidium, which is eaten by a crustacean intermediate host. The coracidium penetrates the intestinal wall of the crustacean and then develops into a procercoid larva. The small crustacean is eaten by a fish, and the procercoid larva migrates through the intestinal wall of the fish into fish muscle, where it changes into a plerocercoid larva. It is this final larval stage that is ingested by a human and that subsequently attaches to the intestine, where it grows into a mature tapeworm.

Classic symptoms include subacute abdominal pain, nausea, vomiting, diarrhea, and weight loss. Proglottids may be passed in the stool. Chronic *D. latum* infestation may induce megaloblastic anemia, as the tapeworm splits the vitamin B_{12}–intrinsic factor complex and prevents absorption of the vitamin.[156] The diagnosis can be made by examination of the stool for typical proglottids or operculate egg forms, which measure 60 to 75 μm in length. Proper identification of the eggs is important in the differentiation from the ova of trematodes endemic in southeast Asia, such as *Paragonimus westermani*, which may be carried by refugees to the United States.[113] For documented *D. latum* infestation, treatment for adults is niclosamide (*N*-[2′-chloro-4′-nitrophenyl]-5-

chloro-salicylamide) 2 g in one dose (pediatric dose 1 g for children 11 to 34 kg and 1.5 g for children 35 to 70 kg), which is provided by the Centers for Disease Control, Parasitic Disease Drug Service, Atlanta, Georgia, or as Niclocide, from Miles Pharmaceuticals, West Haven, Connecticut. The drug uncouples oxidative phosphorylation in the scolex and proximal segments of the adult tapeworm and stimulates ATPase activity of mitochondria, which results in destruction of the scolex, followed by destruction of the remainder of the worm.[333] An alternative therapy is praziquantel 5 to 10 mg/kg in one dose for adults or children. Because a worm may not be identifiable if expulsion is delayed or follows a purge, stool analysis should be repeated at 3 months to confirm successful therapy.

Fish tapeworm infection can be avoided by cooking fish until the parts for consumption reach a temperature of at least 56° C (133° F) for 5 minutes or freezing the fish to −18° C (0° F) for 24 hours or −10° C (14° F) for 72 hours.[451]

Trematodes

Humans can acquire an intestinal infection from the trematode *Nanophyetus salmincola salmincola,* which infests salmonid fishes such as steelhead trout or salmon.[118] Canine infection with this fluke is a well-known phenomenon in the Pacific northwest of the United States.

Humans ingest the flesh of fish infested with the metacercariae, which excyst in the host and attach to the upper small bowel. The worms release eggs that are detected in the stool approximately 1 week after ingestion of infected fish.

Symptoms of nanophyetiasis include diarrhea, peripheral blood eosinophilia, abdominal discomfort, bloating, nausea and vomiting, weight loss, and fatigue. Although symptoms may resolve spontaneously over a period of months, antihelminthic treatment is recommended. Effective regimens have included bithitonol 50 mg/kg orally for two doses, niclosamide 2 g orally for three doses, or mebendazole 100 mg orally bid for 3 days. A similar syndrome has been caused by intestinal infection with *Heterophyes heterophyes,* which was successfully treated with praziquantel 25 mg/kg orally three times a day for 1 day.[5]

Numerous other trematode infections are the cause of enormous morbidity worldwide as the liver and intestinal flukes cause distinct medical syndromes. For instance, in Southeast Asia, opisthorchosis caused by the liver fluke *Opisthorchis viverrini* is quite serious. The cercariae are ubiquitous in cyprinid fish.[151] Clonorchiasis occurs when humans eat raw or undercooked freshwater fish harboring the metacercariae of *Clonorchis sinensis.*[372]

Anisakiasis

Approximately 5000 restaurants serve sushi in the United States. Many of these do so without specific knowledge of the various parasites that can infest their fare. For instance, many serve raw salmon, squid, shrimp, and mackerel.

The first report of acute gastric anisakiasis caused by penetration of the *Anisakis* larvae through the gastric mucosa was by Van Thiel[435] in 1960. It is a rare problem in the United States but increasingly noted in Japan, where raw fish is more commonly eaten.[226,402,432] In a Japanese series the fish consumed included predominantly mackerel; less common perpetrators included horse mackerel, bream, squid, sardines, and bonito.[402] In the United States, anisakine nematodes are present in many commercial fish intended for raw or semiraw consumption, such as Pacific herring (thus "herring worm disease"), sablefish, Pacific cod (thus "codworm disease"), arrowtooth flounder, petrale sole, coho salmon, Pacific ocean perch, silvergray rockfish, yellowtail rockfish, and bocaccio.[320] In rare cases the anisakine worm can be present in tuna or yellowtail. The preservation of marine mammals along the West Coast of the United States has been linked to greater worm burdens in fishes associated with these mammals, such as Pacific rockfish, red snapper, and salmon.[290]

LIFE AND HABITS

Anisakine nematodes, members of the order Ascarida (suborder Ascaridae), are found in great numbers in the viscera and muscles of fish.[320] There are 30 genera in the family Anisakidae, including *Anisakis* and *Pseudoterranova* (or *Phocanema*). Adult worms infest the stomachs of marine mammals (thus "sealworm disease"), burrowing in clusters into the mucosal surface.[137] Eggs passed in the stool embryonate and hatch in seawater to produce second-stage larvae, which are ingested by crustaceans, which are in turn eaten by squid or fish. In these hosts the larvae migrate through the gut wall and encyst in the viscera or musculature.[366] The fish may then pass the parasite to other fish, to humans, or back to another marine mammal. The coiled *Anisakis* larva grows to approximately 2.5 to 3 cm in length and 0.5 to 1 mm in diameter. Thus fish are usually the intermediate (transport) host for larval anisakines. The definitive host for *Phocanema decipiens* is the seal; the *Anisakis* larvae grow to maturity in the whale. Shellfish are not infested. The presence of these roundworms is unappealing from a marketing perspective, and thus they were first examined for commercial reasons in the early 1950s.[319] Only four genera of anisakine nematodes have been implicated in human anisakiasis: *Anisakis, Phocanema, Porrocaecum,* and *Contracaecum.*[200] In the United States, all cases are related to the larval stages of *Anisakis simplex* and *Phocanema decipiens.*[290]

CLINICAL ASPECTS

Symptoms from ingestion of *Anisakis* may begin within 1 hour of ingestion of raw fish and include severe epigastric pain, nausea, and vomiting. The presentation may mimic an acute abdomen. The roentgenographic findings of an upper gastrointestinal series are remarkable. Threadlike gastric filling defects approximately 30 mm in length are typical, with a circular or ringlike shape.[402] Mucosal edema may obscure the diagnosis. Acute gastritis may be clinically classified in accordance with data from upper gastrointestinal series and gastroscopy as edematous, hemorrhagic, or ulcerative.[401] The presence of edema, particularly of the antral folds with irregular marginal indentations, introduces the differential diagnosis of gastric carcinoma. On endoscopy, worms may be found anywhere on the mucosal surface of the stomach. If they are not removed, they die within a few days of implantation into the gastric mucosa. However, microscopic lesions can rapidly progress from diffuse interstitial edema to an eosinophilic abscess or epithelioid granuloma.[137] If the anisakine worms (such as *Phocanema*) do not implant and the infection is luminal without tissue penetration, the worms may be coughed up, vomited, or defecated, generally within 48 hours of the meal.[88,99,213] If the worm is felt in the oropharynx or proximal esophagus, the "tingling throat syndrome" is described.[290]

Intestinal anisakiasis is more often delayed in onset (up to 7 days after ingestion) and marked by abdominal pain, nausea, vomiting, diarrhea, fever, eosinophilia (particularly with gastric anisakiasis), and occult blood in the stool.[99] This may be easily confused with appendicitis, regional enteritis, gastric ulcer, colonic or other gastrointestinal carcinoma, or most commonly, other causes of small bowel inflammation with partial obstruction.[381] Although the worms are usually found in the submucosa, they may penetrate the wall of the intestine.[339] Fourth-stage larvae of *Anisakis simplex* and *Pseudoterranova (Phocanema) decipiens* are found in the intestine and stomach of humans.[227] During surgery the operator may note transudative ascites and that the affected area of the bowel is edematous and covered with a fibrinous exudate. The larva is visible in the mucosa or buried within the submucosa, surrounded by an intense inflammatory granulomatous response.

Scattered anecdotal reports from the Indo-Pacific suggest that parasitic nematodes can invade an open wound. This would be most likely to occur during fish handling, cleaning, or filleting.

DIAGNOSIS AND TREATMENT

The definitive diagnosis of anisakiasis is usually made on the basis of morphologic characteristics of the whole worm when the creature is expectorated by the patient or removed from the stomach after endoscopic examination.[366] If the worms have migrated to extragastric sites, the diagnosis can be difficult. Antibodies to the ileal worm have been detected by RAST, ELISA, and immunofluorescent antibody assay, but these laboratory methods are not widely available.

The larvae of *Anisakis* can be visualized on endoscopy and removed with biopsy forceps. Chemotherapeutic antihelminthic agents and purgatives are not yet proven efficacious in humans, and endoscopic removal is necessary to relieve the pain. Therefore early fiberoptic gastroscopy is recommended for patients in whom acute gastric anisakiasis is suspected and for those who have eaten raw fish within 6 to 12 hours before the onset of gastric symptoms. After removal a comprehensive antacid regimen allows healing of the gastric mucosa.[402] Ulcer formation is rare, but when it occurs, the area of chronic inflammation should be cautiously debrided to eliminate the nidus of organic worm debris that perpetuates the inflammatory response. When laparotomy is performed for presumed appendicitis, the diagnosis is based on identification of the worm in an inflamed segment of appendix, cecum, small intestine, mesentery, or omentum.[290] The only effective therapy for inflamed bowel is resection.

PREVENTION

The larvae are extremely difficult to spot in fish flesh, since they are colorless and normally tightly coiled in a spiral of approximately 3 mm. Only cooked (above 60° C) or previously frozen (to −20° C for 24 hours) fish should be eaten. Smoking (kippering), marinating, pickling, brining, and salting may not kill the worms.[99] Candling is an inadequate method of surveillance, particularly in dark-fleshed fish infested with *Anisakis* larvae.[137] Fish should be gutted as soon as possible after they are caught to limit the migration of worms from the viscera into the muscle.

The irradiation of fish to limit their infectivity is controversial because of potential generation of long-lived free radicals within the fish, as well as germination of spores of *Clostridium botulinum*.[450] To date, this practice is not legal for seafood.

Eustrongylides

Eustrongylides is a genus of roundworms that can invade fish in its larval form and thus be consumed by humans in their quest for sushi and sashimi. *Eustrongylides* may also parasitize bait minnows, which are swallowed whole by fishermen. The worms are released into the human gastrointestinal tract, where they attain lengths of 15 to 30 cm and penetrate the intestinal wall to enter the peritoneal cavity. Symptoms include unexplained abdominal pain, peritonitis, and fever in a live-bait fisherman. Surgical intervention may be required in pursuit of the acute abdomen, at which time the characteristically bright red worm is identified.[451]

Primary Amebic Meningoencephalitis

Amebae of the genera *Naegleria* and *Acanthamoeba* are free-living freshwater organisms found in lakes, ponds, hot springs, swimming pools, and warm coastal waters of the United States.[228,289,373,446] *Acanthamoeba,* but not *Naegleria,* may grow in ocean water. Both genera cause primary amebic meningoencephalitis (PAM), with a predilection for infectious involvement of the frontal areas of the brain and olfactory bulb neuroepithelium.[374] *Naegleria fowleri* is an ameboflagellate more commonly involved with rapidly fatal disease. Victims likely to acquire the organism include those with upper respiratory tract infections or with immunosuppression. However, the majority of reported *Naegleria* infections have been in previously healthy individuals.[100,287] The organisms are reputed to enter the central nervous system through the nasal mucosa, along the olfactory nerve fila, and through the cribriform plate.[67,97,228] The organisms are soon found in the subarachnoid and perivascular spaces.

The interval from swimming to the onset of PAM can range from a few days to over 2 weeks.[80] Symptoms include those of upper respiratory tract infection or allergy, along with nausea, vomiting, headache, and altered taste or smell. Rapid neurologic deterioration caused by *Naegleria,* accompanied by signs of fulminant meningitis, follows within 2 to 3 days. PAM should be suspected in any previously healthy individual who has been exposed to fresh warm water within 7 days of onset of illness and who has clinical findings of bacterial meningitis with basilar distribution of exudate by brain computed tomography.[80]

Acanthamoeba meningoencephalitis may be more indolent, similar to tuberculous meningitis. This disorder has been attributed to several species, including *A. culbertsoni, A. castellani, A. polyphaga,* and *A. astronyxis. Naegleria* infections generally afflict previously healthy individuals; *Acanthamoeba* causes opportunistic infections in victims who are immunocompromised, debilitated, diabetic, or alcoholic.[77,96,228,373] *Acanthamoeba* keratitis has been described, attributed largely to *A. polyphaga.*[77,211,284]

The diagnosis of amebic meningoencephalitis is made by cerebrospinal fluid (CSF) culture and observation of motile trophozoites *(Naegleria,* not *Acanthomoeba)* in fresh CSF. In addition, the CSF has an elevated cell count (predominantly polymorphonuclear leukocytes), elevated protein level, and low glucose level, similar to more common bacterial meningitis.[140] The 10 to 20 μm *Naegleria* trophozoite can be recognized by a flagellum and single nucleus with a central large karyosome surrounded by a clear halo.[68] The CSF should be maintained at a temperature of 30° to 37° C to avoid reducing trophozoite motility.[228] Amebae can be cultured onto *Escherichia coli* or *Enterobacter aerogenes* inoculated onto nonnutrient agar.[97] Dilution of 1 drop of CSF with 1 ml of distilled water allows transformation of the organism within 1 to 20 hours from the ameboid to the biflagellate form.[80] For permanently stained preparations, Masson's trichrome stain is recommended.

Therapy must be aggressive and requires the administration of amphotericin B in combination with miconazole or tetracycline, the first two agents intravenously and intrathecally or intraventricularly.[374] Clotrimazole and rifampin also demonstrate in vitro activity against *Naegleria.*[75,201,423] Delay or lack of treatment culminates in almost certain death. Regardless of the institution of prompt treatment, prognosis is poor. *Acanthamoeba* keratitis usually requires surgical removal of the affected tissue, since medical cure has not yet been published. Promising therapies include corneal grafts in combination with topical clotrimazole, penetrating keratoplasty with cryotherapy, topical propamidine isethionate, topical neomycin, and oral ketoconazole.[77,183,284]

Poisoning by Environmental Contamination

In the process of concentrating fish proteins as a food source, a variety of protein-bound, non-water-soluble, or non-alcohol-soluble toxic compounds may be preserved. These include organic mercurials, hydrocarbons, dioxins, polychlorinated dibenzofurans, chlorinated pesticides, and heavy metals (such as antimony, arsenic, cadmium, chromium, cobalt, lead, phosphorus, mercury, nickel, and zinc).[182,404,444] In California waters, toxic piscine levels of polychlorinated biphenyls and insecticides are encountered in the south and selenium and methyl mercury in the north. Dioxin has been found on Dungeness crabs in Humboldt Bay. It is interesting to note that polychlorinated compounds are excreted in breast milk.

Spills of toxic chemicals and petroleum by-products will certainly continue to expand the list of carcinogens to which humans are becoming exposed through the marine environment. Although radiation exposure is not known to induce production of new marine poisons, the ingestion of radioactive fish poses a potential radiation hazard.[273] Divers are exposed to a variety of environmental contaminants while exploring polluted waters. These hazards include solvents, nuclear wastes, herbicides, chemical effluents, and sewage.

Domoic Acid Intoxication

In late 1987 in eastern Canada an outbreak of gastrointestinal and neurologic symptoms occurred after consumption of mussels found to be contaminated with domoic acid, which is structurally related to the excitatory neurotransmitter glutamate.[335]

The source of the outbreak was traced to three river estuaries in Prince Edward Island, where there was an extensive bloom of the phytoplanktonic diatom *Nitzshia pungens.* The mussels concentrate the toxin in the hepatopancreas.[161] Before the 1987 outbreak, domoic acid had been found in two species of red algae. Domoic acid has also been detected in Gulf shellfish (Gulf coast oyster, *Crassostrea virginica*) and phytoplankton in the Gulf of Mexico, although no outbreaks of amnesic shellfish poisoning have been recorded in this region. The toxic *N. pungens* forma *multiseries* has also been confirmed in Korea, Japan, Oslofjord of Scandinavia, the northeastern and northwestern United States, eastern and western Canada, and eastern South America.[109] Domoic acid is a secondary metabolite of the diatom.

A rapid onset of abnormalities of arousal, confusion, disorientation, and memory loss took place within 24 hours of eating blue mussels *(Mytilus edulis)*.[416] Range of onset of symptoms was from 15 minutes to 38 hours (median 5.5 hours) after ingestion. Other prominent symptoms included headache (severe and debilitating), nausea, vomiting, diarrhea, abdominal cramps, hiccoughs, arrhythmias, hypotension, seizures, ophthalmoplegia, hemiparesis, mutism, grimacing, agitation, emotional lability, coma, copious bronchial secretions, and pulmonary edema.[345] A severe reaction was associated with male sex, chronic disease (particularly chronic renal failure), older age, and quantity of domoic acid ingested. There were a few fatalities. Histologic study of brain tissue taken from the deceased at autopsy showed neuronal necrosis or cell loss and astrocytosis, most prominently in the hippocampus and the amygdaloid nucleus.[416] This is similar to damage seen in animals poisoned with kainic acid. Several months after the primary intoxication, victims still demonstrated chronic residual memory deficits and motor neuronopathy or axonopathy. Nonneurologic illness did not persist.

The mussels were analyzed and showed levels of domoic acid of 31 to 128 mg/100 g of mussel tissue. Domoic acid could not be identified in the blood, serum, or cerebrospinal fluid specimens from any patient, even though it is estimated that 200 to 300 mg was consumed per victim. Domoic acid is a heat-stable neuroexcitatory amino acid with biochemical analogs kainic acid and glutamic acid. Domoic acid binds to the kainate type of glutamate receptor with three times the affinity of kainic acid and is 20 times as powerful. In the presence of glutamate, domoic acid can cause massive cell depolarization with an intracellular rise in calcium ion and cell dysfunction or death.[343] In animal models, domoic acid is more potent than its analogs and produces limbic seizures and memory and gait abnormalities in rats. Seaweeds containing kainic acid and domoic acid have been used in Japanese folk medicine (seaweed *Chondria armata*) to expel intestinal parasites.[343,161]

Therapy for all acute and chronic syndromes to date is supportive and based on symptoms. Since kainic acid neuropathology seems to be nearly entirely seizure mediated, an emphasis should be placed on finding an efficacious anticonvulsant.[343] Diazepam appears to be as effective as any other. Some authorities believe that an electroencephalogram (EEG) to detect seizure activity should be obtained even for a person in a severely depressed mental state. If epileptoid activity is present, an anticonvulsant should be administered until the EEG normalizes.

Mussels can be tested for the presence of domoic acid by mouse bioassay (involuntary scratching of the shoulders with the hind legs, uncoordinated movements, followed by death) and HPLC. The LD_{50} (with intraperitoneal administration) of domoic acid in mice is 3.6 mg/kg.[161]

Red Seaweed (Gracilaria Tsudae)

An outbreak of poisoning affecting 13 individuals related to ingestion of the red algae *Polycavernosa tsudae* (formerly *Gracilaria tsudae* or *edulisi*) in Guam was observed in 1991.[174] Symptoms consisted of diarrhea, abdominal cramping, vomiting, generalized numbness, perioral and extremity paresthesias, numbness of the fingertips, diaphoresis, jaw aching, muscle spasm, and tremors. The onset of symptoms was from less than 2 to several hours after ingestion. Three deaths occurred in individuals who had ingested large quantities of the seaweed.

Preliminary bioassay tests of aqueous extracts of the toxic algae using the standard paralytic shellfish poisoning mouse bioassay test confirmed an unidentified toxic substance, but HPLC confirmation failed to identify any of the ciguatoxin or saxitoxin complexes, so the specific agent or agents) involved remain undetermined. It does not appear to be palytoxin.[45] It is not known if what occurred in Guam is similar to Japanese "ogonuri poisoning," which can be fatal and follow ingestion of the red seaweeds *G. verrucosa* (ogonuri) or *G. chordai* (tsurushiramo).

Botulism

Botulism is a paralytic disease caused by the potent natural toxin elaborated by *Clostridium botulinum.* Seven toxins (A to G) have been identified, but only A, B, E, F, and G cause human illness.[390] Food-borne botulism can be caused by raw, parboiled, salt-cured, or fermented meats from marine mammals (seal, walrus, whale) or fish products (particularly salmon and salmon roe).[178] In the last four decades in the United States, over 10% of outbreaks of food-borne botulism have been related to the consumption of fish. Although the predominant type of botulism is generally considered to be E, types A and B may also be involved. Improperly preserved (smoked, dried, or canned) foods are at high risk for *Clostridium botulinum* toxin proliferation. The technique of "hanging" meat for decomposition (flavor and texture improvement) supports growth of the nonproteolytic, psychrotolerant forms of *C. botulinum,* which may grow at temperatures as low as 4° C.[178] Type E spores are abundant in northern coastal areas and around inland lakes.

Clostridium botulinum spores are encouraged to germinate in an environment of appropriate pH (greater than 4.6), warm temperature (higher than 10° C), sufficient moisture, and an anaerobic environment. The spores are resistant to brief boiling and readily survive haphazard home food preservation techniques. In the food poisoning variety (as distinct from wound or infant botulism), the preformed toxin is ingested.[38a] The toxins are proteins of approximate molecular weight 150,000 daltons, absorbed in the proximal gastrointestinal tract. The lethal dose in the bloodstream is 10^{-9} mg/kg body weight.

CLINICAL ASPECTS

The toxin affects the presynaptic cholinergic neuromuscular junction, where it blocks the release of acetylcholine and causes flaccid paralysis.[38] Signs and symptoms develop within 6 to 72 hours of ingestion and include nausea, vomiting, abdominal pain, and diarrhea, followed by dry mouth, dysphonia (hoarseness), difficulty swallowing, facial weakness, ptosis, nonreactive or sluggishly reactive pupils (third cranial nerve), mydriasis, blurred or double vision (sixth cranial nerve), descending symmetric muscular weakness leading to paralysis, and bulbar and respiratory paralysis. With adequate ventilatory support, mentation frequently remains normal. Death occurs in 10% to 50% of cases, depending on the availability of antitoxin.

If botulism is suspected, a careful food history should be obtained and the suspected food items collected. Stool and serum samples should be procured and refrigerated, since laboratory confirmation of botulism is achieved when botulinal toxin or viable *C. botulinum* is detected in the food, toxin is demonstrated in the patient's serum or stool, or the organism is cultured from the stool. Toxin is detected by intraperitoneal injection of specimens into mice, where lethality is neutralized by the addition of antiserum to the inoculum. Toxin types are distinguished using type-specific antitoxin.[38] To determine the clinical need for botulism antitoxin, a number of tests may be helpful. Electromyography should be performed using repetitive stimulation at 40 Hz or greater; a positive test shows diminished amplitude of the muscle action potential with a single supramaximal stimulus, and facilitation of action potentials using paired or repetitive stimuli.[38] CSF may be examined for white blood cells and protein (to rule out infectious etiologies), and an edrophonium (Tensilon) challenge test may be performed to rule out myasthenia gravis. Vital capacity should be monitored as a sensitive indicator of clinical deterioration.

TREATMENT

Ventilatory support should be provided at the first sign of respiratory inadequacy. Gastric emptying, repeated doses of activated charcoal with cathartics, or both may help to eliminate and adsorb residual toxin in the gastrointestinal tract. Equine trivalent antitoxin A,B,E should be administered as soon as possible to any person with symptoms, before irreversible neural dysfunction.[305,409] Each 8 ml vial of trivalent antitoxin contains 7500 IU type A, 5500 IU type B, and 8500 IU type E antitoxin.[38] Bivalent (A,B) or monovalent (E) antitoxin may be inadequate. A physician who seeks antitoxin should first contact the state health department. If this is unsatisfactory, the Centers for Disease Control and Prevention may be telephoned at 404-329-2888 (24 hours). The trivalent antitoxin is administered as an initial dose of 16 ml (two vials) every 2 to 4 hours for 3 to 5 doses or longer if symptoms persist.[38] Before administration the victim should be skin tested for hypersensitivity to horse serum. If horse serum test material is not available, 0.1 ml of a 1:10 dilution of antitoxin in saline may be used. The antitoxin should not be stored at a temperature greater than 37° C.

An adjunct to therapy may be administration of guanidine, which increases the release of acetylcholine from nerve endings. The dosage is 15 to 50 mg/kg/day orally in four divided doses.

PREVENTION

Prophylaxis with antitoxin is not currently recommended, nor is general pentavalent (A to E) toxoid immunization.[15,176] The best prevention is public health education with respect to food preparation and avoidance of improperly stored food products. Since the spores are frequently detected in fish intestines, it is important to clean fish properly and to avoid consumption of the viscera, even in salt-cured products. To eliminate spores in food, heat or irradiation may be used. Types A and B may survive boiling for several hours (particularly at the lower temperatures associated with higher altitude) and generally require pressure heating at 120° C for 30 minutes; type E spores are killed at 80° C after 30 minutes. Preformed toxin is inactivated after heating for 20 minutes at 80° C or 10 minutes at 90° C. Germination is inhibited by acidification, refrigeration, freezing, drying, or the addition of salt, sugar, or sodium nitrate; however, heating remains the most reliable technique.[38]

Poisoning by Sea Hare Ingestion

Sea hares are marine gastropod mollusks prevalent in certain South Pacific waters, including Fiji. *Aplysia* species have been considered to be toxic since Roman times. *A. juliana* secretes an antibacterial and antineoplastic protein found in the water-soluble fraction of a fetid secretion lethal to crabs.[216] Human poisoning has been reported after ingestion of *Dolabella auricularia* ("veata").[391] The symptoms began approximately 30 minutes after eating and included prickling skin sensation, vomiting, diarrhea, shaking, tremors, fasciculations, arthralgias, dyspnea, visual disorientation, altered sensorium, and fever. The course of illness exceeded a week.

Since sea hares are known to concentrate bromine and because chronic bromine intoxication has clinical features similar to those described previously, it has been suggested that sea hare poisoning in humans might be a form of subacute organobromine intoxication, in which case sodium or ammonium chloride therapy might prove useful.[391]

Chelonintoxication

A variety of tropical Pacific, particularly Japanese, marine turtles are toxic when ingested (see Box 53-5).[393] All portions of the turtle are toxic; the freshness of the meat is irrelevant. Symptoms develop from 1 to 48 hours after ingestion and include ulcerative glossitis and stomatitis, pharyngitis, diaphoresis, hypersalivation, nausea, vomiting, diarrhea, abdominal pain, vertigo, icterus, desquamative dermatitis, hepatosplenomegaly, centrilobular hepatic necrosis with fatty degeneration, renal failure, somnolence, and hypotension. The mortality rate is 28% to 44%. Therapy is supportive and based on symptoms. Prevention includes feeding potential turtle dinners to sacrificial small animals, which are observed for 24 to 48 hours. Survivalists in the Philippines, India, New Guinea, Tahiti, and Japan should be aware of the hazard.

A variety of *Salmonella* serotypes have been isolated from pet turtles *(Pseudemys* [or *Chrysemys*] *scripta elegans)* imported into and from the United States.[85,412] The public health implications remain to be determined.

Polar Bear Liver Poisoning

The ingestion of polar bear *(Thalarctos maritimus)* liver causes a syndrome related to hypervitaminosis A. This also occurs with the ingestion of the livers of certain seals, sea lions, whales, dolphins, walruses, husky dogs, and Pacific sharks. The vitamin A content of shark liver can attain 100,000 IU per gram. A typical ingestion involves the administration of more than 1 million (and occasionally up to 3 to 8 million) IU of vitamin A (the recommended daily allowance is 4000 to 5000 IU) and results in the following symptoms: formication, headache, apathy, drowsiness, giddiness, irritability, photophobia, nausea, vomiting, diarrhea, polyarthralgia, seizures, desquamative dermatitis, ophthalmoplegia, and raised CSF pressure with a pseudotumor cerebri–type presentation (acute or chronic, the latter with headache, lip fissuring, papilledema, decreased visual acuity, and tinnitus).[132,300] Elevated levels of serum glutamic oxaloacetic transaminase and serum vitamin A (markedly in excess of 70 µg%) may be measured. A normal serum β-carotene level excludes the possibility of a plant source (for example carrots or mangoes) for the vitamin.[300] The syndrome is rarely fatal and resolves in 2 to 8 weeks.

BOX 53-5

REPRESENTATIVE MARINE TURTLES HAZARDOUS TO HUMANS

Phylum Chordata
- Class Reptilia
  - Order Chelonia: turtles
    - Family Cheloniidae
      - *Caretta caretta gigas:* Pacific loggerhead turtle
      - *Chelonia mydas:* green turtle
      - *Eretmochelys imbricata:* hawksbill turtle
    - Family Dermochelidae
      - *Dermochelys coriacea:* leathery turtle
    - Family Thioncychidae
      - *Pelochelys bibroni:* soft shell turtle

Blue-Green Algae

Blue-green algae are worldwide freshwater cyanobacteria that may proliferate rapidly in a bloom, discoloring the surface of the water and spoiling its odor and taste.[360] They generate significant toxins that are ingested by animals, resulting in severe illness and death. Typical algal species include *Microcystis aeruginosa, Anabaena flos-aquae, Nodularia spumigena, Nostoc, Oscillatoria agardhii,* and *Aphanizomenon flos-aquae*.[324,359]

During conditions of a bloom (warm stagnant water, frequently enhanced by phosphorus and nitrogen fertilizers), the toxins are concentrated to a degree to become a significant hazard to wild and domestic animals, such as the dogs that drank from Loch Insh, Scotland.[119,129] In most species of toxic cyanobacteria the toxins are cyclic heptapeptides called microcystins or cyanoginosins.[399] More than 40 microcystins have been isolated from blue-green algae.[386] The toxins are of multiple configurations and include alkaloids, polypeptides, and lipopolysaccharides (endotoxins).[395] The rapid-acting "death factors" resemble saxitoxin and tetrodotoxin. Animals may collapse quickly and appear to suffer neuromuscular paralysis, with features of staggering, muscle fasciculations, gasping, and convulsions.[175] A different dominant symptom complex includes gastrointestinal hemorrhage and hepatic failure. The latter can be rapid or delayed. In mice, administration of microcystin-LR causes rapid hepatocellular necrosis with hemorrhagic shock.[98,422] Anatoxin-a and anatoxin-a(s) are both derived from *Anabaena flos-aquae*. The first is a potent nicotinic agonist that acts as a postsynaptic, depolarizing neuromuscular blocking agent; the second is an anticholinesterase that causes demonstrable cholinergic toxicity in animals.[175,280]

Human exposure to blue-green algal blooms has thus far resulted only in allergic reactions, mild liver enzyme elevation, and gastroenteritis.[395] A person who swims through a bloom may suffer local effects, such as conjunctivitis, facial swelling, or papulovesicular dermatitis. Ingestion of contaminated water causes a dysenteric diarrhea, with green slimy stools. This may or may not be associated with elevation of γ-glutamyl-transpeptidase and alanine aminotransferase.

Treatment is supportive in humans and animals. Recently, cyclosporine A has been shown to inhibit the fatal effects of microcystins administered to mice. In humans, no special treatment is recommended other than fluid and electrolyte supplementation as needed, since all related afflictions appear to be self-limited.

REFERENCES

1. Aas K: Studies of hypersensitivity to fish: a clinical study, *Int Arch Appl Immunol* 29:23, 1966.
2. Aas K: Studies of hypersensitivity to fish; allergological and serological differentiation between various species of fish, *Arch Allergy* 30:257, 1966.
3. Acott C: Stonefish envenomation, *S Pacific Undersea Med Soc J* 15:5, 1985.
4. Acres J, Gray J: Paralytic shellfish poisoning, *Can Med Assoc J* 119:1195, 1978.
5. Adams KO et al: Intestinal fluke infection as a result of eating sushi, *Am J Clin Pathol* 86:688, 1986.
6. Adams MJ: An outbreak of ciguatera poisoning in a group of scuba divers, *J Wilderness Med* 4:304, 1993.
7. Agnew WS et al: Purification of the tetrodotoxin-binding component associated with the voltage-sensitive sodium channel from *Electrophorus electricus* electroplax membranes, *Proc Natl Acad Sci USA* 75:2606, 1978.
8. Alcala AC et al: Human fatality due to ingestion of the crab *Demania reynaudii* that contained a palytoxin-like toxin, *Toxicon* 26(1):105, 1988.
9. Alexander JW: Nutrition and infection: new perspectives for an old problem, *Arch Surg* 121:966, 1986.
10. Alexander JW et al: The importance of lipid type in the diet after burn injury, *Ann Surg* 204:1, 1986.
11. Ali MB, Raff MJ: Primary *Vibrio vulnificus* sepsis in Kentucky, *South Med J* 83(3):356, 1990.
12. Ali AE et al: Tetrodotoxin and related substances in a ribbon worm *Cephalothrix linearis* (nemertean), *Toxicon* 28(9):1083, 1990.
13. Anderson BS et al: The epidemiology of ciguatera fish poisoning in Hawaii, 1975-1981, *Hawaii Med J* 42:326, 1983.
14. Anderson JA, Sogn DA, editors: *Adverse reactions to foods,* Bethesda, Md, 1984, Public Health Service, National Institutes of Health, US Department of Health and Human Services.
15. Anderson JH, Lewis GE: Clinical evaluation of botulinum toxoids. In Lewis GE, editor: *Biomedical aspects of botulism,* New York, 1981, Academic Press.
16. Anthoni U et al: Tetramine: occurrence in marine organisms and pharmacology, *Toxicon* 27(7):707, 1989.
17. Anthoni U et al: The toxin tetramine from the "edible" whelk *Neptunea antiqua, Toxicon* 27(7):717, 1989.
18. Anthoni U et al: Poisonings from flesh of the greenland shark *Somniosus microcephalus* may be due to trimethylamine, *Toxicon* 29(10):1205, 1991.
19. Apold J, Elsayad S: The effect of amino acid modification and polymerization on the immunochemical reactivity of cod allergen M, *Mol Immunol* 16:559, 1979.
20. Armstrong CW, Lake JL, Miller GB: Extraintestinal infections due to halophilic vibrios, *South Med J* 76:571, 1983.
21. Arnold SH, Brown WS: Histamine toxicity from fish products, *Adv Food Res* 24:113, 1978.
22. Asakawa M et al: Structure of the toxin isolated from carp *(Cyprinus carpio)* bile, *Toxicon* 28(9):1063, 1990.
23. Auerbach PS: Ciguatera toxin poisoning, *West J Med* 142:380, 1985.
24. Auerbach PS: Persistent headache associated with scombroid poisoning: resolution with cimetidine, *J Wilderness Med* 1(4):279, 1990.
25. Auerbach PS et al: Bacteriology of the marine environment: implications for clinical therapy, *Ann Emerg Med* 16:643, 1987.
26. Auerbach PS et al: Bacteriology of the freshwater environment: implications for clinical therapy, *Ann Emerg Med* 16:1016, 1987.
27. Bachman B et al: Marine noncholera *Vibrio* infections in Florida, *South Med J* 76:296, 1983.
28. Baden DG: Brevetoxins: unique polyether dinoflagellate toxins, *FASEB J* 3:1807, 1989.
29. Baden DG et al: Brevetoxin binding: molecular pharmacology versus immunoassay, *Toxicon* 26(1):97, 1988.
30. Bagnis R: Clinical aspects of ciguatera (fish poisoning) in French Polynesia, *Hawaii Med J* 28:25, 1968.
31. Bagnis R: Concerning a fatal case of ciguatera poisoning in the Tuamoto Islands, *Clin Toxicol* 3:579, 1970.
32. Bagnis R, Kuberski T, Langier S: Clinical observations on 3009 cases of ciguatera fish poisoning in the South Pacific, *Am J Trop Med Hyg* 28:1067, 1979.
33. Bagnis R et al: Problems of toxicants in marine food products, *Bull WHO* 42:69, 1970.
34. Bagnis R et al: Origins of ciguatera fish poisoning: a new dinoflagellate, *Gambierdiscus toxicus* Adachi and Fukuyo, definitively involved as a causal agent, *Toxicon* 18:199, 1980.
35. Baldo BA, Krills S, Taylor KM: IgE-mediated acute asthma following inhalation of a powdered marine sponge, *Clin Allergy* 12:179, 1982.
36. Baldridge HD Jr, Reber LJ: Reaction of sharks to a mammal in distress, *Milit Med* 131:440, 1966.
37. Barker WH Jr: *Vibrio parahaemolyticus* outbreaks in the United States, *Lancet* 1:551, 1974.
38. Bartlett JC: Botulism. In Wyngaarden JB, Smith LH, editors: *Textbook of medicine,* ed 16, Philadelphia, 1982, WB Saunders.

38a. Bartlett JC: Infant botulism in adults, *N Engl J Med* 315:254, 1986.

39. Beckman EN et al: Histopathology of marine vibrio wound infections, *Am J Clin Pathol* 76:765, 1981.
40. Behling AR, Taylor SH: Bacterial histamine production as a function of temperature and time of incubation, *J Food Sci* 47:1311, 1982.
41. Benoit E, Legrand AM, Dubois JM: Effects of ciguatoxin on current and voltage clamped frog myelinated nerve fibre, *Toxicon* 24:357, 1986.
42. Bernhisel-Broadbent J, Scanlon SM, Sampson HA: Fish hypersensitivity. I. In vitro and oral challenge results in fish-allergic patients, *J Allergy Clin Immunol* 89:730, 1992.
43. Bernhisel-Broadbent J, Straus D, Sampson HA: Fish hypersensitivity. II. Clinical relevance of altered fish allergenicity caused by various preparation methods, *J Allergy Clin Immunol* 90:622, 1992.
44. Bernstein M, Day JH, Welsh A: Double-blind food sensitivity in the adult, *J Allergy Clin Immunol* 70:205, 1982.
45. Bignami GS: A rapid and sensitive hemolysis neutralization assay for palytoxin, *Toxicon* 31(6):817, 1993.
46. Blacklow NR et al: Immune response and prevalence of antibody to Norwalk enteritis virus as determined by radioimmunoassay, *J Clin Microbiol* 10:903, 1979.
47. Blake PA: Diseases of humans (other than cholera) caused by vibrios, *Annu Rev Microbiol* 34:341, 1980.
48. Blake PA: Vibrios on the half shell: what the walrus and the carpenter didn't know, *Ann Intern Med* 99:558, 1983.
49. Blake PA, Weaver RE, Hollis DG: Diseases of humans (other than cholera) caused by vibrios, *Annu Rev Microbiol* 34:341, 1980.
50. Blake PA et al: Disease caused by a marine vibrio: clinical characteristics and epidemiology, *N Engl J Med* 300:1, 1979.
51. Blake PA et al: Cholera—a possible endemic focus in the United States, *N Engl J Med* 302:305, 1980.
52. Blankenship JE: Tetrodotoxin: from poison to powerful tool, *Perspect Biol Med* 19:509, 1976.
53. Blythe DF, deSylva DP: Mother's milk turns toxic following fish feast (letter), *JAMA* 264:2074, 1990.

54. Bock SA et al: Proper use of skin tests with food extracts in diagnosis of hypersensitivity reactions to food in children, *Clin Allergy* 7:375, 1977.
55. Bode RB et al: A new *Vibrio* species, *Vibrio cincinnatiensis,* causing meningitis: successful treatment in an adult, *Ann Intern Med* 104:55, 1986.
56. Boland MP et al: A unified bioscreen for the detection of diarrhetic shellfish toxins and microcystins in marine and freshwater environments, *Toxicon* 31(11):1393, 1993.
57. Bonner JR et al: Spectrum of *Vibrio* infections in a Gulf Coast community, *Ann Intern Med* 99:464, 1983.
58. Bowen RE, Potter ME: Ciguatera: effective control of a growing health problem, *J Wilderness Med* 4:237, 1993.
59. Bradley SG, Klika LJ: A fatal poisoning from the Oregon rough-skinned newt *(Taricha granulosa), JAMA* 246:247, 1981.
60. Brayton PR et al: *Purification and characterization of shark serum proteins which agglutinate bacteria of the family Vibrionacea,* Victoria, BC, June 1986, American Elasmobranch Society.
61. Brenner DJ et al: *Vibrio furnissii* (formerly aerogenic biogroup of *Vibrio fluvialis*), a new species isolated from human feces and the environment, *J Clin Microbiol* 18:816, 1983.
62. Brodie ED: Investigations of the skin toxins of the adult rough skinned newt, *Taricha granulosa, Copeia* 1:307, 1968.
63. Brodie ED Jr: Toxic salamanders, *JAMA* 247:1408, 1982.
64. Brodie ED Jr, Hensel JL, Johnson JA: Toxicity of the urodele amphibians, *Taricha, Notophthalmus, Cynops,* and *Paramesotriton salamidridae, Copeia* 2:506, 1974.
65. Buck JD, Spotte S: The occurrence of potentially pathogenic vibrios in marine mammals, *Marine Mammal Sci* 2:319, 1986.
66. Buckley RH, Metcalfe D: Food allergy, *JAMA* 248:2627, 1982.
67. Butt CG: Primary amebic meningoencephalitis, *N Engl J Med* 274:1473, 1966.
68. Callicott JH: Amebic meningoencephalitis due to free-living amebas of the *Hartmanella (Acanthamoeba)-Naegleria* group, *Am J Clin Pathol* 49:84, 1968.
69. Calvert GM, Hryhorczuk DO, Leikin JB: Treatment of ciguatera fish poisoning with amitryptiline and nifedipine, *Clin Toxicol* 25(5):423, 1987.
70. Campbell B, et al: *Gambierdiscus toxicus* in gut content of the surgeonfish *Ctenochaetus strigosus* (herbivore) and its relationship to toxicity, *Toxicon* 25(10):1125, 1987.
71. Cameron J, Flowers AE, Capra MR: Electrophysiological studies on ciguatera poisoning in man (Part II), *J Neurol Sci* 101:93, 1991.
72. Canzonier WJ: Accumulation and elimination of coliphage S-13 by the hard clam, *Mercenaria mercenaria, Appl Microbiol* 21:1024, 1971.
73. Carrillo T et al: Allergy to limpet, *Allergy* 46:515, 1991.
74. Carrillo T et al: Squid hypersensitivity: a clinical and immunologic study, *Ann Allergy* 68:483, 1992.
75. Carter RF: Sensitivity to amphotercin B of a *Naegleria* sp. isolated from a case of primary amoebic meningoencephalitis, *J Clin Pathol* 22:470, 1969.
76. Cartier A et al: Occupational asthma in snow crab–processing workers, *J Allergy Clin Immunol* 74:261, 1984.
77. Case 10-1985, Case Records of the Massachusetts General Hospital, *N Eng J Med* 312:634, 1985.
78. Case records of the Massachusetts General Hospital, *N Engl J Med* 321(15):1029, 1989.
79. Castillo LE, Winslow DL, Pankey GA: Wound infection and septic shock due to *Vibrio vulnificus, Am J Trop Med Hyg* 30:844, 1981.
80. Centers for Disease Control: Primary amebic meningoencephalitis—North Carolina, 1991, *MMWR* 41(25):437, 1992.
81. Chabalko JJ, Rizzo AA, Land LP: Crab lung, *N Engl J Med* 311:1703, 1984.
82. Chagla AH et al: Septicaemia caused by *Vibrio vulnificus, J Infect* 17:135, 1988.
83. Chan DWS, Yeung CK, Chan MK: Acute renal failure after eating raw fish gall bladder, *Br Med J* 290:897, 1985.
84. Chan TYK, Wang AYM: Life-threatening bradycardia and hypotension in a patient with ciguatera fish poisoning, *Trans R Soc Trop Med Hyg* 87:71, 1993.
85. Chassis G et al: *Salmonella* in turtles imported to Israel from Louisiana, *JAMA* 266:1003, 1986.
86. Chen DZK et al: Identification of protein phosphatase inhibitors of the microcystin class in the marine environment, *Toxicon* 31(11):1407, 1993.
87. Chia DGB et al: Localization of toxins in the poisonous mosaic crab, *Lophozozymus pictor* (Fabricius, 1798) (Brachyura, Xanthidae), *Toxicon* 31(7):901, 1993.
88. Chitwood MB: *Phocanema*-type larval nematode coughed up by a boy in California, *Am J Trop Med Hyg* 24:710, 1975.
89. Chungue E et al: Isolation of two toxins from a parrotfish *Scarus gibbus, Toxicon* 15:89, 1977.
90. Clark RB: Biological causes and effects of paralytic shellfish poisoning, *Lancet* 2:770, 1968.
91. Clarke PA: Immediate respiratory hypersensitivity to abalone (letter), *Med J Aust* 1:623, 1979.
92. Clarridge JE, Zighelboim-Daum S: Isolation and characterization of two hemolytic phenotypes of *Vibrio damsela* associated with a fatal wound infection, *J Clin Microbiol* 21:302, 1985.
93. Coffee JA et al: *Vibrio damsela:* another potentially virulent marine vibrio, *J Infect Dis* 153:800, 1986.
94. Cook TM, Goldman CK: Bacteriology of Chesapeake Bay surface waters, *Chesapeake Sci* 17:40, 1976.
95. Craig CP: It's always the big ones that should get away, *JAMA* 244:272, 1980.
96. Culbertson RF: *Naegleria* and *Acanthamoeba (Hartmanella)* infections. In Feigen RD, Cherry JD, editors: *Textbook of pediatric infectious diseases,* Philadelphia, 1981, WB Saunders.
97. Culbertson RF et al: Experimental infection of mice and monkeys by *Acanthamoeba, Am J Pathol* 35:185, 1959.
98. Dabholkar AS, Carmichael WW: Ultrastructural changes in the mouse liver induced by hepatotoxin from the freshwater cyanobacterium *Microcystis aeruginosa* strain 7820, *Toxicon* 25(3):285, 1987.
99. Dailey MD, Jensen LA, Hill BW: Larval anisakine roundworms of marine fishes from southern and central California, with comments on public health significance, *Calif Fish and Game* 67:240, 1981.
100. Darby CP et al: Primary amebic meningoencephalitis, *Am J Dis Child* 133:1025, 1979.
101. Daul CB, Slattery M, Lehrer SB: Shared antigenic/allergenic epitopes between shrimp *Pen a* I and fruit fly extract (abstract), *J Allergy Clin Immunol* 91:341, 1993.
102. Daul CB et al: Immunologic evaluation of shrimp-allergic individuals, *J Allergy Clin Immunol* 80:716, 1987.
103. Daul CB et al: Identification of a common major crustacea allergen (abstract), *J Allergy Clin Immunol* 89:194, 1992.
104. Davis BR et al: Characterization of biochemically atypical *Vibrio cholerae* strains, and designation of a new pathogenic species, *Vibrio mimicus, J Clin Microbiol* 14:631, 1981.
105. De SP et al: Distribution of vibrios in Calcutta environment with particular reference to *V. parahaemolyticus, Indian J Med Res* 65:21, 1977.
106. de Martino M et al: Allergy to different fish species in cod-allergic children: in vivo and in vitro studies, *J Allergy Clin Immunol* 86:909, 1990.
107. Dickey RW, Miller DM, Tindall DR: Extraction of a water-soluble toxin from a dinoflagellate, *Gambierdiscus toxicus.* In Ragelis EP, editor: *Seafood toxins,* Washington, DC, 1984, American Chemical Society.
108. Dickey RW et al: Identification of okadaic acid from a caribbean dinoflagellate, *Prorocentrum concavum, Toxicon* 28(4):371, 1990.
109. Dickey RW et al: Detection of the marine toxins okadaic acid and domoic acid in shellfish and phytoplankton in the Gulf of Mexico, *Toxicon* 30(3):355, 1992.

110. Dickinson G: Scombroid fish poisoning syndrome, *Ann Emerg Med* 11:487, 1982.
111. DiGaetano M, Ball SF, Strauss JG: *Vibrio vulnificus* corneal ulcer, *Arch Ophthalmol* 107:323, 1989.
112. DiGirolamo R, Liston J, Matches JR: Survival of virus in chilled, frozen and processed oysters, *Appl Microbiol* 20:58, 1970.
113. Dooley JR: Diphyllobothriasis in Americans and Asians, *JAMA* 247:2230, 1982.
114. Doty MS, Aguilar-Santos G: Caulerpicin, a toxic constituent of *Caulerpa, Nature* 211:990, 1966.
115. Droszcz W et al: Allergy to fish meal in fish meal factory workers, *Int Arch Occup Environ Health* 49:13, 1981.
116. DuPont HL: Consumption of raw shellfish—is the risk now unacceptable? *N Engl J Med* 314:707, 1986.
117. Earampamoorthy S, Koff RS: Health hazards of bivalve-mollusk ingestion, *Ann Intern Med* 83:107, 1975.
118. Eastburn RL, Fritsche TR, Terhune CA: Human intestinal infection with *Nanophetus salminicola* from salmonid fishes, *Am J Trop Med Hyg* 36(3):586, 1987.
119. Edwards C et al: Identification of anatoxin-A in benthic cyanobacteria (blue-green algae) and in associated dog poisonings at Loch Insh, Scotland, *Toxicon* 30(10):1165, 1992.
120. Elsayad S, Apold J: Immunochemical analysis of cod fish allergen M: locations of the immunoglobulin binding sites as demonstrated by the native and synthetic peptides, *Allergy* 38:449, 1983.
121. Elsayad S, Bennich H: The primary structure of allergen M from cod, *Scand J Immunol* 4:203, 1975.
122. Elsayad S et al: The structural requirements of epitopes with IgE binding capacity demonstrated by three major allergens from fish, egg, and tree pollen, *Scand J Clin Lab Invest* 204(suppl):17, 1991.
123. Emerson DL et al: Preliminary immunologic studies of ciguatera poisoning, *Arch Intern Med* 143:1931, 1983.
124. Endean R et al: Variation in the toxins present in ciguateric narrow-barred Spanish mackerel, *Scomberomorus commersoni, Toxicon* 31(6):723, 1993.
125. Endean R et al: Apparent relationships between toxins elaborated by the cyanobacterium *Trichodesmium erythraeum* and those present in the flesh of the narrow-barred Spanish mackerel *Scomberomorus commersoni, Toxicon* 31(9):1155, 1993.
126. Eng RHK et al: Early diagnosis of overwhelming *Vibrio vulnificus* infections, *South Med J* 81(3):410, 1988.
127. English VL, Lindberg RB: Isolation of *Vibrio alginolyticus* from wounds and blood of a burn patient, *Am J Med Tech* 43:989, 1977.
128. Erikkson NE, Ryden F, Jonsson P: Hypersensitivity to larvae of chironomids (non-biting midges), *Allergy* 44:305, 1989.
129. Eriksson JE et al: Preliminary characterization of a toxin isolated from the cyanobacterium *Nodularia spumigena, Toxicon* 26(2):161, 1988.
130. Farmer JJ: *Vibrio (Beneckae) vulnificus,* the bacterium associated with sepsis, septicaemia, and the sea, *Lancet* 2:903, 1979.
131. Farmer JJ, Hickman-Brenner FW, Kelly MT: *Vibrio.* In Lennette EH et al: *Manual of clinical microbiology,* Washington, DC, 1985, American Society for Microbiology.
132. Farris WA, Erdman JW: Protracted hypervitaminosis A following long-term, low-level intake, *JAMA* 247:1317, 1982.
133. Fasano A et al: Diarrhea in ciguatera fish poisoning: preliminary evaluation of pathophysiological mechanisms, *Gastroenterology* 100:471, 1991.
134. Fernandez CR, Pankey GA: Tissue invasion by unnamed marine vibrios, *JAMA* 233:1173, 1975.
135. Fishbein M, Mehlman IJ, Pitcher J: Isolation of *Vibrio parahaemolyticus* from the processed meat of Chesapeake Bay blue crabs, *Appl Microbiol* 20:176, 1970.
136. Food and Drug Administration: *Med Bul* 23(1):6, 1992.
137. Fontaine RE: Anisakiasis from the American perspective, *JAMA* 253:1024, 1985.
138. Foo LY: Scombroid-type poisoning induced by the ingestion of smoked kahawai, *NZ Med J* 81:476, 1975.
139. Foo LY: Scombroid poisoning: isolation and identification of "saurine," *J Sci Food Agric* 27:807, 1976.
140. Fowler M, Carter RF: Acute pyogenic meningitis probably due to *Acanthamoeba* sp: a preliminary report, *Br Med J* 2:740, 1965.
141. From the NIH: highly invasive new bacterium isolated from U.S. East Coast waters, *JAMA* 251:323, 1984.
142. Fujino T, et al: On the bacterial examination of Shirasu food poisoning, *Med J Osaka Univ* 4:299, 1953.
143. Fukiya S, Matsumura K: Active and passive immunization for tetrodotoxin in mice, *Toxicon* 30(12):1631, 1992.
144. Fukui M et al: Occurrence of palytoxin in the trigger fish *Melichtys vidua, Toxicon* 25(10):1121, 1987.
145. Fusetani N, Hashimoto K: Occurrence of pahutoxin and homopahutoxin in the mucus secretion of the Japanese boxfish, *Toxicon* 25(4):459, 1987.
146. Gaddie J, Legge JS, Friend JAR: Pulmonary hypersensitivity in prawn workers, *Lancet* 2:1350, 1980.
147. Geiger E: Role of histamine in poisoning with spoiled fish, *Science* 121:865, 1955.
148. Geller RJ, Olson KR, Senécal PE: Ciguatera fish poisoning in San Francisco, California, caused by imported barracuda, *West J Med* 155:639, 1991.
149. Gellert GA et al: Scombroid fish poisoning: underreporting and prevention among noncommercial recreational fishers, *West J Med* 157:645, 1992.
150. Gerba CP et al: Failure of indicator bacteria to reflect the occurrence of enteroviruses in marine waters, *Am J Public Health* 69:1116, 1979.
151. Giboda M et al: Human *Opisthorchis* and *Haplorchis* infections in Laos, *Trans R Soc Trop Med Hyg* 85:538, 1991.
152. Giusti G, Gaeta GB: Doctors in the kitchen: experiments with cooking bivalve mollusks, *N Engl J Med* 304:1371, 1981.
153. Glaziouu P, Martin PMV: Study of factors that influence the clinical response to ciguatera fish poisoning, *Toxicon* 31(9):1151, 1993.
154. Glomset JA: Fish, fatty acids, and human health, *N Engl J Med* 312:1253, 1985.
155. Goldberg AS, Duffield AM, Barrow DK: Distribution and chemical composition of the toxic skin secretions from trunkfish (family Ostraciidae), *Toxicon* 26(7):651, 1988.
156. Goldmann DR: Hold the sushi, *JAMA* 253:2495, 1985.
157. Granata AV, Halickman JF, Borak J: Utility of military anti-shock trousers (MAST) in anaphylactic shock—a case report, *J Emerg Med* 2:349, 1984.
158. Grimes DJ et al: *Vibrio* species associated with mortality of sharks held in captivity, *Microb Ecol* 10:271, 1984.
159. Grimes DJ et al: *Vibrio* species as agents of elasmobranch disease, *Helgolander Meeresuntersuchungen* 37:309, 1984.
160. Grimes DJ et al: *Vibrios* as autochthonous flora of neritic sharks, *Syst Appl Microbiol* 6:221, 1985.
161. Grimmelt B et al: Relationship between domoic acid levels in the blue mussel *(Mytilus edulis)* and toxicity in mice, *Toxicon* 28(5):501, 1990.
162. Grohman GS et al: Norwalk virus gastroentritis in volunteers consuming depurated oysters, *Aust J Exp Biol Med Sci* 59:219, 1981.
163. Gudger EW: Poisonous fishes and fish poisonings, with special reference to ciguatera in the West Indies, *Am J Trop Med* 10:43, 1930.
164. Gunn RA et al: Norwalk virus gastroenteritis following raw oyster consumption, *Am J Epidemiol* 115:348, 1982.
165. Habermann E: Palytoxin acts through Na^+, K^+-ATPase, *Toxicon* 27(11):1171, 1989.
166. Haghighi L, Waleh NS: Isolation of *Vibrio parahaemolyticus* from Persian Gulf, *J Trop Med Hyg* 81:255, 1978.
167. Hahn ST, Capra MF, Walsh TP: Ciguatoxin-protein association in skeletal muscle of Spanish mackerel *(Scomberomorus commersoni), Toxicon* 30(8):843, 1992.

168. Hall S, Reichardt PB: Cryptic paralytic shellfish toxins. In Ragelis EP, editor: *Seafood toxins,* Washington, DC, 1984, American Chemical Society.
169. Halmepuro L, Salvaggio JE, Lehrer SB: Crawfish and lobster allergens: identification and structural similarities with other crustacea, *Int Arch Allergy Immunol* 84:165, 1987.
170. Halstead BW: Marine pollution and the pharmaceutical scientist *Am J Pharmacol Ed* 37:267, 1978.
171. Halstead BW: *Dangerous marine animals,* Centreville, Md, 1980, Cornell Maritime Press.
172. Halstead BW: Current status of marine biotoxicology—an overview, Colton, Calif, 1980, International Biotoxicological Center, World Life Research Institute.
173. Halstead BW: Miscellaneous seafood toxicants. In Ragelis EP, editor: *Seafood toxins,* Washington, DC, 1984, American Chemical Society.
174. Halstead BW, Haddock RL: A fatal outbreak of poisoning from the ingestion of red seaweed *Gracilaria tsudae* in Guam—a review of the oral marine biotoxicity problem, *J Nat Toxins* 1(1):87, 1992.
175. Harada K-I et al: A new procedure for the analysis and purification of naturally occurring anatoxin-a from the blue-green alga *Anabaena flos-aquae, Toxicon* 27(12):1289, 1982.
176. Hardegree MC: Bacterial toxoids: perspectives for the future. In Lewis GE, editor: *Biomedical aspects of botulism,* New York, 1981, Academic Press.
177. Hashimoto Y, Kamiya H: Occurrence of a toxic substance in the skin of a sea bass *Pogonoperca punctata, Toxicon* 7:65, 1969.
178. Hauschild AHW, Gauvreau L: Food-borne botulism in Canada, 1971-84, *Can Med Assoc J* 133:1141, 1985.
179. Helfrich P: Fish poisoning in Hawaii, *Hawaii Med J* 22:361, 1963.
180. Helfrich P, Banner AH: Experimental induction of ciguatera toxicity in fish through diet, *Nature* 197:1025, 1963.
181. Henderson R, Ritchie JM, Strichartz GR: Evidence that tetrodotoxin and saxitoxin act at a metal cation binding site in the sodium channels of nerve membrane, *Proc Natl Acad Sci USA* 71:3936, 1974.
182. Hessel DW, Halstead BW, Heckham NH: Marine biotoxins. I. Ciguatera poison: some biological and chemical aspects, *Ann NY Acad Sci* 90:788, 1960.
183. Hirst LW et al: Management of *Acanthamoeba* keratitis: a case report and review of the literature, *Ophthalmology* 91:1105, 1984.
184. Ho AM, Fraser IM, Todd ECD: Ciguatera poisoning: a report of three cases, *Ann Emerg Med* 15:1225, 1986.
185. Hoffman DR, Day ED, Miller JS: The major heat stable allergen of shrimp, *Ann Allergy* 47:17, 1981.
186. Hokama Y: A rapid, simplified enzyme immunoassay stick test for the detection of ciguatoxin and related polyethers from fish tissues, *Toxicon* 23:939, 1985.
187. Hokama Y et al: An enzyme immunoassay for the detection of ciguatoxin and competitive inhibition by related natural polyether toxins. In Ragelis EP, editor: *Seafood toxins,* 1984, American Chemical Society.
188. Hokama Y et al: Evaluation of the stick enzyme immunoassay in *Caranx* sp. and *Seriola dumerili* associated with ciguatera, *J Clin Lab Anal* 4:363, 1990.
189. Hollis DG et al: Halophilic *Vibrio* species isolated from blood cultures, *J Clin Microbiol* 3:425, 1976.
190. Holtzer R, Clary D, Noriel D: Fatal paralytic shellfish poisoning from scallops—a rarity, October 3, 1980, *California Morbidity* 39, Infectious Disease Section, State Department of Health Services, Sacramento, Calif.
191. Hughes JM, Merson MH: Fish and shellfish poisoning, *N Engl J Med* 295:1117, 1976.
192. Hughes JM, Potter ME: Scombroid-fish poisoning: from pathogenesis to prevention, *N Engl J Med* 324(11):766, 1991.
193. Hughes JM et al: Noncholera *Vibrio* infections in the United States, *Ann Intern Med* 88:602, 1978.
194. Huq MI et al: Isolation of *Vibrio*-like group, EF-6, from patients with diarrhea, *J Clin Microbiol* 11:621, 1980.
195. Hwang DF, Chueh CH, Jeng SS: Occurrence of tetrodotoxin in the gastropod mollusk *Natica lineata* (lined moon shell), *Toxicon* 28(1):21, 1990.
196. Hwang DF et al: Tetrodotoxin and derivatives in several species of the gastropod Naticidae, *Toxicon* 2998:1019, 1991.
197. Hwang DF et al: Comparison of paralytic toxins in aquaculture of purple clam in Taiwan, *Toxicon* 30(5/6):669, 1992.
198. Ioannides G, Davis JH: Portuguese man-of-war stinging, *Arch Dermatol* 91:448, 1965.
199. Iwaoka W et al: Analysis of *Acanthurus triostegus* for marine toxins by the stick enzyme immunoassay and mouse bioassay, *Toxicon* 30(12):1575, 1992.
200. Jackson GJ: The new disease status of human anisakiasis and North American cases: a review, *J Food Milk Technol* 38:769, 1975.
201. Jamieson A: Effect of clotrimazole on *Naegleria fowleri, J Clin Pathol* 28:446, 1975.
202. Janda JM et al: Current perspectives on the epidemiology and pathogenesis of clinically significant *Vibrio* spp, *Clin Microbiol Rev* 1(3):245, 1988.
203. Janda JM: A lethal leviathan—*Vibrio vulnificus, West J Med* 155: 421, 1991.
204. Jean-Jacques W et al: *Vibrio metschnikovii* bacteremia in a patient with cholecystitis, *J Clin Microbiol* 14:711, 1981.
205. Jellett JF et al: Paralytic shellfish poison (saxitoxin family) bioassays: automated endpoint determination and standardization of the in vitro tissue culture bioassay, and comparison with the standard mouse bioassay, *Toxicon* 30(10):1143, 1992.
206. Jenkins RD, Johnston JM: Inland presentation of *Vibrio vulnificus* primary septicemia and necrotizing fasciitis, *West J Med* 144:78, 1986.
207. Johnson R, Jong EC: Ciguatera: Caribbean and Indo-Pacific fish poisoning, *West J Med* 138:872, 1983.
208. Johnson RM, Katarski ME, Weisrock WP: Correlation of taxonomic criteria for a collection of marine bacteria, *Appl Microbiol* 16:708, 1968.
209. Johnston JM, Andes A, Glasser G: *Vibrio vulnificus:* a gastronomic hazard, *JAMA* 249:1756, 1983.
210. Johnston JM, Becker SF, McFarland LM: Gastroenteritis in patients with stool isolates of *Vibrio vulnificus, Am J Med* 80:336, 1986.
211. Jones DB, Visvesvara GS, Robinson NM: *Acanthamoeba polyphagia* keratitis and fatal meningoencephalitis, *Trans Ophthalmol Soc UK* 95:221, 1975.
212. Jordan JH, Flynn T: *Vibrio* sepsis in a cirrhotic patient, *South Med J* 82(6):799, 1989.
213. Juels CW et al: Temporary human infection with a *Phocanema* sp. larva, *Am J Trop Med Hyg* 24:942, 1975.
214. Juranovic LR, Park DL: Foodborne toxins of marine origin: ciguatera, *Rev Environ Contam Toxicol* 117:51, 1991.
215. Jyo T et al: Sea squirt asthma—occupational asthma induced by inhalation of antigenic substances contained in the sea squirt body fluid, *Allergy Immunol* 21:425, 1974.
216. Kamiya H et al: Purification and characterization of an antibacterial and antineoplastic protein secretion of a sea hare, *Aplysia juliana, Toxicon* 27(12):1269, 1989.
217. Kan SKP, Singh N, Chan MKC: *Oliva vidua fulminans,* a marine mollusc, responsible for five fatal cases of neurotoxic food poisoning in Sabah, Malaysia, *Trans R Soc Trop Med Hyg* 80:64, 1986.
218. Kaneko I, Colwell R: Ecology of *Vibrio parahaemolyticus* in Chesapeake Bay, *J Bacteriol* 113:24, 1973.
219. Kao CY, Yasumoto T: Tetrodotoxin in "zombie powder," *Toxicon* 28(2):129, 1990.
220. Kao CY, Yeoh PH: Different receptors for saxitoxin and tetrodotoxin, *Proc Physiol Soc* 284:88P, 1982.
221. Karlin JM: Occupational asthma to clam's liver extract (abstract), *J Allergy Clin Immunol* 63:197, 1979.
222. Kasha EE, Norins AL: Scombroid fish poisoning with facial flushing (letter), *J Am Acad Dermatol* 18(6):1363, 1988.

223. Kelly MT, McCormick WF: Acute bacterial myositis caused by *Vibrio vulnificus, JAMA* 246:72, 1981.
224. Kim R: Flushing syndrome due to mahimahi (scombroid fish) poisoning, *Arch Dermatol* 115:963, 1979.
225. Kim YH et al: Tetrodotoxin: occurrence in atelopid frogs of Costa Rica, *Science* 189:151, 1975.
226. Kliks MM: Anisakiasis in the western United States: four new case reports from California, *Am J Trop Med Hyg* 32:526, 1983.
227. Kliks MM: Human anisakiasis: an update, *JAMA* 255:2605, 1986.
228. Kline MW et al: Primary amebic meningoencephalitis, *Pediatr Emerg Care* 2:173, 1986.
229. Klontz KC: Fatalities associated with *Vibrio parahaemolyticus* and *Vibrio cholerae* non-01 infections in Florida (1981 to 1988), *South Med J* 83(5):500, 1990.
230. Knape JTA et al: An anaphylactic reaction to protamine in a patient allergic to fish, *Anaethesiology* 55:324, 1981.
231. Knapp HR et al: In vivo indexes of platelet and vascular function during fish-oil administration in patients with atherosclerosis, *N Engl J Med* 314:937, 1986.
232. Kodama AM, Hokama Y: Variations in symptomatology of ciguatera poisoning, *Toxicon* 27(5):593, 1989.
233. Kodama M et al: Occurrence of saxitoxin and other toxins in the liver of the pufferfish *Takifugu paradalis, Toxicon* 21:897, 1983.
234. Kodama AM et al: Clinical and laboratory findings implicating palytoxin as cause of ciguatera poisoning due to *Decapterus macrosoma* (mackerel), *Toxicon* 27(9):1051, 1989.
235. Kodama M et al: Production of paralytic shellfish toxins by a bacterium *Moraxella* sp. isolated from *Protogonyaulax tamarensis, Toxicon* 28(6):707, 1990.
236. Koenig KL, Mueller J, Rose T: *Vibrio vulnificus:* hazard on the half shell, *West J Med* 155:400, 1991.
237. Koenig MG et al: Clinical and laboratory observations of type E botulism in man, *Medicine* 43:517, 1964.
238. Koff RS, Sear HS: Internal temperature of steamed clams, *N Engl J Med* 276:737, 1967.
239. Koff RS et al: Viral hepatitis in a group of Boston hospitals. III. Importance of exposure to shellfish in a nonepidemic period, *N Engl J Med* 276:703, 1967.
240. Koshte VL, Kagen SL, Aalberse RC: Cross-reactivity of IgE antibodies to caddis fly with arthropoda and mollusca, *J Allergy Clin Immunol* 84:174, 1989.
241. Kothary MH, Kreger AS: Purification and characterization of an extracellular cytolysin produced by *Vibrio damsela, Infect Immun* 49:25, 1985.
242. Kreger AS: Cytolytic activity and virulence of *Vibrio damsela, Infect Immun* 44:326, 1984.
243. Kreger AS, Lockwood D: Detection of extracellular toxin(s) produced by *Vibrio vulnificus, Infect Immun* 33:583, 1981.
244. Kromhout D, Bosschieter EB, Coulander CDL: The inverse relation between fish consumption and 20-year mortality from coronary heart disease, *N Engl J Med* 312:1205, 1985.
245. Lange WR: Severity rating scales for ciguatera fish poisoning, *Toxicon* 31(6):777, 1993.
246. Lange WR, Lipkin KM, Yang GC: Can ciguatera be a sexually transmitted disease? *Clin Toxicol* 27(3):193, 1989.
247. Lange WR et al: Potential benefit of tocainide in the treatment of ciguatera: report of three cases (letter), *Am J Med* 84:1087, 1988.
248. Laobhripatr S et al: Food poisoning due to consumption of the freshwater puffer *Tetraodon fangi* in Thailand, *Toxicon* 28(11):1372, 1990.
249. Lawrence DN et al: *Vibrio parahaemolyticus* gastroenteritis outbreaks aboard two cruise ships, *Am J Epidemiol* 109:71, 1979.
250. Lawrence DN et al: Ciguatera fish poisoning in Miami, *JAMA* 244:254, 1980.
251. Lee JV et al: Taxonomy and description of *Vibrio fluvialis* sp. nov. (synonym group F *vibrios,* group EF6), *J Appl Bacteriol* 50:73, 1981.
252. Lee TH et al: Effect of dietary enrichment with eicosapentaenoic and docosahexaenoic acids on in vitro neutrophil and monocyte leukotriene generation and neutrophil function, *N Engl J Med* 312:1217, 1985.
253. Legrand AM, Bagnis R: Mode of action of ciguatera toxins. In Ragelis EP, editor: *Seafood toxins,* Washington, DC, 1984, American Chemical Society.
254. Lehrer SB: The complex nature of food antigens: studies of cross-reacting crustacea allergens, *Ann Allergy* 57:267, 1986.
255. Lehrer SB, McCants ML: Reactivity of IgE antibodies with crustacea and oyster allergens: evidence for common antigenic structures, *J Allergy Clin Immunol* 80:133, 1987.
256. Lehrer SB, McCants M, Salvaggio J: Identification of crustacea allergens by crossed radioimmunoelectrophoresis, *Int Arch Allergy Appl Immunol* 77:192, 1985.
257. Lemanske RJ Jr, Taylor SL: Standardized extracts, foods, *Clin Rev Allergy* 5:23, 1987.
258. Lennette EH et al, editors: *Manual of clinical microbiology,* Washington, DC, 1985, American Society for Microbiology.
259. Lerke PA: Scombroid poisoning—report of an outbreak, *West J Med* 129:381, 1978.
260. Levine L et al: Production of antibodies and development of a radioimmunoassay for okadaic acid, *Toxicon* 26(12):1123, 1988.
261. Lewis RJ: Ciguatoxins are potent ichthyotoxins, *Toxicon* 30(2):207, 1992.
262. Lewis RJ, Hoy AWW: Comparative action of three major ciguatoxins on guinea-pig atria and ilea, *Toxicon* 31(4):437, 1993.
263. Lewis RJ, Hoy AWW, McGiffin DC: Action of ciguatoxin on human atrial trabeculae, *Toxicon* 30(8):907, 1992.
264. Lewis RJ, Sellin M: Multiple ciguatoxins in the flesh of fish, *Toxicon* 30(8):915, 1992.
265. Lewis RJ, Wong Hoy AW, Sellin M: Ciguatera and mannitol: in vivo and in vitro assessment in mice, *Toxicon* 31(8):1039, 1993.
266. Lewis RJ et al: Purification and characterization of ciguatoxins from moray eel (*Lycodontis javanicus,* Muraenidae), *Toxicon* 29(9):1115, 1991.
267. Lewis RJ et al: Ciguatoxin-2 is a diastereomer of ciguatoxin-3, *Toxicon* 31(5):637, 1993.
268. Llewellyn LE, Endean R: Toxic coral reef crabs from Australian waters, *Toxicon* 26(11):1085, 1988.
269. Llewellyn LE, Endean R: Toxicity and paralytic shellfish toxin profiles of the xanthid crabs, *Lophozozymus pictor* and *Zosimus aeneus,* collected from some Australian coral reefs, *Toxicon* 27(5):596, 1989.
270. Llewellyn LE, Endean R: Toxins extracted from Australian specimens of the crab, *Eriphia sebana* (Xanthidae), *Toxicon* 27(5):579, 1989.
271. Llewellyn LE, Endean R: Paralytic shellfish toxins in the xanthid crab *Atergatis floridus* collected from Australian coral reefs, *J Wilderness Med* 2(2):118, 1991.
272. Li KM: Ciguatera fish poison: a cholinesterase inhibitor, *Science* 147:1580, 1965.
273. Linaweaver PG: Toxic marine life, *Milit Med* 131:437, 1967.
274. Linco SJ, Grohmann GS: The Darwin outbreak of oyster-associated viral gastroenteritis, *Med J Aust* 1:211, 1980.
275. Lipkin KM: Ciguatera poisoning presenting as a psychiatric disorder (letter), *Arch Gen Psychiatry* 46:384, 1989.
276. Lotz MJ, Tamplin ML, Rodrick GE: Thiosulfate–citrate–bile salts–sucrose agar and its selectivity for clinical and marine vibrio organisms, *Ann Clin Lab Sci* 13:45, 1983.
277. Love M et al: *Vibrio damsela,* a marine bacterium, causes skin ulcers on the damselfish *Chromis punctipinnis, Science* 214:1139, 1981.
278. Luu HA et al: Quantification of diarrhetic shellfish toxins and identification of novel protein phosphatase inhibitors in marine phytoplankton and mussels, *Toxicon* 31(1):75, 1993.
279. MacDonnell MT, Colwell RR: Phylogeny of the Vibrionaceae, and recommendation for two new genera, *Listonella* and *Shewanella, Syst Appl Microbiol* 6:171, 1985.

280. MacLeod RA: The question of the existence of specific marine bacteria, *Bacteriol Rev* 29:9, 1965.
281. Maeda S et al: Eleven cases of anaphylaxis caused by grand keyhole limpet (abalone-like shellfish), *Arerugi* 40:1415, 1991.
282. Mahmood NA, Carmichael WW: Anatoxin-a(s), an anticholinesterase from the cyanobacterium *Anabaena flos-aquae* NRC-525-17, *Toxicon* 25(11):1221, 1987.
283. Manowitz NR, Rosenthal RR: Cutaneous-systemic reactions to toxins and venoms of common marine organisms, *Cutis* 23:450, 1979.
284. Margo CE, Brinser JH, Groden L: Exfoliated cytopathology of *Acanthamoeba* keratitis, *JAMA* 255:2216, 1986.
285. Marr JC et al: Detection of new 7-*O*-acyl derivatives of diarrhetic shellfish poisoning toxins by liquid chromatography–mass spectrometry, *Toxicon* 30(12):1621, 1992.
286. Maulitz RM, Pratt DS, Schocket AL: Exercise-induced anaphylactic reaction to shellfish, *J Allergy Clin Immunol* 63:433, 1979.
287. McCabe MJ et al: A fatal brain injury caused by a needlefish, *Neuroradiology* 15:137, 1978.
288. McCollum JPK et al: An epidemic of mussel poisoning in north-east England, *Lancet* 2:767, 1968.
289. McCool JA et al: Primary amebic meningoencephalitis diagnosed in the emergency department, *Ann Emerg Med* 12:35, 1983.
290. McKerrow JH, Sakanari J, Deardorff TL: Anisakiasis: revenge of the sushi parasite (letter), *N Engl J Med* 319:1228, 1988.
291. McSweeney RJ, Forgan-Smith WR: Wound infections in Australia from halophilic vibrios, *Med J Aust* 1:896, 1977.
292. Meadors MC, Pankey GA: *Vibrio vulnificus* wound infection treated successfully with oral ciprofloxacin (letter), *J Infect* 20(1):88, 1990.
293. Mebs D, Schmidt K: Occurrence of tetrodotoxin in the frog *Atelopus oxyrhynchus, Toxicon* 27(7):819, 1989.
294. Mehtar S et al: Adult epiglottitis due to *Vibrio vulnificus, Br Med J* 296:827, 1988.
295. Melton RJ et al: Fatal sardine poisoning: a fatal case of fish poisoning in Hawaii associated with the Marquesan sardine, *Hawaii Med J* 43:114, 1984.
296. Merson MH et al: Scombroid fish poisoning: outbreak traced to commercially canned tuna fish, *JAMA* 228:1268, 1974.
297. Mertens A et al: Halophilic, lactose-positive *Vibrio* in a case of fatal septicemia, *J Clin Microbiol* 9:233, 1979.
298. Miller DM, Dickey RW, Tindall DR: Lipid-extracted toxins from a dinoflagellate, *Gambierdiscus toxicus.* In Ragelis EP, editor: *Seafood toxins,* Washington, DC, 1984, American Chemical Society.
299. Mills AR, Passmore R: Pelagic paralysis, *Lancet* 1:161, 1988.
300. Misbah SA, Peiris JB, Atukorala TMS: Ingestion of shark liver associated with pseudotumor cerebri due to acute hypervitaminosis A, *J Neurol Neurosurg Psychiatry* 47:216, 1984.
301. Miyahara JT, Akau CK, Yasumoto T: Effects of ciguatoxin and maitotoxin on the isolated guinea pig atria, *Res Comm Chem Pathol Pharmacol* 25:177, 1979.
302. Morgan JE et al: Species-specific shrimp allergens: RAST and RAST-inhibition studies, *J Allergy Clin Immunol* 83:1112, 1989.
303. Morris GK et al: Comparison of four plating media for isolating *Vibrio cholerae, J Clin Microbiol* 9:79, 1979.
304. Morris JG: Ciguatera fish poisoning, *JAMA* 244:273, 1980.
305. Morris JG: Current trends in therapy of botulism in the United States. In Lewis GE, editor: *Biomedical aspects of botulism,* New York, 1981, Academic Press.
306. Morris JG Jr: *Vibrio vulnificus*—a new monster of the deep? *Ann Intern Med* 109(4):261, 1988.
307. Morris JG, Black RE: Cholera and other vibrioses in the United States, *N Engl J Med* 310:343, 1985.
308. Morris JG et al: Clinical features of ciguatera fish poisoning: a study of the disease in the US Virgin Islands, *Arch Intern Med* 142:1090, 1982.
309. Morris JG et al: Illness caused by *Vibrio damsela* and *Vibrio hollisae, Lancet* 1:1294, 1982.
310. Morris JG et al: Virulence of *Vibrio vulnificus:* association with utilization of transferrin-bound iron, and lack of correlation with levels of cytotoxin or protease, *FEMS Microbiol Lett* 40:55, 1987.
311. Morris PD, Campbell DS, Freeman JI: Ciguatera fish poisoning: an outbreak associated with fish caught from North Carolina coastal waters, *South Med J* 83(4):379, 1990.
312. Morrow JD et al: Evidence that histamine is the causative toxin of scombroid-fish poisoning, *N Engl J Med* 324(11):716, 1991.
313. Morse DL et al: Widespread outbreaks of clam- and oyster-associated gastroenteritis: association of Norwalk virus, *N Engl J Med* 314:678, 1986.
314. Morse DL et al: Clam-associated gastroenteritis—in reply, *N Engl J Med* 315:583, 1986.
315. Mosher HS, Fuhrman FA: Occurrence and origin of tetrodotoxin. In Ragelis EP, editor: *Seafood toxins,* Washington, DC, 1984, American Chemical Society.
316. Muic V et al: Infection and contamination of some edible animals in the polluted sea area of Pula, *Toxicon* 16:424, 1978.
317. Murakami-Walker A: Fast, simple test for ciguatoxin developed at UH, *Makai* (U Hawaii Sea Grant College Program) 7(9):1, 1985.
318. Murata M et al: Structures and configurations of ciguatoxin from the moray eel *Gymnothorax javanicus* and its likely precursor from the dinoflagellate *Gambierdiscus toxicus, J Am Chem Soc* 112:4380, 1990.
319. Myers BJ: Nematodes transmitted to man by fish and aquatic animals, *J Wildfire Dis* 6:266, 1970.
320. Myers BJ: Anisakine nematodes in fresh commercial fish from waters along the Washington, Oregon and California coasts, *J Food Protection* 42:380, 1979.
321. Nagpal S, Metcalfe DD, Rao PV: Identification of a shrimp-derived allergen as tRNA, *J Immunol* 138:4169, 1987.
322. Nagpal S et al: Isolation and characterization of heat-stable allergens from shrimp *(Penaeus indicus), J Allergy Clin Immunol* 83:26, 1989.
323. Nakashima T: Studies on bronchial asthma observed in culture oyster workers, *Hiroshima J Med Sci* 18:41, 1969.
324. Namikoshi M et al: Isolation and structures of microcystins from a cyanobacterial water bloom (Finland), *Toxicon* 30(11):1473, 1992.
325. Narahashi T, Morre JW, Poston RN: Tetrodotoxin derivatives: chemical structure and blockage of nerve membrane conductance, *Science* 156:976, 1967.
326. Narahashi T: Mechanism of action of tetrodotoxin and saxitoxin on excitable membranes, *Fed Proc* 31:1124, 1972.
327. Ogata T, Sato S, Kodama M: Paralytic shellfish toxins in bivalves which are not associated with dinoflagellates, *Toxicon* 27(11):1241, 1989.
328. Oshima Y et al: Paralytic shellfish toxins in tropical waters. In Ragelis EP, editor: *Seafood toxins,* Washington, DC, 1984, American Chemical Society.
329. Pacy H: Australian catfish injuries with report of a typical case, *Med J Aust* 2:63, 1966.
330. Patel PC, Cockcraft DW: Occupational asthma caused by exposure to cooking lobster in the work environment: a case report, *Ann Allergy* 68:360, 1992.
331. Pearn J: Ciguatera—an early report (letter), *Med J Aust* 151:724, 1989.
332. Pearn JH et al: Ciguatera and mannitol: experience with a new treatment regimen, *Med J Aust* 151:77, 1989.
333. Pearson RD, Hewlett EL: Niclosamide therapy for tapeworm infections, *Ann Intern Med* 102:550, 1985.
334. Pepper SJ, Smith HM: *Toxic fish and mollusks,* Information Bulletin No 12, Maxwell AFB, Alabama, Air Training Command/ Experimental Information Division.
335. Perl TM et al: An outbreak of toxic encephalopathy caused by eating mussels contaminated with domoic acid, *N Engl J Med* 332:1775, 1990.
336. Pettit GR, Ode RH: Antineoplastic agents L: isolation and characterization of sphyrnastatins 1 and 2 from the hammerhead shark *Sphyrna lewini, J Pharm Sci* 66:757, 1977.

337. Pien F, Lee K, Higa, H: *Vibrio alginolyticus* infections in Hawaii, *J Clin Microbiol* 5:670, 1977.
338. Pien FD et al: Bacterial flora of marine penetrating injuries, *Diagn Microbiol Infect Dis* 1:229, 1983.
339. Pinkus GS, Coolidge C, Little MD: Intestinal anisakiasis: first case report from North America, *Am J Med* 59:114, 1975.
340. Pollack SJ et al: *Vibrio vulnificus* septicemia: isolation of organism from stool and demonstration of antibodies by indirect immunofluorescence, *Arch Intern Med* 143:837, 1983.
341. Portnoy BL et al: Oyster-associated hepatitis: failure of shellfish certification programs to prevent outbreaks, *JAMA* 233:1065, 1975.
342. Prescott BD: "Scombroid poisoning" and bluefish: the Connecticut connection, *Conn Med* 48:105, 1984.
343. Proceedings of a Symposium on Domoic Acid Toxicity (suppl), *Can Dis Wkly Rep* 16S1E:1, 1990.
344. Pugno PA, Daufman D, Feder HM: Bluefish: a newly discovered cause of scombroid poisoning, *J Fam Pract* 17:1071, 1983.
345. Quilliam MA, Wright JLC: The amnesic shellfish poisoning mystery, *Analyt Chem* 61(18):1053A, 1989.
346. Ragelis EP: Ciguatera seafood poisoning: overview. In Ragelis EP, editor: *Seafood toxins,* Washington, DC, 1984, American Chemical Society.
347. Rajkovic IA, Williams R: Abnormalities of neutrophil phagocytosis, intracellular killing and metabolic activity in alcoholic cirrhosis and hepatitis, *Hepatology* 6:252, 1986.
348. Randall JE: A review of ciguatera tropical fish poisoning, with a tentative explanation of its cause, *Bull Marine Sci Gulf Caribbean* 8:236, 1958.
349. Rayner MD: Mode of action of ciguatoxin, *Fed Proc* 31:1139, 1972.
350. Rayner MD, Szerkerczes J: Ciguatoxin: effects on the sodium-potassium activated adenosine triphosphatase of human erythrocyte ghosts, *Tox Appl Pharmacocol* 24:489, 1973.
351. Reppun JIF: Ciguatera poisoning in the Pacific, *Hawaii Med J* 47(10):462, 1988.
352. Richards IS et al: Florida red-tide toxins (brevetoxins) produce depolarization of airway smooth muscle, *Toxicon* 28(9):1105, 1990.
353. Roland FP: Leg gangrene and endotoxin shock due to *Vibrio parahaemolyticus:* an infection acquired in New England coastal waters, *N Engl J Med* 282:1306, 1970.
354. Rosen L et al: Studies on eosinophilic meningitis. 3. Epidemiologic and clinical observations on Pacific Islands and the possible etiologic role of *Angiostrongylus cantonensis, Am J Epidemiol* 85:17, 1967.
355. Rubin SJ, Tilton RC: Isolation of *Vibrio alginolyticus* from wound infections, *J Clin Microbiol* 2:556, 1975.
356. Ruff TA: Ciguatera in the Pacific: a link with military activities, *Lancet* 1:201, 1989.
357. Rump S, Rabsztyn T: Effects of some veratrine-like agents on the muscular blocking action of tetrodotoxin, *Toxicon* 15:521, 1977.
358. Runge JW et al: Histamine antagonists in the treatment of acute allergic reactions, *Ann Emerg Med* 21:237, 1992.
359. Runnegar MTC, Jackson ARB, Falconer IR: Toxicity of the cyanobacterium *Nodularia spumigena* Mertens, *Toxicon* 26(2):143, 1988.
360. Runnegar MTC et al: Injury to hepatocytes induced by a peptide toxin from the cyanobacterium *Microcystis aeruginosa, Toxicon* 25(11): 1235, 1987.
361. Russell FE: Comparative pharmacology of some animal toxins, *Fed Proc* 26:1206, 1967.
362. Russell FE: Ciguatera poisoning: a report of 35 cases, *Toxicon* 13:383, 1975.
363. Ruttenber AJ et al: Diphyllobothriasis associated with salmon consumption in Pacific coast states, *Am J Trop Med Hyg* 33:455, 1984.
364. Ryan WJ: Marine vibrios associated with superficial septic lesions, *J Clin Pathol* 29:1014, 1976.
365. Sachs MI: Value of food antigen specific IgE-RAST and immediate reaction skin tests, *Ann Allergy* 51:264, 1983.
366. Sakanari JA et al: Intestinal anisakiasis: a case diagnosed by morphologic and immunologic methods, *Am J Clin Pathol* 90:107, 1988.
367. Sampson HA: Role of immediate food hypersensitivity in the pathogenesis of atopic dermatitis, *J Allergy Clin Immunol* 71:473, 1983.
368. Schandevyl P, Van Dyk E, Piot P: Halophilic *Vibrio* species from seafish in Senegal, *Appl Environ Microbiol* 48:236, 1984.
369. Schantz EJ: Poisons produced by dinoflagellates—a review. In Carmichael WW, editor: *The water environment: algal toxins and health,* New York, 1981, Plenum Press.
370. Schantz EJ: Historical perspective on paralytic shellfish poison. In Ragelis EP, editor: *Seafood toxins,* Washington, DC, 1984, American Chemical Society.
371. Scheuer PJ et al: Ciguatoxin: isolation and chemical nature, *Science* 155:1267, 1967.
372. Scully RE: Case records of the Massachusetts General Hospital, *N Engl J Med* 323(7):467, 1990.
373. Seidel JS: Primary amebic meningoencephalitis, *Pediatr Clin North Am* 32:881, 1985.
374. Seidel JS, et al: Successful treatment of primary amebic meningoencephalitis, *N Engl J Med* 306:346, 1982.
375. Seidler RJ, et al: Biochemical characteristics and virulence of environmental group F bacteria isolated in the United States, *Appl Environ Microbiol* 40:715, 1980.
376. Senecal P-E, Osterloh JD: Normal fetal outcome after maternal ciguateric toxin exposure in the second trimester, *Clin Tox* 29(4):473, 1991.
377. Shandera WX, et al: Disease from infection with *Vibrio mimicus,* a newly recognized *Vibrio* species, *Ann Intern Med* 99:169, 1983.
378. Shaw JFE, et al: Restaurant-associated scombroid fish poisoning—Alabama, Tennessee, *MMWR* 35:264, 1986.
379. Shestowsky WS, Quilliam MA, Sikorska HM: An idiotypic-anti-idiotypic competitive immunoassay for quantitation of okadaic acid, *Toxicon* 30(11):1441, 1992.
380. Shiomi K et al: Occurrence of tetrodotoxin-binding high molecular weight substances in the body fluid of shore crab *(Hemigrapsus sanguineus), Toxicon* 30(12):1529, 1992.
381. Shirahama M et al: Colonic anisakiasis simulating carcinoma of the colon (letter), *AJR* 155:895, 1990.
382. Simpson LM et al: Correlation between virulence and colony morphology in *Vibrio vulnificus, Infect Immun* 55:269, 1987.
383. Sims JK: The diet in ciguatera fish poisoning, *Communicable Dis Rep,* Hawaii State Dept. Health, April, 1985, p 4.
384. Sims JK, Ostman DC: Pufferfish poisoning: emergency diagnosis and management of mild human tetrodotoxication, *Ann Emerg Med* 15:1094, 1986.
385. Sims JK, Young BG: Personal communication, 1985.
386. Sivonen K et al: Isolation and structures of five microcystins from a Russian *Microcystis aeruginosa* strain CALU 972, *Toxicon* 30(11):1481, 1992.
387. Smart DR: Scombroid poisoning: a report of seven cases involving the western Australian salmon, *Arripis truttaceus, Med J Aust* 157:748, 1992.
388. Smith GC, Merkel JR: Collagenolytic activity of *Vibrio vulnificus:* potential contribution to its invasiveness, *Infect Immun* 35:1155, 1982.
389. Smith HM: Toxic fish and mollusks. Information Bulletin No 12. Maxwell Air Force Base, Alabama, 1975, Air Training Command, Environmental Information Division.
390. Sonnabend O et al: Isolation of *Clostridium botulinum* type G and identification of type G botulinal toxin in humans: report of five sudden unexpected deaths, *J Infect Dis* 143:22, 1981.
391. Sorokin M: Human poisoning by ingestion of a sea hare *(Dolabella auricularia), Toxicon* 26(11):1095, 1988.
392. Southcott RV: Human injuries from invertebrate animals in the Australian seas, *Clin Toxicol* 3:617, 1970.
393. Southcott RV: Australian venomous and poisonous fishes, *Clin Toxicol* 10:291, 1977.
394. Spark RP et al: *Vibrio alginolyticus* wound infection: case report and review, *Ann Clin Lab Sci* 9:133, 1979.

395. Spoerke DG, Rumack BH: Blue-green algae poisoning, *J Emerg Med* 2:353, 1985.
396. Steinfeld AD, Steinfeld HJ: Ciguatera and the voyage of Captain Bligh, *JAMA* 228:1270, 1974.
397. Stewart MPM: Ciguatera fish poisoning: treatment with intravenous mannitol, *Trop Doctor* 21:54, 1991.
398. Stommel EW, Parsonnet J, Jenkyn LR: Polymyositis after ciguatera toxin exposure, *Arch Neurol* 48:874, 1991.
399. Stoner RD et al: Cyclosporine A inhibition of microcystin toxins, *Toxicon* 28(5):569, 1990.
400. Suenaga K, Kotoku S: Detection of tetrodotoxin in autopsy material by gas chromatography, *Arch Toxicol* 44:291, 1980.
401. Sugimachi K et al: Acute gastritis clinically classified in accordance with data from both upper GI series and endoscopy, *Scand J Gastroenterol* 19:31, 1984.
402. Sugimachi K et al: Acute gastric anisakiasis: analysis of 178 cases, *JAMA* 253:1012, 1985.
403. Sutherland SK: *Australian animal toxins,* Melbourne, Aust, 1983, Oxford University Press.
404. Svensson B-G et al: Exposure to dioxins and dibenzofurans through the consumption of fish, *N Engl J Med* 324:8, 1991.
405. Swift AEB, Swift TR: The transmission of ciguatera toxicity: another first isn't (letter), *JAMA* 265(18):2339, 1991.
406. Tacket CO et al: Panophthalmitis caused by *Vibrio parahaemolyticus, Clin Microbiol* 16:195, 1982.
407. Tacket CO, Brenner F, Blake PA: Clinical features and an epidemiological study of *Vibrio vulnificus* infections, *J Infect Dis* 149:558, 1984.
408. Tacket CO et al: Diarrhea associated with *Vibrio fluvialis* in the United States, *J Clin Microbiol* 16:991, 1982.
409. Tacket CO, et al: Equine antitoxin use and other factors that predict outcome in type A foodborne botulism, *Am J Med* 76:794, 1984.
410. Tacket CO et al: Wound infections caused by *Vibrio vulnificus,* a marine vibrio, in inland areas of the United States, *J Clin Microbiol* 19:197, 1984.
411. Tamplin M et al: Isolation and characterization of *Vibrio vulnificus* from two Florida estuaries, *Appl Environ Microbiol* 44:1466, 1982.
412. Tauxe RV et al: Turtle-associated salmonellosis in Puerto Rico: hazards of global turtle trade, *JAMA* 254:237, 1985.
413. Taylor FJR: Toxic dinoflagellates: taxonomic and biogeographic aspects with emphasis on *Protogonyaulax.* In Ragelis EP, editor: *Seafood toxins,* Washington, DC, 1984, American Chemical Society.
414. Taylor SL, Hui JY, Lyons DE: Toxicology of scombroid poisoning. In Ragelis EP, editor: *Seafood toxins,* Washington, DC, 1984, American Chemical Society.
415. Taylor SL, Stratton JE, Nordlee JA: Histamine poisoning (scombroid fish poisoning): an allergy-like intoxication, *Clin Toxicol* 27(4&5):225, 1989.
416. Teitelbaum JS et al: Neurologic sequelae of domoic acid intoxication due to the ingestion of contaminated mussels, *N Engl J Med* 322:1781, 1990.
417. Tennessee Department of Health and Environment: *Tennessee Communicable Dis Bull* 18(2):7, 1986.
418. Terao K, Ito E, Yasumoto T: Light and electron microscopic studies of the murine heart after repeated administrations of ciguatoxin or ciguatoxin-4c, *Nat Toxins* 1:19, 1992.
419. Terao K et al: Histopathological studies on experimental marine toxin poisoning. 4. Pathogenesis of experimental maitotoxin poisoning, *Toxicon* 27(9):979, 1989.
420. Terao K et al: Light and electron microscopic studies of pathologic changes induced in mice by ciguatoxin poisoning, *Toxicon* 29(6):633, 1991.
421. Terao K et al: Histopathological studies on experimental marine toxin poisoning. 5. The effects in mice of yessotoxin isolated from *Patinopecten yessoensis* and of a desulfated derivative, *Toxicon* 28(9):1095, 1990.
422. Theiss WC et al: Blood pressure and hepatocellular effects of the cyclic heptapeptide toxin produced by the freshwater cyanobacterium (blue-green alga) *Microcystis aeruginosa* strain PCC-7820, *Toxicon* 26(7):603, 1988.
423. Thong YH et al: Growth inhibition of *Naegleria fowleri* by tetracycline, rifamycin, and miconazole, *Lancet* 2:876, 1977.
424. Thorsteinsson SB, Minuth JN, Musher DM: Clinical manifestations of halophilic non-cholera vibrio infections, *Lancet* 2:1283, 1974.
425. Tindall DR, et al: Ciguatoxigenic dinoflagellates from the Caribbean Sea. In Ragelis EP, editor: *Seafood toxins,* Washington, DC, 1984, American Chemical Society.
426. Tison DL, Kelly MT: *Vibrio vulnificus* endometritis, *J Clin Microbiol* 20:185, 1984.
427. Torda TA, Sinclair E, Ulyatt DB: Puffer fish (tetrodotoxin) poisoning: clinical record and suggested management, *Med J Aust* 1:599, 1973.
428. Tosteson TR, Ballantine DL, Durst D: Seasonal frequency of ciguatoxic barracuda in southwest Puerto Rico, *Toxicon* 26(9):795, 1988.
429. Trainer VL, Baden DG: An enzyme immunoassay for the detection of Florida red tide brevetoxins, *Toxicon* 29(11):1387, 1991.
430. Truwit JD et al: *Vibrio vulnificus* bacteremia with endocarditis, *South Med J* 80(11):1457, 1987.
431. Uragoda CG: Histamine poisoning in tuberculous patients after ingestion of tuna fish, *Am Rev Respir Dis* 121:157, 1980.
432. Valdiserri RO: Intestinal anisakiasis: report of a case and recovery of larvae from market fish, *Am J Clin Pathol* 76:329, 1981.
433. van Egmond HP, Speyers GJA, van den Top HJ: Current situation on worldwide regulations for marine phycotoxins, *J Nat Toxins* 1(1):67, 1992.
434. van Egmond HP et al: Paralytic and diarrhetic shellfish poisons: occurrence in Europe, toxicity, analysis and regulations, *J Nat Toxins* 2(1):41, 1992.
435. Van Thiel PH: A nematode parasitic to herring causing acute abdominal syndromes in man, *Trop Geogr Med* 2:97, 1960.
436. Vietmeyer ND: The preposterous puffer, *Natl Geographic* 166:260, 1984.
437. Vogt RL, Liang AP: Ciguatera fish poisoning—Vermont, *MMWR* 35:263, 1986.
438. Von Graevenitz A, Carrington GO: Halophilic vibrios from extraintestinal lesions in man, *Infection* 1:54, 1973.
439. Wagner KR, Crichton EP: Marine vibrio infections acquired in Canada, *Can Med Assoc J* 124:435, 1981.
440. Wakely JF et al: The occurrence of tetrodotoxin (tarichatoxin) in amphibia and the distribution of the toxin in the organs of newts *(Taricha), Toxicon* 3:195, 1966.
441. Waring N et al: Hypersensitivity reactions to ingested crustacea; clinical evaluation and diagnostic studies in shrimp-sensitive individuals, *J Allergy Clin Immunol* 76:440, 1985.
442. Warpinski JR et al: Fish surface mucin hypersensitivity, *J Wilderness Med* 4:261, 1993.
443. Watabe S et al: Distribution of tritiated tetrodotoxin administered intraperitoneally to pufferfish, *Toxicon* 25(12):1283, 1987.
444. Weber JN: Disaster at Green Island—other outer Pacific Islands may share its fate, *Earth and Mineral Sciences, Penn State University* 38:37, 1969.
445. Weiner BH et al: Inhibition of atherosclerosis by cod-liver oil in a hyperlipidemic swine model, *N Engl J Med* 315:841, 1986.
446. Wellings FM et al: Isolation and identification of pathogenic *Naegleria* from Florida, *Appl Environ Microbiol* 34:661, 1977.
447. White AW: Paralytic shellfish toxins and finfish. In Ragelis EP, editor: *Seafood toxins,* 1984, American Chemical Society.
448. Williams RK, Palafox NA: Treatment of pediatric ciguatera fish poisoning (letter), *Am J Dis Child* 144:747, 1990.
449. Williamson J: Ciguatera and mannitol: a successful treatment (letter), *Med J Aust* 153:306, 1990.
450. Wittner M, Tanowitz HB, Ash LR: Safe sushi (reply) (letter), *N Engl J Med* 321(13):901, 1989.

451. Wittner M et al: Eustrongylidiasis—a parasitic infection acquired by eating sushi, *N Engl J Med* 320(17):1124, 1989.
452. Wongpaitoon V et al: Spontaneous *Vibrio vulnificus* peritonitis and primary sepsis in two patients with alcoholic cirrhosis, *Am J Gastroenterol* 80:706, 1985.
453. Wright AC, Simpson LM, Oliver JD: Role of iron in the pathogenesis of *Vibrio vulnificus* infections, *Infect Immun* 34:503, 1981.
454. Yamashita N et al: Allergenicity of Chironomidae in asthmatic patients, *Ann Allergy* 63:423, 1989.
455. Yasumoto T, Bagnis R, Vernoux JP: Toxicity of the surgeonfishes. II. Properties of the principal water-soluble toxin, *Bull Jpn Soc Sci Fish* 42:359, 1976.
456. Yasumoto T, Kanno K: Occurrence of toxins resembling ciguatoxin, scaritoxin, and maitotoxin in a turban shell, *Bull Jpn Soc Sci Fish* 42:1399, 1976.
457. Yasumoto T, Kao CY: Tetrodotoxin and the Haitian zombie, *Toxicon* 24:747, 1986.
458. Yasumoto T et al: Diarrhetic shellfish poisoning. In Ragelis EP, editor: *Seafood toxins,* Washington, DC, 1984, American Chemical Society.
459. Yentson CM: Paralytic shellfish poisoning: an emerging perspective. In Ragelis EP, editor: *Seafood toxins,* Washington, DC, 1984, American Chemical Society.
460. Yoshida S, Ogawa M, Mizuguchi Y: Relation of capsular materials and colony opacity to virulence of *Vibrio vulnificus, Infect Immun* 47:446, 1985.
461. Yotsu M, Iorizzi M, Yasumoto T: Distribution of tetrodotoxin, 6-epitetrodotoxin, and 11-deoxytetrodotoxin in newts, *Toxicon* 28(2):238, 1990.
462. Yotsu M et al: Production of tetrodotoxin and its derivatives by *Pseudomonas* sp. isolated from the skin of a pufferfish, *Toxicon* 25(2):225, 1987.
463. Yotsu-Yamashita M, Mebs D, Yasumoto T: Tetrodotoxin and its analogues in extracts from the toad *Atelopus oxyrhynchus* (family: Bufonidae), *Toxicon* 30(11):1489, 1992.
464. Yunginger JW: Food antigens in food allergy. In Metcalfe DD, Sampson HA, Simon RA, editors: *Food allergy; adverse reactions to foods and food additives,* Boston, 1991, Blackwell Scientific Publications.
465. Zakaria-Meehan Z et al: Ability of *Vibrio vulnificus* to obtain iron from hemoglobin-haptoglobin complexes, *Infect Immun* 56:275, 1988.

ADDITIONAL RECOMMENDED READINGS

Anderson DM, Sullivan JJ, Reguera B: Paralytic shellfish poisoning in northwest Spain: the toxicity of the dinoflagellate *Gymnodinium catenatum, Toxicon* 27(6):665, 1989.

Benedek C, Rivier L: Evidence for the presence of tetrodotoxin in a powder used in Haiti for zombification, *Toxicon* 27(4):473, 1989.

Endean R et al: Multiple toxins in a specimen of the narrow-barred Spanish mackerel *Scomberomorus commersoni, Toxicon* 31(2):195, 1993.

Kaufman B et al: Protection against tetrodotoxin and saxitoxin intoxication by a cross-protective rabbit anti-tetrodotoxin antiserum, *Toxicon* 29(6):581, 1991.

Miller DM, editor: *Ciguatera seafood toxins,* Boca Raton, Fla, 1991, CRC Press.

Tu AT, editor: *Toxin-related diseases: poisons originating from plants, animals and spoilage,* New Delhi, India, 1993, Oxford & IBH Publishing.

Watanabe MF et al: Toxins contained in *Microcystis* species of cyanobacteria (blue-green algae), *Toxicon* 26(11):1017, 1988.

54 AQUATIC SKIN DISORDERS

Paul S. Auerbach

Physicians now appreciate that dermatitis originating from the aquatic environment merits investigation. In many cases, the toxicity of the plant or animal varies with the location and season. To date, the evolutionary advantage for stinging creatures or plants is not entirely clear. The emergency physician must always consider an aquatic origin for an acute and painful skin irritation or indolent infection.

Dermatitis Caused by Sponges

Dermatitis caused by sponges is discussed in Chapter 52.

Dermatitis Caused by Seaweed

Seaweed dermatitis is divided into two types: the "animal" plant (taxonomy is confusing) variety, including sea moss (mat) dermatitis, and the marine plant variety, including Hawaiian dermatitis caused by algae.[33]

SEA MOSS DERMATITIS (DOGGER BANK ITCH)

Dogger Bank itch is an eczematous dermatitis caused by the sea-chervil, *Alcyondium hirsutum,* a seaweedlike animal colony. North Sea fishermen contact sea mosses, or sea mats, as they are drawn up within fishing nets. Large quantities of sea-chervil are often harvested and then returned to the ocean.

Clinical Aspects

The irritation first appears on the hands and often disappears when the fisherman goes ashore. However, with recurrent exposures the attacks become more severe, characterized by a vesiculated and edematous eruption of the hands, arms, legs, and face. It is not clear whether this is an allergic reaction, a view supported by positive patch test reactions with an extract from the causative marine animals and negative controls, or an irritant dermatitis, supported by the fact that all crew members may acquire the rash, except for the cook.[84] Proper protective clothing may prevent recurrence.

Treatment

Treatment is the same as for mild rhus dermatitis. Depending on the severity of the reaction, the physician may use oral corticosteroids, topical fluorinated corticosteroids, calamine lotion, or oral antihistamines. A dilute (26%) isopropyl alcohol in calamine lotion may be soothing.

SEAWEED DERMATITIS CAUSED BY ALGAE

Seaweed dermatitis is almost always secondary to irritation from algae, of which more than 25,000 species are known. They are loosely defined as chlorophyll-bearing organisms (and colorless species), which are thalloid (without true roots, stems, or leaves). They vary in size, shape, and color. Some are equipped with flagella and propel themselves through water.[118] They range from microscopic diatoms (1 μm in length) to kelp plants (100 m in length).[7] Algae are found in all marine environments and are extremely adaptive to temperature and depth variation. For instance, one form of blue-green algae thrives at hot spring temperatures of 160° F; others dwell in frigid Arctic water. Although sunlight can penetrate only to a depth of 900 feet in the ocean, some blue-green algae exist at depths of up to 12,000 feet.

The blue-green alga *Microcoleus lyngbyaceus* (formerly *Lyngbya majuscula*) has strains of varying toxicity, often within geographic proximity. The stinging seaweed is dark green or olive colored, drab, and finely filamentous, occurring in abundance at depths of up to 100 feet (Color Plate 138).[107] It grows in hairlike masses or mats throughout the Pacific and Indian Oceans and Caribbean Sea, although large epidemics of seaweed dermatitis have been reported only in Hawaii and Okinawa.[54] Outbreaks of *Microcoleus*-induced dermatitis occur from March to September in Florida and June to September in Hawaii. In Hawaii the largest reported series involved windward beaches.[41] The assumption is that strong currents and winds dislodge the alga from its normal habitat, fragment it, and blow the fragments into the surf line.[54]

M. lyngbyaceus produces a dermatonecrotic and potent inflammatory agent called debromoaplysiatoxin, as well as an indole alkaloid dermatitis-producing toxin called lyngbyatoxin A.[19,82,108] An indole stain identifies the presence of lyngbyatoxin A; a radioimmunoassay is under development.[54]

Clinical Aspects

Typically a victim swimming in water infested with plant life (the water may appear turbid) does not remove his or her wet bathing suit for a while after leaving the water. In minutes to hours a pruritic, burning, moist, and erythematous rash develops in a bathing suit distribution, followed by bullous escharotic desquamation in the genital, perineal, and perianal regions. Differentiating this reaction from sea bather's eruption (which is attributed to larval anemone organisms) may be difficult. There have also been occasional outbreaks of similar skin reactions after exposure to freshwater blue-green algae.[22,48] Oral and ocular mucous membrane lesions, facial rash, conjunctivitis, and perhaps interstitial pulmonary edema have been attributed to *M. lyngbyaceus*.[54,107]

Treatment

The treatment is vigorous irrigation with soap and warm water, followed by isopropyl alcohol rinses and topical medium- to high-potency steroid application. Severe cases may require systemic corticosteroids (prednisone, 20 to 60 mg daily tapered over 2 weeks). Prevention is essential. Persons who swim in algae-abundant areas should shower with soap and water and wash all swimwear immediately after leaving the water.

Infections Caused by Achlorophyllic Algae (Protothecosis)

Human and animal infections are caused by achlorophyllic mutants of the green alga *Chlorella*. Species of *Prototheca* can be found in fresh and marine water, trees, animals, soil, and sewage treatment systems.[83,119] Three species of *Prototheca* are recognized: *P. stagnora, P. wickerhamii,* and *P. zopfii*. *P. filamenta* has been reclassified to genus *Fissuricella*.[4,21,83,92] *P. zopfii* and *P. wickerhamii* have been demonstrated as pathogens in humans.[24,68] The condition is most likely to follow barefoot walks in swampy areas, aquarium management, contamination of preexisting wounds with dirty water or soil, or exposure of skin to water from a contaminated supply.[83] Although widespread visceral disease has been noted in animals, infections in humans have been limited to skin, subcutaneous tissue, and regional lymphatics. Most victims cannot identify the portal of entry. Human protothecosis has been reported worldwide.

Clinical Aspects

The disease takes two forms, either a papular or eczematoid dermatitis in immunosuppressed individuals, or a localized infection of the olecranon bursa in individuals with normal immunity.[83] In the former the initial lesion is a nodule or tender red papule, which enlarges, becomes pustular, and ulcerates. A purulent, malodorous, blood-tinged discharge may be present. Satellite lesions usually develop and frequently become confluent. The lesions may become verrucous and resemble chromomycosis. Regional lymph nodes may develop metastatic granulomas. The lesions develop centrifugally and may occasionally disseminate. In the olecranon bursitis form the infection develops several weeks after an injury to the elbow and is localized to the bursa with overlying sinus tracts.[83] At least one case of chlorellosis has occurred, with the report of a granulomatous reaction of the human foot.[61] The diagnosis is made through histologic sections and culture. The organisms are spherical, basophilic, and gram positive, vary in diameter from 3 to 15 μm *(P. wickerhamii)* or 7 to 30 μm *(P. zopfii)*, and stain well with Grocott-Gomori methenamine silver nitrate, colloidal iron for acid mucopolysaccharides, and periodic acid–Schiff. Larger organisms have thick walls and characteristic internal septation. *Prototheca* grows on Sabouraud agar, blood agar, or brain-heart infusion agar at an optimum temperature of 30° to 32° C. The colonies are cream colored and yeastlike. The organisms are microaerophilic and reproduce in 1 to 2 days.[10,63] Antisera for identification of species of *Prototheca* can be used on fresh or formalin-fixed tissues.[117]

Treatment

Unfortunately, the disease is chronic and progressive. Topical medications are unsatisfactory. There is early indication that parenteral therapy with amphotericin B and tetracycline may be effective.[79,91,123,124] Experience with ketoconazole has been variable.[79,89] Early excision (bursectomy) may be curative.

Blue-Green Algae Poisoning

In freshwater environments, warm weather can cause the rapid growth of blue-green algae (group Cyanophyta) in a "bloom."[111] Species such as *Microcystis aeruginosa, Anabaena spiroides,* and *Anabaena flos-aquae* have been implicated in acute poisoning and death in birds and cattle. While ingestion of contaminated water may cause considerable animal mortality, human exposures to date have been limited to reports of local effects, including conjunctivitis, ear infection, lip swelling, papulovesicular dermatitis, and gastroenteritis.[14,71] Therapy is supportive.

Dermatitis Caused by Schistosomes and Other Marine Worms

SCHISTOSOMIASIS

There are two types of human schistosomiasis: (1) a cutaneous affliction (cercarial dermatitis or "swimmer's itch") caused by nonhuman schistosomes for which humans are abnormal hosts, and (2) visceral schistosomiasis (bilharziasis), a serious systemic disorder caused by the human blood flukes *Schistosoma mansoni, S. japonicum,* and *S. haematobium.* This discussion is limited to the cutaneous variety; however, when human blood flukes penetrate the skin during the invasive stage of visceral schistosomiasis, an eruption that mimics the purely cutaneous syndrome is occasionally provoked.

Cercarial Dermatitis

Cercarial dermatitis is an infestation that results from penetration of the skin by the cercariae of avian, rodent, or ungulate schistosomes (of the genera *Trichobilharzia, Ornithobilharzia, Gigantobilharzia, Orientobilharzia, Austrobilharzia,* and *Bilharziella*.[3,51,78,98] A milder and rare variety has also been noted with *S. mansoni* and *S. haematobium,* but not with *S. japonicum.* The cercariae are immature larval forms, usually microscopic, of the parasitic flatworms. The geographic distribution is worldwide, occurring in Arctic, temperate, and tropical zones and in fresh and salt water. Although serious infestation is uncommon in North America, cercarial dermatitis is a vexing problem in certain U.S. locations and has been documented in Massachusetts, Rhode Island, Connecticut, New York, Florida, Louisiana, California, Texas, Oregon, Washington, North Dakota, Nebraska, Iowa, Wisconsin, Minnesota, Michigan, and Ohio.[8] Most commonly, snails and birds that inhabit the lakes of Wisconsin, Michigan, Manitoba, and neighboring north central states are the intermediate hosts for these trematodes.[81]

Various synonyms, including "Pearl Harbor itch," "sawah itch," "el Caribe," "Koganbyo," "lakeside disease," "clam digger's itch," "swimmer's itch," "collector's itch," and "sea bather's eruption," have been used interchangeably with cercarial dermatitis.[8] Many observers insist on a clear distinction between swimmer's itch and sea bather's eruption, limiting the former to eruptions on exposed areas and the latter to dermatitis that results from ocean bathing. Sea bather's eruption is now known to be caused by the larvae of anenomes and thimble jellyfish and probably other coelenterate species. This disorder is fully discussed in Chapter 52. Environmental conditions that may favor human infestation with any cause of marine dermatitis related to floating flora and fauna include areas with abundant submerged vegetation, seaweed in the surf, strong shoreward winds, and hot weather.[8]

Ecologic Cycle

Cercarial dermatitis results when humans become interlopers in the complex life cycle. The adult schistosomes are blood parasites of birds or mammals. The schistosome eggs are excreted in animal feces. Swimming miracidia hatch from these eggs and then infest certain species of snails, which serve as intermediate hosts. After incubation in the snails and passage through two sporocyst stages, approximately 200,000 fork-tailed cercariae (infective larvae) are released into the water.[8] A specific warm-blooded host is entered, and the parasites mature in the vascular system, unless humans accidentally intrude into the life cycle at the cercaria stage. When the adult worms produce eggs, the cycle restarts.

Clinical Aspects

Schistosome cercarial dermatitis is a skin infestation that triggers an immune response in the human, an unnatural host. Although penetration of cercariae may occur in the water, it usually occurs as the film of water evaporates on the skin. The cercariae penetrate the epidermis but cannot travel beyond the papillary dermis. Histologic examination reveals intraepithelial burrows and abscesses surrounded by an infiltrate of eosinophils, polymorphonuclear leukocytes, and lymphocytes.[135] The cercariae are walled off and destroyed within 10 to 20 hours in the epithelial layers of the skin, where they initiate the destructive inflammatory reaction.[8] Cercariae are not seen in serial histologic sections unless the biopsy is taken within 24 hours of penetration.[16] The victim initially experiences a prickling sensation. Itching occurs 4 to 60 minutes after the cercariae penetrate the skin, accompanied by erythema and mild edema. The initial urticarial reaction subsides over 60 minutes, leaving red macules that become papular and more pruritic over the next 10 to 15 hours. Discrete and highly pruritic papules of 3 to 5 mm, surrounded by a zone of erythema, are typical of this disorder. Vesicles, which may become pustules, frequently form within 48 hours. These may persist for 7 to 14 days.[51] The eruption occurs primarily on exposed areas of the body. Excoriation leads to pustulation, crusting, and secondary infection. The inflammatory response peaks within 3 days and subsides slowly over 1 to 2 weeks. The reaction is more severe in persons who have had a previous episode, suggesting sensitization.

Treatment

In mild cases, application of isopropyl alcohol or equal parts of isopropyl alcohol and calamine lotion controls the itching. Severe cases may require systemic corticosteroids (prednisone, 20 to 60 mg daily tapered over 2 weeks). Secondary bacterial infections, which are frequently caused by *Staphylococcus aureus* or *Streptococcus* species, may be managed with topical antibacterial ointments (for example, bacitracin) or systemic antibiotics (such as erythromycin sustained release, 333 mg three times a day for 8 to 10 days).

Some prevention may be obtained by brisk rubbing with a rough, dry towel immediately on leaving the water to remove the water droplets that harbor the cercariae. Washing the skin with rubbing alcohol or soap and water after bathing is not effective.[8] Previously, copper sulfate was used as a molluscicide in cercariae-infested lakes, but this has been recognized as an environmental hazard.[8] Niclosamide does not contain heavy metals and is applied as a molluscicide in 5% granular form to bathing areas. Preliminary experiments indicate that niclosamide applied to the skin prevents penetration of cercariae.[8]

Sea Bather's Eruption

Sea bather's eruption is a dermatitis that results from contact with ocean water but is not traceable to cercarial penetration or seaweed dermatitis, although it resembles both syndromes.[86] It involves covered areas of the body and is caused by the larval form of the sea anemone *Edwardsia leidyi* and related species.[11]

The eruption occurs a few hours after bathing and consists of pruritic, erythematous wheals or papules that persist for 1 to 3 days and then involute spontaneously. The areas involved include the buttocks, genital region, and breasts (women). Individual lesions resemble insect bites. In children with extensive eruptions, fever is common.

The disorder is self-limited and rarely persists beyond 10 days. Treatment is palliative and consists of calamine lotion with 1% menthol. Unlike other marine dermatoses, sea bather's eruption may respond to topical steroids, since the pathology seems to be limited to the epidermis and the superficial dermis. In more severe cases, oral or parenteral antihistamines or systemic corticosteroids may be used. A thorough soap and water scrub after leaving the water provides partial prophylaxis.[11] For a more complete discussion, see Chapter 52.

Leeches

Leeches are members of the phylum Annelida, class Hirudinea, found in fresh water in the midwestern and northeastern United States. Other species are marine or terrestrial. They attach to the skin of the victim with jaws that allow the introduction of an anticoagulant (hirudin), which causes moderate painless bleeding at the site of removal. Leeches feed until they are engorged, then fall off. The usual victims of leech bites are persons walking through streams or marshes. In some areas of the world, leeches are still used medicinally.

Clinical Aspects

The wound bleeds freely and heals slowly in unsensitized individuals. Lesions frequently become secondarily infected. If sensitization has developed, the reaction to the bite may be urticarial, bullous, or necrotic. The bite of a leech can cause a serious allergic reaction, including anaphylaxis.[49]

Treatment

Removal of a leech may be facilitated by application of a few drops of brine, alcohol, or strong vinegar, or a match flame near the site of attachment.[33] The leech should never be ripped off the skin, since the jaws may remain and induce phagedena. After removal of the leech the wound site should be closely inspected for retained mouthparts. Although the bleeding stops with pressure, hemostasis can be hastened by the application of a styptic pencil, topical thrombin solution, or oxidized regenerated cellulose absorbable hemostat. Wounds should be cleansed several times daily with an antiseptic to prevent infection.

Marine Annelid Dermatitis

BRISTLE WORM DERMATITIS

Irritations caused by bristle worms are discussed in Chapter 52.

WORM BITES

Worm bites are discussed in Chapter 52.

Dermatitis Caused by Other Macroscopic Organisms

SEA LOUSE DERMATITIS (CYMOTHOIDISM)

Sea "lice" (cymothoids) are small marine crustaceans of the order Isopoda, suborder Cymothoidra. Water skiers, skin divers, and swimmers who frequent the coastal waters of temperate and tropical seas may encounter these free-swimming crustaceans.[12] The creatures often are buried in the sandy bottom. Equipped with powerful biting parts, they attach to fish, feet, or inquisitive hands.[12] Sea lice bites are common along the coast of southern California. The bite is rapid and sharp, with a noticeable punctate hemorrhage. The injury resolves over 5 to 7 days. It should be cleaned initially with hydrogen peroxide or a brisk soap and water scrub, coated lightly with an antiseptic ointment, and inspected daily for secondary infection.

CUTANEOUS LARVA MIGRANS

Cutaneous larva migrans ("creeping eruption") is a cutaneous eruption caused by the larvae of various nematode parasites for which humans are an abnormal final host. The following are the more common species responsible: *Ancylostoma braziliensis* in the central and southeastern United States, *A. caninum, Uncinaria stenocephala* (hookworm), and *Bunostomum phlebotomum* (hookworm of cattle). A transient creeping eruption also results from the larvae of the human hookworms *Ancylostoma duodenale* and *Necator americanus*.

The ova are deposited in the soil and hatch into larvae, which penetrate human skin. Sandy, warm, and shady areas are favorable soil locations. Persons commonly affected include ocean bathers, children, gardeners, farmers, and those who work under buildings.

In humans, the larvae penetrate the skin but are unable to penetrate the dermis. The larvae migrate between the dermis and the epidermis, producing superficial serpiginous tunnels. The feet and buttocks are most commonly involved. Some larvae remain quiescent for a few weeks or months, after which migration is manifested by a wandering, thin, linear, raised, and tunnel-like lesion 2 to 3 mm in width. Older lesions become dry and crusted. Pruritus may be marked. The larvae move a few millimeters to a few centimeters each day. Larva migrans may be associated with eosinophilia (10% to 35%) and Loeffler's syndrome.

Larva currens is a special form of cutaneous larva migrans caused by *Strongyloides stercoralis*. Usually, the eruption is associated with intestinal strongyloidiasis and begins in the perianal skin. It may involve the buttocks, thighs, back, and shoulders, but the genitalia are spared. Pruritus is intense, and the lesions spread as rapidly as 5 to 10 cm/hr. The larvae leave the skin, enter the bloodstream, and later settle in the intestinal mucosa, while the rash fades.

Treatment of cutaneous larva migrans includes cryotherapy with ethyl chloride for very mild infestations, topical thiabendazole in more refractory cases, and oral thiabendazole (25 to 50 mg/kg) for 2 to 4 days in more severe cases. Secondary infection is not uncommon, which may require incision and drainage of pustules or furuncles and the use of topical and systemic antibiotics.

In endemic areas precautions include (1) avoidance of sitting or lying on damp soil or sand, especially during rainy seasons, (2) not walking barefoot, (3) draping the ground with impenetrable material before crawling in the dirt, and (4) covering sandboxes with a tarpaulin to prevent contamination by prowling cats.

SOAPFISH DERMATITIS

The soapfish (family Grammistidae) *Rypticus saponaceus* receives its name from the soapy mucus it releases when handled or disturbed (Fig. 54-1). Fishermen in the Caribbean know that a soapfish held in a restricted volume of seawater with other fishes often causes death of the other fish.[46] Human contact results in dermatitis. The skin irritant is called grammistin; similar substances have been isolated from boxfishes and sea bass species.[15,46] Treatment consists of cold compresses of Burow's solution to alleviate the burning and itching. In severe cases, topical corticosteroids are beneficial.

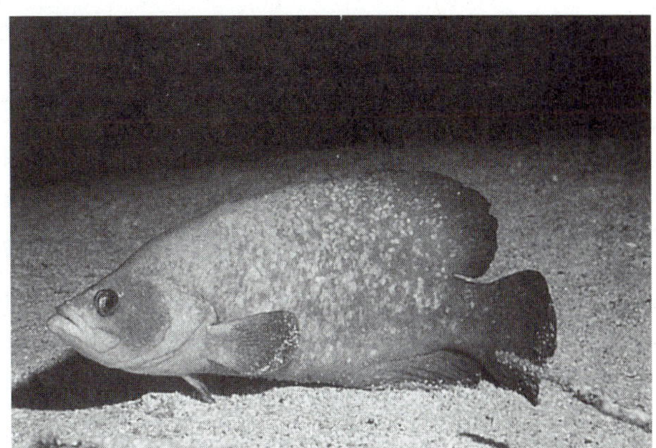

Fig. 54-1 Soapfish *(Rypticus saponaceus).* Skin contact with soapy mucus causes dermatitis. (Photo by Carl Roessler.)

Dermatitis and Infections Caused by Marine Bacteria

MYCOBACTERIUM MARINUM

Skin granulomas ("swimming pool" granulomas) caused by *Mycobacterium marinum* were first described in 1954 by Linell and Norden.[72] The lesions resembled tuberculosis verrucosa cutis.

M. marinum is a so-called atypical (anonymous or unclassified) bacterium. Typical mycobacteria are animal pathogens that cannot multiply outside the animal host, while atypical mycobacteria are free-living soil and water saprophytes, rarely pathogens. *M. marinum* is an acid-fast, rod-shaped bacillus, a Runyon group 1 photochromogen that produces yellow-orange pigment after light exposure. It grows optimally at 31° to 33° C; therefore human infections are limited to the cooler acral skin and rarely involve deeper and warmer lymphatic or lymph node structures. Swimming pool chlorination provides little protection, since the organism is relatively resistant to chlorine.

Infections may occur after exposure to either fresh or salt water in aquariums, fish bites (commercial or captive wild animals), or swimming pools.[7,23,33,36,60] *M. marinum* invades tissue through a preexisting skin lesion. In one variety of presentation, 7 to 10 days after sustaining a puncture wound or laceration, particularly of the cooler distal extremity, a localized area of cellulitis develops that may progress in the absence of appropriate treatment to localized arthritis, bony erosion, formation of subcutaneous nodules, and superficial desquamation.[7,52,133] Aspiration of a joint effusion may reveal the acid-fast bacilli. Alternatively, within 3 to 4 weeks after the primary inoculation, a red papule develops, which slowly increases in size to become a hard purple nodule. This is frequently scaly, ulcerated, and verrucous with a violaceous base, resembling tuberculosis verrucosa cutis.[33,69,74,101,106] The lesion may enlarge to 6 cm in diameter, although 1 to 2 cm is more common. New lesions may develop in a pattern that resembles sporotrichosis, with dermal granulomas in a linear distribution along the superficial lymphatics. The granuloma may become secondarily infected, resulting in cellulitis or lymphangitis. The differential diagnosis should include sporotrichosis, cutaneous leishmaniasis, psoriasis, verrucous lichen planus, verruca vulgaris, iodine and bromine granulomas, sarcoidosis, paratuberculosis, syphilis, gout, other cutaneous mycobacterioses, and chronic pyogenic infections.[58]

The diagnosis of *M. marinum* granuloma is confirmed bacteriologically by isolation of the organism from a homogenized skin biopsy (minimum 4 mm punch) specimen on standard mycobacterial culture medium (Lowenstein-Jensen) at 31° to 33° C, rather than the standard 37° C.[58,132] Acid-fast bacilli are visualized directly in only 10% to 13% of biopsies, and approximately 50% of cultures are positive.[30] Cutaneous intradermal skin tests show cross-reactivity between *Mycobacterium marinum* and *M. tuberculosis.*

Treatment should be conservative, since most lesions heal spontaneously within 2 to 3 years, generally with some scarring and residual pigmentation. Some small lesions are easily excised. Although there have been few reports of prompt diagnosis and successful treatment with antibiotics before surgical biopsy, the astute physician may recognize the initial presentation.[7] Minocycline (100 mg twice a day for 2 to 4 months) or tetracycline (2 g daily for 2 to 4 months) is currently recommended.[58,66,74] Numerous drug combinations, such as ethambutol-ethionamide-cycloserine, may afford symptomatic relief, but before antituberculous chemotherapeutic agents are initiated, drug sensitivities of the isolated organisms should be determined because of the high rate of drug resistance.[33,69,74,101,106] Trimethoprim-sulfamethoxazole has also been recommended. Although the organism is sensitive to heat, heat therapy is no longer recommended. While small lesions are easily excised, excision may be complicated by local recurrences. Intralesional steroids are contraindicated.

ERYSIPELOTHRIX RHUSIOPATHIAE

Erysipeloid is an acute infection of traumatized skin caused by a slender gram-positive bacillus (rod), *Erysipelothrix rhusiopathiae* (formerly *E. insidiosa*). It occurs in fishermen, butchers, and others who handle raw fish, poultry, or meat products. Also called "speck finger," "fish handlers' disease," "blubber finger," and less commonly, "erysipeloid of Rosenbach," the condition is common on the Atlantic coast in workers who handle crabs and live fish.[35,38,43,96,107] The bacillus is facultatively aerobic and nonmotile and does not have spores or capsules. It is hardy enough to survive saltwater or freshwater exposure, drying, salting, pickling, and smoking, and it may be found alive after 12 days in direct sunlight, 4 months in putrefied flesh, and 9 months in a buried carcass.[43]

Erysipelothrix enters the skin through a puncture wound or abrasion, usually on the finger or hand. Within 2 to 7 days a violaceous, raised area appears and enlarges, accompanied by pain and itching. Low-grade fever and malaise are not uncommon; bacteremia, severe generalized cutaneous infections, and endocarditis are rare.[33,43]

Within 1 to 7 days after a puncture wound a hallmark lesion develops. The puncture wound takes on the appearance of a minor purplish red skin irritation or infected paronychia, with edema and a small amount of purulent discharge. This is surrounded by an area of relative central fading or noninvolvement ("clearing"), surrounded by a classical centripetally advancing, raised, well-demarcated, and marginated erythematous or violaceous ring (Color Plate 139). Usually on the finger or hand, the lesion is warm and tender, with characteristic progression up the dorsal edge of the finger into the web space and descent along the adjoining finger.[130] The lesion is painful and often pruritic, and regional lymph nodes may be inflamed. Pitting and suppuration are absent.[43] The infection seldom affects the palm. Although the infection is generally limited to the hand, it may spread to the wrist or forearm.[67] Systemic symptoms such as fever and mild malaise may develop. In the diffuse cutaneous form, the local lesion enlarges and dissemination results in multiple satellite lesions distant from the original site, occasionally with vesiculation or formation of large bullae.[28]

Erysipelothrix may be cultured from the erysipeloid lesion by excising a pinch biopsy or by injecting sterile (not bacteriostatic) saline into the edge of the lesion and then reaspirating without withdrawing the needle.[130] The specimen should be immediately placed for transport into an infusion broth containing 1% glucose. The microbiology laboratory should be alerted to the suspicion for presence of *E. rhusiopathiae,* since it is closely related bacteriologically to *Listeria monocytogenes* and *Corynebacterium* species and may be easily confused with streptococci or diphtheroids.[43] Untreated, erysipeloid usually runs its course within 3 weeks. For isolated skin involvement, penicillin VK (250 to 500 mg orally four times a day), cephalexin (250 mg orally four times a day), or erythromycin (333 mg orally three times a day) are rapidly effective.[9] *E. rhusiopathiae* is resistant to aminoglycoside antibiotics.[105] If arthritis, septicemia, or endocarditis is present, aqueous penicillin G should be administered in a dose of 2 to 4 million units intravenously every 4 hours for 4 to 6 weeks.

VIBRIO SPECIES

Vibrio infections are discussed in Chapter 53.

Dermatitis and Infections Caused by Freshwater Bacteria

AEROMONAS HYDROPHILA

Aeromonas hydrophila is a gram-negative, facultatively anaerobic, polarly flagellated, non-spore-forming, motile rod member of the family Vibrionaceae that commonly inhabits soil, freshwater streams, and lakes.* *Aeromonas* species are widely distributed and found at wide ranges of temperature and pH.[47,126] Three species *(A. hydrophila, A. sobia,* and *A. caviae)* have been associated with human disease; there are seven or more distinct genotypes. Soft tissue and gastroenteric human infections occur predominantly during the period from May to November.[56,126] A wound, particularly of the puncture variety, immersed in contaminated water may become cellulitic within 24 hours, with erythema, edema, and a purulent discharge. The lower extremity is most frequently involved. This usually occurs from stepping on a foreign object or being punctured under water.[102] The appearance may be indistinguishable from a typical streptococcal cellulitis, with localized pain, lymphangitis, fever, and chills.[45,65,127] Untreated or managed with antibiotics to which the organism is not susceptible, this may rarely progress to a severe gas-forming soft tissue reaction, bulla formation, necrotizing myositis, or osteomyelitis.[26,37,64,70] Appearance similar to ecthyma gangrenosum caused by *Pseudomonas aeruginosa* has been reported in *Aeromonas* septicemia.[134] In a manner analogous to the pathogenicity of virulent *Vibrio* species, the chronically ill or immunocompromised host is probably at greater risk of a severe complication, such as meningitis, endocarditis, or septicemia.† Freshwater aspiration may result in *Aeromonas hydrophila* pneumonitis and bacteremia.[93] Infection has followed the bite of an alligator.[97] A 15-year-old boy suffered *A. hydrophila* wound infection after a bite from his pet piranha.[94] For unknown reasons there is a marked preponderance of male patients.[6] This may represent the phenotypic variation of critical bacterial adhesins.

Gram's stain of the purulent discharge may demonstrate gram-negative bacilli. Given the appropriate clinical setting (after a wound acquired in the freshwater environment), this should not be casually attributed to contamination.[65] *Aeromonas hydrophila* is generally sensitive to chloramphenicol, gentamicin, tobramycin, tetracycline, trimethoprim-sulfamethoxazole, cefotaxime, moxalactam, imipenem, ceftazidime, and ciprofloxacin.[5,31,32,64,87] In one case, culture of a severe wound infection demonstrated the presence of two species, *Aeromonas hydophila* and *A. sobia.*[62] Notably, the latter was resistant to tetracycline in vitro. Initial therapy for a severe infection that includes an aminoglycoside provides coverage against concomitant *Pseudomonas* or *Serratia* infection.[45] As has been demonstrated with *Vibrio* species, the first-generation cephalosporins, penicillin, and ampicillin are not efficacious, perhaps because of the production of a β-lactamase by the organism.[5,17,31,32,87] Because of the microbiologic similarity of *Aeromonas* on biochemical testing to members of the Enterobacteriaceae family, such as *Escherichia coli* or *Serratia* species, it is important to alert the laboratory to the clinical setting.

Initial therapy of a severe soft tissue infection related to *Aeromonas* should include aggressive wound debridement to mitigate the potentially invasive nature of the organism.

Curiously, medicinal leeches can harbor *Aeromonas* in their gut flora; soft tissue infections related to this phenomenon have been reported.[128] The genus *Plesiomonas* also belongs to the family Vibrionaceae; it has been definitively linked with aquarium-associated infection complicated by watery diarrhea and fever.[120]

*References 37, 45, 62, 64, 97, 127.

†References 27, 37, 64, 70, 73, 105, 134.

CHROMOBACTERIUM VIOLACEUM

Chromobacterium violaceum is a mesophilic (prefers 20° to 37° C), gram-negative, saprophytic bacterium with both polarly and laterally placed flagella. It shows violet pigmentation (violacein) with oxidative and fermentative glucose use. An abundant inhabitant of tropical and subtropical freshwater rivers and soil, it usually enters the victim through a skin injury.[57,85,112] The skin manifestations are secondary to systemic disease and include suppurative lymphadenitis, lung and liver abscesses, osteomyelitis, and sepsis.[76,112,121,125] Bacteremia leads to a diffuse pustular dermatitis; *C. violaceum* can be cultured from both blood and pustules.[112] Other skin manifestations include vesicles, ecchymotic maculae, maculopapular rash, ulcers, subcutaneous nodules, cellulitis, lymphangitis, and digital gangrene.[76] Persons at particular risk for severe infection are those with chronic granulomatous disease, characterized by the inability of granulocytes and monocytes to convert oxygen into hydrogen peroxide and other oxygen metabolites necessary for microbicidal activity.[40,59,76] The mortality rate is high; as of 1986, only three persons were reported to have survived human infection.[116] The organism is sensitive in vitro to carbenicillin, chloramphenicol, tetracycline, gentamicin, kanamycin, tobramycin, and trimethoprim-sulfamethoxazole. Notably, resistance to cephalothin and ampicillin has been reported.[112,116]

HOT TUB (PSEUDOMONAS AERUGINOSA) DERMATITIS

Numerous cases of "hot tub" or "whirlpool" dermatitis have been described.[20,99,129] The eruptions occurred after the use of motel whirlpools, hot tubs, swimming pools, and even water slides.* *Pseudomonas aeruginosa* (predominantly serotype 0-11), a nonfermentative, obligate aerobic, gram-negative bacillus, has been implicated as the causative agent. *P. aeruginosa* infects healthy moistened skin. The high water temperature, hydrated skin, high concentration of organisms, and chemical irritants in the water all contribute to this dermatitis. Deficiencies in disinfection have been found in several outbreaks.

The folliculitic rash appears within 48 hours of the exposure and resolves within 7 days without treatment. The eruption is most pronounced in areas covered by bathing garments and spares the head and neck (unless they are submerged). Other symptoms include external otitis, conjunctivitis, tender breasts, enlarged tender lymph nodes, fever, and malaise.[100] The erythematous, maculopapular, and vesiculopustular eruption is usually accompanied by pruritus.

Because the eruption is self-limited (7 to 14 days), treatment should be conservative. The pruritus may be managed by drying lotions such as calamine or with oral antihistamines. In severe cases a course of antibiotic therapy may be warranted. Rapid progression to severe skin disease (such as hemorrhagic bullae), pneumonia, or septicemia suggests immunosuppression.[29,39,95,100,109] Showering does not appear to prevent the disorder.[100]

Other infections that have been acquired in closed-cycle recreational water systems include eczema herpeticum and molluscum contagiosum. Whether viral afflictions after water exposure are caused by diminished host resistance from skin hyperhydration or by an unusual presentation of pathogens remains to be determined.

Reactions to Diving Equipment

Allergic reactions to underwater masks and mouthpieces are common dermatologic problems.[2] "Mask burn" may range from a minor reddish imprint of the mask on the face to severe, vesicular, weeping eruption. Mouthpieces to regulators and snorkels similarly may produce severe intraoral inflammation and ulceration. Glossitis is common. Chemical constituents in the equipment may be the causative allergens.[2] Rubber mouthpieces and masks contain antioxidants similar to those that cause contact dermatitis in surgeons who cannot tolerate rubber gloves. Mercaptobenzothiazol, tetramethylthiuram, and isopropyl paraphenylene diamine have been implicated in such reactions.[35] *N*-isopropyl-*N*-phenyl-paraphenylenediamine, a rubber antioxidant, has been demonstrated to cause scuba mask facial dermatitis.[77,122] Both irritant and allergic reactions to diving equipment may occur.[33]

Acute facial dermatitis may be treated with cool compresses of Burow's solution and oral systemic corticosteroids (prednisone, 30 to 50 mg daily tapered over 7 to 10 days). For serious intraoral reactions, a twice daily mouthwash of equal parts of antihistamine elixir (diphenhydramine) and milk of magnesia may be efficacious.[35] Individual sores may be coated twice daily and at bedtime with triamcinolone acetonide (0.1%) dental paste (Kenalog in Orabase) for 5 to 7 days. The problem may be avoided at the outset by using silicone rubber hypoallergenic masks and mouthpieces.

Allergies to wet suits may reflect sensitivity to thiourea, which is used to bond the nylon lining to the rubber diving suit.[1,34,35]

Water-Induced Itching (Aquagenic Pruritus)

Common causes of nonspecific water-induced itching include xerosis or eczema, aquagenic urticaria (described below), cholinergic urticaria, cold urticaria, heat urticaria, vibratory urticaria, symptomatic dermographism, polycythemia rubra vera, aquagenic pruritus of the elderly, and aquagenic pruritus.[113] Water-induced itching (aquagenic pruritus) is a condition in which contact with water at any temperature causes intense itching without visible skin changes.[42] Criteria for the diagnosis of aquagenic pruritus include the following: (1) severe pruritus, prickling, stinging, or burning consistently develops after water contact, regardless of the water temperature; (2) the discomfort develops within minutes after water contact; (3) no visible skin changes occur; (4) no concurrent skin disease, internal disorder, or medication use can explain the discomfort; (5) aquagenic, cholinergic, cold, heat, pressure, and vibratory urticaria, and symptomatic dermographism are excluded; and (6) polycythemia rubra vera is excluded.[113]

The discomfort lasts from 10 to 120 minutes and is usually severe. Commonly the head, palms, and soles are spared.[114] An irritable mood swing often accompanies the itching. Postulated causes have included increased local mast cell degranulation, acetylcholine release, and increased cutaneous fibrinolytic activity.[42,75] There is no consistently effective therapy. Variable success has been reported with systemic antihistamines, ultraviolet B irradiation, protective application of petrolatum ointment, and sodium bicarbonate soaks.[113] Excessive contact with water should be avoided.

Aquagenic Urticaria

Aquagenic urticaria occurs when contact of the skin with water at any temperature causes an immediate urticarial eruption at the sites of contact.[88,103] Patients demonstrate punctate perifollicular wheals 1 to 2 mm in diameter 10 to 30 minutes after exposure to water, usually confined to the neck, upper torso, and arms.[88] Itching commonly precedes the rash. Although local levels of histamine are elevated, dermatographism is not present and serum IgE levels are

*References 44, 53, 55, 80, 90, 99, 100, 110, 129, 137.

normal.[104] Familial aquagenic urticaria has been reported, as has been a combination of aquagenic and cholinergic urticaria.[13,25] Systemic complications do not occur. The syndrome can largely be prevented by the application of petrolatum ointment to the skin.[104] Oral antihistamines may be of some value.

Otitis Externa (Swimmer's Ear)

After sunburn, otitis externa ("swimmer's ear") accounts for the termination of more ocean holidays than any other physical disorder. As the name implies, the affliction affects the external ear canal. As described by Strauss, the adult canal is a cul-de-sac lined with stratified squamous epithelium of approximately 5 mm in diameter and 25 mm in length. The outer third is protected from infection by the production of an acidic waxy mantle, not present to the same degree on the thinner and more delicate epithelium of the inner two thirds.[115] Factors that predispose to the development of an infection include constant moisture (it is difficult to dry the ear), warm (body) temperature, introduction of microorganisms, occlusion of the canal (ecostoses, cerumen plugs, entrapped particles of sand, earplugs), trauma (mechanical attempts to clean the ear canal), intrinsic dermatoses (allergic conditions, eczema, psoriasis, contact and seborrheic dermatitis, neurodermatitis), degradation of cerumen, and variation of pH (normal 4 to 5). The usual bacterial pathogens are *Staphylococcus aureus* and *Pseudomonas aeruginosa*.[50,136] Otitis externa does not appear to be associated with bacterial indicators of recreational water quality such as fecal coliform bacteria, enterococci, or *P. aeruginosa* organisms.[18] The initial symptoms of external otitis are itching, mild pain, and rarely, decreased hearing. There may be a sensation of "fullness" in the affected ear. As the inflammation progresses, the pain worsens, so that the victim complains bitterly and is markedly uncomfortable when the tragus is pressed or the earlobe tugged. Severe infections proceed to cellulitis, with purulent discharge, occlusion of the canal, cervical lymphadenopathy, headache, nausea, fever, and toxemia. Suppuration in the ear canal may discharge toward the surrounding skin, causing a secondary periauricular irritant contact dermatitis. Another complication is cellulitis of the periauricular soft tissues that may include the parotid gland and temperomandibular joint.

Treatment is based on the degree of severity. A mild case (slight pain and discharge) may be treated with ear drops alone. Antibiotics are not generally necessary at this stage. An excellent topical preparation is nonaqueous acetic acid (VoSol Otic). Colistin sulfate has been recommended to directly combat *Pseudomonas*.[13] The use of acetic acid or acetic acid with hydrocortisone 1% (VoSol HC) avoids the issue of sensitization associated with neomycin. Products not currently recommended include antipyrine, benzocaine, camphor, ichthammol, and thymol.[115] The most important issue of topical therapy is reacidification and desiccation of the ear canal, which can be accomplished with a mixture of alcohol and acetic acid (vinegar) or Burow's solution (Domeboro: aluminum sulfate and calcium acetate). Oily solutions should be avoided.

If the ear canal is swollen so that drops do not penetrate the distance, a gauze wick should be placed and kept soaked with the topical solution for 24 to 72 hours. If adenopathy, profuse purulent discharge, or fever is present, oral trimethoprim-sulfamethoxazole or amoxicillin-clavulanate should be administered. If the infection does not resolve or rapidly accelerates, intravenous antibiotics may be necessary.

The most important preventive measure is to diminish moisture retention in the external ear canal (for example, tilt and shake the head to one side, use a hair dryer). Cotton-tipped applicators should not be used to extract moisture because they can damage the ear lining or press cerumen deeply into the canal. Cerumen-softening products do not help because they soften hardened or impacted cerumen without removing it. A trained professional can remove it with irrigations or curettement. Acidifying and desiccating agents (97% absolute alcohol and 3% acetic acid) are effective prophylaxis. External otitis is often prevented by a brief rinse with common rubbing alcohol, household vinegar, or both after each entry into the water. Earplugs should be avoided because they may produce ischemia of the canal lining. Petroleum jelly or other substances aimed to form a watertight seal should be avoided, since they may act as a moisture trap for debris.

REFERENCES

1. Adams RM: Contact allergic dermatitis due to diethylthiourea in a wetsuit, *Contact Dermatitis* 8:277, 1982.
2. Alexander JE: Allergic reactions to mask skirts, regulator mouthpieces, and snorkel mouthpieces, *Pressure* 5:10, 1976.
3. Appleton CC: Schistosome dermatitis: an unrecognized problem in South Africa? *S Afr Med J* 65:467, 1984.
4. Arnold P, Ahearn DG: The systematics of the genus *Prototheca* with a description of a new species *P. filamenta, Mycologia* 64:265, 1972.
5. Auerbach PS et al: Bacteriology of the freshwater environment: implications for clinical therapy, *Ann Emerg Med* 16:1016, 1987.
6. Baddour LM: Extraintestinal *Aeromonas* infections—looking for Mr. Sandbar, *Mayo Clin Proc* 67:496, 1992.
7. Bailey JP et al: *Mycobacterium marinum:* a fishy story, *JAMA* 247:1314, 1982.
8. Baird JK, Wear DJ, Connor DH: Cercarial dermatitis—the swimmer's itch, *Clin Dermatol* 5(3):88, 1987.
9. Barber M, Nellen M, Zoob M: Erysipeloid of Rosenbach: response to penicillin, *Lancet* 1:125, 1946.
10. Berkhoff HA, Connelly MR, Lockett LJ: Differential microbiological diagnosis of protothecosis from nonhuman sources, *Am J Med Technol* 48:609, 1982.
11. Bernhardt MJ, Mandojana RM: Seabather's eruption, *Clin Dermatol* 5(3):101, 1987.
12. Best WC, Sablan RG: Cymothoidism (sea louse dermatitis), *Arch Dermatol* 90:177, 1964.
13. Bonnetblanc JM et al: Familial aquagenic urticaria, *Dermatologica* 158:468, 1979.
14. Bourke ATC, Hawes RB: Freshwater cyanobacteria (blue-green algae) and human health, *Med J Aust* 1:491, 1983.

15. Boylan DB, Scheuer PJ: Pahutoxin: a fish poison, *Science* 155:52, 1967.
16. Brackett S: Pathology of schistosome dermatitis, *Arch Dermatol* 42:410, 1940.
17. Bugler RJ, Sherris JC: The clinical significance of *Aeromonas hydrophila:* a report of two cases, *Arch Intern Med* 118:562, 1966.
18. Calderon R, Mood EW: An epidemiological assessment of water quality and "swimmer's ear," *Arch Environ Health* 37:300, 1982.
19. Cardellina JH, Marner FJ, Moore RE: Seaweed dermatitis: structure of lyngbyatoxin A, *Science* 204:193, 1979.
20. Centers for Disease Control: Pool-associated rash illness—North Carolina, *MMWR* 24:349, 1975.
21. Chandler FW, Kaplan W, Callaway CS: Differentiation between *Prototheca* and morphologically similar green algae in tissue, *Arch Pathol Lab Med* 102:353, 1978.
22. Cohen SG, Reif CB: Cutaneous sensitization to blue-green algae, *J Allergy* 24:452, 1953.
23. Cott RE, Carter DM, Sall T: Cutaneous disease caused by atypical mycobacteria, *Arch Dermatol* 95:259, 1967.
24. Davies RR, Spencer H, Wakelin PO: A case of human protothecosis, *Trans R Soc Trop Med Hyg* 58:448, 1964.
25. Davis RS et al: Evaluation of a patient with both aquagenic and cholinergic urticaria, *J Allergy Clin Immunol* 68:479, 1979.
26. Davis WA, Kane JH, Garagusi VF: Human *Aeromonas* infections: a review of the literature and a case report of endocarditis, *Medicine* 57:267, 1978.
27. Dean HM, Post RM: Fatal infection with *Aeromonas hydrophila* in a patient with acute myelogenous leukemia, *Ann Intern Med* 66:1177, 1967.
28. Ehrlich JC: *Erysipelothrix rhusopathiae* infection in man, *Arch Intern Med* 78:565, 1944.
29. El Baze P et al: *Pseudeomonas aeruginosa* 0-11 folliculitis, *Arch Dermatol* 212:873, 1985.
30. Even-Paz Z et al: *Mycobacterium marinum* skin infections mimicking cutaneous leishmaniasis, *Br J Dermatol* 94:435, 1976.
31. Fainstein V, Weaver S, Bodey GP: In vitro susceptibilities of *Aeromonas hydrophila* against new antibiotics, *Antimicrob Agents Chemother* 22:513, 1982.
32. Fass RJ, Barnishan J: In vitro susceptibilities of *Aeromonas hydrophila* to 32 antimicrobial agents, *Antimicrob Agents Chemother* 19:357, 1981.
33. Fisher AA: *Atlas of aquatic dermatology,* New York, 1978, Grune & Stratton.
34. Fisher AA: Water related dermatoses, *Cutis* 25:132, 1980.
35. Fisher AA: Contact dermatitis to diving equipment, swimming pool chemicals, and other aquatic denizens, *Clin Dermatol* 5(3):36, 1987.
36. Flowers DJ: Human infection due to *Mycobacterium marinum* after a dolphin bite, *J Clin Pathol* 23:475, 1970.
37. Fulghum DD, Linton WR Jr, Taplin D: Fatal *Aeromonas hydrophila* infection of the skin, *South Med J* 71:739, 1978.
38. Gilchrist TC: Erysipeloid, with a record of 322 cases, of which 239 were caused by crab bites or lesions produced by crabs, *J Cut Dis* 22:507, 1904.
39. Goett KD, Fowler V: Hot tub acquired *Pseudomonas* septicemia, *J Assoc Milit Dermatol* 10:40, 1984.
40. Good RA et al: Fatal (chronic) granulomatous disease of childhood: a hereditary defect of leukocyte function, *Semin Hematol* 5:215, 1968.
41. Grauer FH, Arnold HL: Seaweed dermatitis: first report of a dermatitis-producing marine alga, *Arch Dermatol* 84:720, 1961.
42. Greaves MW et al: Aquagenic pruritus, *Br Med J* 282:2008, 1981.
43. Grieco MH, Sheldon C: *Erysipelothrix rhusopathiae, Ann NY Acad Sci* 174:523, 1970.
44. Gustafson TL et al: *Pseudomonas* folliculitis: an outbreak and review, *Rev Infect Dis* 5:1, 1983.
45. Hanson PG et al: Freshwater wound infection due to *Aeromonas hydrophila, JAMA* 238:1053, 1977.
46. Hashimoto Y, Kamiya H: Occurrence of a toxic substance in the skin of a sea bass *Pogonoperca punctata, Toxicon* 7:65, 1969.
47. Hazen TC et al: Prevalence and distribution of *Aeromonas hydrophila* in the United States, *Appl Microbiol* 36:731, 1978.
48. Heise HA: Symptoms of hay fever caused by algae. II. Microcystis: another form of algae producing allergenic reactions, *Ann Allergy* 9:100, 1951.
49. Heldt TJ: Allergy to leeches, *Henry Ford Hosp Med J* 9:498, 1961.
50. Hoadley AF, Knight DE: External otitis among swimmers and nonswimmers, *Arch Environ Health* 30:445, 1975.
51. Hoeffler DF: Cercarial dermatitis: its etiology, epidemiology, and clinical aspects, *Arch Environ Health* 29:225, 1974.
52. Hoffman GS et al: Septic arthritis associated with *Mycobacterium avium:* a case report and literature review, *J Rheumatol* 5:199, 1978.
53. Hopkins RS, Abbott DO, Wallace LE: Follicular dermatitis outbreak caused by *Pseudomonas aeruginosa* associated with a motel's indoor swimming pool, *Public Health Rep* 96:246, 1981.
54. Izumi AK, Moore RE: Seaweed *(Lyngbya majuscula)* dermatitis, *Clin Dermatol* 5(3):92, 1987.
55. Jacobson JA: Pool-associated *Pseudomonas aeruginosa* dermatitis and other bathing-associated infections, *Infect Control* 6:398, 1985.
56. Janda JM, Bottone EJ, Reitano M: *Aeromonas* species in clinical microbiology: significance, epidemiology, and speciation, *Diagn Microbiol Infect Dis* 1:221, 1983.
57. Johnson WM, Disalvo AP, Steuer RR: Fatal *Chromobacterium violaceum* septicemia, *Am J Clin Pathol* 56:400, 1971.
58. Johnston JM, Izumi AK: Cutaneous *Mycobacterium marinum* infection ("swimming pool granuloma"), *Clin Dermatol* 5(3), 1987.
59. Johnston RB, Baehner RL: Chronic granulomatous disease: correlation between pathogenesis and clinical findings, *Pediatrics* 48:730, 1971.
60. Johnston RG, Fung J: Bacterial flora of wild and captive porpoises, *J Occup Med* 11:276, 1969.
61. Jones J et al: Green algal infection in a human, *Am J Clin Pathol* 80:102, 1983.
62. Joseph SW et al: *Aeromonas* primary wound infection of a diver in polluted waters, *J Clin Microbiol* 10:46, 1979.
63. Kapica L: First case of human protothecosis in Canada: laboratory aspects, *Mycopathologia* 73:43, 1981.
64. Karam GH, Ackley AM, Dismukes WE: Posttraumatic *Aeromonas hydrophila* osteomyelitis, *Arch Intern Med* 143:2073, 1983.
65. Katz D, Smith H: *Aeromonas hydrophila* infection of a puncture wound, *Ann Emerg Med* 9:529, 1980.
66. Kim R: Tetracycline therapy for atypical mycobacterial granuloma, *Arch Dermatol* 110:299, 1974.
67. Klauder JV: Erysipeloid as an occupational disease, *JAMA* 111:1345, 1938.
68. Klintworth GK, Fetter BF, Nielson HS Jr: Protothecosis, an algal infection: report of a case in man, *J Med Microbiol* 1:211, 1968.
69. Knox JM et al: Atypical acid-fast organism of the skin, *Arch Dermatol* 84:386, 1961.
70. Levin ML: Gas-forming *Aeromonas hydrophila* in a diabetic, *Postgrad Med* 54:127, 1973.
71. Linell F, Norden A: *Mycobacterium balnei, Acta Tuberc Scand Suppl* 33:1, 1954.
72. Lippy EC, Erb J: Gastrointestinal illness at Sewickley, Pennsylvania, *J Am Water Works Assoc* 68:606, 1976.
73. Lopez JF, Quesada J, Saied A: Bacteremia and osteomyelitis due to *Aeromonas hydrophila, Am J Clin Pathol* 50:587, 1968.
74. Loria PR: Minocycline hydrochloride treatment for atypical acid-fast infection, *Arch Dermatol* 112:517, 1976.
75. Lotti T et al: Increased cutaneous fibrinolytic activity in a case of aquagenic pruritus, *Int J Dermatol* 23:61, 1984.
76. Macher AM, Casale TB, Fauci AS: Chronic granulomatous disease of childhood and *Chromobacterium violaceum* infections in the southeastern United States, *Ann Intern Med* 97:51, 1982.

77. Mahmoud AAF: Schistosomiasis. In Warren KS, Mahmoud AAF, editors: *Tropical and geographical medicine,* New York, 1984, McGraw-Hill.
78. Maibach H: Scuba diver facial dermatitis: allergic contact dermatitis to *N*-isopropyl-*N*-phenylparaphenylenediamine, *Contact Dermatitis* 1:330, 1975.
79. McAnally T, Parry EL: Cutaneous protothecosis presenting as recurrent chromomycosis, *Arch Dermatol* 121:1066, 1985.
80. McCausland WJ, Cox PJ: *Pseudomonas* infection traced to motel whirlpool, *J Environ Sci Health* 37:455, 1975.
81. McMullen DB, Brackett S: Distribution and control of schistosome dermatitis in Wisconsin and Michigan, *Am J Trop Med* 21:725, 1941.
82. Mynderse JS, et al: Antileukemia activity in the Oscillatoriaceae: isolation of debromoaplysiatoxin from *Lyngbya, Science* 196:538, 1977.
83. Nelson AM, Neaflie RC, Connor DH: Cutaneous protothecosis and chlorellosis, extraordinary opportunistic "aquatic-borne" algal infections, *Clin Dermatol* 5(3):76, 1987.
84. Newhouse ML: Dogger Bank itch: survey of trawlermen, *Br Med J* 1:1142, 1966.
85. Ognibene AJ, Thomas E: Fatal infection due to *Chromobacterium violaceum* in Vietnam, *Am J Clin Pathol* 54:607, 1970.
86. Osment LS: Update: seabather's eruption and swimmer's itch, *Cutis* 18:545, 1976.
87. Overman TL: Antimicrobial susceptibility of *Aeromonas hydrophila, Antimicrob Agents Chemother* 17:612, 1980.
88. Panconesi E, Lotti T: Aquagenic urticaria, *Clin Dermatol* 5(3):49, 1987.
89. Pegram PS et al: Successful ketoconazole treatment of protothecosis with ketoconazole-associated hepatotoxicity, *Arch Intern Med* 143:1802, 1983.
90. Perrotta DM et al: An outbreak of *Pseudomonas* folliculitis associated with a waterslide—Utah, *JAMA* 250:1259, 1983.
91. Phair JP et al: Phagocytosis and algacidal activity of human polymorphonuclear neutrophils against *Prototheca wickerhamii, J Infect Dis* 144:72, 1981.
92. Pore RS, D'Amato RF, Ajello L: *Fissuricella gen* Nov.: a new taxon for *Prototheca filamenta, Sabouradia* 15:69, 1977.
93. Reines HD, Cook F: Pneumonia and bacteremia due to *Aeromonas hydrophila, Chest* 30:264, 1981.
94. Revord ME, Goldfarb J, Shurin SB: *Aeromonas hydrophila* wound infection in a patient with cyclic neutropenia following a piranha bite (letter), *Pediatr Infect Dis J* 7(1):70, 1988.
95. Rose HD et al: *Pseudomonas pneumonia* associated with use of a home whirlpool spa, *JAMA* 250:2027, 1983.
96. Rosenbach FJ: Experimentelle morphologische und blinische studie uber die krankheitserregenden microorganismen des schweinrotlaufs, des erysepiloids und der mausesepsis, *Hyg Infectionschr* 63:343, 1909.
97. Rosenthal SG, Bernhardt HE, Phillips JA III: *Aeromonas hydrophila* wound infection, *Plast Reconstr Surg* 53:77, 1974.
98. Sabha GH, Malek EA: Dermatitis caused by cercariae of *Orientobilharzia turkestanicum* in the Caspian Sea area of Iran, *Am J Trop Med Hyg* 28:912, 1979.
99. Sausker WF: *Pseudomonas aeruginosa* folliculitis ("splash rash"), *Clin Dermatol* 5(3):62, 1987.
100. Sausker WF et al: *Pseudomonas* folliculitis acquired from a health spa whirlpool, *JAMA* 239:2362, 1978.
101. Schaeffer WB, Davis CL: A bacteriologic and histopathologic study of skin granuloma due to *Mycobacterium balnei, Am Rev Respir Dis* 84:837, 1961.
102. Semel JD, Trenholme G: *Aeromonas hydrophila* water-associated traumatic wound infections: a review, *J Trauma* 30(3):324, 1990.
103. Shelley WB, Rawnsley HM: Aquagenic urticaria: contact sensitivity reaction to water, *JAMA* 189:895, 1964.
104. Sibbald RG et al: Aquagenic urticaria: evidence of cholinergic and histaminergic basis, *Br J Dermatol* 105:297, 1981.
105. Simerkoff MS, Rahal JJ Jr: Acute and subacute endocarditis due to *Erysipelothrix rhusopathiae, Am J Med Sci* 266:53, 1973.
106. Sims JK: Dangerous marine life. In Shilling CW, Carlston CB, Mathias RA, editors: *The physician's guide to diving medicine,* New York, 1984, Plenum Press.
107. Sims JK, Zandee Van Rilland RD: Escharotic stomatitis caused by the "stinging seaweed" *Microcoleus lyngbyaceus* (formerly *Lyngbya majuscula*)—a case report and review of literature, *Hawaii Med J* 40:243, 1981.
108. Solomon AE, Stoughton RB: Dermatitis from purified sea algae toxin (debromoaplysiatoxin), *Arch Dermatol* 114:1333, 1979.
109. Spiers ASD, Tattersall MHN, Goya H: Indications for systemic antibiotic prophylaxis in neurotropenic patients, *Br Med J* 4:440, 1974.
110. Spitalny KC, Vogt RL, Witherall LE: National survey on outbreaks associated with whirlpool spas, *Am J Public Health* 74:725, 1978.
111. Spoerke DG, Rumack BH: Blue-green algae poisoning, *J Emerg Med* 2:353, 1985.
112. Starr AJ et al: *Chromobacterium violaceum* presenting as a surgical emergency, *South Med J* 74:1137, 1981.
113. Steinman HK: Water-induced pruritus, *Clin Dermatol* 5(3):41, 1987.
114. Steinman HK, Greaves MW: Aquagenic pruritus, *J Am Acad Dermatol* 13:91, 1985.
115. Strauss MB, Dierker RL: Otitis externa associated with aquatic activities (swimmer's ear), *Clin Dermatol* 5(3):103, 1987.
116. Suarez AE et al: Nonfatal chromobacterial sepsis, *South Med J* 79:1146, 1986.
117. Sudman MS, Kaplan W: Identification of *Prototheca* species by immunofluorescence, *Appl Microbiol* 25:981, 1973.
118. Tiffany HL: *Algae, the grass of many waters,* Springfield, Ill, 1968, Charles C Thomas.
119. Tindal JP, Fetter BF: Infection caused by achloric algae (protothecosis), *Arch Dermatol* 104:490, 1911.
120. Tippen PS, Meyer A, Blank EC: Aquarium-associated *Plesiomonas shigelloides* infection—Missouri, *MMWR* 38(36):617, 1989.
121. Tucker RF, Winter WG, Wilson HD: Osteomyelitis associated with *Chromobacterium violaceum* infection, *Bone Joint Surg* 61A:949, 1979.
122. Tyup E, Mitchell JC: Scuba diver facial dermatitis, *Contact Dermatitis* 9:334, 1983.
123. Venezio FR et al: Progressive cutaneous protothecosis, *Am J Clin Pathol* 77:485, 1982.
124. Vernon SE, Goldman LS: Protothecosis in the southeastern United States, *South Med J* 76:949, 1983.
125. Victoria B, Baer H, Ayoub EM: Successful treatment of systemic *Chromobacterium violaceum* infection, *JAMA* 230:580, 1974.
126. Von Graevenitz A: *Aeromonas* and *Plesiomonas.* In Lennett EH et al, editors: *Manual of clinical microbiology,* Washington, DC, 1985, American Society for Microbiology.
127. Von Graevenitz A, Mensch AH: The genus *Aeromonas* in human bacteriology: report of 30 cases and review of the literature, *N Engl J Med* 278:245, 1968.
128. Voss LM, Rhodes KH, Johnson KA: Musculoskeletal and soft tissue *Aeromonas* infection: an environmental disease, *Mayo Clin Proc* 67:422, 1992.
129. Washburn J et al: *Pseudomonas aeruginosa* rash associated with a whirlpool, *JAMA* 235:2205, 1976.
130. Weaver RE: *Erysipelothrix.* In Lennette EH et al, editors: *Manual of clinical microbiology,* Washington, DC, 1985, American Society of Microbiology.
131. Werner SB: *Aeromonas* wound infections associated with outdoor activities—California, *MMWR* 39(20):334, 1990.
132. Williams CS, Riordan DC: *Mycobacterium marinum* (atypical acid-fast bacillus) infections of the hand, *J Bone Joint Surg Am* 55:1042, 1973.

133. Winter FE, Ruyon EH: Prepatellar bursitis caused by *Mycobacterium marinum (balnei), J Bone Joint Surg Am* 47:375, 1965.
134. Wolff RL, Wiseman SL, Kitchens CS: *Aeromonas hydrophila* bacteremia in ambulatory immunocompromised hosts, *Am J Med* 68:238, 1980.
135. Wood MG, Srolovitz H, Schetman D: Schistosomiasis: paraplegia and ectopic skin lesions as admission symptoms, *Arch Dermatol* 112:690, 1976.
136. Wright DN, Alexander JM: Effect of water on the bacterial flora of swimmers' ears, *Arch Otolaryngol* 99:15, 1974.
137. Zacherle BJ, Silver DS: Hot tub folliculitis: a clinical syndrome, *West J Med* 137:191, 1982.

55 MEDICAL LIABILITY AND WILDERNESS EMERGENCIES

Gregory L. Henry
Edward R. Stein

The Problem

Medical emergencies are often not a prominent focus in planning a wilderness excursion. The majority of people who take part in strenuous and potentially hazardous wilderness activities are young and healthy adventurers with a tendency for risk taking. For outdoor activity planners, the potential for liability exists as it does for any planned activity. The location of activity is relatively unimportant. If, for example, an excursion is organized in the United States that eventually travels to Kathmandu, the court system of the United States would be used if a liability question should arise. Activities planned and directed from the United States would be considered a business operation and would fall under the laws of the organizing jurisdiction. Should there be litigants from multiple states or provinces, the federal court system of the United States would handle the matter. No matter where an unexpected medical problem takes place, a U.S. citizen has an arena in which to air grievances.

Trip physicians and organizers should not plan around the possibility of a liability situation. The most reasonable assumption is that a liability situation *will* exist and that proper precautions must be taken to ensure that all involved are protected. The real issues for wilderness organizers revolve around the questions of the extent to which Good Samaritan laws prevail, physician preparedness, physician activities, and organizational liability and activities.

Case Discussion

Physicians involved in the provision of services outside the usual medical settings tend to view the prospects of a liability situation as distant. The presentation of an actual case illustrates the problems that a physician can encounter when acting in what appears to be an innocuous and good-hearted manner. In the case *Boccasile et al, v. Cajun Music Ltd., et al,* all the major elements and problems are brought together.[1] Briefly described, the facts in this case are that an emergency physician had volunteered to serve in the medical tent at a folk music festival in a neighboring state. The physician showed up as promised and received essentially free entry and a T-shirt as compensation. During the presentation, spectators came running to the tent saying that a patron was suffering some type of severe medical reaction in the field. With no emergency transportation available, the physician went out to the scene and found that a young man who was known to be allergic to seafood had consumed some shrimp gumbo and had gone into anaphylactic shock. The patient's airway began to close, and multiple attempts in the field to ventilate the patient were unsuccessful. Another patron was allergic to bee stings and was carrying a bee sting kit. The patient was administered the epinephrine from that kit, but to no avail, and died.

The allegations against the emergency physician were multiple. Besides claims of actual medical malfeasance was a litany of charges against almost everyone involved. The sponsors of the music festival were sued for having inadequate medical personnel, transportation services, and equipment on site. They also had no written emergency response program and no organized system for managing medical problems. The physician was charged not only with acts of medical negligence, but also with not being prepared to manage an emergency. The emergency physician, being out of the emergency department, was not covered by the standard malpractice policy, which was location specific. The insurance company for the music festival had a clause in the contract that specifically provided that they would not cover negligent acts of professionals associated with the festival. They were to be considered subcontractors, not employees.

The emergency physician, using his own attorney, brought a motion for dismissal based on Good Samaritan principles. This case was initially denied at the trial court level because (1) the physician had accepted his responsibilities and therefore had a duty to provide medical care at the festival; (2) the physician had received compensation, although it could be considered minimal, and such compensation further solidified the contract and the duty to provide service; and (3) the physician knew, or should have known, that in his capacity as festival physician he might need to respond to emergencies, and that preparation for such emergencies would lie with the medical personnel present.

This case is actual and ongoing. The issues raised, although not precisely applicable to wilderness expeditions, certainly have all the elements that would prompt any physician to consider the exact burden he or she assumes when agreeing to serve in any type of stand-by physician capacity.

American Legal System and Medical Malpractice

Before understanding the nuances and details of liability with regard to wilderness outfitting, understanding the general legal framework in which all parties must participate is important. The legal system of the United States consists of a gigantic maze of complex rules that purport to regulate almost all phases of human contact. A brief description of the legal system may help to explain how, where, and why law and medicine interact or, as some view it, collide.

Conceptually, the legal system is divided into substantive law, which sets forth rules for people to follow, and procedural law, which governs disputes about compliance with substantive law. For example, a substantive rule permits private ownership of property and another substantive rule proscribes theft of property. The corner grocer owns the apples displayed in front of his store, and it is unlawful for someone to take one of the apples without paying for it. When someone is accused of theft, procedural law dictates how to decide whether the accused is guilty. Procedural law describes how the accused should be charged, his rights, who decides guilt, and what and how information may be used to make that decision.

The legal system is also divided into criminal and civil spheres. Criminal law deals with activities that society has proscribed. When committing a proscribed act, that person may be punished. Proscribed activities include trivial acts (misdemeanors) and more serious acts (felonies). In theory at least, the more serious the act, the more severe the punishment.

Civil law, rather than proscribing certain activities, prescribes what conduct *should* be. When failing to measure up to the law's prescription, a person is not "punished," but anyone damaged by the shortcoming must be compensated.

Confusion arises because the criminal-civil dichotomy is not always clear, since some acts violate both criminal and civil substantive law. For example, when Smith, for no good reason, punches Jones in the nose, Smith has committed a crime and criminal proceedings may be instituted against him. This requires that the government bring charges and prove them beyond a reasonable doubt. If found guilty, Smith may be punished by a fine, imprisonment, or both. In addition, Smith has violated civil law and Jones may institute a civil action against him. In his suit, Jones would be required to prove his case by a preponderance of evidence and, if successful, would be entitled to receive payment (damages) from Smith as compensation for his injuries.

The law pertaining to the conduct of people toward each other is known as the law of "torts." Tort law provides that people should act reasonably toward one another. One person injured because of another person's unreasonable conduct is entitled to compensation. Unreasonable conduct may be intentional or unintentional. Unintentional and unreasonable conduct is considered "negligence."

Although tort law is somewhat different in each of the 50 states, the concept of reasonableness is common to all states. The law provides that each of us is under a duty to act reasonably toward another person in circumstances in which foreseeable unreasonable action could lead to injury. If a person breaches his or her duty to act reasonably, and the breach *causes* injury to another person, the injured person may legally acquire compensation for damages.

When a person charges that another has committed a tort, the trier of fact (a jury or judge) must decide whether the plaintiff has proven, by a preponderance of the evidence, breach of a duty to act reasonably that caused the injury or damage. Where the defendant is accused of acting unreasonably with respect to an everyday activity, a judge or juror can determine reasonableness based on his or her own experience. If the defendant is a professional person engaged in an occupation about which the trier of fact knows little or nothing and cannot make an informed decision about reasonableness, the tort is known as "professional negligence" or "malpractice." The law provides that a professional defendant is held to the standard of reasonableness of his or her own profession (the "standard of practice"). In all states, subject to vagaries of language, a person charged with malpractice is charged with failing to perform at the minimum level of practice that his or her profession considers reasonable.

To prevail in a medical malpractice action, the plaintiff must prove that the defendant physician violated the standard of practice of the medical profession and that the violation resulted in damages to the plaintiff. In almost all instances the plaintiff must prove these elements through expert testimony, because the trier of fact would otherwise have no frame of reference within which to make an informed judgment. The plaintiff is compelled to present the testimony of someone, usually a physician in the same area of practice as the defendant, who by virtue of training, skill, or experience knows what the standard of practice was and can testify that the defendant's conduct violated the standard of practice and caused injury to the plaintiff.

These elements of malpractice law form a very small part of the law of torts, which itself is a relatively small part of the civil-substantive law of the 50 states. The basic principles of tort law were incorporated into American law from English case-made or "common" law. Common law is based on the principle of *stare decisis,* which provides that once a court has decided a controversy in a certain way, it will decide further similar controversies in the same way (legal precedent). Hundreds of years ago, a long forgotten judge first ruled that physicians would be held to a standard of professional reasonableness rather than ordinary reasonableness, a proposition followed until the present day. Lawyers being what they are, 101 exceptions have been grafted onto the rule, but the rule remains "the law."

The common law of each of the 50 states is the product of the appellate courts. The decisions of trial courts are not binding on one another, but the decisions of appellate courts are supposed to be binding on the lower, trial courts. Where a lawyer is confronted with an appellate case that is contrary to his or her position, the lawyer will attempt to "distinguish" the case, that is, to show that the facts of his or her case are so different from the facts of the appellate case that the appellate case has no precedential value. If a judge rules a "distinction without a difference," the appellate case is considered to be a binding precedent.

A case arrives in appellate court when one side, usually the loser, feels that the trial was flawed. Usually a case can be reversed on appeal only if the appellate judge feels that the trial judge misapplied the law. The appellate courts usually publish their decisions, which are the "cases" that form the common law. The cases of the appellate courts of one state are not binding on the courts of another state. Although the laws among the 50 states are similar, many significant differences exist.

In addition to the 50 sets of state common law, a system of federal courts in the United States creates case-made law. The relationship between federal and state law is complex and largely irrelevant to this discussion because substantive tort law is almost always a matter of state concern.

In addition to case-made common law, law may be created by a legislative "statute" from the elected representatives. It is at least of equal importance with and can supersede common law. The change in many states to a no-fault automobile accident reparation system is an example of legislation changing hallowed precepts of common law.

Once a legislature has passed a statute, the courts cannot change that law except by declaring it unconstitutional. The constitution of each state is the supreme law of that state, and the Constitution of the United States is the supreme law of the land. The courts, pursuant to the principle of "judicial review," have the last say on whether a given law is constitutional. In addition to rendering opinions based on the constitutionality of statutes, courts are frequently asked to interpret statutes.

The relationship between common and legislative law is important in the area of medical malpractice. In response to recent "crises" regarding malpractice, some state legislatures have made radical changes in common law tort principles. Presuit screening panels, mandatory arbitration, and caps on damages have been passed by a number of state legislatures. In some instances a state supreme court has ruled such legislation unconstitutional, while another state supreme court has found similar legislation to be constitutional. In these latter cases the legislature has succeeded in significantly changing common law.

Common law can be changed not only by a legislature, but also by the courts pursuant to the principle of "enough is enough." For example, for many years a plaintiff in a medical malpractice action was required to prove that a defendant physician violated the standard of medical practice in the defendant's community. This proved difficult where the defendant was one of two specialists in a community, with the other one his partner. The chances of a plaintiff's finding a specialist who was knowledgeable of the standard of practice in that particular community, and willing to testify against the defendant, were remote. During the 1970s the appellate courts of many states recognized this problem and that the standard of specialty practice is fairly uniform across the United States. The common law was therefore changed so that a plaintiff must prove that a physician violated the standard of practice not of a specific community, but of his or her specialty.[4]

Civil procedural law may come from either judges or legislatures. Each state has its own set of rules of civil procedure, and a separate set exists for the federal courts. Although the great majority of civil procedural rules apply to all civil cases, in recent years attempts have been made to redress physicians' grievances by creating special procedural rules applicable only to medical malpractice cases. Several state legislatures have considered setting specific requirements for expert witnesses testifying in medical malpractice cases. The constitutionality of such malpractice-only rules of procedure is usually challenged.

Good Samaritan Laws and Existing State Statutes

Under common law within the jurisdictions of the United States, a physician has no duty to render aid at the scene of a medical emergency. However, most states have recognized that encouraging physicians and other health care personnel to become involved is good public policy, even when help is not mandated by law. Good Samaritan statutes have been enacted in virtually all jurisdictions but do not totally provide immunity from suit. A physician who undertakes a Good Samaritan activity should understand that he or she can essentially be sued by anyone for anything. However, under most Good Samaritan laws a successful suit requires that the physician be guilty of gross or willful negligence. Attempts made in several jurisdictions to get the acts of physicians who supply services to emergency departments deemed as Good Samaritan activities have universally been rejected. A summation of these decisions would state that three conditions must be met for Good Samaritan immunity to be invoked. The first is that the emergency aid applied must be unscheduled or unplanned; second, that aid must be provided at or near the scene where the illness or injury occurs; and third, that the physician must act without compensation and outside of the legal scope of his or her employment.

Understanding the natural reluctance of physicians to be involved in legal entanglements, Vermont acted under statutory law to compel a physician response and eliminate the filing of malpractice actions, with the Duty to Aid the Endangered Act. This statute requires medical personnel to stop at the scene of an accident and specifically provides immunity from legal actions.

Consent and Abandonment

Even in the emergency out-of-hospital situation, a physician has two other major legal concepts to consider when providing emergency care. These are consent and abandonment.

CONSENT

Consent involves all aspects of medical care. In 1914, Justice Cardozo of the Supreme Court of the State of New York said, "Every human being of adult years and sound mind has the right to determine what shall be done with his own body, and a surgeon who performs an operation without his patient's consent commits an assault for which he is liable in damages."[6] A physician who offers to render aid must obtain the patient's permission. This does not mean, however, that an explicit verbal consent must be obtained from the patient in all situations. Clearly, severely injured or comatose patients may lack capacity to give consent. In such situations the law recognizes the concept of the "reasonable man." That is, the reasonable human being would desire medical care and give consent were he or she in a condition to be able to do so. The physician who approaches a patient with severe altered mental status should have no fear of acting on an implied consent. The reasonable argument that would be put forward in defense is that a normal human being of sound mind would wish competent medical assistance in a potentially life-threatening situation. The patient who has reasonable mental status and the capacity to interact in his or her own defense can accept or reject treatment in a wilderness or hospital setting.

In an emergency, consent is almost always obtained in an implied, as opposed to an expressed, manner. An expressed consent is one in which the physician specifically asks permission to treat. Under implied consent theory the physician begins medical activity and is not resisted by the patient. In Massachusetts the courts held that no basis exists for financial recovery if a patient's behavior indicates that he or she is giving consent.[5] An indication by the patient that medical care can proceed is essentially equivalent to expressed oral or written consent. The situation alone may constitute implied consent, as in the case of the unconscious patient.

Clinical circumstances may be found both in and out of the standard medical setting in which obtaining expressed consent for the treatment of a minor is impossible. On any planned outing far from established medical care, having advance written permission from a parent or guardian for the trip leader or medical personnel to render or obtain medical care that seems to be in the best interest of the minor is advisable. However, failure to obtain expressed consent should never deter emergency medical personnel from rendering immediate care to a minor. A universally recognized "emergency doctrine" comes into effect when such situations arise. This doctrine is the extension of the "reasonable man" assumptions previously noted. That is, a "reasonable parent" would want a child treated if in the opinion of medical personnel a delay in such treatment might result in serious harm or injury. A few states have codified this emergency doctrine into statutory law. In Washington State it is directly stated that "no physician or hospital licensed in this area shall be subject to civil liability, based solely upon failure to obtain consent in rendering emergency medical, surgical, hospital, or health services to any individual regardless of age where its patient is unable to give consent for any reason and there is no other person reasonably available who is legally authorized to consent to the providing of such care; *provided,* that such physician or hospital has acted in good faith and without knowledge of facts negating consent."[7] The basic conclusion from all aspects of the consent issue is that a physician confronted with an emergency situation should never delay reasonable emergency care based on a lack of expressed consent. As of this writing, no physicians have been successfully sued for providing emergency medical care before obtaining expressed consent.

ABANDONMENT

A second major issue is abandonment. Although the common law expresses no duty to render aid, a universally held tenet of the law states that once care is begun, a physician has an obligation to see that it is carried through until the patient is no longer in danger or has been properly placed in a situation where care can be continued.[3] Such decisions are extremely judgmental. If a physician properly splints an upper extremity injury on a wilderness excursion and then turns the victim over to emergency medical services (EMS) personnel for transport to a medical care facility, he or she has provided proper aid and has not abandoned care, although not physically accompanying the victim to the hospital. In the case of a person with a tenuous airway, in which physician intervention might become crucial en route to a proper medical facility, turning a victim over to EMS personnel may constitute abandonment. No current legal cases exist that more clearly define this issue with regard to the wilderness setting. However, assuming that the physician will be held to a standard of ordinary reasonableness is prudent. The physician is not expected to be clairvoyant but is expected to be able to anticipate common complications that a patient may have en route to further medical care, and needs to properly provide for such situations. A physician must understand that when involved, he or she needs not only to provide reasonable emergency care, but also to provide for entry into the health care system. To do less potentially opens the door to gross or willful negligence.

Liability

PHYSICIAN LIABILITY

The liabilities of a physician on a wilderness trip are as varied as the roles that the physician chooses to play. The physician should ask a simple question: "Am I a physician on a trip or the trip physician?" A physician who is on a trip has no more duty to his or her fellow passengers than any other member of the group. The fact that the physician's professional life involves the practice of medicine in no way conveys automatic responsibility. Should the physician choose to act in an emergency situation, his or her actions would certainly be considered under the tenets of Good Samaritan rules. However, if a physician is acting in an official capacity as "trip physician," the entire base of liability and responsibility has changed. In this circumstance, emergency actions fall within the usual scope of medical duties. Payment of money does not have to occur to establish an employment duty. Frequently physicians are given reduced trip fares or other inducements to act in the capacity of trip physician. Such arrangements are viewed as payment for services rendered or expected to be rendered. Trip outfitters and organizers will advertise the fact that a physician's presence is available for medical emergencies. Advertising constitutes agreement with the physician in these activities.

The trip physician is held to a standard of action considerably superior to the Good Samaritan standard should a liability question arise. The physician will be held to a standard related to a familiar interpretation of professional negligence. In a planned activity a trip physician is expected to anticipate usual and customary medical problems and to make contingency plans for immediate treatment and further care. Even at the professional level, "reasonableness" is the key word. A physician accompanying an expedition to climb mountains in Norway is not reasonably expected to provide poisonous snakebite kits. The physician would, however, be reasonably expected to be able to diagnose and manage orthopedic injuries and to arrange for follow-up care. The physician is expected to function up to the level of his or her peers in like or similar circumstances and therefore is required to be able to use customary physician examination and diagnostic skills and to apply first aid measures necessary to reduce the threat to life or limb until further help can be made available.

If a physician is further involved in the planning of such expeditions, he or she needs to have input into the selection of course participants. The reasonable and prudent physician should set minimum physical standard guidelines or requirements for participants to engage in certain activities. The physical requirements for a person to be involved in a bus tour are considerably different from those for a mountain climber on a trek. The trip physician or medical advisor needs to counsel participants not meeting minimum physical requirements and make certain that proper waivers of liability are explained, signed, and witnessed before the event.

Physicians who are involved in search and rescue activities can be considered both the unexpected Good Samaritans and planned wilderness trip physicians. They are generally uncompensated and must provide medical care at the scene of an injury, where the medical condition of the victim may be quite unanticipated. However, unlike improvising at the scene of a roadside accident, the search and rescue physician understands the nature and object of the search mission in advance. The reasonable physician should carry adequate supplies to render initial first aid and properly extricate and transport patients from the rescue scene. To this extent the physician can reasonably be held to standard medical norms. For a physician involved in search and rescue activities on a full-time compensated basis, formal medical standards of professional negligence would certainly be invoked. Such physicians would be considered to be operating within the scope of their employment, and standard medical malpractice policies usually cover such activities. An emergency physician, however, should have a letter on file from the malpractice carrier specifically endorsing any such activities on a prospective basis.

Physicians are frequently asked to serve as medical advisors for excursions and to prepare nonphysician trip leaders to handle on-scene medical problems. Basic and advanced emergency medicine personnel, nursing personnel, and physicians-in-training are all instructed by physicians. The teaching of basic techniques of first aid, such as airway management, compression of hemorrhage, and splinting of injuries, would seem to be so universally recognized and available through multiple sources that it should not constitute liability for the physician educator. Extending this training in a nonorganized system may create problems for both the physician and the person employing the techniques. Training a person with no other medical training to insert a chest tube without proper anatomic and physiologic understanding of its indications, contraindications, and potential hazards might be considered unreasonable. A physician who teaches and provides equipment for such advanced procedures could be construed as expressing consent for their use, and even extending license to another person. If a trip organizer believes that activities are so hazardous that preparation for advanced techniques is necessary, perhaps properly trained medical personnel should accompany the participants.

Prescribing medications for use by nonphysician trip leaders is fraught with danger. A physician is perfectly reasonable in prescribing an individual patient medications that may be required or anticipated, provided the patient is properly instructed in the use of such drugs. Drugs, such as epinephrine, required on an emergency basis for specific medical problems of individual course participants should be prescribed with impunity. However, turning medications over to a nonphysician trip leader carries certain dangers. If the nonphysician trip leader decides to employ a bee sting kit on a patient with minimal symptoms and the patient has an unexpected reaction to the medications, liability may fall back to the prescribing physician. Prescribing physicians should assume that if they order medications, they are extending license and coverage to the person who is dispensing those medications. Whenever an intermediary is given discretion in the use of medications, the physician must instruct this person in drug indications, contraindications, and side effects. In general, few medications are needed on an emergency basis. Rarely are antibiotics needed immediately in a wilderness situation unless extrication will be delayed or prolonged. Even common medications used for "mundane" medical problems, such as diarrhea and sea sickness, have side effects; if a physician desires to write standing orders for such medications to be dispensed, it should be done under a strict protocol situation that is also approved by the physician. In this way physicians can at least partially protect themselves from liability.

OUTFITTER LIABILITY FOR MEDICAL EMERGENCIES

People who outfit and organize any type of trip or activity for others are engaged in a business that carries with it usual and customary business responsibilities and liabilities.[2] The trip organizer who runs summer excursions to London can reasonably expect to rely on services available in a medically sophisticated country. No one would expect such an outfitter to carry splinting materials and bandages in anticipation that someone might break a leg getting off the bus at Trafalgar Square. However, the outfitter planning an expedition to the headwaters of the Amazon River has considerably different responsibilities. The outfitter should anticipate that expedition participants will be a considerable distance from currently acceptable Western medical care. Contingency plans are necessary for immediate medical care, transportation, and entry into the health care system of a foreign country. Under such circumstances the outfitter should have assessed the physical capabilities and limitations of those wishing to participate in the journey and have obtained releases from persons who do not meet minimum standards. If the activity involved carries obvious hazards, the outfitter should make arrangements for reasonable medical personnel to accompany the expedition. This does not necessarily require a physician, but must involve people of sufficient training to provide adequate immediate first aid and medical care until more sophisticated help can be arranged. For an outfitter planning an expedition in a remote area and in particularly hazardous terrain, seeking expert consultation in determining minimum physical requirements for each participant, supplies required, level of medical expertise needed, and system of entry into the local health care system is also reasonable. Any outfitter or trip organizer must make certain that promotional literature specifically addresses all hazards and specifically enumerates minimum physical requirements.

Most important, an outfitter or tour organization needs to make certain that performance matches advertising. If promotional materials state that a physician will be available and emergency medical care will be provided, this must absolutely be true. A liability claim against the outfitter or trip organizer would note that a decision to participate on such an excursion may have been in full or partly based on the fact that medical care would be available. Even if a reasonableness standard were met by persons in attendance, if they did not meet the level of personnel advertised in the literature, a situation of false advertising would constitute a successful claim for business negligence.

TRIP LEADER LIABILITY FOR MEDICAL EMERGENCIES

As with physician liability, a trip leader's liability varies tremendously depending on duties and responsibilities identified in writing or by understanding. A trip leader on an expedition with a physician or other highly trained medical person may be required only to identify a medical emergency and to aid in management. In situations where local medical care is readily accessible, the trip leader's responsibility may be only to activate the local health care system.

In situations where the trip leader is responsible for the immediate management of medical emergencies, a new level of responsibility exists. The organization responsible for the activity will bear the brunt of any actions undertaken by the trip leader, under the doctrine of *respondeat superior,* or "let the master answer." Any activities undertaken by the trip leader that could be reasonably construed as a direct result of the employment refer the responsibility for actions back to the employer. Any individual actions taken, unauthorized equipment used, or unauthorized medical treatments or drugs employed would most likely be construed as acts under personal auspices and would generate personal liability. The trip leader who passes out medications for such illnesses under strict medical protocol as authorized by an employer is probably personally exempt from liability. This does not in any way exempt from liability the organization or physician writing a prescription.

The same logic can be extended to the use of medical equipment and techniques. If oxygen is employed on a high-altitude expedition under strict medical protocol, the trip leader probably bears little personal responsibility. The judicious application of standard first aid techniques, such as fracture immobilization, cleansing and dressing of wounds, and compression of bleeding, seems to constitute such reasonable actions as to incur little or no liability for either the trip leader or the organization. More advanced techniques require proper supervision and training. If suturing is expected, the trip leader should have been properly instructed and should be experienced in suturing technique. Techniques such as intravenous fluid administration, joint relocations, and diagnosis of specific illness should not be undertaken by the trip leader without appropriate training and experience. The greater the likelihood that such advanced techniques will be required, the greater the need for properly trained medical personnel.

REFERENCES

1. Boccasile et al. v. Cajun Music Ltd et al., Dr. Jane Doe et al (Superior Court, Providence County, State of Rhode Island-C.A. No. 92-5233).
2. Colby v. Schwartz and Uriu, 78 Cal App 3d 885 (1978).
3. Hamburger v. Henry Ford Hospital, 284 NW 2d 155 (1979).
4. McKenna v. Cedars of Lebanon Hospitals, 93 Cal App 3d 282 (1979).
5. O'Brien v. Cunard S.S. Co., 154 Mass, 272, 28 NE 266.
6. Schloendorff v. Society of New York Hospital, 211 NY 125, 105 NE 92 (1914).
7. State of Washington—Compiled Laws, Chapter 305, Laws of 1971, 1st Extraordinary Session, effective May 20, 1971.

56 ETHICS OF WILDERNESS MEDICINE

Kenneth V. Iserson

What Is Ethics?

Ethics is the application of rules and principles to guide human action. Bioethics is the area of ethics that specifically speaks to health care providers and biomedical researchers. It involves the patient–health care provider encounter, biomedical research, and health policy. Wilderness medicine, however, is not directly comparable to either the medicine delivered in health care facilities or even to care delivered by common (urban) emergency medical services. Wilderness medicine is unique, and its special attributes provide unique ethical problems (Table 56-1). While a hospital's working environment is rarely a factor considered by the hospital-based practitioner in the determination of what medical care is delivered, the working environment is of major concern in the wilderness. Similarly, while patients are usually known to the hospital practitioner and arrive requesting care, neither is true in the wilderness setting. Even more striking are the differences between the hospital and wilderness setting with regard to equipment availability, personnel training, the need for evacuation or rescue, and the provision for the security of those involved. All potentially lead to unique ethical dilemmas.

This chapter first provides an overview of ethical values in general and those applied to bioethics. It then describes and provides a model for bioethics decision making in general. Next is an adaptation of the model for the bioethics of wilderness medicine, the ethics of wilderness health care providers, researchers, and in some cases, health policymakers. Finally, unique dilemmas in wilderness medicine are discussed.

APPLYING RULES, PRINCIPLES, AND ACTION GUIDES TO HUMAN ACTIVITIES: DERIVING FROM VALUES

The action guidelines of ethics derive from an individual's values that are acquired throughout life from multiple sources. In everyday situations, some individuals may be unaware that their values are guiding their actions. However, when facing situations that are rarely encountered, many people question how these values can be applied to solve practical problems. This is the case in wilderness medicine, since it encompasses both situations and practitioners outside the scope of the usual medical practice.

Both personal and professional values control any patient-clinician encounter. A patient expresses his or her own values, derived from religious and cultural sources. By interacting with the patient, the clinician can glimpse the patient's view of necessary treatment, quality of life, and other complex attitudes that control his or her willingness to seek and accept medical care. Whether these expressions are valid is based on the clinician's "bedside" determination of decision-making capacity. The clinician's own values, both personal and professional, are also part of the relationship and sometimes cause conflict.

Ethical discussions often revolve around applying ethical rules *consistently,* or in a way that they could be applied by all similar practitioners in the same situation *(universalizability.)* Ethical decisions derived from accepted principles, rules, or values should be applied uniformly (consistently) across all scenarios. If an accepted rule is that patients with decision-making capacity may make their own decisions about health care, this rule should be applied to all situations, not just when it is convenient for the health care provider. Likewise, the rule, if truly ethical, must be able to be applied by all health care providers, not just by a privileged or unique group.

Table 56-1 Differences Among Hospital, Emergency Medical Services, and Wilderness Medical Care

	Hospital Practice*	Emergency Medical Services†	Wilderness Medicine
Environment	Controlled, known, static	Semicontrolled, partly known, changeable	Uncontrolled, partly known, changeable
Patient	Known, requests care	Unknown, sometimes requests care	Unknown, sometimes requests care
Equipment	Sophisticated	Adequate	Rudimentary
Security	Safe	Usually safe	Questionable
Personnel	Highly educated, definitive care	Highly educated, basic care	Variable education, basic care
Evacuation	Rare	Built into system	Major concern
Rescue	No	Rare	Common

*The emergency department falls somewhere between hospital practice and emergency medical services.
†Does not include search and rescue, which is a part of wilderness medicine.

Where Do Individuals Get Values?

The basic elements of any ethical discussion are personal values. Values are the guideposts used to structure an individual's actions in life. They signify a person's duties and responsibilities, what is important to that person, and how a person interacts with others. Thomas Aquinas said that the three vital things for each person are "to know what he ought to believe; to know what he ought to desire; and to know what he ought to do."[1]

Personal values derive from many sources: family, society, school, religion, the media, and professional training and interactions. Family and religion generally guide the development of values in the early formative years. For nearly everyone these values form the bedrock on which the rest of their life rests, coloring what they learn and how they act from then on. Emphasizing the importance of early childhood learning is the maxim, "If you control a child's life until the age of six, he is yours forever." Additional significant influences are the media, schooling, and society. In our electronic age, the media begins to influence an individual's values early in life. Secular education broadens a child's experiences and values beyond the small world of the home. Finally, societal pressures continue to influence an individual's value system throughout, at the least, the formative years. Taken as a whole, values of different individuals derived from multiple sources may conflict, leading to the popular concept of a "nation without values."

Professional schooling and interactions often further refine how a person's previously learned values are applied. One reason medical students take anatomy courses is to destroy an ingrained cultural value against mutilating the dead. This allows the professional to accept and acquire the values of beneficial mutilation (surgery), handling the dead (resuscitations, pathology, transplants), and invading another's body (every invasive medical procedure).[9] In addition, when exposed to clinical practice, medical students, nurses, medics, and other health care providers learn to adopt the values of their preceptors. In any residency program the majority of trainees behave just like the faculty. Trainees are there to learn—professional values are one of the intrinsic lessons.

Values in Modern Biomedical Ethics

Another category of values has emerged as an ideal for modern medicine, especially in the United States. This set of values (sometimes referred to as the Georgetown catechism of bioethics) has been generally adopted by biomedical ethicists. These values include autonomy, beneficence, nonmaleficence, and distributive justice.

For the past two decades in the United States, the overriding professional and societal bioethical value has been patient autonomy. *Autonomy* recognizes an adult individual's right to accept or reject recommendations for his or her own medical care (even to the extent of refusing all care) in the presence of appropriate decision-making capacity (see below). This is the counterweight to the long-practiced paternalism of the medical profession, wherein what was "good" for the patient was determined solely by the physician. Coupled with paternalism is coercion, the threat or use of violence to influence behavior or choice. The joining of the august figure in white (or in a medic's uniform) with implied or explicit threats remains a potent force against any potential patient autonomy. Nevertheless, current bioethical opinion demands respect for patient autonomy.

At the patient's bedside, *beneficence,* the act of doing good, and *confidentiality,* the holding of information in confidence, have been long-held and nearly universal tenets of the medical profession. Likewise, *personal integrity,* the adherence to one's own moral and professional standards, is basic to thinking and acting ethically. The basic tenet taught all medical students is *nonmaleficence,* or "First, do no harm." This credo, often stated in the Latin form, *"Primum non nocere,"* derives from the historical knowledge that patients' encounters with physicians can be harmful as well as helpful. This recognizes the physician's fallibility.

The concept of *comparative* or *distributive justice* suggests that comparable individuals and groups in society should share equitably in the benefits and burdens of the society. Many society-wide decisions about the allocation of limited health care resources are based on this principle. Yet it is a fallacy to extrapolate from this valid principle to the idea that simply because a need to limit health care resource expenditures exists, individual clinicians can arbitrarily limit or terminate care on a case-by-case basis at the bedside of individual patients.[12]

Decision-Making Capacity and Consent

A concern in both the health care facility and the wilderness setting is whether a patient has decision-making capacity. Patient autonomy hinges on decision-making capacity. Many ethical dilemmas in emergency medical care revolve around ascertaining a patient's decision-making capacity, often linked with consent to (or more often refusal of) a medical procedure. Since a basic canon of both ethics and law, as stated by Justice Cardozo, is that "Every human being of adult years and sound mind has a right to determine what shall be done with his own body," these decisions about what action to take can often be made clearer by understanding what is meant by decision-making capacity and how it relates to consent.[15] (Note that the term "competence" is often used, when "capacity" is really meant. Competence is a legal term and can be determined only by the court.)

Capacity refers to a patient's decision-making ability and is determined by clinicians. Capacity is always decision relative rather than global. While an inebriated person, for example, can have the capacity to refuse to have stitches put in a small laceration, especially with evidence that he has previously refused similar treatments without remorse, the same individual may not have the capacity either to accept an elective operation of any sort or to refuse an emergency lifesaving procedure or operation. To have adequate decision-making capacity in any one circumstance, a person must understand the options and the consequences of acting on the various options and must be able to assess the costs and benefits of these consequences by relating them to a relatively stable framework of personal values and priorities (see Box 56-1).[2,3] Disagreement with the physician's recommendation is *not* in itself grounds for determining that a patient is incapable of making his or her own decisions. In fact, even the refusal of lifesaving medical care may not prove the person incapable of making valid decisions, if it is made on the basis of firmly held religious beliefs, as in the case of a Jehovah's Witness patient refusing a blood transfusion.

A patient must give consent to any medical intervention if he or she has decision-making capacity for that decision, and if the clinician respects the patient's autonomy. Three general types of consent exist: presumed, implied, and informed. *Presumed consent,* sometimes called emergency consent, covers the necessary lifesaving procedures that any reasonable person would wish to have if lacking decision-making capacity. Controlling hemorrhage and securing an airway in an unconscious fall victim are common examples of this type of consent. *Implied consent* is when a patient with decision-making capacity cooperates with a procedure, such as holding out an arm to donate blood or to allow initiation of an intravenous line. *Informed consent* is when a patient who retains decision-making capacity is given all the pertinent facts regarding the risks and benefits of a particular procedure, understands them, and voluntarily agrees to undergo the procedure.[7]

BOX 56-1

COMPONENTS OF DECISION-MAKING CAPACITY

Knowledge of the options
Awareness of the consequences of each option
Appreciation of personal costs and benefits of options in relation to relatively stable values and preferences

Modified from Buchanan AE: The question of competence. In Iserson KV et al, editors: *Ethics in emergency medicine,* ed 2, Tucson, Ariz, Galen Press, in press.

Questions applying to consent in the wilderness setting can be difficult. Does the patient have the capacity to understand the situation? Will decision-making capacity be questioned only if a person refuses "good" medical care? And, unresolved even in standard medical practice, what procedures require informed, as distinct from implied, consent? The requirement for informed consent varies in practice and law from area to area and even among practitioners and institutions within the same area. Determining decision-making capacity and providing an opportunity to consent to a procedure when appropriate are crucial to respecting a patient's autonomy.

Another Value Applicable to Wilderness Medicine

Given the unique setting of wilderness medicine, the value of security must also be applied. *Security* signifies a measure of responsibility towards oneself, one's companions, and the patient. This responsibility is to avoid risking the safety of the wilderness team. This is a concept far removed from normal medical practice. However, this value is of paramount importance in wilderness medicine. Safety is the responsibility of any wilderness medical provider, even if he or she is not officially designated a provider but must take over in a medical crisis on the basis of special knowledge or skills. Decisions about rescue, evacuation, aborting group travel, or even attempting some medical interventions must include considerations of security.

Security is wilderness medicine's controlling value in most circumstances. Concerns about safety are applied in the following order: oneself, other team members, and then the patient. Ethical theory supports this hierarchy. Beneficence by medical personnel does *not* imply a need to endanger oneself. Indeed, if medical skills are to be useful, medical personnel *must be able* to render care. Additionally inherent in any leadership position is a responsibility to protect one's team. Therefore the team members' safety is the second responsibility. Finally, the patient's security should be assured, but never at the expense of the medical team's safety. This is not to say that in unknown or unknowable circumstances the medical leader may not have to weigh potential risks versus benefits. It does say that the risks must weigh heavily in the calculations, since otherwise these concerns are often ignored. An example is the case in which a badly injured trekker may survive if evacuated by aeromedical transport. The helicopter team is willing to at least attempt a pickup, if requested. Yet the wilderness medical care provider must determine whether local conditions are safe enough, balanced with the chance of benefit to the patient, to make the request.

In the language of ethics, then, utilitarian thinking plays a dominant role in wilderness ethics. Utilitarianism is the philosophy that promotes the greatest good (or happiness) for the greatest number. In wilderness medicine, it promotes the well-being of the many over the well-being of the individual. This can be defended by simply recognizing the unique aspects of wilderness medical practice, such as the uncontrolled environment, unfamiliarity with the patient, rudimentary equipment, and changeable situations—all contributing to safety concerns. Moreover, the majority of people who are in the wilderness have risk-taking personalities, leading them to downplay security in favor of adventure.

Ethical Dilemmas

Health care professionals commonly apply their values without much thought. They act instinctively based on their prior behavior and training. Values are constantly (although not necessarily consistently) applied to everyday decisions. Of course, most decisions are not ethical decisions. Ethical dilemmas arise with conflict between two seemingly equivalent values, represented by different and mutually exclusive possible actions. A graphic depiction of this situation is the picture of a practitioner standing before two doors, each of which is a possible action to take. One is labeled "Damned if you do," the other is labeled "Damned if you don't." The practitioner has a profound decision to make. That is where ethical decision making comes into play.

Another example of a bioethical dilemma in wilderness medicine may help illustrate ethical decision making. A distress call has been received from anxious relatives or by radio from a plane flying over a wilderness area. The victim is in a hazardous area (such as an active volcano), or more commonly the weather is terrible (snow or thunderstorm). The physician directing a search and rescue team must decide how to respond to the call in a setting that would put the team in danger. The standard bioethical value of beneficence directly competes with the wilderness bioethical value of security. Each has a strong pull on the decision maker, with each value providing good arguments for sending or not sending the rescue team. Although the value of security may often be considered paramount in the wilderness setting, the emotional and altruistic pulls of beneficence make this a difficult choice. Considering this case, a word should first be said about rights and duties in relation to health care.

Although the word "rights" is glibly used in many situations in our society, a personal right is present only if another person or society as a whole has an identifiable *duty* to the individual. For example, if all U.S. citizens had a right to health care, the government would have the duty to provide this care. Health care providers would have a corresponding duty to furnish this care. However, except in limited circumstances, such as emergency departments and prisons, no such legal right currently exists. Morally and practically, citizens do not have the right to *health,* and how much health care people are owed is unresolved.[11] Correspondingly, no health care practitioner has a duty to provide all the health care people desire. Practitioners do, however, have a duty to provide security, when possible, for those they direct in wilderness settings. This may provide part of the answer for this case; yet other factors may be involved.

Since the ethical dilemma arises when two or more seemingly "correct" actions appear to have equal benefits, the choice of actions should be examined first. How are these proposed "correct" actions decided upon in the first place? After that, which of these actions is the more ethically acceptable?

Solving the Bioethical Dilemma

Deciding on an action in the standard setting. In the standard clinical paradigm, Jonsen and co-workers have suggested four groups of factors to consider when deciding on a course of action in the face of a bioethical dilemma. These include the medical indications for the action, the patient's (or surrogate's) preferences, consideration of the quality of life, and other contextual factors.[10] These have been seen as an "ethical square," with the top two boxes weighing more heavily (Fig. 56-1).

In a broad sense, *patient wishes* equate to *patient autonomy,* previously discussed. In a growing number of instances, however, especially at the end of life, surrogate decision makers rather than the patient may exercise this autonomy. This may also be true in the wilderness setting, albeit with less legal backing. Many critically ill patients in health care facilities have an advance directive (durable power of attorney for health care) naming a surrogate to make health care decisions if they lack decision-making capacity. Finding such advance directives in the wilderness setting would be rare. Rather, if a person lacks decision-making capacity, a spouse, close friend, or medical care

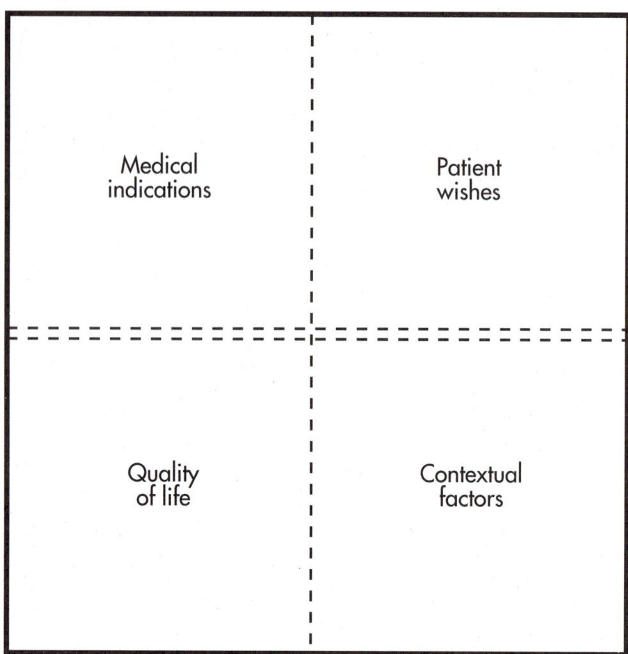

Fig. 56-1 The ethical square. (Modified from Jonsen AR, Siegler M, Winslade WJ: *Clinical ethics,* ed 3, New York, 1992, McGraw-Hill.)

provider makes critical decisions for the patient, acting in his or her "best interest." While parents normally act as decision makers for minor children, a complete discussion of this is beyond the scope of this chapter.[8]

Medical indications are often more straightforward in the wilderness setting than they are in standard health care. In the wilderness, treatment is basic, injuries and illnesses are generally acute, and intervention is normally life preserving rather than death prolonging. Standard clinical algorithms are used by the clinicians for their level of training. In remote areas, of course, questions may arise about whether the ophthalmologist should attempt to reduce a hip dislocation or whether the nurse should attempt to establish a surgical airway. These dilemmas should, when feasible, be decided with input from the patient or surrogate. As a matter of proper planning, behavior in critical scenarios must be decided in advance. Normally, however, medical indications are clear.

Bioethicists normally feel most comfortable helping to resolve cases using only the medical indications and patient (or surrogate) wishes (above the double line in Fig. 56-1). When these factors are ambiguous, however, two other sets of factors must be considered: contextual and quality-of-life. Contextual factors normally include everything from the insurance status of the patient to family circumstances. In the standard medical situation this is admittedly a fuzzy area. Related to these and even more nebulous are quality-of-life factors. These relate to the nature of a patient's current and presumed future existence as viewed by others. (If a patient has decision-making capacity, his or her own view of life is comfortably built into patient autonomy.) In the wilderness setting, time and circumstances do not allow clinicians to make quality-of-life judgments, but contextual factors take on a dominant role in the form of security factors.

Deciding on an action in the wilderness. The importance of security factors in the wilderness setting leads to the altered diagram of decision making for ethical problems in wilderness medicine (Fig. 56-2). This includes three groups of factors to consider when deciding on a course of action in the wilderness setting: patient autonomy, security, and medical indications. Within this decision model, the security factors must be given the most weight.

Security factors include the safety of the medical and rescue personnel, the patient, the proposed procedures, and the evacuation method. As mentioned previously, security of the medical team is a valid consideration because of the inherent risk-taking nature of people in the wilderness. In recent legal actions pertaining to wilderness injuries, the law has recognized a "doctrine of reasonable implied assumption of risk." This implied risk is also part of an acceptable concept of wilderness triage. Wilderness triage takes place when the same injuries or illnesses that would cause only minimal morbidity if they occurred in a medically sophisticated environment inevitably cause death if they happen in the wilderness. The fractured femur in the lone wilderness traveler or the abdominal gunshot wound in a remote area is often a virtual death sentence. This is a risk that wilderness adventurers take, although not always with a clear understanding of the enormity of the risks involved.

Both standard bioethics and wilderness medical ethics often involve difficult situations with no "correct" answer in every situation. Usually more than two possible actions exist. That is the wilderness ethical and standard bioethical dilemma. What should the practitioner do?

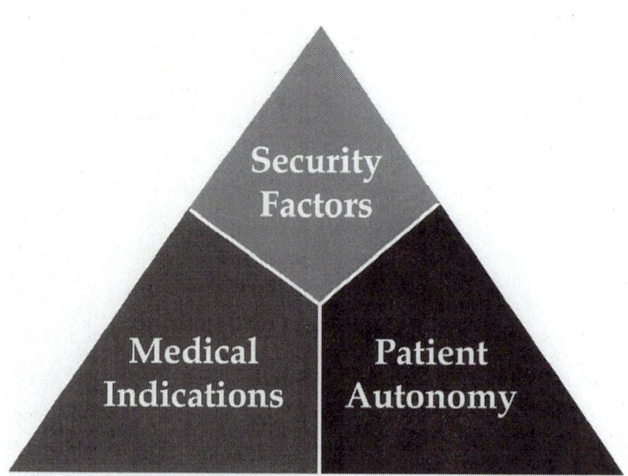

Fig. 56-2 Wilderness medicine's ethical triangle.

Bioethical Decision-Making Process[8]

Using the algorithm as a guide for a decision. In bioethics, while disagreements may arise regarding the optimal course of action using a specific set of values, often general agreement exists as to what constitutes ethically wrong actions. The method of ethical case analysis described in Fig. 56-3 is designed to provide the emergency practitioner with prompt assistance in selecting an ethically correct, although not necessarily a theoretically "best," course of action.[6] This method applies equally well in the wilderness setting and in the normal hospital setting.

The first step in using the algorithm in Fig. 56-3 is to use a known precedent. This is the simplest solution to an ethical dilemma, but it requires planning in advance, including reading and thinking about ethical problems. Many physicians and other health care professionals are not prepared to do this. Just as with any emergency procedure, emergency physicians and health care professionals should be prepared with a course of action for, at the least, the most common ethical dilemmas likely to occur in either the emergency department or the wilderness setting.

With no precedent the second step is to "buy time." What action is not harmful to the patient that provides time for consultation or any information gathering needed to refine the action plan? In a wilderness medical setting, this might mean placing a patient's arm in a sling for comfort while deciding whether an inexperienced provider should attempt to reduce a dislocation or fracture.

With no precedent to rely on and no way to "buy time," the health care professional must select a possible course of action and test it for ethical viability. Three tests, the impartiality test, the universalizability test, and the interpersonal justifiability test, are drawn from three different philosophical theories. First the impartiality test is applied. The practitioner asks whether he or she would have this action performed if in the patient's place. In essence, this is a form of the Golden Rule, "Do unto others as you would have done unto you." According to John Stuart Mill, this espouses "the complete spirit of the ethics of utility."[14] Second, the universalizability test asks if the health care professional would feel comfortable having all practitioners perform this action in all relevantly similar circumstances. This generalizes the action and asks whether developing a universal rule for the contemplated behavior is reasonable. This is merely an application of Kant's categorical imperative. Finally, the interpersonal justifiability test asks if the practitioner can supply good reasons to others for his or her action. Will peers, superiors, or the public be satisfied with the action taken and reasons for it? This test uses David Gauthier's basic theory of consensus values as a final screen for a proposed action.[5] If all three tests can be answered in the affirmative, the health care professional can have reasonable assurance that the proposed action falls within the scope of morally acceptable actions. If, however, the proposed action fails these tests, the algorithm must be applied to another proposed action.

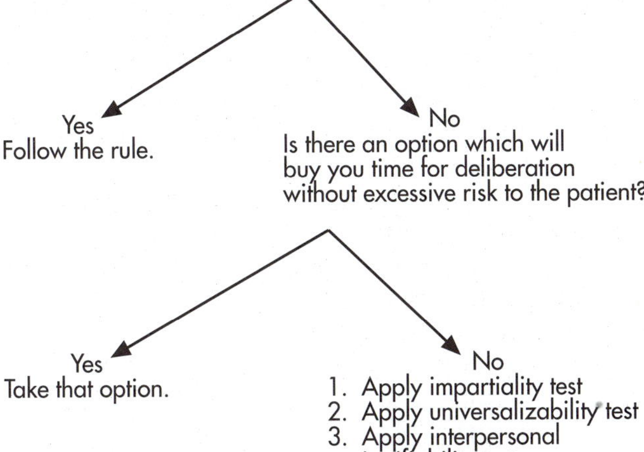

Fig. 56-3 A rapid approach to emergency ethical problems. (Modified from Iserson KV: An approach to ethical problems in emergency medicine. In Iserson KV et al, editors: *Ethics in emergency medicine,* ed 2, Tucson, Ariz, Galen Press, in press.)

Ethical Dilemmas in Wilderness Medicine

With its unique setting and mode of practice, wilderness medicine provides practitioners with ethical dilemmas that are rarely seen by most other providers. These dilemmas can be grouped into three categories: dilemmas involving standards of care, dilemmas with priority in care, and dilemmas with the decision-making process (Box 56-2). As might be expected, some of the issues in each group deal with provider-patient dilemmas, while others have more to do with group or governmental policies. Also, the unusual circumstances found in the wilderness setting may result in ethical decisions that are different from those in the standard medical setting. The ethical decision-making process used to puzzle through these dilemmas, however, is similar to the process in other settings; wilderness medical care's unique setting and issues sometimes obscure this basic truism.

APPLICATION OF VALUES

In wilderness medicine, ethical dilemmas arise and values must be applied to patient-clinician interactions, to group activities, and to public wilderness policies. In this setting the unique position of wilderness medical practitioners must be recognized. These dilemmas have few parallels to other medical practice—perhaps only to battlefield medical practice or medical care during major, widespread dis-

BOX 56-2

ETHICAL DILEMMAS IN WILDERNESS CARE

STANDARD OF CARE DILEMMAS

Limited resources—standard of care differs. What should be brought into the field? How are resources distributed?
Cultural: Are Western standards of care and attitudes appropriate when treating locals in a foreign country?
How much authority is delegated to nontrained personnel?

PRIORITY IN CARE DILEMMAS

Triage choices: Who should be rescued first?
Issues of survival
Issues of direct life-threatening situations for the provider(s)
Motorized vehicle restrictions and environmental protection in wilderness areas

DECISION-MAKING DILEMMAS

No surrogate or family available
Euthanasia
No ethics consultation
Advance directives
No-rescue areas

asters. These dilemmas may include providing euthanasia for nonfatal medical conditions, abandoning patients, and prioritizing medical care between original patients and rescue team members. Each of these deserves significant discussion, but space allows only that the ethical dilemmas be explicated.

STANDARD OF CARE DILEMMAS

Limited Resources

In the wilderness setting, resources are limited. They are usually confined to the supplies that can be carried into the field on foot or in some cases on horseback or by helicopter. Personnel may have limited skills. The combination of limited skills and limited availability of supplies and equipment gives rise to ethical dilemmas. What should be included in wilderness medical kits? Who decides?

While decisions about what goes into medical kits are rarely considered under the rubric of triage, that is exactly what they represent. The individual wilderness traveler usually determines what is brought into the field. However, most individuals fail to realize that this decision identifies the limits on treatment that the traveler is willing to accept for himself or herself. Any traveler into wilderness areas must assume that the contents of the medical kit will be the only resources available for medical treatment. When equipment is selected for organized wilderness excursions or search and rescue teams, the decision may be made by the group, a medical committee, or the medical director or advisor. However, the limit to available care still exists.

While the commercially available standardized medical kits are usually designed on the basis of "medical" criteria, recognizing that some types of treatment and treatment of some types of patients will be implicitly unavailable because of what is excluded from these kits is vital. Decisions must be made concerning what to include in field medical kits; no one is expected to carry a fully stocked emergency department into the field. Clearly identifying the ethical dilemmas entailed in compiling these kits helps team members in their decision.

Explicit triage decisions, while harder to make, are often easier to recognize as ethical dilemmas. These are dealt with in the section on priority in care dilemmas later in the chapter.

Cultural Differences

Many wilderness emergencies occur in places outside of the United States or other Westernized countries. Are Western standards of care and attitudes appropriate when treating locals in a foreign country? Whose values control the treatment and other actions?

Three circumstances may present ethical dilemmas in the delivery of medical care during wilderness expeditions to remote areas. The first is a lack of cultural sensitivity. Aggressive offers to care for disease or injury may frustrate or anger local patients or providers, whose methods of treatment fit within the region's cultural milieu and may be as good as or better than "modern" medicine. Temporarily replacing or upstaging traditional healers and their healing methods may degrade them in the eyes of the local population.

The second situation is when medical problems occur that are beyond the capabilities of an expedition's practitioners. After offering the care they are competent to give, practitioners may feel obligated to attempt treatments beyond their knowledge or abilities. An internist may face treating a gunshot wound to the chest, a pediatrician may encounter a complicated obstetric emergency, or a paramedic may confront an epidemic. Often without any oversight except their own moral compass, these caregivers may be tempted to stretch their abilities beyond the patients' safety limit. The advisability of doing so will be unique in each case. However, cultural ethical concerns should be considered when deciding what course of action to pursue.

The third situation relates to the larger question of the fairness of chance encounters. A woman's life is saved through the luck that a passing trekker could treat her pyelonephritis; a surgeon relocates a hip and a man will continue to provide for his family; a paramedic happens to be on hand to intubate a child with epiglottitis. These situations in themselves rarely encompass ethical issues. The larger question, which may be more philosophic than practical, is how these interventions interfere with the balance of life in the area. Are chance encounters an aberration or simply a part of life?

How Much Authority Is Given to Nontrained Personnel?

Wilderness travelers face ethical dilemmas when they encounter medical situations for which they are untrained. Not only lay persons, but also medics, physician assistants, nurses, and physicians, may quickly find themselves out of their depth in wilderness settings when faced with treating patients who have conditions they would either feel comfortable treating only if in their normal environment or whose illness or injury is beyond the scope of their experience or knowledge. In deciding whether to intervene in such a situation, the person planning to help must weigh the chance of benefiting the patient (value of beneficence) against the chance of doing the patient harm (nonmaleficence).

The following hypothetical case illustrates both the questions raised in this type of dilemma and the application of the rapid decision-making model (Fig. 56-3).

A common scenario revolves around the backcountry excursion with a medical provider unprepared for orthopedic emergencies. When a group member dislocates a shoulder, the provider may be unwilling to go beyond his or her level of training by attempting a reduction, although the patient (as well as the rest of the party) may encourage the attempt. If another member of the party with even less training volunteers to try the reduction, the clinician is in a double-bind, seemingly forced to either overextend his or her skills or to acquiesce to even less accomplished medical care for the patient.

How could this dilemma be resolved using the rapid decision-making model (Fig. 56-3)? The first step would be to anticipate such a situation in advance and plan a course of action. Since orthopedic trauma is common in the wilderness, any medical provider should expect to face such a situation. (Note that preplanning may obviate this ethical dilemma, as it does in many other situations, since the provider may then get the requisite orthopedic knowledge and skills in advance or may abandon plans to take this wilderness medical role.) Whether or not the skill level is unchanged, the provider may also decide on an ethical course of action after discussing in advance the potential problem with knowledgeable peers or getting information from other sources. Perhaps the provider decides to act in such a situation (paradigm case) based on (1) determining the patient's decisional capacity, (2) informing the patient fully and honestly of the apparent situation and options, and (3) acquiescing to the patient's desires, whether trying a reduction or simply securing the arm in place. Honest acceptance of a patient's autonomy to control his or her medical care often resolves a seemingly difficult ethical dilemma. Yet the circumstances in this case may be that the provider believes the "experienced layman" offering help may actually have no knowledge at all. The provider must then decide whether the paradigm case for which he or she prepared a response is similar enough to the current circumstances to use that response. If it is, the dilemma is resolved and that rule should be followed.

If, however, the provider believes that the current situation differs significantly from his or her paradigm case, or from lack of foresight simply failed to decide in advance on an ethical course of action, he or she should go to step two—buying time. In the scenario presented, buying time may consist of making the patient comfortable to obtain time for contacting help or thinking through the problem. Help is usually available to organized wilderness excursions through radio or cellular telephone communications. The assistance may be experienced advice about other actions to resolve the dilemma or orthopedic advice on how to reduce the shoulder. Sometimes, however, no help is available or not enough time can be bought to secure help. The health care provider must make a decision to act—go to step three.

At this stage the provider attempts to choose an action (by applying Fig. 56-2) that is ethically acceptable, even if not the optimal action more time were available to consider the problem. Possible actions in this case might include attempting a reduction, allowing the lay person to attempt a reduction, simply immobilizing the patient's shoulder, leaving the patient and going for help, or ignoring the situation and leaving the decision to someone else. The provider must first choose a course of action (even not deciding is a course of action) and then decide whether it falls within the scope of ethically acceptable behavior. If, for example, the proposed action is immobilization of the shoulder, the three tests of impartiality, universalizability, and interpersonal justifiability should be applied to this action. If the action passes all three tests, it is probably ethically acceptable and may be used if desired. Remember that ethically acceptable actions may differ with the circumstances or the wilderness group involved.

Another aspect of this type of ethical dilemma is caused by health care policy. Wilderness medical care may be limited by restricting medical practitioners from fully using their skills and knowledge. Paramedics, for example, are told that in some jurisdictions, on pain of losing their licenses, they may not reduce fractures, perform cricothyrotomies, or (in a few backward locations) perform endotracheal intubations. Emergency medical technicians, first aiders, first responders, and the like are more severely restricted. Nurses may not know what procedures their licenses allow, and physicians are constantly concerned about liability. In general, many practitioners in wilderness settings feel that the laws and administrative policies under which they work restrict their actions. This attitude and their subsequent behavior may lead to care for victims of wilderness injury or illness far below the standard that is available.

The Wilderness Medical Society and other groups have begun working to overcome these limitations. At present, however, an ethical dilemma may exist when practitioners face a medical situation in the field that they know how to treat but that exceeds their license or official certification. A clear conflict may exist between the law and ethical responsibility. Practitioners have to decide the best course of action—preferably in advance of the problem.

PRIORITY IN CARE DILEMMAS

Ethical dilemmas easily arise when in wilderness settings the health care provider faces not only triage among patients, but critical decisions about whether to help a patient. Triage takes on new dimensions in wilderness settings. These settings also produce situations in which the rescuers or other members of the party may be placed in danger by helping an injured person.

Triage Choices: Whom to Rescue First? How Are Resources Distributed?

Medical practitioners, especially those in surgery and emergency care, are familiar with medical triage in the face of multiple patients needing care, sorting patients by severity of injury, availability of resources, and the possibility of successful treatment. These triage decisions have their own unique set of ethical dilemmas. Wilderness triage is unusual on several counts and may present ethical dilemmas markedly different from those encountered in the nonwilderness environment. Three ethical dilemmas result from wilderness triage questions that are unlikely to occur elsewhere except for battlefield settings.[4]

The first ethical dilemma arises when, providing care for a group, the wilderness practitioner knows all the patients and may have personal ties to one or more of them. This is unlike normal triage scenarios and complicates any decision about who gets treated, especially if resources are limited. For example, in an outbreak of giardiasis in a party of twelve, the provider has only enough metronidazole (Flagyl) to treat five people. Another, more serious example would be the lightning strike in the midst of six people, with only one individual remaining capable of providing assistance. In each case the medical practitioner weighing triage criteria may be torn between medical and personal concerns.

A second ethical triage dilemma arises in what may be termed the "us versus them" situation. Members of both the wilderness party and local population may be in the patient pool to be triaged. To whom does the provider owe primary responsibility? Some may argue that the implicit or explicit contract between the provider and group members warrants treating group members first. If the battlefield is considered analogous, the same contract exists there. The Geneva Convention specifies that patients are always to be triaged for medical care on the basis of medical need and the ability to treat. Whether military caregivers follow this dictum in practice is moot. The wilderness caregiver must carefully consider this issue before venturing into the field.

Finally, ethical dilemmas arise because not all team members are equal. If triage among team members is necessary, treatment on the basis of pure medical necessity is not always realistic. In the giardiasis example, will the sickest patients be treated or will treatment be given to the less sick guide and translator, who are essential to get the party out of the wilderness? The greatest good for the greatest number, or the concept of group safety, must prevail. But this may be neither a comfortable nor an intuitively obvious decision.

An ethical dilemma also arises when rescue teams are called into the field and a rescue team member is injured. The question is asked whether rescue teams should treat their injured team member before, or instead of, victims. Wilderness rescue is an inherently dangerous operation. Although the safety record of some organized and experienced rescue groups has been excellent, this is not universal, particularly with ad hoc rescue attempts. An ethical dilemma arises when rescuers themselves become victims. Where should the team's priorities lie? Again, an analogy can be drawn with triage parameters in emergency care. The principle of triage is that, as long as resources are available, the most seriously injured are treated first. This situation logically and morally prevails in wilderness medical care. However, emotion rather than reason often influence actions, so the wilderness health care provider must ensure that ethical decision making prevails.

Issues of Survival

In some situations the lives of trip members may be put at immediate risk if an injured person receives optimum assistance. When a scuba diver aboard a dive boat loses the ability to move his lower body on surfacing (presumably central nervous system decompression sickness or air embolism), optimum therapy includes immediate transport to a recompression chamber. This poses an ethical dilemma if other divers in the party are still in the water, since in most instances they cannot be easily contacted and retrieved. The longer the wait to get the paralyzed diver to a chamber, the less the chance of recovery. Leaving the area puts the uninjured divers at serious risk. (The level of risk would, among other factors, be based on the divers' experience level, distance from land, time of day, and weather conditions.)

Reviewing the ethical considerations in wilderness medicine's ethical triangle, both medical indications and possibly the patient (patient autonomy) influence the decision toward leaving the area to get the patient to a recompression chamber. This example demonstrates that in the wilderness setting, security factors are the primary factor in making ethical decisions. Unless the safety of the other divers can be guaranteed, the boat should not leave the area until the other divers are on board.

Issues of Direct Life-Threatening Situations for the Provider

Health care providers in a wilderness setting often have the opportunity to literally rescue others, which feeds on their underlying motivation to be of help to others. Situations arise where providing help puts the caregiver (or the entire team) at significant risk. This has already been discussed in the section on safety as a key concern of wilderness medical ethics. Wilderness medical leaders commonly decline to enter a dangerous situation to attempt to rescue a patient. However, a more direct and powerful ethical issue arises when the caregiver must directly and explicitly sacrifice the patient for personal or team safety. (This is somewhat analogous to the difference between passive and active euthanasia, although the differences are clear.) This occurs, for example, when a helicopter hoisting a wilderness patient encounters difficulties endangering the craft. Standard procedure is to cut the hoist line, sacrificing the patient. In the abstract, the safety of the helicopter crew (and possibly rescuers on the ground) outweighs that of the patient. Yet in reality the conflict between safety and beneficence may not be intrinsically clear to the health provider; an answer in favor of safety contradicts all professional education and experiences. This conflict must be resolved in advance or within a few seconds during the event if anyone is to survive. In the analogous scenario of the battlefield, the question is raised, "How many medics do you sacrifice to save one infantryman?" So too with rescuers.

DECISION-MAKING DILEMMAS

Health care decisions are generally the responsibility of the adult patient with decision-making capacity. If a patient lacks the ability to make these decisions, health care providers normally seek out a surrogate decision maker, an advance directive, or the counsel of a bioethics committee or colleague. These resources are rarely available in the wilderness setting. Health care decisions can therefore become more problematic.

No Surrogate or Family Available

When a person needing health care in the wilderness lacks decision-making capacity because of illness or injury, the health care provider must make decisions based on knowledge of the patient's values (often from a relatively brief period of interaction), the values of the group, or the provider's own perceptions of what is in the patient's best interest. When family or close friends are present, they may act as surrogates to make the patient's decisions, but this is much less frequent in the wilderness setting than in the urban environment. The wilderness medical provider therefore must be prepared to make the difficult decisions without this guidance.

Advance Directives

To allay the problems of the absence of surrogate decision makers or knowledge about a patient's wishes, health care providers for organized expeditions, especially those in which significant risk of danger exists, may want to request that team members complete an advance directive. However, the normal forms of advance directive (durable power of attorney for health care and living will) may not suffice in the wilderness setting. Rather, a more specific directive should be used. It should detail how aggressive the individuals would want the team to be in trying to extract them from a dangerous situation if they (1) had a good chance of survival; (2) had a good chance of survival, but with serious physical disability; (3) had a good chance of survival, but with serious brain injury; or (4) had a poor chance of surviving. Any directives given by a team member would of course be tempered by the need to ensure the safety of other team members, but such a directive might give the medical provider a better idea of each team member's desires. Indeed, just discussing these scenarios with the team may be beneficial in elucidating attitudes and health care desires in the wilderness. Some team members might want to use a durable power of attorney, naming a surrogate within the team, for use with or in place of the more specific directive.

Euthanasia

Controversy continues to rage in society and medicine over the concept of active euthanasia (so-called mercy killing). In wilderness medicine, however, euthanasia may be less ethically problematic. Active euthanasia may be an ethically acceptable alternative in the rare situation when a patient will die either because he or she cannot be rescued from the wilderness environment or because group survival would be jeopardized by attempting to evacuate or remain with him or her until help arrives. The seriously injured person on a high-altitude climb with inclement weather quickly approaching and the injured caver in a flooding cave are two examples. In these cases, euthanasia is based on the beneficence of relieving suffering in a doomed individual (although many in the medical profession believe that mercy killing violates professional principles), security for other members of the party, and often patient autonomy (although some psychiatrists might argue that by asking for death a person demonstrates a lack of decision-making capacity). Indeed, a particularly difficult situation is the psychiatric patient who cannot be made to continue out of the wilderness and who will endanger the group and himself or herself if either remains. This has happened at least once in the dual peril of war and wilderness, when British soldiers of the 111th Indian Infantry Brigade in Burma euthanized their own during World War II.[16] In nonwar situations, however, any episodes of active wilderness euthanasia have gone unreported.

Further complicating the preceding scenarios is the question of whether such patients should be simply left to die (passive euthanasia) or should be more humanely killed (active euthanasia). This question should be given serious consideration, since many incidents of passive euthanasia in wilderness settings occur, especially in high-risk or remote areas.

DILEMMAS IN WILDERNESS POLICIES

Ethical decision making also plays a part in policies governing wilderness medicine. The values of beneficence and nonmaleficence make proposed and actual rules for wilderness medical practice untenable. These policies include no-rescue areas, no motorized vehicles in wilderness areas, no environmental destruction, and restriction of medical providers' roles (see earlier discussion).

Motorized Vehicle Restrictions and Environmental Protection in Wilderness Areas

A policy imposed on wilderness medical practice is that of no motorized vehicles in designated wilderness areas. This rule has logical roots and is enforced only intermittently, but when it is used to hinder rescue efforts or delay needed medical care, it defeats a basic purpose of society—the assurance of citizens' welfare.

A related issue is the basic tenet of wilderness travel that the environment should be left at least as pristine as it was found. This presents no problem in most circumstances (except perhaps that some of our most adventurous parties, such as the climbers of Mt. Everest, have left in their wilderness areas great junk piles). Situations arise, however, when preservation of a wilderness area must be weighed against pain and suffering, or life and death. Helicopter pads chopped into the forest or a new entryway blasted into a cave are only two examples. The preservation of wilderness areas is an important goal, but so is the preservation of human virtues, and these should not be overridden to reach a symbolic goal. Human life is a priority.

No-Rescue Areas

Perhaps the most pernicious concept proposed to govern wilderness medical care is that of the "no-rescue area," into which adventurers would go with the foreknowledge that no rescue would be available.[13] Akin to playing Russian roulette, people entering these wilderness areas would put life and limb at risk while society condoned and presumably enforced a requirement not to assist those in need. This macho concept disregards both patient societal beneficence and individual autonomy. Those familiar with advance directives, such as health care powers of attorney or living wills, know that patients in extremis often countermand their preconceived instructions. To prevent wilderness trekkers from doing the same in order to preserve their life contradicts basic ethical values.

REFERENCES

1. Aquinas T: *Two precepts of charity,* 1273.
2. Buchanan AE: The question of competence. In Iserson KV et al, editors: *Ethics in emergency medicine,* Baltimore, 1986, Williams & Wilkins.
3. Drane JF: Competency to give an informed consent, *JAMA* 252 (7): 925, 1984.
4. Frisina ME: Ethical principles and the practice of battlefield health care, *Milit Chaplains Rev,* Spring 1991.
5. Gauthier DP: *Morals by agreement.* Oxford, 1986, Clarendon Press.
6. Iserson KV: An approach to ethical problems in emergency medicine. In Iserson KV et al, editors: *Ethics in emergency medicine,* Tucson, Ariz, Galen Press, in press.
7. Iserson KV: Bioethics. In Rosen P, Barkin RM, editors: *Emergency medicine: concepts and clinical practice,* ed 3, St Louis, 1992, Mosby.
8. Iserson KV: Pediatric bioethics. In Reisdorff EJ, Roberts MR, Wiegenstein JG, editors: *Pediatric emergency medicine,* Philadelphia, 1992, WB Saunders.
9. Iserson KV: *Death to dust: what happens to dead bodies?* Tucson, Ariz, 1994, Galen Press.
10. Jonsen AR, Siegler M, Winslade WJ: *Clinical ethics,* ed 3, New York, 1992, McGraw-Hill.
11. Knopp RK et al: An ethical foundation for health care: an emergency medicine perspective, *Ann Emerg Med* 21:1381, 1992.
12. Landesman BM: Physician attitudes toward patients. In Iserson KV et al, editors: *Ethics in Emergency Medicine,* Baltimore, 1986, Williams & Wilkins.
13. McAvoy L, Dustin D: You're losing your right to be alone, *Backpacker* 12:5:60, 1984.
14. Mill JS: *Utilitarianism* The Great Books, Chicago, 1952, Encyclopaedia Britannica, first published in London in 1861.
15. *Schloendorff v. Society of New York Hospital* (1914) 105 N.E. 92, 93.
16. Swann SW: Euthanasia on the battlefield, *Milit Chaplains Rev,* Spring 1991.

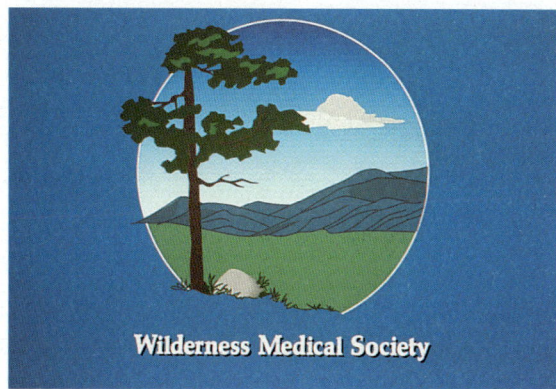

1. **Logo of the Wilderness Medical Society.**

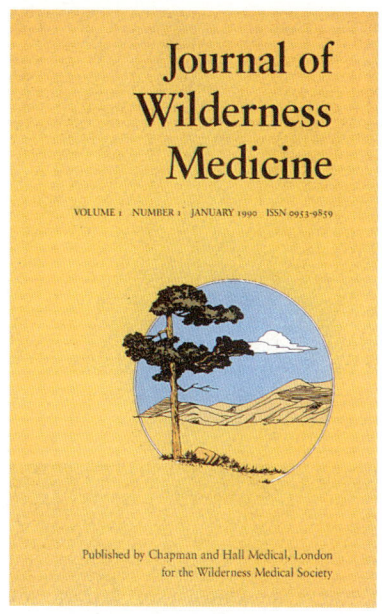

2. **The Journal of Wilderness Medicine.**

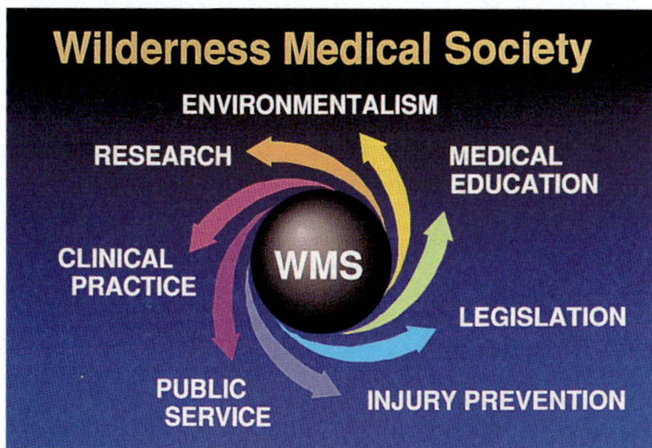

3. **Mission of the Wilderness Medical Society.**

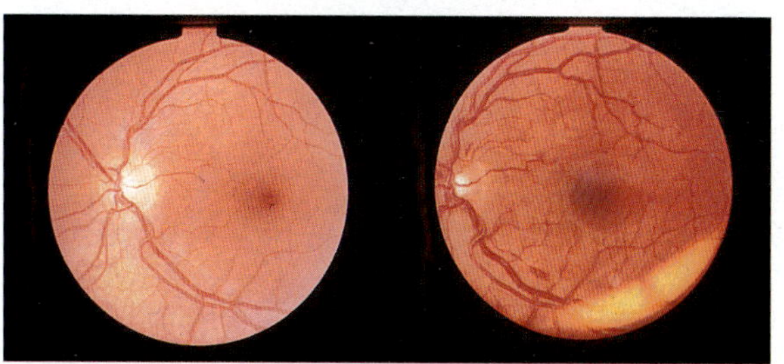

4. **The normal fundus at sea level *(left)*. The same fundus at 5400 meters *(right)*. Note the vascular engorgement and tortuousness at altitude.**

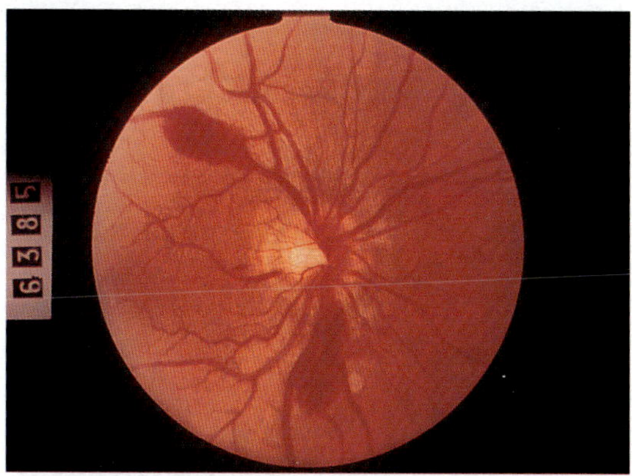

5. **High-altitude retinal hemorrhages.**

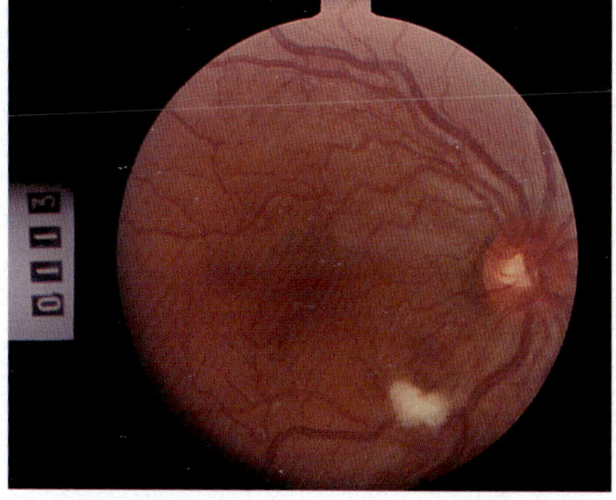

6. **Cotton wool spots seen at 5400 meters. This occurred in a climber after Valsalva maneuver and represents the most severe form of retinopathy.** (Plates 4 through 6 courtesy Dr. M. McFadden, U.B.C., Vancouver, B.C., in association with Dr. C. Houston, Burlington, Vt.; Dr. G. Gray, D.C.I.E.M., Toronto, Ontario; and Drs. J. Sutton and P. Powles, McMaster University, Hamilton, Ontario.)

A

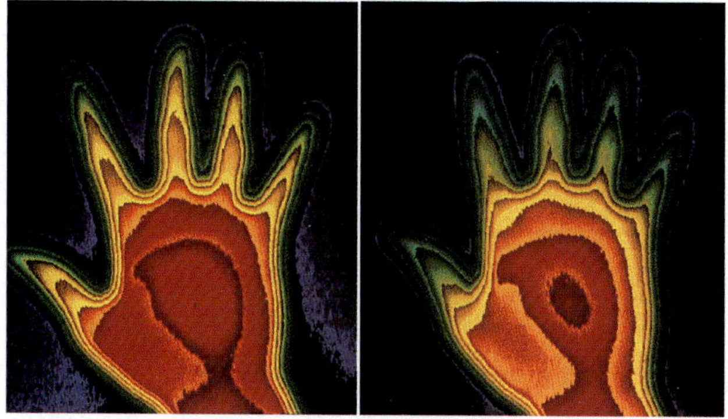

B

7. **Infrared scan of the palmar hand surface. Blue color = 43° C; red color = 68° C.** A, **At room temperature.** B, **After 5 minutes in a cold room, with evidence of vasoconstriction.** (Courtesy Naval Health Research Center, San Diego, Calif.)

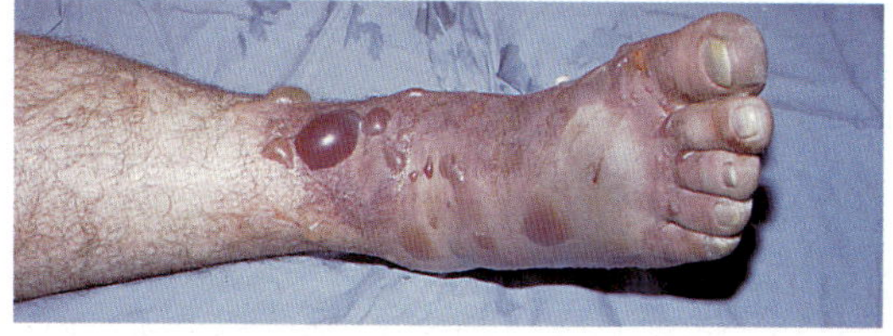

8. **Edema and blister formation 24 hours after frostbite injury occurring in an area covered by a tightly fitted boot.**

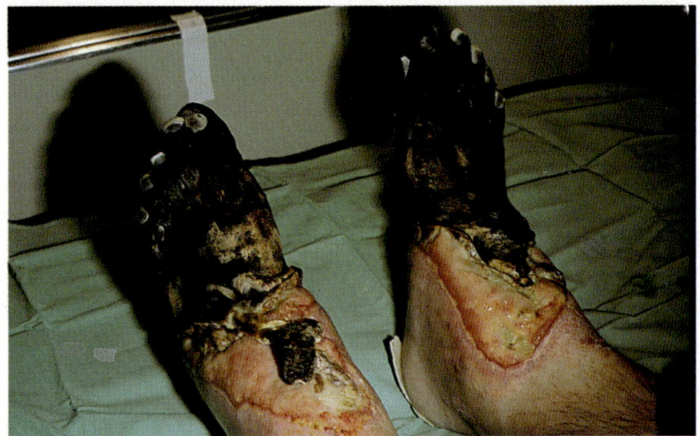

9. Gangrenous necrosis 6 weeks after frostbite injury shown in Plate 8. (Plates 8 and 9 courtesy Cameron Bangs, M.D.)

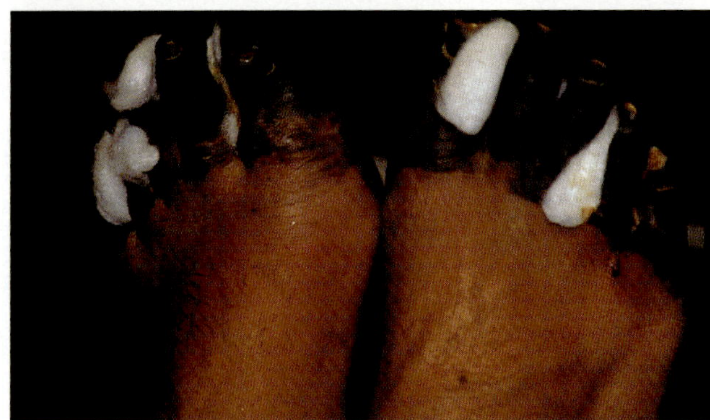

10. Frostbitten toes demarcate 3 weeks after injury. Note the cotton padding between the toes. Minimal tissue loss occurred. (Paul Auerbach, M.D.)

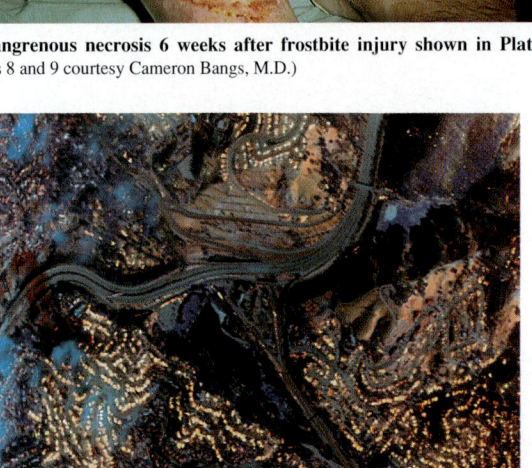

11. More than 2800 homes and apartments were devastated by a wildfire on October 20, 1991, in the hills overlooking Oakland and Berkeley, California. This major wildland/urban interface conflagration killed 25 people.

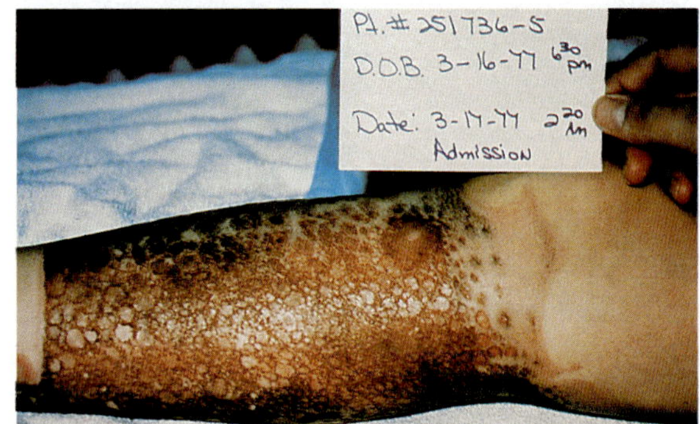

12. Punctate burns from lighting injury. (Courtesy Arthur Kahn, M.D.)

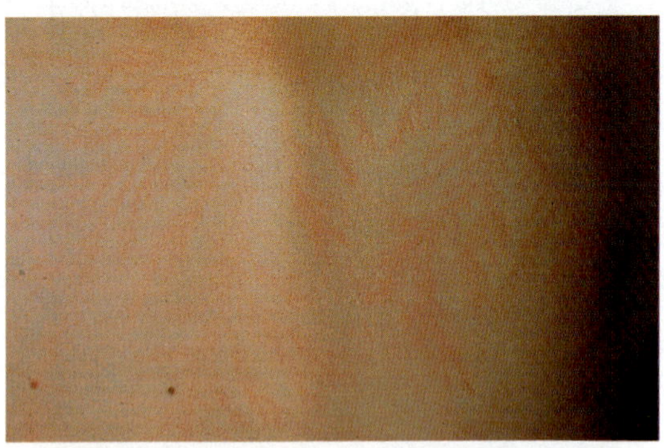

13. Feathering burns from lightning injury. (Mary Ann Cooper, M.D.)

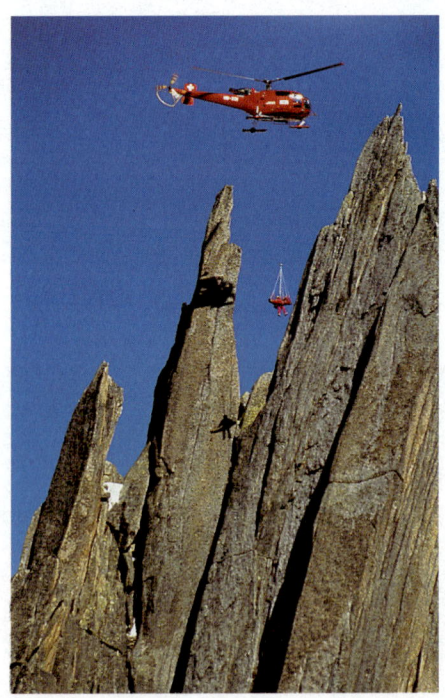

14. A helicopter rescue in extremely difficult terrain. (Courtesy P. Bärtsch, M.D. and the Swiss Alpine Club.)

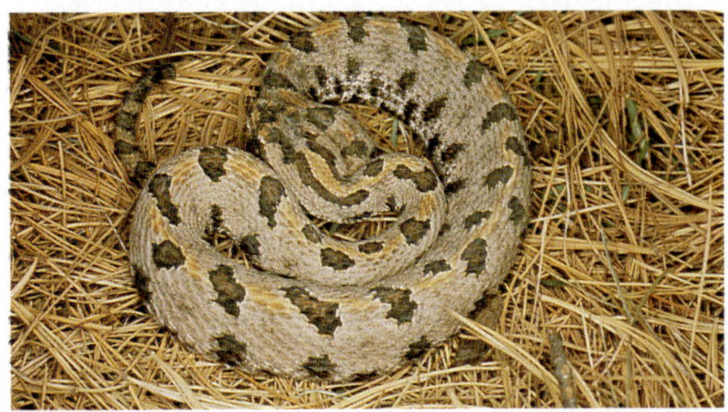

15. Pigmy rattlesnake *(Sistrurus miliaris)*. A common small rattlesnake of the southeastern United States and a frequent cause of snakebites. (Sherman Minton, M.D.)

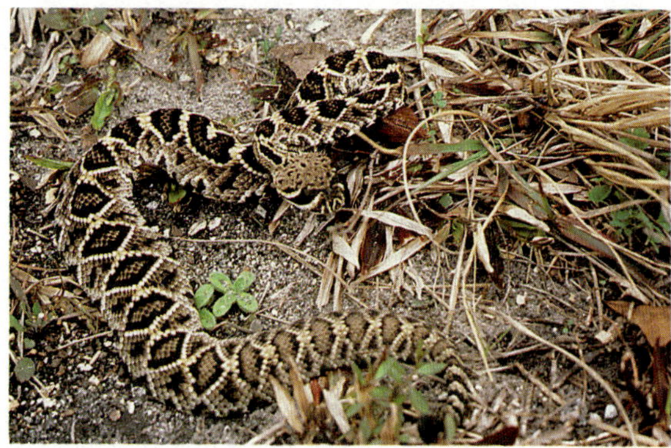

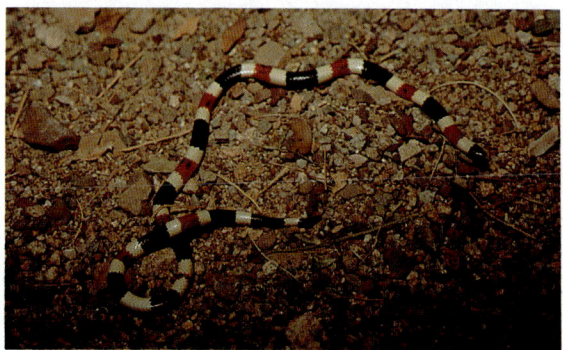

16. **Eastern diamondback rattlesnake *(Crotalus adamanteus)*. This is the largest U.S. rattlesnake, which sometimes attains a length of 7.5 feet. Note the definitive diamond-shaped pattern on the dorsum of the animal.** (Sherman Minton, M.D.)

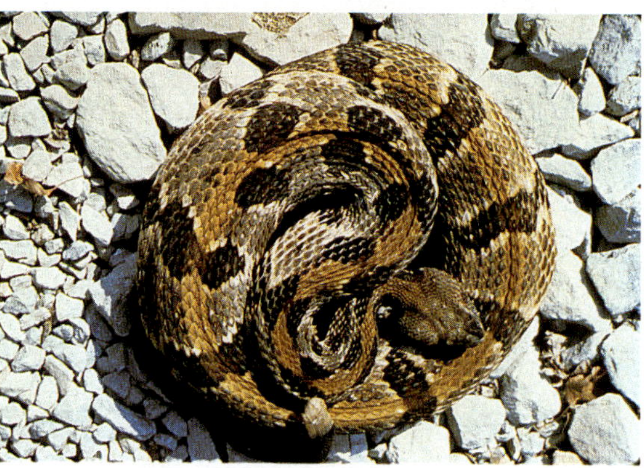

17. **Timber rattlesnake *(Crotalus horridus)*. This is a widely distributed large rattlesnake of the eastern United States.** (Sherman Minton, M.D.)

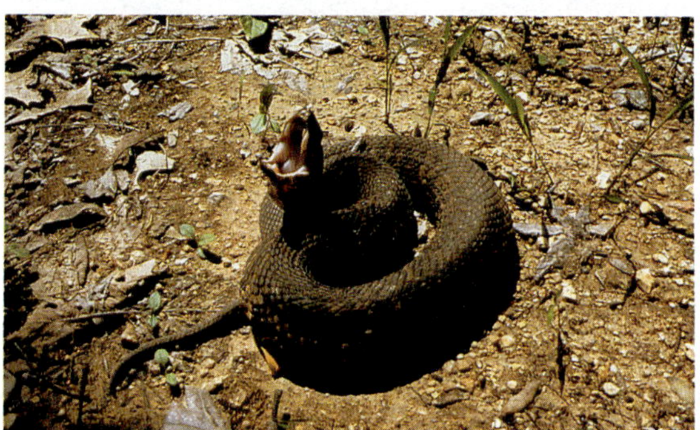

18. **Cottonmouth *(Agkistrodon piscivoris)*. The open-mouthed threat gesture is characteristic of this semiaquatic pit viper.** (Sherman Minton, M.D.)

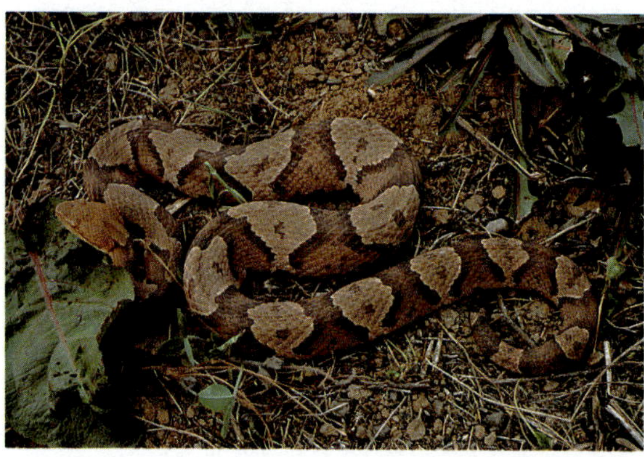

19. **Copperhead *(Agkistrodon contortrix mokasen)*. Copperheads are probably the leading cause of snakebites in the United States, but fatalities from their bites are extremely rare. This specimen is typical of the northeastern variety.** (Sherman Minton, M.D.)

20. **Sonoran coral snake *(Micruroides euryxanthus)*. This small coral snake occurs in southern Arizona and adjacent Mexico.** (Sherman Minton, M.D.)

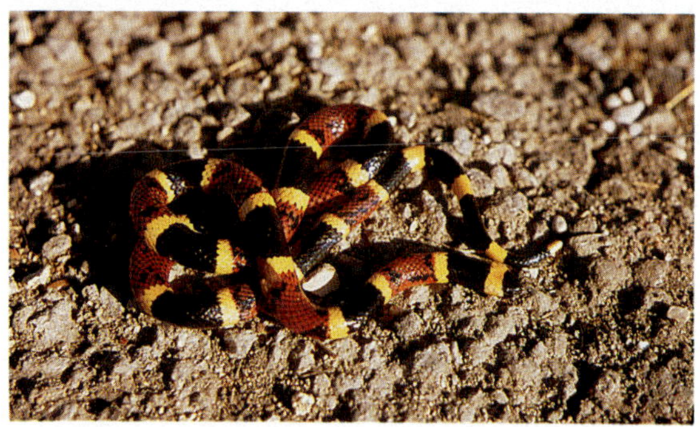

21. **North American coral snake *(Micrurus fulvius)*. Northernmost representative of a tropical American group.** (Sherman Minton, M.D.)

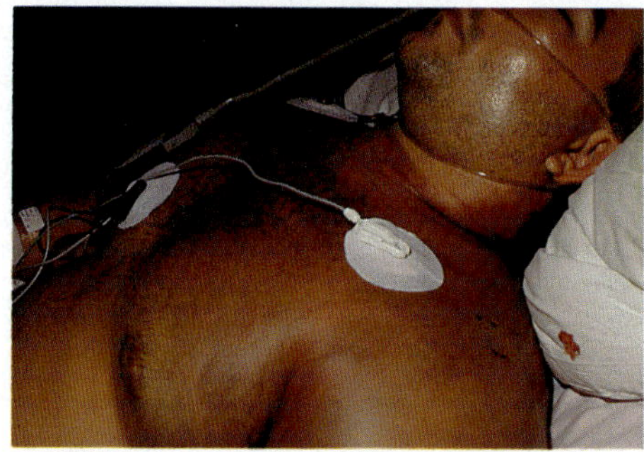

22. **Diffuse hemorrhage associated with thrombocytopenia from a rattlesnake bite.** (Paul Auerbach, M.D.)

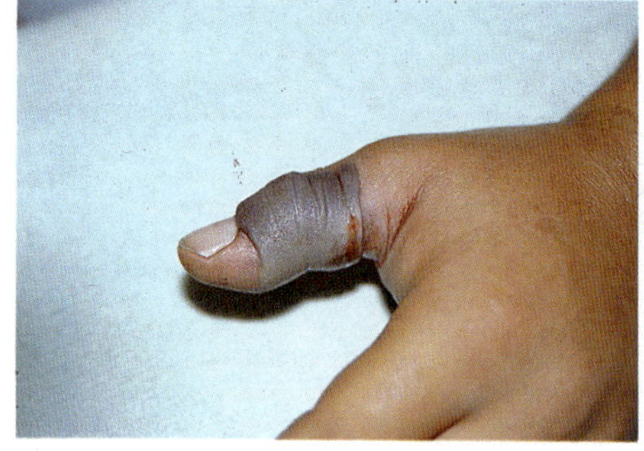

23. **Moderate rattlesnake envenomation.** (Robert Norris, M.D.)

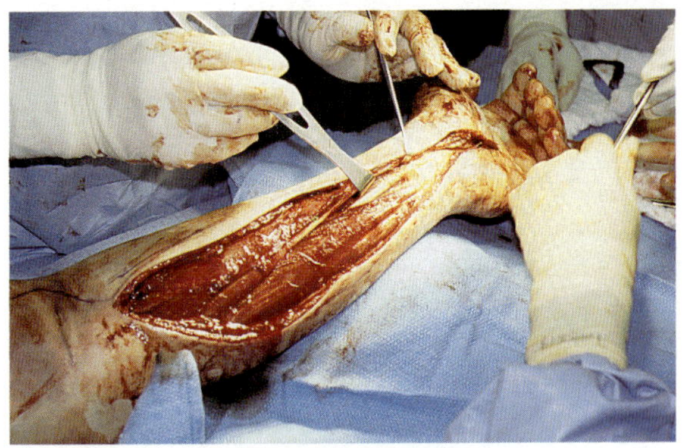

24. Fasciotomy of the upper extremity for elevated compartment pressures following a rattlesnake bite. (Robert Norris, M.D.)

A

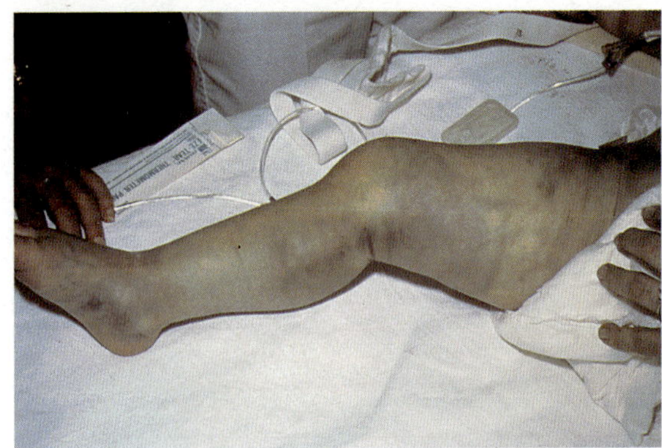

B

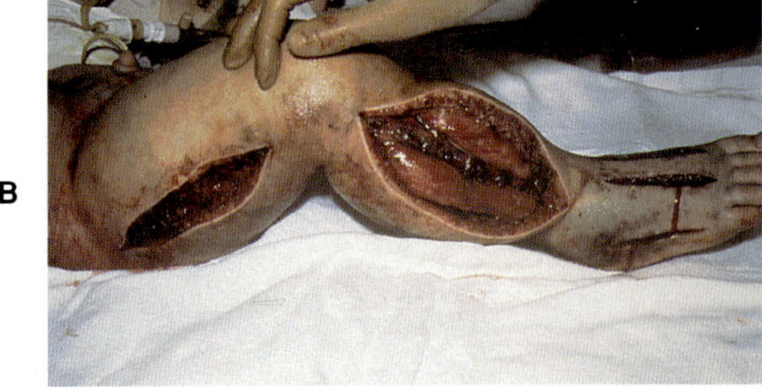

25. Fasciotomy of the severely snakebitten lower extremity for elevated compartment pressures. A, **Before surgery.** B, **After surgery.** (John Sullivan, M.D.)

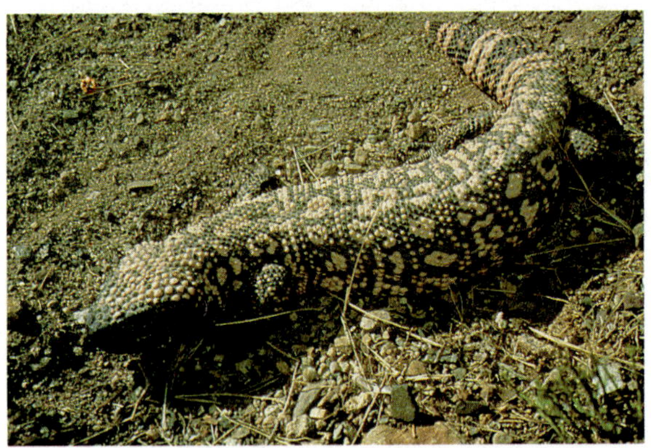

26. Gila monster *(Heloderma suspectum)*. (Willis Wingert, M.D.)

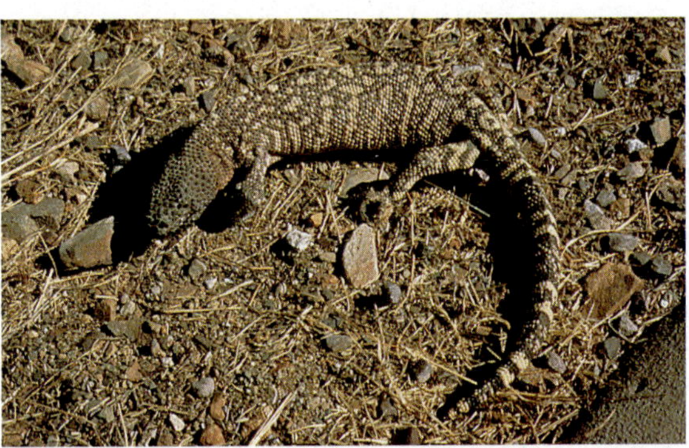

27. Beaded lizard *(Heloderma horridum)*. (Willis Wingert, M.D.)

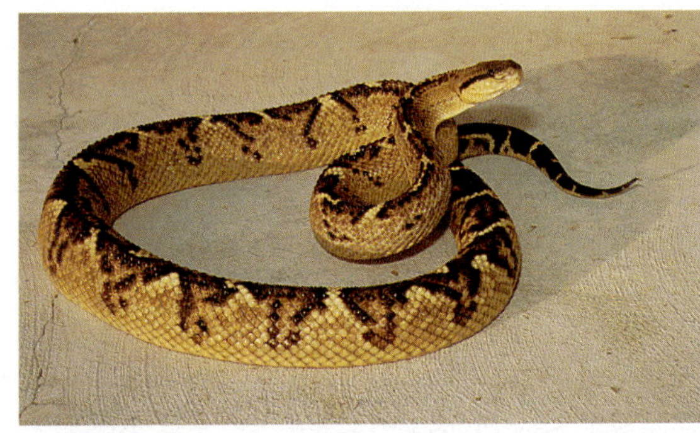

28. Bushmaster *(Lachesis muta)*. These largest of pit vipers reach lengths of 11 feet. The snake is found in southern Central America and northern South America. (Sherman Minton, M.D.)

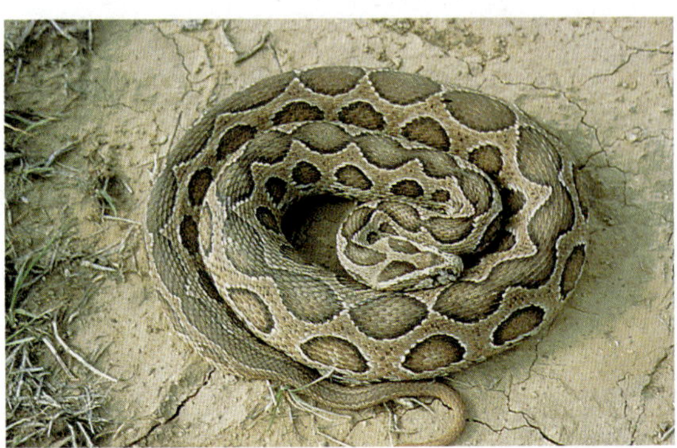

29. Russell's viper *(Vipera russelli)*. Plentiful in agricultural regions of southern Asia, these large vipers are a leading cause of fatal snakebites. (Sherman Minton, M.D.)

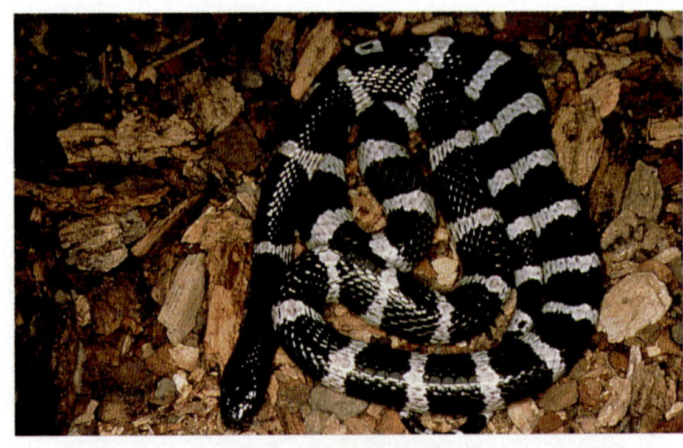

30. Many-banded krait *(Bungarus multicinctus)*. Kraits are widely distributed in southern Asia and have highly lethal neurotoxic venoms. They are nocturnal and rarely aggressive. (Sherman Minton, M.D.)

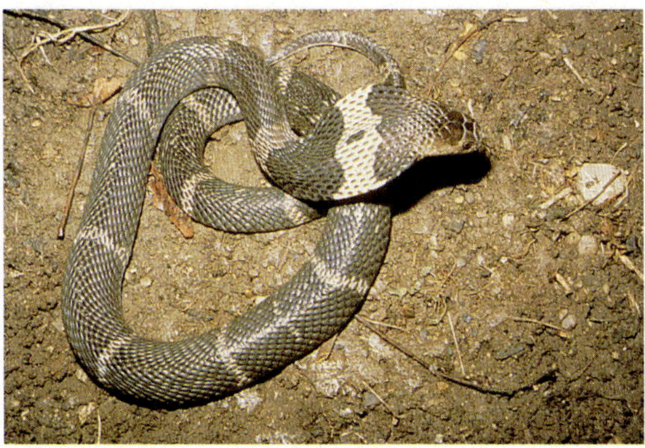

31. **Chinese cobra *(Naja naja atra)*. Cobras are among the world's most venomous snakes, dangerous by virtue of potent venom and distribution in densely populated regions.** (Sherman Minton, M.D.)

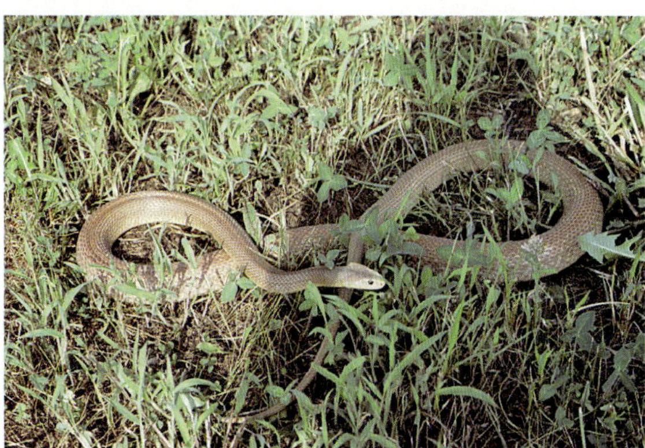

32. **Coastal taipan *(Oxyuranus scutellatus)*. Australia's largest venomous snake sometimes reaches a length of 3 m. Its range is largely in semitropical Queensland. This very dangerous snake can be aggressive.** (Sherman Minton, M.D.)

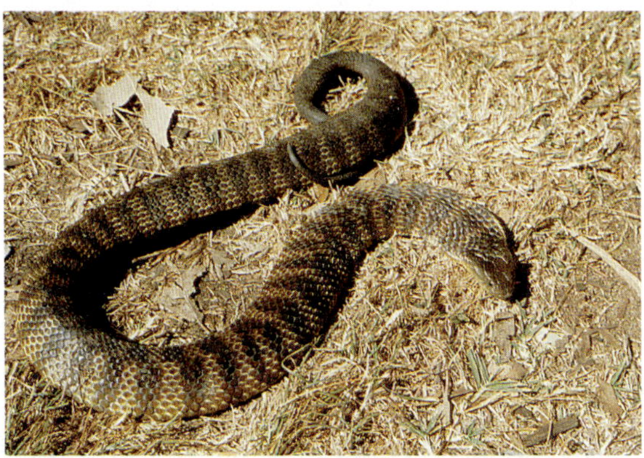

33. **Tiger snake *(Notechis scutatus)*. This highly venomous elapid snake is found in the densely populated eastern part of Australia.** (Sherman Minton, M.D.)

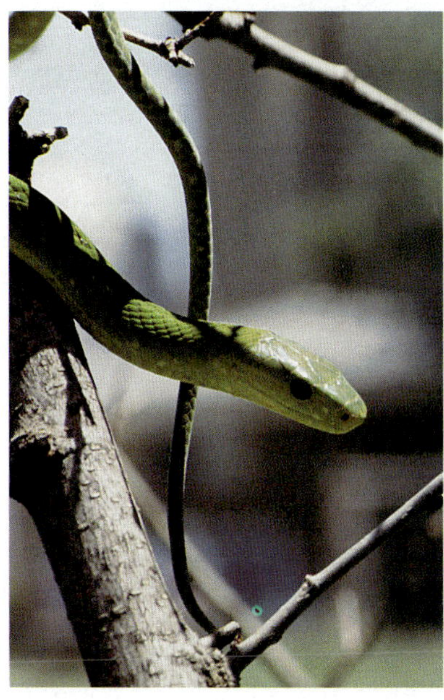

34. **Green mamba *(Dendroaspis angusticeps)*. Mambas are large, slender arboreal African snakes. They are quick, alert, and often dangerous.** (Sherman Minton, M.D.)

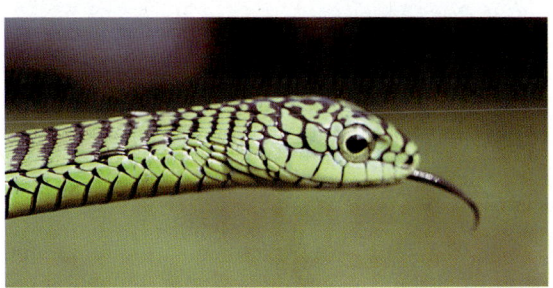

35. **Boomslang *(Dispholidus typus)*. This is the most dangerous of the rear-fanged colubrid snakes. It is an arboreal snake widely distributed in Africa.** (Sherman Minton, M.D.)

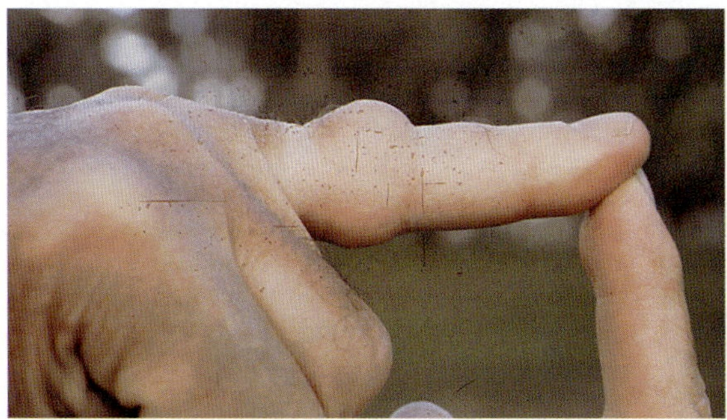

36. **Bite of a small Australian elapid snake *(Hemiaspis signata)* resulting in localized swelling with some discoloration but no systemic symptoms.** (Sherman Minton, M.D.)

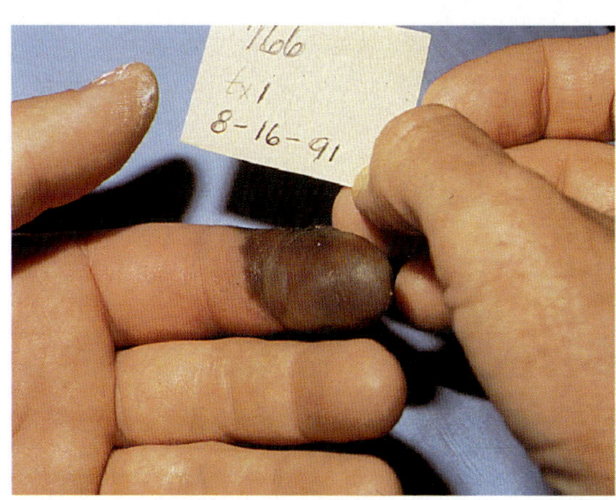

37. **Sharply demarcated necrosis, sometimes extensive, often follows bites by both African and Asian cobras.** (Sherman Minton, M.D.)

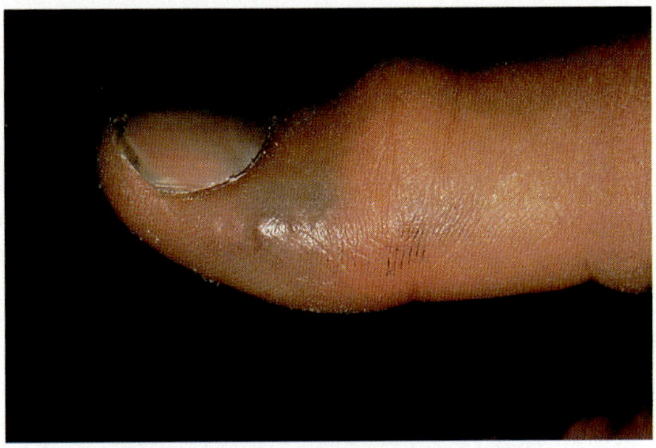

38. **Bite of a southeast Asian water snake *(Enhydrina plumbea),* generally considered to be nonvenomous. Swelling and ecchymosis were still present after 24 hours.** (Sherman Minton, M.D.)

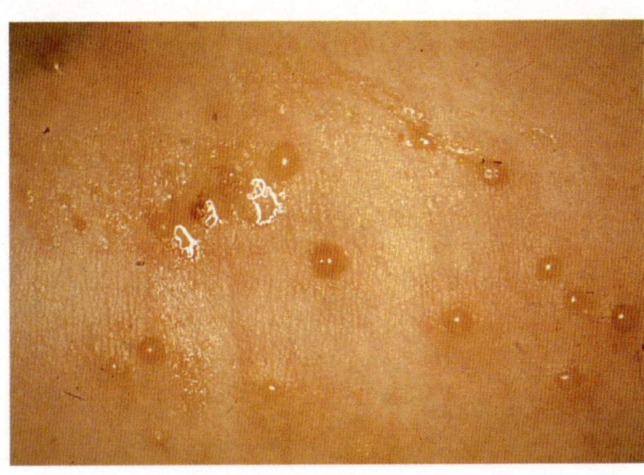

39. **Vesicles produced by fire ant stings approximately 2 hours after the injury. These subsequently became sterile pustules.** (Courtesy Cameron Smith.)

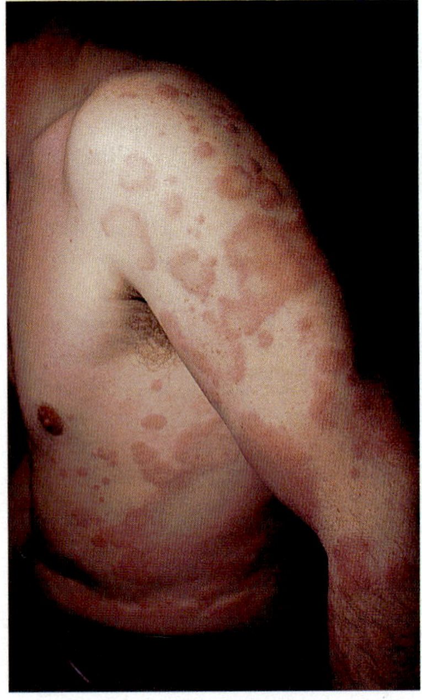

40. **Victim of delayed reaction to a wasp sting. Hymenopteran envenomation should be suspected in any unexplained episode of diffuse urticaria.** (Paul Auerbach, M.D.)

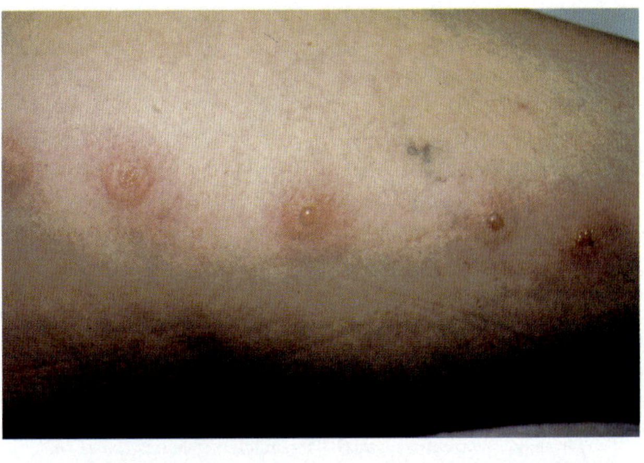

41. **Typical linear pattern of triatomid bites on the forearm.** (Sherman Minton, M.D.)

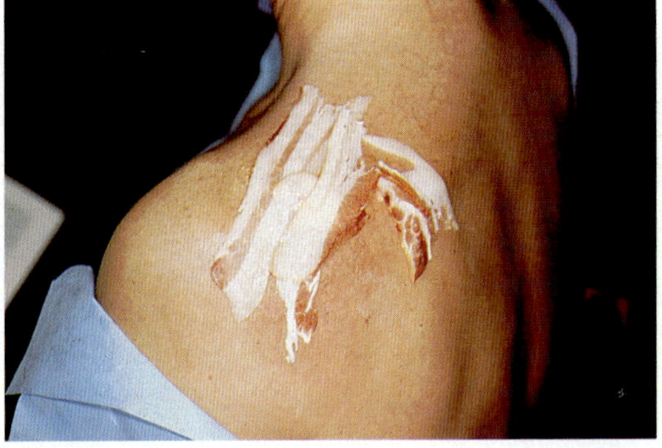

43. **The fatty portion of multiple strips of raw bacon were placed over the larval apertures to obstruct the air supply and encourage the larvae's egress from the skin.**

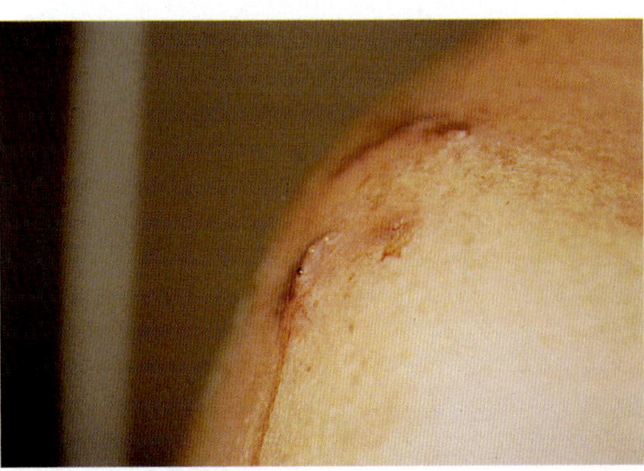

42. **Lateral view of three lesions caused by infestation with *D. hominis* larvae. The nodules were initially assumed to be furunculosis. A central breathing aperture is present in each nodule. Serosanguineous fluid is draining from two of the nodules. Larval spiracles are visible emerging from the uppermost nodule.** (Plates 42 through 44 courtesy Donna Felsenstein, M.D.; Timothy Brewer, M.D.; Ernesto Gonzales, M.D.; and Mary Wilson, M.D. Copyright 1993, AMA-*JAMA* 270[17]:2087-2088.)

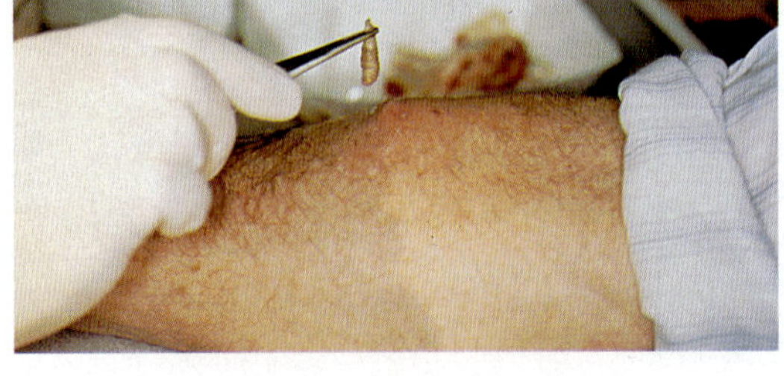

44. **After approximately 2 hours of treatment with bacon therapy, the *D. hominis* larvae have emerged far enough from the subcutaneous tissues to be grasped with forceps. The larva is removed intact.**

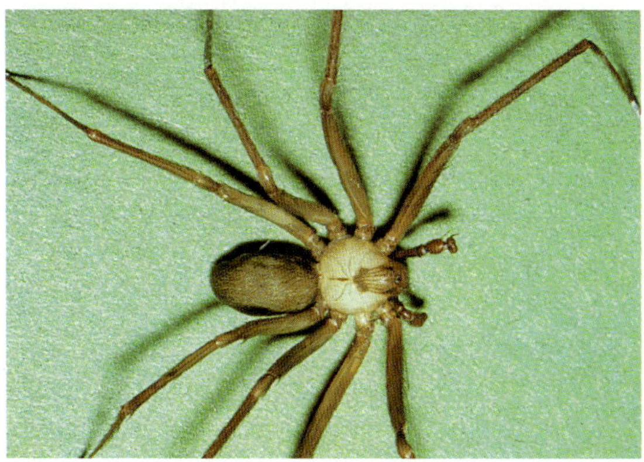

45. **Brown recluse spider *(Loxosceles reclusa)*. This is the most important member of the genus in the United States. The dark violin-shaped mark on the cephalothorax is seen in most North American species.** (Courtesy Indiana University Medical Center.)

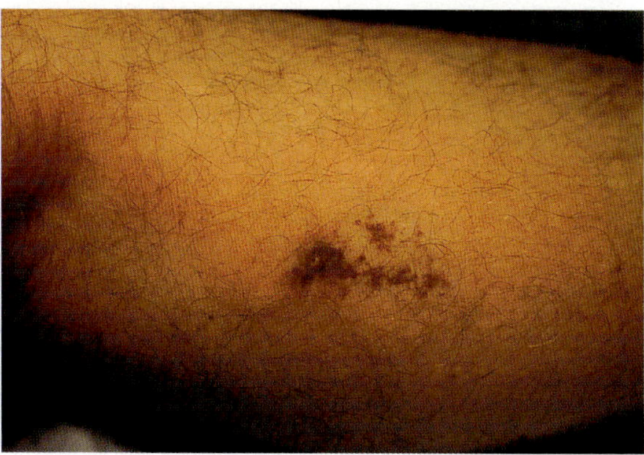

46. **Brown recluse spider bite after 6 hours, with central hemorrhagic vesicle and gravitational pattern spread of venom.** (Paul Auerbach, M.D., and Riley Rees, M.D.)

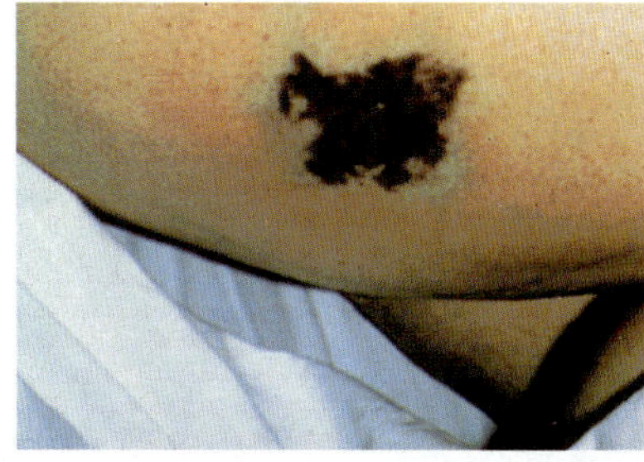

47. **Cutaneous presentation of brown recluse spider bite after 24 hours, with central ischemia and rapidly advancing cellulitis.** (Paul Auerbach, M.D.)

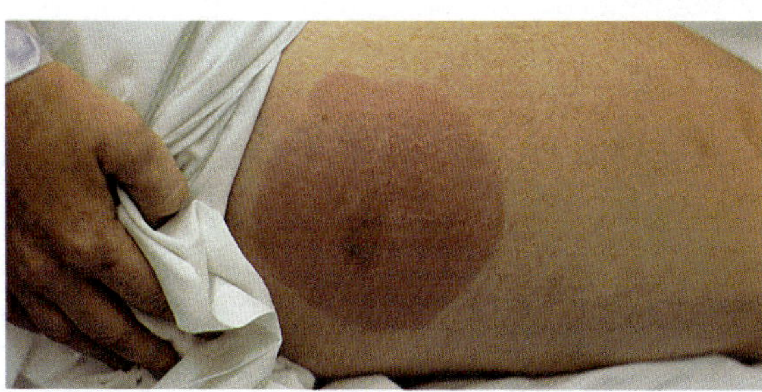

48. **Brown recluse spider bite after 48 hours, with incipient central necrosis.**

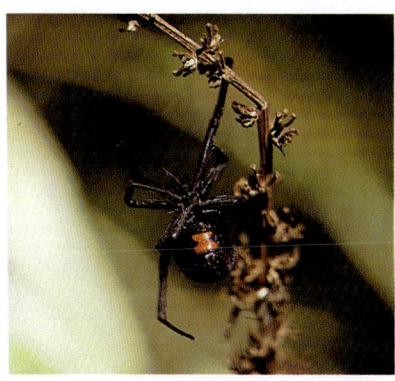

49. **North American black widow spider *(Latrodectus mactans)*.** (Paul Auerbach, M.D.)

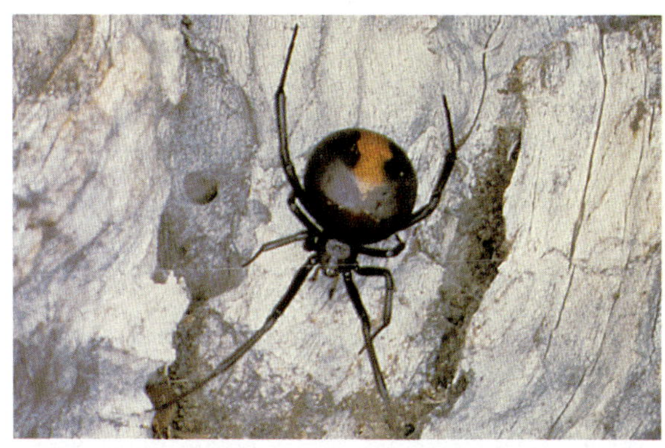

50. **Red-backed spider *(Latrodectus hasselti)*. This spider is related to the North American black widow and is medically important in Australia, New Zealand, and parts of southern Asia.** (Sherman Minton, M.D.)

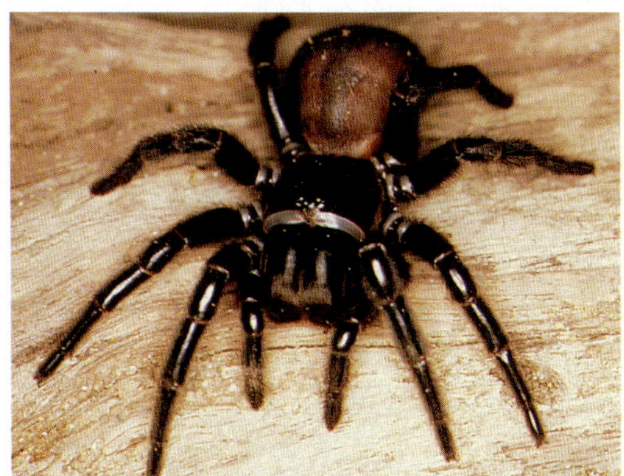

51. **Funnel web spider (*Atrax* species) wearing a wedding ring. This large specimen from New South Wales is typical of the most dangerous mygalomorphs of southeastern Australia.** (Sherman Minton, M.D.)

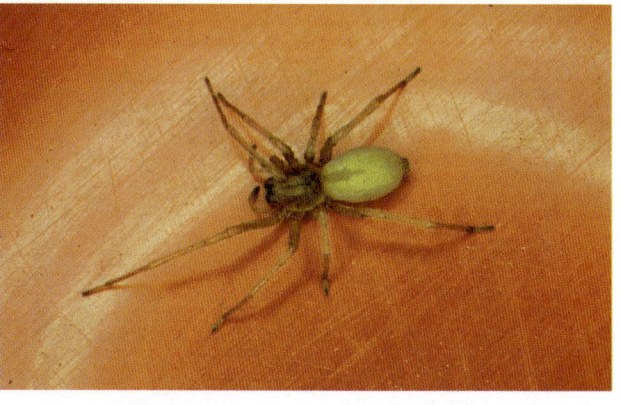

52. ***Chiracanthium inclusum* is the only species of this genus indigenous to the United States.** (Sherman Minton, M.D.)

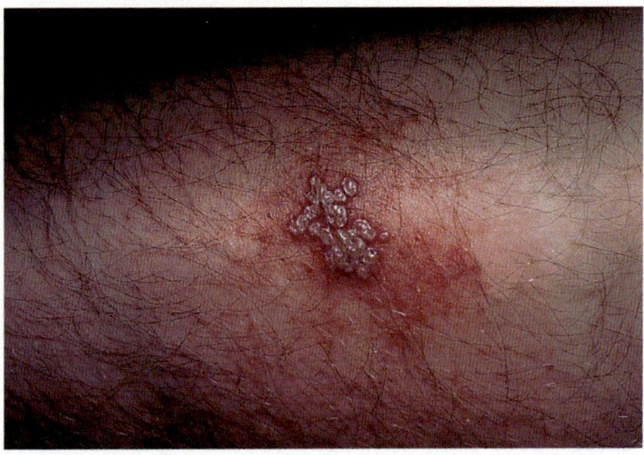

53. Unidentified spider bite. Multiple bites make this unlikely to be the work of a brown recluse. (Paul Auerbach, M.D.)

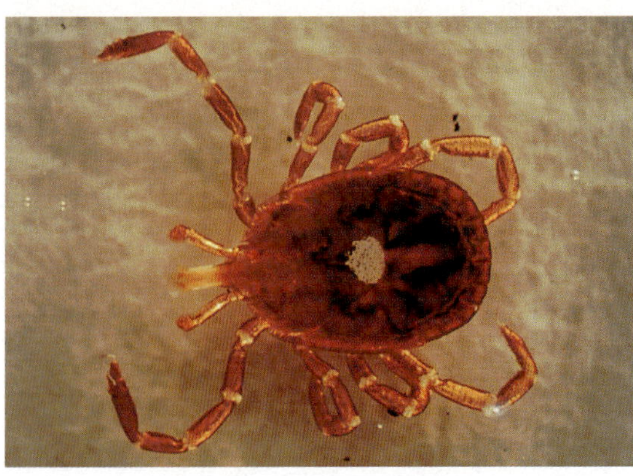

54. Lone star tick *(Amblyomma americanum)*. This tick has been implicated in cases of tick paralysis in North America. (Sherman Minton, M.D.)

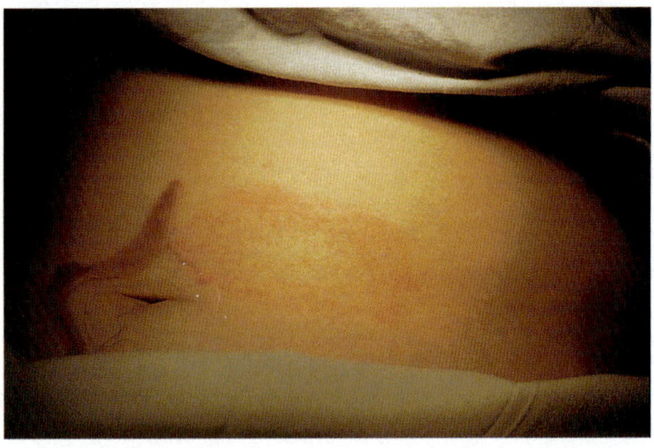

55. Erythema migrans rash of Lyme disease in a pregnant female. (Paul Auerbach, M.D.)

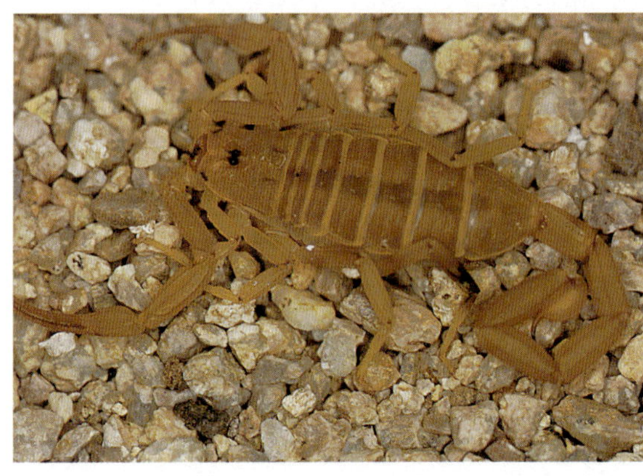

56. Scorpion of the genus *Centruroides* (bark scorpion). (William Banner, M.D.)

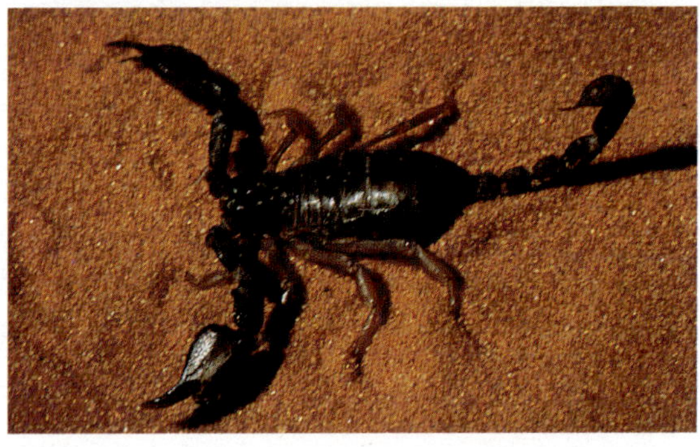

57. *Uroloctonus mordax*, a moderate-sized but comparatively innocuous scorpion of the northwestern United States. (Sherman Minton, M.D.)

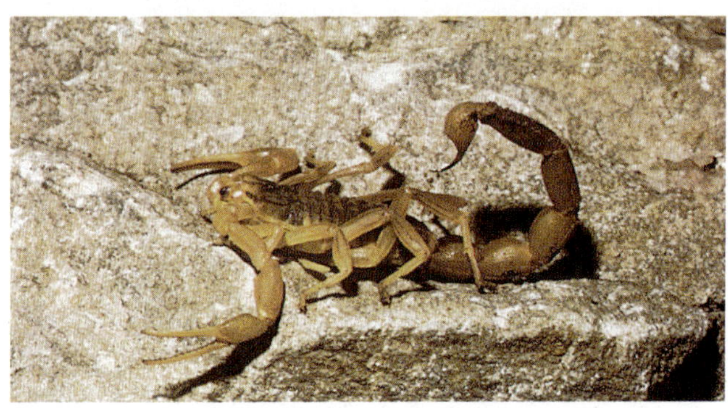

58. *Leiurus quinquestriatus*, one of the most dangerous scorpions in the world. This arachnid lives in Egypt and the Middle East. (Sherman Minton, M.D.)

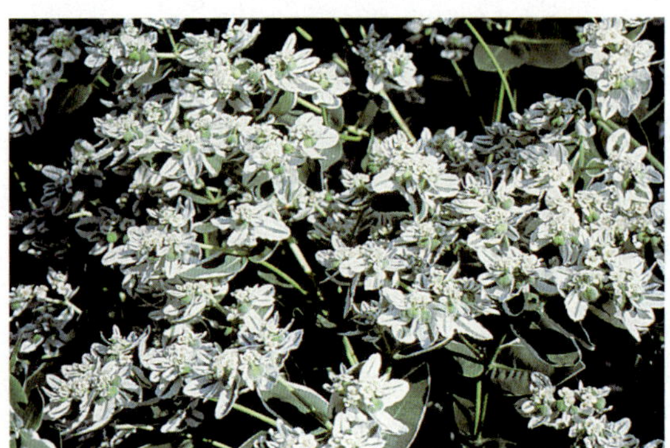

59. Plants that cause primary skin irritation: Snow-on-the-mountain.

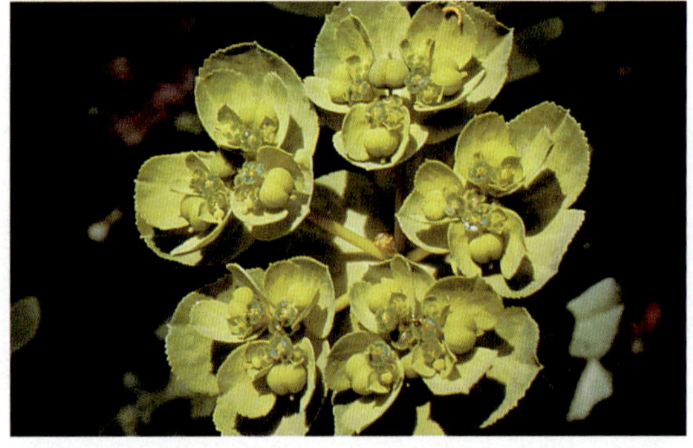

60. Plants that cause primary skin irritation: Wolfsmilk.

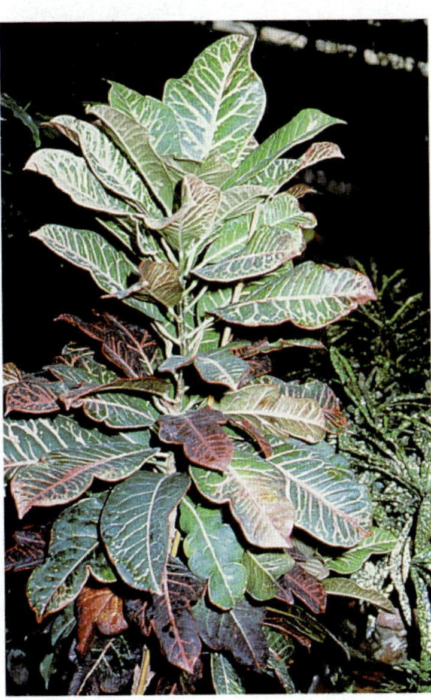

61. Plants that cause primary skin irritation: Croton bush. (Plates 61 and 62 courtesy Professor Yves Sell, Institute of Botany, Louis Pasteur University, Strasbourg.)

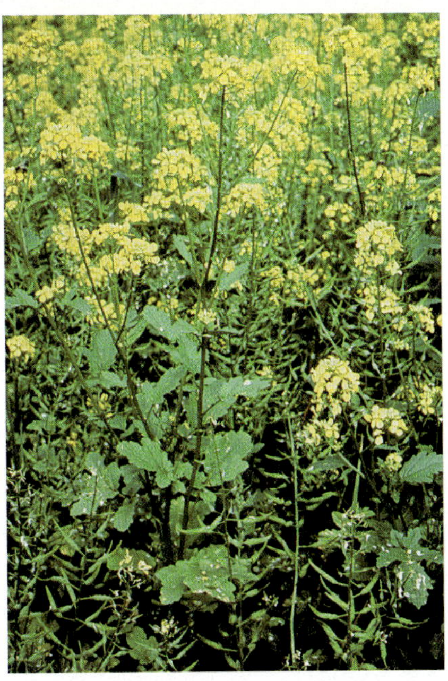

62. White mustard plant, an irritant of the Brassicaceae family.

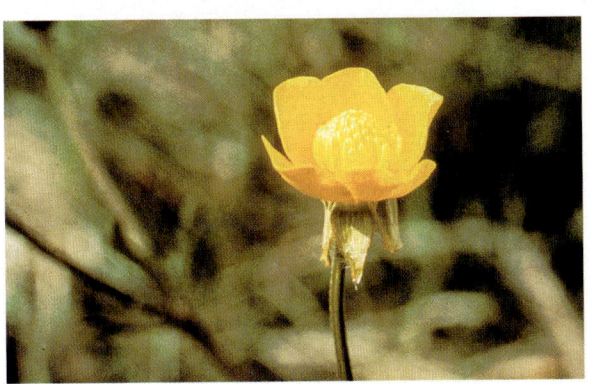

63. Plant of the family Ranunculaceae: Buttercup.

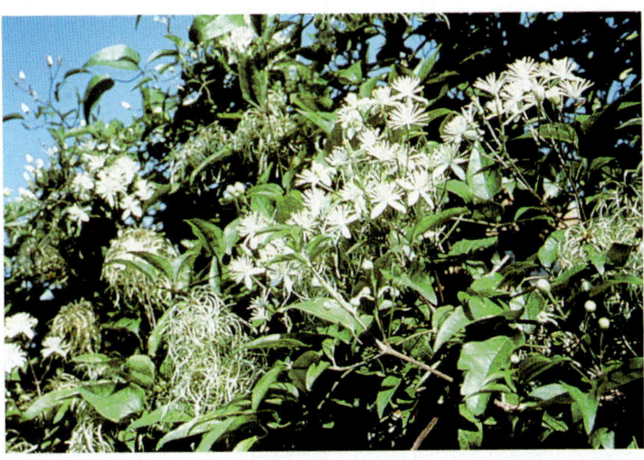

64. Plant of the family Ranunculaceae: Old man's beard. (Courtesy Professor Yves Sell, Institute of Botany, Louis Pasteur University, Strasbourg.)

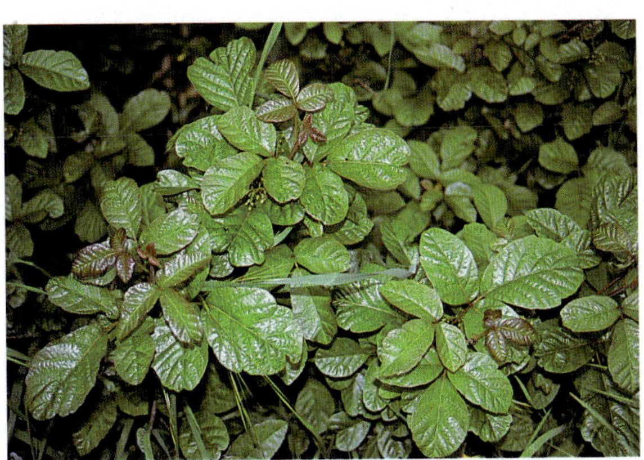

65. Poison oak. (Paul Auerbach, M.D.)

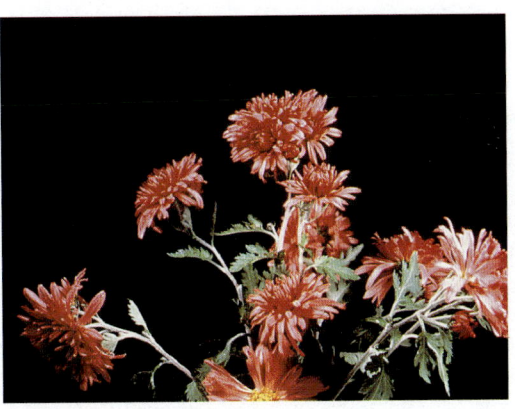

66. Compositae contact sensitizer: Chrysanthemum.

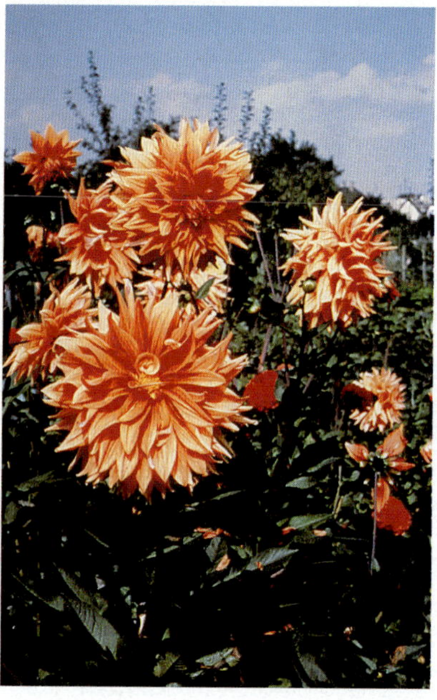

67. Compositae contact sensitizer: Dahlia.

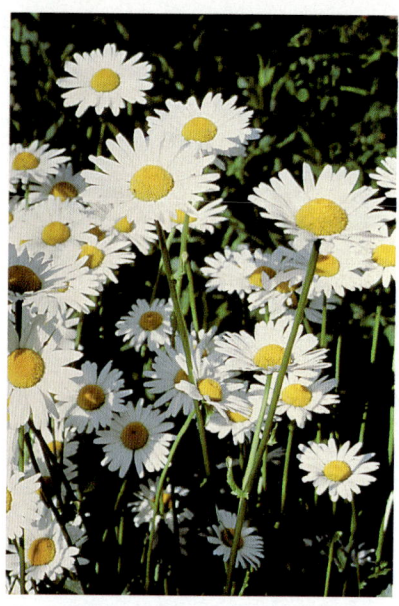

68. Compositae contact sensitizer: Daisy. (Courtesy Professor Yves Sell, Institute of Botany, Louis Pasteur University, Strasbourg.)

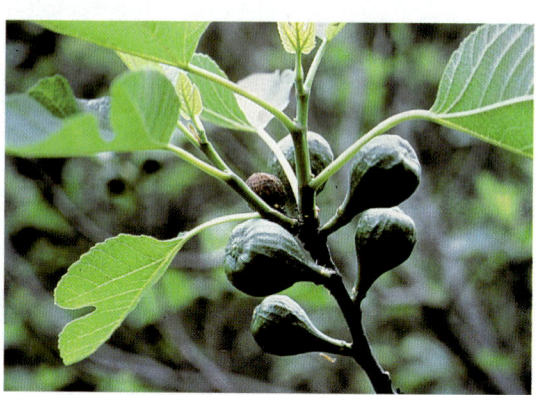

69. Plant that contributes to phototoxicity: Fig tree.

70. Plant that contributes to phototoxicity: Gas plant. (Courtesy Professor Yves Sell, Institute of Botany, Louis Pasteur University, Strasbourg.)

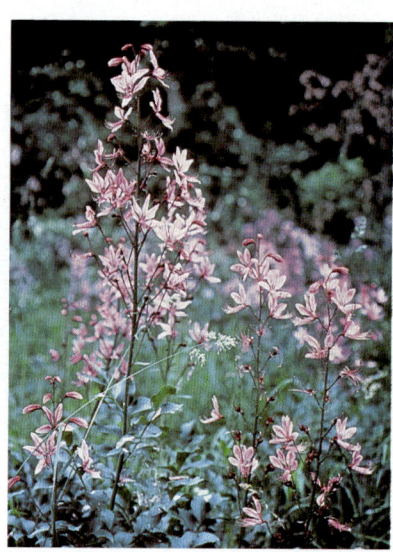

71. Beaver tail cactus (*Opuntia* species). (Courtesy Eric Lewis, M.D.)

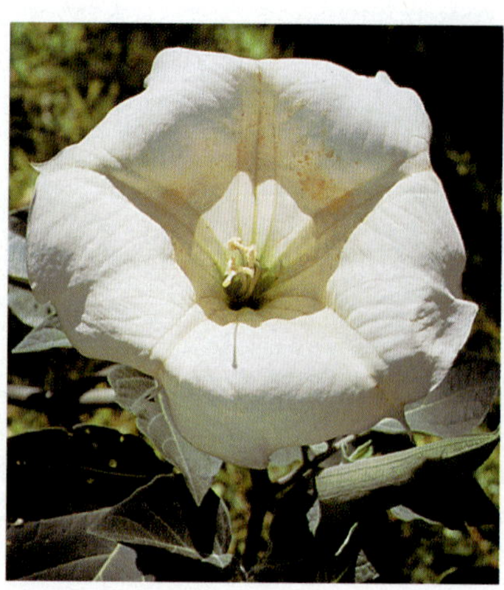

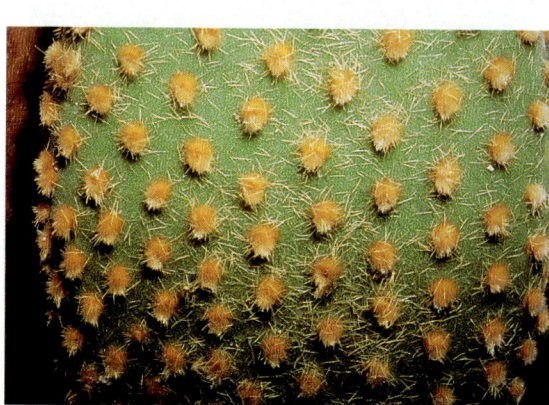

72. Jimson weed (*Datura* species). (Plates 72 through 77 courtesy Donald Kunkel, M.D.)

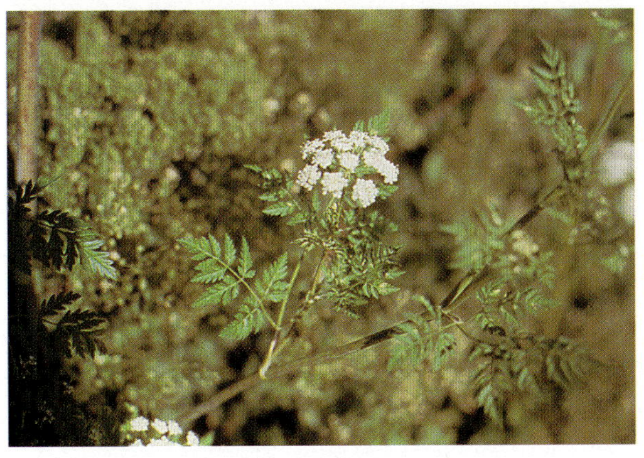

73. Poison hemlock *(Conium maculatum).*

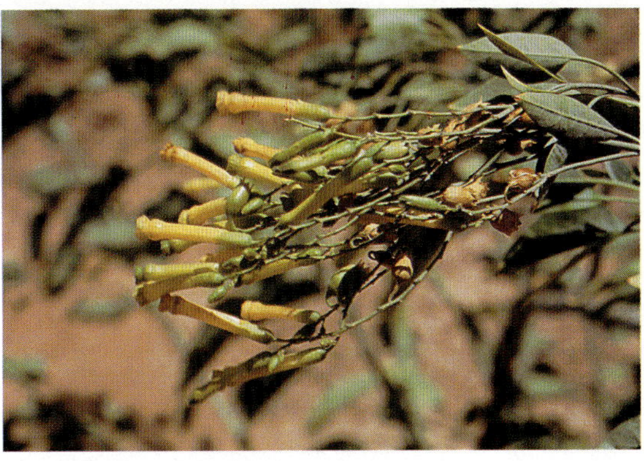

74. Tree tobacco *(Nicotiana glauca).*

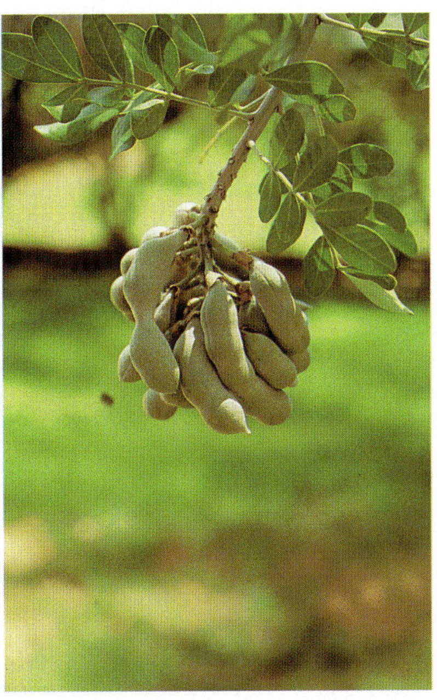

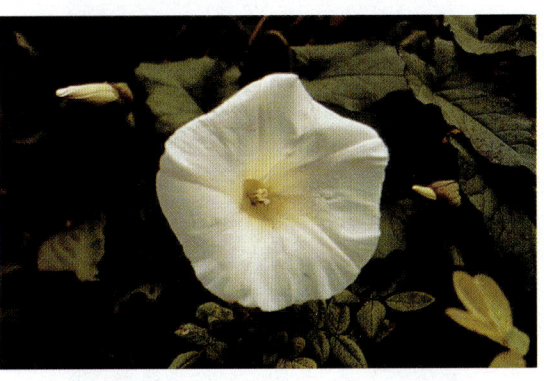

75. Mescal bean bush *(Sophora secundiflora).*

76. Morning glory *(Ipomoea violacea).*

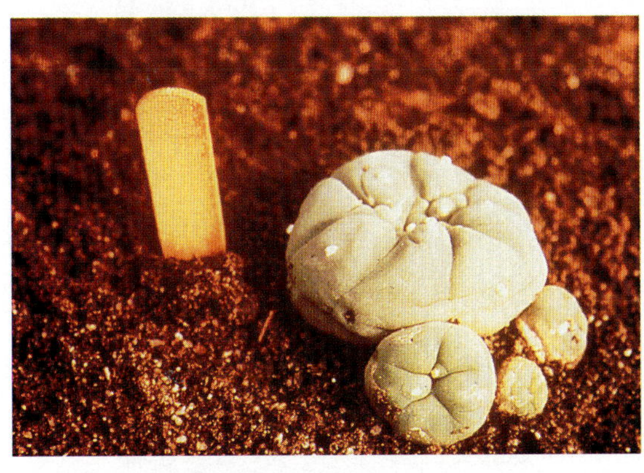

77. Peyote *(Lophophora williamsii).*

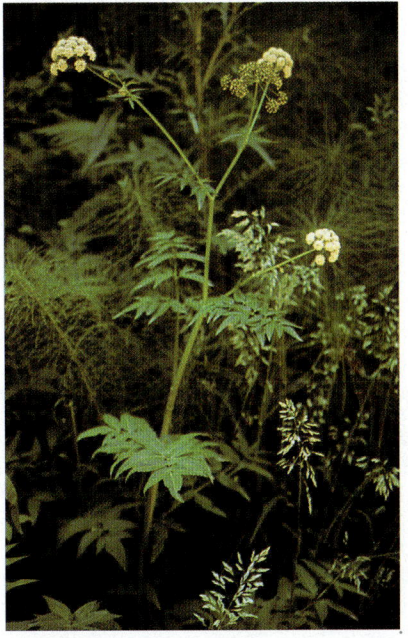

78. Water hemlock *(Cicuta maculata).*

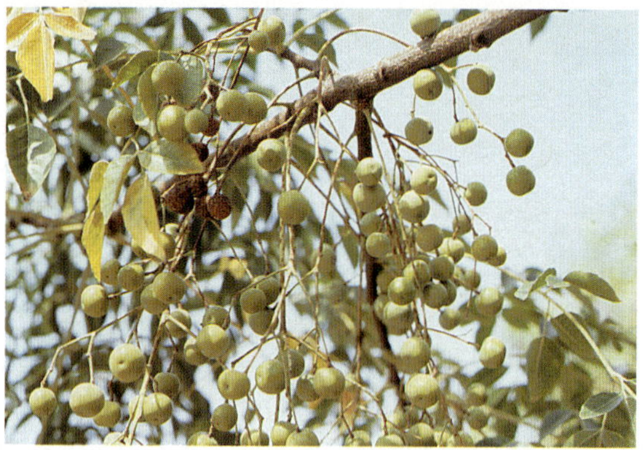

79. Chinaberry *(Melia azedarach).* (Donald Kunkel, M.D.)

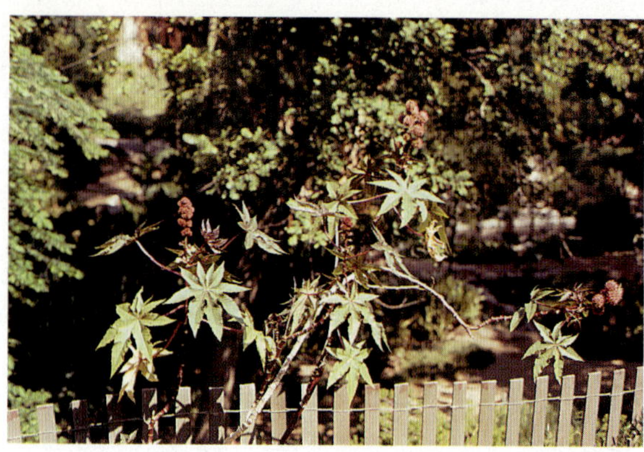

80. Castor bean *(Ricinus communis)* (Edward Geehr, M.D.)

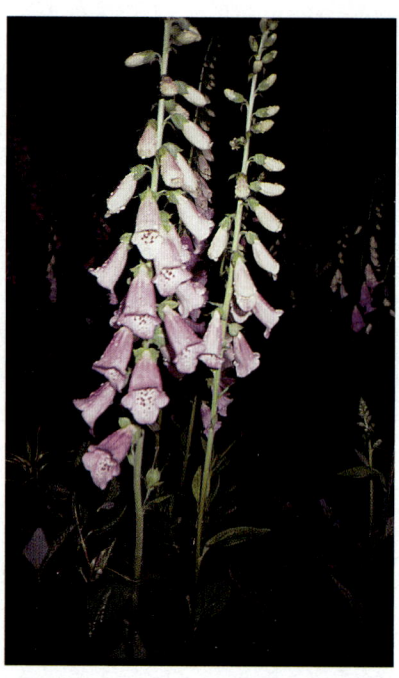

81. Wild foxglove (*Digitalis* species) in the Galapagos Islands. (Paul Auerbach, M.D.)

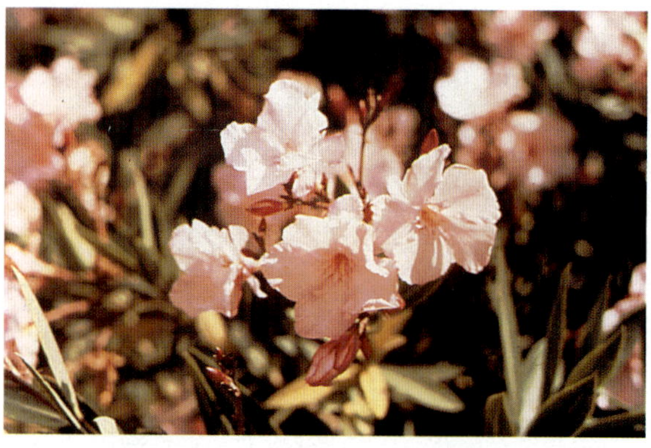

82. Oleander *(Nerium oleander)* flowers. (Edward Geehr, M.D.)

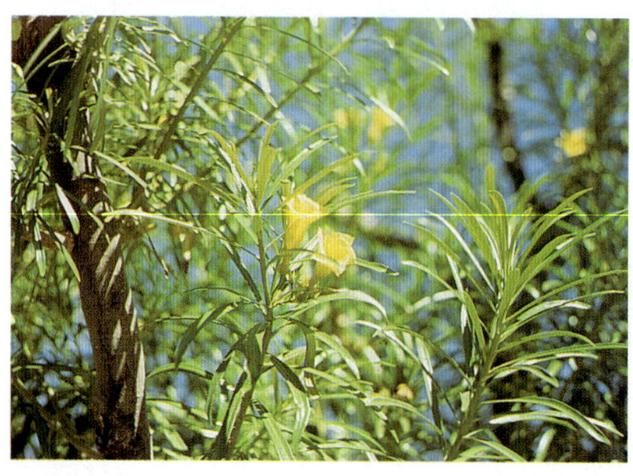

83. Yellow oleander *(Thevetia peruviana).* (Donald Kunkel, M.D.)

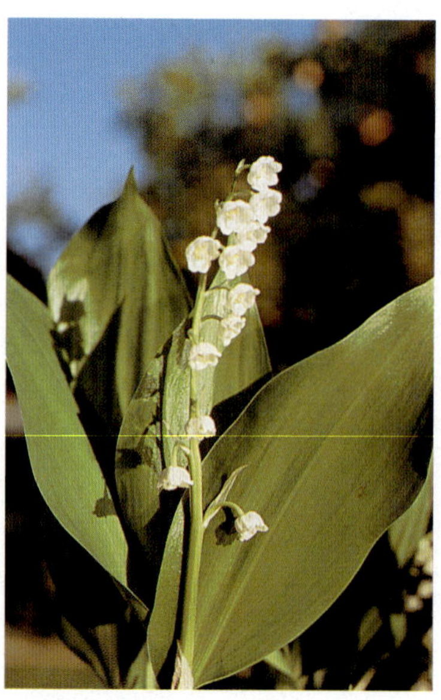

84. Lily of the valley *(Convallaria majalis).* (Donald Kunkel, M.D.)

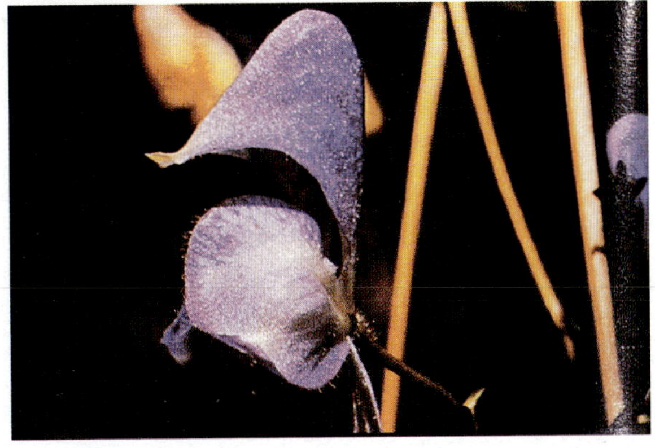

85. **Monkshood (*Aconitum* species).**

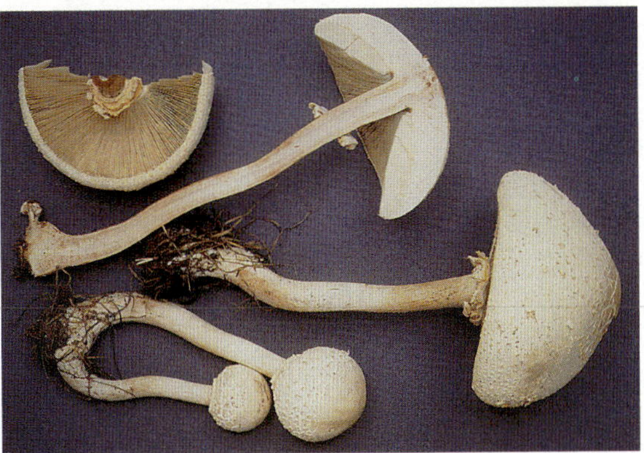

86. ***Chlorophyllum molybdites.*** **A gastrointestinal irritant.** (From Phillips R: *Mushrooms of North America*. Copyright © 1991 by Roger Phillips. By permission of Little, Brown.)

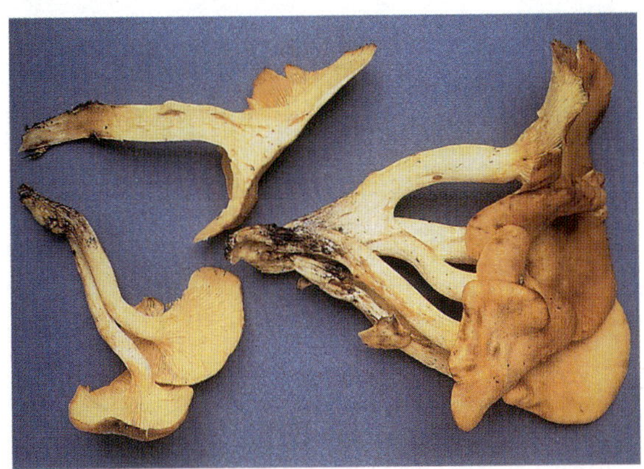

87. ***Omphalotus olearius*** **(Jack O'Lantern mushroom). A gastrointestinal irritant.** (From Phillips R: *Mushrooms of North America*. Copyright © 1991 by Roger Phillips. By permission of Little, Brown.)

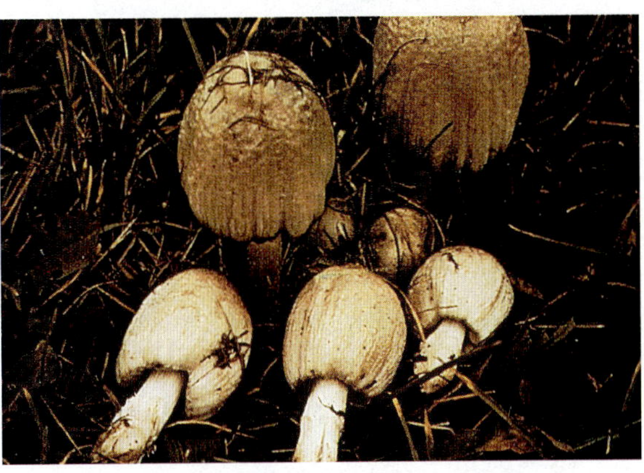

88. **Inky cap *(Coprinus atramentarius).*** (Courtesy Orson J. Miller, Ph.D.)

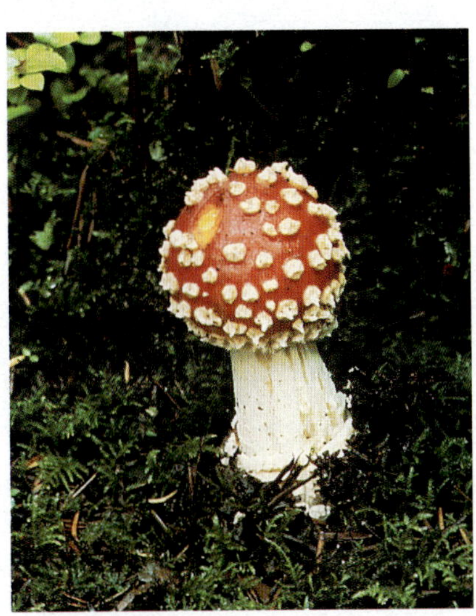

89. ***Amanita muscaria.***

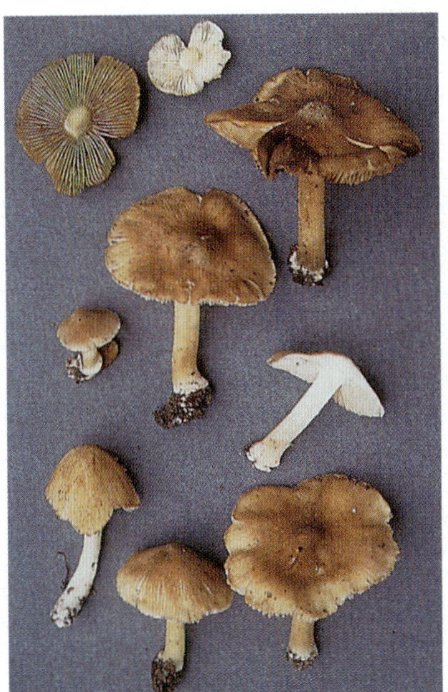

90. ***Inocybe cookei.*** **Contains muscarinic toxins.** (From Phillips R: *Mushrooms of North America*. Copyright © 1991 by Roger Phillips. By permission of Little, Brown.)

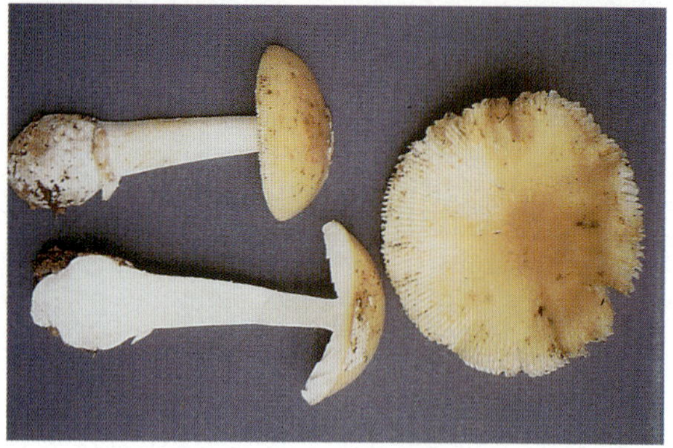

91. ***Amanita pantherina.*** **Contains the neurotoxins ibotenic acid and isozazole derivatives.** (From Phillips R: *Mushrooms of North America.* Copyright © 1992 by Roger Phillips. By permission of Little, Brown.)

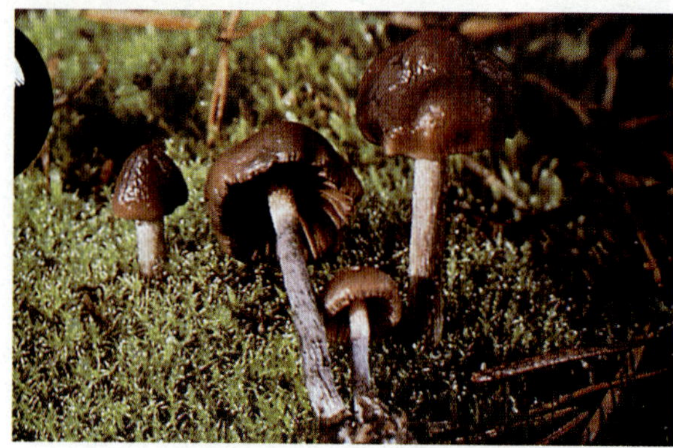

92. ***Psilocybe caerulipes.***

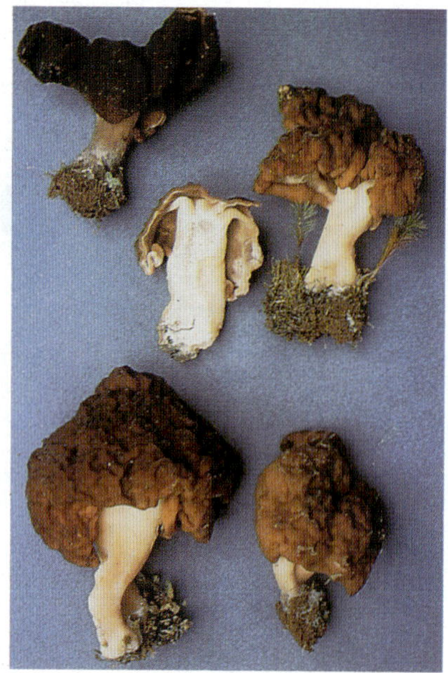

93. ***Gyromitra esculenta.*** **Contains the hepatotoxin gyromitrin.** (From Phillips R: *Mushrooms of North America.* Copyright © 1992 by Roger Phillips. By permission of Little, Brown.)

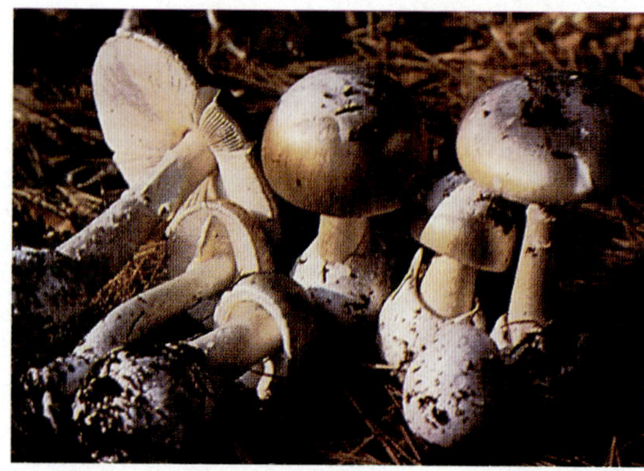

94. **Death cap *(Amanita phalloides).***

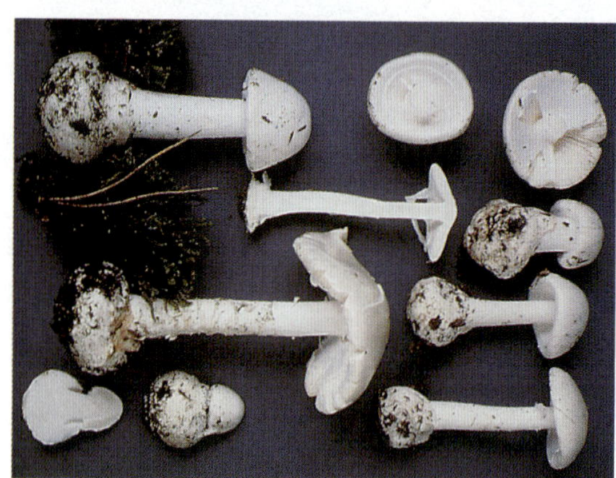

95. ***Amanita virosa.*** **Causes delayed hepatotoxicity.** (From Phillips R: *Mushrooms of North America.* Copyright © 1991 by Roger Phillips. By permission of Little, Brown.)

A

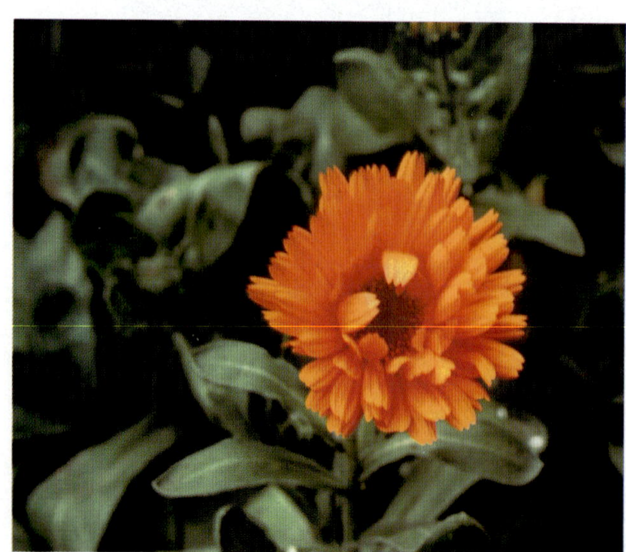

B

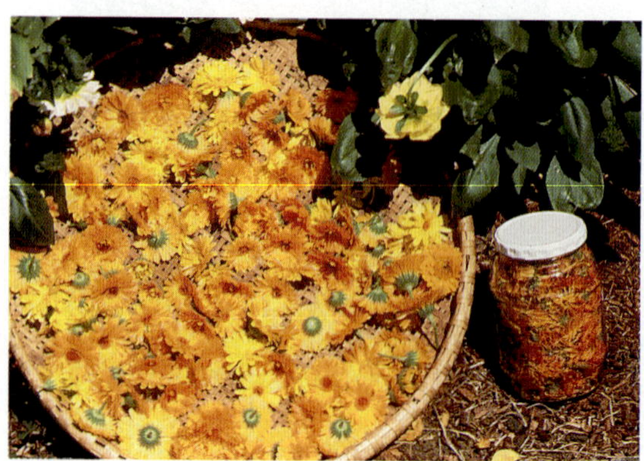

96. A, ***Calendula officinalis.*** B, ***Calendula*** **drying and dried in a jar.** (Plates 96 through 101 courtesy Cascade Anderson Geller.)

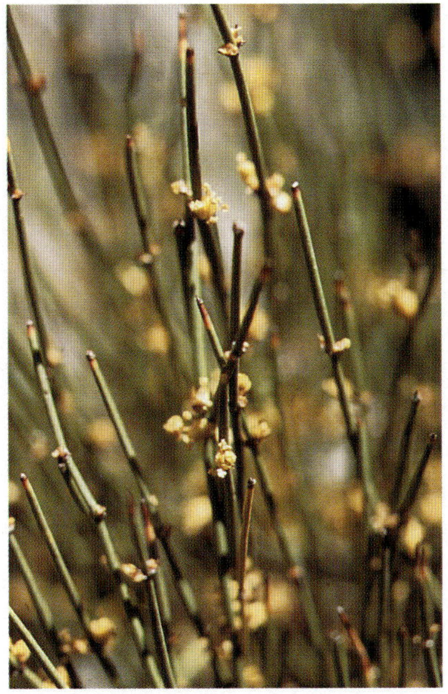

97. ***Ephedra viridis.***

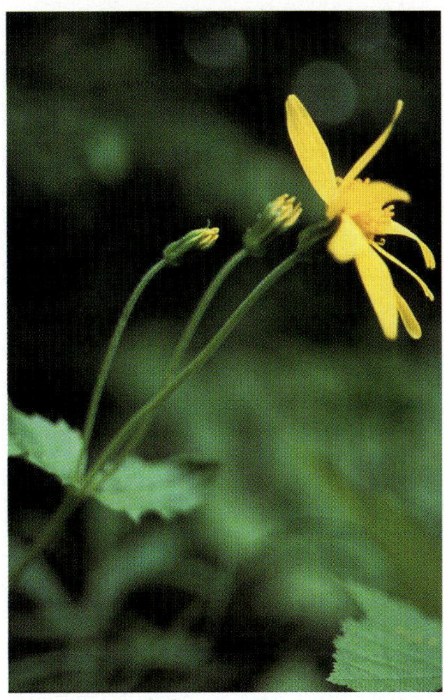

98. ***Arnica latifolia.***

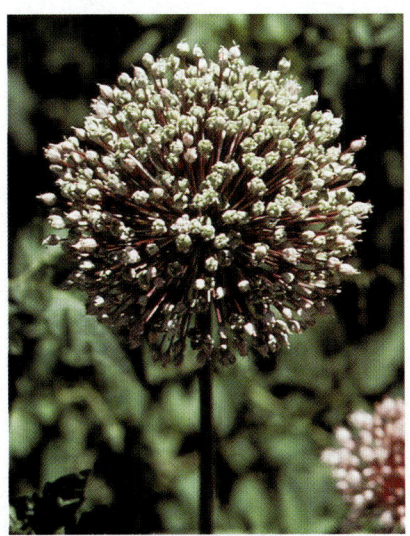

99. Garlic blossom (*Allium* species).

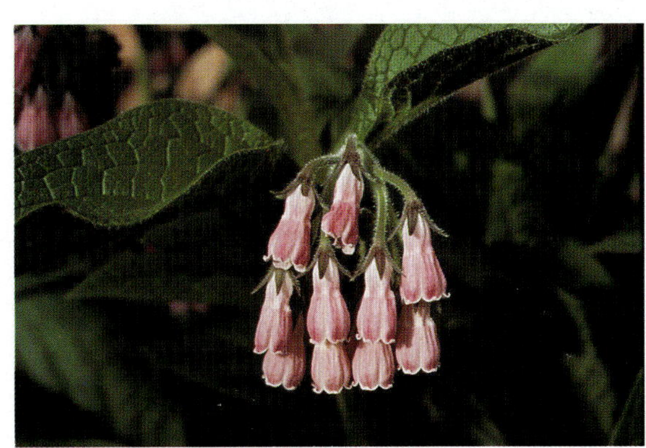

100. Comfrey *(Symphytum officinale)*

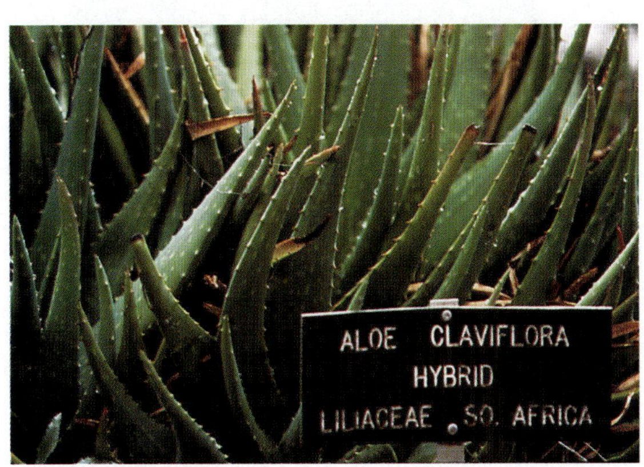

101. ***Aloe claviflora.***

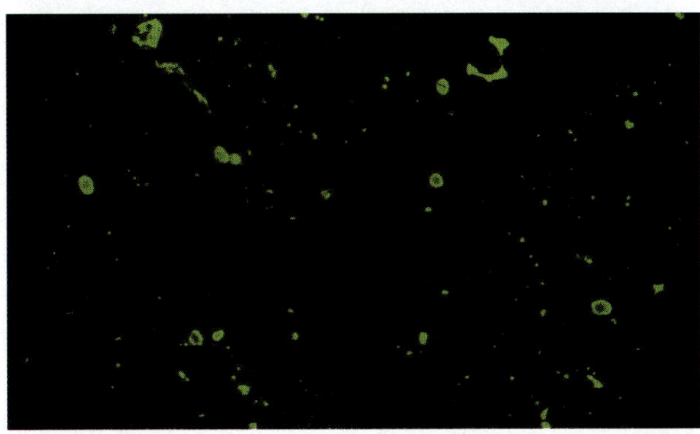

102. Brain impression smear (direct fluorescent antibody preparation) positive for rabies from a Canadian fox. Original magnification 400 x. (Courtesy Centers for Disease Control and Prevention.)

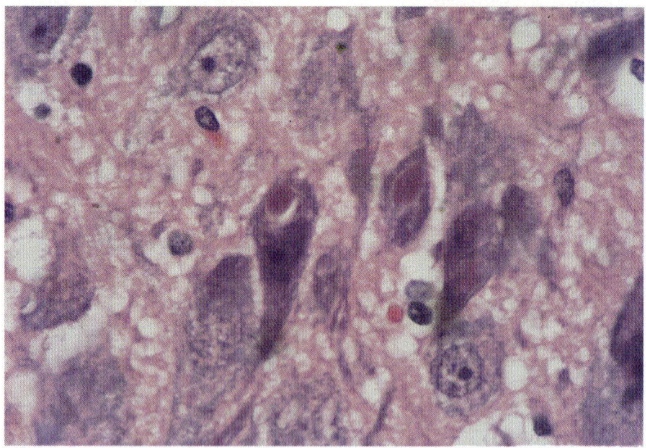

103. **Negri bodies in the cytoplasm of neurons in the hippocampus of a dog. These inclusion bodies show some internal structure. H & E stain, original magnification 1000 x.** (Courtesy Merieux Institute, Inc.)

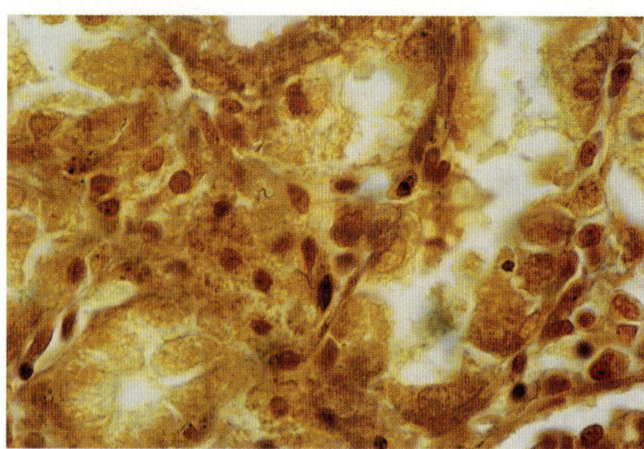

104. ***Leptospira ictohemorrhagiae*** **in the kidney of an experimentally infected dog. The organisms are indicated by the arrows. Warthin-Starry silver stain, original magnification 1000 x.**

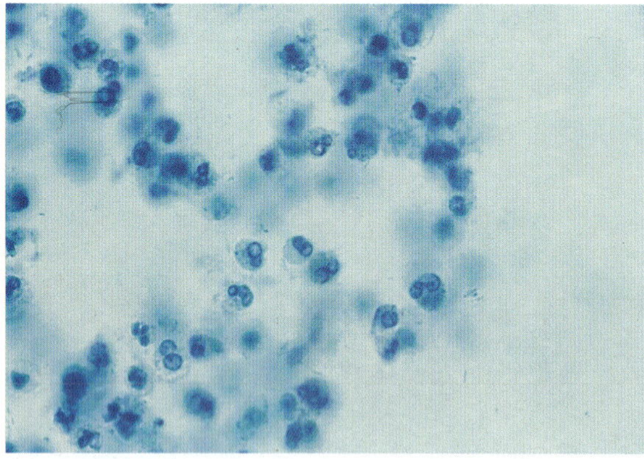

105. **Methylene blue stain of a fecal smear from a patient with bacillary dysentery (400 x). Numerous polymorphonuclear leukocytes are present, which indicates the presence of diffuse colonic inflammation.**

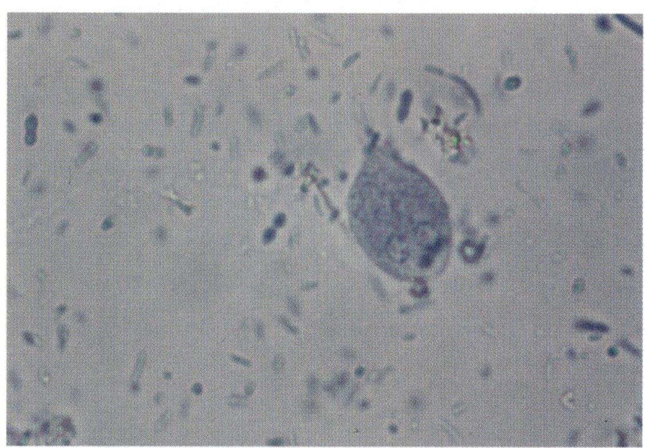

106. ***Giardia lamblia*** **trophozoite seen by methylene blue wet mount staining under oil (1000 x). The finding of cysts or trophozoites in a patient with diarrhea is sufficient to make a tentative diagnosis of giardiasis.**

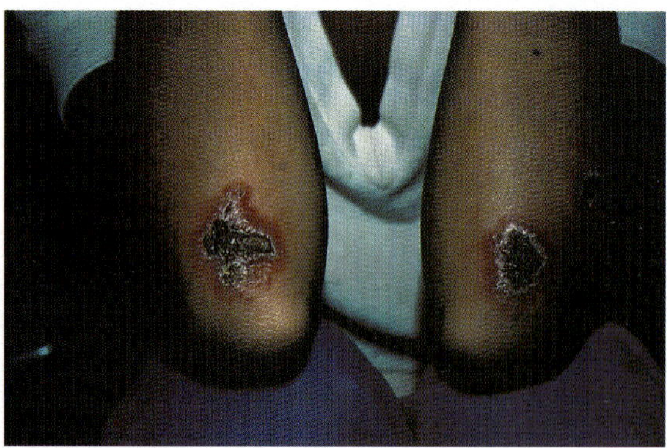

107. Old world leishmaniasis. (Courtesy Richard Kaplan, M.D.)

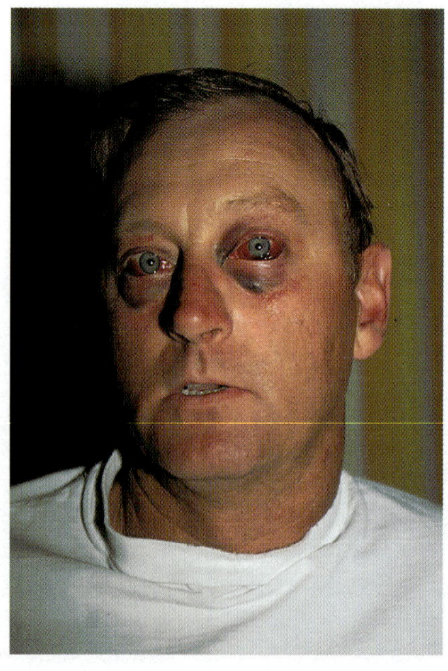

108. Mask squeeze in a diver who descended to 45 FSW without exhaling into his mask. (Kenneth W. Kizer, M.D.)

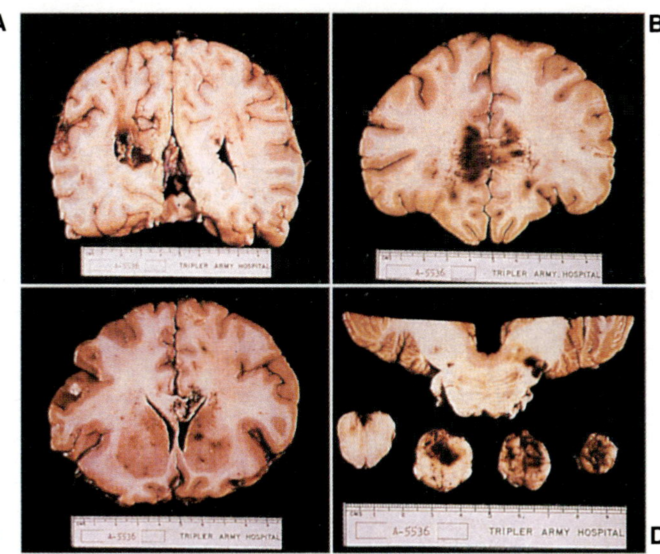

109. (A through D) **Cross sections of the brain of a 31-year-old male sport diver who suffered an arterial gas embolism, dying 4 days after the accident and extended hyperbaric oxygen treatment. Bubble-induced infarcts are found throughout the brain in the distribution of both the carotid and vertebral arteries.** (Kenneth W. Kizer, M.D.)

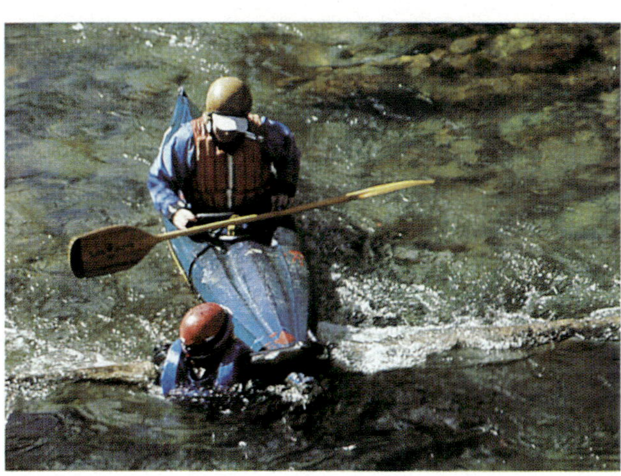

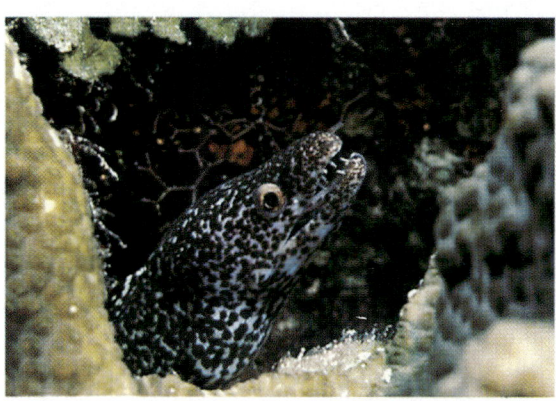

110. River rescue. The plastic kayak has revolutionized whitewater sports. (Paul Auerbach, M.D.)

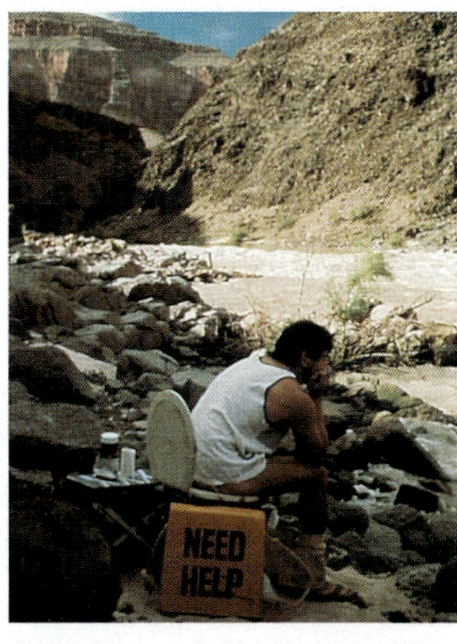

111. The river adventurer who does not properly disinfect his drinking water can suffer inglorious moments. (Eric A. Weiss, M.D.)

112. The moray eel peers out cautiously from a coral crevice. (Paul Auerbach, M.D.)

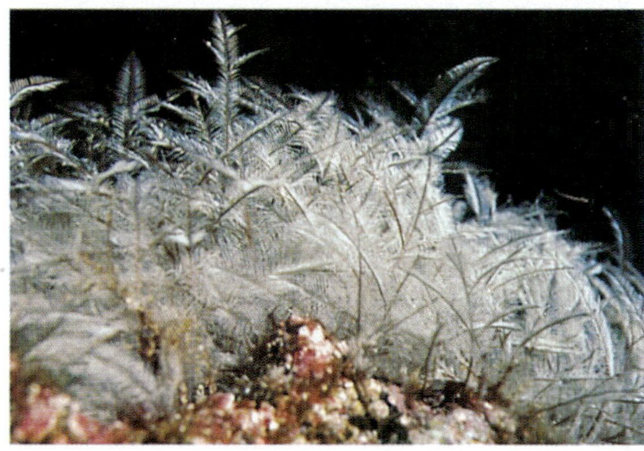

113. Coelenterate hydroid. (Paul Auerbach, M.D.)

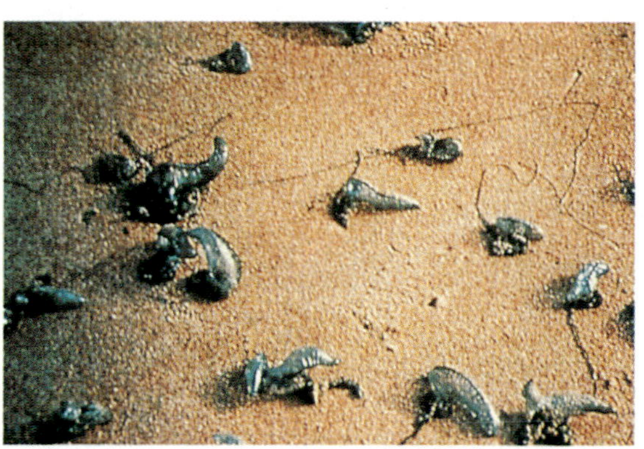

114. Pacific man of war *(Physalia utriculus)* washed ashore may retain their stinging potency for weeks. (Courtesy John Williamson, M.D.)

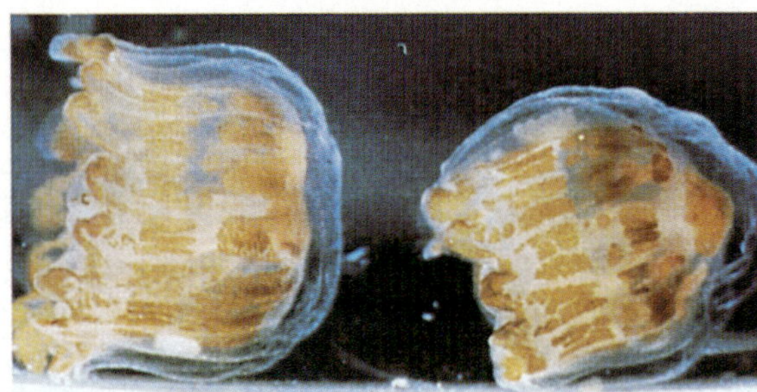

115. **Mature *Linuche unguiculata,* whose juvenile larval forms are the causative agents of seabather's eruption. The planula or larvae of these coelenterates were collected from plankton tows and grown to maturity at the University of Miami Marine School. Slightly smaller than their brethren found in the open ocean, these specimens are approximately 2 cm in diameter when open and 1 cm when contracted.** (Courtesy David Taplin and Terri L. Meinking.)

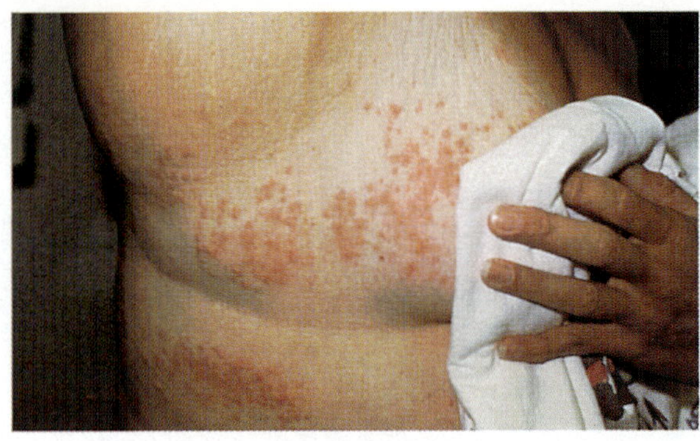

116. **Seabather's eruption.** (Courtesy D.E. Wong, T.L. Meinking, L.B. Rosen, D. Taplin, D. Hogan, and J.W. Burnett. With permission of J Am Acad Dermatol.)

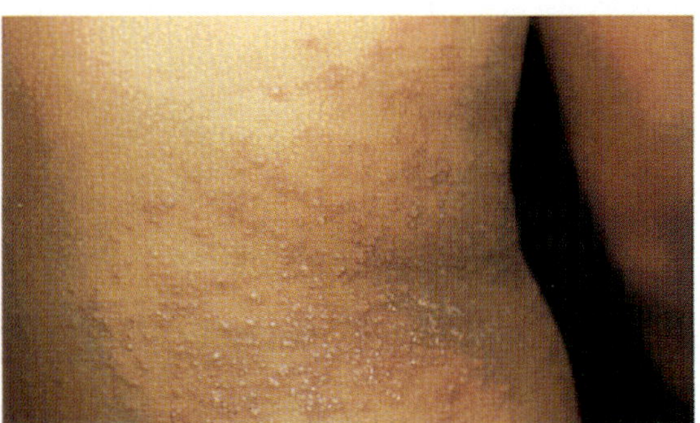

117. **Seabather's eruption in an area under the weight belt.** (Courtesy Doug Wong, M.D.)

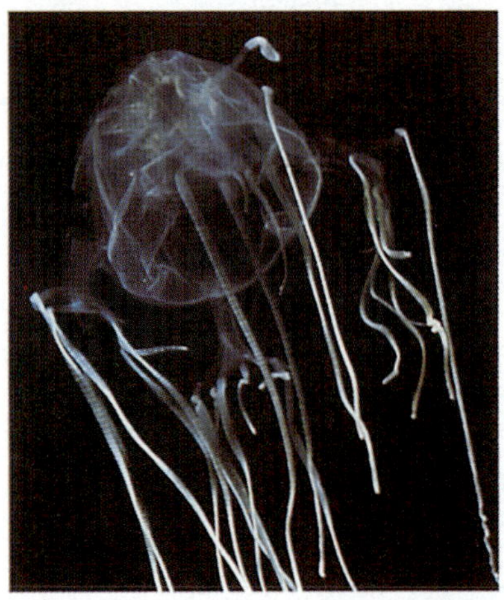

118. ***Chironex fleckeri,* the most toxic marine creature in existence.** (Courtesy Keith Gillett and the World Life Research Institute.)

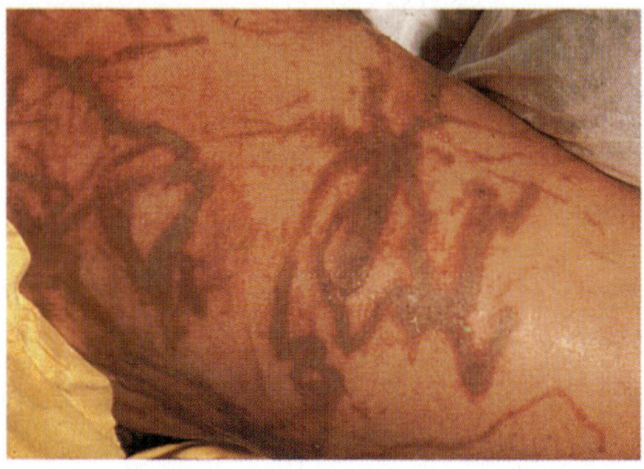

119. **Early intense necrosis is typical of a severe box-jellyfish *(Chironex fleckeri)* sting.** (Courtesy John Williamson, M.D.)

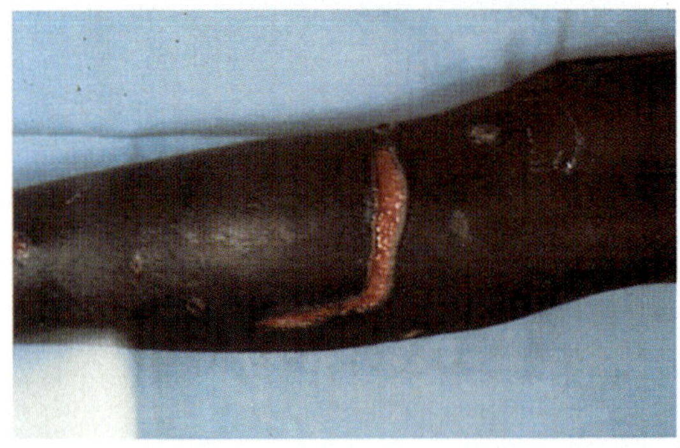

120. **Skin ulcer in the precise configuration of a tentacle print following a box-jellyfish *(Chironex fleckeri)* sting.** (Courtesy John Williamson, M.D.)

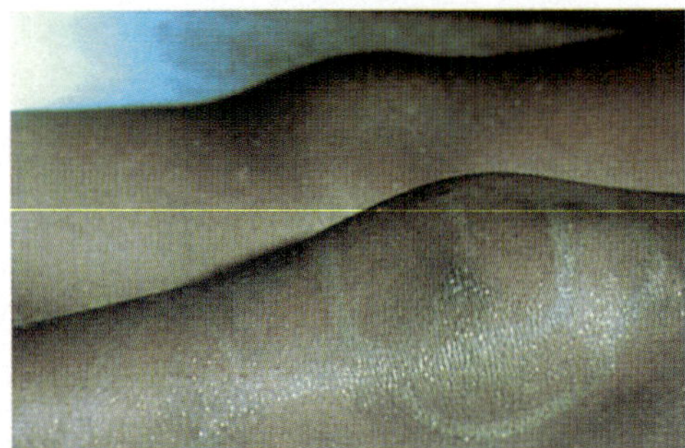

121. **Frosted cross-hatched pattern pathognomonic for a box-jellyfish envenomation. The aboriginal youth rapidly expired following this sting, which occurred in North Queensland waters in 1983.** (Courtesy John Williamson, M.D.)

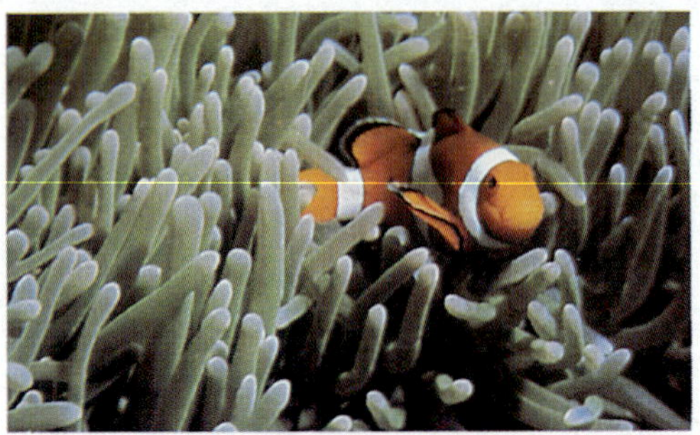

122. **Clownfish in peaceful coexistence with a sea anemone.** (Kenneth W. Kizer, M.D.)

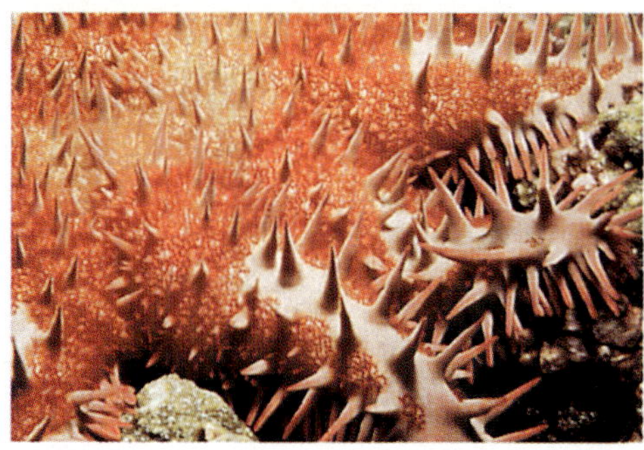

123. Spines of the crown of thorns starfish *(Acanthaster planci).* (Paul Auerbach, M.D.)

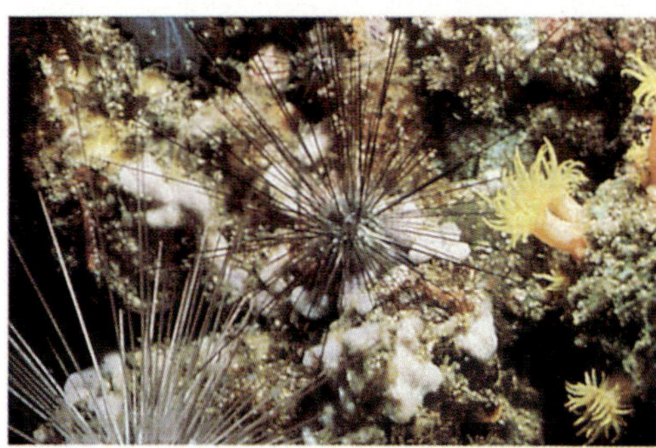

124. Needle-like spines of sea urchins in their natural habitat. (Courtesy Kenneth W. Kizer, M.D.)

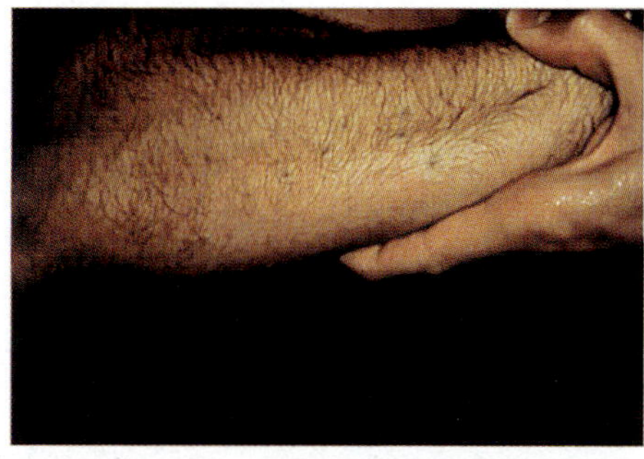

125. The author's forearm immediately after multiple punctures by the spines of black sea urchins. In 24 hours, the darkened discolorations were absent, indicative of spine dye without residual spines. (Kenneth W. Kizer, M.D.)

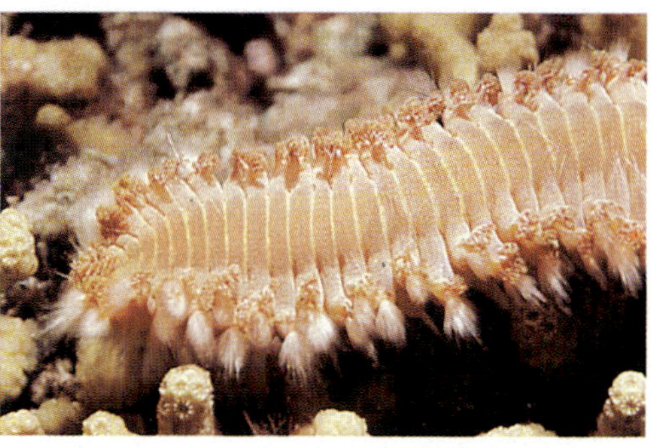

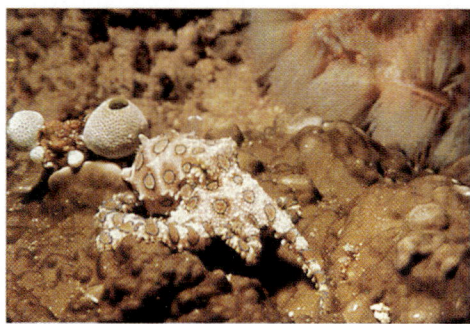

126. The chitinous spines of a bristleworm are easily dislodged into the skin of an unwary diver. (Paul Auerbach, M.D.)

127. The blue-ringed octopus *(Octopus maculosus).* This creature manufactures tetrodotoxin, a potent paralytic agent. (Courtesy Carl Roessler.)

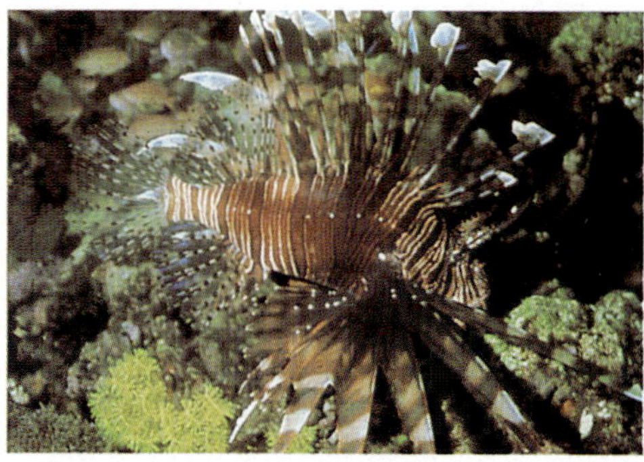

128. The ornate lionfish is the most extravagantly plumed of the venomous scorpionfishes. (Paul Auerbach, M.D.)

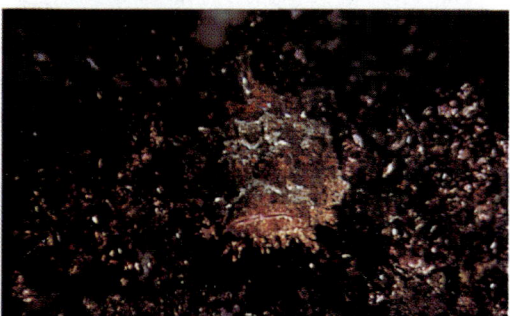

129. The Galapagos scorpionfish conceals itself to await passing prey. (Paul Auerbach, M.D.)

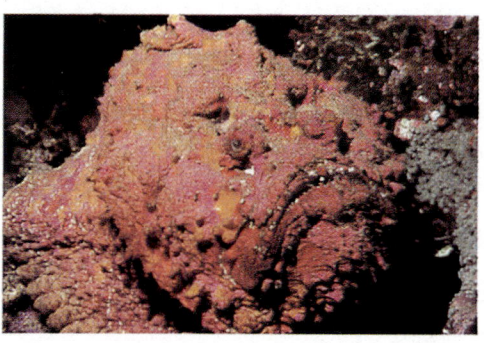

130. The deadly stonefish *(Synanceia horrida).* (Courtesy Carl Roessler.)

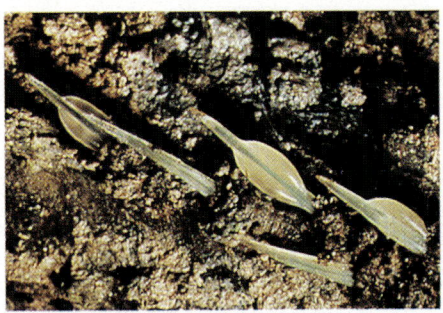

131. Spines of the venomous stonefish, demonstrating the venom glands. (Courtesy John Williamson, M.D.)

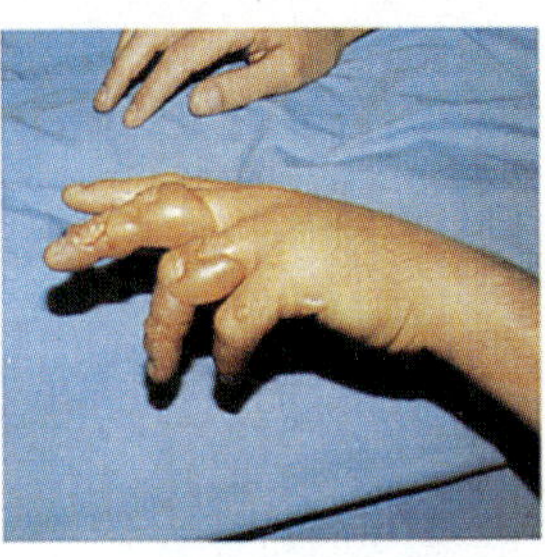

132. Vesiculation of the hand 48 hours after a sting by the lionfish *Pterois volitans*. (Courtesy Howard McKinney, Pharm. D.)

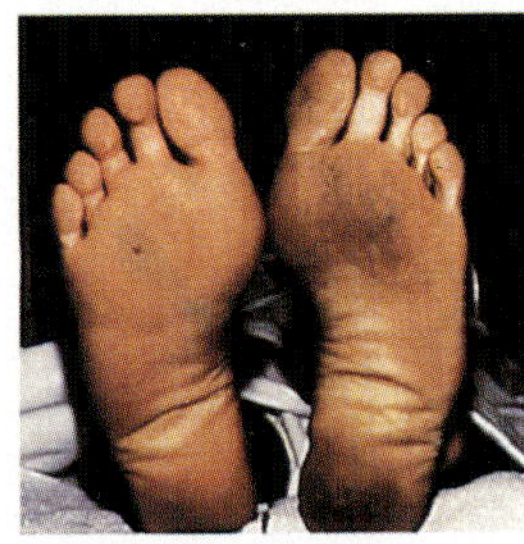

133. The victim sustained a puncture wound to the volar aspect of the right foot from a venomous stonefish. (Courtesy John Williamson, M.D.)

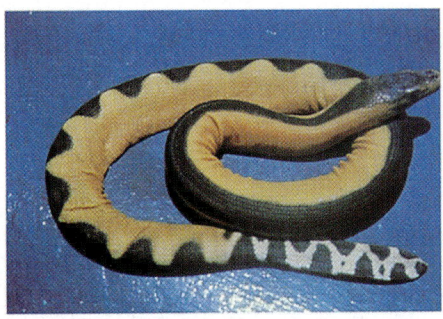

134. Pelagic sea snake *(Pelamis platurus)*. This is the most widely distributed sea snake and the only species found in American waters. (Sherman Minton, M.D.)

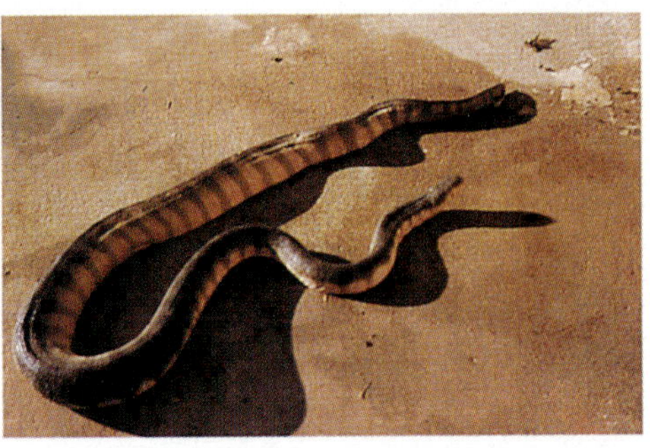

135. Beaked sea snake *(Enhydrina schistosa)*. A common sea snake of southeast Asia, the average length is about 1 meter. This creature inflicts a high proportion of the sea snake bites recorded in Asian coastal waters. (Sherman Minton, M.D.)

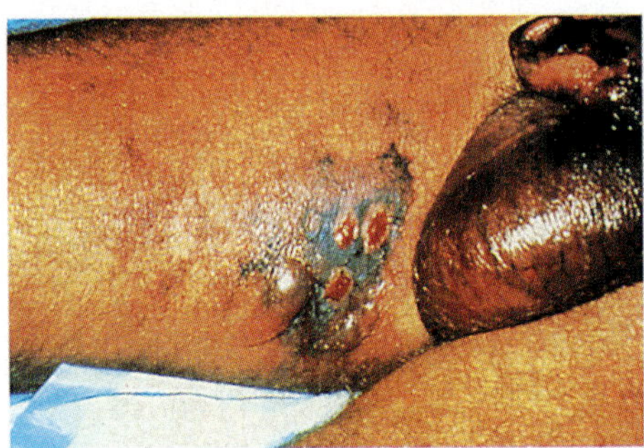

136. Echthyma gangrenosum associated with *Vibrio vulnificus* sepsis. (Courtesy Edward J. Bottone, M.D., Dept. of Microbiology, Mt. Sinai Hospital, N.Y.)

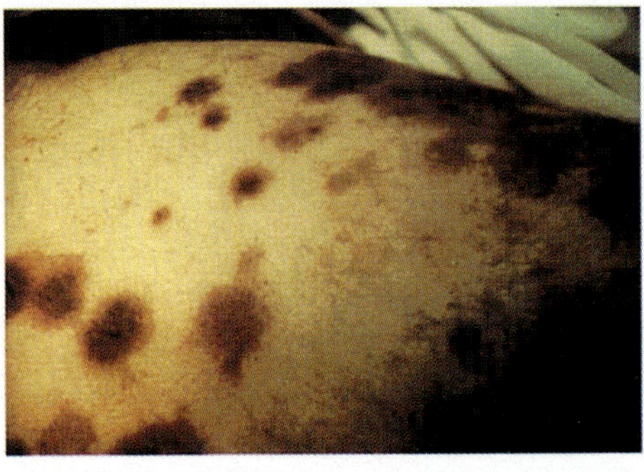

137. Torso of a victim with *Vibrio vulnificus* sepsis.

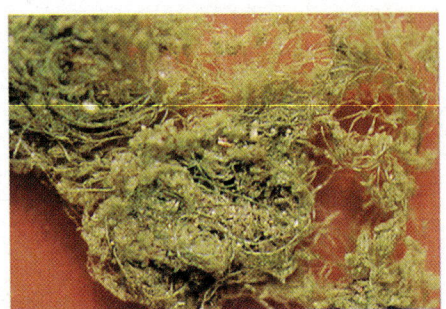

138. *Microcoleus lyngbyaceus*, the causative agent for one form of seaweed dermatitis. (Courtesy Ricardo Mandojana, M.D.)

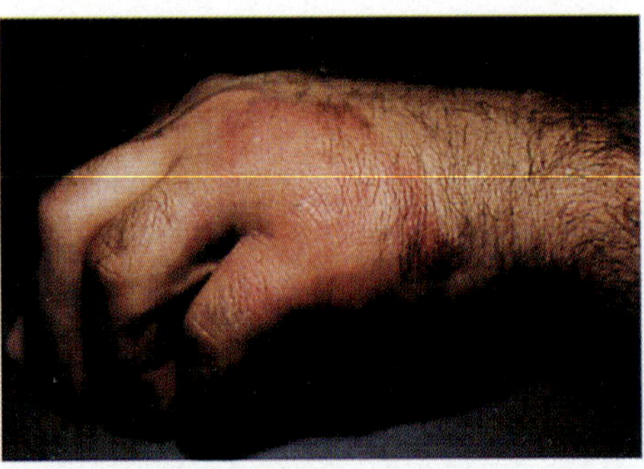

139. Typical appearance of *Erysipelothrix rhusopathiae* skin infection. (Paul Auerbach, M.D.)

INDEX

B

D

E

H

I

M

N

Q

U

W